a LANGE medical book

2017
CURRENT
Medical Diagnosis
& Treatment

FIFTY-SIXTH EDITION

Edited by

Maxine A. Papadakis, MD
Professor of Medicine
Associate Dean of Students
School of Medicine
University of California, San Francisco

Stephen J. McPhee, MD
Professor of Medicine, Emeritus
Division of General Internal Medicine
Department of Medicine
University of California, San Francisco

Associate Editor

Michael W. Rabow, MD
Professor of Medicine and Urology
Division of General Internal Medicine
Department of Medicine
University of California, San Francisco

With Associate Authors

New York   Chicago   San Francisco   Athens   London   Madrid   Mexico City
Milan   New Delhi   Singapore   Sydney   Toronto

1 2 3 4 5 6 7 8 9 0   DOW   21 20 19 18 17 16

ISBN 978-1-25-958511-1
MHID 1-25-958511-5
ISSN 0092-8682

Notice

Medicine is an ever-changing science. As new research and clinical experience broaden our knowledge, changes in treatment and drug therapy are required. The authors and the publisher of this work have checked with sources believed to be reliable in their efforts to provide information that is complete and generally in accord with the standards accepted at the time of publication. However, in view of the possibility of human error or changes in medical sciences, neither the authors nor the publisher nor any other party who has been involved in the preparation or publication of this work warrants that the information contained herein is in every respect accurate or complete, and they disclaim all responsibility for any errors or omissions or for the results obtained from use of the information contained in this work. Readers are encouraged to confirm the information contained herein with other sources. For example and in particular, readers are advised to check the product information sheet included in the package of each medication they plan to administer to be certain that the information contained in this work is accurate and that changes have not been made in the recommended dose or in the contraindications for administration. This recommendation is of particular importance in connection with new or infrequently used medications.

This book was set by Cenveo® Publisher Services.
The editors were Amanda Fielding, Harriet Lebowitz, and Barbara Holton.
The production supervisor was Jeffrey Herzich.
Project management was provided by Yashmita Hota at Cenveo Publisher Services.
The copyeditor was Jennifer Bernstein.
Design modified from original by Alan Barnett.
The index was prepared by Katherine Pitcoff.
RR Donnelley was printer and binder.

This book is printed on acid-free paper.

Contents

Authors   v
Preface   xiii

1. **Disease Prevention & Health Promotion**   1

   Michael Pignone MD, MPH, & René Salazar, MD

2. **Common Symptoms**   19

   Paul L. Nadler, MD, & Ralph Gonzales, MD, MSPH

3. **Preoperative Evaluation & Perioperative Management**   45

   Hugo Q. Cheng, MD

4. **Geriatric Disorders**   55

   G. Michael Harper, MD, C. Bree Johnston, MD, MPH, & C. Seth Landefeld, MD

5. **Palliative Care & Pain Management**   72

   Michael W. Rabow, MD, & Steven Z. Pantilat, MD

6. **Dermatologic Disorders**   95

   Kanade Shinkai, MD, PhD, & Lindy P. Fox, MD

7. **Disorders of the Eyes & Lids**   164

   Paul Riordan-Eva, FRCOphth

8. **Ear, Nose, & Throat Disorders**   200

   Lawrence R. Lustig, MD, & Joshua S. Schindler, MD

9. **Pulmonary Disorders**   241

   Mark S. Chesnutt, MD, & Thomas J. Prendergast, MD

10. **Heart Disease**   322

    Thomas M. Bashore, MD, Christopher B. Granger, MD, Kevin P. Jackson, MD, & Manesh R. Patel, MD

11. **Systemic Hypertension**   439

    Michael Sutters, MD, MRCP (UK)

12. **Blood Vessel & Lymphatic Disorders**   472

    Christopher D. Owens, MD, MSc, Warren J. Gasper, MD, & Meshell D. Johnson, MD

13. **Blood Disorders**   499

    Lloyd E. Damon, MD, & Charalambos Babis Andreadis, MD, MSCE

14. **Disorders of Hemostasis, Thrombosis, & Antithrombotic Therapy**   546

    Andrew D. Leavitt, MD, & Tracy Minichiello, MD

15. **Gastrointestinal Disorders**   578

    Kenneth R. McQuaid, MD

16. **Liver, Biliary Tract, & Pancreas Disorders**   674

    Lawrence S. Friedman, MD

17. **Breast Disorders**   734

    Armando E. Giuliano, MD, & Sara A. Hurvitz, MD

18. **Gynecologic Disorders**   762

    Jason Woo, MD, MPH, FACOG, & Alicia Y. Armstrong, MD, MHSCR

19. **Obstetrics & Obstetric Disorders**   797

    Vanessa L. Rogers, MD, & Kevin C. Worley, MD

20. **Rheumatologic, Immunologic, & Allergic Disorders**   826

    David B. Hellmann, MD, MACP, & John B. Imboden Jr., MD

21. **Electrolyte & Acid-Base Disorders**   884

    Kerry C. Cho, MD

22. **Kidney Disease**   913

    Suzanne Watnick, MD, & Tonja C. Dirkx, MD

23. **Urologic Disorders**   953

    Maxwell V. Meng, MD, FACS, Thomas J. Walsh, MD, MS, & Thomas D. Chi, MD

24. **Nervous System Disorders**   977

    Michael J. Aminoff, MD, DSc, FRCP, & Vanja C. Douglas, MD

25. **Psychiatric Disorders**   1050

    Nolan Williams, MD, & Charles DeBattista, DMH, MD

26. **Endocrine Disorders**   1108

    Paul A. Fitzgerald, MD

27. Diabetes Mellitus & Hypoglycemia 1210

Umesh Masharani, MB, BS, MRCP(UK)

28. Lipid Disorders 1259

Robert B. Baron, MD, MS

29. Nutritional Disorders 1268

Robert B. Baron, MD, MS

30. Common Problems in Infectious Diseases & Antimicrobial Therapy 1287

Peter V. Chin-Hong, MD,
& B. Joseph Guglielmo, PharmD

31. HIV Infection & AIDS 1330

Mitchell H. Katz, MD

32. Viral & Rickettsial Infections 1363

Wayne X. Shandera, MD,
& Natalie J. M. Dailey Garnes, MD, MPH

33. Bacterial & Chlamydial Infections 1441

Brian S. Schwartz, MD

34. Spirochetal Infections 1488

Susan S. Philip, MD, MPH

35. Protozoal & Helminthic Infections 1507

Philip J. Rosenthal, MD

36. Mycotic Infections 1547

Samuel A. Shelburne, III, MD, PhD,
& Richard J. Hamill, MD

37. Disorders Related to Environmental Emergencies 1561

Jacqueline A. Nemer, MD, FACEP,
& Melissa C. Clark, MD

38. Poisoning 1577

Kent R. Olson, MD

39. Cancer 1607

Patricia A. Cornett, MD,
& Tiffany O. Dea, PharmD

40. Inherited Disorders 1676

Reed E. Pyeritz, MD, PhD

41. Sports Medicine & Outpatient Orthopedics 1685

Anthony Luke, MD, MPH, & C. Benjamin Ma, MD

e1. Anti-Infective Chemotherapeutic & Antibiotic Agents Online*

B. Joseph Guglielmo, PharmD

e2. Fundamentals of Human Genetics & Genomics Online*

Reed E. Pyeritz, MD, PhD

e3. Diagnostic Testing & Medical Decision Making Online*

C. Diana Nicoll, MD, PhD, MPA,
& Chuanyi Mark Lu, MD

e4. Information Technology in Patient Care Online*

Russ Cucina, MD, MS

e5. Integrative Medicine Online*

Kevin Barrows, MD, & Sanjay Reddy, MD

e6. Podiatric Disorders Online*

Monara Dini, DPM, & Nina Babu, DPM

e7. Women's Health Issues Online*

Megan McNamara, MD, MSc,
& Judith Walsh, MD, MPH

e8. Lesbian & Bisexual Women's Health Online*

Juno Obedin-Maliver, MD, MPH,
& Patricia A. Robertson, MD

e9. Transgender Health & Disease Prevention Online*

Madeline B. Deutsch, MD, MPH

e10. Appendix: Therapeutic Drug Monitoring, Laboratory Reference Intervals, & Pharmacogenetic Testing Online*

C. Diana Nicoll, MD, PhD, MPA,
& Chuanyi Mark Lu, MD

Index 1719

*Free access to online chapters at www.accessmedicine.com/cmdt

Authors

N. Franklin Adkinson, Jr., MD
Professor of Medicine, Johns Hopkins Asthma & Allergy
Center, Baltimore, Maryland
fadkinso@jhmi.edu
Allergic & Immunologic Disorders (in Chapter 20)

Diana Alba, MD
Fellow, Division of Endocrinology and Metabolism,
University of California, San Francisco
References

Michael J. Aminoff, MD, DSc, FRCP
Distinguished Professor and Executive Vice Chair,
Department of Neurology, University of California,
San Francisco; Attending Physician, University of
California Medical Center, San Francisco
michael.aminoff@ucsf.edu
Nervous System Disorders

Charalambos Babis Andreadis, MD, MSCE
Associate Professor of Clinical Medicine, Division of
Hematology/Oncology, University of California,
San Francisco
Charalambos.Andreadis@ucsf.edu
Blood Disorders

Alicia Y. Armstrong, MD, MHSCR
Medical Officer, Contraceptive Discovery and
Development Branch, Eunice Kennedy Shriver
National Institute for Child Health and Human
Development, National Institutes for Health,
Rockville, Maryland
ayba55@aol.com
Gynecologic Disorders

Nina Babu, DPM
Assistant Clinical Professor, Department
of Orthopaedic Surgery, University of California,
San Francisco
CMDT Online—Podiatric Disorders

David M. Barbour, PharmD, BCPS
Pharmacist, Denver, Colorado
dbarbour99@gmail.com
Drug References

Robert B. Baron, MD, MS
Professor of Medicine; Associate Dean for Graduate and
Continuing Medical Education; Vice Chief, Division of
General Internal Medicine, University of California,
San Francisco
baron@medicine.ucsf.edu
Lipid Disorders; Nutritional Disorders

Kevin Barrows, MD
Clinical Professor of Family and Community Medicine,
Director of Mindfulness Programs, Osher Center for
Integrative Medicine; Department of Family and
Community Medicine, University of California,
San Francisco
Kevin.Barrows@ucsf.edu
CMDT Online—Integrative Medicine

Thomas M. Bashore, MD
Professor of Medicine; Senior Vice Chief, Division of
Cardiology, Duke University Medical Center, Durham,
North Carolina
thomas.bashore@duke.edu
Heart Disease

Brook Calton, MD, MHS
Assistant Professor of Clinical Medicine, Division of
Geriatrics, Department of Medicine, University of
California, San Francisco
References

Amy D. Chen, MD
Clinical Instructor, Division of Hospital Medicine,
University of California, San Francisco
References

Hugo Q. Cheng, MD
Clinical Professor of Medicine, University of California,
San Francisco
quinny.cheng@ucsf.edu
Preoperative Evaluation & Perioperative Management

Mark S. Chesnutt, MD
Clinical Professor, Pulmonary & Critical Care Medicine,
Dotter Interventional Institute, Oregon Health &
Science University, Portland, Oregon; Director, Critical
Care, Portland Veterans Affairs Health Care System
chesnutm@ohsu.edu
Pulmonary Disorders

Thomas D. Chi, MD
Assistant Professor, Department of Urology, University of
California, San Francisco
tom.chi@ucsf.edu
Urologic Disorders

Peter V. Chin-Hong, MD
Professor, Division of Infectious Diseases, Department of
Medicine, University of California, San Francisco
peter.chin-hong@ucsf.edu
*Common Problems in Infectious Diseases & Antimicrobial
Therapy*

Kerry C. Cho, MD
Associate Clinical Professor of Medicine, Division of
Nephrology, University of California, San Francisco
kerry.cho@ucsf.edu
Electrolyte & Acid-Base Disorders

Pelin Cinar, MD, MS
Clinical Assistant Professor of Medicine in Oncology,
University of California San Francisco; Director of
Quality Improvement, UCSF Helen Diller Family
Comprehensive Cancer Center
pelin.cinar@ucsf.edu
Alimentary Tract Cancers (in Chapter 39)

Melissa C. Clark, MD
Assistant Clinical Professor, Department of Emergency
Medicine, University of California, San Francisco,
San Francisco General Hospital
melissa.clark@ucsf.edu
Disorders Related to Environmental Emergencies

Patricia A. Cornett, MD
Professor of Medicine, University of California,
San Francisco; Chief, Hematology/Oncology,
San Francisco Veterans Affairs Health Care System,
San Francisco, California
patricia.cornett@ucsf.edu
Cancer

Russ Cucina, MD, MS
Associate Professor of Hospital Medicine; Chief Health
Information Officer, UCSF Health System; University
of California, San Francisco
russ.cucina@ucsf.edu
*CMDT Online—Information Technology in
Patient Care*

Natalie J. M. Dailey Garnes, MD, MPH
Clinical Postdoctoral Fellow, Division of Pediatric
Infectious Diseases, Department of Pediatrics and
Medicine, Baylor College of Medicine,
Houston, Texas
dailey@bcm.edu
Viral & Rickettsial Infections

Lloyd E. Damon, MD
Professor of Clinical Medicine, Department of Medicine,
Division of Hematology/Oncology; Director of Adult
Hematologic Malignancies and Blood and Marrow
Transplantation, Deputy Chief of the Division of
Hematology and Medical Oncology, University of
California, San Francisco
lloyd.damon@ucsf.edu
Blood Disorders

Tiffany O. Dea, PharmD, BCOP
Oncology Pharmacist, Veterans Affairs Health Care
System, San Francisco, California; Adjunct Professor,
Thomas J. Long School of Pharmacy and Health
Sciences, Stockton, California
tiffany.dea@va.gov
Cancer

Charles DeBattista, DMH, MD
Professor of Psychiatry and Behavioral Sciences, Director:
Depression Clinic and Research Program Director of
Medical Student Education in Psychiatry, Stanford
University School of Medicine, Stanford, California
debattista@stanford.edu
Psychiatric Disorders

Madeline B. Deutsch, MD
Assistant Clinical Professor, Clinical Director, Center of
Excellence for Transgender Health, Department of
Family & Community Medicine, University of
California, San Francisco
Madeline.Deutsch@ucsf.edu
CMDT Online—Transgender Health & Disease Prevention

Monara Dini, DPM
Assistant Clinical Professor, Chief of Podiatric Surgery
Division, Department of Orthopedic Surgery,
University of California, San Francisco
monara.dini@ucsf.edu
CMDT Online—Podiatric Disorders

Tonja C. Dirkx, MD
Associate Professor of Medicine, Division of Nephrology,
Department of Medicine, Oregon Health and Sciences
University, Portland, Oregon; Renal Clinic Director,
Portland Veterans Affairs Health Care System
dirkxt@ohsu.edu
Kidney Disease

Vanja C. Douglas, MD
Sara & Evan Williams Foundation Endowed
Neurohospitalist Chair, Associate Professor of Clinical
Neurology, Department of Neurology, University of
California, San Francisco
Vanja.Douglas@ucsf.edu
Nervous System Disorders

Paul A. Fitzgerald, MD
Clinical Professor of Medicine, Department of Medicine,
Division of Endocrinology, University of California,
San Francisco
paul.fitzgerald@ucsf.edu
Endocrine Disorders

Lindy P. Fox, MD
Associate Professor, Department of Dermatology,
University of California, San Francisco
Lindy.Fox@ucsf.edu
Dermatologic Disorders

Lawrence S. Friedman, MD
Professor of Medicine, Harvard Medical School; Professor
of Medicine, Tufts University School of Medicine,
Boston, Massachusetts; The Anton R. Fried, MD, Chair,
Department of Medicine, Newton-Wellesley Hospital,
Newton, Massachusetts; Assistant Chief of Medicine,
Massachusetts General Hospital, Boston, Massachusetts
lfriedman@partners.org
*Liver, Biliary Tract, & Pancreas Disorders; Hepatobiliary
Cancers (in Chapter 39)*

Warren J. Gasper, MD
Assistant Professor of Clinical Surgery, Division of
Vascular and Endovascular Surgery, Department of
Surgery, University of California,
San Francisco
warren.gasper@ucsf.edu
Blood Vessel & Lymphatic Disorders

Armando E. Giuliano, MD, FACS, FRCSEd
Executive Vice Chair of Surgery, Associate Director of
Surgical Oncology, Cedars-Sinai Medical Center,
Los Angeles, California
armando.giuliano@cshs.org
Breast Disorders

Ralph Gonzales, MD, MSPH
Associate Dean, Clinical Innovation and Chief Innovation
Officer, UCSF Health; Professor of Medicine, Division
of General Internal Medicine, Department of Medicine,
University of California, San Francisco
ralph.gonzales@ucsf.edu
Common Symptoms

Christopher B. Granger, MD
Professor of Medicine; Director, Cardiac Care Unit, Duke
University Medical Center, Duke Clinical Research
Institute, Durham, North Carolina
christopher.granger@dm.duke.edu
Heart Disease

B. Joseph Guglielmo, PharmD
Professor and Dean, School of Pharmacy, University of
California, San Francisco
BJoseph.Guglielmo@ucsf.edu
*Common Problems in Infectious Diseases & Antimicrobial
Therapy; CMDT Online—Anti-Infective
Chemotherapeutic & Antibiotic Agents*

Elan L. Guterman, MD
Neurology Resident, Department of Neurology, University
of California, San Francisco
References

Richard J. Hamill, MD
Professor, Division of Infectious Diseases, Departments of
Medicine and Molecular Virology & Microbiology,
Baylor College of Medicine, Houston, Texas
rhamill@bcm.edu
Mycotic Infections

G. Michael Harper, MD
Professor, Division of Geriatrics, Department of Medicine,
University of California San Francisco School of
Medicine; San Francisco Veterans Affairs Health Care
System, San Francisco, California
michael.harper3@va.gov
Geriatric Disorders

David B. Hellmann, MD, MACP
Aliki Perroti Professor of Medicine; Vice Dean for Johns
Hopkins Bayview; Chairman, Department of Medicine,
Johns Hopkins Bayview Medical Center, Johns Hopkins
University School of Medicine, Baltimore, Maryland
hellmann@jhmi.edu
Rheumatologic, Immunologic, & Allergic Disorders

Sara A. Hurvitz, MD
Associate Professor; Director, Breast Oncology Program,
Division of Hematology/Oncology, Department of
Internal Medicine, University of California, Los Angeles
shurvitz@mednet.ucla.edu
Breast Disorders

John B. Imboden, Jr., MD
Alice Betts Endowed Chair for Arthritis Research;
Professor of Medicine, University of California,
San Francisco; Chief, Division of Rheumatology,
San Francisco General Hospital
John.Imboden@ucsf.edu
Rheumatologic, Immunologic, & Allergic Disorders

Kevin P. Jackson, MD
Assistant Professor of Medicine, Director of
Electrophysiology, Duke Raleigh Hospital, Duke
University Medical Center, Durham, North Carolina
k.j@duke.edu
Heart Disease

Jane Jih, MD, MPH, MAS
Assistant Professor of Medicine, Division of General
Internal Medicine, Department of Medicine, University
of California, San Francisco
jane.jih@ucsf.edu
References

Meshell D. Johnson, MD
Associate Professor of Medicine, Division of Pulmonary
and Critical Care Medicine, Department of Medicine,
University of California, San Francisco
meshell.johnson@ucsf.edu
*Blood Vessel & Lymphatic Disorders; Alcohol Use Disorder
(Alcoholism) (in Chapter 25)*

C. Bree Johnston, MD, MPH
Medical Director of Palliative and Supportive Care,
PeaceHealth St. Joseph Medical Center, Bellingham,
Washington; Clinical Professor of Medicine, University
of Washington
bjohnston@peacehealth.org
Geriatric Disorders

Mitchell H. Katz, MD
Clinical Professor of Medicine, Epidemiology &
Biostatistics, University of California, San Francisco;
Director of Health Services, Los Angeles County
mkatz@dhs.lacounty.gov
HIV Infection & AIDS

C. Seth Landefeld, MD
Professor of Medicine; Chair, Department of Medicine
    and Spencer Chair in Medical Science Leadership,
    University of Alabama at Birmingham
sethlandefeld@uab.edu
Geriatric Disorders

David C. Lange, MD
Clinical Fellow, Division of Cardiology, Department of
    Internal Medicine, Cedars-Sinai Medical Center,
    Los Angeles, California
References

Andrew D. Leavitt, MD
Professor, Departments of Medicine (Hematology) and
    Laboratory Medicine; Medical Director, UCSF Adult
    Hemophilia Treatment Center, University of California,
    San Francisco
andrew.leavitt@ucsf.edu
*Disorders of Hemostasis, Thrombosis, & Antithrombotic
    Therapy*

Chuanyi Mark Lu, MD
Professor, Department of Laboratory Medicine, University
    of California, San Francisco; Chief, Hematology,
    Hematopathology & Molecular Diagnostics,
    Laboratory Medicine Service, Veterans Affairs Health
    Care System, San Francisco, California
mark.lu@va.gov
*CMDT Online—Appendix: Therapeutic Drug Monitoring
    & Laboratory Reference Intervals, & Pharmacogenetic
    Testing; CMDT Online—Diagnostic Testing & Medical
    Decision Making*

Anthony Luke, MD, MPH
Professor of Clinical Orthopaedics, Department of
    Orthopaedics; Director, UCSF Primary Care Sports
    Medicine; Director, Human Performance Center at the
    Orthopaedic Institute, University of California,
    San Francisco
anthony.luke@ucsf.edu
Sports Medicine & Outpatient Orthopedics

Lawrence R. Lustig, MD
Howard W. Smith Professor and Chair, Department of
    Otolaryngology—Head & Neck Surgery, Columbia
    University Medical Center & New York Presbyterian
    Hospital, New York, New York
lrl2125@cumc.columbia.edu
Ear, Nose, & Throat Disorders

C. Benjamin Ma, MD
Associate Professor, Department of Orthopaedic Surgery;
    Chief, Sports Medicine and Shoulder Service,
    University of California, San Francisco
MaBen@orthosurg.ucsf.edu
Sports Medicine & Outpatient Orthopedics

Umesh Masharani, MB, BS, MRCP(UK)
Professor of Medicine, Division of Endocrinology and
    Metabolism, Department of Medicine, University of
    California, San Francisco
umesh.masharani@ucsf.edu
Diabetes Mellitus & Hypoglycemia

Megan McNamara, MD, MSc
Associate Professor of Medicine, Case Western Reserve
    University School of Medicine; Louis Stokes Cleveland
    Veterans Affairs Medical Center
Megan.Mcnamara@va.gov
CMDT Online—Women's Health Issues

Kenneth R. McQuaid, MD
Chief, Gastroenterology and Medical Service,
    San Francisco Veterans Affairs Medical Center;
    Professor of Clinical Medicine, Marvin H. Sleisenger
    Endowed Chair and Vice-Chairman, Department of
    Medicine, University of California,
    San Francisco
Kenneth.Mcquaid@va.gov
*Gastrointestinal Disorders; Alimentary Tract Cancers
    (in Chapter 39)*

Maxwell V. Meng, MD, FACS
Professor, Chief of Urologic Oncology, Department of
    Urology, University of California, San Francisco
max.meng@ucsf.edu
*Urologic Disorders; Cancers of the Genitourinary Tract
    (in Chapter 39)*

Tracy Minichiello, MD
Clinical Professor of Medicine, University of California,
    San Francisco; Chief, Anticoagulation and Thrombosis
    Services, San Francisco Veterans Affairs Medical
    Center
Tracy.Minichiello@ucsf.edu
*Disorders of Hemostasis, Thrombosis, & Antithrombotic
    Therapy*

Paul L. Nadler, MD
Clinical Professor of Medicine; Director, Screening and
    Acute Care Clinic, Division of General Internal
    Medicine, Department of Medicine, University of
    California, San Francisco
nadler@medicine.ucsf.edu
Common Symptoms

Jacqueline A. Nemer, MD, FACEP
Professor of Emergency Medicine, Director of
    Advanced Clinical Skills, Department of Emergency
    Medicine, University of California,
    San Francisco
jacqueline.nemer@ucsf.edu
Disorders Related to Environmental Emergencies

C. Diana Nicoll, MD, PhD, MPA
Clinical Professor and Vice Chair, Department of Laboratory Medicine; Associate Dean, University of California, San Francisco; Chief of Staff and Chief, Laboratory Medicine Service, San Francisco Veterans Affairs Health Care System
diana.nicoll@va.gov
CMDT Online—Appendix: Therapeutic Drug Monitoring & Laboratory Reference Intervals, & Pharmacogenetic Testing; CMDT Online—Diagnostic Testing & Medical Decision Making

Juno Obedin-Maliver, MD, MPH
Clinical Research Fellow, Women's Health, San Francisco Veterans Affairs Medical Center; Clinical Instructor, Department of Obstetrics, Gynecology, and Reproductive Sciences, University of California San Francisco; Founder and Investigator, Lesbian, Gay, Bisexual, and Transgender Medical Education Research Group, Stanford University School of Medicine, Stanford, California
Juno.Obedin-Maliver@ucsf.edu
CMDT Online—Lesbian & Bisexual Women's Health

Kent R. Olson, MD
Clinical Professor of Medicine, Pediatrics, and Pharmacy, University of California, San Francisco; Medical Director, San Francisco Division, California Poison Control System
kent.olson@ucsf.edu
Poisoning

R. Anthony Orden, MD
Clinical Fellow, Division of Allergy & Clinical Immunology, Johns Hopkins Asthma & Allergy Center, Baltimore, Maryland
rorden1@jhmi.edu
Allergic & Immunologic Disorders (in Chapter 20)

Christopher D. Owens, MD, MSc
Associate Professor of Surgery, Division of Vascular and Endovascular Surgery, Department of Surgery, University of California, San Francisco; Chief, Vascular Surgery, San Francisco Veteran's Affairs Medical Center
christopher.owens@ucsfmedctr.org
Blood Vessel & Lymphatic Disorders

Steven Z. Pantilat, MD
Professor of Medicine, Department of Medicine; Kates-Burnard and Hellman Distinguished Professor of Palliative Care; Director, Palliative Care Program, University of California, San Francisco
steve.pantilat@ucsf.edu
Palliative Care & Pain Management

Manesh R. Patel, MD
Associate Professor of Medicine, Division of Cardiology, Department of Medicine; Director of Interventional Cardiology, Duke University Medical Center, Durham, North Carolina
manesh.patel@duke.edu
Heart Disease

Susan S. Philip, MD, MPH
Assistant Clinical Professor, Division of Infectious Diseases, Department of Medicine, University of California, San Francisco; Disease Prevention and Control Branch, Population Health Division, San Francisco Department of Public Health, San Francisco, California
susan.philip@sfdph.org
Spirochetal Infections

Michael Pignone, MD, MPH
Professor of Medicine; Chief, Division of General Internal Medicine, Department of Medicine, University of North Carolina, Chapel Hill
pignone@med.unc.edu
Disease Prevention & Health Promotion

Thomas J. Prendergast, MD
Clinical Professor of Medicine, Oregon Health and Science University; Pulmonary Critical Care Section Chief, Portland Veterans Affairs Health Care System, Portland, Oregon
thomas.prendergast@va.gov
Pulmonary Disorders

Reed E. Pyeritz, MD, PhD
William Smilow Professor of Medicine and Genetics, Raymond and Ruth Perelman School of Medicine of the University of Pennsylvania, Philadelphia
reed.pyeritz@uphs.upenn.edu
Inherited Disorders; CMDT Online—Fundamentals of Human Genetics & Genomics

Michael W. Rabow, MD, FAAHPM
Helen Diller Family Chair in Palliative Care, Professor of Clinical Medicine and Urology, Division of General Internal Medicine, Department of Medicine; Director, Symptom Management Service, Helen Diller Family Comprehensive Cancer Center, University of California, San Francisco
Mike.Rabow@ucsf.edu
Palliative Care & Pain Management

Sanjay Reddy, MD
Assistant Clinical Professor of Medicine, Division of Hospital Medicine, Department of Medicine. University of California, San Francisco
Sanjay.Reddy@ucsf.edu
CMDT Online—Integrative Medicine

Paul Riordan-Eva, FRCOphth
Consultant Ophthalmologist, King's College Hospital, London, United Kingdom
paulreva@doctors.org.uk
Disorders of the Eyes & Lids

Patricia A. Robertson, MD
Professor, Department of Obstetrics, Gynecology, and Reproductive Sciences, University of California, San Francisco
Patricia.Robertson@ucsf.edu
CMDT Online—Lesbian & Bisexual Women's Health

Vanessa L. Rogers, MD
Associate Professor, Obstetrics and Gynecology, University of Texas Southwestern Medical Center, Dallas, Texas
vanessa.rogers@utsouthwestern.edu
Obstetrics & Obstetric Disorders

Philip J. Rosenthal, MD
Professor, Department of Medicine, University of California, San Francisco; Associate Chief, Division of HIV, Infectious Diseases, and Global Health, San Francisco General Hospital
philip.rosenthal@ucsf.edu
Protozoal & Helminthic Infections

René Salazar, MD
Associate Professor of Clinical Medicine, Division of General Internal Medicine, Department of Medicine, University of California, San Francisco
salazarr@medicine.ucsf.edu
Disease Prevention & Health Promotion

Joshua S. Schindler, MD
Associate Professor, Department of Otolaryngology, Oregon Health & Science University, Portland, Oregon; Medical Director, OHSU-Northwest Clinic for Voice and Swallowing
schindlj@ohsu.edu
Ear, Nose, & Throat Disorders

Brian S. Schwartz, MD
Associate Professor, Division of Infectious Diseases, Department of Medicine, University of California, San Francisco
brian.schwartz@ucsf.edu
Bacterial & Chlamydial Infections

Wayne X. Shandera, MD
Assistant Professor, Department of Internal Medicine, Baylor College of Medicine, Houston, Texas
shandera@bcm.tmc.edu
Viral & Rickettsial Infections

Samuel A. Shelburne, III, MD, PhD
Associate Professor, Department of Infectious Diseases and Department of Genomic Medicine, The University of Texas MD Anderson Cancer Center, Houston, Texas
sshelburne@mdanderson.org
Mycotic Infections

Yiwey Shieh, MD
Primary Care Research Fellow, Division of General Internal Medicine, Department of Medicine, University of California, San Francisco
References

Kanade Shinkai, MD, PhD
Associate Professor, Department of Dermatology, University of California, San Francisco
Kanade.Shinkai@ucsf.edu
Dermatologic Disorders

Scott J. Steiger, MD, FACP, FASAM
Assistant Professor of Clinical Medicine, Division of General Internal Medicine, Department of Medicine, University of California, San Francisco
scott.steiger@ucsf.edu
Opioids for Chronic, Noncancer Pain (in Chapter 5)

Michael Sutters, MD, MRCP(UK)
Attending Nephrologist, Virginia Mason Medical Center, Seattle, Washington; Affiliate Assistant Professor of Medicine, Division of Nephrology, University of Washington School of Medicine, Seattle, Washington
michael.sutters@vmmc.org
Systemic Hypertension

Philip Tiso
Principal Editor, Division of General Internal Medicine, University of California, San Francisco
References

Judith Walsh, MD, MPH
Professor of Clinical Medicine, Division of General Internal Medicine, Women's Health Center of Excellence, University of California, San Francisco
Judith.Walsh@ucsf.edu
CMDT Online—Women's Health Issues

Thomas J. Walsh, MD, MS
Associate Professor, Department of Urology, University of Washington School of Medicine, Seattle, Washington
walsht@u.washington.edu
Urologic Disorders

Sunny Wang, MD
Assistant Clinical Professor of Medicine, Division of Hematology and Oncology, University of California, San Francisco; San Francisco Veterans Affairs Health Care System
sunny.wang@ucsf.edu
Lung Cancer (in Chapter 39)

Suzanne Watnick, MD
Professor of Medicine, Division of Nephrology and Hypertension, Oregon Health & Science University, Portland; Portland Veterans Affairs Health Care System, Portland, Oregon
watnicks@ohsu.edu
Kidney Disease

Nolan Williams, MD
Instructor, Department of Psychiatry, Stanford University
  School of Medicine, Stanford, California
nolanw@stanford.edu
Psychiatric Disorders

CAPT Jason Woo, MD, MPH, FACOG
Medical Officer, Office of Generic Drugs, Center for Drug
  Evaluation and Research, U.S. Food and Drug
  Administration, Silver Spring, Maryland
woojjmd@gmail.com
Gynecologic Disorders

Kevin C. Worley, MD
Associate Professor of Obstetrics and Gynecology,
  Department of Obstetrics and Gynecology, Division of
  Maternal-Fetal Medicine, University of Texas
  Southwestern Medical Center, Dallas, Texas
Kevin.Worley@UTSouthwestern.edu
Obstetrics & Obstetric Disorders

Bree Zimmerman, MD
Chief Resident, Department of Dermatology, University
  of California, San Francisco
References

Preface

Current Medical Diagnosis & Treatment 2017 (CMDT 2017) is the 56th edition of this single-source reference for practitioners in both hospital and ambulatory settings. The book emphasizes the practical features of clinical diagnosis and patient management in all fields of internal medicine and in specialties of interest to primary care practitioners and to subspecialists who provide general care.

Our students have inspired us to look at issues of race and justice, which surely impact people's health. We have therefore reviewed the content of our work to ensure that it contains the dignity and equality that every patient deserves.

INTENDED AUDIENCE FOR *CMDT*

House officers, medical students, and all other health professions students will find the descriptions of diagnostic and therapeutic modalities, with citations to the current literature, of everyday usefulness in patient care.

Internists, family physicians, hospitalists, nurse practitioners, physicians' assistants, and all primary care providers will appreciate *CMDT* as a ready reference and refresher text. Physicians in other specialties, pharmacists, and dentists will find the book a useful basic medical reference text. Nurses, nurse-practitioners, and physicians' assistants will welcome the format and scope of the book as a means of referencing medical diagnosis and treatment.

Patients and their family members who seek information about the nature of specific diseases and their diagnosis and treatment may also find this book to be a valuable resource.

NEW IN THIS EDITION OF *CMDT*

- Updated treatment recommendations for direct-acting oral anticoagulants (dabigatran, rivaroxaban, apixaban, and edoxaban)
- New combination therapy (sacubitril plus valsartan) to improve clinical outcome in heart failure with reduced left ventricular ejection fraction
- New information on Zika virus and infection caused by *Elizabethkingia* species
- Alternative, noninvasive diagnostic tests for the diagnosis of cirrhosis
- Diagnosis of *Clostridium difficile* by PCR tests, including newly recognized NAP1 hypervirulent strains
- Treatment of recurrent *C difficile* infections with fidaxomicin
- Revised USPSTF recommendations for cardiovascular prevention methods
- New information on proprotein convertase subtilisin/kexin type 9 (PCSK9) inhibitors for hypercholesterolemia
- Latest antiviral regimens for chronic hepatitis C and treatment of autoimmune hepatitis
- New pneumococcal, meningococcal vaccines
- Update on influenza vaccines
- Update on MMR and HPV vaccines
- New FDA-approved medications for diabetes mellitus
- Update on anti-TNF and immunomodulatory therapies of inflammatory bowel disease
- New pharmacologic treatment for schizophrenia and bipolar disorder
- Updated recommendations regarding appendicitis
- New table summarizing 2015 Revised Jones Criteria for rheumatic fever
- New table outlining European Society of Cardiology guidelines for defining and diagnosing pericarditis
- Latest information on treatment options for obesity
- Updated information on dilated cardiomyopathy and Tako-Tsubo cardiomyopathy
- Extensive revision of Disorders of Hemostasis, Thrombosis, & Antithrombotic Therapy chapter
- Revised treatment recommendations for infective endocarditis
- Information on increasing deaths due to opioid overdose
- Update on predictors of acute coronary syndrome
- Updated and new treatment recommendations for HIV
- Latest treatment recommendations for latent tuberculosis in HIV-positive and HIV-negative patients
- Substantial revision of Nervous System Disorders chapter
- The combination of PET and CT imaging in preoperative staging and role of programmed cell-death-1 (PD-1) inhibitors (nivolumab and pembrolizumab) for non–small cell lung cancers
- Pharmacologic treatment for female hyposexual desire disorder

- Extensively revised section on Alcohol Use Disorder (Alcoholism)
- Updated treatment options for hepatitis C–associated renal disease and focal segmental glomerulosclerosis
- Revised treatment options for Cushing syndrome and hypercortisolism
- Latest revision of recommended adult immunization schedule from the Centers for Disease Control
- Two new online chapters: Lesbian & Bisexual Women's Health and Transgender Health & Disease Prevention
- Expanded online Podiatry chapter

OUTSTANDING FEATURES OF *CMDT*

- Medical advances up to time of annual publication
- Detailed presentation of primary care topics, including gynecology, obstetrics, dermatology, ophthalmology, otolaryngology, psychiatry, neurology, toxicology, urology, geriatrics, orthopedics, women's health, preventive medicine, and palliative care
- Concise format, facilitating efficient use in any practice setting
- More than 1000 diseases and disorders
- Annual update on HIV/AIDS and other newly emerging infections.
- Specific disease prevention information
- Easy access to medication dosages, with trade names indexed and costs updated in each edition
- Recent references, with unique identifiers (PubMed, PMID numbers) for rapid downloading of article abstracts and, in some instances, full-text reference articles

CMDT Online (www.AccessMedicine.com) provides full electronic access to *CMDT 2017* plus expanded basic science information and ten additional chapters. The ten online-only chapters (Anti-Infective Chemotherapeutic & Antibiotic Agents, Fundamentals of Human Genetics & Genomics, Diagnostic Testing & Medical Decision Making, Information Technology in Patient Care, Integrative Medicine, Podiatric Disorders, Women's Health Issues, Lesbian & Bisexual Women's Health, Transgender Health & Disease Prevention, and Appendix: Therapeutic Drug Monitoring & Laboratory Reference Intervals, & Pharmacogenetic Testing) are available at www.AccessMedicine.com/CMDT. CMDT Online is updated throughout the year and includes an expanded, dedicated Media Gallery as well as links to related Web sites. Subscribers also receive access to Diagnosaurus with 1000+ differential diagnoses, *Guide to Diagnostic Tests, Quick Medical Diagnosis & Treatment,* and *CURRENT Practice Guidelines in Primary Care.*

ACKNOWLEDGMENTS

We wish to thank our associate authors for participating once again in the annual updating of this important book. We are especially grateful to Timothy G. Berger, MD, Patrick F. Fogarty, MD, J. Daniel Kelly, MD, Geoffrey A. Kerchner, MD, PhD, and Cynthia A. Luu, DPM who are leaving *CMDT* this year. We have all benefited from their clinical wisdom and commitment.

Many students and physicians also have contributed useful suggestions to this and previous editions, and we are grateful. We continue to welcome comments and recommendations for future editions in writing or via electronic mail. The editors' e-mail addresses are below and author e-mail addresses are included in the Authors section.

Maxine A. Papadakis, MD
Maxine.Papadakis@ucsf.edu
Stephen J. McPhee, MD
smcphee@medicine.ucsf.edu
Michael W. Rabow, MD
Mike.Rabow@ucsf.edu
San Francisco, California

From inability to let alone; from too much zeal for the new and contempt for what is old; from putting knowledge before wisdom, and science before art and cleverness before common sense; from treating patients as cases; and from making the cure of the disease more grievous than the endurance of the same, Good Lord, deliver us.

—Sir Robert Hutchison

Disease Prevention & Health Promotion

Michael Pignone MD, MPH[1]

René Salazar, MD

The medical interview serves several functions. It is used to collect information to assist in diagnosis (the "history" of the present illness), to understand patient values, to assess and communicate prognosis, to establish a therapeutic relationship, and to reach agreement with the patient about further diagnostic procedures and therapeutic options. It also serves as an opportunity to influence patient behavior, such as in motivational discussions about smoking cessation or medication adherence. Interviewing techniques that avoid domination by the clinician increase patient involvement in care and patient satisfaction. Effective clinician-patient communication and increased patient involvement can improve health outcomes.

► Patient Adherence

For many illnesses, treatment depends on difficult fundamental behavioral changes, including alterations in diet, taking up exercise, giving up smoking, cutting down drinking, and adhering to medication regimens that are often complex. Adherence is a problem in every practice; up to 50% of patients fail to achieve full adherence, and one-third never take their medicines. Many patients with medical problems, even those with access to care, do not seek appropriate care or may drop out of care prematurely. Adherence rates for short-term, self-administered therapies are higher than for long-term therapies and are inversely correlated with the number of interventions, their complexity and cost, and the patient's perception of overmedication.

As an example, in HIV-infected patients, adherence to antiretroviral therapy is a crucial determinant of treatment success. Studies have unequivocally demonstrated a close relationship between patient adherence and plasma HIV RNA levels, CD4 cell counts, and mortality. Adherence levels of more than 95% are needed to maintain virologic suppression. However, studies show that over 60% of patients are less than 90% adherent and that adherence tends to decrease over time.

Patient reasons for nonadherence include simple forgetfulness, being away from home, being busy, and changes in daily routine. Other reasons include psychiatric disorders (depression or substance abuse), uncertainty about the effectiveness of treatment, lack of knowledge about the consequences of poor adherence, regimen complexity, and treatment side effects.

Patients seem better able to take prescribed medications than to adhere to recommendations to change their diet, exercise habits, or alcohol intake or to perform various self-care activities (such as monitoring blood glucose levels at home). For short-term regimens, adherence to medications can be improved by giving clear instructions. Writing out advice to patients, including changes in medication, may be helpful. Because low functional health literacy is common (almost half of English-speaking US patients are unable to read and understand standard health education materials), other forms of communication—such as illustrated simple text, videotapes, or oral instructions—may be more effective. For non–English-speaking patients, clinicians and health care delivery systems can work to provide culturally and linguistically appropriate health services.

To help improve adherence to long-term regimens, clinicians can work with patients to reach agreement on the goals for therapy, provide information about the regimen, ensure understanding by using the "teach-back" method, counsel about the importance of adherence and how to organize medication-taking, reinforce self-monitoring, provide more convenient care, prescribe a simple dosage regimen for all medications (preferably one or two doses daily), suggest ways to help in remembering to take doses (time of day, mealtime, alarms) and to keep appointments, and provide ways to simplify dosing (medication boxes). Single-unit doses supplied in foil wrappers can increase adherence but should be avoided for patients who have difficulty opening them. Medication boxes with compartments (eg, Medisets) that are filled weekly are useful. Microelectronic devices can provide feedback to show patients whether they have taken doses as scheduled or to notify patients within a day if doses are skipped. Reminders, including cell phone text messages, are another effective means of encouraging adherence. The clinician can also enlist social support from family and friends, recruit

[1]Dr. Pignone is a member of the US Preventive Services Task Force (USPSTF). The views expressed in this chapter are his and Dr. Salazar's and not necessarily those of the USPSTF.

an adherence monitor, provide a more convenient care environment, and provide rewards and recognition for the patient's efforts to follow the regimen. Collaborative programs that utilize pharmacists to help ensure adherence are also effective.

Adherence is also improved when a trusting doctor-patient relationship has been established and when patients actively participate in their care. Clinicians can improve patient adherence by inquiring specifically about the behaviors in question. When asked, many patients admit to incomplete adherence with medication regimens, with advice about giving up cigarettes, or with engaging only in "safer sex" practices. Although difficult, sufficient time must be made available for communication of health messages.

Medication adherence can be assessed generally with a single question: "In the past month, how often did you take your medications as the doctor prescribed?" Other ways of assessing medication adherence include pill counts and refill records; monitoring serum, urine, or saliva levels of drugs or metabolites; watching for appointment nonattendance and treatment nonresponse; and assessing predictable drug effects, such as weight changes with diuretics or bradycardia from beta-blockers. In some conditions, even partial adherence, as with drug treatment of hypertension and diabetes mellitus, improves outcomes compared with nonadherence; in other cases, such as HIV antiretroviral therapy or treatment of tuberculosis, partial adherence may be worse than complete nonadherence.

▶ Guiding Principles of Care

Ethical decisions are often called for in medical practice, at both the "micro" level of the individual patient-clinician relationship and at the "macro" level of the allocation of resources. Ethical principles that guide the successful approach to diagnosis and treatment are honesty, beneficence, justice, avoidance of conflict of interest, and the pledge to do no harm. Increasingly, Western medicine involves patients in important decisions about medical care, eg, which colorectal screening test to obtain or which modality of therapy for breast cancer or how far to proceed with treatment of patients who have terminal illnesses (see Chapter 5).

The clinician's role does not end with diagnosis and treatment. The importance of the empathic clinician in helping patients and their families bear the burden of serious illness and death cannot be overemphasized. "To cure sometimes, to relieve often, and to comfort always" is a French saying as apt today as it was five centuries ago—as is Francis Peabody's admonition: "The secret of the care of the patient is in caring for the patient." Training to improve mindfulness and enhance patient-centered communication increases patient satisfaction and may also improve clinician satisfaction.

Choudhry NK et al. Improving adherence to therapy and clinical outcomes while containing costs: opportunities from the greater use of generic medications: best practice advice from the Clinical Guidelines Committee of the American College of Physicians. Ann Intern Med. 2016 Jan 5;164(1):41–9. [PMID: 26594818]

O'Connor PJ et al. Randomized trial of telephone outreach to improve medication adherence and metabolic control in adults with diabetes. Diabetes Care. 2014 Dec;37(12):3317–24. [PMID: 25315207]
Zillich AJ et al. A randomized, controlled pragmatic trial of telephonic medication therapy management to reduce hospitalization in home health patients. Health Serv Res. 2014 Oct;49(5):1537–54. [PMID: 24712335]

HEALTH MAINTENANCE & DISEASE PREVENTION

Preventive medicine can be categorized as primary, secondary, or tertiary. Primary prevention aims to remove or reduce disease risk factors (eg, immunization, giving up or not starting smoking). Secondary prevention techniques promote early detection of disease or precursor states (eg, routine cervical Papanicolaou screening to detect carcinoma or dysplasia of the cervix). Tertiary prevention measures are aimed at limiting the impact of established disease (eg, partial mastectomy and radiation therapy to remove and control localized breast cancer).

Tables 1–1 and 1–2 give leading causes of death in the United States and estimates of deaths from preventable causes. Mortality rates continue to decline overall, but recent data suggest increased rates of death, mainly from suicide and substance misuse, among less well-educated middle-aged white adults.

Many effective preventive services are underutilized, and few adults receive all of the most strongly recommended services. Several methods, including the use of provider or patient reminder systems (including interactive patient health records), reorganization of care environments, and possibly provision of financial incentives to clinicians (though this remains controversial), can increase

Table 1–1. Leading causes of death in the United States, 2013.

Category	Estimate
All causes	**2,596,993**
1. Diseases of the heart	611,105
2. Malignant neoplasms	584,881
3. Chronic lower respiratory diseases	149,205
4. Accidents (unintentional injuries)	130,557
5. Cerebrovascular diseases	128,978
6. Alzheimer disease	84,767
7. Diabetes mellitus	75,578
8. Influenza and pneumonia	56,979
9. Nephritis, nephrotic syndrome, and nephrosis	47,112
10. Intentional self-harm (suicide)	41,149

Data from National Center for Health Statistics 2015.

Table 1–2. Deaths from all causes attributable to common preventable risk factors. (Numbers given in the thousands.)

Risk Factor	Male (95% CI)	Female (95% CI)	Both Sexes (95% CI)
Tobacco smoking	248 (226–269)	219 (196–244)	467 (436–500)
High blood pressure	164 (153–175)	231 (213–249)	395 (372–414)
Overweight–obesity (high BMI)	114 (95–128)	102 (80–119)	216 (188–237)
Physical inactivity	88 (72–105)	103 (80–128)	191 (164–222)
High blood glucose	102 (80–122)	89 (69–108)	190 (163–217)
High LDL cholesterol	60 (42–70)	53 (44–59)	113 (94–124)
High dietary salt (sodium)	49 (46–51)	54 (50–57)	102 (97–107)
Low dietary omega-3 fatty acids (seafood)	45 (37–52)	39 (31–47)	84 (72–96)
High dietary trans fatty acids	46 (33–58)	35 (23–46)	82 (63–97)
Alcohol use	45 (32–49)	20 (17–22)	64 (51–69)
Low intake of fruits and vegetables	33 (23–45)	24 (15–36)	58 (44–74)
Low dietary polyunsaturated fatty acids (in place of saturated fatty acids)	9 (6–12)	6 (3–9)	15 (11–20)

BMI, body mass index; CI, confidence interval; LDL, low-density lipoprotein.
Note: Numbers of deaths cannot be summed across categories.
Used, with permission, from Danaei G et al. The preventable causes of death in the United States: comparative risk assessment of dietary, lifestyle, and metabolic risk factors. PLoS Med. 2009 Apr 28;6(4):e1000058.

utilization of preventive services, but such methods have not been widely adopted.

Case A et al. Rising morbidity and mortality in midlife among white non-Hispanic Americans in the 21st century. Proc Natl Acad Sci U S A. 2015 Dec 8;112(49):15078–83. [PMID: 26575631]

Forman-Hoffman VL et al. Disability status, mortality, and leading causes of death in the United States community population. Med Care. 2015 Apr;53(4):346–54. [PMID: 25719432]

Johnson NB et al; Centers for Disease Control and Prevention (CDC). CDC National Health Report: leading causes of morbidity and mortality and associated behavioral risk and protective factors—United States, 2005–2013. MMWR Surveill Summ. 2014 Oct 31;63(Suppl 4):3–27. [PMID: 25356673]

Kochanek KD et al. Mortality in the United States, 2013. NCHS Data Brief. 2014 Dec;(178):1–8. [PMID: 25549183]

Ma J et al. Temporal trends in mortality in the United States, 1969–2013. JAMA. 2015 Oct 27;314(16):1731–9. [PMID: 26505597]

Yoon PW et al; Centers for Disease Control and Prevention (CDC). Potentially preventable deaths from the five leading causes of death—United States, 2008–2010. MMWR Morb Mortal Wkly Rep. 2014 May 2;63(17):369–74. [PMID: 24785982]

PREVENTION OF INFECTIOUS DISEASES

Much of the decline in the incidence and fatality rates of infectious diseases is attributable to public health measures—especially immunization, improved sanitation, and better nutrition.

Immunization remains the best means of preventing many infectious diseases. Recommended immunization schedules for children and adolescents can be found online at http://www.cdc.gov/vaccines/schedules/hcp/child-adolescent.html, and the schedule for adults is outlined in Table 30–7. Substantial vaccine-preventable morbidity and mortality continue to occur among adults from vaccine-preventable diseases, such as hepatitis A, hepatitis B, influenza, and pneumococcal infections.

Evidence suggests annual **influenza vaccination** is safe and effective with potential benefit in all age groups, and the Advisory Committee on Immunization Practices (ACIP) recommends routine influenza vaccination for all persons aged 6 months and older, including all adults. When vaccine supply is limited, certain groups should be given priority, such as adults 50 years and older, individuals with chronic illness or immunosuppression, and pregnant women. An alternative high-dose inactivated vaccine is available for adults 65 years and older. Adults 65 years and older can receive either the standard-dose or high-dose vaccine, whereas those younger than 65 years should receive a standard-dose preparation.

The ACIP recommends two doses of measles, mumps, and rubella (MMR) vaccine in adults at high risk for exposure and transmission (eg, college students, health care workers). Otherwise, one dose is recommended for adults aged 18 years and older. Physician documentation of disease is not acceptable for evidence of MMR immunity.

Routine use of 13-valent pneumococcal conjugate vaccine (PCV13) is recommended among adults aged 65 and older. Individuals 65 years of age or older who have never received a pneumococcal vaccine should first receive PCV13 followed by a dose of 23-valent pneumococcal polysaccharide vaccine (PPSV23) 6–12 months later. Individuals who have received more than one dose of PPSV23 should receive a dose of PCV13 more than 1 year after the last dose of PPSV23 was administered.

The ACIP recommends routine use of a single dose of tetanus, diphtheria, and 5-component acellular pertussis vaccine (Tdap) for adults aged 19–64 years to replace the next booster dose of tetanus and diphtheria toxoids vaccine (Td). Due to increasing reports of pertussis in the United States, clinicians may choose to give Tdap to persons aged 65 years and older (particularly to those who might risk transmission to at-risk infants who are most susceptible to complications, including death), despite limited published data on the safety and efficacy of the vaccine in this age group.

Both **hepatitis A vaccine** and **immune globulin** provide protection against hepatitis A; however, administration of immune globulin may provide a modest benefit over vaccination in some settings. Hepatitis B vaccine administered as a three-dose series is recommended for all children aged 0–18 years and high-risk individuals (ie, health care workers, injection drug users, people with end-stage renal disease). Adults with diabetes are also at increased risk for hepatitis B infection, and in October 2011, the ACIP recommended **vaccination for hepatitis B** in diabetic patients aged 19–59 years. In diabetic persons aged 60 and older, hepatitis B vaccination should be considered.

Human papillomavirus (HPV) virus-like particle (VLP) vaccines have demonstrated effectiveness in preventing persistent HPV infections and thus may impact the rate of cervical intraepithelial neoplasia (CIN) II–III. The ACIP recommends routine HPV vaccination (with three doses of the 9-valent [9vHPV], 4-valent [4vHPV], or 2-valent [2vHPV] vaccine) for girls aged 11–12 years. The ACIP also recommends that all unvaccinated girls and women through age 26 years receive the three-dose HPV vaccination. Studies suggest that one dose of vaccine may be as effective as three. The ACIP recommends the routine vaccination with three doses of the 4vHPV or 9vHPV vaccine for boys aged 11 or 12 years, males through age 21 years, and men who have sex with men and immunocompromised men (including those with HIV infection) through age 26 years. Vaccination of males with HPV may lead to indirect protection of women by reducing transmission of HPV and may prevent anal intraepithelial neoplasia and squamous cell carcinoma in men who have sex with men. The use of HPV vaccine in the United States among women aged 18–26 years increased by 22% between 2008 and 2012; however, rates of immunization are low, especially among Latina women and those with limited access to care. Interventions addressing personal beliefs and system barriers to vaccinations may help address the slow adoption of this vaccine.

Persons traveling to countries where infections are endemic should take the precautions described in Chapter 30 and at http://wwwnc.cdc.gov/travel/destinations/list. Immunization registries—confidential, population-based, computerized information systems that collect vaccination data about all residents of a geographic area—can be used to increase and sustain high vaccination coverage.

The rate of tuberculosis in the United States has been declining since 1992. Two blood tests, which are not confounded by prior bacillus Calmette-Guérin (BCG) vaccination, have been developed to detect tuberculosis infection by measuring in vitro T-cell interferon-gamma release in response to two antigens (one, the enzyme-linked immunospot [ELISpot], [T-SPOT.TB], and the other, a quantitative ELISA [QuantiFERON-TBGold] test). These T-cell–based assays have an excellent specificity that is higher than tuberculin skin testing in BCG-vaccinated populations.

Treatment of tuberculosis poses a risk of hepatotoxicity and thus requires close monitoring of liver transaminases. Alanine aminotransferase (ALT) monitoring during the treatment of latent tuberculosis infection is recommended for certain individuals (preexisting liver disease, pregnancy, chronic alcohol consumption). ALT should be monitored in HIV-infected patients during treatment of tuberculosis disease and should be considered in patients over the age of 35. Symptomatic patients with an ALT elevation three times the upper limit of normal or asymptomatic patients with an elevation five times the upper limit of normal should be treated with a modified or alternative regimen.

The US Preventive Services Task Force (USPSTF) recommends behavioral counseling for adolescents and adults who are sexually active and at increased risk for sexually transmitted infections. Sexually active women aged 24 years or younger and older women who are at increased risk for infection should be screened for chlamydia.

HIV infection remains a major infectious disease problem in the world. The Centers for Disease Control and Prevention (CDC) recommends universal HIV screening of all patients aged 13–64, and the USPSTF recommends that clinicians screen adolescents and adults aged 15 to 65 years. Clinicians should integrate biomedical and behavioral approaches for HIV prevention. In addition to reducing sexual transmission of HIV, initiation of antiretroviral therapy reduces the risk for AIDS-defining events and death among patients with less immunologically advanced disease.

Since sexual contact is a common mode of transmission, primary prevention relies on eliminating high-risk sexual behavior by promoting abstinence, later onset of first sexual activity, decreased number of partners, and use of latex condoms. Daily preexposure prophylaxis with the fixed-dose combination of tenofovir 300 mg and emtricitabine 200 mg should be considered for people who are HIV-negative but at substantial risk for HIV infection. Studies of men who have sex with men suggest preexposure prophylaxis therapy is very effective in reducing the risk of contracting HIV. Patients taking preexposure prophylaxis should be encouraged to use other prevention strategies to maximally reduce their risk, such as consistent condom use and choosing less risky sexual behaviors (eg, oral sex). Postexposure prophylaxis is widely used after occupational and nonoccupational contact, and it has been estimated to reduce the risk of transmission by approximately 80%. Postexposure prophylaxis should be initiated within 72 hours of exposure.

In immunocompromised patients, live vaccines are contraindicated, but many killed or component vaccines are safe and recommended. *Asymptomatic* HIV-infected patients have not shown adverse consequences when given live MMR and influenza vaccinations as well as tetanus, hepatitis B, *H influenza* type b, and pneumococcal vaccinations—all should be given. However, if poliomyelitis immunization is required, the inactivated poliomyelitis vaccine is indicated. In *symptomatic* HIV-infected patients, live-virus vaccines, such as MMR, should generally be avoided, but annual influenza vaccination is safe.

Herpes zoster, caused by reactivation from previous varicella zoster virus infection, affects many older adults and people with immune system dysfunction. It can cause postherpetic neuralgia, a potentially debilitating chronic pain syndrome. A varicella vaccine is available for the prevention of herpes zoster. Several clinical trials have shown that this vaccine (Zostavax) is safe, elevates varicella zoster virus–specific cell-mediated immunity, and significantly reduces the incidence of herpes zoster and postherpetic neuralgia in persons older than 60 years. The ACIP recommends routine zoster vaccination, administered as a one-time subcutaneous dose (0.65 mL), of all persons aged 60 years or older. Persons who report a previous episode of zoster can be vaccinated; however, the vaccine is contraindicated in immunocompromised (primary or acquired) individuals. The durability of vaccine response and whether any booster vaccination is needed are still uncertain. Despite its availability, uptake of the vaccine remains low at 2–7% nationally. Financial barriers (cost, limited knowledge of reimbursement) have had a significant impact on its underutilization.

Centers for Disease Control and Prevention (CDC). Adult Immunization Schedules, United States, 2015. http://www.cdc.gov/vaccines/schedules/hcp/adult.html

Centers for Disease Control and Prevention (CDC). Birth-18 Years & "Catch-up" Immunization Schedules, United States, 2015. http://www.cdc.gov/vaccines/schedules/hcp/child-adolescent.html

Centers for Disease Control and Prevention (CDC). HIV/AIDS, 2015. http://www.cdc.gov/hiv/basics/index.html

Centers for Disease Control and Prevention (CDC). Pertussis outbreak trends, 2015. http://www.cdc.gov/pertussis/outbreaks/trends.html

Centers for Disease Control and Prevention (CDC). HIV/AIDS: preexposure prophylaxis for the prevention of HIV infection in the United States—2014. http://www.cdc.gov/hiv/pdf/guidelines/prepguidelines2014.pdf

Centers for Disease Control and Prevention (CDC). Reported tuberculosis in the United States, 2014. http://www.cdc.gov/tb/statistics/reports/2014/default.htm

Gagliardi AM et al. Vaccines for preventing herpes zoster in older adults. Cochrane Database Syst Rev. 2012 Oct 17; 10:CD008858. [PMID: 23076951]

Grohskopf LA et al. Prevention and control of influenza with vaccines: recommendations of the Advisory Committee on Immunization Practices, United States, 2015–16 Influenza Season. MMWR Morb Mortal Wkly Rep. 2015 Aug 7; 64(30);818–25. [PMID: 26247435]

Halperin BA et al. Universal tetanus, diphtheria, acellular pertussis (Tdap) vaccination of adults: what the Canadian public knows and wants to know. Vaccine. 2015 Nov 27;33(48): 6840–8. [PMID: 26392011]

Kreimer AR et al; Costa Rica Vaccine Trial and PATRICIA study groups. Efficacy of fewer than three doses of an HPV-16/18 AS04-adjuvanted vaccine: combined analysis of data from the Costa Rica Vaccine and PATRICIA trials. Lancet Oncol. 2015 Jul;16(7):775–86. [PMID: 26071347]

LeFevre ML. Behavioral counseling interventions to prevent sexually transmitted infections: U.S. Preventive Services Task Force recommendation statement. Ann Intern Med. 2014 Dec 16;161(12):894–901. [PMID: 25244227]

LeFevre ML. Screening for *Chlamydia* and gonorrhea: U.S. Preventive Services Task Force recommendation statement. Ann Intern Med. 2014 Dec 16;161(12):902–10. [PMID: 25243785]

MacDougall D et al. Universal tetanus, diphtheria, acellular pertussis (Tdap) vaccination of adults: what Canadian health care providers know and need to know. Hum Vaccin Immunother. 2015;11(9):2167–79. [PMID: 26090861]

Markowitz LE et al. Human papillomavirus vaccination: recommendations of the Advisory Committee on Immunization Practices (ACIP). MMWR Morb Mortal Wkly Rep Recomm Rep. 2014 Aug 29;63(RR-05):1–30. Erratum in: MMWR 2014 Dec 12;63(49):1182. [PMID: 25167164]

Marrazzo JM et al. HIV prevention in clinical care settings: 2014 recommendations of the International Antiviral Society-USA Panel. JAMA. 2014 Jul 23–30;312(4):390–409. Erratum in: JAMA. 2014 Aug 13;312(6):652. [PMID: 25038358]

McLean HQ et al; Centers for Disease Control and Prevention. Prevention of measles, rubella, congenital rubella syndrome, and mumps, 2013: summary recommendations of the Advisory Committee on Immunization Practices (ACIP). MMWR Recomm Rep. 2013 Jun 14;62(RR-04):1–34. Erratum in: MMWR Recomm Rep. 2015 Mar 13;64(9):259. [PMID: 23760231]

Moyer VA. Screening for HIV: U.S. Preventive Services Task Force Recommendation Statement. Ann Intern Med. 2013 Jul 2;159(1):51–60. [PMID: 23698354]

Sultan B et al. Current perspectives in HIV post-exposure prophylaxis. HIV AIDS (Auckl). 2014 Oct 24;6:147–58. [PMID: 25368534]

Thillai M et al. Interferon-gamma release assays for tuberculosis: current and future applications. Expert Rev Respir Med. 2014 Feb;8(1):67–78. [PMID: 24308653]

Thompson AE. JAMA patient page. Recognizing measles. JAMA. 2015 Apr 21;313(15):1584. [PMID: 25898066]

Tomczyk S et al; Centers for Disease Control and Prevention (CDC). Use of 13-valent pneumococcal conjugate vaccine and 23-valent pneumococcal polysaccharide vaccine among adults aged ≥ 65 years: recommendations of the Advisory Committee on Immunization Practices (ACIP). MMWR Morb Mortal Wkly Rep. 2014 Sep 19;63(37):822–5. [PMID: 25233284]

Williams WW et al; Centers for Disease Control and Prevention (CDC). Vaccination coverage among adults, excluding influenza vaccination—United States, 2013. MMWR Morb Mortal Wkly Rep. 2015 Feb 6;64(4):95–102. [PMID: 25654611]

Yan S et al. Early versus delayed antiretroviral therapy for HIV and tuberculosis co-infected patients: a systematic review and meta-analysis of randomized controlled trials. PLoS One. 2015 May 22;10(5):e0127645. [PMID: 26000446]

PREVENTION OF CARDIOVASCULAR DISEASE

Cardiovascular diseases, including coronary heart disease (CHD) and stroke, represent two of the most important causes of morbidity and mortality in developed countries. Several risk factors increase the risk for coronary disease and stroke. These risk factors can be divided into those that are modifiable (eg, lipid disorders, hypertension, cigarette smoking) and those that are not (eg, age, sex, family history of early coronary disease). Impressive declines in age-specific mortality rates from heart disease and stroke have been achieved in all age groups in North America during the past two decades, in large part through improvement of modifiable risk factors: reductions in cigarette smoking, improvements in lipid levels, and more

aggressive detection and treatment of hypertension. This section considers the role of screening for cardiovascular risk and the use of effective therapies to reduce such risk. Key recommendations for cardiovascular prevention are shown in Table 1–3. Guidelines encourage regular assessment of global cardiovascular risk in adults 40–79 years of age without known cardiovascular disease.

Table 1–3. Expert recommendations for cardiovascular risk prevention methods: US Preventive Services Task Force (USPSTF).[1]

Prevention Method	Recommendation/[Year Issued]
Screening for abdominal aortic aneurysm (AAA)	Recommends one-time screening for AAA by ultrasonography in men aged 65–75 years who have ever smoked. (B) Selectively offer screening for AAA in men aged 65–75 years who have never smoked. (C) Current evidence is insufficient to assess the balance of benefits and harms of screening for AAA in women aged 65–75 years who have ever smoked. (I) Recommends against routine screening for AAA in women who have never smoked. (D) [2014]
Aspirin use	Recommends the use of aspirin for men aged 45–79 years when the potential benefit due to a reduction in myocardial infarctions outweighs the potential harm due to an increase in gastrointestinal hemorrhage. (A) Recommends the use of aspirin for women aged 55–79 years when the potential benefit of a reduction in ischemic strokes outweighs the potential harm of an increase in gastrointestinal hemorrhage. (A) Current evidence is insufficient to assess the balance of benefits and harms of aspirin for cardiovascular disease prevention in men and women 80 years or older. (I) Recommends against the use of aspirin for stroke prevention in women younger than 55 years and for myocardial infarction prevention in men younger than 45 years. (D) [2009]
Blood pressure screening	Recommends screening for high blood pressure in adults aged 18 years and older. (A) [2015]
Serum lipid screening	Strongly recommends screening men aged 35 years and older for lipid disorders. (A) Recommends screening men aged 20–35 years for lipid disorders if they are at increased risk for coronary heart disease. (B) Strongly recommends screening women aged 45 years and older for lipid disorders if they are at increased risk for coronary heart disease. (A) Recommends screening women aged 20–45 years for lipid disorders if they are at increased risk for coronary heart disease. (B) No recommendation for or against routine screening for lipid disorders in men aged 20–35 years, or in women aged 20 years and older who are not at increased risk for coronary heart disease. (C) [2008]
Counseling about healthful diet and physical activity for cardiovascular disease (CVD) prevention	Recommends offering or referring adults who are overweight or obese and have additional CVD risk factors to intensive behavioral counseling interventions to promote a healthful diet and physical activity for CVD prevention. (B) [2014]
Screening for diabetes mellitus	Recommends screening for abnormal blood glucose as part of cardiovascular risk assessment in adults aged 40–70 years who are overweight or obese. Clinicians should offer or refer patients with abnormal blood glucose to intensive behavioral counseling interventions to promote a healthful diet and physical activity. (B) [2015]
Screening for smoking and counseling to promote cessation	Recommends that clinicians ask all adults about tobacco use, advise them to stop using tobacco, and provide behavioral interventions and US Food and Drug Administration (FDA)–approved pharmacotherapy for cessation to adults who use tobacco. (A) [2015]

[1]**Recommendation A:** The USPSTF strongly recommends that clinicians routinely provide the service to eligible patients. (The USPSTF found good evidence that the service improves important health outcomes and concludes that benefits substantially outweigh harms.)
Recommendation B: The USPSTF recommends that clinicians routinely provide the service to eligible patients. (The USPSTF found at least fair evidence that the service improves important health outcomes and concludes that benefits substantially outweigh harms.)
Recommendation C: The USPSTF makes no recommendation for or against routine provision of the service.
Recommendation D: The USPSTF recommends against routinely providing the service to asymptomatic patients. (The USPSTF found at least fair evidence that the service is ineffective or that harms outweigh benefits.)
Recommendation I: The USPSTF concludes that the evidence is insufficient to recommend for or against routinely providing the service.
http://www.uspreventiveservicestaskforce.org/BrowseRec/Index/browse-recommendations

Goff DC Jr et al. 2013 ACC/AHA Guideline on the assessment of cardiovascular risk: a report of the American College of Cardiology/American Heart Association Task Force on Practice Guidelines. Circulation. 2014 Jun 24;129(25 Suppl 2): S49–73. [PMID: 24222018]

Kavousi M et al. Comparison of application of the ACC/AHA guidelines, Adult Treatment Panel III guidelines, and European Society of Cardiology guidelines for cardiovascular disease prevention in a European cohort. JAMA. 2014 Apr 9; 311(14):1416–23. [PMID: 24681960]

Abdominal Aortic Aneurysm

One-time screening for abdominal aortic aneurysm (AAA) by ultrasonography in men aged 65–75 years is associated with a relative reduction in odds of AAA-related mortality of almost 50% and possibly a reduction in all-cause mortality (OR = 0.98, 95% CI, 0.97, 1.00). Women do not appear to benefit from screening, and most of the benefit in men appears to accrue among current or former smokers. Screening men aged 65 years and older is highly cost effective.

Guirguis-Blake JM et al. Ultrasonography screening for abdominal aortic aneurysms: a systematic evidence review for the U.S. Preventive Services Task Force. Ann Intern Med. 2014 Mar 4;160(5):321–9. [PMID: 24473919]

Søgaard R et al. Cost effectiveness of abdominal aortic aneurysm screening and rescreening in men in a modern context: evaluation of a hypothetical cohort using a decision analytical model. BMJ. 2012 Jul 5;345:e4276. [PMID: 22767630]

Cigarette Smoking

Cigarette smoking remains the most important cause of preventable morbidity and early mortality. In 2010, there were an estimated 6.3 million premature deaths in the world attributable to smoking and tobacco use. Cigarettes are responsible for one in every five deaths in the United States. From 2005 to 2009, more than 480,000 deaths per year (more than 278,000 in men and more than 201,000 in women) were attributable to smoking. Annual cost of smoking-related health care is approximately $130 billion in the United States, with another $150 billion in productivity losses. Fortunately, US smoking rates are declining; in 2014, 16.8% of US adults were smokers.

Nicotine is highly addictive, raises brain levels of dopamine, and produces withdrawal symptoms on discontinuation. Smokers die 5–8 years earlier than never-smokers. They have twice the risk of fatal heart disease; 10 times the risk of lung cancer; and several times the risk of cancers of the mouth, throat, esophagus, pancreas, kidney, bladder, and cervix. In the United States, over 90% of cases of COPD occur among current or former smokers.

In addition, over 41,000 deaths per year in the United States are attributable to environmental tobacco smoke.

Smoking cessation reduces the risks of death and of myocardial infarction in people with coronary artery disease; reduces the rate of death and acute myocardial infarction in patients who have undergone percutaneous coronary revascularization; lessens the risk of stroke; and is associated with improvement of COPD symptoms. On average, women smokers who quit smoking by age 35 add about 3 years to their life expectancy, and men add more than 2 years to theirs. Smoking cessation can increase life expectancy even for those who stop after the age of 65.

Although tobacco use constitutes the most serious common medical problem, it is undertreated. Almost 40% of smokers attempt to quit each year, but only 4% are successful. Persons whose clinicians advise them to quit are 1.6 times as likely to attempt quitting. Over 70% of smokers see a physician each year, but only 20% of them receive any medical quitting advice or assistance.

Factors associated with successful cessation include having a rule against smoking in the home, being older, and having greater education. Several effective interventions are available to promote smoking cessation, including counseling, pharmacotherapy, and combinations of the two. The five steps for helping smokers quit are summarized in Table 1–4.

Common elements of supportive smoking cessation treatments are reviewed in Table 1–5. A system should be implemented to identify smokers, and advice to quit should be tailored to the patient's level of readiness to change. All patients trying to quit should be offered pharmacotherapy except those with medical contraindications, women who are pregnant or breast-feeding, and adolescents. Weight gain occurs in most patients (80%) following smoking cessation. Average weight gain is 2 kg, but for some (10–15%), major weight gain—over 13 kg—may occur. Planning for the possibility of weight gain, and means of mitigating it, may help with maintenance of cessation.

Several pharmacologic therapies have been shown to be effective in promoting cessation. Nicotine replacement therapy doubles the chance of successful quitting. The nicotine patch, gum, and lozenges are available over the counter and nicotine nasal spray and inhalers by prescription. The sustained-release antidepressant drug bupropion (150–300 mg/day orally) is an effective smoking cessation agent and is associated with minimal weight gain, although seizures are a contraindication. It acts by boosting brain levels of dopamine and norepinephrine, mimicking the effect of nicotine. More recently, varenicline, a partial nicotinic acetylcholine-receptor agonist, has been shown to improve cessation rates; however, its adverse effects, particularly its effects on mood, are not completely understood and warrant careful consideration. No single pharmacotherapy is clearly more effective than others, so patient preferences and data on adverse effects should be taken into account in selecting a treatment. Combination therapy is more effective than a single pharmacologic modality. Recently, e-cigarettes have become popular. Their efficacy in smoking cessation, however, has not been well evaluated, and some users may find them addictive.

Clinicians should not show disapproval of patients who failed to stop smoking or who are not ready to make a quit attempt. Thoughtful advice that emphasizes the benefits of cessation and recognizes common barriers to success can increase motivation to quit and quit rates. An intercurrent illness or hospitalization may motivate even the most addicted smoker to quit.

Table 1–4. Actions and strategies for the primary care clinician to help patients quit smoking.

Action	Strategies for Implementation
Step 1. Ask—Systematically Identify All Tobacco Users at Every Visit	
Implement an officewide system that ensures that for *every* patient at *every* clinic visit, tobacco-use status is queried and documented[1]	Expand the vital signs to include tobacco use. Data should be collected by the health care team. The action should be implemented using preprinted progress note paper that includes the expanded vital signs, a vital signs stamp or, for computerized records, an item assessing tobacco-use status. Alternatives to the vital signs stamp are to place tobacco-use status stickers on all patients' charts or to indicate smoking status using computerized reminder systems.
Step 2. Advise—Strongly Urge All Smokers to Quit	
In a clear, strong, and personalized manner, urge every smoker to quit	Advice should be **Clear:** "I think it is important for you to quit smoking now, and I will help you. Cutting down while you are ill is not enough." **Strong:** "As your clinician, I need you to know that quitting smoking is the most important thing you can do to protect your current and future health." **Personalized:** Tie smoking to current health or illness and/or the social and economic costs of tobacco use, motivational level/readiness to quit, and the impact of smoking on children and others in the household. Encourage clinic staff to reinforce the cessation message and support the patient's quit attempt.
Step 3. Attempt—Identify Smokers Willing to Make a Quit Attempt	
Ask every smoker if he or she is willing to make a quit attempt at this time	If the patient is willing to make a quit attempt at this time, provide assistance (see step 4). If the patient prefers a more intensive treatment or the clinician believes more intensive treatment is appropriate, refer the patient to interventions administered by a smoking cessation specialist and follow up with him or her regarding quitting (see step 5). If the patient clearly states he or she is not willing to make a quit attempt at this time, provide a motivational intervention.
Step 4. Assist—Aid the Patient in Quitting	
A. Help the patient with a quit plan	**Set a quit date.** Ideally, the quit date should be within 2 weeks, taking patient preference into account. **Help the patient prepare for quitting.** The patient must: **Inform** family, friends, and coworkers of quitting and request understanding and support. **Prepare the environment** by removing cigarettes from it. Prior to quitting, the patient should avoid smoking in places where he or she spends a lot of time (eg, home, car). **Review** previous quit attempts. What helped? What led to relapse? **Anticipate** challenges to the planned quit attempt, particularly during the critical first few weeks.
B. Encourage nicotine replacement therapy except in special circumstances	Encourage the use of the nicotine patch or nicotine gum therapy for smoking cessation.
C. Give key advice on successful quitting	**Abstinence:** Total abstinence is essential. Not even a single puff after the quit date. **Alcohol:** Drinking alcohol is highly associated with relapse. Those who stop smoking should review their alcohol use and consider limiting or abstaining from alcohol use during the quit process. **Other smokers in the household:** The presence of other smokers in the household, particularly a spouse, is associated with lower success rates. Patients should consider quitting with their significant others and/or developing specific plans to maintain abstinence in a household where others still smoke.
D. Provide supplementary materials	**Source:** Federal agencies, including the National Cancer Institute and the Agency for Health Care Policy and Research; nonprofit agencies (American Cancer Society, American Lung Association, American Heart Association); or local or state health departments. **Selection concerns:** The material must be culturally, racially, educationally, and age appropriate for the patient. **Location:** Readily available in every clinic office.

(continued)

Table 1–4. Actions and strategies for the primary care clinician to help patients quit smoking. (continued)

Action	Strategies for Implementation
Step 5. Arrange—Schedule Follow-Up Contact	
Schedule follow-up contact, either in person or via telephone	**Timing:** Follow-up contact should occur soon after the quit date, preferably during the first week. A second follow-up contact is recommended within the first month. Schedule further follow-up contacts as indicated. **Actions during follow-up:** Congratulate success. If smoking occurred, review the circumstances and elicit recommitment to total abstinence. Remind the patient that a lapse can be used as a learning experience and is not a sign of failure. Identify the problems already encountered and anticipate challenges in the immediate future. Assess nicotine replacement therapy use and problems. Consider referral to a more intense or specialized program.

[1]Repeated assessment is not necessary in the case of the adult who has never smoked or not smoked for many years and for whom the information is clearly documented in the medical record.

Adapted and reproduced, with permission, from The Agency for Health Care Policy and Research. Smoking Cessation Clinical Practice Guideline. JAMA. 1996 Apr 24; 275(16):1270–80. Copyright © 1996 American Medical Association. All rights reserved.

Individualized or group counseling is very cost effective, even more so than in treating hypertension. Smoking cessation counseling by telephone ("quitlines") and text messaging–based interventions have both proved effective. An additional strategy is to recommend that any smoking take place out of doors to limit the effects of passive smoke on housemates and coworkers. This can lead to smoking reduction and quitting.

The clinician's role in smoking cessation is summarized in Tables 1–4 and 1-5. Public policies, including higher cigarette taxes and more restrictive public smoking laws, have also been shown to encourage cessation, as have financial incentives directed to patients.

Table 1–5. Common elements of supportive smoking treatments.

Component	Examples
Encouragement of the patient in the quit attempt	Note that effective cessation treatments are now available. Note that half the people who have *ever* smoked have now quit. Communicate belief in the patient's ability to quit.
Communication of caring and concern	Ask how the patient feels about quitting. Directly express concern and a willingness to help. Be open to the patient's expression of fears of quitting, difficulties experienced, and ambivalent feelings.
Encouragement of the patient to talk about the quitting process	Ask about: Reasons that the patient wants to quit. Difficulties encountered while quitting. Success the patient has achieved. Concerns or worries about quitting.
Provision of basic information about smoking and successful quitting	Inform the patient about: The nature and time course of withdrawal. The addictive nature of smoking. The fact that any smoking (even a single puff) increases the likelihood of full relapse.

Adapted, with permission, from The Agency for Health Care Policy and Research. Smoking Cessation Clinical Practice Guideline. JAMA. 1996 Apr 24; 275(16):1270–80. Copyright © 1996 American Medical Association. All rights reserved.

Cahill K et al. Pharmacological interventions for smoking cessation: an overview and network meta-analysis. Cochrane Database Syst Rev. 2013 May 31;5:CD009329. [PMID: 23728690]

Holford TR et al. Tobacco control and the reduction in smoking-related premature deaths in the United States, 1964–2012. JAMA. 2014 Jan 8;311(2):164–71. [PMID: 24399555]

Jamal A et al. Current cigarette smoking among adults—United States, 2005–2014. MMWR Morb Mortal Wkly Rep. 2015 Nov 13;64(44):1233–40. [PMID: 26562061]

Lindson-Hawley N et al. Reduction versus abrupt cessation in smokers who want to quit. Cochrane Database Syst Rev. 2012 Nov 14;11:CD008033. [PMID: 23152252]

Martín Cantera C et al. Effectiveness of multicomponent interventions in primary healthcare settings to promote continuous smoking cessation in adults: a systematic review. BMJ Open. 2015 Oct 1;5(10):e008807. [PMID: 26428333]

National Center for Chronic Disease Prevention and Health Promotion (US) Office on Smoking and Health. The Health Consequences of Smoking—50 Years of Progress: A Report of the Surgeon General. Atlanta (GA): Centers for Disease Control and Prevention (US); 2014. [PMID: 24455788]

Rahman MA et al. E-cigarettes and smoking cessation: evidence from a systematic review and meta-analysis. PLoS One. 2015 Mar 30;10(3):e0122544. [PMID: 25822251]

Rigotti NA et al. Sustained care intervention and postdischarge smoking cessation among hospitalized adults: a randomized clinical trial. JAMA. 2014 Aug 20;312(7):719–28. [PMID: 25138333]

Rostron BL et al. Estimation of cigarette smoking-attributable morbidity in the United States. JAMA Intern Med. 2014 Dec;174(12):1922–8. [PMID: 25317719]

Stead LF et al. Combined pharmacotherapy and behavioural interventions for smoking cessation. Cochrane Database Syst Rev. 2012 Oct 17;10:CD008286. [PMID: 23076944]

Sugerman DT. JAMA patient page. e-Cigarettes. JAMA. 2014 Jan 8;311(2):212. [PMID: 24399571]

Lipid Disorders (see Chapter 28)

Higher low-density lipoprotein (LDL) cholesterol concentrations and lower high-density lipoprotein (HDL) levels are associated with an increased risk of CHD. Cholesterol-lowering therapy reduces the relative risk of CHD events, with the degree of reduction proportional to the reduction in LDL cholesterol achieved. The absolute benefits of screening for—and treating—abnormal lipid levels depend on the presence and level of other cardiovascular risk factors, including hypertension, diabetes mellitus, smoking, age, and gender. If other risk factors are present, cardiovascular risk is higher and the potential benefits of therapy are greater. Patients with known cardiovascular disease are at higher risk and have larger benefits from reduction in LDL cholesterol.

Evidence for the effectiveness of statin-type drugs is better than for the other classes of lipid-lowering agents or dietary changes specifically for improving lipid levels. Multiple large, randomized, placebo-controlled trials have demonstrated important reductions in total mortality, major coronary events, and strokes with lowering levels of LDL cholesterol by statin therapy for patients with known cardiovascular disease. Statins also reduce cardiovascular events for patients with diabetes mellitus. For patients with no previous history of cardiovascular events or diabetes, meta-analyses have shown important reductions of cardiovascular events.

Guidelines for therapy are discussed in Chapter 28.

Cholesterol Treatment Trialists' (CTT) Collaborators. The effects of lowering LDL cholesterol with statin therapy in people at low risk of vascular disease: meta-analysis of individual data from 27 randomised trials. Lancet. 2012 Aug 11; 380(9841):581–90. [PMID: 22607822]

Mitchell AP et al. Statin cost effectiveness in primary prevention: a systematic review of the recent cost-effectiveness literature in the United States. BMC Res Notes. 2012 Jul 24;5:373. [PMID: 22828389]

Pencina MJ et al. Application of new cholesterol guidelines to a population-based sample. N Engl J Med. 2014 Apr 10;370(15):1422–31. [PMID: 24645848]

Taylor F et al. Statins for the primary prevention of cardiovascular disease. Cochrane Database Syst Rev. 2013 Jan 31; 1:CD004816. [PMID: 23440795]

Hypertension (see Chapter 11)

Over 67 million adults in the United States have hypertension, representing 29% of the adult US population. Hypertension in nearly half of these adults is not controlled (ie, less than 140/90 mm Hg). Among those whose hypertension is not well controlled, nearly 40% are unaware of their elevated blood pressure; almost 16% are aware but not being treated; and 45% are being treated but the hypertension is not controlled. In every adult age group, higher values of systolic and diastolic blood pressure carry greater risks of stroke and heart failure. Systolic blood pressure is a better predictor of morbid events than diastolic blood pressure. Home monitoring is better correlated with target organ damage than clinic-based values. Clinicians can apply specific blood pressure criteria, such as those of the Joint National Committee, along with consideration of the patient's cardiovascular risk and personal values, to decide at what levels treatment should be considered in individual cases. A new trial suggests additional benefit from more intensive blood pressure control (goal systolic blood pressure of 120 mm Hg) in patients at higher risk.

Primary prevention of hypertension can be accomplished by strategies aimed at both the general population and special high-risk populations. The latter include persons with high-normal blood pressure or a family history of hypertension, blacks, and individuals with various behavioral risk factors, such as physical inactivity; excessive consumption of salt, alcohol, or calories; and deficient intake of potassium. Effective interventions for primary prevention of hypertension include reduced sodium and alcohol consumption, weight loss, and regular exercise. Potassium supplementation lowers blood pressure modestly, and a diet high in fresh fruits and vegetables and low in fat, red meats, and sugar-containing beverages also reduces blood pressure. Interventions of unproven efficacy include pill supplementation of potassium, calcium, magnesium, fish oil, or fiber; macronutrient alteration; and stress management.

Improved identification and treatment of hypertension is a major cause of the recent decline in stroke deaths as well as the reduction in incidence of heart failure–related hospitalizations. Because hypertension is usually asymptomatic, screening is strongly recommended to identify patients for treatment. Despite strong recommendations in favor of screening and treatment, hypertension control remains suboptimal. An intervention that included patient education and provider education was more effective than provider education alone in achieving control of hypertension, suggesting the benefits of patient participation; another trial found that home monitoring combined with telephone-based nurse support was more effective than home monitoring alone for blood pressure control. Pharmacologic management of hypertension is discussed in Chapter 11.

Egan BM et al. The growing gap in hypertension control between insured and uninsured adults: National Health and Nutrition Examination Survey 1988 to 2010. Hypertension. 2014 Nov;64(5):997–1004. [PMID: 25185135]

James PA et al. 2014 evidence-based guideline for the management of high blood pressure in adults: report from the panel members appointed to the Eighth Joint National Committee (JNC 8). JAMA. 2014 Feb 5;311(5):507–20. Erratum in: JAMA. 2014 May 7;311(17):1809. [PMID: 24352797]

SPRINT Research Group; Wright JT Jr et al. A randomized trial of intensive versus standard blood-pressure control. N Engl J Med. 2015 Nov 26;373(22):2103–16. [PMID: 26551272]

Yoon SS et al. Trends in blood pressure among adults with hypertension: United States, 2003 to 2012. Hypertension. 2015 Jan;65(1):54–61. [PMID: 25399687]

Chemoprevention

Regular use of low-dose aspirin (81–325 mg) can reduce the incidence of myocardial infarction in men (see Chapter 10). Low-dose aspirin reduces incidence of stroke but not myocardial infarction in middle-aged women (see Chapter 24). Based on its ability to prevent cardiovascular events, aspirin use appears cost-effective for men and women who are at increased cardiovascular risk, which can be defined as a 10-year risk over 10%. Results from a meta-analysis suggest that aspirin may also reduce the risk of death from several common types of cancer (colorectal, esophageal, gastric, breast, prostate, and possibly lung).

Nonsteroidal anti-inflammatory drugs may reduce the incidence of colorectal adenomas and polyps but may also increase heart disease and gastrointestinal bleeding, and thus are not recommended for colon cancer prevention in average-risk patients.

Antioxidant vitamin (vitamin E, vitamin C, and beta-carotene) supplementation produced no significant reductions in the 5-year incidence of—or mortality from—vascular disease, cancer, or other major outcomes in high-risk individuals with coronary artery disease, other occlusive arterial disease, or diabetes mellitus.

Guirguis-Blake JM et al. Aspirin for the primary prevention of cardiovascular events: a systematic evidence review for the U.S. Preventive Services Task Force [Internet]. 2015 Sep. http://www.ncbi.nlm.nih.gov/books/NBK321623/ [PMID: 26491760]

Moyer VA et al. Vitamin, mineral, and multivitamin supplements for the primary prevention of cardiovascular disease and cancer: U.S. Preventive Services Task Force recommendation statement. Ann Intern Med. 2014 Apr 15;160(8):558–64. [PMID: 24566474]

Sutcliffe P et al. Aspirin for prophylactic use in the primary prevention of cardiovascular disease and cancer: a systematic review and overview of reviews. Health Technol Assess. 2013 Sep;17(43):1–253. [PMID: 24074752]

PREVENTION OF OSTEOPOROSIS

See Chapters 26 and 42.

Osteoporosis, characterized by low bone mineral density, is common and associated with an increased risk of fracture. The lifetime risk of an osteoporotic fracture is approximately 50% for women and 30% for men. Osteoporotic fractures can cause significant pain and disability. As such, research has focused on means of preventing osteoporosis and related fractures. Primary prevention strategies include calcium supplementation, vitamin D supplementation, and exercise programs. The effectiveness of calcium and vitamin D for fracture prevention remain controversial, particularly in non-institutionalized individuals.

Screening for osteoporosis on the basis of low bone mineral density is also recommended for women over age 65, based on indirect evidence that screening can identify women with low bone mineral density and that treatment of women with low bone density with bisphosphonates is effective in reducing fractures. However, real-world adherence to pharmacologic therapy for osteoporosis is low: one-third to one-half of patients do not take their medication as directed. The effectiveness of screening for osteoporosis in younger women and in men has not been established. Concern has been raised that bisphosphonates may increase the risk of certain types of fractures and osteonecrosis of the jaw, making consideration of the benefits and risks of therapy important when considering screening.

Crandall CJ et al. Comparative effectiveness of pharmacologic treatments to prevent fractures: an updated systematic review. Ann Intern Med. 2014 Nov 18;161(10):711–23. [PMID: 25199883]

Golob AL et al. Osteoporosis: screening, prevention, and management. Med Clin North Am. 2015 May;99(3):587–606. [PMID: 25841602]

Moyer VA et al. Vitamin D and calcium supplementation to prevent fractures in adults: U.S. Preventive Services Task Force recommendation statement. Ann Intern Med. 2013 May 7;158(9):691–6. [PMID: 23440163]

PREVENTION OF PHYSICAL INACTIVITY

Lack of sufficient physical activity is the second most important contributor to preventable deaths, trailing only tobacco use. A sedentary lifestyle has been linked to 28% of deaths from leading chronic diseases. Worldwide, approximately 30% of adults are physically inactive. Inactivity rates are higher in women, those from high-income countries (such as the Americas), and increase with age. Among teens aged 13–15, 80% report doing fewer than 60 minutes of physical activity of moderate to vigorous intensity per day, and boys are more active than girls.

The US Department of Health and Human Services and the CDC recommend that adults and older adults engage in 150 minutes of moderate-intensity (such as brisk walking) or 75 minutes of vigorous-intensity (such as jogging or running) aerobic activity or an equivalent mix of moderate- and vigorous-intensity aerobic activity each week. In addition to activity recommendations, the CDC recommends activities to strengthen all major muscle groups (abdomen, arms, back, chest, hips, legs, and shoulders) at least twice a week.

Patients who engage in regular moderate to vigorous exercise have a lower risk of myocardial infarction, stroke, hypertension, hyperlipidemia, type 2 diabetes mellitus, diverticular disease, and osteoporosis. Evidence supports the recommended guidelines of 30 minutes of moderate physical activity on most days of the week in both the primary and secondary prevention of CHD.

In longitudinal cohort studies, individuals who report higher levels of leisure-time physical activity are less likely to gain weight. Conversely, individuals who are overweight are less likely to stay active. However, at least 60 minutes of daily moderate-intensity physical activity may be necessary to maximize weight loss and prevent significant weight regain. Moreover, adequate levels of physical activity appear to be important for the prevention of weight gain and the development of obesity. Physical activity also appears to have an independent effect on health-related outcomes, such as development of type 2 diabetes mellitus in patients with impaired glucose tolerance when compared with body weight, suggesting that adequate levels of activity may counteract the negative influence of body weight on health outcomes.

Physical activity can be incorporated into any person's daily routine. For example, the clinician can advise a patient to take the stairs instead of the elevator, to walk or bike instead of driving, to do housework or yard work, to get off the bus one or two stops earlier and walk the rest of the way, to park at the far end of the parking lot, or to walk during the lunch hour. The basic message should be the more the better, and anything is better than nothing.

To be more effective in counseling about exercise, clinicians can also incorporate motivational interviewing techniques, adopt a whole-practice approach (eg, use practice nurses to assist), and establish linkages with community agencies. Clinicians can incorporate the "5 As" approach:

1. Ask (identify those who can benefit).
2. Assess (current activity level).
3. Advise (individualize plan).
4. Assist (provide a written exercise prescription and support material).
5. Arrange (appropriate referral and follow-up).

Such interventions have a moderate effect on self-reported physical activity and cardiorespiratory fitness, even if they do not always help patients achieve a predetermined level of physical activity. In their counseling, clinicians should advise patients about both the benefits and risks of exercise, prescribe an exercise program appropriate for each patient, and provide advice to help prevent injuries and cardiovascular complications.

Behavioral change interventions have been proven effective in increasing physical activity in sedentary older women, although evidence is lacking to support the use of pedometers to increase physical activity in this population. Although primary care providers regularly ask patients about physical activity and advise them with verbal counseling, few providers provide written prescriptions or perform fitness assessments. Tailored interventions may potentially help increase physical activity in individuals. Exercise counseling with a prescription, eg, for walking at either a hard intensity or a moderate intensity with a high frequency, can produce significant long-term improvements in cardiorespiratory fitness. To be effective, exercise prescriptions must include recommendations on type, frequency, intensity, time, and progression of exercise and must follow disease-specific guidelines.

Several factors influence physical activity behavior, including personal, social (eg, family and work), and environmental (eg, access to exercise facilities and well-lit parks). Walkable neighborhoods around workplaces support physical activity such as walking and bicycling. Broad-based interventions targeting various factors are often the most successful, and interventions to promote physical activity are more effective when health agencies work with community partners, such as schools, businesses, and health care organizations. Enhanced community awareness through mass media campaigns, school-based strategies, and policy approaches are proven strategies to increase physical activity.

Adlakha D et al. Home and workplace built environment supports for physical activity. Am J Prev Med. 2015 Jan;48(1): 104–7. [PMID: 25442233]

Centers for Disease Control and Prevention (CDC). How much physical activity do adults need? 2015 Jun 4. http://www.cdc.gov/physicalactivity/basics/adults/index.htm

Hallal PC et al; Lancet Physical Activity Series Working Group. Global physical activity levels: surveillance progress, pitfalls, and prospects. Lancet. 2012 Jul 21;380(9838):247–57. [PMID: 22818937]

Hunter GR et al. Combined aerobic and strength training and energy expenditure in older women. Med Sci Sports Exerc. 2013 Jul;45(7):1386–93. [PMID: 23774582]

Orrow G et al. Effectiveness of physical activity promotion based in primary care: systematic review and meta-analysis of randomised controlled trials. BMJ. 2012 Mar 26;344:e1389. [PMID: 22451477]

PREVENTION OF OVERWEIGHT & OBESITY

Obesity is now a true epidemic and public health crisis that both clinicians and patients must face. Normal body weight is defined as a body mass index (BMI), calculated as the weight in kilograms divided by the height in meters squared, of less than 25; overweight is defined as a BMI = 25.0–29.9, and obesity as a BMI greater than 30. Between 1980 and 2013, there was an 8% increase worldwide in the proportion of men and women with a BMI greater than 25. The most recent national data reveal that one-third of adults in the United States are obese, and prevalence rates are higher in blacks and Hispanics compared to non-Hispanic whites.

Risk assessment of the overweight and obese patient begins with determination of BMI, waist circumference for those with a BMI of 35 or less, presence of comorbid conditions, and a fasting blood glucose and lipid panel. Obesity is clearly associated with type 2 diabetes mellitus, hypertension, hyperlipidemia, cancer, osteoarthritis, cardiovascular disease, obstructive sleep apnea, and asthma. In addition, almost one-quarter of the US population currently has the metabolic syndrome.

Obesity is associated with a higher all-cause mortality rate. Data suggest an increase among those with grades 2 and 3 obesity (BMI more than 35); however, the impact on all-cause mortality among overweight (BMI 25–30) and grade 1 obesity (BMI 30–35) is questionable. Persons with a BMI 40 or higher have death rates from cancers that are 52% higher for men and 62% higher for women than the rates in men and women of normal weight. Significant trends of increasing risk of death with higher BMIs are observed for cancers of the stomach and prostate in men and for cancers of the breast, uterus, cervix, and ovary in women, and for cancers of the esophagus, colon and rectum, liver, gallbladder, pancreas, and kidney, non-Hodgkin lymphoma, and multiple myeloma in both men and women.

Prevention of overweight and obesity involves both increasing physical activity and dietary modification to reduce caloric intake. Adequate levels of physical activity appear to be important for the prevention of weight gain and the development of obesity. Despite this, only 49% of Americans are physically active at a moderate level and 20% at a more vigorous level. In addition, only 3% of Americans meet four of the five USDA recommendations for the intake of grains, fruits, vegetables, dairy products, and meat. Only one of four Americans eats the recommended five or more fruits and vegetables per day.

Clinicians can help guide patients to develop personalized eating plans to reduce energy intake, particularly by recognizing the contributions of fat, concentrated carbohydrates, and large portion sizes (see Chapter 29). Patients typically underestimate caloric content, especially when consuming food away from home. Providing patients with caloric and nutritional information may help address the current obesity epidemic. To prevent the long-term chronic disease sequelae of overweight and obesity, clinicians must work with patients to modify other risk factors, eg, by smoking cessation (see above) and strict blood pressure and glycemic control (see Chapters 11 and 27).

Lifestyle modification, including diet, physical activity, and behavior therapy, has been shown to induce clinically significant weight loss. Other treatment options for obesity include pharmacotherapy and surgery (see Chapter 29). In overweight and obese persons, at least 60 minutes of moderate- to high-intensity physical activity per day may be necessary to maximize weight loss and prevent significant weight regain. Counseling interventions or pharmacotherapy can produce modest (3–5 kg) sustained weight loss over 6–12 months. Counseling appears to be most effective when intensive and combined with behavioral therapy. Pharmacotherapy appears safe in the short term; long-term safety is still not established. Lorcaserin, a selective 5-hydroxytryptamine (5-HT) (2C) agonist, has been shown to reduce body weight through a reduction of energy intake without influencing energy expenditure. It was approved by the US Food and Drug Administration (FDA) for adults with a BMI 30 or higher or adults with a BMI 27 or higher who have at least one obesity-related condition, such as hypertension, type 2 diabetes mellitus, or hypercholesterolemia.

Finally, clinicians seem to share a general perception that almost no one succeeds in long-term maintenance of weight loss. However, research demonstrates that approximately 20% of overweight individuals are successful at long-term weight loss (defined as losing 10% or more of initial body weight and maintaining the loss for 1 year or longer). National Weight Control Registry members who lost an average of 33 kg and maintained the loss for more than 5 years have provided useful information about how to maintain weight loss. Members report engaging in high levels of physical activity (approximately 60 min/day), eating a low-calorie, low-fat diet, eating breakfast regularly, self-monitoring weight, and maintaining a consistent eating pattern from weekdays to weekends.

Clinicians must work to identify and provide the best prevention and treatment strategies for patients who are overweight and obese. Clinician advice on weight loss can have a significant impact on patient attempts to adjust weight-related behaviors. Unfortunately, many clinicians are poorly prepared to address obesity. Clinician bias and lack of training in behavior-change strategies impair the care of obese patients. Strategies to address these issues should be incorporated into innovative treatment and care-delivery strategies.

Dietz WH et al. Management of obesity: improvement of health-care training and systems for prevention and care. Lancet. 2015 Jun 20;385(9986):2521–33. [PMID: 25703112]

Flegal KM et al. Association of all-cause mortality with overweight and obesity using standard body mass index categories: a systematic review and meta-analysis. JAMA. 2013 Jan 2; 309(1):71–82. [PMID: 23280227]

Guth E. JAMA patient page. Healthy weight loss. JAMA. 2014 Sep 3;312(9):974. [PMID: 25182116]

Jin J. JAMA patient page. Obesity and the heart. JAMA. 2013 Nov 20;310(19):2113. [PMID: 24240948]

Ng M et al. Global, regional, and national prevalence of overweight and obesity in children and adults during 1980–2013: a systematic analysis for the Global Burden of Disease Study 2013. Lancet. 2014 Aug 30;384(9945):766–81. Erratum in: Lancet. 2014 Aug 30;384(9945):746. [PMID: 24880830]

Ogden CL et al. Prevalence of childhood and adult obesity in the United States, 2011–2012. JAMA. 2014 Feb 26;311(8):806–14. [PMID: 24570244]

Rose SA et al. Physician weight loss advice and patient weight loss behavior change: a literature review and meta-analysis of survey data. Int J Obes (Lond). 2013 Jan;37(1):118–28. [PMID: 22450855]

CANCER PREVENTION

▶ Primary Prevention

Cancer mortality rates continue to decrease in the United States; part of this decrease results from reductions in tobacco use, since cigarette smoking is the most important preventable cause of cancer. Primary prevention of skin cancer consists of restricting exposure to ultraviolet light by wearing appropriate clothing and use of sunscreens. In the past two decades, there has been a threefold increase in the incidence of squamous cell carcinoma and a fourfold increase in melanoma in the United States. Persons who engage in regular physical exercise and avoid obesity have lower rates of breast and colon cancer. Prevention of occupationally induced cancers involves minimizing exposure to carcinogenic substances, such as asbestos, ionizing radiation, and benzene compounds. Chemoprevention has been widely studied for primary cancer prevention (see above Chemoprevention section and Chapter 39). Use of tamoxifen, raloxifene, and aromatase inhibitors for breast cancer prevention is discussed in Chapters 17 and 39. Hepatitis B vaccination can prevent hepatocellular carcinoma (HCC), and screening and vaccination programs may be cost effective and useful in preventing HCC in high-risk groups, such as Asians and Pacific Islanders. The use of HPV vaccine to prevent cervical and possibly anal cancer is discussed above. In addition to preventing anogenital cancers, HPV vaccines may have a role in the prevention of HPV-related head and neck cancers.

Smith RA et al. Cancer screening in the United States, 2014: a review of current American Cancer Society guidelines and current issues in cancer screening. CA Cancer J Clin. 2014 Jan–Feb;64(1):30–51. [PMID: 24408568]

▶ Screening & Early Detection

Screening prevents death from cancers of the breast, colon, and cervix. Current cancer screening recommendations from the USPSTF are shown in Table 1–6. Despite an increase in rates of screening for breast, cervical, and colon cancer over the last decade, overall screening for these cancers is suboptimal. Interventions including group education, one-on-one education, patient reminders, reduction of structural barriers, reduction of out-of-pocket costs, and provider assessment and feedback are effective in promoting recommended cancer screening.

Evidence from randomized trials suggests that screening mammography has both benefits and downsides. Currently, the appropriate form and frequency of screening for breast cancer remains controversial, and screening guidelines vary. Clinicians should discuss the risks and benefits with each patient and consider individual patient preferences when deciding when to begin screening (see Chapters 17 and 42).

Table 1–6. Cancer screening recommendations for average-risk adults: US Preventive Services Task Force (USPSTF).[1]

Test	USPSTF Recommendation/[Year Issued]
Breast self-examination	Recommends against teaching breast self-examination (D). [2009]
Clinical breast examination	Insufficient evidence to recommend for or against clinical breast examination (I). [2009]
Mammography	Recommends biennial screening mammography for women aged 50–74 years (B). Decision to start biennial screening before the age of 50 should be an individual one and take patient context into account, including the patient's values regarding specific benefits and harms (C). [2009]
Cervical cancer screening	Recommends screening for cervical cancer in women aged 21–65 years with cytology (Pap smear) every 3 years or, for women aged 30–65 years who want to lengthen the screening interval, screening with a combination of cytology and human papillomavirus (HPV) testing every 5 years (A). Recommends against screening for cervical cancer in women younger than 21 years (D). Recommends against screening for cervical cancer in women older than 65 years who have had adequate prior screening and are not otherwise at high risk for cervical cancer (D). Recommends against screening for cervical cancer in women who have had a hysterectomy with removal of the cervix and who do not have a history of a high-grade precancerous lesion (ie, cervical intraepithelial neoplasia [CIN] grade 2 or 3) or cervical cancer (D). Recommends against screening for cervical cancer with HPV testing, alone or in combination with cytology, in women younger than 30 years (D). [2012]
Colorectal cancer (CRC) screening	Recommends CRC screening using fecal occult blood testing,[2] sigmoidoscopy, or colonoscopy in adults beginning at age 50 years and continuing until age 75 years (A). Recommends against routine screening in adults aged 76–85 years (C). Recommends against screening in adults older than aged 85 years (D). [2008]
Lung cancer screening	Recommends annual lung cancer screening using low-dose CT in current smokers age 55–80 years with a 30-pack-year smoking history, or in smokers who quit within the past 15 years (B). Recommends stopping screening once a person has not smoked for 15 years or a health problem that significantly limits life expectancy has developed. [2013]
Prostate cancer screening	Recommends against prostate specific antigen (PSA)-based screening for prostate cancer (D). [2012]
Testicular cancer screening	Recommends against screening for testicular cancer in adolescent or adult males. [2011]

[1]United States Preventive Services Task Force recommendations available at http://www.ahrq.gov/professionals/clinicians-providers/guidelines-recommendations/guide/section2d.html.
[2]Home test with three samples.
Recommendation A: The USPSTF strongly recommends that clinicians routinely provide the service to eligible patients. (The USPSTF found good evidence that the service improves important health outcomes and concludes that benefits substantially outweigh harms.)
Recommendation B: The USPSTF recommends that clinicians routinely provide the service to eligible patients. (The USPSTF found at least fair evidence that the service improves important health outcomes and concludes that benefits substantially outweigh harms.)
Recommendation C: The USPSTF recommends against routinely providing the service. There may be considerations that support providing the service in an individual patient. There is at least moderate certainty that the net benefit is small.
Recommendation D: The USPSTF recommends against routinely providing the service to asymptomatic patients. (The USPSTF found at least fair evidence that the service is ineffective or that harms outweigh benefits.)
Recommendation I: The USPSTF concludes that the evidence is insufficient to recommend for or against routinely providing the service.
http://www.uspreventiveservicestaskforce.org/BrowseRec/Index/browse-recommendations

Digital mammography is more sensitive in women with dense breasts and younger women; however, studies exploring outcomes are lacking. MRI is not currently recommended for general screening, and its impact on breast cancer mortality is uncertain; however, the American Cancer Society recommends it for women at high risk (20–25% or more), including those with a strong family history of breast or ovarian cancer. Screening with both MRI and mammography might be superior to mammography alone in ruling out cancerous lesions in women with an inherited predisposition to breast cancer.

All current recommendations call for cervical and colorectal cancer screening. Screening for testicular cancers among asymptomatic adolescent or adult males is not recommended by the USPSTF. Prostate cancer screening remains controversial, since no completed trials have answered the question of whether early detection and treatment after screen detection produce sufficient benefits to outweigh harms of treatment. A 2013 Cochrane systematic review revealed that prostate cancer screening with PSA testing did not decrease all-cause mortality and may not decrease prostate cancer-specific mortality. Any benefits in terms of reduction in prostate cancer-related mortality would take more than 10 years to become evident. Men with less than 10–15 years' life expectancy should be informed that screening for prostate cancer is unlikely to be beneficial. In May 2012, the USPSTF recommended against PSA-based screening for prostate cancer (Grade D Recommendation).

Annual or biennial fecal occult blood testing reduces mortality from colorectal cancer by 16–33%. Fecal immunochemical tests (FIT) are superior to guaiac-based fecal occult blood tests (gFOBT) in detecting advanced adenomatous polyps and colorectal cancer, and patients are more likely to favor FIT over gFOBTs. Randomized trials using sigmoidoscopy as the screening method found 20–30% reductions in mortality from colorectal cancer. Colonoscopy has also been advocated as a screening examination. It is more accurate than flexible sigmoidoscopy for detecting cancer and polyps, but its value in reducing colon cancer mortality has not been studied directly. CT colonography (virtual colonoscopy) is a noninvasive option in screening for colorectal cancer. It has been shown to have a high safety profile and performance similar to colonoscopy. The American College of Physicians (ACP) recommends clinicians stop screening for colorectal cancer in individuals over the age of 75 years or with a life expectancy of less than 10 years.

The USPSTF recommends screening for cervical cancer in women aged 21–65 years with a Papanicolaou smear (cytology) every 3 years or, for women aged 30–65 years who desire longer intervals, screening with cytology and HPV testing every 5 years. The USPSTF recommends against screening in women younger than 21 years of age and average-risk women over 65 with adequate prior screening. Receipt of HPV vaccination has no impact on screening intervals.

In 2012, the American Cancer Society, the American Society for Colposcopy and Cervical Pathology, and the American Society for Clinical Pathology published updated guidelines for management of abnormal results. Women whose cervical specimen HPV tests are positive but cytology results are otherwise negative should repeat co-testing in 12 months (option 1) or undergo HPV-genotype–specific testing for types 16 or 16/18 (option 2). Colposcopy is recommended in women who test positive for types 16 or 16/18. Women with atypical squamous cells of undetermined significance (ASCUS) on cytology and a negative HPV test result should continue routine screening as per age-specific guidelines.

Evidence suggests that chest CT is significantly more sensitive that chest radiography in identifying small asymptomatic lung cancers; however, controversy exists regarding the efficacy and cost-effectiveness of low-dose CT screening in high-risk individuals. The National Lung Screening Trial (NLST), a randomized clinical trial of over 53,000 individuals at high risk for lung cancer, revealed a 20% relative reduction and 6.7% absolute reduction in lung cancer mortality in those who were screened with annual low-dose CTs for 3 years compared with those who had chest radiographs. There were a greater number of false-positive results in the low-dose CT group compared with those in the radiography group (23.3% vs 6.5%) (see Chapter 39). The Multicentric Italian Lung Detection (MILD) study, a randomized trial of over 4000 participants comparing annual or biennial low-dose CT with observation revealed no evidence of a protective effect with annual or biennial low-dose CT screening.

The USPSTF recommends annual lung cancer screening with low-dose CT in current smokers age 55 to 80 years with a 30-pack-year smoking history or smokers who quit within the past 15 years. Screening should stop once a person has not smoked for 15 years or a health problem that significantly limits life expectancy has developed. Screening should not be viewed as an alternative to smoking cessation.

Goodman DM et al. JAMA patient page: Screening tests. JAMA. 2013 Mar 20;309(11):1185. [PMID: 23512066]

Gøtzsche PC et al. Screening for breast cancer with mammography. Cochrane Database Syst Rev. 2013 Jun 4;6:CD001877. [PMID: 23737396]

Holme Ø et al. Effect of flexible sigmoidoscopy screening on colorectal cancer incidence and mortality: a randomized clinical trial. JAMA. 2014 Aug 13;312(6):606–15. [PMID: 25117129]

Ilic D et al. Screening for prostate cancer. Cochrane Database Syst Rev. 2013 Jan 31;1:CD004720. [PMID: 23440794]

Moyer VA; U.S. Preventive Services Task Force. Screening for cervical cancer: U.S. Preventive Services Task Force recommendation statement. Ann Intern Med. 2012 Jun 19;156(12):880–91. [PMID: 22711081]

Moyer VA; U.S. Preventive Services Task Force. Screening for lung cancer: U.S. Preventive Services Task Force recommendation statement. Ann Intern Med. 2014 Mar 4;160(5):330–8. [PMID: 24378917]

Moyer VA; U.S. Preventive Services Task Force. Screening for prostate cancer: U.S. Preventive Services Task Force recommendation statement. Ann Intern Med. 2012 Jul 17;157(2):120–34. [PMID: 22801674]

Qaseem A et al; Clinical Guidelines Committee of the American College of Physicians. Screening for colorectal cancer: a guidance statement from the American College of Physicians. Ann Intern Med. 2012 Mar 6;156(5):378–86. Erratum in: Ann Intern Med. 2012 Jul 17;157(2):152. [PMID: 22393133]

Roberts H et al; Lung Cancer Screening Guideline Development Group. Screening high-risk populations for lung cancer: guideline recommendations. J Thorac Oncol. 2013 Oct;8(10):1232–7. [PMID: 24457233]

Saslow D et al. American Cancer Society, American Society for Colposcopy and Cervical Pathology, and American Society for Clinical Pathology screening guidelines for the prevention and early detection of cervical cancer. J Low Genit Tract Dis. 2012 Jul;16(3):175–204. [PMID: 22418039]

Tria Tirona M. Breast cancer screening update. Am Fam Physician. 2013 Feb 15;87(4):274–8. [PMID: 23418799]

Wender R et al. American Cancer Society lung cancer screening guidelines. CA Cancer J Clin. 2013 Mar–Apr;63(2):107–17. [PMID: 23315954]

PREVENTION OF INJURIES & VIOLENCE

Injuries remain the most important cause of loss of potential years of life before age 65. Homicide and motor vehicle accidents are a major cause of injury-related deaths among young adults, and accidental falls are the most common cause of injury-related death in the elderly. Approximately one-third of all injury deaths include a diagnosis of traumatic brain injury. Other causes of injury-related deaths include suicide and accidental exposure to smoke, fire, and flames.

Motor vehicle accident deaths per miles driven continue to decline in the United States. Despite this overall decline, evidence suggests that sleeping medications (such as zolpidem) almost double the risk of motor vehicle accidents. Clinicians should discuss this risk when selecting a sleeping medication. Each year in the United States, more than 500,000 people are nonfatally injured while riding bicycles. The rate of helmet use by bicyclists and motorcyclists is significantly increased in states with helmet laws. Young men appear most likely to resist wearing helmets. Clinicians should try to educate their patients about seat belts, safety helmets, the risks of using cellular telephones while driving, drinking and driving—or using other intoxicants or long-acting benzodiazepines and then driving—and the risks of having guns in the home.

Long-term alcohol abuse adversely affects outcome from trauma and increases the risk of readmission for new trauma. Alcohol and illicit drug use are associated with an increased risk of violent death.

Males aged 16–35 are at especially high risk for serious injury and death from accidents and violence, with blacks and Latinos at greatest risk. For 16- and 17-year-old drivers, the risk of fatal crashes increases with the number of passengers. Deaths from firearms have reached epidemic levels in the United States and will soon surpass the number of deaths from motor vehicle accidents. Having a gun in the home increases the likelihood of homicide nearly threefold and of suicide fivefold. Educating clinicians to recognize and treat depression as well as restricting access to lethal methods have been found to reduce suicide rates.

Clinicians have a critical role in the detection, prevention, and management of intimate partner violence (see Chapter 42). The USPSTF recommends screening women of childbearing age for intimate partner violence and providing or referring women to intervention services when needed. Inclusion of a single question in the medical history—"At any time, has a partner ever hit you, kicked you, or otherwise physically hurt you?"—can increase identification of this common problem. Assessment for abuse and offering of referrals to community resources create potential to interrupt and prevent recurrence of domestic violence and associated trauma. Clinicians should take an active role in following up with patients whenever possible, since intimate partner violence screening with passive referrals to services may not be adequate. A randomized controlled trial to assess the impact of intimate partner violence screening on violence reduction and health outcomes in women revealed no difference in violence occurrence between screened and nonscreened women. Evaluation of services for patients *after* identification of intimate partner violence should be a priority.

Physical and psychological abuse, exploitation, and neglect of older adults are serious, underrecognized problems; they may occur in up to 10% of elders. Elder abuse is associated with increased risk of hospitalization. Risk factors for elder abuse include a culture of violence in the family; a demented, debilitated, or depressed and socially isolated victim; and a perpetrator profile of mental illness, alcohol or drug abuse, or emotional and/or financial dependence on the victim. Clues to elder mistreatment include the patient's appearance, recurrent urgent-care visits, missed appointments, suspicious physical findings, and implausible explanations for injuries.

Centers for Disease Control and Prevention (CDC). CDC Grand Rounds: reducing severe traumatic brain injury in the United States. MMWR Morb Mortal Wkly Rep. 2013 Jul 12;62(27):549–52. [PMID: 23842444]

Dong X et al. Elder abuse as a risk factor for hospitalization in older persons. JAMA Intern Med. 2013 May 27;173(10):911–7. [PMID: 23567991]

Hansen RN et al. Sedative hypnotic medication use and the risk of motor vehicle crash. Am J Public Health. 2015 Aug;105(8):e64–9. [PMID: 26066943]

Lachs MS et al. Elder abuse. N Engl J Med. 2015 Nov 12;373(20):1947–56. [PMID: 26559573]

Moyer VA. Screening for intimate partner violence and abuse of elderly and vulnerable adults: U.S. Preventive Services Task Force recommendation statement. Ann Intern Med. 2013 Mar 19;158(6):478–86. [PMID: 23338828]

O'Doherty LJ et al. Screening women for intimate partner violence in healthcare settings: abridged Cochrane systematic review and meta-analysis. BMJ. 2014 May 12;348:g2913. [PMID: 24821132]

Sumner SA et al. Violence in the United States: status, challenges, and opportunities. JAMA. 2015 Aug 4;314(5):478–88. [PMID: 26241599]

PREVENTION OF SUBSTANCE ABUSE: ALCOHOL & ILLICIT DRUGS

Substance abuse is a major public health problem in the United States. In the United States, approximately 51% of adults 18 years and older are current regular drinkers (at least 12 drinks in the past year). Maximum recommended consumption for adult women and those older than 65 years is three or fewer drinks per day (seven per week), and for adult men, four or fewer drinks per day (14 per week).

The spectrum of **alcohol misuse** includes **risky drinking** (alcohol consumption above the recommended daily, weekly, or per-occasion amounts), **harmful use** (a pattern causing damage to health), **alcohol abuse** (a pattern leading to clinically significant impairment or distress), and **alcohol dependence** (includes three or more of the following: tolerance, withdrawal, increased consumption, desire to cut down use, giving up social activities, increased time using alcohol or recovering from use, continued use despite known adverse effects).

As with cigarette use, clinician identification and counseling about alcohol misuse is essential. An estimated 15–30% of hospitalized patients have problems with alcohol abuse or dependence, but the connection between patients' presenting complaints and their alcohol use is often missed. The USPSTF recommends screening adults aged 18 years and older for alcohol misuse. Clinicians should provide those who screen positive for hazardous or risky drinking with brief behavioral counseling interventions to reduce alcohol misuse.

Use of screening procedures and brief intervention methods (see Chapter 25) can produce a 10–30% reduction in long-term alcohol use and alcohol-related problems. The Alcohol Use Disorder Identification Test (AUDIT) consists of questions on the quantity and frequency of alcohol consumption, on alcohol dependence symptoms, and on alcohol-related problems (Table 1–7). The AUDIT questionnaire is a cost-effective and efficient diagnostic tool for routine screening of alcohol use disorders in primary care settings. Brief advice and counseling without regular follow-up and reinforcement cannot sustain significant long-term reductions in unhealthy drinking behaviors.

Time restraints may prevent clinicians from screening patients, but single-question screening tests for unhealthy alcohol use may help increase the frequency of screening in primary care settings. Clinical trials support the use of screening and brief intervention for unhealthy alcohol use in adults. The National Institute on Alcohol Abuse and Alcoholism recommends the following single-question screening test: "How many times in the past year have you had X or more drinks in a day?" (X is 5 for men and 4 for women, and a response of more than 1 is considered positive.) The single-item screening test has been validated in primary care settings.

Several pharmacologic agents are effective in reducing alcohol consumption. In acute alcohol detoxification, standard treatment regimens include long-acting benzodiazepines, the preferred medications for alcohol detoxification, because they can be given on a fixed schedule or through "front-loading" or "symptom-triggered" regimens. Adjuvant sympatholytic medications can be used to treat hyperadrenergic symptoms that persist despite adequate sedation. Three drugs are FDA approved for treatment of alcohol dependence: disulfiram, naltrexone, and acamprosate. Disulfiram, an aversive agent, has significant adverse effects and consequently, compliance difficulties have resulted in no clear evidence that it increases abstinence rates, decreases relapse rates, or reduces cravings. Compared with placebo, naltrexone can lower the risk of

treatment withdrawal in alcohol-dependent patients, and the long-acting intramuscular formulation of naltrexone has been found to be well tolerated and to reduce drinking significantly among treatment-seeking alcoholics over a 6-month period. In a randomized, controlled trial, patients receiving medical management with naltrexone, a combined behavioral intervention, or both, fared better on drinking outcomes, whereas acamprosate showed no evidence of efficacy with or without combined behavioral intervention. Topiramate is a promising treatment for alcohol dependence. A 6-month randomized trial of topiramate versus naltrexone revealed a greater reduction of alcohol intake and cravings in participants receiving topiramate. Topiramate's side effect profile is favorable, and the benefits appear to increase over time. Clinicians should be aware that although topiramate appears to be an effective treatment for alcohol dependence, the manufacturer has not pursued FDA approval for this indication.

Over the last decade, the rate of **prescription drug abuse** has increased dramatically, particularly at both ends of the age spectrum. The most commonly abused classes of medications are pain relievers, tranquilizers, stimulants, and sedatives. Opioid-based prescription drug abuse, misuse, and overdose has reached epidemic proportions in the United States. Deaths due to prescription opioid overdose have dramatically increased. Opioid risk mitigation strategies include use of risk assessment tools, treatment agreements (contracts), and urine drug testing. Additional strategies include establishing and strengthening prescription drug monitoring programs, regulating pain management facilities, and establishing dosage thresholds requiring consultation with pain specialists. Further evaluation is necessary to determine the impact of these strategies on opioid abuse and misuse. (See Chapter 5.)

Use of illegal drugs—including cocaine, methamphetamine, and so-called "designer drugs"—either sporadically or episodically remains an important problem. Lifetime prevalence of drug abuse is approximately 8% and is generally greater among men, young and unmarried individuals, Native Americans, and those of lower socioeconomic status. As with alcohol, drug abuse disorders often coexist with personality, anxiety, and other substance abuse disorders. Abuse of anabolic-androgenic steroids has been associated with use of other illicit drugs, alcohol, and cigarettes and with violence and criminal behavior.

As with alcohol abuse, the lifetime treatment rate for drug abuse is low (8%). The recognition of drug abuse presents special problems and requires that the clinician actively consider the diagnosis. Clinical aspects of substance abuse are discussed in Chapter 25.

Buprenorphine has potential as a medication to ameliorate the symptoms and signs of withdrawal from opioids and has been shown to be effective in reducing concomitant cocaine and opioid abuse. The risk of overdose is lower with buprenorphine than methadone and it is preferred for patients at high risk for methadone toxicity. Evidence does not support the use of naltrexone in maintenance treatment of opioid addiction. Rapid opioid detoxification with opioid antagonist induction using

Table 1–7. Screening for alcohol abuse using the Alcohol Use Disorder Identification Test (AUDIT).[1]

(Scores for response categories are given in parentheses. Scores range from 0 to 40, with a cutoff score of 5 or more indicating hazardous drinking, harmful drinking, or alcohol dependence.)				
1. How often do you have a drink containing alcohol?				
(0) Never	(1) Monthly or less	(2) Two to four times a month	(3) Two or three times a week	(4) Four or more times a week
2. How many drinks containing alcohol do you have on a typical day when you are drinking?				
(0) 1 or 2	(1) 3 or 4	(2) 5 or 6	(3) 7 to 9	(4) 10 or more
3. How often do you have six or more drinks on one occasion?				
(0) Never	(1) Less than monthly	(2) Monthly	(3) Weekly	(4) Daily or almost daily
4. How often during the past year have you found that you were not able to stop drinking once you had started?				
(0) Never	(1) Less than monthly	(2) Monthly	(3) Weekly	(4) Daily or almost daily
5. How often during the past year have you failed to do what was normally expected of you because of drinking?				
(0) Never	(1) Less than monthly	(2) Monthly	(3) Weekly	(4) Daily or almost daily
6. How often during the past year have you needed a first drink in the morning to get yourself going after a heavy drinking session?				
(0) Never	(1) Less than monthly	(2) Monthly	(3) Weekly	(4) Daily or almost daily
7. How often during the past year have you had a feeling of guilt or remorse after drinking?				
(0) Never	(1) Less than monthly	(2) Monthly	(3) Weekly	(4) Daily or almost daily
8. How often during the past year have you been unable to remember what happened the night before because you had been drinking?				
(0) Never	(1) Less than monthly	(2) Monthly	(3) Weekly	(4) Daily or almost daily
9. Have you or has someone else been injured as a result of your drinking?				
(0) No		(2) Yes, but not in the past year		(4) Yes, during the past year
10. Has a relative or friend or a doctor or other health worker been concerned about your drinking or suggested you cut down?				
(0) No		(2) Yes, but not in the past year		(4) Yes, during the past year

[1]Adapted, with permission, from BMJ Publishing Group Ltd. and Piccinelli M et al. Efficacy of the alcohol use disorders identification test as a screening tool for hazardous alcohol intake and related disorders in primary care: a validity study. BMJ. 1997 Feb 8;314 (7078):420–4.

general anesthesia has emerged as an approach to treat opioid dependence. However, a randomized comparison of buprenorphine-assisted rapid opioid detoxification with naltrexone induction and clonidine-assisted opioid detoxification with delayed naltrexone induction found no significant differences in rates of completion of inpatient detoxification, treatment retention, or proportions of opioid-positive urine specimens, and the anesthesia procedure was associated with more potentially life-threatening adverse events. Finally, cognitive-behavior therapy, contingency management, couples, and family therapy, and other types of behavioral treatment have been shown to be effective interventions for drug addiction.

Berger D et al. Primary care management of alcohol misuse. Med Clin North Am. 2015 Sep;99(5):989–1016. [PMID: 26320043]

Garcia AM. State laws regulating prescribing of controlled substances: balancing the public health problems of chronic pain and prescription painkiller abuse and overdose. J Law Med Ethics. 2013 Mar;41(Suppl 1):42–5. [PMID: 23590739]

Moyer VA; Preventive Services Task Force. Screening and behavioral counseling interventions in primary care to reduce alcohol misuse: U.S. Preventive Services Task Force recommendation statement. Ann Intern Med. 2013 Aug 6;159(3): 210–8. [PMID: 23698791]

Nuckols TK et al. Opioid prescribing: a systematic review and critical appraisal of guidelines for chronic pain. Ann Intern Med. 2014 Jan 7;160(1):38–47. [PMID: 24217469]

Common Symptoms

Paul L. Nadler, MD

Ralph Gonzales, MD, MSPH

COUGH

ESSENTIAL INQUIRIES

- ▶ Age, tobacco use history, and duration of cough.
- ▶ Dyspnea (at rest or with exertion).
- ▶ Vital signs (heart rate, respiratory rate, body temperature).
- ▶ Chest examination.
- ▶ Chest radiography when unexplained cough lasts more than 3–6 weeks.

▶ General Considerations

Cough adversely affects personal and work-related interactions, disrupts sleep, and often causes discomfort of the throat and chest wall. Most people seeking medical attention for acute cough desire symptom relief; few are worried about serious illness. Cough results from stimulation of mechanical or chemical afferent nerve receptors in the bronchial tree. Effective cough depends on an intact afferent–efferent reflex arc, adequate expiratory and chest wall muscle strength, and normal mucociliary production and clearance.

▶ Clinical Findings

A. Symptoms

Distinguishing **acute** (less than 3 weeks), **persistent** (3–8 weeks), and **chronic** (more than 8 weeks) cough illness syndromes is a useful first step in evaluation. Postinfectious cough lasting 3–8 weeks has also been referred to as **subacute** cough to distinguish this common, distinct clinical entity from acute and chronic cough.

1. Acute cough—In healthy adults, most acute cough syndromes are due to viral respiratory tract infections. Additional features of infection such as fever, nasal congestion, and sore throat help confirm this diagnosis. Dyspnea (at rest or with exertion) may reflect a more serious condition, and further evaluation should include assessment of oxygenation (pulse oximetry or arterial blood gas measurement), airflow (peak flow or spirometry), and pulmonary parenchymal disease (chest radiography). The timing and character of the cough are not very useful in establishing the cause of acute cough syndromes, although cough-variant asthma should be considered in adults with prominent nocturnal cough, and persistent cough with phlegm increases the likelihood of chronic obstructive pulmonary disease (COPD). The presence of post-tussive emesis or inspiratory whoop modestly increases the likelihood of pertussis, and the absence of paroxysmal cough decreases its likelihood when cough lasts more than 1 week. Uncommon causes of acute cough should be suspected in those with heart disease (heart failure [HF]) or hay fever (allergic rhinitis) and those with environmental risk factors (such as farm workers).

2. Persistent and chronic cough—Cough due to acute respiratory tract infection resolves within 3 weeks in the vast majority (more than 90%) of patients. Pertussis should be considered in adolescents and adults with persistent or severe cough lasting more than 3 weeks, and in selected geographic areas, its prevalence approaches 20% (although its exact prevalence is difficult to ascertain due to the limited sensitivity of diagnostic tests).

When angiotensin-converting enzyme (ACE) inhibitor therapy, acute respiratory tract infection, and chest radiograph abnormalities are absent, most cases of persistent and chronic cough are due to (or exacerbated by) postnasal drip, asthma, or gastroesophageal reflux disease (GERD), or some combination of these three entities. A history of nasal or sinus congestion, wheezing, or heartburn should direct subsequent evaluation and treatment, though these conditions frequently cause persistent cough in the absence of typical symptoms. Dyspnea at rest or with exertion is not commonly reported among patients with persistent cough; dyspnea requires assessment for chronic lung disease, HF, or anemia.

Bronchogenic carcinoma is suspected when cough is accompanied by unexplained weight loss, hemoptysis, and fevers with night sweats, particularly in persons with significant tobacco or occupational exposures (asbestos, radon, diesel exhaust, and metals). Persistent and chronic cough accompanied by excessive mucus secretions increases the likelihood of COPD, particularly among smokers, or of bronchiectasis if accompanied by a history of recurrent or complicated pneumonia; chest radiographs are helpful in diagnosis.

B. Physical Examination

Examination can direct subsequent diagnostic testing for acute cough. Pneumonia is suspected when acute cough is accompanied by vital sign abnormalities (tachycardia, tachypnea, fever). Findings suggestive of airspace consolidation (rales, decreased breath sounds, fremitus, egophony) are significant predictors of community-acquired pneumonia but are present in the minority of cases. Purulent sputum is associated with bacterial infections in patients with structural lung disease (eg, COPD, cystic fibrosis), but it is a poor predictor of pneumonia in the otherwise healthy adult. Wheezing and rhonchi are frequent findings in adults with acute bronchitis and do not indicate consolidation or adult-onset asthma in most cases.

Examination of patients with persistent cough should look for evidence of chronic sinusitis, contributing to postnasal drip syndrome or asthma. Chest and cardiac signs may help distinguish COPD from HF. In patients with cough and dyspnea, a normal match test (ability to blow out a match from 25 cm away) and maximum laryngeal height greater than 4 cm (measured from the sternal notch to the cricoid cartilage at end expiration) substantially decrease the likelihood of COPD. Similarly, normal jugular venous pressure and no hepatojugular reflux decrease the likelihood of biventricular HF.

C. Diagnostic Studies

1. Acute cough—Chest radiography should be considered for any adult with acute cough whose vital signs are abnormal or whose chest examination suggests pneumonia. The relationship between specific clinical findings and the probability of pneumonia is shown in Table 2–1. A large, multicenter randomized clinical trial found that elevated serum C-reactive protein (levels greater than 30 mg/dL) improves diagnostic accuracy of clinical prediction rules for pneumonia in adults with acute cough. In patients with dyspnea, pulse oximetry and peak flow help exclude hypoxemia or obstructive airway disease. However, a normal pulse oximetry value (eg, greater than 93%) does not rule out a significant alveolar–arterial (A–a) gradient when patients have effective respiratory compensation. During documented outbreaks, clinical diagnosis of influenza has a positive predictive value of ~70%; this usually obviates the need for rapid diagnostic tests.

2. Persistent and chronic cough—Chest radiography is indicated when ACE inhibitor therapy–related and postinfectious cough are excluded by history or further diagnostic testing. If pertussis is suspected, polymerase chain reaction testing should be performed on a nasopharyngeal swab or nasal wash specimen—although the ability to detect pertussis decreases as the duration of cough increases. When the chest film is normal, postnasal drip,

Table 2–1. Positive and negative likelihood ratios for history, physical examination, and laboratory findings in the diagnosis of pneumonia.

Finding	Positive Likelihood Ratio	Negative Likelihood Ratio
Medical history		
Fever	1.7–2.1	0.6–0.7
Chills	1.3–1.7	0.7–0.9
Physical examination		
Tachypnea (RR > 25 breaths/min)	1.5–3.4	0.8
Tachycardia (> 100 beats/min in two studies or > 120 beats/min in one study)	1.6–2.3	0.5–0.7
Hyperthermia (> 37.8°C)	1.4–4.4	0.6–0.8
Chest examination		
Dullness to percussion	2.2–4.3	0.8–0.9
Decreased breath sounds	2.3–2.5	0.6–0.8
Crackles	1.6–2.7	0.6–0.9
Rhonchi	1.4–1.5	0.8–0.9
Egophony	2.0–8.6	0.8–1.0
Laboratory findings		
Leukocytosis (> 11 × 10⁹/L in one study or ≥ 10.4 × 10⁹/L in another study)	1.9–3.7	0.3–0.6

RR, respiratory rate.

asthma, or GERD are the most likely causes. The presence of typical symptoms of these conditions directs further evaluation or empiric therapy, though typical symptoms are often absent. Definitive tests for determining the presence of each are available (Table 2–2). However, empiric treatment with a maximum-strength regimen for postnasal drip, asthma, or GERD for 2–4 weeks is one recommended approach since documenting the presence of postnasal drip, asthma, or GERD does not mean they are the cause of the cough. Alternative approaches to identifying patients who have asthma with its

Table 2–2. Empiric treatments or tests for persistent cough.

Suspected Condition	Step 1 (Empiric Therapy)	Step 2 (Diagnostic Testing)
Postnasal drip	Therapy for allergy or chronic sinusitis	ENT referral; sinus CT scan
Asthma	Beta-2-agonist	Spirometry; consider methacholine challenge if normal
GERD	Proton pump inhibitors	Esophageal pH monitoring

ENT, ear, nose, and throat; GERD, gastroesophageal reflux disease.

corticosteroid-responsive cough include examining induced sputum for increased eosinophil counts (greater than 3%) or providing an empiric trial of prednisone, 30 mg daily orally for 2 weeks. Spirometry may help identify large airway obstruction in patients who have persistent cough and wheezing and who are not responding to asthma treatment. When empiric treatment trials are not successful, additional evaluation with pH manometry, endoscopy, barium swallow, sinus CT or high-resolution chest CT may identify the cause.

▶ Differential Diagnosis

A. Acute Cough

Acute cough may be a symptom of acute respiratory tract infection, asthma, allergic rhinitis, and HF, as well as many less common causes.

B. Persistent and Chronic Cough

Causes of persistent cough include environmental exposures (cigarette smoke, air pollution), pertussis, postnasal drip, asthma (including cough-variant asthma), GERD, COPD, bronchiectasis, eosinophilic bronchitis, tuberculosis or other chronic infection, interstitial lung disease, and bronchogenic carcinoma. COPD is a common cause of persistent cough among patients older than 50 years. Persistent cough may also be due to somatic cough syndrome (previously called "psychogenic cough") or tic cough (previously called "habit cough").

▶ Treatment

A. Acute Cough

Treatment of acute cough should target the underlying etiology of the illness, the cough reflex itself, and any additional factors that exacerbate the cough. Cough duration is typically 1–3 weeks, yet patients frequently expect cough to last fewer than 10 days. When influenza is diagnosed (including H1N1 influenza), treatment with oseltamivir or zanamivir is equally effective (1 less day of illness) when initiated within 30–48 hours of illness onset; treatment is recommended regardless of illness duration when patients have severe influenza requiring hospitalization. In *Chlamydophila*- or *Mycoplasma*-documented infection or outbreaks, first-line antibiotics include erythromycin or doxycycline. However, antibiotics do not improve cough severity or duration in patients with uncomplicated acute bronchitis. In some patients with bronchitis, inhaled beta-2-agonist therapy reduces severity and duration of cough. In patients with acute cough, treating the accompanying postnasal drip (with antihistamines, decongestants, or nasal corticosteroids) or GERD (with H_2-blockers or proton-pump inhibitors) can be helpful. Vitamin C and echinacea are not effective in reducing the severity of acute cough after it develops; however, vitamin C (at least 1 g daily) can prevent colds among persons with major physical stressors (eg, post-marathon) or malnutrition. Zinc lozenges, when initiated within 24 hours of symptom onset, can reduce the duration and severity of cold symptoms.

B. Persistent and Chronic Cough

Evaluation and management of persistent cough often require multiple visits and therapeutic trials, which frequently lead to frustration, anger, and anxiety. When pertussis infection is suspected early in its course, treatment with a macrolide antibiotic (see Chapter 33) is appropriate to reduce organism shedding and transmission. When pertussis has lasted more than 7–10 days, antibiotic treatment does not affect the duration of cough, which can last up to 6 months. Early identification, revaccination with Tdap, and treatment of adult patients who work or live with persons at high risk for complications from pertussis (pregnant women, infants [particularly younger than 1 year], and immunosuppressed individuals) are encouraged.

Table 2–2 outlines empiric treatments for persistent cough. There is no evidence to guide how long to continue treatment for persistent cough due to postnasal drip, asthma, or GERD. Studies have not found a consistent benefit of inhaled corticosteroid therapy in adults with persistent cough. Sensory dysfunction of the laryngeal branches of the vagus nerve may contribute to persistent cough syndromes and may help explain the effectiveness of gabapentin in patients with chronic cough. In patients with reflex cough syndrome, therapy aimed at shifting the patient's attentional focus from internal to external can be helpful.

When empiric treatment trials fail, consider other causes of chronic cough such as obstructive sleep apnea, tonsillar enlargement, and environmental fungi. The small percentage of patients with idiopathic chronic cough should be managed in consultation with an otolaryngologist or a pulmonologist; consider a high-resolution CT scan of the lungs. Treatment options include nebulized lidocaine therapy and morphine sulfate, 5–10 mg orally twice daily.

▶ When to Refer

- Failure to control persistent or chronic cough following empiric treatment trials.
- Patients with recurrent symptoms should be referred to an otolaryngologist, pulmonologist, or gastroenterologist.
- Adults needing Tdap vaccination to enable "cocooning" of at-risk individuals (eg, infants aged younger than 1 year).

▶ When to Admit

- Patient at high risk for tuberculosis for whom compliance with respiratory precautions is uncertain.
- Need for urgent bronchoscopy, such as suspected foreign body.
- Smoke or toxic fume inhalational injury.
- Intractable cough despite treatment, when cough impairs gas exchange, or in patients at high risk for barotrauma (eg, recent pneumothorax).

Barrecheguren M et al. The asthma-chronic obstructive pulmonary disease overlap syndrome (ACOS): opportunities and challenges. Curr Opin Pulm Med. 2015 Jan;21(1):74–9. [PMID: 25405671]

Canning BJ et al; CHEST Expert Cough Panel. Anatomy and neurophysiology of cough: CHEST Guideline and Expert Panel report. Chest. 2014 Dec;146(6):1633–48. [PMID: 25188530]

Iyer VN et al. Chronic cough: an update. Mayo Clin Proc. 2013 Oct;88(10):1115–26. [PMID: 24079681]

Johnstone KJ et al. Inhaled corticosteroids for subacute and chronic cough in adults. Cochrane Database Syst Rev. 2013 Mar 28;3:CD009305. [PMID: 23543575]

Kline JM et al. Pertussis: a reemerging infection. Am Fam Physician. 2013 Oct 15;88(8):507–14. Erratum in: Am Fam Physician. 2014 Mar 1;89(5):317. [PMID: 24364571]

Lim KG et al. Long-term safety of nebulized lidocaine for adults with difficult-to-control chronic cough: a case series. Chest. 2013 Apr;143(4):1060–5. [PMID: 23238692]

Rivard G et al. Staying ahead of pertussis. J Fam Pract. 2014 Nov;63(11):658–69. [PMID: 25362496]

Ryan NM. A review on the efficacy and safety of gabapentin in the treatment of chronic cough. Expert Opin Pharmacother. 2015 Jan;16(1):135–45. [PMID: 25380977]

Vertigan AE et al; CHEST Expert Cough Panel. Somatic cough syndrome (previously referred to as psychogenic cough) and tic cough (previously referred to as habit cough) in adults and children: CHEST Guideline and Expert Panel Report. Chest. 2015 Jul;148(1):24–31. [PMID: 25856777]

Xu X et al. Comparison of gastroesophageal reflux disease questionnaire and multichannel intraluminal impedance pH monitoring in identifying patients with chronic cough responsive to antireflux therapy. Chest. 2014 Jun;145(6):1264–70. [PMID: 24457470]

DYSPNEA

ESSENTIAL INQUIRIES

▶ Fever, cough, and chest pain.

▶ Vital sign measurements; pulse oximetry.

▶ Cardiac and chest examination.

▶ Chest radiography and arterial blood gas measurement in selected patients.

General Considerations

Dyspnea is a subjective experience or perception of uncomfortable breathing. However, the relationship between level of dyspnea and the severity of underlying disease varies widely across individuals. Dyspnea can result from conditions that increase the mechanical effort of breathing (eg, COPD, restrictive lung disease, respiratory muscle weakness), conditions that produce compensatory tachypnea (eg, hypoxemia, acidosis), or psychogenic conditions. The following factors play a role in how and when dyspnea presents in patients: rate of onset, previous dyspnea, medications, comorbidities, psychological profile, and severity of underlying disorder.

Clinical Findings

A. Symptoms

The duration, severity, and periodicity of dyspnea influence the tempo of the clinical evaluation. Rapid onset or severe dyspnea in the absence of other clinical features should raise concern for pneumothorax, pulmonary embolism, or increased left ventricular end-diastolic pressure (LVEDP). Spontaneous pneumothorax is usually accompanied by chest pain and occurs most often in thin, young males and in those with underlying lung disease. Pulmonary embolism should always be suspected when a patient with new dyspnea reports a recent history (previous 4 weeks) of prolonged immobilization or hospitalization, estrogen therapy, or other risk factors for deep venous thrombosis (DVT) (eg, previous history of thromboembolism, cancer, obesity, lower extremity trauma) and when the cause of dyspnea is not apparent. Silent myocardial infarction, which occurs more frequently in diabetic persons and women, can result in increased LVEDP, acute heart failure, and dyspnea.

Accompanying symptoms provide important clues to causes of dyspnea. When cough and fever are present, pulmonary disease (particularly infection) is the primary concern; myocarditis, pericarditis, and septic emboli can present in this manner. Chest pain should be further characterized as acute or chronic, pleuritic or exertional. Although acute pleuritic chest pain is the rule in acute pericarditis and pneumothorax, most patients with pleuritic chest pain in the outpatient clinic have pleurisy due to acute viral respiratory tract infection. Periodic chest pain that precedes the onset of dyspnea suggests myocardial ischemia or pulmonary embolism. When associated with wheezing, most cases of dyspnea are due to acute bronchitis; however, other causes include new-onset asthma, foreign body, and vocal cord dysfunction.

When a patient reports prominent dyspnea with mild or no accompanying features, consider noncardiopulmonary causes of impaired oxygen delivery (anemia, methemoglobinemia, cyanide ingestion, carbon monoxide), metabolic acidosis, panic disorder, neuromuscular disorders, and chronic pulmonary embolism.

B. Physical Examination

A focused physical examination should include evaluation of the head and neck, chest, heart, and lower extremities. Visual inspection of the patient can suggest obstructive airway disease (pursed-lip breathing, use of accessory respiratory muscles, barrel-shaped chest), pneumothorax (asymmetric excursion), or metabolic acidosis (Kussmaul respirations). Patients with impending upper airway obstruction (eg, epiglottitis, foreign body) or severe asthma exacerbation sometimes assume a tripod position. Focal wheezing raises the suspicion for a foreign body or other bronchial obstruction. Maximum laryngeal height (the distance between the top of the thyroid cartilage and the suprasternal notch at end expiration) is a measure of hyperinflation. Obstructive airway disease is virtually

Table 2–3. Clinical findings suggesting obstructive airway disease.

	Adjusted Likelihood Ratios	
	Factor Present	Factor Absent
> 40 pack-years smoking	11.6	0.9
Age ≥ 45 years	1.4	0.5
Maximum laryngeal height ≤ 4 cm	3.6	0.7
All three factors	58.5	0.3

Reproduced, with permission, from Straus SE et al. The accuracy of patient history, wheezing, and laryngeal measurements in diagnosing obstructive airway disease. CARE-COAD1 Group. Clinical Assessment of the Reliability of the Examination—Chronic Obstructive Airways Disease. JAMA. 2000 Apr 12;283(14):1853–7. © 2000 American Medical Association. All rights reserved.

nonexistent when a nonsmoking patient younger than 45 years has a maximum laryngeal height greater than 4 cm (Table 2–3). Absent breath sounds suggest a pneumothorax. An accentuated pulmonic component of the second heart sound (loud P2) is a sign of pulmonary hypertension and pulmonary embolism.

Table 2–4 shows clinical predictors of increased LVEDP in dyspneic patients with no prior history of HF. When none is present, there is a very low probability (less than 10%) of increased LVEDP, but when two or more are present, there is a very high probability (greater than 90%) of increased LVEDP.

C. Diagnostic Studies

Causes of dyspnea that can be managed without chest radiography are few: ingestions causing lactic acidosis, anemia, methemoglobinemia, and carbon monoxide poisoning.

Table 2–4. Clinical findings suggesting increased left ventricular end-diastolic pressure.

Tachycardia
Systolic hypotension
Jugular venous distention (> 5–7 cm H_2O)[1]
Hepatojugular reflux (> 1 cm)[2]
Crackles, especially bibasilar
Third heart sound[3]
Lower extremity edema
Radiographic pulmonary vascular redistribution or cardiomegaly[1]

[1]These findings are particularly helpful.
[2]Proper abdominal compression for evaluating hepatojugular reflux requires > 30 seconds of sustained right upper quadrant abdominal compression.
[3]Cardiac auscultation of the patient at 45-degree angle in left lateral decubitus position doubles the detection rate of third heart sounds.
Data from Badgett RG et al. Can the clinical examination diagnose left-sided heart failure in adults? JAMA. 1997 Jun 4;277(21):1712–9.

The diagnosis of pneumonia should be confirmed by chest radiography in most patients. When COPD exacerbation is severe enough to require hospitalization, results of chest radiography can influence management decisions in up to 20% of patients. Chest radiography is fairly sensitive and specific for new-onset HF (represented by redistribution of pulmonary venous circulation) and can help guide treatment of patients with other cardiac disease. End-expiratory chest radiography enhances detection of a small pneumothorax.

A normal chest radiograph has substantial diagnostic value. When there is no physical examination evidence of COPD or HF and the chest radiograph is normal, the major remaining causes of dyspnea include pulmonary embolism, *Pneumocystis jirovecii* infection (initial radiograph may be normal in up to 25%), upper airway obstruction, foreign body, anemia, and metabolic acidosis. If a patient has tachycardia and hypoxemia but a normal chest radiograph and electrocardiogram (ECG), then tests to exclude pulmonary emboli (see Chapter 9), anemia, or metabolic acidosis are warranted. High-resolution chest CT is particularly useful in the evaluation of interstitial and alveolar lung disease. Helical ("spiral") CT is useful to diagnose pulmonary embolism since the images are high resolution and require only one breathhold by the patient, but to minimize unnecessary testing and radiation exposure, the clinician should first use a clinical decision rule (such as the modified Wells criteria or the pulmonary embolism rule-out criteria) to estimate the pretest probability of a pulmonary embolism. For instance, if a patient has fewer than 2 points using the Wells criteria, the mean probability of a pulmonary embolism is only 3.6% (very low).

Table 2–4 shows clinical findings suggesting increased LVEDP. Elevated serum or B-type natriuretic peptide (BNP or NT-proBNP) levels are both sensitive and specific for increased LVEDP in symptomatic persons. BNP has been shown to reliably diagnose severe dyspnea caused by HF and to differentiate it from dyspnea due to other conditions. However, systematic use of BNP in evaluation of dyspnea in the emergency department does not appear to have a clinically significant impact on patient or system outcomes, and it does not conclusively affect hospital mortality rates.

Arterial blood gas measurement may be considered if clinical examination and routine diagnostic testing are equivocal. With two notable exceptions (carbon monoxide poisoning and cyanide toxicity), arterial blood gas measurement distinguishes increased mechanical effort causes of dyspnea (respiratory acidosis with or without hypoxemia) from compensatory tachypnea (respiratory alkalosis with or without hypoxemia or metabolic acidosis) and from psychogenic dyspnea (respiratory alkalosis). An observational study, however, found that arterial blood gas measurement had little value in determining the cause of dyspnea in patients presenting to the emergency department. Carbon monoxide and cyanide impair oxygen delivery with minimal alterations in Po_2; percent carboxyhemoglobin identifies carbon monoxide toxicity.

Cyanide poisoning should be considered in a patient with profound lactic acidosis following exposure to burning vinyl (such as a theater fire or industrial accident). Suspected carbon monoxide poisoning or methemoglobinemia can also be confirmed with venous carboxyhemoglobin or methemoglobin levels.

Because arterial blood gas testing is impractical in most outpatient settings, **pulse oximetry** has assumed a central role in the office evaluation of dyspnea. Oxygen saturation values above 96% almost always correspond with a Po_2 greater than 70 mm Hg, and values less than 94% almost always represent clinically significant hypoxemia. Important exceptions to this rule include carbon monoxide toxicity, which leads to a normal oxygen saturation (due to the similar wavelengths of oxyhemoglobin and carboxyhemoglobin), and methemoglobinemia, which results in an oxygen saturation of about 85% that fails to increase with supplemental oxygen. A delirious or obtunded patient with obstructive lung disease warrants immediate measurement of arterial blood gases to exclude hypercapnia and the need for intubation, regardless of the oxygen saturation. If a patient reports dyspnea with exertion, but resting oximetry is normal, assessment of desaturation with ambulation (eg, a brisk walk around the clinic) can be useful for confirming impaired gas exchange.

Episodic dyspnea can be challenging if an evaluation cannot be performed during symptoms. Life-threatening causes include recurrent pulmonary embolism, myocardial ischemia, and reactive airway disease. When associated with audible wheezing, vocal cord dysfunction should be considered, particularly in a young woman who does not respond to asthma therapy. Spirometry is very helpful in further classifying patients with obstructive airway disease but is rarely needed in the initial or emergent evaluation of patients with acute dyspnea.

Differential Diagnosis

Urgent and emergent conditions causing acute dyspnea include pneumonia, COPD, asthma, pneumothorax, pulmonary embolism, cardiac disease (eg, HF, acute myocardial infarction, valvular dysfunction, arrhythmia, intracardiac shunt), diffuse alveolar hemorrhage, metabolic acidosis, cyanide toxicity, methemoglobinemia, and carbon monoxide poisoning.

Treatment

The treatment of urgent or emergent causes of dyspnea should aim to relieve the underlying cause. Pending diagnosis, patients with hypoxemia should be immediately provided supplemental oxygen unless significant hypercapnia is present or strongly suspected pending arterial blood gas measurement. Dyspnea frequently occurs in patients nearing the end of life. Opioid therapy, anxiolytics, and corticosteroids can provide substantial relief independent of the severity of hypoxemia. However, inhaled opioids are not effective. Oxygen therapy is most beneficial to patients with significant hypoxemia (Pao_2 less than

55 mm Hg) (see Chapter 5). In patients with severe COPD and hypoxemia, oxygen therapy improves mortality and exercise performance. Pulmonary rehabilitation programs are another therapeutic option for patients with moderate to severe COPD or interstitial pulmonary fibrosis. Noninvasive ventilation may be considered for patients with dyspnea caused by an acute COPD exacerbation, but the efficacy of this treatment is still uncertain.

▶ When to Refer

- Following acute stabilization, patients with advanced COPD should be referred to a pulmonologist, and patients with HF or valvular heart disease should be referred to a cardiologist.
- Cyanide toxicity or carbon monoxide poisoning should be managed in conjunction with a toxicologist.

▶ When to Admit

- Impaired gas exchange from any cause or high risk of pulmonary embolism pending definitive diagnosis.
- Suspected cyanide toxicity or carbon monoxide poisoning.

Bausewein C et al. Inhaled nebulized and intranasal opioids for the relief of breathlessness. Curr Opin Support Palliat Care. 2014 Sep;8(3):208–12. [PMID: 25004175]

Jang TB et al. The predictive value of physical examination findings in patients with suspected acute heart failure syndrome. Intern Emerg Med. 2012 Jun;7(3):271–4. [PMID: 22094407]

Junker C et al. Are arterial blood gases necessary in the evaluation of acutely dyspneic patients? Crit Care. 2011 Aug 2; 15(4):176. [PMID: 21892979]

Le Gal et al. D-dimer for pulmonary embolism. JAMA. 2015 Apr 28;313(16):1668–9. [PMID: 25919531]

Mahler DA et al. Recent advances in dyspnea. Chest. 2015 Jan;147(1):232–41. [PMID: 25560861]

Mastandrea P. The diagnostic utility of brain natriuretic peptide in heart failure patients presenting with acute dyspnea: a meta-analysis. Clin Chem Lab Med. 2013 Jun;51(6):1155–65. [PMID: 23152414]

Oelsner EC et al. Noninvasive tests for the diagnostic evaluation of dyspnea among outpatients: the Multi-Ethnic Study of Atherosclerosis lung study. Am J Med. 2015 Feb;128(2): 171–80. [PMID: 25447621]

Parshall MB et al; American Thoracic Society Committee on Dyspnea. An official American Thoracic Society statement: update on the mechanisms, assessment, and management of dyspnea. Am J Respir Crit Care Med. 2012 Feb 15;185(4): 435–52. [PMID: 22336677]

Shreves A et al. Emergency management of dyspnea in dying patients. Emerg Med Pract. 2013 May;15(5):1–20. [PMID: 23967787]

Smith TA et al. The use of non-invasive ventilation for the relief of dyspnoea in exacerbations of chronic obstructive pulmonary disease; a systematic review. Respirology. 2012 Feb;17(2):300–7. [PMID: 22008176]

Uronis HE et al. Oxygen for relief of dyspnoea in people with chronic obstructive pulmonary disease who would not qualify for home oxygen: a systematic review and meta-analysis. Thorax. 2015 May;70(5):492–4. [PMID: 25472664]

HEMOPTYSIS

ESSENTIAL INQUIRIES

- ▶ Fever, cough, and other symptoms of lower respiratory tract infection.
- ▶ Smoking history.
- ▶ Nasopharyngeal or gastrointestinal bleeding.
- ▶ Chest radiography and complete blood count (and, in some cases, INR).

▶ General Considerations

Hemoptysis is the expectoration of blood that originates below the vocal cords. It is commonly classified as trivial, mild, or massive—the latter defined as more than 200–600 mL (about 1–2 cups) in 24 hours. Massive hemoptysis can be usefully defined as any amount that is hemodynamically significant or threatens ventilation. Its in-hospital mortality was 6.5% in one study. The initial goal of management of massive hemoptysis is therapeutic, not diagnostic.

The lungs are supplied with a dual circulation. The pulmonary arteries arise from the right ventricle to supply the pulmonary parenchyma in a low-pressure circuit. The bronchial arteries arise from the aorta or intercostal arteries and carry blood under systemic pressure to the airways, blood vessels, hila, and visceral pleura. Although the bronchial circulation represents only 1–2% of total pulmonary blood flow, it can increase dramatically under conditions of chronic inflammation—eg, chronic bronchiectasis—and is frequently the source of hemoptysis.

The causes of hemoptysis can be classified anatomically. Blood may arise from the airways in COPD, bronchiectasis, and bronchogenic carcinoma; from the pulmonary vasculature in left ventricular failure, mitral stenosis, pulmonary embolism, pulmonary arterial hypertension, and arteriovenous malformations; or from the pulmonary parenchyma in pneumonia, inhalation of crack cocaine, or granulomatosis with polyangiitis (formerly Wegener granulomatosis). Diffuse alveolar hemorrhage—manifested by alveolar infiltrates on chest radiography—is due to small vessel bleeding usually caused by autoimmune or hematologic disorders, or rarely precipitated by warfarin. Most cases of hemoptysis presenting in the outpatient setting are due to infection (eg, acute or chronic bronchitis, pneumonia, tuberculosis, aspergillosis). Hemoptysis due to lung cancer increases with age, accounting for up to 20% of cases among the elderly. Less commonly (less than 10% of cases), pulmonary venous hypertension (eg, mitral stenosis, pulmonary embolism) causes hemoptysis. Most cases of hemoptysis that have no visible cause on CT scan or bronchoscopy will resolve within 6 months without treatment, with the notable exception of patients at high risk for lung cancer (smokers older than 40 years). Iatrogenic hemorrhage may follow transbronchial lung biopsies, anticoagulation, or pulmonary artery rupture due to distal placement of a balloon-tipped catheter. No cause is identified in up to 15–30% of cases.

▶ Clinical Findings

A. Symptoms

Blood-tinged sputum in the setting of an upper respiratory tract infection in an otherwise healthy, young (age under 40 years) nonsmoker does not warrant an extensive diagnostic evaluation if the hemoptysis subsides with resolution of the infection. However, hemoptysis is frequently a sign of serious disease, especially in patients with a high prior probability of underlying pulmonary pathology. Hemoptysis is the only symptom found to be a specific predictor of lung cancer. One should not distinguish between blood-streaked sputum and cough productive of blood alone with regard to the evaluation plan. The goal of the history is to identify patients at risk for one of the disorders listed above. Pertinent features include duration of symptoms, presence of respiratory infection, and past or current tobacco use. Nonpulmonary sources of hemorrhage—from the sinuses or the gastrointestinal tract—must be excluded.

B. Physical Examination

Elevated pulse, hypotension, and decreased oxygen saturation suggest large-volume hemorrhage that warrants emergent evaluation and stabilization. The nares and oropharynx should be carefully inspected to identify a potential upper airway source of bleeding. Chest and cardiac examination may reveal evidence of HF or mitral stenosis.

C. Diagnostic Studies

Diagnostic evaluation should include a chest radiograph and complete blood count. Kidney function tests, urinalysis, and coagulation studies are appropriate in specific circumstances. Hematuria that accompanies hemoptysis may be a clue to Goodpasture syndrome or vasculitis. Flexible bronchoscopy reveals endobronchial cancer in 3–6% of patients with hemoptysis who have a normal (non-lateralizing) chest radiograph. Nearly all of these patients are smokers over the age of 40, and most will have had symptoms for more than 1 week. High-resolution chest CT scan complements bronchoscopy and should be strongly considered in patients with normal chest radiograph and low risk for malignancy. It can visualize unsuspected bronchiectasis and arteriovenous malformations and will show central endobronchial cancers in many cases. It is the test of choice for suspected small peripheral malignancies. Helical CT pulmonary angiography has become the initial test of choice for evaluating patients with suspected pulmonary embolism, although caution should be taken to avoid large contrast loads in patients with even mild chronic kidney disease (serum creatinine greater than 2.0 g/dL or rapidly rising creatinine in normal range). Helical CT scanning can be avoided in patients who are at "unlikely" risk for pulmonary embolism using the Wells score for pulmonary embolism and the sensitive D-dimer test. Echocardiography may reveal evidence of HF or mitral stenosis.

Treatment

Management of mild hemoptysis consists of identifying and treating the specific cause. Massive hemoptysis is life-threatening. The airway should be protected with endotracheal intubation, ventilation ensured, and effective circulation maintained. If the location of the bleeding site is known, the patient should be placed in the decubitus position with the involved lung dependent. Uncontrollable hemorrhage warrants rigid bronchoscopy and surgical consultation. In stable patients, flexible bronchoscopy may localize the site of bleeding, and angiography can embolize the involved bronchial arteries. Embolization is effective initially in 85% of cases, although rebleeding may occur in up to 20% of patients during the following year. The anterior spinal artery arises from the bronchial artery in up to 5% of people, and paraplegia may result if it is inadvertently cannulated and embolized. There is limited evidence that antifibrinolytics may reduce the duration of bleeding.

When to Refer

- Patients should be referred to a pulmonologist when bronchoscopic evaluation of the lower respiratory tract is required.
- Patients should be referred to an otolaryngologist when an upper respiratory tract bleeding source is identified.
- Patients with severe coagulopathy complicating management should be referred to a hematologist.

When to Admit

- To stabilize bleeding process in patients at risk for or experiencing massive hemoptysis.
- To correct disordered coagulation (using clotting factors or platelets, or both).
- To stabilize gas exchange.

Eggeman D et al. Nasal congestion and hemoptysis. JAMA Otolaryngol Head Neck Surg. 2014 Nov;140(11):1081–2. [PMID: 25322081]

Ketai LH et al; Expert Panel on Thoracic Imaging. ACR appropriateness criteria® hemoptysis. J Thorac Imaging. 2014 May;29(3):W19–22. [PMID: 24717602]

Le Gal G et al. D-dimer for pulmonary embolism. JAMA. 2015 Apr 28;313(16):1668–9. [PMID: 25919531]

Shim J et al. A systematic review of symptomatic diagnosis of lung cancer. Fam Pract. 2014 Apr;31(2):137–48. [PMID: 24347594]

Uysal E et al. A life-threatening complication of warfarin therapy in ED: diffuse alveolar hemorrhage. Am J Emerg Med. 2014 Jun;32(6):690.e3–4. [PMID: 24412020]

Worrell SG et al. Thoracic emergencies. Surg Clin North Am. 2014 Feb;94(1):183–91. [PMID: 24267505]

CHEST PAIN

ESSENTIAL INQUIRIES

- Chest pain onset, character, location/size, duration, periodicity, and exacerbators; and shortness of breath.
- Vital signs; chest and cardiac examination.
- Electrocardiography and biomarkers of myocardial necrosis in selected patients.

General Considerations

Chest pain (or chest discomfort) is a common symptom that can occur as a result of cardiovascular, pulmonary, pleural, or musculoskeletal disease, esophageal or other gastrointestinal disorders, herpes zoster, or anxiety states. The frequency and distribution of life-threatening causes of chest pain, such as acute coronary syndrome (ACS), pericarditis, aortic dissection, vasospastic angina, pulmonary embolism, pneumonia, and esophageal perforation, vary substantially between clinical settings. Systemic lupus erythematosus, rheumatoid arthritis, reduced estimated glomerular filtration rate, and HIV are conditions that confer a strong risk of coronary artery disease. Precocious ACS may represent acute thrombosis independent of underlying atherosclerotic disease. In patients aged 35 years or younger, risk factors for ACS are obesity, hyperlipidemia, and smoking.

Chest pain characteristics that can lead to early diagnosis of acute myocardial infarction do not differ in frequency or strength of association between men and women. Because pulmonary embolism can present with a wide variety of symptoms, consideration of the diagnosis and rigorous risk factor assessment for venous thromboembolism (VTE) is critical. Classic VTE risk factors include cancer, trauma, recent surgery, prolonged immobilization, pregnancy, oral contraceptives, and family history and prior history of VTE. Other conditions associated with increased risk of pulmonary embolism include HF and COPD. Sickle cell anemia can cause acute chest syndrome. Patients with this syndrome often have chest pain, fever, and cough.

Clinical Findings

A. Symptoms

Myocardial ischemia is usually described as a dull, aching sensation of "pressure," "tightness," "squeezing," or "gas," rather than as sharp or spasmodic. Ischemic symptoms usually subside within 5–20 minutes but may last longer. Progressive symptoms or symptoms at rest may represent unstable angina. Prolonged chest pain episodes might represent myocardial infarction, although up to one-third of patients with acute myocardial infarction do not report chest pain. When present, pain due to myocardial ischemia is commonly accompanied by a sense of anxiety or uneasiness. The location is usually retrosternal or left precordial. Because the heart lacks somatic innervation, precise localization of pain due to cardiac ischemia is difficult; the pain is commonly referred to the throat, lower jaw, shoulders, inner arms, upper abdomen, or back. Ischemic pain may be precipitated or exacerbated by exertion, cold temperature, meals, stress, or combinations of these factors and is usually relieved by rest. However, many episodes do not conform to these patterns, and atypical presentations of ACS are more common in the elderly, women, and persons with diabetes mellitus. Other symptoms that are associated with ACS include shortness of breath; dizziness; a feeling of impending doom; and vagal symptoms, such as nausea and diaphoresis. In the elderly, fatigue is a common presenting complaint of ACS. Likelihood ratios (LRs) for cardinal symptoms considered in the evaluation of acute myocardial infarction are summarized in Table 2–5.

Table 2–5. Likelihood ratios (LRs) for clinical features associated with acute myocardial infarction.

Clinical Feature	LR+ (95% CI)
History	
Chest pain that radiates to the left arm	2.3 (1.7–3.1)
Chest pain that radiates to the right shoulder	2.9 (1.4–3.0)
Chest pain that radiates to both arms	7.1 (3.6–14.2)
Pleuritic chest pain	0.2 (0.2–0.3)
Sharp or stabbing chest pain	0.3 (0.2–0.5)
Positional chest pain	0.3 (0.2–0.4)
Chest pain reproduced by palpation	0.2–0.41
Nausea or vomiting	1.9 (1.7–2.3)
Diaphoresis	2.0 (1.9–2.2)
Physical examination	
Systolic blood pressure ≤ 80 mm Hg	3.1 (1.8–5.2)
Pulmonary crackles	2.1 (1.4–3.1)
Third heart sound	3.2 (1.6–6.5)
Electrocardiogram	
Any ST segment elevation (≥ 1 mm)	11.2 (7.1–17.8)
Any ST segment depression	3.2 (2.5–4.1)
Any Q wave	3.9 (2.7–7.7)
Any conduction defect	2.7 (1.4–5.4)
New ST segment elevation (≥ 1 mm)	(5.7–53.9)[1]
New ST segment depression	(3.0–5.2)[1]
New Q wave	(5.3–24.8)[1]
New conduction defect	6.3 (2.5–15.7)

[1]Heterogenous studies do not allow for calculation of a point estimate.
Adapted, with permission, from Panju AA et al. The rational clinical examination. Is this patient having a myocardial infarction? JAMA. 1998 Oct 14;280(14):1256–63. © 1998 American Medical Association. All rights reserved.

A meta-analysis found the clinical findings and risk factors most suggestive of ACS were prior abnormal stress test (specificity, 96%; LR, 3.1 [95% confidence interval {CI}, 2.0–4.7]), peripheral arterial disease (specificity, 97%; LR, 2.7 [95% CI, 1.5–4.8]), and pain radiation to both arms (specificity, 96%; LR, 2.6 [95% CI, 1.8–3.7]). The ECG findings associated with ACS were ST-segment depression (specificity, 95%; LR, 5.3 [95% CI, 2.1–8.6]) and any evidence of ischemia (specificity, 91%; LR, 3.6 [95% CI,1.6–5.7]). Risk scores derived from both the History, Electrocardiogram, Age, Risk Factors, Troponin (HEART) and Thrombolysis in Myocardial Infarction (TIMI) trials performed well in detecting ACS (LR, 13 [95% CI, 7.0–24] for HEART score of 7–10, and LR, 6.8 [95% CI, 5.2–8.9] for TIMI score of 5–7).

Hypertrophy of either ventricle or aortic stenosis may also give rise to chest pain with less typical features. Pericarditis produces pain that may be greater when supine than upright and increases with respiration, coughing, or swallowing. Pleuritic chest pain is usually not ischemic, and pain on palpation may indicate a musculoskeletal cause. Aortic dissection classically produces an abrupt onset of tearing pain of great intensity that often radiates to the back; however, this classic presentation occurs in a small proportion of cases. Anterior aortic dissection can also lead to myocardial or cerebrovascular ischemia.

Pulmonary embolism has a wide range of clinical presentations, with chest pain present in about 75% of cases. The chief objective in evaluating patients with suspected pulmonary embolism is to assess the patient's clinical risk for VTE based on medical history and associated signs and symptoms (see above and Chapter 9). Rupture of the thoracic esophagus iatrogenically or secondary to vomiting is another cause of chest pain.

B. Physical Examination

Findings on physical examination can occasionally yield important clues to the underlying cause of chest pain; however, a normal physical examination should never be used as the sole basis for ruling out most diagnoses, particularly ACS and aortic dissection. Vital signs (including pulse oximetry) and cardiopulmonary examination are always the first steps for assessing the urgency and tempo of the subsequent examination and diagnostic work-up.

Findings that increase the likelihood of ACS include diaphoresis, hypotension, S_3 or S_4 gallop, pulmonary crackles, or elevated jugular venous pressure (see Table 2–5). Although chest pain that is reproducible or worsened with palpation strongly suggests a musculoskeletal cause, up to 15% of patients with ACS will have reproducible chest wall tenderness. Pointing to the location of the pain with one finger has been shown to be highly correlated with nonischemic chest pain. Aortic dissection can result in differential blood pressures (greater than 20 mm Hg), pulse amplitude deficits, and new diastolic murmurs. Although hypertension is considered the rule in patients with aortic dissection, systolic blood pressure less than 100 mm Hg is present in up to 25% of patients.

A cardiac friction rub represents pericarditis until proven otherwise. It can best be heard with the patient sitting forward at end-expiration. Tamponade should be excluded in all patients with a clinical diagnosis of pericarditis by assessing pulsus paradoxus (a decrease in systolic blood pressure during inspiration greater than 10 mm Hg) and inspection of jugular venous pulsations. Subcutaneous emphysema is common following cervical esophageal perforation but present in only about one-third of thoracic perforations (ie, those most commonly presenting with chest pain).

The absence of abnormal physical examination findings in patients with suspected pulmonary embolism usually serves to *increase* the likelihood of pulmonary embolism, although a normal physical examination is also compatible with the much more common conditions of panic/anxiety disorder and musculoskeletal disease.

C. Diagnostic Studies

Unless a competing diagnosis can be confirmed, an ECG is warranted in the initial evaluation of most patients with acute chest pain to help exclude ACS. ST segment elevation is the ECG finding that is the strongest predictor of acute myocardial infarction (see Table 2–5); however, up to 20% of patients with ACS can have a normal ECG. In the emergency department, patients with suspected ACS can be safely removed from cardiac monitoring if they are pain-free at initial physician assessment and have a normal or nonspecific ECG. This decision rule had 100% sensitivity for serious arrhythmia (95% CI, 80–100%), but deserves further validation. Clinically stable patients with cardiovascular disease risk factors, normal ECG, normal cardiac biomarkers, and no alternative diagnoses (such as typical GERD or costochondritis) should be followed up with a timely exercise stress test that includes perfusion imaging. The ECG can also provide evidence for alternative diagnoses, such as pericarditis and pulmonary embolism. Chest radiography is often useful in the evaluation of chest pain, and is always indicated when cough or shortness of breath accompanies chest pain. Findings of pneumomediastinum or new pleural effusion are consistent with esophageal perforation.

Diagnostic protocols using a single high-sensitivity troponin assay combined with a standardized clinical assessment have been proposed as an efficient strategy to rapidly determine whether patients with chest pain are at low risk and may be discharged from the emergency department. The TRUST ADP diagnostic protocol identified low-risk patients with suspected ACS using a single measurement of high-sensitivity cardiac troponin T (hs-cTnT), a nonischemic ECG, and a modified Goldman risk score. This protocol identified 40% of patients as low risk after a single hs-cTnT taken at presentation to the emergency department, with a negative predictive value of greater than 99.5%. The Manchester Acute Coronary Syndromes (MACS) decision rule identified 27% of patients who arrived at the emergency department complaining of chest pain as "very low risk" and potentially suitable for discharge; on the other hand, patients were admitted if they were judged to be "high risk" using the following eight variables: high-sensitivity troponin T, high heart-type fatty-acid–binding protein, ischemia on ECG, observed diaphoresis, vomiting, pain radiation to the arm or shoulder, worsening angina, and hypotension.

While some studies of high-sensitivity cardiac troponin suggest that it may be the best cardiac biomarker, it may not outperform conventional troponin assays if an appropriate cut-off is used. Copeptin and heart-type fatty-acid–binding protein may also have a role in increasing diagnostic sensitivity.

Patients who arrive at the emergency department with chest pain of intermediate or high probability for ACS without electrocardiographic or biomarker evidence of a myocardial infarction can be safely discharged from an observation unit after stress cardiac MRI. Sixty-four–slice CT coronary angiography (CTA), an alternative to stress testing in the emergency department, has been studied for detecting ACS among patients with normal or nonspecific ECG and normal biomarkers. A meta-analysis of nine studies found ACS in 10% of patients, and an estimated sensitivity of CTA for ACS of 95%, specificity of 87%, yielding a negative LR of 0.06 and a positive LR of 7.4. One study examined the prognostic implications of CTA during acute chest pain and found very low incidence rates of major adverse cardiac events in persons with normal CTA and in persons with nonobstructing coronary artery disease (0.6% and 1.3%, respectively). Coronary CTA may also have a role in identifying high-risk plaques increasing the likelihood of ACS independent of significant coronary artery disease and clinical risk assessment. However, in symptomatic patients with suspected coronary artery disease who required noninvasive testing, initial CTA did not improve clinical outcomes over a median follow-up of 2 years, and led to more catheterization and revascularization procedures than initial functional testing. Thus, functional testing (such as stress cardiac MRI) appears to be the best initial noninvasive test in symptomatic patients with suspected coronary artery disease.

While multidetector CTA enables diagnosis (or exclusion) of coronary artery disease, ACS, and pulmonary emboli (so-called "triple rule-out"), it involves both radiation and contrast exposure. At most centers, helical CT is the study of choice for evaluating possible aortic dissection and esophageal perforation.

In the evaluation of pulmonary embolism, diagnostic test decisions and results must be interpreted in the context of the clinical likelihood of VTE. A negative D-dimer test is helpful for excluding pulmonary embolism in patients with low clinical probability of VTE (3-month incidence = 0.5%); however, the 3-month risk of VTE among patients with intermediate and high risk of VTE is sufficiently high in the setting of a negative D-dimer test (3.5% and 21.4%, respectively) to warrant further imaging given the life-threatening nature of this condition if left untreated. CT angiography (with helical or multidetector CT imaging) has replaced ventilation-perfusion scanning as the preferred initial diagnostic test, having approximately 90–95% sensitivity and 95% specificity for detecting pulmonary embolism (compared with pulmonary angiography). However, for patients with high clinical probability of VTE, lower extremity ultrasound or pulmonary angiogram may be indicated even with a normal helical CT.

Panic disorder is a common cause of chest pain, accounting for up to 25% of cases that present to emergency departments and a higher proportion of cases presenting in primary care office practices. Features that correlate with an increased likelihood of panic disorder include absence of coronary artery disease, atypical quality of chest pain, female sex, younger age, and a high level of self-reported anxiety.

Treatment

Treatment of chest pain should be guided by the underlying etiology. The term "noncardiac chest pain" is used when a diagnosis remains elusive after patients have undergone an extensive work-up. Almost half reported symptom improvement with high-dose proton-pump inhibitor therapy. A meta-analysis of 15 trials suggested modest to moderate benefit for psychological (especially cognitive-behavioral) interventions. It is unclear whether tricyclic or selective serotonin reuptake inhibitor antidepressants have benefit in noncardiac chest pain. Hypnotherapy may offer some benefit.

When to Refer

- Refer patients with poorly controlled, noncardiac chest pain to a pain specialist.
- Refer patients with sickle cell anemia to a hematologist.

When to Admit

- Failure to adequately exclude life-threatening causes of chest pain, particularly myocardial infarction, dissecting aortic aneurysm, pulmonary embolism, and esophageal rupture.
- High risk of pulmonary embolism and a positive sensitive D-dimer test.
- TIMI score of 1 or more, abnormal electrocardiogram and abnormal 0- and 2-hour troponin tests.
- Pain control for rib fracture that impairs gas exchange.

Atluri DK et al. Systematic review with meta-analysis: selective serotonin reuptake inhibitors for noncardiac chest pain. Aliment Pharmacol Ther. 2015 Jan;41(2):167–76. [PMID: 25412947]

Bandstein N et al. Undetectable high-sensitivity cardiac troponin T level in the emergency department and risk of myocardial infarction. J Am Coll Cardiol. 2014 Jun 17;63(23):2569–78. [PMID: 24694529]

Basra SS et al. Acute coronary syndromes: unstable angina and non-ST elevation myocardial infarction. Cardiol Clin. 2014 Aug;32(3):353–70. [PMID: 25091963]

Beigel R et al. Prognostic implications of nonobstructive coronary artery disease in patients undergoing coronary computed tomographic angiography for acute chest pain. Am J Cardiol. 2013 Apr 1;111(7):941–5. [PMID: 23332596]

Body R et al. The Manchester Acute Coronary Syndromes (MACS) decision rule for suspected cardiac chest pain: derivation and external validation. Heart. 2014 Sep 15; 100(18):1462–8. [PMID: 24780911]

Burgstaller JM et al. Treatment efficacy for non-cardiovascular chest pain: a systematic review and meta-analysis. PLoS One. 2014 Aug 11;9(8):e104722. [PMID: 25111147]

Carlton EW et al. A novel diagnostic protocol to identify patients suitable for discharge after a single high-sensitivity troponin. Heart. 2015 Jul;101(13):1041–6. [PMID: 25691511]

Collinson P et al. Comparison of contemporary troponin assays with the novel biomarkers, heart fatty acid binding protein and copeptin, for the early confirmation or exclusion of myocardial infarction in patients presenting to the emergency department with chest pain. Heart. 2014 Jan;100(2):140–5. [PMID: 24270743]

Davidson L et al. Clinical features of precocious acute coronary syndrome. Am J Med. 2014 Feb;127(2):140–4. [PMID: 24332726]

Douglas PS et al; PROMISE Investigators. Outcomes of anatomical versus functional testing for coronary artery disease. N Engl J Med. 2015 Apr 2;372(14):1291–300. [PMID: 25773919]

Fanaroff AC et al. Does this patient with chest pain have acute coronary syndrome? The Rational Clinical Examination Systematic Review. JAMA. 2015 Nov 10;314(18):1955–65. [PMID: 26547467]

Foy AJ et al. Chest pain evaluation in the emergency department. Med Clin North Am. 2015 Jul;99(4):835–47. [PMID: 26042885]

Hoffmann U et al; ROMICAT-II Investigators. Coronary CT angiography versus standard evaluation in acute chest pain. N Engl J Med. 2012 Jul 26;367(4):299–308. [PMID: 22830462]

Holly J et al. Prospective evaluation of the use of the Thrombolysis In Myocardial Infarction score as a risk stratification tool for chest pain patients admitted to an ED observation unit. Am J Emerg Med. 2013 Jan;31(1):185–9. [PMID: 22944539]

Januzzi JL et al. Sensitive troponin assays in patients with suspected acute coronary syndrome: results from the multicenter Rule Out Myocardial Infarction using Computer Assisted Tomography II trial. Am Heart J. 2015 Apr;169(4):572–8. [PMID: 25819865]

Kosowsky JM. Approach to the ED patient with "low risk" chest pain. Emerg Med Clin North Am. 2011 Nov;29(4):721–7. [PMID: 22040703]

McConaghy JR et al. Outpatient diagnosis of acute chest pain in adults. Am Fam Physician. 2013 Feb 1;87(3):177–82. [PMID: 23418761]

Puchner SB et al. High-risk plaque detected on coronary CT angiography predicts acute coronary syndromes independent of significant stenosis in acute chest pain: results from the ROMICAT-II trial. J Am Coll Cardiol. 2014 Aug 19;64(7): 684–92. [PMID: 25125300]

Schlett CL et al. Cardiac computed tomography for the evaluation of the acute chest pain syndrome: state of the art. Radiol Clin North Am. 2015 Mar;53(2):297–305. [PMID: 25726995]

SCOT-HEART investigators. CT coronary angiography in patients with suspected angina due to coronary heart disease (SCOT-HEART): an open-label, parallel-group, multicentre trial. Lancet. 2015 Jun 13;385(9985):2383–91. Erratum in: Lancet. 2015 Jun 13;385(9985):2354. [PMID: 25788230]

Sethi A et al. Diagnostic accuracy of sensitive or high-sensitive troponin on presentation for myocardial infarction: a meta-analysis and systematic review. Vasc Health Risk Manag. 2014 Jul 21;10:435–50. [PMID: 25092986]

Staniak HL et al. Coronary CT angiography for acute chest pain in the emergency department. J Cardiovasc Comput Tomogr. 2014 Sep–Oct;8(5):359–67. [PMID: 25301041]

Than M et al. 2-Hour accelerated diagnostic protocol to assess patients with chest pain symptoms using contemporary troponins as the only biomarker: the ADAPT trial. J Am Coll Cardiol. 2012 Jun 5;59(23):2091–8. [PMID: 22578923]

Than M et al. A 2-hour diagnostic protocol for possible cardiac chest pain in the emergency department: a randomized clinical trial. JAMA Intern Med. 2014 Jan;174(1):51–8. [PMID: 24100783]

PALPITATIONS

ESSENTIAL INQUIRIES

▸ Forceful, rapid, or irregular beating of the heart.

▸ Rate, duration, and degree of regularity of heart beat; age at first episode.

▸ Factors that precipitate or terminate episodes.

▸ Light-headedness or syncope; neck pounding.

▸ Chest pain.

▶ General Considerations

Palpitations are defined as an unpleasant awareness of the forceful, rapid, or irregular beating of the heart. They are the primary symptom for approximately 16% of patients presenting to an outpatient clinic with a cardiac complaint. Palpitations represent 5.8 of every 1000 emergency department visits, with an admission rate of 24.6%. While palpitations are usually benign, they are occasionally the symptom of a life-threatening arrhythmia. To avoid missing a dangerous cause of the patient's symptom, clinicians sometimes pursue expensive and invasive testing when a conservative diagnostic evaluation is sufficient. The converse is also true; in one study, 54% of patients with supraventricular tachycardia were initially wrongly diagnosed with panic, stress, or anxiety disorder. A disproportionate number of these misdiagnosed patients are women. Table 2–6 lists history, physical examination, and ECG findings suggesting a cardiovascular cause for the palpitations.

▶ Clinical Findings

A. Symptoms

Although described by patients in a myriad of ways, guiding the patient through a careful description of their palpitations may indicate a mechanism and narrow the differential diagnosis. Pertinent questions include the age at first episode; precipitants; and rate, duration, and degree of regularity of the heart beat during the subjective palpitations. Palpitations lasting less than 5 minutes and a family history of panic disorder reduce the likelihood of an arrhythmic cause (LR = 0.38 and LR = 0.26, respectively). To better understand the symptom, the examiner can ask the patient to "tap out" the rhythm with their fingers. The circumstances associated with onset and termination can also be helpful in determining the cause. Palpitations that start and stop abruptly suggest supraventricular or ventricular tachycardias. Termination of palpitations using vagal maneuvers (eg, Valsalva maneuver) suggests supraventricular tachycardia.

Three common descriptions of palpitations are (1) "flip-flopping" (or "stop and start"), often caused by premature contraction of the atrium or ventricle, with the perceived "stop" from the pause following the contraction, and the "start" from the subsequent forceful contraction; (2) rapid "fluttering in the chest," with regular "fluttering" suggesting supraventricular or ventricular arrhythmias (including sinus tachycardia) and irregular "fluttering" suggesting atrial fibrillation, atrial flutter, or tachycardia with variable block; and (3) "pounding in the neck" or neck pulsations, often due to "cannon" A waves in the jugular venous pulsations that occur when the right atrium contracts against a closed tricuspid valve.

Palpitations associated with chest pain suggest ischemic heart disease, or if the chest pain is relieved by leaning forward, pericardial disease is suspected. Palpitations associated with light-headedness, presyncope, or syncope suggest hypotension and may signify a life-threatening cardiac arrhythmia. Palpitations that occur regularly with exertion suggest a rate-dependent bypass tract or hypertrophic cardiomyopathy. If a benign etiology for these concerning symptoms cannot be ascertained at the initial visit, then ambulatory monitoring or prolonged cardiac monitoring in the hospital might be warranted.

Noncardiac symptoms should also be elicited since the palpitations may be caused by a normal heart responding to a metabolic or inflammatory condition. Weight loss suggests hyperthyroidism. Palpitations can be precipitated by vomiting or diarrhea that leads to electrolyte disorders and hypovolemia. Hyperventilation, hand tingling, and nervousness are common when anxiety or panic disorder is the cause of the palpitations.

A family history of palpitations or sudden death suggests an inherited etiology such as long QT syndrome or Brugada syndrome. Chagas disease may cause palpitations and acute myocarditis.

B. Physical Examination

Rarely does the clinician have the opportunity to examine a patient during an episode of palpitations. However, careful cardiovascular examination can find abnormalities that can increase the likelihood of specific cardiac arrhythmias. The midsystolic click of mitral valve prolapse can suggest the diagnosis of a supraventricular arrhythmia. The harsh holosystolic murmur of hypertrophic cardiomyopathy, which occurs along the left sternal border and increases

Table 2–6. Palpitations: Patients at high risk for a cardiovascular cause.

Historical risk factors
Family history of significant arrhythmias
Personal or family history of syncope or resuscitated sudden death
History of myocardial infarction (and likely scarred myocardium)
Physical examination findings
Structural heart disease such as dilated or hypertrophic cardiomyopathies
Valvular disease (stenotic or regurgitant)
ECG findings
Long QT syndrome
Bradycardia
Second- or third-degree heart block
Sustained ventricular arrhythmias

with the Valsalva maneuver, suggests atrial fibrillation or ventricular tachycardia. The presence of dilated cardiomyopathy, suggested on examination by a displaced and enlarged cardiac point-of-maximal impulse, increases the likelihood of ventricular tachycardia and atrial fibrillation. In patients with chronic atrial fibrillation, in-office exercise (eg, a brisk walk in the hallway) may reveal an intermittent accelerated ventricular response as the cause of the palpitations. The clinician should also look for signs of hyperthyroidism (eg, tremulousness, brisk deep tendon reflexes, or fine hand tremor), or signs of stimulant drug use (eg, dilated pupils or skin or nasal septal perforations). Visible neck pulsations (LR, 2.68; 95% CI, 1.25–5.78) in association with palpitations increases the likelihood of atrioventricular nodal reentry tachycardia.

C. Diagnostic Studies

Commonly used studies in the initial evaluation of a patient with palpitations are the 12-lead ECG and ambulatory ECG monitoring devices (eg, the Holter monitor or an event recorder).

A 12-lead ECG should be performed on all patients reporting palpitations because it can provide evidence for a wide variety of causes. Although in most instances a specific arrhythmia will not be detected on the tracing, a careful evaluation of the ECG can help the clinician deduce a likely etiology in certain circumstances.

For instance, bradyarrhythmias and heart block can be associated with ventricular ectopy or escape beats that may be experienced as palpitations by the patient. Evidence of prior myocardial infarction on ECG (eg, Q waves) increases the patient's risk for nonsustained or sustained ventricular tachycardia. Ventricular preexcitation (Wolff-Parkinson-White syndrome) is suggested by a short PR interval (less than 0.20 ms) and delta waves (upsloping PR segments). Left ventricular hypertrophy with deep septal Q waves in I, AVL, and V4 through V6 is seen in patients with hypertrophic obstructive cardiomyopathy. The presence of left atrial enlargement as suggested by a terminal P-wave force in V1 more negative than 0.04 msec and notching in lead II reflects a patient at increased risk for atrial fibrillation. A prolonged QT interval and abnormal T-wave morphology suggest the long-QT syndrome, which puts patients at increased risk for ventricular tachycardia. Persistent ST segment elevations in ECG leads V1–V3 (particularly with a coved or saddle-back pattern) suggest Brugada syndrome.

For high-risk patients (Table 2–6), further diagnostic studies are warranted. A step-wise approach has been suggested—starting with ambulatory monitoring devices (Holter monitoring if the palpitations are expected to occur within the subsequent 72-hour period, event monitoring if less frequent). This is then followed by inpatient continuous monitoring if serious arrhythmias are strongly suspected despite normal findings on the ambulatory monitoring, and by invasive electrophysiologic testing if the ambulatory or inpatient monitor records a worrisome arrhythmia. A single-lead, lightweight, continuously recording ambulatory adhesive patch monitor (Zio Patch) has been shown to be superior to 24-hour Holter monitoring.

In patients with a prior myocardial infarction, ambulatory cardiac monitoring or signal-averaged ECG are appropriate next steps to help exclude ventricular tachycardia. ECG exercise testing is appropriate in patients with suspected coronary artery disease and in patients who have palpitations with physical exertion. Echocardiography is useful when physical examination or ECG suggests structural abnormalities or decreased ventricular function.

▶ Differential Diagnosis

When assessing a patient with palpitations in an urgent care setting, the clinician must ascertain whether the symptoms represent (1) an arrhythmia that is minor and transient, (2) a significant cardiovascular disease, (3) a cardiac manifestation of a systemic disease such as thyrotoxicosis, or (4) a benign somatic symptom that is amplified by the patient's underlying psychological make-up.

Palpitations in patients with known cardiac disease or palpitations that occur during sleep increase the likelihood of a cardiac arrhythmia. A history of panic disorder or palpitations that last less than 5 minutes make a cardiac arrhythmia slightly less likely. Patients with palpitations who seek medical attention in an emergency department instead of a medical clinic are more likely to have a cardiac cause (47% versus 21%), whereas psychiatric causes are more common among those who seek attention in office practices (45% versus 27%). In a study of patients who went to a university medical clinic with the chief complaint of palpitations, causes were cardiac in 43%, psychiatric in 31%, and miscellaneous in 10%.

Cardiac arrhythmias that can result in symptoms of palpitations include sinus bradycardia; sinus, supraventricular, and ventricular tachycardia; premature ventricular and atrial contractions; sick sinus syndrome; and advanced atrioventricular block.

Cardiac nonarrhythmic causes of palpitations include valvular heart diseases, such as aortic regurgitation or stenosis, atrial or ventricular septal defect, cardiomyopathy, congenital heart disease, and pericarditis.

The most common psychiatric causes of palpitations are anxiety and panic disorder. The release of catecholamines during a significant stress or panic attack can trigger an arrhythmia. Asking a single question, "Have you experienced brief periods, for seconds or minutes, of an overwhelming panic or terror that was accompanied by racing heartbeats, shortness of breath, or dizziness?" can help identify patients with panic disorder.

Miscellaneous causes of palpitations include fever, dehydration, hypoglycemia, anemia, thyrotoxicosis, mastocytosis, and pheochromocytoma. Drugs such as cocaine, alcohol, caffeine, pseudoephedrine, and illicit ephedra can precipitate palpitations, as can prescription medications, including digoxin, phenothiazines, theophylline, and beta-agonists.

▶ Treatment

After ambulatory monitoring, most patients with palpitations are found to have benign atrial or ventricular ectopy or nonsustained ventricular tachycardia. In patients with structurally normal hearts, these arrhythmias are not associated with adverse outcomes. Abstention from caffeine and tobacco may help. Often, reassurance suffices. If not, or in very symptomatic patients, a trial of a beta-blocker may be prescribed. A three-session course of cognitive-behavioral therapy that includes some physical activity has proven effective for patients with benign palpitations with or without chest pain. For treatment of specific atrial or ventricular arrhythmias, see Chapter 10.

▶ When to Refer

- For electrophysiologic studies.
- For advice regarding treatment of atrial or ventricular arrhythmias.

▶ When to Admit

- Palpitations associated with syncope or near-syncope, particularly when the patient is aged 75 years or older and has an abnormal ECG, hematocrit less than 30%, shortness of breath, respiratory rate higher than 24/min, or a history of HF.
- Patients with risk factors for a serious arrhythmia.

Barrett PM et al. Comparison of 24-hour Holter monitoring with 14-day novel adhesive patch electrocardiographic monitoring. Am J Med. 2014 Jan;127(1):95.e11–7. [PMID: 24384108]

Helton MR. Diagnosis and management of common types of supraventricular tachycardia. Am Fam Physician. 2015 Nov 1; 92(9):793–800. [PMID: 26554472]

Jamshed N et al. Emergency management of palpitations in the elderly: epidemiology, diagnostic approaches, and therapeutic options. Clin Geriatr Med. 2013 Feb;29(1):205–30. [PMID: 23177608]

Probst MA et al. Analysis of emergency department visits for palpitations (from the National Hospital Ambulatory Medical Care Survey). Am J Cardiol. 2014 May 15;113(10):1685–90. [PMID: 24698469]

Probst MA et al. Emergency physicians' perceptions and decision-making processes regarding patients presenting with palpitations. J Emerg Med. 2015 Aug;49(2):236–43. [PMID: 25943288]

Sedaghat-Yazdi F et al. The teenager with palpitations. Pediatr Clin North Am. 2014 Feb;61(1):63–79. [PMID: 24267458]

LOWER EXTREMITY EDEMA

ESSENTIAL INQUIRIES

- ▶ History of venous thromboembolism.
- ▶ Symmetry of swelling.
- ▶ Pain.
- ▶ Change with dependence.
- ▶ Skin findings: hyperpigmentation, stasis dermatitis, lipodermatosclerosis, atrophie blanche, ulceration.

▶ General Considerations

Acute and chronic lower extremity edema present important diagnostic and treatment challenges. Lower extremities can swell in response to increased venous or lymphatic pressures, decreased intravascular oncotic pressure, increased capillary leak, and local injury or infection. **Chronic venous insufficiency** is by far the most common cause, affecting up to 2% of the population, and the incidence of venous insufficiency has not changed during the past 25 years. Venous insufficiency is a common complication of DVT; however, only a small number of patients with chronic venous insufficiency report a history of this disorder. Venous ulceration commonly affects patients with chronic venous insufficiency, and its management is labor-intensive and expensive. Other causes of lower extremity edema include cellulitis, musculoskeletal disorders (Baker cyst rupture, gastrocnemius tear or rupture, diabetic myonecrosis), lymphedema, lipoedema, HF, cirrhosis, nephrotic syndrome, left common iliac vein compression (May-Thurner syndrome), and medication side effects (eg, calcium channel blockers, minoxidil, or pioglitazone).

▶ Clinical Findings

A. Symptoms and Signs

Normal lower extremity venous pressure (in the erect position: 80 mm Hg in deep veins, 20–30 mm Hg in superficial veins) and cephalad venous blood flow require competent bicuspid venous valves, effective muscle contractions, and normal respirations. When one or more of these components fail, venous hypertension may result. Chronic exposure to elevated venous pressure by the postcapillary venules in the legs leads to leakage of fibrinogen and growth factors into the interstitial space, leukocyte aggregation and activation, and obliteration of the cutaneous lymphatic network. These changes account for the brawny, fibrotic skin changes observed in patients with chronic venous insufficiency, and the predisposition toward skin ulceration, particularly in the medial malleolar area.

Among common causes of lower extremity swelling, DVT is the most life-threatening. Clues suggesting DVT include a history of cancer, recent limb immobilization, or confinement to bed for at least 3 days following major surgery within the past month (Table 2–7). A search for alternative explanations is equally important in excluding DVT. Bilateral involvement and significant improvement upon awakening favor systemic causes (eg, venous insufficiency, HF, and cirrhosis). The sensation of "heavy legs" is the most frequent symptom of chronic venous insufficiency, followed by itching. Pain, particularly if severe, is uncommon in uncomplicated venous insufficiency. Lower extremity swelling and inflammation in a limb recently affected by DVT could represent anticoagulation failure and thrombus recurrence but more often are caused by **postphlebitic syndrome** with valvular incompetence. Other causes of a painful, swollen calf include ruptured popliteal cyst ("pseudothrombophlebitis"), calf strain or trauma, and cellulitis.

Lower extremity swelling is a familiar complication of therapy with calcium channel blockers (particularly

Table 2–7. Risk stratification of adults referred for ultrasound to rule out DVT.

Step 1: Calculate risk factor score		
Score 1 point for each		
Untreated malignancy		
Paralysis, paresis, or recent plaster immobilization		
Recently bedridden for > 3 days due to major surgery within 4 weeks		
Localized tenderness along distribution of deep venous system		
Entire leg swelling		
Swelling of one calf > 3 cm more than the other (measured 10 cm below tibial tuberosity)		
Ipsilateral pitting edema		
Collateral superficial (nonvaricose) veins		
Previously documented DVT		
Alternative diagnosis as likely as or more likely than DVT: subtract 2 points		

	Step 2: Obtain ultrasound	
Score	**Ultrasound Positive**	**Ultrasound Negative**
0	Confirm with venogram	DVT ruled out
1–2	Treat for DVT	Repeat ultrasound in 3–7 days
≥ 3	Treat for DVT	Confirm with venogram

DVT, deep venous thrombosis.

felodipine and amlodipine), pioglitazone, and minoxidil. Bilateral lower extremity edema can be a presenting symptom of nephrotic syndrome or volume overload caused by renal failure or cirrhosis. Prolonged airline flights (longer than 10 hours) are associated with edema. In addition, among those with low to medium risk of thromboembolism (eg, women taking oral contraceptives), long flights are associated with a 2% incidence of asymptomatic popliteal DVT.

B. Physical Examination

Physical examination should include assessment of the heart, lungs, and abdomen for evidence of pulmonary hypertension (primary or secondary to chronic lung disease), HF, or cirrhosis. Some patients with cirrhosis have pulmonary hypertension without lung disease. There is a spectrum of skin findings related to chronic venous insufficiency that depends on the severity and chronicity of the disease, ranging from hyperpigmentation and stasis dermatitis to abnormalities highly specific for chronic venous insufficiency: lipodermatosclerosis (thick, brawny skin; in advanced cases, the lower leg resembles an inverted champagne bottle) and atrophie blanche (small depigmented macules within areas of heavy pigmentation). The size of both calves should be measured 10 cm below the tibial tuberosity and pitting and tenderness elicited. Swelling of the entire leg or of one leg 3 cm more than the other suggests deep venous obstruction. The left calf is normally slightly larger than the right as a result of the left common iliac vein coursing under the aorta.

An ulcer located over the medial malleolus is a hallmark of chronic venous insufficiency but can be due to other causes. Shallow, large, modestly painful ulcers are characteristic of venous insufficiency, whereas small, deep, and more painful ulcers are more apt to be due to arterial insufficiency, vasculitis, or infection (including cutaneous diphtheria). Diabetic vascular ulcers, however, may be painless. When an ulcer is on the foot or above the mid-calf, causes other than venous insufficiency should be considered.

C. Diagnostic Studies

Most causes of lower extremity swelling can be demonstrated with color duplex ultrasonography. Patients without an obvious cause of acute lower extremity swelling (eg, calf strain) should have an ultrasound performed, since DVT is difficult to exclude on clinical grounds. A prediction rule allows a clinician to exclude a lower extremity DVT in patients without an ultrasound if the patient has low pretest probability for DVT and a negative sensitive D-dimer test (the "Wells prediction rule"). Assessment of the ankle-brachial pressure index (ABPI) is important in the management of chronic venous insufficiency, since peripheral arterial disease may be exacerbated by compression therapy. This can be performed at the same time as ultrasound. Caution is required in interpreting the results of ABPI in older patients and diabetics due to the decreased compressibility of their arteries. A urine dipstick test that is strongly positive for protein can suggest nephrotic syndrome, and a serum creatinine can help estimate kidney function.

▶ Treatment

Treatment of lower extremity edema should be guided by the underlying cause. See relevant chapters for treatment of edema in patients with HF (Chapter 10), nephrosis (Chapter 22), cirrhosis (Chapter 16), and lymphedema and venous stasis ulcers (Chapter 12). Edema resulting from calcium channel blocker therapy responds to concomitant therapy with ACE inhibitors or angiotensin receptor blockers.

In patients with chronic venous insufficiency without a comorbid volume overload state (eg, HF), it is best to avoid diuretic therapy. These patients have relatively decreased intravascular volume, and administration of diuretics may first enhance sodium retention through increased secretion of renin and angiotensin and then result in acute kidney injury and oliguria. Instead, the most effective treatment involves (1) leg elevation, above the level of the heart, for 30 minutes three to four times daily, and during sleep; (2) compression therapy; and (3) ambulatory exercise to increase venous return through calf muscle contractions. There is no evidence for benefit or harm of valvuloplasty in the treatment of patients with deep venous insufficiency secondary to primary valvular incompetence.

A wide variety of stockings and devices are effective in decreasing swelling and preventing ulcer formation. They should be put on with awakening, before hydrostatic forces result in edema. To control simple edema, 20–30 mm Hg is usually sufficient, whereas 30–40 mm Hg is usually required to control moderate to severe edema associated with ulcer formation. Patients with decreased ABPI should be managed in concert with a vascular surgeon. Compression stockings (12–18 mm Hg at the ankle) are effective in preventing edema and asymptomatic thrombosis associated with long airline flights in low- to medium-risk persons. For lymphedema, new bandaging systems applied twice weekly can be effective. Short-term manual lymphatic drainage treatment may improve chronic venous insufficiency severity, symptoms, and quality of life.

▶ When to Refer

- Chronic lower extremity ulcerations requiring specialist wound care.
- Refer patients with nephrotic syndrome to a nephrologist.
- Refer patients with coexisting severe arterial insufficiency (claudication) that would complicate treatment with compression stockings to a vascular surgeon.

▶ When to Admit

- Pending definitive diagnosis in patients at high risk for DVT despite normal lower extremity ultrasound.
- Severe, acute swelling raising concern for an impending compartment syndrome.
- Severe edema that impairs ability to ambulate or perform activities of daily living.

Aguilar-Ferrándiz ME et al. Effect of a mixed kinesio taping-compression technique on quality of life and clinical and gait parameters in postmenopausal women with chronic venous insufficiency: double-blinded, randomized controlled trial. Arch Phys Med Rehabil. 2014 Jul;95(7):1229–39. [PMID: 24732169]

Chwała M et al. Varicose veins of lower extremities, hemodynamics and treatment methods. Adv Clin Exp Med. 2015 Jan–Feb;24(1):5–14. [PMID: 25923081]

dos Santos Crisóstomo RS et al. Influence of manual lymphatic drainage on health-related quality of life and symptoms of chronic venous insufficiency: a randomized controlled trial. Arch Phys Med Rehabil. 2015 Feb;96(2):283–91. [PMID: 25308883]

Goel RR et al. Surgery for deep venous incompetence. Cochrane Database Syst Rev. 2015 Feb 23;2:CD001097. [PMID: 25702915]

FEVER & HYPERTHERMIA

ESSENTIAL INQUIRIES

- ▶ Age; injection substance use.
- ▶ Localizing symptoms; weight loss; joint pain.
- ▶ Immunosuppression or neutropenia; history of cancer.
- ▶ Medications.
- ▶ Travel.

▶ General Considerations

The average normal oral body temperature taken in mid-morning is 36.7°C (range 36–37.4°C). This range includes a mean and 2 standard deviations, thus encompassing 95% of a normal population (normal diurnal temperature variation is 0.5–1°C). The normal rectal or vaginal temperature is 0.5°C higher than the oral temperature, and the axillary temperature is 0.5°C lower. Rectal temperature is more reliable than oral temperature, particularly in patients who breathe through their mouth or who are tachypneic.

Fever is a regulated rise to a new "set point" of body temperature in the hypothalamus induced by pyrogenic cytokines. These cytokines include interleukin-1 (IL-1), tumor necrosis factor (TNF), interferon-gamma, and interleukin-6 (IL-6). The elevation in temperature results from either increased heat production (eg, shivering) or decreased heat loss (eg, peripheral vasoconstriction). Body temperature in cytokine-induced fever seldom exceeds 41.1°C unless there is structural damage to hypothalamic regulatory centers.

▶ Clinical Findings

A. Fever

Fever as a symptom provides important information about the presence of illness—particularly infections—and about changes in the clinical status of the patient. The fever pattern, however, is of marginal value for most specific diagnoses except for the relapsing fever of malaria, borreliosis, and occasional cases of lymphoma, especially Hodgkin disease. Furthermore, the degree of temperature elevation does not necessarily correspond to the severity of the illness. In general, the febrile response tends to be greater in children than in adults. In older persons, neonates, and in persons receiving certain medications (eg, NSAIDs, corticosteroids), a normal temperature or even hypothermia may be observed. Markedly elevated body temperature may result in profound metabolic disturbances. High temperature during the first trimester of pregnancy may cause birth defects, such as anencephaly. Fever increases insulin requirements and alters the metabolism and disposition of drugs used for the treatment of the diverse diseases associated with fever.

Fever in the intensive care unit can occur directly from brain injury (called "central fever"). One model predicted "central fever" with 90% probability if a patient met the following criteria: less than 72 hours of neurologic intensive care unit admission, presence of subarachnoid or intraventricular hemorrhage, brain tumor, absence of infiltrate on chest radiograph, blood transfusion, and negative cultures.

B. Hyperthermia

Hyperthermia—not mediated by cytokines—occurs when body metabolic heat production (as in thyroid storm) or environmental heat load exceeds normal heat loss capacity or when there is impaired heat loss; heat stroke is an example. Body temperature may rise to levels (more than 41.1°C) capable of producing irreversible protein denaturation and resultant brain damage; no diurnal variation is observed.

Neuroleptic malignant syndrome is a rare and potentially lethal idiosyncratic reaction to neuroleptic medications, particularly haloperidol and fluphenazine; however, it has also been reported with the atypical neuroleptics (such as olanzapine or risperidone) (see Chapter 25). **Serotonin syndrome** resembles neuroleptic malignant syndrome but occurs within hours of ingestion of agents that increase levels of serotonin in the central nervous system, including serotonin reuptake inhibitors, monoamine oxidase inhibitors, tricyclic antidepressants, meperidine, dextromethorphan, bromocriptine, tramadol, lithium, and psychostimulants (such as cocaine, methamphetamine, and MDMA) (see Chapter 38). Clonus and hyperreflexia are more common in serotonin syndrome, whereas "lead pipe" rigidity is more common in neuroleptic malignant syndrome. Neuroleptic malignant and serotonin syndromes share common clinical and pathophysiologic features with **malignant hyperthermia** of anesthesia (see Chapter 38).

C. Fever of Undetermined Origin

See Fever of Unknown Origin, Chapter 30.

▶ Treatment

Most fever is well tolerated. When the temperature is less than 40°C, symptomatic treatment only is required. A temperature greater than 41°C is likely to be hyperthermia rather than cytokine mediated, and *emergent management is indicated.* (See Heat Stroke, Chapter 37.) The treatment of fever with antipyretics does not appear to affect mortality of critically ill patients.

A. General Measures for Removal of Heat

Regardless of the cause of the fever, alcohol sponges, cold sponges, ice bags, ice-water enemas, and ice baths will lower body temperature (see Chapter 37). They are more useful in hyperthermia, since patients with cytokine-related fever will attempt to override these therapies.

B. Pharmacologic Treatment of Fever

1. Antipyretic drugs—Antipyretic therapy is not needed except for patients with marginal hemodynamic status. Aspirin or acetaminophen, 325–650 mg every 4 hours, is effective in reducing fever. These drugs are best administered around the clock, rather than as needed, since "as needed" dosing results in periodic chills and sweats due to fluctuations in temperature caused by varying levels of drug.

2. Antimicrobial therapy—Antibacterial and antifungal prophylactic regimens are only recommended for

patients expected to have less than 100 neutrophils/mcL for more than 7 days, unless other factors increase risks for complications or mortality. In most febrile patients, empiric antibiotic therapy should be deferred pending further evaluation. However, empiric antibiotic therapy is sometimes warranted. Prompt broad-spectrum antimicrobials are indicated for febrile patients who are clinically unstable, even before infection can be documented. These include patients with hemodynamic instability, those with neutropenia (neutrophils less than 500/mcL), others who are asplenic (surgically or secondary to sickle cell disease) or immunosuppressed (including individuals taking systemic corticosteroids, azathioprine, cyclosporine, or other immunosuppressive medications) (Tables 30–4 and 30–5), and those who are HIV infected (see Chapter 31).

Febrile neutropenic patients should receive initial doses of empiric antibacterial therapy within an hour of triage and should either be monitored for at least 4 hours to determine suitability for outpatient management or be admitted to the hospital. Inpatient treatment is standard to manage febrile neutropenic episodes, although carefully selected patients may be managed as outpatients after systematic assessment beginning with a validated risk index (eg, Multinational Association for Supportive Care in Cancer [MASCC] score or Talcott rules). In the MASCC index calculation, low-risk factors include the following: age under 60 years (2 points), burden of illness (5 points for no or mild symptoms and 3 points for moderate symptoms), outpatient status (3 points), solid tumor or hematologic malignancy with no previous fungal infection (4 points), no COPD (4 points), no dehydration requiring parenteral fluids (3 points), and systolic blood pressure greater than 90 mm Hg (5 points). Patients with MASCC scores 21 or higher or in Talcott group 4 (presentation as an outpatient without significant comorbidity or uncontrolled cancer), and without other risk factors, can be managed safely as outpatients.

The carefully selected outpatients determined to be at low risk by MASCC score (particularly in combination with a normal serum C-reactive protein level) or by Talcott rules can be managed with an oral fluoroquinolone plus amoxicillin/clavulanate (or clindamycin, if penicillin allergic), unless fluoroquinolone prophylaxis was used before fever developed. For treatment of fever during neutropenia following chemotherapy, outpatient parenteral antimicrobial therapy can be provided effectively and safely (in low-risk patients) with a single agent such as cefepime, piperacillin/tazobactam, imipenem, meropenem or doripenem; or (in high-risk patients) with a combination of agents such as an aminoglycoside *plus* one of the following agents: piperacillin/tazobactam, cefepime (or ceftazidime), imipenem, or meropenem (or doripenem); *or* vancomycin *plus* one of the following: either piperacillin/tazobactam, cefepime (or ceftazidime), imipenem, meropenem, or aztreonam *and* an aminoglycoside, or ciprofloxacin *and* an aminoglycoside. If a fungal infection is suspected in patients with prolonged fever and neutropenia, fluconazole is an equally effective but less toxic alternative to amphotericin B.

C. Treatment of Hyperthermia

Discontinuation of the offending agent is mandatory. Treatment of neuroleptic malignant syndrome includes dantrolene in combination with bromocriptine or levodopa (see Chapter 25). Treatment of serotonin syndrome includes administration of a central serotonin receptor antagonist—cyproheptadine or chlorpromazine—alone or in combination with a benzodiazepine (see Chapter 38). In patients for whom it is difficult to distinguish which syndrome is present, treatment with a benzodiazepine may be the safest therapeutic option.

► When to Admit

- Neuroleptic malignant syndrome; serotonin syndrome; malignant hyperthermia of anesthesia.

- Heat stroke.

- For measures to control a temperature higher than 41°C or when fever is associated with seizure or other mental status changes.

Combariza JF et al. C-reactive protein and the MASCC risk index identify high-risk patients with febrile neutropenia and hematologic neoplasms. Support Care Cancer. 2015 Apr;23(4):1009–13. [PMID: 25270070]

Flowers CR et al. Antimicrobial prophylaxis and outpatient management of fever and neutropenia in adults treated for malignancy: American Society of Clinical Oncology clinical practice guideline. J Clin Oncol. 2013 Feb 20;31(6):794–810. [PMID: 23319691]

Hocker SE et al. Indicators of central fever in the neurologic intensive care unit. JAMA Neurol. 2013 Dec;70(12):1499–504. [PMID: 24100963]

Klastersky J et al. The Multinational Association for Supportive Care in Cancer (MASCC) risk index score: 10 years of use for identifying low-risk febrile neutropenic cancer patients. Support Care Cancer. 2013 May;21(5):1487–95. [PMID: 23443617]

Santelli J et al. Heat illness in the emergency department: keeping your cool. Emerg Med Pract. 2014 Aug;16(8):1–22. [PMID: 25422847]

Saxena MK et al. A multicentre audit of temperature patterns after traumatic brain injury. Crit Care Resusc. 2015 Jun;17(2):129–34. [PMID: 26017131]

INVOLUNTARY WEIGHT LOSS

ESSENTIAL INQUIRIES

- ► Age; caloric intake; secondary confirmation (eg, changes in clothing size).
- ► Fever; change in bowel habits.
- ► Substance abuse.
- ► Age-appropriate cancer screening history.

► General Considerations

Body weight is determined by a person's caloric intake, absorptive capacity, metabolic rate, and energy losses. Body weight normally peaks by the fifth or sixth decade and then gradually declines at a rate of 1–2 kg per decade. In NHANES II, a national survey of community-dwelling elders (age 50–80 years), recent involuntary weight loss (more than 5% usual body weight) was reported by 7% of respondents, and this was associated with a 24% higher mortality. In contrast, one study found that a BMI of 33 or less is not associated with an increased mortality in adults aged 65 years or older. In postmenopausal women, unintentional weight loss was associated with increased rates of hip and vertebral fractures.

► Etiology

Involuntary weight loss is regarded as clinically significant when it exceeds 5% or more of usual body weight over a 6- to 12-month period. It often indicates serious physical or psychological illness. Physical causes are usually evident during the initial evaluation. The most common causes are cancer (about 30%), gastrointestinal disorders (about 15%), and dementia or depression (about 15%). When an adequately nourished–appearing patient complains of weight loss, inquiry should be made about exact weight changes (with approximate dates) and about changes in clothing size. Family members can provide confirmation of weight loss, as can old documents such as driver's licenses. A mild, gradual weight loss occurs in some older individuals because of decreased energy requirements. However, rapid involuntary weight loss is predictive of morbidity and mortality. In addition to various disease states, causes in older individuals include loss of teeth and consequent difficulty with chewing, medications interfering with taste or causing nausea, alcoholism, and social isolation.

► Clinical Findings

Once the weight loss is established, the history, medication profile, physical examination, and conventional laboratory and radiologic investigations (eg, complete blood count, serologic tests including HIV, thyroid-stimulating hormone [TSH] level, urinalysis, fecal occult blood test, chest radiography, and upper gastrointestinal series) usually reveal the cause. When these tests are normal, the second phase of evaluation should focus on more definitive gastrointestinal investigation (eg, tests for malabsorption, endoscopy) and cancer screening (eg, Papanicolaou smear, mammography, prostate specific antigen [PSA]). A prospective case study in patients with unintentional weight loss showed that colonoscopy did not find colorectal cancer if weight loss was the sole indication for the test.

If the initial evaluation is unrevealing, follow-up is preferable to further diagnostic testing. Death at 2-year follow-up was not nearly as common in patients with unexplained involuntary weight loss (8%) as in those with weight loss due to malignant (79%) and established nonmalignant diseases (19%). Psychiatric consultation should be considered when there is evidence of depression, dementia, anorexia nervosa, or other emotional problems. Ultimately, in approximately 15–25% of cases, no cause for the weight loss can be found.

Differential Diagnosis

Malignancy, gastrointestinal disorders (poorly fitting dentures, cavities, swallowing or malabsorption disorders, pancreatic insufficiency), psychological problems (dementia, depression, paranoia), endocrine disorders (hyperthyroidism, hypothyroidism, hyperparathyroidism, hypoadrenalism), eating problems (dietary restrictions, lack of money for food), social problems (alcoholism, social isolation), and medication side effects are all established causes.

Treatment

Weight stabilization occurs in most surviving patients with both established and unknown causes of weight loss through treatment of the underlying disorder and caloric supplementation. Nutrient intake goals are established in relation to the severity of weight loss, in general ranging from 30 to 40 kcal/kg/d. In order of preference, route of administration options include oral, temporary nasojejunal tube, or percutaneous gastric or jejunal tube. Parenteral nutrition is reserved for patients with serious associated problems. A variety of pharmacologic agents have been proposed for the treatment of weight loss. These can be categorized into appetite stimulants (corticosteroids, progestational agents, dronabinol, and serotonin antagonists); anabolic agents (growth hormone and testosterone derivatives); and anticatabolic agents (omega-3 fatty acids, pentoxifylline, hydrazine sulfate, and thalidomide). There is no evidence that appetite stimulants decrease mortality, and they may have severe adverse side effects.

When to Refer

- Weight loss caused by malabsorption.
- Persistent nutritional deficiencies despite adequate supplementation.
- Weight loss as a result of anorexia or bulimia.

When to Admit

- Severe protein-energy malnutrition, including the syndromes of kwashiorkor and marasmus.
- Vitamin deficiency syndromes.
- Cachexia with anticipated progressive weight loss secondary to unmanageable psychiatric disease.
- Careful electrolyte and fluid replacement in protein-energy malnutrition and avoidance of "re-feeding syndrome."

Crandall CJ et al. Postmenopausal weight change and incidence of fracture: post hoc findings from Women's Health Initiative Observational Study and Clinical Trials. BMJ. 2015 Jan 27; 350:h25. [PMID: 25627698]

Gaddey HL et al. Unintentional weight loss in older adults. Am Fam Physician. 2014 May 1;89(9):718–22. [PMID: 24784334]

Morley JE. Undernutrition in older adults. Fam Pract. 2012 Apr;29(Suppl 1):i89–i93. [PMID: 22399563]

FATIGUE & CHRONIC FATIGUE SYNDROME

> ## ESSENTIAL INQUIRIES
>
> - Weight loss; fever.
> - Sleep-disordered breathing.
> - Medications; substance use.

General Considerations

Fatigue, as an isolated symptom, accounts for 1–3% of visits to generalists. The symptom of fatigue is often poorly described and less well defined by patients than symptoms associated with specific dysfunction of organ systems. Fatigue or lassitude and the closely related complaints of weakness, tiredness, and lethargy are often attributed to overexertion, poor physical conditioning, sleep disturbance, obesity, undernutrition, and emotional problems. A history of the patient's daily living and working habits may obviate the need for extensive and unproductive diagnostic studies.

The diagnosis of chronic fatigue syndrome remains hotly debated because of the lack of a gold standard. Persons with chronic fatigue syndrome meeting specific criteria (such as those from the CDC) report a greater frequency of childhood trauma and psychopathology and demonstrate higher levels of emotional instability and self-reported stress than persons who do not have chronic fatigue. Neuropsychological and neuroendocrine studies reveal abnormalities in most patients but no consistent pattern. For example, one study found widespread areas of neuroinflammation in the brain of chronic fatigue syndrome patients that were correlated with the severity of neuropsychological symptoms. A longitudinal MRI study showed no abnormal patterns in rate and extent of brain atrophy, ventricle volume, white matter lesions, cerebral blood flow, or aqueductal cerebrospinal fluid flow. Sleep disorders have been reported in 40–80% of patients with chronic fatigue syndrome, but polysomnographic studies have not shown a greater incidence of primary sleep disorders in those with chronic fatigue syndrome than in controls, suggesting that the sleep disorders are comorbid rather than causative. Veterans of the Gulf War show a tenfold greater incidence of chronic fatigue syndrome compared with nondeployed military personnel. Older patients with chronic fatigue syndrome demonstrate a greater disease impact than younger patients, perhaps secondary to their greater autonomic dysfunction, decreased baroreflex sensitivity, and prolonged left ventricular ejection time.

Clinical Findings

A. Fatigue

Clinically relevant fatigue is composed of three major components: generalized weakness (difficulty in initiating activities); easy fatigability (difficulty in completing activities); and mental fatigue (difficulty with concentration and memory). Important diseases that can cause fatigue include hyperthyroidism and hypothyroidism, HF, infections (endocarditis, hepatitis), COPD, sleep apnea, anemia, autoimmune disorders, irritable bowel syndrome, Parkinson disease, and cancer. Solution-focused therapy has a significant initial beneficial effect on the severity of fatigue and quality of life in patients with quiescent inflammatory bowel disease.

Alcoholism, side effects from medications (eg, sedatives and beta-blockers), and psychological conditions (eg, insomnia, depression, anxiety, panic attacks, dysthmia, and somatization disorder) may be the cause. Common outpatient infectious causes include mononucleosis and sinusitis. These conditions are usually associated with other characteristic signs, but patients may emphasize fatigue and not reveal their other symptoms unless directly asked. The lifetime prevalence of significant fatigue (present for at least 2 weeks) is about 25%. Fatigue of unknown cause or related to psychiatric illness exceeds that due to physical illness, injury, alcohol, or medications.

B. Chronic Fatigue Syndrome

A working case definition of chronic fatigue syndrome indicates that it is not a homogeneous abnormality, there is no single pathogenic mechanism (Figure 2–1), and no physical finding or laboratory test can be used to confirm the diagnosis.

The evaluation of chronic fatigue syndrome includes a history and physical examination as well as complete blood count, erythrocyte sedimentation rate, chemistries (blood urea nitrogen [BUN]), serum electrolytes, glucose, creatinine, calcium, liver and thyroid function tests), antinuclear antibody, urinalysis, and tuberculin skin test, and screening questionnaires for psychiatric disorders. Other tests to be performed as clinically indicated are serum cortisol, rheumatoid factor, immunoglobulin levels, Lyme serology in endemic areas, and HIV antibody. More extensive testing is usually unhelpful, including antibody to Epstein-Barr virus. There may be an abnormally high rate of postural hypotension. MRI scans may show brain abnormalities on T_2-weighted images—chiefly small, punctate, subcortical white matter hyperintensities, predominantly in the frontal lobes, although a 2010 study found no such abnormalities, and brain MRI is not routinely recommended.

▶ Treatment

A. Fatigue

Management of fatigue involves identification and treatment of conditions that contribute to fatigue, such as cancer, pain, depression, disordered sleep, weight loss, and anemia. Resistance training and aerobic exercise lessens fatigue and improves performance for a number of chronic conditions associated with a high prevalence of fatigue, including HF, COPD, arthritis, and cancer. Continuous positive airway pressure is an effective treatment for obstructive sleep apnea. Psychostimulants such as methylphenidate have shown inconsistent results in randomized trials of treatment of cancer-related fatigue. Modafinil and armodafinil appear to be effective, well-tolerated agents in

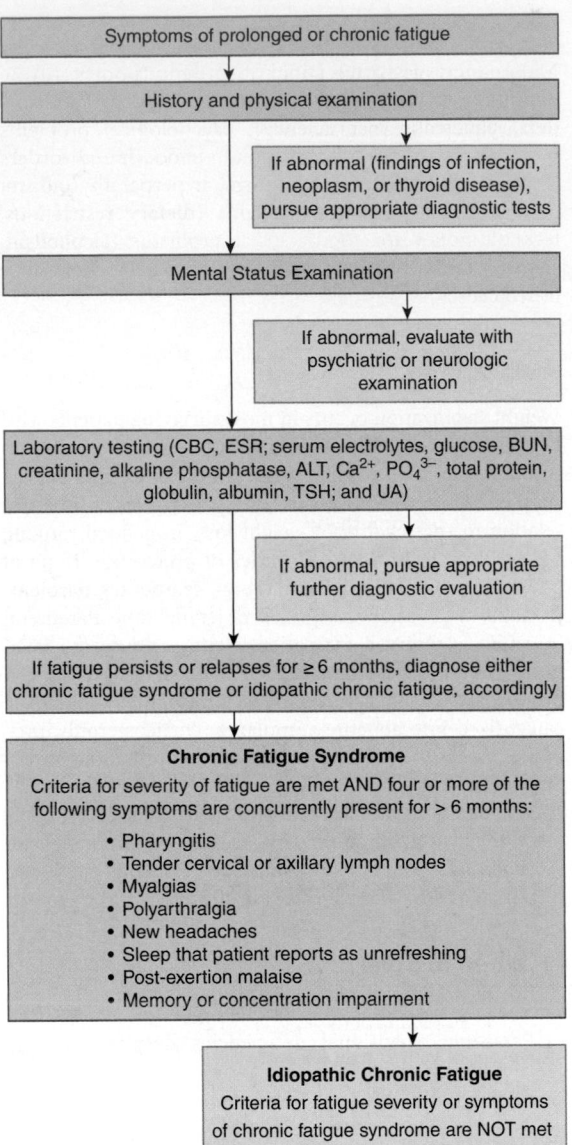

▲ **Figure 2–1.** Classification of chronic fatigue patients. ALT, alanine aminotransferase; BUN, blood urea nitrogen; Ca^{2+}, calcium; CBC, complete blood count; ESR, erythrocyte sedimentation rate; PO_4^{3-}, phosphate; TSH, thyroid-stimulating hormone; UA, urinalysis.

HIV-positive patients with fatigue and as adjunctive agents in patients with depression or bipolar disorder with fatigue.

B. Chronic Fatigue Syndrome

A variety of agents and modalities have been tried for the treatment of chronic fatigue syndrome. Acyclovir, intravenous immunoglobulin, nystatin, clonidine (in adolescent chronic fatigue syndrome), and low-dose hydrocortisone do not improve symptoms. Some patients with postural hypotension report response to increases in dietary sodium as well as fludrocortisone, 0.1 mg orally daily.

There is a greater prevalence of past and current psychiatric diagnoses in patients with this syndrome. Affective disorders are especially common. Patients with chronic fatigue syndrome have benefited from a comprehensive multidisciplinary intervention, including optimal medical management, treating any ongoing affective or anxiety disorder pharmacologically, and implementing a comprehensive cognitive-behavioral treatment program. At present, cognitive-behavioral therapy and graded exercise are the treatments of choice for patients with chronic fatigue syndrome. **Cognitive-behavioral therapy,** a form of nonpharmacologic treatment emphasizing self-help and aiming to change perceptions and behaviors that may perpetuate symptoms and disability, is helpful. Although few patients are cured, the treatment effect is substantial. Response to cognitive-behavioral therapy is not predictable on the basis of severity or duration of chronic fatigue syndrome. Patients with high neuroticism or low acceptance show more improvement in mental quality of life with cognitive-behavioral therapy.

Graded exercise has also been shown to improve functional work capacity and physical function. A 2011 randomized trial (PACE trial) confirmed the independent benefits of cognitive-behavioral therapy and graded exercise; it found no benefit of adaptive pacing therapy. Physiologic studies find an altered immune response to exercise in patients with chronic fatigue syndrome.

In addition, the clinician's sympathetic listening and explanatory responses can help overcome the patient's frustrations and debilitation by this still mysterious illness. All patients should be encouraged to engage in normal activities to the extent possible and should be reassured that full recovery is eventually possible in most cases.

When to Refer

- Infections not responsive to standard treatment.
- Difficult to control hyperthyroidism or hypothyroidism.
- Severe psychological disease.
- Malignancy.

When to Admit

- Failure to thrive.
- Fatigue severe enough to impair activities of daily living.

Kerr CW et al. Effects of methylphenidate on fatigue and depression: a randomized, double-blind, placebo-controlled trial. J Pain Symptom Manage. 2012 Jan;43(1):68–77. [PMID: 22208450]

Larun L et al. Exercise therapy for chronic fatigue syndrome. Cochrane Database Syst Rev. 2015 Feb 10;2:CD003200. [PMID: 25674924]

Nakatomi Y et al. Neuroinflammation in patients with chronic fatigue syndrome/myalgic encephalomyelitis: an ^{11}C-(R)-PK11195 PET study. J Nucl Med. 2014 Jun;55(6):945–50. [PMID: 24665088]

Stocchi F et al; FORTE Study Group. Prevalence of fatigue in Parkinson disease and its clinical correlates. Neurology. 2014 Jul 15;83(3):215–20. [PMID: 24928125]

Sulheim D et al. Disease mechanisms and clonidine treatment in adolescent chronic fatigue syndrome: a combined cross-sectional and randomized clinical trial. JAMA Pediatr. 2014 Apr;168(4):351–60. [PMID: 24493300]

Vogelaar L et al. Fatigue management in patients with IBD: a randomised controlled trial. Gut. 2014 Jun;63(6):911–8. [PMID: 23884638]

Wang XS et al. Prevalence and characteristics of moderate to severe fatigue: a multicenter study in cancer patients and survivors. Cancer. 2014 Feb 1;120(3):425–32. [PMID: 24436136]

Wiborg JF et al. Towards an evidence-based treatment model for cognitive behavioral interventions focusing on chronic fatigue syndrome. J Psychosom Res. 2012 May;72(5):399–404. [PMID: 22469284]

Wright J et al. Fatigue. Med Clin North Am. 2014 May;98(3):597–608. [PMID: 24758963]

ACUTE HEADACHE

ESSENTIAL INQUIRIES

- Age older than 40 years.
- Rapid onset and severe intensity (ie, "thunderclap" headache); trauma, onset during exertion.
- Fever; vision changes, neck stiffness.
- HIV infection.
- Current or past history of hypertension.
- Neurologic findings (mental status changes, motor or sensory deficits, loss of consciousness).

General Considerations

Headache is a common reason that adults seek medical care, accounting for approximately 13 million visits each year in the United States to physicians' offices, urgent care clinics, and emergency departments. It is the fifth most common reason for emergency department visits, and second most common reason for neurologic consultation in the emergency department. A broad range of disorders can cause headache (see Chapter 24). This section deals only with acute nontraumatic headache in adolescents and adults. The challenge in the initial evaluation of acute headache is to identify which patients are presenting with an uncommon but life-threatening condition, approximately 1% of patients seeking care in emergency department settings and considerably less in office practice settings.

Diminution of headache in response to typical migraine therapies (such as serotonin receptor antagonists or ketorolac) does not rule out critical conditions such as subarachnoid hemorrhage or meningitis as the underlying cause.

Clinical Findings

A. Symptoms

A careful history and physical examination should aim to identify causes of acute headache that require immediate treatment. These causes can be broadly classified as imminent or completed **vascular events** (intracranial hemorrhage, thrombosis, cavernous sinus thrombosis, vasculitis, malignant hypertension, arterial dissection, or aneurysm), **infections** (abscess, encephalitis, or meningitis), **intracranial masses** causing intracranial hypertension, **preeclampsia,** and **carbon monoxide poisoning.** Having the patient carefully describe the onset of headache can be helpful in diagnosing a serious cause. Report of a sudden-onset headache that reaches maximal and severe intensity within seconds or a few minutes is the classic description of a "thunderclap" headache; it should precipitate work-up for subarachnoid hemorrhage, since the estimated prevalence of subarachnoid hemorrhage in patients with "thunderclap" headache is 43%. Thunderclap headache during the postpartum period precipitated by the Valsalva maneuver or recumbent positioning may indicate reversible cerebral vasoconstriction syndrome. Other historical features that raise the need for diagnostic testing include headache brought on by the Valsalva maneuver, cough, exertion, or sexual activity.

The medical history can also guide the need for additional work-up. Under most circumstances (including a normal neurologic examination), new headache in a patient older than 50 years or with HIV infection warrants immediate neuroimaging (Table 2–8). When the patient has a history of hypertension—particularly uncontrolled hypertension—a complete search for other features of "malignant hypertension" is appropriate to determine the urgency of control of hypertension (see Chapter 11). Headache and hypertension associated with pregnancy may be due to preeclampsia. Episodic headache associated with the triad of hypertension, heart palpitations, and sweats is suggestive of pheochromocytoma. In the absence of "thunderclap" headache, advanced age, and HIV infection, a careful physical examination and detailed neurologic examination

Table 2–8. Clinical features associated with acute headache that warrant urgent or emergent neuroimaging.

Prior to lumbar puncture
  Abnormal neurologic examination
  Abnormal mental status
  Abnormal funduscopic examination (papilledema; loss of venous pulsations)
  Meningeal signs
Emergent (conduct prior to leaving office or emergency department)
  Abnormal neurologic examination
  Abnormal mental status
  "Thunderclap" headache
Urgent (scheduled prior to leaving office or emergency department)
  HIV-positive patient[1]
  Age > 50 years (normal neurologic examination)

[1]Use CT with or without contrast or MRI if HIV positive.
Data from American College of Emergency Physicians. Clinical policy: critical issues in the evaluation and management of patients presenting to the emergency department with acute headache. Ann Emerg Med. 2002 Jan;39(1):108–22.

Table 2–9. Summary likelihood ratios (LRs) for individual clinical features associated with migraine diagnosis.

Clinical Feature	LR+ (95% CI)	LR– (95% CI)
Nausea	19 (15–25)	0.19 (0.18–0.20)
Photophobia	5.8 (5.1–6.6)	0.24 (0.23–0.26)
Phonophobia	5.2 (4.5–5.9)	0.38 (0.36–0.40)
Exacerbation by physical activity	3.7 (3.4–4.0)	0.24 (0.23–0.26)

will usually determine acuity of the work-up and need for further diagnostic testing.

Symptoms can also be useful for diagnosing migraine headache in the absence of the "classic" migraine pattern of scintillating scotoma followed by unilateral headache, photophobia, and nausea and vomiting (Table 2–9). The presence of three or more of these symptoms (nausea, photophobia, phonophobia, and exacerbation by physical activity) can establish the diagnosis of migraine (in the absence of other clinical features that warrant neuroimaging studies), and one or more symptom (provided it is not nausea) can help rule out migraine.

B. Physical Examination

Critical components of the physical examination of the patient with acute headache include vital signs, neurologic examination, and vision testing with funduscopic examination. The finding of fever with acute headache warrants additional maneuvers to elicit evidence of meningeal inflammation, such as Kernig and Brudzinski signs. The absence of jolt accentuation of headache cannot accurately rule out meningitis. Patients older than 60 years should be examined for scalp or temporal artery tenderness.

Careful assessment of visual acuity, ocular gaze, visual fields, pupillary defects, optic disks, and retinal vein pulsations is crucial. Diminished visual acuity is suggestive of glaucoma, temporal arteritis, or optic neuritis. Ophthalmoplegia or visual field defects may be signs of venous sinus thrombosis, tumor, or aneurysm. Afferent pupillary defects can be due to intracranial masses or optic neuritis. In the setting of headache and hypertension, retinal cotton wool spots, flame hemorrhages, and disk swelling indicate acute severe hypertensive retinopathy. Ipsilateral ptosis and miosis suggest Horner syndrome and in conjunction with acute headache may signify carotid artery dissection. Finally, papilledema or absent retinal venous pulsations are signs of elevated intracranial pressure—findings that should be followed by neuroimaging prior to performing lumbar puncture (Table 2–8). On nonmydriatic fundoscopy, up to 8.5% of patients who arrive at the emergency department complaining of headache had abnormalities; although few had other significant physical examination findings, 59% had abnormal neuroimaging studies.

Complete neurologic evaluations are also critical and should include assessment of mental status, motor and sensory systems, reflexes, gait, cerebellar function, and pronator drift. Any abnormality on neurologic evaluation (especially mental status) warrants emergent neuroimaging (Table 2–8).

C. Diagnostic Studies

Neuroimaging is summarized in Table 2–8. Under most circumstances, a noncontrast head CT is sufficient to exclude intracranial hypertension with impending herniation, intracranial hemorrhage, and many types of intracranial masses (notable exceptions include lymphoma and toxoplasmosis in HIV-positive patients, herpes simplex encephalitis, and brain abscess). When needed, a contrast study can be ordered to follow a normal noncontrast study. A normal neuroimaging study does not exclude subarachnoid hemorrhage and should be followed by lumbar puncture. One study supported a change of practice wherein a lumbar puncture can be withheld when a head CT scan was performed less than 6 hours after headache onset and showed no evidence of subarachnoid hemorrhage (negative predictive value 99.9% [95% CI, 99.3–100.0%]).

In patients for whom there is a high level of suspicion for subarachnoid hemorrhage or aneurysm, a normal CT and lumbar puncture should be followed by angiography within the next few days (provided the patient is medically stable). Lumbar puncture is also indicated to exclude infectious causes of acute headache, particularly in patients with fever or meningeal signs. Cerebrospinal fluid tests should routinely include Gram stain, white blood cell count with differential, red blood cell count, glucose, total protein, and bacterial culture. In appropriate patients, also consider testing cerebrospinal fluid for VDRL (syphilis), cryptococcal antigen (HIV-positive patients), acid-fast bacillus stain and culture, and complement fixation and culture for coccidioidomycosis. Storage of an extra tube with 5 mL of cerebrospinal fluid is also prudent for conducting unanticipated tests in the immediate future. Polymerase chain reaction tests for specific infectious pathogens (eg, herpes simplex 2) should also be considered in patients with evidence of central nervous system infection but no identifiable pathogen.

The Ottawa subarachnoid hemorrhage clinical decision rule had 100% sensitivity (and 15.3% specificity) in predicting subarachnoid hemorrhage. According to it, patients who seek medical attention in an emergency department complaining of an acute nontraumatic headache should be evaluated for subarachnoid hemorrhage if they have the following factors: age 40 years or older, neck pain or stiffness, witnessed loss of consciousness, onset during exertion, thunderclap headache (instantly peaking pain), and limited neck flexion on examination.

In addition to neuroimaging and lumbar puncture, additional diagnostic tests for exclusion of life-threatening causes of acute headache include erythrocyte sedimentation rate (temporal arteritis; endocarditis), urinalysis (malignant hypertension; preeclampsia), and sinus CT (bacterial sinusitis, independently or as a cause of venous sinus thrombosis).

▶ Treatment

Treatment should be directed at the cause of acute headache. In patients in whom migraine or migraine-like

headache has been diagnosed, early treatment with NSAIDs (oral or intramuscular ketorolac) or triptans (oral, nasal, subcutaneous) can often abort or provide significant relief of symptoms (see Chapter 24). Sumatriptan may be less effective as immediate therapy for migraine attacks with aura compared to attacks without aura. In a double-blind, randomized-controlled trial of 100 patients with migraine, ginger powder appeared to be as efficacious as sumatriptan.

High-flow oxygen therapy may also provide effective treatment for all headache types in the emergency department setting. Peripheral nerve blocks for treatment-refractory migraine may be an effective therapeutic option in pregnancy. The oral 5-HT1F receptor agonist, lasmiditan, is currently in clinical trials for the treatment of acute migraine. Other causes of acute headache, such as subarachnoid hemorrhage, intracranial mass, or meningitis, require emergent treatment in the hospital.

▶ When to Refer

- Frequent migraines not responsive to standard therapy.
- Migraines with atypical features.
- Chronic daily headaches due to medication overuse.

▶ When to Admit

- Need for repeated doses of parenteral pain medication.
- To facilitate an expedited work-up requiring a sequence of neuroimaging and procedures.
- To monitor for progression of symptoms and to obtain neurologic consultation when the initial emergency department work-up is inconclusive.
- Pain severe enough to impair activities of daily living or limit participation in follow-up appointments or consultations.
- Patients with subarachnoid hemorrhage, intracranial mass, or meningitis.

Bird S et al. Zolmitriptan for acute migraine attacks in adults. Cochrane Database Syst Rev. 2014 May 21;5:CD008616. [PMID: 24848613]

Blok KM et al. CT within 6 hours of headache onset to rule out subarachnoid hemorrhage in nonacademic hospitals. Neurology. 2015 May 12;84(19):1927–32. [PMID: 25862794]

Chiang CC et al. Treatment of medication-overuse headache: a systematic review. Cephalalgia. 2015 Jun 29. [Epub ahead of print] [PMID: 26122645]

Derry S et al. Ibuprofen for acute treatment of episodic tension-type headache in adults. Cochrane Database Syst Rev. 2015 Jul 31;7:CD011474. [PMID: 26230487]

Easter JS et al. Will neuroimaging reveal a severe intracranial injury in this adult with minor head trauma? The rational clinical examination. JAMA. 2015 Dec 22–29;314(24): 2672–81. [PMID: 26717031]

Freitag FG et al. Medical management of adult headache. Otolaryngol Clin North Am. 2014 Apr;47(2):221–37. [PMID: 24680490]

Govindappagari S et al. Peripheral nerve blocks in the treatment of migraine in pregnancy. Obstet Gynecol. 2014 Dec;124(6):1169–74. [PMID: 25415168]

Hainer BL et al. Approach to acute headache in adults. Am Fam Physician. 2013 May 15;87(10):682–7. [PMID: 23939446]

Hale N et al. Diagnosis and treatment of headache in the ambulatory care setting: a review of classic presentations and new considerations in diagnosis and management. Med Clin North Am. 2014 May;98(3):505–27. [PMID: 24758958]

Hansen JM et al. Reduced efficacy of sumatriptan in migraine with aura vs without aura. Neurology. 2015 May 5; 84(18):1880–5. [PMID: 25841032]

Lenger SM et al. Recumbent thunderclap headache in the postpartum period. Obstet Gynecol. 2014 Feb;123(2 Pt 2 Suppl 2): 477–9. [PMID: 24413232]

Malem A et al. Headache, flashing lights, and blurred vision. BMJ. 2015 Feb 2;350:h446. [PMID: 25645460]

Marmura MJ et al. The acute treatment of migraine in adults: the American Headache Society Evidence Assessment of Migraine Pharmacotherapies. Headache. 2015 Jan;55(1): 3–20. [PMID: 25600718]

McMillan-Persaud B et al. Headache · fatigue · blurred vision · Dx? J Fam Pract. 2015 Apr;64(4):228–30. [PMID: 25973449]

Minen MT et al. Evaluation and treatment of migraine in the emergency department: a review. Headache. 2014 Jul–Aug; 54(7):1131–45. [PMID: 24898930]

Perry JJ et al. Clinical decision rules to rule out subarachnoid hemorrhage for acute headache. JAMA. 2013 Sep 25;310(12): 1248–55. [PMID: 24065011]

Reuter U et al. The pharmacological profile and clinical prospects of the oral 5-HT1F receptor agonist lasmiditan in the acute treatment of migraine. Ther Adv Neurol Disord. 2015 Jan;8(1):46–54. [PMID: 25584073]

Rivara FP et al. Use of clinical prediction rules for guiding use of computed tomography in adults with head trauma. JAMA. 2015 Dec 22–29;314(24):2629–31. [PMID: 26717029]

Sakaida H et al. Cavernous sinus thrombosis: linking a swollen red eye and headache. Lancet. 2014 Sep 6;384(9946):928. [PMID: 25209492]

Yancey JR et al. Chronic daily headache: diagnosis and management. Am Fam Physician. 2014 Apr 15;89(8):642–8. [PMID: 24784123]

DYSURIA

 ESSENTIAL INQUIRIES

- ▶ Fever; new back or flank pain; nausea or vomiting.
- ▶ Vaginal discharge.
- ▶ Pregnancy risk.
- ▶ Structural abnormalities.
- ▶ Instrumentation of urethra or bladder.

▶ General Considerations

Dysuria (painful urination) is a common reason for adolescents and adults to seek urgent medical attention. An inflammatory process (eg, infection, autoimmune disorder) underlies most causes of dysuria. In women, cystitis will be diagnosed in up to 50–60% of cases. Cystitis has an incidence of 0.5–0.7% per year in sexually active young women. The key objective in evaluating women with dysuria is to exclude serious upper urinary tract disease, such as acute pyelonephritis, and sexually transmitted diseases. In elderly men, dysuria may be a symptom of prostatitis.

In contrast, in younger men, urethritis accounts for the vast majority of cases of dysuria.

▶ Clinical Findings

A. Symptoms

Well-designed cohort studies have shown that some women can be reliably diagnosed with uncomplicated cystitis without a physical examination or urinalysis, and randomized controlled trials show that telephone management of uncomplicated cystitis is safe and effective. An increased likelihood of cystitis is present when women report multiple irritative voiding symptoms (dysuria, urgency, frequency), fever, or back pain (LRs = 1.6–2.0). Inquiring about symptoms of vulvovaginitis is imperative. When women report dysuria and urinary frequency, and deny vaginal discharge and irritation, the LR for culture-confirmed cystitis is 24.5. In contrast, when vaginal discharge or irritation is present, as well as dysuria or urinary frequency, the LR is 0.7. Gross hematuria in women with voiding symptoms usually represents hemorrhagic cystitis but can also be a sign of bladder cancer (particularly in older patients) or upper tract disease. Failure of hematuria to resolve with antibiotic treatment should prompt further evaluation of the bladder and kidneys. Chlamydial infection should be strongly considered among women age 25 years or younger who are sexually active and seeking medical attention for a suspected urinary tract infection for the first time or who have a new partner.

Because fever and back pain, as well as nausea and vomiting, are considered harbingers of (or clinical criteria for) acute pyelonephritis, women with these symptoms should usually be examined by a clinician prior to treatment in order to exclude coexistent urosepsis, hydronephrosis, or nephrolithiasis. Other major risk factors for acute pyelonephritis (among women 18–49 years of age) relate to sexual behaviors (frequent sexual intercourse 3 times per week or more, new sexual partner in previous year, recent spermicide use), as well as diabetes mellitus and recent urinary tract infection or incontinence. Finally, pregnancy, underlying structural factors (polycystic kidney disease, nephrolithiasis, neurogenic bladder), immunosuppression, diabetes mellitus, and a history of recent bladder or urethral instrumentation usually alter the treatment regimen (antibiotic choice or duration of treatment, or both) of cystitis.

B. Physical Examination

Fever, tachycardia, or hypotension suggests the possibility of urosepsis and potential need for hospitalization. A focused examination in women, in uncomplicated circumstances, could be limited to ascertainment of costovertebral angle tenderness and to a lower abdominal and pelvic examination if the history suggests vulvovaginitis or cervicitis.

C. Diagnostic Studies

1. Urinalysis—Urinalysis is probably overutilized in the evaluation of dysuria. The probability of culture-confirmed urinary tract infection among women with a history and physical examination compatible with uncomplicated cystitis is about 70–90%. Urinalysis is most helpful in atypical presentations of cystitis. Dipstick detection (greater than trace) of leukocytes, nitrites, or blood supports a diagnosis of cystitis. When both leukocyte and nitrite tests are positive, the LR is 4.2, and when both are negative, the LR is 0.3. The negative predictive value of urinalysis is not sufficient to exclude culture-confirmed urinary tract infection in women with multiple and typical symptoms; and randomized trial evidence shows that antibiotic treatment is beneficial to women with typical symptoms and negative urinalysis dipstick tests. Microscopy of unspun urine may also be helpful in diagnosis and reduce unnecessary use of antibiotics. The combination of urgency, dysuria, and pyuria, assessed with the high-power objective (40 ×) for pus cells (more than 1 pus cell/7 high-power fields) had a positive predictive value of 71.71 and LR of 2.97. Because older patients frequently have asymptomatic bacteriuria, a positive urine dipstick test should be interpreted cautiously if urinary tract infection symptoms are absent. A negative dipstick result for leukocyte esterase and nitrites excludes infection in older patients with equivocal cystitis symptoms.

2. Urine culture—Urine culture should be considered for all women with upper tract symptoms (prior to initiating antibiotic therapy), as well as those with dysuria and a negative urine dipstick test. In symptomatic women, a clean-catch urine culture is considered positive when 10^2–10^3 colony-forming units/mL of a uropathogenic organism is detected.

3. Renal imaging—When severe flank or back pain is present, the possibility of complicated kidney infection (perinephric abscess, nephrolithiasis) or of hydronephrosis should be considered. Renal ultrasound or CT scanning should be done to rule out abscess and hydronephrosis. To exclude nephrolithiasis, noncontrast helical CT scanning is more accurate than intravenous urography and has become the diagnostic test of choice. In a meta-analysis, the positive and negative LRs of helical CT scanning for diagnosis of nephrolithiasis were 23.2 and 0.05, respectively.

Differential Diagnosis

The differential diagnosis of dysuria in women includes acute cystitis, acute pyelonephritis, vaginitis (*Candida*, bacterial vaginosis, *Trichomonas*, herpes simplex), urethritis/cervicitis (*Chlamydia*, gonorrhea), and interstitial cystitis/painful bladder syndrome. Nucleic acid amplification tests from first-void urine or vaginal swab specimens are highly sensitive for detecting chlamydial infection. Other infectious pathogens associated with dysuria and urethritis in men include *Mycoplasma genitalium* and Enterobacteriaceae.

Treatment

Definitive treatment is directed to the underlying cause of the dysuria. An evidence-informed algorithm for managing suspected urinary tract infection in women is shown in Figure 2–2. This algorithm supports antibiotic treatment of most women with multiple and typical symptoms of urinary tract infection without performing urinalysis or urine culture. Antibiotic selection should be guided by local resistance patterns; major options for uncomplicated cystitis include nitrofurantoin, cephalosporins, ciprofloxacin,

fosfomycin, and trimethoprim-sulfamethoxazole. According to The American Academy of Pediatrics' Committee on Drugs, antibiotics that are usually acceptable when treating women who are breastfeeding include trimethoprim-sulfamethoxazole (unless G6PD deficiency is present), amoxicillin, nitrofurantoin, ciprofloxacin, and ofloxacin.

Prolonged treatment of urinary tract infections (more than 7 days) in men does not appear to reduce early or late recurrences. Symptomatic relief can be provided with phenazopyridine, a urinary analgesic that is available over the counter; it is used in combination with antibiotic therapy (when a urinary tract infection has been confirmed) but for no more than 2 days. Patients should be informed that phenazopyridine will cause orange/red discoloration of their urine and other bodily fluids (eg, some contact lens wearers have reported discoloration of their lenses). Rare cases of methemoglobinemia and hemolytic anemia have been reported, usually with overdoses or underlying renal dysfunction. If a broad-spectrum antibiotic was initially prescribed empirically for urinary tract infection, and urine culture results return establishing efficacy of a narrow-spectrum antibiotic, treatment should be "de-escalated" to the narrow-spectrum antimicrobial.

In cases of interstitial cystitis/painful bladder syndrome (see Chapter 23), patients will often respond to a multimodal approach that may include urethral/vesicular dilation, biofeedback, cognitive-behavioral therapy, antidepressants, dietary changes, vaginal emollients, and other supportive measures. Vaginal estrogen effectively relieves urinary urgency and frequency as well as recurrent UTIs related to vulvovaginal atrophy of menopause (also known as genitourinary syndrome of menopause).

When to Refer

- Anatomic abnormalities leading to repeated urinary infections.
- Infections associated with nephrolithiasis.
- Persistent interstitial cystitis/painful bladder syndrome.

When to Admit

- Severe pain requiring parenteral medication or impairing ambulation or urination (such as severe primary herpes simplex genitalis).
- Dysuria associated with urinary retention or obstruction.
- Pyelonephritis with ureteral obstruction.

Best J et al. Diagnosis and management of urinary tract infections in the emergency department. Emerg Med Pract. 2014 Jul;16(7):1–24. [PMID: 25379602]

Cooper M et al. Clinical inquiry: how best to treat UTIs in women who breastfeed? J Fam Pract. 2014 Feb;63(2):102–3. [PMID: 24527473]

Drekonja DM et al. Urinary tract infection in male veterans: treatment patterns and outcomes. JAMA Intern Med. 2013 Jan 14;173(1):62–8. [PMID: 23212273]

Grigoryan L et al. Diagnosis and management of urinary tract infections in the outpatient setting: a review. JAMA. 2014 Oct 22–29;312(16):1677–84. [PMID: 25335150]

¹In women who have risk factors for sexually transmitted diseases, consider testing for *Chlamydia*. The US Preventive Services Task Force recommends screening for *Chlamydia* for all women 25 years or younger and women of any age with more than one sexual partner, a history of sexually transmitted disease, or inconsistent use of condoms.

²A complicated UTI is one in an individual with a functional or anatomic abnormality of the urinary tract, including a history of polycystic renal disease, nephrolithiasis, neurogenic bladder, diabetes mellitus, immunosuppression, pregnancy, indwelling urinary catheter, or recent urinary tract instrumentation.

³The only physical examination finding that increases the likelihood of UTI is costovertebral angle tenderness, and clinicians may consider not performing this test in patients with typical symptoms of acute uncomplicated UTI (as in telephone management).

▲ **Figure 2–2.** Proposed algorithm for evaluating women with symptoms of acute urinary tract infection (UTI). (Modified and reproduced, with permission, from Bent S et al. Does this woman have an acute uncomplicated urinary tract infection? JAMA. 2002 May 22–29;287(20):2701–10.) © 2002 American Medical Association. All rights reserved.

Juthani-Mehta M et al. Tests for urinary tract infection in nursing home residents. JAMA. 2014 Oct 22–29;312(16):1687–8. [PMID: 25335152]

Michels TC et al. Dysuria: evaluation and differential diagnosis in adults. Am Fam Physician. 2015 Nov 1;92(9):778–86. [PMID: 26554471]

Mishra B et al. Symptom-based diagnosis of urinary tract infection in women: are we over-prescribing antibiotics? Int J Clin Pract. 2012 May;66(5):493–8. [PMID: 22512608]

Mody L et al. JAMA patient page. Urinary tract infections in older women. JAMA. 2014 Feb 26;311(8):874. [PMID: 24570259]

Mody L et al. Urinary tract infections in older women: a clinical review. JAMA. 2014 Feb 26;311(8):844–54. [PMID: 24570248]

Ninan S et al. Investigation of suspected urinary tract infection in older people. BMJ. 2014 Jul 3;349:g4070. [PMID: 24994808]

Rahn DD et al; Society of Gynecologic Surgeons Systematic Review Group. Vaginal estrogen for genitourinary syndrome of menopause: a systematic review. Obstet Gynecol. 2014 Dec;124(6):1147–56. [PMID: 25415166]

Rowe TA et al. Diagnosis and management of urinary tract infection in older adults. Infect Dis Clin North Am. 2014 Mar;28(1):75–89. [PMID: 24484576]

Weiskopf J et al. Asymptomatic bacteriuria, what are you treating? JAMA Intern Med. 2015 Mar;175(3):344–5. [PMID: 25581848]

Preoperative Evaluation & Perioperative Management

Hugo Q. Cheng, MD

EVALUATION OF THE ASYMPTOMATIC PATIENT

Patients without significant medical problems—especially those under age 50—are at very low risk for perioperative complications. Their preoperative evaluation should include a history and physical examination. Special emphasis is placed on obtaining a careful pharmacologic history and assessment of functional status, exercise tolerance, and cardiopulmonary symptoms and signs in an effort to reveal previously unrecognized disease that may require further evaluation prior to surgery. In addition, a directed bleeding history (Table 3–1) should be taken to uncover coagulopathy that could contribute to excessive surgical blood loss. **Routine preoperative laboratory tests in asymptomatic healthy patients under age 50 have not been found to help predict or prevent complications.** Even elderly patients undergoing minor or minimally invasive procedures (such as cataract surgery) are unlikely to benefit from preoperative screening tests.

Czoski-Murray C et al. What is the value of routinely testing full blood count, electrolytes and urea, and pulmonary function tests before elective surgery in patients with no apparent clinical indication and in subgroups of patients with common comorbidities: a systematic review of the clinical and cost-effective literature. Health Technol Assess. 2012 Dec;16(50): i–xvi, 1–159. [PMID: 23302507]

Oresanya LB et al. Preoperative assessment of the older patient: a narrative review. JAMA. 2014 May;311(20):2110–20. [PMID: 24867014]

CARDIAC RISK ASSESSMENT & REDUCTION IN NONCARDIAC SURGERY

The most important perioperative cardiac complications are myocardial infarction (MI) and cardiac death. Other complications include heart failure (HF), arrhythmias, and unstable angina. The principal patient-specific risk factor is the presence of end-organ cardiovascular disease. This includes not only coronary artery disease and HF but also cerebrovascular disease and chronic kidney disease. Diabetes mellitus, especially if treated with insulin, is considered a cardiovascular disease equivalent and has also been shown to increase the risk of cardiac complications. Major abdominal, thoracic, and vascular surgical procedures (especially abdominal aortic aneurysm repair) carry a higher risk of postoperative cardiac complications, likely due to their associated major fluid shifts, hemorrhage, and hypoxemia. These risk factors were identified in a validated, multifactorial risk prediction tool: The Revised Cardiac Risk Index (RCRI) (Table 3–2). Another risk prediction tool, derived from the American College of Surgeons' National Surgical Quality Improvement Program (NSQIP) patient database, identified patient age, the location or type of operation, serum creatinine greater than 1.5 mg/dL (132.6 mcmol/L), dependency in activities of daily living, and the patient's American Society of Anesthesiologists physical status classification as predictors for postoperative MI or cardiac arrest. An online risk calculator using the NSQIP tool can be found at http://www.qxmd.com/calculate-online/cardiology/gupta-perioperative-cardiac-risk. The American College of Cardiology and American Heart Association endorse both prediction tools. Patients with two or more RCRI predictors or a cardiac risk in excess of 1% as calculated by the NSQIP prediction tool are deemed to be at elevated risk for cardiac complications.

Limited exercise capacity (eg, the inability to walk for two blocks at a normal pace or climb a flight of stairs without resting) also predicts higher cardiac risk. Emergency operations are also associated with greater cardiac risk. However, emergency operations should not be delayed by extensive cardiac evaluation. Instead, patients facing emergency surgery should be medically optimized for surgery as quickly as possible and closely monitored for cardiac complications during the perioperative period.

► Role of Preoperative Noninvasive Ischemia Testing

Most patients can be accurately risk-stratified by history and physical examination. A resting electrocardiogram (ECG) should also be obtained in patients with at least one RCRI predictor prior to major surgery. Additional noninvasive stress testing rarely improves risk stratification or management, especially in patients without cardiovascular disease, undergoing minor operations, or who have at least fair functional capacity. Patients with poor functional

Table 3–1. Findings suggestive of a bleeding disorder.

Unprovoked bruising on the trunk of > 5 cm in diameter
Frequent unprovoked epistaxis or gingival bleeding
Menorrhagia with iron deficiency
Hemarthrosis with mild trauma
Prior excessive surgical blood loss or reoperation for bleeding
Family history of abnormal bleeding
Presence of severe kidney or liver disease
Use of medications that impair coagulation, including nutritional
  supplements and herbal remedies

capacity or a high RCRI score are much more likely to suffer cardiac complications. Stress testing prior to vascular surgery in these patients can stratify them into low-risk and high-risk subgroups. The absence of ischemia on dipyridamole scintigraphy or dobutamine stress echocardiography is reassuring. In contrast, extensive inducible ischemia in this population predicts a very high risk of cardiac complications, which may not be modifiable by either medical management or coronary revascularization. The predictive value of an abnormal stress test result for nonvascular surgery patients is less well established. An approach to perioperative cardiac risk assessment and management in patients with known or suspected stable coronary artery disease is shown in Figure 3–1.

▶ **Perioperative Management of Patients with Coronary Artery Disease**

Patients with acute coronary syndromes require immediate management of their cardiac disease prior to any

Table 3–2. Revised Cardiac Risk Index.

Independent Predictors of Postoperative Cardiac Complications
1. Intrathoracic, intraperitoneal, or suprainguinal vascular surgery
2. History of ischemic heart disease
3. History of heart failure
4. Insulin treatment for diabetes mellitus
5. Serum creatinine level > 2 mg/dL [> 176.8 mcmol/L]
6. History of cerebrovascular disease

Scoring (Number of Predictors Present)	Risk of Major Cardiac Complications[1]
None	0.4%
One	1%
Two	2.4%
More than two	5.4%

[1]Cardiac death, myocardial infarction, or nonfatal cardiac arrest. Data from Devereaux PJ et al. Perioperative cardiac events in patients undergoing noncardiac surgery: a review of the magnitude of the problem, the pathophysiology of the events and methods to estimate and communicate risk. CMAJ. 2005 Sept 13; 173(6):627–34.

preoperative evaluation (see Chapter 10). In a large cohort study, postoperative MI typically occurred within 3 days of surgery and was associated with a 30-day mortality rate of 11.6%. Postoperative MI often presents without chest pain. Symptoms and signs that should prompt consideration of postoperative MI include unexplained hypotension, hypoxemia, and delirium. Screening asymptomatic patients for postoperative MI through the use of ECG or cardiac enzyme monitoring remains controversial, since it has not yet been demonstrated to improve outcomes.

A. Medications

Preoperative antianginal medications, including beta-blockers, calcium channel blockers, and nitrates, should be continued throughout the perioperative period. Numerous trials and meta-analyses have investigated whether **beta-blockers** should be used to prevent perioperative cardiac complications. These agents appear to reduce the risk of nonfatal myocardial infarction in patients at elevated cardiac risk. However, in the largest of these trials, a high, fixed dose of metoprolol succinate increased total mortality and the risk of stroke. Because of the uncertain benefit-to-risk ratio of perioperative beta-blockade, it should only be considered in patients with a high risk of cardiac complications. Possible indications and starting doses for prophylactic beta-blockade are presented in Table 3–3. Ideally, beta-blockers should be started well in advance of surgery, to allow time to gradually titrate up the dose without causing excessive bradycardia or hypotension, and they should not be started on the day of surgery. The dose should be adjusted to maintain a heart rate between 50 and 70 beats per minute while keeping systolic blood pressure above 100 mm Hg. If beta-blockers are started, they should be continued for at least 3–7 days after surgery.

A meta-analysis of randomized trials found that the use of **HMG-CoA reductase inhibitors (statins)** prevents MI in patients undergoing noncardiac surgery. Safety concerns, such as liver failure or rhabdomyolysis, have not materialized in these studies. **Statins should be considered in all patients undergoing vascular surgery and other patients deemed to be at high risk for cardiac complications, regardless of lipid levels.** Patients already taking statins should continue these agents during the perioperative period. A trial of **aspirin and clonidine** found that neither agent prevented cardiac complications. Aspirin increased the bleeding risk, while clonidine was associated with hypotension and bradycardia.

B. Coronary Revascularization

Patients who have previously had coronary artery bypass grafting (CABG) surgery or percutaneous coronary interventions (PCI) have a relatively low risk of cardiac complications when undergoing subsequent noncardiac surgery. However, a trial that randomized over 500 patients with angiographically proven coronary artery disease to either coronary revascularization (with either CABG or PCI) or medical management alone before vascular surgery found no difference in postoperative MI, 30-day mortality, and long-term mortality. Thus, **preoperative CABG or PCI**

▲ **Figure 3–1.** Assessment and management of patients with known or suspected stable coronary artery disease (CAD) undergoing major elective noncardiac surgery. (OR, operating room; RCRI, Revised Cardiac Risk Index [Table 3–2]; NSQIP, National Surgical Quality Improvement Program: http://www.qxmd.com/calculate-online/cardiology/gupta-perioperative-cardiac-risk)

should only be performed on patients who have indications for the procedure independent of the planned noncardiac operation. In addition, the perioperative cardiac mortality rate may be very high in patients who have

Table 3–3. Indications for prophylactic perioperative beta-blockade.[1]

Strong indications	Patient already taking beta-blocker to treat ischemia, arrhythmia, or hypertension
Possible indications	Patient with myocardial ischemia detected on preoperative stress testing
	Patient with 3 or more Revised Cardiac Risk Index predictors (see Table 3–2)

[1]Initial dose recommendations: atenolol 25 mg orally daily, bisoprolol 2.5 mg orally daily, or metoprolol 25 mg orally twice daily. The dose of beta-blocker should be carefully titrated to keep heart rate < 70 beats per minute and systolic blood pressure > 100 mm Hg.

undergone recent intracoronary stenting, especially if antiplatelet therapy is stopped prematurely. The presumed mechanism of this increased mortality is acute stent thrombosis. Therefore, elective surgery should be deferred for at least 4–6 weeks after placement of a bare-metal stent and for a full year after placement of a drug-eluting stent. A retrospective analysis showed that cardiac complication rates level off 6 months after PCI. Thus, surgery could be considered 6 months after implantation of a drug-eluting stent if further delay poses significant risks, such as in patients undergoing surgery for cancer.

▶ Heart Failure & Left Ventricular Dysfunction

Decompensated HF, manifested by an elevated jugular venous pressure, an audible third heart sound, or evidence of pulmonary edema on physical examination or chest radiography, significantly increases the risk of perioperative cardiac complications. **Elective surgery should be** postponed in patients with decompensated HF until it can be evaluated and brought under control.

The risk of perioperative cardiac complications is similar in patients with ischemic or nonischemic cardiomyopathy. HF with reduced ejection fraction likely confers more risk that HF with preserved ejection fraction. Patients with a history of symptomatic HF are at higher risk than those with asymptomatic left ventricular systolic dysfunction. Guidelines recommend preoperative echocardiography in patients without known HF with unexplained dyspnea and in patients with known HF with clinical deterioration. A small observational study found that routine echocardiography in patients with suspected heart disease or those aged 65 years or older prior to emergency noncardiac surgery frequently led to a change in diagnosis or management plan. While this is not an established practice, preoperative echocardiography should be considered when there is uncertainty about the patient's cardiac status.

Patients receiving diuretics and digoxin should have serum electrolyte and digoxin levels measured prior to surgery because abnormalities in these levels may increase the risk of perioperative arrhythmias. Clinicians must be cautious not to give too much diuretic, since the volume-depleted patient will be much more susceptible to intraoperative hypotension. The surgeon and anesthesiologist should be made aware of the presence and severity of left ventricular dysfunction so that appropriate decisions can be made regarding perioperative fluid management and intraoperative monitoring.

Valvular Heart Disease

If the severity of valvular lesions is unknown, or if there has been a recent change in clinical status, echocardiography should be performed prior to noncardiac surgery. Candidates for valve replacement surgery or valvuloplasty independent of the planned noncardiac surgery should have the valve correction procedure performed first. Patients with uncorrected severe or symptomatic aortic stenosis are at particular risk for cardiac complications. They should only undergo surgery after consultation with a cardiologist and anesthesiologist. Patients with asymptomatic aortic stenosis appeared to be at lower risk than patients with symptomatic aortic stenosis and may be reasonable candidates for major surgery with appropriate intraoperative and postoperative monitoring. Patients with mitral stenosis require heart rate control to prolong diastolic filling time. Regurgitant valvular lesions are generally less problematic during surgery because the vasodilatory effect of anesthetics promotes forward flow. Patients with aortic regurgitation likely benefit from afterload reduction and careful attention to volume status.

Arrhythmias

The finding of a rhythm disturbance on preoperative evaluation should prompt consideration of further cardiac evaluation, particularly when the finding of structural heart disease would alter perioperative management. **Patients with a rhythm disturbance without evidence of** underlying heart disease are at low risk for perioperative cardiac complications. There is no evidence that the use of antiarrhythmic medications to suppress an asymptomatic arrhythmia alters perioperative risk.

Patients with symptomatic arrhythmias should not undergo elective surgery until their cardiac condition has been addressed. Thus, in patients with atrial fibrillation or other supraventricular arrhythmias, adequate rate control should be established prior to surgery. Symptomatic ventricular tachycardia must be thoroughly evaluated and controlled prior to surgery. Patients who have independent indications for a permanent pacemaker or implanted defibrillator should have it placed prior to noncardiac surgery. The anesthesiologist must be notified that a patient has an implanted pacemaker or defibrillator so that steps may be taken to prevent device malfunction caused by electromagnetic interference from the intraoperative use of electrocautery.

Hypertension

Mild to moderate hypertension (systolic blood pressure below 180 mm Hg and diastolic blood pressure below 110 mm Hg) does not appear to be an independent risk factor for postoperative MI or cardiac death. No evidence supports delaying surgery in order to better control mild to moderate hypertension. Most medications for chronic hypertension should generally be continued up to and including the day of surgery. Consideration should be given to holding angiotensin-converting enzyme inhibitors and angiotensin receptor blockers on the day of surgery in the absence of HF, since these agents may increase the risk of intraoperative hypotension and potentiate postoperative acute kidney injury. Diuretic agents are also frequently held on the day of surgery to prevent hypovolemia and electrolyte disorders if they are not needed to control HF; however, the benefit of this practice is uncertain.

Severe hypertension, defined as a systolic pressure greater than 180 mm Hg or diastolic pressure greater than 110 mm Hg, does appear to be an independent predictor of perioperative cardiac complications, including MI and HF. It is reasonable to consider delaying surgery in patients with such severe hypertension until blood pressure can be controlled, although it is not known whether the risk of cardiac complications is reduced with this approach.

Berwanger O et al; VISION Investigators. Association between pre-operative statin use and major cardiovascular complications among patients undergoing non-cardiac surgery: the VISION study. Eur Heart J. 2016 Jan 7;37(2):177–85. [PMID: 26330424]

Bouri S et al. Meta-analysis of secure randomised controlled trials of β-blockade to prevent perioperative death in non-cardiac surgery. Heart. 2014 Mar;100(6):456–64. [PMID: 23904357]

Fleisher LA et al. 2014 ACC/AHA Guideline on Perioperative Cardiovascular Evaluation and Management of Patients Undergoing Noncardiac Surgery: A Report of the American College of Cardiology/American Heart Association Task Force on Practice Guidelines. J Am Coll Cardiol. 2014 Dec 9; 64(22):e77–137. [PMID: 25091544]

PULMONARY EVALUATION IN NON–LUNG RESECTION SURGERY

Pneumonia and respiratory failure requiring prolonged mechanical ventilation are the most important postoperative pulmonary complications. The occurrence of these complications has been associated with a significant increase in mortality and hospital length of stay. Pulmonary thromboembolism is another serious complication; prophylaxis against venous thromboembolic disease is described in Chapter 14.

▶ Risk Factors for the Development of Postoperative Pulmonary Complications

The risk of developing a pulmonary complication is highest in patients undergoing cardiac, thoracic, and upper abdominal surgery, with reported complication rates ranging from 9% to 19%. The risk in patients undergoing lower abdominal or pelvic procedures ranges from 2% to 5%, and for extremity procedures, the range is less than 1% to 3%. **The pulmonary complication rate for laparoscopic procedures appears to be much lower than that for open procedures.** In one series of over 1500 patients who underwent laparoscopic cholecystectomy, the pulmonary complication rate was less than 1%. Other procedure-related risk factors include prolonged anesthesia time, need for general anesthesia, and emergency operations.

It remains unclear which of the many patient-specific risk factors that have been identified are independent predictors. Advanced age appears to confer increased risk. Surgical patients in their seventh decade had a fourfold higher risk of pulmonary complications compared with patients under age 50. The presence and severity of systemic disease of any type is associated with pulmonary complications. In particular, patients with chronic obstructive pulmonary disease (COPD) or HF have at least twice the risk compared with patients without these conditions. A risk calculator for assessing the risk of postoperative respiratory failure was derived from the NSQIP patient database (http://www.qxmd.com/calculate-online/respirology/postoperative-respiratory-failure-risk-calculator). Predictors in this model include the type of surgery, emergency surgery, preoperative sepsis, dependency in activities of daily living, and the patient's American Society of Anesthesiologists physical status classification.

Patients with well-controlled asthma at the time of surgery are not at increased risk for pulmonary complications. Obesity causes restrictive pulmonary physiology, which may increase pulmonary risk in surgical patients. Obstructive sleep apnea has been associated with a variety of postoperative complications, particularly in patients undergoing bariatric surgery. The STOP screening questionnaire asks whether a patient has *s*noring, *t*iredness during the day, *o*bserved apnea, and high blood *p*ressure. The presence of two or more of these findings had a 78% positive predictive value for obstructive sleep apnea and was associated with a doubled risk for postoperative pulmonary complications. A summary of risk factors for pulmonary complications is presented in Table 3–4.

Table 3–4. Clinical risk factors for postoperative pulmonary complications.

Upper abdominal or cardiothoracic surgery
Prolonged anesthesia time (> 4 hours)
Emergency surgery
Age > 60 years
Chronic obstructive pulmonary disease
Heart failure
Severe systemic disease
Tobacco use (> 20 pack-years)
Impaired cognition or sensorium
Functional dependency or prior stroke
Preoperative sepsis
Low serum albumin level
Obstructive sleep apnea

▶ Pulmonary Function Testing & Laboratory Studies

The main role for preoperative pulmonary function tests (PFTs) is to characterize pulmonary disease in patients with unexplained symptoms prior to major abdominal or cardiothoracic surgery. **In patients with diagnosed lung disease, PFTs often add little information above clinical assessment.** Furthermore, there is no clear degree of PFT abnormality that can be used as an absolute contraindication to non–lung resection surgery. **Chest radiographs in unselected patients also rarely add clinically useful information.** In one study, only 0.1% of routine preoperative chest radiographs changed clinical management. They may be more useful in patients who are undergoing abdominal or thoracic surgery, who are over age 50, or who have known cardiopulmonary disease. Some experts have also advocated polysomnography to diagnose obstructive sleep apnea prior to bariatric surgery, but the benefits of this approach are unproven. Abnormally low or high blood urea nitrogen levels (indicating malnutrition or kidney disease, respectively) and hypoalbuminemia predict higher risk of pulmonary complications and mortality, although the added value of laboratory testing over clinical assessment is uncertain. Arterial blood gas measurement is not routinely recommended except in patients with known lung disease and suspected hypoxemia or hypercapnia.

▶ Perioperative Management

Retrospective studies have shown that smoking cessation reduced the incidence of pulmonary complications, but only if it was initiated at least 1–2 months before surgery. A meta-analysis of randomized trials found that preoperative smoking cessation programs reduced both pulmonary and surgical wound complications, especially if smoking cessation was initiated at least 4 weeks prior to surgery. **The preoperative period may be an optimal time to initiate smoking cessation efforts.** A systematic review found that smoking cessation programs started in a preoperative evaluation clinic increased the odds of abstinence at 3–6 months by nearly 60%.

The incidence of postoperative pulmonary complications in patients with COPD or asthma may be reduced by preoperative optimization of pulmonary function. Patients who are wheezing should receive preoperative therapy with bronchodilators and, in certain cases, corticosteroids. Antibiotics may be beneficial for patients with COPD with increased sputum production or purulence. Patients receiving oral theophylline should continue taking the medication perioperatively. A serum theophylline level should be measured to rule out toxicity.

Postoperative risk reduction strategies have centered on promoting lung expansion through the use of incentive spirometry, continuous positive airway pressure (CPAP), intermittent positive-pressure breathing (IPPB), and deep breathing exercises. Although trial results have been mixed, all these techniques have been shown to reduce the incidence of postoperative atelectasis and, in a few studies, to reduce the incidence of postoperative pulmonary complications. In most comparative trials, these methods were equally effective. **Given the higher cost of CPAP and IPPB, incentive spirometry and deep breathing exercises are the preferred methods for most patients.**

Taylor A et al. Prevention of postoperative pulmonary complications. Surg Clin North Am. 2015 Apr;95(2):237–54. [PMID: 25814104]

Thomsen T et al. Interventions for preoperative smoking cessation. Cochrane Database Syst Rev. 2014 Mar 27;3:CD002294. [PMID: 24671929]

Weingarten TN et al. Predicting postoperative pulmonary complications in high-risk populations. Curr Opin Anaesthesiol. 2013 Apr;26(2):116–25. [PMID: 23407151]

EVALUATION OF THE PATIENT WITH LIVER DISEASE

Patients with serious liver disease are at increased risk for perioperative morbidity and demise. Appropriate preoperative evaluation requires consideration of the effects of anesthesia and surgery on postoperative liver function and of the complications associated with anesthesia and surgery in patients with preexisting liver disease.

▶ The Effects of Anesthesia & Surgery on Liver Function

Postoperative elevation of serum aminotransferase levels is a relatively common finding after major surgery. Most of these elevations are transient and not associated with hepatic dysfunction. While direct hepatotoxicity is rare with modern anesthetics agents, these medications may cause deterioration of hepatic function via intraoperative reduction in hepatic blood flow leading to ischemic injury. Intraoperative hypotension, hemorrhage, and hypoxemia may also contribute to liver injury.

▶ Risk Assessment in Surgical Patients with Liver Disease

Screening unselected patients with liver function tests has a low yield and is not recommended. Patients with suspected or known liver disease based on history or physical examination, however, should have measurement of liver enzyme levels as well as tests of hepatic synthetic function performed prior to surgery.

Acute hepatitis increases surgical mortality risk. In three small series of patients with acute viral hepatitis who underwent abdominal surgery, the mortality rate was roughly 10%. Similarly, patients with undiagnosed alcoholic hepatitis had high mortality rates when undergoing abdominal surgery. Thus, elective surgery in patients with acute viral or alcoholic hepatitis should be delayed until the acute episode has resolved. In the absence of cirrhosis or synthetic dysfunction, chronic viral hepatitis is unlikely to increase risk significantly. A large cohort study of hepatitis C seropositive patients who underwent surgery found a mortality rate of less than 1%. Similarly, nonalcoholic fatty liver disease without cirrhosis probably does not pose a serious risk in surgical patients.

In patients with cirrhosis, postoperative complication rates correlate with the severity of liver dysfunction. Traditionally, severity of dysfunction has been assessed with the Child-Turcotte-Pugh score (see Chapter 16). Patients with Child-Turcotte-Pugh class C cirrhosis who underwent portosystemic shunt surgery, biliary surgery, or trauma surgery during the 1970s and 1980s had a 50–85% mortality rate. Patients with Child-Turcotte-Pugh class A or B cirrhosis who underwent abdominal surgery during the 1990s, however, had relatively low mortality rates (hepatectomy 0–8%, open cholecystectomy 0–1%, laparoscopic cholecystectomy 0–1%). A conservative approach would be to avoid elective surgery in patients with Child-Turcotte-Pugh class C cirrhosis and pursue it with great caution in class B patients. The Model for End-stage Liver Disease (MELD) score, based on serum bilirubin and creatinine levels, and the prothrombin time expressed as the International Normalized Ratio, also predicted surgical mortality and outperformed the Child-Turcotte-Pugh classification in some studies. A web-based risk assessment calculator incorporating age and MELD score can predict both perioperative and long-term mortality (http://www.mayoclinic.org/medical-professionals/model-end-stage-liver-disease/post-operative- mortality-risk-patients-cirrhosis).

In addition, when surgery is elective, it is prudent to attempt to reduce the severity of ascites, encephalopathy, and coagulopathy preoperatively. Ascites is a particular problem in abdominal operations, where it can lead to wound dehiscence or hernias. Great care should be taken when using analgesics and sedatives, as these can worsen hepatic encephalopathy. In general, short-acting agents and lower doses should be used. Patients with coagulopathy should receive vitamin K (if there is concern for concomitant malnutrition) and may need fresh frozen plasma transfusion at the time of surgery.

Im GY et al. Surgery in patients with portal hypertension: a preoperative checklist and strategies for attenuating risk. Clin Liver Dis. 2014 May;18(2):477–505. [PMID: 24679507]

Nicoll A. Surgical risk in patients with cirrhosis. J Gastroenterol Hepatol. 2012 Oct;27(10):1569–75. [PMID: 22694313]

PREOPERATIVE HEMATOLOGIC EVALUATION

Three of the more common clinical situations faced by the medical consultant are the patient with anemia, the assessment of bleeding risk, and the perioperative management of long-term anticoagulation.

Preoperative anemia is common, with a prevalence of 43% in a large cohort of elderly veterans undergoing surgery. The main goals of the preoperative evaluation of the anemic patient are to determine the need for preoperative diagnostic evaluation and the need for transfusion. **When feasible, the diagnostic evaluation of the patient with previously unrecognized anemia should be done prior to surgery because certain types of anemia (particularly those due to sickle cell disease, hemolysis, and acute blood loss) have implications for perioperative management.** These types of anemia are typically associated with an elevated reticulocyte count. While preoperative anemia is associated with higher perioperative morbidity and mortality, it is not known whether correction of preoperative anemia with transfusions or erythropoiesis-stimulating agents will improve postoperative outcomes. Determination of the need for preoperative transfusion in an individual patient must consider factors other than the absolute hemoglobin level, including the presence of cardiopulmonary disease, the type of surgery, and the likely severity of surgical blood loss. The few studies that have compared different postoperative transfusion thresholds failed to demonstrate improved outcomes with a more aggressive transfusion strategy. One trial randomized hip fracture patients, most of whom had cardiovascular disease, to either transfusion to maintain a hemoglobin level greater than 10 g/dL (100 g/L) or transfusion for symptomatic anemia. Patients receiving symptom-triggered transfusion received far fewer units of packed red blood cells without increased mortality or complication rates.

The most important component of the bleeding risk assessment is a **directed bleeding history** (see Table 3–1). Patients who provide a reliable history of no abnormal bleeding on directed bleeding history and have no suggestion of abnormal bleeding on physical examination are at very low risk for having an occult bleeding disorder. Laboratory tests of hemostatic parameters in these patients are generally not needed. When the directed bleeding history is unreliable or incomplete, or when abnormal bleeding is suggested, a formal evaluation of hemostasis should be done prior to surgery and should include measurement of the prothrombin time, activated partial thromboplastin time, and platelet count (see Chapter 13).

Patients receiving long-term oral anticoagulation are at risk for thromboembolic complications when an operation requires interruption of this therapy. **"Bridging" anticoagulation, where unfractionated or low-molecular-weight heparin is administered parenterally while oral anticoagulants are held, is commonly practiced, but its benefit is unproven and there is the potential for harm.** A randomized trial of bridging anticoagulation in surgical patients taking warfarin for atrial fibrillation demonstrated no difference in thromboembolism. Bleeding complications were twice as common in patients who received bridging anticoagulation. Most experts recommend bridging therapy only in patients at high risk for thromboembolism. An approach to perioperative anticoagulation management is shown in Table 3–5, but the recommendations must be considered in the context of patient preference and hemorrhagic risk. The newer oral anticoagulants should be withheld several days prior to surgery, based on the patient's renal function (Table 3–6). There are only limited options to reverse the anticoagulant effect of these medications, so they should only be restarted after surgery when adequate hemostasis is assured. These agents take effect

Table 3–5. Recommendations for perioperative anticoagulation management.

Thromboembolic Risk without Anticoagulation	Recommendation
Low (eg, atrial fibrillation with no more than two other stroke risk factors,[1] mechanical bileaflet aortic valve prosthesis with no other stroke risk factors, or single venous thromboembolism > 3 months ago without hypercoagulability condition[2])	1. Stop warfarin 5 days before surgery 2. Measure INR the day before surgery to confirm that it is acceptable (< 1.6 for most operations) 3. Resume warfarin when hemostasis permits 4. No bridging with parenteral anticoagulants before or after surgery
High (eg, atrial fibrillation or mechanical heart valve with stroke < 3 months prior, mechanical mitral valve prosthesis, caged-ball or tilting disk valve prosthesis, or venous thrombosis < 3 months ago or associated with hypercoagulability condition[2])	1. Stop warfarin 5 days before surgery 2. Begin bridging with therapeutic dose UFH infusion or LMWH 2 days after stopping oral anticoagulation 3. Administer last dose of LMWH 24 hours before surgery; discontinue UFH 4–6 hours before surgery 4. Measure INR the day before surgery to confirm that it is acceptable (< 1.6 for most operations) 5. Resume warfarin when hemostasis permits 6. If hemostasis permits, resume bridging with therapeutic dose UFH infusion or LMWH beginning 48–72 hours after surgery and continuing until the INR is therapeutic

[1]Heart failure, hypertension, diabetes mellitus, age > 75 years.
[2]Patients should receive venous thromboembolism prophylaxis after surgery (see Chapter 14).
INR, international normalized ratio; LMWH, low-molecular-weight heparin; UFH, unfractionated heparin.

Table 3–6. Recommendations for preoperative management of direct acting oral anticoagulants.[1]

Creatinine Clearance	Dabigatran	Rivaroxaban	Apixaban	Edoxaban
>50 mL/min/1.73 m² (0.83 mL/s/m²)	Hold 4-6 doses	Hold 2 doses	Hold 4 doses	Hold 2 doses
30-50 mL/min/1.73 m² (0.5-0.83 mL/s/m²)	Hold 6-8 doses	Hold 2 doses	Hold 6 doses	Hold 2 doses

[1]Recommendations are for the number of doses to hold before the day of surgery for complete reversal of anticoagulant effect. If mild to moderate anticoagulant effect at time of procedure is desired, the number of held doses should be reduced by 50%.

immediately, and no bridging is required when they are restarted (see Chapter 14).

Clevenger B et al. Pre-operative anaemia. Anaesthesia. 2015 Jan;70(Suppl 1):2–8, e6–8. [PMID: 25440391]

Douketis JD et al; BRIDGE Investigators. Perioperative bridging anticoagulation in patients with atrial fibrillation. N Engl J Med. 2015 Aug 27;373(9):823–33. [PMID: 26095867]

Douketis JD et al. Perioperative management of antithrombotic therapy: Antithrombotic Therapy and Prevention of Thrombosis, 9th ed: American College of Chest Physicians Evidence-Based Clinical Practice Guidelines. Chest. 2012 Feb;141(2 Suppl):e326S–50S. Erratum in: Chest. 2012 Apr;141(4):1129. [PMID: 22315266]

Lai A et al. Perioperative management of patients on new oral anticoagulants. Br J Surg. 2014 Jun;101(7):742–9. [PMID: 24777590]

NEUROLOGIC EVALUATION

Delirium can occur after any major operation but is particularly common after hip fracture repair and cardiovascular surgery, where the incidence is 30–60%. Postoperative delirium has been associated with higher rates of major postoperative cardiac and pulmonary complications, poor functional recovery, increased length of hospital stay, increased risk of subsequent dementia and functional decline, and increased mortality. Several preoperative and postoperative factors have been associated with the development of postoperative delirium. Delirium occurred in half of the patients with at least three of the risk factors listed in Table 3–7.

Two types of intervention to prevent delirium have been evaluated: focused geriatric care and psychotropic medications. In a randomized trial of hip fracture surgery patients, those who received daily visits and targeted recommendations from a geriatrician had a lower risk of postoperative delirium (32%) than the control patients (50%). **Common interventions to prevent delirium were minimizing the use of benzodiazepines and anticholinergic medications, maintenance of regular bowel function, and early discontinuation of urinary catheters.** Other studies comparing postoperative care in specialized geriatrics units with standard wards have shown similar reductions in the incidence of delirium. Limited data support the effectiveness of using low doses of neuroleptics to prevent postoperative delirium, but this practice is uncommon.

Only a minority of patients with postoperative delirium will have a single, reversible etiology for their condition. Evaluation of delirious patients should exclude electrolyte derangements, occult urinary tract infection, and adverse effects from psychotropic medications. Opioids, benzodiazepines, anticholinergic agents, and antispasmodics are often implicated in postoperative delirium. Conservative management includes reassuring and reorienting the patient; eliminating unneeded psychotropic medication, intravenous lines, and urinary catheters; and keeping the patient active during the day while allowing uninterrupted sleep at night. In situations where delirium jeopardizes patient or provider safety, low doses of neuroleptic agents are preferred over the use of benzodiazepines.

Stroke complicates less than 1% of all surgical procedures but may occur in 1–6% of patients undergoing cardiac or carotid artery surgery. Most of the strokes in cardiac surgery patients are embolic in origin, and about half occur within the first postoperative day. Stroke after cardiac surgery is associated with significantly increased mortality, up to 22% in some studies. A retrospective analysis found that patients who had previously suffered a stroke had an 18% risk of MI, recurrent stroke, or cardiac death if they underwent noncardiac surgery within 3 months of the stroke. This risk declined over time and reached a plateau 9 months after the stroke, suggesting a benefit to delaying elective surgery.

Symptomatic carotid artery stenosis is associated with a high risk of stroke in patients undergoing cardiac surgery. In general, symptomatic carotid lesions should be treated prior to elective cardiac surgery. In contrast, most studies suggest that **asymptomatic carotid bruits and asymptomatic carotid stenosis are associated with little or no increased risk of stroke in surgical patients.** Prophylactic carotid endarterectomy or stenting in patients with asymptomatic carotid artery disease is unlikely to be beneficial in most patients, as the stroke risk of the carotid procedure

Table 3–7. Risk factors for the development of postoperative delirium.

Preoperative factors
Age > 70 years
Alcohol abuse
Cognitive impairment
Poor physical function status
Markedly abnormal serum sodium, potassium, or glucose level
Aortic, thoracic, hip fracture, or emergency surgery

Postoperative factors
Use of meperidine or benzodiazepines, anticholinergics, antihistamines
Postoperative hematocrit < 30%
Use of urinary catheters

likely outweighs any risk reduction it provides in a subsequent operation. On the other hand, patients with independent indications for such procedures (see Chapter 12) should probably have the carotid operation prior to the elective surgery.

Javedan H et al. Management of common postoperative complications: delirium. Clin Geriatr Med. 2014 May;30(2):271–8. [PMID: 24721366]

Mashour GA et al. Neurological complications of surgery and anaesthesia. Br J Anaesth. 2015 Feb;114(2):194–203. [PMID: 25204699]

van Meenen LC et al. Risk prediction models for postoperative delirium: a systematic review and meta-analysis. J Am Geriatr Soc. 2014 Dec;62(12):2383–90. [PMID: 25516034]

MANAGEMENT OF ENDOCRINE DISEASES

▶ Diabetes Mellitus

The most challenging issue in diabetic patients is the maintenance of glucose control during the perioperative period. The increased secretion of cortisol, epinephrine, glucagon, and growth hormone during surgery is associated with insulin resistance and hyperglycemia in diabetic patients. **The goal of management is the prevention of severe hyperglycemia or hypoglycemia in the perioperative period.**

Cohort studies demonstrate that poor preoperative glycemic control, as indicated by an elevated hemoglobin A_{1c} level, is associated with a greater risk of surgical complications, particularly infections. However, a strategy of delaying surgery until glycemic control improves has not been rigorously studied. The ideal postoperative blood glucose level is not known. Trials have demonstrated that tighter perioperative glycemic control leads to better clinical outcomes in cardiac surgery patients in a critical care unit. This finding is not generally applicable to other surgical patients, however, as a subsequent trial demonstrated **increased** mortality with tight control in surgical patients in an intensive care unit. Data are lacking on risks and benefits of tight control in patients outside of intensive care units. The American College of Physicians recommends maintaining serum glucose between 140 mg/dL and 200 mg/dL (7.8–11.1 mmol/L), whereas the British National Health Service guidelines recommend a range of 108–180 mg/dL (6–10 mmol/L).

The specific pharmacologic management of diabetes during the perioperative period depends on the type of diabetes (insulin-dependent or not), the level of glycemic control, and the type and length of surgery. Oral hypoglycemic agents should be held on the day of surgery. They should not be restarted after surgery until oral intake is adequate and unlikely to be interrupted. For patients taking insulin, a common practice is to reduce the last preoperative dose of long-acting, basal insulin by 50% and hold short-acting nutritional insulin. Most patients with type 1 diabetes and some with type 2 diabetes will need an intravenous insulin infusion perioperatively. **Consultation with an endocrinologist should be strongly considered when patients with type 1 diabetes mellitus undergo major surgery.** All diabetic patients require frequent blood glucose monitoring to prevent hypoglycemia and to ensure prompt treatment of hyperglycemia. Perioperative use of corticosteroids, common in neurosurgical and organ transplant procedures, increases glucose intolerance. Patients receiving corticosteroids often require additional short-acting insulin with meals, while their fasting glucose levels and basal insulin requirements may remain relatively unchanged.

▶ Corticosteroid Replacement

Perioperative complications (predominantly hypotension) resulting from primary or secondary adrenocortical insufficiency are rare. The common practice of administering high-dose corticosteroids during the perioperative period in patients at risk for adrenocortical insufficiency has not been rigorously studied. While definitive recommendations regarding perioperative corticosteroid therapy cannot be made, a conservative approach would be to consider any patient who has received the equivalent of at least 7.5 mg of prednisone daily for 3 weeks within the past year to be at risk for having adrenocortical insufficiency. Patients who have been taking less than 5 mg of prednisone daily and those receiving alternate-day corticosteroid dosing are unlikely to require supplemental coverage. A commonly used regimen is 100 mg of hydrocortisone given intravenously daily, divided every 8 hours, beginning before induction of anesthesia and continuing for 24–48 hours. Tapering the dose is not necessary. Patients receiving long-term maintenance corticosteroid therapy should also continue their usual dose throughout the perioperative period.

▶ Thyroid Disease

Severe symptomatic hypothyroidism has been associated with perioperative complications, including intraoperative hypotension, HF, cardiac arrest, and death. Elective surgery should be delayed in patients with severe hypothyroidism until adequate thyroid hormone replacement can be achieved. Similarly, patients with symptomatic hyperthyroidism are at risk for perioperative thyroid storm and should not undergo elective surgery until their thyrotoxicosis is controlled. An endocrinologist should be consulted if emergency surgery is needed in such patients. Conversely, patients with asymptomatic or mild hypothyroidism generally tolerate surgery well, with only a slight increase in the incidence of intraoperative hypotension; surgery need not be delayed for the month or more required to ensure adequate thyroid hormone replacement.

Njoku MJ. Patients with chronic endocrine disease. Med Clin North Am. 2013 Nov;97(6):1123–37. [PMID: 24182723]

Sebranek JJ et al. Glycaemic control in the perioperative period. Br J Anaesth. 2013 Dec;111(Suppl 1):i18–34. [PMID: 24335396]

KIDNEY DISEASE

Approximately 1% of patients suffer a significant reduction in kidney function after major surgery. The risk is

Table 3–8. Risk factors for the development of postoperative acute kidney failure.

Preoperative chronic kidney disease
Aortic and major peripheral vascular surgery
Cardiac surgery
Severe heart failure
Preoperative jaundice
Age > 70 years
Diabetes mellitus
COPD requiring daily bronchodilator therapy
ACE inhibitor or ARB therapy

ACE, angiotensin-converting enzyme; ARB, angiotensin receptor blocker; COPD, chronic obstructive pulmonary disease.

much higher, however, in patients undergoing cardiac operations, where 10–30% of patients develop acute kidney injury. **The development of acute kidney injury is an independent predictor of mortality, even if renal dysfunction resolves.** The mortality associated with the development of perioperative acute kidney injury that requires dialysis exceeds 50%. Risk factors associated with postoperative deterioration in kidney function are shown in Table 3–8. Several medications, including "renal-dose" dopamine, mannitol, N-acetylcysteine, and clonidine, have been evaluated in an attempt to preserve kidney function during the perioperative period. None of these has proved effective in clinical trials and generally should not be used for this indication. **Maintenance of adequate intravascular volume is likely to be the most effective method to reduce the risk of perioperative deterioration in kidney function.** Exposure to renal-toxic agents, such as nonsteroidal anti-inflammatory drugs and intravenous contrast, should be minimized or avoided. Angiotensin-converting enzyme inhibitors and angiotensin receptor blockers reduce renal perfusion and may increase the risk of perioperative acute kidney injury. Although firm evidence is lacking, it may be useful to temporarily discontinue these medications in patients at risk for perioperative acute kidney injury.

Although the mortality rate for elective major surgery is low (1–4%) in patients with dialysis-dependent chronic kidney disease, the risk for perioperative complications, including postoperative hyperkalemia, pneumonia, fluid overload, and bleeding, is substantially increased. Postoperative hyperkalemia requiring emergent hemodialysis has been reported to occur in 20–30% of patients. Patients should undergo dialysis preoperatively within 24 hours before surgery, and their serum electrolyte levels should be measured just prior to surgery and monitored closely during the postoperative period.

Ng SY et al. Prediction of acute kidney injury within 30 days of cardiac surgery. J Thorac Cardiovasc Surg. 2014 Jun; 147(6): 1875–83. [PMID: 23993316]
Romagnoli S et al. Postoperative acute kidney injury. Minerva Anestesiol. 2015 Jun;81(6):684–96. [PMID: 25057935]

ANTIBIOTIC PROPHYLAXIS OF SURGICAL SITE INFECTIONS

Surgical site infection is estimated to occur in roughly 4% of general or vascular operations. Although the type of procedure is the main factor determining the risk of developing a surgical site infection, certain patient factors have been associated with increased risk, including diabetes mellitus, older age, obesity, heavy alcohol consumption, admission from a long-term care facility, and multiple medical comorbidities. **For most major procedures, the use of prophylactic antibiotics has been demonstrated to reduce the incidence of surgical site infections significantly.** Multiple studies have evaluated the effectiveness of different antibiotic regimens for various surgical procedures. Several general conclusions can be drawn from these data. First, substantial evidence suggests that a single dose of an appropriate intravenous antibiotic—or combination of antibiotics—is as effective as multiple-dose regimens that extend into the postoperative period. For longer procedures, the dose should be repeated every 3–4 hours to ensure maintenance of a therapeutic serum level. Second, for most procedures, a first-generation cephalosporin is as effective as later-generation agents. Third, prophylactic antibiotics should be given intravenously at induction of anesthesia or roughly 30–60 minutes prior to the skin incision.

Other strategies to prevent surgical site infections have proven to be controversial. Evidence suggests that nasal carriage with Staphylococcus aureus is associated with a twofold to ninefold increased risk of surgical site and catheter-related infections in surgical patients. Treatment of nasal carriers of S aureus with 2% mupirocin ointment (twice daily intranasally for 3 days) prior to cardiac surgery decreases the risk of surgical site infections. However, in a cohort study, universal screening for methicillin-resistant S aureus in surgical patients failed to reduce infection rates from this pathogen. High-concentration oxygen delivered in the immediate postoperative period may reduce surgical site infections in patients undergoing colorectal surgery or operations requiring general anesthesia. Preoperative bathing with antiseptic agents and preoperative hair removal are common practices but have not demonstrated a reduction in surgical site infections in randomized trials. The use of razors for hair removal actually seems to increase the risk of surgical site infections and is therefore specifically not recommended. If preoperative hair removal is indicated, the use of clippers is preferred.

Guidelines for antibiotic prophylaxis against infective endocarditis in patients undergoing invasive procedures are presented in Chapter 33. The American Association of Orthopaedic Surgeons recommends consideration of prophylactic antibiotics in patients with prosthetic joints on a case-by-case basis. More definitive or evidence-based guidelines for antibiotic prophylaxis against prosthetic joint infection are lacking.

Najjar PA et al. Prophylactic antibiotics and prevention of surgical site infections. Surg Clin North Am. 2015 Apr;95(2): 269–83. [PMID: 25814106]

Geriatric Disorders

G. Michael Harper, MD
C. Bree Johnston, MD, MPH
C. Seth Landefeld, MD

GENERAL PRINCIPLES OF GERIATRIC CARE

The following principles help in caring for older adults:

1. Many disorders are multifactorial in origin and are best managed by multifactorial interventions.
2. Diseases often present atypically.
3. Not all abnormalities require evaluation and treatment.
4. Complex medication regimens, adherence problems, and polypharmacy are common challenges.

ASSESSMENT OF THE OLDER ADULT

In addition to conventional assessment of symptoms and diseases, comprehensive assessment addresses three topics: prognosis, values and preferences, and ability to function independently. Comprehensive assessment is warranted before major clinical decisions are made.

▶ Assessment of Prognosis

When an older person's life expectancy is longer than 10 years (ie, 50% of similar persons live longer than 10 years), it is reasonable to consider effective tests and treatments much as they are considered in younger persons. When life expectancy is less than 10 years (and especially when it is much less), choices of tests and treatments should be made on the basis of their ability to improve that particular patient's prognosis and quality of life given that patient's shorter life expectancy. The relative benefits and harms of tests and treatments often change as prognosis worsens.

When an older patient's clinical situation is dominated by a single disease process (eg, lung cancer metastatic to brain), prognosis can be estimated well with a disease-specific instrument. Even in this situation, however, prognosis generally worsens with age (especially age over 90 years) and with the presence of serious age-related conditions, such as dementia, malnutrition, or impaired ability to walk.

When an older patient's clinical situation is not dominated by a single disease process, prognosis can be estimated initially by considering basic demographic and health elements (Figure 4–1). For example, less than 25% of

men aged 95 will live 5 years, whereas nearly 75% of women aged 70 will live 10 years. The prognosis of older persons living at home can be estimated by considering age, sex, comorbid conditions, and function (Table 4–1). The prognosis of older persons discharged from the hospital is worse than that of those living at home and can be estimated by considering sex, comorbid conditions, and function at discharge (Table 4–2).

▶ Assessment of Values & Preferences

Although patients vary in their values and preferences, most frail older patients prioritize maintaining their independence over prolonging survival. Values and preferences are determined by speaking directly with a patient or, when the patient cannot express preferences reliably, with the patient's surrogate. The clinician might ask a patient considering a hip replacement, "How would you like your hip pain and function to be different? Tell me about the risk and discomfort you are willing to go through to achieve that improvement."

In assessing values and preferences, it is important to keep in mind the following:

1. Patients are experts about their preferences for outcomes and experiences; however, they often do not have adequate information to express informed preferences for specific tests or treatments.
2. Patients' preferences often change over time. For example, some patients find living with a disability more acceptable than they thought before experiencing it.

▶ Assessment of Function

People often lose function in multiple domains as they age, with the result that they may not be able to do some activities as quickly or capably and may need assistance with other activities. Assessment of function improves prognostic estimates. **Assessment of function is essential to determining an individual's needs in the context of their values and preferences and the possible effects of prescribed treatment.**

About one-fourth of patients over age 65 and half of persons older than 85 have impairments in their **basic**

Women

Men

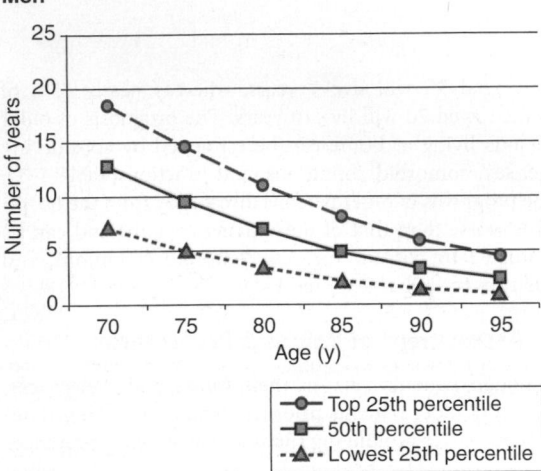

- ● Top 25th percentile
- ■ 50th percentile
- ▲ Lowest 25th percentile

▲ **Figure 4–1.** Median life expectancy of older women and men. (Adapted, with permission, from Walter LC et al. Screening for colorectal, breast, and cervical cancer in the elderly: a review of the evidence. Am J Med. 2005 Oct;118(10):1078–86. Copyright © Elsevier.)

Table 4–1. Prognostic factors, "risk points," and 4-year mortality rates for older persons living at home.

Prognostic Factor	Risk Points
Age	
60–64 years	1
65–69 years	2
70–74 years	3
75–79 years	4
80–84 years	5
85 years and older	7
Male sex	2
Comorbid conditions reported by patients	
Diabetes mellitus	1
Cancer	2
Lung disease	2
Heart failure	2
Body mass index < 25	1
Current smoker	2
Function	
Bathing difficulty	2
Difficulty handling finances	2
Difficulty walking several blocks	2
Sum of Risk Points	**4-year Mortality Rate**
1–2	2%
3–6	7%
7–10	19%
> 10	53%

Reprinted, with permission, from Lee SJ et al. Development and validation of a prognostic index for 4-year mortality in older adults. JAMA. 2006 Feb 15;295(7):801–8. Copyright © 2006 American Medical Association. All rights reserved.

activities of daily living (ADLs): bathing, dressing, eating, transferring from bed to chair, continence, toileting, or instrumental activities of daily living (IADLs): transportation, shopping, cooking, using the telephone, managing money, taking medications, housecleaning, laundry.

▶ Functional Screening Instrument

Functional screening should include assessment of ADLs and IADLs and questions to detect weight loss, falls, incontinence, depressed mood, self-neglect, fear for personal safety, and common serious impairments (eg, hearing, vision, cognition, and mobility). Standard functional screening measures may not be useful in capturing subtle impairments in highly functional independent elders. One technique for these patients is to identify and regularly ask about a target activity, such as bowling or gardening. If the patient begins to have trouble with or discontinues such an "advanced" ADL, it may indicate early impairment, such as onset of cognitive impairment, incontinence, or worsening hearing loss, which additional gentle questioning or assessment may uncover.

▶ Frailty

Frailty is a syndrome characterized by multisystem dysregulation that usually includes chronic inflammation, sarcopenia (age-related loss of muscle mass, strength, or function), neuroendocrine function alterations, and loss of functional reserve. **Persons with frailty are at increased risk for functional decline and death.** There is not one universally agreed upon definition or assessment tool for frailty, although several are in use. Elements of the frailty syndrome include slow gait speed, low hand grip strength, weight loss, low energy expenditure, and in some persons, cognitive decline. The ideal strategies for preventing and treating the frailty syndrome are unknown. At present, treatment is largely supportive, multifactorial, and individualized based on patient goals, life expectancy, and

Table 4–2. Prognostic factors, "risk points," and 1-year mortality rates for older patients discharged from the hospital after an acute medical illness.

Prognostic Factor	Risk Points
Male sex	1
Comorbid conditions reported by patients	
Cancer, metastatic	8
Cancer, not metastatic	3
Serum creatinine > 3 mg/dL	2
Albumin < 3 mg/dL	2
Albumin 3.0–3.4 mg/dL	1
Function	
Dependent in 1–4 ADL[1]	2
Dependent in 5 ADL[1]	5
Sum of Risk Points	**1-year Mortality Rate**
0–1	4%
2–3	19%
4–6	34%
> 6	64%

[1]ADL refers to five activities of daily living: bathing, dressing, transferring, using the toilet, and eating.

Reprinted, with permission, from Walter LC et al. Development and validation of a prognostic index for 1-year mortality in older adults after hospitalization. JAMA. 2001 Jun 20;285(23):2987–94. Copyright © 2001 American Medical Association. All rights reserved.

comorbidities. Exercise, particularly strength and resistance training, is the intervention with the strongest evidence for benefit. Sometimes, transitioning a patient to a palliative care–only approach or a hospice program is the most appropriate clinical intervention when efforts to prevent functional decline fail.

Butler M et al. Decision aids for advance care planning: an overview of the state of the science. Ann Intern Med. 2014 Sep 161(6):408–18. [PMID: 25069709]

Clegg A et al. Frailty in elderly people. Lancet. 2013 Mar 2; 381(9868):752–62. Erratum in: Lancet. 2013 Oct 19; 382(9901):1328. [PMID: 23395245]

Fried TR et al. The effects of comorbidity on the benefits and harms of treatment for chronic disease: a systematic review. PLoS One. 2014 Nov 17;9(11):e112593. [PMID: 25402463]

Piers RD et al. Advance Care Planning in terminally ill and frail older persons. Patient Educ Couns. 2013 Mar;90(3):323–9. [PMID: 21813261]

Ward KT et al. Do internal medicine residents know enough about skilled nursing facilities to orchestrate a good care transition? J Am Med Dir Assoc. 2014;15(11):841–3. [PMID: 25282630]

Yourman LC et al. Prognostic indices for older adults: a systematic review. JAMA. 2012 Jan 11;307(2):182–92. [PMID: 22235089]

MANAGEMENT OF COMMON GERIATRIC PROBLEMS

1. Dementia

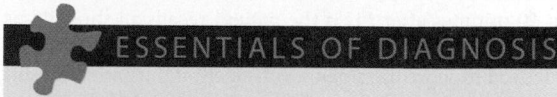

> ESSENTIALS OF DIAGNOSIS

- ► Progressive decline of intellectual function.
- ► Loss of short-term memory and at least one other cognitive deficit.
- ► Deficit severe enough to cause impairment of function.
- ► Not delirious.

► General Considerations

Dementia is an acquired, persistent, and progressive impairment in intellectual function, with compromise of memory and at least one other cognitive domain, most commonly aphasia (typically, word-finding difficulty), apraxia (inability to perform motor tasks, such as cutting a loaf of bread, despite intact motor function), agnosia (inability to recognize objects), and impaired executive function (poor abstraction, mental flexibility, planning, and judgment). The diagnosis of dementia requires a significant decline in function that is severe enough to interfere with work or social life.

Dementia has a prevalence that doubles every 5 years in the older population, reaching 30–50% at age 85. Alzheimer disease accounts for roughly two-thirds of dementia cases in the United States, with vascular dementia (either alone or combined with Alzheimer disease) and dementia with Lewy bodies accounting for much of the rest.

Depression and delirium are also common in elders, may coexist with dementia, and may also present with cognitive impairment. Depression is a common concomitant of early dementia. A patient with depression and cognitive impairment whose intellectual function improves with treatment of the mood disorder has an almost fivefold greater risk of suffering irreversible dementia later in life. Delirium, characterized by acute confusion, occurs much more commonly in patients with underlying dementia.

► Clinical Findings

A. Screening

1. Cognitive impairment—The Medicare Annual Wellness Visit mandates that clinicians assess patients for cognitive impairment. However, according to the US Preventive Services Task Force, there is insufficient evidence to recommend for or against screening all older adults for cognitive impairment. While there is logic in the argument that early detection may improve future planning and patient outcomes, empiric evidence that demonstrates a clear benefit for either patients or caregivers is lacking.

When there is suspicion of cognitive impairment, the combination of **a three-item word recall** with **a clock** drawing task (also known as the "mini-cog") is a simple, quick screening test. The clinician asks the patient to repeat three items followed by instructions to draw the face of a clock, or pre-draws a four-inch circle on a sheet of paper and instructs the patient to "draw a clock" with the time set at 10 minutes after 11. If the patient recalls all three items after 3 minutes, the test is considered normal, and there is no need to score the clock. Conversely, if the patient recalls zero items, the test is considered abnormal, and there is no need to score the clock. When the patient recalls one or two items, the test is normal when the clock is drawn correctly (numbers in the proper position and the time accurately portrayed). When a patient fails this simple screen, further cognitive evaluation with a standardized instrument is warranted. The **Montreal Cognitive Assessment (MoCA©)** is a 30-point test that takes about 10 minutes to administer and examines several areas of cognitive function. A score below 26 is considered abnormal. Free downloadable versions in multiple languages are available at http://www.mocatest.org.

2. Decision-making capacity—Cognitively impaired elders commonly face serious medical decisions, and the clinicians involved in their care must ascertain whether the capacity exists to make medical decisions. The following five elements should be considered in a thorough assessment: (1) ability to express a choice; (2) understanding relevant information about the risks and benefits of planned therapy and the alternatives (including no treatment), in the context of one's values; (3) comprehension of the problem and its consequences; (4) ability to reason; and (5) consistency of choice. A patient's choice should follow from an understanding of the consequences.

Sensitivity must be used in applying these five components to people of various cultural backgrounds. Decision-making capacity varies over time. Furthermore, the capacity to make a decision is a function of the decision in question. A woman with mild dementia may lack the capacity to consent to coronary artery bypass grafting yet retain the capacity to designate a surrogate decision-maker.

B. Symptoms and Signs

The clinician can gather important information about the type of dementia by asking about (1) the rate of progression of the deficits as well as their nature (including any personality or behavioral change); (2) the presence of other neurologic symptoms, particularly motor problems; (3) risk factors for HIV; (4) family history of dementia; and (5) medications, with particular attention to recent changes.

Work-up is directed at identifying any potentially reversible causes of dementia. However, such cases are rare. For a detailed description of the symptoms and signs of different forms of dementia, see Chapter 24.

C. Physical Examination

The neurologic examination emphasizes assessment of mental status but should also include evaluation for sensory deficits, previous strokes, parkinsonism, or peripheral neuropathy. The remainder of the physical examination should focus on identifying comorbid conditions that may aggravate the individual's disability. For a detailed description of the neuropsychological assessment, see Chapter 24.

D. Laboratory Findings

Laboratory studies should include a complete blood count and serum electrolytes, calcium, creatinine, glucose, thyroid-stimulating hormone (TSH), and vitamin B_{12} levels. While hypothyroidism or vitamin B_{12} deficiency may contribute to the cognitive impairment, treating these conditions typically does not completely reverse the dementia. HIV and rapid plasma reagin (RPR) tests, a heavy metal screen, and liver tests may be informative in selected patients but are not part of routine testing. For a detailed description of laboratory findings, see Chapter 24.

E. Imaging

Most patients should receive neuroimaging as part of the work-up to rule out subdural hematoma, tumor, previous stroke, and hydrocephalus (usually normal pressure). Those who are younger; those who have focal neurologic symptoms or signs, seizures, or gait abnormalities; and those with an acute or subacute onset are most likely to have positive findings and most likely to benefit from MRI scanning. In older patients with a more classic picture of Alzheimer disease for whom neuroimaging is desired, a noncontrast CT scan is sufficient. For a detailed description of imaging, see Chapter 24.

► Differential Diagnosis

Older individuals experience occasional difficulty retrieving items from memory (usually word-finding difficulty) and experience a slowing in their rate of information processing. In **mild cognitive impairment,** a patient complains of memory problems, demonstrates mild deficits (most commonly in short-term memory) on formal testing, but does not meet criteria for dementia. **Annual dementia conversion rates vary between less than 5% to 20%.** No medications have been demonstrated to delay the progression of mild cognitive impairment to Alzheimer disease. An elderly patient with intact cognition but with severe impairments in vision or hearing commonly becomes confused in an unfamiliar medical setting and consequently may be falsely labeled as demented.

Delirium can be distinguished from dementia by its acute onset, fluctuating course, and deficits in attention rather than memory. Because delirium and dementia often coexist, it may not be possible to determine how much impairment is attributable to each condition until the patient has resolved the delirium and is back in their usual setting. Many medications have been associated with delirium and other types of cognitive impairment in older patients. Anticholinergic agents, hypnotics, neuroleptics, opioids, nonsteroidal anti-inflammatory drugs (NSAIDs), antihistamines (both H_1- and H_2-antagonists), and corticosteroids are just some of the medications that have been associated with cognitive impairment in elders.

▶ Treatment

Patients and families should be made aware of the Alzheimer's Association (http://www.alz.org) as well as the wealth of helpful community and online resources and publications available. Caregiver support, education, and counseling may prevent or delay nursing home placement. Education should include the manifestations and natural history of dementia as well as the availability of local support services, such as respite care. Even under the best of circumstances, caregiver stress can be substantial.

A. Cognitive Impairment

1. Acetylcholinesterase inhibitors—Many experts recommend a trial of acetylcholinesterase inhibitors (eg, donepezil, galantamine, rivastigmine) in most patients with mild to moderate Alzheimer disease. These medications produce a modest improvement in cognitive function that is not likely to be detected in routine clinical encounters. However, acetylcholinesterase inhibitors have not convincingly been shown to delay functional decline or institutionalization. There is insufficient evidence to recommend their use in mild cognitive impairment to slow the progression toward dementia.

Starting (and maximum) doses are donepezil, 5 mg orally once daily (maximum 10 mg once daily); galantamine, 4 mg orally twice daily (maximum 12 mg twice daily); and rivastigmine, 1.5 mg orally twice daily (maximum 6 mg twice daily). Dosages are increased gradually as tolerated. The most bothersome side effects include diarrhea, nausea, anorexia, weight loss, and syncope. Some patients with moderate to severe cognitive impairment experience benefits from acetylcholinesterase inhibitors, but the medication should be discontinued in those patients who have had no apparent benefit, who experience side effects, or for whom the financial outlay is a burden. While there are no published guidelines that describe what constitutes an adequate treatment trial, evaluation after 2 months at the highest tolerated dose is reasonable.

2. Memantine—In clinical trials, patients with more advanced disease have been shown to have statistical benefit from the use of memantine (5 mg orally daily to 10 mg twice daily), an N-methyl-D-aspartate (NMDA) antagonist, with or without concomitant use of an acetylcholinesterase inhibitor. Long-term and meaningful functional outcomes have yet to be demonstrated.

B. Behavioral Problems

1. Nonpharmacologic approaches—Behavioral problems in demented patients are often best managed nonpharmacologically. Initially, it should be established that the problem is not unrecognized delirium, pain, urinary obstruction, or fecal impaction. Determining whether the caregiver or institutional staff can tolerate the behavior is also helpful, since it is often easier to find ways to accommodate the behavior than to modify it. If not, the caregiver should keep a brief log in which the behavior is described along with antecedent events and consequences. Recurring precipitants of the behavior are often delineated or perhaps the behavior is being rewarded. Caregivers are taught to use simple language when communicating with the patient, to break down activities into simple component tasks, and to use a "distract, not confront" approach when the patient seems disturbed by a troublesome issue. Additional steps to address behavioral problems include providing structure and routine, discontinuing all medications except those considered absolutely necessary, and correcting, if possible, sensory deficits.

2. Pharmacologic approaches—There is no clear consensus about pharmacologic approaches to the treatment of behavioral problems in patients who have not benefited from nonpharmacologic therapies. The patient's target symptoms—depression, anxiety, psychosis, mood lability, or pain—may suggest which class of medications might be most helpful, eg, antidepressant therapy for depression symptoms. Patients with dementia with Lewy bodies have shown clinically significant improvement in behavioral symptoms when treated with rivastigmine (3–6 mg orally twice daily).

Despite the lack of strong evidence, antipsychotic medications have remained a mainstay for the treatment of behavioral disturbances, particularly agitation and aggression, largely because of the lack of alternatives. The "atypical" antipsychotic agents (eg, risperidone, olanzapine, quetiapine, aripiprazole, clozapine, ziprasidone) are reported to be better tolerated than older ("typical") agents (eg, haloperidol) but should be avoided in patients with vascular risk factors due to an increased risk of stroke; they can cause weight gain and are also associated with hyperglycemia in diabetic patients and are considerably more expensive. **In several short-term trials and one long-term trial, both typical and atypical antipsychotics increased mortality compared with placebo when used to treat elderly demented patients with behavioral disturbances.** Starting and target dosages should be much lower than those used in schizophrenia (eg, haloperidol, 0.5–2 mg orally; risperidone, 0.25–2 mg orally).

A randomized placebo-controlled trial in patients with Alzheimer disease showed that citalopram (30 mg orally daily) improves symptoms of agitation. However, during the study, the US Food and Drug Administration issued a warning against using doses greater than 40 mg daily because of the risk of dysrhythmia from QT interval prolongation. For patients older than age 60, the maximum recommended dose is 20 mg daily (a dose not specifically evaluated in the study). In addition, while no serious cardiac events were observed, QT prolongation did occur, as did a small but measurable decline in cognitive function. Thus, while citalopram may be used to treat agitation, safe and effective dosing for patients older than age 60 has not been established.

C. Driving

Although drivers with dementia are at an increased risk for motor vehicle accidents, many patients continue to drive safely well beyond the time of initial diagnosis, making the timing of when to recommend that a patient stop driving particularly challenging.

There is no clear-cut evidence to suggest a single best approach to determining an individual patient's capability, and there is no accepted "gold-standard" test. The result is that clinicians must consider several factors upon which to base their judgment. For example, determining the severity of dementia can be useful. Patients with very mild or mild dementia according to the Clinical Dementia Rating Scale were able to pass formal road tests at rates of 88% and 69%, respectively. Experts agree that patients with moderately severe or more advanced dementia should be counseled to stop driving. Although not well studied, clinicians should also consider the effects of comorbid conditions and medications and the role each may play in contributing to the risk of driving by a patient with dementia. Assessment of the ability to carry out IADLs may also assist in the determination of risk. Finally, in some cases of mild dementia, referral may be needed to a **driver rehabilitation specialist** for evaluation. Although not standardized, this evaluation often consists of both off- and on-road testing. The cost for this assessment can be substantial, and it is typically not covered by health insurance. Experts recommend such an evaluation for patients with mild dementia, for those with dementia for whom new impairment in driving skills is observed, and for those with significant deficits in cognitive domains, such as attention, executive function, and visuospatial skills.

Clinicians must also be aware of the reporting requirements in their individual jurisdictions. Some states have mandatory reporting laws for clinicians, but in other states, the decision to report an unsafe driver with dementia is voluntary. When a clinician has made the decision to report an unsafe driver to the Department of Motor Vehicles, he or she must consider the impact of a potential breach in confidentiality and must weigh and address, in advance when possible, the consequences of the loss of driving independence.

D. Advance Financial Planning

Difficulty in managing financial affairs often develops early in the course of dementia. Although expertise is not expected, clinicians should have some proficiency to address financial concerns. Just as clinicians counsel patients and families about advance care planning, the same should be done to educate about the need for advance financial planning and to recommend that patients complete a durable power of attorney for finance matters (DPOAF) when the capacity to do so still exists. In most states, the DPOAF can be executed with or without the aid of an attorney. Other options to assist in managing and monitoring finances include online banking, automatic bill payments, direct deposits, and joint bank accounts.

No gold-standard test is available to identify when a patient with dementia no longer has financial capacity. However, the clinician should be on the lookout for signs that a patient is either at risk for or actually experiencing financial incapacity. **Because financial impairment can occur when dementia is mild, making that diagnosis should alone be enough to warrant further investigation.** Questioning patients and caregivers about late, missed, or repeated bill payments, unusual or uncharacteristic

purchases or gifts, overdrawn bank accounts, or reports of missing funds can provide evidence of suspected financial impairment. Patients with dementia are also at increased risk for becoming victims of financial abuse, and some answers to these same questions might also be signs of potential financial abuse. When financial abuse is suspected, clinicians should be aware of the reporting requirements in their local jurisdictions.

▶ Prognosis

Life expectancy after a diagnosis of Alzheimer disease is typically 3–15 years; it may be shorter than previously reported. Other neurodegenerative dementias, such as dementia with Lewy bodies, show more rapid decline. Hospice care is often appropriate for patients with end-stage dementia.

▶ When to Refer

Referral for neuropsychological testing may be helpful to distinguish dementia from depression, to diagnose dementia in persons of very poor education or very high premorbid intellect, and to aid diagnosis when impairment is mild.

Howard R et al. Donepezil and memantine for moderate-to-severe Alzheimer's disease. N Engl J Med. 2012 Mar 8; 366(10):893–903. [PMID: 22397651]

Jin J. JAMA patient page. Alzheimer disease. JAMA. 2015 Apr 14; 313(14):1488. [PMID: 25871685]

Langa KM et al. The diagnosis and management of mild cognitive impairment: a clinical review. JAMA. 2014 Dec 17; 312(23):2551–61. [PMID: 25514304]

Lin JS et al. Screening for cognitive impairment in older adults: a systematic review for the U.S. Preventive Services Task Force Ann Intern Med. 2013 November 5;159(9):601–12. [PMID: 24145578]

Porsteinsson AP et al. Effect of citalopram on agitation in Alzheimer disease: the CitAD randomized clinical trial. JAMA. 2014 Feb 19;311(7):682–91. [PMID: 24549548]

Russ TC et al. Cholinesterase inhibitors for mild cognitive impairment. Cochrane Database Syst Rev. 2012 Sep 12; 9:CD009132. [PMID: 22972133]

2. Depression

 ESSENTIALS OF DIAGNOSIS

▶ Depressed elders may not admit to depressed mood.

▶ Depression screening in elders should include a question about anhedonia.

▶ General Considerations

Major depressive disorder occurs in up to 5% of community-dwelling older adults, whereas clinically significant depressive symptoms—often related to loss, disease, and life changes—are present in up to 16% of older adults. Depression rates rise as illness burden increases. Depression is particularly common among hospitalized and institutionalized elders. **Older single men have the highest suicide rate of any demographic group.**

Older patients with depression are more likely to have somatic complaints, less likely to report depressed mood, and more likely to experience psychotic features than younger patients. In addition, depression may be an early symptom of dementia. Depressed patients who have comorbid conditions (eg, heart failure) are at higher risk for hospitalization, tend to have longer hospital stays, and have worse outcomes than their nondepressed counterparts.

Clinical Findings

A simple two-question screen—which consists of asking "During the past 2 weeks, have you felt down, depressed, or hopeless?" and "During the past 2 weeks, have you felt little interest or pleasure in doing things?"—is highly sensitive for detecting major depression in persons over age 65. Positive responses should be followed up with more comprehensive, structured interviews, such as the Geriatric Depression Scale (http://www.stanford.edu/~yesavage/GDS.html) or the nine items regarding depression on the Patient Health Questionnaire (PHQ-9).

Elderly patients with depressive symptoms should be questioned about use of alcohol and medications (eg, benzodiazepines, corticosteroids), since these may contribute to the clinical picture. Similarly, many medical problems can cause fatigue, lethargy, or hypoactive delirium, all of which may be mistaken for depression.

Treatment

Treatment may involve psychosocial interventions, increased physical activity, problem-solving therapy, cognitive-behavioral therapy, reduction of alcohol or medication intake, antidepressant medications, or a combination approach. In older patients with depressive symptoms who do not meet criteria for major depressive disorder, nonpharmacologic treatment approaches should be used.

Choice of antidepressant agent is usually based on side-effect profile, cost, and patient-specific factors, such as presenting symptoms and comorbidities. Selective serotonin reuptake inhibitors (SSRIs), particularly sertraline, are often used as first-line agents because of their relatively benign side-effect profile (see Table 25–7). Mirtazapine is often used for patients with weight loss, anorexia, or insomnia. Duloxetine is useful in patients who also have neuropathic pain and is better tolerated than venlafaxine among older adults. Adding methylphenidate to an SSRI appears to enhance clinical response rates. Regardless of the medication chosen, many experts recommend **starting elders at a relatively low dose, titrating to full dose slowly, and continuing for a longer trial (at least 8 weeks) before trying a different medication.** For patients experiencing their first episode of depression, pharmacologic treatment should continue for at least 6 months after remission of the depression. Recurrence of major depression is common enough among elders that long-term maintenance medication therapy should be considered.

For patients with major depression, problem-solving therapy and cognitive-behavioral therapy can be effective alone or in combination with antidepressant medication. Depressed elders may do better with a collaborative or multidisciplinary care model that includes socialization and other support elements than with usual care.

When to Refer

Consider psychiatric referral for patients who have mania or psychosis or have not responded to an initial trial of medication.

When to Admit

Consider psychiatric evaluation and admission for patients who are psychotic, suicidal, homicidal, catatonic, or gravely disabled.

Lavretsky H et al. Citalopram, methylphenidate, or their combination in geriatric depression: a randomized, double-blind, placebo controlled trial. Am J Psychiatry. 2015 Jun;172(6):561–9. [PMID: 25677354]
Mojtabai R. Diagnosing depression in older adults in primary care. N Engl J Med. 2014 Mar 27;370(13):1180–2. [PMID: 24670164]
Taylor WD. Clinical practice. Depression in the elderly. N Engl J Med. 2014 Sep 25;371(13):1228–36. [PMID: 25251617]
Thorlund K et al. Comparative efficacy and safety of selective serotonin reuptake inhibitors and serotonin-norepinephrine reuptake inhibitors in older adults: a network meta-analysis. J Am Geriatr Soc. 2015 May;63(5):1002–9. [PMID: 25945410]

3. Delirium

ESSENTIALS OF DIAGNOSIS

▸ Rapid onset and fluctuating course.
▸ Primary deficit in attention rather than memory.
▸ May be hypoactive or hyperactive.
▸ Dementia frequently coexists.

General Considerations

Delirium is an acute, fluctuating disturbance of consciousness, associated with a change in cognition or development of perceptual disturbances (see also Chapter 25). It is the pathophysiologic consequence of an underlying general medical condition, such as infection, coronary ischemia, hypoxemia, or metabolic derangement. Delirium persists in up to 25% of hospitalized patients and is associated with worse clinical outcomes (higher in-hospital and postdischarge mortality, longer lengths of stay, greater probability of placement in a nursing facility).

Although the acutely agitated elderly patient often comes to mind when considering delirium, many episodes are more subtle. **Such quiet, or hypoactive, delirium may be suspected only if one notices new cognitive slowing or inattention.**

Cognitive impairment is an important risk factor for delirium. Other risk factors include severe illness, polypharmacy, use of psychoactive medications, sensory impairment, depression, and alcoholism.

Clinical Findings

A number of bedside instruments are available for the assessment of delirium (http://www.hospitalelderlifeprogram.org/delirium-instruments/). The **confusion assessment method (CAM),** available as the Long CAM, Short CAM, and 3D CAM (3-minute diagnostic CAM), requires (1) acute onset and fluctuating course and (2) inattention and *either* (3) disorganized thinking *or* (4) altered level of consciousness. All three instruments perform well; the Short CAM and 3D CAM are particularly useful for clinical assessment of delirium. Two variations, the CAM-ICU and the CAM-S, are useful for the intensive care unit setting and in assessing delirium severity, respectively.

A key component of a delirium work-up is review of medications because many medications, the addition of a new medication, or the discontinuation of a medication known to cause withdrawal symptoms are all associated with the development of delirium. Medications that are particularly likely to increase the risk of delirium include sedative/hypnotics, anticholinergics, opioids, benzodiazepines, and H_1- and H_2-antihistamines.

Evaluation of most patients should include a complete blood count; blood urea nitrogen (BUN); serum electrolyte, creatinine, glucose, calcium, albumin, and liver tests; urinalysis; and ECG. In selected cases, serum magnesium, medication levels, arterial blood gas measurements, blood cultures, chest radiography, urinary toxin screen, head CT scan, and lumbar puncture may be helpful.

Prevention

Prevention is the best approach in the management of delirium. Measures include improving cognition (frequent reorientation, activities, socialization with family and friends when possible), sleep (massage, noise reduction, minimizing interruptions at night), mobility, vision (visual aids and adaptive equipment), hearing (portable amplifiers, cerumen disimpaction), and hydration status (volume repletion). No medications have been consistently shown to prevent delirium.

Treatment

Management of established episodes of delirium is largely supportive and includes reassurance and reorientation, treatment of underlying causes, eliminating unnecessary medications, and avoidance of indwelling catheters and restraints. Antipsychotic agents (such as haloperidol, 0.5–1 mg orally, or quetiapine, 25 mg orally, at bedtime or twice daily) are considered the medications of choice. As with dementia, caution should be used when prescribing antipsychotic medications, including checking the QTc interval on the ECG, eliminating other QTc-prolonging medications, and correcting any electrolyte abnormalities.

Benzodiazepines should be avoided except in the circumstance of alcohol or benzodiazepine withdrawal. In ventilated patients in the intensive care unit setting, dexmedetomidine or propofol (or both) may also be useful alternatives or adjuncts to antipsychotic therapy in patients with delirium.

Most episodes of delirium clear in a matter of days after correction of the precipitant, but some patients suffer episodes of much longer duration, and a significant percentage never return to their former baseline level of functioning.

When to Refer

If an initial evaluation does not reveal the cause of delirium or if entities other than delirium are in the differential diagnosis, referral to a neuropsychologist, neurologist, or geropsychiatrist should be considered.

When to Admit

Patients with delirium of unknown cause should be admitted for an expedited work-up if consistent with the patient's goals of care.

Inouye SK et al. The CAM-S: development and validation of a new scoring system for delirium severity in 2 cohorts. Ann Intern Med. 2014 Apr 15;160(8):526–3. [PMID: 24733193]

Inouye SK et al; American Geriatrics Society Expert Panel on Postoperative Delirium in Older Adults. American Geriatrics Society abstracted clinical practice guideline for postoperative delirium in older adults. J Am Geriatr Soc. 2015 Jan;63(1):142–50. [PMID: 25495432]

Marcantonio ER. 3D-CAM: derivation and validation of a 3-minute diagnostic interview for CAM-defined delirium: a cross-sectional diagnostic test study. Ann Intern Med. 2014 Oct 21;161(8):554–61. [PMID: 25329203]

Vidal EI et al. Delirium in older adults. BMJ. 2013 Apr 9;346:f2031. [PMID: 23571740]

4. Immobility

Mobility limitation is common in older adults and is associated with increased rates of morbidity, hospitalization, disability, and mortality. Structured physical activity programs may help reduce mobility-related disability among community-dwelling elders. Hospital-associated bed rest is a common precipitant of immobility and functional decline. Among hospitalized medical patients over age 70, about 10% experience a decline in function, and those who experience critical illness are at particularly high risk.

The hazards of bed rest in older adults are multiple, serious, quick to develop, and slow to reverse. Within days after being confined to bed, deconditioning of the cardiovascular system occurs and involves fluid shifts, decreased cardiac output, decreased peak oxygen uptake, increased resting heart rate, and postural hypotension. More striking changes occur in skeletal muscle, with loss of strength. Pressure ulcers, deep venous thrombosis, pulmonary embolism, and falls are additional serious risks. Recovery from these changes usually takes weeks to months.

▶ Prevention & Treatment

Physical activity should be encouraged for all elders, particularly sedentary elders. Protocols for hospitalized elders that promote walking two to three times daily and sitting upright for much of the day can minimize unnecessary immobility. When immobilization cannot be avoided, several measures can be used to minimize its consequences. To reduce the risks of contracture and weakness, range-of-motion and strengthening exercises should be started immediately and continued as long as the patient is in bed. Avoiding restraints and discontinuing intravenous lines and urinary catheters will increase opportunities for early mobility. Graduated ambulation should begin as soon as it is feasible. Prior to discharge, physical therapists can recommend appropriate exercises and assistive devices; after discharge, they can recommend safety modifications and maintenance exercises.

Brown CJ et al. Mobility limitation in the older patient: a clinical review. JAMA. 2013 Sep 18;310(11):1168–77. [PMID: 24045741]
Pahor M et al. Effect of structured physical activity on prevention of major mobility disability in older adults: the LIFE study randomized clinical trial. JAMA. 2014 Jun 18; 311(23):2387–96. [PMID: 24866862]

5. Falls & Gait Disorders

About one-third of people over age 65 fall each year, and the frequency of falls increases markedly with advancing age. About 10% of falls result in serious injuries, such as fractures, soft-tissue injuries, and traumatic brain injuries. Complications from falls are the leading cause of death from injury in persons over age 65. Hip fractures are common precursors to functional impairment, nursing home placement, and death.

Every older person should be asked about falls. Assessment of patients who fall should include postural blood pressure and pulse; cardiac examination; evaluations of strength, range of motion, cognition, and proprioception; and examination of feet and footwear. A thorough gait assessment should be performed in all older people. Gait and balance can be readily assessed by the **"Up and Go Test,"** in which the patient is asked to stand up from a sitting position without use of hands, walk 10 feet, turn around, walk back, and sit down. Patients who take less than 10 seconds are usually normal, patients who take longer than 30 seconds tend to need assistance with many mobility tasks, and those in between tend to vary widely with respect to gait, balance, and function. The ability to recognize common patterns of gait disorders is an extremely useful clinical skill to develop. Examples of gait abnormalities and their causes are listed in Table 4–3.

▶ Causes of Falls

Balance and ambulation require a complex interplay of cognitive, neuromuscular, and cardiovascular function. With age, balance mechanisms can become compromised and postural sway increases. These changes predispose the older person to a fall when challenged by an additional insult to any of these systems.

A fall may be the clinical manifestation of an occult problem, such as pneumonia or myocardial infarction, but much more commonly, falls are due to the interaction between an impaired patient and an environmental risk factor. **Falls in older people are rarely due to a single cause, and effective intervention entails a comprehensive assessment of the patient's intrinsic deficits (eg, diseases and medications), the activity engaged in at the time of the fall, and environmental obstacles.**

Table 4–3. Evaluation of gait abnormalities.

Gait Abnormality	Possible Cause
Inability to stand without use of hands	Deconditioning Myopathy (hyperthyroidism, alcohol, statin-induced) Hip or knee pain
Unsteadiness upon standing	Orthostatic hypotension Balance problem (peripheral neuropathy, vision problem, vestibular, other central nervous system causes) Generalized weakness
Stagger with eyes closed	Often indicates that vision is compensating for another deficit
Short steps	Weakness Parkinson disease or related condition
Asymmetry	Cerebrovascular accident Focal pain or arthritis
Wide-based gait	Fear, balance problems
Flexed knees	Contractures, quadriceps weakness
Slow gait	Fear of falling, weakness, deconditioning, peripheral vascular disease, chronic obstructive pulmonary disease, heart failure, angina pectoris

Intrinsic deficits are those that impair sensory input, judgment, blood pressure regulation, reaction time, and balance and gait. Dizziness may be closely related to the deficits associated with falls and gait abnormalities. While it may be impossible to isolate a sole "cause" or a "cure" for falls, gait abnormalities, or dizziness, it is often possible to identify and ameliorate some of the underlying contributory conditions and improve the patient's overall function.

Medication use is one of the most common, significant, and reversible causes of falling. A meta-analysis found that sedative/hypnotics, antidepressants, and benzodiazepines were the classes of medications most likely to be associated with falling. The use of multiple medications simultaneously has also been associated with an increased fall risk. Other often overlooked but treatable contributors include postural hypotension (including postprandial, which peaks 30–60 minutes after a meal), insomnia, use of multifocal lenses, and urinary urgency.

Since most falls occur in or around the home, a visit by a visiting nurse, physical therapist, or health care provider for a home safety evaluation reaps substantial benefits in identifying environmental obstacles and is generally reimbursed by third-party payers, including Medicare.

▶ Complications of Falls

The most common fractures resulting from falls are of the wrist, hip, and vertebrae. There is a high mortality rate (approximately 20% in 1 year) in elderly women with hip fractures, particularly if they were debilitated prior to the time of the fracture.

Fear of falling again is a common, serious, but treatable factor in the elderly person's loss of confidence and independence. Referral to a physical therapist for gait training with special devices is often all that is required.

Chronic subdural hematoma is an easily overlooked complication of falls that must be considered in any elderly patient presenting with new neurologic symptoms or signs. Headache and known history of trauma may both be absent.

Patients who are unable to get up from a fall are at risk for dehydration, electrolyte imbalance, pressure sores, rhabdomyolysis, and hypothermia.

▶ Prevention & Management

The risk of falling and consequent injury, disability, and potential institutionalization can be reduced by modifying the factors outlined in Table 4–4. Emphasis is placed on treating all contributory medical conditions (eg, cataracts), minimizing environmental hazards, and eliminating medications where the harms may outweigh the benefits—particularly those that induce orthostasis and parkinsonism (eg, alpha-blockers, nitrates, antipsychotics). Also important are strength, balance, and gait training as well as screening and treatment for osteoporosis, if present. Some evidence suggests falls may be prevented by prescribing vitamin D at a dose of 800 international units daily or higher.

Assistive devices, such as canes and walkers, are useful for many older adults but are often used incorrectly. Canes should be used on the "good" side. The height of walkers and canes should generally be about the level of the wrist. Physical therapists are invaluable in assessing the need for an assistive device, selecting the best device, and training a patient in its correct use.

Table 4–4. Fall risk factors and targeted interventions and best evidence for fall prevention.

Risk Factor	Targeted Intervention
Postural hypotension (> 20 mm Hg drop in systolic blood pressure, or systolic blood pressure < 90 mm Hg)	Behavioral recommendations, such as hand clenching, elevation of head of bed; discontinuation or substitution of high-risk medications
Use of benzodiazepine or sedative/hypnotic agent	Education about sleep hygiene; discontinuation or substitution of medications
Use of multiple prescription medications	Review of medications
Environmental hazards	Appropriate changes; installation of safety equipment (eg, grab bars)
Gait impairment	Gait training, assistive devices, balance or strengthening exercises
Impairment in transfer or balance	Balance exercises, training in transfers, environmental alterations (eg, grab bars)
Impairment in leg or arm muscle strength or limb range of motion	Exercise with resistance bands or putty, with graduated increases in resistance
Best Evidence for Fall Prevention[1]	**Number of Trials and Risk Ratios (RR)**
Exercise or physical therapy	16 randomized controlled trials RR for falls = 0.87 (95% confidence interval [CI], 0.81–0.94)
Vitamin D supplementation	9 randomized controlled trials RR for falls = 0.83 (95% CI, 0.77–0.89)
Multifactorial intervention	19 randomized controlled trials RR for falls = 0.94 (95% CI, 0.87–1.02)

[1]Adapted from Michael YL et al. Primary care-relevant interventions to prevent falling in older adults: a systematic evidence review for the U.S. Preventive Services Task Force. Ann Intern Med. 2010 Dec 21;153(12):815–25. [PMID: 21173416]

Early surgery for patients with cataracts may reduce falls, but eyeglasses, particularly bifocal or graduated lenses, may actually increase the risk of falls, particularly in the early weeks of use. Patients should be counseled about the need to take extra care when new eyeglasses are being used.

Patients with repeated falls are often reassured by the availability of telephones at floor level, a mobile telephone on their person, or a lightweight radio call system. Their therapy should also include training in techniques for arising after a fall.

▶ When to Refer

Patients with a recent history of falls should be referred for physical therapy, eye examination, and home safety evaluation.

▶ When to Admit

If the patient has new falls that are unexplained, particularly in combination with a change in the physical examination or an injury requiring surgery, hospitalization should be considered.

LeBlanc ES et al. Screening for vitamin D deficiency: a systematic review for the U.S. Preventive Services Task Force. Ann Intern Med. 2015 Jan 20;162(2):109–22. [PMID: 25419719]

Moyer VA. Prevention of falls in community-dwelling older adults: U.S. Preventive Health Services Task Force recommendation statement. Ann Intern Med. 2012 Aug 7;157(3):197–204. [PMID: 22868837]

Uusi-Rasi K et al. Exercise and vitamin D in fall prevention among older women: a randomized clinical trial. JAMA Intern Med. 2015 May;175(5):703–11. [PMID: 25799402]

6. Urinary Incontinence

ESSENTIALS OF DIAGNOSIS

▶ Involuntary loss of urine.

▶ *Stress* incontinence: leakage of urine upon coughing, sneezing, or standing.

▶ *Urge* incontinence: urgency and inability to delay urination.

▶ *Overflow* incontinence: variable presentation.

▶ General Considerations

Urinary incontinence in older adults is common, and interventions can improve most patients. Many patients fail to tell their providers about it. A simple question about involuntary leakage of urine is a reasonable annual screen: "Do you have a problem with urine leaks or accidents?"

▶ Classification

A. Transient Causes

Use of the mnemonic "DIAPPERS" may be helpful in remembering the categories of "transient" urinary incontinence.

1. Delirium—A clouded sensorium impedes recognition of both the need to void and the location of the nearest toilet. Delirium is the most common cause of incontinence in hospitalized patients; once it clears, incontinence usually resolves.

2. Infection—Symptomatic urinary tract infection commonly causes or contributes to urgency and incontinence. Asymptomatic bacteriuria does not.

3. Atrophic urethritis and vaginitis—Atrophic urethritis and vaginitis can usually be diagnosed presumptively by the presence of vaginal mucosal telangiectasia, petechiae, erosions, erythema, or friability. Urethral inflammation, if symptomatic, may contribute to incontinence in some women. Some experts suggest a trial of topical estrogen in these cases.

4. Pharmaceuticals—Medications are one of the most common causes of transient incontinence. Typical offending agents include potent diuretics, anticholinergics, psychotropics, opioid analgesics, alpha-blockers (in women), alpha-agonists (in men), and calcium channel blockers.

5. Psychological factors—Severe depression with psychomotor retardation may impede the ability or motivation to reach a toilet.

6. Excess urinary output—Excess urinary output may overwhelm the ability of an older person to reach a toilet in time. In addition to diuretics, common causes include excess fluid intake; metabolic abnormalities (eg, hyperglycemia, hypercalcemia, diabetes insipidus); and disorders associated with peripheral edema, with its associated heavy nocturia when previously dependent legs assume a horizontal position in bed.

7. Restricted mobility—(See Immobility, above.) If mobility cannot be improved, access to a urinal or commode (eg, at the bedside) may improve continence.

8. Stool impaction—This is a common cause of urinary incontinence in hospitalized or immobile patients. Although the mechanism is still unknown, a clinical clue to its presence is the onset of both urinary and fecal incontinence. Disimpaction usually restores urinary continence.

B. Established Causes

Causes of "established" incontinence should be addressed after the "transient" causes have been uncovered and managed appropriately.

1. Detrusor overactivity (urge incontinence)—Detrusor overactivity refers to uninhibited bladder contractions that cause leakage. It is the most common cause of established geriatric incontinence, accounting for two-thirds of cases, and is usually idiopathic. Women will complain of urinary leakage after the onset of an intense urge to urinate that cannot be forestalled. In men, the symptoms are similar, but detrusor overactivity commonly coexists with urethral obstruction from benign prostatic hyperplasia. **Because detrusor overactivity also may be due to bladder stones or tumor, the abrupt onset of otherwise unexplained urge incontinence—especially if accompanied**

by perineal or suprapubic discomfort or sterile hematuria—should be investigated by cystoscopy and cytologic examination of a urine specimen.

2. Urethral incompetence (stress incontinence)—Urethral incompetence is the second most common cause of established urinary incontinence in older women. Stress incontinence is most commonly seen in men after radical prostatectomy. Stress incontinence is characterized by instantaneous leakage of urine in response to a stress maneuver. It commonly coexists with detrusor overactivity. Typically, urinary loss occurs with laughing, coughing, or lifting heavy objects. Leakage is worse or occurs only during the day, unless another abnormality (eg, detrusor overactivity) is also present. To test for stress incontinence, have the patient relax her perineum and cough vigorously (a single cough) while standing with a full bladder. Instantaneous leakage indicates stress incontinence if urinary retention has been excluded by postvoiding residual determination using ultrasound. A delay of several seconds or persistent leakage suggests that the problem is instead caused by an uninhibited bladder contraction induced by coughing.

3. Urethral obstruction—Urethral obstruction (due to prostatic enlargement, urethral stricture, bladder neck contracture, or prostatic cancer) is a common cause of established incontinence in older men but is rare in older women. It can present as dribbling incontinence after voiding, urge incontinence due to detrusor overactivity (which coexists in two-thirds of cases), or overflow incontinence due to urinary retention.

4. Detrusor underactivity (overflow incontinence)—Detrusor underactivity is the least common cause of incontinence. It may be idiopathic or due to sacral lower motor nerve dysfunction. When it causes incontinence, detrusor underactivity is associated with urinary frequency, nocturia, and frequent leakage of small amounts. The elevated postvoiding residual urine (generally over 450 mL) distinguishes it from detrusor overactivity and stress incontinence, but only urodynamic testing differentiates it from urethral obstruction in men. Such testing usually is not required in women, in whom obstruction is rarely present.

▶ **Treatment**

A. Transient Causes

Each identified transient cause should be treated regardless of whether an established cause coexists. For patients with urinary retention induced by an anticholinergic agent, discontinuation of the medication should first be considered. If this is not feasible, substituting a less anticholinergic agent may be useful.

B. Established Causes

1. Detrusor overactivity—The cornerstone of treatment is **bladder training**. Patients start by voiding on a schedule based on the shortest interval recorded on a bladder record. They then gradually lengthen the interval between

voids by 30 minutes each week using relaxation techniques to postpone the urge to void. Lifestyle modifications, including weight loss and caffeine reduction, may also improve incontinence symptoms. For cognitively impaired patients and nursing home residents who are unable to manage on their own, timed and prompted voiding initiated by caregivers is effective. Pelvic floor muscle ("Kegel") exercises can reduce the frequency of incontinence episodes when performed correctly and sustained.

If behavioral approaches prove insufficient, antimuscarinic agents may provide additional benefit. The two oral medications for which there is the most experience are tolterodine and oxybutynin. Available regimens of these agents include short-acting tolterodine, 1–2 mg orally twice a day; long-acting tolterodine, 2–4 mg orally daily; short-acting oxybutynin, 2.5–5 mg orally twice or three times a day; long-acting oxybutynin, 5–15 mg orally daily; and oxybutynin transdermal patch, 3.9 mg/day applied twice weekly. All of these agents can produce delirium, dry mouth, or urinary retention; long-acting preparations may be better tolerated. Agents such as fesoterodine (4–8 mg orally once daily), trospium chloride (20 mg orally once or twice daily), long-acting trospium chloride (60 mg orally daily), darifenacin (7.5–15 mg orally daily), and solifenacin (5–10 mg orally daily) appear to have similar efficacy, and only fesoterodine has been demonstrated to have tolerability in medically complex older adults that is comparable to younger adults.

The beta-3-agonist mirabegron, 25–50 mg orally daily, is approved for overactive bladder symptoms, which include urge urinary incontinence. In trials comparing mirabegron with antimuscarinic agents, the efficacy and safety profiles have been comparable, with less dry mouth reported in persons who received mirabegron. However, because of its potential cardiac effects and the relatively small number of adults over the age of 70 who have been studied in trials, mirabegron's role in the treatment of urge urinary incontinence in frail older adults or those with hypertension or cardiac conditions remains to be determined.

An alternative to oral agents is an injection of onabotulinum toxin A into the detrusor muscle. In a head-to-head comparison of onabotulinum toxin A with antimuscarinic medications, patients had similar rates of reduction of incontinence episodes. Persons who received onabotulinum toxin A had higher rates of complete resolution of incontinence and lower rates of dry mouth but were more likely to experience urinary retention and urinary tract infections than those who did not receive onabotulinum toxin A.

The combination of behavioral therapy and antimuscarinics appears to be more effective than either alone, although one study in a group of younger women showed that adding behavioral therapy to individually titrated doses of extended-release oxybutynin was no better than with medication treatment alone.

In men with both benign prostatic hyperplasia and detrusor overactivity and with postvoiding residual volumes of 150 mL or less, an antimuscarinic agent added to an alpha-blocker may provide additional relief of lower urinary tract symptoms.

2. Urethral incompetence (stress incontinence)—
Lifestyle modifications, including limiting caffeine intake
and timed voiding, may be helpful for some women, particularly women with mixed stress/urge incontinence. Pelvic floor muscle exercises are effective for women with
mild to moderate stress incontinence; the exercises can be
combined, if necessary, with biofeedback or electrical
stimulation. Instruct the patient to pull in the pelvic floor
muscles and hold for 6–10 seconds and to perform three
sets of 8–12 contractions daily. Benefits may not be seen for
6 weeks. Pessaries or vaginal cones may be helpful in some
women but should only be prescribed by providers who are
experienced with using these modalities.

Pharmacologic therapy is limited, and a clinical practice
guideline from the American College of Physicians recommends against pharmacologic treatment. Although a last
resort, surgery is the most effective treatment for stress
incontinence; cure rates as high as 96% can result, even in
older women.

3. Urethral obstruction—Surgical decompression is the
most effective treatment for obstruction, especially in the
setting of urinary retention due to benign prostatic hyperplasia. A variety of nonsurgical techniques make decompression feasible even for frail men. For the nonoperative
candidate with urinary retention, intermittent or indwelling catheterization is used. For a man with prostatic
obstruction who does not require or desire immediate
surgery, treatment with alpha-blocking agents (eg, terazosin, 1–10 mg orally daily; prazosin, 1–5 mg orally twice
daily; tamsulosin, 0.4–0.8 mg orally daily) can improve
symptoms and delay obstruction. Finasteride, 5 mg orally
daily, can provide additional benefit to an alpha-blocking
agent in men with an enlarged prostate.

4. Detrusor underactivity—For the patient with a poorly
contractile bladder, augmented voiding techniques (eg,
double voiding, suprapubic pressure) often prove effective.
If further emptying is needed, intermittent or indwelling
catheterization is the only option. Antibiotics should be
used only for symptomatic upper urinary tract infection
or as prophylaxis against recurrent symptomatic infections in a patient using intermittent catheterization; they
should not be used as prophylaxis in a patient with an
indwelling catheter.

When to Refer

- Men with urinary obstruction who do not respond to
  medical therapy should be referred to a urologist.
- Women who do not respond to medical and behavioral
  therapy should be referred to a urogynecologist or
  urologist.

Chapple CR et al. Randomized double-blind, active-controlled
phase 3 study to assess 12-month safety and efficacy of mirabegron, a β₃-adrenoreceptor agonist, in overactive bladder.
Eur Urol. 2013 Feb;63(2):296–305. [PMID: 23195283]
Dubeau CE et al. Effect of fesoterodine in vulnerable elderly subjects with urgency incontinence: a double-blind, placebo controlled trial. J Urol. 2014 Feb;191(2):395–404. [PMID: 23973522]

Qaseem A et al. Nonsurgical management of urinary incontinence in women: a clinical practice guideline from the American
College of Physicians. Ann Intern Med. 2014 Sep 16;161(6):
429–40. [PMID: 25222388]
Visco AG et al. Anticholinergic therapy vs. onabotulinumtoxinA
for urgency urinary incontinence. N Engl J Med. 2012 Nov 8;
367(19):1803–13. [PMID: 23036134]

7. Weight Loss

General Considerations

Weight loss affects substantial numbers of elders. The
degree of unintended weight loss that deserves evaluation
is not agreed upon, although a reasonable threshold is loss
of 5% of body weight in 1 month or 10% of body weight in
6 months.

Clinical Findings

Useful laboratory and radiologic studies for the patient
with weight loss include complete blood count, serum
chemistries (including glucose, TSH, creatinine, calcium,
and in men, testosterone), urinalysis, and chest radiograph.
These studies are intended to uncover an occult metabolic
or neoplastic cause but are not exhaustive. **Exploring the
patient's social situation, cognition, mood, and dental
health are at least as important as looking for a purely
medical cause of weight loss.**

Treatment

Oral nutritional supplements of 200–1000 kcal/day can
increase weight and improve outcomes in malnourished
hospitalized elders. Sodium-containing flavor enhancers
(eg, iodized salt) can improve food intake without adverse
health effects when there is no contraindication to their
use. Megestrol acetate as an appetite stimulant has not been
shown to increase body mass or lengthen life among elders
and has significant side effects. For those who have lost the
ability to feed themselves, assiduous hand feeding may
allow maintenance of weight. Although liquid artificial
nutrition and hydration ("tube feeding") may seem a more
convenient alternative, it deprives the patient of the enjoyment associated with eating as well as the social milieu
typically associated with mealtime; before this option is
chosen, the patient or his or her surrogate should be
offered the opportunity to review the benefits and burdens
of the treatment in light of overall goals of care. If liquid
artificial nutrition is initiated and the patient makes
repeated attempts to pull out the tube, its utility should be
reconsidered. Liquid artificial nutrition is not recommended for patients with end-stage dementia.

Bautista EN et al. Effect of flavor enhancers on the nutritional
status of older persons. J Nutr Health Aging. 2013
Apr;17(4):390–2. [PMID: 23538664]

8. Pressure Ulcers

▶ Examine at-risk patients on admission to the hospital and daily thereafter.

▶ Pressure ulcers are classified into one of six categories:

- Non-blanchable hyperemia (stage I).

- Extension through epidermis (stage II).

- Full-thickness skin loss (stage III).

- Full-thickness wounds with extension into muscle, bone, or supporting structures (stage IV).

- Area of discolored or blistered skin (suspected deep tissue injury).

- Slough or eschar overlies the wound (unstageable).

General Considerations

The majority of pressure ulcers develop during a hospital stay for an acute illness. Incidence ranges from 12% to 16%. The primary risk factor for pressure ulcers is immobility. Other contributing risk factors include reduced sensory perception, moisture (urinary and fecal incontinence), poor nutritional status, and friction and shear forces.

"Suspected deep-tissue injury" and "unstageable" are included in the six pressure ulcer categories. An area of purple or maroon discolored intact skin or blood-filled blister is characteristic of suspected deep-tissue injury. The area may be preceded by tissue that is painful, firm, mushy, boggy, warmer, or cooler compared with adjacent tissue. Ulcers in which the base is covered by slough (yellow, tan, gray, green, or brown) or eschar (tan, brown, or black) are considered unstageable.

A number of risk assessment instruments including the Braden Scale and the Norton score can be used to assess the risk of developing pressure ulcers; both have reasonable performance characteristics. These instruments can be used to identify the highest-risk patients who might benefit most from scarce resources, such as alternating pressure air mattresses that reduce or relieve pressure.

While Medicare does not reimburse for hospital-acquired pressure ulcers, there is a higher reimbursement for pressure ulcers present on admission. Clinicians should include a full skin assessment on every admission evaluation.

Prevention

Using specialized support surfaces (including mattresses, beds, and cushions), patient repositioning, optimizing nutritional status, and moisturizing sacral skin are strategies that have been shown to reduce pressure ulcers. For moderate- to high-risk patients, mattresses or overlays that reduce tissue pressure below a standard mattress appear to be superior to standard mattresses. The literature comparing specific products is sparse and inconclusive.

Evaluation

Evaluation of pressure ulcers should include patient's risk factors and goals of care; wound stage, size, and depth; absence or presence (and type) of exudate; appearance of the wound bed and possible surrounding infection; and sinus tracking, or cellulitis.

Treatment

Treatment is aimed toward removing necrotic debris and maintaining a moist wound bed that will promote healing and formation of granulation tissue. The type of dressing that is recommended depends on the location and depth of the wound, whether necrotic tissue or dead space is present, and the amount of exudate (Table 4–5). Pressure-reducing devices (eg, air-fluid beds and low-air-loss beds) are associated with improved healing rates. **Although poor nutritional status is a risk factor for the development of pressure ulcers, the results of trials of nutritional supplementation in the treatment of pressure ulcers have been disappointing.**

Providers can become easily overwhelmed by the array of products available for the treatment of established pressure ulcers. Most institutions should designate a wound care expert or team to select a streamlined wound care product line that has simple guidelines. In a patient with end-stage disease who is receiving end-of-life care, appropriate treatment might be directed toward palliation

Table 4–5. Treatment of pressure ulcers.

Ulcer Type	Dressing Type and Considerations
Stage I and suspected deep tissue injury	Polyurethane film Hydrocolloid wafer Semipermeable foam dressing
Stage II	Hydrocolloid wafers Semipermeable foam dressing Polyurethane film
Stage III/IV	For highly exudative wounds, use highly absorptive dressing or packing, such as calcium alginate Wounds with necrotic debris must be debrided Debridement can be autolytic, enzymatic, or surgical Shallow, clean wounds can be dressed with hydrocolloid wafers, semipermeable foam, or polyurethane film Deep wounds can be packed with gauze; if the wound is deep and highly exudative, an absorptive packing should be used
Heel ulcer	Do not remove eschar on heel ulcers because it can help promote healing (eschar in other locations should be debrided)
Unstageable	Debride before deciding on further therapy

(including minimizing dressing changes and odors) rather than efforts directed at healing.

Complications

Pressure ulcers are associated with increased mortality rates, although a causal link has not been proven. Complications include pain, cellulitis, osteomyelitis, systemic sepsis, and prolongation of lengths of stay in the hospital or nursing home.

When to Refer

Ulcers that are large or nonhealing should be referred to a plastic or general surgeon or dermatologist for biopsy, debridement, and possible skin grafting.

When to Admit

Patients with pressure ulcers should be admitted if the primary residence is unable to provide adequate wound care or pressure reduction, or if the wound is infected or requires complex or surgical care.

Chou R et al. Pressure ulcer risk assessment and prevention: a systematic comparative effectiveness review. Ann Intern Med. 2013 Jul 2;159(1):28–38. [PMID: 23817702]
Smith ME et al. Pressure ulcer treatment strategies: a systematic comparative effectiveness review. Ann Intern Med. 2013 July;159(1):39–50. [PMID: 23817703]

9. Pharmacotherapy & Polypharmacy

There are several reasons for the greater incidence of iatrogenic drug reactions in the elderly population, the most important of which is the large number of medications that elders take. Drug metabolism is often impaired in elders due to a decrease in glomerular filtration rate as well as reduced hepatic clearance. Older individuals often have varying responses to a given serum drug level. Thus, they are more sensitive to some medications (eg, opioids) and less sensitive to others (eg, beta-blocking agents). Most emergency hospitalizations for recognized adverse drug events among older persons result from only a few medications used alone or in combination; examples include antianxiety medications, sedative/hypnotics, warfarin, antiplatelet agents, insulins, oral hypoglycemics, opioids, and digoxin.

Precautions in Administering Medications

Nonpharmacologic interventions can often be a first-line alternative to medications (eg, diet for mild hypertension or type 2 diabetes mellitus). Pharmacologic therapy is begun with less than the medication's usual adult dosage, and the dosage increased slowly, consistent with its pharmacokinetics in older patients. However, age-related changes in drug distribution and clearance are variable among individuals, and some require full doses. After determining acceptable measures of success and toxicity, the dose is increased until one or the other is reached.

Despite the importance of beginning new medications in a slow, measured fashion, all too often an inadequate

trial is attempted (in terms of duration or dose) before discontinuation. Antidepressants, in particular, are frequently stopped before therapeutic dosages are reached for sufficient durations.

A number of simple interventions can help improve adherence to the prescribed medical regimen. When possible, the clinician should keep the dosing schedule simple, the number of pills low, the medication changes as infrequent as possible, and encourage the patient to use a single pharmacy. Pillboxes or "medi-sets" help some patients with adherence.

Having the patient or caregiver bring in all medications at each visit can help the clinician perform medication reconciliation and reinforce reasons for medication use, dosage, frequency of administration, and possible adverse effects. Medication reconciliation is particularly important if the patient sees multiple providers.

The risk of toxicity goes up with the number of medications prescribed. Certain combinations of medications (eg, warfarin and many types of antibiotics, angiotensin-converting enzyme inhibitors and NSAIDs) are particularly likely to cause drug-drug interactions and should be watched carefully.

Trials of individual medication discontinuation should be considered (including sedative/hypnotics, antipsychotic medications, digoxin, proton pump inhibitors, and NSAIDs) when the original indication is unclear, the goals of care have changed, or the patient might be experiencing side effects. Clinical tools such as "STOPP/START" and the Beers Criteria can help guide clinicians in appropriate medication prescribing for older adults.

When to Refer

Patients with poor or uncertain adherence may benefit from referral to a pharmacist or a home health nurse.

Frankenthal D et al. Intervention with the screening tool of older persons potentially inappropriate prescriptions/screening tool to alert doctors to right treatment criteria in elderly residents of a chronic geriatric facility: a randomized clinical trial. J Am Geriatr Soc. 2014 Sep;62(9):1658–65. [PMID: 25243680]
Fried TR et al. Health outcomes associated with polypharmacy in community-dwelling older adults: a systematic review. J Am Geriatr Soc. 2014 Dec;62(12):2261–72. [PMID: 25516023]
Patterson SM et al. Interventions to improve the appropriate use of polypharmacy for older people. Cochrane Database Syst Rev. 2014 Oct 7;10:CD008165. [PMID: 25288041]

10. Vision Impairment

Visual impairment due to age-related refractive error ("presbyopia"), macular degeneration, cataracts, glaucoma, and diabetic retinopathy is associated with significant physical and mental health comorbidities, falls, mobility impairment, and reduced quality of life. **The prevalence of serious and correctable visual disorders in elders is sufficient to warrant a complete eye examination by an ophthalmologist or optometrist annually or biannually for most elders.** Many patients with visual loss benefit from a referral to a low-vision program.

Court H et al. Visual impairment is associated with physical and mental comorbidities in older adults: a cross-sectional study. BMC Med. 2014 Oct 17;12:181. [PMID: 25603915]

Swenor BK et al. Visual impairment and incident mobility limitations: the health, aging and body composition study. J Am Geriatr Soc. 2015 Jan;63(1):46–54. [PMID: 25536849]

11. Hearing Impairment

Over one-third of persons over age 65 and half of those over age 85 have some hearing loss. Hearing loss is associated with social isolation, depression, disability, cognitive impairment, and excess risk of hospitalization and nursing home placement. A reasonable screen is to ask patients if they have hearing impairment. Those who answer "yes" should be referred for audiometry. Those who answer "no" may still have hearing impairment and can be screened by a handheld audioscope or the whispered voice test. The whispered voice test is administered by standing 2 feet behind the subject, whispering three random numbers while simultaneously rubbing the external auditory canal of the non-tested ear to mask the sound. If the patient is unable to identify all three numbers, the test should be repeated with different numbers, and if still abnormal, a referral should be made for an audiogram. To determine the degree to which hearing impairment interferes with functioning, the provider may ask if the patient becomes frustrated when conversing with family members, is embarrassed when meeting new people, has difficulty watching TV, or has problems understanding conversations. Caregivers or family members often have important information on the impact of hearing loss on the patient's social interactions.

Hearing amplification can improve hearing-related quality of life in patients with hearing loss. However, compliance with hearing amplification can be a challenge because of dissatisfaction with performance; stigma associated with hearing aid use; and cost, since hearing amplification is not paid for under most Medicare plans. Newer digital devices may perform better but are considerably more expensive. Special telephones, amplifiers for the television, and other devices are helpful to many patients. Portable amplifiers are pager-sized units with earphones attached; they can be purchased inexpensively at many electronics stores and can be useful in health care settings for improving communication with hearing-impaired patients. In general, facing the patient and speaking slowly in a low tone is a more effective communication strategy than shouting.

Chen DS et al; Health ABC study. Association of hearing impairment with declines in physical functioning and the risk of disability in older adults. J Gerontol A Biol Sci Med Sci. 2015 May;70(5):654–61. [PMID: 25477427]

Genther DJ et al; Health, Aging and Body Composition Study. Association between hearing impairment and risk of hospitalization in older adults. J Am Geriatr Soc. 2015 Jun;63(6):1146–52. [PMID: 26096388]

Lin FR et al; Health ABC Study Group. Hearing loss and cognitive decline in older adults. JAMA Intern Med. 2013 Feb 25;173(4):293–9. [PMID: 23337978]

Pacala JT et al. Hearing deficits in the older patient: "I didn't notice anything". JAMA. 2012 Mar 21;307(11):1185–94. [PMID: 22436959]

12. Elder Mistreatment & Self-Neglect

Elder mistreatment is defined as "actions that cause harm or create a serious risk of harm to an older adult by a caregiver or other person who stands in a trust relationship to the older adult, or failure by a caregiver to satisfy the elder's basic needs or to protect the elder from harm." **Self-neglect is the most common form of elder mistreatment and occurs among all demographic strata of the aging population.** According to the best available estimates, the prevalence of potential neglect and psychological and financial abuse is about 5% each, with other forms of abuse being less common.

Clues to the possibility of elder abuse include behavioral changes in the presence of the caregiver, delays between occurrences of injuries and when treatment was sought, inconsistencies between an observed injury and its associated explanation, lack of appropriate clothing or hygiene, and not filling prescriptions. Many elders with cognitive impairment become targets of financial abuse. Both elder abuse and self-neglect are associated with an increased risk of mortality.

It is helpful to observe and talk with every older person alone for at least part of a visit in order to ask questions directly about possible abuse and neglect (Table 4–6). When self-neglect is suspected, it is critical to establish whether a patient has decision-making capacity in order to determine what course of action needs to be taken. A patient who has full decision-making capacity should be provided with help and support but can choose to live in conditions of self-neglect, providing that the public is not endangered by the actions of the person. In contrast, a patient who lacks decision-making capacity who lives in conditions of self-neglect will require more aggressive intervention, which may include guardianship, in-home help, or placement in a supervised setting. Mental state

Table 4–6. Phrases and actions that may be helpful in situations of suspected abuse or neglect.

Questions for the Elder
1. Has anyone hurt you?
2. Are you afraid of anybody?
3. Is anyone taking or using your money without your permission?

Questions for the Caregiver
1. Are your relative's needs more than you can handle?
2. Are you worried that you might hit your relative?
3. Have you hit your relative?

If abuse is suspected

Tell the patient that you are concerned, want to help, and will call Adult Protective Services to see if there is anything that they can do to help

Document any injuries

Document the patient's words

Document whether or not the patient has decision-making capacity using a tool such as "Aid to Capacity Evaluation" scores, such as the MoCA, may provide some insight into the patient's cognitive status but are not designed to assess decision-making capacity. A standardized tool, such as the "Aid to Capacity Evaluation," is easy to administer, has good performance characteristics for determining decision-making capacity, and is available free online at www.jointcentreforbioethics.ca/tools/ace_download.shtml.

▶ When to Refer

- Refer elders with suspected abuse or self-neglect to Adult Protective Services, as required by law in most states (consult the National Center on Elder Abuse at http://www.ncea.aoa.gov).
- Refer elders to a mental health professional when it is unclear whether they have decision-making capacity

after an initial assessment or whether an untreated mental health disorder is contributing to their problem.

▶ When to Admit

Admit elders who would be unsafe in the community when an alternative plan cannot be put into place in a timely manner.

Burnett J et al. Prevention and early identification of elder abuse. Clin Geriatr Med. 2014 Nov;30(4):743–59. [PMID: 25439639]

Hoover RM et al. Detecting elder abuse and neglect: assessment and intervention. Am Fam Physician. 2014 Mar 15;89(6):453–60. [PMID: 24695564]

Smith AK et al. Elder self-neglect—how can a physician help? N Engl J Med. 2013 Dec 26;369(26):2476–9. [PMID: 24369074]

Palliative Care & Pain Management

Michael W. Rabow, MD
Steven Z. Pantilat, MD

DEFINITION & SCOPE OF PALLIATIVE CARE

The focus of palliative care is to improve symptoms and quality of life at any stage of any serious illness, to support patients' families and loved ones, and to help align patients' care with their preferences and goals. At the end of life, palliative care often becomes the sole focus of care, but **palliative care alongside cure-focused treatment is beneficial throughout the course of a serious illness, regardless of prognosis, whether the goal is to cure disease or manage it.**

Palliative care includes management of physical symptoms, such as pain, dyspnea, nausea and vomiting, constipation, and agitation; emotional distress, such as depression, anxiety, and interpersonal strain; and existential distress, such as spiritual crisis. While palliative care is a medical subspecialty recognized by the American Board of Medical Specialties ("specialty palliative care"), all clinicians routinely should provide "primary palliative care" and possess the basic skills to be able to manage pain; treat dyspnea; identify possible depression; communicate about important issues, such as prognosis and patient preferences for care; and help address spiritual distress.

During any stage of illness, symptoms that cause significant suffering are a medical emergency that should be managed aggressively with frequent elicitation and reassessment as well as individualized treatment. While patients at the end of life may experience a host of distressing symptoms, pain, dyspnea, and delirium are among the most feared and burdensome. Management of these common symptoms is described later in this chapter. The principles of palliative care dictate that properly informed patients or their surrogates may decide to pursue aggressive symptom relief at the end of life even if, as a known but unintended consequence, the treatments preclude further unwanted curative interventions or even hasten death, although increasingly, palliative care has been shown to prolong life.

Bakitas MA et al. Early versus delayed initiation of concurrent palliative oncology care: patient outcomes in the ENABLE III randomized controlled trial. J Clin Oncol. 2015 May 1; 33(13):1438–45. [PMID: 25800768]

Davis MP et al. A review of the trials which examine early integration of outpatient and home palliative care for patients with serious illnesses. Ann Palliat Med. 2015 Jul;4(3):99–121. [PMID: 26231807]
Epstein RM et al. A piece of my mind. Responding to suffering. JAMA. 2015 Dec 22–29;314(24):2623–4. [PMID: 26720023]
Hui D et al. Impact of timing and setting of palliative care referral on quality of end-of-life care in cancer patients. Cancer. 2014 Jun 1;120(11):1743–9. [PMID: 24967463]
Institute of Medicine. Dying in America: improving quality and honoring individual preferences near the end of life. National Academies Press, 2014.
Kelley AS et al. Palliative care for the seriously ill. N Engl J Med. 2015 Aug 20;373(8):747–55. [PMID: 26287850]

PAIN MANAGEMENT

PRINCIPLES OF PAIN MANAGEMENT

The experience of pain includes the patient's emotional reaction to it and is influenced by many factors, including the patient's prior experiences with pain, meaning given to the pain, emotional stresses, and family and cultural influences. Pain is a subjective phenomenon, and clinicians cannot reliably detect its existence or quantify its severity without asking the patient directly. A useful means of assessing pain and evaluating the effectiveness of analgesia is to ask the patient to rate the degree of pain along a numeric or visual pain scale (Table 5–1).

General guidelines for management of pain are recommended for the treatment of all patients with pain. Clinicians should ask about the nature, severity, timing, location, quality, and aggravating and relieving factors of the pain. Distinguishing between neuropathic and nociceptive (somatic or visceral) pain is essential to proper treatment. The goal of pain management is properly decided by the patient. Some patients may wish to be completely free of pain even at the cost of significant sedation, while others will wish to control pain to a level that still allows maximal functioning.

Chronic severe pain should be treated continuously. For ongoing pain, a long-acting analgesic can be given around the clock with a short-acting medication as needed for "breakthrough" pain. Whenever possible, the oral route of administration is preferred because it is easier to administer

Table 5–1. Pain assessment scales.

A. Numeric Rating Scale

No pain   Worst pain

0 1 2 3 4 5 6 7 8 9 10

B. Numeric Rating Scale Translated into Word and Behavior Scales

Pain Intensity	Word Scale	Nonverbal Behaviors
0	No pain	Relaxed, calm expression
1–2	Least pain	Stressed, tense expression
3–4	Mild pain	Guarded movement, grimacing
5–6	Moderate pain	Moaning, restless
7–8	Severe pain	Crying out
9–10	Excruciating pain	Increased intensity of above

C. Wong Baker FACES Pain Rating Scale[1]

0 No hurt	1 Hurts Little Bit	2 Hurts Little More	3 Hurts Even More	4 Hurts Whole Lot	5 Hurts Worst

[1]Especially useful for patients who cannot read English and for pediatric patients.
© 1983 Wong-Baker FACES Foundation. www.WongBakerFACES.org. Used with permission. Originally published in Whaley & Wong's Nursing Care of Infants and Children.

at home, is not painful, and imposes no risk from needle exposure.

The underlying cause of pain should be diagnosed and treated, balancing the burden of diagnostic tests or therapeutic interventions with the patient's suffering. For example, single-fraction radiation therapy for painful bone metastases or nerve blocks for neuropathic pain may obviate the need for ongoing treatment with analgesics and their side effects. Regardless of decisions about seeking and treating the underlying cause of pain, every patient should be offered prompt relief.

PAIN MANAGEMENT FOR PATIENTS WITH SERIOUS & END-STAGE ILLNESS

Definition & Prevalence

Pain is what many people say they fear most about dying, and it is consistently undertreated. Up to 75% of patients dying of cancer, heart failure, chronic obstructive pulmonary disease (COPD), or other diseases experience pain. In the United States, the Joint Commission reviews of health care organizations include pain management standards.

Barriers to Good Care

One barrier to good pain control is that many clinicians have limited training and clinical experience with pain management and thus are reluctant to attempt to manage severe pain. Lack of knowledge about the proper selection and dosing of analgesic medications carries with it attendant and typically exaggerated fears about the side effects of pain medications, including the possibility of respiratory depression from opioids. Most clinicians, however, can develop good pain management skills, and nearly all pain, even at the end of life, can be managed without hastening death through respiratory depression. In rare instances, palliative sedation may be necessary to control intractable suffering as an intervention of last resort.

A misunderstanding of the physiologic effects of opioids can lead to unfounded concerns on the part of clinicians, patients, or family members that patients will become addicted to opioids. While physiologic **tolerance** (requiring increasing dosage to achieve the same analgesic effect) and **dependence** (requiring continued dosing to prevent symptoms of medication withdrawal) are expected with regular opioid use, the use of opioids at the end of life for relief of pain and dyspnea is not generally associated with a risk of psychological **addiction** (misuse of a substance for purposes other than the one for which it was prescribed and despite negative consequences in health, employment, or legal and social spheres). The risk for problematic use of pain medications is higher, however, in patients with a history of addiction or substance abuse. Yet even patients with such a history need pain relief, albeit with closer monitoring. Some patients who demonstrate behaviors associated with addiction (demand for specific medications and doses, anger and irritability, poor cooperation or disturbed interpersonal reactions) may have **pseudo-addiction,** defined as exhibiting behaviors associated with addiction but only because their pain is inadequately treated. Once pain is relieved, these behaviors cease. In all cases, clinicians must be prepared to use appropriate doses of opioids in order to relieve distressing symptoms for patients at the end of life.

Harms from the use of opioid analgesics, including medication diversion or death from accidental or intentional overdose, are known and significant risks. Some clinicians fear legal repercussions from prescribing the high doses of opioids sometimes necessary to control pain at the end of life. The US Food and Drug Administration (FDA) offers a Risk Evaluation and Management Strategy for long-acting and extended-release opioids to inform clinicians about appropriate prescribing and to promote safe use of opioids for patients who require them (http://www.fda.gov/Drugs/DrugSafety/InformationbyDrugClass/ucm163647.htm). Some states have special training, licensing, and documentation requirements for opioid prescribing. However, governmental and professional medical groups, regulators (including the FDA), and the US Supreme Court have made it clear that appropriate treatment of pain is the right of the patient and a fundamental responsibility of the clinician. Although clinicians may feel trapped between consequences of over- or under-prescribing opioids, there remains a wide range of practice in which clinicians can safely and appropriately treat pain. Referral to pain management or palliative care experts is appropriate whenever pain cannot be controlled expeditiously or safely by other clinicians. In the field of chronic noncancer pain (CNCP) management and increasingly in palliative care earlier in the course of serious illness, many clinicians are using pain medication agreements and urine drug testing to help monitor for and limit the potential for abuse and diversion (see "Opioids for Chronic, Noncancer Pain").

PHARMACOLOGIC PAIN MANAGEMENT STRATEGIES

In the palliative care setting, pain generally can be well controlled with opioid and nonopioid analgesic medications. For mild to moderate pain, acetaminophen, aspirin, and nonsteroidal anti-inflammatory drugs (NSAIDs) may be sufficient. For moderate to severe pain, opioids often are necessary. In all cases, the choice of analgesic must be guided by a careful consideration of the physiology of the pain and the benefits and risks of the particular analgesic being considered.

▶ Acetaminophen & NSAIDs

Appropriate doses of acetaminophen may be just as effective an analgesic and antipyretic as NSAIDs but without the risk of gastrointestinal bleeding or ulceration. Acetaminophen can be given at a dosage of 500–1000 mg orally every 6 hours, not to exceed 4000 mg/day maximum for short-term use. Total acetaminophen doses should not exceed 3000 mg/day for long-term use or 2000 mg/day for older patients and for those with liver disease. Hepatotoxicity

is of particular concern because of how commonly acetaminophen is also an ingredient in various over-the-counter medications and because of failure to account for the acetaminophen dose in combination acetaminophen-opioid medications such as Vicodin or Norco. The FDA has limited the amount of acetaminophen available in combination analgesics.

Aspirin (325–650 mg orally every 4 hours) is an effective analgesic, antipyretic, and anti-inflammatory medication. Gastrointestinal irritation and bleeding are side effects that are lessened with enteric-coated formulations of aspirin and concomitant use of proton-pump inhibitor medication. Bleeding, allergy, and an association with Reye syndrome in children and teenagers further limit its use.

Commonly used NSAIDs and their dosages are listed in Table 5–2. NSAIDs are antipyretic, analgesic, and anti-inflammatory. NSAIDs increase the risk of gastrointestinal bleeding 1.5 times. The risks of bleeding and nephrotoxicity from NSAIDs are both increased in elders. Gastrointestinal bleeding and ulceration may be prevented with the concurrent use of proton pump inhibitors (eg, omeprazole, 20–40 mg orally daily) or with celecoxib (100 mg orally daily to 200 mg orally twice daily), the only cyclooxygenase (COX)-2 inhibitor available. NSAIDs, including celecoxib, can lead to fluid retention, kidney injury, and exacerbations of heart failure and should be used with caution in patients with that condition. Topical formulations of NSAIDs (such as diclofenac 1.3% patch or 1% gel), placed over the painful body part for treatment of musculoskeletal pain, are associated with less systemic absorption and fewer side effects than oral administration and are likely underutilized in patients at risk for gastrointestinal bleeding.

▶ Opioids for Palliative Treatment of Pain from Cancer & Other Serious Illnesses

A. Formulations and Regimens

For many patients, opioids are the mainstay of pain management. Opioids are appropriate for managing severe pain due to any cause, including the following: neuropathic pain, pain from cancer, pain from other serious illnesses, and pain associated with end of life. Opioid medications are listed in Table 5–3. Full opioid agonists such as morphine, hydromorphone, oxycodone, methadone, fentanyl, hydrocodone, and codeine are used most commonly. Hydrocodone and codeine are typically combined with acetaminophen or an NSAID, although acetaminophen in these combinations is restricted to 325 mg per unit dose due to the risk of toxicity. Extended-release hydrocodone without acetaminophen is FDA approved. **Short-acting formulations** of oral morphine sulfate (starting dosage 4–8 mg orally every 3–4 hours), hydromorphone (1–2 mg orally every 3–4 hours), or oxycodone (5 mg orally every 3–4 hours) are useful for acute pain not controlled with other analgesics. These same oral medications, or oral transmucosal fentanyl (200 mcg oralet dissolved in the mouth) or buccal fentanyl (100 mcg dissolved in the mouth), can be used for "rescue" or "breakthrough" treatment for patients experiencing pain that breaks through

Table 5–2. Acetaminophen and useful nonsteroidal anti-inflammatory drugs.

Medication	Usual Oral Dose for Adults ≥ 50 kg	Usual Oral Dose for Adults < 50 kg[1]	Cost per Unit	Cost for 30 Days[2]	Comments[3]
Acetaminophen or paracetamol[4] (Tylenol, Datril, etc)	325–500 mg every 4 hours or 750 mg every 6 hours, up to 2000–3000 mg/day	10–15 mg/kg every 4 hours (oral); 15–20 mg/kg every 4 hours (rectal), up to 2000–3000 mg/day	$0.02/500 mg (oral) OTC; $0.71/650 mg (rectal) OTC	$3.60 (oral); $127.80 (rectal)	Not an NSAID because it lacks peripheral anti-inflammatory effects. Equivalent to aspirin as analgesic and antipyretic agent. Limit dose to 3000 mg/day and to 2000 mg/day in older patients and those with liver disease. Be mindful of multiple sources of acetaminophen as in combination analgesics, cold remedies, and sleep aids.
Aspirin[5]	650 mg every 4 hours or 975 mg every 6 hours	10–15 mg/kg every 4 hours (oral); 15–20 mg/kg every 4 hours (rectal)	$0.02/325 mg OTC; $1.51/600 mg (rectal) OTC	$7.20 (oral); $271.80 (rectal)	Available also in enteric-coated form that is more slowly absorbed but better tolerated.
Celecoxib[4] (Celebrex)	200 mg once daily (osteoarthritis); 100–200 mg twice daily (RA)	100 mg once or twice daily	$4.62/100 mg; $7.58/200 mg	$227.40 OA; $454.80 RA	Cyclooxygenase-2 inhibitor. No antiplatelet effects. Lower doses for elderly who weigh < 50 kg. Lower incidence of endoscopic gastrointestinal ulceration. Not known if true lower incidence of gastrointestinal bleeding. Possible link to cardiovascular toxicity. Celecoxib is contraindicated in sulfonamide allergy.
Choline magnesium salicylate[6] (Trilasate, others)	1000–1500 mg three times daily	25 mg/kg three times daily	$0.46/500 mg	$124.20	Salicylates cause less gastrointestinal distress and kidney impairment than NSAIDs but are probably less effective in pain management than NSAIDs.
Diclofenac (Voltaren, Cataflam, others)	50–75 mg orally two or three times daily; 1% gel 2–4 g four times daily; 1.3% patch two times daily		$1.47/50 mg; $1.77/75 mg	$132.30; $159.30	May impose higher risk of hepatotoxicity. Enteric-coated product; slow onset. Topical formulations may result in fewer side effects than oral formulations.
Diclofenac sustained release (Voltaren-XR, others)	100–200 mg once daily		$2.81/100 mg	$168.60	
Diflunisal[7] (Dolobid, others)	500 mg every 12 hours		$2.07/500 mg	$124.20	Fluorinated acetylsalicylic acid derivative.
Etodolac (Lodine, others)	200–400 mg every 6–8 hours		$1.32/400 mg	$158.40	
Fenoprofen calcium (Nalfon, others)	300–600 mg every 6 hours		$3.40/600 mg	$408.00	Perhaps more side effects than others, including tubulointerstitial nephritis.
Flurbiprofen (Ansaid)	50–100 mg three or four times daily		$0.83/50 mg; $1.25/100 mg	$99.60; $150.00	Adverse gastrointestinal effects may be more common among elderly.
Ibuprofen (Motrin, Advil, Rufen, others)	400–800 mg every 6 hours	10 mg/kg every 6–8 hours	$0.28/600 mg Rx; $0.05/200 mg OTC	$33.60; $9.00	Relatively well tolerated and inexpensive.
Indomethacin (Indocin, Indometh, others)	25–50 mg two to four times daily		$0.38/25 mg; $0.64/50 mg	$45.60; $76.80	Higher incidence of dose-related toxic effects, especially gastrointestinal and bone marrow effects.

(continued)

Table 5–2. Acetaminophen and useful nonsteroidal anti-inflammatory drugs. (continued)

Medication	Usual Oral Dose for Adults ≥ 50 kg	Usual Oral Dose for Adults < 50 kg[1]	Cost per Unit	Cost for 30 Days[2]	Comments[3]
Ketoprofen (Orudis, Oruvail, others)	25–75 mg every 6–8 hours (max 300 mg/day)		$1.07/50 mg Rx; $1.17/75 mg Rx	$128.40; $140.40	Lower doses for elderly.
Ketorolac tromethamine (Toradol)	10 mg every 4–6 hours to a maximum of 40 mg/day orally		$2.16/10 mg	Not recommended	Short-term use (< 5 days) only; otherwise, increased risk of gastrointestinal side effects.
Ketorolac tromethamine[8] (Toradol)	60 mg intramuscularly or 30 mg intravenously initially, then 30 mg every 6 hours intramuscularly or intravenously		$1.45/30 mg	Not recommended	Intramuscular or intravenous NSAID as alternative to opioid. Lower doses for elderly. Short-term use (< 5 days) only.
Magnesium salicylate (various)	467–934 mg every 6 hours		$0.23/467 mg OTC	$55.20	
Meclofenamate sodium[9] (Meclomen)	50–100 mg every 6 hours		$5.07/100 mg	$608.40	Diarrhea more common.
Mefenamic acid (Ponstel)	250 mg every 6 hours		$17.41/250 mg	$2089.20	
Nabumetone (Relafen)	500–1000 mg once daily (max dose 2000 mg/day)		$1.30/500 mg; $1.53/750 mg	$78.00; $91.80	May be less ulcerogenic than ibuprofen, but overall side effects may not be less.
Naproxen (Naprosyn, Anaprox, Aleve [OTC], others)	250–500 mg every 6–8 hours	5 mg/kg every 8 hours	$1.29/500 mg Rx; $0.08/220 mg OTC	$154.80; $7.20 OTC	Generally well tolerated. Lower doses for elderly.
Oxaprozin (Daypro, others)	600–1200 mg once daily		$1.50/600 mg	$90.00	Similar to ibuprofen. May cause rash, pruritus, photosensitivity.
Piroxicam (Feldene, others)	20 mg daily		$2.64/20 mg	$79.20	Not recommended in the elderly due to high adverse drug reaction rate. Single daily dose convenient. Long half-life. May cause higher rate of gastrointestinal bleeding and dermatologic side effects.
Sulindac (Clinoril, others)	150–200 mg twice daily		$0.98/150 mg; $1.21/200 mg	$58.80; $72.60	May cause higher rate of gastrointestinal bleeding. May have less nephrotoxic potential.
Tolmetin (Tolectin)	200–600 mg four times daily		$0.75/200 mg; $3.98/600 mg	$90.00; $477.60	Perhaps more side effects than others, including anaphylactic reactions.

[1]Acetaminophen and NSAID dosages for adults weighing < 50 kg should be adjusted for weight.
[2]Average wholesale price (AWP, for AB-rated generic when available) for quantity listed. Source: *Red Book* (electronic version), Truven Health Analytics Information, http://www.micromedexsolutions.com, accessed March 1, 2016. AWP may not accurately represent the actual pharmacy cost because wide contractual variations exist among institutions.
[3]The adverse effects of headache, tinnitus, dizziness, confusion, rashes, anorexia, nausea, vomiting, gastrointestinal bleeding, diarrhea, nephrotoxicity, visual disturbances, etc, can occur with any of these drugs. Tolerance and efficacy are subject to great individual variations among patients. Note: All NSAIDs can increase serum lithium levels.
[4]Acetaminophen and celecoxib lack antiplatelet effects.
[5]May inhibit platelet aggregation for 1 week or more and may cause bleeding.
[6]May have minimal antiplatelet activity.
[7]Administration with antacids may decrease absorption.
[8]Has the same gastrointestinal toxicities as oral NSAIDs.
[9]Coombs-positive autoimmune hemolytic anemia has been associated with prolonged use.
OA, osteoarthritis; RA, rheumatoid arthritis; OTC, over the counter; Rx, prescription.
Data from Jacox AK et al. *Management of Cancer Pain: Quick Reference Guide for Clinicians No. 9.* AHCPR Publication No. 94–0593. Rockville, MD: Agency for Health Care Policy and Research, Public Health Service, U.S. Department of Health and Human Services. March 1994.

Table 5–3. Useful opioid agonist analgesics.

Medication	Approximate Equianalgesic Dose (compared to morphine 30 mg orally or 10 mg IV/SC)[1]		Usual Starting Dose				Potential Advantages	Potential Disadvantages
			Adults ≥ 50 kg Body Weight		Adults < 50 kg Body Weight			
	Oral	Parenteral	Oral	Parenteral	Oral	Parenteral		
Opioid Agonists[2]								
Buprenorphine	Sublingual formulation approved for opioid use disorder	0.38 mg	Sublingual formulation approved for opioid use disorder	300 mcg IV; 600 mcg IM every 6–8 hours; $11.84/300 mcg	Sublingual formulation approved for opioid use disorder	Not available	Less suppression of testosterone than methadone.	Restricted distribution for opioid use disorder. Use for analgesia is not FDA approved. Concomitant use of other opioids for acute pain could be difficult due to strong receptor binding of buprenorphine, although this is often not found in clinical practice. QT prolongation.
Buprenorphine transdermal	Not available	Not available	Not available orally. Transdermal doses available: 5, 10, and 20 mcg/h. Initiate 5 mcg/h patch for opioid-naive patients (may currently be using nonopioid analgesics); $92.01/10 mcg/h	Not available	Not available	Not available	7-day analgesia; may be initiated in opioid-naïve patients with 5 mcg/h. Can titrate up dose by 5 mcg/h after 72 hours, to a maximum dose of 20 mcg/h.	Concomitant use of other opioids for acute pain could be difficult due to strong receptor binding of buprenorphine, although this is often not found in clinical practice. QT prolongation.
Fentanyl	Not available	100 mcg every hour	Not available	50–100 mcg IV/IM every hour or 0.5–1.5 mcg/kg/h IV infusion $1.03/100 mcg	Not available	0.5–1 mcg/kg IV every 1–4 hours or 1–2 mcg/kg IV × 1, then 0.5–1 mcg/kg/h infusion	Possibly less neuroexcitatory effects, including in kidney failure.	
Fentanyl oral transmucosal (Actiq); buccal (Fentora)	Not available	Not available	200 mcg transmucosal; 100 mcg buccal; $18.80/200 mcg transmucosal; $64.97/200 mcg buccal	Not available	Not available	Not available	For pain breaking through long-acting opioid medication.	Transmucosal and buccal formulations are not bio-equivalent; there is higher bioavailability in buccal formulation.

(continued)

Table 5–3. Useful opioid agonist analgesics. (continued)

Medication	Approximate Equianalgesic Dose (compared to morphine 30 mg orally or 10 mg IV/SC)[1]		Usual Starting Dose				Potential Advantages	Potential Disadvantages
			Adults ≥ 50 kg Body Weight		Adults < 50 kg Body Weight			
	Oral	Parenteral	Oral	Parenteral	Oral	Parenteral		
Fentanyl transdermal	Conversion to fentanyl patch is based on total daily dose of oral morphine:[2] morphine 60–134 mg/day orally = fentanyl 25 mcg/h patch; morphine 135–224 mg/day orally = fentanyl 50 mcg/h patch; morphine 225–314 mg/day orally = fentanyl 75 mcg/h patch; and morphine 315–404 mg/day orally = fentanyl 100 mcg/h patch	Not available	Not available orally 12.5–25 mcg/h patch every 72 hours; $14.43/25 mcg/h	Not available	12.5–25 mcg/h patch every 72 hours	Not available	Stable medication blood levels.	Not for use in opioid-naïve patients. Minimum starting dose is 25 mcg/h patch in patients who have been taking stable dose of opioids for at least 1 week at the equivalent of at least 60 mg/day of oral morphine.
Hydrocodone, extended release (Zohydro ER)	20 mg[1]	Not available	10 mg every 12 hours; $8.10/10 mg	Not available	Not available	Not available	Available as an extended-release formulation without acetaminophen.	
Hydromorphone[3] (Dilaudid)	7.5 mg every 3–4 hours	1.5 mg every 3–4 hours	1–2 mg every 3–4 hours; $0.45/2 mg	1.5 mg every 3–4 hours; $2.73/2 mg	0.06 mg/every 3–4 hours	0.015 mg/kg every 3–4 hours	Similar to morphine. Available in injectable high-potency preparation, rectal suppository.	Short duration.
Hydromorphone extended release (Exalgo)	45–60 mg every 24 hours	Not available	8 mg every 24 hours; $15.21/8 mg	Not available	Not available	Not available	Similar to morphine.	
Levorphanol (Levo-Dromoran)	4 mg every 6–8 hours	2 mg every 6–8 hours	4 mg every 6–8 hours; $46.50/2 mg	Not available	0.04 mg/kg every 6–8 hours	Not available	Longer-acting than morphine sulfate.	Taper dose 25–50% every 2–3 days to 8 mg/day to discontinue.

Drug							
Meperidine[4] (Demerol)	300 mg every 2–3 hours; usual dose 50–150 mg every 3–4 hours	100 mg every 3 hours	Not recommended	100 mg every 3 hours; $6.34/100 mg	Not recommended	0.75 mg/kg every 2–3 hours	Use only when single-dose, short-duration analgesia is needed, as for outpatient procedures like colonoscopy. Not recommended for chronic pain or for repeated dosing.	Short duration. Normeperidine metabolite accumulates in kidney failure and other situations, and in high concentrations may cause irritability and seizures.
Methadone (Dolophine, others)	10–20 mg every 6–8 hours (when converting from < 100 mg long-term daily oral morphine[5])	5–10 mg every 6–8 hours	5–20 mg every 6–8 hours; $0.44/10 mg	2.5–10 mg every 6–8 hours; $15.45/10 mg	0.2 mg/kg every 6–8 hours	0.1 mg/kg every 6–8 hours	Somewhat longer acting than morphine. Useful in cases of intolerance to morphine. May be particularly useful for neuropathic pain. Available in liquid formulation.	Analgesic duration shorter than plasma duration. May accumulate, requiring close monitoring during first weeks of treatment. Equianalgesic ratios vary with opioid dose. Risk of QT prolongation at doses >100–150 mg/day. Baseline ECG recommended.
Morphine[3] immediate release (Morphine sulfate tablets, Roxanol liquid)	30 mg every 3–4 hours (around-the-clock dosing); 60 mg every 3–4 hours (single or intermittent dosing)	10 mg every 3–4 hours	4–8 mg every 3–4 hours; used for breakthrough pain in patients already taking controlled-release preparations; $0.41/15 mg tab; $0.69/20 mg liquid	10 mg every 3–4 hours; $12.90/10 mg	0.3 mg/kg every 3–4 hours	0.1 mg/kg every 3–4 hours	Standard of comparison; multiple dosage forms available.	No unique problems when compared with other opioids. Active metabolite accumulates in renal insufficiency.
Morphine controlled release[3] (MS Contin, Oramorph)	90–120 mg every 12 hours	Not available	15–60 mg every 12 hours; $3.17/30 mg	Not available	Not available	Not available		
Morphine extended release (Kadian, Avinza)	180–240 mg every 24 hours	Not available	20–30 mg every 24 hours; $5.69/30 mg	Not available	Not available	Not available	Once-daily dosing possible.	
Oxycodone (Roxicodone, OxyIR)	20–30 mg every 3–4 hours	Not available	5–10 mg every 3–4 hours; $0.48/5 mg	Not available	0.2 mg/kg every 3–4 hours	Not available	Similar to morphine.	
Oxycodone controlled release (Oxycontin)	40 mg every 12 hours	Not available	20–40 mg every 12 hours; $6.86/20 mg	Not available	Not available	Not available		Physical and chemical pill formulation to deter misuse (injection or intranasal administration).

(continued)

Table 5–3. Useful opioid agonist analgesics. (continued)

Medication	Approximate Equianalgesic Dose (compared to morphine 30 mg orally or 10 mg IV/SC)[1]		Usual Starting Dose				Potential Advantages	Potential Disadvantages
			Adults ≥ 50 kg Body Weight		Adults < 50 kg Body Weight			
	Oral	Parenteral	Oral	Parenteral	Oral	Parenteral		
Oxymorphone[6] oral, immediate release (Opana)	10 mg every 6 hours	Not available	5–10 mg every 6 hours; $3.24/5 mg	Not available				Taking with food can increase serum levels by 50%. Equianalgesic dosing conversion range is wide.
Oxymorphone[6] extended release (Opana ER)	30–40 mg every 12 hours	Not available	15–30 mg every 12 hours; $3.48/10 mg	Not available				Taking with food can increase serum levels by 50%. Equianalgesic dosing conversion range is wide.
Combination Opioid–Nonopioid Preparations								
Codeine[7,8] (with aspirin or acetaminophen)[9]	180–200 mg every 3–4 hours; commonly available dose in combination with acetaminophen, 15–60 mg of codeine every 4–6 hours	130 mg every 3–4 hours	60 mg every 4–6 hours; $0.54/60 mg	60 mg every 2 hours (IM/SC); price not available in the United States	0.5–1 mg/kg every 3–4 hours	Not recommended	Similar to morphine.	Closely monitor for efficacy as patients vary in their ability to convert the prodrug codeine to morphine.
Hydrocodone[6] (in Lorcet, Lortab, Vicodin, others)[9]	30 mg every 3–4 hours	Not available	10 mg every 3–4 hours; $0.54/5 mg	Not available	0.2 mg/kg every 3–4 hours	Not available		Combination with acetaminophen limits dosage titration.
Oxycodone[7] (in Percocet, Percodan, Tylox, others)[9]	30 mg every 3–4 hours	Not available	10 mg every 3–4 hours; $1.04/5 mg	Not available	0.2 mg/kg every 3–4 hours	Not available	Similar to morphine.	Combination with acetaminophen and aspirin limits dosage titration.
Opioid Agonists, Norepinephrine Reuptake Inhibitors								
Tapentadol (Nucynta)	Not known	Not known	Start 50–100 mg once, may repeat dose in 1 hour. Can increase to 50–100 mg every 4 hours. Maximum daily dose 600 mg; $8.18/100 mg	Not available		Not available		Avoid in severe kidney or liver impairment.

Tapentadol, extended release (Nucynta ER)	Not known	Not known	Start 50 mg orally every 12 hours. Can increase by 50-mg increments twice daily every 3 days to dose of 100–250 mg twice daily; $10.46/100 mg	Not available	Not available	Not available	Avoid in severe kidney or liver impairment.
Tramadol (Ultram)	Not known	Not known	Start 25 mg orally daily. Can increase by 25 mg every 3 days to 25 mg orally 4 times daily, then may increase by 50 mg/day every 3 days to 100 mg orally 4 times daily. Limit of 300 mg/day in patients > 75 years old; $0.84/50 mg	Not available	Not available	Not available	If creatinine clearance less than 30, limit to 200 mg/day; with cirrhosis, limit to 100 mg/day.

[1] Published tables vary in the suggested doses that are equianalgesic to morphine. Clinical response is the criterion that must be applied for each patient; titration to clinical efficacy is necessary. Because there is not complete cross-tolerance among these drugs, it is usually necessary to use a lower than equianalgesic dose initially when changing drugs and to retitrate to response.

[2] Conversion is conservative; therefore, do not use these equianalgesic doses for converting back from fentanyl patch to other opioids because they may lead to inadvertent overdose. Patients may require breakthrough doses of short-acting opioids during conversion to transdermal fentanyl.

[3] Caution: For morphine, hydromorphone, and oxymorphone, rectal administration is an alternative route for patients unable to take oral medications. Equianalgesic doses may differ from oral and parenteral doses. A short-acting opioid should normally be used for initial therapy.

[4] Not recommended for chronic pain. Doses listed are for brief therapy of acute pain only. Switch to another opioid for long-term therapy.

[5] Methadone conversion varies depending on the equivalent total daily dose of morphine. Consult with a pain management or palliative care expert for conversion.

[6] Caution: Recommended doses do not apply for adult patients with kidney or liver impairment or other conditions affecting drug metabolism.

[7] Caution: Doses of aspirin and acetaminophen in combination products must also be adjusted to the patient's body weight.

[8] Caution: Doses of codeine above 60 mg often are not appropriate because of diminishing incremental analgesia with increasing doses but continually increasing nausea, constipation, and other side effects.

[9] Caution: Monitor total acetaminophen dose carefully, including any OTC use. Total acetaminophen dose maximum 3 g/day. If liver impairment or heavy alcohol use, maximum is 2 g/day. Available dosing formulations of these combination medications are being adjusted to reflect increased caution about acetaminophen toxicity. Acetaminophen doses in a single combination tablet or capsule will be limited to no more than 325 mg.

Note: Average wholesale price (AWP, generic when available) for quantity listed. Source: Red Book (electronic version), Truven Health Analytics Information, http://www.micromedexsolutions.com, accessed March 1, 2016. AWP may not accurately represent the actual pharmacy cost because wide contractual variations exist among institutions. Data from Jacox AK et al. Management of Cancer Pain: Quick Reference Guide for Clinicians No. 9. AHCPR Publication No. 94–0593. Rockville, MD. Agency for Health Care Policy and Research, Public Health Service, U.S. Department of Health and Human Services. March 1994, and from Erstad BL. A rational approach to the management of acute pain states. Hosp Formul 1994;29 (8 Part 2):586.

long-acting medications or before activity known to cause more pain. Distribution of opioid agonist-antagonists, such as buprenorphine, for opioid use disorder is restricted in the United States, and management issues are complex. The use of buprenorphine as a short-acting analgesic generally should be reserved for specialists.

For chronic stable pain, **long-acting medications** are preferred, such as oral sustained-release formulations of morphine (one to three times a day), oxycodone (two or three times a day), or hydrocodone (two times a day), or the long-acting medication methadone (three or four times a day) (Table 5–3). Buprenorphine is available as a transdermal patch. Clinicians prescribing opioids must understand the concept of **equianalgesic dosing** (Table 5–3). The dosages of any full opioid agonists used to control pain can be converted into an equivalent dose of any other opioid. This approach is helpful in estimating the appropriate dose of a long-acting opioid based on the amount of short-acting opioid required over the preceding days. For example, 24-hour opioid requirements established using short-acting opioid medications can be converted into equivalent dosages of long-acting medications or formulations. Cross-tolerance is often incomplete, however, so generally only two-thirds to three-quarters of the full, calculated equianalgesic dosage is administered initially when switching between opioid formulations.

Methadone deserves special consideration among the long-acting opioids because it is inexpensive, available in a liquid formulation, and may have added efficacy for neuropathic pain. However, equianalgesic dosing is complex because it varies with the patient's opioid dose, and caution must be used at higher methadone doses (generally more than 100–150 mg/day) because of the risk of QT prolongation. Baseline ECG is recommended before starting methadone and repeated up to monthly except at the end of life where comfort is the only goal. Given the complexities of management and the increasing prevalence of methadone overdose in the United States, consultation with a palliative medicine or pain specialist may be appropriate.

Transdermal fentanyl is appropriate for patients already tolerant to other opioids for at least 1 week at a dose equivalent to at least 60 mg/day of oral morphine (equivalent to transdermal fentanyl 25 mcg/h every 72 hours) and therefore should not be used in the postoperative setting or be the first opioid used. Medications that inhibit cytochrome P450 3A4, such as ritonavir, ketoconazole, itraconazole, troleandomycin, clarithromycin, nelfinavir, nefazodone, amiodarone, amprenavir, aprepitant, diltiazem, erythromycin, fluconazole, fosamprenavir, and verapamil, as well as grapefruit juice can cause increased levels and duration of transdermal fentanyl. Since transdermal fentanyl can require 24–48 hours to achieve pharmacologic "steady state," patients should be weaned off their current opioid and given short-acting opioids while awaiting the full analgesic effect of transdermal fentanyl, and changes in dose of transdermal fentanyl should be made no more frequently than every 6 days.

While some clinicians and patients inexperienced with the management of severe pain may feel more comfortable with combined nonopioid-opioid agents, full agonist opioids are typically a better choice in patients with severe pain because the dose of opioid is not limited by the toxicities of the acetaminophen, aspirin, or NSAID component of combination preparations. There is no maximal allowable or effective dose for full opioid agonists. The dose can be gradually increased to whatever is necessary to relieve pain, remembering that not all pain is opioid sensitive and that certain types of pain, such as neuropathic pain, may respond better to agents other than opioids, or to combinations of opioids with co-analgesics.

While physiologic tolerance is possible with opioids, failure of a previously effective opioid dose to adequately relieve pain is usually due to worsening of the underlying condition causing pain, such as tumor growth or new metastasis in a patient with cancer. In this case, for moderate unrelieved pain, the dose of opioid can be increased by 25–50%. For severe unrelieved pain, a dose increase of 50–100% may be appropriate. The frequency of dosing should be adjusted so that pain control is continuous. Long-term dosing may then be adjusted by adding the average daily amount of short-acting opioid necessary for breakthrough pain over the preceding 72–96 hours to the long-acting medication dose. In establishing or reestablishing adequate dosing, frequent reassessment of the patient's pain and medication side effects is necessary.

B. Opioid Adverse Effects

As opioids are titrated upward, increasing difficulty with the side effects can be expected. Constipation is common at any dose of opioid, and tolerance to this side effect does not develop over time. **Opioid-induced constipation should be anticipated and prevented in all patients.**

Sedation can be expected with opioids, although tolerance to this effect and to side effects other than constipation typically develops within 24–72 hours at a stable dose. Sedation typically appears well before significant respiratory depression. If treatment for sedation is desired, dextroamphetamine (2.5–7.5 mg orally at 8 AM and noon) or methylphenidate (2.5–10 mg orally at 8 AM and noon) may be helpful. Caffeinated beverages can also ameliorate minor opioid sedation.

Opioid-induced neurotoxicity—including myoclonus, hyperalgesia, delirium with hallucinosis, and seizures—may develop in patients who take high doses of opioids for a prolonged period. Opioid-induced hyperalgesia appears to be a result of changes in both the peripheral and central nervous systems leading to sensitivity to pain. Typically benign or even soothing stimuli (eg, light massage) may be perceived as painful (allodynia), and increasing opioid dose may exacerbate the problem. These symptoms may resolve after lowering the dose or switching opioids ("opioid rotation"), especially to ones like fentanyl or methadone that do not have active metabolites. While waiting for the level of the offending opioid to fall, low doses of lorazepam, baclofen, or gabapentin may be helpful for treating myoclonus; haloperidol may be useful for treating delirium. Avoiding or correcting dehydration may be helpful for prevention and treatment of opioid-induced neurotoxicity.

Nausea due to opioids may occur with initiation of therapy and resolve after a few days. Notably, unrelieved constipation may be a more likely cause of nausea in the setting of opioid use than opioid-induced nausea. Severe or persistent nausea despite treatment of constipation can be managed by switching opioids or by giving haloperidol, 0.5–4 mg orally, subcutaneously, or intravenously every 6 hours; prochlorperazine, 10 mg orally or intravenously or 25 mg rectally every 6 hours; or metoclopramide, 5–20 mg orally, subcutaneously, or intravenously before meals and bed. Ondansetron, 4–8 mg orally or intravenously every 6 hours, also relieves nausea but can contribute to constipation. Mirtazapine and medical cannabis may each have a role in treating opioid-induced nausea. Most antiemetic treatments can contribute to sedation.

Although clinicians may worry about respiratory depression with opioids, this side effect is uncommon when a low dose is given initially and titrated upward slowly. Patients at particular risk for respiratory depression include those with chronic obstructive pulmonary disease, obstructive sleep apnea, and baseline CO_2 retention; those with liver or kidney or combined liver-kidney failure; and those with adrenal insufficiency or frank myxedema. Yet, even patients with severe pulmonary disease and obstructive sleep apnea can tolerate low-dose opioids, but they should be monitored carefully. Hospitalized patients with these conditions who require increased doses of opioids should be monitored with continuous pulse oximetry. Clinicians should not allow unfounded concerns about respiratory depression to prevent them from treating pain adequately.

▶ Medications for Neuropathic Pain

It is essential when taking a patient's history to listen for descriptions such as burning, shooting, pins and needles, or electricity, and for pain associated with numbness. Such a history suggests neuropathic pain, which is treated with some medications not typically used for other types of pain. While opioids are effective for neuropathic pain, a number of nonopioid medications also have been found to be effective in randomized trials (Table 5–4). Successful management of neuropathic pain often requires the use of more than one effective medication.

The tricyclic antidepressants (TCAs) are good first-line therapy. Nortriptyline and desipramine are preferred because they cause less orthostatic hypotension and have fewer anticholinergic effects than amitriptyline. Start with a low dosage (10–25 mg orally daily) and titrate upward in 10-mg increments every 4 or 5 days aiming to use the lowest effective dose and titrating up to 100 mg daily. It may take several weeks for a TCA to have its full effect as a neuropathic pain analgesic.

Table 5–4. Pharmacologic management of neuropathic pain.

Medication[1]	Starting Dose	Typical Dose
Antidepressants[2]		
Nortriptyline	10 mg orally at bedtime	10–150 mg orally at bedtime
Desipramine	10 mg orally at bedtime	10–150 mg orally at bedtime
Calcium-channel Alpha2-delta Ligands		
Gabapentin[3]	100–300 mg orally once to three times daily	300–1200 mg orally three times daily
Pregabalin[4]	50 mg orally three times daily	100 mg orally three times daily
Selective Serotonin Norepinephrine Reuptake Inhibitors		
Duloxetine	60 mg orally daily or 20 mg orally twice daily in elders	60–120 mg orally daily
Venlafaxine[5]	75 mg orally daily divided into two or three doses	150–225 mg orally daily divided into two or three doses
Opioids	(see Table 5–3)	(see Table 5–3)
Other Medications		
Lidocaine transdermal	5% patch applied daily, for a maximum of 12 hours	1–3 patches applied daily for a maximum of 12 hours
Tramadol hydrochloride[6]	50 mg orally four times daily	100 mg orally two to four times daily

[1]Begin at the starting dose and titrate up every 4 or 5 days. Within each category, drugs listed in order of prescribing preference.
[2]Begin with a low dose. Use the lowest effective dose. Pain relief may be achieved at doses below antidepressant doses, thereby minimizing adverse side effects.
[3]Common side effects include nausea, somnolence, and dizziness. Take medication on a full stomach. Do not combine with serotonin or norepinephrine uptake inhibitors, or with tricyclic antidepressants.
[4]Common side effects include dizziness, somnolence, peripheral edema, and weight gain. Must adjust dose for kidney impairment.
[5]*Caution:* Can cause hypertension and ECG changes. Obtain baseline ECG and monitor.
[6]Tramadol is classified by the DEA as a Schedule IV controlled substance.

The calcium channel alpha2-delta ligands gabapentin and pregabalin are also first-line therapies for neuropathic pain. Both medications can cause sedation, dizziness, ataxia, and gastrointestinal side effects but have no significant medication interactions. Both medications require dose adjustments in patients with kidney dysfunction. Gabapentin should be started at low dosages of 100–300 mg orally three times a day and titrated upward by 300 mg/day every 4 or 5 days with a typical effective dose of 1800–3600 mg/day. Pregabalin should be started at 150 mg/day in two or three divided doses. If necessary, the dose of pregabalin can be titrated upward to 300–600 mg/day in two or three divided doses. Both medications are relatively safe in accidental overdose and may be preferred over TCAs for a patient with a history of heart failure or arrhythmia or if there is a risk of suicide. Prescribing both gabapentin and an opioid for neuropathic pain may provide better analgesia at lower doses than if each is used as a single agent.

The selective serotonin norepinephrine reuptake inhibitors (SSNRIs), duloxetine and venlafaxine, are also first-line treatments for neuropathic pain. Patients should be advised to take duloxetine on a full stomach because nausea is a common side effect. Duloxetine may provide increased benefit for neuropathic pain up to a total daily dose of 120 mg, beyond the 60 mg limit used for depression. Duloxetine generally should not be combined with other serotonin or norepinephrine uptake inhibitors, but it can be combined with gabapentin or pregabalin. Because venlafaxine can cause hypertension and induce ECG changes, patients with cardiovascular risk factors should be carefully monitored when starting this medication.

Other medications effective for neuropathic pain include tramadol, tapentadol, and the 5% lidocaine patch. The 5% lidocaine patch is effective in postherpetic neuralgia and may be effective in other types of localized neuropathic pain that causes hypesthesia. The 5% lidocaine patch is not effective for other causes of pain. Medical cannabis strains high in cannabidiol (CBD) have proven efficacy for some types of neuropathic pain.

▶ Adjuvant Pain Medications & Treatments

If pain cannot be controlled without uncomfortable medication side effects, clinicians should consider using lower doses of multiple medications, as is done commonly for neuropathic pain, rather than larger doses of one or two medications. For metastatic bone pain, the anti-inflammatory effect of NSAIDs can be particularly helpful. Radiation therapy (including single-fraction treatments), bisphosphonates, and receptor activator of NF-kappa-B ligand (RANKL) inhibitors may also relieve bone pain. For some patients, a nerve block can provide substantial relief, such as a celiac plexus block for pain from pancreatic cancer. Intrathecal pumps may be useful for patients with severe pain responsive to opioids but who require such large doses that systemic side effects (eg, sedation and constipation) become limiting.

Corticosteroids, such as dexamethasone and prednisone, can be helpful for patients with headache due to increased intracranial pressure, pain from spinal cord compression, metastatic bone pain, and neuropathic pain due to invasion or infiltration of nerves by tumor. Because of the side effects of long-term corticosteroid administration, they are most appropriate for short-term use and in patients with end-stage disease. Low-dose intravenous, oral, and nasal ketamine has been used successfully for neuropathic and other pain syndromes refractory to opioids, although research data are limited.

OPIOIDS FOR CHRONIC, NONCANCER PAIN
Scott J. Steiger, MD

The potential harms and benefits of daily opioid therapy for patients with chronic, noncancer pain (CNCP) may be different than for patients receiving opioids in the setting of palliative and end-of-life care. CNCP is often the primary disease rather than a symptom of another process.

CNCP is common, with the World Health Organization estimating worldwide prevalence at 20%. The Institute of Medicine estimates 100 million US adults suffer from CNCP, and the disease costs $635 billion annually in treatment and lost productivity. In an effort to more aggressively treat CNCP, US providers dramatically increased the prescription of opioids beginning in the mid-1990s. Hydrocodone has been the most commonly prescribed medication in the United States since at least 2008, and the United States consumes 99% of the global supply. Methadone prescriptions for pain increased 1300% between 1997 and 2006. The total amount of opioid prescriptions filled in 2007 would have been enough for each adult in the United States to receive 700 mg of morphine.

The increased attention to treating CNCP has undoubtedly improved the lives of many patients, but the increase in prescribing opioids has had a deleterious effect on the health of the population as a whole. From 1991 to 2008, the number of deaths from opioid overdose quadrupled, and the number of patients admitted to treatment for addiction to opioids has quintupled. The Centers for Disease Control and Prevention has named prescription drug abuse an epidemic in the United States.

A. Assessing Benefits of Opioids

Research demonstrates that **the beneficial effect of opioids for CNCP is modest at best, and no measures have been identified to predict a good response**. The improvements are generally measured in terms of a reduction in the analog pain score of 2–3 points on a 10-point scale or in improvements in the important but less precise outcome of *function*. Prior to considering a trial of daily opioids, clinicians should discuss these modest possible benefits with patients in order to help set realistic goals of therapy (eg, moving from an average pain of 7 to a 4). Clinicians should also set a deadline for reaching the patient's goals. Since the published trials have generally lasted less than 16 weeks, it is reasonable to set a deadline before that, with some experts advocating a 90-day trial period. Limiting the time of a trial will also help prevent dose escalation to levels associated with increased risk of adverse effects, including overdose.

Many experts recommend developing a specific goal of improved function, and tracking the patient's progress toward achieving this goal over time. But for the many patients who do not have specific, measurable goals—or who come to the clinician already on daily opioid medication—monitoring response to treatment over time can be difficult. A useful tracking measure is asking about **pain, energy, and general activity (PEG)**, which directs patients to quantify on a scale of 0–10 the following three outcomes: **pain** intensity on average over the last week; how the pain has affected their **energy** level; and how much pain has impacted their **general activity.** Patients who do not progress toward their goal or whose PEG scores remain high over time may have pain that is unresponsive to opioids, and clinicians should reconsider the original diagnosis and use other modalities (both pharmacologic and nonpharmacologic) to provide analgesia. **Without a clear analgesic benefit from opioids for CNCP, the risks may predominate, and the ineffective therapy should be discontinued.**

B. Risks of Long-Term Opioid Therapy

The risks of opioids are different from those of most other medications. One of the most attractive features of opioids is the absence of specific organ toxicity attendant to most other kinds of medications. However, not every patient with CNCP is a good candidate for long-term opioid therapy. In addition to the grave risks of addiction and death and the common side effects of sedation and constipation, long-term opioid use leads to increased risk of many problems, including hypogonadism, fracture, hyperalgesia, psychosocial problems, and fraught interactions with the health care system. When considering whether to initiate or continue opioids for CNCP, clinicians should delineate these specific risks for patients so an informed decision can be made.

In addition to overdose, the biggest concern of many patients and clinicians is addiction. The level of risk to the individual patient with CNCP is uncertain. While physical opioid *dependence* has been demonstrated with daily use in virtually all patients, the published risk of *addiction* in patients prescribed opioids for CNCP varies between less than 1% to more than 20%, with the lowest frequencies observed in studies that excluded patients with a history of substance abuse or addiction. Survey data found that nearly 80% of people in the United States who tried heroin for the first time in 2012 had already abused opioid medications.

Importantly, **diversion** of medication from patients to whom they are prescribed into other hands is another risk that must be considered when prescribing long-term opioids for CNCP. Diversion can represent opportunism, as when a patient sells medication in order to make money. Family members (including children), acquaintances, or strangers may steal or extort medication for their own use or gain.

C. Limiting Risks

A number of interventions have been used in an effort to limit the risks of opioids for patients with CNCP. Data

demonstrating the effectiveness of such measures are limited, but nearly all medical society consensus panels and expert guidelines recommend using a risk assessment tool, patient–provider agreements, urine drug testing, dose limitations, and limits on the use of some medications:

1. Risk assessment tool—Although there are no highly predictive models for who will benefit from long-term opioids for CNCP, some models can identify patients most likely to exhibit aberrant or addictive behaviors. Most published guidelines recommend using an instrument like the Opioid Risk Tool (available at http://www.opioidrisk.com/node/884) to determine how tightly to monitor patients who are receiving opioids long term, or whether to offer long-term opioids at all.

2. Patient–provider agreements—Also known as "pain contracts," these agreements have a modest effect, with 7–23% reduction in aberrant behaviors reported. They do represent an opportunity for the clinician to discuss explicitly the risks and benefits of opioids for CNCP, protocols and procedures for refills and monitoring, and consequences of worrisome behaviors.

3. Urine drug testing—Toxicology testing is a tool borrowed from addiction treatment with goals of limiting diversion and identifying risky secondary drug use. Guidelines recommend increasing frequency of testing with increased risk as determined by dose, risk assessment tool, or recent behavior. It is imperative that clinicians choose their tests appropriately and understand the limitations of toxicology testing when using this tool. **Universal testing is recommended,** given provider inability to judge misuse of medication and documented racial differences in monitoring.

4. Dose limitations—No published data support the use of daily doses of opioids above approximately 200 mg of morphine for CNCP, while risk of overdose increases approximately linearly with dose in observational studies. This has led some guideline experts to impose limits on the amount of opioid a prescriber can offer. Clinicians must be cautious when tapering a patient's dose to meet these limits. Tapering too quickly may result in acutely risky behavior, like extramedical use of prescription drugs or heroin.

5. Special medication limitations—The FDA requires companies making extended-release opioid formulations to provide trainings for prescribers. Many guidelines recommend that the prescription of methadone and fentanyl be limited to specialists, and some recommend against *concurrent* prescription of opioids and benzodiazepines.

6. Antidote to overdose—Distributing naloxone—a quick-onset opioid-receptor antagonist—has long been known to reduce overdose deaths in people who use heroin and, more recently, prescribing naloxone to patients taking opioids for CNCP has been demonstrated to reduce rates of opioid overdose. Educating both patients and their caregivers on the use of rescue naloxone is an important consideration, since those experiencing sedation and respiratory suppression from opioid overdose will not be able to self-administer. In addition to pre-loaded needle-tipped syringes, intranasal and an intramuscular auto-injector have been approved for sale in the United States, where an increasing number of states authorize pharmacies to dispense naloxone in the absence of a prescription.

D. A Shared Decision-Making Approach

Prescribing opioids for patients with CNCP is fraught with challenges for clinicians, but taking the approach of carefully evaluating risks and benefits allows the opportunity for shared decision making in individual cases. **Clinical trials do not suggest that the majority of people with CNCP will benefit significantly from daily opioid therapy, and the dramatic increase in morbidity and mortality witnessed with the increased availability of these medications warrants very careful patient selection.** It is incumbent upon the clinician to provide frank advice to patients prescribed long-term opioids for CNCP and offer safer alternatives when the benefit is insufficient or the risks too high.

Albert S et al. Project Lazarus: community-based overdose prevention in rural North Carolina. Pain Med. 2011 Jun;12(Suppl 2): S77–85. [PMID: 21668761]
Bohnert AS et al. Association between opioid prescribing patterns and opioid overdose-related deaths. JAMA. 2011 Apr 6; 305(13):1315–21. [PMID: 21467284]
Chou R et al. The effectiveness and risks of long-term opioid therapy for chronic pain: a systematic review for a National Institutes of Health Pathways to Prevention Workshop. Ann Intern Med. 2015 Feb 17;162(4):276–86. [PMID: 25581257]
Noble M et al. Long-term opioid management for chronic non-cancer pain. Cochrane Database Syst Rev. 2010 Jan 20; (1):CD006605. [PMID: 20091598]
Nuckols TK et al. Opioid prescribing: a systematic review and critical appraisal of guidelines for chronic pain. Ann Intern Med. 2014 Jan 7;160(1):38–47. [PMID: 24217469]
Warner M et al. Drug poisoning deaths in the United States, 1980–2008. NCHS Data Brief. 2011 Dec;(81):1–8. [PMID: 22617462]

NONPHARMACOLOGIC TREATMENTS

Nonpharmacologic therapies are valuable in treating pain. Hot or cold packs, massage, and physical therapy can be helpful for musculoskeletal pain. Similarly, biofeedback, acupuncture, chiropractic, meditation, music therapy, cognitive-behavioral therapy, guided imagery, cognitive distraction, and framing may be of help in treating pain. Because mood and psychological issues play an important role in the patient's perception of and response to pain, psychotherapy, support groups, prayer, and pastoral counseling can also help in the management of pain. Depression, which may be instigated by chronic pain or may alter the response to pain, should be treated aggressively.

▶ When to Refer

- Pain not responding to opioids at typical doses.
- Neuropathic pain not responding to first-line treatments.
- Complex methadone management issues.
- Intolerable side effects from oral opioids.

- Severe pain from bone metastases.
- For a surgical or anesthesia-based procedure, intrathecal pump, or nerve block.

▶ When to Admit

- Severe exacerbation of pain that is not responsive to previous stable oral opioid around the clock plus breakthrough doses.
- Patients whose pain is so severe that they cannot be cared for at home.
- Uncontrollable side effects from opioids, including nausea, vomiting, myoclonus, and altered mental status.

Paulsen O et al. Efficacy of methylprednisolone on pain, fatigue, and appetite loss in patients with advanced cancer using opioids: a randomized, placebo-controlled, double-blind trial. J Clin Oncol. 2014 Oct 10;32(29):3221–8. [PMID: 25002731]
Salpeter SR et al. The use of very-low-dose methadone for palliative pain control and the prevention of opioid hyperalgesia. J Palliat Med. 2013 Jun;16(6):616–22. [PMID: 23556990]

▼ PALLIATION OF OTHER COMMON SYMPTOMS CONSTIPATION

CONSTIPATION

Given the frequent use of opioids, poor dietary intake, and physical inactivity, constipation is a common problem in the seriously ill or dying. Clinicians must inquire about any difficulty with hard or infrequent stools. Constipation is an easily preventable and treatable cause of discomfort, distress, and nausea and vomiting (see Chapter 15).

Constipation may be prevented or relieved if patients can increase their activity and their intake of fluids. Simple considerations, such as privacy, undisturbed toilet time, and a bedside commode rather than a bedpan may be important for some patients.

For patients taking opioids, anticipating and preventing constipation is key. A prophylactic bowel regimen with a stimulant laxative (senna or bisacodyl) should be started when opioid treatment is begun. Table 15–4 lists other agents (including osmotic laxatives such as polyethylene glycol) that can be added as needed. Docusate, a stool softener, is not recommended. Naloxegol, an oral peripherally acting receptor antagonist, and lubiprostone are FDA approved to treat opioid-induced constipation in patients with CNCP. Methylnaltrexone, a subcutaneous medication, is a peripherally acting mu-receptor antagonist and is available for severe, unrelieved, opioid-induced constipation.

DYSPNEA

Dyspnea is the subjective experience of difficulty breathing and may be characterized by patients as tightness in the chest, shortness of breath, or a feeling of suffocation. Up to 50% of terminally ill patients may experience severe dyspnea. Treatment of dyspnea is usually first directed at the cause (see Chapter 9). At the end of life, dyspnea is often treated nonspecifically with opioids. **Immediate-release**

morphine given orally (2–4 mg every 4 hours) or intravenously (1–2 mg every 4 hours) treats dyspnea effectively. Doses are typically lower than would be necessary for the relief of moderate pain. **Sustained-release morphine** given orally at 10 mg daily appears to be safe and effective for most patients with dyspnea. Supplemental oxygen may be useful for the dyspneic patient *who is hypoxic.* However, a nasal cannula and face mask are sometimes not well tolerated, and fresh air from a window or fan may provide relief. Judicious use of noninvasive ventilation as well as nonpharmacologic relaxation techniques, such as meditation and guided imagery may be beneficial for some patients. Benzodiazepines may be useful adjuncts for treatment of dyspnea-related agitation. Nonpharmacologic treatments, including acupuncture, may be effective.

NAUSEA & VOMITING

Nausea and vomiting are common and distressing symptoms. As with pain, the management of nausea may be maximized by regular dosing and often requires multiple medications. An understanding of the four major inputs to the vomiting center may help direct treatment (see Chapter 15).

Vomiting associated with opioids is discussed above. Nasogastric suction may provide rapid, short-term relief for vomiting associated with constipation (in addition to laxatives), gastroparesis, or gastric outlet or bowel obstruction. Prokinetic agents, such as metoclopramide (5–20 mg orally or intravenously four times a day), can be helpful in the setting of partial bowel obstruction. Transdermal scopolamine (1.5-mg patch every 3 days) can reduce peristalsis and cramping pain, and ranitidine (50 mg intravenously every 6 hours) can reduce gastric secretions. Octreotide (starting at 50–100 mcg subcutaneously every 8 hours or as continuous intravenous or subcutaneous infusion, beginning at 10–20 mcg/h) can reduce gastric secretions and may have a role in relieving nausea and vomiting from malignant bowel obstruction. High-dose corticosteroids (eg, dexamethasone, 20 mg orally or intravenously daily in divided doses) can be used in refractory cases of nausea or vomiting or when it is due to bowel obstruction or increased intracranial pressure.

Vomiting due to disturbance of the vestibular apparatus may be treated with anticholinergic and antihistaminic agents (including diphenhydramine, 25 mg orally or intravenously every 8 hours, or scopolamine, 1.5-mg patch every 3 days).

Benzodiazepines can be effective in preventing the *anticipatory* nausea associated with chemotherapy. There is strong evidence that olanzapine can be effective for chemotherapy-induced nausea and vomiting. Finally, medical cannabis or dronabinol (2.5–20 mg orally every 4–6 hours) can be helpful in the management of nausea and vomiting.

FATIGUE

Fatigue is a distressing symptom and is the most common complaint among cancer patients. Specific abnormalities that can contribute to fatigue, including anemia, hypothyroidism, hypogonadism, cognitive and functional impairment, and malnutrition, should be corrected. Because pain, depression, and fatigue often coexist in patients with cancer, pain and depression should be managed adequately in patients with fatigue. Fatigue from medication adverse effects and polypharmacy is common and should be addressed. For nonspecific fatigue, exercise and physical rehabilitation may be most effective. Although commonly used, evidence for psychostimulants, such as methylphenidate, 5–10 mg orally in the morning and afternoon, or modafinil, 200 mg orally in the morning, for cancer-related fatigue is lacking. American Ginseng (*Panax quinquefolius*) has been shown to be effective for cancer-related fatigue. Corticosteroids may have a short-term benefit.

DELIRIUM & AGITATION

Many patients die in a state of delirium—a disturbance of consciousness and a change in cognition that develops over a short time and is manifested by misinterpretations, illusions, hallucinations, disturbances in the sleep-wake cycle, psychomotor disturbances (eg, lethargy, restlessness), and mood disturbances (eg, fear, anxiety). Delirium may be hyperactive, hypoactive, or mixed. Agitated delirium at the end of life has been called **terminal restlessness.**

Careful attention to patient safety and nonpharmacologic strategies to help the patient remain oriented (clocks, calendars, a familiar environment, reassurance and redirection from caregivers) may be sufficient to prevent or manage mild delirium. Some delirious patients may be "pleasantly confused," although it is difficult to know the patient's experience, and a decision by the patient's family and the clinician not to treat delirium may be considered.

More commonly, however, delirium at the end of life is distressing to patients and family and requires treatment. Delirium may interfere with the family's ability to feel comforting to the patient and may prevent a patient from being able to recognize and report important symptoms. While there are many reversible causes of delirium (see Chapter 25), identifying and correcting the underlying cause at the end of life is often complex because a patient may have many possible causes. When the cause of delirium cannot be identified, treated, or corrected rapidly enough, it may be treated symptomatically with neuroleptic agents, such as haloperidol (1–10 mg orally, subcutaneously, intramuscularly, or intravenously twice or three times a day) or risperidone (1–3 mg orally twice a day). The benefits of neuroleptic agents in the treatment of agitation must be weighed carefully against potential harms, based on evidence showing an association between antipsychotic medications and increased mortality for older adults with dementia. There is no evidence that hydration relieves or dehydration causes delirium. Ramelteon, a melatonin agonist, at 8 mg/day orally has been shown to prevent delirium in seriously ill, older hospitalized patients. It should be avoided in patients with severe liver disease. When delirium is refractory to treatment and remains intolerable, sedation may be required to provide relief and may be achieved rapidly with midazolam (0.5–5 mg/h subcutaneously or intravenously) or barbiturates (especially useful in the outpatient setting).

Bruera E et al. Parenteral hydration in patients with advanced cancer: a multicenter, double-blind, placebo-controlled randomized trial. J Clin Oncol. 2013 Jan 1;31(1):111–8. [PMID: 23169523]

Candy B et al. Laxatives or methylnaltrexone for the management of constipation in palliative care patients. Cochrane Database Syst Rev. 2011 Jan 19;(1):CD003448. [PMID: 21249653]

Hatta K et al; DELIRIA-J Group. Preventive effects of ramelteon on delirium: a randomized placebo-controlled trial. JAMA Psychiatry. 2014 Apr;71(4):397–403. [PMID: 24554232]

Mitchell GK et al. The effect of methylphenidate on fatigue in advanced cancer: an aggregated N-of-1 Trial. J Pain Symptom Manage. 2015 Sep;50(3):289–96. [PMID: 25896104]

Singer AE et al. Symptom trends in the last year of life from 1998 to 2010: a cohort study. Ann Intern Med. 2015 Feb 3; 162(3):175–83. [PMID: 25643305]

Spathis A et al. Modafinil for the treatment of fatigue in lung cancer: results of a placebo-controlled, double-blind, randomized trial. J Clin Oncol. 2014 Jun 20;32(18):1882–8. [PMID: 24778393]

Suzuki M et al. A randomized, placebo-controlled trial of acupuncture in patients with chronic obstructive pulmonary disease (COPD): the COPD-acupuncture trial (CAT). Arch Intern Med. 2012 Jun 11;172(11):878–86. [PMID: 22905352]

Tarumi Y et al. Randomized, double-blind, placebo-controlled trial of oral docusate in the management of constipation in hospice patients. J Pain Symptom Manage. 2013 Jan;45(1): 2–13. [PMID: 22889861]

CARE OF PATIENTS AT THE END OF LIFE

In the United States, nearly 2.5 million people die each year. Caring for patients at the end of life is an important responsibility and a rewarding opportunity for clinicians. From the medical perspective, the end of life may be defined as that time when death—whether due to terminal illness or acute or chronic illness—is expected within weeks to months and can no longer be reasonably forestalled by medical intervention. Palliative care at the end of life focuses on relieving distressing symptoms and promoting quality of life (as with all other stages of illness). For patients at the end of life, palliative care may become the sole focus of care.

Prognosis at the End of Life

Clinicians must help patients understand when they are approaching the end of life. Most patients (and their family caregivers) want prognostic information. This information influences patients' treatment decisions and may change how they spend their remaining time and does not negatively impact patient survival. One-half or more of cancer patients do not understand that many treatments they might be offered are palliative and not curative. Patients require support for distress that may accompany discussions of prognostic information.

While certain diseases, such as cancer, are more amenable to prognostic estimates regarding the time course to death, the other common causes of mortality in the United States—including heart disease, stroke, chronic lung disease, and dementia—have more variable trajectories and difficult-to-predict prognoses. Even for patients with cancer, clinician estimates of prognosis are often inaccurate

and generally overly optimistic. Nonetheless, clinical experience, epidemiologic data, guidelines from professional organizations (eg, the National Hospice and Palliative Care Organization), and computer modeling and prediction tools (eg, the Palliative Performance Scale or www.eprognosis.org) may be used to help patients identify the end period of their lives. Clinicians can also ask themselves "Would I be surprised if this patient died in the next year?" to determine whether a discussion of prognosis would be appropriate. If the answer is "no," then the clinician should initiate a discussion. Recognizing that patients may have different levels of comfort with prognostic information, clinicians can introduce the topic by simply saying, "I have information about the likely time course of your illness. Would you like to talk about it?"

Expectations About the End of Life

Death is often regarded by clinicians, patients, and families as a failure of medical science. This attitude can create or heighten a sense of guilt about the failure to prevent dying. Both the general public and clinicians often are complicit in denying death, treating dying persons merely as patients and death as an enemy to be battled furiously in hospitals rather than as an inevitable outcome to be experienced as a part of life at home. As a result, approximately 75–80% of people in the United States die in hospitals or long-term care facilities.

Even when the clinician and patient continue to pursue cure of potentially reversible disease, relieving suffering, providing support, and helping the patient prepare for death should be foremost considerations. Patients at the end of life and their families identify a number of elements as important to quality end-of-life care: managing pain and other symptoms adequately, avoiding inappropriate prolongation of dying, communicating clearly, preserving dignity, preparing for death, achieving a sense of control, relieving the burden on others, and strengthening relationships with loved ones.

Communication & Care of the Patient

Caring for patients at the end of life requires the same skills clinicians use in other tasks of medical care: diagnosing treatable conditions, providing patient education, facilitating decision making, and expressing understanding and caring. Higher-quality communication is associated with greater satisfaction and awareness of patient wishes. Clinicians must become proficient at delivering serious news and then dealing with its consequences (Table 5–5). Smartphone and Internet communication resources are available to support clinicians, and preliminary evidence suggests that communication checklists can be effective. When the clinician and patient do not share a common language, the use of a professional interpreter is needed to facilitate clear communication and help broker cultural issues.

Three further obligations are central to the clinician's role at this time. First, he or she must work to identify, understand, and relieve physical, psychological, social, and spiritual distress or suffering. Second, clinicians can serve as facilitators or catalysts for hope. While hope for a

Table 5–5. Suggestions for the delivery of serious news.

Prepare an appropriate place and time.
Address basic information needs.
Be direct; avoid jargon and euphemisms.
Allow for silence and emotional ventilation.
Assess and validate patient reactions.
Respond to immediate discomforts and risks.
Listen actively and express empathy.
Achieve a common perception of the problem.
Reassure about pain relief.
Ensure basic follow-up and make specific plans for the future.

Table 5–6. Clinician interventions helpful to families of dying patients.

Excellent communication, including clinician willingness to talk about death, timely and clear information, proactive guidance, listening, and empathic responses

Advance care planning and clear decision-making, including culturally sensitive communication, achieving consensus among family members and an understanding that surrogate decision makers are trying to determine what the *patient* would have wanted, not what the surrogate would want

Support for home care, including orienting family members to the scope and details of family caregiving, providing clear direction about how to contact professional caregivers, and informing patients and families of the benefits of hospice care

Empathy for family emotions and relationships, including recognizing and validating common positive and negative feelings

Attention to grief and bereavement, including support for anticipatory grief and follow-up with the family after the patient's death

Data from Rabow MW et al. Supporting family caregivers at the end of life: "they don't know what they don't know." JAMA. 2004 Jan 28;291(4):483–91.

particular outcome may fade, it can be redefined by the patient's belief of what is *still* possible. Although expecting a "miraculous cure" may be simplistic, hope for relief of pain, for reconciliation with loved ones, for discovery of meaning, and for spiritual growth is realistic at the end of life. With such questions as "What is still possible now for you?", "When you look to the future, what do you hope for?", and "What good might come of this?" clinicians can help patients uncover hope, explore meaningful and realistic goals, and develop strategies to achieve them.

Finally, dying patients' feelings of isolation and fear demand that clinicians assert that they will care for the patient throughout the final stage of life. The promise of nonabandonment is perhaps the central principle of end-of-life care and is a clinician's pledge to an individual patient to serve as a caring partner, a resource for creative problem solving and relief of suffering, a guide during uncertain times, and a witness to the patient's experiences—no matter what happens. Clinicians can say to a patient, "I will care for you whatever happens."

Caring for the Family

In caring for patients at the end of life, clinicians must appreciate the central role played by family, friends, and partners and often must deal with strong emotions of fear, anger, shame, sadness, and guilt experienced by those individuals. While significant others may support and comfort a patient at the end of life, the threatened loss of a loved one may also create or reveal dysfunctional or painful family dynamics. Furthermore, clinicians must be attuned to the potential impact of illness on the patient's family: substantial physical caregiving responsibilities and financial burdens as well as increased rates of anxiety, depression, chronic illness, and even mortality. Family caregivers, typically women, commonly provide the bulk of care for patients at the end of life, yet their work is often not acknowledged, supported, or compensated.

Clinicians can help families confront the imminent loss of a loved one (Table 5–6) and often must negotiate amid complex and changing family needs. Identifying a spokesperson for the family, conducting family meetings, allowing all to be heard, and providing time for consensus may help the clinician work effectively with the family. Providing good palliative care to the patient can reduce the risk of depression and complicated grief in loved ones after the

patient's death. Palliative care support directly for caregivers improves caregiver depression.

Clinician Self-Care

Many clinicians find caring for patients at the end of life to be one of the most rewarding aspects of practice. However, working with the dying requires tolerance of uncertainty, ambiguity, and existential challenges. Clinicians must recognize and respect their own limitations and attend to their own needs in order to avoid being overburdened, overly distressed, or emotionally depleted.

Candy B et al. Interventions for supporting informal caregivers of patients in the terminal phase of a disease. Cochrane Database Syst Rev. 2011 Jun 15;(6):CD007617. [PMID: 21678368]

Dionne-Odom JN et al. Benefits of early versus delayed palliative care to informal family caregivers of patients with advanced cancer: outcomes from the ENABLE III randomized controlled trial. J Clin Oncol. 2015 May 1;33(13):1446–52. [PMID: 25800762]

El-Jawahri A et al. Associations among prognostic understanding, quality of life, and mood in patients with advanced cancer. Cancer. 2014 Jan 15;120(2):278–85. [PMID: 24122784]

Goyal M et al. Meditation programs for psychological stress and well-being: a systematic review and meta-analysis. JAMA Intern Med. 2014 Mar;174(3):357–68. [PMID: 24395196]

Jin J. JAMA patient page. Caregiver support. JAMA. 2014 Mar 12; 311(10):1082. [PMID: 24618980]

Kearney MK et al. Self-care of physicians caring for patients at the end of life: "Being connected. . . a key to my survival". JAMA. 2009 Mar 18;301(11):1155–64. [PMID: 19293416]

Lennes IT et al. Predictors of newly diagnosed cancer patients' understanding of the goals of their care at initiation of chemotherapy. Cancer. 2013 Feb 1;119(3):691–9. [PMID: 23011902]

Moon JR et al. Short- and long-term associations between widowhood and mortality in the United States: longitudinal analyses. J Public Health (Oxf). 2014 Sep;36(3):382–9. [PMID: 24167198]

Pantilat SZ. Communicating with seriously ill patients: better words to say. JAMA. 2009 Mar 25;301(12):1279–81. [PMID: 19318656]

Weeks JC et al. Patients' expectations about effects of chemotherapy for advanced cancer. N Engl J Med. 2012 Oct 25; 367(17):1616–25. [PMID: 23094723]

▶ Decision-Making, Advance Care Planning & Advance Directives

The idea that patients must choose between quality and length of life is an outmoded concept that presents patients with a false choice. Clinicians should discuss with patients that an approach that provides concurrent palliative and disease-focused care is the one most likely to achieve improvements in both quality and quantity of life. Patients deserve to have their health care be consistent with their values, preferences, and goals of care. Well-informed, competent adults have a right to refuse life-sustaining interventions even if this is likely to result in death. In order to promote patient autonomy, clinicians are obligated to inform patients about the risks, benefits, alternatives, and expected outcomes of medical interventions, such as cardiopulmonary resuscitation (CPR), mechanical ventilation, hospitalization and ICU care, and artificial nutrition and hydration. **Advance directives** are oral or written statements made by patients when they are competent that project their autonomy into the future and are intended to guide care should they lose the ability to make and communicate their own decisions. Advance directives are an important part of **advance care planning**—a process whereby clinicians help patients ensure that treatments and care match their goals and values. Advance directives take effect when the patient can no longer communicate his or her preferences directly. While oral statements about these matters are ethically binding, they are not legally binding in all states. State-specific advance directive forms are available from a number of sources, including http://www.caringinfo.org.

Clinicians should facilitate the process for all patients—ideally, well before the end of life—to consider their preferences, to appoint a surrogate, to talk to that person about their preferences, and to complete a formal advance directive. Most patients with a serious illness have already thought about end-of-life issues, want to discuss them with their clinician, want the clinician to bring up the subject, and feel better for having had the discussion. Patients who have such discussions with their clinicians are perceived by their family as having a better quality of life at the end of life, are less likely to die in the hospital, and more likely to utilize hospice care. With advance care planning discussions, patients' loved ones are less likely to suffer from depression during bereavement. Beginning in 2016 in the United States Medicare provides payment to clinicians for having advance care planning discussions with patients.

One type of advance directive is the **Durable Power of Attorney for Health Care (DPOA-HC)** that allows the patient to designate a surrogate decision maker. The DPOA-HC is particularly useful because it is often difficult to anticipate what decisions will need to be made.

The responsibility of the surrogate is to provide "substituted judgment"—to decide as the *patient* would, not as the *surrogate* wants. Clinicians should encourage patients to talk with their surrogates about their preferences generally and about scenarios that are likely to arise, such as the need for mechanical ventilation in a patient with end-stage emphysema. Clear clinician communication is important to correct misunderstandings and address biases. In the absence of a designated surrogate, clinicians usually turn to family members or next of kin. Regulations require health care institutions to inform patients of their rights to formulate an advance directive, and 72% of Americans older than 60 years have completed an advance directive. Some communities have achieved nearly universal completion with concerted efforts. **Physician (or Medical) Orders for Life-Sustaining Treatment (POLST or MOLST)** forms are clinician orders that accompany patients wherever they are cared for—home, hospital, or nursing home—and are increasingly widely used to complement advance directives for patients at the end of life.

▶ Do Not Attempt Resuscitation Orders

As part of advance care planning, clinicians can elicit patient preferences about CPR. Most patients and many clinicians overestimate the chances of success of CPR. Only about 17% of all patients who undergo CPR in the hospital survive to hospital discharge. Moreover, among certain populations—especially those with multisystem organ failure, metastatic cancer, and sepsis—the likelihood of survival to hospital discharge following CPR is virtually nil. Patients may ask their clinician to write an order that CPR not be attempted on them.

For some patients at the end of life, decisions about CPR may not be about *whether* they will live but about *how* they will die. Clinicians should correct the misconception that withholding CPR in appropriate circumstances is tantamount to "not doing everything" or "just letting someone die." While respecting the patient's right ultimately to make the decision—and keeping in mind their own biases and prejudices—clinicians should offer explicit recommendations about Do Not Attempt Resuscitation (DNAR) orders and protect dying patients and their families from feelings of guilt and from the sorrow associated with vain hopes. Clinicians should discuss what interventions will be continued and started to promote quality of life rather than focusing only on what is *not* to be done. For patients with implantable cardioverter defibrillators (ICDs), clinicians must also address issues of turning off these devices as death approaches to prevent them from discharging during the dying process.

▶ Hospice & Other Palliative Care Institutions

In the United States, hospice is a specific type of palliative care service focused on comprehensively addressing the needs of the dying. In the United States, about 45% of people who die use hospice, and about 66% of hospice patients die at home where they can be cared for by their family and visiting hospice staff. Hospice care can also be provided in hospitals and institutional residences. As is true of all types of palliative care, hospice emphasizes individualized attention, human contact, and an interdisciplinary team approach. Hospice care can include arranging for respite for family caregivers and assisting with referrals for legal, financial, and other services. Patients in hospice require a physician who is responsible for their care. Primary care clinicians are strongly encouraged to fulfill this role.

Hospice care is highly rated by families and has been shown to increase patient satisfaction, to reduce costs (depending on when patients are referred to hospice care), and to decrease family caregiver mortality. Despite evidence that suggests that hospice care does not increase mortality and may even extend life, hospice care tends to be used very near the end of life. The average length of stay in hospices in the United States is 72 days, the median length of stay is 18.7 days, with 36% of patients dying within 7 days of beginning hospice care.

In the United States, most hospice organizations require clinicians to estimate the patient's prognosis to be less than 6 months, since this is a criterion for eligibility under the Medicare hospice benefit that is typically the same for other insurance coverage. Regrettably, the hospice benefit can be difficult to provide to people who are homeless or isolated.

▶ Cultural Issues

The individual patient's experience of dying occurs in the context of a complex interaction of personal, philosophic, and cultural influences. Various religious, ethnic, gender, class, and cultural traditions help determine patients' styles of communication, comfort in discussing particular topics, expectations about dying and medical interventions, and attitudes about the appropriate disposition of dead bodies. While each patient is an individual, being sensitive to a person's cultural beliefs and respecting traditions are important responsibilities of the clinician caring for a patient at the end of life, especially when the cultures of origin of the clinician and patient differ. A clinician may ask a patient, "What do I need to know about you and your beliefs that will help me take care of you?"

Bischoff KE et al. Advance care planning and the quality of end-of-life care in older adults. J Am Geriatr Soc. 2013 Feb;61(2):209–14. [PMID: 23350921]
Houben CH et al. Efficacy of advance care planning: a systematic review and meta-analysis. J Am Med Dir Assoc. 2014 Jul;15(7):477–89. [PMID: 24598477]
Tang ST et al. Associations between accurate prognostic understanding and end-of-life care preferences and its correlates among Taiwanese terminally ill cancer patients surveyed in 2011–2012. Psychooncology. 2014 Jul;23(7):780–7. [PMID: 24470441]
Teno JM et al. Change in end-of-life care for Medicare beneficiaries: site of death, place of care, and health care transitions in 2000, 2005, and 2009. JAMA. 2013 Feb 6;309(5):470–7. [PMID: 23385273]
Thompson AE. JAMA patient page. Advance directives. JAMA. 2015 Feb 24;313(8):868. [PMID: 25710673]
Torpy JM et al. JAMA patient page. Hospice care. JAMA. 2012 Jul 11;308(2):200. [PMID: 22782425]

▶ Nutrition & Hydration

People approaching the end of life often lose their appetite and most stop eating and drinking in their last days. The anorexia-cachexia syndrome frequently occurs in patients with advanced cancer, and cachexia is a common and poor prognostic sign in patients with heart failure. Ill people often have no hunger with total caloric deprivation, and the associated ketonemia produces a sense of well-being, analgesia, and mild euphoria. Although it is unclear to what extent withholding hydration at the end of life creates an uncomfortable sensation of thirst, any such sensation is usually relieved by simply moistening the dry mouth. Ice chips, hard candy, swabs, popsicles, or minted mouthwash may be effective. Although this normal process of diminishing oral intake and accompanying weight loss is very common, it can be distressing to patients and families who may associate the offering of food with compassion and love and lack of eating with distressing images of starvation. In response, patients and families often ask about supplemental enteral or parenteral nutrition.

Unfortunately supplemental, artificial nutrition and hydration offer little benefit to those at the end of life and rarely achieve patient and family goals. For example, although tube feedings are often considered in patients with advanced dementia who aspirate, they do not prevent aspiration pneumonia, and there is debate about whether artificial nutrition prolongs life in the terminally ill. Furthermore, force feeding may cause nausea and vomiting in ill patients, and eating can lead to diarrhea in the setting of malabsorption. Artificial nutrition and hydration may increase oral and airway secretions as well as increase the risk of choking, aspiration, and dyspnea; ascites, edema, and effusions may be worsened. Nasogastric and gastrostomy tube feeding and parenteral nutrition impose risks of infection, epistaxis, pneumothorax, electrolyte imbalance, and aspiration—as well as the need to physically restrain the delirious patient to prevent dislodgment of catheters and tubes.

Individuals at the end of life have a right to refuse all nutrition and hydration. Because they may have deep social and cultural significance for patients, families, and clinicians themselves, decisions about artificial nutrition and hydration are not simply medical. Eliciting perceived goals of artificial nutrition and hydration and correcting misperceptions can help patients and families make clear decisions.

▶ Withdrawal of Curative Efforts

Requests from appropriately informed and competent patients or their surrogates for withdrawal of life-sustaining interventions must be respected. Limitation of life-sustaining interventions prior to death is an increasingly common practice in intensive care units. The withdrawal of life-sustaining interventions, such as mechanical ventilation, must be approached carefully to avoid needless patient suffering and distress for those in attendance. Clinicians should educate the patient and family about the expected course of events and the difficulty of determining the precise timing of death after withdrawal of

Table 5–7. Guidelines for withdrawal of mechanical ventilation.

1. Stop neuromuscular blocking agents.
2. Administer opioids or sedatives to eliminate distress. If not already sedated, begin with fentanyl 100 mcg (or morphine sulfate 10 mg). Provide repeated boluses as needed during the process of withdrawing mechanical ventilation. Patients who require repeated boluses may benefit from a continuous infusion of fentanyl 100 mcg/h intravenously (or morphine sulfate 10 mg/h intravenously). Distress is indicated by RR > 24, nasal flaring, use of accessory muscles of respiration, HR increase > 20%, MAP increase > 20%, grimacing, clutching.
3. Discontinue vasoactive agents and other agents unrelated to patient comfort, such as antibiotics, intravenous fluids, and diagnostic procedures.
4. Decrease Fio_2 to room air and PEEP to 0 cm H_2O.
5. Observe patient for distress. If patient is distressed, increase opioids by repeating bolus dose and increasing hourly infusion rate by 50 mcg fentanyl (or 5 mg morphine sulfate),[1] then return to observation. If patient is not distressed, place on T piece and observe. If patient continues without distress, extubate patient and continue to observe for distress.

[1]Ventilatory support may be increased until additional opioids have effect.
RR, respiratory rate; HR, heart rate; MAP, mean airway pressure; Fio_2, fraction of inspired oxygen; PEEP, positive end-expiratory pressure.
Adapted, with permission, from San Francisco General Hospital Guidelines for Withdrawal of Mechanical Ventilation/Life Support.

interventions. Sedative and analgesic agents should be administered to ensure patient comfort even at the risk of respiratory depression or hypotension. While "death rattle," the sound of air flowing over airway secretions, is common in actively dying patients and can be distressing to families, it is doubtful that it causes discomfort to the patient. Turning the patient can decrease the sound of death rattle. There is no evidence that antimuscarinic medications reduce death rattle, and suctioning should be avoided as it can cause patient discomfort. A guideline for withdrawal of mechanical ventilation is provided in Table 5–7.

▶ **Psychological, Social, & Spiritual Issues**

Dying is not exclusively or even primarily a biomedical event. It is an intimate personal experience with profound psychological, interpersonal, and existential meanings. For many people at the end of life, the prospect of impending death stimulates a deep and urgent assessment of their identity, the quality of their relationships, the meaning and purpose of their existence, and their legacy.

A. Psychological Challenges

In 1969, Elisabeth Kübler-Ross identified five psychological reactions or patterns of emotions that patients at the end of life may experience: denial and isolation, anger, bargaining, depression, and acceptance. Not every patient will experience all these emotions, and typically not in an orderly progression. In addition to these five reactions are the perpetual challenges of anxiety and fear of the

unknown. Simple information, listening, assurance, and support may help patients with these psychological challenges. In fact, patients and families rank emotional support as one of the most important aspects of good end-of-life care. Psychotherapy and group support may be beneficial as well.

Despite the significant emotional stress of facing death, clinical depression is not normal at the end of life and should be treated. Cognitive and affective signs of depression (such as hopelessness or helplessness) may help distinguish depression from the low energy and other vegetative signs common with end-stage illness. Although traditional antidepressant treatments such as selective serotonin reuptake inhibitors are effective, more rapidly acting medications, such as dextroamphetamine or methylphenidate (in doses used for sedation described earlier in this chapter), may be particularly useful when the end of life is near or while waiting for other antidepressant medication to take effect. Oral ketamine is being explored as a rapid-onset treatment for anxiety and depression at the end of life. Some research suggests a mortality benefit from treating depression in the setting of serious illness.

B. Social Challenges

At the end of life, patients should be encouraged to discharge personal, professional, and business obligations. These tasks include completing important work or personal projects, distributing possessions, writing a will, and making funeral and burial arrangements. The prospect of death often prompts patients to examine the quality of their interpersonal relationships and to begin the process of saying goodbye (Table 5–8). Concern about estranged relationships or "unfinished business" with significant others and interest in reconciliation may become paramount at this time.

C. Spiritual Challenges

Spirituality is the attempt to understand or accept the underlying meaning of life, one's relationships to oneself and other people, one's place in the universe, one's legacy, and the possibility of a "higher power" in the universe. Spirituality is distinguished from particular religious practices or beliefs.

Unlike physical ailments, such as infections and fractures, which usually require a clinician's intervention to be treated, the patient's spiritual concerns often require only a clinician's attention, listening, and witness. Clinicians can inquire about the patient's spiritual concerns and ask

Table 5–8. Five statements often necessary for the completion of important interpersonal relationships.

1. "Forgive me."	(An expression of regret)
2. "I forgive you."	(An expression of acceptance)
3. "Thank you."	(An expression of gratitude)
4. "I love you."	(An expression of affection)
5. "Goodbye."	(Leave-taking)

Reprinted, with permission, from Byock I. *Dying Well: Peace and Possibilities at the End of Life.* New York: Riverhead Books, an imprint of Penguin Group (USA) LLC 1997.

Table 5–9. An existential review of systems.

Intrapersonal
What does your illness/dying mean to you?
What do you think caused your illness?
How have you been healed in the past?
What do you think is needed for you to be healed now?
What is right with you now?
What do you hope for?
Are you at peace?

Interpersonal
Who is important to you?
To whom does your illness/dying matter?
Do you have any unfinished business with significant others?

Transpersonal
What is your source of strength, help, or hope?
Do you have spiritual concerns or a spiritual practice?
If so, how does your spirituality relate to your illness/dying, and how can I help integrate your spirituality into your health care?
What do you think happens after we die?
What purpose might your illness/dying serve?
What do you think is trying to happen here?

whether the patient wishes to discuss them. For example, asking, "How are you within yourself?" or "Are you at peace?" communicates that the clinician is interested in the patient's whole experience and provides an opportunity for the patient to share perceptions about his or her inner life. Questions that might constitute an existential "review of systems" are presented in Table 5–9. Formal legacy work and dignity therapy have been shown to be effective in improving quality of life and spiritual well-being.

The end of life offers an opportunity for psychological, interpersonal, and spiritual development. Individuals may grow—even achieve a heightened sense of well-being or transcendence—in the process of dying. Through listening, support, and presence, clinicians may help foster this learning and be a catalyst for this transformation. Rather than thinking of dying simply as the termination of life, clinicians and patients may be guided by a developmental model of life that recognizes a series of lifelong developmental tasks and landmarks and allows for growth at the end of life.

Balboni TA et al. Provision of spiritual support to patients with advanced cancer by religious communities and associations with medical care at the end of life. JAMA Intern Med. 2013 Jun 24;173(12):1109–17. [PMID: 23649656]
Chochinov HM et al. Effect of dignity therapy on distress and end-of-life experience in terminally ill patients: a randomised controlled trial. Lancet Oncol. 2011 Aug;12(8):753–62. [PMID: 21741309]
Rayner L et al. Antidepressants for the treatment of depression in palliative care: systematic review and meta-analysis. Palliat Med. 2011 Jan;25(1):36–51. [PMID: 20935027]

TASKS AFTER DEATH

After the death of a patient, the clinician is called upon to perform a number of tasks, both required and recommended. The clinician must plainly and directly inform the family of the death, complete a death certificate, contact an organ procurement organization, and request an autopsy. Providing words of sympathy and reassurance, time for questions and initial grief and, for people who die in the hospital or other health care facility, a quiet private room for the family is appropriate and much appreciated.

The Pronouncement & Death Certificate

In the United States, state policies direct clinicians to confirm the death of a patient in a formal process called "pronouncement." The diagnosis of death is typically easy to make, and the clinician need only verify the absence of spontaneous respirations and cardiac activity. Attempting to elicit pain in a patient who has died is unnecessary and disrespectful and should be avoided. A note describing these findings, the time of death, and that the family has been notified is entered in the patient's medical record. In many states, when a patient whose death is expected dies outside of the hospital (at home or in prison, for example), nurses may be authorized to report the death over the telephone to a physician who assumes responsibility for signing the death certificate within 24 hours. For traumatic deaths, some states allow emergency medical technicians to pronounce a patient dead at the scene based on clearly defined criteria and with physician telephonic or radio supervision.

While the pronouncement may often seem like an awkward and unnecessary formality, clinicians may use this time to reassure the patient's loved ones at the bedside that the patient died peacefully and that all appropriate care had been given. Both clinicians and families may use the ritual of the pronouncement as an opportunity to begin to process emotionally the death of the patient.

Physicians are legally required to report certain deaths to the coroner and to accurately report the underlying cause of death on the death certificate. This reporting is important both for patients' families (for insurance purposes and the need for an accurate family medical history) and for the epidemiologic study of disease and public health. The physician should be specific about the major cause of death being the condition without which the patient would not have died (eg, "decompensated cirrhosis") and its contributory cause (eg, "hepatitis B and hepatitis C infections, chronic alcoholic hepatitis, and alcoholism") as well as any associated conditions (eg, "acute kidney injury")—and not simply put down "cardiac arrest" as the cause of death.

Autopsy & Organ Donation

Discussing the options and obtaining consent for autopsy and organ donation with patients prior to death is usually the best practice. This approach advances the principle of patient autonomy and lessens the responsibilities of distressed family members during the period immediately following the death. In the case of brain death, designated organ transplant personnel are more successful than treating clinicians at obtaining consent for organ donation from surviving family members. Federal regulations require that a designated representative of an organ procurement organization approach the family about organ donation if the organs are appropriate for transplantation. Most people in the United States support the donation of organs for transplants. Currently, however, organ transplantation is severely limited by the availability of donor organs. Many potential donors and the families of actual donors experience a sense of reward in contributing, even through death, to the lives of others.

Clinicians must be sensitive to ethnic and cultural differences in attitudes about autopsy and organ donation. Patients or their families should be reminded of their right to limit autopsy or organ donation in any way they choose, although such restriction may limit the utility of autopsy. Pathologists can perform autopsies without interfering with funeral plans or the appearance of the deceased.

The results of an autopsy may help surviving family members and clinicians understand the exact cause of a patient's death and foster a sense of closure. A clinician–family conference to review the results of the autopsy provides a good opportunity for clinicians to assess how well families are grieving and to answer questions.

▶ Follow-up & Grieving

Proper care of patients at the end of life includes following up with surviving family members after the patient has died. Following up by telephone enables the clinician to assuage any guilt about decisions the family may have made, assess how families are grieving, reassure them about the nature of normal grieving, and identify complicated grief or depression. Clinicians can recommend support groups and counseling as needed. A card or telephone call from the clinician to the family days to weeks after the patient's death (and perhaps on the anniversary of the death) allows the clinician to express concern for the family and the deceased.

After a patient dies, the clinician also may need to grieve. Although clinicians may be relatively unaffected by the deaths of some patients, other deaths may cause feelings of sadness, loss, and guilt. These emotions should be recognized as the first step toward processing and healing them. Each clinician may find personal or communal resources that help with the process of grieving. Shedding tears, the support of colleagues, time for reflection, and traditional or personal mourning rituals all may be effective. Attending the funeral of a patient who has died can be a satisfying personal experience that is almost universally appreciated by families and that may be the final element in caring well for people at the end of life.

Morris SE et al. Adding value to palliative care services: the development of an institutional bereavement program. J Palliat Med. 2015 Nov;18(11):915–22. [PMID: 26275079]

Dermatologic Disorders

Kanade Shinkai, MD, PhD

Lindy P. Fox, MD

Dermatologic diseases are diagnosed by the types of lesions they cause. To make a diagnosis: (1) identify the type of lesion(s) the patient exhibits by morphology establishing a differential diagnosis (Table 6–1); and (2) obtain the elements of the history, physical examination, and appropriate laboratory tests to confirm the diagnosis. Specific clinical situations, such as an immunocompromised or critically ill patient, lead to different diagnostic considerations.

PRINCIPLES OF DERMATOLOGIC THERAPY

▶ Frequently Used Treatment Measures

A. Bathing

Soap should be used only in the axillae and groin and on the feet by persons with dry or inflamed skin. Soaking in water for 10–15 minutes before applying topical corticosteroids enhances their efficacy (Soak and Smear). Bath oils can be used, but add little above the use of moisturizers, and may make the tub slippery, increasing the risk of falling.

B. Topical Therapy

Nondermatologists should become familiar with a representative agent in each category for each indication (eg, topical corticosteroid, topical retinoid, etc).

1. Corticosteroids—Topical corticosteroid creams, lotions, ointments, gels, foams, and sprays are presented in Table 6–2. Topical corticosteroids are divided into classes based on potency. Agents within the same class are equivalent therapies; however, prices of even generic topical corticosteroids vary dramatically. **For a given agent, an ointment is more potent than a cream.** The potency of a topical corticosteroid may be dramatically increased by occlusion (covering with a water-impermeable barrier) for at least 4 hours. Depending on the location of the skin condition, gloves, plastic wrap, moist pajamas covered by dry pajamas (wet wraps), or plastic occlusive suits for patients can be used. Caution should be used in applying topical corticosteroids to areas of thin skin (face, scrotum, vulva, skin folds). Topical corticosteroid use on the eyelids may result in glaucoma or cataracts. One may estimate the amount of topical corticosteroid needed by using the "rule of nines"

(as in burn evaluation; see Figure 37–2). Approximately 20–30 g is needed to cover the entire body surface of an adult. Systemic absorption does occur, but adrenal suppression, diabetes mellitus, hypertension, osteoporosis, and other complications of systemic corticosteroids are very rare with topical corticosteroid therapy.

2. Emollients for dry skin ("moisturizers")—Dry skin is not related to water intake but to abnormal function of the epidermis. Many types of emollients are available. Petrolatum, mineral oil, Aquaphor, CeraVe, Cetaphil, and Eucerin cream are the heaviest and best. **Emollients are most effective when applied to wet skin.** If the skin is too greasy after application, pat dry with a damp towel. Vanicream is relatively allergen-free and can be used if allergic contact dermatitis to topical products is suspected.

The scaly appearance of dry skin may be improved by keratolytics including urea, lactic acid, or glycolic acid–containing products provided no inflammation (erythema or pruritus) is present.

3. Drying agents for weepy dermatoses—If the skin is weepy from infection or inflammation, drying agents may be beneficial. The best drying agent is water, applied as repeated compresses for 15–30 minutes, alone or with aluminum salts (Burow solution, Domeboro tablets).

4. Topical antipruritics—Lotions that contain 0.5% each of camphor and menthol (Sarna) or pramoxine hydrochloride 1% (with or without 0.5% menthol, eg, Prax, PrameGel, Aveeno Anti-Itch lotion) are effective antipruritic agents. Hydrocortisone, 1% or 2.5%, may be incorporated for its anti-inflammatory effect (Pramosone cream, lotion, or ointment). Doxepin cream 5% may reduce pruritus but may cause drowsiness. Pramoxine and doxepin are most effective when applied with topical corticosteroids. Topical capsaicin can be effective in some forms of neuropathic itch.

C. Systemic Antipruritic Drugs

1. Antihistamines—H_1-blockers are the agents of choice for pruritus when due to histamine, such as in urticaria. Otherwise, they appear to benefit itchy patients only by their sedating effects. Hydroxyzine 25–50 mg nightly is a typical dose. **Sedating and nonsedating antihistamines are of**

Table 6–1. Morphologic categorization of skin lesions and diseases.

Pigmented	Freckle, lentigo, seborrheic keratosis, nevus, blue nevus, halo nevus, atypical nevus, melanoma
Scaly	Psoriasis, dermatitis (atopic, stasis, seborrheic, chronic allergic contact or irritant contact), xerosis (dry skin), lichen simplex chronicus, tinea, tinea versicolor, secondary syphilis, pityriasis rosea, discoid lupus erythematosus, exfoliative dermatitis, actinic keratoses, Bowen disease, Paget disease, drug eruption
Vesicular	Herpes simplex, varicella, herpes zoster, pompholyx (vesicular dermatitis of palms and soles), vesicular tinea, autoeczematization, dermatitis herpetiformis, miliaria crystallina, scabies, photosensitivity, acute contact allergic dermatitis, drug eruption
Weepy or encrusted	Impetigo, acute contact allergic dermatitis, any vesicular dermatitis
Pustular	Acne vulgaris, acne rosacea, folliculitis, candidiasis, miliaria pustulosa, pustular psoriasis, any vesicular dermatitis, drug eruption
Figurate ("shaped") erythema	Urticaria, erythema multiforme, erythema migrans, cellulitis, erysipelas, erysipeloid, arthropod bites
Bullous	Impetigo, blistering dactylitis, pemphigus, pemphigoid, porphyria cutanea tarda, drug eruptions, erythema multiforme, toxic epidermal necrolysis, or other drug eruption
Papular	Hyperkeratotic: warts, corns, seborrheic keratoses Purple-violet: lichen planus, drug eruptions, Kaposi sarcoma, lymphoma cutis, Sweet syndrome Flesh-colored, umbilicated: molluscum contagiosum Pearly: basal cell carcinoma, intradermal nevi Small, red, inflammatory: acne, rosacea, miliaria rubra, candidiasis, scabies, folliculitis
Pruritus[1]	Xerosis, scabies, pediculosis, lichen planus, lichen simplex chronicus, bites, systemic causes, anogenital pruritus
Nodular, cystic	Erythema nodosum, furuncle, cystic acne, follicular (epidermal) inclusion cyst, metastatic tumor to skin
Photodermatitis (photodistributed rashes)	Drug eruption, polymorphic light eruption, lupus erythematosus
Morbilliform	Drug eruption, viral infection, secondary syphilis
Erosive	Any vesicular dermatitis, impetigo, aphthae, lichen planus, erythema multiforme, intertrigo
Ulcerated	Decubiti, herpes simplex, skin cancers, parasitic infections, syphilis (chancre), chancroid, vasculitis, stasis, arterial disease, pyoderma gangrenosum

[1]Not a morphologic class but included because it is one of the most common dermatologic presentations.

Table 6–2. Useful topical dermatologic therapeutic agents.

Agent	Formulations, Strengths, and Prices[1]	Frequency of Application	Potency Class	Common Indications	Comments
Corticosteroids					
Hydrocortisone acetate	Cream 1%: $1.38/30 g Ointment 1%: $3.99/30 g Lotion 1%: $5.84/120 mL	Twice daily	Low	Seborrheic dermatitis Pruritus ani Intertrigo	Not the same as hydrocortisone butyrate or valerate Not for poison oak, OTC lotion (Aquinil HC), OTC solution (Scalpicin, T Scalp)
	Cream 2.5%: $33.85/30 g			As for 1% hydrocortisone	Perhaps better for pruritus ani Not clearly better than 1% More expensive Not OTC
Alclometasone dipropionate (Aclovate)	Cream 0.05%: $48.07/15 g Ointment 0.05%: $20.00/15 g	Twice daily	Low	As for hydrocortisone	More efficacious than hydrocortisone Perhaps causes less atrophy
Desonide	Cream 0.05%: $80.29/15 g Ointment 0.05%: $240.40/60 g Lotion 0.05%: $296.10/60 mL	Twice daily	Low	As for hydrocortisone For lesions on face or body folds resistant to hydrocortisone	More efficacious than hydrocortisone Can cause rosacea or atrophy Not fluorinated

(continued)

Table 6–2. Useful topical dermatologic therapeutic agents. (continued)

Agent	Formulations, Strengths, and Prices[1]	Frequency of Application	Potency Class	Common Indications	Comments
Clocortolone (Cloderm)	Cream 0.1%: $260.38/30 g	Three times daily	Medium	Contact dermatitis Atopic dermatitis	Does not cross-react with other corticosteroids chemically and can be used in patients allergic to other corticosteroids
Prednicarbate (Dermatop)	Emollient cream 0.1%: $137.10/60 g Ointment 0.1%: $30.00/15 g	Twice daily	Medium	As for triamcinolone	May cause less atrophy No generic formulations Preservative-free
Triamcinolone acetonide	Cream 0.1%: $5.57/15 g Ointment 0.1%: $5.57/15 g Lotion 0.1%: $42.42/60 mL	Twice daily	Medium	Eczema on extensor areas Used for psoriasis with tar Seborrheic dermatitis and psoriasis on scalp	Caution in body folds, face Economical in 0.5-lb and 1-lb sizes for treatment of large body surfaces Economical as solution for scalp
	Cream 0.025%: $4.45/15 g Ointment 0.025%: $10.11/80 g	Twice daily	Medium	As for 0.1% strength	Possibly less efficacy and few advantages over 0.1% formulation
Fluocinolone acetonide	Cream 0.025%: $33.77/15 g Ointment 0.025%: $33.77/15 g	Twice daily	Medium	As for triamcinolone	
	Solution 0.01%: $180.00/60 mL	Twice daily	Medium	As for triamcinolone solution	
Mometasone furoate (Elocon)	Cream 0.1%: $26.75/15 g Ointment 0.1%: $24.30/15 g Lotion 0.1%: $55.45/60 mL	Once daily	Medium	As for triamcinolone	Often used inappropriately on the face or on children Not fluorinated
Diflorasone diacetate	Cream 0.05%: $209.68/15 g Ointment 0.05%: $419.35/30 g	Twice daily	High	Nummular dermatitis Allergic contact dermatitis Lichen simplex chronicus	
Fluocinonide (Lidex)	Cream 0.05%: $3.66/15 g Gel 0.05%: $59.56/15 g Ointment 0.05%: $6.54/15 g Solution 0.05%: $97.19/60 mL	Twice daily	High	As for betamethasone Gel useful for poison oak	Economical generics Lidex cream can cause stinging on eczema Lidex emollient cream preferred
Betamethasone dipropionate (Diprolene)	Cream 0.05%: $41.60/15 g Ointment 0.05%: $43.22/15 g Lotion 0.05%: $45.00/60 mL	Twice daily	Ultra-high	For lesions resistant to high-potency corticosteroids Lichen planus Insect bites	Economical generics available
Clobetasol propionate (Temovate)	Cream 0.05%: $128.23/15 g Ointment 0.05%: $155.45/15 g Lotion 0.05%: $288.96/60 mL	Twice daily	Ultra-high	As for betamethasone dipropionate	Somewhat more potent than diflorasone Limited to 2 continuous weeks of use Limited to 50 g or less per week Cream may cause stinging; use "emollient cream" formulation Generic available
Halobetasol propionate (Ultravate)	Cream 0.05%: $79.58/15 g Ointment 0.05%: $79.58/15 g	Twice daily	Ultra-high	As for clobetasol	Same restrictions as clobetasol Cream does not cause stinging Compatible with calcipotriene (Dovonex)

(continued)

Table 6–2. Useful topical dermatologic therapeutic agents. (continued)

Agent	Formulations, Strengths, and Prices[1]	Frequency of Application	Potency Class	Common Indications	Comments
Desoximetasone	Cream 0.05: $62.43/15 g 0.25%: $58.28/15 g Gel 0.05: $280.20/60 g Ointment 0.25%: $88.69/15 g	Twice daily	High	As for triamcinolone	Suggested for use when allergic contact dermatitis to topical corticosteroid is suspected; ointment useful when allergic contact dermatitis to propylene glycol is suspected
Flurandrenolide (Cordran)	Tape: $295.50/24" × 3" roll Lotion 0.05%: $394.68/60 mL	Every 12 hours	Ultra-high	Lichen simplex chronicus	Protects the skin and prevents scratching
Nonsteroidal anti-inflammatory agents					
Tacrolimus[2] (Protopic)	Ointment 0.1%: $277.81/30 g Ointment 0.03%: $277.81/30 g	Twice daily	N/A	Atopic dermatitis	Steroid substitute not causing atrophy or striae Burns in ≥ 40% of patients with eczema
Pimecrolimus[2] (Elidel)	Cream 1%: $296.83/30 g	Twice daily	N/A	Atopic dermatitis	Steroid substitute not causing atrophy or striae
Antibiotics (for acne)					
Clindamycin phosphate	Solution 1%: $40.81/30 mL Gel 1%: $86.38/30 mL Lotion 1%: $120.18/60 mL Pledget 1%: $46.40/60	Twice daily	N/A	Mild papular acne	Lotion is less drying for patients with sensitive skin
Dapsone	Gel 5%: $310.68/30 g	Once daily	N/A	Mild papulopustular acne	More expensive, well tolerated
Erythromycin	Solution 2%: $47.63/60 mL Gel 2%: $149.20/30 g Pledget 2%: $94.55/60	Twice daily	N/A	As for clindamycin	Many different manufacturers Economical
Erythromycin/ Benzoyl peroxide (Benzamycin)	Gel: $199.08/23.3 g Gel: $398.18/46.6 g	Twice daily	N/A	As for clindamycin Can help treat comedonal acne	No generics More expensive More effective than other topical antibiotics Main jar requires refrigeration
Clindamycin/ Benzoyl peroxide (BenzaClin)	Gel: $204.19/25 g Gel: $408.35/50 g	Twice daily	N/A	As for benzamycin	No generic More effective than either agent alone
Antibiotics (for impetigo)					
Mupirocin (Bactroban)	Ointment 2%: $42.75/22 g Cream 2%: $124.93/15 g	Three times daily	N/A	Impetigo, folliculitis	Because of cost, use limited to tiny areas of impetigo Used in the nose twice daily for 5 days to reduce staphylococcal carriage
Antifungals: Imidazoles					
Clotrimazole	Cream 1%: $5.29/15 g OTC Solution 1%: $45.13/10 mL	Twice daily	N/A	Dermatophyte and *Candida* infections	Available OTC Inexpensive generic cream available
Econazole (Spectazole)	Cream 1%: $104.40/15 g	Once daily	N/A	As for clotrimazole	Somewhat more effective than clotrimazole and miconazole
Ketoconazole	Cream 2%: $30.90/15 g	Once daily	N/A	As for clotrimazole	Somewhat more effective than clotrimazole and miconazole
Miconazole	Cream 2%: $5.50/30 g OTC	Twice daily	N/A	As for clotrimazole	As for clotrimazole

(continued)

Table 6–2. Useful topical dermatologic therapeutic agents. (continued)

Agent	Formulations, Strengths, and Prices[1]	Frequency of Application	Potency Class	Common Indications	Comments
Oxiconazole (Oxistat)	Cream 1%: $655.72/30 g Lotion 1%: $655.72/30 mL	Twice daily	N/A	As for clotrimazole	
Sertaconazole (Ertaczo)	Cream 2%: $908.52/60 g	Twice daily	N/A	Refractory tinea pedis	By prescription More expensive
Sulconazole (Exelderm)	Cream 1%: $62.05/15 g Solution 1%: $353.73/30 mL	Twice daily	N/A	As for clotrimazole	No generic Somewhat more effective than clotrimazole and miconazole
Other antifungals					
Butenafine (Mentax)	Cream 1%: $112.66/15 g	Once daily	N/A	Dermatophytes	Fast response; high cure rate; expensive Available OTC
Ciclopirox (Loprox) (Penlac)	Cream 0.77%: $51.10/30 g Lotion 0.77%: $96.15/60 mL Solution 8%: $52.95/6.6 mL	Twice daily	N/A	As for clotrimazole	No generic Somewhat more effective than clotrimazole and miconazole
Naftifine (Naftin)	Cream 1%: $375.38/60 g Gel 1%: $331.37/60 mL	Once daily	N/A	Dermatophytes	No generic Somewhat more effective than clotrimazole and miconazole
Terbinafine (Lamisil)	Cream 1%: $8.72/12 g OTC	Once daily	N/A	Dermatophytes	Fast clinical response OTC
Efinaconazole (Jublia)	Solution 10%: $645.43/4 mL	Once daily for 48 weeks	N/A	Onychomycosis	No generic; more effective than ciclopirox for nail disease
Tavaborole (Kerydin)	Solution 5%: $645.43/4 mL	Once daily for 48 weeks	N/A	Onychomycosis	No generic available
Antipruritics					
Camphor/ menthol (Sarna)	Lotion 0.5%/0.5%: $7.80/222 mL	Two to three times daily	N/A	Mild eczema, xerosis, mild contact dermatitis	
Pramoxine hydrochloride (Prax)	Lotion 1%: $17.86/120 mL OTC	Four times daily	N/A	Dry skin, varicella, mild eczema, pruritus ani	OTC formulations (Prax, Aveeno Anti-Itch Cream or Lotion; Itch-X Gel) By prescription mixed with 1% or 2% hydrocortisone
Doxepin (Zonalon)	Cream 5%: $568.46/30 g	Four times daily	N/A	Topical antipruritic, best used in combination with appropriate topical corticosteroid to enhance efficacy	Can cause sedation
Capsaicin (various)	Cream 0.025–0.1% 0.025%: $11.55/ 56.6 g 0.075%: $14.18/ 56.6 g	Three to four times daily	N/A	Topical antipruritic, best used for neuropathic itching	Burning/stinging with initial application that subsides with consistent ongoing use
Emollients					
Aveeno	Cream, lotion, others	Once to three times daily	N/A	Xerosis, eczema	Choice of emollient is most often based on personal preference by patient
Aqua glycolic	Cream, lotion, shampoo, others	Once to three times daily	N/A	Xerosis, ichthyosis, keratosis pilaris Mild facial wrinkles Mild acne or seborrheic dermatitis	Contains 8% glycolic acid Available from other makers, eg, Alpha Hydrox, or generic 8% glycolic acid lotion May cause stinging on eczematous skin

(continued)

Table 6–2. Useful topical dermatologic therapeutic agents. (continued)

Agent	Formulations, Strengths, and Prices[1]	Frequency of Application	Potency Class	Common Indications	Comments
Aquaphor	Ointment: $17.68/39.6	Once to three times daily	N/A	Xerosis, eczema For protection of area in pruritus ani	Not as greasy as petrolatum
Complex 15	Lotion: $6.48/240 mL Cream: $4.82/75 g	Once to three times daily	N/A	Xerosis Lotion or cream recommended for split or dry nails	Active ingredient is a phospholipid
DML	Cream, lotion, facial moisturizer: $5.95/240 mL	Once to three times daily	N/A	As for Complex 15	Face cream has sunscreen
Eucerin	Cream: $7.37/240 g Lotion: $5.10/240 mL	Once to three times daily	N/A	Xerosis, eczema	Many formulations made Eucerin Plus contains alphahydroxy acid and may cause stinging on eczematous skin Facial moisturizer has SPF 25 sunscreen
Lac-Hydrin-Five	Lotion: $11.37/226 g OTC	Twice daily	N/A	Xerosis, ichthyosis, keratosis pilaris	Prescription strength is 12% May sting on eczematous skin
Lubriderm	Lotion: $6.13/473 mL	Once to three times daily	N/A	Xerosis, eczema	Unscented usually preferred
Neutrogena	Cream, lotion, facial moisturizer: $7.58/240 mL	Once to three times daily	N/A	Xerosis, eczema	Face cream has titanium-based sunscreen
Ceratopic Cream	Cream: $60.00/6 oz	Twice daily	N/A	Xerosis, eczema	Contains ceramide; anti-inflammatory and nongreasy moisturizer
U-Lactin	Lotion: $14.00/480 mL OTC	Once daily	N/A	Hyperkeratotic heels	Moisturizes and removes keratin May sting on eczematous skin
Urea (various)	Cream 20%: $12.00/85 g Lotion 10%: $9.85/240 mL	Twice daily	N/A	Xerosis	Contains urea as humectant Nongreasy hydrating agent (10%); debrides keratin (20%)

[1]Average wholesale price (AWP, for AB-rated generic when available) for quantity listed. AWP may not accurately represent the actual pharmacy cost because wide contractual variations exist among institutions. Source: *Red Book Online, Truven Health Analytics Information*, http://www.micromedexsolutions.com, March 1, 2016.
[2]Topical tacrolimus and pimecrolimus should only be used when other topical treatments are ineffective. Treatment should be limited to an area and duration to be as brief as possible. Treatment with these agents should be avoided in persons with known immunosuppression, HIV infection, bone marrow and organ transplantation, lymphoma, at high risk for lymphoma, and those with a prior history of lymphoma. N/A, not applicable; OTC, over-the-counter.

limited value for the treatment of pruritus associated with inflammatory skin disease. Cumulative use of anticholinergics may be associated with increased risk of dementia. Agents that may treat pruritus better include antidepressants (such as doxepin, mirtazapine, and paroxetine) as well as agents that may act either centrally or peripherally directly on the neurons that perceive or modulate pruritus (such as gabapentin, pregabalin, and duloxetine). Aprepitant and opioid antagonists, such as naltrexone and butorphanol, can be very effective in select patients, but their exact role in the management of the pruritic patient is not yet defined.

2. Systemic corticosteroids—(See Chapter 26.)

American Academy of Dermatology. Medical student core curriculum. http://www.aad.org/education-and-quality-care/medical-student-core-curriculum

Gray SL et al. Cumulative use of strong anticholinergics and incident dementia: a prospective cohort study. JAMA Intern Med. 2015 Mar;175(3):401–7. [PMID: 25621434]
Skojec A et al. Variation in the cost of generic topical corticosteroids. JAMA Dermatol. 2015 Nov 1;151(11):1255–6. [PMID: 26288382]
van Zuuren EJ et al. No high level evidence to support the use of oral H₁ antihistamines as monotherapy for eczema: a summary of a Cochrane systematic review. Syst Rev. 2014 Mar 13; 3:25. [PMID: 24625301]
Yosipovitch G et al. Clinical practice. Chronic pruritus. N Engl J Med. 2013 Apr 25;368(17):1625–34. [PMID: 23614588]

▶ Sunscreens

Protection from ultraviolet light should begin at birth and will reduce the incidence of actinic keratoses, melanoma, and some nonmelanoma skin cancers when initiated at

any age. The best protection is shade, but protective clothing, avoidance of direct sun exposure during the peak hours of the day, and daily use of sunscreens are important.

Fair-complexioned persons should use a sunscreen with a sun protective factor (SPF) of at least 30 every day. Clinicians should reinforce regular sunscreen use. Sunscreens with SPF values greater than 30 usually afford some protection against UVA as well as UVB and are helpful in managing photosensitivity disorders. The actual SPF achieved is about one-quarter or less than that listed on the product due to insufficient application compared with the amount used in tests to determine the listed SPF. Repeated daily applications enhance sunscreen efficacy. Aggressive sunscreen use should be accompanied by vitamin D supplementation in persons at risk for osteopenia.

Agbai ON et al. Skin cancer and photoprotection in people of color: a review and recommendations for physicians and the public. J Am Acad Dermatol. 2014 Apr;70(4):748–62. [PMID: 24485530]

Akamine KL et al. Trends in sunscreen recommendation among US physicians. JAMA Dermatol. 2014 Jan;150(1):51–5. [PMID: 24005847]

Jansen R et al. Photoprotection by naturally occurring, physical, and systemic agents. J Am Acad Dermatol. 2013 Dec;69(6): 853.e1–12. [PMID: 24238179]

Jansen R et al. Photoprotection: part II. Sunscreen: development, efficacy, and controversies. J Am Acad Dermatol. 2013 Dec;69 (6):867.e1–14. [PMID: 24238180]

► Complications of Topical Dermatologic Therapy

Complications of topical therapy can be largely avoided. They fall into several categories: allergy, irritation, and other side effects.

A. Allergy

Of the topical antibiotics, neomycin and bacitracin have the greatest potential for sensitization. Diphenhydramine, benzocaine, vitamin E, aromatic oils, preservatives, fragrances, tea tree oil, and even the topical corticosteroids themselves can cause allergic contact dermatitis.

B. Irritation

Preparations of tretinoin, benzoyl peroxide, and other acne medications should be applied sparingly to the skin.

C. Other Side Effects

Topical corticosteroids may induce acne-like lesions on the face (steroid rosacea) and atrophic striae in body folds.

COMMON DERMATOSES

PIGMENTED LESIONS

MELANOCYTIC NEVI (NORMAL MOLES)

In general, **a benign mole is a small (less than 6 mm) macule or papule with a well-defined border and**

▲ **Figure 6–1.** Benign, flat and macular compound nevus on the arm. (Used, with permission, from Richard P. Usatine, MD in Usatine RP, Smith MA, Mayeaux EJ Jr, Chumley H, Tysinger J. *The Color Atlas of Family Medicine.* McGraw-Hill, 2009.)

homogeneous beige or pink to dark brown pigment. They represent benign melanocytic growths.

Moles have a typical natural history. Early in life, moles often appear as flat, small, brown lesions and are termed "junctional nevi" because the nevus cells are at the junction of the epidermis and dermis. Over time, these moles enlarge and often become raised, reflecting the appearance of a dermal component, giving rise to compound nevi (Figure 6–1). Moles may darken and grow during pregnancy. As white patients enter their eighth decade, most moles have lost their junctional component and dark pigmentation. At every stage of life, normal moles should be well demarcated, symmetric, and uniform in contour and color. Regular mole screening is not an evidence-based recommendation for all adults although rates of screening continue to rise.

Enamandram M et al. Delivering value in dermatology: insights from skin cancer detection in routine clinical visits. J Am Acad Dermatol. 2015 Feb;72(2):310–3. [PMID: 25484266]

Lakhani NA et al. Total body skin examination for skin cancer screening among U.S. adults from 2000 to 2010. Prev Med. 2014 Apr;61:75–80. [PMID: 24418263]

Mayer JE et al. Screening, early detection, education, and trends for melanoma: current status (2007–2013) and future directions: Part I. Epidemiology, high-risk groups, clinical strategies, and diagnostic technology. J Am Acad Dermatol. 2014 Oct;71(4):599.e1–599.e12. [PMID: 25219716]

Mayer JE et al. Screening, early detection, education, and trends for melanoma: current status (2007–2013) and future directions: Part II. Screening, education, and future directions. J Am Acad Dermatol. 2014 Oct;71(4):611.e1–611.e10. [PMID: 25219717]

Puig S et al. Monitoring patients with multiple nevi. Dermatol Clin. 2013 Oct;31(4):565–77. [PMID: 24075545]

Watts CG et al. Clinical practice guidelines for identification, screening and follow-up of individuals at high risk of primary cutaneous melanoma: a systematic review. Br J Dermatol. 2015 Jan;172(1):33–47. [PMID: 25204572]

Duffy K et al. The dysplastic nevus: from historical perspective to management in the modern era: part I. Historical, histologic, and clinical aspects. J Am Acad Dermatol. 2012 Jul;67 (1):1.e1–16. [PMID: 22703915]

Duffy K et al. The dysplastic nevus: from historical perspective to management in the modern era: part II. Molecular aspects and clinical management. J Am Acad Dermatol. 2012 Jul;67 (1):19.e1–12. [PMID: 22703916]

Kim CC et al. Addressing the knowledge gap in clinical recommendations for management and complete excision of clinically atypical nevi/dysplastic nevi: Pigmented Lesion Subcommittee consensus statement. JAMA Dermatol. 2015 Feb 1;151(2): 212–8. [PMID: 25409291]

Marghoob AA et al. Dermoscopy for the family physician. Am Fam Physician. 2013 Oct 1;88(7):441–50. [PMID: 24134084]

ATYPICAL NEVI

The term "atypical nevus" or "atypical mole" has supplanted "dysplastic nevus." The diagnosis of atypical moles is made clinically and not histologically, and moles should be removed only if they are suspected to be melanomas. Dermoscopy by a trained clinician may be a useful tool in the evaluation of atypical nevi. Clinically, these moles are large (6 mm or more in diameter), with an ill-defined, irregular border and irregularly distributed pigmentation (Figure 6–2). It is estimated that 5–10% of the white population in the United States has one or more atypical nevi, and **recreational sun exposure is a primary risk for the development of atypical nevi in nonfamilial settings**. Studies have defined an increased risk of melanoma in the following populations: patients with 50 or more nevi with one or more atypical moles and one mole at least 8 mm or larger, and patients with any number of definitely atypical moles. These patients should be educated in how to recognize changes in moles and be monitored regularly (every 6–12 months) by a clinician. Kindreds with familial melanoma (numerous atypical nevi and a family history of two first-degree relatives with melanoma) deserve even closer attention, as the risk of developing single or even multiple melanomas in these individuals approaches 50% by age 50.

BLUE NEVI

Blue nevi are small, slightly elevated, blue-black lesions (Figure 6–3) that favor the dorsal hands. They are common in persons of Asian descent, and an individual patient may have several of them. If the lesion has remained unchanged for years, it may be considered benign, since malignant blue nevi are rare. However, blue-black papules and nodules that are new or growing must be evaluated to rule out nodular melanoma.

▲ **Figure 6–3.** Blue nevus on the left cheek, with some resemblance to a melanoma. (Used, with permission, from Richard P. Usatine, MD in Usatine RP, Smith MA, Mayeaux EJ Jr, Chumley H, Tysinger J. *The Color Atlas of Family Medicine.* McGraw-Hill, 2009.)

▲ **Figure 6–2.** Atypical (dysplastic) nevus on the chest. (Used, with permission, from Richard P. Usatine, MD in Usatine RP, Smith MA, Mayeaux EJ Jr, Chumley H, Tysinger J. *The Color Atlas of Family Medicine.* McGraw-Hill, 2009.)

Cabral ES et al. Acquired blue nevi in older individuals: retrospective case series from a Veterans Affairs population, 1991 to 2013. JAMA Dermatol. 2014 Aug;150(8):873–6. [PMID: 24788980]

Longo C et al. Blue lesions. Dermatol Clin. 2013 Oct;31(4): 637–47. [PMID: 24075551]

FRECKLES & LENTIGINES

Freckles (ephelides) and lentigines are flat brown macules, typically between 3 mm and 5 mm in diameter. Freckles first appear in young children, darken with ultraviolet exposure, and fade with cessation of sun exposure. They are determined by genetic factors. In adults, lentigines gradually appear in sun-exposed areas, particularly the face, dorsal hands, upper back, and upper chest, starting in the fourth to fifth decade of life, and are associated with photoaging as well as estrogen and progesterone use. On the upper back, they may have a very irregular border (inkspot lentigines). They do not fade with cessation of sun exposure. They should be evaluated like all pigmented lesions: if the pigmentation is homogeneous and they are symmetric and flat, they are most likely benign. They can be treated with topical 0.1% tretinoin, 0.1% tazarotene, 2% 4-hydroxyanisole with 0.01% tretinoin, hydroquinone laser/light therapy, or cryotherapy.

Hexsel D et al. Triple combination as adjuvant to cryotherapy in the treatment of solar lentigines: investigator-blinded, randomized clinical trial. J Eur Acad Dermatol Venereol. 2015 Jan;29(1):128–33. [PMID: 24684165]

Praetorius C et al. Sun-induced freckling: ephelides and solar lentigines. Pigment Cell Melanoma Res. 2014 May;27(3): 339–50. [PMID: 24517859]

SEBORRHEIC KERATOSES

Seborrheic keratoses are benign papules and plaques, beige to brown or even black, 3–20 mm in diameter, with a velvety or warty surface (Figure 6–4). They appear to be stuck or pasted onto the skin. They are extremely common—especially in the elderly—and may be mistaken for melanomas or other types of cutaneous neoplasms. Although they may be frozen with liquid nitrogen or curetted if they itch or are inflamed, no treatment is needed.

Choi JW et al. Differentiation of benign pigmented skin lesions with the aid of computer image analysis: a novel approach. Ann Dermatol. 2013 Aug;25(3):340–7. [PMID: 24003278]

MALIGNANT MELANOMA

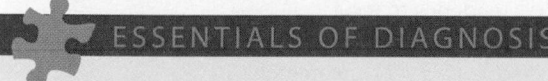

ESSENTIALS OF DIAGNOSIS

► May be flat or raised.

► Should be suspected in any pigmented skin lesion with recent change in appearance.

► Examination with good light may show varying colors, including red, white, black, and blue.

► Borders typically irregular.

▲ **Figure 6–4.** Seborrheic keratosis with "stuck-on appearance" but irregular borders and color variation suspicious for possible melanoma. (Used, with permission, from Richard P. Usatine, MD in Usatine RP, Smith MA, Mayeaux EJ Jr, Chumley H, Tysinger J. *The Color Atlas of Family Medicine.* McGraw-Hill, 2009.)

► General Considerations

Malignant melanoma is the leading cause of death due to skin disease. The reported incidence of melanoma has doubled over the past 30 years. In 2015, approximately 73,870 new melanomas were diagnosed in the United States, with 42,670 cases in men and 31,200 in women. Each year melanoma causes an estimated 9940 deaths (two-thirds in men). One in four cases of melanoma occurs before the age of 40. Increased detection of early melanomas has led to increased survival, but melanoma fatalities continue to increase, especially in men older than 70 years. The lifetime risk of melanoma is 2% in whites, and 0.1–0.5% in nonwhites.

Tumor thickness is the single most important prognostic factor. Ten-year survival rates—related to thickness in millimeters—are as follows: less than 1 mm, 95%; 1–2 mm, 80%; 2–4 mm, 55%; and greater than 4 mm, 30%. With lymph node involvement, the 5-year survival rate is 62%; with distant metastases, it is 16%.

► Clinical Findings

Primary malignant melanomas may be classified into various clinicohistologic types, including lentigo maligna melanoma (arising on chronically sun-exposed skin of older individuals); superficial spreading malignant melanoma (two-thirds of all melanomas arising on intermittently sun-exposed skin); nodular malignant melanoma; acral-lentiginous melanomas (arising on palms, soles, and nail beds); ocular melanoma; and malignant melanomas on mucous membranes. These different clinical types of melanoma appear to have different oncogenic mutations, which may be important in the treatment of patients with advanced disease. Clinical features of pigmented lesions suspicious for melanoma are an **irregular notched border where the pigment appears to be spreading into the**

▲ **Figure 6–5.** Malignant melanoma, with multiple colors and classic "ABCD" features. (Used, with permission, from Berger TG, Dept Dermatology, UCSF.)

normal surrounding skin; surface topography that may be irregular, ie, partly raised and partly flat (Figure 6–5). Color variegation is present and is an important indication for referral. A useful mnemonic is the ABCD rule: "ABCD = Asymmetry, Border irregularity, Color variegation, and Diameter greater than 6 mm." "E" for Evolution can be added. **The history of a changing mole (evolution) is the single most important historical reason for close evaluation and possible referral.** Bleeding and ulceration are ominous signs. A mole that appears distinct from the patient's other moles deserves special scrutiny—the "ugly duckling sign." A patient with a large number of moles is statistically at increased risk for melanoma and deserves annual total body skin examination by a primary care clinician or dermatologist, particularly if the lesions are atypical. Referral of suspicious pigmented lesions is always appropriate.

While superficial spreading melanoma is largely a disease of whites, persons of other races are still at risk for this and other types of melanoma, particularly acral lentiginous melanomas. These occur as dark, irregularly shaped lesions on the palms and soles and as new, often broad and solitary, darkly pigmented, longitudinal streaks in the nails, typically with involvement of the proximal nail fold. Acral lentiginous melanoma may be a difficult diagnosis because benign pigmented lesions of the hands, feet, and nails occur commonly in more darkly pigmented persons, and clinicians may hesitate to biopsy the palms, soles, and nail beds. As a result, the diagnosis is often delayed until the tumor has become clinically obvious and histologically thick. Clinicians should give special attention to new or changing lesions in these areas.

 Treatment

Treatment of melanoma consists of excision. After histologic diagnosis, reexcision is recommended with margins dictated by the thickness of the tumor. Thin low-risk and intermediate-risk tumors require margins of 1–3 cm.

Surgical margins of 0.5–1 cm for melanoma in situ and 1 cm for lesions less than 1 mm in thickness are recommended.

Sentinel lymph node biopsy (selective lymphadenectomy) using preoperative lymphoscintigraphy and intraoperative lymphatic mapping is effective for staging melanoma patients with intermediate risk without clinical adenopathy and is recommended for all patients with lesions over 1 mm in thickness or with high-risk histologic features (ulceration, high mitotic index). This procedure may not confer a survival advantage. Referral of intermediate-risk and high-risk patients to centers with expertise in melanoma is strongly recommended. Identifying the oncogenic mutations in patients with advanced melanoma may be important because many new treatments targeting oncogenic mutations and immunotherapy now exist.

Durham AB et al. Sentinel lymph node biopsy in melanoma: controversies and current guidelines. Future Oncol. 2014 Feb;10(3):429–42. [PMID: 24559449]

Eggermont AM et al. Cutaneous melanoma. Lancet. 2014 Mar 1; 383(9919):816–27. [PMID: 24054424]

Fox MC et al. Management options for metastatic melanoma in the era of novel therapies: a primer for the practicing dermatologist: Part I: management of stage III disease. J Am Acad Dermatol. 2013 Jan;68(1):1.e1–9. [PMID: 23244383]

Fox MC et al. Management options for metastatic melanoma in the era of novel therapies: a primer for the practicing dermatologist: Part II: management of stage IV disease. J Am Acad Dermatol. 2013 Jan;68(1):13.e1–13. [PMID: 23244384]

Watts CG et al. Clinical practice guidelines for identification, screening and follow-up of individuals at high risk of primary cutaneous melanoma: a systematic review. Br J Dermatol. 2015 Jan;172(1):33–47. [PMID: 25204572]

SCALING DISORDERS

ATOPIC DERMATITIS

ESSENTIALS OF DIAGNOSIS

► Pruritic, xerotic, exudative, or lichenified eruption on face, neck, upper trunk, wrists, and hands and in the antecubital and popliteal folds.

► Personal or family history of allergic manifestations (eg, asthma, allergic rhinitis, atopic dermatitis).

► Tendency to recur.

► Onset in childhood in most patients. Onset after age 30 is very uncommon.

General Considerations

Atopic dermatitis has distinct presentations in people of different ages and races. Diagnostic criteria for atopic dermatitis must include pruritus, typical morphology and distribution (flexural lichenification, hand eczema, nipple eczema, and eyelid eczema in adults), onset in childhood, and chronicity. Also helpful are: (1) a personal or family history of atopy (asthma, allergic rhinitis, atopic dermatitis), (2) xerosis-ichthyosis, (3) facial pallor with infraorbital darkening, (4) elevated serum IgE, and (5) repeated skin infections.

▶ Clinical Findings

A. Symptoms and Signs

Itching is a key clinical feature and may be severe and prolonged. Ill-defined, scaly, red plaques affect the face, neck, and upper trunk. The flexural surfaces of elbows and knees are often involved. In chronic cases, the skin is dry and lichenified. In dark-skinned patients with severe disease, pigmentation may be lost in lichenified areas. During acute flares, widespread redness with weeping, either diffusely or in discrete plaques, is common.

B. Laboratory Findings

Food allergy is an uncommon cause of flares of atopic dermatitis in adults. Eosinophilia and increased serum IgE levels may be present.

▶ Differential Diagnosis

Atopic dermatitis must be distinguished from seborrheic dermatitis (less pruritic, frequent scalp and central face involvement, greasy and scaly lesions, and quick response to therapy). Psoriasis is marked by sharply demarcated thickly scaled plaques on elbows, knees, scalp, and intergluteal cleft. Secondary staphylococcal or herpetic infections may exacerbate atopic dermatitis and should be considered during hyperacute, weeping flares of atopic dermatitis. An infra-auricular fissure is a cardinal sign of secondary infection. **Since virtually all patients with atopic dermatitis have skin disease before age 5, a new diagnosis of atopic dermatitis in an adult over age 30 should be made only after consultation.**

▶ Treatment

Patient education regarding gentle skin care and exactly how to use medications is critical to successful management of atopic dermatitis.

A. General Measures

Atopic patients have hyperirritable skin. Anything that dries or irritates the skin will potentially trigger dermatitis. Atopic individuals are sensitive to low humidity and often flare in the winter. Adults with atopic disorders should not bathe more than once daily. Soap should be confined to the armpits, groin, scalp, and feet. Washcloths and brushes should not be used. After rinsing, the skin should be patted dry (not rubbed) and then immediately—within minutes—covered with a thin film of an emollient or a corticosteroid as needed. Vanicream can be used if contact dermatitis resulting from additives in medication is suspected. Atopic patients may be irritated by rough fabrics, including wools and acrylics. Cottons are preferable, but synthetic blends also are tolerated. Other triggers of eczema in some patients include sweating, ointments, and heat.

B. Local Treatment

Corticosteroids should be applied sparingly to the dermatitis once or twice daily and rubbed in well. Their potency should be appropriate to the severity of the dermatitis. In general, for treatment of lesions on the body (excluding genitalia, axillary or crural folds), one should begin with triamcinolone 0.1% or a stronger corticosteroid then taper to hydrocortisone or another slightly stronger mild corticosteroid (alclometasone, desonide). It is vital that patients taper off corticosteroids and substitute emollients as the dermatitis clears to avoid side effects of corticosteroids. Tapering is also important to avoid rebound flares of the dermatitis that may follow their abrupt cessation. Tacrolimus ointment (Protopic 0.03% or 0.1%) and pimecrolimus cream (Elidel 1%) can be effective in managing atopic dermatitis when applied twice daily. Burning on application occurs in about 50% of patients using Protopic and in 10–25% of Elidel users, but it may resolve with continued treatment. These medications do not cause skin atrophy or striae, avoiding the complications of long-term topical corticosteroid use. They are safe for application on the face and even the eyelids but are more expensive than generic topical corticosteroids.

The US Food and Drug Administration (FDA) has issued a black box warning for both topical tacrolimus and pimecrolimus due to concerns about the development of T-cell lymphoma. The agents should be used sparingly and only in locations where less expensive corticosteroids cannot be used. They should be avoided in patients at high risk for lymphoma (ie, those with HIV, iatrogenic immunosuppression, or prior lymphoma).

The treatment of atopic dermatitis is dictated by the pattern and stage of the dermatitis—acute/weepy, subacute/scaly, or chronic/lichenified.

1. Acute weeping lesions— Staphylococcal or herpetic superinfection should be formally excluded. Use water or aluminum subacetate solution (Domeboro tablets, one in a pint of cool water), or colloidal oatmeal (Aveeno; dispense one box, and use as directed on box) as soothing or astringent soaks, baths, or wet dressings for 10–30 minutes two to four times daily. Lesions on extremities particularly may be bandaged for protection at night. Use high-potency corticosteroids after soaking, but spare the face and body folds. Tacrolimus is usually not tolerated at this stage. Systemic corticosteroids may be required.

2. Subacute or scaly lesions— At this stage, the lesions are dry but still red and pruritic. Mid- to high-potency corticosteroids in ointment form should be continued until scaling and elevated skin lesions are cleared and itching is decreased substantially. At that point, patients should begin a 2- to 4-week taper from twice-daily to daily dosing with topical corticosteroids to reliance on emollients, with occasional use of corticosteroids only to inflamed areas. It is preferable to switch to daily use of a low-potency corticosteroid instead of further tapering the frequency of usage of a more potent corticosteroid. Tacrolimus and pimecrolimus may be substituted if corticosteroids cannot be stopped completely.

3. Chronic, dry, lichenified lesions—Thickened and usually well demarcated, they are best treated with high-potency to ultra–high-potency corticosteroid ointments. Nightly occlusion for 2–6 weeks may enhance the initial response. Adding tar preparations, such as liquor carbonis detergens (LCD) 10% in Aquaphor or 2% crude coal tar may be beneficial.

4. Maintenance treatment—Once symptoms have improved, constant application of effective moisturizers is recommended to prevent flares. In patients with moderate disease, use of topical anti-inflammatories only on weekends or three times weekly can prevent flares.

C. Systemic and Adjuvant Therapy

Systemic corticosteroids are indicated only for severe acute exacerbations. Oral prednisone dosages should be high enough to suppress the dermatitis quickly, usually starting with 1 mg/kg daily for adults. The dosage is then tapered off over a period of 2–4 weeks. Owing to the chronic nature of atopic dermatitis and the side effects of long-term systemic corticosteroids, ongoing use of these agents is not recommended for maintenance therapy. Bedtime doses of hydroxyzine, diphenhydramine, or doxepin may be helpful via their sedative properties to mitigate perceived pruritus. Fissures, crusts, erosions, or pustules indicate staphylococcal or herpetic infection clinically. Systemic antistaphylococcal antibiotics—such as a first-generation cephalosporin or doxycycline if methicillin-resistant *Staphylococcus aureus* is suspected—should be given only if indicated and guided by bacterial culture. Cultures to exclude methicillin-resistant *S aureus* are recommended. In this setting, continuing and augmenting the topical anti-inflammatory treatment often improves the dermatitis despite the presence of infection. Oral cyclosporine, mycophenolate mofetil, methotrexate, interferon gamma, dupilumab (undergoing phase III trials), tofacitinib, or azathioprine may be used for the most severe and recalcitrant cases.

▶ Complications of Treatment

The clinician should monitor for skin atrophy. Eczema herpeticum, a generalized herpes simplex infection manifested by monomorphic vesicles, crusts, or scalloped erosions superimposed on atopic dermatitis or other extensive eczematous processes, is treated successfully with oral

acyclovir, 200 mg five times daily, or intravenous acyclovir in a dose of 10 mg/kg intravenously every 8 hours (500 mg/m^2 every 8 hours).

▶ Prognosis

Atopic dermatitis runs a chronic or intermittent course. Affected adults may have only hand dermatitis. Poor prognostic factors for persistence into adulthood in atopic dermatitis include generalized disease or onset early in childhood and asthma. Only 40–60% of these patients have lasting remissions.

Coenraads PJ. Eczema. N Engl J Med. 2012 Nov8;367(19): 1829–37. [PMID: 23134383]

Eichenfield LF et al. Guidelines of care for the management of atopic dermatitis: section 1. Diagnosis and assessment of atopic dermatitis. J Am Acad Dermatol. 2014 Feb;70(2): 338–51. [PMID: 24290431]

Eichenfield LF et al. Guidelines of care for the management of atopic dermatitis: section 2. Guidelines of care for the management and treatment of atopic dermatitis with topical therapies. J Am Acad Dermatol. 2014 Jul;71(1):116–32. [PMID: 24813302]

Sidbury R et al. Guidelines of care for the management of atopic dermatitis: section 3. Management and treatment with phototherapy and systemic agents. J Am Acad Dermatol. 2014 Aug;71(2):327–49. [PMID: 24813298]

Sidbury R et al. Guidelines of care for the management of atopic dermatitis: section 4. Prevention of disease flares and use of adjunctive therapies and approaches. J Am Acad Dermatol. 2014 Dec;71(6):1218–33. [PMID: 25264237]

Sugerman DT. JAMA patient page. Atopic eczema. JAMA. 2014 Feb 12;311(6):636. [PMID: 24519314]

PSORIASIS

 ESSENTIALS OF DIAGNOSIS

▶ Silvery scales on bright red, well-demarcated plaques, usually on the knees, elbows, and scalp.

▶ Nail findings including pitting and onycholysis (separation of the nail plate from the bed).

▶ Mild itching (usually).

▶ May be associated with psoriatic arthritis.

▶ Psoriasis patients are at increased risk for cardiovascular events, type 2 diabetes mellitus, metabolic syndrome, and lymphoma.

▶ Histopathology can be helpful to exclude clinical mimics.

▶ General Considerations

Psoriasis is a common benign, chronic inflammatory skin disease with both a genetic basis and known environmental triggers. Injury or irritation of normal skin tends to induce lesions of psoriasis at the site (Koebner phenomenon). Obesity worsens psoriasis, and significant weight loss in obese persons may lead to substantial improvement of their psoriasis. Psoriasis has several variants—the most common is the plaque type. Eruptive (guttate) psoriasis consisting of myriad lesions 3–10 mm in diameter occurs occasionally after streptococcal pharyngitis. Rarely, grave, occasionally life-threatening forms (generalized pustular and erythrodermic psoriasis) may occur.

▶ Clinical Findings

There are often no symptoms, but itching may occur and be severe. Favored sites include the scalp, elbows, knees, palms and soles, and nails. The lesions are red, sharply defined plaques covered with silvery scales (Figure 6–6). The glans penis and vulva may be affected. Occasionally, only the flexures (axillae, inguinal areas) are involved (termed **inverse psoriasis**). Fine stippling ("pitting") in the nails is highly suggestive of psoriasis (Figure 6–7). Patients with psoriasis often have a pink or red intergluteal fold (Figure 6–6). Not all patients have findings in all locations, but the occurrence of a few may help make the diagnosis when other lesions are not typical. Some patients have mainly hand or foot dermatitis and only

▲ **Figure 6–7.** Nail pitting due to psoriasis. (Used, with permission, from Richard P. Usatine, MD in Usatine RP, Smith MA, Mayeaux EJ Jr, Chumley H, Tysinger J. *The Color Atlas of Family Medicine.* McGraw-Hill, 2009.)

minimal findings elsewhere. There may be associated arthritis that is most commonly distal and oligoarticular, although the rheumatoid variety with a negative rheumatoid factor may occur. The psychosocial impact of psoriasis is a major factor in determining the treatment of the patient.

▶ Differential Diagnosis

The combination of red plaques with silvery scales on elbows and knees, with scaliness in the scalp or nail findings, is diagnostic. Psoriasis lesions are well demarcated and affect extensor surfaces—in contrast to atopic dermatitis, with poorly demarcated plaques in flexural distribution. In body folds, scraping and culture for *Candida* and examination of scalp and nails will distinguish "inverse psoriasis" from intertrigo and candidiasis. Dystrophic changes in nails may mimic onychomycosis, and a potassium hydroxide (KOH) preparation or fungal culture is valuable in diagnosis. The cutaneous features of reactive arthritis, pityriasis rosea, systemic lupus erythematosus, and syphilis mimic psoriasis.

▲ **Figure 6–6.** Plaque psoriasis in the sacral region and intergluteal fold. (Used, with permission, from Richard P. Usatine, MD in Usatine RP, Smith MA, Mayeaux EJ Jr, Chumley H, Tysinger J. *The Color Atlas of Family Medicine.* McGraw-Hill, 2009.)

▶ Treatment

There are many therapeutic options in psoriasis to be chosen according to the extent (body surface area [BSA] affected) and the presence of other findings (for example, arthritis). Certain medications, such as beta-blockers, antimalarials, statins, and lithium, may flare or worsen psoriasis. Even tiny doses of systemic corticosteroids given to patients with psoriasis may lead to severe rebound flares of their disease when they are tapered. **Systemic corticosteroids should never be used to treat flares of psoriasis.** Patients with moderate to severe psoriasis should be managed by or in conjunction with a dermatologist.

A. Limited Disease

High- to ultra–high-potency topical corticosteroids are the mainstay for limited disease (less than 10% BSA). For patients with numerous small plaques, phototherapy is the best therapy. For patients with large plaques and less than 10% of the BSA involved, the easiest regimen is to use a high-potency to ultra–high-potency topical corticosteroid cream or ointment. It is best to restrict the ultra–high-potency corticosteroids to 2–3 weeks of twice-daily use and then use them in a pulse fashion three or four times on weekends or switch to a mid-potency corticosteroid. Topical corticosteroids rarely induce a lasting remission. Additional measures are therefore commonly added to topical corticosteroid therapy. Calcipotriene ointment 0.005% or calcitriol ointment 0.003%, both vitamin D analogs, are used twice daily for plaque psoriasis. Initially, patients are treated with twice-daily corticosteroids plus a vitamin D analog twice daily. This rapidly clears the lesions. Calcipotriene usually cannot be applied to the groin or face because of irritation. Treatment of extensive psoriasis with vitamin D analogs may result in hypercalcemia, so that the maximum dose for calcipotriene is 100 g/week and for calcitriol is 200 g/week. Calcipotriene is incompatible with many topical corticosteroids (but not halobetasol), so if used concurrently, it must be applied at a different time.

For the scalp, start with a tar shampoo, used daily if possible. For thick scales, use 6% salicylic acid gel (eg, Keralyt), P & S solution (phenol, mineral oil, and glycerin), or fluocinolone acetonide 0.01% in oil (Derma-Smoothe/FS) under a shower cap at night, and shampoo in the morning. In order of increasing potency, triamcinolone 0.1%, fluocinolone, betamethasone dipropionate, amcinonide, and clobetasol are available in solution form for use on the scalp twice daily. For psoriasis in the body folds, treatment is difficult, since potent corticosteroids cannot be used and other agents are poorly tolerated. Tacrolimus ointment 0.1% or 0.03% or pimecrolimus cream 1% may be effective in intertriginous, genital, and facial psoriasis.

B. Moderate Disease

Psoriasis affecting 10–30% of the patient's BSA is frequently treated with UV phototherapy, either in a medical office or via a home light unit. Systemic agents listed below may also be used.

C. Generalized Disease

If psoriasis involves more than 30% of the body surface, it is difficult to treat with topical agents. The treatment of choice is outpatient narrowband UVB (NB-UVB) three times weekly. Clearing occurs in an average of 7 weeks, and maintenance may be required. Severe psoriasis unresponsive to outpatient ultraviolet light may be treated in a psoriasis day care center with the Goeckerman regimen, which involves use of crude coal tar for many hours and exposure to UVB light. Such treatment may offer the best chance for prolonged remissions.

Psoralen plus UVA (PUVA) photochemotherapy may be effective even in patients who have not responded to standard NB-UVB treatment. Long-term use of PUVA (greater than 250 doses) is associated with an increased risk of skin cancer (especially squamous cell carcinoma and perhaps melanoma) in persons with fair complexions. Thus, periodic examination (every 3–6 months) of the skin is imperative. Atypical lentigines are a common complication. There can be rapid aging of the skin in fair individuals. Cataracts have not been reported with proper use of protective glasses. PUVA may be used in combination with other therapy, such as acitretin or methotrexate.

Methotrexate is very effective for severe psoriasis in doses up to 25 mg once weekly. It should be used according to published protocols. Long-term methotrexate use may be associated with cirrhosis. After receiving a 3.5–4-g cumulative dose, the patient should be referred to a hepatologist for consideration of a liver biopsy. Administration of folic acid, 1–2 mg daily, can eliminate nausea caused by methotrexate without compromising efficacy.

Acitretin, a synthetic retinoid, is most effective for pustular psoriasis in dosages of 0.5–0.75 mg/kg/day. Liver enzymes and serum lipids must be checked periodically. Because acitretin is a teratogen and persists for 2–3 years in fat, women of childbearing age must wait at least 3 years after completing acitretin treatment before considering pregnancy. When used as single agents, retinoids will flatten psoriatic plaques, but will rarely result in complete clearing. Retinoids find their greatest use when combined with phototherapy—either UVB or PUVA, with which they are synergistic.

Cyclosporine dramatically improves psoriasis and may be used to control severe cases. Rapid relapse (rebound) is the rule after cessation of therapy, so another agent must be added if cyclosporine is stopped. The tumor necrosis factor (TNF) inhibitors etanercept (Enbrel), infliximab (Remicade), and adalimumab (Humira) are effective in pustular and chronic plaque psoriasis and are also effective for the associated arthritis. Infliximab provides the most rapid response and can be used for severe pustular or erythrodermic flares. Etanercept is used more frequently for long-term treatment at a dose of 50 mg twice weekly for 3 months, then 50 mg once weekly. All three TNF inhibitors can also induce or worsen psoriasis. IL-12/23 monoclonal antibodies (ustekinumab [Stelara], guselkumab), Janus kinase inhibitors (tofacitinib, undergoing phase III clinical trials), and IL-17 monoclonal antibodies (secukinumab, as well as the medications in clinical trials brodalumab and ixekizumab) are showing promise as alternative treatments. The phosphodiesterase 4 inhibitor apremilast is an approved option for plaque-type psoriasis with minimal immunosuppressive effects. Given the large number of psoriasis treatments available, consultation with a dermatologist is recommended when considering systemic treatment for moderate to severe psoriasis.

▶ Prognosis

The course tends to be chronic and unpredictable, and the disease may be refractory to treatment. Patients (especially those older than 40 years) should be monitored for metabolic syndrome, which correlates with the severity of their skin disease.

Armstrong AW et al. Combining biologic therapies with other systemic treatments in psoriasis: evidence-based, best-practice recommendations from the Medical Board of the National Psoriasis Foundation. JAMA Dermatol. 2015 Apr;151(4): 432–8. [PMID: 25517130]

Boehncke WH et al. Psoriasis. Lancet. 2015 Sep 5;386(9997): 983–94. [PMID: 26025581]

Lynch M et al. Treating moderate to severe psoriasis—best use of biologics. Expert Rev Clin Immunol. 2014 Feb;10(2):269–79. [PMID: 24372444]

Mason A et al. Topical treatments for chronic plaque psoriasis: an abridged Cochrane Systematic Review. J Am Acad Dermatol. 2013 Nov;69(5):799–807. [PMID: 24124809]

Signorovitch JE et al. Comparative efficacy of biological treatments for moderate-to-severe psoriasis: a network meta-analysis adjusting for cross-trial differences in reference arm response. Br J Dermatol. 2015 Feb;173(2):504–12. [PMID: 25288183]

PITYRIASIS ROSEA

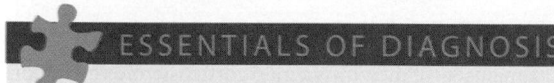

ESSENTIALS OF DIAGNOSIS

▶ Oval, fawn-colored, scaly eruption following cleavage lines of trunk.

▶ Herald patch precedes eruption by 1–2 weeks.

▶ Occasional pruritus.

▶ General Considerations

This is a common mild, acute inflammatory disease that is 50% more common in females. Young adults are principally affected, mostly in the spring or fall. Concurrent household cases have been reported.

▶ Clinical Findings

Itching is common but is usually mild. The diagnosis is made by finding one or more classic lesions. The lesions consist of oval, fawn-colored plaques up to 2 cm in diameter. The centers of the lesions have a crinkled or "cigarette paper" appearance and a collarette scale, ie, a thin bit of scale that is bound at the periphery and free in the center. Only a few lesions in the eruption may have this characteristic appearance, however. Lesions follow cleavage lines on the trunk (so-called Christmas tree pattern, Figure 6–8), and the proximal portions of the extremities are often involved. A variant that affects the flexures (axillae and groin), so-called "inverse pityriasis rosea," and a papular variant, especially in black patients, also occur. An initial lesion ("herald patch") that is often larger than the later lesions often precedes the general eruption by 1–2 weeks. The eruption usually lasts 6–8 weeks and heals without scarring.

▲ **Figure 6–8.** Pityriasis rosea with scaling lesions following skin lines and resembling a Christmas tree. (From EJ Mayeaux, MD; used, with permission, from Usatine RP, Smith MA, Mayeaux EJ Jr, Chumley H, Tysinger J. *The Color Atlas of Family Medicine.* McGraw-Hill, 2009.)

▶ Differential Diagnosis

A serologic test for syphilis, such as a rapid plasma reagin (RPR) test, should be performed if at least a few perfectly typical lesions are not present and especially if there are palmar and plantar or mucous membrane lesions or adenopathy, features that are suggestive of secondary syphilis. Tinea corporis may present with red, slightly scaly plaques, but rarely are there more than a few lesions of tinea corporis compared to the many lesions of pityriasis rosea. A potassium hydroxide examination should be performed to exclude a fungal cause. Seborrheic dermatitis on occasion presents on the body with poorly demarcated patches over the sternum, in the pubic area, and in the axillae. Tinea versicolor lacks the typical collarette rimmed lesions. Certain medications (eg, angiotensin-converting enzyme [ACE] inhibitors and metronidazole) and immunizations rarely may induce a skin eruption mimicking pityriasis rosea.

▶ Treatment

Pityriasis rosea often requires no treatment. In darker-skinned individuals, in whom lesions may remain hyperpigmented for some time, more aggressive management may be indicated. Treatment is, otherwise, indicated only if the patient is symptomatic. While adequately controlled and reproduced trials have not demonstrated widely effective treatments, most dermatologists recommend UVB treatments or a short course of prednisone for severe or severely symptomatic cases. For mild to moderate cases, topical corticosteroids of medium strength (triamcinolone 0.1%) and oral antihistamines may also be used if pruritus is bothersome. The role of macrolide antibiotics is controversial.

Prognosis

Pityriasis rosea is usually an acute self-limiting illness that typically disappears in about 6 weeks although prolonged variants have been reported.

Drago F et al. Persistent pityriasis rosea: an unusual form of pityriasis rosea with persistent active HHV-6 and HHV-7 infection. Dermatology. 2015;230(1):23–6. [PMID: 25612842]
Sinha S et al. Coexistence of two atypical variants of pityriasis rosea: a case report and review of literature. Pediatr Dermatol. 2012 Jul–Aug;29(4):538–40. [PMID: 21906158]

SEBORRHEIC DERMATITIS

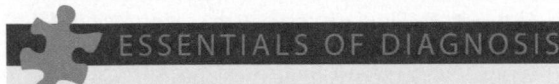

ESSENTIALS OF DIAGNOSIS

► Dry scales and underlying erythema.
► Scalp, central face, presternal, interscapular areas, umbilicus, and body folds.

General Considerations

Seborrheic dermatitis is an acute or chronic papulosquamous dermatitis that often coexists with psoriasis.

Clinical Findings

The scalp, face, chest, back, umbilicus, eyelid margins, genitalia, and body folds have dry scales (dandruff) or oily yellowish scurf (Figure 6–9). Pruritus is a variable

▲ **Figure 6–9.** Seborrheic dermatitis. (Used, with permission, from Berger TG, Dept Dermatology, UCSF.)

finding. Patients with Parkinson disease, HIV infection, and patients who become acutely ill often have seborrheic dermatitis.

Differential Diagnosis

There is a spectrum from seborrheic dermatitis to scalp psoriasis. Extensive seborrheic dermatitis may simulate intertrigo in flexural areas, but scalp, face, and sternal involvement suggests seborrheic dermatitis.

Treatment

A. Seborrhea of the Scalp

Shampoos that contain zinc pyrithione or selenium are used daily if possible. These may be alternated with ketoconazole shampoo (1% or 2%) used twice weekly. A combination of shampoos is used in refractory cases. Tar shampoos are also effective for milder cases and for scalp psoriasis. Topical corticosteroid solutions or lotions are then added if necessary and are used twice daily. (See treatment for scalp psoriasis, above.)

B. Facial Seborrheic Dermatitis

The mainstay of therapy is a mild corticosteroid (hydrocortisone 1%, alclometasone, desonide) used intermittently and not near the eyes. If the disorder cannot be controlled with intermittent use of a mild topical corticosteroid alone, ketoconazole (Nizoral) 2% cream is added twice daily. Topical tacrolimus (Protopic) and pimecrolimus (Elidel) are steroid-sparing alternatives.

C. Seborrheic Dermatitis of Nonhairy Areas

Low-potency corticosteroid creams—ie, 1% or 2.5% hydrocortisone, desonide, or alclometasone dipropionate—are highly effective.

D. Seborrhea of Intertriginous Areas

Apply low-potency corticosteroid lotions or creams twice daily for 5–7 days and then once or twice weekly for maintenance as necessary. Selenium lotion, ketoconazole, or clotrimazole gel or cream may be a useful adjunct. Tacrolimus or pimecrolimus topically may avoid corticosteroid atrophy in chronic cases.

E. Involvement of Eyelid Margins

"Marginal blepharitis" usually responds to gentle cleaning of the lid margins nightly as needed, with undiluted Johnson & Johnson Baby Shampoo using a cotton swab.

Prognosis

The tendency is for lifelong recurrences. Individual outbreaks may last weeks, months, or years.

Dessinioti C et al. Seborrheic dermatitis: etiology, risk factors, and treatments: facts and controversies. Clin Dermatol. 2013 Jul–Aug;31(4):343–51. [PMID: 23806151]

Gupta AK et al. Systematic review of oral treatments for sebor-rheic dermatitis. J Eur Acad Dermatol Venereol. 2014 Jan;28(1):16–26. [PMID: 23802806]

FUNGAL INFECTIONS OF THE SKIN

Mycotic infections are traditionally divided into two prin-cipal groups—superficial and deep. In this chapter, only the superficial infections are discussed: tinea corporis and tinea cruris; dermatophytosis of the feet and dermatophy-tid of the hands; tinea unguium (onychomycosis); and tinea versicolor. See Chapter 36 for discussion of deep mycoses.

The diagnosis of fungal infections of the skin is usually based on the location and characteristics of the lesions and on the following laboratory examinations: (1) Direct dem-onstration of fungi in 10% KOH evaluation of suspected lesions. **"If it's scaly, scrape it" is a time-honored maxim** (Figure 6–10). (2) Cultures of organisms from skin scrap-ings. (3) Histologic sections of biopsies stained with peri-odic acid-Schiff technique may be diagnostic if scrapings and cultures are falsely negative.

Principles of Treatment

A diagnosis should always be confirmed by KOH prepara-tion, culture, or biopsy. Many other diseases cause scaling,

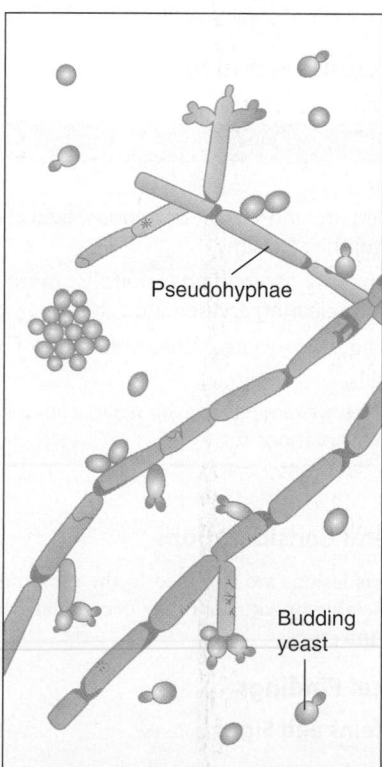

▲ **Figure 6–10.** KOH preparation of fungus demon-strating pseudohyphae and budding yeast forms. (Reproduced, with permission, from Nicoll D et al. *Pocket Guide to Diagnostic Tests*, 6th ed. McGraw-Hill, 2012.)

and use of an antifungal agent without a firm diagnosis makes subsequent diagnosis more difficult. In general, fun-gal infections are treated topically except for those with extensive involvement or involving the nails or hair follicles. In these situations, oral agents may be useful, with special attention to their side effects and complications, including hepatic toxicity.

General Measures & Prevention

Since moist skin favors the growth of fungi, dry the skin carefully after bathing or after perspiring heavily. Talc or other drying powders may be useful with the exception of powders containing corn starch, which may exacerbate fungal infections. The use of topical corticosteroids for other diseases may be complicated by intercurrent tinea or candidal infection, and topical antifungals are often used in intertriginous areas with corticosteroids to prevent this.

1. Tinea Corporis or Tinea Circinata

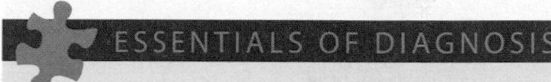

ESSENTIALS OF DIAGNOSIS

► Ring-shaped lesions with an advancing scaly bor-der and central clearing or scaly patches with a distinct border.
► Microscopic examination of scrapings or culture confirms the diagnosis.

General Considerations

The lesions are often on exposed areas of the body such as the face and arms. A history of exposure to an infected pet may occasionally be obtained, usually indicating *Microspo-rum* infection. *Trichophyton rubrum* is the most common pathogen, usually representing extension onto the trunk or extremities of tinea cruris, pedis, or manuum.

Clinical Findings

A. Symptoms and Signs

Itching may be present. In classic lesions, rings of ery-thema have an advancing scaly border and central clear-ing (Figure 6–11).

B. Laboratory Findings

The diagnosis should be confirmed by KOH preparation or culture.

Differential Diagnosis

Positive fungal studies distinguish tinea corporis from other skin lesions with annular configuration, such as the annular lesions of psoriasis, lupus erythematosus, syphilis, granuloma annulare, and pityriasis rosea. Psoriasis has typical lesions on elbows, knees, scalp, and nails.

▲ **Figure 6–11.** Tinea pedis and corporis. (Used, with permission, from Berger TG, Dept Dermatology, UCSF.)

Secondary syphilis is often manifested by characteristic palmar, plantar, and mucous membrane lesions. Tinea corporis rarely has the large number of symmetric lesions seen in pityriasis rosea. Granuloma annulare lacks scale.

► Complications

Complications include extension of the disease down the hair follicles (which presents as papules and pustules and is more difficult to cure) and pyoderma.

► Prevention

Treat infected household pets (*Microsporum* infections). To prevent recurrences, the use of foot powder and keeping feet dry by wearing sandals, or changing socks can be useful.

► Treatment

A. Local Measures

Tinea corporis responds to most topical antifungals, including econazole, miconazole, clotrimazole, butenafine, and terbinafine, most of which are available over the counter in the United States (see Table 6–2). Terbinafine and butenafine require shorter courses and lead to the most rapid response. **Treatment should be continued for 1–2 weeks after clinical clearing.** Betamethasone dipropionate with clotrimazole (Lotrisone) is not recommended. Long-term improper use may result in side effects from the high-potency corticosteroid component, especially in body folds.

B. Systemic Measures

Itraconazole as a single week-long pulse of 200 mg daily is also effective in tinea corporis. Terbinafine, 250 mg daily for 1 month, is an alternative.

► Prognosis

Tinea corporis usually responds promptly to conservative topical therapy or to an oral agent within 4 weeks.

El-Gohary M et al. Topical antifungal treatments for tinea cruris and tinea corporis. Cochrane Database Syst Rev. 2014 Aug 4; 8:CD009992. [PMID: 25090020]

2. Tinea Cruris (Jock Itch)

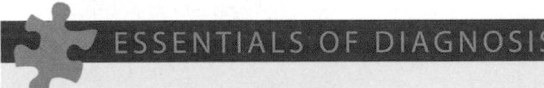

ESSENTIALS OF DIAGNOSIS

- ▶ Marked itching in intertriginous areas, usually sparing the scrotum.
- ▶ Peripherally spreading, sharply demarcated, centrally clearing erythematous lesions.
- ▶ May have associated tinea infection of feet or toenails.
- ▶ Laboratory examination with microscope or culture confirms diagnosis.

► General Considerations

Tinea cruris lesions are confined to the groin and gluteal cleft. Intractable pruritus ani may occasionally be caused by a tinea infection.

► Clinical Findings

A. Symptoms and Signs

Itching may be severe, or the rash may be asymptomatic. The lesions have sharp margins, cleared centers, and active, spreading scaly peripheries. Follicular pustules are sometimes encountered. The area may be hyperpigmented on resolution.

B. Laboratory Findings

Hyphae can be demonstrated microscopically in KOH preparations or skin biopsy. The organism may be cultured.

Differential Diagnosis

Tinea cruris must be distinguished from other lesions involving the intertriginous areas, such as candidiasis, seborrheic dermatitis, intertrigo, psoriasis of body folds ("inverse psoriasis"), and erythrasma. Candidiasis is generally bright red and marked by satellite papules and pustules outside of the main border of the lesion. *Candida* typically involves the scrotum. Seborrheic dermatitis also often involves the face, sternum, and axillae. Intertrigo tends to be more red, less scaly, and present in obese individuals in moist body folds with less extension onto the thigh. "Inverse psoriasis" is characterized by distinct plaques. Other areas of typical psoriatic involvement should be checked, and the KOH examination will be negative. Erythrasma is best diagnosed with Wood (ultraviolet) light—a brilliant coral-red fluorescence is seen.

Treatment

A. General Measures

Drying powder (eg, miconazole nitrate [Zeasorb-AF]) can be dusted into the involved area in patients with excessive perspiration or occlusion of skin due to obesity.

B. Local Measures

Any of the topical antifungal preparations listed in Table 6–2 may be used. Terbinafine cream is curative in over 80% of cases after once-daily use for 7 days.

C. Systemic Measures

One week of either itraconazole, 200 mg daily, or terbinafine, 250 mg daily, can be effective.

Prognosis

Tinea cruris usually responds promptly to topical or systemic treatment but often recurs.

3. Tinea Manuum & Tinea Pedis (Dermatophytosis, Tinea of Palms & Soles, "Athlete's Foot")

ESSENTIALS OF DIAGNOSIS

▶ Most often presents with asymptomatic scaling.

▶ May progress to fissuring or maceration in toe web spaces.

▶ May be a portal of entry for bacteria causing lower extremity cellulitis.

▶ Itching, burning, and stinging of interdigital web; scaling palms and soles; vesicles of soles in inflammatory cases.

▶ The fungus is shown in skin scrapings examined microscopically or by culture of scrapings.

General Considerations

Tinea of the feet is an extremely common acute or chronic dermatosis. Most infections are caused by *Trichophyton* species.

Clinical Findings

A. Symptoms and Signs

The presenting symptom may be itching, burning, or stinging. Pain may indicate secondary infection with complicating cellulitis. **Interdigital tinea pedis is the most common predisposing cause of lower extremity cellulitis in healthy individuals.** Regular examination of the feet of diabetic patients for evidence of scaling and fissuring and treatment of any identified tinea pedis may prevent complications. Tinea pedis has several presentations that vary with the location. On the sole and heel, tinea may appear as chronic noninflammatory scaling, occasionally with thickening and fissuring. This may extend over the sides of the feet in a "moccasin" distribution. The KOH preparation is usually positive. Tinea pedis often appears as a scaling or fissuring of the toe webs, often with maceration (Figure 6–12). As the web spaces become more macerated, the KOH preparation and fungal culture are less often positive because bacterial species begin to dominate. Finally, there may also be vesicles, bullae, or generalized exfoliation of the skin of the soles, or nail involvement in the form of discoloration, friability, and thickening of the nail plate.

B. Laboratory Findings

KOH and culture do not always demonstrate pathogenic fungi from macerated areas.

Differential Diagnosis

Differentiate from other skin conditions involving the same areas, such as interdigital erythrasma (use Wood light).

▲ **Figure 6–12.** Tinea pedis in the interdigital space between fourth and fifth digits. (Used, with permission, from Richard P. Usatine, MD in Usatine RP, Smith MA, Mayeaux EJ Jr, Chumley H, Tysinger J. *The Color Atlas of Family Medicine.* McGraw-Hill, 2009.)

Psoriasis may be a cause of chronic scaling on the palms or soles and may cause nail changes. Repeated fungal cultures should be negative, and the condition will not respond to antifungal therapy. Contact dermatitis will often involve the dorsal surfaces and will respond to topical or systemic corticosteroids. Vesicular lesions should be differentiated from pompholyx (dyshidrosis) and scabies by proper scraping of the roofs of individual vesicles. Rarely, gram-negative organisms may cause toe web infections, manifested as an acute erosive flare of interdigital disease. This entity is treated with aluminum salts and imidazole antifungal agents or ciclopirox. *Candida* may also cause erosive interdigital disease.

▶ Prevention

The essential factor in prevention is personal hygiene. Wear open-toed sandals if possible. Use of sandals in community showers and bathing places is often recommended, though the effectiveness of this practice has not been studied. Careful drying between the toes after showering is essential. A hair dryer used on low setting may be used. Socks should be changed frequently, and absorbent non-synthetic socks are preferred. Apply dusting and drying powders as necessary. The use of powders containing antifungal agents (eg, Zeasorb-AF) or long-term use of antifungal creams may prevent recurrences of tinea pedis.

▶ Treatment

A. Local Measures

1. Macerated stage—Treat with aluminum subacetate solution soaks for 20 minutes twice daily. Broad-spectrum antifungal creams and solutions (containing imidazoles or ciclopirox) will help combat diphtheroids and other gram-positive organisms present at this stage and alone may be adequate therapy. If topical imidazoles fail, 1 week of once-daily topical allylamine treatment (terbinafine or butenafine) will often result in clearing.

2. Dry and scaly stage—Use any of the antifungal agents listed in Table 6–2. The addition of urea 10–20% lotion or cream may increase the efficacy of topical treatments in thick ("moccasin") tinea of the soles.

B. Systemic Measures

Itraconazole, 200 mg daily for 2 weeks or 400 mg daily for 1 week, or terbinafine, 250 mg daily for 2–4 weeks, may be used in refractory cases. If the infection is cleared by systemic therapy, the patient should be encouraged to begin maintenance with topical therapy, since recurrence is common.

▶ Prognosis

For many individuals, tinea pedis is a chronic affliction, temporarily cleared by therapy only to recur.

Bell-Syer SE et al. Oral treatments for fungal infections of the skin of the foot. Cochrane Database Syst Rev. 2012 Oct 17; 10:CD003584. [PMID: 23076898]

Canavan TN et al. Identifying signs of tinea pedis: a key to understanding clinical variables. J Drugs Dermatol. 2015 Oct;14(10):s42–7. [PMID: 26461834]

4. Tinea Versicolor (Pityriasis Versicolor)

ESSENTIALS OF DIAGNOSIS

▶ Velvety, tan, or pink macules or white macules that do not tan with sun exposure.

▶ Fine scales that are not visible but are seen by scraping the lesion.

▶ Central upper trunk the most frequent site.

▶ Yeast and short hyphae observed on microscopic examination of scales.

▶ General Considerations

Tinea versicolor is a mild, superficial *Malassezia* infection of the skin (usually of the upper trunk). This yeast is a colonizer of all humans, which accounts for the high recurrence rate after treatment. The eruption is often called to patients' attention by the fact that the involved areas will not tan, and the resulting hypopigmentation may be mistaken for vitiligo. A hyperpigmented form is not uncommon.

▶ Clinical Findings

A. Symptoms and Signs

Lesions are asymptomatic, but a few patients note itching. The lesions are velvety, tan, pink, or white macules that vary from 4 mm to 5 mm in diameter to large confluent areas. The lesions initially do not look scaly, but scales may be readily obtained by scraping the area. Lesions may appear on the trunk, upper arms, neck, and groin.

B. Laboratory Findings

Large, blunt hyphae and thick-walled budding spores ("spaghetti and meatballs") are seen on KOH. Fungal culture is not useful.

▶ Differential Diagnosis

Vitiligo usually presents with larger periorificial and acral lesions and is also characterized by total (not partial) depigmentation. Vitiligo does not scale. Pink and red-brown lesions on the chest are differentiated from seborrheic dermatitis of the same areas by the KOH preparation.

▶ Treatment & Prognosis

Topical treatments include selenium sulfide lotion, which may be applied from neck to waist daily and left on for 5–15 minutes for 7 days; this treatment is repeated weekly for a month and then monthly for maintenance. Ketoconazole shampoo, 1% or 2%, lathered on the chest and back and left on for 5 minutes may also be used weekly for treatment and to prevent recurrence. Clinicians must stress to the patient that the raised and scaly aspects of the rash are being treated; the alterations in pigmentation may take months to fade or fill in.

Ketoconazole, 200 mg daily orally for 1 week or 400 mg as a single oral dose, with exercise to the point of sweating after ingestion, results in short-term cure of 90% of cases. Patients should be instructed not to shower for 8–12 hours after taking ketoconazole, because it is delivered in sweat to the skin. The single dose may not work in more hot and humid areas, and more protracted therapy carries a small risk of drug-induced hepatitis. Two doses of oral fluconazole, 300 mg, 14 days apart, has similar efficacy. Without maintenance therapy, recurrences will occur in over 80% of "cured" cases over the subsequent 2 years. Imidazole creams, solutions, and lotions are quite effective for localized areas but are too expensive for use over large areas such as the chest and back.

Gupta AK et al. Systematic review of systemic treatments for tinea versicolor and evidence-based dosing regimen recommendations. J Cutan Med Surg. 2014 Mar–Apr;18(2):79–90. [PMID: 24636433]

DISCOID & SUBACUTE LUPUS ERYTHEMATOSUS (Chronic Cutaneous Lupus Erythematosus)

ESSENTIALS OF DIAGNOSIS

▶ Localized violaceous red plaques, usually on the face and scalp.

▶ Scaling, follicular plugging, atrophy, dyspigmentation, and telangiectasia of involved areas.

▶ Distinctive histology.

▶ Photosensitivity.

General Considerations

The two most common forms of chronic cutaneous lupus erythematosus (CCLE) are chronic scarring (discoid) lesions (DLE) and erythematous non-scarring red plaques (subacute cutaneous LE) (SCLE). Both occur most frequently in photoexposed areas. Permanent hair loss and loss of pigmentation are common sequelae of discoid lesions. Systemic lupus erythematosus (SLE) is discussed in Chapter 20. Patients with SLE may have DLE or SCLE lesions.

Clinical Findings

A. Symptoms and Signs

Symptoms are usually mild. The lesions consist of violaceous red, well-localized, single or multiple plaques, 5–20 mm in diameter, usually on the head in DLE and the trunk in SCLE. In DLE, the scalp, face, and external ears (conchal

bowl) may be involved. In discoid lesions, there is atrophy, telangiectasia, depigmentation, and follicular plugging. On the scalp, significant permanent hair loss may occur in lesions of DLE. In SCLE, the lesions are erythematous annular or psoriasiform plaques up to several centimeters in diameter and favor the upper chest and back.

B. Laboratory Findings

In patients with DLE, the possibility of SLE should be considered if the following findings are present: positive antinuclear antibody (ANA), other positive serologic studies (eg, anti-double-stranded DNA or anti-Smith antibody), high erythrocyte sedimentation rate, arthralgias/arthritis, presence of hypocomplementemia, widespread lesions (not localized to the head), or nail changes. Patients with marked photosensitivity and a picture otherwise suggestive of lupus may have negative ANA tests but are positive for antibodies against Ro/SSA or La/SSB (SCLE).

▶ Differential Diagnosis

The diagnosis is based on the clinical appearance confirmed by skin biopsy in all cases. In DLE, the scales are dry and "thumbtack-like" and can thus be distinguished from those of seborrheic dermatitis and psoriasis. Older lesions that have left depigmented scarring or areas of hair loss will also differentiate lupus from these diseases. Ten percent of patients with SLE have discoid skin lesions, and 5% of patients with discoid lesions have SLE. Medications (most commonly, hydrochlorothiazide, calcium channel blockers, H_2-blockers and proton pump inhibitors, ACE inhibitors, TNF inhibitors, and terbinafine) may induce SCLE with a positive Ro/SSA.

▶ Treatment

A. General Measures

Protect from sunlight. Use high-SPF (more than 50) sunblock with UVB and UVA coverage daily. **Caution:** do not use any form of radiation therapy. Avoid using medications that are potentially photosensitizing when possible.

B. Local Treatment

For limited lesions, the following should be tried before systemic therapy: high-potency corticosteroid creams applied each night and covered with airtight, thin, pliable plastic film (eg, Saran Wrap); Cordran tape; or ultra–high-potency corticosteroid cream or ointment applied twice daily without occlusion.

C. Local Infiltration

Triamcinolone acetonide suspension, 2.5–10 mg/mL, may be injected into the lesions of DLE once a month.

D. Systemic Treatment

1. Antimalarials—Caution: these medications should be used only when the diagnosis is secure because they have been associated with flares of psoriasis, which may be in the differential diagnosis.

A. Hydroxychloroquine sulfate—0.2–0.4 g orally daily for several months may be effective and is often used prior to chloroquine. A minimum 3-month trial is recommended.

B. Chloroquine sulfate—250 mg daily may be effective in some cases where hydroxychloroquine is not.

C. Quinacrine (atabrine)—100 mg daily may be the safest of the antimalarials, since eye damage has not been reported. It colors the skin yellow and is therefore not acceptable to some patients. It may be added to the other antimalarials for patients with incomplete responses.

2. Isotretinoin—Isotretinoin, 1 mg/kg/day, is effective in hypertrophic DLE lesions.

3. Thalidomide—Thalidomide is effective in refractory cases in doses of 50–300 mg daily. Monitor for neuropathy.

Both isotretinoin and thalidomide are teratogens and should be used with appropriate contraception and monitoring in women of childbearing age.

Prognosis

The disease is persistent but not life-endangering unless systemic lupus is present. Treatment with one or more antimalarials is effective in more than half of cases. **Although the only morbidity may be cosmetic, this can be of overwhelming significance in more darkly pigmented patients with widespread disease.** Scarring alopecia can be prevented or lessened with close attention and aggressive therapy. Over years, DLE tends to become inactive. Drug-induced SCLE usually resolves over months when the inciting medication is stopped.

Grönhagen CM et al. Subacute cutaneous lupus erythematosus and its association with drugs: a population-based matched case-control study of 234 patients in Sweden. Br J Dermatol. 2012 Aug;167(2):296–305. [PMID: 22458771]
Merola JF et al. Association of discoid lupus erythematosus with other clinical manifestations among patients with systemic lupus erythematosus. J Am Acad Dermatol. 2013 Jul;69(1):19–24. [PMID: 23541758]
Okon LG et al. Cutaneous lupus erythematosus: diagnosis and treatment. Best Pract Res Clin Rheumatol. 2013 Jun;27(3):391–404. [PMID: 24238695]
Wieczorek IT et al. Systemic symptoms in the progression of cutaneous to systemic lupus erythematosus. JAMA Dermatol. 2014 Mar;150(3):291–6. [PMID: 24477339]

CUTANEOUS T-CELL LYMPHOMA (Mycosis Fungoides)

ESSENTIALS OF DIAGNOSIS

► Localized or generalized erythematous scaling patches that progress to plaques and nodules.
► Pruritus.
► Lymphadenopathy.
► Distinctive histology.

General Considerations

Mycosis fungoides is a cutaneous T-cell lymphoma that begins on the skin and may involve only the skin for years or decades. It may progress to systemic disease, including **Sézary syndrome** (erythroderma with circulating malignant T cells).

Clinical Findings

A. Symptoms and Signs

Localized or generalized erythematous scaly patches or plaques are present usually on the trunk. Plaques are almost always over 5 cm in diameter. Pruritus is a frequent complaint and can be severe. The lesions often begin as nondescript or nondiagnostic patches, and it is not unusual for the patient to have skin lesions for more than a decade before the diagnosis can be confirmed. Follicular involvement with hair loss is characteristic of mycosis fungoides, and its presence should raise the suspicion of mycosis fungoides for any pruritic eruption. In more advanced cases, tumors appear. Lymphadenopathy may occur locally or widely. Lymph node enlargement may be due to benign expansion of the node (dermatopathic lymphadenopathy) or by specific involvement with mycosis fungoides.

B. Laboratory Findings

The skin biopsy remains the basis of diagnosis, though at times numerous biopsies are required before the diagnosis can be confirmed. In more advanced disease, circulating malignant T cells (Sézary cells) can be detected in the blood (T-cell gene rearrangement test). Eosinophilia may be present.

Differential Diagnosis

Mycosis fungoides may be confused with psoriasis, a drug eruption (including to serotonin reuptake inhibitors), photoallergy, an eczematous dermatitis, or tinea corporis. Histologic examination can distinguish these conditions.

Treatment

The treatment of mycosis fungoides is complex. Early and aggressive treatment has not been proven to cure or prevent disease progression. Skin-directed therapies, including topical corticosteroids, topical mechlorethamine, bexarotene gel, and UV phototherapy, are used initially. If the disease progresses, PUVA plus retinoids, PUVA plus interferon, extracorporeal photophoresis, bexarotene, alpha-interferon with or without retinoids, interleukin 12, denileukin, and total skin electron beam treatment are used.

Prognosis

Mycosis fungoides is usually slowly progressive (over decades). Prognosis is better in patients with patch or plaque stage disease and worse in patients with erythroderma, tumors, and lymphadenopathy. Survival is not reduced in patients with limited patch disease. Elderly patients with limited patch and plaque stage disease commonly die of other causes. Overly aggressive treatment may lead to complications and premature demise.

Ai WZ et al. Outcomes after diagnosis of mycosis fungoides and Sézary syndrome before 30 years of age: a population-based study. JAMA Dermatol. 2014 Jul;150(7):709–15. [PMID: 24718769]

DeSimone JA et al. Recent advances in primary cutaneous T-cell lymphoma. Curr Opin Oncol. 2015 Mar;27(2):128–33. [PMID: 25594623]

Jawed SI et al. Primary cutaneous T-cell lymphoma (mycosis fungoides and Sézary syndrome): part I. Diagnosis: clinical and histopathologic features and new molecular and biologic markers. J Am Acad Dermatol. 2014 Feb;70(2):205.e1–16. [PMID: 24438969]

Jawed SI et al. Primary cutaneous T-cell lymphoma (mycosis fungoides and Sézary syndrome): part II. Prognosis, management, and future directions. J Am Acad Dermatol. 2014 Feb;70(2):223.e1–17. [PMID: 24438970]

EXFOLIATIVE DERMATITIS (Exfoliative Erythroderma)

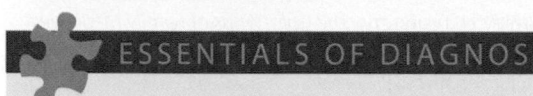

ESSENTIALS OF DIAGNOSIS

▶ Scaling and erythema over most of the body.
▶ Itching, malaise, fever, chills, weight loss.

General Considerations

Erythroderma describes generalized redness and scaling of the skin of more than 30% BSA. A preexisting dermatosis is the cause of exfoliative dermatitis in two-thirds of cases, including psoriasis, atopic dermatitis, contact dermatitis, pityriasis rubra pilaris, and seborrheic dermatitis. Reactions to topical or systemic medications account for about 15% of cases, cancer (underlying lymphoma, solid tumors and, most commonly, cutaneous T-cell lymphoma) for about 10%, and 10% are idiopathic. Widespread scabies is an important diagnostic consideration since patients with erythrodermic presentation are highly contagious. At the time of acute presentation, without a clear-cut prior history of skin disease or medication exposure, it may be impossible to make a specific diagnosis of the underlying condition, and diagnosis may require continued observation.

Clinical Findings

A. Symptoms and Signs

Symptoms may include itching, weakness, malaise, fever, and weight loss. Chills are prominent. Erythema and scaling are widespread. Loss of hair and nails can occur. Generalized lymphadenopathy may be due to lymphoma or leukemia or may be reactive. The mucosae are typically spared.

B. Laboratory Findings

A skin biopsy is required and may show changes of a specific inflammatory dermatitis or cutaneous T-cell lymphoma. Peripheral leukocytes may show clonal rearrangements of the T-cell receptor in Sézary syndrome.

Differential Diagnosis

It may be impossible to identify the cause of exfoliative erythroderma early in the course of the disease, so careful follow-up is necessary.

Complications

Protein and electrolyte loss as well as dehydration may develop in patients with generalized inflammatory exfoliative erythroderma; or sepsis may occur.

Treatment

A. Topical Therapy

Home treatment is with cool to tepid baths and application of mid-potency corticosteroids under wet dressings or with the use of an occlusive plastic suit. If the exfoliative erythroderma becomes chronic and is not manageable in an outpatient setting, the patient should be hospitalized. Keep the room at a constant warm temperature and provide the same topical treatment as for an outpatient.

B. Specific Measures

Stop all medications, if possible. Systemic corticosteroids may provide spectacular improvement in severe or fulminant exfoliative dermatitis, but long-term therapy should be avoided (see Chapter 26). In addition, systemic corticosteroids must be used with caution because some patients with erythroderma have psoriasis and could develop pustular flare. For cases of psoriatic erythroderma and pityriasis rubra pilaris, acitretin, methotrexate, cyclosporine, or a TNF inhibitor may be indicated. Erythroderma secondary to lymphoma or leukemia requires specific topical or systemic chemotherapy. Suitable antibiotic medications with coverage for *Staphylococcus* should be given when there is evidence of bacterial infection.

Prognosis

Most patients recover completely or improve greatly over time but may require long-term therapy. Deaths are rare in the absence of cutaneous T-cell lymphoma. A minority of patients will suffer from undiminished erythroderma for indefinite periods.

Li J et al. Erythroderma: a clinical and prognostic study. Dermatology. 2012;225(2):154–62. [PMID: 23037884]
Zattra E et al. Erythroderma in the era of biological therapies. Eur J Dermatol. 2012 Mar–Apr;22(2):167–71. [PMID: 22321651]

MISCELLANEOUS SCALING DERMATOSES

Isolated scaly patches may represent actinic (solar) keratoses, nonpigmented seborrheic keratoses, or Bowen or Paget disease.

1. Actinic Keratoses

Actinic keratoses are small (0.2–0.6 cm) macules or papules—flesh-colored, pink, or slightly hyperpigmented—that **feel like sandpaper** and are tender when the finger is drawn over them. They occur on sun-exposed parts of the body in persons of fair complexion. Actinic keratoses are considered premalignant, but only 1:1000 lesions per year progress to become squamous cell carcinomas.

Application of liquid nitrogen is a rapid method of eradication. The lesions crust and disappear in 10–14 days. "Field treatment" with a topical agent to the anatomic area where the actinic keratoses are most prevalent (eg, forehead, dorsal hands, etc) can be considered in patients with multiple lesions in one region. The topical agents used for field treatment include fluorouracil, imiquimod, and ingenol mebutate. Photodynamic therapy can be effective in cases refractory to topical treatment. Any lesions that persist should be evaluated for possible biopsy.

Patel G et al. Efficacy of photodynamic therapy vs other interventions in randomized clinical trials for the treatment of actinic keratoses: a systematic review and meta-analysis. JAMA Dermatol. 2014 Dec;150(12):1281–8. [PMID: 25162181]

Werner RN et al. Evidence- and consensus-based (S3) guidelines for the treatment of actinic keratosis – International League of Dermatological Societies in cooperation with the European Dermatology Forum – short version. J Eur Acad Dermatol Venereol. 2015 Nov;29(11):2069–79. [PMID: 26370093]

Werner RN et al. The natural history of actinic keratosis: a systematic review. Br J Dermatol. 2013 Sep;169(3):502–18. [PMID: 23647091]

2. Bowen Disease & Paget Disease

Bowen disease (intraepidermal squamous cell carcinoma) can develop on both sun-exposed and non–sun-exposed skin. The lesion is usually a small (0.5–3 cm), well-demarcated, slightly raised, pink to red, scaly plaque and may resemble psoriasis or a large actinic keratosis. These lesions may progress to invasive squamous cell carcinoma. Excision or other definitive treatment is indicated.

Extramammary Paget disease, a manifestation of intraepidermal carcinoma or underlying genitourinary or gastrointestinal cancer, resembles chronic eczema and usually involves apocrine areas such as the genitalia. **Mammary Paget disease of the nipple**, a unilateral or rarely bilateral red scaling plaque that may ooze, is associated with an underlying intraductal mammary carcinoma (Figure 6–13). While these lesions appear as red patches and plaques in fair-skinned persons, in darker-skinned individuals, hyperpigmentation may be prominent.

Bath-Hextall FJ et al. Interventions for cutaneous Bowen's disease. Cochrane Database Syst Rev. 2013 Jun 24;6:CD007281. [PMID: 23794286]

Edey KA et al. Interventions for the treatment of Paget's disease of the vulva. Cochrane Database Syst Rev. 2013 Oct 26; 10:CD009245. [PMID: 24163070]

Morton CA et al. British Association of Dermatologists' guidelines for the management of squamous cell carcinoma in situ (Bowen's disease) 2014. Br J Dermatol. 2014 Feb;170(2): 245–60. [PMID: 24313974]

INTERTRIGO

Intertrigo is caused by the macerating effect of heat, moisture, and friction. It is especially likely to occur in obese persons and in humid climates. The symptoms are

▲ **Figure 6–13.** Paget disease of the breast surrounding the nipple. (From the University of Texas Health Sciences Center, Division of Dermatology; used, with permission, from Usatine RP, Smith MA, Mayeaux EJ Jr, Chumley H, Tysinger J. *The Color Atlas of Family Medicine.* McGraw-Hill, 2009.)

itching, stinging, and burning. The body folds develop fissures, erythema, and sodden epidermis, with superficial denudation. Candidiasis may complicate intertrigo. "Inverse psoriasis," seborrheic dermatitis, tinea cruris, erythrasma, and candidiasis must be ruled out.

Maintain hygiene in the area, and keep it dry. Compresses may be useful acutely. Hydrocortisone 1% cream plus an imidazole or clotrimazole 1% cream is effective. Recurrences are common.

Kalra MG et al. Intertrigo and secondary skin infections. Am Fam Physician. 2014 Apr 1;89(7):569–73. [PMID: 24695603]

VESICULAR DERMATOSES

HERPES SIMPLEX (Cold or Fever Sore; Genital Herpes)

 ESSENTIALS OF DIAGNOSIS

▶ Recurrent small grouped vesicles on an erythematous base, especially in the orolabial and genital areas.

▶ May follow minor infections, trauma, stress, or sun exposure; regional lymph nodes may be swollen and tender.

▶ Viral cultures and direct fluorescent antibody tests are positive.

▶ General Considerations

Over 85% of adults have serologic evidence of herpes simplex type 1 (HSV-1) infections, most often acquired asymptomatically in childhood. Occasionally, primary infections may be manifested as severe gingivostomatitis. Thereafter, the patient may have recurrent self-limited attacks, provoked by sun exposure, orofacial surgery, fever, or a viral infection.

About 25% of the United States population has serologic evidence of infection with herpes simplex type 2 (HSV-2). HSV-2 causes lesions whose morphology and natural history are similar to those caused by HSV-1 but are typically located on the genitalia of both sexes. The infection is acquired by sexual contact. In monogamous heterosexual couples where one partner has HSV-2 infection, **seroconversion of the noninfected partner occurs in 10% over a 1-year period. Up to 70% of such infections appeared to be transmitted during periods of asymptomatic shedding.** Genital herpes may also be due to HSV-1.

▶ Clinical Findings

A. Symptoms and Signs

The principal symptoms are burning and stinging. Neuralgia may precede or accompany attacks. The lesions consist of small, grouped vesicles that can occur anywhere but which most often occur on the vermilion border of the lips (Figure 6–14), the penile shaft, the labia, the perianal skin, and the buttocks. Any erosion or fissure in the anogenital region can be due to herpes simplex. Regional lymph nodes may be swollen and tender. The lesions usually crust and heal in 1 week. Immunosuppressed patients may have unusual variants, including verrucous or nodular herpes lesions at typical sites of involvement.

B. Laboratory Findings

Lesions of herpes simplex must be distinguished from chancroid, syphilis, pyoderma, or trauma. Direct fluorescent antibody slide tests offer rapid, sensitive diagnosis. Viral culture may also be helpful. Herpes serology is not used in the diagnosis of an acute genital ulcer. However, specific HSV-2 serology by Western blot assay or enzyme-linked immunosorbent assay (ELISA) can determine who is HSV-infected and potentially infectious. Such testing is very useful in couples in which only one partner reports a history of genital herpes.

▶ Complications

Complications include pyoderma, eczema herpeticum, herpetic whitlow, herpes gladiatorum (epidemic herpes in wrestlers transmitted by contact), proctitis, esophagitis, neonatal infection, keratitis, and encephalitis.

▶ Treatment

A. Systemic Therapy

Three systemic agents are available for the treatment of herpes infections: acyclovir, its valine analog valacyclovir, and famciclovir. All three agents are very effective, and when used properly, virtually nontoxic. Only acyclovir is available for intravenous administration. In the immunocompetent, with the exception of severe orolabial herpes, only genital disease is treated. For first clinical episodes of herpes simplex, the dosage of acyclovir is 400 mg orally five times daily (or 800 mg three times daily); of valacyclovir, 1000 mg twice daily; and of famciclovir, 250 mg three times daily. The duration of treatment is from 7 to 10 days depending on the severity of the outbreak.

Most cases of recurrent herpes are mild and do not require therapy. In addition, pharmacotherapy of recurrent HSV is of limited benefit, with studies finding a reduction in the average outbreak by only 12–24 hours. **To be effective, the treatment must be initiated by the patient at the first sign of recurrence.** If treatment is desired, recurrent genital herpes outbreaks may be treated with 3 days of valacyclovir, 500 mg twice daily, 5 days of acyclovir, 200 mg five times a day, or 5 days of famciclovir, 125 mg twice daily. Valacyclovir, 2 g twice daily for 1 day, or famciclovir, 1 g once or twice in 1 day, are equally effective short-course alternatives and can abort impending recurrences of both orolabial and genital herpes. The addition of a potent topical corticosteroid three times daily reduces the duration, size, and pain of orolabial herpes treated with an oral antiviral agent.

In patients with frequent or severe recurrences, suppressive therapy may be effective in controlling disease. Suppressive treatment will reduce outbreaks by 85% and reduces viral shedding by more than 90%. This results in about a 50% reduced risk of transmission. The recommended suppressive doses, taken continuously, are acyclovir, 400 mg twice daily; valacyclovir, 500 mg once daily; or famciclovir, 125–250 mg twice daily. Long-term suppression appears very safe, and after 5–7 years a substantial proportion of patients can discontinue treatment.

The use of latex condoms and patient education have proved effective in reducing genital herpes transmission in some studies but have not proved beneficial in others. No single or combination intervention absolutely prevents transmission. Sunscreens are useful adjuncts in preventing sun-induced HSV-1 recurrences. A preventive antiviral medication should be started beginning 24 hours prior to ultraviolet light exposure, dental surgery, or orolabial cosmetic surgery.

▲ **Figure 6–14.** Herpes simplex type 1 vesicles at the vermillion border of the lip. (Used, with permission, from Richard P. Usatine, MD in Usatine RP, Smith MA, Mayeaux EJ Jr, Chumley H, Tysinger J. *The Color Atlas of Family Medicine.* McGraw-Hill, 2009.)

B. Local Measures

In general, topical therapy has only limited efficacy and is generally not recommended because evidence shows that it only minimally reduces skin healing time.

► Prognosis

Aside from the complications described above, recurrent attacks last several days, and patients recover without sequelae.

Hofstetter AM et al. Current thinking on genital herpes. Curr Opin Infect Dis. 2014 Feb;27(1):75–83. [PMID: 24335720]
Le Cleach L et al. Oral antiviral therapy for prevention of genital herpes outbreaks in immunocompetent and nonpregnant patients. Cochrane Database Syst Rev. 2014 Aug 3;8: CD009036. [PMID: 25086573]
Richardson VN et al. Patterns of disease and treatment of cold sores. J Dermatolog Treat. 2013 Dec;24(6):439–43. [PMID: 23541214]

HERPES ZOSTER (Shingles)

ESSENTIALS OF DIAGNOSIS

- ► Pain along the course of a nerve followed by grouped vesicular lesions.

- ► Involvement is unilateral; some lesions (fewer than 20) may occur outside the affected dermatome.

- ► Lesions are usually on face or trunk.

- ► Direct fluorescent antibody positive, especially in vesicular lesions.

▲ **Figure 6–15.** Herpes zoster. (Used, with permission, from Berger TG, Dept Dermatology, UCSF.)

► General Considerations

Herpes zoster is an acute vesicular eruption due to the varicella-zoster virus. It usually occurs in adults and incidence rises with age. With rare exceptions, patients suffer only one attack. While dermatomal herpes zoster is common, generalized disease raises the suspicion of an associated immunosuppressive disorder, such as HIV infection. HIV-infected patients are 20 times more likely to develop zoster, often before other clinical findings of HIV disease are present. A history of HIV risk factors and HIV testing when appropriate should be considered, especially in patients with zoster who are younger than 55 years.

► Clinical Findings

Pain usually precedes the eruption by 48 hours or more and may persist after the lesions have disappeared. The lesions consist of grouped, tense, deep-seated vesicles distributed unilaterally along a dermatome (Figure 6–15). The most common distributions are on the trunk or face. Up to 20 lesions may be found outside the affected dermatomes, even in immune-competent persons. Regional lymph nodes may be tender and swollen.

► Differential Diagnosis

Since poison oak and poison ivy dermatitis can occur unilaterally, they must be differentiated at times from herpes zoster. Allergic contact dermatitis is pruritic; zoster is painful. One must differentiate herpes zoster from lesions of herpes simplex, which rarely occurs in a dermatomal distribution. Doses of antivirals appropriate for zoster should be used in the absence of a clear diagnosis. Facial zoster may simulate erysipelas initially, but zoster is unilateral and shows vesicles after 24–48 hours. Depending on the dermatome involved, the pain of preeruptive herpes zoster may lead the clinician to diagnose migraine, myocardial infarction, acute abdomen, herniated disk, etc.

► Complications

Sacral zoster may be associated with bladder and bowel dysfunction. Persistent neuralgia, anesthesia or scarring of the affected area, facial or other nerve paralysis, and encephalitis may occur. Postherpetic neuralgia is most common after involvement of the trigeminal region and in patients over the age of 55. **Early (within 72 hours after onset) and aggressive antiviral treatment of herpes zoster reduces the severity** and duration of postherpetic neuralgia. Zoster ophthalmicus (V1) can result in visual impairment. Increased risk of transient ischemic attack and stroke has been demonstrated.

► Prevention

An effective live herpes zoster vaccine (Zostavax) is available and recommended to prevent both herpes zoster and postherpetic neuralgia. It is approved for persons over the age of 50 and recommended in persons aged 60 and older, even in those who have had zoster.

► Treatment

A. General Measures

1. Immunocompetent host—Antiviral treatment within 72 hours of rash decreases the duration and severity of acute herpes zoster. Since such treatment also reduces postherpetic neuralgia, those with a risk of developing this complication should be treated (ie, those over age 50 and those with nontruncal eruption). In addition, patients with acute moderate to severe pain or rash may benefit from antiviral therapy. Treatment can be given with oral acyclovir, 800 mg five times daily; famciclovir, 500 mg three times daily; or valacyclovir, 1 g three times daily—all for 7 days (see Chapter 32). For reasons of increased bioavailability and ease of dosing schedule, the preferred agents are those given three times daily. Patients should maintain good hydration. The dose of antiviral should be adjusted for kidney function as recommended. Nerve blocks may be used in the management of initial severe pain. Ophthalmologic consultation is vital for involvement of the first branch of the trigeminal nerve, even if the patient has no ocular symptoms.

Systemic corticosteroids are effective in reducing acute pain, improving quality of life, and returning patients to normal activities much more quickly. They do not increase the risk of dissemination in immunocompetent hosts. If not contraindicated, a tapering 3-week course of prednisone, starting at 60 mg/day, should be considered for its adjunctive benefit in immunocompetent patients. **Oral corticosteroids do not reduce the prevalence, severity, or duration of postherpetic neuralgia beyond that achieved by effective antiviral therapy.** Adequate analgesia, including the use of opioids, tricyclic antidepressants, and gabapentin as necessary, should be given for zoster-associated pain.

2. Immunocompromised host—Given the safety and efficacy of currently available antivirals, most immunocompromised patients with herpes zoster are candidates for antiviral therapy. The dosage schedule is as listed above, but treatment should be continued until the lesions have completely crusted and are healed or almost healed (up to 2 weeks). **Because corticosteroids increase the risk of dissemination in immunosuppressed patients, they should not be used in these patients.** Progression of disease may necessitate intravenous therapy with acyclovir, 10 mg/kg intravenously, three times daily. After 3–4 days, oral therapy may be substituted if there has been a good response to intravenous therapy. Adverse effects include decreased kidney function from crystallization, nausea and vomiting, and abdominal pain.

Foscarnet, administered in a dosage of 40 mg/kg two or three times daily intravenously, is indicated for treatment of acyclovir-resistant varicella-zoster virus infections.

B. Local Measures

Calamine or aluminum salt compresses (Domeboro, Burow soaks) may be helpful for dry weeping lesions.

C. Postherpetic Neuralgia Therapy

The most effective treatment is prevention with vaccination of those at risk for developing zoster and early and aggressive antiviral therapy once zoster has occurred. Once established, postherpetic neuralgia may be treated with capsaicin ointment, 0.025–0.075%, or lidocaine (Lidoderm) topical patches. Chronic postherpetic neuralgia may be relieved by regional blocks (stellate ganglion, epidural, local infiltration, or peripheral nerve), with or without corticosteroids added to the injections. Tricyclic antidepressants, such as amitriptyline, 25–75 mg orally as a single nightly dose, are the first-line therapy beyond simple analgesics. Gabapentin, up to 3600 mg orally daily (starting at 300 mg orally three times daily), or duloxetine, up to 60–120 mg orally daily (starting at 30–60 mg orally daily) may be added for additional pain relief. Long-acting opioids may be appropriate. Referral to a pain management clinic should be considered in moderate to severe cases and in those who do not respond to the above treatments.

► Prognosis

The eruption persists 2–3 weeks and usually does not recur. Motor involvement in 2–3% of patients may lead to temporary palsy.

Gagliardi AM et al. Vaccines for preventing herpes zoster in older adults. Cochrane Database Syst Rev. 2012 Oct 17; 10:CD008858. [PMID: 23076951]

Johnson RW et al. Clinical practice. Postherpetic neuralgia. N Engl J Med. 2014 Oct 16;371(16):1526–33. [PMID: 25317872]

Kawai K et al. Systematic review of incidence and complications of herpes zoster: towards a global perspective. BMJ Open. 2014 Jun 10;4(6):e004833. [PMID: 24916088]

Lal H et al. Efficacy of an adjuvanted herpes zoster subunit vaccine in older adults. N Engl J Med. 2015 May 28;372(22): 2087–96. [PMID: 25916341]

O'Connor KM et al. Herpes zoster. Med Clin North Am. 2013 Jul;97(4):503–22. [PMID: 23809711]

POMPHOLYX; VESICULOBULLOUS HAND ECZEMA (Formerly Known as Dyshidrosis, Dyshidrotic Eczema)

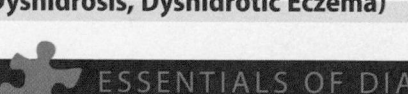

ESSENTIALS OF DIAGNOSIS

► Pruritic "tapioca" vesicles of 1–2 mm on the palms, soles, and sides of fingers.

► Vesicles may coalesce to form multiloculated blisters.

► Scaling and fissuring may follow drying of the blisters.

► Appearance in the third decade, with lifelong recurrences.

General Considerations

This is an extremely common form of hand dermatitis, preferably called pompholyx (Gr "bubble") or vesiculobullous dermatitis of the palms and soles. About half of patients have an atopic background, and many patients report flares with stress. Patients with widespread dermatitis due to any cause may develop pompholyx-like eruptions as a part of an autoeczematization response.

Clinical Findings

Small clear vesicles stud the skin at the sides of the fingers and on the palms (Figure 6–16) or soles. They look like the grains in tapioca. They may be associated with intense itching. Later, the vesicles dry and the area becomes scaly and fissured.

Differential Diagnosis

Unroofing the vesicles and examining the blister roof with a KOH preparation will reveal hyphae in cases of bullous tinea. Always examine the feet of a patient with a hand eruption because patients with inflammatory tinea pedis may have a vesicular autoeczematization of the palms.

▲ **Figure 6–16.** Pompholyx (acute vesiculobullous hand eczema). (Used, with permission, from Berger TG, Dept Dermatology, UCSF.)

Nonsteroidal anti-inflammatory drugs (NSAIDs) may produce an eruption very similar to that of dyshidrosis on the hands.

Prevention

There is no known way to prevent attacks if the condition is idiopathic. About one-third to one-half of patients with vesiculobullous hand dermatitis have a relevant contact allergen, especially nickel. Patch testing and avoidance of identified allergens can lead to improvement.

Treatment

Topical and systemic corticosteroids help some patients dramatically. Since this is a chronic problem, systemic corticosteroids are generally not appropriate therapy. A high-potency topical corticosteroid used early in the attack may help abort the flare and ameliorate pruritus. Topical corticosteroids are also important in treating the scaling and fissuring that are seen after the vesicular phase. It is essential that patients avoid anything that irritates the skin; they should wear cotton gloves inside vinyl gloves when doing dishes or other wet chores, use long-handled brushes instead of sponges, and use a hand cream after washing the hands. Patients respond to PUVA therapy and injection of botulinum toxin into the palms as for hyperhidrosis.

Prognosis

For most patients, the disease is an inconvenience. For some, vesiculobullous hand eczema can be incapacitating.

Apfelbacher C et al. Characteristics and provision of care in patients with chronic hand eczema: updated data from the CARPE Registry. Acta Derm Venereol. 2014 Feb 26;94(2): 163–7. [PMID: 23995048]

Golden S et al. Hand dermatitis: review of clinical features and treatment options. Semin Cutan Med Surg. 2013 Sep;32(3): 147–57. [PMID: 24175402]

Wold L et al. Hand dermatitis: an allergist's nightmare. Curr Allergy Asthma Rep. 2014 Nov;14(11):474. [PMID: 25228264]

PORPHYRIA CUTANEA TARDA

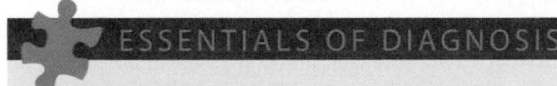

ESSENTIALS OF DIAGNOSIS

▶ Noninflammatory blisters on sun-exposed sites, especially the dorsal surfaces of the hands.

▶ Hypertrichosis, skin fragility.

▶ Associated liver disease.

▶ Elevated urine porphyrins.

General Considerations

Porphyria cutanea tarda is the most common type of porphyria. Cases are sporadic or hereditary. The disease is associated with ingestion of certain medications (eg,

▲ **Figure 6–17.** Porphyria cutanea tarda. (From Lewis Rose, MD; used, with permission, from Usatine RP, Smith MA, Mayeaux EJ Jr, Chumley H, Tysinger J. *The Color Atlas of Family Medicine.* McGraw-Hill, 2009.)

estrogens) and liver disease from alcoholism, hemochromatosis, or hepatitis C.

► Clinical Findings

A. Symptoms and Signs

Patients complain of painless blistering and fragility of the skin of the dorsal surfaces of the hands (Figure 6–17). Facial hypertrichosis and hyperpigmentation are common.

B. Laboratory Findings

Urinary uroporphyrins are elevated twofold to fivefold above coproporphyrins. Patients may also have abnormal liver function tests, evidence of hepatitis C infection, increased liver iron stores, and hemochromatosis gene mutations.

► Differential Diagnosis

Skin lesions identical to those of porphyria cutanea tarda may be seen in patients who undergo dialysis and in those who take certain medications (tetracyclines, voriconazole, and NSAIDs, especially naproxen). In this so-called **pseudoporphyria,** the biopsy results are identical to those associated with porphyria cutanea tarda, but urine porphyrins are normal.

► Prevention

Barrier sun protection with clothing is required. Although the lesions are triggered by sun exposure, the wavelength of light triggering the lesions is beyond that absorbed by sunscreens.

► Treatment

Stopping all triggering medications and substantially reducing or stopping alcohol consumption may alone lead to improvement. Phlebotomy without oral iron supplementation at a rate of 1 unit every 2–4 weeks will gradually lead to

improvement. Very low-dose antimalarial medication (as low as 200 mg of hydroxychloroquine twice weekly), alone or in combination with phlebotomy, will increase the excretion of porphyrins, improving the skin disease. Deferasirox, an iron chelator can also improve porphyria cutanea tarda. Treatment is continued until the patient is asymptomatic. Urine porphyrins may be monitored.

► Prognosis

Most patients improve with treatment. Sclerodermoid skin lesions may develop on the trunk, scalp, and face.

Schulenburg-Brand D et al. The cutaneous porphyrias. Dermatol Clin. 2014 Jul;32(3):369–84. [PMID: 24891059]
Singal AK et al. Low-dose hydroxychloroquine is as effective as phlebotomy in treatment of patients with porphyria cutanea tarda. Clin Gastroenterol Hepatol. 2012 Dec;10(12):1402–9. [PMID: 22985607]

DERMATITIS HERPETIFORMIS

Dermatitis herpetiformis is an uncommon disease manifested by pruritic papules, vesicles, and papulovesicles mainly on the elbows, knees, buttocks, posterior neck, and scalp. It appears to have its highest prevalence in Northern Europe and is associated with HLA antigens -B8, -DR3, and -DQ2. The histopathology is distinctive. Circulating antibodies to tissue transglutaminase are present in 90% of cases. NSAIDs may cause flares. **Patients have gluten-sensitive enteropathy, but it is subclinical in the great majority.** However, ingestion of gluten is the cause of the disease, and strict long-term avoidance of dietary gluten has been shown to decrease the dose of dapsone (usually 100–200 mg daily) required to control the disease and may even eliminate the need for treatment. Patients with dermatitis herpetiformis are at increased risk for development of gastrointestinal lymphoma, and this risk is reduced by a gluten-free diet.

Cardones AR et al. Management of dermatitis herpetiformis. Immunol Allergy Clin North Am. 2012 May;32(2):275–81. [PMID: 22560140]
Clarindo MV et al. Dermatitis herpetiformis: pathophysiology, clinical presentation, diagnosis and treatment. An Bras Dermatol. 2014 Nov–Dec;89(6):865–75. [PMID: 25387490]
Jakes AD et al. Dermatitis herpetiformis. BMJ. 2014 Apr 16; 348:g2557. [PMID: 24740905]

WEEPING OR CRUSTED LESIONS

IMPETIGO

 ESSENTIALS OF DIAGNOSIS

► Superficial blisters filled with purulent material that rupture easily.
► Crusted superficial erosions.
► Positive Gram stain and bacterial culture.

▲ **Figure 6–18.** Bullous impetigo. (Used, with permission, from Berger TG, Dept Dermatology, UCSF.)

General Considerations

Impetigo is a contagious and autoinoculable infection of the skin (epidermis) caused by staphylococci or streptococci.

Clinical Findings

A. Symptoms and Signs

The lesions consist of macules, vesicles, bullae, pustules, and honey-colored crusts that when removed leave denuded red areas (Figure 6–18). The face and other exposed parts are most often involved. **Ecthyma** is a deeper form of impetigo caused by staphylococci or streptococci, with ulceration and scarring that occurs frequently on the extremities.

B. Laboratory Findings

Gram stain and culture confirm the diagnosis. In temperate climates, most cases are associated with *S aureus* infection. *Streptococcus* species are more common in tropical infections.

Differential Diagnosis

The main differential diagnoses are acute allergic contact dermatitis and herpes simplex. Contact dermatitis may be suggested by the history or by linear distribution of the lesions, and culture should be negative for staphylococci and streptococci. Herpes simplex infection usually presents with grouped vesicles or discrete erosions and may be associated with a history of recurrences. Viral cultures are positive.

Treatment

Soaks and scrubbing can be beneficial, especially in unroofing lakes of pus under thick crusts. Topical agents, such as bacitracin, mupirocin, and retapamulin, are first-line treatment options for infections limited to small areas. In widespread cases, systemic antibiotics are indicated. Cephalexin, 250 mg four times daily, is usually effective. Doxycycline, 100 mg twice daily, is a reasonable alternative. Community-associated methicillin-resistant *S aureus* (CA-MRSA) may

cause impetigo, and initial coverage for MRSA could include doxycycline or trimethoprim-sulfamethoxazole (TMP-SMZ). About 50% of CA-MRSA cases are quinolone resistant. Recurrent impetigo is associated with nasal carriage of *S aureus* and is treated with rifampin, 600 mg daily for 5 days. Intranasal mupirocin ointment twice daily for 5 days clears the carriage of 40% of MRSA strains. Bleach baths (¼ to ½ cup per 20 liters of bathwater for 15 minutes 3–5 times weekly) for all family members, and the use of dilute household bleach to clean showers and other bath surfaces may help reduce the spread. Individuals should not share towels if there is a case of impetigo in the household.

Hartman-Adams H et al. Impetigo: diagnosis and treatment. Am Fam Physician. 2014 Aug 15;90(4):229–35. [PMID: 25250996]
Koning S et al. Interventions for impetigo. Cochrane Database Syst Rev. 2012 Jan 18;1:CD003261. [PMID: 22258953]

CONTACT DERMATITIS

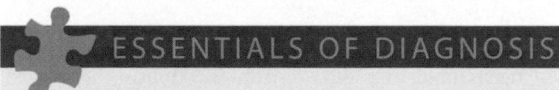

ESSENTIALS OF DIAGNOSIS

► Erythema and edema, with pruritus, often followed by vesicles, bullae, weeping or crusting in an area of contact with a suspected agent.

► A history of previous reaction to suspected contactant.

► Positive patch test (in allergic contact dermatitis).

General Considerations

Contact dermatitis (irritant or allergic) is an acute or chronic dermatitis that results from direct skin contact with chemicals or allergens. Eighty percent of cases are due to excessive exposure to or additive effects of universal irritants (eg, soaps, detergents, organic solvents) and are called **irritant contact dermatitis**. This appears red and scaly but not vesicular and occurs only in the direct sites of contact with the irritant. The most common causes of **allergic contact dermatitis** are poison ivy or poison oak, topically applied antimicrobials (especially bacitracin and neomycin), anesthetics (benzocaine), hair-care products, preservatives, jewelry (nickel), rubber, essential oils, propolis (from bees), vitamin E, and adhesive tape. Occupational exposure is an important cause of allergic contact dermatitis. Weeping and crusting are typically due to allergic and not irritant dermatitis; lesions may also occur slightly outside of contact sites, distinguishing it from irritant dermatitis.

Clinical Findings

A. Symptoms and Signs

In allergic contact dermatitis, the acute phase is characterized by tiny vesicles and weepy and crusted lesions, whereas resolving or chronic contact dermatitis presents

▲ **Figure 6–19.** Contact dermatitis with linear pattern due to poison ivy. (Used, with permission, from Berger TG, Dept Dermatology, UCSF.)

with scaling, erythema, and possibly thickened skin. Itching, burning, and stinging may be severe. The lesions, distributed on exposed parts or in bizarre asymmetric patterns, consist of erythematous macules, papules, and vesicles. The affected area is often hot and swollen, with exudation and crusting, simulating—and at times complicated by—infection. The pattern of the eruption may be diagnostic (eg, typical linear streaked vesicles on the extremities in poison oak or ivy dermatitis [Figure 6–19]). The location will often suggest the cause: Scalp involvement suggests hair dyes or shampoos; face involvement, creams, cosmetics, soaps, shaving materials, nail polish; and neck involvement, jewelry, hair dyes.

B. Laboratory Findings

Gram stain and culture will rule out impetigo or secondary infection (impetiginization). If itching is generalized, then scabies should be considered. After the episode of allergic contact dermatitis has cleared, patch testing may be useful if the triggering allergen is not known.

▶ Differential Diagnosis

Asymmetric distribution, blotchy erythema around the face, linear lesions, and a history of exposure help distinguish acute contact dermatitis from other skin lesions. The most commonly mistaken diagnosis is impetigo or cellulitis. Chronic allergic contact dermatitis must be differentiated from scabies, atopic dermatitis, and pompholyx.

▶ Prevention

Prompt and thorough removal of the causative oil by washing with liquid soap may be effective if done within 30 minutes after exposure to poison oak or ivy. Goop and Tecnu are also effective but much more costly without increased efficacy. The three most effective over-the-counter barrier creams that are applied prior to exposure and prevent/reduce the severity of the dermatitis are Stokogard, Hollister Moisture Barrier, and Hydropel.

The mainstay of prevention is identification of the agent causing the dermatitis and avoidance of exposure or use of protective clothing and gloves. In industry-related cases, prevention may be accomplished by moving or retraining the worker.

▶ Treatment

A. Overview

While local measures are important, severe or widespread involvement is difficult to manage without systemic corticosteroids because even the highest-potency topical corticosteroids seem not to work well on vesicular and weepy lesions. Localized involvement (except on the face) can often be managed solely with topical agents. Irritant contact dermatitis is treated by protection from the irritant and use of topical corticosteroids as for atopic dermatitis (described above). The treatment of allergic contact dermatitis is detailed below.

B. Local Measures

1. Acute weeping dermatitis—Compresses are most often used. Gentle cleansing is recommended. Calamine lotion or zinc oxide paste may be used between wet dressings, especially for involvement of intertriginous areas or when oozing is not marked. Lesions on the extremities may be bandaged with wet dressings for 30–60 minutes several times a day. High-potency topical corticosteroids in gel or cream form (eg, fluocinonide, clobetasol, or halobetasol) may help suppress acute contact dermatitis and relieve itching. This treatment should be followed by tapering of the number of applications per day or use of a mid-potency corticosteroid, such as triamcinolone 0.1% cream to prevent rebound of the dermatitis. A soothing formulation is 2 oz of 0.1% triamcinolone acetonide cream in 7.5 oz Sarna lotion (0.5% camphor, 0.5% menthol, 0.5% phenol) mixed by the patient.

2. Subacute dermatitis (subsiding)—Mid-potency (triamcinolone 0.1%) to high-potency corticosteroids (clobetasol, fluocinonide, desoximetasone) are the mainstays of therapy.

3. Chronic dermatitis (dry and lichenified)—High-potency to superpotency corticosteroids are used in ointment form. Occlusion may be helpful on the hands.

C. Systemic Therapy

For acute severe cases, prednisone may be given orally for 12–21 days. Prednisone, 60 mg for 4–7 days, 40 mg for 4–7 days, and 20 mg for 4–7 days without a further taper is one useful regimen. Another is to dispense seventy-eight 5-mg pills to be taken 12 the first day, 11 the second day, and so on. **The key is to use enough corticosteroid (and as early as possible) to achieve a clinical effect and to taper slowly enough to avoid rebound.** A Medrol Dosepak (methylprednisolone) with 5 days of medication is inappropriate on both counts. (See Chapter 26.)

▶ Prognosis

Allergic contact dermatitis is self-limited if reexposure is prevented but often takes 2–3 weeks for full resolution. Removal of the causative agent is paramount to avoid recurrences.

Fonacier LS et al. Allergic contact dermatitis. Ann Allergy Asthma Immunol. 2014 Jul;113(1):9–12. [PMID: 24950843]

Holness DL. Occupational skin allergies: testing and treatment (the case of occupational allergic contact dermatitis). Curr Allergy Asthma Rep. 2014 Feb;14(2):410. [PMID: 24408535]

Tan CH et al. Contact dermatitis: allergic and irritant. Clin Dermatol. 2014 Jan–Feb;32(1):116–24. [PMID: 24314385]

Wolf R et al. Patch testing: facts and controversies. Clin Dermatol. 2013 Jul–Aug;31(4):479–86. [PMID: 23806165]

PUSTULAR DISORDERS

ACNE VULGARIS

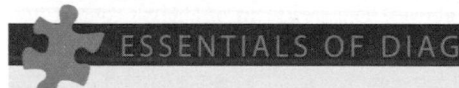

ESSENTIALS OF DIAGNOSIS

▶ The most common of all skin conditions.

▶ Almost universal in puberty, though onset may begin in premenarchal girls and present or persist into the fourth or fifth decade.

▶ Comedones are the hallmark of acne vulgaris. Severity varies from purely comedonal to papular or pustular inflammatory acne to cysts or nodules.

▶ Face and upper trunk may be affected.

▶ Scarring may be a sequela of the disease or picking by the patient.

▶ General Considerations

Acne vulgaris is polymorphic. Open and closed comedones, papules, pustules, and cysts are found.

In younger persons, acne vulgaris is more common and more severe in males. It does not always clear spontaneously when maturity is reached. Twelve percent of women and 3%

of men over age 25 have acne vulgaris. This rate does not decrease until the fourth or fifth decade of life. The skin lesions parallel sebaceous activity. Pathogenic events include plugging of the infundibulum of the follicles, retention of sebum, overgrowth of the acne bacillus (*Propionibacterium acnes*) with resultant release of and irritation by accumulated fatty acids, and foreign-body reaction to extrafollicular sebum. The mechanism of antibiotics in controlling acne is not clearly understood, but they may work because of their antibacterial or anti-inflammatory properties.

When a resistant case of acne is encountered in a woman, hyperandrogenism may be suspected. This may or may not be accompanied by hirsutism, irregular menses, or signs of virilism. Polycystic ovary syndrome (PCOS) is the most common identifiable cause.

▶ Clinical Findings

There may be mild tenderness, pain, or itching. The lesions occur mainly over the face, neck, upper chest, back, and shoulders. **Comedones (tiny, flesh-colored, white or black noninflamed superficial papules that give the skin a rough texture or appearance) are the hallmark of acne vulgaris.** Inflammatory papules, pustules, ectatic pores, acne cysts, and scarring are also seen (Figure 6–20).

Acne may have different presentations at different ages. Preteens often present with comedones as their first lesions. Inflammatory lesions in young teenagers are often

▲ **Figure 6–20.** Acne vulgaris, severe nodular cystic form with scarring. (Used, with permission, from Richard P. Usatine, MD in Usatine RP, Smith MA, Mayeaux EJ Jr, Chumley H, Tysinger J. *The Color Atlas of Family Medicine.* McGraw-Hill, 2009.)

found in the middle of the face, extending outward as the patient becomes older. Women in their third and fourth decades (often with no prior history of acne) commonly present with papular lesions on the chin and jawline.

Differential Diagnosis

In adults, rosacea presents with papules and pustules in the middle third of the face, but absence of truncal involvement, telangiectasia, flushing, and the absence of comedones distinguish rosacea from acne vulgaris. A pustular eruption on the face in patients receiving antibiotics or with otitis externa should be investigated with culture to rule out an uncommon gram-negative folliculitis. Acne may develop in patients who use systemic corticosteroids or topical fluorinated corticosteroids on the face. Acne may be exacerbated or caused by cosmetic creams or oils. Pustules on the face can also be caused by tinea infections. Lesions on the back are more problematic. When they occur alone, staphylococcal folliculitis, miliaria ("heat rash") or, uncommonly, *Malassezia (Pityrosporum)* folliculitis should be suspected. Bacterial culture, trial of an antistaphylococcal antibiotic, and observing the response to therapy will help in the differential diagnosis. In patients with HIV infection, folliculitis is common and may be either staphylococcal folliculitis or eosinophilic folliculitis (typically pruritic tumid papules on the face and neck).

Complications

Cyst formation, pigmentary changes, scarring, and poor quality of life may result.

Treatment

A. General Measures

1. Education of the patient—Education on proper use of medications and cosmetics is paramount. **Because lesions take 4–6 weeks to improve, clinical improvement should be measured by the number of new lesions forming after 6–8 weeks of therapy.** Additional time (3–4 months) will be required to see improvement on the back and chest, as these areas are slowest to respond. Avoid topical exposure to oils, cocoa butter (theobroma oil), and greases in cosmetics, including hair products. When scarring seems out of proportion to the severity of the lesions, clinicians must suspect that the patient is manipulating the lesions. It is essential that the patient be educated in a supportive way about this complication. Anxiety and depression are common in patients with excoriated acne.

2. Diet—A low glycemic diet has been associated with improvement and lower incidence of acne. This improvement was associated with a reduction in insulin resistance. Hyperinsulinemia has also been associated with acne in both eumenorrheic women and individuals with PCOS. This finding suggests a possible common pathogenic mechanism for acne in both adult women and men.

B. Comedonal Acne

Treatment of acne is based on the type and severity of lesions. Comedones require treatment different from that

of pustules and cystic lesions. In assessing severity, take the sequelae of the lesions into account. An individual who gets only a few new lesions per month that scar or leave postinflammatory hyperpigmentation must be treated much more aggressively than a comparable patient whose lesions clear without sequelae. **Hygiene plays little role in acne treatment**, and a mild soap is almost always recommended. The agents effective in comedonal acne are listed below in the order in which they should be tried.

1. Topical retinoids—Tretinoin is very effective for comedonal acne or for treatment of the comedonal component of more severe acne, but its usefulness is limited by irritation. Start with 0.025% cream (not gel) and have the patient use it at first twice weekly at night, increasing frequency to nightly as tolerated. A few patients cannot use even this low-strength preparation more than three times weekly but even that may cause improvement. A lentil-sized amount is sufficient to cover the entire face. To avoid irritation, have the patient wait 20 minutes after washing to apply. Adapalene gel 0.1% and reformulated tretinoin (Renova, Retin A Micro, Avita) are other options for patients irritated by standard tretinoin preparations. Although the absorption of tretinoin is minimal, its use during pregnancy is contraindicated. Patients should be warned that their acne may flare in the first 4 weeks of treatment.

2. Benzoyl peroxide—Benzoyl peroxide products are available in concentrations of 2.5%, 4%, 5%, 8%, and 10%, but 2.5% is as effective as 10% and less irritating. In general, water-based and not alcohol-based gels should be used to decrease irritation. Benzoyl peroxide in combination with several other topical agents, including adapalene and topical antibiotics (erythromycin, clindamycin phosphate), are available as a single formulation.

C. Papular or Cystic Inflammatory Acne

Brief treatment (3 weeks to 3 months) with topical or oral antibiotics is the mainstay for treatment of inflammatory acne that does not respond to topical therapy with retinoids or benzoyl peroxide. Topical clindamycin phosphate and erythromycin are used only for mild papular acne that can be controlled by topicals alone or for patients who refuse or cannot tolerate oral antibiotics. To decrease resistance, benzoyl peroxide should be used in combination with the topical antibiotic.

1. Mild acne—The first choice of topical antibiotics in terms of efficacy and relative lack of induction of resistant *P acnes* is the combination of erythromycin or clindamycin with benzoyl peroxide topical gel or wash. These may be used once or twice daily. The addition of tretinoin cream or gel at night may increase improvement, since it works via a different mechanism. Topical retinoids ideally are used after acne clearance is achieved as a long-term maintenance therapy.

2. Moderate acne—Common oral antibiotics used for acne include doxycycline (100 mg twice daily), minocycline (50–100 mg once or twice daily), TMP-SMZ (one double-strength tablet twice daily), or a cephalosporin (cefadroxil or cephalexin 500 mg twice daily) may be used in combination with benzoyl peroxide to minimize development of antibiotic resistance. Once the patient's skin is clear, instructions should be given for tapering the dose by 50% every 6–8 weeks—while treating with topicals—to arrive at the lowest systemic dose needed to maintain clearing. In general, discontinuing antibiotics immediately without adjunctive topical therapy results in prompt recurrence. Topical retinoids are excellent for long-term maintenance following antibiotics. Combination oral contraceptives or spironolactone (50–200 mg/day) may be added in women with treatment-resistant acne. Tetracycline, minocycline, and doxycycline are contraindicated in pregnancy, but certain oral erythromycins or cephalosporins may be used.

3. Severe acne

A. Isotretinoin—A vitamin A analog, isotretinoin is used for the treatment of severe acne that has not responded to conventional therapy. A dosage of 0.5–1 mg/kg/day for 20 weeks for a cumulative dose of at least 120 mg/kg is usually adequate for severe cystic acne. Patients should be offered isotretinoin therapy before they experience significant scarring if they are not promptly and adequately controlled by antibiotics. **The medication is absolutely contraindicated during pregnancy because of its teratogenicity;** two serum pregnancy tests should be obtained before starting the drug in women and every month thereafter. Sufficient medication for only 1 month can be dispensed. Two forms of effective contraception must be used; abstinence is an acceptable first option. Informed consent must be obtained before its use, and patients must be enrolled in a monitoring program (iPledge). In addition to its teratogenicity, isotretinoin has numerous serious side effects and should only be prescribed by clinicians (usually dermatologists) well aware of these issues. Consider ordering laboratory tests, including complete blood cell count (CBC), cholesterol levels, triglyceride levels, and liver function studies, in patients before treatment and after 4 weeks on therapy; monitoring through the entire treatment may not be high value.

Abnormal laboratory tests, especially elevated liver enzymes and triglyceride levels, return to normal quickly upon conclusion of therapy. The medication may induce long-term remissions in 40–60%, or acne may recur that is more easily controlled with conventional therapy. Occasionally, a second course is needed if acne does not respond or recurs.

B. Intralesional injection—Intralesional injection of dilute suspensions of triamcinolone acetonide (2.5 mg/mL, 0.05 mL per lesion) will often hasten the resolution of deeper papules and occasional cysts.

C. Laser dermabrasion—Cosmetic improvement may be achieved by excision and punch-grafting of deep scars and by physical or chemical abrasion of inactive acne lesions, particularly flat, superficial scars. Corrective surgery within 12 months after isotretinoin therapy may not be advisable.

Prognosis

Acne vulgaris eventually remits spontaneously, but when this will occur cannot be predicted. The condition may persist throughout adulthood and may lead to severe scarring if left untreated. Patients treated with antibiotics continue to improve for the first 3–6 months of therapy. Relapse during treatment may suggest the emergence of resistant *P acnes*. The disease is chronic and tends to flare intermittently in spite of treatment. Remissions following systemic treatment with isotretinoin may be lasting in up to 60% of cases. Relapses after isotretinoin usually occur within 3 years and require a second course in up to 20% of patients. Immediate relapse after isotretinoin discontinuation may suggest hyperandrogenism or other underlying hormonal disorders in a female patient.

Arowojolu AO et al. Combined oral contraceptive pills for treatment of acne. Cochrane Database Syst Rev. 2012 Jul 11; 7:CD004425. [PMID: 22786490]

Das S et al. Recent advances in acne pathogenesis: implications for therapy. Am J Clin Dermatol. 2014 Dec;15(6):479–88. [PMID: 25388823]

Dréno B et al; Global Alliance to Improve Outcomes in Acne. Antibiotic stewardship in dermatology: limiting antibiotic use in acne. Eur J Dermatol. 2014 May–Jun;24(3):330–4. [PMID: 24721547]

Dréno B et al; Global Alliance to Improve Outcomes in Acne. Large-scale international study enhances understanding of an emerging acne population: adult females. J Eur Acad Dermatol Venereol. 2015 Jun;29(6):1096–106. [PMID: 25296739]

Thompson AE. JAMA patient page. Acne. JAMA. 2015 Feb 10; 313(6):640. [PMID: 25668279]

Williams HC et al. Acne vulgaris. Lancet. 2012 Jan 28;379(9813): 361–72. [PMID: 21880356]

ROSACEA

ESSENTIALS OF DIAGNOSIS

▶ A chronic disorder affecting the face.

▶ A neurovascular component (erythema and telangiectasis and a tendency to flush easily).

▶ An acneiform component (papules and pustules) may also be present.

▶ A glandular component accompanied by hyperplasia of the soft tissue of the nose (rhinophyma).

General Considerations

Rosacea is a common condition that presents in adulthood. The pathogenesis of this chronic disorder is not known. Topical corticosteroids applied to the face can induce rosacea-like conditions.

Clinical Findings

Patients frequently report flushing or exacerbation of their rosacea due to heat, hot drinks, spicy food, sunlight,

▲ **Figure 6–21.** Rosacea. (Used, with permission, from Berger TG, Dept Dermatology, UCSF.)

exercise, alcohol, emotions, or menopausal flushing. The cheeks, nose, and chin—at times the entire face—may be affected. **No comedones are seen.** In its mildest form, erythema and dilated vessels are seen on the cheeks. Inflammatory papules may be superimposed on this background and may evolve to pustules (Figure 6–21). Associated seborrhea may be found. The patient often complains of burning or stinging with episodes of flushing and extremely cosmetic-intolerant skin. Patients may have associated ophthalmic disease, including blepharitis and keratitis, which often requires topical or systemic antibiotic or immunosuppressive therapy.

▶ Differential Diagnosis

Rosacea is distinguished from acne by the presence of the neurovascular component and the absence of comedones. The rosy hue of rosacea and telangiectasis will pinpoint the diagnosis. Lupus is often misdiagnosed, but the presence of pustules excludes that diagnosis.

▶ Treatment

Educating patients to avoid the factors they know to produce exacerbations is important. Patients should wear a broad-spectrum sunscreen with UVA coverage; however, exquisite sensitivity to topical preparations may limit patient options. Zinc- or titanium-based sunscreens are tolerated best. Medical management is most effective for the inflammatory papules and pustules and the erythema that surrounds them. Rosacea is usually a lifelong condition, so maintenance therapy is required.

A. Local Therapy

Avoidance of triggers (especially alcohol and spicy or hot foods) and drinking ice water may be effective in reducing facial erythema and flushing. Metronidazole (available as creams, gels, or lotions), 0.75% applied twice daily or 1% applied once daily, and ivermectin 1% cream applied once daily are effective topical treatments. Another effective treatment includes topical clindamycin (solution, gel, or lotion) 1% applied twice daily. Response is noted in 4–8 weeks. Sulfur-sodium sulfacetamide-containing topicals are helpful in patients only partially responsive to topical antibiotics. Topical retinoids can be carefully added for maintenance. Topical brimonidine tartrate gel 0.33% can temporarily reduce the flush/redness of rosacea patients.

B. Systemic Therapy

Oral tetracyclines should be used when topical therapy is inadequate. Minocycline or doxycycline, 50–100 mg orally once or twice daily, is effective. Metronidazole or amoxicillin, 250–500 mg orally twice daily, or rifaximin, 400 mg orally three times daily (for 10 days), may be used in refractory cases. Side effects are few, although metronidazole may produce a disulfiram-like effect when the patient ingests alcohol, and it may cause neuropathy with long-term use. Long-term maintenance with subantimicrobial dosing of minocycline or doxycycline is recommended once the initial flare of rosacea has resolved. Isotretinoin may succeed where other measures fail. A dosage of 0.5 mg/kg/d orally for 12–28 weeks is recommended. See precautions above. Telangiectases are benefitted by laser therapy, and phymatous overgrowth of the nose can be treated by surgical reduction.

▶ Prognosis

Rosacea tends to be a persistent process. With the regimens described above, it can usually be controlled adequately.

Taieb A et al; The ivermectin Phase III study group. Superiority of ivermectin 1% cream over metronidazole 0.75% cream in treating inflammatory lesions of rosacea: a randomized, investigator-blinded trial. Br J Dermatol. 2015 Apr;172(4): 1103–10. [PMID: 25228137]

Two AM et al. Rosacea: part I. Introduction, categorization, histology, pathogenesis, and risk factors. J Am Acad Dermatol. 2015 May;72(5):749–58. [PMID: 25890455]

Two AM et al. Rosacea: part II. Topical and systemic therapies in the treatment of rosacea. J Am Acad Dermatol. 2015 May;72(5):761–70. [PMID: 25890456]

Van Zuuren EJ et al. Interventions for rosacea: abridged updated Cochrane systematic review including GRADE assessments. Br J Dermatol. 2015 Sep;173(3):651–62. [PMID: 26099423]

Webster G et al. Ocular rosacea: a dermatologic perspective. J Am Acad Dermatol. 2013 Dec;69(6 Suppl 1):S42–3. [PMID: 24229636]

Weinstock LB et al. Rosacea and small intestinal bacterial overgrowth: prevalence and response to rifaximin. J Am Acad Dermatol. 2013 May;68(5):875–6. [PMID: 23602178]

FOLLICULITIS (Including Sycosis)

► Itching and burning in hairy areas.
► Pustules in the hair follicles.

General Considerations

Folliculitis has multiple causes. It is frequently caused by staphylococcal infection and may be more common in the diabetic patient. When the lesion is deep-seated, chronic, and recalcitrant on the head and neck, it is called **sycosis.**

Gram-negative folliculitis, which may develop during antibiotic treatment of acne, may present as a flare of acne pustules or nodules. *Klebsiella, Enterobacter, Escherichia coli,* and *Proteus* have been isolated from these lesions.

Hot tub folliculitis (*Pseudomonas* folliculitis), caused by *Pseudomonas aeruginosa,* is characterized by pruritic or tender follicular, pustular lesions occurring within 1–4 days after bathing in a contaminated hot tub, whirlpool, or swimming pool. Systemic flu-like symptoms may accompany cutaneous lesions. Rarely, systemic infections may result. Neutropenic patients should avoid these exposures.

Nonbacterial folliculitis may also be caused by friction and oils. Occlusion, perspiration, and rubbing, such as that resulting from tight jeans and other heavy fabrics on the upper legs can worsen this type of folliculitis.

Steroid acne may be seen during topical or systemic corticosteroid therapy and presents as eruptive monomorphous papules and papulopustules on the face and trunk. It responds to topical benzoyl peroxide.

Eosinophilic folliculitis is a sterile folliculitis that presents with urticarial papules with prominent eosinophilic infiltration. It is common in patients with AIDS. It may appear first with institution of highly active antiretroviral therapy (ART) and be mistaken for a drug eruption.

Pseudofolliculitis is caused by ingrowing hairs in the beard area. It occurs in men and women with tightly curled beard hair. In this entity, the papules and pustules are located at the side of and not in follicles. It may be treated by growing a beard, by using chemical depilatories, or by shaving with a foil-guard razor. Laser hair removal is dramatically beneficial in patients with pseudofolliculitis, requires limited maintenance, and can be done on patients of any skin color. Pseudofolliculitis is a true medical indication for such a procedure and should not be considered cosmetic.

Malassezia (Pityrosporum) **folliculitis** presents as 1–2-mm pruritic pink papulopustules on the upper trunk and arms. It is often pruritic and tends to develop during periods of excessive sweating.

Clinical Findings

The symptoms range from slight burning and tenderness to intense itching. The lesions consist of pustules of hair follicles (Figure 6–22).

▲ **Figure 6–22.** Bacterial folliculitis. (Used, with permission, from Berger TG, Dept Dermatology, UCSF.)

Differential Diagnosis

It is important to differentiate bacterial from nonbacterial folliculitis. The history is important for pinpointing the causes of nonbacterial folliculitis, and a Gram stain and culture are indispensable. One must differentiate folliculitis from acne vulgaris or pustular miliaria (heat rash) and from infections of the skin, such as impetigo or fungal infections, especially *Malassezia (Pityrosporum)* folliculitis. *Pseudomonas* folliculitis is often suggested by the history of hot tub use. Eosinophilic folliculitis in AIDS often requires biopsy for diagnosis.

Complications

Abscess formation is the major complication of bacterial folliculitis.

Prevention

Correct any predisposing local causes, such as oils or friction. Be sure that the water in hot tubs and spas is treated properly. If staphylococcal folliculitis is persistent, treatment of nasal or perineal carriage with rifampin, 600 mg daily for 5 days, or with topical mupirocin ointment 2% twice daily for 5 days, may help. Prolonged oral clindamycin, 150–300 mg/day for 4–6 weeks, or oral TMP-SMZ given 1 week per month for 6 months can be effective in preventing recurrent staphylococcal folliculitis and furunculosis. Bleach baths (¼ to ½ cup per 20 liters of bathwater for 15 minutes 3–5 times weekly) may reduce cutaneous staphylococcal carriage and not contribute to antibiotic resistance. Control of blood glucose in diabetes may reduce the number of these infections.

Treatment

A. Local Measures

Anhydrous ethyl alcohol containing 6.25% aluminum chloride (Xerac AC), applied three to seven times weekly to lesions and environs, may be helpful, especially for chronic frictional folliculitis of the buttocks. **Topical antibiotics are generally ineffective if bacteria have invaded the hair follicle** but may be prophylactic if used as an aftershave in patients with recurrent folliculitis after shaving.

B. Specific Measures

Pseudomonas folliculitis will clear spontaneously in non-neutropenic patients if the lesions are superficial. It may be treated with ciprofloxacin, 500 mg twice daily for 5 days.

Systemic antibiotics are recommended for bacterial folliculitis due to other organisms. Extended periods of treatment (4–8 weeks or more) with antistaphylococcal antibiotics are required if infection has involved the scalp or densely hairy areas, such as the axilla, beard, or groin.

Gram-negative folliculitis in acne patients may be treated with isotretinoin in compliance with all precautions discussed above (see Acne Vulgaris).

Eosinophilic folliculitis may be treated initially by the combination of potent topical corticosteroids and oral antihistamines. In more severe cases, treatment is with one of the following: topical permethrin (application for 12 hours every other night for 6 weeks); itraconazole, 200–400 mg daily; UVB or PUVA phototherapy; or isotretinoin, 0.5 mg/kg/day for up to 5 months. A remission may be induced by some of these therapies, but long-term treatment may be required.

Malassezia (Pityrosporum) folliculitis is treated with topical sulfacetamide lotion twice a day, alone or in combination with itraconazole or fluconazole.

Prognosis

Bacterial folliculitis is occasionally stubborn and persistent, requiring prolonged or intermittent courses of antibiotics.

Laureano AC et al. Facial bacterial infections: folliculitis. Clin Dermatol. 2014 Nov–Dec;32(6):711–4. [PMID: 25441463]
Pedrosa AF et al. Malassezia infections: a medical conundrum. J Am Acad Dermatol. 2014 Jul;71(1):170–6. [PMID: 24569116]
Weingartner JS et al. What is your diagnosis? Demodex folliculitis. Cutis. 2012 Aug;90(2): 62, 65–6, 69. [PMID: 22988646]

MILIARIA (Heat Rash)

ESSENTIALS OF DIAGNOSIS

- Burning, itching, superficial aggregated small vesicles, papules, or pustules on covered areas of the skin, usually the trunk.
- More common in hot, moist climates.
- Rare forms associated with fever and even heat prostration.

General Considerations

Miliaria occurs most commonly on the trunk and intertriginous areas. A hot, moist environment is the most frequent cause. Occlusive clothing required for certain occupations may increase the risk. Bedridden febrile patients are susceptible. Plugging of the ostia of sweat ducts occurs, with ultimate rupture of the sweat duct, producing an irritating, stinging reaction. Increase in numbers of resident aerobes, notably cocci, plays a role. Medications that enhance sweat gland function (eg, clonidine, beta-blockers, opioids) may contribute.

Clinical Findings

The usual symptoms are burning and itching. The histologic depth of sweat gland obstruction determines the clinical presentation: **miliaria crystallina** in the superficial (subcorneal) epidermis, **miliaria rubra** in the deep epidermis, and **miliaria profunda** in the dermis. The lesions consist of small (1–3 mm) nonfollicular lesions. Subcorneal thin-walled, discrete clear fluid-filled vesicles are termed "miliaria crystallina." When fluid is turbid and lesions present as vesicopustules or pustules, they are called **miliaria pustulosa**. Miliaria rubra (prickly heat) presents as pink papules. Miliaria profunda presents as nonfollicular skin-colored papules that develop after multiple bouts of miliaria rubra. In a hospitalized patient, the reaction virtually always affects the back.

Differential Diagnosis

Miliaria is to be distinguished from drug eruption and folliculitis.

Prevention

Use of an antibacterial preparation, such as chlorhexidine, prior to exposure to heat and humidity may help prevent the condition. Frequent turning or sitting of the hospitalized patient may reduce miliaria on the back.

Treatment

The patient should keep cool and wear light clothing. Triamcinolone acetonide, 0.1% in Sarna lotion, or a mid-potency corticosteroid in a lotion or cream may be applied two to four times daily. Secondary infections (superficial pyoderma) are treated with appropriate antistaphylococcal antibiotics. Anticholinergic medications (eg, glycopyrrolate 1 mg orally twice a day) may be helpful in severe cases

Prognosis

Miliaria is usually a mild disorder, but severe forms (tropical anhidrosis and asthenia) result from interference with the heat-regulating mechanism.

Carvalho R et al. sQUIZ your knowledge! "Water-drop" lesions in a febrile patient. Miliaria crystalline (MC). Eur J Dermatol. 2012 Jan–Feb;22(1):160–1. [PMID: 22370171]
Tey HL et al. In vivo imaging of miliaria profunda using high-definition optical coherence tomography: diagnosis, pathogenesis, and treatment. JAMA Dermatol. 2015 Mar 1;151(3): 346–8. [PMID: 25390622]

MUCOCUTANEOUS CANDIDIASIS

ESSENTIALS OF DIAGNOSIS

► Severe pruritus of vulva, anus, or body folds.

► Superficial denuded, beefy-red areas with or without satellite vesicopustules.

► Whitish curd-like concretions on the oral and vaginal mucous membranes.

► Yeast and pseudohyphae on microscopic examination of scales or curd.

▲ **Figure 6–23.** Oral mucosal candidiasis. (Used with permission from Sol Silverman, Jr, DDS, Public Health Image Library, CDC.)

► General Considerations

Mucocutaneous candidiasis is a superficial fungal infection that may involve almost any cutaneous or mucous surface of the body. It is particularly likely to occur in diabetics, during pregnancy, and in obese persons. Systemic antibiotics, oral corticosteroids, and oral contraceptive agents may be contributory. Oral and interdigital candidiasis may be the first sign of HIV infection (see Chapter 31). Denture use predisposes the elderly to infection. The Th-17 pathway is important in maintaining host defense against *Candida* infections, and mutations that interfere with normal Th-17 function predispose to *Candida* infection of the skin and mucous membranes.

► Clinical Findings

A. Symptoms and Signs

Itching may be intense. Burning is reported, particularly around the vulva and anus. The lesions consist of superficially denuded, beefy-red areas in the depths of the body folds, such as in the groin and the intergluteal cleft, beneath the breasts, at the angles of the mouth, in the webspaces of digits, and in the umbilicus. The peripheries of these denuded lesions are superficially undermined, and there may be satellite vesicopustules. Whitish, curd-like concretions may be present on mucosal lesions (Figure 6–23). Paronychia may occur (Figure 6–24).

B. Laboratory Findings

Clusters of budding yeast and pseudohyphae can be seen under high power (400×) when skin scales or curd-like lesions are mounted in 10% KOH. Culture can confirm the diagnosis.

► Differential Diagnosis

Intertrigo, seborrheic dermatitis, tinea cruris, "inverse psoriasis", and erythrasma involving the same areas may mimic mucocutaneous candidiasis.

► Complications

Systemic invasive candidiasis with candidemia may be seen with immunosuppression and in patients receiving broad-spectrum antibiotic and hypertonic glucose solutions, as in hyperalimentation. There may or may not be clinically evident mucocutaneous candidiasis.

► Treatment

A. General Measures

Affected parts should be kept dry and exposed to air as much as possible. Water immersion should be minimized and gloves should be worn for those with infected nails or digital skin. If possible, discontinue systemic antibiotics. For treatment of systemic invasive candidiasis, see Chapter 36.

▲ **Figure 6–24.** Acute paronychia. (From EJ Mayeaux, MD; used, with permission, from Usatine RP, Smith MA, Mayeaux EJ Jr, Chumley H, Tysinger J. *The Color Atlas of Family Medicine.* McGraw-Hill, 2009.)

B. Local Measures

1. Nails and paronychia—Apply clotrimazole solution 1% twice daily. Thymol 4% in ethanol applied once daily is an alternative.

2. Skin—Apply nystatin ointment or clotrimazole cream 1%, either with hydrocortisone cream 1%, twice daily. Gentian violet 0.5% solution is economical and highly effective in treating mucocutaneous candidiasis, but the purple discoloration may represent a cosmetic issue. Severe or widespread cutaneous disease responds to fluconazole, 100–200 mg daily, for 1 week.

3. Vulvar and anal mucous membranes—For vaginal candidiasis, single-dose fluconazole (150 mg orally) is effective. Intravaginal clotrimazole, miconazole, terconazole, or nystatin may also be used. Long-term suppressive therapy may be required for recurrent or "intractable" cases. Non-albicans candidal species may be identified by culture in some refractory cases and may respond to oral itraconazole, 200 mg twice daily for 2–4 weeks.

4. Balanitis—This is most frequent in uncircumcised men, and *Candida* usually plays a role. Topical nystatin ointment is the initial treatment if the lesions are mildly erythematous or superficially erosive. Soaking with dilute aluminum acetate for 15 minutes twice daily may quickly relieve burning or itching. Chronicity and relapses, especially after sexual contact, suggest reinfection from a sexual partner who should be treated. Severe purulent balanitis is usually due to bacteria. If it is so severe that phimosis occurs, oral antibiotics—some with activity against anaerobes—are required; if rapid improvement does not occur, urologic consultation is indicated.

5. Mastitis—Lancinating breast pain and nipple dermatitis in breast-feeding women may be a manifestation of *Candida* colonization/infection of the breast ducts. Topical nystatin cream and clotrimazole 0.1% cream are safe during lactation. Topical gentian violet 0.5% daily for 7 days is also useful. Oral fluconazole, 200 mg daily can be dramatically effective.

▶ Prognosis

Cases of cutaneous candidiasis range from the easily cured to the intractable and prolonged.

Barrett ME et al. Dermatoses of the breast in lactation. Dermatol Ther. 2013 Jul–Aug;26(4):331–6. [PMID: 23914890]

Coronado-Castellote L et al. Clinical and microbiological diagnosis of oral candidiasis. J Clin Exp Dent. 2013 Dec 1;5(5): e279–86. [PMID: 24455095]

Nenoff P et al. Mycology—an update part 2: dermatomycoses: clinical picture and diagnostics. J Dtsch Dermatol Ges. 2014 Sep;12(9):749–77. [PMID: 25176455]

Pichard DC et al. Primary immunodeficiency update: Part II. Syndromes associated with mucocutaneous candidiasis and noninfectious cutaneous manifestations. J Am Acad Dermatol. 2015 Sep;73(3):367–81. [PMID: 26282795]

Singh A et al. Oral candidiasis: An overview. J Oral Maxillofac Pathol. 2014 Sep;18(Suppl 1):S81–5. [PMID: 25364186]

ERYTHEMAS

REACTIVE ERYTHEMAS

1. Urticaria & Angioedema

ESSENTIALS OF DIAGNOSIS

▶ Eruptions of evanescent wheals or hives.

▶ Itching is usually intense but may, on rare occasions, be absent.

▶ Special forms of urticaria have special features (dermatographism, cholinergic urticaria, solar urticaria, or cold urticaria).

▶ Most incidents are acute and self-limited over a period of 1–2 weeks.

▶ Chronic urticaria (episodes lasting longer than 6 weeks) may have an autoimmune basis.

▶ General Considerations

Urticaria can result from many different stimuli on an immunologic or nonimmunologic basis. The most common immunologic mechanism is mediated by IgE, as seen in the majority of patients with acute urticaria; another involves activation of the complement cascade. Some patients with chronic urticaria demonstrate autoantibodies directed against mast cell IgE receptors. ACE inhibitor and angiotensin receptor blocker therapy may be complicated by urticaria or angioedema. **In general, extensive costly workups are not indicated in patients who have urticaria.** A careful history and physical examination are more helpful.

▶ Clinical Findings

A. Symptoms and Signs

Lesions are itchy, red swellings of a few millimeters to many centimeters (Figure 6–25). The morphology of the lesions may vary over a period of minutes to hours, resulting in geographic or bizarre patterns. Individual lesions in true urticaria last less than 24 hours, and often only 2–4 hours. Angioedema is involvement of deeper subcutaneous tissue with swelling of the lips, eyelids, palms, soles, and genitalia. **Angioedema is no more likely than urticaria to be associated with systemic complications, such as laryngeal edema or hypotension.** In cholinergic urticaria, triggered by a rise in core body temperature (hot showers, exercise), wheals are 2–3 mm in diameter with a large surrounding red flare. Cold urticaria is acquired or inherited and triggered by exposure to cold and wind (see Chapter 37).

B. Laboratory Findings

The most common causes of acute urticaria are foods, infections, and medications. The cause of chronic urticaria

▲ **Figure 6–25.** Urticaria. (Used, with permission, from Berger TG, Dept Dermatology, UCSF.)

is often not found. Laboratory studies are not likely to be helpful in the evaluation of acute or chronic urticaria. In patients with individual lesions that persist past 24 hours, skin biopsy may confirm neutrophilic urticaria or urticarial vasculitis. A functional ELISA test looking for antibodies against the high-affinity receptor for IgE (Fc-Epislon RI) can detect patients with an autoimmune basis for their chronic urticaria.

▶ Differential Diagnosis

Papular urticaria resulting from insect bites persists for days. A central punctum can usually be seen. Streaked urticarial lesions may be seen in the 24–48 hours before blisters appear in acute allergic plant dermatitis, eg, poison ivy, oak, or sumac. Urticarial responses to heat, sun, water, and pressure are quite rare. Urticarial vasculitis may be seen as part of serum sickness, associated with fever and arthralgia. In this setting, a low serum complement level may be associated with severe systemic disease.

In hereditary angioedema, there is generally a positive family history and gastrointestinal or respiratory symptoms. Urticaria is not part of the syndrome, and lesions are not pruritic.

▶ Treatment

A. General Measures

A detailed search by history for a cause of acute urticaria should be undertaken, and treatment may then be tailored to include the provocative condition. The chief causes are medications—eg, aspirin, NSAIDs, morphine, and codeine; arthropod bites—eg, insect bites and bee stings (though the latter may cause anaphylaxis as well as angioedema); physical factors, such as heat, cold, sunlight, and pressure; and, presumably, neurogenic factors, as in cholinergic urticaria induced by exercise, excitement, hot showers, etc. Other causes may include penicillins and other medications; inhalants such as feathers and animal danders; ingestion of shellfish, tomatoes, or strawberries; infections, such as viral hepatitis (causing urticarial vasculitis); and in selected patients salicylates and tartrazine dyes.

B. Systemic Treatment

The mainstay of treatment initially includes H_1-antihistamines. Initial therapy is hydroxyzine, 10 mg twice daily to 25 mg three times daily, or as a single nightly dose of 50–75 mg to reduce daytime sedation. Cyproheptadine, 4 mg four times daily, may be especially useful for cold urticaria. "Nonsedating" or less sedating antihistamines are added if the generic sedating antihistamines are not effective. Options include fexofenadine, 180 mg once daily; or cetirizine or loratadine, 10 mg daily. **Higher doses of these second-generation antihistamines may be required to suppress urticaria (up to four times the standard recommended dose) than are required for allergic rhinitis.** These high doses are safe and can be used in refractory cases. Montelukast (10 mg daily) in combination with antihistamines appears to have a therapeutic benefit.

Doxepin (a tricyclic antidepressant with potent antihistaminic properties), 10–75 mg at bedtime, can be very effective in chronic urticaria. It has anticholinergic side effects.

H_2-antihistamines in combination with H_1-blockers may be helpful in patients with symptomatic dermatographism and to a lesser degree in chronic urticaria. UVB phototherapy can suppress some cases of chronic urticaria. If a skin biopsy of a lesion of chronic urticaria identifies neutrophils as a significant component of the inflammatory infiltrate, dapsone or colchicine (or both) may be useful.

A few patients with chronic urticaria may respond to elimination of salicylates and tartrazine (a coloring agent). Asymptomatic foci of infection—sinusitis, vaginal candidiasis, cholecystitis, and intestinal parasites—may rarely cause chronic urticaria. Although systemic corticosteroids in a dose of about 40 mg daily will usually suppress acute and chronic urticaria, the use of corticosteroids is rarely indicated and, once withdrawn, the urticaria virtually always returns. Instead of instituting systemic corticosteroids, consultation should be sought from a dermatologist or an allergist with experience in managing severe urticaria. Cyclosporine (3–5 mg/kg/day), mycophenolate mofetil, and other immunosuppressives may be effective in severe cases of chronic urticaria. Omalizumab is approved for the treatment of refractory chronic urticaria and should be considered when severe chronic urticaria fails to respond to high-dose antihistamines.

C. Local Treatment

Local treatment is rarely rewarding.

Prognosis

Acute urticaria usually lasts only a few days to weeks. Half of patients whose urticaria persists for longer than 6 weeks will have it for years. Patients in whom angioedema develops with an ACE inhibitor may be switched to an angiotensin receptor blocker with caution (estimated cross-reaction about 10%).

Asero R et al. Treatment of refractory chronic urticaria: current and future therapeutic options. Am J Clin Dermatol. 2013 Dec;14(6):481–8. [PMID: 24085572]

Carr TF et al. Chapter 21: Urticaria and angioedema. Allergy Asthma Proc. 2012 May–Jun;33(Suppl 1):S70–2. [PMID: 22794694]

Saini SS et al. Efficacy and safety of omalizumab in patients with chronic idiopathic/spontaneous urticaria who remain symptomatic on H_1 antihistamines: a randomized, placebo-controlled study. J Invest Dermatol. 2015 Mar;135(3):925. [PMID: 25501032]

Sharma M et al. H_1-antihistamines for chronic spontaneous urticaria. Cochrane Database Syst Rev. 2014 Nov 14;11:CD006137. [PMID: 25397904]

2. Erythema Multiforme/Stevens-Johnson Syndrome/Toxic Epidermal Necrolysis

ESSENTIALS OF DIAGNOSIS

▸ Sudden onset of symmetric erythematous skin lesions with history of recurrence.

▸ May be macular, papular, urticarial, bullous, or purpuric.

▸ "Target" lesions with clear centers and concentric erythematous rings or "iris" lesions may be noted in erythema multiforme minor. Well-defined target lesions are rare in drug-associated Stevens-Johnson syndrome.

▸ Erythema multiforme minor presents on the extensor surfaces, palms, soles, or mucous membranes. Stevens-Johnson syndrome favors the trunk.

▸ Herpes simplex is the most common cause of erythema multiforme minor.

▸ Medications are the most common cause of Stevens-Johnson syndrome in adults.

General Considerations

Erythema multiforme is an acute inflammatory skin disease that was traditionally divided clinically into minor and major types based on the clinical findings. Approximately 90% of cases of erythema multiforme minor follow outbreaks of herpes simplex, and so is preferably termed **herpes-associated erythema multiforme.** The term "erythema multiforme major" has been replaced by three terms: **Stevens-Johnson syndrome** (SJS), with less than 10% BSA detachment; **toxic epidermal necrolysis** (TEN) when there is greater than 30% BSA detachment; and **SJS/TEN overlap** for cases with between 10% and 30% BSA detachment.

The abbreviation SJS/TEN is often used to refer to these three variants of what is considered one syndrome. All these clinical scenarios are characterized by toxicity and involvement of two or more mucosal surfaces (often oral and conjunctival). They are most often caused by medications, especially sulfonamides, NSAIDs, allopurinol, and anticonvulsants. In certain races, polymorphisms of antigen-presenting major histocompatibility (MHC) loci increase the risk for the development of SJS/TEN. *Mycoplasma pneumoniae* may trigger a mucocutaneous reaction with skin and oral lesions closely resembling Stevens-Johnson syndrome in up to 50% of children/young adults in some series. The exposure to medications associated with SJS/TEN may be systemic or topical (eg, eyedrops).

Clinical Findings

A. Symptoms and Signs

A classic target lesion, found most commonly in herpes-associated erythema multiforme, consists of three concentric zones of color change, most often found acrally on the hands and feet. Medication-associated bullous eruptions in the SJS/TEN spectrum present with raised purpuric target-like lesions, with only two zones of color change and a central blister, or nondescript reddish or purpuric macules favoring the trunk and proximal upper extremities (Figure 6–26). Pain on eating, swallowing, and urination can occur if the appropriate mucosae are involved.

B. Laboratory Findings

Blood tests are not useful for diagnosis. Skin biopsy is diagnostic. Direct immunofluorescence studies are negative.

Differential Diagnosis

Urticaria and drug eruptions are the chief entities that must be differentiated from erythema multiforme minor. In true urticaria, lesions are not purpuric or bullous, last less than 24 hours, and respond to antihistamines. The differential diagnosis of SJS/TEN includes autoimmune bullous diseases (eg, pemphigus, pemphigoid, and linear IgA

▲ **Figure 6–26.** Stevens-Johnson syndrome. (Used, with permission, from Berger TG, Dept Dermatology, UCSF.)

bullous dermatosis), acute systemic lupus erythematosus, vasculitis, and Sweet syndrome. The presence of a blistering eruption requires biopsy and consultation for appropriate diagnosis and treatment.

► Complications

The tracheobronchial mucosa, conjunctiva, and urethral mucosa may be involved in severe cases with resultant scarring. **Ophthalmologic consultation is required if ocular involvement is present because vision loss is the major consequence of SJS/TEN.**

► Treatment

A. General Measures

Toxic epidermal necrolysis is best treated in an acute care environment, which may include an ICU or a burn unit. Patients should be admitted if mucosal involvement interferes with hydration and nutrition or extensive blistering develops. Open lesions should be managed like second-degree burns. Immediate discontinuation of the inciting medication (before blistering occurs) is a significant predictor of outcome. Delay in establishing the diagnosis and inadvertently continuing the offending medication results in higher morbidity and mortality.

B. Specific Measures

The most important aspect of treatment is to stop the offending medication and to move patients with greater than 25–30% BSA involvement to an appropriate acute care environment. Nutritional and fluid support and high vigilance for infection are the most important aspects of care. Reviews of systemic treatments for SJS and TEN have been conflicting. Some data support the use of high-dose corticosteroids. If corticosteroids are to be tried, they should be used early, before blistering occurs, and in moderate to high doses (prednisone, 1–2 mg/kg/day) and stopped within days if there is no dramatic response. Intravenous immunoglobulin (IVIG) (1 g/kg/day for 4 days) has become standard of care at some centers for toxic epidermal necrolysis cases. IVIG used early in the course and at a total dose of at least 2 g/kg may result in decreased mortality, although not all studies support this finding. Cyclosporine (3–5 mg/kg/day for 7 days) may also be effective. Tumor necrosis factor inhibitors are used at some centers as well. Oral and topical corticosteroids are useful in the oral variant of erythema multiforme. Oral acyclovir prophylaxis of herpes simplex infections may be effective in preventing recurrent herpes-associated erythema multiforme minor.

C. Local Measures

Topical therapy is not very effective in this disease.

► Prognosis

Erythema multiforme minor usually lasts 2–6 weeks and may recur. SJS/TEN may be serious with a mortality of about 30% in cases with greater than 30% BSA involvement. SCORTEN (a severity of illness scale) predicts mortality in SJS/TEN.

Barron SJ et al. Intravenous immunoglobulin in the treatment of Stevens-Johnson syndrome and toxic epidermal necrolysis: a meta-analysis with meta-regression of observational studies. Int J Dermatol. 2015 Jan;54(1):108–15. [PMID: 24697283]

Canavan TN et al. *Mycoplasma pneumoniae*-induced rash and mucositis as a syndrome distinct from Stevens-Johnson syndrome and erythema multiforme: a systematic review. J Am Acad Dermatol. 2015 Feb;72(2):239–45. [PMID: 25592340]

Huang YC et al. The efficacy of intravenous immunoglobulin for the treatment of toxic epidermal necrolysis: a systematic review and meta-analysis. Br J Dermatol. 2012 Aug;167(2):424–32. [PMID: 22458671]

Kirchhof MG et al. Retrospective review of Stevens-Johnson syndrome/toxic epidermal necrolysis treatment comparing intravenous immunoglobulin with cyclosporine. J Am Acad Dermatol. 2014 Nov;71(5):941–7. [PMID: 25087214]

Mockenhaupt M. Stevens-Johnson syndrome and toxic epidermal necrolysis: clinical patterns, diagnostic considerations, etiology, and therapeutic management. Semin Cutan Med Surg. 2014 Mar;33(1):10–6. [PMID: 25037254]

Paradisi A et al. Etanercept therapy for toxic epidermal necrolysis. J Am Acad Dermatol. 2014 Aug;71(2):278–83. [PMID: 24928706]

Sokumbi O et al. Clinical features, diagnosis, and treatment of erythema multiforme: a review for the practicing dermatologist. Int J Dermatol. 2012 Aug;51(8):889–902. [PMID: 22788803]

Zhu QY et al. Toxic epidermal necrolysis: performance of SCORTEN and the score-based comparison of the efficacy of corticosteroid therapy and intravenous immunoglobulin combined therapy in China. J Burn Care Res. 2012 Nov;33(6):e295–308. [PMID: 22955159]

3. Erythema Migrans (See also Chapter 34)

Erythema migrans is a unique cutaneous eruption that characterizes the localized or generalized early stage of Lyme disease (caused by *Borrelia burgdorferi*) (Figure 6–27).

INFECTIOUS ERYTHEMAS

1. Erysipelas

ESSENTIALS OF DIAGNOSIS

► Edematous, raised, circumscribed, hot, erythematous area, with or without vesicles or bullae.

► Central face or lower extremity frequently involved.

► Pain, chills, fever, and systemic toxicity may be striking.

► General Considerations

Erysipelas is a superficial form of cellulitis that is caused by beta-hemolytic streptococci.

► Clinical Findings

A. Symptoms and Signs

The symptoms are pain, malaise, chills, and moderate fever. A bright red spot appears and then spreads to form a tense, sharply demarcated, glistening, smooth, hot plaque.

▲ **Figure 6–27.** Erythema migrans due to *Borrelia burgdorferi* (Lyme disease). (Used, with permission, from James Gathany, Public Health Image Library, CDC.)

The margin characteristically makes noticeable advances in days or even hours. The lesion is edematous with a raised edge and may pit slightly with the finger. Vesicles or bullae occasionally develop on the surface. The lesion does not usually become pustular or gangrenous and heals without scar formation. The disease may complicate any break in the skin that provides a portal of entry for the organism. On the face, erysipelas begins near a fissure at the angle of the nose. On the lower extremity, tinea pedis with interdigital fissuring is a common portal of entry.

B. Laboratory Findings

Leukocytosis is almost invariably present; blood cultures may be positive.

▶ Differential Diagnosis

Erysipeloid is a benign bacillary infection producing cellulitis of the skin of the fingers or the backs of the hands in fishermen and meat handlers.

▶ Complications

Unless erysipelas is promptly treated, death may result from extension of the process and systemic toxicity, particularly in the elderly.

▶ Treatment

Intravenous antibiotics effective against group A beta-hemolytic streptococci and staphylococci should be considered, but outpatient treatment with oral antibiotics has demonstrated equal efficacy. Oral regimens include a 7-day course with penicillin VK (250 mg), dicloxacillin (250 mg), or a first-generation cephalosporin (250 mg) orally four times a day. Alternatives in penicillin-allergic patients are clindamycin (250 mg twice daily orally for 7–14 days) or erythromycin (250 mg four times daily orally for 7–14 days), the latter only if the infection is known to be due to streptococci.

▶ Prognosis

With appropriate treatment, rapid improvement is expected. The presence of lymphedema carries the greatest risk of recurrence.

2. Cellulitis

> ### ESSENTIALS OF DIAGNOSIS
>
> ▶ Edematous, expanding, erythematous, warm plaque with or without vesicles or bullae.
>
> ▶ Lower leg is frequently involved.
>
> ▶ Pain, chills, and fever are commonly present.
>
> ▶ Septicemia may develop.

▶ General Considerations

Cellulitis, a diffuse spreading infection of the dermis and subcutaneous tissue, is usually on the lower leg (Figure 6–28) and most commonly due to gram-positive cocci, especially group A beta-hemolytic streptococci and *S aureus*. Rarely, gram-negative rods or even fungi can produce a similar picture. **In otherwise healthy persons, the most common portal of entry for lower leg cellulitis is toe web intertrigo with fissuring, usually a complication of interdigital tinea pedis.** Other diseases that predispose to cellulitis are prior episodes of cellulitis, chronic edema, venous insufficiency with secondary edema, lymphatic obstruction, saphenectomy, and other perturbations of the skin barrier. **Bacterial cellulitis is almost never bilateral.**

▶ Clinical Findings

A. Symptoms and Signs

Cellulitis begins as a tender small patch. Swelling, erythema, and pain are often present. The lesion expands over hours, so that from onset to presentation is usually 6 to 36 hours. As the lesion grows, the patient becomes more ill with progressive chills, fever, and malaise. Lymphangitis and lymphadenopathy are often present. If septicemia develops, hypotension may develop, followed by shock.

▲ **Figure 6–28.** Cellulitis. (Used, with permission, from Berger TG, Dept Dermatology, UCSF.)

B. Laboratory Findings

Leukocytosis or at least a neutrophilia (left shift) is present from early in the course. Blood cultures may be positive. If a central ulceration, pustule, or abscess is present, culture may be of value. Aspiration of the advancing edge has a low yield (20%) and is usually not performed. In immunosuppressed patients, or if an unusual organism is suspected and there is no loculated site to culture, a full thickness skin biopsy taken before antibiotics are given can be useful. Either two specimens or one divided in half should be sent for routine histologic evaluation and for culture. Skin biopsy is particularly important in the immunocompromised patient in whom cellulitis may be due to an uncommon organism. If a primary source for the infection is identified (wound, leg ulcer, toe web intertrigo), cultures from these sites isolate the causative pathogen in half of cases and can be used to guide antibiotic therapy.

▶ Differential Diagnosis

Two potentially life-threatening entities that can mimic cellulitis (ie, present with a painful, red, swollen lower extremity) include deep venous thrombosis and necrotizing fasciitis. The diagnosis of necrotizing fasciitis should be suspected in a patient who has a very toxic appearance, bullae, crepitus or anesthesia of the involved skin, overlying skin necrosis, and laboratory evidence of rhabdomyolysis (elevated creatine kinase [CK]) or disseminated intravascular coagulation. While these findings may be present with severe cellulitis and bacteremia, it is essential to rule out necrotizing fasciitis because rapid surgical debridement is essential. Other skin lesions that may resemble cellulitis include **sclerosing panniculitis**, an acute, exquisitely tender red plaque on the medial lower legs above the malleolus in patients with venous stasis or varicosities, and **acute severe contact dermatitis** on a limb, which produces erythema, vesiculation, and edema, as seen in cellulitis, but with itching instead of pain. **Bilateral lower leg bacterial cellulitis is exceedingly rare, and other diagnoses, especially severe stasis dermatitis (see Figure 12–1), should be considered in this setting.** Severe lower extremity stasis dermatitis usually develops over days to weeks rather than the hours of cellulitis. It is also not as tender to palpation as cellulitis. Cryptococcal cellulitis in the organ transplant recipient is often bilateral.

▶ Treatment

Intravenous or parenteral antibiotics may be required for the first 2–5 days, with adequate coverage for *Streptococcus* and *Staphylococcus*. Methicillin-susceptible *S aureus* (MSSA) can be treated with nafcillin, cefazolin, clindamycin, dicloxacillin, cephalexin, doxycycline, or TMP-SMZ. If MRSA is suspected or proven, treatment options include vancomycin, linezolid, clindamycin, daptomycin, doxycycline, or TMP-SMZ. In mild cases or following the initial parenteral therapy, dicloxacillin or cephalexin, 250–500 mg four times daily for 5–10 days, is usually adequate. In patients in whom intravenous treatment is not instituted, the first dose of oral antibiotic can be doubled to achieve high blood levels rapidly. In patients with recurrent lower leg cellulitis (3–4 episodes per year), oral penicillin 250 mg twice daily or erythromycin can delay the appearance of the next episode. Prior episodes of cellulitis, lymphedema, chronic venous insufficiency, peripheral vascular disease, and deep venous thrombosis are associated with an increased risk of recurrent cellulitis.

▶ When to Admit

- Severe local symptoms and signs.
- Systemic inflammatory response syndrome (SIRS) criteria are met.
- Elevated white blood cell count with marked left shift.
- Failure to respond to oral antibiotics.

Oh CC et al. Antibiotic prophylaxis for preventing recurrent cellulitis: a systematic review and meta-analysis. J Infect. 2014 Jul;69(1):26–34. [PMID: 24576824]

Stevens DL et al. Practice guidelines for the diagnosis and management of skin and soft tissue infections: 2014 update by the Infectious Diseases Society of America. Clin Infect Dis. 2014 Jul 15;59(2):147–59. [PMID: 24947530]

Strazzula L et al. Inpatient dermatology consultation aids diagnosis of cellulitis among hospitalized patients: a multi-institutional analysis. J Am Acad Dermatol. 2015 Jul;73(1): 70–5. [PMID: 26089048]

Tay EY et al. Cellulitis Recurrence Score: a tool for predicting recurrence of lower limb cellulitis. J Am Acad Dermatol. 2015 Jan;72(1):140–5. [PMID: 25443627]

BLISTERING DISEASES

PEMPHIGUS

ESSENTIALS OF DIAGNOSIS

▶ Relapsing crops of bullae, often fragile and leading to erosions.

▶ Often preceded by mucous membrane bullae, erosions, and ulcerations.

▶ Superficial detachment of the skin after pressure or trauma variably present (Nikolsky sign).

▶ Acantholysis on biopsy.

▶ Immunofluorescence studies and serum ELISA for pathogenic antibodies are confirmatory.

▶ General Considerations

Pemphigus is an uncommon intraepidermal blistering disease occurring on skin and mucous membranes. It is caused by autoantibodies to adhesion molecules expressed in the skin and mucous membranes. The cause is unknown, and in the preantibiotic, presteroid era, the condition was usually fatal within 5 years. The bullae appear spontaneously and are tender and painful when they rupture. Drug-induced pemphigus from penicillamine, captopril, and others has been reported. There are several forms of pemphigus: **pemphigus vulgaris** and its variant, **pemphigus vegetans**; and the more superficially blistering **pemphigus foliaceus** and its variant, **pemphigus erythematosus.** All forms may occur at any age, but most present in middle age. The vulgaris form begins in the mouth in over 50% of cases. The foliaceus form is especially apt to be associated with other autoimmune diseases, or it may be drug-induced. **Paraneoplastic pemphigus,** a unique form of the disorder, is associated with numerous types of benign and malignant neoplasms but most frequently non-Hodgkin lymphoma.

▶ Clinical Findings

A. Symptoms and Signs

Pemphigus is characterized by an insidious onset of flaccid bullae, crusts, and erosions in crops or waves (Figure 6–29). In pemphigus vulgaris, lesions often appear first on the oral mucous membranes. These rapidly become erosive. The scalp is another site of early involvement. Rubbing a cotton swab or finger laterally on the surface of

▲ **Figure 6–29.** Pemphigus. (Used, with permission, from Berger TG, Dept Dermatology, UCSF.)

uninvolved skin may cause easy separation of the epidermis (**Nikolsky sign**).

B. Laboratory Findings

The diagnosis is made by light microscopy and by direct and indirect immunofluorescence (IIF) microscopy. Autoantibodies to intercellular adhesion molecules (desmoglien 3 and 1) can be detected with ELISA assays and have replaced the use of IIF in some centers.

▶ Differential Diagnosis

Blistering diseases include erythema multiforme, SJS/TEN, drug eruptions, bullous impetigo, contact dermatitis, dermatitis herpetiformis, and bullous pemphigoid, but flaccid blisters are not typical of these diseases, and acantholysis is not seen on biopsy. All of these diseases have clinical characteristics and different immunofluorescence test results that distinguish them from pemphigus.

Paraneoplastic pemphigus is clinically, histologically, and immunologically distinct from other forms of the disease. Oral erosions and erythematous plaques resembling erythema multiforme are seen. Survival rates are low because of the underlying malignancy.

▶ Complications

Secondary infection commonly occurs; this is a major cause of morbidity and mortality. Disturbances of fluid, electrolyte, and nutritional intake can occur as a result of painful oral ulcers.

▶ Treatment

A. General Measures

When the disease is severe, hospitalize the patient at bed rest and provide antibiotics and intravenous feedings as indicated. Anesthetic troches used before eating ease painful oral lesions.

B. Systemic Measures

Pemphigus requires systemic therapy as early in its course as possible. However, the main morbidity in this disease is due to the side effects of such therapy. Initial therapy is with systemic corticosteroids: prednisone, 60–80 mg daily. In all but the mildest cases, a steroid-sparing agent is added from the beginning, since the course of the disease is long and the steroid-sparing agents take several weeks to exert their activity. Azathioprine (100–200 mg daily) or mycophenolate mofetil (1–1.5 g twice daily) are used most frequently. Rituximab treatment (1 g intravenously on days 1 and 15), especially early in the course, appears to be associated with therapeutic induction of a complete remission and is increasingly being used as first-line therapy. Repeated courses are efficacious and well tolerated in patients who do not achieve complete remission or relapse. Monthly IVIG at 2 g/kg intravenously over 3–4 days frequently is beneficial. In refractory cases, cyclophosphamide, pulse intravenous corticosteroids, and plasmapheresis can be used. Increased risk of thromboembolism is associated with IVIG therapy at these doses.

C. Local Measures

In patients with limited disease, skin and mucous membrane lesions should be treated with topical corticosteroids. Complicating infection requires appropriate systemic and local antibiotic therapy.

► Prognosis

The course tends to be chronic in most patients, though about one-third appear to experience remission. Infection is the most frequent cause of death, usually from *S aureus* septicemia.

Heelan K et al. Durable remission of pemphigus with a fixed-dose rituximab protocol. JAMA Dermatol. 2014 Jul;150(7): 703–8. [PMID: 24500264]

Ingen-Housz-Oro S et al. First-line treatment of pemphigus vulgaris with a combination of rituximab and high-potency topical corticosteroids. JAMA Dermatol. 2015 Feb;151(2): 200–3. [PMID: 25354242]

Ishii K. Importance of serological tests in diagnosis of autoimmune blistering diseases. J Dermatol. 2015 Jan;42(1):3–10. [PMID: 25558946]

Jonkman MF. JAMA Dermatology Patient Page. Pemphigus. JAMA Dermatol. 2014 Jun;150(6):680. [PMID: 24919519]

Venugopal SS et al. Diagnosis and clinical features of pemphigus vulgaris. Immunol Allergy Clin North Am. 2012 May;32(2): 233–43. [PMID: 22560136]

BULLOUS PEMPHIGOID

Many other autoimmune skin disorders are characterized by formation of bullae, or blisters. These include bullous pemphigoid, cicatricial pemphigoid, dermatitis herpetiformis, and pemphigoid gestationis.

Bullous pemphigoid is a relatively benign pruritic disease characterized by tense blisters in flexural areas, usually remitting in 5 or 6 years, with a course characterized by exacerbations and remissions. Most affected persons are over the age of 60 (often in their 70s or 80s), and men are affected twice as frequently as women. The appearance of blisters may be preceded by pruritic urticarial or edematous lesions for months. Oral lesions are present in about one-third of affected persons. The disease may occur in various forms, including localized, vesicular, vegetating, erythematous, erythrodermic, and nodular.

The diagnosis is made by biopsy and direct immunofluorescence examination. Light microscopy shows a subepidermal blister. With direct immunofluorescence, IgG and C3 are found at the dermal-epidermal junction. When ELISA testing for bullous pemphigoid antibodies BP 180 or BP 230 is performed, positivity of either will be found in 97% of patients. If the patient has mild disease, ultrapotent corticosteroids may be adequate. Prednisone at a dosage of 0.75 mg/kg daily is often used to achieve rapid control of more widespread disease. Tetracycline (500 mg three times daily), alone or combined with nicotinamide—not nicotinic acid or niacin—(up to 1.5 g/day), may control the disease in patients who cannot use corticosteroids or may allow decreasing or eliminating corticosteroids after control is achieved. Dapsone is particularly effective in mucous membrane pemphigoid. If these medications are not effective, methotrexate, 5–25 mg weekly, azathioprine, 50 mg one to three times daily, or mycophenolate mofetil (1–1.5 g twice daily) may be used as steroid-sparing agents. Intravenous immunoglobulin, rituximab, and omalizumab have been used with success in refractory cases.

Cho YT et al. First-line combination therapy with rituximab and corticosteroids provides a high complete remission rate in moderate-to-severe bullous pemphigoid. Br J Dermatol. 2015 Jul;173(1):302–4. [PMID: 25529394]

Gaitanis G et al. High-dose intravenous immunoglobulin in the treatment of adult patients with bullous pemphigoid. Eur J Dermatol. 2012 May–Jun;22(3):363–9. [PMID: 22548754]

Ishii K. Importance of serological tests in diagnosis of autoimmune blistering diseases. J Dermatol. 2015 Jan;42(1):3–10. [PMID: 25558946]

Schmidt E et al. Pemphigoid diseases. Lancet. 2013 Jan 26; 381(9863):320–32. [PMID: 23237497]

Yu KK et al. Omalizumab therapy for bullous pemphigoid. J Am Acad Dermatol. 2014 Sep;71(3):468–74. [PMID: 24954907]

PAPULES

WARTS

 ESSENTIALS OF DIAGNOSIS

► Verrucous papules anywhere on the skin or mucous membranes, usually no larger than 1 cm in diameter.

► Prolonged incubation period (average 2–18 months).

► Spontaneous "cures" are frequent in common warts (50% at 2 years).

► "Recurrences" (new lesions) are frequent.

General Considerations

Warts (common, plantar, and genital) are caused by human papillomaviruses (HPVs). Typing of HPV lesions is not a part of standard medical evaluation except in the case of anogenital dysplasia.

Clinical Findings

There are usually no symptoms. Tenderness on pressure occurs with plantar warts; itching occurs with anogenital warts (Figure 6–30). Flat warts are most evident under oblique illumination. Periungual warts may be dry, fissured, and hyperkeratotic and may resemble hangnails. Plantar warts resemble plantar corns or calluses.

Differential Diagnosis

Some warty-looking lesions are actually hypertrophic actinic keratoses or squamous cell carcinomas. Some genital warty lesions may be due to secondary syphilis (condylomata lata). The lesions of molluscum contagiosum are pearly with a central dell. In AIDS, wart-like lesions may be caused by varicella zoster virus.

Prevention

Administration of a vaccine against certain anogenital HPV types (including 6, 11, 16, 18) can prevent infection with these wart types and reduce anogenital, oropharyngeal, and cervical cancer. It is recommended for teenagers and young adults (see Chapters 1 and 18).

Treatment

Treatment is aimed at inducing "wart-free" intervals for as long as possible without scarring, since no treatment can guarantee a remission or prevent recurrences. In immunocompromised patients, the goal is even more modest, ie, to control the size and number of lesions present.

▲ **Figure 6–30.** Condylomata acuminata, or genital warts, of the anal region due to human papillomavirus. (Public Health Image Library, CDC.)

A. Removal

For common warts of the hands, patients are usually offered liquid nitrogen or keratolytic agents. The former may work in fewer treatments but requires office visits and is painful.

1. Liquid nitrogen—Liquid nitrogen is applied to achieve a thaw time of 30–45 seconds. Two freeze-thaw cycles are given every 2–4 weeks for several visits. Scarring will occur if it is used incorrectly. Liquid nitrogen may cause permanent depigmentation in pigmented individuals. Cryotherapy is first-line physician-applied surgical treatment for genital warts (**condyloma acuminata**).

2. Keratolytic agents and occlusion—Salicylic acid products may be used against common warts or plantar warts. They are applied, then occluded. Plantar warts may be treated by applying a 40% salicylic acid plaster after paring. The plaster may be left on for 5–6 days, then removed, the lesion pared down, and another plaster applied. Although it may take weeks or months to eradicate the wart, the method is safe and effective with almost no side effects. Chronic occlusion alone with water-impermeable tape (duct tape, adhesive tape) is less effective than cryotherapy.

3. Podophyllum resin—For genital warts, the purified active component of the podophyllum resin, podofilox, is applied by the patient twice daily 3 consecutive days a week for cycles of 4–6 weeks. It is less irritating and more effective than "physician-applied" podophyllum resin. After a single 4-week cycle, 45% of patients were wart-free; but of these, 60% relapsed at 6 weeks. Thus, multiple cycles of treatment are often necessary. Patients unable to obtain the take-home podofilox may be treated in the clinician's office by painting each wart carefully (protecting normal skin) every 2–3 weeks with 25% podophyllum resin (podophyllin) in compound tincture of benzoin. Podophyllin is ineffective for common warts and plantar warts and should not be used in pregnant women (pregnancy category X).

4. Imiquimod—A 5% cream of this local interferon inducer has moderate activity in clearing external genital warts. Treatment is once daily on 3 alternate days per week. Response may be slow, with patients who eventually cleared having responses at 8 weeks (44%) or 12 weeks (69%). There is a marked difference between the sexes with respect to response, with 77% of women and 40% of men having complete clearing of their lesions. Once cleared, about 13% have recurrences in the short term.

   Although imiquimod is considerably more expensive than podophyllotoxin, its high rate of response in women and its safety (pregnancy category B) make it the "patient-administered" treatment of choice for external genital warts in women. In men, the more rapid response, lower cost, and similar efficacy make podophyllotoxin the initial treatment of choice, with imiquimod used for recurrences or refractory cases. Imiquimod has no demonstrated efficacy for—and should not be used to treat—plantar or common warts.

5. Operative removal—Plantar warts may be removed by blunt dissection. For genital warts, snip biopsy (scissors) removal followed by light electrocautery is more effective than cryotherapy, especially for patients with pedunculated or large lesions.

6. Laser therapy—The CO_2 laser can be effective for treating recurrent warts, periungual warts, plantar warts, and condylomata acuminata. It leaves open wounds that must fill in with granulation tissue over 4–6 weeks and is best reserved for warts resistant to all other modalities. Lasers with emissions of 585, 595, or 532 nm may also be used every 3–4 weeks to gradually ablate common or plantar warts. This is no more effective than cryotherapy in controlled trials. For genital warts, it has not been shown that laser therapy is more effective than electrosurgical removal. Photodynamic therapy can be considered in refractory widespread flat and genital warts.

7. Other agents—Bleomycin diluted to 1 unit/mL may be injected into common and plantar warts. It has been shown to have a high cure rate. It should be used with caution on digital warts because of the potential complications of Raynaud phenomenon, nail loss, and terminal digital necrosis. 5-Fluorouracil 5% cream applied once or twice daily, usually with occlusion, may be applied to warts with the similar efficacy to other treatment methods.

B. Immunotherapy

Squaric acid dibutylester may be applied in a concentration of 0.2–2% directly to the warts from once weekly to five times weekly to induce a mild contact dermatitis. Between 60% and 80% of warts clear over 10–20 weeks. Injection of *Candida* antigen starting at 1:50 dilution and repeated every 3–4 weeks may be similarly effective in stimulating immunologic regression of common and plantar warts.

C. Physical Modalities

Soaking warts in hot (42.2°C) water for 10–30 minutes daily for 6 weeks has resulted in involution in some cases.

▶ Prognosis

There is a striking tendency to develop new lesions. Warts may disappear spontaneously or may be unresponsive to treatment.

Alikhan A et al. Use of *Candida* antigen injections for the treatment of verruca vulgaris: a two-year mayo clinic experience. J Dermatolog Treat. 2015 Nov 11:1–4. [Epub ahead of print] [PMID: 26558635]

Grillo-Ardila CF et al. Imiquimod for anogenital warts in non-immunocompromised adults. Cochrane Database Syst Rev. 2014 Nov 1;11:CD010389. [PMID: 25362229]

Kwok CS et al. Topical treatments for cutaneous warts. Cochrane Database Syst Rev. 2012 Sep 12;9:CD001781. [PMID: 22972052]

Patel H et al. Systematic review of the incidence and prevalence of genital warts. BMC Infect Dis. 2013 Jan 25;13:39. [PMID: 23347441]

MOLLUSCUM CONTAGIOSUM

Molluscum contagiosum, caused by a poxvirus, presents as single or multiple dome-shaped, waxy papules 2–5 mm in

▲ **Figure 6–31.** Molluscum contagiosum lesion on the back. (Used, with permission, from Richard P. Usatine, MD in Usatine RP, Smith MA, Mayeaux EJ Jr, Chumley H, Tysinger J. *The Color Atlas of Family Medicine.* McGraw-Hill, 2009.)

diameter that are umbilicated (Figure 6–31). Lesions at first are firm, solid, and flesh-colored but upon reaching maturity become soft, whitish, or pearly gray and may suppurate. The principal sites of involvement are the face, lower abdomen, and genitals.

The lesions are autoinoculable and spread by wet skin-to-skin contact. In sexually active individuals, they may be confined to the penis, pubis, and inner thighs and are considered a sexually transmitted infection.

Molluscum contagiosum is common in patients with AIDS, usually with a helper T-cell count less than 100/mcL. Extensive lesions tend to develop over the face and neck as well as in the genital area.

The diagnosis is easily established in most instances because of the distinctive central umbilication of the dome-shaped lesion. It has been estimated that time to remission is 13 months. The best treatment is by curettage or applications of liquid nitrogen as for warts—but more briefly. When lesions are frozen, the central umbilication often becomes more apparent. Light electrosurgery with a fine needle is also effective. Ten percent potassium hydroxide solution applied twice daily until lesions clear is emerging as a viable treatment option. They are difficult to eradicate in patients with AIDS unless immunity improves. However, in AIDS, with highly effective antiretroviral treatment, molluscum do not need to be treated because they usually spontaneously clear.

Chen X et al. Molluscum contagiosum virus infection. Lancet Infect Dis. 2013 Oct;13(10):877–88. [PMID: 23972567]

Handjani F et al. Comparison of 10% potassium hydroxide solution versus cryotherapy in the treatment of molluscum contagiosum: an open randomized clinical trial. J Dermatolog Treat. 2014 Jun;25(3):249–50. [PMID: 23924070]

Olsen JR et al. Time to resolution and effect on quality of life of molluscum contagiosum in children in the UK: a prospective community cohort study. Lancet Infect Dis. 2015 Feb;15(2):190–5. [PMID: 25541478]

BASAL CELL CARCINOMA

> ## ESSENTIALS OF DIAGNOSIS
>
> ▶ Pearly papule, erythematous patch greater than 6 mm, or nonhealing ulcer in sun-exposed areas (face, trunk, lower legs).
>
> ▶ History of bleeding.
>
> ▶ Fair-skinned person with a history of sun exposure (often intense, intermittent).

General Considerations

Basal cell carcinomas are the most common form of cancer. They occur on sun-exposed skin in otherwise normal, fair-skinned individuals; ultraviolet light is the cause. The most common presentation is a papule or nodule that may have a central scab or erosion (Figure 6–32). Occasionally the nodules have stippled pigment (pigmented basal cell carcinoma). Intradermal nevi without pigment on the face of older white individuals may resemble basal cell carcinomas. Basal cell carcinomas grow slowly, attaining a size of 1–2 cm or more in diameter, usually only after years of growth. There is a **waxy, "pearly" appearance,** with telangiectatic vessels easily visible. It is the pearly or translucent quality of these lesions that is most diagnostic, a feature best appreciated if the skin is stretched. On the back and chest, basal cell carcinomas appear as reddish, somewhat shiny, scaly patches. Basal cell carcinomas are more common and more likely to recur in immunosuppressed patients, including those with non-Hodgkin lymphoma and those who have undergone solid organ or allogeneic hematopoietic stem cell transplantation.

▶ Treatment

Lesions suspected to be basal cell carcinomas should be biopsied, by shave or punch biopsy. Therapy is then aimed at eradication with minimal cosmetic deformity, often by excision and suturing with recurrence rates of 5% or less. The technique of three cycles of curettage and electrodesiccation depends on the skill of the operator and is not recommended for head and neck lesions. After 4–6 weeks of healing, it leaves a broad, hypopigmented, at times hypertrophic scar. Radiotherapy is effective and sometimes appropriate for older individuals (over age 65), but recurrent tumors after radiation therapy are more difficult to treat and may be more aggressive. Radiation therapy is the most expensive method to treat basal cell carcinoma and should only be used if other treatment options are not appropriate. **Mohs surgery**—removal of the tumor followed by immediate frozen section histopathologic examination of margins with subsequent reexcision of tumor-positive areas and final closure of the defect—gives the highest cure rates (98%) and results in least tissue loss. It is an appropriate therapy for tumors of the eyelids, nasolabial folds, canthi, external ear, and temple; for recurrent lesions; or where tissue sparing is needed for cosmesis. Vismodegib is reserved for the treatment of advanced or metastatic basal cell carcinoma or in patients with extensive tumor burden (eg, basal cell nevus syndrome). Imiquimod may be appropriate for select patients with superficial basal cell carcinomas, but the treated area must be observed for evidence of complete cure. Since a second lesion will develop in up to half of patients with a basal cell carcinoma, **patients with basal cell carcinomas must be monitored at least yearly to detect new or recurrent lesions.**

Ad Hoc Task Force; Connolly SM et al. AAD/ACMS/ASDSA/ASMS 2012 appropriate use criteria for Mohs micrographic surgery: a report of the American Academy of Dermatology, American College of Mohs Surgery, American Society for Dermatologic Surgery Association, and the American Society for Mohs Surgery. J Am Acad Dermatol. 2012 Oct;67(4):531–50. [PMID: 22959232]

Basset-Seguin N et al. Vismodegib in patients with advanced basal cell carcinoma (STEVIE): a pre-planned interim analysis of an international, open-label trial. Lancet Oncol. 2015 Jun;16(6):729–36. [PMID: 25981813]

Brewer JD et al. Increased incidence and recurrence rates of nonmelanoma skin cancer in patients with non-Hodgkin lymphoma: a Rochester Epidemiology Project population-based study in Minnesota. J Am Acad Dermatol. 2015 Feb;72(2):302–9. [PMID: 25479909]

Flohil SC et al. Trends in basal cell carcinoma incidence rates: a 37-Year Dutch observational study. J Invest Dermatol. 2013 Apr;133(4):913–8. [PMID: 23190883]

Kauvar AN et al; American Society for Dermatologic Surgery. Consensus for nonmelanoma skin cancer treatment: basal cell carcinoma, including a cost analysis of treatment methods. Dermatol Surg. 2015 May;41(5):550–71. [PMID: 25868035]

Omland SH et al. Skin cancer risk in hematopoietic stem-cell transplant recipients compared with background population and renal transplant recipients: a population-based cohort study. JAMA Dermatol. 2015 Oct 10:1–7. [PMID: 26454261]

▲ **Figure 6–32.** Nodular basal cell carcinoma of the nose. (Used, with permission, from Richard P. Usatine, MD in Usatine RP, Smith MA, Mayeaux EJ Jr, Chumley H, Tysinger J. *The Color Atlas of Family Medicine.* McGraw-Hill, 2009.)

SQUAMOUS CELL CARCINOMA

▶ Nonhealing ulcer or warty nodule.

▶ Skin damage due to long-term sun exposure.

▶ Common in fair-skinned organ transplant recipients.

Squamous cell carcinoma usually occurs subsequent to prolonged sun exposure on exposed parts in fair-skinned individuals who sunburn easily and tan poorly. It may arise from an actinic keratosis. The lesions appear as small red, conical, hard nodules that occasionally ulcerate (Figure 6–33). In actinically induced squamous cell cancers, rates of metastasis are estimated from retrospective studies to be 3–7%. Squamous cell carcinomas of the ear, temple, lip, oral cavity, tongue, and genitalia have much higher rates of recurrence or metastasis and require special management.

Examination of the skin and therapy are essentially the same as for basal cell carcinoma. The preferred treatment of squamous cell carcinoma is excision. Electrodesiccation and curettage and x-ray radiation may be used for some lesions, and fresh tissue microscopically controlled excision (Mohs) is recommended for high-risk lesions (lips, temples, ears, nose) and for recurrent tumors. **Follow-up for** squamous cell carcinoma must be more frequent and thorough than for basal cell carcinoma, starting at every 3 months, with careful examination of lymph nodes for 1 year, then twice yearly thereafter. In addition, palpation of the lips is essential to detect hard or indurated areas that represent early squamous cell carcinoma. All such cases must be biopsied. Multiple squamous cell carcinomas are very common on the sun-exposed skin of organ transplant patients. The intensity of immunosuppression, not the use of any particular immunosuppressive agent, is the primary risk factor in determining the development of skin cancer after transplant. The tumors begin to appear after 5 years of immunosuppression. Voriconazole treatment appears to increase the risk of development of squamous cell carcinoma, especially in lung transplant patients. **Regular dermatologic evaluation in at-risk organ transplant recipients is recommended.** Biologic behavior of skin cancer in organ transplant recipients may be aggressive, and careful management is required. Other forms of immunosuppression, such as allogeneic hematopoietic stem cell transplants, chronic lymphocytic leukemia, HIV/AIDS, and chronic iatrogenic immunosuppression, may also increase skin cancer risk and be associated with more aggressive skin cancer behavior.

Kauvar AN et al. Consensus for nonmelanoma skin cancer treatment, part II: squamous cell carcinoma, including a cost analysis of treatment methods. Dermatol Surg. 2015 Nov;41(11): 1214–40. [PMID: 26445288]

Lansbury L et al. Interventions for non-metastatic squamous cell carcinoma of the skin: systematic review and pooled analysis of observational studies. BMJ. 2013 Nov 4;347:f6153. [PMID: 24191270]

Schmults CD et al. Factors predictive of recurrence and death from cutaneous squamous cell carcinoma: a 10-year, single-institution cohort study. JAMA Dermatol. 2013 May;149(5): 541–7. [PMID: 23677079]

Tessari G et al. Nonmelanoma skin cancer in solid organ transplant recipients: update on epidemiology, risk factors, and management. Dermatol Surg. 2012 Oct;38(10):1622–30. [PMID: 22805312]

Williams K et al. Voriconazole-associated cutaneous malignancy: a literature review on photocarcinogenesis in organ transplant recipients. Clin Infect Dis. 2014 Apr;58(7):997–1002. [PMID: 24363331]

VIOLACEOUS TO PURPLE PAPULES & NODULES

LICHEN PLANUS

▶ Pruritic, violaceous, flat-topped papules with fine white streaks and symmetric distribution.

▶ Lacy or erosive lesions of the buccal, vulvar, and vaginal mucosa; nail dystrophy.

▶ Commonly seen along linear scratch marks (Koebner phenomenon) on anterior wrists, penis, and legs.

▶ Histopathologic examination is diagnostic.

▲ **Figure 6–33.** Squamous cell carcinoma. (Used, with permission, from Berger TG, Dept Dermatology, UCSF.)

General Considerations

Lichen planus is an inflammatory pruritic disease of the skin and mucous membranes characterized by distinctive papules with a predilection for the flexor surfaces and trunk. **The three cardinal findings are typical skin lesions, mucosal lesions, and histopathologic features of band-like infiltration of lymphocytes in the upper dermis.** The most common medications causing lichen planus-like reactions include sulfonamides, tetracyclines, quinidine, NSAIDs, beta-blockers, and hydrochlorothiazide. Lichenoid drug eruptions can resemble lichen planus clinically and histologically. Hepatitis C infection is found with greater frequency in lichen planus patients than in controls. Allergy to mercury and other metal-containing amalgams can trigger oral lesions identical to lichen planus.

Clinical Findings

Itching is mild to severe. The lesions are violaceous, flat-topped, angulated papules, up to 1 cm in diameter, discrete or in clusters, with very fine white streaks (Wickham striae) on the flexor surfaces of the wrists and on the penis, lips, tongue as well as buccal, vulvar, vaginal, esophageal, and anorectal mucous membranes. The papules may become bullous or eroded. The disease may be generalized (Figure 6–34). Mucous membrane lesions have a lacy white network overlying them that may be confused with leukoplakia. The presence of oral and vulvo-vaginal lichen planus in the same patient is common. Patients with both these mucous membranes involved are at much higher risk for esophageal lichen planus. The **Koebner phenomenon** (appearance of lesions in areas of trauma) may be seen.

A special form of lichen planus is the erosive or ulcerative variety, a major problem in the mouth or genitalia. Squamous cell carcinoma develops in up to 5% of patients with erosive oral or genital lichen planus and may occur in esophageal lichen planus. There is also an increased risk of squamous cell carcinoma developing in lesions of hypertrophic lichen on the lower extremities.

Differential Diagnosis

Lichen planus must be distinguished from similar lesions produced by medications and other papular lesions, such as psoriasis, lichen simplex chronicus, graft-versus-host disease, and syphilis. Lichen planus on the mucous membranes must be differentiated from leukoplakia. Erosive oral lesions require biopsy and often direct immunofluorescence for diagnosis since lichen planus may simulate other erosive diseases.

Treatment

A. Topical Therapy

Superpotent topical corticosteroids applied twice daily are most helpful for localized disease in nonflexural areas. Alternatively, high-potency corticosteroid cream or ointment may be used nightly under thin pliable plastic film.

Topical tacrolimus appears effective in oral and vaginal erosive lichen planus, but long-term therapy is required to prevent relapse. If tacrolimus is used, lesions must be

▲ **Figure 6–34.** Lichen planus. (Used, with permission, from Berger TG, Dept Dermatology, UCSF.)

observed carefully for development of cancer. Since absorption can occur through mucous membranes, serum tacrolimus levels should be checked at least once if widespread mucosal application (more than 5–10 cm²) is used. If the erosive oral lichen planus lesions are adjacent to a metal-containing amalgam, removal of the amalgam may result in clearing of the erosions.

B. Systemic Therapy

Corticosteroids (see Chapter 26) may be required in severe cases or in circumstances where the most rapid response to treatment is desired. Unfortunately, relapse almost always occurs as the corticosteroids are tapered, making systemic corticosteroid therapy an impractical option for the management of chronic lichen planus. NB-UVB, bath PUVA, oral PUVA, and the combination of an oral retinoid plus PUVA (re-PUVA) are all forms of phototherapy that can improve lichen planus. Hydroxychloroquine, 200 mg orally twice daily, acitretin 10–25 mg daily, and cyclosporine 3–5 mg/kg can also be effective in mucosal and cutaneous lichen planus.

Prognosis

Lichen planus is a benign disease, but it may persist for months or years and may be recurrent. Hypertrophic lichen planus and oral lesions tend to be especially persistent, and neoplastic degeneration has been described in chronically eroded lesions.

Cheng S et al. Interventions for erosive lichen planus affecting mucosal sites. Cochrane Database Syst Rev. 2012 Feb 15;2: CD008092. [PMID: 22336835]

Davari P et al. Mucosal lichen planus: an evidence-based treatment update. Am J Clin Dermatol. 2014 Jul;15(3):181–95. [PMID: 24781705]

Gorouhi F et al. Cutaneous and mucosal lichen planus: a comprehensive review of clinical subtypes, risk factors, diagnosis, and prognosis. Scientific World Journal. 2014 Jan 30;2014: 742826. [PMID: 24672362]

Knackstedt TJ et al. Squamous cell carcinoma arising in hypertrophic lichen planus: a review and analysis of 38 cases. Dermatol Surg. 2015 Dec;41(12):1411–8. [PMID: 26551772]

Le Cleach L et al. Clinical practice. Lichen planus. N Engl J Med. 2012 Feb 23;366(8):723–32. [PMID: 22356325]

KAPOSI SARCOMA

▶ General Considerations

Human herpes virus 8 (HHV-8), or Kaposi sarcoma–associated herpes virus, is the cause of all forms of Kaposi sarcoma.

Before 1980 in the United States, this rare, malignant skin lesion was seen mostly in elderly men, had a chronic clinical course, and was rarely fatal. Kaposi sarcoma occurs endemically in an often aggressive form in young black men of equatorial Africa, but it is rare in American blacks. Kaposi sarcoma continues to occur largely in homosexual men with HIV infection as an AIDS-defining illness. Kaposi sarcoma may complicate immunosuppressive therapy, and stopping the immunosuppression may result in improvement.

Red or purple plaques or nodules on cutaneous or mucosal surfaces are characteristic. Marked edema may occur with few or no skin lesions. Kaposi sarcoma commonly involves the gastrointestinal tract and can be screened for by fecal occult blood testing. In asymptomatic patients, these lesions are not sought or treated. Pulmonary Kaposi sarcoma can present with shortness of breath, cough, hemoptysis, or chest pain; it may be asymptomatic, appearing only on chest radiograph. Bronchoscopy may be indicated. The incidence of AIDS-associated Kaposi sarcoma is diminishing; however, chronic Kaposi sarcoma can develop in patients with HIV infection, high CD4 counts, and low viral loads. In this setting, the Kaposi sarcoma usually resembles the endemic form, being indolent and localized. At times, however, it can be clinically aggressive. The presence of Kaposi sarcoma at the time of antiretroviral initiation is associated with Kaposi sarcoma–immune reconstitution inflammatory syndrome (KS-IRIS), which has an especially aggressive course in patients with visceral disease.

▶ Treatment

For Kaposi sarcoma in the elderly, palliative local therapy with intralesional chemotherapy or radiation is usually all that is required. In the setting of iatrogenic immunosuppression, the treatment of Kaposi sarcoma is primarily reduction of doses of immunosuppressive medications. In AIDS-associated Kaposi sarcoma, the patient should first be given ART. Other therapeutic options include cryotherapy or intralesional vinblastine (0.1–0.5 mg/mL) for cosmetically objectionable lesions; radiation therapy for accessible and space-occupying lesions; and laser surgery for certain intraoral and pharyngeal lesions. Systemic therapy is indicated in patients with rapidly progressive skin disease (more than 10 new lesions per month), with edema or pain, and with symptomatic visceral disease or pulmonary disease. ART plus chemotherapy appears to be more effective than ART alone. Liposomal doxorubicin is highly effective in severe cases and may be used alone or in combination with bleomycin and vincristine. Alpha-interferon may also be used. Paclitaxel and other taxanes can be effective even in patients who do not respond to anthracycline treatment.

Achenbach CJ et al. Paradoxical immune reconstitution inflammatory syndrome in HIV-infected patients treated with combination antiretroviral therapy after AIDS-defining opportunistic infection. Clin Infect Dis. 2012 Feb 1;54(3): 424–33. [PMID: 22095568]

Gbabe OF et al. Treatment of severe or progressive Kaposi's sarcoma in HIV-infected adults. Cochrane Database Syst Rev. 2014 Aug 13;8:CD003256. [PMID: 25221796]

Luu HN et al. Age patterns of Kaposi's sarcoma incidence in a cohort of HIV-infected men. Cancer Med. 2014 Dec;3(6): 1635–43. [PMID: 25139791]

Régnier-Rosencher E et al. Treatments for classic Kaposi sarcoma: a systematic review of the literature. J Am Acad Dermatol. 2013 Feb;68(2):313–31. [PMID: 22695100]

Stiller CA et al. Descriptive epidemiology of Kaposi sarcoma in Europe. Report from the RARECARE project. Cancer Epidemiol. 2014 Dec;38(6):670–8. [PMID: 25454979]

PRURITUS (ITCHING)

Pruritus is the sensation that provokes a desire to scratch. It is modulated by multiple factors, including anxiety, depression, and amphetamine and cocaine use. Pruritus as a medical complaint is 40% as common as low back pain. Elderly Asian men are most significantly affected with 20% of all health care visits in Asian men over the age of 65 involving the complaint of itch. The quality of life of a patient with chronic pruritus is the same as a patient on hemodialysis. Most cases of pruritus are not mediated by histamine, hence the poor response of many pruritic patients to antihistamines. Neuropathic disease, especially in diabetics, is associated with pruritus, making neurally acting agents attractive new approaches to the management of pruritus. Evidence suggests that increased interleukin-31 (IL-31) signalling through the IL-31 receptor on epithelial cells and keratinocytes is associated with itch, especially in allergic skin disease.

Dry skin is the first cause of itch that should be sought, since it is common and easily treated. Primary cutaneous diseases with associated pruritus include scabies, atopic dermatitis, insect bites, pediculosis, contact dermatitis, drug reactions, urticaria, psoriasis, lichen planus, and fiberglass dermatitis. Theses conditions all present with recognizable cutaneous morphologies, and the treatment of the skin condition usually results in control of the associated pruritus.

Persistent pruritus not explained by cutaneous disease or association with a primary skin eruption should prompt a staged work-up for systemic causes. Perhaps the most common cause of pruritus associated with systemic disease is uremia in conjunction with hemodialysis. This condition and to a lesser degree the pruritus of liver disease may be helped by phototherapy with ultraviolet B or PUVA. Naltrexone and nalmefene have been shown to relieve the pruritus of liver disease. Naltrexone is not effective in pruritus associated with advanced chronic kidney disease, but gabapentin may be effective. Endocrine disorders, such as hypothyroidism, hyperthyroidism, or hyperparathyroidism, psychiatric disturbances, lymphoma, leukemia, and other internal malignant disorders, iron deficiency anemia, and certain neurologic disorders may also cause pruritus. Calcium channel blockers can cause pruritus with or without eczema, even years after they have been started, and it may take up to 1 year for the pruritus to resolve after the calcium channel blocker has been stopped. The treatment of chronic pruritus can be frustrating. Combinations of antihistamines, sinequan, gabapentin, mirtazapine, and opioid antagonists can be attempted in refractory cases. In cancer-associated and other forms of pruritus, aprepitant (Emend) 80 mg daily for several days can be dramatically effective. Il-31 blockade may represent a future target of itch therapy.

► Prognosis

Elimination of external factors and irritating agents may give complete relief. Pruritus accompanying a specific skin disease will subside when the skin disease is controlled. Pruritus accompanying serious internal disease may not respond to any type of therapy.

Berger TG et al. Pruritus in the older patient: a clinical review. JAMA. 2013 Dec 11;310(22):2443–50. [PMID: 24327039]

Ko MJ et al. Interleukin-31 is associated with uremic pruritus in patients receiving hemodialysis. J Am Acad Dermatol. 2014 Dec;71(6):11519.e1. [PMID: 25270263]

Leslie TA et al. Current topical and systemic therapies for itch. Handb Exp Pharmacol. 2015;226:337–56. [PMID: 25861788]

Nemoto O et al. The first trial of CIM331, a humanized anti-human IL-31 receptor A antibody, for healthy volunteers and patients with atopic dermatitis to evaluate safety, tolerability and pharmacokinetics of a single dose in a randomised, double-blind, placebo-controlled study. Br J Dermatol. 2015 Sep 26. [Epub ahead of print] [PMID: 26409172]

Shive M et al. Itch as a patient-reported symptom in ambulatory care visits in the United States. J Am Acad Dermatol. 2013 Oct;69(4):550–6. [PMID: 23870201]

Summers EM et al. Chronic eczematous eruptions in the aging: further support for an association with exposure to calcium channel blockers. JAMA Dermatol. 2013 Jul;149(7):814–8. [PMID: 23636109]

ANOGENITAL PRURITUS

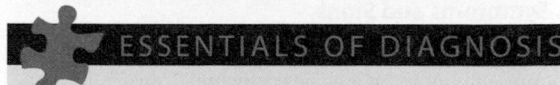

ESSENTIALS OF DIAGNOSIS

► Itching, chiefly nocturnal, of the anogenital area.

► Examination is highly variable, ranging from no skin findings to excoriations and inflammation of any degree, including lichenification.

► General Considerations

Anogenital pruritus may be due to a primary inflammatory skin disease (intertrigo, psoriasis, lichen simplex chronicus, seborrheic dermatitis, lichen sclerosus), contact dermatitis (soaps, colognes, douches, and topical treatments), irritating secretions (diarrhea, leukorrhea, or trichomoniasis), infections (candidiasis, dermatophytosis, erythrasma), or oxyuriasis (pinworms). Erythrasma (Figure 6–35) is diagnosed by coral-red fluorescence with Wood light and cured with erythromycin. Squamous cell carcinoma of the anus and extramammary Paget disease are rare causes of genital pruritus.

In pruritus ani, hemorrhoids are often found, and leakage of mucus and bacteria from the distal rectum onto the perianal skin may be important in cases in which no other skin abnormality is found.

Many women experience pruritus vulvae. Pruritus vulvae does not usually involve the anal area, though anal itching may spread to the vulva. In men, pruritus of the scrotum is most commonly seen in the absence of pruritus ani. **Up to one-third of causes of anogenital pruritus may be due to nerve impingements of the lumbosacral spine**, so referral for evaluation of lumbosacral spine disease is appropriate if no skin disorder is identified and topical therapy is ineffective.

▲ **Figure 6–35.** Erythrasma of the axilla. (Used, with permission, from Richard P. Usatine, MD in Usatine RP, Smith MA, Mayeaux EJ Jr, Chumley H, Tysinger J. *The Color Atlas of Family Medicine.* McGraw-Hill, 2009.)

Clinical Findings

A. Symptoms and Signs

The only symptom is itching. Physical findings are usually not present, but there may be erythema, fissuring, maceration, lichenification, excoriations, or changes suggestive of candidiasis or tinea.

B. Laboratory Findings

Microscopic examination or culture of tissue scrapings may reveal yeasts or fungi. Stool examination may show pinworms. Radiologic studies may demonstrate spinal disease.

Differential Diagnosis

The etiologic differential diagnosis consists of *Candida* infection, parasitosis, local irritation from contactants or irritants, nerve impingement and other primary skin disorders of the genital area, such as psoriasis, seborrhea, intertrigo, or lichen sclerosus.

Prevention

Instruct the patient in proper anogenital hygiene after treating systemic or local conditions. If appropriate, physical therapy and exercises to support the lower spine are recommended.

Treatment

A. General Measures

Treating constipation, preferably with high-fiber management (psyllium), may help. Instruct the patient to use very soft or moistened tissue or cotton after bowel movements and to clean the perianal area thoroughly with cool water if possible. Women should use similar precautions after urinating. Avoid "baby wipes" as they frequently contain preservatives that cause allergic contact dermatitis.

B. Local Measures

Pramoxine cream or lotion or hydrocortisone-pramoxine (Pramosone), 1% or 2.5% cream, lotion, or ointment, is helpful for anogenital pruritus and should be applied after a bowel movement. Topical doxepin cream 5% is similarly effective, but it may be sedating. Topical calcineurin inhibitors (tacrolimus 0.03%) improve pruritus ani in patients with atopic dermatitis. Underclothing should be changed daily, and in men, the seam of their "boxers" should not rub against or contact the scrotum. Balneol Perianal Cleansing Lotion or Tucks premoistened pads, ointment, or cream may be very useful for pruritus ani. About one-third of patients with scrotal or anal pruritus will respond to capsaicin cream 0.006%. Treatment for underlying spinal neurologic disease may be required. The use of high-potency topical corticosteroids should be avoided in the genital area.

Prognosis

Although benign, anogenital pruritus is often persistent and recurrent.

Guerrero A et al. Inflammatory vulvar dermatoses. Clin Obstet Gynecol. 2015 Sep;58(3):464–75. [PMID: 26125955]
Ucak H et al. Efficacy of topical tacrolimus for the treatment of persistent pruritus ani in patients with atopic dermatitis. J Dermatolog Treat. 2013 Dec;24(6):454–7. [PMID: 23638997]

SCABIES

ESSENTIALS OF DIAGNOSIS

▶ Generalized very severe itching.

▶ Burrows, vesicles, and pustules, especially on finger webs and in wrist creases.

▶ Mites, ova, and brown dots of feces (scybala) visible microscopically.

▶ Red papules or nodules on the scrotum and on the penile glans and shaft are pathognomonic.

General Considerations

Scabies is caused by infestation with *Sarcoptes scabiei*. The infestation usually spares the head and neck (though these areas may be involved in infants, the elderly, and patients with AIDS). Close physical contact for 15–20 minutes with an infected person is the typical mode of transmission. However, scabies may be acquired by contact with the bedding of an infested individual. Facility-associated scabies is increasingly common, primarily in long-term care facilities. Index patients are usually elderly and immunosuppressed. When these patients are hospitalized, hospital-based epidemics can occur. These epidemics are difficult to eradicate since many health care workers become infected and spread the infestation to other patients.

Clinical Findings

A. Symptoms and Signs

Itching is almost always present and can be severe. The lesions consist of more or less generalized excoriations with small pruritic vesicles, pustules, and "burrows" in the interdigital spaces of the hands and feet, on the heels of the palms, wrists (Figure 6–36), elbows, umbilicus, around the

▲ **Figure 6–36.** Scabies. (Used, with permission, from Berger TG, Dept Dermatology, UCSF.)

axillae, on the areolae in women, or on the penile shaft and scrotum in men. The burrow appears as a short irregular mark, 2–3 mm long and the width of a hair. Characteristic nodular lesions may occur on the scrotum or penis and along the posterior axillary line.

Hyperkeratotic or crusted scabies presents as thick flaking scale. These areas contain millions of mites, and these patients are highly infectious. Patients with widespread hyperkeratotic scabies are at risk for superinfection with *S aureus*, which in some cases progresses to sepsis if left untreated.

B. Laboratory Findings

The diagnosis should be confirmed by microscopic demonstration of the organism, ova, or feces in a mounted specimen, examined with tap water, mineral oil, or KOH. Best results are obtained when multiple lesions are scraped, choosing the best unexcoriated lesions from interdigital webs, wrists, elbows, or feet. A No. 15 blade is used to scrape each lesion until it is flat. **Patients with crusted/hyperkeratotic scabies must be evaluated for immunosuppression (especially HIV and HTLV-1 infections) if no iatrogenic cause of immunosuppression is present.** Patients with hyperkeratotic scabies and associated bacterial superinfection may have laboratory findings consistent with infection and, if severe, sepsis.

▶ Differential Diagnosis

Scabies must be distinguished from the various forms of pediculosis, from bedbug and flea bites, and from other causes of pruritus.

▶ Treatment & Prognosis

Treatment is aimed at killing scabies mites and controlling the dermatitis, which can persist for months after effective eradication of the mites. Bedding and clothing should be laundered or cleaned or set aside for 14 days in plastic bags. High heat (60°C) is required to kill the mites and ova. Unless treatment is aimed at all infected persons in a family or institutionalized group, reinfestations will likely occur.

Permethrin 5% cream is highly effective and safe in the management of scabies. Treatment consists of a single application from the neck down for 8–12 hours, repeated in 1 week.

Pregnant patients should be treated only if they have documented scabies themselves. Permethrin 5% cream once for 12 hours—or 5% or 6% sulfur in petrolatum applied nightly for 3 nights from the collarbones down—may be used.

Patients will continue to itch for several weeks after treatment. Use of triamcinolone 0.1% cream will help resolve the dermatitis.

Scabies in nursing home patients, institutionalized or mentally impaired (especially Down syndrome) patients, and AIDS patients may be much more difficult to treat.

Most failures in normal persons are related to incorrect use or incomplete treatment of the housing unit. In these cases, repeat treatment with permethrin once weekly for 2 weeks, with reeducation regarding the method and extent

of application, is suggested. In immunocompetent individuals, ivermectin in a dose of 200 mcg/kg is effective in about 75% of cases with a single dose and 95% of cases with two doses 2 weeks apart.

In immunosuppressed hosts and those with crusted (hyperkeratotic) scabies, multiple doses of ivermectin (every 2 weeks for two or three doses) plus topical therapy with permethrin every 3 days to once weekly, depending on degree of involvement, may be effective when topical treatment and oral therapy alone fail. A topical keratolytic (urea) should be used to help remove the scale, thereby decreasing the mite load, of hyperkeratotic scabies.

Oral ivermectin can be very beneficial in mass treatment to eradicate infections in institutions or villages.

If secondary pyoderma is present, it is treated with systemic antibiotics. Staphylococcal superinfection may lead to sepsis. In areas where nephritogenic streptococcal strains are prevalent, infestation with scabies or exposure to scabies-infested dogs may be followed by acute poststreptococcal glomerulonephritis.

Persistent pruritic postscabietic papules may be treated with mid- to high-potency corticosteroids or with intralesional triamcinolone acetonide (2.5–5 mg/mL).

Gunning K et al. Pediculosis and scabies: treatment update. Am Fam Physician. 2012 Sep 15;86(6):535–41. [PMID: 23062045]

Monsel G et al. Management of scabies. Skin Therapy Lett. 2012 Mar;17(3):1–4. [PMID: 22446818]

Panahi Y et al. The efficacy of topical and oral ivermectin in the treatment of human scabies. Ann Parasitol. 2015;61(1):11–6. [PMID: 25911032]

Shimose L et al. Diagnosis, prevention, and treatment of scabies. Curr Infect Dis Rep. 2013 Oct;15(5):426–31. [PMID: 23904181]

PEDICULOSIS

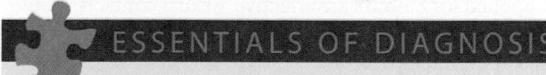

ESSENTIALS OF DIAGNOSIS

▶ Pruritus with excoriation.

▶ Nits on hair shafts; lice on skin or clothes.

▶ Occasionally, sky-blue macules (maculae ceruleae) on the inner thighs or lower abdomen in pubic louse infestation.

▶ General Considerations

Pediculosis is a parasitic infestation of the skin of the scalp, trunk, or pubic areas. Body lice usually occur among people who live in overcrowded dwellings with inadequate hygiene facilities. Pubic lice may be sexually transmitted. Head lice may be transmitted by shared use of hats or combs. Adults in contact with children with head lice frequently acquire the infestation.

There are three different varieties: (1) **pediculosis pubis,** caused by *Phthirus pubis* (pubic louse, "crabs"); (2) **pediculosis corporis**, caused by *Pediculus humanus* var *corporis* (body louse); and (3) **pediculosis capitis**, caused by *Pediculus humanus* var *capitis* (head louse).

Head and body lice are similar in appearance and are 3–4 mm long. The body louse can seldom be found on the body, because the insect comes onto the skin only to feed and must be looked for in the seams of the clothing. Trench fever, relapsing fever, and typhus are transmitted by the body louse in countries where those diseases are endemic. In the United States, *Bartonella quintana*, the organism that causes trench fever, has been found in lice infesting the homeless population.

Clinical Findings

Itching may be very intense in body louse infestations, and scratching may result in deep excoriations, especially over the upper shoulders, posterior flanks, and neck. In some cases, only itching is present, with few excoriations seen. Pyoderma may be the presenting sign. Head lice can be found on the scalp or may be manifested as small nits resembling pussy willow buds on the scalp hairs close to the skin. They are easiest to see above the ears and at the nape of the neck. Pubic louse infestations are occasionally generalized, particularly in hairy individuals; the lice may even be found on the eyelashes and in the scalp.

Differential Diagnosis

Head louse infestation must be distinguished from seborrheic dermatitis, body louse infestation from scabies and bedbug bites, and pubic louse infestation from anogenital pruritus and eczema.

Treatment

Body lice are treated by disposing of the infested clothing and addressing the patient's social situation. For pubic lice, permethrin rinse 1% for 10 minutes and permethrin cream 5% applied for 8 hours are effective. Sexual contacts should be treated. Clothes and bedclothes should be washed and dried at high temperature.

Permethrin 1% cream rinse (Nix) is a topical over-the-counter pediculicide and ovicide. It is applied to the scalp and hair and left on for 8 hours before being rinsed off. Although it is the treatment of choice for head lice, permethrin resistance is common. Malathion lotion 1% (Ovide) is very effective, but it is highly volatile and flammable, so application must be done in a well-ventilated room or out of doors. Topical ivermectin 0.5% lotion, benzyl alcohol 5%, or spinosad 0.9% suspension are additional agents that appear to have efficacy against pediculosis capitis; of these agents, topical ivermectin is the most effective. All infested persons in a household, school, or other facility should ideally be treated at the same time. Other than topical ivermectin, topical therapies should be repeated 7–9 days after the initial treatment. For involvement of eyelashes, petrolatum is applied thickly twice daily for 8 days, and remaining nits are then plucked off. Oral ivermectin can be used in children older than 5 years and more than 15 kg.

Devore CD et al; Council on School Health and Committee on Infectious Diseases, American Academy of Pediatrics. Head lice. Pediatrics. 2015 May;135(5):e1355–65. [PMID: 25917986]

Feldmeier H. Treatment of pediculosis capitis: a critical appraisal of the current literature. Am J Clin Dermatol. 2014 Oct;15(5):401–12. [PMID: 25223568]

SKIN LESIONS DUE TO OTHER ARTHROPODS

ESSENTIALS OF DIAGNOSIS

- ▶ Localized grouped urticarial papules with pruritus.
- ▶ Lesions in linear groups of three ("breakfast, lunch, and dinner") is characteristic of bed bugs.
- ▶ Furuncle-like lesions containing live arthropods.
- ▶ Tender erythematous patches that migrate ("larva migrans").

General Considerations

Some arthropods (eg, mosquitoes and biting flies) are readily detected as they bite. Many others are not because they are too small, because there is no immediate reaction, or because they bite during sleep. Reactions are allergic and may be delayed for hours to days. Patients are most apt to consult a clinician when the lesions are multiple and pruritus is intense.

Many persons will react severely only to their earliest contacts with an arthropod, thus presenting pruritic lesions when traveling, moving into new quarters, etc. Body lice, fleas, bedbugs, and mosquitoes should be considered. Bedbug exposure typically occurs in hotels and in housing with inadequate hygiene but also may occur in stable domiciles. Spiders are often incorrectly believed to be the source of bites; they rarely attack humans, though the brown recluse spider (*Loxosceles laeta*, *L reclusa*) may cause severe necrotic reactions and death due to intravascular hemolysis, and the black widow spider (*Latrodectus mactans*) may cause severe systemic symptoms and death. (See also Chapter 38.) The majority of patient-diagnosed, physician-diagnosed, and even published cases of brown recluse spider bites (or loxoscelism) are incorrect, especially if made in areas where these spiders are not endemic. Many of these lesions are actually due to CA-MRSA.

In addition to arthropod bites, the most common lesions are venomous stings (wasps, hornets, bees, ants, scorpions) or bites (centipedes), furuncle-like lesions due to fly maggots or sand fleas in the skin, and a linear creeping eruption due to a migrating larva.

Clinical Findings

The diagnosis may be difficult when the patient has not noticed the initial attack but suffers a delayed reaction. Individual bites are often in clusters and tend to occur either on exposed parts (eg, midges and gnats) or under clothing, especially around the waist or at flexures (eg, small mites or insects in bedding or clothing). The reaction is often delayed for 1–24 hours or more. Pruritus is almost always present and may be all but intolerable once the patient starts to scratch. Secondary infection may follow scratching. Urticarial wheals are common. Papules may become vesicular. The diagnosis is aided by searching for exposure to arthropods and by considering the patient's occupation and recent activities.

The principal arthropods are as follows:

1. **Fleas:** Fleas are bloodsucking ectoparasites that feed on dogs, cats, humans, and other species. Flea saliva produces papular urticaria in sensitized individuals. To break the life cycle of the flea, one must treat the home and pets, using quick-kill insecticides, residual insecticides, and a growth regulator.

2. **Bedbugs:** In crevices of beds or furniture; bites tend to occur in lines or clusters. Papular urticaria is a characteristic lesion of bedbug (*Cimex lectularius*) bites. Bedbugs are not restricted to any socioeconomic group and are a major health problem in some major metropolitan areas, especially in commercial and residential hotels.

3. **Ticks:** Usually picked up by brushing against low vegetation.

4. **Chiggers or red bugs:** These are larvae of trombiculid mites. A few species confined to particular regions and locally recognized habitats (eg, berry patches, woodland edges, lawns, brush turkey mounds in Australia, poultry farms) attack humans, often around the waist, on the ankles, or in flexures, raising intensely itching erythematous papules after a delay of many hours. The red chiggers may sometimes be seen in the center of papules that have not yet been scratched.

5. **Bird and rodent mites:** Larger than chiggers, bird mites infest birds and their nests. Bites are multiple anywhere on the body. Room air conditioning units may suck in bird mites and infest the inhabitants of the room. Rodent mites from mice or rats may cause similar effects. If the domicile has evidence of rodent activity, then rodent mite dermatitis should be suspected, as the mites are rarely found. Pet rodents or birds may be infested with mites, maintaining the infestation.

6. **Mites in stored products:** These are white and almost invisible and infest products, such as copra, vanilla pods, sugar, straw, cottonseeds, and cereals. Persons who handle these products may be attacked, especially on the hands and forearms and sometimes on the feet.

7. **Caterpillars of moths with urticating hairs:** The hairs are blown from cocoons or carried by emergent moths, causing severe and often seasonally recurrent outbreaks after mass emergence. The gypsy moth is a cause in the eastern United States.

8. **Tungiasis:** Tungiasis is due to the burrowing flea known as *Tunga penetrans* and is found in Africa, the West Indies, and South and Central America. The female burrows under the skin, sucks blood, swells to 0.5 cm, and then ejects her eggs onto the ground. Ulceration, lymphangitis, gangrene, and septicemia may result, in some cases with lethal effect. Simple surgical removal is usually performed.

Prevention

Arthropod infestations are best prevented by avoidance of contaminated areas, personal cleanliness, and disinfection of clothing, bedclothes, and furniture as indicated. Chiggers and mites can be repelled by permethrin applied to the head and clothing. (It is not necessary to remove clothing.) Bedbugs are no longer repelled by permethrin and can survive for up to 1 year without feeding. Aggressive cleaning, usually requiring removal of the affected occupant from the domicile, may be necessary to eradicate bedbug infestation in a residence.

Treatment

Living arthropods should be removed carefully with tweezers after application of alcohol and preserved in alcohol for identification. In endemic Rocky Mountain spotted fever areas, ticks should not be removed with the bare fingers.

Corticosteroid lotions or creams are helpful. Topical antibiotics may be applied if secondary infection is suspected. Localized persistent lesions may be treated with intralesional corticosteroids.

Stings produced by many arthropods may be alleviated by applying papain powder (Adolph's Meat Tenderizer) mixed with water, or aluminum chloride hexahydrate (Xerac AC).

Extracts from venom sacs of bees, wasps, yellow jackets, and hornets are available for immunotherapy of patients at risk for anaphylaxis.

Bernardeschi C et al. Bed bug infestation. BMJ. 2013 Jan 22;346:f138. Erratum in: BMJ. 2013;346:F1044. [PMID: 23341545]

Juckett G. Arthropod bites. Am Fam Physician. 2013 Dec 15; 88(12):841–7. [PMID: 24364549]

INFLAMMATORY NODULES

ERYTHEMA NODOSUM

ESSENTIALS OF DIAGNOSIS

▶ Painful nodules without ulceration on anterior aspects of legs.

▶ Slow regression over several weeks to resemble contusions.

▶ Women are predominantly affected by a ratio of 10:1 compared to men.

▶ Some cases associated with infection, inflammatory bowel disease, or drug exposure.

General Considerations

Erythema nodosum is a symptom complex characterized by tender, erythematous nodules that appear most commonly on the extensor surfaces of the lower legs. It usually lasts about 6 weeks and may recur. The disease may be associated with various infections—streptococcosis, primary coccidioidomycosis, other deep fungal infections, tuberculosis, *Yersinia pseudotuberculosis* and *Y enterocolitica* infection, diverticulitis, or syphilis. It may accompany sarcoidosis, Behçet disease, and inflammatory bowel disease. Erythema nodosum may be associated with pregnancy or with use of oral contraceptives.

► Clinical Findings

A. Symptoms and Signs

The subcutaneous swellings are exquisitely tender and may be preceded by fever, malaise, and arthralgia. They are most often located on the anterior surfaces of the legs below the knees but may occur on the arms, trunk, and face. The lesions, 1–10 cm in diameter, are at first pink to red; with regression, all the various hues seen in a contusion can be observed (Figure 6–37) but the lesions do not ulcerate.

B. Laboratory Findings

Evaluation of patients presenting with acute erythema nodosum should include a careful history (including medication exposures) and physical examination for prior upper respiratory infection or diarrheal illness, symptoms of any deep fungal infection endemic to the area, a chest radiograph, a PPD, and two consecutive ASO/DNAse B titers at 2- to 4-week intervals. If no underlying cause is found, only a small percentage of patients will go on to develop a significant underlying illness (usually sarcoidosis) over the next year.

► Differential Diagnosis

Erythema induratum from tuberculosis is seen on the posterior surfaces of the legs and may ulcerate. Lupus panniculitis presents as tender nodules in fatty areas of the buttocks and posterior arms and heals with depressed scars. In polyarteritis nodosa, the subcutaneous nodules are often associated with fixed livedo reticularis. In its late stages, erythema nodosum must be distinguished from simple bruises and contusions.

► Treatment

First, the underlying cause should be identified and treated. Primary therapy is with NSAIDs in usual doses. Saturated solution of potassium iodide, 5–15 drops three times daily, results in prompt involution in many cases. Complete bed rest may be advisable if the lesions are painful. Systemic therapy directed against the lesions themselves may include corticosteroid therapy (see Chapter 26) (unless contraindicated by associated infection), dapsone, colchicine, or hydroxychloroquine.

► Prognosis

The lesions usually disappear after about 6 weeks, but they may recur.

Blake T et al. Erythema nodosum—a review of an uncommon panniculitis. Dermatol Online J. 2014 Apr 16;20(4):22376. [PMID: 24746312]

Chen S et al. *Mycobacterium tuberculosis* infection is associated with the development of erythema nodosum and nodular vasculitis. PLoS One. 2013 May 1;8(5):e62653. [PMID: 23650522]

Eimpunth S et al. Tender cutaneous nodules of the legs: diagnosis and clinical clues to diagnosis. Int J Dermatol. 2013 May;52(5):560–6. [PMID: 22928517]

Passarini B et al. Erythema nodosum. G Ital Dermatol Venereol. 2013 Aug;148(4):413–7. [PMID: 23900162]

FURUNCULOSIS (Boils) & CARBUNCLES

ESSENTIALS OF DIAGNOSIS

► Extremely painful inflammatory swelling based on a hair follicle that forms an abscess.

► Predisposing condition (diabetes mellitus, HIV disease, injection drug use) sometimes present.

► Coagulase-positive *S aureus* is the causative organism.

▲ **Figure 6–37.** Erythema nodosum. (Used, with permission, from Berger TG, Dept Dermatology, UCSF.)

General Considerations

A **furuncle (boil)** is a deep-seated infection (abscess) caused by *S aureus* and involving the entire hair follicle and adjacent subcutaneous tissue. The most common sites of occurrence are the hairy parts exposed to irritation and friction, pressure, or moisture. Because the lesions are autoinoculable, they are often multiple. Diabetes mellitus (especially if using insulin injections), injection drug use, allergy injections, and HIV disease all increase the risk of staphylococcal infections by increasing the rate of carriage. Certain other exposures including hospitalization, athletic teams, prisons, military service, and homelessness may also increase the risk of infection.

A **carbuncle** consists of several furuncles developing in adjoining hair follicles and coalescing to form a conglomerate, deeply situated mass with multiple drainage points.

Recurrent furunculosis (three or more episodes in 12 months) tends to occur in those with direct contact with other infected individuals, especially family members.

Clinical Findings

A. Symptoms and Signs

Pain and tenderness may be prominent. The abscess is either rounded or conical. It gradually enlarges, becomes fluctuant, and then softens and opens spontaneously after a few days to 1–2 weeks to discharge a core of necrotic tissue and pus. The inflammation occasionally subsides before necrosis occurs. Infection of the soft tissue around the nails (paronychia) may be due to staphylococci when it is acute.

B. Laboratory Findings

There may be slight leukocytosis, but a white blood cell count is rarely required. Pus can be cultured to rule out MRSA or other bacteria. Culture of the anterior nares and anogenital area (including the rectum to test for gastrointestinal carriage) may identify chronic staphylococcal carriage in cases of recurrent cutaneous infection.

Differential Diagnosis

The most common entity in the differential is an inflamed epidermal inclusion cyst that suddenly becomes red, tender, and expands greatly in size over one to a few days. The history of a prior cyst in the same location, the presence of a clearly visible cyst orifice, and the extrusion of malodorous cheesy rather than purulent material helps in the diagnosis. Tinea profunda (deep dermatophyte infection of the hair follicle) may simulate recurrent furunculosis. Furuncle is also to be distinguished from deep mycotic infections, such as sporotrichosis; from other bacterial infections, such as anthrax and tularemia (rare); from atypical mycobacterial infections; and from acne cysts. Hidradenitis suppurativa (acne inversa) presents with recurrent tender sterile abscesses in the axillae and groin, on the buttocks, or below the breasts. The presence of old scars or sinus tracts plus negative cultures suggests this diagnosis.

Complications

Serious and sometimes fatal complications of staphylococcal infection such as septicemia can occur.

Prevention

Identifying and eliminating the source of infection is critical to prevent recurrences after treatment. The source individual may have chronic dermatitis or be an asymptomatic carrier. Nasal carriage of MRSA and the number of children in a household are risk factors for transmission between household members. Local measures, such as meticulous handwashing; no sharing of towels and clothing; aggressive scrubbing of showers, bathrooms, and surfaces with bleach; bleach baths (¼–½ cup per 20 liters of bathwater for 15 minutes 3–5 times weekly), 4% chlorhexidine washes, and isolation of infected patients who reside in institutions to prevent spread are all effective measures.

Treatment

A. Specific Measures

Incision and drainage is recommended for all loculated suppurations and is the mainstay of therapy. Systemic antibiotics are usually given, although they offer little beyond adequate incision and drainage. Sodium dicloxacillin or cephalexin, 1 g daily in divided doses by mouth for 10 days, is usually effective. Doxycycline 100 mg twice daily, TMP-SMZ double-strength one tablet twice daily, clindamycin 150–300 mg twice daily, and linezolid 400 mg twice daily are effective in treating MRSA. Recurrent furunculosis may be effectively treated with a combination of cephalexin (250–500 mg four times daily) or doxycycline (100 mg twice daily) for 2–4 weeks plus either rifampin (300 mg twice daily for 5 days for 2–4 weeks) or long-term clindamycin (150–300 mg daily for 1–2 months). Shorter courses of antibiotics (7–14 days) plus longer-term daily 4% chlorhexidine whole body washing and intranasal, axilla, and anogenital mupirocin may also cure recurrent furunculosis. Oral vancomycin (1 g twice daily for 5 days) can treat gastrointestinal carriage of *S aureus*. Family members, pets, and intimate contacts may need evaluation for staphylococcal carrier state and perhaps concomitant treatment. Stopping high-risk behavior, such as injection drug use, can also prevent recurrence of furunculosis.

B. Local Measures

Immobilize the part and avoid overmanipulation of inflamed areas. Use moist heat to help larger lesions "localize." Use surgical incision and drainage after the lesions are "mature." To incise and drain an acute staphylococcal paronychia, insert a flat metal spatula or sharpened hardwood stick into the nail fold where it adjoins the nail. This will release pus from a mature lesion.

Prognosis

Recurrent crops may harass the patient for months or years.

Davido B et al. Recurrent furunculosis: Efficacy of the CMC regimen—skin disinfection (chlorhexidine), local nasal antibiotic (mupirocin), and systemic antibiotic (clindamycin). Scand J Infect Dis. 2013 Nov;45(11):837–41. [PMID: 23848409]

Demos M et al. Recurrent furunculosis: a review of the literature. Br J Dermatol. 2012 Oct;167(4):725–32. [PMID: 22803835]

Ibler KS et al. Recurrent furunculosis—challenges and management: a review. Clin Cosmet Investig Dermatol. 2014 Feb 18; 7:59–64. [PMID: 24591845]

Knox J et al. Community-associated methicillin-resistant *Staphylococcus aureus* transmission in households of infected cases: a pooled analysis of primary data from three studies across international settings. Epidemiol Infect. 2015 Jan;143(2): 354–65. [PMID: 24763185]

Mun JH et al. Importance of keen observation for the diagnosis of epidermal cysts: dermoscopy can be a useful adjuvant tool. J Am Acad Dermatol. 2014 Oct;71(4):e138–40. [PMID: 25219733]

EPIDERMAL INCLUSION CYST

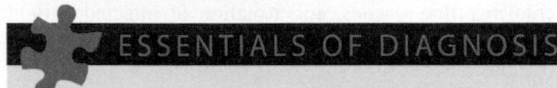

- Firm dermal papule or nodule.
- Overlying black comedone or "punctum."
- Expressible foul-smelling cheesy material.
- May become red and drain, mimicking an abscess.

General Considerations

Epidermal inclusion cysts (EICs) are common, benign growths of the upper portion of the hair follicle. They are common in Gardner syndrome and may be the first stigmata of the condition.

EICs favor the face and trunk and may complicate nodulocystic acne vulgaris. Individual lesions range in size from 0.3 cm to several centimeters. **An overlying pore or punctum is characteristic.** Dermoscopy can aid in observing a tiny punctum when not visible to the naked eye. Lateral pressure may lead to extrusion of a foul-smelling, cheesy material.

Differential Diagnosis

EICs are distinguished from lipomas by being more superficial (in the dermis, not the subcutaneous fat) and by their overlying punctum. Many other benign and malignant tumors may superficially resemble EICs, but all lack the punctum.

Complications

EICs may rupture, creating an acute inflammatory nodule very similar to an abscess. Cultures of the expressed material will be sterile.

Treatment

Treatment is not required if asymptomatic. Inflamed lesions may be treated with incision and drainage or intralesional triamcinolone acetomide 5–10 mg/mL. For large or symptomatic cysts, surgical excision is curative.

PHOTODERMATITIS

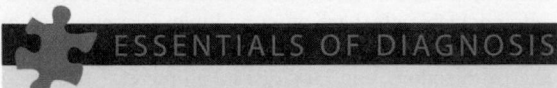

- Painful or pruritic erythema, edema, or vesiculation on sun-exposed surfaces: the face, neck, hands, and "V" of the chest.
- Inner upper eyelids spared, as is the area under the chin.

General Considerations

Photodermatitis is a cutaneous reaction to ultraviolet radiation. Photodermatitis is classified into four groups: **primary photodermatoses** that are immunologically mediated but are idiopathic in etiology, **drug- or chemical-induced photodermatoses**, dermatoses that are worsened or aggravated by **ultraviolet exposure**, and **genetic diseases** with mutations predisposing to photodermatitis.

Primary photodermatoses include polymorphic light eruption, chronic actinic dermatitis, and actinic prurigo. Drug- or chemical-induced photodermatitis may be either exogenous or endogenous in origin. Porphyria cutanea tarda and pellagra are examples of endogenous phototoxic dermatoses. Exogenous drug- or chemical-induced photodermatitis manifests either as phototoxicity (a tendency for the individual to sunburn more easily than expected) or as photoallergy (a true immunologic reaction that presents with dermatitis). Drug-induced phototoxicity is triggered by UVA. Contact photosensitivity may occur with plants, perfumes, and sunscreens. The sunscreen oxybenzone (a benzophenone) is a common cause of photoallergic dermatitis. Dermatoses that are worsened or aggravated by ultraviolet exposure include systemic lupus erythematosus and dermatomyositis. Three percent of persons with atopic dermatitis, especially middle-aged women, are photosensitive.

Clinical Findings

A. Symptoms and Signs

The acute inflammatory phase of phototoxicity, if severe enough, is accompanied by pain, fever, gastrointestinal symptoms, malaise, and even prostration. Signs include erythema, edema, and possibly vesiculation and oozing on exposed surfaces. Peeling of the epidermis and pigmentary changes often result. The key to diagnosis is localization of the rash to photoexposed areas, though these eruptions may become generalized with time to involve even photoprotected areas. The lower lip may be affected.

B. Laboratory Findings

Blood and urine tests are generally not helpful unless porphyria cutanea tarda is suggested by the presence of blistering, scarring, milia (white cysts 1–2 mm in diameter) and skin fragility of the dorsal hands, and facial hypertrichosis. Eosinophilia may be present in chronic photoallergic responses.

Differential Diagnosis

The differential diagnosis is long. If a clear history of the use of a topical or systemic photosensitizer is not available and if the eruption is persistent, then a work-up including biopsy and light testing may be required. Photodermatitis must be differentiated from contact dermatitis that may develop from one of the many substances in suntan lotions and oils, as these may often have a similar distribution. Sensitivity to actinic rays may also be part of a more serious condition, such as porphyria cutanea tarda or lupus erythematosus. These disorders are diagnosed by appropriate blood or urine tests. Phenothiazines, quinine or quinidine, griseofulvin, sulfonamides (especially hydrochlorothiazide), NSAIDs, antibiotics (eg, some tetracyclines, quinolones, TMP-SMZ), voriconazole, eculizumab, topical and systemic retinoids (tretinoin, isotretinoin, acitretin), quinolones, and calcium channel blockers are all potential photosensitizers. Polymorphous light eruption (PMLE) is a very common idiopathic photodermatitis and often has its onset in the third to fourth decades, except in Native Americans and Latinos, in whom it may present in childhood. PMLE is chronic in nature. Transitory periods of spontaneous remission do occur.

Complications

Some individuals continue to be chronic light reactors even when they apparently are no longer exposed to photosensitizing medications.

Prevention

While sunscreens are useful agents in general and should be used by persons with photosensitivity, patients may react to such low amounts of energy that sunscreens alone may not be sufficient. Sunscreens with an SPF of 30–60 and broad UVA coverage, containing dicamphor sulfonic acid (Mexoryl SX), avobenzone (Parasol 1789), titanium dioxide, and micronized zinc oxide, are especially useful in patients with photoallergic dermatitis. Photosensitivity due to porphyria is not prevented by sunscreens and requires barrier protection (clothing) to prevent outbreaks.

Treatment

A. Specific Measures

Medications should be suspected in cases of photosensitivity even if the particular medication (such as hydrochlorothiazide) has been used for months.

B. Local Measures

When the eruption is vesicular or weepy, treatment is similar to that of any acute dermatitis, using cooling and soothing wet dressing.

Sunscreens should be used as described above. Mid-potency to high-potency topical corticosteroids are of limited benefit in sunburn reactions but may help in PMLE and photoallergic reactions. Since the face is often involved, close monitoring for corticosteroid side effects is recommended.

C. Systemic Measures

Aspirin may have some value for fever and pain of acute sunburn. Systemic corticosteroids in doses as described for acute contact dermatitis may be required for severe photosensitivity reactions. Otherwise, different photodermatoses are treated in specific ways.

Patients with severe photoallergy may require immunosuppressives, such as azathioprine, in the range of 50–300 mg/day, or cyclosporine, 3–5 mg/kg/day.

Prognosis

The most common phototoxic sunburn reactions are usually benign and self-limited. PMLE and some cases of photoallergy can persist for years.

Choi D et al. Evaluation of patients with photodermatoses. Dermatol Clin. 2014 Jul;32(3):267–75. [PMID: 24891050]
Dawe RS et al. Drug-induced photosensitivity. Dermatol Clin. 2014 Jul;32(3):363–8. [PMID: 24891058]
Kutlubay Z et al. Photodermatoses, including phototoxic and photoallergic reactions (internal and external). Clin Dermatol. 2014 Jan–Feb;32(1):73–9. [PMID: 24314379]

ULCERS

LEG ULCERS SECONDARY TO VENOUS INSUFFICIENCY

ESSENTIALS OF DIAGNOSIS

▶ Past history of varicosities, thrombophlebitis, or postphlebitic syndrome.

▶ Irregular ulceration, often on the medial aspect of the lower legs above the malleolus.

▶ Edema of the legs, varicosities, hyperpigmentation, red and scaly areas (stasis dermatitis), and scars from old ulcers support the diagnosis.

General Considerations

Patients at risk may have a history of venous insufficiency, either with obvious varicosities or with a past history of thrombophlebitis, or with immobility of the calf muscle group (paraplegics, etc). Red, pruritic patches of stasis dermatitis often precede ulceration. Because venous insufficiency plays a role in between 75% and 90% of lower leg ulcerations, **testing of venous competence is a required part of a leg ulcer evaluation even when no changes of venous insufficiency are present.** The left leg is usually more severely affected than the right.

▲ **Figure 6–38.** Venous stasis ulcer near the medial malleolus. (From Maureen Sheehan, MD; used, with permission, from Usatine RP, Smith MA, Mayeaux EJ Jr, Chumley H, Tysinger J. *The Color Atlas of Family Medicine.* McGraw-Hill, 2009.)

▶ Clinical Findings

A. Symptoms and Signs

Classically, chronic edema is followed by a dermatitis, which is often pruritic. These changes are followed by hyperpigmentation, skin breakdown, and eventually sclerosis of the skin of the lower leg (Figure 6–38). The ulcer base may be clean, but it often has a yellow fibrin eschar that may require surgical removal. Ulcers that appear on the feet, toes, or above the knees should be approached with other diagnoses in mind.

B. Laboratory Findings

Thorough evaluation of the patient's vascular system (including measurement of the ankle/brachial index [ABI]) is essential. If the ABI is less than 0.7, the patient should be referred to a vascular surgeon for surgical evaluation. Doppler and light rheography examinations as office procedures are usually sufficient (except in the diabetic) to elucidate the cause of most vascular cases of lower leg ulceration.

▶ Differential Diagnosis

The differential includes vasculitis, pyoderma gangrenosum, arterial ulcerations, infection, trauma, skin cancer, arachnid bites, and sickle cell anemia. When the diagnosis is in doubt, a punch biopsy from the border (not base) of the lesion may be helpful.

▶ Prevention

Compression stockings to reduce edema are the most important means of prevention. Compression should achieve a pressure of 30 mm Hg below the knee and 40 mm Hg at the ankle. The stockings should not be used in patients with arterial insufficiency with an ABI less than 0.7. Pneumatic sequential compression devices may be of great benefit when edema is refractory to standard compression dressings.

▶ Treatment

A. Local Measures

Clean the base of the ulcer with saline or cleansers, such as Saf-Clens. A curette or small scissors can be used to remove the yellow fibrin eschar; local anesthesia may be used if the areas are very tender.

Overall, there is little evidence to support topical antibiotics other than cadexomer iodine for the treatment of venous insufficiency ulcerations. In dermatology clinics, metronidazole gel is used to reduce bacterial growth and odor. Red dermatitic skin is treated with a medium- to high-potency corticosteroid ointment. The ulcer is then covered with an occlusive hydroactive dressing (DuoDerm or Cutinova) or a polyurethane foam (Allevyn) followed by an Unna zinc paste boot. This is changed weekly. The ulcer should begin to heal within weeks, and healing should be complete within 4–6 months. If the patient is diabetic, becaplermin (Regranex) may be applied to those ulcers that are not becoming smaller or developing a granulating base. Some ulcerations require grafting. Full- or split-thickness grafts often do not take, and pinch grafts (small shaves of skin laid onto the bed) may be effective. Cultured epidermal cell grafts may accelerate wound healing, but they are very expensive. They should be considered in refractory ulcers, especially those that have not healed after a year or more of conservative therapy.

No topical intervention has evidence to suggest that it will improve healing of arterial leg ulcers.

B. Systemic Therapy

Pentoxifylline, 400 mg three times daily administered with compression dressings, is beneficial in accelerating healing of venous insufficiency leg ulcers. Zinc supplementation is occasionally beneficial in patients with low serum zinc levels. In the absence of cellulitis, there is no role for systemic antibiotics in the treatment of venous insufficiency ulcers. The diagnosis of cellulitis in the setting of a venous insufficiency ulcer can be very difficult. Surface cultures are of limited value. **The diagnosis of cellulitis should be considered in the following settings: 1) expanding warmth and erythema surrounding the ulceration with or without 2) increasing pain of the ulceration.** The patient may also report increased exudate from the ulceration, but this without the other cardinal findings of cellulitis does not confirm the diagnosis of cellulitis. If cellulitis accompanies the ulcer, systemic antibiotics are recommended: dicloxacillin, 250 mg orally four times a day, or levofloxacin, 500 mg once daily for 1–2 weeks, is usually adequate. Routine use of antibiotics and treating bacteria isolated from a chronic ulcer without clinical evidence of infection is discouraged. If the ulcer fails to heal or there is a persistent draining tract in the ulcer, an underlying osteomyelitis should be sought.

Prognosis

The combination of limited debridement, compression dressings or stockings, and newer moist dressings will heal the majority of venous stasis ulcers within an average of 18 months. These need to be applied at least 80% of the time to optimize ulcer healing. Topical growth factors, antibiotics, debriding agents, and xenografts and autografts can be considered in recalcitrant cases, but they are usually not required in most patients. The failure of venous insufficiency ulcerations to heal is most often related to not using the basic treatment methods consistently, rather than failure to use these specific modalities. Ongoing control of edema is essential to prevent recurrent ulceration. The use of compression stockings following ulcer healing is critical to prevent recurrence, with recurrence rates 2–20 times higher if patients do not comply with compression stocking use. If the ABI is less than 0.5, the prognosis for healing is poor. Patients with an ABI below 0.5 or refractory ulcerations (or both) should be considered for surgical procedure (artery-opening procedures or ablation of the incompetent superficial vein).

Broussard KC et al. Wound dressings: selecting the most appropriate type. Am J Clin Dermatol. 2013 Dec;14(6):449–59. [PMID: 24062083]

Chaby G et al; Angio-Dermatology Group of the French Society of Dermatology. Prognostic factors associated with healing of venous leg ulcers: a multicentre, prospective, cohort study. Br J Dermatol. 2013 Nov;169(5):1106–13. [PMID: 23909381]

Eberhardt RT et al. Chronic venous insufficiency. Circulation. 2014 Jul 22;130(4):333–46. [PMID: 25047584]

O'Meara S et al. Antibiotics and antiseptics for venous leg ulcers. Cochrane Database Syst Rev. 2014 Jan 10;1:CD003557. [PMID: 24408354]

MISCELLANEOUS DERMATOLOGIC DISORDERS[1]

PIGMENTARY DISORDERS

Although the color of skin may be altered by many diseases and agents, the vast majority of patients have either an increase or decrease in pigment secondary to an inflammatory disease, such as acne or atopic dermatitis.[1]

Other pigmentary disorders include those resulting from exposure to exogenous pigments, such as carotenemia, argyria, and tattooing. Other endogenous pigmentary disorders are attributable to metabolic substances (eg, hemosiderin [iron]) in purpuric processes, to homogentisic acid in ochronosis, and bile pigments.

Classification

First, determine whether the disorder is hyperpigmentation or hypopigmentation, ie, an increase or decrease in normal skin colors. Each may be considered to be primary or to be secondary to other disorders. Depigmentation, the absence of all pigment, should also be differentiated from hypopigmentation, in which the affected skin is lighter than baseline skin color, but not completely devoid of pigment.

The evaluation of pigmentary disorders is helped by Wood light, which accentuates epidermal pigmentation in hyperpigmented disorders and highlights depigmentation. Depigmentation, as seen in vitiligo, enhances with Wood light examination, whereas postinflammatory hypopigmentation does not.

A. Primary Pigmentary Disorders

1. Hyperpigmentation—The disorders in this category are nevoid, congenital or acquired, and include pigmented nevi, ephelides (juvenile freckles), and lentigines (senile freckles). Hyperpigmentation occurs also in arsenical melanosis or in association with Addison disease. **Melasma (chloasma)** occurs as patterned hyperpigmentation of the face, usually as a direct effect of estrogens. It occurs not only during pregnancy but also in 30–50% of women taking oral contraceptives, and rarely in men.

2. Hypopigmentation and depigmentation—The disorders in this category are vitiligo, albinism, and piebaldism. In **vitiligo**, pigment cells (melanocytes) are destroyed (Figure 6–39). Vitiligo, present in approximately 1% of the population, may be associated with other autoimmune disorders, such as autoimmune thyroid disease, pernicious anemia, diabetes mellitus, and Addison disease.

B. Secondary Pigmentary Disorders

Any damage to the skin (irritation, allergy, infection, excoriation, burns, or dermatologic therapy, such as chemical peels and freezing with liquid nitrogen) may result in hyperpigmentation or hypopigmentation. Several disorders of clinical importance are described below.

1. Hyperpigmentation—The most common type of secondary hyperpigmentation occurs after another inflammatory dermatologic condition, such as acne, lichen planus,

▲ **Figure 6–39.** Vitiligo of the hands. (Used, with permission, from Richard P. Usatine, MD in Usatine RP, Smith MA, Mayeaux EJ Jr, Chumley H, Tysinger J. *The Color Atlas of Family Medicine.* McGraw-Hill, 2009.)

---

[1] Hirsutism is discussed in Chapter 26.

or eczema, and is most commonly seen in moderately complexioned persons (Asians, Hispanics, and light-skinned African Americans). It is called post-inflammatory hyperpigmentation.

Pigmentation may be produced by certain medications, eg, chloroquine, chlorpromazine, minocycline, and amiodarone. Fixed drug eruptions to phenolphthalein (in laxatives), TMP-SMZ, NSAIDs, and tetracyclines also lead to hyperpigmentation, typically in annular patches.

2. Hypopigmentation—Hypopigmentation may complicate atopic dermatitis, lichen planus, psoriasis, discoid lupus, and lichen simplex chronicus. It may also be post-traumatic. **Practitioners must exercise special care in using liquid nitrogen on any patient with olive or darker complexions, since doing so may result in hypopigmentation or depigmentation, at times permanent.** Intralesional or intra-articular injections of high concentrations of corticosteroids may also cause localized temporary hypopigmentation.

▶ Complications

Actinic keratoses and skin cancers are more likely to develop in persons with vitiligo. Severe emotional trauma may occur in extensive vitiligo and other types of hypopigmentation and hyperpigmentation, particularly in naturally dark-skinned persons.

▶ Treatment & Prognosis

A. Hyperpigmentation

Therapeutic bleaching preparations generally contain hydroquinone. Hydroquinone has occasionally caused unexpected hypopigmentation, hyperpigmentation, or even secondary ochronosis and pigmented milia, particularly with prolonged use.

The role of exposure to ultraviolet light cannot be overstressed as a factor promoting or contributing to most disorders of hyperpigmentation, and such exposure should be minimized. Melasma, ephelides, and postinflammatory hyperpigmentation may be treated with varying success with 4% hydroquinone and a sunscreen containing UVA photoprotectants (Avobenzone, Mexoryl, zinc oxide, titanium dioxide). Tretinoin cream, 0.025–0.05%, may be added. Superficial melasma responds well, but if there is predominantly dermal deposition of pigment (does not enhance with Wood light), the prognosis is poor. Response to therapy may take months and requires avoidance of sunlight. Hyperpigmentation often recurs after treatment if the skin is exposed to ultraviolet light. Acne with postinflammatory hyperpigmentation responds well to azelaic acid and tretinoin, as both address both acne and hyperpigmentation. Solar lentigines respond to liquid nitrogen application. Tretinoin, 0.1% cream and tazarotene 0.1% used over 10 months, will fade solar lentigines (liver spots), hyperpigmented facial macules in Asians, and postinflammatory hyperpigmentation in blacks. Lasers are available for the removal of epidermal and dermal pigment, and referral should be considered for patients whose responses to medical treatment are inadequate.

B. Hypopigmentation

In secondary hypopigmentation, repigmentation may occur spontaneously. Cosmetics such as Covermark and Dermablend are highly effective for concealing disfiguring patches. Therapy of vitiligo is long and tedious, and the patient must be strongly motivated. If less than 20% of the skin is involved (most cases), topical tacrolimus 0.1% twice daily is the first-line therapy. A superpotent corticosteroid may also be used, but local skin atrophy from prolonged use may ensue. With 20–25% involvement, narrowband UVB or oral PUVA is the best option. Severe phototoxic response (sunburn) may occur with PUVA. The face and upper chest respond best, and the fingertips and the genital areas do not respond as well to treatment. Years of treatment may be required.

Ezzedine K et al. Vitiligo. Lancet. 2015 Jul 4;386(9988):74–84. [PMID: 25596811]

Handel AC et al. Melasma: a clinical and epidemiological review. An Bras Dermatol. 2014 Sep–Oct;89(5):771–82. [PMID: 25184917]

Nicolaidou E et al. Pigmentation disorders: hyperpigmentation and hypopigmentation. Clin Dermatol. 2014 Jan–Feb;32(1):66–72. [PMID: 24314378]

Passeron T. Melasma pathogenesis and influencing factors—an overview of the latest research. J Eur Acad Dermatol Venereol. 2013 Jan;27(Suppl 1):5–6. [PMID: 23205539]

Rivas S et al. Treatment of melasma with topical agents, peels and lasers: an evidence-based review. Am J Clin Dermatol. 2013 Oct;14(5):359–76. [PMID: 23881551]

Whitton ME et al. Interventions for vitiligo. Cochrane Database Syst Rev. 2015 Feb 24;2:CD003263. [PMID: 25710794]

ALOPECIA

▶ Classification

Alopecias are divided into scarring and nonscarring forms. When first evaluating a patient who complains of hair loss, it is most important on physical examination to determine if follicular markings (the opening where hair exits the skin) are present or absent. **Present follicular markings suggest a nonscarring alopecia; absent follicular markings suggest a scarring alopecia.**

▶ Nonscarring Alopecia

Nonscarring alopecia may occur in association with various systemic diseases, such as SLE, secondary syphilis, hyperthyroidism or hypothyroidism, iron deficiency anemia, vitamin D deficiency, and pituitary insufficiency. The only treatment necessary is prompt and adequate control of the underlying disorder, which usually leads to regrowth of the hair.

Androgenetic alopecia, the most common form of alopecia, is of genetic predetermination. In men, the earliest changes occur at the anterior portions of the calvarium on either side of the "widow's peak" and on the crown (vertex). The extent of hair loss is variable and unpredictable. Minoxidil 5% is available over the counter and can be specifically recommended for persons with recent onset (less than 5 years) and smaller areas of alopecia.

Approximately 40% of patients treated twice daily for a year will have moderate to dense growth. Finasteride (Propecia), 1 mg orally daily, has similar efficacy and may be additive to minoxidil.

Androgenetic alopecia also occurs in women. Classically, there is retention of the anterior hairline while there is diffuse thinning of the vertex scalp hair and a widening of the part. Treatment includes topical minoxidil and, in women not of childbearing potential, finasteride at doses up to 2.5 mg/day. A work-up consisting of determination of serum testosterone, DHEAS, iron, total iron-binding capacity, thyroid function tests, vitamin D level, and a complete blood count will identify most other causes of hair thinning in premenopausal women. Women who complain of thin hair but show little evidence of alopecia need follow-up, because more than 50% of the scalp hair can be lost before the clinician can perceive it.

Telogen effluvium is a transitory increase in the number of hairs in the telogen (resting) phase of the hair growth cycle. This may occur spontaneously, may appear at the termination of pregnancy, may be precipitated by "crash dieting," high fever, stress from surgery or shock, malnutrition, or may be provoked by hormonal contraceptives. Whatever the cause, telogen effluvium usually has a latent period of 4 months. The prognosis is generally good. The condition is diagnosed by the presence of large numbers of hairs with white bulbs coming out upon gentle tugging of the hair. Counts of hairs lost by the patient on combing or shampooing often exceed 150 per day, compared to an average of 70–100. In one study, a major cause of telogen effluvium was found to be iron deficiency, and the hair counts bore a clear relationship to serum iron levels. If iron deficiency is suspected, a serum ferritin should be obtained, and the value followed with supplementation.

Alopecia areata is of unknown cause but is believed to be an immunologic process. Typically, there are patches that are perfectly smooth and without scarring. Tiny hairs 2–3 mm in length, called "exclamation hairs," may be seen. Telogen hairs are easily dislodged from the periphery of active lesions. The beard, brows, and lashes may be involved. Involvement may extend to all of the scalp hair (**alopecia totalis**) or to all scalp and body hair (**alopecia universalis**). Severe forms may be treated by systemic corticosteroid therapy, although recurrences follow discontinuation of therapy. Alopecia areata is occasionally associated with autoimmune disorders, including Hashimoto thyroiditis, pernicious anemia, Addison disease, and vitiligo. Additional comorbidities may include SLE, atopy, and mental health disease.

Intralesional corticosteroids are frequently effective for alopecia areata. Triamcinolone acetonide in a concentration of 2.5–10 mg/mL is injected in aliquots of 0.1 mL at approximately 1- to 2-cm intervals, not exceeding a total dose of 30 mg per month for adults. Alopecia areata is usually self-limiting, with complete regrowth of hair in 80% of patients with focal disease. Some mild cases are resistant to treatment, as are the extensive totalis and universalis types. Support groups for patients with extensive alopecia areata are very beneficial. Evidence suggests that interleukin-2 (upregulates T regulatory cells) or JAK inhibitors

(ruxolitinib, baricitinib) may be future therapeutic options for patients with highly morbid disease.

In **trichotillomania** (the pulling out of one's own hair), the patches of hair loss are irregular, with short, growing hairs almost always present, since they cannot be pulled out until they are long enough. The patches are often unilateral, occurring on the same side as the patient's dominant hand. The patient may be unaware of the habit.

Scarring (Cicatricial) Alopecia

Cicatricial alopecia may occur following any type of trauma or inflammation that may scar hair follicles. Examples include chemical or physical trauma, lichen planopilaris, bacterial or fungal infections, severe herpes zoster, chronic discoid lupus erythematosus (DLE), scleroderma, and excessive ionizing radiation. The specific cause is often suggested by the history, the distribution of hair loss, and the appearance of the skin, as in DLE. Biopsy is useful in the diagnosis of scarring alopecia, but specimens must be taken from the active border and not from the scarred central zone. **Scarring alopecias are irreversible and permanent. It is important to diagnose and treat the scarring process as early in its course as possible.**

Castela E et al. Effects of low-dose recombinant interleukin 2 to promote T-regulatory cells in alopecia areata. JAMA Dermatol. 2014 Jul;150(7):748–51. [PMID: 24872229]

Ertas R et al. Androgenetic alopecia as an indicator of metabolic syndrome and cardiovascular risk. Blood Press. 2015 Nov 20: 1–8. [Epub ahead of print] [PMID: 26585114]

Islam N et al. The autoimmune basis of alopecia areata: A comprehensive review. Autoimmun Rev. 2015 Feb;14(2):81–9. [PMID: 25315746]

Su LH et al. Association of androgenetic alopecia with mortality from diabetes mellitus and heart disease. JAMA Dermatol. 2013 May;149(5):601–6. [PMID: 23677087]

Varothai S et al. Androgenetic alopecia: an evidence-based treatment update. Am J Clin Dermatol. 2014 Jul;15(3):217–30. [PMID: 24848508]

Xing L et al. Alopecia areata is driven by cytotoxic T lymphocytes and is reversed by JAK inhibition. Nat Med. 2014 Sep;20(9):1043–9. [PMID: 25129481]

NAIL DISORDERS

1. Morphologic Abnormalities of the Nails

Classification

Acquired nail disorders may be classified as local or those associated with systemic or generalized skin diseases.

A. Local Nail Disorders

1. Onycholysis (distal separation of the nail plate from the nail bed, usually of the fingers) is caused by excessive exposure to water, soaps, detergents, alkalies, and industrial cleaning agents. Candidal infection of the nail folds and subungual area, nail hardeners, drug-induced photosensitivity, hyperthyroidism, hypothyroidism, and psoriasis may cause onycholysis.

2. Distortion of the nail occurs as a result of chronic inflammation or infiltration of the nail matrix underlying

the eponychial fold. Such changes may be caused by impingement on the nail matrix by inflammatory diseases (eg, psoriasis, lichen planus, eczema), warts, tumors, or cysts.

3. Discoloration and crumbly thickened nails are noted in dermatophyte infection and psoriasis.

4. Allergic reactions (to resins in undercoats and polishes or to nail glues) are characterized by onycholysis or by grossly distorted, hypertrophic, and misshapen nails.

B. Nail Changes Associated with Systemic or Generalized Skin Diseases

1. Beau lines (transverse furrows) affect all nails and classically develop after a serious systemic illness.

2. Atrophy of the nails may be related to trauma or to vascular or neurologic disease.

3. Clubbed fingers may be due to the prolonged hypoxemia associated with cardiopulmonary disorders (Figure 6–40) (See Chapter 9).

4. Spoon nails may be seen in anemic patients.

5. Stippling or pitting of the nails is seen in psoriasis, alopecia areata, and hand eczema.

6. Nail hyperpigmentation may be caused by many chemotherapeutic agents, but especially the taxanes.

▶ Differential Diagnosis

Onychomycosis may cause nail changes identical to those seen in psoriasis. Careful examination for more characteristic lesions elsewhere on the body is essential to the diagnosis of the nail disorders. **Cancer should be suspected (eg, Bowen disease or squamous cell carcinoma) as the cause of any persistent solitary subungual or periungual lesion.**

▲ **Figure 6–40.** Clubbing of the fingers in congenital heart disease. (Used, with permission, from Richard P. Usatine, MD in Usatine RP, Smith MA, Mayeaux EJ Jr, Chumley H, Tysinger J. *The Color Atlas of Family Medicine.* McGraw-Hill, 2009.)

▶ Complications

Toenail changes may lead to an ingrown nail—in turn often complicated by bacterial infection and occasionally by exuberant granulation tissue. Poor manicuring and poorly fitting shoes may contribute to this complication. Cellulitis may result.

▶ Treatment & Prognosis

Treatment consists usually of careful debridement and manicuring and, above all, reduction of exposure to irritants (soaps, detergents, alkali, bleaches, solvents, etc). Longitudinal grooving due to temporary lesions of the matrix, such as warts, synovial cysts, and other impingements, may be cured by removal of the offending lesion.

2. Tinea Unguium (Onychomycosis)

Tinea unguium is a trichophyton infection of one or more (but rarely all) fingernails or toenails. The species most commonly found is *T rubrum.* "Saprophytic" fungi may rarely cause onychomycosis (less than 5% of cases).

The nails are lusterless, brittle, and hypertrophic, and the substance of the nail is friable. **Laboratory diagnosis is mandatory since only 50% of dystrophic nails are due to dermatophytosis.** Portions of the nail should be clipped, digested with 10% KOH and examined under the microscope for hyphae. Fungi may also be cultured from debris collected from underneath the nail plate. Periodic acid-Schiff stain of a histologic section of the nail plate will also demonstrate the fungus readily. Each technique is positive in only 50% of cases so several different tests may need to be performed.

Onychomycosis is difficult to treat because of the long duration of therapy required and the frequency of recurrences. Fingernails respond more readily than toenails. **For toenails, treatment is indicated for patients with discomfort, inability to exercise, diabetes, and immune compromise.**

In general, systemic therapy is required to effectively treat nail onychomycosis. Although historically topical therapy has had limited value, efinaconazole 10% has been approved as a topical therapy; preliminary evidence suggests that it performs better than prior topical treatment options. Tavaborole 5% solution has also been approved for the treatment of onychomycosis, but its clearance rates do not appear to be as good as those of efinaconazole. Adjunctive value of surgical procedures is unproven, and the efficacy of laser treatments is lacking, especially with regard to long-term cures.

Fingernails can virtually always be cured, and toenails are cured 35–50% of the time and are clinically improved about 75% of the time. In all cases, before treatment, the diagnosis should be confirmed. The costs of the various treatment options should be known and the most cost-effective treatment chosen. Drug interactions must be avoided. **Ketoconazole, due to its higher risk for hepatotoxicity, is not recommended to treat any form of onychomycosis.** For fingernails, ultramicronized griseofulvin 250 mg orally three times daily for 6 months can be effective. Alternative treatments are (in order of preference) oral terbinafine 250 mg daily for 6 weeks, oral itraconazole 400 mg daily for 7 days each month for 2 months, and oral itraconazole 200 mg daily for 2 months. Off-label use of fluconazole, 400 mg once weekly for 6 months, can also be effective, but there is limited evidence for this option. Once clear, fingernails usually remain free of disease for some years.

Onychomycosis of the toenails does not respond to griseofulvin therapy. The best treatment, which is also FDA approved, is oral terbinafine 250 mg daily for 12 weeks. Liver function tests and a complete blood count with platelets are performed monthly during treatment. Pulse oral itraconazole 200 mg twice daily for 1 week per month for 3 months is inferior to standard terbinafine treatments, but it is an acceptable alternative for those unable to take terbinafine. The courses of terbinafine or itraconazole may need to be repeated 6 months after the first treatment cycle if fungal cultures of the nail are still positive.

Dehesa L et al. Treatment of inflammatory nail disorders. Dermatol Ther. 2012 Nov–Dec;25(6):525–34. [PMID: 23210751]

Gupta AK et al. Topical therapy for toenail onychomycosis: an evidence-based review. Am J Clin Dermatol. 2014 Dec;15(6): 489–502. [PMID: 25257931]

Shemer A. Update: medical treatment of onychomycosis. Dermatol Ther. 2012 Nov;25(6):582–93. [PMID: 23210757]

DERMATITIS MEDICAMENTOSA (Drug Eruption)

ESSENTIALS OF DIAGNOSIS

▶ Usually, abrupt onset of widespread, symmetric erythematous eruption.

▶ May mimic any inflammatory skin condition.

▶ Constitutional symptoms (malaise, arthralgia, headache, and fever) may be present.

General Considerations

Only a minority of cutaneous drug reactions result from allergy. Rashes are among the most common adverse reactions to medications and occur in 2–3% of hospitalized patients. Amoxicillin, TMP-SMZ, and ampicillin or penicillin are the most common causes of urticarial and maculopapular reactions. SJS and TEN are most commonly produced by sulfonamides, anticonvulsants, allopurinol, and NSAIDs. Drug-induced hypersensitivity reaction (DIHS) (also known as drug eruption with eosinophilia and systemic symptoms [DRESS]) is most often caused by anticonvulsants, allopurinol, and sulfonamides. Phenolphthalein, pyrazolone derivatives, tetracyclines, NSAIDs, TMP-SMZ, and barbiturates are the major causes of fixed drug eruptions. Calcium channel blockers are a common cause of pruritus and eczemas in the elderly.

Certain genetic polymorphisms of antigen-presenting major histocompatibility (MHC) loci increase the risk for the development of severe drug eruptions, including SJS/TEN and DIHS. Pharmacogenetic testing is becoming increasingly utilized to predict who is at risk for and therefore should avoid certain medication exposures. For example, in Han Chinese, HLA typing is indicated before institution of carbamazepine treatment.

Clinical Findings

A. Symptoms and Signs

Drug eruptions are generally classified as "simple" or "complex," referring to the risk of morbidity and mortality associated with the specific eruption. Simple drug eruptions involve an exanthem, usually appear in the second week of medication therapy, and have no associated constitutional or laboratory findings. Antibiotics, including the penicillins and quinolones, are the most common causes. Complex drug eruptions include DIHS and SJS/TEN.

DIHS occurs later than the simple morbilliform drug eruptions with signs and symptoms developing 2–6 weeks after the medication has been started and has associated constitutional and laboratory findings. These may include fevers, chills, hematologic abnormalities (especially eosinophilia), and abnormal liver or kidney function. The most common causes are sulfonamides, allopurinol, and anticonvulsants. Coexistent reactivation of certain viruses, such as Epstein-Barr virus, cytomegalovirus, and especially HHV-6, is often present and may be important in the pathogenesis of these complex drug eruptions. Table 6–3 summarizes the types of skin reactions, their appearance and distribution, and the common offenders in each case.

B. Laboratory Findings

Routinely ordered blood work is of no value in the diagnosis of simple drug eruptions. In complex drug eruptions, the CBC, liver biochemical tests, and renal function tests should be monitored. Skin biopsies may be helpful in making the diagnosis. Serum PCR for HHV-6, Epstein-Barr virus, and cytomegalovirus are routinely performed in some centers.

Differential Diagnosis

Observation after discontinuation, which may be a slow process, helps establish the diagnosis. Rechallenge, though of theoretical value, may pose a danger to the patient and is best avoided.

Complications

Some cutaneous drug reactions may be associated with visceral involvement. The organ systems involved depend on the individual medication or drug class. Most common is an infectious mononucleosis-like illness and hepatitis associated with administration of anticonvulsants. Myocarditis may be a serious complication of drug-induced hypersensitivity syndrome. Months after recovering from DIHS patients may suffer hypothyroidism.

Table 6–3. Skin reactions due to systemic medications.

Reaction	Appearance	Distribution and Comments	Common Offenders
Drug exanthem	Morbilliform, maculopapular, exanthematous reactions.	The most common skin reaction to medications. Initially begins on trunk 7–10 days after the medication has been started. Spreads to extremities and begins to clear on the trunk over 3-5 days. In previously exposed patients, the rash may start in 2–3 days. Fever may be present.	Antibiotics (especially ampicillin and TMP-SMZ), sulfonamides and related compounds (including thiazide diuretics, furosemide, and sulfonylurea hypoglycemic agents), and barbiturates.
SJS/TEN	Target-like lesions. Bullae may occur. Mucosal involvement.	Usually trunk and proximal extremities.	Sulfonamides, anticonvulsants, allopurinol, NSAIDs, lamotrigine.
Erythema nodosum	Inflammatory cutaneous nodules.	Usually limited to the extensor aspects of the legs. May be accompanied by fever, arthralgias, and pain.	Oral contraceptives.
Allergic vasculitis	The primary lesion is typically a 2–3 mm purpuric papule. Other morphologies include urticaria that lasts over 24 hours, vesicles, bullae, or necrotic ulcers.	Most severe on the legs.	Sulfonamides, phenytoin, propylthiouracil.
Exfoliative dermatitis and erythroderma	Red and scaly.	Entire skin surface. Typically associated with elevated liver function tests, eosinophilia, and acute kidney injury Eruption begins between 2 and 6 weeks after first dose of medication.	Allopurinol, sulfonamides, isoniazid, anticonvulsants, or carbamazepine.
Photosensitivity: increased sensitivity to light, often of ultraviolet A wavelengths, but may be due to UVB or visible light as well	Sunburn, vesicles, papules in photodistributed pattern.	Exposed skin of the face, the neck, and the backs of the hands and, in women, the lower legs. Exaggerated response to ultraviolet light.	Sulfonamides and sulfonamide-related compounds (thiazide diuretics, furosemide, sulfonylureas), tetracyclines, phenothiazines, sulindac, amiodarone, voriconazole, and NSAIDs.
Drug-related subacute cutaneous lupus erythematosus (Drug-induced SLE rarely produces a skin reaction)	May present with a photosensitive rash, annular lesions, or psoriasis on upper trunk.	Less severe than SLE, sparing the kidneys and central nervous system. Recovery often follows medication withdrawal.	Diltiazem, etanercept, hydrochlorothiazide, infliximab, lisinopril, terbinafine.
Lichenoid and lichen planus–like eruptions	Pruritic, erythematous to violaceous polygonal papules that coalesce or expand to form plaques.	May be in photo- or nonphotodistributed pattern.	Carbamazepine, furosemide, hydroxychloroquine, phenothiazines, beta-blockers, quinidine, quinine, sulfonylureas, tetracyclines, thiazides, and triprolidine.
Fixed drug eruptions	Single or multiple demarcated, round, erythematous plaques that often become hyperpigmented.	Recur at the same site when the drug is repeated. Hyperpigmentation, if present, remains after healing.	Antimicrobials, analgesics, barbiturates, cardiovascular drugs, heavy metals, antiparasitic agents, antihistamines, phenolphthalein, ibuprofen, and naproxen.
Urticaria	Red, itchy wheals that vary in size from less than 1 cm to many centimeters. May be accompanied by angioedema.	Chronic urticaria is rarely caused by medications.	Acute urticaria: penicillins, NSAIDs, sulfonamides, opioids, and salicylates. Angioedema is common in patients receiving ACE inhibitors and angiotensin receptor blockers.

(continued)

Table 6–3. Skin reactions due to systemic medications. (continued)

Reaction	Appearance	Distribution and Comments	Common Offenders
Pigmentary changes	Flat hyperpigmented areas.	Forehead and cheeks (chloasma, melasma). The most common pigmentary disorder associated with drug ingestion. Improvement is slow despite stopping the drug.	Oral contraceptives are the usual cause. Diltiazem causes facial hyperpigmentation that may be difficult to distinguish from melasma.
	Blue-gray discoloration.	Light-exposed areas.	Chlorpromazine and related phenothiazines.
	Brown or blue-gray pigmentation.	Generalized.	Heavy metals (silver, gold, bismuth, and arsenic).
	Yellow color.	Generalized.	Quinacrine.
	Blue-black patches on the shins.		Minocycline, chloroquine.
	Blue-black pigmentation of the nails and palate and depigmentation of the hair.		Chloroquine.
	Slate-gray color.	Primarily in photoexposed areas.	Amiodarone.
	Brown discoloration of the nails.	Especially in more darkly pigmented patients.	Hydroxyurea.
Psoriasiform eruptions	Scaly red plaques.	May be located on trunk and extremities. Palms and soles may be hyperkeratotic. May cause psoriasiform eruption or worsen psoriasis.	Antimalarials, lithium, beta-blockers, and TNF inhibitors.
Pityriasis rosea–like eruptions	Oval, red, slightly raised patches with central scale.	Mainly on the trunk.	Barbiturates, bismuth, captopril, clonidine, methopromazine, metoprolol, metronidazole, and tripelennamine.

ACE, angiotensin-converting enzyme; NSAIDs, nonsteroidal anti-inflammatory drugs; SJS/TEN, Stevens-Johnson syndrome/toxic epidermal necrolysis; SLE, systemic lupus erythematosus; TMP-SMZ, trimethorim-sulfamethoxazole; TNF, tumor necrosis factor.

► Treatment

A. General Measures

Systemic manifestations are treated as they arise (eg, anemia, icterus, purpura). Antihistamines may be of value in urticarial and angioneurotic reactions. Epinephrine 1:1000, 0.5–1 mL intravenously or subcutaneously, should be used as an emergency measure. In DIHS, systemic corticosteroids are typically required, starting at about 1–1.5 mg/kg/day and tapering very slowly over a minimum of 6 weeks, since rapid taper leads to rebound and more recalcitrant disease.

B. Local Measures

SJS/TEN with extensive blistering eruptions resulting in erosions and superficial ulcerations demands hospitalization and nursing care as for burn patients.

► Prognosis

Drug rash usually disappears upon withdrawal of the medication and proper treatment. DIHS may be associated with autoimmune phenomena, including abnormal thyroid function. This can occur months after the hypersensitivity syndrome has resolved.

Ahronowitz I et al. Severe drug-induced dermatoses. Semin Cutan Med Surg. 2014 Mar;33(1):49–58. [PMID: 25037258]

Bourgeois GP et al. A review of DRESS-associated myocarditis. J Am Acad Dermatol. 2012 Jun;66(6):e229–36. [PMID: 21658796]

Cheng CY et al. HLA associations and clinical implications in T-cell mediated drug hypersensitivity reactions: an updated review. J Immunol Res. 2014;2014:565320. [PMID: 24901010]

Dodiuk-Gad RP et al. Epidemiology of severe drug hypersensitivity. Semin Cutan Med Surg. 2014 Mar;33(1):2–9. [PMID: 25037253]

Harp JL et al. Severe cutaneous adverse reactions: impact of immunology, genetics, and pharmacology. Semin Cutan Med Surg. 2014 Mar;33(1):17–27. [PMID: 25037255]

Husain Z et al. DRESS syndrome: Part II. Management and therapeutics. J Am Acad Dermatol. 2013 May;68(5):709.e1–9. [PMID: 23602183]

7

Disorders of the Eyes & Lids

Paul Riordan-Eva, FRCOphth

REFRACTIVE ERRORS

Refractive errors are the most common cause of reduced clarity of vision (visual acuity) and may be a readily treatable component of poor vision in patients with other diagnoses.

Use of a pinhole will overcome most refractive errors and thus allows their identification as a cause of reduced visual acuity.

▶ Treatment

A. Contact Lenses

An estimated 40.9 million US adults wear contact lenses, mostly for correction of refractive errors, for which they provide better optical correction than glasses. Drug-eluting lenses are used to treat diseases of the cornea, conjunctiva, or lids. Colored contact lenses are being used increasingly for cosmesis.

The major risk from contact lens wear is bacterial, amebic, or fungal corneal infection, potentially a blinding condition. Such infections occur more commonly with soft lenses, particularly extended wear, for which there is at least a fivefold increase in risk of corneal ulceration compared with daily wear. Contact lens wearers, especially those using lenses for cosmesis, should be made aware of the risks they face and ways to minimize them, such as avoiding overnight wear or use of lenses past their replacement date and maintaining meticulous lens hygiene, including not using tap water or saliva for lens cleaning. Contact lenses should be removed whenever there is ocular discomfort or redness. Ophthalmologic care should be sought if symptoms persist.

B. Surgery

Various surgical techniques are available to reduce refractive errors, particularly nearsightedness. Laser corneal refractive surgery reshapes the middle layer (stroma) of the cornea with an excimer laser. Other refractive surgery techniques are extraction of the clear crystalline lens with insertion of a single vision, multifocal, or accommodative intraocular lens; insertion of an intraocular lens without removal of the crystalline lens (phakic intraocular lens); intrastromal corneal ring segments (INTACS); collagen cross-linking; laser thermal keratoplasty; and conductive keratoplasty (CK).

C. Reduction of Rate of Progression of Nearsightedness

Topical atropine and pirenzepine, a selective muscarinic antagonist; rigid contact lens wear during sleep (orthokeratology); and various types of soft contact lenses and spectacles reduce the rate of progression of nearsightedness but their long-term efficacy and safety are uncertain.

Walline JJ. Myopia control: a review. Eye Contact Lens. 2016 Jan;42(1):3–8. [PMID: 26513719]

▶ When to Refer

Any contact lens wearer with an acute painful red eye must be referred emergently to an ophthalmologist.

Collier SA et al. Estimated burden of keratitis—United States, 2010. MMWR Morb Mortal Wkly Rep. 2014 Nov 14; 63(45):1027–30. [PMID: 25393221]
Cope JR et al. Contact lens wearer demographics and risk behaviors for contact lens-related eye infections—United States, 2014. MMWR Morb Mortal Wkly Rep. 2015 Aug 21; 64(32):865–70. [PMID: 26292204]
Razmaria AA. JAMA patient page. Proper care of contact lenses. JAMA. 2015 Oct 13;314(14):1534. [PMID: 26462011]

DISORDERS OF THE LIDS & LACRIMAL APPARATUS

1. Hordeolum

Hordeolum is a common staphylococcal abscess that is characterized by a localized red, swollen, acutely tender area on the upper or lower lid. Internal hordeolum is a meibomian gland abscess that usually points onto the conjunctival surface of the lid; external hordeolum or sty usually is smaller and on the margin.

Warm compresses are helpful. Incision may be indicated if resolution does not begin within 48 hours. An antibiotic ointment (bacitracin or erythromycin) applied to the eyelid every 3 hours may be beneficial during the acute stage. Internal hordeolum may lead to generalized cellulitis of the lid.

2. Chalazion

Chalazion is a common granulomatous inflammation of a meibomian gland that may follow an internal hordeolum. It is characterized by a hard, nontender swelling on the upper or lower lid with redness and swelling of the adjacent conjunctiva. If the chalazion is large enough to impress the cornea, vision will be distorted. Treatment is usually by incision and curettage but corticosteroid injection may also be effective.

3. Blepharitis

Blepharitis is a common chronic bilateral inflammatory condition of the lid margins. **Anterior blepharitis** involves the eyelid skin, eyelashes, and associated glands. It may be ulcerative, because of infection by staphylococci, or seborrheic in association with seborrhea of the scalp, brows, and ears. **Posterior blepharitis** results from inflammation of the meibomian glands. There may be bacterial infection, particularly with staphylococci, or primary glandular dysfunction, in which there is a strong association with acne rosacea.

► Clinical Findings

Symptoms are irritation, burning, and itching. In **anterior blepharitis,** the eyes are "red-rimmed" and scales or granulations can be seen clinging to the lashes. In **posterior blepharitis,** the lid margins are hyperemic with telangiectasias, and the meibomian glands and their orifices are inflamed. The lid margin is frequently rolled inward to produce a mild entropion, and the tears may be frothy or abnormally greasy.

Blepharitis is a common cause of recurrent conjunctivitis. Both anterior and, more particularly, posterior blepharitis may be complicated by hordeola or chalazia; abnormal lid or lash positions, producing trichiasis; epithelial keratitis of the lower third of the cornea; marginal corneal infiltrates; and inferior corneal vascularization and thinning.

► Treatment

Anterior blepharitis is usually controlled by cleanliness of the lid margins, eyebrows, and scalp. Scales should be removed from the lids daily with a hot wash cloth or a damp cotton applicator and baby shampoo. In acute exacerbations, an antistaphylococcal antibiotic eye ointment, such as bacitracin or erythromycin, is applied daily to the lid margins. Antibiotic sensitivity studies may be helpful in severe cases.

In mild **posterior blepharitis,** regular meibomian gland expression may be sufficient to control symptoms. Inflammation of the conjunctiva and cornea indicates a need for more active treatment, including long-term low-dose oral antibiotic therapy, usually with tetracycline (250 mg twice daily), doxycycline (100 mg daily), minocycline (50–100 mg daily), or erythromycin (250 mg three times daily), and possibly short-term topical corticosteroids, eg, prednisolone, 0.125% twice daily. Topical therapy with antibiotics, such as

▲ **Figure 7–1.** Involutional ectropion of right lower eyelid. (From M. Reza Vagefi and John H Sullivan. Reproduced, with permission, from Riordan-Eva P, Cunningham ET Jr. *Vaughan & Asbury's General Ophthalmology,* 18th edition, McGraw-Hill, 2011.)

ciprofloxacin 0.3% ophthalmic solution twice daily, may be helpful but should be restricted to short courses.

Carlisle RT et al. Differential diagnosis of the swollen red eyelid. Am Fam Physician. 2015 Jul 15;92(2):106–12. [PMID: 26176369]
Duncan K et al. Medical management of blepharitis. Curr Opin Ophthalmol. 2015 Jul;26(4):289–94. [PMID: 26058027]

4. Entropion & Ectropion

Entropion (inward turning of usually the lower lid) occurs occasionally in older people as a result of degeneration of the lid fascia, or may follow extensive scarring of the conjunctiva and tarsus. Surgery is indicated if the lashes rub on the cornea. Botulinum toxin injections may also be used for temporary correction of the involutional lower eyelid entropion of older people.

Ectropion (outward turning of the lower lid) is common with advanced age (Figure 7–1). Surgery is indicated if there is excessive tearing, exposure keratitis, or a cosmetic problem.

Marcet MM et al. Involutional entropion: risk factors and surgical remedies. Curr Opin Ophthalmol. 2015 Jul;26(5):416–21. [PMID: 26154839]

5. Tumors

Eyelid tumors are usually benign. Basal cell carcinoma is the most common malignant tumor. Squamous cell carcinoma, meibomian gland carcinoma, and malignant melanoma also occur. Surgery for any lesion involving the lid margin should be performed by an ophthalmologist or suitably trained plastic surgeon to avoid deformity of the lid. Otherwise, small lesions can often be excised by the nonophthalmologist. Histopathologic examination of eyelid tumors should be routine, since 2% of lesions thought to be benign clinically are found to be malignant. The Mohs technique of intraoperative examination of excised tissue is particularly valuable in ensuring complete excision so that the risk of recurrence is reduced. Vismodegib, which is an oral inhibitor of the hedgehog pathway, is effective in advanced eyelid basal cell carcinoma unsuitable for surgery and imiquimod cream, an immunodoulator, may be helpful.

Iglesias ME et al. Oncologic surgery of the eyelid and orbital region. Actas Dermosifiliogr. 2015 Jun;106(5):365–75. [PMID: 25701895]

Leung C et al. Identifying predictive morphologic features of malignancy in eyelid lesions. Can Fam Physician. 2015 Jan; 61(1):e43–9. [PMID: 25756148]

Yin VT et al. Eyelid and ocular surface carcinoma: diagnosis and management. Clin Dermatol. 2015 Mar–Apr;33(2):159–69. [PMID: 25704936]

6. Dacryocystitis

Dacryocystitis is infection of the lacrimal sac usually due to congenital or acquired obstruction of the nasolacrimal system. It may be acute or chronic and occurs most often in infants and in persons over 40 years. It is usually unilateral. The usual infectious organisms are *Staphylococcus aureus* and streptococci in acute dacryocystitis and *Staphylococcus epidermidis*, streptococci, or gram-negative bacilli in chronic dacryocystitis.

Acute dacryocystitis is characterized by pain, swelling, tenderness, and redness in the tear sac area; purulent material may be expressed. In chronic dacryocystitis, tearing and discharge are the principal signs, and mucus or pus may also be expressed.

Acute dacryocystitis responds well to systemic antibiotic therapy. Surgical relief of the underlying obstruction is usually done electively but may be performed urgently in acute cases. The chronic form may be kept latent with antibiotics, but relief of the obstruction is the only cure. In adults, the standard procedure for obstruction of the lacrimal drainage system is dacryocystorhinostomy, which involves

surgical exploration of the lacrimal sac and formation of a fistula into the nasal cavity; if necessary, the procedure can be supplemented by nasolacrimal intubation. Congenital nasolacrimal duct obstruction is common and often resolves spontaneously. It can be treated by probing of the nasolacrimal system and supplemented by nasolacrimal intubation or balloon catheter dilation, if necessary. Dacryocystorhinostomy is rarely required.

Ali MJ et al. Clinical profile and management outcome of acute dacryocystitis: two decades of experience in a tertiary eye care center. Semin Ophthalmol. 2015 Mar;30(2):118–23. [PMID: 24171807]

CONJUNCTIVITIS

Conjunctivitis is the most common eye disease. It may be acute or chronic. Most cases are due to viral or bacterial (including gonococcal and chlamydial) infection. Other causes include keratoconjunctivitis sicca, allergy, chemical irritants, and deliberate self-harm. The mode of transmission of infectious conjunctivitis is usually direct contact via fingers, towels, handkerchiefs, etc, to the fellow eye or to other persons. It may be through contaminated eye drops.

Conjunctivitis must be differentiated from acute uveitis, acute glaucoma, and corneal disorders (Table 7–1).

Alfonso SA et al. Conjunctivitis. Prim Care. 2015 Sep;42(3): 325–45. [PMID: 26319341]

1. Viral Conjunctivitis

Adenovirus is the most common cause of viral conjunctivitis. There is usually bilateral disease with copious watery discharge, often with marked foreign body sensation, and a follicular conjunctivitis. Infection spreads easily. Eye clinics

Table 7–1. The inflamed eye: Differential diagnosis of common causes.

	Acute Conjunctivitis	Acute Anterior Uveitis (Iritis)	Acute Angle-Closure Glaucoma	Corneal Trauma or Infection
Incidence	Extremely common	Common	Uncommon	Common
Discharge	Moderate to copious	None	None	Watery or purulent
Vision	No effect on vision	Often blurred	Markedly blurred	Usually blurred
Pain	Mild	Moderate	Severe	Moderate to severe
Conjunctival injection	Diffuse; more toward fornices	Mainly circumcorneal	Mainly circumcorneal	Mainly circumcorneal
Cornea	Clear	Usually clear	Cloudy	Clarity change related to cause
Pupil size	Normal	Small	Moderately dilated	Normal or small
Pupillary light response	Normal	Poor	None	Normal
Intraocular pressure	Normal	Usually normal but may be low or elevated	Markedly elevated	Normal
Smear	Causative organisms	No organisms	No organisms	Organisms found only in corneal infection

and contaminated swimming pools are sometimes the source of infection. Epidemic keratoconjunctivitis, which may result in visual loss due to corneal subepithelial infiltrates, is usually caused by adenovirus types 8, 19, and 37. The disease lasts at least 2 weeks. Infection with adenovirus types 3, 4, 7, and 11 is typically associated with pharyngitis, fever, malaise, and preauricular adenopathy (pharyngoconjunctival fever). The disease usually lasts 10 days. Viral conjunctivitis may also be due to herpes simplex virus (HSV), when it is usually unilateral and may be associated with lid vesicles, and enterovirus 70 or coxsackievirus A24 that characteristically cause acute hemorrhagic conjunctivitis (see Chapter 32).

Except for HSV infection for which treatment with topical (eg, ganciclovir 0.15% gel) and/or systemic (eg, oral acyclovir) antivirals is recommended, there is no specific treatment. Cold compresses reduce discomfort and topical sulfonamides (or oral antibiotics) can be prescribed to prevent secondary bacterial infection. The value of weak topical corticosteroids or topical cyclosporine for corneal infiltrates due to adenoviral infection is uncertain.

Jhanji V et al. Adenoviral keratoconjunctivitis. Surv Ophthalmol. 2015 Sep–Oct;60(5):435–43. [PMID: 26077630]

2. Bacterial Conjunctivitis

The organisms isolated most commonly in bacterial conjunctivitis are staphylococci, including methicillin-resistant *S aureus* (MRSA); streptococci, particularly *S pneumoniae*; *Haemophilus* species; *Pseudomonas;* and *Moraxella*. All may produce a copious purulent discharge. There is no blurring of vision and only mild discomfort. In severe (hyperpurulent) cases, examination of stained conjunctival scrapings and cultures is recommended, particularly to identify gonococcal infection.

The disease is usually self-limited, lasting about 10–14 days if untreated. A topical sulfonamide or oral antibiotic will usually clear the infection in 2–3 days. Except in special circumstances, the use of topical fluoroquinolones is rarely justified for treatment of a generally self-limiting, benign infection.

A. Gonococcal Conjunctivitis

Gonococcal conjunctivitis, usually acquired through contact with infected genital secretions, typically causes copious purulent discharge. It is an ophthalmologic emergency because corneal involvement may rapidly lead to perforation. The diagnosis should be confirmed by stained smear and culture of the discharge. A single 1-g dose of intramuscular ceftriaxone is usually adequate. (Fluoroquinolone resistance is common.) Topical antibiotics such as erythromycin and bacitracin may be added. Other sexually transmitted diseases, including chlamydiosis, syphilis, and HIV infection, should be considered. Routine treatment for chlamydial infection is recommended.

McAnena L et al. Prevalence of gonococcal conjunctivitis in adults and neonates. Eye (Lond). 2015 Jul;29(7):875–80. [PMID: 25907207]

B. Chlamydial Keratoconjunctivitis

1. Trachoma—Trachoma is the most common infectious cause of blindness worldwide, with approximately 40 million people affected and 1.3 million with profound vision loss. Recurrent episodes of infection in childhood manifest as bilateral follicular conjunctivitis, epithelial keratitis, and corneal vascularization (pannus). Scarring (cicatrization) of the tarsal conjunctiva leads to entropion and trichiasis in adulthood, with secondary central corneal scarring.

Immunologic tests or polymerase chain reaction on conjunctival samples will confirm the diagnosis but treatment should be started on the basis of clinical findings. A single 1-g dose of oral azithromycin is the preferred drug for mass treatment campaigns, but improvements in hygiene and living conditions probably have contributed more to the marked reduction in the prevalence of trachoma during the past 25 years. Local treatment is not necessary. Surgical treatment includes correction of eyelid deformities and corneal transplantation.

Taylor HR et al. Trachoma. Lancet. 2014 Dec 13;384(9960):2142–52. [PMID: 25043452]
West SK et al. Trachoma control: 14 years later. Ophthalmic Epidemiol. 2015;22(3):145–7. [PMID: 26158571]

2. Inclusion conjunctivitis—Inclusion conjunctivitis is usually associated with genital infection, the eye being involved following contact with genital secretions. The disease starts with acute redness, discharge, and irritation. The eye findings consist of follicular conjunctivitis with mild keratitis. A nontender preauricular lymph node can often be palpated. Healing usually leaves no sequelae. Diagnosis can be rapidly confirmed by immunologic tests or polymerase chain reaction on conjunctival samples. Treatment is with a single dose of azithromycin, 1 g orally. Before treatment, all cases should be assessed for genital tract infection and other sexually transmitted diseases.

Mohamed-Noriega K et al. Conjunctival infection with *Chlamydia trachomatis* in sexual partners of patients with adult inclusion conjunctivitis. Int Ophthalmol. 2015 Apr;35(2):179–85. [PMID: 24643518]
Petrovay F et al. Chlamydial conjunctivitis: prevalence and serovar distribution of *Chlamydia trachomatis* in adults. J Med Microbiol. 2015 Sep;64(9):967–70. [PMID: 26297635]

3. Dry Eyes (Keratoconjunctivitis Sicca)

This is a common disorder, affecting around 50% of older women. Hypofunction of the lacrimal glands, causing loss of the aqueous component of tears, may be due to aging, hereditary disorders, systemic disease (eg, Sjögren syndrome), or systemic drugs. Excessive evaporation of tears may be due to environmental factors (eg, a hot, dry, or windy climate) or abnormalities of the lipid component of the tear film, as in blepharitis. Mucin deficiency may be due to vitamin A deficiency, or conjunctival scarring from trachoma, Stevens-Johnson syndrome and related conditions, mucous membrane pemphigoid, burns, or topical drugs or their preservatives.

Clinical Findings

The patient complains of dryness, redness, or foreign body sensation. In severe cases, there is persistent marked discomfort, with photophobia, difficulty in moving the eyelids, and often excessive mucus secretion. In many cases, inspection reveals no abnormality, but on slit-lamp examination there are subtle abnormalities of tear film stability and reduced volume of the tear film meniscus along the lower lid. In more severe cases, damaged corneal and conjunctival cells stain with 1% rose bengal. In the most severe cases, there is marked conjunctival injection, loss of the normal conjunctival and corneal luster, epithelial keratitis that may progress to frank ulceration, and mucous strands. The Schirmer test, which measures the rate of production of the aqueous component of tears, may be helpful.

Treatment

Aqueous deficiency can be treated with various types of artificial tears. The simplest preparations are physiologic (0.9%) or hypo-osmotic (0.45%) solutions of sodium chloride, which can be used as frequently as every half-hour, but in most cases are needed only three or four times a day. More prolonged duration of action can be achieved with drop preparations containing a mucomimetic such as methylcellulose, polyvinyl alcohol, or polyacrylic acid (carbomers), or by using petrolatum ointment or a hydroxypropyl cellulose (Lacrisert) insert. Sodium hyaluronate or autologous serum eye drops may be used in severe cases. All these mucomimetics are particularly indicated when there is mucin deficiency. If there is tenacious mucus, mucolytic agents (eg, acetylcysteine 10% or 20%, one drop six times daily) may be helpful.

Artificial tear preparations are generally very safe and without side effects. However, preservatives included in some preparations to maintain sterility are potentially toxic and allergenic and may cause keratitis and cicatrizing conjunctivitis in frequent users. The development of such reactions may be misinterpreted as a worsening of the dry eye state requiring more frequent use of the artificial tears and leading in turn to further deterioration, rather than being recognized as a need to change to a preservative-free preparation.

Disease modification can be achieved with topical anti-inflammatory agents such as corticosteroids, of which loteprednol (Lotemax) is favored because of its low risk of intraocular adverse effects, or calcineurin inhibitors, of which cyclosporine 0.05% ophthalmic emulsion (Restasis) twice a day has been used most widely. Diquafosol eye drops, which also promote water transfer, and rebamipide eye drops increase mucin secretion. Increased dietary intake of omega-3 fatty acids has been reported to be beneficial.

Lacrimal punctal occlusion by canalicular plugs or cautery is useful in severe cases. Blepharitis is treated as described above. Associated blepharospasm may benefit from botulinum toxin injections.

Foulks GN et al. Clinical guidelines for management of dry eye associated with Sjögren disease. Ocul Surf. 2015 Apr;13(2):118–32. [PMID: 25881996]

Sharma A et al. Aging: a predisposition to dry eyes. J Ophthalmol. 2014;2014:781683. [PMID: 25197560]

Torpy JM et al. JAMA patient page. Dry eye. JAMA. 2012 Aug 8; 308(6):632. [PMID: 22871877]

4. Allergic Eye Disease

Allergic eye disease is common and takes a number of different forms but all are expressions of atopy, which may also manifest as atopic asthma, atopic dermatitis, or allergic rhinitis.

Clinical Findings

Symptoms include itching, tearing, redness, stringy discharge, and occasionally, photophobia and visual loss.

Allergic conjunctivitis is a benign disease, occurring usually in late childhood and early adulthood. It may be seasonal (hay fever), developing usually during the spring or summer, or perennial. Clinical signs are limited to conjunctival hyperemia and edema (chemosis), the latter at times being marked and sudden in onset. **Vernal keratoconjunctivitis** also tends to occur in late childhood and early adulthood. It is usually seasonal, with a predilection for the spring. Large "cobblestone" papillae are noted on the upper tarsal conjunctiva. There may be lymphoid follicles at the limbus. **Atopic keratoconjunctivitis** is a more chronic disorder of adulthood. Both the upper and the lower tarsal conjunctivas exhibit a fine papillary conjunctivitis with fibrosis, resulting in forniceal shortening and entropion with trichiasis. Staphylococcal blepharitis is a complicating factor. Corneal involvement, including refractory ulceration, is frequent during exacerbations of both vernal and atopic keratoconjunctivitis. The latter may be complicated by herpes simplex keratitis.

Treatment

A. Mild and Moderately Severe Allergic Eye Disease

Topical treatments include emedastine and levocabastine, which are antihistamines; cromolyn, lodoxamide, nedocromil, and pemirolast, which are mast cell stabilizers; alcaftadine, azelastine, bepotastine, epinastine, ketotifen, and olopatadine, which are combined antihistamines and mast cell stabilizers; and bromfenac, diclofenac, flurbiprofen, indomethacin, ketorolac, and nepafenac, which are nonsteroidal anti-inflammatory drugs (Table 7–2). Mast cell stabilization takes longer to act than antihistamine and nonsteroidal anti-inflammatory effects but is useful for prophylaxis. Topical vasoconstrictors such as ephedrine, naphazoline, tetrahydrozoline, and phenylephrine, alone or in combination with antihistamines such as antazoline and pheniramine, are available as over-the-counter medications but are of limited efficacy in allergic eye disease and may produce rebound hyperemia and follicular conjunctivitis. Systemic antihistamines (eg, loratadine 10 mg orally daily)

Table 7–2. Topical ophthalmic agents.

Agent	Cost/Size[1]	Recommended Regimen	Indications
Antibacterial Agents[2]			
Azithromycin (AzaSite)	$194.19/2.5 mL	1 drop two times daily for 2 days, then once daily for 5 days	Bacterial conjunctivitis
Bacitracin 500 units/g ointment (various)[3]	$37.60/1 g	Refer to package insert (instructions vary)	
Bacitracin/Polymyxin ointment (Polysporin, AK-Poly)	$28.65/3.5 g	Refer to package insert (instructions vary)	
Besifloxacin ophthalmic suspension, 0.6% (Besivance)	$168.10/5 mL	1 drop three times daily for 7 days	Bacterial conjunctivitis
Cefazolin 10% (fortified) solution	Compounding pharmacy		
Chloramphenicol 1% ointment[4]	Compounding pharmacy		
Chloramphenicol 0.5% solution[4]	Compounding pharmacy		
Ciprofloxacin HCl 0.3% solution (Ciloxan)	$47.31/5 mL	1–2 drops every 2 hours while awake for 2 days, then every 4 hours for 5 days	Bacterial conjunctivitis
Ciprofloxacin HCl 0.3% ointment	$210.30/3.5 g	Apply small amount (0.5 inch) into lower conjunctival sac three times daily for 2 days, then two times daily for 5 days	Bacterial conjunctivitis
Erythromycin 0.5% ointment (various)[5]	$17.95/3.5 g	1 cm ribbon up to six times daily (depending on severity of infection)	Bacterial infection of the eye
Fusidic acid 1% (Fucithalmic)	Not available in United States	1 drop two times daily	Bacterial conjunctivitis, blepharitis, sty, keratitis
Gatifloxacin 0.5% solution (Zymaxid)	$118.16/2.5 mL	1 drop every 2 hours while awake, up to eight times on day 1, then two to four times daily while awake, days 2–7	
Gentamicin sulfate 0.3% solution (various)	$17.93/5 mL	1–2 drops every 4 hours up to 2 drops every hour for severe infections	Ocular surface infection
Gentamicin sulfate 0.3% ointment (various)	$19.67/3.5 g	Apply small amount (0.5 inch) into lower conjunctival sac two to three times daily	Ocular surface infection
Levofloxacin 0.5% solution (various)	$78.12/5 mL	1–2 drops every 2 hours while awake for 2 days (maximum eight times per day), then every 4 hours for 5 days (maximum four times per day)	Bacterial conjunctivitis
Moxifloxacin 0.5% solution (Vigamox)	$178.80/3 mL	1 drop three times daily for 7 days	Bacterial conjunctivitis
Neomycin/Polymyxin B/Gramicidin (Neosporin)	$55.74/10 mL	1–2 drops every 4 hours for 7–10 days or more frequently, as required	Ocular surface infection
Norfloxacin 0.3% solution	Compounding pharmacy		Ocular surface infection
Ofloxacin 0.3% solution (Ocuflox)	$20.94/5 mL	1–2 drops every 2–4 hours for 2 days, then four times daily for 5 days	Bacterial conjunctivitis
Polymyxin B/Trimethoprim sulfate 10,000 U/mL/1 mg/mL (Polytrim)[6]	$12.87/10 mL	1 drop every 3 hours for 7–10 days (maximum of 6 doses per day)	Ocular surface infection
Propamidine isetionate 0.1% solution	Not available in the United States	1–2 drops every 2–4 hours for 2 days, then four times daily for 5 days	Ocular surface infection (including *Ancathamoeba* keratitis)
Propamidine isetionate 0.1% ointment	Not available in the United States	Apply small amount (0.5 inch) into lower conjunctival sac up to four times daily	
Sulfacetamide sodium 10% solution (various)	$55.65/15 mL	1 or 2 drops every 2–3 hours initially; taper by increasing time intervals as condition responds; usual duration 7–10 days	Bacterial infection of the eye

(continued)

Table 7–2. Topical ophthalmic agents. (continued)

Agent	Cost/Size[1]	Recommended Regimen	Indications
Sulfacetamide sodium 10% ointment (various)	$65.86/3.5 g	Apply small amount (0.5 inch) into lower conjunctival sac once every 3–4 hours and at bedtime; taper by increasing time intervals as condition responds; usual duration 7–10 days	Bacterial infections of the eye
Tobramycin 0.3% solution (various)	$14.56/5 mL	1–2 drops every 4 hours for a mild to moderate infection or hourly until improvement (then reduce prior to discontinuation) for a severe infection	
Tobramycin 1.5% (fortified) solution	Compounding pharmacy		
Tobramycin 0.3% ointment (Tobrex)	$210.30/3.5 g	Apply small amount (0.5 inch) into lower conjunctival sac two to three times daily for a mild to moderate infection or every 3–4 hours until improvement (then reduce prior to discontinuation) for a severe infection	
Antifungal Agents			
Amphotericin 0.1–0.5% solution	Compounding pharmacy		
Natamycin 5% suspension (Natacyn)	$354.90/15 mL	1 drop every 1–2 hours initially; see prescribing information for further recommendations	Fungal blepharitis, conjunctivitis, keratitis
Voriconazole 1% solution	Compounding pharmacy		
Antiviral Agents			
Acyclovir 3% ointment (Zovirax)	Not available in United States	Five times daily	Herpes simplex virus keratitis
Ganciclovir 0.15% gel (Zirgan)	$348.65/5 g	Five times daily	Herpetic keratitis
Trifluridine 1% solution (Viroptic)	$178.28/7.5 mL	1 drop onto cornea every 2 hours while awake for a maximum daily dose of 9 drops until resolution occurs; then an additional 7 days of 1 drop every 4 hours while awake (minimum five times daily)	Herpes simplex virus keratitis
Anti-Inflammatory Agents			
Antihistamines[7]			
Bepotastine besilate 1.5% solution (Bepreve)	$412.09/10 mL	1 drop twice daily	Allergic eye disease
Emedastine difumarate 0.05% solution (Emadine)	$122.76/5 mL	1 drop four times daily	
Levocabastine (Livostin)	Not available in United States	1 drop twice daily	
Mast cell stabilizers			
Cromolyn sodium 4% solution (Crolom)	$28.12/10 mL	1 drop four to six times daily	Allergic eye disease
Lodoxamide tromethamine 0.1% solution (Alomide)	$167.82/10 mL	1 or 2 drops four times daily (up to 3 months)	
Nedocromil sodium 2% solution (Alocril)	$214.00/5 mL	1 drop twice daily	
Pemirolast potassium 0.1% solution (Alamast)	Not available in the United States	1 drop four times daily	
Combined antihistamines and mast cell stabilizers			
Alcaftadine 0.25% ophthalmic solution (Lastacaft)	$215.04/3 mL	1 drop once daily	Allergic eye disease
Azelastine HCl 0.05% ophthalmic solution (Optivar)	$102.90/6 mL	1 drop two to four times daily (up to 6 weeks)	

(continued)

Table 7–2. Topical ophthalmic agents. (continued)

Agent	Cost/Size[1]	Recommended Regimen	Indications
Epinastine hydrochloride 0.05% ophthalmic solution (Elestat)	$106.99/5 mL	1 drop twice daily (up to 8 weeks)	Allergic eye disease
Ketotifen fumarate 0.025% solution (Zaditor)	OTC $11.70/5 mL	1 drop two to four times daily	
Olopatadine hydrochloride 0.1% solution (Patanol)	$256.50/5 mL	1 drop twice daily	
Nonsteroidal anti-inflammatory agents[8]			
Bromfenac 0.09% solution (Xibrom)	$144.54/2.5 mL	1 drop to operated eye twice daily beginning 24 hours after cataract surgery and continuing through first 2 postoperative weeks	Treatment of postoperative inflammation following cataract extraction
Diclofenac sodium 0.1% solution (Voltaren)	$73.00/5 mL	1 drop to operated eye four times daily beginning 24 hours after surgery and continuing through first 2 postoperative weeks.	Treatment of postoperative inflammation following cataract extraction and laser corneal surgery
Flurbiprofen sodium 0.03% solution (various)	$8.14/2.5 mL	1 drop every half hour beginning 2 hours before surgery; 1 drop to operated eye four times daily beginning 24 hours after cataract surgery	Inhibition of intraoperative miosis. Treatment of cystoid macular edema and inflammation after cataract surgery
Ketorolac tromethamine 0.5% solution (Acular)	$105.50/5 mL	1 drop four times daily	Treatment of allergic eye disease, postoperative inflammation following cataract extraction and laser corneal surgery
Nepafenac 0.1% suspension (Nevanac)	$270.00/3 mL	1 drop to operated eye three times daily beginning 24 hours after cataract surgery and continuing through first 2 postoperative weeks	Treatment of postoperative inflammation following cataract extraction
Corticosteroids[9]			
Dexamethasone sodium phosphate 0.1% solution (various)	$21.10/5 mL	1 or 2 drops as often as indicated by severity; use every hour during the day and every 2 hours during the night in severe inflammation; taper off as inflammation decreases	Treatment of steroid-responsive inflammatory conditions
Dexamethasone sodium phosphate 0.05% ointment	Compounding pharmacy	Apply thin coating on lower conjunctival sac three or four times daily	
Fluorometholone 0.1% suspension (various)[10]	$148.26/10 mL	1 or 2 drops as often as indicated by severity; use every hour during the day and every 2 hours during the night in severe inflammation; taper off as inflammation decreases	
Fluorometholone 0.25% suspension (FML Forte)[10]	$291.49/10 mL	1 drop two to four times daily	
Fluorometholone 0.1% ointment (FML S.O.P.)	$145.74/3.5 g	Apply thin coating on lower conjunctival sac three or four times daily	
Loteprednol etabopate 0.5% (Lotemax)	$471.85/10 mL	1 or 2 drops four times daily	
Prednisolone acetate 0.12% suspension (Pred Mild)	$277.61/10 mL	1 or 2 drops as often as indicated by severity of inflammation; use every hour during the day and every 2 hours during the night in severe inflammation; taper off as inflammation decreases	

(continued)

Table 7–2. Topical ophthalmic agents. (continued)

Agent	Cost/Size[1]	Recommended Regimen	Indications
Prednisolone sodium phosphate 0.125% solution	Compounding pharmacy		
Prednisolone acetate 1% suspension (various)	$105.60/10 mL	2 drops four times daily	
Prednisolone sodium phosphate 1% solution (various)	$57.55/10 mL	1–2 drops two to four times daily	
Rimexolone 1% suspension (Vexol)	$140.64/10 mL	1–2 drops four times daily for 2 weeks	Treatment of postoperative inflammation
Immunomodulators			
Cyclosporine 0.05% emulsion (Restasis) 0.4 mL/container	$256.04/30 containers	1 drop twice daily	Dry eyes and severe allergic eye disease
Tacrolimus 0.1% ointment	$250.03/30 g tube	Not yet established (no label to support)	Severe allergic eye disease; no indication in United States
Agents for Glaucoma and Ocular Hypertension			
Sympathomimetics			
Apraclonidine HCl 0.5% solution (Iopidine)	$86.77/5 mL	1 drop three times daily	Reduction of intraocular pressure; expensive; reserve for treatment of resistant cases
Apraclonidine HCl 1% solution (Iopidine)	$27.20/unit dose	1 drop 1 hour before and immediately after anterior segment laser surgery	To control or prevent elevations of intraocular pressure after laser trabeculoplasty or iridotomy
Brimonidine tartrate 0.2% solution (Alphagan, Alphagan P [benzalkonium chloride-free])	$37.60/5 mL	1 drop two or three times daily	Reduction of intraocular pressure
Beta-adrenergic blocking agents			
Betaxolol HCl 0.5% solution (Betoptic) and 0.25% suspension (Betoptic S)[11]	0.5%: $123.28/10 mL 0.25%: $327.18/10 mL	1 drop twice daily	Reduction of intraocular pressure
Carteolol HCl 1% and 2% solution (Various, Teoptic)[12]	1%: $37.07/10 mL	1 drop twice daily	
Levobunolol HCl 0.25% and 0.5% solution (Betagan)[13]	0.5%: $41.80/10 mL	1 drop once or twice daily	
Metipranolol HCl 0.3% solution (OptiPranolol)[13]	$50.17/10 mL	1 drop twice daily	
Timolol 0.25% and 0.5% solution (Betimol)[13]	0.5%: $155.40/10 mL	1 drop once or twice daily	
Timolol maleate 0.25% and 0.5% solution (Istalol, Ocudose [preservative-free], Timoptic) and 0.1%, 0.25% and 0.5% gel (Timoptic-XE, Timoptic GFS)[13]	0.5% solution: $32.35/10 mL 0.5% gel: $164.10/5 mL	1 drop once or twice daily	
Miotics			
Pilocarpine HCl (various)[14] 1–4%, 6%, 8%, and 10% solution	2%: $100.81/15 mL	1 drop three or four times daily	Reduction of intraocular pressure, treatment of acute or chronic angle-closure glaucoma, and pupillary constriction
Pilocarpine HCl 4% gel (Pilopine HS)	$109.50/4 g	Apply 0.5-inch ribbon in lower conjunctival sac at bedtime	

(continued)

Table 7–2. Topical ophthalmic agents. (continued)

Agent	Cost/Size[1]	Recommended Regimen	Indications
Carbonic anhydrase inhibitors			
Brinzolamide 1% suspension (Azopt)	$300.00/10 mL	1 drop three times daily	Reduction of intraocular pressure
Dorzolamide HCl 2% solution (Trusopt)	$45.89/10 mL	1 drop three times daily	
Prostaglandin analogs			
Bimatoprost 0.03% solution (Lumigan)	$114.48/3 mL	1 drop once daily at night	Reduction of intraocular pressure
Latanoprost 0.005% solution (Xalatan, Monopost [preservative-free])	$21.60/2.5 mL (Monopost not available in United States)	1 drop once or twice daily at night	
Tafluprost 0.0015% solution (Saflutan [preservative-free], Zioptan [preservative-free])	$200.59/30 units (Saflutan not available in United States)	1 drop once daily at night	
Travoprost 0.004% solution (Travatan, Travatan Z [benzalkonium chloride-free])	$104.05/2.5 mL	1 drop once daily at night	
Unoprostone isopropyl 0.15% solution (Rescula)	$153.84/5 mL	1 drop twice daily	
Combined preparations			
Brimonidine 0.2% and timolol 0.5% (Combigan)	$322.34/10 mL	1 drop twice daily	Reduction of intraocular pressure
Brimonidine 0.2% and brinzolamide 1% (Simbrinza)	$158.16/8 mL	1 drop three times a day	
Brinzolamide 1% and timolol 0.5% (Azarga)	Not available in United States	1 drop twice daily	
Dorzolamide 2% and timolol 0.5% (Cosopt, Cosopt PF [preservative-free])	$238.41/10 mL	1 drop twice daily	
Bimatoprost 0.03% and timolol 0.5% (Ganfort)	Not available in United States	1 drop daily in the morning	
Latanoprost 0.005% and timolol 0.5% (Xalacom)	Not available in United States	1 drop daily in the morning	
Tafluprost 0.0015% and timolol 0.5% (Taptiqom [preservative-free])	Not available in United States	1 drop daily	
Travoprost 0.004% and timolol 0.5% (DuoTrav)	Not available in United States	1 drop daily	

[1]Average wholesale price (AWP, for AB-rated generic when available) for quantity listed. Source: *Red Book Online, Truven Health Analytics Information,* http://www.micromedexsolutions.com, March 1, 2016. AWP may not accurately represent the actual pharmacy cost because wide contractual variations exist among institutions.
[2]Many combination products containing antibacterials or antibacterials and corticosteroids are available.
[3]Little efficacy against gram-negative organisms (except *Neisseria*).
[4]Aplastic anemia has been reported with prolonged ophthalmic use.
[5]Also indicated for prophylaxis of neonatal conjunctivitis due to *Neisseria gonorrhoeae* or *Chlamydia trachomatis.*
[6]No gram-positive coverage.
[7]May produce rebound hyperemia and local reactions.
[8]Cross-sensitivity to aspirin and other nonsteroidal anti-inflammatory drugs.
[9]Long-term use increases intraocular pressure, causes cataracts, and predisposes to bacterial, herpes simplex virus, and fungal keratitis.
[10]Less likely to elevate intraocular pressure.
[11]Cardioselective (beta-1) beta-blocker.
[12]Teoptic is not available in the United States.
[13]Nonselective (beta-1 and beta-2) beta-blocker. Monitor all patients for systemic side effects, particularly exacerbation of asthma.
[14]Decreased night vision and headaches possible.

may be useful in prolonged atopic keratoconjunctivitis. In allergic conjunctivitis, specific allergens may be avoidable. In vernal keratoconjunctivitis, a cooler climate often provides significant benefit.

B. Acute Exacerbations and Severe Allergic Eye Disease

Topical corticosteroids (Table 7–2) are essential to control acute exacerbations of both vernal and atopic keratoconjunctivitis. Corticosteroid-induced side effects, including cataracts, glaucoma, and exacerbation of herpes simplex keratitis, are major problems but may be attenuated by the ester corticosteroid, loteprednol. Topical cyclosporine or tacrolimus is also effective. Systemic corticosteroid or other immunosuppressant therapy and even plasmapheresis may be required in severe atopic keratoconjunctivitis.

Castillo M et al. Topical antihistamines and mast cell stabilisers for treating seasonal and perennial allergic conjunctivitis. Cochrane Database Syst Rev. 2015 Jun 1;6:CD009566. [PMID: 26028608]
Jalbert I et al. Environmental aeroallergens and allergic rhinoconjunctivitis. Curr Opin Allergy Clin Immunol. 2015 Oct; 15(5):476–81. [PMID: 26258925]

PINGUECULA & PTERYGIUM

Pinguecula is a yellow, elevated conjunctival nodule, more commonly on the nasal side, in the area of the palpebral fissure. It is common in persons over age 35 years. Pterygium is a fleshy, triangular encroachment of the conjunctiva onto the nasal side of the cornea and is usually associated with prolonged exposure to wind, sun, sand, and dust. Pinguecula and pterygium are often bilateral.

Pingueculae rarely grow but may become inflamed (pingueculitis). Pterygia become inflamed and may grow. No treatment is usually required for inflammation of pinguecula or pterygium, but artificial tears are often beneficial, and short courses of topical nonsteroidal anti-inflammatory agents or weak corticosteroids (loteprednol or fluorometholone four times a day) may be necessary.

The indications for excision of pterygium are growth that threatens vision by encroaching on the visual axis, marked induced astigmatism, or severe ocular irritation. Recurrence is common and often more aggressive than the primary lesion.

Chan TC et al. Twelve-year outcomes of pterygium excision with conjunctival autograft versus intraoperative mitomycin C in double-head pterygium surgery. J Ophthalmol. 2015;2015: 891582. [PMID: 25810921]
Masters JS et al. Low recurrence rate of pterygium after excision with conjunctival limbal autograft: a retrospective study with long-term follow-up. Cornea. 2015 Dec;34(12):1569–72. [PMID: 26382900]

CORNEAL ULCER

Corneal ulcers are most commonly due to infection by bacteria, viruses, fungi, or amebas. Noninfectious causes— all of which may be complicated by infection—include neurotrophic keratitis (resulting from loss of corneal sensation), exposure keratitis (due to inadequate eyelid closure), severe dry eye, severe allergic eye disease, and various inflammatory disorders that may be purely ocular or part of a systemic vasculitis. Delayed or ineffective treatment of corneal ulceration may lead to devastating consequences with corneal scarring or intraocular infection. Prompt referral is essential.

Patients complain of pain, photophobia, tearing, and reduced vision. The eye is red, with predominantly circumcorneal injection, and there may be purulent or watery discharge. The corneal appearance varies according to the underlying cause.

When to Refer

Any patient with an acute painful red eye and corneal abnormality should be referred emergently to an ophthalmologist.

Gomes BA et al. Corneal involvement in systemic inflammatory diseases. Eye Contact Lens. 2015 May;41(3):141–4. [PMID: 25794330]

INFECTIOUS KERATITIS

1. Bacterial Keratitis

Bacterial keratitis usually pursues an aggressive course. Precipitating factors include contact lens wear—especially overnight wear—and corneal trauma, including refractive surgery. The pathogens most commonly isolated are *Pseudomonas aeruginosa*, *Moraxella* species, and other gram-negative bacilli; staphylococci, including MRSA; and streptococci. The cornea is hazy, with an ulcer and adjacent stromal abscess. Hypopyon is often present. The ulcer is scraped to recover material for Gram stain and culture prior to starting treatment with high-concentration topical antibiotic drops applied hourly day and night for at least the first 48 hours. Fluoroquinolones, such as levofloxacin 0.5%, ofloxacin 0.3%, norfloxacin 0.3%, or ciprofloxacin 0.3%, are commonly used as first-line agents as long as local prevalence of resistant organisms is low (Table 7–2). The fourth-generation fluoroquinolones (moxifloxacin 0.5% and gatifloxacin 0.3%) may be preferable because they are also active against mycobacteria. Gram-positive cocci can also be treated with a cephalosporin, such as fortified cefazolin 10%, but vancomycin may be required for MRSA; and gram-negative bacilli can be treated with an aminoglycoside, such as fortified tobramycin 1.5%. If no organisms are seen on Gram stain, these two agents can be used together in areas where resistance to fluoroquinolones is common. Although early adjunctive topical corticosteroid therapy may improve visual outcome, it should be prescribed only by an ophthalmologist.

When to Refer

Any patient with suspected bacterial keratitis must be referred emergently to an ophthalmologist.

Mascarenhas J et al. *Acanthamoeba*, fungal, and bacterial keratitis: a comparison of risk factors and clinical features. Am J Ophthalmol. 2014 Jan;157(1):56–62. [PMID: 24200232]

McDonald EM et al. Topical antibiotics for the management of bacterial keratitis: an evidence-based review of high quality randomised controlled trials. Br J Ophthalmol. 2014 Nov;98(11):1470–7. [PMID: 24729078]

2. Herpes Simplex Keratitis

Herpes simplex keratitis is an important cause of ocular morbidity. The ability of the virus to colonize the trigeminal ganglion leads to recurrences that may be precipitated by fever, excessive exposure to sunlight, or immunodeficiency.

Primary infection may manifest as eyelid, conjunctival, and corneal ulceration. The dendritic (branching) corneal ulcer is the most characteristic manifestation of recurrent ocular disease. More extensive ("geographic") ulcers also occur, particularly if topical corticosteroids have been used. The corneal ulcers are most easily seen after instillation of fluorescein and examination with a blue light. Such corneal epithelial disease in itself does not lead to corneal scarring. It responds well to simple debridement and patching. More rapid healing can be achieved by the addition of topical antivirals, such as trifluridine drops, ganciclovir gel, or acyclovir ointment (Table 7–2), or oral antivirals, such as acyclovir, 400 mg five times daily. Long-term oral acyclovir, 400 mg twice daily, or valacyclovir, 500 mg once daily, reduces the rate of recurrent epithelial disease, particularly in atopic individuals.

Stromal herpes simplex keratitis produces increasingly severe corneal opacity with each recurrence. Topical antivirals alone are insufficient to control stromal disease, so topical corticosteroids are used as well but they may enhance viral replication, exacerbating epithelial disease, and steroid dependence is common. Oral acyclovir, 200–400 mg five times a day, is often helpful in the treatment of severe herpetic keratitis. Severe stromal scarring may require corneal grafting, but the overall outcome is relatively poor. **Caution:** For patients with known or possible herpetic disease, topical corticosteroids should be prescribed only with ophthalmologic supervision.

▶ When to Refer

Any patient with a history of herpes simplex keratitis and an acute red eye should be referred urgently to an ophthalmologist.

Njoya JM et al. Herpetic epithelial keratitis. QJM. 2015 Jul;108(7):595. [PMID: 25524905]

Prakash G et al. The three faces of herpes simplex epithelial keratitis: a steroid-induced situation. BMJ Case Rep. 2015 Apr 2;2015. pii: bcr2014209197. [PMID: 25837655]

Wilhelmus KR. Antiviral treatment and other therapeutic interventions for herpes simplex virus epithelial keratitis. Cochrane Database Syst Rev. 2015 Jan 9;1:CD002898. [PMID: 25879115]

3. Herpes Zoster Ophthalmicus

Herpes zoster frequently involves the ophthalmic division of the trigeminal nerve. It presents with malaise, fever, headache, and periorbital burning and itching. These symptoms may precede the eruption by a day or more. The rash is initially vesicular, quickly becoming pustular and then crusting. Involvement of the tip of the nose or the lid margins predicts involvement of the eye. Ocular signs include conjunctivitis, keratitis, episcleritis, and anterior uveitis, often with elevated intraocular pressure. Recurrent anterior segment inflammation, neurotrophic keratitis, and posterior subcapsular cataract are long-term complications. Optic neuropathy, cranial nerve palsies, acute retinal necrosis, and cerebral angiitis occur infrequently. HIV infection is an important risk factor for herpes zoster ophthalmicus and increases the likelihood of complications.

High-dose oral acyclovir (800 mg five times a day), valacyclovir (1 g three times a day), or famciclovir (250–500 mg three times a day) started within 72 hours after the appearance of the rash reduces the incidence of ocular complications but not of postherpetic neuralgia. Keratitis can be treated with a topical antiviral such as ganciclovir 0.15% gel. Anterior uveitis requires treatment with topical corticosteroids and cycloplegics. Neurotrophic keratitis is an important cause of long-term morbidity. Whether varicella vaccination alters the incidence or severity of herpes zoster remains uncertain.

▶ When to Refer

Any patient with herpes zoster ophthalmicus and ocular symptoms or signs should be referred urgently to an ophthalmologist.

Cohen EJ. Management and prevention of herpes zoster ocular disease. Cornea. 2015 Oct;34(Suppl 10):S3–8. [PMID: 26114827]

Johnson JL et al. Herpes zoster ophthalmicus. Prim Care. 2015 Sep;42(3):285–303. [PMID: 26319339]

4. Fungal Keratitis

Fungal keratitis tends to occur after corneal injury involving plant material or in an agricultural setting, in eyes with chronic ocular surface disease, and increasingly in contact lens wearers. It is usually an indolent process, with the cornea characteristically having multiple stromal abscesses and relatively little epithelial loss. Intraocular infection is common. Corneal scrapings should be cultured on media suitable for fungi whenever the history or corneal appearance is suggestive of fungal disease. Diagnosis is often delayed and treatment is difficult. Natamycin 5%, amphotericin 0.1–0.5%, and voriconazole 1% are the most commonly used topical agents. Systemic imidazoles may be helpful. Corneal grafting is often required.

FlorCruz NV et al. Medical interventions for fungal keratitis. Cochrane Database Syst Rev. 2015 Apr 9;4:CD004241. [PMID: 25855311]

5. *Acanthamoeba* Keratitis

Acanthamoeba infection is an important cause of keratitis in contact lens wearers. Although severe pain with perineural and ring infiltrates in the corneal stroma is characteristic, it is not specific and earlier forms with changes confined to the corneal epithelium are identifiable. Diagnosis is facilitated by confocal microscopy. Culture requires specialized media. Long-term treatment is required because of the organism's ability to encyst within the corneal stroma. Intensive topical biguanide (polyhexamethylene or chlorhexidine) and diamidine (propamidine or hexamidine) is the standard initial treatment with addition of a triazole (voriconazole) if necessary. Delayed diagnosis and prior treatment with topical steroids adversely affect the visual outcome. Corneal grafting may be required after resolution of infection to restore vision. If there is scleral involvement, monotherapy or combination therapy with systemic anti-inflammatory and immunosuppressive medication is helpful but the prognosis is poor.

Alkharashi M et al. Medical interventions for acanthamoeba keratitis. Cochrane Database Syst Rev. 2015 Feb 24;2: CD010792. [PMID: 25710134]

Jiang C et al. *Acanthamoeba* keratitis: clinical characteristics and management. Ocul Surf. 2015 Apr;13(2):164–8. [PMID: 25881999]

ACUTE ANGLE-CLOSURE GLAUCOMA

> ### ESSENTIALS OF DIAGNOSIS
>
> ► Older age group, particularly farsighted individuals.
> ► Rapid onset of severe pain and profound visual loss with "halos around lights."
> ► Red eye, cloudy cornea, dilated pupil.
> ► Hard eye on palpation.

▶ General Considerations

Primary acute angle-closure glaucoma (acute angle-closure crisis) results from closure of a preexisting narrow anterior chamber angle. The factors predisposing to the narrow angle are shallow anterior chamber, which may be associated with farsightedness or short stature (or both); enlargement of the crystalline lens with age causing further shallowing; and inheritance, being particularly prevalent among Inuits and Asians. Closure of the angle is precipitated by pupillary dilation and thus can occur from sitting in a darkened theater, during times of stress, following nonocular administration of anticholinergic or sympathomimetic agents (eg, nebulized bronchodilators, atropine for preoperative medication, antidepressants, bowel or bladder antispasmodics, nasal decongestants, or tocolytics) or, rarely, from pharmacologic mydriasis (see Precautions in Management of Ocular Disorders, below). Secondary acute angle-closure glaucoma, which does not require a preexisting narrow angle, may occur in anterior uveitis or dislocation of the lens or due to various drugs (see Table 7–3). Symptoms are the same as in primary acute angle-closure glaucoma, but differentiation is important because of differences in management. Acute glaucoma, for which the mechanism may not be the same in all cases, can occur in

association with hemodialysis. (Chronic angle-closure glaucoma presents in the same way as chronic open-angle glaucoma.)

▶ Clinical Findings

Patients with acute glaucoma usually seek treatment immediately because of extreme pain and blurred vision, though there are subacute cases. Typically, the blurred vision is associated with halos around lights. Nausea and abdominal pain may occur. The eye is red, the cornea cloudy, and the pupil moderately dilated and nonreactive to light. Intraocular pressure is usually over 50 mm Hg, producing a hard eye on palpation.

▶ Differential Diagnosis

Acute glaucoma must be differentiated from conjunctivitis, acute uveitis, and corneal disorders (Table 7–1).

▶ Treatment

Initial treatment in acute glaucoma is reduction of intraocular pressure. A single 500-mg intravenous dose of acetazolamide, followed by 250 mg orally four times a day, together with topical medications is usually sufficient. Osmotic diuretics, such as oral glycerin and intravenous urea or mannitol—the dosage of all three being 1–2 g/kg—may be necessary if there is no response to acetazolamide.

A. Primary

In primary acute angle-closure glaucoma, once the intraocular pressure has started to fall, topical 4% pilocarpine, 1 drop every 15 minutes for 1 hour and then four times a day, is used to reverse the underlying angle closure. The definitive treatment is laser peripheral iridotomy or surgical peripheral iridectomy. Cataract extraction is a possible alternative. If it is not possible to control the intraocular pressure medically, the angle closure may be overcome by corneal indentation, laser treatment (argon laser peripheral iridoplasty), cyclodiode laser treatment, or paracentesis; or by glaucoma drainage surgery as for uncontrolled open-angle glaucoma.

All patients with primary acute angle-closure should undergo prophylactic laser peripheral iridotomy to the unaffected eye, unless that eye has already undergone cataract or glaucoma surgery. Whether prophylactic laser peripheral iridotomy should be undertaken in asymptomatic patients with narrow anterior chamber angles is uncertain and mainly influenced by the risk of the more common chronic angle-closure.

B. Secondary

In secondary acute angle-closure glaucoma, additional treatment is determined by the cause.

▶ Prognosis

Untreated acute angle-closure glaucoma results in severe and permanent visual loss within 2–5 days after onset of symptoms. Affected patients need to be monitored for development of chronic glaucoma.

Table 7–3. Adverse ophthalmic effects of systemic drugs.

Drug	Possible Side Effects
Ophthalmic drugs	
Carbonic anhydrase inhibitors (eg, acetazolamide, methazolamide)	Stevens-Johnson syndrome, nearsightedness, angle-closure glaucoma due to ciliary body swelling
Respiratory drugs	
Anticholinergic bronchodilators (eg, ipratropium)	Angle-closure glaucoma due to mydriasis, blurring of vision due to cycloplegia, dry eyes
Oxygen	Retinopathy of prematurity
Sympathomimetic bronchodilators (eg, salbutamol) and decongestants (eg, ephedrine)	Angle-closure glaucoma due to mydriasis
Cardiovascular system drugs	
Amlodipine	Chemosis (conjunctival edema)
Amiodarone	Corneal deposits (vortex keratopathy), optic neuropathy, thyroid ophthalmopathy
Digitalis	Disturbance of color vision, photopsia
Phosphodiesterase type 5 inhibitors (eg, sildenafil, tadalafil, vardenafil)	Disturbance of color vision, ischemic optic neuropathy
Statins	Extraocular muscle paralysis (myasthenic syndrome)
Thiazides (eg, indapamide)	Angle-closure glaucoma due to ciliary body swelling, nearsightedness, xanthopsia (yellow vision)
Gastrointestinal drugs	
Anticholinergic agents	Angle-closure glaucoma due to mydriasis, blurring of vision due to cycloplegia, dry eyes
Urinary tract drugs	
Alpha-2-antagonists (eg, alfuzosin, doxazosin, tamsulosin, terazosin, silodosin)	Complications during (floppy-iris syndrome) and after cataract surgery
Anticholinergic agents	Angle-closure glaucoma due to mydriasis, blurring of vision due to cycloplegia, dry eyes
Central nervous system drugs	
Amphetamines	Widening of palpebral fissure, blurring of vision due to mydriasis, elevated intraocular pressure
Anticholinergic agents including preoperative medications	Angle-closure glaucoma due to mydriasis, blurring of vision due to cycloplegia, dry eyes
Diazepam	Nystagmus
Haloperidol	Capsular cataract
Lithium carbonate	Proptosis, oculogyric crisis, nystagmus
Monoamine oxidase inhibitors	Nystagmus
Morphine	Miosis
Neostigmine	Nystagmus, miosis
Olanzapine	Angle-closure glaucoma due to mydriasis
Phenothiazines	Pigmentary deposits in conjunctiva, cornea, lens, and retina, oculogyric crisis
Phenytoin	Nystagmus
Retigabine	Ocular pigmentation and retinopathy
Risperidone, paliperidone	Complications during (floppy-iris syndrome) and after cataract surgery
Selective serotonin reuptake inhibitors (SSRIs) (eg, paroxetine, sertraline)	Angle-closure glaucoma, optic neuropathy
Serotonin and noradrenaline reuptake inhibitors (eg, venlafaxine)	Angle-closure glaucoma
Thioridazine	Corneal and lens deposits, retinopathy, oculogyric crisis

(continued)

Table 7–3. Adverse ophthalmic effects of systemic drugs. (continued)

Drug	Possible Side Effects
Topiramate	Angle-closure glaucoma due to ciliary body swelling, nearsightedness, macular folds, anterior uveitis
Tricyclic agents (eg, imipramine)	Angle-closure glaucoma due to mydriasis, blurring of vision due to cycloplegia
Vigabatrin	Visual field constriction
Zonisamide	Angle-closure glaucoma due to ciliary body swelling, nearsightedness
Obstetric drugs	
Sympathomimetic tocolytics	Angle-closure glaucoma due to mydriasis
Hormonal agents	
Aromatase inhibitors (eg, anastozole)	Dry eye, vitreo-retinal traction, retinal hemorrhages
Cabergoline	Angle-closure glaucoma
Female sex hormones	Retinal artery occlusion, retinal vein occlusion, papilledema, cranial nerve palsies, ischemic optic neuropathy
Tamoxifen	Crystalline retinal and corneal deposits, altered color perception, cataract, optic neuropathy
Immunomodulators	
Alpha-interferon	Retinopathy, keratoconjunctivitis, dry eyes, optic neuropathy
Corticosteroids	Cataract (posterior subcapsular); susceptibility to viral (herpes simplex), bacterial, and fungal infections; steroid-induced glaucoma
Cyclosporine	Posterior reversible leukoencephalopathy
Fingolimod	Macular edema
Tacrolimus	Optic neuropathy, posterior reversible leukoencephalopathy
Antibacterials	
Chloramphenicol	Optic neuropathy
Ethambutol	Optic neuropathy
Fluoroquinolones	Diplopia, retinal detachment
Isoniazid	Optic neuropathy
Linezolid	Optic neuropathy
Rifabutin	Uveitis
Streptomycin	Optic neuropathy, Stevens-Johnson syndrome
Sulfonamides	Stevens-Johnson syndrome, nearsightedness, angle-closure glaucoma due to ciliary body swelling
Tetracycline, doxycycline, minocycline	Papilledema
Antivirals	
Cidofovir	Uveitis
Antimalarial agents	
Chloroquine, hydroxychloroquine	Retinal degeneration principally involving the macula, keratopathy
Quinine	Retinal toxicity, pupillary abnormalities
Amebicides	
Iodochlorhydroxyquin	Optic neuropathy
Chemotherapeutic agents	
Chlorambucil	Optic neuropathy
Cisplatin	Optic neuropathy
Docetaxel	Lacrimal (canalicular) obstruction
Fluorouracil	Lacrimal (canalicular) obstruction
Vincristine	Optic neuropathy

(continued)

Table 7–3. Adverse ophthalmic effects of systemic drugs.(continued)

Drug	Possible Side Effects
Chelating agents	
Deferoxamine, deferasirox	Retinopathy, optic neuropathy, lens opacity
Penicillamine	Ocular pemphigoid, optic neuropathy, extraocular muscle paralysis (myasthenic syndrome)
Oral hypoglycemic agents	
Chlorpropamide	Refractive error, Stevens-Johnson syndrome, optic neuropathy
Thiazolidinediones (glitazones)	Increase in diabetic macular edema
Vitamins	
Vitamin A	Papilledema
Vitamin D	Band-shaped keratopathy
Antirheumatic agents	
Chloroquine, hydroxychloroquine	Retinal degeneration principally involving the macula, keratopathy
Allopurinol	Stevens-Johnson syndrome
Gold salts	Deposits in the cornea, conjunctiva, and lens
Indomethacin	Corneal deposits
Penicillamine	Ocular pemphigoid, optic neuropathy, extraocular muscle paralysis (myasthenic syndrome)
Phenylbutazone	Retinal hemorrhages
Salicylates	Subconjunctival and retinal hemorrhages, nystagmus
Dermatologic agents	
Retinoids (eg, isotretinoin, tretinoin, acitretin, and etretinate)	Papilledema, blepharoconjunctivitis, corneal opacities, decreased contact lens tolerance, decreased dark adaptation, teratogenic ocular abnormalities
Bisphosphonates	
Alendronate, pamidronate	Scleritis, episcleritis, uveitis

► When to Refer

Any patient with suspected acute angle-closure glaucoma must be referred emergently to an ophthalmologist.

Emanuel ME et al. Evidence-based management of primary angle closure glaucoma. Curr Opin Ophthalmol. 2014 Mar;25(2):89–92. [PMID: 24463418]
Gracitelli CP et al. Ability of non-ophthalmologist doctors to detect eyes with occludable angles using the flashlight test. Int Ophthalmol. 2014 Jun; 34(3):557–61. [PMID: 24081914]
Weinreb RN et al. The pathophysiology and treatment of glaucoma: a review. JAMA. 2014 May 14;311(18):1901–11. [PMID: 24825645]

CHRONIC GLAUCOMA

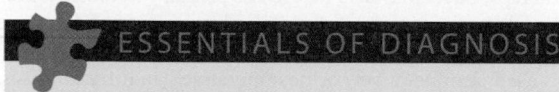

ESSENTIALS OF DIAGNOSIS

► No symptoms in early stages.

► Insidious progressive bilateral loss of peripheral vision, resulting in tunnel vision but preserved visual acuities until advanced disease.

► Pathologic cupping of the optic disks.

► Intraocular pressure is usually elevated.

► General Considerations

Chronic glaucoma is characterized by gradually progressive excavation ("cupping") and corresponding pallor of the optic disk with loss of vision progressing from slight visual field loss to complete blindness. In chronic open-angle glaucoma, primary or secondary, the intraocular pressure is elevated due to reduced drainage of aqueous fluid through the trabecular meshwork. In chronic angle-closure glaucoma, which is particularly common in Inuits and eastern Asians, flow of aqueous fluid into the anterior chamber angle is obstructed. In normal-tension glaucoma, intraocular pressure is not elevated but the same pattern of optic nerve damage occurs.

Primary (chronic) open-angle glaucoma is usually bilateral. There is an increased prevalence in first-degree relatives of affected individuals and in diabetic patients. In Afro-Caribbeans and Africans, and probably in Hispanics, it is more frequent, occurs at an earlier age, and results in more severe optic nerve damage. Secondary open-angle glaucoma may result from ocular disease, eg, pigment dispersion, pseudoexfoliation, uveitis, or trauma; or corticosteroid therapy, whether it is intraocular, topical, systemic, inhaled, or administered by nasal spray.

In the United States, it is estimated that 2% of people over 40 years of age have glaucoma, affecting over 2.5 million individuals. At least 25% of cases are undetected. Over 90%

of cases are of the open-angle type. Worldwide, about 45
million people have open-angle glaucoma, of whom
about 4.5 million are bilaterally blind. About 4 million
people, of whom approximately 50% live in China, are
bilaterally blind from chronic angle-closure glaucoma.

► Clinical Findings

Because initially there are no symptoms, chronic glaucoma
is often first suspected at a routine eye test. Diagnosis
requires consistent and reproducible abnormalities in at
least two of three parameters—optic disk or retinal nerve
fiber layer (or both), visual field, and intraocular pressure.
Optic disk cupping is identified as an absolute increase or
an asymmetry between the two eyes of the ratio of the
diameter of the optic cup to the diameter of the whole optic
disk (cup-disk ratio). (Cup-disk ratio greater than 0.5 or
0.2 or more asymmetry between eyes is suggestive.) Detection of optic disk cupping and associated abnormalities of
the retinal nerve fiber layer is facilitated by optical coherence tomography scans. Visual field abnormalities initially
develop in the paracentral region, followed by constriction
of the peripheral visual field. Central vision remains good
until late in the disease. The normal range of intraocular
pressure is 10–21 mm Hg.

In many individuals (about 4.5 million in the United States),
elevated intraocular pressure is not associated with optic
disk or visual field abnormalities (**ocular hypertension**).
Treatment to reduce intraocular pressure is justified if
there is a moderate to high risk of progression to glaucoma,
determined by several factors, including age, optic disk
appearance, level of intraocular pressure, and corneal
thickness, but monitoring for development of glaucoma is
required in all cases. A significant proportion of eyes with
primary open-angle glaucoma have normal intraocular
pressure when it is first measured, and only repeated measurements identify the abnormally high pressure. In normal-tension glaucoma, intraocular pressure is always
within the normal range.

► Prevention

There are many causes of optic disk abnormalities or visual
field changes that mimic glaucoma and visual field testing
may prove unreliable in some patients, particularly in the
older age group. The diagnosis of glaucoma is not always
straightforward and screening programs need to involve
ophthalmologists.

Although all persons over age 50 years may benefit
from intraocular pressure measurement and optic disk
examination every 3–5 years, population-based screening
for glaucoma is not cost-effective. Screening for chronic
open-angle glaucoma should be targeted at individuals
with an affected first-degree relative, at persons who have
diabetes mellitus, and at older individuals with African or
Hispanic ancestry. Screening may also be warranted in
patients taking long-term oral or combined intranasal and
inhaled corticosteroid therapy. Screening for chronic
angle-closure glaucoma should be targeted at Inuits and
Asians.

► Treatment

A. Medications (Table 7–2)

Prostaglandin analog eye drops are commonly used as first-
line therapy because of their efficacy, their lack of systemic
side effects, and the convenience of once-daily dosing
(except unoprostone) (Table 7–2). All may produce conjunctival hyperemia, permanent darkening of the iris and eyebrow color, increased eyelash growth, and reduction of
periorbital fat (prostaglandin-associated periorbitopathy).
Topical beta-adrenergic blocking agents may be used alone
or in combination with a prostaglandin analog. They may be
contraindicated in patients with reactive airway disease or
heart failure. Betaxolol is theoretically safer in reactive airway disease but less effective at reducing intraocular pressure. Brimonidine 0.2%, a selective alpha-2-agonist, and
topical carbonic anhydrase inhibitors also can be used in
addition to a prostaglandin analog or a beta-blocker (twice
daily) or as initial therapy when prostaglandin analogs and
beta-blockers are contraindicated (brimonidine twice daily,
carbonic anhydrase inhibitors three times daily). All three
are associated with allergic reactions. Brimonidine may
cause uveitis. Apraclonidine, 0.5–1%, another alpha-2-agonist,
can be used three times a day to postpone the need for surgery in patients receiving maximal medical therapy, but
long-term use is limited by drug reactions. It is more commonly used to control acute rises in intraocular pressure,
such as after laser therapy. Pilocarpine 1–4%, epinephrine,
0.5–1%, and the prodrug dipivefrin, 0.1%, are rarely used
because of adverse effects. Oral carbonic anhydrase inhibitors (acetazolamide [Diamox], methazolamide [Neptazane],
dichlorphenamide [Daranide]) may still be used on a long-
term basis if topical therapy is inadequate and surgical or
laser therapy is inappropriate.

Various eye drop preparations combining two agents
out of the prostaglandin analogs, beta-adrenergic blocking
agents, brimonidine and topical carbonic anhydrase inhibitors are available to improve compliance when multiple
medications are required. Formulations of one or two
agents without preservative or not including benzalkonium
chloride as the preservative are increasingly used to reduce
adverse effects on the ocular surface.

B. Laser Therapy and Surgery

Laser trabeculoplasty is used as an adjunct to topical therapy to defer surgery and is also advocated as primary treatment. Surgery is generally undertaken when intraocular
pressure is inadequately controlled by medical and laser
therapy, but it may also be used as primary treatment. Trabeculectomy remains the standard procedure. Adjunctive
treatment with subconjunctival mitomycin or fluorouracil
is used perioperatively or postoperatively in difficult cases.
Viscocanalostomy, deep sclerectomy with collagen implant
and Trabectome—alternative procedures that avoid a full-
thickness incision into the eye—are associated with fewer
complications but are less effective than trabeculectomy
and more difficult to perform.

In chronic angle-closure glaucoma, laser peripheral
iridotomy or surgical peripheral iridectomy may be helpful. In patients with asymptomatic narrow anterior

chamber angles, which includes about 10% of Chinese adults, prophylactic laser peripheral iridotomy can be performed to reduce the risk of acute and chronic angle-closure glaucoma. However, there are concerns about the efficacy of such treatment and the risk of cataract progression and corneal decompensation. In the United States, about 1% of people over age 35 years have narrow anterior chamber angles, but acute and chronic angle-closure are sufficiently uncommon that prophylactic therapy is not generally advised.

▶ Prognosis

Untreated chronic glaucoma that begins at age 40–45 years will probably cause complete blindness by age 60–65. Early diagnosis and treatment can preserve useful vision throughout life. In primary open-angle glaucoma—and if treatment is required in ocular hypertension—the aim is to reduce intraocular pressure to a level that will adequately reduce progression of visual field loss. In eyes with marked visual field or optic disk changes, intraocular pressure must be reduced to less than 16 mm Hg. In normal-tension glaucoma with progressive visual field loss, it is necessary to achieve even lower intraocular pressure such that surgery is often required.

▶ When to Refer

All patients with suspected chronic glaucoma should be referred to an ophthalmologist.

Jin J. JAMA patient page. Glaucoma. JAMA. 2014 May 14; 311(18):1934. [PMID: 24825657]

Li T et al. Comparative effectiveness of first-line medications for primary open-angle glaucoma: a systematic review and network meta-analysis. Ophthalmology. 2016 Jan;123(1):129–40. [PMID: 26526633]

Mantravadi AV et al. Glaucoma. Prim Care. 2015 Sep;42(3): 437–49. [PMID: 26319348]

Moyer VA et al. Screening for glaucoma: U.S. Preventive Services Task Force Recommendation Statement. Ann Intern Med. 2013 Oct 1;159(7):484–9. [PMID: 24325017]

Shaikh Y et al. Burden of undetected and untreated glaucoma in the United States. Am J Ophthalmol. 2014 Dec;158(6):1121–9.e1. [PMID: 25152501]

Stone JS et al. Glaucoma blindness at a tertiary eye care center. N C Med J. 2015 Sep–Oct;76(4):211–8. [PMID: 26509509]

Weinreb RN et al. The pathophysiology and treatment of glaucoma: a review. JAMA. 2014 May 14;311(18):1901–11. [PMID: 24825645]

UVEITIS

▶ ESSENTIALS OF DIAGNOSIS

- ▶ Usually immunologic but possibly infective or neoplastic.
- ▶ Acute nongranulomatous anterior uveitis: pain, redness, photophobia, and visual loss.
- ▶ Granulomatous anterior uveitis: blurred vision in a mildly inflamed eye.
- ▶ Posterior uveitis: gradual loss of vision in a quiet eye.

▶ General Considerations

Intraocular inflammation (uveitis) is classified as acute or chronic, nongranulomatous or granulomatous, according to the clinical signs, or by its distribution—involving the anterior, intermediate, or posterior segments of the eye or panuveitis (in which all segments are affected). The common types are acute nongranulomatous anterior uveitis, granulomatous anterior uveitis, and posterior uveitis.

In most cases, the pathogenesis of uveitis is primarily immunologic, but infection may be the cause, particularly in immunodeficiency states. The systemic disorders associated with acute nongranulomatous anterior uveitis are the HLA-B27-related conditions (ankylosing spondylitis, reactive arthritis, psoriasis, ulcerative colitis, and Crohn disease). Chronic nongranulomatous anterior uveitis occurs in juvenile idiopathic arthritis. Behçet syndrome produces both anterior uveitis, with recurrent hypopyon but little discomfort, and posterior uveitis, characteristically with branch retinal vein occlusions. Both herpes simplex and herpes zoster infections may cause nongranulomatous anterior uveitis as well as retinitis (acute retinal necrosis), which has a very poor prognosis.

Diseases producing granulomatous anterior uveitis also tend to be causes of posterior uveitis. These include sarcoidosis, toxoplasmosis, tuberculosis, syphilis, Vogt-Koyanagi-Harada syndrome (bilateral uveitis associated with alopecia, poliosis [depigmented eyelashes, eyebrows, or hair], vitiligo, and hearing loss), and sympathetic ophthalmia that occurs after penetrating ocular trauma. In toxoplasmosis there may be evidence of previous episodes of retinochoroiditis. Syphilis characteristically produces a "salt and pepper" fundus but may present with a wide variety of clinical manifestations. The other principal pathogens responsible for ocular inflammation in HIV infection are cytomegalovirus (CMV), herpes simplex and herpes zoster viruses, mycobacteria, *Cryptococcus, Toxoplasma,* and *Candida.*

Retinal vasculitis and intermediate uveitis predominantly manifest as posterior uveitis with central or peripheral retinal abnormalities in retinal vasculitis and far peripheral retinal abnormalities (pars planitis) in intermediate uveitis. Retinal vasculitis can be caused by a wide variety of infectious agents and noninfectious systemic conditions but also may be idiopathic. Intermediate uveitis is often idiopathic but can be due to multiple sclerosis or sarcoidosis.

▶ Clinical Findings

Anterior uveitis is characterized by inflammatory cells and flare within the aqueous. In severe cases there may be hypopyon (layered collection of white cells) and fibrin within the anterior chamber. Cells may also be seen on the corneal endothelium as keratic precipitates (KPs). In granulomatous uveitis there are large "mutton-fat" KPs (Figure 7–2), and iris nodules may be seen. In nongranulomatous uveitis the KPs are smaller and iris nodules are not seen. The pupil is usually small, and with the development of posterior synechiae (adhesions between the iris and anterior lens capsule) it also becomes irregular.

▲ **Figure 7–2.** Granulomatous keratic precipitates located on the inferior corneal endothelium. (From Emmett T Cunningham, Jr. Reproduced, with permission, from Riordan-Eva P, Cunningham ET Jr. *Vaughan & Asbury's General Ophthalmology,* 18th ed. McGraw-Hill, 2011.)

Nongranulomatous anterior uveitis tends to present acutely with unilateral pain, redness, photophobia, and visual loss. In juvenile idiopathic arthritis there tends to be an indolent, often initially asymptomatic process with a high risk of sight-threatening complications. Granulomatous anterior uveitis is usually indolent, causing blurred vision in a mildly inflamed eye.

In **posterior uveitis** there are cells in the vitreous. Inflammatory lesions may be present in the retina or choroid. Fresh lesions are yellow with indistinct margins and there may be retinal hemorrhages, whereas older lesions have more definite margins and are commonly pigmented. Retinal vessel sheathing may occur adjacent to such lesions or more diffusely. In severe cases, vitreous opacity precludes visualization of retinal details.

Posterior uveitis tends to present with gradual visual loss in a relatively quiet eye. Bilateral involvement is common. Visual loss may be due to vitreous haze and opacities, inflammatory lesions involving the macula, macular edema, retinal vein occlusion, or rarely associated optic neuropathy.

▶ Differential Diagnosis

Retinal detachment, intraocular tumors, and central nervous system lymphoma may all masquerade as uveitis.

▶ Treatment

Anterior uveitis usually responds to topical corticosteroids. Occasionally periocular corticosteroid injections or even systemic corticosteroids are required. Dilation of the pupil is important to relieve discomfort and prevent posterior synechiae. **Posterior uveitis** more commonly requires systemic, periocular or intravitreal corticosteroid therapy and occasionally systemic immunosuppression with agents such as azathioprine, tacrolimus, cyclosporine, mycophenolate, or methotrexate, of which the last also can be administered by intraocular injection. The use of biologic therapies is increasing. Pupillary dilation is not usually necessary.

If an infectious cause is identified, specific antimicrobial therapy may be indicated. In general, the prognosis for anterior uveitis, particularly the nongranulomatous type, is better than for posterior uveitis.

▶ When to Refer

- Any patient with suspected acute uveitis should be referred urgently to an ophthalmologist or emergently if visual loss or pain is severe.

- Any patient with suspected chronic uveitis should be referred to an ophthalmologist, urgently if there is more than mild visual loss.

▶ When to Admit

Patients with severe uveitis, particularly those requiring intravenous therapy, may require hospital admission.

Dunn JP. Uveitis. Prim Care. 2015 Sep;42(3):305–23. [PMID: 26319340]

Harman LE et al. Uveitis: the collaborative diagnostic evaluation. Am Fam Physician. 2014 Nov 15;90(10):711–6. [PMID: 25403035]

Kempen JH et al. Factors predicting visual acuity outcome in intermediate, posterior, and panuveitis: the Multicenter Uveitis Steroid Treatment (MUST) Trial. Am J Ophthalmol. 2015 Dec; 160(6):1133–41. [PMID: 26386159]

Khan MA et al. Acute anterior uveitis and spondyloarthritis: more than meets the eye. Curr Rheumatol Rep. 2015 Sep; 17(9):59. [PMID: 26233598]

CATARACT

ESSENTIALS OF DIAGNOSIS

- ▶ Gradually progressive blurred vision.
- ▶ No pain or redness.
- ▶ Lens opacities (may be grossly visible).

▶ General Considerations

Cataracts are opacities of the crystalline lens and are usually bilateral. They are the leading cause of blindness worldwide. They may be congenital (owing to intrauterine infections, such as rubella and CMV, or inborn errors of metabolism, such as galactosemia); traumatic; secondary to systemic disease (diabetes mellitus, myotonic dystrophy, atopic dermatitis); systemic or inhaled corticosteroid treatment, uveitis, or radiation exposure; or associated with other drugs, including statins; but age-related cataract is by far the most common type. Most persons over age 60 have some degree of lens opacity. Cigarette smoking increases the risk of cataract formation. Multivitamin/mineral supplements and high dietary antioxidants may prevent the development of age-related cataract.

Clinical Findings

The predominant symptom is progressive blurring of vision. Glare, especially in bright light or when driving at night; change of focusing, particularly development of nearsightedness; and monocular double vision may also occur.

Even in its early stages, a cataract can be seen through a dilated pupil with an ophthalmoscope or slit lamp. As the cataract matures, the retina will become increasingly difficult to visualize, until finally the fundus reflection is absent and the pupil is white.

Treatment

Functional visual impairment is the prime criterion for surgery. The cataract is usually removed by one of the techniques in which the posterior lens capsule remains (extracapsular), thus providing support for a prosthetic intraocular lens. Laser treatment may be used during surgery and may be required subsequently if the posterior capsule opacifies. Ultrasonic fragmentation (phacoemulsification) of the lens nucleus and foldable intraocular lenses allow cataract surgery to be performed through a small incision without the need for sutures, thus reducing the postoperative complication rate and accelerating visual rehabilitation. Multifocal and accommodative intraocular lenses reduce the need for both distance and near vision correction. In the developing world, manual small-incision surgery, in which the lens nucleus is removed intact, is popular because less equipment is required.

Prognosis

Cataract surgery is cost-effective in improving survival and quality of life. In the developed world, it improves visual acuity in 95% of cases. In the other 5%, there is preexisting retinal damage or operative or postoperative complications. In less developed areas, the improvement in visual acuity is not as high, in part due to uncorrected refractive error postoperatively. Treatment with an alpha-1-antagonist, such as tamsulosin, alfuzosin, doxazosin, or silodosin for benign prostatic hyperplasia; prazosin for systemic hypertension; or risperidone or paliperidone for psychiatric disease increases the risk of complications during surgery (floppy iris syndrome) and in the early postoperative period. Nasolacrimal duct obstruction increases the risk of intraocular infection (endophthalmitis).

When to Refer

Patients with cataracts should be referred to an ophthalmologist when their visual impairment adversely affects their everyday activities.

Grewal DS et al. Femtosecond laser assisted cataract surgery—current status and future directions. Surv Ophthalmol. 2016 Mar-Apr;61(2):103–31. [PMID: 26409902]

Gupta VB et al. Etiopathogenesis of cataract: an appraisal. Indian J Ophthalmol. 2014 Feb;62(2):103–10. [PMID: 24618482]

Thompson J et al. Cataracts. Prim Care. 2015 Sep;42(3):409–23. [PMID: 26319346]

RETINAL DETACHMENT

 ESSENTIALS OF DIAGNOSIS

▶ Loss of vision in one eye that is usually rapid, possibly with "curtain" spreading across field of vision.

▶ No pain or redness.

▶ Detachment seen by ophthalmoscopy.

General Considerations

Most cases of retinal detachment are due to development of one or more peripheral retinal tears or holes or both (rhegmatogenous retinal detachment). This is usually spontaneous, related to degenerative changes in the vitreous, and generally occurs in persons over 50 years of age. Nearsightedness and cataract extraction are the two most common predisposing causes. It may also be caused by penetrating or blunt ocular trauma.

Tractional retinal detachment occurs when there is preretinal fibrosis, such as in proliferative retinopathy due to diabetic retinopathy or retinal vein occlusion or as a complication of rhegmatogenous retinal detachment. Serous retinal detachment results from accumulation of subretinal fluid, such as in neovascular age-related macular degeneration or secondary to choroidal tumor.

Clinical Findings

Rhegmatogenous retinal detachment usually starts in the superior temporal area, spreading rapidly to cause visual field loss that starts inferiorly and expands upwards. Premonitory symptoms of the predisposing vitreous degeneration and vitreo-retinal traction are recent onset of or increase in floaters (moving spots or streaks in the visual field) and photopsias (flashes of light). Central vision remains intact until the macula becomes detached. On ophthalmoscopic examination, the retina is seen hanging in the vitreous like a gray cloud. One or more retinal tears or holes (or both) will usually be found on further examination. In traction retinal detachment, there is irregular retinal elevation. In serous retinal detachment, the retina is dome-shaped and the subretinal fluid shifts position with changes in posture. Ocular ultrasonography assists the detection and characterization of retinal detachment.

Treatment

Treatment of rhegmatogenous retinal detachments is directed at closing all of the retinal tears and holes by forming a permanent adhesion between the neurosensory retina, the retinal pigment epithelium, and the choroid with laser photocoagulation to the retina or cryotherapy to the sclera. The following may be required to achieve apposition of the neurosensory retina to the retinal pigment epithelium while the adhesion is developing: indentation of the sclera with a silicone sponge or buckle, subretinal fluid drainage via an incision in the sclera, or injection of an expansile gas or silicone oil into the vitreous cavity following intraocular surgery to remove the vitreous (pars plana vitrectomy). Certain types of uncomplicated retinal detachment may be treated by pneumatic retinopexy, in which an expansile gas is injected into the vitreous cavity followed by positioning of the patient's head to facilitate reattachment of the retina. Once the retina is repositioned, the defects are sealed by laser photocoagulation or cryotherapy; these two methods are also used to seal retinal defects without associated detachment. Intravitreal injection of ocriplasmin (Jetrea), a serine protease, may release vitreo-macular traction to avoid the need for vitrectomy.

In complicated retinal detachments, particularly traction retinal detachments, retinal reattachment can be accomplished only by pars plana vitrectomy, direct manipulation of the retina, and internal tamponade of the retina with air, expansile gas, or silicone oil. (The presence of an expansile gas within the eye is a contraindication to air travel, mountaineering at high altitude, and nitrous oxide anesthesia. Such gases persist in the globe for weeks after surgery.) Treatment of serous retinal detachments is determined by the underlying cause.

▶ Prognosis

About 90% of uncomplicated rhegmatogenous retinal detachments can be cured with one operation. The visual prognosis is worse if the macula is detached or if the detachment is of long duration.

▶ When to Refer

All cases of retinal detachment must be referred urgently to an ophthalmologist, emergently if central vision is good because this indicates that the macula has not detached. During transportation the patient's head is positioned so that the detached portion of the retina will fall back with the aid of gravity.

Daien V et al. Incidence, risk factors, and impact of age on retinal detachment after cataract surgery in France: a national population study. Ophthalmology. 2015 Nov;122(11):2179–85. [PMID: 26278859]

Farioli A et al. Vascular risk factors and rhegmatogenous retinal detachment: a follow-up of a national cohort of Swedish men. Br J Ophthalmol. 2015 Oct 15. [Epub ahead of print] [PMID: 26472402]

Goh YW et al. The incidence of retinal breaks in the presenting and fellow eyes in patients with acute symptomatic posterior vitreous detachment and their associated risk factors. Asia Pac J Ophthalmol (Phila). 2015 Jan–Feb;4(1):5–8. [PMID: 26068606]

Hatef E et al. Pneumatic retinopexy versus scleral buckle for repairing simple rhegmatogenous retinal detachments. Cochrane Database Syst Rev. 2015 May 7;5:CD008350. [PMID: 25950286]

Kikushima W et al. Quick referral and urgent surgery to preempt foveal detachment in retinal detachment repair. Asia Pac J Ophthalmol (Phila). 2014 May–Jun;3(3):141–5. [PMID: 26107583]

Kwon OW et al. Retinal detachment and proliferative vitreoretinopathy. Dev Ophthalmol. 2016;55:154–62. [PMID: 26501375]

Parravano M et al. Vitrectomy for idiopathic macular hole. Cochrane Database Syst Rev. 2015 May 12;5:CD009080. [PMID: 25965055]

Smretschnig E et al. Vision-related quality of life and visual function after retinal detachment surgery. Retina. 2015 Oct 27. [Epub ahead of print] [PMID: 26509221]

van Bussel EM et al. Impact of duration of macula-off retinal detachment on visual outcome: a systematic review and meta-analysis of the literature. Retina. 2014 Oct;34(10):1917–25. [PMID: 25121930]

Zvorničanin J et al. The diagnostic accuracy of bedside ocular ultrasonography for the diagnosis of retinal detachment: a systematic review and meta-analysis. Ann Emerg Med. 2015 Sep; 66(3):342–3. [PMID: 26304260]

VITREOUS HEMORRHAGE

Patients with vitreous hemorrhage complain of sudden visual loss, abrupt onset of floaters that may progressively increase in severity, or occasionally, "bleeding within the eye." Visual acuity ranges from 20/20 (6/6) to light perception. The eye is not inflamed, and clues to diagnosis are inability to see fundal details or localized collection of blood in front of the retina (Figure 7–3). Causes of vitreous hemorrhage include retinal tear (with or without detachment), diabetic or sickle cell retinopathy, retinal vein occlusion, retinal vasculitis, neovascular age-related macular degeneration, blood dyscrasia, therapeutic anticoagulation, trauma, subarachnoid hemorrhage, and severe straining.

▶ When to Refer

All patients with suspected vitreous hemorrhage must be referred urgently to an ophthalmologist.

Jun JH et al. Association of rivaroxaban anticoagulation and spontaneous vitreous hemorrhage. JAMA Ophthalmol. 2015 Oct 1;133(10):1184–6. [PMID: 26111247]

▲ **Figure 7–3.** Large preretinal hemorrhage. (Reproduced, with permission, from Riordan-Eva P, Cunningham ET Jr. *Vaughan & Asbury's General Ophthalmology*, 18th ed. McGraw-Hill, 2011.)

Kim DY et al. Acute-onset vitreous hemorrhage of unknown origin before vitrectomy: causes and prognosis. J Ophthalmol. 2015;2015:429251. [PMID: 26504593]

Melamud A et al. Early vitrectomy for spontaneous, fundus-obscuring vitreous hemorrhage. Am J Ophthalmol. 2015 Nov; 160(5):1073–7.e1. [PMID: 26209230]

AGE-RELATED MACULAR DEGENERATION

ESSENTIALS OF DIAGNOSIS

- ▶ Older age group.
- ▶ Acute or chronic deterioration of central vision in one or both eyes.
- ▶ Distortion or abnormal size of images.
- ▶ No pain or redness.
- ▶ Macular abnormalities seen by ophthalmoscopy.

General Considerations

In developed countries, age-related macular degeneration is the leading cause of permanent visual loss in the older population. Its prevalence increases with each decade over age 50 years (to almost 30% by age 75). Its occurrence and response to treatment are influenced by genetically determined variations in the complement pathway and in lipoprotein metabolism. Other associated factors are race (usually white), sex (slight female predominance), family history, cigarette smoking, and possibly regular aspirin use.

Age-related macular degeneration is classified into dry ("atrophic," "geographic") and wet ("neovascular," "exudative"). Although both are progressive and usually bilateral, they differ in manifestations, prognosis, and management.

Clinical Findings

The precursor to age-related macular degeneration is age-related maculopathy that is characterized by retinal drusen. Hard drusen appear ophthalmoscopically as discrete yellow deposits. Soft drusen are larger, paler, and less distinct. Large, confluent soft drusen are particularly associated with neovascular (wet) age-related macular degeneration. Age-related macular degeneration results in loss of central field vision only. Peripheral fields, and hence navigational vision, are maintained.

"Dry" age-related macular degeneration is characterized by gradually progressive bilateral visual loss of moderate severity due to atrophy and degeneration of the outer retina and retinal pigment epithelium. In **"wet" age-related macular degeneration,** choroidal new vessels grow between the retinal pigment epithelium and Bruch membrane, leading to accumulation of serous fluid, hemorrhage, and fibrosis. The onset of visual loss is more rapid and more severe than in atrophic degeneration. The two eyes are frequently affected sequentially over a period of a few years. Although "dry" age-related macular degeneration is much more common, "wet" age-related macular degeneration accounts for about 90% of all cases of legal blindness due to age-related macular degeneration.

Treatment

No dietary modification has been shown to prevent the development of age-related maculopathy. In patients with age-related maculopathy, oral treatment with antioxidants (vitamins C and E), zinc, copper, and carotenoids (lutein and zeaxanthin, rather than vitamin A [beta-carotene]) is recommended to reduce the risk of progression to age-related macular degeneration. Oral omega-3 fatty acids do not provide additional benefit.

Inhibitors of vascular endothelial growth factors (VEGF), such as ranibizumab (Lucentis), pegaptanib (Macugen), bevacizumab (Avastin), and aflibercept (VEGF Trap-Eye, Eylea), reverse choroidal neovascularization, resulting in stabilization and, less frequently, improvement in vision in neovascular degeneration. They have to be administered repeatedly by intraocular injection, possibly long term. Treatment is well tolerated with minimal adverse effects, but there is a risk of intraocular complications. Long-term outcome studies show up to one-third of eyes have a poor outcome even with prolonged treatment. In bilateral severe disease, macular surgery may be beneficial.

There is no specific treatment for atrophic degeneration, but—as with the neovascular form—patients may benefit from low-vision aids.

When to Refer

Older patients developing sudden visual loss due to macular disease—particularly paracentral distortion or scotoma with preservation of central acuity—should be referred urgently to an ophthalmologist.

Broadhead GK et al. Dietary modification and supplementation for the treatment of age-related macular degeneration. Nutr Rev. 2015 Jul;73(7):448–62. [PMID: 26081455]

Brown MM et al. Societal costs associated with neovascular age-related macular degeneration in the United States. Retina. 2016 Feb;36(2):285–98. [PMID: 26428606]

Buckle M et al. Long-term outcomes of intravitreal ranibizumab for neovascular age-related macular degeneration in a well defined region of the UK. Br J Ophthalmol. 2016 Jan;123(1):70–7. [PMID: 26124462]

Chakravarthy U et al. A randomised controlled trial to assess the clinical effectiveness and cost-effectiveness of alternative treatments to Inhibit VEGF in Age-related choroidal Neovascularisation (IVAN). Health Technol Assess. 2015 Oct; 19(78):1–298. [PMID: 26445075]

Gillies MC et al; Fight Retinal Blindness Study Group. Long-term outcomes of treatment of neovascular age-related macular degeneration: data from an observational study. Ophthalmology. 2015 Sep;122(9):1837–45. [PMID: 26096346]

Hanus J et al. Current therapeutic development for atrophic age-related macular degeneration. Br J Ophthalmol. 2016 Jan; 100(1):122–7. [PMID: 26553922]

Joachim N et al. The incidence and progression of age-related macular degeneration over 15 years: The Blue Mountains Eye Study. Ophthalmology. 2015 Dec;122(12):2482–9. [PMID: 26383995]

Lai K et al. Current choice of treatments for neovascular AMD. Expert Rev Clin Pharmacol. 2015 Jan;8(1):135–40. [PMID: 25487081]

Mehta S. Age-related macular degeneration. Prim Care. 2015 Sep;42(3):377–91. [PMID: 26319344]

Michels S et al. Nonneovascular age-related macular degeneration. Dev Ophthalmol. 2016;55:112–24. [PMID: 26502209]

Schmitz-Valckenberg S et al. Natural history of geographic atrophy progression secondary to age-related macular degeneration (Geographic Atrophy Progression Study). Ophthalmology. 2016 Feb;123(2):361–8. [PMID: 26545317]

Schmucker CM et al. Treatment as required versus regular monthly treatment in the management of neovascular age-related macular degeneration: a systematic review and meta-analysis. PLoS One. 2015 Sep 14;10(9):e0137866. [PMID: 26368921]

Solomon SD et al. Intravitreal bevacizumab versus ranibizumab for treatment of neovascular age-related macular degeneration: findings from a Cochrane Systematic Review. Ophthalmology. 2016 Jan;123(1):70–7. [PMID: 26477843]

Virgili G et al. Laser treatment of drusen to prevent progression to advanced age-related macular degeneration. Cochrane Database Syst Rev. 2015 Oct 23;10:CD006537. [PMID: 26493180]

Wong WL et al. Global prevalence of age-related macular degeneration and disease burden projection for 2020 and 2040: a systematic review and meta-analysis. Lancet Glob Health. 2014 Feb;2(2):e106–16. [PMID: 25104651]

Wu J et al. Intakes of lutein, zeaxanthin, and other carotenoids and age-related macular degeneration during 2 decades of prospective follow-up. JAMA Ophthalmol. 2015 Dec 1;133(12):1415–24. [PMID: 26447482]

Yonekawa Y et al. Age-related macular degeneration: advances in management and diagnosis. J Clin Med. 2015 Feb 12;4(2):343–59. [PMID: 26239130]

CENTRAL & BRANCH RETINAL VEIN OCCLUSIONS

ESSENTIALS OF DIAGNOSIS

▶ Sudden monocular loss of vision.

▶ No pain or redness.

▶ Widespread or sectoral retinal hemorrhages.

▶ General Considerations

Central and branch retinal vein occlusion are common causes of acute loss of vision with branch being four times more common. The major predisposing factors are the etiologic factors associated with arteriosclerosis.

▶ Clinical Findings

A. Symptoms and Signs

The visual impairment in **central retinal vein occlusion** is commonly first noticed upon waking. Ophthalmoscopic signs include widespread retinal hemorrhages, retinal venous dilation and tortuosity, retinal cotton-wool spots, and optic disk swelling.

Branch retinal vein occlusion may present in a variety of ways. Sudden loss of vision may occur at the time of occlusion if the fovea is involved or some time afterward from vitreous hemorrhage due to retinal new vessels. More gradual visual loss may occur with development of macular edema. In acute branch retinal vein occlusion, the retinal abnormalities (hemorrhages, venous dilation and tortuosity, and cotton-wool spots) are confined to the area drained by the obstructed vein.

To assess possible reversible risk factors, check blood pressure and ask about tobacco smoking in all patients and ask women about estrogen therapy (including combined oral contraceptives).

B. Laboratory Findings

Obtain screening laboratory studies for diabetes mellitus, hyperlipidemia, and hyperviscosity (especially in simultaneous bilateral disease), including serum protein electrophoresis for paraproteinemia. Particularly in younger patients, consider obtaining antiphospholipid antibodies, lupus anticoagulant, tests for inherited thrombophilia, and plasma homocysteine levels.

▶ Complications

If central retinal vein occlusion is associated with widespread retinal ischemia, manifesting as poor visual acuity (20/200 [6/60] or worse), florid retinal abnormalities, and extensive areas of capillary closure on fluorescein angiography, there is a high risk of development of neovascular (rubeotic) glaucoma, typically within the first 3 months.

Branch retinal vein occlusion may be complicated by peripheral retinal neovascularization or chronic macular edema.

▶ Treatment

Eyes at risk for neovascular glaucoma following ischemic central retinal vein occlusion can be treated by panretinal laser photocoagulation prophylactically or as soon as there is evidence of neovascularization, the latter approach necessitating frequent monitoring. Regression of **iris neovascularization** has been achieved with intravitreal injections of bevacizumab, an inhibitor of VEGF. In branch retinal vein occlusion complicated by **retinal neovascularization,** the ischemic retina should be laser photocoagulated.

Intravitreal injection of a VEGF inhibitor, such as ranibizumab (Lucentis), pegaptanib (Macugen), bevacizumab (Avastin), or aflibercept (VEGF Trap-Eye, Eylea), is beneficial in **chronic macular edema** due to either branch or nonischemic central retinal vein occlusion. Intravitreal triamcinolone improves vision in chronic macular edema due to nonischemic central retinal vein occlusion, whereas an intravitreal implant containing dexamethasone is beneficial in both central and branch retinal vein occlusion. Retinal laser photocoagulation may be indicated in chronic macular edema due to branch, but not central, retinal vein occlusion.

Prognosis

In central retinal vein occlusion, severity of visual loss initially is a good guide to visual outcome. Initial visual acuity of 20/60 (6/18) or better indicates a good prognosis. Visual prognosis is poor for eyes with neovascular glaucoma.

Visual outcome in branch retinal vein occlusion is determined by the severity of macular damage from hemorrhage, ischemia, or edema.

When to Refer

All patients with retinal vein occlusion should be referred urgently to an ophthalmologist.

Ford JA et al. Drug treatment of macular oedema secondary to central retinal vein occlusion: a network meta-analysis. BMJ Open. 2014 Jul 23;4(7):e005292. [PMID: 25056974]

Kolar P. Risk factors for central and branch retinal vein occlusion: a meta-analysis of published clinical data. J Ophthalmol. 2014;2014:724780. [PMID: 25009743]

Macdonald D. The ABCs of RVO: A review of retinal venous occlusion. Clin Exp Optom. 2014 Jul;97(4):311–23. [PMID: 24256639]

Rajagopal R et al. Seeing through thick and through thin: retinal manifestations of thrombophilic and hyperviscosity syndromes. Surv Ophthalmol. 2015 Oct 28. [Epub ahead of print] [PMID: 26519860]

Schockman S et al. Diagnostic ramifications of ocular vascular occlusion as a first thrombotic event associated with factor V Leiden and prothrombin gene heterozygosity. Clin Ophthalmol. 2015 Apr 3;9:591–600. [PMID: 25897198]

CENTRAL & BRANCH RETINAL ARTERY OCCLUSIONS

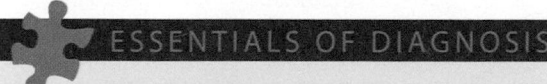

ESSENTIALS OF DIAGNOSIS

► Sudden monocular loss of vision.

► No pain or redness.

► Widespread or sectoral retinal pallid swelling.

General Considerations

In patients 50 years of age or older with central retinal artery occlusion, giant cell arteritis must be considered (see Ischemic Optic Neuropathy and Chapter 20). Otherwise, even if no retinal emboli are identified on ophthalmoscopy, urgent investigation for carotid and cardiac sources of emboli must be undertaken in central and particularly in branch retinal artery occlusion, so that timely treatment can be given to reduce the risk of stroke (see Chapters 12, 14, and 24). Diabetes mellitus, hyperlipidemia, and systemic hypertension are common etiologic factors. Migraine, oral contraceptives, systemic vasculitis, congenital or acquired thrombophilia, and hyperhomocysteinemia are also causes, particularly in young patients. Internal carotid artery dissection should be considered especially when there is neck pain or a recent history of neck trauma.

Multiple branch retinal artery occlusions, which may be asymptomatic, along with encephalopathy and hearing loss are the characteristic features of Susac syndrome.

Clinical Findings

A. Symptoms and Signs

Central retinal artery occlusion presents as sudden profound monocular visual loss. Visual acuity is usually reduced to counting fingers or worse, and visual field is restricted to an island of vision in the temporal field. Ophthalmoscopy reveals pallid swelling of the retina with a cherry-red spot at the fovea (Figure 7–4). The retinal arteries are attenuated, and "box-car" segmentation of blood in the veins may be seen. Occasionally, emboli are seen in the central retinal artery or its branches. The retinal swelling subsides over a period of 4–6 weeks, leaving a pale optic disk and attenuated arterioles.

Branch retinal artery occlusion may also present with sudden loss of vision if the fovea is involved, but more commonly sudden loss of visual field is the presenting complaint. Fundal signs of retinal swelling and adjacent cotton-wool spots are limited to the area of retina supplied by the occluded artery.

Identify risk factors for cardiac source of emboli including arrhythmia, particularly atrial fibrillation, and cardiac valvular disease, and check the blood pressure. Clinical features of giant cell arteritis include age 50 years or older, jaw claudication (which is very specific), headache, scalp tenderness, general malaise, weight loss, symptoms of polymyalgia rheumatica, and tenderness, thickening, or absence of pulse of the superficial temporal arteries. Table 20–12 lists the clinical manifestations of vasculitis.

▲ **Figure 7–4.** Acute central retinal artery occlusion with cherry-red spot (arrow) and preserved retina (arrowheads) adjacent to the optic disk due to cilioretinal artery supply. (From Esther Posner. Reproduced, with permission, from Riordan-Eva P, Cunningham ET Jr. *Vaughan & Asbury's General Ophthalmology*, 18th ed. McGraw-Hill, 2011.)

B. Laboratory Findings

Erythrocyte sedimentation rate and C-reactive protein are usually markedly elevated in giant cell arteritis but one or both may be normal. Consider screening for other types of vasculitis (see Table 20–13). Screen for diabetes mellitus and hyperlipidemia in all patients. Particularly in younger patients, consider testing for antiphospholipid antibodies, lupus anticoagulant, inherited thrombophilia, and elevated plasma homocysteine.

C. Imaging

To identify carotid and cardiac sources of emboli, obtain duplex ultrasonography of the carotid arteries, ECG, and echocardiography, with transesophageal studies (if necessary). When indicated, obtain CT or MR studies for internal carotid artery dissection.

▶ Treatment

If the patient is seen within a few hours after onset, emergency treatment—including laying the patient flat, ocular massage, high concentrations of inhaled oxygen, intravenous acetazolamide, and anterior chamber paracentesis—may influence the visual outcome. Studies of early thrombolysis, particularly by local intra-arterial injection but also intravenously, have shown good results in central retinal artery occlusion not due to giant cell arteritis, but the former method has a high incidence of adverse effects and may be difficult to accomplish within the required time.

In giant cell arteritis there is risk—highest in the first few days—of involvement of the other eye. When the diagnosis is suspected, high-dose corticosteroids (oral prednisolone 1–1.5 mg/kg/day, if necessary preceded by intravenous hydrocortisone 250–500 mg immediately or, especially in patients with bilateral visual loss, methylprednisolone 0.5–1 g/day for 1–3 days) must be instituted immediately, possibly together with low-dose aspirin (~81 mg/day orally). The patient must be monitored closely to ensure that treatment is adequate. A temporal artery biopsy should be performed promptly, and if necessary, assistance should be sought from a rheumatologist.

Patients with embolic retinal artery occlusion and 70–99% ipsilateral carotid artery stenosis and possibly those with 50–69% stenosis should be considered for carotid endarterectomy or possibly angioplasty with stenting to be performed within 2 weeks (see Chapters 12 and 24). Retinal embolization due to cardiac disease such as atrial fibrillation or a hypercoagulable state usually requires anticoagulation. Cardiac valvular disease and patent foramen ovale may require surgical treatment.

▶ When to Refer

• Patients with central retinal artery occlusion should be referred emergently to an ophthalmologist.
• Patients with branch retinal artery occlusion should be referred urgently.

▶ When to Admit

Patients with visual loss due to giant cell arteritis may require emergency admission for high-dose corticosteroid therapy and close monitoring to ensure that treatment is adequate.

Cugati S et al. Treatment options for central retinal artery occlusion. Curr Treat Options Neurol. 2013 Feb;15(1):63–77. [PMID: 23070637]
Hayreh SS. Ocular vascular occlusive disorders: natural history of visual outcome. Prog Retin Eye Res. 2014 Jul;41:1–25. [PMID: 24769221]
Park SJ et al. Risk and risk periods for stroke and acute myocardial infarction in patients with central retinal artery occlusion. Ophthalmology. 2015 Nov;122(11):2336–43.e2. [PMID: 26298716]
Pielen A et al. Predictors of prognosis and treatment outcome in central retinal artery occlusion: local intra-arterial fibrinolysis vs. conservative treatment. Neuroradiology. 2015 Oct;57(10):1055–62. [PMID: 26349479]
Stoffelns BM et al. Cilioretinal artery occlusion. Klin Monbl Augenheilkd. 2015 Apr;232(4):519–24. [PMID: 25902112]
Varma DD et al. A review of central retinal artery occlusion: clinical presentation and management. Eye (Lond). 2013 Jun;27(6):688–97. [PMID: 23470793]

TRANSIENT MONOCULAR VISUAL LOSS

 ESSENTIALS OF DIAGNOSIS

▶ Monocular loss of vision usually lasting a few minutes with complete recovery.

Transient monocular visual loss ("ocular transient ischemic attack [TIA]") is usually caused by a retinal embolus from ipsilateral carotid disease or the heart. The visual loss is characteristically described as a curtain passing vertically across the visual field with complete monocular visual loss lasting a few minutes and a similar curtain effect as the episode passes (amaurosis fugax; also called "fleeting blindness"). An embolus is rarely seen on ophthalmoscopy. Other causes of transient, often recurrent, visual loss due to ocular ischemia are giant cell arteritis, hypercoagulable state (such as antiphospholipid syndrome), hyperviscosity, and severe occlusive carotid disease. More transient visual loss, lasting only a few seconds to 1 minute, usually recurrent, and affecting one or both eyes, occurs in patients with optic disk swelling, for example in those with raised intracranial pressure. In young patients, there is a benign form of transient recurrent visual loss that has been ascribed to choroidal or retinal vascular spasm.

▶ Diagnostic Studies

In most cases, clinical assessment and investigations are much the same as for retinal artery occlusion with emphasis on identifying a source of emboli. Optic disk swelling requires different investigations.

► Treatment

All patients with possible embolic transient visual loss should be treated immediately with oral aspirin (at least 81 mg daily), or another antiplatelet drug, until the cause has been determined. Affected patients with 70–99% (and possibly those with 50–69%) ipsilateral carotid artery stenosis should be considered for urgent carotid endarterectomy or possibly angioplasty with stenting (see Chapters 12 and 24). In all patients, vascular risk factors (eg, hypertension) need to be controlled. Retinal embolization due to cardiac arrhythmia, such as atrial fibrillation, or hypercoagulable state usually requires anticoagulation. Cardiac valvular disease and patent foramen ovale may require surgical treatment. In younger patients with the benign variant of transient monocular blindness, calcium channel blockers, such as slow-release nifedipine, 60 mg/day, may be effective.

► When to Refer

In all cases of episodic visual loss, early ophthalmologic consultation is advisable.

► When to Admit

Hospital admission is advisable in embolic transient visual loss if there have been two or more episodes in the preceding week ("crescendo TIA") or the underlying cause is cardiac or hypercoagulable state.

Bagheri N et al. Acute vision loss. Prim Care. 2015 Sep;42(3):347–61. [PMID: 26319342]

Georgalas I et al. Images in clinical medicine. Amaurosis fugax caused by a branch retinal artery embolus. N Engl J Med. 2015 Nov 26;373(22):e26. [PMID: 26605943]

Lauda F et al. Acute silent brain infarction in monocular visual loss of ischemic origin. Cerebrovasc Dis. 2015;40(3–4):151–6. [PMID: 26278894]

Weinberg DV et al. Amaurosis fugax captured during fluorescein angiography. Retina. 2015 Dec;35(12):2669–71. [PMID: 26049618]

RETINAL DISORDERS ASSOCIATED WITH SYSTEMIC DISEASES

1. Diabetic Retinopathy

 ESSENTIALS OF DIAGNOSIS

- ► Present in about 35% of all diagnosed diabetic patients.
- ► Present in about 20% of type 2 diabetic patients at diagnosis.
- ► Background retinopathy: mild retinal abnormalities without visual loss.
- ► Maculopathy: macular edema, exudates, or ischemia.
- ► Proliferative retinopathy: new retinal vessels.

► General Considerations

Diabetic retinopathy is broadly classified as **nonproliferative,** which is subclassified as mild, moderate, or severe, or **proliferative,** which is less common but causes more severe visual loss. Diabetic retinopathy is present in about one-third of patients in whom diabetes has been diagnosed, and about one-third of those have sight-threatening disease. In the United States, it affects about 4 million people; it is the leading cause of new blindness among adults aged 20–65 years; and the number of affected individuals aged 65 years or older is increasing. Worldwide, there are approximately 93 million people with diabetic retinopathy, including 28 million with vision-threatening disease. Retinopathy increases in prevalence and severity with increasing duration and poorer control of diabetes. In type 1 diabetes, retinopathy is not detectable for at least 3 years after diagnosis. In type 2 diabetes, retinopathy is present in about 20% of patients at diagnosis and may be the presenting feature.

► Clinical Findings

Clinical assessment comprises visual acuity testing, stereoscopic examination of the retina, retinal imaging with optical coherence tomography, and sometimes fluorescein angiography.

Nonproliferative retinopathy manifests as microaneurysms, retinal hemorrhages, venous beading, retinal edema, and hard exudates (Figure 7–5). Reduction of

▲ **Figure 7–5.** Moderate nonproliferative diabetic retinopathy with multiple microaneurysms and hemorrhages, mild macular hard exudates, and two cotton-wool spots in the superior retina. (Reproduced, with permission, from Riordan-Eva P, Cunningham ET Jr. *Vaughan & Asbury's General Ophthalmology,* 18th ed. McGraw-Hill, 2011.)

vision is most commonly due to **diabetic macular edema,** which may be focal or diffuse, but it can also be due to macular ischemia. Macular involvement is the most common cause of legal blindness in type 2 diabetes. Macular edema may be associated with treatment with thiazolidinediones (glitazones).

Proliferative retinopathy is characterized by neovascularization, arising from either the optic disk or the major vascular arcades. Vitreous hemorrhage is a common sequela. Proliferation into the vitreous of blood vessels, with their associated fibrous component, may lead to tractional retinal detachment.

▶ Screening

Visual symptoms and visual acuity are poor guides to the presence of diabetic retinopathy. Adult and adolescent patients with diabetes mellitus should undergo at least yearly screening by fundal photography, commonly with centralized screening that may involve computer detection software programs, or slit-lamp examination. (Failure to identify diabetic retinopathy by direct ophthalmoscopy is common, particularly if the pupils are not dilated.) More frequent monitoring is required in women during pregnancy and in those planning pregnancy. Patients with type 2 diabetes mellitus should be screened shortly after diagnosis. Diabetic retinopathy may worsen after bariatric surgery.

▶ Treatment

Treatment includes optimizing blood glucose, blood pressure, kidney function, and serum lipids, although such measures are probably more important in preventing the development of retinopathy than in influencing its subsequent course. Fenofibrate and renin-angiotensin system inhibitors are beneficial even in established retinopathy.

Macular edema and exudates, but not ischemia, may respond to laser photocoagulation; to intravitreal administration of a VEGF inhibitor (ranibizumab [Lucentis], pegaptanib [Macugen], bevacizumab [Avastin], or aflibercept [VEGF Trap-Eye, Eylea]) or corticosteroid (triamcinolone, dexamethasone implant [Ozurdex], or fluocinolone implant [Retisert, Iluvien]); to vitrectomy; or to intravitreal injection of a serine protease (ocriplasmin [Jetrea]) to release vitreo-retinal traction.

Proliferative retinopathy is usually treated by panretinal laser photocoagulation, preferably before vitreous hemorrhage or tractional detachment has occurred. Regression of neovascularization can also be achieved by intravitreal injection of a VEGF inhibitor. In patients with severe **nonproliferative retinopathy,** fluorescein angiography can help determine whether panretinal laser photocoagulation should be undertaken prophylactically by visualizing the extent of retinal ischemia. Vitrectomy is necessary for removal of persistent vitreous hemorrhage, to improve vision and allow panretinal laser photocoagulation for the underlying retinal neovascularization, for treatment of tractional retinal detachment involving the macula, and for management of rapidly progressive proliferative disease.

Proliferative diabetic retinopathy, especially after successful laser treatment, is not a contraindication to treatment with thrombolytic agents, aspirin, or warfarin unless there has been recent vitreous or pre-retinal hemorrhage.

▶ When to Refer

- All diabetic patients with sudden loss of vision or retinal detachment should be referred emergently to an ophthalmologist.
- Proliferative retinopathy or macular involvement requires urgent referral to an ophthalmologist.
- Severe nonproliferative retinopathy or unexplained reduction of visual acuity requires early referral to an ophthalmologist.

Cheung D et al. The impact of bariatric surgery on diabetic retinopathy: a systematic review and meta-analysis. Obes Surg. 2015 Sep;25(9):1604–9. [PMID: 25515499]

Do DV et al. Blood pressure control for diabetic retinopathy. Cochrane Database Syst Rev. 2015 Jan 31;1:CD006127. [PMID: 25637717]

Gilbert MP. Screening and treatment by the primary care provider of common diabetes complications. Med Clin North Am. 2015 Jan;99(1):201–19. [PMID: 25456651]

Hendrick AM et al. Diabetic retinopathy. Prim Care. 2015 Sep;42(3):451–64. [PMID: 26319349]

National Collaborating Centre for Women's and Children's Health (UK). Diabetes in pregnancy: management of diabetes and its complications from preconception to the postnatal period. 2015 Feb. [PMID: 25950069] http://www.ncbi.nlm.nih.gov/pubmed/25950069

Nentwich MM et al. Diabetic retinopathy—ocular complications of diabetes mellitus. World J Diabetes. 2015 Apr 15;6(3):489–99. [PMID: 25897358]

2. Hypertensive Retinochoroidopathy

Systemic hypertension affects both the retinal and choroidal circulations. The clinical manifestations vary according to the degree and rapidity of rise in blood pressure and the underlying state of the ocular circulation. The most florid ocular changes occur in young patients with abrupt elevations of blood pressure, such as may occur in pheochromocytoma, malignant hypertension, or preeclampsia-eclampsia. Hypertensive retinopathy can be a surrogate marker for current and future nonocular end-organ damage. Its detection is aided by nonmydriatic fundal photography.

Chronic hypertension accelerates the development of atherosclerosis. The retinal arterioles become more tortuous and narrow and develop abnormal light reflexes ("silver-wiring" and "copper-wiring"). There is increased venous compression at the retinal arteriovenous crossings ("arteriovenous nicking"), predisposing to branch retinal vein occlusions. Flame-shaped hemorrhages occur in the nerve fiber layer of the retina.

Acute elevations of blood pressure result in loss of autoregulation in the retinal circulation, leading to breakdown of endothelial integrity and occlusion of precapillary arterioles and capillaries that manifest as cotton-wool spots, retinal hemorrhages, retinal edema, and retinal exudates, often in a stellate appearance at the macula (Figure 7–6).

▲ **Figure 7–6.** Accelerated hypertension in a young woman manifesting as marked optic disk edema, macular star of hard exudates, serous retinal detachment, retinal hemorrhages, and cotton-wool spots. (Reproduced, with permission, from Riordan-Eva P, Cunningham ET Jr. *Vaughan & Asbury's General Ophthalmology,* 18th ed. McGraw-Hill, 2011.)

Vasoconstriction and ischemia in the choroid result in serous retinal detachments and retinal pigment epithelial infarcts that later develop into pigmented lesions that may be focal, linear, or wedge-shaped. The abnormalities in the choroidal circulation may also affect the optic nerve head, producing ischemic optic neuropathy with optic disk swelling. Fundal abnormalities are the hallmark of hypertensive crisis with retinopathy (previously known as malignant hypertension) that requires emergency treatment. Marked fundal abnormalities are likely to be associated with permanent retinal, choroidal, or optic nerve damage. Precipitous reduction of blood pressure may exacerbate such damage.

Akal A et al. Papilledema in a hypertensive adult with grade 4 retinopathy. J Clin Hypertens (Greenwich). 2015 Sep;17(9): 740. [PMID: 25884103]

Cremer A et al. From malignant hypertension to hypertension-MOD: a modern definition for an old but still dangerous emergency. J Hum Hypertens. 2015 Nov 19. [Epub ahead of print] [PMID: 26582411]

Henderson AD et al. Grade III or grade IV hypertensive retinopathy with severely elevated blood pressure. West J Emerg Med. 2012 Dec;13(6):529–34. [PMID: 23359839]

3. Blood Dyscrasias

Severe **thrombocytopenia** or **anemia** may result in various types of retinal or choroidal hemorrhages, including white centered retinal hemorrhages (Roth spots) that occur in leukemia and other situations besides bacterial endocarditis. Involvement of the macula may result in permanent visual loss.

Sickle cell retinopathy is particularly common in hemoglobin SC disease but may also occur with other hemoglobin S variants. Manifestations include "salmon-patch" preretinal/intraretinal hemorrhages, "black sunbursts" resulting from intraretinal hemorrhage, and new vessels. Severe visual loss is rare but more common in patients with pulmonary hypertension. Retinal laser photocoagulation reduces the frequency of vitreous hemorrhage from new vessels. Surgery is occasionally needed for persistent vitreous hemorrhage or tractional retinal detachment.

Gualandro SF et al. Cohort study of adult patients with haemoglobin SC disease: clinical characteristics and predictors of mortality. Br J Haematol. 2015 Nov;171(4):631–7. [PMID: 26255986]

Myint KT et al. Laser therapy for retinopathy in sickle cell disease. Cochrane Database Syst Rev. 2015 Oct 9;10:CD010790. [PMID: 26451693]

Yawn BP et al. Management of sickle cell disease: summary of the 2014 evidence-based report by expert panel members. JAMA. 2014 Sep 10;312(10):1033–48. Erratum in: JAMA. 2014 Nov 12;312(18):1932. [PMID: 25203083]

4. HIV Infection/AIDS

HIV retinopathy manifests clinically as cotton-wool spots, retinal hemorrhages, and microaneurysms but may also lead to reduced contrast sensitivity and retinal nerve fiber layer and outer retinal damage (HIV neuroretinal disorder).

CMV retinitis has become less common with the availability of antiretroviral therapy (ART) but continues to be prevalent where resources are limited. It usually occurs when CD4 counts are below 50/mcL (or 0.05×10^9/L) and is characterized by progressively enlarging yellowish-white patches of retinal opacification, accompanied by retinal hemorrhages and usually beginning adjacent to the major retinal vascular arcades. Patients are often asymptomatic until there is involvement of the fovea or optic nerve, or until retinal detachment develops. Choices for initial therapy are (1) valganciclovir 900 mg orally twice daily for 3 weeks; (2) ganciclovir 5 mg/kg intravenously twice a day, foscarnet 60 mg/kg intravenously three times a day, or cidofovir 5 mg/kg intravenously once weekly, for 2–3 weeks; or (3) local administration, using either intravitreal injection of ganciclovir or foscarnet, or the sustained-release ganciclovir intravitreal implant. All available agents are virostatic. Maintenance therapy can be achieved with lower-dose therapy (oral valganciclovir 900 mg once daily, intravenous ganciclovir 5 mg/kg/day, intravenous foscarnet 90 mg/kg/day, or intravenous cidofovir 5 mg/kg once every 2 weeks) or with intravitreal therapy. Systemic therapy has a greater risk of nonocular adverse effects but reduces mortality, incidence of nonocular CMV disease (but this is less common with ART), and incidence of retinitis in the fellow eye and avoids intraocular complications of intravitreal administration. Pharmacologic prophylaxis against CMV retinitis in patients with low CD4 counts or high CMV burdens has not been found to be worthwhile. In all patients with CMV retinitis, ART needs to be instituted or adjusted. This may lead to the immune reconstitution inflammatory syndrome (IRIS), of which the immune recovery uveitis may lead to visual loss, predominantly due to cystoid macular edema. If the CD4 count is maintained above 100/mcL (0.1×10^9/L), it may be possible to discontinue maintenance anti-CMV therapy.

Other ophthalmic manifestations of opportunistic infections occurring in AIDS patients include herpes simplex retinitis, which usually manifests as acute retinal necrosis; toxoplasmic and candidal chorioretinitis possibly progressing to endophthalmitis; herpes zoster ophthalmicus and herpes zoster retinitis, which can manifest as acute retinal necrosis or progressive outer retinal necrosis; and various entities due to syphilis, tuberculosis, or cryptococcosis. Kaposi sarcoma of the conjunctiva (see Chapter 31) and orbital lymphoma may also be seen on rare occasions. Chronic HIV infection is associated with increased prevalence of age-related macular degeneration.

Demirkaya N et al. Neuroretinal degeneration in HIV patients without opportunistic ocular infections in the cART era. AIDS Patient Care STDS. 2015 Oct;29(10):519–32. [PMID: 26258992]

Jabs DA et al. Incidence and long-term outcomes of the human immunodeficiency virus neuroretinal disorder in patients with AIDS. Ophthalmology. 2015 Apr;122(4):760–8. [PMID: 25600199]

Jabs DA et al. Prevalence of intermediate-stage age-related macular degeneration in patients with acquired immunodeficiency syndrome. Am J Ophthalmol. 2015 Jun;159(6):1115–22.e1. [PMID: 25769246]

ISCHEMIC OPTIC NEUROPATHY

ESSENTIALS OF DIAGNOSIS

▶ Sudden painless visual loss with signs of optic nerve dysfunction.

▶ Optic disk swelling in anterior ischemic optic neuropathy.

Anterior ischemic optic neuropathy—due to inadequate perfusion of the posterior ciliary arteries that supply the anterior portion of the optic nerve—produces sudden visual loss, usually with an altitudinal field defect, and optic disk swelling. In older patients it may be caused by giant cell arteritis (arteritic anterior ischemic optic neuropathy). The predominant factor predisposing to nonarteritic anterior ischemic optic neuropathy, which subsequently affects the fellow eye in around 20% of cases, is a congenitally crowded optic disk. Other causative factors include systemic hypertension, diabetes mellitus, hyperlipidemia, systemic vasculitis, inherited or acquired thrombophilia, interferon-alpha therapy, obstructive sleep apnea, and possibly ingestion of phosphodiesterase type 5 inhibitors. Diabetic papillopathy is a cause of chronic (possibly ischemic) optic disk swelling that generally has a better visual outcome. Rarely, an optic neuropathy that can be difficult to differentiate from nonarteritic anterior optic neuropathy, but typically affecting both eyes simultaneously and having a more chronic course, develops in patients taking amiodarone.

Ischemic optic neuropathy, usually involving the retrobulbar optic nerve and thus not causing any optic disk swelling (**posterior ischemic optic neuropathy**), may occur with severe blood loss; nonocular surgery, particularly prolonged lumbar spine surgery in the prone position; severe burns; or in association with dialysis. In all such situations there may be several contributory factors.

▶ Treatment

Arteritic anterior ischemic optic neuropathy necessitates emergency high-dose systemic corticosteroid treatment to prevent visual loss in the other eye. (See Central & Branch Retinal Artery Occlusions, above, and Polymyalgia Rheumatica & Giant Cell Arteritis, Chapter 20.) Similar treatment is required in anterior ischemic optic neuropathy due to systemic vasculitis, which may also be classified as arteritic anterior ischemic optic neuropathy. It is uncertain whether systemic or intravitreal corticosteroid therapy influences the outcome in nonarteritic anterior ischemic optic neuropathy or whether oral low-dose (~81 mg daily) aspirin reduces the risk of fellow eye involvement. In ischemic optic neuropathy after nonocular surgery, treatment of marked anemia by blood transfusion may be beneficial.

▶ When to Refer

Patients with ischemic optic neuropathy should be referred urgently to an ophthalmologist.

▶ When to Admit

Patients with ischemic optic neuropathy due to giant cell arteritis may require emergency admission for high-dose corticosteroid therapy and close monitoring to ensure that treatment is adequate.

Bansal S et al. Hypotension-induced blindness in haemodialysis patients. Clin Kidney J. 2014 Aug;7(4):387–90. [PMID: 25852914]

Bernstein SL et al. Ischemic optic neuropathies and their models: disease comparisons, model strengths and weaknesses. Jpn J Ophthalmol. 2015 May;59(3):135–47. [PMID: 25690987]

Biousse V et al. Ischemic optic neuropathies. N Engl J Med. 2015 Jun 18;372(25):2428–36. [PMID: 26083207]

Katz DM et al. Is there treatment for nonarteritic anterior ischemic optic neuropathy? Curr Opin Ophthalmol. 2015 Nov;26(6):458–63. [PMID: 26367094]

Lemos J et al. Neuro-ophthalmological emergencies. Neurohospitalist. 2015 Oct;5(4):223–33. [PMID: 26425250]

Wu Y et al. The association between obstructive sleep apnea and nonarteritic anterior ischemic optic neuropathy: a systematic review and meta-analysis. Curr Eye Res. 2015 Oct 7:1–6. [Epub ahead of print] [PMID: 26443989]

OPTIC NEURITIS

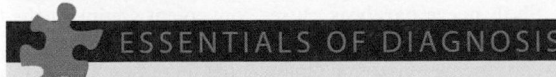

ESSENTIALS OF DIAGNOSIS

▸ Subacute unilateral visual loss with signs of optic nerve dysfunction.

▸ Pain exacerbated by eye movements.

▸ Optic disk usually normal in acute stage but subsequently develops pallor.

▸ General Considerations

Inflammatory optic neuropathy (optic neuritis) is strongly associated with demyelinating disease, particularly multiple sclerosis but also acute disseminated encephalomyelitis. It also occurs in sarcoidosis; in neuromyelitis optica spectrum disorder, which is characterized by serum antibodies to aquaporin-4; in association with serum antibodies to myelin oligodendrocyte glycoprotein; following viral infection (usually in children); in varicella zoster virus infection; in various autoimmune disorders, particularly systemic lupus erythematosus; during treatment with biologics; and by spread of inflammation from the meninges, orbital tissues, or paranasal sinuses.

▸ Clinical Findings

Optic neuritis in demyelinating disease is characterized by unilateral loss of vision developing over a few days. Visual acuity ranges from 20/30 (6/9) to no perception of light, with more severe visual loss being associated with low serum vitamin D. In almost all cases there is pain behind the eye, exacerbated by eye movements. Field loss is usually central. There is particular loss of color vision and a relative afferent pupillary defect. In about two-thirds of cases, the optic nerve is normal during the acute stage (retrobulbar optic neuritis). In the remainder, the optic disk is swollen (papillitis) with occasional flame-shaped peripapillary hemorrhages. Visual acuity usually improves within 2–3 weeks and returns to 20/40 (6/12) or better in 95% of previously unaffected eyes. Optic atrophy subsequently develops if there has been destruction of sufficient optic nerve fibers. Any patient with presumed demyelinating optic neuritis in which visual recovery does not occur or there are other atypical features, including continuing deterioration of vision or persisting pain after 2 weeks, should undergo further investigation, including CT or MRI of the head and orbits to exclude a lesion compressing the optic nerve.

▸ Treatment

In acute demyelinating optic neuritis, intravenous methylprednisolone (1 g daily for 3 days followed by a tapering course of oral prednisolone) has been shown to accelerate visual recovery, although in clinical practice, the oral taper is not often prescribed and oral methylprednisolone may be used. Use in an individual patient is determined by the degree of visual loss, the state of the fellow eye, and the patient's visual requirements.

Optic neuritis due to sarcoidosis, neuromyelitis optica, herpes zoster, or systemic lupus erythematosus generally has a poorer prognosis, requires more prolonged corticosteroid therapy, may require plasma exchange in neuromyelitis optica, and may necessitate long-term immunosuppression.

▸ Prognosis

Among patients with a first episode of clinically isolated optic neuritis, multiple sclerosis will develop in 50% within 15 years but the visual and neurologic prognoses are good. The major risk factors are female sex and multiple white matter lesions on brain MRI. Various disease-modifying drugs, including interferon (Avonex, Rebif, Betaseron, Extavia), glatiramer acetate (Copaxone), mitoxantrone (Novantrone), natazilumab (Tysabri), alemtuzumab (Lemtrada, Campath), fingolimod (Gilenya), teriflunomide (Aubagio), and dimethyl fumarate (Tecfidera), are available to reduce the risk of further neurologic episodes and potentially the accumulation of disability, but each has its own range of adverse effects that in some instances are life-threatening. Fingolimod is associated with macular edema. In addition, laquinimod (Nerventra), daclizumab (Zenapax), and ocrelizumab are being investigated.

▸ When to Refer

All patients with optic neuritis should be referred urgently for ophthalmologic or neurologic assessment.

Balcer LJ et al. Vision and vision-related outcome measures in multiple sclerosis. Brain. 2015 Jan;138(Pt 1):11–27. [PMID: 25433914]

Gaier ED et al. Atypical optic neuritis. Curr Neurol Neurosci Rep. 2015 Dec;15(12):76. [PMID: 26467052]

Gal RL et al. Corticosteroids for treating optic neuritis. Cochrane Database Syst Rev. 2015 Aug 14;8:CD001430. [PMID: 26273799]

Mackay DD. Should patients with optic neuritis be treated with steroids? Curr Opin Ophthalmol. 2015 Nov;26(6):439–44. [PMID: 26367086]

Saguil A et al. Multiple sclerosis: a primary care perspective. Am Fam Physician. 2014 Nov 1;90(9):644–52. [PMID: 25368924]

Torkildsen Ø et al. Disease-modifying treatments for multiple sclerosis—a review of approved medications. Eur J Neurol. 2016 Jan;23(Suppl 1):18–27. [PMID: 26563094]

Tur C et al. Early accurate diagnosis crucial in multiple sclerosis. Practitioner. 2015 Sep;259(1785):21–7. [PMID: 26591653]

Wilhelm H et al. The diagnosis and treatment of optic neuritis. Dtsch Arztebl Int. 2015 Sep 11;112(37):616–26. [PMID: 26396053]

OPTIC DISK SWELLING

Optic disk swelling may result from intraocular disease, orbital and optic nerve lesions, severe hypertensive retinochoroidopathy, or raised intracranial pressure, the last necessitating urgent imaging to exclude an intracranial mass or cerebral venous sinus occlusion. Intraocular causes include central retinal vein occlusion, posterior uveitis, and posterior scleritis. Optic nerve lesions causing disk swelling include anterior ischemic optic neuropathy; optic neuritis; optic nerve sheath meningioma; and infiltration by sarcoidosis, leukemia, or lymphoma. Any orbital lesion causing nerve compression may produce disk swelling.

Papilledema (optic disk swelling due to raised intracranial pressure) is usually bilateral and most commonly produces enlargement of the blind spot without loss of acuity. Chronic papilledema, as in idiopathic intracranial hypertension and cerebral venous sinus occlusion, or severe acute papilledema may be associated with visual field loss and occasionally with profound loss of acuity. All patients with chronic papilledema must be monitored carefully—especially their visual fields—and cerebrospinal fluid shunt or optic nerve sheath fenestration should be considered in those with progressive visual failure not controlled by medical therapy (weight loss where appropriate and acetazolamide).

Optic disk drusen and congenitally crowded optic disks, which are associated with farsightedness, cause optic disk elevation that may be mistaken for swelling (pseudopapilledema). Exposed optic disk drusen may be obvious clinically or can be demonstrated by their autofluorescence. Buried drusen are best detected by orbital ultrasound or CT scanning. Other family members may be similarly affected.

Piper RJ et al. Interventions for idiopathic intracranial hypertension. Cochrane Database Syst Rev. 2015 Aug 7;8:CD003434. [PMID: 26250102]
Raj C. Papilledema: a case of bilateral blurred vision caused by idiopathic intracranial hypertension. Aust Fam Physician. 2015 Mar;44(3):117–20. [PMID: 25770576]

OCULAR MOTOR PALSIES

In complete **third nerve paralysis,** there is ptosis with a divergent and slightly depressed eye. Extraocular movements are restricted in all directions except laterally (preserved lateral rectus function). Intact fourth nerve (superior oblique) function is detected by the presence of inward rotation on attempted depression of the eye. Pupillary involvement (relatively dilated pupil that does not constrict normally to light) is an important sign differentiating "surgical," including traumatic, from "medical" causes of isolated third nerve palsy. Compressive lesions of the third nerve—eg, aneurysm of the posterior communicating artery and uncal herniation due to a supratentorial mass lesion—characteristically have pupillary involvement. Patients with painful acute isolated third nerve palsy and pupillary involvement should be assumed to have a posterior communicating artery aneurysm until this has been excluded. Pituitary apoplexy is a rarer cause. Medical causes of isolated third nerve palsy include diabetes mellitus, hypertension, giant cell arteritis, and herpes zoster.

Fourth nerve paralysis causes upward deviation of the eye with failure of depression on adduction. In acquired cases, there is vertical and torsional diplopia that is most apparent on looking down. Trauma is a major cause of acquired—particularly bilateral—fourth nerve palsy, but posterior fossa tumor and medical causes, such as in third nerve palsies, should also be considered. Similar clinical features are seen in congenital cases due to developmental anomaly of the nerve, muscle, or tendon.

Sixth nerve paralysis causes convergent squint in the primary position with failure of abduction of the affected eye, producing horizontal diplopia that increases on gaze to the affected side and on looking into the distance. It is an important sign of raised intracranial pressure. Sixth nerve palsy may also be due to trauma, neoplasms, brainstem lesions, or medical causes, such as in third nerve palsy.

An intracranial or intraorbital mass lesion should be considered in any patient with an isolated ocular motor palsy. In patients with isolated ocular motor nerve palsies presumed to be due to medical causes, brain MRI is generally only necessary if recovery has not begun within 3 months, although some authors suggest that it should be undertaken in all cases.

Ocular motor nerve palsies occurring in association with other neurologic signs may be due to lesions in the brainstem, cavernous sinus, or orbit. Lesions around the cavernous sinus involve the upper divisions of the trigeminal nerve, the ocular motor nerves, and occasionally the optic chiasm. Orbital apex lesions involve the optic nerve and the ocular motor nerves.

Myasthenia gravis and Graves ophthalmopathy (thyroid eye disease) should also be considered in the differential diagnosis of disordered extraocular movements.

▶ When to Refer

- Any patient with recent onset isolated third nerve palsy, particularly if there is pupillary involvement or pain, must be referred emergently for neurologic assessment and possibly CT, MRI, or catheter angiography for intracranial aneurysm.

- All patients with recent onset double vision should be referred urgently to an ophthalmologist or neurologist, particularly if there is multiple cranial nerve dysfunction or other neurologic abnormalities.

▶ When to Admit

Patients with double vision due to giant cell arteritis may require emergency admission for high-dose corticosteroid therapy and close monitoring to ensure that treatment is adequate. (See Central & Branch Retinal Artery Occlusions and Chapter 20.)

Kontzialis M et al. High resolution 3D magnetic resonance imaging of the sixth cranial nerve: anatomic and pathologic considerations by segment. J Neuroophthalmol. 2015 Dec; 35(4):412–25. [PMID: 26576019]
Kung NH et al. Isolated ocular motor nerve palsies. Semin Neurol. 2015 Oct;35(5):539–48. [PMID: 26444399]
Lemos J et al. Neuro-ophthalmological emergencies. Neurohospitalist. 2015 Oct;5(4):223–33. [PMID: 26425250]

THYROID EYE DISEASE (GRAVES OPHTHALMOPATHY)

Thyroid eye disease is a syndrome of clinical and orbital imaging abnormalities caused by deposition of mucopolysaccharides and infiltration with chronic inflammatory cells of the orbital tissues, particularly the extraocular muscles. It usually occurs in association with autoimmune hyperthyroidism. Clinical or laboratory evidence of thyroid dysfunction and thyroid antibodies may not be detectable at presentation or even on long-term follow-up, but their absence requires consideration of other disease entities. Radioiodine therapy, possibly indirectly due to induction of hypothyroidism, and cigarette smoking increase the severity of thyroid eye disease and ethanol injection of thyroid nodules has been reported to be followed by severe disease. Ocular myasthenia and thyroid eye disease are associated and may coexist, the presence of ptosis rather than eyelid retraction being a characteristic of the former.

▶ Clinical Findings

The primary clinical features are proptosis, lid retraction and lid lag, conjunctival chemosis and episcleral inflammation, and extraocular muscle dysfunction. Resulting symptoms are cosmetic abnormalities, surface irritation, which usually responds to artificial tears, and diplopia, which should be treated conservatively (eg, with prisms) in the active stages of the disease and only by surgery when the disease has been static for at least 6 months. The important complications are corneal exposure and optic nerve compression, both of which may lead to marked visual loss. The primary imaging features are enlargement of the extraocular muscles, usually affecting both orbits. The clinical and imaging abnormalities of thyroid eye disease may be mimicked by dural carotico-cavernous sinus fistula.

▶ Treatment

Treatment options for optic nerve compression or severe corneal exposure are intravenous pulse methylprednisolone therapy (eg, 1 g daily for 3 days, repeated weekly for 3 weeks), oral prednisolone 80–100 mg/day, radiotherapy, or surgery (usually consisting of extensive removal of bone from the medial, inferior, and lateral walls of the orbit), either singly or in combination. The role of systemic or orbital rituximab is uncertain.

The optimal management of moderately severe thyroid eye disease without visual loss is controversial. Systemic corticosteroids and radiotherapy may be beneficial. Peribulbar corticosteroid injections have been advocated. Surgical decompression may be justified in patients with marked proptosis. Lateral tarsorrhaphy may be used for moderately severe corneal exposure. Other procedures are particularly useful for correcting lid retraction but should not be undertaken until the orbital disease is quiescent and any orbital decompression and/or extraocular muscle surgery has been completed. Oral selenium seems to be beneficial in mild disease. Establishing and maintaining euthyroidism are important in all cases.

▶ When to Refer

All patients with thyroid eye disease should be referred to an ophthalmologist, urgently if there is reduced vision.

Hsu HJ et al. Thyroid eye disease. QJM. 2016 Jan;109(1):67–8. [PMID: 26450988]

Mitchell AL et al. Diagnosis of Graves' orbitopathy (DiaGO): results of a pilot study to assess the utility of an office tool for practicing endocrinologists. J Clin Endocrinol Metab. 2015 Mar;100(3):E458–62. [PMID: 25485725]

Perros P et al. Management of patients with Graves' orbitopathy: initial assessment, management outside specialised centres and referral pathways. Clin Med. 2015 Apr;15(2):173–8. [PMID: 25824071]

Phelps PO et al. Thyroid eye disease for the primary care physician. Dis Mon. 2014 Jun;60(6):292–8. [PMID: 24906675]

Pillar AJ et al. Treatment options for thyroid eye disease. Curr Treat Options Neurol. 2014 Aug;16(8):303. [PMID: 24928251]

Rao R et al. Current trends in the management of thyroid eye disease. Curr Opin Ophthalmol. 2015 Nov;26(6):484–90. [PMID: 26397888]

ORBITAL CELLULITIS

Orbital cellulitis is characterized by fever, proptosis, restriction of extraocular movements, and swelling with redness of the lids. Immediate treatment with intravenous antibiotics is necessary to prevent optic nerve damage and spread of infection to the cavernous sinuses, meninges, and brain. Infection of the paranasal sinuses is the usual underlying cause; examples of infecting organisms include *S pneumoniae*, the incidence of which has been reduced by the administration of pneumococcal vaccine, other streptococci, such as the anginosus group, *H influenzae* and, less commonly, *S aureus*. Penicillinase-resistant penicillin, such as nafcillin, is recommended, possibly together with metronidazole or clindamycin to treat anaerobic infections. If trauma is the underlying cause, a cephalosporin, such as cefazolin or ceftriaxone, should be added to ensure coverage for *S aureus* and group A beta-hemolytic streptococci. Vancomycin or clindamycin may be required if there is concern about MRSA, which is infrequently associated with paranasal sinus infection. MRSA may cause multiple orbital abscesses, and delay in the institution of vancomycin or clindamycin frequently necessitates surgery with a poor visual outcome. For patients with penicillin hypersensitivity, vancomycin, levofloxacin, and metronidazole are recommended. The response to antibiotics is usually excellent, but surgery may be required to drain the paranasal sinuses or orbital abscess. In immunocompromised patients, zygomycosis must be considered.

▶ When to Refer

All patients with suspected orbital cellulitis must be referred emergently to an ophthalmologist.

Atfeh MS et al. Orbital infections: five-year case series, literature review and guideline development. J Laryngol Otol. 2015 Jul; 129(7):670–6. [PMID: 26059425]

Carlisle RT et al. Differential diagnosis of the swollen red eyelid. Am Fam Physician. 2015 Jul 15;92(2):106–12. [PMID: 26176369]

Erickson BP et al. Orbital cellulitis and subperiosteal abscess: a 5-year outcomes analysis. Orbit. 2015 Jun;34(3):115–20. [PMID: 25867948]

Marchiano E et al. Characteristics of patients treated for orbital cellulitis: an analysis of inpatient data. Laryngoscope. 2016 Mar;126(3):554–9. [PMID: 26307941]

OCULAR TRAUMA

Ocular trauma, which occurs in many different circumstances and by a variety of mechanisms, is an important cause of severe visual impairment at all ages but particularly in young adult males and is the leading cause of monocular blindness in the United States. Thorough but safe clinical assessment, supplemented when necessary by imaging, is crucial to effective management. Ocular trauma and the possible need for early assessment by an ophthalmologist need to be borne in mind in the assessment of any patient with mid-facial injuries.

Cai M et al. Epidemiological characteristics of work-related ocular trauma in Southwest region of China. Int J Environ Res Public Health. 2015 Aug 19;12(8):9864–75. [PMID: 26295403]

Haring RS et al. Ocular injury in the United States: emergency department visits from 2006–2011. Injury. 2016 Jan;47(1):104–8. [PMID: 26275512]

Kong Y et al. Six-year clinical study of firework-related eye injuries in North China. Postgrad Med J. 2015 Jan;91(1071):26–9. [PMID: 25583736]

Lipke KJ et al. Emergency treatment of ocular trauma. Facial Plast Surg. 2015 Aug;31(4):345–50. [PMID: 26372708]

Welman T et al. Assessment of emergency department eye examinations in patients presenting with mid-face injury. J Emerg Med. 2016 Mar;15(3):422–6. [PMID: 26443644]

Zhou J et al. Ocular trauma in a rural population of North China: The Handan Eye Study. Biomed Environ Sci. 2015 Jul; 28(7):495–501. [PMID: 26248733]

1. Conjunctival & Corneal Foreign Bodies

If a patient complains of "something in my eye" and gives a consistent history, a foreign body is usually present on the cornea or under the upper lid even though it may not be visible. Visual acuity should be tested before treatment is instituted, to assess the severity of the injury and as a basis for comparison in the event of complications.

After a local anesthetic (eg, proparacaine, 0.5%) is instilled, the eye is examined with a slit-lamp or with a hand flashlight, using oblique illumination, and loupe. Corneal foreign bodies may be made more apparent by the instillation of sterile fluorescein. They are then removed with a sterile wet cotton-tipped applicator or hypodermic needle. Bacitracin-polymyxin ophthalmic ointment should be instilled. It is not necessary to patch the eye. All patients need to be advised to return promptly for reassessment if there is any increase in pain, redness, or impairment of vision.

Iron foreign bodies usually leave a diffuse rust ring (Figure 7–7). This requires excision of the affected tissue and is best done under local anesthesia using a slit lamp. **Caution:** Anesthetic drops should not be given to the patient for self-administration.

If there is no infection, a layer of corneal epithelial cells will line the crater within 24 hours. The intact corneal epithelium forms an effective barrier to infection, but once it is disturbed the cornea becomes extremely susceptible to infection. Early infection is manifested by a white necrotic area around the crater and a small amount of gray exudate.

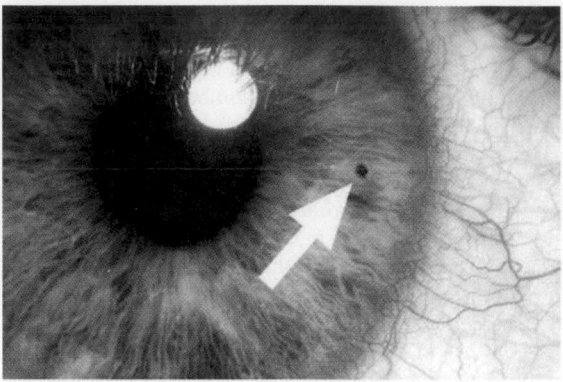

▲ **Figure 7–7.** Corneal rust stain from iron foreign body (arrow). (From James J Augsburger and Zélia M Corrêa. Reproduced, with permission, from Riordan-Eva P, Cunningham ET Jr. *Vaughan & Asbury's General Ophthalmology,* 18th ed. McGraw-Hill, 2011.)

In the case of a foreign body under the upper lid, a local anesthetic is instilled and the lid is everted by grasping the lashes gently and exerting pressure on the mid portion of the outer surface of the upper lid with an applicator. If a foreign body is present, it can easily be removed by passing a wet sterile cotton-tipped applicator across the conjunctival surface.

▶ When to Refer

Urgent referral to an ophthalmologist should be arranged if a corneal foreign body cannot be removed or if there is suspicion of corneal infection.

Ahmed F et al. Corneal abrasions and corneal foreign bodies. Prim Care. 2015 Sep;42(3):363–75. [PMID: 26319343]

Brissette A et al. Evaluating the need for close follow-up after removal of a noncomplicated corneal foreign body. Cornea. 2014 Nov;33(11):1193–6. [PMID: 25090166]

2. Intraocular Foreign Body

Intraocular foreign body requires emergency treatment by an ophthalmologist. Patients giving a history of "something hitting the eye"—particularly while hammering on metal or using grinding equipment—must be assessed for this possibility, especially when no corneal foreign body is seen, a corneal or scleral wound is apparent, or there is marked visual loss or media opacity. Such patients must be treated as for corneal laceration and referred without delay. Intraocular foreign bodies significantly increase the risk of intraocular infection.

▶ When to Refer

Patients with suspected intraocular foreign body must be referred emergently to an ophthalmologist.

Lin TC et al. Management and clinical outcomes of intraocular foreign bodies with the aid of orbital computed tomography. J Chin Med Assoc. 2014 Aug;77(8):433–6. [PMID: 25028294]

3. Corneal Abrasions

A patient with a corneal abrasion complains of severe pain and photophobia. There is often a history of trauma to the eye, commonly involving a fingernail, piece of paper, or contact lens. Visual acuity is recorded, and the cornea and conjunctiva are examined with a light and loupe to rule out a foreign body. If an abrasion is suspected but cannot be seen, sterile fluorescein is instilled into the conjunctival sac: the area of corneal abrasion will stain a deeper green than the surrounding cornea.

Treatment includes bacitracin-polymyxin ophthalmic ointment, mydriatic (cyclopentolate 1%), and analgesics either topical or oral nonsteroidal anti-inflammatory agents. Padding the eye is probably not helpful for small abrasions. Corneal abrasions heal more slowly in persons who smoke cigarettes. Recurrent corneal erosion may follow corneal abrasions.

Although topical tetracaine for 24 hours in the treatment of corneal abrasion has been reported to be safe and effective, there is a risk of severe corneal disease from misuse of topical anesthetics.

Ahmed F et al. Corneal abrasions and corneal foreign bodies. Prim Care. 2015 Sep;42(3):363–75. [PMID: 26319343]
Saccomano SJ et al. Managing corneal abrasions in primary care. Nurse Pract. 2014 Sep 18;39(9):1–6. [PMID: 25140844]
Tok OY et al. Toxic keratopathy associated with abuse of topical anesthetics and amniotic membrane transplantation for treatment. Int J Ophthalmol. 2015 Oct 18;8(5):938–44. [PMID: 26558205]

4. Contusions

Contusion injuries of the eye (closed globe injuries) and surrounding structures may cause ecchymosis ("black eye"), subconjunctival hemorrhage, edema or rupture of the cornea, hemorrhage into the anterior chamber (hyphema), rupture of the root of the iris (iridodialysis), paralysis of the pupillary sphincter, paralysis of the muscles of accommodation, cataract, dislocation of the lens, vitreous hemorrhage, retinal hemorrhage and edema (most common in the macular area), detachment of the retina, rupture of the choroid, fracture of the orbital floor ("blowout fracture"), or optic nerve injury. Many of these injuries are immediately obvious; others may not become apparent for days or weeks. The possibility of globe injury must always be considered in patients with facial injury, particularly if there is an orbital fracture. Patients with moderate to severe contusions should be seen by an ophthalmologist.

Any injury causing hyphema involves the danger of secondary hemorrhage, which may cause intractable glaucoma with permanent visual loss. The patient should be advised to rest until complete resolution has occurred. Frequent ophthalmologic assessment is essential. Aspirin and any drugs inhibiting coagulation increase the risk of secondary hemorrhage and are to be avoided. Sickle cell anemia or trait adversely affects outcome.

▶ When to Refer

Patients with moderate or severe ocular contusion should be referred to an ophthalmologist, emergently if there is hyphema.

Alhamdani F et al. Diplopia and ocular motility in orbital blow-out fractures: 10-year retrospective study. J Craniomaxillofac Surg. 2015 Sep;43(7):1010–6. [PMID: 26133790]
Boyette JR et al. Management of orbital fractures: challenges and solutions. Clin Ophthalmol. 2015 Nov 17;9:2127–37. [PMID: 26604678]
Cockerham GC et al. Closed-globe injuries of the ocular surface associated with combat blast exposure. Ophthalmology. 2014 Nov;121(11):2165–72. [PMID: 25124272]

5. Lacerations

A. Lids

If the lid margin is lacerated, the patient should be referred for specialized care, since permanent notching may result. Lacerations of the lower eyelid near the inner canthus often sever the lower canaliculus, for which canalicular intubation is likely to be required. Lid lacerations not involving the margin may be sutured like any skin laceration.

Örge FH et al. Canalicular laceration repair using a viscoelastic injection to locate and dilate the proximal torn edge. J AAPOS. 2015 Jun;19(3):217–9. [PMID: 26059664]

B. Conjunctiva

In lacerations of the conjunctiva, sutures are not necessary. To prevent infection, topical sulfonamide or antibiotic is used until the laceration is healed.

C. Cornea or Sclera

Patients with suspected corneal or scleral lacerations (open globe injuries) must be seen promptly by an ophthalmologist (Figure 7–8). Manipulation is kept to a minimum, since pressure may result in extrusion of the intraocular contents. The eye is bandaged lightly and covered with a shield that rests on the orbital bones above and below. The patient should be instructed not to squeeze the eye shut

▲ **Figure 7–8.** Corneoscleral laceration inferonasally with pupil displaced toward the laceration and iris incarcerated in wound. (From James J Augsburger and Zélia M Corrêa. Reproduced, with permission, from Riordan-Eva P, Cunningham ET Jr. *Vaughan & Asbury's General Ophthalmology*, 18th ed. McGraw-Hill, 2011.)

and to remain still. The eye is routinely imaged by radiography, and CT scanning if necessary, to identify and localize any metallic intraocular foreign body. MRI is contraindicated because of the risk of movement of the foreign body in the magnetic field. Endophthalmitis occurs in over 5% of open globe injuries.

▶ When to Refer

Patients with suspected globe laceration must be referred emergently to an ophthalmologist.

Agrawal R et al. Prognostic factors for open globe injuries and correlation of ocular trauma score at a tertiary referral eye care centre in Singapore. Indian J Ophthalmol. 2013 Sep; 61(9):502–6. [PMID: 24104709]

Nicoară SD et al. Intraocular foreign bodies extracted by pars plana vitrectomy: clinical characteristics, management, outcomes and prognostic factors. BMC Ophthalmol. 2015 Nov 2; 15(1):151. [PMID: 26526732]

ULTRAVIOLET KERATITIS (ACTINIC KERATITIS)

Ultraviolet burns of the cornea are usually caused by use of a sunlamp without eye protection, exposure to a welding arc, or exposure to the sun when skiing ("snow blindness"). There are no immediate symptoms, but about 6–12 hours later the patient complains of agonizing pain and severe photophobia. Slit-lamp examination after instillation of sterile fluorescein shows diffuse punctate staining of both corneas.

Treatment consists of binocular patching and instillation of 1–2 drops of 1% cyclopentolate (to relieve the discomfort of ciliary spasm). All patients recover within 24–48 hours without complications. Local anesthetics should not be prescribed because they delay corneal epithelial healing.

CHEMICAL CONJUNCTIVITIS & KERATITIS

Chemical burns are treated by copious irrigation of the eyes with tap water, saline solution, or buffering solution if available as soon as possible after exposure. Neutralization of an acid with an alkali or vice versa generates heat and may cause further damage. Alkali injuries are more serious and require prolonged irrigation, since alkalies are not precipitated by the proteins of the eye as are acids. It is important to remove any retained particulate matter, such as is typically present in injuries involving cement and building plaster. This may require double eversion of the upper lid. The pupil should be dilated with 1% cyclopentolate, 1 drop twice a day, to relieve discomfort, and prophylactic topical antibiotics should be started. In moderate to severe injuries, intensive topical corticosteroids and topical and systemic vitamin C are also necessary. Complications include mucus deficiency, scarring of the cornea and conjunctiva, symblepharon (adhesions between the tarsal and bulbar conjunctiva), tear duct obstruction, and secondary infection. It can be difficult to assess severity of chemical burns without slit-lamp examination.

Cabalag MS et al. Early and late complications of ocular burn injuries. J Plast Reconstr Aesthet Surg. 2015 Mar;68(3):356–61. [PMID: 25465150]

Movahedan A et al. Long-term management of severe ocular surface injury due to methamphetamine production accidents. Cornea. 2015 Apr;34(4):433–7. [PMID: 25642642]

Scott WJ et al. Emergency eye rinse for chemical injuries: new considerations. JAMA Ophthalmol. 2015 Mar;133(3):245. [PMID: 25474079]

Tschopp M et al. Incidence and causative agents of chemical eye injuries in Switzerland. Clin Toxicol (Phila). 2015 Dec;53(10):957–61. [PMID: 26479216]

Wang BZ et al. Characteristics, management and outcomes of chemical eye injuries in Victoria. Med J Aust. 2015 Feb 2; 202(2):79–80. [PMID: 25627737]

TREATMENT OF OCULAR DISORDERS

Table 7–2 lists commonly used ophthalmic drugs and their indications and costs.

PRECAUTIONS IN MANAGEMENT OF OCULAR DISORDERS

1. Use of Local Anesthetics

Unsupervised self-administration of local anesthetics is dangerous because they are toxic to the corneal epithelium and the patient may further injure an anesthetized eye without knowing it.

Erdem E et al. Topical anesthetic eye drops abuse: are we aware of the danger? Cutan Ocul Toxicol. 2013 Sep;32(3):189–93. [PMID: 23410261]

Patel M et al. Toxicity of topical ophthalmic anesthetics. Expert Opin Drug Metab Toxicol. 2013 Aug;9(8):983–8. [PMID: 23617273]

Tok OY et al. Toxic keratopathy associated with abuse of topical anesthetics and amniotic membrane transplantation for treatment. Int J Ophthalmol. 2015 Oct 18;8(5):938–44. [PMID: 26558205]

2. Pupillary Dilation

Dilating the pupil can very occasionally precipitate acute glaucoma if the patient has a narrow anterior chamber angle and should be undertaken with caution if the anterior chamber is obviously shallow (readily determined by oblique illumination of the anterior segment of the eye). A short-acting mydriatic, such as tropicamide, should be used and the patient warned to report immediately if ocular discomfort or redness develops. Angle closure is more likely to occur if pilocarpine is used to overcome pupillary dilation than if the pupil is allowed to constrict naturally.

Ah-Kee EY et al. A review of drug-induced acute angle closure glaucoma for non-ophthalmologists. Qatar Med J. 2015 May 10;2015(1):6. [PMID: 26535174]

3. Corticosteroid Therapy

Repeated use of local corticosteroids presents several hazards: herpes simplex (dendritic) and fungal keratitis, open-angle glaucoma, and cataract formation. Furthermore, perforation of the cornea may occur when corticosteroids are used for herpes simplex keratitis. Topical nonsteroidal anti-inflammatory agents are being used increasingly. The potential for causing or exacerbating systemic hypertension, diabetes mellitus, gastritis, osteoporosis, or glaucoma must always be borne in mind when systemic corticosteroids are prescribed, such as for uveitis or giant cell arteritis.

4. Contaminated Eye Medications

Ophthalmic solutions are prepared with the same degree of care as fluids intended for intravenous administration, but once bottles are opened there is always a risk of contamination, particularly with solutions of tetracaine, proparacaine, fluorescein, and any preservative-free preparations. The most dangerous is fluorescein, as this solution is frequently contaminated with *P aeruginosa*, which can rapidly destroy the eye. Single-use fluorescein eye drops or sterile fluorescein filter paper strips are recommended for use in place of multiple-use fluorescein solutions.

Whether in plastic or glass containers, eye solutions should not remain in use for long periods after the bottle is opened. Four weeks after opening is an absolute maximal time to use a solution containing preservatives before discarding. Preservative-free preparations should be kept refrigerated and discarded within 1 week after opening. Single-use products should not be reused.

If the eye has been injured accidentally or by surgical trauma, it is of the greatest importance to use freshly opened bottles of sterile medications or single-use products.

5. Toxic & Hypersensitivity Reactions to Topical Therapy

In patients receiving long-term topical therapy, local toxic or hypersensitivity reactions to the active agent or preservatives may develop, especially if there is inadequate tear secretion. Preservatives in contact lens cleaning solutions may produce similar problems. Burning and soreness are exacerbated by drop instillation or contact lens insertion; occasionally, fibrosis and scarring of the conjunctiva and cornea may occur. Preservative-free topical medication, increasingly used in the treatment of glaucoma, and contact lens solutions are available.

An antibiotic instilled into the eye can sensitize the patient to that drug and cause an allergic reaction upon subsequent systemic administration. Potentially fatal anaphylaxis is known to occur in up to 0.3% of patients after intravenous fluorescein for fluorescein angiography. Anaphylaxis also has been reported after topical fluorescein.

6. Systemic Effects of Ocular Drugs

The systemic absorption of certain topical drugs (through the conjunctival vessels and lacrimal drainage system) must be considered when there is a systemic medical contraindication to the use of the drug. Ophthalmic solutions of the nonselective beta-blockers, eg, timolol, may worsen bradycardia, heart failure, or asthma. Phenylephrine eye drops may precipitate hypertensive crises and angina. Also to be considered are adverse interactions between systemically administered and ocular drugs. Using only 1 or 2 drops at a time and a few minutes of nasolacrimal occlusion or eyelid closure ensure maximum efficacy and decrease systemic side effects of topical agents.

ADVERSE OCULAR EFFECTS OF SYSTEMIC DRUGS

Systemically administered drugs produce a wide variety of adverse effects on the visual system. Table 7–3 lists the major examples. Repeated screening for toxic retinopathy is recommended in patients receiving long-term chloroquine or hydroxychloroquine therapy.

Fraunfelder FW. Ocular & systemic side effects of drugs. In: *Vaughan & Asbury's General Ophthalmology*, 18th ed. Riordan-Eva P et al (editors). McGraw-Hill, 2011.

Melles RB et al. The risk of toxic retinopathy in patients on long-term hydroxychloroquine therapy. JAMA Ophthalmol. 2014 Dec 1;132(12):1453–60. [PMID: 25275721]

8

Ear, Nose, & Throat Disorders

Lawrence R. Lustig, MD
Joshua S. Schindler, MD

DISEASES OF THE EAR

HEARING LOSS

ESSENTIALS OF DIAGNOSIS

► Three main types of hearing loss: conductive, sensory, and neural.

► Most commonly due to cerumen impaction, transient eustachian tube dysfunction associated with upper respiratory tract infection, or age-related hearing loss.

► Classification & Epidemiology

Table 8–1 categorizes hearing loss as normal, mild, moderate, severe, and profound and outlines the vocal equivalent as well as the decibel range.

A. Conductive Hearing Loss

Conductive hearing loss results from dysfunction of the external or middle ear. There are four mechanisms, each resulting in impairment of the passage of sound vibrations to the inner ear: (1) obstruction (eg, cerumen impaction), (2) mass loading (eg, middle ear effusion), (3) stiffness effect (eg, otosclerosis), and (4) discontinuity (eg, ossicular disruption). Conductive losses in adults are most commonly due to cerumen impaction or transient eustachian tube dysfunction associated with upper respiratory tract infection. Persistent conductive losses usually result from chronic ear infection, trauma, or otosclerosis. Conductive hearing loss is often correctable with medical or surgical therapy—or in some cases both.

B. Sensory Hearing Loss

Sensory and neural causes of hearing loss are difficult to differentiate due to testing methodology, thus often referred to as "sensorineural." Sensory hearing loss results from deterioration of the cochlea, usually due to loss of hair cells from the organ of Corti. Sensorineural losses in adults are common. The most common form is a gradually progressive, predominantly high-frequency loss with advancing age (presbyacusis). Additional common causes include excessive noise exposure, head trauma, and systemic diseases. An individual's genetic make-up influences all of these causes of hearing loss. Sensory hearing loss is usually not correctable with medical or surgical therapy but often may be prevented or stabilized. An exception is a sudden sensory hearing loss, which may respond to corticosteroids if delivered within several weeks of onset.

Yamasoba T et al. Current concepts in age-related hearing loss: epidemiology and mechanistic pathways. Hear Res. 2013 Sep;303:30–8. [PMID: 23422312]

C. Neural Hearing Loss

Neural hearing loss occurs with lesions involving the eighth nerve, auditory nuclei, ascending tracts, or auditory cortex. It is the least common clinically recognized cause of hearing loss. Causes include acoustic neuroma, multiple sclerosis, and auditory neuropathy.

Ouda L et al. Age-related changes in the central auditory system. Cell Tissue Res. 2015 Jul;361(1):337–58. [PMID: 25630878]

► Evaluation of Hearing (Audiology)

In a quiet room, the hearing level may be estimated by having the patient repeat aloud words presented in a soft whisper, a normal spoken voice, or a shout. A 512-Hz tuning fork is useful in differentiating conductive from sensorineural losses. In the **Weber test,** the tuning fork is placed on the forehead or front teeth. In conductive losses, the sound appears louder in the poorer-hearing ear, whereas in sensorineural losses it radiates to the better side. In the **Rinne test,** the tuning fork is placed alternately on the mastoid bone and in front of the ear canal. In conductive losses greater than 25 dB, bone conduction exceeds air conduction; in sensorineural losses, the opposite is true.

Formal audiometric studies are performed in a sound-proofed room. Pure-tone thresholds in decibels (dB) are obtained over the range of 250–8000 Hz for both air and

Table 8–1. Hearing loss classification.

Classification	Vocal Equivalent	Decibel (dB) Range
Normal	Soft whisper	0–20 dB
Mild	Soft spoken voice	20–40 dB
Moderate	Normal spoken voice	40–60 dB
Severe	Loud spoken voice	60–80 dB
Profound	Shout	> 80 dB

bone conduction. Conductive losses create a gap between the air and bone thresholds, whereas in sensorineural losses, both air and bone thresholds are equally diminished. Speech discrimination measures the clarity of hearing, reported as percentage correct (90–100% is normal). The site of the lesion responsible for sensorineural loss (cochlea versus central auditory system) may be determined with auditory brainstem-evoked responses; however, an MRI scan is preferred for its better sensitivity and specificity in the evaluation of central lesions.

Every patient who complains of a hearing loss should be referred for audiologic evaluation unless the cause is easily remediable (eg, cerumen impaction, otitis media). Because idiopathic sudden sensorineural hearing loss requires treatment (corticosteroids) within a limited several-week time period, any new-onset hearing loss without obvious ear pathology needs an immediate audiometric referral. Routine audiologic screening is recommended for adults who have been exposed to potentially injurious levels of noise or in those who have reached the age of 65, after which screening evaluations may be done every few years.

Lasak JM et al. Hearing loss: diagnosis and management. Prim Care. 2014 Mar;41(1):19–31. [PMID: 24439878]

▶ **Hearing Amplification**

Patients with hearing loss not correctable by medical therapy may benefit from hearing amplification. Contemporary hearing aids are comparatively free of distortion and have been miniaturized to the point where they often may be contained entirely within the ear canal or lie inconspicuously behind the ear.

For patients with conductive loss or unilateral profound sensorineural loss, bone-conducting hearing aids directly stimulate the ipsilateral cochlea (for conductive losses) or contralateral ear (profound unilateral sensorineural loss).

For patients with severe to profound sensory hearing loss, the cochlear implant—an electronic device that is surgically implanted into the cochlea to stimulate the auditory nerve—offers socially beneficial auditory rehabilitation to most adults with acquired deafness and children with congenital or genetic deafness. New trends in cochlear implantation include its use for patients with only partial deafness, preserving residual hearing and allowing both acoustic and electrical hearing in the same ear.

Gaylor JM et al. Cochlear implantation in adults: a systematic review and meta-analysis. JAMA Otolaryngol Head Neck Surg. 2013 Mar;139(3):265–72. [PMID: 23429927]

DISEASES OF THE AURICLE

Disorders of the auricle are for the most part dermatologic. Skin cancers due to sun exposure are common and may be treated with standard techniques. Traumatic auricular hematoma must be recognized and drained to prevent significant cosmetic deformity (cauliflower ear) or canal blockage resulting from dissolution of supporting cartilage. Similarly, cellulitis of the auricle must be treated promptly to prevent development of perichondritis and its resultant deformity. Relapsing polychondritis is a rheumatologic disorder often associated with recurrent, frequently bilateral, painful episodes of auricular erythema and edema. Treatment with corticosteroids may help forestall cartilage dissolution. Respiratory compromise may occur as a result of progressive involvement of the cartilaginous tracheobronchial tree. Chondritis and perichondritis may be differentiated from auricular cellulitis by sparing of involvement of the lobule, which does not contain cartilage.

Moitri MO et al. Red ear syndrome: literature review and a pediatric case report. Int J Pediatr Otorhinolaryngol. 2015 Mar;79(3):281–5. [PMID: 25583087]
Shakeel M et al. Open surgical management of auricular haematoma: incision, evacuation and mattress sutures. J Laryngol Otol. 2015 May;129(5):496–501. [PMID: 25994384]

DISEASES OF THE EAR CANAL

1. Cerumen Impaction

Cerumen is a protective secretion produced by the outer portion of the ear canal. In most persons, the ear canal is self-cleansing. Recommended hygiene consists of cleaning the external opening with a washcloth over the index finger without entering the canal itself. In most cases, cerumen impaction is self-induced through ill-advised attempts at cleaning the ear. It may be relieved with detergent ear drops (eg, 3% hydrogen peroxide; 6.5% carbamide peroxide), mechanical removal, suction, or irrigation. Irrigation is performed with water at body temperature to avoid a vestibular caloric response. The stream should be directed at the posterior ear canal wall adjacent to the cerumen plug. Irrigation should be performed only when the tympanic membrane is known to be intact.

Use of jet irrigators designed for cleaning teeth (eg, WaterPik) for wax removal should be avoided since they may result in tympanic membrane perforations. Following professional irrigation, the ear canal should be thoroughly dried (eg, by instilling isopropyl alcohol or using a hair blow-dryer on low-power setting) to reduce the likelihood of inducing external otitis. Specialty referral for cleaning under microscopic guidance is indicated when the impaction is frequently recurrent, has not responded to routine measures, or if the patient has a history of chronic otitis media or tympanic membrane perforation.

2. Foreign Bodies

Foreign bodies in the ear canal are more frequent in children than in adults. Firm materials may be removed with a loop or a hook, taking care not to displace the object medially toward the tympanic membrane; microscopic guidance is helpful. Aqueous irrigation should not be performed for organic foreign bodies (eg, beans, insects), because water may cause them to swell. Living insects are best immobilized before removal by filling the ear canal with lidocaine.

3. External Otitis

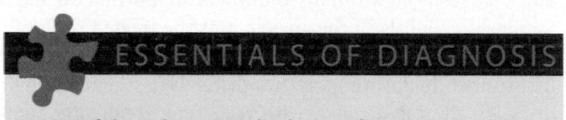

ESSENTIALS OF DIAGNOSIS

▶ Painful erythema and edema of the ear canal skin.

▶ Often with purulent exudate.

▶ May evolve into osteomyelitis of the skull base, often called malignant external otitis, particularly in the diabetic or immunocompromised patient.

▶ General Considerations

External otitis presents with otalgia, frequently accompanied by pruritus and purulent discharge. There is often a history of recent water exposure (ie, swimmer's ear) or mechanical trauma (eg, scratching, cotton applicators). External otitis is usually caused by gram-negative rods (eg, *Pseudomonas, Proteus*) or fungi (eg, *Aspergillus*), which grow in the presence of excessive moisture. Persistent external otitis in the diabetic or immunocompromised patient may evolve into osteomyelitis of the skull base, often called **malignant external otitis.** Usually caused by *Pseudomonas aeruginosa*, osteomyelitis begins in the floor of the ear canal and may extend into the middle fossa floor, the clivus, and even the contralateral skull base.

▶ Clinical Findings

Examination reveals erythema and edema of the ear canal skin, often with a purulent exudate. Manipulation of the auricle often elicits pain. Because the lateral surface of the tympanic membrane is ear canal skin, it is often erythematous. However, in contrast to acute otitis media, it moves normally with pneumatic otoscopy. When the canal skin is very edematous, it may be impossible to visualize the tympanic membrane. **Malignant external otitis,** which usually occurs in patients with immune compromise or diabetes mellitus, typically presents with persistent foul aural discharge, granulations in the ear canal, deep otalgia, and in advanced cases, progressive cranial nerve palsies involving nerves VI, VII, IX, X, XI, or XII. Diagnosis is confirmed by the demonstration of osseous erosion on CT and radionuclide scanning.

▶ Treatment

Fundamental to the treatment of external otitis is protection of the ear from additional moisture and avoidance of

further mechanical injury by scratching. In cases of swimmer's ear, acidification with a drying agent (ie, a 50/50 mixture of isopropyl alcohol/white vinegar) after getting moisture into the ear is often helpful. When infected, acidic otic antibiotic drops that contain either an aminoglycoside or fluoroquinolone antibiotic, with or without corticosteroids, are usually effective (eg, neomycin sulfate, polymyxin B sulfate, and hydrocortisone). Purulent debris filling the ear canal should be gently removed to permit entry of the topical medication. Drops should be used abundantly (five or more drops three or four times a day) to penetrate the depths of the canal. When substantial edema of the canal wall prevents entry of drops into the ear canal, a wick is placed to facilitate entry of the medication. In recalcitrant cases—particularly when cellulitis of the periauricular tissue has developed—oral fluoroquinolones (eg, ciprofloxacin, 500 mg twice daily for 1 week) are the drugs of choice because of their effectiveness against *Pseudomonas* species. Any case of persistent otitis externa in an immunocompromised or diabetic individual must be referred for specialty evaluation.

Treatment of **malignant external otitis** is medical, requiring prolonged antipseudomonal antibiotic administration, often for several months. Although intravenous therapy is often required (eg, ciprofloxacin 200–400 mg every 12 hours), selected patients may be treated with oral ciprofloxacin (500–1000 mg twice daily), which has proved effective against many of the causative *Pseudomonas* strains. To avoid relapse, antibiotic therapy should be continued, even in the asymptomatic patient, until gallium scanning indicates a marked reduction in the inflammatory process. Surgical debridement of infected bone is reserved for cases of deterioration despite medical therapy.

Hobson CE et al. Malignant otitis externa: evolving pathogens and implications for diagnosis and treatment. Otolaryngol Head Neck Surg. 2014 Mar 26;151(1):112–6. [PMID: 24675790]

Rosenfeld RM et al; American Academy of Otolaryngology—Head and Neck Surgery Foundation. Clinical practice guideline: acute otitis externa executive summary. Otolaryngol Head Neck Surg. 2014 Feb;150(2):161–8. [PMID: 24492208]

4. Pruritus

Pruritus of the external auditory canal, particularly at the meatus, is a common problem. While it may be associated with external otitis or with dermatologic conditions, such as seborrheic dermatitis and psoriasis, most cases are self-induced, either from excoriation or by overly zealous ear cleaning. To permit regeneration of the protective cerumen blanket, patients should be instructed to avoid use of soap and water or cotton swabs in the ear canal and avoid any scratching. Patients with excessively dry canal skin may benefit from application of mineral oil, which helps counteract dryness and repel moisture. When an inflammatory component is present, topical application of a corticosteroid (eg, 0.1% triamcinolone) may be beneficial.

5. Exostoses & Osteomas

Bony overgrowths of the ear canal are a frequent incidental finding and occasionally have clinical significance.

Clinically, they present as skin-covered bony mounds in the medial ear canal obscuring the tympanic membrane to a variable degree. Solitary osteomas are of no significance as long as they do not cause obstruction or infection. Multiple exostoses, which are generally acquired from repeated exposure to cold water (eg, "surfer's ear") may progress and require surgical removal.

Mudry A et al. Birth and evolution of chiselling and drilling techniques for removing ear canal exostoses. Otol Neurotol. 2016 Jan;37(1):109–114. [PMID: 26649611]

6. Neoplasia

The most common neoplasm of the ear canal is squamous cell carcinoma. When an apparent otitis externa does not resolve on therapy, a malignancy should be suspected and biopsy performed. This disease carries a very high 5-year mortality rate because the tumor tends to invade the lymphatics of the cranial base and must be treated with wide surgical resection and radiation therapy. Adenomatous tumors, originating from the ceruminous glands, generally follow a more indolent course.

Lionello M et al. Temporal bone carcinoma. Current diagnostic, therapeutic, and prognostic concepts. J Surg Oncol. 2014 Sep; 110(4):383–92. [PMID: 24962035]
Zanoletti E et al. A critical look at persistent problems in the diagnosis, staging and treatment of temporal bone carcinoma. Cancer Treat Rev. 2015 Dec;41(10):821–6. [PMID: 26549119]

DISEASES OF THE EUSTACHIAN TUBE

1. Eustachian Tube Dysfunction

ESSENTIALS OF DIAGNOSIS

▶ Aural fullness.

▶ Fluctuating hearing.

▶ Discomfort with barometric pressure change.

▶ At risk for serous otitis media.

The tube that connects the middle ear to the nasopharynx—the eustachian tube—provides ventilation and drainage for the middle ear cleft. It is normally closed, opening only during swallowing or yawning. When eustachian tube function is compromised, air trapped within the middle ear becomes absorbed and negative pressure results. The most common causes of eustachian tube dysfunction are diseases associated with edema of the tubal lining, such as viral upper respiratory tract infections and allergy. The patient usually reports a sense of fullness in the ear and mild to moderate impairment of hearing. When the tube is only partially blocked, swallowing or yawning may elicit a popping or crackling sound. Examination may reveal retraction of the tympanic membrane and decreased mobility on pneumatic otoscopy. Following a viral illness,

this disorder is usually transient, lasting days to weeks. Treatment with systemic and intranasal decongestants (eg, pseudoephedrine, 60 mg orally every 4 hours; oxymetazoline, 0.05% spray every 8–12 hours) combined with autoinflation by forced exhalation against closed nostrils may hasten relief. Autoinflation should not be recommended to patients with active intranasal infection, since this maneuver may precipitate middle ear infection. Allergic patients may also benefit from desensitization or intranasal corticosteroids (eg, beclomethasone dipropionate, two sprays in each nostril twice daily for 2–6 weeks). Air travel, rapid altitudinal change, and underwater diving should be avoided during an active phase of the disease.

Conversely, an overly patent eustachian tube, termed "patulous eustachian tube," is a relatively uncommon problem though may be quite distressing. Typical complaints include fullness in the ear and autophony, an exaggerated ability to hear oneself breathe and speak. A patulous eustachian tube may develop during rapid weight loss, or it may be idiopathic. In contrast to a hypofunctioning eustachian tube, the aural pressure is often made worse by exertion and may diminish during an upper respiratory tract infection. Although physical examination is usually normal, respiratory excursions of the tympanic membrane may occasionally be detected during vigorous breathing. Treatment includes avoidance of decongestant products, insertion of a ventilating tube to reduce the outward stretch of the eardrum during phonation and, rarely, surgical procedure in the eustachian tube.

Norman G et al. Systematic review of the limited evidence base for treatments of Eustachian tube dysfunction: a health technology assessment. Clin Otolaryngol. 2014 Feb;39(1):6–21. [PMID: 24438176]
Randrup TS et al. Balloon eustachian tuboplasty: a systematic review. Otolaryngol Head Neck Surg. 2015 Mar;152(3):383–92. [PMID: 25605694]

2. Serous Otitis Media

ESSENTIALS OF DIAGNOSIS

▶ Blocked eustachian tube remains for a prolonged period.

▶ Resultant negative pressure will result in transudation of fluid.

Prolonged eustachian tube dysfunction with resultant negative middle ear pressure may cause a transudation of fluid. This condition, known as serous otitis media, is especially common in children because their eustachian tubes are narrower and more horizontal in orientation than those in adults. Serous otitis media is less common in adults, in whom it usually occurs after an upper respiratory tract infection, with barotrauma, or with chronic allergic rhinitis. In any adult with persistent unilateral serous otitis media, nasopharyngeal carcinoma must be excluded. The tympanic membrane in serous otitis media is dull and hypomobile, occasionally accompanied by air bubbles in the middle ear and conductive hearing loss. The treatment of serous otitis media is similar to that for eustachian tube dysfunction. A short course of oral corticosteroids (eg, prednisone, 40 mg/day for 7 days) has been advocated by some clinicians, as have oral antibiotics (eg, amoxicillin, 250 mg three times daily for 7 days)—or even a combination of the two. The role of these regimens remains controversial, but they are probably of little lasting benefit. When medication fails to bring relief after several months, a ventilating tube placed through the tympanic membrane may restore hearing and alleviate the sense of aural fullness. Endoscopically guided laser expansion of the nasopharyngeal orifice of the eustachian tube may improve function in recalcitrant cases.

Bhutta MF. Epidemiology and pathogenesis of otitis media: construction of a phenotype landscape. Audiol Neurootol. 2014;19(3):210–23. [PMID: 24819621]
Wallace IF et al. Surgical treatments for otitis media with effusion: a systematic review. Pediatrics. 2014 Feb;133(2):296–311. [PMID: 24394689]

3. Barotrauma

Persons with poor eustachian tube function (eg, congenital narrowness or acquired mucosal edema) may be unable to equalize the barometric stress exerted on the middle ear by air travel, rapid altitudinal change, or underwater diving. The problem is generally most acute during airplane descent, since the negative middle ear pressure tends to collapse and block the eustachian tube. Several measures are useful to enhance eustachian tube function and avoid otic barotrauma. The patient should be advised to swallow, yawn, and autoinflate frequently during descent, which may be painful if the eustachian tube collapses. Oral decongestants (eg, pseudoephedrine, 60–120 mg) should be taken several hours before anticipated arrival time so that they will be maximally effective during descent. Topical decongestants such as 1% phenylephrine nasal spray should be administered 1 hour before arrival.

For acute negative middle ear pressure that persists on the ground, treatment includes decongestants and attempts at autoinflation. Myringotomy (creation of a small eardrum perforation) provides immediate relief and is appropriate in the setting of severe otalgia and hearing loss. Repeated episodes of barotrauma in persons who must fly frequently may be alleviated by insertion of ventilating tubes.

Underwater diving may represent an even greater barometric stress to the ear than flying. The problem occurs most commonly during the descent phase, when pain develops within the first 15 feet if inflation of the middle ear via the eustachian tube has not occurred. Divers must descend slowly and equilibrate in stages to avoid the development of severely negative pressures in the tympanum that may result in hemorrhage (hemotympanum) or perilymphatic fistula. In the latter, the oval or round window ruptures, resulting in sensory hearing loss and acute vertigo. Sensory hearing loss or vertigo, which develops during the ascent phase of a saturation dive, may be the first (or only) symptom of decompression sickness. Immediate

recompression will return intravascular gas bubbles to solution and restore the inner ear microcirculation. Patients should be warned to avoid diving when they have upper respiratory infections or episodes of nasal allergy. Tympanic membrane perforation is an absolute contraindication to diving, as the patient will experience an unbalanced thermal stimulus to the semicircular canals and may experience vertigo, disorientation, and even emesis.

Lynch JH et al. Barotrauma with extreme pressures in sport: from scuba to skydiving. Curr Sports Med Rep. 2014 Mar–Apr;13(2):107–12. [PMID: 24614424]

DISEASES OF THE MIDDLE EAR

1. Acute Otitis Media

ESSENTIALS OF DIAGNOSIS

▶ Otalgia, often with an upper respiratory tract infection.
▶ Erythema and hypomobility of tympanic membrane.

▶ General Considerations

Acute otitis media is a bacterial infection of the mucosally lined air-containing spaces of the temporal bone. Purulent material forms not only within the middle ear cleft but also within the pneumatized mastoid air cells and petrous apex. Acute otitis media is usually precipitated by a viral upper respiratory tract infection that causes eustachian tube obstruction. This results in accumulation of fluid and mucus, which becomes secondarily infected by bacteria. The most common pathogens are *Streptococcus pneumoniae,* *Haemophilus influenzae,* and *Streptococcus pyogenes.*

▶ Clinical Findings

Acute otitis media is most common in infants and children, although it may occur at any age. Presenting symptoms and signs include otalgia, aural pressure, decreased hearing, and often fever. The typical physical findings are erythema and decreased mobility of the tympanic membrane. Occasionally, bullae will be seen on the tympanic membrane.

Rarely, when middle ear empyema is severe, the tympanic membrane can bulge outward. In such cases, tympanic membrane rupture is imminent. Rupture is accompanied by a sudden decrease in pain, followed by the onset of otorrhea. With appropriate therapy, spontaneous healing of the tympanic membrane occurs in most cases. When perforation persists, chronic otitis media may evolve. Mastoid tenderness often accompanies acute otitis media and is due to the presence of pus within the mastoid air cells. This alone does not indicate suppurative (surgical) mastoiditis. Frank swelling over the mastoid bone or the association of cranial neuropathies or central findings indicates severe disease requiring urgent care.

Treatment

The treatment of acute otitis media is specific antibiotic therapy, often combined with nasal decongestants. The first-choice oral antibiotic treatment is amoxicillin (80–90 mg/kg/day divided twice daily) (*or* erythromycin [50 mg/kg/day]) plus sulfonamide (150 mg/kg/day) for 10 days. Alternatives useful in resistant cases are cefaclor (20–40 mg/kg/day) or amoxicillin-clavulanate (20–40 mg/kg/day) combinations.

Tympanocentesis for bacterial (aerobic and anaerobic) and fungal culture may be performed by any experienced physician. A 20-gauge spinal needle bent 90 degrees to the hub attached to a 3-mL syringe is inserted through the inferior portion of the tympanic membrane. Interposition of a pliable connecting tube between the needle and syringe permits an assistant to aspirate without inducing movement of the needle. Tympanocentesis is useful for otitis media in immunocompromised patients and when infection persists or recurs despite multiple courses of antibiotics.

Surgical drainage of the middle ear (myringotomy) is reserved for patients with severe otalgia or when complications of otitis (eg, mastoiditis, meningitis) have occurred.

Recurrent acute otitis media may be managed with long-term antibiotic prophylaxis. Single daily oral doses of sulfamethoxazole (500 mg) or amoxicillin (250 or 500 mg) are given over a period of 1–3 months. Failure of this regimen to control infection is an indication for insertion of ventilating tubes.

Atkinson H et al. Acute otitis media. Postgrad Med. 2015 May; 127(4):386–90. [PMID: 25913598]

2. Chronic Otitis Media

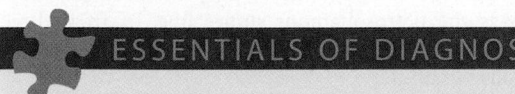

ESSENTIALS OF DIAGNOSIS

▶ Chronic otorrhea with or without otalgia.

▶ Tympanic membrane perforation with conductive hearing loss.

▶ Often amenable to surgical correction.

General Considerations

Chronic infection of the middle ear and mastoid generally develops as a consequence of recurrent acute otitis media, although it may follow other diseases and trauma. Perforation of the tympanic membrane is usually present. The bacteriology of chronic otitis media differs from that of acute otitis media. Common organisms include *P aeruginosa*, *Proteus* species, *Staphylococcus aureus*, and mixed anaerobic infections.

Clinical Findings

The clinical hallmark of chronic otitis media is purulent aural discharge. Drainage may be continuous or intermittent, with increased severity during upper respiratory tract infection or following water exposure. Pain is uncommon except during acute exacerbations. Conductive hearing loss results from destruction of the tympanic membrane or ossicular chain, or both.

Treatment

The medical treatment of chronic otitis media includes regular removal of infected debris, use of earplugs to protect against water exposure, and topical antibiotic drops (ofoxacin 0.3% or ciprofloxacin with dexamethasone) for exacerbations. The activity of ciprofloxacin against *Pseudomonas* may help dry a chronically discharging ear when given in a dosage of 500 mg orally twice a day for 1–6 weeks.

Definitive management is surgical in most cases. Successful reconstruction of the tympanic membrane may be achieved in about 90% of cases, often with elimination of infection and significant improvement in hearing. When the mastoid air cells are involved by irreversible infection, they should be exenterated at the same time through a mastoidectomy.

Harris AS et al. Why are ototopical aminoglycosides still first-line therapy for chronic suppurative otitis media? A systematic review and discussion of aminoglycosides versus quinolones. J Laryngol Otol. 2016 Jan;130(1):2–7. [PMID: 26584651]
Wallis S et al. Chronic otitis media. Postgrad Med. 2015 May; 127(4):391–5. [PMID: 25913599]

Complications of Otitis Media

A. Cholesteatoma

Cholesteatoma is a special variety of chronic otitis media (Figure 8–1). The most common cause is prolonged

▲ **Figure 8–1.** Cholesteatoma. (From Vladimir Zlinksy, MD, in Roy F. Sullivan, PhD: Audiology Forum: Video Otoscopy, www.RCSullivan.com; used with permission from Usatine RP, Smith MA, Mayeaux EJ Jr, Chumley H, Tysinger J. *The Color Atlas of Family Medicine*. McGraw-Hill, 2009.)

eustachian tube dysfunction, with inward migration of the upper flaccid portion of the tympanic membrane. This creates a squamous epithelium-lined sac, which—when its neck becomes obstructed—may fill with desquamated keratin and become chronically infected. Cholesteatomas typically erode bone, with early penetration of the mastoid and destruction of the ossicular chain. Over time they may erode into the inner ear, involve the facial nerve, and on rare occasions spread intracranially. Otoscopic examination may reveal an epitympanic retraction pocket or a marginal tympanic membrane perforation that exudes keratin debris, or granulation tissue. The treatment of cholesteatoma is surgical marsupialization of the sac or its complete removal. This may require the creation of a "mastoid bowl" in which the ear canal and mastoid are joined into a large common cavity that must be periodically cleaned.

Jackler RK et al. A new theory on the pathogenesis of acquired cholesteatoma: mucosal traction. Laryngoscope. 2015 Aug; 125(Suppl 4):S1–14. [PMID: 26013635]

B. Mastoiditis

Acute suppurative mastoiditis usually evolves following several weeks of inadequately treated acute otitis media. It is characterized by postauricular pain and erythema accompanied by a spiking fever. CT scan reveals coalescence of the mastoid air cells due to destruction of their bony septa. Initial treatment consists of intravenous antibiotics (eg, cefazolin 0.5–1.5 g every 6–8 hours) directed against the most common offending organisms (*S pneumoniae, H influenzae,* and *S pyogenes),* and myringotomy for culture and drainage. Failure of medical therapy indicates the need for surgical drainage (mastoidectomy).

C. Petrous Apicitis

The medial portion of the petrous bone between the inner ear and clivus may become a site of persistent infection when the drainage of its pneumatic cell tracts becomes blocked. This may cause foul discharge, deep ear and retro-orbital pain, and sixth nerve palsy (Gradenigo syndrome); meningitis may be a complication. Treatment is with prolonged antibiotic therapy (based on culture results) and surgical drainage via petrous apicectomy.

Sharma N et al. Complications of chronic suppurative otitis media and their management: a single institution 12 years experience. Indian J Otolaryngol Head Neck Surg. 2015 Dec; 67(4):353–60. [PMID: 26693451]

D. Facial Paralysis

Facial palsy may be associated with either acute or chronic otitis media. In the acute setting, it results from inflammation of the seventh nerve in its middle ear segment, perhaps mediated through bacterially secreted neurotoxins. Treatment consists of myringotomy for drainage and culture, followed by intravenous antibiotics (based on culture results). The use of corticosteroids is controversial. The prognosis is excellent, with complete recovery in most cases.

Facial palsy associated with chronic otitis media usually evolves slowly due to chronic pressure on the seventh nerve in the middle ear or mastoid by cholesteatoma. Treatment requires surgical correction of the underlying disease. The prognosis is less favorable than for facial palsy associated with acute otitis media.

Choi JW et al. Facial nerve paralysis in patients with chronic ear infections: surgical outcomes and radiologic analysis. Clin Exp Otorhinolaryngol. 2015 Sep;8(3):218–23. [PMID: 26330915]

E. Sigmoid Sinus Thrombosis

Trapped infection within the mastoid air cells adjacent to the sigmoid sinus may cause septic thrombophlebitis. This is heralded by signs of systemic sepsis (spiking fevers, chills), at times accompanied by signs of increased intracranial pressure (headache, lethargy, nausea and vomiting, papilledema). Diagnosis can be made noninvasively by magnetic resonance venography. Primary treatment is with intravenous antibiotics (based on culture results). Surgical drainage with ligation of the internal jugular vein may be indicated when embolization is suspected.

Ulanovski D et al. Pediatric otogenic sigmoid sinus thrombosis: 12-Year experience. Int J Pediatr Otorhinolaryngol. 2014 Jun; 78(6):930–3. [PMID: 24735608]

F. Central Nervous System Infection

Otogenic meningitis is by far the most common intracranial complication of ear infection. In the setting of acute suppurative otitis media, it arises from hematogenous spread of bacteria, most commonly *H influenzae* and *S pneumoniae.* In chronic otitis media, it results either from passage of infections along preformed pathways, such as the petrosquamous suture line, or from direct extension of disease through the dural plates of the petrous pyramid.

Epidural abscesses arise from direct extension of disease in the setting of chronic infection. They are usually asymptomatic but may present with deep local pain, headache, and low-grade fever. They are often discovered as an incidental finding at surgery. Brain abscess may arise in the temporal lobe or cerebellum as a result of septic thrombophlebitis adjacent to an epidural abscess. The predominant causative organisms are *S aureus, S pyogenes,* and *S pneumoniae.* Rupture into the subarachnoid space results in meningitis and often death. (See Chapter 30.)

Sharma N et al. Complications of chronic suppurative otitis media and their management: a single institution 12 years experience. Indian J Otolaryngol Head Neck Surg. 2015 Dec; 67(4):353–60. [PMID: 26693451]

3. Otosclerosis

Otosclerosis is a progressive disease with a marked familial tendency that affects the bony otic capsule. Lesions involving the footplate of the stapes result in increased impedance to the passage of sound through the ossicular chain, producing conductive hearing loss. This may be treated either through the use of a hearing aid or surgical replacement of the stapes with a prosthesis (stapedectomy). When otosclerotic lesions impinge on the cochlea ("cochlear otosclerosis"), permanent sensory hearing loss occurs.

Rudic M et al. The pathophysiology of otosclerosis: review of current research. Hear Res. 2015 Dec;330(Pt A):51–6. [PMID: 26276418]

Wegner I et al. A systematic review of the diagnostic value of CT imaging in diagnosing otosclerosis. Otol Neurotol. 2016 Jan; 37(1):9–15. [PMID: 26649602]

4. Trauma to the Middle Ear

Tympanic membrane perforation may result from impact injury or explosive acoustic trauma (Figure 8–2). Spontaneous healing occurs in most cases. Persistent perforation may result from secondary infection brought on by exposure to water. Patients should be advised to wear earplugs while swimming or bathing during the healing period. Hemorrhage behind an intact tympanic membrane (hemotympanum) may follow blunt trauma or extreme barotrauma. Spontaneous resolution over several weeks is the usual course. When a conductive hearing loss greater than 30 dB persists for more than 3 months following trauma, disruption of the ossicular chain should be suspected. Middle ear exploration with reconstruction of the ossicular chain, combined with repair of the tympanic membrane when required, will usually restore hearing.

Shah A et al. Otologic assessment of blast and nonblast injury in returning Middle East-deployed service members. Laryngoscope. 2014 Jan;124(1):272–7. [PMID: 23686673]

▲ **Figure 8–2.** Traumatic perforation of the left tympanic membrane. (From William Clark, MD; reproduced, with permission, from Usatine RP, Smith MA, Mayeaux EJ Jr, Chumley H, Tysinger J. *The Color Atlas of Family Medicine.* McGraw-Hill, 2009.)

5. Middle Ear Neoplasia

Primary middle ear tumors are rare. Glomus tumors arise either in the middle ear (glomus tympanicum) or in the jugular bulb with upward erosion into the hypotympanum (glomus jugulare). They present clinically with pulsatile tinnitus and hearing loss. A vascular mass may be visible behind an intact tympanic membrane. Large glomus jugulare tumors are often associated with multiple cranial neuropathies, especially involving nerves VII, IX, X, XI, and XII. Treatment usually requires surgery, radiotherapy, or both. Pulsatile tinnitus thus warrants magnetic resonance angiography and venography to rule out a vascular mass.

Pelosi S et al. Adenomatous tumors of the middle ear. Otolaryngol Clin North Am. 2015 Apr;48(2):305–15. [PMID: 25769353]

Sweeney AD et al. Glomus tympanicum tumors. Otolaryngol Clin North Am. 2015 Apr;48(2):293–304. [PMID: 25659513]

EARACHE

Earache can be caused by a variety of otologic problems, but external otitis and acute otitis media are the most common. Differentiation of the two should be apparent by pneumatic otoscopy (see relevant sections on otitis externa and otitis media). Pain out of proportion to the physical findings may be due to herpes zoster oticus, especially when vesicles appear in the ear canal or concha. Persistent pain and discharge from the ear suggest osteomyelitis of the skull base or cancer, and patients with these complaints should be referred for specialty evaluation.

Nonotologic causes of otalgia are numerous. The sensory innervation of the ear is derived from the trigeminal, facial, glossopharyngeal, vagal, and upper cervical nerves. Because of this rich innervation, referred otalgia is quite frequent. Temporomandibular joint dysfunction is a common cause of referred ear pain. Pain is exacerbated by chewing or psychogenic grinding of the teeth (bruxism) and may be associated with dental malocclusion. Repeated episodes of severe lancinating otalgia may occur in glossopharyngeal neuralgia. Infections and neoplasia that involve the oropharynx, hypopharynx, and larynx frequently cause otalgia. Persistent earache demands specialty referral to exclude cancer of the upper aerodigestive tract.

DISEASES OF THE INNER EAR

1. Sensory Hearing Loss

Diseases of the cochlea result in sensory hearing loss, a condition that is usually irreversible. Most cochlear diseases result in bilateral symmetric hearing loss. The presence of unilateral or asymmetric sensorineural hearing loss suggests a lesion proximal to the cochlea. Lesions affecting the eighth cranial nerve and central auditory system are discussed in the section on neural hearing loss. The primary goals in the management of sensory hearing loss are prevention of further losses and functional improvement with amplification and auditory rehabilitation.

A. Presbyacusis

Presbyacusis, or age-related hearing loss, is the most frequent cause of sensory hearing loss and is progressive, predominantly high-frequency, and symmetrical. It is difficult to separate the various etiologic factors (eg, noise trauma, drug exposure) that may contribute to presbyacusis, but genetic predisposition and prior noise exposure appear to play an important role. Most patients notice a loss of speech discrimination that is especially pronounced in noisy environments. About 25% of people between the ages of 65 and 75 years and almost 50% of those over 75 experience hearing difficulties.

Roth TN. Aging of the auditory system. Handb Clin Neurol. 2015;129:357–73. [PMID: 25726279]
Uchida Y et al. Progress and prospects in human genetic research into age-related hearing impairment. Biomed Res Int. 2014;2014:390601. [PMID: 25140308]

B. Noise Trauma

Noise trauma is the second most common cause of sensory hearing loss. Sounds exceeding 85 dB are potentially injurious to the cochlea, especially with prolonged exposures. The loss typically begins in the high frequencies (especially 4000 Hz) and progresses to involve the speech frequencies with continuing exposure. Among the more common sources of injurious noise are industrial machinery, weapons, and excessively loud music. Personal music devices (eg, MP3 and CD players) used at excessive loudness levels may also be potentially injurious. Monitoring noise levels in the workplace by regulatory agencies has led to preventive programs that have reduced the frequency of occupational losses. Individuals of all ages, especially those with existing hearing losses, should wear earplugs when exposed to moderately loud noises and specially designed earmuffs when exposed to explosive noises.

Lie A et al. Occupational noise exposure and hearing: a systematic review. Int Arch Occup Environ Health. 2015 Aug 7. [Epub ahead of print] [PMID: 26249711]

C. Physical Trauma

Head trauma has effects on the inner ear similar to those of severe acoustic trauma. Some degree of sensory hearing loss may occur following simple concussion and is frequent after skull fracture. Deployment of air bags during an automobile accident has also been associated with hearing loss.

Pfannenstiel TJ. Noise-induced hearing loss: a military perspective. Curr Opin Otolaryngol Head Neck Surg. 2014 Oct;22(5):384–7. [PMID: 25188428]

D. Ototoxicity

Ototoxic substances may affect both the auditory and vestibular systems. The most commonly used ototoxic medications are aminoglycosides; loop diuretics; and several antineoplastic agents, notably cisplatin. These medications may cause irreversible hearing loss even when administered in therapeutic doses. When using these medications, it is important to identify high-risk patients, such as those with preexisting hearing losses or kidney disease. Patients simultaneously receiving multiple ototoxic agents are at particular risk owing to ototoxic synergy. Useful measures to reduce the risk of ototoxic injury include serial audiometry, monitoring of serum peak and trough levels, and substitution of equivalent nonototoxic drugs whenever possible.

It is possible for topical agents that enter the middle ear to be absorbed into the inner ear via the round window. When the tympanic membrane is perforated, use of potentially ototoxic ear drops (eg, neomycin, gentamicin) is best avoided.

Crundwell G et al. Ototoxicity (cochleotoxicity) classifications: a review. Int J Audiol. 2016 Feb;55(2):65–74. [PMID: 26618898]
Santabarbara G et al. Pharmacotherapeutic options for treating adverse effects of cisplatin chemotherapy. Expert Opin Pharmacother. 2015 Dec 17:1–10. [PMID: 26581586]

E. Sudden Sensory Hearing Loss

Idiopathic sudden loss of hearing in one ear may occur at any age, but typically, it occurs in persons over age 20 years. The cause is unknown; however, one hypothesis is that it results from a viral infection or a sudden vascular occlusion of the internal auditory artery. Prognosis is mixed, with many patients suffering permanent deafness in the involved ear, while others have complete recovery. Prompt treatment with corticosteroids has been shown to improve the odds of recovery. A common regimen is oral prednisone, 1 mg/kg/day, followed by a tapering dose over a 10-day period. Intratympanic administration of corticosteroids alone or in association with oral corticosteroids has been associated with an equal or more favorable prognosis in some reports. Because treatment appears to be most effective as close to the onset of the loss as possible, and appears not to be effective after 6 weeks, a prompt audiogram should be obtained in all patients who present with sudden hearing loss without obvious middle ear pathology.

Li H et al. Intratympanic steroid therapy as a salvage treatment for sudden sensorineural hearing loss after failure of conventional therapy: a meta-analysis of randomized, controlled trials. Clin Ther. 2015 Jan 1;37(1):178–87. [PMID: 25542075]
Yang HC et al. Efficacy of concomitant intratympanic steroid injection for sudden deafness according to initial hearing loss. Otol Neurotol. 2015 Dec;36(10):1604–9. [PMID: 26485600]

F. Hereditary Hearing Loss

Sensory hearing loss with onset during adult life often runs in families. The mode of inheritance may be either autosomal dominant or recessive. The age at onset, the rate of progression of hearing loss, and the audiometric pattern (high-frequency, low-frequency, or flat) can often be predicted by studying family members. The connexin-26 mutation, the most common cause of genetic deafness, may be tested clinically, as can most other single gene mutations known to cause hearing loss.

Abou Tayoun AN et al. Improving hearing loss gene testing: a systematic review of gene evidence toward more efficient next-generation sequencing-based diagnostic testing and interpretation. Genet Med. 2015 Nov 12. [Epub ahead of print] [PMID: 26562227]

Jayawardena AD et al. Sensorineural hearing loss: a changing paradigm for its evaluation. Otolaryngol Head Neck Surg. 2015 Nov;153(5):843–50. [PMID: 26216887]

G. Autoimmune Hearing Loss

Sensory hearing loss may be associated with a wide array of systemic autoimmune disorders, such as systemic lupus erythematosus, granulomatosis with polyangiitis (formerly Wegener granulomatosis), and Cogan syndrome (hearing loss, keratitis, aortitis). The loss is most often bilateral and progressive. The hearing level often fluctuates, with periods of deterioration alternating with partial or even complete remission. The tendency is for the gradual evolution of permanent hearing loss, which usually stabilizes with some remaining auditory function but occasionally proceeds to complete deafness. Vestibular dysfunction, particularly dysequilibrium and postural instability, may accompany the auditory symptoms. A syndrome resembling Ménière disease may also occur with intermittent attacks of severe vertigo.

In many cases, the autoimmune pattern of audiovestibular dysfunction presents in the absence of recognized systemic autoimmune disease. Use of laboratory tests to screen for autoimmune disease (eg, antinuclear antibody, rheumatoid factor, erythrocyte sedimentation rate) may be informative. Specific tests of immune reactivity against inner ear antigens (anticochlear antibodies, lymphocyte transformation tests) are current research tools and have limited clinical value to date. Responsiveness to oral corticosteroid treatment is helpful in making the diagnosis and constitutes first-line therapy. If stabilization of hearing becomes dependent on long-term corticosteroid use, steroid-sparing immunosuppressive regimens may become necessary.

Vambutas A et al. Early efficacy trial of anakinra in corticosteroid-resistant autoimmune inner ear disease. J Clin Invest. 2014 Sep 2;124(9):4115–22. [PMID: 25133431]

Zhai SQ. Review of experimental and clinical studies on autoimmune sensorineural hearing loss. Minerva Med. 2015 Jun; 106(3):177–80. [PMID: 25532537]

2. Tinnitus

ESSENTIALS OF DIAGNOSIS

► Perception of abnormal ear or head noises.

► Persistent tinnitus often, though not always, indicates the presence of sensory hearing loss.

► Intermittent periods of mild, high-pitched tinnitus lasting seconds to minutes are common in normal-hearing persons.

► General Considerations

Tinnitus is defined as the sensation of sound in the absence of an exogenous sound source. Tinnitus can accompany any form of hearing loss, and its presence provides no diagnostic value in determining the cause of a hearing loss. Approximately 15% of the general population experience some type of tinnitus, with prevalence beyond 20% in aging populations.

► Clinical Findings

A. Symptoms and Signs

Though tinnitus is commonly associated with hearing loss, tinnitus severity correlates poorly with the degree of hearing loss. About one in seven tinnitus sufferers experience severe annoyance, and 4% are severely disabled. When severe and persistent, tinnitus may interfere with sleep and the ability to concentrate, resulting in considerable psychological distress.

Pulsatile tinnitus—often described by the patient as listening to one's own heartbeat—should be distinguished from tonal tinnitus. Although often ascribed to conductive hearing loss, pulsatile tinnitus may be far more serious and may indicate a vascular abnormality, such as glomus tumor, venous sinus stenosis, carotid vaso-occlusive disease, arteriovenous malformation, or aneurysm. In contrast, a staccato "clicking" tinnitus may result from middle ear muscle spasm, sometimes associated with palatal myoclonus. The patient typically perceives a rapid series of popping noises, lasting seconds to a few minutes, accompanied by a fluttering feeling in the ear.

B. Diagnostic Testing

For routine, nonpulsatile tinnitus, audiometry should be ordered to rule out an associated hearing loss. For unilateral tinnitus, particularly associated with hearing loss in the absence of an obvious causative factor (ie, noise trauma), an MRI should be obtained to rule out a retrocochlear lesion, such as vestibular schwannoma. Magnetic resonance angiography and venography should be considered for patients who have pulsatile tinnitus to rule out a vascular lesion as causative.

► Treatment

The most important treatment of tinnitus is avoidance of exposure to excessive noise, ototoxic agents, and other factors that may cause cochlear damage. Masking the tinnitus with music or through amplification of normal sounds with a hearing aid may also bring some relief. Among the numerous drugs that have been tried, oral antidepressants (eg, nortriptyline at an initial dosage of 50 mg orally at bedtime) have proved to be the most effective. Habituation techniques, such as tinnitus retraining therapy, and masking techniques may prove beneficial in those with refractory symptoms. Transcranial magnetic stimulation of the central auditory system has been shown to improve symptoms in some patients.

Langguth B. Treatment of tinnitus. Curr Opin Otolaryngol Head Neck Surg. 2015 Oct;23(5):361–8. [PMID: 26261868]
Plein CT et al. A systematic review of eligibility and outcomes in tinnitus trials: reassessment of tinnitus guideline. Otolaryngol Head Neck Surg. 2016 Jan;154(1):24–32. [PMID: 26459245]

3. Hyperacusis

Excessive sensitivity to sound may occur in normal-hearing individuals, either in association with ear disease, following noise trauma, in patients susceptible to migraines, or for psychological reasons. Patients with cochlear dysfunction commonly experience "recruitment," an abnormal sensitivity to loud sounds despite a reduced sensitivity to softer ones. Fitting hearing aids and other amplification devices to patients with recruitment requires use of compression circuitry to avoid uncomfortable overamplification. For normal-hearing individuals with hyperacusis, use of an earplug in noisy environments may be beneficial, though attempts should be made at habituation.

Jastreboff PJ et al. Decreased sound tolerance: hyperacusis, misophonia, diplacousis, and polyacousis. Handb Clin Neurol. 2015;129:375–87. [PMID: 25726280]

4. Vertigo

ESSENTIALS OF DIAGNOSIS

▶ Either a sensation of motion when there is no motion or an exaggerated sense of motion in response to movement.

▶ Duration of vertigo episodes and association with hearing loss are the key to diagnosis.

▶ Must differentiate peripheral from central etiologies of vestibular dysfunction.

▶ **Peripheral:** Onset is sudden; often associated with tinnitus and hearing loss; horizontal nystagmus may be present.

▶ **Central:** Onset is gradual; no associated auditory symptoms.

▶ Evaluation includes audiogram and electronystagmography (ENG) or videonystagmography (VNG) and MRI.

▶ General Considerations

Vertigo can be caused by either a peripheral or central etiology, or both (Table 8–2).

▶ Clinical Findings

A. Symptoms and Signs

Vertigo is the cardinal symptom of vestibular disease. While vertigo is typically experienced as a distinct "spinning" sensation, it may also present as a sense of tumbling or of falling forward or backward. It should be

Table 8–2. Causes of vertigo.

Peripheral causes
Vestibular neuritis/labyrinthitis
Ménière disease
Benign positional vertigo
Ethanol intoxication
Inner ear barotraumas
Semicircular canal dehiscence
Central causes
Seizure
Multiple sclerosis
Wernicke encephalopathy
Chiari malformation
Cerebellar ataxia syndromes
Mixed central and peripheral causes
Migraine
Stroke and vascular insufficiency
Posterior inferior cerebellar artery stroke
Anterior inferior cerebellar artery stroke
Vertebral artery insufficiency
Vasculitides
Cogan syndrome
Susac syndrome
Granulomatosis with polyangiitis (formerly Wegener granulomatosis)
Behçet disease
Cerebellopontine angle tumors
Vestibular schwannoma
Meningioma
Infections
Lyme disease
Syphilis
Vascular compression
Hyperviscosity syndromes
Waldenström macroglobulinemia
Endocrinopathies
Hypothyroidism
Pendred syndrome

distinguished from imbalance, light-headedness, and syncope, all of which are nonvestibular in origin (Table 8–3).

1. Peripheral vestibular disease—Peripheral vestibulopathy usually causes vertigo of sudden onset, may be so severe that the patient is unable to walk or stand, and is frequently accompanied by nausea and vomiting. Tinnitus and hearing loss may be associated and provide strong support for a peripheral (ie, otologic) origin.

Table 8–3. Common vestibular disorders: differential diagnosis based on classic presentations.

Duration of Typical Vertiginous Episodes	Auditory Symptoms Present	Auditory Symptoms Absent
Seconds	Perilymphatic fistula	Positioning vertigo (cupulolithiasis), vertebrobasilar insufficiency, migraine-associated vertigo
Hours	Endolymphatic hydrops (Ménière syndrome, syphilis)	Migraine-associated vertigo
Days	Labyrinthitis, labyrinthine concussion, autoimmune inner ear disease	Vestibular neuronitis, migraine-associated vertigo
Months	Acoustic neuroma, ototoxicity	Multiple sclerosis, cerebellar degeneration

A thorough history will often narrow down, if not confirm the diagnosis. Critical elements of the history include the duration of the discrete vertiginous episodes (seconds, minutes to hours, or days), and associated symptoms. Triggers should also be sought, including diet (eg, high salt in the case of Ménière disease), stress, fatigue, and bright lights (eg, migraine-associated dizziness).

The physical examination of the patient with vertigo includes evaluation of the ears, eye motion in response to head turning and observation for nystagmus, cranial nerve examination, and Romberg testing. In acute peripheral lesions, nystagmus is usually horizontal with a rotatory component; the fast phase usually beats away from the diseased side. Visual fixation tends to inhibit nystagmus except in very acute peripheral lesions or with central nervous system disease. Dix-Hallpike testing (quickly lowering the patient to the supine position with the head extending over the edge and placed 30 degrees lower than the body, turned either to the left or right) will elicit a delayed onset (~10 sec) fatiguable nystagmus in cases of benign positional vertigo. Nonfatigable nystagmus in this position indicates a central etiology for the dizziness.

Since visual fixation often suppresses observed nystagmus, many of these maneuvers are performed with Frenzel goggles, which prevent visual fixation, and often bring out subtle forms of nystagmus. The Fukuda test can demonstrate vestibular asymmetry when the patient steps in place with eyes closed and consistently rotates.

2. Central disease—In contrast to peripheral forms of vertigo, dizziness arising from central etiologies (Table 8–2) tends to develop gradually and then becomes progressively more severe and debilitating. Nystagmus is not always present but can occur in any direction and may be dissociated in the two eyes. The associated nystagmus is often nonfatigable, vertical rather than horizontal in orientation, without latency, and unsuppressed by visual fixation. ENG is useful in documenting these characteristics. The evaluation of central audiovestibular dysfunction requires imaging of the brain with MRI.

Episodic vertigo can occur in patients with diplopia from external ophthalmoplegia and is maximal when the patient looks in the direction where the separation of images is greatest. Cerebral lesions involving the temporal cortex may also produce vertigo, which is sometimes the initial symptom of a seizure. Finally, vertigo may be a feature of a number of systemic disorders and can occur as a side effect of certain anticonvulsant, antibiotic, hypnotic, analgesic, and tranquilizing drugs or of alcohol.

B. Laboratory Findings

Laboratory investigations, such as audiologic evaluation, caloric stimulation, ENG, VNG, vestibular-evoked myogenic potentials (VEMPs), and MRI, are indicated in patients with persistent vertigo or when central nervous system disease is suspected. These studies will help distinguish between central and peripheral lesions and identify causes requiring specific therapy. ENG consists of objective recording of the nystagmus induced by head and body movements, gaze, and caloric stimulation. It is helpful in quantifying the degree of vestibular hypofunction. Computer-driven rotatory chairs and posturography platforms offer additional diagnostic modalities from specialized centers.

Curthoys IS et al. Neural basis of new clinical vestibular tests: otolithic neural responses to sound and vibration. Clin Exp Pharmacol Physiol. 2014 May;41(5):371–80. [PMID: 24754528]
Welgampola MS et al. Bedside assessment of acute dizziness and vertigo. Neurol Clin. 2015 Aug;33(3):551–64. [PMID: 26231271]

▶ Vertigo Syndromes Due to Peripheral Lesions

A. Endolymphatic Hydrops (Ménière Syndrome)

The cause of Ménière syndrome is unknown. Distention of the endolymphatic compartment of the inner ear is a pathologic finding and thought to be part of the pathogenesis of the disorder. Although a precise cause of hydrops cannot be established in most cases, two known causes are syphilis and head trauma. The classic syndrome consists of episodic vertigo, with discrete vertigo spells lasting 20 minutes to several hours in association with fluctuating low-frequency sensorineural hearing loss, tinnitus (usually low-tone and "blowing" in quality), and a sensation of unilateral aural pressure (Table 8–3). These symptoms in the absence of hearing fluctuations suggest migraine-associated dizziness. Symptoms wax and wane as the endolymphatic pressure rises and falls. Caloric testing commonly reveals loss or impairment of thermally induced nystagmus on the involved side. Primary treatment involves a low-salt diet and diuretics (eg, acetazolamide). For symptomatic relief of acute vertigo attacks, oral meclizine (25 mg) or valium (5 mg) can be used. In refractory cases, patients may undergo intratympanic corticosteroid injections, endolymphatic sac decompression, or vestibular ablation, either through transtympanic gentamicin, vestibular nerve section, or surgical labyrinthectomy.

Ishiyama G et al. Meniere's disease: histopathology, cytochemistry, and imaging. Ann N Y Acad Sci. 2015 Apr;1343:49–57. [PMID: 25766597]

McRackan TR et al. Intratympanic dexamethasone as a symptomatic treatment for Ménière's disease. Otol Neurotol. 2014 Oct; 35(9):1638–40. [PMID: 25188506]

B. Labyrinthitis

Patients with labyrinthitis suffer from acute onset of continuous, usually severe vertigo lasting several days to a week, accompanied by hearing loss and tinnitus. During a recovery period that lasts for several weeks, the vertigo gradually improves. Hearing may return to normal or remain permanently impaired in the involved ear. The cause of labyrinthitis is unknown. Treatment consists of antibiotics if the patient is febrile or has symptoms of a bacterial infection, and supportive care. Vestibular suppressants are useful during the acute phase of the attack (eg, diazepam or meclizine) but should be discontinued as soon as feasible to avoid long-term dysequilibrium from inadequate compensation.

C. Benign Paroxysmal Positioning Vertigo

Patients suffering from recurrent spells of vertigo, lasting a few minutes per spell, associated with changes in head position (often provoked by rolling over in bed), usually have benign paroxysmal positioning vertigo (BPPV). The term "positioning vertigo" is more accurate than "positional vertigo" because it is provoked by changes in head position rather than by the maintenance of a particular posture.

The typical symptoms of positioning vertigo occur in clusters that persist for several days. There is a brief (10–15 sec) latency period following a head movement before symptoms develop, and the acute vertigo subsides within 10–60 seconds, though the patient may remain imbalanced for several hours. Constant repetition of the positional change leads to habituation. Since some central nervous system disorders can mimic BPPV (eg, vertebrobasilar insufficiency), recurrent cases warrant MRI scanning of the head. In central lesions, there is no latent period, fatigability, or habituation of the symptoms and signs. Treatment of BPPV involves physical therapy protocols (eg, the Epley maneuver or Brandt-Daroff exercises), based on the theory that peripheral positioning vertigo results from free-floating otoconia within a semicircular canal.

Hilton MP et al. The Epley (canalith repositioning) manoeuvre for benign paroxysmal positional vertigo. Cochrane Database Syst Rev. 2014 Dec 8;12:CD003162. [PMID: 25485940]

Kim JS et al. Clinical practice. Benign paroxysmal positional vertigo. N Engl J Med. 2014 Mar 20;370(12):1138–47. [PMID: 24645946]

D. Vestibular Neuronitis

In vestibular neuronitis, a paroxysmal, usually single attack of vertigo occurs without accompanying impairment of auditory function and will persist for several days to a week before gradually clearing. During the acute phase, examination reveals nystagmus and absent responses to caloric stimulation on one or both sides. The cause of the disorder is unclear though presumed to be viral. Treatment consists of supportive care, including oral diazepam (5 mg) or meclizine (25 mg) during the acute phases of the vertigo only, followed by vestibular therapy if the patient does not completely compensate.

Jeong SH et al. Vestibular neuritis. Semin Neurol. 2013 Jul; 33(3):185–94. [PMID: 24057821]

E. Traumatic Vertigo

The most common cause of vertigo following head injury is labyrinthine concussion. Symptoms generally diminish within several days but may linger for a month or more. Basilar skull fractures that traverse the inner ear usually result in severe vertigo lasting several days to a week and deafness in the involved ear. Chronic posttraumatic vertigo may result from cupulolithiasis. This occurs when traumatically detached statoconia (otoconia) settle on the ampulla of the posterior semicircular canal and cause an excessive degree of cupular deflection in response to head motion. Clinically, this presents as episodic positioning vertigo. Treatment consists of supportive care and vestibular suppressant medication (diazepam or meclizine) during the acute phase of the attack, and vestibular therapy.

Fife TD et al. Persistent vertigo and dizziness after mild traumatic brain injury. Ann N Y Acad Sci. 2015 Apr;1343:97–105. [PMID: 25728715]

F. Perilymphatic Fistula

Leakage of perilymphatic fluid from the inner ear into the tympanic cavity via the round or oval window is a rare cause of vertigo and sensory hearing loss. Most cases result from either physical injury (eg, blunt head trauma, hand slap to ear); extreme barotrauma during airflight, scuba diving, etc; or vigorous Valsalva maneuvers (eg, during weight lifting). Treatment may require middle ear exploration and window sealing with a tissue graft; however, this is seldom indicated without a clear-cut history of a precipitating traumatic event.

Alzahrani M et al. Perilymphatic fistulas: can we predict the diagnosis? Eur Arch Otorhinolaryngol. 2015 Aug;272(8):1885–91. [PMID: 24652117]

G. Cervical Vertigo

Position receptors located in the facets of the cervical spine are important physiologically in the coordination of head and eye movements. Cervical proprioceptive dysfunction is a common cause of vertigo triggered by neck movements. This disturbance often commences after neck injury, particularly hyperextension. An association also exists with degenerative cervical spine disease. Although symptoms vary, vertigo may be triggered by assuming a particular head position as opposed to moving to a new head position (the latter typical of labyrinthine dysfunction). Diagnosis may often be confused with migraine-associated vertigo, which is also associated with head movement. Management consists of neck movement exercises to the extent permitted by orthopedic considerations.

Hain TC. Cervicogenic causes of vertigo. Curr Opin Neurol. 2015 Feb;28(1):69–73. [PMID: 25502050]

H. Migrainous Vertigo

Episodic vertigo is frequently associated with a migraine type of headache. Head trauma may also be a precipitating feature. The vertigo may be temporally related to the headache and last up to several hours, although the vertigo may also occur in the absence of any headache. It may appear identical to Ménière disease but without associated hearing loss or tinnitus. Accompanying symptoms may include head pressure, visual and motion sensitivity, auditory sensitivity, and photosensitivity. Symptoms typically worsen with lack of sleep and anxiety or stress. There is often a history of motion intolerance (easily carsick as a child) and there may be a familial tendency. Food triggers may also be common, including caffeine, chocolate, and alcohol among others. Treatment includes dietary and lifestyle changes (improved sleep pattern, avoidance of stress) and antimigraine prophylactic medication.

Furman JM et al. Vestibular migraine. Ann N Y Acad Sci. 2015 Apr; 1343:90–6. [PMID: 25728541]

I. Superior Semicircular Canal Dehiscence

Deficiency in the bony covering of the superior semicircular canal may be associated with vertigo triggered by loud noise exposure, straining, and an apparent conductive hearing loss. Diagnosis is with coronal high-resolution CT scan and VEMPs. Surgically sealing the dehiscent canal can improve symptoms.

Lookabaugh S et al. Radiologic classification of superior canal dehiscence: implications for surgical repair. Otol Neurotol. 2015 Jan;36(1):118–25. [PMID: 25122602]

▶ Vertigo Syndromes Due to Central Lesions

Central nervous system causes of vertigo include brainstem vascular disease, arteriovenous malformations, tumor of the brainstem and cerebellum, multiple sclerosis, and vertebrobasilar migraine (Table 8–2). Vertigo of central origin often becomes unremitting and disabling. The associated nystagmus is often nonfatigable, vertical rather than horizontal in orientation, without latency, and unsuppressed by visual fixation. ENG is useful in documenting these characteristics. There are commonly other signs of brainstem dysfunction (eg, cranial nerve palsies; motor, sensory, or cerebellar deficits in the limbs) or of increased intracranial pressure. Auditory function is generally spared. The underlying cause should be treated.

Saber Tehrani AS et al. Small strokes causing severe vertigo: frequency of false-negative MRIs and nonlacunar mechanisms. Neurology. 2014 Jul 8;83(2):169–73. [PMID: 24920847]

DISEASES OF THE CENTRAL AUDITORY & VESTIBULAR SYSTEMS (Table 8–3)

Lesions of the eighth cranial nerve and central audiovestibular pathways produce neural hearing loss and vertigo. One characteristic of neural hearing loss is deterioration of speech discrimination out of proportion to the decrease in pure tone thresholds. Another is auditory adaptation, wherein a steady tone appears to the listener to decay and eventually disappear. Auditory evoked responses are useful in distinguishing cochlear from neural losses and may give insight into the site of lesion within the central pathways.

The evaluation of central audiovestibular disorders usually requires imaging of the internal auditory canal, cerebellopontine angle, and brain with enhanced MRI.

1. Vestibular Schwannoma (Acoustic Neuroma)

Eighth cranial nerve schwannomas are among the most common intracranial tumors. Most are unilateral, but about 5% are associated with the hereditary syndrome neurofibromatosis type 2, in which bilateral eighth nerve tumors may be accompanied by meningiomas and other intracranial and spinal tumors. These benign lesions arise within the internal auditory canal and gradually grow to involve the cerebellopontine angle, eventually compressing the pons and resulting in hydrocephalus. Their typical auditory symptoms are unilateral hearing loss with a deterioration of speech discrimination exceeding that predicted by the degree of pure tone loss. Nonclassic presentations, such as sudden unilateral hearing loss, are fairly common. Any individual with a unilateral or asymmetric sensorineural hearing loss should be evaluated for an intracranial mass lesion. Vestibular dysfunction more often takes the form of continuous dysequilibrium than episodic vertigo. Diagnosis is made by enhanced MRI. Treatment consists of observation, microsurgical excision, or stereotactic radiotherapy, depending on such factors as patient age, underlying health, and size of the tumor at presentation. Bevacizumab (vascular endothelial growth factor blocker) has shown promise for treatment of tumors in patients with neurofibromatosis type 2.

Gao X et al. Anti-VEGF treatment improves neurological function and augments radiation response in NF2 schwannoma model. Proc Natl Acad Sci U S A. 2015 Nov 24;112(47):14676–81. [PMID: 26554010]

Lim SH et al. Systemic therapy in neurofibromatosis type 2. Cancer Treat Rev. 2014 Aug;40(7):857–61. [PMID: 24877986]

2. Vascular Compromise

Vertebrobasilar insufficiency is a common cause of vertigo in the elderly. It is often triggered by changes in posture or extension of the neck. Reduced flow in the vertebrobasilar system may be demonstrated noninvasively through magnetic resonance angiography. Empiric treatment is with vasodilators and aspirin.

Kim JH et al. Audiovestibular impairment presenting as a portent of vertebrobasilar infarction. Br J Hosp Med (Lond). 2014 Jan; 75(1):48–9. [PMID: 24401972]
Lee H. Isolated vascular vertigo. J Stroke. 2014 Sep;16(3):124–30. [PMID: 25328871]

3. Multiple Sclerosis

Patients with multiple sclerosis may suffer from episodic vertigo and chronic imbalance. Hearing loss in this disease is most commonly unilateral and of rapid onset. Spontaneous recovery may occur.

Mostafa BE et al. Central vestibular dysfunction in an otorhinolaryngological vestibular unit: incidence and diagnostic strategy. Int Arch Otorhinolaryngol. 2014 Jul;18(3):235–8. [PMID: 25992098]

OTOLOGIC MANIFESTATIONS OF AIDS

The otologic manifestations of AIDS are protean. The pinna and external auditory canal may be affected by Kaposi sarcoma as well as persistent and potentially invasive fungal infections, particularly due to *Aspergillus fumigatus.* The most common middle ear manifestation of AIDS is serous otitis media due to eustachian tube dysfunction arising from adenoidal hypertrophy (HIV lymphadenopathy), recurrent mucosal viral infections, or an obstructing nasopharyngeal tumor (eg, lymphoma). For middle ear effusions, ventilating tubes are seldom helpful and may trigger profuse watery otorrhea. Acute otitis media is usually caused by the typical bacterial organisms that occur in the nonimmunocompromised, including *Proteus, Staphylococcus,* and *Pseudomonas,* although *Pneumocystis jirovecii* otitis has been reported. Sensorineural hearing loss is common and in some cases appears to result from viral central nervous system infection. In cases of progressive hearing loss, it is important to evaluate for cryptococcal meningitis and syphilis. Acute facial paralysis due to herpes zoster infection (Ramsay Hunt syndrome) is quite common and follows a clinical course similar to that in nonimmunocompromised patients. Treatment is primarily with high-dose acyclovir (see Chapters 6 and 32). Corticosteroids may also be effective.

Palacios GC et al. Audiologic and vestibular findings in a sample of human immunodeficiency virus type-1-infected Mexican children under highly active antiretroviral therapy. Int J Pediatr Otorhinolaryngol. 2008 Nov;72(11):1671–81. [PMID: 18814921]

DISEASES OF THE NOSE & PARANASAL SINUSES

INFECTIONS OF THE NOSE & PARANASAL SINUSES

1. Acute Viral Rhinosinusitis (Common Cold)

> ### ESSENTIALS OF DIAGNOSIS
>
> ▶ Clear rhinorrhea, hyposmia, and nasal congestion.
> ▶ Associated symptoms, including malaise, headache, and cough.
> ▶ Erythematous, engorged nasal mucosa on examination without intranasal purulence.
> ▶ Symptoms last less than 4 weeks and typically less than 10 days.
> ▶ Symptoms are self-limited.

▶ Clinical Findings

The nonspecific symptoms of the ubiquitous common cold are present in the early phases of many diseases that affect the upper aerodigestive tract. Because there are numerous serologic types of rhinoviruses, adenoviruses, and other viruses, patients remain susceptible throughout life. These infections, while generally quite benign and self-limited, have been implicated in the development or exacerbation of more serious conditions, such as acute bacterial sinusitis, acute otitis media, asthma and cystic fibrosis exacerbation, and bronchitis. Nasal congestion, decreased sense of smell, watery rhinorrhea, and sneezing, accompanied by general malaise, throat discomfort and, occasionally, headache are typical in viral infections. Nasal examination usually shows erythematous, edematous mucosa and a watery discharge. The presence of purulent nasal discharge suggests bacterial rhinosinusitis.

▶ Treatment

Even though there are no effective antiviral therapies for either the prevention or treatment of viral rhinitis, there is a common misperception among patients that antibiotics are helpful. Zinc for the treatment of viral rhinitis has been controversial. A 2011 meta-analysis of randomized controlled trials demonstrated no benefit in five studies that used less than 75 mg of zinc acetate daily, but significant reduction in duration of cold symptoms was noted in all three studies that used zinc acetate in daily doses of over 75 mg. The effect with zinc salts other than acetate was also significant at doses greater than 75 mg/day, but not as high as the zinc acetate lozenge studies (20% vs 42% reduction in cold duration). Buffered hypertonic saline (3–5%) nasal irrigation has been shown to improve symptoms and reduce the need for nonsteroidal anti-inflammatory drugs. Other supportive measures, such as oral decongestants (pseudoephedrine, 30–60 mg every 4–6 hours or 120 mg twice daily), may provide some relief of rhinorrhea and nasal obstruction. Nasal sprays, such as oxymetazoline or phenylephrine, are rapidly effective but should not be used for more than a few days to prevent rebound congestion. Withdrawal of the drug after prolonged use leads to **rhinitis medicamentosa,** an almost addictive need for continuous usage. Treatment of rhinitis medicamentosa requires mandatory cessation of the sprays, and this is often extremely frustrating for patients. Topical intranasal corticosteroids (eg, flunisolide, 2 sprays in each nostril twice daily), intranasal anticholinergic (ipratropium 0.06% nasal spray, 2–3 sprays every 8 hours as needed), or a short tapering course of oral prednisone may help during the process of withdrawal.

▶ Complications

Other than mild eustachian tube dysfunction or transient middle ear effusion, complications of viral rhinitis are unusual. Secondary acute bacterial rhinosinusitis may occur and is suggested by persistence of symptoms beyond 10 days, accompanied both by purulent green or yellow nasal secretions and unilateral facial or tooth pain. (See Acute Bacterial Rhinosinusitis below.)

Hemilä H. Zinc lozenges may shorten the duration of colds: a systematic review. Open Respir Med J. 2011;5:51–8. [PMID: 21769305]

2. Acute Bacterial Rhinosinusitis (Sinusitis)

ESSENTIALS OF DIAGNOSIS

▶ Purulent yellow-green nasal discharge or expectoration.

▶ Facial pain or pressure over the affected sinus or sinuses.

▶ Nasal obstruction.

▶ Acute onset of symptoms (between 1 and 4 weeks' duration).

▶ Associated symptoms, including cough, malaise, fever, and headache.

▶ General Considerations

Acute sinus infections are uncommon compared with viral rhinitis, but they still affect nearly 20 million Americans annually, accounting for over 2 billion dollars in health care expenditures for sinusitis annually. Such infections are often associated with inflammation of the nasal cavity mucosa near the drainage pores of the sinuses. To acknowledge this inflammation as a major component of the disease and to differentiate it from such processes as allergic or acute viral rhinitis, otolaryngologists prefer the term "bacterial rhinosinusitis."

Acute bacterial rhinosinusitis usually is a result of impaired mucociliary clearance and obstruction of the ostiomeatal complex, or sinus "pore." Edematous mucosa causes obstruction of the complex, resulting in the accumulation of mucous secretion in the sinus cavity that becomes secondarily infected by bacteria. The largest of these ostiomeatal complexes is deep to the middle turbinate in the middle meatus. This complex is actually a confluence of complexes draining the maxillary, ethmoid, and frontal sinuses. The sphenoid drains from a separate complex between the septum and superior turbinate.

The typical pathogens of bacterial sinusitis are the same as those that cause acute otitis media: *S pneumoniae,* other streptococci, *H influenzae,* and less commonly, *S aureus* and *Moraxella catarrhalis.* Pathogens vary regionally in both prevalence and drug resistance; about 25% of healthy asymptomatic individuals may, if sinus aspirates are cultured, harbor such bacteria as well. Understanding of the anatomy, pathogenesis, and microbiology of acute bacterial rhinosinusitis can help the clinician make the most expeditious and cost-effective diagnosis and treatment while avoiding serious complications.

▶ Clinical Findings

A. Symptoms and Signs

There are no agreed-upon criteria for the diagnosis of acute bacterial rhinosinusitis in adults. All study groups note a number of major symptoms, including purulent nasal drainage, nasal obstruction or congestion, facial pain/pressure, altered smell, cough, and fever. Minor symptoms include headache, otalgia, halitosis, dental pain, and fatigue. Many of the more specific signs and symptoms may be related to the affected sinuses. It is important to note that studies have demonstrated no correlation between patient reports of "sinus headache" and presence of sinusitis on CT scan. Bacterial rhinosinusitis can be distinguished from viral rhinitis by persistence of symptoms more than 10 days after onset or worsening of symptoms within 10 days after initial improvement. Acute infections are defined as those lasting less than 4 weeks, with subacute infections lasting between 4 weeks and 12 weeks.

Acute maxillary sinusitis is the most common form of acute bacterial rhinosinusitis because the maxillary is the largest sinus with a single drainage pathway that is easily obstructed. Unilateral facial fullness, pressure, and tenderness over the cheek are common symptoms, but may not be present in many cases. Pain may refer to the upper incisor and canine teeth via branches of the trigeminal nerve, which traverse the floor of the sinus. Purulent nasal drainage should be noted with nasal airway obstruction or facial pain (pressure). Maxillary sinusitis may result from dental infection, and teeth that are tender should be carefully examined for signs of abscess. Removal of the diseased tooth or drainage of the periapical abscess typically resolves the sinus infection.

Acute ethmoiditis in adults is often accompanied by maxillary sinusitis, and symptoms are similar to those described above. Localized ethmoid sinusitis may present with pain and pressure over the high lateral wall of the nose between the eyes that may radiate to the orbit.

Sphenoid sinusitis is usually seen in the setting of pansinusitis or infection of all the paranasal sinuses on at least one side. The patient may complain of a headache "in the middle of the head" and often points to the vertex.

Acute frontal sinusitis may cause pain and tenderness of the forehead. This is most easily elicited by palpation of the orbital roof just below the medial end of the eyebrow.

Hospital-associated sinusitis is a form of acute bacterial rhinosinusitis that may present without any symptoms in the head and neck. It is a common source of fever in critically ill patients and is often associated with prolonged presence of a nasogastric or, rarely, nasotracheal tube causing inflammation of the nasal mucosa and ostiomeatal complex obstruction. Pansinusitis on the side of the tube is common on imaging studies.

B. Imaging

It is usually possible to make the diagnosis of acute bacterial rhinosinusitis on clinical grounds alone. Although more sensitive than clinical examination, routine radiographs are not cost-effective and are not recommended by the Agency for Health Care Policy and Research or American Association of Otolaryngology Guidelines in the routine diagnosis of acute bacterial rhinosinusitis. Consensus guidelines report that imaging may be helpful when clinically based criteria are difficult to evaluate, when the patient does not respond to appropriate therapy, when patients have been treated repeatedly with antibiotics for presumed sinusitis, when intracranial involvement or cerebrospinal fluid rhinorrhea is suspected, when complicated dental infection is suspected, or when symptoms of more serious infection are noted.

When necessary, noncontrast screening coronal CT scans are more cost-effective and provide more information than conventional sinus films. CT provides a rapid and effective means to assess all of the paranasal sinuses, identify areas of greater concern (such as bony dehiscence, periosteal elevation or maxillary tooth root exposure within the sinus), and speed appropriate therapy.

CT scans are reasonably sensitive but are not specific. Swollen soft tissue and fluid may be difficult to distinguish when opacification of the sinus is present from other conditions, such as chronic rhinosinusitis, nasal polyposis, or mucus retention cysts. Sinus abnormalities can be seen in most patients with an upper respiratory infection, while bacterial rhinosinusitis develops in only 2%.

If malignancy, intracranial extension, or opportunistic infection is suspected, MRI with gadolinium should be ordered instead of, or in addition to, CT. MRI will distinguish tumor from fluid, inflammation, and inspissated mucus far better than CT, as well as better delineating tumor extent with respect to adjacent structures, such as the orbit, skull base, and palate. Bone destruction can be demonstrated as well by MRI as by CT.

▶ Treatment

All patients with acute bacterial rhinosinusitis should have careful evaluation of pain. Nonsteroidal anti-inflammatory drugs are generally recommended. Sinus symptoms may be improved with oral or nasal decongestants (or both)—eg, oral pseudoephedrine, 30–120 mg per dose, up to 240 mg/day; nasal oxymetazoline, 0.05%; or xylometazoline, 0.05–0.1%, one or two sprays in each nostril every 6–8 hours for up to 3 days. All clinical practice guidelines recommend using intranasal corticosteroids (high-dose mometasone furoate 200 mcg each nostril twice daily for 21 days) from the initiation of symptoms that could be acute bacterial rhinosinusitis or acute viral rhinitis since meta-analysis demonstrates a small, but significant, reduction in facial pain and congestion scores with use.

Between 40% and 69% of patients with acute bacterial rhinosinusitis improve symptomatically within 2 weeks without antibiotic therapy. Antibiotic treatment is controversial in uncomplicated cases of clinically diagnosed acute bacterial rhinosinusitis because only 5% of patients will note a shorter duration of illness with treatment, and antibiotic treatment is associated with nearly twice the number of adverse events compared with placebo. Antibiotics may be considered when symptoms last more than 10 days or when symptoms (including fever, facial pain, and swelling of the face) are severe or when cases are complicated (such as immunodeficiency). In these patients, administration of antibiotics does reduce the incidence of clinical failure by 50% and represents the most cost-effective treatment strategy. Double-blinded studies exist to support numerous antibiotic choices. A summary of national guidelines for the treatment of acute sinusitis can be found in Table 8–4. Selection of antibiotics is usually empiric and based on a number of factors, including regional patterns of antibiotic resistance, antibiotic allergy, cost, and patient tolerance. Unless the patient is allergic to penicillin, amoxicillin should be used as the first-line agent. Treatment is usually for 7–10 days, although longer courses are sometimes required to prevent relapses. Macrolide therapy has been recommended as first-line therapy in patients with penicillin allergy, and tetracyclines have also been used.

Multidrug-resistant *S pneumoniae* prevalence is growing in many urban areas of the United States, as are beta-lactamase beta-lactam inhibitor–producing strains of *H influenza* and *M catarrhalis*. In such regions, guidelines call for empiric use of amoxicillin-clavulanate or second- or third-generation cephalosporins. Fluoroquinolones are reserved for treatment failures or for patients with a recent history of antibiotic therapy for another infection. Recurrent sinusitis or sinusitis that does not appear to respond clinically warrants CT imaging and evaluation by a specialist.

Hospital-associated infections in critically ill patients are treated differently from community-acquired infections. Broad-spectrum antibiotic coverage for bacteria, including *P aeruginosa*, *S aureus* (including methicillin-resistant strains), and anaerobes must be considered. Removal of the nasogastric tube and improved nasal hygiene (nasal saline sprays, humidification of supplemental nasal oxygen, and nasal decongestants) are critical interventions and often curative in mild cases without aggressive antibiotic use. Endoscopic or transantral cultures may help direct medical therapy in complicated cases.

Table 8–4. Oral antibiotic regimens for acute sinusitis.

Drug	Dose	Duration	Notes
First-line therapy			
Amoxicillin	1000 mg three times daily	7–10 days	
Trimethoprim-sulfamethoxazole	160 mg–800 mg twice daily	7–10 days	Suitable in penicillin allergy
Doxycycline	200 mg once daily × 1 day, 100 mg twice daily thereafter	7–10 days	Suitable in penicillin allergy
Amoxicillin-clavulanate[1]	1000/62.5 mg ER 2 tablets twice daily	10 days	
First-line therapy after recent antibiotic use (within 4–6 weeks)			
Levofloxacin	500 mg once daily	10 days	
Amoxicillin-clavulanate	875/125 mg twice daily	10 days	
Second-line therapy			
Amoxicillin-clavulanate	1000/62.5 mg ER 2 tablets twice daily	10 days	If no improvement after 3 days on first-line therapy
Moxifloxacin	400 mg once daily	10 days	If no improvement after 3 days on first-line therapy

[1]In communities where there is multidrug-resistant *S pneumoniae* and beta-lactamase beta-lactam inhibitor–producing strains of *H influenza* and *M catarrhalis*.

Adapted, with permission, from Marple BF et al. Acute bacterial rhinosinusitis: a review of US treatment guidelines. Otolaryngol Head Neck Surg. 2006 Sep;135(3):341–8. Copyright © 2006 Sage Publications. Reprinted by permission of Sage Publications.

Complications

Local complications of acute bacterial rhinosinusitis include orbital cellulitis and abscess, osteomyelitis, intracranial extension, and cavernous sinus thrombosis.

Any change in the ocular examination in a patient with acute bacterial rhinosinusitis necessitates immediate CT imaging. Orbital complications typically occur by extension of ethmoid sinusitis through the lamina papyracea, a thin layer of bone that comprises the medial orbital wall. Extension in this area may cause orbital cellulitis leading to proptosis, gaze restriction, and orbital pain. Select cases are responsive to intravenous antibiotics, with or without corticosteroids, and should be managed in close conjunction with an ophthalmologist or otolaryngologist, or both. Extension through the lamina papyracea can also lead to subperiosteal abscess formation (orbital abscess). Such abscesses cause marked proptosis, ophthalmoplegia, and pain with medial gaze. While some of these abscesses will respond to antibiotics, such findings should prompt an immediate referral to a specialist for consideration of decompression and evacuation. Failure to intervene quickly may lead to permanent visual impairment and a "frozen globe."

Osteomyelitis requires prolonged antibiotics as well as removal of necrotic bone. The frontal sinus is most commonly affected, with bone involvement suggested by a tender swelling of the forehead (Pott puffy tumor). Following treatment, secondary cosmetic reconstructive procedures may be necessary.

Intracranial complications of sinusitis can occur either through hematogenous spread, as in cavernous sinus thrombosis and meningitis, or by direct extension, as in epidural and intraparenchymal brain abscesses. Fortunately, they are rare today. Cavernous sinus thrombosis is heralded by ophthalmoplegia, chemosis, and visual loss. The diagnosis is most commonly confirmed by MRI, and when identified early, it typically responds to intravenous antibiotics. Frontal epidural and intracranial abscesses are often clinically silent, but may present with altered mental status, persistent fever, or severe headache.

When to Refer

Failure of acute bacterial rhinosinusitis to resolve after an adequate course of oral antibiotics may necessitate referral to an otolaryngologist for evaluation. Endoscopic cultures may direct further treatment choices. Nasal endoscopy and CT scan are indicated when symptoms persist longer than 4–12 weeks. Any patients with suspected extension of disease outside the sinuses should be evaluated urgently by an otolaryngologist and imaging should be obtained.

When to Admit

- Facial swelling and erythema indicative of facial cellulitis.
- Proptosis.
- Vision change or gaze abnormality indicative of orbital cellulitis.
- Abscess or cavernous sinus involvement.
- Mental status changes suggestive of intracranial extension.
- Immunocompromised status.
- Failure to respond to appropriate first-line treatment for acute bacterial rhinosinusitis or symptoms persisting longer than 4 weeks.

Hayward G et al. Intranasal corticosteroids in management of acute sinusitis: a systematic review and meta-analysis. Ann Fam Med. 2012 May–Jun;10(3):241–9. [PMID: 22585889]
Lemiengre MB et al. Antibiotics for clinically diagnosed acute rhinosinusitis in adults. Cochrane Database Syst Rev. 2012 Oct 17; 10:CD006089. [PMID: 23076918]

3. Nasal Vestibulitis & *S aureus* Nasal Colonization

Inflammation of the nasal vestibule may result from folliculitis of the hairs that line this orifice and is usually the result of nasal manipulation or hair trimming. Systemic antibiotics effective against *S aureus* (such as dicloxacillin, 250 mg orally four times daily for 7–10 days) are indicated. Topical mupirocin or bacitracin (applied two or three times daily) may be a helpful addition and may prevent future occurrences. If recurrent, the addition of rifampin (10 mg/kg orally twice daily for the last 4 days of treatment) may eliminate the *S aureus* carrier state. If a furuncle exists, it should be incised and drained, preferably intranasally. Adequate treatment of these infections is important to prevent retrograde spread of infection through valveless veins into the cavernous sinus and intracranial structures.

S aureus is the leading nosocomial pathogen in the world, and nasal carriage is a well-defined risk factor in the development and spread of nosocomial infections. Nasal and extranasal methicillin-resistant *S aureus* (MRSA) colonization are associated with a 30% risk of developing an invasive MRSA infection during hospital stays. While the vast majority of patients with nasal colonization have no vestibulitis symptoms, screening methods (including nasal swabs and PCR-based assays) have demonstrated rates of *S aureus* nasal colonization at around 30% and methicillin-resistant *S aureus* colonization in patients in the intensive care unit to be as high as 11%. Elimination of the carrier state is challenging, but studies of mupirocin (2% topical nasal application) with chlorhexidine facial washing (40 mg/mL) twice daily for 5 days have demonstrated decolonization in 39% of patients.

Sai N et al. Efficacy of the decolonization of methicillin-resistant *Staphylococcus aureus* carriers in clinical practice. Antimicrob Resist Infect Control. 2015 Dec 18;4:56. [PMID: 26688720]

4. Invasive Fungal Sinusitis

Invasive fungal sinusitis is rare and includes both rhinocerebral mucormycosis (*Mucor, Absidia,* and *Rhizopus sp.*) and other invasive fungal infections, such as *Aspergillus.* The fungus spreads rapidly through vascular channels and may be lethal if not detected early. Patients with mucormycosis almost invariably have a contributing factor that results in some degree of immunocompromise, such as diabetes mellitus, long-term corticosteroid therapy, or end-stage renal disease. Mucormycosis is more common, however, in patients who are profoundly immunocompromised for the treatment of hematologic malignancies. Occasional cases have been reported in patients with AIDS, though *Aspergillus sp.* is more common in this setting. The initial symptoms may be similar to those of acute bacterial rhinosinusitis, although facial pain is often more severe. Nasal drainage is typically clear or straw-colored, rather than purulent, and visual symptoms may be noted at presentation in the absence of significant nasal findings. On examination, the classic finding of mucormycosis is a black eschar on the middle turbinate. This finding is not universal and may be inapparent if the infection is deep or high within the nasal bones. Often the mucosa appears normal or simply pale and dry. Early diagnosis requires suspicion of the disease and nasal biopsy with silver stains, revealing broad nonseptate hyphae within tissues and necrosis with vascular occlusion. Because CT or MRI may initially show only soft tissue changes, biopsy and ultimate debridement should be based on the clinical setting rather than radiographic demonstration of bony destruction or intracranial changes.

Invasive fungal sinusitis represents a medical and surgical emergency. Once recognized, prompt wide surgical debridement and amphotericin B by intravenous infusion are indicated for patients with reversible immune deficiency. Lipid-based amphotericin B (Ambisome) may be used in patients who have kidney disease or in those in whom it develops secondary to nephrotoxic doses of nonlipid amphotericin. Other antifungals, including voriconazole and caspofungin, may be appropriate therapy depending on the speciation of the organism. There is evidence that suggests that iron chelator therapy may also be a useful adjunct. While necessary for any possibility of cure, surgical management often results in tremendous disfigurement and functional deficits. Even with early diagnosis and immediate appropriate intervention, the prognosis is guarded and often results in the loss of at least one eye. In persons with diabetes, the mortality rate is about 20%. If kidney disease is present or develops, mortality is over 50%; in the setting of AIDS or hematologic malignancy with neutropenia, mortality approaches 100%. Aggressive management with surgery should be considered carefully, since the disease-specific survival is only about 57%; because many patients are gravely ill at the time of diagnosis, the overall survival is about 18%.

Monroe MM et al. Invasive fungal rhinosinusitis: a 15-year experience with 29 patients. Laryngoscope. 2013 Jul;123(7):1583–7. [PMID: 23417294]

ALLERGIC RHINITIS

ESSENTIALS OF DIAGNOSIS

▶ Clear rhinorrhea, sneezing, tearing, eye irritation, and pruritus.

▶ Associated symptoms, including cough, bronchospasm, and eczematous dermatitis.

▶ Environmental allergen exposure with presence of allergen-specific IgE.

▶ General Considerations

Allergic rhinitis is very common in the United States. Population studies have reported the prevalence as between

14% and 40% among Americans, with most consensus panels agreeing on 20%. Allergic rhinitis adversely affects school and work performance, costing about $6 billion annually in the United States. These costs may be underestimated as epidemiology studies consistently show an association with asthma. Seasonal allergic rhinitis is most commonly caused by pollens and spores. Flowering shrub and tree pollens are most common in the spring, flowering plants and grasses in the summer, and ragweed and molds in the fall. Dust, household mites, air pollution, and pet dander may produce year-round symptoms, termed "perennial rhinitis."

Clinical Findings

The symptoms of "hay fever" are similar to those of viral rhinitis but are usually persistent and may show seasonal variation. Nasal symptoms are often accompanied by eye irritation, pruritus, conjunctival erythema, and excessive tearing. Many patients will note a strong family history of atopy or allergy.

The clinician should be careful to distinguish allergic rhinitis from nonallergic or vasomotor rhinitis. **Vasomotor rhinitis** is caused by increased sensitivity of the vidian nerve and is a common cause of clear rhinorrhea in the elderly. Often patients will report that they have troubling rhinorrhea in response to numerous nasal stimuli, including warm or cold air, odors or scents, light, or particulate matter.

On physical examination, the mucosa of the turbinates is usually pale or violaceous because of venous engorgement. This is in contrast to the erythema of viral rhinitis. Nasal polyps, which are yellowish boggy masses of hypertrophic mucosa, are associated with long-standing allergic rhinitis.

Treatment

A. Intranasal Corticosteroids

Intranasal corticosteroid sprays have revolutionized the treatment of allergic rhinitis. Evidence-based literature reviews show that these are more effective—and frequently less expensive—than nonsedating antihistamines. Patients should be reminded that there may be a delay in onset of relief of 2 or more weeks. Corticosteroid sprays may also shrink hypertrophic nasal mucosa and nasal polyps, thereby providing an improved nasal airway and ostiomeatal complex drainage. Because of this effect, intranasal corticosteroids are critical in treating allergy in patients prone to recurrent acute bacterial rhinosinusitis or chronic rhinosinusitis. There are many available preparations, including beclomethasone (42 mcg/spray twice daily per nostril), flunisolide (25 mcg/spray twice daily per nostril), mometasone furoate (200 mcg once daily per nostril), budesonide (100 mcg twice daily per nostril), and fluticasone propionate (200 mcg once daily per nostril). All intranasal corticosteroids are considered equally effective. Probably the most critical factors are compliance with regular use and proper introduction into the nasal cavity. In order to deliver medication to the region of the middle meatus, proper application involves holding the bottle straight up with the head tilted forward and pointing the bottle toward the ipsilateral ear when spraying. Side effects are limited and the most annoying is epistaxis. Some experts believe that this is related to incorrect delivery of the drug to the nasal septum.

B. Antihistamines

Antihistamines offer temporary, but immediate, control of many of the most troubling symptoms of allergic rhinitis. Effective antihistamines include nonsedating loratadine (10 mg orally once daily), desloratadine (5 mg once daily), and fexofenadine (60 mg twice daily or 120 mg once daily), and minimally sedating cetirizine (10 mg orally once daily). Brompheniramine or chlorpheniramine (4 mg orally every 6–8 hours, or 8–12 mg orally every 8–12 hours as a sustained-release tablet) and clemastine (1.34–2.68 mg orally twice daily) may be less expensive although usually associated with some drowsiness. The H_1-receptor antagonist nasal spray azelastine (1–2 sprays per nostril daily) has also been shown to be effective in a randomized trial, although many patients object to its bitter taste. Topical nasal sprays are particularly useful in patients who experience side effects, mostly xerostomia and sedation, of oral antihistamines. Many patients who find initial benefit from an antihistamine complain that allergy symptoms eventually return after several months of use. In such patients, typically with perennial allergy problems, antihistamine tolerance seems to develop, and alternating effective antihistamines periodically can control symptoms over the long term.

C. Adjunctive Treatment Measures

In addition to intranasal corticosteroid sprays and antihistamines, including H_1-receptor antagonists, the literature supports the use of antileukotriene medications, such as montelukast (10 mg/day orally), alone or with cetirizine (10 mg/day orally), or loratadine (10 mg/day orally). Improved nasal rhinorrhea, sneezing, and congestion are seen with the use of leukotriene receptor antagonists, often in conjunction with antihistamines. Cromolyn sodium and sodium nedocromil are also useful adjunct agents for allergic rhinitis. They work by stabilizing mast cells and preventing proinflammatory mediator release. They are not absorbed by the gastrointestinal tract but do function topically and have very few side effects. The most useful form of cromolyn is probably the ophthalmologic preparation; the nasal preparation is not nearly as effective as inhaled corticosteroids. Intranasal cromolyn is cleared rapidly and must be administered four times daily for continued relief of symptoms.

Intranasal anticholinergic agents, such as ipratropium bromide 0.03% or 0.06% sprays (42–84 mcg per nostril three times daily), may be helpful adjuncts when rhinorrhea is a major symptom. Ipratropium nasal sprays are not as effective as intranasal corticosteroids for treating allergic rhinitis but are particularly useful for treating **vasomotor rhinitis**.

Avoiding or reducing exposure to airborne allergens is the most effective means of alleviating symptoms of allergic rhinitis. Depending on the allergen, this can be extremely difficult. Maintaining an allergen-free environment by covering pillows and mattresses with plastic covers, substituting synthetic materials (foam mattress, acrylics) for animal products (wool, horsehair), and removing dust-collecting household fixtures (carpets, drapes, bedspreads, wicker) is worth the attempt to help more troubled patients. Air purifiers and dust filters may also aid in maintaining an allergen-free environment. Nasal saline irrigations are a useful adjunct in the treatment of allergic rhinitis to mechanically flush the allergens from the nasal cavity. Though debated, there is no clear benefit to hypertonic saline over commercially available normal saline preparations (eg, Ayr or Ocean Spray). When symptoms are extremely bothersome, a search for offending allergens may prove helpful. This can either be done by serum radioallergosorbent test (RAST) testing or skin testing by an allergist.

In some cases, allergic rhinitis symptoms are inadequately relieved by medication and avoidance measures. Often, such patients have a strong family history of atopy and may also have lower respiratory manifestations, such as allergic asthma. Referral to an allergist may be appropriate for consideration of immunotherapy. This treatment course is quite involved, with proper identification of offending allergens, progressively increasing doses of allergen(s), and eventual maintenance dose administration over a period of 3–5 years. Immunotherapy has been proven to reduce circulating IgE levels in patients with allergic rhinitis and reduce the need for allergy medications. Both subcutaneous and sublingual immunotherapy have been shown to be effective in the long-term treatment of refractory allergic rhinitis. Treatments are given at a suitable medical facility with monitoring following treatment because of the risk of anaphylaxis during dose escalation. Local reactions from injections are common and usually self-limited.

Caimmi D et al. Allergen immunotherapy outcomes and unmet needs: a critical review. Immunol Allergy Clin North Am. 2016 Feb;36(1):181–9. [PMID: 26617234]

Hoyte FC et al. Recommendations for the pharmacologic management of allergic rhinitis. Allergy Asthma Proc. 2014 May–Jun; 35(Suppl 1):S20–7. [PMID: 25582158]

Nankervis H et al. House dust mite reduction and avoidance measures for treating eczema. Cochrane Database Syst Rev. 2015 Jan 19;1:CD008426. [PMID: 25598014]

OLFACTORY DYSFUNCTION

 ESSENTIALS OF DIAGNOSIS

► Subjective diminished smell or taste sensation.

► Lack of objective nasal obstruction.

► Objective decrease in olfaction demonstrated by testing.

► General Considerations

Anatomic blockage of the nasal cavity with subsequent airflow disruption is the most common cause of olfactory dysfunction (hyposmia or anosmia). Polyps, septal deformities, and nasal tumors may be the cause. Transient olfactory dysfunction often accompanies the common cold, nasal allergies, and perennial rhinitis through changes in the nasal and olfactory epithelium. About 20% of olfactory dysfunction is idiopathic, although it often follows a viral illness. Central nervous system neoplasms, especially those that involve the olfactory groove or temporal lobe, may affect olfaction and must be considered in patients with no other explanation for their hyposmia or other neurologic signs. Head trauma is a rare but severe cause of olfactory dysfunction. Shearing of the olfactory neurites accounts for less than 5% of cases of hyposmia but is more commonly associated with anosmia. Absent, diminished, or distorted smell or taste has been reported in a wide variety of endocrine, nutritional, and nervous disorders. In particular, olfactory dysfunction in Parkinson disease and Alzheimer disease has been the subject of research as neurofibrillary tangles and Lewy bodies are found throughout the olfactory system. Quantitation of olfactory dysfunction may serve as a useful marker of disease progression and response to specific treatment.

► Clinical Findings

Evaluation of olfactory dysfunction should include a thorough history of systemic illnesses and medication use as well as a physical examination focusing on the nose and nervous system. Nasal obstruction (from polyps, trauma, foreign bodies, or nasal masses) can cause functional hyposmia and should be excluded before concluding that the disruption of olfaction is primary. Most clinical offices are not set up to test olfaction, but such tests may at times be worthwhile if only to assess whether a patient possesses any sense of smell at all. The University of Pennsylvania Smell Identification Test (UPSIT) is available commercially and is a simple, self-administered "scratch-and-sniff" test that is useful in differentiating hyposmia, anosmia, and malingering. Odor threshold can be tested at regional specialty centers using increasing concentrations of various odorants.

► Treatment

Hyposmia secondary to nasal polyposis, obstruction, and chronic rhinosinusitis may respond to endoscopic sinus surgery. Unfortunately, there is no specific treatment for primary disruption of olfaction. While some disturbances spontaneously resolve, little evidence supports the use of large doses of vitamin A and zinc in patients with transient olfactory dysfunction. The degree of hyposmia is the greatest predictor of recovery, with less severe hyposmia recovering at a much higher rate. In permanent hyposmia, counseling should be offered about seasoning foods with spices (eg, pepper) that stimulate the trigeminal as well as olfactory chemoreceptors, abuse of table salt as a seasoning, and safety issues, such as the use of smoke alarms and electric rather than gas home appliances.

Coelho DH et al. Posttraumatic olfactory dysfunction. Auris Nasus Larynx. 2015 Oct 1. [Epub ahead of print] [PMID: 26441369]

Franks KH et al. Connectivity of pathology: the olfactory system as a model for network-driven mechanisms of Alzheimer's disease pathogenesis. Front Aging Neurosci. 2015 Dec 15; 7:234. [PMID: 26696886]

EPISTAXIS

ESSENTIALS OF DIAGNOSIS

▶ Bleeding from the unilateral anterior nasal cavity most commonly.

▶ Most cases may be successfully treated by direct pressure on the bleeding site for 15 minutes. When this is inadequate, topical sympathomimetics and various nasal tamponade methods are usually effective.

▶ Posterior, bilateral, or large-volume epistaxis should be triaged immediately to a specialist in a critical care setting.

▶ General Considerations

Epistaxis is an extremely common problem in the primary care setting. Predisposing factors include nasal trauma (nose picking, foreign bodies, forceful nose blowing), rhinitis, drying of the nasal mucosa from low humidity or supplemental nasal oxygen, deviation of the nasal septum, atherosclerotic disease, hereditary hemorrhagic telangiectasia (Osler-Weber-Rendu syndrome), inhaled nasal cocaine or other drug use, and alcohol use. Poorly controlled hypertension has traditionally been associated with epistaxis, although confounding factors during bleeding events make establishing a causal relationship impossible. Anticoagulation or antiplatelet medications may be associated with a higher incidence of epistaxis, more frequent recurrence of epistaxis, and greater difficulty controlling bleeding, but they do not cause epistaxis. Bleeding is most common in the anterior septum where a confluence of veins creates a superficial venous plexus (Kiesselbach plexus).

▶ Clinical Findings

It is important in all patients with epistaxis to consider underlying causes of the bleeding. Laboratory assessment of bleeding parameters may be indicated, especially in recurrent cases. Once the acute episode has passed, careful examination of the nose and paranasal sinuses to rule out neoplasia and hereditary hemorrhagic telangiectasia is wise.

Patients presenting with epistaxis often have higher blood pressures than control patients, but in many cases, blood pressure returns to normal following treatment of acute bleeding. Repeat evaluation for clinically significant hypertension and treatment should be performed following control of epistaxis and removal of any packing.

▶ Treatment

Most cases of anterior epistaxis may be successfully treated by direct pressure on the site by compression of the nares continuously for 15 minutes. Venous pressure is reduced in the sitting position, and slight leaning forward lessens the swallowing of blood. Short-acting topical nasal decongestants (eg, phenylephrine, 0.125–1% solution, one or two sprays), which act as vasoconstrictors, may also be helpful. When the bleeding does not readily subside, the nose should be examined, using good illumination and suction, in an attempt to locate the bleeding site. Topical 4% cocaine applied either as a spray or on a cotton strip serves both as an anesthetic and a vasoconstrictor. If cocaine is unavailable, a topical decongestant (eg, oxymetazoline) and a topical anesthetic (eg, tetracaine or lidocaine) provide similar results. When visible, the bleeding site may be cauterized with silver nitrate, diathermy, or electrocautery. A supplemental patch of Surgicel or Gelfoam may be helpful with a moisture barrier, such as petroleum-based ointment, to prevent drying and crusting.

Occasionally, a site of bleeding may be inaccessible to direct control, or attempts at direct control may be unsuccessful. In such cases there are a number of alternatives. When the site of bleeding is anterior, a hemostatic sealant, pneumatic nasal tamponade, or anterior packing may suffice. There are a number of ways to do this, such as with several feet of lubricated iodoform packing systematically placed in the floor of the nose and then the vault of the nose, or with various manufactured products designed for nasal tamponade.

About 5% of nasal bleeding originates in the **posterior nasal cavity**. Such bleeds are more commonly associated with atherosclerotic disease and hypertension. If an anteriorly placed pneumatic nasal tamponade is unsuccessful, it may be necessary to consult an otolaryngologist for a pack to occlude the choana before placing a pack anteriorly. In emergency settings, double balloon packs (Epistat) may facilitate rapid control of bleeding with little or no mucosal trauma. Because such packing is uncomfortable, bleeding may persist, and vasovagal syncope is quite possible, hospitalization for monitoring and stabilization is indicated. Opioid analgesics are needed to reduce the considerable discomfort and elevated blood pressure caused by a posterior pack.

Surgical management of epistaxis, through ligation of the nasal arterial supply (internal maxillary artery and ethmoid arteries) is an alternative to posterior nasal packing. Endovascular embolization of the internal maxillary artery or facial artery is also quite effective and can allow very specific control of hemorrhage. Such alternatives are necessary when packing fails to control life-threatening hemorrhage. On very rare occasions, ligation of the external carotid artery may be necessary.

After control of epistaxis, the patient is advised to avoid straining and vigorous exercise for several days. Nasal saline should be applied to the packing frequently to keep the packing moist. Avoidance of hot or spicy foods and tobacco is also advisable, since these may cause nasal vasodilation. Avoiding nasal trauma, including nose picking, is an obvious necessity. Lubrication with petroleum jelly or bacitracin ointment and increased home humidity may also be useful ancillary measures. Finally, antistaphylococcal antibiotics (eg, cephalexin, 500 mg orally four times daily, or clindamycin, 150 mg orally four times daily) are indicated to reduce the risk of toxic shock syndrome developing while the packing remains in place (at least 5 days).

When to Refer

- Patients with recurrent epistaxis, large-volume epistaxis, and episodic epistaxis with associated nasal obstruction should be referred to an otolaryngologist for endoscopic evaluation and possible imaging.
- Those with ongoing bleeding beyond 15 minutes should be taken to a local emergency department if the clinician is not prepared to manage acute epistaxis.

Barnes ML et al. Epistaxis: a contemporary evidence based approach. Otolaryngol Clin North Am. 2012 Oct;45(5):1005–17. [PMID: 22980681]
Kikidis D et al. Is epistaxis associated with arterial hypertension? A systematic review of the literature. Eur Arch Otorhinolaryngol. 2014 Feb;271(2):237–43. [PMID: 23539411]

NASAL TRAUMA

The nasal pyramid is the most frequently fractured bone in the body. Fracture is suggested by crepitance or palpably mobile bony segments. Epistaxis and pain are common, as are soft-tissue hematomas ("black eye"). It is important to make certain that there is no palpable step-off of the infraorbital rim, which would indicate the presence of a zygomatic complex fracture. Radiologic confirmation may at times be helpful but is not necessary in uncomplicated nasal fractures. It is also important to assess for possible concomitant additional facial, pulmonary, or intracranial injuries when the circumstances of injury are suggestive, as in the case of automobile and motorcycle accidents.

Treatment is aimed at maintaining long-term nasal airway patency and cosmesis. Closed reduction can be performed under local or general anesthesia. A recent meta-analysis suggests that in spite of the decreased cost associated with local procedures, closed reduction under general anesthesia afforded better patient satisfaction and decreased need for subsequent revision septoplasty or rhinoplasty.

Intranasal examination should be performed in all cases to rule out septal hematoma, which appears as a widening of the anterior septum, visible just posterior to the columella. The septal cartilage receives its only nutrition from its closely adherent mucoperichondrium. An untreated subperichondrial hematoma will result in loss of the nasal cartilage with resultant saddle nose deformity. Septal hematomas may become infected, with *S aureus*

most commonly, and should be drained with an incision in the inferior mucoperichondrium on both sides.

Packing for 2–5 days is often helpful to help prevent reformation of the hematoma. Antibiotics with antistaphylococcal efficacy (eg, cephalexin, 500 mg four times daily, or clindamycin, 150 mg four times daily) should be given for 3–5 days or the duration of the packing to reduce the risk of toxic shock syndrome and the drained fluid sent for culture.

Al-Moraissi EA et al. Local versus general anesthesia for the management of nasal bone fractures: a systematic review and meta-analysis. J Oral Maxillofac Surg. 2015 Apr;73(4):606–15. [PMID: 25577456]

TUMORS & GRANULOMATOUS DISEASE

1. Benign Nasal Tumors

A. Nasal Polyps

Nasal polyps are pale, edematous, mucosally covered masses commonly seen in patients with allergic rhinitis, but compelling evidence argues against a purely allergic pathogenesis. They may result in chronic nasal obstruction and a diminished sense of smell. In patients with nasal polyps and a history of asthma, aspirin should be avoided as it may precipitate a severe episode of bronchospasm, known as **triad asthma** (Samter triad). Such patients may have an immunologic salicylate sensitivity. The presence of polyps in children should suggest the possibility of cystic fibrosis.

Use of topical intranasal corticosteroids improves the quality of life in patients with nasal polyposis and chronic rhinosinusitis. Initial treatment with topical nasal corticosteroids (see Allergic Rhinitis section for specific drugs) for 1–3 months is usually successful for small polyps and may reduce the need for operation. A short course of oral corticosteroids (eg, prednisone, 6-day course using 21 [5-mg] tablets: 30 mg on day 1 and tapering by 5 mg each day) may also be of benefit. When polyps are massive or medical management is unsuccessful, polyps may be removed surgically. In healthy persons, this is a minor outpatient procedure. In recurrent cases or when surgery itself is associated with increased risk (such as in patients with asthma), a more complete procedure, such as ethmoidectomy, may be advisable. In recurrent polyposis, it may be necessary to remove polyps from the ethmoid, sphenoid, and maxillary sinuses to provide longer-lasting relief. Intranasal corticosteroids should be continued following polyp removal to prevent recurrence, and the clinician should consider allergen testing to determine the offending allergen and avoidance measures.

Martinez-Devesa P et al. Oral steroids for nasal polyps. Cochrane Database Syst Rev. 2011 Jul 6;(7):CD005232. [PMID: 21735400]
Rudmik L et al. Impact of topical nasal steroid therapy on symptoms of nasal polyposis: a meta-analysis. Laryngoscope. 2012 Jul; 122(7):1431–7. [PMID: 22410935]

B. Inverted Papilloma

Inverted papillomas are benign tumors caused by human papillomavirus (HPV) that usually arise on the lateral nasal wall. They present with unilateral nasal obstruction and occasionally hemorrhage. They are often easily seen on anterior rhinoscopy as cauliflower-like growths in or around the middle meatus. Because squamous cell carcinoma is seen in about 10% of inverted or schneiderian papillomas, complete excision is strongly recommended. This usually requires a medial maxillectomy, but in selected cases an endoscopic approach may be possible. Because recurrence rates for inverted papilloma are reported to be as high as 20%, subsequent clinical and radiologic follow-up is imperative. All excised tissue (not just a portion) should be carefully reviewed by the pathologist to be sure no carcinoma is present.

Govindaraj S et al. Does human papilloma virus play a role in sinonasal inverted papilloma? Curr Opin Otolaryngol Head Neck Surg. 2014 Feb;22(1):47–51. [PMID: 24322658]
Syrjänen K et al. Detection of human papillomavirus in sinonasal papillomas: systematic review and meta-analysis. Laryngoscope. 2013 Jan;123(1):181–92. [PMID: 23161522]

2. Malignant Nasopharyngeal & Paranasal Sinus Tumors

Though rare, malignant tumors of the nose, nasopharynx, and paranasal sinuses are quite problematic because they tend to remain asymptomatic until late in their course. Squamous cell carcinoma is the most common cancer found in the sinuses and nasopharynx. It is especially common in the nasopharynx, where it obstructs the eustachian tube and results in serous otitis media. Nasopharyngeal carcinoma (nonkeratinizing squamous cell carcinoma or lymphoepithelioma) is usually associated with elevated IgA antibody to the viral capsid antigen of the Epstein-Barr virus (EBV). It is particularly common in patients of southern Chinese descent and has a weaker association with tobacco exposure than other head and neck squamous cell carcinomas. Adenocarcinomas, mucosal melanomas, sarcomas, and non-Hodgkin lymphomas are less commonly encountered neoplasms of this area.

Early symptoms are nonspecific, mimicking those of rhinitis or sinusitis. Unilateral nasal obstruction, otitis media, and discharge are common, with pain and recurrent hemorrhage often clues to the diagnosis of cancer. Any adult with persistent unilateral nasal symptoms or new otitis media should be thoroughly evaluated with nasal endoscopy and nasopharyngoscopy. A high index of suspicion remains a key to early diagnosis of these tumors. Patients often present with advanced symptoms, such as proptosis, expansion of a cheek, or ill-fitting maxillary dentures. Malar hypesthesia, due to involvement of the infraorbital nerve, is common in maxillary sinus tumors. Biopsy is necessary for definitive diagnosis, and MRI is the best imaging study to delineate the extent of disease and plan appropriate surgery and radiation.

Treatment depends on the tumor type and the extent of disease. Very early stage disease may be treated with megavoltage radiation therapy alone, but advanced

nasopharyngeal carcinoma is best treated with concurrent radiation and cisplatin followed by adjuvant chemotherapy with cisplatin and fluorouracil. This chemoradiation therapy protocol significantly decreases local, nodal, and distant failures and increases progression-free and overall survival in advanced stage disease. Locally recurrent nasopharyngeal carcinoma may in selected cases be treated with repeat irradiation protocols or surgery with moderate success and a high degree of concern about local wound healing. Other squamous cell carcinomas are best treated—when resectable—with a combination of surgery and irradiation. Cranial base surgery, which can be done endoscopically using image navigation, appears to be an effective modality in improving the overall prognosis in paranasal sinus malignancies eroding the ethmoid roof. Although the prognosis is poor for advanced tumors, the results of treating resectable tumors of paranasal sinus origin have improved with the wider use of skull base resections and intensity-modulated radiation therapy. Cure rates are often 45–60%.

Lee AW et al. Management of nasopharyngeal carcinoma: current practice and future perspective. J Clin Oncol. 2015 Oct 10;33(29):3356–64. [PMID: 26351355]

3. Sinonasal Inflammatory Disease (Granulomatosis with Polyangiitis & Sarcoidosis)

The nose and paranasal sinuses are involved in over 90% of cases of **granulomatosis with polyangiitis**. It is often not realized that involvement at these sites is more common than involvement of lungs or kidneys. Examination shows bloodstained crusts and friable mucosa. Biopsy, when positive, shows necrotizing granulomas and vasculitis. Other recognized sites of granulomatosis with polyangiitis in the head and neck include the subglottis and the middle ear.

Sarcoidosis commonly involves the paranasal sinuses and is clinically similar to other chronic sinonasal inflammatory processes. Sinonasal symptoms, including rhinorrhea, nasal obstruction, and hyposmia or anosmia may precede diagnosis of sarcoidosis in other organ systems. Clinically, the turbinates appear engorged with small white granulomas. Biopsy shows classic noncaseating granulomas. Notably, patients with sinonasal involvement generally have more trouble managing sarcoidosis in other organ systems.

Polymorphic reticulosis (midline malignant reticulosis, idiopathic midline destructive disease, lethal midline granuloma)—as the multitude of apt descriptive terms suggest—is not well understood but appears to be a nasal T-cell or NK-cell lymphoma. In contrast to granulomatosis with polyangiitis, involvement is limited to the mid-face, and there may be extensive bone destruction. Many destructive lesions of the mucosa and nasal structures labeled as polymorphic reticulosis are in fact non-Hodgkin lymphoma of either NK-cell or T-cell origin. Immunophenotyping, especially for CD56 expression, is essential in the histologic evaluation. Even when apparently localized, these lymphomas have a poor prognosis, with progression and death within a year the rule.

For treatment of granulomatosis with polyangiitis, see Chapter 20.

Gulati S et al. Sinonasal involvement in sarcoidosis: a report of seven cases and review of literature. Eur Arch Otorhinolaryngol. 2012 Mar;269(3):891–6. [PMID: 21947433]

Taylor SC et al. Progression and management of Wegener's granulomatosis in the head and neck. Laryngoscope. 2012 Aug; 122(8):1695–700. [PMID: 22674560]

▼ DISEASES OF THE ORAL CAVITY & PHARYNX

LEUKOPLAKIA, ERYTHROPLAKIA, ORAL LICHEN PLANUS & ORAL CANCER

 ESSENTIALS OF DIAGNOSIS

► **Leukoplakia**—A white lesion that cannot be removed by rubbing the mucosal surface.

► **Erythroplakia**—Similar to leukoplakia except that it has a definite erythematous component.

► **Oral Lichen Planus**—Most commonly presents as lacy leukoplakia but may be erosive; definitive diagnosis requires biopsy.

► **Oral Cancer**—Early lesions appear as leukoplakia or erythroplakia; more advanced lesions will be larger, with invasion into the tongue such that a mass lesion is palpable. Ulceration may be present.

Leukoplakic regions range from small to several centimeters in diameter (Figure 8–3). Histologically, they are often hyperkeratoses occurring in response to chronic irritation (eg, from dentures, tobacco, lichen planus); about 2–6%, however, represent either dysplasia or early invasive squamous cell carcinoma. Distinguishing

▲ **Figure 8–3.** Leukoplakia with moderate dysplasia on the lateral border of the tongue. (From Ellen Eisenberg, DMD; reproduced, with permission, from Usatine RP, Smith MA, Mayeaux EJ Jr, Chumley H, Tysinger J. *The Color Atlas of Family Medicine.* McGraw-Hill, 2009.)

between **erythroplakia** and **leukoplakia** is important because about 90% of cases of erythroplakia are either dysplasia or carcinoma. **Squamous cell carcinoma** accounts for 90% of oral cancer. Alcohol and tobacco use are the major epidemiologic risk factors.

The differential diagnosis may include oral candidiasis, necrotizing sialometaplasia, pseudoepitheliomatous hyperplasia, median rhomboid glossitis, and vesiculoerosive inflammatory disease, such as erosive lichen planus. This should not be confused with the brown-black gingival melanin pigmentation—diffuse or speckled—common in nonwhites, blue-black embedded fragments of dental amalgam, or other systemic disorders associated with general pigmentation (neurofibromatosis, familial polyposis, Addison disease). Intraoral melanoma is extremely rare and carries a dismal prognosis.

Any area of **erythroplakia**, enlarging area of **leukoplakia**, or a lesion that has submucosal depth on palpation should have an incisional biopsy or an exfoliative cytologic examination. Ulcerative lesions are particularly suspicious and worrisome. Specialty referral should be sought early both for diagnosis and treatment. A systematic intraoral examination—including the lateral tongue, floor of the mouth, gingiva, buccal area, palate, and tonsillar fossae—and palpation of the neck for enlarged lymph nodes should be part of any general physical examination, especially in patients over the age of 45 who smoke tobacco or drink immoderately. Indirect or fiberoptic examination of the nasopharynx, oropharynx, hypopharynx, and larynx by an otolaryngologist, head and neck surgeon, or radiation oncologist should also be considered for such patients when there is unexplained or persistent throat or ear pain, oral or nasal bleeding, or oral erythroplakia. Fine-needle aspiration (FNA) biopsy may expedite the diagnosis if an enlarged lymph node is found. To date, there are no approved therapies for reversing or stabilizing leukoplakia or erythroplakia.

Oral lichen planus is a relatively common (0.5–2% of the population) chronic inflammatory autoimmune disease that may be difficult to diagnose clinically because of its numerous distinct phenotypic subtypes. For example, the reticular pattern may mimic candidiasis or hyperkeratosis, while the erosive pattern may mimic squamous cell carcinoma. Management begins with distinguishing it from other oral lesions. Exfoliative cytology or a small incisional or excisional biopsy is indicated, especially if squamous cell carcinoma is suspected. Therapy is aimed at managing pain and discomfort. Corticosteroids have been used widely both locally and systemically. Cyclosporines and retinoids have also been used. Many think there is a low rate (1%) of squamous cell carcinoma arising within lichen planus (in addition to the possibility of clinical misdiagnosis).

Hairy leukoplakia occurs on the lateral border of the tongue and is a common early finding in HIV infection (see Chapter 31). It often develops quickly and appears as slightly raised leukoplakic areas with a corrugated or "hairy" surface (Figure 8–4). Clinical response following administration of zidovudine or acyclovir has been reported, and treatment is under active investigation.

▲ **Figure 8–4.** Oral hairy leukoplakia on the side of the tongue in AIDS. (Used, with permission, from Richard P. Usatine, MD, in Usatine RP, Smith MA, Mayeaux EJ Jr, Chumley H, Tysinger J. *The Color Atlas of Family Medicine.* McGraw-Hill, 2009.)

Early detection of **squamous cell carcinoma** is the key to successful management (Figure 8–5). Lesions less than 4 mm in depth have a low propensity to metastasize. Most patients in whom the tumor is detected before it is 2 cm in diameter are cured by local resection. Radiation is an alternative but not generally used as first-line therapy for small lesions. Large tumors are usually treated with a combination of resection, neck dissection, and external beam radiation. Reconstruction, if required, is done at the time of resection and can involve the use of myocutaneous flaps or vascularized free flaps with or without bone.

Clinical trials have suggested a role for beta-carotene, cyclooxygenase (COX)-2 inhibitors, vitamin E, and retinoids in producing regression of leukoplakia and reducing the incidence of recurrent squamous cell carcinomas. Retinoids suppress head and neck and lung carcinogenesis in animal models and inhibit carcinogenesis in individuals with premalignant lesions. They also seem to reduce the incidence of second primary cancers in head and neck and lung cancer patients previously treated for a primary cancer.

García-García V et al. New perspectives on the dynamic behaviour of oral lichen planus. Eur J Dermatol. 2012 Mar–Apr; 22(2):172–7. [PMID: 22381396]

ORAL CANDIDIASIS

 ESSENTIALS OF DIAGNOSIS

► Fluctuating throat or mouth discomfort.

► Systemic or local immunosuppression, such as recent corticosteroid, chemotherapy, or antibiotic use.

► Erythema of the oral cavity or oropharynx with fluffy, white patches.

► Rapid resolution of symptoms with appropriate treatment.

► **Clinical Findings**

A. Symptoms and Signs

Oral candidiasis (thrush) is usually painful and looks like creamy-white curd-like patches overlying erythematous mucosa (see Figure 6–23). Because these white areas are easily rubbed off (eg, by a tongue depressor)—unlike leukoplakia or lichen planus—only the underlying irregular erythema may be seen. Oral candidiasis is commonly associated with the following risk factors: (1) use of dentures, (2) debilitated state with poor oral hygiene, (3) diabetes, (4) anemia, (5) chemotherapy or local irradiation, and (6) corticosteroid use (oral or systemic) or broad-spectrum antibiotics. Angular cheilitis is another manifestation of candidiasis, although it is also seen in nutritional deficiencies (Figure 8–6).

▲ **Figure 8–5.** Squamous cell carcinoma of the palate. (From Frank Miller, MD; reproduced, with permission, from Usatine RP, Smith MA, Mayeaux EJ Jr, Chumley H, Tysinger J. *The Color Atlas of Family Medicine.* McGraw-Hill, 2009.)

▲ **Figure 8–6.** Severe angular cheilitis in HIV-positive man with oral thrush. (Used, with permission, from Richard P. Usatine, MD, in Usatine RP, Smith MA, Mayeaux EJ Jr, Chumley H, Tysinger J. *The Color Atlas of Family Medicine.* McGraw-Hill, 2009.)

B. Diagnostic Studies

The diagnosis is made clinically. A wet preparation using potassium hydroxide will reveal spores and may show non-septate mycelia. Biopsy will show intraepithelial pseudo-mycelia of *Candida albicans*.

Candidiasis is often the first manifestation of HIV infection, and HIV testing should be considered in patients with no known predisposing cause for *Candida* over-growth (see also Chapter 31). The US Department of Health Services Clinical Practice Guideline for Evaluation and Management of Early HIV Infection recommends examination of the oral mucosa with each clinician visit as well as at a dental examination every 6 months for individuals infected with HIV.

► Treatment

Effective antifungal therapy may be achieved with any of the following: fluconazole (100 mg orally daily for 7 days), ketoconazole (200–400 mg orally with breakfast [requires acidic gastric environment for absorption] for 7–14 days), clotrimazole troches (10 mg dissolved orally five times daily), or nystatin mouth rinses (500,000 units [5 mL of 100,000 units/mL] held in the mouth before swallowing three times daily). In patients with HIV infection, however, longer courses of therapy with fluconazole may be needed, and oral itraconazole (200 mg/day) may be indicated in fluconazole-refractory cases. Many of the *Candida* species in these patients are resistant to first-line azoles and may require newer drugs, such as voriconazole. In addition, 0.12% chlorhexidine or half-strength hydrogen peroxide mouth rinses may provide local relief. Nystatin powder (100,000 units/g) applied to dentures three or four times daily and rinsed off for several weeks may help denture wearers.

Pienaar ED et al. Interventions for the prevention and management of oropharyngeal candidiasis associated with HIV infection in adults and children. Cochrane Database Syst Rev. 2010 Nov 10;11:CD003940. [PMID: 21069679]
Singh A et al. Oral candidiasis: an overview. J Oral Maxillofac Pathol. 2014 Sep;18(Suppl 1):S81–5. [PMID: 25364186]

GLOSSITIS, GLOSSODYNIA, DYSGEUSIA & BURNING MOUTH SYNDROME

Inflammation of the tongue with loss of filiform papillae leads to a red, smooth-surfaced tongue (glossitis). Rarely painful, it may be secondary to nutritional deficiencies (eg, niacin, riboflavin, iron, or vitamin E), drug reactions, dehydration, irritants, or foods and liquids, and possibly to autoimmune reactions or psoriasis. If the primary cause cannot be identified and corrected, empiric nutritional replacement therapy may be of value.

Glossodynia is burning and pain of the tongue, which may occur with or without glossitis. In the absence of any clinical findings, it has been termed "burning mouth syndrome." Glossodynia with glossitis has been associated with diabetes mellitus, drugs (eg, diuretics), tobacco, xerostomia, and candidiasis as well as the listed causes of glossitis. Periodontal disease is not apt to be a factor.

The burning mouth syndrome typically has no identifiable associated risk factors and seems to be most common in postmenopausal women. Treating possible underlying causes, changing long-term medications to alternative ones, and smoking cessation may resolve symptoms of glossitis. Both glossodynia and the burning mouth syndrome are benign, and reassurance that there is no infection or tumor is likely to be appreciated. Effective treatments for the burning mouth syndrome include alpha-lipoic acid and clonazepam. Clonazepam is most effective as a rapid-dissolving tablet placed on the tongue in doses from 0.25 mg to 0.5 mg every 8–12 hours. Behavioral therapy has also been shown to be effective. Unilateral symptoms, symptoms that cannot be related to a specific medication, and symptoms and signs involving regions supplied by other cranial nerves all may suggest neuropathology, and imaging of the brain, brainstem, and skull base with MRI should be considered.

Minor JS et al. Burning mouth syndrome and secondary oral burning. Otolaryngol Clin North Am. 2011 Feb;44(1):205–19. [PMID: 21093630]

INTRAORAL ULCERATIVE LESIONS

1. Necrotizing Ulcerative Gingivitis (Trench Mouth, Vincent Angina)

Necrotizing ulcerative gingivitis, often caused by an infection of both spirochetes and fusiform bacilli, is common in young adults under stress (classically in students at examination time). Underlying systemic diseases may also predispose to this disorder. Clinically, there is painful acute gingival inflammation and necrosis, often with bleeding, halitosis, fever, and cervical lymphadenopathy. Warm half-strength peroxide rinses and oral penicillin (250 mg three times daily for 10 days) may help. Dental gingival curettage may prove necessary.

Atout RN et al. Managing patients with necrotizing ulcerative gingivitis. J Can Dent Assoc. 2013;79:d46. [PMID: 23763733]

2. Aphthous Ulcer (Canker Sore, Ulcerative Stomatitis)

Aphthous ulcers are very common and easy to recognize. Their cause remains uncertain, although an association with human herpesvirus 6 has been suggested. Found on freely moving, nonkeratinized mucosa (eg, buccal and labial mucosa and not attached gingiva or palate), they may be single or multiple, are usually recurrent, and appear as painful small round ulcerations with yellow-gray fibrinoid centers surrounded by red halos (Figure 8–7). Minor aphthous ulcers are less than 1 cm in diameter and generally heal in 10–14 days. Major aphthous ulcers are greater than 1 cm in diameter and can be disabling due to the degree of associated oral pain. Stress seems to be a major predisposing factor to the eruptions of aphthous ulcers. A study found that the frequency of viral rhinitis and bedtime after 11 pm were independent predictors of aphthous ulcer frequency and severity in college students.

▲ **Figure 8–7.** Aphthous stomatitis. (From Ellen Eisenberg, MD and Dr. Joanna Douglas; reproduced, with permission, from Usatine RP, Smith MA, Mayeaux EJ Jr, Chumley H, Tysinger J. *The Color Atlas of Family Medicine.* McGraw-Hill, 2009.)

Treatment is challenging because no single systemic treatment has proven effective. Topical corticosteroids (triamcinolone acetonide, 0.1%, or fluocinonide ointment, 0.05%) in an adhesive base (Orabase Plain) do appear to provide symptomatic relief in many patients. Other topical therapies shown to be effective in controlled studies include diclofenac 3% in hyaluronan 2.5%, doxymycine-cyanoacrylate, mouthwashes containing the enzymes amyloglucosidase and glucose oxidase, and amlexanox 5% oral paste. A 1-week tapering course of prednisone (40–60 mg/day) has also been used successfully. Cimetidine maintenance therapy may be useful in patients with recurrent aphthous ulcers. Thalidomide has been used selectively in recurrent aphthous ulcerations in HIV-positive patients.

Large or persistent areas of ulcerative stomatitis may be secondary to erythema multiforme or drug allergies, acute herpes simplex, pemphigus, pemphigoid, epidermolysis bullosa acquisita, bullous lichen planus, Behçet disease, or inflammatory bowel disease. Squamous cell carcinoma may occasionally present in this fashion. When the diagnosis is not clear, incisional biopsy is indicated.

Brocklehurst P et al. Systemic interventions for recurrent aphthous stomatitis (mouth ulcers). Cochrane Database Syst Rev. 2012 Sep 12;9: CD005411. [PMID: 22972085]
Ma R et al. Effect of bedtime on recurrent aphthous stomatitis in college students. Oral Surg Oral Med Oral Pathol Oral Radiol. 2015 Feb;119(2):196–201.e2. [PMID: 25577415]

3. Herpes Stomatitis

Herpes gingivostomatitis is common, mild, and short-lived and requires no intervention in most adults. In immunocompromised persons, however, reactivation of herpes simplex virus infection is frequent and may be severe. Clinically, there is initial burning, followed by typical small vesicles that rupture and form scabs. Lesions are most commonly found on the attached gingiva and mucocutaneous junction of the lip, but lesions can also form on the tongue, buccal mucosa, and soft palate. Acyclovir (200–800 mg orally five times daily for 7–10 days) or valacyclovir (1000 mg orally twice daily for 7–10 days) may shorten the course and reduce postherpetic pain. These treatments may be effective only when started within 24–48 hours of the onset of initial symptoms (pain, itching, burning) and are not effective once vesicles have erupted. Differential diagnosis includes aphthous stomatitis, erythema multiforme, syphilitic chancre, and carcinoma. Coxsackievirus-caused lesions (grayish-white tonsillar plaques and palatal ulcers of herpangina or buccal and lip ulcers in hand-foot-and-mouth disease) are seen more commonly in children under age 6.

Balasubramaniam R et al. Update on oral herpes virus infections. Dent Clin North Am. 2014 Apr;58(2):265–80. [PMID: 24655522]

PHARYNGITIS & TONSILLITIS

ESSENTIALS OF DIAGNOSIS

- ▶ Sore throat.
- ▶ Fever.
- ▶ Anterior cervical adenopathy.
- ▶ Tonsillar exudate.
- ▶ Focus is to treat group A beta-hemolytic streptococcus infection to prevent rheumatic sequelae.

▶ General Considerations

Pharyngitis and tonsillitis account for over 10% of all office visits to primary care clinicians and 50% of outpatient antibiotic use. The main concern is determining who is likely to have a group A beta-hemolytic streptococcal (GABHS) infection, as this can lead to subsequent complications, such as rheumatic fever and glomerulonephritis. A second public health policy concern is reducing the extraordinary cost (both in dollars and in the development of antibiotic-resistant *S pneumoniae*) in the United States associated with unnecessary antibiotic use. Questions being asked: Have the rapid antigen tests supplanted the need to culture a throat under most circumstances? Are clinical criteria alone a sufficient basis for decisions about which patients should be given antibiotics? Should any patient receive any antibiotic other than penicillin (or erythromycin if penicillin-allergic)? For how long should treatment be continued? Numerous well-done studies and experience with rapid laboratory tests for detection of streptococci (eliminating the delay caused by culturing) informed a consensus experience.

▲ **Figure 8–8.** Streptococcal pharyngitis showing tonsillar exudate and erythema. (From Michael Nguyen, MD; reproduced, with permission, from Usatine RP, Smith MA, Mayeaux EJ Jr, Chumley H, Tysinger J. *The Color Atlas of Family Medicine.* McGraw-Hill, 2009.)

▶ Clinical Findings

A. Symptoms and Signs

The clinical features most suggestive of GABHS pharyngitis include fever over 38°C, tender anterior cervical adenopathy, lack of a cough, and a pharyngotonsillar exudate (Figures 8–8 and 8–9). These four features (the Centor criteria), when present, strongly suggest GABHS. When two or three of the four are present, there is an intermediate likelihood of GABHS. When only one criterion is present, GABHS is unlikely. Sore throat may be severe, with odynophagia, tender adenopathy, and a scarlatiniform rash. An elevated white count and left shift are also possible. Hoarseness, cough, and coryza are not suggestive of this disease.

▲ **Figure 8–9.** Pharyngeal inflammation and petechiae of the soft palate caused by group A streptococcus. (Used, with permission, from Dr. Heinz F. Eichenwald, Public Health Image Library, CDC.)

Marked lymphadenopathy and a shaggy, white-purple tonsillar exudate, often extending into the nasopharynx, suggest mononucleosis, especially if present in a young adult. With about 90% sensitivity, lymphocyte-to-white-blood-cell ratios of greater than 35% suggest EBV infection and not tonsillitis. Hepatosplenomegaly and a positive heterophil agglutination test or elevated anti-EBV titer are corroborative. However, about one-third of patients with infectious mononucleosis have secondary streptococcal tonsillitis, requiring treatment. Ampicillin should routinely be avoided if mononucleosis is suspected because it induces a rash that might be misinterpreted by the patient as a penicillin allergy. Diphtheria (extremely rare but described in the alcoholic population) presents with low-grade fever and an ill patient with a gray tonsillar pseudomembrane.

The most common pathogens other than GABHS in the differential diagnosis of "sore throat" are viruses, *Neisseria gonorrhoeae*, *Mycoplasma*, and *Chlamydia trachomatis*. Rhinorrhea and lack of exudate would suggest a virus, but in practice it is not possible to confidently distinguish viral upper respiratory infection from GABHS on clinical grounds alone. Infections with *Corynebacterium diphtheria*, anaerobic streptococci, and *Corynebacterium haemolyticum* (which responds better to erythromycin than penicillin) may also mimic pharyngitis due to GABHS.

B. Laboratory Findings

A single-swab throat culture is 90–95% sensitive and the rapid antigen detection testing (RADT) is 90–99% sensitive for GABHS. Results from the RADT are available in about 15 minutes.

▶ Treatment

Given the availability of many well-documented studies in recent years, one would think that a consensus might develop as to the most appropriate way to treat a sore throat. The Infectious Diseases Society of America recommends laboratory confirmation of the clinical diagnosis by means of either throat culture or RADT of the throat swab. The American College of Physicians–American Society of Internal Medicine (ACP-ASIM), in collaboration with the Centers for Disease Control and Prevention, advocates use of a clinical algorithm alone—in lieu of microbiologic testing—for confirmation of the diagnosis in adults for whom the suspicion of streptococcal infection is high. Others examine the assumptions of the ACP-ASIM guideline for using a clinical algorithm alone and question whether those recommendations will achieve the stated objective of dramatically decreasing excess antibiotic use. A reasonable strategy to follow is that patients with zero or one Centor criteria are at very low risk for GABHS and therefore do not need throat cultures or RADT of the throat swab and should not receive antibiotics. Patients with two or three Centor criteria need throat cultures or RADT of the throat swab, since positive results would warrant antibiotic treatment. Patients who have four Centor criteria are likely to have GABHS and can receive empiric therapy without throat culture or RADT.

Forty years ago, a single intramuscular injection of benzathine penicillin or procaine penicillin, 1.2 million units once, was the standard antibiotic treatment. This remains effective, but the injection is painful. It is now used for patients if compliance with an oral regimen is an issue. Currently, oral treatment is effective and preferred. Antibiotic choice aims to reduce the already low (10–20%) incidence of treatment failures (positive culture after treatment despite symptomatic resolution) and recurrences. Penicillin V potassium (250 mg orally three times daily or 500 mg twice daily for 10 days) or cefuroxime axetil (250 mg orally twice daily for 5–10 days) are both effective. The efficacy of a 5-day regimen of penicillin V potassium appears to be similar to that of a 10-day course, with a 94% clinical response rate and an 84% streptococcal eradication rate. Erythromycin (also active against *Mycoplasma* and *Chlamydia*) is a reasonable alternative to penicillin in allergic patients. Cephalosporins are somewhat more effective than penicillin in producing bacteriologic cures; 5-day administration has been successful for cefpodoxime and cefuroxime. The macrolide antibiotics have also been reported to be successful in shorter-duration regimens. Azithromycin (500 mg once daily), because of its long half-life, need be taken for only 3 days.

Adequate antibiotic treatment usually avoids the streptococcal complications of scarlet fever, glomerulonephritis, rheumatic myocarditis, and local abscess formation.

Antibiotics for treatment failures are also somewhat controversial. Surprisingly, penicillin-tolerant strains are not isolated more frequently in those who fail treatment than in those treated successfully with penicillin. The reasons for failure appear to be complex, and a second course of treatment with the same drug is reasonable. Alternatives to penicillin include cefuroxime and other cephalosporins, dicloxacillin (which is beta-lactamase–resistant), and amoxicillin with clavulanate. When there is a history of penicillin allergy, alternatives should be used, such as erythromycin. Erythromycin resistance—with failure rates of about 25%—is an increasing problem in many areas. In cases of severe penicillin allergy, cephalosporins should be avoided as the cross-reaction is common (8% or more).

Ancillary treatment of pharyngitis includes analgesics and anti-inflammatory agents, such as aspirin, acetaminophen, and corticosteroids. In meta-analysis, corticosteroids increased the likelihood of complete pain resolution at 24 hours by threefold without an increase in recurrence or adverse events. Some patients find that salt water gargling is soothing. In severe cases, anesthetic gargles and lozenges (eg, benzocaine) may provide additional symptomatic relief. Occasionally, odynophagia is so intense that hospitalization for intravenous hydration and antibiotics is necessary. (See Chapter 33.)

Patients who have had rheumatic fever should be treated with a continuous course of antimicrobial prophylaxis (erythromycin, 250 mg twice daily orally, or penicillin G, 500 mg once daily orally) for at least 5 years.

Hayward G et al. Corticosteroids as standalone or add-on treatment for sore throat. Cochrane Database Syst Rev. 2012 Oct 17; 10:CD008268. [PMID: 23076943]
Hildreth AF et al. Evidence-based evaluation and management of patients with pharyngitis in the emergency department. Emerg Med Pract. 2015 Sep;17(9):1–16. [PMID: 26276908]

PERITONSILLAR ABSCESS & CELLULITIS

When infection penetrates the tonsillar capsule and involves the surrounding tissues, peritonsillar cellulitis results. Peritonsillar abscess (**quinsy**) and cellulitis present with severe sore throat, odynophagia, trismus, medial deviation of the soft palate and peritonsillar fold, and an abnormal muffled ("hot potato") voice. Following therapy, peritonsillar cellulitis usually either resolves over several days or evolves into peritonsillar abscess. The existence of an abscess may be confirmed by aspirating pus from the peritonsillar fold just superior and medial to the upper pole of the tonsil. A 19-gauge or 21-gauge needle should be passed medial to the molar and no deeper than 1 cm, because the internal carotid artery may lie more medially than its usual location and pass posterior and deep to the tonsillar fossa. Most commonly, patients with peritonsillar abscess present to the emergency department and receive a dose of parenteral amoxicillin (1 g), amoxicillin-sulbactam (3 g), or clindamycin (600–900 mg). Less severe cases and patients who are able to tolerate oral intake may be treated for 7–10 days with oral antibiotics, including amoxicillin, 500 mg three times a day; amoxicillin-clavulanate, 875 mg twice a day; or clindamycin, 300 mg four times daily. Although antibiotic treatment is generally undisputed, there is controversy regarding the surgical management of peritonsillar abscess. Methods include needle aspiration, incision and drainage, and tonsillectomy. Some clinicians incise and drain the area and continue with parenteral antibiotics, whereas others aspirate only and monitor as an outpatient. To drain the abscess and avoid recurrence, it may be appropriate to consider immediate tonsillectomy (quinsy tonsillectomy). About 10% of patients with peritonsillar abscess exhibit relative indications for tonsillectomy. All three approaches are effective and have support in the literature. Regardless of the method used, one must be sure the abscess is adequately treated, since complications such as extension to the retropharyngeal, deep neck, and posterior mediastinal spaces are possible. Bacteria may also be aspirated into the lungs, resulting in pneumonia. There is controversy about whether a single abscess is a sufficient indication for tonsillectomy; about 30% of patients aged 17–30 who do not undergo early planned tonsillectomy following peritonsillar abscess ultimately undergo surgery, and only about 13% of those over 30 have their tonsils removed.

Tagliareni JM et al. Tonsillitis, peritonsillar and lateral pharyngeal abscesses. Oral Maxillofac Surg Clin North Am. 2012 May;24(2):197–204. [PMID: 22503067]
Wikstén J et al. Who ends up having tonsillectomy after peritonsillar infection? Eur Arch Otorhinolaryngol. 2012 Apr; 269(4):1281–4. [PMID: 22037720]

DEEP NECK INFECTIONS

- Marked acute neck pain and swelling.
- Abscesses are emergencies because rapid airway compromise may occur.
- May spread to the mediastinum or cause sepsis.

General Considerations

Ludwig angina is the most commonly encountered neck space infection. It is a cellulitis of the sublingual and submaxillary spaces, often arising from infection of the mandibular dentition. **Deep neck abscesses** most commonly originate from odontogenic infections. Other causes include suppurative lymphadenitis, direct spread of pharyngeal infection, penetrating trauma, pharyngoesophageal foreign bodies, cervical osteomyelitis, and intravenous injection of the internal jugular vein, especially in drug abusers. Recurrent deep neck infection may suggest an underlying congenital lesion, such as a branchial cleft cyst. Suppurative lymphadenopathy in middle-aged persons who smoke and drink alcohol regularly should be considered a manifestation of malignancy (typically metastatic squamous cell carcinoma) until proven otherwise.

Clinical Findings

Patients with **Ludwig angina** have edema and erythema of the upper neck under the chin and often of the floor of the mouth. The tongue may be displaced upward and backward by the posterior spread of cellulitis, and coalescence of pus is often present in the floor of mouth. This may lead to occlusion of the airway. Microbiologic isolates include streptococci, staphylococci, *Bacteroides,* and *Fusobacterium.*

Patients with **deep neck abscesses** usually present with marked neck pain and swelling. Fever is common but not always present. *Deep neck abscesses are emergencies because they may rapidly compromise the airway.* Untreated or inadequately treated, they may spread to the mediastinum or cause sepsis.

Contrast-enhanced CT usually augments the clinical examination in defining the extent of the infection. It often will distinguish inflammation and phlegmon (requiring antibiotics) from abscess (requiring drainage) and define for the surgeon the extent of an abscess. CT with MRI may also identify thrombophlebitis of the internal jugular vein secondary to oropharyngeal inflammation. This condition, known as **Lemierre syndrome**, is rare and usually associated with severe headache. The presence of pulmonary infiltrates consistent with septic emboli in the setting of a neck abscess should lead one to suspect Lemierre syndrome.

Treatment

Usual doses of penicillin plus metronidazole, ampicillin-sulbactam, clindamycin, or selective cephalosporins are good initial choices for treatment of **Ludwig angina**. Culture and sensitivity data are then used to refine the choice. Dental consultation is advisable to address the offending tooth or teeth. External drainage via bilateral submental incisions is required if the airway is threatened or when medical therapy has not reversed the process.

Treatment of **deep neck abscesses** includes securing the airway, intravenous antibiotics, and incision and drainage. When the infection involves the floor of the mouth, base of the tongue, or the supraglottic or paraglottic space, the airway may be secured either by intubation or tracheotomy. Tracheotomy is preferable in the patients with substantial pharyngeal edema, since attempts at intubation may precipitate acute airway obstruction. Bleeding in association with a deep neck abscess is very rare but suggests carotid artery or internal jugular vein involvement and requires prompt neck exploration both for drainage of pus and for vascular control.

Patients with **Lemierre syndrome** require prompt institution of antibiotics appropriate for *Fusobacterium necrophorum* as well as the more usual upper airway pathogens. The use of anticoagulation in treatment is debated and of no proven benefit.

Horváth T et al. Severe neck infections that require wide external drainage: clinical analysis of 17 consecutive cases. Eur Arch Otorhinolaryngol. 2015 Nov;272(11):3469–74. [PMID: 25359195]

SNORING

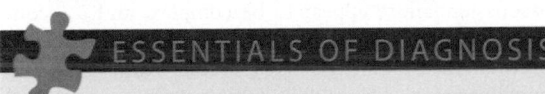

- Noise produced on inspiration during sleep.
- Snoring is associated with obstructive sleep apnea (OSA) but has no disruption of sleep by clinical sleep evaluation.

General Considerations

Ventilation disorders during sleep are extremely common. While OSA occurs in 5–10% of Americans, clinically relevant snoring may occur in as many as 59%. In general, sleep-disordered breathing problems are attributed to narrowing of the upper aerodigestive tract during sleep due to changes in position, muscle tone, and soft tissue hypertrophy or laxity. The most common sites of obstruction are the oropharynx and the base of the tongue. The spectrum of the problem ranges from simple snoring without cessation of airflow to OSA with long periods of apnea and life-threatening physiologic sequelae. OSA is discussed in Chapter 9. In contrast to OSA, snoring is almost exclusively a social problem, and despite its prevalence and association with OSA, there is comparatively little known about the management of this problem.

Clinical Findings

A. Symptoms and Signs

All patients who complain of snoring should be evaluated for OSA as discussed in Chapter 9. Symptoms of OSA (including snoring, excessive daytime somnolence, daytime headaches, and weight gain) may be present in as many as 30% of patients without demonstrable apnea or hypopnea on formal testing. Clinical examination should include examination of the nasal cavity, nasopharynx, oropharynx, and larynx to help exclude other causes of dynamic airway obstruction. In many cases of isolated snoring, the palate and uvula appear enlarged and elongated with excessive mucosa hanging below the muscular portion of the soft palate.

B. Imaging and Diagnostic Testing

Sleep examination with polysomnography is strongly advised in the evaluation of a patient with complaints of snoring. Radiographic imaging of the head or neck is generally not necessary for management of primary snoring.

Treatment

Expeditious and inexpensive management solutions of snoring are sought, often with little or no benefit. Diet modification and a regimen of physical exercise can lead to improvement in snoring through weight loss and the improvement in pharyngeal tone that accompanies overall physical conditioning. Position change during sleep can be effective, and time-honored treatments, such as taping or sewing a tennis ball to the back of a shirt worn during sleep may satisfactorily eliminate symptoms by ensuring recumbency on one side.

Anatomic management of snoring can be challenging. As with OSA, snoring can come from a number of sites in the upper aerodigestive tract. While medical or surgical correction of nasal obstruction may help alleviate snoring problems, most interventions aim to improve airflow through the nasopharynx and oropharynx. Nonsurgical options include mandibular advancement appliances designed to pull the base of the tongue forward and continuous positive airway pressure via face or nasal mask. Compliance with both of these treatment options is problematic because snorers without OSA do not notice the physiologic benefits of these devices noted by patients with sleep apnea.

Surgical correction of snoring is most commonly directed at the soft palate. Historical approaches involved resection of redundant mucosa and the uvula similar to uvulopalatopharyngoplasty that is used for OSA. Regardless of how limited the procedure or what technique was used, postoperative pain, the expense of general anesthesia, and high recurrence rates limit the utility of these procedures. Office-based approaches are more widely used because of these limitations. Most of these procedures aim to stiffen the palate to prevent vibration rather than remove it. A series of procedures, including injection snoreplasty, radiofrequency thermal fibrosis, and an implantable palatal device have been used with variable success and patient tolerance. The techniques can be technically challenging. Persistent symptoms may occur following initial treatment necessitating costly (and sometimes painful) repeat procedures. The durability of these procedures in alleviating symptoms is also poorly understood, and late failures can lead to patient and clinician frustration.

Bratton DJ et al. CPAP vs mandibular advancement devices and blood pressure in patients with obstructive sleep apnea: a systematic review and meta-analysis. JAMA. 2015 Dec 1; 314(21):2280–93. [PMID: 26624827]

Rivas M et al. Obstructive sleep apnea and its effects on cardiovascular diseases: a narrative review. Anatol J Cardiol. 2015 Nov; 15(11):944–50. [PMID: 26574763]

DISEASES OF THE SALIVARY GLAND

ACUTE INFLAMMATORY SALIVARY GLAND DISORDERS

1. Sialadenitis

Acute bacterial sialadenitis most commonly affects either the parotid or submandibular gland. It typically presents with acute swelling of the gland, increased pain and swelling with meals, and tenderness and erythema of the duct opening. Pus often can be massaged from the duct. Sialadenitis often occurs in the setting of dehydration or in association with chronic illness. Underlying Sjögren syndrome may contribute. Ductal obstruction, often by an inspissated mucous plug, is followed by salivary stasis and secondary infection. The most common organism recovered from purulent draining saliva is *S aureus*. Treatment consists of intravenous antibiotics, such as nafcillin (1 g intravenously every 4–6 hours), measures to increase salivary flow, including hydration, warm compresses, sialagogues (eg, lemon drops), and massage of the gland. Treatment can usually then be switched to an oral agent based on clinical and microbiologic improvement to complete a 10-day treatment course. Less severe cases can often be treated with oral antibiotics with similar spectrum. Complete resolution of parotid swelling and pain can take 2–3 weeks. Failure of the process to improve and ultimately resolve on this regimen suggests abscess formation, ductal stricture, stone, or tumor causing obstruction. Ultrasound or CT scan may be helpful in establishing the diagnosis. In the setting of acute illness, a severe and potentially life-threatening form of sialadenitis, sometimes called **suppurative sialadenitis**, may develop. The causative organism is usually *S aureus*, but often no pus will drain from Stensen papilla. These patients often do not respond to rehydration and intravenous antibiotics and thus may require operative incision and drainage to resolve the infection.

2. Sialolithiasis

Calculus formation is more common in Wharton duct (draining the submandibular glands) than in Stensen duct (draining the parotid glands). Clinically, a patient may note postprandial pain and local swelling, often with a history of recurrent acute sialadenitis. Stones in Wharton duct are usually large and radiopaque, whereas those in Stensen duct are usually radiolucent and smaller. Those very close to the orifice of Wharton duct may be palpated manually in the anterior floor of the mouth and removed intraorally by dilating or incising the distal duct. Those more than 1.5–2 cm from the duct are too close to the lingual nerve to be removed safely in this manner. Similarly, dilation of Stensen duct, located on the buccal surface opposite the second maxillary molar, may relieve distal stricture or allow a small stone to pass. Sialoendoscopy for the management of chronic sialolithiasis is superior to extracorporeal shock-wave lithotripsy and fluoroscopically guided basket retrieval. Repeated episodes of sialadenitis are usually associated with stricture and chronic infection. If the obstruction cannot be safely removed or dilated, excision of the gland may be necessary to relieve recurrent symptoms.

Atienza G et al. Management of obstructive salivary disorders by sialendoscopy: a systematic review. Br J Oral Maxillofac Surg. 2015 Jul;53(6):507–19. [PMID: 25823614]
Harrison JD. Causes, natural history, and incidence of salivary stones and obstructions. Otolaryngol Clin North Am. 2009 Dec; 42(6):927–47. [PMID: 19962002]

CHRONIC INFLAMMATORY & INFILTRATIVE DISORDERS OF THE SALIVARY GLANDS

Numerous infiltrative disorders may cause unilateral or bilateral parotid gland enlargement. Sjögren syndrome and sarcoidosis are examples of lymphoepithelial and granulomatous diseases that may affect the salivary glands. Metabolic disorders, including alcoholism, diabetes mellitus, and vitamin deficiencies, may also cause diffuse enlargement. Several drugs have been associated with parotid enlargement, including thioureas, iodine, and drugs with cholinergic effects (eg, phenothiazines), which stimulate salivary flow and cause more viscous saliva.

SALIVARY GLAND TUMORS

Approximately 80% of salivary gland tumors occur in the parotid gland. In adults, about 80% of these are benign. In the submandibular triangle, it is sometimes difficult to distinguish a primary submandibular gland tumor from a metastatic submandibular space node. Only 50–60% of primary submandibular tumors are benign. Tumors of the minor salivary glands are most likely to be malignant, with adenoid cystic carcinoma predominating, and may be found throughout the oral cavity or oropharynx.

Most parotid tumors present as an asymptomatic mass in the superficial part of the gland. Their presence may have been noted by the patient for months or years. Facial nerve involvement correlates strongly with malignancy. Tumors may extend deep to the plane of the facial nerve or may originate in the parapharyngeal space. In such cases, medial deviation of the soft palate is visible on intraoral examination. MRI and CT scans have largely replaced sialography in defining the extent of tumor.

When the clinician encounters a patient with an otherwise asymptomatic salivary gland mass where tumor is the most likely diagnosis, the choice is whether to simply excise the mass via a parotidectomy with facial nerve dissection or submandibular gland excision or to first obtain an FNA biopsy. Although the accuracy of FNA biopsy for malignancy has been reported to be quite high, results vary among institutions. If a negative FNA biopsy would lead to a decision not to proceed to surgery, then it should be considered. Poor overall health of the patient and the possibility of inflammatory disease as the cause of the mass are situations where FNA biopsy might be helpful. In otherwise straightforward nonrecurrent cases, excision is indicated. In benign and small, low-grade malignant tumors, no additional treatment is needed. Postoperative irradiation is indicated for larger and high-grade cancers.

Adelstein DJ et al. Biology and management of salivary gland cancers. Semin Radiat Oncol. 2012 Jul;22(3):245–53. [PMID: 22687949]

DISEASES OF THE LARYNX

DYSPHONIA, HOARSENESS & STRIDOR

The primary symptoms of laryngeal disease are hoarseness and stridor. Hoarseness is caused by an abnormal vibration of the vocal folds. The voice is breathy when too much air passes incompletely apposed vocal folds, as in unilateral vocal fold paralysis or vocal fold mass. The voice is harsh when the vocal folds are stiff and vibrate irregularly, as is the case in laryngitis or malignancy. Heavy, edematous vocal folds produce a rough, low-pitched vocal quality. Stridor (a high-pitched, typically inspiratory, sound) is the result of turbulent airflow from a narrowed upper airway. Airway narrowing at or above the vocal folds produces inspiratory stridor. Airway narrowing below the vocal fold level produces either expiratory or biphasic stridor. The timing and rapidity of onset of stridor are critically important in determining the seriousness of the airway problem. *All cases of stridor should be evaluated by a specialist and rapid-onset stridor should be evaluated emergently.*

Evaluation of an abnormal voice begins with obtaining a history of the circumstances preceding its onset and an examination of the airway.

Any patient with hoarseness that has persisted beyond 2 weeks should be evaluated by an otolaryngologist with laryngoscopy. Especially when the patient has a history of tobacco use, laryngeal cancer or lung cancer (leading to paralysis of a recurrent laryngeal nerve) must be strongly considered. In addition to structural causes of dysphonia, laryngoscopy can help identify functional problems with the voice, including vocal fold paralysis, muscle tension dysphonia, and spasmodic dysphonia.

Johns MM 3rd et al. Shortfalls of the American Academy of Otolaryngology-Head and Neck Surgery's Clinical practice guideline: Hoarseness (Dysphonia). Otolaryngol Head Neck Surg. 2010 Aug;143(2):175–7. [PMID: 20647114]

Schwartz SR et al. Clinical practice guideline: hoarseness (dysphonia). Otolaryngol Head Neck Surg. 2009 Sep;141(3 Suppl 2):S1–S31. [PMID: 19729111]

COMMON LARYNGEAL DISORDERS

1. Acute Laryngitis

Acute laryngitis is probably the most common cause of hoarseness, which may persist for a week or so after other symptoms of an upper respiratory infection have cleared. The patient should be warned to avoid vigorous use of the voice (singing, shouting) until their voice returns to normal, since persistent use may lead to the formation of traumatic vocal fold hemorrhage, polyps, and cysts. Although thought to be usually viral in origin, both *M catarrhalis* and *H influenzae* may be isolated from the nasopharynx at higher than expected frequencies. Despite this finding, a meta-analysis has failed to demonstrate any convincing evidence that antibiotics significantly alter the natural resolution of acute laryngitis. Erythromycin may speed subjective perception of hoarseness and cough. Oral or intramuscular corticosteroids may be used in highly selected cases of professional vocalists to speed recovery and allow scheduled performances. Examination of the vocal folds and assessment of vocal technique are mandatory prior to corticosteroid initiation, since inflamed vocal folds are at greater risk for hemorrhage and the subsequent development of traumatic vocal fold pathology.

Reveiz L et al. Antibiotics for acute laryngitis in adults. Cochrane Database Syst Rev. 2013 Mar 28;3:CD004783. [PMID: 23543536]

Schomacker H et al. Pathogenesis of acute respiratory illness caused by human parainfluenza viruses. Curr Opin Virol. 2012 Jun;2(3):294–9. [PMID: 22709516]

2. Laryngopharyngeal Reflux

ESSENTIALS OF DIAGNOSIS

► Commonly associated with hoarseness, throat irritation, and chronic cough.

► Symptoms typically occur when upright, and half of patients do not experience heartburn.

► Laryngoscopy is critical to exclude other causes of hoarseness.

► Diagnosis is made based on response to proton pump inhibitor therapy.

► Treatment failure with proton pump inhibitors is common and may suggest other etiologies.

Gastroesophageal reflux into the larynx (laryngopharyngeal reflux) is considered a cause of chronic hoarseness when other causes of abnormal vocal fold vibration (such as tumor or nodules) have been excluded by laryngoscopy. Gastroesophageal reflux disease (GERD) has also been suggested as a contributing factor to other symptoms, such as throat clearing, throat discomfort, chronic cough, a sensation of postnasal drip, esophageal spasm, and some cases of asthma. Since less than half of patients with laryngeal acid exposure have typical symptoms of heartburn and regurgitation, the lack of such symptoms should not be construed as eliminating this cause. Indeed, most patients with symptomatic laryngopharyngeal reflux, as it is now called, do not meet criteria for GERD by pH probe testing and these entities must be considered separately. The prevalence of this condition is hotly debated in the literature, and laryngopharyngeal reflux may not be as common as once thought.

Evaluation should initially exclude other causes of dysphonia through laryngoscopy; consultation with an otolaryngologist is advisable. Many clinicians opt for an empiric trial of a proton pump inhibitor since no gold standard exists for diagnosing this condition. Such an empiric trial should not precede visualization of the vocal folds to exclude other causes of hoarseness. When used, the American Academy of Otolaryngology—Head and Neck Surgery recommends twice-daily therapy with full-strength proton pump inhibitor (eg, omeprazole 40 mg orally twice daily, or equivalent) for a minimum of 3 months. Patients may note improvement in symptoms after 3 months, but the changes in the larynx often take 6 months to resolve. If symptoms improve and cessation of therapy leads to symptoms again, then a proton pump inhibitor is resumed at the lowest dose effective for remission, usually daily but at times on a demand basis. Although H_2-receptor antagonists are an alternative to proton pump inhibitors, they are generally both less clinically effective and less cost-effective. Nonresponders should undergo pH testing and manometry. Twenty-four-hour pH monitoring of the pharynx should best document laryngopharyngeal reflux and is advocated by some as the initial management step, but it is costly, more difficult, and less available than lower esophageal monitoring alone. Double pH probe (proximal and distal esophageal probes) testing is the best option for evaluation, since lower esophageal pH monitoring alone does not correlate well with laryngopharyngeal reflux symptoms. Oropharyngeal pH probe testing is available, but its ability to predict response to reflux treatment in patients with laryngopharyngeal reflux is not known.

Altman KW et al. The challenge of protocols for reflux disease: a review and development of a critical pathway. Otolaryngol Head Neck Surg. 2011 Jul;145(1):7–14. [PMID: 21493264]

Ford CN. GERD-related chronic laryngitis: pro. Arch Otolaryngol Head Neck Surg. 2010 Sep;136(9):910–3. [PMID: 20855685]

Vaezi MF. Gastroesophageal reflux-related chronic laryngitis: con. Arch Otolaryngol Head Neck Surg. 2010 Sep;136(9):908–9. [PMID: 20855684]

3. Recurrent Respiratory Papillomatosis

Papillomas are common lesions of the larynx and other sites where ciliated and squamous epithelia meet. Unlike oral papillomas, recurrent respiratory papillomatosis typically becomes symptomatic, with hoarseness that occasionally progresses over weeks to months. These papillomas are almost always due to HPV types 6 and 11. The disease is more common in children where it causes hoarseness and stridor. Repeated laser vaporizations or cold knife resections via operative laryngoscopy are the mainstay of treatment. Severe cases can cause airway compromise even in adults and may require treatment as often as every 6 weeks to maintain airway patency. Extension can occur into the trachea and lungs. Tracheotomy should be avoided, if possible, since it introduces an additional squamociliary junction for which papillomas appear to have an affinity. Interferon treatment has been under investigation for many years but is only indicated in severe cases with pulmonary involvement. Rarely, cases of malignant transformation have been reported (often in smokers), but recurrent respiratory papillomatosis should generally be thought of as a benign condition. Cidofovir (a cytosine nucleotide analog in use to treat cytomegalovirus retinitis) has been used with success as intralesional therapy for recurrent respiratory papillomatosis. Because cidofovir causes adenocarcinomas in laboratory animals, its potential for carcinogenesis is being monitored. The quadrivalent and new 9 serotype recombinant human HPV vaccines (Gardasil and Gardasil 9) offer hope for the eventual eradication of this benign, but terribly morbid, disease.

Bonagura VR et al. Recurrent respiratory papillomatosis: a complex defect in immune responsiveness to human papillomavirus-6 and -11. APMIS. 2010 Jun;118(6–7):455–70. [PMID: 20553528]
Carvalho CM et al. Prognostic factors of recurrent respiratory papillomatosis from a registry of 72 patients. Acta Otolaryngol. 2009 Apr;129(4):462–70. [PMID: 19235575]

4. Epiglottitis

Epiglottitis (or, more correctly, supraglottitis) should be suspected when a patient presents with a rapidly developing sore throat or when odynophagia (pain on swallowing) is out of proportion to apparently minimal oropharyngeal findings on examination. It is more common in diabetic patients and may be viral or bacterial in origin. Rarely in the era of *H influenzae* type b vaccine is this bacterium isolated in adults. Unlike in children, indirect laryngoscopy is generally safe and may demonstrate a swollen, erythematous epiglottis. Lateral plain radiographs may demonstrate an enlarged epiglottis (the epiglottis "thumb sign"). Initial treatment is hospitalization for intravenous antibiotics—eg, ceftizoxime, 1–2 g intravenously every 8–12 hours; or cefuroxime, 750–1500 mg intravenously every 8 hours; and dexamethasone, usually 4–10 mg as initial bolus, then 4 mg intravenously every 6 hours—and observation of the airway. Corticosteroids may be tapered as symptoms and signs resolve. Similarly, substitution of oral antibiotics may be appropriate to complete a 10 day course. Less than 10% of adults require intubation. Indications for intubation are dyspnea, rapid pace of sore throat (where progression to airway compromise may occur before the effects of corticosteroids and antibiotics), and endolaryngeal abscess noted on CT imaging. If the patient is not intubated, prudence suggests monitoring oxygen saturation with continuous pulse oximetry and initial admission to a monitored unit.

Verbruggen K et al. Epiglottitis and related complications in adults. Case reports and review of the literature. B-ENT. 2012;8(2):143–8. [PMID: 22896936]

MASSES OF THE LARYNX

1. Traumatic Lesions of the Vocal Folds

Vocal fold nodules are smooth, paired lesions that form at the junction of the anterior one-third and posterior two-thirds of the vocal folds. They are a common cause of hoarseness resulting from vocal abuse. In adults, they are referred to as "singer's nodules" and in children as "screamer's nodules." Treatment requires modification of voice habits, and referral to a speech therapist is indicated. While nearly all true nodules will resolve with behavior modification, recalcitrant nodules may require surgical excision. Often, additional pathology, such as a polyp or cyst, may be encountered.

Vocal fold polyps are unilateral masses that form within the superficial lamina propria of the vocal fold. They are related to vocal trauma and seem to follow resolution of vocal fold hemorrhage. Small, sessile polyps may resolve with conservative measures, such as voice rest and corticosteroids, but larger polyps are often irreversible and require operative removal to restore normal voice.

Vocal fold cysts are also considered traumatic lesions of the vocal folds and are either true cysts with an epithelial lining or pseudocysts. They typically form from mucus-secreting glands on the inferior aspect of the vocal folds. Cysts may fluctuate in size from week to week and cause a variable degree of hoarseness. They rarely, if ever, resolve completely and may leave behind a sulcus, or vocal fold scar, if they decompress or are marsupialized. Such scarring can be a frustrating cause of permanent dysphonia.

Polypoid corditis is different from vocal fold polyps and may form from loss of elastin fibers and loosening of the intracellular junctions within the lamina propria. This loss allows swelling of the gelatinous matrix of the superficial lamina propria (called **Reinke edema**). These changes in the vocal folds are strongly associated with smoking, but also with vocal abuse, chemical industrial irritants, and hypothyroidism. While this problem is common in both male and female smokers, women seem more troubled by the characteristic decline in modal pitch caused by the increased mass of the vocal folds. If the patient stops smoking or the lesions cause stridor and airway obstruction, surgical resection of the hyperplastic vocal fold mucosa may be indicated to improve the voice or airway, or both.

A common but often unrecognized cause of hoarseness and odynophonia are **contact ulcers** or their close relatives, **granulomas**. Both lesions form on the vocal processes of the arytenoid cartilages, and patients often can correctly inform the clinician which side is affected. The cause of these ulcers and granulomas is disputed, but they are clearly related to trauma and may be related to exposure of the underlying perichondrium. They are common following intubation and generally resolve quite quickly. Chronic ulceration or granuloma formation has been associated with gastroesophageal reflux but is also common in patients with muscle tension dysphonia. Treatment is often multimodal, and an inhaled corticosteroid (eg, fluticasone 440 mcg twice daily) may be the most effective pharmacologic therapy. Adjunct treatment measures include proton pump inhibitor therapy (omeprazole 40 mg orally twice daily, or equivalent) and voice therapy with special attention to vocal hygiene. Rare cases can be quite stubborn and persistent without adequate therapy. Surgical removal is rarely, if ever, required for nonobstructive lesions.

Gökcan KM et al. Vascular lesions of the vocal fold. Eur Arch Otorhinolaryngol. 2009 Apr;266(4):527–33. [PMID: 18704472]

2. Laryngeal Leukoplakia

Leukoplakia of the vocal folds is commonly found in association with hoarseness in smokers. Direct laryngoscopy with biopsy is advised in almost all cases. Histologic examination usually demonstrates mild, moderate, or severe dysplasia. In some cases, invasive squamous cell carcinoma is present in the initial biopsy specimen. Cessation of smoking may reverse or stabilize mild or moderate dysplasia. Some patients—estimated to be less than 5% of those with mild dysplasia and about 35–60% of those with severe dysplasia—will subsequently develop squamous cell carcinoma. Treatment options include close follow-up with laryngovideostroboscopy, serial resection, and external beam radiation therapy. Despite their cost and the lack of any evidence for their use in the treatment of leukoplakia, proton pump inhibitors have become the mainstay of treatment for these lesions.

Isenberg JS et al. Institutional and comprehensive review of laryngeal leukoplakia. Ann Otol Rhinol Laryngol. 2008 Jan; 117(1):74–9. [PMID: 18254375]

3. Squamous Cell Carcinoma of the Larynx

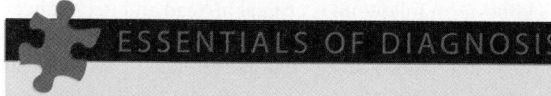

ESSENTIALS OF DIAGNOSIS

- ▶ New and persistent (more than 2 weeks' duration) hoarseness in a smoker.
- ▶ Persistent throat or ear pain, especially with swallowing.
- ▶ Neck mass.
- ▶ Hemoptysis.
- ▶ Stridor or other symptoms of a compromised airway.

▶ General Considerations

Squamous cell carcinoma of the larynx, the most common malignancy of the larynx, occurs almost exclusively in patients with a history of significant tobacco use. Squamous cell carcinoma is usually seen in men aged 50–70 years; about 13,000 new cases are seen in United States each year. There may be an association between laryngeal cancer and HPV type 16 or 18 infection, but this association is much less strong than that between HPV 16 or 18 and oropharyngeal cancer. In both cancer types, the association with HPV seems to be strongest in nonsmokers. Laryngeal cancer is very treatable and early detection is the key to maximizing posttreatment voice, swallowing, and breathing function.

▶ Clinical Findings

A. Symptoms and Signs

A change in voice quality is most often the presenting complaint, although throat or ear pain, hemoptysis, dysphagia, weight loss, and airway compromise may occur. Because of their early impact on vocal quality, glottic cancers are among the smallest detectable human malignancies and treatment success is very high with early lesions. Neck metastases are not common in early glottic (true vocal fold) cancer in which the vocal folds are mobile, but a third of patients in whom there is impaired fold mobility will also have involved lymph nodes at neck dissection. Supraglottic carcinoma (false vocal folds, aryepiglottic folds, epiglottis), on the other hand, often metastasizes to both sides of the neck early in the disease. Complete head and neck examination, including laryngoscopy, by an experienced clinician is mandated for any person with the concerning symptoms listed under Essentials of Diagnosis.

B. Imaging and Laboratory Studies

Radiologic evaluation by CT or MRI is helpful in assessing tumor extent. Imaging evaluates neck nodes, tumor volume, and cartilage sclerosis or destruction. A chest CT scan is indicated if there are level VI enlarged nodes (around the trachea and the thyroid gland) or level IV enlarged nodes (inferior to the cricoid cartilage along the internal jugular vein), or if a chest film is concerning for a second primary lesion or metastases. Laboratory evaluation includes complete blood count and liver function tests. Formal cardiopulmonary evaluation may be indicated, especially if partial laryngeal surgery is being considered. All partial laryngectomy candidates should have good to excellent lung function and exercise tolerance because chronic microaspiration may be expected following the procedure. A positron emission tomography (PET) scan or CT-PET scan may be indicated to assess for distant metastases when there appears to be advanced local or regional disease.

C. Biopsy

Diagnosis is made by biopsy at the time of laryngoscopy when true fold mobility and arytenoid fixation, as well as surface tumor extent, can be evaluated. Most otolaryngologists recommend esophagoscopy and bronchoscopy at the same time to exclude synchronous primary tumor. Although an FNA biopsy of an enlarged neck node may have already been done, it is generally acceptable to assume radiographically enlarged neck nodes (greater than

1–1.5 cm) or nodes with necrotic centers are neck metastases. Open biopsies of nodal metastases should be discouraged because they may lead to higher rates of tumor treatment failure.

D. Tumor Staging

The American Joint Committee on Cancer (AJCC) staging of laryngeal cancers uses the TNM system to describe tumor extent and can be used for prognosis. Early laryngeal cancers, T1 and T2 (stage I and II) lesions, involve 1–2 laryngeal subsites locally and have no nodal metastases or profound functional abnormalities. T3 and T4 lesions may involve multiple laryngeal subsites with limitation of laryngeal mobility. These locally advanced lesions are stage III or IV cancers, and any size tumor with regional nodal metastases is at least a stage III tumor. Stage I and II lesions are generally treated with single-modality therapy (surgery or radiation), while multimodality therapy, usually including chemotherapy with radiation therapy, is reserved for more advanced stage III and IV lesions.

▶ Treatment

Treatment of laryngeal carcinoma has four goals: cure, preservation of safe and effective swallowing, preservation of useful voice, and avoidance of a permanent tracheostoma. For early glottic and supraglottic cancers, radiation therapy is the standard of care since cure rates are greater than 95% and 80%, respectively. That said, radiation therapy carries substantial morbidity, and many early tumors (T1 and T2 lesions, without involved nodes) and selected advanced tumors (T3 and T4) may be treated with partial laryngectomy if at least one cricoarytenoid unit can be preserved. Five-year locoregional cure rates exceed 80–90% with surgery, and patient-reported satisfaction is excellent. In supraglottic tumors, even when clinically N0, elective limited neck dissection is indicated following surgical resection because of the high risk of neck node involvement.

Advanced stage III and IV tumors represent a challenging and ever-changing treatment dilemma. Twenty-five years ago, total laryngectomy was often recommended for such patients. However, the 1994 VA study (with induction cisplatin and 5-fluorouracil followed by irradiation alone in responders) demonstrated that two-thirds of patients could preserve their larynx. Subsequent studies have further defined multimodal therapy. Cisplatin-based chemotherapy concomitant with radiation therapy has been shown to be superior to either irradiation alone or induction chemotherapy followed by radiation. The same benefits have been demonstrated with the epidermal growth factor receptor blocker cetuximab with lower overall systemic toxicity and better patient tolerance. However, chemoradiation using either cetuximab or cisplatin is associated with prolonged gastrostomy-dependent dysphagia.

The high rate of dysphagia and morbidity associated with severe laryngeal stenosis following chemoradiation has prompted a reevaluation of the role of extended, but less-than-total, laryngeal resection for selected advanced laryngeal carcinoma in which at least one cricoarytenoid unit is intact (organ preservation surgery). In addition to the late complications, clinicians have noted that the overall success in the treatment of larynx cancer has declined in parallel with the increase in organ preservation chemoradiation therapy over the past 20 years. Some experts have proposed that this decline is the direct result of the shift in management of advanced laryngeal cancer away from surgery. Organ preservation surgery should be considered and discussed as an alternative to chemoradiation but may require referral to an appropriate regional center where such techniques are offered. After thorough evaluation of candidacy and discussion of the treatment options, patient choice plays a critical role in the ultimate decision to pursue surgery or chemoradiation as a definitive treatment modality. The patient and treating clinicians must carefully consider *different* early and late side effects and complications associated with different treatment modalities.

The presence of malignant adenopathy in the neck affects the prognosis greatly. Supraglottic tumors metastasize early and bilaterally to the neck, and this must be included in the treatment plans even when the neck is apparently uninvolved. Glottic tumors in which the true vocal folds are mobile (T1 or T2) have less than a 5% rate of nodal involvement; when a fold is immobile, the rate of ipsilateral nodal involvement climbs to about 30%. An involved neck is treated by surgery or chemoradiation, or both. This decision will depend on the treatment chosen for the larynx and the extent of neck involvement.

Total laryngectomy is largely reserved for patients with advanced resectable tumors with extralaryngeal spread or cartilage involvement, for those with persistent tumor following chemoradiation, and for patients with recurrent or second primary tumor following previous radiation therapy. Voice rehabilitation via a primary (or at times secondary) tracheoesophageal puncture produces intelligible and serviceable speech in about 75–85% of patients. Indwelling prostheses that are changed every 3–6 months are a common alternative to patient-inserted prostheses, which need changing more frequently.

Long-term follow-up is critical in head and neck cancer patients. In addition to the 3–4% annual rate of second tumors and monitoring for recurrence, psychosocial aspects of treatment are common. Dysphagia, impaired communication, and altered appearance may result in patient difficulties adapting to the workplace and to social interactions. In addition, smoking cessation and alcohol abatement are common challenges. Nevertheless, about 65% of patients with larynx cancer are cured, most have useful speech, and many resume their prior livelihoods with adaptations.

Bonner JA et al. Radiotherapy plus cetuximab for locoregionally advanced head and neck cancer: 5-year survival data from a phase 3 randomised trial, and relation between cetuximab-induced rash and survival. Lancet Oncol. 2010 Jan;11(1):21–8. [PMID: 19897418]

Suárez C et al. Transoral microsurgery for treatment of laryngeal and pharyngeal cancers. Curr Oncol Rep. 2013 Apr;15(2):134–41. [PMID: 23275183]

Wang CJ et al. Current concepts of organ preservation in head and neck cancer. Eur Arch Otorhinolaryngol. 2011 Apr; 268(4):481–7. [PMID: 21107854]

VOCAL FOLD PARALYSIS

Vocal fold paralysis can result from a lesion or damage to either the vagus or recurrent laryngeal nerve and usually results in breathy dysphonia and effortful voicing. Common causes of **unilateral recurrent laryngeal nerve** involvement include thyroid surgery (and occasionally thyroid cancer), other neck surgery (anterior discectomy and carotid endarterectomy), and mediastinal or apical involvement by lung cancer. Skull base tumors often involve or abut upon lower cranial nerves and may affect the vagus nerve directly, or the vagus nerve may be damaged during surgical management of the lesion. While iatrogenic injury is the most common cause of unilateral vocal fold paralysis, the second most common cause is idiopathic. However, before deciding whether the paralysis is due to iatrogenic injury or is idiopathic, the clinician must exclude other causes, such as malignancy. In the absence of other cranial neuropathies, a CT scan with contrast from the skull base to the aorto-pulmonary window (the span of the recurrent laryngeal nerve) should be performed. If other cranial nerve deficits or high vagal weakness with palate paralysis is noted, an MRI scan of the brain and brainstem is warranted.

Unlike unilateral fold paralysis, **bilateral fold paralysis** usually causes inspiratory stridor with deep inspiration. If the onset of bilateral fold paralysis is insidious, it may be asymptomatic at rest, and the patient may have a normal voice. However, the acute onset of bilateral vocal fold paralysis with inspiratory stridor at rest should be managed by a specialist immediately in a critical care environment. Causes of bilateral fold paralysis include thyroid surgery, esophageal cancer, and ventricular shunt malfunction. Unilateral or bilateral fold immobility may also be seen in cricoarytenoid arthritis secondary to advanced rheumatoid arthritis, intubation injuries, glottic and subglottic stenosis, and, of course, laryngeal cancer. The goal of intervention is the creation of a safe airway with minimal reduction in voice quality and airway protection from aspiration. A number of fold lateralization procedures for bilateral paralysis have been advocated as a means of removing the tracheotomy tube.

Unilateral vocal fold paralysis is occasionally temporary and may take over a year to resolve spontaneously. Surgical management of persistent or irrecoverable symptomatic unilateral vocal fold paralysis has evolved over the last several decades. The primary goal is medialization of the paralyzed fold in order to create a stable platform for vocal fold vibration. Additional goals include improving pulmonary toilet by facilitating of cough and advancing diet. Success has been reported for years with injection laryngoplasty using Teflon, Gelfoam, fat, and collagen. Teflon is the only permanent injectable material, but its use is discouraged because of granuloma formation within the vocal folds of some patients. Temporary injectable materials, such as collagen or fat, provide excellent temporary restoration of voice and can be placed under local or general anesthesia. Once the paralysis is determined to be permanent, formal medialization thyroplasty may be performed by creating a small window in the thyroid cartilage and placing an implant between the thyroarytenoid muscle and inner table of the thyroid cartilage. This procedure moves the vocal fold medially and creates a stable platform for bilateral, symmetric mucosal vibration.

Gardner GM et al. The cost of vocal fold paralysis after thyroidectomy. Laryngoscope. 2013 Jun;123(6):1455–63. [PMID: 23703383]
Misono S et al. Evidence-based practice: evaluation and management of unilateral vocal fold paralysis. Otolaryngol Clin North Am. 2012 Oct;45(5):1083–108. [PMID: 22980687]

TRACHEOSTOMY & CRICOTHYROTOMY

There are two primary indications for tracheotomy: airway obstruction at or above the level of the larynx and respiratory failure requiring prolonged mechanical ventilation. In an acute emergency, cricothyrotomy secures an airway more rapidly than tracheotomy, with fewer potential immediate complications, such as pneumothorax and hemorrhage. Percutaneous dilatational tracheotomy as an elective bedside (or intensive care unit) procedure has undergone scrutiny in recent years as an alternative to tracheotomy. In experienced hands, the various methods of percutaneous tracheotomy have been documented to be safe in carefully selected patients. Simultaneous videobronchoscopy can reduce the incidence of major complications. The major cost reduction comes from avoiding the operating room. Bedside tracheotomy (in the intensive care unit) achieves similar cost reduction and is advocated by some experts as slightly less costly than the percutaneous procedures.

The most common indication for elective tracheotomy is the need for prolonged mechanical ventilation. There is no firm rule about how many days a patient must be intubated before conversion to tracheotomy should be advised. The incidence of serious complications, such as subglottic stenosis increases with extended endotracheal intubation. As soon as it is apparent that the patient will require protracted ventilatory support, tracheotomy should replace the endotracheal tube. Less frequent indications for tracheostomy are life-threatening aspiration pneumonia, the need to improve pulmonary toilet to correct problems related to insufficient clearing of tracheobronchial secretions, and sleep apnea.

Posttracheotomy care requires humidified air to prevent secretions from crusting and occluding the inner cannula of the tracheotomy tube. The tracheotomy tube should be cleaned several times daily. The most frequent early complication of tracheotomy is dislodgment of the tracheotomy tube. Surgical creation of an inferiorly based tracheal flap sutured to the inferior neck skin may make reinsertion of a dislodged tube easier. It should be recalled that the act of swallowing requires elevation of the larynx, which is limited by tracheotomy. Therefore, frequent tracheal and bronchial suctioning is often required to clear the aspirated saliva as well as the increased tracheobronchial secretions. Care of the skin around the stoma is important to prevent maceration and secondary infection.

Halum SL et al. A multi-institutional analysis of tracheotomy complications. Laryngoscope. 2012 Jan;122(1):38–45. [PMID: 22183627]

FOREIGN BODIES IN THE UPPER AERODIGESTIVE TRACT

FOREIGN BODIES OF THE TRACHEA & BRONCHI

Aspiration of foreign bodies occurs much less frequently in adults than in children. The elderly and denture wearers appear to be at greatest risk. Wider familiarity with the Heimlich maneuver has reduced deaths. If the maneuver is unsuccessful, cricothyrotomy may be necessary. Plain chest radiographs may reveal a radiopaque foreign body. Detection of radiolucent foreign bodies may be aided by inspiration-expiration films that demonstrate air trapping distal to the obstructed segment. Atelectasis and pneumonia may occur later.

Tracheal and bronchial foreign bodies should be removed under general anesthesia with rigid bronchoscopy by a skilled endoscopist working with an experienced anesthesiologist.

ESOPHAGEAL FOREIGN BODIES

Foreign bodies in the esophagus create urgent but not life-threatening situations as long as the airway is not compromised. There is probably time to consult an experienced clinician for management. It is a useful diagnostic sign of complete obstruction if the patient is drooling or cannot handle secretions. Patients may often point to the exact level of the obstruction. Indirect laryngoscopy often shows pooling of saliva at the esophageal inlet. Plain films may detect radiopaque foreign bodies, such as chicken bones. Coins tend to align in the coronal plane in the esophagus and sagittally in the trachea. If a foreign body is suspected, a barium swallow may help make the diagnosis.

The treatment of an esophageal foreign body depends very much on identification of its nature. In children, swallowed nonfood objects are common. In adults, however, food foreign bodies are more common, and there is the greater possibility of underlying esophageal pathology. Endoscopic removal and examination is usually best via flexible esophagoscopy or rigid laryngoscopy and esophagoscopy. If there is nothing sharp, such as a bone, some clinicians advocate a hospitalized 24-hour observation period prior to esophagoscopy, noting that spontaneous passage of the foreign body will occur in 50% of adult patients. In the management of meat obstruction, the use of papain (meat tenderizer) should be discouraged because it can damage the esophageal mucosa and lead to stenosis or perforation.

Weissberg D et al. Foreign bodies in the esophagus. Ann Thorac Surg. 2007 Dec;84(6):1854–7. [PMID: 18036898]

DISEASES PRESENTING AS NECK MASSES

The differential diagnosis of neck masses is heavily dependent on the location in the neck, the age of the patient, and the presence of associated disease processes. Rapid growth and tenderness suggest an inflammatory process, while firm, painless, and slowly enlarging masses are often neoplastic. In young adults, most neck masses are benign (branchial cleft cyst, thyroglossal duct cyst, reactive lymphadenitis), although malignancy should always be considered (lymphoma, metastatic thyroid carcinoma). Lymphadenopathy is common in HIV-positive persons, but a growing or dominant mass may well represent lymphoma. In adults over age 40, cancer is the most common cause of persistent neck mass. A metastasis from squamous cell carcinoma arising within the mouth, pharynx, larynx, or upper esophagus should be suspected, especially if there is a history of tobacco or significant alcohol use. Especially among patients younger than 30 or older than 70, lymphoma should be considered. In any case, a comprehensive otolaryngologic examination is needed. Cytologic evaluation of the neck mass via FNA biopsy is likely to be the next step if an obvious primary tumor is not obvious on physical examination.

CONGENITAL LESIONS PRESENTING AS NECK MASSES IN ADULTS

1. Branchial Cleft Cysts

Branchial cleft cysts usually present as a soft cystic mass along the anterior border of the sternocleidomastoid muscle. These lesions are usually recognized in the second or third decades of life, often when they suddenly swell or become infected. To prevent recurrent infection and possible carcinoma, they should be completely excised, along with their fistulous tracts.

First branchial cleft cysts present high in the neck, sometimes just below the ear. A fistulous connection with the floor of the external auditory canal may be present. Second branchial cleft cysts, which are far more common, may communicate with the tonsillar fossa. Third branchial cleft cysts, which may communicate with the piriform sinus, are rare and present low in the neck.

Magdy EA et al. First branchial cleft anomalies: presentation, variability and safe surgical management. Eur Arch Otorhinolaryngol. 2013 May;270(6):1917–25. [PMID: 23192665]

2. Thyroglossal Duct Cysts

Thyroglossal duct cysts occur along the embryologic course of the thyroid's descent from the tuberculum impar of the tongue base to its usual position in the low neck. Although they may occur at any age, they are most common before age 20. They present as a midline neck mass, often just below the hyoid bone, which moves with swallowing. Surgical excision is recommended to prevent recurrent infection. This requires removal of the entire fistulous tract along with the middle portion of the hyoid bone through which many of the fistulas pass. Preoperative evaluation should include a thyroid ultrasound to confirm anatomic position of the thyroid.

Oomen KP et al. Thyroglossal duct cyst and ectopic thyroid: surgical management. Otolaryngol Clin North Am. 2015 Feb; 48(1):15–27. [PMID: 25439547]

INFECTIOUS & INFLAMMATORY NECK MASSES

1. Reactive Cervical Lymphadenopathy

Normal lymph nodes in the neck are usually less than 1 cm in length. Infections involving the pharynx, salivary glands, and scalp often cause tender enlargement of neck nodes. Enlarged nodes are common in HIV-infected persons. Except for the occasional node that suppurates and requires incision and drainage, treatment is directed against the underlying infection. An enlarged node (larger than 1.5 cm) or node with a necrotic center that is not associated with an obvious infection should be further evaluated, especially if the patient has a history of smoking, alcohol use, or prior cancer. Other common indications for FNA biopsy of a node include its persistence or continued enlargement. Common causes of cervical adenopathy include tumor (squamous cell carcinoma, lymphoma, occasional metastases from non-head and neck sites) and infection (eg, reactive nodes, mycobacteria, and cat-scratch disease). Rare causes of adenopathy include Kikuchi disease (histiocytic necrotizing lymphadenitis) and autoimmune adenopathy.

Leung AK et al. Cervical lymphadenitis: etiology, diagnosis, and management. Curr Infect Dis Rep. 2009 May;11(3):183–9. [PMID: 19366560]

2. Tuberculous & Nontuberculous Mycobacterial Lymphadenitis

Granulomatous neck masses are not uncommon. The differential diagnosis includes mycobacterial adenitis, sarcoidosis, and cat-scratch disease due to *Bartonella henselae*. Mycobacterial lymphadenitis is on the rise both in immunocompromised and immunocompetent individuals. The usual presentation of granulomatous disease in the neck is simply single or matted nodes. Although mycobacterial adenitis can extend to the skin and drain externally (as described for atypical mycobacteria and referred to as scrofula), this late presentation is no longer common.

FNA biopsy is usually the best initial diagnostic approach: cytology, smear for acid-fast bacilli, culture, and a sensitivity test can all be done. PCR from FNA (or from excised tissue) is the most sensitive test and is particularly useful when conventional methods have not been diagnostic but clinical impression remains consistent for tuberculous infection. While FNA has a high sensitivity (about 88%), its specificity is low (49%), often requiring an excisional biopsy to confirm the diagnosis.

See Table 9–16 for current recommended treatment of tuberculous lymphadenopathy. For atypical (nontuberculous) lymphadenopathy, treatment depends on the sensitivity results of culture, but antibiotics likely to be useful include 6 months of isoniazid and rifampin and, for at least the first 2 months, ethambutol—all in standard dosages. Some would totally excise the involved nodes prior to chemotherapy, depending on location and other factors, but this can lead to chronic draining fistulas.

Abdissa K et al. Bacteriological methods as add on tests to fine-needle aspiration cytology in diagnosis of tuberculous lymphadenitis: can they reduce the diagnostic dilemma? BMC Infect Dis. 2014 Dec 31;14(1):3850. [PMID: 25551280]
Fontanilla JM et al. Current diagnosis and management of peripheral tuberculous lymphadenitis. Clin Infect Dis. 2011 Sep; 53(6):555–62. [PMID: 21865192]

3. Lyme Disease

Lyme disease, caused by the spirochete *Borrelia burgdorferi* and transmitted by ticks of the *Ixodes* genus, may have protean manifestation, but over 75% of patients have symptoms involving the head and neck. Facial paralysis, dysesthesias, dysgeusia, or other cranial neuropathies are most common. Headache, pain, and cervical lymphadenopathy may occur. See Chapter 34 for a more detailed discussion.

Ljøstad U et al. Chronic Lyme; diagnostic and therapeutic challenges. Acta Neurol Scand Suppl. 2013;(196):38–47. [PMID: 23190290]

TUMOR METASTASES

In older adults, 80% of firm, persistent, and enlarging neck masses are metastatic in origin. The great majority of these arise from squamous cell carcinoma of the upper aerodigestive tract. A complete head and neck examination may reveal the tumor of origin, but examination under anesthesia with direct laryngoscopy, esophagoscopy, and bronchoscopy is usually required to fully evaluate the tumor and exclude second primaries.

It is often helpful to obtain a cytologic diagnosis if initial head and neck examination fails to reveal the primary tumor. An open biopsy should be done only when neither physical examination by an experienced clinician specializing in head and neck cancer nor FNA biopsy performed by an experienced cytopathologist yields a diagnosis. In such a setting, one should strongly consider obtaining an MRI or PET scan prior to open biopsy, as these methods may yield valuable information about a possible presumed primary site or another site for FNA.

With the exception of papillary thyroid carcinoma, non–squamous cell metastases to the neck are infrequent. While tumors that are not primary in the head or neck seldom metastasize to the cervical lymph nodes, the supraclavicular lymph nodes are quite often involved by lung, gastroesophageal, and breast tumors. Infradiaphragmatic tumors, with the exception of renal cell carcinoma and testicular cancer, rarely metastasize to the neck.

Barzilai G et al. Pattern of regional metastases from cutaneous squamous cell carcinoma of the head and neck. Otolaryngol Head Neck Surg. 2005 Jun;132(6):852–6. [PMID: 15944554]

LYMPHOMA

About 10% of lymphomas present in the head and neck. Multiple rubbery nodes, especially in young adults or in patients who have AIDS, are suggestive of this disease. A thorough physical examination may demonstrate other sites of nodal or organ involvement. FNA biopsy may be diagnostic, but open biopsy is often required to determine architecture and an appropriate treatment course.

Bryson TC et al. Cervical lymph node evaluation and diagnosis. Otolaryngol Clin North Am. 2012 Dec;45(6):1363–83. [PMID: 23153753]

Pulmonary Disorders

Mark S. Chesnutt, MD
Thomas J. Prendergast, MD

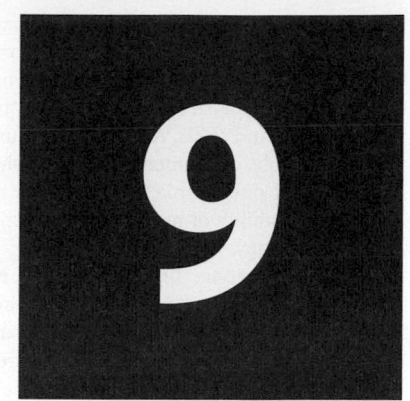

9

DISORDERS OF THE AIRWAYS

Airway disorders have diverse causes but share certain common pathophysiologic and clinical features. Airflow limitation is characteristic and frequently causes dyspnea and cough. Other symptoms are common and typically disease-specific. Disorders of the airways can be classified as those that involve the upper airways—loosely defined as those above and including the vocal folds—and those that involve the lower airways.

DISORDERS OF THE UPPER AIRWAYS

Acute upper airway obstruction can be immediately life-threatening and must be relieved promptly to avoid asphyxia. Causes of acute upper airway obstruction include trauma to the larynx or pharynx, foreign body aspiration, laryngospasm, laryngeal edema from thermal injury or angioedema, infections (acute epiglottitis, Ludwig angina, pharyngeal or retropharyngeal abscess), and acute allergic laryngitis.

Chronic obstruction of the upper airway may be caused by carcinoma of the pharynx or larynx, laryngeal or subglottic stenosis, laryngeal granulomas or webs, or bilateral vocal fold paralysis. Laryngeal or subglottic stenosis may become evident weeks or months after translaryngeal endotracheal intubation. Inspiratory stridor, intercostal retractions on inspiration, a palpable inspiratory thrill over the larynx, and wheezing localized to the neck or trachea on auscultation are characteristic findings. Flow-volume loops may show flow limitations characteristic of obstruction. Soft-tissue radiographs of the neck may show supraglottic or infraglottic narrowing. CT and MRI scans can reveal exact sites of obstruction. Flexible endoscopy may be diagnostic, but caution is necessary to avoid exacerbating upper airway edema and precipitating critical airway narrowing.

Vocal fold dysfunction syndrome is characterized by paradoxical vocal fold adduction, resulting in both acute and chronic upper airway obstruction. It can cause dyspnea and wheezing that may be distinguished from asthma or exercise-induced asthma by the lack of response to bronchodilator therapy, normal spirometry immediately after an attack, spirometric evidence of upper airway obstruction, a negative bronchial provocation test, or direct visualization of adduction of the vocal folds on both inspiration and expiration. The condition appears to be psychogenic in nature. Bronchodilators are of no therapeutic benefit. Treatment consists of speech therapy, which uses breathing, voice, and neck relaxation exercises to abort the symptoms.

Hoyte FC. Vocal cord dysfunction. Immunol Allergy Clin North Am. 2013 Feb;33(1):1–22. [PMID: 23337061]
Idrees M et al. Vocal cord dysfunction in bronchial asthma. A review article. J Asthma. 2015 May;52(4):327–35. [PMID: 25365113]

DISORDERS OF THE LOWER AIRWAYS

Tracheal obstruction may be intrathoracic (below the suprasternal notch) or extrathoracic. Fixed tracheal obstruction may be caused by acquired or congenital tracheal stenosis, primary or secondary tracheal neoplasms, extrinsic compression (tumors of the lung, thymus, or thyroid; lymphadenopathy; congenital vascular rings; aneurysms; etc), foreign body aspiration, tracheal granulomas and papillomas, and tracheal trauma. Tracheomalacia, foreign body aspiration, and retained secretions may cause variable tracheal obstruction.

Acquired **tracheal stenosis** is usually secondary to previous tracheotomy or endotracheal intubation. Dyspnea, cough, and inability to clear pulmonary secretions occur weeks to months after tracheal decannulation or extubation. Physical findings may be absent until tracheal diameter is reduced 50% or more, when wheezing, a palpable tracheal thrill, and harsh breath sounds may be detected. The diagnosis is usually confirmed by plain films or CT of the trachea. Complications include recurring pulmonary infection and life-threatening respiratory failure. Management is directed toward ensuring adequate ventilation and oxygenation and avoiding manipulative procedures that may increase edema of the tracheal mucosa. Surgical reconstruction, endotracheal stent placement, or laser photoresection may be required.

Bronchial obstruction may be caused by retained pulmonary secretions, aspiration, foreign bodies, bronchomalacia, bronchogenic carcinoma, compression by extrinsic masses, and tumors metastatic to the airway. Clinical and radiographic findings vary depending on the location of the obstruction and the degree of airway narrowing. Symptoms include dyspnea, cough, wheezing, and, if infection is present, fever and chills. A history of recurrent pneumonia in the same lobe or segment or slow resolution (more than 3 months) of pneumonia on successive radiographs suggests the possibility of bronchial obstruction and the need for bronchoscopy.

Roentgenographic findings include **atelectasis** (local parenchymal collapse), postobstructive infiltrates, and air trapping caused by unidirectional expiratory obstruction. CT scanning may demonstrate the nature and exact location of obstruction of the central bronchi. MRI may be superior to CT for delineating the extent of underlying disease in the hilum, but it is usually reserved for cases in which CT findings are equivocal. Bronchoscopy is the definitive diagnostic study, particularly if tumor or foreign body aspiration is suspected. The finding of bronchial breath sounds on physical examination or an air bronchogram on chest radiograph in an area of atelectasis rules out complete airway obstruction. Bronchoscopy is unlikely to be of therapeutic benefit in this situation.

Al-Qadi MO et al. The "forgotten zone": acquired disorders of the trachea in adults. Respir Med. 2013 Sep;107(9):1301–13. [PMID: 23669413]

ASTHMA

ESSENTIALS OF DIAGNOSIS

► Episodic or chronic symptoms of airflow obstruction.

► Reversibility of airflow obstruction, either spontaneously or following bronchodilator therapy.

► Symptoms frequently worse at night or in the early morning.

► Prolonged expiration and diffuse wheezes on physical examination.

► Limitation of airflow on pulmonary function testing or positive bronchoprovocation challenge.

▶ General Considerations

Asthma is a common disease, affecting approximately 8–10% of the population. It is slightly more common in male children (younger than 14 years) and in female adults. There is a genetic predisposition to asthma. Prevalence, hospitalizations, and fatal asthma have all increased in the United States over the past 20 years. Each year, approximately 1.75 million emergency department visits, 480,000 hospital admissions, and more than 3000 deaths in the United States are attributed to asthma. Hospitalization rates have been highest among blacks and children, and death rates are consistently highest among blacks aged 15–24 years.

▶ Definition & Pathogenesis

Asthma is a chronic inflammatory disorder of the airways. No single histopathologic feature is pathognomonic but common findings include inflammatory cell infiltration with eosinophils, neutrophils, and lymphocytes (especially T lymphocytes); goblet cell hyperplasia, sometimes with plugging of small airways with thick mucus; collagen deposition beneath the basement membrane; hypertrophy of bronchial smooth muscle; airway edema; mast cell activation; and denudation of airway epithelium. This airway inflammation underlies disease chronicity and contributes to airway hyper-responsiveness and airflow limitation.

The strongest identifiable predisposing factor for the development of asthma is atopy, but obesity is increasingly recognized as a risk factor. Exposure of sensitive patients to inhaled allergens increases airway inflammation, airway hyper-responsiveness, and symptoms. Symptoms may develop immediately (immediate asthmatic response) or 4–6 hours after allergen exposure (late asthmatic response). Common allergens include house dust mites (often found in pillows, mattresses, upholstered furniture, carpets, and drapes), cockroaches, cat dander, and seasonal pollens. Substantially reducing exposure reduces pathologic findings and clinical symptoms.

Nonspecific precipitants of asthma include exercise, upper respiratory tract infections, rhinosinusitis, postnasal drip, aspiration, gastroesophageal reflux, changes in the weather, and stress. Exposure to **products of combustion** (eg, from tobacco, crack cocaine, methamphetamines, and other agents) increases asthma symptoms and the need for medications and reduces lung function. **Air pollution** (increased air levels of respirable particles, ozone, SO_2, and NO_2) precipitate asthma symptoms and increase emergency department visits and hospitalizations. Selected individuals may experience asthma symptoms after exposure to aspirin, nonsteroidal anti-inflammatory drugs, or tartrazine dyes. Other **medications** may precipitate asthma symptoms (see Table 9–24). **Occupational asthma** is triggered by various agents in the workplace and may occur weeks to years after initial exposure and sensitization. Women may experience **catamenial asthma** at predictable times during the menstrual cycle. **Exercise-induced bronchoconstriction** begins during exercise or within 3 minutes after its end, peaks within 10–15 minutes, and then resolves by 60 minutes. This phenomenon is thought to be a consequence of the airways' attempt to warm and humidify an increased volume of expired air during exercise. "Cardiac asthma" is wheezing precipitated by decompensated heart failure.

▶ Clinical Findings

Symptoms and signs vary widely among patients as well as individually over time. General clinical findings in stable asthma patients are listed in Figure 9–1 and Table 9–1; Table 9–2 lists findings seen during asthma exacerbations.

A. Symptoms and Signs

Asthma is characterized by episodic wheezing, difficulty in breathing, chest tightness, and cough. Excess sputum

Components of Severity		Classification of Asthma Severity ≥12 years of age			
			Persistent		
		Intermittent	Mild	Moderate	Severe
Impairment Normal FEV_1/FVC: 8–19 yr 85% 20–39 yr 80% 40–59 yr 75% 60–80 yr 70%	Symptoms	≤ 2 days/week	> 2 days/week but not daily	Daily	Throughout the day
	Nighttime awakenings	≤ 2x/month	3–4x/month	> 1x/week but not nightly	Often 7x/week
	Short-acting β_2-agonist use for symptom control (not prevention of EIB)	≤ 2 days/week	> 2 days/week but not daily, and not more than 1x on any day	Daily	Several times per day
	Interference with normal activity	None	Minor limitation	Some limitation	Extremely limited
	Lung function	• Normal FEV_1 between exacerbations • FEV_1 > 80% predicted • FEV_1/FVC normal	• FEV_1 > 80% predicted • FEV_1/FVC normal	• FEV_1 > 60% but < 80% predicted • FEV_1/FVC reduced 5%	• FEV_1 < 60% predicted • FEV_1/FVC reduced > 5%
Risk	Exacerbations requiring oral systemic corticosteroids	0–1/year (see note)	≥ 2/year (see note) ⟶		
		⟵ Consider severity and interval since last exacerbation. ⟶ Frequency and severity may fluctuate over time for patients in any severity category. Relative annual risk of exacerbations may be related to FEV_1.			
Recommended Step for Initiating Treatment (See Figure 9–2 for treatment steps.)		Step 1	Step 2	Step 3 and consider short course of oral systemic corticosteroids	Step 4 or 5
		In 2–6 weeks, evaluate level of asthma control that is achieved and adjust therapy accordingly.			

EIB, exercise-induced bronchospasm; FEV_1, forced expiratory volume in 1 second; FVC, forced vital capacity; ICU, intensive care unit.

Notes:

- The stepwise approach is meant to assist, not replace, the clinical decision-making required to meet individual patient needs.

- Level of severity is determined by assessment of both impairment and risk. Assess impairment domain by patient's/caregiver's recall of previous 2–4 weeks and spirometry. Assign severity to the most severe category in which any feature occurs.

- At present, there are inadequate data to correspond frequencies of exacerbations with different levels of asthma severity. In general, more frequent and intense exacerbations (eg, requiring urgent, unscheduled care, hospitalization, or ICU admission) indicate greater underlying disease severity. For treatment purposes, patients who had ≥ 2 exacerbations requiring oral systemic corticosteroids in the past year may be considered the same as patients who have persistent asthma, even in the absence of impairment levels consistent with persistent asthma.

▲ **Figure 9–1. Classifying asthma severity and initiating treatment.** (Adapted from National Asthma Education and Prevention Program. Expert Panel Report 3: Guidelines for the Diagnosis and Management of Asthma. National Institutes of Health Pub. No. 08-4051. Bethesda, MD, 2007. http://www.nhlbi.nih.gov/guidelines/asthma/asthgdln.htm.)

production is common. The frequency of asthma symptoms is highly variable. Some patients have infrequent, brief attacks of asthma while others may suffer nearly continuous symptoms. Asthma symptoms may occur spontaneously or be precipitated or exacerbated by many different triggers as discussed above. Asthma symptoms are frequently worse at

night; circadian variations in bronchomotor tone and bronchial reactivity reach their nadir between 3 AM and 4 AM, increasing symptoms of bronchoconstriction.

Some physical examination findings increase the probability of asthma. Nasal mucosal swelling, secretion increases, and polyps are often seen in patients with

Table 9–1. Assessing asthma control.

Components of Control		Classification of Asthma Control (≥ 12 years of age)		
		Well Controlled	**Not Well Controlled**	**Very Poorly Controlled**
Impairment	Symptoms	≤ 2 days/week	> 2 days/week	Throughout the day
	Nighttime awakenings	≤ 2×/month	1–3×/week	≥ 4×/week
	Interference with normal activity	None	Some limitation	Extremely limited
	Short-acting beta-2-agonist use for symptom control (not prevention of EIB)	≤ 2 days/week	> 2 days/week	Several times/day
	FEV$_1$ or peak flow Validated Questionnaires	> 80% predicted/ personal best	60–80% predicted/ personal best	< 60% predicted/ personal best
	ATAQ	0	1–2	3–4
	ACQ	≤ 0.75[1]	≥ 1.5	N/A
	ACT	≥ 20	16–19	≤ 15
Risk	Exacerbations requiring oral system corticosteroids	0–1/year	≥ 2/year (see note)	
		Consider severity and interval since last exacerbation		
	Progressive loss of lung function	Evaluation requires long-term follow-up care		
	Treatment-related adverse effects	Medication side effects can vary in intensity from none to very troublesome and worrisome. The level of intensity does not correlate to specific levels of control but should be considered in the overall assessment of risk.		
Recommended Action for Treatment (see Figure 9–2 for steps)		• Maintain current step • Regular follow-ups every 1–6 months to maintain control. • Consider step down if well controlled for at least 3 months.	• Step up 1 step and • Reevaluate in 2–6 weeks. • For side effects, consider alternative treatment options.	• Consider short course of oral systemic corticosteroids, • Step up 1–2 steps, and • Reevaluate in 2 weeks. • For side effects, consider alternative treatment options.

[1]ACQ values of 0.76–1.4 are indeterminate regarding well-controlled asthma.

EIB, exercise-induced bronchospasm; FEV$_1$, forced expiratory volume in 1 second; ICU, intensive care unit.

Notes:

- The stepwise approach is meant to assist, not replace, the clinical decision-making required to meet individual patient needs.
- The level of control is based on the most severe impairment or risk category. Assess impairment domain by patient's recall of previous 2–4 weeks and by spirometry or peak flow measures. Symptom assessment for longer periods should reflect a global assessment, such as inquiring whether the patient's asthma is better or worse since the last visit.
- At present, there are inadequate data to correspond frequencies of exacerbations with different levels of asthma control. In general, more frequent and intense exacerbations (eg, requiring urgent, unscheduled care, hospitalization, or ICU admission) indicate poorer disease control. For treatment purposes, patients who had ≥ 2 exacerbations requiring oral systemic corticosteroids in the past year may be considered the same as patients who have not-well-controlled asthma, even in the absence of impairment levels consistent with not-well-controlled asthma.
- Validated Questionnaires for the impairment domain (the questionnaire did not assess lung function or the risk domain).
  ATAQ = Asthma Therapy Assessment Questionnaire©
  ACQ = Asthma Control Questionnaire© (user package may be obtained at www.qoltech.co.uk)
  ACT = Asthma Control Test™
Minimal Importance Difference: 1.0 for the ATAQ; 0.5 for the ACQ; not determined for the ACT.
- Before step up in therapy:
  —Review adherence to medication, inhaler.
  —If an alternative treatment option was used in a step, discontinue and use the preferred treatment for that step.

Adapted from National Asthma Education and Prevention Program. Expert Panel Report 3: Guidelines for the Diagnosis and Management of Asthma. National Institutes of Health Pub. No. 08-4051. Bethesda, MD, 2007. http://www.nhlbi.nih.gov/guidelines/asthma/-guidelines/fullreport.

Table 9–2. Evaluation and classification of severity of asthma exacerbations.

	Mild	Moderate	Severe	Respiratory Arrest Imminent
Symptoms				
Breathlessness	While walking	At rest, limits activity	At rest, interferes with conversation	While at rest, mute
Talks in	Sentences	Phrases	Words	Silent
Alertness	May be agitated	Usually agitated	Usually agitated	Drowsy or confused
Signs				
Respiratory rate	Increased	Increased	Often > 30/minute	> 30/minute
Body position	Can lie down	Prefers sitting	Sits upright	Unable to recline
Use of accessory muscles; suprasternal retractions	Usually not	Commonly	Usually	Paradoxical thoracoabdominal movement
Wheeze	Moderate, often only end expiratory	Loud; throughout exhalation	Usually loud; throughout inhalation and exhalation	Absent
Pulse/minute	< 100	100–120	> 120	Bradycardia
Pulsus paradoxus	Absent < 10 mm Hg	May be present 10–25 mm Hg	Often present > 25 mm Hg	Absence suggests respiratory muscle fatigue
Functional Assessment				
PEF or FEV_1 % predicted or % personal best	≥ 70%	40–69%	< 40%	< 25%
Pao_2 (on air, mm Hg)	Normal[1]	≥ 60[1]	< 60: possible cyanosis	< 60: possible cyanosis
Pco_2 (mm Hg)	< 42 mm Hg[1]	< 42 mm Hg[1]	≥ 42[1]	≥ 42[1]
Sao_2 (on air, %)	> 95%[1]	90–95%[1]	< 90%[1]	< 90%[1]

[1]Test not usually necessary.
FEV_1, forced expiratory volume in 1 second; PEF, peak expiratory flow; Sao_2, oxygen saturation.
Adapted from National Asthma Education and Prevention Program. Expert Panel Report 3: Guidelines for the Diagnosis and Management of Asthma. National Institutes of Health Pub. No. 08-4051. Bethesda, MD, 2007. http://www.nhlbi.nih.gov/healthpro/guidelines/current/asthma-guidelines/fullreport.

allergic asthma. Eczema, atopic dermatitis, or other allergic skin disorders may also be present. Wheezing or a prolonged expiratory phase during normal breathing correlates well with the presence of airflow obstruction. (Wheezing during forced expiration does not.) Chest examination may be normal between exacerbations in patients with mild asthma. During severe asthma exacerbations, airflow may be too limited to produce wheezing, and the only diagnostic clue on auscultation may be globally reduced breath sounds with prolonged expiration. Hunched shoulders and use of accessory muscles of respiration suggest an increased work of breathing.

B. Laboratory Findings

Arterial blood gas measurements may be normal during a mild asthma exacerbation, but respiratory alkalosis and an increase in the alveolar-arterial oxygen difference (A–a–Do_2) are common. During severe exacerbations, hypoxemia develops and the $Paco_2$ returns to normal. The combination of an increased $Paco_2$ and respiratory acidosis may indicate impending respiratory failure and the need for mechanical ventilation.

C. Pulmonary Function Testing

Clinicians are able to identify airflow obstruction on examination, but they have limited ability to assess its severity or to predict whether it is reversible. The evaluation for asthma should therefore include **spirometry** (forced expiratory volume in 1 second [FEV_1], forced vital capacity [FVC], FEV_1/FVC) before and after the administration of a short-acting bronchodilator. These measurements help determine the presence and extent of airflow obstruction and whether it is immediately reversible. Airflow obstruction is indicated by a reduced FEV_1/FVC ratio. Significant reversibility of airflow obstruction is defined by an increase of 12% or more and 200 mL in FEV_1 or FVC after inhaling a short-acting bronchodilator. **A positive bronchodilator response strongly confirms the diagnosis of asthma but a lack of responsiveness in the pulmonary function laboratory does not preclude success in a clinical trial of bronchodilator therapy.** Severe airflow obstruction results in significant air trapping, with an increase in residual volume and consequent reduction in FVC, resulting in a pattern that may mimic a restrictive ventilatory defect.

Bronchial provocation testing with inhaled histamine or methacholine may be useful when asthma is suspected but spirometry is nondiagnostic. Bronchial provocation is not recommended if the FEV_1 is less than 65% of predicted. A positive methacholine test is defined as a fall in the FEV_1 of 20% or more at exposure to a concentration of 16 mg/mL or less. A negative test has a negative predictive value for asthma of 95%. Exercise challenge testing may be useful in patients with symptoms of exercise-induced bronchospasm.

Peak expiratory flow (PEF) meters are handheld devices designed as personal monitoring tools. PEF monitoring can establish peak flow variability, quantify asthma severity, and provide both patient and clinician with objective measurements on which to base treatment decisions. There are conflicting data about whether measuring PEF improves asthma outcomes, but doing so is recommended to help confirm the diagnosis of asthma, to improve asthma control in patients with poor perception of airflow obstruction, and to identify environmental and occupational causes of symptoms. Predicted values for PEF vary with age, height, and gender but are poorly standardized. **Comparison with reference values is less helpful than comparison with the patient's own baseline.** PEF shows diurnal variation. It is generally lowest on first awakening and highest several hours before the midpoint of the waking day. PEF should be measured in the morning before the administration of a bronchodilator and in the afternoon after taking a bronchodilator. A 20% change in PEF values from morning to afternoon or from day to day suggests inadequately controlled asthma. PEF values less than 200 L/min indicate severe airflow obstruction.

D. Additional Testing

Routine chest radiographs in patients with asthma are usually normal or show only hyperinflation. Other findings may include bronchial wall thickening and diminished peripheral lung vascular shadows. Chest imaging is indicated when pneumonia, another disorder mimicking asthma, or a complication of asthma such as pneumothorax is suspected.

Skin testing or in vitro testing to assess sensitivity to environmental allergens can identify atopy in patients with persistent asthma who may benefit from therapies directed at their allergic diathesis. Evaluations for paranasal sinus disease or gastroesophageal reflux should be considered in patients with pertinent, severe, or refractory asthma symptoms.

▶ Complications

Complications of asthma include exhaustion, dehydration, airway infection, and tussive syncope. Pneumothorax occurs but is rare. Acute hypercapnic and hypoxemic respiratory failure occurs in severe disease.

▶ Differential Diagnosis

Patients who have atypical symptoms or poor response to therapy may have a condition that mimics asthma. These disorders typically fall into one of four categories: upper airway disorders, lower airway disorders, systemic vasculitides, and psychiatric disorders. **Upper airway disorders** that mimic asthma include vocal fold paralysis, vocal fold dysfunction syndrome, foreign body aspiration, laryngotracheal masses, tracheal narrowing, tracheobronchomalacia, and airway edema (eg, angioedema or inhalation injury). **Lower airway disorders** include nonasthmatic chronic obstructive pulmonary disease (COPD) (chronic bronchitis or emphysema), bronchiectasis, allergic bronchopulmonary mycosis, cystic fibrosis, eosinophilic pneumonia, and bronchiolitis obliterans. **Systemic vasculitides** with pulmonary involvement may have an asthmatic component, such as eosinophilic granulomatosis with polyangiitis. **Psychiatric causes** include conversion disorders ("functional" asthma), emotional laryngeal wheezing, vocal fold dysfunction, or episodic laryngeal dyskinesis. Rarely, Münchausen syndrome or malingering may explain a patient's complaints.

▶ NAEPP 3 Diagnosis & Management Guidelines

The third Expert Panel Report of the National Asthma Education and Prevention Program (NAEPP), in conjunction with the Global Initiative for Asthma (GINA), a collaboration between the National Institutes of Health (NIH)/National Heart, Lung, and Blood Institute (NHLBI) and the World Health Organization (WHO), provides guidelines for diagnosis and management of asthma (NAEPP 3) (Figure 9–2). This report identifies four components of chronic asthma diagnosis and management: (1) assessing and monitoring asthma severity and asthma control, (2) patient education designed to foster a partnership for care, (3) control of environmental factors and comorbid conditions that affect asthma, and (4) pharmacologic agents for asthma.

1. Assessing and monitoring asthma severity and asthma control—**Severity** is the intrinsic intensity of the disease process. **Control** is the degree to which symptoms and limitations on activity are minimized by therapy. **Responsiveness** is the ease with which control is achieved with therapy. NAEPP 3 guidelines emphasize control over classifications of severity, since the latter is variable over time and in response to therapy. A measure of severity on initial presentation (Figure 9–1) is helpful, however, in guiding the initiation of therapy. Control of asthma is assessed in terms of **impairment** (frequency and intensity of symptoms and functional limitations) and **risk** (the likelihood of acute exacerbations or chronic decline in lung function). A key insight is that these two domains of control may respond differently to treatment: some patients may have minimal impairment yet remain at risk for severe exacerbations, for example, in the setting of an upper respiratory tract infection. Table 9–1 is used to assess the adequacy of asthma control and is used in conjunction with Figure 9–2 to guide adjustments in therapy based on the level of control.

2. Patient education designed to foster a partnership for care—Active self-management reduces urgent care visits

Intermittent Asthma	Persistent Asthma: Daily Medication Consult with asthma specialist if step 4 care or higher is required. Consider consultation at step 3.

Step 1

Preferred:

SABA PRN

Step 2

Preferred:

Low-dose ICS

Alternative:

Cromolyn, LTRA, nedocromil, or theophylline

Step 3

Preferred:

Low-dose ICS + LABA
OR
Medium-dose ICS

Alternative:

Low-dose ICS + either LTRA, theophylline, or zileuton

Step 4

Preferred:

Medium-dose ICS + LABA

Alternative:

Low-dose ICS + either LTRA, theophylline, or zileuton

Step 5

Preferred:

High-dose ICS + LABA

AND

Consider omalizumab for patients who have allergies

Step 6

Preferred:

High-dose ICS + LABA + oral corticosteroid

AND

Consider omalizumab for patients who have allergies

Step up if needed

(first, check adherence, environmental control, and comorbid conditions)

Assess control

Step down if possible

(and asthma is well controlled at least 3 months)

Each step: Patient education, environmental control, and management of comorbidities.

Steps 2–4: Consider subcutaneous allergen immunotherapy for patients who have allergic asthma (see notes).

Quick-Relief Medication for All Patients

- SABA as needed for symptoms. Intensity of treatment depends on severity of symptoms: up to three treatments at 20-minute intervals as needed. Short course of oral systemic corticosteroids may be needed.
- Use of SABA > 2 days a week for symptom relief (not prevention of EIB) generally indicates inadequate control and the need to step up treatment.

Key: *Alphabetical order is used when more than one treatment option is listed within either preferred or alternative therapy.* EIB, exercise-induced bronchospasm; ICS, inhaled corticosteroid; LABA, inhaled long-acting beta-2-agonist; LTRA, leukotriene receptor antagonist; SABA, inhaled short-acting beta-2-agonist

Notes:

- The stepwise approach is meant to assist, not replace, the clinical decision-making required to meet individual patient needs.

- If alternative treatment is used and response is inadequate, discontinue it and use the preferred treatment before stepping up.

- Zileuton is a less desirable alternative as adjunctive therapy due to limited studies and the need to monitor liver function. Theophylline requires monitoring of serum concentration levels.

- In step 6, before oral systemic corticosteroids are introduced, a trial of high-dose ICS + LABA + either LTRA, theophylline, or zileuton may be considered, although this approach has not been studied in clinical trials.

- Step 1, 2, and 3 preferred therapies are based on Evidence A; step 3 alternative therapy is based on Evidence A for LTRA, Evidence B for theophylline, and Evidence D for zileuton. Step 4 preferred therapy is based on Evidence B, and alternative therapy is based on Evidence B for LTRA and theophylline and Evidence D for zileuton. Step 5 preferred therapy is based on Evidence B. Step 6 preferred therapy is based on NAEPP Expert Panel Report 2, 1997 and Evidence B for omalizumab.

- Immunotherapy for steps 2–4 is based on Evidence B for house-dust mites, animal danders, and pollens; evidence is weak or lacking for molds and cockroaches. Evidence is strongest for immunotherapy with single allergens. The role of allergy in asthma is greater in children than in adults.

- Clinicians who administer immunotherapy or omalizumab should be prepared and equipped to identify and treat anaphylaxis that may occur.

▲ **Figure 9–2.** Stepwise approach to managing asthma. (Adapted from National Asthma Education and Prevention Program. Expert Panel Report 3: Guidelines for the Diagnosis and Management of Asthma. National Institutes of Health Pub. No. 08-4051. Bethesda, MD, 2007. http://www.nhlbi.nih.gov/guidelines/asthma/asthgdln.htm.)

and hospitalizations and improves perceived control of asthma. Therefore, an outpatient preventive approach that includes self-management education is an integral part of effective asthma care.

All patients, but particularly those with poorly controlled symptoms or history of severe exacerbations, should have a written **asthma action plan** that includes instructions for daily management and measures to take in response to specific changes in status. Patients should be taught to recognize symptoms—especially patterns indicating inadequate asthma control or predicting the need for additional therapy.

3. Control of environmental factors and comorbid conditions that affect asthma—Significant reduction in exposure to nonspecific airway irritants or to inhaled allergens in atopic patients may reduce symptoms and medication needs. Comorbid conditions that impair asthma management, such as rhinosinusitis, gastroesophageal reflux, obesity, and obstructive sleep apnea, should be identified and treated. This search for complicating conditions is particularly crucial in the initial evaluation of new asthma, and in patients who have difficult-to-control symptoms or frequent exacerbations.

4. Pharmacologic agents for asthma—Asthma medications can be divided into two categories: quick-relief (**reliever**) medications that act principally by direct relaxation of bronchial smooth muscle, thereby promoting prompt reversal of acute airflow obstruction to relieve accompanying symptoms, and long-term control (**controller**) medications that act primarily to attenuate airway inflammation and that are taken daily independent of symptoms to achieve and maintain control of persistent asthma.

Most asthma medications are administered orally or by inhalation. Inhalation of an appropriate agent results in a more rapid onset of pulmonary effects as well as fewer systemic effects compared with oral administration of the same dose. Proper inhaler technique and the use of an inhalation chamber (a "spacer") with metered-dose inhalers (MDIs) decrease oropharyngeal deposition and improve drug delivery to the lung. Nebulizer therapy is reserved for acutely ill patients and those who cannot use inhalers because of difficulties with coordination, understanding, or cooperation.

► **Treatment**

The goals of asthma therapy are to minimize chronic symptoms that interfere with normal activity (including exercise), to prevent recurrent exacerbations, to reduce or eliminate the need for emergency department visits or hospitalizations, and to maintain normal or near-normal pulmonary function. These goals should be met while providing pharmacotherapy with the fewest adverse effects and while satisfying patients' and families' expectations of asthma care. **NAEPP 3 recommendations emphasize daily anti-inflammatory therapy with inhaled corticosteroids as the cornerstone of treatment of persistent asthma.**

A. Long-Term Control Medications

Anti-inflammatory agents, long-acting bronchodilators, and leukotriene modifiers comprise the important long-term control medications (Tables 9–3 and 9–4). Other classes of agents are mentioned briefly below as well.

1. Anti-inflammatory agents—Corticosteroids are the most potent and consistently effective anti-inflammatory agents currently available. They reduce both acute and chronic inflammation, resulting in improved airflow, decreased airway hyper-responsiveness, and fewer asthma exacerbations. These agents may also potentiate the action of beta-adrenergic agonists.

Inhaled corticosteroids are preferred, first-line agents for all patients with persistent asthma. Patients with persistent symptoms or asthma exacerbations who are not taking an inhaled corticosteroid should be started on one. The most important determinants of agent selection and appropriate dosing are the patient's status and response to treatment. Dosages for inhaled corticosteroids vary depending on the specific agent and delivery device. For most patients, twice-daily dosing provides adequate control of asthma. Once-daily dosing may be sufficient in selected patients. Maximum responses from inhaled corticosteroids may not be observed for months. The use of an inhalation chamber coupled with mouth washing after inhaled corticosteroid use decreases local side effects (cough, dysphonia, oropharyngeal candidiasis) and systemic absorption. Dry powder inhalers (DPIs) are not used with an inhalation chamber. Systemic effects (adrenal suppression, osteoporosis, skin thinning, easy bruising, and cataracts) may occur with high-dose inhaled corticosteroid therapy.

Systemic corticosteroids (oral or parenteral) are most effective in achieving prompt control of asthma during exacerbations or when initiating long-term asthma therapy in patients with severe symptoms. In patients with refractory, poorly controlled asthma, systemic corticosteroids may be required for the long-term suppression of symptoms. Repeated efforts should be made to reduce the dose to the minimum needed to control symptoms. Alternate-day treatment is preferred to daily treatment. Concurrent treatment with calcium supplements and vitamin D should be initiated to prevent corticosteroid-induced bone mineral loss in long-term administration. Bone mineral density testing after 3 or more months of systemic corticosteroid lifetime use can guide the use of bisphosphonates for treatment of steroid-induced osteoporosis. Rapid discontinuation of systemic corticosteroids after long-term use may precipitate adrenal insufficiency.

2. Long-acting bronchodilators

A. MEDIATOR INHIBITORS—Cromolyn sodium and nedocromil are long-term control medications that prevent asthma symptoms and improve airway function in patients with mild persistent or exercise-induced asthma. These agents modulate mast cell mediator release and eosinophil recruitment and inhibit both early and late asthmatic responses to allergen challenge and exercise-induced bronchospasm. They can be effective when taken before an exposure or exercise but do not relieve asthmatic

Table 9–3. Long-term control medications for asthma.

Medication	Dosage Form	Adult Dose	Comments
Inhaled Corticosteroids			(See Table 9–4)
Systemic Corticosteroids			(Applies to all three corticosteroids)
Methylprednisolone	2, 4, 6, 8, 16, 32 mg tablets	7.5–60 mg	• Administer single dose in AM either daily or on alternate days (alternate-day therapy may produce less adrenal suppression) as needed for control. • Short courses or "bursts" as single or 2 divided doses for 3–10 days are effective for establishing control when initiating therapy or during a period of gradual deterioration. • There is no evidence that tapering the dose following improvement in symptom control and pulmonary function prevents relapse.
Prednisolone	5 mg tablets; 5 mg/5 mL, 15 mg/5 mL	40–60 mg	
Prednisone	1, 2.5, 5, 10, 20, 50 mg tablets; 5 mg/mL		
Inhaled Long-Acting Beta-2-Agonists			Should not be used for symptom relief or exacerbations. Use with inhaled corticosteroids.
Salmeterol	DPI 50 mcg/actuation	1 blister every 12 hours	• Decreased duration of protection against EIB may occur with regular use. • Additional doses should not be administered for at least 12 hours. • Agents should be used only with their specific inhaler and should not be taken orally.
Formoterol	DPI 12 mcg/single-use capsule	1 capsule every 12 hours	
Combined Medication			
Fluticasone/Salmeterol	DPI 100 mcg/50 mcg 250 mcg/50 mcg, or 500 mcg/50 mcg HFA 45 mcg/21 mcg 115 mcg/21 mcg 230 mcg/21 mcg	1 inhalation twice daily; dose depends on severity of asthma	• 100/50 DPI or 45/21 HFA for patient not controlled on low- to medium-dose inhaled corticosteroids • 250/50 DPI or 115/21 HFA for patients not controlled on medium- to high-dose inhaled corticosteroids
Budesonide/Formoterol	HFA MDI 80 mcg/4.5 mcg 160 mcg/4.5 mcg	2 inhalations twice daily; dose depends on severity of asthma	• 80/4.5 for asthma not controlled on low- to medium-dose inhaled corticosteroids • 160/4.5 for asthma not controlled on medium- to high-dose inhaled corticosteroids
Cromolyn and Nedocromil			
Cromolyn	MDI 0.8 mg/puff	2 puffs four times daily	• 4–6 week trial may be needed to determine maximum benefit.
	Nebulizer 20 mg/ampule	1 ampule four times daily	• Dose by MDI may be inadequate to affect hyperresponsiveness.
Nedocromil	MDI 1.75 mg/puff	2 puffs four times daily	• One dose before exercise or allergen exposure provides effective prophylaxis for 1–2 hours. Not as effective for EIB as SABA. • Once control is achieved, the frequency of dosing may be reduced.
Inhaled Long-Acting Anticholinergic			Should not be used for symptom relief or exacerbations. Use with inhaled corticosteroids.
Tiotropium	DPI 18 mcg/blister	1 blister daily	
Leukotriene Modifiers			
Leukotriene Receptor Antagonists			
Montelukast	4 mg or 5 mg chewable tablet; 10 mg tablet	10 mg daily at bedtime	• Exhibits a flat dose-response curve. Doses > 10 mg will not produce a greater response in adults.

(continued)

Table 9–3. Long-term control medications for asthma. (continued)

Medication	Dosage Form	Adult Dose	Comments
Zafirlukast	10 or 20 mg tablet	20 mg tablet twice daily	• Administration with meals decreases bioavailability; take at least 1 hour before or 2 hours after meals. • Monitor for symptoms and signs of hepatic dysfunction.
5-Lipoxygenase Inhibitor			
Zileuton	600-mg tablet	600 mg four times daily	• Monitor hepatic enzyme (ALT).
Methylxanthines			
Theophylline	Liquids, sustained-release tablets, and capsules	Starting dose 10 mg/kg/day up to 300 mg maximum; usual maximum dose 800 mg/day	• Adjust dose to achieve serum concentration of 5–15 mcg/mL after at least 48 hours on same dose. • Due to wide interpatient variability in theophylline metabolic clearance, routine serum theophylline level monitoring is important.
Immunomodulators			
Omalizumab	Subcutaneous injection, 150 mg/1.2 mL following reconstitution with 1.4 mL sterile water for injection	150–375 mg subcutaneously every 2–4 weeks, depending on body weight and pretreatment serum IgE level	• Do not administer more than 150 mg per injection site. • Monitor for anaphylaxis for 2 hours following at least the first 3 injections.

Table 9–4. Estimated comparative daily dosages for inhaled corticosteroids for asthma.

Medication	Low Daily Dose Adult	Medium Daily Dose Adult	High Daily Dose Adult
Beclomethasone HFA 40 or 80 mcg/puff	80–240 mcg	> 240–480 mcg	> 480 mcg
Budesonide DPI 90, 180, or 200 mcg/inhalation	180–600 mcg	> 600–1200 mcg	> 1200 mcg
Flunisolide 250 mcg/puff	500–1000 mcg	> 1000–2000 mcg	> 2000 mcg
Flunisolide HFA 80 mcg/puff	320 mcg	> 320–640 mcg	> 640 mcg
Fluticasone **HFA/MDI:** 44, 110, or 220 mcg/puff **DPI:** 50, 100, or 250 mcg/inhalation	88–264 mcg 100–300 mcg	> 264–440 mcg > 300–500 mcg	> 440 mcg > 500 mcg
Mometasone DPI 200 mcg/puff	200 mcg	400 mcg	> 400 mcg
Triamcinolone acetonide 75 mcg/puff	300–750 mcg	> 750–1500 mcg	> 1500 mcg

DPI, dry powder inhaler; EIB, exercise-induced bronchospasm; HFA, hydrofluoroalkaline; MDI, metered-dose inhaler; SABA, short-acting beta-2-agonist.
Notes:
• The most important determinant of appropriate dosing is the clinician's judgment of the patient's response to therapy.
• Potential drug interactions:
  A number of the inhaled corticosteroids, including fluticasone, budesonide, and mometasone, are metabolized in the gastrointestinal tract and liver by CYP 3A4 isoenzymes. Potent inhibitors of CYP 3A4, such as ritonavir and ketoconazole, have the potential for increasing systemic concentrations of these inhaled corticosteroids by increasing oral availability and decreasing systemic clearance. Some cases of clinically significant Cushing syndrome and secondary adrenal insufficiency have been reported.
Adapted from National Asthma Education and Prevention Program. Expert Panel Report 3: Guidelines for the Diagnosis and Management of Asthma. National Institutes of Health Pub. No. 08-4051. Bethesda, MD, 2007. http://www.nhlbi.nih.gov/health-pro/guidelines/current/asthma-guidelines/full-report.

symptoms once present. The clinical response to these agents is less predictable than to inhaled corticosteroids. Nedocromil may help reduce the dose requirements for inhaled corticosteroids. Both agents have excellent safety profiles.

B. Beta-adrenergic agonists—Long-acting beta-2-agonists provide bronchodilation for up to 12 hours after a single dose. Salmeterol and formoterol are the two long-acting beta-2-agonists available for asthma in the United States. They are administered via dry powder delivery devices. They are indicated for long-term prevention of asthma symptoms, nocturnal symptoms, and for prevention of exercise-induced bronchospasm. When added to low and medium daily doses of inhaled corticosteroids (Table 9–4), long-acting beta-2-agonists provide control equivalent to what is achieved by doubling the inhaled corticosteroid dose. Side effects are minimal at standard doses. **Long-acting beta-2-agonists should not be used as monotherapy** since they have no anti-inflammatory effect and since monotherapy with long-acting beta-2-agonists has been associated in two large studies with a small but statistically significant increased risk of severe or fatal asthma attacks. This increased risk has not been fully explained but may relate to genetic variation in the beta-adrenergic receptor and remains an area of controversy. The efficacy of combined inhaled corticosteroid and long-acting beta-2-agonist therapy has led to the marketing of combination medications that deliver both agents simultaneously (Table 9–3). Combination inhalers containing formoterol and budesonide have shown efficacy in both maintenance and rescue, given formoterol's short time to onset.

C. Anticholinergics—The long-acting anticholinergic tiotropium has been studied as add-on therapy for patients who have either a bronchodilator response or a positive methacholine challenge that is not adequately controlled with a low-dose inhaled corticosteroid. After 14 weeks of treatment, the addition of tiotropium resulted in improvements in PEF, FEV_1, and symptom control; the improvements were greater than those achieved by doubling the dose of the inhaled corticosteroid for the same period of time. The addition of tiotropium was not inferior to the addition of salmeterol. In patients with asthma receiving inhaled corticosteroids and long-acting beta-2-agonists who suffered at least one exacerbation in the preceding year, the addition of tiotropium resulted in a small improvement in peak FEV_1 as well as a modest increase in time to next exacerbation.

D. Phosphodiesterase inhibitors—Theophylline provides mild bronchodilation in asthmatic patients. Theophylline also has anti-inflammatory and immunomodulatory properties, enhances mucociliary clearance, and strengthens diaphragmatic contractility. Sustained-release theophylline preparations are effective in controlling nocturnal symptoms and as added therapy in patients with moderate or severe persistent asthma whose symptoms are inadequately controlled by inhaled corticosteroids. When added to inhaled corticosteroids, theophylline may allow equivalent control at lower corticosteroid doses.

Theophylline serum concentrations need to be monitored closely owing to the medication's narrow toxic-therapeutic range, individual differences in metabolism, and the effects of many factors on drug absorption and metabolism. At therapeutic doses, potential adverse effects include insomnia, aggravation of dyspepsia and gastroesophageal reflux, and urination difficulties in men with prostatic hyperplasia. Dose-related toxicities include nausea, vomiting, tachyarrhythmias, headache, seizures, hyperglycemia, and hypokalemia.

3. Leukotriene modifiers—Leukotrienes are potent biochemical mediators that contribute to airway obstruction and asthma symptoms by contracting airway smooth muscle, increasing vascular permeability and mucus secretion, and attracting and activating airway inflammatory cells. Zileuton is a 5-lipoxygenase inhibitor that decreases leukotriene production, and zafirlukast and montelukast are cysteinyl leukotriene receptor antagonists. In randomized controlled trials (RCTs), these agents caused modest improvements in lung function and reductions in asthma symptoms and lessened the need for beta-2-agonist rescue therapy. These agents are alternatives to low-dose inhaled corticosteroids in patients with mild persistent asthma, although, as monotherapy, their effect is generally less than inhaled corticosteroids. In real-life community trials, leukotriene receptor antagonists were equivalent in efficacy to an inhaled corticosteroid as first-line long-term controller medication or to a long-acting beta-2-agonist as add-on therapy. Zileuton can cause reversible elevations in plasma aminotransferase levels. Eosinophilic granulomatosis with polyangiitis has been diagnosed in a small number of patients who have taken montelukast or zafirlukast, perhaps due to corticosteroid withdrawal rather than a direct drug effect.

4. Desensitization—Immunotherapy for specific allergens may be considered in selected asthma patients who have exacerbations when exposed to allergens to which they are sensitive and when unresponsive to environmental control measures or other therapies. Studies show a reduction in asthma symptoms in patients treated with single-allergen immunotherapy. Because of the risk of immunotherapy-induced bronchoconstriction, it should be administered only in a setting where such complications can be immediately treated.

5. Omalizumab and reslizumab—Omalizumab is a recombinant antibody that binds IgE without activating mast cells. In clinical trials in patients with moderate to severe asthma and elevated IgE levels, omalizumab reduced the need for corticosteroids. In 2016, the FDA approved reslizumab (Cinqair) for treatment of severe asthma in patients age 18 years and older.

6. Vaccination—Patients with asthma should receive pneumococcal vaccination (Pneumovax) and annual influenza (both seasonal and epidemic influenza A [H1N1]) vaccinations. Inactive vaccines (Pneumovax) are associated with few side effects, but the use of the live attenuated influenza vaccine intranasally may be associated with asthma exacerbations in young children.

7. Oral sustained-release beta-2-agonists—These agents are reserved for patients with bothersome nocturnal asthma symptoms or moderate to severe persistent asthma who do not respond to other therapies.

B. Quick-Relief Medications

Short-acting bronchodilators and systemic corticosteroids are the important quick-relief medications (Table 9–5).

1. Beta-adrenergic agonists—Short-acting inhaled beta-2-agonists, including albuterol, levalbuterol, bitolterol, pirbuterol, and terbutaline, are the most effective bronchodilators during exacerbations. All patients with acute symptoms should have immediate access to one of these agents. There is no convincing evidence to support the use of one agent over another. Beta-2-agonists relax airway smooth muscle and cause a prompt increase in airflow and decrease in symptoms. Administration before exercise effectively prevents exercise-induced bronchoconstriction. Beta-2-selective agents may produce less cardiac stimulation than those with mixed beta-1 and beta-2 activities, although clinical trials have not consistently demonstrated this finding.

Inhaled beta-adrenergic therapy is as effective as oral or parenteral therapy in relaxing airway smooth muscle and improving acute asthma and offers the advantages of rapid onset of action (less than 5 minutes) with fewer systemic side effects. Repetitive administration produces incremental bronchodilation. One or two inhalations of a short-acting inhaled beta-2-agonist from an MDI are usually sufficient for mild to moderate symptoms. Severe exacerbations frequently require higher doses: **6–12 puffs every 30–60 minutes of albuterol by MDI with an inhalation chamber or 2.5 mg by nebulizer provide equivalent bronchodilation.** Administration by nebulization does not offer more effective delivery than MDIs used correctly but does provide higher doses. With most beta-2-agonists, the recommended dose by nebulizer for acute asthma (albuterol, 2.5 mg) is 25–30 times that delivered by a single activation of the MDI (albuterol, 0.09 mg). This difference suggests that **standard dosing of inhalations from an MDI will often be insufficient in the setting of an acute exacerbation.** Independent of dose, nebulizer therapy may be more effective in patients who are unable to coordinate inhalation of medication from an MDI because of age, agitation, or severity of the exacerbation.

Scheduled daily use of short-acting beta-2-agonists is not recommended. Increased use (more than one canister a month) or lack of expected effect indicates diminished asthma control and the need for additional long-term control therapy.

2. Anticholinergics—Anticholinergic agents reverse vagally mediated bronchospasm but not allergen- or exercise-induced bronchospasm. They may decrease mucus gland hypersecretion. Ipratropium bromide, a quaternary derivative of atropine free of atropine's side effects, is less effective than beta-2-agonists for relief of acute bronchospasm, but it is the inhaled drug of choice for patients with intolerance to beta-2-agonists or with bronchospasm due to beta-blocker medications. Ipratropium bromide reduces the rate of hospital admissions when added to inhaled short-acting beta-2-agonists in patients with moderate to severe asthma exacerbations.

3. Corticosteroids—Systemic corticosteroids are effective primary treatment for patients with moderate to severe asthma exacerbations and for patients with exacerbations who do not respond promptly and completely to inhaled beta-2-agonist therapy. These medications speed the resolution of airflow obstruction and reduce the rate of relapse. Delays in administering corticosteroids may result in delayed benefits from these important agents. **Therefore, oral corticosteroids should generally be prescribed for early administration at home** in patients with moderate to severe asthma. The minimal effective dose of systemic corticosteroids for asthma patients has not been identified. Outpatient prednisone "burst" therapy is 0.5–1 mg/kg/day (typically 40–60 mg) in 1–2 doses for 3–10 days. Severe exacerbations requiring hospitalization typically require 1 mg/kg of prednisone or methylprednisolone every 6–12 hours for 48 hours or until the FEV_1 (or PEF rate) returns to 50% of predicted (or 50% of baseline). The dose is then decreased to 60–80 mg/day until the PEF reaches 70% of predicted or personal best. No clear advantage has been found for higher doses of corticosteroids. It may be prudent to administer corticosteroids intravenously to critically ill patients to avoid concerns about altered gastrointestinal absorption.

4. Antimicrobials—Multiple studies suggest that infections with viruses (rhinovirus) and bacteria (*Mycoplasma pneumoniae, Chlamydophila pneumoniae*) predispose to acute exacerbations of asthma and may underlie chronic, severe asthma. **The use of empiric antibiotics is, however, not recommended in routine asthma exacerbations because there is no consistent evidence to support improved clinical outcomes.** Antibiotics should be considered when there is a high likelihood of acute bacterial respiratory tract infection, such as for patients with fever or purulent sputum and evidence of pneumonia or bacterial sinusitis.

▶ Treatment of Asthma Exacerbations

NAEPP 3 asthma treatment algorithms begin with an assessment of the severity of a patient's baseline asthma. Adjustments to that algorithm follow a stepwise approach based on a careful assessment of asthma control. Most instances of uncontrolled asthma are mild and can be managed successfully by patients at home with the telephone assistance of a clinician (Figure 9–3). More severe exacerbations require evaluation and management in an urgent care or emergency department setting (Figure 9–4).

A. Mild Exacerbations

Mild asthma exacerbations are characterized by only minor changes in airway function (PEF more than 80%) and minimal symptoms and signs of airway dysfunction (see Table 9–2). Many such patients respond quickly and fully to an inhaled short-acting beta-2-agonist alone. However, an inhaled short-acting beta-2-agonist may need to be continued at increased doses, eg, every 3–4 hours for 24–48 hours.

Table 9–5. Quick-relief medications for asthma.

Medication	Dosage Form	Adult Dose	Comments
Inhaled Short-Acting Beta-2-Agonists			
	MDI		
Albuterol CFC	90 mcg/puff, 200 puffs/canister	2 puffs 5 minutes before exercise	• An increasing use or lack of expected effect indicates diminished control of asthma.
Albuterol HFA	90 mcg/puff, 200 puffs/canister	2 puffs every 4–6 hours as needed	• Not recommended for long-term daily treatment. Regular use exceeding 2 days/week for symptom control (not prevention of EIB) indicates the need to step up therapy.
Pirbuterol CFC	200 mcg/puff, 400 puffs/canister		• Differences in potency exist, but all products are essentially comparable on a per-puff basis.
Levalbuterol HFA	45 mcg/puff, 200 puffs/canister		• May double usual dose for mild exacerbations. • Prime the inhaler by releasing four actuations prior to use. • Periodically clean HFA activator, as drug may block/plug orifice.
	Nebulizer solution		
Albuterol	0.63 mg/3 mL 1.25 mg/3 mL 2.5 mg/3 mL 5 mg/mL (0.5%)	1.25–5 mg in 3 mL of saline every 4–8 hours as needed	• May mix with budesonide inhalant suspension, cromolyn or ipratropium nebulizer solutions. • May double dose for severe exacerbations.
Levalbuterol (R-albuterol)	0.31 mg/3 mL 0.63 mg/3 mL 1.25 mg/0.5 mL 1.25 mg/3 mL	0.63 mg–1.25 mg every 8 hours as needed	• Compatible with budesonide inhalant suspension. The product is a sterile-filled, preservative-free, unit dose vial.
Anticholinergics			
	MDI		
Ipratropium HFA	17 mcg/puff, 200 puffs/canister	2–3 puffs every 6 hours	• Evidence is lacking for anticholinergics producing added benefit to beta-2-agonists in long-term control asthma therapy.
	Nebulizer solution		
	0.25 mg/mL (0.025%)	0.25 mg every 6 hours	
	MDI		
Ipratropium with albuterol	18 mcg/puff of ipratropium bromide and 90 mcg/puff of albuterol, 200 puffs/canister	2–3 puffs every 6 hours	
	Nebulizer solution		
	0.5 mg/3 mL ipratropium bromide and 2.5 mg/3 mL albuterol	3 mL every 4–6 hours	• Contains EDTA to prevent discolorations of the solution. This additive does not induce bronchospasm.
Systemic Corticosteroids			
Methylprednisolone	2, 4, 6, 8, 16, 32 mg tablets	40–60 mg/day as single or 2 divided doses	• Short courses or "bursts" are effective for establishing control when initiating therapy or during a period of gradual deterioration. • The burst should be continued until symptoms resolve and the PEF is at least 80% of personal best. This usually requires 3–10 days but may require longer. There is no evidence that tapering the dose following improvements prevents relapse.
Prednisolone	5 mg tablets, 5 mg/5 mL, 15 mg/5 mL		
Prednisone	1, 2.5, 5, 10, 20, 50 mg tablets; 5 mg/mL		

(continued)

Table 9–5. Quick-relief medications for asthma. (continued)

Medication	Dosage Form	Adult Dose	Comments
	Repository injection		
Methylprednisolone acetate	40 mg/mL 80 mg/mL	240 mg intramuscularly once	May be used in place of a short burst of oral corticosteroids in patients who are vomiting or if adherence is a problem.

CFC, chlorofluorocarbon; EIB, exercise-induced bronchospasm; HFA, hydrofluoroalkane; MDI, metered-dose inhaler; PEF, peak expiratory flow.
Adapted from National Asthma Education and Prevention Program. Expert Panel Report 3: Guidelines for the Diagnosis and Management of Asthma. National Institutes of Health Pub. No. 08-4051. Bethesda, MD, 2007. http://www.nhlbi.gov/health-pro/guidelines/current/asthma-guidelines/full-report

In patients not taking an inhaled corticosteroid, initiating one should be considered during the mild exacerbation. In patients already taking an inhaled corticosteroid, a 7-day course of oral corticosteroids (0.5–1.0 mg/kg/day) may be necessary. Doubling the dose of inhaled corticosteroid is not effective and is not recommended in the NAEPP 3 guidelines.

B. Moderate Exacerbations

The principal goals of treatment of moderate asthma exacerbations are correction of hypoxemia, reversal of airflow obstruction, and reduction of the likelihood of recurrence of obstruction. Early intervention may lessen the severity and shorten the duration of an exacerbation. **Of paramount importance is the correction of hypoxemia through the use of supplemental oxygen.** Airflow obstruction is treated with continuous administration of an inhaled short-acting beta-2-agonist and the early administration of systemic corticosteroids. Serial measurements of lung function to quantify the severity of airflow obstruction and its response to treatment are useful. The improvement in FEV_1 after 30 minutes of treatment correlates significantly with the severity of the asthma exacerbation. Serial measurement of airflow in the emergency department may reduce the rate of hospital admissions for asthma exacerbations. The post-exacerbation care plan is important. **Regardless of the severity, all patients should be provided with necessary medications and education in how to use them, instruction in self-assessment, a follow-up appointment, and an action plan for managing recurrence.**

C. Severe Exacerbations

Severe exacerbations of asthma can be life-threatening, so treatment should be started immediately. All patients with a severe exacerbation should immediately receive oxygen, high doses of an inhaled short-acting beta-2-agonist, and systemic corticosteroids. A brief history pertinent to the exacerbation can be completed while such treatment is being initiated. More detailed assessments, including laboratory studies, usually add little early on and so should be postponed until after therapy is instituted.

Oxygen therapy is very important because asphyxia is a common cause of asthma deaths. Supplemental oxygen should be given to maintain an SaO_2 greater than 90% or a PaO_2 greater than 60 mm Hg. Oxygen-induced hypoventilation is extremely rare, and concern for hypercapnia should never delay correction of hypoxemia.

Frequent high-dose delivery of an **inhaled short-acting beta-2-agonist** is indicated and usually well tolerated in severe airway obstruction. Some studies suggest that continuous therapy is more effective than intermittent administration of these agents, but there is no clear consensus as long as similar doses are administered. At least three MDI or nebulizer treatments should be given in the first hour of therapy. Thereafter, the frequency of administration varies according to the improvement in airflow and symptoms and the occurrence of side effects. Ipratropium bromide reduces the rate of hospital admissions when added to inhaled short-acting beta-2-agonists in patients with moderate to severe asthma exacerbations.

Systemic corticosteroids are administered as detailed above. **Intravenous magnesium sulfate** (2 g intravenously over 20 minutes) produces a detectable improvement in airflow and may reduce hospitalization rates in acute severe asthma (FEV_1 less than 25% of predicted on presentation or failure to respond to initial treatment).

Mucolytic agents (eg, acetylcysteine, potassium iodide) may worsen cough or airflow obstruction. Anxiolytic and hypnotic drugs are generally contraindicated in severe asthma exacerbations because of their potential respiratory depressant effects.

In the **emergency department setting, repeat assessment** of patients with severe exacerbations should be done after the initial dose of inhaled bronchodilator and again after three doses of inhaled bronchodilators (60–90 minutes after initiating treatment). The response to initial treatment is a better predictor of the need for hospitalization than is the severity of an exacerbation on presentation. The decision to hospitalize a patient should be based on the duration and severity of symptoms, severity of airflow obstruction, arterial blood gas results (if available), course and severity of prior exacerbations, medication use at the time of the exacerbation, access to medical care and medications, adequacy of social support and home conditions, and presence of psychiatric illness. In general, discharge to home is appropriate if the PEF or FEV_1 has returned to 60% or more of predicted or personal best and symptoms are minimal or absent. Patients with a rapid response to treatment should be observed for 30 minutes after the most

Assess Severity

- **Patients at high risk for a fatal attack require immediate medical attention after initial treatment.**

- Symptoms and signs suggestive of a more serious exacerbation, such as marked breathlessness, inability to speak more than short phrases, use of accessory muscles, or drowsiness (see Table 9–2) should result in initial treatment while immediately consulting with a clinician.

- Less severe symptoms and signs can be treated initially with assessment of response to therapy and further steps as listed below.

- If available, measure PEF—values of 50–79% predicted or personal best indicate the need for quick-relief medication. Depending on the response to treatment, contact with a clinician may also be indicated. Values below 50% indicate the need for immediate medical care.

Initial Treatment

- Inhaled SABA: up to two treatments 20 minutes apart of 2–6 puffs by MDI or nebulizer treatments.

- Note: Medication delivery is highly variable. Children and individuals who have exacerbations of lesser severity may need fewer puffs than suggested above.

Good Response

No wheezing or dyspnea (assess tachypnea in young children).

PEF ≥ 80% predicted or personal best.

- Contact clinician for follow-up instructions and further management.
- May continue inhaled SABA every 3–4 hours for 24–48 hours.
- Consider short course of oral systemic corticosteroids.

Incomplete Response

Persistent wheezing and dyspnea (tachypnea).

PEF 50–79% predicted or personal best.

- Add oral systemic corticosteroid.
- Continue inhaled SABA.
- Contact clinician urgently (this day) for further instruction.

Poor Response

Marked wheezing and dyspnea.

PEF < 50% predicted or personal best.

- Add oral systemic corticosteroid.
- Repeat inhaled SABA immediately.
- If distress is severe and nonresponsive to initial treatment:

  —Call your doctor AND
  —**PROCEED TO ED;**
  —Consider calling 9–1–1 (ambulance transport).

- To ED.

ED, emergency department; MDI, metered-dose inhaler; PEF, peak expiratory flow; SABA short-acting beta-2-agonist (quick-relief inhaler).

▲ **Figure 9–3.** Management of asthma exacerbations: home treatment. (Adapted from National Asthma Education and Prevention Program. Expert Panel Report 3: Guidelines for the Diagnosis and Management of Asthma. National Institutes of Health Pub. No. 08-4051. Bethesda, MD, 2007. http://www.nhlbi.nih.gov/health-pro/guidelines/current/asthma-guidelines/full-report.)

recent dose of bronchodilator to ensure stability of response before discharge.

In the **intensive care setting,** a small subset of patients will not respond to treatment and will progress to impending respiratory failure due to a combination of worsening airflow obstruction and respiratory muscle fatigue (see Table 9–2). Since such patients can deteriorate rapidly, they must be monitored in a critical care setting. Intubation of an acutely ill asthma patient is technically difficult and is best done semi-electively, before the crisis of a respiratory arrest. At the time of intubation, the patient's intravascular volume should be closely monitored because hypotension commonly follows the administration of sedative medications and the initiation of positive-pressure ventilation; these

FEV$_1$, forced expiratory volume in 1 second; ICS, inhaled corticosteroid; MDI, metered-dose inhaler; PEF, peak expiratory flow; SABA, short-acting beta-2-agonist; SaO$_2$, oxygen saturation.

▲ **Figure 9–4.** Management of asthma exacerbations: emergency department and hospital-based treatment. (Adapted from National Asthma Education and Prevention Program. Expert Panel Report 3: Guidelines for the Diagnosis and Management of Asthma. National Institutes of Health Pub. No. 08-4051. Bethesda, MD, 2007. http://www.nhlbi.nih.gov/health-pro/guidelines/current/asthma-guidelines/full-report.)

patients are often dehydrated due to poor recent oral intake and high insensible losses.

The main goals of mechanical ventilation are to ensure adequate oxygenation and to avoid barotrauma. Controlled hypoventilation with permissive hypercapnia is often required to limit airway pressures. Frequent high-dose delivery of inhaled short-acting beta-2-agonists should be continued along with anti-inflammatory agents as discussed above. Many questions remain regarding the optimal delivery of inhaled beta-2-agonists to intubated, mechanically ventilated patients.

When to Refer

- Atypical presentation or uncertain diagnosis of asthma, particularly if additional diagnostic testing is required (bronchoprovocation challenge, allergy skin testing, rhinoscopy, consideration of occupational exposure).

- Complicating comorbid problems, such as rhinosinusitis, tobacco use, multiple environmental allergies, suspected allergic bronchopulmonary mycosis.

- Suboptimal response to therapy.

- Patient not meeting goals of asthma therapy after 3–6 months of treatment.

- Requires high-dose inhaled corticosteroids for control.

- More than two courses of oral prednisone therapy in the past 12 months.

- Any life-threatening asthma exacerbation or exacerbation requiring hospitalization in the past 12 months.

- Presence of social or psychological issues interfering with asthma management.

Albertson TE et al. The acute management of asthma. Clin Rev Allergy Immunol. 2015 Feb;48(1):114–25. [PMID: 25213370]

Bel EH. Clinical Practice. Mild asthma. N Engl J Med. 2013 Aug 8; 369(6):549–57. Erratum in: N Engl J Med. 2013 Nov 14;369(20): 1970. [PMID: 23924005]

Chung KF et al. International ERS/ATS guidelines on definition, evaluation and treatment of severe asthma. Eur Respir J. 2014 Feb; 43(2):343–73. Erratum in: Eur Respir J. 2014 Apr;43(4): 1216. Dosage error in article text. [PMID: 24337046]

Lenaeus MJ et al. Primary care of the patient with asthma. Med Clin North Am. 2015 Sep;99(5):953–67. [PMID: 26320041]

National Asthma Education and Prevention Program. https://www.nhlbi.nih.gov/about/org/naepp

Rodrigo GJ. Advances in acute asthma. Curr Opin Pulm Med. 2015 Jan;21(1):22–6. [PMID: 25405669]

CHRONIC OBSTRUCTIVE PULMONARY DISEASE

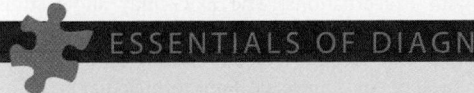

ESSENTIALS OF DIAGNOSIS

- History of cigarette smoking.
- Chronic cough, dyspnea, and sputum production.
- Rhonchi, decreased intensity of breath sounds, and prolonged expiration on physical examination.
- Airflow limitation on pulmonary function testing that is not fully reversible and is most often progressive.

General Considerations

The American Thoracic Society defines COPD as a disease state characterized by the presence of airflow obstruction due to chronic bronchitis or emphysema; the airflow obstruction is generally progressive, may be accompanied by airway hyperreactivity, and may be partially reversible. The NHLBI estimates that 15 million Americans have been diagnosed with COPD; an equal number are thought to be afflicted but remain undiagnosed. Grouped together, COPD and asthma now represent the fourth leading cause of death in the United States, with over 140,000 deaths reported annually. The death rate from COPD is increasing rapidly, especially among elderly men.

Most patients with COPD have features of both emphysema and chronic bronchitis. **Chronic bronchitis** is a clinical diagnosis defined by excessive secretion of bronchial mucus and is manifested by daily productive cough for 3 months or more in at least 2 consecutive years. **Emphysema** is a pathologic diagnosis that denotes abnormal permanent enlargement of air spaces distal to the terminal bronchiole, with destruction of their walls and without obvious fibrosis.

Cigarette smoking is clearly the most important cause of COPD in North America and Western Europe. Nearly all smokers suffer an accelerated decline in lung function that is dose- and duration-dependent. Fifteen percent develop progressively disabling symptoms in their 40s and 50s. Approximately 80% of patients seen for COPD have significant exposure to tobacco smoke. The remaining 20% frequently have a combination of exposures to environmental tobacco smoke, occupational dusts and chemicals, and indoor air pollution from biomass fuel used for cooking and heating in poorly ventilated buildings. Outdoor air pollution, airway infection, familial factors, and allergy have also been implicated in chronic bronchitis, and hereditary factors (deficiency of alpha-1-antiprotease [alpha-1-antitrypsin]) have been implicated. Atopy and the tendency for bronchoconstriction to develop in response to nonspecific airway stimuli may be important risks.

Clinical Findings

A. Symptoms and Signs

Patients with COPD characteristically present in the fifth or sixth decade of life complaining of excessive cough, sputum production, and shortness of breath. Symptoms have often been present for 10 years or more. Dyspnea is noted initially only on heavy exertion, but as the condition progresses it occurs with mild activity. In severe disease, dyspnea occurs at rest. As the disease progresses, two symptom patterns tend to emerge, historically referred to as "pink puffers" and "blue bloaters" (Table 9–6). Most COPD patients have pathologic evidence of both disorders, and their clinical course may involve other factors, such as central control of ventilation and concomitant sleep-disordered breathing.

Pneumonia, pulmonary hypertension, cor pulmonale, and chronic respiratory failure characterize the late stage of COPD. **A hallmark of COPD is the periodic exacerbation**

Table 9–6. Patterns of disease in advanced COPD.

	Type A: Pink Puffer (Emphysema Predominant)	Type B: Blue Bloater (Bronchitis Predominant)
History and physical examination	Major complaint is dyspnea, often severe, usually presenting after age 50. Cough is rare, with scant clear, mucoid sputum. Patients are thin, with recent weight loss common. They appear uncomfortable, with evident use of accessory muscles of respiration. Chest is very quiet without adventitious sounds. No peripheral edema.	Major complaint is chronic cough, productive of mucopurulent sputum, with frequent exacerbations due to chest infections. Often presents in late 30s and 40s. Dyspnea usually mild, though patients may note limitations to exercise. Patients frequently overweight and cyanotic but seem comfortable at rest. Peripheral edema is common. Chest is noisy, with rhonchi invariably present; wheezes are common.
Laboratory studies	Hemoglobin usually normal (12–15 g/dL). PaO_2 normal to slightly reduced (65–75 mm Hg) but SaO_2 normal at rest. $PaCO_2$ normal to slightly reduced (35–40 mm Hg). Chest radiograph shows hyperinflation with flattened diaphragms. Vascular markings are diminished, particularly at the apices.	Hemoglobin usually elevated (15–18 g/dL). PaO_2 reduced (45–60 mm Hg) and $PaCO_2$ slightly to markedly elevated (50–60 mm Hg). Chest radiograph shows increased interstitial markings ("dirty lungs"), especially at bases. Diaphragms are not flattened.
Pulmonary function tests	Airflow obstruction ubiquitous. Total lung capacity increased, sometimes markedly so. DL_{CO} reduced. Static lung compliance increased.	Airflow obstruction ubiquitous. Total lung capacity generally normal but may be slightly increased. DL_{CO} normal. Static lung compliance normal.
Special Evaluations		
$\dot{V}/\dot{Q}$ matching	Increased ventilation to high $\dot{V}/\dot{Q}$ areas, ie, high dead space ventilation.	Increased perfusion to low $\dot{V}/\dot{Q}$ areas.
Hemodynamics	Cardiac output normal to slightly low. Pulmonary artery pressures mildly elevated and increase with exercise.	Cardiac output normal. Pulmonary artery pressures elevated, sometimes markedly so, and worsen with exercise.
Nocturnal ventilation	Mild to moderate degree of oxygen desaturation not usually associated with obstructive sleep apnea.	Severe oxygen desaturation, frequently associated with obstructive sleep apnea.
Exercise ventilation	Increased minute ventilation for level of oxygen consumption; PaO_2 tends to fall; $PaCO_2$ rises slightly.	Decreased minute ventilation for level of oxygen consumption. PaO_2 may rise; $PaCO_2$ may rise significantly.

DL_{CO}, single-breath diffusing capacity for carbon monoxide; $\dot{V}/\dot{Q}$, ventilation-perfusion.

of symptoms beyond normal day-to-day variation, often including increased dyspnea, an increased frequency or severity of cough, and increased sputum volume or change in sputum character. These exacerbations are commonly precipitated by infection (more often viral than bacterial) or environmental factors. Exacerbations of COPD vary widely in severity but typically require a change in regular therapy.

B. Laboratory Findings

Spirometry provides objective information about pulmonary function and assesses the response to therapy. Pulmonary function tests early in the course of COPD reveal only evidence of abnormal closing volume and reduced midexpiratory flow rate. Reductions in FEV_1 and in the ratio of forced expiratory volume to vital capacity (FEV_1% or FEV_1/FVC ratio) (Table 9–6) occur later. In severe disease, the FVC is markedly reduced. Lung volume measurements reveal a marked increase in residual volume (RV), an increase in total lung capacity (TLC), and an elevation of the RV/TLC ratio, indicative of air trapping, particularly in emphysema.

Arterial blood gas measurements characteristically show no abnormalities early in COPD other than an increased $A–a–DO_2$. Indeed, measurement is unnecessary unless (1) hypoxemia or hypercapnia is suspected, (2) the FEV_1 is less than 40% of predicted, or (3) there are clinical signs of right heart failure. Hypoxemia occurs in advanced disease, particularly when chronic bronchitis predominates. Compensated respiratory acidosis occurs in patients with chronic respiratory failure, particularly in chronic bronchitis, with worsening of acidemia during acute exacerbations.

Positive sputum cultures are poorly correlated with acute exacerbations, and research techniques demonstrate evidence of preceding viral infection in a majority of patients with exacerbations. The ECG may show sinus tachycardia and, in advanced disease, chronic pulmonary hypertension may produce electrocardiographic abnormalities typical of cor pulmonale. Supraventricular arrhythmias (multifocal atrial tachycardia, atrial flutter, and atrial fibrillation) and ventricular irritability also occur.

C. Imaging

Radiographs of patients with chronic bronchitis typically show only nonspecific peribronchial and perivascular markings. Plain radiographs are insensitive for the diagnosis of emphysema; they show hyperinflation with flattening of the diaphragm or peripheral arterial deficiency in about half of cases. CT of the chest, particularly using high-resolution CT, is more sensitive and specific than plain radiographs for its diagnosis. In advanced disease, pulmonary hypertension may be suggested by enlargement of central pulmonary arteries on radiographs, and Doppler echocardiography provides an estimate of pulmonary artery pressure.

▶ Differential Diagnosis

Clinical, imaging, and laboratory findings should enable the clinician to distinguish COPD from other obstructive pulmonary disorders, such as asthma, bronchiectasis, cystic fibrosis, bronchopulmonary mycosis, and central airflow obstruction. Asthma is characterized by complete or near-complete reversibility of airflow obstruction. Bronchiectasis is distinguished from COPD by recurrent pneumonia and hemoptysis, digital clubbing, and characteristic imaging abnormalities. Patients with severe alpha-1-antitrypsin deficiency have a family history of the disorder and the finding of panacinar bibasilar emphysema early in life, usually in the third or fourth decade; hepatic cirrhosis and hepatocellular carcinoma may develop. Cystic fibrosis occurs in children, adolescents, and young adults. Mechanical obstruction of the central airways can be distinguished from COPD by flow-volume loops.

▶ Complications

Acute bronchitis, pneumonia, pulmonary thromboembolism, atrial dysrhythmias (such as atrial fibrillation, atrial flutter, and multifocal atrial tachycardia), and concomitant left ventricular failure may worsen otherwise stable COPD. Pulmonary hypertension, cor pulmonale, and chronic respiratory failure are common in advanced COPD. Spontaneous pneumothorax occurs in a small fraction of patients with emphysema. Hemoptysis may result from chronic bronchitis or may signal bronchogenic carcinoma.

▶ Prevention

COPD is largely preventable through elimination of long-term exposure to tobacco smoke or other inhaled toxins. Smokers with early evidence of airflow limitation can significantly alter their disease by smoking cessation. Smoking cessation slows the decline in FEV_1 in middle-aged smokers with mild airways obstruction. Vaccination against seasonal and epidemic influenza A (H1N1) and pneumococcal infection may also be of benefit.

▶ Treatment

The treatment of COPD is guided by the severity of symptoms or the presence of an exacerbation of stable symptoms. Standards for the management of patients with stable COPD and COPD exacerbations from the American Thoracic Society and the Global Initiative for Obstructive Lung Disease (GOLD), a joint expert committee of the NHLBI and the WHO, are incorporated in the recommendations below. See Chapter 37 for a discussion of air travel in patients with lung disease.

A. Ambulatory Patients

1. Smoking cessation—The single most important intervention in smokers with COPD is to encourage smoking cessation (discussed further in Chapter 1). Simply telling a patient to quit succeeds 5% of the time. Behavioral approaches, ranging from clinician advice to intensive group programs, may improve cessation rates. Pharmacologic therapy includes bupropion, nicotine replacement (transdermal patch, gum, lozenge, inhaler, or nasal spray), varenicline (a partial agonist of nicotinic acetylcholine receptors), and cytisine. Combined pharmacotherapies (two forms of nicotine replacement, or nicotine replacement and bupropion), with or without behavioral approaches, have been recommended. Varenicline is effective but use has been limited by concerns of neuropsychiatric side effects. Electronic cigarettes are being aggressively marketed as an aid for tobacco cigarette cessation. One RCT showed electronic cigarettes to be noninferior to nicotine transdermal patches. Most pulmonologists do not recommend electronic cigarettes as a tobacco cessation aid, based on safety concerns (they are not regulated and contain a variety of chemicals), and limited clinical trial data, although some clinicians will not discourage motivated smokers who refuse to consider standard approaches from trying electronic cigarettes.

2. Oxygen therapy—Supplemental oxygen for patients with resting hypoxemia is the only therapy with evidence of improvement in the natural history of COPD. Proved benefits of home oxygen therapy in hypoxemic patients include longer survival, reduced hospitalizations, and better quality of life. Survival in hypoxemic patients with COPD treated with supplemental oxygen therapy is directly proportionate to the number of hours per day oxygen is administered: in COPD hypoxemic patients treated with continuous oxygen for 24 hours daily, the survival after 36 months is about 65%—significantly better than the survival rate of about 45% in those treated with only nocturnal oxygen. Oxygen by nasal prongs must be given for at least 15 hours a day unless therapy is specifically intended only for exercise or sleep. In COPD patients with borderline low-normal resting oxygen levels (Pao_2 between 56 mm Hg and 69 mm Hg), however, several studies of supplemental oxygen therapy showed no survival benefit. COPD patients with normal or low-normal resting oxygen levels who desaturate with exertion improve their exercise tolerance and shorten recovery from dyspnea when supplemental oxygen therapy is used during activity, but there is no evidence of a mortality benefit. Requirements for US Medicare coverage for a patient's home use of oxygen and oxygen equipment are listed in Table 9–7. Arterial blood gas analysis is preferred over oximetry to guide initial oxygen therapy. Hypoxemic patients with pulmonary hypertension, chronic cor pulmonale, erythrocytosis, impaired cognitive function, exercise intolerance, nocturnal restlessness, or morning headache are particularly likely to benefit from home oxygen therapy.

Home oxygen may be supplied by liquid oxygen systems, compressed gas cylinders, or oxygen concentrators. Most patients benefit from having both stationary and portable systems. For most patients, a flow rate of 1–3 L/min

Table 9–7. Home oxygen therapy: Requirements for Medicare coverage.[1]

Group I (any of the following):
1. $PaO_2 \le 55$ mm Hg or $SaO_2 \le 88\%$ taken while awake, at rest, breathing room air.
2. During sleep (prescription for nocturnal oxygen use only):
   a. $PaO_2 \le 55$ mm Hg or $SaO_2 \le 88\%$ for a patient whose awake, resting, room air PaO_2 is ≥ 56 mm Hg or $SaO_2 \ge 89\%$, *or*
   b. Decrease in $PaO_2 > 10$ mm Hg or decrease in $SaO_2 > 5\%$ associated with symptoms or signs reasonably attributed to hypoxemia (eg, impaired cognitive processes, nocturnal restlessness, insomnia).
3. During exercise (prescription for oxygen use only during exercise):
   a. $PaO_2 \le 55$ mg Hg or $SaO_2 \le 88\%$ taken during exercise for a patient whose awake, resting, room air PaO_2 is ≥ 56 mm Hg or $SaO_2 \ge 89\%$, *and*
   b. There is evidence that the use of supplemental oxygen during exercise improves the hypoxemia that was demonstrated during exercise while breathing room air.

Group II[2]:
$PaO_2 = 56–59$ mm Hg or $SaO_2 = 89\%$ if there is evidence of any of the following:
1. Dependent edema suggesting heart failure.
2. P pulmonale on ECG (P wave > 3 mm in standard leads II, III, or aVF).
3. Hematocrit > 56%.

[1]Centers for Medicare & Medicaid Services, 2003.
[2]Patients in this group must have a second oxygen test 3 months after the initial oxygen set-up.

achieves a PaO_2 greater than 55 mm Hg. The monthly cost of home oxygen therapy ranges from $300 to $500 or more, higher for liquid oxygen systems. Medicare covers approximately 80% of home oxygen expenses. **Transtracheal oxygen** is an alternative method of delivery and may be useful for patients who require higher flows of oxygen than can be delivered via the nose or who are experiencing troublesome side effects from nasal delivery, such as nasal drying or epistaxis. Reservoir nasal cannulas or "pendants" and demand (pulse) oxygen delivery systems are also available to conserve oxygen.

3. Inhaled bronchodilators—Bronchodilators do not alter the inexorable decline in lung function that is a hallmark of COPD, but they improve symptoms, exercise tolerance, and overall health status. Aggressiveness of bronchodilator therapy should be matched to the severity of the patient's disease. In patients who experience no symptomatic improvement, bronchodilators should be discontinued.

The most commonly prescribed short-acting bronchodilators are the anticholinergic ipratropium bromide and beta-2-agonists (eg, albuterol, metaproterenol), delivered by MDI or as an inhalation solution by nebulizer. **Ipratropium bromide is generally preferred to the short-acting beta-2-agonists as a first-line agent because of its longer duration of action and absence of sympathomimetic side effects.** Some studies have suggested that ipratropium

achieves superior bronchodilation in COPD patients. Typical doses are two to four puffs (36–72 mcg) every 6 hours. Short-acting beta-2-agonists are less expensive and have a more rapid onset of action, commonly leading to greater patient satisfaction. At maximal doses, beta-2-agonists have bronchodilator action equivalent to that of ipratropium but may cause tachycardia, tremor, or hypokalemia. **There does not appear to be any advantage of scheduled use of short-acting beta-2-agonists compared with as-needed administration.** Use of both short-acting beta-2-agonists and anticholinergics at submaximal doses leads to improved bronchodilation compared with either agent alone but does not improve dyspnea.

Long-acting beta-2-agonists (eg, formoterol, salmeterol, indacaterol, arformoterol, vilanterol) and anticholinergics (tiotropium, aclidinium, and umeclidinium) appear to achieve bronchodilation that is equivalent or superior to what is experienced with ipratropium, in addition to similar improvements in health status. Although more expensive than short-acting agents, long-acting bronchodilators may have superior clinical efficacy in persons with advanced disease. One RCT of long-term administration of tiotropium added to standard therapy reported fewer exacerbations or hospitalizations, and improved dyspnea scores, in the tiotropium group. Tiotropium had no effect on long-term decline in lung function, however. Another RCT comparing the effects of tiotropium with those of salmeterol-fluticasone over 2 years reported no difference in the risk of COPD exacerbation. The incidence of pneumonia was higher in the salmeterol-fluticasone group, yet dyspnea scores were lower and there was a mortality benefit compared with tiotropium.

The symptomatic benefits of long-acting bronchodilators are firmly established. Increased exacerbations and mortality in patients treated with salmeterol have not been observed in COPD patients, and several studies report a trend toward lower mortality in patients treated with salmeterol alone, compared with placebo. In addition, a 4-year tiotropium trial reported fewer cardiovascular events in the intervention group. Subsequent meta-analyses that include the 4-year tiotropium trial did not find an increase in cardiovascular events in treated patients. Most practitioners believe that the documented benefits of anticholinergic therapy outweigh any potential risks.

4. Corticosteroids—Multiple large clinical trials have reported a reduction in the frequency of COPD exacerbations and an increase in self-reported functional status in COPD patients treated with inhaled corticosteroids. These same trials demonstrate no effect of inhaled corticosteroids on mortality or the characteristic decline in lung function experienced by COPD patients. Thus, inhaled corticosteroids alone should not be considered first-line therapy in stable COPD patients.

However, combination therapy with an inhaled corticosteroid and a long-acting beta-2-agonist reduces the frequency of exacerbations and improves self-reported functional status in COPD patients, compared with placebo or with sole use of inhaled corticosteroids, long-acting beta-2-agonists, or anticholinergics. In one RCT, addition of an inhaled corticosteroid/long-acting beta-2-agonist to tiotropium therapy in COPD patients did not reduce the frequency of exacerbations but did improve hospitalization rates and functional status.

Apart from acute exacerbations, COPD is not generally responsive to oral corticosteroid therapy. Compared with patients receiving placebo, only 10–20% of stable outpatients with COPD given oral corticosteroids will have a greater than 20% increase in FEV_1. **There may be a subset of steroid-responsive COPD patients more likely to benefit from long-term oral or inhaled corticosteroids.** Since there are no clinical predictors to identify such responders, empiric trials of oral corticosteroids are common. If an empiric trial of oral corticosteroid is conducted, a baseline FEV_1 should be documented when the patient is stable (ie, not measured during an exacerbation), on maximal long-term bronchodilator therapy, and obtained immediately after a bronchodilator administration. After a 3- to 4-week trial of 0.25–0.5 mg/kg oral prednisone, the corticosteroid should only be continued if there is a 20% or greater increase in FEV_1 over this baseline value. Responders to oral corticosteroids are usually switched to inhaled agents, but there are few data to guide this practice. Oral corticosteroids have well-recognized adverse effects, so it is prudent to minimize cumulative exposure. It is rare for a patient to be truly "corticosteroid-dependent" when all other available therapies are optimized.

5. Theophylline—Oral theophylline is a fourth-line agent for treating COPD patients who do not achieve adequate symptom control with inhaled anticholinergic, beta-2-agonist, and corticosteroid therapies. Sustained-release theophylline improves hemoglobin saturation during sleep in COPD patients and is a first-line agent for those with sleep-related breathing disorders. Theophylline improves dyspnea ratings, exercise performance, and pulmonary function in many patients with stable COPD. Its benefits result from bronchodilation; anti-inflammatory properties; and extrapulmonary effects on diaphragm strength, myocardial contractility, and kidney function. Theophylline toxicity is a significant concern due to the medication's narrow therapeutic window, and long-term administration requires careful monitoring of serum levels. Despite potential for adverse effects, theophylline continues to have a beneficial role in carefully selected patients.

6. Antibiotics—Antibiotics are commonly prescribed to outpatients with COPD for the following indications: (1) to treat an acute exacerbation, (2) to treat acute bronchitis, and (3) to prevent acute exacerbations of chronic bronchitis (prophylactic antibiotics). In patients with COPD, antibiotics appear to improve outcomes slightly in all three situations. **Patients with a COPD exacerbation associated with increased sputum purulence accompanied by dyspnea or an increase in the quantity of sputum are thought to benefit the most from antibiotic therapy.** The choice of antibiotic depends on local bacterial resistance patterns and individual risk of *Pseudomonas aeruginosa* infection (history of *Pseudomonas* isolation, FEV_1 less than 50% of predicted, recent hospitalization [2 or more days in the past 3 months], more than three courses of antibiotics within the past year, use of systemic corticosteroids). Oral antibiotic options include doxycycline (100 mg every

12 hours), trimethoprim-sulfamethoxazole (160/800 mg every 12 hours), a cephalosporin (eg, cefpodoxime 200 mg every 12 hours or cefprozil 500 mg every 12 hours), a macrolide (eg, azithromycin 500 mg followed by 250 mg daily for 5 days), a fluoroquinolone (eg, ciprofloxacin 500 mg every 12 hours), and amoxicillin-clavulanate (875/125 mg every 12 hours). Suggested duration of therapy is 3–7 days and depends on response to therapy; some studies suggest that 5 days is as effective as 7 days but with fewer adverse effects. There are few controlled trials of antibiotics in severe COPD exacerbations, but prompt administration is appropriate, particularly in persons with risk factors for poor outcomes (age older than 65 years, FEV_1 less than 50% of predicted, three or more exacerbations in the past year, antibiotic therapy within the past 3 months, comorbid conditions, such as cardiac disease). In COPD patients subject to frequent exacerbations despite optimal medical therapy, azithromycin (daily or three times weekly) and moxifloxacin (a 5-day course 1 week in 8 over 48 weeks) were modestly effective in clinical trials at reducing the frequency of exacerbations.

7. Pulmonary rehabilitation—Graded aerobic physical exercise programs (eg, walking 20 minutes three times weekly or bicycling) are helpful to prevent deterioration of physical condition and to improve patients' ability to carry out daily activities. Training of inspiratory muscles by inspiring against progressively larger resistive loads reduces dyspnea and improves exercise tolerance, health status, and respiratory muscle strength in some but not all patients. Pursed-lip breathing to slow the rate of breathing and abdominal breathing exercises to relieve fatigue of accessory muscles of respiration may reduce dyspnea in some patients. Many patients undergo these exercise and educational interventions in a structured rehabilitation program. In a number of studies, pulmonary rehabilitation has been shown to improve exercise capacity, decrease hospitalizations, and enhance quality of life. Referral to a comprehensive rehabilitation program is recommended in patients who have severe dyspnea, reduced quality of life, or frequent hospitalizations despite optimal medical therapy.

8. Other measures—In patients with chronic bronchitis, increased mobilization of secretions may be accomplished through the use of adequate systemic hydration, effective cough training methods, or the use of a hand-held flutter device and postural drainage, sometimes with chest percussion or vibration. Postural drainage and chest percussion should be used only in selected patients with excessive amounts of retained secretions that cannot be cleared by coughing and other methods; these measures are of no benefit in pure emphysema. Expectorant-mucolytic therapy has generally been regarded as unhelpful in patients with chronic bronchitis. Cough suppressants and sedatives should be avoided.

Human alpha-1-antitrypsin is available for replacement therapy in emphysema due to congenital deficiency (PiZZ or null genotype) of alpha-1-antiprotease (alpha-1-antitrypsin). Patients over 18 years of age with airflow obstruction by spirometry and serum levels less than 11 mcmol/L (~50 mg/dL) are potential candidates for replacement therapy. Alpha-1-antitrypsin is administered intravenously in a dose of 60 mg/kg body weight once weekly. Severe dyspnea in spite of optimal medical management may warrant a clinical trial of an opioid (eg, morphine 5–10 mg orally every 3–4 hours, oxycodone 5–10 mg orally every 4–6 hours, sustained-release morphine 10 mg orally once daily). Sedative-hypnotic drugs (eg, diazepam, 5 mg three times daily) marginally improve intractable dyspnea but cause significant drowsiness; they may benefit very anxious patients. Transnasal positive-pressure ventilation at home to rest the respiratory muscles is an approach to improve respiratory muscle function and reduce dyspnea in patients with severe COPD.

B. Hospitalized Patients

Management of the hospitalized patient with an acute exacerbation of COPD includes (1) supplemental oxygen (titrated to maintain Sao_2 between 90% and 94% or Pao_2 between 60 mm Hg and 70 mm Hg), (2) inhaled ipratropium bromide (500 mcg by nebulizer, or 36 mcg by MDI with spacer, every 4 hours as needed) plus beta-2-agonists (eg, albuterol 2.5 mg diluted with saline to a total of 3 mL by nebulizer, or MDI, 90 mcg per puff, four to eight puffs via spacer, every 1–4 hours as needed), (3) corticosteroids (prednisone 30–40 mg orally per day for 7–10 days is usually sufficient, even 5 days may be adequate), (4) broad-spectrum antibiotics, and (5) in selected cases, chest physiotherapy.

For patients without risk factors for *Pseudomonas*, management options include a fluoroquinolone (eg, levofloxacin 750 mg orally or intravenously per day, or moxifloxacin 400 mg orally or intravenously every 24 hours) or a third-generation cephalosporin (eg, ceftriaxone 1 g intravenously per day, or cefotaxime 1 g intravenously every 8 hours).

For patients with risk factors for *Pseudomonas*, therapeutic options include piperacillin-tazobactam (4.5 g intravenously every 6 hours), ceftazidime (1 g intravenously every 8 hours), cefepime (1 g intravenously every 12 hours), or levofloxacin (750 mg orally or intravenously per day for 3–7 days).

Theophylline should not be initiated in the acute setting, but patients taking theophylline prior to acute hospitalization should have their theophylline serum levels measured and maintained in the therapeutic range. **Oxygen therapy should not be withheld for fear of worsening respiratory acidemia; hypoxemia is more detrimental than hypercapnia.** Cor pulmonale usually responds to measures that reduce pulmonary artery pressure, such as supplemental oxygen and correction of acidemia; bed rest, salt restriction, and diuretics may add some benefit. Cardiac dysrhythmias, particularly multifocal atrial tachycardia, usually respond to aggressive treatment of COPD itself. Atrial flutter may require DC cardioversion after initiation of the above therapy. If progressive respiratory failure ensues, tracheal intubation and mechanical ventilation are necessary. In clinical trials of COPD patients with hypercapnic acute respiratory failure, **noninvasive positive-pressure ventilation (NIPPV)** delivered via face mask reduced the need for intubation and shortened lengths of stay in the intensive care unit (ICU). Other studies have suggested a lower risk of nosocomial infections and less use of antibiotics in COPD patients treated with NIPPV. These benefits do not appear to extend to hypoxemic respiratory failure or to patients with acute lung injury or acute respiratory distress syndrome (ARDS).

C. Surgery for COPD

1. Lung transplantation— Requirements for lung transplantation are severe lung disease, limited activities of daily living, exhaustion of medical therapy, ambulatory status, potential for pulmonary rehabilitation, limited life expectancy without transplantation, adequate function of other organ systems, and a good social support system. Average total charges for lung transplantation through the end of the first postoperative year exceed $250,000. The 2-year survival rate after lung transplantation for COPD is 75%. Complications include acute rejection, opportunistic infection, and obliterative bronchiolitis. Substantial improvements in pulmonary function and exercise performance have been noted after transplantation.

2. Lung volume reduction surgery—Lung volume reduction surgery (LVRS), or reduction pneumoplasty, is a surgical approach to relieve dyspnea and improve exercise tolerance in patients with advanced diffuse emphysema and lung hyperinflation. Bilateral resection of 20–30% of lung volume in selected patients results in modest improvements in pulmonary function, exercise performance, and dyspnea. The duration of any improvement as well as any mortality benefit remains uncertain. Prolonged air leaks occur in up to 50% of patients postoperatively. Mortality rates in centers with the largest experience with LVRS range from 4% to 10%.

The National Emphysema Treatment Trial compared LVRS with medical treatment in a randomized, multicenter clinical trial of 1218 patients with severe emphysema. Overall, surgery improved exercise capacity but not mortality when compared with medical therapy. The persistence of this benefit remains to be defined. Subgroup analysis suggested that patients with upper lobe–predominant emphysema and low exercise capacity might have improved survival, while other groups suffered excess mortality when randomized to surgery.

3. Bullectomy—Bullectomy is an older surgical procedure for palliation of dyspnea in patients with severe bullous emphysema. Bullectomy is most commonly pursued when a single bulla occupies at least 30–50% of the hemithorax.

▶ Prognosis

The outlook for patients with clinically significant COPD is poor. The degree of pulmonary dysfunction at the time the patient is first seen is an important predictor of survival: median survival of patients with FEV_1 1 L or less is about 4 years. A multidimensional index (the BODE index), which includes body mass index (BMI), airway obstruction (FEV_1), dyspnea (Medical Research Council dyspnea score), and exercise capacity is a tool that predicts death and hospitalization better than FEV_1 alone.

Comprehensive care programs, cessation of smoking, and supplemental oxygen may reduce the rate of decline of pulmonary function, but therapy with bronchodilators and other approaches probably has little, if any, impact on the natural course of COPD.

Dyspnea at the end of life can be extremely uncomfortable and distressing to the patient and family. As patients near the end of life, meticulous attention to palliative care is essential to effectively manage dyspnea (see Chapter 5).

When to Refer

- COPD onset occurs before the age of 40.
- Frequent exacerbations (two or more a year) despite optimal treatment.
- Severe or rapidly progressive COPD.
- Symptoms disproportionate to the severity of airflow obstruction.
- Need for long-term oxygen therapy.
- Onset of comorbid illnesses (eg, bronchiectasis, heart failure, or lung cancer).

When to Admit

- Severe symptoms or acute worsening that fails to respond to outpatient management.
- Acute or worsening hypoxemia, hypercapnia, peripheral edema, or change in mental status.
- Inadequate home care, or inability to sleep or maintain nutrition/hydration due to symptoms.
- The presence of high-risk comorbid conditions.

Aaron SD. Management and prevention of exacerbations of COPD. BMJ. 2014 Sep 22;349:g5237. [PMID: 25245156]

Herath SC et al. Prophylactic antibiotic therapy for chronic obstructive pulmonary disease (COPD). Cochrane Database Syst Rev. 2013 Nov 28;11:CD009764. [PMID: 24288145]

Klooster K et al. Endobronchial valves for emphysema without interlobar collateral ventilation. N Engl J Med 2015 Dec 10; 373(24):2325–35. [PMID: 26650153]

Laue J et al. When should acute exacerbations of COPD be treated with systemic corticosteroids and antibiotics in primary care: a systematic review of current COPD guidelines. NPJ Prim Care Respir Med. 2015 Feb 19;25:15002. [PMID: 25695630]

Leuppi JD et al. Short-term vs conventional glucocorticoid therapy in acute exacerbations of chronic obstructive pulmonary disease: the REDUCE randomized clinical trial. JAMA. 2013 Jun 5;309(21):2223–31. [PMID: 23695200]

Stefan MS et al. Comparative effectiveness of noninvasive and invasive ventilation in critically ill patients with acute exacerbation of chronic obstructive pulmonary disease. Crit Care Med. 2015 Jul;43(7):1386–94. [PMID: 25768682]

Torpy JM et al. JAMA patient page. Chronic obstructive pulmonary disease. JAMA. 2012 Sep 26;308(12):1281. [PMID: 23011720]

Walters JA et al. Different durations of corticosteroid therapy for exacerbations of chronic obstructive pulmonary disease. Cochrane Database Syst Rev. 2014 Dec 10;12:CD006897. [PMID: 25491891]

Walters JA et al. Systemic corticosteroids for acute exacerbations of chronic obstructive pulmonary disease. Cochrane Database Syst Rev. 2014 Sep 1;9:CD001288. [PMID: 25178099]

Wilson R et al. Antibiotics for treatment and prevention of exacerbations of chronic obstructive pulmonary disease. J Infect. 2013 Dec;67(6):497–515. [PMID: 23973659]

BRONCHIECTASIS

 ESSENTIALS OF DIAGNOSIS

- ► Chronic productive cough with dyspnea and wheezing.
- ► Radiographic findings of dilated, thickened airways and scattered, irregular opacities.

General Considerations

Bronchiectasis is a congenital or acquired disorder of the large bronchi characterized by permanent, abnormal dilation and destruction of bronchial walls. It may be caused by recurrent inflammation or infection of the airways and may be localized or diffuse. Cystic fibrosis causes about half of all cases of bronchiectasis. Other causes include lung infection (tuberculosis, fungal infections, lung abscess, pneumonia), abnormal lung defense mechanisms (humoral immunodeficiency, alpha-1-antiprotease [alpha-1-antitrypsin] deficiency with cigarette smoking, mucociliary clearance disorders, rheumatic diseases), and localized airway obstruction (foreign body, tumor, mucoid impaction). Immunodeficiency states that may lead to bronchiectasis include congenital or acquired panhypogammaglobulinemia; common variable immunodeficiency; selective IgA, IgM, and IgG subclass deficiencies; and acquired immunodeficiency from cytotoxic therapy, AIDS, lymphoma, multiple myeloma, leukemia, and chronic kidney and liver diseases. Most patients with bronchiectasis have panhypergammaglobulinemia, however, presumably reflecting an immune system response to chronic airway infection. Acquired primary bronchiectasis is now uncommon in the United States because of improved control of bronchopulmonary infections.

Clinical Findings

A. Symptoms and Signs

Symptoms of bronchiectasis include chronic cough with production of copious amounts of purulent sputum, hemoptysis, and pleuritic chest pain. Dyspnea and wheezing occur in 75% of patients. Weight loss, anemia, and other systemic manifestations are common. Physical findings are nonspecific, but persistent crackles at the lung bases are common. Clubbing is infrequent in mild cases but is common in severe disease (Figure 6–40). Copious, foul-smelling, purulent sputum is characteristic. Obstructive pulmonary dysfunction with hypoxemia is seen in moderate or severe disease.

B. Imaging

Radiographic abnormalities include dilated and thickened bronchi that may appear as "tram tracks" or as ring-like markings. Scattered irregular opacities, atelectasis, and focal consolidation may be present. High-resolution CT is the diagnostic study of choice.

C. Microbiology

Haemophilus influenzae is the most common organism recovered from non–cystic fibrosis patients with bronchiectasis. *P aeruginosa, S pneumoniae,* and *Staphylococcus aureus* are commonly identified. Nontuberculous mycobacteria are seen less commonly. Patients with *Pseudomonas* infection experience an accelerated course, with more frequent exacerbations and more rapid decline in lung function.

▶ Treatment

Treatment of acute exacerbations consists of antibiotics, daily chest physiotherapy with postural drainage and chest percussion, and inhaled bronchodilators. Hand-held flutter valve devices may be as effective as chest physiotherapy in clearing secretions. Antibiotic therapy should be guided by sputum smears and cultures. If a specific bacterial pathogen cannot be isolated, then empiric oral antibiotic therapy for 10–14 days is appropriate. Common regimens include amoxicillin or amoxicillin-clavulanate (500 mg every 8 hours), ampicillin or tetracycline (250–500 mg four times daily), trimethoprim-sulfamethoxazole (160/800 mg every 12 hours), or ciprofloxacin (500–750 mg twice daily). It is important to screen patients for infection with nontuberculous mycobacteria because these organisms may underlie a lack of treatment response. Preventive or suppressive treatment is sometimes given to stable outpatients with bronchiectasis who have copious purulent sputum. Prolonged macrolide therapy (azithromycin 500 mg three times a week for 6 months or 250 mg daily for 12 months) has been found to decrease the frequency of exacerbations compared to placebo. High-dose amoxicillin (3 g/day) or alternating cycles of the antibiotics listed above given orally for 2–4 weeks are also used, although this practice is not supported by clinical trial data. In patients with underlying cystic fibrosis, inhaled aerosolized aminoglycosides reduce colonization by *Pseudomonas* species, improve FEV_1, and reduce hospitalizations. Complications of bronchiectasis include hemoptysis, cor pulmonale, amyloidosis, and secondary visceral abscesses at distant sites (eg, brain). Bronchoscopy is sometimes necessary to evaluate hemoptysis, remove retained secretions, and rule out obstructing airway lesions. Massive hemoptysis may require embolization of bronchial arteries or surgical resection. Surgical resection is otherwise reserved for the few patients with localized bronchiectasis and adequate pulmonary function in whom conservative management fails.

Altenburg J et al. Effect of azithromycin maintenance treatment on infectious exacerbations among patients with non–cystic fibrosis bronchiectasis: the BAT randomized controlled trial. JAMA. 2013 Mar 27;309(12):1251–9. [PMID: 23532241]

McShane PJ et al. Non-cystic fibrosis bronchiectasis. Am J Respir Crit Care Med. 2013 Sep 15;188(6):647–56. [PMID: 23898922]

Wilkinson M et al. Mucolytics for bronchiectasis. Cochrane Database Syst Rev. 2014 May 2;5:CD001289. [PMID: 24789119]

Wong C et al. Azithromycin for prevention of exacerbations in non–cystic fibrosis bronchiectasis (EMBRACE): a randomised, double-blind, placebo-controlled trial. Lancet. 2012 Aug 18; 380(9842):660–7. [PMID: 22901887]

ALLERGIC BRONCHOPULMONARY MYCOSIS

Allergic bronchopulmonary mycosis is a pulmonary hypersensitivity disorder caused by allergy to fungal antigens that colonize the tracheobronchial tree. It usually occurs in atopic asthmatic individuals who are 20–40 years of age, in response to antigens of *Aspergillus* species. For this reason, the disorder is commonly referred to as allergic bronchopulmonary aspergillosis (ABPA). Primary criteria for the diagnosis of ABPA include (1) a clinical history of asthma, (2) peripheral eosinophilia, (3) immediate skin reactivity to *Aspergillus* antigen, (4) precipitating antibodies to *Aspergillus* antigen, (5) elevated serum IgE levels, (6) pulmonary infiltrates (transient or fixed), and (7) central bronchiectasis. If the first six of these seven primary criteria are present, the diagnosis is almost certain. Secondary diagnostic criteria include identification of *Aspergillus* in sputum, a history of brown-flecked sputum, and late skin reactivity to *Aspergillus* antigen. High-dose prednisone (0.5–1 mg/kg orally per day) for at least 2 months is the treatment of choice, and the response in early disease is usually excellent. Depending on the overall clinical situation, prednisone can then be cautiously tapered. Relapses are frequent, and protracted or repeated treatment with corticosteroids is not uncommon. Patients with corticosteroid-dependent disease may benefit from itraconazole (200 mg orally three times a day with food for 3 days, followed by twice daily for at least 16 weeks) without added toxicity. Bronchodilators (see Table 9–5) are also helpful. Complications include hemoptysis, severe bronchiectasis, and pulmonary fibrosis.

Agarwal R et al; ABPA complicating asthma ISHAM working group. Allergic bronchopulmonary aspergillosis: review of literature and proposal of new diagnostic and classification criteria. Clin Exp Allergy. 2013 Aug;43(8):850–73. [PMID: 23889240]

Agbetile J et al. Effectiveness of voriconazole in the treatment of *Aspergillus fumigatus*-associated asthma (EVITA3 study). J Allergy Clin Immunol. 2014 Jul;134(1):33–9. [PMID: 24290286]

Bains SN et al. Allergic bronchopulmonary aspergillosis. Clin Chest Med. 2012 Jun;33(2):265–81. [PMID: 22640845]

Mahdavinia M et al. Management of allergic bronchopulmonary aspergillosis: a review and update. Ther Adv Respir Dis. 2012 Jun;6(3):173–87. [PMID: 22547692]

CYSTIC FIBROSIS

 ESSENTIALS OF DIAGNOSIS

▶ Chronic or recurrent productive cough, dyspnea, and wheezing.

▶ Recurrent airway infections or chronic colonization of the airways with *H influenzae, P aeruginosa, S aureus,* or *Burkholderia cepacia.* Bronchiectasis and scarring on chest radiographs.

► Airflow obstruction on spirometry.

► Pancreatic insufficiency, recurrent pancreatitis, distal intestinal obstruction syndrome, chronic hepatic disease, nutritional deficiencies, or male urogenital abnormalities.

► Sweat chloride concentration greater than 60 mEq/L on two occasions or gene mutation known to cause cystic fibrosis.

General Considerations

Cystic fibrosis is the most common cause of severe chronic lung disease in young adults and the most common fatal hereditary disorder of whites in the United States. It is an autosomal-recessive disorder affecting about 1 in 3200 whites; 1 in 25 is a carrier. Cystic fibrosis is caused by abnormalities in a membrane chloride channel (the cystic fibrosis transmembrane conductance regulator [CFTR] protein) that results in altered chloride transport and water flux across the apical surface of epithelial cells. Almost all exocrine glands produce an abnormal mucus that obstructs glands and ducts and leads to tissue damage. In the respiratory tract, inadequate hydration of the tracheobronchial epithelium impairs mucociliary function. High concentration of extracellular DNA in airway secretions (due to chronic airway inflammation and autolysis of neutrophils) increases sputum viscosity.

Over one-third of the nearly 30,000 cystic fibrosis patients in the United States are adults. Patients with cystic fibrosis have an increased risk of malignancies of the gastrointestinal tract, osteopenia, and arthropathies.

Clinical Findings

A. Symptoms and Signs

Cystic fibrosis should be suspected in a young adult with a history of chronic lung disease (especially bronchiectasis), pancreatitis, or infertility. Cough, sputum production, decreased exercise tolerance, and recurrent hemoptysis are typical complaints. Patients also often complain of chronic rhinosinusitis symptoms, steatorrhea, diarrhea, and abdominal pain. Patients with cystic fibrosis are often malnourished with low body mass index. Digital clubbing, increased anteroposterior chest diameter, hyperresonance to percussion, and apical crackles are noted on physical examination. Sinus tenderness, purulent nasal secretions, and nasal polyps may also be seen. Nearly all men with cystic fibrosis have congenital bilateral absence of the vas deferens with azoospermia. Biliary cirrhosis and gallstones may occur.

B. Laboratory Findings

Arterial blood gas studies often reveal hypoxemia and, in advanced disease, a chronic, compensated respiratory acidosis. Pulmonary function studies show a mixed obstructive and restrictive pattern. There is a reduction in FVC, airflow rates, and TLC. Air trapping (high ratio of RV to TLC) and reduction in pulmonary diffusing capacity are common.

C. Imaging

Hyperinflation is seen early in the disease process. Peribronchial cuffing, mucus plugging, bronchiectasis (ring shadows and cysts), increased interstitial markings, small rounded peripheral opacities, and focal atelectasis are common findings. Pneumothorax can also be seen. Thin-section CT scanning often confirms the presence of bronchiectasis.

D. Diagnosis

The **quantitative pilocarpine iontophoresis sweat test** reveals elevated sodium and chloride levels (greater than 60 mEq/L) in the sweat of patients with cystic fibrosis. Two tests on different days performed in experienced laboratories are required for accurate diagnosis. A normal sweat chloride test does not exclude the diagnosis, in which case genotyping or other alternative diagnostic studies (such as measurement of nasal membrane potential difference, semen analysis, or assessment of pancreatic function) should be pursued, especially if there is a high clinical suspicion of cystic fibrosis.

Treatment

Early recognition and comprehensive multidisciplinary therapy improve symptom control and the chances of survival. Referral to a regional cystic fibrosis center is strongly recommended. Conventional treatment programs focus on the following areas: clearance and reduction of lower airway secretions, reversal of bronchoconstriction, treatment of respiratory tract infections and airway bacterial burden, pancreatic enzyme replacement, and nutritional and psychosocial support (including genetic and occupational counseling). The Pulmonary Therapies Committee, established by the Cystic Fibrosis Foundation, has issued evidenced-based recommendations regarding long-term use of medications for maintenance of lung function and reduction of exacerbations in patients with cystic fibrosis.

Clearance of lower airway secretions can be promoted by postural drainage, chest percussion or vibration techniques, positive expiratory pressure (PEP) or flutter valve breathing devices, directed cough, and other breathing techniques; these approaches require detailed patient instruction by experienced personnel. Inhaled recombinant human deoxyribonuclease (rhDNase, dornase alpha) cleaves extracellular DNA in sputum, decreasing sputum viscosity; when administered long-term at a daily nebulized dose of 2.5 mg, this therapy leads to improved FEV_1 and reduces the risk of cystic fibrosis–related respiratory exacerbations and the need for intravenous antibiotics. Inhalation of hypertonic saline twice daily has been associated with small improvements in pulmonary function and fewer pulmonary exacerbations. The beneficial effects of hypertonic saline may derive from improved airway mucous clearance.

Short-term antibiotics are used to treat active airway infections based on results of culture and susceptibility testing of sputum. S aureus (including methicillin-resistant strains) and a mucoid variant of *P aeruginosa* are commonly present. *H influenzae, Stenotrophomonas maltophilia,* and *B cepacia* (a highly drug-resistant organism) are occasionally isolated. **Long-term antibiotic therapy** is helpful in slowing disease progression and reducing exacerbations in patients with sputum cultures positive for *P aeruginosa.* These antibiotics include azithromycin 500 mg orally three times a week, which has immunomodulatory properties, and various inhaled antibiotics (eg, tobramycin, aztreonam, colistin, and levofloxacin) taken two to three times a day. The length of therapy depends on the persistent presence of *P aeruginosa* in the sputum. The incidence of atypical mycobacterial colonization is higher in cystic fibrosis patients, and directed antibiotic treatment is recommended for frequent exacerbations, progressive decline in lung function, or failure to thrive. Yearly screening with sputum acid-fast bacilli cultures is advised.

Inhaled bronchodilators (eg, albuterol, two puffs every 4 hours as needed) should be considered in patients who demonstrate an increase of at least 12% in FEV_1 after an inhaled bronchodilator. An inhaled corticosteroid should be added to the treatment regimen for patients who have cystic fibrosis with persistent asthma or allergic bronchopulmonary mycosis.

Ivacaftor is an oral medication, available for the 5% of cystic fibrosis patients with a G551D mutation. Ivacaftor is a potentiator of the CFTR channel that works by increasing the time the channel remains open after being activated; it has been found to improve lung function by 10% within 2 weeks of treatment, decrease pulmonary exacerbations by 55%, and decrease sweat chloride into the indeterminate range. CFTR corrector therapy for the most common mutation (DeltaF508) is under trial.

Lung transplantation is the only definitive treatment for advanced cystic fibrosis. Double-lung or heart-lung transplantation is required. A few transplant centers offer living lobar lung transplantation to selected patients. The 3-year survival rate following transplantation for cystic fibrosis is about 55%.

Vaccination against pneumococcal infection and annual influenza vaccination are advised. **Screening** of family members and genetic counseling are suggested.

▶ Prognosis

The longevity of patients with cystic fibrosis is increasing, and the median survival age is over 36 years. Death occurs from pulmonary complications (eg, pneumonia, pneumothorax, or hemoptysis) or as a result of terminal chronic respiratory failure and cor pulmonale.

Mogayzel PJ Jr et al; Cystic Fibrosis Foundation Pulmonary Clinical Practice Guidelines Committee. Cystic Fibrosis Foundation pulmonary guideline. Pharmacologic approaches to prevention and eradication of initial *Pseudomonas aeruginosa* infection. Ann Am Thorac Soc. 2014 Dec;11(10):1640–50. [PMID: 25549030]

Mogayzel PJ Jr et al; Pulmonary Clinical Practice Guidelines Committee. Cystic fibrosis pulmonary guidelines. Chronic medications for maintenance of lung health. Am J Respir Crit Care Med. 2013 Apr 1;187(7):680–9. [PMID: 23540878]

Stoltz DA et al. Origins of cystic fibrosis lung disease. N Engl J Med. 2015 Jan 22;372(4):351–62. [PMID: 25607428]

Weill D et al. A consensus document for the selection of lung transplant candidates: 2014—an update from the Pulmonary Transplantation Council of the International Society for Heart and Lung Transplantation. J Heart Lung Transplant. 2015 Jan;34(1):1–15. [PMID: 25085497]

BRONCHIOLITIS

ESSENTIALS OF DIAGNOSIS

- ▶ Insidious onset of cough and dyspnea.
- ▶ Irreversible airflow obstruction on pulmonary function testing.
- ▶ Minimal findings on chest radiograph.
- ▶ Relevant exposure or risk factors: toxic fumes, viral infections, organ transplantation, connective tissue disease.

▶ General Considerations

Bronchiolitis is a generic term applied to varied inflammatory processes that affect the bronchioles, which are small conducting airways less than 2 mm in diameter. In infants and children, bronchiolitis is common and usually caused by respiratory syncytial virus or adenovirus infection. In adults, bronchiolitis is less common but is encountered in multiple clinical settings. Disorders associated with bronchiolitis include organ transplantation, connective tissue diseases, and hypersensitivity pneumonitis. Inhalational injuries as well as postinfectious and drug-induced causes are identified by association with a known exposure or illness prior to the onset of symptoms. Idiopathic cases are characterized by the insidious onset of dyspnea or cough and include cryptogenic organizing pneumonitis (COP).

▶ Clinical Findings

Acute bronchiolitis is most commonly seen following viral infection in children.

Constrictive bronchiolitis (also referred to as obliterative bronchiolitis, or bronchiolitis obliterans) is relatively infrequent although it is the most common finding following inhalation injury. It may also be seen in rheumatoid arthritis; medication reactions; and chronic rejection following heart-lung, lung, or bone marrow transplant. Patients with constrictive bronchiolitis have airflow obstruction on spirometry; minimal radiographic abnormalities; and a progressive, deteriorating clinical course.

Proliferative bronchiolitis is associated with diverse pulmonary disorders, including infection, aspiration, ARDS, hypersensitivity pneumonitis, connective tissue diseases, and organ transplantation. Compared with constrictive bronchiolitis, proliferative bronchiolitis is more likely to have an abnormal chest radiograph.

Cryptogenic organizing pneumonitis (COP) formally referred to as **bronchiolitis obliterans with organizing pneumonia** (BOOP) affects men and women between the ages of 50 and 70 years, typically with a dry cough, dyspnea, and constitutional symptoms that may be present for weeks to months prior to seeking medical attention. A history of a preceding viral illness is present in half of cases. Pulmonary function testing typically reveals a restrictive ventilatory defect and impaired oxygenation. The chest radiograph frequently shows bilateral patchy, ground-glass or alveolar infiltrates, although other patterns have been described.

Follicular bronchiolitis is most commonly associated with connective tissue disease, especially rheumatoid arthritis and Sjögren syndrome, and with immunodeficiency states.

Respiratory bronchiolitis usually occurs without symptoms or physiologic evidence of lung impairment.

Diffuse panbronchiolitis is most frequently diagnosed in Japan. Men are affected about twice as often as women, two-thirds are nonsmokers, and most patients have a history of chronic pansinusitis. Patients complain of dyspnea, cough, and sputum production, and chest examination shows crackles and rhonchi. Pulmonary function tests reveal obstructive abnormalities, and the chest radiograph shows a distinct pattern of diffuse, small, nodular shadows with hyperinflation.

▶ **Treatment**

Constrictive bronchiolitis is relatively unresponsive to corticosteroids and is frequently progressive. Corticosteroids are effective in two-thirds of patients with **proliferative bronchiolitis,** and improvement can be prompt. Therapy is initiated with prednisone at 1 mg/kg/day orally for 1–3 months. The dose is then tapered slowly to 20–40 mg/day, depending on the response, and weaned over the subsequent 3–6 months as tolerated. Relapses are common if corticosteroids are stopped prematurely or tapered too quickly. Most patients with COP recover following corticosteroid treatment. Diffuse panbronchiolitis is effectively treated with azithromycin.

Barker AF et al. Obliterative bronchiolitis. N Engl J Med. 2014 May 8;370(19):1820–8. [PMID: 24806161]

Bergeron A et al. Budesonide/formoterol for bronchiolitis obliterans after hematopoietic stem cell transplantation. Am J Respir Crit Care Med. 2015 Jun 1;191(11):1242–9. [PMID: 25835160]

Meyer KC et al. An international ISHLT/ATS/ERS clinical practice guideline: diagnosis and management of bronchiolitis obliterans syndrome. Eur Respir J. 2014 Dec;44(6):1479–503. [PMID: 25359357]

Weigt SS et al. Bronchiolitis obliterans syndrome: the Achilles' heel of lung transplantation. Semin Respir Crit Care Med. 2013 Jun;34(3):336–51. [PMID: 23821508]

PULMONARY INFECTIONS

PNEUMONIA

Pneumonia has classically been considered in terms of the infecting organism (Table 9–8). This approach facilitates discussion of characteristic clinical presentations but is a limited guide to patient management since specific microbiologic information is rarely available at initial presentation. More recent classification schemes emphasize epidemiologic factors that predict etiology and guide initial therapy. Pneumonia may be classified as community-acquired (CAP) or nosocomial and, within the latter, as health care–associated (HCAP), hospital-acquired (HAP), or ventilator-associated (VAP). These categories are based on differing settings and infectious agents and require different diagnostic and therapeutic interventions. Anaerobic pneumonia and lung abscess can occur in both hospital and community settings and warrant separate consideration.

This section sets forth the evaluation and management of pulmonary infiltrates in immunocompetent persons separately from the approach to immunocompromised persons—defined as those with HIV disease, absolute neutrophil counts less than 1000/mcL (1.0×10^9/L), current or recent exposure to myelosuppressive or immunosuppressive medications, or those currently taking prednisone in a dosage greater than 5 mg/day.

1. Community-Acquired Pneumonia

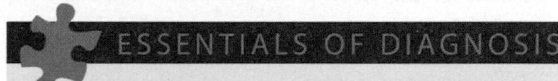

ESSENTIALS OF DIAGNOSIS

▶ Fever or hypothermia, tachypnea, cough with or without sputum, dyspnea, chest discomfort, sweats or rigors (or both).

▶ Bronchial breath sounds or inspiratory crackles on chest auscultation.

▶ Parenchymal opacity on chest radiograph.

▶ Occurs outside of the hospital or within 48 hours of hospital admission in a patient not residing in a long-term care facility.

▶ **General Considerations**

Community-acquired pneumonia (CAP) is a common disorder, with approximately 4–5 million cases diagnosed each year in the United States, 25% of which require hospitalization. It is the deadliest infectious disease in the United States and the eighth leading cause of death. Mortality in milder cases treated as outpatients is less than 1%. Among patients hospitalized for CAP, in-hospital mortality is approximately 10–12% and 1-year mortality (in those over age 65) is greater than 40%. Risk factors for the development of CAP include advanced age; alcoholism; tobacco use; comorbid medical conditions, especially asthma or COPD; and immunosuppression.

The patient's history, physical examination, and imaging studies are essential to establishing a diagnosis of CAP. None of these efforts identifies a specific microbiologic cause, however. Sputum examination may be helpful in selected patients but 40% of patients cannot produce an evaluable sputum sample and Gram stain and culture lack sensitivity for the most common causes of pneumonia. Since patient outcomes improve when the initial antibiotic

Table 9–8. Characteristics of selected pneumonias.

Organism; Appearance on Smear of Sputum	Clinical Setting	Complications
Streptococcus pneumoniae (pneumococcus). Gram-positive diplococci.	Chronic cardiopulmonary disease; follows upper respiratory tract infection	Bacteremia, meningitis, endocarditis, pericarditis, empyema
Haemophilus influenzae. Pleomorphic gram-negative coccobacilli.	Chronic cardiopulmonary disease; follows upper respiratory tract infection	Empyema, endocarditis
Staphylococcus aureus. Plump gram-positive cocci in clumps.	Residence in chronic care facility, healthcare–associated, influenza epidemics, cystic fibrosis, bronchiectasis, injection drug use	Empyema, cavitation
Klebsiella pneumoniae. Plump gram-negative encapsulated rods.	Alcohol abuse, diabetes mellitus; health care–associated	Cavitation, empyema
Escherichia coli. Gram-negative rods.	Health care–associated; rarely, community-acquired	Empyema
Pseudomonas aeruginosa. Gram-negative rods.	Health care–associated; cystic fibrosis, bronchiectasis	Cavitation
Anaerobes. Mixed flora.	Aspiration, poor dental hygiene	Necrotizing pneumonia, abscess, empyema
Mycoplasma pneumoniae. PMNs and monocytes; no bacteria.	Young adults; summer and fall	Skin rashes, bullous myringitis; hemolytic anemia
Legionella species. Few PMNs; no bacteria.	Summer and fall; exposure to contaminated construction site, water source, air conditioner; community-acquired or health care-associated	Empyema, cavitation, endocarditis, pericarditis
Chlamydophila pneumoniae. Nonspecific.	Clinically similar to *M pneumoniae*, but prodromal symptoms last longer (up to 2 weeks). Sore throat with hoarseness common. Mild pneumonia in teenagers and young adults.	Reinfection in older adults with underlying COPD or heart failure may be severe or even fatal
Moraxella catarrhalis. Gram-negative diplococci.	Preexisting lung disease; elderly; corticosteroid or immunosuppressive therapy	Rarely, pleural effusions and bacteremia
Pneumocystis jirovecii. Nonspecific.	AIDS, immunosuppressive or cytotoxic drug therapy, cancer	Pneumothorax, respiratory failure, ARDS, death

ARDS, acute respiratory distress syndrome; COPD, chronic obstructive pulmonary disease; PMN, polymorphonuclear leukocyte.

choice is appropriate for the infecting organism, the American Thoracic Society and the Infectious Diseases Society of America recommend empiric treatment based on epidemiologic data (Table 9–9). Such treatment improves initial antibiotic coverage, reduces unnecessary hospitalization, and appears to improve 30-day survival.

Decisions regarding hospitalization and ICU care should be based on prognostic criteria.

Definition & Pathogenesis

CAP is diagnosed outside of the hospital in ambulatory patients who are not residents of nursing homes or other long-term care facilities. It may also be diagnosed in a previously ambulatory patient within 48 hours after admission to the hospital.

Pulmonary defense mechanisms (cough reflex, mucociliary clearance system, immune responses) normally prevent the development of lower respiratory tract infections following aspiration of oropharyngeal secretions containing bacteria or inhalation of infected aerosols. CAP occurs when there is a defect in one or more of these normal defense mechanisms or when a large infectious inoculum or a virulent pathogen overwhelms the immune response.

Prospective studies fail to identify the cause of CAP in 40–60% of cases; two or more causes are identified in up to 5% of cases. Bacteria are more commonly identified than viruses. The most common bacterial pathogen identified in most studies of CAP is *S pneumoniae*, accounting for approximately two-thirds of bacterial isolates. Other common bacterial pathogens include *H influenzae*, *M pneumoniae*, *C pneumoniae*, *S aureus*, *Neisseria meningitidis*, *M catarrhalis*, *Klebsiella pneumoniae*, other gram-negative rods, and *Legionella* species. Common viral causes of CAP include influenza virus, respiratory syncytial virus, adenovirus, and parainfluenza virus. A detailed assessment of epidemiologic risk factors may aid in diagnosing pneumonias due to the following uncommon causes: *Chlamydophila psittaci* (psittacosis), *Coxiella burnetii* (Q fever), *Francisella tularensis* (tularemia), endemic fungi (*Blastomyces*, *Coccidioides*, *Histoplasma*), and sin nombre virus (hantavirus pulmonary syndrome).

Clinical Findings

A. Symptoms and Signs

Most patients with CAP experience an acute or subacute onset of fever, cough with or without sputum production,

Table 9–9. Recommended empiric antibiotics for community-acquired pneumonia.

Outpatient management

1. For previously healthy patients who have not taken antibiotics within the past 3 months:
   a. A macrolide (clarithromycin, 500 mg orally twice a day; or azithromycin, 500 mg orally as a first dose and then 250 mg orally daily for 4 days, or 500 mg orally daily for 3 days), *or*
   b. Doxycycline, 100 mg orally twice a day.
2. For patients with such comorbid medical conditions as chronic heart, lung, liver, or renal disease; diabetes mellitus; alcoholism; malignancy; asplenia; immunosuppressant conditions or use of immunosuppressive drugs; or use of antibiotics within the previous 3 months (in which case, an alternative from a different antibiotic class should be selected):
   a. A respiratory fluoroquinolone (moxifloxacin, 400 mg orally daily; gemifloxacin, 320 mg orally daily; levofloxacin, 750 mg orally daily) *or*
   b. A macrolide (as above) *plus* a beta-lactam (amoxicillin, 1 g orally three times a day; amoxicillin-clavulanate, 2 g orally twice a day are preferred to cefpodoxime, 200 mg orally twice a day; cefuroxime, 500 mg orally twice a day).
3. In regions with a high rate (> 25%) of infection with high level (MIC ≥ 16 mcg/mL) macrolide-resistant *Streptococcus pneumoniae*, consider use of alternative agents listed above in (2) for patients with comorbidities.

Inpatient management not requiring intensive care

1. A respiratory fluoroquinolone. See above for oral therapy. For intravenous therapy, moxifloxacin, 400 mg daily; levofloxacin, 750 mg daily; ciprofloxacin, 400 mg every 8–12 hours *or*
2. A macrolide *plus* a beta-lactam. See above for oral therapy. For intravenous therapy, ampicillin, 1–2 g every 4–6 hours; cefotaxime, 1–2 g every 4–12 hours; ceftriaxone, 1–2 g every 12–24 hours.

Inpatient intravenous management requiring intensive care

1. Azithromycin (500 mg orally as a first dose and then 250 mg orally daily for 4 days, or 500 mg orally daily for 3 days) or a respiratory fluoroquinolone plus an antipneumococcal beta-lactam (cefotaxime, ceftriaxone, or ampicillin-sulbactam, 1.5–3 g every 6 hours).
2. For patients allergic to beta-lactam antibiotics, a fluoroquinolone *plus* aztreonam (1–2 g every 6–12 hours).
3. For patients at risk for *Pseudomonas* infection:
   a. An antipneumococcal, antipseudomonal beta-lactam (piperacillin-tazobactam, 3.375–4.5 g every 6 hours; cefepime, 1–2 g twice a day; imipenem, 0.5–1 g every 6–8 hours; meropenem, 1 g every 8 hours) *plus* ciprofloxacin (400 mg every 8–12 hours) or levofloxacin, *or*
   b. The above beta-lactam *plus* an aminoglycoside (gentamicin, tobramycin, amikacin, all weight-based dosing administered daily adjusted to appropriate trough levels) *plus* azithromycin or a respiratory fluoroquinolone.
4. For patients at risk for methicillin-resistant *Staphylococcus* aureus infection, add vancomycin (interval dosing based on renal function to achieve serum trough concentration 15–20 mcg/mL) *or* linezolid (600 mg twice a day).

MIC, minimum inhibitory concentration.
Recommendations assembled from Mandell LA et al. Infectious Diseases Society of America/American Thoracic Society consensus guidelines on the management of community-acquired pneumonia in adults. Clin Infect Dis. 2007;44:S27–72. [PMID: 17278083]

and dyspnea. Other common symptoms include sweats, chills, rigors, chest discomfort, pleurisy, hemoptysis, fatigue, myalgias, anorexia, headache, and abdominal pain.

Common physical findings include fever or hypothermia, tachypnea, tachycardia, and arterial oxygen desaturation. Many patients appear acutely ill. Chest examination often reveals inspiratory crackles and bronchial breath sounds. Dullness to percussion may be observed if lobar consolidation or a parapneumonic pleural effusion is present. **The clinical evaluation is less than 50% sensitive compared to chest imaging for the diagnosis of CAP** (see Imaging section below). In most patients, therefore, a chest radiograph is essential to the evaluation of suspected CAP.

B. Diagnostic Testing

Diagnostic testing for a specific infectious cause of CAP is not generally indicated in ambulatory patients treated as outpatients because empiric antibiotic therapy is almost always effective in this population. In ambulatory outpatients whose presentation (travel history, exposure) suggests an etiology not covered by standard therapy (eg, *Coccidioides)* or public health concerns (eg, *Mycobacterium tuberculosis*, influenza), diagnostic testing is appropriate. Diagnostic testing is recommended in hospitalized CAP

patients for multiple reasons: the likelihood of an infectious cause unresponsive to standard therapy is higher in more severe illness, the inpatient setting allows narrowing of antibiotic coverage as specific diagnostic information is available, and the yield of testing is improved in more acutely ill patients.

Diagnostic testing results are used to guide initial antibiotic therapy, permit adjustment of empirically chosen therapy to a specific infectious cause or resistance pattern, and facilitate epidemiologic analysis. There are three widely available, rapid point-of-care diagnostic tests that may guide initial therapy: the sputum Gram stain, urinary antigen tests for *S pneumonia* and *Legionella* species, and rapid antigen detection tests for influenza. Sputum Gram stain is neither sensitive nor specific for *S pneumonia*, the most common cause of CAP. The usefulness of a sputum Gram stain lies in broadening initial coverage in patients to be hospitalized for CAP, most commonly to cover *S aureus* (including community-acquired methicillin-resistant strains, CA-MRSA) or gram-negative rods. Urinary antigen assays for *Legionella pneumophilia* and *S pneumoniae* are at least as sensitive and specific as sputum Gram stain and culture. Results are available immediately and are not affected by early initiation of antibiotic therapy. Positive tests may allow narrowing of initial antibiotic coverage.

Urinary antigen assay for *S pneumoniae* should be ordered for patients with leukopenia, asplenia, active alcohol use, chronic severe liver disease, pleural effusion, and those requiring ICU admission. Urinary antigen assay for *L pneumophilia* should be ordered for patients with active alcohol use, travel within previous 2 weeks, pleural effusion, and those requiring ICU admission. Rapid influenza testing has intermediate sensitivity but high specificity. Positive tests may reduce unnecessary antibacterial use and direct isolation of hospitalized patients.

Additional microbiologic testing including pre-antibiotic sputum and blood cultures (at least two sets with needle sticks at separate sites) has been standard practice for patients with CAP who require hospitalization. The yield of blood and sputum cultures is low; however, false-positive results are common, and the impact of culture results on patient outcomes is small. As a result, targeted testing based on specific indications is recommended. Culture results are not available prior to initiation of antibiotic therapy. Their role is to allow narrowing of initial empiric antibiotic coverage, adjustment of coverage based on specific antibiotic resistance patterns, to identify unsuspected pathogens not covered by initial therapy, and to provide information for epidemiologic analysis.

Apart from microbiologic testing, hospitalized patients should undergo complete blood count with differential and a chemistry panel (including serum glucose, electrolytes, urea nitrogen, creatinine, bilirubin, and liver enzymes). Hypoxemic patients should have arterial blood gases sampled. Test results help assess severity of illness and guide evaluation and management. HIV testing should be considered in all adult patients, and performed in those with risk factors.

C. Imaging

A pulmonary opacity on chest radiography or CT scan is required to establish a diagnosis of CAP. Chest CT scan is more sensitive and specific than chest radiography and may be indicated in selected cases. Radiographic findings range from patchy airspace opacities to lobar consolidation with air bronchograms to diffuse alveolar or interstitial opacities. Additional findings can include pleural effusions and cavitation. Chest imaging cannot identify a specific microbiologic cause of CAP, however. No pattern of radiographic abnormalities is pathognomonic of any infectious cause.

Chest imaging may help assess severity and response to therapy over time. Progression of pulmonary opacities during antibiotic therapy or lack of radiographic improvement over time are poor prognostic signs and also raise concerns about secondary or alternative pulmonary processes. **Clearing of pulmonary opacities in patients with CAP can take 6 weeks or longer.** Clearance is usually quickest in younger patients, nonsmokers, and those with only single-lobe involvement.

D. Special Examinations

Patients with CAP who have significant pleural fluid collections may require diagnostic thoracentesis (glucose, lactate dehydrogenase [LD], and total protein levels;

leukocyte count with differential; pH determination) with pleural fluid Gram stain and culture. Positive pleural cultures indicate the need for tube thoracostomy drainage.

Patients with cavitary opacities should have sputum fungal and mycobacterial cultures.

Sputum induction and fiberoptic bronchoscopy to obtain samples of lower respiratory secretions are indicated in patients who cannot provide expectorated sputum samples or who may have *Pneumocystis jirovecii* or *M tuberculosis* pneumonia.

Serologic assays, polymerase chain reaction tests, specialized culture tests, and other diagnostic tests for organisms such as viruses, *Legionella*, *M pneumoniae*, and *C pneumoniae* may be performed when these diagnoses are suspected.

▶ Differential Diagnosis

The differential diagnosis of lower respiratory tract infection is extensive and includes upper respiratory tract infections, reactive airway diseases, heart failure, cryptogenic organizing pneumonitis, lung cancer, pulmonary vasculitis, pulmonary thromboembolic disease, and atelectasis.

▶ Treatment

Two general principles guide antibiotic therapy once the diagnosis of CAP is established: **prompt** initiation of a medication to which the etiologic pathogen is **susceptible.**

In patients who require specific diagnostic evaluation, sputum and blood culture specimens should be obtained prior to initiation of antibiotics. Since early administration of antibiotics to acutely ill patients is associated with improved outcomes, **obtaining other diagnostic specimens or test results should not delay the initial dose of antibiotics.**

Optimal antibiotic therapy would be pathogen directed, but a definitive microbiologic diagnosis is rarely available on or within 6 hours of presentation. A syndromic approach to therapy, based on clinical presentation and chest imaging, does not reliably predict the microbiology of CAP. Therefore, initial antibiotic choices are typically empiric, based on acuity (treatment as an outpatient, inpatient, or in the ICU), patient risk factors for specific pathogens, and local antibiotic resistance patterns (Table 9–9).

Since *S pneumoniae* remains a common cause of CAP in all patient groups, local prevalence of drug-resistant *S pneumoniae* significantly affects initial antibiotic choice. Prior treatment with one antibiotic in a pharmacologic class (eg, beta-lactam, macrolide, fluoroquinolone) predisposes the emergence of drug-resistant *S pneumoniae*, with resistance developing against that class of antibiotics to which the pathogen was previously exposed. Definitions of resistance have shifted based on observations of continued clinical efficacy at achievable serum levels. In CAP, for parenteral penicillin G or oral amoxicillin, susceptible strains have a minimum inhibitory concentration (MIC) 2 mcg/mL or less; intermediate resistance is defined as an MIC between 2 mcg/mL and 4 mcg/mL because treatment failures are uncommon with MIC 4 mcg/mL or less. Macrolide resistance has increased; approximately one-third of *S pneumoniae* isolates now show in vitro resistance to macrolides. Treatment failures have been reported but remain rare compared to the number of patients treated; current in vivo efficacy appears to justify maintaining macrolides as first-line therapy except in areas where there is a high prevalence of resistant strains. S pneumoniae resistant to fluoroquinolones is rare in the United States (1% to levo-floxacin, 2% to ciprofloxacin) but is increasing.

Community-acquired methicillin-resistant S aureus (CA-MRSA) is genetically and phenotypically different from hospital-acquired MRSA strains. CA-MRSA is a rare cause of necrotizing pneumonia, empyema, respiratory failure, and shock; it appears to be associated with prior influenza infection. Linezolid may be preferred to vancomycin in treatment of CA-MRSA pulmonary infection. For expanded discussions of specific antibiotics, see Chapter 30.

A. Treatment of Outpatients

See Table 9–9 for specific medication dosages. The most common etiologies of CAP in outpatients who do not require hospitalization are S pneumoniae; M pneumoniae; C pneumoniae; and respiratory viruses, including influenza. For previously healthy patients with no recent (90 days) use of antibiotics, the recommended treatment is a macrolide (clarithromycin or azithromycin) or doxycycline.

In patients at risk for drug resistance (antibiotic therapy within the past 90 days, age greater than 65 years, comorbid illness, immunosuppression, exposure to a child in daycare), the recommended treatment is a respiratory fluoroquinolone (moxifloxacin, gemifloxacin, or levofloxacin) or a macrolide plus a beta-lactam (high-dose amoxicillin and amoxicillin-clavulanate are preferred to cefpodoxime and cefuroxime).

In regions where there is a high incidence of macrolide-resistant S pneumoniae, initial therapy in patients with no comorbidities may include a respiratory fluoroquinolone or the combination of a beta-lactam added to a macrolide.

There are limited data to guide recommendations for duration of treatment. The decision should be influenced by the severity of illness, etiologic pathogen, response to therapy, other medical problems, and complications. Most experts recommend administering a minimum of 5 days of therapy and continuing antibiotics until the patient is afebrile for 48–72 hours.

B. Treatment of Hospitalized and ICU Patients

The most common etiologies of CAP in patients who require hospitalization but not intensive care are S pneumoniae, M pneumoniae, C pneumoniae, H influenza, Legionella species, and respiratory viruses. Some patients have aspiration as an immediate precipitant to the CAP without a specific bacterial etiology. First-line therapy in hospitalized patients is a respiratory fluoroquinolone (eg, moxifloxacin, gemifloxacin, or levofloxacin) or the combination of a macrolide (clarithromycin or azithromycin) plus a beta-lactam (cefotaxime, ceftriaxone, or ampicillin) (see Table 9–9).

Almost all patients admitted to a hospital for treatment of CAP receive intravenous antibiotics. However, no studies in hospitalized patients demonstrated superior outcomes with intravenous antibiotics compared with oral antibiotics, as long as patients were able to tolerate the oral therapy and

the medication was well absorbed. Duration of inpatient antibiotic treatment is the same as for outpatients.

The most common etiologies of CAP in patients who require admission to intensive care are S pneumoniae, Legionella species, H influenza, Enterobacteriaceae species, S aureus, and Pseudomonas species. First-line therapy in ICU patients with CAP is either azithromycin or a respiratory fluoroquinolone (moxifloxacin, gemifloxacin, or levofloxacin) combined with an antipneumococcal beta-lactam (cefotaxime, ceftriaxone, or ampicillin-sulbactam). In patients at risk for Pseudomonas infection, one of two following regimens can be used: an antipneumococcal, antipseudomonal beta-lactam (piperacillin-tazobactam, cefepime, imipenem, meropenem) plus ciprofloxacin or levofloxacin **or** the above antipneumococcal beta-lactam plus an aminoglycoside (gentamicin, tobramycin, amikacin) plus either azithromycin or a respiratory fluoroquinolone (moxifloxacin, gemifloxacin, or levofloxacin).

▶ Prevention

Pneumococcal vaccines have the potential to prevent or lessen the severity of pneumococcal infections in immunocompetent patients. Two pneumococcal vaccines for adults are available and approved for use in the United States: one containing capsular polysaccharide antigens of 23 common strains of S pneumoniae in use for many years (Pneumovax 23) and a conjugate vaccine containing 13 common strains approved for adult use in 2011 (Prevnar-13). Current recommendations are for sequential administration of the two vaccines in those age 65 years or older and in immunocompromised persons. Adults with chronic illness that increases the risk of CAP (see Chapter 30) should receive the 23-valent vaccine regardless of age. Immunocompromised patients and those at highest risk for fatal pneumococcal infections should receive a single revaccination of the 23-valent vaccine 6 years after the first vaccination regardless of age. Immunocompetent persons 65 years of age or older should receive a second dose of the 23-valent vaccine if the patient first received the vaccine 6 or more years previously and was under 65 years old at the time of first vaccination.

The seasonal influenza vaccine is effective in preventing severe disease due to influenza virus with a resulting positive impact on both primary influenza pneumonia and secondary bacterial pneumonias. The seasonal influenza vaccine is administered annually to persons at risk for complications of influenza infection (age 65 years or older, residents of long-term care facilities, patients with pulmonary or cardiovascular disorders, patients recently hospitalized with chronic metabolic disorders) as well as health care workers and others who are able to transmit influenza to high-risk patients.

Hospitalized patients who would benefit from pneumococcal and influenza vaccines should be vaccinated during hospitalization. The vaccines can be given simultaneously, and may be administered as soon as the patient has stabilized.

▶ When to Admit

Once a diagnosis of CAP is made, the first management decision is to determine the site of care: Is it safe to treat the patient at home or does he or she require hospital or intensive care admission? There are two widely used clinical prediction rules available to guide admission and triage decisions, the **Pneumonia Severity Index (PSI)** and the **CURB-65.**

A. Hospital Admission Decision

The PSI is a validated prediction model that uses 20 items from demographics, medical history, physical examination, laboratory results, and imaging to stratify patients into five risk groups. The PSI is weighted toward discrimination at low predicted mortality. In conjunction with clinical judgment, it facilitates safe decisions to treat CAP in the outpatient setting. An online PSI risk calculator is available at http://internalmedicine.osu.edu/pulmonary/cap/10849.cfm. The CURB-65 assesses five simple, independent predictors of increased mortality (**c**onfusion, **u**remia, **r**espiratory rate, **b**lood pressure, and age greater than **65**) to calculate a 30-day predicted mortality (http://www.mdcalc.com/curb-65-severity-score-community-acquired-pneumonia/). Compared with the PSI, the simpler CURB-65 is less discriminating at low mortality but excellent at identifying patients with high mortality who may benefit from ICU-level care. A modified version (CRB-65) dispenses with serum blood urea nitrogen and eliminates the need for laboratory testing. Both have the advantage of simplicity: Patients with zero CRB-65 predictors have a low predicted mortality (less than 1%) and usually do not need hospitalization; hospitalization should be considered for those with one or two predictors, since they have an increased risk of death; and urgent hospitalization (with consideration of ICU admission) is required for those with three or four predictors.

B. Intensive Care Unit Admission Decision

Expert opinion has defined major and minor criteria to identify patients at high risk for death. Major criteria are septic shock with need for vasopressor support and respiratory failure with need for mechanical ventilation. Minor criteria are respiratory rate 30 breaths or more per minute, hypoxemia (defined as Pao_2/Fio_2 250 or less), hypothermia (core temperature less than 36.0°C), hypotension requiring aggressive fluid resuscitation, confusion/disorientation, multilobar pulmonary opacities, leukopenia due to infection with WBC less than 4000/mcL (less than 4.0×10^9/L), thrombocytopenia with platelet count less than 100,000/mcL (less than 100×10^9/L), uremia with blood urea nitrogen 20 mg/dL or more (7.1 mmol/L or more), metabolic acidosis, or elevated lactate level. Either one major criterion or three or more minor criteria of illness severity generally require ICU-level care.

In addition to pneumonia-specific issues, good clinical practice always makes an admission decision in light of the whole patient. Additional factors suggesting need for inpatient hospitalization include the following:

- Exacerbations of underlying disease (eg, heart failure) that would benefit from hospitalization.

- Other medical or psychosocial needs (such as cognitive dysfunction, psychiatric disease, homelessness, drug abuse, lack of outpatient resources, or poor overall functional status).

- Failure of outpatient therapy, including inability to maintain oral intake and medications.

Moran GJ et al. Emergency management of community-acquired bacterial pneumonia: what is new since the 2007 Infectious Diseases Society of America/American Thoracic Society guidelines. Am J Emerg Med. 2013 Mar;31(3):602–12. [PMID: 23380120]

Musher DM et al. Community-acquired pneumonia. N Engl J Med. 2014 Oct 23;371(17):1619–28. [PMID: 25337751]

National Clinical Guideline Centre (UK). Pneumonia: diagnosis and management of community- and hospital-acquired pneumonia in adults. London: National Institute for Health and Care Excellence (UK); 2014 Dec. [PMID: 25520986]

Prina E et al. Community-acquired pneumonia. Lancet. 2015 Sep 12;386(9998):1097–108. [PMID: 26277247]

Siemieniuk RA et al. Corticosteroid therapy for patients hospitalized with community-acquired pneumonia: a systematic review and meta-analysis. Ann Intern Med. 2015 Oct 6; 163(7):519–28. [PMID: 26258555]

Wunderink RG et al. Clinical practice. Community-acquired pneumonia. N Engl J Med. 2014 Feb 6;370(6):543–51. [PMID: 24499212]

2. Nosocomial Pneumonia (Hospital-Acquired, Ventilator-Associated, and Health Care–Associated)

ESSENTIALS OF DIAGNOSIS

▶ **Hospital-acquired pneumonia (HAP)** occurs more than 48 hours after admission to the hospital or other health care facility and excludes any infection present at the time of admission.

▶ **Health care–associated pneumonia (HCAP)** occurs in community members whose extensive contact with healthcare has changed their risk for virulent and drug-resistant organisms.

▶ **Ventilator-associated pneumonia (VAP)** develops following endotracheal intubation and mechanical ventilation.

▶ At least two of the following: fever, leukocytosis, purulent sputum.

▶ New or progressive parenchymal opacity on chest radiograph.

▶ Especially common in patients requiring intensive care or mechanical ventilation.

 General Considerations

Hospitalized patients carry different flora with different resistance patterns than healthy patients in the community, and their health status may place them at higher risk for more severe infection. The diagnostic approach and antibiotic treatment of patients with hospital-acquired pneumonia (HAP) is, therefore, different from patients with CAP. Similarly, management of patients in whom pneumonia develops following endotracheal intubation and mechanical ventilation (ventilator-associated pneumonia or VAP)

should address issues specific to this group of patients. Some community members have extensive contact with the healthcare system and carry flora that more closely resemble hospitalized patients than healthy community residents. When pneumonia develops in these persons, the infection is referred to as health care–associated pneumonia (HCAP). Initial management and antibiotic therapy should be targeted to the common flora and specific risk factors for severe disease.

Considered together, these nosocomial pneumonias (HAP/VAP/HCAP) represent an important cause of morbidity and mortality despite widespread use of preventive measures, advances in diagnostic testing, and potent new antimicrobial agents. HAP is the second most common cause of infection among hospital inpatients and is the leading cause of death due to infection with mortality rates ranging from 20% to 50%. While a minority of cases occurs in ICU patients, the highest-risk patients are those in ICUs or who are being mechanically ventilated; these patients also experience higher morbidity and mortality from HAP. As management of more chronic illnesses shifts to the outpatient setting, more cases of HCAP are caused by unusual organisms, and there is a high frequency of drug resistance. Definitive identification of the infectious cause of a lower respiratory infection is rarely available on presentation, thus, rather than pathogen-directed antibiotic treatment, the choice of empiric therapy is informed by epidemiologic and patient data.

▶ Definition & Pathogenesis

HAP develops more than 48 hours after admission to the hospital and VAP develops in a mechanically ventilated patient more than 48 hours after endotracheal intubation. HCAP is defined as pneumonia that occurs in a non-hospitalized patient with extensive healthcare contact (Table 9–10).

Three factors distinguish nosocomial pneumonia from CAP: (1) different infectious causes; (2) different antibiotic susceptibility patterns, specifically, a higher incidence of

drug resistance; and (3) poorer underlying health status of patients putting them at risk for more severe infections. Since access to the lower respiratory tract occurs primarily through microaspiration, nosocomial pneumonia starts with a change in upper respiratory tract flora. Colonization of the pharynx and possibly the stomach with bacteria is the most important step in the pathogenesis of nosocomial pneumonia. Pharyngeal colonization is promoted by exogenous factors (eg, instrumentation of the upper airway with nasogastric and endotracheal tubes; contamination by dirty hands, equipment, and contaminated aerosols; and treatment with broad-spectrum antibiotics that promote the emergence of drug-resistant organisms) and patient factors (eg, malnutrition, advanced age, altered consciousness, swallowing disorders, and underlying pulmonary and systemic diseases). Within 48 hours of admission, 75% of seriously ill hospitalized patients have their upper airway colonized with organisms from the hospital environment.

Impaired cellular and mechanical defense mechanisms in the lungs of hospitalized patients raise the risk of infection after aspiration has occurred.

Gastric acid may play a role in protection against nosocomial pneumonias. Observational studies have suggested that elevation of gastric pH due to antacids, H_2-receptor antagonists, proton pump inhibitors (PPIs), or enteral feeding is associated with gastric microbial overgrowth, tracheobronchial colonization, and HAP/VAP. Sucralfate, a cytoprotective agent that does not alter gastric pH, is associated with a trend toward a lower incidence of VAP. The Infectious Diseases Society of America and other professional organizations recommend that acid-suppressive medications (H_2-receptor antagonists and PPIs) only be given to patients at high risk for stress gastritis.

The microbiology of the nosocomial pneumonias differs from CAP but is substantially the same among HAP, VAP, and HCAP (Table 9–11). The most common organisms responsible for HAP include *S aureus* (both methicillin-sensitive *S aureus* and MRSA), *P aeruginosa*, gram-negative rods, including non-extended spectrum beta-lactamase (non-ESBL)–producing and ESBL-producing (*Enterobacter* species, *K pneumoniae*, and *Escherichia coli*) organisms. VAP patients may be infected with *Acinetobacter species* and *Stenotrophomonas maltophilia*. HCAP patients may have common organisms (*S pneumoniae, H influenzae*) that are more likely to be

Table 9–10. Risk factors for health care–associated pneumonia.

- Antibiotic therapy in the preceding 90 days.
- Acute care hospitalization for at least 2 days in the preceding 90 days.
- Residence in a nursing home or extended care facility.
- Home infusion therapy, including chemotherapy, within the past 30 days.
- Long-term dialysis within the past 30 days.
- Home wound care.
- Family member with an infection involving a multiple drug-resistant pathogen.
- Immunosuppressive disease or immunosuppressive therapy.

Adapted with permission of the American Thoracic Society. Copyright © American Thoracic Society. American Thoracic Society, Infectious Diseases Society of America. Guidelines for the management of adults with hospital-acquired, ventilator-associated and healthcare-associated pneumonia. Am J Respir Crit Care Med. 2005;171(4):388-416. [PMID: 15699079]

Table 9–11. Organisms prevalent in nosocomial pneumonias.[1]

- *Streptococcus pneumonia*, often drug-resistant, in HCAP
- *Staphylococcus aureus*, methicillin-sensitive (MSSA)
- *S aureus*, methicillin-resistant (MRSA)
- Gram-negative rods, non-ESBL
- ESBL-producing gram-negative rods, including *Klebsiella pneumonia, Escherichia coli,* and *Enterobacter* species
- *Pseudomonas aeruginosa*
- *Acinetobacter* species

ESBL, extended-spectrum beta-lactamase.
[1]Nosocomial pneumonias include hospital-associated pneumonia (HAP), ventilator-associated pneumonia (VAP), and health care–associated pneumonia (HCAP).

drug-resistant, or flora that resemble HAP. Anaerobic organisms (bacteroides, anaerobic streptococci, fusobacterium) may also cause pneumonia in the hospitalized patient; when isolated, they are commonly part of a polymicrobial flora. Mycobacteria, fungi, chlamydiae, viruses, rickettsiae, and protozoal organisms are uncommon causes of nosocomial pneumonias.

► Clinical Findings

A. Symptoms and Signs

The symptoms and signs associated with nosocomial pneumonias are nonspecific; however, two or more clinical findings (fever, leukocytosis, purulent sputum) in the setting of a new or progressive pulmonary opacity on chest radiograph were approximately 70% sensitive and 75% specific for the diagnosis of VAP in one study. Other findings include those listed above for CAP.

The differential diagnosis of new lower respiratory tract symptoms and signs in hospitalized patients includes heart failure, atelectasis, aspiration, ARDS, pulmonary thromboembolism, pulmonary hemorrhage, and medication reactions.

B. Laboratory Findings

Diagnostic evaluation for suspected nosocomial pneumonia includes blood cultures from two different sites. Blood cultures can identify the pathogen in up to 20% of all patients with nosocomial pneumonias; positivity is associated with increased risk of complications and other sites of infection. Blood counts and clinical chemistry tests do not establish a specific diagnosis of HCAP; however, they help define the severity of illness and identify complications. The assessment of oxygenation by an arterial blood gas or pulse oximetry determination helps define the severity of illness and determines the need for assisted ventilation. Thoracentesis for pleural fluid analysis should be considered in patients with pleural effusions.

Examination of sputum is attended by the same disadvantages as in CAP. Gram stains and cultures of sputum are neither sensitive nor specific in the diagnosis of nosocomial pneumonias. The identification of a bacterial organism by culture of sputum does not prove that the organism is a lower respiratory tract pathogen. However, it can be used to help identify bacterial antibiotic sensitivity patterns and as a guide to adjusting empiric therapy.

C. Imaging

Radiographic findings in HAP/VAP are nonspecific and often confounded by other processes that led initially to hospitalization or ICU admission. (See CAP above.)

D. Special Examinations

Endotracheal aspiration using a sterile suction catheter and fiberoptic bronchoscopy with bronchoalveolar lavage or a protected specimen brush can be used to obtain lower respiratory tract secretions for analysis, most commonly in patients with VAP. Endotracheal aspiration cultures have significant negative predictive value but limited positive predictive value in the diagnosis of specific infectious causes of HAP/VAP. An invasive diagnostic approach using quantitative culture of bronchoalveolar lavage samples or protected specimen brush samples in patients in whom VAP is suspected leads to significantly less antibiotic use, earlier attenuation of organ dysfunction, and fewer deaths at 14 days.

► Treatment

Treatment of the nosocomial pneumonias, like treatment of CAP, is usually empiric (Table 9–12). Because of the high mortality rate, therapy should be started as soon as pneumonia is suspected. There is no consensus on the best regimens because this patient population is heterogeneous and local flora and resistance patterns must be taken into account.

After results of sputum, blood, and pleural fluid cultures are available, it may be possible to de-escalate initially broad therapy. Duration of antibiotic therapy should be individualized based on the pathogen, severity of illness, response to therapy, and comorbid conditions. Data from one large trial assessing treatment outcomes in VAP suggested that 8 days of antibiotics is as effective as 15 days, except in cases caused by *P aeruginosa*.

For expanded discussions of specific antibiotics, see Chapter 30.

Barbier F et al. Hospital-acquired pneumonia and ventilator-associated pneumonia: recent advances in epidemiology and management. Curr Opin Pulm Med. 2013 May;19(3):216–28. [PMID: 23524477]

Chalmers JD et al. Healthcare-associated pneumonia does not accurately identify potentially resistant pathogens: a systematic review and meta-analysis. Clin Infect Dis. 2014 Feb;58(3):330–9. Erratum in: Clin Infect Dis. 2015 Apr 1;60(7):1143. [PMID: 24270053]

Madaras-Kelly KJ et al. Guideline-based antibiotics and mortality in healthcare-associated pneumonia. J Gen Intern Med. 2012 Jul;27(7):845–52. [PMID: 22396110]

Quartin AA et al. A comparison of microbiology and demographics among patients with healthcare-associated, hospital-acquired, and ventilator-associated pneumonia: a retrospective analysis of 1184 patients from a large, international study. BMC Infect Dis. 2013 Nov 27;13:561. [PMID: 24279701]

Vallés J et al. Epidemiology, antibiotic therapy and clinical outcomes of healthcare-associated pneumonia in critically ill patients: a Spanish cohort study. Intensive Care Med. 2014 Apr; 40(4):572–81. [PMID: 24638939]

3. Anaerobic Pneumonia & Lung Abscess

ESSENTIALS OF DIAGNOSIS

► History of or predisposition to aspiration.

► Indolent symptoms, including fever, weight loss, and malaise.

► Poor dentition.

► Foul-smelling purulent sputum (in many patients).

► Infiltrate in dependent lung zone, with single or multiple areas of cavitation or pleural effusion.

Table 9–12. Recommended empiric antibiotics for nosocomial pneumonias.[1]

When there is low risk for multiple drug–resistant pathogens, use **one** of the following:
  Ceftriaxone, 1–2 g intravenously every 12–24 hours
  Gemifloxacin, 320 mg orally daily
  Moxifloxacin, 400 mg orally or intravenously daily
  Levofloxacin, 750 mg orally or intravenously daily
  Ciprofloxacin, 400 mg intravenously every 8–12 hours
  Ampicillin-sulbactam, 1.5–3 g intravenously every 6 hours
  Piperacillin-tazobactam 3.375–4.5 g intravenously every 6 hours
  Ertapenem, 1 g intravenously daily

When there is higher risk for multiple drug–resistant pathogens, use **one** agent from **each** of the following categories:
1. Antipseudomonal coverage
   a. Cefepime, 1–2 g intravenously twice a day *or* ceftazidime, 1–2 g intravenously every 8 hours
   b. Imipenem, 0.5–1 g intravenously every 6–8 hours *or* meropenem, 1 g intravenously every 8 hours
   c. Piperacillin-tazobactam, 3.375–4.5 g intravenously every 6 hours
   d. For penicillin-allergic patients, aztreonam, 1–2 g intravenously every 6–12 hours
2. A second antipseudomonal agent
   a. Levofloxacin, 750 mg intravenously daily *or* ciprofloxacin, 400 mg intravenously every 8–12 hours
   b. Intravenous gentamicin, tobramycin, amikacin, all weight-based dosing administered daily adjusted to appropriate trough levels
3. Coverage for MRSA if appropriate with either
   a. Intravenous vancomycin (interval dosing based on renal function to achieve serum trough concentration 15–20 mcg/mL) *or*
   b. Linezolid, 600 mg intravenously twice a day

[1]Nosocomial pneumonias includes hospital-acquired pneumonia (HAP), ventilator-associated pneumonia (VAP), and health care–associated pneumonia (HCAP).
MRSA, methicillin-resistant *Staphylococcus aureus*.
Modified with permission from the American Thoracic Society. Copyright © American Thoracic Society. American Thoracic Society, Infectious Diseases Society of America. Guidelines for the management of adults with hospital-acquired, ventilator-associated and healthcare-associated pneumonia. Am J Respir Crit Care Med. 2005;171(4):388–416. [PMID: 15699079]

General Considerations

Aspiration of small amounts of oropharyngeal secretions occurs during sleep in normal individuals but rarely causes disease. Sequelae of aspiration of larger amounts of material include nocturnal asthma, chemical pneumonitis, mechanical obstruction of airways by particulate matter, bronchiectasis, and pleuropulmonary infection. Individuals predisposed to disease induced by aspiration include those with depressed levels of consciousness due to drug or alcohol use, seizures, general anesthesia, or central nervous system disease; those with impaired deglutition due to esophageal disease or neurologic disorders; and those with tracheal or nasogastric tubes, which disrupt the mechanical defenses of the airways.

Periodontal disease and poor dental hygiene, which increase the number of anaerobic bacteria in aspirated material, are associated with a greater likelihood of anaerobic pleuropulmonary infection. Aspiration of infected oropharyngeal contents initially leads to pneumonia in dependent lung zones, such as the posterior segments of the upper lobes and superior and basilar segments of the lower lobes. Body position at the time of aspiration determines which lung zones are dependent. The onset of symptoms is insidious. By the time the patient seeks medical attention, necrotizing pneumonia, lung abscess, or empyema may be apparent.

In most cases of aspiration and necrotizing pneumonia, lung abscess, and empyema, multiple species of anaerobic bacteria are causing the infection. Most of the remaining cases are caused by infection with both anaerobic and aerobic bacteria. *Prevotella melaninogenica*, *Peptostreptococcus*, *Fusobacterium nucleatum*, and *Bacteroides* species are commonly isolated anaerobic bacteria.

Clinical Findings

A. Symptoms and Signs

Patients with anaerobic pleuropulmonary infection usually present with constitutional symptoms, such as fever, weight loss, and malaise. Cough with expectoration of foul-smelling purulent sputum suggests anaerobic infection, though the absence of productive cough does not rule out such an infection. Dentition is often poor. Patients are rarely edentulous; if so, an obstructing bronchial lesion is usually present.

B. Laboratory Findings

Expectorated sputum is inappropriate for culture of anaerobic organisms because of contaminating mouth flora. Representative material for culture can be obtained only by transthoracic aspiration, thoracentesis, or bronchoscopy with a protected brush. Transthoracic aspiration is rarely indicated, because drainage occurs via the bronchus and anaerobic pleuropulmonary infections usually respond well to empiric therapy.

C. Imaging

The different types of anaerobic pleuropulmonary infection are distinguished on the basis of their radiographic appearance. **Lung abscess** appears as a thick-walled solitary cavity surrounded by consolidation. An air-fluid level is usually present. Other causes of cavitary lung disease (tuberculosis, mycosis, cancer, infarction, granulomatosis with polyangiitis [formerly Wegener granulomatosis]) should be excluded. **Necrotizing pneumonia** is distinguished by multiple areas of cavitation within an area of consolidation. **Empyema** is characterized by the presence of purulent pleural fluid and may accompany either of the other two radiographic findings. Ultrasonography is of value in locating fluid and may also reveal pleural loculations.

► Treatment

Medications of choice are clindamycin (600 mg intravenously every 8 hours until improvement, then 300 mg orally every 6 hours) or amoxicillin-clavulanate (875 mg/ 125 mg orally every 12 hours). Penicillin (amoxicillin, 500 mg every 8 hours, or penicillin G, 1–2 million units intravenously every 4–6 hours) plus metronidazole (500 mg orally or intravenously every 8–12 hours) is another option. Penicillin alone is inadequate treatment for anaerobic pleuropulmonary infections because an increasing number of anaerobic organisms produce beta-lactamases, and up to 20% of patients do not respond to penicillins. Antibiotic therapy for anaerobic pneumonia should be continued until the chest radiograph improves, a process that may take a month or more; patients with lung abscesses should be treated until radiographic resolution of the abscess cavity is demonstrated. Anaerobic pleuropulmonary disease requires adequate drainage with tube thoracostomy for the treatment of empyema. Open pleural drainage is sometimes necessary because of the propensity of these infections to produce loculations in the pleural space.

Bartlett JG. Anaerobic bacterial infection of the lung. Anaerobe. 2012 Apr;18(2):235–9. [PMID: 22209937]
Desai H et al. Pulmonary emergencies: pneumonia, acute respiratory distress syndrome, lung abscess, and empyema. Med Clin North Am. 2012 Nov;96(6):1127–48. [PMID: 23102481]
DiBardino DM et al. Aspiration pneumonia: a review of modern trends. J Crit Care. 2015 Feb;30(1):40–8. [PMID: 25129577]

PULMONARY INFILTRATES IN THE IMMUNOCOMPROMISED HOST

Pulmonary infiltrates in immunocompromised patients (patients with HIV disease, absolute neutrophil counts less than 1000/mcL [less than 1.0×10^9/L], current or recent exposure to myelosuppressive or immunosuppressive medications, or those currently taking more than 5 mg/day of prednisone) may arise from infectious or noninfectious causes. Infection may be due to bacterial, mycobacterial, fungal, protozoal, helminthic, or viral pathogens. Noninfectious processes, such as pulmonary edema, alveolar hemorrhage, medication reactions, pulmonary thromboembolic disease, malignancy, and radiation pneumonitis may mimic infection.

Although almost any pathogen can cause pneumonia in an immunocompromised host, two clinical tools help the clinician narrow the differential diagnosis. The first is knowledge of the underlying immunologic defect. Specific immunologic defects are associated with particular infections. Defects in humoral immunity predispose to bacterial infections; defects in cellular immunity lead to infections with viruses, fungi, mycobacteria, and protozoa. Neutropenia and impaired granulocyte function predispose to infections from *S aureus*, *Aspergillus*, gram-negative bacilli, and *Candida*. Second, the time course of infection also provides clues to the etiology of pneumonia in immunocompromised patients. A fulminant pneumonia is often caused by bacterial infection, whereas an insidious pneumonia is more apt to be caused by viral, fungal, protozoal, or mycobacterial infection. Pneumonia occurring within 2–4 weeks after organ transplantation is usually bacterial, whereas several months or more after transplantation *P jirovecii*, viruses (eg, cytomegalovirus) and fungi (eg, *Aspergillus*) are encountered more often.

► Clinical Findings

Chest radiography is rarely helpful in narrowing the differential diagnosis. Examination of expectorated sputum for bacteria, fungi, mycobacteria, *Legionella*, and *P jirovecii* is important and may preclude the need for expensive, invasive diagnostic procedures. Sputum induction is often necessary for diagnosis. The sensitivity of induced sputum for detection of *P jirovecii* depends on institutional expertise, number of specimens analyzed, and detection methods.

Routine evaluation frequently fails to identify a causative organism. The clinician may begin empiric antimicrobial therapy before proceeding to invasive procedures, such as bronchoscopy, transthoracic needle aspiration, or open lung biopsy. The approach to management must be based on the severity of the pulmonary infection, the underlying disease, the risks of empiric therapy, and local expertise and experience with diagnostic procedures. Bronchoalveolar lavage using the flexible bronchoscope is a safe and effective method for obtaining representative pulmonary secretions for microbiologic studies. It involves less risk of bleeding and other complications than bronchial brushing and transbronchial biopsy. Bronchoalveolar lavage is especially suitable for the diagnosis of *P jirovecii* pneumonia in patients with AIDS when induced sputum analysis is negative. Surgical lung biopsy, now often performed by video-assisted thoracoscopy, provides the definitive option for diagnosis of pulmonary infiltrates in the immunocompromised host. However, a specific diagnosis is obtained in only about two-thirds of cases, and the information obtained may not affect the outcome.

Godbole G et al. Respiratory tract infections in the immunocompromised. Curr Opin Pulm Med. 2013 May;19(3):244–50. [PMID: 23508112]
Letourneau AR et al. Pneumonia in the immunocompromised host. Curr Opin Pulm Med. 2014 May;20(3):272–9. [PMID: 24626236]

PULMONARY TUBERCULOSIS

► General Considerations

Tuberculosis is one of the world's most widespread and deadly illnesses. *M tuberculosis*, the organism that causes tuberculosis infection and disease, infects one-third of the world's population. In 2013, there were 9 million new cases of tuberculosis worldwide with 1.5 million people dying of the disease. In the United States, an estimated 11 million people are infected with *M tuberculosis* and in 2013 there were 9582 active cases. By 2015, the number of cases of tuberculosis increased for the first time in 23 years in 29 US states, particularly in Texas, California, Florida, and New York. Tuberculosis occurs disproportionately among disadvantaged populations, such as the malnourished, homeless, and those living in overcrowded and substandard housing. There is an increased occurrence of tuberculosis among HIV-positive individuals.

Infection with *M tuberculosis* begins when a susceptible person inhales airborne droplet nuclei containing viable organisms. Tubercle bacilli that reach the alveoli are ingested by alveolar macrophages. Infection follows if the inoculum escapes alveolar macrophage microbicidal activity. Once infection is established, lymphatic and hematogenous dissemination of tuberculosis typically occurs before the development of an effective immune response. This stage of infection, **primary tuberculosis,** is usually clinically and radiographically silent. In most persons with intact cell-mediated immunity, T-cells and macrophages surround the organisms in granulomas that limit their multiplication and spread. The infection is contained but not eradicated, since viable organisms may lie dormant within granulomas for years to decades.

Individuals with **latent tuberculosis infection** do not have active disease and cannot transmit the organism to others. However, reactivation of disease may occur if the host's immune defenses are impaired. **Active tuberculosis will develop in approximately 6% of individuals with latent tuberculosis infection who are not given preventive therapy;** half of these cases occur in the 2 years following primary infection. Diverse conditions such as gastrectomy, silicosis, diabetes mellitus, and an impaired immune response (eg, HIV infection; therapy with corticosteroids, tumor necrosis factor inhibitors or other immunosuppressive drugs) are associated with an increased risk of reactivation.

In approximately 5% of cases, the immune response is inadequate to contain the primary infection and **progressive primary tuberculosis** develops, accompanied by both pulmonary and constitutional symptoms as described below. The clinical presentation does not definitively distinguish primary disease from reactivation of latent tuberculosis infection. Standard teaching has held that 90% of tuberculosis in adults represents activation of latent disease. However, DNA fingerprinting of the bacillus suggests that as many as one-third of new cases of tuberculosis in urban populations are primary infections resulting from person-to-person transmission.

The prevalence of drug-resistant strains is increasing worldwide; however, in the United States, the rate of drug-resistant isolates has fallen to less than 1%. Risk factors for drug resistance include immigration from countries with a high prevalence of drug-resistant tuberculosis, close and prolonged contact with individuals with drug-resistant tuberculosis, unsuccessful previous therapy, and nonadherence to treatment. Drug resistance may be single or multiple. **Drug-resistant tuberculosis** is resistant to one first-line antituberculous drug, either isoniazid or rifampin. **Multidrug-resistant tuberculosis** is resistant to isoniazid and rifampin, and possibly additional agents. **Extensively drug-resistant tuberculosis** is resistant to isoniazid, rifampin, fluoroquinolones, and either aminoglycosides or capreomycin or both. Outcomes of drug-resistant tuberculosis treatment are worse than when the isolate is drug-sensitive, but outcomes appear to vary with HIV status. In a review of extensively drug-resistant tuberculosis cases in the United States, mortality was 10% and 68% in HIV-negative and HIV-positive patients, respectively.

► Clinical Findings

A. Symptoms and Signs

The patient with pulmonary tuberculosis typically presents with slowly progressive constitutional symptoms of malaise, anorexia, weight loss, fever, and night sweats. Chronic cough is the most common pulmonary symptom. It may be dry at first but typically becomes productive of purulent sputum as the disease progresses. Blood-streaked sputum is common, but significant hemoptysis is rarely a presenting symptom; life-threatening hemoptysis may occur in advanced disease. Dyspnea is unusual unless there is extensive disease. Rarely, the patient is asymptomatic. On physical examination, the patient appears chronically ill and malnourished. On chest examination, there are no physical findings specific for tuberculosis infection. The examination may be normal or may reveal classic findings such as posttussive apical rales.

B. Laboratory Findings

Definitive diagnosis depends on recovery of *M tuberculosis* from cultures or identification of the organism by DNA or RNA amplification techniques. Three consecutive morning sputum specimens are advised. Fluorochrome staining with rhodamine-auramine of concentrated, digested sputum specimens is performed initially as a screening method, with confirmation by the Kinyoun or Ziehl-Neelsen stains. Demonstration of acid-fast bacilli on sputum smear does not establish a diagnosis of *M tuberculosis*, since nontuberculous mycobacteria may colonize the airways and are increasingly recognized to cause clinical illness in patients with underlying structural lung disease.

In patients thought to have tuberculosis who cannot produce satisfactory specimens or when the smear of the spontaneously expectorated sputum is negative for acid-fast bacilli, sputum induction with 3% hypertonic saline should be performed. Flexible bronchoscopy with bronchial washings has similar diagnostic yield to induced sputum; transbronchial lung biopsies do not significantly increase the diagnostic yield but may lead to earlier diagnosis by identifying tissue granulomas. Post-bronchoscopy expectorated sputum specimens should be collected. Early morning aspiration of gastric contents after an overnight fast is suitable only for culture and not for stained smear because nontuberculous mycobacteria may be present in the stomach in the absence of tuberculous infection. Positive blood cultures for *M tuberculosis* are uncommon in patients with normal CD4 cell counts, but the organism may be cultured from blood in up to 50% of HIV-seropositive patients with tuberculosis whose CD4 cell counts are less than 100/mcL (less than 0.1×10^9/L).

Traditional light-microscopic examination of stained sputum for acid-fast bacilli and culture of sputum specimens remain the mainstay of tuberculosis diagnosis. The slow rate of mycobacterial growth, the urgency to provide early, appropriate treatment to patients to improve their outcomes and limit community spread, and concerns about potential drug toxicities in patients treated empirically who do not have tuberculosis infection have fostered interest in rapid diagnostic techniques (Table 9–13). Molecular diagnostics offer multiple options and many advantages at significantly increased expense. Nucleic acid amplification testing not only detects *M tuberculosis* (NAAT-TB) but it also identifies resistance markers (NAAT-R). NAAT-TB can identify *M tuberculosis* within hours of sputum processing, allowing early isolation and treatment, but the negative predictive value is low in smear-negative patients. NAAT-R allows rapid identification of primary drug resistance and is indicated in the following patients: (1) those treated previously for tuberculosis, (2) those born (or who lived for more than 1 year) in a country with moderate tuberculosis incidence or a high incidence of multiple drug-resistant isolates, (3) contacts of patients with multidrug-resistant tuberculosis, or (4) those

Table 9–13. Essential laboratory tests for the detection of *Mycobacterium tuberculosis*.[1]

Test	Time to Result	Test Characteristics
Acid-fast bacilli light microscopy	1 day	Three morning specimens recommended. Combined sensitivity of 70% (54% for the first specimen, 11% for the second specimen, and 5% for the third specimen). First morning specimen increased yield by 12% compared to spot specimen.
Nucleic acid amplification test, detection (NAAT-TB)	1 day	Sensitivity/specificity high for smear-positive specimens, 85–97% for both, but sensitivity falls in smear-negative specimens to ~66%. Therefore, a positive NAAT in smear-negative patients with intermediate to high (> 30%) pretest probability of *M tuberculosis* infection is helpful while a negative NAAT is not. Should not be ordered in patients with low pretest probability of *M tuberculosis* infection.
Nucleic acid amplification test, resistance markers (NAAT-R)	1–2 days	Multiple assays for rifampin and isoniazid are available. Specificity uniformly high, > 98%. Sensitivity varies from about 84% to 96%, increases with multiple specimens. See text for indications for testing.
Mycobacterial growth detection Liquid (broth based) medium Solid (agar or egg based) medium	Up to 6–8 weeks Avg 10–14 days Avg 3–4 weeks	Liquid culture methods are more sensitive (~90% and 76%, respectively) with shorter time to detection but higher contamination with bacterial growth than solid culture methods. Specificity exceeds 99% for all methods.
Identification of *M tuberculosis* complex by DNA probe or high performance liquid chromatography	1 day[1]	May be useful in areas of low *M tuberculosis* incidence where nontuberculous mycobacteria are commonly isolated.
First-line drug susceptibility testing (liquid medium)	1–2 weeks[1]	Gold standard. Should be performed routinely on the initial isolate.
Second-line and novel compound drug susceptibility testing Liquid (broth based) medium Solid (agar or egg based) medium	1–2 weeks[1] 3–4 weeks[1]	

[1]Following detection of mycobacterial growth.
Adapted, with permission, from Diagnostic Standards and Classification of Tuberculosis in Adults and Children. This official statement of the American Thoracic Society and the Centers for Disease Control and Prevention was adopted by the ATS Board of Directors, July 1999. This statement was endorsed by the Council of the Infectious Disease Society of America, September 1999. Am J Respir Crit Care Med. 2000 Apr; 161(4 Pt 1):1376-95.

who are HIV seropositive. Clinical suspicion remains the critical factor in interpreting all these studies. Standard drug susceptibility testing of culture isolates is considered routine for the first isolate of *M tuberculosis*, when a treatment regimen is failing, and when sputum cultures remain positive after 2 months of therapy.

Needle biopsy of the pleura reveals granulomatous inflammation in approximately 60% of patients with pleural effusions caused by *M tuberculosis*. Pleural fluid cultures are positive for *M tuberculosis* in less than 23–58% of cases of pleural tuberculosis. Culture of three pleural biopsy specimens combined with microscopic examination of a pleural biopsy yields a diagnosis in up to 90% of patients with pleural tuberculosis. Tests for pleural fluid adenosine deaminase (approximately 90% sensitivity and specificity for pleural tuberculosis at levels greater than 70 units/L) and interferon-gamma (89% sensitivity, 97% specificity in a recent meta-analysis) can be extremely helpful diagnostic aids, particularly in making decisions to pursue invasive testing in complex cases.

C. Imaging

Contrary to traditional teaching, molecular analysis demonstrates that radiographic abnormalities in pulmonary tuberculosis do not distinguish primary disease from reactivation of latent tuberculosis (Figure 9–5). The only independent predictor of an atypical pattern on chest radiograph—that is, not associated with upper lobe or cavitary disease—is an impaired host immune response. In elderly patients, lower lobe infiltrates with or without pleural effusion are frequently encountered. Lower lung tuberculosis may masquerade as pneumonia or lung cancer. A "miliary" pattern (diffuse small nodular densities)

▲ **Figure 9–5. Pulmonary tuberculosis.** Chest CT scan showing biapical noncavitary consolidation consistent with pulmonary tuberculosis and associated right axillary lymphadenopathy.

can be seen with hematologic or lymphatic dissemination of the organism. Immunocompromised patients—particularly those with late-stage HIV infection—often display lower lung zone, diffuse, or miliary infiltrates; pleural effusions; and involvement of hilar, and, in particular, mediastinal lymph nodes.

Resolution of active tuberculosis leaves characteristic radiographic findings. Dense nodules in the pulmonary hila, with or without obvious calcification, upper lobe fibronodular scarring, and bronchiectasis with volume loss are common findings. Ghon (calcified primary focus) and Ranke (calcified primary focus and calcified hilar lymph node) complexes are seen in a minority of patients.

D. Special Examinations

Testing for latent tuberculosis infection is used to evaluate an asymptomatic person in whom *M tuberculosis* infection is suspected (eg, following contact exposure) or to establish the prevalence of tuberculosis infection in a population. Testing may be used in a person with symptoms of active tuberculosis, but a positive test does not distinguish between active and latent infection. Routine testing of individuals at low risk for tuberculosis is not recommended.

The traditional approach to testing for latent tuberculosis infection is the **tuberculin skin test.** The Mantoux test is the preferred method: 0.1 mL of purified protein derivative (PPD) containing 5 tuberculin units is injected intradermally on the volar surface of the forearm using a 27-gauge needle on a tuberculin syringe. The **transverse width in millimeters of induration** at the skin test site is measured after 48–72 hours. To optimize test performance, criteria for determining a positive reaction vary depending on the likelihood of infection. Table 9–14 summarizes the criteria established by the Centers for Disease Control and Prevention (CDC) for interpretation of the Mantoux tuberculin skin test. Sensitivity and specificity of the tuberculin skin test are high: 77% and 97%, respectively. Specificity falls to 59% in populations previously vaccinated with bacillus Calmette-Guérin (BCG, an attenuated form of *Mycobacterium bovis*). False-negative tuberculin skin test reactions may result from improper testing technique; concurrent infections, including fulminant tuberculosis; malnutrition; advanced age; immunologic disorders; malignancy; corticosteroid therapy; chronic kidney disease; and HIV infection. Some individuals with latent tuberculosis infection may have a negative tuberculin skin test when tested many years after exposure. **Anergy testing is not recommended for routine use to distinguish a true-negative result from anergy.** Poor anergy test standardization and lack of outcome data limit the evaluation of its effectiveness. Interpretation of the tuberculin skin test in persons who have previously received BCG vaccination is the same as in those who have not had BCG.

Interferon gamma release assays (including the QuantiFERON and T-SPOT tests) are in vitro assays of CD4+ T-cell–mediated interferon gamma release in response to stimulation by specific *M tuberculosis* antigens. The antigens are absent from all BCG strains and most nontuberculous mycobacteria; therefore, in whole blood, the specificity of interferon gamma release assays is superior to

Table 9–14. Classification of positive tuberculin skin test reactions.[1]

Induration Size	Group
≥ 5 mm	1. HIV-positive persons. 2. Recent contacts of individuals with active tuberculosis. 3. Persons with fibrotic changes on chest films suggestive of prior tuberculosis. 4. Patients with organ transplants and other immunosuppressed patients (receiving the equivalent of > 15 mg/day of prednisone for 1 month or more).
≥ 10 mm	1. Recent immigrants (< 5 years) from countries with a high prevalence of tuberculosis (eg, Asia, Africa, Latin America). 2. HIV-negative injection drug users. 3. Mycobacteriology laboratory personnel. 4. Residents of and employees[2] in the following high-risk congregate settings: correctional institutions; nursing homes and other long-term facilities for the elderly; hospitals and other health care facilities; residential facilities for AIDS patients; and homeless shelters. 5. Persons with the following medical conditions that increase the risk of tuberculosis: gastrectomy, ≥ 10% below ideal body weight, jejunoileal bypass, diabetes mellitus, silicosis, advanced chronic kidney disease, some hematologic disorders, (eg, leukemias, lymphomas), and other specific malignancies (eg, carcinoma of the head or neck and lung). 6. Children younger than 4 years or infants, children, and adolescents exposed to adults at high risk.
≥ 15 mm	1. Persons with no risk factors for tuberculosis.

[1]A tuberculin skin test reaction is considered positive if the transverse diameter of the *indurated* area reaches the size required for the specific group. All other reactions are considered negative.
[2]For persons who are otherwise at low risk and are tested at entry into employment, a reaction of greater than 15 mm induration is considered positive.
Data from Screening for tuberculosis and tuberculosis infection in high-risk populations: recommendations of the Advisory Council for the Elimination of Tuberculosis. MMWR Morb Mortal Wkly Rep 1995 Sep 8;44(RR-11):19–34. [PMID: 7565540]

the tuberculin skin test in BGC-vaccinated individuals. Sensitivity is comparable to the tuberculin skin test: 60–90% depending on the specific assay and study population. Sensitivity is reduced by HIV infection, particularly in patients with low CD4 counts. Specificity is high, greater than 95%. Potential advantages of interferon gamma release assay testing include fewer false-positive results from prior BCG vaccination, better discrimination of positive responses due to nontuberculous mycobacteria, and the requirement for only one patient contact (ie, no need for the patient to return to have the tuberculin skin test read 48–72 hours later). Disadvantages include the need for specialized laboratory equipment and personnel, and the substantially increased cost compared to the tuberculin skin test.

In endemic areas, interferon gamma release assays are no more sensitive than the tuberculin skin test in active tuberculosis (20–40% false-negative rate) and cannot distinguish active from latent disease. Interferon gamma release assays should not be used to exclude active tuberculosis.

Guidelines established by the CDC allow interferon gamma release assays to be used interchangeably with the tuberculin skin testing in the diagnosis of latent tuberculosis infection. Interferon gamma release assays are preferred in patients with prior BCG vaccination; the tuberculin skin test is preferred in children under 5 years old. Routine use of both tests is not recommended. In individuals with a positive tuberculin skin test but a low prior probability of latent tuberculosis infection and low risk for progression to active disease, the interferon gamma release assay may be helpful as a confirmatory test to exclude a false-positive tuberculin skin test.

▶ **Treatment**

A. General Measures

The goals of therapy are to eliminate all tubercle bacilli from an infected individual while avoiding the emergence of clinically significant drug resistance. The basic principles of antituberculous treatment are (1) to administer multiple medications to which the organisms are susceptible; (2) to add at least two new antituberculous agents to a regimen when treatment failure is suspected; (3) to provide the safest, most effective therapy in the shortest period of time; and (4) to ensure adherence to therapy.

All suspected and confirmed cases of tuberculosis should be reported promptly to local and state public health authorities. Public health departments will perform case investigations on sources and patient contacts to determine if other individuals with untreated, infectious tuberculosis are present in the community. They can identify infected contacts eligible for treatment of latent tuberculous infection and ensure that a plan for monitoring adherence to therapy is established for each patient with tuberculosis. Patients with tuberculosis should be treated by clinicians who are skilled in the management of this infection. Clinical expertise is especially important in cases of drug-resistant tuberculosis.

Nonadherence to antituberculous treatment is a major cause of treatment failure, continued transmission of tuberculosis, and the development of medication resistance. Adherence to treatment can be improved by providing detailed patient education about tuberculosis and its treatment in addition to a case manager who oversees all aspects of an individual patient's care. **Directly**

observed therapy (DOT), which requires that a health care worker physically observe the patient ingest antituberculous medications in the home, clinic, hospital, or elsewhere, also improves adherence to treatment. The importance of direct observation of therapy cannot be overemphasized. The CDC recommends DOT for all patients with drug-resistant tuberculosis and for those receiving intermittent (twice- or thrice-weekly) therapy.

Hospitalization for initial therapy of tuberculosis is not necessary for most patients. It should be considered if a patient is incapable of self-care or is likely to expose new, susceptible individuals to tuberculosis. Hospitalized patients with active disease require a private room with negative-pressure ventilation until tubercle bacilli are no longer found in their sputum ("smear-negative") on three consecutive smears taken on separate days.

Characteristics of antituberculous drugs are provided in Table 9–15. Additional treatment considerations can be found in Chapter 33. More complete information can be obtained from the CDC's Division of Tuberculosis Elimination Web site at http://www.cdc.gov/tb/.

B. Treatment of Tuberculosis in HIV-Negative Persons

Most patients with previously untreated pulmonary tuberculosis can be effectively treated with either a 6-month or a 9-month regimen, though the 6-month regimen is preferred. The initial phase of a 6-month regimen consists of 2 months of daily isoniazid, rifampin, pyrazinamide, and ethambutol. Once the isolate is determined to be isoniazid-sensitive, ethambutol may be discontinued. If the

Table 9–15. Characteristics of antituberculous medications.

Medication	Most Common Side Effects	Tests for Side Effects	Drug Interactions	Remarks
Isoniazid	Peripheral neuropathy, hepatitis, rash, mild CNS effects.	AST and ALT; neurologic examination.	Phenytoin (synergistic); disulfiram.	Bactericidal to both extracellular and intracellular organisms. Pyridoxine, 10 mg orally daily as prophylaxis for neuritis; 50–100 mg orally daily as treatment.
Rifampin	Hepatitis, fever, rash, flu-like illness, gastrointestinal upset, bleeding problems, kidney failure.	CBC, platelets, AST and ALT.	Rifampin inhibits the effect of oral contraceptives, quinidine, corticosteroids, warfarin, methadone, digoxin, oral hypoglycemics; aminosalicylic acid may interfere with absorption of rifampin. Significant interactions with protease inhibitors and nonnucleoside reverse transcriptase inhibitors.	Bactericidal to all populations of organisms. Colors urine and other body secretions orange. Discoloring of contact lenses.
Rifapentine	Bone marrow suppression, hematuria/pyuria, hepatitis, gastrointestinal upset, flu-like illness.	CBC, platelets, AST and ALT.	Strong cytochrome P450 inducer with multiple drug interactions. Use in HIV patients receiving antiretroviral therapy should be limited to experts in antiretroviral therapy.	Bactericidal to both extracellular and intracellular organisms. Colors urine and other body secretions orange. Long half-life, can be administered weekly in LTBI prophylaxis. Not for use in induction phase of therapy.
Pyrazinamide	Hyperuricemia, hepatotoxicity, rash, gastrointestinal upset, joint aches.	Uric acid, AST, ALT.	Rare.	Bactericidal to intracellular organisms.
Ethambutol	Optic neuritis (reversible with discontinuance of drug; rare at 15 mg/kg); rash.	Red-green color discrimination and visual acuity.	Rare.	Bacteriostatic to both intracellular and extracellular organisms. Mainly used to inhibit development of resistant mutants. Use with caution in kidney disease or when ophthalmologic testing is not feasible.
Streptomycin	Eighth nerve damage, nephrotoxicity.	Vestibular function (audiograms); BUN and creatinine.	Neuromuscular blocking agents may be potentiated and cause prolonged paralysis.	Bactericidal to extracellular organisms. Use with caution in older patients or those with kidney disease.

ALT, alanine aminotransferase; AST, aspartate aminotransferase; BUN, blood urea nitrogen; CBC, complete blood count; LTBI, latent tuberculosis infection.

M tuberculosis isolate is susceptible to isoniazid and rifampin, the second phase of therapy consists of isoniazid and rifampin for a minimum of 4 additional months, with treatment to extend at least 3 months beyond documentation of conversion of sputum cultures to negative for *M tuberculosis*. If DOT is used, medications may be given intermittently using one of three regimens: (1) Daily isoniazid, rifampin, pyrazinamide, and ethambutol for 2 months, followed by isoniazid and rifampin two or three times each week for 4 months if susceptibility to isoniazid and rifampin is demonstrated. (2) Daily isoniazid, rifampin, pyrazinamide, and ethambutol for 2 weeks, then administration of the same agents twice a week for 6 weeks followed by administration of isoniazid and rifampin twice each week for 4 months if susceptibility to isoniazid and rifampin is demonstrated. (3) Isoniazid, rifampin, pyrazinamide, and ethambutol three times a week for 6 months.

Patients who cannot or should not (eg, pregnant women) take pyrazinamide should receive daily isoniazid and rifampin along with ethambutol for 4–8 weeks. If susceptibility to isoniazid and rifampin is demonstrated or drug resistance is unlikely, ethambutol can be discontinued and isoniazid and rifampin may be given twice a week for a total of 9 months of therapy. If drug resistance is a concern, patients should receive isoniazid, rifampin, and ethambutol for 9 months. Patients with smear- and culture-negative disease (eg, pulmonary tuberculosis diagnosed on clinical grounds) and patients for whom drug susceptibility testing is not available can be treated with 6 months of isoniazid and rifampin combined with pyrazinamide for the first 2 months. This regimen assumes low prevalence of drug resistance. Previous guidelines have used streptomycin interchangeably with ethambutol. Increasing worldwide streptomycin resistance has made this medication less useful as empiric therapy.

When a twice-weekly or thrice-weekly regimen is used instead of a daily regimen, the dosages of isoniazid, pyrazinamide, and ethambutol or streptomycin must be increased. Recommended dosages for the initial treatment of tuberculosis are listed in Table 9–16. Fixed-dose combinations of isoniazid and rifampin (Rifamate) and of isoniazid, rifampin, and pyrazinamide (Rifater) are available to simplify treatment. Single tablets improve compliance but are more expensive than the individual medications purchased separately.

C. Treatment of Tuberculosis in HIV-Positive Persons

Management of tuberculosis is complex in patients with concomitant HIV disease. Experts in the management of both tuberculosis and HIV disease should be involved in the care of such patients. The CDC has published detailed recommendations for the treatment of tuberculosis in HIV-positive patients (http://www.cdc.gov/tb/topic/tbhiv-coinfection/default.htm).

The basic approach to HIV-positive patients with tuberculosis is similar to that detailed above for patients without HIV disease. Additional considerations in HIV-positive patients include: (1) longer duration of therapy and (2) drug interactions between rifamycin derivatives such as rifampin and rifabutin used to treat tuberculosis and some of the protease inhibitors and nonnucleoside reverse transcriptase inhibitors (NNRTIs) used to treat HIV (see http://www.cdc.gov/tb/topic/tbhivcoinfection/default.htm). DOT should be used for all HIV-positive tuberculosis patients. Pyridoxine (vitamin B_6), 25–50 mg orally each day, should be administered to all HIV-positive patients being treated with isoniazid to reduce central and peripheral nervous system side effects.

D. Treatment of Drug-Resistant Tuberculosis

Patients with drug-resistant *M tuberculosis* infection require careful supervision and management. Clinicians who are unfamiliar with the treatment of drug-resistant tuberculosis should seek expert advice. Tuberculosis resistant only to isoniazid can be successfully treated with a 6-month regimen of rifampin, pyrazinamide, and

Table 9–16. Recommended dosages for the initial treatment of tuberculosis.

Medication	Daily	Cost[1]	Twice a Week[2]	Cost[1]/wk	Three Times a Week[2]	Cost[1]/wk
Isoniazid	5 mg/kg Max: 300 mg/dose	$0.15/300 mg	15 mg/kg Max: 900 mg/dose	$0.90	15 mg/kg Max: 900 mg/dose	$1.35
Rifampin	10 mg/kg Max: 600 mg/dose	$4.02/600 mg	10 mg/kg Max: 600 mg/dose	$8.04	10 mg/kg Max: 600 mg/dose	$12.06
Pyrazinamide	18.2–26.3 mg/kg Max: 2 g/dose	$11.44/2 g	Weight-based dosing: see references below.[3]	—	Weight-based dosing: see references below.[3]	—
Ethambutol	14.5–21.1 mg/kg Max: 1.6 g/dose	$8.38/2.5 g	Weight-based dosing: see references below.[3]	—	Weight-based dosing: see references below.[3]	—

[1]Average wholesale price (AWP, for AB-rated generic when available) for quantity listed. Source: *Red Book Online, Truven Health Analytics* Information, http://www.micromedexsolutions.com, March 1,2016., *Inc*. AWP may not accurately represent the actual pharmacy cost because wide contractual variations exist among institutions.
[2]All intermittent dosing regimens should be used with directly observed therapy.
[3]American Thoracic Society; CDC; Infectious Diseases Society of America. Treatment of tuberculosis. MMWR Recomm Rep. 2003 Jun 20; 52(RR-11):1–77. Erratum in: MMWR Recomm Rep. 2005 Jan 7; 53(51):1203. Dosage error in article text. [PMID: 12836625] Also available at http://www.cdc.gov/tb/publications/guidelines/Treatment.htm

ethambutol or streptomycin or a 12-month regimen of rifampin and ethambutol. When isoniazid resistance is documented during a 9-month regimen without pyrazinamide, isoniazid should be discontinued. If ethambutol was part of the initial regimen, rifampin and ethambutol should be continued for a minimum of 12 months. If ethambutol was not part of the initial regimen, susceptibility tests should be repeated and two other medications to which the organism is susceptible should be added. Treatment of *M tuberculosis* isolates resistant to agents other than isoniazid and treatment of drug resistance in HIV-infected patients require expert consultation.

Multidrug-resistant tuberculosis and extensively drug-resistant tuberculosis call for an individualized daily DOT plan under the supervision of an experienced clinician. Treatment regimens are based on the patient's overall status and the results of susceptibility studies. Most drug-resistant isolates are resistant to at least isoniazid and rifampin and require a minimum of three drugs to which the organism is susceptible. These regimens are continued until culture conversion is documented, and then a two-drug regimen is continued for at least another 12 months. Some experts recommend at least 18–24 months of a three-drug regimen.

E. Treatment of Extrapulmonary Tuberculosis

In most cases, regimens that are effective for treating pulmonary tuberculosis are also effective for treating extrapulmonary disease. However, many experts recommend 9 months of therapy when miliary, meningeal, or bone and joint disease is present. Treatment of skeletal tuberculosis is enhanced by early surgical drainage and debridement of necrotic bone. Corticosteroid therapy has been shown to help prevent constrictive pericarditis from tuberculous pericarditis and to reduce neurologic complications from tuberculous meningitis (Chapter 33).

F. Treatment of Pregnant or Lactating Women

Tuberculosis in pregnancy is usually treated with isoniazid, rifampin, and ethambutol for 2 months, followed by isoniazid and rifampin for an additional 7 months. Ethambutol can be stopped after the first month if isoniazid and rifampin susceptibility is confirmed. Since the risk of teratogenicity with pyrazinamide has not been clearly defined, pyrazinamide should be used only if resistance to other drugs is documented and susceptibility to pyrazinamide is likely. Streptomycin is contraindicated in pregnancy because it may cause congenital deafness. Pregnant women taking isoniazid should receive pyridoxine (vitamin B_6), 10–25 mg orally once a day, to prevent peripheral neuropathy.

Small concentrations of antituberculous drugs are present in breast milk. First-line therapy is not known to be harmful to nursing newborns at these concentrations. Therefore, breastfeeding is not contraindicated while receiving first-line antituberculous therapy. Lactating women receiving other agents should consult a tuberculosis expert.

G. Treatment Monitoring

Adults should have measurements of a complete blood count (including platelets) and serum bilirubin, hepatic enzymes, urea nitrogen, and creatinine before starting therapy for tuberculosis. Visual acuity and red-green color vision tests are recommended before initiation of ethambutol and serum uric acid before starting pyrazinamide. Audiometry should be performed if streptomycin therapy is initiated.

Routine monitoring of laboratory tests for evidence of medication toxicity during therapy is not recommended, unless baseline results are abnormal or liver disease is suspected. Monthly questioning for symptoms of medication toxicity is advised. Patients should be educated about common side effects of antituberculous medications and instructed to seek medical attention should these symptoms occur. Monthly follow-up of outpatients is recommended, including sputum smear and culture for *M tuberculosis*, until cultures convert to negative. Patients with negative sputum cultures after 2 months of treatment should have at least one additional sputum smear and culture performed at the end of therapy. Patients with drug-resistant isolates should have sputum cultures performed monthly during the entire course of treatment. A chest radiograph at the end of therapy provides a useful baseline for any future films.

Patients whose cultures do not become negative or whose symptoms do not resolve despite 3 months of therapy should be evaluated for nonadherence to the regimen and for drug-resistant organisms. DOT is required for the remainder of the treatment regimen, and the addition of at least two drugs not previously given should be considered pending repeat drug susceptibility testing. The clinician should seek expert assistance if drug resistance is newly found, if the patient remains symptomatic, or if smears or cultures remain positive.

Patients with only a clinical diagnosis of pulmonary tuberculosis (smears and cultures negative for *M tuberculosis*) whose symptoms and radiographic abnormalities are unchanged after 3 months of treatment usually either have another process or have had tuberculosis in the past.

H. Treatment of Latent Tuberculosis

Treatment of latent tuberculous infection is essential to controlling and eliminating tuberculosis. Treatment of latent tuberculous infection substantially reduces the risk that infection will progress to active disease. Targeted testing with the tuberculin skin test or interferon gamma release assays is used to identify persons who are at high risk for tuberculosis and who stand to benefit from treatment of latent infection. Table 9–14 gives the tuberculin skin test criteria for treatment of latent tuberculous infection. In general, patients with a positive tuberculin skin test or interferon gamma release assay who are at increased risk for exposure or disease are treated. It is essential that each person who meets the criteria for treatment of latent tuberculous infection undergo a careful assessment to exclude active disease. A history of past treatment for tuberculosis and contraindications to treatment should be sought. All patients at risk for HIV infection should be tested for HIV. Patients suspected of having tuberculosis should receive one of the recommended multidrug regimens for active disease until the diagnosis is confirmed or excluded.

Some close contacts of persons with active tuberculosis should be evaluated for treatment of latent tuberculous infection despite a negative tuberculin skin test reaction (less than 5 mm induration). These include immunosuppressed persons and those who may develop disease quickly after tuberculous infection. Close contacts who have a negative tuberculin skin test reaction on initial testing should be retested 10–12 weeks later.

Several treatment regimens for both HIV-negative and HIV-positive persons are available for the treatment of latent tuberculous infection: (1) **Isoniazid:** A 9-month oral regimen (minimum of 270 doses administered within 12 months) is preferable to 6 months of therapy. Dosing options include a daily dose of 300 mg or twice-weekly doses of 15 mg/kg. Persons at risk for developing isoniazid-associated peripheral neuropathy (diabetes mellitus, uremia, malnutrition, alcoholism, HIV infection, pregnancy, seizure disorder) may be given supplemental pyridoxine (vitamin B_6), 10–50 mg/day. (2) **Isoniazid and rifampin:** A 3-month oral regimen of daily isoniazid (300 mg) and rifampin (600 mg). (3) **Isoniazid and rifapentine:** A 3-month oral regimen of once weekly isoniazid at 15 mg/kg and rifapentine at 15–30 mg/kg. (4) **Rifampin:** Patients who cannot tolerate isoniazid can be considered for a 4-month oral regimen of rifampin at 600 mg daily. HIV-positive patients receiving protease inhibitors or NNRTIs who are given rifampin or rifapentine require management by experts in both tuberculosis and HIV disease (see Treatment of Tuberculosis in HIV-Positive Persons, above).

Contacts of persons with isoniazid-resistant, rifampin-sensitive tuberculosis should receive a 2-month regimen of rifampin and pyrazinamide or a 4-month regimen of daily rifampin alone. Contacts of persons with drug-resistant tuberculosis should receive two drugs to which the infecting organism has demonstrated susceptibility. Contacts in whom the tuberculin skin test or interferon gamma release assay is negative and contacts who are HIV seronegative may be observed without treatment or treated for 6 months. HIV-positive contacts should be treated for 12 months. All contacts of persons with multidrug-resistant tuberculosis or extensively drug-resistant tuberculosis should have 2 years of follow-up regardless of treatment.

Persons with a positive tuberculin skin test (5 mm or more of induration) and fibrotic lesions suggestive of old tuberculosis on chest radiographs who have no evidence of active disease and no history of treatment for tuberculosis should receive 9 months of isoniazid or 4 months of rifampin (with or without isoniazid). Pregnant or breastfeeding women with latent tuberculosis should receive either daily or twice-weekly isoniazid with pyridoxine (vitamin B_6).

Baseline laboratory testing is indicated for patients at risk for liver disease, patients with HIV infection, women who are pregnant or within 3 months of delivery, and persons who use alcohol regularly. Patients receiving treatment for latent tuberculous infection should be evaluated once a month to assess for symptoms and signs of active tuberculosis and hepatitis and for adherence to their treatment regimen. Routine laboratory testing during treatment is indicated for those with abnormal baseline laboratory tests and for those at risk for developing liver disease.

Vaccine BCG is an antimycobacterial vaccine developed from an attenuated strain of *M bovis*. Millions of individuals worldwide have been vaccinated with BCG. However, it is not generally recommended in the United States because of the low prevalence of tuberculous infection, the vaccine's interference with the ability to determine latent tuberculous infection using tuberculin skin test reactivity, and its variable effectiveness in prophylaxis of pulmonary tuberculosis. BCG vaccination in the United States should only be undertaken after consultation with local health officials and tuberculosis experts. Vaccination of health care workers should be considered on an individual basis in settings in which a high percentage of tuberculosis patients are infected with strains resistant to both isoniazid and rifampin, in which transmission of such drug-resistant *M tuberculosis* and subsequent infection are likely, and in which comprehensive tuberculous infection-control precautions have been implemented but have not been successful. The BCG vaccine is contraindicated in persons with impaired immune responses due to disease or medications.

▶ Prognosis

Almost all properly treated immunocompetent patients with tuberculosis can be cured. Relapse rates are less than 5% with current regimens. The main cause of treatment failure is nonadherence to therapy.

Dorman SE et al; Tuberculosis Trials Consortium. Daily rifapentine for treatment of pulmonary tuberculosis. A randomized, dose-ranging trial. Am J Respir Crit Care Med. 2015 Feb 1; 191(3):333–43. Erratum in: Am J Respir Crit Care Med. 2015 May 15;191(10):1210. [PMID: 25489785]

Getahun H et al. Latent *Mycobacterium tuberculosis* infection. N Engl J Med. 2015 May 28;372(22):2127–35. [PMID: 26017823]

Horsburgh CR Jr et al. Treatment of tuberculosis. N Engl J Med. 2015 Nov 26;373(22):2149–60. [PMID: 26605929]

Punnoose AR et al. JAMA patient page. Tuberculosis. JAMA. 2013 Mar 6;309(9):938. [PMID: 23462792]

Salgame P et al. Latent tuberculosis infection—revisiting and revising concepts. Tuberculosis (Edinb). 2015 Jul;95(4):373–84. [PMID: 26038289]

Salinas JL et al. Leveling of tuberculosis incidence United States, 2013-2015. MMWR Morb Mortal WKLY Rep. 2016 March; 65(11): 273–8.

PULMONARY DISEASE CAUSED BY NONTUBERCULOUS MYCOBACTERIA

 ESSENTIALS OF DIAGNOSIS

- ▶ Chronic cough, sputum production, and fatigue; less commonly: malaise, dyspnea, fever, hemoptysis, and weight loss.
- ▶ Parenchymal opacities on chest radiograph, most often thin-walled cavities or multiple small nodules associated with bronchiectasis.
- ▶ Isolation of nontuberculous mycobacteria in a sputum culture.

General Considerations

Mycobacteria other than *M tuberculosis*—nontuberculous mycobacteria (NTM), sometimes referred to as "atypical" mycobacteria—are ubiquitous in water and soil and have been isolated from tap water. Marked geographic variability exists, both in the NTM species responsible for disease and in the prevalence of disease. These organisms are not considered communicable from person to person, have distinct laboratory characteristics, and are often resistant to most antituberculous medications (Chapter 33). Long-term epidemiologic data suggest that NTM disease has been increasing in the United States.

Definition & Pathogenesis

The diagnosis of lung disease caused by NTM is based on a combination of clinical, radiographic, and bacteriologic criteria and the exclusion of other diseases that can resemble the condition. Specific diagnostic criteria are discussed below. Complementary data are important for diagnosis because NTM organisms can reside in or colonize the airways without causing clinical disease.

Mycobacterium avium complex (MAC) is the most frequent cause of NTM pulmonary disease in humans in the United States. *Mycobacterium kansasii* is the next most frequent pulmonary pathogen. Other NTM causes of pulmonary disease include *Mycobacterium abscessus, Mycobacterium xenopi,* and *Mycobacterium malmoense;* the list of more unusual etiologic NTM species is long. Most NTM cause a chronic pulmonary infection that resembles tuberculosis but tends to progress more slowly. Disseminated disease is rare in immunocompetent hosts; however, disseminated MAC disease is common in patients with AIDS.

Clinical Findings

A. Symptoms and Signs

NTM infection among immunocompetent hosts frequently presents in one of three prototypical patterns: cavitary, upper lobe lesions in older male smokers that may mimic *M tuberculosis*; nodular bronchiectasis affecting the mid lung zones in middle-aged women with chronic cough; and hypersensitivity pneumonitis following environmental exposure. Most patients with NTM infection experience a chronic cough, sputum production, and fatigue. Less common symptoms include malaise, dyspnea, fever, hemoptysis, and weight loss. Symptoms from coexisting lung disease (COPD, bronchiectasis, previous mycobacterial disease, cystic fibrosis, and pneumoconiosis) may confound the evaluation. In patients with bronchiectasis, coinfection with NTM and *Aspergillus* is a negative prognostic factor. New or worsening infiltrates as well as adenopathy or pleural effusion (or both) are described in HIV-positive patients with NTM infection as part of the immune reconstitution inflammatory syndrome following institution of antiretroviral therapy.

B. Laboratory Findings

The diagnosis of NTM infection rests on recovery of the pathogen from cultures. **Sputum cultures positive for atypical mycobacteria do not prove infection because NTM may exist as saprophytes colonizing the airways or may be environmental contaminants.** Bronchial washings are considered to be more sensitive than expectorated sputum samples; however, their specificity for clinical disease is not known.

Bacteriologic criteria have been proposed based on studies of patients with cavitary disease with MAC or *M kansasii*. Diagnostic criteria in immunocompetent persons include the following: positive culture results from at least two separate expectorated sputum samples; or positive culture from at least one bronchial wash; or a positive culture from pleural fluid or any other normally sterile site. The diagnosis can also be established by demonstrating NTM cultured from a lung biopsy, bronchial wash, or sputum plus histopathologic changes, such as granulomatous inflammation in a lung biopsy. Rapid species identification of some NTM is possible using DNA probes or high-pressure liquid chromatography.

Diagnostic criteria are less stringent for patients with severe immunosuppression. HIV-infected patients may show significant MAC growth on culture of bronchial washings without clinical infection; therefore, HIV patients being evaluated for MAC infection must be considered individually.

Medication susceptibility testing on cultures of NTM is recommended for the following NTM: (1) *Mycobacterium avium intracellulare* to macrolides only (clarithromycin and azithromycin); (2) *M kansasii* to rifampin; and (3) rapid growers (such as *Mycobacterium fortuitum, Mycobacterium chelonae, and M abscessus*) to amikacin, doxycycline, imipenem, fluoroquinolones, clarithromycin, cefoxitin, and sulfonamides.

C. Imaging

Chest radiographic findings include infiltrates that are progressive or persist for at least 2 months, cavitary lesions, and multiple nodular densities. The cavities are often thin-walled and have less surrounding parenchymal infiltrate than is commonly seen with MTB infections. Evidence of contiguous spread and pleural involvement is often present. High-resolution CT of the chest may show multiple small nodules with or without multifocal bronchiectasis. Progression of pulmonary infiltrates during therapy or lack of radiographic improvement over time are poor prognostic signs and also raise concerns about secondary or alternative pulmonary processes. Clearing of pulmonary infiltrates due to NTM is slow.

Treatment

Establishing NTM infection does not mandate treatment in all cases, for two reasons. First, clinical disease may never develop in some patients, particularly asymptomatic patients with few organisms isolated from single specimens. Second, the spectrum of clinical disease severity is very wide; in patients with mild or slowly progressive symptoms, traditional chemotherapeutic regimens using a combination of agents may lead to drug-induced side effects worse than the disease itself.

Specific treatment regimens and responses to therapy vary with the species of NTM. HIV-seronegative patients with MAC pulmonary disease usually receive a combination of daily clarithromycin or azithromycin, rifampin or rifabutin, and ethambutol (Table 9–16). For patients with severe fibrocavitary disease, streptomycin or amikacin is added for the first 2 months. The optimal duration of treatment is unknown, but therapy should be continued for 12 months after sputum conversion. Medical treatment is initially successful in about two-thirds of cases, but relapses after treatment are common; long-term benefit is demonstrated in about half of all patients. Those who do not respond favorably generally have active but stable disease. Surgical resection is an alternative for the patient with progressive disease that responds poorly to chemotherapy; the success rate with surgical therapy is good. Disease caused by M kansasii responds well to drug therapy. A daily regimen of rifampin, isoniazid, and ethambutol for at least 18 months with a minimum of 12 months of negative cultures is usually successful. Rapidly growing mycobacteria (M abscessus, M fortuitum, M chelonae) are generally resistant to standard antituberculous therapy.

▶ When to Refer

Patients with rapidly growing mycobacteria infection should be referred for expert management.

Henkle E et al. Nontuberculous mycobacteria infections in immunosuppressed hosts. Clin Chest Med. 2015 Mar;36(1):91–9. [PMID: 25676522]

Honda JR et al. Pathogenesis and risk factors for nontuberculous mycobacterial lung disease. Clin Chest Med. 2015 Mar;36(1):1–11. [PMID: 25676515]

Johnson MM et al. Nontuberculous mycobacterial pulmonary infections. J Thorac Dis. 2014 Mar;6(3):210–20. [PMID: 24624285]

Mitchell JD. Surgical approach to pulmonary nontuberculous mycobacterial infections. Clin Chest Med. 2015 Mar;36(1):117–22. [PMID: 25676524]

Prevots DR et al. Epidemiology of human pulmonary infection with nontuberculous mycobacteria: a review. Clin Chest Med. 2015 Mar;36(1):13–34. [PMID: 25676516]

van Ingen J. Microbiological diagnosis of nontuberculous mycobacterial pulmonary disease. Clin Chest Med. 2015 Mar;36 (1):43–54. [PMID: 25676518]

Wu UI et al. Host susceptibility to non-tuberculous mycobacterial infections. Lancet Infect Dis. 2015 Aug;15(8):968–80. [PMID: 26049967]

▼ PULMONARY NEOPLASMS

See Chapter 39 for discussions of Lung Cancer, Secondary Lung Cancer, and Mesothelioma.

SCREENING FOR LUNG CANCER

Two large RCTs reported findings in 2011 that clarify the utility of lung cancer screening. The Prostate, Lung, Colorectal and Ovarian Randomized Trial (PLCO) randomized 154,901 adults (52% current or former smokers) between the ages of 55 and 74 years to receive either no screening or annual posterior-anterior chest radiographs for 4 consecutive years. The investigators monitored the participants after screening for an average of 12 years. Results showed no mortality benefit from four annual chest radiographs either in the whole cohort or in a subset of heavy smokers who met the entry criteria for the other major trial, the National Lung Screening Trial (NLST). The NLST enrolled 53,454 current or former smokers (minimum 30-pack year exposure history) between the ages of 55 and 74 years who were randomly assigned to one of two screening modalities: three annual posterior-anterior chest radiographs or three annual low-dose chest CT scans. They were monitored for an additional 6.5 years after screening. Compared with chest radiography, low-dose chest CT detected more early-stage lung cancers and fewer advanced-stage lung cancers, indicating that CT screening systematically shifted the time of diagnosis to earlier stages, thereby providing more persons the opportunity for effective treatment. Furthermore, compared with chest radiographs, the cohort that received three annual CT scans had a statistically significant mortality benefit, with reductions in both lung cancer deaths (20.0%) and all-cause mortality (6.7%). This is the first time that evidence from an RCT demonstrated that lung cancer screening reduces all-cause mortality.

Additional information from PLCO, the NLST, and multiple other ongoing randomized trials is available. Salient issues that temper enthusiasm for widespread screening at this time include the following: (1) Generalizability to community practice: NLST-participating institutions demonstrated a high level of expertise in imaging interpretation and diagnostic evaluation. Ninety-six percent of findings on CT were false positives but the vast majority of patients were monitored with serial imaging. Invasive diagnostic evaluations were uncommon and were associated with a low complication rate (1.4%). (2) Duration of screening: The rate of detection of new lung cancers did not fall with each subsequent annual screening over 3 years. Since each year lung cancers first become detectable during that screening interval, the optimal number of annual CT scans is unknown as is the optimal screening interval. (3) Overdiagnosis: After 6.4 years of post-screening observation, there were more lung cancers in the NLST CT cohort than the chest radiography cohort (1089 and 969, respectively). Since the groups were randomized and well matched, lung cancer incidence should have been identical. Therefore, 18.5% of the lung cancers detected by CT remained clinically silent and invisible on chest radiograph for 6.4 years. Many, perhaps most, of these lung cancers will never cause clinical disease and represent overdiagnosis. (4) Cost effectiveness: The number needed to screen with three annual chest CT scans to prevent one death from lung cancer was 320.

Clear evidence exists showing the benefit of screening with low-dose chest CT in high-risk individuals and, since late 2013, screening has been recommended by the US Preventive Services Task Force. There is no evidence of benefit in a mixed population screened with chest radiography.

Aberle DR et al; National Lung Screening Trial Research Team. Results of the two incidence screenings in the National Lung Screening Trial. N Engl J Med. 2013 Sep 5;369(10):920–31. [PMID: 24004119]

Humphrey LL et al. Screening for lung cancer with low-dose computed tomography: a systematic review to update the US Preventive Services Task Force Recommendation. Ann Intern Med. 2013 Sep 17;159(6):411–20. [PMID: 23897166]

Kovalchik SA et al. Targeting of low-dose CT screening according to the risk of lung-cancer death. N Engl J Med. 2013 Jul 18; 369(3):245–54. [PMID: 23863051]

Infante M et al; DANTE Study Group. Long-term follow-up results of the DANTE trial, a randomized study of lung cancer screening with spiral computed tomography. Am J Respir Crit Care Med. 2015 May 15;191(10):1166–75. [PMID: 25760561]

Moyer VA. Screening for Lung Cancer: U.S. Preventive Services Task Force Recommendation Statement. Ann Intern Med. 2014 Mar 4;160(5):330–8. [PMID: 24378917]

Patz EF Jr et al. Overdiagnosis in low-dose computed tomography screening for lung cancer. JAMA Intern Med. 2014 Feb 1; 174(2):269–74. [PMID: 24322569]

Tanoue LT et al. Lung cancer screening. Am J Respir Crit Care Med. 2015 Jan 1;191(1):19–33. [PMID: 25369325]

SOLITARY PULMONARY NODULE

A solitary pulmonary nodule, sometimes referred to as a "coin lesion," is a less-than-3-cm isolated, rounded opacity on chest imaging outlined by normal lung and not associated with infiltrate, atelectasis, or adenopathy. Most are asymptomatic and represent an unexpected finding on chest radiography or CT scanning. The finding is important because it carries a significant risk of malignancy. The frequency of malignancy in surgical series ranges from 10% to 68% depending on patient population. **Benign neoplasms,** such as hamartomas, account for less than 5% of solitary nodules. Most benign nodules are infectious granulomas.

The goals of evaluation are to identify and resect malignant tumors in patients who will benefit from resection while avoiding invasive procedures in benign disease. The task is to identify nodules with a sufficiently high probability of malignancy to warrant biopsy or resection or a sufficiently low probability of malignancy to justify observation.

Symptoms alone rarely establish the cause, but clinical and imaging data can be used to assess the probability of malignancy. Malignant nodules are rare in persons under age 30. Above age 30, the likelihood of malignancy increases with age. Smokers are at increased risk, and the likelihood of malignancy increases with the number of cigarettes smoked daily. Patients with a prior malignancy have a higher likelihood of having a malignant solitary nodule.

The first and most important step in the imaging evaluation is to review old imaging studies. Comparison with prior studies allows estimation of *doubling time*, which is an important marker for malignancy. Rapid progression (doubling time less than 30 days) suggests infection while long-term stability (doubling time greater than 465 days) suggests benignity. Certain radiographic features help in estimating the probability of malignancy. *Size* is correlated with malignancy. A study of solitary nodules identified by CT scan showed a 1% malignancy rate in those measuring 2–5 mm, 24% in 6–10 mm, 33% in 11–20 mm, and 80% in 21–45 mm. The appearance of a *smooth, well-defined edge*

is characteristic of a benign process. *Ill-defined margins* or a *lobular* appearance suggest malignancy. A high-resolution CT finding of *spiculated margins* and a *peripheral halo* are both highly associated with malignancy. *Calcification and its pattern* are also helpful clues. Benign lesions tend to have dense calcification in a central or laminated pattern. Malignant lesions are associated with sparser calcification that is typically stippled or eccentric. *Cavitary* lesions with thick (greater than 16 mm) walls are much more likely to be malignant. High-resolution CT offers better resolution of these characteristics than chest radiography and is more likely to detect lymphadenopathy or the presence of multiple lesions. Chest CT is indicated in any suspicious solitary pulmonary nodule.

▶ Treatment

Based on clinical and radiologic data, the clinician should assign a specific probability of malignancy to the lesion. The decision whether to recommend a biopsy or surgical excision depends on the interpretation of this probability in light of the patient's unique clinical situation. The probabilities in parentheses below represent guidelines only and should not be interpreted as prescriptive.

In the case of solitary pulmonary nodules, a continuous probability function may be grouped into three categories. In patients with a **low probability (less than 5%) of malignancy** (eg, age under 30, lesions stable for more than 2 years, characteristic pattern of benign calcification), watchful waiting is appropriate. Management consists of serial imaging studies (CT scans or chest radiographs) at intervals that identify growth suggestive of malignancy. Three-dimensional reconstruction of high-resolution CT images provides a more sensitive test for growth.

Patients with a **high probability (greater than 60%) of malignancy** should proceed directly to resection following staging, provided the surgical risk is acceptable. Biopsies rarely yield a specific benign diagnosis and are not indicated.

Optimal management of patients with an **intermediate probability of malignancy (5–60%)** remains controversial. The traditional approach is to obtain a diagnostic biopsy, either through transthoracic needle aspiration (TTNA) or bronchoscopy. Bronchoscopy yields a diagnosis in 10–80% of procedures depending on the size of the nodule and its location. In general, the bronchoscopic yield for nodules that are less than 2 cm and peripheral is low, although complications are generally rare. Newer bronchoscopic modalities, such as electromagnetic navigation and ultrathin bronchoscopy are being studied, although their impact upon diagnostic yield remains uncertain. TTNA has a higher diagnostic yield, reported to be between 50% and 97%. The yield is strongly operator-dependent, however, and is affected by the location and size of the lesion. Complications are higher than bronchoscopy, with pneumothorax occurring in up to 30% of patients, with up to one-third of these patients requiring placement of a chest tube.

Disappointing diagnostic yields and a high false-negative rate (up to 20–30% in TTNA) have prompted alternative approaches. **Positron emission tomography (PET)** detects increased glucose metabolism within malignant lesions with high sensitivity (85–97%) and specificity (70–85%). Many diagnostic algorithms have incorporated PET into the assessment of patients with inconclusive high-resolution CT findings. A positive PET increases the likelihood of malignancy, and a negative PET correctly excludes cancer in most cases. False-negative PET scans can occur with tumors with low metabolic activity (well-differentiated adenocarcinomas, carcinoids, and bronchioloalveolar tumors), and follow-up CT imaging is typically performed at discrete intervals to ensure absence of growth. PET has several drawbacks, however: resolution below 1 cm is poor, the test is expensive, and availability remains limited.

Sputum cytology is highly specific but lacks sensitivity. It is used in central lesions and in patients who are poor candidates for invasive diagnostic procedures.

Some centers recommend **video-assisted thoracoscopic surgery (VATS)** resection of all solitary pulmonary nodules with intermediate probability of malignancy. In some cases, the surgeon will remove the nodule and evaluate it in the operating room with frozen section. If the nodule is malignant, he or she will proceed to lobectomy and lymph node sampling, either thoracoscopically or through conversion to standard thoracotomy. This approach is less common when PET scanning is available.

All patients should be provided with an estimate of the likelihood of malignancy, and their preferences should be used to help guide diagnostic and therapeutic decisions. A strategy that recommends observation may not be preferred by a patient who desires a definitive diagnosis. Similarly, a surgical approach may not be agreeable to all patients unless the presence of cancer is definitive. Patient preferences should be elicited, and patients should be well informed regarding the specific risks and benefits associated with the recommended approach as well as the alternative strategies.

Alpert JB et al. Imaging the solitary pulmonary nodule. Clin Chest Med. 2015 Jun;36(2):161–78. [PMID: 26024598]

Álvarez Martínez CJ et al. Guideline on management of solitary pulmonary nodule. Arch Bronconeumol. 2014 Jul;50(7): 285–93. [PMID: 24630316]

Krochmal R et al. Diagnosis and management of pulmonary nodules. Expert Rev Respir Med. 2014 Dec;8(6):677–91. [PMID: 25152306]

RIGHT MIDDLE LOBE SYNDROME

Right middle lobe syndrome is recurrent or persistent atelectasis of the right middle lobe. This collapse is related to the relatively long length and narrow diameter of the right middle lobe bronchus and the oval ("fish mouth") opening to the lobe, in the setting of impaired collateral ventilation. Fiberoptic bronchoscopy or CT scan is often necessary to rule out obstructing tumor. Foreign body or other benign causes are common.

Gudbjartsson T et al. Middle lobe syndrome: a review of clinicopathological features, diagnosis and treatment. Respiration. 2012;84(1):80–6. [PMID: 22377566]

BRONCHIAL CARCINOID TUMORS

Carcinoid and bronchial gland tumors are sometimes termed "bronchial adenomas." This term should be avoided because it implies that the lesions are benign when, in fact, carcinoid tumors and bronchial gland carcinomas are low-grade malignant neoplasms.

Carcinoid tumors are about six times more common than bronchial gland carcinomas, and most of them occur as pedunculated or sessile growths in central bronchi. Men and women are equally affected. Most patients are under 60 years of age. Common symptoms of bronchial carcinoid tumors are hemoptysis, cough, focal wheezing, and recurrent pneumonia. Peripherally located bronchial carcinoid tumors are rare and present as asymptomatic solitary pulmonary nodules. **Carcinoid syndrome** (flushing, diarrhea, wheezing, hypotension) is rare. Fiberoptic bronchoscopy may reveal a pink or purple tumor in a central airway. These lesions have a well-vascularized stroma, and biopsy may be complicated by significant bleeding. CT scanning is helpful to localize the lesion and to follow its growth over time. Octreotide scintigraphy is also available for localization of these tumors.

Bronchial carcinoid tumors grow slowly and rarely metastasize. Complications involve bleeding and airway obstruction rather than invasion by tumor and metastases. Surgical excision of clinically symptomatic lesions is often necessary, and the prognosis is generally favorable. Most bronchial carcinoid tumors are resistant to radiation and chemotherapy (see Chapter 39).

Caplin ME et al; ENETS consensus conference participants. Pulmonary neuroendocrine (carcinoid) tumors: European Neuroendocrine Tumor Society expert consensus and recommendations for best practice for typical and atypical pulmonary carcinoids. Ann Oncol. 2015 Aug;26(8):1604–20. [PMID: 25646366]

Detterbeck FC. Clinical presentation and evaluation of neuroendocrine tumors of the lung. Thorac Surg Clin. 2014 Aug;24 (3):267–76. [PMID: 25065927]

Filosso PL et al; European Society of Thoracic Surgeons Lung Neuroendocrine Tumors Working-Group Steering Committee. Multidisciplinary management of advanced lung neuroendocrine tumors. J Thorac Dis. 2015 Apr;7(Suppl 2):S163–71. [PMID: 25984363]

Marquez-Medina D et al. Systemic therapy for pulmonary carcinoids. Lung Cancer. 2015 Nov;90(2):139–47. [PMID: 26371699]

MEDIASTINAL MASSES

Various developmental, neoplastic, infectious, traumatic, and cardiovascular disorders may cause masses that appear in the mediastinum on chest radiograph. A useful convention arbitrarily divides the mediastinum into three compartments—anterior, middle, and posterior—in order to classify mediastinal masses and assist in differential diagnosis. Specific mediastinal masses have a predilection for one or more of these compartments; most are located in the anterior or middle compartment. The differential diagnosis of an **anterior mediastinal mass** includes thymoma, teratoma, thyroid lesions, lymphoma, and mesenchymal tumors (lipoma, fibroma). The differential diagnosis of a **middle mediastinal mass** includes lymphadenopathy, pulmonary artery enlargement, aneurysm of the aorta or innominate artery, developmental cyst (bronchogenic, enteric, pleuropericardial), dilated azygous or hemiazygous vein, and foramen of Morgagni hernia. The differential diagnosis of a **posterior mediastinal mass** includes hiatal hernia, neurogenic tumor, meningocele, esophageal tumor, foramen of Bochdalek hernia, thoracic spine disease, and extramedullary hematopoiesis. The neurogenic tumor group includes neurilemmoma, neurofibroma, neurosarcoma, ganglioneuroma, and pheochromocytoma.

Symptoms and signs of mediastinal masses are nonspecific and are usually caused by the effects of the mass on surrounding structures. Insidious onset of retrosternal chest pain, dysphagia, or dyspnea is often an important clue to the presence of a mediastinal mass. In about half of cases, symptoms are absent, and the mass is detected on routine chest radiograph. Physical findings vary depending on the nature and location of the mass.

CT scanning is helpful in management; additional radiographic studies of benefit include barium swallow if esophageal disease is suspected, Doppler sonography or venography of brachiocephalic veins and the superior vena cava, and angiography. MRI is useful; its advantages include better delineation of hilar structures and distinction between vessels and masses. MRI also allows imaging in multiple planes, whereas CT permits only axial imaging. Tissue diagnosis is necessary if a neoplastic disorder is suspected. Treatment and prognosis depend on the underlying cause of the mediastinal mass.

Carter BW et al. Approaching the patient with an anterior mediastinal mass: a guide for clinicians. J Thorac Oncol. 2014 Sep;9(9 Suppl 2):S102–9. [PMID: 25396306]

Gubens MA. Treatment updates in advanced thymoma and thymic carcinoma. Curr Treat Options Oncol. 2012 Dec;13(4):527–34. [PMID: 22961051]

Mikhail M et al. Thymic neoplasms: a clinical update. Curr Oncol Rep. 2012 Aug;14(4):350–8. [PMID: 22639107]

Ruffini E et al. Management of thymic tumors: a European perspective. J Thorac Dis. 2014 May;6(Suppl 2):S228–37. [PMID: 24868441]

INTERSTITIAL LUNG DISEASE (DIFFUSE PARENCHYMAL LUNG DISEASE)

ESSENTIALS OF DIAGNOSIS

▶ Insidious onset of progressive dyspnea and nonproductive chronic cough; extrapulmonary findings may accompany specific diagnoses.

▶ Tachypnea, small lung volumes, bibasilar dry rales; digital clubbing and right heart failure with advanced disease.

▶ Chest radiographs with low lung volumes and patchy distribution of ground glass, reticular, nodular, reticulonodular, or cystic opacities.

▶ Reduced lung volumes, pulmonary diffusing capacity and 6-minute walk distance; hypoxemia with exercise.

Interstitial lung disease, or diffuse parenchymal lung disease, comprises a heterogeneous group of disorders that share common presentations (dyspnea), physical findings (late inspiratory crackles), and chest radiographs (septal thickening and reticulonodular changes).

The term "interstitial" is misleading since the pathologic process usually begins with injury to the alveolar epithelial or capillary endothelial cells (alveolitis). Persistent alveolitis may lead to obliteration of alveolar capillaries and reorganization of the lung parenchyma, accompanied by irreversible fibrosis. The process does not affect the airways proximal to the respiratory bronchioles. At least 180 disease entities may present as interstitial lung disease. Table 9–17 outlines a selected list of differential diagnoses of interstitial lung disease. **In most patients, no specific cause can be identified. In the remainder, medications and a variety of organic and inorganic dusts are the principal causes.** The history—particularly the occupational and medication history—may provide evidence of a specific cause.

The connective tissue diseases are a group of immunologically mediated inflammatory disorders including rheumatoid arthritis, systemic lupus erythematosus, scleroderma, polymyositis-dermatomyositis, Sjögren syndrome, and other overlap conditions. The presence of diffuse parenchymal lung disease in the setting of an established connective tissue disease is suggestive of the etiology. In some cases, lung disease precedes the more typical manifestations of the underlying connective tissue disease by months or years.

Known causes of interstitial lung disease are dealt with in their specific sections. The important idiopathic forms are discussed below.

DIFFUSE INTERSTITIAL PNEUMONIAS

ESSENTIALS OF DIAGNOSIS

▶ Important to identify specific fibrosing disorders.

▶ Idiopathic disease may require biopsy for diagnosis.

▶ Accurate diagnosis identifies patients most likely to benefit from therapy.

▶ General Considerations

The most common diagnosis among patients with diffuse interstitial lung disease is one of the interstitial pneumonias, including all the entities described in Table 9–18. Historically, a diagnosis of interstitial lung disease was based on clinical and radiographic criteria with only a small number of patients undergoing surgical lung biopsy. When biopsies were obtained, the common element of fibrosis led to the grouping together of several histologic patterns under the category of interstitial pneumonia or idiopathic pulmonary fibrosis (IPF). Distinct histopathologic features are now understood to represent different

Table 9–17. Differential diagnosis of interstitial lung disease.

Medication-related
Antiarrhythmic agents (amiodarone)
Antibacterial agents (nitrofurantoin, sulfonamides)
Antineoplastic agents (bleomycin, cyclophosphamide, methotrexate, nitrosoureas)
Antirheumatic agents (gold salts, penicillamine)
Phenytoin
Environmental and occupational (inhalation exposures)
Dust, inorganic (asbestos, silica, hard metals, beryllium)
Dust, organic (thermophilic actinomycetes, avian antigens, *Aspergillus* species)
Gases, fumes, and vapors (chlorine, isocyanates, paraquat, sulfur dioxide)
Ionizing radiation
Talc (injection drug users)
Infections
Fungus, disseminated (*Coccidioides immitis, Blastomyces dermatitidis, Histoplasma capsulatum*)
Mycobacteria, disseminated
Pneumocystis jirovecii
Viruses
Primary pulmonary disorders
Cryptogenic organizing pneumonia (COP)
Idiopathic interstitial pneumonia: Acute interstitial pneumonia, desquamative interstitial pneumonia, nonspecific interstitial pneumonia, usual interstitial pneumonia, respiratory bronchiolitis-associated interstitial lung disease
Pulmonary alveolar proteinosis
Systemic disorders
Acute respiratory distress syndrome
Amyloidosis
Ankylosing spondylitis
Autoimmune disease: Dermatomyositis, polymyositis, rheumatoid arthritis, systemic sclerosis (scleroderma), systemic lupus erythematosus
Chronic eosinophilic pneumonia
Goodpasture syndrome
Idiopathic pulmonary hemosiderosis
Inflammatory bowel disease
Langerhans cell histiocytosis (eosinophilic granuloma)
Lymphangitic spread of cancer (lymphangitic carcinomatosis)
Lymphangioleiomyomatosis
Pulmonary edema
Pulmonary venous hypertension, chronic
Sarcoidosis
Granulomatosis polyangiitis (formerly Wegener granulomatosis)

natural histories and responses to therapy (Table 9–18). Therefore, in the evaluation of patients with diffuse interstitial lung disease, clinicians should attempt to identify specific disorders.

Patients with diffuse interstitial pneumonia may have any of the histologic patterns described in Table 9–18. The first step in evaluation is to identify patients whose disease is truly *idiopathic*. As indicated in Table 9–17, most identifiable causes of diffuse interstitial pneumonia are infectious, medication-related, or environmental or occupational agents. Interstitial lung diseases associated with other medical conditions (pulmonary-renal syndromes, collagen-vascular disease) may be identified through a careful

medical history. Apart from acute interstitial pneumonia, the clinical presentations of the diffuse interstitial pneumonias are sufficiently similar to preclude a specific diagnosis. Chest radiographs and high-resolution CT scans are diagnostic in some patients. Ultimately, many patients with apparently idiopathic disease require surgical lung biopsy to make a definitive diagnosis. The importance of accurate diagnosis is twofold. First, it allows the clinician to provide accurate information about the cause and natural history of the illness. Second, accurate diagnosis helps distinguish patients most likely to benefit from therapy.

▶ **Clinical Findings**

A. Symptoms, Signs, and Imaging

The most common of the diffuse interstitial pneumonias is pulmonary fibrosis associated with the histopathologic pattern of **usual interstitial pneumonia (UIP).** When no associated cause is evident, this is **IPF.** A diagnosis of IPF/UIP can be made with 90% confidence in patients over 65 years of age who have (1) idiopathic disease by history and who demonstrate inspiratory crackles on physical examination; (2) restrictive physiology on pulmonary function testing; (3) characteristic radiographic evidence of progressive fibrosis over several years; and (4) diffuse, patchy fibrosis with pleural-based honeycombing on high-resolution CT scan (Figure 9–6). Such patients do not need surgical lung biopsy.

B. Special Studies

Three diagnostic techniques are in common use: bronchoalveolar lavage, transbronchial biopsy, and surgical lung biopsy, either through an open procedure or using VATS.

Bronchoalveolar lavage may provide a specific diagnosis in cases of infection, particularly with *P jirovecii* or mycobacteria, or when cytologic examination reveals the presence of malignant cells. The findings may be suggestive and sometimes diagnostic of eosinophilic pneumonia, Langerhans cell histiocytosis, or alveolar proteinosis. Analysis of the cellular constituents of lavage fluid may suggest a specific disease, but these findings are not diagnostic.

Transbronchial biopsy through the flexible bronchoscope is easily performed in most patients. The risks of pneumothorax (5%) and hemorrhage (1–10%) are low. However, the tissue specimens recovered are small, sampling error is common, and crush artifact may complicate diagnosis. Transbronchial biopsy can make a definitive diagnosis of sarcoidosis, lymphangitic spread of carcinoma, pulmonary alveolar proteinosis, miliary tuberculosis, and Langerhans cell histiocytosis. Note that the diagnosis of IPF cannot be confirmed on transbronchial lung biopsy since the histologic diagnosis requires a pattern of changes rather than a single pathognomonic finding. Transbronchial biopsy may exclude IPF by confirming a specific alternative diagnosis. Transbronchial biopsy also cannot establish a specific diagnosis of idiopathic interstitial pneumonia. These patients generally require surgical lung biopsy.

Surgical lung biopsy is the standard for diagnosis of diffuse interstitial lung disease. Two or three biopsies taken

Table 9–18. Idiopathic interstitial pneumonias.

Name and Clinical Presentation	Histopathology	Radiographic Pattern	Response to Therapy and Prognosis
Usual interstitial pneumonia (UIP) Age 55–60, slight male predominance. Insidious dry cough and dyspnea lasting months to years. Clubbing present at diagnosis in 25–50%. Diffuse fine late inspiratory crackles on lung auscultation. Restrictive ventilatory defect and reduced diffusing capacity on pulmonary function tests. ANA and RF positive in ~25% in the absence of documented collagen-vascular disease.	Patchy, temporally and geographically nonuniform distribution of fibrosis, honeycomb change, and normal lung. Type I pneumocytes are lost, and there is proliferation of alveolar type II cells. "Fibroblast foci" of actively proliferating fibroblasts and myofibroblasts. Inflammation is generally mild and consists of small lymphocytes. Intra-alveolar macrophage accumulation is present but is not a prominent feature.	Diminished lung volume. Increased linear or reticular bibasilar and subpleural opacities. Unilateral disease is rare. High-resolution CT scanning shows minimal ground-glass and variable honeycomb change. Areas of normal lung may be adjacent to areas of advanced fibrosis. Between 2% and 10% have normal chest radiographs and high-resolution CT scans on diagnosis.	No randomized study has demonstrated improved survival compared with untreated patients. Inexorably progressive. Median survival approximately 3 years, depending on stage at presentation. Nintedanib and pirfenidone reduce rate of decline in lung function.
Respiratory bronchiolitis-associated interstitial lung disease (RB-ILD)[1] Age 40–45. Presentation similar to that of UIP though in younger patients. Similar results on pulmonary function tests, but less severe abnormalities. Patients with respiratory bronchiolitis are invariably heavy smokers.	Increased numbers of macrophages evenly dispersed within the alveolar spaces. Rare fibroblast foci, little fibrosis, minimal honeycomb change. In RB-ILD the accumulation of macrophages is localized within the peribronchiolar air spaces; in DIP[1], it is diffuse. Alveolar architecture is preserved.	May be indistinguishable from UIP. More often presents with a nodular or reticulonodular pattern. Honeycombing rare. High-resolution CT more likely to reveal diffuse ground-glass opacities and upper lobe emphysema.	Spontaneous remission occurs in up to 20% of patients, so natural history unclear. Smoking cessation is essential. Prognosis clearly better than that of UIP: median survival greater than 10 years. Corticosteroids thought to be effective, but there are no randomized clinical trials to support this view.
Acute interstitial pneumonia (AIP) Clinically known as Hamman-Rich syndrome. Wide age range, many young patients. Acute onset of dyspnea followed by rapid development of respiratory failure. Half of patients report a viral syndrome preceding lung disease. Clinical course indistinguishable from that of idiopathic ARDS.	Pathologic changes reflect acute response to injury within days to weeks. Resembles organizing phase of diffuse alveolar damage. Fibrosis and minimal collagen deposition. May appear similar to UIP but more homogeneous and there is no honeycomb change—though this may appear if the process persists for more than a month in a patient on mechanical ventilation.	Diffuse bilateral airspace consolidation with areas of ground-glass attenuation on high-resolution CT scan.	Supportive care (mechanical ventilation) critical but effect of specific therapies unclear. High initial mortality: Fifty to 90 percent die within 2 months after diagnosis. Not progressive if patient survives. Lung function may return to normal or may be permanently impaired.
Nonspecific interstitial pneumonia (NSIP) Age 45–55. Slight female predominance. Similar to UIP but onset of cough and dyspnea over months, not years.	Nonspecific in that histopathology does not fit into better-established categories. Varying degrees of inflammation and fibrosis, patchy in distribution but uniform in time, suggesting response to single injury. Most have lymphocytic and plasma cell inflammation without fibrosis. Honeycombing present but scant. Some have advocated division into cellular and fibrotic subtypes.	May be indistinguishable from UIP. Most typical picture is bilateral areas of ground-glass attenuation and fibrosis on high-resolution CT. Honey combing is rare.	Treatment thought to be effective, but no prospective clinical studies have been published. Prognosis overall good but depends on the extent of fibrosis at diagnosis. Median survival greater than 10 years.
Cryptogenic organizing pneumonia (COP, formerly bronchiolitis obliterans organizing pneumonia [BOOP]) Typically age 50–60 but wide variation. Abrupt onset, frequently weeks to a few months following a flu-like illness. Dyspnea and dry cough prominent, but constitutional symptoms are common: fatigue, fever, and weight loss. Pulmonary function tests usually show restriction, but up to 25% show concomitant obstruction.	Included in the idiopathic interstitial pneumonias on clinical grounds. Buds of loose connective tissue (Masson bodies) and inflammatory cells fill alveoli and distal bronchioles.	Lung volumes normal. Chest radiograph typically shows interstitial and parenchymal disease with discrete, peripheral alveolar and ground-glass infiltrates. Nodular opacities common. High-resolution CT shows subpleural consolidation and bronchial wall thickening and dilation.	Rapid response to corticosteroids in two-thirds of patients. Long-term prognosis is generally good for those who respond. Relapses are common.

[1]Includes desquamative interstitial pneumonia (DIP).

ANA, antinuclear antibody; ARDS, acute respiratory distress syndrome; RF, rheumatoid factor; UIP, usual interstitial pneumonia.

▲ **Figure 9–6.** Idiopathic pulmonary fibrosis. CT scan of the lungs showing the typical radiographic pattern of idiopathic pulmonary fibrosis, with a predominantly basilar, peripheral pattern of traction bronchiectasis, reticulation, and early honeycombing.

from multiple sites in the same lung, including apparently normal tissue, may yield a specific diagnosis as well as prognostic information regarding the extent of fibrosis versus active inflammation. Patients under age 60 without a specific diagnosis generally should undergo surgical lung biopsy. In older and sicker patients, the risks and benefits must be weighed carefully for three reasons: (1) the morbidity of the procedure can be significant; (2) a definitive diagnosis may not be possible even with surgical lung biopsy; and (3) when a specific diagnosis is made, there may be no effective treatment. Empiric therapy or no treatment may be preferable to surgical lung biopsy in some patients.

▶ **Treatment**

Clinical experience suggests that patients with RB-ILD, nonspecific interstitial pneumonia (NSIP), or COP (Table 9–18) frequently respond to corticosteroids and should be given a trial of therapy—typically prednisone, 1–2 mg/kg/day for a minimum of 2 months. The same therapy is ineffective in patients with IPF. Since this therapy carries significant morbidity, experts do not recommend routine use of corticosteroids in patients with IPF. A number of antifibrotic (interferon gamma 1b) and immunomodulator/immunosuppressant (cyclosporine A, azathioprine, etanercept) agents have been investigated and are not recommended for the treatment of IPF, either in monotherapy or combination therapy. In 2014, two agents, nintedanib and pirfenidone, were approved for the treatment of IPF based on controlled trials showing a significant reduction in the rate of decline in lung function in the population studied. Neither agent improved survival or quality of life compared with no treatment, however. Both agents will cost approximately $100,000 per patient per year in the United States. The only definitive treatment for IPF is lung transplantation, with a 5-year survival rate estimated at 50%.

Hobbs S et al. The idiopathic interstitial pneumonias: an update and review. Radiol Clin North Am. 2014 Jan;52(1):105–20. [PMID: 24267713]
Loomis-King H et al. Pathogenesis, current treatments and future directions for idiopathic pulmonary fibrosis. Curr Opin Pharmacol. 2013 Jun;13(3):377–85. [PMID: 23602652]
Raghu G et al. An official ATS/ERS/JRS/ALAT statement: idiopathic pulmonary fibrosis: evidence-based guidelines for diagnosis and management. Am J Respir Crit Care Med. 2011 Mar 15;183(6):788–824. [PMID: 21471066]
Ryu JH et al. Idiopathic pulmonary fibrosis: evolving concepts. Mayo Clin Proc. 2014 Aug;89(8):1130–42. [PMID: 24867394]

SARCOIDOSIS

 ESSENTIALS OF DIAGNOSIS

▶ Symptoms related to the lung, skin, eyes, peripheral nerves, liver, kidney, heart, and other tissues.
▶ Demonstration of noncaseating granulomas in a biopsy specimen.
▶ Exclusion of other granulomatous disorders.

▶ **General Considerations**

Sarcoidosis is a systemic disease of unknown etiology characterized in about 90% of patients by granulomatous inflammation of the lung. The incidence is highest in North American blacks and northern European whites; among blacks, women are more frequently affected than men. Onset of disease is usually in the third or fourth decade.

▶ **Clinical Findings**

A. Symptoms and Signs

Patients may have malaise, fever, and dyspnea of insidious onset. Symptoms from skin involvement (erythema nodosum, lupus pernio [Figure 9–7]), iritis, peripheral neuropathy, arthritis (Chapter 20), or cardiomyopathy may also cause the patient to seek care. Some individuals are asymptomatic and come to medical attention after abnormal findings (typically bilateral hilar and right paratracheal lymphadenopathy) on chest radiographs. Physical findings are atypical of interstitial lung disease in that crackles are uncommon on chest examination. Other symptoms and findings may include parotid gland enlargement, hepatosplenomegaly, and lymphadenopathy.

B. Laboratory Findings

Laboratory tests may show leukopenia, an elevated erythrocyte sedimentation rate, and hypercalcemia (about 5% of patients) or hypercalciuria (20%). Angiotensin-converting enzyme (ACE) levels are elevated in 40–80% of patients

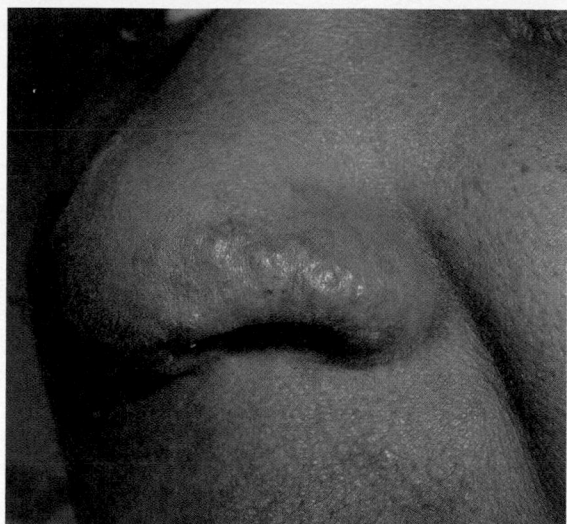

▲ **Figure 9-7.** Skin involvement in sarcoidosis (lupus pernio), here involving the nasal rim. (Used, with permission, from Richard P. Usatine, MD in Usatine RP, Smith MA, Mayeaux EJ Jr, Chumley H, Tysinger J. *The Color Atlas of Family Medicine.* McGraw-Hill, 2009.)

with active disease. This finding is neither sensitive nor specific enough to have diagnostic significance. Physiologic testing may reveal evidence of airflow obstruction, but restrictive changes with decreased lung volumes and diffusing capacity are more common. Skin test anergy is present in 70%. ECG may show conduction disturbances and dysrhythmias.

C. Imaging

Radiographic findings are variable and include bilateral hilar adenopathy alone (radiographic stage I), hilar adenopathy and parenchymal involvement (radiographic stage II), or parenchymal involvement alone (radiographic stage III). Parenchymal involvement is usually manifested radiographically by diffuse reticular infiltrates, but focal infiltrates, acinar shadows, nodules, and, rarely, cavitation may be seen. Pleural effusion is noted in less than 10% of patients. Stage IV disease refers to advanced fibrotic changes principally in the upper lobes.

D. Special Examinations

The diagnosis of sarcoidosis generally requires histologic demonstration of noncaseating granulomas in biopsies from a patient with other typical associated manifestations. Other granulomatous diseases (eg, berylliosis, tuberculosis, fungal infections) and lymphoma must be excluded. Biopsy of easily accessible sites (eg, palpable lymph nodes, skin lesions, or salivary glands) is likely to be positive. Transbronchial lung biopsy has a high yield (75–90%) as well, especially in patients with radiographic evidence of parenchymal involvement. Some clinicians believe that tissue biopsy is not necessary when stage I radiographic findings are detected in a clinical situation that strongly favors

the diagnosis of sarcoidosis (eg, a young black woman with erythema nodosum). Biopsy is essential whenever clinical and radiographic findings suggest the possibility of an alternative diagnosis, such as lymphoma. Bronchoalveolar lavage fluid in sarcoidosis is usually characterized by an increase in lymphocytes and a high CD4/CD8 cell ratio. Bronchoalveolar lavage does not establish a diagnosis but may be useful in following the activity of sarcoidosis in selected patients. All patients require a complete ophthalmologic evaluation.

▶ Treatment

Indications for treatment with oral corticosteroids (prednisone, 0.5–1.0 mg/kg/day) include disabling constitutional symptoms, hypercalcemia, iritis, uveitis, arthritis, central nervous system involvement, cardiac involvement, granulomatous hepatitis, cutaneous lesions other than erythema nodosum, and progressive pulmonary lesions. Long-term therapy is usually required over months to years. Immunosuppressive medications, most commonly methotrexate, azathioprine, or infliximab, are used in patients who are intolerant of corticosteroids or who have corticosteroid-refractory disease, but sound clinical research to support specific agents is lacking.

▶ Prognosis

The outlook is best for patients with hilar adenopathy alone; radiographic involvement of the lung parenchyma is associated with a worse prognosis. Erythema nodosum portends a good outcome. About 20% of patients with lung involvement suffer irreversible lung impairment, characterized by progressive fibrosis, bronchiectasis, and cavitation. Pneumothorax, hemoptysis, mycetoma formation in lung cavities, and respiratory failure often complicate this advanced stage. Myocardial sarcoidosis occurs in about 5% of patients, sometimes leading to restrictive cardiomyopathy, cardiac dysrhythmias, and conduction disturbances. Death from respiratory insufficiency occurs in about 5% of patients.

Patients require long-term follow-up: at a minimum, yearly physical examination, pulmonary function tests, chemistry panel, ophthalmologic evaluation, chest radiograph, and ECG.

Baughman RP et al. Medical therapy of sarcoidosis. Semin Respir Crit Care Med. 2014 Jun;35(3):391–406. [PMID: 25007090]

Baughman RP et al. New treatment strategies for pulmonary sarcoidosis: antimetabolites, biological drugs, and other treatment approaches. Lancet Respir Med. 2015 Oct;3(10):813–22. [PMID: 26204816]

Judson MA. Corticosteroids in sarcoidosis. Rheum Dis Clin North Am. 2016 Feb;42(1):119–35. [PMID: 26611555]

Valeyre D et al. Clinical presentation of sarcoidosis and diagnostic work-up. Semin Respir Crit Care Med. 2014 Jun;35(3): 336–51. [PMID: 25007086]

Valeyre D et al. Pulmonary sarcoidosis. Clin Chest Med. 2015 Dec;36(4):631–41. [PMID: 26593138]

Valeyre D et al. Sarcoidosis. Lancet. 2014 Mar 29;383(9923): 1155–67. [PMID: 24090799]

Wijsenbeek MS et al. Treatment of sarcoidosis. Clin Chest Med. 2015 Dec;36(4):751–67. [PMID: 26593147]

PULMONARY ALVEOLAR PROTEINOSIS

Pulmonary alveolar proteinosis is a rare disease in which phospholipids accumulate within alveolar spaces. The condition may be primary (idiopathic) or secondary (occurring in immunodeficiency; hematologic malignancies; inhalation of mineral dusts; or following lung infections, including tuberculosis and viral infections). Progressive dyspnea is the usual presenting symptom, and chest radiograph shows bilateral alveolar infiltrates suggestive of pulmonary edema. The diagnosis is based on demonstration of characteristic findings on bronchoalveolar lavage (milky appearance and PAS-positive lipoproteinaceous material) in association with typical clinical and radiographic features. In secondary disease, an elevated anti-GM-CSF titer in serum or bronchoalveolar lavage fluid is highly sensitive and specific. In some cases, transbronchial or surgical lung biopsy (revealing amorphous intra-alveolar phospholipid) is necessary.

The course of the disease varies. Some patients experience spontaneous remission; others develop progressive respiratory insufficiency. Pulmonary infection with *Nocardia* or fungi may occur. Therapy for alveolar proteinosis consists of periodic whole-lung lavage. Patients who cannot tolerate whole lung lavage or who fail to respond may benefit from inhalational or subcutaneous GM-CSF.

Ben-Dov I et al. Autoimmune pulmonary alveolar proteinosis: clinical course and diagnostic criteria. Autoimmun Rev. 2014 Apr–May;13(4–5):513–7. [PMID: 24424195]
Chaulagain CP et al. Secondary pulmonary alveolar proteinosis in hematologic malignancies. Hematol Oncol Stem Cell Ther. 2014 Dec;7(4):127–35. [PMID: 25300566]
Patel SM et al. Pulmonary alveolar proteinosis. Can Respir J. 2012 Jul–Aug;19(4):243–5. [PMID: 22891182]

EOSINOPHILIC PULMONARY SYNDROMES

Eosinophilic pulmonary syndromes are a diverse group of disorders typically characterized by eosinophilic pulmonary infiltrates, dyspnea, and cough. Many patients have constitutional symptoms, including fever. Common causes include exposure to medications (nitrofurantoin, phenytoin, ampicillin, acetaminophen, ranitidine) or infection with helminths (eg, *Ascaris*, hookworms, *Strongyloides*) or filariae (eg, *Wuchereria bancrofti, Brugia malayi*, tropical pulmonary eosinophilia). **Löffler syndrome** refers to acute eosinophilic pulmonary infiltrates in response to transpulmonary passage of helminth larvae. Pulmonary eosinophilia can also be a feature of other illnesses, including allergic bronchopulmonary mycosis, eosinophilic granulomatosis with polyangiitis, systemic hypereosinophilic syndromes, eosinophilic granuloma of the lung (properly referred to as pulmonary Langerhans cell histiocytosis), neoplasms, and numerous interstitial lung diseases. If an extrinsic cause is identified, therapy consists of removal of the offending medication or treatment of the underlying parasitic infection.

One-third of cases are idiopathic, and there are two common syndromes. **Chronic eosinophilic pneumonia** is seen predominantly in women and is characterized by fever, night sweats, weight loss, and dyspnea. Asthma is present in half of cases. Chest radiographs often show peripheral infiltrates, the "photographic negative" of pulmonary edema. Bronchoalveolar lavage typically has a marked eosinophilia; peripheral blood eosinophilia is present in greater than 80%. Therapy with oral prednisone (1 mg/kg/day for 1–2 weeks, followed by a gradual taper over many months) usually results in dramatic improvement; however, most patients require at least 10–15 mg of prednisone every other day for a year or more (sometimes indefinitely) to prevent relapses. **Acute eosinophilic pneumonia** is an acute, febrile illness characterized by cough and dyspnea, sometimes rapidly progressing to respiratory failure. The chest radiograph is abnormal but nonspecific. Bronchoalveolar lavage frequently shows eosinophilia but peripheral blood eosinophilia is rare at the onset of symptoms. The response to corticosteroids is usually dramatic.

Cottin V et al. Eosinophilic lung diseases. Immunol Allergy Clin North Am. 2012 Nov;32(4):557–86. [PMID: 23102066]
Rose DM et al. Primary eosinophilic lung diseases. Allergy Asthma Proc. 2013 Jan–Feb;34(1):19–25. [PMID: 23406932]

DISORDERS OF THE PULMONARY CIRCULATION

PULMONARY VENOUS THROMBOEMBOLISM

ESSENTIALS OF DIAGNOSIS

- ► Predisposition to venous thrombosis, usually of the lower extremities.
- ► One or more of the following: dyspnea, chest pain, hemoptysis, syncope.
- ► Tachypnea and a widened alveolar-arterial P_{O_2} difference.
- ► Elevated rapid D-dimer and characteristic defects on CT arteriogram of the chest, ventilation-perfusion lung scan, or pulmonary angiogram.

 General Considerations

Pulmonary venous thromboembolism, often referred to as pulmonary embolism (PE), is a common, serious, and potentially fatal complication of thrombus formation within the deep venous circulation. PE is the third leading cause of death among hospitalized patients. Despite this prevalence, most cases are not recognized antemortem, and less than 10% of patients with fatal emboli have received specific treatment for the condition. Management demands a vigilant systematic approach to diagnosis and an understanding of risk factors so that appropriate preventive therapy can be given.

Many substances can embolize to the pulmonary circulation, including air (during neurosurgery, from central venous catheters), amniotic fluid (during active labor), fat (long bone fractures), foreign bodies (talc in injection drug users), parasite eggs (schistosomiasis), septic emboli (acute infectious endocarditis), and tumor cells (renal cell carcinoma). The most common embolus is thrombus, which may arise anywhere in the venous circulation or heart but most often originates in the deep veins of the lower extremities. Thrombi confined to the calf rarely embolize to the pulmonary circulation. However, about 20% of calf vein thrombi propagate proximally to the popliteal and ileofemoral veins, at which point they may break off and embolize to the pulmonary circulation. Pulmonary emboli will develop in 50–60% of patients with proximal deep venous thrombosis (DVT); half of these embolic events will be asymptomatic. **Approximately 50–70% of patients who have symptomatic pulmonary emboli will have lower extremity DVT when evaluated.**

PE and DVT are two manifestations of the same disease. The risk factors for PE are the risk factors for thrombus formation within the venous circulation: venous stasis, injury to the vessel wall, and hypercoagulability (Virchow triad). Venous stasis increases with immobility (bed rest—especially postoperative—obesity, stroke), hyperviscosity (polycythemia), and increased central venous pressures (low cardiac output states, pregnancy). Vessels may be damaged by prior episodes of thrombosis, orthopedic surgery, or trauma. Hypercoagulability can be caused by medications (oral contraceptives, hormonal replacement therapy) or disease (malignancy, surgery) or may be the result of inherited gene defects. The most common inherited cause in white populations is resistance to activated protein C, also known as factor V Leiden. The trait is present in approximately 3% of healthy American men and in 20–40% of patients with idiopathic venous thrombosis. Other major risks for hypercoagulability include the following: deficiencies or dysfunction of protein C, protein S, and antithrombin; prothrombin gene mutation; hyperhomocysteinemia and the presence of antiphospholipid antibodies (lupus anticoagulant and anticardiolipin antibody).

PE has multiple physiologic effects. Physical obstruction of the vascular bed and vasoconstriction from neurohumoral reflexes both increase pulmonary vascular resistance. Massive thrombus may cause right ventricular failure. Vascular obstruction increases physiologic dead space (wasted ventilation) and leads to hypoxemia through right-to-left shunting, decreased cardiac output, and surfactant depletion causing atelectasis. Reflex bronchoconstriction promotes wheezing and increased work of breathing.

▶ Clinical Findings

A. Symptoms and Signs

The clinical diagnosis of PE is notoriously difficult for two reasons. First, the clinical findings depend on both the size of the embolus and the patient's preexisting cardiopulmonary status. Second, common symptoms and signs of pulmonary emboli are not specific to this disorder (Table 9–19).

Indeed, no single symptom or sign or combination of clinical findings is specific to PE. Some findings are fairly sensitive: dyspnea and pain on inspiration occur in 75–85% and 65–75% of patients, respectively. Tachypnea is the only sign reliably found in more than half of patients. A common clinical strategy is to use combinations of clinical findings to identify patients' risk for PE. For example, 97% of patients in the original Prospective Investigation of Pulmonary Embolism Diagnosis (PIOPED I) study with angiographically proved pulmonary emboli had one or more of three findings: dyspnea, chest pain with breathing, or tachypnea. Wells and colleagues have published and validated a simple clinical decision rule that quantifies and dichotomizes this clinical risk assessment, allowing diversion of patients deemed unlikely to have PE to a simpler diagnostic algorithm (see Integrated Approach to Diagnosis of Pulmonary Embolism).

B. Laboratory Findings

The **ECG** is abnormal in 70% of patients with PE. However, the most common abnormalities are sinus tachycardia and nonspecific ST and T wave changes, each seen in approximately 40% of patients. Five percent or less of patients in the PIOPED I study had P pulmonale, right ventricular hypertrophy, right axis deviation, and right bundle branch block.

Arterial blood gases usually reveal acute respiratory alkalosis due to hyperventilation. The arterial Po_2 and the alveolar-arterial oxygen difference ($A-a-Do_2$) are usually abnormal in patients with PE compared with healthy, age-matched controls. However, arterial blood gases are not diagnostic: among patients who were evaluated in the PIOPED I study, neither the Po_2 nor the $A-a-Do_2$ differentiated between those with and those without pulmonary emboli. Profound hypoxia with a normal chest radiograph in the absence of preexisting lung disease is highly suspicious for PE.

Plasma levels of **D-dimer,** a degradation product of cross-linked fibrin, are elevated in the presence of thrombus. Using a D-dimer threshold between 300 and 500 ng/mL (300 and 500 mcg/L), a rapid quantitative enzyme-linked immunosorbent assay (ELISA) has shown a sensitivity for venous thromboembolism of 95–97% and a specificity of 45%. Therefore, a D-dimer less than 500 ng/mL (less than 500 mcg/L) using a rapid quantitative ELISA provides strong evidence against venous thromboembolism, with a likelihood ratio of 0.11–0.13. Appropriate diagnostic thresholds have not been established for patients in whom D-dimer is elevated.

Serum troponin I, troponin T, and plasma B-type natriuretic peptide (BNP) levels are typically higher in patients with PE compared with those without embolism; the presence and magnitude of the elevation are not useful in diagnosis, but correlate with adverse outcomes, including mechanical ventilation, prolonged hospitalization, and death.

C. Imaging and Special Examinations

1. Chest radiography—The chest radiograph is necessary to exclude other common lung diseases and to permit interpretation of the ventilation-perfusion ($\dot{V}/\dot{Q}$) scan, but

Table 9–19. Frequency of specific symptoms and signs in patients at risk for pulmonary thromboembolism.

	UPET[1] PE+ (n = 327)	PIOPEDI[2] PE+ (n = 117)	PIOPEDI[2] PE– (n = 248)
Symptoms			
Dyspnea	84%	73%	72%
Respirophasic chest pain	74%	66%	59%
Cough	53%	37%	36%
Leg pain	NR	26%	24%
Hemoptysis	30%	13%	8%
Palpitations	NR	10%	18%
Wheezing	NR	9%	11%
Anginal pain	14%	4%	6%
Signs			
Respiratory rate ≥ 16 UPET, ≥ 20 PIOPED I	92%	70%	68%
Crackles (rales)	58%	51%	40%[3]
Heart rate ≥ 100/min	44%	30%	24%
Fourth heart sound (S_4)	NR	24%	13%[3]
Accentuated pulmonary component of second heart sound (S_2P)	53%	23%	13%[3]
T ≥ 37.5°C UPET, ≥ 38.5°C PIOPED	43%	7%	12%
Homans sign	NR	4%	2%
Pleural friction rub	NR	3%	2%
Third heart sound (S_3)	NR	3%	4%
Cyanosis	19%	1%	2%

[1]Data from the Urokinase-Streptokinase Pulmonary Embolism Trial (UPET), as reported in Bell WR et al. The clinical features of submassive and massive pulmonary emboli. Am J Med. 1977 Mar;62(3):355–60. [PMID: 842555]
[2]Data from patients enrolled in the PIOPED I study, as reported in Stein PD et al. Clinical, laboratory, roentgenographic, and electrocardiographic findings in patients with acute pulmonary embolism and no preexisting cardiac or pulmonary disease. Chest. 1991 Sep; 100(3): 598–603. [PMID: 1909617]
[3]$P < 0.05$ comparing patients in the PIOPED I study.
PE+, confirmed diagnosis of pulmonary embolism; PE–, diagnosis of pulmonary embolism ruled out; NR, not reported.

it does not establish the diagnosis by itself. The chest radiograph was normal in only 12% of patients with confirmed PE in the PIOPED I study. The most frequent findings were atelectasis, parenchymal infiltrates, and pleural effusions. However, the prevalence of these findings was the same in hospitalized patients without PE. A prominent central pulmonary artery with local oligemia (Westermark sign) or pleural-based areas of increased opacity that represent intraparenchymal hemorrhage (Hampton hump) are uncommon. Paradoxically, the chest radiograph may be most suggestive of PE when normal in the setting of hypoxemia.

2. CT—Helical CT pulmonary angiography is used as the initial diagnostic study in North America for suspected PE (Figure 9–8). Helical CT pulmonary angiography requires administration of intravenous radiocontrast dye but is otherwise noninvasive. A high-quality study is very sensitive for the detection of thrombus in the proximal pulmonary arteries but less so in more distal arteries where it may miss

as many as 75% of subsegmental defects, compared with pulmonary angiography. Comparing helical CT pulmonary angiography to the V̇/Q̇ scan as the initial test for PE, detection of thrombi is roughly comparable, although more alternative pulmonary diagnoses are made with CT scanning.

Test characteristics of helical CT pulmonary angiography vary widely by study and facility. Factors influencing results include patient size and cooperation, the type and quality of the scanner, the imaging protocol, and the experience of the interpreting radiologist. The 2006 PIOPED II study, using multidetector (four-row) helical CT and excluding the 6% of patients whose studies were "inconclusive," reported sensitivity of 83% and specificity of 96%.

A 15–20% false-negative rate is high for a screening test, and raises the practical question whether it is safe to withhold anticoagulation in patients with a negative helical CT. Research data provide two complementary answers. The insight of PIOPED I, that the clinical assessment of pretest probability improves the performance of the V̇/Q̇ scan, was

▲ **Figure 9–8.** Pulmonary emboli. Pulmonary CT angiogram demonstrating multiple segmental and subsegmental pulmonary emboli (arrows) in the right lung in a patient with a spontaneous upper extremity deep venous thrombosis.

confirmed with helical CT pulmonary angiography in PIOPED II, where positive and negative predictive values were highest in patients with concordant clinical assessments but poor with conflicting assessments. The negative predictive value of a normal helical CT in patients with a high pretest probability was only 60%. Therefore, a normal helical CT alone does not exclude PE in high-risk patients, and either empiric therapy or further testing is indicated.

A large, prospective trial, the Christopher Study, incorporated objective, validated pretest clinical assessment into diagnostic algorithms using D-dimer measurement. In this study, patients with a high pretest probability and a negative helical CT pulmonary angiogram who were not receiving anticoagulation had a low (less than 2%) 3-month incidence of subsequent PE. This low rate of complications supports the contention that many false-negative studies represent clinically insignificant, small distal thrombi and provides support for monitoring most patients with a high-quality negative helical CT pulmonary angiogram off therapy (see Integrated Approach to Diagnosis of Pulmonary Embolism below). The rate of false-positive helical CT pulmonary angiograms and overtreatment of PE has not been as well studied to date.

3. Ventilation-perfusion lung scanning—A perfusion scan is performed by injecting radiolabeled microaggregated albumin into the venous system, allowing the particles to embolize to the pulmonary capillary bed. To perform a ventilation scan, the patient breathes a radioactive gas or aerosol while the distribution of radioactivity in the lungs is recorded. A defect on perfusion scanning represents diminished blood flow to that region of the lung. This finding is not specific for PE. Defects in the perfusion scan are interpreted in conjunction with the ventilation

scan to give a high, low, or intermediate (indeterminate) probability that PE is the cause of the abnormalities. Criteria for the combined interpretation of ventilation and perfusion scans (commonly referred to as a single test, the $\dot{V}/\dot{Q}$ scan) are complex, confusing, and not completely standardized. A normal perfusion scan excludes the diagnosis of clinically significant PE (negative predictive value of 91% in the PIOPED I study). A high-probability $\dot{V}/\dot{Q}$ scan is most often defined as having two or more segmental perfusion defects in the presence of normal ventilation and is sufficient to make the diagnosis of PE in most instances (positive predictive value of 88% among PIOPED I patients). $\dot{V}/\dot{Q}$ scans are most helpful when they are either normal or indicate a high probability of PE. Such readings are reliable—interobserver agreement is best for normal and high-probability scans—and they carry predictive power. The likelihood ratios associated with normal and high-probability scans are 0.10 and 18, respectively, indicating significant and frequently conclusive changes from pretest to posttest probability.

However, 75% of PIOPED I $\dot{V}/\dot{Q}$ scans were nondiagnostic, ie, of low or intermediate probability. At angiography, these patients had an overall incidence of PE of 14% and 30%, respectively.

One of the most important findings of PIOPED I was that the clinical assessment of pretest probability could be used to aid the interpretation of the $\dot{V}/\dot{Q}$ scan. For patients with low-probability $\dot{V}/\dot{Q}$ scans and a low (20% or less) clinical pretest probability of PE, the diagnosis was confirmed in only 4%. Such patients may reasonably be observed off therapy without angiography. All other patients with nondiagnostic $\dot{V}/\dot{Q}$ scans require further testing to determine the presence of venous thromboembolism.

4. Venous thrombosis studies—Seventy percent of patients with PE will have DVT on evaluation, and approximately half of patients with DVT will have PE on angiography. Since the history and physical examination are neither sensitive nor specific for PE and since the results of $\dot{V}/\dot{Q}$ scanning are frequently equivocal, documentation of DVT in a patient with suspected PE establishes the need for treatment and may preclude further testing.

Commonly available diagnostic techniques include venous ultrasonography, impedance plethysmography, and contrast venography. In most centers, **venous ultrasonography** is the test of choice to detect proximal DVT. Inability to compress the common femoral or popliteal veins in symptomatic patients is diagnostic of first-episode DVT (positive predictive value of 97%); full compressibility of both sites excludes proximal DVT (negative predictive value of 98%). The test is less accurate in distal thrombi, recurrent thrombi, or in asymptomatic patients. Impedance plethysmography relies on changes in electrical impedance between patent and obstructed veins to determine the presence of thrombus. Accuracy is comparable though not quite as high as ultrasonography. Both ultrasonography and impedance plethysmography are useful in the serial examination of patients with high clinical suspicion of venous thromboembolism but negative leg studies. In patients with suspected first-episode DVT and a negative ultrasound or impedance plethysmography examination, multiple studies have confirmed the safety of withholding anticoagulation while conducting two sequential studies on days 1–3 and 7–10. Similarly, patients with nondiagnostic V̇/Q̇ scans and an initial negative venous ultrasound or impedance plethysmography examination may be monitored off therapy with serial leg studies over 2 weeks. When serial examinations are negative for proximal DVT, the risk of subsequent venous thromboembolism over the following 6 months is less than 2%.

Contrast venography remains the reference standard for the diagnosis of DVT. An intraluminal filling defect is diagnostic of venous thrombosis. However, venography has significant shortcomings and has been replaced by venous ultrasound as the diagnostic procedure of choice. Venography may be useful in complex situations where there is discrepancy between clinical suspicion and noninvasive testing.

5. Pulmonary angiography—Pulmonary angiography remains the reference standard for the diagnosis of PE. An intraluminal filling defect in more than one projection establishes a definitive diagnosis. Secondary findings highly suggestive of PE include abrupt arterial cutoff, asymmetry of blood flow—especially segmental oligemia—or a prolonged arterial phase with slow filling. Pulmonary angiography was performed in 755 patients in the PIOPED I study. A definitive diagnosis was established in 97%; in 3% the studies were nondiagnostic. Four patients (0.8%) with negative angiograms subsequently had pulmonary thromboemboli at autopsy. Serial angiography has demonstrated minimal resolution of thrombus prior to day 7 following presentation. Thus, negative angiography within 7 days of presentation excludes the diagnosis.

Pulmonary angiography is a safe but invasive procedure with well-defined morbidity and mortality data. Minor complications occur in approximately 5% of patients. Most are allergic contrast reactions, transient kidney injury, or percutaneous catheter–related injuries; cardiac perforation and arrhythmias are reported but rare. Among the PIOPED I patients who underwent angiography, there were five deaths (0.7%) directly related to the procedure.

The appropriate role of pulmonary angiography in the diagnosis of PE remains a subject of ongoing debate. There is wide agreement that angiography is indicated in any patient in whom the diagnosis is in doubt when there is a high clinical pretest probability of PE or when the diagnosis of PE must be established with certainty, as when anticoagulation is contraindicated or placement of an inferior vena cava filter is contemplated.

Integrated Approach to Diagnosis of Pulmonary Embolism

An integrated approach to the diagnosis of PE uses the clinical likelihood of venous thromboembolism derived from a clinical prediction rule (Table 9–20) along with the results of diagnostic tests to come to one of three decision points: to establish venous thromboembolism (PE or DVT) as the diagnosis, to exclude venous thromboembolism with sufficient confidence to follow the patient off anticoagulation, or to refer the patient for additional testing. An ideal diagnostic

Table 9–20. Clinical prediction rule for pulmonary embolism (PE).

Variable	Points
Clinical symptoms and signs of deep venous thrombosis (DVT) (leg swelling and pain with palpation of deep veins)	3.0
Alternative diagnosis less likely than PE	3.0
Heart rate > 100 beats/min	1.5
Immobilization for more than 3 days or surgery in previous 4 weeks	1.5
Previous PE or DVT	1.5
Hemoptysis	1.0
Cancer (with treatment within past 6 months or palliative care)	1.0
Three-tiered clinical probability assessment	**Score**
High	> 6.0
Moderate	2.0 to 6.0
Low	< 2.0
Dichotomous clinical probability assessment	**Score**
PE likely	> 4.0
PE unlikely	< or = 4.0

Data from Wells PS et al. Derivation of a simple clinical model to categorize patients' probability of pulmonary embolism: increasing the models' utility with the SimpliRED D-dimer. Thromb Haemost. 2000 Mar;83(3):416–20. [PMID: 10744147]

algorithm would proceed in a cost-effective, stepwise fashion to come to these decision points at minimal risk to the patient. Most North American centers use a rapid D-dimer and helical CT pulmonary angiography based diagnostic algorithm (Figure 9–9). The standard V̇/Q̇ scan based algorithm (Table 9–21) remains useful in many patients, especially those who are not able to undergo CT pulmonary angiography (eg, those with advanced chronic kidney disease). In the rigorously conducted Christopher Study, the incidence of venous thromboembolism was only 1.3% and fatal PE occurred in just 0.5% of persons monitored for 3 months off anticoagulation therapy after objective, validated tools for clinical assessment, quantitative rapid D-dimer assays and a negative helical CT pulmonary angiography. The incidence of PE following a negative evaluation by these three means is comparable to that seen following negative pulmonary angiography.

Prevention

Venous thromboembolism is often clinically silent until it presents with significant morbidity or mortality. It is a prevalent disease, clearly associated with identifiable risk factors. For example, the incidence of proximal DVT, PE, and fatal PE in untreated patients undergoing hip fracture surgery is reported to be 10–20%, 4–10%, and 0.2–5%,

▲ **Figure 9–9.** D-dimer and helical CT-PA based diagnostic algorithm for PE. CT-PA, CT pulmonary angiogram; PE, pulmonary embolism; ELISA, enzyme-linked immunosorbent assay; VTE, venous thromboembolic disease; LE US, lower extremity venous ultrasound for deep venous thrombosis; PA, pulmonary angiogram. (Reproduced, with permission, from van Belle A et al. Effectiveness of managing suspected pulmonary embolism using an algorithm combining clinical probability, D-dimer testing, and computed tomography. JAMA. 2006 Jan 11;295(2):172–9.)

Table 9–21. Pulmonary ventilation-perfusion scan based diagnostic algorithm for PE.

Clinical concern for PE:

1. Analyze by three-tiered clinical probability assessment (Table 9–20)

2. Obtain scan

3. Match results in the following table

	Clinical suspicion for PE by clinical probability assessment		
	HIGH	**MODERATE**	**LOW**
High Probability scan	STOP. Diagnosis established. Treat for PE.	STOP. Diagnosis established. Treat for PE.	Diagnosis likely (56% in PIOPED I, but small number of patients). Treat for PE or evaluate further with LE US or CT-PA.
Indeterminate Probability scan	Diagnosis highly likely (66% in PIOPED I). Treat for PE or evaluate further with LE US or CT-PA.	Uncertain diagnosis. Evaluate further with LE US or CT-PA.	Uncertain diagnosis. Evaluate further with LE US or CT-PA.
Low Probability scan	Uncertain diagnosis. Evaluate further with LE US or CT-PA.	Uncertain diagnosis. Evaluate further with LE US or CT-PA.	STOP. Diagnosis excluded; monitor off anticoagulation. Consider alternative diagnoses.
Normal scan	STOP. Diagnosis excluded; monitor off anticoagulation. Consider alternative diagnoses.	STOP. Diagnosis excluded; monitor off anticoagulation. Consider alternative diagnoses.	STOP. Diagnosis excluded; monitor off anticoagulation. Consider alternative diagnoses.

Data from The PIOPED Investigators. Value of the ventilation/perfusion scan in acute pulmonary embolism: results of the Prospective Investigation of Pulmonary Embolism Diagnosis (PIOPED). JAMA. 1990 May 23–30;263(20):2753–9. [PMID: 2332918]
CT-PA, helical CT pulmonary angiography; LE US, lower extremity venous ultrasound for DVT; PE, pulmonary embolism.

respectively. There is unambiguous evidence of the efficacy of prophylactic therapy in this and other clinical situations, yet it remains underused. Only about 50% of surgical deaths from PE had received any form of preventive therapy. Discussion of strategies for the prevention of venous thromboembolism can be found in Chapter 14.

► Treatment

A. Anticoagulation

Anticoagulation is not definitive therapy but a form of secondary prevention. Heparin binds to and accelerates the ability of antithrombin to inactivate thrombin, factor Xa, and factor IXa. It thus retards additional thrombus formation, allowing endogenous fibrinolytic mechanisms to lyse existing clot. The standard regimen of heparin followed by 6 months of oral warfarin results in an 80–90% reduction in the risk of both recurrent venous thrombosis and death from PE (see Tables 14–16, 14–19, 14–20). LMWHs are as effective as unfractionated heparin in the treatment of venous thromboembolism. Newer agents, such as factor Xa inhibitors and direct thrombin inhibitors, are alternatives for oral anticoagulation (see Table 14–11).

The optimal duration of anticoagulation therapy for venous thromboembolism is unknown. There appears to be a protective benefit to continued anticoagulation in first-episode venous thromboembolism (twice the rate of recurrence in 6 weeks compared with 6 months of therapy) and recurrent disease (eightfold risk of recurrence in 6 months compared with 4 years of therapy). These studies did not distinguish patients with reversible risk factors, such as surgery or transient immobility, from patients who have a nonreversible hypercoagulable state, such as factor V Leiden, inhibitor deficiency, antiphospholipid syndrome, or malignancy. An RCT of low-dose warfarin (INR 1.5–2.0) versus no therapy following 6 months of standard therapy in patients with idiopathic DVT was stopped early. The protective benefits of continued anticoagulation include fewer DVTs in addition to a trend toward lower mortality despite more hemorrhage in the warfarin group. Risk reductions were consistent across groups with and without inherited thrombophilia.

For many patients, venous thrombosis is a recurrent disease, and continued therapy results in a lower rate of recurrence at the cost of an increased risk of hemorrhage. Therefore, the appropriate duration of therapy needs to take into consideration the patient's age, potentially reversible risk factors, likelihood and potential consequences of hemorrhage, and preferences for continued therapy. The current American College of Chest Physician Guidelines recommend 3 months of anticoagulation after a first episode provoked by a surgery or a transient nonsurgical risk factor. Extended therapy (6–12 months) is recommended for unprovoked or recurrent episode with a low to moderate risk of bleeding. For patients with cancer, extended therapy is recommended regardless of bleeding risk and LMWH is preferred over vitamin K antagonists. It is reasonable to continue therapy for 6 months after a first episode when there is a reversible risk factor, 12 months after a first episode of idiopathic thrombosis, and 6–12 months

to indefinitely in patients with nonreversible risk factors or recurrent disease. D-dimer testing has been suggested to identify those who may benefit from continued anticoagulation after 3 months of therapy but clinical data have not supported its utility in this regard.

The major complication of anticoagulation is hemorrhage. Risk factors for hemorrhage include the intensity of the anticoagulation; duration of therapy; concomitant administration of medications, such as aspirin, that interfere with platelet function; and patient characteristics, particularly increased age, previous gastrointestinal hemorrhage, and coexistent chronic kidney disease.

The reported incidence of major hemorrhage following intravenous administration of unfractionated heparin is nil to 7%; that of fatal hemorrhage is nil to 2%. The incidence with LMWHs is not statistically different. There is no information comparing hemorrhage rates at different doses of heparin. The risk of death from another pulmonary embolism during subtherapeutic heparin administration in the first 24–48 hours after diagnosis is significant; it appears to outweigh the risk of short-term supratherapeutic heparin levels. The incidence of hemorrhage during therapy with warfarin is reported to be between 3% and 4% per patient year. The frequency varies with the target INR and is consistently higher when the INR exceeds 4.0. There is no apparent additional antithrombotic benefit in venous thromboembolism with a target INR above 2.0–3.0 (see Chapter 14).

B. Thrombolytic Therapy

Streptokinase, urokinase, and recombinant tissue plasminogen activator (rt-PA; alteplase) increase plasmin levels and thereby directly lyse intravascular thrombi. In patients with established PE, thrombolytic therapy accelerates resolution of emboli within the first 24 hours compared with standard heparin therapy. This is a consistent finding using angiography, $\dot{V}/\dot{Q}$ scanning, echocardiography, and direct measurement of pulmonary artery pressures. However, at 1 week and 1 month after diagnosis, these agents show no difference in outcome compared with heparin and warfarin. There is no evidence that thrombolytic therapy improves mortality. Subtle improvements in pulmonary function, including improved single-breath diffusing capacity and a lower incidence of exercise-induced pulmonary hypertension, have been observed. The reliability and clinical importance of these findings is unclear. The major disadvantages of thrombolytic therapy compared with heparin are its greater cost and significant increase in major hemorrhagic complications. The incidence of intracranial hemorrhage in patients with PE treated with alteplase is 2.1% compared with 0.2% in patients treated with heparin.

Current evidence supports thrombolytic therapy for PE in patients at high risk for death in whom the more rapid resolution of thrombus may be lifesaving. Such patients are usually hemodynamically unstable despite heparin therapy. Absolute contraindications to thrombolytic therapy include active internal bleeding and stroke within the past 2 months. Major contraindications include uncontrolled hypertension and surgery or trauma within the past 6 weeks. The role of thrombolysis in patients who are hemodynamically stable but with echocardiographic evidence of right heart strain from acute pulmonary embolism is unclear and is subject to considerable practice variation.

C. Additional Measures

Interruption of the inferior vena cava may be indicated in patients with a major contraindication to anticoagulation who have or are at high risk for development of proximal DVT or PE. Placement of an inferior vena cava filter is also recommended for recurrent thromboembolism despite adequate anticoagulation, for chronic recurrent embolism with a compromised pulmonary vascular bed (eg, in pulmonary hypertension), and with the concurrent performance of surgical pulmonary embolectomy or pulmonary thromboendarterectomy. Percutaneous transjugular placement of a mechanical filter is the preferred mode of inferior vena cava interruption. These devices reduce the short-term incidence of PE in patients presenting with proximal lower extremity DVT. However, they are associated with **a twofold increased risk of recurrent DVT in the first 2 years following placement** so plans must be usually made for their subsequent removal.

In rare critically ill patients for whom thrombolytic therapy is contraindicated or unsuccessful, mechanical or surgical extraction of thrombus may be indicated. Pulmonary embolectomy is an emergency procedure of last resort with a very high mortality rate. It is performed only in a few specialized centers.

▶ Prognosis

PE is estimated to cause more than 50,000 deaths annually. **In the majority of deaths, PE is not recognized antemortem or death occurs before specific treatment can be initiated.** These statistics highlight the importance of preventive therapy in high-risk patients (Chapter 14). The outlook for patients with diagnosed and appropriately treated PE is generally good. Overall prognosis depends on the underlying disease rather than the PE itself. Death from recurrent thromboemboli is uncommon, occurring in less than 3% of cases. Perfusion defects resolve in most survivors. Chronic thromboembolic pulmonary hypertension develops in approximately 1% of patients. Selected patients may benefit from pulmonary endarterectomy.

Couturaud F et al; PADIS-PE Investigators. Six months vs extended oral anticoagulation after a first episode of pulmonary embolism: the PADIS-PE randomized clinical trial. JAMA. 2015 Jul 7;314(1):31–40. [PMID: 26151264]

Jaff MR et al; American Heart Association Council on Cardiopulmonary, Critical Care, Perioperative and Resuscitation; American Heart Association Council on Peripheral Vascular Disease; American Heart Association Council on Arteriosclerosis, Thrombosis and Vascular Biology. Management of massive and submassive pulmonary embolism, iliofemoral deep vein thrombosis, and chronic thromboembolic pulmonary hypertension: a scientific statement from the American Heart Association. Circulation. 2011 Apr 26;123(16):1788–830. [PMID: 21422387]

Kearon C et al. Antithrombotic therapy for VTE disease: Antithrombotic Therapy and Prevention of Thrombosis, 9th ed: American College of Chest Physicians Evidence-Based Clinical Practice Guideline. Chest. 2012 Feb;141(2 Suppl): e419S–94S. [PMID: 22315268]

Merrigan JM et al. JAMA patient page. Pulmonary embolism. JAMA. 2013 Feb 6;309(5):504. [PMID: 23385279]

Raja AS et al. Evaluation of patients with suspected acute pulmonary embolism: best practice advice from the Clinical Guidelines Committee of the American College of Physicians. Ann Intern Med. 2015 Nov 3;163(9):701–11. [PMID: 26414967]

Righini M et al. Age-adjusted D-dimer cutoff levels to rule out pulmonary embolism: the ADJUST-PE study. JAMA. 2014 Mar 19;311(11):1117–24. [PMID: 24643601]

PULMONARY HYPERTENSION

 ESSENTIALS OF DIAGNOSIS

▶ Dyspnea, fatigue, chest pain, and syncope on exertion.

▶ Narrow splitting of second heart sound with loud pulmonary component; findings of right ventricular hypertrophy and heart failure in advanced disease.

▶ Electrocardiographic evidence of right ventricular strain or hypertrophy and right atrial enlargement.

▶ Enlarged central pulmonary arteries on chest radiograph.

▶ Elevated right ventricular systolic pressure on two-dimensional echocardiography with Doppler flow studies.

▶ General Considerations

Pulmonary hypertension is a complex problem characterized by pathologic elevation in pulmonary arterial pressure. Normal pulmonary artery systolic pressure at rest is 15–30 mm Hg, with a mean pressure between 10 mm Hg and 18 mm Hg. The pulmonary circulation is a low-pressure, low-resistance system due to its large cross-sectional area, and it can accommodate significant increase in blood flow during exercise. The primary pathologic mechanism in pulmonary hypertension is an increase in pulmonary vascular resistance that leads to an increase in the pulmonary systolic pressure greater than 30 mm Hg or the mean pressure greater than 20 mm Hg.

The World Health Organization currently classifies pulmonary hypertension based on similarities in pathologic mechanisms and includes the following five groups.

Group 1 (pulmonary arterial hypertension secondary to various disorders): This group gathers diseases that localize directly to the pulmonary arteries leading to structural changes, smooth muscle hypertrophy, and endothelial dysfunction. This group includes idiopathic (formerly primary) pulmonary arterial hypertension, heritable pulmonary arterial hypertension, HIV infection, portal hypertension, drugs and toxins, connective tissue disorders, congenital heart disease, schistosomiasis, primary veno-occlusive disease, and pulmonary capillary hemangiomatosis.

Group 2 (pulmonary venous hypertension secondary to left heart disease): Often referred to as pulmonary venous hypertension or "post-capillary" pulmonary hypertension, this group includes left ventricular systolic or diastolic dysfunction and valvular heart disease.

Group 3 (pulmonary hypertension secondary to lung disease or hypoxemia): This group is caused by advanced obstructive and restrictive lung disease, including COPD, interstitial lung disease, pulmonary fibrosis, bronchiectasis, as well as other causes of chronic hypoxemia, such as sleep-disordered breathing, alveolar hypoventilation syndromes, and high altitude exposure.

Group 4 (pulmonary hypertension secondary to chronic thromboembolism): This group consists of patients with pulmonary hypertension due to thromboembolic occlusion of the proximal and distal pulmonary arteries. (This classification no longer includes patients with nonthrombotic occlusion, such as tumors or foreign objects.)

Group 5 (pulmonary arterial hypertension secondary to hematologic, systemic, metabolic, or miscellaneous causes): These patients have pulmonary hypertension secondary to hematologic disorders (eg, chronic hemolytic anemia, myeloproliferative disorders, splenectomy), systemic disorders (eg, sarcoidosis, vasculitis, pulmonary Langerhans cell histiocytosis, neurofibromatosis type 1), metabolic disorders (eg, glycogen storage disease, Gaucher disease, thyroid disease), and miscellaneous causes (tumor embolization, external compression of the pulmonary vasculature, end-stage renal disease on dialysis).

The clinical severity of pulmonary hypertension is classified according to the New York Heart Association (NYHA) classification system, which was originally developed for heart failure but subsequently modified by the World Health Organization; it is based primarily on symptoms and functional status.

Class I: Pulmonary hypertension without limitation of physical activity. No dyspnea, fatigue, chest pain, or near syncope with exertion.

Class II: Pulmonary hypertension resulting in slight limitation of physical activity. No symptoms at rest but ordinary physical activity causes dyspnea, fatigue, chest pain, or near syncope.

Class III: Pulmonary hypertension resulting in marked limitation of physical activity. No symptoms at rest but less than ordinary activity causes dyspnea, fatigue, chest pain, or near syncope.

Class IV: Pulmonary hypertension with inability to perform any physical activity without symptoms. Evidence of right heart failure. Dyspnea and fatigue at rest and worsening of symptoms with any activity.

▶ Clinical Findings

A. Symptoms and Signs

There are no specific symptoms or signs but patients with pulmonary hypertension typically experience dyspnea with exertion and even, with advanced disease, at rest.

Anginal pain, nonproductive cough, malaise, and fatigue may be present. Syncope occurs with exertion when there is insufficient cardiac output or if there is an arrhythmia. Hemoptysis is a rare but life-threatening event in pulmonary hypertension usually caused by the rupture of a pulmonary artery.

Findings on physical examination can include jugular venous distention, accentuated pulmonary valve component of the second heart sound, right-sided third heart sound, tricuspid regurgitation murmur, hepatomegaly, and lower extremity edema. Cyanosis can occur in patients with an open patent foramen ovale and right-to-left shunt due to increased right atrial pressure.

B. Laboratory Findings

Routine blood work is often normal; any abnormalities noted are usually related to the underlying disease in secondary pulmonary hypertension. On arterial blood gas analysis, patients with idiopathic pulmonary arterial hypertension often have normal Pao_2 at rest but show evidence of hyperventilation with a decrease in $Paco_2$. All patients should be screened for HIV and collagen vascular disease.

The ECG is typically normal except in advanced disease, where right ventricular hypertrophy (right axis deviation, incomplete right bundle branch block) and right atrial enlargement (peaked P wave in the inferior and right-sided leads) can be noted.

C. Imaging and Special Examinations

Radiographs and CT scans of the chest are useful in diagnosis. Enlargement of the right and left main pulmonary arteries is common; right ventricular and right atrial enlargement is seen in advanced disease. Chest imaging and pulmonary function testing are also useful in determining the cause of pulmonary hypertension for patients in Group 3 (pulmonary hypertension due to lung disease). On pulmonary function testing, the combination of decreased single-breath diffusing capacity, normal FVC on spirometry, normal TLC on lung volume measurement, and increased wasted ventilation on cardiopulmonary exercise testing is suggestive of pathologically increased pulmonary arterial pressures.

Patients in whom pulmonary hypertension is suspected should undergo echocardiography with Doppler flow. The echocardiogram is useful in the assessment of underlying cardiac disease while Doppler flow can estimate the right ventricular systolic pressure. Right ventricular systolic pressure can be estimated based on tricuspid jet velocity and right atrial pressure. The severity of pulmonary hypertension can also be assessed based on the right ventricular size and function. Right-sided cardiac catheterization remains the gold standard for the diagnosis and quantification of pulmonary hypertension and should be performed prior to initiation of advanced therapies. Estimated pressures on echocardiogram correlate with right heart catheterization measurement but can vary by at least 10 mm Hg in more than 50% of cases so should not be used to direct therapy. Cardiac catheterization is particularly helpful in differentiating pulmonary arterial hypertension from pulmonary venous hypertension by assessment of the drop in pressure across the pulmonary circulation, also known as the transpulmonary gradient. Vasodilator challenge is often performed during right heart catheterization and for a significant acute vasodilator response consists of a drop in mean pulmonary pressure of greater than 10 mm Hg (or 20%) to less than 40 mm Hg.

In patients with unexplained pulmonary hypertension who have a history of PE or risk factors for thromboembolic disease, chronic thromboembolic disease (Group 4 pulmonary hypertension) should be excluded prior to diagnosing idiopathic pulmonary hypertension. V/Q lung scanning is a very sensitive test that can differentiate chronic thromboembolic pulmonary hypertension from idiopathic pulmonary arterial hypertension. Currently, pulmonary angiography is considered the most definitive diagnostic procedure for defining the distribution and extent of disease in chronic thromboembolic pulmonary hypertension.

▶ **Treatment**

Primary therapy refers to treatment directed at the underlying cause of pulmonary hypertension. Currently, there are no primary therapies available targeting the underlying lesion for patients in Group 1 (pulmonary arterial hypertension) but advanced therapies are available directly targeting the pulmonary hypertension itself. The advanced therapy chosen is typically based on patient symptoms and functional status according to the NYHA/WHO classification. Based on observational studies showing improved functional status and possible decreased mortality, first-line therapy consists of oral calcium channel blockers. However, these medications should only be given to patients with positive acute vasodilator response when tested in the cardiac catheterization laboratory because they may be harmful to nonresponders. Preferred treatments for Group 1 patients in functional class II include oral endothelin receptor antagonists (ambrisentan, bosentan), and phosphodiesterase inhibitors (sildenafil, tadalafil). RCTs using either endothelin receptor antagonists or phosphodiesterase inhibitors have shown improvement in symptoms, 6-minute walk distance, WHO functional status, and hemodynamic measurements. For Group 1 patients in functional classes III and IV or Group 1 patients who are not responsive to previous therapies, prostanoid agents are available. Continuous long-term intravenous epoprostenol infusion improved mortality in a prospective RCT. Limitations to intravenous prostacyclins (epoprostenol, treprostinil) include short medication half-life requiring a reliable continuous infusion, difficulty in titration, and high cost of therapy. Inhaled prostanoids (iloprost, treprostinil) and subcutaneous prostanoids (treprostinil) are available for patients unable to tolerate continuous intravenous infusion. One oral formulation of prostacyclin analogs has been approved for Group 1 disease based on a clinical trial that demonstrated a small increase in 6-minute walk distance.

Treatment of patients with Group 2 pulmonary hypertension (secondary to left heart failure) is discussed in Chapter 10. The main goal is to decrease pulmonary venous pressure by treating heart failure and volume overload.

Patients with Group 3 pulmonary hypertension (due to lung disease) and hypoxemia at rest or with physical activity should receive supplemental oxygen. In patients with COPD and hypoxemia, administration of supplemental oxygen for 15 hours or more per day has been shown to slow the progression of pulmonary hypertension.

For patients with Group 1 pulmonary hypertension and Group 4 pulmonary hypertension (due to thromboembolic disease), long-term anticoagulation is recommended and generally accepted, based solely on observational studies suggesting improvement in survival. For Group 4 patients in functional class IV and no response to other advanced therapies, thromboendarterectomy is recommended. Only patients with surgically accessible lesions and acceptable perioperative risk should undergo this procedure.

Lung transplantation is a treatment option for selected patients with pulmonary hypertension when medical therapy is no longer effective. Double-lung transplant is the preferred method, although single-lung transplant is routinely done as well. In some cases, transplantation of the heart and both lungs is needed.

▶ **Prognosis**

The prognosis of idiopathic (some Group 1) pulmonary hypertension is poor and is not affected by therapies primarily used to treat symptoms. Conversely, the prognosis for patients with secondary pulmonary hypertension (some Group 1 and Groups 2–5) depends on the underlying disease and its response to treatment. In all cases, right ventricular function is one of the most important prognostic factors. The presence of cor pulmonale carries a poor survival outcome regardless of the underlying cause.

▶ **When to Refer**

Patients with pulmonary arterial hypertension and symptoms of dyspnea, fatigue, chest pain, or near syncope should be referred to a pulmonologist or cardiologist at a specialized center for expert management.

▶ **When to Admit**

- Patients with pulmonary hypertension, severe symptoms, and evidence of decompensated right heart failure with volume overload should be admitted to the hospital for aggressive diuresis.
- Patients with Group 1 pulmonary hypertension and functional class IV symptoms should be admitted to a specialized center for initiation of advanced therapies, such as intravenous prostacyclins.

Galiè N et al. 2015 ESC/ERS Guidelines for the diagnosis and treatment of pulmonary hypertension: The Joint Task Force for the Diagnosis and Treatment of Pulmonary Hypertension of the European Society of Cardiology (ESC) and the European Respiratory Society (ERS) Endorsed by: Association for European Paediatric and Congenital Cardiology (AEPC), International Society for Heart and Lung Transplantation (ISHLT). Eur Heart J. 2016 Jan 1;37(1):67–119. [PMID: 26320113]

Humbert M et al. Advances in therapeutic interventions for patients with pulmonary arterial hypertension. Circulation. 2014 Dec 9;130(24):2189–208. [PMID: 25602947]

Taichman DB et al. Pharmacologic therapy for pulmonary arterial hypertension in adults: CHEST guideline and expert panel report. Chest. 2014 Aug;146(2):449–75. [PMID: 24937180]

PULMONARY VASCULITIS

Granulomatosis with polyangiitis (formerly referred to as **Wegener granulomatosis**) is an idiopathic disease manifested by a combination of glomerulonephritis, necrotizing granulomatous vasculitis of the upper and lower respiratory tracts, and varying degrees of small-vessel vasculitis. Chronic sinusitis, arthralgias, fever, skin rash, and weight loss are frequent presenting symptoms. Specific pulmonary complaints occur less often. The most common sign of lung disease is nodular pulmonary infiltrates, often with cavitation, seen on chest radiography. Tracheal stenosis and endobronchial disease are sometimes seen. The diagnosis is most often based on serologic testing and biopsy of lung, sinus tissue, or kidney with demonstration of necrotizing granulomatous vasculitis (Chapter 20).

Eosinophilic granulomatosis with polyangiitis (formerly referred to as **Churg-Strauss syndrome**) is an idiopathic multisystem vasculitis of small and medium-sized arteries that occurs in patients with asthma. The skin and lungs are most often involved, but other organs, including the paranasal sinuses, the heart, gastrointestinal tract, liver, and peripheral nerves, may also be affected. Peripheral eosinophilia greater than 1500 cells/mcL (greater than 1.5 $\times$ 10^9/L) or greater than 10% of peripheral WBCs is the rule. Abnormalities on chest radiographs range from transient opacities to multiple nodules. This illness may be part of a spectrum that includes polyarteritis nodosa. The diagnosis requires demonstration of histologic features, including fibrinoid necrotizing epithelioid and eosinophilic granulomas.

▶ Treatment

Treatment of pulmonary vasculitis usually requires corticosteroids and cyclophosphamide. Oral prednisone (1 mg/kg ideal body weight per day initially, tapering slowly to alternate-day therapy over 3–6 months) is the corticosteroid of choice; in granulomatosis with polyangiitis, some clinicians may use cyclophosphamide alone. For fulminant vasculitis, therapy may be initiated with intravenous methylprednisolone (up to 1 g intravenously per day) for several days. Cyclophosphamide (1–2 mg/kg ideal body weight orally per day initially, with dosage adjustments to avoid neutropenia) is given until complete remission is obtained and then is slowly tapered, and often replaced with methotrexate or azathioprine for maintenance therapy.

▶ Prognosis

Five-year survival rates in patients with these vasculitis syndromes have been improved by combination therapy. Complete remission can be achieved in over 90% of patients with granulomatosis with polyangiitis. The addition of trimethoprim-sulfamethoxazole (one double-strength tablet by mouth twice daily) to standard therapy may help prevent relapses.

Greco A et al. Churg-Strauss syndrome. Autoimmun Rev. 2015 Apr;14(4):341–8. [PMID: 25500434]

Lally L et al. Pulmonary vasculitis. Rheum Dis Clin North Am. 2015 May;41(2):315–31. [PMID: 25836645]

ALVEOLAR HEMORRHAGE SYNDROMES

Diffuse alveolar hemorrhage may occur in a variety of immune and nonimmune disorders. Hemoptysis, alveolar infiltrates on chest radiograph, anemia, dyspnea, and occasionally fever are characteristic. Rapid clearing of diffuse lung infiltrates within 2 days is a clue to the diagnosis of diffuse alveolar hemorrhage. Pulmonary hemorrhage can be associated with an increased single-breath diffusing capacity for carbon monoxide (DL$_{CO}$).

Causes of **immune alveolar hemorrhage** have been classified as anti-basement membrane antibody disease (Goodpasture syndrome), vasculitis and collagen vascular disease (systemic lupus erythematosus, granulomatosis with polyangiitis, systemic necrotizing vasculitis, and others), and pulmonary capillaritis associated with idiopathic rapidly progressive glomerulonephritis. **Nonimmune causes** of diffuse hemorrhage include coagulopathy, mitral stenosis, necrotizing pulmonary infection, drugs (penicillamine), toxins (trimellitic anhydride), and idiopathic pulmonary hemosiderosis.

Goodpasture syndrome is idiopathic recurrent alveolar hemorrhage and rapidly progressive glomerulonephritis. The disease is mediated by anti-glomerular basement membrane antibodies. Goodpasture syndrome occurs mainly in men who are in their 30s and 40s. Hemoptysis is the usual presenting symptom, but pulmonary hemorrhage may be occult. Dyspnea, cough, hypoxemia, and diffuse bilateral alveolar infiltrates are typical features. Iron deficiency anemia and microscopic hematuria are usually present. The diagnosis is based on characteristic linear IgG deposits detected by immunofluorescence in glomeruli or alveoli and on the presence of anti-glomerular basement membrane antibody in serum. Combinations of immunosuppressive drugs (initially methylprednisolone, 30 mg/kg intravenously over 20 minutes every other day for three doses, followed by daily oral prednisone, 1 mg/kg/day, with cyclophosphamide, 2 mg/kg orally per day) and plasmapheresis have yielded excellent results.

Idiopathic pulmonary hemosiderosis is a disease of children or young adults characterized by recurrent pulmonary hemorrhage; in contrast to Goodpasture syndrome, renal involvement and anti-glomerular basement membrane antibodies are absent, but iron deficiency is typical. It is frequently associated with celiac disease. Treatment of acute episodes of hemorrhage with corticosteroids may be useful. Recurrent episodes of pulmonary hemorrhage may result in interstitial fibrosis and pulmonary failure.

de Prost N et al. Diffuse alveolar hemorrhage in immunocompetent patients: etiologies and prognosis revisited. Respir Med. 2012 Jul;106(7):1021–32. [PMID: 22541718]

Krause ML et al. Update on diffuse alveolar hemorrhage and pulmonary vasculitis. Immunol Allergy Clin North Am. 2012 Nov;32(4):587–600. [PMID: 23102067]

Lichtenberger JP 3rd et al. Diffuse pulmonary hemorrhage: clues to the diagnosis. Curr Probl Diagn Radiol. 2014 May–Jun; 43(3):128–39. [PMID: 24791616]

ENVIRONMENTAL & OCCUPATIONAL LUNG DISORDERS

SMOKE INHALATION

The inhalation of products of combustion may cause serious respiratory complications. As many as one-third of patients admitted to burn treatment units have pulmonary injury from smoke inhalation. **Morbidity and mortality due to smoke inhalation may exceed those attributed to the burns themselves.** The death rate of patients with both severe burns and smoke inhalation exceeds 50%.

All patients in whom significant smoke inhalation is suspected must be assessed for three consequences of smoke inhalation: impaired tissue oxygenation, thermal injury to the upper airway, and injury to the lower airways and lung parenchyma. Impaired tissue oxygenation may result from inhalation of a hypoxemia gas mixture, carbon monoxide or cyanide, or from alterations in $\dot{V}/\dot{Q}$ matching, and is an immediate threat to life. Immediate treatment with 100% oxygen is essential. The management of patients with carbon monoxide and cyanide poisoning is discussed in Chapter 38. The clinician must recognize that patients with carbon monoxide poisoning display a normal partial pressure of oxygen in arterial blood (Pa_{O_2}) but have a low *measured* (ie, not oximetric) hemoglobin saturation (Sa_{O_2}). Treatment with 100% oxygen should be continued until the measured carboxyhemoglobin level falls to less than 10% and concomitant metabolic acidosis has resolved.

Thermal injury to the mucosal surfaces of the upper airway occurs from inhalation of super-heated gases. Complications, including mucosal edema, upper airway obstruction, and impaired ability to clear oral secretions, usually become evident by 18–24 hours and produce inspiratory stridor. Respiratory failure occurs in severe cases. Early management (Chapter 37) includes the use of a high-humidity face mask with supplemental oxygen, gentle suctioning to evacuate oral secretions, elevation of the head 30 degrees to promote clearing of secretions, and topical epinephrine to reduce edema of the oropharyngeal mucous membrane. Helium-oxygen gas mixtures (Heliox) may reduce labored breathing due to critical upper airway narrowing. Close monitoring with arterial blood gases and later with oximetry is important. Examination of the upper airway with a fiberoptic laryngoscope or bronchoscope is superior to routine physical examination. Endotracheal intubation is often necessary to establish airway patency and is likely to be necessary in patients with deep facial burns or oropharyngeal or laryngeal edema. Tracheotomy should be avoided if possible because of an increased risk of pneumonia and death from sepsis.

Injury to the lower airways and lung parenchyma results from inhalation of toxic gases and products of combustion, including aldehydes and organic acids. The site of lung injury depends on the solubility of the gases inhaled, the duration of exposure, and the size of inhaled particles that transport noxious gases to distal lung units. Bronchorrhea and bronchospasm are seen early after exposure along with dyspnea, tachypnea, and tachycardia. Labored breathing and cyanosis may follow. Physical examination at this stage reveals diffuse wheezing and rhonchi. Bronchiolar and alveolar edema (eg, ARDS) may develop within 1–2 days after exposure. Sloughing of the bronchiolar mucosa may occur within 2–3 days, leading to airway obstruction, atelectasis, and worsening hypoxemia. Bacterial colonization and pneumonia are common by 5–7 days after the exposure.

Treatment of smoke inhalation consists of supplemental oxygen, bronchodilators, suctioning of mucosal debris and mucopurulent secretions via an indwelling endotracheal tube, chest physical therapy to aid clearance of secretions, and adequate humidification of inspired gases. Positive end-expiratory pressure (PEEP) has been advocated to treat bronchiolar edema. Judicious fluid management and close monitoring for secondary bacterial infection with daily sputum Gram stains round out the management protocol.

The routine use of corticosteroids for lung injury from smoke inhalation has been shown to be ineffective and may even be harmful. Routine or prophylactic use of antibiotics is not recommended.

Patients who survive should be watched for the late development of bronchiolitis obliterans.

Albright JM et al. The acute pulmonary inflammatory response to the graded severity of smoke inhalation injury. Crit Care Med. 2012 Apr;40(4):1113–21. [PMID: 22067627]

Dries DJ et al. Inhalation injury: epidemiology, pathology, treatment strategies. Scand J Trauma Resusc Emerg Med. 2013 Apr 19;21:31. [PMID: 23597126]

PULMONARY ASPIRATION SYNDROMES

Aspiration of material into the tracheobronchial tree results from various disorders that impair normal deglutition, especially disturbances of consciousness and esophageal dysfunction.

1. Acute Aspiration of Gastric Contents (Mendelson Syndrome)

Acute aspiration of gastric contents may be catastrophic. The pulmonary response depends on the characteristics and amount of gastric contents aspirated. The more acidic the material, the greater the degree of chemical pneumonitis. Aspiration of pure gastric acid (pH less than 2.5) causes extensive desquamation of the bronchial epithelium, bronchiolitis, hemorrhage, and pulmonary edema. **Acute gastric aspiration is one of the most common causes of ARDS.** The clinical picture is one of abrupt onset of respiratory distress, with cough, wheezing, fever, and tachypnea. Crackles may be audible at the bases of the lungs. Hypoxemia may be noted immediately after aspiration occurs. Radiographic abnormalities, consisting of patchy alveolar opacities in dependent lung zones, appear within a few hours. If particulate food matter has been aspirated along with gastric acid, radiographic features of bronchial obstruction may be observed. Fever and leukocytosis are common even in the absence of infection.

Treatment of acute aspiration of gastric contents consists of supplemental oxygen, measures to maintain the airway, and the usual measures for treatment of acute respiratory failure. **There is no evidence to support the routine use of prophylactic antibiotics or corticosteroids after gastric aspiration.** Secondary pulmonary infection, which occurs in about one-fourth of patients, typically appears 2–3 days after aspiration. Management of infection depends on the observed flora of the tracheobronchial tree. Hypotension secondary to alveolar capillary membrane injury and intravascular volume depletion is common and is managed with the judicious administration of intravenous fluids.

2. Chronic Aspiration of Gastric Contents

Chronic aspiration of gastric contents may result from primary disorders of the larynx or the esophagus, such as achalasia, esophageal stricture, systemic sclerosis (scleroderma), esophageal carcinoma, esophagitis, and gastroesophageal reflux. In the last condition, relaxation of the tone of the lower esophageal sphincter allows reflux of gastric contents into the esophagus and predisposes to chronic pulmonary aspiration, especially at night. Cigarette smoking, consumption of alcohol or caffeine, and use of theophylline are known to relax the lower esophageal sphincter. Pulmonary disorders linked to gastroesophageal reflux and chronic aspiration include asthma, chronic cough, bronchiectasis, and pulmonary fibrosis. Even in the absence of aspiration, acid in the esophagus may trigger bronchospasm or bronchial hyperreactivity through reflex mechanisms.

The diagnosis and management of gastroesophageal reflux and chronic aspiration is challenging. A discussion of strategies for the evaluation, prevention, and management of extraesophageal reflux manifestations can be found in Chapter 15.

3. "Café Coronary"

Acute obstruction of the upper airway by food is associated with difficulty swallowing, old age, dental problems that impair chewing, and use of alcohol and sedative drugs. The Heimlich procedure is lifesaving in many cases.

4. Retention of an Aspirated Foreign Body

Retention of an aspirated foreign body in the tracheobronchial tree may produce both acute and chronic conditions, including atelectasis, postobstructive hyperinflation, both acute and recurrent pneumonia, bronchiectasis, and lung abscess. Occasionally, a misdiagnosis of asthma, COPD, or lung cancer is made in adult patients who have aspirated a foreign body. The plain chest radiograph usually suggests the site of the foreign body. In some cases, an expiratory film, demonstrating regional hyperinflation due to a check-valve effect, is helpful. Bronchoscopy is usually necessary

to establish the diagnosis and attempt removal of the foreign body.

5. Aspiration of Inert Material

Most patients suffer no serious sequelae from aspiration of inert material. However, it may cause asphyxia if the amount aspirated is massive and if cough is impaired, in which case immediate tracheobronchial suctioning is necessary.

6. Aspiration of Toxic Material

Aspiration of toxic material into the lung usually results in clinically evident pneumonia. **Hydrocarbon pneumonitis** is caused by aspiration of ingested petroleum distillates, eg, gasoline, kerosene, furniture polish, and other household petroleum products. Lung injury results mainly from vomiting of ingested products and secondary aspiration. Therapy is supportive. The lung should be protected from repeated aspiration with a cuffed endotracheal tube if necessary. **Lipoid pneumonia** is a chronic syndrome related to the repeated aspiration of oily materials, eg, mineral oil, cod liver oil, and oily nose drops; it usually occurs in elderly patients with impaired swallowing. Patchy opacities in dependent lung zones and lipid-laden macrophages in expectorated sputum are characteristic findings.

DiBardino DM et al. Aspiration pneumonia: a review of modern trends. J Crit Care. 2015 Feb;30(1):40–8. [PMID: 25129577]
Prather AD et al. Aspiration-related lung diseases. J Thorac Imaging. 2014 Sep;29(5):304–9. [PMID: 24911122]

OCCUPATIONAL PULMONARY DISEASES

Many acute and chronic pulmonary diseases are directly related to inhalation of noxious substances encountered in the workplace. Disorders that are linked to occupational exposures may be classified as follows: (1) pneumoconioses, (2) hypersensitivity pneumonitis, (3) obstructive airway disorders, (4) toxic lung injury, (5) lung cancer, (6) pleural diseases, and (7) other occupational pulmonary diseases.

1. Pneumoconioses

Pneumoconioses are chronic fibrotic lung diseases caused by the inhalation of inorganic dusts. Pneumoconioses due to inhalation of inert dusts may be asymptomatic disorders with diffuse nodular opacities on chest radiograph or may be severe, symptomatic, life-shortening disorders. Clinically important pneumoconioses include coal worker's pneumoconiosis, silicosis, and asbestosis (Table 9–22). Treatment for each is supportive.

A. Coal Worker's Pneumoconiosis

In coal worker's pneumoconiosis, ingestion of inhaled coal dust by alveolar macrophages leads to the formation of coal macules, usually 2–5 mm in diameter, that appear on chest radiograph as diffuse small opacities that are especially prominent in the upper lung. Simple coal worker's pneumoconiosis is usually asymptomatic; pulmonary function

Table 9–22. Selected pneumoconioses.

Disease	Agent	Occupations
Metal dusts		
Siderosis	Metallic iron or iron oxide	Mining, welding, foundry work
Stannosis	Tin, tin oxide	Mining, tin-working, smelting
Baritosis	Barium salts	Glass and insecticide manufacturing
Coal dust		
Coal worker's pneumoconiosis	Coal dust	Coal mining
Inorganic dusts		
Silicosis	Free silica (silicon dioxide)	Rock mining, quarrying, stone cutting, tunneling, sandblasting, pottery, diatomaceous earth
Silicate dusts		
Asbestosis	Asbestos	Mining, insulation, construction, shipbuilding
Talcosis	Magnesium silicate	Mining, insulation, construction, shipbuilding
Kaolin pneumoconiosis	Sand, mica, aluminum silicate	Mining of china clay; pottery and cement work
Shaver disease	Aluminum powder	Manufacture of corundum

abnormalities are unimpressive. Cigarette smoking does not increase the prevalence of coal worker's pneumoconiosis but may have an additive detrimental effect on ventilatory function. In complicated coal worker's pneumoconiosis (**"progressive massive fibrosis"**), conglomeration and contraction in the upper lung zones occur, with radiographic features resembling complicated silicosis. **Caplan syndrome** is a rare condition characterized by the presence of necrobiotic rheumatoid nodules (1–5 cm in diameter) in the periphery of the lung in coal workers with rheumatoid arthritis.

B. Silicosis

In silicosis, extensive or prolonged inhalation of free silica (silicon dioxide) particles in the respirable range (0.3–5 mcm) causes the formation of small rounded opacities (silicotic nodules) throughout the lung. Calcification of the periphery of hilar lymph nodes ("eggshell" calcification) is an unusual radiographic finding that strongly suggests silicosis. Simple silicosis is usually asymptomatic and has no effect on routine pulmonary function tests; in complicated silicosis, large conglomerate densities appear in the upper lung and are accompanied by dyspnea and obstructive and

restrictive pulmonary dysfunction. The incidence of pulmonary tuberculosis is increased in patients with silicosis. All patients with silicosis should have a tuberculin skin test and a current chest radiograph. If old, healed pulmonary tuberculosis is suspected, multidrug treatment for tuberculosis (not single-agent preventive therapy) should be instituted.

C. Asbestosis

Asbestosis is a nodular interstitial fibrosis occurring in workers exposed to asbestos fibers (shipyard and construction workers, pipe fitters, insulators) over many years (typically 10–20 years). Patients with asbestosis usually first seek medical attention at least 15 years after exposure with the following symptoms and signs: progressive dyspnea, inspiratory crackles, and in some cases, clubbing and cyanosis. The radiographic features of asbestosis include linear streaking at the lung bases, opacities of various shapes and sizes, and honeycomb changes in advanced cases. The presence of pleural calcifications may be a clue to diagnosis. High-resolution CT scanning is the best imaging method for asbestosis because of its ability to detect parenchymal fibrosis and define the presence of coexisting pleural plaques. Cigarette smoking in asbestos workers increases the prevalence of radiographic pleural and parenchymal changes and markedly increases the incidence of lung carcinoma. It may also interfere with the clearance of short asbestos fibers from the lung. Pulmonary function studies show restrictive dysfunction and reduced diffusing capacity. The presence of a ferruginous body in tissue suggests significant asbestos exposure; however, other histologic features must be present for diagnosis. There is no specific treatment.

Banks DE. Clinical aspects of asbestos-related diseases—what are the unresolved topics? J Occup Environ Med. 2014 Oct; 56(Suppl 10):S8–12. [PMID: 25285978]

Karkhanis VS et al. Pneumoconioses. Indian J Chest Dis Allied Sci. 2013 Jan–Mar;55(1):25–34. [PMID: 23798087]

Laney AS et al. Respiratory diseases caused by coal mine dust. J Occup Environ Med. 2014 Oct;56(Suppl 10):S18–22. [PMID: 25285970]

Leung CC et al. Silicosis. Lancet. 2012 May 26;379(9830): 2008–18. [PMID: 22534002]

2. Hypersensitivity Pneumonitis

Hypersensitivity pneumonitis (also called extrinsic allergic alveolitis) is a nonatopic, nonasthmatic inflammatory pulmonary disease. It is manifested mainly as an occupational disease (Table 9–23), in which exposure to inhaled organic antigens leads to an acute illness. Prompt diagnosis is essential since symptoms are usually reversible if the offending antigen is removed from the patient's environment early in the course of illness. Continued exposure may lead to progressive disease. The histopathology of acute hypersensitivity pneumonitis is characterized by interstitial infiltrates of lymphocytes and plasma cells, with noncaseating granulomas in the interstitium and air spaces.

Table 9–23. Selected causes of hypersensitivity pneumonitis.

Disease	Antigen	Source
Farmer's lung	*Micropolyspora faeni, Thermoactinomyces vulgaris*	Moldy hay
"Humidifier" lung	Thermophilic actinomycetes	Contaminated humidifiers, heating systems, or air conditioners
Bird fancier's lung ("pigeon-breeder's disease")	Avian proteins	Bird serum and excreta
Bagassosis	*Thermoactinomyces sacchari* and *T vulgaris*	Moldy sugar cane fiber (bagasse)
Sequoiosis	Graphium, Aureobasidium, and other fungi	Moldy redwood sawdust
Maple bark stripper's disease	*Cryptostroma (Coniosporium) corticale*	Rotting maple tree logs or bark
Mushroom picker's disease	Same as farmer's lung	Moldy compost
Suberosis	*Penicillium frequentans*	Moldy cork dust
Detergent worker's lung	*Bacillus subtilis* enzyme	Enzyme additives

▶ Clinical Findings

A. Acute Illness

The symptoms are characterized by sudden onset of malaise, chills, fever, cough, dyspnea, and nausea 4–8 hours after exposure to the offending antigen. This may occur after the patient has left work or even at night and thus may mimic paroxysmal nocturnal dyspnea. Bibasilar crackles, tachypnea, tachycardia, and (occasionally) cyanosis are noted. Small nodular densities sparing the apices and bases of the lungs are noted on chest radiograph. Laboratory studies reveal an increase in the white blood cell count with a shift to the left, hypoxemia, and the presence of precipitating antibodies to the offending agent in serum. Hypersensitivity pneumonitis antibody panels against common offending antigens are available; positive results, while supportive, do not establish a definitive diagnosis. Pulmonary function studies reveal restrictive dysfunction and reduced diffusing capacity.

B. Subacute Illness

A subacute hypersensitivity pneumonitis syndrome (15% of cases) is characterized by the insidious onset of chronic cough and slowly progressive dyspnea, anorexia, and

weight loss. Chronic exposure leads to progressive respiratory insufficiency and the appearance of pulmonary fibrosis on chest imaging. Surgical lung biopsy may be necessary for the diagnosis of subacute and chronic hypersensitivity pneumonitis. Even with surgical lung biopsy, however, chronic hypersensitivity pneumonitis may be difficult to diagnose because histopathologic patterns overlap with several idiopathic interstitial pneumonias.

▶ Treatment

Treatment of acute hypersensitivity pneumonitis consists of identification of the offending agent and avoidance of further exposure. In severe acute or protracted cases, oral corticosteroids (prednisone, 0.5 mg/kg daily as a single morning dose for 2 weeks, tapered to nil over 4–6 weeks) may be given. Change in occupation is often unavoidable.

Nowicka U et al. Pulmonary function abnormalities in regard to age at the time of diagnosis of hypersensitivity pneumonitis. Adv Exp Med Biol. 2015;861:75–84. [PMID: 26017728]

Spagnolo P et al. Hypersensitivity pneumonitis: a comprehensive review. J Investig Allergol Clin Immunol. 2015;25(4):237–50. [PMID: 26310038]

3. Obstructive Airway Disorders

Occupational pulmonary diseases manifested as obstructive airway disorders include occupational asthma, industrial bronchitis, and byssinosis.

A. Occupational Asthma

It has been estimated that from 2% to 5% of all cases of asthma are related to occupation. Offending agents in the workplace are numerous; they include grain dust, wood dust, tobacco, pollens, enzymes, gum arabic, synthetic dyes, isocyanates (particularly toluene diisocyanate), rosin (soldering flux), inorganic chemicals (salts of nickel, platinum, and chromium), trimellitic anhydride, phthalic anhydride, formaldehyde, and various pharmaceutical agents. Diagnosis of occupational asthma depends on a high index of suspicion, an appropriate history, spirometric studies before and after exposure to the offending substance, and peak flow rate measurements in the workplace. Bronchial provocation testing may be helpful in some cases. Treatment consists of avoidance of further exposure to the offending agent and bronchodilators, but symptoms may persist for years after workplace exposure has been terminated.

B. Industrial Bronchitis

Industrial bronchitis is chronic bronchitis found in coal miners and others exposed to cotton, flax, or hemp dust. Chronic disability from industrial bronchitis is infrequent.

C. Byssinosis

Byssinosis is an asthma-like disorder in textile workers caused by inhalation of cotton dust. The pathogenesis is obscure. Chest tightness, cough, and dyspnea are characteristically worse on Mondays or the first day back at work, with symptoms subsiding later in the week. Repeated exposure leads to chronic bronchitis.

4. Toxic Lung Injury

Toxic lung injury from inhalation of irritant gases is discussed in the section on smoke inhalation. **Silo-filler's disease** is acute toxic high-permeability pulmonary edema caused by inhalation of nitrogen dioxide encountered in recently filled silos. Bronchiolitis obliterans is a common late complication, which may be prevented by early treatment of the acute reaction with corticosteroids. Extensive exposure to silage gas may be fatal. Inhalation of the compound diacetyl, a constituent of butter-flavoring, has been linked to the development of bronchiolitis obliterans among microwave popcorn production workers.

5. Lung Cancer

Many industrial pulmonary carcinogens have been identified, including asbestos, radon gas, arsenic, iron, chromium, nickel, coal tar fumes, petroleum oil mists, isopropyl oil, mustard gas, and printing ink. Cigarette smoking acts as a cocarcinogen with asbestos and radon gas to cause bronchogenic carcinoma. Asbestos alone causes malignant mesothelioma. Almost all histologic types of lung cancer have been associated with these carcinogens. Chloromethyl methyl ether specifically causes small-cell carcinoma of the lung.

6. Pleural Diseases

Occupational diseases of the pleura may result from exposure to asbestos or talc. Inhalation of talc causes pleural plaques that are similar to those caused by asbestos. Benign asbestos pleural effusion occurs in some asbestos workers and may cause chronic blunting of the costophrenic angle on chest radiograph.

7. Other Occupational Pulmonary Diseases

Occupational agents are also responsible for other pulmonary disorders. These include exposure to beryllium, which now occurs in machining and handling of beryllium products and alloys. Beryllium miners are not at risk for berylliosis and beryllium is no longer used in fluorescent lamp production, which was a source of exposure before 1950. **Berylliosis,** an acute or chronic pulmonary disorder, occurs from absorption of beryllium through the lungs or skin and wide dissemination throughout the body. Acute berylliosis is a toxic, ulcerative tracheobronchitis and chemical pneumonitis following intense and severe exposure to beryllium. Chronic berylliosis, a systemic disease closely resembling sarcoidosis, is more common. Chronic pulmonary beryllium disease is an alveolitis mediated by the proliferation of beryllium-specific CD4 T-cells in the lung.

Balmes JR et al; ATS Ad Hoc Committee on Beryllium Sensitivity and Chronic Beryllium Disease. An official American Thoracic Society statement: diagnosis and management of beryllium sensitivity and chronic beryllium disease. Am J Respir Crit Care Med. 2014 Nov 15;190(10):e34–59. [PMID: 25398119]

Lai PS et al. Long-term respiratory health effects in textile workers. Curr Opin Pulm Med. 2013 Mar;19(2):152–7. [PMID: 23361196]

Muñoz X et al. Work-related asthma: diagnosis and prognosis of immunological occupational asthma and work-exacerbated asthma. J Investig Allergol Clin Immunol. 2014;24(6):396–405. [PMID: 25668891]

Omland O et al. Occupational chronic obstructive pulmonary disease: a systematic literature review. Scand J Work Environ Health. 2014 Jan;40(1):19–35. [PMID: 24220056]

Reid PA et al. Occupational lung disease. J R Coll Physicians Edinb. 2013;43(1):44–8. [PMID: 23516692]

Tarlo S. Clinical aspects of work-related asthma: past achievements, persistent challenges, and emerging triggers. J Occup Environ Med. 2014 Oct;56(Suppl 10):S40–4. [PMID: 25285975]

MEDICATION-INDUCED LUNG DISEASE

Typical patterns of pulmonary response to medications implicated in medication-induced respiratory disease are summarized in Table 9–24. Pulmonary injury due to medications occurs as a result of allergic reactions, idiosyncratic reactions, overdose, or undesirable side effects. In most patients, the mechanism of pulmonary injury is unknown.

Precise diagnosis of medication-induced pulmonary disease is often difficult because results of routine laboratory studies are not helpful and radiographic findings are not specific. A high index of suspicion and a thorough history of medication usage are critical to establishing the diagnosis of medication-induced lung disease. The clinical response to cessation of the suspected offending agent is also helpful. Acute episodes of medication-induced pulmonary disease usually disappear 24–48 hours after the medication has been discontinued, but chronic syndromes may take longer to resolve. Challenge tests to confirm the diagnosis are risky and rarely performed.

Treatment of medication-induced lung disease consists of discontinuing the offending agent immediately and managing the pulmonary symptoms appropriately.

Inhalation of crack cocaine may cause a spectrum of acute pulmonary syndromes, including pulmonary infiltration with eosinophilia, pneumothorax and pneumomediastinum, bronchiolitis obliterans, and acute respiratory failure associated with diffuse alveolar damage and alveolar hemorrhage. Corticosteroids have been used with variable success to treat alveolar hemorrhage.

Matsuno O. Drug-induced interstitial lung disease: mechanisms and best diagnostic approaches. Respir Res. 2012 May 31; 13: 39. [PMID: 22651223]

RADIATION LUNG INJURY

The lung is an exquisitely radiosensitive organ that can be damaged by external beam radiation therapy. The degree of pulmonary injury is determined by the volume of lung irradiated, the dose and rate of exposure, and potentiating factors (eg, concurrent chemotherapy, previous radiation therapy in the same area, and simultaneous withdrawal of corticosteroid therapy). Symptomatic radiation lung injury occurs in about 10% of patients treated for carcinoma of the breast, 5–15% of patients treated for carcinoma of the lung, and 5–35% of patients treated for lymphoma. Two

Table 9–24. Pulmonary manifestations of selected medication toxicities.

Asthma	Pulmonary edema
Beta-blockers	Noncardiogenic
Aspirin	Aspirin
Nonsteroidal anti-inflammatory drugs	Chlordiazepoxide
	Cocaine
Histamine	Ethchlorvynol
Methacholine	Heroin
Acetylcysteine	Cardiogenic
Aerosolized pentamidine	Beta-blockers
Any nebulized medication	**Pleural effusion**
Chronic cough	Bromocriptine
Angiotensin-converting enzyme inhibitors	Nitrofurantoin
	Any drug inducing systemic lupus erythematosus
Pulmonary infiltration	
Without eosinophilia	Methysergide
Amitriptyline	Chemotherapeutic agents (eg, carmustine, cyclophosphamide, dasatinib, docetaxel, GM-CSF, methotrexate)
Azathioprine	
Amiodarone	
With eosinophilia	
Sulfonamides	
L-Tryptophan	**Mediastinal widening**
Nitrofurantoin	Phenytoin
Penicillin	Corticosteroids
Methotrexate	Methotrexate
Crack cocaine	**Respiratory failure**
Drug-induced systemic lupus erythematosus	Neuromuscular blockade
Hydralazine	Aminoglycosides
Procainamide	Succinylcholine
Isoniazid	Gallamine
Chlorpromazine	Dimethyltubocurarine (metocurine)
Phenytoin	
Interstitial pneumonitis/fibrosis	Central nervous system depression
Nitrofurantoin	Sedatives
Bleomycin	Hypnotics
Busulfan	Opioids
Cyclophosphamide	Alcohol
Methysergide	Tricyclic antidepressants
Phenytoin	Oxygen

GM-CSF, granulocyte-macrophage colony-stimulating factor.

phases of the pulmonary response to radiation are apparent: an acute phase (radiation pneumonitis) and a chronic phase (radiation fibrosis).

1. Radiation Pneumonitis

Acute radiation pneumonitis usually occurs 2–3 months (range 1–6 months) after completion of radiotherapy and is characterized by insidious onset of dyspnea, intractable dry cough, chest fullness or pain, weakness, and fever. Late radiation pneumonitis may develop 6–12 months after completion of radiation. The pathogenesis of acute radiation pneumonitis is unknown, but there is speculation that hypersensitivity mechanisms are involved. The dominant histopathologic findings are a lymphocytic interstitial pneumonitis progressing to an exudative alveolitis. Inspiratory crackles may be heard in the involved area. In severe disease, respiratory distress and cyanosis occur that are characteristic of ARDS. An increased white blood cell count and elevated sedimentation rate are common. Pulmonary function studies reveal reduced lung volumes, reduced lung compliance, hypoxemia, reduced diffusing capacity, and reduced maximum voluntary ventilation. Chest radiography, which correlates poorly with the presence of symptoms, usually demonstrates alveolar or nodular opacities limited to the irradiated area. Air bronchograms are often observed. Sharp borders of an opacity may help distinguish radiation pneumonitis from other conditions, such as infectious pneumonia, lymphangitic spread of carcinoma, and recurrent tumor; however, the opacity may extend beyond the radiation field. No specific therapy is proved to be effective in radiation pneumonitis, but prednisone (1 mg/kg/day orally) is commonly given immediately for about 1 week. The dose is then reduced and maintained at 20–40 mg/day for several weeks, then slowly tapered. Radiation pneumonitis may improve in 2–3 weeks following onset of symptoms as the exudative phase resolves. Acute respiratory failure, if present, is treated supportively. Death from ARDS is unusual in radiation pneumonitis.

2. Pulmonary Radiation Fibrosis

Radiation fibrosis may occur with or without antecedent radiation pneumonitis. Cor pulmonale and chronic respiratory failure are rare. Radiographic findings include obliteration of normal lung markings, dense interstitial and pleural fibrosis, reduced lung volumes, tenting of the diaphragm, and sharp delineation of the irradiated area. No specific therapy is proven effective, and corticosteroids have no value. Pulmonary fibrosis may develop after an intervening period (6–12 months) of well-being in patients who experience radiation pneumonitis. Pulmonary radiation fibrosis occurs in most patients who receive a full course of radiation therapy for cancer of the lung or breast. Most patients are asymptomatic, although slowly progressive dyspnea may occur.

3. Other Complications of Radiation Therapy

Other complications of radiation therapy directed to the thorax include pericardial effusion, constrictive pericarditis, tracheoesophageal fistula, esophageal candidiasis, radiation dermatitis, and rib fractures. Small pleural effusions, radiation pneumonitis outside the irradiated area, spontaneous pneumothorax, and complete obstruction of central airways are unusual occurrences.

Westbury CB et al. Radiation fibrosis—current clinical and therapeutic perspectives. Clin Oncol (R Coll Radiol). 2012 Dec; 24(10):657–72. [PMID: 22608361]

Yamashita H et al. Radiation pneumonitis after stereotactic radiation therapy for lung cancer. World J Radiol. 2014 Sep 28; 6(9):708–15. [PMID: 25276313]

PLEURAL DISEASES

PLEURITIS

Pain due to acute pleural inflammation is caused by irritation of the parietal pleura. Such pain is localized, sharp, and fleeting; it is made worse by coughing, sneezing, deep breathing, or movement. When the central portion of the diaphragmatic parietal pleura is irritated, pain may be referred to the ipsilateral shoulder. There are numerous causes of pleuritis. The setting in which pleuritic pain develops helps narrow the differential diagnosis. In young, otherwise healthy individuals, pleuritis is usually caused by viral respiratory infections or pneumonia. The presence of pleural effusion, pleural thickening, or air in the pleural space requires further diagnostic and therapeutic measures. Simple rib fracture may cause severe pleurisy.

Treatment of pleuritis consists of treating the underlying disease. Analgesics and anti-inflammatory medications (eg, indomethacin, 25 mg orally two or three times daily) are often helpful for pain relief. Codeine (30–60 mg orally every 8 hours) or other opioids may be used to control cough associated with pleuritic chest pain if retention of airway secretions is not a likely complication. Intercostal nerve blocks are sometimes helpful but the benefit is usually transient.

PLEURAL EFFUSION

ESSENTIALS OF DIAGNOSIS

▶ May be asymptomatic; chest pain frequently seen in the setting of pleuritis, trauma, or infection; dyspnea is common with large effusions.

▶ Dullness to percussion and decreased breath sounds over the effusion.

▶ Radiographic evidence of pleural effusion.

▶ Diagnostic findings on thoracentesis.

General Considerations

There is constant movement of fluid from parietal pleural capillaries into the pleural space at a rate of 0.01 mL/kg body weight/h. Absorption of pleural fluid occurs through parietal pleural lymphatics. The resultant homeostasis leaves 5–15 mL of fluid in the normal pleural space. A pleural effusion is an abnormal accumulation of fluid in the pleural space. Pleural effusions may be classified by differential diagnosis (Table 9–25) or by underlying pathophysiology. Five pathophysiologic processes account for most pleural effusions: increased production of fluid in the setting of normal capillaries due to increased hydrostatic or decreased oncotic pressures (**transudates**); increased production of fluid due to abnormal capillary permeability (**exudates**); decreased lymphatic clearance of fluid from the pleural space (**exudates**); infection in the pleural space

Table 9–25. Causes of pleural fluid transudates and exudates.

Transudates	Exudates
Heart failure (> 90% of cases)	Pneumonia (parapneumonic effusion)
Cirrhosis with ascites	Cancer
Nephrotic syndrome	Pulmonary embolism
Peritoneal dialysis	Bacterial infection
Myxedema	Tuberculosis
Atelectasis (acute)	Connective tissue disease
Constrictive pericarditis	Viral infection
Superior vena cava obstruction	Fungal infection
Pulmonary embolism	Rickettsial infection
	Parasitic infection
	Asbestos
	Meigs syndrome
	Pancreatic disease
	Uremia
	Chronic atelectasis
	Trapped lung
	Chylothorax
	Sarcoidosis
	Drug reaction
	Post-myocardial injury syndrome

(**empyema**); and bleeding into the pleural space (**hemothorax**). **Parapneumonic pleural effusions** are exudates that accompany bacterial pneumonias.

Diagnostic thoracentesis should be performed whenever there is a new pleural effusion and no clinically apparent cause. Observation is appropriate in some situations (eg, symmetric bilateral pleural effusions in the setting of heart failure), but an atypical presentation or failure of an effusion to resolve as expected warrants thoracentesis. Sampling allows visualization of the fluid in addition to chemical and microbiologic analyses to identify the underlying pathophysiologic process.

Clinical Findings

A. Symptoms and Signs

Patients with pleural effusions most often report dyspnea, cough, or respirophasic chest pain. Symptoms are more common in patients with existing cardiopulmonary disease. Small pleural effusions are less likely to be symptomatic than larger effusions. Physical findings are usually absent in small effusions. Larger effusions may present with dullness to percussion and diminished or absent breath sounds over the effusion. Compressive atelectasis may cause bronchial breath sounds and egophony just above the effusion. A massive effusion with increased intrapleural pressure may cause contralateral shift of the trachea and bulging of the intercostal spaces. A pleural friction rub indicates infarction or pleuritis.

B. Laboratory Findings

The gross appearance of pleural fluid helps identify several types of pleural effusion. Grossly purulent fluid signifies empyema. Milky white pleural fluid should be centrifuged. A clear supernatant above a pellet of white cells indicates empyema, whereas a persistently turbid supernatant suggests a **chylous effusion;** analysis of this supernatant reveals chylomicrons and a high triglyceride level (greater than 100 mg/dL [1 mmol/L]), often from disruption of the thoracic duct. **Hemorrhagic pleural effusion** is a mixture of blood and pleural fluid. Ten thousand red cells per microliter create blood-tinged pleural fluid; 100,000 red cells/mcL create grossly bloody pleural fluid. **Hemothorax** is the presence of gross blood in the pleural space, usually following chest trauma or instrumentation. It is defined as a ratio of pleural fluid hematocrit to peripheral blood hematocrit greater than 0.5.

Pleural fluid samples should be sent for measurement of protein, glucose, and LD in addition to total and differential white blood cell counts. Chemistry determinations are used to classify effusions as transudates or exudates. This classification is important because the differential diagnosis and subsequent evaluation for each entity is vastly different (Table 9–25). A **pleural exudate** is an effusion that has one or more of the following laboratory features: (1) ratio of pleural fluid protein to serum protein greater than 0.5; (2) ratio of pleural fluid LD to serum LD greater than 0.6; (3) pleural fluid LD greater than two-thirds the upper limit of normal serum LD. **Pleural transudates** occur in the setting of normal capillary integrity and demonstrate none of the laboratory features of exudates. A transudate suggests the absence of local pleural disease; characteristic laboratory findings include a glucose equal to serum glucose, pH between 7.40 and 7.55, and fewer than 1000 white blood cells/mcL (1.0×10^9/L) with a predominance of mononuclear cells.

Heart failure accounts for 90% of transudates. Bacterial pneumonia and cancer are the most common causes of exudative effusion. Other causes of exudates with characteristic laboratory findings are summarized in Table 9–26.

Pleural fluid pH is useful in the assessment of parapneumonic effusions. A pH below 7.30 suggests the need for drainage of the pleural space. An elevated amylase level in pleural fluid suggests pancreatitis, pancreatic pseudocyst, adenocarcinoma of the lung or pancreas, or esophageal rupture.

Suspected tuberculous pleural effusion should be evaluated by thoracentesis with culture along with pleural biopsy, since pleural fluid culture positivity for *M tuberculosis* is low (less than 23–58% of cases). Closed pleural biopsy reveals granulomatous inflammation in approximately 60% of patients, and culture of three pleural biopsy specimens combined with histologic examination of a pleural biopsy for granulomas yields a diagnosis in up to 90% of patients. Tests for pleural fluid adenosine deaminase (approximately 90% sensitivity and specificity for pleural tuberculosis at levels greater than 70 units/L) and interferon-gamma (89% sensitivity, 97% specificity in a meta-analysis) can be extremely helpful diagnostic aids, particularly in making decisions to pursue invasive testing in complex patients.

Between 40% and 80% of exudative pleural effusions are malignant, while over 90% of malignant pleural effusions are exudative. Almost any form of cancer may cause effusions, but the most common causes are lung cancer (one-third of cases) and breast cancer. In 5–10% of malignant pleural effusions, no primary tumor is identified. The term **"paramalignant"** pleural effusion refers to an effusion in a patient with cancer when repeated attempts to identify tumor cells in the pleura or pleural fluid are nondiagnostic but when there is a presumptive relation to the underlying malignancy. For example, superior vena cava syndrome with elevated systemic venous pressures causing a transudative effusion would be "paramalignant."

Pleural fluid specimens should be sent for cytologic examination in all cases of exudative effusions in patients suspected of harboring an underlying malignancy. The diagnostic yield depends on the nature and extent of the underlying malignancy. Sensitivity is between 50% and 65%. A negative cytologic examination in a patient with a high prior probability of malignancy should be followed by one repeat thoracentesis. If that examination is negative, thoracoscopy is preferred to closed pleural biopsy. The sensitivity of thoracoscopy is 92–96%.

C. Imaging

The lung is less dense than water and floats on pleural fluid that accumulates in dependent regions. Subpulmonary fluid may appear as lateral displacement of the apex of the diaphragm with an abrupt slope to the costophrenic sulcus or a greater than 2 cm separation between the gastric air bubble and the lung. On a standard upright chest radiograph, approximately 75–100 mL of pleural fluid must accumulate in the posterior costophrenic sulcus to be visible on the lateral view, and 175–200 mL must be present in the lateral costophrenic sulcus to be visible on the frontal view. Chest CT scans may identify as little as 10 mL of fluid. At least 1 cm of fluid on the decubitus view is necessary to permit blind thoracentesis. Ultrasonography is useful to guide thoracentesis in the setting of smaller effusions.

Pleural fluid may become trapped (loculated) by pleural adhesions, thereby forming unusual collections along the lateral chest wall or within lung fissures. Round or oval fluid collections in fissures that resemble intraparenchymal masses are called pseudotumors. Massive pleural effusion causing opacification of an entire hemithorax is most commonly caused by cancer but may be seen in tuberculosis and other diseases.

▶ Treatment

A. Transudative Pleural Effusion

Transudative pleural effusions characteristically occur in the absence of pleural disease. Therefore, treatment is directed at the underlying condition. Therapeutic thoracentesis for severe dyspnea typically offers only transient benefit. Pleurodesis and tube thoracostomy are rarely indicated.

B. Malignant Pleural Effusion

Chemotherapy or radiation therapy or both offer temporary control in some malignant effusions but are generally

Table 9–26. Characteristics of important exudative pleural effusions.

Etiology or Type of Effusion	Gross Appearance	White Blood Cell Count (cells/mcL)	Red Blood Cell Count (cells/mcL)	Glucose	Comments
Malignancy	Turbid to bloody; occasionally serous	1000 to < 100,000 M	100 to several hundred thousand	Equal to serum levels; < 60 mg/dL in 15% of cases	Eosinophilia uncommon; positive results on cytologic examination
Uncomplicated parapneumonic	Clear to turbid	5000–25,000 P	< 5000	Equal to serum levels	Tube thoracostomy unnecessary
Empyema	Turbid to purulent	25,000–100,000 P	< 5000	Less than serum levels; often very low	Drainage necessary; putrid odor suggests anaerobic infection
Tuberculosis	Serous to serosanguineous	5000–10,000 M	< 10,000	Equal to serum levels; occasionally < 60 mg/dL	Protein > 4.0 g/dL and may exceed 5 g/dL; eosinophils (> 10%) or mesothelial cells (> 5%) make diagnosis unlikely; see text for discussion of additional diagnostic tests
Rheumatoid	Turbid; greenish yellow	1000–20,000 M or P	< 1000	< 40 mg/dL	Secondary empyema common; high LD, low complement, high rheumatoid factor, cholesterol crystals are characteristic
Pulmonary infarction	Serous to grossly bloody	1000–50,000 M or P	100 to > 100,000	Equal to serum levels	Variable findings; no pathognomonic features
Esophageal rupture	Turbid to purulent; red-brown	< 5000 to > 50,000 P	1000–10,000	Usually low	High amylase level (salivary origin); pneumothorax in 25% of cases; effusion usually on left side; pH < 6.0 strongly suggests diagnosis
Pancreatitis	Turbid to serosanguineous	1000–50,000 P	1000–10,000	Equal to serum levels	Usually left-sided; high amylase level

LD, lactate dehydrogenase; M, mononuclear cell predominance; P, polymorphonuclear leukocyte predominance.

ineffective in lung cancer in the pleural space except for small-cell lung cancer. Asymptomatic malignant effusions usually do not require specific treatment. Symptomatic patients should have a therapeutic thoracentesis. If symptoms are relieved but the effusion returns, the options are serial thoracenteses, attempted pleurodesis, or placement of an indwelling drainage catheter that the patient can access at home. Choice among these options depends on the rate of reaccumulation in addition to the functional status, tolerance for discomfort, and life expectancy of the patient. Consultation with a thoracic specialist is advised. (Chapter 39.)

C. Parapneumonic Pleural Effusion

Parapneumonic pleural effusions are divided into three categories: simple or uncomplicated, complicated, and empyema. **Uncomplicated parapneumonic effusions** are free-flowing sterile exudates of modest size that resolve quickly with antibiotic treatment of pneumonia. They do not need drainage. **Empyema** is gross infection of the pleural space indicated by positive Gram stain or culture. Empyema should always be drained by tube thoracostomy

to facilitate clearance of infection and to reduce the probability of fibrous encasement of the lung, causing permanent pulmonary impairment.

Complicated parapneumonic effusions present the most difficult management decisions. They tend to be larger than simple parapneumonic effusions and to show more evidence of inflammatory stimuli, such as low glucose level, low pH, or evidence of loculation. Inflammation probably reflects ongoing bacterial invasion of the pleural space despite rare positive bacterial cultures. The morbidity associated with complicated effusions is due to their tendency to form a fibropurulent pleural "peel," trapping otherwise functional lung and leading to permanent impairment. Tube thoracostomy is indicated when pleural fluid glucose is less than 60 mg/dL (less than 3.3 mmol/L) or the pH is less than 7.2. These thresholds have not been prospectively validated and should not be interpreted strictly. The clinician should consider drainage of a complicated effusion if the pleural fluid pH is between 7.2 and 7.3 or the LD is greater than 1000 units/L (greater than 20 mckat/L). Pleural fluid cell count and protein have little diagnostic value in this setting.

Tube thoracostomy drainage of empyema or complicated parapneumonic effusions is frequently complicated by loculation that prevents adequate drainage. Intrapleural instillation of fibrinolytic agents has not been shown in controlled trials to improve drainage. The combination of intrapleural tissue plasminogen activator and deoxyribonuclease (DNase), an enzyme that catalyses extracellular DNA and degrades biofilm formation within the pleural cavity, has been found to improve clinical outcome (increased drainage, decreased length of stay and surgical referral) compared with placebo or either agent alone.

D. Hemothorax

A small-volume hemothorax that is stable or improving on chest radiographs may be managed by close observation. In all other cases, hemothorax is treated by immediate insertion of a large-bore thoracostomy tube to: (1) drain existing blood and clot, (2) quantify the amount of bleeding, (3) reduce the risk of fibrothorax, and (4) permit apposition of the pleural surfaces in an attempt to reduce hemorrhage. Thoracotomy may be indicated to control hemorrhage, remove clot, and treat complications such as bronchopleural fistula formation.

Azzopardi M et al. Current controversies in the management of malignant pleural effusions. Semin Respir Crit Care Med. 2014 Dec;35(6):723–31. [PMID: 25463163]

Fortin M et al. Pleural controversies: indwelling pleural catheter vs. pleurodesis for malignant pleural effusions. J Thorac Dis. 2015 Jun;7(6):1052–7. [PMID: 26150918]

Kummerfeldt CE et al. Improving the predictive accuracy of identifying exudative effusions. Chest. 2014 Mar 1;145(3): 586–92. [PMID: 24008773]

Light RW. Pleural effusions. Med Clin North Am. 2011 Nov;95 (6):1055–70. [PMID: 22032427]

Vorster MJ et al. Tuberculous pleural effusions: advances and controversies. J Thorac Dis. 2015 Jun;7(6):981–91. [PMID: 26150911]

Wilcox ME et al. Does this patient have an exudative pleural effusion? The Rational Clinical Examination systematic review. JAMA. 2014 Jun 18;311(23):2422–31. [PMID: 24938565]

SPONTANEOUS PNEUMOTHORAX

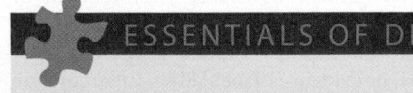

ESSENTIALS OF DIAGNOSIS

► Acute onset of unilateral chest pain and dyspnea.

► Minimal physical findings in mild cases; unilateral chest expansion, decreased tactile fremitus, hyperresonance, diminished breath sounds, mediastinal shift, cyanosis and hypotension in tension pneumothorax.

► Presence of pleural air on chest radiograph.

► General Considerations

Pneumothorax, or accumulation of air in the pleural space, is classified as spontaneous (primary or secondary) or traumatic. Primary spontaneous pneumothorax occurs in the absence of an underlying lung disease, whereas secondary spontaneous pneumothorax is a complication of preexisting pulmonary disease. Traumatic pneumothorax results from penetrating or blunt trauma. Iatrogenic pneumothorax may follow procedures such as thoracentesis, pleural biopsy, subclavian or internal jugular vein catheter placement, percutaneous lung biopsy, bronchoscopy with transbronchial biopsy, and positive-pressure mechanical ventilation. Tension pneumothorax usually occurs in the setting of penetrating trauma, lung infection, cardiopulmonary resuscitation, or positive-pressure mechanical ventilation. In tension pneumothorax, the pressure of air in the pleural space exceeds ambient pressure throughout the respiratory cycle. A check-valve mechanism allows air to enter the pleural space on inspiration and prevents egress of air on expiration.

Primary pneumothorax affects mainly tall, thin boys and men between the ages of 10 and 30 years. It is thought to occur from rupture of subpleural apical blebs in response to high negative intrapleural pressures. Family history and cigarette smoking may also be important factors.

Secondary pneumothorax occurs as a complication of COPD, asthma, cystic fibrosis, tuberculosis, *Pneumocystis* pneumonia, menstruation (catamenial pneumothorax), and a wide variety of interstitial lung diseases, including sarcoidosis, lymphangioleiomyomatosis, Langerhans cell histiocytosis, and tuberous sclerosis. Aerosolized pentamidine and a prior history of *Pneumocystis* pneumonia are considered risk factors for the development of pneumothorax. One-half of patients with pneumothorax in the setting of recurrent (but not primary) *Pneumocystis* pneumonia will develop pneumothorax on the contralateral side. The mortality rate of pneumothorax in *Pneumocystis* pneumonia is high.

► Clinical Findings

A. Symptoms and Signs

Chest pain ranging from minimal to severe on the affected side and dyspnea occur in nearly all patients. Symptoms usually begin during rest and usually resolve within 24 hours even if the pneumothorax persists. Alternatively, pneumothorax may present with life-threatening respiratory failure if underlying COPD or asthma is present.

If pneumothorax is small (less than 15% of a hemithorax), physical findings, other than mild tachycardia, are normal. If pneumothorax is large, diminished breath sounds, decreased tactile fremitus, and decreased movement of the chest are often noted. Tension pneumothorax should be suspected in the presence of marked tachycardia, hypotension, and mediastinal or tracheal shift.

B. Laboratory Findings

Arterial blood gas analysis is often unnecessary but reveals hypoxemia and acute respiratory alkalosis in most patients. Left-sided primary pneumothorax may produce QRS axis and precordial T-wave changes on the ECG that may be misinterpreted as acute myocardial infarction.

C. Imaging

Demonstration of a visceral pleural line on chest radiograph is diagnostic and may be seen only on an expiratory film. A few patients have secondary pleural effusion that demonstrates a characteristic air-fluid level on chest radiography. In supine patients, pneumothorax on a conventional chest radiograph may appear as an abnormally radiolucent costophrenic sulcus (the "deep sulcus" sign). In patients with tension pneumothorax, chest radiographs show a large amount of air in the affected hemithorax and contralateral shift of the mediastinum.

► Differential Diagnosis

If the patient is a young, tall, thin, cigarette-smoking man, the diagnosis of primary spontaneous pneumothorax is usually obvious and can be confirmed by chest radiograph. In secondary pneumothorax, it is sometimes difficult to distinguish loculated pneumothorax from an emphysematous bleb. Occasionally, pneumothorax may mimic myocardial infarction, pulmonary embolism, or pneumonia.

► Complications

Tension pneumothorax may be life-threatening. Pneumomediastinum and subcutaneous emphysema may occur as complications of spontaneous pneumothorax. If pneumomediastinum is detected, rupture of the esophagus or a bronchus should be considered.

► Treatment

Treatment depends on the severity of the pneumothorax and the nature of the underlying disease. In a reliable patient with a small (less than 15% of a hemithorax), stable, spontaneous primary pneumothorax, observation alone may be appropriate. Many small pneumothoraces resolve spontaneously as air is absorbed from the pleural space; supplemental oxygen therapy may increase the rate of reabsorption. Simple aspiration drainage of pleural air with a small-bore catheter (eg, 16-gauge angiocatheter or larger drainage catheter) can be performed for spontaneous primary pneumothoraces that are large or progressive. Placement of a small-bore chest tube (7F to 14F) attached to a one-way Heimlich valve provides protection against development of tension pneumothorax and may permit observation from home. The patient should be treated symptomatically for cough and chest pain, and followed with serial chest radiographs every 24 hours.

Patients with secondary pneumothorax, large pneumothorax, tension pneumothorax, or severe symptoms or those who have a pneumothorax on mechanical ventilation should undergo chest tube placement (tube thoracostomy). The chest tube is placed under water-seal drainage, and suction is applied until the lung expands. The chest tube can be removed after the air leak subsides.

All patients who smoke should be advised to discontinue smoking and warned that the risk of recurrence is 50% if cigarette smoking is continued. Future exposure to high altitudes, flying in unpressurized aircraft, and scuba diving should be avoided.

Indications for thoracoscopy or open thoracotomy include recurrences of spontaneous pneumothorax, any occurrence of bilateral pneumothorax, and failure of tube thoracostomy for the first episode (failure of lung to reexpand or persistent air leak). Surgery permits resection of blebs responsible for the pneumothorax and pleurodesis by mechanical abrasion and insufflation of talc.

Management of pneumothorax in patients with *Pneumocystis* pneumonia is challenging because of a tendency toward recurrence, and there is no consensus on the best approach. Use of a small chest tube attached to a Heimlich valve has been proposed to allow the patient to leave the hospital. Some clinicians favor its insertion early in the course.

► Prognosis

An average of 30% of patients with spontaneous pneumothorax experience recurrence of the disorder after either observation or tube thoracostomy for the first episode. Recurrence after surgical therapy is less frequent. Following successful therapy, there are no long-term complications.

Ashby M et al. Conservative versus interventional management for primary spontaneous pneumothorax in adults. Cochrane Database Syst Rev. 2014 Dec 18;12:CD010565. [PMID: 25519778]

Bintcliffe OJ et al. Spontaneous pneumothorax: time to rethink management? Lancet Respir Med. 2015 Jul;3(7):578–88. [PMID: 26170077]

Visouli AN et al. Catamenial pneumothorax. J Thorac Dis. 2014 Oct;6(Suppl 4):S448–60. [PMID: 25337402]

DISORDERS OF CONTROL OF VENTILATION

The principal influences on ventilatory control are arterial P_{CO_2}, pH, P_{O_2}, and brainstem tissue pH. These variables are monitored by peripheral and central chemoreceptors. Under normal conditions, the ventilatory control system maintains arterial pH and P_{CO_2} within narrow limits; arterial P_{O_2} is more loosely controlled.

Abnormal control of ventilation can be seen with a variety of conditions ranging from rare disorders, such as central alveolar hypoventilation, Ondine curse, neuromuscular disorders, myxedema, starvation, and carotid body resection to more common disorders, such as asthma, COPD, obesity, heart failure, and sleep-related breathing disorders. A few of these disorders will be discussed in this section.

Annane D et al. Nocturnal mechanical ventilation for chronic hypoventilation in patients with neuromuscular and chest wall disorders. Cochrane Database Syst Rev. 2014 Dec 13; 12: CD001941. [PMID: 25503955]

Böing S et al. Chronic hypoventilation syndromes and sleep-related hypoventilation. J Thorac Dis. 2015 Aug;7(8):1273–85. [PMID: 26380756]

OBESITY-HYPOVENTILATION SYNDROME (PICKWICKIAN SYNDROME)

In obesity-hypoventilation syndrome, alveolar hypoventilation appears to result from a combination of blunted ventilatory drive and increased mechanical load imposed upon the chest by obesity. Voluntary hyperventilation returns the P_{CO_2} and the P_{O_2} toward normal values, a correction not seen in lung diseases causing chronic respiratory failure, such as COPD. Most patients with obesity-hypoventilation syndrome also suffer from obstructive sleep apnea, which must be treated aggressively if identified as a comorbid disorder. Therapy of obesity-hypoventilation syndrome consists mainly of weight loss, which improves hypercapnia and hypoxemia as well as the ventilatory responses to hypoxia and hypercapnia. NIPPV is helpful in some patients. Respiratory stimulants may be helpful and include theophylline, acetazolamide, and medroxyprogesterone acetate, 10–20 mg every 8 hours orally. Improvement in hypoxemia, hypercapnia, erythrocytosis, and cor pulmonale are goals of therapy.

Chau EH et al. Obesity hypoventilation syndrome: a review of epidemiology, pathophysiology, and perioperative considerations. Anesthesiology. 2012 Jul;117(1):188–205. [PMID: 22614131]

Pierce AM et al. Obesity hypoventilation syndrome: current theories of pathogenesis. Curr Opin Pulm Med. 2015 Nov;21(6):557–62. [PMID: 26390338]

Verbraecken J et al. Respiratory mechanics and ventilatory control in overlap syndrome and obesity hypoventilation. Respir Res. 2013 Nov 20;14:132. [PMID: 24256627]

HYPERVENTILATION SYNDROMES

Hyperventilation is an increase in alveolar ventilation that leads to hypocapnia. It may be caused by a variety of conditions, such as pregnancy, hypoxemia, obstructive and infiltrative lung diseases, sepsis, hepatic dysfunction, fever, and pain. The term "central neurogenic hyperventilation" denotes a monotonous, sustained pattern of rapid and deep breathing seen in comatose patients with brainstem injury of multiple causes. Functional hyperventilation may be acute or chronic. **Acute hyperventilation** presents with hyperpnea, paresthesias, carpopedal spasm, tetany, and anxiety. **Chronic hyperventilation** may present with various nonspecific symptoms, including fatigue, dyspnea, anxiety, palpitations, and dizziness. The diagnosis of chronic hyperventilation syndrome is established if symptoms are reproduced during voluntary hyperventilation. Once organic causes of hyperventilation have been excluded, treatment of acute hyperventilation consists of breathing through pursed lips or through the nose with one nostril pinched, or rebreathing expired gas from a paper bag held over the face in order to decrease respiratory alkalemia and its associated symptoms. Anxiolytic drugs may also be useful.

Jones M et al. Breathing exercises for dysfunctional breathing/hyperventilation syndrome in adults. Cochrane Database Syst Rev. 2013 May 31;5:CD009041. [PMID: 23728685]

SLEEP-RELATED BREATHING DISORDERS

Abnormal ventilation during sleep is manifested by apnea (breath cessation for at least 10 seconds) or hypopnea (decrement in airflow with drop in hemoglobin saturation of at least 4%). Episodes of apnea are **central** if ventilatory effort is absent for the duration of the apneic episode, **obstructive** if ventilatory effort persists throughout the apneic episode but no airflow occurs because of transient obstruction of the upper airway, and **mixed** if absent ventilatory effort precedes upper airway obstruction during the apneic episode. Pure central sleep apnea is uncommon; it may be an isolated finding or may occur in patients with primary alveolar hypoventilation or with lesions of the brainstem. Obstructive and mixed sleep apneas are more common and may be associated with life-threatening cardiac arrhythmias, severe hypoxemia during sleep, daytime somnolence, pulmonary hypertension, cor pulmonale, systemic hypertension, and secondary erythrocytosis.

OBSTRUCTIVE SLEEP APNEA

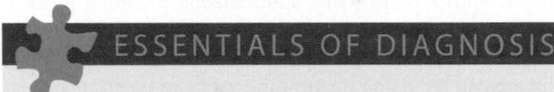

ESSENTIALS OF DIAGNOSIS

▶ Daytime somnolence or fatigue.

▶ A history of loud snoring with witnessed apneic events.

▶ Overnight polysomnography demonstrating apneic episodes with hypoxemia.

▶ General Considerations

Upper airway obstruction during sleep occurs when loss of normal pharyngeal muscle tone allows the pharynx to collapse passively during inspiration. Patients with anatomically narrowed upper airways (eg, micrognathia, macroglossia, obesity, tonsillar hypertrophy) are predisposed to the development of obstructive sleep apnea. Ingestion of alcohol or sedatives before sleeping or nasal obstruction of any type, including the common cold, may precipitate or worsen the condition. Hypothyroidism and cigarette smoking are additional risk factors for obstructive sleep apnea. Before making the diagnosis of obstructive sleep apnea, a drug history should be obtained and a seizure disorder, narcolepsy, and depression should be excluded.

▶ Clinical Findings

A. Symptoms and Signs

Most patients with obstructive or mixed sleep apnea are obese, middle-aged men. Arterial hypertension is common. Patients may complain of excessive daytime somnolence, morning sluggishness and headaches, daytime fatigue, cognitive impairment, recent weight gain, and impotence. Bed partners usually report loud cyclical snoring, breath cessation, witnessed apneas, restlessness, and thrashing movements of the extremities during sleep. Personality changes, poor judgment, work-related problems, depression, and intellectual deterioration (memory impairment, inability to concentrate) may also be observed.

Physical examination may be normal or may reveal systemic and pulmonary hypertension with cor pulmonale. The patient may appear sleepy or even fall asleep during the evaluation. The oropharynx is frequently found to be narrowed by excessive soft tissue folds, large tonsils, pendulous uvula, or prominent tongue. Nasal obstruction by a deviated nasal septum, poor nasal airflow, and a nasal twang to the speech may be observed. A "bull neck" appearance is common.

B. Laboratory Findings

Erythrocytosis is common. Thyroid function tests (serum, TSH, FT_4) should be obtained to exclude hypothyroidism.

C. Other Studies

Observation of the sleeping patient may reveal loud snoring interrupted by episodes of increasingly strong ventilatory effort that fail to produce airflow. A loud snort often accompanies the first breath following an apneic episode. Definitive diagnostic evaluation for suspected sleep apnea includes otorhinolaryngologic examination and overnight polysomnography (the monitoring of multiple physiologic factors during sleep). Screening may be performed using home nocturnal pulse oximetry, which when normal has a high negative predictive value in ruling out significant sleep apnea. A complete **polysomnography** examination includes electroencephalography, electro-oculography, electromyography, ECG, pulse oximetry, and measurement of respiratory effort and airflow. Polysomnography reveals apneic episodes lasting as long as 60 seconds. Oxygen saturation falls, often to very low levels. Bradydysrhythmias, such as sinus bradycardia, sinus arrest, or atrioventricular block, may occur. Tachydysrhythmias, including paroxysmal supraventricular tachycardia, atrial fibrillation, and ventricular tachycardia, may be seen once airflow is reestablished.

▶ Treatment

Weight loss and strict avoidance of alcohol and hypnotic medications are the first steps in management. Weight loss may be curative, but most patients are unable to lose the 10–20% of body weight required. **Nasal continuous positive airway pressure (nasal CPAP)** at night is curative in many patients. Polysomnography is frequently necessary to determine the level of CPAP (usually 5–15 cm H_2O) necessary to abolish obstructive apneas. Unfortunately, **only about 75% of patients continue to use nasal CPAP after 1 year.** Pharmacologic therapy for obstructive sleep apnea is disappointing. Supplemental oxygen may lessen the severity of nocturnal desaturation but may also lengthen apneas; it should not be routinely prescribed without polysomnography to assess the effects of oxygen therapy. Mechanical devices inserted into the mouth at bedtime to hold the jaw forward and prevent pharyngeal occlusion have modest effectiveness in relieving apnea; however, patient compliance is not optimal.

Uvulopalatopharyngoplasty (UPPP), a procedure consisting of resection of pharyngeal soft tissue and amputation of approximately 15 mm of the free edge of the soft palate and uvula, is helpful in approximately 50% of selected patients. It is more effective in eliminating snoring than apneic episodes. UPPP may be performed on an outpatient basis with a laser. **Nasal septoplasty** is performed if gross anatomic nasal septal deformity is present. **Tracheostomy** relieves upper airway obstruction and its physiologic consequences and represents the definitive treatment for obstructive sleep apnea. However, it has numerous adverse effects, including granuloma formation, difficulty with speech, and stoma and airway infection. Furthermore, the long-term care of the tracheostomy, especially in obese patients, can be difficult. Tracheostomy and other maxillofacial surgery approaches are reserved for patients with life-threatening arrhythmias or severe disability who have not responded to conservative therapy. A randomized trial of adaptive servo-ventilation in sleep apnea patients with predominant central apnea and impaired left ventricular ejection fraction (less than 45%) reported increased cardiovascular and all-cause mortality in the treatment group.

Aurora RN et al. The treatment of central sleep apnea syndromes in adults: practice parameters with an evidence-based literature review and meta-analyses. Sleep. 2012 Jan 1;35(1):17–40. [PMID: 22215916]
Basner RC. Cardiovascular morbidity and obstructive sleep apnea. N Engl J Med. 2014 Jun 12;370(24):2339–41. Erratum in: N Engl J Med. 2014 Jul 10;371(2):189. [PMID: 24918377]
Bratton DJ et al. CPAP vs. mandibular advancement devices and blood pressure in patient with obstructive sleep apnea: a systematic review and meta-analysis. JAMA. 2015 Dec 1; 314(21):2280–93. [PMID: 26624827]
Cowie MR et al. Adaptive servo-ventilation for central sleep apnea in systolic heart failure. N Engl J Med. 2015 Sep 17; 373(12):1095–105. [PMID: 26323938]
Jordan AS et al. Adult obstructive sleep apnoea. Lancet. 2014 Feb 22;383(9918):736–47. [PMID: 23910433]
Qaseem A et al. Diagnosis of obstructive sleep apnea in adults: a clinical practice guideline from the American College of Physicians. Ann Intern Med. 2014 Aug 5;161(3):210–20. [PMID: 25089864]

▼ ACUTE RESPIRATORY FAILURE

Respiratory failure is defined as respiratory dysfunction resulting in abnormalities of oxygenation or ventilation (CO_2 elimination) severe enough to threaten the function of vital organs. Arterial blood gas criteria for respiratory failure are not absolute but may be arbitrarily established as a Po_2 under 60 mm Hg (7.8 kPa) or a Pco_2 over 50 mm Hg (6.5 kPa). Acute respiratory failure may occur in a variety of pulmonary and nonpulmonary disorders (Table 9–27). Only a few selected general principles of management will be reviewed here.

▶ Clinical Findings

Symptoms and signs of acute respiratory failure are those of the underlying disease combined with those of hypoxemia or hypercapnia. The chief symptom of hypoxemia is dyspnea, though profound hypoxemia may exist in the absence of complaints. Signs of hypoxemia include cyanosis, restlessness, confusion, anxiety, delirium, tachypnea, bradycardia or tachycardia, hypertension, cardiac dysrhythmias, and tremor. Dyspnea and headache are the cardinal symptoms of hypercapnia. Signs of hypercapnia include peripheral and conjunctival hyperemia, hypertension, tachycardia, tachypnea, impaired consciousness,

Table 9–27. Selected causes of acute respiratory failure in adults.

Airway disorders	Neuromuscular and related disorders
Asthma	Primary neuromuscular
Acute exacerbation of chronic bronchitis or emphysema	diseases
Obstruction of pharynx, larynx, trachea, main stem bronchus, or lobar bronchus by edema, mucus, mass, or foreign body	Guillain-Barré syndrome
	Myasthenia gravis
	Poliomyelitis
Pulmonary edema	Polymyositis
Increased hydrostatic pressure	Drug- or toxin-induced
Left ventricular dysfunction (eg, myocardial ischemia, heart failure)	Botulism
	Organophosphates
	Neuromuscular blocking agents
Mitral regurgitation	Aminoglycosides
Left atrial outflow obstruction (eg, mitral stenosis)	Spinal cord injury
	Phrenic nerve injury or dysfunction
Volume overload states	
Increased pulmonary capillary permeability	Electrolyte disturbances: hypokalemia, hypophosphatemia
Acute respiratory distress syndrome	
Acute lung injury	Myxedema
Unclear etiology	Central nervous system disorders
Neurogenic	
Negative pressure (inspiratory airway obstruction)	Drugs: sedative, hypnotic, opioid, anesthetics
Reexpansion	Brainstem respiratory center disorders: trauma, tumor, vascular disorders, hypothyroidism
Tocolytic-associated	
Parenchymal lung disorders	
Pneumonia	
Interstitial lung diseases	Intracranial hypertension
Diffuse alveolar hemorrhage syndromes	Central nervous system infections
Aspiration	Increased CO$_2$ production
Lung contusion	Fever
Pulmonary vascular disorders	Infection
Thromboembolism	Hyperalimentation with excess caloric and carbohydrate intake
Air embolism	
Amniotic fluid embolism	
Chest wall, diaphragm, and pleural disorders	Hyperthyroidism
	Seizures
Rib fracture	Rigors
Flail chest	Drugs
Pneumothorax	
Pleural effusion	
Massive ascites	
Abdominal distention and abdominal compartment syndrome	

papilledema, and asterixis. The symptoms and signs of acute respiratory failure are both insensitive and nonspecific; therefore, the clinician must maintain a high index of suspicion and obtain arterial blood gas analysis if respiratory failure is suspected.

▶ **Treatment**

Treatment of the patient with acute respiratory failure consists of: (1) specific therapy directed toward the underlying disease; (2) respiratory supportive care directed toward the maintenance of adequate gas exchange; and (3) general supportive care. Only the last two aspects are discussed below.

A. Respiratory Support

Respiratory support has both nonventilatory and ventilatory aspects.

1. Nonventilatory aspects—The main therapeutic goal in acute hypoxemic respiratory failure is to ensure adequate oxygenation of vital organs. Inspired oxygen concentration should be the lowest value that results in an arterial hemoglobin saturation of 90% or more (Po$_2$ 60 mm Hg or more [7.8 kPa or more]). Higher arterial oxygen tensions are of no proven benefit and may be deleterious. Restoration of normoxia may rarely cause hypoventilation in patients with chronic hypercapnia; however, **oxygen therapy should not be withheld for fear of causing progressive respiratory acidemia.** Hypoxemia in patients with obstructive airway disease is usually easily corrected by administering low-flow oxygen by nasal cannula (1–3 L/min) or Venturi mask (24–40%). Higher concentrations of oxygen are necessary to correct hypoxemia in patients with ARDS, pneumonia, and other parenchymal lung diseases.

2. Ventilatory aspects—Ventilatory support consists of maintaining patency of the airway and ensuring adequate alveolar ventilation. Mechanical ventilation may be provided via mask (noninvasive) or through tracheal intubation.

A. NONINVASIVE POSITIVE-PRESSURE VENTILATION— NIPPV delivered via a full face mask or nasal mask is first-line therapy in COPD patients with hypercapnic respiratory failure who can protect and maintain the patency of their airway, handle their own secretions, and tolerate the mask apparatus. Several studies have demonstrated the effectiveness of this therapy in reducing intubation rates and ICU stays in patients with ventilatory failure. A bilevel positive-pressure ventilation mode is preferred for most patients. Patients with acute lung injury or ARDS or those who suffer from severely impaired oxygenation are less likely to benefit and should be intubated if they require mechanical ventilation.

B. TRACHEAL INTUBATION—Indications for tracheal intubation include: (1) hypoxemia despite supplemental oxygen, (2) upper airway obstruction, (3) impaired airway protection, (4) inability to clear secretions, (5) respiratory acidosis, (6) progressive general fatigue, tachypnea, use of accessory respiratory muscles, or mental status deterioration, and (7) apnea. Patients in respiratory failure who undergo a trial of NIPPV and do not improve within 30–90 minutes should be intubated. In general, orotracheal intubation is preferred to nasotracheal intubation in urgent or emergency situations because it is easier, faster, and less traumatic. The tip of the endotracheal tube should be positioned 2–4 cm above the carina and be verified by chest radiograph immediately following intubation. Only tracheal tubes with high-volume, low-pressure air-filled cuffs should be used. Cuff inflation pressure should be kept below 20 mm Hg if possible to minimize tracheal mucosal injury.

c. Mechanical ventilation—Indications for mechanical ventilation include: (1) apnea, (2) acute hypercapnia that is not quickly reversed by appropriate specific therapy, (3) severe hypoxemia, and (4) progressive patient fatigue despite appropriate treatment.

Several modes of positive-pressure ventilation are available. Controlled mechanical ventilation (CMV; also known as assist-control [A-C]) and synchronized intermittent mandatory ventilation (SIMV) are ventilatory modes in which the ventilator delivers a minimum number of breaths of a specified tidal volume each minute. In both CMV and SIMV, the patient may trigger the ventilator to deliver additional breaths. In CMV, the ventilator responds to breaths initiated by the patient above the set rate by delivering additional full tidal volume breaths. In SIMV, additional breaths are not supported by the ventilator unless the pressure support mode is added. Numerous alternative modes of mechanical ventilation now exist, the most popular being pressure support ventilation (PSV), pressure control ventilation (PCV), and CPAP.

PEEP is useful in improving oxygenation in patients with diffuse parenchymal lung disease, such as ARDS. It should be used cautiously in patients with localized parenchymal disease, emphysema, hyperinflation, or very high airway pressure requirements during mechanical ventilation.

d. Complications of mechanical ventilation—Potential complications of mechanical ventilation are numerous. Migration of the tip of the endotracheal tube into a main bronchus can cause atelectasis of the contralateral lung and overdistention of the intubated lung. Barotrauma refers to rupture and loss of integrity of the alveolar space secondary to high transmural pressures applied during positive pressure ventilation. Barotrauma is manifested by subcutaneous emphysema, pneumomediastinum, subpleural air cysts, pneumothorax, or systemic gas embolism. Volutrauma is sometimes used to refer to subtle parenchymal injury due to overdistention of alveoli from excessive tidal volumes without alveolar rupture, mediated through inflammatory rather than physical mechanisms. The principal strategy to avoid volutrauma is the use of low tidal volume ventilation.

Acute respiratory alkalosis caused by overventilation is common. Hypotension induced by elevated intrathoracic pressure that results in decreased return of systemic venous blood to the heart may occur in patients treated with PEEP, particularly those with intravascular volume depletion, and in patients with severe airflow obstruction at high respiratory rates that promote "breath stacking" (dynamic hyperinflation). Ventilator-associated pneumonia is another serious complication of mechanical ventilation.

B. General Supportive Care

Hypokalemia and hypophosphatemia may worsen hypoventilation due to respiratory muscle weakness. Sedative-hypnotics and opioid analgesics should be titrated carefully to avoid oversedation, leading to prolongation of intubation. Temporary paralysis with a nondepolarizing neuromuscular blocking agent is used to facilitate mechanical ventilation and to lower oxygen consumption.

Prolonged muscle weakness due to an acute myopathy is a potential complication of these agents. Myopathy is more common in patients with kidney injury and in those given concomitant corticosteroids.

Psychological and emotional support of the patient and family, skin care to avoid pressure ulcers, and meticulous avoidance of health care–associated infection and complications of tracheal tubes are vital aspects of comprehensive care for patients with acute respiratory failure.

Attention must also be paid to preventing complications associated with serious illness. Stress gastritis and ulcers may be avoided by administering sucralfate (1 g orally twice a day), histamine H_2-receptor antagonists, or PPIs. There is some concern that the latter two agents, which raise gastric pH, may permit increased growth of gram-negative bacteria in the stomach, predisposing to pharyngeal colonization and ultimately HCAP; many clinicians therefore prefer sucralfate. The risk of DVT and PE may be reduced by subcutaneous administration of heparin (5000 units every 12 hours), the use of LMWH (see Table 14–14), or placement of sequential compression devices on the lower extremities.

▶ Course & Prognosis

The course and prognosis of acute respiratory failure vary and depend on the underlying disease. The prognosis of acute respiratory failure caused by uncomplicated sedative or opioid overdose is excellent. Acute respiratory failure in patients with COPD who do not require intubation and mechanical ventilation has a good immediate prognosis. On the other hand, ARDS and respiratory failure associated with sepsis have a poor prognosis.

Cabrini L et al. Noninvasive ventilation and survival in acute care settings: a comprehensive systematic review and meta-analysis of randomized controlled trials. Crit Care Med. 2015 Apr;43(4):880–8. [PMID: 25565461]

ACUTE RESPIRATORY DISTRESS SYNDROME

 ESSENTIALS OF DIAGNOSIS

▶ Onset of respiratory distress, often progressing to respiratory failure, within 7 days of a known clinical insult.

▶ New, bilateral radiographic pulmonary opacities not explained by pleural effusion, atelectasis, or nodules.

▶ Respiratory failure not fully explained by heart failure or volume overload.

▶ Impaired oxygenation, with ratio of partial pressure of oxygen in arterial blood (PaO_2) to fractional concentration of inspired oxygen (FiO_2) less than 300 mm Hg, with PEEP 5 cm H_2O or more.

General Considerations

Acute respiratory distress syndrome (ARDS) as a clinical syndrome is based on three inclusion criteria plus one exclusion criterion, as detailed above. The severity of ARDS is based on the level of oxygenation impairment: **mild,** Pao_2/Fio_2 ratio between 200 and 300 mm Hg; **moderate,** Pao_2/Fio_2 ratio between 100 and 200 mm Hg; and **severe,** Pao_2/Fio_2 ratio less than 100 mm Hg.

ARDS may follow a wide variety of clinical events (Table 9–28). Common risk factors for ARDS include sepsis, aspiration of gastric contents, shock, infection, lung contusion, nonthoracic trauma, toxic inhalation, near-drowning, and multiple blood transfusions. About one-third of ARDS patients initially have sepsis syndrome. Damage to capillary endothelial cells and alveolar epithelial cells is common to ARDS regardless of cause or mechanism of lung injury, resulting in increased vascular permeability and decreased production and activity of surfactant; these abnormalities lead to interstitial and alveolar pulmonary edema, alveolar collapse, and hypoxemia.

Clinical Findings

ARDS is marked by the rapid onset of profound dyspnea that usually occurs 12–48 hours after the initiating event. Labored breathing, tachypnea, intercostal retractions, and crackles are noted on physical examination. Chest radiography shows diffuse or patchy bilateral infiltrates that rapidly become confluent; these characteristically spare the costophrenic angles. Air bronchograms occur in about 80% of cases. Heart size is usually normal, and pleural

Table 9–28. Selected disorders associated with ARDS.

Systemic Insults	Pulmonary Insults
Trauma	Aspiration of gastric contents
Sepsis	Embolism of thrombus, fat, air, or amniotic fluid
Pancreatitis	
Shock	Miliary tuberculosis
Multiple transfusions	Diffuse pneumonia (eg, SARS)
Disseminated intravascular coagulation	Acute eosinophilic pneumonia
	Cryptogenic organizing pneumonitis
Burns	
Drugs and drug overdose	Upper airway obstruction
Opioids	Free-base cocaine smoking
Aspirin	Near-drowning
Phenothiazines	Toxic gas inhalation
Tricyclic antidepressants	Nitrogen dioxide
Amiodarone	Chlorine
Chemotherapeutic agents	Sulfur dioxide
Nitrofurantoin	Ammonia
Protamine	Smoke
Thrombotic thrombocytopenic purpura	Oxygen toxicity
	Lung contusion
Cardiopulmonary bypass	Radiation exposure
Head injury	High-altitude exposure
Paraquat	Lung reexpansion or reperfusion

ARDS, acute respiratory distress syndrome; SARS, severe acute respiratory syndrome.

effusions are small or nonexistent. Marked hypoxemia occurs that is refractory to treatment with supplemental oxygen. Many patients with ARDS demonstrate multiple organ failure, particularly involving the kidneys, liver, gut, central nervous system, and cardiovascular system.

Differential Diagnosis

Since ARDS is a physiologic and radiographic syndrome rather than a specific disease, the concept of differential diagnosis does not strictly apply. Normal-permeability ("cardiogenic" or hydrostatic) pulmonary edema must be excluded, however, because specific therapy is available for that disorder. Emergent echocardiogram or measurement of pulmonary capillary wedge pressure by means of a flow-directed pulmonary artery catheter may be required in selected patients with suspected cardiac dysfunction; routine use in ARDS is discouraged.

Prevention

No measures that effectively prevent ARDS have been identified; specifically, prophylactic use of PEEP in patients at risk for ARDS has not been shown to be effective. Intravenous methylprednisolone does not prevent ARDS when given early to patients with sepsis syndrome or septic shock.

Treatment

The first principle in management is to identify and treat the primary condition that has led to ARDS. Meticulous supportive care must then be provided to compensate for the severe dysfunction of the respiratory system associated with ARDS and to prevent complications.

Treatment of the hypoxemia seen in ARDS usually requires tracheal intubation and positive-pressure mechanical ventilation. The lowest levels of PEEP (used to recruit atelectatic alveoli) and supplemental oxygen required to maintain the Pao_2 above 55 mm Hg (7.13 kPa) or the Sao_2 above 88% should be used. Efforts should be made to decrease Fio_2 as soon as possible in order to avoid oxygen toxicity. PEEP can be increased as needed as long as cardiac output and oxygen delivery do not decrease and airway pressures do not increase excessively. Prone positioning frequently improves oxygenation by helping recruit atelectatic alveoli and may have a mortality benefit in severe ARDS. In one placebo-controlled randomized trial, neuromuscular blockade (by continuous infusion of cisatracurium at 37.5 mg/h) for 48 hours upon initiation of mechanical ventilation was associated with improved mortality and more ventilator-free days in patients with Pao_2/Fio_2 ratio less than 120 mm Hg.

A variety of mechanical ventilation strategies are available. The most significant advance in the treatment of ARDS over the past 20 years has been the recognition of the potential for excessive alveolar stretch to cause lung injury, and the widespread adoption of low tidal volume ventilation. A multicenter study of 800 patients demonstrated that a protocol using volume-control ventilation with low tidal volumes (6 mL/kg of ideal body weight) resulted in a 10% absolute mortality reduction over therapy with standard tidal volumes (defined as 12 mL/kg of ideal body weight).

Approaches to hemodynamic monitoring and fluid management in patients with acute lung injury have been carefully studied. A prospective RCT comparing hemodynamic management guided either by a pulmonary artery catheter or a central venous catheter using an explicit management protocol demonstrated that a pulmonary artery catheter should not be routinely used for the management of acute lung injury. A subsequent randomized, prospective clinical study of restrictive fluid intake and diuresis as needed to maintain central venous pressure less than 4 mm Hg or pulmonary artery occlusion pressure less than 8 mm Hg (conservative strategy group) versus a fluid management protocol to target a central venous pressure of 10–14 mm Hg or a pulmonary artery occlusion pressure 14–18 mm Hg (liberal strategy group), showed that patients in the conservative strategy group experienced faster improvement in lung function and spent significantly fewer days on mechanical ventilation and in the ICU without an improvement in death by 60 days or worsening nonpulmonary organ failure at 28 days. Oxygen delivery can be increased in anemic patients by ensuring that hemoglobin concentrations are at least 7 g/dL (70 g/L); patients are not likely to benefit from higher levels. Increasing oxygen delivery to supranormal levels through the use of inotropes and high hemoglobin concentrations is not clinically useful and may be harmful. Strategies to decrease oxygen consumption include the appropriate use of sedatives, analgesics, and antipyretics.

A large number of innovative therapeutic interventions to improve outcomes in ARDS patients have been or are being investigated. Unfortunately, to date, none have consistently shown benefit in clinical trials. Systemic corticosteroids have been studied extensively with variable and inconsistent results. While a few small studies suggest some specific improved outcomes when given within the first 2 weeks after the onset of ARDS, mortality appears increased when corticosteroids are started more than 2 weeks after the onset of ARDS. Therefore, routine use of corticosteroids is not recommended.

▶ **Course & Prognosis**

Overall, ARDS mortality with low tidal volume ventilation is around 30% in ARDSnet studies. The major causes of death are the primary illness and secondary complications, such as multiple organ system failure or sepsis. Many patients who die of ARDS and its complications die after withdrawal of mechanical ventilation (see Chapter 5). One troubling aspect of ARDS care is that the actual mortality of ARDS in community hospitals continues to be higher than at academic hospitals. This may reflect the fact that a significant number of community hospital–based clinicians have not adopted low lung volume ventilation.

Different clinical syndromes that lead to ARDS carry different prognoses. For example, patients with trauma-associated ARDS have better prognosis, with a mortality rate close to 20%, whereas those with end-stage liver disease have an 80% mortality rate. This presumably reflects the effect of significant comorbidities (trauma patients tend to be younger and healthier) but may also represent different types/severities of inflammation associated with different precipitants of ARDS.

Failure to improve in the first week of treatment is a poor prognostic sign. Survivors tend to be young and pulmonary function generally recovers over 6–12 months, although residual abnormalities often remain, including mild restrictive or obstructive defects, low diffusion capacity, and impaired gas exchange with exercise. Survivors of ARDS also have diminished health-related and pulmonary disease–specific quality of life as well as systemic effects, such as muscle wasting, weakness, and fatigue.

Fanelli V et al. Acute respiratory distress syndrome: new definition, current and future therapeutic options. J Thorac Dis. 2013 Jun;5(3):326–34. [PMID: 23825769]

Hager DN. Recent advances in the management of the acute respiratory distress syndrome. Clin Chest Med. 2015 Sep; 36(3):481–96. [PMID: 26304285]

The ARDS Definition Task Force; Ranieri VM et al. Acute respiratory distress syndrome: the Berlin Definition. JAMA. 2012 Jun 20;307(23):2526–33. [PMID: 22797452]

Heart Disease

Thomas M. Bashore, MD

Christopher B. Granger, MD

Kevin P. Jackson, MD

Manesh R. Patel, MD

CONGENITAL HEART DISEASE

In the United States, there are many more adults with congenital heart disease than children, with an estimated 2 million adults in the United States surviving with congenital heart disease.

Baumgartner H et al; Task Force on the Management of Grown-up Congenital Heart Disease of the European Society of Cardiology (ESC); Association for European Paediatric Cardiology (AEPC); ESC Committee for Practice Guidelines (CPG). ESC Guidelines for the management of grown-up congenital heart disease (new version 2010). Eur Heart J. 2010 Dec;31 (23):2915–57. [PMID: 20801927]

Bhatt AB et al. Congenital heart disease in the older adult: a scientific statement from the American Heart Association. Circulation. 2015 May 26;131(21):1884–931. [PMID: 25896865]

Warnes CA et al. ACC/AHA 2008 Guidelines for the Management of Adults With Congenital Heart Disease. A Report of the American College of Cardiology/American Heart Association Task Force on Practice Guidelines. Circulation. 2008 Dec 2;118(23):e714–833. [PMID: 18997169]

PULMONARY VALVE STENOSIS

 ESSENTIALS OF DIAGNOSIS

▶ Severe cases may present with right-sided heart failure.

▶ P_2 delayed and soft or absent.

▶ Ejection click often present and decreases with inspiration—the only right heart sound that decreases with inspiration; all other right heart sounds increase.

▶ Echocardiography/Doppler is diagnostic.

▶ Patients with peak pulmonic valve gradients greater than 60 mm Hg or a mean of 40 mm Hg by echocardiography/Doppler should undergo intervention regardless of symptoms. Otherwise, operate for symptoms.

▶ General Considerations

Stenosis of the pulmonary valve or right ventricular (RV) infundibulum increases the resistance to RV outflow, raises the RV pressure, and limits pulmonary blood flow. Pulmonic stenosis is often congenital and associated with other cardiac lesions. Pulmonary blood flow preferentially goes to the left lung in valvular pulmonic stenosis. In the absence of associated shunts, arterial saturation is normal. Infundibular stenosis may be so severe that the RV is divided into a low-pressure and high-pressure chamber (double-chambered RV). Peripheral pulmonic stenosis can accompany valvular pulmonic stenosis and may be part of a variety of clinical syndromes, including the congenital rubella syndrome. Patients who have had the Ross procedure for aortic valve disease (transfer of the pulmonary valve to the aortic position with a homograft pulmonary valve placed in the pulmonary position) may experience noncongenital postoperative pulmonic stenosis due to an immune response in the homograft. RV outflow obstructions can also occur when there is a conduit from the RV to the pulmonary artery (PA) that becomes stenotic from degenerative changes over time.

▶ Clinical Findings

A. Symptoms and Signs

Mild cases of pulmonic stenosis are asymptomatic; moderate to severe pulmonic stenosis may cause symptoms of dyspnea on exertion, syncope, chest pain, and eventually RV failure.

On examination, there is often a palpable parasternal lift due to right ventricular hypertrophy (RVH) and the pulmonary outflow tract may be palpable if it is enlarged. A loud, harsh systolic murmur and occasionally a prominent thrill are present in the left second and third interspaces parasternally. The murmur radiates toward the left shoulder due to the flow pattern and increases with inspiration. In mild to moderate pulmonic stenosis, a loud ejection click can be heard to precede the murmur; this sound decreases with inspiration as the increased RV filling from inspiration prematurely opens the valve during atrial systole. This is the only right-sided auscultatory event that decreases with inspiration because the valve excursion in systole is less with inspiration than with expiration due to premature opening of the pulmonary valve with the atrial kick into the RV. The second sound is obscured by the murmur in severe cases; the pulmonary component of S_2 may be diminished, delayed, or absent. A right-sided S_4 and a prominent *a* wave in the venous pulse are present when there is RV diastolic dysfunction or a *c-v* wave may be observed in the JVP if tricuspid regurgitation is present. Pulmonary valve regurgitation is relatively uncommon in primary pulmonic stenosis and may be very difficult to hear, as the gradient between the reduced PA diastolic pressure and the elevated RV diastolic pressure may be quite small (low-pressure pulmonary valve regurgitation).

B. ECG and Chest Radiography

Right axis deviation or RVH is noted; peaked P waves provide evidence of right atrial (RA) overload. Heart size may be normal on radiographs, or there may be a prominent RV and RA or gross cardiac enlargement, depending on the severity. There is often poststenotic dilation of the main and left pulmonary arteries. Pulmonary vascularity is usually normal.

C. Diagnostic Studies

Echocardiography/Doppler is the diagnostic tool of choice, can provide evidence for a doming valve versus a dysplastic valve, can determine the gradient across the valve, and can provide information regarding subvalvular obstruction and the presence or absence of tricuspid or pulmonic valvular regurgitation. Mild pulmonic stenosis is present if the peak gradient by echocardiography/Doppler is less than 30 mm Hg, moderate pulmonic stenosis is present if the peak gradient is between 30 mm Hg and 60 mm Hg, and severe pulmonic stenosis is present if the peak gradient is greater than 60 mm Hg or the mean gradient is greater than 40 mm Hg. Catheterization is usually unnecessary for the diagnosis; it should be used only if the data are unclear or in preparation for either a percutaneous intervention or surgery.

▶ Prognosis & Treatment

Patients with mild pulmonic stenosis have a normal life span with no intervention. Moderate stenosis may be asymptomatic in childhood and adolescence, but symptoms often appear as patients grow older. The degree of stenosis does worsen with time in many patients, so serial follow-up is important. Severe stenosis is rarely associated with sudden death but can cause right heart failure in patients as early as in their 20s and 30s. Pregnancy and exercise tend to be well tolerated except in severe stenosis.

Class I (definitive) indications for intervention include all symptomatic patients and all those with a resting peak gradient greater than 60 mm Hg or a mean greater than 40

mm Hg, regardless of symptoms. Percutaneous balloon valvuloplasty is highly successful in domed valve patients and is the treatment of choice. Surgical commissurotomy can also be done, or pulmonary valve replacement (with either a bioprosthetic valve or homograft) when pulmonary valve regurgitation is too severe or the valve is dysplastic. Pulmonary outflow tract obstruction due to RV to PA conduit obstruction or to homograft pulmonary valve stenosis can be relieved with a percutaneously implanted pulmonary valve. The applicability of this approach to primary pulmonic valve stenosis remains under investigation.

Endocarditis prophylaxis is unnecessary for native valves even after valvuloplasty unless there has been prior pulmonary valve endocarditis (a very rare entity) (see Table 33–4).

▶ When to Refer

All symptomatic patients (regardless of gradient) and all asymptomatic patients whose peak pulmonary valve gradient is greater than 60 mm Hg or whose mean gradient is greater than 40 mm Hg should be referred to a cardiologist with expertise in adult congenital heart disease.

Cuypers JA et al. Pulmonary stenosis: update on diagnosis and therapeutic options. Heart. 2013 Mar;99(5):339–47. [PMID: 23303481]
Warnes CA et al. ACC/AHA 2008 Guidelines for the Management of Adults With Congenital Heart Disease. A Report of the American College of Cardiology/American Heart Association Task Force on Practice Guidelines. Circulation. 2008 Dec 2;118(23):e714–833. [PMID: 18997169]

COARCTATION OF THE AORTA

ESSENTIALS OF DIAGNOSIS

▶ Usual presentation is systemic hypertension.

▶ Echocardiography/Doppler is diagnostic; a gradient of more than 20 mm Hg may be significant due to collaterals around the coarctation reducing gradient despite severe obstruction.

▶ Associated bicuspid aortic valve (in 50–80% of patients).

▶ Systolic pressure is higher in upper extremities than in lower extremities; diastolic pressures are similar.

▶ General Considerations

Coarctation of the aorta consists of localized narrowing of the aortic arch just distal to the origin of the left subclavian artery. Collateral circulation develops around the coarctation site through the intercostal arteries and the branches of the subclavian arteries and can result in a lower transcoarctation gradient by enabling blood flow to bypass the obstruction. **Coarctation is a cause of secondary hypertension and should be considered in young patients with elevated blood pressure (BP).** The renin-angiotensin system is reset, however, and contributes to the hypertension occasionally seen even after coarctation repair. A bicuspid valve is seen in over 50–80% of the cases, and there is an increased incidence of cerebral berry aneurysms.

▶ Clinical Findings

A. Symptoms and Signs

If cardiac failure does not occur in infancy, there are usually no symptoms until the hypertension produces left ventricular (LV) failure. Cerebral hemorrhage, though rare, may occur. Strong arterial pulsations are seen in the neck and suprasternal notch. Hypertension is present in the arms, but the pressure is normal or low in the legs. This difference is exaggerated by exercise. Femoral pulsations are weak and are delayed in comparison with the brachial or radial pulse. Patients may have severe coarctation, but with large collateral blood vessels that course around the obstruction, the gradient across the coarctation may be relatively low. A continuous murmur heard superiorly and midline in the back or over the left anterior chest may be present when these large collaterals are present and is a clue that the coarctation is severe. The coarctation itself may result in systolic ejection murmurs heard in the left upper lung field anteriorly and near the spine on the left side posteriorly. There may be an aortic regurgitation or stenosis murmur due to an associated bicuspid aortic valve.

B. ECG and Chest Radiography

The ECG usually shows LV hypertrophy (LVH). Radiography may show scalloping of the inferior portion of the ribs due to enlarged collateral intercostal arteries, dilation of the left subclavian artery and poststenotic aortic dilation, and LV enlargement. The coarctation region and the poststenotic dilation of the descending aorta may result in a "3" sign along the aortic shadow on the PA chest radiograph (the notch in the "3" representing the area of coarctation).

C. Diagnostic Studies

Echocardiography/Doppler is usually diagnostic and may provide additional evidence for a bicuspid aortic valve. Both MRI and CT can provide excellent images of the coarctation anatomy and one or the other should be done in all patients to define the coarctation anatomic structure. MRI and echocardiography/Doppler can also provide estimates of the gradient across the lesion. Cardiac catheterization provides definitive gradient information and is necessary if percutaneous stenting is to be considered.

▶ Prognosis & Treatment

Cardiac failure is common in infancy and in older untreated patients; it is uncommon in late childhood and young adulthood. Patients with a demonstrated peak gradient of greater than 20 mm Hg should be considered for intervention, especially if there is evidence of collateral blood vessels. Many untreated patients with severe coarctation die of hypertension, rupture of the aorta, infective endarteritis, or cerebral hemorrhage before the age of 50. Aortic dissection also occurs with increased frequency. Coarctation of any significance may be poorly tolerated in pregnancy because of the inability to support the placental flow.

Resection of the coarctation site has a surgical mortality rate of 1–4% and includes risk of spinal cord injury. The percutaneous interventional procedure of choice is endovascular stenting when anatomically feasible; self-expanding and balloon-expandable covered stents have been shown to be advantageous over bare metal stents. Otherwise, surgical resection (usually with end-to-end anastomosis) should be performed. About 25% of surgically corrected patients continue to be hypertensive years after surgery because of permanent changes in the renin-angiotensin system, endothelial dysfunction, aortic stiffness, altered arch morphology, and increased ventricular stiffness. Recurrence of the coarctation stenosis following intervention requires long-term follow-up.

▶ When to Refer

All patients with coarctation and a detectable gradient should be referred to a cardiologist with expertise in adult congenital heart disease.

Brown ML et al. Coarctation of the aorta: lifelong surveillance is mandatory following surgical repair. J Am Coll Cardiol. 2013 Sep 10;62(11):1020–5. [PMID: 23850909]

O'Sullivan J. Late hypertension in patients with repaired aortic coarctation. Curr Hypertens Rep. 2014 Mar;16(3):421. [PMID: 24488485]

Vergales JE et al. Coarctation of the aorta—the current state of surgical and transcatheter therapies. Curr Cardiol Rev. 2013 Aug;9(3):211–9. [PMID: 23909637]

Warnes CA et al. ACC/AHA 2008 Guidelines for the Management of Adults With Congenital Heart Disease. A Report of the American College of Cardiology/American Heart Association Task Force on Practice Guidelines. Circulation. 2008 Dec 2;118(23):e714–833. [PMID: 18997169]

ATRIAL SEPTAL DEFECT & PATENT FORAMEN OVALE

ESSENTIALS OF DIAGNOSIS

▶ Often asymptomatic and discovered on routine physical examination.

▶ RV lift; S_2 widely split and fixed.

▶ Echocardiography/Doppler is diagnostic.

▶ All atrial septal defects (ASD) should be closed if there is any evidence of an RV volume overload regardless of symptoms.

▶ A patent foramen ovale (PFO), present in 25% of the population, rarely can lead to paradoxic emboli. Suspicion should be highest in patients who have cryptogenic stroke before age 55 years.

General Considerations

The most common form of ASD (80% of cases) is **persistence of the ostium secundum** in the mid-septum. A less common abnormality is **persistence of the ostium primum** (low in the septum). In most patients with an ostium primum defect, there are mitral or tricuspid valve "clefts" as well as a ventricular septal defect (VSD) as part of the atrioventricular (AV) septal defect. A third form of ASD is the **sinus venosus defect,** a hole usually at of the upper or (rarely) the lower part of the atrial septum due to failure of the embryonic superior vena cava or the inferior vena cava to merge with the atria properly. An inferior vena cava sinus venosus defect is uncommon. The superior vena cava sinus venosus defect is usually associated with an anomalous connection of the right upper pulmonary vein into the superior vena cava. The **coronary sinus ASD** is rare and is basically an unroofed coronary sinus. In all cases, normally oxygenated blood from the higher-pressure LA passes into the RA, increasing RV output and pulmonary blood flow. In children, the degree of shunting across these defects may be quite large (pulmonary to systemic blood flow ratios of 3:1 or so). As the RV diastolic pressure rises from the chronic volume overload, the RA pressure may rise and the degree of left-to-right shunting may decrease over time. Eventually, if the RA pressure exceeds the LA, the shunt may reverse and be primarily right-to-left and systemic cyanosis appears. The major factor in the direction of shunt flow is thus the compliance of the respective atrial chambers.

The pulmonary pressures are modestly elevated in most patients with an ASD due to the high pulmonary blood flow, but severe pulmonary hypertension with cyanosis (Eisenmenger physiology) is actually unusual, occurring in only about 15% of the patients with an ASD alone. Increased pulmonary vascular resistance (PVR) and pulmonary hypertension secondary to pulmonary vascular disease rarely occur in childhood or young adult life in secundum defects and are more common in primum defects. Eventual RV failure may occur though with any atrial shunt of significant size, and most shunts should be corrected unless they are quite small (less than 1.5:1 left-to-right shunt). In adults, a large left-to-right shunt may have begun to reverse, so the absolute left-to-right shunt measurement (Qp/Qs, where Qp = pulmonary flow and Qs = systemic flow) at the time the patient is studied may underestimate the original shunt size. In addition, in most people the LV and LA compliance normally declines more over time than the RV and RA compliance, and the natural history of small atrial septal shunts is to increase the left-to-right shunt as the patient ages.

ASDs predispose to atrial fibrillation due to RA enlargement, and paradoxic right-to-left emboli do occur. Interestingly, paradoxic emboli may be more common in patients with a PFO than a true ASD. An **aneurysm of the atrial septum** is not a true aneurysm but rather simply a redundancy of the atrial septum. When present with a PFO, the back and forth swinging of the redundant atrial septum ("jump rope septum") tends to pull open the PFO. This helps explain why more right-to-left shunting occurs in patients with an atrial septal aneurysm and PFO than in those with a PFO alone and creates the anatomic substrate for the occurrence of paradoxical emboli. Other factors may distort the atrial septum (such as an enlarged aorta) and increase shunting in patients with a PFO. Right-to-left PFO shunting may be more prominent upright, creating orthostatic hypoxemia (**platypnea orthodeoxia**).

Clinical Findings

A. Symptoms and Signs

Patients with a small or moderate ASD or with a PFO are asymptomatic unless a complication occurs. There is only trivial shunting in a PFO unless the RA pressure increases for some other reason or the atrial septum is distorted. Shunting in a PFO is more common if an atrial septal aneurysm is present. The increased RA pressure during sleep apnea may result in increased right-to-left shunting and worsen hypoxemia. With larger ASD shunts, exertional dyspnea or heart failure may develop, most commonly in the fourth decade of life or later. Prominent RV and PA pulsations are then readily visible and palpable. A moderately loud systolic ejection murmur can be heard in the second and third interspaces parasternally as a result of increased flow through the pulmonary valve. S_2 is widely split and does not vary with breathing because the left-to-right shunt decreases as the RA pressure increases with inspiration and the RV stroke volume is held relatively constant in inspiration and expiration ("fixed" splitting of the second sound results). In very large left-to-right shunts, a tricuspid rumble may be heard due to the high flow across the tricuspid valve.

B. ECG and Chest Radiography

Right axis deviation or RVH may be present depending on the size of the RV volume overload. Incomplete or complete right bundle branch block is present in nearly all cases of ASD, and superior axis deviation is noted in the complete AV septal defect, where complete heart block is often seen as well. With sinus venosus defects, the P axis is leftward of $+15°$ due to abnormal atrial activation with loss of the upper RA tissue from around the sinus node. The chest radiograph shows large pulmonary arteries, increased pulmonary vascularity, an enlarged RA and RV, and a small aortic knob as with all pre-tricuspid valve cardiac left-to-right shunts. The LA is not traditionally enlarged due to an ASD shunt because the chamber is being decompressed.

C. Diagnostic Studies

Echocardiography demonstrates evidence of RA and RV volume overload. The atrial defect is usually observed by echocardiography, although sinus venosus defects may be elusive since they are high in the atrial septum. Many patients with a PFO also have an atrial septal aneurysm (defined as greater than 10 mm excursion of the septum from the static position). Echocardiography with saline injection (bubble contrast) can demonstrate the right-to-left component of the shunt, and both pulsed and color flow Doppler flow studies can demonstrate shunting in either direction. In platypnea orthodeoxia, the shunt may primarily result from inferior vena cava blood, and a femoral vein saline injection may be required to demonstrate the shunt. Transesophageal echocardiography (TEE) is helpful when transthoracic echocardiography quality is not optimal because it improves the sensitivity for detection of small shunts and provides a better assessment of PFO or ASD anatomy. Both CT and MRI can elucidate the atrial septal anatomy, better detect multiple fenestrations, and demonstrate associated lesions such as anomalous pulmonary venous connections. Atrial septal anatomy can be complex, and MRI, TEE, or CT can reveal whether there is an adequate rim around the defect to allow for safe positioning of an atrial septal occluder device. Cardiac catheterization can define the size and location of the shunt and determine the pulmonary pressure and PVR.

▶ Prognosis & Treatment

Patients with small atrial shunts live a normal life span with no intervention. Large shunts usually cause disability by age 40 years. Because left-to-right shunts and RV overload tend to increase with normal age-related reduction in LV (and subsequently LA) compliance, guidelines suggest that closure of all left-to-right shunts over 1.5:1 should be accomplished either by a percutaneous device or by surgery. This situation always results in RV volume overload if the lesion is left untreated. If the pulmonary systolic pressure is more than two-thirds the systemic systolic pressure, the pulmonary hypertension may preclude ASD closure. Testing with transient balloon occlusion of the shunt and with pulmonary vasodilators may be required in the presence of pulmonary hypertension. After age 40 years, cardiac arrhythmias (especially atrial fibrillation) and heart failure occur with increased frequency due to the chronic right heart volume overload. Paradoxical systemic arterial embolization also becomes more of a concern as RV compliance is lost and the left-to-right shunt begins to reverse.

PFOs are usually not associated with significant shunting, and therefore the patients are hemodynamically asymptomatic and the heart size is normal. However, PFOs can be responsible for paradoxical emboli and are one of the most common causes of cryptogenic strokes in patients under age 55 years. An associated atrial septal aneurysm increases the risk of right-to-left shunting. Interestingly, the risk of recurrent paradoxical emboli is low, and that observation has reduced the value of closing these defects in cryptogenic stroke. Further confounding the advantage of PFO closure for cryptogenic stroke/TIA has been the discovery of frequent bouts of paroxysmal atrial fibrillation using 30-day monitoring in these patients.

Occasionally, a PFO that has not been pathologic may become responsible for cyanosis, especially if the RA pressure is elevated from pulmonary or RV hypertension or from severe tricuspid regurgitation.

Surgery involves stitching or patching of the foramen. For ostium secundum ASDs, percutaneous closure by use of a variety of devices is preferred over surgery when the anatomy is appropriate (usually this means there is enough atrial septal rim around the defect to secure the occluder device).

Patients who have hypoxemia (especially upon standing) should have the PFO closed if no other cause for hypoxia is evident and there is right-to-left shunting demonstrated through the PFO. For patients with cryptogenic stroke or transient ischemic attack, it remains uncertain whether closure of the PFO, either by open surgical or percutaneous techniques, has any advantage over anticoagulation with either warfarin, one of the direct-acting oral anticoagulants, or aspirin. There have been three major trials evaluating the advantage of PFO closure in cryptogenic stroke. None proved the concept valid because of the low rate of recurrent neurologic events. From a practical standpoint, patients younger than 55 years with cryptogenic stroke/transient ischemic attack and no other identifiable cause except for the presence of a PFO should still be considered for PFO closure, albeit the data suggest medical therapy remains an equally viable option. A workup for any causes for hypercoagulability and a 30-day monitor should also be part of the clinical assessment to exclude other potential causes for cryptogenic stroke/transient ischemic attack.

PFO closure is also occasionally recommended for deep sea divers to help prevent the "bends" due to nitrous oxide shunting. Despite much fanfare from small studies suggesting an advantage, there are no strong data to confirm an advantage in PFO closure for patients suffering from migraine headaches. One randomized, placebo-controlled trial did not show a lessening of migraine events with PFO closure.

▶ When to Refer

- All patients with an ASD should be evaluated by a cardiologist with expertise in adult congenital disease to ensure no other structural disease is present and to investigate whether the RV is enlarged.

- If the RA and RV sizes remain normal, serial echocardiography should be performed every 3–5 years.

- If the RA and RV volumes are increased, then referral to a cardiologist who performs percutaneous closure is warranted.

- Patients younger than 55 years with cryptogenic stroke when no other source is identified except for a PFO with right-to-left shunting should be considered for PFO closure.

- Patients with cyanosis and a PFO with evidence of a right-to-left shunt by agitated saline bubble contrast on echocardiography, especially if the cyanosis is worsened upon assuming the upright posture.

Gladstone DJ et al; EMBRACE Investigators and Coordinators. Atrial fibrillation in patients with cryptogenic stroke. N Engl J Med. 2014 Jun 26;370(26):2467–77. [PMID: 24963566]

Katsanos AH et al. Recurrent stroke and patent foramen ovale: a systematic review and meta-analysis. Stroke. 2014 Nov; 45(11):3352–9. [PMID: 25293664]

Lau EM et al. Prevalence of patent foramen ovale and its impact on oxygen desaturation in obstructive sleep apnea. Int J Cardiol. 2013 Apr 30;165(1):35–40. [PMID: 21816494]

Rizvi AA et al. PFO and ASD closure in adulthood: Where do we stand? Curr Treat Options Cardiovasc Med. 2014 Apr;16(4):295. [PMID: 24574109]

Warnes CA et al. ACC/AHA 2008 Guidelines for the Management of Adults With Congenital Heart Disease. A Report of the American College of Cardiology/American Heart Association Task Force on Practice Guidelines. Circulation. 2008 Dec 2;118(23):e714–833. [PMID: 18997169]

VENTRICULAR SEPTAL DEFECT

ESSENTIALS OF DIAGNOSIS

▸ A restrictive VSD is small and makes a louder murmur than an unrestricted one, often with an accompanying thrill. The higher the gradient across the septum, the smaller the left-to-right shunt.

▸ Small defects may be asymptomatic.

▸ Larger defects result in pulmonary hypertension (Eisenmenger physiology) if not repaired or the pulmonary circuit is not protected by RV outflow tract obstruction.

▸ Echocardiography/Doppler is diagnostic.

General Considerations

Congenital VSDs occur in various parts of the ventricular septum. Four types are often described: in **type A,** the outflow tract VSD lies underneath the semilunar valves; in **type B,** the membranous VSD has three variations; in **type C,** the inlet VSD is present below the tricuspid valve and often part of the AV septal defect; and **type D** is the muscular VSD. Membranous and muscular septal defects may spontaneously close in childhood as the septum grows and hypertrophies. A left-to-right shunt is present, the degree depending on associated RV hypertension. The smaller the defect, the greater the gradient from the LV to the RV and the louder the murmur. The presentation in adults depends on the size of the shunt and whether there is associated pulmonic or subpulmonic stenosis that has protected the lung from the systemic pressure and volume. Unprotected lungs with large shunts invariably lead to pulmonary vascular disease and severe pulmonary hypertension (Eisenmenger physiology). VSD sizes are defined by comparison to the aortic root size; a small or restrictive VSD diameter is less than 25% of the aortic root diameter, a moderately restrictive VSD diameter is 25–50% of the aorta, and an unrestricted VSD size is greater than 50% of the aortic diameter.

Clinical Findings

A. Symptoms and Signs

The clinical features depend on the size of the defect and the presence or absence of RV outflow obstruction or increased PVR. Small shunts are associated with loud, harsh holosystolic murmurs in the left third and fourth interspaces along the sternum. A systolic thrill is common.

Larger shunts may create RV volume and pressure overload. If pulmonary hypertension occurs, high-pressure pulmonary valve regurgitation may result. Right heart failure may gradually become evident late in the course, and the shunt will begin to balance or reverse as RV and LV systolic pressures equalize with the advent of pulmonary hypertension. Cyanosis from right-to-left shunting may then occur. Cyanosis with pulmonary hypertension and an intracardiac shunt define the **Eisenmenger syndrome.**

B. ECG and Chest Radiography

The ECG may be normal or may show right, left, or biventricular hypertrophy, depending on the size of the defect and the PVR. With large shunts, the LV, the LA, and the pulmonary arteries are enlarged and pulmonary vascularity is increased on chest radiographs. The RV is often normal until late in the process. If an increased PVR (pulmonary hypertension) evolves, an enlarged PA with pruning of the distal pulmonary vascular bed is seen. In rare cases of a VSD high in the ventricular septum, an aortic cusp (right coronary cusp) may prolapse into the VSD and reduce the VSD shunt but result in acute aortic regurgitation and acute heart failure.

C. Diagnostic Studies

Echocardiography can demonstrate the size of the overloaded chambers and can usually define the defect anatomy. Doppler can qualitatively assess the magnitude of shunting by noting the gradient from LV to RV and, if some tricuspid regurgitation is present, the RV systolic pressure can be estimated. The septal leaflet of the tricuspid valve may be part of the VSD anatomy and the complex appears as a ventricular septal "aneurysm." These membranous septal aneurysms resemble a "windsock" and may fenestrate and result in a VSD shunt being present or may remain intact. Color flow Doppler helps delineate the shunt severity and the presence of valvular regurgitation. MRI and cardiac CT can often visualize the defect and describe any other anatomic abnormalities. MRI can provide quantitative shunt data as well. Cardiac catheterization is usually reserved for those with at least moderate shunting to determine the PVR and the degree of pulmonary hypertension. A PVR of greater than 7.0 absolute units or a PVR/systemic vascular resistance ratio or a systolic PA pressure/systolic aortic pressure ratio greater than 0.67 (two-thirds) generally means the patient's VSD is inoperable. The vasoreactivity of the pulmonary circuit may be tested at catheterization using agents such as inhaled nitric oxide, and if the pulmonary pressures can be lowered enough that the above ratios fall below the two-thirds value, then repair is reasonable as long as the left-to-right VSD shunt is greater than 1.5:1.

Prognosis & Treatment

Patients with a small VSD have a normal life expectancy except for the small risk of infective endocarditis. Antibiotic prophylaxis after dental work is recommended only when the VSD is residual from a prior patch closure or when there is associated pulmonary hypertension and cyanosis (see Tables 33–4, 33–5, and 33–6). With large VSD shunts, heart failure may develop early in life, and survival beyond age 40 years is unusual without intervention.

The ACC/AHA guidelines for the management of patients with VSD include the following:

1. Medical management (Class 2b recommendation [benefit exceeds risk and may be considered]): Pulmonary vasodilatory therapy is appropriate for adults with a VSD and severe pulmonary hypertension. The response to inhaled nitric oxide is used to guide which agent would be the best option.

2. Surgical management (Class 1 recommendation): Closure is indicated when the left-to-right shunt ratio is greater than 2.0 or there is clinical LV volume overload. In addition, closure is recommended if there has been a history of infective endocarditis.

3. Surgical management (Class 2b recommendation): Closure is reasonable if the left-to-right shunt is greater than 1.5 and pulmonary systolic pressure and PVR are less than two-thirds systemic systolic pressure and systemic vascular resistance. Closure is also reasonable if the shunt ratio is greater than 1.5 with evidence of heart failure.

Small shunts (pulmonary-to-systemic flow ratio less than 1.5) in asymptomatic patients do not require surgery or other intervention. The presence of RV infundibular stenosis or pulmonary valve stenosis may protect the pulmonary circuit such that some patients even with a large VSD may still be operable as adults.

Surgical repair of a VSD is generally a low-risk procedure unless there is significant Eisenmenger physiology. Devices for nonsurgical closure of muscular VSDs are approved and those for membranous VSDs are being implanted with promising results; however, conduction disturbance is a major complication. The percutaneous devices are also approved for closure of a VSD related to acute myocardial infarction, although the results in this very high-risk patient population have not been encouraging. The medications used to treat pulmonary hypertension secondary to VSD are similar to those used to treat idiopathic ("primary") pulmonary hypertension and at times can be quite effective.

When to Refer

All patients with a VSD should be referred to a cardiologist with expertise in adult congenital disease to decide if long-term follow-up is warranted.

Anderson BR et al. Contemporary outcomes of surgical ventricular septal defect closure. J Thorac Cardiovasc Surg. 2013 Mar; 145(3):641–7. [PMID: 23414985]

Penny DJ et al. Ventricular septal defect. Lancet. 2011 Mar 26;377(9771):1103–12. [PMID: 21349577]

Warnes CA et al. ACC/AHA 2008 Guidelines for the Management of Adults With Congenital Heart Disease. A Report of the American College of Cardiology/American Heart Association Task Force on Practice Guidelines. Circulation. 2008 Dec 2; 118(23):e714–833. [PMID: 18997169]

Yang J et al. Transcatheter versus surgical closure of perimembranous ventricular septal defects in children: a randomized controlled trial. J Am Coll Cardiol. 2014 Apr 1;63(12):1159–68. [PMID: 24509270]

TETRALOGY OF FALLOT

 ESSENTIALS OF DIAGNOSIS

► Five features are characteristic:
 – VSD.
 – RVH.
 – RV outflow obstruction from infundibular stenosis.
 – Overriding aorta in half (requires less than 50% of the aorta overriding the septum).
 – A right-sided aortic arch in 25%.

► Most adult patients with tetralogy of Fallot have been operated upon, usually with an RV outflow patch and VSD closure.

► Physical examination may be deceptive after classic tetralogy repair, with wide-open pulmonary valve regurgitation often present if a transannular patch was used.

► Echocardiography/Doppler may underestimate significant pulmonary valve regurgitation. Be wary if the RV is enlarged.

► Arrhythmias are common; periodic Holter monitoring is recommended.

► Serious arrhythmias and sudden death may occur if the QRS width is greater than 180 msec or the RV becomes quite large.

General Considerations

Patients with tetralogy of Fallot have a VSD, RV infundibular stenosis, RVH, and a dilated aorta (in about 50% of patients it overrides the septum). If there is an associated ASD, the complex is referred to as pentalogy of Fallot. There may or may not be pulmonary valve stenosis as well, usually due to a bicuspid pulmonary valve or RV outflow hypoplasia. The aorta can be quite enlarged and aortic regurgitation may occur. If more than 50% of the aorta overrides into the RV outflow tract, the anatomy is referred to as a double outlet RV. Two vascular abnormalities are common: a right-sided aortic arch (in 25%) and an anomalous left anterior descending coronary artery from the right cusp (7–9%). The latter is important in that surgical correction must avoid injuring the coronary artery when repairing the RV outflow obstruction.

Most adult patients have undergone prior surgery. If significant RV outflow obstruction is present in the neonatal period, a systemic arterial to pulmonary artery shunt may be the initial surgical procedure to improve pulmonary blood flow, though most infants undergo repair without this first step. Most adults will have had this initial palliative repair, however. The palliative procedure enables blood to reach the underperfused lung either by directly attaching one of the subclavian arteries to a main PA branch (**classic Blalock shunt**) or by creating a conduit between the two (**modified Blalock shunt**). Other types of systemic to pulmonary shunts no longer in use include a window between the right PA and the aorta (**Waterston-Cooley shunt**) or a window between the left PA and the descending aorta (**Potts shunt**). In the adult, there may be a reduced upper extremity pulse on the side used for the classic Blalock procedure. **Total repair** of the tetralogy of Fallot generally includes a VSD patch and usually an enlarging RV outflow tract patch, as well as a take-down of the arterial-pulmonary artery shunt. Often the RV outflow tract patch extends through the pulmonary valve into the PA (**transannular patch**), and the patient is left with varying degrees of pulmonary valve regurgitation (although great effort is made to avoid pulmonary valve regurgitation if at all possible). **Over the years, the volume overload from severe pulmonary valve regurgitation becomes the major hemodynamic problem seen in adults.** Ventricular arrhythmias can also originate from the edge of the patch, and tend to increase with the size of the RV.

▶ Clinical Findings

Most adult patients in whom tetralogy of Fallot has been repaired are relatively asymptomatic unless right heart failure occurs or arrhythmias become an issue. Patients can be active and generally require no specific therapy.

A. Symptoms and Signs

Physical examination should include checking both arms for any loss of pulse from a prior shunt procedure in infancy. The jugular venous pulsations (JVP) may reveal an increased *a* wave from poor RV compliance or rarely a *c-v* wave due to tricuspid regurgitation. The right-sided arch has no consequence. The precordium may be active, often with a persistent pulmonary outflow murmur. P_2 may or may not be audible. A right-sided gallop may be heard. A residual VSD or aortic regurgitation murmur may be present. At times, the insertion site of a prior Blalock or other shunt may create a stenotic area in the branch PA and a continuous murmur occurs as a result.

B. ECG and Chest Radiography

The ECG reveals RVH and right axis deviation; in repaired tetralogy, there is often a right bundle branch block pattern. The chest radiograph shows a classic boot-shaped heart with prominence of the RV and a concavity in the RV outflow tract. This may be less impressive following repair. The aorta may be enlarged and right-sided. Importantly, the width of the QRS should be examined yearly because persons at greatest risk for sudden death are those with a QRS width of more than 180 msec. Most experts recommend Holter monitoring periodically as well, especially if the patient experiences palpitations. The width of the QRS corresponds to the RV size, and in some patients, the QRS width actually decreases following relief of the

pulmonary valve regurgitation with use of a prosthetic pulmonary valve.

C. Diagnostic Studies

Echocardiography/Doppler usually establishes the diagnosis by noting the unrestricted (large) VSD, the RV infundibular stenosis, and the enlarged aorta. In patients who have had tetralogy of Fallot repaired, echocardiography/Doppler also provides data regarding the amount of pulmonary valve regurgitation, RV and LV function, and the presence of aortic regurgitation.

Cardiac MRI and CT can quantitate both the pulmonary insufficiency and the RV volumes. In addition, cardiac MRI and CT can identify whether there is either a native pulmonary arterial branch stenosis or a stenosis at the distal site of a prior arterial-to-PA shunt or other anomalies, such as an ASD. Cardiac catheterization may be required to document the degree of pulmonary valve regurgitation because noninvasive studies depend on velocity gradients. Pulmonary angiography demonstrates the degree of pulmonary valve regurgitation, and RV angiography helps assess any postoperative outflow tract aneurysm.

▶ Prognosis & Treatment

A few patients with "just the right amount" of subpulmonic stenosis enter adulthood without having had surgical correction. However, most adult patients have had surgical repair, including VSD closure, resection of infundibular muscle, and insertion of an outflow tract patch to relieve the subpulmonic obstruction. Many have a transannular patch resulting in pulmonary valve regurgitation. Patients should be monitored to ensure the RV volume does not progressively increase. Low-pressure pulmonary valve regurgitation is difficult to diagnose due to the fact that the RV diastolic pressures tend to be high and the pulmonary arterial diastolic pressure low. This means there is little gradient between the PA and the RV in diastole, so that there may be little murmur or evidence of turbulence on color flow Doppler. If the RV begins to enlarge, it must be assumed that this is due to pulmonary valve regurgitation until proven otherwise. Early surgical pulmonary valve replacement is increasingly being favored. A percutaneous approach to pulmonary valve regurgitation is under investigation.

If an anomalous coronary artery is present, then an extracardiac conduit around it from the RV to the PA may be necessary. By 20-year follow-up, reoperation of the common tetralogy repair is needed in about 10–15%, not only for severe pulmonary valve regurgitation but also for residual infundibular stenosis. Usually the pulmonary valve is replaced with a pulmonary homograft, although a porcine bioprosthetic valve is also suitable. Cryoablation of tissue giving rise to arrhythmias is sometimes performed at the time of reoperation. Branch pulmonary stenosis may be percutaneously opened by stenting. If a conduit has been used already for repair of the RV outflow obstruction, a percutaneous approach with a stented pulmonary valve may be possible. **All patients require endocarditis** prophylaxis (see Tables 33–4, 33–5, and 33–6). Most adults with stable hemodynamics can be quite active, and most women can carry a pregnancy adequately if RV function is preserved.

Atrial fibrillation and ventricular ectopy are common, especially after the age of 45. Left heart disease appears to cause these arrhythmias more often than right heart disease. Biventricular dysfunction is not an uncommon consequence as the patient ages. The cause of associated LV dysfunction is often multifactorial and frequently unclear. Similarly, the aorta may enlarge with accompanying aortic regurgitation, and these lesions can become severe enough to warrant surgical intervention. Patients with RV or LV dysfunction or with dysfunction of both ventricles may require a prophylactic defibrillator.

▶ When to Refer

All patients with tetralogy of Fallot should be referred to a cardiologist with expertise in adult congenital heart disease.

Aboulhosn JA et al; Alliance for Adult Research in Congenital Cardiology (AARCC). Left and right ventricular diastolic function in adults with surgically repaired tetralogy of Fallot: a multi-institutional study. Can J Cardiol. 2013 Jul;29(7):866–72. [PMID: 23369488]

Downing TE et al. Tetralolgy of Fallot: General principles of management. Cardiol Clin. 2015 Nov;33(4):531–41. [PMID: 26471818]

Weinberg CR et al. Pulmonary valve replacement in tetralogy of Fallot. Circulation. 2014 Aug 26;130(9):795–8. [PMID: 25156915]

PATENT DUCTUS ARTERIOSUS

ESSENTIALS OF DIAGNOSIS

▸ Rare in adults.

▸ Adults with a small or moderate size patent ductus arteriosus are usually asymptomatic, at least until middle age.

▸ The lesion is best visualized by MRI, CT, or contrast angiography.

▶ General Considerations

The embryonic ductus arteriosus allows shunting of blood from the PA to the aorta in utero (thus bypassing the lungs). The ductus arteriosus normally closes immediately after birth so that all right heart blood flows to the pulmonary arteries. Failure to close results in a persistent left-to-right shunt connecting the left PA and aorta, usually near the origin of the left subclavian artery. Prior to birth, the ductus is kept patent by the effect of circulating prostaglandins; in the neonate, a patent ductus can often be closed by administration of a prostaglandin inhibitor, such as indomethacin. The effect of the persistent left-to-right shunt on the pulmonary circuit is dependent on the size of the ductus. If large enough, pulmonary hypertension (Eisenmenger physiology) may occur. A small ductus may be well tolerated until adulthood.

▶ Clinical Findings

A. Symptoms and Signs

There are no symptoms unless LV failure or pulmonary hypertension develops. The heart is of normal size or slightly enlarged, with a hyperdynamic apical impulse. The pulse pressure is wide, and diastolic pressure is low. A continuous rough "machinery" murmur, accentuated in late systole at the time of S_2, is heard best in the left first and second interspaces at the left sternal border. Thrills are common. If pulmonary hypertension is present (Eisenmenger physiology), the shunt may reverse and the lower body receives desaturated blood, while the upper body receives saturated blood. Thus, the hands appear normal while the toes are cyanotic and clubbed (differential cyanosis).

B. ECG and Chest Radiography

A normal ECG tracing or LVH is found, depending on the magnitude of shunting. On chest radiographs, the heart is normal in size and contour, or there may be LV and LA enlargement. The PA, aorta, and LA are prominent because they all are in the shunt pathway.

C. Diagnostic Studies

Echocardiography/Doppler can determine LV, RV, and atrial dimensions. Color flow Doppler allows visualization of the high-velocity shunt jet into the proximal left PA. Cardiac MRI and CT, however, are the best noninvasive modalities to demonstrate the ductus size and shape and to assess the size of the pulmonary arteries. Cardiac catheterization can establish the shunt size and direction and also defines the size and anatomic features of the ductus. Invasive hemodynamic testing defines pulmonary pressures and vasodilatory testing can be performed to see if the pulmonary hypertension is reactive.

▶ Prognosis & Treatment

Large shunts cause a high mortality rate from cardiac failure early in life. Smaller shunts are compatible with long-term survival, heart failure being the most common late complication. Infective endocarditis or endarteritis may rarely occur, and antibiotic prophylaxis for dental procedures continues to be recommended (see Tables 33–4, 33–5, and 33–6).

Surgical ligation of the patent ductus can be accomplished with excellent results. If the ductus has a "neck" and is of small enough size, percutaneous approaches using occluder devices are the preferred therapy; there is a high success rate at a very low risk. Patients with Eisenmenger physiology may benefit from pulmonary vasodilator therapy. To monitor these latter patients, serial assessment of toe oxygen saturation as a marker of improvement in the right-to-left shunt is important because of the reversal in flow in the ductus. On rare occasions, the ductus may become aneurysmal and require surgical repair.

Table 10–1 outlines the current recommendations for intervention in adult patients with a patent ductus arteriosus.

Table 10–1. Recommendations for interventions in patients with patent ductus arteriosus.[1]

Class I

A. Closure of a patent ductus arteriosus either percutaneously or surgically is indicated for the following:
   1. Presence of left atrial or left ventricular enlargement, pulmonary artery hypertension, or net left-to-right shunting (level of evidence: C).
   2. Prior endarteritis (level of evidence: C).
B. Consultation with adult congenital heart disease interventional cardiologists is recommended before surgical closure is selected as the method of repair for patients with a calcified patent ductus arteriosus (level of evidence: C).
C. Surgical repair by a surgeon experienced in coronary heart disease surgery is recommended when:
   1. The patent ductus arteriosus is too large for device closure (level of evidence: C).
   2. Distorted ductal anatomy precludes device closure (eg, aneurysm or endarteritis) (level of evidence: B).

Class IIa

A. It is reasonable to close an asymptomatic small patent ductus arteriosus by catheter device (level of evidence: C).
B. Patent ductus arteriosus closure is reasonable for patients with pulmonary artery hypertension with a net left-to-right shunt (level of evidence: C).

Class III

Patent ductus arteriosus closure is not indicated for patients with pulmonary artery hypertension and net right-to-left shunt (level of evidence: C).

[1]Class I indicates treatment is useful and effective, class IIa indicates weight of evidence is in favor of usefulness/efficacy, class IIb indicates weight of evidence is less well established, and class III indicates intervention is not useful/effective and may be harmful. Type A recommendations are based on data derived from multiple randomized clinical trials or meta-analyses. Type B recommendations are based on data derived from a single randomized clinical trial or large nonrandomized studies. Type C recommendations are based on consensus of opinion of the experts or on data derived from small studies, retrospective studies, or registries. ACC/AHA, American College of Cardiology/American Heart Association.

Note it is the only cardiac lesion for which treatment decisions depend on auscultation; if the murmur is audible and there is evidence of any volume overload, it should be closed regardless of symptoms.

► When to Refer

All patients with patent ductus arteriosus should be referred to a cardiologist with expertise in adult congenital disease.

Song S et al. Hybrid approach for aneurysm of patent ductus arteriosus in an adult. Ann Thorac Surg. 2013 Jan;95(1):e15–7. [PMID: 23272885]

Wardle AJ et al. Patent ductus arteriosus: an analysis of management. Cardiol Young. 2014 Oct;24(5):941–3. [PMID: 24153161]

Warnes CA et al. ACC/AHA 2008 Guidelines for the Management of Adults With Congenital Heart Disease. A Report of the American College of Cardiology/American Heart Association Task Force on Practice Guidelines. Circulation. 2008 Dec 2;118(23):e714–833. [PMID: 18997169]

▼ VALVULAR HEART DISEASE

The 2014 AHA/ACC guidelines provide current information on valvular heart disease diagnosis and treatment. The typical findings of each native valve lesion are described in Table 10–2. Table 10–3 outlines bedside maneuvers to distinguish among the various systolic murmurs.

The 2014 update of the AHA/ACC valvular guidelines suggests all lesions may be best classified clinically into one of six categories:

Stage A: Patients at risk for valvular heart disease (VHD).

Stage B: Patients with progressive VHD (mild to moderate severity) and asymptomatic.

Stage C: Asymptomatic patients who have reached criteria for severe VHD.

   C1: Normal LV function.

   C2: Abnormal LV function.

Stage D: Symptomatic patients as a result of VHD.

Nishimura RA et al. 2014 AHA/ACC guideline for the management of patients with valvular heart disease: executive summary: a report of the American College of Cardiology/American Heart Association Task Force on Practice Guidelines. J Am Coll Cardiol. 2014 Jun 10;63(22):2438–88. Erratum in: J Am Coll Cardiol. 2014 Jun 10;63(22):2489. [PMID: 24603192]

MITRAL STENOSIS

 ESSENTIALS OF DIAGNOSIS

► Fatigue, exertional dyspnea, and orthopnea when the stenosis becomes severe.

► Symptoms often precipitated by onset of atrial fibrillation or pregnancy.

► Echocardiography/Doppler is diagnostic.

► Intervention indicated for symptoms, atrial fibrillation, or evidence of pulmonary hypertension. Most symptomatic patients have a mitral valve area of less than 1.5 cm^2.

► General Considerations

Most patients with mitral stenosis are presumed to have underlying rheumatic heart disease, although a history of rheumatic fever is noted in only about one-third. Rheumatic mitral stenosis results in thickening of the leaflets, fusion of the mitral commissures, retraction, thickening and fusion of the chordae, and calcium deposition in the valve. Mitral stenosis can also occur due to congenital disease with chordal fusion or papillary muscle malposition. The papillary muscles may be abnormally close together, sometimes so close that they merge into a single papillary muscle (the parachute mitral valve). In these patients, the

Table 10–2. Differential diagnosis of valvular heart disease.

	Mitral Stenosis	Mitral Regurgitation	Aortic Stenosis	Aortic Regurgitation	Tricuspid Stenosis	Tricuspid Regurgitation
Inspection	Malar flush, precordial bulge, and diffuse pulsation in young patients.	Usually prominent and hyperdynamic apical impulse to left of MCL.	Sustained PMI, prominent atrial filling wave.	Hyperdynamic PMI to left of MCL and downward. Visible carotid pulsations. Pulsating nailbeds (Quincke), head bob (deMusset).	Giant a wave in jugular pulse with sinus rhythm. Peripheral edema or ascites, or both.	Large v wave in jugular pulse; time with carotid pulsation. Peripheral edema or ascites, or both.
Palpation	"Tapping" sensation over area of expected PMI. Right ventricular pulsation in left third to fifth ICS parasternally when pulmonary hypertension is present. P_2 may be palpable.	Forceful, brisk PMI; systolic thrill over PMI. Pulse normal, small, or slightly collapsing.	Powerful, heaving PMI to left and slightly below MCL. Systolic thrill over aortic area, sternal notch, or carotid arteries in severe disease. Small and slowly rising carotid pulse. If bicuspid AS, check for delay at femoral artery to exclude coarctation.	Apical impulse forceful and displaced significantly to left and downward. Prominent carotid pulses. Rapidly rising and collapsing pulses (Corrigan pulse).	Pulsating, enlarged liver in ventricular systole.	Right ventricular pulsation. Systolic pulsation of liver.
Heart sounds, rhythm, and blood pressure	S_1 loud if valve mobile. Opening snap following S_2. The worse the disease, the closer the S_2-opening snap interval.	S_1 normal or buried in early part of murmur (exception in mitral prolapse where murmur may be late). Prominent third heart sound when severe MR. Atrial fibrillation common. Blood pressure normal. Midsystolic clicks may be present and may be multiple.	A_2 normal, soft, or absent. Prominent S_4. Blood pressure normal, or systolic pressure normal with high diastolic pressure.	S_1 normal or reduced, A_2 loud. Wide pulse pressure with diastolic pressure < 60 mm Hg. When severe, gentle compression of femoral artery with diaphragm of stethoscope may reveal diastolic flow (Duroziez) and pressure in leg on palpation > 40 mm Hg than arm (Hill).	S_1 often loud.	Atrial fibrillation maybe present.
Murmurs						
Location and transmission	Localized at or near apex. Diastolic rumble best heard in left lateral position; may be accentuated by having patient do sit-ups. Rarely, short diastolic murmur along lower left sternal border (Graham Steell) in severe pulmonary hypertension.	Loudest over PMI; posteriorly directed jets (ie, anterior mitral prolapse) transmitted to left axilla, left infrascapular area; anteriorly directed jets (ie, posterior mitral prolapse) heard over anterior precordium. Murmur unchanged after premature beat.	Right second ICS parasternally or at apex, heard in carotid arteries and occasionally in upper interscapular area. May sound like MR at apex (Gallaverdin phenomenon), but murmur occurs after S_1 and stops before S_2.	Diastolic: louder along left sternal border in third to fourth interspace. Heard over aortic area and apex. May be associated with low-pitched middiastolic murmur at apex (Austin Flint) due to functional mitral stenosis. If due to an enlarged aorta, murmur may radiate to right sternal border.	Third to fifth ICS along left sternal border out to apex. Murmur increases with inspiration.	Third to fifth ICS along left sternal border. Murmur hard to hear but increases with inspiration. Sit-ups can increase cardiac output and accentuate murmur.

Timing	Relation of opening snap to A_2 important. The higher the LA pressure, the earlier the opening snap. Presystolic accentuation before S_1 if in sinus rhythm. Graham Steell begins with P_2 (early diastole) if associated pulmonary hypertension.	Pansystolic: begins with S_1 and ends at or after A_2. May be late systolic in mitral valve prolapse.	Begins after S_1, ends before A_2. The more severe the stenosis, the later the murmur peaks.	Begins immediately after aortic second sound and ends before first sound (blurring both); helps distinguish from MR.	Rumble often follows opening snap.	At times, hard to hear. Begins with S_1 and fills systole. Increases with inspiration.
Character	Low-pitched, rumbling; presystolic murmur merges with loud S_1.	Blowing, high-pitched; occasionally harsh or musical.	Harsh, rough.	Blowing, often faint.	As for mitral stenosis.	Blowing, coarse, or musical.
Optimum auscultatory conditions	After exercise, left lateral recumbency. Bell chest piece lightly applied.	After exercise; use diaphragm chest piece. In prolapse, findings may be more evident while standing.	Use stethoscope diaphragm. Patient resting, leaning forward, breath held in full expiration.	Use stethoscope diaphragm. Patient leaning forward, breath held in expiration.	Use stethoscope bell. Murmur usually louder and at peak during inspiration. Patient recumbent.	Use stethoscope diaphragm. Murmur usually becomes louder during inspiration.
Radiography	Straight left heart border from enlarged LA appendage. Elevation of left mainstem bronchus. Large right ventricle and pulmonary artery if pulmonary hypertension is present. Calcification in mitral valve in rheumatic mitral stenosis or in annulus in calcific mitral stenosis.	Enlarged left ventricle and LA.	Concentric left ventricular hypertrophy. Prominent ascending aorta. Calcified aortic valve common.	Moderate to severe left ventricular enlargement. Aortic root often dilated.	Enlarged right atrium with prominent SVC and azygous shadow.	Enlarged right atrium and right ventricle.
ECG	Broad P waves in standard leads; broad negative phase of diphasic P in V_1. If pulmonary hypertension is present, tall peaked P waves, right axis deviation, or right ventricular hypertrophy appears.	Left axis deviation or frank left ventricular hypertrophy. P waves broad, tall, or notched in standard leads. Broad negative phase of diphasic P in V_1.	Left ventricular hypertrophy.	Left ventricular hypertrophy.	Tall, peaked P waves. Possible right ventricular hypertrophy.	Right axis usual.

(continued)

Table 10–2. Differential diagnosis of valvular heart disease. (continued)

	Mitral Stenosis	Mitral Regurgitation	Aortic Stenosis	Aortic Regurgitation	Tricuspid Stenosis	Tricuspid Regurgitation
Echocardiography						
Two-dimensional echocardiography	Thickened, immobile mitral valve with anterior and posterior leaflets moving together. "Hockey stick" shape to opened anterior leaflet in rheumatic mitral stenosis. Annular calcium with thin leaflets in calcific mitral stenosis. LA enlargement, normal to small left ventricle. Orifice can be traced to approximate mitral valve orifice area.	Thickened mitral valve in rheumatic disease; mitral valve prolapse; flail leaflet or vegetations may be seen. Dilated left ventricle in volume overload. Operate for left ventricular end-systolic dimension < 4.5 cm.	Dense persistent echoes from the aortic valve with poor leaflet excursion. Left ventricular hypertrophy late in the disease. Bicuspid valve in younger patients.	Abnormal aortic valve or dilated aortic root. Diastolic vibrations of the anterior leaflet of the mitral valve and septum. In acute aortic regurgitation, premature closure of the mitral valve before the QRS. When severe, dilated left ventricle with normal or decreased contractility. Operate when left ventricular end-systolic dimension > 5.0 cm.	In rheumatic disease, tricuspid valve thickening, decreased early diastolic filling slope of the tricuspid valve. In carcinoid, leaflets fixed, but no significant thickening.	Enlarged right ventricle with paradoxical septal motion. Tricuspid valve often pulled open by displaced chordae.
Continuous and color flow Doppler and TEE	Prolonged pressure half-time across mitral valve allows estimation of gradient. MVA estimated from pressure half-time. Indirect evidence of pulmonary hypertension by noting elevated right ventricular systolic pressure measured from the tricuspid regurgitation jet.	Regurgitant flow mapped into LA. Use of PISA helps assess MR severity. TEE important in prosthetic mitral valve regurgitation.	Increased transvalvular flow velocity; severe AS when peak jet > 4 m/sec (64 mm Hg). Valve area estimate using continuity equation is poorly reproducible.	Demonstrates regurgitation and qualitatively estimates severity based on percentage of left ventricular outflow filled with jet and distance jet penetrates into left ventricle. TEE important in aortic valve endocarditis to exclude abscess. Mitral inflow pattern describes diastolic dysfunction.	Prolonged pressure half-time across tricuspid valve can be used to estimate mean gradient. Severe tricuspid stenosis present when mean gradient > 5 mm Hg.	Regurgitant flow mapped into right atrium and venae cavae. Right ventricular systolic pressure estimated by tricuspid regurgitation jet velocity.

A$_2$, aortic second sound; AS, aortic stenosis; ICS, intercostal space; LA, left atrial; MCL, midclavicular line; MR, mitral regurgitation; MVA, measured valve area; P$_2$, pulmonary second sound; PISA, proximal isovelocity surface area; PMI, point of maximal impulse; S$_1$, first heart sound; S$_2$, second heart sound; S$_4$, fourth heart sound; SVC, superior vena cava; TEE, transesophageal echocardiography; V$_1$, chest ECG lead 1.

Table 10–3. Effect of various interventions on systolic murmurs.

Intervention	Hypertrophic Cardiomyopathy	Aortic Stenosis	Mitral Regurgitation	Mitral Prolapse
Valsalva	↑	↓	↓ or ×	↑ or ↓
Standing	↑	↑ or ×	↓ or ×	↑
Handgrip or squatting	↓	↓ or ×	↑	↓
Supine position with legs elevated	↓	↑ or ×	×	↓
Exercise	↑	↑ or ×	↓	↑

↑, increased; ↓, decreased; ×, unchanged.
Modified, with permission, from Paraskos JA. Combined valvular disease. In: *Valvular Heart Disease, 3e.* Dalen JE, Alpert JS, Rahimtoola SH (editors). Philadelphia: Lippincott Williams & Wilkins, 2000.

chordae or valvular tissue (or both) may also be fused. In older patients and in those undergoing dialysis, mitral annular calcification may stiffen the mitral valve and reduce its motion to the point where a mitral gradient is present. Calcium in the mitral annulus virtually invades the mitral leaflet from the annulus inward as opposed to the calcium buildup in the leaflets and commissures as seen in rheumatic heart disease. Mitral valve obstruction may also develop in patients who have had mitral valve repair with a mitral annular ring that is too small, or in patients who have had a surgical valve replacement (prosthetic valve-patient mismatch or degeneration of the valve over time).

► **Clinical Findings**

A. Symptoms and Signs

Two clinical syndromes classically occur in patients with mitral stenosis. In **mild** to **moderate mitral stenosis,** LA pressure and cardiac output may be essentially normal, and the patient is either asymptomatic or symptomatic only with extreme exertion. The measured valve area is usually between 1.5 cm^2 and 1.0 cm^2. In **severe mitral stenosis** (valve area less than 1.0 cm^2), severe pulmonary hypertension develops due to a "secondary stenosis" of the pulmonary vasculature. In this condition, pulmonary edema is uncommon, but symptoms of low cardiac output and right heart failure predominate.

A characteristic finding of rheumatic mitral stenosis is an opening snap following A$_2$ due to the stiff mitral valve. The interval between the opening snap and aortic closure sound is long when the LA pressure is low but shortens as the LA pressure rises and approaches the aortic diastolic pressure. As mitral stenosis worsens, there is a localized diastolic murmur low in pitch whose duration increases with the severity of the stenosis as the mitral gradient continues throughout more of diastole. The diastolic murmur is best heard at the apex with the patient in the left lateral position (Table 10–2). Mitral regurgitation may be present as well.

Paroxysmal or chronic atrial fibrillation eventually develops in 50–80% of patients. Any increase in the heart rate reduces diastolic filling time and increases the mitral gradient. A sudden increase in heart rate may precipitate

pulmonary edema. Therefore, heart rate control is important, with slow heart rates allowing for more diastolic filling of the LV.

B. Diagnostic Studies

Echocardiography is the most valuable technique for assessing mitral stenosis (Table 10–2). A scoring system is helpful in defining which patients are eligible for percutaneous valvuloplasty. One to four points are assigned to each of four observed parameters, with 1 being the least involvement and 4 the greatest: mitral leaflet thickening, mitral leaflet mobility, submitral scarring, and commissural calcium. Patients with a total valve score of 8 or less respond best to balloon valvuloplasty as long as there is no significant mitral regurgitation. LA size can also be determined by echocardiography; increased size denotes an increased likelihood of atrial fibrillation and thrombus formation.

Because echocardiography and careful symptom evaluation provide most of the needed information, cardiac catheterization is used primarily to detect associated coronary or myocardial disease—usually after the decision to intervene has been made.

► **Treatment & Prognosis**

In most cases, there is a long asymptomatic phase after the initial rheumatic infection, followed by subtle limitation of activity. Pregnancy and its associated increase in stroke volume results in an increased transmitral pressure gradient and may precipitate symptoms. Toward the end of pregnancy, the cardiac output continues to be maintained by an increase in heart rate, further increasing the mitral gradient by shortening diastolic time. Patients with moderate to severe mitral stenosis should have the condition corrected prior to becoming pregnant if possible. Pregnant patients who become symptomatic can undergo successful surgery, preferably in the third trimester, although balloon valvuloplasty is the treatment of choice if the echocardiography valve score is low enough.

The onset of atrial fibrillation often precipitates symptoms, which improve with control of the ventricular rate or restoration of sinus rhythm. Conversion to and subsequent maintenance of sinus rhythm are most commonly successful when the duration of atrial fibrillation is brief (less than 6–12 months) and the LA is not severely dilated (diameter less than 4.5 cm). Once atrial fibrillation occurs, the patient should receive warfarin anticoagulation therapy even if sinus rhythm is restored, since atrial fibrillation often recurs even with antiarrhythmic therapy and 20–30% of these patients will have systemic embolization if untreated. Systemic embolization in the presence of only mild to moderate disease is not an indication for surgery but should be treated with warfarin anticoagulation. Direct-acting oral anticoagulants (DOACs), also known as new (or novel) oral anticoagulants or as target-specific oral anticoagulants (dabigatran, apixaban, rivaroxaban, edoxaban), have not been studied for the prevention of stroke and non–central nervous system embolism in patients with moderate or severe mitral stenosis and atrial fibrillation, and they are not approved for these patients.

Indications for intervention focus on symptoms such as an episode of pulmonary edema, a decline in exercise capacity, or any evidence of pulmonary hypertension (peak systolic pulmonary pressure greater than 50 mm Hg). Some experts believe that the presence of atrial fibrillation

should also be a consideration for an intervention. Most interventions are not pursued until the patient is symptomatic (stage D) (Figure 10–1). In some patients, symptoms develop with calculated mitral valve areas between 1.5 cm² and 1.0 cm². **Symptoms or evidence of pulmonary hypertension should drive the decision to intervene in these patients, not the estimated valve area.**

Open mitral commissurotomy is now rarely performed and has given way to percutaneous balloon valvuloplasty. Ten-year follow-up data comparing surgery to balloon valvuloplasty suggest no real difference in outcome between the two modalities. Replacement of the valve is indicated when combined stenosis and regurgitation are present or when the mitral valve echo score is greater than 8–10. Percutaneous balloon valvuloplasty has a very low mortality rate (less than 0.5%) and a low morbidity rate (3–5%). Operative mortality rates are also low: 1–3% in most institutions. Repeat balloon valvuloplasty can be done if the morphology of the valve remains suitable. At surgery, a Maze procedure may be done at the same time to reduce recurrent atrial arrhythmias. It involves a number of endocardial incisions across the right and left atria to disrupt the electrical activity that sustains atrial arrhythmias.

AF, atrial fibrillation; LA, left atrial; MR, mitral regurgitation; MS, mitral stenosis; MVA, mitral valve area; MVH, mitral valve replacement; NYHA, New York Heart Association; PBMC, percutaneous balloon mitral commissurotomy; PCWP, pulmonary capillary wedge pressure; ΔP$_{mean}$, mean pressure gradient; T$^{1}/_{2}$, half-life.

▲ **Figure 10–1.** The 2014 AHA/ACC guidelines for intervention in mitral stenosis. (Reproduced with permission from Nishimura RA et al. 2014 AHA/ACC Guideline for the Management of Patients With Valvular Heart Disease: A Report of the American College of Cardiology/American Heart Association Task Force on Practice Guidelines. Circulation. 2014 Jun 10; 129(23):e521–643. © 2014 American Heart Association, Inc. [PMID: 24589853])

Mechanical mitral prosthetic valves are more prone to thrombosis than mechanical aortic prosthetic valves. The recommended INR range is thus higher (INR 2.5–3.5) and low-dose aspirin should be used in conjunction. Bioprosthetic valves tend to degenerate after about 10–15 years. Percutaneous balloon valvuloplasty is not effective when bioprosthetic valve stenosis occurs, but stented valve-in-valve procedures have been successful and will likely be used more often. Younger patients and those with end-stage kidney disease are generally believed to do least well with bioprosthetic heart valves, although data have questioned the role of chronic kidney disease as a major risk factor. Endocarditis prophylaxis is indicated for patients with prosthetic heart valves but is not indicated in native valve disease (see Tables 33–4, 33–5, and 33–6).

► When to Refer

- Patients with mitral stenosis should be monitored with yearly examinations, and echocardiograms should be performed more frequently as the severity of the obstruction increases.

- All patients should initially be seen by a cardiologist, who can then decide how often the patient needs cardiology follow-up.

Nishimura RA et al. 2014 AHA/ACC guideline for the management of patients with valvular heart disease: executive summary: a report of the American College of Cardiology/American Heart Association Task Force on Practice Guidelines. J Am Coll Cardiol. 2014 Jun 10;63(22):2438–88. Erratum in: J Am Coll Cardiol. 2014 Jun 10;63(22):2489. [PMID: 24603192]

Vahanian A et al; Joint Task Force on the Management of Valvular Heart Disease of the European Society of Cardiology (ESC); European Association for Cardio-Thoracic Surgery (EACTS). Guidelines on the management of valvular heart disease (version 2012). Eur Heart J. 2012 Oct;33(19):2451–96. [PMID: 22922415]

MITRAL REGURGITATION
(Mitral Insufficiency)

ESSENTIALS OF DIAGNOSIS

- ► May be asymptomatic for years (or for life).

- ► Severe mitral regurgitation may cause left-sided heart failure.

- ► For chronic primary mitral regurgitation, surgery is indicated for symptoms or when the LV ejection fraction (LVEF) is less than 60% or the echocardiographic LV end-systolic dimension is greater than 4.0 cm.

- ► In patients with mitral prolapse and severe mitral regurgitation, earlier surgery is indicated if mitral repair can be performed.

- ► Patients with functional mitral regurgitation may improve with biventricular pacing. Some may require surgical intervention.

► General Considerations

Mitral regurgitation places a volume load on the heart (increases preload) but reduces afterload. The result is an enlarged LV with an increased EF. Over time, the stress of the volume overload reduces myocardial contractile function; when this occurs, there is a drop in EF and a rise in end-systolic volume.

► Clinical Findings

A. Symptoms and Signs

In acute mitral regurgitation, the LA size is not large, and LA pressure rises abruptly, leading to pulmonary edema if severe. When chronic, the LA enlarges progressively and the increased volume can be handled without a major rise in the LA pressure; the pressure in pulmonary veins and capillaries may rise only during exertion. Exertional dyspnea and fatigue progress gradually over many years.

Mitral regurgitation leads to chronic LA and LV enlargement and may result in subsequent atrial fibrillation and eventually LV dysfunction. Clinically, mitral regurgitation is characterized by a pansystolic murmur maximal at the apex, radiating to the axilla and occasionally to the base. The murmur does not change in intensity after a premature beat. In addition, a hyperdynamic LV impulse and a brisk carotid upstroke may be present, and a prominent third heart sound due to the increased volume returning to the LV in early diastole may be heard (Tables 10–2 and 10–3). The mitral regurgitation murmur due to mitral valve prolapse tends to radiate anteriorly in the presence of posterior leaflet prolapse and posteriorly when the prolapse is primarily of the anterior leaflet. Mitral regurgitation may not be pansystolic but occur only after the mitral click in patients with mitral valve prolapse (until late in the disease process when it becomes progressively more holosystolic).

B. Diagnostic Studies

Echocardiographic information demonstrating the underlying pathologic process (rheumatic, calcific, prolapse, flail leaflet, endocarditis, cardiomyopathy), LV size and function, LA size, PA pressure, and RV function can be invaluable in planning treatment as well as in recognizing associated lesions. The 2014 guidelines for VHD from the AHA/ACC provide details of the classification of primary and secondary mitral valve regurgitation. Doppler techniques provide qualitative and semiquantitative estimates of the severity of mitral regurgitation. TEE may help reveal the cause of regurgitation and is especially useful in patients who have had mitral valve replacement, in suspected endocarditis, and in identifying candidates for valvular repair. Echocardiographic dimensions and measures of systolic function are critical in deciding the timing of surgery. Patients with severe mitral regurgitation (stage C1) but preserved LV dimensions should undergo at least yearly echocardiography. Exercise hemodynamics with either Doppler echocardiography or cardiac catheterization may be useful when the symptoms do not fit the anatomic severity of mitral regurgitation. B-type natriuretic peptide (BNP) is useful in the early identification of LV dysfunction in the presence of mitral regurgitation and asymptomatic patients and appears to have some prognostic importance.

Cardiac MRI is occasionally useful, if specific myocardial causes are being sought (such as amyloid or myocarditis) or if myocardial viability assessment is needed prior to deciding whether to add coronary artery bypass grafting to mitral valve surgery.

Cardiac catheterization provides a further assessment of regurgitation and its hemodynamic impact along with LV function, resting cardiac output, and PA pressure. The 2014 AHA/ACC guidelines recommend coronary angiography to determine the presence of coronary artery disease (CAD) prior to valve surgery in all men over age 40 years and in menopausal women with coronary risk factors. In younger patients, cardiac multidetector CT may be adequate to screen patients with VHD for asymptomatic CAD. A normal CT angiogram identifies normal or insignificant disease in a very high percentage of patients.

▶ Treatment & Prognosis

A. Primary Mitral Regurgitation

The degree of LV enlargement reflects the severity and chronicity of regurgitation. LV volume overload may ultimately lead to LV failure and reduced cardiac output. LA enlargement may be considerable in **chronic mitral regurgitation** and a large amount of mitral regurgitation regurgitant volume may be tolerated. Patients with chronic lesions may thus remain asymptomatic for many years. Surgery is necessary when symptoms develop or when there is evidence for LV dysfunction, since progressive and irreversible deterioration of LV function can occur prior to the onset of symptoms. Early surgery is indicated even in asymptomatic patients with a reduced EF (less than 60%) or marked LV dilation with reduced contractility (end-systolic dimension greater than 4.0 cm) (Figure 10–2). Pulmonary hypertension development suggests the mitral regurgitation is severe and should prompt intervention.

¹Mitral valve repair preferred over MVR when possible.
AF, atrial fibrillation; CAD, coronary artery disease; CRT, cardiac resynchronization therapy; ERO, effective regurgitant orifice; HF, heart failure; LV, left ventricular; LVEF, left ventricular ejection fraction; LVESD, left ventricular end-systolic dimension; MR, mitral regurgitation, MV, mitral valve; MVR, mitral valve replacement; NYHA, New York Heart association; PASP, pulmonary artery systolic pressure; RF, regurgitant fraction; R Vol, regurgitant volume; Rx, prescription.

▲ **Figure 10–2.** The 2014 AHA/ACC guidelines for intervention in mitral regurgitation. (Reproduced with permission from Nishimura RA et al. 2014 AHA/ACC Guideline for the Management of Patients With Valvular Heart Disease: A Report of the American College of Cardiology/American Heart Association Task Force on Practice Guidelines. Circulation. 2014 Jun 10;129(23):e521–643. © 2014 American Heart Association, Inc. [PMID: 24589853])

Acute mitral regurgitation may develop abruptly, such as with papillary muscle dysfunction following myocardial infarction, valve perforation in infective endocarditis, in patients with hypertrophic cardiomyopathy, or when there are ruptured chordae tendineae in patients with mitral valve prolapse. Emergency surgery may be required for acute nonrheumatic mitral regurgitation.

Some patients may become hemodynamically unstable and can be initially treated with vasodilators or intra-aortic balloon counterpulsation, which reduce the amount of retrograde regurgitant flow by lowering systemic vascular resistance. There is controversy regarding the role of afterload reduction in chronic mitral regurgitation, since the lesion inherently results in a reduction in afterload, and there are no data that chronic afterload reduction is effective. A heightened sympathetic state has led some experts to suggest that beta-blockade be considered routinely. The mitral regurgitation in patients with tachycardia-related cardiomyopathy may also improve with normalization of the heart rate.

B. Myocardial Disease and Mitral Regurgitation

When mitral regurgitation is due to papillary dysfunction, it may subside as the infarction heals or LV dilation diminishes. The cause of the regurgitation in most of these situations is displacement of the papillary muscles and an enlarged mitral annulus rather than papillary muscle ischemia. The fundamental problem is the lack of leaflet coaptation during systole (due to either leaflet prolapse or retraction). In acute infarction, rupture of the papillary muscle may occur with catastrophic results. Transient—but sometimes severe—mitral regurgitation may occur during episodes of myocardial ischemia and contribute to flash pulmonary edema. Patients with dilated cardiomyopathies of any origin may have **secondary mitral regurgitation** due to the papillary muscle displacement or dilation of the mitral annulus, or both. If mitral valve replacement is performed, preservation of the chordae to the native valve helps prevent further ventricular dilation following surgery. Several groups have reported good results with mitral valve repair in patients with LVEF less than 30% and secondary mitral regurgitation. The 2014 AHA/ACC guidelines (Figure 10–2) advise that mitral valve repair/replacement can be attempted in severe mitral regurgitation patients with an EF less than 30% or an LV end-systolic dimension greater than 5.5 cm, or both, as long as repair and preservation of the chordae are possible. There may also be a role for cardiac resynchronization therapy with biventricular pacemaker insertion, which has been found to reduce mitral regurgitation related to cardiomyopathy in many patients. Guidelines recommend biventricular pacing prior to surgical repair in those patients who have functional mitral regurgitation.

There are several ongoing trials of percutaneous approaches to reducing mitral regurgitation. These approaches include the use of a mitral clip device to create a double orifice mitral valve, various coronary catheter devices to reduce the mitral annular area, and devices to reduce the septal-lateral ventricular size and consequent mitral orifice size. Of these devices, some success has been noted with the mitral clip device. The device, however, is reserved for patients in whom surgical risk is considered excessive and in those with primary mitral valve disease. Its role continues to be defined. In addition, vascular plugging and occluder devices are being used in selected patients to occlude perivalvular leaks around prosthetic mitral valves. A transcatheter stented valve, which is used as a transcatheter aortic valve replacement (TAVR) device, can be used to open a degenerated mitral bioprosthetic valve in any position (aortic, mitral, tricuspid, or pulmonary). Finally, the first reported cases of the stented mitral valve prosthesis to replace the mitral valve have been reported.

▶ When to Refer

- All patients with more than mild mitral regurgitation should be referred to a cardiologist for an evaluation.
- Serial examinations and echocardiograms should be obtained and surgical referral made if there is an increase in the LV end-systolic dimensions, a fall in the LVEF to less than 60%, symptoms, evidence for pulmonary hypertension or the new onset of atrial fibrillation.
- There is growing evidence that mitral valve repair should be done early in the course of the disease to improve mortality and morbidity.

Ahmed MI et al. A randomized controlled phase IIb trial of beta(1)-receptor blockade for chronic degenerative mitral regurgitation. J Am Coll Cardiol. 2012 Aug 28;60(9):833–8. [PMID: 22818065]

De Backer O et al. Percutaneous transcatheter mitral valve replacement: an overview of devices in preclinical and early clinical evaluation. Circ Cardiovasc Interv. 2014 Jun;7(3):400–9. [PMID: 24944303]

Mauri L et al; EVEREST II Investigators. 4-year results of a randomized controlled trial of percutaneous repair versus surgery for mitral regurgitation. J Am Coll Cardiol. 2013 Jul 23;62(4):317–28. [PMID: 23665364]

Nishimura RA et al. 2014 AHA/ACC guideline for the management of patients with valvular heart disease: executive summary: a report of the American College of Cardiology/American Heart Association Task Force on Practice Guidelines. J Am Coll Cardiol. 2014 Jun 10;63(22):2438–88. Erratum in: J Am Coll Cardiol. 2014 Jun 10;63(22):2489. [PMID: 24603192]

Suri RM et al. Association between early surgical intervention vs watchful waiting and outcomes for mitral regurgitation due to flail mitral valve leaflets. JAMA. 2013 Aug 14;310(6):609–16. [PMID: 23942679]

MITRAL VALVE PROLAPSE SYNDROME

ESSENTIALS OF DIAGNOSIS

- ▶ Single or multiple mid-systolic clicks often heard on auscultation.
- ▶ Murmur may be pansystolic or only late in systole.
- ▶ Often associated with skeletal changes (straight back, pectus excavatum, and scoliosis) or hyperflexibility of joints.
- ▶ Echocardiography is confirmatory with prolapse of mitral leaflets in systole into the LA.
- ▶ Chest pain and palpitations are common symptoms in the young adult.

General Considerations

The significance of mild mitral valve prolapse ("floppy" or myxomatous mitral valve), also commonly referred to as "degenerative" mitral valve disease, has been in dispute because of the frequency with which it is diagnosed by echocardiography even in healthy young women (up to 10%). A controversial hyperadrenergic syndrome has also been described (especially in young females) that may be responsible for some of the noncardiac symptoms observed. Fortunately, this hyperadrenergic component attenuates with age. Some patients with mitral prolapse have findings of a systemic collagen abnormality (Marfan or Ehlers-Danlos syndrome). In these conditions, a dilated aortic root and aortic regurgitation may coexist. In many persons, the "degenerative" myxomatous mitral valve clearly leads to long-term sequelae and is the most common cause of mitral regurgitation in developing countries.

Patients who have only a mid-systolic click usually have no immediate clinical issues, but significant mitral regurgitation may develop, occasionally suddenly due to rupture of chordae tendineae (flail leaflet) or gradually due to progressive annular and LV dilation. The need for valve repair or replacement increases with age, so that approximately 2% per year of patients with clinically significant regurgitation over age 60 years will eventually require surgery.

Clinical Findings

A. Symptoms and Signs

Mitral valve prolapse without significant mitral regurgitation is usually asymptomatic but may be associated with a syndrome of nonspecific chest pain, dyspnea, fatigue, or palpitations. Most patients are female, many are thin, and some have skeletal deformities, such as pectus excavatum or scoliosis. On auscultation, there are characteristic mid-systolic clicks that may be multiple and emanate from the chordae or redundant valve tissue. If leaflets fail to come together properly, the clicks will be followed by a late systolic murmur. As the mitral regurgitation worsens, the murmur is heard more and more throughout systole. The smaller the LV chamber, the greater the degree of leaflet prolapse, and thus auscultatory findings are often accentuated in the standing position or during the Valsalva maneuver. Whether sudden cardiac death presumably due to ventricular arrhythmias is more frequent in patients with mitral valve prolapse remains controversial.

B. Diagnostic Studies

The diagnosis is primarily clinical and confirmed echocardiographically. Mitral prolapse is often associated with aortic root disease, and any evidence for a dilated aorta by chest radiography should prompt either CT or MRI angiography. If palpitations are an issue, an ambulatory monitor is often helpful to distinguish atrial from ventricular tachyarrhythmias.

Treatment

Beta-blockers in low doses are used to treat the hyperadrenergic state when present and are usually satisfactory for treatment of arrhythmias (see Table 11–6). Selective serotonin reuptake inhibitors have also been used, especially if orthostatic hypotension or anxiety is associated with mitral valve prolapse; results have been mixed. Afterload reduction has not been shown to change prognosis when mitral regurgitation is present.

Mitral valve repair is strongly favored over valve replacement, and its efficacy has led many to recommend intervention earlier and earlier in the course of the disease process. Mitral repair may include shortening of chordae, chordae transfers, wedge resection of redundant valve tissue, or the insertion of a mitral annular ring to reduce the annular size, or some combination of these techniques. Stitching of the leaflets together to create a double-orifice mitral valve is also used at times (Alfieri procedure) and can be performed percutaneously. Mitral repair or replacement can be achieved through a right minithoracotomy with or without the use of a robotic device. Endocarditis prophylaxis is no longer recommended for most patients with mitral valve prolapse regardless of the degree of mitral regurgitation. A variety of percutaneous techniques and devices have been tried with some success (notably in the mitral clip trials), although results suggest that surgical repair may be more durable.

When to Refer

- All patients with mitral valve prolapse and audible mitral regurgitation should be seen at least once by a cardiologist.
- Periodic echocardiography is warranted to assess LV size (especially end-systolic dimensions) and EF when mitral regurgitation is present. If only mitral clicks are audible, then serial echocardiography is not warranted.

Basso C et al. Arrhythmic mitral valve prolapse and sudden cardiac death. Circulation. 2015 Aug 18;132(7):556–66. [PMID: 26160859]

Delling FN et al. Epidemiology and pathophysiology of mitral valve prolapse: new insights into disease progression, genetics, and molecular basis. Circulation. 2014 May 27;129(21):2158–70. [PMID: 24867995]

Theofilogiannakos EK et al. Floppy mitral valve/mitral valve prolapse syndrome: beta-adrenergic receptor polymorphism may contribute to the pathogenesis of symptoms. J Cardiol. 2015 May;65(5):434–8. [PMID: 25172623]

AORTIC STENOSIS

ESSENTIALS OF DIAGNOSIS

- ► Congenital bicuspid aortic valve, usually asymptomatic until middle or old age.
- ► "Degenerative" or calcific aortic stenosis; same risk factors as atherosclerosis.

- Visual observation of immobile aortic valve plus a valve area of less than 1.0 cm² define severe disease; low gradient but severe aortic stenosis can thus be recognized.
- Echocardiography/Doppler is diagnostic.
- Surgery typically indicated for symptoms.
- Surgery considered for asymptomatic patients with severe aortic stenosis (mean gradient greater than 55 mm Hg) or when undergoing heart surgery for other reasons (eg, coronary artery bypass grafting [CABG]).
- BNP is a marker of early LV myocardial failure, and high levels suggest poor prognosis.

General Considerations

There are two common clinical scenarios in which aortic stenosis is prevalent. The first is due to a congenitally abnormal **unicuspid** or **bicuspid valve,** rather than tricuspid. Symptoms occur in young or adolescent individuals if the stenosis is severe, but more often emerge at age 50–65 years when calcification and degeneration of the valve become manifest. A dilated ascending aorta, primarily due to an intrinsic defect in the aortic root media, may accompany the bicuspid valve in about half of these patients. Coarctation of the aorta is also seen in a number of patients with congenital aortic stenosis. Offspring of patients with a bicuspid valve have a much higher incidence of the disease in either the valve, the aorta, or both (up to 30% in some series).

A second pathologic process, **degenerative** or **calcific aortic stenosis**, is thought to be related to calcium deposition due to processes similar to what occurs in atherosclerotic vascular disease. Approximately 25% of patients over age 65 years and 35% of those over age 70 years have echocardiographic evidence of aortic valve thickening (sclerosis). About 10–20% of these will progress to hemodynamically significant aortic stenosis over a period of 10–15 years. Certain genetic markers are associated with aortic stenosis (most notably Notch 1), so a genetic component appears a likely contributor, at least in some patients. Other associated genetic markers have also been described.

Aortic stenosis has become the most common surgical valve lesion in developed countries, and many patients are elderly. The risk factors include hypertension, hypercholesterolemia, and smoking. Hypertrophic cardiomyopathy (HCM) may also coexist with valvular aortic stenosis.

Clinical Findings

A. Symptoms and Signs

Slightly narrowed, thickened, or roughened valves (aortic sclerosis) or aortic dilation may contribute to the typical ejection murmur of aortic stenosis. In mild or moderate cases where the valve is still pliable, an ejection click may precede the murmur and the closure of the valve (S_2) is preserved. The characteristic systolic ejection murmur is heard at the aortic area and is usually transmitted to the neck and apex. In severe aortic stenosis, a palpable LV heave or thrill, a weak to absent aortic second sound, or reversed splitting of the second sound is present (see Table 10–2). In some cases, only the high-pitched components of the murmur are heard at the apex, and the murmur may sound like mitral regurgitation (the so-called Gallaverdin phenomenon). When the valve area is less than 0.8–1.0 cm² (normal, 3–4 cm²), ventricular systole becomes prolonged and the typical carotid pulse pattern of delayed upstroke and low amplitude is present. A delayed upstroke, though, is an unreliable finding in older patients with extensive arteriosclerotic vascular disease and a stiff aorta. LVH increases progressively due to the pressure overload, eventually resulting in elevation of ventricular end-diastolic pressure. Cardiac output is maintained until the stenosis is severe. LV failure, angina pectoris, or syncope may be presenting symptoms of significant aortic stenosis; importantly, all symptoms tend to occur with exertion.

B. Redefining Severe Aortic Stenosis

There are four different anatomic syndromes that occur in patients with severe aortic stenosis. The common underlying measure of severe aortic stenosis is an aortic valve area of less than 1.0 cm² and echocardiographic evidence of an immobile aortic valve. In patients with a normal LVEF and normal cardiac output, the threshold for intervention is a peak aortic gradient of greater than 64 mm Hg and mean aortic gradient of greater than 40 mm Hg. In the same situation, "**super-severe aortic stenosis**" is defined as a mean gradient of greater than 55 mm Hg or peak aortic velocity greater than 5 m/sec by Doppler.

In some patients with an aortic valve area of less than 1.0 cm² with a low cardiac output and stroke volume, the mean gradient may be less than 40 mm Hg. This can occur when the LV systolic function is poor (**low-gradient severe aortic stenosis with low EF**) or when the LV systolic function is normal (**"paradoxical" low-flow severe aortic stenosis).** Low flow (low output) in these situations is defined by an echocardiographic stroke volume index of less than 35 mL/min/m². Prognosis in patients with **low gradient, low valve area, low output, and a normal LVEF aortic stenosis** may actually be worse than in patients with the traditional high gradient, low valve area, normal output, and normal LVEF aortic stenosis. If low-flow severe aortic stenosis is present, provocative testing with dobutamine or nitroprusside is warranted to increase the stroke volume to discover if a mean aortic valve gradient of at least 40 mm Hg can be demonstrated without increasing the aortic valve area. If the aortic valve area can be made to increase and a mean gradient of greater than 40 mm Hg cannot be demonstrated by inotropic challenge, the presumption is that the low gradient is due to an associated cardiomyopathy and not the aortic valve stenosis. In this latter situation intervention is not indicated. The 2014 AHA/ACC guidelines acknowledge these four situations (Table 10–4).

Table 10–4. Summary of 2014 AHA/ACC guideline definitions of symptomatic severe aortic stenosis.

Category of Severe Aortic Stenosis[1]	Properties
High gradient	> 4.0 m/sec Doppler jet velocity > 40 mm Hg mean gradient
Super-severe	> 5.0 m/sec Doppler jet velocity > 55 mm Hg mean gradient
Low flow	Reduced LVEF (< 50%) Normal LVEF (> 50%)

[1]All categories of severe aortic stenosis have abnormal systolic opening of the aortic valve and an aortic valve area < 1.0 cm². LVEF, left ventricular ejection fraction.

Symptoms of LV failure may be sudden in onset or may progress gradually. Angina pectoris frequently occurs in aortic stenosis due to underperfusion of the endocardium. Of patients with calcific aortic stenosis and angina, half have significant associated CAD. Syncope, a late finding, occurs with exertion as the LV pressure rises, stimulating the LV baroreceptors to cause peripheral vasodilation. This vasodilation results in the need for an increase in stroke volume, which increases the LV systolic pressure again, creating a cycle of vasodilation and stimulation of the baroreceptors that eventually results in a drop in BP, as the stenotic valve prevents further increase in stroke volume. Less commonly, syncope may be due to arrhythmias (usually ventricular tachycardia but sometimes AV block as calcific invasion of the conduction system from the aortic valve may occur).

C. Diagnostic Studies

The ECG reveals LVH or secondary repolarization changes in most patients but can be normal in up to 10%. The chest radiograph may show a normal or enlarged cardiac silhouette, calcification of the aortic valve, and dilation and calcification of the ascending aorta. The echocardiogram provides useful data about aortic valve calcification and opening and the severity of LV wall thickness and overall ventricular function, while Doppler can provide an excellent estimate of the aortic valve gradient. Valve area estimation by echocardiography is less reliable but is a critical component of the diagnosis of aortic stenosis due to issues such as paradoxical low flow aortic stenosis (low gradient, low flow, normal LVEF patients). Likewise, the echocardiography/Doppler can estimate the stroke volume index used to define low flow when the valve area is small but the gradient is less than 40 mm Hg. Cardiac catheterization mostly provides an assessment of the hemodynamic consequence of the aortic stenosis, and the anatomy of the coronary arteries. Catheterization data can be important when there is a discrepancy between symptoms and the echocardiography/Dopper information of aortic stenosis severity. In younger patients and in patients with high aortic gradients, the aortic valve need not be crossed at catheterization. Aortic regurgitation can be semiquantified by aortic root angiography. Some authors have suggested the use of BNP (or N-terminal proBNP [NT-proBNP]) may provide additional prognostic data in the setting of poor LV function and aortic stenosis. A BNP greater than 550 pg/mL has been associated with a poor outcome in these patients regardless of the results of dobutamine testing.

▶ Prognosis & Treatment

Table 10–5 outlines the 2014 guidelines for surgical intervention in aortic stenosis. Valve intervention is warranted in all patients who have **symptomatic severe aortic stenosis.** There are also times when asymptomatic aortic stenosis should undergo intervention. **Asymptomatic patients with severe aortic stenosis** (aortic valve area less than 1.0 cm²) should generally undergo intervention according to the following guidelines: (1) they are undergoing other cardiac surgery (ie, CABG), (2) there is evidence for a reduced LVEF (less than 50%), (3) when the mean gradient exceeds 55 mm Hg (peak velocity greater than 5 m/sec), (4) when there is failure of the BP to rise more than 20 mm Hg with exercise, (5) when there is severe valvular calcium, or (6) when there is evidence of a rapid increase in the peak aortic gradient (more than 0.3 m/sec/year). Following the onset of heart failure, angina, or syncope, the prognosis without surgery is poor (50% 3-year mortality rate). Medical treatment may stabilize patients in heart failure, but intervention is indicated for all symptomatic patients with evidence of significant aortic stenosis.

The surgical mortality rate for valve replacement is low, even in the elderly, and ranges from 2% to 5%. This low risk is due to the dramatic hemodynamic improvement that occurs with relief of the increased afterload. Mortality rates are substantially higher when there is an associated ischemic cardiomyopathy. Severe coronary lesions are usually bypassed at the same time as aortic valve replacement (AVR), although there are little data to suggest this practice affects outcome. In some cases, a staged procedure with stenting of the coronaries prior to surgery may be considered. Around one-third to one-half of all patients with aortic stenosis have significant CAD, so this is a common concern. With the advent of transcatheter valve replacement, the procedure is being used in patients for whom surgery is not an option. For this reason, a Heart Valve Team approach bringing together invasive and noninvasive cardiologists, radiologists, anesthesiologists, and cardiac surgeons is mandatory; clinical factors (such as frailty) and anatomic features (such as a calcified aorta, vascular access, etc) can affect the decision making.

Statins have not been shown to be beneficial in preventing the progression of aortic stenosis despite the association of aortic stenosis with atherosclerosis, but longer-term studies are pending in patients who have early disease. If patients with aortic stenosis have concomitant CAD, the guidelines for the use of statins should be followed. Control of systemic hypertension is also an important adjunct, and inadequate systemic BP control is common due to unreasonable concerns about providing too much afterload reduction in patients with aortic stenosis. Normal systemic BP is important to maintain.

The interventional options in patients with aortic valve stenosis has expanded with the use of TAVR and depend on the patient's lifestyle and age. The algorithm to decide

Table 10–5. 2014 AHA/ACC guidelines for surgical indications in aortic stenosis.

Recommendations	COR	LOE
AVR is recommended in symptomatic patients with severe AS (stage D)	I	B
AVR is recommended for asymptomatic patients with severe AS (stage C2 or D) and LVEF < 50%	I	B
AVR is indicated for patients with severe AS (stage C or D) when undergoing other cardiac surgery	I	B
AVR is reasonable for asymptomatic patients with very severe AS (aortic velocity ≥ 5 m/s) (stage C2) and low surgical risk	IIa	B
AVR is reasonable in asymptomatic patients (stage C1) with severe AS and an abnormal exercise test	IIa	B
AVR is reasonable in symptomatic patients with low-flow/low-gradient severe AS with reduced LVEF (stage S1) with a low-dose dobutamine stress study that shows an aortic velocity ≥ 4 m/s (or mean gradient ≥ 40 mm Hg) with a valve area ≤ 1.0 cm^2 at any dobutamine dose	IIa	B
AVR is reasonable for patients with moderate AS (stage B) (velocity 3.0–3.9 m/s) who are undergoing other cardiac surgery	IIa	C
AVR may be considered for asymptomatic patients with severe AS (stage C1) and rapid disease progression and low surgical risk	IIb	C
AVR may be considered in symptomatic patients who have low-flow/low-gradient severe AS (stage S2) who are normotensive and have an LVEF ≥ 50% if clinical, hemodynamic, and anatomic data support valve obstruction as the most likely cause of symptoms	IIb	C

AS, aortic stenosis, AVR, aortic valve replacement; COR, class of recommendation; LOE, level of evidence; LVEF, left ventricular ejection fraction.
Reproduced, with permission, from Nishimura RA et al. 2014 AHA/ACC Guideline for the Management of Patients With Valvular Heart Disease: A Report of the American College of Cardiology/American Heart Association Task Force on Practice Guidelines. Circulation. 2014 Jun 10;129(23):e521–643. © 2014 American Heart Association, Inc. [PMID: 24589853]

when an intervention is appropriate in various situations is outlined in Figure 10–3.

In young and adolescent patients, percutaneous balloon valvuloplasty still has a small role. Balloon valvuloplasty is associated with early restenosis in the elderly, and thus is rarely used except as a temporizing measure. Data suggest aortic balloon valvuloplasty in the elderly has an advantage only in those with preserved LV function, and such patients are usually excellent candidates for surgical AVR. Middle-aged adults generally can tolerate the anticoagulation therapy necessary for the use of mechanical aortic valves, so patients younger than 60 years generally undergo AVR with a bileaflet mechanical valve. If the aortic root is severely dilated as well (greater than 4.5 cm), then the valve may be housed in a Dacron sheath (Bentall procedure) and the root replaced along with the aortic valve. Alternatively, a human homograft root and valve replacement can be used. In patients older than 60 years, bioprosthetic (either porcine or bovine pericardial) valves with a life expectancy of about 10–15 years are routinely used instead of mechanical valves to avoid need for anticoagulation. Data favor the bovine pericardial valve over the porcine aortic valve. As it is becoming clearer that bioprosthetic valve degeneration can be repaired by percutaneous valve-in-valve stented valve replacement, it is likely that the use of mechanical valves will continue to decline. If the aortic annulus is small, a bioprosthetic valve with a short sheath can be sewn to the aortic wall (the stentless AVR) rather than sewing the prosthetic annulus to the aortic annulus. (Annulus is a relative term when speaking of the aortic valve, since there is no true annulus.) Another popular surgical option if the

aorta is enlarged is the Wheat procedure; it involves aortic root replacement above the coronary arteries and aortic valve. The coronary arteries thus remain attached to the native aorta between the new graft and prosthetic valve rather than being reimplanted onto an artificial sheath or homograft.

In patients with a bicuspid aortic valve, there is an associated ascending aortic aneurysm in about half. If the maximal dimension of the aortic root is greater than 5.5 cm, it is recommended to proceed with root replacement regardless of the severity of the aortic valve disease. It is appropriate to intervene when the maximal aortic root size is greater than 5.0 cm in diameter if there is a family history of aortic dissection or the aortic root size increases by more than 0.5 cm in 1 year. The aortic valve may be replaced at the same time if at least moderate aortic stenosis is present or may be either left alone or repaired (valve sparing operation).

Anticoagulation is required with the use of mechanical valves, and the international normalized ratio (INR) should be maintained between 2.0 and 3.0 for bileaflet valves. In general, mechanical aortic valves are less subject to thrombosis than mechanical mitral valves. Low-dose aspirin is recommended as well. Some newer bileaflet mechanical valves (On-X) allow for a lower INR range from 1.5 to 2.0.

The use of TAVR has grown dramatically, with over 75,000 implants reported. In the United States, the Food and Drug Administration (FDA) has granted limited approval for two devices, the Edwards SAPIEN and the Medtronic CoreValve, in high-risk patients. These devices are fundamentally stents with a trileaflet bioprosthetic

Class I

Class IIa

Class IIb

Abnormal aortic valve with reduced systolic opening

$V_{max} \geq 4$ m/s
$\Delta P_{mean} \geq 40$ mm Hg

V_{max} 3 m/s–3.9 m/s
ΔP_{mean} 20–39 mm Hg

$V_{max} < 3$ m/s
$\Delta P_{mean} < 30$ mm Hg

Symptomatic (stage D)

Asymptomatic (stage C)

Asymptomatic (stage B)

Symptomatic

LVEF < 50% (stage C2)

Other cardiac surgery

Abnormal ETT

$V_{max} \geq 5$ m/s
$\Delta P_{mean} \geq 60$ mm Hg
low-surgical risk

$\Delta V_{max} > 0.3$ m/s/y

LVEF < 50%

Yes — No

Stage S1: DSE with AVA ≤ 1.0 cm² and $V_{max} \geq 4.0$ m/s

Stage S2*
AVA ≤ 1.0 cm² and LVEF ≥ 50%

Other cardiac surgery

AS likely cause of symptoms

Yes — No

AVR (I)   AVR (IIa)   AVR (IIb)   Periodic monitoring

*AVR should be considered with stage S2 AS only if valve obstruction is the most likely cause of symptoms, stroke volume index is < 35 mL/m², indexed AVA is ≤ 0.6 cm²/m² and data are recorded when the patient is normotensive (systolic BP < 140 mm Hg).

AS, aortic stenosis; AVA, aortic valve area; AVR, aortic valve replacement; BP, blood pressure; DSE, dobutamine stress echocardiography; ETT, exercise treadmill test; LVEF, left ventricular ejection fraction; ΔP_{mean}, mean pressure gradient; V_{max}, maximum velocity.

▲ **Figure 10–3.** Algorithm for the management of aortic valve stenosis. (Reproduced, with permission from Nishimura RA et al. 2014 AHA/ACC Guideline for the Management of Patients With Valvular Heart Disease: A Report of the American College of Cardiology/American Heart Association Task Force on Practice Guidelines. Circulation. 2014 Jun 10;129(23): e521–643. © 2014 American Heart Association, Inc. [PMID: 24589853])

valve constructed within them. There are a variety of implantation approaches, though most valves are placed via a femoral artery approach. Other options include an antegrade approach via transseptal across the atrial septum, via the LV apex with a small surgical incision, via the subclavian arteries, or via a minithoracotomy. The Edwards SAPIEN valve is a balloon-expandable valvular stent, while the CoreValve is a valvular stent that self-expands when pushed out of the catheter sheath. Multiple other devices are in trials. These devices will allow for a wider range of aortic valve sizes to be treated; can be delivered with smaller catheters, eliminating the need for femoral artery cutdowns; will allow for repositioning before permanent implantation; and appear to result in less paravalvular regurgitation and less injury to the conduction system.

Cost remains a major issue. All of the professional societies stress the importance of a Heart Valve Team when considering aortic stenosis intervention. This is critically important because many patients referred for TAVR have serious comorbid conditions that will not improve with alleviation of the aortic stenosis.

Table 10–6 outlines the suggested indications for TAVR based on the 2014 AHA/ACC guidelines. TAVR is also being used more frequently in "valve-in-valve" procedures to reduce the gradient in patients with prosthetic valve dysfunction (regardless of whether in the aortic, mitral, tricuspid, or pulmonary position). The excellent results in very high-risk and very elderly patients have triggered studies regarding the use of TAVR in lower-risk populations as an alternative to surgical AVR.

Table 10–6. Recommendations for use of TAVR.

Recommendations	COR	LOE
Surgical AVR is recommended in patients who meet indication for AVR with low or intermediate surgical risk	I	A
TAVR is recommended in patients who meet an indication for AVR for AS who have a prohibitive surgical risk and a predicted post-TAVR surival > 12 mo	I	B
For patient in whom TAVR or high-risk surgical AVR is being considered, members of a Heart Valve Team should collaborate closely to provide optimal patient care	I	C
TAVR is a reasonable alternative to surgical AVR for AS in patients who meet indication for AVR and who have high surgical risk	IIa	B
Percutaneous aortic balloon dilation may be considered as a bridge to surgical or transcatheter AVR in severely symptomatic patients (NYHA class III-IV) with severe AS	IIb	C
TAVR is not recommended in patients in whom the existing comorbidities would preclude the expected benefit from correction of AS	III: No Benefit	B

AS, aortic stenosis; AVR, aortic valve replacement; COR, class of recommendation; LOE, level of evidence; NYHA, New York Heart Association; TAVR, transcatheter aortic valve replacement.
Reproduced, with permission, from Nishimura RA et al. 2014 AHA/ACC Guideline for the Management of Patients With Valvular Heart Disease: A Report of the American College of Cardiology/American Heart Association Task Force on Practice Guidelines. Circulation. 2014 Jun 10;129(23):e521–643. [PMID: 24589853]

► When to Refer

• All patients with echocardiographic evidence for mild-to-moderate aortic stenosis (estimated peak valve gradient greater than 30 mm Hg by echocardiography/Doppler) should be referred to a cardiologist for evaluation and to determine the frequency of follow-up.

• Any patients with symptoms suggestive of aortic stenosis (ie, exertional symptoms of chest pressure, shortness of breath, or presyncope) should be seen by a cardiologist.

Babaliarois V. Innovation in intervention: transcatheter aortic valve replacement focus issue. JACC Cardiol Interv. 2015 Apr 27;8(5):758–9. [PMID: 25946454]
Goel SS et al. Severe aortic stenosis and coronary artery disease—implications for management in the transcatheter aortic valve replacement era: a comprehensive review. J Am Coll Cardiol. 2013 Jul 2;62(1):1–10. [PMID: 23644089]
Herrmann HC et al. Predictors of mortality and outcomes of therapy in low-flow severe aortic stenosis: a Placement of Aortic Transcatheter Valves (PARTNER) trial analysis. Circulation. 2013 Jun 11;127(23):2316–26. [PMID: 23661722]
Holmes DR Jr et al. 2012 ACCF/AATS/SCAI/STS expert consensus document on transcatheter aortic valve replacement. J Am Coll Cardiol. 2012 Mar 27;59(13):1200–54. [PMID: 22300974]
Kapadia SR et al. 5-year outcomes of transcatheter aortic valve replacement for patients with inoperable aortic stenosis (PARTNER 1): a randomised controlled trial. Lancet. 2015 Jun 20;385(9986):2485–91. [PMID: 25788231]
Nishimura RA et al. 2014 AHA/ACC guideline for the management of patients with valvular heart disease: executive summary: a report of the American College of Cardiology/American Heart Association Task Force on Practice Guidelines. J Am Coll Cardiol. 2014 Jun 10;63(22):2438–88. Erratum in: J Am Coll Cardiol. 2014 Jun 10;63(22):2489. [PMID: 24603192]
Puskas J et al; PROACT Investigators. Reduced anticoagulation after mechanical aortic valve replacement: interim results from the prospective randomized on-X valve anticoagulation clinical trial randomized Food and Drug Administration investigational device exemption trial. J Thorac Cardiovasc Surg. 2014 Apr;147(4):1202–10. [PMID: 24512654]

Waksman R et al. Will TAVR become the default treatment for patients with severe aortic stenosis? J Am Coll Cardiol. 2015 Jul 14;66(2):122–4. [PMID: 26055948]
Webb JG et al. Transcatheter aortic valve replacement for bioprosthetic aortic valve failure: the valve-in-valve procedure. Circulation. 2013 Jun 25;127(25):2542–50. [PMID: 23797741]

AORTIC REGURGITATION

 ESSENTIALS OF DIAGNOSIS

► Usually asymptomatic until middle age; presents with left-sided failure or rarely chest pain.

► Echocardiography/Doppler is diagnostic.

► Surgery for symptoms, EF less than 50%, LV end-systolic dimension greater than 50 mm or LV end-diastolic dimension greater than 65 mm.

► General Considerations

Rheumatic aortic regurgitation has become much less common than in the preantibiotic era, and nonrheumatic causes now predominate. These include congenitally bicuspid valves, infective endocarditis, and hypertension. Many patients have aortic regurgitation secondary to aortic root diseases, such as that associated with Marfan syndrome or aortic dissection. Rarely, inflammatory diseases, such as ankylosing spondylitis or reactive arthritis, may be implicated.

► Clinical Findings

A. Symptoms and Signs

The clinical presentation is determined by the rapidity with which regurgitation develops. In **chronic aortic**

regurgitation, the only sign for many years may be a soft aortic diastolic murmur. As the severity of the aortic regurgitation increases, diastolic BP falls, and the LV progressively enlarges. Most patients remain asymptomatic for long periods even at this point. LV failure is a late event and may be sudden in onset. Exertional dyspnea and fatigue are the most frequent symptoms, but paroxysmal nocturnal dyspnea and pulmonary edema may also occur. Angina pectoris or atypical chest pain may occasionally be present. Associated CAD and presyncope or syncope are less common than in aortic stenosis.

Hemodynamically, because of compensatory LV dilation, patients eject a large stroke volume, which is adequate to maintain forward cardiac output until late in the course of the disease. LV diastolic pressure may rise when heart failure occurs. Abnormal LV systolic function (as manifested by reduced EF less than 50%) and increasing end-systolic LV volume (greater than 5.0 cm) are signs that surgical intervention is warranted.

The major physical findings in chronic aortic regurgitation relate to the high stroke volume being ejected into the systemic vascular system with rapid runoff as the regurgitation takes place (see Table 10–2). This results in a wide arterial pulse pressure. The pulse has a rapid rise and fall (water-hammer pulse or Corrigan pulse), with an elevated systolic and low diastolic pressure. The large stroke volume is also responsible for characteristic findings, such as Quincke pulses (nailbed capillary pulsations), Duroziez sign (to-and-fro murmur over a partially compressed femoral peripheral artery), and Musset sign (head bob with each pulse). In younger patients, the increased stroke volume may summate with the pressure wave reflected from the periphery and create a higher than expected systolic pressure in the lower extremities compared with the central aorta. Since the peripheral bed is much larger in the leg than the arm, the BP in the leg may be over 40 mm Hg higher than in the arm (Hill sign) in severe aortic regurgitation. The apical impulse is prominent, laterally displaced, usually hyperdynamic, and may be sustained. A systolic flow murmur is usually present and may be quite soft and localized; the aortic diastolic murmur is usually high-pitched and decrescendo. A mid or late diastolic low-pitched mitral murmur (Austin Flint murmur) may be heard in advanced aortic regurgitation, owing to relative obstruction of mitral inflow produced by partial closure of the mitral valve by the rapidly rising LV diastolic pressure due to the aortic regurgitation.

In acute aortic regurgitation (usually from aortic dissection or infective endocarditis), LV failure is manifested primarily as pulmonary edema and may develop rapidly; surgery is urgently required in such cases. Patients with acute aortic regurgitation do not have the dilated LV of chronic aortic regurgitation and the extra LV volume is handled poorly. For the same reason, the diastolic murmur is shorter, may be minimal in intensity, and the pulse pressure may not be widened—making clinical diagnosis difficult. The mitral valve may close prematurely even before LV systole has been initiated (preclosure) due to the rapid rise in the LV diastolic pressure, and the first heart sound is thus diminished or inaudible. Preclosure of the mitral valve can be readily detected on echocardiography and is considered an indication for urgent surgical intervention.

B. Diagnostic Studies

The ECG usually shows moderate to severe LVH. Radiographs show cardiomegaly with LV prominence and sometimes a dilated aorta.

Echocardiography demonstrates the major diagnostic features, including whether the lesion includes the proximal aortic root and what valvular pathology is present. Annual assessments of LV size and function are critical in determining the timing for valve replacement when the aortic regurgitation is severe. The 2014 AHA/ACC valvular guideline provides criteria for assessing the severity of aortic regurgitation. Cardiac MRI and CT can estimate aortic root size, particularly when there is concern for an ascending aneurysm. MRI can provide a regurgitant fraction to help confirm severity. Cardiac catheterization may be unnecessary in younger patients, particularly those with acute aortic regurgitation, but can help define hemodynamics, aortic root abnormalities, and associated CAD preoperatively in older patients. Increasing data are emerging that serum BNP or NT-pro BNP may be an early sign of LV dysfunction, and it is possible that these data will be added to recommendations for surgical intervention in the future.

▶ Treatment & Prognosis

Aortic regurgitation that appears or worsens during or after an episode of infective endocarditis or aortic dissection may lead to acute severe LV failure or subacute progression over weeks or months. The former usually presents as pulmonary edema; surgical replacement of the valve is indicated even during active infection. These patients may be transiently improved or stabilized by vasodilators.

Chronic aortic regurgitation may be tolerated for many years, but the prognosis without surgery becomes poor when symptoms occur. Since aortic regurgitation places both a preload (volume) and afterload increase on the LV, medications that decrease afterload can reduce regurgitation severity, although there are no convincing data that afterload reduction alters mortality. Current recommendations advocate afterload reduction in aortic regurgitation only when there is associated systolic hypertension (systolic BP greater than 140 mm Hg). Afterload reduction in normotensive patients does not appear warranted. Angiotensin receptor blockers (ARBs), rather than beta-blockers, are the preferred additions to the medical therapy in patients with an enlarged aorta, such as in Marfan syndrome, because of the theoretical ability of an ARB to reduce aortic stiffness (by blocking TGF-beta) and to slow the rate of aortic dilation. However, clinical trials evaluating the efficacy of ARBs to reduce aortic stiffness and slow the rate of aortic dilation have not yielded a positive outcome.

Surgery is indicated once symptoms emerge or for any evidence of LV dysfunction (as exhibited by a reduction in the LVEF or increase in the LV end-systolic diameter).

Table 10–7. When to operate in chronic severe aortic regurgitation (AR).

Indication for Surgery	Class and Level of Evidence (LOE)
Symptomatic	Class 1 LOE B
Asymptomatic	
Abnormal LVEF < 50%	CLASS 1 LOE B
Undergoing other heart surgery	CLASS 1 LOE C
Normal LVEF, but LVESD > 50 mm	CLASS 2a LOE B
Moderate AR and other heart surgery	CLASS 2a LOE C
Normal LVEF, but LVEDD > 65 mm	CLASS 2b LOE C

LVEF, left ventricular ejection fraction; LVEDD, left ventricular end-diastolic dimension; LVESD, left ventricular end-systolic dimension.

In addition, it is suggested that surgery should be considered when the LV becomes excessively enlarged (LV end-diastolic diameter greater than 65 mm) (Table 10–7).

The issues with AVR covered in the above section concerning aortic stenosis pertain here. Currently, however, there are no percutaneous approaches that specifically address aortic regurgitation when the cause is an enlarged aortic root. Aortic regurgitation due to a paravalvular prosthetic valve defect can occasionally be occluded with percutaneous occluder devices. The choice of prosthetic valve for AVR depends on the patient's age and compatibility with warfarin anticoagulation similar to the choices for AVR in aortic stenosis.

The operative mortality for AVR is usually in the 3–5% range. Aortic regurgitation due to aortic root disease requires repair or replacement of the root as well as surgical treatment of the aortic valve. Though valve-sparing operations have improved recently, most patients with root replacement undergo valve replacement at the same time. Root replacement in association with valve replacement may require reanastomosis of the coronary arteries, and thus the procedure is more complex than valve replacement alone. The Wheat procedure replaces the aortic root but spares the area where the coronaries attach to avoid the necessity for their reimplantation. Following surgery, LV size usually decreases and LV function generally improves even when the baseline EF is depressed.

The AHA/ACC 2014 valvular guidelines suggest the "cutoff" diameter value for repair of the aortic root in patients with a bicuspid valve should be 5.5 cm. There are data that dissection is much more prevalent when the aortic root diameter exceeds 6.0 cm, and the general sense is not to let it approach that size. Patients with risk factors (family history of dissection or an increase in the diameter of the root greater than 0.5 cm in 1 year) should have the aorta repaired when the maximal dimension exceeds 5.0 cm. The following classifications summarize when to operate on the aortic root in patients with a bicuspid aortic valve based on the guidelines:

Class 1 indication (LOE C): aortic root diameter at sinuses or ascending aorta greater than 5.5 cm (regardless of need for AVR).

Class 2a indication (LOE C): aortic root diameter at sinuses or ascending aorta greater than 5.0 cm when there are associated risk factors (family history of dissection or increase in size more than 0.5 cm in 1 year).

Class 2a indication (LOE C): aortic root diameter greater than 4.5 cm if patient undergoing AVR for valvular reasons.

▶ When to Refer

- Patients with audible aortic regurgitation should be seen, at least initially, by a cardiologist who can determine whether the patient needs follow-up.

- Patients with a dilated aortic root should be monitored by a cardiologist, since imaging studies other than the chest radiograph or echocardiogram may be required to decide surgical timing.

Bonow RO. Chronic mitral regurgitation and aortic regurgitation: have indications for surgery changed? J Am Coll Cardiol. 2013 Feb 19;61(7):693–701. [PMID: 23265342]

Nishimura RA et al. 2014 AHA/ACC guideline for the management of patients with valvular heart disease: executive summary: a report of the American College of Cardiology/American Heart Association Task Force on Practice Guidelines. J Am Coll Cardiol. 2014 Jun 10;63(22):2438–88. Erratum in: J Am Coll Cardiol. 2014 Jun 10;63(22):2489. [PMID: 24603192]

Vahanian A et al; Joint Task Force on the Management of Valvular Heart Disease of the European Society of Cardiology (ESC); European Association for Cardio-Thoracic Surgery (EACTS). Guidelines on the management of valvular heart disease (version 2012). Eur Heart J. 2012 Oct;33(19):2451–96. [PMID: 22922415]

TRICUSPID STENOSIS

 ESSENTIALS OF DIAGNOSIS

▶ Female predominance.

▶ History of rheumatic heart disease most likely. Carcinoid disease and prosthetic valve degeneration are the most common etiologies in the United States.

▶ Echocardiography/Doppler is diagnostic; mean valve gradient greater than 5 mm Hg or tricuspid valve area less than 1.0 cm² indicates severe tricuspid stenosis.

▶ General Considerations

Tricuspid valve stenosis is usually rheumatic in origin, although in the United States, tricuspid stenosis is more commonly due to prior tricuspid valve repair or replacement or to the carcinoid syndrome. Tricuspid regurgitation frequently accompanies the lesion. It should be suspected when "right heart failure" appears in the course of mitral valve disease or in the postoperative period after tricuspid valve repair or replacement. Congenital forms of tricuspid stenosis may also be rarely observed, as have case reports of multiple pacemaker leads creating RV inflow obstruction at the tricuspid valve.

▶ **Clinical Findings**

A. Symptoms and Signs

Tricuspid stenosis is characterized by right heart failure with hepatomegaly, ascites, and dependent edema. In sinus rhythm, a giant **a** wave is seen in the JVP, which is elevated (see Table 10–2). The typical diastolic rumble along the lower left sternal border mimics mitral stenosis, though in tricuspid stenosis the rumble increases with inspiration. In sinus rhythm, a presystolic liver pulsation may be found. It should be considered when patients exhibit signs of carcinoid syndrome.

B. Diagnostic Studies

In the absence of atrial fibrillation, the ECG reveals RA enlargement. The chest radiograph may show marked cardiomegaly with a normal PA size. A dilated superior vena cava and azygous vein may be evident.

The normal valve area of the tricuspid valve is 10 cm², so significant stenosis must be present to produce a gradient. Hemodynamically, a mean diastolic pressure gradient greater than 5 mm Hg is considered significant, although even a 2 mm Hg gradient can be considered abnormal. This can be demonstrated by echocardiography or cardiac catheterization. The 2014 AHA/ACC guidelines suggest a tricuspid valve area of less than 1.0 cm² should be considered significant.

▶ **Treatment & Prognosis**

Tricuspid stenosis may be progressive, eventually causing severe right-sided heart failure. Initial therapy is directed at reducing the fluid congestion, with diuretics the mainstay (see Treatment, Heart Failure). When there is considerable bowel edema, torsemide or bumetanide may have an advantage over other loop diuretics, such as furosemide, because they are better absorbed from the gut. Aldosterone inhibitors also help, particularly if there is liver engorgement or ascites. Neither surgical nor percutaneous valvuloplasty is particularly effective for relief of tricuspid stenosis, as residual tricuspid regurgitation is common. Tricuspid valve replacement is the preferred surgical approach. Mechanical tricuspid valve replacement is rarely done because the low flow predisposes to thrombosis and because the mechanical valve cannot be crossed should the need arise for right heart catheterization or pacemaker implantation. Therefore, bioprosthetic valves are almost always preferred. Often tricuspid valve replacement is performed in conjunction with mitral valve replacement for rheumatic mitral stenosis or regurgitation. Percutaneous transcatheter valve replacement (stented valve) has been used in degenerative prosthetic valve stenosis. The indications for valve replacement in severe tricuspid stenosis are straightforward:

> **Class 1** indication (LOE C): at time of operation for left-sided valve disease.
>
> **Class 1** indication (LOE C): if symptomatic.
>
> **Class 2b** indication (LOE C): rarely percutaneous balloon commissurotomy for isolated tricuspid stenosis in high-risk patients with no significant tricuspid regurgitation.

Al-Hijii M et al. The forgotten valve: Isolated severe tricuspid valve stenosis. Circulation. 2015 Aug 18;132(7):e123–5. [PMID: 26283605]

Petit CJ et al. Melody valve implantation in the pulmonary and tricuspid position. Catheter Cardiovasc Interv. 2013 Dec 1;82(7):E944–6. [PMID: 23197462]

TRICUSPID REGURGITATION

 ESSENTIALS OF DIAGNOSIS

▶ Frequently occurs in patients with pulmonary or cardiac disease with pressure or volume overload on the right ventricle.

▶ Tricuspid valve regurgitation from pacemaker lead placement is becoming more common.

▶ Echocardiography useful in determining cause (low- or high-pressure tricuspid regurgitation).

▶ **General Considerations**

Tricuspid valvular regurgitation often occurs whenever there is RV dilation from any cause. As tricuspid regurgitation increases, the RV size increases further pulling the valve open due to chordal and papillary muscle displacement. This, in turn, worsens the severity of the tricuspid regurgitation. **In most cases, the cause of the tricuspid regurgitation is the RV geometry and not primary tricuspid valve disease.** An enlarged, dilated RV may be present if there is RV systolic hypertension from valvular or subvalvular pulmonary valve stenosis, pulmonary hypertension for any reason, in severe pulmonary valve regurgitation, or in cardiomyopathy. The RV may also be injured from myocardial infarction or may be inherently dilated due to infiltrative diseases (RV dysplasia or sarcoidosis). RV dilation often occurs secondary to left heart failure. Inherent abnormalities of the tricuspid valve include Ebstein anomaly (displacement of the septal and posterior, but not the anterior, leaflets into the RV), tricuspid valve prolapse, carcinoid plaque formation, collagen disease inflammation, valvular tumors, or tricuspid endocarditis. In addition, pacemaker lead valvular injury is becoming an increasingly recognized iatrogenic cause.

Clinical Findings

A. Symptoms and Signs

The symptoms and signs of tricuspid regurgitation are identical to those resulting from RV failure due to any cause. As a generality, the diagnosis can be made by careful inspection of the JVP (see Table 10–2). The JVP waveform should decline during ventricular systole (the x descent). The timing of this decline can be observed by palpating the opposite carotid artery. As tricuspid regurgitation worsens, more and more of this x descent valley in the JVP is filled with the regurgitant wave until all of the x descent is obliterated and a positive systolic waveform will be noted in the JVP. An associated tricuspid regurgitation murmur may or may not be audible and can be distinguished from mitral regurgitation by the left parasternal location and increase with inspiration (Carvallo sign). An S_3 may accompany the murmur and is related to the high flow returning to the RV from the RA. Cyanosis may be present if the increased RA pressure stretches the atrial septum and opens a PFO or there is a true ASD (eg, in about 50% of patients with Ebstein anomaly). Severe tricuspid regurgitation results in hepatomegaly, edema, and ascites.

B. Diagnostic Studies

The ECG is usually nonspecific, though atrial flutter or atrial fibrillation is not uncommon. The chest radiograph may reveal evidence of an enlarged RA or dilated azygous vein and pleural effusion. The echocardiogram helps assess severity of tricuspid regurgitation (see the 2014 AHA/ACC valvular heart disease guidelines for definitions). In addition, echocardiography/Doppler provides RV systolic pressure as well as RV size and function. A paradoxically moving interventricular septum may be present due to the volume overload on the RV. Catheterization confirms the presence of the regurgitant wave in the RA and elevated RA pressures. If the PA or RV systolic pressure is less than 40 mm Hg, primary valvular tricuspid regurgitation should be suspected.

Treatment & Prognosis

Mild tricuspid regurgitation is common and generally can be well managed with diuretics. When severe tricuspid regurgitation is present, bowel edema may reduce the effectiveness of diuretics, such as furosemide, and intravenous diuretics should initially be used. Torsemide or bumetanide is better absorbed in this situation when oral diuretics are added. Aldosterone antagonists have a role as well, particularly if ascites is present. At times, the efficacy of loop diuretics can be enhanced by adding a thiazide diuretic (see Treatment, Heart Failure). Aquapheresis has also been proven helpful to reduce the edema in marked right heart failure, although results have been inconsistent.

Since most tricuspid regurgitation is secondary, definitive treatment usually requires elimination of the cause of the RV dysfunction. If the problem is left heart disease, then treatment of the left heart issues may lower pulmonary pressures, reduce RV size, and resolve the tricuspid regurgitation. Treatment for primary and secondary causes of pulmonary hypertension will generally reduce the tricuspid regurgitation. It is a class I recommendation that tricuspid annuloplasty be performed when significant tricuspid regurgitation is present and mitral valve replacement or repair is being performed for mitral regurgitation. Annuloplasty without insertion of a prosthetic ring (DeVega annuloplasty) may also be effective in reducing the tricuspid annular dilation. The valve leaflet itself can occasionally be primarily repaired in tricuspid valve endocarditis. In years past, tricuspid regurgitation due to endocarditis in substance-use patients was treated temporarily with removal of the entire valve, although it had to be replaced eventually (usually by 3–6 months); this practice is rarely done now. If there is an inherent defect in the tricuspid valve apparatus that cannot be repaired, then replacement of the tricuspid valve is warranted. Almost always, a bioprosthetic valve, and not a mechanical valve, is used. Anticoagulation is not required for bioprosthetic valves unless there is associated atrial fibrillation or flutter. Tricuspid regurgitation due to bioprosthetic degeneration has been shown to respond to transcatheter valve replacement in experienced centers. There are early reports of percutaneous tricuspid valve replacement for native valve tricuspid regurgitation being successful, so this may emerge soon as a treatment option.

When to Refer

- Anyone with moderate or severe tricuspid regurgitation should be seen at least once by a cardiologist to determine whether studies and intervention are needed.

- Severe tricuspid regurgitation requires regular follow-up by a cardiologist.

Eicken A et al. Percutaneous tricuspid valve implantation: two center experience with mid-term results. Circ Cardiovasc Interv. 2015;8(4):e002155. [PMID: 25873731]

Nishimura RA et al. 2014 AHA/ACC guideline for the management of patients with valvular heart disease: executive summary: a report of the American College of Cardiology/American Heart Association Task Force on Practice Guidelines. J Am Coll Cardiol. 2014 Jun 10;63(22):2438–88. Erratum in: J Am Coll Cardiol. 2014 Jun 10;63(22):2489. [PMID: 24603192]

Vahanian A et al; Joint Task Force on the Management of Valvular Heart Disease of the European Society of Cardiology (ESC); European Association for Cardio-Thoracic Surgery (EACTS). Guidelines on the management of valvular heart disease (version 2012). Eur Heart J. 2012 Oct;33(19):2451–96. [PMID: 22922415]

PULMONARY VALVE REGURGITATION

ESSENTIALS OF DIAGNOSIS

► Most cases are due to pulmonary hypertension resulting in high-pressure pulmonary valve regurgitation.

► Echocardiogram is definitive in high-pressure, but may be less definitive in low-pressure pulmonary valve regurgitation.

► Low-pressure pulmonary valve regurgitation is well tolerated.

General Considerations

Pulmonary valve regurgitation can be divided into **high-pressure causes** (due to pulmonary hypertension) and **low-pressure causes** (usually due to a dilated pulmonary annulus, to a congenitally abnormal [bicuspid or dysplastic] pulmonary valve, or to plaque from carcinoid disease). It may also follow surgical repair, eg, frequently occurring after repair of tetralogy of Fallot with a transannular patch or after surgical pulmonary valve replacement. Because the RV tolerates a volume load better than a pressure load, it tends to tolerate low pressure pulmonary valve regurgitation for long periods of time without dysfunction.

Clinical Findings

Most patients are asymptomatic. Others show symptoms of right heart volume overload. On examination, a hyperdynamic RV can usually be palpated (RV lift). If the PA is enlarged, it may be palpated along the left sternal border. P_2 will be palpable in pulmonary hypertension and both systolic and diastolic thrills are occasionally noted. On auscultation, the second heart sound may be widely split due to prolonged RV systole or associated right bundle branch block. A pulmonary valve systolic click may be noted as well as a right-sided gallop. If pulmonic stenosis is also present, the ejection click may decline with inspiration, while any associated systolic pulmonary murmur will increase. In high-pressure pulmonary valve regurgitation, the pulmonary diastolic (Graham Steell) murmur is readily audible. It is often contributed to by a dilated pulmonary annulus. The murmur increases with inspiration and diminishes with the Valsalva maneuver. In low-pressure pulmonary valve regurgitation, the PA diastolic pressure may be only a few mm Hg higher than the RV diastolic pressure, and there is little diastolic gradient to produce a murmur or characteristic echocardiography/Doppler findings. At times, only contrast angiography or MRI of the main PA will show the free flowing pulmonary valve regurgitation in low-pressure pulmonary valve regurgitation. This situation is common in patients following repair of tetralogy of Fallot where, despite little murmur, there may effectively be no pulmonary valve present. This can be suspected by noting an enlarging right ventricle.

The ECG is generally of little value, although right bundle branch block is common, and there may be ECG criteria for RVH. The chest radiograph may show only the enlarged RV and PA. Echocardiography may demonstrate evidence of RV volume overload (paradoxic septal motion and an enlarged RV), and Doppler can determine peak systolic RV pressure and reveal any associated tricuspid regurgitation. The interventricular septum may appear flattened if there is pulmonary hypertension. The size of the main PA can be determined and color flow Doppler can demonstrate the pulmonary valve regurgitation, particularly in the high-pressure situation. Cardiac MRI and CT can be useful for assessing the size of the PA, for estimating regurgitant flow, for excluding other causes of pulmonary hypertension (eg, thromboembolic disease, peripheral PA stenosis), and for evaluating RV function. Cardiac catheterization is confirmatory only.

Treatment & Prognosis

Pulmonary valve regurgitation rarely needs specific therapy other than treatment of the primary cause. In low-pressure pulmonary valve regurgitation due to surgical transannular patch repair of tetralogy of Fallot, pulmonary valve replacement may be indicated if RV enlargement or dysfunction is present. In tetralogy of Fallot, the QRS will widen as RV function declines (a QRS greater than 180 msec suggests a higher risk for sudden death) and increasing RV volumes should trigger an evaluation for potential severe pulmonary valve regurgitation. In carcinoid heart disease, pulmonary valve replacement with a porcine bioprosthesis may be undertaken, though the plaque from this disorder eventually covers the prosthetic pulmonary valve, which tends to limit the lifespan of these valves. In high-pressure pulmonary valve regurgitation, treatment to control the cause of the pulmonary hypertension is key. High-pressure pulmonary valve regurgitation is poorly tolerated and is a serious condition that needs a thorough evaluation for cause and therapy. Pulmonary valve replacement requires a bioprosthetic valve in most cases. Pulmonary valve regurgitation due to an RV to PA conduit or due to a pulmonary autograft replacement as part of the Ross procedure can be repaired with a percutaneous pulmonary valve (Melody valve). Bioprosthetic pulmonary valve regurgitation has also been treated using a percutaneous valve (Edwards Sapien).

When to Refer

Patients with pulmonary valve regurgitation that results in RV enlargement should be referred to a cardiologist regardless of the estimated pulmonary pressures.

McElhinney DB et al. Short- and medium-term outcomes after transcatheter pulmonary valve replacement in the expanded multicenter US Melody valve trial. Circulation. 2010 Aug 3;122(5):507–16. [PMID: 20644013]
Warnes CA et al. ACC/AHA 2008 Guidelines for the Management of Adults With Congenital Heart Disease. A Report of the American College of Cardiology/American Heart Association Task Force on Practice Guidelines. Circulation. 2008 Dec 2;118(23):e714–833. [PMID: 18997169]

MANAGEMENT OF ANTICOAGULATION FOR PROSTHETIC HEART VALVES DURING PREGNANCY & NONCARDIAC SURGERY OR PROCEDURES

The risk of thromboembolism is much lower with bioprosthetic valves than mechanical prosthetic valves. Mechanical mitral valve prostheses pose a greater risk for thrombosis than mechanical aortic valves. For that reason, the INR should be kept between 2.5 and 3.5 for mechanical mitral prosthetic valves but can be kept between 2.0 and 2.5 for most mechanical aortic prosthetic valves. In 2013, the On-X bileaflet aortic valve prosthesis trial confirmed that with the On-X bileaflet AVR, an INR range as low as 1.5–2.0 may be considered safe. Most guidelines recommend that anticoagulation with a vitamin K antagonist (VKA) is reasonable for the first 3 months after a bioprosthetic mitral valve replacement or repair, although many experts do not feel that is necessary without atrial fibrillation. Enteric-coated aspirin (81 mg once daily) is recommended for both types of mechanical valves. Clopidogrel is recommended for the first 6 months after transcatheter valve replacement in addition to lifelong aspirin.

In 2015 the European Registry of Pregnancy and Cardiac Disease (ROPAC) reported on a registry that compared pregnant women who had undergone mechanical and bioprosthetic valve replacement to pregnant women who had not. Maternal mortality was similar between the mechanical and bioprosthetic valve patients (1.5% and 1.4%, respectively) but was much higher than those without an artificial valve (0.2%). When the mechanical versus the bioprosthetic patients were further assessed, it was found that pregnant women with mechanical valves were more likely to suffer negative events than women with bioprosthetic valves. Hemorraghic events occurred in 23.1% versus 9.2%, miscarriage on warfarin occurred in 28.6% versus 9.2%, and late fetal death was noted in 7.1% versus 0.7%, respectively. These data suggest **a high risk for mortality and morbidity for pregnant patients with mechanical heart valves.**

Stoppage of warfarin for noncardiac surgery is likewise dependent on which mechanical valve is involved, the patient-specific risk factors, and the procedure contemplated. The risk of thromboembolism is highest in the first few months after valve replacement. While the interruption of warfarin therapy is generally safe, most cases of valve thrombosis occur during periods of inadequate anticoagulation, so the time interval without coverage should be kept as short as possible. High-risk features include atrial fibrillation, a prior history of thromboembolism, heart failure or low LVEF, a hypercoagualable state, a mechanical valve in the mitral position, a known high-risk valve (ball-in-cage), or concomitant cancer. The use of bridging vitamin K antagonists (VKAs), unfractionated heparin, low-molecular-weight heparin (LMWH) and antifibrinolytics in various clinical situations in patients with VHD is summarized in Table 10–8 and the issues are covered in more depth in both the 2012 European Society of Cardiology (ESC) and the 2014 AHA/ACC VHD guidelines. In general, some procedures (eg, pacemaker implantation and routine dental work) require no stoppage of VKAs, while in other situations the warfarin can be stopped 3 days ahead of the procedure and resumed the night after the procedure (ie, in patients with bileaflet aortic valves) without any bridging unfractionated heparin or LMWH. In high-risk patients, though, the warfarin should be stopped and bridging with either unfractionated heparin or LMWH begun once the INR falls below therapeutic levels. Fresh frozen plasma or prothrombin complex concentrate is reasonable in an emergency situation for acute reversal. Most patients with a mechanical valve should not have the warfarin reversed with vitamin K if it can be avoided because this can result in a transient hypercoagualable state and it may take many days to reach a therapeutic INR once vitamin K has been administered.

Warfarin causes fetal skeletal abnormalities in up to 2% of women who become pregnant while taking the medication, so every effort is made to defer valve replacement in women until after childbearing age. However, if a woman with a mechanical valve becomes pregnant while taking warfarin, the risk of stopping warfarin may be higher for the mother than the risk of continuing warfarin for the fetus. The risk of warfarin to the fetal skeleton is greatest during the first trimester and, remarkably, is **more related to dose than to the INR level.** Guidelines suggest it is reasonable to continue warfarin for the first trimester if the dose is 5 mg/day or less. If the dose is more than 5 mg/day, it is appropriate to consider either LMWH (as long as the anti-Xa is being monitored [range: 0.8 units/mL to 1.2 units/mL]) or unfractionated heparin (if the activated partial thromboplastin time [aPTT] can be monitored and is at least two times control). Guidelines suggest warfarin and low-dose aspirin are safe during the second and third trimester and then should be stopped at time of delivery. At time of vaginal delivery, unfractionated intravenous heparin with aPTT at least two times control is desirable. DOACs (antithrombin or Xa inhibitors) should not be used in place of warfarin for mechanical prosthetic valves. This is based on the RE-ALIGN trial that showed that carefully dosed dabigatran had both more thrombotic complications and more bleeding than warfarin. Because of questions regarding compliance in this trial though, other studies are ongoing to further define whether the DOACs may have any role in patients with mechanical heart valves.

Management of suspected mechanical valve thrombosis depends on whether a left-sided or right-sided valve is involved, the size of the thrombus, and the patient's clinical condition. Simple fluoroscopy can help assess mechanical valve motion, although a TEE is often indicated to assess thrombus size. Therapeutic unfractionated heparin should be given to all patients, and this is generally effective. Fibrinolytic therapy is indicated if heparin therapy is ineffective and the clinical onset has been less than 2 weeks, the thrombus is smaller than 0.8 cm^2, NYHA class symptoms are mild (FC 1 or 2) or the valve is right-sided. Surgery is rarely indicated, and reserved for those with left-sided mechanical valves in NYHA FC 3 or 4 or in whom TEE demonstrates a mobile thrombus larger than 0.8 cm^2.

Eikelboom JW et al; RE-ALIGN Investigators. Dabigatran versus warfarin in patients with mechanical heart valves. N Engl J Med. 2013 Sep 26;369(13):1206–14. [PMID: 23991661]

Holbrook A et al. Evidence-based management of anticoagulant therapy: Antithrombotic Therapy and Prevention of Thrombosis, 9th ed: American College of Chest Physicians Evidence-Based Clinical Practice Guidelines. Chest. 2012 Feb;141(2 Suppl):e152S–84S. [PMID: 22315259]

Nishimura RA et al. 2014 AHA/ACC guideline for the management of patients with valvular heart disease: executive summary: a report of the American College of Cardiology/American Heart Association Task Force on Practice Guidelines. J Am Coll Cardiol. 2014 Jun 10;63(22):2438–88. Erratum in: J Am Coll Cardiol. 2014 Jun 10;63(22):2489. [PMID: 24603192]

Van Hagen IM et al. Pregnancy in women with a mechanical heart valve: data from the ESC Registry of Pregnancy and Cardiac Diseases (ROPAC). Circulation. 2015 Jul 14;132(2): 132–42. [PMID: 26100109]

Table 10–8. Recommendations for administering vitamin K antagonist (VKA) therapy in patients undergoing procedures or patients with certain clinical conditions.

Procedures	Recommendations
General	Stop VKA 5 days prior and resume 12–24 hours after procedure
Bridging for mechanical heart valves	Required only for those at high risk for thromboembolism Bridge with UFH or LMWH and stop UFH 4–6 hours before procedure or stop LMWH 24 hours before procedure Resume 48–72 hours after the procedure

Clinical Situations	Recommendations
Atrial fibrillation and moderate or severe mitral stenosis	VKA (target INR 2.0–3.0) If patient refuses, aspirin (50–100 mg) plus clopidogrel (75 mg)
Sinus rhythm and mitral stenosis	If left atrial size > 5.5 cm, then consider VKA (target 2.0–3.0)
Intermittent atrial fibrillation or history of systemic embolus and mitral stenosis	VKA (target INR 2.0–3.0)

Endocarditis
  Native valve or bioprosthetic valve endocarditis
  Mechanical valve endocarditis
	No anticoagulation recommended
	Hold VKA until "safe to resume" (generally when mycotic aneurysm is ruled out or there is no need for urgent surgery)

First 3 months following valve replacement
  Bioprosthetic aortic valve replacement
  Transcatheter valve replacement
  Mitral or aortic repair
  Bioprosthetic mitral valve
	
	Aspirin (50–100 mg)
	Aspirin (50–100 mg) plus clopidogrel (75 mg)
	Aspirin (50–100 mg)
	VKA (target INR 2.0–3.0)

Long-term anticoagulation after valve replacement
  Bioprosthetic valve in normal sinus rhythm
  Mechanical valve replacement
	
	Aspirin (50–100 mg)
	VKA (target INR 2.0–3.0 for aortic, target INR 2.5–3.5 for mitral) plus aspirin (50–100 mg)

Prosthetic valve thrombosis
  Right sided valve
  Left sided valve
	
	Fibrinolytic therapy
	Early surgery if thrombus large (> 0.8 cm^2 area), otherwise either fibrinolytic therapy or UFH

Pregnancy and a mechanical heart valve	Add aspirin (50–100 mg) for high risk Adjusted dose LMWH twice daily throughout pregnancy (follow anti-Xa 4 hours after dose) *or* Adjusted dose UFH every 12 hours throughout pregnancy (aPTT > 2 times control or anti-Xa between 0.35 and 0.70) *or* Adjusted dose UFH or LMWH until 13th week of pregnancy then VKA until close to delivery, then resume UFH or LMWH

aPTT, activated partial thromboplastin time; INR, international normalized ratio; LMWH, low-molecular-weight heparin; UFH, unfractionated heparin.

Data from Holbrook A et al. Evidence-based management of anticoagulant therapy: Antithrombotic Therapy and Prevention of Thrombosis, 9th ed: American College of Chest Physicians Evidence-Based Clinical Practice Guidelines. Chest 2012;141: (Suppl 2:e152S–e184S).

CORONARY HEART DISEASE (ATHEROSCLEROTIC CAD, ISCHEMIC HEART DISEASE)

Coronary heart disease (CHD), or atherosclerotic CAD, is the number one cause of death in the United States and worldwide. Every minute, an American dies of CHD. About 37% of people who experience an acute coronary event, either angina or myocardial infarction, will die of it in the same year. Death rates of CHD have declined every year since 1968, with about half of the decline from 1980 to 2000 due to treatments and half due to improved risk factors. CHD is still responsible for approximately one of five

deaths and over 600,000 deaths per year in the United States. CHD afflicts nearly 16 million Americans and the prevalence rises steadily with age; thus, the aging of the US population promises to increase the overall burden of CHD.

▶ Risk Factors for CAD

Most patients with CHD have some identifiable risk factor. These include a positive family history (the younger the onset in a first-degree relative, the greater the risk), male sex, blood lipid abnormalities, diabetes mellitus, hypertension, physical inactivity, abdominal obesity, and cigarette smoking, psychosocial factors, consumption of too few fruits and vegetables, and too much alcohol. Many of these risk factors are modifiable. **Smoking** remains the number one preventable cause of death and illness in the United States. Although smoking rates have declined in the United States in recent decades, 18% of women and 21% of men still smoke. According to the World Health Organization, 1 year after quitting, the risk of CHD decreases by 50%. Various interventions have been shown to increase the likelihood of successful smoking cessation (see Chapter 1).

Hypercholesterolemia is an important modifiable risk factor for CHD. Risk increases progressively with higher levels of low-density lipoprotein (LDL) cholesterol and declines with higher levels of high-density lipoprotein (HDL) cholesterol. Composite risk scores, such as the Framingham score and the 10-year atherosclerotic cardiovascular disease risk calculator (http://my.americanheart.org/cvriskcalculator), provide estimates of the 10-year probability of development of CHD that can guide primary prevention strategies. The 2013 ACC/AHA Guideline on the Treatment of Blood Cholesterol to Reduce Atherosclerotic Cardiovascular Risk in Adults suggests statin therapy in four populations: patients with (1) clinical atherosclerotic disease, (2) LDL cholesterol 190 mg/dL or higher, (3) diabetes who are aged 40–75 years, and (4) an estimated 10-year atherosclotic risk of 7.5% or more aged 40–75 years (Figure 10–4). Importantly, the updated guidelines do not recommend treating to a target LDL cholesterol, an approach that has never been shown to be effective in randomized trials. Patients in these categories should be treated with moderate or high intensity statin, with high intensity statin for the higher risk populations (Table 10–9). The ACC/AHA atherosclerotic cardiovascular disease risk estimator allows clinicians to determine the 10-year CHD risk to determine treatment decisions (http://tools.cardiosource.org/ASCVD-Risk-Estimator/). The predominant therapy recommended based on patient risk is either moderate- or high-intensity statin therapy.

The **metabolic syndrome** is defined as a constellation of three or more of the following: abdominal obesity, triglycerides 150 mg/dL or higher, HDL cholesterol less than 40 mg/dL for men and less than 50 mg/dL for women, fasting glucose 110 mg/dL or higher, and hypertension. This syndrome is increasing in prevalence at an alarming rate. Related to the metabolic syndrome, the epidemic of **obesity** in the United States is likewise a major factor contributing to CHD risk.

Myocardial Hibernation & Stunning

Areas of myocardium that are persistently underperfused but still viable may develop sustained contractile dysfunction. This phenomenon, which is termed **myocardial hibernation,** appears to represent an adaptive response that may be associated with depressed LV function. It is important to recognize this phenomenon, since this form of dysfunction is reversible following coronary revascularization. Hibernating myocardium can be identified by radionuclide testing, positron emission tomography (PET), contrast-enhanced MRI, or its retained response to inotropic stimulation with dobutamine. A related phenomenon, termed **myocardial stunning,** is the occurrence of persistent contractile dysfunction following prolonged or repetitive episodes of myocardial ischemia. Clinically, myocardial stunning is often seen after reperfusion of acute myocardial infarction and is defined with improvement following revascularization.

Stone NJ et al. 2013 ACC/AHA Guideline on the Treatment of Blood Cholesterol to Reduce Atherosclerotic Cardiovascular Risk in Adults: a report of the American College of Cardiology/ American Heart Association Task Force on Practice Guidelines. Circulation. 2014 Jun 24;129(25 Suppl 2):S1–45. [PMID: 24222016]

Primary & Secondary Prevention of CHD

Although many risk factors for CHD are not modifiable, it is now clear that interventions, such as smoking cessation, treatment of dyslipidemia, and lowering of BP can both prevent coronary disease and delay its progression and complications after it is manifest.

Lowering LDL levels delays the progression of atherosclerosis and in some cases may produce regression. Even in the absence of regression, fewer new lesions develop, endothelial function may be restored, and coronary event rates are markedly reduced in patients with clinical evidence of vascular disease.

A series of clinical trials has demonstrated the efficacy of hydroxymethylglutaryl coenzyme A (HMG-CoA) reductase inhibitors (statins) in preventing death, coronary events, and strokes. Beneficial results have been found in patients who have already experienced coronary events (secondary prevention), in those at particularly high risk for events (patients with diabetes and patients with peripheral artery disease), and those with elevated cholesterol without multiple risk factors, and those without vascular disease or diabetes with elevated hsCRP with normal LDL levels. The benefits of statin therapy at moderate and high doses (Table 10–9) are recommended by the cholesterol treatment guidelines. The IMPROVE-IT study showed that ezetimibe, 10 mg daily, combined with simvastatin was superior to simvastatin alone in reducing LDL cholesterol and in reducing the risk of myocardial infarction and ischemic stroke, but not mortality, in stabilized patients following an acute coronary syndrome. This was associated with a reduction of LDL to 53.7 mg/dL compared to 69.7 mg/dL.

Novel monoclonal antibodies that inhibit proprotein convertase subtilisin/kexin type 9 (PCSK9) have been developed and have shown to reduce LDL cholesterol levels significantly beyond levels associated with traditional statin therapy. These therapies have been studied in initial randomized trials of patients with maximally tolerated statin therapy (and for patients with statin intolerance) and have lowered LDL with signals of improved cardiovascular outcomes, but with ongoing trials to test whether clinical outcomes are actually improved. Two such medications—alirocumab and evolocumab—have been approved by the FDA for patients on maximally tolerated statin therapy with familial hypercholesterolemia and atherosclerotic vascular disease, or both, and who require additional lowering of LDL. These medications cost approximately $14,000 per year in the United States.

ASCVD statin benefit groups
Heart healthy lifestyle habits are the foundation of ASCVD prevention.
In individuals not receiving cholesterol-lowering drug therapy, recalculate estimated 10-y ASCVD risk every 4–6 y in individuals aged 40–75 y without clinical ASCVD or diabetes and with LDL–C 70–189 mg/dL.

Adults age > 21 y and a candidate for statin therapy —Yes→ Clinical ASCVD

—Yes→ Age ≤ 75 y
High-intensity statin
(Moderate-intensity statin if not candidate for high-intensity statin)

—Yes→ Age > 75 y OR if not candidate for high-intensity statin
Moderate-intensity statin

No ↓

Definitions of high- and moderate-intensity statin therapy
(See Table 10–9)

High	Moderate
Daily dose lowers LDL–C by appox. ≥ 50%	Daily dose lowers LDL–C by appox. 30% to < 50%

LDL–C ≥ 190 mg/dL —Yes→ **High-intensity statin**
(Moderate-intensity statin if not candidate for high-intensity statin)

No ↓

Diabetes
Type 1 or 2
age 40–75 y

—Yes→ **Moderate-intensity statin**

—Yes→ Estimated 10-y ASCVD risk ≥ 7.5%[1]
High-intensity statin

No ↓

Estimate 10-y ASCVD risk
with pooled cohort equations[2]

↓

≥ 7.5% estimated 10-y ASCVD risk and age 40–75 y —Yes→ Moderate-to-high intensity statin

No ↓

ASCVD prevention benefit of statin therapy may be less clear in other groups.
In selected individuals, consider additional factors influencing ASCVD risk[3] and potential ASCVD risk benefits and adverse effects, drug-drug interactions, and patient preferences for statin treatment.

[1]Percent reduction in LDL–C can be used as an indication of response and adherence to therapy but is not in itself a treatment goal.

[2]The Pooled Cohort Equations can be used to estimate 10-year ASCVD risk in individuals with and without diabetes. A downloadable spreadsheet enabling estimation of 10-year and lifetime risk for ASCVD and a web-based calculator are available at http://my.americanheart.org/cvriskcalculator and http://www.cardiosource.org/science-and-quality/practice-guidelines-and-quality-standards/2013-prevention-guideline-tools.aspx.

[3]Primary LDL–C ≥ 160 mg/dL or other evidence of genetic hyperlipidemias, family history of premature ASCVD with onset < 55 years of age in a first-degree male relative or < 65 years of age in a first-degree female relative, high-sensitivity C-reactive protein > 2 mg/L, CAC score ≥ 300 Agatston units or ≥ 75 percentile for age, sex, and ethnicity, ankle-brachial index < 0.9, or elevated lifetime risk of ASCVD.

ASCVD, atherosclerotic cardiovascular disease; CAC, coronary artery calcium; LDL–C, low-density lipoprotein cholesterol.

▲ **Figure 10–4.** Major recommendation for statin therapy for ASCVD prevention. (Adapted from Stone NJ et al. 2013 ACC/AHA Guideline on the Treatment of Blood Cholesterol to Reduce Atherosclerotic Cardiovascular Risk in Adults: A Report of the American College of Cardiology/American Heart Association Task Force on Practice Guidelines. Circulation. 2014 Jun 24;129(25 Suppl 2):S1–45. [PMID: 24222016])

Table 10–9. High-, moderate-, and low-intensity statin therapy (used in the RCTs reviewed by the expert panel).[1,2]

High-Intensity Statin Therapy	Moderate-Intensity Statin Therapy	Low-Intensity Statin Therapy
Daily dose lowers LDL-C on average by approximately ≥ 50%	Daily dose lowers LDL-C on average by approximately 30% to < 50%	Daily dose lowers LDL-C on average by < 30%
Atorvastatin (40[3])–80 mg **Rosuvastatin 20** (40) **mg**	**Atorvastatin 10** (20) **mg** **Rosuvastatin** (5) **10 mg** **Simvastatin 20–40 mg**[4] **Pravastatin 40** (80) **mg** **Lovastatin 40 mg** *Fluvastatin XL 80 mg* **Fluvastatin 40 mg twice daily** **Pitavastatin 2–4 mg**	*Simvastatin 10 mg* **Pravastatin 10–20 mg** **Lovastatin 20 mg** *Fluvastatin 20–40 mg* *Pitavastatin 1 mg*

[1]Statins and doses in boldface were evaluated in RCTs; all demonstrated a reduction in major cardiovascular events. Statins and doses that are approved by the US FDA but were not tested in the RCTs reviewed are listed in italics.
[2]Individual responses to statin therapy varied in the RCTs and should be expected to vary in clinical practice. There might be a biologic basis for a less-than-average response.
[3]Evidence from one RCT only: down-titration if unable to tolerate atorvastatin 80 mg in IDEAL.
[4]Although simvastatin 80 mg was evaluated in RCTs, initiation of simvastatin 80 mg or titration to 80 mg is not recommended by the FDA due to the increased risk of myopathy, including rhabdomyolysis.
FDA, Food and Drug Administration; IDEAL, Incremental Decrease through Aggressive Lipid Lowering study; LDL–C, low-density lipoprotein cholesterol; RCTs, randomized controlled trials.
Modified, with permission, from Stone NJ et al. 2013 ACC/AHA Guideline on the Treatment of Blood Cholesterol to Reduce Atherosclerotic Cardiovascular Risk in Adults: A Report of the American College of Cardiology/American Heart Association Task Force on Practice Guidelines. Circulation. 2014 Jul 1;63(25 Pt B):2889–934.

Treatment to raise HDL levels has failed to show benefit. The AIM High trial found no benefit from the addition of niacin in patients with vascular disease and a serum LDL near 70 mg/dL who were receiving statin therapy. The HPS2-THRIVE trial found no benefit but rather substantial harm of extended-release niacin (2 g) plus laropiprant (an antiflushing agent) for preventing vascular events in a population of over 25,000 patients with vascular disease who were taking simvastatin.

Antiplatelet therapy is another very effective preventive measure. Aspirin (325 mg every other day) in men over the age of 50 years reduces the incidence of myocardial infarction. A similar approach (100 mg every other day), however, did not prevent myocardial infarction in women age 45 years or older, although stroke did appear to be reduced. Thus, the role of aspirin in primary prevention, including the dose, remains controversial. A prudent approach would be to administer 81–325 mg daily to men with multiple coronary risk factors or concomitant diabetes starting at age 45–50 years if no contraindication is present. While clopidogrel was found to be effective at preventing vascular events for 9–12 months after acute coronary syndromes, it was not found to be effective at preventing vascular events with longer-term treatment in the CHARISMA trial. This trial included patients with clinically evident stable atherothrombosis or with multiple risk factors; all were treated with aspirin and observed for a median of 28 months. The previously mentioned GISSI Prevention Trial found a significant but modest reduction in mortality with administration of omega-3 fatty acid (850 mg daily) in postinfarction patients.

The HOPE and the EUROPA trials demonstrated that ACE inhibitors (ramipril 10 mg/day and perindopril 8 mg/day, respectively) reduced fatal and nonfatal vascular events (cardiovascular deaths, nonfatal myocardial infarctions, and nonfatal strokes) by 20–25% in patients at high risk, including patients with diabetes with additional risk factors or patients with clinical coronary, cerebral, or peripheral arterial atherosclerotic disease.

Cannon CP et al; IMPROVE-IT Investigators. Ezetimibe added to statin therapy after acute coronary syndromes. N Engl J Med. 2015 Jun 18;372(25):2387–97. [PMID: 26039521]

Kohno T. Report of the American Heart Association (AHA) Scientific Sessions 2014, Chicago. Circ J. 2015;79(1):34–40. [PMID: 25502168]

Robinson JG et al; ODYSSEY LONG TERM Investigators. Efficacy and safety of alirocumab in reducing lipids and cardiovascular events. N Engl J Med. 2015 Apr 16;372(16):1489–99. [PMID: 25773378]

Sabatine MS et al; Open-Label Study of Long-Term Evaluation against LDL Cholesterol (OSLER) Investigators. Efficacy and safety of evolocumab in reducing lipids and cardiovascular events. N Engl J Med. 2015 Apr 16;372(16):1500–9. [PMID: 25773607]

CHRONIC STABLE ANGINA PECTORIS

ESSENTIALS OF DIAGNOSIS

▶ Precordial chest pain, usually precipitated by stress or exertion, relieved rapidly by rest or nitrates.

▶ ECG or scintigraphic evidence of ischemia during pain or stress testing.

▶ Angiographic demonstration of significant obstruction of major coronary vessels.

General Considerations

Angina pectoris is usually due to atherosclerotic heart disease. Coronary vasospasm may occur at the site of a lesion or, less frequently, in apparently normal vessels. Other unusual causes of coronary artery obstruction, such as congenital anomalies, emboli, arteritis, or dissection may cause ischemia or infarction. Angina may also occur in the absence of coronary artery obstruction as a result of severe myocardial hypertrophy, severe aortic stenosis or regurgitation, or in response to increased metabolic demands, as in hyperthyroidism, marked anemia, or paroxysmal tachycardias with rapid ventricular rates.

Clinical Findings

A. Symptoms

The diagnosis of angina pectoris depends principally upon the history, which should specifically include the following information: circumstances that precipitate and relieve angina, characteristics of the discomfort, location and radiation, duration of attacks, and effect of nitroglycerin.

1. Circumstances that precipitate and relieve angina— Angina occurs most commonly during activity and is relieved by resting. Patients may prefer to remain upright rather than lie down, as increased preload in recumbency increases myocardial work. The amount of activity required to produce angina may be relatively consistent under comparable physical and emotional circumstances or may vary from day to day. The threshold for angina is usually lower after meals, during excitement, or on exposure to cold. It is often lower in the morning or after strong emotion; the latter can provoke attacks in the absence of exertion. In addition, discomfort may occur during sexual activity, at rest, or at night as a result of coronary spasm.

2. Characteristics of the discomfort—Patients often do not refer to angina as "pain" but as a sensation of tightness, squeezing, burning, pressing, choking, aching, bursting, "gas," indigestion, or an ill-characterized discomfort. It is often characterized by clenching a fist over the mid chest. The distress of angina is rarely sharply localized and is not spasmodic.

3. Location and radiation—The distribution of the distress may vary widely in different patients but is usually the same for each patient unless unstable angina or myocardial infarction supervenes. In most cases, the discomfort is felt behind or slightly to the left of the mid sternum. When it begins farther to the left or, uncommonly, on the right, it characteristically moves centrally substernally. Although angina may radiate to any dermatome from C8 to T4, it radiates most often to the left shoulder and upper arm, frequently moving down the inner volar aspect of the arm to the elbow, forearm, wrist, or fourth and fifth fingers. It may also radiate to the right shoulder or arm, the lower jaw, the neck, or even the back.

4. Duration of attacks—Angina is generally of short duration and subsides completely without residual discomfort. If the attack is precipitated by exertion and the patient promptly stops to rest, it usually lasts under 3 minutes. Attacks following a heavy meal or brought on by anger often last 15–20 minutes. Attacks lasting more than 30 minutes are unusual and suggest the development of an acute coronary syndrome with unstable angina, myocardial infarction, or an alternative diagnosis.

5. Effect of nitroglycerin—The diagnosis of angina pectoris is supported if sublingual nitroglycerin promptly and invariably shortens an attack and if prophylactic nitrates permit greater exertion or prevent angina entirely.

B. Signs

Examination during angina frequently reveals a significant elevation in systolic and diastolic BP, although hypotension may also occur, and may reflect more severe ischemia or inferior ischemia (especially with bradycardia) due to a Bezold-Jarisch reflex. Occasionally, a gallop rhythm and an apical systolic murmur due to transient mitral regurgitation from papillary muscle dysfunction are present during pain only. Supraventricular or ventricular arrhythmias may be present, either as the precipitating factor or as a result of ischemia.

It is important to detect signs of diseases that may contribute to or accompany atherosclerotic heart disease, eg, diabetes mellitus (retinopathy or neuropathy), xanthelasma tendinous xanthomas, hypertension, thyrotoxicosis, myxedema, or peripheral artery disease. Aortic stenosis or regurgitation, hypertrophic cardiomyopathy, and mitral valve prolapse should be sought, since they may produce angina or other forms of chest pain.

C. Laboratory Findings

Other than standard laboratory tests to evaluate for acute coronary syndrome (troponin and CK-MB), factors contributing to ischemia (such as anemia), and to screen for risk factors that may increase the probability of true CHD (such as hyperlipidemia and diabetes mellitus), blood tests are not helpful to diagnose chronic angina.

D. ECG

The resting ECG is often normal in patients with angina. In the remainder, abnormalities include old myocardial infarction, nonspecific ST–T changes, and changes of LVH. During anginal episodes, as well as during asymptomatic ischemia, the characteristic ECG change is horizontal or downsloping ST-segment depression that reverses after the ischemia disappears. T wave flattening or inversion may also occur. Less frequently, transient ST-segment elevation is observed; this finding suggests severe (transmural) ischemia from coronary occlusion, and it can occur with coronary spasm.

E. Pretest Probability

The history as detailed above, the physical examination findings, and laboratory and ECG findings are used to develop a pretest probability of CAD as the cause of the clinical symptoms. Other important factors to include in calculating the pretest probability of CAD are patient age, sex, and clinical symptoms. Patients with low to intermediate pretest probability for CAD should undergo noninvasive stress testing whereas patients with high pretest probability are generally referred for cardiac catheterization.

F. Exercise ECG

Exercise ECG testing is the most commonly used noninvasive procedure for evaluating for inducible ischemia in the patient with angina. Exercise ECG testing is often combined with imaging studies (nuclear or echocardiography), but in low-risk patients without baseline ST segment abnormalities or in whom anatomic localization is not necessary, the exercise ECG remains the recommended initial procedure because of considerations of cost, convenience, and longstanding prognostic data.

Exercise testing can be done on a motorized treadmill or with a bicycle ergometer. A variety of exercise protocols are utilized, the most common being the **Bruce protocol,** which increases the treadmill speed and elevation every 3 minutes until limited by symptoms. At least two ECG leads should be monitored continuously.

1. Precautions and risks—The risk of exercise testing is about one infarction or death per 1000 tests, but individuals who have pain at rest or minimal activity are at higher risk and should not be tested. **Many of the traditional exclusions, such as recent myocardial infarction or heart failure, are no longer used if the patient is stable and ambulatory, but symptomatic aortic stenosis remains a relative contraindication.**

2. Indications—Exercise testing is used (1) to confirm the diagnosis of angina; (2) to determine the severity of limitation of activity due to angina; (3) to assess prognosis in patients with known coronary disease, including those recovering from myocardial infarction, by detecting groups at high or low risk; and (4) to evaluate responses to therapy. Because false-positive tests often exceed true positives, leading to much patient anxiety and self-imposed or mandated disability, exercise testing of asymptomatic individuals should be done only for those whose occupations place them or others at special risk (eg, airline pilots) and older individuals commencing strenuous activity.

3. Interpretation—The usual ECG criterion for a positive test is 1 mm (0.1 mV) horizontal or downsloping ST-segment depression (beyond baseline) measured 80 msec after the J point. By this criterion, 60–80% of patients with anatomically significant coronary disease will have a positive test, but 10–30% of those without significant disease will also be positive. False positives are uncommon when a 2-mm depression is present. Additional information is inferred from the time of onset and duration of the ECG changes, their magnitude and configuration, BP and heart rate changes, the duration of exercise, and the presence of associated symptoms. In general, patients exhibiting more severe ST-segment depression (more than 2 mm) at low workloads (less than 6 minutes on the Bruce protocol) or heart rates (less than 70% of age-predicted maximum)—especially when the duration of exercise and rise in BP are limited or when hypotension occurs during the test—have more severe disease and a poorer prognosis. Depending on symptom status, age, and other factors, such patients should be referred for coronary arteriography and possible revascularization. On the other hand, less impressive positive tests in asymptomatic patients are often "false positives." Therefore, exercise testing results that do not conform to the clinical suspicion should be confirmed by stress imaging.

G. Myocardial Stress Imaging

Myocardial stress imaging (scintigraphy, echocardiography, or MRI) is indicated (1) when the resting ECG makes an exercise ECG difficult to interpret (eg, left bundle branch block, baseline ST–T changes, low voltage); (2) for confirmation of the results of the exercise ECG when they are contrary to the clinical impression (eg, a positive test in an asymptomatic patient); (3) to localize the region of ischemia; (4) to distinguish ischemic from infarcted myocardium; (5) to assess the completeness of revascularization following bypass surgery or coronary angioplasty; or (6) as a prognostic indicator in patients with known coronary disease. Published criteria summarize these indications for stress testing.

1. Myocardial perfusion scintigraphy—This test, also known as radionuclide imaging, provides images in which radionuclide uptake is proportionate to blood flow at the time of injection.

Stress imaging is positive in about 75–90% of patients with anatomically significant coronary disease and in 20–30% of those without it. Occasionally, other conditions, including infiltrative diseases (sarcoidosis, amyloidosis), left bundle branch block, and dilated cardiomyopathy, may produce resting or persistent perfusion defects. False-positive radionuclide tests may occur as a result of diaphragmatic attenuation or, in women, attenuation through breast tissue. Tomographic imaging (single-photon emission computed tomography, SPECT) can reduce the severity of artifacts.

2. Radionuclide angiography—This procedure, also known as Multi-Gated Acquisition Scan, or MUGA scan, uses radionuclide tracers to image the LV and measures its EF and wall motion. In coronary disease, resting abnormalities usually represent infarction, and those that occur only with exercise usually indicate stress-induced ischemia. Exercise radionuclide angiography has approximately the same sensitivity as myocardial perfusion scintigraphy, but it is less specific in older individuals and those with other forms of heart disease. In addition, because of the precision around LVEF, the test is also used for monitoring patients exposed to cardiotoxic therapies (such as chemotherapeutic agents).

3. Stress echocardiography—Echocardiograms performed during supine exercise or immediately following upright exercise may demonstrate exercise-induced segmental wall motion abnormalities as an indicator of ischemia. In experienced laboratories, the test accuracy is comparable to that obtained with scintigraphy—though a higher proportion of tests is technically inadequate. While exercise is the preferred stress because of other information derived, pharmacologic stress with high-dose dobutamine (20–40 mcg/kg/min) can be used as an alternative to exercise.

H. Other Imaging

1. Positron emission tomography—PET and SPECT scanning can accurately distinguish transiently dysfunctional ("stunned") myocardium from scar tissue.

2. CT and MRI scanning—CT scanning can image the heart and, with contrast medium and multislice technology, the coronary arteries. Multislice CT angiography may be useful in evaluating patients with low likelihood of significant CAD to rule out disease. With similar radiation exposure as radionuclide SPECT imaging, CT angiography may also be useful for evaluating chest pain and suspected acute coronary syndrome. In the large randomized comparative effectiveness PROMISE trial, patients with stable chest pain undergoing anatomic imaging with CT angiography had similar outcomes to patients undergoing functional testing (stress ECG, stress radionuclide, or stress echocardiography). CT angiography with noninvasive functional assessment of coronary stenosis (fractional flow reserve), termed "CT-FFR," has also been evaluated in patients with low-intermediate likelihood of CAD. CT-FFR has been shown to reduce the number of patients without coronary disease requiring invasive angiography.

Electron beam CT (EBCT) can quantify coronary artery calcification, which is highly correlated with atheromatous plaque and has high sensitivity, but low specificity, for obstructive coronary disease. Thus, although this test can stratify patients into lower and higher risk groups, the appropriate management of individual patients with asymptomatic coronary artery calcification—beyond aggressive risk factor modification—is unclear. This test has not traditionally been used in symptomatic patients. According to the American Heart Association, persons who are at low risk (less than 10% 10-year risk) or at high risk (greater than 20% 10-year risk) for obstructive coronary disease do not benefit from coronary calcium assessment (class III, level of evidence: B) (see Table 28–1). However, in clinically selected, intermediate-risk patients, it may be reasonable to determine the atherosclerosis burden using EBCT in order to refine clinical risk prediction and to select patients for more aggressive target values for lipid-lowering therapies (class IIb, level of evidence: B).

Cardiac MRI using gadolinium provides high-resolution images of the heart and great vessels without radiation exposure or use of iodinated contrast media. Gadolinium has been associated with a rare but fatal complication in patients with severe kidney disease, called necrotizing systemic fibrosis. Gadolinium can demonstrate perfusion using dobutamine or adenosine to produce pharmacologic stress. Advances have been made in imaging the proximal coronary arteries, but this application remains investigational. Perhaps the most clinically used indication of cardiac MRI is for identification of myocardial fibrosis, either from myocardial infarction or infiltration. This allows high resolution imaging of myocardial viability.

I. Ambulatory ECG Monitoring

Ambulatory ECG recorders can monitor for ischemic ST-segment depression but this modality is rarely used for ischemia detection.

J. Coronary Angiography

Selective coronary arteriography is the definitive diagnostic procedure for CAD. It can be performed with low mortality (about 0.1%) and morbidity (1–5%), but due to the invasive nature and cost, it is recommended only in patients with a high pretest probability of CAD.

Coronary arteriography should be performed in the following circumstances if percutaneous transluminal coronary angioplasty or bypass surgery is a consideration:

1. Life-limiting stable angina despite an adequate medical regimen.
2. Clinical presentation (unstable angina, postinfarction angina, etc) or noninvasive testing suggests high-risk disease (see Indications for Revascularization).
3. Concomitant aortic valve disease and angina pectoris, to determine whether the angina is due to accompanying coronary disease.
4. Asymptomatic older patients undergoing valve surgery so that concomitant bypass may be done if the anatomy is propitious.
5. Recurrence of symptoms after coronary revascularization to determine whether bypass grafts or native vessels are occluded.
6. Cardiac failure where a surgically correctable lesion, such as LV aneurysm, mitral regurgitation, or reversible ischemic dysfunction, is suspected.
7. Survivors of sudden death, symptomatic, or life-threatening arrhythmias when CAD may be a correctable cause.
8. Chest pain of uncertain cause or cardiomyopathy of unknown cause.
9. Emergently performed cardiac catheterization with intention to perform primary PCI in patients with suspected acute myocardial infarction.

A narrowing of more than 50% of the luminal diameter is considered hemodynamically (and clinically) significant, although most lesions producing ischemia are associated with narrowing in excess of 70%. In those with strongly positive exercise ECGs or scintigraphic studies, three-vessel or left main disease may be present in 75–95% depending on the criteria used. **Intravascular ultrasound** (IVUS) is useful when the angiogram is equivocal as well as for assessing the results of angioplasty or stenting. In addition, IVUS is the invasive diagnostic method of choice for ostial left main lesions and coronary dissections. In fractional flow reserve (FFR), a pressure wire is used to measure the relative change in pressure across a coronary lesion after adenosine-induced hyperemia. Revascularization based on abnormal FFR improves clinical outcomes compared to revascularization of all angiographically stenotic lesions. FFR is an important invasive tool to aid with ischemia-driven revascularization and has become the standard tool to evaluate borderline lesions in cases in which the clinical team is evaluating the clinical and hemodynamic significance of a coronary stenosis.

LV angiography is usually performed at the same time as coronary arteriography. Global and regional LV function are visualized, as well as mitral regurgitation if present. LV function is a major determinant of prognosis in CHD.

▶ Differential Diagnosis

When atypical features are present—such as prolonged duration (hours or days) or darting, or knifelike pains at the apex or over the precordium—ischemia is less likely.

Anterior chest wall syndrome is characterized by a sharply localized tenderness of the intercostal muscles. Inflammation of the chondrocostal junctions may result in diffuse chest pain that is also reproduced by local pressure (Tietze syndrome). Intercostal neuritis (due to herpes zoster or diabetes mellitus, for example) also mimics angina.

Cervical or thoracic spine disease involving the dorsal roots produces sudden sharp, severe chest pain suggesting angina in location and "radiation" but related to specific movements of the neck or spine, recumbency, and straining or lifting. Pain due to cervical or thoracic disk disease involves the outer or dorsal aspect of the arm and the thumb and index fingers rather than the ring and little fingers.

Reflux esophagitis, peptic ulcer, chronic cholecystitis, esophageal spasm, and functional gastrointestinal disease may produce pain suggestive of angina pectoris. The picture may be especially confusing because ischemic pain may also be associated with upper gastrointestinal symptoms, and esophageal motility disorders may be improved by nitrates and calcium channel blockers. Assessment of esophageal motility may be helpful.

Degenerative and inflammatory lesions of the left shoulder and thoracic outlet syndromes may cause chest pain due to nerve irritation or muscular compression; the symptoms are usually precipitated by movement of the arm and shoulder and are associated with paresthesias.

Pneumonia, pulmonary embolism, and spontaneous pneumothorax may cause chest pain as well as dyspnea. Dissection of the thoracic aorta can cause severe chest pain that is commonly felt in the back; it is sudden in onset, reaches maximum intensity immediately, and may be associated with changes in pulses. Other cardiac disorders, such as mitral valve prolapse, hypertrophic cardiomyopathy, myocarditis, pericarditis, aortic valve disease, or RVH may cause atypical chest pain or even myocardial ischemia.

▶ Treatment

Sublingual nitroglycerin is the drug of choice for acute management; it acts in about 1–2 minutes. As soon as the attack begins, one fresh tablet is placed under the tongue. This may be repeated at 3- to 5-minute intervals, but if pain is not relieved or improving after 5 minutes, the patient should call 9-1-1; pain not responding to three tablets or lasting more than 20 minutes may represent evolving infarction. The dosage (0.3, 0.4, or 0.6 mg) and the number of tablets to be used before seeking further medical attention must be individualized. Nitroglycerin buccal spray is also available as a metered (0.4 mg) delivery system. It has the advantage of being more convenient for patients who have difficulty handling the pills and of being more stable.

▶ Prevention of Further Attacks

A. Aggravating Factors

Angina may be aggravated by hypertension, LV failure, arrhythmia (usually tachycardias), strenuous activity, cold temperatures, and emotional states. These factors should be identified and treated when possible.

B. Nitroglycerin

Nitroglycerin, 0.3–0.6 mg sublingually or 0.4–0.8 mg translingually by spray, should be taken 5 minutes before any activity likely to precipitate angina. Sublingual isosorbide dinitrate (2.5–5 mg) is only slightly longer-acting than sublingual nitroglycerin.

C. Long-Acting Nitrates

Longer-acting nitrate preparations include isosorbide dinitrate, 10–40 mg orally three times daily; isosorbide mononitrate, 10–40 mg orally twice daily or 60–120 mg once daily in a sustained-release preparation; oral sustained-release nitroglycerin preparations, 6.25–12.5 mg two to four times daily; nitroglycerin ointment, ointment 2%, 0.5 to 2 inches (7.5 to 30 mg in the morning and six hours later); and transdermal nitroglycerin patches that deliver nitroglycerin at rates of 0.2, 0.4, and 0.6 mg/h rate (0.1–0.8 mg/h), and should be taken off after 12–14 hours of use for a 10–12 hour patch-free interval daily. The main limitation to long-term nitrate therapy is tolerance, which can be limited by using a regimen that includes a minimum 8- to 10-hour period per day without nitrates. Isosorbide dinitrate can be given three times daily, with the last dose after dinner, or longer-acting isosorbide mononitrate once daily. Transdermal nitrate preparations should be removed overnight in most patients.

Nitrate therapy is often limited by headache. Other side effects include nausea, light-headedness, and hypotension.

D. Beta-Blockers

Beta-blockers are the only antianginal agents that have been demonstrated to prolong life in patients with coronary disease (post-myocardial infarction). Beta-blockers should be considered for first-line therapy in most patients with chronic angina and are recommended as such by the Stable Ischemic Heart disease guidelines (Figure 10–5).

Beta-blockers with intrinsic sympathomimetic activity, such as pindolol, are less desirable because they may

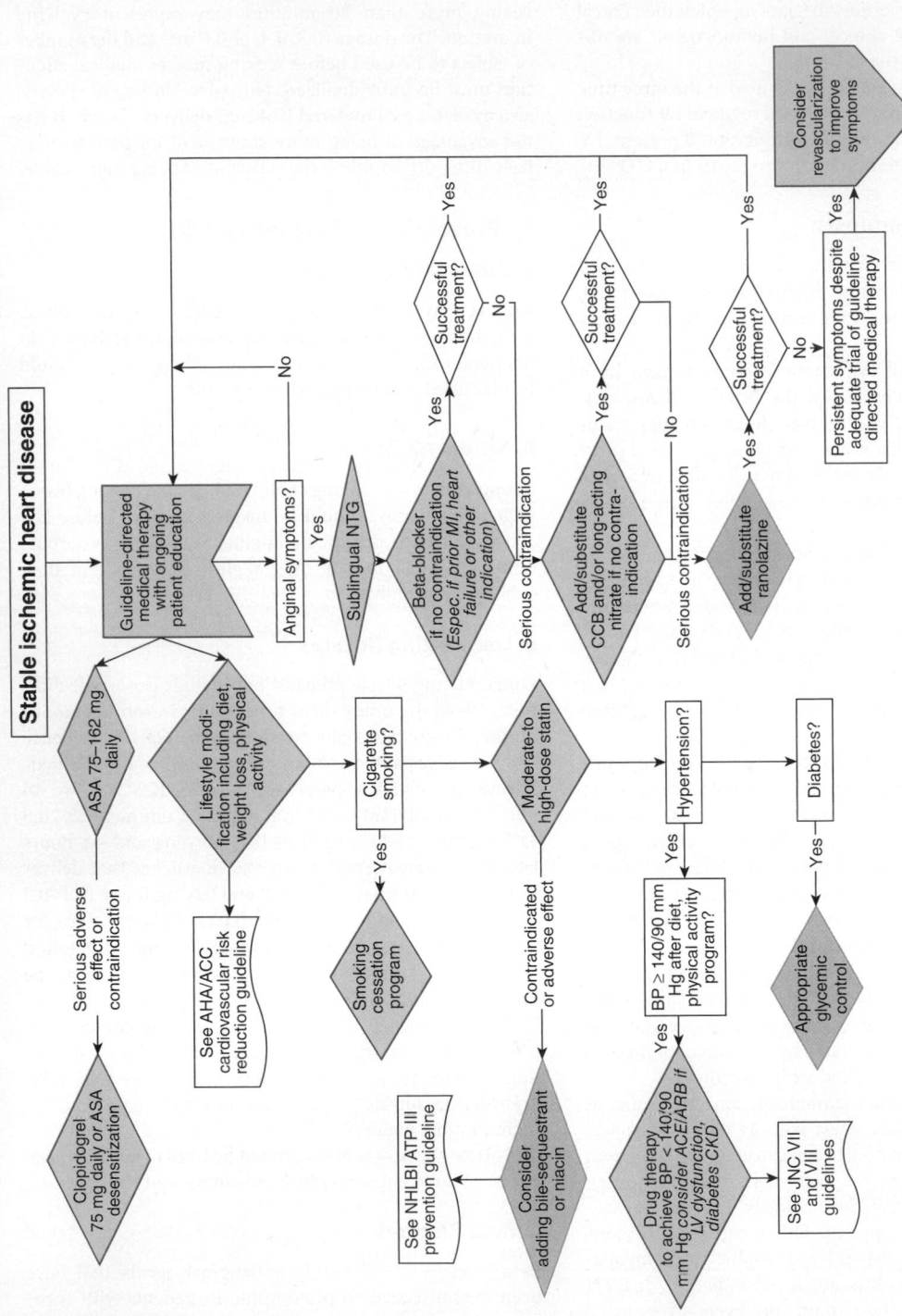

▲ **Figure 10–5.** Algorithm for guideline-directed medical therapy for patients with stable ischemic heart disease. The use of bile acid sequestrant is relatively contraindicated when triglycerides are 200 mg/dL or higher and contraindicated when triglycerides are 500 mg/dL or higher. Dietary supplement niacin must not be used as a substitute for prescription niacin. (Reproduced, with permission, from Fihn SD et al; American College of Cardiology Foundation/American Heart Association Task Force. 2012 ACCF/AHA/ACP/AATS/PCNA/SCAI/STS guideline for the diagnosis and management of patients with stable ischemic heart disease. Circulation. 2012 Dec 18;126(25):e354-471.) © 2012 American Heart Association, Inc.

ACE/ARB, angiotensin-converting enzyme; AHA/ACC, American Heart Association/American College of Cardiology; ASA, aspirin; BP, blood pressure; CCB, calcium channel blocker; CKD, chronic kidney disease; MI, myocardial infarction; NTG, nitroglycerin.

exacerbate angina in some individuals and have not been effective in secondary prevention trials. The pharmacology and side effects of the beta-blockers are discussed in Chapter 11 (see Table 11–6). The dosages of all these medications when given for angina are similar. The major contraindications are severe bronchospastic disease, brady-arrhythmias, and decompensated heart failure.

E. Ranolazine

Ranolazine is indicated as first-line use for chronic angina. Ranolazine has no effect on heart rate and BP, and it has been shown in clinical trials to prolong exercise duration and time to angina, both as monotherapy and when administered with conventional antianginal therapy. It is safe to use with erectile dysfunction drugs. The usual dose is 500 mg orally twice a day. Because it can cause QT pro-longation, it is contraindicated in patients with existing QT prolongation; in patients taking QT prolonging medica-tions, such as class I or III antiarrhythmics (eg, quinidine, dofetilide, sotalol); and in those taking potent and moder-ate CYP450 3A inhibitors (eg, clarithromycin and rifampin). Of interest, in spite of the QT prolongation, there is a significantly lower rate of ventricular arrhythmias with its use following acute coronary syndromes, as shown in the MERLIN trial. It also decreases occurrence of atrial fibrillation and results in a small decrease in HbA_{1c}. It is contraindicated in patients with significant liver and kid-ney disease. Ranolazine is not to be used for treatment of acute anginal episodes. Ranolazine does not improve out-comes of patients who do not get complete coronary revascularization.

F. Calcium Channel Blocking Agents

Unlike the beta-blockers, calcium channel blockers have not been shown to reduce mortality postinfarction and in some cases have increased ischemia and mortality rates. This appears to be the case with some dihydropyridines (eg, nifedipine) and with diltiazem and verapamil in patients with clinical heart failure or moderate to severe LV dysfunction. Meta-analyses have suggested that short-act-ing nifedipine in moderate to high doses causes an increase in mortality. It is uncertain whether these findings are rel-evant to longer-acting dihydropyridines. Nevertheless, considering the uncertainties and the lack of demonstrated favorable effect on outcomes, calcium channel blockers should be considered third-line anti-ischemic drugs in the postinfarction patient. Similarly, these agents, with the exception of amlodipine (which proved safe in patients with heart failure in the PRAISE-2 trial), should be avoided in patients with heart failure or low EFs.

The pharmacologic effects and side effects of the cal-cium channel blockers are discussed in Chapter 11 and summarized in Table 11–8. Diltiazem, amlodipine, and verapamil are preferable because they produce less reflex tachycardia and because the former, at least, may cause fewer side effects. Nifedipine, nicardipine, and amlodipine are also approved agents for angina. Isradipine, felodipine, and nisoldipine are not approved for angina but probably are as effective as the other dihydropyridines.

G. Ivabradine

Ivabradine selectively blocks the I_f current and specifically lowers heart rate. It has been shown to reduce angina in patients with chronic stable angina and is approved in Europe. However, the SIGNIFY trial found that there may have been harm for patients with significant angina with regard to out-comes of cardiovascular death and myocardial infarction, thus raising concerns regarding its use for this indication.

H. Alternative and Combination Therapies

Patients who do not respond to one class of antianginal medication often respond to another. It may, therefore, be worthwhile to use an alternative agent before progressing to combinations. The stable ischemic heart disease guide-lines recommend starting with a beta-blocker as initial therapy, followed by calcium channel blockers, long-acting nitrates, or ranolazine. A few patients will have further response to a regimen including all four agents.

I. Platelet-Inhibiting Agents

Several studies have demonstrated the benefit of antiplate-let drugs for patients with stable and unstable vascular disease. Therefore, unless contraindicated, aspirin (81–325 mg orally daily) should be prescribed for all patients with angina. Clopidogrel, 75 mg orally daily, reduces vascular events in patients with stable vascular disease (as an alter-native to aspirin) and in patients with acute coronary syn-dromes (in addition to aspirin). Thus, it is also a good alternative in aspirin-intolerant patients. Clopidogrel in addition to aspirin did not reduce myocardial infarction, stroke, or cardiovascular death in the CHARISMA trial of patients with cardiovascular disease or multiple risk factors, with about a 50% increase in bleeding. However, it might be reasonable to use combination clopidogrel and aspirin for certain high-risk patients with established coronary disease. Specifically, prolonged used of dual antiplatelet therapy with aspirin and clopidogrel may be beneficial in patients post-percutaneous stenting with drug-eluting stents.

Ticagrelor, a P2Y12 inhibitor, has been shown to reduce cardiovascular events in patients with acute coronary syn-dromes. Additionally, in patients with prior myocardial infarction, long-term treatment with ticagrelor plus aspirin reduced cardiovascular events compared to aspirin alone.

The latest antiplatelet agent to be approved by the FDA, vorapaxar, is an inhibitor of the protease-activated recep-tor-1. It was shown to reduce cardiovascular events for patients with stable atherosclerosis with a history of myo-cardial infarction or peripheral artery disease in the TRA 2P trial. It is contraindicated for patients with a history of stroke or transient ischemic attack due to increased risk of intracranial hemorrhage.

J. Risk Reduction

Patients with coronary disease should undergo aggressive risk factor modification. This approach, with a particular focus on statin treatment, treating hypertension, stopping smoking, and exercise and weight control (especially for patients with metabolic syndrome or at risk for diabetes), may markedly improve outcomes. For patients with diabetes and cardiovascular disease, there is uncertainty about the optimal target blood sugar control. The ADVANCE trial suggested some benefit for tight blood sugar control with target HbA_{1C} of 6.5% or less but the ACCORD trial found that routine aggressive targeting for blood sugar control to HbA_{1C} to less than 6.0% in patients with diabetes and coronary disease was associated with increased mortality. Therefore, tight blood sugar control should be avoided particularly in patients with a history of severe hypoglycemia, long-standing diabetes, and advanced vascular disease. Aggressive BP control (target systolic BP less than 120 mm Hg) in the ACCORD trial was not associated with reduction in CHD events, although stroke was reduced.

K. Revascularization

1. Indications—There is general agreement that otherwise healthy patients in the following groups should undergo revascularization: (1) Patients with unacceptable symptoms despite medical therapy to its tolerable limits. (2) Patients with left main coronary artery stenosis greater than 50% with or without symptoms. (3) Patients with three-vessel disease with LV dysfunction (EF less than 50% or previous transmural infarction). (4) Patients with unstable angina who after symptom control by medical therapy continue to exhibit ischemia on exercise testing or monitoring. (5) Post-myocardial infarction patients with continuing angina or severe ischemia on noninvasive testing. The use of revascularization for patients with acute coronary syndromes and acute ST elevation myocardial infarction is discussed below.

Data from the COURAGE trial have shown that for patients with chronic angina and disease suitable for PCI, PCI in addition to stringent guideline-directed medical therapy aimed at both risk reduction and anti-anginal care offers no mortality benefit beyond excellent medical therapy alone, and relatively moderate long-term symptomatic improvement. Therefore, for patients with mild to moderate CAD and limited symptoms, revascularization may not provide significant functional status quality-of-life benefit. For patients with moderate to significant coronary stenosis, such as those who have two-vessel disease associated with underlying LV dysfunction, anatomically critical lesions (greater than 90% proximal stenoses, especially of the proximal left anterior descending artery), or physiologic evidence of severe ischemia (early positive exercise tests, large exercise-induced thallium scintigraphic defects, or frequent episodes of ischemia on ambulatory monitoring), a Heart Team consisting of revascularization physicians (interventional cardiologists and surgeons) may be required to review and provide patients with the best revascularization options.

2. Type of procedure

A. PERCUTANEOUS CORONARY INTERVENTION INCLUDING STENTING—PCI, including balloon angioplasty and coronary stenting, can effectively open stenotic coronary arteries. Coronary stenting, with either bare metal stents or drug-eluting stents, has substantially reduced restenosis. Stenting can also be used selectively for left main coronary stenosis, particularly when CABG is contraindicated or deemed high risk.

PCI is possible but often less successful in bypass graft stenoses. Experienced operators are able to successfully dilate more than 90% of lesions attempted. The major early complication is intimal dissection with vessel occlusion, although this is rare with coronary stenting. The use of intravenous platelet glycoprotein IIb/IIIa inhibitors (abciximab, eptifibatide, tirofiban) substantially reduces the rate of periprocedural myocardial infarction, and placement of intracoronary stents markedly improves initial and long-term angiographic results, especially with complex and long lesions. After percutaneous coronary intervention, all patients should have CK-MB and troponin measured. The definition of a periprocedural infarction has been debated, with many experts advocating for a clinical definition that incorporates different enzyme cutpoints, angiographic findings, and electrocardiographic evidence. Acute thrombosis after stent placement can largely be prevented by aggressive antithrombotic therapy (long-term aspirin, 81–325 mg, plus clopidogrel, 300–600 mg loading dose followed by 75 mg daily, for between 30 days and 1 year, and with acute use of platelet glycoprotein IIb/IIIa inhibitors).

A major limitation with PCI has been **restenosis,** which occurs in the first 6 months in less than 10% of vessels treated with drug-eluting stents, 15–30% of vessels treated with bare metal stents, and 30–40% of vessels without stenting. Factors associated with higher restenosis rates include diabetes, small luminal diameter, longer and more complex lesions, and lesions at coronary ostia or in the left anterior descending coronary artery. Drug-eluting stents that elute antiproliferative agents, such as sirolimus, everolimus, zotarolimus, or paclitaxel, have substantially reduced restenosis. In-stent restenosis is often treated with restenting with drug-eluting stents, and rarely with brachytherapy. The nearly 2 million PCIs performed worldwide per year far exceed the number of CABG operations, but the rationale for many of the procedures performed in patients with stable angina should be for angina symptom reduction. The COURAGE trial has confirmed earlier studies in showing that even for patients with moderate anginal symptoms and positive stress tests PCI provides no benefit over medical therapy with respect to death or myocardial infarction. PCI was more effective at relieving angina, although most patients in the medical group had improvement in symptoms. Thus, **in patients with mild or moderate stable symptoms, aggressive lipid-lowering and antianginal therapy may be a preferable initial strategy, reserving PCI for patients with significant and refractory symptoms or for those who are unable to take the prescribed medicines.**

Several studies of PCI, including those with drug-eluting stents, versus CABG in patients with multivessel disease have been reported. The SYNTAX trial as well as previously performed trials with drug-eluting stent use in PCI patients show comparable mortality and infarction rates over follow-up periods of 1–3 years but a high rate (approximately 40%) of repeat procedures following PCI. Stroke rates are higher with CABG. As a result, the choice of revascularization procedure may depend on details of coronary anatomy and is often a matter of patient preference. However, it should be noted that less than 20% of patients with multivessel disease meet the entry criteria for the clinical trials, so these results cannot be generalized to all multivessel disease patients. Outcomes with percutaneous revascularization in patients with diabetes have generally been inferior to those with CABG. The FREEDOM trial demonstrated that CABG surgery was superior to PCI with regards to death, myocardial infarction, and stroke for patients with diabetes and multivessel coronary disease at 5 years across all subgroups of SYNTAX score anatomy.

B. CORONARY ARTERY BYPASS GRAFTING—CABG can be accomplished with a very low mortality rate (1–3%) in otherwise healthy patients with preserved cardiac function. However, the mortality rate of this procedure rises to 4–8% in older individuals and in patients who have had a prior CABG.

Grafts using one or both internal mammary arteries (usually to the left anterior descending artery or its branches) provide the best long-term results in terms of patency and flow. Segments of the saphenous vein (or, less optimally, other veins) or the radial artery interposed between the aorta and the coronary arteries distal to the obstructions are also used. One to five distal anastomoses are commonly performed.

Minimally invasive surgical techniques may involve a limited sternotomy, lateral thoracotomy (MIDCAB), or thoracoscopy (port-access). They are more technically demanding, usually not suitable for more than two grafts, and do not have established durability. Bypass surgery can be performed both on circulatory support (on-pump) and without direct circulatory support (off-pump). Randomized trial data have not shown a benefit with off-pump bypass surgery but minimally invasive surgical techniques allow earlier postoperative mobilization and discharge.

The operative mortality rate is increased in patients with poor LV function (LVEF less than 35%) or those requiring additional procedures (valve replacement or ventricular aneurysmectomy). Patients over 70 years of age, patients undergoing repeat procedures, or those with important noncardiac disease (especially chronic kidney disease and diabetes) or poor general health also have higher operative mortality and morbidity rates, and full recovery is slow. Thus, CABG should be reserved for more severely symptomatic patients in this group. Early (1–6 months) graft patency rates average 85–90% (higher for internal mammary grafts), and subsequent graft closure rates are about 4% annually. Early graft failure is common in vessels with poor distal flow, while late closure is more frequent in patients who continue smoking and those with untreated hyperlipidemia. Antiplatelet therapy with aspirin improves graft patency rates. Smoking cessation and vigorous treatment of blood lipid abnormalities (particularly with statins) are necessary. Repeat revascularization may be necessitated because of recurrent symptoms due to progressive native vessel disease and graft occlusions. Reoperation is technically demanding and less often fully successful than the initial operation. In addition, in patients with ischemic mitral regurgitation, mitral repair at the time of a CABG does not offer any clinical benefit.

L. Mechanical Extracorporeal Counterpulsation

Extracorporeal counterpulsation entails repetitive inflation of a high-pressure chamber surrounding the lower half of the body during the diastolic phase of the cardiac cycle for daily 1-hour sessions over a period of 7 weeks. Randomized trials have shown that extracorporeal counterpulsation reduces angina thus it may be considered for relief of refractory angina in patients with stable coronary disease.

M. Neuromodulation

Spinal cord stimulation can be used to relieve chronic refractory angina. Spinal cord stimulators are subcutaneously implantable via a minimally invasive procedure under local anesthesia.

▶ Prognosis

The prognosis of angina pectoris has improved with development of therapies aimed at secondary prevention. Mortality rates vary depending on the number of vessels diseased, the severity of obstruction, the status of LV function, and the presence of complex arrhythmias. Mortality rates are progressively higher in patients with one-, two-, and three-vessel disease and those with left main coronary artery obstruction (ranging from 1% per year to 25% per year). The outlook in individual patients is unpredictable, and nearly half of the deaths are sudden. Therefore, risk stratification is attempted. Patients with accelerating symptoms have a poorer outlook. Among stable patients, those whose exercise tolerance is severely limited by ischemia (less than 6 minutes on the Bruce treadmill protocol) and those with extensive ischemia by exercise ECG or scintigraphy have more severe anatomic disease and a poorer prognosis. The Duke Treadmill Score, based on a standard Bruce protocol exercise treadmill test, provides an estimate of risk of death at 1 year. The score uses time on the treadmill, amount of ST-segment depression, and presence of angina (Table 10–10).

Table 10–10. Duke treadmill score: Calculation and interpretation.

Time in minutes on Bruce protocol		= _____
−5 × amount of depression (in mm)		− _____
−4 × angina index 0 = no angina on test 1 = angina, not limiting 2 = limiting angina		= _____
Total Summed Score	**Risk Group**	**Annual Mortality**
≥ 5	Low	0.25%
−10 to 4	Intermediate	1.25%
≤ −11	High	5.25%

When to Refer

All patients with new or worsening symptoms believed to represent progressive angina or a positive stress test for myocardial ischemia with continued angina despite medical therapy (or both) should be referred to a cardiologist.

When to Admit

- Patients with elevated cardiac biomarkers, ischemic ECG findings, or hemodynamic instability.

- Patients with new or worsened symptoms, possibly thought to be ischemic, but who lack high-risk features can be observed with serial ECGs and biomarkers, and discharged if stress testing shows low-risk findings.

Boden WE et al; COURAGE Trial Research Group. Optimal medical therapy with or without PCI for stable coronary disease. N Engl J Med. 2007 Apr 12;356(15):1503–16. [PMID: 17387127]

Douglas PS et al; PLATFORM Investigators. Clinical outcomes of fractional flow reserve by computed tomographic angiography-guided diagnostic strategies vs. usual care in patients with suspected coronary artery disease: the prospective longitudinal trial of FFRCT: outcome and resource impacts study. Eur Heart J. 2015 Dec 14;36(47):3359–67. [PMID: 26330417]

Douglas PS et al; PROMISE Investigators. Outcomes of anatomical versus functional testing for coronary artery disease. N Engl J Med. 2015 Apr 2;372(14):1291–300. [PMID: 25773919]

Fihn SD et al. 2012 ACCF/AHA/ACP/AATS/PCNA/SCAI/STS Guideline for the Diagnosis and Management of Patients With Stable Ischemic Heart Disease: a report of the American College of Cardiology Foundation/American Heart Association task force on practice guidelines, and the American College of Physicians, American Association for Thoracic Surgery, Preventive Cardiovascular Nurses Association, Society for Cardiovascular Angiography and Interventions, and Society of Thoracic Surgeons. Circulation. 2012 Dec 18;126(25):e354–471. [PMID: 23166211]

Fox K et al; SIGNIFY Investigators. Ivabradine in stable coronary artery disease without clinical heart failure. N Engl J Med. 2014 Sep 18;371(12):1091–9. [PMID: 25176136]

Levine GN et al. 2011 ACCF/AHA/SCAI Guideline for Percutaneous Coronary Intervention: a report of the American College of Cardiology Foundation/American Heart Association Task Force on Practice Guidelines and the Society for Cardiovascular Angiography and Interventions. Circulation. 2011 Dec 6;124(23):e574–651. [PMID: 22064601]

Mauri L et al; DAPT Study Investigators. Twelve or 30 months of dual antiplatelet therapy after drug-eluting stents. N Engl J Med. 2014 Dec 4;371(23):2155–66. [PMID: 25399658]

Morrow DA et al; TRA 2P–TIMI 50 Steering Committee and Investigators. Vorapaxar in the secondary prevention of atherothrombotic events. N Engl J Med. 2012 Apr 12;366(15):1404–13. [PMID: 22443427]

Moussa ID et al. Consideration of a new definition of clinically relevant myocardial infarction after coronary revascularization: an expert consensus document from the Society for Cardiovascular Angiography and Interventions (SCAI). J Am Coll Cardiol. 2013 Oct 22;62(17):1563–70. [PMID: 24135581]

Patel MR et al. ACCF/SCAI/STS/AATS/AHA/ASNC 2009 Appropriateness Criteria for Coronary Revascularization: a report by the American College of Cardiology Foundation Appropriateness Criteria Task Force, Society for Cardiovascular Angiography and Interventions, Society of Thoracic Surgeons, American Association for Thoracic Surgery, American Heart Association, and the American Society of Nuclear Cardiology Endorsed by the American Society of Echocardiography, the Heart Failure Society of America, and the Society of Cardiovascular Computed Tomography. J Am Coll Cardiol. 2009 Feb 10;53(6):530–53. [PMID: 19195618]

Patel MR et al. ACCF/SCAI/AATS/AHA/ASE/ASNC/HFSA/HRS/SCCM/SCCT/SCMR/STS 2012 appropriate use criteria for diagnostic catheterization: a report of the American College of Cardiology Foundation Appropriate Use Criteria Task Force, Society for Cardiovascular Angiography and Interventions, American Association for Thoracic Surgery, American Heart Association, American Society of Echocardiography, American Society of Nuclear Cardiology, Heart Failure Society of America, Heart Rhythm Society, Society of Critical Care Medicine, Society of Cardiovascular Computed Tomography, Society for Cardiovascular Magnetic Resonance, and Society of Thoracic Surgeons. J Am Coll Cardiol. 2012 May 29;59(22):1995–2027. [PMID: 22578925]

Patel MR et al. Low diagnostic yield of elective coronary angiography. N Engl J Med. 2010 Mar 11;362(10):886–95. [PMID: 20220183]

Skyler JS et al. Intensive glycemic control and the prevention of cardiovascular events: implications of the ACCORD, ADVANCE, and VA Diabetes Trials: a position statement of the American Diabetes Association and a Scientific Statement of the American College of Cardiology Foundation and the American Heart Association. J Am Coll Cardiol. 2009 Jan 20;53(3):298–304. [PMID: 19147051]

Smith PK et al; Cardiothoracic Surgical Trials Network Investigators. Surgical treatment of moderate ischemic mitral regurgitation. N Engl J Med. 2014 Dec 4;371(23):2178–88. [PMID: 25405390]

Weisz G et al; RIVER-PCI investigators. Ranolazine in patients with incomplete revascularisation after percutaneous coronary intervention (RIVER-PCI): a multicentre, randomised, double-blind, placebo-controlled trial. Lancet. 2016 Jan 9; 387(10014):136–45.

CORONARY VASOSPASM & ANGINA WITH NORMAL CORONARY ARTERIOGRAMS

 ESSENTIALS OF DIAGNOSIS

▶ Precordial chest pain, often occurring at rest during stress or without known precipitant, relieved rapidly by nitrates.

▶ ECG evidence of ischemia during pain, sometimes with ST-segment elevation.

▶ Angiographic demonstration of:

– No significant obstruction of major coronary vessels.

– Coronary spasm that responds to intra-coronary nitroglycerin or calcium channel blockers.

General Considerations

Although most symptoms of myocardial ischemia result from fixed stenosis of the coronary arteries, intraplaque hemorrhage, or thrombosis at the site of lesions, some ischemic events may be precipitated or exacerbated by coronary vasoconstriction.

Spasm of the large coronary arteries with resulting decreased coronary blood flow may occur spontaneously or may be induced by exposure to cold, emotional stress, or vasoconstricting medications, such as ergot-derivative medications. Spasm may occur both in normal and in stenosed coronary arteries. Even myocardial infarction may occur as a result of spasm in the absence of visible obstructive CHD, although most instances of such coronary spasm occur in the presence of coronary stenosis.

Cocaine can induce myocardial ischemia and infarction by causing coronary artery vasoconstriction or by increasing myocardial energy requirements. It also may contribute to accelerated atherosclerosis and thrombosis. The ischemia in **Prinzmetal (variant) angina** usually results from coronary vasoconstriction. It tends to involve the right coronary artery and there may be no fixed stenoses. Myocardial ischemia may also occur in patients with normal coronary arteries as a result of disease of the coronary microcirculation or abnormal vascular reactivity. This has been termed "syndrome X."

▶ Clinical Findings

Ischemia may be silent or result in angina pectoris.

Prinzmetal (variant) angina is a clinical syndrome in which chest pain occurs without the usual precipitating factors and is associated with ST-segment elevation rather than depression. It often affects women under 50 years of age. It characteristically occurs in the early morning, awakening patients from sleep, and is apt to be associated with arrhythmias or conduction defects. It may be diagnosed by challenge with ergonovine (a vasoconstrictor), although the results of such provocation are not specific and it entails risk.

▶ Treatment

Patients with chest pain associated with ST-segment elevation should undergo coronary arteriography to determine whether fixed stenotic lesions are present. If they are, aggressive medical therapy or revascularization is indicated, since this may represent an unstable phase of the disease. If significant lesions are not seen and spasm is suspected, avoidance of precipitants, such as cigarette smoking and cocaine, is the top priority. Episodes of coronary spasm generally respond well to nitrates, and both nitrates and calcium channel blockers (including long-acting nifedipine, diltiazem, or amlopidine [see Table 11–8]) are effective prophylactically. By allowing unopposed alpha-1-mediated vasoconstriction, beta-blockers have exacerbated coronary vasospasm, but they may have a role in management of patients in whom spasm is associated with fixed stenoses.

▶ When to Refer

All patients with persistent symptoms of chest pain that may represent spasm should be referred to a cardiologist.

ACUTE CORONARY SYNDROMES WITHOUT ST-SEGMENT ELEVATION

ESSENTIALS OF DIAGNOSIS

▶ Distinction in acute coronary syndrome between patients with and without ST-segment elevation at presentation is essential to determine need for reperfusion therapy.

▶ Fibrinolytic therapy is harmful in acute coronary syndrome without ST-segment elevation, unlike with ST-segment elevation, where acute reperfusion saves lives.

▶ Antiplatelet and anticoagulation therapies and coronary intervention are mainstays of treatment.

▶ General Considerations

Acute coronary syndromes comprise the spectrum of unstable cardiac ischemia from unstable angina to acute myocardial infarction. Acute coronary syndromes are classified based on the presenting ECG as either "ST-segment elevation" (STEMI) or "non–ST-segment elevation" (NSTEMI). This allows for immediate classification and guides determination of whether patients should be considered for acute reperfusion therapy. The evolution of cardiac biomarkers then allows determination of whether myocardial infarction has occurred.

Acute coronary syndromes represent a dynamic state in which patients frequently shift from one category to another, as new ST elevation can develop after presentation and cardiac biomarkers can become abnormal with recurrent ischemic episodes.

▶ Clinical Findings

A. Symptoms and Signs

Patients with acute coronary syndromes generally have symptoms and signs of myocardial ischemia either at rest or with minimal exertion. These symptoms and signs are similar to the chronic angina symptoms described above, consisting of substernal chest pain or discomfort that may radiate to the jaw, left shoulder or arm. Dyspnea, nausea, diaphoresis, or syncope may either accompany the chest discomfort or may be the only symptom of acute coronary syndrome. **About one-third of patients with myocardial infarction have no chest pain per se—these patients tend to be older, female, have diabetes, and be at higher risk for subsequent mortality.** Patients with acute coronary syndromes have signs of heart failure in about 10% of cases, and this is also associated with higher risk of death.

Many hospitals have developed **chest pain observation units** to provide a systematic approach toward serial risk stratification to improve the triage process. In many cases, those who have not experienced new chest pain and have insignificant ECG changes and no cardiac biomarker elevation undergo treadmill exercise tests or imaging procedures to exclude ischemia at the end of an 8- to 24-hour period and are discharged directly from the emergency department if these tests are negative.

B. Laboratory Findings

Depending on the time from symptom onset to presentation, initial laboratory findings may be normal. The markers of cardiac myocyte necrosis, myoglobin, CK-MB, and troponin I and T may all be used to identify acute myocardial infarction. These markers have a well-described pattern of release over time in patients with myocardial infarction (see Laboratory Findings, Acute Myocardial Infarction with ST-Segment Elevation, below). In patients with STEMI, these initial markers are often within normal limits as the patient is being rushed to immediate reperfusion. In patients without ST-segment elevation, it is the presence of abnormal CK-MB or troponin values that are associated with myocyte necrosis and the diagnosis of myocardial infarction. **The universal definition of myocardial infarction** is a rise of cardiac biomarkers with at least one value above the 99th percentile of the upper reference limit together with evidence of myocardial ischemia with at least one of the following: symptoms of ischemia, ECG changes of new ischemia, new Q waves, or imaging evidence of new loss of viable myocardium or new wall motion abnormality.

Serum creatinine is an important determinant of risk, and estimated creatinine clearance is important to guide dosing of certain antithrombotics, including eptifibatide and enoxaparin.

C. ECG

Many patients with acute coronary syndromes will exhibit ECG changes during pain—either ST-segment elevation, ST-segment depression, or T wave flattening or inversion. Dynamic ST segment shift is the most specific for acute coronary syndrome. ST-segment elevation in lead AVR suggests left main or three vessel disease.

▶ Treatment

A. General Measures

Treatment of acute coronary syndromes without ST elevation should be multifaceted. Patients who are at medium or high risk should be hospitalized, maintained at bed rest or at very limited activity for the first 24 hours, monitored, and given supplemental oxygen. Sedation with a benzodiazepine agent may help if anxiety is present.

B. Specific Measures

Figure 10–6 provides an algorithm for initial management of non–ST-segment myocardial infarction.

C. Antiplatelet and Anticoagulation Therapy

Patients should receive a combination of antiplatelet and anticoagulant agents on presentation. **Fibrinolytic therapy should be avoided in patients without** ST-segment elevation since they generally do not have an acute coronary occlusion, and the risk of such therapy appears to outweigh the benefit.

1. Antiplatelet therapy

A. Aspirin—Aspirin, 162–325 mg loading dose, then 81–325 mg daily, should be commenced immediately and continued for the first month. The 2012 ACC/AHA guidelines for longer-term aspirin treatment recommend aspirin 75–162 mg/day as preferable to higher doses with or without coronary stenting.

B. P2Y$_{12}$ Inhibitors—ACC/AHA guidelines call for either a P2Y$_{12}$ inhibitor (clopidogrel, prasugrel [at the time of PCI], or ticagrelor) as a class I recommendation. The ESC guidelines provide a stronger recommendation for a P2Y$_{12}$ inhibitor up-front, as a class IA recommendation for all patients. Both sets of guidelines recommend postponing elective CABG surgery for at least 5 days after the last dose of clopidogrel or ticagrelor and at least 7 days after the last dose of prasugrel, due to risk of bleeding.

The Clopidogrel in Unstable Angina to Prevent Recurrent Events (CURE) trial demonstrated a 20% reduction in the composite end point of cardiovascular death, myocardial infarction, and stroke with the addition of clopidogrel (300 mg loading dose, 75 mg/day for 9–12 months) to aspirin in patients with non–ST-segment elevation acute coronary syndromes. The large CURRENT trial showed that "double-dose" clopidogrel (600 mg initial oral loading dose, followed by 150 mg orally daily) for 7 days reduced stent thrombosis with a modest increase in major (but not fatal) bleeding and, therefore, it is an option for patients with acute coronary syndrome undergoing PCI.

The ESC guidelines recommend **ticagrelor** for all patients at moderate to high risk for acute coronary syndrome (class 1 recommendation). **Prasugrel** is recommended for patients who have not yet received another P2Y$_{12}$ inhibitor, for whom a PCI is planned, and who are not at high risk for life-threatening bleeding. Clopidogrel is reserved for patients who cannot receive either ticagrelor or prasugrel. Some studies have shown an association between assays of residual platelet function and thrombotic risk during P2Y$_{12}$ inhibitor therapy, and both the European and the US guidelines do not recommend routine platelet function testing to guide therapy (class IIb recommendation).

Prasugrel is both more potent and has a faster onset of action than clopidogrel. The TRITON trial compared prasugrel with clopidogrel in patients with STEMI or NSTEMI in whom PCI was planned; prasugrel resulted in a 19% relative reduction in death from cardiovascular causes, myocardial infarction, or stroke, at the expense of an increase in serious bleeding (including fatal bleeding). Stent thrombosis was reduced by half. Because patients with prior stroke or transient ischemic attack had higher risk of intracranial hemorrhage, prasugrel is contraindicated in such patients. Bleeding was also higher in patients with low body weight (less than 60 kg) and age 75 years or older, and caution should be used in these populations. For patients with STEMI treated with PCI, prasugrel appears to

▲ **Figure 10–6.** Flowchart for class 1 and class IIa recommendations for initial management of unstable angina/non–ST-segment elevation myocardial infarction (UA/NS TEMI). ASA, aspirin; CABG, coronary artery bypass grafting; GP IIb/IIIa, glycoprotein IIb/IIIa; LOE, level of evidence; UFH, unfractionated heparin. (Reproduced, with permission, from Wright RS et al. 2011 ACCF/AHA Focused Update of the Guidelines for the Management of Patients With Unstable Angina/ Non-ST-Elevation Myocardial Infarction (Updating the 2007 Guideline): a report of the American College of Cardiology Foundation/American Heart Association Task Force on Practice Guidelines. Circulation. 2011 May 10;123(18):2022–60. Erratum in: Circulation. 2011 Sep 20;124(12):e337–40; Circulation. 2011 Jun 7;123(22):e625–6. © 2011 American Heart Association, Inc. [PMID: 21444889])

be especially effective without a substantial increase in bleeding. For patients who will not receive revascularization, prasugrel, when compared to clopidogrel, had no overall benefit in the TRILOGY trial (the dose of prasugrel was lowered for the elderly).

Ticagrelor has a faster onset of action than clopidogrel and a more consistent and potent effect. The PLATO trial showed that when ticagrelor was started at the time of presentation in acute coronary syndrome patients (UA/NSTEMI and STEMI), it reduced cardiovascular death, myocardial infarction, and stroke by 16% when compared with clopidogrel. In addition, there was a 22% relative risk reduction

in mortality with ticagrelor. The overall rates of bleeding were similar between ticagrelor and clopidogrel, although non-CABG related bleeding was modestly higher. The finding of a lesser treatment effect in the United States may have been related to use of higher-dose aspirin, and thus when using ticagrelor, low-dose aspirin (81 mg/day) is recommended.

C. **Glycoprotein IIb/IIIa inhibitors**—Small-molecule inhibitors of the platelet glycoprotein IIb/IIIa receptor are useful adjuncts in high-risk patients (usually defined by fluctuating ST-segment depression or positive biomarkers) with acute coronary syndromes, particularly when they are undergoing PCI. **Tirofiban,** 25 mcg/kg over 3 minutes, followed by 0.15 mcg/kg/min, and **eptifibatide,** 180 mcg/kg bolus followed by a continuous infusion of 2 mcg/kg/min, have both been shown to be effective. Downward dose adjustments of the infusions are required in patients with reduced kidney function. The bolus or loading dose remains unadjusted. For example, if the estimated creatinine clearance is below 50 mL/min, the eptifibatide infusion should be cut in half to 1 mcg/kg/min. The ISAR-REACT 2 trial showed that for patients undergoing PCI with high-risk acute coronary syndrome, especially with elevated troponin, intravenous **abciximab** (added to a 600-mg loading dose of clopidogrel) reduces ischemic events by about 25%. The EARLY-ACS trial in over 10,000 patients with high-risk acute coronary syndrome found no benefit from eptifibatide started at the time of admission and higher rates of bleeding compared with eptifibatide treatment started at the time of invasive coronary angiography.

2. Anticoagulant therapy

A. Heparin—Several trials have shown that **LMWH** (enoxaparin 1 mg/kg subcutaneously every 12 hours) is somewhat more effective than **unfractionated heparin** in preventing recurrent ischemic events in the setting of acute coronary syndromes. However, the SYNERGY trial showed that unfractionated heparin and enoxaparin had similar rates of death or (re)infarction in the setting of frequent early coronary intervention.

B. Fondaparinux—Fondaparinux, a specific factor Xa inhibitor given in a dose of 2.5 mg subcutaneously once a day, was found in the OASIS-5 trial to be equally effective as enoxaparin among 20,000 patients at preventing early death, myocardial infarction, and refractory ischemia, and resulted in a 50% reduction in major bleeding. This reduction in major bleeding translated into a significant reduction in mortality (and in death or myocardial infarction) at 30 days. While catheter-related thrombosis was more common during coronary intervention procedures with fondaparinux, the FUTURA trial found that it can be controlled by adding unfractionated heparin (in a dose of 85 units/kg without glycoprotein IIb/IIIa inhibitors, and 60 units/kg with glycoprotein IIb/IIIa inhibitors) during the procedure. Guidelines recommend fondaparinux, describing it as especially favorable for patients who are initially treated medically and who are at high risk for bleeding, such as the elderly.

C. Direct thrombin inhibitors—The ACUITY trial showed that **bivalirudin** appears to be a reasonable alternative to heparin (unfractionated heparin or enoxaparin) plus a glycoprotein IIb/IIIa antagonist for many patients with acute coronary syndromes who are undergoing early coronary intervention. Bivalirudin (without routine glycoprotein IIb/IIIa inhibitor) is associated with substantially less bleeding than heparin plus glycoprotein IIb/IIIa inhibitor. The ISAR REACT-4 trial showed that bivalirudin has similar efficacy compared to abciximab but better bleeding outcomes in NSTEMI patients. Bivalrudin does

not currently have an FDA-approved indication for NSTEMI care.

D. Temporary Discontinuation of Antiplatelet Therapy for Procedures

Patients who have had recent coronary stents are at risk for thrombotic events, including **stent thrombosis,** if $P2Y_{12}$ inhibitors are discontinued for procedures (eg, dental procedures or colonoscopy). If possible, these procedures should be delayed until the end of the necessary treatment period with $P2Y_{12}$ inhibitors, which generally is at least 1 month with bare metal stents and 3–6 months with drug-eluting stents. Before that time, if a procedure is necessary, risk and benefit of continuing the antiplatelet therapy through the time of the procedure should be assessed. Aspirin should generally be continued throughout the period of the procedure. A cardiologist should be consulted before temporary discontinuation of these agents.

E. Nitroglycerin

Nitrates are first-line therapy for patients with acute coronary syndromes presenting with chest pain. Nonparenteral therapy with sublingual or oral agents or nitroglycerin ointment is usually sufficient. If pain persists or recurs, intravenous nitroglycerin should be started. The usual initial dosage is 10 mcg/min. The dosage should be titrated upward by 10–20 mcg/min (to a maximum of 200 mcg/min) until angina disappears or mean arterial pressure drops by 10%. Careful—usually continuous—BP monitoring is required when intravenous nitroglycerin is used. Avoid hypotension (systolic BP less than 100 mm Hg). Tolerance to continuous nitrate infusion is common.

F. Beta-Blockers

Beta-blockers are an important part of the initial treatment of unstable angina unless otherwise contraindicated. The pharmacology of these agents is discussed in Chapter 11 and summarized in Table 11–6. Use of agents with intrinsic sympathomimetic activity should be avoided in this setting. Oral medication is adequate in most patients, but intravenous treatment with metoprolol, given as three 5-mg doses 5 minutes apart as tolerated and in the absence of heart failure, achieves a more rapid effect. Oral therapy should be titrated upward as BP permits.

G. Calcium Channel Blockers

Calcium channel blockers have not been shown to favorably affect outcome in unstable angina, and they should be used primarily as third-line therapy in patients with continuing symptoms on nitrates and beta-blockers or those who are not candidates for these medications. In the presence of nitrates and without accompanying beta-blockers, diltiazem or verapamil is preferred, since nifedipine and the other dihydropyridines are more likely to cause reflex tachycardia or hypotension. The initial dosage should be low, but upward titration should proceed steadily (see Table 11–8).

H. Statins

The PROVE-IT trial provides evidence for starting a statin in the days immediately following an acute coronary syndrome. In this trial, more intensive therapy with atorvastatin 80 mg/day, regardless of total or LDL cholesterol level, improved outcome compared to pravastatin 40 mg/day, with the curves of death or major cardiovascular event separating as early as 3 months after starting therapy. High-dose statins are recommended for all patients with acute coronary syndromes (see Table 10–9).

► Indications for Coronary Angiography

For patients with acute coronary syndrome, including non–ST-segment elevation myocardial infarction, risk stratification is important for determining intensity of care. Several therapies, including glycoprotein IIb/IIIa inhibitors, LMWH heparin, and early invasive catheterization, have been shown to have the greatest benefit in higher-risk patients with acute coronary syndrome. As outlined in the ACC/AHA guidelines, patients with any high-risk feature (Table 10–11) generally warrant an early invasive strategy with catheterization and revascularization. For patients without these high-risk features, either an invasive or non-invasive approach, using exercise (or pharmacologic stress for patients unable to exercise) stress testing to identify patients who have residual ischemia and/or high risk, can be used. Moreover, based on the ICTUS trial, a strategy based on selective coronary angiography and revascularization for instability or inducible ischemia, or both, even for patients with positive troponin, is acceptable (ACC/AHA class IIb recommendation).

Two risk-stratification tools are available that can be used at the bedside, the GRACE Risk Score (http://www.outcomes-umassmed.org/grace) and the TIMI Risk Score (available for download at http://www.timi.org). The **GRACE Risk Score,** which applies to patients with or without ST elevation, was developed in a more generalizable registry population and includes Killip class, BP, ST-segment deviation, cardiac arrest at presentation, serum creatinine, elevated creatine kinase (CK)-MB or troponin, and heart rate. The **TIMI Risk Score** includes seven variables: age 65 years or older, three or more cardiac risk factors, prior coronary stenosis 50% or more, ST-segment deviation, two anginal events in prior 24 hours, aspirin in prior 7 days, and elevated cardiac markers.

► When to Refer

- All patients with acute myocardial infarction should be referred to a cardiologist.
- Patients who are taking a $P2Y_{12}$ inhibitor following coronary stenting should consult a cardiologist before discontinuing treatment for nonemergency procedures.

Gurbel PA et al. Platelet function during extended prasugrel and clopidogrel therapy for patients with ACS treated without revascularization: the TRILOGY ACS Platelet Function Substudy. JAMA. 2012 Nov 7;308(17):1785–94. [PMID: 23124119]

Table 10–11. Indications for catheterization and percutaneous coronary intervention.[1]

Acute coronary syndromes (unstable angina and non-ST elevation MI)	
Class I	Early invasive strategy for any of the following high-risk indicators:
	Recurrent angina/ischemia at rest or with low-level activity
	Elevated troponin
	ST-segment depression
	Recurrent ischemia with evidence of HF
	High-risk stress test result
	EF < 40%
	Hemodynamic instability
	Sustained ventricular tachycardia
	PCI within 6 months
	Prior CABG
	In the absence of these findings, either an early conservative or early invasive strategy
Class IIa	Early invasive strategy for patients with repeated presentations for ACS despite therapy
Class III	Extensive comorbidities in patients in whom benefits of revascularization are not likely to outweigh the risks
	Acute chest pain with low likelihood of ACS
Acute MI after fibrinolytic therapy	
Class I	Cardiogenic shock or acute severe heart failure that develops after initial presentation
	Intermediate or high-risk findings on predischarge noninvasive ischemia testing
	Spontaneous or easily provoked myocardial ischemia
Class IIa	Failed reperfusion or reocclusion after fibrinolytic therapy
	Stable[2] patients after successful fibrinolysis, before discharge and ideally between 3 and 24 hours

[1]Class I indicates treatment is useful and effective, IIa indicates weight of evidence is in favor of usefulness/efficacy, class IIb indicates weight of evidence is less well established, and class III indicates intervention is not useful/effective and may be harmful. Level of evidence A recommendations are derived from large-scale randomized trials, and B recommendations are derived from smaller randomized trials or carefully conducted observational analyses.

[2]Although individual circumstances will vary, clinical stability is defined by the absence of low output, hypotension, persistent tachycardia, apparent shock, high-grade ventricular or symptomatic supraventricular tachyarrhythmias, and spontaneous recurrent ischemia.

ACCF/AHA, American College of Cardiology Foundation/American Heart Association; ACS, acute coronary syndrome; CABG, coronary artery bypass grafting; EF, ejection fraction; HF, heart failure; MI, myocardial infarction; PCI, percutaneous coronary intervention.

Data from O'Gara PT et al. 2013 ACCF/AHA guideline for the management of ST-elevation myocardial infarction: a report of the American College of Cardiology Foundation/American Heart Association Task Force on Practice Guidelines. Circulation. 2013;127.

Hamm CW et al. ESC Guidelines for the management of acute coronary syndromes in patients presenting without persistent ST-segment elevation: The Task Force for the management of acute coronary syndromes (ACS) in patients presenting without persistent ST-segment elevation of the European Society of Cardiology (ESC). Eur Heart J. 2011 Dec;32(23): 2999–3054. [PMID: 21873419]

Jneid H et al. 2012 ACCF/AHA focused update of the guideline for the management of patients with unstable angina/non–ST-elevation myocardial infarction (updating the 2007 guideline and replacing the 2011 focused update): a report of the American College of Cardiology Foundation/American Heart Association Task Force on Practice Guidelines. Circulation. 2012 Aug 14;126(7):875–910. [PMID: 22800849]

Levine GN et al. 2011 ACCF/AHA/SCAI Guideline for Percutaneous Coronary Intervention: a report of the American College of Cardiology Foundation/American Heart Association Task Force on Practice Guidelines and the Society for Cardiovascular Angiography and Interventions. Circulation. 2011 Dec 6;124(23):e574–651. [PMID: 22064601]

Thygesen K et al. Third universal definition of myocardial infarction. Circulation. 2012 Oct 16;126(16):2020–35. [PMID: 22923432]

ACUTE MYOCARDIAL INFARCTION WITH ST-SEGMENT ELEVATION

ESSENTIALS OF DIAGNOSIS

▶ Sudden but not instantaneous development of prolonged (more than 30 minutes) anterior chest discomfort (sometimes felt as "gas" or pressure).

▶ Sometimes painless, masquerading as acute heart failure, syncope, stroke, or shock.

▶ ECG: ST-segment elevation or left bundle branch block.

▶ Immediate reperfusion treatment is warranted.

▶ Primary PCI within 90 minutes of first medical contact is the goal and is superior to fibrinolytic therapy.

▶ Fibrinolytic therapy within 30 minutes of hospital presentation is the goal, and reduces mortality if given within 12 hours of onset of symptoms.

General Considerations

STEMI results, in most cases, from an occlusive coronary thrombus at the site of a preexisting (though not necessarily severe) atherosclerotic plaque. More rarely, infarction may result from prolonged vasospasm, inadequate myocardial blood flow (eg, hypotension), or excessive metabolic demand. Very rarely, myocardial infarction may be caused by embolic occlusion, vasculitis, aortic root or coronary artery dissection, or aortitis. Cocaine, a cause of infarction, should be considered in young individuals without risk factors. A condition that may mimic STEMI is stress cardiomyopathy (also referred to as tako-tsubo or apical ballooning syndrome).

ST elevation connotes an acute coronary occlusion and warrants immediate reperfusion therapy.

Clinical Findings

A. Symptoms

1. Premonitory pain—There is usually a worsening in the pattern of angina preceding the onset of symptoms of myocardial infarction; classically the onset of angina occurs with minimal exertion or at rest.

2. Pain of infarction—Unlike anginal episodes, most infarctions occur at rest, and more commonly in the early morning. The pain is similar to angina in location and radiation but it may be more severe, and it builds up rapidly or in waves to maximum intensity over a few minutes or longer. Nitroglycerin has little effect; even opioids may not relieve the pain.

3. Associated symptoms—Patients may break out in a cold sweat, feel weak and apprehensive, and move about, seeking a position of comfort. They prefer not to lie quietly. Light-headedness, syncope, dyspnea, orthopnea, cough, wheezing, nausea and vomiting, or abdominal bloating may be present singly or in any combination.

4. Painless infarction—One-third of patients with acute myocardial infarction present without chest pain, and these patients tend to be undertreated and have poor outcomes. Older patients, women, and patients with diabetes mellitus are more likely to present without chest pain. As many as 25% of infarctions are detected on routine ECG without any recallable acute episode.

5. Sudden death and early arrhythmias—Of all deaths from myocardial infarction, about 50% occur before the patients arrive at the hospital, with death presumably caused by ventricular fibrillation.

B. Signs

1. General—Patients may appear anxious and sometimes are sweating profusely. The heart rate may range from marked bradycardia (most commonly in inferior infarction) to tachycardia, low cardiac output, or arrhythmia. The BP may be high, especially in former hypertensive patients, or low in patients with shock. Respiratory distress usually indicates heart failure. Fever, usually low grade, may appear after 12 hours and persist for several days.

2. Chest—The **Killip classification** is the standard way to classify heart failure in patients with acute myocardial infarction and has powerful prognostic value. Killip class I is absence of rales and S_3, class II is rales that do not clear with coughing over one-third or less of the lung fields or presence of an S_3, class III is rales that do not clear with coughing over more than one-third of the lung fields, and class IV is cardiogenic shock (rales, hypotension, and signs of hypoperfusion).

3. Heart—The cardiac examination may be unimpressive or very abnormal. Jugular venous distention reflects RA hypertension, and a Kussmaul sign (failure of decrease of jugular venous pressure with inspiration) is suggestive of RV infarction. Soft heart sounds may indicate LV dysfunction. Atrial gallops (S_4) are the rule, whereas ventricular gallops (S_3) are less common and indicate significant LV dysfunction. Mitral regurgitation murmurs are not uncommon and may indicate papillary muscle dysfunction or, rarely, rupture. Pericardial friction rubs are uncommon in the first 24 hours but may appear later.

4. Extremities—Edema is usually not present. Cyanosis and cold temperature indicate low output. The peripheral pulses should be noted, since later shock or emboli may alter the examination.

C. Laboratory Findings

Cardiac-specific markers of myocardial damage include quantitative determinations of CK-MB, highly sensitive and conventional troponin I, and troponin T. Each of these tests may become positive as early as 4–6 hours after the onset of a myocardial infarction and should be abnormal by 8–12 hours. Troponins are more sensitive and specific than CK-MB. "Highly sensitive" or "fourth-generation" troponin assays, which are not yet widely used in the United States but are the standard assays in most of Europe, have a 10- to 100-fold lower limit of detection, allowing myocardial infarction to be detected earlier, using the change in value over 3 hours.

Circulating levels of troponins may remain elevated for 5–7 days or longer and therefore are generally not useful for evaluating suspected early reinfarction. Elevated CK-MB generally normalizes within 24 hours, thus being more helpful for evaluation of reinfarction. Low-level elevations of troponin in patients with severe chronic kidney disease may not be related to acute coronary disease but rather a function of the physiologic washout of the marker. While many conditions including chronic heart failure are associated with elevated levels of the high-sensitivity troponin assays, these assays may be especially useful when negative to exclude myocardial infarction in patients reporting chest pain.

D. ECG

The extent of the ECG abnormalities, especially the sum of the total amount of ST-segment deviation, is a good indicator of the extent of acute infarction and risk of subsequent adverse events. The classic evolution of changes is from peaked ("hyperacute") T waves, to ST-segment elevation, to Q wave development, to T wave inversion. This may occur over a few hours to several days. The evolution of new Q waves (longer than 30 msec in duration and 25% of the R wave amplitude) is diagnostic, but Q waves do not occur in 30–50% of acute infarctions (non-Q wave infarctions). Left bundle branch block, especially when new (or not known to be old), in a patient with symptoms of an acute myocardial infarction, is considered to be a "**STEMI equivalent**"; reperfusion therapy is indicated for the affected patient. Concordant ST elevation (ie, ST elevation in leads with an overall positive QRS complex) with left bundle branch block is a specific finding indicating STEMI.

E. Chest Radiography

The chest radiograph may demonstrate signs of heart failure, but these changes often lag behind the clinical findings. Signs of aortic dissection, including mediastinal widening, should be sought as a possible alternative diagnosis.

F. Echocardiography

Echocardiography provides convenient bedside assessment of LV global and regional function. This can help with the diagnosis and management of infarction; echocardiography has been used successfully to make judgments about admission and management of patients with suspected infarction, including in patients with ST-segment elevation or left bundle branch block of uncertain significance, since normal wall motion makes an infarction unlikely. Doppler echocardiography is generally the most convenient procedure for diagnosing postinfarction mitral regurgitation or VSD.

G. Other Noninvasive Studies

Diagnosis of myocardial infarction and extent of myocardial infarction can be assessed by various imaging studies in addition to echocardiography. **MRI with gadolinium contrast enhancement** is the most sensitive test to detect and quantitate extent of infarction, with the ability to detect as little as 2 g of myocardial infarction. **Technetium-99m pyrophosphate scintigraphy,** when injected at least 18 hours postinfarction, complexes with calcium in necrotic myocardium to provide a "hot spot" image of the infarction. This test is insensitive to small infarctions, and false-positive studies occur, so its use is limited to patients in whom the diagnosis by ECG and enzymes is not possible—principally those who present several days after the event or have intraoperative infarctions. **Scintigraphy with thallium-201** or technetium-based perfusion tracers will demonstrate "cold spots" in regions of diminished perfusion, which usually represent infarction when the radiotracer is administered at rest, but abnormalities do not distinguish recent from old damage. All of these tests may be considered after the patient has had revascularization.

H. Hemodynamic Measurements

These can be helpful in managing the patient with suspected cardiogenic shock. Use of PA catheters, however, has generally not been associated with better outcomes and should be limited to patients with severe hemodynamic compromise for whom the information would be anticipated to change management.

▶ Treatment

A. Aspirin, P2Y₁₂ Inhibitors (Prasugrel, Ticagrelor, and Clopidogrel)

All patients with definite or suspected acute myocardial infarction should receive aspirin at a dose of 162 mg or 325 mg at once regardless of whether fibrinolytic therapy is being considered or the patient has been taking aspirin.

Chewable aspirin provides more rapid blood levels. Patients with a definite aspirin allergy should be treated with a P2Y$_{12}$ inhibitor (clopidogrel, prasugrel, or ticagrelor).

P2Y$_{12}$ inhibitors, *in combination with aspirin,* have been shown to provide important benefits in patients with acute STEMI. **Thus, guidelines call for a P2Y$_{12}$ inhibitor to be added to aspirin for all patients with STEMI, regardless of whether reperfusion is given, and continued for at least 14 days, and generally for 1 year.** The preferred P2Y$_{12}$ inhibitors are prasugrel (60 mg orally on day 1, then 10 mg daily) or ticagrelor (180 mg orally on day 1, then 90 mg twice daily). Both of these medications demonstrated superior outcomes to clopidogrel in clinical studies of primary PCI. Clopidogrel should be administered as a loading dose of 300–600 mg orally for faster onset of action than the 75 mg maintenance dose. With fibrinolytic therapy, there are no randomized trial data regarding when the early use of prasugrel or ticagrelor and clopidogrel is

indicated (with a 300-mg loading dose for patients younger than 75 years and no loading dose for patients older than 75 years). Prasugrel is contraindicated in patients with history of stroke or who are older than 75 years.

B. Reperfusion Therapy

Patients with STEMI who seek medical attention within 12 hours of the onset of symptoms should be treated with reperfusion therapy, either primary PCI or fibrinolytic therapy. Patients without ST-segment elevation (previously labeled "non-Q wave" infarctions) do not benefit, and may derive harm, from thrombolysis (Figure 10–7).

1. Primary percutaneous coronary intervention—Immediate coronary angiography and **primary PCI (including stenting) of the infarct-related artery have been shown to be superior to thrombolysis** when done by experienced operators in high-volume centers with rapid time from first

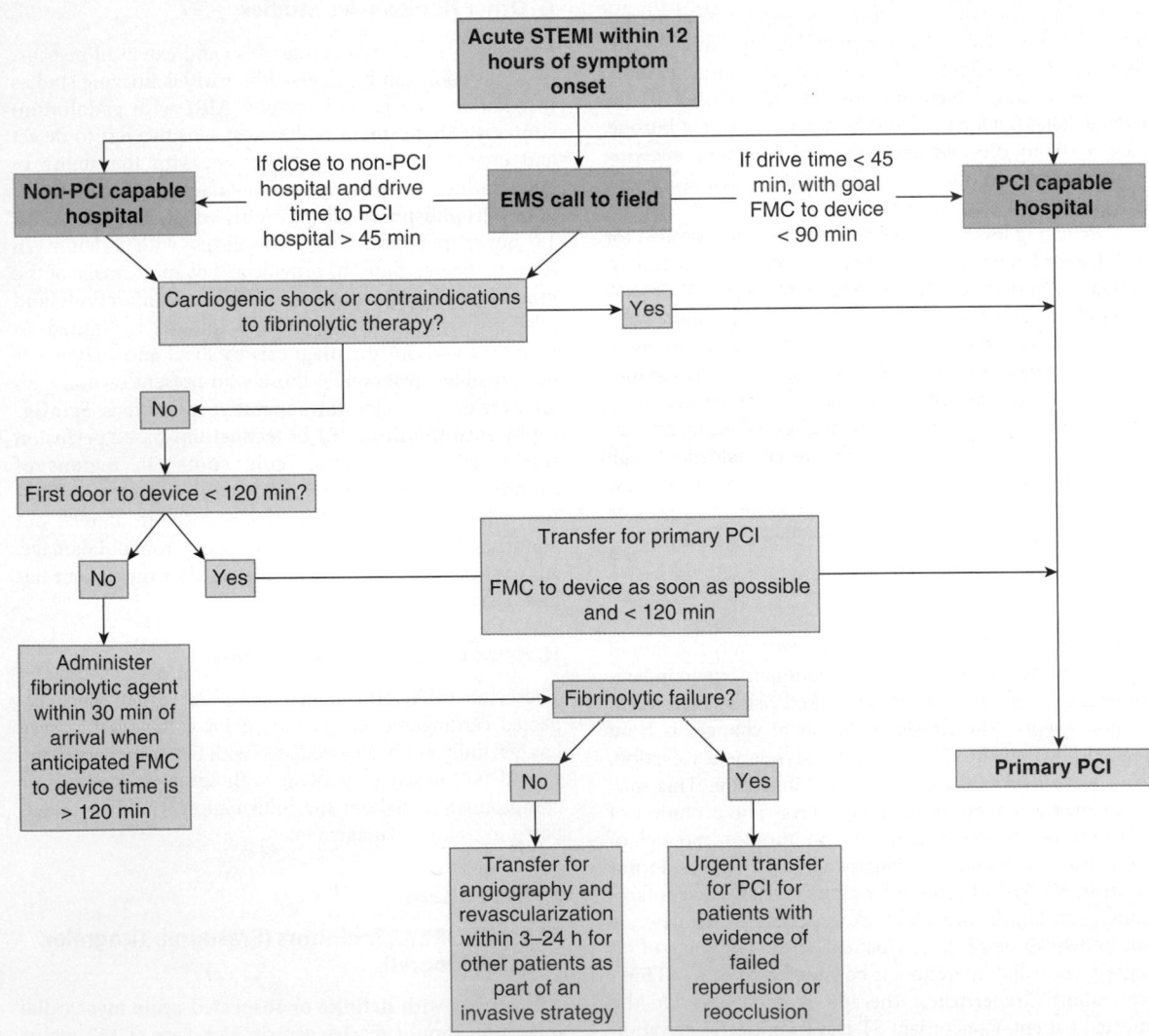

▲ **Figure 10–7.** Summary of 2013 guidelines for reperfusion managment of myocardial infarction with ST-segment elevation (STEMI). FMC, first medical contact.

medical contact to intervention ("door-to-balloon"). US and European guidelines call for first medical contact or "door-to-balloon" times of 90 minutes or less. Several trials have shown that if efficient transfer systems are in place, transfer of patients with acute myocardial infarction from hospitals without primary PCI capability to hospitals with primary PCI capability with first door-to-device times of 120 minutes or less can improve outcome compared with fibrinolytic therapy at the presenting hospital, although this requires sophisticated systems to ensure rapid identification, transfer, and expertise in PCI. Because PCI also carries a lower risk of hemorrhagic complications, including intracranial hemorrhage, it may be the preferred strategy in many older patients and others with contraindications to fibrinolytic therapy (see Table 10–12 for factors to consider in choosing fibrinolytic therapy or primary PCI).

A. Stenting—PCI with stenting is standard for patients with acute myocardial infarction. Primary PCI stenting is done with bivalirudin, a direct thrombin inhibitor, or unfractionated heparin with or without glycoprotein IIb/IIIa inhibitors. Although randomized trials have shown a benefit with regard to fewer repeat interventions for restenosis with the use of drug-eluting stents in STEMI patients, bare metal stents are still used for patients without the ability to obtain and comply with P2Y$_{12}$ inhibitor therapy, which is often not known at the time of PCI. In the subgroup of patients with cardiogenic shock, early catheterization and percutaneous or surgical revascularization are the preferred management and have been shown to reduce mortality.

The Heat PPCI trial showed increased stent thrombosis and more adverse cardiovascular events with bivalirudin compared to unfractionated heparin.

"Facilitated" PCI, whereby a combination of medications (full- or reduced-dose fibrinolytic agents, with or without glycoprotein IIb/IIIa inhibitors) is given followed by immediate PCI is not recommended. Patients should be treated either with primary PCI or with fibrinolytic agents (and immediate rescue PCI for reperfusion failure), if it can be done promptly as outlined in the ACC/AHA and European guidelines. Timely access to most appropriate reperfusion, including primary PCI, can be expanded with development of regional systems of care, including emergency medical systems and networks of hospitals. Patients treated with fibrinolytic therapy appear to have improved outcomes if transferred for routine coronary angiography and PCI within 24 hours. The American Heart Association has a program called "Mission: Lifeline" to support the development of regional systems of care (see http://www.heart.org/missionlifeline).

Table 10–12. Fibrinolytic therapy for acute myocardial infarction.

	Alteplase; Tissue Plasminogen Activator (t-PA)	Reteplase	Tenecteplase (TNK-t-PA)	Streptokinase
Source	Recombinant DNA	Recombinant DNA	Recombinant DNA	Group C streptococcus
Half-life	5 minutes	15 minutes	20 minutes	20 minutes
Usual dose	100 mg	20 units	40 mg	1.5 million units
Administration	Initial bolus of 15 mg, followed by 50 mg infused over the next 30 minutes and 35 mg over the following 60 minutes	10 units as a bolus over 2 minutes, repeated after 30 minutes	Single weight-adjusted bolus, 0.5 mg/kg	750,000 units over 20 minutes followed by 750,000 units over 40 minutes
Anticoagulation after infusion	Aspirin, 325 mg daily; heparin, 5000 units as bolus, followed by 1000 units per hour infusion, subsequently adjusted to maintain PTT 1.5–2 times control	Aspirin, 325 mg; heparin as with t-PA	Aspirin, 325 mg daily	Aspirin, 325 mg daily; there is no evidence that adjunctive heparin improves outcome following streptokinase
Clot selectivity	High	High	High	Low
Fibrinogenolysis	+	+	+	+++
Bleeding	+	+	+	+
Hypotension	+	+	+	+++
Allergic reactions	+	+	+	++
Reocclusion	10–30%	—	5–20%	5–20%
Approximate cost[1]	$6712.54	$5211.86	$4194.30	Not available in the United States

[1]Average wholesale price (AWP, for AB-rated generic when available) for quantity listed.
PTT, partial thromboplastin time.
Source: *Red Book Online, 2014, Truven Health Analytics, Inc.* AWP may not accurately represent the actual pharmacy cost because wide contractual variations exist among institutions.

B. Antiplatelet therapy after drug-eluting or bare metal stents—In patients with an acute coronary syndrome, **dual antiplatelet therapy is indicated for 1 year in all patients (including those with medical therapy and those patients undergoing revascularization irrespective of stent type).** For patients undergoing elective or stable PCI, the duration of dual antiplatelet therapy is recommended for at least 1 month for patients receiving bare metal stents. For patients receiving drug-eluting stents, dual antiplatelet therapy is recommended for at least 1 year by the ACC/AHA PCI guidelines. These recommendations are based both on the durations of therapies during the studies evaluating the stents, and the pathophysiologic understanding of the timing of endothelialization following bare metal versus drug-eluting stent implantation. The DAPT (dual antiplatelet therapy) study showed fewer death, myocardial infarction, and stroke events with longer (up to 30 months) dual antiplatelet therapy for patients who had received drug-eluting stents, but it also showed more bleeding and a tendency for higher mortality. Treatment with clopidogrel for longer than 1 year after drug-eluting stents, therefore, should be individualized based on thrombotic and bleeding risks.

2. Fibrinolytic therapy

A. Benefit—Fibrinolytic therapy reduces mortality and limits infarct size in patients with STEMI (defined as 0.1 mV or more in two inferior or lateral leads or two contiguous precordial leads), or with left bundle branch block (not known to be old). The greatest benefit occurs if treatment is initiated within the first 3 hours after the onset of presentation, when up to a 50% reduction in mortality rate can be achieved. The magnitude of benefit declines rapidly thereafter, but a 10% relative mortality reduction can be achieved up to 12 hours after the onset of chest pain. The survival benefit is greatest in patients with large—usually anterior—infarctions. Primary PCI (including stenting) of the infarct-related artery, however, is superior to thrombolysis when done by experienced operators with rapid time from first medical contact to intervention ("door-to-balloon").

B. Contraindications—Major bleeding complications occur in 0.5–5% of patients, the most serious of which is intracranial hemorrhage. The major risk factors for intracranial bleeding are age 75 years or older, hypertension at presentation (especially over 180/110 mm Hg), low body weight (less than 70 kg), and the use of fibrin-specific fibrinolytic agents (alteplase, reteplase, tenecteplase). Although patients over age 75 years have a much higher mortality rate with acute myocardial infarction and therefore may derive greater benefit, the risk of severe bleeding is also higher, particularly among patients with risk factors for intracranial hemorrhage, such as severe hypertension or recent stroke. Patients presenting more than 12 hours after the onset of chest pain may also derive a small benefit, particularly if pain and ST-segment elevation persist, but rarely does this benefit outweigh the attendant risk.

Absolute contraindications to fibrinolytic therapy include previous hemorrhagic stroke, other strokes or cerebrovascular events within 1 year, known intracranial neoplasm, recent head trauma (including minor trauma), active internal bleeding (excluding menstruation), or suspected aortic dissection. **Relative contraindications** are BP greater than 180/110 mm Hg at presentation, other intracerebral pathology not listed above as a contraindication, known bleeding diathesis, trauma within 2–4 weeks, major surgery within 3 weeks, prolonged (more than 10 minutes) or traumatic cardiopulmonary resuscitation, recent (within 2–4 weeks) internal bleeding, noncompressible vascular punctures, active diabetic retinopathy, pregnancy, active peptic ulcer disease, a history of severe hypertension, current use of anticoagulants (INR greater than 2.0–3.0), and (for streptokinase) prior allergic reaction or exposure to streptokinase or anistreplase within 2 years.

C. Fibrinolytic agents—The following fibrinolytic agents are available for acute myocardial infarction and are characterized in Table 10–12.

Alteplase (recombinant tissue plasminogen activator; t-PA) results in about a 50% reduction in circulating fibrinogen. In the first GUSTO trial, which compared a 90-minute dosing of t-PA (with unfractionated heparin) with streptokinase, the 30-day mortality rate with t-PA was one absolute percentage point lower (one additional life saved per 100 patients treated), though there was also a small *increase* in the rate of intracranial hemorrhage. An angiographic substudy confirmed a higher 90-minute patency rate and a higher rate of normal (TIMI grade 3) flow in patients.

Reteplase is a recombinant deletion mutant of t-PA that is slightly less fibrin specific. In comparative trials, it appeared to have efficacy similar to that of alteplase, but it has a longer duration of action and can be administered as two boluses 30 minutes apart.

Tenecteplase (TNK-t-PA) is a genetically engineered substitution mutant of native t-PA that has reduced plasma clearance, increased fibrin sensitivity, and increased resistance to plasminogen activator inhibitor-1. It can be given as a single weight-adjusted bolus. In the ASSENT 2 trial, this agent was equivalent to t-PA with regard to efficacy and resulted in significantly less noncerebral bleeding.

Streptokinase, commonly used outside of the United States, is somewhat less effective at opening occluded arteries and less effective at reducing mortality. It is non–fibrin-specific, causes depletion of circulating fibrinogen, and has a tendency to induce hypotension, particularly if infused rapidly. This can be managed by slowing or interrupting the infusion and administering fluids. There is controversy as to whether adjunctive heparin is beneficial in patients given streptokinase, unlike its administration with the more clot-specific agents. Allergic reactions, including anaphylaxis, occur in 1–2% of patients, and this agent should generally not be administered to patients with prior exposure.

(1) Selection of a fibrinolytic agent—In the United States, most patients are treated with alteplase, reteplase, or tenecteplase. The differences in efficacy between them are small compared with the potential benefit of treating a greater proportion of appropriate candidates in a more prompt manner. The principal objective should be to administer a thrombolytic agent within 30 minutes of presentation—or even during transport. The ability to administer tenecteplase as a single bolus is an attractive feature

that may facilitate earlier treatment. The combination of a reduced-dose thrombolytic given with a platelet glycoprotein IIb/IIIa inhibitor does not reduce mortality but does cause a modest increase in bleeding complications.

(2) Postfibrinolytic management—After completion of the fibrinolytic infusion, aspirin (81–325 mg/day) and anticoagulation should be continued until revascularization or for the duration of the hospital stay (or up to 8 days). Anticoagulation with LMWH (enoxaparin or fondaparinux) is preferable to unfractionated heparin.

(A) LOW-MOLECULAR-WEIGHT HEPARIN—In the EXTRACT trial, enoxaparin significantly reduced death and myocardial infarction at day 30 (compared with unfractionated heparin), at the expense of a modest increase in bleeding. In patients younger than age 75, enoxaparin was given as a 30-mg intravenous bolus and 1 mg/kg subcutaneously every 12 hours; in patients age 75 years and older, it was given with no bolus and 0.75 mg/kg subcutaneously every 12 hours. This appeared to attenuate the risk of intracranial hemorrhage in the elderly that had been seen with full-dose enoxaparin. Another antithrombotic option is fondaparinux, given at a dose of 2.5 mg subcutaneously once a day. There is no benefit of fondaparinux among patients undergoing primary PCI, and fondaparinux is not recommended as a sole anticoagulant during PCI due to risk of catheter thrombosis.

(B) UNFRACTIONATED HEPARIN—Anticoagulation with intravenous heparin (initial dose of 60 units/kg bolus to a maximum of 4000 units, followed by an infusion of 12 units/kg/h to a maximum of 1000 units/hour, then adjusted to maintain an aPTT of 50–75 seconds beginning with an aPTT drawn 3 hours after thrombolytic) is continued for at least 48 hours after alteplase, reteplase, or tenecteplase, and with continuation of an anticoagulant until revascularization (if performed) or until hospital discharge (or day 8).

(C) PROPHYLACTIC THERAPY AGAINST GASTROINTESTINAL BLEEDING—For all patients with STEMI treated with intensive antithrombotic therapy, prophylactic treatment with proton pump inhibitors, or antacids and an H$_2$-blocker, is advisable, although certain proton pump inhibitors, such as omeprazole and esomeprazole, decrease the effect of clopidogrel.

3. Assessment of myocardial reperfusion, recurrent ischemic pain, reinfarction—Myocardial reperfusion can be recognized clinically by the early cessation of pain and the resolution of ST-segment elevation. Although at least 50% resolution of ST-segment elevation by 90 minutes may occur without coronary reperfusion, ST resolution is a strong predictor of better outcome. Even with anticoagulation, 10–20% of reperfused vessels will reocclude during hospitalization, although reocclusion and reinfarction appear to be reduced following intervention. Reinfarction, indicated by recurrence of pain and ST-segment elevation, can be treated by readministration of a thrombolytic agent or immediate angiography and PCI.

C. General Measures

Cardiac care unit monitoring should be instituted as soon as possible. Patients without complications can be transferred to a telemetry unit after 24 hours. Activity should initially be limited to bed rest but can be advanced within 24 hours. Progressive ambulation should be started after 24–72 hours if tolerated. For patients without complications, discharge by day 4 appears to be appropriate. Low-flow oxygen therapy (2–4 L/min) should be given if oxygen saturation is reduced.

D. Analgesia

An initial attempt should be made to relieve pain with sublingual nitroglycerin. However, if no response occurs after two or three tablets, intravenous opioids provide the most rapid and effective analgesia and may also reduce pulmonary congestion. Morphine sulfate, 4–8 mg, or meperidine, 50–75 mg, should be given. Subsequent small doses can be given every 15 minutes until pain abates.

Nonsteroidal anti-inflammatory agents, other than aspirin, should be avoided during hospitalization for STEMI due to increased risk of mortality, myocardial rupture, hypertension, heart failure, and kidney injury with their use.

E. Beta-Adrenergic Blocking Agents

Trials have shown modest short-term benefit from beta-blockers started during the first 24 hours after acute myocardial infarction if there are no contraindications (metoprolol 25–50 mg orally twice daily). Aggressive beta-blockade can increase shock, with overall harm in patients with heart failure. Thus, early beta-blockade should be avoided in patients with any degree of heart failure, evidence of low output state, increased risk of cardiogenic shock, or other relative contraindications to beta-blockade. Carvedilol (beginning at 6.25 mg twice a day, titrated to 25 mg twice a day) was shown to be beneficial in the CAPRICORN trial following the acute phase of large myocardial infarction.

F. Nitrates

Nitroglycerin is the agent of choice for continued or recurrent ischemic pain and is useful in lowering BP or relieving pulmonary congestion. However, routine nitrate administration is not recommended, since no improvement in outcome has been observed in the ISIS-4 or GISSI-3 trials. Nitrates should be avoided in patients who received phosphodiesterase inhibitors (sildenafil, vardenafil, and tadalafil) in the prior 24 hours.

G. Angiotensin-Converting Enzyme (ACE) Inhibitors

A series of trials (SAVE, AIRE, SMILE, TRACE, GISSI-III, and ISIS-4) have shown both short- and long-term improvement in survival with ACE inhibitor therapy. The benefits are greatest in patients with an EF of 40% or less, large infarctions, or clinical evidence of heart failure. Because substantial amounts of the survival benefit occur on the first day, ACE inhibitor treatment should be commenced early in patients without hypotension, especially patients with large or anterior myocardial infarction. Given the benefits of ACE inhibitors for patients with vascular disease, it is reasonable to use **ACE inhibitors for all patients following STEMI who do not have contraindications** (see Table 11–4).

H. Angiotensin Receptor Blockers

Although there has been inconsistency in the effects of different ARBs on mortality for patients post-myocardial infarction with heart failure and/or LV dysfunction, the VALIANT trial showed that valsartan 160 mg orally twice a day is equivalent to captopril in reducing mortality. Thus, valsartan should be used for all patients with ACE inhibitor intolerance, and is a reasonable, albeit more expensive, alternative to captopril. The combination of captopril and valsartan (at a reduced dose) was no better than either agent alone and resulted in more side effects.

I. Aldosterone Antagonists

The RALES trial showed that 25 mg spironolactone can reduce the mortality rate of patients with advanced heart failure, and the EPHESUS trial showed a 15% relative risk reduction in mortality with eplerenone 25 mg daily for patients post-myocardial infarction with LV dysfunction (LVEF of 40% or less) and either clinical heart failure or diabetes. Kidney dysfunction or hyperkalemia are contraindications, and patients must be monitored carefully for development of hyperkalemia.

J. Calcium Channel Blockers

There are no studies to support the routine use of calcium channel blockers in most patients with acute myocardial infarction—and indeed, they have the potential to exacerbate ischemia and cause death from reflex tachycardia or myocardial depression. Long-acting calcium channel blockers should generally be reserved for management of hypertension or ischemia as second- or third-line medications after beta-blockers and nitrates.

K. Long-Term Antithrombotic Therapy

Discharge on aspirin, 81–325 mg/day, since it is highly effective, inexpensive, and well tolerated, is a key quality indicator of myocardial infarction care. Patients who received a coronary stent should also receive a $P2Y_{12}$ inhibitor (see Antiplatelet therapy after drug-eluting or bare metal stents, above).

Patients who have received a coronary stent and who require warfarin anticoagulation present a particular challenge, since "triple therapy" with aspirin, clopidogrel, and warfarin has a high risk of bleeding. Triple therapy should be (1) limited to patients with a clear indication for warfarin (such as $CHADS_2$ score of 2 or more or a mechanical prosthetic valve), (2) used for the shortest period of time (such as 1 month after placement of bare metal stent; drugeluting stents that would require longer clopidogrel duration should be avoided if possible), (3) used with low-dose aspirin and with strategies to reduce risk of bleeding (eg, proton pump inhibitors for patients with a history of gastrointestinal bleeding), and (4) used with consideration of

a lower target anticoagulation intensity (INR 2.0 to 2.5, at least for the indication of atrial fibrillation) during the period of concomitant treatment with aspirin and $P2Y_{12}$ therapy. Several ongoing studies are evaluating the DOACs in this area.

L. Coronary Angiography

For patients who do not reperfuse based on lack of at least 50% resolution of ST elevation, rescue angioplasty should be performed and has been shown to reduce the composite risk of death, reinfarction, stroke, or severe heart failure. According to the evidence in the 2012 European and ACC/AHA guidelines, patients treated with coronary angiography and PCI 3–24 hours after fibrinolytic therapy showed improved outcomes. Patients with recurrent ischemic pain prior to discharge should undergo catheterization and, if indicated, revascularization. PCI of a totally occluded infarct-related artery more than 24 hours after STEMI should generally not be performed in asymptomatic patients with one or two vessel disease without evidence of severe ischemia.

▶ When to Refer

All patients with acute myocardial infarction should be referred to a cardiologist.

Armstrong PW et al; STREAM Investigative Team. Fibrinolysis or primary PCI in ST-segment elevation myocardial infarction. N Engl J Med. 2013 Apr 11;368(15):1379–87. [PMID: 23473396]

O'Gara PT et al. 2013 ACCF/AHA guideline for the management of ST-elevation myocardial infarction: executive summary: a report of the American College of Cardiology Foundation/American Heart Association Task Force on Practice Guidelines: developed in collaboration with the American College of Emergency Physicians and Society for Cardiovascular Angiography and Interventions. Catheter Cardiovasc Interv. 2013 Jul 1;82(1):E1–27. [PMID: 23299937]

Shahzad A et al; HEAT-PPCI trial investigators. Unfractionated heparin versus bivalirudin in primary percutaneous coronary intervention (HEAT-PPCI): an open-label, single centre, randomised controlled trial. Lancet. 2014 Nov 22; 384(9957):1849–58. [PMID: 25002178]

Steg PG et al. ESC Guidelines for the management of acute myocardial infarction in patients presenting with ST-segment elevation: The Task Force on the management of ST-segment elevation acute myocardial infarction of the European Society of Cardiology (ESC). Eur Heart J. 2012 Oct;33(20):2569–619. [PMID: 22922416]

Tamis-Holland JE et al. Highlights from the 2013 ACCF/AHA guidelines for the management of ST-elevation myocardial infarction and beyond. Clin Cardiol. 2014 Apr;37(4):252–9. [PMID: 24523153]

▶ Complications

A variety of complications can occur after myocardial infarction even when treatment is initiated promptly.

A. Postinfarction Ischemia

In clinical trials of thrombolysis, recurrent ischemia occurred in about one-third of patients, was more common following non–ST elevation myocardial infarction than after STEMI, and had important short- and long-term prognostic implications. Vigorous medical therapy should be instituted, including nitrates and beta-blockers as well as aspirin 81–325 mg/day, anticoagulant therapy (unfractionated heparin, enoxaparin, or fondaparinux) and clopidogrel (75 mg orally daily). Most patients with postinfarction angina—and all who are refractory to medical therapy—should undergo early catheterization and revascularization by PCI or CABG.

B. Arrhythmias

Abnormalities of rhythm and conduction are common.

1. Sinus bradycardia—This is most common in inferior infarctions or may be precipitated by medications. Observation or withdrawal of the offending agent is usually sufficient. If accompanied by signs of low cardiac output, atropine intravenously is usually effective. Temporary pacing is rarely required.

2. Supraventricular tachyarrhythmias—Sinus tachycardia is common and may reflect either increased adrenergic stimulation or hemodynamic compromise due to hypovolemia or pump failure. In the latter, beta-blockade is contraindicated. Supraventricular premature beats are common and may be premonitory for atrial fibrillation. Electrolyte abnormalities and hypoxia should be corrected and causative agents (especially aminophylline) stopped. Atrial fibrillation should be rapidly controlled or converted to sinus rhythm. Intravenous beta-blockers, such as metoprolol (2.5–5 mg intravenously every 2–5 minutes, maximum 15 mg over 10–minutes) or short-acting esmolol (50–200 mcg/kg/min) are the agents of choice if cardiac function is adequate. Intravenous diltiazem (5–15 mg/h) may be used if beta-blockers are contraindicated or ineffective. Electrical cardioversion (commencing with 100 J) may be necessary if atrial fibrillation is complicated by hypotension, heart failure, or ischemia, but the arrhythmia often recurs. Amiodarone (150 mg intravenous bolus and then 15–30 mg/h intravenously, or rapid oral loading dose for cardioversion of 400 mg three times daily) may be helpful to restore or maintain sinus rhythm.

3. Ventricular arrhythmias—Ventricular arrhythmias are most common in the first few hours after infarction and are a marker of high risk. Ventricular premature beats may be premonitory for ventricular tachycardia or fibrillation but generally should not be treated in the absence of frequent or sustained ventricular tachycardia. Lidocaine is *not* recommended as a prophylactic measure.

Sustained ventricular tachycardia should be treated with a 1 mg/kg bolus of lidocaine if the patient is stable or by electrical cardioversion (100–200 J) if not. If the arrhythmia cannot be suppressed with lidocaine, procainamide (100 mg boluses over 1–2 minutes every 5 minutes to a cumulative dose of 750–1000 mg) or intravenous amiodarone (150 mg over 10 minutes, which may be repeated as needed, followed by 360 mg over 6 hours and then 540 mg over 18 hours) should be initiated, followed by an infusion of 0.5 mg/min (720 mg/24 hours). Ventricular fibrillation is treated electrically (300–400 J). All patients taking antiarrhythmics should be monitored with telemetry or ECGs during initiation. Unresponsive ventricular fibrillation should be treated with additional amiodarone and repeat cardioversion while cardiopulmonary resuscitation (CPR) is administered.

Accelerated idioventricular rhythm is a regular, wide-complex rhythm at a rate of 70–100/min. It may occur with or without reperfusion and should not be treated with antiarrhythmics, which could cause asystole.

4. Conduction disturbances—All degrees of AV block may occur in the course of acute myocardial infarction. Block at the level of the AV node is more common than infranodal block and occurs in approximately 20% of inferior myocardial infarctions. First-degree block is the most common and requires no treatment. Second-degree block is usually of the Mobitz type I form (Wenckebach), is often transient, and requires treatment only if associated with a heart rate slow enough to cause symptoms. Complete AV block occurs in up to 5% of acute inferior infarctions, usually is preceded by Mobitz I second-degree block, and generally resolves spontaneously, though it may persist for hours to several weeks. The escape rhythm originates in the distal AV node or AV junction and hence has a narrow QRS complex and is reliable, albeit often slow (30–50 beats/min). Treatment is often necessary because of resulting hypotension and low cardiac output. Intravenous atropine (1 mg) usually restores AV conduction temporarily, but if the escape complex is wide or if repeated atropine treatments are needed, temporary ventricular pacing is indicated. The prognosis for these patients is only slightly worse than for patients in whom AV block does not develop.

In anterior infarctions, the site of block is distal, below the AV node, and usually a result of extensive damage of the His-Purkinje system and bundle branches. New first-degree block (prolongation of the PR interval) is unusual in anterior infarction; Mobitz type II AV block or complete heart block may be preceded by intraventricular conduction defects or may occur abruptly. The escape rhythm, if present, is an unreliable wide-complex idioventricular rhythm. *Urgent ventricular pacing is mandatory*, but even with successful pacing, morbidity and mortality are high because of the extensive myocardial damage. New conduction abnormalities, such as right or left bundle branch block or fascicular blocks, may presage progression, often sudden, to second- or third-degree AV block. Temporary ventricular pacing is recommended for new-onset alternating bilateral bundle branch block, bifascicular block, or bundle branch block with worsening first-degree AV block. Patients with anterior infarction who progress to second- or third-degree block even transiently should be considered for insertion of a prophylactic permanent ventricular pacemaker before discharge.

C. Myocardial Dysfunction

Persons with hypotension not responsive to fluid resuscitation or refractory heart failure or cardiogenic shock should be considered for urgent echocardiography to assess left and right ventricular function and for mechanical complications, right heart catheterization, and continuous measurements of arterial pressure. These measurements permit the accurate assessment of volume status and may facilitate decisions about volume resuscitation, selective use of pressors and inotropes, and mechanical support.

1. Acute LV failure—Dyspnea, diffuse rales, and arterial hypoxemia usually indicate LV failure. General measures include supplemental oxygen to increase arterial saturation to above 95% and elevation of the trunk. Diuretics are usually the initial therapy unless RV infarction is present. Intravenous furosemide (10–40 mg) or bumetanide (0.5–1 mg) is preferred because of the reliably rapid onset and short duration of action of these medications. Higher dosages can be given if an inadequate response occurs. Morphine sulfate (4 mg intravenously followed by increments of 2 mg) is valuable in acute pulmonary edema.

Diuretics are usually effective; however, because most patients with acute infarction are not volume overloaded, the hemodynamic response may be limited and may be associated with hypotension. In mild heart failure, sublingual isosorbide dinitrate (2.5–10 mg every 2 hours) or nitroglycerin ointment (6.25–25 mg every 4 hours) may be adequate to lower PCWP. In more severe failure, especially if cardiac output is reduced and BP is normal or high, sodium nitroprusside may be the preferred agent. It should be initiated only with arterial pressure monitoring; the initial dosage should be low (0.25 mcg/kg/min) to avoid excessive hypotension, but the dosage can be increased by increments of 0.5 mcg/kg/min every 5–10 minutes up to 5–10 mcg/kg/min until the desired hemodynamic response is obtained. Excessive hypotension (mean BP less than 65–75 mm Hg) or tachycardia (greater than 10/min increase) should be avoided.

Intravenous nitroglycerin (starting at 10 mcg/min) also may be effective but may lower PCWP with less hypotension. Oral or transdermal vasodilator therapy with nitrates or ACE inhibitors is often necessary after the initial 24–48 hours.

Inotropic agents should be avoided if possible, because they often increase heart rate and myocardial oxygen requirements and worsen clinical outcomes. Dobutamine has the best hemodynamic profile, increasing cardiac output and modestly lowering PCWP, usually without excessive tachycardia, hypotension, or arrhythmias. The initial dosage is 2.5 mcg/kg/min, and it may be increased by similar increments up to 15–20 mcg/kg/min at intervals of 5–10 minutes. Dopamine is more useful in the presence of hypotension, since it produces peripheral vasoconstriction, but it has a less beneficial effect on PCWP. Digoxin has not been helpful in acute infarction except to control the ventricular response in atrial fibrillation, but it may be beneficial if chronic heart failure persists.

2. Hypotension and shock—Patients with hypotension (systolic BP less than 90 mm Hg, individualized depending on prior BP) and signs of diminished perfusion (low urinary output, confusion, cold extremities) that does not respond to fluid resuscitation should be presumed to have cardiogenic shock and should be considered for urgent catheterization and revascularization as well as selective

use of intra-aortic balloon pump (IABP) support and hemodynamic monitoring with a PA catheter, although these later measures have not been shown to improve outcome. Up to 20% will have findings indicative of intravascular hypovolemia (due to diaphoresis, vomiting, decreased venous tone, medications—such as diuretics, nitrates, morphine, beta-blockers, calcium channel blockers, and thrombolytic agents—and lack of oral intake). These should be treated with successive boluses of 100 mL of normal saline until PCWP reaches 15–18 mm Hg to determine whether cardiac output and BP respond. Pericardial tamponade due to hemorrhagic pericarditis (especially after thrombolytic therapy or cardiopulmonary resuscitation) or ventricular rupture should be considered and excluded by echocardiography if clinically indicated. RV infarction, characterized by a normal PCWP but elevated RA pressure, can produce hypotension. This is discussed below.

Most patients with cardiogenic shock will have moderate to severe LV systolic dysfunction, with a mean EF of 30% in the SHOCK trial. If hypotension is only modest (systolic pressure higher than 90 mm Hg) and the PCWP is elevated, diuretics should be administered. If the BP falls, inotropic support will need to be added. A large randomized trial showed no benefit of IABP support in cardiogenic shock.

Dopamine is generally considered to be the most appropriate pressor for cardiogenic hypotension. It should be initiated at a rate of 2–4 mcg/kg/min and increased at 5-minute intervals to the appropriate hemodynamic end point. At dosages lower than 5 mcg/kg/min, it improves renal blood flow; at intermediate dosages (2.5–10 mcg/kg/min), it stimulates myocardial contractility; at higher dosages (greater than 8 mcg/kg/min), it is a potent alpha-1-adrenergic agonist. In general, BP and cardiac index rise, but PCWP does not fall. Dopamine may be combined with nitroprusside or dobutamine (see above for dosing), or the latter may be used in its place if hypotension is not severe. Norepinephrine (0.1–0.5 mcg/kg/min) is generally reserved for failure of other vasopressors, since epinephrine produces less vasoconstriction and does not increase coronary perfusion pressure (aortic diastolic pressure), but it does tend to worsen the balance between myocardial oxygen delivery and utilization.

Patients with cardiogenic shock not due to hypovolemia have a poor prognosis, with 30-day mortality rates of 40–80%. The IABP-SHOCK II trial found that the use of an IABP does not offer a mortality benefit at 30 days or 1 year, compared with routine care with rapid revascularization, and is likely not helpful. Surgically implanted (or percutaneous) ventricular assist devices may be used in refractory cases. Emergent cardiac catheterization and coronary angiography followed by percutaneous or surgical revascularization offer the best chance of survival.

D. RV Infarction

RV infarction is present in one-third of patients with inferior wall infarction but is clinically significant in less than 50% of these. It presents as hypotension with relatively preserved LV function and should be considered whenever patients with inferior infarction exhibit low BP, raised venous pressure, and clear lungs. Hypotension is often exacerbated by medications that decrease intravascular volume or produce venodilation, such as diuretics, nitrates, and opioids. RA pressure and JVP are high, while PCWP is normal or low and the lungs are clear. The diagnosis is suggested by ST-segment elevation in right-sided anterior chest leads, particularly RV_4. The diagnosis can be confirmed by echocardiography or hemodynamic measurements. Treatment consists of fluid loading beginning with 500 mL of 0.9% saline over 2 hours to improve LV filling, and inotropic agents only if necessary.

E. Mechanical Defects

Partial or complete rupture of a papillary muscle or of the interventricular septum occurs in less than 1% of acute myocardial infarctions and carries a poor prognosis. These complications occur in both anterior and inferior infarctions, usually 3–7 days after the acute event. They are detected by the appearance of a new systolic murmur and clinical deterioration, often with pulmonary edema. The two lesions are distinguished by the location of the murmur (apical versus parasternal) and by Doppler echocardiography. Hemodynamic monitoring is essential for appropriate management and demonstrates an increase in oxygen saturation between the RA and PA in VSD and, often, a large *v* wave with mitral regurgitation. Treatment by nitroprusside and, preferably, intra-aortic balloon counterpulsation (IABC) reduces the regurgitation or shunt, but surgical correction is mandatory. In patients remaining hemodynamically unstable or requiring continuous parenteral pharmacologic treatment or counterpulsation, early surgery is recommended, though mortality rates are high (15% to nearly 100%, depending on residual ventricular function and clinical status). Patients who are stabilized medically can have delayed surgery with lower risks (10–25%), although this may be due to the death of sicker patients, some of whom may have been saved by earlier surgery.

F. Myocardial Rupture

Complete rupture of the LV free wall occurs in less than 1% of patients and usually results in immediate death. It occurs 2–7 days postinfarction, usually involves the anterior wall, and is more frequent in older women. Incomplete or gradual rupture may be sealed off by the pericardium, creating a **pseudoaneurysm**. This may be recognized by echocardiography, radionuclide angiography, or LV angiography, often as an incidental finding. It demonstrates a narrow-neck connection to the LV. Early surgical repair is indicated, since delayed rupture is common.

G. LV Aneurysm

An LV aneurysm, a sharply delineated area of scar that bulges paradoxically during systole, develops in 10–20% of patients surviving an acute infarction. This usually follows anterior Q wave infarctions. Aneurysms are recognized by persistent ST-segment elevation (beyond 4–8 weeks), and a

wide neck from the LV can be demonstrated by echocardiography, scintigraphy, or contrast angiography. They rarely rupture but may be associated with arterial emboli, ventricular arrhythmias, and heart failure. Surgical resection may be performed for these indications if other measures fail. The best results (mortality rates of 10–20%) are obtained when the residual myocardium contracts well and when significant coronary lesions supplying adjacent regions are bypassed.

H. Pericarditis

The pericardium is involved in approximately 50% of infarctions, but pericarditis is often not clinically significant. Twenty percent of patients with Q wave infarctions will have an audible friction rub if examined repetitively. Pericardial pain occurs in approximately the same proportion after 2–7 days and is recognized by its variation with respiration and position (improved by sitting). Often, no treatment is required, but aspirin (650 mg every 4–6 hours) will usually relieve the pain. Indomethacin and corticosteroids can cause impaired infarct healing and predispose to myocardial rupture, and therefore should generally be avoided in the early post-myocardial infarction period. Likewise, anticoagulation should be used cautiously, since hemorrhagic pericarditis may result.

One week to 12 weeks after infarction, Dressler syndrome (post-myocardial infarction syndrome) occurs in less than 5% of patients. This is an autoimmune phenomenon and presents as pericarditis with associated fever, leukocytosis and, occasionally, pericardial or pleural effusion. It may recur over months. Treatment is the same as for other forms of pericarditis. A short course of nonsteroidal agents or corticosteroids may help relieve symptoms.

I. Mural Thrombus

Mural thrombi are common in large anterior infarctions but not in infarctions at other locations. Arterial emboli occur in approximately 2% of patients with known infarction, usually within 6 weeks. Anticoagulation with heparin followed by short-term (3-month) warfarin therapy prevents most emboli and should be considered in all patients with large anterior infarctions. Mural thrombi can be detected by echocardiography or cardiac MRI, but these procedures should not be relied upon for determining the need for anticoagulation.

Thiele H et al; IABP-SHOCK II Trial Investigators. Intraaortic balloon support for myocardial infarction with cardiogenic shock. N Engl J Med. 2012 Oct 4;367(14):1287–96. [PMID: 22920912]

▶ **Postinfarction Management**

After the first 24 hours, the focus of patient management is to prevent recurrent ischemia, improve infarct healing and prevent remodeling, and prevent recurrent vascular events. Patients with hemodynamic compromise, who are at high risk for death, need careful monitoring and management of volume status.

A. Risk Stratification

Risk stratification is important for the management of STEMI. GRACE and TIMI risk scores can be helpful tools. The GRACE risk score is available for web access and/or download at http://gracescore.org, and the TIMI Risk Score is available at http://www.timi.org. Patients with recurrent ischemia (spontaneous or provoked), hemodynamic instability, impaired LV function, heart failure, or serious ventricular arrhythmias should undergo cardiac catheterization (see Table 10–11). ACE inhibitor (or ARB) therapy is indicated in patients with clinical heart failure or LVEF of 40% or less. Aldosterone blockade is indicated for patients with an LVEF of 40% or less and either heart failure or diabetes mellitus.

For patients not undergoing cardiac catheterization, submaximal exercise (or pharmacologic stress testing for patients unable to exercise) before discharge or a maximal test after 3–6 weeks (the latter being more sensitive for ischemia) helps patients and clinicians plan the return to normal activity. Imaging in conjunction with stress testing adds additional sensitivity for ischemia and provides localizing information. Both exercise and pharmacologic stress imaging have successfully predicted subsequent outcome. One of these tests should be used prior to discharge in patients who have received thrombolytic therapy as a means of selecting appropriate candidates for coronary angiography.

B. Secondary Prevention

Postinfarction management should begin with identification and modification of risk factors. Treatment of hyperlipidemia and smoking cessation both prevent recurrent infarction and death. Statin therapy should be started before the patient is discharged from the hospital to reduce recurrent atherothrombotic events. BP control and cardiac rehabilitation or exercise are also recommended.

Beta-blockers improve survival rates, primarily by reducing the incidence of sudden death in high-risk subsets of patients, though their value may be less in patients without complications with small infarctions and normal exercise tests. While a variety of beta-blockers have been shown to be beneficial, for patients with LV dysfunction managed with contemporary treatment, carvedilol titrated to 25 mg orally twice a day has been shown to reduce mortality. Beta-blockers with intrinsic sympathomimetic activity have not proved beneficial in postinfarction patients.

Antiplatelet agents are beneficial; aspirin (81–325 mg daily, with 81 mg daily the preferred long-term dose) is recommended, and adding clopidogrel (75 mg daily) has been shown to provide additional short-term benefit after STEMI. Prasugrel provides further reduction in thrombotic outcomes compared with clopidogrel, at the cost of more bleeding. Likewise, ticagrelor provides benefit over clopidogrel but should be used with low-dose aspirin (81 mg/day). Warfarin anticoagulation for 3 months reduces the incidence of arterial emboli after large anterior infarctions and, according to the results of at least one study, it improves long-term prognosis; however, these studies were done before the routine use of aspirin and clopidogrel. An advantage to combining low-dose aspirin and warfarin has not been demonstrated, except perhaps in patients with atrial fibrillation.

Calcium channel blockers have not been shown to improve prognoses overall and should not be prescribed purely for secondary prevention. Antiarrhythmic therapy other than with beta-blockers has not been shown to be effective except in patients with symptomatic arrhythmias. Amiodarone has been studied in several trials of postinfarct patients with either LV dysfunction or frequent ventricular ectopy. Although survival was not improved, amiodarone was not harmful—unlike other agents in this setting. Therefore, it is the agent of choice for individuals with symptomatic postinfarction supraventricular arrhythmias. While implantable defibrillators improve survival for patients with postinfarction LV dysfunction and heart failure, the DINAMIT trial found no benefit to implantable defibrillators implanted in the 40 days following acute myocardial infarction.

Cardiac rehabilitation programs and exercise training can be of considerable psychological benefit and appear to improve prognosis.

C. ACE Inhibitors and ARBs in Patients with LV Dysfunction

Patients who sustain substantial myocardial damage often experience subsequent progressive LV dilation and dysfunction, leading to clinical heart failure and reduced long-term survival. **In patients with EFs less than 40%, long-term ACE inhibitor (or ARB) therapy prevents LV dilation and the onset of heart failure and prolongs survival.** The HOPE trial, as well as an overview of trials of ACE inhibitors for secondary prevention, also demonstrated a reduction of approximately 20% in mortality rates and the occurrence of nonfatal myocardial infarction and stroke with ramipril treatment of patients with coronary or peripheral vascular disease and without confirmed LV systolic dysfunction. Therefore, ACE inhibitor therapy should be strongly considered in this broader group of patients—and especially in patients with diabetes and those with even mild systolic hypertension, in whom the greatest benefit was observed (see Table 11–7).

D. Revascularization

Postinfarction patients not treated with primary PCI who appear likely to benefit from early revascularization with CABG if the anatomy is appropriate are (1) those who have undergone fibrinolytic therapy, especially if they have high-risk features (including systolic BP of less than 100 mm Hg, heart rate of greater than 100 bpm, Killip class II or III, and ST-segment depression of 2 mm or more in the anterior leads); (2) patients with LV dysfunction (EF less than 30–40%); (3) patients with NSTEMI and high-risk features; and (4) patients with markedly positive exercise tests and multi-vessel disease. The value of revascularization in patients not treated with acute reperfusion therapy with preserved LV function who have mild ischemia and are not symptom limited is less clear. In general, patients without high-risk features who survive infarctions without complications, have preserved LV function (EF greater than 50%), and have no exercise-induced ischemia have an excellent prognosis and do not require invasive evaluation.

Smaller randomized trials have demonstrated that patients with noninfarct-related artery disease may benefit from revascularization strategies at the time of acute myocardial infarction care.

O'Gara PT et al. 2013 ACCF/AHA guideline for the management of ST-elevation myocardial infarction: a report of the American College of Cardiology Foundation/American Heart Association Task Force on Practice Guidelines. Circulation. 2013 Jan 29;127(4):e362–425. Erratum in: Circulation. 2013 Dec 24;128(25):e481. [PMID: 23247304]

Wald DS et al; PRAMI Investigators. Randomized trial of preventive angioplasty in myocardial infarction. N Engl J Med. 2013 Sep 19;369(12):1115–23. [PMID: 23991625]

DISORDERS OF RATE & RHYTHM

Abnormalities of cardiac rhythm and conduction can be symptomatic (syncope, near syncope, dizziness, fatigue, or palpitations), or asymptomatic. In addition, they can be lethal (sudden cardiac death) or dangerous to the extent that they reduce cardiac output, so that perfusion of the brain and myocardium is impaired. Stable supraventricular tachycardia is generally well tolerated in patients without underlying heart disease but may lead to myocardial ischemia or heart failure in patients with coronary disease, valvular abnormalities, and systolic or diastolic myocardial dysfunction. Ventricular tachycardia, if prolonged (lasting more than 10–30 seconds), often results in hemodynamic compromise and may deteriorate into ventricular fibrillation if left untreated.

Whether slow heart rates produce symptoms at rest or with exertion depends on whether cerebral and peripheral perfusion can be maintained, which is generally a function of whether the patient is upright or supine and whether LV function is adequate to maintain stroke volume. If the heart rate abruptly slows, as with the onset of complete heart block or sinus arrest, syncope or convulsions (or both) may result.

Arrhythmias are detected either because they produce symptoms or because they are detected during monitoring. Arrhythmias causing sudden death, syncope, or near syncope require further evaluation and treatment unless they are related to conditions that are reversible or immediately treatable (eg, electrolyte abnormalities or acute myocardial infarction). In contrast, there is controversy over when and how to evaluate and treat rhythm disturbances that are not symptomatic but are possible markers for more serious abnormalities (eg, nonsustained ventricular tachycardia [NSVT]). This uncertainty reflects two issues: (1) the difficulty of reliably stratifying patients into high-risk and low-risk groups; and (2) the lack of treatments that are both effective and safe. Thus, screening patients for these so-called "premonitory" abnormalities is often not productive.

A number of procedures are used to evaluate patients with symptoms who are believed to be at risk for life-threatening arrhythmias, including in-hospital and ambulatory ECG monitoring, event recorders (instruments that can be used for prolonged periods to record or transmit rhythm tracings when infrequent episodes occur), exercise testing, catheter-based electrophysiologic studies (to assess sinus node function, AV conduction, and inducibility of arrhythmias), and tests of autonomic nervous system function (tilt-table testing).

Treatment of arrhythmias varies and can include modalities such as antiarrhythmic medications and more invasive techniques such as catheter ablation.

▶ Antiarrhythmic Medications (Table 10–13)

Antiarrhythmic medications are frequently used to treat arrhythmias, but have variable efficacy and produce frequent side effects. They are often divided into classes based on their electropharmacologic actions and many of these medications have multiple actions. The most frequently used classification scheme is the Vaughan-Williams, which consists of four classes.

Class I agents block membrane sodium channels. Three subclasses are further defined by the effect of the agents on the Purkinje fiber action potential. Class Ia medications (ie, quinidine, procainamide, disopyramide) slow the rate of rise of the action potential (V_{max}) and prolong its duration, thus slowing conduction and increasing refractoriness (moderate depression of phase 0 upstroke of the action potential). Class Ib agents (ie, lidocaine, mexiletine) shorten action potential duration; they do not affect conduction or refractoriness (minimal depression of phase 0 upstroke of the action potential). Class Ic agents (ie, flecainide, propafenone) prolong V_{max} and slow repolarization, thus slowing conduction and prolonging refractoriness, but more so than class Ia drugs (maximal depression of phase 0 upstroke of the action potential).

Class II agents are the beta-blockers, which decrease automaticity, prolong AV conduction, and prolong refractoriness.

Class III agents (ie, amiodarone, dronedarone, sotalol, dofetilide, ibutilide) block potassium channels and prolong repolarization, widening the QRS and prolonging the QT interval. They decrease automaticity and conduction and prolong refractoriness. Dronedarone has been shown to reduce cardiovascular hospitalizations when used in patients with paroxysmal atrial fibrillation in the absence of heart failure; however, the PALLAS trial found an *increase* in cardiovascular events when dronedarone was used in patients with permanent atrial fibrillation.

Class IV agents are the calcium channel blockers, which decrease automaticity and AV conduction.

There are some antiarrhythmic agents that do not fall into one of these categories. The most frequently used are digoxin and adenosine. Digoxin inhibits the Na+, K+-ATPase pump. Digoxin prolongs AV nodal conduction and the AV nodal refractory period, but it shortens the action potential and decreases the refractoriness of the ventricular myocardium and Purkinje fibers. Adenosine can block AV nodal conduction and shortens atrial refractoriness.

Although the in vitro electrophysiologic effects of most of these agents have been defined, their use remains largely empiric. **All can exacerbate arrhythmias (proarrhythmic effect), and many depress LV function.**

Table 10–13. Antiarrhythmic medications.

Agent	Intravenous Dosage	Oral Dosage	Therapeutic Plasma Level	Route of Elimination	Side Effects
Class Ia: Action: Sodium channel blockers: Depress phase 0 depolarization; slow conduction; prolong repolarization.					
Indications: Supraventricular tachycardia, ventricular tachycardia, prevention of ventricular fibrillation, symptomatic ventricular premature beats.					
Quinidine	6–10 mg/kg (intramuscularly or intravenously) over 20 min (rarely used parenterally)	200–400 mg every 4–6 h or every 8 h (long-acting)	2–5 mg/mL	Hepatic	GI, ↓ LVF, ↑ Dig
Procainamide	100 mg/1–3 min to 500–1000 mg; maintain at 2–6 mg/min	50 mg/kg/d in divided doses every 3–4 h or every 6 h (long-acting)	4–10 mg/mL; NAPA (active metabolite), 10–20 mcg/mL	Renal	SLE, hypersensitivity, ↓ LVF
Disopyramide		100–200 mg every 6–8 h	2–8 mg/mL	Renal	Urinary retention, dry mouth, markedly ↓ LVF
Class Ib: Action: Shorten repolarization.					
Indications: Ventricular tachycardia, prevention of ventricular fibrillation, symptomatic ventricular beats.					
Lidocaine	1–2 mg/kg at 50 mg/min; maintain at 1–4 mg/min		1–5 mg/mL	Hepatic	CNS, GI
Mexiletine		100–300 mg every 6–12 h; maximum: 1200 mg/day	0.5–2 mg/mL	Hepatic	CNS, GI, leukopenia
Class Ic: Action: Depress phase 0 repolarization; slow conduction. (Propafenone is a weak calcium channel blocker and beta-blocker and prolongs action potential and refractoriness.)					
Indications: Life-threatening ventricular tachycardia or fibrillation, refractory supraventricular tachycardia.					
Flecainide		50–150 mg twice daily	0.2–1 mg/mL	Hepatic	CNS, GI, AFL with 1:1 conduction, ventricular pro-arrhythmia
Propafenone		150–300 mg every 8–12 h	**Note:** Active metabolites	Hepatic	CNS, GI, AFL with 1:1 conduction, ventricular pro-arrhythmia
Class II: Action: Beta-blocker, slows AV conduction.					
Indications: Supraventricular tachycardia; may prevent ventricular fibrillation.					
Esmolol	500 mcg/kg over 1–2 min; maintain at 25–200 mcg/kg/min	Other beta-blockers may be used concomitantly	Not established	Hepatic	↓ LVF, bronchospasm
Propranolol	1–5 mg at 1 mg/min	40–320 mg in 1–4 doses daily (depending on preparation)	Not established	Hepatic	↓ LVF, bradycardia, AV block, bronchospasm
Metoprolol	2.5–5 mg	50–200 mg daily	Not established	Hepatic	↓ LVF, bradycardia, AV block
Class III: Action: Prolong action potential.					
Indications: *Amiodarone:* refractory ventricular tachycardia, supraventricular tachycardia, prevention of ventricular tachycardia, atrial fibrillation, ventricular fibrillation; *Dofetilide:* atrial fibrillation and flutter; *Sotalol:* ventricular tachycardia, atrial fibrillation; *Ibutilide:* conversion of atrial fibrillation and flutter.					
Amiodarone	150–300 mg infused rapidly, followed by 1-mg/min infusion for 6 h (360 mg) and then 0.5 mg/min	800–1600 mg/day for 7–21 days; maintain at 100–400 mg/day (higher doses may be needed)	1–5 mg/mL	Hepatic	Pulmonary fibrosis, hypothyroidism, hyperthyroidism, photosensitivity, corneal and skin deposits, hepatitis, ↑ Dig, neurotoxicity, GI

(continued)

Table 10–13. Antiarrhythmic medications. (continued)

Agent	Intravenous Dosage	Oral Dosage	Therapeutic Plasma Level	Route of Elimination	Side Effects
Dronedarone		400 mg twice daily		Hepatic (contraindicated in severe impairment)	QTc prolongation, HF. Contraindicated in HF (NYHA class IV and class II and III if recent decompensation)
Sotalol		80–160 mg every 12 h (higher doses may be used for life-threatening arrhythmias)		Renal (dosing interval should be extended if creatinine clearance is < 60 mL/min)	Early incidence of torsades de pointes, LVF, bradycardia, fatigue (and other side effects associated with beta-blockers)
Dofetilide		125–500 mcg every 12 h		Renal (dose must be reduced with kidney dysfunction)	Torsades de pointes in 3%; interaction with cytochrome P-450 inhibitors
Ibutilide	1 mg over 10 min, followed by a second infusion of 0.5–1 mg over 10 min			Hepatic and renal	Torsades de pointes in up to 5% of patients within 3 h after administration; patients must be monitored with defibrillator nearby
Class IV: Action: Slow calcium channel blockers.					
Indications: Supraventricular tachycardia.					
Verapamil	2.5 mg bolus followed by additional boluses of 2.5–5 mg every 1–3 min; total 20 mg over 20 min; maintain at 5 mg/kg/min	80–120 mg every 6–8 h; 240–360 mg once daily with sustained-release preparation	0.1–0.15 mg/mL	Hepatic	↓ LVF, constipation, ↑ Dig, hypotension
Diltiazem	0.25 mg/kg over 2 min; second 0.35-mg/kg bolus after 15 min if response is inadequate; infusion rate, 5–15 mg/h	180–360 mg daily in 1–3 doses depending on preparation (oral forms not approved for arrhythmias)		Hepatic metabolism, renal excretion	Hypotension, ↓ LVF
Miscellaneous: Indications: Supraventricular tachycardia.					
Adenosine	6 mg rapidly followed by 12 mg after 1–2 min if needed; use half these doses if administered via central line			Adenosine receptor stimulation, metabolized in blood	Transient flushing, dyspnea, chest pain, AV block, sinus bradycardia; effect ↓ by theophylline, ↑ by dipyridamole
Digoxin	0.5 mg over 20 min followed by increment of 0.25 or 0.125 mg to 1–1.5 mg over 24 h	1–1.5 mg over 24–36 h in 3 or 4 doses; maintenance, 0.125–0.5 mg/day	0.7–2 mg/mL	Renal	AV block, arrhythmias, GI, visual changes

AFL, atrial flutter; AV, atrioventricular; CNS, central nervous system; Dig, elevation of serum digoxin level; GI, gastrointestinal (nausea, vomiting, diarrhea); HF, heart failure; ↓LVF, reduced left ventricular function; NAPA, N-acetylprocainamide; NYHA, New York Heart Association; SLE, systemic lupus erythematosus; VT, ventricular tachycardia.

The risk of antiarrhythmic agents has been highlighted by many studies, most notably the Coronary Arrhythmia Suppression Trial (CAST), in which two class Ic agents (flecainide, encainide) and a class Ia agent (moricizine) increased mortality rates in patients with asymptomatic ventricular ectopy after myocardial infarction. A similar result has been reported in the Mortality in the Survival With Oral D-sotalol (SWORD) study with d-sotalol, a class III agent without the beta-blocking activity of the currently marketed formulation d,l-sotalol. Class 1c antiarrhythmic agents should therefore not be used in patients with prior myocardial infarction or structural heart disease.

The use of antiarrhythmic agents for specific arrhythmias is discussed below.

▶ Catheter Ablation for Cardiac Arrhythmias

Catheter ablation has become the primary modality of therapy for many symptomatic supraventricular arrhythmias, including AV nodal reentrant tachycardia, tachycardias involving accessory pathways, paroxysmal atrial tachycardia, and atrial flutter. Catheter ablation of atrial fibrillation is more complex and usually involves complete electrical isolation of the pulmonary veins (which are often the sites of initiation of atrial fibrillation) or placing linear lesions within the atria to prevent propagation throughout the atrial chamber. This technique is considered a reasonable second-line therapy (after pharmacologic treatment) for certain patients with symptomatic medication-refractory atrial fibrillation. Catheter ablation of ventricular arrhythmias has proved more difficult, but experienced centers have demonstrated reasonable success with all types of ventricular tachycardias including bundle-branch reentry, tachycardia originating in the ventricular outflow tract or papillary muscles, tachycardias originating in the specialized conduction system (fascicular ventricular tachycardia), and ventricular tachycardias occurring in patients with ischemic or dilated cardiomyopathy. Ablation of many of these arrhythmias can be performed from the endocardial surface via endovascular catheter placement or on the epicardial surface of the heart via a percutaneous subxiphoid approach.

Catheter ablation has also been successfully performed for the treatment of ventricular fibrillation when a uniform premature ventricular contraction (PVC) can be identified. In addition, patients with symptomatic PVCs or PVCs occurring at a high enough burden to result in a cardiomyopathy (usually more than 10,000/day) are often referred for catheter ablation as well.

Catheter ablation procedures are generally safe, with an overall major complication rate ranging from 1% to 5%. Major vascular damage during catheter insertion occurs in less than 2% of patients. There is a low incidence of perforation of the myocardial wall resulting in pericardial tamponade. Sufficient damage to the AV node to require permanent cardiac pacing occurs in less than 1% of patients. When transseptal access through the interatrial septum or retrograde LV catheterization is required, additional potential complications include damage to the heart valves, damage to a coronary artery, or systemic emboli. A rare but potentially fatal complication after catheter ablation of atrial fibrillation is the development of an atrio-esophageal fistula resulting from ablation on the posterior wall of the LA just overlying the esophagus, estimated to occur in less than 0.1% of procedures.

Deshmukh A et al. In-hospital complications associated with catheter ablation of atrial fibrillation in the United States between 2000 and 2010: analysis of 93 801 procedures. Circulation. 2013 Nov 5;128(19):2104–12. [PMID: 24061087]
January CT et al. 2014 AHA/ACC/HRS guideline for the management of patients with atrial fibrillation: a report of the American College of Cardiology/American Heart Association Task Force on Practice Guidelines and the Heart Rhythm Society. J Am Coll Cardiol. 2014 Dec 2;64(21):e1–76. [PMID: 24685669]

SINUS ARRHYTHMIA, BRADYCARDIA, & TACHYCARDIA

Sinus arrhythmia is a cyclic increase in normal heart rate with inspiration and decrease with expiration. It results from reflex changes in vagal influence on the normal pacemaker and disappears with breath holding or increase of heart rate. It is common in both the young and the elderly and is not a pathologic arrhythmia.

Sinus bradycardia is a heart rate slower than 60 beats/min due to increased vagal influence on the normal pacemaker or organic disease of the sinus node. The rate usually increases during exercise or administration of atropine. In healthy individuals, and especially in patients who are in excellent physical condition, sinus bradycardia to rates of 50 beats/min or even lower is a normal finding. However, severe sinus bradycardia (less than 45 beats/min) may be an indication of sinus node pathology, especially in elderly patients and individuals with heart disease. It may cause weakness, confusion, or syncope if cerebral perfusion is impaired. Atrial, junctional and ventricular ectopic rhythms are more apt to occur with slow sinus rates. Pacing may be required if symptoms correlate with the bradycardia.

Sinus tachycardia is defined as a heart rate faster than 100 beats/min that is caused by rapid impulse formation from the sinoatrial node; it occurs with fever, exercise, emotion, pain, anemia, heart failure, shock, thyrotoxicosis, or in response to many medications. Alcohol and alcohol withdrawal are common causes of sinus tachycardia and other supraventricular arrhythmias. The onset and termination are usually gradual, in contrast to paroxysmal supraventricular tachycardia due to reentry. The rate infrequently exceeds 160 beats/min but may reach 180 beats/min in young persons. The rhythm is generally regular, but serial 1-minute counts of the heart rate indicate that it varies five or more beats per minute with changes in position, with breath holding, or with sedation. In rare instances, otherwise healthy individuals may present with "inappropriate" sinus tachycardia where persistently elevated basal heart rates are not in-line with physiologic demands. Long-term consequences of this disorder are few. While the exact mechanism underlying "inappropriate" sinus tachycardia is unclear, pharmacologic agents, such as beta-blockers or ivabradine (which selectively blocks the I_f current within the sinus node), have been shown to have varying success in improving symptoms. Catheter ablation aimed at modifying the sinus node to lower mean heart rate has been reported; however, recurrence rates are high.

When to Refer

Patients with symptoms related to bradycardia or tachycardia when reversible etiologies have been excluded.

When to Admit

Patients with bradycardia and recent or recurrent syncope.

ATRIAL PREMATURE BEATS
(Atrial Extrasystoles)

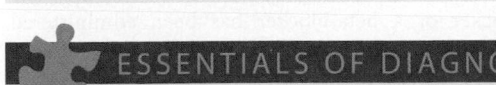

ESSENTIALS OF DIAGNOSIS

- ► Usually asymptomatic.
- ► Isolated interruption in regular rhythm.
- ► P-wave morphology on ECG usually differs from sinus P-wave morphology.
- ► Can be harbinger of future development of atrial fibrillation.

Atrial premature beats occur when an ectopic focus in the atria fires before the next sinus node impulse. The contour of the P wave usually differs from the patient's normal complex, unless the ectopic focus is near the sinus node. Such premature beats occur frequently in normal hearts. Acceleration of the heart rate by any means usually abolishes most premature beats. Treatment of this arrhythmia is rarely indicated. Early atrial premature beats may cause aberrant QRS complexes (left or right bundle branch block) or may not be conducted to the ventricles because the AV node or ventricles are still refractory.

Making the distinction between aberrantly conducted supraventricular beats and ventricular beats can be very difficult in patients with a wide QRS complex; it is important because of the differing prognostic and therapeutic implications of each type. Findings favoring a ventricular origin include (1) AV dissociation; (2) a QRS duration exceeding 0.14 second; (3) capture or fusion beats (infrequent); (4) left axis deviation with right bundle branch block morphology; (5) monophasic (R) or biphasic (qR, QR, or RS) complexes in V_1; and (6) a qR or QS complex in V_6. Supraventricular origin is favored by (1) a triphasic QRS complex, especially with initial negativity in leads I and V_6; (2) ventricular rates exceeding 170 beats/min; (3) QRS duration longer than 0.12 second but not longer than 0.14 second; and (4) the presence of preexcitation syndrome.

The relationship of the P waves to the tachycardia complex is helpful. A 1:1 relationship usually means a supraventricular origin, except in the case of ventricular tachycardia with retrograde atrial activation.

PAROXYSMAL SUPRAVENTRICULAR TACHYCARDIA

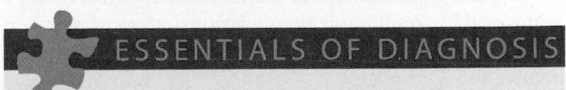

ESSENTIALS OF DIAGNOSIS

- ► Frequently associated with palpitations.
- ► Abrupt onset/offset.
- ► Rapid, regular rhythm.
- ► Most commonly seen in young adults.
- ► Rarely causes syncope.
- ► Usually have a narrow QRS complex on ECG.
- ► Often responsive to vagal maneuvers, AV nodal blockers, or adenosine.

General Considerations

This is a common paroxysmal tachycardia and often occurs in patients without structural heart disease. The most common mechanism for paroxysmal supraventricular tachycardia is **reentry**, which may be initiated or terminated by a fortuitously timed atrial or ventricular premature beat. The reentrant circuit most commonly involves dual pathways (a slow and a fast pathway) within the AV node. This is referred to as AV nodal reentrant tachycardia (AVNRT). Less commonly, reentry is due to an accessory pathway between the atria and ventricles, referred to as atrioventricular reciprocating tachycardia (AVRT). Approximately one-third of patients with supraventricular tachycardia have accessory pathways to the ventricles. The pathophysiology and management of arrhythmias due to accessory pathways differ in important ways and are discussed separately below.

Clinical Findings

A. Symptoms and Signs

Patients may be asymptomatic except for awareness of rapid heart action, but some experience mild chest pain, shortness of breath, diaphoresis or faintness especially when episodes are prolonged, even in the absence of associated cardiac abnormalities. Episodes begin and end abruptly and may last a few seconds to several hours or longer.

B. ECG

The heart rate may be 140–280 beats/min (usually 160–220 beats/min) and is regular (despite exercise or change in position). The P wave usually differs in contour from sinus beats and is often simultaneous with the QRS complex.

Treatment

In the absence of structural heart disease, serious effects are rare, and most episodes resolve spontaneously. Particular effort should be made to terminate the episode quickly if cardiac failure, syncope, or anginal pain develops or if there is underlying cardiac or (particularly) coronary disease. Because reentry is the most common mechanism for paroxysmal supraventricular tachycardia, effective therapy requires that conduction be interrupted at some point in the reentry circuit and the vast majority of these circuits involve the AV node.

A. Mechanical Measures

A variety of maneuvers have been used to interrupt episodes, and patients may learn to perform these themselves. These maneuvers result in an acute increase in vagal tone and include the Valsalva maneuver, lowering the head between the knees, coughing, splashing cold water on the face, and breath holding. The **Valsalva maneuver** is performed with the patient semirecumbent (45 degrees), exerting around 40 mm Hg of intrathoracic pressure (by blowing through a 10 mL syringe) for at least 15 seconds. Moving the patient supine immediately following the strain maneuver and passively raising their legs for an additional 15 seconds may increase effectiveness of the maneuver. **Carotid sinus massage** is an additional technique often performed by physicians but should be avoided if the patient has carotid bruits or a history of transient cerebral ischemic attacks. Firm but gentle pressure and massage are applied first over the right carotid sinus for 10–20 seconds and, if unsuccessful, then over the left carotid sinus. Pressure should not be exerted on both sides at the same time. **Facial contact with cold water** may cause transient bradycardia and termination of sustained ventricular tachycardia, a phenomenon known as the diving reflex. When performed properly, these maneuvers result in abrupt termination of the arrhythmia in 20–50% of cases.

B. Medication Therapy

If mechanical measures fail to terminate the arrhythmia, pharmacologic agents should be tried. Intravenous **adenosine is recommended as the first-line agent due to its** brief duration of action and minimal negative inotropic activity (Table 10–13). Because the half-life of adenosine is less than 10 seconds, the medication is given rapidly (in 1–2 seconds) as a 6 mg bolus followed by 20 mL of fluid. If this regimen is unsuccessful at terminating the arrhythmia, a second higher dose (12 mg) may be given. Adenosine causes block of electrical conduction through the AV node and results in termination of SVT in approximately 90% of cases. Minor side effects are common and include transient flushing, chest discomfort, nausea, and headache. Adenosine may excite both atrial and ventricular tissue causing atrial fibrillation (in up to 12% of patients) or rarely ventricular arrhythmias and therefore administration should be performed with continuous cardiac monitoring and availability of an external defibrillator. Adenosine must also be used with caution in patients with reactive airways disease because it can promote bronchospasm.

When adenosine fails to terminate the arrhythmia or if a contraindication to its use is present, intravenous calcium channel blockers, including **verapamil** and **diltiazem,** may be used (Table 10–13). Verapamil in particular has been shown to be as effective at terminating SVT in the acute setting (approximately 90%) as adenosine. Calcium channel blockers should be used with caution in patients with heart failure due to their negative inotropic effects. Their longer half-life compared to adenosine may result in prolonged hypotension despite restoration of normal rhythm.

Intravenous beta-blockers include **esmolol** (a very short-acting beta-blocker), propranolol, and metoprolol. All may be effective for virtually any type of supraventricular tachycardia and cause less myocardial depression than the calcium channel blockers. If the tachycardia is believed to be mediated by an accessory pathway, intravenous **procainamide** may terminate the tachycardia by prolonging refractoriness in the accessory pathway; however, because it facilitates AV conduction and an initial increase in rate may occur, it is usually not given until after a calcium channel blocker or a beta-blocker has been administered. Although intravenous amiodarone is safe, it is usually not required and often ineffective for treatment of these arrhythmias.

C. Cardioversion

If the patient is hemodynamically unstable or if adenosine, beta-blockers, and calcium channel blockers are contraindicated or ineffective, synchronized electrical cardioversion (beginning at 100 J) should be performed.

▶ Prevention

A. Catheter Ablation

Because of concerns about the safety and the intolerability of antiarrhythmic medications, radiofrequency ablation is the preferred approach to patients with recurrent symptomatic reentrant supraventricular tachycardia, whether it is due to dual pathways within the AV node or to accessory pathways.

B. Medications

AV nodal blocking agents are the medications of choice as first-line medical therapy (Table 10–13). Beta-blockers or non-dihydropyridine calcium channel blockers, such as diltiazem and verapamil, are typically used first. Patients who do not respond to agents that increase refractoriness of the AV node may be treated with antiarrhythmics. The class Ic agents (flecainide, propafenone) can be used in patients without underlying structural heart disease. In patients with evidence of structural heart disease, class III agents, such as sotalol or amiodarone, should be used because of the lower incidence of ventricular proarrhythmia during long-term therapy.

Appelboam A et al. Postural modification to the standard Valsalva manoeuvre for emergency treatment of supraventricular tachycardias (REVERT): a randomised controlled trial. Lancet. 2015 Oct 31;386(10005):1747–53. [PMID: 26314489]

Link MS. Clinical practice. Evaluation and initial treatment of supraventricular tachycardia. N Engl J Med. 2012 Oct 11; 367(15): 1438–48. [PMID: 23050527]

Smith GD et al. Effectiveness of the Valsalva Manoeuvre for reversion of supraventricular tachycardia. Cochrane Database Syst Rev. 2013 Mar 28;3:CD009502. [PMID: 23543578]

SUPRAVENTRICULAR TACHYCARDIAS DUE TO ACCESSORY AV PATHWAYS (Preexcitation Syndromes)

ESSENTIALS OF DIAGNOSIS

- ▶ Frequently associated with palpitations.
- ▶ Can be associated with syncope.
- ▶ Rapid, regular rhythm.
- ▶ May have narrow or wide QRS complex on ECG.
- ▶ Often have preexcitation (delta wave) on baseline ECG.

General Considerations

Accessory pathways or bypass tracts between the atrium and the ventricle bypass the compact AV node and can predispose to reentrant arrhythmias, such as AV reciprocating tachycardia (AVRT) and atrial fibrillation. These may be wholly or partly within the node (eg, Mahaim fibers), yielding a short PR interval and normal QRS morphology. More commonly, they make direct connections between the atrium and ventricle through Kent bundles (**Wolff-Parkinson-White syndrome**). This often produces a short PR interval with a delta wave (preexcitation) at the onset of the wide, slurred QRS complex owing to early ventricular depolarization of the region adjacent to the pathway. Although the morphology and polarity of the delta wave can suggest the location of the pathway, mapping by intracardiac recordings is required for precise anatomic localization.

Accessory pathways occur in 0.1–0.3% of the population and facilitate reentrant arrhythmias owing to the disparity in refractory periods of the AV node and accessory pathway. Whether the tachycardia is associated with a narrow or wide QRS complex is frequently determined by whether antegrade conduction is through the node (narrow) or the bypass tract (wide). Some bypass tracts only conduct in a retrograde direction. In these cases, the bypass tract is termed "concealed" because it is not readily apparent on a baseline (sinus) ECG. **Orthodromic** reentrant tachycardia is a reentrant rhythm that conducts antegrade down the AV node and retrograde up the accessory pathway, resulting in a narrow QRS complex unless an underlying bundle branch block or interventricular conduction delay is present. **Antidromic** reentrant tachycardia conducts antegrade down the accessory pathway and retrograde through the AV node, resulting in a wide and often bizarre appearing QRS complex which may be mistaken for ventricular tachycardia. Accessory pathways often have shorter refractory periods than specialized conduction tissue and thus tachycardias involving accessory pathways have the potential to be more rapid. Up to 30% of patients with Wolff-Parkinson-White syndrome will develop atrial fibrillation or flutter with antegrade conduction down the accessory pathway and a rapid ventricular response. If this conduction is very rapid, it can potentially degenerate to ventricular fibrillation.

▶ Clinical Findings & Treatment

Some patients have a delta wave found incidentally on ECG (Wolff-Parkinson-White pattern). Even in the absence of palpitations, light-headedness, or syncope, these patients are at higher risk for sudden cardiac death than the general population. Risk factors include younger than age 30, male sex, history of atrial fibrillation and associated congenital heart disease. Multiple risk stratification strategies have been proposed to identify asymptomatic patients with Wolff-Parkinson-White pattern ECG who may be at higher risk for lethal cardiac arrhythmias. A sudden loss of preexcitation during exercise testing likely indicates an accessory pathway with poor conduction properties and therefore low risk for rapid anterograde conduction. In the absence of this finding or other signs of weak anterograde properties (intermittent preexcitation on resting ECG or Holter monitoring), patients may be referred for invasive electrophysiology testing. During the study, patients found to have the shortest preexcited R-R interval (SPERRI) during atrial fibrillation of 250 msec or less or inducible supraventricular tachycardia are at increased risk for sudden cardiac death and should undergo catheter ablation.

A. Catheter Ablation

As with AVNRT, radiofrequency catheter ablation has become the procedure of choice in patients with accessory pathways and recurrent symptoms or asymptomatic patients with Wolff-Parkinson-White pattern ECG and high risk features at baseline or during electrophysiology study. Success rates for ablation of accessory pathways with radiofrequency catheters exceed 95% in appropriate patients. Major complications from catheter ablation are rare but include AV block, cardiac tamponade, and thromboembolic events. Minor complications, including hematoma at the catheter access site, occur in 1–2% of procedures.

B. Pharmacologic Therapy

Narrow-complex reentrant rhythms involving a bypass tract can be managed as discussed for AVNRT. Atrial fibrillation with a concomitant antegrade conducting bypass tract presents as an irregular, wide-complex arrhythmia and must be managed differently. Agents such as calcium channel blockers and beta-blockers may increase the refractoriness of the AV node with minimal or no effect on the accessory pathway, often leading to faster ventricular rates and increasing the risk of ventricular fibrillation. Therefore, these agents should be avoided. Intravenous class Ia (procainamide) and class III (amiodarone) antiarrhythmic agents will increase the refractoriness of the bypass tract and are the medications of choice for wide-complex tachycardias involving accessory pathways. If hemodynamic compromise is present, electrical cardioversion is warranted.

Long-term therapy often involves a combination of agents that increase refractoriness in the bypass tract (class Ia or Ic agents) and in the AV node (calcium channel blockers and beta-blockers), provided that atrial fibrillation or flutter with short RR cycle lengths is not present. The class III agent, amiodarone, can be effective in refractory cases. Patients who are difficult to manage should undergo expert consultation with a cardiac electrophysiologist.

▶ When to Refer

- Patients with an incidental finding of Wolff-Parkinson-White pattern on ECG without evidence of loss of pre-excitation spontaneously or during exercise testing.
- Patients with recurrent symptoms or episodes despite treatment with AV nodal blocking agents.
- Patients with preexcitation and a history of atrial fibrillation.

▶ When to Admit

- Patients with paroxysmal supraventricular tachycardia and syncope.
- Patients with a history of syncope and preexcitation identified on an ECG.

Cohen MI et al. PACES/HRS expert consensus statement on the management of the asymptomatic young patient with a Wolff-Parkinson-White (WPW, ventricular preexcitation) electro-cardiographic pattern: developed in partnership between the Pediatric and Congenital Electrophysiology Society (PACES) and the Heart Rhythm Society (HRS). Endorsed by the governing bodies of PACES, HRS, the American College of Cardiology Foundation (ACCF), the American Heart Association (AHA), the American Academy of Pediatrics (AAP), and the Canadian Heart Rhythm Society (CHRS). Heart Rhythm. 2012 Jun;9(6):1006–24. [PMID: 22579340]
Czosek RJ et al. Cost-effectiveness of various risk stratification methods for asymptomatic ventricular pre-excitation. Am J Cardiol. 2013 Jul 15;112(2):245–50. [PMID: 23587276]
Obeyesekere MN et al. Risk of arrhythmia and sudden death in patients with asymptomatic preexcitation: a meta-analysis. Circulation. 2012 May 15;125(19):2308–15. [PMID: 22532593]

ATRIAL FIBRILLATION

ESSENTIALS OF DIAGNOSIS

- ▶ Irregularly irregular heart rhythm.
- ▶ Usually tachycardic.
- ▶ Often associated with palpitations (acute onset) or fatigue (chronic).
- ▶ ECG shows erratic atrial activity with irregular ventricular response.
- ▶ High risk for thromboembolism: common cause of stroke.
- ▶ High incidence and prevalence in the elderly population.

▶ General Considerations

Atrial fibrillation is the most common chronic arrhythmia, with an incidence and prevalence that rise with age, so that it affects approximately 9% of individuals over age 65 years. It occurs in rheumatic and other forms of VHD, dilated cardiomyopathy, ASD, hypertension, and CHD as well as in patients with no apparent cardiac disease; it may be the initial presenting sign in thyrotoxicosis, and this condition should be excluded with the initial episode. The atrial activity may be very fine and difficult to detect on the ECG, or quite coarse and often mistaken for atrial flutter. Atrial fibrillation often appears in a paroxysmal fashion before becoming the established rhythm. Pericarditis, chest trauma, thoracic or cardiac surgery, thyroid disorders, obstructive sleep apnea, or pulmonary disease (pneumonia, pulmonary embolism) as well as medications such as theophylline and beta-adrenergic agonists may cause attacks in patients with normal hearts. Acute alcohol excess and alcohol withdrawal—and, in predisposed individuals, even consumption of small amounts of alcohol—may precipitate atrial fibrillation. This latter presentation, which is often termed "holiday heart," is usually transient and self-limited. Short-term rate control usually suffices as treatment.

Atrial fibrillation, particularly when the ventricular rate is uncontrolled, can lead to LV dysfunction, heart failure or myocardial ischemia (when underlying CAD is present). Perhaps the most serious consequence of atrial fibrillation is the propensity for thrombus formation due to stasis in the atria (particularly the left atrial appendage) and consequent embolization, most devastatingly to the cerebral circulation. Untreated, the rate of stroke is approximately 5% per year. However, patients with significant obstructive valvular disease, chronic heart failure or LV dysfunction, diabetes mellitus, hypertension, or age over 75 years and those with a history of prior stroke or other embolic events are at substantially higher risk (up to nearly 20% per year in patients with multiple risk factors) (Table 10–14). A substantial portion of the aging population with hypertension has asymptomatic or "subclinical" atrial fibrillation that is also associated with increased risk of stroke.

▶ Clinical Findings

A. Symptoms and Signs

Atrial fibrillation itself is rarely life-threatening; however, it can have serious consequences if the ventricular rate is sufficiently rapid to precipitate hypotension, myocardial ischemia, or tachycardia-induced myocardial dysfunction. Moreover, particularly in patients with risk factors, **atrial fibrillation is a major preventable cause of stroke**. Although many patients—particularly older or inactive individuals—have relatively few symptoms if the rate is controlled, some patients are aware of the irregular rhythm and may find it very uncomfortable. Most patients will complain of fatigue whether they experience other symptoms or not. The heart rate may range from quite slow to extremely rapid, but is uniformly irregular unless underlying complete heart block with junctional escape rhythm or a permanent ventricular pacemaker is in place. **Atrial**

Table 10–14. CHADS$_2$ Risk Score for assessing risk of stroke and for selecting antithrombotic therapy for patients with atrial fibrillation.

	Condition	Points
C	Congestive heart failure	1
H	Hypertension (current or treated)	1
A	Age ≥ 75 years	1
D	Diabetes mellitus	1
S$_2$	Stroke or transient ischemic attack	2
CHADS$_2$ Score	Adjusted Stroke Rate, %/year (95% Confidence Interval)	Patients[1] (n = 1733)
0	1.9 (1.2 to 3.0)	120
1	2.8 (2.0 to 3.8)	463
2	4.0 (3.1 to 5.1)	523
3	5.9 (4.6 to 7.3)	337
4	8.5 (6.3 to 11)	220
5	12.5 (8.2 to 17.5)	65

[1]Validation performed in a population of Medicare beneficiaries aged 65 to 95 years who were not prescribed warfarin at hospital discharge.
Reproduced, with permission, from Gage BF et al. Validation of clinical classification schemes for predicting stroke: results from the National Registry of Atrial Fibrillation. JAMA. 2001;285(22):2864–70. © 2001 American Medical Association. Al rights reserved.

fibrillation is the only common arrhythmia in which the ventricular rate is rapid and the rhythm very irregular. Because of the varying stroke volumes resulting from fluctuating periods of diastolic filling, not all ventricular beats produce a palpable peripheral pulse. The difference between the apical rate and the pulse rate is the "pulse deficit"; this deficit is greater when the ventricular rate is high.

B. ECG

The surface ECG typically demonstrates erratic, disorganized atrial activity between discrete QRS complexes occurring in an irregular pattern. The atrial activity may be very fine and difficult to detect on the ECG, or quite coarse and often mistaken for atrial flutter.

▶ Treatment

A. Newly Diagnosed Atrial Fibrillation

1. Initial management

A. Hemodynanmicaliy unstable patient—If the patient is hemodynamically unstable—usually as a result of a rapid ventricular rate or associated cardiac or noncardiac conditions—hospitalization and immediate treatment of atrial fibrillation are required. Intravenous beta-blockers (esmolol, propranolol, and metoprolol) or calcium channel blockers (diltiazem and verapamil) are usually effective at rate control in the acute setting. Urgent electrical cardioversion is only indicated in patients with shock or severe hypotension, pulmonary edema, or ongoing myocardial infarction

or ischemia. There is a potential risk of thromboembolism in patients undergoing cardioversion who have not received anticoagulation therapy if atrial fibrillation has been present for more than 48 hours or is of unknown duration; however, in hemodynamically unstable patients the need for immediate rate control outweighs that risk. An initial shock with 100–200 J is administered in synchrony with the R wave. If sinus rhythm is not restored, an additional attempt with 360 J is indicated. If this fails, cardioversion may be successful after loading with intravenous **ibutilide** (1 mg over 10 minutes, repeated in 10 minutes if necessary).

B. Hemodynamicaliy stable patient—If the patient has no symptoms, hemodynamic instability, or evidence of important precipitating conditions (such as silent myocardial infarction or ischemia, decompensated heart failure, pulmonary embolism, or hemodynamically significant valvular disease), hospitalization is usually not necessary. In most of these cases, atrial fibrillation is an unrecognized chronic or paroxysmal condition and should be managed accordingly (see Subsequent Management, below). For new onset atrial fibrillation, thyroid function tests and echocardiography to assesss for occult valvular or myocardial disease should be performed.

In stable patients with atrial fibrillation, a strategy of rate control and anticoagulation is appropriate. This is true whether the conditions that precipitated atrial fibrillation are likely to persist (such as following cardiac or noncardiac surgery, with respiratory failure, or with pericarditis) or might resolve spontaneously over a period of hours to days (such as atrial fibrillation due to excessive alcohol intake, electrolyte imbalance or atrial fibrillation due to exposure to excessive theophylline or sympathomimetic agents). The choice of agent is guided by the hemodynamic status of the patient, associated conditions, and the urgency of achieving rate control. In the stable patient with atrial fibrillation, a beta-blocker or calcium channel blocker (orally or intravenously) is usually the first-line agent for ventricular rate control. In the setting of myocardial infarction or ischemia, beta-blockers are the preferred agent. The most frequently used agents are either metoprolol (administered as a 5 mg intravenous bolus, repeated twice at intervals of 5 minutes and then given as needed by repeat boluses or orally at total daily doses of 50–400 mg) or, in unstable patients, esmolol (0.5 mg/kg intravenously, repeated once if necessary, followed by a titrated infusion of 0.05–0.2 mg/kg/min). If beta-blockers are contraindicated, calcium channel blockers are immediately effective. Diltiazem (20 mg bolus, repeated after 15 minutes if necessary, followed by a maintenance infusion of 5–15 mg/h) is the preferred calcium blocker if hypotension or LV dysfunction is present. Otherwise, verapamil (5–10 mg intravenously over 2–3 minutes, repeated after 30 minutes if necessary) may be used. Rate control using digoxin is slow (onset of action more than 1 hour with peak effect at 6 hours) and may be inadequate and is usually not indicated for use in the acute setting. Similarly, amiodarone, even when administered intravenously, has a relatively slow onset and is most useful as an adjunct when rate control with the previously cited agents is incomplete or contraindicated or when cardioversion is planned in the near future. Care should be taken in patients with hypotension or heart failure because the rapid intravenous administration of amiodarone may worsen hemodynamics.

If the onset of atrial fibrillation was more than 48 hours prior to presentation (or unknown) and early cardioversion is considered necessary due to inability to adequately rate control, a transesophageal echocardiogram should be performed prior to cardioversion to exclude left atrial thrombus. If thrombus is present, the cardioversion is delayed until after a 4-week period of therapeutic anticoagulation. In any case, because atrial contractile activity may not recover for several weeks after restoration of sinus rhythm in patients who have been in atrial fibrillation for more than several days, cardioversion should be followed by anticoagulation for at least 1 month unless there is a strong contraindication.

2. Subsequent management—Up to two-thirds of patients experiencing a first episode of atrial fibrillation will spontaneously revert to sinus rhythm within 24 hours. In the absence of VHD, diabetes, hypertension or other risk factors for stroke, these patients may not require long-term anticoagulation beyond aspirin. If atrial fibrillation persists or has been present for more than a week, spontaneous conversion is unlikely. In most cases immediate cardioversion is not required and management consists of rate control and anticoagulation whether or not the patient has been admitted to the hospital. Rate control is usually relatively easy to achieve with beta-blockers, rate-slowing calcium blockers and, occasionally, digoxin used in combination with other agents. In older patients, who often have diminished AV nodal function and relatively limited activity, modest rate control can often be achieved with a single agent. Many younger or more active individuals require a combination of two agents. Choice of the initial medication is best based on the presence of accompanying conditions: Hypertensive patients should be given beta-blockers or calcium blockers (see Tables 11–6 and 11–8); patients with CHD should receive a beta-blocker; and patients with heart failure should be given a beta-blocker with consideration of adding digoxin. Adequacy of rate control should be evaluated by recording the apical pulse rate both at rest and with an appropriate level of activity (such as after brisk walking around the corridor or climbing stairs).

A. Anticoagulation—For patients with atrial fibrillation, even when it is paroxysmal or occurs rarely, the need for oral anticoagulation should be evaluated and treatment initiated for those without strong contraindication. Patients with "**lone atrial fibrillation**" (eg, no evidence of associated heart disease, hypertension, atherosclerotic vascular disease, diabetes mellitus, or history of stroke or TIA) under age 65 years need no antithrombotic treatment. Patients with **transient atrial fibrillation**, such as in the setting of acute myocardial infarction or pneumonia, but no prior history of arrhythmia, are at high risk for future development of atrial fibrillation and appropriate anticoagulation should be initiated based on risk factors (Table 10–14). If the cause is **reversible**, such as after coronary artery bypass surgery or associated with hyperthyroidism, then long term anticoagulation is not necessary.

In addition to the traditional five risk factors that comprise the CHADS$_2$ score (heart failure, hypertension, age 75 years or older, diabetes mellitus, and [2 points for] history of stroke or transient ischemic attack), the European and American guidelines recommend that three additional factors included in the CHA$_2$DS$_2$-VASc score be considered: age 65–74 years, female sex, and presence of vascular disease (Table 10–15). The CHA$_2$DSv-VASc score is

Table 10–15. CHA$_2$DS$_2$-VASc Risk Score for assessing risk of stroke and for selecting antithrombotic therapy for patients with atrial fibrillation.

CHA$_2$DS$_2$-VASc Risk Score	
Heart failure or LVEF ≤ 40%	1
Hypertension	1
Age ≥ 75 years	2
Diabetes mellitus	1
Stroke, transient ischemic attack, or thromboembolism	2
Vascular disease (previous myocardial infarction, peripheral artery disease, or aortic plaque)	1
Age 65–74 years	1
Female sex (but not a risk factor if female sex is the only factor)	1
Maximum score	9

Adjusted stroke rate according to CHA$_2$DS$_2$-VASc score		
CHA$_2$DS$_2$-VASc Score	Patients (n = 7329)	Adjusted stroke rate (%/year)
0	1	0%
1	422	1.3%
2	1230	2.2%
3	1730	3.2%
4	1718	4.0%
5	1159	6.7%
6	679	9.8%
7	294	9.6%
8	82	6.7%
9	14	15.2%

CHA$_2$DS$_2$-VASc score = 0: recommend no antithrombotic therapy

CHA$_2$DS$_2$-VASc score = 1: recommend antithrombotic therapy with oral anticoagulation or antiplatelet therapy but preferably oral anticoagulation.

CHA$_2$DS$_2$-VASc score = 2: recommend oral anticoagulation

CHA$_2$DS$_2$-VASc, Cardiac failure, Hypertension, Age ≥ 75 years (doubled), Diabetes, Stroke (doubled), Vascular disease, Age 65–74, and Sex category (female); LVEF, left ventricular ejection fraction. Data from Camm AJ et al. 2012 focused update of the ESC Guidelines for the management of atrial fibrillation: an update of the 2010 ESC Guidelines for the management of atrial fibrillation. Developed with the special contribution of the European Heart Rhythm Association. Eur Heart J. 2012 Nov;33(21) 2719–47. [PMID: 22922413] especially relevant for patients who have a CHADS$_2$ score of 0 or 1; if the CHA$_2$DS$_2$-VASc score is greater than or equal to 2, oral anticoagulation is recommended, and if CHA$_2$DS$_2$-VASc score is 1, oral anticoagulation, aspirin, or no anticoagulation can be used, with a preference for oral anticoagulation, taking into account risk, benefit, and patient preferences. (The use of warfarin is discussed in the section on Selecting Appropriate Anticoagulant Therapy in Chapter 14.) Unfortunately, studies show that only about half of patients with atrial fibrillation and an indication for oral anticoagulation are receiving it, and even when treated with warfarin, they are out of the target INR range nearly half the time. Cardioversion, if planned, should be performed after at least 3–4 weeks of anticoagulation at a therapeutic level (or after exclusion of left atrial appendage thrombus by transesophageal echocardiogram as discussed above). Anticoagulation clinics with systematic management of warfarin dosing and adjustment have been shown to result in better maintenance of target anticoagulation.

Four DOACs—dabigatran, rivaroxaban, apixaban, and edoxaban—have been shown to be at least as effective as warfarin for stroke prevention in patients with atrial fibrillation and have been approved by the FDA for this indication (Table 10–16). These medications have not been studied in patients with moderate or severe mitral stenosis (called "valvular atrial fibrillation"), and they should not be used for patients with mechanical prosthetic valves.

Dabigatran (studied in the RE-LY trial) is superior to warfarin at preventing stroke at the 150 mg twice daily dose, and it is noninferior at the 110 mg twice daily dose, although this dose is not approved in the United States. Both doses result in less intracranial hemorrhage than warfarin but also in more gastrointestinal bleeding than warfarin. Neither dabigatran nor any of the DOACs should be used in patients with mechanical prosthetic heart valves where the medications are less effective and riskier.

Rivaroxaban is noninferior to warfarin for stroke prevention in atrial fibrillation (in the ROCKET-AF trial). Rivaroxaban is dosed at 20 mg once daily, with a reduced dose (15 mg/day) for patients with creatinine clearances between 15 and 50 mL/min. It should be administered with food, since that results in a 40% higher drug absorption. Similar to dabigatran, there is substantially less intracranial hemorrhage with rivaroxaban than warfarin.

Apixaban is more effective than warfarin at stroke prevention while having a substantially lower risk of major bleeding (in the ARISOTLE trial) and a lower risk of all-cause mortality. The apixaban dosage is 5 mg twice daily or 2.5 mg twice daily for patients with two of three high-risk criteria (age 80 years or older, body weight 60 kg or less, and serum creatinine of 1.5 mg/dL or more). Apixaban is associated with less intracranial hemorrhage and is well tolerated. Apixaban was also shown to be superior to aspirin (and better tolerated) in the AVERROES trial of patients deemed not suitable for warfarin.

Edoxaban, 60 mg once a day, is noninferior to warfarin for stroke prevention with lower rates of major bleeding and lower rates of hemorrhagic stroke (studied in the ENGAGE-AF trial). Edoxaban carries a boxed warning in FDA labellleling that it should not be used in patients whose creatinine clearance is more than 95 mL/min because it is less effective in this population. The dose is decreased to 30 mg/day for patients whose creatinine clearance is less than or equal to 50 mL/min.

These four DOACs have important advantages over warfarin, and therefore they are recommended preferentially over VKAs in the European Guidelines (Figure 10–8). In practice, these medications are often underdosed. They should be used at the doses shown to be effective in the clinical trials as shown in Table 10–16. Even though labeled for "nonvalvular" atrial fibrillation, the DOACs are safe and effective for patients with moderate or severe valvular

Table 10–16. Direct-acting oral anticoagulants for stroke prevention in patients with nonvalvular atrial fibrillation.

	Dabigatran	Rivaroxaban	Apixaban	Edoxaban
Class	Antithrombin	Factor Xa inhibitor	Factor Xa inhibitor	Factor Xa inhibitor
Bleeding risk compared to warfarin	Less intracranial bleeding Higher incidence of gastrointestinal bleeding	Less intracranial bleeding Higher incidence of gastrointestinal bleeding	Substantially lower risk of major bleeding Less intracranial bleeding	Lower risk of major bleeding Less intracranial bleeding
Dosage	110 mg twice daily 150 mg twice daily	20 mg once daily (give with food)	5 mg twice daily	60 mg once daily
Dosage adjustments	75 mg twice daily for creatinine clearance[1] 15–30 mL/min (approved in the United States but not tested in clinical trials)	15 mg once daily for creatinine clearance[1] < 50 mL/min	2.5 mg twice daily for patients with at least two of three risk factors: 1. Age ≥ 80 years 2. Body weight ≤ 60 kg 3. Serum creatinine ≥ 1.5 mg/dL	30 mg once daily for creatinine clearance[1] ≤ 50 mL/min FDA recommends not to use if creatinine clearance[1] > 95 mL/min

[1]Creatinine clearance calculated by Cockcroft-Gault equation.
Data from Nishimura RA et al. 2014 AHA/ACC Guideline for the Management of Patients With Valvular Heart Disease: A Report of the American College of Cardiology/American Heart Association Task Force on Practice Guidelines. Circulation. 2014 Jun 10;129(23):e521–643. [PMID: 24589853]

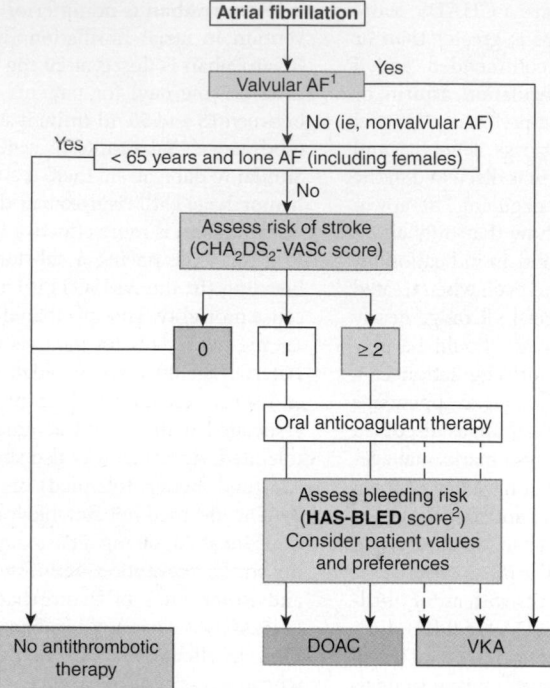

Figure 10–8. Choice of anticoagulant. (Reproduced, with permission, from Camm AJ et al. 2012 focused update of the ESC Guidelines for the management of atrial fibrillation: an update of the 2010 ESC Guidelines for the management of atrial fibrillation. Developed with the special contribution of the European Heart Rhythm Association. Eur Heart J. 2012 Nov;33(21):2719–47.)

abnormalities, with the exception of moderate or severe mitral stenosis.

There are some patients with atrial fibrillation, however, who should be treated with VKAs. These patients include those who have mechanical prosthetic valves, advanced kidney disease (creatinine clearance less than 30 mL/min), moderate or severe mitral stenosis, and those who cannot afford the newer medications. Patients who have been stable while receiving warfarin for a long time, with a high time in target INR range, and who are at lower risk for intracranial hemorrhage will have relatively less benefit with a switch to a newer medication.

There are some important practical issues with using the DOACs. It is important to monitor kidney function at baseline and at least once a year, or more often for those with impaired kidney function. Each of the medications interacts with other medications affecting the P-glycoprotein pathway, like oral ketoconazole, verapamil, dronederone, and phenytoin. To transition patients from warfarin to a DOAC, wait until the INR decreases to about 2.0. Each of the medications has a half-life of about 10 hours for patients with normal kidney function. For elective procedures, stop the medications two to three half-lives (usually 24–48 hours) before procedures with low to moderate bleeding risk (ie, colonoscopy, dental extraction, cardiac catheterization), and five half-lives before procedures like major surgery. Discontinuation times should be extended in patients with impaired renal function, particularly with dabigatran. There are no practical tests to immediately measure the effect of the medications, although a normal aPTT suggests little effect with dabigatran, and a normal prothrombin suggests little effect with rivaroxaban. For rivaroxaban and apixaban, chromogenic Xa assays will measure the effect, but may not be readily available. For bleeding, standard measures (eg, diagnosing and controlling the source, stopping antithrombotic agents, and replacing blood products) should be taken. If the direct-acting medication was taken in the prior 2–4 hours, use activated oral charcoal to reduce absorption. If the patient is taking aspirin, consider platelet transfusion. For life-threatening bleeding, prothrombin complex concentrate may have an effect, but this should generally be used in consultation with a hematologist. For cardioversion, the target specific medications appear to have similar rates of subsequent stroke as warfarin, as long as patients have been taking the medications and adherent for at least several weeks. Like with warfarin, there appears to be a 1.5- to 2-fold increased rate of bleeding associated with the use of aspirin, which therefore should not be used with the DOACs unless there is a clear indication, like acute coronary syndrome within the prior year.

A patient with severe bleeding while taking dabigatran may be treated with the reversal agent idarucizumab, which is a humanized monoclonal antibody approved by the FDA for rapid reversal of the anticoagulation effects, generally in the event of severe bleeding or the need for an urgent procedure. Reversal agents are in development for the other DOACs. Until then, preliminary data suggest that administration of four-factor prothrombin complex concentrate may partially reverse the effects of these agents. Due to the short half-life of the DOACs (10–12 hours with normal kidney function), supportive measures (local control, packed red blood cells, platelets) may suffice until the medication has cleared.

Each of the DOACs appears to be safe and effective around the time of electrical cardioversion. In each of these trials, and in one modest-sized prospective randomized trial of rivaroxaban that specifically addressed cardioversion, the rates of stroke were low (and similar to warfarin) with the DOACs when given for at least 3–4 weeks prior to cardioversion. An advantage of the DOACs is that when stable anticoagulation is desired before elective cardioversion, it is achieved faster than with warfarin.

Devices to exclude the left atrial appendage have been shown to provide protection against stroke compared to warfarin in patients with atrial fibrillation, although their role in clinical practice is still being defined.

B. RATE CONTROL OR ELECTIVE CARDIOVERSION—Two large randomized controlled trials (the 4060-patient Atrial Fibrillation Follow-up Investigation of Rhythm Management, or AFFIRM trial; and the Rate Control Versus Electrical Cardioversion for Persistent Atrial Fibrillation, or RACE trial) compared strategies of rate control and rhythm control. In both, a strategy of rate control and long-term anticoagulation was associated with no higher rates of death or stroke—**both, if anything, favored rate control—and only a modestly increased risk of hemorrhagic events over a strategy of restoring sinus rhythm and maintaining it with antiarrhythmic drug therapy**. Of note is that exercise tolerance and quality of life were not significantly better in the rhythm control group. Nonetheless, the decision of whether to attempt to restore sinus rhythm following the initial episode remains controversial. Elective cardioversion following an appropriate period of anticoagulation is generally recommended for the initial episode in patients in whom atrial fibrillation is thought to be of recent onset and when there is an identifiable precipitating factor. Similarly, cardioversion is appropriate in patients who remain symptomatic from the rhythm despite efforts to achieve rate control.

In cases in which elective cardioversion is required, it may be accomplished electrically or pharmacologically. A number of factors influence the success of electrical cardioversion, including energy, waveform, and electrode placement. Biphasic energy waveform and anteroposterior electrode placement provide superior effectiveness. Pharmacologic cardioversion with **intravenous ibutilide** may be used as described above in a setting in which the patient can undergo continuous ECG monitoring for at least 4–6 hours following administration. Pretreatment with intravenous magnesium (1–2 g) may prevent rare episodes of torsades de pointes associated with ibutilide administration. In patients in whom a decision has been made to continue antiarrhythmic therapy to maintain sinus rhythm (see next paragraph), cardioversion can be attempted with an agent that is being considered for long-term use. For instance, after therapeutic anticoagulation has been established, amiodarone can be initiated on an outpatient basis (400 mg twice daily for 2 weeks, followed by 200 mg twice daily for at least 2–4 weeks and then a maintenance dose of 200 mg daily). Because amiodarone increases the prothrombin time in patients taking warfarin and increases digoxin levels, careful monitoring of anticoagulation and medication levels is required.

Other agents that may be used for both cardioversion and maintenance therapy include dofetilide, propafenone, flecainide, and sotalol. **Dofetilide** (125–500 mcg twice daily orally) must be initiated in hospital due to the potential risk of torsades de pointes and the downward dose adjustment that is required for patients with renal impairment. Propafenone (150–300 mg orally every 8 hours) should be avoided in patients with structural heart disease (CAD, systolic dysfunction, or significant LVH). **Flecainide** (50–150 mg twice daily orally) should be used in conjunction with an AV nodal blocking medication if there is a history of atrial flutter and should be avoided in patients with structural heart disease. **Sotalol** (80–160 mg orally twice daily) should be initiated in the hospital in patients with structural heart disease due to a risk of torsades de pointes; it is not very effective for converting atrial fibrillation but can be used to maintain sinus rhythm following cardioversion.

In patients treated long-term with an antiarrhythmic agent, sinus rhythm will persist in 30–50%. The most commonly used medications are amiodarone, dronedarone, sotalol, propafenone, flecainide, and dofetilide, but the latter four agents are associated with a clear risk of proarrhythmia in certain populations; dronedarone has less efficacy than amiodarone, and amiodarone frequently causes other adverse effects. Therefore, after an initial presentation of atrial fibrillation, it may be prudent to determine whether atrial fibrillation recurs during a period of 6 months without antiarrhythmic medications (during which anticoagulation is maintained). If it does recur, the decision to restore sinus rhythm and initiate long-term antiarrhythmic therapy can be based on how well the patient tolerates atrial fibrillation. The decision to maintain long-term anticoagulation should be based on risk factors (CHADS$_2$ or CHA$_2$DSv-VASc score, Tables 10–14 and 10–15) and not on the perceived presence or absence of atrial fibrillation as future episodes may be asymptomatic.

B. Recurrent and Refractory Atrial Fibrillation

1. Recurrent paroxysmal atrial fibrillation—Patients with recurrent paroxysmal atrial fibrillation are at similar stroke risk as those who are in atrial fibrillation chronically. Although these episodes may be apparent to the patient, many are not recognized and may be totally asymptomatic. Thus, extended continuous ambulatory monitoring or event recorders are indicated in those in whom paroxysmal atrial fibrillation is suspected. Long-term anticoagulation should be considered for all patients except in those who are under 65 years of age and have no additional stroke risk factors. Antiarrhythmic agents are first-line therapy for recurrent, symptomatic atrial fibrillation; however, they are not often successful in preventing all paroxysmal atrial fibrillation episodes.

2. Refractory atrial fibrillation—Atrial fibrillation should generally be considered refractory if it causes persistent symptoms or limits activity despite attempts at rate control. This is much more likely in younger individuals and those who are active or engage in strenuous exercise. Even in such individuals, two-medication or three-medication combinations of a beta-blocker, rate-slowing calcium blocker, and digoxin usually can prevent excessive ventricular rates, though in some cases they are associated with excessive bradycardia during sedentary periods.

If antiarrhythmic or rate-control medications fail to improve the symptoms of atrial fibrillation, catheter ablation of foci in and around the pulmonary veins that initiate atrial fibrillation may be considered. Pulmonary vein isolation is a reasonable second-line therapy for individuals with symptomatic atrial fibrillation that is refractory to pharmacologic therapy. Ablation is successful about 70% of the time but more than one procedure may be required. The procedure is routinely performed in the electrophysiology laboratory using a catheter-based approach and can also be performed via a subxiphoid approach thorascopically, via thoracotomy, or via median sternotomy in the operating room by experienced surgeons. In symptomatic patients with poor rate-control and deemed inappropriate for pulmonary vein isolation, radiofrequency ablation of the AV node and permanent pacing ensure rate control and may facilitate a more physiologic rate response to activity, but this is used only as a last resort.

▶ When to Refer

- Symptomatic atrial fibrillation with or without rate control.
- Asymptomatic atrial fibrillation with poor rate control despite AV nodal blockers.
- Patients at risk for stroke who have not tolerated oral anticoagulants.

▶ When to Admit

- Atrial fibrillation with rapid ventricular response resulting in hemodynamic compromise.
- Atrial fibrillation resulting in acute heart failure.

January CT et al. 2014 AHA/ACC/HRS Guideline for the Management of Patients With Atrial Fibrillation: A Report of the American College of Cardiology/American Heart Association Task Force on Practice Guidelines and the Heart Rhythm Society. J Am Coll Cardiol. 2014 Dec 2;64(21):e1–76. [PMID: 24685669]

ATRIAL FLUTTER

ESSENTIALS OF DIAGNOSIS

- ▶ Usually regular heart rhythm.
- ▶ Often tachycardic (100–150 beats/min).
- ▶ Often associated with palpitations (acute onset) or fatigue (chronic).
- ▶ ECG shows "sawtooth" pattern of atrial activity in leads II, III, and AVF.
- ▶ Often seen in conjunction with structural heart disease or chronic obstructive pulmonary disease (COPD).

Atrial flutter is less common than fibrillation. It may occur in patients with structurally normal hearts, but is more commonly seen in patients with COPD, rheumatic or CHD, heart failure, ASD, or surgically repaired congenital heart disease. The reentrant circuit generates atrial rates of 250–350 beats/min, usually with transmission of every second, third, or fourth impulse through the AV node to the ventricles. The ECG typically demonstrates a "sawtooth" pattern of atrial activity in the inferior leads (II, III, and AVF).

▶ Treatment

Ventricular rate control is accomplished using the same agents used in atrial fibrillation, but it is much more difficult with atrial flutter than with atrial fibrillation. Conversion of atrial flutter to sinus rhythm with class I antiarrhythmic agents is also difficult to achieve, and administration of these medications has been associated with slowing of the atrial flutter rate to the point at which 1:1 AV conduction can occur at rates in excess of 200 beats/min, with subsequent hemodynamic collapse. The intravenous class III antiarrhythmic agent ibutilide has been significantly more successful in converting atrial flutter (see Table 10–13). About 50–70% of patients return to sinus rhythm within 60–90 minutes following the infusion of 1–2 mg of this agent. Electrical cardioversion is also very effective for atrial flutter, with approximately 90% of patients converting following synchronized shocks of as little as 25–50 J.

Although the organization of atrial contractile function in this arrhythmia may provide some protection against thrombus formation, **the risk of thromboembolism should be considered equivalent to atrial fibrillation due to the common coexistence of these arrhythmias**. Precardioversion anticoagulation is not necessary for atrial flutter of less than 48 hours duration except in the setting of mitral valve disease. As with atrial fibrillation, anticoagulation should be continued for at least 4 weeks after electrical or chemical cardioversion and chronically in patients with risk factors for thromboembolism.

Chronic atrial flutter is often a difficult management problem, as rate control is difficult. If pharmacologic therapy is chosen, amiodarone and dofetilide are the antiarrhythmics of choice (see Table 10–13). Dofetilide is often given in conjunction with an AV nodal blocker (other than verapamil). Atrial flutter can follow a typical or atypical reentry circuit around the atrium. The anatomy of the typical circuit has been well defined and allows for catheter ablation within the atrium to interrupt the circuit and eliminate atrial flutter. **Catheter ablation is a highly successful treatment that has become the preferred approach for recurrent typical atrial flutter**. Due to frequent coexistence of atrial flutter with atrial fibrillation, patients may require catheter ablation of both arrhythmias.

When to Refer

- Symptomatic atrial flutter with or without rate control.
- Asymptomatic atrial flutter with poor rate control despite AV nodal blockers.

When to Admit

- Atrial flutter with 1:1 conduction resulting in hemodynamic compromise.
- Atrial flutter resulting in acute heart failure.

Mohanty S et al. Results from a single-blind, randomized study comparing the impact of different ablation approaches on long-term procedure outcome in coexistent atrial fibrillation and flutter (APPROVAL). Circulation. 2013 May 7;127 (18):1853–60. [PMID: 23572499]
Scheuermeyer FX et al. Emergency department management and 1-year outcomes of patients with atrial flutter. Ann Emerg Med. 2011 Jun;57(6):564–71. [PMID: 21257230]

MULTIFOCAL ATRIAL TACHYCARDIA

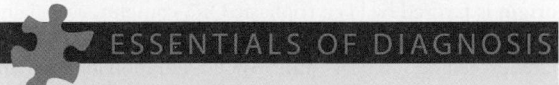
ESSENTIALS OF DIAGNOSIS

- ► ECG reveals three or more distinct P-wave morphologies.
- ► Often associated with palpitations.
- ► Associated with severe COPD.
- ► Treatment of the underlying lung disease is the most effective therapy.

This is a rhythm characterized by varying P wave morphology (by definition, three or more foci) and markedly irregular PP intervals. The rate is usually between 100 and 140 beats/min. Most patients have concomitant severe COPD. Treatment of the underlying condition is the most effective approach; verapamil, 240–480 mg orally daily in divided doses is also of value in some patients. This arrhythmia may progress to atrial fibrillation in some patients.

Yokoshiki H et al. Swallowing-induced multifocal atrial tachycardia originating from right pulmonary veins. J Electrocardiol. 2011 May-Jun;44(3):395. [PMID: 21353237]

AV JUNCTIONAL RHYTHM

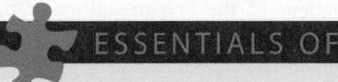
ESSENTIALS OF DIAGNOSIS

- ► Regular heart rhythm.
- ► Can have wide or narrow QRS complex.
- ► Often seen in digitalis toxicity.

The atrial-nodal junction or the nodal-His bundle junction may assume pacemaker activity for the heart, usually at a rate of 35–60 beats/min. This may occur in patients with myocarditis, CAD, and digitalis toxicity as well as in individuals with normal hearts. The rate responds normally to exercise, and the diagnosis is often an incidental finding on ECG monitoring, but it can be suspected if the jugular venous pulse shows cannon *a* waves. Junctional rhythm is often an escape rhythm because of depressed sinus node function with sinoatrial block or delayed conduction in the AV node. **Nonparoxysmal junctional tachycardia** results from increased automaticity of the junctional tissues in digitalis toxicity or ischemia and is associated with a narrow QRS complex and a rate usually less than 120–130 beats/min. It is usually considered benign when it occurs in acute myocardial infarction, but the ischemia that induces it may also cause ventricular tachycardia and ventricular fibrillation.

VENTRICULAR PREMATURE BEATS (Ventricular Extrasystoles)

Ventricular premature beats, also called PVCs, are typically isolated beats originating from ventricular tissue. Sudden death occurs more frequently (presumably as a result of ventricular fibrillation) when ventricular premature beats occur in the presence of organic heart disease but not in individuals with no known cardiac disease.

Clinical Findings

The patient may or may not sense the irregular beat, usually as a skipped beat. Exercise generally abolishes premature beats in normal hearts, and the rhythm becomes regular. Ventricular premature beats are characterized by wide QRS complexes that differ in morphology from the patient's normal beats. They are usually not preceded by a

P wave, although retrograde ventriculoatrial conduction may occur. Bigeminy and trigeminy are arrhythmias in which every second or third beat is premature; these patterns confirm a reentry mechanism for the ectopic beat. Ambulatory ECG monitoring or monitoring during graded exercise may reveal more frequent and complex ventricular premature beats than occur in a single routine ECG. An increased frequency of ventricular premature beats during exercise is associated with a higher risk of cardiovascular mortality and should be investigated further.

Treatment

If no associated cardiac disease is present and if the ectopic beats are asymptomatic, no therapy is indicated. Mild symptoms or anxiety from palpitations may be allayed with reassurance to the patient of the benign nature of this arrhythmia. If PVCs are frequent, electrolyte abnormalities (especially hypokalemia or hyperkalemia and hypomagnesemia), hyperthyroidism, and occult heart disease should be excluded. In addition, an echocardiogram should be performed in patients in whom a burden of PVCs of greater than 10,000 per day has been documented by Holter monitoring. Pharmacologic treatment is indicated only for patients who are symptomatic or who develop cardiomyopathy thought due to high burden PVCs (generally greater than 10% of daily heart beats). Beta-blockers or non-dihydropyridine calcium channel blockers are appropriate as first-line therapy. The class I and III agents (see Table 10–13) may be effective in reducing ventricular premature beats but are often poorly tolerated and can be proarrhythmic in up to 5% of patients. Catheter ablation is a well-established therapy for symptomatic individuals who do not respond to medication or for those patients whose burden of ectopic beats has resulted in a tachycardia-induced cardiomyopathy.

Chen T et al. Ventricular ectopy in patients with left ventricular dysfunction: should it be treated? J Card Fail. 2013 Jan;19(1):40–9. [PMID: 23273593]
Yokokawa M et al. Recovery from left ventricular dysfunction after ablation of frequent premature ventricular complexes. Heart Rhythm. 2013 Feb;10(2):172–5. [PMID: 23099051]

VENTRICULAR TACHYCARDIA

 ESSENTIALS OF DIAGNOSIS

- ► Fast, wide QRS complex on ECG.
- ► Often associated with structural heart disease.
- ► Frequently associated with syncope.
- ► In the absence of reversible cause, implantable cardioverter defibrillator (ICD) is recommended.

General Considerations

Ventricular tachycardia is defined as three or more consecutive ventricular premature beats. The usual rate is 160–240 beats/min and is moderately regular but less so than atrial tachycardia. The usual mechanism is reentry, but abnormally triggered rhythms occur.

Ventricular tachycardia is a frequent complication of acute myocardial infarction and dilated cardiomyopathy but may occur in chronic coronary disease, hypertrophic cardiomyopathy, mitral valve prolapse, myocarditis, and in most other forms of myocardial disease. It can also be a consequence of atypical forms of cardiomyopathies, such as arrhythmogenic right ventricular cardiomyopathy. However, ventricular tachycardia can also occur in patients with structurally normal hearts. **Torsades de pointes**, a form of ventricular tachycardia in which QRS morphology twists around the baseline, may occur in the setting of severe hypokalemia, hypomagnesemia, or after administration of a medication that prolongs the QT interval. In nonacute settings, most patients with ventricular tachycardia have known or easily detectable cardiac disease, and the finding of ventricular tachycardia is an unfavorable prognostic sign.

Clinical Findings

A. Symptoms and Signs

Patients may be asymptomatic or experience syncope or milder symptoms of impaired cerebral perfusion.

B. Laboratory Findings

Ventricular tachycardia can occur in the setting of hypokalemia and hypomagnesemia. Cardiac markers may be elevated when ventricular tachycardia presents in the setting of acute myocardial infarction or as a consequence of underlying coronary disease and demand ischemia.

C. Differentiation of Aberrantly Conducted Supraventricular Beats from Ventricular Beats

Ventricular tachycardia is either nonsustained (three or more consecutive beats lasting less than 30 seconds and terminating spontaneously) or sustained. The distinction from aberrant conduction of supraventricular tachycardia may be difficult in patients with a wide QRS complex; it is important because of the differing prognostic and therapeutic implications of each type. Findings favoring a **ventricular origin** include (1) AV dissociation; (2) a QRS duration exceeding 0.14 second; (3) capture or fusion beats (infrequent); (4) left axis deviation with right bundle branch block morphology; (5) monophasic (R) or biphasic (qR, QR, or RS) complexes in V_1; and (6) a qR or QS complex in V_6. **Supraventricular origin** is favored by (1) a triphasic QRS complex, especially if there was initial negativity in leads I and V_6; (2) ventricular rates exceeding 170 beats/min; (3) QRS duration longer than 0.12 second but not longer than 0.14 second; and (4) the presence of preexcitation syndrome.

Treatment

A. Acute Ventricular Tachycardia

The treatment of acute ventricular tachycardia is determined by the degree of hemodynamic compromise and the duration of the arrhythmia. In patients with structurally normal hearts, the prognosis is generally benign and syncope is uncommon. The etiology is often triggered activity from the right or left ventricular outflow tract and acute treatment with a short-acting intravenous beta-blocker may terminate the episode. The management of ventricular tachycardia in acute myocardial infarction is discussed in the Complications section of Acute Myocardial Infarction with ST-Segment Elevation, above. In other patients, if ventricular tachycardia causes hypotension, heart failure, or myocardial ischemia, synchronized DC cardioversion with 100–360 J should be performed immediately. If the patient is tolerating the rhythm, amiodarone 150 mg as a slow intravenous bolus over 10 minutes, followed by an infusion of 1 mg/min for 6 hours and then a maintenance infusion of 0.5 mg/min for an additional 18–42 hours can be used. Significant hyoptension can occur with rapid infusions of amiodarone. Lidocaine, 1 mg/kg as an intravenous bolus injection, can also be used. If the ventricular tachycardia recurs, supplemental amiodarone infusions of 150 mg over 10 minutes can be given. If the patient is stable, intravenous procainamide, 20 mg/min intravenously (up to 1000 mg), followed by an infusion of 20–80 mcg/kg/min could also be tried. Empiric magnesium replacement (1–2 g intravenously) may help especially for polymorphic ventricular tachycardia. If polymorphic VT recurs, increasing the heart rate with isoproterenol infusion (up to 20 mcg/min) or atrial pacing with a temporary pacemaker (at 90–120 bpm) will effectively shorten the QT interval to prevent further episodes.

B. Chronic Recurrent Ventricular Tachycardia

1. Sustained ventricular tachycardia—Patients with symptomatic or sustained ventricular tachycardia in the absence of a reversible precipitating cause (acute myocardial infarction or ischemia, electrolyte imbalance, medication toxicity, etc) are at high risk for recurrence. In patients with structurally normal hearts and ventricular tachycardia with typical outflow tract (left bundle branch block with inferior axis) or left posterior fascicle (right bundle branch block with superior axis) appearance on ECG, medical treatment with beta-blocker or a non-dihydropyridine calcium channel blocker may be tried. Catheter ablation has a high success rate in these patients who fail initial medical treatment. In patients with significant LV dysfunction, subsequent sudden death is common and ICD implantation is recommended. Beta-blockers are the mainstay for medical treatment of ventricular tachycardia in patients with structural heart disease. Antiarrhythmic medications have not been shown to lower mortality in these patients, but may decrease subsequent episodes and reduce the number of ICD shocks. Amiodarone is generally preferred in patients with structural heart disease but sotalol may be considered as well. Catheter ablation can be used as a palliative therapy for those patients with recurrent tachycardia who receive ICD shocks despite medical therapy; however, recurrence rates are high.

2. Nonsustained ventricular tachycardia (NSVT)—NSVT is defined as runs of three or more ventricular beats lasting less than 30 seconds and terminating spontaneously. These may be symptomatic (usually experienced as lightheadedness) or asymptomatic. In individuals without heart disease, NSVT is generally associated with a benign prognosis. In patients with structural heart disease, NSVT is associated with an increased risk of subsequent symptomatic ventricular tachycardia and sudden death, especially when seen more than 48 hours after myocardial infarction. In general, treatment of the underlying cardiac disease is indicated rather than treatment of the arrhythmia itself. In patients with chronic heart failure and reduced EF who do not otherwise meet the indications for ICD implantation (EF less than 35%), the presence of NSVT may prompt electrophysiology study. Inducibility of sustained ventricular tachycardia in this situation warrants ICD implantation.

When to Admit

Any sustained ventricular tachycardia.

Pedersen CT et al. EHRA/HRS/APHRS expert consensus on ventricular arrhythmias. Europace. 2014 Sep;16(9):1257–83. [PMID: 25172618]

VENTRICULAR FIBRILLATION & DEATH

Sudden cardiac death is defined as unexpected nontraumatic death in clinically well or stable patients who die within 1 hour after onset of symptoms. The causative rhythm in most cases is ventricular fibrillation, which is usually preceded by ventricular tachycardia except in the setting of acute ischemia or infarction. Complete heart block and sinus node arrest may also cause sudden death. A disproportionate number of sudden deaths occur in the early morning hours and this suggests that there is a strong interplay with the autonomic nervous system. Over 75% of victims of sudden cardiac death have severe CAD. Many have old myocardial infarctions. Sudden death may be the initial manifestation of coronary disease in up to 20% of patients and accounts for approximately 50% of deaths from coronary disease. Other conditions that predispose to sudden death include severe LVH, hypertrophic cardiomyopathy, congestive cardiomyopathy, aortic stenosis, pulmonic stenosis, primary pulmonary hypertension, cyanotic congenital heart disease, atrial myxoma, mitral valve prolapse, hypoxia, electrolyte abnormalities, prolonged QT interval syndrome, the Brugada syndrome, arrhythmogenic right ventricular cardiomyopathy, catecholaminergic polymorphic ventricular tachycardia, and conduction system disease.

Treatment

Unless ventricular fibrillation occurs shortly after myocardial infarction, is associated with ischemia, or is seen with a correctable process (such as an electrolyte abnormality or medication toxicity), surviving patients require evaluation and intervention since recurrences are frequent. Ventricular function should be evaluated with echocardiography. Coronary arteriography should be performed to exclude coronary disease as the underlying cause, since revascularization may prevent recurrence. When ventricular fibrillation occurs in the initial 24 hours after infarction, long-term management is no different from that of other patients with acute infarction. Conduction disturbances should be managed as described in the next section. Survivors of ventricular fibrillation or cardiac arrest have improved long-term outcomes if a hypothermia protocol is rapidly initiated and continued for 24–36 hours after cardiac arrest.

If myocardial infarction or ischemia, bradyarrhythmias and conduction disturbances or other identifiable and correctable precipitating causes of ventricular fibrillation are not found to be the cause of the sudden death episode, an ICD is the treatment of choice. In addition, evidence from the MADIT II study and Sudden Cardiac Death in Heart Failure Trial (SCD-HeFT) suggest that patients with severe LV dysfunction—whether due to an ischemic cause such as a remote myocardial infarction or a nonischemic cause of advanced heart failure—have a reduced risk of death with the prophylactic implantation of an ICD. However, the DINAMIT study demonstrated that implanting prophylactic ICDs in patients early after myocardial infarction is associated with a trend toward worse outcomes. These patients may be managed with a wearable defibrillator vest until recovery of ventricular function can be assessed by echocardiogram at a later date.

Nielsen N et al; TTM Trial Investigators. Targeted temperature management at 33 degrees C versus 36 degrees C after cardiac arrest. N Engl J Med. 2013 Dec 5;369(23):2197–206. [PMID: 24237006]

Olashansky B et al. Sudden death risk in syncope: the role of the implantable cardioverter defibrillator. Prog Cardiovasc Dis. 2013 Jan-Feb;55(4):443–53. [PMID: 23472783]

ACCELERATED IDIOVENTRICULAR RHYTHM

Accelerated idioventricular rhythm is a regular wide complex rhythm with a rate of 60–120 beats/min, usually with a gradual onset. Because the rate is often similar to the sinus rate, fusion beats and alternating rhythms are common. Two mechanisms have been invoked: (1) an escape rhythm due to suppression of higher pacemakers resulting from sinoatrial and AV block or from depressed sinus node function; and (2) slow ventricular tachycardia due to increased automaticity or, less frequently, reentry. It occurs commonly in acute infarction and following reperfusion with thrombolytic medications. The incidence of associated ventricular fibrillation is much less than that of ventricular tachycardia with a rapid rate, and treatment is not indicated unless there is hemodynamic compromise or more serious arrhythmias. This rhythm also is common in digitalis toxicity.

Accelerated idioventricular rhythm must be distinguished from the idioventricular or junctional rhythm with rates less than 40–45 beats/min that occurs in the presence of complete AV block. AV dissociation—where ventricular rate exceeds sinus—but not AV block occurs in most cases of accelerated idioventricular rhythm.

LONG QT SYNDROME

Congenital long QT syndrome is an uncommon disease that is characterized by recurrent syncope, a long QT interval (usually 0.5–0.7 second), documented ventricular arrhythmias, and sudden death. It may occur in the presence (Jervell-Lange-Nielsen syndrome) or absence (Romano-Ward syndrome) of congenital deafness. Inheritance may be autosomal recessive or autosomal dominant (Romano-Ward). Specific genetic mutations affecting membrane potassium and sodium channels have been identified and help delineate the mechanisms and susceptibility to arrhythmia.

Because this is a primary electrical disorder usually with no evidence of structural heart disease or LV dysfunction, the long-term prognosis is excellent if arrhythmia is controlled. Long-term treatment with beta-blockers (particularly nadolol) has been shown to be effective. ICD implantation is recommended for patients in whom recurrent syncope, sustained ventricular arrhythmias, or sudden cardiac death occurs despite medical therapy. An ICD should be considered as primary therapy in certain patients, such as those in whom aborted sudden cardiac death is the initial presentation of the long-QT syndrome, when there is a strong family history of sudden cardiac death, or when compliance or intolerance to medications is a concern.

Acquired long QT interval secondary to use of antiarrhythmic agents, methadone, antidepressant medications, or certain antibiotics; electrolyte abnormalities; myocardial ischemia; or significant bradycardia may result in ventricular tachycardia (particularly torsades de pointes). Notably, many antiarrhythmic medications that are effective for the treatment of atrial and ventricular arrhythmias may significantly prolong the QT interval (sotalol, dofetilide). If a medication is found to prolong the QT interval beyond 500 ms or 15% longer than the baseline QT, it should be discontinued.

The management of torsades de pointes differs from that of other forms of ventricular tachycardia. Class Ia, Ic, or III antiarrhythmics, which prolong the QT interval, should be avoided—or withdrawn immediately if being used. Intravenous beta-blockers may be effective, especially in congenital forms of long-QT syndrome; intravenous magnesium should be given acutely. Increasing the heart rate, whether by infusion of beta-agonist (dopamine or isoproterenol) or temporary atrial or ventricular pacing, is an effective approach that can both break and prevent the rhythm.

Abrams DJ et al. Long QT syndrome. Circulation. 2014 Apr 8;129(14):1524–9. [PMID: 24709866]

Moskovitz JB et al. Electrocardiographic implications of the prolonged QT interval. Am J Emerg Med. 2013 May; 31(5):866–71. [PMID: 23602761]

BRADYCARDIAS & CONDUCTION DISTURBANCES

SICK SINUS SYNDROME

 ESSENTIALS OF DIAGNOSIS

- ▶ Most patients are asymptomatic.
- ▶ More common in elderly population.
- ▶ May have recurrent supraventricular arrhythmia and bradyarrhythmia.
- ▶ Frequently seen in patients with concomitant atrial fibrillation.
- ▶ Often chronotropically incompetent.
- ▶ May be caused by medications.

▶ General Considerations

This broad diagnosis is applied to patients with sinus arrest, sinoatrial exit block (recognized by a pause equal to a multiple of the underlying PP interval or progressive shortening of the PP interval prior to a pause), or persistent sinus bradycardia. These rhythms are often caused or exacerbated by medications (digitalis, calcium channel blockers, beta-blockers, sympatholytic agents, antiarrhythmics), and agents that may be responsible should be withdrawn prior to making the diagnosis. Another presentation is of recurrent supraventricular tachycardias (paroxysmal reentry tachycardias, atrial flutter, and atrial fibrillation), associated with bradyarrhythmias ("tachy-brady syndrome"). The long pauses that often follow the termination of tachycardia cause the associated symptoms.

Sick sinus syndrome occurs most commonly in elderly patients and is frequently seen in patients with concomitant atrial fibrillation. The pathologic changes are usually nonspecific, characterized by patchy fibrosis of the sinus node and cardiac conduction system. Sick sinus syndrome may rarely be caused by other conditions, including sarcoidosis, amyloidosis, Chagas disease, and various cardiomyopathies. Coronary disease is an uncommon cause.

▶ Clinical Findings

Most patients with ECG evidence of sick sinus syndrome are asymptomatic, but rare individuals may experience syncope, dizziness, confusion, palpitations, heart failure, or angina. Because these symptoms are either nonspecific or are due to other causes, it is essential that they be demonstrated to coincide temporally with arrhythmias. This may require prolonged ambulatory monitoring or the use of an event recorder.

▶ Treatment

Most symptomatic patients will require permanent pacing (see AV block). Treatment of associated tachyarrhythmias is often difficult without first instituting pacing, since

beta-blockers, calcium-channel blockers, digoxin, and other antiarrhythmic agents may exacerbate the bradycardia. Unfortunately, symptomatic relief following pacing has not been consistent, largely because of inadequate documentation of the etiologic role of bradyarrhythmias in producing the symptom. Furthermore, some of these patients may have associated ventricular arrhythmias that may require treatment. Permanent pacing does not reduce mortality but may alleviate symptoms and improve quality of life in carefully selected patients.

Semelka M et al. Sick sinus syndrome: a review. Am Fam Physician. 2013 May 15;87(10):691–6. [PMID: 23939447]

AV BLOCK

AV block is categorized as **first-degree** (PR interval greater than 0.21 seconds with all atrial impulses conducted), **second-degree** (intermittent blocked beats), or **third-degree** (complete heart block, in which no supraventricular impulses are conducted to the ventricles).

Second-degree block is further subclassified. In **Mobitz type I (Wenckebach)** AV block, the AV conduction time (PR interval) progressively lengthens, with the RR interval shortening before the blocked beat; this phenomenon is almost always due to abnormal conduction within the AV node. In **Mobitz type II** AV block, there are intermittently nonconducted atrial beats not preceded by lengthening AV conduction. It is usually due to block within the His bundle system. The classification as Mobitz type I or Mobitz type II is difficult when only 2:1 AV block is present on the ECG. If the width of the QRS complex is narrow (less than 0.12 second), the block is usually nodal; if the QRS complex is wide (greater than or equal to 0.12 second), the block is more likely infranodal. In addition, the presence of PR prolongation (greater than 0.21 second) during 2:1 AV block suggests nodal disease and therefore Mobitz type I AV block. Electrophysiologic studies may be necessary for accurate localization. Management of AV block in acute myocardial infarction has already been discussed.

First-degree and **Mobitz type I block** may occur in normal individuals with heightened vagal tone. They may also occur as a medication effect (especially digitalis, calcium channel blockers, beta-blockers, or other sympatholytic agents), often superimposed on organic disease. These disturbances also occur transiently or chronically due to ischemia, infarction, inflammatory processes (including Lyme disease), fibrosis, calcification, or infiltration. The prognosis is usually good, since reliable alternative pacemakers arise from the AV junction below the level of block if higher degrees of block occur.

Mobitz type II block is almost always due to organic disease involving the infranodal conduction system. In the event of progression to complete heart block, alternative pacemakers are not reliable. Thus, prophylactic ventricular pacing is usually required.

Complete (third-degree) heart block is a more advanced form of block often due to a lesion distal to the His bundle and associated with bilateral bundle branch block. The QRS is wide and the ventricular rate is slower, usually less than 50 beats/min. Transmission of atrial impulses through the AV node is completely blocked, and a ventricular pacemaker maintains a slow, regular ventricular rate, usually less than 45 beats/min. Exercise does not increase the rate. Patients may be asymptomatic or may complain of weakness or dyspnea if the rate is less than 35 beats/min; symptoms may occur at higher rates if the left ventricle cannot increase its stroke output. During periods of transition from partial to complete heart block, some patients have ventricular asystole that lasts several seconds or longer. Syncope occurs abruptly.

Patients with episodic or chronic infranodal complete heart block require permanent pacing, and temporary pacing is indicated if implantation of a permanent pacemaker is delayed.

▶ **Treatment**

The indications for **permanent pacing** are symptomatic bradyarrhythmias, asymptomatic Mobitz II AV block, or complete heart block. A standardized nomenclature for pacemaker generators is used, usually consisting of four letters. The first letter refers to the chamber that is stimulated (A = atrium, V = ventricle, D = dual, for both). The second letter refers to the chamber in which sensing occurs (also A, V, or D). The third letter refers to the sensory mode (I = inhibition by a sensed impulse, T = triggering by a sensed impulse, D = dual modes of response). The fourth letter refers to the programmability or rate modulation capacity (usually P for programming for two functions, M for programming more than two, and R for rate modulation).

A dual-chamber multiple programmable pacemaker that senses and paces in both chambers is the most physiologic approach to pacing patients who remain in sinus rhythm. AV synchrony is particularly important in patients in whom atrial contraction produces a substantial increment in stroke volume and in those in whom sensing the atrial rate to provide rate-responsive ventricular pacing is useful. In patients with single-chamber ventricular pacemakers, the lack of an atrial kick may lead to the so-called pacemaker syndrome, in which the patient experiences signs of low cardiac output while upright. In patients with complete heart block with left ventricular systolic dysfunction, implantation of a pacemaker capable of simultaneous left and right ventricular pacing (CRT-P) may be indicated.

Pulse generators are also available that can increase their rate in response to motion or respiratory rate when the intrinsic atrial rate is inappropriately low. These are most useful in active individuals. Follow-up after pacemaker implantation, usually by telephonic monitoring, is essential. All pulse generators and lead systems have an early failure rate that is now well below 1% and an expected battery life varying from 6 to 10 years.

Epstein AE et al. 2012 ACCF/AHA/HRS focused update incorporated into the ACCF/AHA/HRS 2008 guidelines for device-based therapy of cardiac rhythm abnormalities: a report of the American College of Cardiology Foundation/American Heart Association Task Force on Practice Guidelines and the Heart Rhythm Society. Circulation. 2013 Jan 22;127(3):e283–352. [PMID: 23255456]

AV DISSOCIATION

When a ventricular pacemaker is firing at a rate faster than or close to the sinus rate (accelerated idioventricular rhythm, ventricular premature beats, or ventricular tachycardia), atrial impulses arriving at the AV node when it is refractory may not be conducted. This phenomenon is AV dissociation but does not necessarily indicate AV block. No treatment is required aside from management of the causative arrhythmia.

INTRAVENTRICULAR CONDUCTION DEFECTS

Intraventricular conduction defects, including bundle branch block, are common in individuals with otherwise normal hearts and in many disease processes, including ischemic heart disease, inflammatory disease, infiltrative disease, cardiomyopathy, and postcardiotomy.

The prognosis of intraventricular block is generally related to the underlying myocardial process. Patients with no apparent heart disease have an overall survival rate similar to that of matched controls. However, left bundle branch block—but not right—is associated with a higher risk of development of overt cardiac disease and cardiac mortality. In patients with underlying CHD, both right and left bundle branch block are associated with higher cardiovascular and all-cause mortality.

In asymptomatic patients with bifascicular block (block in two of three infranodal components—right bundle, left anterior, and left posterior fascicle), the incidence of occult complete heart block or progression to it is low and pacing is not usually warranted. However, in patients with bifascicular block that present with syncope where no other readily identifiable cause is found, early pacemaker implantation has been shown to reduce further episodes.

Santini M et al. Prevention of syncope through permanent cardiac pacing in patients with bifascicular block and syncope of unexplained origin: the PRESS study. Circ Arrhythm Electrophysiol. 2013 Feb;6(1):101–7. [PMID: 23390123]

SYNCOPE

ESSENTIALS OF DIAGNOSIS

▶ Transient loss of consciousness and postural tone from vasodepressor or cardiogenic causes.

▶ Prompt recovery without resuscitative measures.

▶ High risk features on presentation include history of structural heart disease, abnormal ECG findings and age older than 60 years.

▶ **General Considerations**

Syncope is a symptom defined as a transient, self-limited loss of consciousness, usually leading to a fall. Thirty percent of the adult population will experience at least one episode of syncope. It accounts for approximately 3% of emergency department visits. A specific cause of syncope is identified in about 50% of cases during the initial evaluation. The prognosis is relatively favorable except when accompanying cardiac disease is present. In many patients with recurrent syncope or near syncope, arrhythmias are not the cause. This is particularly true when the patient has no evidence of associated heart disease by history, examination, standard ECG, or noninvasive testing. **The history is the most important component of the evaluation to identify the cause of syncope**.

Vasodepressor syncope may be due to excessive vagal tone or impaired reflex control of the peripheral circulation. The most frequent type of vasodepressor syncope is vasovagal hypotension or the "common faint," which is often initiated by a stressful, painful, or claustrophobic experience, especially in young women. Enhanced vagal tone with resulting hypotension is the cause of syncope in carotid sinus hypersensitivity and postmicturition syncope; vagal-induced sinus bradycardia, sinus arrest, and AV block are common accompaniments and may themselves be the cause of syncope.

Orthostatic (postural) hypotension is another common cause of vasodepressor syncope, especially in the elderly; in diabetic patients or others with autonomic neuropathy; in patients with blood loss or hypovolemia; and in patients taking vasodilators, diuretics, and adrenergic-blocking medications. In addition, a syndrome of chronic idiopathic orthostatic hypotension exists primarily in older men. In most of these conditions, the normal vasoconstrictive response to assuming upright posture, which compensates for the abrupt decrease in venous return, is impaired.

Cardiogenic syncope can occur on a mechanical or arrhythmic basis. There is usually no prodrome; thus, injury secondary to falling is common. Mechanical problems that can cause syncope include aortic stenosis (where syncope may occur from autonomic reflex abnormalities or ventricular tachycardia), pulmonary stenosis, HCM, congenital lesions associated with pulmonary hypertension or right-to-left shunting, and LA myxoma obstructing the mitral valve. Episodes are commonly exertional or postexertional. More commonly, cardiac syncope is due to disorders of automaticity (sick sinus syndrome), conduction disorders (AV block), or tachyarrhythmias (especially ventricular tachycardia and supraventricular tachycardia with rapid ventricular rate).

► Clinical Findings

A. Symptoms and Signs

Syncope is characteristically abrupt in onset, often resulting in injury, transient (lasting for seconds to a few minutes), and followed by prompt recovery of full consciousness.

Vasodepressor premonitory symptoms, such as nausea, diaphoresis, tachycardia, and pallor, are usual in the "common faint." Episodes can be aborted by lying down or removing the inciting stimulus. In **orthostatic (postural) hypotension,** a greater than normal decline (20 mm Hg) in BP immediately upon arising from the supine to the standing position is observed, with or without tachycardia depending on the status of autonomic (baroreceptor) function.

B. Diagnostic Tests

The evaluation for syncope depends on findings from the history and physical examination (especially orthostatic BP evaluation, auscultation of carotid arteries, and cardiac examination).

1. ECG—A resting ECG is recommended for all patients undergoing evaluation for syncope. High-risk findings on ECG include non-sinus rhythm and complete or partial left bundle branch block. Patients with normal sinus rhythm on ECG should undergo continuous cardiac telemetry monitoring or Holter monitoring to exclude transient or intermittent arrhythmia. Event recorder and transtelephone ECG monitoring may be helpful in patients with infrequent presyncopal episodes. Caution is required before attributing a patient's symptom to rhythm or conduction abnormalities observed during monitoring without concomitant symptoms. In many cases, the symptoms are due to a different arrhythmia or to noncardiac causes. For instance, dizziness or syncope in older patients may be unrelated to concomitantly observed bradycardia, sinus node abnormalities, or ventricular ectopy.

2. Autonomic testing—Orthostatic hypotension from autonomic function can be diagnosed with more certainty by observing BP and heart rate responses to Valsalva maneuver and by tilt testing.

Carotid sinus massage in patients who do *not* have carotid bruits or a history of cerebral vascular disease can precipitate sinus node arrest or AV block in patients with carotid sinus hypersensitivity. **Head-up tilt-table testing** can identify patients whose syncope may be on a vasovagal basis. In older patients, vasoconstrictor abnormalities and autonomic insufficiency are perhaps the most common causes of syncope. Thus, tilt testing should be done before proceeding to invasive studies unless clinical and ambulatory ECG evaluation suggests a cardiac abnormality. Although different testing protocols are used, passive tilting to at least 70 degrees for 10–40 minutes—in conjunction with isoproterenol infusion or sublingual nitroglycerin, if necessary—is typical. Syncope due to bradycardia, hypotension, or both will occur in approximately one-third of patients with recurrent syncope. With more aggressive protocols, false-positive responses may occur.

3. Electrophysiologic studies—Electrophysiologic studies to assess sinus node function, AV conduction and to induce supraventricular or ventricular tachycardia are indicated in patients with recurrent episodes, nondiagnostic ambulatory ECGs, and negative autonomic testing (if vasomotor syncope is a consideration). Electrophysiologic studies reveal an arrhythmic cause in 20–50% of patients, depending on the study criteria, and are most often diagnostic when the patient has had multiple episodes and has identifiable cardiac abnormalities.

► Treatment

In patients with vasodepressor syncope, treatment consists largely of counseling patients to avoid predisposing situations and maintaining adequate hydration. Although neurally mediated syncope is distressing for the patient and affects quality of life, mortaliy rate is low and evaluation and treatment can generally be initiated on an outpatient basis. Beta-blockers have been used in patients with altered autonomic function uncovered by head-up tilt testing but generally provide minimal benefit. Volume expanders, such as fludrocortisone, or vasoconstrictors, such as midodrine, may also be tried. Selective serotonin reuptake inhibitors have shown some benefit in select patients.

If symptomatic bradyarrhythmias or supraventricular tachyarrhythmias are detected and felt to be the cause of syncope, therapy can usually be initiated without additional diagnostic studies. Permanent pacing is indicated in patients with syncope and documented severe pauses (greater than 3 seconds), bradycardia, or high-degree AV block (second-degree Mobitz type II or complete heart block).

▶ When to Admit

- Patients with syncope and underlying structural heart disease.
- Bradyarrhythmia or tachyarrhythmia associated with symptoms.
- Unclear etiology of syncope with high-risk features (heart failure, abnormal ECG findings, advanced age, multiple unexplained episodes).

Benditt DG. Syncope risk assessment in the emergency department and clinic. Prog Cardiovasc Dis. 2013 Jan–Feb;55(4): 376–81. [PMID: 23472774]
Krahn AD et al. Selecting appropriate diagnostic tools for evaluating the patient with syncope/collapse. Prog Cardiovasc Dis. 2013 Jan–Feb;55(4):402–9. [PMID: 23472778]

RECOMMENDATIONS FOR RESUMPTION OF DRIVING

An important management problem in patients who have experienced syncope, symptomatic ventricular tachycardia, or aborted sudden death is to provide recommendations concerning automobile driving. Patients with syncope or aborted sudden death thought to have been due to temporary factors (acute myocardial infarction, bradyarrhythmias subsequently treated with permanent pacing, medication effect, electrolyte imbalance) should be advised after recovery not to drive for at least 1 week. Other patients with symptomatic ventricular tachycardia or aborted sudden death, whether treated pharmacologically, with antitachycardia devices, or with ablation therapy, should not drive for at least 6 months. Longer restrictions are warranted in these patients if spontaneous arrhythmias persist. The clinician should comply with local reporting and driving restriction regulations and consult local authorities concerning individual cases where required.

Sakaguchi S et al. Syncope and driving, flying and vocational concerns. Prog Cardiovasc Dis. 2013 Jan–Feb;55(4):454–63. [PMID: 23472784]

HEART FAILURE

ESSENTIALS OF DIAGNOSIS

- ▶ **LV failure:** Either due to systolic or diastolic dysfunction. Predominant symptoms are those of low cardiac output and congestion, including dyspnea.
- ▶ **RV failure:** Symptoms of fluid overload predominate; usually RV failure is secondary to LV failure.
- ▶ Assessment of LV function is a crucial part of diagnosis and management.
- ▶ Optimal management of chronic heart failure includes combination medical therapies, such as ACE inhibitors, aldosterone antagonists, and beta-blockers.

▶ General Considerations

Heart failure is a common syndrome that is increasing in incidence and prevalence. Approximately 5 million patients in the United States have heart failure, and there are around 800,000 new cases each year. Each year in the United States, over 1 million patients are discharged from the hospital with a diagnosis of heart failure. **It is primarily a disease of aging,** with over 75% of existing and new cases occurring in individuals over 65 years of age. Seventy-five percent of heart failure patients have antecedent hypertension. The prevalence of heart failure rises from less than 1% in individuals below 60 years to nearly 10% in those over 80 years of age.

Heart failure may be right sided or left sided (or both). Patients with **left heart failure** may have symptoms of low cardiac output and elevated pulmonary venous pressure; dyspnea is the predominant feature. Signs of fluid retention predominate in **right heart failure**. Most patients exhibit symptoms or signs of both right- and left-sided failure, and **LV dysfunction is the primary cause of RV failure.** Approximately half of patients with heart failure have **preserved LV systolic function** and usually have some degree of diastolic dysfunction. Patients with reduced or preserved systolic function may have similar symptoms and it may be difficult to distinguish clinically between the two based on signs and symptoms. In developed countries, CAD with resulting myocardial infarction and loss of functioning myocardium **(ischemic cardiomyopathy)** is the most common cause of **systolic heart failure.** Systemic hypertension remains an important cause of heart failure and, even more commonly in the United States, an exacerbating factor in patients with cardiac dysfunction due to other causes, such as CAD. Several processes may present with **dilated or congestive cardiomyopathy,** which is characterized by LV or biventricular dilation and generalized systolic dysfunction. These are discussed elsewhere in this chapter, but the most common are alcoholic cardiomyopathy, viral myocarditis (including infections by HIV), and dilated cardiomyopathies with no obvious underlying cause (idiopathic cardiomyopathy). Rare causes of dilated cardiomyopathy include infiltrative diseases (hemochromatosis, sarcoidosis, amyloidosis, etc), other infectious agents, metabolic disorders, cardiotoxins, and medication toxicity. VHDs—particularly degenerative aortic stenosis and chronic aortic or mitral regurgitation—are not infrequent causes of heart failure. Persistent tachycardia, often related to atrial arrhythmias, can cause systolic dysfunction that may be reversible with controlling the rate. **Diastolic cardiac dysfunction** is associated with aging and related myocardial stiffening, as well as LVH, commonly resulting from hypertension. Conditions such as hypertrophic or restrictive cardiomyopathy, diabetes, and pericardial disease can produce the same clinical picture. Atrial fibrillation with or without rapid ventricular response may contribute to impaired left ventricular filling.

Heart failure is often preventable by early detection of patients at risk and by early intervention. The importance of these approaches is emphasized by US guidelines that have incorporated a classification of heart failure that includes four stages. **Stage A** includes patients at risk for developing heart failure (such as patients with hypertension). In the majority of these patients, development of heart failure can be prevented with interventions such as the aggressive treatment of hypertension, modification of coronary risk factors, and reduction of excessive alcohol intake. **Stage B** includes patients who have structural heart disease but no current or previously recognized symptoms of heart failure. Examples include patients with previous myocardial infarction, other causes of reduced systolic function, LVH, or asymptomatic valvular disease. Both ACE inhibitors and beta-blockers prevent heart failure in the first two of these conditions, and more aggressive treatment of hypertension and early surgical intervention are effective in the latter two. **Stages C** and **D** include patients with clinical heart failure and the relatively small group of patients that has become refractory to the usual therapies, respectively. These are discussed below.

▶ **Clinical Findings**

A. Symptoms

The most common symptom of patients with **left heart failure** is shortness of breath, chiefly exertional dyspnea at first and then progressing to orthopnea, paroxysmal nocturnal dyspnea, and rest dyspnea. Chronic nonproductive cough, which is often worse in the recumbent position, may occur. Nocturia due to excretion of fluid retained during the day and increased renal perfusion in the recumbent position is a common nonspecific symptom of heart failure, as is fatigue and exercise intolerance. These symptoms correlate poorly with the degree of cardiac dysfunction. Patients with **right heart failure** have predominate signs of fluid retention, with the patient exhibiting edema, hepatic congestion and, on occasion, loss of appetite and nausea due to edema of the gut or impaired gastrointestinal perfusion and ascites. **Surprisingly, some individuals with severe LV dysfunction will display few signs of left heart failure and appear to have isolated right heart failure.** Indeed, they may be clinically indistinguishable from patients with cor pulmonale, who have right heart failure secondary to pulmonary disease.

Patients with acute heart failure from myocardial infarction, myocarditis, and acute valvular regurgitation due to endocarditis or other conditions usually present with pulmonary edema. Patients with episodic symptoms may be having LV dysfunction due to intermittent ischemia. Patients may also present with acute exacerbations of chronic, stable heart failure. Exacerbations are usually caused by alterations in therapy (or patient noncompliance), excessive salt and fluid intake, arrhythmias, excessive activity, pulmonary emboli, intercurrent infection, or progression of the underlying disease.

Patients with heart failure are often categorized by the NYHA classification as **class I** (asymptomatic), **class II** (symptomatic with moderate activity), **class III** (symptomatic with mild activity), or **class IV** (symptomatic at rest). This classification is important since some of the treatments are indicated based on NYHA classification.

B. Signs

Many patients with heart failure, including some with severe symptoms, appear comfortable at rest. Others will be dyspneic during conversation or minor activity, and those with long-standing severe heart failure may appear cachectic or cyanotic. The vital signs may be normal, but tachycardia, hypotension, and reduced pulse pressure may be present. Patients often show signs of increased sympathetic nervous system activity, including cold extremities and diaphoresis. Important peripheral signs of heart failure can be detected by examination of the neck, the lungs, the abdomen, and the extremities. RA pressure may be estimated through the height of the pulsations in the jugular venous system. In addition to the height of the venous pressure, abnormal pulsations, such as regurgitant v waves, should be sought. Examination of the carotid pulse may allow estimation of pulse pressure as well as detection of aortic stenosis. Thyroid examination may reveal occult hyperthyroidism or hypothyroidism, which are readily treatable causes of heart failure. Crackles at the lung bases reflect transudation of fluid into the alveoli. Pleural effusions may cause bibasilar dullness to percussion. Expiratory wheezing and rhonchi may be signs of heart failure. Patients with severe right heart failure may have hepatic enlargement—tender or nontender—due to passive congestion. Systolic pulsations may be felt in tricuspid regurgitation. Sustained moderate pressure on the liver may increase jugular venous pressure (a positive hepatojugular reflux is an increase of greater than 1 cm). Ascites may also be present. Peripheral pitting edema is a common sign in patients with right heart failure and may extend into the thighs and abdominal wall.

Cardinal cardiac examination signs are a parasternal lift, indicating pulmonary hypertension; an enlarged and sustained LV impulse, indicating LV dilation and hypertrophy; a diminished first heart sound, suggesting impaired contractility; and an S_3 gallop originating in the LV and sometimes the RV. An S_4 is usually present in diastolic heart failure. Murmurs should be sought to exclude primary valvular disease; secondary mitral regurgitation and tricuspid regurgitation murmurs are common in patients with dilated ventricles. In chronic heart failure, many of the expected signs of heart failure may be absent despite markedly abnormal cardiac function and hemodynamic measurements.

C. Laboratory Findings

A blood count may reveal anemia and a high red-cell distribution width (RDW), both of which are associated with poor prognosis in chronic heart failure through poorly understood mechanisms. Kidney function tests can determine whether cardiac failure is associated with impaired kidney function that may reflect poor kidney perfusion. Chronic kidney disease is another poor prognostic factor in heart failure and may limit certain treatment options. Serum electrolytes may disclose hypokalemia, which increases the risk of arrhythmias; hyperkalemia, which may limit the use of inhibitors of the renin–angiotensin system; or hyponatremia, an indicator of marked activation of the renin–angiotensin system and a poor prognostic sign. Thyroid function should be assessed to detect occult thyrotoxicosis or myxedema, and iron studies should be checked to test for hemochromatosis. In unexplained cases, appropriate biopsies may lead to a diagnosis of amyloidosis. Myocardial biopsy may exclude specific causes of dilated cardiomyopathy but rarely reveals specific reversible diagnoses.

Serum BNP is a powerful prognostic marker that adds to clinical assessment in differentiating dyspnea due to heart failure from noncardiac causes. Two markers—BNP and NT-proBNP—provide similar diagnostic and prognostic information. BNP is expressed primarily in the ventricles and is elevated when ventricular filling pressures are high. It is quite sensitive in patients with symptomatic heart failure—whether due to systolic or to diastolic dysfunction—but less specific in older patients, women, and patients with COPD. Studies have shown that BNP can help in emergency department triage in the diagnosis of acute decompensated heart failure, such that an NT-proBNP less than 300 pg/mL or BNP less than 100 pg/mL, combined with a normal ECG, makes heart failure unlikely. BNP is less sensitive and specific to diagnose heart failure in the chronic setting. BNP may be helpful in guiding the intensity of diuretic and a more consistent use of disease-modifying therapies, such as ACE inhibitors and beta-blockers, for the management of chronic heart failure. Worsening breathlessness or weight associated with a rising BNP (or both) might prompt increasing the dose of diuretics. However, to date, in spite of evidence from a meta-analysis of randomized trials showing benefit from using BNP to guide therapy, particularly for patients younger than 75 years, practice guidelines have not yet recommended this strategy. Elevation of serum troponin, and especially of high-sensitivity troponin, is common in both chronic and acute heart failure, and it is associated with higher risk of adverse outcomes.

D. ECG and Chest Radiography

ECG may indicate an underlying or secondary arrhythmia, myocardial infarction, or nonspecific changes that often include low voltage, intraventricular conduction defects, LVH, and nonspecific repolarization changes. Chest radiographs provide information about the size and shape of the cardiac silhouette. Cardiomegaly is an important finding and is a poor prognostic sign. Evidence of pulmonary venous hypertension includes relative dilation of the upper lobe veins, perivascular edema (haziness of vessel outlines), interstitial edema, and alveolar fluid. In acute heart failure, these findings correlate moderately well with pulmonary venous pressure. However, patients with chronic heart failure may show relatively normal pulmonary vasculature despite markedly elevated pressures. Pleural effusions are common and tend to be bilateral or right-sided.

E. Additional Studies

Many studies have indicated that the clinical diagnosis of systolic myocardial dysfunction is often inaccurate. The primary confounding conditions are diastolic dysfunction of the heart with decreased relaxation and filling of the LV (particularly in hypertension and in hypertrophic states) and pulmonary disease. Because patients with heart failure usually have significant resting ECG abnormalities, stress imaging procedures, such as perfusion scintigraphy or dobutamine echocardiography, are often indicated.

The most useful test is the echocardiogram because it can differentiate heart failure with and without preserved LV systolic function. The echocardiogram can define the size and function of both ventricles and of the atria. It will also allow detection of pericardial effusion, valvular abnormalities, intracardiac shunts, and segmental wall motion abnormalities suggestive of old myocardial infarction as opposed to more generalized forms of dilated cardiomyopathy.

Radionuclide angiography as well as cardiac MRI also measure LVEF and permit analysis of regional wall motion. These tests are especially useful when echocardiography is technically suboptimal, such as in patients with severe pulmonary disease. When myocardial ischemia is suspected as a cause of LV dysfunction, stress testing should be performed.

F. Cardiac Catheterization

In most patients with heart failure, clinical examination and noninvasive tests can determine LV size and function and valve function to confirm the diagnosis. Left heart catheterization may be helpful to define the presence and extent of CAD, although CT angiography may also be appropriate, especially when the likelihood of coronary disease is low. Evaluation for coronary disease is particularly important when LV dysfunction may be partially reversible by revascularization. The combination of angina or noninvasive evidence of significant myocardial ischemia with symptomatic heart failure is often an indication for coronary angiography if the patient is a potential candidate for revascularization. Right heart catheterization may be useful to select and monitor therapy in patients refractory to standard therapy.

▶ Treatment: Heart Failure with Reduced EF

The treatment of heart failure is aimed at relieving symptoms, improving functional status, and preventing death and hospitalizations. Figure 10–9 outlines the role of the major pharmacologic and device therapies for chronic

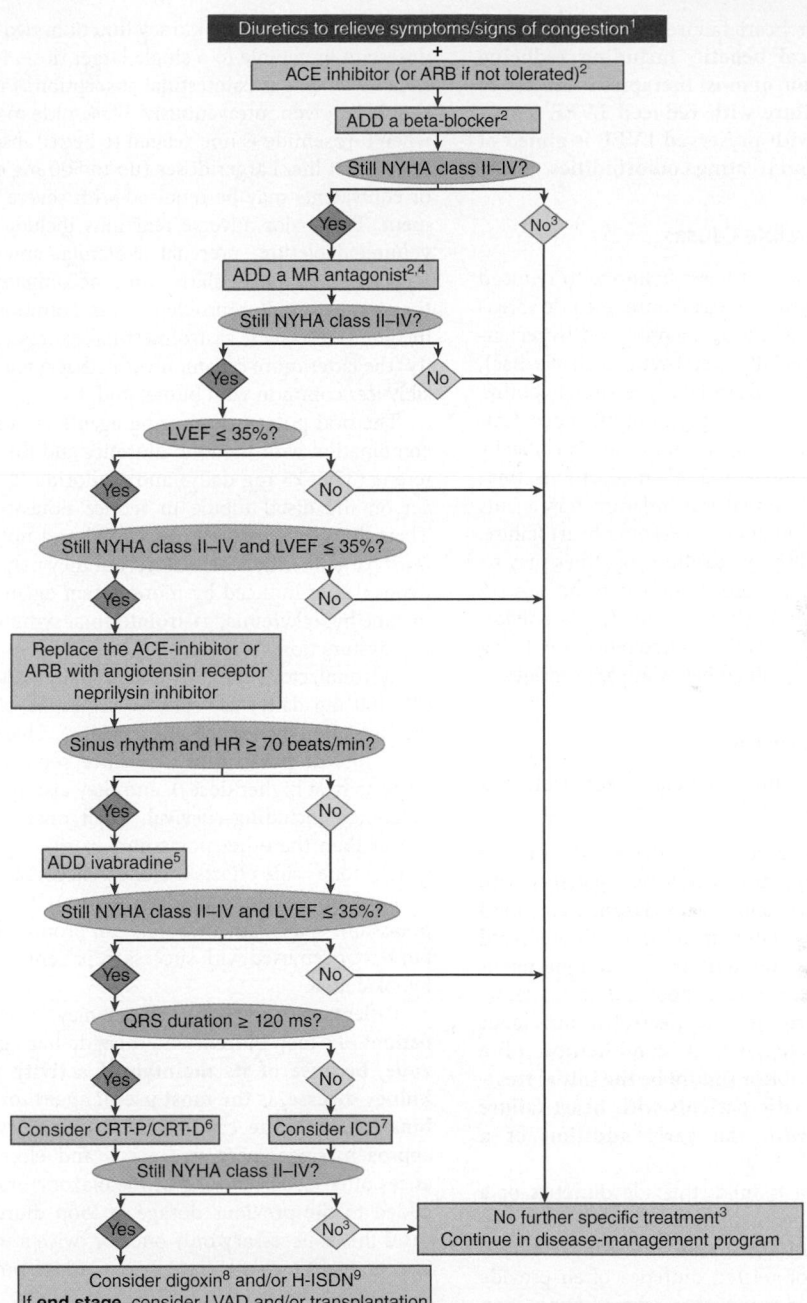

▲ **Figure 10–9.** Treatment options for patients with chronic symptomatic systolic heart failure. ACE, angiotensin-converting enzyme; ARB, angiotensin receptor blocker; CRT-D, cardiac resynchronization therapy defibrillator; CRT-P, cardiac resynchronization therapy pacemaker; H-ISDN, hydralazine and isosorbide dinitrate; HR, heart rate; ICD, implantable cardioverter defibrillator; LBBB, left bundle branch block; LVAD, left ventricular assist device; LVEF, left ventricular ejection fraction; MR antagonist, mineralocorticoid receptor antagonist; NYHA, New York Heart Association. (Modified, with permission, from McMurray JJ et al. ESC guidelines for the diagnosis and treatment of acute and chronic heart failure 2012: the Task Force for the Diagnosis and Treatment of Acute and Chronic Heart Failure 2012 of the European Society of Cardiology. Eur J Heart Fail. 2012 Aug;14(8):803–69. [PMID: 22828712])

systolic heart failure (or heart failure with reduced EF). **The evidence of clinical benefit, including reducing death and hospitalization, of most therapies is limited to patients with heart failure with reduced LVEF. Treatment of heart failure with preserved LVEF is aimed at improving symptoms and treating comorbidities.**

A. Correction of Reversible Causes

The major reversible causes of heart failure with reduced EF, also called chronic systolic heart failure, include valvular lesions, myocardial ischemia, uncontrolled hypertension, arrhythmias (especially persistent tachycardias), alcohol- or drug-induced myocardial depression, hypothyroidism, intracardiac shunts, and high-output states. Calcium channel blockers with negative inotropy (specifically verapamil or diltiazem), antiarrhythmic medications, thiazolidinediones, and nonsteroidal anti-inflammatory agents may be important contributors to worsening heart failure. Some metabolic and infiltrative cardiomyopathies may be partially reversible, or their progression may be slowed; these include hemochromatosis, sarcoidosis, and amyloidosis. Once possible reversible components are being addressed, the measures outlined below are appropriate.

B. Pharmacologic Treatment

See also the following section on Acute Heart Failure & Pulmonary Edema.

1. Diuretic therapy—Diuretics are the most effective means of providing symptomatic relief to patients with moderate to severe heart failure with dyspnea and fluid overload, for heart failure with reduced and with preserved LVEF. Few patients with symptoms or signs of fluid retention can be optimally managed without a diuretic. However, excessive diuresis can lead to electrolyte imbalance and neurohormonal activation. **A combination of a diuretic and an ACE inhibitor should be the initial treatment in most symptomatic patients with heart failure and reduced LVEF, with the early addition of a beta-blocker.**

When fluid retention is mild, thiazide diuretics or a similar type of agent (hydrochlorothiazide, 25–100 mg; metolazone, 2.5–5 mg; chlorthalidone, 25–50 mg; etc) may be sufficient. Thiazide or related diuretics often provide better control of hypertension than short-acting loop agents. The thiazides are generally ineffective when the glomerular filtration rate falls below 30–40 mL/min, a not infrequent occurrence in patients with severe heart failure. Metolazone maintains its efficacy down to a glomerular filtration rate of approximately 20–30 mL/min. Adverse reactions include hypokalemia and intravascular volume depletion with resulting prerenal azotemia, skin rashes, neutropenia and thrombocytopenia, hyperglycemia, hyperuricemia, and hepatic dysfunction.

Patients with more severe heart failure should be treated with one of the oral loop diuretics. These include furosemide (20–320 mg daily), bumetanide (1–8 mg daily), and torsemide (20–200 mg daily). These agents have a rapid onset and a relatively short duration of action. In patients with preserved kidney function, two or more daily doses are preferable to a single larger dose. In acute situations or when gastrointestinal absorption is in doubt, they should be given intravenously. Torsemide may be effective when furosemide is not, related to better absorption and a longer half life. Larger doses (up to 500 mg of furosemide or equivalent) may be required with severe renal impairment. The major adverse reactions include intravascular volume depletion, prerenal azotemia, and hypotension. Hypokalemia, particularly with accompanying digitalis therapy, is a major problem. Less common side effects include skin rashes, gastrointestinal distress, and ototoxicity (the latter more common with ethacrynic acid and possibly less common with bumetanide).

The oral potassium-sparing agents are often useful in combination with the loop diuretics and thiazides. Triamterene (37.5–75 mg daily) and amiloride (5–10 mg daily) act on the distal tubule to reduce potassium secretion. Their diuretic potency is only mild and not adequate for most patients with heart failure, but they may minimize the hypokalemia induced by more potent agents. Side effects include hyperkalemia, gastrointestinal symptoms, and kidney dysfunction.

Spironolactone (12.5–100 mg daily) and eplerenone (25–100 mg daily) are specific inhibitors of aldosterone, which is often increased in heart failure. These medications spare loss of potassium, they have some diuretic effect (especially at higher doses), and they also improve clinical outcomes, including survival. Their onsets of action are slower than the other potassium-sparing agents, and spironolactone's side effects include gynecomastia. Combinations of potassium supplements or ACE inhibitors and potassium-sparing medications can produce hyperkalemia but have been used with success in patients with persistent hypokalemia.

Patients with refractory edema may respond to combinations of a loop diuretic and thiazide-like agents. **Metolazone, because of its maintained activity with chronic kidney disease, is the most useful agent for such a combination.** Extreme caution must be observed with this approach, since massive diuresis and electrolyte imbalances often occur; 2.5 mg of metolazone orally should be added to the previous dosage of loop diuretic. In many cases this is necessary only once or twice a week, but dosages up to 10 mg daily have been used in some patients.

2. Inhibitors of the renin–angiotensin–aldosterone system—Inhibition of the renin–angiotensin–aldosterone system with ACE inhibitors should be part of the initial therapy of this syndrome based on their mortality benefits.

A. ACE INHIBITORS—At least seven ACE inhibitors have been shown to be effective for the treatment of heart failure or the related indication of postinfarction LV dysfunction (see Table 11–7). ACE inhibitors reduce mortality by approximately 20% in patients with symptomatic heart failure and have also been shown to prevent hospitalizations, increase exercise tolerance, and reduce symptoms in these patients. As a result, **ACE inhibitors generally should be part of first-line treatment of patients with symptomatic LV systolic dysfunction (EF less than 40%),**

usually in combination with a diuretic. They are also indicated for the management of patients with reduced EFs without symptoms because they prevent the progression to clinical heart failure.

Because ACE inhibitors may induce significant hypotension, particularly following the initial doses, they must be started with caution. Hypotension is most prominent in patients with already low BPs (systolic pressure less than 100 mm Hg), hypovolemia, prerenal azotemia (especially if it is diuretic induced), and hyponatremia (an indicator of activation of the renin–angiotensin system). These patients should generally be started at low dosages (captopril 6.25 mg orally three times daily, enalapril 2.5 mg orally daily, or the equivalent), but other patients may be started at twice these dosages. Within several days (for those with the markers of higher risk) or at most 2 weeks, patients should be questioned about symptoms of hypotension, and both kidney function and potassium levels should be monitored.

ACE inhibitors should be titrated to the dosages proved effective in clinical trials (captopril 50 mg three times daily, enalapril 10 mg twice daily, ramipril 10 mg daily, lisinopril 20 mg daily, or the equivalent) over a period of 1–3 months. Most patients will tolerate these doses. Asymptomatic hypotension is not a contraindication to up-titrating or continuing ACE inhibitors. Some patients exhibit increases in serum creatinine or potassium, but they do not require discontinuation if the levels stabilize—even at values as high as 3 mg/dL and 5.5 mEq/L, respectively. Kidney dysfunction is more frequent in patients with diabetes, older patients, and those with low systolic pressures, and these groups should be monitored more closely. The most common side effects of ACE inhibitors in heart failure patients are dizziness (often not related to the level of BP) and cough, though the latter is often due as much to heart failure or intercurrent pulmonary conditions as to the ACE inhibitor. ACE inhibitor–induced cough is more common in women than in men.

B. Angiotensin II receptor blockers—Another approach to inhibiting the renin–angiotensin–aldosterone system is the use of specific ARBs (see Table 11–7), which will decrease adverse effects of angiotensin II by blocking the AT$_1$ receptor. In addition, because there are alternative pathways of angiotensin II production in many tissues, the receptor blockers may provide more complete blockade of the AT$_1$ receptor.

However, these agents do not share the effects of ACE inhibitors on other potentially important pathways that produce increases in bradykinin, prostaglandins, and nitric oxide in the heart, blood vessels, and other tissues. **ARBs, specifically candesartan or valsartan, provide important benefits as an alternative to, and in addition to, ACE inhibitors in chronic heart failure with reduced LVEF.** (A large trial of patients with chronic heart failure and preserved LVEF found no benefit from the ARB irbesartan.)

C. Spironolactione and eplerenone—Inhibiting aldosterone has become a mainstay of management of symptomatic heart failure with reduced LVEF. The RALES trial compared spironolactone 25 mg daily with placebo in patients with advanced heart failure (current or recent class IV) already receiving ACE inhibitors and diuretics and showed a 29% reduction in mortality as well as similar decreases in other clinical end points. Based on the EMPHASIS-HF trial, **the efficacy and safety of aldosterone antagonism—in the form of eplerenone, 25–50 mg orally daily—is established for patients with mild or moderate heart failure.** Hyperkalemia was uncommon in severe heart failure clinical trial patients who received high doses of diuretic as maintenance therapy; however, hyperkalemia in patients taking spironolactone appears to be common in general practice. **Potassium levels must be monitored closely during initiation of spironolactone (after 1 and 4 weeks of therapy) and periodically thereafter, particularly for patients with even mild degrees of kidney injury, and in patients receiving ACE inhibitors.**

D. Combination sacubitril and valsartan—The most recently approved medication to improve clinical outcome in patients with heart failure and reduced LVEF is the combination neprilysin inhibitor sacubitril and angiotensin II receptor blocker valsartan. Compared to the ACE inhibitor enalapril, the angiotensin-neprilysin inhibitor was shown to reduce cardiovascular death and hospitalization for heart failure by 20% for patients with heart failure and reduced LVEF in a large randomized trial (PARADIGM-HF) of patients already taking an ACE inhibitor or ARB.

3. Beta-blockers—Beta-blockers are part of the foundation of care of chronic heart failure based on their life-saving benefits. The mechanism of this benefit remains unclear, but it is likely that chronic elevations of catecholamines and sympathetic nervous system activity cause progressive myocardial damage, leading to worsening LV function and dilation. The primary evidence for this hypothesis is that over a period of 3–6 months, beta-blockers produce consistent substantial rises in EF (averaging 10% absolute increase) and reductions in LV size and mass.

Three medications have strong evidence of reducing mortality: **carvedilol** (a nonselective beta-1- and beta-2-receptor blocker), the beta-1-selective **extended-release agent metoprolol succinate** (but not short-acting metoprolol tartrate), and **bisoprolol** (beta-1-selective agent). This has led to a strong recommendation that *stable patients (defined as having no recent deterioration or evidence of volume overload) with mild, moderate, and even severe heart failure should be treated with a beta-blocker unless there is a noncardiac contraindication.* In the COPERNICUS trial, carvedilol was both well tolerated and highly effective in reducing both mortality and heart failure hospitalizations in a group of patients with severe (NYHA class III or IV) symptoms, but care was taken to ensure that they were free of fluid retention at the time of initiation. In this study, one death was prevented for every 13 patients treated for 1 year—as dramatic an effect as has been seen with a pharmacologic therapy in the history of cardiovascular medicine. One trial comparing carvedilol and (short-acting) metoprolol tartrate (COMET) found significant reductions in all-cause mortality and cardiovascular mortality with carvedilol. Thus, patients with chronic heart failure should be treated with extended-release metoprolol succinate, bisoprolol, or carvedilol but *not* short-acting metoprolol tartrate.

Because even apparently stable patients may deteriorate when beta-blockers are initiated, initiation must be done gradually and with great care. Carvedilol is initiated at a dosage of 3.125 mg orally twice daily and may be increased to 6.25, 12.5, and 25 mg twice daily at intervals of approximately 2 weeks. The protocols for sustained-release metoprolol use were started at 12.5 or 25 mg orally daily and doubled at intervals of 2 weeks to a target dose of 200 mg daily (using the Toprol XL sustained-release preparation). Bisoprolol was administered at a dosage of 1.25, 2.5, 3.75, 5, 7.5, and 10 mg orally daily, with increments at 1- to 4-week intervals. More gradual up-titration is often more convenient and may be better tolerated. The SENIORS trial of 2135 patients found that nebivolol was effective in elderly patients (70 years and older) with chronic heart failure, although the evidence of degree of benefit was not as strong as with the three proven beta-blockers carvedilol, metoprolol succinate, or bisoprolol.

Patients should be instructed to monitor their weights at home as an indicator of fluid retention and to report any increase or change in symptoms immediately. Before each dose increase, patients should be seen and examined to ensure that there has not been fluid retention or worsening of symptoms. If heart failure worsens, this can usually be managed by increasing diuretic doses and delaying further increases in beta-blocker doses, though downward adjustments or discontinuation is sometimes required. Carvedilol, because of its beta-blocking activity, may cause dizziness or hypotension. This can usually be managed by reducing the doses of other vasodilators and by slowing the pace of dose increases.

4. Digitalis glycosides—The efficacy of digitalis glycosides in reducing the symptoms of heart failure has been established in at least four multicenter trials that have demonstrated that digoxin withdrawal is associated with worsening symptoms and signs of heart failure, more frequent hospitalizations for decompensation, and reduced exercise tolerance. **Digoxin should be considered for patients who remain symptomatic when taking diuretics and ACE inhibitors as well as for patients with heart failure who are in atrial fibrillation and require rate control.**

Digoxin has a half-life of 24–36 hours and is eliminated almost entirely by the kidneys. The oral maintenance dose may range from 0.125 mg three times weekly to 0.5 mg daily. It is lower in patients with kidney dysfunction, in older patients, and in those with smaller lean body mass. Although an oral loading dose of 0.75–1.25 mg (depending primarily on lean body size) over 24–48 hours may be given if an early effect is desired, in most patients with chronic heart failure it is sufficient to begin with the expected maintenance dose (usually 0.125–0.25 mg daily). Amiodarone, quinidine, propafenone, and verapamil are among the medications that may increase digoxin levels up to 100%. It is prudent to measure a blood level after 7–14 days (and at least 6 hours after the last dose was administered). Optimum serum digoxin levels are 0.7–1.2 ng/mL, though clinically evident toxicity is rare with levels less than 1.8 ng/mL. Digoxin may induce ventricular arrhythmias, especially when hypokalemia or myocardial ischemia is present. Once an appropriate maintenance dose is established, subsequent levels are usually not indicated unless there is a change in kidney function or medications that affects digoxin levels or a significant deterioration in cardiac status that may be associated with reduced clearance. Digoxin toxicity is discussed in Chapter 38.

5. Nitrates and hydralazine—Although ACE inhibitors, which have vasodilating properties, improve prognosis, such a benefit is not established with the direct-acting vasodilators. The combination of hydralazine and isosorbide dinitrate has been shown to improve outcome in African Americans, but the effect is less clear than the well-established benefits of ACE inhibitors. The 2012 European guidelines give hydralazine and isosorbide dinitrate a modest class IIb recommendation for patients with reduced LVEF who are unable to tolerate ACE inhibitor and ARB therapy or who have persistent symptoms despite treatment with a beta-blocker, ACE inhibitor, and aldosterone antagonist.

See section on Acute Myocardial Infarction earlier in this chapter for a discussion on the intravenous vasodilating drugs and their dosages.

A. NITRATES—Intravenous vasodilators (sodium nitroprusside or nitroglycerin) are used primarily for acute or severely decompensated chronic heart failure, especially when accompanied by hypertension or myocardial ischemia. If neither of the latter is present, therapy is best initiated and adjusted based on hemodynamic measurements. The starting dosage for nitroglycerin is generally about 10 mcg/min, which is titrated upward by 10–20 mcg/min (to a maximum of 200 mcg/min) until mean arterial pressure drops by 10%. Hypotension (BP less than 100 mm Hg systolic) should be avoided. For sodium nitroprusside, the starting dosage is 5–10 mcg/min, with upward titration to a maximum dose of 400 mcg/min.

Isosorbide dinitrate, 20–40 mg orally three times daily, and nitroglycerin ointment, 2%, 15–16 mg (1.4 inches; 1 inch = 15 mg) every 6–8 hours, appears to be equally effective, although the ointment is generally reserved for inpatient use only. The nitrates are moderately effective in relieving shortness of breath, especially in patients with mild to moderate symptoms, but less successful—probably because they have little effect on cardiac output—in advanced heart failure. Nitrate therapy is generally well tolerated, but headaches and hypotension may limit the dose of all agents. The development of tolerance to long-term nitrate therapy occurs. This is minimized by intermittent therapy, especially if a daily 8- to 12-hour nitrate-free interval is used, but probably develops to some extent in most patients receiving these agents. Transdermal nitroglycerin patches have no sustained effect in patients with heart failure and should not be used for this indication.

B. HYDRALAZINE—Oral hydralazine is a potent arteriolar dilator; when used as a single agent, it has not been shown to improve symptoms or exercise tolerance during long-term treatment. The combination of nitrates and oral hydralazine produces greater hemodynamic effects.

Hydralazine therapy is frequently limited by side effects. Approximately 30% of patients are unable to tolerate the relatively high doses required to produce hemodynamic improvement in heart failure (200–400 mg daily in divided doses). The major side effect is gastrointestinal distress, but headaches, tachycardia, and hypotension are relatively common. ARBs have largely supplanted the use of the hydralazine–isosorbide dinitrate combination in ACE-intolerant patients.

6. Ivabradine—Ivabradine inhibits the I_f channel in the sinus node and has the specific effect of slowing sinus rate. Ivabradine is approved by the FDA for use in stable patients with heart failure and heart rate of 70 beats per minute who are taking the maximally tolerated dose of beta-blockers or in patients in whom beta-blockers are contraindicated. It is approved by the European Medicines Agency for use in patients with a heart rate of 75 beats per minute or more. The European guidelines give it a class IIa recommendation for patients in sinus rhythm with a heart rate of 70 beats per minute or more with an EF of 35% or less, and persisting symptoms despite treatment with an evidence-based dose of beta-blocker (or a maximum tolerated dose below that), ACE inhibitor (or ARB), and an aldosterone antagonist (or ARB). In a trial of patients with chronic angina, ivabradine did not reduce cardiovascular events, and there may have been more events with ivabradine (than placebo) in patients with symptomatic angina.

7. Combination of medical therapies—Optimal management of chronic heart failure involves using combinations of proven life-saving therapies. In addition to ACE inhibitors and beta-blockers, patients who remain symptomatic should be considered for additional therapy, in the form of ARBs (best proven in class II–III heart failure), mineralocorticoid (aldosterone) receptor antagonists, or hydralazine and isosorbide dinitrate (with some evidence of benefit in African Americans). However, combination of ACE inhibitor, ARB, and mineralocorticoid receptor antagonists should generally be avoided due to risk of hyperkalemia.

8. Treatments that may cause harm in heart failure with reduced LVEF—Several therapies should be avoided, when possible, in patients with systolic heart failure. These include thiazoladinediones (glitazones) that cause worsening heart failure, most calcium channel blockers (with the exception of amlodipine and felodipine), nonsteroidal anti-inflammatory medications, and cyclooxygenase-2 inhibitors that cause sodium and water retention and renal impairment, and the combination of an ACE inhibitor, ARB, and aldosterone blocker that increases the risk of hyperkalemia.

9. Anticoagulation—Patients with LV failure and reduced EF are at somewhat increased risk for developing intracardiac thrombi and systemic arterial emboli. However, this risk appears to be primarily in patients who are in atrial fibrillation, who have had thromboemboli, or who have had a large recent anterior myocardial infarction. In general, these patients should receive warfarin for 3 months following the myocardial infarction. Other patients with heart failure have embolic rates of approximately two per 100 patient-years of follow-up, which approximates the rate of major bleeding, and routine anticoagulation does not appear warranted except in patients with prior embolic events or mobile LV thrombi.

10. Antiarrhythmic therapy—Patients with moderate to severe heart failure have a high incidence of both symptomatic and asymptomatic arrhythmias. Although less than 10% of patients have syncope or presyncope resulting from ventricular tachycardia, ambulatory monitoring reveals that up to 70% of patients have asymptomatic episodes of NSVT. These arrhythmias indicate a poor prognosis independent of the severity of LV dysfunction, but many of the deaths are probably not arrhythmia related. Beta-blockers, because of their marked favorable effect on prognosis in general and on the incidence of sudden death specifically, should be initiated in these as well as all other patients with heart failure (see Beta-Blockers, above). Empiric antiarrhythmic therapy with amiodarone did not improve outcome in the SCD-HeFT trial, and most other agents are contraindicated because of their proarrhythmic effects in this population and their adverse effect on cardiac function. For patients with systolic heart failure and atrial fibrillation, a rhythm control strategy has not been shown to improve outcome compared to a rate control strategy and thus should be reserved for patients with a reversible cause of atrial fibrillation or refractory symptoms. Then, amiodarone is the drug of choice.

11. Statin therapy—Even though vascular disease is present in many patients with chronic heart failure, the role of statins has not been well defined in the heart failure population. The CORONA and the GISSI-HF trials show no benefits of statins in the chronic heart failure population.

C. Nonpharmacologic Treatment

1. Implantable cardioverter defibrillators—Indications for ICDs include not only patients with symptomatic or asymptomatic arrhythmias but also patients with chronic heart failure and LV systolic dysfunction who are receiving contemporary heart failure treatments, including beta-blockers. In the second Multicenter Automatic Defibrillator Implantation Trial (MADIT II), 1232 patients with prior myocardial infarction and an EF less than 30% were randomized to an ICD or a control group. Mortality was 31% lower in the ICD group, which translated into 9 lives saved for each 100 patients who received a device and were monitored for 3 years. The United States Centers for Medicare and Medicaid Services provides reimbursement coverage to include patients with **chronic heart failure and ischemic or nonischemic cardiomyopathy with an EF of 35% or less.**

2. Biventricular pacing (resynchronization)—Many patients with heart failure due to systolic dysfunction have abnormal intraventricular conduction that results in dyssynchronous and hence inefficient contractions. Several studies have evaluated the efficacy of "multisite" pacing, using leads that stimulate the RV from the apex and the LV from the lateral wall via the coronary sinus. Patients with wide QRS complexes (generally 120 msec or more), reduced EFs, and moderate to severe symptoms have been evaluated. Results from trials with up to 2 years of follow-up have shown an increase in EF, improvement in symptoms and exercise tolerance, and reduction in death and hospitalization. The best responders to cardiac resynchronization therapy are patients with wider QRS, left bundle branch block, and nonischemic cardiomyopathy, and the lowest responders are those with narrow QRS and non–left bundle branch block pattern. Thus, as recommended in the 2013 European guidelines, **resynchronization therapy is indicated for patients with class II, III, and ambulatory class IV heart failure, EF of 35% or less, and left bundle branch block pattern with QRS duration of 120 msec or more.** Patients with non–left bundle branch block pattern and prolonged QRS duration may be considered for treatment.

3. Case management, diet, and exercise training—Thirty to 50 percent of heart failure patients who are hospitalized will be readmitted within 3–6 months. **Strategies to prevent clinical deterioration, such as case management, home monitoring of weight and clinical status, and patient adjustment of diuretics, can prevent rehospitalizations and should be part of the treatment regimen of advanced heart failure.** Involvement of a multidisciplinary team (rather than a single physician) and in-person (rather than telephonic) communication appear to be important features of successful programs.

Patients should routinely practice moderate salt restriction (2–2.5 g sodium or 5–6 g salt per day). More severe sodium restriction is usually difficult to achieve and unnecessary because of the availability of potent diuretic agents.

Exercise training improves activity tolerance in significant part by reversing the peripheral abnormalities associated with heart failure and deconditioning. In severe heart failure, restriction of activity may facilitate temporary recompensation. A large trial showed no significant benefit (nor harm) from a structured exercise training program on death or hospitalization, although functional status and symptoms were improved. Thus, in stable patients, a prudent increase in activity or a regular exercise regimen can be encouraged. Indeed, a gradual exercise program is associated with diminished symptoms and substantial increases in exercise capacity.

4. Coronary revascularization—Since underlying CAD is the cause of heart failure in the majority of patients, coronary revascularization has been thought to be able to both improve symptoms and prevent progression. However, the STITCH trial failed to show an overall survival benefit from CABG among patients with multivessel coronary disease who were candidates for CABG but who also had heart failure and an LVEF of 35% or less. Revascularization does appear warranted for some patients with heart failure, including those with more severe angina or left main coronary disease (excluded from the STITCH trial), or selected patients with less severe symptoms.

5. Cardiac transplantation—Because of the poor prognosis of patients with advanced heart failure, cardiac transplantation is widely used. Many centers have 1-year

survival rates exceeding 80–90%, and 5-year survival rates above 70%. Infections, hypertension and kidney dysfunction caused by cyclosporine, rapidly progressive coronary atherosclerosis, and immunosuppressant-related cancers have been the major complications. The high cost and limited number of donor organs require careful patient selection early in the course.

6. Other surgical treatment options—Externally powered and implantable ventricular assist devices can be used in patients who require ventricular support either to allow the heart to recover or as a bridge to transplantation. The latest generation devices are small enough to allow patients unrestricted mobility and even discharge from the hospital. Continuous flow devices appear to be more effective than pulsatile flow devices. However, complications are frequent, including bleeding, thromboembolism, and infection, and the cost is very high, exceeding $200,000 in the initial 1–3 months.

Although 1-year survival was improved in the REMATCH randomized trial, all 129 patients died by 26 months. Newer-generation continuous flow pump ventricular assist devices have been shown to result in better survival than the first-generation pulsatile flow device used in REMATCH.

7. Palliative care—Despite the technologic advances of recent years, it should be remembered that many patients with chronic heart failure are elderly and have multiple comorbidities. Many of them will not experience meaningful improvements in survival with aggressive therapy. The goal of management for these patients and all those with serious illness should include symptomatic improvement and palliation (see Chapter 5).

▶ **Treatment: Heart Failure with Preserved EF**

Although half of all heart failure occurs among patients with normal LVEF, often with diastolic dysfunction, **no therapies have been shown to improve survival in this population.** The mainstay of management of patients with heart failure with preserved EF is to manage fluid overload with diuretic therapy and to treat comorbidities like hypertension.

A. Correction of Reversible Causes

Hypertension, pericardial disease, and atrial tachycardias are potentially reversible factors that can contribute to heart failure with preserved EF. Since tachycardia is associated with shorter overall diastolic filling time, controlling accelerated heart rate may be important.

B. Pharmacologic Treatment

1. Diuretic therapy—Diuretics are important to control symptoms of fluid overload in patients with heart failure with preserved EF, similar to symptoms from systolic heart failure.

2. Inhibitors of the renin-angiotensin-aldosterone system—ACE inhibitors and ARBs have *not* been shown to improve outcome in patients with heart failure and preserved EF, despite being good therapies for the comorbidity of hypertension. Spironolactone has not shown to improve outcome in a large trial of patients with heart failure and preserved EF, but there may have been some benefit in patients enrolled in the Americas who had more clearly defined heart failure. Spironolactone should remain a therapeutic option, especially for patients who also have hypertension.

C. Nonpharmacologic Treatment

Unlike in patients with heart failure and reduced EF, ICD and resynchronization device treatments do not have a role in patients with preserved EF. Revascularization for patients with heart failure and preserved EF should be guided by the same considerations as for patients with heart failure with reduced EF.

▶ Prognosis

Once manifest, heart failure with reduced EF carries a poor prognosis. Even with modern treatment, the 5-year mortality is approximately 50%. Mortality rates vary from less than 5% per year in those with no or few symptoms to greater than 30% per year in those with severe and refractory symptoms. These figures emphasize the critical importance of early detection and intervention. Higher mortality is related to older age, lower LVEF, more severe symptoms, chronic kidney disease, and diabetes. The prognosis of heart failure has improved in the past two decades, probably at least in part because of the more widespread use of ACE inhibitors and beta-blockers, which markedly improve survival in those with heart failure with reduced EF.

▶ When to Refer

Patients with new symptoms of heart failure not explained by an obvious cause should be referred to a cardiologist. Patients with continued symptoms of heart failure and reduced LVEF (35% or less) should be referred to a cardiologist for consideration of placement of an ICD or cardiac resynchronization therapy (if QRS duration is 120 msec or more, especially with left bundle branch block pattern).

▶ When to Admit

- Patients with unexplained new or worsened symptoms or positive cardiac biomarkers concerning for acute myocardial necrosis.
- Patients with hypoxia, fluid overload, or pulmonary edema not readily resolved in an outpatient setting.

Brignole M et al. 2013 ESC Guidelines on cardiac pacing and cardiac resynchronization therapy: the Task Force on cardiac pacing and resynchronization therapy of the European Society of Cardiology (ESC). Developed in collaboration with the European Heart Rhythm Association (EHRA). Eur Heart J. 2013 Aug;34(29):2281–329. [PMID: 23801822]

Hunt SA et al. 2009 focused update incorporated into the ACC/AHA 2005 Guidelines for the Diagnosis and Management of Heart Failure in Adults: a report of the American College of Cardiology Foundation/American Heart Association Task Force on Practice Guidelines: developed in collaboration with the International Society for Heart and Lung Transplantation. Circulation. 2009 Apr 14;119(14):e391–479. [PMID: 19324966]

McMurray JJ et al. ESC guidelines for the diagnosis and treatment of acute and chronic heart failure 2012: the Task Force for the Diagnosis and Treatment of Acute and Chronic Heart Failure 2012 of the European Society of Cardiology. Eur J Heart Fail. 2012 Aug;14(8):803–69. [PMID: 22828712]

McMurray JJ et al; PARADIGM-HF Investigators and Committees. Angiotensin-neprilysin inhibition versus enalapril in heart failure. N Engl J Med. 2014 Sep 11;371(11):993–1004. [PMID: 25176015]

Pfeffer MA et al. Regional variation in patients and outcomes in the Treatment of Preserved Cardiac Function Heart Failure With an Aldosterone Antagonist (TOPCAT) trial. Circulation. 2015 Jan 6;131(1):34–42. [PMID: 25406305]

Pitt B et al; TOPCAT Investigators. Spironolactone for heart failure with preserved ejection fraction. N Engl J Med. 2014 Apr 10;370(15):1383–92. [PMID: 24716680]

Troughton RW et al. Effect of B-type natriuretic peptide-guided treatment of chronic heart failure on total mortality and hospitalization: an individual patient meta-analysis. Eur Heart J. 2014 Jun 14;35(23):1559–67. [PMID: 24603309]

Velazquez EJ et al; STICH Investigators. Coronary-artery bypass surgery in patients with left ventricular dysfunction. N Engl J Med. 2011 Apr 28;364(17):1607–16. [PMID: 21463150]

ACUTE HEART FAILURE & PULMONARY EDEMA

ESSENTIALS OF DIAGNOSIS

- ▶ Acute onset or worsening of dyspnea at rest.
- ▶ Tachycardia, diaphoresis, cyanosis.
- ▶ Pulmonary rales, rhonchi; expiratory wheezing.
- ▶ Radiograph shows interstitial and alveolar edema with or without cardiomegaly.
- ▶ Arterial hypoxemia.

▶ General Considerations

Typical causes of acute cardiogenic pulmonary edema include acute myocardial infarction or severe ischemia, exacerbation of chronic heart failure, acute severe hypertension, acute kidney injury, acute volume overload of the LV (valvular regurgitation), and mitral stenosis. By far the most common presentation in developed countries is one of acute or subacute deterioration of chronic heart failure, precipitated by discontinuation of medications, excessive salt intake, myocardial ischemia, tachyarrhythmias (especially rapid atrial fibrillation), or intercurrent infection. Often in the latter group, there is preceding volume overload with worsening edema and progressive shortness of breath for which earlier intervention can usually avoid the need for hospital admission.

▶ Clinical Findings

Acute pulmonary edema presents with a characteristic clinical picture of severe dyspnea, the production of pink, frothy sputum, and diaphoresis and cyanosis. Rales are present in all lung fields, as are generalized wheezing and rhonchi. Pulmonary edema may appear acutely or subacutely in the setting of chronic heart failure or may be the first manifestation of cardiac disease, usually acute myocardial infarction, which may be painful or silent. Less severe decompensations usually present with dyspnea at rest, rales, and other evidence of fluid retention but without severe hypoxia.

Noncardiac causes of pulmonary edema include intravenous opioids, increased intracerebral pressure, high altitude, sepsis, medications, inhaled toxins, transfusion reactions, shock, and disseminated intravascular coagulation. These are distinguished from cardiogenic pulmonary edema by the clinical setting, history, and physical examination. Conversely, in most patients with cardiogenic pulmonary edema, an underlying cardiac abnormality can usually be detected clinically or by ECG, chest radiograph, or echocardiogram.

The chest radiograph reveals signs of pulmonary vascular redistribution, blurriness of vascular outlines, increased interstitial markings, and, characteristically, the butterfly pattern of distribution of alveolar edema. The heart may be enlarged or normal in size depending on whether heart failure was previously present. Assessment of cardiac function by echocardiography is important, since a substantial proportion of patients has normal EFs with elevated atrial pressures due to diastolic dysfunction. In cardiogenic pulmonary edema, BNP is elevated, and the PCWP is invariably elevated, usually over 25 mm Hg. In noncardiogenic pulmonary edema, the wedge pressure may be normal or even low.

► **Treatment**

In full-blown pulmonary edema, the patient should be placed in a sitting position with legs dangling over the side of the bed; this facilitates respiration and reduces venous return. Oxygen is delivered by mask to obtain an arterial PO_2 greater than 60 mm Hg. Noninvasive pressure support ventilation may improve oxygenation and prevent severe CO_2 retention while pharmacologic interventions take effect. However, if respiratory distress remains severe, endotracheal intubation and mechanical ventilation may be necessary.

Morphine is highly effective in pulmonary edema and may be helpful in less severe decompensations when the patient is uncomfortable. The initial dosage is 2–8 mg intravenously (subcutaneous administration is effective in milder cases) and may be repeated after 2–4 hours. Morphine increases venous capacitance, lowering LA pressure, and relieves anxiety, which can reduce the efficiency of ventilation. However, morphine may lead to CO_2 retention by reducing the ventilatory drive. It should be avoided in patients with opioid-induced pulmonary edema, who may improve with opioid antagonists, and in those with neurogenic pulmonary edema.

Intravenous diuretic therapy (furosemide, 40 mg, or bumetanide, 1 mg—or higher doses if the patient has been receiving long-term diuretic therapy) is usually indicated even if the patient has not exhibited prior fluid retention. These agents produce venodilation prior to the onset of diuresis. The DOSE trial has shown that, for acute decompensated heart failure, bolus doses of furosemide are of similar efficacy as continuous intravenous infusion, and that higher-dose furosemide (2.5 times the prior daily dose) resulted in more rapid fluid removal without a substantially higher risk of kidney impairment.

Nitrate therapy accelerates clinical improvement by reducing both BP and LV filling pressures. Sublingual nitroglycerin or isosorbide dinitrate, topical nitroglycerin, or intravenous nitrates will ameliorate dyspnea rapidly prior to the onset of diuresis, and these agents are particularly valuable in patients with accompanying hypertension.

Intravenous nesiritide, a recombinant form of human BNP, is a potent vasodilator that reduces ventricular filling pressures and improves cardiac output. Its hemodynamic effects resemble those of intravenous nitroglycerin with a more predictable dose–response curve and a longer duration of action. In clinical studies, nesiritide (administered as 2 mcg/kg by intravenous bolus injection followed by an infusion of 0.01 mcg/kg/min, which may be up-titrated if needed) produced a rapid improvement in both dyspnea and hemodynamics. The primary adverse effect is hypotension, which may be symptomatic and sustained. Because most patients with acute heart failure respond well to conventional therapy, the role of nesiritide may be primarily in patients who continue to be symptomatic after initial treatment with diuretics and nitrates.

A randomized placebo-controlled trial of 950 patients evaluating intravenous milrinone in patients admitted for decompensated heart failure who had no definite indications for inotropic therapy showed no benefit in increasing survival, decreasing length of admission, or preventing readmission. In addition, rates of sustained hypotension and atrial fibrillation were significantly increased. Thus, the role of positive inotropic agents appears to be limited in patients with refractory symptoms and signs of low cardiac output, particularly if life-threatening vital organ hypoperfusion (such as deteriorating kidney function) is present. In some cases, dobutamine or milrinone may help maintain patients who are awaiting cardiac transplantation.

Bronchospasm may occur in response to pulmonary edema and may itself exacerbate hypoxemia and dyspnea. Treatment with inhaled beta-adrenergic agonists or intravenous aminophylline may be helpful, but both may also provoke tachycardia and supraventricular arrhythmias.

In most cases, pulmonary edema responds rapidly to therapy. When the patient has improved, the cause or precipitating factor should be ascertained. In patients without prior heart failure, evaluation should include echocardiography and, in many cases, cardiac catheterization and coronary angiography. Patients with acute decompensation of chronic heart failure should be treated to achieve a euvolemic state and have their medical regimen optimized. Generally, an oral diuretic and an ACE inhibitor should be initiated, with efficacy and tolerability confirmed prior to discharge. In selected patients, early but careful initiation of beta-blockers in low doses should be considered.

Felker GM et al; NHLBI Heart Failure Clinical Research Network. Diuretic strategies in patients with acute decompensated heart failure. N Engl J Med. 2011 Mar 3;364(9):797–805. [PMID: 21366472]

MYOCARDITIS & THE CARDIOMYOPATHIES

INFECTIOUS MYOCARDITIS

ESSENTIALS OF DIAGNOSIS

▶ Often follows an upper respiratory infection.

▶ May present with chest pain (pleuritic or nonspecific) or signs of heart failure.

▶ Echocardiogram documents cardiomegaly and contractile dysfunction.

▶ Myocardial biopsy, though not sensitive, may reveal a characteristic inflammatory pattern. MRI now has a role in diagnosis.

▶ General Considerations

Cardiac dysfunction due to primary myocarditis is presumedly caused by either an acute viral infection or a postviral immune response. Secondary myocarditis is the result of inflammation caused by nonviral pathogens, medications, chemicals, physical agents, or inflammatory diseases (such as systemic lupus erythematosus). The list of both infectious and noninfectious causes of myocarditis is extensive (Table 10–17).

Early-phase myocarditis is initiated by infection of cardiac tissue. Injury can be fulminant. Both cellular and humoral inflammatory processes contribute to the progression to chronic injury, and there are subgroups that might benefit from immunosuppression.

Genetic predisposition is a likely factor in at least a few cases. Autoimmune myocarditis (eg, giant cell myocarditis) may occur with no identifiable viral infection.

▶ Clinical Findings

A. Symptoms and Signs

Patients may present several days to a few weeks after the onset of an acute febrile illness or a respiratory infection or they may present with heart failure without antecedent symptoms. The onset of heart failure may be gradual or may be abrupt and fulminant. Pulmonary and systemic emboli may occur. Pleural-pericardial chest pain is common. Examination reveals tachycardia, a gallop rhythm, and other evidence of heart failure or conduction defects. Many acute infections are subclinical, though they may present later as idiopathic cardiomyopathy or with ventricular arrhythmias. At times, the presentation may mimic an acute myocardial infarction with ST changes, positive cardiac markers, and regional wall motion abnormalities despite normal coronaries. Microaneurysms may also occur and may be associated with serious ventricular arrhythmias. Patients may present in a variety of ways with fulminant, subacute, or chronic myocarditis. In the European Study of Epidemiology and Treatment of Inflammatory Heart Disease, 72% had dyspnea, 32% had chest pain, and 18% had arrhythmias.

Table 10–17. Causes of myocarditis.

1. **INFECTIOUS CAUSES**

   RNA viruses: Picornaviruses (coxsackie A and B, echovirus, poliovirus, hepatitis virus), orthomyxovirus (influenza), paramyxoviruses (respiratory syncytial virus, mumps), togaviruses (rubella), flaviviruses (dengue fever, yellow fever)

   DNA viruses: Adenovirus (A1, 2, 3, and 5), erythrovirus (Bi9V and 2), herpesviruses (human herpes virus 6 A and B, cytomegalovirus, Epstein-Barr virus, varicella-zoster), retrovirus (HIV)

   Bacteria: Chlamydia (*Chlamydophila pneumoniae, C psittaci*), *Haemophilus influenzae, Legionella, Pneumophilia, Brucella, Clostridium, Francisella tularensis, Neisseria meningitis, Mycobacterium* (tuberculosis), *Salmonella, Staphylococcus,* streptococcus A, *Streptococcus pneumoniae,* tularemia, tetanus, syphilis, *Vibrio cholera*

   Spirocheta: *Borrelia recurrentis,* leptospira, *Treponema pallidum*

   Rickettsia: *Coxiella burnetti, R rickettsii, R prowazekii*

   Fungi: *Actinomyces, Aspergillus, Candida, Cryptococcus, Histoplasma, Nocardia*

   Protozoa: *Entamoeba histolytica, Plasmodium falciparum, Trypanosoma cruzi, T burcei, T gondii, Leishmania*

   Helminthic: *Ascaris, Echinococcus granulosus, Schistosoma, Trichenella spiralis, Wuchereria bancrofti*

2. **NONINFECTIOUS CAUSES**

   Autoimmune diseases: Dermatomyositis, inflammatory bowel disease, rheumatoid arthritis, Sjögren syndrome, systemic lupus erythematosus, granulomatosis with polyangiitis (formerly Wegener granulomatosis), giant cell myocarditis

   Drugs: Aminophylline, amphetamine, anthracyclin, catecholamines, chloramphenicol, cocaine, cyclophosphamide, doxorubicin, 5-FU, mesylate, methysergide, phenytoin, trastuzumab, zidovudine

   Hypersensitivity reactions due to drugs: Azithromycin, benzodiazepines, clozapine, cephalosporins, dapsone, dobutamine, lithium, diuretics, thiazide, methyldopa, mexiletine, streptomycin, sulfonamides, nonsteroidal anti-inflammatory drugs, tetanus toxoid, tetracycline, tricyclic antidepressants

   Hypersensitivity reactions due to venoms: Bee, wasp, black widow spider, scorpion, snake

   Systemic diseases: Eosinophilic granulomatosis with polyangiitis (formerly known as Churg-Strauss syndrome), collagen diseases, sarcoidosis, Kawasaki disease, scleroderma

   Other: Heat stroke, hypothermia, transplant rejection, radiation injury

Modified, with permission, from Schultheiss HP et al. The management of myocarditis. Eur Heart J. 2011;32:2616–25.

B. ECG and Chest Radiography

ECG may show sinus tachycardia, other arrhythmias, nonspecific repolarization changes, and intraventricular conduction abnormalities. The presence of Q waves or left bundle branch block portends a higher rate of death or cardiac transplantation. Ventricular ectopy may be the initial and only clinical finding. The chest radiograph is nonspecific, but cardiomegaly is frequent, though not universal. Evidence for pulmonary venous hypertension is common and frank pulmonary edema may be present.

C. Diagnostic Studies

There is no specific laboratory study that is consistently present, though the white blood cell count is usually elevated and the sedimentation rate and CRP may be increased. Troponin I levels are elevated in about one-third of patients, but CK-MB is elevated in only 10%. Echocardiography provides the most convenient way of evaluating cardiac function and can exclude many other processes. MRI with gadolinium enhancement reveals spotty areas of injury throughout the myocardium, but both T2- and T1-weighted images are needed to achieve optimal results; correlation with endomyocardial biopsy results has been poor.

D. Endomyocardial Biopsy

Confirmation of myocarditis still requires histologic evidence. The AHA/ACC/ESC class 1 recommendations for biopsy are (1) in patients with heart failure, a normal-sized or dilated LV less than 2 weeks after onset of symptoms, and hemodynamic compromise; or (2) in patients with a dilated LV 2 weeks to 3 months after onset of symptoms, new ventricular arrhythmias or AV nodal block (Mobitz II or complete heart block) or who do not respond to usual care after 1–2 weeks. In some cases, the identification of inflammation without viral genomes by PCR suggests that immunosuppression might be useful.

Treatment & Prognosis

Patients with fulminant myocarditis may present with acute cardiogenic shock. Acute myocarditis has been implicated as a cause of sudden death in 5–22% of such cases in athletes younger than 35 years. The ventricles are usually not dilated, but thickened (possibly due to myoedema). There is a high death rate, but if the patients recover, they are often left with no residual cardiomyopathy. Patients with subacute disease have a dilated cardiomyopathy and generally make an incomplete recovery. Those who present with chronic disease tend to have only mild dilation of the LV and eventually present with a more restrictive cardiomyopathy. Treatment is directed toward the clinical scenario with ACE inhibitors and beta-blockers if LVEF is less than 40%. Nonsteroidal anti-inflammatory medications should be used if myopericarditis-related chest pain occurs. Colchicine has been suggested if pericarditis predominates. Arrhythmias should be suppressed. Corticosteroids have not proved effective.

Specific antimicrobial therapy is indicated when an infecting agent is identified. Exercise should be limited during the recovery phase. Some experts believe digoxin should be avoided, and it likely has little value in this setting anyway. Controlled trials of immunosuppressive therapy with corticosteroids and intravenous immunoglobulin (IVIG) have not suggested a benefit, though some recommend IVIG given at 2 g/kg over 24 hours in proven cases. Uncontrolled trials suggest that interferon might have a supportive role. Studies are lacking as to when to discontinue the chosen therapy if the patient improves. Patients with fulminant myocarditis require aggressive short-term

support, including an IABP or an LV assist device. If severe pulmonary infiltrates accompany the fulminant myocarditis, extracorporeal membrane oxygenation (ECMO) support may be temporarily required and has had notable success. Ongoing studies are addressing whether patients with giant cell myocarditis may be responsive to immunosuppressive agents, as a special case. A 2013 review suggested that two-thirds of patients with giant cell myocarditis reach at least a partial remission (characterized by freedom from severe heart failure and need for a transplant), although they were prone to ventricular arrhythmias. Overall, if improvement does not occur, many patients may be eventual candidates for cardiac transplantation or long-term use of the newer LV assist devices.

When to Refer

Patients in whom myocarditis is suspected should be seen by a cardiologist at a tertiary care center where facilities are available for diagnosis and therapies available should a fulminant course ensue. The facility should have ventricular support devices and transplantation options available.

Kanolin R et al. Diagnosis, treatment, and outcome of giant-cell myocarditis in the era of combined immunotherapy. Circ Heart Fail. 2013 Jan;6(1):15–22. [PMID: 23149495]
Schultheiss HP et al. The management of myocarditis. Eur Heart J. 2011 Nov;32(21):2616–25. [PMID: 21705357]

DRUG-INDUCED & TOXIC MYOCARDITIS

A variety of medications, illicit drugs, and toxic substances can produce acute or chronic myocardial injury; the clinical presentation varies widely. The phenothiazines, lithium, chloroquine, disopyramide, antimony-containing compounds, and arsenicals can also cause ECG changes, arrhythmias, or heart failure. Hypersensitivity reactions to sulfonamides, penicillins, and aminosalicylic acid as well as other medications can result in cardiac dysfunction. Radiation can cause an acute inflammatory reaction as well as a chronic fibrosis of heart muscle, usually in conjunction with pericarditis.

Cardiotoxicity from cocaine may occur from coronary artery spasm, myocardial infarction, arrhythmias, and myocarditis. Because many of these processes are believed to be mediated by cocaine's inhibitory effect on norepinephrine reuptake by sympathetic nerves, beta-blockers have been used in patients with fixed stenosis. In documented coronary spasm, calcium channel blockers and nitrates may be effective. Usual therapy for heart failure or conduction system disease is warranted when symptoms occur. Other illicit drug use has been associated with myocarditis in various case reports.

The problem of cardiovascular side effects from cancer chemotherapy agents is a growing one. Anthracyclines remain the cornerstone of treatment of many malignancies. Heart failure can be expected in 5% of patients treated with a cumulative dose of 400–450 mg/m^2, and this rate is doubled if the patient is over age 65. The major mechanism of cardiotoxicity is thought to be due to oxidative stress inducing both apoptosis and necrosis of myocytes. There is also disruption of the sarcomere. This is the rationale behind the superoxide dismutase mimetic and iron-chelating agent, dexrazoxane, to protect from the injury. The use of trastuzumab in combination with anthracyclines increases the risk of cardiac dysfunction up to 28%; this has been an issue since combined use of these agents is particularly effective in HER 2-positive breast cancer.

In patients receiving chemotherapy, it is important to look for subtle signs of cardiovascular compromise. Echocardiography, cardiac MRI, and serial MUGA studies can provide concrete data regarding LV function. Multiple biomarkers may appear early in the course of myocardial injury (especially troponin and myeloperoxidase) and may allow for early detection of cardiotoxicity before other signs become evident. There is some evidence that beta-blocker therapy may reduce the negative effects on myocardial function.

When to Refer

Many patients with myocardial injury from toxic agents can be monitored safely if ventricular function remains relatively preserved (EF greater than 40%) and no heart failure symptoms occur. Diastolic dysfunction may be subtle.

Once heart failure becomes evident or significant conduction system disease becomes manifest, the patient should be evaluated and monitored by a cardiologist in case myocardial dysfunction worsens and further intervention becomes warranted.

Caforio AL et al. Clinical presentation and diagnosis of myocarditis. Heart. 2015 Aug;101(16):1332–44. [PMID: 26109587]

Chaudhry MA et al. Modern day management of giant cell myocarditis. Int J Cardiol. 2015 Jan 15;178:82–4. [PMID: 25464225]

Eschenhagen T et al. Cardiovascular side effects of cancer therapies: a position statement from the Heart Failure Association of the European Society of Cardiology. Eur J Heart Fail. 2011 Jan;13(1):1–10. [PMID: 21169385]

Ky B et al. Early increases in multiple biomarkers predict subsequent cardiotoxicity in patients with breast cancer treated with doxorubicin, taxanes, and trastuzumab. J Am Coll Cardiol. 2014 Mar 4;63(8):809–16. [PMID: 24291281]

Lal H et al. Cancer genetics and the cardiotoxicity of the therapeutics. J Am Coll Cardiol. 2013 Jan 22;61(3):267–74. [PMID: 23328609]

Nohria A. Beta-adrenergic blockade for anthracycline- and trastuzumab-induced cardiotoxicity: is prevention better than cure? Circ Heart Fail. 2013 May;6(3):358–61. [PMID: 23694770]

DILATED CARDIOMYOPATHY

ESSENTIALS OF DIAGNOSIS

► Symptoms and signs of heart failure.

► Echocardiogram confirms LV dilation, thinning, and global dysfunction.

► Severity of RV dysfunction critical in long-term prognosis.

General Considerations

Heart failure definitions have changed over the years and patients with a dilated cardiomyopathy are generally placed into the category of heart failure with reduced ejection fraction where the LVEF is defined as less than or equal to 40%. In about half of the patients in this category there is LV enlargement and it is this group that defines dilated cardiomyopathy. This is a large group of heterogeneous myocardial disorders characterized by reduced myocardial contractility in the absence of abnormal loading conditions such as with hypertension or valvular disease. The prevalence averages 36 cases/100,000 in the United States and accounts for approximately 10,000 deaths annually. Blacks are afflicted three times as often as whites. The prognosis is poor with 50% mortality at 5 years once symptoms emerge.

The causes are multiple and diverse. Up to 20–35% have a familial etiology. Endocrine and metabolic causes include obesity, diabetes, thyroid disease, acromegaly, and growth hormone deficiency. Toxic, drug-induced, and inflammatory causes are listed in the prior section. Dilated cardiomyopathy may also be caused by prolonged tachycardia and right ventricular pacing. Dilated cardiomyopathy is also associated with HIV, Chagas disease, rheumatologic disorders, iron overload, amyloidosis, and sarcoidosis. Peripartum cardiomyopathy and stress-induced disease (tako-tsubo) are discussed separately.

Clinical Findings

A. Symptoms and Signs

In most patients, symptoms of heart failure develop gradually. It is important to seek out a history of familial dilated cardiomyopathy and to identify behaviors that might predispose patients to the disease. The physical examination reveals rales, an elevated JVP, cardiomegaly, S₃ gallop rhythm, often the murmurs of functional mitral or tricuspid regurgitation, peripheral edema, or ascites. In severe heart failure, Cheyne-Stokes breathing, pulsus alternans, pallor, and cyanosis may be present.

B. ECG and Chest Radiography

The major findings are listed in Table 10–18. Sinus tachycardia is common. Other common abnormalities include left bundle branch block and ventricular or atrial arrhythmias. The chest radiograph reveals cardiomegaly, evidence for left and/or right heart failure, and pleural effusions (right more than left).

C. Diagnostic Studies

In the 2013 AHA/ACCF heart failure guidelines, patients with dyspnea should have a BNP or N-terminal pro-BNP measured to help establish prognosis and disease severity (Class 1, LOE A). Other biomarkers, such as troponin I or T and measures that reflect inflammation, oxidative stress, neurohormonal disarray and myocardial or matrix remodeling are under investigation for their ability to guide therapy.

Table 10–18. Classification of the cardiomyopathies.

	Dilated	Hypertrophic	Restrictive
Frequent causes	Idiopathic, alcoholic, major catecholamine discharge, myocarditis, postpartum, doxorubicin, endocrinopathies, genetic diseases	Hereditary syndrome, possibly chronic hypertension in the elderly	Amyloidosis, post-radiation, post-open heart surgery, diabetes, endomyocardial fibrosis
Symptoms	Left or biventricular heart failure	Dyspnea, chest pain, syncope	Dyspnea, fatigue, right-sided heart failure > left heart failure
Physical examination	Cardiomegaly, S_3, elevated jugular venous pressure, rales	Sustained point of maximal impulse, S_4, variable systolic murmur, bisferiens carotid pulse	Elevated jugular venous pressure, Kussmaul sign
Electrocardiogram	ST–T changes, conduction abnormalities, ventricular ectopy	Left ventricular hypertrophy, exaggerated septal Q waves	ST–T changes, conduction abnormalities, low voltage
Chest radiograph	Enlarged heart, pulmonary congestion	Mild cardiomegaly	Mild to moderate cardiomegaly
Echocardiogram, nuclear studies, MRI	Left ventricular dilation and dysfunction	Left ventricular hypertrophy, asymmetric septal hypertrophy, small left ventricular size, normal or supranormal function, systolic anterior mitral motion, diastolic dysfunction	Small or normal left ventricular size, normal or mildly reduced left ventricular function. Gadolinium-hyperenhancement on MRI.
Cardiac catheterization	Left ventricular dilation and dysfunction, high diastolic pressures, low cardiac output. Coronary angiography important to exclude ischemic cause.	Small, hypercontractile left ventricle, dynamic outflow gradient, diastolic dysfunction	High diastolic pressure, "square root" sign, normal or mildly reduced left ventricular function

An echocardiogram is indicated to exclude unsuspected valvular or other lesions and confirm the presence of ventricular dilatation, reduced LV systolic function and associated RV systolic dysfunction, or pulmonary hypertension. Mitral Doppler inflow patterns also help in the diagnosis of concomitant diastolic dysfunction. Color flow Doppler can reveal tricuspid or mitral regurgitation, and continuous Doppler can estimate PA pressures. Intracavitary thrombosis is occasionally seen. Exercise or pharmacologic stress myocardial perfusion imaging may uncover underlying coronary disease. Radionuclide ventriculography provides a noninvasive measure of the EF and both RV and LV wall motion, though its use has been supplanted by cardiac MRI in most institutions. Cardiac MRI is particularly helpful in inflammatory or infiltrative processes, such as sarcoidosis or hemochromatosis, and is the diagnostic study of choice for RV dysplasia where there is fatty infiltration. MRI can also help define an ischemic etiology by noting gadolinium hyperenhancement consistent with myocardial scar. Cardiac catheterization is seldom of specific value unless myocardial ischemia or LV aneurysm is suspected, although right heart catheterization should be considered to help guide therapy when the clinical syndrome is not clear cut (Class 1 indication, LOE C). Myocardial biopsy is rarely useful in establishing the diagnosis, although occasionally the underlying cause (eg, sarcoidosis, hemochromatosis) can be discerned. Its use is considered a Class 2a indication with LOE of C. It should not be used routinely. Biopsy is most useful in transplant rejection.

▶ **Treatment**

The management of heart failure is outlined in the section on heart failure. Standard therapy includes control of abnormal lipids and BP and contributing factors such as obesity, smoking, diabetes or potentially cardiotoxic agents. All patients with a remote history of myocardial infarction or acute coronary syndrome and reduced LVEF should be given ACE inhibitors or ARBs. Beta-blockers and statins should be included in this population as well. All patients with dilated cardiomyopathy regardless of etiology should be treated with beta-blockers and ACE inhibitors. The use of combined ACE inhibition, ARB, and aldosterone antagonists can create harm, though, and is discouraged. A few beta-blockers, including bisoprolol, carvedilol, and sustained-release metoprolol, have been shown to reduce mortality and should be preferentially used if possible. Calcium channel blockers should be avoided except as necessary to control ventricular response in atrial fibrillation or flutter. If congestive symptoms are present, diuretics and an aldosterone antagonist should be added. In patients with Class 2–4 heart failure symptoms, an aldosterone receptor antagonist should be added when the LVEF is less than 35% (unless contraindicated). Care in the use of aldosterone antagonists is warranted when the glomerular filtration rate is less than 30 mL/min/1.73 m^2 or when the potassium is elevated. All patients with diabetes should be taking aldosterone antagonists if the LVEF is less than or equal to 40%. Systemic BP control is extremely important.

Digoxin is a second-line medication but remains favored as an adjunct by some clinicians; digoxin may be beneficial to reduce recurrent hospitalizations and to control the ventricular response in atrial fibrillation in sedentary patients. Given the question of abnormal nitric oxide utilization in blacks, the use of hydralazine-nitrate combination therapy is recommended in this population. Sodium restriction is helpful, especially in acute heart failure. Continuous positive airway pressure can improve LV function in patients with sleep apnea.

When atrial fibrillation is present, heart rate control is vital if sinus rhythm cannot be established or maintained. There are little data, however, to suggest an advantage of sinus rhythm over atrial fibrillation on long-term outcomes. Many patients may be candidates for cardiac synchronization therapy with biventricular pacing if there is significant mitral regurgitation and the QRS width is greater than 150 msec. To help prevent sudden death, an ICD is reasonable (Class 2a, LOE B) in asymptomatic ischemic cardiomyopathy patients with an LVEF of less than 30% on appropriate medical therapy (at least 40 days post-myocardial infarction). Cardiac rehabilitation and exercise training have consistently been found to improve clinical status.

Few cases of cardiomyopathy are amenable to specific therapy for the underlying cause. Alcohol use should be discontinued, since there is often marked recovery of cardiac function following a period of abstinence in alcoholic cardiomyopathy. Endocrine causes (hyperthyroidism or hypothyroidism, acromegaly, and pheochromocytoma) should be treated. Immunosuppressive therapy is not indicated in chronic dilated cardiomyopathy. There are some patients who may benefit from implantable LV assist devices either as a bridge to transplantation or as a temporary measure until cardiac function returns. LV assist devices can be considered as destination therapy in patients who are not candidates for cardiac transplantation. Arterial and pulmonary emboli are more common in dilated cardiomyopathy than in ischemic cardiomyopathy. Suitable candidates may benefit from long-term anticoagulation, and all patients with atrial fibrillation should be so treated. The newer targeted antithrombotic agents are appropriate unless there is associated mitral stenosis. Either warfarin or a targeted antithrombotic agent should be considered when a mobile LV thrombus is observed on the echocardiogram.

▶ Prognosis

The prognosis of dilated cardiomyopathy without clinical heart failure is variable, with some patients remaining stable, some deteriorating gradually, and others declining rapidly. Once heart failure is manifest, the natural history is similar to that of other causes of heart failure, with an annual mortality rate of around 11–13%. In a 2000 review of survival in dilated cardiomyopathy, the underlying cause of heart failure has prognostic value in patients with unexplained cardiomyopathy. Patients with peripartum cardiomyopathy or stress-induced cardiomyopathy appear to have a better prognosis than those with other forms of cardiomyopathy. Patients with cardiomyopathy due to

infiltrative myocardial diseases, HIV infection, or doxorubicin therapy have an especially poor prognosis.

▶ When to Refer

Patients with new or worsened symptoms of heart failure with dilated cardiomyopathy should be referred to a cardiologist. Patients with continued symptoms of heart failure and reduced LVEF (35% or less) should be referred to a cardiologist for consideration of placement of an ICD or cardiac resynchronization therapy (if QRS duration is 120 msec or more, especially with a left bundle branch block pattern). Patients with advanced refractory symptoms should be referred for consideration of heart transplant or LV assist device therapy.

▶ When to Admit

Patients with hypoxia, fluid overload, or pulmonary edema not readily resolved in an outpatient setting should be admitted.

McNally EM et al. Genetic mutations and mechanisms in dilated cardiomyopathy. J Clin Invest. 2013 Jan 2;123(1):19–26. [PMID: 23281406]

Yancy CW et al; American College of Cardiology Foundation/ American Heart Association Task Force on Practice Guidelines. 2013 ACCF/AHA guideline for the management of heart failure. Circulation. 2013 Oct 15;128(16):e240–327. [PMID: 23741058]

TAKO-TSUBO CARDIOMYOPATHY

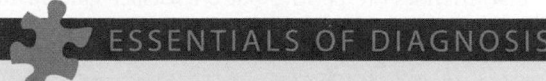
ESSENTIALS OF DIAGNOSIS

▶ Occurs after a major catecholamine discharge.

▶ Acute chest pain or shortness of breath.

▶ Predominately affects postmenopausal women.

▶ Presents as an acute anterior myocardial infarction, but coronaries normal at cardiac catheterization.

▶ Imaging reveals apical left ventricular ballooning due to anteroapical stunning of the myocardium.

▶ Most patients recover completely.

▶ General Considerations

LV apical ballooning (Tako-Tsubo syndrome) follows a high catecholamine surge. It is sometimes referred to as stress cardiomyopathy. The resulting shape of the LV acutely suggests a rounded ampulla form similar to a Japanese octopus pot (tako-tsubo pot). Mid-ventricular ballooning has also been described. The key feature is that the myocardial stunning that occurs does not follow the pattern suggestive of coronary ischemia (even though about 15% of patients will have coexisting CAD). It has been described following some stressful event, such as hypoglycemia, lightning strikes, earthquakes, postventricular tachycardia, during alcohol withdrawal, following surgery, during hyperthyroidism, after stroke, and following emotional stress ("broken-heart syndrome"). Virtually any event that triggers excess catecholamines has been implicated in a wide number of case reports. Pericarditis and even tamponade have been described in isolated cases. Recurrences have also been described. First described in 1990, it predominantly affects women (up to 90%), primarily postmenopausal. Among patients with tako-tsubo cardiomyopathy, compared to patients with ACS, there are more neurologic and psychiatric disorders.

▶ Clinical Findings

A. Symptoms and Signs

The symptoms are similar to any acute coronary syndrome. Typical angina and dyspnea are usually present. Syncope is rare, although arrhythmias are not uncommon.

B. ECG and Chest Radiography

The ECG reveals ST-segment elevation as well as deep anterior T-wave inversion. The chest radiograph is either normal or reveals pulmonary congestion. The dramatic T-wave inversions gradually resolve over time.

C. Diagnostic Studies

The echocardiogram reveals LV apical dyskinesia usually not consistent with any particular coronary distribution. The urgent cardiac catheterization reveals the LV apical ballooning in association with normal coronaries. Initial cardiac enzymes are positive but often taper quickly. In almost all cases, MRI hyperenhancement studies reveal no long-term scarring.

▶ Treatment

Immediate therapy is similar to any acute myocardial infarction. Initiation of long-term therapy depends on whether LV dysfunction persists. Most patients receive aspirin, beta-blockers, and ACE inhibitors until the LV fully recovers. Despite the presumed association with high catecholamines, the use of ACE inhibitors or ARBs, but not beta-blockers has been associated with improved long-term survival. See Treatment of Heart Failure.

▶ Prognosis

In a 2015 registry of 1759 patients, the rate of severe in-hospital complications, including shock and death were similar between those with an acute coronary syndrome and tako-tsubo. Physical triggers, acute neurologic or psychiatric disease, high troponin levels and a low EF were independent predictors of in-hospital complications. Men appear to be at higher risk for major adverse cardiac and cerebrovascular events during the first 30 days following the event. During long-term follow-up the rate of major adverse cardiac and cerebrovascular events was 9.95% per patient year with a death rate of 5.6% per patient year. In this registry it was reported that 32.5% of patients were

taking beta-blockers with the first event and 29/57 (51%) at the time of a second event, suggesting beta-blockers are ineffective in preventing the clinical syndrome. Overall, prognosis is good unless there is a serious complication (such as mitral regurgitation, ventricular rupture, or ventricular tachycardia). Recovery of the LVEF is expected in most cases after a period of weeks to months. At times, the LV function recovers fully in a few days.

Templin C et al. Clinical features and outcome of takotsubo (stress) cardiomyopathy. N Engl J Med. 2015 Sep 3;373(10): 929–38. [PMID: 26332547]

HYPERTROPHIC CARDIOMYOPATHY

ESSENTIALS OF DIAGNOSIS

- ▶ May present with dyspnea, chest pain, syncope.
- ▶ Though LV outflow gradient is classic, symptoms are primarily related to diastolic dysfunction.
- ▶ Echocardiogram is diagnostic. Any wall thickness greater than 1.5 cm defines the disease.
- ▶ Increased risk of sudden death.

▶ General Considerations

Hypertrophic cardiomyopathy (HCM) is noted when there is LVH unrelated to any pressure or volume overload. The definition has evolved over time; while it traditionally has been defined by LV outflow obstruction due to septal hypertrophy, now it is considered present any time that any LV wall is measured at more than 1.5 cm thick on an echocardiogram. This allows for many forms to be considered that do not create LV outflow obstruction. The increased wall thickness reduces LV systolic stress, increases the EF, and can result in an "empty ventricle" at end-systole. The interventricular septum may be disproportionately involved (asymmetric septal hypertrophy), but in some cases the hypertrophy is localized to the mid-ventricle or to the apex. The LV outflow tract is usually narrowed during systole due to the hypertrophied septum and systolic anterior motion of the mitral valve occurs as the anterior mitral valve leaflet is pulled into the LV outflow. The obstruction is worsened by factors that increase myocardial contractility (sympathetic stimulation, digoxin, and postextrasystolic beat) or that decrease LV filling (Valsalva maneuver, peripheral vasodilators). The amount of obstruction is preload and afterload dependent and can vary from day to day. **The consequence of the hypertrophy is elevated LV diastolic pressures rather than systolic dysfunction.** Rarely, systolic dysfunction develops late in the disease. The LV is usually more involved than the RV, and the atria are frequently significantly enlarged.

HCM is inherited as an autosomal-dominant trait with variable penetrance and is caused by mutations of one of a large number of genes, most of which code for myosin heavy chains or proteins regulating calcium handling. The prognosis is related to the specific gene mutation. Patients usually present in early adulthood. Elite athletes may demonstrate considerable hypertrophy that can be confused with HCM, but generally diastolic dysfunction is not present in the athlete and this finding helps separate pathologic disease from athletic hypertrophy. The apical variety is particularly common in those of Asian descent. A midventricular obstructive form is also known where there is contact between the septum and papillary muscles. A hypertrophic cardiomyopathy in the elderly (usually in association with hypertension) has also been defined as a distinct entity (often a sigmoid interventricular septum is noted). Mitral annular calcification is often present. Mitral regurgitation is variable and often dynamic, depending on the degree of outflow tract obstruction.

▶ Clinical Findings

A. Symptoms and Signs

The most frequent symptoms are dyspnea and chest pain (see Table 10–18). Syncope is also common and is typically postexertional, when diastolic filling diminishes due to fluid loss and tachycardia increasing LV outflow tract obstruction. Residual circulating catecholamines accentuate the changes. Arrhythmias are an important problem. Atrial fibrillation is a long-term consequence of chronically elevated LA pressures and is a poor prognostic sign. Ventricular arrhythmias are also common, and sudden death may occur, often after extraordinary exertion.

Features on physical examination include a bisferiens carotid pulse, triple apical impulse (due to the prominent atrial filling wave and early and late systolic impulses), and a loud S_4. The JVP may reveal a prominent a wave due to reduced RV compliance. In cases with LV outflow obstruction, a loud systolic murmur is present along the left sternal border that increases with upright posture or Valsalva maneuver and decreases with squatting. These maneuvers help differentiate the murmur of HCM from that of aortic stenosis, since in HCM, reducing the LV volume increases the outflow obstruction and the murmur intensity; whereas in valvular aortic stenosis, reducing the stroke volume across the valve decreases the murmur. Mitral regurgitation is frequently present as well.

B. ECG and Chest Radiography

LVH is nearly universal in symptomatic patients, though entirely normal ECGs are present in up to 25%, usually in those with localized hypertrophy. Exaggerated septal Q waves inferolaterally may mimic myocardial infarction. The chest radiograph is often unimpressive. Unlike aortic stenosis, the ascending aorta is not dilated.

C. Diagnostic Studies

The echocardiogram is diagnostic, revealing LVH (involving the septum more commonly than the posterior walls), systolic anterior motion of the mitral valve, early closing followed by reopening of the aortic valve, a small and hypercontractile LV, and delayed relaxation and filling of the LV during diastole. The septum is usually 1.3–1.5 times the thickness of the posterior wall. Septal motion tends to be reduced. Doppler ultrasound reveals turbulent flow and a dynamic gradient in the LV outflow tract and, commonly, mitral regurgitation. Abnormalities in the diastolic filling pattern are present in 80% of patients. Echocardiography can usually differentiate the disease from ventricular noncompaction, a congenital myocardial disease pattern with marked trabeculation that partially fills the LV cavity. Myocardial perfusion imaging may suggest septal ischemia in the presence of normal coronary arteries. Cardiac MRI confirms the hypertrophy and contrast enhancement frequently reveals evidence of scar at the junction of the RV attachment to the interventricular septum. Cardiac catheterization confirms the diagnosis and defines the presence or absence of CAD. Frequently, coronary arterial bridging (squeezing of the coronary in systole) occurs, especially in the septal arteries. Exercise studies are recommended to assess for ventricular arrhythmias and to document the BP response. Holter monitoring is recommended for determination of ventricular ectopy.

▶ Treatment

Beta-blockers should be the initial medication in symptomatic individuals, especially when dynamic outflow obstruction is noted on the echocardiogram. The resulting slower heart rates assist with diastolic filling of the stiff LV. Dyspnea, angina, and arrhythmias respond in about 50% of patients. Calcium channel blockers, especially verapamil, have also been effective in symptomatic patients. Their effect is due primarily to improved diastolic function; however, their vasodilating actions can also increase outflow obstruction and cause hypotension. Disopyramide is also effective because of its negative inotropic effects; it is usually used as an addition to the medical regimen rather than as primary therapy or to help control atrial arrhythmias. Diuretics are frequently necessary due to the high LV diastolic pressure and elevated LA pressures. Patients do best in sinus rhythm, and atrial fibrillation should be aggressively treated with antiarrhythmics or radiofrequency ablation. Dual-chamber pacing may help prevent the progression of hypertrophy and obstruction. There appears to be an advantage to the use of short-AV delay biventricular pacing.

Nonsurgical septal ablation has been performed by injection of alcohol into septal branches of the left coronary artery to create a controlled myocardial infarct in the regions of greatest wall thickness. Good results in small series of patients with significant outflow tract gradients have been reported. Patients with malignant ventricular arrhythmias and unexplained syncope in the presence of a positive family history for sudden death, with or without an abnormal BP response to exercise, are probably best managed with an implantable defibrillator. Excision of part of the outflow myocardial septum (myotomy–myomectomy) by experienced surgeons has been successful in patients with severe symptoms unresponsive to medical therapy. A few surgeons advocate mitral valve replacement, since this results in resolution of the gradient and prevents associated mitral regurgitation. In some cases, myomectomy has been combined with an Alfieri stitch on the mitral valve (a stitch that binds the midportion of the anterior and posterior mitral valve leaflets together). Rare cases of progression to LV dilation or patients with intractable symptoms can be considered for cardiac transplantation. Figure 10–10 provides an algorithm for the treatment of HCM as defined in the 2011 AHA/ACC guidelines.

Pregnancy results in an increased risk in patients with symptoms or outflow tract gradients of greater than 50 mm Hg. Genetic counseling is indicated before planned conception. In pregnant patients with HCM, continuation of beta-blocker therapy is recommended.

▶ Prognosis

The natural history of HCM is highly variable. Several specific mutations are associated with a higher incidence of early malignant arrhythmias and sudden death, and definition of a genetic abnormality provides the best estimate of prognosis. Genetic testing is recommended if first-degree relatives are available to participate.

Some patients remain asymptomatic for many years or for life. Sudden death, especially during exercise, may be the initial event. The highest risk patients are those with (1) a personal history of serious ventricular arrhythmias or survival of a sudden death episode; (2) a family history of sudden death; (3) unexplained syncope; (4) documented

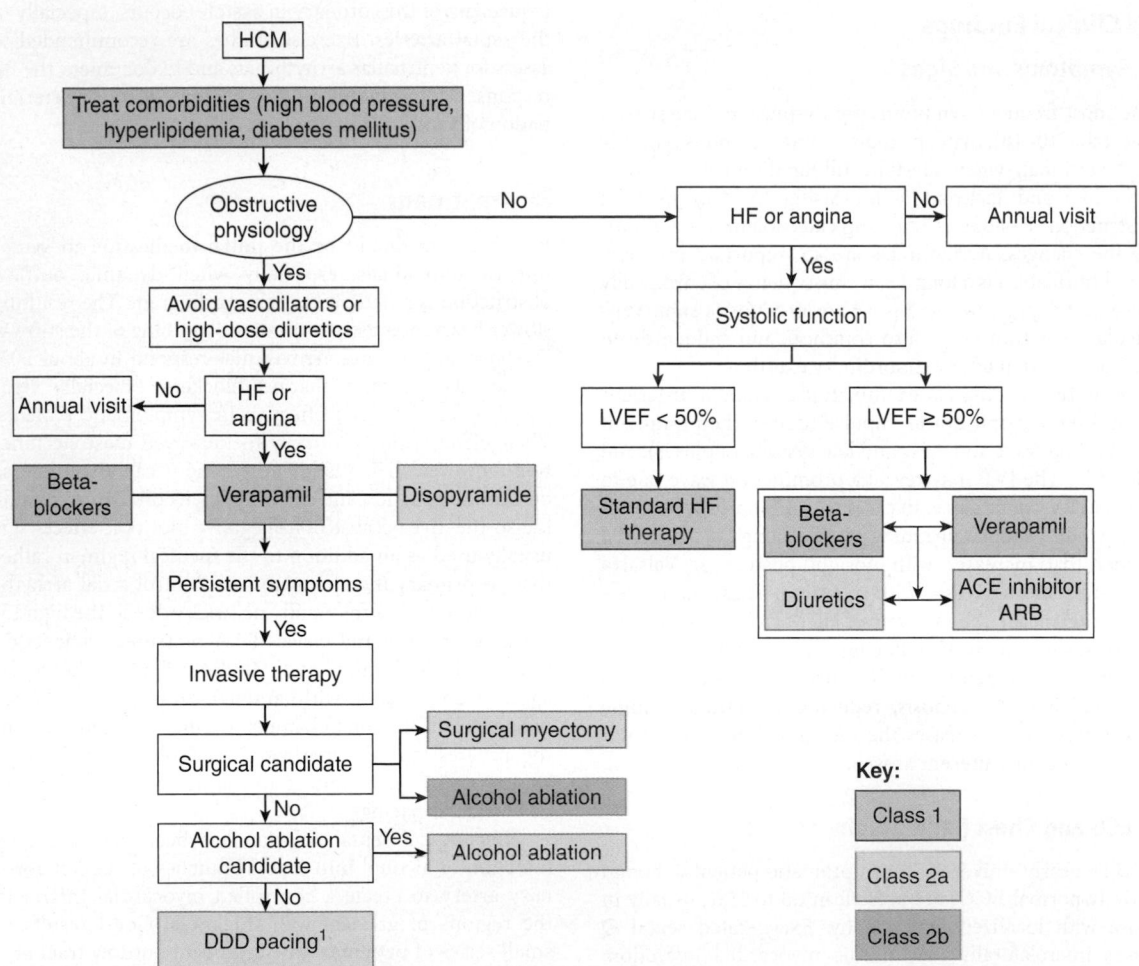

^{1}See section on AV Block in the text.

▲ **Figure 10–10.** Recommended therapeutic approach to the patient with hypertrophic cardiomyopathy (HCM). ACE, angiotensin-converting enzyme; ARB, angiotensin receptor blockers; HF, heart failure; LVEF, left ventricular ejection fraction. (Reproduced, with permission, from Gersh BJ et al. 2011 ACCF/AHA Guideline for the Diagnosis and Treatment of Hypertrophic Cardiomyopathy A Report of the American College of Cardiology Foundation/ American Heart Association Task Force on Practice Guidelines Developed in Collaboration With the American Association for Thoracic Surgery, American Society of Echocardiography, American Society of Nuclear Cardiology, Heart Failure Society of America, Heart Rhythm Society, Society for Cardiovascular Angiography and Interventions, and Society of Thoracic Surgeons. J Am Coll Cardiol. 2011 Dec 13;58(25):e212–60.)

NSVT, defined as three or more beats of ventricular tachycardia at 120 beats per minute or more on ambulatory Holter monitoring; and (5) maximal LV wall thickness of 30 mm or more. In addition, patients in whom the systolic BP does not increase more than 20 mm Hg during treadmill stress testing are also at risk, as are those with double and compound genetic mutations and those with marked LV outflow tract obstruction. MRI data suggest that the extent of scarring on hyperenhancement may also be predictive of adverse events. HCM is the pathologic feature most frequently associated with sudden death in athletes. Endocarditis prophylaxis is not indicated. A final stage may be a transition into dilated cardiomyopathy in 5–10% of patients due to the long-term effects of LV remodeling; treatment at that stage is similar to that for dilated cardiomyopathy.

▶ When to Refer

Patients should be referred to a cardiologist when symptoms are difficult to control, syncope has occurred, or there are any of the high-risk features present, which may denote the need for a prophylactic defibrillator.

Gersh BJ et al. 2011 ACCF/AHA guideline for the treatment of hypertrophic cardiomyopathy. J Am Coll Cardiol. 2011 Dec 13; 58(25):e212–60. [PMID: 22075469]
Maron BJ et al. Hypertrophic cardiomyopathy. Lancet. 2013 Jan 19; 381(9862):242–55. [PMID: 22874472]

RESTRICTIVE CARDIOMYOPATHY

ESSENTIALS OF DIAGNOSIS

- ▶ Right heart failure tends to dominate over left heart failure.
- ▶ Pulmonary hypertension is present.
- ▶ Amyloidosis is the most common cause.
- ▶ Echocardiography is key to diagnosis.
- ▶ Myocardial biopsy or cardiac MRI can confirm amyloid.

▶ General Considerations

Restrictive cardiomyopathy is characterized by impaired diastolic filling with reasonably preserved contractile function. The condition is relatively uncommon, with the most frequent cause being amyloidosis. **Cardiac amyloidosis** is more common in men than in women and rarely manifests before the age of 40. While light-chain amyloid proteins can be toxic to cardiomyocytes, they may also internalize into many cell types and this may explain some of the cardiac dysfunction observed. The AL (light-chain) type is the most common, with cardiac involvement in 50%. Other forms include mutated transthyretin (ATTR) in familial amyloidosis (usually manifested in the elderly black population) and a wild-type transthyretin in senile amyloidosis. Transthyretin is produced almost entirely in the liver. Secondary (AA) amyloidosis due to fragments of serum amyloid A protein associated with chronic inflammatory disorders is a rare cause of cardiac disease. An isolated atrial amyloid form is also recognized.

In Africa, endomyocardial fibrosis, a specific entity in which there is severe fibrosis of the endocardium, often with eosinophilia (Löffler syndrome) is seen. Other causes of restrictive cardiomyopathy include infiltrative cardiomyopathies (eg, hemochromatosis, sarcoidosis) and connective tissue diseases (eg, scleroderma).

▶ Clinical Findings

A. Symptoms and Signs

Restrictive cardiomyopathy must be distinguished from constrictive pericarditis (see Table 10–18). **The key feature is that ventricular interaction is accentuated with respiration in constrictive pericarditis and that interaction is absent in restrictive cardiomyopathy.** In addition, the pulmonary arterial pressure is invariably elevated in restrictive cardiomyopathy due to the high PCWP and is normal in uncomplicated constrictive pericarditis. Symptoms may include angina, syncope, stroke, and peripheral neuropathy. Periorbital purpura, a thickened tongue, or hepatomegaly are all suggestive physical findings of amyloidosis.

B. Diagnostic Studies

Conduction disturbances are frequently present. Low voltage on the ECG combined with ventricular hypertrophy on the echocardiogram is suggestive of disease. Cardiac MRI presents a distinctive pattern of diffuse hyperenhancement of the gadolinium image in amyloidosis and is a useful screening test. The echocardiogram reveals a small, thickened LV with bright myocardium (speckled), rapid early diastolic filling revealed by the mitral inflow Doppler, and biatrial enlargement. The LV chamber size is usually normal with a reduced LVEF. Atrial septal thickening may be evident. Rectal, abdominal fat, or gingival biopsies can confirm systemic involvement, but myocardial involvement may still be present if these are negative and requires endomyocardial biopsy for the confirmation that cardiac amyloid is present. Demonstration of tissue infiltration on biopsy specimens using special stains followed by immunohistochemical studies and genetic testing are essential to define which specific protein is involved. Mass spectroscopy on all tissue in question and TTR gene sequencing in patients in whom the TTR wild type or TTR mutant variant is suspected is recommended.

▶ Treatment

Unfortunately, little useful therapy is available for either the causative conditions or the restrictive cardiomyopathy physiology. As a result of evolving chemotherapeutic regimens and novel monoclonal antibodies, outcomes in AL amyloidosis are improving. In immunoglobin light chain amyloidosis, standard- or high-dose chemotherapy with stem cell rescue is often pursued. In ATTR, therapies that decrease protein production, prevent dissociation, and promote clearance have the potential to slow or even halt the disease. Medications being investigated for this purpose include diflunisal or tafamidis, and there are multiple alternative antibody therapies being developed.

In acute cases, diuretics can help, but excessive diuresis can produce worsening kidney dysfunction. As with most patients with severe right heart failure, loop diuretics, thiazides, and aldosterone antagonists are all useful. Ultrafiltration devices may improve diuresis, although it is not clear if prognosis is improved. Atrial thrombi are not uncommon, although the role of anticoagulation in amyloidosis remains ill defined. Digoxin may precipitate arrhythmias and should not be used. Beta-blockers help slow heart rates and improve filling by increasing diastolic time. Corticosteroids may be helpful in sarcoidosis but they are more effective for conduction abnormalities than heart failure. In amyloidosis, the therapeutic strategy depends on the characterization of the type of amyloid protein and extent of disease and may include chemotherapy or bone marrow transplantation. In familial amyloidosis with transthyretin deposition, liver transplantation may be an option. Cardiac transplantation has also been used in patients with primary cardiac amyloidosis and no evidence of systemic involvement.

▶ When to Refer

All patients with the diagnosis of a restrictive cardiomyopathy should be referred to a cardiologist to decide etiology and plan appropriate treatment. This is especially true if amyloidosis is suspected given its poor prognosis.

Gertz MA et al. Pathophysiology and treatment of cardiac amyloidosis. Nat Rev Cardiol. 2015 Feb;12(2):91–102. [PMID: 25311231]
Ruberg FL et al. Cardiovascular magnetic resonance visualization of cardiac amyloid infiltration: challenges and opportunities. Circulation. 2015 Oct 20;132(16):1525–27. [PMID: 26362630]
Sharma N et al. Current state of cardiac amyloidosis. Curr Opin Cardiol. 2013 Mar;28(2):242–8. [PMID: 23324855]

RHEUMATIC FEVER

ESSENTIALS OF DIAGNOSIS

▶ More common in developing countries (100 cases/100,000 population) than in the United States (~2 cases/100,000 population).

▶ Peak incidence between ages 5 and 15 years.

▶ Revision of Jones criteria in 2015 includes echocardiographic findings.

▶ May involve mitral and other valves acutely, rarely leading to heart failure.

▶ General Considerations

Rheumatic fever is a systemic immune process that is a sequela of a beta-hemolytic streptococcal infection of the pharynx. It is a major scourge in developing countries and

responsible for 250,000 deaths in young people worldwide each year. Over 15 million people have evidence for rheumatic heart disease. Signs of acute rheumatic fever usually commence 2–3 weeks after infection but may appear as early as 1 week or as late as 5 weeks. The disease has become quite uncommon in the United States, except in immigrants; however, there have been reports of new outbreaks in several regions of the United States. The peak incidence is between ages 5 and 15 years; rheumatic fever is rare before age 4 years or after age 40 years. Rheumatic carditis and valvulitis may be self-limited or may lead to slowly progressive valvular deformity. The characteristic lesion is a perivascular granulomatous reaction with vasculitis. The mitral valve is acutely attacked in 75–80% of cases, the aortic valve in 30% (but rarely as the sole valve involved), and the tricuspid and pulmonary valves in under 5% of cases.

The clinical profile of the infection includes carditis in 50–70% and arthritis in 35–66%, followed by chorea (10–30% and predominantly in girls) then subcutaneous nodules (0–10%) and erythema marginatum (in less than 6%). Echocardiography has been found to be superior to auscultation, and the 2015 guidelines introduced **subclinical carditis** to the Jones criteria to represent abnormal echocardiographic findings when auscultatory findings were either not present or not recognized.

Chronic rheumatic heart disease results from single or repeated attacks of rheumatic fever that produce rigidity and deformity of valve cusps, fusion of the commissures, or shortening and fusion of the chordae tendineae. Valvular stenosis or regurgitation results, and the two often coexist. In chronic rheumatic heart disease, the mitral valve alone is abnormal in 50–60% of cases; combined lesions of the aortic and mitral valves occur in 20%; pure aortic lesions are less common. Tricuspid involvement occurs in about 10% of cases but only in association with mitral or aortic disease and is thought to be more common when recurrent infections have occurred. The pulmonary valve is rarely affected long term. A history of rheumatic fever is obtainable in only 60% of patients with rheumatic heart disease.

▶ Clinical Findings

The presence of two major criteria—or one major and two minor criteria—establishes the diagnosis. While India, New Zealand, and Australia have all published revised guidelines since 2001, the recommendations have led to the latest revision of the Jones criteria as a scientific statement from the AHA where subclinical carditis is recognized. In the review, subclinical carditis was evident in 16.8% of the 10 studies used by the World Health Organization. The revised criteria also recognize that a lower threshold should be used to diagnosis acute rheumatic fever in high-risk populations. The Revised Jones Criteria are outlined in their entirety in Table 10–19.

A. Major Criteria

1. Carditis—Carditis is most likely to be evident in children and adolescents. Any of the following suggests the presence of carditis: (1) pericarditis; (2) cardiomegaly, detected by physical signs, radiography, or echocardiography; (3) heart

Table 10–19. The 2015 Revised Jones Criteria.[1]

Population	Criteria	
	Major	Minor
Low risk	Carditis (clinical or subclinical)	Polyarthralgia
	Arthritis (polyarthritis only)	Fever (≥ 38.5°C)
	Chorea	ESR ≥ 60 mm/h or CRP ≥ 3.0 mg/dL (or both)
	Erythema marginatum	Prolonged PR interval (unless carditis is major criterion)
	Subcutaneous nodules	
Moderate and high risk	Carditis (clinical or subclinical)	Monoarthralgia
	Arthritis (monoarthritis, polyarthritis, polyarthalgia)	Fever (≥ 38°C)
	Chorea	ESR ≥ 30 mm/h or CRP ≥ 3.0 mg/dL (or both)
	Erythema marginatum	Prolonged PR interval (unless carditis is a major criterion)
	Subcutaneous nodules	

[1]For all patients with evidence of preceding group A streptococcal pharyngitis: initial acute rheumatic fever can be diagnosed when 2 major criteria or 1 major plus 2 minor criteria are met. Recurrent acute rheumatic fever can be diagnosed when 2 major or 1 major plus 2 minor or 3 minor criteria are met.
ESR, erythrocyte sedimentation rate; CRP, C-reactive protein.
Modified with permission from Gewitz, MH et al; American Heart Association Committee on Rheumatic Fever, Endocarditis, and Kawasaki Disease of the Council on Cardiovascular Disease in the Young. Revision of the Jones Criteria for the diagnosis of acute rheumatic fever in the era of Doppler echocardiography. A scientific statement from the American Heart Association. Circulation. 2015 May 19;131(20):1806–18. © 2015 American Heart Association, Inc. [PMID: 25908771]

failure, right- or left-sided—the former perhaps more prominent in children, with painful liver engorgement due to tricuspid regurgitation; and (4) mitral or aortic regurgitation murmurs, indicative of dilation of a valve ring with or without associated valvulitis or morphologic findings on echocardiography of rheumatic valvulitis. The Carey–Coombs short mid-diastolic mitral murmur may be present due to inflammation of the mitral valve. It is a Class 1 (LOE B) indication to perform echocardiography/Doppler studies on all cases of suspected or confirmed acute rheumatic fever.

2. Erythema marginatum and subcutaneous nodules— Erythema marginatum begins as rapidly enlarging macules that assume the shape of rings or crescents with clear centers. They may be raised, confluent, and either transient or persistent and usually on the trunk or proximal extremities. Subcutaneous nodules are uncommon except in children. They are small (2 cm or less in diameter), firm, and nontender and are attached to fascia or tendon sheaths over bony prominences. They persist for days or weeks, are recurrent, and are indistinguishable from rheumatoid nodules. Neither the rash nor nodules ever occur as the sole manifestation of acute rheumatic fever.

3. Sydenham chorea—This is the most definitive manifestation of acute rheumatic fever. Defined as involuntary choreoathetoid movements primarily of the face, tongue, and upper extremities, Sydenham chorea may be the sole manifestation of rheumatic fever. Girls are more frequently affected than boys, and occurrence in adults is rare.

4. Polyarthritis—This is a migratory polyarthritis that involves the large joints sequentially. In adults and in

certain moderate- to high-risk populations, only a single joint may be affected. The arthritis lasts 1–5 weeks and subsides without residual deformity. Prompt response of arthritis to therapeutic doses of salicylates or nonsteroidal agents is characteristic.

B. Minor Criteria

These include fever, polyarthralgias, reversible prolongation of the PR interval, and an elevated erythrocyte sedimentation rate or CRP. A lower threshold is set for patients at high risk (Table 10–19). The 2015 guidelines stipulate that evidence for a preceding streptococcal infection can be defined by an increase or rising anti-streptolysin O titer or streptococcal antibodies (anti-DNAase B), a positive throat culture for group A beta-hemolytic streptococcal or a positive rapid group A streptococcal carbohydrate antigen test in a child with a high pretest probability of streptococcal pharyngitis.

▶ **Treatment**

A. General Measures

The patient should be kept at strict bed rest until the temperature returns to normal (without the use of antipyretic medications) and the sedimentation rate, plus the resting pulse rate, and the ECG have all returned to baseline.

B. Medical Measures

1. Salicylates—The salicylates markedly reduce fever and relieve joint pain and swelling. They have no effect on the natural course of the disease. Adults may require large doses of aspirin, 0.6–0.9 g every 4 hours; children are treated with lower doses.

2. Penicillin—Penicillin (benzathine penicillin, 1.2 million units intramuscularly once, or procaine penicillin, 600,000 units intramuscularly daily for 10 days) is used to eradicate streptococcal infection if present. Erythromycin may be substituted (40 mg/kg/day).

3. Corticosteroids—There is no proof that cardiac damage is prevented or minimized by corticosteroids. A short course of corticosteroids (prednisone, 40–60 mg orally daily, with tapering over 2 weeks) usually causes rapid improvement of the joint symptoms and is indicated when response to salicylates has been inadequate.

► Prevention of Recurrent Rheumatic Fever

Improvement in socioeconomic conditions and public health are critical to reducing bouts of rheumatic fever. The initial episode of rheumatic fever can usually be prevented by early treatment of streptococcal pharyngitis with penicillin (see Chapter 33). Prevention of recurrent episodes of rheumatic fever is critical. Recurrences of rheumatic fever are most common in patients who have had carditis during their initial episode and in children, 20% of whom will have a second episode within 5 years. The preferred method of prophylaxis is with benzathine penicillin G, 1.2 million units intramuscularly every 4 weeks. Oral penicillin (250 mg twice daily) is less reliable.

If the patient is allergic to penicillin, sulfadiazine (or sulfisoxazole), 1 g daily, or erythromycin, 250 mg orally twice daily, may be substituted. The macrolide azithromycin is similarly effective against group A streptococcal infection. If the patient has not had an immediate hypersensitivity (anaphylactic-type) reaction to penicillin, then cephalosporin may also be used.

Recurrences are uncommon after 5 years following the first episode and in patients over 21 years of age. Prophylaxis is usually discontinued after these times except in groups with a high risk of streptococcal infection—parents or teachers of young children, nurses, military recruits, etc. Secondary prevention of rheumatic fever depends on whether carditis has occurred. Current guidelines suggest that if there is no evidence for carditis, preventive therapy can be stopped at age 21 years. If carditis has occurred but there is no residual valvular disease, it can be stopped at 10 years after the acute rheumatic fever episode. If carditis has occurred with residual valvular involvement, it should be continued for 10 years after the last episode or until age 40 years if the patient is in a situation in which reexposure would be expected.

► Prognosis

Initial episodes of rheumatic fever may last months in children and weeks in adults. The immediate mortality rate is 1–2%. Persistent rheumatic carditis with cardiomegaly, heart failure, and pericarditis implies a poor prognosis; 30% of children thus affected die within 10 years after the initial attack. After 10 years, two-thirds of patients will have detectable valvular abnormalities (usually thickened valves with limited mobility), but significant symptomatic VHD or persistent cardiomyopathy occurs in less than 10% of patients with a single episode. In developing countries, acute rheumatic fever occurs earlier in life and recurs more frequently, thus the evolution to chronic valvular disease is both accelerated and more severe.

Gewitz MH et al; American Heart Association Committee on Rheumatic Fever, Endocarditis, and Kawasaki Disease of the Council on Cardiovascular Disease in the Young. Revision of the Jones Criteria for the diagnosis of acute rheumatic fever in the era of Doppler echocardiography. A scientific statement from the American Heart Association. Circulation. 2015 May 19; 131(20):1806–18. [PMID: 25908771]

Marijon E et al. Rheumatic heart disease. Lancet. 2012 Mar 10; 379(9819):953–64. [PMID: 22405798]

Roberts K et al. Screening for rheumatic heart disease: current approaches and controversies. Nat Rev Cardiol. 2013 Jan;10(1):49–58. [PMID: 23149830]

DISEASES OF THE PERICARDIUM

ACUTE INFLAMMATORY PERICARDITIS

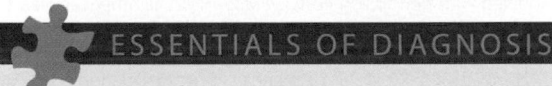

ESSENTIALS OF DIAGNOSIS

- ► Anterior pleuritic chest pain that is worse supine than upright.
- ► Pericardial rub.
- ► Fever common.
- ► Erythrocyte sedimentation rate usually elevated.
- ► ECG reveals diffuse ST-segment elevation with associated PR depression.

► General Considerations

Acute (less than 2 weeks) inflammation of the pericardium may be infectious in origin or may be due to systemic diseases (autoimmune syndromes, uremia), neoplasm, radiation, drug toxicity, hemopericardium, postcardiac surgery, or contiguous inflammatory processes in the myocardium or lung. In many of these conditions, the pathologic process involves both the pericardium and the myocardium. Overall pericarditis accounts for 0.2% of hospital admissions and about 5% of patients with nonischemic chest pain seen in the emergency department. The ESC in 2015 proposed four definitions for pericarditis and elucidated diagnostic criteria for each (Table 10–20). **Viral infections** (especially infections with coxsackieviruses and echoviruses but also influenza, Epstein-Barr, varicella, hepatitis, mumps, and HIV viruses) are the most common cause of acute pericarditis and probably are responsible for many cases classified as idiopathic. Males—usually under age 50 years—are most commonly affected. The differential diagnosis primarily requires exclusion of acute myocardial infarction. **Tuberculous pericarditis** is rare in developed countries but remains common in certain areas of the

Table 10–20. Definitions and diagnostic criteria for pericarditis.

Pericarditis	Definition and Diagnosis
Acute	At least two of the following four listed findings: 1. Pericardial chest pain 2. Pericardial rub 3. New widespread ST-elevation or PR depression 4. Pericardial effusion (new or worsening)
	Additional supportive findings: 1. Elevated inflammatory markers (CRP, ESR, WBC) 2. Evidence for pericardial inflammation (CT or MRI)
Incessant	Pericarditis lasting longer than 4–6 weeks but less than 3 months without remission
Recurrent	Recurrence after a documented first espisode and a symptom-free interval of 4–6 weeks or longer.
Chronic	Pericarditis lasting longer than 3 months

CRP, C-reactive protein; CT, computed tomography; ESR, erythrocyte sedimentation rate; MRI, magnetic resonance imaging; WBC, white blood count.

Modified with permission from Adler Y et al. 2015 ESC guidelines for the diagnosis and management of pericardial diseases: The Task Force for the Diagnosis and Management of Pericardial Diseases of the European Society of Cardiology (ESC) Endorsed by: The European Association for Cardio-Thoracic Surgery (EACTS). Eur Heart J. 2015 Nov 7;36(42):2921–64. [PMID: 26320112]

world. It results from direct lymphatic or hematogenous spread; clinical pulmonary involvement may be absent or minor, although associated pleural effusions are common. **Bacterial pericarditis** is equally rare and usually results from direct extension from pulmonary infections. Pneumococci, though, can cause a primary pericardial infection. *Borrelia burgdorferi,* the organism responsible for Lyme disease, can also cause myopericarditis (and occasionally heart block). **Uremic pericarditis** is a common complication of chronic kidney disease. The pathogenesis is uncertain; it occurs both with untreated uremia and in otherwise stable dialysis patients. Spread of adjacent lung cancer as well as invasion by breast cancer, renal cell carcinoma, Hodgkin disease, and lymphomas are the most common **neoplastic processes** involving the pericardium and have become the most frequent causes of pericardial tamponade in many countries. Pericarditis may occur 2–5 days after infarction due to an inflammatory reaction to transmural myocardial necrosis (**postmyocardial infarction** or **postcardiotomy pericarditis [Dressler syndrome]**). **Radiation** can initiate a fibrinous and fibrotic process in the pericardium, presenting as subacute pericarditis or constriction. Radiation pericarditis usually follows treatments of more than 4000 cGy delivered to ports including more than 30% of the heart.

Other causes of pericarditis include connective tissue diseases, such as lupus erythematosus and rheumatoid arthritis, drug-induced pericarditis (minoxidil, penicillins, clozapine), and myxedema. In addition, pericarditis may result from **pericardial injury** from invasive cardiac procedures (such as cardiac pacemaker and defibrillator perforation and intracardiac ablation, especially atrial fibrillation ablation), and the implantation of intracardiac devices (such as ASD occluder devices).

Pericarditis and myocarditis may coexist in 20–30% of patients. Myocarditis is often suspected when there is an elevation of serum troponins, although there are no data that suggest troponin elevations are associated with a poor prognosis.

▶ Clinical Findings

A. Symptoms and Signs

The presentation and course of inflammatory pericarditis depend on its cause, but most syndromes have associated chest pain, which is usually pleuritic and postural (relieved by sitting). The pain is substernal but may radiate to the neck, shoulders, back, or epigastrium. Dyspnea may also be present and the patient is often febrile. A pericardial friction rub is characteristic, with or without evidence of fluid accumulation or constriction. The presentation of **tuberculous pericarditis** tends to be subacute, but nonspecific symptoms (fever, night sweats, fatigue) may be present for days to months. Pericardial involvement develops in 1–8% of patients with pulmonary tuberculosis. Symptoms and signs of **bacterial pericarditis** are similar to those of other types of inflammatory pericarditides, but patients appear toxic and are often critically ill. **Uremic pericarditis** can present with or without symptoms; fever is absent. Often **neoplastic pericarditis** is painless, and the presenting symptoms relate to hemodynamic compromise or the primary disease. At times the pericardial effusion is very large, consistent with its chronic nature. **Postmyocardial infarction** or **postcardiotomy pericarditis (Dressler syndrome)** usually presents as a recurrence of pain with pleural-pericardial features. A rub is often audible, and repolarization changes on the ECG may be confused with ischemia. Large effusions are uncommon, and spontaneous resolution usually occurs in a few days. Dressler syndrome occurs days to weeks to several months after myocardial infarction or open heart surgery, may be recurrent, and probably represents an autoimmune syndrome. Patients present with typical pain, fever, malaise, and leukocytosis. Rarely, other symptoms of an autoimmune disorder, such as joint pain and fever, may occur. Tamponade is rare with Dressler syndrome after myocardial infarction but not when it occurs postoperatively. The clinical onset of **radiation pericarditis** is usually within the first year but may be delayed for many years; often a full decade or more may pass before constriction becomes evident.

B. Laboratory Findings and Diagnostic Studies

The diagnosis of **viral pericarditis** is usually clinical, and leukocytosis is often present. Rising viral titers in paired sera may be obtained for confirmation but are rarely done. Cardiac enzymes may be slightly elevated, reflecting an epicardial myocarditis component. The echocardiogram is often normal or reveals only a trivial amount of extra fluid during the acute inflammatory process. The diagnosis of **tuberculous pericarditis** can be inferred if acid-fast bacilli are found elsewhere. The tuberculous pericardial effusions are usually small or moderate but may be large when chronic. The yield of organisms by pericardiocentesis is low; pericardial biopsy has a higher yield but may also be negative, and pericardiectomy may be required. If **bacterial pericarditis** is suspected on clinical grounds, diagnostic pericardiocentesis can be confirmatory. In **uremic patients** not on dialysis, the incidence of pericarditis correlates roughly with the level of blood urea nitrogen (BUN) and creatinine. The pericardium is characteristically "shaggy" in uremic pericarditis, and the effusion is hemorrhagic and exudative. The diagnosis of **neoplastic pericarditis** can occasionally be made by cytologic examination of the effusion or by pericardial biopsy, but it may be difficult to establish clinically if the patient has received mediastinal radiation within the previous year. Neoplastic pericardial effusions develop over a long period of time and may become quite huge (more than 2 L). The sedimentation rate is high in **postmyocardial infarction** or **postcardiotomy pericarditis** and can help confirm the diagnosis. Large pericardial effusions and accompanying pleural effusions are frequent. Myxedema pericardial effusions due to hypothyroidism usually are characterized by the presence of cholesterol crystals within the fluid.

C. Other Studies

The ECG usually shows generalized ST and T wave changes and may manifest a characteristic progression beginning with diffuse ST elevation, followed by a return to baseline and then to T-wave inversion. Atrial injury is often present and manifested by PR depression, especially in the limb leads. The chest radiograph is frequently normal but may show cardiac enlargement (if pericardial fluid is present), as well as signs of related pulmonary disease. Mass lesions and enlarged lymph nodes may suggest a neoplastic process. About 60% of patients have a pericardial effusion (usually mild) detectable by echocardiography. MRI and CT scan can visualize neighboring tumor in neoplastic pericarditis. A screening chest CT or MRI is often recommended to ensure there are no extracardiac diseases contiguous to the pericardium. A consensus statement from the American Society of Echocardiography proposes adding an elevated CRP and late gadolinium enhancement of the pericardium to confirmatory criteria for the diagnosis of pericarditis.

► Treatment

For acute pericarditis, experts suggest a restriction in activity until symptom resolution. For athletes the duration of exercise restriction should be until resolution of symptoms and normalization of all laboratory tests (generally 3 months). The 2015 ESC guidelines recommend aspirin 750–1000 mg every 8 hours for 1–2 weeks with a taper by decreasing the dose 250–500 mg every 1–2 weeks or ibuprofen 600 mg every 8 hours for 1–2 weeks with a taper by decreasing the dose by 200–400 mg every 1–2 weeks.

Gastroprotection should be included. Studies support initial treatment of the acute episode with colchicine to prevent recurrences. Colchicine should be added to the nonsteroidal anti-inflammatory medication at 0.5–0.6 mg once (for patients less than 70 kg) or twice (for patients more than 70 kg) daily and continued for at least 3 months. Tapering of colchicine is not mandatory; however, in the last week of treatment, the dosage can be reduced every other day for patients less than 70 kg or once a day for those more than 70 kg. Aspirin and colchicine should be used instead of nonsteroidal anti-inflammatory medications in postmyocardial infarction pericarditis (Dressler syndrome), since nonsteroidal anti-inflammatory medications and corticosteroids may have an adverse effect on myocardial healing. Aspirin in doses of 750–1000 mg three times daily for 1–2 weeks plus 3 months of colchicine is the recommended treatment.

Colchicine should be used for at least 6 months as therapy in all refractory cases and in recurrent pericarditis. At times longer therapy is required. The CRP is used to assess the effectiveness of treatment, and once it is normalized, tapering is initiated. Indomethacin in doses of 25–50 mg every 8 hours can also be considered in recurrent pericarditis in place of ibuprofen. Systemic corticosteroids can be added in patients with severe symptoms, in refractory cases, or in patients with immune-mediated etiologies, but such therapy may entail a higher risk of recurrence and may actually prolong the illness. Colchicine is recommended in addition to corticosteroids, again for at least 3 months, to help prevent recurrences. Prednisone in doses of 0.25–0.5 mg/kg/day orally is generally suggested with tapering over a 4–6 week period.

As a rule, symptoms subside in several days to weeks. The major early complication is tamponade, which occurs in less than 5% of patients. There may be recurrences in the first few weeks or months. Rarely, when colchicine therapy alone fails or cannot be tolerated (usually do to gastrointestinal symptoms), the pericarditis may require more significant immunosuppression, such as cyclophosphamide, azathioprine, intravenous human immunoglobulins, interleukin-1 receptor antagonists (anakinra), or methotrexate. If colchicine plus more significant immunosuppression fails, surgical pericardial stripping may be considered in recurrent cases even without clinical evidence for constrictive pericarditis.

Standard antituberculous drug therapy is usually successful for **tuberculous pericarditis** (see Chapter 9), but constrictive pericarditis can occur. **Uremic pericarditis** usually resolves with the institution of—or with more aggressive—dialysis. Tamponade is fairly common, and partial pericardiectomy (pericardial window) may be necessary. Whereas anti-inflammatory agents may relieve the pain and fever associated with uremic pericarditis, indomethacin and systemic corticosteroids do not affect its natural history. The prognosis with **neoplastic effusion** is poor, with only a small minority surviving 1 year. If it is compromising the clinical comfort of the patient, the effusion is initially drained percutaneously. A pericardial window, either by a subxiphoid approach or via video-assisted thoracic surgery, allows for partial pericardiectomy.

Instillation of chemotherapeutic agents or tetracycline may be used to reduce the recurrence rate. Symptomatic therapy is the initial approach to **radiation pericarditis,** but recurrent effusions and constriction often require surgery.

► When to Refer

Patients who do not respond initially to conservative management, who have recurrences, or who appear to be developing constrictive pericarditis should be referred to a cardiologist for further assessment.

Adler Y et al. 2015 ESC guidelines for the diagnosis and management of pericardial diseases: The Task Force for the Diagnosis and Management of Pericardial Diseases of the European Society of Cardiology (ESC) Endorsed by: The European Association for Cardio-Thoracic Surgery (EACTS). Eur Heart J. 2015 Nov 7;36(42):2921–64. [PMID: 26320112]

Imazio M et al. Evaluation and treatment of pericarditis. A systematic review. JAMA. 2015 Oct 13;314(14):1498–506. [PMID: 26461998]

Imazio M et al; ICAP Investigators. A randomized trial of colchicine for acute pericarditis. N Engl J Med. 2013 Oct 17; 369(16):1522–8. [PMID: 23992557]

Klein AL et al. American Society of Echocardiography clinical recommendations for multimodality cardiovascular imaging of patients with pericardial disease: endorsed by the Society for Cardiovascular Magnetic Resonance and Society of Cardiovascular Computed Tomography. J Am Soc Echocardiogr. 2013 Sep;26(9):965–1012. [PMID: 23998693]

PERICARDIAL EFFUSION & TAMPONADE

ESSENTIALS OF DIAGNOSIS

Pericardial Effusion

► Clinical impact determined by the speed of accumulation.

► May or may not cause pain.

Tamponade

► Tachycardia with an elevated JVP and either hypotension or a paradoxical pulse.

► Low voltage or electrical alternans on ECG.

► Echocardiography is diagnostic.

Pericardial effusion can develop during any of the acute pericarditis processes. Because the pericardium covers the ascending aorta and arch, aortic dissection and/or rupture can lead to tamponade as well. The speed of accumulation determines the physiologic importance of the effusion. Because of pericardial compliance, effusions larger than 1000 mL that develop slowly may produce no hemodynamic effects. Conversely, smaller effusions that appear rapidly can cause tamponade due to the curvilinear relationship between the volume of fluid and the intrapericardial pressure. Tamponade is characterized by elevated intrapericardial pressure (greater than 15 mm Hg), which restricts venous return and ventricular filling. As a result, the stroke volume and arterial pulse pressure fall, and the heart rate and venous pressure rise. Shock and death may result.

► Clinical Findings

A. Symptoms and Signs

Pericardial effusions may be associated with pain if they occur as part of an acute inflammatory process or may be painless, as is often the case with neoplastic or uremic effusion. Dyspnea and cough are common, especially with tamponade. Cardiac tamponade can be a life-threatening syndrome evidenced by tachycardia, hypotension, pulsus paradoxicus, raised JVP, muffled heart sounds, and decreased ECG voltage or electrical alternans. Other symptoms may result from the primary disease. The prognosis is a function of the cause. Large idiopathic chronic effusions (over 3 months) have a 30–35% risk of progression to cardiac tamponade.

A pericardial friction rub may be present even with large effusions. In cardiac tamponade, tachycardia, tachypnea, a narrow pulse pressure, and a relatively preserved systolic pressure are characteristic. Pulsus paradoxus is defined as a decline of greater than 10 mm Hg in systolic pressure during inspiration. Since the RV and LV share the same pericardium, when there is significant pericardial effusion, as the RV enlarges with inspiratory filling, septal motion toward the LV chamber reduces LV filling and results in an accentuated drop in the stroke volume and systemic BP with inspiration (the paradoxical pulse). Central venous pressure is elevated and, since the intrapericardial, and thus intracardiac, pressures are high even at the initiation of diastole, there is no evident y descent in the RA, RV, or LV hemodynamic tracings. This differs from constriction where most of the initial filling of the RV and LV occurs during early diastole (rapid y descent), and it is only in mid to late diastole that the ventricles can no longer fill. Edema or ascites are rarely present in tamponade; these signs favor a more chronic process.

B. Laboratory Findings

Laboratory tests tend to reflect the underlying processes (see causes of pericarditis above).

C. Diagnostic Studies

Chest radiograph can suggest chronic effusion by an enlarged cardiac silhouette with a globular configuration but may appear normal in acute situations. The ECG often reveals nonspecific T-wave changes and reduced QRS voltage. Electrical alternans is present only occasionally but is pathognomonic and is believed to be due to the heart swinging within the large effusion. Echocardiography is the primary method for demonstrating pericardial effusion and is quite sensitive. If tamponade is present, the high intrapericardial pressure may collapse lower pressure cardiac structures, such as the RA and RV. Cardiac CT and MRI also demonstrate pericardial fluid, pericardial thickening, and any associated contiguous lesions. Diagnostic pericardiocentesis or biopsy is often indicated for microbiologic and cytologic studies; a pericardial biopsy may be performed relatively simply through a small subxiphoid incision or by use of a video-assisted thoracoscopic surgical procedure. Unfortunately, the quality of the pericardial fluid itself rarely leads to a diagnosis, and any type of fluid (serous, serosanguinous, bloody, etc) can be seen in most diseases. Pericardial fluid analysis is most useful in excluding a bacterial cause and is occasionally helpful in malignancies. Effusions due to hypothyroidism or lymphatic obstruction may contain cholesterol or be chylous in nature, respectively.

► Treatment

Small effusions can be followed clinically by careful observations of the JVP and by testing for a change in the paradoxical pulse. Serial echocardiograms are indicated if no intervention is immediately contemplated. Vasodilators and diuretics should be avoided. When tamponade is present, urgent pericardiocentesis or cardiac surgery is required. Because the pressure–volume relationship in the pericardial fluid is curvilinear and upsloping, removal of a small amount of fluid often produces a dramatic fall in the intrapericardial pressure and immediate hemodynamic benefit; but complete drainage with a catheter is preferable. Continued or repeat drainage may be indicated, especially in malignant effusions. Pericardial windows via video-assisted thoracoscopy have been particularly effective in preventing recurrences. Effusions related to recurrent inflammatory pericarditis can be treated as noted above (see Acute Inflammatory Pericarditis).

Additional therapy is determined by the nature of the primary process. Recurrent effusion in neoplastic disease and uremia, in particular, may require partial pericardiectomy.

► When to Refer

- Any unexplained pericardial effusion should be referred to a cardiologist.
- Trivial pericardial effusions are common, especially in heart failure, and need not be referred unless symptoms of pericarditis are evident.
- Hypotension or a paradoxical pulse suggesting the pericardial effusion is hemodynamically compromising the patient is a medical emergency and requires immediate drainage.
- Any echocardiographic signs of tamponade.

Adler Y et al. 2015 ESC guidelines for the diagnosis and management of pericardial diseases: The Task Force for the Diagnosis and Management of Pericardial Diseases of the European Society of Cardiology (ESC) Endorsed by: The European Association for Cardio-Thoracic Surgery (EACTS). Eur Heart J. 2015 Nov 7;36(42):2921–64. [PMID: 26320112]

CONSTRICTIVE PERICARDITIS

ESSENTIALS OF DIAGNOSIS

- ► Evidence of right heart failure.
- ► No fall or an elevation of the JVP with inspiration (Kussmaul sign).
- ► Echocardiographic evidence for septal bounce and reduced mitral inflow velocities with inspiration.
- ► At times may be difficult to differentiate from restrictive cardiomyopathy.
- ► Cardiac catheterization may be necessary when clinical and echocardiographic features are equivocal.

► General Considerations

Inflammation can lead to a thickened, fibrotic, adherent pericardium that restricts diastolic filling and produces chronically elevated venous pressures. In the past, tuberculosis was the most common cause of constrictive pericarditis, but while it remains so in underdeveloped countries, it is otherwise rare now. Constrictive pericarditis rarely occurs following recurrent pericarditis. The risk of constrictive pericarditis due to viral or idiopathic pericarditis is less than 1%. Its occurrence increases following immune-mediated or neoplastic pericarditis (2–5%) and is highest after purulent bacterial pericarditis (20–30%). Other causes include post cardiac surgery, radiation therapy, and connective tissue disorders. A small number of cases are drug-induced or secondary to trauma, asbestosis, sarcoidosis, or uremia. At times, both pericardial tamponade and constrictive pericarditis may coexist, a condition referred to as **effusive-constrictive pericarditis**. The only definitive way to diagnose this condition is to reveal the underlying constrictive physiology once the pericardial fluid is drained.

► Clinical Findings

A. Symptoms and Signs

The principal symptoms are slowly progressive dyspnea, fatigue, and weakness. Chronic edema, hepatic congestion, and ascites are usually present. Ascites often seems out of proportion to the degree of peripheral edema. The examination reveals these signs and a characteristically elevated jugular venous pressure with a rapid *y* descent. This can be detected at bedside by careful observation of the jugular pulse and noting an apparent increased pulse wave at the end of ventricular systole (due to the relative accentuation of the *v* wave by the rapid *y* descent). **Kussmaul sign**—a failure of the JVP to fall with inspiration—is also a frequent finding. The apex may actually retract with systole and a pericardial "knock" may be heard in early diastole. Pulsus paradoxus is unusual. Atrial fibrillation is common.

B. Diagnostic Studies

At times constrictive pericarditis is extremely difficult to differentiate from restrictive cardiomyopathy and the two may coexist. When unclear, the use of both noninvasive testing and cardiac catheterization is required to sort out the difference.

1. Radiographic findings—The chest radiograph may show normal heart size or cardiomegaly. Pericardial calcification is best seen on the lateral view and is uncommon. It rarely involves the LV apex, and finding of calcification at the LV apex is more consistent with LV aneurysm.

2. Echocardiography—Echocardiography rarely demonstrates a thickened pericardium. A septal "bounce" reflecting the rapid early filling is common, though. RV/LV interaction may be demonstrated by an inspiratory reduction in the mitral inflow Doppler pattern of greater than 25%, much as in tamponade. Usually the initial mitral inflow into the LV is very rapid and this can be demonstrated as well by the Doppler inflow (E wave) pattern.

3. Cardiac CT and MRI—These imaging tests are only occasionally helpful. Pericardial thickening of more than 4 mm must be present to establish the diagnosis, but no pericardial thickening is demonstrable in 20–25% of patients with constrictive pericarditis. Some MRI techniques demonstrate the septal bounce and can provide further evidence for ventricular interaction.

4. Cardiac catheterization—This procedure is often confirmatory or can be diagnostic in difficult cases where the echocardiographic features are unclear or mixed. As a generality, the pulmonary pressure is low in constriction (as opposed to restrictive cardiomyopathy). In constrictive pericarditis, because of the need to demonstrate RV/LV interaction, cardiac catheterization should include simultaneous measurement of both the LV and RV pressure tracings with inspiration and expiration. Hemodynamically, patients with constriction have equalization of end-diastolic pressures throughout their cardiac chambers, there is rapid early filling then an abrupt increase in diastolic pressure ("square-root" sign), the RV end-diastolic pressure is more than one-third the systolic pressure, simultaneous measurements of RV and LV systolic pressure reveal a discordance with inspiration (the RV rises as the LV falls), and there is usually a Kussmaul sign (failure of the RA pressure to fall with inspiration).

Treatment

Therapy should be aimed at the specific etiology initially. If there is laboratory evidence of ongoing inflammation, then anti-inflammatory medications may have a role. Once the hemodynamics are evident, the mainstay of treatment is diuresis. As in other disorders of right heart failure, the diuresis should be aggressive, using loop diuretics (oral torsemide or bumetanide if bowel edema is suspected or intravenous furosemide), thiazides, and aldosterone antagonists (especially in the presence of ascites and liver congestion). At times, aquaphoresis may be of value. Surgical pericardiectomy should be recommended when diuretics are unable to control symptoms. Pericardiectomy removes only the pericardium between the phrenic nerve pathways, however, and most patients still require diuretics after the procedure, though symptoms are usually dramatically improved. Morbidity and mortality after pericardiectomy are high (up to 15%) and are greatest in those with the most disability prior to the procedure. Poor prognostic predictors include prior radiation, renal dysfunction, higher pulmonary systolic pressures, abnormal LV systolic function, a lower serum sodium level, liver dysfunction, and older age. Pericardial calcium has no impact on survival.

When to Refer

If the diagnosis of constrictive pericarditis is unclear or the symptoms of fluid retention resist medical therapy, then referral to a cardiologist is warranted to both establish the diagnosis and recommend therapy.

Adler Y et al. 2015 ESC guidelines for the diagnosis and management of pericardial diseases: The Task Force for the Diagnosis and Management of Pericardial Diseases of the European Society of Cardiology (ESC) Endorsed by: The European Association for Cardio-Thoracic Surgery (EACTS). Eur Heart J. 2015 Nov 7;36(42):2921–64. [PMID: 26320112]

Imazio M. Contemporary management of pericardial diseases. Curr Opin Cardiol. 2012 May;27(3):308–17. [PMID: 22450720]

Syed FF et al. Constrictive pericarditis—a curable diastolic heart failure. Nat Rev Cardiol. 2014 Sep;11(9):530–44. [PMID: 25072910]

PULMONARY HYPERTENSION

ESSENTIALS OF DIAGNOSIS

- ▶ Mean PA pressure of 25 mm Hg or more with normal PCWP.
- ▶ Dyspnea, and often cyanosis, with no evidence of left heart disease.
- ▶ Enlarged pulmonary arteries on chest radiograph.
- ▶ Elevated JVP and RV heave.
- ▶ Echocardiography is often diagnostic.

General Considerations

The normal pulmonary bed offers about one-tenth as much resistance to blood flow as the systemic arterial system. Experts recommend that a diagnosis of idiopathic pulmonary hypertension should be firmly based on a mean PA pressure of 25 mm Hg or more in association with a PCWP of less than 16 mm Hg at rest.

The clinical classification of pulmonary hypertension by the Fourth World Symposium on Pulmonary Hypertension is outlined in Table 10–21. It is a complex disorder due to multiple causes.

Group 1 includes pulmonary arterial hypertension (PAH) related to an underlying pulmonary vasculopathy.

Table 10–21. Clinical classification of pulmonary hypertension.

I. Pulmonary arterial hypertension from pulmonary vasculopathy
Idiopathic pulmonary arterial hypertension
Heritable gene mutations
BMPR2 (bone morphogenic protein receptor type 2)
ALK1 (activin A receptor type II-like kinase-1), *endoglin* (with or without hereditary hemorrhagic telangiectasia)
Unknown
Drug and toxin-induced
Associated with
Connective tissue diseases
HIV infection
Portal hypertension
Congenital heart disease
Schistosomiasis
Chronic hemolytic anemia
Persistent pulmonary hypertension of the newborn
Pulmonary veno-occlusive disease and/or pulmonary capillary hemangiomatosis
II. Pulmonary hypertension due to left heart disease
Systolic dysfunction
Diastolic dysfunction
III. Pulmonary hypertension due to lung disease and/or hypoxia
Chronic obstructive pulmonary disease
Interstitial lung disease
Other pulmonary disease with mixed restrictive and obstructive pattern
IV. Chronic thromboembolic pulmonary hypertension
V. Pulmonary hypertension with unclear multifactorial mechanisms
Hematologic disorders: myeloproliferative disorders, lenectomy
Systemic disorders: sarcoidosis, pulmonary Langerhans cell histiocytosis: lymphangioleimyomatosis, neurofibromatosis, vasculitis
Metabolic disorders: glycogen storage disease, Gaucher disease, thyroid disorders
Others: tumoral obstruction, fibrosing mediastinitis, chronic renal failure on dialysis

Modified, with permission, from Simonneau G et al. Updated clinical classification of pulmonary hypertension. J Am Coll Cardiol. 2009 Jun 30;54(1 Suppl):S43–54.

It includes the former "primary" pulmonary hypertension under the term "idiopathic pulmonary hypertension" and is defined as pulmonary hypertension and elevated PVR in the absence of other disease of the lungs or heart. Its cause is unknown. About 6–10% have heritable PAH. Drug and toxic pulmonary hypertension have been described as associated with the use of anorexigenic agents that increase serotonin release and block its uptake. These include aminorex fumarate, fenfluramine, and dexfenfluramine. In some cases, there is epidemiologic linkage to ingestion of rapeseed oil or L-tryptophan and use of illicit drugs, such as amphetamines. Pulmonary hypertension associated with connective tissue disease includes cases associated with scleroderma—up to 8–12% of patients with

scleroderma may be affected. Pulmonary hypertension has also been associated with HIV infection, portal hypertension, congenital heart disease (Eisenmenger syndrome), schistosomiasis, and chronic hemolytic anemia (eg, sickle cell anemia). In rare instances, obstruction of the pulmonary venous circulation may occur (pulmonary veno-occlusive disease and capillary hemangiomatosis).

Group 2 includes all cases related to left heart disease. **Group 3** includes cases due to parenchymal lung disease, impaired control of breathing, or living at high altitude. This group encompasses those with idiopathic pulmonary fibrosis and COPD. **Group 4** represents patients with chronic thromboemboli. **Group 5** includes multifactorial cases.

In recognition that the causes and treatment options may differ in children, the AHA and the American Thoracic Society published guidelines in 2015 regarding pulmonary hypertension in children. These guidelines cover persistent pulmonary hypertension in the newborn, diaphragmatic hernia in the young child, and bronchopulmonary dyplasia in children. Idiopathic pulmonary hypertension is not covered because it is uncommon in children. Because of the complexity of treating pulmonary hypertension in children, a multi-disciplinary team approach is critical.

▶ **Clinical Findings**

A. Symptoms and Signs

Common to all is exertional dyspnea, chest pain, fatigue, and lightheadedness as early symptoms; later symptoms include syncope, abdominal distention, ascites, and peripheral edema as RV function worsens. **Chronic lung disease, especially sleep apnea, often is overlooked as a cause for pulmonary hypertension as is chronic thromboembolic disease.** Patients with idiopathic pulmonary hypertension are characteristically young women who have evidence of right heart failure that is usually progressive, leading to death in 2–8 years without therapy. This is a decidedly different prognosis than patients with Eisenmenger physiology due to a left-to-right shunt; 40% of patients with Eisenmenger physiology are alive 25 years after the diagnosis has been made. Patients have manifestations of low cardiac output, with weakness and fatigue, as well as edema and ascites as right heart failure advances. Peripheral cyanosis is present, and syncope on effort may occur.

B. Diagnostic Studies

The laboratory evaluation of idiopathic pulmonary hypertension must exclude a secondary cause. A hypercoagulable state should be sought by measuring protein C and S levels, the presence of a lupus anticoagulant, the level of factor V Leiden, prothrombin gene mutations, and D-dimer. Chronic pulmonary emboli must be excluded (usually by ventilation-perfusion lung scan or contrast spiral CT); the ventilation-perfusion scan is the more sensitive test but not specific. If it is normal, then chronic thromboembolic pulmonary hypertension (CTEPH) is very unlikely. The chest radiograph helps exclude a primary pulmonary etiology—evidence for patchy pulmonary edema may raise the suspicion of pulmonary veno-occlusive disease due to localized obstruction in pulmonary venous drainage. A sleep study may be warranted if sleep apnea is suspected. The ECG is generally consistent with RVH and RA enlargement. Echocardiography with Doppler helps exclude an intracardiac shunt and usually demonstrates an enlarged RV and RA—at times they may be huge and hypocontractile. Severe pulmonic or tricuspid regurgitation may be present. Septal flattening seen on the echocardiogram is consistent with pulmonary hypertension. Doppler interrogation of the tricuspid regurgitation jet provides an estimate of RV systolic pressure. Pulmonary function tests help exclude other disorders, though primary pulmonary hypertension may present with a reduced carbon monoxide diffusing capacity of the lung (DL_{CO}) and severe desaturation (particularly if a PFO has been stretched open and a right-to-left shunt is present). A declining DL_{CO} in a scleroderma patient may precede the development of pulmonary hypertension. Chest CT demonstrates enlarged pulmonary arteries and excludes other causes (such as emphysema or interstitial lung disease). Pulmonary angiography (or magnetic resonance angiography or CT angiography) reveals loss of the smaller acinar pulmonary vessels and tapering of the larger ones. Catheterization allows measurement of pulmonary pressures and testing for vasoreactivity using a variety of agents, including 100% oxygen, adenosine, epoprostenol, and nitric oxide. Nitric oxide is preferred due to its ease of use and short half-life. A positive response is defined as one that decreases the pulmonary mean pressure by 10 mm Hg, with the final mean PA pressure less than 40 mm Hg. More and more, a 6-minute walk test is done to provide both clinical assessment of disease progression and prognosis. Cardiopulmonary testing provides a more sophisticated measure by assessing BP and oxygen consumption with stress.

▶ Treatment & Prognosis

The testing results described can be used to help define low- and high-risk patients. Table 10–22 outlines the 2013 recommendations of the determination of the risk of an adverse outcome in patients with pulmonary hypertension based on the clinical testing described above.

The treatment of PAH has evolved considerably over the last few years as more and more targeted therapies have been made available. The latest algorithm for the treatment of PAH as suggested by the 2013 World Symposium on Pulmonary Hypertension in Nice, France, is shown in Figure 10–11.

Counseling and patient education are also important. Aerobic exercise is recommended but no heavy physical exertion or isometric exercise. Routine immunizations are advised. Pregancy should be strongly discouraged and preventive measures taken to ensure it does not occur. Maternal mortality in severe PAH may be up to 50%.

Warfarin anticoagulation is recommended in all patients with idiopathic PAH and no contraindication. Diuretics are useful for the management of right-sided heart failure; clinical experience suggests loop diuretics (torsemide or butmetanide), which are absorbed if bowel edema is present, plus spironolactone are preferable. Oxygen should be used to maintain oxygen saturation greater than 90%. Acute vasodilator testing (generally with nitric oxide) should be performed in all patients with idiopathic PAH who may be potential candidates for long-term therapy with calcium channel blockers. Patients with PAH caused by conditions other than idiopathic PAH respond poorly to oral calcium channel blockers, and there is little value of acute vasodilator testing in these patients. Calcium channel blockers are primarily indicated for patients who have a positive acute vasodilator response. For patients who do not have a positive acute vasodilatory testing and are considered to be at lower risk based on clinical assessment, oral therapy with an endothelin receptor antagonist or phosphodiesterase-5 inhibitor is considered first-line of therapy. If an oral regimen is not appropriate, consideration of the other treatments would need to be based on the patient's profile, side effects, and the risk associated with each therapy. For patients who are considered high risk based on the clinical assessment, continuous treatment with an intravenous prostacyclin (epoprostenol or treprostinil) is considered

Table 10–22. 2013 recommendations about risk assessment for adverse outcomes in pulmonary hypertension.

Determinants of Risk	Lower Risk (Good Prognosis)	Higher Risk (Poor Prognosis)
Clinical evidence of RV failure	No	Yes
Progression of symptoms	Gradual	Rapid
WHO class	II, III	IV
6 minute walking distance	Longer (> 400 meters)	Shorter (< 300 meters)
Cardiopulmary stress		
Echocardiography	Minimal RV dysfunction	Pericardial effusion, significant RV enlargement/dysfunction, right atrial enlargement
Hemodynamics	RAP < 10 mm Hg, CI > 2.5 L/min/m²	RAP > 20 mm Hg, CI < 2.0 L/min/m²
BNP	Minimally elevated	Significantly elevated

[1]Most data available pertain to idiopathic pulmonary hypertension, with little data available for other forms of pulmonary artery hypertension. One should not rely on any single factor to make risk predictions.
BNP, B-type natriuretic peptide; RAP, right atrial pressure; RV, right ventricular; WHO, World Health Organization.

Supervised exercise training (I-A)	General measures and	Oral anticoagulants:
Psychosocial support (I-C)	supportive therapy	IPAH, heritable PAH, and PAH
Avoid strenuous physical activity (I-C)		due to anorexigens (IIa-C)
Avoid pregnancy (I-C)	Expert referral (I-C)	APAH (IIb-C)
Influenza and pneumococcal		Diuretics (I-C)
immunization (I-C)	Acute vasoreactivity test	Oxygen (I-C)
	(I-C for IPAH; IIb-C for APAH)	Digoxin (IIb-C)

VASOREACTIVE

NONVASOREACTIVE

WHO-FC I-II

CCB (I-C)

Sustained response (WHO-FC I-II)

Continue CCB ← Yes   No

INITIAL THERAPY WITH PAH-APPROVED DRUGS

Red: Morbidity and mortality as primary endpoint in randomized controlled study or reduction in all-cause mortality (prospectively defined)
* Level of evidence is based on the WHO-FC of most of the patients in the studies
† Approved only in the United States (treprostinil inhaled), in New Zealand (iloprost intravenously), in Japan and South Korea (beraprost)
‡ Drugs under regulatory approval

Recommendation	Evidence*	WHO-FC II	WHO-FC III	WHO-FC intravenously
I	A or B	Ambrisentan, Bosentan Macitentan‡ Riociguat‡ Sildenafil Tadalafil	Ambrisentan, Bosentan, Epoprostenol intravenously Iloprost inhaled Macitentan‡ Riociguat‡ Sildenafil Tadalafil Treprostinil subcutaneously, inhaled†	Epoprostenol intravenously
IIa	C		Iloprost intravenously† Treprostinil intravenously	Ambrisentan, bosentan Iloprost inhaled and intravenously† Macitentan‡ Riociguat‡ Sildenafil, tadalafil Treprostinil subcutaneously, intravenously, inhaled†
IIb	B		Beraprost†	
	C		Initial combination therapy	Initial combination therapy

Inadequate clinical response → Consider eligibilty for lung transplantation

Sequential combination therapy (I-A)
ERAs
† †
Prostanoids — † — PDE5-I or GCS‡

Inadequate clinical response on maximal therapy → Referral for lung transplantation (I-C)

BAS (IIa-C)

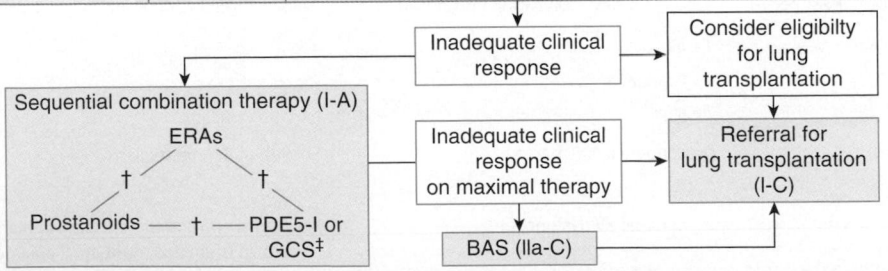

▲ **Figure 10–11.** The 2013 updated guideline treatment algorithm for pulmonary hypertension. In parentheses are the guideline recommendation classification and the level of evidence for specific therapies. APAH, associated pulmonary hypertension; BAS, balloon atrial septostomy; CCB, calcium channel blockers; ERA, endothelin receptor antagonists; GSC, guanylate cyclase stimulator (riociguat); IPAH, idiopathic pulmonary hypertension; PDE5-I, phosphodiesterase-5 inhibitors; WHO-FC, World Health Organization functional class. (Reproduced with permission from Galiè N et al. Updated treatment algorithm of pulmonary arterial hypertension. J Am Coll Cardiol 2013;62:D60.)

first-line of therapy. Epoprostenol improves exercise capacity, hemodynamics, and survival in patients with idiopathic PAH and is the preferred treatment option for the most critically ill patients. Combination therapy should be considered when patients are not responding adequately to initial monotherapy.

In patients with chronic thromboembolic disease, surgical or catheter thrombectomy or the use of a guanylate cyclase stimulator (riociquat) can be considered.

► **When to Refer**

All patients with suspected pulmonary hypertension should be referred to either a cardiologist or pulmonologist who specializes in pulmonary hypertension.

Abman SH et al. Pediatric pulmonary hypertension: Guidelines from the American Heart Association and American Thoracic Society. Circulation. 2015 Nov 24;132(21):2037–99. [PMID: 26534956]

Galiè N et al. Updated treatment algorithm of pulmonary arterial hypertension. J Am Coll Cardiol. 2013 Dec 24;62 (25 Suppl):D60–72. [PMID: 24355643]

Ghofrani HA et al; PATENT-1 Study Group. Riociguat for the treatment of pulmonary arterial hypertension. N Engl J Med. 2013 Jul 25;369(4):330–40. [PMID: 23883378]

Pulido T et al; SERAPHIN Investigators. Macitentan and morbidity and mortality in pulmonary arterial hypertension. N Engl J Med. 2013;369(9):809–18. [PMID: 23984728]

Simonneau G et al. Updated clinical classification of pulmonary hypertension. J Am Coll Cardiol. 2013 Dec 24;62 (25 Suppl):D34–41. Erratum in: J Am Coll Cardiol. 2014 Feb 25;63(7):746. [PMID: 24355639]

NEOPLASTIC DISEASES OF THE HEART

PRIMARY CARDIAC TUMORS

Primary cardiac tumors are rare and constitute only a small fraction of all tumors that involve the heart or pericardium. The most common primary tumor is **atrial myxoma**; it comprises about 50% of all tumors in adult case series. It is generally attached to the atrial septum and is more likely grow on the LA side of the septum rather than the RA. Patients with myxoma can rarely present with the characteristics of a systemic illness, with obstruction of blood flow at the mitral valve level or with signs of peripheral embolization. The syndrome includes fever, malaise, weight loss, leukocytosis, elevated sedimentation rate, and emboli (peripheral or pulmonary, depending on the location of the tumor). This is often confused with infective endocarditis, lymphoma, other cancers, or autoimmune diseases. In other cases, the tumor may grow to considerable size and produce symptoms by simply obstructing mitral inflow. Episodic pulmonary edema (classically occurring when an upright posture is assumed) and signs of low output may result. Physical examination may reveal a diastolic sound related to motion of the tumor ("tumor plop") or a diastolic murmur similar to that of mitral stenosis. Right-sided myxomas may cause symptoms of right-sided failure. Familial myxomas occur as part of the **Carney complex**, which consists of myxomas, pigmented skin lesions, and endocrine neoplasia.

The diagnosis is established by echocardiography or by pathologic study of embolic material. Cardiac MRI is useful as an adjunct. Contrast angiography is frequently unnecessary, although it may demonstrate a "tumor blush" when the mass is vascular. Surgical excision is usually curative, though recurrences do occur and serial echocardiographic follow-up is recommended.

The second most common primary cardiac tumors are **valvular papillary fibroelastomas** and **atrial septal lipomas.** These tend to be benign and usually require no therapy, although large papillary fibroelastomas may embolize or cause valvular dysfunction. Other primary cardiac tumors include rhabdomyomas (that often appear multiple in both the RV and LV), fibrous histiocytomas, hemangiomas, and a variety of unusual sarcomas. Some sarcomas may be of considerable size before discovery. Primary pericardial tumors, such as mesotheliomas related to asbestos exposure, may also occur. The diagnosis may be supported by an abnormal cardiac contour on radiograph. Echocardiography is usually helpful but may miss tumors infiltrating the ventricular wall. Cardiac MRI is emerging as the diagnostic procedure of choice.

SECONDARY CARDIAC TUMORS

Metastases from malignant tumors can also affect the heart. Most often this occurs in malignant melanoma, but other tumors that are known to metastasize to the heart include bronchogenic carcinoma, carcinoma of the breast, the lymphomas, renal cell carcinoma and, in patients with AIDS, Kaposi sarcoma. These are often clinically silent but may lead to pericardial tamponade, arrhythmias and conduction disturbances, heart failure, and peripheral emboli. The ECG may reveal regional Q waves. The diagnosis is often made by echocardiography, but cardiac MRI and CT scanning can often better delineate the extent of involvement. Metastatic tumors, especially lung or breast, may invade the pericardium and result in very large pericardial effusions as they result in slow accumulation of fluid. The prognosis is poor for all secondary cardiac tumors as treatment is generally palliative. On rare occasions, surgical resection for debulking or removal and chemotherapy may be effective.

Many primary tumors may be resectable. Atrial myxomas should be removed surgically due to the high incidence of embolization from these friable tumors. Papillary fibroelastomas are usually benign but they should be removed if they appear mobile and are larger than 10 mm in size or if there is evidence of embolization at the time of discovery. Large pericardial effusions from metastatic tumors may be drained for comfort, but the fluid invariably recurs. Rhabdomyomas may be surgically cured if the tumor is accessible and can be removed while still leaving enough functioning myocardium intact.

► **When to Refer**

All patients with suspected cardiac tumors should be referred to a cardiologist or cardiac surgeon for evaluation and possible therapy.

Burnside N et al. Malignant primary cardiac tumours. Interact Cardiovasc Thorac Surg. 2012 Dec;15(6):1004–6. [PMID: 22922450]

TRAUMATIC HEART DISEASE

Trauma is the leading cause of death in patients aged 1–44 years; **cardiac and vascular trauma is second only to neurologic injury as the reason for these deaths**. Penetrating wounds to the heart are often lethal unless surgically repaired. In a 20-year review of penetrating trauma at a single institution, it was found that gunshot wounds were fatal 13 times more often than stab wounds and that factors such as hypotension, Glasgow Coma Score less than 8, Revised Trauma Score less than 7.84, associated injuries and the more severe the injuries (Injury Severity Score greater than 25) all added to the mortality and morbidity risk.

Blunt trauma is a more frequent cause of cardiac injuries, particularly outside of the emergency department setting. This type of injury is common in motor vehicle accidents and may occur with any form of chest trauma, including CPR efforts. The most common injuries are myocardial contusions or hematomas. Other forms of nonischemic cardiac injury include metabolic injury due to burns, electrical current, or sepsis. These may be asymptomatic (particularly in the setting of more severe injuries) or may present with chest pain of a nonspecific nature or, not uncommonly, with a pericardial component. Elevations of cardiac enzymes are frequent but the levels do not correlate with prognosis. There are some data that the presence of certain other cardiac biomarkers, such as NT-proBNP, correlate better with significant myocardial injury. Echocardiography may reveal an akinetic segment or pericardial effusion. Cardiac MRI may also suggest acute injury. Coronary CTA or angiography can reveal a coronary dissection or acute occlusion if that is a concern. Pericardiocentesis is warranted if tamponade is evident. Heart failure is uncommon if there are no associated cardiac or pericardial injuries, and conservative management is usually sufficient. As noted above, tako-tsubo transient myocardial dysfunction can occur due to the accompanying stress.

Severe trauma may also cause myocardial or valvular rupture. Cardiac rupture can involve any chamber, but survival is most likely if injury is to one of the atria or the RV. Hemopericardium or pericardial tamponade is the usual clinical presentation, and surgery is almost always necessary. Mitral and aortic valve rupture may occur during severe blunt trauma—the former presumably if the impact occurs during systole and the latter if during diastole. Patients reach the hospital in shock or severe heart failure. Immediate surgical repair is essential. The same types of injuries may result in transection of the aorta, either at the level of the arch or distal to the takeoff of the left subclavian artery. Transthoracic echocardiography and TEE are the most helpful and immediately available diagnostic techniques.

Blunt trauma may also result in damage to the coronary arteries. Acute or subacute coronary thrombosis is the most common presentation. The clinical syndrome is one of acute myocardial infarction with attendant ECG, enzymatic, and contractile abnormalities. Emergent revascularization is sometimes feasible, either by the percutaneous route or by coronary artery bypass surgery. LV aneurysms are common outcomes of traumatic coronary occlusions, likely due to sudden occlusion with no collateral vascular support. Coronary artery dissection or rupture may also occur in the setting of blunt cardiac trauma.

As expected, patients with severe preexisting conditions fare the least well after cardiac trauma. Data from ReCO-NECT, a trauma consortium, reveal that mortality is linked to volume of cases seen at various centers, preexisting coronary disease or heart failure, intubation, age, and a severity scoring index.

Bock JS et al. Blunt cardiac injury. Cardiol Clin. 2012 Nov;30(4):545–55. [PMID: 23102031]

Clancy K et al. Screening for blunt cardiac injury: an Eastern Association for the Surgery of Trauma practice management guideline. J Trauma Acute Care Surg. 2012 Nov;73(5 Suppl 4): S301–6. [PMID: 23114485]

HEART DISEASE & PREGNANCY

The management of cardiac disease in pregnancy is discussed in the references listed below, including the available scoring systems to assess risk. The substantial risks inherent in mechanical heart valve patients who become pregnant are discussed in the valvular heart disease section. Only a few major points are covered in this brief section.

General principles to discuss with the patient include preconceptual counseling, pregnancy risk assessment, genetic risks, environmental risks, and pregnancy management. For some patients, it may also include a discussion regarding contraception, termination of a pregnancy, and a conversation about not only the delivery but what will happen post-pregnancy (including issues such as an eventual need for heart surgery or transplantation).

The Cardiac Disease in Pregnancy Investigation (CAR-PREG) scoring system for risk from cardiac events for women with heart disease noted four major risk factors: **(1)** NYHA FC III or IV heart failure, **(2)** prior cardiac events, **(3)** mitral or aortic obstruction, and **(4)** LVEF less than 40%. One point is assigned to each. Patients with no points had a 5% risk, those with 1 point had a complication rate of 27%, while for those with 2 or more points, the risk was 74%. Other reviews have suggested that the major risk for adverse outcomes or death to either the mother or fetus include pulmonary hypertension (with pulmonary pressure greater than three-quarters of systemic pressure), maternal cyanosis, systemic ventricular dysfunction, poor maternal functional class, severe left-sided valvular obstruction, aortic coarctation, significantly dilated aortic root, significant unrepaired heart defects, and warfarin therapy in patients with mechanical valves. In 2011, the World Health Organization outlined guidelines for the management of pregnancy in patients with congenital heart disease.

Medication usage during pregnancy is always a difficult decision, since most have not been studied. ACE inhibitors and amiodarone should not be used, but beta-blockers (including sotalol), digoxin, and calcium channel blockers are generally well tolerated. Labetalol has been found to be particularly useful for treating hypertension as have hydralazine and methyldopa. Diuretics can generally be given safely as well. For many patients, the most common potential complication is an atrial arrhythmia.

CARDIOVASCULAR COMPLICATIONS OF PREGNANCY

Pregnancy-related hypertension (eclampsia and preeclampsia) is discussed in Chapter 19.

1. Cardiomyopathy of Pregnancy (Peripartum Cardiomyopathy)

In approximately 1 in 3000 to 4000 live births, dilated cardiomyopathy develops in the mother in the final month of pregnancy or within 6 months after delivery. Risk factors include preeclampsia, twin pregnancies, and African ethnicity. It has been postulated that the problem is due to a cathepsin-D cleavage product of the hormone prolactin (16kDa fragment), suggesting blockage of prolactin may be a potential therapeutic strategy; clinical trials studying the role of bromocriptine are underway. Immune and viral causes have also been postulated. Small studies have suggested some improvement with the use of intravenous immunoglobulin and pentoxifylline. The disease occurs more frequently in women over age 30 years, is usually related to the first or second pregnancy, and there has been some association with gestational hypertension and medications used to stop uterine contractions.

The course of the disease is variable; most cases improve or resolve completely over several months, but others progress to refractory heart failure. About 60% of patients make a complete recovery. Serum BNP levels are routinely elevated in pregnancy, but serial values may be useful in predicting who may be at increased risk for a worse outcome. Beta-blockers have been administered judiciously to these patients, with at least anecdotal success. Diuretics, hydralazine, and nitrates help treat the heart failure with minimal risk to the fetus. Sotalol is acceptable for ventricular or atrial arrhythmias if other beta-blockers are ineffective. Some experts advocate anticoagulation because of an increased risk of thrombotic events, and both warfarin and heparin have their proponents. In severe cases, transient use of extracorporeal oxygenation (ECMO) has been lifesaving. Recurrence in subsequent pregnancies is common, particularly if cardiac function has not completely recovered, and subsequent pregnancies are to be discouraged if the EF remains less than 55%. The risk of recurrent heart failure in a subsequent pregnancy has been estimated to be about 1 in 5 (21%).

Givertz MM. Cardiology patient page: peripartum cardiomyopathy. Circulation. 2013 May 21;127(20):e622–6. [PMID: 23690457]

Hilfiker-Kleiner D et al. Pathophysiology and epidemiology of peripartum cardiomyopathy. Nat Rev Cardiol. 2014 Jun; 11(6):364–70. [PMID: 24686946]

Johnson-Coyle L et al; American College of Cardiology Foundation; American Heart Association. Peripartum cardiomyopathy: review and practice guidelines. Am J Crit Care. 2012 Mar; 21(2):89–98. Erratum in: Am J Crit Care. 2012 May;21(3):155. Dosage error in article text. [PMID: 22381985]

Shah T et al. Peripartum cardiomyopathy: a contemporary review. Methodist Debakey Cardiovasc J. 2013 Jan–Mar;9(1): 38–43. [PMID: 23519269]

2. Coronary Artery & Other Vascular Abnormalities During Pregnancy

There have been a number of reports of myocardial infarction during pregnancy. It is known that pregnancy predisposes to dissection of the aorta and other arteries, perhaps because of the accompanying connective tissue changes. The risk may be particularly high in patients with Marfan, Ehlers-Danlos, or Loeys-Dietz syndromes. However, coronary artery dissection is responsible for only a minority of the infarctions; most are caused by atherosclerotic CAD or coronary emboli. The majority of the events occur near term or shortly following delivery, and paradoxical emboli through a PFO have been implicated in a few instances. Clinical management is essentially similar to that of other patients with acute infarction, unless there is a connective tissue disorder. If nonatherosclerotic dissection is present, coronary intervention may be risky, as further dissection can be aggravated. In most instances, conservative management is warranted. At times, extensive aortic dissection requires surgical intervention. The 2011 European guidelines suggest Marfan patients are particularly susceptible to further aortic expansion during pregnancy when the aortic diameter is more than 4.5 cm (greater or equal to 27 mm/m^2) and pregnancy be discouraged in these situations. Some data, however, suggest that there is an increased risk of dissection during pregnancy even when the aortic root is at 4.0 cm, since pregnancy appears to have a small, but significant, influence on aortic growth even at this size. The earlier 2010 ACC/AHA/AATS guidelines suggest elective repair is reasonable when the aortic root is greater than 4.0 cm in women with Marfan syndrome contemplating pregnancy; as the review notes, half of women with Marfan syndrome and this large an aorta will need surgery since they are at risk for rupture or life-threatening aortic root growth during pregnancy.

Donnelly RT et al. The immediate and long-term impact of pregnancy on aortic growth rate and mortality in women with Marfan syndrome. J Am Coll Cardiol. 2012 Jul 17;60(3):224–9. [PMID: 22789886]

El-Deeb M et al. Acute coronary syndrome in pregnant women. Expert Rev Cardiovasc Ther. 2011 Apr;9(4):505–15. [PMID: 21517733]

European Society of Gynecology (ESG); Association for European Paediatric Cardiology (AEPC); German Society for Gender Medicine (DGesGM); Regitz-Zagrosek V et al. ESC Guidelines on the management of cardiovascular diseases during pregnancy: the Task Force on the Management of Cardiovascular Diseases during Pregnancy of the European Society of Cardiology (ESC). Eur Heart J. 2011 Dec;32(24):3147–97. [PMID: 21873418]

Hiratzka LF et al; American College of Cardiology Foundation/ American Heart Association Task Force on Practice

Guidelines; American Association for Thoracic Surgery; American College of Radiology; American Stroke Association; Society of Cardiovascular Anesthesiologists; Society for Cardiovascular Angiography and Interventions; Society of Interventional Radiology; Society of Thoracic Surgeons; Society for Vascular Medicine. 2010 ACCF/AHA/AATS/ACR/ ASA/SCA/SCAI/SIR/STS/SVM guidelines for the diagnosis and management of patients with Thoracic Aortic Disease: a report of the American College of Cardiology Foundation/ American Heart Association Task Force on Practice Guidelines, American Association for Thoracic Surgery, American College of Radiology, American Stroke Association, Society of Cardiovascular Anesthesiologists, Society for Cardiovascular Angiography and Interventions, Society of Interventional Radiology, Society of Thoracic Surgeons, and Society for Vascular Medicine. Circulation. 2010 Apr 6;121(13):e266–369. Erratum in Circulation. 2010 Jul 27;122(4):e410. [PMID: 20233780]

Mulder BJ et al. Pregnancy and Marfan syndrome: an ongoing discussion. J Am Coll Cardiol. 2012 Jul 17;60(3):230–1. [PMID: 22789887]

3. Prophylaxis for Infective Endocarditis During Pregnancy & Delivery

The 2007 ACC/AHA Task Force addressing adults with congenital heart disease has formulated guidelines outlining recommendations for pregnant women during labor and delivery. Pregnancy itself is not considered a risk for endocarditis. Since vaginal delivery might include bacteremia, the guidelines advocate endocarditis prophylaxis to cover the same high-risk groups as in the traditional endocarditis recommendations from the ACC/AHA, acknowledging that data are lacking to support this approach. Antibiotic prophylaxis against infective endocarditis is considered reasonable (Class 2a, LOE C) in select patients with the highest risk of adverse outcomes before vaginal delivery at the time of membrane rupture. Indications for antibiotic use include (1) prosthetic cardiac valve or prosthetic material used for cardiac valve repair, and (2) unrepaired and palliated cyanotic congenital heart disease, including surgically constructed palliative shunt conduits.

Brickner ME. Cardiovascular management in pregnancy: congenital heart disease. Circulation. 2014 Jul 15;130(3):273–82. [PMID: 25024123]

Warnes CA et al. ACC/AHA 2008 Guidelines for the Management of Adults With Congenital Heart Disease. A Report of the American College of Cardiology/American Heart Association Task Force on Practice Guidelines. Circulation. 2008 Dec 2;118(23):e714–833. [PMID: 18997169]

▶ Management of Labor

Although vaginal delivery is usually well tolerated, unstable patients (including patients with severe hypertension and worsening heart failure) should have planned cesarean section. Spinal anesthesia results in a large drop in the systemic vascular resistant and can worsen right-to-left shunting. An increased risk of aortic rupture has been noted during delivery in patients with coarctation of the aorta and severe aortic root dilation with Marfan syndrome, and vaginal delivery should be avoided in these conditions. For most patients, even those with complex congenital heart disease, vaginal delivery is the preferred method however. Following delivery, there are numerous fluid shifts that occur with the initial blood-reducing preload accompanied by the loss of the afterload reduction provided by the placenta. Venous return increases as the uterus is no longer compressing the inferior vena cava and there is an infusion of fluid into the vascular system as the uterus quickly shrinks back toward its normal size. The sudden increase in preload and loss of afterload following delivery can result in heart failure during the first 48–72 hours after the delivery and that remains the high-risk time for susceptible patients.

▼ CARDIOVASCULAR SCREENING OF ATHLETES

The sudden death of a competitive athlete inevitably becomes an occasion for local, if not national, publicity. On each occasion, the public and the medical community ask whether such events could be prevented by more careful or complete screening. Although each event is tragic, it must be appreciated that there are approximately 5 million competitive athletes at the high school level or above in any given year in the United States. The number of cardiac deaths occurring during athletic participation is unknown, but estimates at the high school level range from one in 300,000 to one in 100,000 participants. Death rates among more mature athletes increase as the prevalence of CAD rises. These numbers highlight the problem of how best to screen individual participants. Even an inexpensive test such as an ECG would generate an enormous cost if required of all athletes, and it is likely that only a few at-risk individuals would be detected. Echocardiography, either as a routine test or as a follow-up examination for abnormal ECGs, would be prohibitively expensive except for the elite professional athlete. Thus, the most feasible approach is that of a careful medical history and cardiac examination performed by personnel aware of the conditions responsible for most sudden deaths in competitive athletes.

It is important to point out that sudden death is much more common in the older than the younger athlete. Older athletes will generally seek advice regarding their fitness for participation. These individuals should recognize that strenuous exercise is associated with an increase in risk of sudden cardiac death and that appropriate training substantially reduces this risk. Preparticipation screening for risk of sudden death in the older athlete is a complex issue and at present is largely focused on identifying inducible ischemia due to significant coronary disease.

In a series of 158 athletic deaths in the United States between 1985 and 1995, **HCM** (36%) and **coronary anomalies** (19%) were by far the most frequent underlying conditions. LVH was present in another 10%, ruptured aorta (presumably due to Marfan syndrome or cystic medial necrosis) in 6%, myocarditis or dilated cardiomyopathy in 6%, aortic stenosis in 4%, and arrhythmogenic RV dysplasia in 3%. In addition, commotio cordis, or sudden death due to direct myocardial injury, may occur. More common in children, ventricular tachycardia or ventricular fibrillation may occur even after a minor direct blow to the heart; it is thought to be due to the precipitation of a PVC just prior to the peak of the T wave on ECG.

A careful family and medical history and cardiovascular examination will identify most individuals at risk (Table 10–22). An update in 2014 recommends that all middle school and higher athletes undergo a medical screen questionnaire and examination. The 12 elements in the examination are outlined in Table 10–23.

A family history of premature sudden death or cardiovascular disease, or of any of these predisposing conditions should mandate further work-up, including an ECG and echocardiogram. Symptoms of unexplained fatigue or dyspnea, exertional chest pain, syncope, or near-syncope also warrant further evaluation. A Marfan-like appearance, significant elevation of BP, abnormalities of heart rate or rhythm, and pathologic heart murmurs or heart sounds should also be investigated before clearance for athletic participation is given. Such an evaluation is recommended before participation at the high school and college levels and every 2 years during athletic competition.

Stress-induced syncope or chest pressure may be the first clue to an anomalous origin of a coronary artery. Anatomically, this lesion occurs most often when the left anterior descending artery or left main coronary arises from the right coronary cusp and traverses between the aorta and pulmonary trunks. The "slit-like" orifice that results from the angulation at the vessel origin is thought to cause ischemia when the aorta and pulmonary arteries enlarge during rigorous exercise and tension is placed on the coronary.

The toughest distinction may be in sorting out the healthy athlete with LVH from the athlete with hypertrophic cardiomyopathy. In general, the healthy athlete's heart is *less* likely to have an unusual pattern of LVH (such as asymmetric septal hypertrophy), or to have LA enlargement, an abnormal ECG, an LV cavity less than 45 mm in diameter at end-diastole, an abnormal diastolic filling pattern, or a family history of hypertrophic cardiomyopathy. The athlete is more likely to be male than the individual with hypertrophic cardiomyopathy, where women are equally at risk. Increased risk is also evident in patients with the Wolff-Parkinson-White syndrome, a prolonged QTc interval, or the Brugada syndrome on their ECG.

Selective use of routine ECG and stress testing is recommended in men above age 40 years and women above age 50 years who continue to participate in vigorous exercise and at earlier ages when there is a positive family history for premature CAD, HCM, or multiple risk factors. Because at least some of the risk features (long QT, LVH, Brugada syndrome, Wolff-Parkinson-White syndrome) may be evident on routine ECG screening, several cost-effectiveness studies have been done. Most suggest that pre-participation ECGs are of potential value, though what to do when the QTc is mildly increased is unclear. Many experts feel the high incidence of false-positive ECG studies make it very ineffective as a screening tool. With the low prevalence of cardiac anomalies in the general public, it has been estimated that 200,000 individual athletes would need to be screened to identify the single individual who would die suddenly. The issue of routine screening, therefore, remains controversial.

Once a high-risk individual has been identified, guidelines from the Bethesda conference and the ESC can be used to help determine whether the athlete may continue to participate in sporting events. Table 10–24 summarizes these recommendations.

Table 10–23. 12-element AHA recommendations for preparticipation cardiovascular screening of competitive athletes.

Medical History
Personal History
1. Exertional chest pain/discomfort
2. Unexplained syncope/near-syncope
3. Excessive exertional and unexplained dyspnea/fatigue
4. Prior recognition of a heart murmur
5. Elevated systemic blood pressure

Family History
6. Premature death (sudden and unexpected, or otherwise) before age of 50 years due to heart disease in one or more relatives
7. Disability from heart disease in a close relative before age of 50 years
8. Specific knowledge of certain cardiac conditions in family members: hypertrophic cardiomyopathy, dilated cardiomyopathy, long QT syndrome or other ion channelopathies, Marfan syndrome, or other important arrhythmias

Physical Examination
9. Heart murmur
10. Diminished femoral pulse (to exclude coarctation)
11. Phenotype of Marfan syndrome
12. Brachial artery blood pressure (sitting position)

Reproduced, with permission, from Lawless CE et al. Protecting the heart of the American athlete: proceedings of the American College of Cardiology Sports and Exercise Cardiology Think Tank, October 18, 2012, Washington, DC. J Am Coll Cardiol. 2014 Nov 18–25;64(20):2146–71. [PMID: 25306533]

Budts W et al. Physical activity in adolescents and adults with congenital heart defects: individualized exercise prescriptions. Eur Heart J. 2013 Dec;34(47):3669–74. [PMID: 24204010]

Chandra N et al. Sudden cardiac death in young athletes: practical challenges and diagnostic dilemmas. J Am Coll Cardiol. 2013 Mar 12;61(10):1027–40. [PMID: 23473408]

Chugh SS et al. Sudden cardiac death in the older athlete. J Am Coll Cardiol. 2015 Feb 10;65(5):493–502. [PMID: 25660928]

Higgins JP et al. Sudden cardiac death in young athletes: preparticipation screening for underlying cardiovascular abnormalities and approaches to prevention. Phys Sportsmed. 2013 Feb; 41(1):81–93. [PMID: 23445863]

Lawless CE et al. Protecting the heart of the American athlete: proceedings of the American College of Cardiology Sports and Exercise Cardiology Think Tank, October 18, 2012, Washington, DC. J Am Coll Cardiol. 2014 Nov 18–25;64(20):2146–71. [PMID: 25306533]

Schoenbaum M et al. Economic evaluation of strategies to reduce sudden cardiac death in young athletes. Pediatrics. 2012 Aug;130(2):e380–9. [PMID: 22753553]

Table 10–24. Recommendations for competitive sports participation among athletes with potential causes of SCD.

Condition	36th Bethesda Conference	European Society of Cardiology
Structural cardiac abnormalities		
HCM	Exclude athletes with a probable or definitive clinical diagnosis from all competitive sports. Genotype-positive/phenotype-negative athletes may still compete.	Exclude athletes with a probable or definitive clinical diagnosis from all competitive sports. Exclude genotype-positive/phenotype-negative individuals from competitive sports.
ARVC	Exclude athletes with a probable or definitive diagnosis from competitive sports.	Exclude athletes with a probable or definitive diagnosis from competitive sports.
CCAA	Exclude from competitive sports. Participation in all sports 3 months after successful surgery would be permitted for an athlete with ischemia, ventricular arrhythmia or tachyarrhythmia, or LV dysfunction during maximal exercise testing.	Not applicable.
Electrical cardiac abnormalities		
WPW	Athletes without structural heart disease, without a history of palpitations, or without tachycardia can participate in all competitive sports. In athletes with symptoms, electrophysiological study and ablation are recommended. Return to competitive sports is allowed after corrective ablation, provided that the ECG has normalized.	Athletes without structural heart disease, without a history of palpitations, or without tachycardia can participate in all competitive sports. In athletes with symptoms, electrophysiological study and ablation are recommended. Return to competitive sport is allowed after corrective ablation, provided that the ECG has normalized.
LQTS	Exclude any athlete with a previous cardiac arrest or syncopal episode from competitive sports. Asymptomatic patients restricted to competitive low-intensity sports. Genotype-positive/phenotype-negative athletes may still compete.	Exclude any athlete with a clinical or genotype diagnosis from competitive sports.
BrS	Exclude from all competitive sports except those of low intensity.	Exclude from all competitive sports.
CPVT	Exclude all patients with a clinical diagnosis from competitive sports. Genotype-positive/phenotype-negative patients may still compete in low-intensity sports.	Exclude all patients with a clinical diagnosis from competitive sports. Genotype-positive/phenotype-negative patients are also excluded.
Acquired cardiac abnormalities		
Commotio cordis	Eligibility for returning to competitive sport in survivors is a matter of individual clinical judgment. Survivors must undergo a thorough cardiovascular workup including 12-lead electrocardiography, ambulatory Holter monitoring, and echocardiography	Not applicable.
Myocarditis	Exclude from all competitive sports. Convalescent period of 6 months. Athletes may return to competitive when test results normalize.	Exclude from all competitive sports. Convalescent period of 6 months. Athletes may return to competition when test results normalize.

ARVC, arrhythmogenic right ventricular cardiomyopathy; BrS, Brugada syndrome; CCAA, congenital coronary artery anomalies; CPVT, cathecholaminergic polymorphic ventricular tachycardia; ECG, electrocardiogram; HCM, hypertrophic cardiomyopathy; LQTS, long QT syndrome; LV, left ventricular; SCD, sudden cardiac death; WPW, Wolff-Parkinson-White syndrome.
Reproduced, with permission, from Chandra N et al. Sudden cardiac death in young athletes: practical challenges and diagnostic dilemmas. J Am Coll Cardiol. 2013 Mar 12;61(10):1027–40.

Systemic Hypertension

Michael Sutters, MD, MRCP (UK)

Based on data from the 2011–2012 NHANES survey, about one-third of adults in the United States are hypertensive. Hypertension is uncontrolled in almost half of these 71 million people, and of those with uncontrolled hypertension, about 36% or 13 million are unaware of the diagnosis. Even in patients in whom hypertension is diagnosed and treated, control is attained in only 60%. By convention, hypertension is categorized based on office measurements as stage 1 (140–159/90–99 mm Hg) and stage 2 (greater than 160/100 mm Hg). Cardiovascular morbidity and mortality increase as both systolic and diastolic blood pressures rise, but in individuals over age 50 years, the systolic pressure and pulse pressure are better predictors of complications than diastolic pressure. The prevalence of hypertension increases with age, and it is more common in blacks than in whites. Adequate blood pressure control reduces the incidence of acute coronary syndrome by 20–25%, stroke by 30–35%, and heart failure by 50%.

HOW IS BLOOD PRESSURE MEASURED & HYPERTENSION DIAGNOSED?

Blood pressure should be measured with a well-calibrated sphygmomanometer. The bladder width within the cuff should encircle at least 80% of the arm circumference. Readings should be taken after the patient has been resting comfortably, back supported in the sitting or supine position, for at least 5 minutes and at least 30 minutes after smoking or coffee ingestion. Office-based devices that permit multiple automated measurements after a preprogrammed rest period produce blood pressure readings that are independent of the "white coat" phenomenon (where blood pressure is elevated in the clinic but normal at home) and digit preference bias. Blood pressure measurements taken outside the office environment, either by intermittent self monitoring (home blood pressure) or with an automated device programmed to take measurements at regular intervals (ambulatory blood pressure) are more powerful predictors of outcomes and are increasingly advocated in clinical guidelines. Home measurements are also helpful in differentiating "white coat" hypertension from hypertension that is resistant to treatment, and in diagnosis of "masked hypertension" (where blood pressure

is normal in the clinic but elevated at home). The cardiovascular risk associated with masked hypertension is similar to that observed in sustained hypertension.

A single elevated blood pressure reading is not sufficient to establish the diagnosis of hypertension. The major exceptions to this rule are hypertensive presentations with unequivocal evidence of life-threatening end-organ damage, as seen in hypertensive emergency, or in hypertensive urgency where blood pressure is greater than 220/125 mm Hg but life-threatening end-organ damage is absent. In less severe cases, the diagnosis of hypertension depends on a series of measurements of blood pressure, since readings can vary and tend to regress toward the mean with time. Patients whose initial blood pressure is in the hypertensive range exhibit the greatest fall toward the normal range between the first and second encounters. However, the concern for diagnostic precision needs to be balanced by an appreciation of the importance of establishing the diagnosis of hypertension as quickly as possible, since a 3-month delay in treatment of hypertension in high-risk patients is associated with a twofold increase in cardiovascular morbidity and mortality. The Canadian Hypertension Education Program provides an algorithm designed to expedite the diagnosis of hypertension (Figure 11–1). To this end, these guidelines recommend short intervals between initial office visits and stress the importance of early identification of target organ damage or diabetes mellitus, which, if present, justifies pharmacologic intervention if blood pressure remains above 140/90 mm Hg after just two visits. The Canadian guidelines suggest the use of ambulatory and home blood pressure measurements as complements to office-based evaluations. Guidelines from the United Kingdom go further in suggesting that ambulatory or home BP measurements should be used in preference to office-based measurements in the diagnosis of hypertension. When measured by automated office devices, manual home cuffs, or daytime ambulatory equipment, stage 1 hypertension is diagnosed at an average blood pressure greater than 135/85 mm Hg; for 24-hour ambulatory measurement, the diagnostic threshold for stage 1 hypertension is still lower at 130/80 mm Hg.

Ambulatory blood pressure readings are normally lowest at night and the loss of this nocturnal dip is a dominant

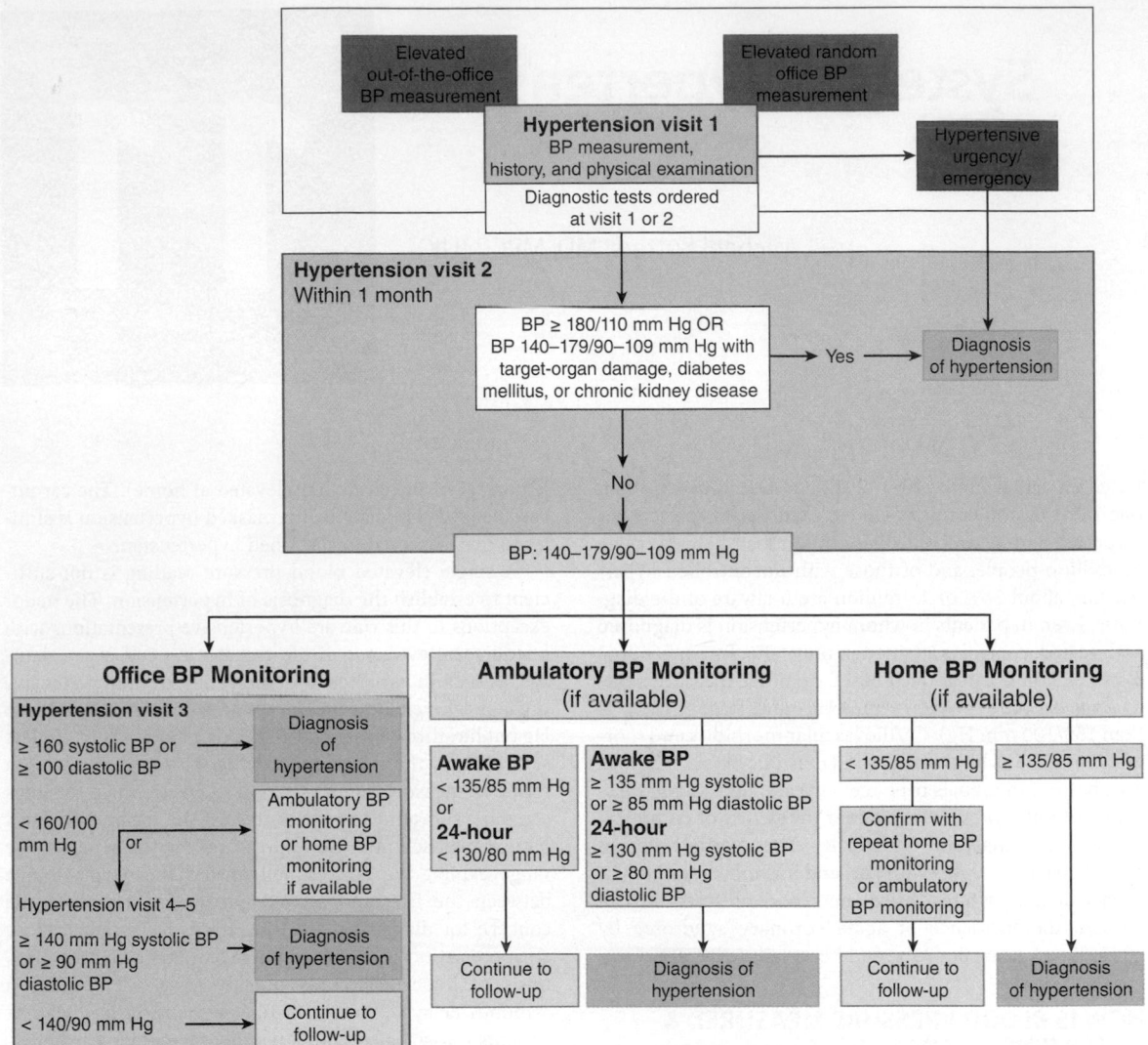

▲ **Figure 11–1.** The Canadian Hypertension Education Program expedited assessment and diagnosis of patients with hypertension: Focus on validated technologies for blood pressure (BP) assessment. (Reprinted, with permission, from the Canadian Hypertension Education Program. The 2012 Canadian Hypertension Education Program recommendations for the management of hypertension: blood pressure management, diagnosis, assessment of risk, and therapy.)

predictor of cardiovascular risk, particularly risk of thrombotic stroke. An accentuation of the normal morning increase in blood pressure is associated with increased likelihood of cerebral hemorrhage. Furthermore, variability of systolic blood pressure predicts cardiovascular events independently of mean systolic blood pressure. It is becoming increasingly clear that in diagnosing and monitoring hypertension, there should be a move away from isolated office readings and toward a more integrated view based on repeated measurements in a more "real world" environment.

It is important to recognize that the diagnosis of hypertension does not automatically entail drug treatment; this decision depends on the clinical setting, as discussed below.

PREHYPERTENSION

Data from the Framingham cohort indicate that blood pressure bears a linear relationship with cardiovascular risk down to a systolic blood pressure of 115 mm Hg; based on these data, it has been suggested that individuals with blood pressures in the gray area of 120–139/80–89 mm Hg be categorized as having "prehypertension." Because prehypertension often develops into hypertension (50% of affected individuals do so within 4 years), prehypertensive patients should be monitored annually.

Egan BM et al. Prehypertension—prevalence, health risks, and management strategies. Nat Rev Cardiol. 2015 May;12(5): 289–300. [PMID: 25687779]

Mancia G et al. Clinical value of ambulatory blood pressure: evidence and limits. Circ Res. 2015 Mar 13;116(6):1034–45. [PMID: 25767288]

McCormack T et al. Management of hypertension in adults in primary care: NICE guideline. Br J Gen Pract. 2012 Mar;62(596): 163–4. [PMID: 22429432]

Sidney S et al; National Forum for Heart Disease and Stroke Prevention. The "heart disease and stroke statistics—2013 update" and the need for a national cardiovascular surveillance system. Circulation. 2013 Jan 1;127(1):21–3. [PMID: 23239838]

Stern HR. The new hypertension guidelines. J Clin Hypertens (Greenwich). 2013 Oct;15(10):748–51. [PMID: 24088284]

Yoon SS et al. Trends in blood pressure among adults with hypertension: United States, 2003 to 2012. Hypertension. 2015 Jan;65(1):54–61. [PMID: 25399687]

APPROACH TO HYPERTENSION

▶ Etiology & Classification

A. Primary Essential Hypertension

Essential hypertension is the term applied to the 95% of hypertensive patients in which elevated blood pressure results from complex interactions between multiple genetic and environmental factors. The proportion regarded as "essential" will diminish with improved detection of clearly defined secondary causes and with better understanding of pathophysiology. Essential hypertension occurs in 10–15% of white adults and 20–30% of black adults in the United States. The onset is usually between ages 25 and 50 years; it is uncommon before age 20 years. The best understood endogenous and environmental determinants of blood pressure include overactivation of the sympathetic nervous and renin-angiotensin-aldosterone systems, blunting of the pressure-natriuresis relationship, variation in cardiovascular and renal development, and elevated intracellular sodium and calcium levels.

Exacerbating factors include obesity, sleep apnea, increased salt intake, excessive alcohol use, cigarette smoking, polycythemia, nonsteroidal anti-inflammatory (NSAID) therapy, and low potassium intake. **Obesity** is associated with an increase in intravascular volume, elevated cardiac output, activation of the renin-angiotensin system, and, probably, increased sympathetic outflow. Weight reduction lowers blood pressure modestly. In patients with **sleep apnea,** treatment with continuous positive airway pressure (CPAP) has been associated with improvements in blood pressure. **Increased salt intake** probably elevates blood pressure in some individuals so dietary salt restriction is recommended in patients with hypertension. Excessive use of **alcohol** also raises blood pressure, perhaps by increasing plasma catecholamines. Hypertension can be difficult to control in patients who consume more than 40 g of ethanol (two drinks) daily or drink in "binges." **Cigarette smoking** raises blood pressure by increasing plasma norepinephrine. Although the long-term effect of smoking on blood pressure is less clear, the synergistic effects of smoking and high blood pressure on cardiovascular risk are well documented. The relationship of **exercise** to hypertension is variable. Aerobic exercise lowers blood pressure in previously sedentary individuals,

but increasingly strenuous exercise in already active subjects has less effect. The relationship between stress and hypertension is not established. **Polycythemia,** whether primary, drug-induced, or due to diminished plasma volume, increases blood viscosity and may raise blood pressure. **NSAIDs** produce increases in blood pressure averaging 5 mm Hg and are best avoided in patients with borderline or elevated blood pressures. **Low potassium intake** is associated with higher blood pressure in some patients; an intake of 90 mmol/day is recommended.

The complex of abnormalities termed the **"metabolic syndrome"** (upper body obesity, insulin resistance, and hypertriglyceridemia) is associated with both the development of hypertension and an increased risk of adverse cardiovascular outcomes. Affected patients usually also have low high-density lipoprotein (HDL) cholesterol levels and elevated catecholamines and inflammatory markers such as C-reactive protein.

B. Secondary Hypertension

Approximately 5% of patients have hypertension secondary to identifiable specific causes (Table 11–1). Secondary hypertension should be suspected in patients in whom hypertension develops at an early age or after the age of 50 years, and in those previously well controlled who become refractory to treatment. Hypertension resistant to three medications is another clue, although multiple medications are usually required to control hypertension in persons with diabetes. Secondary causes include genetic syndromes; kidney disease; renal vascular disease; primary hyperaldosteronism; Cushing syndrome; pheochromocytoma; coarctation of the aorta and hypertension associated with pregnancy, estrogen use, hypercalcemia, and medications.

1. Genetic causes—Hypertension can be caused by mutations in single genes, inherited on a Mendelian basis. Although rare, these conditions provide important insight into blood pressure regulation and possibly the genetic basis of essential hypertension. **Glucocorticoid remediable aldosteronism** is an autosomal dominant cause of early-onset hypertension with normal or high aldosterone and low renin levels. It is caused by the formation of a

Table 11–1. Identifiable causes of hypertension.

Sleep apnea
Drug-induced or drug-related
Chronic kidney disease
Primary aldosteronism
Renovascular disease
Long-term corticosteroid therapy and Cushing syndrome
Pheochromocytoma
Coarctation of the aorta
Thyroid or parathyroid disease

Data from Chobanian AV et al. The Seventh Report of the Joint National Committee on Prevention, Detection, Evaluation, and Treatment of High Blood Pressure: the JNC 7 report. JAMA. 2003 May 21;289(19):2560–72.

chimeric gene encoding both the enzyme responsible for the synthesis of aldosterone (transcriptionally regulated by angiotensin II) and an enzyme responsible for synthesis of cortisol (transcriptionally regulated by ACTH). As a consequence, aldosterone synthesis becomes driven by ACTH, which can be suppressed by exogenous cortisol. In the **syndrome of apparent mineralocorticoid excess,** early-onset hypertension with hypokalemic metabolic alkalosis is inherited on an autosomal recessive basis. Although plasma renin is low and plasma aldosterone level is very low in these patients, aldosterone antagonists are effective in controlling hypertension. This disease is caused by loss of the enzyme 11beta-hydroxysteroid dehydrogenase, which normally metabolizes cortisol and thus protects the otherwise "promiscuous" mineralocorticoid receptor in the distal nephron from inappropriate glucocorticoid activation. Similarly, glycyrrhetinic acid, found in licorice, causes increased blood pressure through inhibition of 11beta-hydroxysteroid dehydrogenase. The syndrome of **hypertension exacerbated in pregnancy** is inherited as an autosomal dominant trait. In these patients, a mutation in the mineralocorticoid receptor makes it abnormally responsive to progesterone and, paradoxically, to spironolactone. **Liddle syndrome** is an autosomal dominant condition characterized by early-onset hypertension, hypokalemic alkalosis, low renin, and low aldosterone levels. This is caused by a mutation that results in constitutive activation of the epithelial sodium channel of the distal nephron, with resultant unregulated sodium reabsorption and volume expansion.

2. Renal disease—Renal parenchymal disease is the most common cause of secondary hypertension and is related to increased intravascular volume or increased activity of the renin–angiotensin–aldosterone system.

3. Renal vascular hypertension—Renal artery stenosis is present in 1–2% of hypertensive patients. The most common cause is atherosclerosis, but fibromuscular dysplasia should be suspected in women under 50 years of age. The mechanisms of hypertension relate to excessive renin release due to reduction in renal perfusion pressure, while attenuation of pressure natriuresis contributes to hypertension in patients with a single kidney or bilateral lesions. Activation of the renal sympathetic nerves may also be important.

Renal vascular hypertension should be suspected in the following circumstances: (1) if the documented onset is before age 20 or after age 50 years, (2) hypertension is resistant to three or more drugs, (3) if there are epigastric or renal artery bruits, (4) if there is atherosclerotic disease of the aorta or peripheral arteries (15–25% of patients with symptomatic lower limb atherosclerotic vascular disease have renal artery stenosis), (5) if there is an abrupt increase (more than 25%) in the level of serum creatinine after administration of angiotensin-converting enzyme (ACE) inhibitors, or (6) if episodes of pulmonary edema are associated with abrupt surges in blood pressure. There is no ideal screening test for renal vascular hypertension. If suspicion is sufficiently high and endovascular intervention is a viable option, renal arteriography, the definitive

diagnostic test, is the best approach. Renal arteriography is not recommended as a routine adjunct to coronary studies. Where suspicion is moderate to low, noninvasive angiography using magnetic resonance (MR) or CT are reasonable approaches. Doppler sonography has good specificity but lacks sensitivity and is operator dependent. Gadolinium, a contrast agent used in MR angiography, is contraindicated in patients with an estimated glomerular filtration rate (eGFR) of less than 30 mL/min because it might precipitate nephrogenic systemic fibrosis in patients with advanced kidney disease. In young patients with fibromuscular disease, angioplasty is very effective, but there is controversy regarding the best approach to the treatment of atheromatous renal artery stenosis. Correction of the stenosis in selected patients might reduce the number of medications required to control blood pressure and could protect kidney function, but the extent of preexisting parenchymal damage to the affected and contralateral kidney has a significant influence on both blood pressure and kidney function outcomes following revascularization. Angioplasty and stenting may prove to be superior to medical therapy in a subset of patients, but identifying this group remains a challenge. A reasonable approach advocates medical therapy as long as hypertension can be well controlled and there is no progression of kidney disease. The addition of a statin should be considered. Endovascular intervention might be considered in patients with uncontrollable hypertension, progressive kidney disease, or episodic pulmonary edema attributable to the lesion. Angioplasty might also be warranted when progression of stenosis is either demonstrated or is predicted by a constellation of risk factors, including systolic blood pressure greater than 160 mm Hg, advanced age, diabetes mellitus, or high-grade stenosis (more than 60%) at the time of diagnosis. However, multiple studies have failed to identify an overall advantage of stenting over medical management in patients with atherosclerotic renal artery stenosis. The CORAL study utilized a distal capture device to prevent embolization into the kidney, but the conclusion was once again that stenting is not superior to medical therapy (incorporating a statin) in the management of atherosclerotic renal artery stenosis. Although drugs modulating the renin-angiotensin system have improved the success rate of medical therapy of hypertension due to renal artery stenosis, they may trigger hypotension and (usually reversible) kidney dysfunction in individuals with bilateral disease.

4. Primary hyperaldosteronism—Hyperaldosteronism is suggested when the plasma aldosterone concentration is elevated (normal: 1–16 ng/dL) in association with suppression of plasma renin activity (normal: 1–2.5 ng/mL/h). However, the plasma aldosterone/renin ratio (normal less than 30) is not highly specific as a screening test. This is because "bottoming out" of renin assays leads to exponential increases in the plasma aldosterone/renin ratio even when aldosterone levels are normal. Hence, an elevated plasma aldosterone/renin ratio should probably not be taken as evidence of hyperaldosteronism unless the aldosterone level is actually supranormal. The lesion responsible for hyperaldosteronism is an adrenal adenoma or bilateral adrenal hyperplasia. Approximately 50% of aldosterone-secreting adenomas arise as a consequence of somatic mutations in genes encoding glomerulosa cell membrane ion transporters, with resultant elevation of intracellular calcium concentration. Screening is appropriate in patients with resistant hypertension (needing more than three drugs for control) and those with spontaneous or thiazide-induced hypokalemia, incidentaloma, or family history of primary hyperaldosteronism.

During the workup for hyperaldosteronism, medications that alter renin and aldosterone levels, including ACE inhibitors, angiotensin receptor blockers (ARBs), diuretics, beta-blockers, and clonidine, should be discontinued for 2 weeks before sampling; spironolactone and eplerenone should be held for 4 weeks. Calcium channel and alpha-receptor blockers can be used to control blood pressure during this drug washout period. Patients with a plasma aldosterone level greater than 16 ng/dL and an aldosterone/renin ratio of 30 or more might require further evaluation for primary hyperaldosteronism.

5. Cushing syndrome—Hypertension occurs in about 80% of patients with spontaneous Cushing syndrome. Excess glucocorticoid may act through salt and water retention (via mineralocorticoid effects), increased angiotensinogen levels, or permissive effects in the regulation of vascular tone.

Diagnosis and treatment of Cushing syndrome are discussed in Chapter 26.

6. Pheochromocytoma—Pheochromocytomas are uncommon; they are probably found in less than 0.1% of all patients with hypertension and in approximately two individuals per million population. However, autopsy studies indicate that pheochromocytomas are very often undiagnosed in life. The blood pressure elevation caused by the catecholamine excess results mainly from alpha-receptor–mediated vasoconstriction of arterioles, with a contribution from beta-1-receptor-mediated increases in cardiac output and renin release. Chronic vasoconstriction of the arterial and venous beds leads to a reduction in plasma volume and predisposes to postural hypotension. Glucose intolerance develops in some patients. Hypertensive crisis in pheochromocytoma may be precipitated by a variety of drugs, including tricyclic antidepressants, antidopaminergic agents, metoclopramide, and naloxone. The diagnosis and treatment of pheochromocytoma are discussed in Chapter 26.

7. Coarctation of the aorta—This uncommon cause of hypertension is discussed in Chapter 10. Evidence of radial-femoral delay should be sought in all younger patients with hypertension.

8. Hypertension associated with pregnancy—Hypertension occurring de novo or worsening during pregnancy, including preeclampsia and eclampsia, is one of the most common causes of maternal and fetal morbidity and mortality (see Chapter 19). Autoantibodies with the potential to activate the angiotensin II type 1 receptor have been causally implicated in preeclampsia, in resistant hypertension, and in progressive systemic sclerosis.

9. Estrogen use—A small increase in blood pressure occurs in most women taking oral contraceptives. However, a more significant increase above 140/90 mm Hg is noted in about 5% of women, mostly in obese individuals older than age 35 who have been treated for more than 5 years. This is caused by increased hepatic synthesis of angiotensinogen. Postmenopausal estrogen does not generally cause hypertension but rather maintains endothelium-mediated vasodilation.

10. Other causes of secondary hypertension—Hypertension has also been associated with hypercalcemia, acromegaly, hyperthyroidism, hypothyroidism, baroreceptor denervation, compression of the rostral ventrolateral medulla, and increased intracranial pressure. A number of medications may cause or exacerbate hypertension—most importantly cyclosporine, tacrolimus, angiogenesis inhibitors, and erythrocyte-stimulating agents (such as erythropoietin, decongestants, and NSAIDs); cocaine and alcohol should also be considered. Over-the-counter products should also be considered, eg, a dietary supplement currently marketed to enhance libido contains yohimbine, an alpha-2–antagonist, which can produce severe rebound hypertension in patients taking clonidine.

▶ When to Refer

Referral to a hypertension specialist should be considered in cases of severe, resistant or early-/late-onset hypertension or when secondary hypertension is suggested by screening.

Textor SC et al. Paradigm shifts in atherosclerotic renovascular disease: where are we now? J Am Soc Nephrol. 2015 Sep;26(9): 2074–80. [PMID: 25868641]

Xia Y et al. Angiotensin receptor agonistic autoantibodies and hypertension: preeclampsia and beyond. Circ Res. 2013 Jun 21; 113(1):78–87. [PMID: 23788505]

Zennaro MC et al. An update on novel mechanisms of primary aldosteronism. J Endocrinol. 2015 Feb;224(2):R63–R77. [PMID: 25424518]

▶ Complications of Untreated Hypertension

Elevated blood pressure results in structural and functional changes in the vasculature and heart. Most of the adverse outcomes in hypertension are associated with thrombosis rather than bleeding, possibly because increased vascular shear stress converts the normally anticoagulant endothelium to a prothrombotic state. The excess morbidity and mortality related to hypertension approximately doubles for each 6 mm Hg increase in diastolic blood pressure. However, target-organ damage varies markedly between individuals with similar levels of office hypertension; home and ambulatory pressures are superior to office readings in the prediction of end-organ damage and variability in blood pressure from visit to visit predicts cardiovascular endpoints independently of mean office-based systolic blood pressure.

A. Hypertensive Cardiovascular Disease

Cardiac complications are the major causes of morbidity and mortality in primary (essential) hypertension. For any level of blood pressure, left ventricular hypertrophy is associated with incremental cardiovascular risk in association with heart failure (through systolic or diastolic dysfunction), ventricular arrhythmias, myocardial ischemia, and sudden death.

The occurrence of heart failure is reduced by 50% with antihypertensive therapy. Hypertensive left ventricular hypertrophy regresses with therapy and is most closely related to the degree of systolic blood pressure reduction. Diuretics have produced equal or greater reductions of left ventricular mass when compared with other drug classes. Conventional beta-blockers are less effective in reducing left ventricular hypertrophy but play a specific role in patients with established coronary artery disease or impaired left ventricular function.

B. Hypertensive Cerebrovascular Disease and Dementia

Hypertension is the major predisposing cause of hemorrhagic and ischemic stroke. Cerebrovascular complications are more closely correlated with systolic than diastolic blood pressure. The incidence of these complications is markedly reduced by antihypertensive therapy. Preceding hypertension is associated with a higher incidence of subsequent dementia of both vascular and Alzheimer types. Home and ambulatory blood pressure may be a better predictor of cognitive decline than office readings in older people. Effective blood pressure control may reduce the risk of development of cognitive dysfunction later in life, but once cerebral small-vessel disease is established, low blood pressure might exacerbate this problem.

C. Hypertensive Kidney Disease

Chronic hypertension is associated with nephrosclerosis, which accounts for about 25% of end-stage renal disease. Whether hypertension causes nephrosclerosis or results from kidney disease driven by other factors (such as diabetes mellitus, age, obesity, and smoking) remains uncertain. Nephrosclerosis is particularly prevalent in blacks, in whom susceptibility is linked to *APOL1* mutations and hypertension results from renal disease rather than causing it.

D. Aortic Dissection

Hypertension is a contributing factor in many patients with dissection of the aorta. Its diagnosis and treatment are discussed in Chapter 12.

E. Atherosclerotic Complications

Most Americans with hypertension die of complications of atherosclerosis, but antihypertensive therapy seems to have a lesser impact on atherosclerotic complications compared with the other effects of treatment outlined above. Prevention of cardiovascular outcomes related to atherosclerosis probably requires control of multiple risk factors, of which hypertension is only one.

Freedman BI et al. Hypertension-attributed nephropathy: what's in a name? Nat Rev Nephrol. 2016 Jan;12(1):27–36. [PMID: 26553514]

White WB et al. Average daily blood pressure, not office blood pressure, is associated with progression of cerebrovascular disease and cognitive decline in older people. Circulation. 2011 Nov 22;124(21):2312–9. [PMID: 22105196]

▶ Clinical Findings

The clinical and laboratory findings are mainly referable to involvement of the target organs: heart, brain, kidneys, eyes, and peripheral arteries.

A. Symptoms

Mild to moderate primary (essential) hypertension is largely asymptomatic for many years. The most frequent symptom, headache, is also very nonspecific. Accelerated hypertension is associated with somnolence, confusion, visual disturbances, and nausea and vomiting (hypertensive encephalopathy).

Hypertension in patients with **pheochromocytomas** that secrete predominantly norepinephrine is usually sustained but may be episodic. The typical attack lasts from minutes to hours and is associated with headache, anxiety, palpitation, profuse perspiration, pallor, tremor, and nausea and vomiting. Blood pressure is markedly elevated, and angina or acute pulmonary edema may occur. In **primary aldosteronism,** patients may have muscular weakness, polyuria, and nocturia due to hypokalemia; malignant hypertension is rare. **Chronic hypertension** often leads to left ventricular hypertrophy and diastolic dysfunction, which can present with exertional and paroxysmal nocturnal dyspnea. Cerebral involvement causes stroke due to thrombosis or hemorrhage from microaneurysms of small penetrating intracranial arteries. **Hypertensive encephalopathy** is probably caused by acute capillary congestion and exudation with cerebral edema, which is reversible.

B. Signs

Like symptoms, physical findings depend on the cause of hypertension, its duration and severity, and the degree of effect on target organs.

1. Blood pressure—Blood pressure is taken in both arms and, if lower extremity pulses are diminished or delayed, in the legs to exclude coarctation of the aorta. An orthostatic drop of at least 20/10 mm Hg is often present in pheochromocytoma. Older patients may have falsely elevated readings by sphygmomanometry because of noncompressible vessels. This may be suspected in the presence of Osler sign—a palpable brachial or radial artery when the cuff is inflated above systolic pressure. Occasionally, it may be necessary to make direct measurements of intra-arterial pressure, especially in patients with apparent severe hypertension who do not tolerate therapy.

2. Retinas—Narrowing of arterial diameter to less than 50% of venous diameter, copper or silver wire appearance, exudates, hemorrhages, or hypertensive retinopathy are associated with a worse prognosis. The typical changes of hypertensive retinopathy are shown in Figure 11–2.

▲ Figure 11–2. Severe acute hypertensive retinopathy with disk edema, intraretinal hemorrhages, nerve fiber layer infarcts (cotton-wool spots) and arteriovenous nicking. Retinal arteries show irregular narrowing. (Used, with permission, from Courtney Francis, MD, Department of Ophthalmology, University of Washington School of Medicine.)

3. Heart—A left ventricular heave indicates severe or long-standing hypertrophy. Aortic regurgitation may be auscultated in up to 5% of patients, and hemodynamically insignificant aortic regurgitation can be detected by Doppler echocardiography in 10–20%. A presystolic (S_4) gallop due to decreased compliance of the left ventricle is quite common in patients in sinus rhythm.

4. Pulses—Radial-femoral delay suggests coarctation of the aorta; loss of peripheral pulses occurs due to atherosclerosis, less commonly aortic dissection, and rarely Takayasu arteritis, all of which can involve the renal arteries.

C. Laboratory Findings

Recommended testing includes the following: hemoglobin; urinalysis and serum creatinine; fasting blood sugar level (hypertension is a risk factor for the development of diabetes, and hyperglycemia can be a presenting feature of pheochromocytoma); plasma lipids (necessary to calculate cardiovascular risk and as a modifiable risk factor); serum uric acid (hyperuricemia is a relative contraindication to diuretic therapy); and serum electrolytes.

D. Electrocardiography and Chest Radiographs

Electrocardiographic criteria are highly specific but not very sensitive for left ventricular hypertrophy. The "strain" pattern of ST–T wave changes is a sign of more advanced disease and is associated with a poor prognosis. A chest radiograph is not necessary in the workup for uncomplicated hypertension.

E. Echocardiography

The primary role of echocardiography should be to evaluate patients with clinical symptoms or signs of cardiac disease.

F. Diagnostic Studies

Additional diagnostic studies are indicated only if the clinical presentation or routine tests suggest secondary or complicated hypertension. These may include 24-hour urine free cortisol, urine or plasma metanephrines and plasma aldosterone and renin concentrations to screen for endocrine causes of hypertension. Renal ultrasound will detect structural changes (such as polycystic kidneys, asymmetry and hydronephrosis) as well as echogenicity and reduced cortical volume, which are reliable indicators of advanced chronic kidney disease. Evaluation for renal artery stenosis should be undertaken in concert with subspecialist consultation.

G. Summary

Since most hypertension is essential or primary, few studies are necessary beyond those listed above. If conventional therapy is unsuccessful or if secondary hypertension is suspected, further studies and perhaps referral to a hypertension specialist are indicated.

Katsi V et al. Impact of arterial hypertension on the eye. Curr Hypertens Rep. 2012 Dec;14(6):581–90. [PMID: 22673879]

▶ Nonpharmacologic Therapy

Lifestyle modification may have an impact on morbidity and mortality. A diet rich in fruits, vegetables, and low-fat dairy foods and low in saturated and total fats (DASH diet) has been shown to lower blood pressure. Additional measures, listed in Table 11–2, can prevent or mitigate hypertension or its cardiovascular consequences.

All patients with high-normal or elevated blood pressures, those who have a family history of cardiovascular complications of hypertension, and those who have multiple coronary risk factors should be counseled about nonpharmacologic approaches to lowering blood pressure. Approaches of proved but modest value include weight reduction, reduced alcohol consumption, and, in some patients, reduced salt intake (less than 5 g salt or 2 g sodium). Gradually increasing activity levels should be encouraged in previously sedentary patients, but strenuous exercise training programs in already active individuals may have less benefit. Alternative approaches that may be modestly effective include relaxation techniques and biofeedback. Calcium and potassium supplements have been advocated, but their ability to lower blood pressure is limited. Smoking cessation will reduce cardiovascular risk. Overall, the effects of lifestyle modification on blood pressure are modest.

Aburto NJ et al. Effect of lower sodium intake on health: systematic review and meta-analyses. BMJ. 2013 Apr 3;346:f1326. [PMID: 23558163]

Brook RD et al; American Heart Association Professional Education Committee of the Council for High Blood Pressure Research, Council on Cardiovascular and Stroke Nursing, Council on Epidemiology and Prevention, and Council on Nutrition, Physical Activity. Beyond medications and diet: alternative approaches to lowering blood pressure: a scientific statement from the American Heart Association. Hypertension. 2013 Jun;61(6):1360–83. [PMID: 23608661]

Table 11–2. Lifestyle modifications to manage hypertension.[1]

Modification	Recommendation	Approximate Systolic BP Reduction, Range
Weight reduction	Maintain normal body weight (BMI, 18.5–24.9)	5–20 mm Hg/10 kg weight loss
Adopt DASH eating plan	Consume a diet rich in fruits, vegetables, and low-fat dairy products with a reduced content of saturated fat and total fat	8–14 mm Hg
Dietary sodium reduction	Reduce dietary sodium intake to no more than 100 mEq/day (2.4 g sodium or 6 g sodium chloride)	2–8 mm Hg
Physical activity	Engage in regular aerobic physical activity such as brisk walking (at least 30 minutes per day, most days of the week)	4–9 mm Hg
Moderation of alcohol consumption	Limit consumption to no more than two drinks per day (1 oz or 30 mL ethanol [eg, 24 oz beer, 10 oz wine, or 3 oz 80-proof whiskey]) in most men and no more than one drink per day in women and lighter-weight persons	2–4 mm Hg

[1]For overall cardiovascular risk reduction, stop smoking. The effects of implementing these modifications are dose- and time-dependent and could be higher for some individuals.
BMI, body mass index calculated as weight in kilograms divided by the square of height in meters; BP, blood pressure; DASH, Dietary Approaches to Stop Hypertension.
Data from Chobanian AV et al. The Seventh Report of the Joint National Committee on Prevention, Detection, Evaluation, and Treatment of High Blood Pressure: the JNC 7 report. JAMA. 2003 May 21;289(19):2560–72.

Hedayati SS et al. Non-pharmacological aspects of blood pressure management: what are the data? Kidney Int. 2011 May;79(10):1061–70. [PMID: 21389976]
Jin J et al. JAMA patient page. Salt in the diet. JAMA. 2014 Mar 26;311(12):1265. [PMID: 24668117]

Who Should Be Treated with Medications?

Treatment should ideally be offered to all persons in whom blood pressure reduction, irrespective of initial blood pressure levels, will appreciably reduce overall cardiovascular risk with an acceptably low rate of medication-associated adverse effects. Outcomes data indicate that patients with office-based blood pressure measurements that consistently exceed 160/100 mm Hg (stage 2 hypertension) will benefit from antihypertensive therapy irrespective of cardiovascular risk. Several international guidelines suggest that treatment thresholds evaluated by home-based measurements should be lower, perhaps 150/95 mm Hg using home blood pressure or daytime ambulatory measurements. However, prospective outcomes data for treatment based on measurements taken outside the clinic are lacking. As outlined in Figure 11–3, treatment should be offered at lower thresholds in those with elevated cardiovascular risk or in the presence of existing end-organ damage. The corollary of this is that treatment thresholds might reasonably be set higher for young people with extremely low cardiovascular risk; the Canadian guidelines suggest a threshold of greater than 160/100 mm Hg. However, since risk may be underestimated in this population, specialist referral should be considered in younger people with stage 1 hypertension to exclude end-organ damage and to screen for secondary causes.

Since evaluation of total cardiovascular risk (Table 11–3) is important in deciding who to treat with antihypertensive medications, risk calculators are becoming essential clinical tools. QRisk2 is a reliable and regularly updated online calculator. Free smart phone applications are also available to estimate coronary heart disease risk. In general, a 20% total cardiovascular risk (which includes stroke) is equivalent to a 15% coronary heart disease risk.

Goals of Treatment

The blood pressure target in most patients with hypertension is less than 140/90 mm Hg. Observational studies suggest that there does not seem to be a blood pressure level below which decrements in risk taper off. However, this may not be true with respect to pharmacologically modulated blood pressure. In fact, over-enthusiastic treatment may have adverse consequences in certain settings. There is an association between lower blood pressure and cognitive decline in elderly patients subjected to intensification of antihypertensive treatment later in life. Antihypertensive treatment in those who are both very elderly and frail may paradoxically increase mortality. Excessive lowering of diastolic pressure, perhaps below 70 mm Hg, should be avoided in patients with coronary artery disease. The SPRINT study suggests that outcomes may improve in nondiabetic patients with elevated cardiovascular risk when treatment lowers systolic pressures to less than 120 mm Hg compared to less than 140 mm Hg.

However, in the ACCORD study, treatment of systolic pressures to below 130–135 mm Hg in diabetic patients significantly increased the risk of serious adverse effects with no additional gain in terms of cardiac, renal, or retinal disease. On the other hand, reducing systolic pressure below 130 mm Hg in this study seemed to further lower the risk of stroke, so lower targets might be justified in patients at high risk for cerebrovascular events.

Similarly, in the SPS3 trial in patients recovering from a lacunar stroke indicated that treating the systolic blood

Thresholds for intervention based on
initial blood pressure (mm Hg)

> 180/110

Unless malignant phase of hypertensive emergency, confirm over 1–2 weeks then treat

160–179
100–109

If cardiovascular complications, target-organ damage, or diabetes is present, confirm over 3–4 weeks then treat; if absent, remeasure weekly and treat if blood pressure persists at these levels over 4–12 weeks

140–159
90–99

If cardiovascular complications, target-organ damage, or diabetes is present, confirm over 12 weeks then treat; if absent, remeasure monthly and treat if these levels are maintained and if estimated 10-year CVD risk is ≥ 20%

130–139
85–89

< 130/85

≥ 160/100

140–159
90–99

< 140/90

Target-organ damage
or
cardiovascular complications
or
diabetes
or
10-year CVD risk[1] ≥ 20%

No target-organ damage
and
no cardiovascular complications
and
no diabetes
and
10-year CVD risk[1] < 20%

Reassess
in 5 years

Treat   Treat   Treat   Observe, reassess CVD risk yearly   Reassess yearly

[1]Assessed with CVD risk chart.

▲ **Figure 11–3.** British Hypertension Society algorithm for diagnosis and treatment of hypertension, incorporating total cardiovascular risk in deciding which "prehypertensive" patients to treat. Cardiovascular disease (CVD) risk chart available at qrisk.org. (Reproduced, with permission, from Guidelines for management of hypertension: report of the Fourth Working Party of the British Hypertension Society, 2004-BHS IV. J Hum Hypertens. 2004 Mar;18(3):139–85.)

pressure to less than 130 mm Hg (mean systolic blood pressure of 127 mm Hg among treated versus mean systolic blood pressure 138 mm Hg among untreated patients) probably reduced the risk of recurrent stroke (and with an acceptably low rate of adverse effects from treatment).

Large-scale trials in hypertension have focused on discrete end points occurring over relatively short intervals, thereby placing the emphasis on the prevention of catastrophic events in advanced disease. There is an ongoing shift in emphasis in viewing hypertension in the context of lifelong cardiovascular risk. Accordingly, treatment of persons with hypertension should focus on comprehensive risk reduction with more careful consideration of the possible long-term adverse effects of antihypertensive medications, which include the metabolic derangements linked to conventional beta-blockers and thiazide diuretics.

Statins should be more widely used. The Anglo-Scandinavian Cardiac Outcomes Trial (ASCOT) showed that statins can significantly improve outcomes in persons with hypertension (with modest background cardiovascular risk) whose total cholesterol is less than 250 mg/dL (6.5 mmol/L). Notably, the effect of statins appeared to be synergistic with calcium channel blocker/ACE inhibitor regimens but not beta-blocker/diuretic regimens. The British Hypertension Society guidelines recommend that statins be offered as secondary prevention to patients whose total cholesterol exceeds 135 mg/dL (3.5 mmol/L) if they have documented coronary artery disease or a history of ischemic stroke. In addition, statins should be considered as primary prevention in patients with long-standing type 2 diabetes or in those with type 2 diabetes who are older than age 50 years, and perhaps in all persons with type 2 diabetes. Low-dose aspirin (81 mg/day) is likely to be beneficial in patients older than age 50 with either target-organ damage or elevated total cardiovascular risk (greater than 20–30%). Care should be taken to ensure that blood pressure is controlled to the recommended levels before starting aspirin to minimize the risk of intracranial hemorrhage.

ACCORD Study Group; Cushman WC et al. Effects of intensive blood-pressure control in type 2 diabetes mellitus. N Engl J Med. 2010 Apr 29;362(17):1575–85. [PMID: 20228401]

Table 11–3. Cardiovascular risk factors.

Major risk factors
Hypertension[1]
Cigarette smoking
Obesity (BMI ≥ 30)[1]
Physical inactivity
Dyslipidemia[1]
Diabetes mellitus[1]
Microalbuminuria or estimated GFR < 60 mL/min
Age (> 55 years for men, > 65 years for women)
Family history of premature cardiovascular disease
    (men < 55 years or women < 65 years)
Target-organ damage
Heart
    Left ventricular hypertrophy
    Angina or prior myocardial infarction
    Prior coronary revascularization
    Heart failure
Brain
    Stroke or transient ischemic attack
Chronic kidney disease
Peripheral arterial disease
Retinopathy

[1]Components of the metabolic syndrome.
BMI indicates body mass index calculated as weight in kilograms divided by the square of height in meters; GFR, glomerular filtration rate.
Data from Chobanian AV et al. The Seventh Report of the Joint National Committee on Prevention, Detection, Evaluation, and Treatment of High Blood Pressure: the JNC 7 report. JAMA. 2003 May 21; 289(19):2560–72.

Jin J. JAMA patient page. New guideline for treatment of high blood pressure in adults. JAMA. 2014 Feb 5;311(5):538. [PMID: 24496549]

McInnes G. Pre-hypertension: how low to go and do drugs have a role? Br J Clin Pharmacol. 2012 Feb;73(2):187–93. [PMID: 21883385]

SPRINT Research Group; Wright JT Jr et al. A randomized trial of intensive versus standard blood-pressure control. N Engl J Med. 2015 Nov 26;373(22):2103–16. [PMID: 26551272]

SPS3 Study Group; Benavente OR et al. Blood-pressure targets in patients with recent lacunar stroke: the SPS3 randomised trial. Lancet. 2013 Aug 10;382(9891):507–15. Erratum in: Lancet. 2013 Aug 10;382(9891):506. [PMID: 23726159]

Working Group on the Summit on Combination Therapy for CVD; Yusuf S et al. Combination pharmacotherapy to prevent cardiovascular disease: present status and challenges. Eur Heart J. 2014 Feb;35(6):353–64. [PMID: 24288261]

DRUG THERAPY: CURRENT ANTIHYPERTENSIVE AGENTS

There are many classes of antihypertensive drugs of which six (diuretics, beta-blockers, renin inhibitors, ACE inhibitors, calcium channel blockers, and ARBs) are suitable for initial therapy based on efficacy and tolerability (Table 11–4). A number of considerations enter into the selection of the initial regimen for a given patient. These include the weight of evidence for beneficial effects on clinical outcomes, the safety and tolerability of the drug, its cost, demographic differences in response, concomitant medical conditions, and lifestyle issues. The specific classes of antihypertensive medications are discussed below, and guidelines for the choice of initial medications are offered.

A. Diuretics

Thiazide diuretics (Table 11–5) are the antihypertensives that have been most extensively studied and most consistently effective in clinical trials. They lower blood pressure initially by decreasing plasma volume, but during long-term therapy, their major hemodynamic effect is reduction of peripheral vascular resistance. Most of the antihypertensive effect of these agents is achieved at lower dosages than used previously (typically, 12.5 mg of hydrochlorothiazide or equivalent), but their biochemical and metabolic effects are dose related. Chlorthalidone has the advantage of better 24-hour blood pressure control than hydrochlorothiazide in clinical trials. Thiazides may be used at higher doses if plasma potassium is above 4.5 mmol/L. The loop diuretics (such as furosemide) may lead to electrolyte and volume depletion more readily than the thiazides and have short durations of action. Because of these adverse effects, loop diuretics should be reserved for use in patients with kidney dysfunction (serum creatinine greater than 2.5 mg/dL [208.3 mcmol/L]; eGFR less than 30 mL/min) in which case they are more effective than thiazides. Relative to beta-blockers and ACE inhibitors, diuretics are more potent in blacks, older individuals, the obese, and other subgroups with increased plasma volume or low plasma renin activity (or both). They are relatively more effective in smokers than in nonsmokers. Long-term thiazide administration also mitigates the loss of bone mineral content in older women at risk for osteoporosis.

Overall, diuretics administered alone control blood pressure in 50% of patients with mild to moderate hypertension and can be used effectively in combination with all other agents. They are also useful for lowering isolated or predominantly systolic hypertension. The adverse effects of diuretics relate primarily to the metabolic changes listed in Table 11–5. Erectile dysfunction, skin rashes, and photosensitivity are less frequent. Hypokalemia has been a concern but is uncommon at the recommended dosages. The risk can be minimized by limiting dietary salt or increasing dietary potassium; potassium replacement is not usually required to maintain serum K[+] at greater than 3.5 mmol/L. Higher serum K[+] levels are prudent in patients at special risk from intracellular potassium depletion, such as those taking digoxin or with a history of ventricular arrhythmias in which case a potassium-sparing agent could be used. Compared with ACE inhibitors and ARBs, diuretic therapy is associated with a slightly higher incidence of mild new-onset diabetes. Diuretics also increase serum uric acid and may precipitate gout. Increases in blood glucose, triglycerides, and LDL cholesterol may occur but are relatively minor during long-term low-dose therapy. The potential for worsening of diabetes is outweighed by the advantages of blood pressure control, and diuretics should not be withheld from diabetic patients.

Table 11–4. Clinical trial and guideline basis for compelling indications for individual drug classes.[1]

High-Risk Conditions with Compelling Indication[2]	Recommended Drugs						Clinical Trial Basis
	Diuretic	Beta-Blockers	ACE Inhibitors	ARB	CCB	Aldosterone Antagonist	
Heart failure	•	•	•	•		•	ACC/AHA Heart Failure Guideline, MERIT-HF, COPERNICUS, CIBIS, SOLVD, AIRE, TRACE, ValHEFT, RALES
Post-myocardial infarction		•	•			•	ACC/AHA Post-MI Guideline, BHAT, SAVE, Capricorn, EPHESUS
High coronary disease risk	•	•	•		•		ALLHAT, HOPE, ANBP2, LIFE, CONVINCE
Diabetes mellitus	•	•	•	•	•		NKF-ADA Guideline, UKPDS, ALLHAT
Chronic kidney disease			•	•			NKF Guideline, Captopril Trial, RENAAL, IDNT, REIN, AASK
Recurrent stroke prevention	•		•				PROGRESS

[1]Compelling indications for antihypertensive drugs are based on benefits from outcome studies or existing clinical guidelines; the compelling indication is managed in parallel with the blood pressure.
[2]Conditions for which clinical trials demonstrate benefit of specific classes of antihypertensive drugs.

AASK, African American Study of Kidney Disease and Hypertension; ACC/AHA, American College of Cardiology/American Heart Association; ACE, angiotensin converting enzyme; AIRE, Acute Infarction Ramipril Efficacy; ALLHAT, Antihypertensive and Lipid-Lowering Treatment to Prevent Heart Attack Trial; ANBP2, Second Australian National Blood Pressure Study; ARB, angiotensin receptor blocker; BHAT, Beta-Blocker Heart Attack Trial; CCB, calcium channel blocker; CIBIS, Cardiac Insufficiency Bisoprolol Study; CONVINCE, Controlled Onset Verapamil Investigation of Cardiovascular End Points; COPERNICUS, Carvedilol Prospective Randomized Cumulative Survival Study; EPHESUS, Eplerenone Post-Acute Myocardial Infarction Heart Failure Efficacy and Survival Study; HOPE, Heart Outcomes Prevention Evaluation Study; IDNT, Irbesartan Diabetic Nephropathy Trial; LIFE, Losartan Intervention For Endpoint Reduction in Hypertension Study; MERIT-HF, Metoprolol CR/XL Randomized Intervention Trial in Congestive Heart Failure; NKF-ADA, National Kidney Foundation–American Diabetes Association; PROGRESS, Perindopril Protection Against Recurrent Stroke Study; RALES, Randomized Aldactone Evaluation Study; REIN, Ramipril Efficacy in Nephropathy Study; RENAAL, Reduction of Endpoints in Non-Insulin-Dependent Diabetes Mellitus with the Angiotensin II Antagonist Losartan Study; SAVE, Survival and Ventricular Enlargement Study; SOLVD, Studies of Left Ventricular Dysfunction; TRACE, Trandolapril Cardiac Evaluation Study; UKPDS, United Kingdom Prospective Diabetes Study; ValHEFT, Valsartan Heart Failure Trial.

Data from Chobanian AV et al. The Seventh Report of the Joint National Committee on Prevention, Detection, Evaluation, and Treatment of High Blood Pressure: the JNC 7 report. JAMA. 2003 May 21;289(19): 2560–72.

B. Beta-Adrenergic Blocking Agents

These drugs are effective in hypertension because they decrease the heart rate and cardiac output. Even after continued use of beta-blockers, cardiac output remains lower and systemic vascular resistance higher with agents that do not have intrinsic sympathomimetic or alpha-blocking activity. The beta-blockers also decrease renin release and are more efficacious in populations with elevated plasma renin activity, such as younger white patients. They neutralize the reflex tachycardia caused by vasodilators and are especially useful in patients with associated conditions that benefit from the cardioprotective effects of these agents. These include individuals with angina pectoris, previous myocardial infarction, and stable heart failure as well as those with migraine headaches and somatic manifestations of anxiety.

Although all beta-blockers appear to be similar in antihypertensive potency, they differ in a number of pharmacologic properties (these differences are summarized in Table 11–6), including specificity to the cardiac beta-1-receptors (cardioselectivity) and whether they also block the beta-2-receptors in the bronchi and vasculature; at higher dosages, however, all agents are nonselective. The beta-blockers also differ in their pharmacokinetics, lipid solubility—which determines whether they cross the blood-brain barrier and affects the incidence of central nervous system side effects—and route of metabolism. Unlike the traditional beta-blockers, carvedilol and nebivolol also diminish peripheral vascular resistance through concomitant alpha-blockade and increased nitric oxide release, respectively. The implications of this distinction are discussed below.

The side effects of beta-blockers include inducing or exacerbating bronchospasm in predisposed patients; sinus node dysfunction and atrioventricular (AV) conduction depression (resulting in bradycardia or AV block); nasal congestion; Raynaud phenomenon; and central nervous system symptoms with nightmares, excitement, depression, and confusion. Fatigue, lethargy, and erectile dysfunction may occur. The traditional beta-blockers (but not the

Table 11–5. Antihypertensive drugs: Diuretics. (In descending order of preference.)

Drugs	Proprietary Names	Initial Oral Doses	Dosage Range	Cost per Unit	Cost of 30 Days Treatment[1] (Average Dosage)	Adverse Effects	Comments
Thiazides and Related Diuretics							
HCTZ	Esidrix, Microzide	12.5 or 25 mg once daily	12.5–50 mg once daily	$0.08/25 mg	$2.40	$\downarrow$K+, $\downarrow$Mg^{2+}, $\uparrow$Ca^{2+}, $\uparrow$uric acid, $\downarrow$Na+, $\uparrow$glucose, $\uparrow$LDL cholesterol, $\uparrow$triglycerides; rash, erectile dysfunction.	Low dosages effective in many patients without associated metabolic abnormalities; metolazone more effective with concurrent kidney disease; indapamide does not alter serum lipid levels.
Chlorthalidone	Thalitone	12.5 or 25 mg once daily	12.5–50 mg once daily	$1.21/25 mg	$36.30		
Metolazone	Zaroxolyn	1.25 or 2.5 mg once daily	1.25–5 mg once daily	$1.48/5 mg	$44.40		
Indapamide	Lozol	2.5 mg once daily	2.5–5 mg once daily	$0.83/2.5 mg	$24.90		
Loop Diuretics							
Furosemide	Lasix	20 mg twice daily	40–320 mg in 2 or 3 doses	$0.16/40 mg	$9.60	Same as thiazides, but higher risk of excessive diuresis and electrolyte imbalance. Increases calcium excretion.	Furosemide: Short duration of action a disadvantage; should be reserved for patients with kidney disease or fluid retention. Poor antihypertensive.
Ethacrynic acid	Edecrin	50 mg once daily	50–100 mg once or twice daily	$26.91/25 mg	$807.30		
Bumetanide	(generic)	0.25 mg twice daily	0.5–10 mg in 2 or 3 doses	$0.45/1 mg	$27.00		
Torsemide	Demadex	5 mg once daily	5–10 mg once daily	$0.70/10 mg	$21.00		Torsemide: Effective blood pressure medication at low dosage.
Aldosterone Receptor Blockers							
Spironolactone	Aldactone	12.5 or 25 mg once daily	12.5–100 mg once daily	$0.46/25 mg	$13.80	Hyperkalemia, metabolic acidosis, gynecomastia.	Can be useful add-on therapy in patients with refractory hypertension.
Amiloride	(generic)	5 mg once daily	5–10 mg once daily	$1.28/5 mg	$38.40		
Eplerenone	Inspra	25 mg once daily	25–100 mg once daily	$4.34/25 mg	$130.20		

Combination Products

Drug	Brand (strength)	Dosage	Cost (generic)	Cost/month (AWP)	Adverse Effects	Comments
HCTZ and triamterene	Dyazide, Maxzide-25 (25/37.5 mg)	1 tab once daily; 1 or 2 tabs once daily	$0.39	$11.70	Same as thiazides plus GI disturbances, hyperkalemia rather than hypokalemia, headache; triamterene can cause kidney stones and kidney dysfunction; spironolactone causes gynecomastia. Hyperkalemia can occur if this combination is used in patients with advanced kidney disease or those taking ACE inhibitors.	Use should be limited to patients with demonstrable need for a potassium-sparing agent.
HCTZ and amiloride	(generic) (50/5 mg)	½ tab once daily; 1 or 2 tabs once daily	$1.16	$34.80		
HCTZ and spironolactone	Aldactazide (25/25 mg; 50/50 mg)	1 tab (25/25 mg) once daily; 1–4 tabs once daily	$1.24	$37.20		

[1]Average wholesale price (AWP, for AB-rated generic when available) for quantity listed.

Source: *Red Book Online*, Truven Health Analytics, Information, http://www.micromedexsolutions.com, March 1, 2016. AWP may not accurately represent the actual pharmacy cost because wide contractual variations exist among institutions.

ACE, angiotensin-converting enzyme; GI, gastrointestinal; HCTZ, hydrochlorothiazide; LDL, low-density lipoprotein.

Table 11–6. Antihypertensive drugs: Beta-adrenergic blocking agents.

Drug	Proprietary Name	Initial Oral Dosage	Dosage Range	Cost per Unit	Cost of 30 Days Treatment (Based on Average Dosage)[1]	Special Properties					Comments[5]
						Beta-1 Selectivity[2]	ISA[3]	MSA[4]	Lipid Solubility	Renal vs Hepatic Elimination	
Acebutolol	Sectral	400 mg once daily	200–1200 mg in 1 or 2 doses	$1.34/400 mg	$40.20	+	+	+	+	H > R	Positive ANA; rare LE syndrome; also indicated for arrhythmias. Doses > 800 mg have beta-1 and beta-2 effects.
Atenolol	Tenormin	25 mg once daily	25–100 mg once daily	$0.83/50 mg	$24.90	+	0	0	0	R	Also indicated for angina pectoris and post-MI. Doses > 100 mg have beta-1 and beta-2 effects.
Atenolol/chlorthalidone	Tenoretic	50 mg/25 mg once daily	50 mg/25 mg–100 mg/25 mg once daily	$1.88/50 mg/25 mg	$56.40	+	0	0	0	R	
Betaxolol	Kerlone	10 mg once daily	10–40 mg once daily	$0.78/10 mg	$23.40	+	0	0	+	H > R	
Bisoprolol	Zebeta	5 mg once daily	5–20 mg once daily	$1.22/10 mg	$36.60	+	0	0	0	R = H	Bisoprolol also effective for heart failure.
Bisoprolol and HCTZ	Ziac	2.5 mg/6.25 mg once daily	2.5 mg/6.25 mg–10 mg/6.25 mg once daily	$1.14/2.5/6.25 mg	$34.20	+	0	0	0	R = H	Low-dose combination approved for initial therapy.
Carvedilol	Coreg Coreg CR	6.25 mg twice daily 20 mg ER once daily	12.5–50 mg in 2 doses 20–80 mg ER once daily	$2.13/25 mg $10.10/any tablet	$127.80 (25 mg twice a day) $303.00	0	0	0	+++	H > R	Alpha:beta blocking activity 1:9; may cause orthostatic symptoms; effective for heart failure. Nitric oxide potentiating vasodilatory activity.
Labetalol	Trandate	100 mg twice daily	200–2400 mg in 2 doses	$0.73/200 mg	$43.80	0	0/+	0	++	H	Alpha:beta blocking activity 1:3; more orthostatic hypotension, fever, hepatotoxicity.

Drug	Proprietary Name	Initial Dosage	Dosage Range	Cost per Unit	Cost per 30 Days [1]	Beta-1 Selectivity [2]	ISA [3]	MSA [4]	Lipid Solubility	Renal vs Hepatic Elimination	Comments [5]
Metoprolol	Lopressor Toprol-XL (SR preparation)	50 mg twice daily 25 mg once daily	50–200 mg twice daily 25–400 mg once daily	$0.56/50 mg $1.58/100 mg	$33.60 $47.40	+	0	+	+++	H	Also indicated for angina pectoris and post-MI. Approved for heart failure. Doses > 100 mg have beta-1 and beta-2 effects.
Metoprolol and HCTZ	Lopressor HCT	50 mg/12.5 mg twice daily	50 mg/25 mg – 200 mg/50 mg	$1.63/100 mg/25 mg	$48.90	+	0	+	+++	H	
Nadolol	Corgard	20 mg once daily	20–320 mg once daily	$4.01/40 mg	$120.30	0	0	0	0	R	
Nadolol and bendroflumethiazide	Corzide	40 mg/5 mg once daily	40 mg/5 mg – 80 mg/5 mg once daily	$2.46/40 mg/5 mg	$73.80						
Nebivolol	Bystolic	5 mg once daily	40 mg once daily	$4.02/5 mg	$120.60	+	0	0	++	H	Nitric oxide potentiating vasodilatory activity.
Penbutolol	Levatol	20 mg once daily	20–80 mg once daily	$4.07/20 mg	$122.10	0	+	0	++	R > H	
Pindolol	Visken	5 mg twice daily	10–60 mg in 2 doses	$1.10/5 mg	$66.60	0	++	+	+	H > R	In adults, 35% renal clearance.
Propranolol	Inderal Inderal LA InnoPran XL	20 mg twice daily 80 mg ER once daily 80 mg ER once nightly	40–640 mg in 2 doses 120–640 mg ER once daily 80–120 mg ER once nightly	$0.72/40 mg $1.92/120 mg $25.05/120 mg	$43.20 $57.60 $751.50	0	0	++	+++	H	Also indicated for angina pectoris and post-MI.
Propranolol and HCTZ	(generic)	40 mg/25 mg twice daily	80 mg/25 mg twice daily	$1.41/80 mg/25 mg	$84.60	0	0	++	+++	H	
Timolol	(generic)	5 mg twice daily	10–60 mg in 2 doses	$1.70/10 mg	$102.00	0	0	0	++	H > R	Also indicated for post-MI; 80% hepatic clearance.

[1] Average wholesale price (AWP, for AB-rated generic when available) for quantity listed. Source: Red Book Online, Truven Health Analytics, Information, http://www.micromedexsolutions.com, March 1, 2016. AWP may not accurately represent the actual pharmacy cost because wide contractual variations exist among institutions.

[2] Agents with beta-1 selectivity are less likely to precipitate bronchospasm and decreased peripheral blood flow in low doses, but selectivity is only relative.

[3] Agents with ISA cause less resting bradycardia and lipid changes.

[4] MSA generally occurs at concentrations greater than those necessary for beta-adrenergic blockade. The clinical importance of MSA by beta-blockers has not been defined.

[5] Adverse effects of all beta-blockers: bronchospasm, fatigue, sleep disturbance and nightmares, bradycardia and atrioventricular block, worsening of heart failure, cold extremities, gastrointestinal disturbances, erectile dysfunction, ↑ triglycerides, ↓ HDL cholesterol, rare blood dyscrasias.

ANA, antinuclear antibody; HCTZ, hydrochlorothiazide; ISA, intrinsic sympathomimetic activity; LE, lupus erythematosus; MI, myocardial infarction; MSA, membrane-stabilizing activity; SR, sustained release; 0, no effect; +, some effect; ++, moderate effect; +++, most effect.

vasodilator beta-blockers carvedilol and nebivolol) have an adverse effect on lipids and glucose metabolism. Metoprolol reduces mortality and morbidity in patients with chronic stable heart failure with reduced ejection fraction (see Chapter 10). Carvedilol and nebivolol, which maintain cardiac output, are also beneficial in patients with systolic left ventricular dysfunction. Beta-blockers are used cautiously in patients with type 1 diabetes, since they can mask the symptoms of hypoglycemia and prolong these episodes by inhibiting gluconeogenesis. These drugs should also be used with caution in patients with advanced peripheral vascular disease associated with rest pain or nonhealing ulcers, but they are generally well tolerated in patients with mild claudication. Nebivolol can be safely used in patients with stage II claudication (claudication at 200 m).

In treatment of pheochromocytoma, beta-blockers should not be administered until alpha-blockade has been established. Otherwise, blockade of vasodilatory beta-2-adrenergic receptors will allow unopposed vasoconstrictor alpha-adrenergic receptor activation with worsening of hypertension. *For the same reason, beta-blockers should not be used to treat hypertension arising from cocaine use.*

In addition to adverse metabolic changes associated with their use, some experts have suggested that the therapeutic shortcomings of traditional beta-blockers are the consequence of the particular hemodynamic profile associated with these drugs. Pressure peaks in the aorta are augmented by reflection of pressure waves from the peripheral circulation. These reflected waves are delayed in patients taking ACE inhibitors and thiazide diuretics, resulting in decreased central systolic and pulse pressures. By contrast, traditional beta-blockers appear to potentiate reflection of pressure waves, possibly because peripheral resistance vessels are a reflection point and peripheral resistance is increased by these drugs. This might explain why the traditional beta-blockers are less effective at controlling systolic and pulse pressure.

Because of the lack of efficacy in primary prevention of myocardial infarction and inferiority compared with other drugs in prevention of stroke and left ventricular hypertrophy, traditional beta-blockers should not be regarded as ideal first-line agents in the treatment of hypertension without specific compelling indications (such as active coronary artery disease). It might be that vasodilating beta-blockers will emerge as alternative first-line antihypertensives, but this possibility has yet to be rigorously tested in outcomes studies.

Great care should be exercised if the decision is made, in the absence of compelling indications, to remove beta-blockers from the treatment regimen because abrupt withdrawal can precipitate acute coronary events and severe increases in blood pressure.

C. Renin Inhibitors

Since renin cleavage of angiotensinogen is the rate-limiting step in the renin-angiotensin cascade, the most efficient inactivation of this system would be expected with renin inhibition. Conventional ACE inhibitors and ARBs probably offer incomplete blockade, even in combination. Aliskiren, a renin inhibitor, binds the proteolytic site of renin, thereby preventing cleavage of angiotensinogen. As a consequence, levels of angiotensins I and II are reduced and renin concentration is increased. Aliskiren effectively lowers blood pressure, reduces albuminuria, and limits left ventricular hypertrophy but it has yet to be established as a first-line drug based on outcomes data. The combination of aliskiren with ACE inhibitors or ARBs in persons with type 2 diabetes mellitus certainly offers no advantage and might even increase the risk of adverse cardiac or renal consequences.

D. Angiotensin-Converting Enzyme Inhibitors

ACE inhibitors are commonly used as the initial medication in mild to moderate hypertension (Table 11–7). Their primary mode of action is inhibition of the renin–angiotensin–aldosterone system, but they also inhibit bradykinin degradation, stimulate the synthesis of vasodilating prostaglandins, and can reduce sympathetic nervous system activity. These latter actions may explain why they exhibit some effect even in patients with low plasma renin activity. ACE inhibitors appear to be more effective in younger white patients. They are relatively less effective in blacks and older persons and in predominantly systolic hypertension. Although as single therapy they achieve adequate antihypertensive control in only about 40–50% of patients, the combination of an ACE inhibitor and a diuretic or calcium channel blocker is potent.

ACE inhibitors are the agents of choice in persons with type 1 diabetes with frank proteinuria or evidence of kidney dysfunction because they delay the progression to end-stage kidney disease. Many authorities have expanded this indication to include persons with type 1 and type 2 diabetics with microalbuminuria who do not meet the usual criteria for antihypertensive therapy. ACE inhibitors may also delay the progression of nondiabetic kidney disease. The Heart Outcomes Prevention Evaluation (HOPE) trial demonstrated that the ACE inhibitor ramipril reduced the number of cardiovascular deaths, nonfatal myocardial infarctions, and nonfatal strokes and also reduced the incidence of new-onset heart failure, kidney dysfunction, and new-onset diabetes in a population of patients at high risk for vascular events. Although this was not specifically a hypertensive population, the benefits were associated with a modest reduction in blood pressure, and the results inferentially support the use of ACE inhibitors in similar hypertensive patients. ACE inhibitors are a drug of choice (usually in conjunction with a diuretic and a beta-blocker) in patients with heart failure with reduced ejection fraction and are indicated also in asymptomatic patients with reduced ejection fraction. An advantage of the ACE inhibitors is their relative freedom from troublesome side effects. Severe hypotension can occur in patients with bilateral renal artery stenosis; sudden increases in creatinine may ensue but are usually reversible with discontinuation of ACE inhibition. Hyperkalemia may develop in patients with kidney disease and type IV renal tubular acidosis (commonly seen in patients with diabetes) and in the elderly. A chronic dry cough is common, seen in 10% of patients or more, and may require stopping the drug. Skin rashes are observed with any ACE inhibitor. Angioedema

Table 11–7. Antihypertensive drugs: Renin and ACE inhibitors and angiotensin II receptor blockers.

Drug	Proprietary Name	Initial Oral Dosage	Dosage Range	Cost per Unit	Cost of 30 Days Treatment (Average Dosage)[1]	Adverse Effects	Comments
Renin Inhibitors							
Aliskiren	Tekturna	150 mg once daily	150–300 mg once daily	$6.01/150 mg	$180.30	Angioedema, hypotension, hyperkalemia. Contraindicated in pregnancy.	Probably metabolized by CYP3A4. Absorption is inhibited by high-fat meal.
Aliskiren and HCTZ	Tekturna HCT	150 mg/12.5 mg once daily	150 mg/12.5 mg–300 mg/ 25 mg once daily	$6.01/150 mg/12.5 mg	$180.30		
ACE Inhibitors							
Benazepril	Lotensin	10 mg once daily	5–40 mg in 1 or 2 doses	$1.05/20 mg	$31.50	Cough, hypotension, dizziness, kidney dysfunction, hyperkalemia, angioedema; taste alteration and rash (may be more frequent with captopril); rarely, proteinuria, blood dyscrasia. Contraindicated in pregnancy.	More fosinopril is excreted by the liver in patients with renal dysfunction (dose reduction may or may not be necessary). Captopril and lisinopril are active without metabolism. Captopril, enalapril, lisinopril, and quinapril are approved for heart failure.
Benazepril and HCTZ	Lotensin HCT	5 mg/6.25 mg once daily	5 mg/6.25 mg–20 mg/ 25 mg	$2.07/any dose	$62.10		
Benazepril and amlodipine	Lotrel	10 mg/2.5 mg once daily	10 mg/2.5 mg–40 mg/ 10 mg	$3.32/20 mg/10 mg	$99.60		
Captopril	Capoten	25 mg twice daily	50–450 mg in 2 or 3 doses	$1.67/25 mg	$100.20		
Captopril and HCTZ	Capozide	25 mg/15 mg twice daily	25 mg/15 mg–50 mg/ 25 mg	$0.72/25 mg/15 mg	$43.20		
Enalapril	Vasotec	5 mg once daily	5–40 mg in 1 or 2 doses	$2.77/20 mg	$83.10		
Enalapril and HCTZ	Vaseretic	5 mg/12.5 mg once daily	5 mg/12.5 mg–10 mg/ 25 mg	$1.19/10 mg/25 mg	$35.70		
Fosinopril	Monopril	10 mg once daily	10–80 mg in 1 or 2 doses	$1.19/20 mg	$35.70		

(continued)

Table 11–7. Antihypertensive drugs: Renin and ACE inhibitors and angiotensin II receptor blockers. (continued)

Drug	Proprietary Name	Initial Oral Dosage	Dosage Range	Cost per Unit	Cost of 30 Days Treatment (Average Dosage)[1]	Adverse Effects	Comments
Fosinopril and HCTZ	Monopril-HCT	10 mg/12.5 mg once daily	10 mg/12.5 mg–20 mg/ 12.5 mg	$1.26/any dose	$37.80		
Lisinopril	Prinivil, Zestril	5–10 mg once daily	5–40 mg once daily	$1.06/20 mg	$31.80		
Lisinopril and HCTZ	Prinzide or Zestoretic	10 mg/12.5 mg once daily	10 mg/12.5 mg–20 mg/ 12.5 mg	$1.20/20 mg/12.5 mg	$36.00		
Moexipril	Univasc	7.5 mg once daily	7.5–30 mg in 1 or 2 doses	$1.39/7.5 mg	$41.70		
Moexipril and HCTZ	Uniretic	7.5 mg/12.5 mg once daily	7.5 mg/12.5 mg–15 mg/ 25 mg	$1.34/7.5 mg/12.5 mg	$40.20		
Perindopril	Aceon	4 mg once daily	4–16 mg in 1 or 2 doses	$2.80/8 mg	$84.00		
Perindopril and amlodipine	Prestalia	3.5 mg/2.5 mg once daily	14 mg/10 mg once daily	$5.87/7 mg/5 mg	$176.10		
Quinapril	Accupril	10 mg once daily	10–80 mg in 1 or 2 doses	$1.22/20 mg	$36.60		
Quinapril and HCTZ	Accuretic	10 mg/12.5 mg once daily	10 mg/12.5 mg–20 mg/ 25 mg	$1.22/20 mg/12.5 mg	$36.60		
Ramipril	Altace	2.5 mg once daily	2.5–20 mg in 1 or 2 doses	$1.89/5 mg	$56.70		
Trandolapril	Mavik	1 mg once daily	1–8 mg once daily	$1.24/4 mg	$37.20		
Trandolapril and verapamil	Tarka	2 mg/180 mg ER once daily	2 mg/180 mg ER–8 mg/ 480 mg ER	$5.29/any dose	$158.70		

Angiotensin II Receptor Blockers

Drug	Trade Name	Initial Dose	Dosage Range	Cost per Unit	Cost	Adverse Effects	Comments
Azilsartan	Edarbi	40 mg once daily	40–80 mg once daily	$6.83/80 mg	$204.90		
Azilsartan and chlorthalidone	Edarbychlor	40 mg/12.5 mg once daily	40 mg/12.5–40 mg/25 mg once daily	$6.45/any dose	$193.50	Hyperkalemia, kidney dysfunction, rare angioedema. Combinations have additional side effects. Contraindicated in pregnancy.	Losartan has a very flat dose-response curve. Valsartan and irbesartan have wider dose-response ranges and longer durations of action. Addition of low-dose diuretic (separately or as combination pills) increases the response.
Candesartan cilexitil	Atacand	16 mg once daily	8–32 mg once daily	$3.17/16 mg	$95.10		
Candesartan cilexitil and HCTZ	Atacand HCT	16 mg/12.5 mg once daily	32 mg/12.5 mg once daily	$4.09/16 mg/12.5 mg	$122.70		
Eprosartan	Teveten	600 mg once daily	400–800 mg in 1–2 doses	$11.42/600 mg	$342.60		
Eprosartan/HCTZ	Teveten HCT	600 mg/12.5 mg once daily	600 mg/12.5 mg–600 mg/25 mg once daily	$5.63/600 mg/12.5 mg	$168.90		
Irbesartan	Avapro	150 mg once daily	150–300 mg once daily	$3.07/150 mg	$92.10		
Irbesartan and HCTZ	Avalide	150 mg/12.5 mg once daily	150–300 mg irbesartan once daily	$3.71/150 mg	$111.30		
Losartan	Cozaar	50 mg once daily	25–100 mg in 1 or 2 doses	$2.26/50 mg	$67.80		
Losartan and HCTZ	Hyzaar	50 mg/12.5 mg once daily	50 mg/12.5 mg–100 mg/25 mg tablets once daily	$2.50/50 mg/12.5 mg/ tablet	$75.00		
Olmesartan	Benicar	20 mg once daily	20–40 mg once daily	$6.34/20 mg	$190.20		
Olmesartan and HCTZ	Benicar HCT	20 mg/12.5 mg once daily	20 mg/12.5 mg–40 mg/25 mg once daily	$6.35/20 mg/12.5 mg	$190.50		
Olmesartan and amlodipine	Azor	20 mg/5 mg once daily	20 mg/5 mg–40 mg/10 mg once daily	$7.92/20 mg/5 mg	$237.60		
Olmesartan and amlodipine and HCTZ	Tribenzor	20 mg/5 mg/ 12.5 mg once daily	20 mg/5 mg/12.5 mg–40 mg/10 mg/25 mg once daily	$7.92/20 mg/5 mg/ 12.5 mg	$237.60		
Telmisartan	Micardis	40 mg once daily	20–80 mg once daily	$4.34/40 mg	$130.20		
Telmisartan and HCTZ	Micardis HCT	40 mg/12.5 mg once daily	40 mg/12.5 mg–80 mg/12.5 mg once daily	$4.83/40 mg/12.5 mg	$144.90		

(continued)

Table 11–7. Antihypertensive drugs: Renin and ACE inhibitors and angiotensin II receptor blockers. (continued)

Drug	Proprietary Name	Initial Oral Dosage	Dosage Range	Cost per Unit	Cost of 30 Days Treatment (Average Dosage)[1]	Adverse Effects	Comments
Telmisartan and amlodipine	Twynsta	40 mg/5 mg once daily	40 mg/5 mg–80 mg/10 mg once daily	$5.20/any dose	$156.00	Hyperkalemia, kidney dysfunction, rare angioedema. Combinations have additional side effects. Contraindicated in pregnancy.	Losartan has a very flat dose-response curve. Valsartan and irbesartan have wider dose-response ranges and longer durations of action. Addition of low-dose diuretic (separately or as combination pills) increases the response.
Valsartan	Diovan	80 mg once daily	80–320 mg once daily	$5.00/160 mg	$150.00		
Valsartan and HCTZ	Diovan HCT	80 mg/12.5 mg once daily	80–320 mg valsartan once daily	$4.27/160 mg/12.5 mg	$128.10		
Valsartan and amlodipine	Exforge	160 mg/5 mg once daily	160 mg/5 mg–320 mg/10 mg once daily	$1.71/160 mg/10 mg	$51.30		
Other Combination Products							
Amlodipine and valsartan and HCTZ	Exforge HCT	5 mg/160 mg/12.5 mg once daily	10 mg/320 mg/25 mg up to once daily	$6.20/160 mg valsartan	$186.00		

[1] Average wholesale price (AWP, for AB-rated generic when available) for quantity listed.

Source: *Red Book Online*, Truven Health Analytics, Information, http://www.micromedexsolutions.com, March 1, 2016. AWP may not accurately represent the actual pharmacy cost because contractual variations exist among institutions.

ACE, angiotensin-converting enzyme; HCTZ, hydrochlorothiazide.

is an uncommon but potentially dangerous side effect of all agents of this class because of their inhibition of kininase. Exposure of the fetus to ACE inhibitors during the second and third trimesters of pregnancy has been associated with a variety of defects due to hypotension and reduced renal blood flow.

E. Angiotensin II Receptor Blockers

ARBs can improve cardiovascular outcomes in patients with hypertension as well as in patients with related conditions such as heart failure and type 2 diabetes with nephropathy. ARBs have not been compared with ACE inhibitors in randomized controlled trials in patients with hypertension, but two trials comparing losartan with captopril in heart failure and post-myocardial infarction left ventricular dysfunction showed trends toward worse outcomes in the losartan group. By contrast, valsartan seems as effective as ACE inhibitors in these settings. Within group heterogeneity of antihypertensive potency and duration of action might explain such observations. The Losartan Intervention for Endpoints (LIFE) trial in nearly 9000 hypertensive patients with electrocardiographic evidence of left ventricular hypertrophy—comparing losartan with the beta-blocker atenolol as initial therapy—demonstrated a significant reduction in stroke with losartan. Of note is that in diabetic patients, death and myocardial infarction were also reduced, and there was a lower occurrence of new-onset diabetes. In this trial, as in the Antihypertensive and Lipid-Lowering Treatment to Prevent Heart Attack Trial (ALLHAT), blacks treated with renin-angiotensin-aldosterone system (RAAS) inhibitors exhibited less blood pressure reduction and less benefit with regard to clinical end points. In the treatment of hypertension, combination therapy with an ACE inhibitor and an ARB is not advised because it generally offers no advantage over monotherapy at maximum dose with addition of a complementary class where necessary.

Unlike ACE inhibitors, the ARBs do not cause cough and are less likely to be associated with skin rashes or angioedema. However, as seen with ACE inhibitors, hyperkalemia can be a problem, and patients with bilateral renal artery stenosis may exhibit hypotension and worsened kidney function. Olmesartan has been linked to a sprue-like syndrome, presenting with abdominal pain, weight loss, and nausea, which subsides upon drug discontinuation.

F. Aldosterone Receptor Antagonists

Spironolactone and eplerenone are natriuretic in sodium-retaining states, such as heart failure and cirrhosis, but only very weakly so in hypertension. These drugs have reemerged in the treatment of hypertension, particularly in resistant patients and are helpful additions to most other antihypertensive medications. Consistent with the increasingly appreciated importance of aldosterone in essential hypertension, the aldosterone receptor blockers are effective at lowering blood pressure in all hypertensive patients regardless of renin level, and are also effective in blacks. Aldosterone plays a central role in target-organ damage, including the development of ventricular and vascular

hypertrophy and renal fibrosis. Aldosterone receptor antagonists ameliorate these consequences of hypertension, to some extent independently of effects on blood pressure. Spironolactone can cause breast pain and gynecomastia in men through activity at the progesterone receptor, an effect not seen with the more specific eplerenone. Hyperkalemia is a problem with both drugs, chiefly in patients with chronic kidney disease. Hyperkalemia is more likely if the pretreatment plasma potassium exceeds 4.5 mmol/L.

G. Calcium Channel Blocking Agents

These agents act by causing peripheral vasodilation but with less reflex tachycardia and fluid retention than other vasodilators. They are effective as single-drug therapy in approximately 60% of patients in all demographic groups and all grades of hypertension (Table 11–8). For these reasons, they may be preferable to beta-blockers and ACE inhibitors in blacks and older persons. Verapamil and diltiazem should be combined cautiously with beta-blockers because of their potential for depressing AV conduction and sinus node automaticity as well as contractility.

Initial concerns about possible adverse cardiac effects of calcium channel blockers have been convincingly allayed by several subsequent large studies that have demonstrated that calcium channel blockers are equivalent to ACE inhibitors and thiazide diuretics in prevention of coronary heart disease, major cardiovascular events, cardiovascular death, and total mortality. A protective effect against stroke with calcium channel blockers is well established, and in two trials (ALLHAT and the Systolic Hypertension in Europe trial), these agents appeared to be more effective than diuretic-based therapy.

The most common side effects of calcium channel blockers are headache, peripheral edema, bradycardia, and constipation (especially with verapamil in the elderly). The dihydropyridine agents—nifedipine, nicardipine, isradipine, felodipine, nisoldipine, and amlodipine—are more likely to produce symptoms of vasodilation, such as headache, flushing, palpitations, and peripheral edema. Edema is minimized by coadministration of an ACE inhibitor or ARB. Calcium channel blockers have negative inotropic effects and should be used cautiously in patients with cardiac dysfunction. Amlodipine is the only calcium channel blocker with established safety in patients with severe heart failure.

H. Alpha-Adrenoceptor Antagonists

Prazosin, terazosin, and doxazosin (Table 11–9) block postsynaptic alpha-receptors, relax smooth muscle, and reduce blood pressure by lowering peripheral vascular resistance. These agents are effective as single-drug therapy in some individuals, but tachyphylaxis may appear during long-term therapy and side effects are relatively common. These include marked hypotension after the first dose which, therefore, should be small and given at bedtime. Post-dosing palpitations, headache, and nervousness may continue to occur during long-term therapy; these symptoms may be less frequent or severe with doxazosin

Table 11–8. Antihypertensive drugs: Calcium channel blocking agents.

Drug	Proprietary Name	Initial Oral Dosage	Dosage Range	Cost of 30 Days Treatment (Average Dosage)[1]	Special Properties			Adverse Effects	Comments
					Peripheral Vasodilation	Cardiac Automaticity and Conduction	Contractility		
Nondihydropyridine Agents									
Diltiazem	Cardizem SR	90 mg twice daily	180–360 mg in 2 doses	$246.60 (120 mg twice daily)	++	↓↓	↓↓	Edema, headache, bradycardia, GI disturbances, dizziness, AV block, heart failure, urinary frequency.	Also approved for angina.
	Cardizem CD	180 mg ER once daily	180–360 mg ER once daily						
	Cartia XT	180 or 240 mg ER once daily	180–480 mg ER once daily	$61.50 (240 mg once daily)					
	Dilacor XR	180 or 240 mg ER once daily	180–540 mg ER once daily						
	Dilt-CD	180 or 240 mg ER once daily	180–480 mg ER once daily						
	Diltia XT	180 or 240 mg ER once daily	180–540 mg ER once daily						
	Tiazac	120 or 240 mg ER once daily	120–540 mg ER once daily						
	Taztia XT	120 or 180 mg ER once daily	120–540 mg ER once daily						
Verapamil	Calan	80 mg three times daily	80–480 mg in 3 divided doses		++	↓↓↓	↓↓↓	Same as diltiazem but more likely to cause constipation and heart failure.	Also approved for angina and arrhythmias.
	Calan SR	180 mg ER once daily	180–480 mg ER in 1 or 2 doses						
	Verelan	120 or 240 mg ER once daily	240–480 mg ER once daily	$68.40 (240 mg once daily)					
	Verelan PM	100 or 200 mg ER once daily	100–400 mg ER once daily	$240.00 (200 mg once daily)					

Dihydropyridines									
Amlodipine	Norvasc	2.5 mg once daily	2.5–10 mg once daily	$71.10 (10 mg once daily)	+++	↓/0	↓/0	Edema, dizziness, palpitations, flushing, headache, hypotension, tachycardia, GI disturbances, urinary frequency, worsening of heart failure (may be less common with felodipine and amlodipine.)	Amlodipine, nicardipine, and nifedipine also approved for angina.
Amlodipine and atorvastatin	Caduet	2.5 mg/10 mg once daily	10 mg/80 mg once daily	$281.10 (10 mg/40 mg daily)	+++	↓/0	↓/0	Myopathy, hepatotoxicity, edema with amlodipine and atorvastatin.	
Felodipine	Plendil	5 mg ER once daily	5–10 mg ER once daily	$81.60 (10 mg ER daily)	+++	↓/0	↓/0		
Isradipine	DynaCirc	2.5 mg twice daily	2.5–5 mg twice daily	$120.00 (5 mg twice daily)	+++	↓/0	→		
Nicardipine	Cardene	20 mg three times daily	20–40 mg three times daily	$196.20 (20 mg three times daily)	+++	↓/0	→		
Nifedipine	Adalat CC	30 mg ER once daily	30–90 mg ER once daily	$90.60/60 mg daily	+++	→	↓↓		
	Afeditab CR	30 mg ER once daily	30–90 mg ER once daily						
	Nifediac CC	30 mg ER once daily	30–90 ER mg once daily						
	Nifedical XL	30 mg ER once daily	30–120 mg ER once daily						
	Procardia XL	30 or 60 mg ER once daily	30–120 mg ER once daily						
Nisoldipine	Sular	17 mg daily	17–34 mg daily	$251.70 (34 mg once daily)	+++	↓/0	→		

¹Average wholesale price (AWP, for AB-rated generic when available) for quantity listed.
Source: *Red Book Online,* Truven Health Analytics, Information, http://www.micromedexsolutions.com, March 1, 2016. AWP may not accurately represent the actual pharmacy cost because wide contractual variations exist among institutions.
AV, atrioventricular; GI, gastrointestinal.

Table 11–9. Alpha-adrenoceptor blocking agents, sympatholytics, and vasodilators.

Drug	Proprietary Names	Initial Dosage	Dosage Range	Cost per Unit	Cost of 30 Days Treatment (Average Dosage)[1]	Adverse Effects	Comments
Alpha-Adrenoceptor Blockers							
Doxazosin	Cardura Cardura XL	1 mg at bedtime 4 mg ER once daily	1–16 mg once daily 4–8 mg ER once daily	$1.42/4 mg $4.38/4 mg ER	$42.60 (4 mg once daily) $131.40 (4 mg ER once daily)	Syncope with first dose; postural hypotension, dizziness, palpitations, headache, weakness, drowsiness, sexual dysfunction, anticholinergic effects, urinary incontinence; first-dose effects may be less with doxazosin.	May ↑ HDL and ↓ LDL cholesterol. May provide short-term relief of obstructive prostatic symptoms. Less effective in preventing cardiovascular events than diuretics.
Prazosin	Minipress	1 mg at bedtime	2–20 mg in 2 or 3 doses	$2.18/5 mg	$130.80 (5 mg twice daily)		
Terazosin	Hytrin	1 mg at bedtime	1–20 mg in 1 or 2 doses	$1.60/1, 2, 5, 10 mg	$48.00 (5 mg once daily)		
Central Sympatholytics							
Clonidine	Catapres Catapres TTS (transdermal patch)	0.1 mg twice daily 0.1 mg/day patch weekly	0.2–0.6 mg in 2 doses 0.1–0.3 mg/day patch weekly	$0.23/0.1 mg $55.77/0.2 mg patch	$19.20 (0.1 mg twice daily) $223.08 (0.2 mg weekly)	Sedation, dry mouth, sexual dysfunction, headache, bradyarrhythmias; side effects may be less with guanfacine. Contact dermatitis with clonidine patch. Methyldopa also causes hepatitis, hemolytic anemia, fever.	"Rebound" hypertension may occur even after gradual withdrawal.
Clonidine and chlorthalidone	Clorpres	0.1 mg/15 mg one to three times daily	0.1 mg/15 mg– 0.3 mg/15 mg	$2.77/0.1 mg/ 15 mg	$166.20/0.1 mg/15 mg twice daily		
Guanfacine	Tenex	1 mg once daily	1–3 mg once daily	$4.72/1 mg	$141.60 (1 mg once daily)		
Methyldopa	Aldochlor	250 mg twice daily	500–2000 mg in 2 doses	$0.70/500 mg	$42.00 (500 mg twice daily)		Methyldopa should be avoided in favor of safer agents.

Peripheral Neuronal Antagonists				
Reserpine	(generic)	0.05 mg once daily	0.05–0.25 mg once daily	$1.19/0.1 mg	$35.70 (0.1 mg once daily)	Depression (less likely at low dosages, ie, < 0.25 mg), night terrors, nasal stuffiness, drowsiness, peptic disease, gastrointestinal disturbances, bradycardia.	
Direct Vasodilators				
Hydralazine	Apresoline	25 mg twice daily	50–300 mg in 2–4 doses	$0.51/25 mg	$30.60 (25 mg twice daily)	GI disturbances, tachycardia, headache, nasal congestion, rash, LE-like syndrome.	May worsen or precipitate angina.
Minoxidil	(generic)	5 mg once daily	10—40 mg once daily	$1.29/10 mg	$38.70 (10 mg once daily)	Tachycardia, fluid retention, headache, hirsutism, pericardial effusion, thrombocytopenia.	Should be used in combination with beta-blocker and diuretic.

[1]Average wholesale price (AWP, for AB-rated generic when available) for quantity listed.
Source: *Red Book Online*, Truven Health Analytics, Information, http://www.micromedexsolutions.com, March 1, 2016. AWP may not accurately represent the actual pharmacy cost because wide contractual variations exist among institutions.
GI, gastrointestinal; LE, lupus erythematosus.

because of its more gradual onset of action. Cataractectomy in patients exposed to alpha-blockers can be complicated by the floppy iris syndrome, even after discontinuation of the drug, so the ophthalmologist should be alerted that the patient has been taking the drug prior to surgery.

Unlike beta-blockers and diuretics, alpha-blockers have no adverse effect on serum lipid levels—in fact, they increase HDL cholesterol while reducing total cholesterol. Whether this is beneficial in the long term has not been established. In ALLHAT, persons receiving doxazosin as initial therapy had a significant increase in heart failure hospitalizations and a higher incidence of stroke relative to those receiving diuretics, prompting discontinuation of this arm of the study. To summarize, alpha-blockers should generally not be used as initial agents to treat hypertension—except perhaps in men with symptomatic prostatism or nightmares linked to posttraumatic stress disorder.

I. Drugs with Central Sympatholytic Action

Methyldopa, clonidine, guanabenz, and guanfacine (Table 11–9) lower blood pressure by stimulating alpha-adrenergic receptors in the central nervous system, thus reducing efferent peripheral sympathetic outflow. These agents are effective as single therapy in some patients, but they are usually used as second- or third-line agents because of the high frequency of drug intolerance, including sedation, fatigue, dry mouth, postural hypotension, and erectile dysfunction. An important concern is rebound hypertension following withdrawal. Methyldopa also causes hepatitis and hemolytic anemia and is avoided except in individuals who have already tolerated long-term therapy. There is considerable experience with methyldopa in pregnant women, and it is still used for this population. Clonidine is available in patches, which may have particular value in patients in whom compliance is a troublesome issue.

J. Arteriolar Dilators

Hydralazine and minoxidil (Table 11–9) relax vascular smooth muscle and produce peripheral vasodilation. When given alone, they stimulate reflex tachycardia, increase myocardial contractility, and cause headache, palpitations, and fluid retention. They are usually given in combination with diuretics and beta-blockers in resistant patients. Hydralazine produces frequent gastrointestinal disturbances and may induce a lupus-like syndrome. Minoxidil causes hirsutism and marked fluid retention; this agent is reserved for the most refractory of cases.

K. Peripheral Sympathetic Inhibitors

These agents are now used infrequently and usually in refractory hypertension. Reserpine remains a cost-effective antihypertensive agent (Table 11–9). Its reputation for inducing mental depression and its other side effects—sedation, nasal stuffiness, sleep disturbances, and peptic ulcers—has made it unpopular, though these problems are uncommon at low dosages. Guanethidine and guanadrel inhibit catecholamine release from peripheral neurons but frequently cause orthostatic hypotension (especially in the morning or after exercise), diarrhea, and fluid retention.

▶ Developing an Antihypertensive Regimen

Historically, data from a number of large trials support the overall conclusion that antihypertensive therapy with diuretics and beta-blockers has a major beneficial effect on a broad spectrum of cardiovascular outcomes, reducing the incidence of stroke by 30–50% and of heart failure by 40–50%, and halting progression to accelerated hypertension syndromes. The decreases in fatal and nonfatal coronary heart disease and cardiovascular and total mortality were less dramatic, ranging from 10% to 15%. Similar placebo-controlled data pertaining to the newer agents are generally lacking, except for stroke reduction with the calcium channel blocker nitrendipine in the Systolic Hypertension in Europe trial. However, there is substantial evidence that ACE inhibitors, and to a lesser extent ARBs, reduce adverse cardiovascular outcomes in other related populations (eg, patients with diabetic nephropathy, heart failure, or postmyocardial infarction and individuals at high risk for cardiovascular events). Most large clinical trials that have compared outcomes in relatively unselected patients have failed to show a difference between newer agents—such as ACE inhibitors, calcium channel blockers, and ARBs—and the older diuretic-based regimens with regard to survival, myocardial infarction, and stroke. Where differences have been observed, they have mostly been attributable to subtle asymmetries in blood pressure control rather than to any inherent advantages of one agent over another. Recommendations for initial treatment identify ACE inhibitors, ARBs, and calcium channel blockers as valid choices. Because of their adverse metabolic profile, initial therapy with thiazides might best be restricted to older patients. Thiazides are acceptable as first-line therapy in blacks because of specific efficacy in this group. Exceptions to these recommendations are appropriate for individuals who have specific (or "compelling") indications for another class of agent, as outlined in Table 11–4.

As discussed above, beta-blockers are not ideal first-line drugs in the treatment of hypertension without compelling indications for their use. Vasodilator beta-blockers (such as carvedilol and nebivolol) may produce better outcomes than traditional beta-blockers; however, this possibility remains a theoretical consideration.

The American Diabetes Association has advocated evening dosing of one or more antihypertensive medications to restore nocturnal blood pressure dipping. Outcomes data to support this proposal are limited. The Spanish MAPEC study of such nocturnal antihypertensive dosing showed a significant reduction in a range of major cardiovascular events in 2156 participants over 5.6 years. However, there are concerns that ischemic optic neuropathy may be triggered by profound nocturnal hypotension. Thus, larger studies are necessary before this approach can be firmly recommended.

For the purpose of devising an optimal treatment regimen, drugs can be divided into two complementary groups easily remembered as **A** and **C** and **D**. **A** refers to drugs that interrupt the renin-angiotensin system (**A**CE/ARB/renin inhibitor) and **C** and **D** refer to those that do not (**c**alcium channel blockers and thiazide **d**iuretics). Combinations of drugs between these groups are likely to be more potent in lowering blood pressure than combinations within a group. Drugs that interrupt the renin-angiotensin cascade are more effective in young, white persons, in whom renin tends to be higher, and drugs **C** and **D** are more effective in older or black persons, in whom renin levels are generally lower. Figure 11–4 illustrates guidelines for initiating antihypertensive therapy established by the United Kingdom's National Institute for Health and Care Excellence (NICE). In trials that include patients with systolic hypertension, most patients require two or more medications and even then a substantial proportion fail to achieve the goal blood pressure. In diabetic patients, three or four drugs are usually required to reduce systolic blood pressure to less than 140 mm Hg. In many patients, blood pressure

cannot be adequately controlled with any combination. As a result, debating the appropriate first-line agent is less relevant than determining the most appropriate combinations of agents. This has led many experts and practitioners to recommend the use of fixed-dose combination antihypertensive agents as first-line therapy in patients with substantially elevated systolic pressures (greater than 160/100 mm Hg) or difficult-to-control hypertension (which is often associated with diabetes or kidney dysfunction). In light of unwanted metabolic effects, calcium channel blockers might be preferable to thiazides in the younger hypertensive patient requiring a second antihypertensive drug. Furthermore, based on the results from the ACCOMPLISH trial, a combination of ACE inhibitor and calcium channel blocker may also prove optimal for patients at high risk for cardiovascular events. The initial use of low-dose combinations allows faster blood pressure reduction without substantially higher intolerance rates and is likely to be better accepted by patients. Data from the ALTITUDE study (in patients with type 2 diabetes and chronic kidney disease or cardiovascular disease or both), indicate that the addition of aliskiren to either ARB or ACE inhibitor was associated with worse outcomes and cannot be recommended, at least in this population. A suggested approach to treatment, tailored to patient demographics, is outlined in Table 11–10.

In sum, as a prelude to treatment, the patient should be informed of common side effects and the need for diligent compliance. In patients with mild or stage 1 hypertension (less than 160/90 mm Hg) in whom pharmacotherapy is indicated, treatment should start with a single agent at a low dose. Follow-up visits should usually be at 4- to 6-week intervals to allow for full medication effects to be established (especially with diuretics) before further titration or adjustment. If, after titration to usual doses, the patient has shown a discernible but incomplete response and a good tolerance of the initial drug, a second medication should be added. The goal of treatment in patients without other risk factors for vascular disease is an office reading of less than 140/90 mm Hg. As a rule of thumb, a blood pressure reduction of 10 mm Hg can be expected for each antihypertensive agent added to the regimen and titrated to the optimum dose. In those with more severe hypertension (stage 2), or with comorbidities (such as diabetes) that are likely to render them resistant to treatment, initiation with combination therapy is advised and more frequent follow-up is indicated.

Patients who are compliant with their medications and who do not respond to conventional combination regimens should usually be evaluated for secondary hypertension before proceeding to more complex regimens.

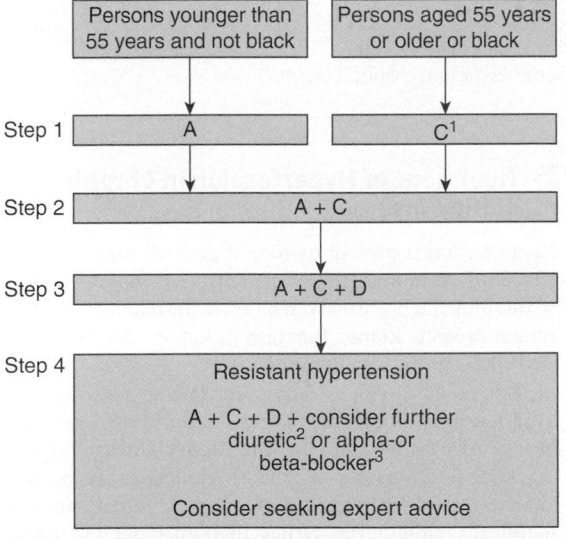

Step 1

Step 2

Step 3

Step 4

[1]A CCB is preferred but consider a thiazide-like diuretic if a CCB is not tolerated or the person has edema, evidence of heart failure or a high risk of heart failure.

[2]Consider a low dose of spironolactone or higher doses of a thiazide-like diuretic.

[3]Consider an alpha- or beta-blocker if further diuretic therapy is not tolerated, or is contraindicated or ineffective.

▲ **Figure 11–4.** Hypertension treatment guidelines from the United Kingdom's National Institute for Health and Care Excellence. Guidelines identify angiotensin-converting enzyme (ACE) inhibitors, angiotensin receptor blockers (ARBs), or calcium channel blockers (CCBs) as first-line medications and suggest a sequence of escalating drug therapy depending on blood pressure response. As noted, the choice of the initial agent is influenced by patient demographics. In step 4, higher doses of thiazide-type diuretics may be used as long as serum potassium levels exceed 4.5 mmol/L. Key: A, ACE inhibitor or ARB; C, calcium-channel blocker; D, diuretic, thiazide-like. (Modified, with permission, from the 2013 hypertension guidelines published by the National Institute for Health and Care Excellence. https://www.nice.org.uk/guidance/cg127/evidence/cg127-hypertension-full-guideline3)

▶ **Medication Nonadherence**

Adherence to antihypertensive treatment is alarmingly poor. In one European study of patients' antihypertensive medication compliance, there was a 40% discontinuation rate at 1 year after initiation. Only 39% of patients were found to be taking their medications continuously over a 10-year period. Collaborative care, utilizing physicians, pharmacists, social workers, and nurses to encourage

Table 11–10. Choice of antihypertensive agent based on demographic considerations.[1,2]

	Black, All Ages	All Others, Age < 55 Years	All Others, Age > 55 Years
First-line	CCB or diuretic	ACE or ARB[3] or CCB or diuretic[4]	CCB or diuretic[5]
Second-line	ACE or ARB[3] or vasodilating beta-blocker[6]	Vasodilating beta-blocker[6]	ACE or ARB or vasodilating beta-blocker[6]
Alternatives	Alpha-agonist or alpha-antagonist[7]	Alpha-agonist or alpha-antagonist	Alpha-agonist or alpha-antagonist[7]
Resistant hypertension	Aldosterone receptor blocker	Aldosterone receptor blocker	Aldosterone receptor blocker

[1]Compelling indications may alter the selection of an antihypertensive drug.
[2]Start with full dose of one agent, or lower doses of combination therapy. In stage 2 hypertension, consider initiating therapy with a fixed dose combination.
[3]Women of childbearing age should avoid ACE and ARB or discontinue as soon as pregnancy is diagnosed.
[4]The adverse metabolic effects of thiazide diuretics and beta-blockers should be considered in younger patients but may be less important in the older patient.
[5]For patients with significant renal impairment, use loop diuretic instead of thiazide.
[6]There are theoretical advantages in the use of vasodilating beta-blockers such as carvedilol and nebivolol.
[7]Alpha-antagonists may precipitate or exacerbate orthostatic hypotension in the elderly.
ACE, angiotensin-converting enzyme; ARB, angiotensin II receptor blocker; CCB, calcium channel blocker.

compliance has had a variable and often rather modest effect on blood pressure control. Adherence is enhanced by patient education and by use of home blood pressure measurement. The choice of antihypertensive medication is important. Better compliance has been reported for patients whose medications could be taken once daily or as combination pills. Adherence is best with ACE inhibitors and ARBs, and worse with beta-blockers and diuretics.

Special Considerations in the Treatment of Diabetic Hypertensive Patients

Hypertensive patients with diabetes are at particularly high risk for cardiovascular events. Data from the ACCORD study of diabetics demonstrated that most of the benefits of blood pressure lowering were seen with a systolic target of less than 140 mm Hg; in fact, except for a reduction in stroke risk, there was an *increased* risk of serious adverse events in diabetics with a systolic target of less than 120/70 mm Hg. Most US and international guidelines suggest a therapeutic systolic blood pressure goal of either less than 130 mm Hg or less than 140 mm Hg in the diabetic population. Because of the beneficial effects of ACE inhibitors in diabetic nephropathy, they should be part of the initial treatment regimen. ARBs or perhaps renin inhibitors may be substituted in those intolerant of ACE inhibitors. While the ONTARGET study showed that combinations of ACE inhibitors and ARBs in persons with atherosclerosis or type 2 diabetes with end-organ damage appeared to minimize proteinuria, this strategy slightly increased the risks of progression to dialysis and of death; thus, it is not recommended. Most diabetic patients require combinations of three to five agents to achieve target blood pressure, usually including a diuretic and a calcium channel blocker or beta-blocker. In addition to rigorous blood pressure control, treatment of persons with diabetes should include aggressive treatment of other risk factors.

Treatment of Hypertension in Chronic Kidney Disease

Hypertension is present in 40% of patients with a GFR of 60–90 mL/min, and 75% of patients with a GFR less than 30 mL/min. It is likely that inhibition of the renin-angiotensin system protects kidney function in kidney disease associated with significant proteinuria.

The blood pressure target in treating patients with hypertension and chronic kidney disease should generally be less than 140/90 mm Hg. The Kidney Disease Improving Global Outcomes (KDIGO) guidelines advocate a lower target of less than 130/80 mm Hg in patients with significant proteinuria. Drugs that interrupt the renin-angiotensin cascade are preferred for initial therapy. Transition from thiazide to loop diuretic is often necessary to control volume expansion as the eGFR falls below 30 mL/min. Evidence has demonstrated that ACE inhibitors remain protective and safe in kidney disease associated with significant proteinuria and serum creatinine as high as 5 mg/dL (380 mcmol/L). However, in patients with significant renal artery stenosis, ACE inhibitor therapy would likely worsen kidney function; therefore, kidney function and electrolytes should be monitored carefully in such patients. Persistence with ACE inhibitor or ARB therapy in the face of hyperkalemia is probably not warranted, since other antihypertensive medications are renoprotective as long as goal blood pressures are maintained.

Hypertension Management in Blacks

Substantial evidence indicates that blacks are not only more likely to become hypertensive and more susceptible to the cardiovascular and renal complications of hypertension—they also respond differently to many antihypertensive medications. The REGARDS study illustrates these disparities. At systolic blood pressures less than 120 mm Hg, black and white participants between 45 and 64 years of age had equal risk of stroke. For a 10 mm Hg increase in systolic blood pressure, the risk of stroke was threefold higher in black participants. At the level of stage 1 hypertension, the hazard ratio for stroke in black compared to white participants between 45 and 64 years of age was 2.35. This increased susceptibility may reflect genetic differences in the cause of hypertension or the subsequent responses to it, differences in occurrence of comorbid conditions such as diabetes or obesity, or environmental factors such as diet, activity, stress, or access to health care services. In any case, as in all persons with hypertension, a multifaceted program of education and lifestyle modification is warranted. Early introduction of combination therapy has been advocated, but there is no clinical trial data to support a lower than usual blood pressure goal (less than 140/90 mm Hg) in blacks. Because it appears that ACE inhibitors and ARBs—in the absence of concomitant diuretics—are less effective in blacks than in whites, initial therapy should generally be a diuretic or a diuretic in combination with a calcium channel blocker.

▶ Treating Hypertension in the Elderly

Several studies in persons over 60 years of age have confirmed that antihypertensive therapy prevents fatal and nonfatal myocardial infarction and reduces overall cardiovascular mortality. These trials placed the focus on control of systolic blood pressure (the hypertension affecting the majority of those over age 60 is predominantly systolic)—in contrast to the historical emphasis on diastolic blood pressure. The most recent US Joint National Committee Panel Report (JNC8) adopted a rigorous outcomes-based position in recommending a treatment goal of less than 150/90 mm Hg in persons older than 60 years of age. However, most clinical guidelines suggest that treatment targets for older people (age 60–80 years) should be the same as those for younger individuals (less than 140/90 mm Hg). In initiating therapy in older patients, pressure should be reduced more gradually with a safe intermediate systolic blood pressure goal of 160 mm Hg. In the very elderly, over age 80 years, the HYVET study indicated that a reasonable ultimate systolic blood pressure goal would be 150/80 mm Hg, reflected by the Canadian and European guidelines target of less than 150/90 mm Hg in this population. The same medications are used in older patients, but at 50% lower doses. As treatment is initiated, older patients should be carefully monitored for orthostasis, altered cognition, and electrolyte disturbances. The HYVET trial recruited individuals who were relatively well; by contrast, there appears to be a loss of the usual relationship between blood pressure and morbidity/mortality in the very elderly who are also frail (as defined by a walking speed of less than 0.8 m/sec over 6 m). In the very frail (those unable to walk 6 m), blood pressure below 140/90 mm Hg was paradoxically associated with worse outcomes. A less aggressive approach to the treatment of hypertension would therefore seem appropriate in the very elderly who are also frail.

▶ Follow-Up of Patients Receiving Hypertension Therapy

Once blood pressure is controlled on a well-tolerated regimen, follow-up visits can be infrequent and laboratory testing limited to those appropriate for the patient and the medications used. Yearly monitoring of blood lipids is recommended, and an electrocardiogram could be repeated at 2- to 4-year intervals depending on whether initial abnormalities are present, the presence of coronary risk factors, and age. Patients who have had excellent blood pressure control for several years, especially if they have lost weight and initiated favorable lifestyle modifications, might be considered for a trial of reduced antihypertensive medications.

ALLHAT Officers and Coordinators for the ALLHAT Collaborative Research Group. Major outcomes in high-risk hypertensive patients randomized to angiotensin-converting enzyme inhibitor or calcium channel blocker vs diuretic. The Antihypertensive and Lipid-Lowering Treatment to Prevent Heart Attack Trial (ALLHAT). JAMA. 2002 Dec 18;288(23):2981–97. [PMID: 12479763]

Burnier M et al. State-of-the-art treatment of hypertension: established and new drugs. Eur Heart J. 2014 Mar;35(9):557–62. [PMID: 24216391]

Carter BL et al. Efficacy and safety of nighttime dosing of antihypertensives: review of the literature and design of a pragmatic clinical trial. J Clin Hypertens (Greenwich). 2014 Feb;16(2):115–21. [PMID: 24373519]

Dasgupta K et al. The 2014 Canadian Hypertension Education Program recommendations for blood pressure measurement, diagnosis, assessment of risk, prevention, and treatment of hypertension. Can J Cardiol. 2014 May;30(5):485–501. [PMID: 24786438]

Howard G et al. Racial differences in the impact of elevated systolic blood pressure on stroke risk. JAMA Intern Med. 2013 Jan 14;173(1):46–51. [PMID: 23229778]

James PA et al. 2014 Evidence-Based Guideline for the Management of High Blood Pressure in Adults: Report From the Panel Members Appointed to the Eighth Joint National Committee (JNC 8). JAMA. 2014 Feb 5;311(5):507–20. [PMID: 24352797]

Kountz DS. Hypertension in black patients: an update. Postgrad Med. 2013 May;125(3):127–35. [PMID: 23748513]

Lipsitz LA. A 91-year-old woman with difficult-to-control hypertension: a clinical review. JAMA. 2013 Sep 25;310(12):1274–80. [PMID: 24065014]

Wiysonge CS et al. Beta-blockers for hypertension. Cochrane Database Syst Rev. 2012 Nov 14;11:CD002003. [PMID: 23152211]

RESISTANT HYPERTENSION

Resistant hypertension is defined in JNC 7 as the failure to reach blood pressure control in patients who are adherent to full doses of an appropriate three-drug regimen (including a diuretic). Adherence is a major issue: the rate of partial or complete noncompliance probably approaches 50% in this group of patients; doxazosin, spironolactone, and hydrochlorothiazide were particularly unpopular in one study based on drug assay in Eastern Europe. In the approach to resistant hypertension, the clinician should first confirm compliance and rule out "white coat hypertension." Exacerbating factors should be considered (as outlined above). Finally, identifiable causes of hypertension should be sought (Table 11–11). The clinician should pay particular attention to the type of diuretic being used in relation to the patient's kidney function. Aldosterone may play an important role in resistant hypertension and aldosterone receptor blockers can be very useful. If goal blood

Table 11–11. Causes of resistant hypertension.

Improper blood pressure measurement
Volume overload and pseudotolerance
Excess sodium intake
Volume retention from kidney disease
Inadequate diuretic therapy
Drug-induced or other causes
Nonadherence
Inadequate doses
Inappropriate combinations
Nonsteroidal anti-inflammatory drugs; cyclooxygenase-2 inhibitors
Cocaine, amphetamines, other illicit drugs
Sympathomimetics (decongestants, anorectics)
Oral contraceptives
Adrenal steroids
Cyclosporine and tacrolimus
Erythropoietin
Licorice (including some chewing tobacco)
Selected over-the-counter dietary supplements and medicines (eg, ephedra, ma huang, bitter orange)
Associated conditions
Obesity
Excess alcohol intake
Identifiable causes of hypertension (see Table 11–1)

Data from Chobanian AV et al. The Seventh Report of the Joint National Committee on Prevention, Detection, Evaluation, and Treatment of High Blood Pressure: the JNC 7 report. JAMA. 2003 May 21;289(19):2560–72.

pressure cannot be achieved following completion of these steps, consultation with a hypertension specialist should be considered. The Symplicity HTN 3 study failed to show that renal sympathetic ablation improved blood pressure compared to a sham-operated control group.

Burnier M et al. Ambulatory blood pressure and adherence monitoring: diagnosing pseudoresistant hypertension. Semin Nephrol. 2014;34(5):498–505. [PMID: 25416658]

Burnier M et al. Measuring, analyzing, and managing drug adherence in resistant hypertension. Hypertension. 2013 Aug;62(2):218–25. [PMID: 23753412]

Ghofrani H et al. Resistant hypertension: medical management and alternative therapies. Cardiol Clin. 2015 Feb;33(1):75–87. [PMID: 25439332]

Lobo MD et al. Joint UK Societies' 2014 consensus statement on renal denervation for resistant hypertension. Heart. 2015 Jan 1; 101(1):10–6. [PMID: 25431461]

HYPERTENSIVE URGENCIES & EMERGENCIES

Hypertensive emergencies have become less frequent in recent years but still require prompt recognition and aggressive but careful management. A spectrum of urgent presentations exists, and the appropriate therapeutic approach varies accordingly.

Hypertensive urgencies are situations in which blood pressure must be reduced within a few hours. These include patients with asymptomatic severe hypertension (systolic blood pressure greater than 220 mm Hg or diastolic pressure greater than 125 mm Hg that persists after a period of observation) and those with optic disk edema, progressive target-organ complications, and severe perioperative hypertension. Elevated blood pressure levels alone—in the absence of symptoms or new or progressive target-organ damage—rarely require emergency therapy. Parenteral drug therapy is not usually required, and partial reduction of blood pressure with relief of symptoms is the goal.

Hypertensive emergencies require substantial reduction of blood pressure within 1 hour to avoid the risk of serious morbidity or death. Although blood pressure is usually strikingly elevated (diastolic pressure greater than 130 mm Hg), the correlation between pressure and end-organ damage is often poor. It is the presence of critical multiple end organ injury that determines the seriousness of the emergency and the approach to treatment. Emergencies include hypertensive encephalopathy (headache, irritability, confusion, and altered mental status due to cerebrovascular spasm), hypertensive nephropathy (hematuria, proteinuria, and acute kidney injury due to arteriolar necrosis and intimal hyperplasia of the interlobular arteries), intracranial hemorrhage, aortic dissection, preeclampsia-eclampsia, pulmonary edema, unstable angina, or myocardial infarction. Encephalopathy or nephropathy accompanying hypertensive retinopathy has historically been termed **malignant hypertension,** but the therapeutic approach is identical to that used in other hypertensive emergencies.

Parenteral therapy is indicated in most hypertensive emergencies, especially if encephalopathy is present. The initial goal in hypertensive emergencies is to reduce the pressure by no more than 25% (within minutes to 1 or 2 hours) and then toward a level of 160/100 mm Hg within 2–6 hours. Excessive reductions in pressure may precipitate coronary, cerebral, or renal ischemia. To avoid such declines, the use of agents that have a predictable, dose-dependent, transient, and progressive antihypertensive effect is preferable (Table 11–12). In that regard, the use of sublingual or oral fast-acting nifedipine preparations is best avoided.

Acute ischemic stroke is often associated with marked elevation of blood pressure, which will usually fall spontaneously. In such cases, antihypertensives should only be used if the systolic blood pressure exceeds 180–200 mm Hg, and blood pressure should be reduced cautiously by 10–15% (Table 11–12). If thrombolytics are to be given, blood pressure should be maintained at less than 185/110 mm Hg during treatment and for 24 hours following treatment.

In hemorrhagic stroke, the aim is to minimize bleeding with a target mean arterial pressure of less than 130 mm Hg. In acute subarachnoid hemorrhage, as long as the bleeding source remains uncorrected, a compromise must be struck between preventing further bleeding and maintaining cerebral perfusion in the face of cerebral vasospasm. In this situation, blood pressure goals depend on the patient's usual blood pressure. In normotensive patients, the target should be a systolic blood pressure of 110–120 mm Hg; in hypertensive patients, blood pressure should be treated to 20% below baseline pressure. In the treatment of hypertensive emergencies complicated by (or precipitated by) central nervous system injury, labetalol or nicardipine

Table 11–12. Treatment of hypertensive emergency depending on primary site of end-organ damage. See Table 11–13 for dosages.

Type of Hypertensive Emergency	Recommended Drug Options and Combinations	Drugs to Avoid
Myocardial ischemia and infarction	Nicardipine plus esmolol[1] Nitroglycerin plus labetalol Nitroglycerin plus esmolol[1]	Hydralazine, diazoxide, minoxidil, nitroprusside
Acute kidney injury	Fenoldopam Nicardipine Clevidipine	
Aortic dissection	Esmolol plus nicardipine Esmolol plus clevidipine Labetalol Esmolol plus nitroprusside	Hydralazine, diazoxide, minoxidil
Acute pulmonary edema, LV systolic dysfunction	Nicardipine plus nitroglycerin[2] plus a loop diuretic Clevidipine plus nitroglycerin[2] plus a loop diuretic	Hydralazine, diazoxide, beta-blockers
Acute pulmonary edema, diastolic dysfunction	Esmolol plus low-dose nitroglycerin plus a loop diuretic Labetalol plus low-dose nitroglycerin plus a loop diuretic	
Ischemic stroke (systolic blood pressure > 180–200 mm Hg)	Nicardipine Clevidipine Labetalol	Nitroprusside, methyldopa, clonidine, nitroglycerin
Intracerebral hemorrhage (systolic blood pressure > 140–160 mm Hg)	Nicardipine Clevidipine Labetalol	Nitroprusside, methyldopa, clonidine, nitroglycerin
Hyperadrenergic states, including cocaine use	Nicardipine plus a benzodiazepine Clevidipine plus a benzodiazepine Phentolamine Labetalol	Beta-blockers
Preeclampsia, eclampsia	Labetalol Nicardipine	Diuretics, ACE inhibitors

[1]Avoid if LV systolic dysfunction.
[2]Drug of choice if LV systolic dysfunction is associated with ischemia.
ACE, angiotensin-converting enzyme; LV, left ventricular.

are good choices, since they are nonsedating and do not appear to cause significant increases in cerebral blood flow or intracranial pressure in this setting. In hypertensive emergencies arising from catecholaminergic mechanisms, such as pheochromocytoma or cocaine use, beta-blockers can worsen the hypertension because of unopposed peripheral vasoconstriction; nicardipine, clevidipine, or phentolamine are better choices. Labetalol is useful in these patients if the heart rate must be controlled. Table 11–12 summarizes treatment recommendations in hypertensive emergency.

Pharmacologic Management

A. Parenteral Agents

Sodium nitroprusside is no longer the treatment of choice for acute hypertensive problems; in most situations, appropriate control of blood pressure is best achieved using combinations of nicardipine or clevidipine plus labetalol or esmolol. (Table 11–13 lists drugs, dosages, and adverse effects.)

1. Nicardipine—Intravenous nicardipine is the most potent and the longest acting of the parenteral calcium

channel blockers. As a primarily arterial vasodilator, it has the potential to precipitate reflex tachycardia, and for that reason it should not be used without a beta-blocker in patients with coronary artery disease.

2. Clevidipine—Intravenous clevidipine is an L-type calcium channel blocker with a 1-minute half-life, which facilitates swift and tight control of severe hypertension. It acts on arterial resistance vessels and is devoid of venodilatory or cardiodepressant effects.

3. Labetalol—This combined beta- and alpha-blocking agent is the most potent adrenergic blocker for rapid blood pressure reduction. Other beta-blockers are far less potent. Excessive blood pressure drops are unusual. Experience with this agent in hypertensive syndromes associated with pregnancy has been favorable.

4. Esmolol—This rapidly acting beta-blocker is approved only for treatment of supraventricular tachycardia but is often used for lowering blood pressure. It is less potent than labetalol and should be reserved for patients in whom there is particular concern about serious adverse events related to beta-blockers.

Table 11–13. Drugs for hypertensive emergencies and urgencies in descending order of preference.

Agent	Action	Dosage	Onset	Duration	Adverse Effects	Comments
Hypertensive Emergencies						
Nicardipine (Cardene)	Calcium channel blocker	5 mg/h; may increase by 1–2.5 mg/h every 15 minutes to 15 mg/h	1–5 minutes	3–6 hours	Hypotension, tachycardia, headache.	May precipitate myocardial ischemia.
Clevidipine (Cleviprex)	Calcium channel blocker	1–2 mg/h initially; double rate every 90 seconds until near goal, then by smaller amounts every 5–10 minutes to a maximum of 32 mg/h	2–4 minutes	5–15 minutes	Headache, nausea, vomiting.	Lipid emulsion: contraindicated in patients with allergy to soy or egg.
Labetalol (Trandate)	Beta- and alpha-blocker	20–40 mg every 10 minutes to 300 mg; 2 mg/min infusion	5–10 minutes	3–6 hours	GI, hypotension, bronchospasm, bradycardia, heart block.	Avoid in acute LV systolic dysfunction, asthma. May be continued orally.
Esmolol (Brevibloc)	Beta-blocker	Loading dose 500 mcg/kg over 1 minute; maintenance, 25–200 mcg/kg/min	1–2 minutes	10–30 minutes	Bradycardia, nausea.	Avoid in acute LV systolic dysfunction, asthma. Weak antihypertensive.
Fenoldopam (Corlopam)	Dopamine receptor agonist	0.1–1.6 mcg/kg/min	4–5 minutes	< 10 minutes	Reflex tachycardia, hypotension, increased intraocular pressure.	May protect kidney function.
Enalaprilat (Vasotec)	ACE inhibitor	1.25 mg every 6 hours	15 minutes	6 hours or more	Excessive hypotension.	Additive with diuretics; may be continued orally.
Furosemide (Lasix)	Diuretic	10–80 mg	15 minutes	4 hours	Hypokalemia, hypotension.	Adjunct to vasodilator.
Hydralazine (Apresoline)	Vasodilator	5–20 mg intravenously or intramuscularly (less desirable); may repeat after 20 minutes	10–30 minutes	2–6 hours	Tachycardia, headache, GI.	Avoid in coronary artery disease, dissection. Rarely used except in pregnancy.
Nitroglycerin	Vasodilator	0.25–5 mcg/kg/min	2–5 minutes	3–5 minutes	Headache, nausea, hypotension, bradycardia.	Tolerance may develop. Useful primarily with myocardial ischemia.
Nitroprusside (Nitropress)	Vasodilator	0.25–10 mcg/kg/min	Seconds	3–5 minutes	GI, CNS; thiocyanate and cyanide toxicity, especially with renal and hepatic insufficiency; hypotension. Coronary steal, decreased cerebral blood flow, increased intracranial pressure.	No longer the first-line agent.
Hypertensive Urgencies						
Clonidine (Catapres)	Central sympatholytic	0.1–0.2 mg initially; then 0.1 mg every hour to 0.8 mg	30–60 minutes	6–8 hours	Sedation.	Rebound may occur.
Captopril (Capoten)	ACE inhibitor	12.5–25 mg	15–30 minutes	4–6 hours	Excessive hypotension.	
Nifedipine (Adalat, Procardia)	Calcium channel blocker	10 mg initially; may be repeated after 30 minutes	15 minutes	2–6 hours	Excessive hypotension, tachycardia, headache, angina, myocardial infarction, stroke.	Response unpredictable.

ACE, angiotensin-converting enzyme; CNS, central nervous system; GI, gastrointestinal; LV, left ventricular.

5. Fenoldopam—Fenoldopam is a peripheral dopamine-1 (DA$_1$) receptor agonist that causes a dose-dependent reduction in arterial pressure without evidence of tolerance, rebound, withdrawal, or deterioration of kidney function. In higher dosage ranges, tachycardia may occur. This drug is natriuretic, which may simplify volume management in acute kidney injury.

6. Enalaprilat—This is the active form of the oral ACE inhibitor enalapril. The onset of action is usually within 15 minutes, but the peak effect may be delayed for up to 6 hours. Thus, enalaprilat is used primarily as an adjunctive agent.

7. Diuretics—Intravenous loop diuretics can be very helpful when the patient has signs of heart failure or fluid retention, but the onset of their hypotensive response is slow, making them an adjunct rather than a primary agent for hypertensive emergencies. Low dosages should be used initially (furosemide, 20 mg, or bumetanide, 0.5 mg). They facilitate the response to vasodilators, which often stimulate fluid retention.

8. Hydralazine—Hydralazine can be given intravenously or intramuscularly, but its effect is less predictable than that of other drugs in this group. It produces reflex tachycardia and should not be given without beta-blockers in patients with possible coronary disease or aortic dissection. Hydralazine is used primarily in pregnancy and in children, but even in these situations, it is not a first-line drug.

9. Nitroglycerin, intravenous—This agent should be reserved for patients with accompanying acute coronary ischemic syndromes.

10. Nitroprusside sodium—This agent is given by controlled intravenous infusion gradually titrated to the desired effect. It lowers the blood pressure within seconds by direct arteriolar and venous dilation. Monitoring with an intra-arterial line avoids hypotension. Nitroprusside—in combination with a beta-blocker—is useful in patients with aortic dissection.

B. Oral Agents

Patients with less severe acute hypertensive syndromes can often be treated with oral therapy. Suitable drugs will reduce the blood pressure over a period of hours. In those presenting as a consequence of noncompliance, it is usually sufficient to restore the patient's previously established oral regimen.

1. Clonidine—Clonidine, 0.2 mg orally initially, followed by 0.1 mg every hour to a total of 0.8 mg, will usually lower blood pressure over a period of several hours. Sedation is frequent, and rebound hypertension may occur if the drug is stopped.

2. Captopril—Captopril, 12.5–25 mg orally, will also lower blood pressure in 15–30 minutes. The response is variable and may be excessive. Captopril is the drug of choice in the management of scleroderma hypertensive crisis.

3. Nifedipine—The effect of fast-acting nifedipine capsules is unpredictable and may be excessive, resulting in hypotension and reflex tachycardia. Because myocardial infarction and stroke have been reported in this setting, the use of sublingual nifedipine is not advised. Nifedipine retard, 20 mg orally, appears to be safe and effective.

C. Subsequent Therapy

When the blood pressure has been brought under control, combinations of oral antihypertensive agents can be added as parenteral drugs are tapered off over a period of 2–3 days.

Cremer A et al. From malignant hypertension to hypertension-MOD: a modern definition for an old but still dangerous emergency. J Hum Hypertens. 2015 Nov 19. [Epub ahead of print] [PMID: 26582411]

van den Born BJ et al. Dutch guideline for the management of hypertensive crisis—2010 revision. Neth J Med. 2011 May;69(5): 248–55. [PMID: 21646675]

12

Blood Vessel & Lymphatic Disorders

Christopher D. Owens, MD, MSc

Warren J. Gasper, MD

Meshell D. Johnson, MD

ATHEROSCLEROTIC PERIPHERAL VASCULAR DISEASE

OCCLUSIVE DISEASE: AORTA & ILIAC ARTERIES

ESSENTIALS OF DIAGNOSIS

▶ Claudication: cramping pain or tiredness in the calf, thigh, or hip while walking.

▶ Diminished femoral pulses.

▶ Tissue loss (ulceration, gangrene) or rest pain.

▶ General Considerations

Occlusive atherosclerotic lesions developing in the extremities, or peripheral arterial disease (PAD), is evidence of a systemic atherosclerotic process. The prevalence of PAD is 30% in patients who are 50 years old who have either diabetes mellitus or a history of tobacco use or in patients who are 70 years old without those risk factors. Pathologic changes of atherosclerosis may be diffuse, but flow-limiting stenoses occur segmentally. In the lower extremities, they classically occur in three anatomic segments: the aortoiliac segment, femoral-popliteal segment, and the infrapopliteal or tibial segment of the arterial tree. Each with its own population demographic, lesions in the distal aorta and proximal common iliac arteries classically occur in white male smokers aged 50–60 years. Disease progression may lead to complete occlusion of one or both common iliac arteries, which can precipitate occlusion of the entire abdominal aorta to the level of the renal arteries. Atherosclerosis of the femoral-popliteal segment usually occurs about a decade after the development of aortoiliac disease, has an even gender distribution, and commonly affects blacks and Hispanic patients. Disease in tibial arteries commonly occurs in patients with diabetes mellitus.

▶ Clinical Findings

A. Symptoms and Signs

Approximately two-thirds of patients with PAD are either asymptomatic or do not have classic symptoms. Pain occurs because blood flow cannot keep up with the increased demand of exercise. This pain, termed "claudication," is typically described as severe and cramping and primarily occurs in the calf muscles. The pain from aortoiliac lesions may extend into the thigh and buttocks with continued exercise and erectile dysfunction may occur from bilateral common iliac disease. Although generally reproducible, there is day-to-day variation in severity, thus the term, "intermittent claudication." Rarely, patients complain only of weakness in the legs when walking, or simply extreme limb fatigue. The symptoms are relieved with rest. Femoral pulses are absent or very weak as are the distal pulses. A bruit may be heard over the aorta, iliac, or femoral arteries or over all three arteries.

B. Doppler and Vascular Findings

The ratio of systolic blood pressure detected by Doppler examination at the ankle compared with the brachial artery (referred to as the ankle-brachial index [ABI]) is reduced to below 0.9 (normal ratio is 1.0–1.2); this difference is exaggerated by exercise. Both the dorsalis pedis and the posterior tibial arteries are measured and the higher of the two artery pressures is used for calculation. Segmental waveforms or pulse volume recordings obtained by strain gauge technology through blood pressure cuffs demonstrate blunting of the arterial inflow throughout the lower extremity.

C. Imaging

CT angiography (CTA) and magnetic resonance angiography (MRA) have largely replaced invasive angiography to determine the anatomic location of disease. Imaging is only required when symptoms require intervention, since a history and physical examination with vascular testing should appropriately identify the involved levels of the arterial tree.

▶ Treatment

A. Conservative Care

The cornerstones of PAD treatment are risk factor reduction, medical optimization, and exercise program. A program that includes smoking cessation, lipid and blood pressure management and weight loss is essential. Nicotine replacement therapy, bupropion, and varenicline have established benefits in smoking cessation. A strategy to motivate individuals to quit smoking uses "5Rs"; *Relevance* of smoking cessation to the patient, discussing the *Risk* of smoking, *Rewards* of quitting (eg, cost savings, health benefits, sense of well-being), identification of *Roadblocks*, and importance of *Repetition* of a motivational intervention at all subsequent visits. All patients with PAD should receive a statin to treat hypercholesterolemia and inflammation. A trial of phosphodiesterase inhibitors, such as cilostazol 100 mg orally twice a day, may be beneficial in approximately two-thirds of patients. Antiplatelet agents, such as aspirin, 81 mg daily, reduce overall cardiovascular morbidity but do not ameliorate symptoms.

B. Endovascular Techniques

When the atherosclerotic lesions are focal, they can be effectively treated with angioplasty and stenting. This approach matches the results of surgery for single stenoses but both effectiveness and durability decrease with longer or multiple stenoses.

C. Surgical Intervention

A prosthetic aorto-femoral bypass graft that bypasses the diseased segments of the aortoiliac system is a highly effective and durable treatment for this disease. Patients may be treated with a graft from the axillary artery to the femoral arteries (axillo-femoral bypass graft) or with a graft from the contralateral femoral artery (fem-fem bypass) when iliac disease is limited to one side. The axillo-femoral and femoral-to-femoral grafts are extra-anatomic bypasses because the abdominal cavity is not entered and the aorta is not cross-clamped; the operative risk is less than with aorto-bifemoral bypass, but the grafts are less durable.

▶ Complications

The complications of the aorto-femoral bypass are those of any major abdominal reconstruction in a patient population that has a high prevalence of cardiovascular disease. Mortality is low (2–3%), but morbidity is higher and includes a 5–10% rate of myocardial infarction. While endovascular approaches are safer and the complication rate is 1% to 3%, they are less durable with extensive disease.

▶ Prognosis

Patients with isolated aortoiliac disease may have a further reduction in walking distance without intervention, but symptoms rarely progress to rest pain or threatened limb loss. Life expectancy is limited by their attendant cardiac disease with a mortality rate of 25–40% at 5 years.

Symptomatic relief is generally excellent after intervention. After aorto-femoral bypass, a patency rate of 90% at 5 years is common. Endovascular patency rates and symptom relief for patients with short stenoses are also good with 20% symptom return at 3 years. Recurrence rates following endovascular treatment of extensive disease are 30–50%.

▶ When to Refer

Patients with progressive reduction in walking distance in spite of risk factor modification and consistent walking programs and those with limitations that interfere with their activities of daily living should be referred for consultation to a vascular surgeon.

ACCF/AHA focused update of the guideline for the management of patients with peripheral artery disease (updating the 2005 guideline): a report of the American College of Cardiology Foundation/American Heart Association Task Force on practice guidelines. Circulation. 2011 Nov 1;124(18):2020–45. [PMID: 21959305]

Alonso-Coello P et al. Antithrombotic therapy in peripheral artery disease: Antithrombotic Therapy and Prevention of Thrombosis, 9th ed: American College of Chest Physicians Evidence-Based Clinical Practice Guidelines. Chest. 2012 Feb;141(2 Suppl):e669S–90S. [PMID: 22315275]

Murphy TP et al; CLEVER Study Investigators. Supervised exercise versus primary stenting for claudication resulting from aortoiliac peripheral artery disease: six-month outcomes from the claudication: exercise versus endoluminal revascularization (CLEVER) study. Circulation. 2012 Jan 3;125(1): 130–9. [PMID: 22090168]

Stoekenbroek RM et al; Incremental Decrease in End Points Through Aggressive Lipid Lowering Study Group. High-dose atorvastatin is superior to moderate-dose simvastatin in preventing peripheral arterial disease. Heart. 2015 Mar;101(5): 356–62. [PMID: 25595417]

OCCLUSIVE DISEASE: FEMORAL & POPLITEAL ARTERIES

 ESSENTIALS OF DIAGNOSIS

▶ Cramping pain or tiredness in the calf with exercise.

▶ Reduced popliteal and pedal pulses.

▶ Foot pain at rest, relieved by dependency.

▶ Foot gangrene or ulceration.

▶ General Considerations

The superficial femoral artery is the peripheral artery most commonly occluded by atherosclerosis. The disease frequently occurs where the superficial femoral artery passes through the abductor magnus tendon in the distal thigh (Hunter canal). The common femoral artery and the popliteal artery are less commonly diseased but lesions in these vessels are debilitating, resulting in short-distance claudication.

▶ Clinical Findings

A. Symptoms and Signs

Symptoms of intermittent claudication caused by lesions of the common femoral artery, superficial femoral artery, and popliteal artery are confined to the calf. Occlusion or stenosis of the superficial femoral artery at the adductor canal when the patient has good collateral vessels from the profunda femoris will cause claudication at approximately 2–4 blocks. However, with concomitant disease of the profunda femoris or the popliteal artery, much shorter distances may trigger symptoms. With short-distance claudication, dependent rubor of the foot with blanching on elevation may be present. Chronic low blood flow states will also cause atrophic changes in the lower leg and foot with loss of hair, thinning of the skin and subcutaneous tissues, and disuse atrophy of the muscles. With segmental occlusive disease of the superficial femoral artery, the common femoral pulsation is normal, but the popliteal and pedal pulses are reduced.

B. Doppler and Vascular Findings

ABI values less than 0.9 are diagnostic of PAD and levels below 0.4 suggest critical limb ischemia. ABI readings depend on arterial compression. Since the vessels may be calcified in diabetes mellitus, chronic kidney disease, and the elderly, ABIs can be misleading. In such patients, the toe brachial index is usually reliable with a value less than 0.7 considered diagnostic of PAD. Pulse volume recordings with cuffs placed at the high thigh, mid-thigh, calf, and ankle will delineate the levels of obstruction with reduced pressures and blunted waveforms.

C. Imaging

Angiography, CTA, or MRA all adequately show the anatomic location of the obstructive lesions and are done only if revascularization is planned.

▶ Treatment

A. Conservative Care

As with aortoiliac disease, risk factor reduction, medical optimization, and exercise treatment are the cornerstone of therapy. Revascularization is reserved for patients who remain significantly disabled after failure of this conservative regimen.

B. Surgical Intervention

1. Bypass surgery—Intervention is indicated if claudication is progressive, incapacitating, or interferes significantly with essential daily activities or employment. Intervention is mandatory if there is rest pain or threatened tissue loss of the foot. The most effective and durable treatment for lesions of the superficial femoral artery is a femoral-popliteal bypass with autogenous saphenous vein. Synthetic material, usually polytetrafluoroethylene (PTFE), can be used, but these grafts do not have the durability of vein bypass.

2. Endovascular surgery—Endovascular techniques are often used for lesions of the superficial femoral artery. Angioplasty may be combined with stenting. These techniques have lower morbidity than bypass surgery but also have lower rates of durability.

Endovascular therapy is most effective when the lesions are less than 10 cm long and performed in patients who are undergoing aggressive risk factor modification. Paclitaxel-eluting stents or paclitaxel-coated balloons offer modest improvement over bare metal stents and noncoated balloons. However, the success of local drug delivery in peripheral arteries is not as robust as that in the coronary arteries. The 1-year patency rate is 50% for balloon angioplasty, 70% for drug-coated balloons, and 80% for stents. It is much harder, however, to treat restenosis in stents than vessels that have undergone angioplasty. Ongoing investigation will determine which therapy is best.

3. Thromboendarterectomy—Removal of the atherosclerotic plaque is limited to the lesions of the common femoral and the profunda femoris arteries where bypass grafts and endovascular techniques have a more limited role.

▶ Complications

Open surgical procedures of the lower extremities, particularly long bypasses with vein harvest, have a risk of wound infection that is higher than in other areas of the body. Wound infection or seroma can occur in as many as 10–15% of cases. Myocardial infarction rates after open surgery are 5–10%, with a 1–4% mortality rate. Complication rates of endovascular surgery are 1–5%, making these therapies attractive despite their lower durability.

▶ Prognosis

The prognosis for motivated patients with isolated superficial femoral artery disease is excellent, and surgery is not recommended for mild or moderate claudication in these patients. However, when claudication significantly limits daily activity and undermines quality of life as well as overall cardiovascular health, intervention may be warranted. All interventions require close postprocedure follow-up with repeated ultrasound surveillance so that any recurrent narrowing can be treated promptly to prevent complete occlusion. The reported patency rate of bypass grafts of the femoral artery, superficial femoral artery, and popliteal artery is 65–70% at 3 years, whereas the patency of angioplasty is less than 50% at 3 years.

Because of the extensive atherosclerotic disease, including associated coronary lesions, 5-year mortality among patients with lower extremity disease can be as high as 50%, particularly with involvement of the infrapopliteal vessels. However, with aggressive risk factor modification, substantial improvement in longevity has been reported.

▶ When to Refer

Patients with progressive symptoms, short-distance claudication, rest pain, or any ulceration should be referred to a peripheral vascular specialist.

Dake MD et al; Zilver PTX Investigators. Sustained safety and effectiveness of paclitaxel-eluting stents for femoropopliteal lesions: 2-year follow-up from the Zilver PTX randomized and single-arm clinical studies. J Am Coll Cardiol. 2013 Jun 18;61(24):2417–27. Erratum in: J Am Coll Cardiol. 2013 Aug 13;62(7):666. [PMID: 23583245]

Rosenfield K et al; LEVANT 2 Investigators. Trial of a paclitaxel-coated balloon for femoropopliteal artery disease. N Engl J Med. 2015 Jul 9;373(2):145–53. [PMID: 26106946]

Siracuse JJ et al. Results for primary bypass versus primary angioplasty/stent for intermittent claudication due to superficial femoral artery occlusive disease. J Vasc Surg. 2012 Apr;55(4):1001–7. [PMID: 22301210]

Tepe G et al. Drug-coated balloon versus standard percutaneous transluminal angioplasty for the treatment of superficial femoral and/or popliteal peripheral artery disease: 12-month results from the IN.PACT SFA randomized trial. Circulation. 2015 Feb 3;131(5):495–502. [PMID: 25472980]

OCCLUSIVE DISEASE: TIBIAL & PEDAL ARTERIES

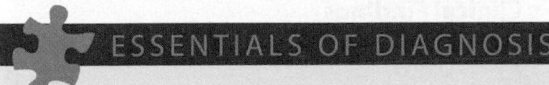
ESSENTIALS OF DIAGNOSIS

▸ Severe pain of the forefoot that is relieved by dependency.

▸ Pain or numbness of the foot with walking.

▸ Ulceration or gangrene of the foot or toes.

▸ Pallor when the foot is elevated.

▸ General Considerations

Occlusive processes of the tibial arteries of the lower leg and pedal arteries in the foot occur primarily in patients with diabetes. There often is extensive calcification of the artery wall. While claudication is a common initial symptom of ischemia, it may not be present. The first manifestation of ischemia is frequently an ulcer or gangrene rather than claudication.

▸ Clinical Findings

A. Symptoms and Signs

Unless there are associated lesions in the aortoiliac or femoral/superficial femoral artery segments, claudication may not occur. The gastrocnemius and soleus muscles may be supplied from collateral vessels from the popliteal artery; therefore, when disease is isolated to the tibial vessels, there may be foot ischemia without attendant claudication, and rest pain or ulceration may be the first sign of severe vascular insufficiency. The presence of rest pain or ulcerations is termed **critical limb ischemia** and is associated with the highest rate of amputation. Classically, ischemic rest pain is confined to the dorsum of the foot and is relieved with dependency; the pain does not occur with standing or sitting. It is severe and burning in character, and because it is only present when recumbent, it may awaken the patient from sleep. Because of the high incidence of neuropathy in these patients, it is important to differentiate rest pain from diabetic neuropathic dysesthesia. If the pain is relieved by simply dangling the foot over the edge of the bed, which increases blood flow to the foot, then the pain is due to vascular insufficiency. Leg night cramps (not related to ischemia) occur often in patients with PAD and should not be confused with rest pain.

On examination, depending on whether associated proximal disease is present, there may or may not be femoral and popliteal pulses, but the pedal pulses will be absent. Dependent rubor may be prominent with pallor on elevation. The skin of the foot is generally cool, atrophic, and hairless.

B. Doppler and Vascular Findings

The ABI may be quite low (in the range of 0.4 or lower). ABIs, however, may be falsely elevated when the medial layer of the arterial wall of the tibial vessels calcify (Mönckeberg medial calcific sclerosis) and are not compressible. Toe brachial indexes should be used if noncompressible vessels are encountered.

C. Imaging

Digital subtraction angiography is the gold standard method to delineate the anatomy of the tibial-popliteal segment. MRA or CTA is less helpful for detection of lesions in this location due to the small vasculature and other technical issues related to image resolution.

▸ Treatment

Good foot care may avoid ulceration, and most diabetic patients will do well with a conservative regimen. However, if ulcerations appear and there is no significant healing within 2–3 weeks and studies indicate poor blood flow, revascularization will be required. Poor blood flow or infrequent rest pain without ulceration is not an indication for revascularization. However, rest pain occurring nightly with monophasic waveforms requires revascularization to prevent threatened tissue loss.

A. Bypass and Endovascular Techniques

Bypass with vein to the distal tibial or pedal arteries has been shown to be an effective mechanism to treat rest pain and heal gangrene or ischemic ulcerations of the foot. Because the foot often has relative sparing of vascular disease, these bypasses have had adequate patency rates (70% at 3 years). Fortunately, in nearly all series, limb salvage rates are much higher than patency rates.

Bypass grafting remains the primary technique of revascularization. Drug-coated balloons have not been successful in the tibial vessels. Coronary drug-eluting stents are associated with the best success when used in short lesions.

B. Amputation

Patients with rest pain and tissue loss are at high risk for amputation, particularly if revascularization cannot be done. Patients with diabetes and PAD have a fourfold risk of critical limb ischemia compared with nondiabetic patients with PAD and have a risk of amputation up to 20-fold when compared to an age-matched population. Many patients who have below-the-knee or above-the-knee amputations due to vascular insufficiency never attain independent ambulatory status and often need assisted-living facilities. These factors combine to demand revascularization whenever possible to preserve the limb.

Complications

The complications of intervention are similar to those listed for superficial femoral artery disease with evidence that the overall cardiovascular risk of intervention increases with decreasing ABI. The patients with critical limb ischemia require aggressive risk factor modification. Wound infection rates after bypass are higher if there is an open wound in the foot.

Prognosis

Patients with tibial atherosclerosis have extensive atherosclerotic burden and a high prevalence of diabetes. Their prognosis without intervention is poor and complicated by the risk of amputation.

When to Refer

Patients with diabetes and foot ulcers should be referred for a formal vascular evaluation. Intervention may not be necessary but the severity of the disease will be quantified, which has implications for future symptom development. Any patient with a diabetic foot infection should be treated emergently with operative incision and drainage. Broad-spectrum antibiotics should be given to cover gram-positive, gram-negative, and anaerobic organisms. Centers that have a multidisciplinary limb preservation center staffed with vascular surgeons, podiatrists, plastic and orthopedic surgeons, prosthetics and orthotic specialists, and diabetes specialists should be sought.

Hinchliffe RJ et al. A systematic review of the effectiveness of revascularization of the ulcerated foot in patients with diabetes and peripheral arterial disease. Diabetes Metab Res Rev. 2012 Feb;28(Suppl 1):179–217. [PMID: 22271740]
Scheinert D. A prospective randomized multicenter comparison of balloon angioplasty and infrapopliteal stenting with the sirolimus-eluting stent in patients with ischemic peripheral artery disease: 1-year results from the ACHILLES trial. J Am Coll Cardiol. 2012 Dec 4;60(22):2290–5. [PMID: 23194941]
Torpy JM et al. JAMA patient page. Peripheral arterial disease. JAMA. 2009 Jan 14;301(2):236. [PMID: 19141772]

ACUTE ARTERIAL OCCLUSION OF A LIMB

ESSENTIALS OF DIAGNOSIS

► Sudden pain in an extremity.
► Usually some neurologic dysfunction with numbness, weakness, or complete paralysis.
► Absent extremity pulses.

General Considerations

Acute occlusion may be due to an embolus or to thrombosis of a diseased atherosclerotic segment. Emboli large enough to occlude proximal arteries in the lower extremities are almost always from the heart. Over 50% of the emboli from the heart go to the lower extremities, 20% to the cerebrovascular circulation, and the remainder to the upper extremities and mesenteric and renal circulation. Atrial fibrillation is the most common cause of cardiac thrombus formation; other causes are valvular disease or thrombus formation on the ventricular surface of a large anterior myocardial infarct.

Emboli from arterial sources such as arterial ulcerations or calcified excrescences are usually small and go to the distal arterial tree (toes).

The typical patient with primary thrombosis has had a history of claudication and now has an acute occlusion. If the stenosis has developed over time, collateral blood vessels will develop, and the resulting occlusion may only cause a minimal increase in symptoms.

Clinical Findings

A. Symptoms and Signs

The sudden onset of extremity pain, with loss or reduction in pulses, is diagnostic of acute arterial occlusion. This often will be accompanied by neurologic dysfunction, such as numbness or paralysis in extreme cases. With popliteal occlusion, symptoms may only affect the foot. With proximal occlusions, the whole leg may be affected. Signs of severe arterial ischemia include pallor, coolness of the extremity, and mottling. Impaired neurologic function progressing to anesthesia accompanied with paralysis suggests a poor prognosis.

B. Doppler and Laboratory Findings

There will be little or no flow found with Doppler examination of the distal vessels. Imaging, if done, may show an abrupt cutoff of contrast with embolic occlusion. Blood work may show myoglobin and metabolic acidosis.

C. Imaging

Whenever possible, imaging should be done in the operating room because obtaining angiography, MRA, or CTA may delay revascularization and jeopardize the viability of the extremity. However, in cases with only modest symptoms and where light touch of the extremity is maintained, imaging may be helpful in planning the revascularization procedure.

Treatment

Immediate revascularization is required in all cases of symptomatic acute arterial thrombosis. Evidence of neurologic injury, including loss of light touch sensation, indicates that collateral flow is inadequate to maintain limb viability and revascularization should be accomplished within 3 hours. Longer delays carry a significant risk of irreversible tissue damage. This risk approaches 100% at 6 hours.

A. Heparin

As soon as the diagnosis is made, unfractionated heparin should be administered (5000–10,000 units) intravenously, followed by a heparin infusion to maintain the activated partial thromboplastin time (aPTT) in the therapeutic range (60–85 seconds) (12–18 units/kg/h). This helps prevent clot propagation and may also help relieve associated vessel spasm. Anticoagulation may improve symptoms, but revascularization will still be required.

B. Endovascular Techniques

Catheter-directed chemical thrombolysis into the clot with tissue plasminogen activator (TPA) may be done but often requires 24 hours or longer to fully lyse the thrombus. This approach can be taken only in patients with an intact neurologic examination who do not have absolute contraindications such as bleeding diathesis, gastrointestinal bleeding, intracranial trauma, or neurosurgery within the past 3 months. A sheath is used to advance a TPA-infusing catheter through the clot. Heparin is administered systemically to prevent thrombus formation around the sheath. Frequent vascular and access site examinations are required during the thrombolytic procedure to assess for improved vascular perfusion and to guard against the development of a hematoma.

C. Surgical Intervention

General anesthesia is usually indicated; local anesthesia may be used in extremely high-risk patients if the exploration is to be limited to the common femoral artery. In extreme cases, it may be necessary to perform thromboembolectomy from the femoral, popliteal and even the pedal vessels to revascularize the limb. The combined use of devices that pulverize and aspirate clot and intraoperative thrombolysis with TPA improves outcomes.

► Complications

Complications of revascularization of an acutely ischemic limb can include severe metabolic acidosis, hyperkalemia, and cardiac arrest. In cases where several hours have elapsed but recovery of viable tissue may still be possible, significant levels of lactic acid, potassium, and other harmful agents may be released into the circulation during revascularization. Pretreatment of the patient with sodium bicarbonate prior to reestablishing arterial flow is required. Surgery in the presence of thrombolytic agents and heparin carries a high risk of postoperative wound hematoma.

► Prognosis

There is a 10–25% risk of amputation with an acute arterial embolic occlusion, and a 25% or higher in-hospital mortality rate. Prognosis for acute thrombotic occlusion of an atherosclerotic segment is generally better because the collateral flow can maintain extremity viability. The longer-term survival reflects the overall condition of the patient. In high-risk patients, an acute arterial occlusion is associated with a dismal prognosis.

OCCLUSIVE CEREBROVASCULAR DISEASE

ESSENTIALS OF DIAGNOSIS

- ► Sudden onset of weakness and numbness of an extremity, aphasia, dysarthria, or unilateral blindness (amaurosis fugax).
- ► Bruit heard loudest in the mid neck.

► General Considerations

Unlike the other vascular territories, symptoms of occlusive cerebrovascular disease are predominantly due to emboli. Transient ischemic attacks (TIAs) are the result of small emboli, and the risk of additional emboli causing permanent deficits is high. One-third of all ischemic strokes may be due to arterial emboli. In the absence of atrial fibrillation, approximately 90% of these emboli originate from the proximal internal carotid artery, an area uniquely prone to the development of atherosclerosis. Lesions in the proximal great vessels of the aortic arch and the common carotid are far less common. Intracranial atherosclerotic lesions are less uncommon in the West but are the most common location of cerebrovascular disease in China.

► Clinical Findings

A. Symptoms and Signs

Generally, the symptoms of a TIA last only a few seconds to minutes but may continue up to 24 hours. The most common lesions are in the cortex with both motor and sensory involvement. Emboli to the retinal artery cause unilateral blindness, which, when transient, is termed "amaurosis fugax." Posterior circulation symptoms referable to the brainstem, cerebellum, and visual regions of the brain are due to atherosclerosis of the vertebral basilar systems and are much less common.

Signs of cerebrovascular disease include carotid artery bruits. However, there is poor correlation between the degree of stenosis and the presence of the bruit. Furthermore, absence of a bruit does not exclude the possibility of carotid stenosis. Nonfocal symptoms, such as dizziness and unsteadiness, seldom are related to cerebrovascular atherosclerosis.

B. Imaging

Duplex ultrasonography is the imaging modality of choice with high specificity and sensitivity for detecting and grading the degree of stenosis at the carotid bifurcation: greater than 50% stenosis in a symptomatic patient and 80% in an asymptomatic patient require intervention. Mild to moderate disease (30–50% stenosis) indicates the need for ongoing surveillance and aggressive risk factor modification.

Excellent depiction of the full anatomy of the cerebrovascular circulation from arch to cranium can be obtained with either MRA or CTA. Each of these modalities may have false-positive or false-negative findings. Since the decision to intervene in cases of carotid stenosis depends on an accurate assessment of the degree of stenosis, it is recommended that at least two modalities be used to confirm the degree of stenosis. Diagnostic cerebral angiography is reserved for cases that cannot be resolved by MRA or CTA.

► Treatment

See Chapter 24 for a discussion of the medical management of occlusive cerebrovascular disease.

A. Asymptomatic Patients

Large studies have shown a 5-year reduction in stroke rate from 11.5% to 5.0% with surgical treatment of greater than

60% asymptomatic carotid stenosis. Patients, therefore, with no neurologic symptoms but with carotid stenosis on imaging will benefit from carotid intervention if they are considered to be at low risk for intervention and their expected survival is longer than 5 years. The usual practice, however, is to treat only patients who have greater than 80% stenosis. Recommendation for intervention also presumes that the treating institution has a stroke rate in asymptomatic patients that is acceptable (less than 3%). Patients with carotid stenosis that suddenly worsens are thought to have an unstable plaque and are at particularly high risk for embolic stroke.

B. Symptomatic Patients

Large randomized trials have shown that patients with TIAs or strokes from which they have completely or nearly completely recovered will benefit from carotid intervention if the ipsilateral carotid artery has a stenosis of more than 70% (Figure 12–1), and they are likely to derive benefit if the artery has a stenosis of 50–69%. In these situations, carotid endarterectomy (CEA) has been shown to have a durable effect in preventing further events.

▶ Complications

The most common complication from carotid intervention is cutaneous sensory or cranial nerve injury. However, the most dreaded complication is stroke due to embolization of plaque material during the procedure. The American Heart Association has recommended upper limits of acceptable combined morbidity and mortality for these interventions: 3% for asymptomatic, 5% for those with

▲ **Figure 12–1.** High-grade (90%) stenosis of internal carotid artery, with ulceration (arrow). (Used, with permission, from Dean SM, Satiani B, Abraham WT. *Color Atlas and Synopsis of Vascular Diseases.* McGraw-Hill, 2014.)

TIAs, and 7% for patients with previous stroke. Results that do not match these guidelines will jeopardize the therapeutic benefit of carotid intervention. In symptomatic patients, intervention should be planned as soon as possible. Delays increase the risk of a second event.

A. Carotid Endarterectomy

In addition to stroke risk, CEA carries an 8% risk of transient cranial nerve injury (usually the vagus or hypoglossal nerve) and a 1–2% risk of permanent deficits. There is also the risk of postoperative neck hematoma, which can cause acute compromise of the airway. Coronary artery disease exists as a comorbidity in most of these patients. Myocardial infarction rates after CEA are approximately 5%.

B. Angioplasty and Stenting

Compared with CEA, the advantage of carotid angioplasty and stenting is the avoidance of both cranial nerve injury and neck hematoma. However, emboli are more common during carotid angioplasty and stenting in spite of the use of embolic protection devices during the procedure. The International Carotid Stenting Study showed increased stroke rates with carotid angioplasty and stenting in symptomatic patients while the Carotid Revascularization Endarterectomy versus Stent Trial (CREST) showed similar overall morbidity with higher myocardial infarction rates with CEA and higher stroke rates with carotid angioplasty and stenting. In cases of restenosis after previous carotid intervention, carotid angioplasty and stenting is an excellent choice since the risk of embolization is low and the risk of cranial nerve injury with surgery is high.

▶ Prognosis

Prognosis for patients with carotid stenosis who have had a TIA or small stroke is poor without treatment; 25% of these patients will have a stroke with most of the events occurring within the first 6 months. Patients with carotid stenosis without symptoms have an annual stroke rate of just over 2% even with risk factor modification and antiplatelet agents. Prospective ultrasound screening is recommended in asymptomatic patients with known carotid stenosis because approximately 10% of asymptomatic patients have evidence of plaque progression in a given year. Concomitant coronary artery disease is common and is an important factor in these patients both for perioperative risk and long-term prognosis. Aggressive risk factor modification should be prescribed for patients with cerebrovascular disease regardless of planned intervention.

▶ When to Refer

Asymptomatic patients with a carotid stenosis of more than 80% and patients with carotid stenosis of more than 50% stenosis with symptoms of a TIA or stroke should be referred to a vascular specialist.

Brott TG et al; CREST Investigators. Stenting versus endarterectomy for treatment of carotid-artery stenosis. N Engl J Med. 2010 Jul 1;363(1):11–23. [PMID: 20505173]

Jalbert JJ et al. Outcomes after carotid artery stenting in medicare beneficiaries, 2005 to 2009. JAMA Neurol. 2015 Mar;72(3): 276–86. [PMID: 25580726]

Zaidat OO et al; VISSIT Trial Investigators. Effect of a balloon-expandable intracranial stent vs medical therapy on risk of stroke in patients with symptomatic intracranial stenosis: the VISSIT randomized clinical trial. JAMA. 2015 Mar 24–31; 313(12):1240–8. [PMID: 25803346]

VISCERAL ARTERY INSUFFICIENCY (Intestinal Angina)

 ESSENTIALS OF DIAGNOSIS

▶ Severe postprandial abdominal pain.

▶ Weight loss with a "fear of eating."

▶ Acute mesenteric ischemia: severe abdominal pain yet minimal findings on physical examination.

▶ General Considerations

Acute visceral artery insufficiency results from either embolic occlusion or primary thrombosis of at least one major mesenteric vessel. Ischemia can also result from **nonocclusive mesenteric vascular insufficiency,** which is generally seen in patients with low flow states, such as heart failure, or hypotension. A **chronic syndrome** occurs when there is adequate perfusion for the viscera at rest but ischemia occurs with severe abdominal pain when flow demands increase with feeding. Because of the rich collateral network in the mesentery, generally at least two of the three major visceral vessels (celiac, superior mesenteric, inferior mesenteric arteries) are affected before symptoms develop. **Ischemic colitis,** a variant of mesenteric ischemia, usually occurs in the distribution of the inferior mesenteric artery. The intestinal mucosa is the most sensitive to ischemia and will slough if underperfused. The clinical presentation is similar to inflammatory bowel disease. Ischemic colitis can occur after aortic surgery, particularly aortic aneurysm resection or aortofemoral bypass for occlusive disease, when there is a sudden reduction in blood flow to the inferior mesenteric artery.

▶ Clinical Findings

A. Symptoms and Signs

1. Acute intestinal ischemia—Patients with primary visceral arterial thrombosis often give an antecedent history consistent with chronic intestinal ischemia. The key finding with acute intestinal ischemia is severe, steady epigastric and periumbilical pain with minimal or no findings on physical examination of the abdomen because the visceral peritoneum is severely ischemic or infarcted and the parietal peritoneum is not involved. A high white cell count, lactic acidosis, hypotension, and abdominal distention may aid in the diagnosis.

2. Chronic intestinal ischemia—Patients are generally over 45 years of age and may have evidence of atherosclerosis in other vascular beds. Symptoms consist of epigastric or periumbilical postprandial pain lasting 1–3 hours. To avoid the pain, patients limit food intake and may develop a fear of eating. Weight loss is universal.

3. Ischemic colitis—Characteristic symptoms are left lower quadrant pain and tenderness, abdominal cramping, and mild diarrhea, which is often bloody.

B. Imaging and Colonoscopy

Contrast-enhanced CT is highly accurate at determining the presence of ischemic intestine. In patients with **acute** or **chronic intestinal ischemia,** a CTA or MRA can demonstrate narrowing of the proximal visceral vessels. In acute intestinal ischemia from a nonocclusive low flow state, angiography is needed to display the typical "pruned tree" appearance of the distal visceral vascular bed. Ultrasound scanning of the mesenteric vessels may show proximal obstructing lesions in laboratories that have experience with this technique.

In patients with **ischemic colitis,** colonoscopy may reveal segmental ischemic changes, most often in the rectal sigmoid and splenic flexure where collateral circulation may be poor.

▶ Treatment

A high suspicion of **acute intestinal ischemia** dictates immediate exploration to determine bowel viability. If the bowel remains viable, bypass can be done either from the supra-celiac aorta or common iliac artery to the celiac and the superior mesentery artery. In cases where bowel viability is questionable or bowel resection will be required, the bypass can be done with autologous vein, or with cryopreserved allografts in order to avoid the use of prosthetic conduits in a potentially contaminated field.

In **chronic intestinal ischemia,** angioplasty and stenting of the proximal vessel may be beneficial depending on the anatomy of the stenosis. Should an endovascular solution not be available, an aorto-visceral artery bypass is the preferred management. The long-term results are highly durable. Visceral artery endarterectomy is reserved for cases with multiple lesions where bypass would be difficult.

The mainstay of treatment of **ischemic colitis** is maintenance of blood pressure and perfusion until collateral circulation becomes well established. The patient must be monitored closely for evidence of perforation, which will require resection.

▶ Prognosis

The combined morbidity and mortality rates are 10–15% from surgical intervention in these debilitated patients. However, without intervention both acute and chronic intestinal ischemia are uniformly fatal. Adequate collateral circulation usually develops in those who have ischemic colitis, and the prognosis for this entity is better than chronic intestinal ischemia.

When to Refer

Any patient in whom there is a suspicion of intestinal ischemia should be urgently referred for imaging and possible intervention.

Acosta S. Epidemiology of mesenteric vascular disease: clinical implications. Semin Vasc Surg. 2010 Mar;23(1):4–8. [PMID: 20298944]
Cangemi JR et al. Intestinal ischemia in the elderly. Gastroenterol Clin North Am. 2009 Sep;38(3):527–40. [PMID: 19699412]
Gupta PK et al. Morbidity and mortality after bowel resection for acute mesenteric ischemia. Surgery. 2011 Oct;150(4):779–87. [PMID: 22000191]

ACUTE MESENTERIC VEIN OCCLUSION

The hallmarks of acute mesenteric vein occlusion are postprandial pain and evidence of a hypercoagulable state. Acute mesenteric vein occlusion presents similarly to the arterial occlusive syndromes but is much less common. Patients at risk include those with paroxysmal nocturnal hemoglobinuria; protein C, protein S, or antithrombin deficiencies; or the *JAK2* mutation. These lesions are difficult to treat surgically, and thrombolysis is the mainstay of therapy. Aggressive long-term anticoagulation is required for these patients.

NONATHEROSCLEROTIC VASCULAR DISEASE

THROMBOANGIITIS OBLITERANS (Buerger Disease)

ESSENTIALS OF DIAGNOSIS

▶ Typically occurs in male cigarette smokers.
▶ Distal extremities involved with severe ischemia, progressing to tissue loss.
▶ Thrombosis of the superficial veins may occur.
▶ Amputation will be necessary unless the patient stops smoking.

General Considerations

Buerger disease is a segmental, inflammatory, and thrombotic process of the distal-most arteries and occasionally veins of the extremities. Pathologic examination reveals arteritis in the affected vessels. The cause is not known but it is rarely seen in nonsmokers. Arteries most commonly affected are the plantar and digital vessels of the foot and lower leg. In advanced stages, the fingers and hands may become involved. While Buerger disease was once common, its incidence has decreased dramatically.

Clinical Findings

A. Symptoms and Signs

Buerger disease may be initially difficult to differentiate from routine peripheral vascular disease, but in most cases,

the lesions are on the toes and the patient is younger than 40 years of age. The observation of superficial thrombophlebitis may aid the diagnosis. Because the distal vessels are usually affected, intermittent claudication is not common with Buerger disease, but rest pain, particularly pain in the distal most extremity (ie, toes), is frequent. This pain often progresses to tissue loss and amputation, unless the patient stops smoking. The progression of the disease seems to be intermittent with acute and dramatic episodes followed by some periods of remission.

B. Imaging

MRA or invasive angiography can demonstrate the obliteration of the distal arterial tree typical of Buerger disease.

Differential Diagnosis

In atherosclerotic peripheral vascular disease, the onset of tissue ischemia tends to be less dramatic than in Buerger disease, and symptoms of proximal arterial involvement, such as claudication, predominate.

Symptoms of Raynaud disease may be difficult to differentiate from Buerger disease. Repetitive atheroemboli may also mimic Buerger disease and may be difficult to differentiate. It may be necessary to image the proximal arterial tree to rule out sources of arterial microemboli.

Treatment

Smoking cessation is the mainstay of therapy and will halt the disease in most cases. As the distal arterial tree is occluded, revascularization is not possible. Sympathectomy is rarely effective.

Prognosis

If smoking cessation can be achieved, the outlook for Buerger disease may be better than in patients with premature peripheral vascular disease. If smoking cessation is not achieved, then the prognosis is generally poor, with amputation of both lower and upper extremities the eventual outcome.

Dargon PT et al. Buerger's disease. Ann Vasc Surg. 2012 Aug;26 (6):871–80. [PMID: 22284771]

ARTERIAL ANEURYSMS

ABDOMINAL AORTIC ANEURYSMS

ESSENTIALS OF DIAGNOSIS

▶ Most aortic aneurysms are asymptomatic until rupture.
▶ Abdominal aortic aneurysms measuring 5 cm are palpable in 80% of patients.
▶ Back or abdominal pain with aneurysmal tenderness may precede rupture.
▶ Rupture is catastrophic; hypotension; excruciating abdominal pain that radiates to the back.

General Considerations

Dilatation of the infrarenal aorta is a normal part of aging. The aorta of a healthy young man measures approximately 2 cm. An aneurysm is considered present when the aortic diameter exceeds 3 cm, but aneurysms rarely rupture until their diameter exceeds 5 cm. Abdominal aortic aneurysms are found in 2% of men over 55 years of age; the male to female ratio is 4:1. Ninety percent of abdominal atherosclerotic aneurysms originate below the renal arteries. The aneurysms usually involve the aortic bifurcation and often involve the common iliac arteries.

Inflammatory aneurysms are an unusual variant. These have an inflammatory peel (similar to the inflammation seen with retroperitoneal fibrosis) that surrounds the aneurysm and encases adjacent retroperitoneal structures, such as the duodenum and, occasionally, the ureters.

Clinical Findings

A. Symptoms and Signs

1. Asymptomatic—Although 80% of 5-cm infrarenal aneurysms are palpable on routine physical examination, most aneurysms are discovered as incidental findings on ultrasound or CT imaging during the evaluation of unrelated abdominal symptoms.

2. Symptomatic—

A. Pain—Aneurysmal expansion may be accompanied by pain that is mild to severe midabdominal discomfort often radiating to the lower back. The pain may be constant or intermittent and is exacerbated by even gentle pressure on the aneurysm sack. Pain may also accompany inflammatory aneurysms. Most aneurysms have a thick layer of thrombus lining the aneurysmal sac, but embolization to the lower extremities is rarely seen.

B. Rupture—The sudden escape of blood into the retroperitoneal space causes severe pain, a palpable abdominal mass, and hypotension. Free rupture into the peritoneal cavity is a lethal event.

B. Laboratory Findings

In acute cases of a contained rupture, the hematocrit may be normal, since there has been no opportunity for hemodilution.

Patients with aneurysms may also have such cardiopulmonary diseases as coronary artery disease, carotid disease, renal impairment, and emphysema, which are typically seen in elderly men who smoke. Preoperative testing may indicate the presence of these comorbid conditions, which increase the risk of intervention.

C. Imaging

Abdominal ultrasonography is the diagnostic study of choice for initial screening for the presence of an aneurysm. In approximately three-quarters of patients with aneurysms, curvilinear calcifications outlining portions of the aneurysm wall may be visible on plain films of the abdomen or back. CT scans provide a more reliable assessment of aneurysm diameter and should be done when the aneurysm nears the diameter threshold (5.5 cm) for treatment. Contrast-enhanced CT scans show the arteries above and below the aneurysm. The visualization of this vasculature is essential for planning repair.

Once an aneurysm is identified, routine follow-up with ultrasound will determine size and growth rate. The frequency of imaging depends on aneurysm size ranging from every 2 years for aneurysms smaller than 4 cm to every 6 months for aneurysms at or approaching 5 cm. When an aneurysm measures approximately 5 cm, a CTA with contrast should be done to more accurately assess the size of the aneurysm and define the anatomy.

Screening

Data support the use of abdominal ultrasound to screen 65- to 74-year-old men, but not women, who are current or past smokers. Guidelines do not recommend repeated screening if the aorta shows no enlargement.

Treatment

A. Elective Repair

In general, elective repair is indicated for aortic aneurysms larger than 5.5 cm in diameter or aneurysms that have undergone rapid expansion (more than 0.5 cm in 6 months). Symptoms such as pain or tenderness may indicate impending rupture and require urgent repair regardless of the aneurysm's diameter.

B. Aneurysmal Rupture

A ruptured aneurysm is a lethal event. Approximately half the patients exsanguinate prior to reaching a hospital. In the remainder, bleeding may be temporarily contained in the retroperitoneum (contained rupture), allowing the patient to undergo emergent surgery. However, only half of those patients will survive. Endovascular repair is available for ruptured aneurysm repair in most major vascular centers, with the results offering some improvement over open repair for these critically ill patients.

C. Inflammatory Aneurysm

The presence of periaortic inflammation (inflammatory aneurysm) is not an indication for surgical treatment, unless there is associated compression of retroperitoneal structures, such as the ureter or pain upon palpation of the aneurysm. Interestingly, the inflammation that encases an inflammatory aneurysm recedes after either endovascular or open surgical aneurysm repair.

D. Assessment of Operative Risk

Aneurysms appear to be a variant of systemic atherosclerosis. Patients with aneurysms have a high rate of coronary disease. A 2004 trial demonstrated minimal value in addressing stable coronary artery disease prior to aneurysm resection. However, in patients with significant symptoms of coronary disease, the coronary disease should be treated first. Aneurysm resection should follow shortly thereafter because there is a slightly increased risk of aneurysm rupture after the coronary procedures.

E. Open Surgical Resection versus Endovascular Repair

In open surgical aneurysm repair, a graft is sutured to the non-dilated vessels above and below the aneurysm. This involves an abdominal incision, extensive dissection, and interruption of aortic blood flow. The mortality rate is low (2–5%) in centers that have a high volume for this procedure and when it is performed in good-risk patients. Older, sicker patients may not tolerate the cardiopulmonary stresses of the operation. With endovascular repair, a stent-graft is used to line the aorta and exclude the aneurysm. The stent must be able to seal securely against the wall of the aorta above and below the aneurysm, thereby excluding blood from flowing into the aneurysm sac. The anatomic requirements to securely achieve aneurysm exclusion vary according to the performance characteristics of the specific stent-graft device. Most studies have found that endovascular aneurysm repair offers patients reduced operative morbidity and mortality as well as shorter recovery periods. Long-term survival is equivalent between the two techniques. Patients who undergo endovascular repair, however, require more repeat interventions and need to be monitored postoperatively, since there is a 10–15% incidence of continued aneurysm growth post–endovascular repair.

F. Thrombus in an Aneurysm

The presence of thrombus within the aneurysm is not an indication for anticoagulation.

► Complications

Myocardial infarction, the most common complication, occurs in up to 10% of patients who undergo open aneurysm repair. The incidence of myocardial infarction is substantially lower with endovascular repair. For routine infrarenal aneurysms, renal injury is unusual; however, when it does occur, or if the baseline creatinine is elevated, it is a significant complicating factor in the postoperative period. Respiratory complications are similar to those seen in most major abdominal surgery. Gastrointestinal hemorrhage, even years after aortic surgeries, suggests the possibility of **graft enteric fistula,** most commonly between the aorta and the distal duodenum; the incidence of this complication is higher when the initial surgery is performed on an emergency basis.

► Prognosis

The mortality rate for an open elective surgical resection is 1–5%, and the mortality rate for endovascular therapy is 0.5–2%. Of those who survive surgery, approximately 60% are alive at 5 years; myocardial infarction is the leading cause of death. The decision to repair aneurysms in high-risk patients is easier with the reduced perioperative morbidity and mortality of the endovascular approach.

Mortality rates of untreated aneurysms vary with aneurysm diameter. The mortality rate among patients with large aneurysms has been defined as follows: 12% annual risk of rupture with an aneurysm larger than 6 cm in diameter and a 25% annual risk of rupture in aneurysms of more than 7 cm diameter. In general, a patient with an aortic aneurysm larger than 5.5 cm has a threefold greater chance of dying of a consequence of rupture of the aneurysm than of dying of the surgical resection.

At present, endovascular aneurysm repair may be less definitive than open surgical repair and requires close follow up with an imaging procedure. Device migration, component separation, and graft limb thrombosis or kinking are common reasons for repeat intervention. With complete exclusion of blood from the aneurysm sac, the pressure is lowered, which causes the aneurysm to shrink. An "endoleak" from the top or bottom seal zones (type 1) or through a graft defect (type 3) is associated with a persistent risk of rupture. Indirect leakage of blood through lumbar and inferior mesenteric branches of the aneurysm (endoleak, type 2) produces an intermediate picture with somewhat reduced pressure in the sac, slow shrinkage, and low rupture risk. However, type 2 endoleak warrants close observation because aneurysm dilatation and rupture can occur.

► When to Refer

- Any patient with a 4-cm aortic aneurysm or larger should be referred for imaging and assessment by a vascular specialist.
- Urgent referrals should be made if the patient complains of pain and gentle palpation of the aneurysm confirms that it is the source, regardless of the aneurysmal size.

► When to Admit

Patients with a tender aneurysm to palpation or signs of aortic rupture require emergent hospital admission.

De Bruin JL et al. Long-term outcome of open or endovascular repair of abdominal aortic aneurysm. N Engl J Med. 2010 May 20;362(20):1881–9. [PMID: 20484396]

Jackson RS et al. Comparison of long-term survival after open vs endovascular repair of intact abdominal aortic aneurysm among Medicare beneficiaries. JAMA. 2012 Apr 18;307(15):1621–8. [PMID: 22511690]

Kent KC. Clinical practice. Abdominal aortic aneurysms. N Engl J Med. 2014 Nov 27;371(22):2101–8. [PMID: 25427112]

United Kingdom EVAR Trial Investigators; Greenhalgh RM et al. Endovascular versus open repair of abdominal aortic aneurysm. N Engl J Med. 2010 May 20;362(20):1863–71. [PMID: 20382983]

Wallace GA et al. Favorable discharge disposition and survival after successful endovascular repair of ruptured abdominal aortic aneurysm. J Vasc Surg. 2013 Jun;57(6):1495–502. [PMID: 23719035]

THORACIC AORTIC ANEURYSMS

ESSENTIALS OF DIAGNOSIS

► Widened mediastinum on chest radiograph.
► With rupture, sudden onset of chest pain radiating to the back.

General Considerations

Most thoracic aortic aneurysms are due to atherosclerosis; syphilis is a rare cause. Disorders of connective tissue and Ehlers-Danlos and Marfan syndromes also are rare causes but have important therapeutic implications. Traumatic, false aneurysms, caused by partial tearing of the aortic wall with deceleration injuries, may occur just beyond the origin of the left subclavian artery. Less than 10% of aortic aneurysms occur in the thoracic aorta.

Clinical Findings

A. Symptoms and Signs

Most thoracic aneurysms are asymptomatic. When symptoms occur, they depend largely on the size and the position of the aneurysm and its rate of growth. Substernal back or neck pain may occur. Pressure on the trachea, esophagus, or superior vena cava can result in the following symptoms and signs: dyspnea, stridor, or brassy cough; dysphagia; and edema in the neck and arms as well as distended neck veins. Stretching of the left recurrent laryngeal nerve causes hoarseness. With aneurysms of the ascending aorta, aortic regurgitation may be present due to dilation of the aortic valve annulus. Rupture of a thoracic aneurysm is catastrophic because bleeding is rarely contained, allowing no time for emergent repair.

B. Imaging

The aneurysm may be diagnosed on chest radiograph by the calcified outline of the dilated aorta. CT scanning is the modality of choice to demonstrate the anatomy and size of the aneurysm and to exclude lesions that can mimic aneurysms, such as neoplasms or substernal goiter. MRI can also be useful. Cardiac catheterization and echocardiography may be required to describe the relationship of the coronary vessels to an aneurysm of the ascending aorta.

Treatment

Indications for repair depend on the location of dilation, rate of growth, associated symptoms, and overall condition of the patient. Aneurysms measuring 6 cm or larger may be considered for repair. Aneurysms of the **descending thoracic aorta** are treated routinely by endovascular grafting. Repair of **arch aneurysms** should be undertaken only if there is a skilled surgical team with an acceptable record of outcomes for these complex procedures. The availability of thoracic aortic endograft technique for descending thoracic aneurysms or experimental branched endovascular reconstructions for aneurysms involving the arch or visceral aorta (custom-made grafts with branches to the vessels involved in the aneurysm) does not change the indications for aneurysm repair. Aneurysms that involve the proximal aortic arch or ascending aorta represent particularly challenging problems. Open surgery is usually required; however, it carries substantial risk of morbidity (including stroke, diffuse neurologic injury, and intellectual impairment) because interruption of arch blood flow is required.

Complications

With the exception of endovascular repair for discrete saccular aneurysms of the descending thoracic aorta, the morbidity and mortality of thoracic repair is considerably higher than that for infra-renal abdominal aortic aneurysm repair. Paraplegia remains a devastating complication. Most large series report approximately 4–10% rate of paraplegia following endovascular repair of thoracic aortic aneurysms. The spinal arterial supply is segmental through intercostal branches of the aorta with variable degrees of intersegmental connection. Therefore, the more extensive the aneurysm, the greater is the risk of paraplegia with resection. Prior infrarenal abdominal aortic surgery, subclavian or internal iliac artery stenosis, and hypotension all increase the paraplegia risk. Involvement of the aortic arch also increases the risk of stroke, even when the aneurysm does not directly affect the carotid artery.

Prognosis

Generally, degenerative aneurysms of the thoracic aorta will enlarge and require repair to prevent death from rupture. However, stable aneurysms can be followed with CT scanning. Saccular aneurysms, particularly those distal to the left subclavian artery and the descending thoracic aorta, have had good results with endovascular repair. Resection of large complex aneurysms of the aortic arch requires a skilled surgical team for the major technical issues and should be attempted only in low-risk patients. Branched or fenestrated technology for endovascular grafting holds promise for reduced morbidity and mortality.

When to Refer

Patients who are deemed to have a reasonable surgical risk with a 5–6 cm aneurysm should be considered for repair, particularly if the aneurysm involves the descending thoracic aorta.

When to Admit

Any patient with chest or back pain with a known or suspected thoracic aorta aneurysm must be admitted to the hospital and undergo imaging studies to rule out the aneurysm as a cause of the pain.

Booher AM et al. Diagnosis and management issues in thoracic aortic aneurysm. Am Heart J. 2011 Jul;162(1):38–46.e1. [PMID: 21742088]

Gasper WJ et al. Assessing the anatomic applicability of the multibranched endovascular repair of thoracoabdominal aortic aneurysm technique. J Vasc Surg. 2013 Jun;57(6):1553–8. [PMID: 23395201]

PERIPHERAL ARTERY ANEURSYMS

ESSENTIALS OF DIAGNOSIS

- ▶ Widened, prominent pulses.
- ▶ Acute leg or foot pain and paresthesias with loss of distal pulses.
- ▶ High association of popliteal aneurysms with abdominal aortic aneurysms.

General Considerations

Like aortic aneurysms, peripheral artery aneurysms are silent until critically symptomatic. However, unlike aortic aneurysms, the presenting manifestations are due to peripheral embolization and thrombosis. Popliteal artery aneurysms account for 70% of peripheral arterial aneurysms. Popliteal aneurysms may embolize repetitively over time and occlude distal arteries. Due to the redundant parallel arterial supply to the foot, ischemia does not occur until a final embolus occludes flow.

Primary femoral artery aneurysms are much less common. However, pseudoaneurysms of the femoral artery following arterial punctures for arteriography and cardiac catheterization occur with an incidence ranging from 0.05% to 6% of arterial punctures.

Clinical Findings

A. Symptoms and Signs

The patient may be aware of a pulsatile mass when the aneurysm is in the groin, but popliteal aneurysms are often undetected by the patient and clinician. Rarely, peripheral aneurysms may produce symptoms by compressing the local vein or nerve. The first symptom may be due to ischemia of acute arterial occlusion. The symptoms range from sudden onset pain and paralysis to short-distance claudication that slowly lessens as collateral circulation develops. Symptoms from recurrent embolization to the leg are often transient, if they occur at all. Sudden ischemia may appear in a toe or part of the foot, followed by slow resolution, and the true diagnosis may be elusive. The onset of recurrent episodes of pain in the foot, particularly if accompanied by cyanosis, suggests embolization and requires investigation of the heart and proximal arterial tree.

Because popliteal pulses are somewhat difficult to palpate even in normal individuals, a particularly prominent or easily felt pulse is suggestive of aneurysm and should be investigated by ultrasound. Since popliteal aneurysms are bilateral in 60% of cases, the diagnosis of thrombosis of a popliteal aneurysm is often aided by the palpation of a pulsatile aneurysm in the contralateral popliteal space. Approximately 50% of patients with popliteal aneurysms have an aneurysmal abdominal aorta.

B. Imaging Studies

Duplex color ultrasound is the most efficient investigation to confirm the diagnosis of peripheral aneurysm, measure its size and configuration, and demonstrate mural thrombus. MRA or CTA are required to define the aneurysm and local arterial anatomy for reconstruction. Arteriography is not recommended because mural thrombus reduces the apparent diameter of the lumen on angiography. Patients with popliteal aneurysms should undergo ultrasonography to determine whether an abdominal aortic aneurysm is also present.

Treatment

To prevent limb loss from thrombosis or embolization, surgery is indicated when an aneurysm is associated with

any peripheral embolization, is smaller than 2 cm, or a mural thrombus is present. Immediate or urgent surgery is indicated when acute embolization or thrombosis has caused acute ischemia. Intra-arterial thrombolysis may be done in the setting of acute ischemia, if examination (light touch) remains intact, suggesting that immediate surgery is not imperative. Bypass is generally performed. Endovascular exclusion of the aneurysm can be done but is reserved for high-risk patients. Acute pseudoaneurysms of the femoral artery due to arterial punctures can be successfully treated using ultrasound-guided compression. Open surgery with prosthetic interposition grafting is preferred for primary aneurysms of the femoral artery.

Prognosis

Approximately one-third of untreated patients will require an amputation. The long-term patency of bypass grafts for femoral and popliteal aneurysms is generally excellent but depends on the adequacy of the outflow tract. Late graft occlusion is less common than in similar surgeries for occlusive disease.

When to Refer

In addition to patients with symptoms of ischemia, any patient with a peripheral arterial aneurysm measuring 2 cm or with ultrasound evidence of thrombus within the aneurysm should be referred to prevent progression to limb-threatening ischemia.

Cross JE et al. Nonoperative versus surgical management of small (less than 3 cm), asymptomatic popliteal artery aneurysms. J Vasc Surg. 2011 Apr;53(4):1145–8. [PMID: 21439460]

AORTIC DISSECTION

ESSENTIALS OF DIAGNOSIS

- ► Sudden searing chest pain with radiation to the back, abdomen, or neck in a hypertensive patient.
- ► Widened mediastinum on chest radiograph.
- ► Pulse discrepancy in the extremities.
- ► Acute aortic regurgitation may develop.

General Considerations

Aortic dissection occurs when a spontaneous intimal tear develops and blood dissects into the media of the aorta. The tear probably results from the repetitive torque applied to the ascending and proximal descending aorta during the cardiac cycle; hypertension is an important component of this disease process. **Type A dissection** involves the arch proximal to the left subclavian artery, and **type B dissection** occurs in the proximal descending thoracic aorta typically just beyond the left subclavian artery. Dissections may occur in the absence of hypertension but abnormalities of smooth muscle, elastic tissue, or collagen are more common in these patients. Pregnancy, bicuspid aortic valve, and coarctation also are associated with increased risk of dissection.

Blood entering the intimal tear may extend the dissection into the abdominal aorta, the lower extremities, the carotid arteries or, less commonly, the subclavian arteries. Both absolute pressure levels and the pulse pressure are important in propagation of dissection. The aortic dissection is a true emergency and requires immediate control of blood pressure to limit the extent of the dissection. With type A dissection, which has the worse prognosis, death may occur within hours due to rupture of the dissection into the pericardial sac or dissection into the coronary arteries, resulting in myocardial infarction. Rupture into the pleural cavity is also possible. The intimal/medial flap of the aortic wall created by the dissection may occlude major aortic branches, resulting in ischemia of the brain, intestines, kidney, or extremities. Patients whose blood pressure is controlled and who survive the acute episode without complications may have long-term survival without surgical treatment.

▶ Clinical Findings

A. Symptoms and Signs

Severe persistent chest pain of sudden onset radiating down the back or possibly into the anterior chest is characteristic. Radiation of the pain into the neck may also occur. The patient is usually hypertensive. Syncope, hemiplegia, or paralysis of the lower extremities may occur. Intestinal ischemia or renal insufficiency may develop. Peripheral pulses may be diminished or unequal. A diastolic murmur may develop as a result of a dissection in the ascending aorta close to the aortic valve, causing valvular regurgitation, heart failure, and cardiac tamponade.

B. Electrocardiographic Findings

Left ventricular hypertrophy from long-standing hypertension is often present. Acute changes suggesting myocardial ischemia do not develop unless dissection involves the coronary artery ostium. Classically, inferior wall abnormalities predominate since dissection leads to compromise of the right rather than the left coronary artery. In some patients, the ECG may be completely normal.

C. Imaging

A multiplanar CT scan is the immediate diagnostic imaging modality of choice; clinicians should have a low threshold for obtaining a CT scan in any hypertensive patient with chest pain and equivocal findings on ECG.

The CT scan should include both the chest and abdomen to fully delineate the extent of the dissected aorta. MRI is an excellent imaging modality for chronic dissections, but in the acute situation, the longer imaging time and the difficulty of monitoring patients in the MRI scanner make the CT scan preferable. Chest radiographs may reveal an abnormal aortic contour or widened superior mediastinum. Although transesophageal echocardiography (TEE) is an excellent diagnostic imaging method, it is generally not readily available in the acute setting.

▶ Differential Diagnosis

Aortic dissection is most commonly misdiagnosed as myocardial infarction or other causes of chest pain such as pulmonary embolization. Dissections may occur with minimal pain; branch vessel occlusion of the lower extremity can mimic arterial embolus.

▶ Treatment

A. Medical

Aggressive measures to lower blood pressure should occur when an aortic dissection is suspected, even before the diagnostic studies have been completed. Treatment requires a simultaneous reduction of the systolic blood pressure to 100–120 mm Hg and pulse pressure. Beta-blockers have the most desirable effect of reducing the left ventricular ejection force that continues to weaken the arterial wall and should be first-line therapy. Labetalol, both an alpha- and beta-blocker, lowers pulse pressure and achieves rapid blood pressure control. Give 20 mg over 2 minutes by intravenous injection. Additional doses of 40–80 mg intravenously can be given every 10 minutes (maximum dose 300 mg) until the desired blood pressure has been reached. Alternatively, 2 mg/min may be given by intravenous infusion, titrated to desired effect. In patients who have asthma, bradycardia, or other conditions that necessitate the patient's reaction to beta-blockers be tested, esmolol is a reasonable choice because of its short half-life. Give a loading dose of esmolol, 0.5 mg/kg intravenously over 1 minute, followed by an infusion of 0.0025–0.02 mg/kg/min. Titrate the infusion to a goal heart rate of 60–70 beats/min. If beta-blockade alone does not control the hypertension, nitroprusside may be added as follows: 50 mg of nitroprusside in 1000 mL of 5% dextrose and water, infused at a rate of 0.5 mL/min for a 70-kg person (0.3 mcg/kg/min); the infusion rate is increased by 0.5 mL every 5 minutes until adequate control of the pressure has been achieved. In patients with bronchial asthma, while there are no data supporting the use of the calcium-channel antagonists, diltiazem and verapamil are potential alternatives to treatment with beta-blocking drugs. Morphine sulfate is the appropriate drug to use for pain relief. Long-term medical care of patients should include beta-blockers in their antihypertensive regimen.

B. Surgical Intervention

Urgent surgical intervention is required for all type A dissections. If a skilled cardiovascular team is not available, the patient should be transferred to an appropriate facility. The procedure involves grafting and replacing the diseased portion of the arch and brachiocephalic vessels as necessary. Replacement of the aortic valve may be required with reattachment of the coronary arteries.

Urgent surgery is required for **type B dissections** if there is aortic branch compromise resulting in malperfusion of the renal, visceral, or extremity vessels. The immediate goal of surgical therapy is to restore flow to the ischemic tissue, which is most commonly accomplished via a bypass. Endovascular stenting of the entry tear at the level of the subclavian artery may result in obliteration of the false lumen and restore flow into the branch vessel from the true lumen. The results, however, are unpredictable and should only be attempted by an experienced team. For acute type B dissections without malperfusion, evidence is emerging that long-term aortic-specific survival and delayed disease progression are improved with early thoracic stent graft repair.

Prognosis & Follow-up

The mortality rate for untreated type A dissections is approximately 1% per hour for 72 hours and over 90% at 3 months. Mortality is also extremely high for untreated complicated type B dissections. The surgical and endovascular options for these patients also have significant morbidity and mortality. They are technically demanding and require an experienced team to achieve perioperative mortalities of less than 10%. Patients with uncomplicated type B dissections whose blood pressure is controlled and who survive the acute episode without complications may have long-term survival without surgical treatment. Aneurysmal enlargement of the false lumen may develop in these patients despite adequate antihypertensive therapy. Yearly CT scans are required to monitor the size of the aneurysm. Indications for repair are determined by size (≥ 6 cm), similar to undissected thoracic aneurysms. Endovascular covering of the intimal tear in the acute setting may prevent this complication, but initial trials on the routine endovascular treatment of type B dissections have not shown an advantage for early intervention and therefore cannot be widely endorsed at this time.

When to Admit

All patients with an acute dissection should be hospitalized. Any dissection involving the aortic arch (type A) should be immediately repaired. Acute type B dissections require repair only when there is evidence of rupture or major branch occlusion.

Nienaber CA et al. Endovascular repair of type B aortic dissection: long-term results of the randomized investigation of stent grafts in aortic dissection trial. Circ Cardiovasc Interv. 2013 Aug;6(4):407–16. [PMID: 23922146]

Suzuki T et al; IRAD Investigators. Type-selective benefits of medications in treatment of acute aortic dissection (from the International Registry of Acute Aortic Dissection [IRAD]). Am J Cardiol. 2012 Jan 1;109(1):122–7. [PMID: 21944678]

VENOUS DISEASES

VARICOSE VEINS

ESSENTIALS OF DIAGNOSIS

▶ Dilated, tortuous superficial veins in the lower extremities.

▶ May be asymptomatic or associated with aching discomfort or pain.

▶ Often hereditary.

▶ Increased frequency after pregnancy.

General Considerations

Varicose veins develop in the lower extremities. Periods of high venous pressure related to prolonged standing or heavy lifting are contributing factors, but the highest incidence occurs in women after pregnancy. Varicosities develop in over 20% of all adults.

This combination of progressive venous reflux and venous hypertension is the hallmark of chronic venous disease. The superficial veins are involved, typically the great saphenous vein and its tributaries, but the short saphenous vein (posterior lower leg) may also be affected. Distention of the vein prevents the valve leaflets from coapting, creating incompetence and reflux of blood toward the foot. Focal venous dilation and reflux leads to increased pressure and distention of the vein segment below that valve, which in turn causes progressive failure of the next lower valve. Perforating veins that connect the deep and superficial systems may become incompetent, allowing blood to reflux into the superficial veins from the deep system, increasing venous pressure and distention.

Secondary varicosities can develop as a result of obstructive changes and valve damage in the deep venous system following thrombophlebitis, or rarely as a result of proximal venous occlusion due to neoplasm or fibrosis. Congenital or acquired arteriovenous fistulas or venous malformations are also associated with varicosities and should be considered in young patients with varicosities.

Clinical Findings

A. Symptoms and Signs

Symptom severity is not correlated with the number and size of the varicosities; extensive varicose veins may produce no subjective symptoms, whereas minimal varicosities may produce many symptoms. Dull, aching heaviness or a feeling of fatigue of the legs brought on by periods of standing is the most common complaint. Itching from venous eczema may occur either above the ankle or directly overlying large varicosities.

Dilated, tortuous veins of the thigh and calf are visible and palpable when the patient is standing. Longstanding varicose veins may progress to chronic venous insufficiency with associated ankle edema, brownish skin hyperpigmentation, and chronic skin induration or fibrosis. A bruit or thrill is never found with primary varicose veins and when found, alerts the clinician to the presence of an arteriovenous fistula or malformation.

B. Imaging

The identification of the source of venous reflux that feeds the symptomatic veins is necessary for effective surgical treatment. Duplex ultrasonography by a technician experienced in the diagnosis and localization of venous reflux is the test of choice for planning therapy. In most cases, reflux will arise from the greater saphenous vein.

Differential Diagnosis

Varicose veins due to primary superficial venous reflux should be differentiated from those secondary to previous or ongoing obstruction of the deep veins (post-thrombotic syndrome). Pain or discomfort secondary to neuropathy should be distinguished from symptoms associated with coexistent varicose veins. Similarly, vein symptoms should be distinguished from pain due to intermittent claudication, which occurs after a predictable amount of exercise and resolves with rest. In adolescent patients with varicose veins, imaging of the deep venous system is obligatory to exclude a congenital malformation or atresia of the deep veins. Surgical treatment of varicose veins in these patients is contraindicated because the varicosities may play a significant role in venous drainage of the limb.

► Complications

Superficial thrombophlebitis of varicose veins is uncommon. The typical presentation is acute localized pain with tender, firm veins. The process is usually self-limiting, resolving within several weeks. The risk of deep venous thrombosis (DVT) or embolization is very low unless the thrombophlebitis extends into the great saphenous vein in the upper medial thigh. Predisposing conditions include pregnancy, local trauma, or prolonged periods of sitting.

In older patients, superficial varicosities may bleed with even minor trauma. The amount of bleeding can be alarming as the pressure in the varicosity is high.

► Treatment

A. Nonsurgical Measures

Nonsurgical treatment is effective. Elastic graduated compression stockings (20–30 mm Hg pressure) reduce the venous pressure in the leg and may prevent the progression of disease. Good control of symptoms can be achieved when stockings are worn daily during waking hours and legs are elevated, especially at night. Compression stockings are well-suited for elderly patients or patients who do not want surgery.

B. Sclerotherapy

Direct injection of a sclerosing agent induces permanent fibrosis and obliteration of the target veins. Chemical irritants (eg, glycerin) or hypertonic saline are often used for small, less-than-4-mm reticular veins or telangiectasias. Foam sclerotherapy is used to treat the great saphenous vein, varicose veins larger than 4 mm, and perforating veins often with no more than local anesthesia. Foam sclerotherapy has similar clinical results as saphenous vein thermal ablation or stripping, although the long-term success rate may be lower and systemic embolization remains a concern. Complications such as phlebitis, tissue necrosis, or infection may occur with any sclerosing agent.

C. Surgical Measures

Treatment with endovenous thermal ablation (with either radiofrequency or laser) or, less commonly, with great saphenous vein stripping is effective for reflux arising from the great saphenous vein. Less common sources of reflux include the small saphenous vein (for varicosities in the posterior calf) and incompetent perforator veins arising

directly from the deep venous system. Correction of reflux is performed at the same time as excision of the symptomatic varicose veins. Phlebectomy without correction of reflux results in a high rate of recurrent varicosities, as the uncorrected reflux progressively dilates adjacent veins. Concurrent reflux detected by ultrasonography in the deep system is not a contraindication to treatment of superficial reflux because the majority of deep vein dilatation is secondary to volume overload in this setting, which will resolve with correction of the superficial reflux.

► Prognosis

Surgical treatment of superficial vein reflux and excision of varicose veins provide excellent results. The 5-year success rate (as defined as lack of pain and recurrent varicosities) is 85–90%. Simple excision (phlebectomy) or injection sclerotherapy without correction of reflux is associated with higher rates of recurrence. Even after adequate treatment, secondary tissue changes may persist.

► When to Refer

- Absolute indications for referral for saphenous ablation include thrombophlebitis and bleeding.
- Pain and cosmetic concerns are responsible for the majority of referrals for ablation.

Brittenden J et al. A randomized trial comparing treatments for varicose veins. N Engl J Med. 2014 Sep 25;371(13):1218–27. [PMID: 25251616]

Gloviczki P et al. The care of patients with varicose veins and associated chronic venous diseases: clinical practice guidelines of the Society for Vascular Surgery and the American Venous Forum. J Vasc Surg. 2011 May;53(5 Suppl):2S–48S. [PMID: 21536172]

Hamdan A et al. JAMA patient page. Treatment of varicose veins. JAMA. 2013 Mar 27;309(12):1306. [PMID: 23532249]

SUPERFICIAL VENOUS THROMBOPHLEBITIS

ESSENTIALS OF DIAGNOSIS

- ► Induration, redness, and tenderness along a superficial vein.
- ► Induration, redness, and tenderness at the site of a recent intravenous line.
- ► Significant swelling of the extremity may not be seen.

► General Considerations

Short-term venous catheterization of superficial arm veins as well as the use of longer-term peripherally inserted central catheter (PICC) lines are the most common cause of superficial thrombophlebitis. Intravenous catheter sites should be observed daily for signs of local inflammation and should be removed if a local reaction develops in the vein. Serious thrombotic or septic complications can occur if this policy is not followed.

Superficial thrombophlebitis may occur spontaneously, often in pregnant or postpartum women or in individuals with varicose veins, or it may be associated with trauma, as with a blow to the leg or following intravenous therapy with irritating solutions. It also may be a manifestation of systemic hypercoagulability secondary to abdominal cancer such as carcinoma of the pancreas and may be the earliest sign of these conditions. Superficial thrombophlebitis may be associated with occult DVT in about 20% of cases. Pulmonary emboli are exceedingly rare and occur from an associated DVT. (See Chapters 9 and 14 for discussion on deep venous thrombosis.)

Clinical Findings

In spontaneous superficial thrombophlebitis, the great saphenous vein is most often involved. The patient usually experiences a dull pain in the region of the involved vein. Local findings consist of induration, redness, and tenderness along the course of a vein. The process may be localized, or it may involve most of the great saphenous vein and its tributaries. The inflammatory reaction generally subsides in 1–2 weeks; a firm cord may remain for a much longer period. Edema of the extremity is uncommon.

Localized redness and induration at the site of a recent intravenous line requires urgent attention. Proximal extension of the induration and pain with chills and high fever suggest septic phlebitis and requires urgent treatment.

Differential Diagnosis

The linear rather than circular nature of the lesion and the distribution along the course of a superficial vein serve to differentiate superficial phlebitis from cellulitis, erythema nodosum, erythema induratum, panniculitis, and fibrositis. Lymphangitis and deep thrombophlebitis must also be considered.

Treatment

For spontaneous thrombophlebitis if the process is well localized and not near the saphenofemoral junction, local heat and nonsteroidal anti-inflammatory medications are usually effective in limiting the process. If the induration is extensive or is progressing toward the saphenofemoral junction (leg) or cephalo-axillary junction (arm), ligation and division of the vein at the junction of the deep and superficial veins is indicated.

Anticoagulation therapy is usually not required for focal processes. Prophylactic dose low-molecular-weight heparin or fondaparinux is recommended for 5 cm or longer superficial thrombophlebitis of the lower limb veins and full anticoagulation is reserved for disease that is rapidly progressing or if there is concern for extension into the deep system.

Septic superficial thrombophlebitis is an intravascular abscess and requires urgent treatment with heparin (see Table 14–16) to limit additional thrombus formation as well as removal of the offending catheter in catheter-related infections (see Chapter 30). *Staphylococcus aureus* is the most common pathogen. Treat with antibiotics (eg, vancomycin, 15 mg/kg intravenously every 12 hours plus ceftriaxone, 1 g intravenously every 24 hours). If cultures are positive, therapy should be continued for 7–10 days or for 4–6 weeks if complicating endocarditis cannot be excluded. Other organisms, including fungi, may also be responsible. Surgical excision of the involved vein may also be necessary to control the infection.

Prognosis

With spontaneous thrombophlebitis, the course is generally benign and brief. The prognosis depends on the underlying pathologic process. In patients with phlebitis secondary to varicose veins, recurrent episodes are likely unless correction of the underlying venous reflux and excision of varicosities is done. In contrast, the mortality from septic thrombophlebitis is 20% or higher and requires aggressive treatment. However, if the involvement is localized, the mortality is low and prognosis is excellent with early treatment.

Decousus H et al; CALISTO Study Group. Fondaparinux for the treatment of superficial-vein thrombosis in the legs. N Engl J Med. 2010 Sep 23;363(13):1222–32. [PMID: 20860504]

Decousus H et al; POST (Prospective Observational Superficial Thrombophlebitis) Study Group. Superficial venous thrombosis and venous thromboembolism: a large, prospective epidemiologic study. Ann Intern Med. 2010 Feb 16;152(4):218–24. [PMID: 20157136]

Di Nisio M et al. Treatment for superficial thrombophlebitis of the leg. Cochrane Database Syst Rev. 2012 Mar 14;3:CD004982. [PMID: 22419302]

Stevens SM. ACP Journal Club: review: fondaparinux reduces VTE and recurrence in superficial thrombophlebitis of the leg. Ann Intern Med. 2012 Aug 21;157(4):JC2–4. [PMID: 22910958]

CHRONIC VENOUS INSUFFICIENCY

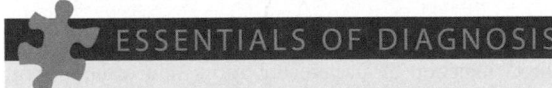

ESSENTIALS OF DIAGNOSIS

► History of prior DVT or leg injury.

► Edema, (brawny) skin hyperpigmentation, subcutaneous lipodermosclerosis in the lower leg.

► Large ulcerations at or above the ankle are common (venous ulcers).

General Considerations

Chronic venous insufficiency is a severe manifestation of venous hypertension. One of the most common etiologies is prior deep venous thrombophlebitis (see Chapter 14), although about 25% of patients do not have a known history of DVT. In these cases, there may be a history of leg trauma or surgery; obesity is often a complicating factor. Progressive superficial venous reflux is also a common cause. Other causes include congenital or neoplastic obstruction of the pelvic veins or a congenital or acquired arteriovenous fistula.

The basic pathology is caused by valve leaflets that do not coapt because they are either thickened and scarred (post-thrombotic syndrome) or in a dilated vein and are therefore functionally inadequate. Proximal venous obstruction due to chronic thrombus or scarring compounds the problem. With the valves unable to stop venous blood from returning to the foot (venous reflux), the leg develops venous hypertension and an abnormally high hydrostatic force is transmitted to the subcutaneous veins and tissues of the lower leg. The resulting edema results in dramatic and deleterious secondary changes. The stigmata of chronic venous insufficiency include fibrosis of the subcutaneous tissue and skin, pigmentation of skin (hemosiderin taken up by the dermal macrophages), and, later, ulceration, which is extremely slow to heal. Itching may precipitate the formation of ulceration or local wound cellulitis. Dilation of the superficial veins may occur, leading to varicosities. Although surgical treatment for venous reflux can improve symptoms, controlling edema and the secondary skin changes usually require life-long compression therapy.

Clinical Findings

A. Symptoms and Signs

Progressive pitting edema of the leg (particularly the lower leg) is the primary presenting symptom. Secondary changes in the skin and subcutaneous tissues develop over time (Figure 12–2). The usual symptoms are itching, a dull discomfort made worse by periods of standing, and pain if an ulceration is present. The skin at the ankle is usually taut from swelling, shiny, and a brownish pigmentation (hemosiderin) often develops. If the condition is long-standing,

▲ **Figure 12–3.** Varicose veins, manifested as blue, subcutaneous, tortuous veins more than 3 mm in diameter. (Used, with permission, from Dean SM, Satiani B, Abraham WT. *Color Atlas and Synopsis of Vascular Diseases.* McGraw-Hill, 2014.)

the subcutaneous tissues become thick and fibrous. Ulcerations may occur, usually just above the ankle, on the medial or anterior aspect of the leg. Healing results in a thin scar on a fibrotic base that often breaks down with minor trauma or further bouts of leg swelling. Varicosities may appear (Figure 12–3) that are associated with incompetent perforating veins. Cellulitis, which is often difficult to distinguish from the hemosiderin pigmentation, may be diagnosed by blanching erythema with pain.

B. Imaging

Patients with post-thrombotic syndrome or signs of chronic venous insufficiency should undergo duplex ultrasonography to determine whether superficial reflux is present and to evaluate the degree of deep reflux and obstruction.

Differential Diagnosis

Patients with heart failure, chronic kidney disease, or decompensated liver disease may have bilateral edema of the lower extremities. Many medications can cause edema (eg, calcium channel blockers, nonsteroidal anti-inflammatory agents, thiazolidinediones). Swelling from lymphedema involves the feet and may be unilateral, but varicosities are absent. Edema from these causes pits easily and brawny discoloration is rare. Lipedema is a disorder of

▲ **Figure 12–2.** Bilateral pretibial edema and erythema consistent with stasis dermatitis (sometimes mimicking cellulitis) in chronic venous insufficiency. (Used, with permission, from Dean SM, Satiani B, Abraham WT. *Color Atlas and Synopsis of Vascular Diseases.* McGraw-Hill, 2014.)

adipose tissue that occurs almost exclusively in women, is bilateral and symmetric, and is characterized by stopping at a distinct line just above the ankles.

Primary varicose veins may be difficult to differentiate from the secondary varicosities of post-thrombotic syndrome or venous obstruction.

Other conditions associated with chronic ulcers of the leg include neuropathic ulcers usually from diabetes mellitus, arterial insufficiency (often very painful with absent pulses), autoimmune diseases (eg, Felty syndrome), sickle cell anemia, erythema induratum (bilateral and usually on the posterior aspect of the lower part of the leg), and fungal infections.

▶ Prevention

Irreversible tissue changes and associated complications in the lower legs can be minimized through early and aggressive anticoagulation of acute DVT to minimize the valve damages and by prescribing compression stockings if chronic edema develops after the DVT has resolved. Catheter-directed thrombolysis or mechanical thrombectomy of acute iliofemoral DVT may be of greater value than simple anticoagulants in preventing post-thrombotic syndrome and chronic venous insufficiency.

▶ Treatment

A. General Measures

Fitted, graduated compression stockings (20–30 mm Hg pressure or higher) worn from the foot to just below the knee during the day and evening are the mainstays of treatment and are usually sufficient. When they are not, additional measures, such as avoidance of long periods of sitting or standing, intermittent elevations of the involved leg, and sleeping with the legs kept above the level of the heart, may be necessary to control the swelling. Pneumatic compression of the leg, which can pump the fluid out of the leg, is used in cases refractory to the above measures.

B. Ulceration

As the primary pathology is edema and venous hypertension, healing of the ulcer will not occur until the edema is controlled and compression is applied. Circumferential nonelastic bandages on the lower leg enhance the pumping action of the calf muscles on venous blood flow out of the calf. A lesion can often be treated on an ambulatory basis by means of a semi-rigid gauze boot made with Unna paste (Gelocast, Medicopaste) or a multi-layer compression dressing (eg, Profore). Initially, the ulcer needs to be debrided and the boot changed every 2–3 days to control ulcer drainage. As the edema and drainage subside, optimal healing is achieved when the boot is kept in place for 5–7 days. The ulcer, tendons, and bony prominences must be adequately padded. Alternatively, knee-high graduated compression stockings with an absorbent dressing may be used, although the wounds can leak large volumes of fluid. Home compression therapy with a pneumatic compression device is used in cases refractory to the above measures, but many patients have severe pain with the "milking"

action of the pump device. Some patients will require admission for complete bed rest and leg elevation to achieve ulcer healing. After the ulcer has healed, daily graduated compression stocking therapy is mandatory to prevent ulcer recurrence.

C. Correction of Superficial Reflux

Compression and treatment of superficial vein reflux has been shown to decrease the recurrence rate of venous ulcers. Incompetent (refluxing) perforator veins that feed the area of ulceration can be treated with percutaneous thermal ablation (radiofrequency or laser) to help decrease the venous pressure in the area of ulceration and promote healing. Where there is substantial obstruction of the deep venous system, superficial varicosities supply the venous return and they should not be removed.

▶ Prognosis

Individuals with chronic venous insufficiency often have recurrent problems, particularly if they do not consistently wear support stockings that have at least 20–30 mm Hg compression.

▶ When to Refer

- Patients with significant saphenous reflux should be evaluated for ablation.
- Patients with ulcers should be monitored by a wound care team so that these challenging wounds receive aggressive care.

Carradice D et al. A comparison of the effectiveness of treating those with and without the complications of superficial venous insufficiency. Ann Surg. 2014 Aug;260(2):396–401. [PMID: 24424141]
Eberhardt RT et al. Chronic venous insufficiency. Circulation. 2014 Jul 22;130(4):333–46. [PMID: 25047584]
O'Donnell TF Jr et al. Management of venous leg ulcers: clinical practice guidelines of the Society for Vascular Surgery and the American Venous Forum. J Vasc Surg. 2014 Aug;60(2 Suppl): 3S–59S. [PMID: 24974070]

SUPERIOR VENA CAVAL OBSTRUCTION

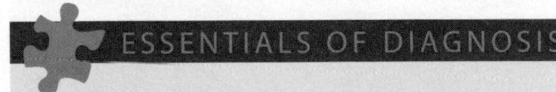
ESSENTIALS OF DIAGNOSIS

- ▶ Swelling of the neck, face, and upper extremities.
- ▶ Dilated veins over the upper chest and neck.

▶ General Considerations

Partial or complete obstruction of the superior vena cava is a relatively rare condition that is usually secondary to neoplastic or inflammatory processes in the superior mediastinum. The most frequent causes are (1) neoplasms, such as lymphomas, primary malignant mediastinal tumors, or carcinoma of the lung with direct extension (over 80%); (2) chronic fibrotic mediastinitis, either of unknown origin or secondary to tuberculosis, histoplasmosis, pyogenic infections, or drugs, especially methysergide; (3) DVT, often by extension of the process from the axillary or subclavian vein into the innominate vein and vena cava associated with catheterization of these veins for dialysis or for hyperalimentation; (4) aneurysm of the aortic arch; and (5) constrictive pericarditis.

Clinical Findings

A. Symptoms and Signs

The onset of symptoms is acute or subacute. Symptoms include swelling of the neck and face and upper extremities. Symptoms are often perceived as congestion and present as headache, dizziness, visual disturbances, stupor, syncope, or cough. There is progressive obstruction of the venous drainage of the head, neck, and upper extremities. The cutaneous veins of the upper chest and lower neck become dilated, and flushing of the face and neck develops. Brawny edema of the face, neck, and arms occurs later, and cyanosis of these areas then appears. Cerebral and laryngeal edema ultimately result in impaired function of the brain as well as respiratory insufficiency. Bending over or lying down accentuates the symptoms; sitting quietly is generally preferred. The manifestations are more severe if the obstruction develops rapidly and if the azygos junction or the vena cava between that vein and the heart is obstructed.

B. Laboratory Findings

The venous pressure is elevated (often more than 20 cm of water) in the arm and is normal in the leg. Since lung cancer is a common cause, bronchoscopy is often performed; transbronchial biopsy, however, is relatively contraindicated because of venous hypertension and the risk of bleeding.

C. Imaging

Chest radiographs and a CT scan will define the location and often the nature of the obstructive process, and contrast venography or magnetic resonance venography (MRV) will map out the extent and degree of the venous obstruction and the collateral circulation. Brachial venography or radionuclide scanning following intravenous injection of technetium Tc-99m pertechnetate demonstrates a block to the flow of contrast material into the right heart and enlarged collateral veins. These techniques also allow estimation of blood flow around the occlusion as well as serial evaluation of the response to therapy.

Treatment

Conservative measures, such as elevation of the head of the bed and lifestyle modification to avoid bending over, are useful. Balloon angioplasty of the obstructed caval segment combined with stent placement provides prompt relief of symptoms and is the procedure of choice for all etiologies. Occasionally, anticoagulation is needed, while thrombolysis is rarely needed.

Urgent treatment for neoplasm consists of (1) cautious use of intravenous diuretics and (2) mediastinal irradiation, starting within 24 hours, with a treatment plan designed to give a high daily dose but a short total course of therapy to rapidly shrink the local tumor. Intensive combined therapy will palliate the process in up to 90% of patients. In patients with a subacute presentation, radiation therapy alone usually suffices. Chemotherapy is added if lymphoma or small-cell carcinoma is diagnosed.

Long-term outcome is complicated by risk of re-occlusion from either thrombosis or further growth of the neoplasm. Surgical procedures to bypass the obstruction are complicated by bleeding relating to high venous pressure. In cases where the thrombosis is secondary to an indwelling catheter, thrombolysis may be attempted. Clinical judgment is required since a long-standing clot may be fibrotic and the risk of bleeding will outweigh the potential benefit.

Prognosis

The prognosis depends on the nature and degree of obstruction and its speed of onset. Slowly developing forms secondary to fibrosis may be tolerated for years. A high degree of obstruction of rapid onset secondary to cancer is often fatal in a few days or weeks because of increased intracranial pressure and cerebral hemorrhage, but treatment of the tumor with radiation and chemotherapeutic drugs may result in significant palliation. Balloon angioplasty and stenting provide good relief but may require re-treatment for recurrent symptoms secondary to thrombosis or restenosis.

When to Refer

Referral should occur with any patient with progressive head and neck swelling to rule out superior vena cava syndrome.

When to Admit

Any patient with acute edema of the head and neck or any patient in whom signs and symptoms of airway compromise, such as hoarseness or stridor, develop should be admitted.

Lepper PM et al. Superior vena cava syndrome in thoracic malignancies. Respir Care. 2011 May;56(5):653–66. [PMID: 21276318]

Watkinson AF et al. Endovascular stenting to treat obstruction of the superior vena cava. BMJ. 2008 Jun 21;336(7658):1434–7. [PMID: 18566082]

DISEASES OF THE LYMPHATIC CHANNELS

LYMPHANGITIS & LYMPHADENITIS

ESSENTIALS OF DIAGNOSIS

- Red streak from wound or area of cellulitis toward regional lymph nodes, which are usually enlarged and tender.
- Chills, fever, and malaise may be present.

General Considerations

Lymphangitis and lymphadenitis are common manifestations of a bacterial infection that is usually caused by hemolytic streptococci or *S aureus* (or by both organisms) and usually arises from the site of an infected wound. The wound may be very small or superficial, or an established abscess may be present, feeding bacteria into the lymphatics. The involvement of the lymphatics is often manifested by a red streak in the skin extending in the direction of the regional lymph nodes, which are, in turn, generally tender and engorged. Systemic manifestations include fever, chills, and malaise. The infection may progress rapidly, often in a matter of hours, and may lead to septicemia and even death.

Clinical Findings

A. Symptoms and Signs

Throbbing pain is usually present in the area of cellulitis at the site of bacterial invasion. Malaise, anorexia, sweating, chills, and fever of 38–40°C develop rapidly. The red streak, when present, may be definite or may be very faint and easily missed, especially in dark-skinned patients. It is usually tender or indurated in the area of cellulitis. The involved regional lymph nodes may be significantly enlarged and are usually quite tender. The pulse is often rapid.

B. Laboratory Findings

Leukocytosis with a left shift is usually present. Blood cultures may be positive, most often for staphylococcal or streptococcal species. Culture and sensitivity studies of the wound exudate or pus may be helpful in treatment of the more severe or refractory infections but are often difficult to interpret because of skin contaminants.

Differential Diagnosis

Lymphangitis may be confused with superficial thrombophlebitis, but the erythema and induration of thrombophlebitis is localized in and around the thrombosed vein. Venous thrombosis is not associated with lymphadenitis, and a wound of entrance with secondary cellulitis is generally absent.

Cat-scratch fever *(Bartonella henselae)* should be considered when lymphadenitis is present; the nodes, though often very large, are relatively nontender. Exposure to cats is common, but the patient may have forgotten about the scratch.

It is extremely important to differentiate cellulitis from acute streptococcal hemolytic gangrene or necrotizing fasciitis. These are deeper infections that may be extensive and are potentially lethal. Patients appear more seriously ill; there may be redness due to leakage of red cells, creating a non-blanching erythema; and subcutaneous crepitus may be palpated or auscultated using the diaphragm with light pressure over the involved area. Immediate wide debridement of all involved deep tissues should be done if these signs are present.

Treatment

A. General Measures

Prompt treatment should include heat (hot, moist compresses or heating pad), elevation when feasible, and immobilization of the infected area. Analgesics may be prescribed for pain.

B. Specific Measures

Empiric antibiotic therapy for hemolytic streptococci or *S aureus* (or by both organisms) should always be instituted when local infection becomes invasive, as manifested by cellulitis and lymphangitis. Cephalosporins or extended-spectrum penicillins are commonly used (eg, cephalexin, 0.5 g orally four times daily for 7–10 days; see Table 30–6). Trimethoprim-sulfamethoxazole (two double-strength tablets twice daily for 7–10 days) should be considered when there is concern that the pathogen is methicillin-resistant *S aureus* (MRSA) (see Tables 30–4 and 30–6).

C. Wound Care

Any wound that is the initiating site of lymphangitis should be treated aggressively. Any necrotic tissue must be debrided and loculated pus drained.

Prognosis

With proper therapy including an antibiotic effective against the invading bacteria, control of the infection can usually be achieved in a few days. Delayed or inadequate therapy can lead to overwhelming infection with septicemia.

When to Admit

Infections causing lymphangitis should be treated in the hospital with intravenous antibiotics. Debridement may be required.

LYMPHEDEMA

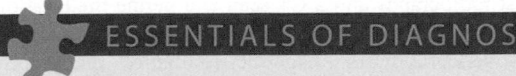

ESSENTIALS OF DIAGNOSIS

► Painless persistent edema of one or both lower extremities, primarily in young women.

► Pitting edema without ulceration, varicosities, or stasis pigmentation.

► There may be episodes of lymphangitis and cellulitis.

General Considerations

When lymphedema is due to congenital developmental abnormalities consisting of hypoplastic or hyperplastic involvement of the proximal or distal lymphatics, it is referred to as the **primary form**. The obstruction may be in the pelvic or lumbar lymph channels and nodes when the disease is extensive and progressive. The **secondary**

form of lymphedema involves inflammatory or mechanical lymphatic obstruction from trauma, regional lymph node resection or irradiation, or extensive involvement of regional nodes by malignant disease or filariasis. Lymphedema may occur following surgical removal of the lymph nodes in the groin or axillae. Secondary dilation of the lymphatics that occurs in both forms leads to incompetence of the valve system, disrupts the orderly flow along the lymph vessels, and results in progressive stasis of a protein-rich fluid. Episodes of acute and chronic inflammation may be superimposed, with further stasis and secondary fibrosis.

Clinical Findings

Hypertrophy of the limb results, with markedly thickened and fibrotic skin and subcutaneous tissue (Figure 12–4) in very advanced cases.

Lymphangiography and radioactive isotope studies may identify focal defects in lymph flow but are of little value in planning therapy. T_2–weighted MRI has been used to identify lymphatics and proximal obstructing masses.

Treatment

Since there is no effective cure for lymphedema, the treatment strategies are designed to control the problem and allow normal activity and function. Most patients can be treated with some of the following measures: (1) The flow of lymph out of the extremity can be aided through intermittent elevation of the extremity, especially during the sleeping hours (foot of bed elevated 15–20 degrees, achieved by placing pillows beneath the mattress); the constant use of graduated elastic compression stockings; and massage toward the trunk—either by hand or by means of pneumatic pressure devices designed to milk edema out of an extremity. Wound care centers specializing in the care of patients with lymphedema may be helpful. (2) Secondary

▲ **Figure 12–4.** Lymphedema with a dorsal pedal hump and exaggerated skin folds near the ankle. (Used, with permission, from Dean SM, Satiani B, Abraham WT. *Color Atlas and Synopsis of Vascular Diseases.* McGraw-Hill, 2014.)

cellulitis in the extremity should be avoided by means of good hygiene and treatment of any trichophytosis of the toes. Once an infection starts, it should be treated by periods of elevation and antibiotic therapy that covers *Staphylococcus* and *Streptococcus* organisms (see Table 30–6). Infections can be a serious and recurring problem and are often difficult to control. Prophylactic antibiotics have not been shown to be of benefit. (3) Intermittent courses of diuretic therapy, especially in those with premenstrual or seasonal exacerbations, are rarely helpful. (4) Amputation is used only for the rare complication of lymphangiosarcoma in the extremity.

Prognosis

With aggressive treatment, including pneumatic compression devices, good relief of symptoms can be achieved. The long-term outlook is dictated by the associated conditions and avoidance of recurrent cellulitis.

Finnane A et al. Review of the evidence of lymphedema treatment effect. Am J Phys Med Rehabil. 2015 Jun;94(6):483–98. [PMID: 25741621]

SHOCK

ESSENTIALS OF DIAGNOSIS

▸ Hypotension, tachycardia, oliguria, altered mental status.

▸ Peripheral hypoperfusion and impaired oxygen delivery.

General Considerations

Shock occurs when the rate of arterial blood flow is inadequate to meet tissue metabolic needs. This results in regional hypoxia and subsequent lactic acidosis from anaerobic metabolism in peripheral tissues as well as eventual end-organ damage and failure.

Classification (Table 12–1)

A. Hypovolemic Shock

Hypovolemic shock results from decreased intravascular volume secondary to loss of blood or fluids and electrolytes. The etiology may be suggested by the clinical setting (eg, trauma) or by signs and symptoms of blood loss (eg, gastrointestinal bleeding) or dehydration (eg, vomiting or diarrhea). Compensatory vasoconstriction may transiently maintain the blood pressure but unreplaced losses of over 15% of the intravascular volume can result in hypotension and progressive tissue hypoxia.

B. Cardiogenic Shock

Cardiogenic shock results from cardiac failure with the resultant inability of the heart to maintain adequate tissue

Table 12–1. Classification of shock by mechanism and common causes.

Hypovolemic shock
  Loss of blood (hemorrhagic shock)
    External hemorrhage
      Trauma
      Gastrointestinal tract bleeding
    Internal hemorrhage
      Hematoma
      Hemothorax or hemoperitoneum
  Loss of plasma
    Burns
    Exfoliative dermatitis
  Loss of fluid and electrolytes
    External losses
      Vomiting
      Diarrhea
      Excessive sweating
      Hyperosmolar states (diabetic ketoacidosis, hyperosmolar nonketotic coma)
    Internal losses (third spacing)
      Pancreatitis
      Ascites
      Bowel obstruction
Cardiogenic shock
  Dysrhythmia (tachyarrhythmia, bradyarrhythmia)
  "Pump failure" (secondary to myocardial infarction or other cardiomyopathy)
  Acute valvular dysfunction (especially regurgitant lesions)
  Rupture of ventricular septum or free ventricular wall
Obstructive shock
  Tension pneumothorax
  Pericardial disease (tamponade, constriction)
  Disease of pulmonary vasculature (massive pulmonary emboli, pulmonary hypertension)
  Cardiac tumor (atrial myxoma)
  Left atrial mural thrombus
  Obstructive valvular disease (aortic or mitral stenosis)
Distributive shock
  Septic shock
  Anaphylactic shock
  Neurogenic shock
  Vasodilator drugs
  Acute adrenal insufficiency

Reproduced, with permission, from Stone CK, Humphries RL (editors). *Current Emergency Diagnosis & Treatment*, 5th ed. p. 193. McGraw-Hill, 2004.

perfusion. The clinical definition of cardiogenic shock is evidence of tissue hypoxia due to decreased cardiac output (cardiac index less than 2.2 L/min/m^2) in the presence of adequate intravascular volume. This is most often caused by myocardial infarction but can also be due to cardiomyopathy, myocardial contusion, valvular incompetence or stenosis, or arrhythmias. See Chapter 10.

C. Obstructive Shock

Cardiac tamponade, tension pneumothorax, and massive pulmonary embolism can cause an acute decrease in cardiac output resulting in shock. These are medical emergencies requiring prompt diagnosis and treatment.

D. Distributive Shock

Distributive or vasodilatory shock has many causes including sepsis, anaphylaxis, systemic inflammatory response syndrome (SIRS) produced by severe pancreatitis or burns, traumatic spinal cord injury, or acute adrenal insufficiency. The reduction in systemic vascular resistance results in inadequate cardiac output and tissue hypoperfusion despite normal circulatory volume.

1. Septic shock—Sepsis is the most common cause of distributive shock and carries a mortality rate of 20–50%. Sepsis is defined as the presence of infection (either documented or suspected) in conjunction with systemic manifestations of infection. Septic shock is diagnosed when hypotension from sepsis persists despite adequate fluid resuscitation. The most common cause of septic shock in hospitalized patients is infection with gram-positive or gram-negative organisms, with a growing incidence of infection from multidrug-resistant organisms. Sepsis from fungal organisms is increasing but remains less than that for bacterial infections. Risk factors for septic shock include bacteremia, extremes of age, diabetes, cancer, immunosuppression, and history of a recent invasive procedure.

2. Systemic inflammatory response syndrome (SIRS)—Defined as a systemic response to a nonspecific infectious or noninfectious insult—such as from burns, pancreatitis, an autoimmune disorder, ischemia, or trauma—the presence of two or more of the following clinical criteria help establish the diagnosis of SIRS: (1) body temperature higher than 38°C (100.4°F) or lower than 36°C (96.8°F), (2) heart rate faster than 90 beats per minute, (3) respiratory rate more than 20 breaths per minute or hyperventilation with an arterial carbon dioxide tension ($Paco_2$) less than 32 mm Hg, or (4) abnormal white blood cell count (greater than 12,000/mcL or less than 4000/mcL or greater than 10% immature [band] forms). When a source of infection is confirmed, SIRS is categorized as sepsis.

3. Neurogenic shock—Neurogenic shock is caused by traumatic spinal cord injury or effects of an epidural or spinal anesthetic. This results in loss of sympathetic tone with a reduction in systemic vascular resistance and hypotension without a compensatory tachycardia. Reflex vagal parasympathetic stimulation evoked by pain, gastric dilation, or fright may simulate neurogenic shock, producing hypotension, bradycardia, and syncope.

▶ Clinical Findings

A. Symptoms and Signs

Hypotension is traditionally defined as a systolic blood pressure of 90 mm Hg or less or a mean arterial pressure of less than 60–65 mm Hg but must be evaluated relative to the patient's normal blood pressure. A drop in systolic pressure of greater than 10–20 mm Hg or an increase in pulse of more than 15 beats per minute with positional change suggests depleted intravascular volume. However, blood pressure is often not the best indicator of end-organ perfusion because compensatory mechanisms, such as increased heart rate, increased cardiac contractility, and vasoconstriction can occur to prevent hypotension. Patients with hypotension often have cool or mottled extremities and weak or thready peripheral pulses. Splanchnic vasoconstriction may lead to oliguria, bowel ischemia, and hepatic dysfunction, which can ultimately result in multi-organ failure. Mentation may be normal or patients may become restless, agitated, confused, lethargic, or comatose as a result of inadequate perfusion of the brain.

Hypovolemic shock is evident when signs of hypoperfusion, such as oliguria, altered mental status, and cool extremities, are present. Jugular venous pressure is low, and there is a narrow pulse pressure indicative of reduced stroke volume. Rapid replacement of fluids can restore tissue perfusion. In **cardiogenic shock,** there are also signs of global hypoperfusion with oliguria, altered mental status, and cool extremities. Jugular venous pressure is elevated and there may be evidence of pulmonary edema with respiratory compromise in the setting of left-sided heart failure. A transthoracic echocardiogram (TTE) or a transesophageal echocardiogram (TEE) is an effective diagnostic tool to differentiate hypovolemic from cardiogenic shock. In hypovolemic shock, the left ventricle will be small because of decreased filling, but contractility is often preserved. Cardiogenic shock results from cardiac failure with a resultant decrease in left ventricular contractility. In some cases, the left ventricle may appear dilated and full because of the inability of the left ventricle to eject a sufficient stroke volume.

In **obstructive shock**, the central venous pressure may be elevated but the TTE or TEE may show reduced left ventricular filling, a pericardial effusion in the case of tamponade, or thickened pericardium in the case of pericarditis. Pericardiocentesis or pericardial window for pericardial tamponade, chest tube placement for tension pneumothorax, or catheter-directed thrombolytic therapy for massive pulmonary embolism can be life-saving in cases of obstructive shock.

In **distributive shock,** signs include hyperdynamic heart sounds, warm extremities initially, and a wide pulse pressure indicative of large stroke volume. The echocardiogram may show a hyperdynamic left ventricle. Fluid resuscitation may have little effect on blood pressure, urinary output, or mentation. **Septic shock** is diagnosed when there is clinical evidence of infection in the setting of persistent hypotension and evidence of organ hypoperfusion, such as lactic acidosis, decreased urinary output, or altered mental status despite adequate volume resuscitation. **Neurogenic shock** is diagnosed when there is evidence of central nervous system injury and persistent hypotension despite adequate volume resuscitation.

B. Laboratory Findings and Imaging

Blood specimens should be evaluated for complete blood count, electrolytes, glucose, arterial blood gas determinations, coagulation parameters, lactate levels, typing and cross-matching, and bacterial cultures. An electrocardiogram and chest radiograph should also be part of the initial assessment. A transthoracic echocardiogram can help assess right- and left-sided filling pressures and cardiac output.

▶ Treatment

A. General Measures

Treatment depends on prompt diagnosis and an accurate appraisal of inciting conditions. Initial management consists of basic life support with an assessment of the patient's circulation, airway, and breathing. This may entail airway intubation and mechanical ventilation. Ventilatory failure should be anticipated in patients with severe metabolic acidosis in association with shock. Mechanical ventilation along with sedation can decrease the oxygen demand of the respiratory muscles and allow improved oxygen delivery to other hypoperfused tissues. Intravenous access and fluid resuscitation should be instituted along with cardiac monitoring and assessment of hemodynamic parameters such as blood pressure and heart rate. Cardiac monitoring can detect myocardial ischemia or malignant arrhythmias, which can be treated by standard advanced cardiac life support (ACLS) protocols.

Unresponsive or minimally responsive patients should have their glucose checked immediately and if their glucose levels are low, 1 ampule of **50% dextrose** intravenously should be given. An arterial line should be placed for continuous blood pressure measurement, and a Foley catheter should be inserted to monitor urinary output.

B. Central Venous Pressure

Early consideration is given to placement of a central venous catheter (CVC) for infusion of fluids and medications and for hemodynamic pressure measurements. A CVC can provide measurements of the central venous pressure (CVP) and the central venous oxygen saturation ($ScvO_2$), both of which can be used to manage sepsis and septic shock. Pulmonary artery catheters (PACs) allow measurement of the pulmonary artery pressure, left-sided filling pressure or the pulmonary capillary wedge pressure (PCWP), the mixed venous oxygen saturation (SvO_2) and cardiac output. Meta-analyses of multiple studies, including randomized controlled trials, suggest that PACs do not increase overall mortality or length of hospital stay, but are associated with higher use of inotropes and intravenous vasodilators in critically ill patients from different patient populations (including those with sepsis, myocardial ischemia, and those who were postsurgical). Thus, the routine use of PACs cannot be recommended. However, in some complex situations, PACs may be useful in distinguishing between cardiogenic and septic shock. The attendant risks associated with PACs (such as infection, arrhythmias, vein thrombosis, and pulmonary artery rupture) can be as high as 4–9%; therefore, the value of the information they might provide must be carefully weighed in each patient. TTE is a noninvasive alternative to the PAC. TTE can provide information about the pulmonary artery pressure and current cardiac function, including cardiac output. The $ScvO_2$, which is obtained through the CVC, can be used as a surrogate for the SvO_2, which is obtained through the PAC. Pulse pressure variation, as determined by arterial waveform analysis, or stroke volume variation are much more sensitive than CVP as a measure of fluid responsiveness in volume resuscitation, but these measurements are only valid in patients who are mechanically ventilated and in normal sinus rhythm.

A CVP less than 5 mm Hg suggests hypovolemia, and a CVP greater than 18 mm Hg suggests volume overload, cardiac failure, tamponade, or pulmonary hypertension. A cardiac index lower than 2 L/min/m² indicates a need for inotropic support. A cardiac index higher than 4 L/min/m² in a hypotensive patient is consistent with early septic shock. The systemic vascular resistance is low (less than 800 dynes · s/cm⁻⁵) in sepsis and neurogenic shock and high (greater than 1500 dynes · s/cm⁻⁵) in hypovolemic and cardiogenic shock. Treatment is directed at maintaining a CVP of 8–12 mm Hg, a mean arterial pressure of 65 mm Hg or higher, a cardiac index of 2–4 L/min/m², and a $ScvO_2$ greater than 70%.

C. Volume Replacement

Volume replacement is critical in the initial management of shock. **Hemorrhagic shock** is treated with immediate efforts to achieve hemostasis and rapid infusions of blood substitutes, such as type-specific or type O negative packed red blood cells (PRBCs) or whole blood, which also provides extra volume and clotting factors. Each unit of PRBC or whole blood is expected to raise the hematocrit by 3%. **Hypovolemic shock** secondary to dehydration is managed with rapid boluses of isotonic crystalloid (0.9% saline or lactated Ringer solution) usually in 1-liter increments. **Cardiogenic shock** in the absence of fluid overload requires smaller fluid challenges, usually in increments of 250 mL. **Septic shock** usually requires large volumes of fluid for resuscitation (usually more than 2 L) as the associated capillary leak releases fluid into the extravascular space. Caution must be used with large-volume resuscitation with unwarmed fluids because this can produce hypothermia, which can lead to hypothermia-induced coagulopathy. Warming of fluids before administration can avoid this complication.

Meta-analyses of studies of heterogenous critically ill populations comparing crystalloid and colloid resuscitation (with albumin) indicate no benefit of colloid over crystalloid solutions except in trauma patients with traumatic brain injury, who had a higher mortality if volume resuscitated with albumin. Furthermore, in patients with severe sepsis, the addition of albumin to crystalloid solutions did not alter mortality when compared to the administration of crystalloid alone. Clinical trials and meta-analyses have also found no difference in mortality between trauma patients receiving hypertonic saline (7.5%) and those receiving isotonic crystalloid. When compared to isotonic saline, the use of hypertonic saline plus dextran has been found to increase survival, particularly in patients with traumatic brain injury.

D. Early Goal-Directed Therapy

Compensated shock can occur in the setting of normalized hemodynamic parameters with ongoing global tissue hypoxia. Traditional endpoints of resuscitation such as blood pressure, heart rate, urinary output, mental status, and skin perfusion can therefore be misleading. Early goal-directed therapy (EGDT) following set protocols for the treatment of septic shock by adjusting the use of fluids, vasopressors, ionotropes and blood transfusions to meet hemodynamic targets (mean arterial pressure 65 mm Hg or higher, CVP 8–12 mm Hg, $ScvO_2$ greater than 70%) provided significant mortality benefits when introduced in 2001. Lactate clearance of more than 10% can be used as a substitute for $ScvO_2$ criteria if $ScvO_2$ monitoring is not available.

Since its introduction, there have been data to suggest that portions of EGDT, such as transfusing to a hematocrit of 30% if the $ScvO_2$ was less than 70%, may do more harm than good. Two large randomized trials published in 2014 (ProCESS and ARISE) demonstrated no mortality benefit from the institution of EGDT, but this may have been due to earlier administration of antibiotics, components of EGDT becoming part of the "usual care" that clinicians deliver, and the effectiveness of education about detecting and treating sepsis in a timely fashion since the inception of EGDT in 2001. A meta-analysis of hemodynamic optimization trials has also suggested that early treatment before the development of organ failure results in improved survival, and patients who respond well to initial efforts demonstrate a survival advantage over nonresponders. The Surviving Sepsis Campaign guidelines from 2012 recommend using EGDT in patients with severe sepsis and septic shock (see www.survivingsepsis.org).

E. Medications

1. Vasoactive therapy—Vasopressors and inotropic agents are administered only after adequate fluid resuscitation. Choice of vasoactive therapy depends on the presumed etiology of shock as well as cardiac output. If there is continued hypotension with evidence of high cardiac output after adequate volume resuscitation, then vasopressor support is needed to improve vasomotor tone. If there is evidence of low cardiac output with high filling pressures, inotropic support is needed to improve contractility.

For **vasodilatory shock** when increased vasoconstriction is required to maintain an adequate perfusion pressure, alpha-adrenergic catecholamine agonists (such as norepinephrine and phenylephrine) are generally used. Although **norepinephrine** is both an alpha-adrenergic and beta-adrenergic agonist, it preferentially increases mean arterial pressure over cardiac output. The initial dose is 1–2 mcg/min as an intravenous infusion, titrated to maintain the mean arterial blood pressure at 65 mm Hg or higher. The usual maintenance dose is 2–4 mcg/min intravenously (maximum dose is 30 mcg/min). Patients with refractory shock may require dosages of 10–30 mcg/min intravenously. **Epinephrine,** also with both alpha-adrenergic and beta-adrenergic effects, may be used in severe shock and during acute resuscitation. It is the vasopressor of choice for anaphylactic shock. For severe shock, give 1 mcg/min as a continuous intravenous infusion initially and titrate to hemodynamic response; the usual dosage range is 1–10 mcg/min intravenously.

Dopamine has variable effects according to dosage. At low doses (2–5 mcg/kg/min intravenously), stimulation of dopaminergic and beta-adrenergic receptors produces increased glomerular filtration, heart rate, and contractility. At doses of 5–10 mcg/kg/min, beta-1-adrenergic effects predominate, resulting in an increase in heart rate and cardiac contractility. At higher doses (greater than 10 mcg/kg/min), alpha-adrenergic effects predominate, resulting in peripheral vasoconstriction. The maximum dose is typically 50 mcg/kg/min.

There is no evidence documenting a survival benefit from, or the superiority of, a particular vasopressor in **septic shock**. Norepinephrine is the initial vasopressor of choice in septic shock to maintain the mean arterial pressure at 65 mm Hg or higher. Phenylephrine can be used as a first-line agent for hyperdynamic septic shock if (1) there is low systemic venous resistance but high cardiac output, which can manifest as hypotension with *warm* extremities or (2) dysrhythmias or tachycardias prevent the use of agents with beta-adrenergic activity. In meta-analyses, the use of dopamine as a first-line vasopressor in septic shock resulted in an increase in 28-day mortality and a higher incidence of arrhythmic events. Dopamine should only be used as an alternative to norepinephrine in select patients with septic shock, including patients with significant bradycardia or low potential for tachyarrhythmias.

Vasopressin (antidiuretic hormone or ADH) is often used as an adjunctive therapy to catecholamine vasopressors in the treatment of **distributive** or **vasodilatory shock**. Vasopressin causes peripheral vasoconstriction via V1 receptors located on smooth muscle cells and attenuation of nitric oxide (NO) synthesis and cGMP, the second messenger of NO. The rationale for using low-dose vasopressin in the management of septic shock includes the relative deficiency of vasopressin in late shock. Vasopressin also potentiates the effects of catecholamines on the vasculature and stimulates cortisol production. Some studies have reported reduced catecholamine requirements with vasopressin administration. Intravenous infusion of vasopressin at a low dose (0.01–0.04 units/min) may be safe and beneficial in septic patients with hypotension that is refractory to fluid resuscitation and conventional catecholamine vasopressors. Higher doses of vasopressin decrease cardiac output and may put patients at greater risk for splanchnic and coronary artery ischemia. Studies do not favor the use of vasopressin as first-line therapy. In the Vasopressin and Septic Shock Trial (VASST), low doses of vasopressin did not reduce mortality compared with norepinephrine in patients with septic shock who were being treated with catecholamine vasopressors.

There is insufficient evidence to recommend a specific vasopressor to use in cardiogenic shock, but expert opinion suggests that either norepinephrine or dopamine be used as a first-line agent. Dobutamine, a predominantly beta-adrenergic agonist, increases contractility and decreases afterload. It is used for patients with low cardiac output and high PCWP but who do not have hypotension. Dobutamine can be added to a vasopressor if there is reduced myocardial function (decreased cardiac output and elevated PCWP), or if there are signs of hypoperfusion despite adequate volume resuscitation and an adequate mean arterial pressure. The initial dose is 0.1–0.5 mcg/kg/min as a continuous intravenous infusion, which can be titrated every few minutes to hemodynamic effect; the usual dosage range is 2–20 mcg/kg/min intravenously. Tachyphylaxis can occur after 48 hours secondary to the down-regulation of beta-adrenergic receptors. Amrinone and milrinone are phosphodiesterase inhibitors that can be substituted for dobutamine. These drugs increase cyclic AMP levels and increase cardiac contractility, bypassing the beta-adrenergic receptor. Vasodilation is a side effect of both amrinone and milrinone.

2. Corticosteroids—Corticosteroids are the treatment of choice in patients with shock secondary to adrenal insufficiency but studies do not support their use in patients with shock from sepsis or other etiologies. Trials where either high or low doses of corticosteroids were administered to patients in septic shock did not show improved survival; rather, some worse outcomes were observed from increased rates of secondary infections, even in patients who had relative adrenal insufficiency, defined by a cortisol response of 9 mcg/dL or less after one injection of 250 mcg of corticotropin. Meta-analyses of multiple smaller trials of steroids in septic shock have demonstrated that in patients in shock that is poorly responsive to fluid resuscitation and vasopressors, low-dose hydrocortisone (300 mg/day or less in divided doses) increased the mean arterial pressure but did not show a mortality benefit.

3. Antibiotics—Definitive therapy for septic shock includes early initiation of empiric broad-spectrum antibiotics after appropriate cultures have been obtained and within 1 hour of recognition of septic shock. Imaging studies may prove useful to attempt localization of sources of infection. Surgical management may also be necessary if necrotic tissue or loculated infections are present (see Table 30–5).

4. Sodium bicarbonate—For patients with sepsis of any etiology and lactic acidosis, clinical studies have failed to show any hemodynamic benefit from bicarbonate therapy, either in increasing cardiac output or in decreasing the vasopressor requirement, even in patients with severe acidemia.

F. Other Treatment Modalities

Cardiac failure may require use of transcutaneous or transvenous pacing or placement of an intra-arterial balloon pump. Emergent revascularization by percutaneous angioplasty or coronary artery bypass surgery appears to improve long-term outcome with increased survival compared with initial medical stabilization for patients with myocardial ischemia leading to cardiogenic shock. Urgent hemodialysis or continuous venovenous hemofiltration may be indicated for maintenance of fluid and electrolyte balance during acute kidney injury resulting in shock from multiple modalities.

Asfar P et al; SEPSISPAM Investigators. High versus low blood-pressure target in patients with septic shock. N Engl J Med. 2014 Apr 24;370(17):1583–93. [PMID: 24635770]
Caironi P et al; ALBIOS Study Investigators. Albumin replacement in patients with severe sepsis or septic shock. N Engl J Med. 2014 Apr 10;370(15):1412–21. [PMID: 24635772]

Dellinger RP et al; Surviving Sepsis Campaign Guidelines Committee including the Pediatric Subgroup. Surviving Sepsis Campaign: international guidelines for management of severe sepsis and septic shock: 2012. Crit Care Med. 2013 Feb;41(2): 580–637. [PMID: 23353941]

Myburgh JA et al. Resuscitation fluids. N Engl J Med. 2013 Sep 26;369(13):1243–51. [PMID: 24066745]

Peake SL et al; ARISE Investigators; ANZICS Clinical Trials Group. Goal-directed resuscitation for patients with early septic shock. N Engl J Med. 2014 Oct 16;371(16):1496–506. [PMID: 25272316]

Raghunathan K et al. What is the ideal crystalloid? Curr Opin Crit Care. 2015 Aug;21(4):309–14. [PMID: 26103144]

Seymour CW et al. Septic Shock: Advances in Diagnosis and Treatment. JAMA. 2015 Aug 18;314(7):708–17. [PMID: 26284722]

Yealy DM et al; ProCESS Investigators. A randomized trial of protocol-based care for early septic shock. N Engl J Med. 2014 May 1;370(18):1683–93. [PMID: 24635773]

Blood Disorders

Lloyd E. Damon, MD
Charalambos Babis Andreadis, MD, MSCE

ANEMIAS

▶ General Approach to Anemias

Anemia is present in adults if the hematocrit is below 41% (hemoglobin less than 13.5 g/dL [135 g/L]) in males or below 36% (hemoglobin less than 12 g/dL [120 g/L]) in females. Congenital anemia is suggested by the patient's personal and family history. The most common cause of anemia is iron deficiency. Poor diet may result in folic acid deficiency and contribute to iron deficiency, but bleeding is the most common cause of iron deficiency in adults. Physical examination demonstrates pallor. Attention to physical signs of primary hematologic diseases (lymphadenopathy; hepatosplenomegaly; or bone tenderness, especially in the sternum or anterior tibia) is important. Mucosal changes such as a smooth tongue suggest megaloblastic anemia.

Anemias are classified according to their pathophysiologic basis, ie, whether related to diminished production (relative or absolute reticulocytopenia) or to increased production due to accelerated loss of red blood cells (reticulocytosis) (Table 13–1), and according to red blood cell size (Table 13–2). A reticulocytosis occurs in one of three pathophysiologic states: acute blood loss, recent replacement of a missing erythropoietic nutrient, or reduced red blood cell survival (ie, hemolysis). A severely microcytic anemia (mean corpuscular volume [MCV] less than 70 fL) is due either to iron deficiency or thalassemia, while a severely macrocytic anemia (MCV less than 125 fL) is almost always due to either megaloblastic anemia or to cold agglutinins in blood analyzed at room temperature. A bone marrow biopsy is generally needed to complete the evaluation of anemia when the laboratory evaluation fails to reveal an etiology, when there are additional cytopenias present, or when an underlying primary or secondary bone marrow process is suspected.

IRON DEFICIENCY ANEMIA

- ▶ Iron deficiency is present if serum ferritin is less than 12 ng/mL (27 pmol/L) or less than 30 ng/mL (67 pmol/L) if also anemic.
- ▶ Caused by bleeding unless proved otherwise.
- ▶ Responds to iron therapy.

▶ General Considerations

Iron deficiency is the most common cause of anemia worldwide. The causes are listed in Table 13–3. Aside from circulating red blood cells, the major location of iron in the body is the storage pool as ferritin or as hemosiderin in macrophages.

The average American diet contains 10–15 mg of iron per day. About 10% of this amount is absorbed in the stomach, duodenum, and upper jejunum under acidic conditions. Dietary iron present as heme is efficiently absorbed (10–20%) but nonheme iron less so (1–5%), largely because of interference by phosphates, tannins, and other food constituents. The major iron transporter from the diet across the intestinal lumen is ferroportin, which also facilitates the transport of iron to apotransferrin in macrophages for delivery to erythroid cells prepared to synthesize hemoglobin. Hepcidin, which is increasingly produced during inflammation, negatively regulates iron transport by promoting the degradation of ferroportin. Small amounts of iron—approximately 1 mg/day—are normally lost through exfoliation of skin and mucosal cells.

Table 13–1. Classification of anemia by pathophysiology.

Decreased red blood cell production (relative or absolute reticulocytopenia)
Hemoglobin synthesis lesion: iron deficiency, thalassemia, anemia of chronic disease, hypoerythropoietinemia
DNA synthesis lesion: megaloblastic anemia, DNA synthesis inhibitor drugs
Hematopoietic stem cell lesion: aplastic anemia, leukemia
Bone marrow infiltration: carcinoma, lymphoma, fibrosis, sarcoidosis, Gaucher disease, others
Immune-mediated inhibition: aplastic anemia, pure red cell aplasia
Increased red blood cell destruction or accelerated red blood cell loss (reticulocytosis)
Acute blood loss
Hemolysis (intrinsic)
Membrane lesion: hereditary spherocytosis, elliptocytosis
Hemoglobin lesion: sickle cell, unstable hemoglobin
Glycolysis abnormality: pyruvate kinase deficiency
Oxidation lesion: glucose-6-phosphate dehydrogenase deficiency
Hemolysis (extrinsic)
Immune: warm antibody, cold antibody
Microangiopathic: thrombotic thrombocytopenic purpura, hemolytic-uremic syndrome, mechanical cardiac valve, paravalvular leak
Infection: *Clostridium perfringens*, malaria
Hypersplenism

With hemorrhage, there is decreased oxygen delivery to the kidneys resulting in stabilization of a hypoxia-inducible factor in the kidneys and increased erythropoietin generation in the kidneys and liver. Erythropoietin stimulates

Table 13–2. Classification of anemia by mean red blood cell volume (MCV).

Microcytic
Iron deficiency
Thalassemia
Anemia of chronic disease
Lead toxicity
Zinc deficiency
Macrocytic (Megaloblastic)
Vitamin B_{12} deficiency
Folate deficiency
DNA synthesis inhibitors
Macrocytic (Nonmegaloblastic)
Myelodysplasia
Liver disease
Reticulocytosis
Hypothyroidism
Bone marrow failure state (eg, aplastic anemia, marrow infiltrative disorder, etc)
Copper deficiency
Normocytic
Kidney disease
Non-thyroid endocrine gland failure
Copper deficiency
Mild form of most acquired microcytic or macrocytic etiologies of anemia

Table 13–3. Causes of iron deficiency.

Deficient diet
Decreased absorption
Autoimmune gastritis
Celiac sprue
Helicobacter pylori gastritis
Hereditary iron-refractory iron deficiency anemia
Zinc deficiency
Increased requirements
Pregnancy
Lactation
Blood loss (chronic)
Gastrointestinal
Menstrual
Blood donation
Hemoglobinuria
Iron sequestration
Pulmonary hemosiderosis
Idiopathic

erythropoiesis, leading to an increased synthesis of erythroferrone. In turn, erythroferrone suppresses hepcidin synthesis leading to ferroportin stability and enhanced iron transport across the gastrointestinal lumen.

Menstrual blood loss plays a major role in iron metabolism. The average monthly menstrual blood loss is approximately 50 mL but may be five times greater in some individuals. Women with heavy menstrual losses must absorb 3–4 mg of iron from the diet each day to maintain adequate iron stores, which is not commonly achieved. Women with menorrhagia of this degree will almost always become iron deficient without iron supplementation.

In general, iron metabolism is balanced between absorption of 1 mg/day and loss of 1 mg/day. Pregnancy and lactation upset the iron balance, since requirements increase to 2–5 mg of iron per day. Normal dietary iron cannot supply these requirements, and medicinal iron is needed during pregnancy and lactation. Decreased iron absorption can also cause iron deficiency, such as in people affected by celiac disease, and it also commonly occurs after gastric resection or jejunal bypass surgery.

The most important cause of iron deficiency anemia in adults is chronic blood loss, especially menstrual and gastrointestinal blood loss. Iron deficiency demands a search for a source of gastrointestinal bleeding if other sites of blood loss (menorrhagia, other uterine bleeding, and repeated blood donations) are excluded. Prolonged aspirin or nonsteroidal anti-inflammatory drug use may cause it even without a documented structural lesion. Celiac disease (gluten enteropathy), even when asymptomatic, is an occult cause of iron deficiency through poor absorption in the gastrointestinal tract. Zinc deficiency is another cause of poor iron absorption. Chronic hemoglobinuria may lead to iron deficiency, but this is uncommon. Traumatic hemolysis due to a prosthetic cardiac valve and other causes of intravascular hemolysis (eg, paroxysmal nocturnal hemoglobinuria) should also be considered. The cause of iron deficiency is not found in up to 5% of cases.

Pure iron deficiency might prove refractory to oral iron replacement. Refractoriness is defined as a hemoglobin increment of less than 1 g/dL (10 g/L) after 4–6 weeks of 100 mg/day of elemental oral iron. The differential diagnosis in these cases (Table 13–3) includes malabsorption from autoimmune gastritis, *Helicobacter pylori* gastric infection, celiac disease, and hereditary iron-refractory iron deficiency anemia. Iron-refractory iron deficiency anemia is a rare autosomal recessive disorder due to mutations in the transmembrane serine protease 6 (*TMPRSS6*) gene, which normally down-regulates hepcidin. In iron-refractory iron deficiency anemia, hepcidin levels are normal to high and ferritin levels are high despite the iron deficiency.

▶ Clinical Findings

A. Symptoms and Signs

The primary symptoms of iron deficiency anemia are those of the anemia itself (easy fatigability, tachycardia, palpitations, and dyspnea on exertion). Severe deficiency causes skin and mucosal changes, including a smooth tongue, brittle nails, spooning of nails (koilonychia), and cheilosis. Dysphagia due to the formation of esophageal webs (Plummer-Vinson syndrome) may occur in severe iron deficiency. Many iron-deficient patients develop pica, craving for specific foods (ice chips, etc) often not rich in iron.

B. Laboratory Findings

Iron deficiency develops in stages. The first is depletion of iron stores without anemia followed by anemia with a normal red blood cell size (normal MCV) followed by anemia with reduced red blood cell size (low MCV). The reticulocyte count is low or inappropriately normal. Ferritin is a measure of total body iron stores. A ferritin value less than 12 ng/mL (27 pmol/L) (in the absence of scurvy) is a highly reliable indicator of depletion of iron stores. Note that the lower limit of normal for ferritin generally is below 12 ng/mL (27 pmol/L) in women due to the fact that the normal ferritin range is generated by including healthy menstruating women who are iron deficient but not anemic. However, because serum ferritin levels may rise in response to inflammation or other stimuli, a normal or elevated ferritin level does not exclude a diagnosis of iron deficiency. A ferritin level less than 30 ng/mL (67 pmol/L) almost always indicates iron deficiency in anyone who is anemic. As iron deficiency progresses, serum iron values decline to less than 30 mcg/dL (67 pmol/L) and transferrin levels rise to compensate, leading to transferrin saturations of less than 15%. Low transferrin saturation is also seen in anemia of inflammation, so caution in the interpretation of this test is warranted. Isolated iron deficiency anemia has a low hepcidin level, not yet a clinically available test. As the MCV falls (ie, microcytosis), the blood smear shows hypochromic microcytic cells. With further progression, anisocytosis (variations in red blood cell size) and poikilocytosis (variation in shape of red cells) develop. Severe iron deficiency will produce a bizarre peripheral blood smear, with severely hypochromic cells, target cells, and pencil-shaped or cigar-shaped cells. Bone marrow biopsy for evaluation of iron stores is rarely performed. If the biopsy is done, it shows the absence of iron in erythroid progenitor cells by Prussian blue staining. The platelet count is commonly increased, but it usually remains under 800,000/mcL (800 × 10⁹/L).

▶ Differential Diagnosis

Other causes of microcytic anemia include anemia of chronic disease (specifically, anemia of inflammation), thalassemia, lead poisoning, and congenital X-linked sideroblastic anemia. Anemia of chronic disease is characterized by normal or increased iron stores in bone marrow macrophages and a normal or elevated ferritin level; the serum iron and transferrin saturation are low, often drastically so, and the total iron-binding capacity (TIBC) and transferrin are either normal or low. Thalassemia produces a greater degree of microcytosis for any given level of anemia than does iron deficiency and, unlike virtually every other cause of anemia, has a normal or elevated (rather than a low) red blood cell count as well as a reticulocytosis. In thalassemia, red blood cell morphology on the peripheral smear resembles severe iron deficiency.

▶ Treatment

The diagnosis of iron deficiency anemia can be made either by the laboratory demonstration of an iron-deficient state or by evaluating the response to a therapeutic trial of iron replacement. Since the anemia itself is rarely life-threatening, the most important part of management is identification of the cause—especially a source of occult blood loss.

A. Oral Iron

Ferrous sulfate, 325 mg one to three times daily on an empty stomach, is a standard approach for replenishing iron stores. As oral iron stimulates hepcidin production, once daily dosing maximizes iron absorption compared to multiple daily dosing, and with fewer side effects. Nausea and constipation limit compliance with ferrous sulfate. Extended-release ferrous sulfate with mucoprotease is a well tolerated oral preparation. Taking ferrous sulfate with food reduces side effects but also its absorption. An appropriate response is a return of the hematocrit level halfway toward normal within 3 weeks with full return to baseline after 2 months. Iron therapy should continue for 3–6 months after restoration of normal hematologic values to replenish iron stores. Failure of response to iron therapy is usually due to noncompliance, although occasional patients may absorb iron poorly, particularly if the stomach is achlorhydric. Such patients may benefit from concomitant administration of oral ascorbic acid. Other reasons for failure to respond include incorrect diagnosis (anemia of chronic disease, thalassemia), celiac disease, and ongoing gastrointestinal blood loss that exceeds the rate of new erythropoiesis. Treatment of *H pylori* infection, in appropriate cases, can improve oral iron absorption.

B. Parenteral Iron

The indications are intolerance of or refractoriness to oral iron (including those with iron-refractory iron deficiency anemia), gastrointestinal disease (usually inflammatory bowel disease) precluding the use of oral iron, and continued blood loss that cannot be corrected, such as chronic hemodialysis. Parenteral iron preparations coat the iron in protective carbohydrate shells. Historical parenteral iron preparations, such as iron dextran, were problematic due to long infusion times (hours), polyarthralgia, and hypersensitivity reactions, including anaphylaxis. Current preparations are safe and can be infused in less than 5 minutes. Iron oxide coated with polyglucose sorbitol carboxymethyl-ether can be given in doses up to 510 mg by intravenous bolus over 15 minutes, with no test dose required.

The iron deficit is calculated by determining the decrement in red cell volume from normal, recognizing there is 1 mg of iron in each milliliter of red blood cells. Total body iron ranges between 2 g and 4 g: approximately 50 mg/kg in men and 35 mg/kg in women. Most (70–95%) of the iron is present in hemoglobin in circulating red blood cells. In men, red blood cell volume is approximately 30 mL/kg; in women, it is about 27 mL/kg. Thus, a 50-kg woman whose hemoglobin is 9 g/dL (75% of normal) has an iron deficit of 0.25×27 mL/kg $\times$ 50 kg = 337.5 mL of red blood cells (or 337.5 mg of iron). The parenteral iron dose is the iron deficit plus (usually) 1 extra gram to replenish iron stores and anticipate further iron loses, so in this case 1.4 g.

Ferric pyrophosphate citrate (Triferic), approved by the FDA in 2015 to replace the 5–7 mg of iron CKD patients tend to lose to each hemodialysis, is added to the dialysate. It appears to be able to deliver sufficient iron to the marrow to maintain hemoglobin and not increase iron stores; it may obviate the need for intravenous iron in hemodialysis patients.

► When to Refer

Patients should be referred to a hematologist if the suspected diagnosis is not confirmed or if they are not responsive to oral iron therapy.

Avni T et al. The safety of intravenous iron preparations: systematic review and meta-analysis. Mayo Clin Proc. 2015 Jan;90(1): 12–23. [PMID: 25572192]

Cancelo-Hildago MJ et al. Tolerability of different oral iron supplements: a systematic review. Curr Med Res Opin. 2013 Apr;29(4):291–303. [PMID: 23252877]

Donker AE et al. Practice guidelines for the diagnosis and management of microcytic anemias due to genetic disorders of iron metabolism or heme synthesis. Blood. 2014 Jun 19; 123(25):3873–86. [PMID: 24665134]

Heeney MM et al. Iron-refractory iron deficiency anemia (IRIDA). Hematol Oncol Clin North Am. 2014 Aug;28(4): 637–52. [PMID: 25064705]

Larson DS et al. Update on intravenous iron choices. Curr Opin Nephrol Hypertens. 2014 Mar;23(2):186–91. [PMID: 24401789]

Moretti D et al. Oral iron supplements increase hepcidin and decrease iron absorption from daily or twice-daily doses in iron-depleted young women. Blood. 2015 Oct 22;126(17): 1981–9. [PMID: 26289639]

Powers JM et al. Diagnosis and management of iron deficiency anemia. Hematol Oncol Clin North Am. 2014 Aug;28(4): 729–45. [PMID: 25064710]

Wang C et al. Comparative risk of anaphylactic reactions associated with intravenous iron products. JAMA. 2015 Nov 17; 314(19):2062–8. [PMID: 26575062]

ANEMIA OF CHRONIC DISEASE

▼ ESSENTIALS OF DIAGNOSIS

► Mild or moderate normocytic or microcytic anemia.

► Normal or increased ferritin and normal or reduced transferrin.

► Underlying chronic disease.

► General Considerations

Many chronic systemic diseases are associated with mild or moderate anemia. The anemias of chronic disease are characterized according to etiology and pathophysiology. First, the **anemia of inflammation** is associated with chronic inflammatory states (such as inflammatory bowel disease, rheumatoid arthritis, chronic infections, and malignancy) and is mediated through hepcidin (a negative regulator of ferroportin), resulting in reduced iron uptake in the gut and reduced iron transfer from macrophages to erythroid progenitor cells in the bone marrow. This is referred to as iron-restricted erythropoiesis since the patient is iron replete. There is also reduced responsiveness to erythropoietin, the elaboration of hemolysins that shorten red blood cell survival, and the production of inflammatory cytokines that dampen red cell production. The serum iron is low in the anemia of inflammation. Second, the **anemia of organ failure** can occur with kidney disease, hepatic failure, and endocrine gland failure. Erythropoietin is reduced and the red blood cell mass decreases in response to the diminished signal for red blood cell production; the serum iron is normal (except in chronic kidney disease where it is low due to the reduced hepcidin clearance and subsequent enhanced degradation of ferroportin). Third, the **anemia of the elderly** is present in up to 20% of individuals over age 85 years in whom a thorough evaluation for an explanation of anemia is negative. It is a consequence of a relative resistance to red blood cell production in response to erythropoietin, a decrease in erythropoietin production relative to the nephron mass, and a negative erythropoietic influence of low levels of chronic inflammatory cytokines in older adults; the serum iron is normal.

► Clinical Findings

A. Symptoms and Signs

The clinical features are those of the causative condition. The diagnosis should be suspected in patients with known chronic diseases. In cases of significant anemia, coexistent iron deficiency or folic acid deficiency should be suspected. Decreased dietary intake of iron or folic acid is common in chronically ill patients, many of whom will also have ongoing gastrointestinal blood losses. Patients undergoing hemodialysis regularly lose both iron and folic acid during dialysis.

B. Laboratory Findings

The hematocrit rarely falls below 60% of baseline (except in kidney failure). The MCV is usually normal or slightly reduced. Red blood cell morphology is usually normal, and the reticulocyte count is mildly decreased or normal. In the anemia of inflammation, serum iron and transferrin values are low, and the transferrin saturation may be extremely low, leading to an erroneous diagnosis of iron deficiency. In contrast to iron deficiency, serum ferritin values should be normal or increased. A serum ferritin value less than 30 ng/mL (67 pmol/L) indicates coexistent iron deficiency. Classic anemia of inflammation has elevated hepcidin levels; however, no clinical test is yet available. In the anemias of organ failure and of the elderly, the iron studies are generally normal. The anemia of the elderly is a diagnosis of exclusion in a patient with anemia who is over age 65 years.

A particular challenge is the diagnosis of iron deficiency in the setting of the anemia of inflammation in which the serum ferritin can be as high as 200 ng/mL (450 pmol/L). The diagnosis is established by a bone marrow biopsy with iron stain. Absent iron staining indicates iron deficiency, whereas iron localized in marrow macrophages indicates pure anemia of inflammation. However, bone marrow biopsies are rarely done for this purpose. Three other tests all support iron deficiency in the setting of inflammation: a reticulocyte hemoglobin concentration of less than 28 pg; a normal hepcidin level; or a soluble serum transferrin receptor (units: mg/L) to log ferritin (units: mcg/L) ratio of 1–8 (a ratio of less than 1 is virtually diagnostic of pure anemia of chronic disease). A functional test is hemoglobin response to oral or parenteral iron in the setting of inflammation when iron deficiency is suspected. A note of caution: certain circumstances of iron-restricted erythropoiesis (such as malignancy) will partially respond to parenteral iron infusion even when the iron stores are replete due to the immediate distribution of iron to erythropoietic progenitor cells after the infusion.

Treatment

In most cases, no treatment of the anemia is necessary and the primary management is to address the condition causing the anemia of chronic disease. When the anemia is severe or is adversely affecting the quality of life or functional status, then treatment involves either red blood cell transfusions or parenteral recombinant erythropoietin (epoetin alfa or darbepoetin). The indications for recombinant erythropoietin are hemoglobin less than 10 g/dL and anemia due to rheumatoid arthritis, inflammatory bowel disease, hepatitis C, zidovudine therapy in HIV-infected patients, myelosuppressive chemotherapy of solid malignancy (treated with palliative intent only), or chronic kidney disease (estimated glomerular filtration rate of less than 60 mL/min). The dosing and schedule of recombinant erythropoietin are individualized to maintain the hemoglobin between 10 g/dL (100 g/L) and 12 g/dL (120 g/L). The use of recombinant erythropoietin is associated with an increased risk of venothromboembolism and arterial thrombotic episodes, especially if the hemoglobin rises to greater than 12 g/dL (120 g/L). There is concern that recombinant erythropoietin is associated with reduced survival in patients with malignancy. For patients with end-stage renal disease receiving recombinant erythropoietin who are on hemodialysis, the anemia of chronic kidney disease can be more effectively corrected by adding soluble ferric pyrophosphate to their dialysate than by administering intravenous iron supplementation.

▶ When to Refer

Referral to a hematologist is not necessary.

Ganz T et al. Hepcidin and disorders of iron metabolism. Annu Rev Med. 2011;62:347–60. [PMID: 20887198]

Gaspar BL et al. Anemia in malignancies: pathogenetic and diagnostic considerations. Hematology. 2015 Jan;20(1): 18–25. [PMID: 24666207]

Nemeth E et al. Anemia of inflammation. Hematol Oncol Clin North Am. 2014 Aug;28(4):671–81. [PMID: 25064707]

Pang WW et al. Anemia in the elderly. Curr Opin Hematol. 2012 May;19(3):133–40. [PMID: 22495692]

Poggiali E et al. Anemia of chronic disease: a unique defect of iron recycling for many different chronic diseases. Eur J Intern Med. 2014 Jan;25(1):12–7. [PMID: 23988263]

Vanasse GJ et al. Anemia in elderly patients: an emerging problem for the 21st century. Hematology Am Soc Hematol Educ Program. 2010;2010:271–5. [PMID: 21239805]

THE THALASSEMIAS

ESSENTIALS OF DIAGNOSIS

▶ Microcytosis disproportionate to the degree of anemia.

▶ Positive family history.

▶ Lifelong personal history of microcytic anemia.

▶ Normal or elevated red blood cell count.

▶ Abnormal red blood cell morphology with microcytes, hypochromia, acanthocytes, and target cells.

▶ In beta-thalassemia, elevated levels of hemoglobin A_2 or F.

▶ General Considerations

The thalassemias are hereditary disorders characterized by reduction in the synthesis of globin chains (alpha or beta). Reduced globin chain synthesis causes reduced hemoglobin synthesis and a hypochromic microcytic anemia because of defective hemoglobinization of red blood cells. Thalassemias can be considered among the hyperproliferative hemolytic anemias, the anemias related to abnormal hemoglobin, and the hypoproliferative anemias, since all of these factors play a role in pathogenesis. The hallmark laboratory features are small (low MCV) and pale (low mean corpuscular hemoglobin [MCH]) red blood cells, anemia, and a normal to elevated red blood cell count (ie, a large number of the small and pale red blood cells are being produced). Although patients often exhibit an elevated reticulocyte count, generally the degree of reticulocyte output is inadequate to meet the degree of red blood cell destruction (hemolysis) occurring in the bone marrow and the patients remain anemic.

Normal adult hemoglobin is primarily hemoglobin A, which represents approximately 98% of circulating hemoglobin. Hemoglobin A is formed from a tetramer of two alpha chains and two beta chains—and is designated alpha-2beta2. Two copies of the alpha-globin gene are located on each chromosome 16, and there is no substitute for alpha-globin in the formation of adult hemoglobin. One copy of the beta-globin gene resides on each chromosome 11 adjacent to genes encoding the beta-like globins delta and gamma (the so-called beta-globin gene cluster region). The tetramer of alpha2delta2 forms hemoglobin A_2, which normally comprises 1–3% of adult hemoglobin. The tetramer alpha2gamma2 forms hemoglobin F, which is the major hemoglobin of fetal life but which comprises less than 1% of normal adult hemoglobin.

The thalassemias are described as **"trait"** when there are laboratory features without significant clinical impact, **"intermedia"** when there is an occasional red blood cell transfusion requirement or other moderate clinical impact, and **"major"** when the disorder is life-threatening and the patient is transfusion-dependent. Most patients with thalassemia major die of the consequences of iron overload from RBC transfusions.

Alpha-thalassemia is due primarily to gene deletions causing reduced alpha-globin chain synthesis (Table 13–4). Each alpha-globin gene produces one-quarter of the total alpha-globin quantity, so there is a predictable proportionate decrease in alpha-globin output with each lost alpha-globin gene. Since all adult hemoglobins are alpha containing, alpha-thalassemia produces no change in the proportions of hemoglobins A, A_2, and F on hemoglobin electrophoresis. In severe forms of alpha-thalassemia, excess beta chains may form a beta-4 tetramer called hemoglobin H. In the presence of reduced alpha chains, the excess beta chains are unstable and precipitate, leading to damage of red blood cell membranes. This leads to both intramedullary (bone marrow) and peripheral blood hemolysis.

Beta-thalassemias are usually caused by point mutations rather than deletions (Table 13–5). These mutations result in premature chain termination or in problems with transcription of RNA and ultimately result in reduced or absent beta-globin chain synthesis. The molecular defects leading to beta-thalassemia are numerous and heterogeneous. Defects that result in absent beta-globin chain expression are termed beta[0], whereas those causing reduced but not absent synthesis are termed beta[+]. In beta[+] thalassemia, the degree of reduction of beta-globin synthesis is consistent within families but is quite variable between families. The reduced beta-globin chain synthesis in beta-thalassemia results in a relative increase in the proportions of hemoglobins A_2 and F compared to hemoglobin A on hemoglobin electrophoresis, as the beta-like globins (delta and gamma) substitute for the missing beta chains. In the presence of reduced beta chains, the excess alpha chains are unstable and precipitate, leading to damage of red blood cell membranes. This leads to both intramedullary (bone marrow) and peripheral blood hemolysis. The bone marrow demonstrates erythroid hyperplasia under the stimuli of anemia and ineffective erythropoiesis (intramedullary destruction of the developing erythroid cells). In cases of severe thalassemia, the marked expansion of the erythroid compartment in the bone marrow may cause severe bony deformities, osteopenia, and pathologic bone fractures.

Table 13–4. Alpha-thalassemia syndromes.

Number of Alpha-globin Genes Transcribed	Syndrome	Hematocrit	MCV
4	Normal	Normal	Normal
3	Silent carrier	Normal	Normal
2	Thalassemia minor (or trait)	28–40%	60–75 fL
1	Hemoglobin H disease	22–32%	60–70 fL
0	Hydrops fetalis[1]	< 18%	< 60 fL

[1]Die in utero.
MCV, mean corpuscular volume.

Table 13–5. Beta-thalassemia syndromes.

	Beta-Globin Genes Transcribed	Hb A	Hb A_2	Hb F	Transfusions
Normal	Homozygous beta	97–99%	1–3%	< 1%	
Thalassemia minor	Heterozygous beta[0]	80–95%	4–8%	1–5%	None
	Heterozygous beta[+]	80–95%	4–8%	1–5%	None
Thalassemia intermedia	Homozygous beta[+] (mild)	0–30%	0–10%	6–100%	Occasional
Thalassemia major	Homozygous beta[0]	0%	4–10%	90–96%	Dependent
Thalassemia major	Homozygous beta[+]	0–10%	4–10%	90–96%	Dependent

Hb, hemoglobin.

▶ Clinical Findings

A. Symptoms and Signs

The **alpha-thalassemia** syndromes are seen primarily in persons from southeast Asia and China, and, less commonly, in blacks and persons of Mediterranean origin (Table 13–4). Normally, adults have four copies of the alpha-globin chain. When three alpha-globin genes are present, the patient is hematologically normal (silent carrier). When two alpha-globin genes are present, the patient is said to have alpha-thalassemia trait, a form of thalassemia minor. In alpha-thalassemia-1 trait, the alpha gene deletion is heterozygous (alpha –/alpha –) and affects mainly those of Asian descent. In alpha-thalassemia-2 trait, the alpha gene deletion is homozygous (alpha alpha/– –) and affects mainly blacks. These patients are clinically normal and have a normal life expectancy and performance status, with a mild microcytic anemia. When only one alpha globin chain is present (alpha –/– –), the patient has hemoglobin H disease (alpha-thalassemia-3). This is a chronic hemolytic anemia of variable severity (thalassemia minor or intermedia). Physical examination might reveal pallor and splenomegaly. Affected individuals usually do not need transfusions; however, they may be required during transient periods of hemolytic exacerbation caused by infection or other stressors or during periods of erythropoietic shutdown caused by certain viruses ("aplastic crisis"). When all four alpha-globin genes are deleted, no normal hemoglobin is produced and the affected fetus is stillborn (hydrops fetalis). In hydrops fetalis, the only hemoglobin species gamma made is called hemoglobin Bart's (gamma4).

Beta-thalassemia primarily affects persons of Mediterranean origin (Italian, Greek) and to a lesser extent Asians and blacks (Table 13–5). Patients homozygous for beta-thalassemia (beta⁰/beta⁰ or some with beta⁺/beta⁺) have thalassemia major (Cooley anemia). Affected children are normal at birth but after 6 months, when hemoglobin synthesis switches from hemoglobin F to hemoglobin A, severe anemia requiring transfusion develops. Numerous clinical problems ensue, including stunted growth, bony deformities (abnormal facial structure, pathologic bone fractures), hepatosplenomegaly, jaundice (due to gallstones, hepatitis-related cirrhosis, or both), and thrombophilia. The clinical course is modified significantly by transfusion therapy, but transfusional iron overload (hemosiderosis) results in a clinical picture similar to hemochromatosis, with heart failure, cardiac arrhythmias, cirrhosis, endocrinopathies, and pseudoxanthoma elasticum (calcification and fragmentation of the elastic fibers of the skin, retina, and cardiovascular system), usually after more than 100 units of red blood cells have been transfused. Iron overloading occurs because the human body has no active iron excretory mechanism. Before the application of allogeneic stem cell transplantation and the development of more effective forms of iron chelation, death from iron overload usually occurred between the ages of 20 and 30 years.

Patients homozygous for a milder form of beta-thalassemia (beta⁺/beta⁺, but allowing a higher rate of beta-globin synthesis) have thalassemia intermedia. These patients have chronic hemolytic anemia but do not require transfusions except under periods of stress or during aplastic crises. They also may develop iron overload because of periodic transfusion. They survive into adult life but with hepatosplenomegaly and bony deformities. Patients heterozygous for beta-thalassemia (beta/beta⁰ or beta/beta⁺) have thalassemia minor and a clinically insignificant microcytic anemia.

Prenatal diagnosis is available, and genetic counseling should be offered and the opportunity for prenatal diagnosis discussed.

B. Laboratory Findings

1. Alpha-thalassemia trait—These patients have mild anemia, with hematocrits between 28% and 40%. The MCV is strikingly low (60–75 fL) despite the modest anemia, and the red blood count is normal or increased. The peripheral blood smear shows microcytes, hypochromia, occasional target cells, and acanthocytes (cells with irregularly spaced spiked projections). The reticulocyte count and iron parameters are normal. Hemoglobin electrophoresis is normal. Alpha-thalassemia trait is thus usually diagnosed by exclusion. Genetic testing to demonstrate alpha-globin gene deletion is available only in a limited number of laboratories.

2. Hemoglobin H disease—These patients have a more marked anemia, with hematocrits between 22% and 32%. The MCV is remarkably low (60–70 fL) and the peripheral blood smear is markedly abnormal, with hypochromia, microcytosis, target cells, and poikilocytosis. The reticulocyte count is elevated and the red blood cell count is normal or elevated. Hemoglobin electrophoresis will show a fast migrating hemoglobin (hemoglobin H), which comprises 10–40% of the hemoglobin. A peripheral blood smear can be stained with supravital dyes to demonstrate the presence of hemoglobin H.

3. Beta-thalassemia minor—These patients have a modest anemia with hematocrit between 28% and 40%. The MCV ranges from 55 fL to 75 fL, and the red blood cell count is normal or increased. The reticulocyte count is normal or slightly elevated. The peripheral blood smear is mildly abnormal, with hypochromia, microcytosis, and target cells. In contrast to alpha-thalassemia, basophilic stippling is present. Hemoglobin electrophoresis shows an elevation of hemoglobin A₂ to 4–8% and occasional elevations of hemoglobin F to 1–5%.

4. Beta-thalassemia intermedia—These patients have a modest anemia with hematocrit between 17% and 33%. The MCV ranges from 55 fL to 75 fL, and the red blood cell count is normal or increased. The reticulocyte count is elevated. The peripheral blood smear is abnormal with hypochromia, microcytosis, basophilic stippling, and target cells. Hemoglobin electrophoresis shows up to 30% hemoglobin A, an elevation of hemoglobin A₂ up to 10%, and elevation of hemoglobin F from 6% to 100%.

5. Beta-thalassemia major—These patients have severe anemia, and without transfusion the hematocrit may fall to less than 10%. The peripheral blood smear is bizarre, showing severe poikilocytosis, hypochromia, microcytosis, target cells, basophilic stippling, and nucleated red blood cells.

Little or no hemoglobin A is present. Variable amounts of hemoglobin A$_2$ are seen, and the predominant hemoglobin present is hemoglobin F.

▶ Differential Diagnosis

Mild forms of thalassemia must be differentiated from iron deficiency. Compared to iron deficiency anemia, patients with thalassemia have a lower MCV, a normal or elevated red blood cell count (rather than low), a more abnormal peripheral blood smear at modest levels of anemia, and usually a reticulocytosis. Iron studies are normal or the transferrin saturation or ferritin (or both) are elevated. Severe forms of thalassemia may be confused with other hemoglobinopathies. The diagnosis of beta-thalassemia is made by the above findings and hemoglobin electrophoresis showing elevated levels of hemoglobins A$_2$ and F (provided the patient is replete in iron), but the diagnosis of alpha-thalassemia is made by exclusion since there is no change in the proportion of the normal adult hemoglobin species. The only other microcytic anemia with a normal or elevated red blood cell count is iron deficiency in a patient with polycythemia vera.

▶ Treatment

Patients with mild thalassemia (alpha-thalassemia trait or beta-thalassemia minor) require no treatment and should be identified so that they will not be subjected to repeated evaluations and treatment for iron deficiency. Patients with hemoglobin H disease should take folic acid supplementation (1 mg/day orally) and avoid medicinal iron and oxidative drugs such as sulfonamides. Patients with severe thalassemia are maintained on a regular transfusion schedule (in part to suppress endogenous erythropoiesis and therefore bone marrow expansion) and receive folic acid supplementation. Splenectomy is performed if hypersplenism causes a marked increase in the transfusion requirement or refractory symptoms. Patients with regular transfusion requirements should be treated with iron chelation (oral or parenteral) in order to prevent life-limiting organ damage from iron overload.

Allogeneic stem cell transplantation is the treatment of choice for beta-thalassemia major and the only available cure. Children who have not yet experienced organ damage from iron overload do well, with long-term survival in more than 80% of cases.

▶ When to Refer

All patients with severe thalassemia should be referred to a hematologist. Any patient with an unexplained microcytic anemia should be referred to help establish a diagnosis. Patients with thalassemia minor or intermedia should be referred for genetic counseling because offspring of thalassemic couples are at risk for inheriting thalassemia major.

Fisher SA et al. Desferrioxamine mesylate for managing transfusional iron overload in people with transfusion-dependent thalassemia. Cochrane Database Syst Rev. 2013 Aug 21; 8:CD004450. [PMID: 23963793]

Goss C et al. Red blood cell transfusions for thalassemia: results of a survey assessing current practice and proposal of evidence-based guidelines. Transfusion. 2014 Jul;54(7):1773–81. [PMID: 24611697]

King A et al. Evidence-based focused review of the status of hematopoietic stem cell transplantation as treatment of sickle cell disease and thalassemia. Blood. 2014 May 15;123(20): 3089–94. [PMID: 24511087]

Mathews V et al. Allogeneic stem cell transplantation for thalassemia major. Hematol Oncol Clin North Am. 2014 Dec;28(6): 1187–200. [PMID: 25459187]

Piel FB et al. The α-thalassemias. N Engl J Med. 2014 Nov 3; 371(20):1908–16. [PMID: 25390741]

VITAMIN B$_{12}$ DEFICIENCY

▶ ESSENTIALS OF DIAGNOSIS

- ▶ Macrocytic anemia.
- ▶ Megaloblastic blood smear (macro-ovalocytes and hypersegmented neutrophils).
- ▶ Low serum vitamin B$_{12}$ level.

▶ General Considerations

Vitamin B$_{12}$ belongs to the family of cobalamins and serves as a cofactor for two important reactions in humans. As methylcobalamin, it is a cofactor for methionine synthetase in the conversion of homocysteine to methionine, and as adenosylcobalamin for the conversion of methylmalonyl-coenzyme A (CoA) to succinyl-CoA. These enzymatic steps are critical for annealing Okazaki fragments during DNA synthesis, particularly in erythroid progenitor cells. Vitamin B$_{12}$ comes from the diet and is present in all foods of animal origin. The daily absorption of vitamin B$_{12}$ is 5 mcg.

The liver contains 2–5 mg of stored vitamin B$_{12}$. Since daily utilization is 3–5 mcg, the body usually has sufficient stores of vitamin B$_{12}$ so that it takes more than 3 years for vitamin B$_{12}$ deficiency to occur if all intake or absorption immediately ceases.

Since vitamin B$_{12}$ is present in foods of animal origin, dietary vitamin B$_{12}$ deficiency is extremely rare but is seen in vegans—strict vegetarians who avoid all dairy products, meat, and fish (Table 13–6). Pernicious anemia is an autoimmune illness whereby autoantibodies destroy gastric parietal cells (that produce intrinsic factor) and cause atrophic gastritis or bind to and neutralize intrinsic factor, or both. Abdominal surgery may lead to vitamin B$_{12}$ deficiency in several ways. Gastrectomy will eliminate the site of intrinsic factor production; blind loop syndrome will cause competition for vitamin B$_{12}$ by bacterial overgrowth in the lumen of the intestine; and surgical resection of the ileum will eliminate the site of vitamin B$_{12}$ absorption. Rare causes of vitamin B$_{12}$ deficiency include fish tapeworm (*Diphyllobothrium latum*) infection, in which the parasite uses luminal vitamin B$_{12}$; pancreatic insufficiency (with failure to inactivate competing cobalamin-binding proteins

Table 13–6. Causes of vitamin B_{12} deficiency.

Dietary deficiency (rare)
Decreased production or neutralization of intrinsic factor
   Pernicious anemia (autoimmune)
   Gastrectomy
   Helicobacter pylori infection
Competition for vitamin B_{12} in gut
   Blind loop syndrome
   Fish tapeworm (rare)
Pancreatic insufficiency
Decreased ileal absorption of vitamin B_{12}
   Surgical resection
   Crohn disease
Transcobalamin II deficiency (rare)

[R-factors]); and severe Crohn disease, causing sufficient destruction of the ileum to impair vitamin B_{12} absorption.

▶ Clinical Findings

A. Symptoms and Signs

Vitamin B_{12} deficiency causes a moderate to severe anemia of slow onset; patients may have few symptoms relative to the degree of anemia. In advanced cases, the anemia may be severe, with hematocrits as low as 10–15%, and may be accompanied by leukopenia and thrombocytopenia. The deficiency also produces changes in mucosal cells, leading to glossitis, as well as other vague gastrointestinal disturbances such as anorexia and diarrhea. Vitamin B_{12} deficiency also leads to a complex neurologic syndrome. Peripheral nerves are usually affected first, and patients complain initially of paresthesias. As the posterior columns of the spinal cord become impaired, patients complain of difficulty with balance or proprioception, or both. In more advanced cases, cerebral function may be altered as well, and on occasion dementia and other neuropsychiatric abnormalities may be present. It is critical to recognize that the non-hematologic manifestations of vitamin B_{12} deficiency can be manifest despite a completely normal complete blood count.

Patients are usually pale and may be mildly icteric or sallow. Typically later in the disease course, neurologic examination may reveal decreased vibration and position sense or memory disturbance (or both).

B. Laboratory Findings

The diagnosis of vitamin B_{12} deficiency is made by finding a low serum vitamin B_{12} (cobalamin) level. Whereas the normal vitamin B_{12} level is greater than 210 pg/mL (155 pmol/L), most patients with overt vitamin B_{12} deficiency have serum levels less than 170 pg/mL (126 pmol/L), with symptomatic patients usually having levels less than 100 pg/mL (74 pmol/L). The diagnosis of vitamin B_{12} deficiency in low or low-normal values (level of 170–210 pg/mL [126–155 pmol/L]) is best confirmed by finding an elevated level of serum methylmalonic acid (greater than 1000 nmol/L) or homocysteine. Of note, elevated levels of serum methylmalonic acid can be due to kidney disease.

The anemia of vitamin B_{12} deficiency is typically moderate to severe with the MCV quite elevated (110–140 fL). However, it is possible to have vitamin B_{12} deficiency with a normal MCV from coexistent thalassemia or iron deficiency; in other cases, the reason is obscure. Patients with neurologic symptoms and signs that suggest possible vitamin B_{12} deficiency should be evaluated for that deficiency despite a normal MCV or the absence of anemia. The peripheral blood smear is megaloblastic, defined as red blood cells that appear as macro-ovalocytes, (although other shape changes are usually present) and neutrophils that are hypersegmented (six [or greater]-lobed neutrophils or mean neutrophil lobe counts greater than four). The reticulocyte count is reduced. Because vitamin B_{12} deficiency can affect all hematopoietic cell lines, the white blood cell count and the platelet count are reduced in severe cases.

Other laboratory abnormalities include elevated serum lactate dehydrogenase (LD) and a modest increase in indirect bilirubin. These two findings are a reflection of intramedullary destruction of developing abnormal erythroid cells and are similar to those observed in peripheral hemolytic anemias.

Bone marrow morphology is characteristically abnormal. Marked erythroid hyperplasia is present as a response to defective red blood cell production (ineffective erythropoiesis). Megaloblastic changes in the erythroid series include abnormally large cell size and asynchronous maturation of the nucleus and cytoplasm—ie, cytoplasmic maturation continues while impaired DNA synthesis causes retarded nuclear development. In the myeloid series, giant bands and meta-myelocytes are characteristically seen.

▶ Differential Diagnosis

Vitamin B_{12} deficiency should be differentiated from folic acid deficiency, the other common cause of megaloblastic anemia, in which red blood cell folic acid is low while vitamin B_{12} levels are normal. The bone marrow findings of vitamin B_{12} deficiency are sometimes mistaken for a myelodysplastic syndrome or even acute erythrocytic leukemia. The distinction between vitamin B_{12} deficiency and myelodysplasia is based on the characteristic morphology and the low vitamin B_{12} and elevated methylmalonic acid levels.

▶ Treatment

Patients with vitamin B_{12} deficiency are usually treated with parenteral therapy. Intramuscular or subcutaneous injections of 100 mcg of vitamin B_{12} are adequate for each dose. Replacement is usually given daily for the first week, weekly for the first month, and then monthly for life. The vitamin deficiency will recur if patients discontinue their therapy. Oral or sublingual methylcobalamin (1 mg/day) may be used instead of parenteral therapy once initial correction of the deficiency has occurred. Oral or sublingual replacement is effective, even in pernicious anemia, since approximately 1% of the dose is absorbed in the intestine via passive diffusion in the absence of active transport. It must be continued indefinitely and serum vitamin B_{12}

levels must be monitored to ensure adequate replacement. For patients with neurologic symptoms caused by vitamin B_{12} deficiency, long-term parenteral vitamin B_{12} therapy is prudent. Because many patients are concurrently folic acid deficient from intestinal mucosal atrophy, simultaneous folic acid replacement (1 mg daily) is recommended for the first several months of vitamin B_{12} replacement.

Patients respond to therapy with an immediate improvement in their sense of well-being. Hypokalemia may complicate the first several days of therapy, particularly if the anemia is severe. A brisk reticulocytosis occurs in 5–7 days, and the hematologic picture normalizes in 2 months. Central nervous system symptoms and signs are reversible if they are of relatively short duration (less than 6 months) but are likely permanent if of longer duration. Red blood cell transfusions are rarely needed despite the severity of anemia, but when given, diuretics are also recommended to avoid heart failure because this anemia develops slowly and the plasma volume is increased.

▶ When to Refer

Referral to a hematologist is not usually necessary.

Bunn HF. Vitamin B_{12} and pernicious anemia—the dawn of molecular medicine. N Engl J Med. 2014 Feb 20;370(8): 773–6. [PMID: 24552327]

Shipton MJ et al. Vitamin B_{12} deficiency—a 21st century perspective. Clin Med (Lond). 2015 Apr;15(2):145–50. [PMID: 25824066]

Stabler SP. Clinical practice. Vitamin B_{12} deficiency. N Engl J Med. 2013 Jan 10;368(2):149–60. [PMID: 23301732]

FOLIC ACID DEFICIENCY

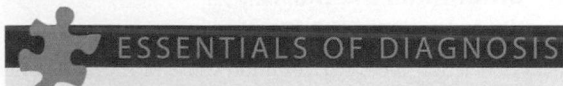

ESSENTIALS OF DIAGNOSIS

▶ Macrocytic anemia.

▶ Megaloblastic blood smear (macro-ovalocytes and hypersegmented neutrophils).

▶ Reduced folic acid levels in red blood cells or serum.

▶ Normal serum vitamin B_{12} level.

▶ General Considerations

Folic acid is the term commonly used for pteroylmonoglutamic acid. Folic acid is present in most fruits and vegetables (especially citrus fruits and green leafy vegetables). Daily dietary requirements are 50–100 mcg. Total body stores of folic acid are approximately 5 mg, enough to supply requirements for 2–3 months.

The most common cause of folic acid deficiency is inadequate dietary intake (Table 13–7). Alcoholic or anorectic patients, persons who do not eat fresh fruits and vegetables, and those who overcook their food are candidates for folic acid deficiency. Reduced folic acid absorption is rarely seen, since absorption occurs from the entire gastrointestinal tract. However, drugs such as phenytoin,

Table 13–7. Causes of folic acid deficiency.

Dietary deficiency
Decreased absorption
Tropical sprue
Drugs: phenytoin, sulfasalazine, trimethoprim-sulfamethoxazole
Concurrent vitamin B_{12} deficiency
Increased requirement
Chronic hemolytic anemia
Pregnancy
Exfoliative skin disease
Excess loss: hemodialysis
Inhibition of reduction to active form
Methotrexate

trimethoprim-sulfamethoxazole, or sulfasalazine may interfere with its absorption. Folic acid absorption is poor in some patients with vitamin B_{12} deficiency due to gastrointestinal mucosal atrophy. Folic acid requirements are increased in pregnancy, hemolytic anemia, and exfoliative skin disease, and in these cases the increased requirements (five to ten times normal) may not be met by a normal diet.

▶ Clinical Findings

A. Symptoms and Signs

The clinical features are similar to those of vitamin B_{12} deficiency. However, isolated folic acid deficiency does not result in the neurologic abnormalities of vitamin B_{12} deficiency.

B. Laboratory Findings

Megaloblastic anemia is identical to anemia resulting from vitamin B_{12} deficiency. A red blood cell folic acid level below 150 ng/mL (340 nmol/L) is diagnostic of folic acid deficiency. Whether to order a serum or a red blood cell folate level remains unsettled since there are few, if any, data to support one test over the other. Usually the serum vitamin B_{12} level is normal, and it should always be measured when folic acid deficiency is suspected. In some instances, folic acid deficiency is a consequence of the gastrointestinal mucosal megaloblastosis from vitamin B_{12} deficiency.

▶ Differential Diagnosis

The megaloblastic anemia of folic acid deficiency should be differentiated from vitamin B_{12} deficiency by the finding of a normal vitamin B_{12} level and a reduced red blood cell (or serum) folic acid level. Alcoholic patients, who often have nutritional deficiency, may also have anemia of liver disease. Anemia of liver disease causes a macrocytic anemia but does not produce megaloblastic morphologic changes in the peripheral blood; rather, target cells are present. Hypothyroidism is associated with mild macrocytosis and also with pernicious anemia.

▶ Treatment

Folic acid deficiency is treated with daily oral folic acid (1 mg). The response is similar to that seen in the treatment of vitamin B_{12} deficiency, with rapid improvement and a sense of well-being, reticulocytosis in 5–7 days, and total correction of hematologic abnormalities within 2 months. Large doses of folic acid may produce hematologic responses in cases of vitamin B_{12} deficiency but permit neurologic damage to progress; hence, obtaining a serum vitamin B_{12} level in suspected folic acid deficiency is paramount.

► When to Refer

Referral to a hematologist is not usually necessary.

Farrell CJ et al. Red cell or serum folate: what to do in clinical practice. Clin Chem Lab Med. 2013 Mar 1;51(3):555–69. [PMID: 23449524]

Gilfix BM. Utility of measuring serum or red blood cell folate in the era of folate fortification of flour. Clin Biochem. 2014 May;47(7–8):533–8. [PMID: 24486651]

Green R. Indicators for assessing folate and vitamin B-12 status and for monitoring the efficacy of intervention strategies. Am J Clin Nutr. 2011 Aug;94(2):666S–72S. [PMID: 21733877]

HEMOLYTIC ANEMIAS

The hemolytic anemias are a group of disorders in which red blood cell survival is reduced, either episodically or continuously. The bone marrow has the ability to increase erythroid production up to eightfold in response to reduced red cell survival, so anemia will be present only when the ability of the bone marrow to compensate is outstripped. This will occur when red cell survival is extremely short or when the ability of the bone marrow to compensate is impaired.

Hemolytic disorders are generally classified according to whether the defect is intrinsic to the red cell or due to some external factor (Table 13–8). Intrinsic defects have been described in all components of the red blood cell, including the membrane, enzyme systems, and hemoglobin; most of these disorders are hereditary. Hemolytic anemias due to external factors are immune and microangiopathic hemolytic anemias and infections of red blood cells.

Certain laboratory features are common to all hemolytic anemias. Haptoglobin, a normal plasma protein that binds and clears free hemoglobin released into plasma, may be depressed in hemolytic disorders. However, the haptoglobin level is influenced by many factors and is not always a reliable indicator of hemolysis, particularly in end-stage liver disease (its site of synthesis). When intravascular hemolysis occurs, transient hemoglobinemia ensues. Hemoglobin is filtered through the glomerulus and is usually reabsorbed by tubular cells. Hemoglobinuria will be present only when the capacity for reabsorption of hemoglobin by renal tubular cells is exceeded. In the absence of hemoglobinuria, evidence for prior intravascular hemolysis is the presence of hemosiderin in shed renal tubular cells (positive urine hemosiderin). With severe intravascular hemolysis, hemoglobinemia and methemalbuminemia may be present. Hemolysis increases the indirect bilirubin, and the total bilirubin may rise to 4 mg/dL (68 mcmol/L). Bilirubin levels higher than this may indicate some degree of hepatic dysfunction. Serum LD levels are strikingly elevated in cases of microangiopathic hemolysis (thrombotic thrombocytopenic purpura, hemolytic-uremic syndrome) and may be elevated in other hemolytic anemias.

PAROXYSMAL NOCTURNAL HEMOGLOBINURIA

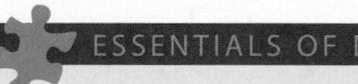
ESSENTIALS OF DIAGNOSIS

► Episodic hemoglobinuria.

► Thrombosis is common.

► Suspect in confusing cases of hemolytic anemia or pancytopenia.

► Flow cytometry demonstrates deficiencies of CD55 and CD59.

► General Considerations

Paroxysmal nocturnal hemoglobinuria (PNH) is a rare acquired clonal hematopoietic stem cell disorder that results in abnormal sensitivity of the red blood cell membrane to lysis by complement. Free hemoglobin is released into the blood that scavenges nitric oxide and promotes esophageal spasms, male erectile dysfunction, renal damage, and thrombosis. Patients with significant PNH live about 10–15 years following diagnosis; thrombosis is the primary cause of death.

► Clinical Findings

A. Symptoms and Signs

Classically, patients report episodic hemoglobinuria resulting in reddish-brown urine. Hemoglobinuria is most often

Table 13–8. Classification of hemolytic anemias.

Intrinsic
  Membrane defects: hereditary spherocytosis, hereditary elliptocytosis, paroxysmal nocturnal hemoglobinuria
  Glycolytic defects: pyruvate kinase deficiency, severe hypophosphatemia
  Oxidation vulnerability: glucose-6-phosphate dehydrogenase deficiency, methemoglobinemia
  Hemoglobinopathies: sickle cell syndromes, thalassemia, unstable hemoglobins, methemoglobinemia

Extrinsic
  Immune: autoimmune, lymphoproliferative disease, drug-induced
  Microangiopathic: thrombotic thrombocytopenic purpura, hemolytic-uremic syndrome, disseminated intravascular coagulation, valve hemolysis, metastatic adenocarcinoma, vasculitis, copper overload
  Infection: *Plasmodium*, *Clostridium*, *Borrelia*
  Hypersplenism
  Burns

noticed in the first morning urine due to the drop in blood pH while sleeping that facilitates this hemolysis. Besides anemia, these patients are prone to thrombosis, especially within mesenteric and hepatic veins, central nervous system veins (sagittal vein), and skin vessels (with formation of painful nodules). As this is a hematopoietic stem cell disorder, PNH may appear de novo or arise in the setting of aplastic anemia with possible progression to myelodysplasia or acute myeloid leukemia (AML).

B. Laboratory Findings

Anemia is of variable severity and frequency, so reticulocytosis may or may not be present at any given time. Abnormalities on the blood smear are nondiagnostic and may include macro-ovalocytes and polychromasia. Since the episodic hemolysis is mainly intravascular, urine hemosiderin is a useful test. Serum LD is characteristically elevated. Iron deficiency is commonly present, related to chronic iron loss from hemoglobinuria.

The white blood cell count and platelet count may be decreased and are always decreased in the setting of aplastic anemia. The best screening test is flow cytometry of blood granulocytes to demonstrate deficiency of CD55 and CD59. The FLAER assay (fluorescein-labeled proaerolysin) by flow cytometry is even more sensitive. Bone marrow morphology is variable and may show either generalized hypoplasia or erythroid hyperplasia or both. The bone marrow karyotype may be either normal or demonstrate a clonal abnormality.

▶ Treatment

Most patients with PNH have mild disease not requiring intervention. In severe cases and in those occurring in the setting of aplastic anemia or myelodysplasia, allogeneic hematopoietic stem cell transplantation has been used. In patients with severe hemolysis (usually requiring red cell transfusions), or thrombosis, treatment with eculizumab is warranted. Eculizumab is a humanized monoclonal antibody against complement protein C5—binding C5 prevents its cleavage so the membrane attack complex cannot assemble. Eculizumab improves quality of life and reduces hemolysis, transfusion requirements, and thrombosis risk. Eculizumab is expensive and increases the risk of *Neisseria meningitidis* infections; patients receiving the antibody must undergo meningococcal vaccination. Iron replacement is indicated for treatment of iron deficiency when present, which may improve the anemia while also causing a transient increase in hemolysis. For unclear reasons, corticosteroids are effective in decreasing hemolysis.

▶ When to Refer

Most patients with PNH should be under the care of a hematologist.

Brodsky RA. Paroxysmal nocturnal hemoglobinuria. Blood. 2014 Oct 30;124(18):2804–11. [PMID: 25237200]
Hill A et al. Thrombosis in paroxysmal nocturnal hemoglobinuria. Blood. 2013 Jan 20;121(25):4985–96. [PMID: 23610373]

Keating GM et al. Eculizumab: a guide to its use in paroxysmal nocturnal hemoglobinuria. BioDrugs. 2012 Apr 1;26(2):125–30. [PMID: 22350448]
Martí-Carvajal AJ et al. Eculizumab for treating patients with paroxysmal nocturnal hemoglobinuria. Cochrane Database Syst Rev. 2014 Oct 30;10:CD010340. [PMID: 25356860]
Parker CJ. Paroxysmal nocturnal hemoglobinuria. Curr Opin Hematol. 2012 May;19(3):141–8. [PMID: 22395662]

GLUCOSE-6-PHOSPHATE DEHYDROGENASE DEFICIENCY

ESSENTIALS OF DIAGNOSIS

- ▶ X-linked recessive disorder seen commonly in American black men.
- ▶ Episodic hemolysis in response to oxidant drugs or infection.
- ▶ Bite cells and blister cells on the peripheral blood smear.
- ▶ Reduced levels of glucose-6-phosphate dehydrogenase between hemolytic episodes.

▶ General Considerations

Glucose-6-phosphate dehydrogenase (G6PD) deficiency is a hereditary enzyme defect that causes episodic hemolytic anemia because of the decreased ability of red blood cells to deal with oxidative stresses. G6PD deficiency leads to excess oxidized glutathione (hence, inadequate levels of reduced glutathione) that forces hemoglobin to denature and form precipitants called Heinz bodies. Heinz bodies cause red blood cell membrane damage, which leads to premature removal of these red blood cells by reticuloendothelial cells within the spleen (extravascular hemolysis).

Numerous G6PD isoenzymes have been described. The usual isoenzyme found in whites is designated G6PD-B and that in American blacks is designated G6PD-A, both of which have normal function and stability and therefore no hemolytic anemia. Ten to 15 percent of American blacks have the variant G6PD isoenzyme designated A–, in which there is both a reduction in normal enzyme activity and a reduction in stability. The A– isoenzyme activity declines rapidly as the red blood cell ages past 40 days, a fact that explains the clinical findings in this disorder. More than 150 G6PD isoenzyme variants have been described, including some Mediterranean, Ashkenazi Jewish, and Asian variants with very low enzyme activity, episodic hemolysis, and exacerbations due to oxidizing substances including fava beans (class II G6PD activity). The other classes of G6PD isoenzyme activity are class I, extremely low activity with associated chronic, severe hemolysis; class III, 10–60% activity with episodic hemolysis (includes the American black A– isoform); class IV, 60–150% activity (normal); and class V, greater than 150% activity. Patients with G6PD deficiency seem to be protected from malaria parasitic infection, have less coronary artery disease, and possibly have fewer cancers and greater longevity.

► Clinical Findings

G6PD deficiency is an X-linked disorder affecting 10–15% of American hemizygous black males and rare female homozygotes. Female carriers are rarely affected—only when an unusually high percentage of cells producing the normal enzyme are X-inactivated.

A. Symptoms and Signs

Patients are usually healthy, without chronic hemolytic anemia or splenomegaly. Hemolysis occurs episodically as a result of oxidative stress on the red blood cells, generated either by infection or exposure to certain drugs. Medications initiating hemolysis that should be avoided include dapsone, methylene blue, phenazopyridine, primaquine, rasburicase, toluidine blue, nitrofurantoin, trimethoprim/sulfamethoxazole, sulfadiazine, and quinolones. Other medications, such as chloroquine, quinine, high-dose aspirin, and isoniazid, have been implicated but are less certain as offenders since they are often given during infections. Even with continuous use of the offending medication, the hemolytic episode is self-limited because older red blood cells (with low enzyme activity) are removed and replaced with a population of young red blood cells (reticulocytes) with adequate functional levels of G6PD. Severe G6PD deficiency (as in Mediterranean variants) may produce a chronic hemolytic anemia.

B. Laboratory Findings

Between hemolytic episodes, the blood is normal. During episodes of hemolysis, the hemoglobin rarely falls below 8 g/dL (80 g/L), and there is reticulocytosis and increased serum indirect bilirubin. The peripheral blood cell smear often reveals a small number of "bite" cells—cells that appear to have had a bite taken out of their periphery, or "blister" cells. This indicates pitting of precipitated membrane hemoglobin aggregates by the spleen. Heinz bodies may be demonstrated by staining a peripheral blood smear with cresyl violet; they are not visible on the usual Wright-Giemsa–stained blood smear. Specific enzyme assays for G6PD reveal a low level but may be falsely normal if they are performed during or shortly after a hemolytic episode during the period of reticulocytosis. In these cases, the enzyme assays should be repeated weeks after hemolysis has resolved. In severe cases of G6PD deficiency, enzyme levels are always low.

► Treatment

No treatment is necessary except to avoid known oxidant drugs.

Luzzatto L et al. G6PD deficiency: a classic example of pharmacogenetics with on-going clinical implications. Br J Haematol. 2014 Feb;164(4):469–80. [PMID: 24372186]
Manganelli G et al. Glucose-6-phosphate dehydrogenase deficiency: disadvantages and possible benefits. Cardiovasc Hematol Disord Drug Targets. 2013 Mar 1;13(1):73–82. [PMID: 23534950]

SICKLE CELL ANEMIA & RELATED SYNDROMES

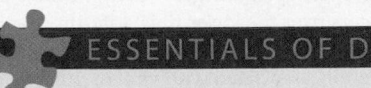

ESSENTIALS OF DIAGNOSIS

► Recurrent pain episodes.
► Positive family history and lifelong history of hemolytic anemia.
► Irreversibly sickled cells on peripheral blood smear.
► Hemoglobin S is the major hemoglobin seen on electrophoresis.

► General Considerations

Sickle cell anemia is an autosomal recessive disorder in which an abnormal hemoglobin leads to chronic hemolytic anemia with numerous clinical consequences. A single DNA base change leads to an amino acid substitution of valine for glutamine in the sixth position on the beta-globin chain. The abnormal beta chain is designated beta^s and the tetramer of alpha-2beta^s-2 is designated hemoglobin S. Hemoglobin S is unstable and polymerizes in the setting of various stressors, including hypoxemia and acidosis, leading to the formation of sickled red blood cells. Sickled cells result in hemolysis and the release of ATP, which is converted to adenosine. Adenosine binds to its receptor (A2B) resulting in the production of 2,3-biphosphoglycerate and the induction of more sickling and to its receptor (A2A) on natural killer cells resulting in pulmonary inflammation. The free hemoglobin from hemolysis scavenges nitric oxide causing endothelial dysfunction, vascular injury, and pulmonary hypertension.

The rate of sickling is influenced by the intracellular concentration of hemoglobin S and by the presence of other hemoglobins within the cell. Hemoglobin F cannot participate in polymer formation, and its presence markedly retards sickling. Factors that increase sickling are red cell dehydration and factors that lead to formation of deoxyhemoglobin S, eg, acidosis and hypoxemia, either systemic or local in tissues. Hemolytic crises may be related to splenic sequestration of sickled cells (primarily in childhood before the spleen has been infarcted as a result of repeated sickling) or with coexistent disorders such as G6PD deficiency.

The beta^s gene is carried in 8% of American blacks, and 1 of 400 American black children will be born with sickle cell anemia. Prenatal diagnosis is available for couples at risk for producing a child with sickle cell anemia. Genetic counseling should be made available to such couples.

► Clinical Findings

A. Symptoms and Signs

The disorder has its onset during the first year of life, when hemoglobin F levels fall as a signal is sent to switch from production of gamma-globin to beta-globin. Chronic hemolytic anemia produces jaundice, pigment (calcium bilirubinate) gallstones, splenomegaly (early in life), and poorly healing ulcers over the lower tibia. Life-threatening severe anemia can occur during hemolytic or aplastic crises, the latter generally associated with viral or other infection or by folic acid deficiency causing reduced erythropoiesis.

Acute painful episodes due to acute vaso-occlusion from clusters of sickled red cells may occur spontaneously or be provoked by infection, dehydration, or hypoxia. Common sites of acute painful episodes include the bones (especially the back and long bones) and the chest. These episodes last hours to days and may produce low-grade fever. Acute vaso-occlusion may cause strokes due to sagittal sinus thrombosis or to bland or hemorrhagic central nervous system arterial ischemia and may also cause priapism. Vaso-occlusive episodes are not associated with increased hemolysis.

Repeated episodes of vascular occlusion especially affect the heart, lungs, and liver. Ischemic necrosis of bone occurs, rendering the bone susceptible to osteomyelitis due to salmonellae and (somewhat less commonly) staphylococci. Infarction of the papillae of the renal medulla causes renal tubular concentrating defects and gross hematuria, more often encountered in sickle cell trait than in sickle cell anemia. Retinopathy similar to that noted in diabetes mellitus is often present and may lead to visual impairment. Pulmonary hypertension may develop and is associated with a poor prognosis. These patients are prone to delayed puberty. An increased incidence of infection is related to hyposplenism as well as to defects in the alternate complement pathway.

On examination, patients are often chronically ill and jaundiced. There is hepatomegaly, but the spleen is not palpable in adult life. The heart is enlarged, with a hyperdynamic precordium and systolic murmurs. Nonhealing ulcers of the lower leg and retinopathy may be present.

Sickle cell anemia becomes a chronic multisystem disease, with death from organ failure. With improved supportive care, average life expectancy is now between 40 and 50 years of age.

B. Laboratory Findings

Chronic hemolytic anemia is present. The hematocrit is usually 20–30%. The peripheral blood smear is characteristically abnormal, with irreversibly sickled cells comprising 5–50% of red cells. Other findings include reticulocytosis (10–25%), nucleated red blood cells, and hallmarks of hyposplenism such as Howell-Jolly bodies and target cells. The white blood cell count is characteristically elevated to 12,000–15,000/mcL, and reactive thrombocytosis may occur. Indirect bilirubin levels are high.

The diagnosis of sickle cell anemia is confirmed by hemoglobin electrophoresis (Table 13–9). Hemoglobin S will usually comprise 85–98% of hemoglobin. In homozygous S disease, no hemoglobin A will be present. Hemoglobin F levels are variably increased, and high hemoglobin F levels are associated with a more benign clinical course. Patients with S-beta$^+$-thalassemia and SS alpha-thalassemia also have a more benign clinical course than sickle cell anemia (SS) patients.

▶ Treatment

When allogeneic hematopoietic stem cell transplantation is performed before the onset of significant end-organ damage, it can cure more than 80% of children with sickle cell anemia who have suitable HLA-matched donors. Transplantation remains investigational in adults. Other therapies modulate disease severity: cytotoxic agents, such as hydroxyurea, increase hemoglobin F levels epigenetically. Hydroxyurea (500–750 mg orally daily) reduces the frequency of painful crises in patients whose quality of life is disrupted by frequent pain crises (three or more per year). Long-term follow-up of patients taking hydroxyurea demonstrates it improves overall survival and quality of life with little evidence for secondary malignancy. The use of omega-3 (n-3) fatty acid supplementation may reduce vaso-occlusive episodes and reduce transfusion needs in patients with sickle cell anemia.

Supportive care is the mainstay of treatment for sickle cell anemia. Patients are maintained on folic acid supplementation (1 mg orally daily) and given transfusions for aplastic or hemolytic crises. When acute painful episodes

Table 13–9. Hemoglobin distribution in sickle cell syndromes.

Genotype	Clinical Diagnosis	Hb A	Hb S	Hb A$_2$	Hb F
AA	Normal	97–99%	0%	1–2%	< 1%
AS	Sickle trait	60%	40%	1–2%	< 1%
AS, alpha-thalassemia	Sickle trait, alpha-thalassemia	70–75%	25–30%	1–2%	< 1%
SS	Sickle cell anemia	0%	86–98%	1–3%	5–15%
SS, alpha-thalassemia (3 genes)	SS alpha-thalassemia, silent	0%	90%	3%	7–9%
SS, alpha-thalassemia (2 genes)	SS alpha-thalassemia, trait	0%	80%	3%	11–21%
S, beta^0-thalassemia	Sickle beta^0-thalassemia	0%	70–80%	3–5%	10–20%
S, beta$^+$-thalassemia	Sickle beta$^+$-thalassemia	10–20%	60–75%	3–5%	10–20%

Hb, hemoglobin.

occur, precipitating factors should be identified and infections treated if present. The patient should be kept well hydrated, given generous analgesics, and supplied oxygen if hypoxic. Pneumococcal vaccination reduces the incidence of infections with this pathogen. Angiotensin-converting enzyme inhibitors are recommended in patients with microalbuminuria.

Exchange transfusions are indicated for the treatment of severe acute vaso-occlusive crises, intractable pain crises, acute chest syndrome, priapism, and stroke. Long-term transfusion therapy has been shown to be effective in reducing the risk of recurrent stroke in children. It has been recommended that children with SS who are aged 2–16 years have annual transcranial ultrasounds and, if the Doppler velocity is abnormal (200 cm/s or greater), the clinician should strongly consider beginning transfusions to prevent stroke. Iron chelation is needed for those on chronic transfusion therapy.

▶ When to Refer

Patients with sickle cell anemia should have their care coordinated with a hematologist and should be referred to a Comprehensive Sickle Cell Center, if one is available.

▶ When to Admit

Patients should be admitted for management of acute chest crises, for aplastic crisis, or for painful episodes that do not respond to outpatient care.

Kassim AA et al. Sickle cell disease, vasculopathy, and therapeutics. Annu Rev Med. 2013;64:451–66. [PMID: 23190149]
Kim HC. Red cell exchange: special focus on sickle cell disease. Hematology Am Soc Hematol Educ Program. 2014 Dec 5; 2014(1):450–6. [PMID: 25696893]
King A et al. Evidence-based focused review of the status of hematopoietic stem cell transplantation as treatment of sickle cell disease and thalassemia. Blood. 2014 May 15;123(20): 3089–94. [PMID: 24511087]
McGann PT et al. Hydroxyurea therapy for sickle cell anemia. Expert Opin Drug Saf. 2015 Nov;14(11):1749–58. [PMID: 26366626]
Yawn BP et al. Management of sickle cell disease: summary of the 2014 evidence-based report by expert panel members. JAMA. 2014 Sep 10;312(10):1033–48. Erratum in: JAMA. 2014 Nov 12;312(18):1932. [PMID: 25203083]

SICKLE CELL TRAIT

People with the heterozygous genotype (AS) have sickle cell trait. These persons are hematologically normal, with no anemia and normal red blood cells on peripheral blood smear. Hemoglobin electrophoresis will reveal that approximately 40% of hemoglobin is hemoglobin S (Table 13–9). People with sickle cell trait may experience sudden cardiac death and rhabdomyolysis during vigorous exercise, especially at high altitudes. They may be at increased risk for venous thromboembolism. Chronic sickling of red blood cells in the acidotic renal medulla results in microscopic and gross hematuria, hyposthenuria (poor urine concentrating ability), and possibly chronic kidney disease.

No treatment is necessary. Genetic counseling is recommended.

Ojodu J et al. Incidence of sickle cell trait—United States, 2010. MMWR Morb Mortal Wkly Rep. 2014 Dec 12;63(49):1155–8. [PMID: 25503918]
Thoreson CK et al. Sickle cell trait from a metabolic, renal, and vascular perspective: linking history, knowledge, and health. J Racial Ethn Health Disparities. 2015 Sep;2(3):330–5. [PMID: 26322267]
Tripette J et al. Exercise-related complications in sick cell trait. Clin Hemorheol Microcirc. 2013 Jan 1;55(1):29–37. [PMID: 23478224]

SICKLE THALASSEMIA

Patients with homozygous sickle cell anemia and alpha-thalassemia have less vigorous hemolysis and run higher hemoglobins than SS patients due to reduced red blood cell sickling related to a lower hemoglobin concentration within the red blood cell and higher hemoglobin F levels (Table 13–9). The MCV is low, and the red cells are hypochromic.

Patients who are compound heterozygotes for beta^s and beta-thalassemia are clinically affected with sickle cell syndromes. Sickle beta^0-thalassemia is clinically very similar to homozygous SS disease. Vaso-occlusive crises may be somewhat less severe, and the spleen is not always infarcted. The MCV is low, in contrast to the normal MCV of sickle cell anemia. Hemoglobin electrophoresis reveals no hemoglobin A but will show an increase in hemoglobins A_2 and F (Table 13–9).

Sickle beta$^+$-thalassemia is a milder disorder than homozygous SS disease, with fewer crises. The spleen is usually palpable. The hemolytic anemia is less severe, and the hematocrit is usually 30–38%, with reticulocytes of 5–10%. Hemoglobin electrophoresis shows the presence of some hemoglobin A and elevated hemoglobins A_2 and F (Table 13–9). The MCV is low.

Angelucci E et al; EBMT Inborn Error and EBMT Paediatric Working Parties. Hematopoietic stem cell transplantation in thalassemia major and sickle cell disease: indications and management recommendations from an international expert panel. Haematologica. 2014 May;99(5):811–20. [PMID: 24790059]
Marsella M et al. Transfusional iron overload and iron chelation therapy in thalassemia major and sickle cell disease. Hematol Oncol Clin North Am. 2014 Aug;28(4):703–27. [PMID: 25064709]
Yacobovich J et al. Thalassemia major and sickle cell disease in adolescents and young adults. Acta Haematol. 2014;132(3–4): 340–7. [PMID: 25228560]

AUTOIMMUNE HEMOLYTIC ANEMIA

 ESSENTIALS OF DIAGNOSIS

▶ Acquired hemolytic anemia caused by IgG autoantibody.

▶ Spherocytes and reticulocytosis on peripheral blood smear.

▶ Positive antiglobulin (Coombs) test.

► General Considerations

Autoimmune hemolytic anemia is an acquired disorder in which an IgG autoantibody is formed that binds to the red blood cell membrane and does so most avidly at body temperature (ie, a "warm" autoantibody). The antibody is most commonly directed against a basic component of the Rh system present on most human red blood cells. When IgG antibodies coat the red blood cell, the Fc portion of the antibody is recognized by macrophages present in the spleen and other portions of the reticuloendothelial system. The interaction between splenic macrophages and the antibody-coated red blood cell results in removal of red blood cell membrane and the formation of a spherocyte due to the decrease in surface-to-volume ratio of the surviving red blood cell. These spherocytic cells have decreased deformability and are unable to squeeze through the 2-mcm fenestrations of splenic sinusoids and become trapped in the red pulp of the spleen. When large amounts of IgG are present on red blood cells, complement may be fixed. Direct complement lysis of cells is rare, but the presence of C3b on the surface of red blood cells allows Kupffer cells in the liver to participate in the hemolytic process via C3b receptors. The destruction of red blood cells in the spleen and liver designates this as extravascular hemolysis.

Approximately one-half of all cases of autoimmune hemolytic anemia are idiopathic. The disorder may also be seen in association with systemic lupus erythematosus, chronic lymphocytic leukemia (CLL), or lymphomas. It must be distinguished from drug-induced hemolytic anemia. When penicillin (or other drugs, especially cefotetan, ceftriaxone, and piperacillin) coats the red blood cell membrane, the autoantibody is directed against the membrane-drug complex. Fludarabine, an antineoplastic, causes autoimmune hemolytic anemia through its immunosuppression effects resulting in defective self-versus non-self immune surveillance permitting the escape of a B-cell clone, which produces the offending autoantibody.

► Clinical Findings

A. Symptoms and Signs

Autoimmune hemolytic anemia typically produces an anemia of rapid onset that may be life threatening. Patients complain of fatigue and dyspnea and may present with angina pectoris or heart failure. On examination, jaundice and splenomegaly are usually present.

B. Laboratory Findings

The anemia is of variable degree but may be very severe, with hematocrit of less than 10%. Reticulocytosis is present, and spherocytes are seen on the peripheral blood smear. In cases of severe hemolysis, the stressed bone marrow may also release nucleated red blood cells. As with other hemolytic disorders, the serum indirect bilirubin is increased and the haptoglobin is low. Approximately 10% of patients with autoimmune hemolytic anemia have coincident immune thrombocytopenia (Evans syndrome).

The antiglobulin (Coombs) test (DAT) forms the basis for diagnosis. The Coombs reagent is a rabbit IgM antibody raised against human IgG or human complement. The direct antiglobulin (Coombs) test is performed by mixing the patient's red blood cells with the Coombs reagent and looking for agglutination, which indicates the presence of antibody or complement or both on the red blood cell surface. The indirect antiglobulin (Coombs) test is performed by mixing the patient's serum with a panel of type O red blood cells. After incubation of the test serum and panel red blood cells, the Coombs reagent is added. Agglutination in this system indicates the presence of free antibody (autoantibody or alloantibody) in the patient's serum.

The direct antiglobulin test is positive (for IgG, complement, or both) in about 90% of patients with autoimmune hemolytic anemia. The indirect antiglobulin test may or may not be positive. A positive indirect antiglobulin test indicates the presence of a large amount of autoantibody that has saturated binding sites in the red blood cell and consequently appears in the serum. Because the patient's serum usually contains the autoantibody, it may be difficult to obtain a "compatible" cross-match with homologous red blood cells for transfusions since the crossmatch indicates the possible presence (true or false) of a red blood cell "alloantibody."

► Treatment

Initial treatment consists of prednisone, 1–2 mg/kg/day orally in divided doses. Patients with DAT-negative and DAT-positive autoimmune hemolysis respond equally well to corticosteroids. Transfused red blood cells will survive similarly to the patient's own red blood cells. Because of difficulty in performing the cross-match, possible "incompatible" blood may need to be given. Decisions regarding transfusions should be made in consultation with a hematologist and a blood bank specialist. If prednisone is ineffective or if the disease recurs on tapering the dose, splenectomy should be considered. Splenectomy may cure the disorder. Death from cardiovascular collapse can occur in the setting of rapid hemolysis. In patients with rapid hemolysis, therapeutic plasmapheresis should be performed early in management to remove autoantibodies. Patients with autoimmune hemolytic anemia refractory to prednisone and splenectomy may be treated with a variety of agents. Treatment with rituximab, a monoclonal antibody against the B cell antigen CD20, is effective in some cases. The suggested dose is 375 mg/m^2 intravenously weekly for 4 weeks. Rituximab is used in conjunction with corticosteroids as initial therapy in some patients with severe disease. Danazol, 400–800 mg/day orally, is less often effective than in immune thrombocytopenia but is well suited for long-term use because of its low toxicity profile. Immunosuppressive agents, including cyclophosphamide, vincristine, azathioprine, mycophenolate mofetil, alemtuzumab (an anti-CD52 antibody), or cyclosporine, may also be used. High-dose intravenous immune globulin (1 g/kg daily for 2 days) may be effective in controlling hemolysis. The benefit is short-lived (1–3 weeks), and the drug is very expensive. The long-term prognosis for patients with this disorder is good, especially if there is no other underlying autoimmune disorder or lymphoproliferative disorder. Treatment of an associated lymphoproliferative disorder will also treat the hemolytic anemia.

When to Refer

Patients with autoimmune hemolytic anemia should be referred to a hematologist for confirmation of the diagnosis and subsequent care.

When to Admit

Patients should be hospitalized for symptomatic anemia or rapidly falling hemoglobin levels.

Arndt PA. Drug-induced immune hemolytic anemia: the last 30 years of changes. Immunohematology. 2014;30(2):44–54. [PMID: 25247622]

Bass GF et al. Diagnosis and classification of autoimmune hemolytic anemia. Autoimmun Rev. 2014 Apr–May;13(4–5):560–4. [PMID: 24418298]

Dierickx D et al. The role of rituximab in adults with warm antibody autoimmune hemolytic anemia. Blood. 2015 May 21; 125(21):3223–9. [PMID: 25827833]

Jaime-Pérez JC et al. Current approaches for the treatment of autoimmune hemolytic anemia. Arch Immunol Ther Exp (Warsz). 2013 Oct;61(5):385–95. [PMID: 23689532]

Kamesaki T et al. Characterization of direct antiglobulin test-negative autoimmune hemolytic anemia: a study of 154 cases. Am J Hematol. 2013 Feb;88(2):93–6. [PMID: 23169533]

Zanella A et al. Treatment of autoimmune hemolytic anemias. Haematologica. 2014 Oct;99(10):1547–54. [PMID: 25271314]

Zeerleder S. Autoimmune haemolytic anaemia—a practical guide to cope with a diagnostic and therapeutic challenge. Neth J Med. 2011 Apr;69(4):177–84. [PMID: 21527804]

COLD AGGLUTININ DISEASE

ESSENTIALS OF DIAGNOSIS

- ▶ Increased reticulocytes on peripheral blood smear.
- ▶ Antiglobulin (Coombs) test positive only for complement.
- ▶ Positive cold agglutinin titer.

General Considerations

Cold agglutinin disease is an acquired hemolytic anemia due to an IgM autoantibody (called a cold agglutinin) usually directed against the I/i antigen on red blood cells. These IgM autoantibodies characteristically will react poorly with cells at 37°C but avidly at lower temperatures, usually at 0–4°C (ie, "cold" autoantibody). Since the blood temperature (even in the most peripheral parts of the body) rarely goes lower than 20°C, only cold autoantibodies reactive at relatively higher temperatures will produce clinical effects. Hemolysis results indirectly from attachment of IgM, which in the cooler parts of the circulation (fingers, nose, ears) binds and fixes complement. When the

red blood cell returns to a warmer temperature, the IgM antibody dissociates, leaving complement on the cell. Lysis of red blood cells rarely occurs. Rather, C3b, present on the red blood cells, is recognized by Kupffer cells (which have receptors for C3b), and red blood cell sequestration and destruction in the liver ensues (extravascular hemolysis). In some cases, the complement membrane attack complex forms, lysing the red blood cells (intravascular hemolysis).

Most cases of chronic cold agglutinin disease are idiopathic. Others occur in association with Waldenström macroglobulinemia, lymphoma, or CLL, in which a monoclonal IgM paraprotein is produced. Acute postinfectious cold agglutinin disease occurs following mycoplasmal pneumonia or viral infection (infectious mononucleosis, measles, mumps, or cytomegalovirus [CMV] with autoantibody directed against antigen i rather than I).

Clinical Findings

A. Symptoms and Signs

In chronic cold agglutinin disease, symptoms related to red blood cell agglutination occur on exposure to cold, and patients may complain of mottled or numb fingers or toes, acrocyanosis, episodic low back pain, and dark-colored urine. Hemolytic anemia is rarely severe, but episodic hemoglobinuria may occur on exposure to cold. The hemolytic anemia in acute postinfectious syndromes is rarely severe.

B. Laboratory Findings

Mild anemia is present with reticulocytosis and rarely spherocytes. The blood smear made at room temperature shows agglutinated red blood cells (there is no agglutination on a blood smear made at body temperature). The direct antiglobulin (Coombs) test will be positive for complement only. Serum cold agglutinin titer will semiquantitate the autoantibody. A monoclonal IgM is often found on serum protein electrophoresis and confirmed by serum immunoelectrophoresis. There is indirect hyperbilirubinemia and the haptoglobin is low during periods of hemolysis.

Treatment

Treatment is largely symptomatic, based on avoiding exposure to cold. Splenectomy and prednisone are usually ineffective (except when associated with a lymphoproliferative disorder) since hemolysis takes place in the liver and blood stream. Rituximab is the treatment of choice. The dose is 375 mg/m² intravenously weekly for 4 weeks. Relapses may be effectively re-treated. High-dose intravenous immunoglobulin (2 g/kg) may be effective temporarily, but it is rarely used because of the high cost and short duration of benefit. Patients with severe disease may be treated with cytotoxic agents, such as cyclophosphamide, fludarabine, or bortezomib, or with immunosuppressive agents, such as cyclosporine. As in warm IgG-mediated autoimmune hemolysis, it may be difficult to find compatible blood for transfusion. Red blood cells should be transfused through an in-line blood warmer.

Barcellini W. Immune hemolysis: diagnosis and treatment recommendations. Semin Hematol. 2015 Oct;52(4):304–12. [PMID: 26404442]

Berentsen S et al. Cold agglutinin-mediated autoimmune hemolytic anemia. Hematol Oncol Clin North Am. 2015 Jun;29(3):455–71. [PMID: 26043385]

Swiecicki PL et al. Cold agglutinin disease. Blood. 2013 Aug 15;122(7):1114–21. [PMID: 23757733]

APLASTIC ANEMIA

ESSENTIALS OF DIAGNOSIS

- ► Pancytopenia.
- ► No abnormal hematopoietic cells seen in blood or bone marrow.
- ► Hypocellular bone marrow.

General Considerations

Aplastic anemia is a condition of bone marrow failure that arises from suppression of, or injury to, the hematopoietic stem cell. The bone marrow becomes hypoplastic, fails to produce mature blood cells, and pancytopenia develops.

There are a number of causes of aplastic anemia (Table 13–10). Direct hematopoietic stem cell injury may be caused by radiation, chemotherapy, toxins, or pharmacologic agents. Systemic lupus erythematosus may rarely cause suppression of the hematopoietic stem cell by an IgG autoantibody directed against the hematopoietic stem cell. However, the most common pathogenesis of aplastic anemia appears to be autoimmune suppression of hematopoiesis by a T-cell-mediated cellular mechanism, so called "idiopathic" aplastic anemia. In some cases of "idiopathic" aplastic anemia, defects in maintenance of the hematopoietic stem cell telomere length (dyskeratosis congenita) or in DNA repair pathways (Fanconi anemia) have been identified and are likely linked to both the initiation of bone marrow failure and the propensity to later progress to myelodysplasia, PNH, or AML. Complex detrimental immune responses to viruses can also cause aplastic anemia.

Table 13–10. Causes of aplastic anemia.

Autoimmune: idiopathic, systemic lupus erythematosus
Congenital: defects in telomere length maintenance or DNA repair (rare)
Chemotherapy, radiotherapy
Toxins: benzene, toluene, insecticides
Drugs: chloramphenicol, gold salts, sulfonamides, phenytoin, carbamazepine, quinacrine, tolbutamide
Post-viral hepatitis (A, B, C, E, G, non-A through -G)
Non-hepatitis viruses (EBV, parvovirus, CMV, echovirus 3, others)
Pregnancy
Paroxysmal nocturnal hemoglobinuria

EBV, Epstein-Barr Virus; CMV, cytomegalovirus.

Clinical Findings

A. Symptoms and Signs

Patients come to medical attention because of the consequences of bone marrow failure. Anemia leads to symptoms of weakness and fatigue, neutropenia causes vulnerability to bacterial or fungal infections, and thrombocytopenia results in mucosal and skin bleeding. Physical examination may reveal signs of pallor, purpura, and petechiae. Other abnormalities such as hepatosplenomegaly, lymphadenopathy, or bone tenderness should *not* be present, and their presence should lead to questioning the diagnosis.

B. Laboratory Findings

The hallmark of aplastic anemia is pancytopenia. However, early in the evolution of aplastic anemia, only one or two cell lines may be reduced.

Anemia may be severe and is always associated with reticulocytopenia. Red blood cell morphology is unremarkable, but there may be mild macrocytosis (increased MCV). Neutrophils and platelets are reduced in number, and no immature or abnormal forms are seen on the blood smear. The bone marrow aspirate and the bone marrow biopsy appear hypocellular, with only scant amounts of morphologically normal hematopoietic progenitors. The bone marrow karyotype should be normal (or germline if normal variant).

Differential Diagnosis

Aplastic anemia must be differentiated from other causes of pancytopenia (Table 13–11). Hypocellular forms of myelodysplasia or acute leukemia may occasionally be confused with aplastic anemia. These are differentiated by the presence of cellular morphologic abnormalities, increased percentage of blasts, or abnormal karyotype in bone marrow cells. Hairy cell leukemia has been misdiagnosed as aplastic anemia and should be recognized by the presence of splenomegaly and by abnormal lymphoid cells

Table 13–11. Causes of pancytopenia.

Bone marrow disorders
Aplastic anemia
Myelodysplasia
Acute leukemia
Chronic idiopathic myelofibrosis
Infiltrative disease: lymphoma, myeloma, carcinoma, hairy cell leukemia, etc
Non–bone marrow disorders
Hypersplenism (with or without portal hypertension)
Systemic lupus erythematosus
Infection: tuberculosis, HIV infection, leishmaniasis, brucellosis, CMV, parvovirus B19
Nutritional deficiency (megaloblastic anemia)
Medications
Cytotoxic chemotherapy
Ionizing radiation

CMV, cytomegalovirus.

in a hypocellular bone marrow biopsy. Pancytopenia with a normocellular bone marrow may be due to systemic lupus erythematosus, disseminated infection, hypersplenism, nutritional (eg, vitamin B$_{12}$ or folate) deficiency, or myelodysplasia. Isolated thrombocytopenia may occur early as aplastic anemia develops and may be confused with immune thrombocytopenia.

► Treatment

Mild cases of aplastic anemia may be treated with supportive care, including erythropoietic (epoetin or darbepoetin) or myeloid (filgrastim or sargramostim) growth factors, or both. Red blood cell transfusions and platelet transfusions are given as necessary, and antibiotics are used to treat infections.

Severe aplastic anemia is defined by a neutrophil count of less than 500/mcL, platelets less than 20,000/mcL, reticulocytes less than 1%, and bone marrow cellularity less than 20%. The treatment of choice for young adults (under age 40 years) who have an HLA-matched sibling is allogeneic bone marrow transplantation. Children or young adults may also benefit from allogeneic bone marrow transplantation using an unrelated donor. Because of the increased risks associated with unrelated donor allogeneic bone marrow transplantation relative to sibling donors, this treatment is usually reserved for patients who have not responded to immunosuppressive therapy.

For adults over age 40 years or those without HLA-matched hematopoietic stem cell donors, the treatment of choice for severe aplastic anemia is immunosuppression with equine antithymocyte globulin (ATG) plus cyclosporine. Equine ATG is given in the hospital in conjunction with transfusion and antibiotic support. A proven regimen is equine ATG 40 mg/kg/day intravenously for 4 days in combination with cyclosporine, 6 mg/kg orally twice daily. Equine ATG is superior to rabbit ATG, resulting in a higher response rate and better survival. ATG should be used in combination with corticosteroids (prednisone or methylprednisolone 1–2 mg/kg/day orally for 1 week, followed by a taper over 2 weeks) to avoid ATG infusion reactions and serum sickness. Responses usually occur in 1–3 months and are usually only partial, but the blood counts rise high enough to give patients a safe and transfusion-free life. The full benefit of immunosuppression is generally assessed at 4 months post-equine ATG. Cyclosporine is maintained at full dose for 6 months and then stopped in responding patients. Androgens (such as fluoxymesterone 10–20 mg/day orally in divided doses) have been widely used in the past, with a low response rate, and may be considered in mild cases. Androgens appear to partially correct telomere length maintenance defects and increase the production of endogenous erythropoietin. The thrombopoietin mimetic, eltrombopag, may help increase platelets (and also red blood cells and white blood cells) in patients with refractory aplastic anemia.

► Course & Prognosis

Patients with severe aplastic anemia have a rapidly fatal illness if left untreated. Allogeneic bone marrow transplant

from a HLA-matched sibling donor produces survival rates of over 80% in recipients under 20 years old and of about 65–70% in those 20- to 50-years-old. Respective survival rates drop 10–15% when the donor is HLA-matched but unrelated. Equine ATG-cyclosporine immunosuppressive treatment leads to a response in approximately 70% of patients (including those with hepatitis virus–associated aplastic anemia). Up to one-third of patients will relapse with aplastic anemia after ATG-based therapy. Clonal hematologic disorders, such as PNH, AML, or myelodysplasia, may develop in one-quarter of patients treated with immunosuppressive therapy after 10 years of follow-up. Factors that predict response to ATG-cyclosporine therapy are patient's age, reticulocyte count, lymphocyte count, and age-adjusted telomere length of leukocytes at the time of diagnosis.

► When to Refer

All patients should be referred to a hematologist.

► When to Admit

Admission is necessary for treatment of neutropenic infection, the administration of ATG, or allogeneic bone marrow transplantation.

Bacigalupo A. Bone marrow transplantation for acquired severe aplastic anemia. Hematol Oncol Clin North Am. 2014 Dec;28(6):1145–55. [PMID: 25459184]

McCormack PL. Eltrombopag: a review of its use in patients with severe aplastic anaemia. Drugs. 2015 Apr;75(5):525–31. [PMID: 25700916]

Willis L et al. Recent developments in drug therapy for aplastic anemia. Ann Pharmacother. 2014 Nov;48(11):1469–78. [PMID: 25184310]

NEUTROPENIA

ESSENTIALS OF DIAGNOSIS

- ► Neutrophils less than 1800/mcL (1.8 × 10^9/L).
- ► Severe neutropenia if neutrophils below 500/mcL (0.5 × 10^9/L).

► General Considerations

Neutropenia is present when the absolute neutrophil count is less than 1800/mcL (1.8 × 10^9/L), although blacks, Asians, and other specific ethnic groups may have normal neutrophil counts as low as 1200/mcL (1.2 × 10^9/L). The neutropenic patient is increasingly vulnerable to infection by gram-positive and gram-negative bacteria and by fungi. The risk of infection is related to the severity of neutropenia. The risk of serious infection rises sharply with neutrophil counts below 500/mcL (0.5 × 10^9/L), and a high risk of infection within days occurs with neutrophil counts below 100/mcL (0.1 × 10^9/L) ("profound neutropenia"). Patients with "chronic benign neutropenia" are free of infection despite very low stable neutrophil levels; they seem to respond adequately to infections and inflammatory stimuli with an appropriate neutrophil release from the bone marrow. In contrast, the neutrophil count of patients with cyclic neutropenia periodically oscillate (usually in 21-day cycles) between normal and low, with infections occurring during the nadirs. Both cyclic neutropenia and congenital neutropenia represent problems in mutations in the neutrophil elastase gene *ELANE* (also called *ELA-2*).

A variety of bone marrow disorders and nonmarrow conditions may cause neutropenia (Table 13–12). All of the causes of aplastic anemia (Table 13–10) and pancytopenia (Table 13–11) may cause neutropenia. The new onset of an isolated neutropenia is most often due to an idiosyncratic reaction to a drug, and agranulocytosis (complete absence of neutrophils in the peripheral blood) is almost always due to a drug reaction. In these cases, examination of the bone marrow shows an almost complete absence of granulocyte precursors with other cell lines undisturbed. This marrow finding is also seen in pure white blood cell aplasia, an autoimmune attack on marrow granulocyte precursors. Neutropenia in the presence of a normal bone marrow may be due to immunologic peripheral destruction (autoimmune neutropenia), sepsis, or hypersplenism. The presence in the serum of antineutrophil antibodies supports the diagnosis of autoimmune neutropenia. Felty syndrome is an immune neutropenia associated with seropositive nodular rheumatoid arthritis and splenomegaly. Severe neutropenia may be associated with clonal disorders of T lymphocytes, often with the morphology of large granular lymphocytes, referred to as CD3-positive T-cell large granular lymphoproliferative disorder. Isolated neutropenia is an uncommon presentation of hairy cell

leukemia or a myelodysplastic syndrome. By its nature, myelosuppressive cytotoxic chemotherapy causes neutropenia in a predictable manner.

▶ Clinical Findings

Neutropenia results in stomatitis and in infections due to gram-positive or gram-negative aerobic bacteria or to fungi such as *Candida* or *Aspergillus*. The most common infections are septicemia, cellulitis, pneumonia, and neutropenic fever of unknown origin. Fever in neutropenic patients should always be initially assumed to be of infectious origin until proven otherwise (Chapter 30).

▶ Treatment

Treatment of neutropenia depends on its cause. Potential causative drugs should be discontinued. Myeloid growth factors (filgrastim or sargramostim) help facilitate neutrophil recovery after offending drugs are stopped. Chronic myeloid growth factor administration (daily or every other day) is effective at dampening the neutropenia seen in cyclic or congenital neutropenia. When Felty syndrome leads to repeated bacterial infections, splenectomy has been the treatment of choice, but sustained use of myeloid growth factors is effective and provides a nonsurgical alternative. Patients with autoimmune neutropenia often respond briefly to immunosuppression with corticosteroids and are best managed with intermittent doses of myeloid growth factors. Splenectomy is held in reserve for failure to respond to corticosteroids and myeloid growth factors. Patients with true pure white blood cell aplasia need immunosuppression with ATG and cyclosporine, as in aplastic anemia and pure red blood cell aplasia. The neutropenia associated with large granular lymphoproliferative disorder may respond to therapy with either low-dose methotrexate or cyclosporine.

Fevers during neutropenia should be considered as infectious until proven otherwise. Febrile neutropenia is a life-threatening circumstance. Enteric gram-negative bacteria are of primary concern and often empirically treated with fluoroquinolones or third- or fourth-generation cephalosporins. For protracted neutropenia, fungal infections are problematic and empiric coverage with azoles (fluconazole for yeast and voriconazole, itraconazole, or posaconazole for molds) or echinocandins is recommended. The neutropenia following myelosuppressive chemotherapy is predictable and is partially ameliorated by the use of myeloid growth factors. For patients with acute leukemia undergoing intense chemotherapy or patients with solid cancer undergoing high-dose chemotherapy, the prophylactic use of antimicrobial agents and myeloid growth factors is recommended.

▶ When to Refer

Refer to a hematologist if neutrophils are persistently and unexplainably less than 1000/mcL (1.0×10^9/L).

▶ When to Admit

Neutropenia by itself is not an indication for hospitalization. However, most patients with severe neutropenia have a serious underlying disease that may require inpatient

Table 13–12. Causes of neutropenia.

Bone marrow disorders
Congenital
Dyskeratosis congenita
Fanconi anemia
Cyclic neutropenia
Large granular lymphoproliferative disorder
Hairy cell leukemia
Myelodysplasia
Non–bone marrow disorders
Drugs: sulfonamides, chlorpromazine, procainamide, penicillin, cephalosporins, cimetidine, methimazole, phenytoin, chlorpropamide, antiretroviral medications, rituximab
Aplastic anemia
Myelosuppressive cytotoxic chemotherapy
Benign chronic neutropenia
Pure white cell aplasia
Hypersplenism
Sepsis
Other immune
Autoimmune (idiopathic)
Felty syndrome
Systemic lupus erythematosus
HIV infection

treatment. Most patients with febrile neutropenia require hospitalization to treat infection.

Autrel-Moignet A et al. Autoimmune neutropenia. Presse Med. 2014 Apr;43(4 Pt 2):e105–18. [PMID: 24680423]
Flowers CR et al. Antimicrobial prophylaxis and outpatient management of fever and neutropenia in adults treated for malignancy: American Society of Clinical Oncology clinical practice guideline. J Clin Oncol. 2013 Feb 20;31(6):794–810. [PMID: 23319691]
Newberger PE et al. Evaluation and management of patients with isolated neutropenia. Semin Hematol. 2013 Jul;50(3):198–206. [PMID: 23953336]
Penack O et al. Management of sepsis in neutropenic patients: 2014 updated guidelines from the Infectious Diseases Working Party of the German Society of Hematology and Medical Oncology (AGIHO). Ann Hematol. 2014 Jul;93(7):1083–95. [PMID: 24777705]

LEUKEMIAS & OTHER MYELOPROLIFERATIVE NEOPLASMS

Myeloproliferative disorders are due to acquired clonal abnormalities of the hematopoietic stem cell. Since the stem cell gives rise to myeloid, erythroid, and platelet cells, qualitative and quantitative changes are seen in all of these cell lines. Classically, the myeloproliferative disorders produce characteristic syndromes with well-defined clinical and laboratory features (Tables 13–13 and 13–14). However, these disorders are grouped together because they may evolve from one into another and because hybrid disorders are commonly seen. All of the myeloproliferative disorders may progress to AML.

The Philadelphia chromosome seen in chronic myeloid leukemia (CML) was the first recurrent cytogenetic abnormality to be described in a human malignancy. Since that time, there has been tremendous progress in elucidating the genetic nature of these disorders, with identification of mutations in JAK2, MPL, CALR, CSF3R, and other genes.

Meier B et al. Myeloproliferative disorders. Emerg Med Clin North Am. 2014 Aug;32(3):597–612. [PMID: 25060252]

POLYCYTHEMIA VERA

ESSENTIALS OF DIAGNOSIS

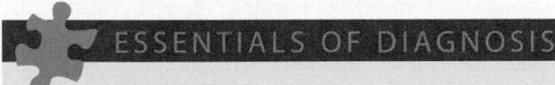

- JAK2 (V617F) mutation.
- Increased red blood cell mass.
- Splenomegaly.
- Normal arterial oxygen saturation.
- Usually elevated white blood count and platelet count.

General Considerations

Polycythemia vera is an acquired myeloproliferative disorder that causes overproduction of all three hematopoietic

Table 13–13. Classification of myeloproliferative disorders.

Myeloproliferative neoplasms
Polycythemia vera
Primary myelofibrosis
Essential thrombocytosis
Chronic myeloid leukemia
Myelodysplastic syndromes
Acute myeloid leukemia

cell lines, most prominently the red blood cells. Erythroid production is independent of erythropoietin, and the serum erythropoietin level is low. A mutation in exon 14 of JAK2 (V617F), a signaling molecule, has been demonstrated in 95% of cases. Additional JAK2 mutations have been identified (exon 12) and suggest that JAK2 is involved in the pathogenesis of this disease and is a potential therapeutic target.

True erythrocytosis, with an elevated red blood cell mass, should be distinguished from spurious erythrocytosis caused by a constricted plasma volume. Primary polycythemia (polycythemia vera) is a bone marrow disorder characterized by autonomous overproduction of erythroid cells.

Clinical Findings

A. Symptoms and Signs

Headache, dizziness, tinnitus, blurred vision, and fatigue are common complaints related to expanded blood volume and increased blood viscosity. Generalized pruritus, especially following a warm shower or bath, is related to histamine release from the basophilia. Epistaxis is probably related to engorgement of mucosal blood vessels in combination with abnormal hemostasis due to qualitative abnormalities in platelet function. Sixty percent of patients are men, and the median age at presentation is 60 years. Polycythemia rarely occurs in persons under age 40 years.

Physical examination reveals plethora and engorged retinal veins. The spleen is palpable in 75% of cases but is nearly always enlarged when imaged. Thrombosis is the most common complication of polycythemia vera and the major cause of morbidity and death in this disorder. Thrombosis appears to be related both to increased blood viscosity and abnormal platelet function. Uncontrolled polycythemia leads to a very high incidence of thrombotic complications of surgery, and elective surgery should be deferred until the condition has been treated. Paradoxically, in addition to thrombosis, increased bleeding can also occur. There is a high incidence of peptic ulcer disease.

B. Laboratory Findings

The hallmark of polycythemia vera is a hematocrit (at sea level) that exceeds 54% in males or 51% in females. Red blood cell morphology is normal (Table 13–14). The white blood count is usually elevated to 10,000–20,000/mcL and the platelet count is variably increased, sometimes to counts exceeding 1,000,000/mcL. Platelet morphology is

Table 13–14. Laboratory features of myeloproliferative neoplasms.

	White Count	Hematocrit	Platelet Count	Red Cell Morphology
Polycythemia vera	N or ↑	↑	N or ↑	N
Essential thrombocytosis	N or ↑	N	↑↑	N
Primary myelofibrosis	N or ↓ or ↑	↓	↓ or N or ↑	Abn
Chronic myeloid leukemia	↑↑	N	N or ↑	N

Abn, abnormal; N, normal.

usually normal. White blood cells are usually normal, but basophilia and eosinophilia are frequently present. Erythropoietin levels are suppressed and are usually low. The diagnosis should be confirmed with *JAK2* mutation screening. The absence of a mutation should lead the clinician to question the diagnosis.

The bone marrow is hypercellular, with panhyperplasia of all hematopoietic elements, but bone marrow examination is not necessary to establish the diagnosis. Iron stores are usually absent from the bone marrow, having been transferred to the increased circulating red blood cell mass. Iron deficiency may also result from chronic gastrointestinal blood loss. Bleeding may lower the hematocrit to the normal range (or lower), creating diagnostic confusion, and may lead to a situation with significant microcytosis with a normal hematocrit.

Vitamin B$_{12}$ levels are strikingly elevated because of increased levels of transcobalamin III (secreted by white blood cells). Overproduction of uric acid may lead to hyperuricemia.

Although red blood cell morphology is usually normal at presentation, microcytosis, hypochromia, and poikilocytosis may result from iron deficiency following treatment by phlebotomy. Progressive hypersplenism may also lead to elliptocytosis.

Differential Diagnosis

Spurious polycythemia, in which an elevated hematocrit is due to contracted plasma volume rather than increased red cell mass, may be related to diuretic use or may occur without obvious cause.

A secondary cause of polycythemia should be suspected if splenomegaly is absent and the high hematocrit is not accompanied by increases in other cell lines. Secondary causes of polycythemia include hypoxia and smoking; carboxyhemoglobin levels may be elevated in smokers (Table 13–15). A renal CT scan or sonogram may be considered to look for an erythropoietin-secreting cyst or

Table 13–15. Causes of polycythemia.

Spurious polycythemia
Secondary polycythemia
　Hypoxia: cardiac disease, pulmonary disease, high altitude
　Carboxyhemoglobin: smoking
　Kidney lesions
　Erythropoietin-secreting tumors (rare)
　Abnormal hemoglobins (rare)
Polycythemia vera

tumor. A positive family history should lead to investigation for congenital high-oxygen-affinity hemoglobin. An absence of a mutation in *JAK2* suggests a different diagnosis. However, *JAK2* mutations are also commonly found in other myeloproliferative disorders, essential thrombocytosis, and myelofibrosis.

Polycythemia vera should be differentiated from other myeloproliferative disorders (Table 13–14). Marked elevation of the white blood count (above 30,000/mcL) suggests CML. Abnormal red blood cell morphology and nucleated red blood cells in the peripheral blood are seen in myelofibrosis. Essential thrombocytosis is suggested when the platelet count is strikingly elevated.

Treatment

The treatment of choice is phlebotomy. One unit of blood (approximately 500 mL) is removed weekly until the hematocrit is less than 45%; the hematocrit is maintained at less than 45% by repeated phlebotomy as necessary. Patients for whom phlebotomy is problematic (because of poor venous access or logistical reasons) may be managed primarily with hydroxyurea. Because repeated phlebotomy intentionally produces iron deficiency, the requirement for phlebotomy should gradually decrease. It is important to avoid medicinal iron supplementation, as this can thwart the goals of a phlebotomy program. A diet low in iron also is not necessary but will increase the intervals between phlebotomies. Maintaining the hematocrit at normal levels has been shown to decrease the incidence of thrombotic complications.

Occasionally, myelosuppressive therapy is indicated. Indications include a high phlebotomy requirement, thrombocytosis, and intractable pruritus. There is evidence that reduction of the platelet count to less than 600,000/mcL will reduce the risk of thrombotic complications. Alkylating agents have been shown to increase the risk of conversion of this disease to acute leukemia and should be avoided. Hydroxyurea is widely used when myelosuppressive therapy is indicated. The usual dose is 500–1500 mg/day orally, adjusted to keep platelets less than 500,000/mcL without reducing the neutrophil count to less than 2000/mcL. The *JAK2* inhibitor, ruxolitinib, has been FDA approved in the United States for patients resistant or intolerant to hydroxyurea. In a randomized study comparing best available therapy with ruxolitinib, treatment with ruxolitinib was associated with greater benefit for both hematocrit control without phlebotomy (60%) and splenic volume reduction (38%). Symptom burden improved by greater than 50% in 49% of patients. Studies of pegylated alfa-2 interferon have demonstrated considerable efficacy, with hematologic responses in greater than 80%, as well as molecular responses in 20% (as measured by *JAK2* mutations). Patients in whom molecular responses were not achieved had a higher frequency of mutations outside the *JAK2* pathway and were more likely to acquire new mutations during therapy. Side effects were generally acceptable and much less significant than with nonpegylated forms of interferon.

Low-dose aspirin (75–81 mg/day orally) has been shown to reduce the risk of thrombosis without excessive bleeding, and should be part of therapy for all patients without contraindications to aspirin. Allopurinol 300 mg orally daily may be indicated for hyperuricemia. Antihistamine therapy with diphenhydramine or other H_1-blockers and, rarely, selective serotonin reuptake inhibitors are used to manage pruritus.

Prognosis

Polycythemia is an indolent disease with median survival of over 15 years. The major cause of morbidity and mortality is arterial thrombosis. Over time, polycythemia vera may convert to myelofibrosis or to CML. In approximately 5% of cases, the disorder progresses to AML, which is usually refractory to therapy.

When to Refer

Patients with polycythemia vera should be referred to a hematologist.

When to Admit

Inpatient care is rarely required.

Barbui T et al. Rethinking the diagnostic criteria of polycythemia vera. Leukemia. 2014 Jun;28(6):1191–5. [PMID: 24352199]
Lee G et al. The clinical and laboratory evaluation of the patient with erythrocytosis. Eur J Intern Med. 2015 Jun;26(5): 297–302. [PMID: 25837692]
Stein BL et al. Polycythemia vera: an appraisal of the biology and management 10 years after the discovery of *JAK2 V617F*. J Clin Oncol. 2015 Nov 20;33(33):3953–60. [PMID: 26324368]

ESSENTIAL THROMBOCYTOSIS

ESSENTIALS OF DIAGNOSIS

▶ Elevated platelet count in absence of other causes.
▶ Normal red blood cell mass.
▶ Absence of *bcr/abl* gene (Philadelphia chromosome).

General Considerations

Essential thrombocytosis is an uncommon myeloproliferative disorder of unknown cause in which marked proliferation of the megakaryocytes in the bone marrow leads to elevation of the platelet count. As with polycythemia vera, the finding of a high frequency of mutations of *JAK2* and others in these patients promises to advance the understanding of this disorder.

Clinical Findings

A. Symptoms and Signs

The median age at presentation is 50–60 years, and there is a slightly increased incidence in women. The disorder is often suspected when an elevated platelet count is found. Less frequently, the first sign is thrombosis, which is the most common clinical problem. The risk of thrombosis rises with age. Venous thromboses may occur in unusual sites such as the mesenteric, hepatic, or portal vein. Some patients experience erythromelalgia, painful burning of the hands accompanied by erythema; this symptom is reliably relieved by aspirin. Bleeding, typically mucosal, is less common and is related to a concomitant qualitative platelet defect. Splenomegaly is present in at least 25% of patients.

B. Laboratory Findings

An elevated platelet count is the hallmark of this disorder, and may be over 2,000,000/mcL (2000 × 10^9/L) (Table 13–14). The white blood cell count is often mildly elevated, usually not above 30,000/mcL (30 × 10^9/L), but with some immature myeloid forms. The hematocrit is normal. The peripheral blood smear reveals large platelets, but giant degranulated forms seen in myelofibrosis are not observed. Red blood cell morphology is normal.

The bone marrow shows increased numbers of megakaryocytes but no other morphologic abnormalities. The Philadelphia chromosome is absent but should be assayed by molecular testing of peripheral blood for the *bcr/abl* fusion gene in all suspected cases to differentiate the disorder from CML.

Differential Diagnosis

Essential thrombocytosis must be distinguished from secondary causes of an elevated platelet count. In reactive thrombocytosis, the platelet count seldom exceeds 1,000,000/mcL (1000 × 10^9/L). Inflammatory disorders such as rheumatoid arthritis and ulcerative colitis cause significant elevations of the platelet count, as may chronic infection. The thrombocytosis of iron deficiency is observed only when anemia is significant. The platelet count is temporarily elevated after splenectomy. *JAK2* mutations are found in 50% of cases. *MPL, CALR,* and *TET2* mutations have also been described in a subset of patients with *JAK2*-negative essential thrombocytosis.

Regarding other myeloproliferative disorders, the lack of erythrocytosis distinguishes it from polycythemia vera. Unlike myelofibrosis, red blood cell morphology is normal, nucleated red blood cells are absent, and giant degranulated platelets are not seen. In CML, the Philadelphia chromosome (or *bcr/abl* by molecular testing) establishes the diagnosis.

Treatment

Patients are considered at high risk for thrombosis if they are older than 60 years, have a leukocyte count of 11 × 10^9/L or higher, or have a previous history of thrombosis. They also have a higher risk for bleeding. The risk of thrombosis can be reduced by control of the platelet count, which should be kept under 500,000/mcL (500 × 10^9/L).

The treatment of choice is oral hydroxyurea in a dose of 500–1000 mg/day. In cases in which hydroxyurea is not well tolerated because of anemia, low doses of anagrelide, 1–2 mg/day orally, may be added. Higher doses of anagrelide can be complicated by headache, peripheral edema, and heart failure. As with polycythemia vera, trials of pegylated interferon alfa-2 have demonstrated significant hematologic responses, but its role in management has not yet been established. Strict control of coexistent cardiovascular risk factors is mandatory for all patients.

Vasomotor symptoms such as erythromelalgia and paresthesias respond rapidly to aspirin, and its long-term low-dose use (81 mg/day orally) may reduce the risk of thrombotic complications in low-risk patients. In the unusual event of severe bleeding, the platelet count can be lowered rapidly with plateletpheresis.

▶ Course & Prognosis

Essential thrombocytosis is an indolent disorder and allows long-term survival. Average survival is longer than 15 years from diagnosis, and the survival of patients younger than 50 years does not appear different from matched controls. The major source of morbidity—thrombosis—can be reduced by appropriate platelet control. Late in the course of the disease, the bone marrow may become fibrotic, and massive splenomegaly may occur, sometimes with splenic infarction. There is a 10–15% risk of progression to myelofibrosis after 15 years, and a 1–5% risk of transformation to acute leukemia over 20 years.

▶ When to Refer

Patients with essential thrombocytosis should be referred to a hematologist.

Kreher S et al. Prophylaxis and management of venous thromboembolism in patients with myeloproliferative neoplasms: consensus statement of the Haemostasis Working Party of the German Society of Hematology and Oncology (DGHO), the Austrian Society of Hematology and Oncology (ÖGHO) and Society of Thrombosis and Haemostasis Research (GTH e.V.). Ann Hematol. 2014 Dec;93(12):1953–63. [PMID: 25307456]
Tefferi A et al. Polycythemia vera and essential thrombocythemia: 2015 update on diagnosis, risk-stratification and management. Am J Hematol. 2015 Feb;90(2):162–73. Erratum in: Am J Hematol. 2015 Sep;90(9):849. [PMID: 25611051]
Tefferi A et al. Polycythemia vera and essential thrombocythemia: 2015 update on diagnosis, risk-stratification and management. Am J Hematol. 2015 Feb;90(2):162–73. [PMID: 25611051]

PRIMARY MYELOFIBROSIS

ESSENTIALS OF DIAGNOSIS

- ▶ Striking splenomegaly.
- ▶ Teardrop poikilocytosis on peripheral smear.
- ▶ Leukoerythroblastic blood picture; giant abnormal platelets.
- ▶ Initially hypercellular, then hypocellular bone marrow with reticulin or collagen fibrosis.

▶ General Considerations

Primary myelofibrosis (myelofibrosis with myeloid metaplasia, agnogenic myeloid metaplasia, idiopathic myelofibrosis) is a myeloproliferative disorder characterized by fibrosis of the bone marrow, splenomegaly, and a leukoerythroblastic peripheral blood picture with teardrop poikilocytosis. Myelofibrosis can also occur as a secondary process following the other myeloproliferative disorders (eg, polycythemia vera, essential thrombocytosis). It is believed that fibrosis occurs in response to increased secretion of platelet-derived growth factor (PDGF) and possibly other cytokines. In response to bone marrow fibrosis, extramedullary hematopoiesis takes place in the liver, spleen, and lymph nodes. In these sites, mesenchymal cells responsible for fetal hematopoiesis can be reactivated. As with other myeloproliferative diseases, abnormalities of *JAK2* and *MPL* may be involved in the pathogenesis.

▶ Clinical Findings

A. Symptoms and Signs

Primary myelofibrosis develops in adults over age 50 years and is usually insidious in onset. Patients most commonly present with fatigue due to anemia or abdominal fullness related to splenomegaly. Uncommon presentations include bleeding and bone pain. On examination, splenomegaly is almost invariably present and is commonly massive. The liver is enlarged in more than 50% of cases.

Later in the course of the disease, progressive bone marrow failure takes place as it becomes increasingly more fibrotic. Progressive thrombocytopenia leads to bleeding. The spleen continues to enlarge, which leads to early satiety. Painful episodes of splenic infarction may occur. The patient becomes cachectic and may experience severe bone pain, especially in the upper legs. Hematopoiesis in the liver leads to portal hypertension with ascites, esophageal varices, and occasionally transverse myelitis caused by myelopoiesis in the epidural space.

B. Laboratory Findings

Patients are almost invariably anemic at presentation. The white blood count is variable—either low, normal, or elevated—and may be increased to 50,000/mcL (50 × 10⁹/L). The platelet count is variable. The peripheral blood smear is dramatic, with significant poikilocytosis and numerous teardrop forms in the red cell line. Nucleated red blood cells are present and the myeloid series is shifted, with immature forms including a small percentage of promyelocytes or myeloblasts. Platelet morphology may be bizarre, and giant degranulated platelet forms (megakaryocyte fragments) may be seen. The triad of teardrop poikilocytosis, leukoerythroblastic blood, and giant abnormal platelets is highly suggestive of myelofibrosis.

The bone marrow usually cannot be aspirated (dry tap), though early in the course of the disease it is hypercellular, with a marked increase in megakaryocytes. Fibrosis at this stage is detected by a silver stain demonstrating increased reticulin fibers. Later, biopsy reveals more severe fibrosis, with eventual replacement of hematopoietic precursors by collagen. There is no characteristic chromosomal abnormality. *JAK2* is mutated in ~65% of cases, and *MPL* is mutated in ~40% of cases. The majority of the *JAK2/MPL*-negative cases were recently found to have a *CALR* mutation.

Differential Diagnosis

A leukoerythroblastic blood picture from other causes may be seen in response to severe infection, inflammation, or infiltrative bone marrow processes. However, teardrop poikilocytosis and giant abnormal platelet forms will not be present. Bone marrow fibrosis may be seen in metastatic carcinoma, Hodgkin lymphoma, and hairy cell leukemia. These disorders are diagnosed by characteristic morphology of involved tissues.

Of the other myeloproliferative disorders, CML is diagnosed when there is marked leukocytosis, normal red blood cell morphology, and the presence of the *bcr/abl* fusion gene. Polycythemia vera is characterized by an elevated hematocrit. Essential thrombocytosis shows predominant platelet count elevations.

Treatment

Patients with mild forms of the disease may require no therapy or occasional transfusion support. Anemic patients are supported with transfusion. Anemia can also be controlled with androgens, prednisone, thalidomide, or lenalidomide. First-line therapy for myelofibrosis-associated splenomegaly is hydroxyurea, which is effective in reducing spleen size by half in approximately 40% of patients. Both thalidomide and lenalidomide may improve splenomegaly and thrombocytopenia in some patients. Splenectomy is not routinely performed but is indicated for medication-refractory splenic enlargement causing recurrent painful episodes, severe thrombocytopenia, or an unacceptable transfusion requirement. Perioperative complications can occur in 28% of patients and include infections, abdominal vein thrombosis, and bleeding. Radiation therapy has a role for painful sites of extramedullary hematopoiesis, pulmonary hypertension, or severe bone pain. Transjugular intrahepatic portosystemic shunt might also be considered to alleviate symptoms of portal hypertension.

Several newer agents have shown activity in this disease. The immunomodulatory medications, lenalidomide and pomalidomide, result in control of anemia in 25% and thrombocytopenia in ~58% of cases, without significant reduction in splenic size. There are several *JAK2* inhibitors in development. Ruxolitinib, the first *JAK2* inhibitor to be FDA approved, results in reduction of spleen size, improvement of constitutional symptoms, and perhaps an overall survival benefit in patients with an intermediate- or high-risk disease. However, ruxolitinib can exacerbate cytopenias. The investigational agent pacritinib is a kinase inhibitor with specificity for *JAK2, FLT3, IRAK1,* and *CFSR1* kinases and has demonstrated activity compared to best available therapy, with 19% of patients achieving a significant splenic volume reduction regardless of underlying platelet count. It is also better tolerated in terms of cytopenias. FDA approval is still pending. The only potentially curative option for this disease is allogeneic stem cell

transplantation in selected patients, especially those with a matched sibling donor.

Course & Prognosis

The median survival from time of diagnosis is approximately 5 years. The Dynamic International Prognostic Scoring system is associated with overall survival. Therapies with biologic agents and the application of reduced-intensity allogeneic stem cell transplantation appear to offer the possibility of improving the outcome for many patients. End-stage myelofibrosis is characterized by generalized asthenia liver failure and bleeding from thrombocytopenia, with some cases terminating in AML.

When to Refer

Patients in whom myelofibrosis is suspected should be referred to a hematologist.

When to Admit

Admission is not usually necessary.

Alimam S et al. The use of *JAK* inhibitors for low-risk myelofibrosis. Expert Rev Hematol. 2015 Oct;8(5):551–3. [PMID: 26343888]

Beauverd Y et al. Pacritinib: a new agent for the management of myelofibrosis? Expert Opin Pharmacother. 2015;16(15): 2381–90. [PMID: 26389774]

Davis KL et al. Real-world assessment of clinical outcomes in patients with lower-risk myelofibrosis receiving treatment with ruxolitinib. Adv Hematol. 2015;2015:848473. [PMID: 26635878]

Ho PJ et al. Practical management of myelofibrosis with ruxolitinib. Intern Med J. 2015 Dec;45(12):1221–30. [PMID: 26648193]

CHRONIC MYELOID LEUKEMIA

ESSENTIALS OF DIAGNOSIS

► Elevated white blood count.
► Markedly left-shifted myeloid series but with a low percentage of promyelocytes and blasts.
► Presence of *bcr/abl* gene (Philadelphia chromosome).

General Considerations

CML is a myeloproliferative disorder characterized by overproduction of myeloid cells. These myeloid cells continue to differentiate and circulate in increased numbers in the peripheral blood.

CML is characterized by a specific chromosomal abnormality and specific molecular abnormality. The Philadelphia chromosome is a reciprocal translocation between the long arms of chromosomes 9 and 22. The portion of 9q that is translocated contains *abl*, a protooncogene that is the cellular homolog of the Ableson murine leukemia virus. The *abl* gene is received at a specific site on 22q, the break point cluster (bcr). The fusion gene *bcr/abl* produces a novel protein that differs from the normal transcript of the *abl* gene in that it possesses tyrosine kinase activity. This disorder is the first example of tyrosine kinase "addiction" by cancer cells.

Early CML ("chronic phase") does not behave like a malignant disease. Normal bone marrow function is retained, white blood cells differentiate and, despite some qualitative abnormalities, the neutrophils combat infection normally. However, untreated CML is inherently unstable, and without treatment the disease progresses to an accelerated and then acute blast phase, which is morphologically indistinguishable from acute leukemia. Remarkable advances in therapy have changed the natural history of the disease, and the relentless progression to more advanced stages of disease is at least greatly delayed, if not eliminated.

Clinical Findings

A. Symptoms and Signs

CML is a disorder of middle age (median age at presentation is 55 years). Patients usually complain of fatigue, night sweats, and low-grade fevers related to the hypermetabolic state caused by overproduction of white blood cells. Patients may also complain of abdominal fullness related to splenomegaly. In some cases, an elevated white blood count is discovered incidentally. Rarely, the patient will present with a clinical syndrome related to leukostasis with blurred vision, respiratory distress, or priapism. The white blood count in these cases is usually greater than 100,000/mcL (100×10^9/L) but less than 500,000/mcL (500×10^9/L). On examination, the spleen is enlarged (often markedly so), and sternal tenderness may be present as a sign of marrow overexpansion. In cases discovered during routine laboratory monitoring, these findings are often absent. Acceleration of the disease is often associated with fever in the absence of infection, bone pain, and splenomegaly.

B. Laboratory Findings

CML is characterized by an elevated white blood count; the median white blood count at diagnosis is 150,000/mcL (150×10^9/L), although in some cases the white blood cell count is only modestly increased (Table 13–14). The peripheral blood is characteristic. The myeloid series is left shifted, with mature forms dominating and with cells usually present in proportion to their degree of maturation. Blasts are usually less than 5%. Basophilia and eosinophilia may be present. At presentation, the patient is usually not anemic. Red blood cell morphology is normal, and nucleated red blood cells are rarely seen. The platelet count may be normal or elevated (sometimes to strikingly high levels). The bone marrow is hypercellular, with left-shifted myelopoiesis. Myeloblasts comprise less than 5% of marrow cells.

The hallmark of the disease is that the *bcr/abl* gene is detected by the polymerase chain reaction (PCR) test in the peripheral blood. A bone marrow examination is not necessary for diagnosis, although it is useful for prognosis and for detecting other chromosomal abnormalities in addition to the Philadelphia chromosome.

With progression to the accelerated and blast phases, progressive anemia and thrombocytopenia occur, and the percentage of blasts in the blood and bone marrow increases. Blast phase CML is diagnosed when blasts comprise more than 20% of bone marrow cells.

Differential Diagnosis

Early CML must be differentiated from the reactive leukocytosis associated with infection. In such cases, the white blood count is usually less than 50,000/mcL (50×10^9/L), splenomegaly is absent, and the *bcr/abl* gene is not present.

CML must be distinguished from other myeloproliferative disease (Table 13–14). The hematocrit should not be elevated, the red blood cell morphology is normal, and nucleated red blood cells are rare or absent. Definitive diagnosis is made by finding the *bcr/abl* gene.

Treatment

Treatment is usually not emergent even with white blood counts over 200,000/mcL (200×10^9/L), since the majority of circulating cells are mature myeloid cells that are smaller and more deformable than primitive leukemic blasts. In the rare instances in which symptoms result from extreme hyperleukocytosis (priapism, respiratory distress, visual blurring, altered mental status), emergent leukapheresis is performed in conjunction with myelosuppressive therapy.

In chronic-phase CML, the goal of therapy is normalization of the hematologic abnormalities and suppression of the malignant *bcr/abl*-expressing clone. The treatment of choice consists of a tyrosine kinase inhibitor (eg, imatinib, nilotinib, dasatinib) targeting the aberrantly active *abl* kinase. It is expected that a hematologic complete remission, with normalization of blood counts and splenomegaly will occur within 3 months of treatment initiation. Second, a major cytogenetic response should be achieved, ideally within 3 months but certainly within 6 months. A major cytogenetic response is identified when less than 35% of metaphases contain the Philadelphia chromosome. Lastly, a major molecular response is desired within 12 months and is defined as a 3-log reduction of the *bcr/abl* transcript as measured by quantitative PCR. This roughly corresponds to a *bcr/abl* ratio (compared to *abl*) of less than 0.01. Patients who achieve this level of molecular response have an excellent prognosis, with 100% of them remaining progression-free at 8 years. On the other hand, patients have a worse prognosis if these targets are not achieved, cytogenetic or molecular response is subsequently lost, or new mutations or cytogenetic abnormalities develop.

Imatinib mesylate was the first tyrosine kinase inhibitor to be approved and it results in nearly universal (98%) hematologic control of chronic phase disease at a dose of 400 mg/day. The rate of a major molecular response with imatinib in chronic-phase disease is ~30% at 1 year. The second-generation tyrosine kinase inhibitors, nilotinib and dasatinib, have also been approved for use as front-line therapy and have been shown to significantly increase the rate of a major molecular response compared to imatinib (71% for nilotinib at 300–400 mg twice daily by 2 years, 64%

for dasatinib at 100 mg/day by 2 years) and result in a lower rate of progression to advanced-stage disease. However, these agents can also salvage 90% of patients who do not respond to treatment with imatinib and may therefore be reserved for use in that setting. A dual *bcr/abl* tyrosine kinase inhibitor, bosutinib, was approved for patients who are resistant or intolerant to the other tyrosine kinase inhibitors. The complete cytogenetic response rate to bosutinib is 25% but it is not active against the *T315I* mutation.

Patients taking tyrosine kinase inhibitors should be monitored with a quantitative PCR assay. Those with a consistent increase in *bcr/abl* transcript or those with a suboptimal molecular response as defined above should undergo *abl* mutation testing and then be switched to an alternative tyrosine kinase inhibitor. The *T315I* mutation in *abl* is specifically resistant to therapy with imatinib, dasatinib, nilotinib, and bosutinib but appears to be sensitive to the third-generation agent ponatinib. However, ponatinib is associated with a high rate of vascular thrombotic complications. Patients who cannot achieve a good molecular response to any of these agents or who progress following therapy should be considered for treatment with allogeneic stem cell transplantation.

Patients with advanced-stage disease (accelerated phase or myeloid/lymphoid blast crisis) should be treated with a tyrosine kinase inhibitor alone or in combination with myelosuppressive chemotherapy. The doses of tyrosine kinase inhibitors in that setting are usually higher than those appropriate for chronic-phase disease. Since the duration of response to tyrosine kinase inhibitors in this setting is limited, patients who have accelerated or blast phase disease should ultimately be considered for allogeneic stem cell transplantation.

Course & Prognosis

Since the introduction of imatinib therapy in 2001, and with the development of molecular-targeted agents, more than 80% of patients remain alive and without disease progression at 9 years. Patients with good molecular responses to tyrosine kinase inhibitor therapy have an excellent prognosis, with essentially 100% survival at 9 years, and it is likely that some fraction of these patients will be cured. Small studies suggest that some patients with complete molecular responses (undetectable *bcr/abl*) lasting more than 2 years can stop drug therapy without disease recurrence, but these findings are being confirmed in prospective studies.

When to Refer

All patients with CML should be referred to a hematologist.

When to Admit

Hospitalization is rarely necessary and should be reserved for symptoms of leukostasis at diagnosis or for transformation to acute leukemia.

Baccarani M et al. A review of the European LeukemiaNet recommendations for the management of CML. Ann Hematol. 2015 Apr;94(Suppl 2):S141–7. [PMID: 25814080]

Barrett AJ et al. The role of stem cell transplantation for chronic myelogenous leukemia in the 21st century. Blood. 2015 May 21;125(21):3230–5. [PMID: 25852053]
Erba HP. Molecular monitoring to improve outcomes in patients with chronic myeloid leukemia in chronic phase: importance of achieving treatment-free remission. Am J Hematol. 2015 Mar;90(3):242–9. [PMID: 25410137]
Rea D. Management of adverse events associated with tyrosine kinase inhibitors in chronic myeloid leukemia. Ann Hematol. 2015 Apr;94(Suppl 2):S149–58. [PMID: 25814081]

MYELODYSPLASTIC SYNDROMES

 ESSENTIALS OF DIAGNOSIS

► Cytopenias with a hypercellular bone marrow.
► Morphologic abnormalities in two or more hematopoietic cell lines.

General Considerations

The myelodysplastic syndromes are a group of acquired clonal disorders of the hematopoietic stem cell. They are characterized by the constellation of cytopenias, a usually hypercellular marrow, and a number of morphologic and cytogenetic abnormalities. The disorders are usually idiopathic but may be caused by prior exposure to cytotoxic chemotherapy or radiation or both. Ultimately, the disorder may evolve into AML, and the term "preleukemia" has been used in the past to describe these disorders.

Myelodysplasia encompasses several heterogeneous syndromes. Those without excess bone marrow blasts are termed "refractory anemia," with or without ringed sideroblasts. Patients with the 5q– syndrome, which is characterized by the cytogenetic finding of loss of part of the long arm of chromosome 5, comprise an important subgroup of patients with refractory anemia. The diagnosis "refractory anemia with excess blasts" (RAEB 1 with 5–9% blasts and RAEB 2 with 10–19% blasts) is made in those with excess blasts. Patients with a proliferative syndrome including sustained peripheral blood monocytosis more than 1000/mcL (1.0×10^9/L) are termed "chronic myelomonocytic leukemia" (CMML), a disorder that shares features of myelodysplastic and myeloproliferative disorders. An International Prognostic Scoring System (IPSS) classifies patients by risk status based on the percentage of bone marrow blasts, cytogenetics, and severity of cytopenias. The IPSS is associated with the rate of progression to AML and with overall survival, which can range from a median of 6 years for the low-risk group to 5 months for the high-risk patients.

Clinical Findings

A. Symptoms and Signs

Patients are usually over age 60 years. Many patients are asymptomatic when the diagnosis is made because of the finding of abnormal blood counts. Fatigue, infection, or bleeding related to bone marrow failure are usually the presenting symptoms and signs. The course may be indolent, and the disease may present as a wasting illness with fever, weight loss, and general debility. On examination, splenomegaly may be present in combination with pallor, bleeding, and various signs of infection. Myelodysplastic syndromes can also be accompanied by a variety of paraneoplastic syndromes prior to or following this diagnosis.

B. Laboratory Findings

Anemia may be marked with the MCV normal or increased, and transfusion support may be required. On the peripheral blood smear, macro-ovalocytes may be seen. The white blood cell count is usually normal or reduced, and neutropenia is common. The neutrophils may exhibit morphologic abnormalities, including deficient numbers of granules or deficient segmentation of the nucleus, especially a bilobed nucleus (Pelger-Huet abnormality). The myeloid series may be left shifted, and small numbers of promyelocytes or blasts may be seen. The platelet count is normal or reduced, and hypogranular platelets may be present.

The bone marrow is characteristically hypercellular but occasionally may be hypocellular. Erythroid hyperplasia is common, and signs of abnormal erythropoiesis include megaloblastic features, nuclear budding, or multinucleated erythroid precursors. The Prussian blue stain may demonstrate ringed sideroblasts. In the marrow, too, the myeloid series is often left shifted, with variable increases in blasts. Deficient or abnormal granules may be seen. A characteristic abnormality is the presence of dwarf megakaryocytes with a unilobed nucleus. Although no single specific chromosomal abnormality is seen in myelodysplasia, there are frequently abnormalities involving the long arm of chromosome 5 as well as deletions of chromosomes 5 and 7. Some patients with an indolent form of the disease have an isolated partial deletion of chromosome 5 (5q– syndrome). The presence of other abnormalities such as monosomy 7 or complex abnormalities is associated with more aggressive disease.

▶ Differential Diagnosis

Myelodysplastic syndromes should be distinguished from megaloblastic anemia, aplastic anemia, myelofibrosis, HIV-associated cytopenias, and acute or chronic drug effect. In subtle cases, cytogenetic evaluation of the bone marrow may help distinguish this clonal disorder from other causes of cytopenias. As the number of blasts increases in the bone marrow, myelodysplasia is arbitrarily separated from AML by the presence of less than 20% blasts.

▶ Treatment

Myelodysplasia is a very heterogeneous disease, and the appropriate treatment depends on a number of factors. For patients with anemia who have a low serum erythropoietin level (500 milliunits/mL or less), erythropoiesis-stimulating agents may raise the hematocrit and reduce the red cell transfusion requirement in 40%. Addition of intermittent granulocyte colony-stimulating factor (G-CSF) therapy may augment the erythroid response to epoetin.

Unfortunately, the patients with the highest transfusion requirements are the least likely to respond. Patients who remain dependent on red blood cell transfusion and who do not have immediately life-threatening disease should receive iron chelation in order to prevent serious iron overload; the dose of oral agent deferasirox is 20 mg/kg/day. Patients affected primarily with severe neutropenia may benefit from the use of myeloid growth factors such as filgrastim. Oral thrombopoietin analogues such as romiplostim and eltrombopag that stimulate platelet production by binding the thrombopoietin receptor have shown effectiveness in raising the platelet count in myelodysplasia. Finally, occasional patients can benefit from immunosuppressive therapy including ATG. Predictors of response to ATG include age younger than 60 years, absence of 5q–, and presence of HLA DR15.

For patients who do not respond to these interventions, there are several therapeutic options available. Lenalidomide is approved for the treatment of transfusion-dependent anemia due to myelodysplasia. It is the treatment of choice in patients with the 5q– syndrome, with significant responses in 70% of patients, and responses typically lasting longer than 2 years. In addition, nearly half of these patients enter a cytogenetic remission with clearing of the abnormal 5q– clone, leading to the hope that lenalidomide may change the natural history of the disease. The recommended initial dose is 10 mg/day orally. The most common side effects are neutropenia and thrombocytopenia, but venous thrombosis occurs and warrants prophylaxis with aspirin, 325 mg/day orally. For patients with high-risk myelodysplasia, azacitidine is the treatment of choice. It can improve both symptoms and blood counts and prolong both overall survival and the time to conversion to acute leukemia. It is used at a dose of 75 mg/m^2 daily for 5–7 days every 28 days and six cycles of therapy may be required to achieve a response. A related hypomethylating agent, decitabine, can produce similar hematologic responses but has not demonstrated a benefit in overall survival compared to supportive care alone. Combination therapy of azacitidine with either lenalidomide or vorinostat, the histone deacetylase inhibitor, has shown preliminary promise in patients with high-risk disease and is being tested in a large prospective clinical trial. Allogeneic stem cell transplantation is the only curative therapy for myelodysplasia, but its role is limited by the advanced age of many patients and the indolent course of disease in some subsets of patients. The optimal use and timing of allogeneic transplantation are controversial, but the use of reduced-intensity preparative regimens for transplantation has expanded the role of this therapy, using both family and matched unrelated donors.

▶ Course & Prognosis

Myelodysplasia is an ultimately fatal disease, and allogeneic transplantation is the only curative therapy, with cure rates of 30–60% depending primarily on the risk status of the disease. Patients most commonly die of infections or bleeding. Patients with 5q– syndrome have a favorable prognosis, with 5-year survival over 90%. Other patients with low-risk disease (with absence of both excess blasts and adverse cytogenetics) may also do well, with similar survival. Those with excess blasts or CMML have a higher (30–50%) risk of developing acute leukemia, and short survival (less than 2 years) without allogeneic transplantation.

► When to Refer

All patients with myelodysplasia should be referred to a hematologist.

► When to Admit

Hospitalization is needed only for specific complications, such as severe infection.

Adès L et al. Myelodysplastic syndromes. Lancet. 2014 Jun 28; 383(9936):2239–52. [PMID: 24656536]

Kröger N. Allogeneic stem cell transplantation for elderly patients with myelodysplastic syndrome. Blood. 2012 Jun 14; 119(24):5632–9. [PMID: 22504927]

Sekeres MA et al. Established and novel agents for myelodysplastic syndromes. Hematology Am Soc Hematol Educ Program. 2014 Dec 5;2014(1):82–9. [PMID: 25696839]

ACUTE LEUKEMIA

ESSENTIALS OF DIAGNOSIS

► Short duration of symptoms, including fatigue, fever, and bleeding.

► Cytopenias or pancytopenia.

► More than 20% blasts in the bone marrow.

► Blasts in peripheral blood in 90% of patients.

► General Considerations

Acute leukemia is a malignancy of the hematopoietic progenitor cell. These cells proliferate in an uncontrolled fashion and replace normal bone marrow elements. Most cases arise with no clear cause. However, radiation and some toxins (benzene) are leukemogenic. In addition, a number of chemotherapeutic agents (especially cyclophosphamide, melphalan, other alkylating agents, and etoposide) may cause leukemia. The leukemias seen after toxin or chemotherapy exposure often develop from a myelodysplastic prodrome and are often associated with abnormalities in chromosomes 5 and 7. Those related to etoposide may have abnormalities in chromosome 11q23 (MLL locus).

Most of the clinical findings in acute leukemia are due to replacement of normal bone marrow elements by the malignant cells. Less common manifestations result from organ infiltration (skin, gastrointestinal tract, meninges). Acute leukemia is potentially curable with combination chemotherapy.

The myeloblastic subtype, AML, is primarily an adult disease with a median age at presentation of 60 years and an increasing incidence with advanced age. Acute promyelocytic leukemia (APL) is characterized by chromosomal translocation t(15;17), which produces the fusion gene

PML-RAR-alpha, which interacts with the retinoic acid receptor to produce a block in differentiation that can be overcome with pharmacologic doses of retinoic acid. The lymphoblastic subtype of acute leukemia, ALL, comprises 80% of the acute leukemias of childhood. The peak incidence is between 3 and 7 years of age. It is also seen in adults, causing approximately 20% of adult acute leukemias.

► Classification of the Leukemias

A. Acute Myeloid Leukemia (AML)

AML is primarily categorized based on recurrent structural chromosomal and molecular abnormalities. The cytogenetic abnormalities can be identified on traditional karyotyping or metaphase FISH and the molecular abnormalities are identified by either targeted or genome-wide sequencing of tumor DNA. Favorable cytogenetics such as t(8;21) producing a chimeric RUNX1/RUNX1T1 protein and inv(16)(p13;q22) are seen in 15% of cases and are termed the "core-binding factor" leukemias. These patients have a higher chance of achieving both short- and long-term disease control. Unfavorable cytogenetics confer a very poor prognosis. These consist of isolated monosomy 5 or 7, the presence of two or more other monosomies, or three or more separate cytogenetic abnormalities. The majority of cases of AML are of intermediate risk by traditional cytogenetics and have either a normal karyotype or chromosomal abnormalities that do not confer strong prognostic significance. However, there are several recurrent gene mutations with prognostic significance in this subgroup. On the one hand, internal tandem duplication in the gene FLT3 occurs in ~30% of AML and is associated with a very poor prognosis. Other mutations conferring a poor prognosis occur in TET2, ASXL1, MLL-PTD, PHF6, and DNMT3A. On the other hand, a relatively favorable group of patients has been identified that lacks FLT3-ITD mutations and includes mutations of nucleophosmin 1 (NPM1) and IDH1 or IDH2.

B. Acute Promyelocytic Leukemia (APL)

In considering the various types of AML, APL is discussed separately because of its unique biologic features and response to non-chemotherapy treatments. APL is characterized by the cytogenetic finding of t(15;17) and the fusion gene PML-RAR-alpha. It is a highly curable form of leukemia (over 90%) with integration of all-trans-retinoic acid (ATRA) and arsenic trioxide (ATO) in induction, consolidation, and maintenance regimens.

C. Acute Lymphoblastic Leukemia (ALL)

ALL is most usefully classified by immunologic phenotype as follows: common, early B lineage, and T cell. Hyperdiploidy (with more than 50 chromosomes), especially of chromosomes 4, 10 and 17, and translocation t(12;21) (TEL-AML1), is associated with a better prognosis. Unfavorable cytogenetics are hypodiploidy (less than 44 chromosomes), the Philadelphia chromosome t(9;22), the t(4;11) translocation (which has fusion genes involving the MLL gene at 11q23), and a complex karyotype with more than five chromosomal abnormalities.

D. Mixed Phenotype Acute Leukemias

These leukemias consist of blasts that lack differentiation along the lymphoid or myeloid lineage or blasts that express both myeloid and lymphoid lineage-specific antigens. This group is considered very high risk and has a poor prognosis. The limited available data suggest that an "acute lymphoblastic leukemia–like" regimen followed by allogeneic stem cell transplant may be advisable; addition of a tyrosine kinase inhibitor in patients with t(9;22) translocation is recommended.

▶ Clinical Findings

A. Symptoms and Signs

Most patients have been ill only for days or weeks. Bleeding (usually due to thrombocytopenia) occurs in the skin and mucosal surfaces, with gingival bleeding, epistaxis, or menorrhagia. Less commonly, widespread bleeding is seen in patients with disseminated intravascular coagulation (DIC) (in APL and monocytic leukemia). Infection is due to neutropenia, with the risk of infection rising as the neutrophil count falls below 500/mcL (0.5×10^9/L). Common presentations include cellulitis, pneumonia, and perirectal infections; death within a few hours may occur if treatment with appropriate antibiotics is delayed. Fungal infections are also commonly seen.

Patients may also seek medical attention because of gum hypertrophy and bone and joint pain. The most dramatic presentation is hyperleukocytosis, in which a markedly elevated circulating blast count (total white blood count greater than 100,000/mcL) leads to impaired circulation, presenting as headache, confusion, and dyspnea. Such patients require emergent chemotherapy with adjunctive leukapheresis as mortality approaches 40% in the first 48 hours.

On examination, patients appear pale and have purpura and petechiae; signs of infection may not be present. Stomatitis and gum hypertrophy may be seen in patients with monocytic leukemia, as may rectal fissures. There is variable enlargement of the liver, spleen, and lymph nodes. Bone tenderness may be present, particularly in the sternum, tibia, and femur.

B. Laboratory Findings

The hallmark of acute leukemia is the combination of pancytopenia with circulating blasts. However, blasts may be absent from the peripheral smear in as many as 10% of cases ("aleukemic leukemia"). The bone marrow is usually hypercellular and dominated by blasts. More than 20% marrow blasts are required to make a diagnosis of acute leukemia.

Hyperuricemia may be seen. If DIC is present, the fibrinogen level will be reduced, the prothrombin time prolonged, and fibrin degradation products or fibrin D-dimers present. Patients with ALL (especially T cell) may have a mediastinal mass visible on chest radiograph. Meningeal leukemia will have blasts present in the spinal fluid, seen in approximately 5% of cases at diagnosis; it is more common in monocytic types of AML and can be seen with ALL.

The Auer rod, an eosinophilic needle-like inclusion in the cytoplasm, is pathognomonic of AML and, if seen, secures the diagnosis. The phenotype of leukemia cells is usually demonstrated by flow cytometry or immunohistochemistry. AML cells usually express myeloid antigens such as CD13 or CD33 and myeloperoxidase. ALL cells of B lineage will express CD19, and most cases will express CD10, formerly known as the "common ALL antigen." ALL cells of T lineage will usually not express mature T-cell markers, such as CD3, CD4, or CD8, but will express some combination of CD2, CD5, and CD7 and will not express surface immunoglobulin. Almost all ALL cells express terminal deoxynucleotidyl transferase (TdT). The uncommon Burkitt type of ALL has a "lymphoma" phenotype, expressing CD19, CD20, and surface immunoglobulin but not TdT and is best treated with aggressive lymphoma regimens.

▶ Differential Diagnosis

AML must be distinguished from other myeloproliferative disorders, CML, and myelodysplastic syndromes. Acute leukemia may also resemble a left-shifted bone marrow recovering from a previous toxic insult. If the diagnosis is in doubt, a bone marrow study should be repeated in several days to see if maturation has taken place. ALL must be separated from other lymphoproliferative disease such as CLL, lymphomas, and hairy cell leukemia. It may also be confused with the atypical lymphocytosis of mononucleosis and pertussis.

▶ Treatment

Most patients up to age 60 with acute leukemia are treated with the objective of cure. The first step in treatment is to obtain complete remission, defined as normal peripheral blood with resolution of cytopenias, normal bone marrow with no excess blasts, and normal clinical status. The type of initial chemotherapy depends on the subtype of leukemia.

1. AML—Most patients with AML are treated with a combination of an anthracycline (daunorubicin or idarubicin) plus cytarabine, either alone or in combination with other agents. This therapy will produce complete remissions in 80–90% of patients under age 60 years and in 50–60% of older patients (see Table 39–4). Older patients with AML who are not candidates for traditional chemotherapy may be given 5-azacitidine, decitabine, or clofarabine initially with acceptable outcomes.

Once a patient has entered remission, post-remission therapy should be given with curative intent whenever possible. Options include standard chemotherapy and allogeneic stem cell transplantation. The optimal treatment strategy depends on the patient's age and clinical status, and the genetic risk factor profile of the leukemia. Patients with a favorable genetic profile can be treated with chemotherapy alone or with autologous transplant with cure rates of 60–80%. Patients who do not enter remission (primary induction failure) or those with high-risk genetics have cure rates of less than 10% with chemotherapy alone and are referred for allogeneic stem cell transplantation. For intermediate-risk patients with AML, cure rates are 35–40% with chemotherapy and 40–60% with allogeneic transplantation. Addition of the investigational FLT3 kinase inhibitor midostaurin to the induction, consolidation, and maintenance therapy of AML patients with *FLT3* mutation has been shown to prolong event-free and overall survival. Patients over age 60 have had a poor prognosis, even in first remission, when treated with standard chemotherapy approaches, and only 10–20% become long-term survivors. The use of reduced-intensity allogeneic transplant appears to be improving the outcome for such patients, with initial studies suggesting that up to 40% of selected patients may be cured.

Once leukemia has recurred after initial chemotherapy, the prognosis is poor. For patients in second remission, transplantation offers a 20–30% chance of cure. Targeted therapies directed at recurrent genetic mutations (*FLT3, IDH1/ IDH2*) have shown promising activity in this setting.

2. ALL—Adults with ALL are treated with combination chemotherapy, including daunorubicin, vincristine, prednisone, and asparaginase. This treatment produces complete remissions in 90% of patients. Those patients with Philadelphia chromosome-positive ALL (or *bcr-abl*-positive ALL) should have a tyrosine kinase inhibitor, such as dasatinib, added to their initial chemotherapy. Older patients (over age 60) may be treated with a tyrosine kinase inhibitor–based regimen, and 90% can enter initial remission.

Remission induction therapy for ALL is less myelosuppressive than treatment for AML and does not necessarily produce marrow aplasia. After achieving complete remission, patients receive central nervous system prophylaxis so that meningeal sequestration of leukemic cells does not develop. As with AML, patients may be treated with either additional cycles of chemotherapy or high-dose chemotherapy and stem cell transplantation. Treatment decisions are made based on patient age and disease risk factors. Adults younger than 39 years have uniformly better outcomes when treated under pediatric protocols. Low-risk patients with ALL may be treated with chemotherapy alone with a 70% chance of cure. Intermediate-risk patients have a 30–50% chance of cure with chemotherapy, and high-risk patients are rarely cured with chemotherapy alone. High-risk patients with adverse cytogenetics or poor responses to chemotherapy are best treated with allogeneic transplantation. Minimal residual disease testing will guide treatment decisions following induction therapy in the future. For patients with relapsed disease, the bispecific antibody blinatumomab has shown remarkable response rates as a bridge to transplantation and was approved for this indication in 2014. Autologous T cells engineered to express an anti-CD-19 antigen receptor (CART-19) are showing promise in both pediatric and adult patients with relapsed B-ALL.

Prognosis

Approximately 70–80% of adults with **AML** under age 60 years achieve complete remission and ~50% are cured using risk-adapted post-remission therapy. Older adults with

AML achieve complete remission in up to 50% of instances. The cure rates for older patients with AML have been very low (approximately 10–20%) even if they achieve remission and are able to receive post-remission chemotherapy. Reduced-intensity allogeneic transplantation is increasingly being utilized in order to improve on these outcomes.

Patients younger than 39 years with **ALL** have excellent outcomes after undergoing chemotherapy followed by risk-adapted intensification and transplantation (cure rates of 60–80%). Patients with adverse cytogenetics, poor response to chemotherapy, or older age have a much lower chance of cure (cure rates of 20–40%).

► When to Refer

All patients should be referred to a hematologist.

► When to Admit

Most patients with acute leukemia will be admitted for treatment.

Curran E et al. How I treat acute lymphoblastic leukemia in older adolescents and young adults. Blood. 2015 Jun 11; 125(24):3702–10. [PMID: 25805810]

Döhner K et al. Intermediate-risk acute myeloid leukemia therapy: current and future. Hematology Am Soc Hematol Educ Program. 2014 Dec 5;2014(1):34–43. [PMID: 25696832]

Gupta V et al. Allogeneic hematopoietic cell transplantation for adults with acute myeloid leukemia: myths, controversies, and unknowns. Blood. 2011 Feb 24;117(8):2307–18. [PMID: 21098397]

Lo-Coco F et al. Retinoic acid and arsenic trioxide for acute promyelocytic leukemia. N Engl J Med. 2013 Jul 11;369(2): 111–21. [PMID: 23841729]

Ossenkoppele G et al. How I treat the older patient with acute myeloid leukemia. Blood. 2015 Jan 29;125(5):767–74. [PMID: 25515963]

CHRONIC LYMPHOCYTIC LEUKEMIA

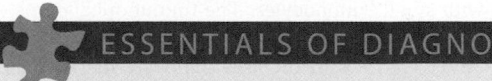

ESSENTIALS OF DIAGNOSIS

▸ B-cell lymphocytosis greater than 5000/mcL.
▸ Coexpression of CD19, CD5 on lymphocytes.

► General Considerations

CLL is a clonal malignancy of B lymphocytes. The disease is usually indolent, with slowly progressive accumulation of long-lived small lymphocytes. These cells are immune-incompetent and respond poorly to antigenic stimulation.

CLL is manifested clinically by immunosuppression, bone marrow failure, and organ infiltration with lymphocytes. Immunodeficiency is also related to inadequate antibody production by the abnormal B cells. With advanced disease, CLL may cause damage by direct tissue infiltration.

Information about CLL is evolving rapidly, with new findings in biology and new treatment options, and outcomes are improving significantly.

► Clinical Findings

A. Symptoms and Signs

CLL is a disease of older patients, with 90% of cases occurring after age 50 years and a median age at presentation of 70 years. Many patients will be incidentally discovered to have lymphocytosis. Others present with fatigue or lymphadenopathy. On examination, 80% of patients will have lymphadenopathy and 50% will have enlargement of the liver or spleen.

The long-standing Rai classification system remains prognostically useful: stage 0, lymphocytosis only; stage I, lymphocytosis plus lymphadenopathy; stage II, organomegaly (spleen, liver); stage III, anemia; stage IV, thrombocytopenia. These stages can be collapsed into low risk (stages 0–I), intermediate risk (stage II), and high risk (stages III–IV).

CLL usually pursues an indolent course, but some subtypes behave more aggressively; a variant, prolymphocytic leukemia, is more aggressive. The morphology of the latter is different, characterized by larger and more immature cells. In 5–10% of cases, CLL may be complicated by autoimmune hemolytic anemia or autoimmune thrombocytopenia. In approximately 5% of cases, while the systemic disease remains stable, an isolated lymph node transforms into an aggressive large cell lymphoma (**Richter syndrome**).

B. Laboratory Findings

The hallmark of CLL is isolated lymphocytosis. The white blood count is usually greater than 20,000/mcL (20 × 10^9/L) and may be markedly elevated to several hundred thousand. Usually 75–98% of the circulating cells are lymphocytes. Lymphocytes appear small and mature, with condensed nuclear chromatin, and are morphologically indistinguishable from normal small lymphocytes, but smaller numbers of larger and activated lymphocytes may be seen. The hematocrit and platelet count are usually normal at presentation. The bone marrow is variably infiltrated with small lymphocytes. The immunophenotype of CLL demonstrates coexpression of the B lymphocyte lineage marker CD19 with the T lymphocyte marker CD5; this finding is commonly observed only in CLL and mantle cell lymphoma. CLL is distinguished from mantle cell lymphoma by the expression of CD23, low expression of surface immunoglobulin and CD20, and the absence of a translocation or overexpression of cyclin D1. Patients whose CLL cells have mutated forms of the immunoglobulin gene (IgVH somatic mutation) have a more indolent form of disease; these cells typically express low levels of the surface antigen CD38 and do not express the zeta-associated protein (ZAP-70). Conversely, patients whose cells have unmutated IgVH genes and high levels of ZAP-70 expression do less well and require treatment sooner. The assessment of genomic changes by fluorescence in-situ hybridization (FISH) provides important prognostic information. The finding of deletion of chromosome 17p (TP53) confers the worst prognosis, while deletion of 11q (ATM) confers an inferior prognosis to the average genotype, and isolated deletion of 13q has a more favorable outcome.

Hypogammaglobulinemia is present in 50% of patients and becomes more common with advanced disease. In some, a small amount of IgM paraprotein is present in the serum.

► Differential Diagnosis

Few syndromes can be confused with CLL. Viral infections producing lymphocytosis should be obvious from the presence of fever and other clinical findings; however, fever may occur in CLL from concomitant bacterial infection. Pertussis may cause a particularly high total lymphocyte count. Other lymphoproliferative diseases such as Waldenström macroglobulinemia, hairy cell leukemia, or lymphoma (especially mantle cell) in the leukemic phase are distinguished on the basis of the morphology and immunophenotype of circulating lymphocytes and bone marrow. Monoclonal B-cell lymphocytosis is a disorder characterized by fewer than 5000/mcL B-cells and is considered a precursor to B-CLL.

► Treatment

Most cases of early indolent CLL require no specific therapy, and the standard of care for early-stage disease has been observation. Indications for treatment include progressive fatigue, symptomatic lymphadenopathy, anemia, or thrombocytopenia. These patients have either symptomatic and progressive Rai stage II disease or stage III/IV disease. Initial treatment choices for patients younger than age 70 years without significant comorbidities include the combination of fludarabine with cyclophosphamide and rituximab or the combination of bendamustine with rituximab. The latter combination is better tolerated and associated with fewer adverse events but results in a shorter time to progression (see Table 39–11).

For older patients or young patients with significant comorbidities, chlorambucil, 0.6–1 mg/kg, a well-tolerated agent given orally every 3 weeks for approximately 6 months, has been the standard therapy. The novel monoclonal antibody obinutuzumab, in combination with chlorambucil produces a significant number of responses (75%) including elimination of disease at the molecular level (in 17%) and offers another well-tolerated choice in this patient population. Lastly, the oral agent ibrutinib, an inhibitor of Bruton tyrosine kinase, a key component in the B-cell receptor signaling pathway, has shown remarkable activity at a dose of 420 mg daily as a first-line agent in older patients, with an overall response rate of 71%, and an estimated progression-free survival rate of 75% at 26 months. The most common nonhematologic adverse events were diarrhea (50%), fatigue (32%), and nausea (18%). Caution should be exercised when this agent is used in conjunction with CYP3A inhibitors or inducers. In addition, there is a potential for serious bleeding when it is used in patients taking warfarin.

For patients with relapsed or refractory disease, both ibrutinib and idelalisib (a PI3 kinase delta inhibitor) demonstrate significant activity, even for patients with high-risk genetics. Both of these agents can be associated with marked lymphocytosis due to release of tumor cells from the lymph nodes into the peripheral blood. This results in a significant early reduction in lymphadenopathy but a potentially misleading, more delayed clearance of peripheral blood and bone marrow. In patients with deletion of chromosome 17p, treatment with ibrutinib can result in a sustained duration of response (85% at 2 years), a breakthrough in this disease. Idelalisib at 150 mg orally twice a day in combination with rituximab has shown similar activity in the relapsed setting across genetic risk groups. Adverse events with idelalisib include fever (29%), fatigue (24%), nausea (24%), and elevations in liver enzymes (35%).

Associated autoimmune hemolytic anemia or immune thrombocytopenia may require treatment with rituximab, prednisone, or splenectomy. Fludarabine should be avoided in patients with autoimmune hemolytic anemia since it may exacerbate it. Rituximab should be used with caution in patients with past HBV infection since HBV reactivation, fulminant hepatitis, and, rarely, death can occur without anti-HBV agent prophylaxis. Patients with recurrent bacterial infections and hypogammaglobulinemia benefit from prophylactic infusions of gamma globulin (0.4 g/kg/month), but this treatment is very expensive and can be justified only when these infections are severe. Patients undergoing therapy with a nucleoside analogue (fludarabine, pentostatin) should receive anti-infective prophylaxis for *Pneumocystis jirovecii* pneumonia, herpes viruses, and invasive fungal infections until there is evidence of T-cell recovery.

Allogeneic transplantation offers potentially curative treatment for patients with CLL, but it should be used only in patients whose disease cannot be controlled by standard therapies. Nonmyeloablative allogeneic transplant has produced encouraging results in CLL. Some subtypes of CLL with genomic abnormalities such as chromosome 17p deletions have a sufficiently poor prognosis with standard therapies that early intervention with allogeneic transplant is being studied to assess whether it can improve outcomes.

▶ **Prognosis**

Therapies have changed the prognosis of CLL. In the past, median survival was approximately 6 years, and only 25% of patients lived more than 10 years. Patients with stage 0 or stage I disease have a median survival of 10–15 years, and these patients may be reassured that they can live a normal life for many years. Patients with stage III or stage IV disease had a median survival of less than 2 years in the past, but with current therapies, 2-year survival is now more than 90% and the long-term outlook appears to be substantially changed. For patients with high-risk and resistant forms of CLL, there is evidence that allogeneic transplantation can overcome risk factors and lead to long-term disease control.

▶ **When to Refer**

All patients with CLL should be referred to a hematologist.

▶ **When to Admit**

Hospitalization is rarely needed.

Gupta NK et al. New meets old: a case study and review of novel therapeutics for the treatment of CLL in older patients. J Natl Compr Canc Netw. 2014 Oct;12(10):1371–5. [PMID: 25313177]

Mato A et al. Management of chronic lymphocytic leukemia (CLL) in the era of B-cell receptor signal transduction inhibitors. Am J Hematol. 2015 Jul;90(7):657–64. [PMID: 25808792]

McClanahan F et al. Transplantation in chronic lymphocytic leukemia: does it still matter in the era of novel targeted therapies? Hematol Oncol Clin North Am. 2014 Dec;28(6): 1055–71. [PMID: 25459179]

Parikh SA et al. Risk factors for Richter syndrome in chronic lymphocytic leukemia. Curr Hematol Malig Rep. 2014 Sep;9(3):294–9. [PMID: 25218362]

Whitaker JA et al. Room for improvement: immunizations for patients with monoclonal B-cell lymphocytosis or chronic lymphocytic leukemia. Clin Adv Hematol Oncol. 2014 Jul;12(7):440–50. [PMID: 25322324]

▼ LYMPHOMAS

NON-HODGKIN LYMPHOMAS

ESSENTIALS OF DIAGNOSIS

▶ Often present with painless lymphadenopathy.

▶ Pathologic diagnosis of lymphoma is made by pathologic examination of tissue.

▶ **General Considerations**

The non-Hodgkin lymphomas are a heterogeneous group of cancers of lymphocytes usually presenting as enlarged lymph nodes. The disorders vary in clinical presentation and course from indolent to rapidly progressive.

Molecular biology has provided clues to the pathogenesis of these disorders, often a matter of balanced chromosomal translocations whereby an oncogene becomes juxtaposed next to either an immunoglobulin gene (B-cell lymphoma) or the T-cell receptor gene or related gene (T-cell lymphoma). The net result is oncogene overexpression and development of lymphoma. The best-studied example is Burkitt lymphoma, in which a characteristic cytogenetic abnormality of translocation between the long arms of chromosomes 8 and 14 has been identified. The protooncogene c-*myc* is translocated from its normal position on chromosome 8 to the immunoglobulin heavy chain locus on chromosome 14. Overexpression of c-*myc* is related to malignant transformation through excess B-cell proliferation. In the follicular lymphomas, the t(14;18) translocation is characteristic and *bcl-2* is overexpressed, resulting in protection against apoptosis, the usual mechanism of B-cell death.

Classification of the lymphomas is a dynamic area still undergoing evolution. The most recent grouping (Table 13–16) separates diseases based on both clinical and pathologic features. Eighty-five percent of non-Hodgkin lymphomas are B-cell and 15% are T-cell or NK-cell in origin. Even though non-Hodgkin lymphomas represent a very diverse group of diseases, they are historically divided

Table 13–16. World Health Organization classification of non-Hodgkin lymphomas (most common).

Precursor B-cell lymphoblastic lymphoma
Mature B-cell lymphomas
Diffuse large B-cell lymphoma
Mediastinal large B-cell lymphoma
Follicular lymphoma
Small lymphocytic lymphoma
Lymphoplasmacytic lymphoma (Waldenström macroglobulinemia)
Mantle cell lymphoma
Burkitt lymphoma
Marginal zone lymphoma
MALT type
Nodal type
Splenic type
Precursor T-cell lymphoblastic lymphoma
Mature T (and NK cell) lymphomas
Anaplastic T-cell lymphoma
Angioimmunoblastic
Peripheral T-cell lymphoma, NOS
Cutaneous T-cell lymphoma (mycosis fungoides)
Extranodal T/NK-cell lymphoma
Adult T-cell leukemia/lymphoma

MALT, mucosa-associated lymphoid tissue; NOS, not otherwise specified.

in two categories based on clinical behavior and pathology: the indolent (low-grade) and the aggressive (intermediate- or high-grade).

⏵ Clinical Findings

A. Symptoms and Signs

Patients with non-Hodgkin lymphomas usually present with lymphadenopathy, which may be isolated or widespread. Involved lymph nodes may be present peripherally or centrally (in the retroperitoneum, mesentery, and pelvis). The indolent lymphomas are usually disseminated at the time of diagnosis, and bone marrow involvement is frequent. Many patients with lymphoma have constitutional symptoms such as fever, drenching night sweats, and weight loss of greater than 10% of prior body weight (referred to as "B" symptoms).

On examination, lymphadenopathy may be isolated or diffuse, and extranodal sites of disease (such as the skin, gastrointestinal tract, liver, and bone marrow) may be found. Patients with Burkitt lymphoma are noted to have abdominal pain or abdominal fullness because of the predilection of the disease for the abdomen.

Once a pathologic diagnosis is established, staging is done using a whole body PET/CT scan, a bone marrow biopsy, and, in patients with high-grade lymphoma or intermediate-grade lymphoma with high-risk features, a lumbar puncture.

B. Laboratory Findings

The peripheral blood is usually normal even with extensive bone marrow involvement by lymphoma. Circulating lymphoma cells in the blood are not commonly seen.

Bone marrow involvement is manifested as paratrabecular monoclonal lymphoid aggregates. In some high-grade lymphomas, the meninges are involved and malignant cells are found with cerebrospinal fluid cytology. The serum LD has been shown to be a useful prognostic marker and is now incorporated in risk stratification of treatment.

The diagnosis of lymphoma is made by tissue biopsy. Needle aspiration may yield evidence for non-Hodgkin lymphoma, but a lymph node biopsy (or biopsy of involved extranodal tissue) is required for accurate diagnosis and classification.

⏵ Treatment

A. Indolent Lymphomas

The most common lymphomas in this group are follicular lymphoma, marginal zone lymphomas, and small lymphocytic lymphoma (CLL). The treatment of **indolent lymphomas** depends on the stage of disease and the clinical status of the patient. A small number of patients have limited disease with only one or two contiguous abnormal lymph node groups and may be treated with localized irradiation with curative intent. However, most patients (85%) with indolent lymphoma have disseminated disease at the time of diagnosis and are not considered curable. Historically, treatment of these patients has not affected overall survival; therefore, treatment is only offered when symptoms develop or for high tumor bulk. Following each treatment response, patients will experience a relapse at traditionally shorter intervals. Some patients will have temporary spontaneous remissions (8%). There are an increasing number of reasonable treatment options for indolent lymphomas, but no consensus has emerged on the best strategy. Treatment with rituximab (375 mg/m^2 intravenously weekly for 4 weeks) is commonly used either alone or in combination with chemotherapy and may be the only agent to affect overall survival in these disorders. Patients should be screened for hepatitis B because rare cases of fatal fulminant hepatitis have been described with the use of anti-CD20 monoclonal therapies without anti-HBV agent prophylaxis. Rituximab is added to chemotherapy regimens including bendamustine; cyclophosphamide, vincristine, and prednisone (R-CVP); and cyclophosphamide, doxorubicin, vincristine, and prednisone (R-CHOP) (see Table 39–11). Radioimmunoconjugates that fuse anti-B cell monoclonal antibodies with radioactive nuclides produce higher response rates compared to antibody alone, and two such agents (yttrium-90 ibritumomab tiuxetan and iodine-131 tositumomab) are in use. Some patients with clinically aggressive low-grade lymphomas may be appropriate candidates for allogeneic stem cell transplantation with curative intent. The role of autologous hematopoietic stem cell transplantation remains uncertain, but some patients with recurrent disease appear to have prolonged remissions without the expectation of cure.

Patients with mucosal-associated lymphoid tumors of the stomach may be appropriately treated with combination antibiotics directed against *H pylori* and with acid blockade but require frequent endoscopic monitoring. Alternatively, MALT confined to the stomach can also be cured with whole-stomach radiotherapy.

B. Aggressive Lymphomas

Patients with **diffuse large B-cell lymphoma** are treated with curative intent. Those with localized disease may receive short-course immunochemotherapy (such as three courses of R-CHOP) plus localized involved-field radiation or six cycles of immunochemotherapy without radiation. Most patients who have more advanced disease are treated with six cycles of immunochemotherapy such as R-CHOP (see Table 39–11). Patients with diffuse large B-cell lymphoma who relapse after initial chemotherapy can still be cured by autologous hematopoietic stem cell transplantation if their disease remains responsive to chemotherapy. A subtype of diffuse large B-cell lymphoma with chromosomal translocations affecting *MYC*, such as t(8;14), and affecting *BCL2*, such as t(14;18), is called "double-hit lymphoma" and has a very aggressive course. Patients with this disease may do better with dose-adjusted R-EPOCH therapy. More recently, about 25% of patients with diffuse large B-cell lymphoma have been identified as "double-protein expressors" with overexpression of *MYC* and *BCL2* by immunohistochemistry. While the outcomes with R-CHOP are inferior, no definitive alternative treatment recommendations can be made at this time.

Mantle cell lymphoma is not effectively treated with standard immunochemotherapy regimens. Intensive initial immunochemotherapy including autologous hematopoietic stem cell transplantation has been shown to improve outcomes. Reduced-intensity allogeneic stem cell transplantation offers curative potential for selected patients. Ibrutinib is active in relapsed or refractory patients with mantle cell lymphoma. For **primary central nervous system lymphoma,** repetitive cycles of high-dose intravenous methotrexate with rituximab early in the treatment course produce better results than whole-brain radiotherapy and with less cognitive impairment.

Patients with **high-grade lymphomas** (Burkitt or lymphoblastic) require urgent, intense, cyclic chemotherapy in the hospital similar to that given for ALL, and they also require intrathecal chemotherapy as central nervous system prophylaxis.

Patients with **peripheral T-cell lymphomas** usually have advanced stage nodal and extranodal disease and typically have inferior response rates to therapy compared to patients with aggressive B-cell disease. Autologous stem cell transplantation is often incorporated in first-line therapy. The antibody-drug conjugate brentuximab vedotin has significant activity in patients with relapsed CD30 positive peripheral T-cell lymphomas, such as anaplastic large-cell lymphoma.

Prognosis

The median survival of patients with indolent lymphomas is 10–15 years. These diseases ultimately become refractory to chemotherapy. This often occurs at the time of histologic progression of the disease to a more aggressive form of lymphoma.

The International Prognostic Index is widely used to categorize patients with aggressive lymphoma into risk groups. Factors that confer adverse prognosis are age over 60 years, elevated serum LD, stage III or stage IV disease, more than one extranodal site of disease, and poor performance status. Cure rates range from more than 80% for low-risk patients (zero risk factors) to less than 50% for high-risk patients (four or more risk factors).

For patients who relapse after initial chemotherapy, the prognosis depends on whether the lymphoma is still responsive to chemotherapy. If the lymphoma remains responsive to chemotherapy, autologous hematopoietic stem cell transplantation offers a 50% chance of long-term lymphoma-free survival.

The treatment of older patients with lymphoma has been difficult because of poorer tolerance of aggressive chemotherapy. The use of myeloid growth factors and prophylactic antibiotics to reduce neutropenic complications may improve outcomes.

Molecular profiling techniques using gene array technology and immunophenotyping have defined subsets of lymphomas with different biologic features and prognoses are being studied in clinical trials to determine choice of therapy.

When to Refer

All patients with lymphoma should be referred to a hematologist or an oncologist.

When to Admit

Admission is necessary only for specific complications of lymphoma or its treatment and for the treatment of all high-grade lymphomas.

Campo E et al. Mantle cell lymphoma: evolving management strategies. Blood. 2015 Jan 1;125(1):48–55. [PMID: 25499451]
Kritharis A et al. Current therapeutic strategies and new treatment paradigms for follicular lymphoma. Cancer Treat Res. 2015;165:197–226. [PMID: 25655611]
Kubuschok B et al. Management of diffuse large B-cell lymphoma (DLBCL). Cancer Treat Res. 2015;165:271–88. [PMID: 25655614]

HODGKIN LYMPHOMA

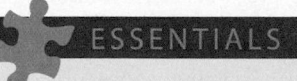 ESSENTIALS OF DIAGNOSIS

► Often painless lymphadenopathy.
► Constitutional symptoms may or may not be present.
► Pathologic diagnosis by lymph node biopsy.

General Considerations

Hodgkin lymphoma is characterized by lymph node biopsy showing Reed-Sternberg cells in an appropriate reactive cellular background. The malignant cell is derived from B lymphocytes of germinal center origin.

Clinical Findings

There is a bimodal age distribution, with one peak in the 20s and a second over age 50 years. Most patients seek medical attention because of a painless mass, commonly in the neck. Others may seek medical attention because of constitutional symptoms such as fever, weight loss, or drenching night sweats, or because of generalized pruritus. An unusual symptom of Hodgkin lymphoma is pain in an involved lymph node following alcohol ingestion.

An important feature of Hodgkin lymphoma is its tendency to arise within single lymph node areas and spread in an orderly fashion to contiguous areas of lymph nodes. Late in the course of the disease, vascular invasion leads to widespread hematogenous dissemination.

Hodgkin lymphoma is divided into two subtypes: classic Hodgkin (nodular sclerosis, mixed cellularity, lymphocyte rich, and lymphocyte depleted) and non-classic Hodgkin (nodular lymphocyte predominant). Hodgkin lymphoma should be distinguished pathologically from other malignant lymphomas and may occasionally be confused with reactive lymph nodes seen in infectious mononucleosis, cat-scratch disease, or drug reactions (eg, phenytoin).

Patients undergo a staging evaluation to determine the extent of disease, including serum chemistries, whole-body PET/CT scan, and bone marrow biopsy. The staging nomenclature (Ann Arbor) is as follows: stage I, one lymph node region involved; stage II, involvement of two or more lymph node regions on one side of the diaphragm; stage III, lymph node regions involved on both sides of the diaphragm; and stage IV, disseminated disease with extranodal involvement. Disease staging is further categorized as "A" if patients lack constitutional symptoms or as "B" if patients have 10% weight loss over 6 months, fever, or drenching night sweats (or some combination thereof).

Treatment

Chemotherapy is the mainstay of treatment for Hodgkin lymphoma and ABVD (doxorubicin, bleomycin, vinblastine, dacarbazine) remains the standard first-line regimen. Even though others such as Stanford V or escalated BEACOPP (bleomycin, etoposide, doxorubicin, cyclophosphamide, vincristine, procarbazine, prednisone) may improve response rates and reduce the need for consolidative radiotherapy, they are usually associated with increased toxicity and lack a definitive overall survival advantage. Low-risk patients are those with stage I or II disease without bulky lymphadenopathy or evidence of systemic inflammation. They traditionally receive a combination of short-course chemotherapy with involved-field radiotherapy or a full course of chemotherapy alone (see Table 39–11). However, ongoing studies are aiming to eliminate the radiotherapy or to abbreviate the chemotherapy in patients who achieve an interim negative PET/CT scan. High-risk patients are those with stage III or IV disease or with stage II disease and a large mediastinal or other bulky mass. These patients are treated with a full course of ABVD for six cycles. End-of-treatment PET/CT scan may identify patients with stage II bulky disease who

can avoid traditional involved-field radiotherapy. Pulmonary toxicity can unfortunately occur following either chemotherapy (bleomycin) or radiation and should be treated aggressively in these patients, since it can lead to permanent fibrosis and death.

Classic Hodgkin lymphoma relapsing after initial treatment may be treatable with high-dose chemotherapy and autologous hematopoietic stem cell transplantation. This offers a 35–50% chance of cure when disease is still chemotherapy responsive. The antibody-drug conjugate brentuximab vedotin has shown impressive activity in patients relapsing after autologous stem cell transplantation (ORR: 75%; CR: 34%) and has been approved by the US Food and Drug Administration for this indication. It is now being studied in front-line therapy, replacing the bleomycin in ABVD.

Prognosis

All patients should be treated with curative intent. Prognosis in advanced stage Hodgkin lymphoma is influenced by seven features: stage, age, gender, hemoglobin, albumin, white blood count, and lymphocyte count. The cure rate is 75% if zero to two risk features are present and 55% when three or more risk features are present. The prognosis of patients with stage IA or IIA disease is excellent, with 10-year survival rates in excess of 90%. Patients with advanced disease (stage III or IV) have 10-year survival rates of 50–60%. Poorer results are seen in patients who are older, those who have bulky disease, and those with lymphocyte depletion or mixed cellularity on histologic examination. Non-classic Hodgkin lymphoma (nodular lymphocyte predominant) is highly curable with radiotherapy alone for early-stage disease; however, for high-stage disease, it is characterized by long survival with repetitive relapses after chemotherapy.

When to Refer

- All patients should be sent to an oncologist or hematologist.
- Secondary referral to a radiation oncologist might be appropriate.

When to Admit

Patients should be admitted for complications of the disease or its treatment.

Connors JM. Risk assessment in the management of newly diagnosed classical Hodgkin lymphoma. Blood. 2015 Mar 12;125(11):1693–702. [PMID: 25575542]

Evens AM et al. The role of FDG-PET in defining prognosis of Hodgkin lymphoma for early-stage disease. Blood. 2014 Nov 27; 124(23):3356–64. [PMID: 25428223]

Meyer RM et al. ABVD alone versus radiation-based therapy in limited-stage Hodgkin's lymphoma. N Engl J Med. 2012 Feb 2;366(5):399–408. [PMID: 22149921]

Rashidi A et al. Biologic agents in the management of Hodgkin lymphoma. J Natl Compr Canc Netw. 2015 May;13(5): 587–96. [PMID: 25964642]

MULTIPLE MYELOMA

ESSENTIALS OF DIAGNOSIS

▸ Bone pain, often in the spine, ribs, or proximal long bones.

▸ Monoclonal paraprotein by serum or urine protein electrophoresis or immunofixation.

▸ Clonal plasma cells in the bone marrow or in a tissue biopsy, or both.

▸ Organ damage due to plasma cells (eg, bones, kidneys, hypercalcemia, anemia).

► General Considerations

Multiple myeloma is a malignancy of hematopoietic stem cells terminally differentiated as plasma cells characterized by infiltration of the bone marrow, bone destruction, and paraprotein formation. The diagnosis is established when monoclonal plasma cells (either kappa or lambda light chain restricted) in the bone marrow (any percentage) or as a tumor (plasmacytoma), or both, are associated with end-organ damage (such as bone disease [lytic lesions, osteopenia], anemia [hemoglobin less than 10 g/dL {100 g/L}], hypercalcemia [calcium greater than 11.5 mg/dL {2.9 mmol/L}], or kidney injury [creatinine greater than 2 mg/dL {176.8 mcmol/L}]) with or without paraprotein elaboration. Sixty percent or more clonal plasma cells in the bone marrow or a serum free kappa to lambda ratio of greater than 100 or less than 0.01 (both criteria regardless of end-organ damage) is also diagnostic of multiple myeloma. Smoldering myeloma is defined as 10% or more clonal plasma cells in the bone marrow, a serum paraprotein level of 3 g/dL (30 g/L) or higher, or both, without plasma cell–related end-organ damage.

Malignant plasma cells can form tumors (plasmacytomas) that may cause spinal cord compression or other soft-tissue problems. Bone disease is common and due to excessive osteoclast activation mediated largely by the interaction of the receptor activator of NF-kappa-B (RANK) with its ligand (RANKL). In multiple myeloma, osteoprotegerin (a decoy receptor for RANKL) is underproduced, thus promoting the binding of RANK with RANKL with consequent excessive bone resorption. Other soluble factors contributing to osteoclast hyperactivation include interleukin-1, interleukin-6, tissue necrosis factor-alpha, macrophage inhibitor protein-1-alpha, and macrophage colony stimulating factor, all of which might prove eventual therapeutic targets.

The paraproteins (monoclonal immunoglobulins) secreted by the malignant plasma cells may cause problems in their own right. Very high paraprotein levels (either IgG or IgA) may cause hyperviscosity, although this is more common with the IgM paraprotein in Waldenström macroglobulinemia. The light chain component of the immunoglobulin, when produced in excess, often leads to kidney failure (frequently aggravated by hypercalcemia or hyperuricemia, or both). Light chain components may be deposited in tissues as amyloid, resulting in kidney failure with albuminuria and a vast array of systemic symptoms.

Myeloma patients are prone to recurrent infections for a number of reasons, including neutropenia, the underproduction of normal immunoglobulins and the immunosuppressive effects of chemotherapy. Myeloma patients are especially prone to infections with encapsulated organisms such as *Streptococcus pneumoniae* and *Haemophilus influenzae*.

► Clinical Findings

A. Symptoms and Signs

Myeloma is a disease of older adults (median age, 65 years). The most common presenting complaints are those related to anemia, bone pain, kidney disease, and infection. Bone pain is most common in the back, hips, or ribs or may present as a pathologic fracture, especially of the femoral neck or vertebrae. Patients may also come to medical attention because of spinal cord compression from a plasmacytoma or the hyperviscosity syndrome (mucosal bleeding, vertigo, nausea, visual disturbances, alterations in mental status, hypoxia). Many patients are diagnosed because of laboratory findings of hypercalcemia, proteinuria, elevated sedimentation rate, or abnormalities on serum protein electrophoresis obtained for symptoms or in routine screening studies. A few patients come to medical attention because of organ dysfunction due to amyloidosis.

Examination may reveal pallor, bone tenderness, and soft tissue masses. Patients may have neurologic signs related to neuropathy or spinal cord compression. Fever occurs mainly with infection. Acute oliguric or nonoliguric kidney failure may be present due to hypercalcemia, hyperuricemia, light-chain cast injury, or primary amyloidosis.

B. Laboratory Findings

Anemia is nearly universal. Red blood cell morphology is normal, but rouleaux formation is common and may be marked. The absence of rouleaux formation, however, excludes neither multiple myeloma nor the presence of a serum paraprotein. The neutrophil and platelet counts are usually normal at presentation. Only rarely will plasma cells be visible on peripheral blood smear (plasma cell leukemia).

The hallmark of myeloma is the finding of a paraprotein on serum or urine protein electrophoresis (PEP) or immunofixation electrophoresis (IFE). The majority of patients will have a monoclonal spike visible in the gamma- or beta-globulin region of the PEP. The semi-quantification of the paraprotein on the PEP is referred to as the M-protein, and IFE will reveal this to be a monoclonal immunoglobulin. Approximately 15% of patients will have no demonstrable paraprotein in the serum because their myeloma cells produce only light chains and not intact immunoglobulin, and the light chains pass rapidly through the glomerulus into the urine. Urine PEP and IFE will demonstrate the light chain paraprotein in this setting. The free light chain assay will sometimes demonstrate excess monoclonal light chains in serum and urine, and in a small proportion of patients, will be the only means to identify and quantify the paraprotein being produced. Overall, the paraprotein is IgG (60%), IgA (20%), or light chain only (15%) in multiple myeloma, with the remainder being rare cases of IgD, IgM, or biclonal gammopathy. In sporadic cases, no paraprotein is present ("nonsecretory myeloma"); these patients have particularly aggressive disease.

The bone marrow will be infiltrated by variable numbers of monoclonal plasma cells. The plasma cells may be morphologically abnormal often demonstrating multinucleation and vacuolization. The plasma cells will display marked skewing of the normal kappa-to-lambda light chain ratio, which will indicate their clonality. Many benign processes can result in bone marrow plasmacytosis, but the presence of atypical plasma cells, light chain restriction, and effacement of normal bone marrow elements helps distinguish myeloma.

C. Imaging

Bone radiographs are important in establishing the diagnosis of myeloma. Lytic lesions are most commonly seen in the axial skeleton: skull, spine, proximal long bones, and ribs. At other times, only generalized osteoporosis is seen. The radionuclide bone scan is not useful in detecting bone lesions in myeloma, since there is usually no osteoblastic component. In the evaluation of patients with known or suspected multiple myeloma, magnetic resonance imaging (MRI) and positron emission tomography (PET) scans visualize disease more effectively than plain radiographs.

▶ Differential Diagnosis

When a patient is discovered to have a paraprotein, the distinction between multiple myeloma or another lymphoproliferative malignancy with a paraprotein (CLL, Waldenström macroglobulinemia, non-Hodgkin lymphoma, primary amyloid, cryoglobulinemia) and monoclonal gammopathy of undetermined significance (MGUS) must be made. MGUS is present in 1% of all adults, (3% of those over age 50 years and more than 5% of those over age 70 years). Thus, among all patients with paraproteins, MGUS is far more common than multiple myeloma. MGUS is defined as bone marrow monoclonal plasma cells less than 10% in the setting of a paraprotein (serum M-protein less than 3 g/dL [30 g/L]) and the absence of end-organ damage. In approximately one quarter of cases, MGUS progresses to overt malignant disease in a median of one decade. The transformation of MGUS to multiple myeloma is approximately 1% per year. Multiple myeloma, smoldering multiple myeloma, and MGUS must be distinguished from reactive (benign) polyclonal hypergammaglobulinemia (which is commonly seen in cirrhosis).

▶ Treatment

Patients with MGUS are observed without treatment. Patients with smoldering myeloma treated with lenalidomide (an immunomodulatory agent) and dexamethasone take longer to progress to symptomatic myeloma and live longer than when simply observed. Most patients with multiple myeloma require treatment at diagnosis because of bone pain or other symptoms and complications related to the disease. The initial treatment generally involves at a minimum an immunomodulatory agent, such as thalidomide or lenalidomide, or a proteasome inhibitor, such as bortezomib, in combination with moderate- or high-dose dexamethasone. The major side effects of lenalidomide are neutropenia and thrombocytopenia, venous thromboembolism, and peripheral neuropathy. Bortezomib has the advantages of producing rapid responses and of being effective in poor-prognosis myeloma. The major side effect of bortezomib is neuropathy (both peripheral and autonomic), which is largely ameliorated when given subcutaneously rather than intravenously. A common regimen for initial treatment is lenalidomide, bortezomib, and dexamethasone. The combinations of bortezomib, dexamethasone, and liposomal doxorubicin and bortezomib, cyclophosphamide, and dexamethasone are also effective. Carfilzomib, a second-generation proteasome inhibitor, produces responses in patients for whom bortezomib treatment fails and does not cause neuropathy. An oral proteasome inhibitor, ixazomib, is available for relapsed disease. Pomalidomide, a new immunomodulatory agent, is effective as salvage therapy.

After initial therapy, many patients under age 80 years are consolidated with autologous hematopoietic stem cell transplantation following high-dose melphalan. Autologous stem cell transplantation prolongs both duration of remission and overall survival, and has the advantage of providing long treatment-free intervals. Lenalidomide or thalidomide prolong remission and survival when given as posttransplant maintenance therapy but at the expense of an elevated rate of second malignancies. Allogeneic stem cell transplantation is potentially curative in multiple myeloma, but its role has been limited because of the unusually high treatment-related mortality rate (40–50%) in myeloma patients. Many new agents are available for relapsed disease, including panobinostat (a histone deacetylase inhibitor) and daratumumab (an anti-CD28 monoclonal antibody).

Localized radiotherapy may be useful for palliation of bone pain or for eradicating tumor at the site of pathologic fracture. Vertebral collapse with its attendant pain and mechanical disturbance can be treated with vertebroplasty or kyphoplasty. Hypercalcemia and hyperuricemia should be treated aggressively and immobilization and dehydration avoided. The bisphosphonates (pamidronate 90 mg or zoledronic acid 4 mg intravenously monthly) reduce pathologic fractures in patients with bone disease and are an important adjunct in this subset of patients. The bisphosphonates are also used to treat malignant hypercalcemia. However, long-term bisphosphonates, especially zoledronic acid, have been associated with a risk of osteonecrosis of the jaw and other bony areas, so treated patients must be monitored for this complication. Myeloma patients with oliguric or anuric renal failure at diagnosis should be treated aggressively with chemotherapy and considered for plasma exchange (to reduce the paraprotein burden), as return of renal function can commonly occur.

Prognosis

The outlook for patients with myeloma has been steadily improving for the past decade. The median survival of patients is more than 7 years. Patients with low-stage disease who lack high-risk genomic changes respond very well to treatment and derive significant benefit from autologous hematopoietic stem cell transplantation and have survivals approaching a decade. The **International Staging System** for myeloma relies on two factors: beta-2-microglobulin and albumin. Stage 1 patients have both beta-2-microglobulin less than 3.5 mg/L and albumin greater than 3.5 g/dL (survival more than 5 years). Stage 3 is established when beta-2-microglobulin is greater than 5.5 mg/L (survival less than 2 years). Stage 2 is established with values in between stage 1 and 3. The other laboratory finding of important adverse prognostic significance on a bone marrow sample is genetic abnormalities established by FISH involving the immunoglobulin heavy chain locus at chromosome 14q32 (such as the finding of t[4;14] or t[14;16]) or multiple copies of the 1q21-23 locus. Abnormalities of chromosome 17p also confer a particularly poor prognosis.

When to Refer

All patients with multiple myeloma should be referred to a hematologist or an oncologist.

When to Admit

Hospitalization is indicated for treatment of acute kidney failure, hypercalcemia, or suspicion of spinal cord compression, for certain chemotherapy regimens, or for hematopoietic stem cell transplantation.

Alegre A et al. Zoledronic acid in the management of bone disease as a consequence of multiple myeloma: a review. Eur J Haematol. 2014 Mar;92(3):181–8. [PMID: 24330023]

Broijl A et al. An update in treatment options for multiple myeloma in nontransplant eligible patients. Expert Opin Pharmacother. 2015;16(13):1945–57. [PMID: 26245702]

Festuccia M et al. Allogeneic stem cell transplantation in multiple myeloma: immunotherapy and new drugs. Expert Opin Biol Ther. 2015 Jun;15(6):857–72. [PMID: 25865214]

Lonial S et al; ELOQUENT-2 Investigators. Elotuzumab therapy for relapsed or refractory multiple myeloma. N Engl J Med. 2015 Aug 13;373(7):621–31. [PMID: 26035255]

Mimura N et al. Novel therapeutic strategies for multiple myeloma. Exp Hematol. 2015 Aug;43(8):732–41. [PMID: 26118499]

Moreau P et al. Frontline therapy of multiple myeloma. Blood. 2015 May 14;125(20):3076–84. [PMID: 25838345]

Nooka AK et al. Treatment options for relapsed and refractory multiple myeloma. Blood. 2015 May 14;125(20):3085–99. [PMID: 25838342]

Rajkumar SV et al. Smoldering multiple myeloma. Blood. 2015 May 14;125(20):3069–75. [PMID: 25838344]

van de Donk NW et al. The clinical relevance and management of monoclonal gammopathy of undetermined significance and related disorders: recommendations from the European Myeloma Network. Haematologica. 2014 Jun;99(6):984–96. [PMID: 24658815]

Zagouri F et al. An update on the use of lenalidomide for the treatment of multiple myeloma. Expert Opin Pharmacother. 2015;16(12):1865–77. [PMID: 26165832]

WALDENSTRÖM MACROGLOBULINEMIA

ESSENTIALS OF DIAGNOSIS

▶ Monoclonal IgM paraprotein.
▶ Infiltration of bone marrow by plasmacytic lymphocytes.
▶ Absence of lytic bone disease.

General Considerations

Waldenström macroglobulinemia is a syndrome of IgM hypergammaglobulinemia that occurs in the setting of a low-grade non-Hodgkin lymphoma characterized by B cells that are morphologically a hybrid of lymphocytes and plasma cells. These cells characteristically secrete the IgM paraprotein, and many clinical manifestations of the disease are related to this macroglobulin.

Clinical Findings

A. Symptoms and Signs

This disease characteristically develops insidiously in patients in their 60s or 70s. Patients usually present with fatigue related to anemia. Hyperviscosity of serum may be manifested in a number of ways. Mucosal and gastrointestinal bleeding is related to engorged blood vessels and platelet dysfunction. Other complaints include nausea, vertigo, and visual disturbances. Alterations in consciousness vary from mild lethargy to stupor and coma. The IgM paraprotein may also cause symptoms of cold agglutinin disease (hemolysis) or chronic demyelinating peripheral neuropathy.

On examination, there may be hepatosplenomegaly or lymphadenopathy. The retinal veins are engorged. Purpura may be present. There should be no bone tenderness.

B. Laboratory Findings

Anemia is nearly universal, and rouleaux formation is common, although the red blood cells are agglutinated when the blood smear is prepared at room temperature. The anemia is related in part to expansion of the plasma volume by 50–100% due to the presence of the paraprotein. Other blood counts are usually normal. The abnormal plasmacytic lymphocytes may appear in small numbers on the peripheral blood smear. The bone marrow is characteristically infiltrated by the plasmacytic lymphocytes.

The hallmark of macroglobulinemia is the presence of a monoclonal IgM spike seen on serum PEP in the beta-globulin region. The serum viscosity is usually increased above the normal of 1.4–1.8 times that of water. Symptoms of hyperviscosity usually develop when the serum viscosity is over four times that of water, and marked symptoms usually arise when the viscosity is over six times that of water. Because paraproteins vary in their physicochemical properties, there is no strict correlation between the concentration of paraprotein and serum viscosity.

The IgM paraprotein may cause a positive antiglobulin (Coombs) test for complement and have cold agglutinin or cryoglobulin properties. If macroglobulinemia is suspected but the serum PEP shows only hypogammaglobulinemia, the test should be repeated while taking special measures to maintain the blood at 37°C, since the paraprotein may precipitate out at room temperature. Bone radiographs are normal, and there is no evidence of kidney failure.

Differential Diagnosis

Waldenström macroglobulinemia is differentiated from MGUS by the finding of bone marrow infiltration with monoclonal malignant cells. It is distinguished from CLL by bone marrow morphology, the absence of CD5 expression and the absence of lymphocytosis and from multiple myeloma by bone marrow morphology, the finding of the characteristic IgM paraprotein, and the absence of bone disease.

Treatment

Patients with marked hyperviscosity syndrome (stupor, coma, pulmonary edema) should be treated on an emergency basis with plasmapheresis. On a chronic basis, some patients can be managed with periodic plasmapheresis alone. As with other indolent malignant lymphoid diseases, rituximab (375 mg/m² intravenously weekly for 4–8 weeks) has significant activity. However, a word of caution: the IgM often rises first after rituximab therapy before it falls. Combination therapy is recommended for advanced disease (see Table 39–11). *MYD88* is commonly mutated in Waldenström macroglobulinemia, and in patients with relapsed or refractory disease, the BTK inhibitor ibrutinib, at a dose of 420 mg daily, has shown significant activity with a 90% response rate and a 73% major response rate that can result in durable remissions. Bortezomib, thalidomide, lenalidomide, and bendamustine have also been shown to have activity in this disease. Autologous hematopoietic stem cell transplantation is reserved for relapsed or refractory patients.

Prognosis

Waldenström macroglobulinemia is an indolent disease with a median survival rate of 5 years, and 10% of patients are alive at 15 years.

When to Refer

All patients should be referred to a hematologist or an oncologist.

When to Admit

Patients should be admitted for treatment of hyperviscosity syndrome.

Castillo JJ et al. Overall survival and competing risks of death in patients with Waldenström macroglobulinaemia: an analysis of the Surveillance, Epidemiology and End Results database. Br J Haematol. 2015 Apr;169(1):81–9. [PMID: 25521528]
Oza A et al. Waldenstrom macroglobulinemia: prognosis and management. Blood Cancer J. 2015 Mar 27;5:e296. [PMID: 25815903]
Stone MJ. Waldenström's macroglobulinemia: hyperviscosity syndrome and cryoglobulinemia. Clin Lymphoma Myeloma. 2009 Mar;9(1):97–9. [PMID: 19362986]
Treon SP et al. Ibrutinib in previously treated Waldenström's macroglobulinemia. N Engl J Med. 2015 Apr 9;372(15):1430–40. [PMID: 25853747]

PRIMARY AMYLOIDOSIS

ESSENTIALS OF DIAGNOSIS

▶ Congo red positive amyloid protein on tissue biopsy.
▶ Amyloid protein is kappa or lambda immunoglobulin light chain.
▶ Serum or urine (or both) light chain paraprotein.

General Considerations

Amyloidosis is an uncommon condition whereby a protein abnormally deposits in tissue resulting in organ dysfunction. The propensity of a protein to be amyloidogenic is a consequence of disturbed translational or posttranslational protein folding. The input of amyloid protein into tissues far exceeds its output, so amyloid build up inexorably proceeds to organ dysfunction and ultimately organ failure and premature death.

Amyloidosis is classified according to the type of amyloid protein deposited. The five main categories are **primary** (immunoglobulin light chain [AL]), **secondary** (serum protein A, produced in inflammatory conditions [AA]), **hereditary** (mutated transthyretin [TTR]; others), **senile** (wild-type TTR; atrial natriuretic peptide; others), and **renal failure type** (beta-2-microglobulin, not filtered out by dialysis membranes [Abeta-2M]). Amyloidosis is further classified as **localized** (amyloid deposits only in a single tissue type or organ) or, most common, **systemic** (widespread amyloid deposition).

Clinical Findings

A. Symptoms and Signs

Patients with **localized amyloidosis** have symptoms and signs related to the affected single organ, such as hoarseness (vocal cords) or proptosis and visual disturbance (orbits). Patients with **systemic amyloidosis** have symptoms and signs of unexplained medical syndromes, including heart failure (infiltrative/restrictive cardiomyopathy), nephrotic syndrome, malabsorption and weight loss, hepatic dysfunction, autonomic insufficiency, carpal tunnel syndrome (often bilateral), and sensorimotor peripheral neuropathy. Other symptoms and signs include an enlarged tongue; waxy, rough plaques on skin; contusions (including the periorbital areas); cough or dyspnea; and disturbed deglutition. These symptoms and signs arise insidiously, and the diagnosis of amyloidosis is generally made late in the disease process.

B. Laboratory Findings

The diagnosis of amyloid protein requires a tissue biopsy that demonstrates deposition of a pink substance in the tissue with the H&E stain. This protein stains red with Congo Red and becomes an apple-green color when the light is polarized. Amyloid is a triple-stranded fibril composed of the amyloid protein, amyloid protein P, and glycosaminoglycan. The amyloid fibrils form beta-pleated sheets as demonstrated by electron microscopy. In primary amyloidosis, the amyloid protein is either the kappa or lambda immunoglobulin light chain.

When systemic amyloidosis is suspected, a blind aspiration of the abdominal fat pad will reveal amyloid two-thirds of the time. If the fat pad aspiration is unrevealing, then the affected organ needs biopsy. In 90% of patients with primary amyloidosis, analysis of the serum and urine will reveal a kappa or lambda light chain paraprotein by PEP, IFE, or free light chain assay; in the remainder, mass spectroscopy demonstrates light chain in the tissue biopsy. Lambda amyloid is more common than kappa amyloid, a relative proportion opposite from normal B-cell stoichiometry. Most patients with primary amyloidosis have a small excess of kappa-or lambda-restricted plasma cells in the bone marrow. The bone marrow may or may not demonstrate interstitial amyloid deposition or amyloid in the blood vessels.

Patients with primary cardiac amyloidosis have an infiltrative cardiomyopathy with thick ventricular walls on echocardiogram that sometimes shows a unique speckling pattern. Paradoxically, QRS voltages are low on ECG. With renal amyloid, albuminuria is present, which can be in the nephrotic range. Late in renal involvement, kidney function decreases.

▶ Differential Diagnosis

Primary amyloidosis must be distinguished from MGUS and multiple myeloma or other malignant lymphoproliferative disorders. Of note, 12% of patients with MGUS will convert to primary amyloidosis in a median of 9 years. One-fifth of patients who have primary amyloidosis will meet the diagnostic criteria for multiple myeloma; conversely, 5% of patients with multiple myeloma will have amyloid deposition of the paraprotein at diagnosis.

▶ Treatment

The treatment approach to primary amyloidosis closely resembles that of multiple myeloma. Prospective, randomized trials of multiple myeloma chemotherapy versus colchicine have demonstrated a survival benefit to chemotherapy. The goal is reduction of light chain production and deposition as a means to arrest progressive end-organ dysfunction. Active agents in primary amyloidosis include melphalan, cyclophosphamide, dexamethasone, lenalidomide, and bortezomib (see Table 39–11). As in multiple myeloma, autologous hematopoietic stem cell transplantation after high-dose melphalan is used in patients with reasonable organ function and a good performance status. The treatment-related mortality, however, is higher in patients with primary amyloidosis than in myeloma (8% vs 1%). Some patients will demonstrate end-organ improvement after therapy. Agents are being developed that facilitate amyloid dissolution or correct protein folding abnormalities in the amyloid protein.

▶ Prognosis

Untreated primary amyloidosis is associated with progressive end-organ failure and premature death. There is no known cure for primary amyloidosis. Although virtually every tissue examined at autopsy will contain amyloid, patients with primary amyloidosis will have one or two primary organs failing that clinically drive the presentation and prognosis. The cardiac biomarkers, B-type natriuretic peptide (BNP), n-terminal pro-BNP, and troponins T and I are prognostic in this disease regardless of overt clinical cardiac involvement. Historically, patients with predominantly cardiac or autonomic nerve presentations had survivals of 3–9 months, and those with carpal tunnel syndrome or nephrosis, 1.5–3 years, and those with peripheral neuropathy, 5 years. These survivals are roughly doubled with multiple myeloma-like treatment. In those patients able to undergo autologous hematopoietic stem cell transplantation, the median survival now approaches 5 years (and approaches 10 years for those achieving a complete hematologic remission).

▶ When to Refer

- All patients who have primary amyloidosis or in whom it is suspected should be referred to a hematologist or oncologist.
- All patients with hereditary amyloidosis should be referred to a hepatologist for consideration of liver transplantation.

▶ When to Admit

- Patients with systemic amyloidosis require hospitalization to treat exacerbations of end-organ failure, such as heart failure or liver failure.
- Patients with primary amyloidosis require hospitalization to undergo autologous hematopoietic stem cell transplantation.

Dispenzieri A et al. Treatment of immunoglobulin light chain amyloidosis: Mayo Stratification of Myeloma and Risk-Adapted Therapy (mSMART) consensus statement. Mayo Clin Proc. 2015 Aug;90(8):1054–81. [PMID: 26250727]

Gertz MA. Immunoglobulin light chain amyloidosis: 2014 update on diagnosis, prognosis, and treatment. Am J Hematol. 2014 Dec;89(12):1132–40. [PMID: 25407896]

Rosenzweig M et al. Light-chain amyloidosis: SCT, novel agents and beyond. Bone Marrow Transplant. 2013 Aug;48(8):1022–7. [PMID: 23103675]

Hematopoietic stem cell transplantation is an extremely valuable treatment for a variety of hematologic malignancies and is also used in a few non-hematologic cancers and some nonmalignant conditions. In many cases, stem cell transplantation offers the only curative option for some types of cancer and can be a life-saving procedure.

The basis of treatment with stem cell transplantation is the ability of the hematopoietic stem cell to completely restore bone marrow function and formation of all blood components, as well as the ability to re-form the immune system. Hematopoietic stem cells were once collected from the bone marrow but are now more commonly collected from the peripheral blood after administration of stimulants such as filgrastim (G-CSF) to mobilize them from the bone marrow into the blood.

The dose-limiting toxicity of almost all cancer chemotherapy has been myelosuppression from damage to the bone marrow. It is typical during the administration of chemotherapy for blood counts to be transiently suppressed and to have to wait for recovery of the blood in order to safely give the next treatment. However, if too high a dose of chemotherapy is given, it is possible to damage the bone marrow beyond recovery, and for the blood counts to never return to within normal ranges. For cancers for which there is a dose-response relationship, that is, a relationship between the dose of chemotherapy administered and the number of cancer cells killed, the limits placed on the allowable dose of chemotherapy can make the difference between cure and failure to cure. In stem cell transplantation, the limit placed on the allowable dose of chemotherapy by the risks of permanent bone marrow damage is eliminated and much higher doses of chemotherapy can be given, since reinfusion of hematopoietic stem cells can completely restore the bone marrow.

AUTOLOGOUS STEM CELL TRANSPLANTATION

Autologous stem cell transplantation is a treatment in which hematopoietic stem cells are collected from the patient and then re-infused after chemotherapy. Therefore, autologous stem cell transplantation relies solely for its effectiveness on the ability to give much higher doses of chemotherapy than would otherwise be possible. In this procedure, the hematopoietic stem cells are usually collected from the patient's peripheral blood after they are mobilized from the bone marrow into the blood by a variety of techniques, most commonly the use of myeloid growth factors such as filgrastim either alone or in combination with chemotherapy (eg, the CXCR4 antagonist plerixafor can help mobilize these cells into the blood). Then, during a leukapheresis, the patient's blood is centrifuged into layers of different densities and the hematopoietic stem cells are collected from the appropriate layer while the remainder of the blood elements are returned unchanged to the patient. After collection, these autologous hematopoietic stem cells are frozen and cryopreserved for later use. Autologous stem cell transplantation

involves administration of high-dose chemotherapy (the "preparative regimen") followed, after clearance of the chemotherapy out of the patient's system, by intravenous reinfusion of the thawed autologous hematopoietic stem cells. The hematopoietic stem cells home to the bone marrow and grow into new bone marrow cells.

During the autologous stem cell transplantation, there is a period of severe pancytopenia between the myelosuppression caused by the chemotherapy and the recovery produced by the new bone marrow derived from the infused stem cells. This period of pancytopenia typically lasts 7–10 days and requires support with red blood cell and platelet transfusions as well as antibiotics. Hospitalization to receive such treatment usually lasts 2–3 weeks. The morbidity of such a treatment varies according to the type of chemotherapy used, and the chance of fatal treatment-related complications is between 1% and 4%.

Autologous stem cell transplantation has the potential to cure cancers that would otherwise be fatal. For example, it is the treatment of choice for some cancers that have recurred after initial chemotherapy but are still responsive to chemotherapy, such as lymphomas (recurrent diffuse large B-cell lymphomas and relapsed Hodgkin lymphomas) and recurrent testicular germ cell cancers. Based on the aggressive clinical course of peripheral T-cell lymphomas, autologous stem cell transplantation is often used following chemotherapy as first-line therapy. Autologous stem cell transplantation can be used, and is potentially curative, in the treatment of AML in both first and second remission. Autologous stem cell transplantation is currently part of standard care for the treatment of mantle cell lymphoma and multiple myeloma, based not on curative potential, but the prolongation of remission and overall survival.

ALLOGENEIC STEM CELL TRANSPLANTATION

In allogeneic stem cell transplantation, the source of the hematopoietic stem cells to restore bone marrow and immune function is derived, not from the patient, but from a different donor. Initially allogeneic stem cell transplantation was thought to derive its effectiveness from the "preparative regimen" of high-dose chemotherapy (or radiation plus chemotherapy). However, it is now known that in allogeneic stem cell transplantation, there is an alloimmune graft-versus-malignancy (GVM) effect derived from the donor immune system. In some cases, this GVM effect can be more important than the chemotherapy in producing a cure of disease. This understanding has led to the development of less myelotoxic preparative regimens, referred to as reduced-intensity or non-myeloablative.

To perform an allogeneic stem cell transplantation, an appropriate donor of hematopoietic stem cells must be located. The donor must be matched with the patient (recipient) at the HLA loci (HLA A, B, C, DR) that specify major histocompatibility antigens. These donors may be full siblings or haploidentical donors (eg, other children of the parents of the prospective recipient), or unrelated donors recruited from a large panel of anonymous volunteer donors through the National Marrow Donor Program (NMDP). Alternatively, cells derived from umbilical cord blood may be used. The hematopoietic stem cells are collected from the donor either from the bone marrow or, more commonly, through leukapheresis of the blood after mobilizing hematopoietic stem cells from the bone marrow with filgrastim (G-CSF).

In the allogeneic stem cell transplantation procedure, the patient is treated with a "preparative regimen" with two purposes: to treat the underlying cancer and to sufficiently suppress the patient's immune system so that the hematopoietic stem cells from the donor will not be rejected. As with autologous stem cell transplantation, after the preparative chemotherapy has been given to the recipient and has cleared from the body, the hematopoietic stem cells are infused intravenously (either fresh or after cryopreservation and thawing), and the stem cells home to the bone marrow and start to grow.

As with autologous stem cell transplantation, there is a period of severe pancytopenia between the myelosuppression caused by the chemotherapy and the recovery produced by the new bone marrow derived from the infused stem cells, lasting 10–14 days and usually requiring red blood cell and platelet transfusions as well as antibiotics.

A major difference between autologous and allogeneic stem cell transplantation is that in the allogeneic setting, the patient becomes a "chimera," that is, a mixture of self and non-self. In allogeneic stem cell transplantation, the infused cells contain mature cells of the donor immune system, and the infused hematopoietic stem cells will grow into bone marrow and blood cells as well as cells of the new immune system. Unless the donor is an identical twin (called a "syngeneic transplant"), the donor's immune system will recognize the patient's tissues as foreign and initiate the "graft-versus-host" (GVH) reaction, the graft from the donor reacting against the patient (host). This GVH reaction is the major cause of morbidity and mortality from allogeneic stem cell transplantation. Immunosuppression must be given to reduce its incidence and severity. The most common regimen used for GVH prophylaxis is a combination of cyclosporine or tacrolimus plus methotrexate. However, in contrast to the experience with solid organ transplantation in which life-long immunosuppression is required to prevent rejection of the transplanted organ, in most cases of allogeneic stem cell transplantation, the immunosuppression can be tapered and discontinued 6 or more months after transplantation.

There is an important positive aspect to the alloimmune reaction of the donor against the host. If there are residual cancer cells present in the patient that have survived the high-dose chemoradiotherapy preparative regimen, these residual cancer cells can be recognized as foreign by the donor immune system and killed in the GVM effect. Even cells that are resistant to chemotherapy may not be resistant to killing through the immune system. Depending on the type of cancer cell, this can be a highly effective mechanism of long-term cancer control. Based on the understanding of how important GVM can be, the allogeneic stem cell transplantation procedure can be modified by reducing the intensity of the preparative regimen, relying for cure more on the GVM effect and less on the high-dose chemotherapy. In these "reduced-intensity"

allogeneic stem cell transplantation procedures, the preparative regimen still has to suppress the patient's immune system enough to avoid rejection of the donor hematopoietic stem cells, but these transplants can be far less toxic than full-dose transplants. Based on this greatly reduced short-term toxicity, the potential benefits of allogeneic stem cell transplantation have been extended to older adults (age 60–75) and to those with comorbid conditions that would have been a contraindication to standard full-dose stem cell transplantation.

Allogeneic stem cell transplantation is the treatment of choice, and in many cases the only potentially curative treatment, for high-risk acute leukemias, for myelodysplasia, and for most cases of severe aplastic anemia. It has also been used for CML, although its use in CML has been greatly curtailed based on the effectiveness of imatinib and related tyrosine kinase inhibitors. Reduced-intensity allogeneic stem cell transplantation is also being explored in the management of difficult cases of CLL, follicular lymphoma, AML, and myelodysplasia.

Arnaout K et al. Complications of allogeneic hematopoietic stem cell transplantation. Cancer Invest. 2014 Aug;32(7):349–62. [PMID: 24902046]

Bejanyan N et al. Alternative donor transplantation for acute myeloid leukemia. J Clin Med. 2015 Jun 9;4(6):1240–68. [PMID: 26239557]

Kharfan-Dabaja M et al. Mycophenolate mofetil versus methotrexate for prevention of graft-versus-host disease in people receiving allogeneic hematopoietic stem cell transplantation. Cochrane Database Syst Rev. 2014 Jul 25;7:CD010280. [PMID: 25061777]

Majhail NS et al; Center for International Blood and Marrow Transplant Research (CIBMTR); American Society for Blood and Marrow Transplantation (ASBMT); European Group for Blood and Marrow Transplantation (EBMT); Asia-Pacific Blood and Marrow Transplantation Group (APBMT); Bone Marrow Transplant Society of Australia and New Zealand (BMTSANZ); East Mediterranean Blood and Marrow Transplantation Group (EMBMT); Sociedade Brasileira de Transplante de Medula Ossea (SBTMO). Recommended screening and preventive practices for long-term survivors after hematopoietic cell transplantation. Hematol Oncol Stem Cell Ther. 2012;5(1):1–30. [PMID: 22446607]

Spellman SR et al; National Marrow Donor Program; Center for International Blood and Marrow Transplant Research. A perspective on the selection of unrelated donors and cord blood units for transplantation. Blood. 2012 Jul 12;120(2):259–65. [PMID: 22596257]

Tewari P et al. Hematopoietic stem cell transplantation in adolescents and young adults. Acta Haematol. 2014;132(3–4): 313–25. [PMID: 25228557]

Tzannou I et al. Accelerating immune reconstitution after hematopoietic stem cell transplantation. Clin Transl Immunology. 2014 Feb 28;3(2):e11. [PMID: 25505959]

BLOOD TRANSFUSIONS

RED BLOOD CELL TRANSFUSIONS

Red blood cell transfusions are given to raise the hemoglobin levels in patients with anemia or to replace losses after acute bleeding episodes.

Preparations of Red Cells for Transfusion

Several types of preparations containing red blood cells are available.

A. Fresh Whole Blood

The advantage of whole blood for transfusion is the simultaneous presence of red blood cells, plasma, and fresh platelets. Fresh whole blood is never absolutely necessary, since all the above components are available separately. The major indications for use of whole blood are cardiac surgery or massive hemorrhage when more than 10 units of blood is required in a 24-hour period.

B. Packed Red Blood Cells

Packed red cells are the component most commonly used to raise the hemoglobin. Each unit has a volume of about 300 mL, of which approximately 200 mL consists of red blood cells. One unit of packed red cells will usually raise the hemoglobin by approximately 1 g/dL. Current guidelines recommend a transfusion "trigger" hemoglobin threshold of 7–8 g/dL (70–80 g/L) for hospitalized critically ill patients, those undergoing cardiothoracic surgery or repair of a hip fracture, those with upper gastrointestinal bleeding, and those with hematologic malignancy undergoing chemotherapy.

C. Leukocyte-Poor Blood

Most blood products are leukoreduced in-line during acquisition and are thus prospectively leukocyte-poor. Leukoreduced blood products reduce the incidence of leukoagglutination reactions, platelet alloimmunization, transfusion-related acute lung injury, and CMV exposure.

D. Frozen Packed Red Blood Cells

Packed red blood cells can be frozen and stored for up to 10 years, but the technique is cumbersome and expensive and should be used sparingly. The major application is for the purpose of maintaining a supply of rare blood types. Patients with such types may donate units for autologous transfusion should the need arise. Frozen red cells are also occasionally needed for patients with severe leukoagglutinin reactions or anaphylactic reactions to plasma proteins, since frozen blood has essentially all white blood cells and plasma components removed.

E. Autologous Packed Red Blood Cells

Patients scheduled for elective surgery may donate blood for autologous transfusion. These units may be stored for up to 35 days before freezing is necessary.

Compatibility Testing

Before transfusion, the recipient's and the donor's blood are typed and cross-matched to avoid hemolytic transfusion reactions. Although many antigen systems are present on red blood cells, only the ABO and Rh systems are specifically tested prior to all transfusions. The A and B antigens are the most important, because everyone who lacks one or both red cell antigens has IgM isoantibodies (called isoagglutinins) in his or her plasma against the missing antigen(s). The isoagglutinins activate complement and can cause rapid intravascular lysis of the incompatible red blood cells. In emergencies, type O/Rh-negative blood can be given to any recipient, but only packed cells should be given to minimize transfusion of donor plasma containing anti-A and anti-B antibodies.

The other important antigen routinely tested for is the D antigen of the Rh system. Approximately 15% of the population lacks this antigen. In patients lacking the antigen, anti-D antibodies are not naturally present, but the antigen is highly immunogenic. A recipient whose red cells lack D and who receives D-positive blood may develop anti-D antibodies that can cause severe lysis of subsequent transfusions of D-positive red cells.

Blood typing includes a crossmatch assay of recipient serum for unusual alloantibodies directed against donor red blood cells by mixing recipient serum with panels of red blood cells representing commonly occurring minor red cell antigens. The screening is particularly important if the recipient has had previous transfusions or pregnancy.

Hemolytic Transfusion Reactions

The most severe hemolytic transfusion reactions are acute (temporally related to the transfusion), involving incompatible mismatches in the ABO system and are isoagglutinin-mediated. Most of these cases are due to clerical errors and mislabeled specimens. With current compatibility testing and double-check clerical systems, the risk of an acute hemolytic reaction is 1 in 76,000 transfused units of red blood cells. Death from acute hemolytic reaction occurs in 1 in 1.8 million transfused units. Hemolysis is rapid and intravascular, releasing free hemoglobin into the plasma. The severity of these reactions depends on the dose of red blood cells given. The most severe reactions are those seen in surgical patients under anesthesia.

Delayed hemolytic transfusion reactions are caused by minor red blood cell antigen discrepancies and are typically less severe. The hemolysis usually takes place at a slower rate and is mediated by IgG alloantibodies causing extravascular red blood cell destruction. These transfusion reactions may be delayed for 5–10 days after transfusion. In such cases, the recipient has received red blood cells containing an immunogenic antigen, and in the time since transfusion, a new alloantibody has formed. The most common antigens involved in such reactions are Duffy, Kidd, Kell, and C and E loci of the Rh system. The current risk of a delayed hemolytic transfusion reaction is 1 in 6000 transfused units of red blood cells.

A. Symptoms and Signs

Major acute hemolytic transfusion reactions cause fever and chills, with backache and headache. In severe cases, there may be apprehension, dyspnea, hypotension, and cardiovascular collapse. Patients under general anesthesia will not manifest such symptoms, and the first indication may be tachycardia, generalized bleeding, or oliguria. *The transfusion must be stopped immediately.* In severe cases, acute DIC, acute kidney injury from tubular necrosis, or both can occur. Death occurs in 4% of acute hemolytic reactions due to ABO incompatibility.

Delayed hemolytic transfusion reactions are usually without symptoms or signs.

B. Laboratory Findings

When an acute hemolytic transfusion episode is suspected, the identification of the recipient and of the transfusion product bag label should be rechecked. The transfusion product bag with its pilot tube must be returned to the blood bank, and a fresh sample of the recipient's blood must accompany the bag for retyping and re–cross-matching of donor and recipient blood samples. The hemoglobin will fail to rise by the expected amount. Coagulation studies may reveal evidence of acute kidney injury or acute DIC. The plasma-free hemoglobin in the recipient will be elevated resulting in hemoglobinuria.

In cases of delayed hemolytic reactions, there will be an unexpected drop in hemoglobin and an increase in the total and indirect bilirubins. The new offending alloantibody is easily detected in the patient's serum.

C. Treatment

If an acute hemolytic transfusion reaction is suspected, the transfusion should be stopped at once. The patient should be vigorously hydrated to prevent acute tubular necrosis. Forced diuresis with mannitol may help prevent or minimize acute kidney injury.

► Leukoagglutinin Reactions

Most transfusion reactions are not hemolytic but represent reactions to antigens present on transfused passenger leukocytes in patients who have been sensitized to leukocyte antigens through previous transfusions or pregnancy. Transfusion products relatively rich in leukocyte-rich plasma, especially platelets, are most likely to cause this. Moderate to severe leukoagglutinin reactions occur in 1% of red blood cell transfusions and 2% of platelet transfusions. Most commonly, fever and chills develop in patients within 12 hours after transfusion. In severe cases, cough and dyspnea may occur and the chest radiograph may show transient pulmonary infiltrates. Because no hemolysis is involved, the hemoglobin rises by the expected amount despite the reaction.

Leukoagglutinin reactions may respond to acetaminophen (500–650 mg) and diphenhydramine (25 mg); corticosteroids, such as hydrocortisone (1 mg/kg), are also of value. Overall, leukoagglutination reactions are diminishing through the routine use of in-line leukotrapping during blood donation (ie, leukoreduced blood). Patients experiencing severe leukoagglutination episodes despite receiving leukoreduced blood transfusions should receive leukopoor or washed blood products.

► Hypersensitivity Reactions

Urticaria or bronchospasm may develop during or soon after a transfusion. These reactions are almost always due to exposure to allogeneic plasma proteins rather than to leukocytes. The risk is low enough that the routine use of antihistamine premedications has been eliminated before PRBC transfusions. A hypersensitivity reaction, including anaphylactic shock, may develop in patients who are IgA deficient because of antibodies to IgA in the patient's plasma directed against the IgA in the transfused blood product. Patients with such reactions may require transfusion of washed or even frozen red blood cells to avoid future severe reactions.

► Contaminated Blood

Blood products can be contaminated with bacteria. Platelets are especially prone to bacterial contamination because they cannot be refrigerated. Bacterial contamination occurs in 1 of every 30,000 red blood cell donations and 1 of every 5000 platelet donations. Receipt of a blood product contaminated with gram-positive bacteria will cause fever and bacteremia but rarely causes a sepsis syndrome. Receipt of a blood product contaminated with gram-negative bacteria often causes septic shock, acute DIC, and acute kidney injury due to the transfused endotoxin and is usually fatal. Strategies to reduce bacterial contamination include enhanced venipuncture site skin cleansing, diverting of the first few milliliters of donated blood, use of single-donor blood products (as opposed to pooled-donor products), and point-of-care rapid bacterial screening in order to discard questionable units. The current risk of a septic transfusion reaction from a culture-negative unit of single-donor platelets is 1 in 60,000. In any patient who may have received contaminated blood, the recipient and the donor blood bag should both be cultured, and antibiotics should be given immediately to the recipient.

► Infectious Diseases Transmitted Through Transfusion

Despite the use of only volunteer blood donors and the routine screening of blood, transfusion-associated viral diseases remain a problem. All blood products (red blood cells, platelets, plasma, cryoprecipitate) can transmit viral diseases. All blood donors are screened with questionnaires designed to detect (and therefore reject) donors at high risk for transmitting infectious diseases. All blood is screened for hepatitis B surface antigen, antibody to hepatitis B core antigen, syphilis, p24 antigen and antibody to HIV, antibody to hepatitis C virus (HCV), antibody to human T-cell lymphotropic/leukemia virus (HTLV), and nucleic acid testing for West Nile virus. Clinical trials are examining the value of screening blood donors for *Trypanosoma cruzi*, the infectious agent that causes Chagas disease.

With improved screening, the risk of posttransfusion hepatitis has steadily decreased after the receipt of screened 'negative' blood products. The risk of acquiring hepatitis B is about 1 in 200,000 transfused units in the United States (versus about 1 in 21,000 to 1 in 600 transfused units in Asia). The risk of hepatitis C acquisition is 1 in 1.5 to 2 million transfused units in the United States. The risk of HIV acquisition is 1 in 2 million transfused units. Unscreened leukoreduced blood products appear to be equivalent to CMV screened-negative blood products in terms of the risk of CMV transmission to a CMV-seronegative recipient.

Transfusion Graft-Versus-Host Disease

Allogeneic passenger lymphocytes within transfused blood products will engraft in some recipients and mount an alloimmune attack against tissues expressing discrepant HLA antigens causing graft-versus-host disease (GVHD). The symptoms and signs of transfusion-associated GVHD include fever, rash, diarrhea, hepatitis, lymphadenopathy, and severe pancytopenia. The outcome is usually fatal. Transfusion-associated GVHD occurs most often in recipients with immune defects, malignant lymphoproliferative disorders, solid tumors being treated with chemotherapy or immunotherapy, treatment with immunosuppressive medications (especially purine analogs such as fludarabine), or older patients undergoing cardiac surgery. HIV infection alone does not seem to increase the risk. The use of leukoreduced blood products is inadequate to prevent transfusion-associated GVHD. This complication can be avoided by irradiating blood products (25 Gy or more) to prevent lymphocyte proliferation in recipients at high risk for transfusion-associated GVHD.

Transfusion-Related Acute Lung Injury

Transfusion-related acute lung injury (TRALI) occurs in 1 in every 5000 transfused units of blood products. It has been associated with allogeneic antibodies in the donor plasma component that bind to recipient leukocyte antigens, including HLA antigens and other granulocyte- and monocyte-specific antigens (such as HNA-1a, -1b, -2a, and -3a). In 20% of cases, no antileukocyte antibodies are identified raising the concern that bioactive lipids or other substances that accumulate while the blood product is in storage can also mediate TRALI in susceptible recipients. TRALI is clinically defined as noncardiogenic pulmonary edema after a blood product transfusion without other explanation, and transfused surgical and critically ill patients seem most susceptible. Ten to 20% of female blood donors and 1–5% of male blood donors have antileukocyte antibodies in their serum. The risk of TRALI is reduced through the use of male-only plasma donors, when possible. There is no specific treatment for TRALI, only supportive care.

PLATELET TRANSFUSIONS

Platelet transfusions are indicated in cases of thrombocytopenia due to decreased platelet production. They are of some use in immune thrombocytopenia when active bleeding is evident, but the clearance of transfused platelets is rapid as they are exposed to the same pathophysiologic forces as the recipient's endogenous platelets. The risk of spontaneous bleeding rises when the platelet count falls to less than 80,000/mcL (80 × 10⁹/L), and the risk of life-threatening spontaneous bleeding increases when the platelet count is less than 5000/mcL (5 × 10⁹/L). Because of

this, prophylactic platelet transfusions are often given at these very low levels, usually when less than 10,000/mcL (10 × 10⁹/L). Platelet transfusions are also given prior to invasive procedures or surgery in thrombocytopenic patients, and the goal is often to raise the platelet count to 50,000/mcL (50 × 10⁹/L) or more.

Platelets for transfusion are most commonly derived from single-donor apheresis collections (roughly the equivalent to the platelets recovered from six donations of whole blood). A single donor unit of platelets should raise the platelet count by 50,000 to 60,000 platelets per mcL (50–60 × 10⁹/L) in a transfusion-naïve recipient without hypersplenism or ongoing platelet consumptive disorder. Transfused platelets typically last for 2 or 3 days. Platelet transfusion responses may be suboptimal with poor platelet increments and short platelet survival times. This may be due to one of several causes, including fever, sepsis, hypersplenism, DIC, large body habitus, low platelet dose in the transfusion, or platelet alloimmunization (from prior transfusions, prior pregnancy or prior organ transplantation). Many, but not all, alloantibodies causing platelet destruction are directed at HLA antigens. Patients requiring long periods of platelet transfusion support should be monitored to document adequate responses to transfusions so that the most appropriate product can be used. Patients requiring ongoing platelet transfusions who become alloimmunized may benefit from HLA-matched platelets derived from either volunteer donors or family members. Techniques of cross-matching platelets have been developed and appear to identify suitable volunteer platelet donors (nonreactive with the patient's serum) without the need for HLA typing. Leukocyte reduction of platelets has been shown to delay or prevent the onset of alloimmunization in multiply transfused recipients.

TRANSFUSION OF PLASMA COMPONENTS

Fresh-frozen plasma (FFP) is available in units of approximately 200 mL. FFP contains normal levels of all coagulation factors (about 1 unit/mL of each factor). FFP is used to correct coagulation factor deficiencies and to treat thrombotic thrombocytopenia purpura or hemolytic-uremic syndrome. FFP is also used to correct or prevent coagulopathy in trauma patients receiving massive transfusion of PRBC. A FFP:PRBC ratio of 1:2 or more is associated with improved survival in trauma patients receiving massive transfusions, regardless of the presence of a coagulopathy.

Cryoprecipitate is made from fresh plasma by cooling the plasma to 4°C and collecting the precipitate. One unit of cryoprecipitate has a volume of approximately 15–20 mL and contains approximately 250 mg of fibrinogen and between 80 and 100 units of factor VIII and von Willebrand factor. Cryoprecipitate is used to supplement fibrinogen in cases of acquired hypofibrinogenemia (eg, DIC) or in rare instances of congenital hypofibrinogenemia.

One unit of cryoprecipitate will raise the fibrinogen level by about 8 mg/dL (0.24 mcmol/L). Cryoprecipitate is sometimes used to temporarily correct the acquired platelet dysfunction associated with kidney disease.

El Kenz H et al. Transfusion-related acute lung injury. Eur J Anaesthesiol. 2014 Jul;31(7):345–50. [PMID: 24892308]

Goodnough LT et al. Concepts of blood transfusion in adults. Lancet. 2013 May 25;381(9880):1845–54. [PMID: 23706801]

Holst LB et al. Restrictive versus liberal transfusion strategy for red blood cell transfusion: systematic review of randomised trials with meta-analysis and trial sequential analysis. BMJ. 2015 Mar 24;350:h1354. [PMID: 25805204]

Kumar A et al; AABB Platelet Transfusion Guidelines Panel. Platelet transfusion: a systematic review of the clinical evidence. Transfusion. 2015 May;55(5):1116–275. [PMID: 25387589]

Marfin AA et al. Granulocyte transfusion therapy. J Intensive Care Med. 2015 Feb;30(2):79–88. [PMID: 23920161]

Stanworth SJ et al; TOPPS Investigators. A no-prophylaxis platelet-transfusion strategy for hematologic cancers. N Engl J Med. 2013 May 9;368(19):1771–80. [PMID: 23656642]

Storch EK et al. Spotlight on pathogenesis of TRALI: HNA-3a (CTL2) antibodies. Blood. 2014 Sep;124(12):1868–72. [PMID: 25006121]

Thiagarajan P et al. Platelet transfusion therapy. Hematol Oncol Clin North Am. 2013 Jun;27(3):629–43. [PMID: 23714315]

14

Disorders of Hemostasis, Thrombosis, & Antithrombotic Therapy

Andrew D. Leavitt, MD

Tracy Minichiello, MD

In evaluating patients for defects of hemostasis, the clinical context must be considered carefully (Table 14–1). Heritable defects are suggested by bleeding that begins in infancy or childhood, is recurrent, and occurs at multiple anatomic sites, although many other patterns of presentation are possible. Acquired disorders of hemostasis more typically are associated with bleeding that begins later in life and may be relatable to introduction of medications (eg, agents that affect platelet activity) or to onset of underlying medical conditions (such as kidney disease, liver disease, myelodysplasia), or may be idiopathic. Importantly, however, a sufficient hemostatic challenge (such as major trauma) may produce excessive bleeding even in individuals with completely normal hemostasis. A personal history for hemostatic challenges (eg, circumcision, trauma, injury during youth sports, tooth extractions, motor vehicle accidents, prior surgery, and pregnancy and delivery) is critical for evaluating a patient for a possible bleeding disorder.

PLATELET DISORDERS

THROMBOCYTOPENIA

Selected causes of thrombocytopenia are shown in Table 14–2. The age of the patient and presence of any comorbid conditions may help direct the diagnostic work-up.

The risk of spontaneous bleeding (including petechial hemorrhage and bruising) does not typically increase appreciably until the platelet count falls below 10,000–20,000/mcL, although patients with dysfunctional platelets may bleed with higher platelet counts. Suggested platelet counts to prevent spontaneous bleeding or to provide adequate hemostasis around the time of invasive procedures are found in Table 14–3. However, most medical centers develop their own local guidelines to have a consistent approach to such complex situations.

DECREASED PLATELET PRODUCTION

1. Thrombocytopenia due to Bone Marrow Failure

ESSENTIALS OF DIAGNOSIS

► Bone marrow failure states may be congenital or acquired.
► Most congenital marrow failure disorders present in childhood.

► General Considerations

Congenital conditions that cause thrombocytopenia include amegakaryocytic thrombocytopenia, the thrombocytopenia-absent radius syndrome, and Wiskott-Aldrich syndrome; these disorders usually feature isolated thrombocytopenia, whereas patients with Fanconi anemia and dyskeratosis congenita typically include cytopenias in other blood cell lineages.

Acquired causes of bone marrow failure (see Chapter 13) leading to thrombocytopenia include acquired aplastic anemia, myelodysplastic syndrome (MDS), and acquired amegakaryocytic thrombocytopenia (albeit a rare disorder). Unlike aplastic anemia, MDS is more common among older patients.

► Clinical Findings

Acquired **aplastic anemia** typically presents with reductions in multiple blood cell lineages, and the CBC reveals pancytopenia. A bone marrow biopsy is required for diagnosis and reveals marked hypocellularity. **Myelodysplastic syndrome** (MDS) also presents as cytopenias and can have

Table 14–1. Evaluation of the bleeding patient.

Necessary Component of Evaluation	Diagnostic Correlate
Location	
Mucocutaneous (bruises, petechiae, gingivae, nosebleeds, GI, GU)	Suggests qualitative/quantitative platelet defects
Joints, soft tissue	Suggests disorders of coagulation factors
Onset	
Infancy/childhood	Suggests heritable condition
Adulthood	Suggests milder heritable condition or acquired defect of hemostasis (eg, ITP, medication related)
Clinical Context	
Postsurgical	Anatomic/surgical defect must be ruled out
Pregnancy	vWD, HELLP syndrome, ITP, acquired factor VIII inhibitor
Sepsis	May indicate DIC
Exposure to anticoagulants	Rule out excessive anticoagulation
Personal History[1]	
Absent	Suggests acquired rather than congenital defect, or anatomic/surgical defect (if applicable)
Present	Suggests established acquired defect or congenital disorder
Family History	
Absent	Suggests acquired defect or no defect of hemostasis
Present	May signify hemophilia A or B, vWD, other heritable bleeding disorders

[1]Includes evaluation of prior spontaneous bleeding, as well as excessive bleeding with circumcision, menses, dental extractions, trauma, minor procedures (eg, endoscopy, biopsies), and major procedures (surgery).
DIC, disseminated intravascular coagulation; GI, gastrointestinal; GU, genitourinary; HELLP, hemolysis, elevated liver enzymes, low platelets; ITP, immune thrombocytopenia; vWD, von Willebrand disease.

pancytopenia, but the marrow cellularity is not decreased; the marrow typically demonstrates hypercellularity. The presence of macrocytosis, ringed sideroblasts on iron staining of the bone marrow aspirate, dysplasia of hematopoietic elements, or cytogenetic abnormalities (especially monosomy 5 or 7, and trisomy 8) are more suggestive of MDS.

► Differential Diagnosis

Adult patients with acquired amegakaryocytic thrombocytopenia (rare) have isolated thrombocytopenia and reduced or absent megakaryocytes in the bone marrow, which (along with failure to respond to immunomodulatory regi-

Table 14–2. Selected causes of thrombocytopenia.

Decreased production of platelets
  Congenital bone marrow failure (eg, Fanconi anemia, Wiskott-Aldrich syndrome)
  Acquired bone marrow failure (eg, aplastic anemia, myelodysplasia, leukemia)
  Exposure to chemotherapy, irradiation
  Marrow infiltration (neoplastic, infectious)
  Nutritional (deficiency of vitamin B_{12}, folate, iron; alcohol)
Increased destruction of platelets
  Immune thrombocytopenia (primary)
  Immune thrombocytopenia (secondary), including hepatitis C virus, HIV-related, and drug-induced
  Heparin-induced thrombocytopenia
  Thrombotic microangiopathy
  Disseminated intravascular coagulation
  Posttransfusion purpura
  Neonatal alloimmune thrombocytopenia
  Mechanical (aortic valvular dysfunction; extracorporeal bypass)
  von Willebrand disease, type 2B
  Hemophagocytosis
Increased sequestration of platelets
  Hypersplenism (eg, related to cirrhosis, myeloproliferative disorders, lymphoma)
Other conditions causing thrombocytopenia
  Gestational thrombocytopenia
  Bernard-Soulier syndrome, gray platelet syndrome, May-Hegglin anomaly
  Pseudothrombocytopenia

mens typically administered in immune thrombocytopenia [ITP]) distinguishes them from patients with ITP.

► Treatment

A. Congenital Conditions

Treatment is varied but may include blood product support, blood cell growth factors, androgens and, in some cases, allogeneic hematopoietic stem cell transplantation.

B. Acquired Conditions

Patients with severe aplastic anemia are treated with immunosuppressive therapy or allogeneic hematopoietic

Table 14–3. Desired platelet count ranges.

Clinical Scenario	Platelet Count (/mcL)
Prevention of spontaneous mucocutaneous bleeding	> 10,000–20,000
Insertion of central venous catheters	> 20,000–50,000[1]
Administration of therapeutic anticoagulation	> 30,000–50,000
Minor surgery and selected invasive procedures[2]	> 50,000–80,000
Major surgery	> 80,000–100,000

[1]A platelet target within the higher range of the reference is required for tunneled catheters.
[2]Such as endoscopy with biopsy.

stem cell transplantation. Allogeneic hematopoietic stem cell transplantation is the preferred therapy for patients younger than age 40 who have an HLA-matched sibling donor (see Chapter 13), and immunosuppressive therapy is preferred for older patients and those who lack an HLA-matched sibling donor. Eltrombopag has been shown to induce multilineage responses (some of which are durable after discontinuing the medication) in selected patients with severe aplastic anemia that is unresponsive to immunosuppressive therapy.

Treatment of thrombocytopenia due to MDS, if clinically significant bleeding is present or if the risk of bleeding is high, is limited to chronic transfusion of platelets in most instances (Table 14–3). Immunomodulatory agents such as lenalidomide do not produce increases in the platelet count in most patients. The thrombopoietin receptor agonists eltrombopag and romiplostim have shown efficacy as an adjunct to hypomethylating agents in low-risk MDS in clinical trials. However, these agents are typically avoided in moderate- and high-risk MDS patients due to concerns regarding possibly accelerating leukemic transformation.

Desmond R et al. Eltrombopag in aplastic anemia. Semin Hematol. 2015 Jan;52(1):31–7. [PMID: 25578417]
Desmond R et al. Eltrombopag restores trilineage hematopoiesis in refractory severe aplastic anemia that can be sustained on discontinuation of drug. Blood. 2014 Mar 20;123(12):1818–25. [PMID: 24345753]
Greenberg PL et al. A randomized controlled trial of romiplostim in patients with low- or intermediate-risk myelodysplastic syndrome receiving decitabine. Leuk Lymphoma. 2013 Feb; 54(2):321–8. [PMID: 22906162]
Marsh JC et al. Management of the refractory aplastic anemia patient: what are the options? Blood. 2013 Nov 21;122(22): 3561–7. [PMID: 24052548]'
Sekeres MA et al. Development and validation of a model to predict platelet response to romiplostim in patients with lower-risk myelodysplastic syndromes. Br J Haematol. 2014 Nov; 167(3):337–45. [PMID: 25039607]

2. Bone Marrow Infiltration

Replacement of the normal bone marrow elements by leukemic cells, myeloma, lymphoma, or other nonhematologic tumors, or by infections (such as mycobacterial disease or ehrlichiosis) may cause thrombocytopenia; however, abnormalities in other blood cell lines are also usually present. These entities are easily diagnosed after examining the bone marrow biopsy and aspirate or determining the infecting organism from an aspirate specimen, and they often lead to a leukoerythroblastic peripheral blood smear (left-shifted myeloid lineage, nucleated red blood cells, and teardrop–shaped red blood cells). Treatment of thrombocytopenia is directed at eradication of the underlying infiltrative disorder, but platelet transfusion may be required if clinically significant bleeding is present.

3. Chemotherapy & Irradiation

Chemotherapeutic agents and irradiation may lead to thrombocytopenia by direct toxicity to megakaryocytes, hematopoietic progenitor cells, or both. The severity and duration of chemotherapy-induced depressions in the

platelet count are determined by the specific regimen used, although the platelet count typically resolves more slowly following a chemotherapeutic insult than does neutropenia or anemia, especially if multiple cycles of treatment have been given. Until recovery occurs, patients may be supported with transfused platelets if bleeding is present or the risk of bleeding is high (Table 14–3). Clinical trials to determine the role of the platelet growth factors eltrombopag and romiplostim in the treatment of chemotherapy-induced thrombocytopenia have not shown clinically significant responses in the majority of treated patients.

4. Nutritional Deficiencies

Thrombocytopenia, typically in concert with anemia, may be observed when a deficiency of folate (that may accompany alcoholism) or vitamin B_{12} is present (concomitant neurologic findings may be manifest). In addition, thrombocytopenia rarely can occur in very severe iron deficiency, but thrombocytosis is more common. Replacing the deficient vitamin or mineral results in improvement in the platelet count.

Briani C et al. Cobalamin deficiency: clinical picture and radiological findings. Nutrients. 2013 Nov 15;5(11):4521–39. [PMID: 24248213]

5. Cyclic Thrombocytopenia

Cyclic thrombocytopenia is a very rare disorder that produces cyclic oscillations of the platelet count, usually with a periodicity of 3–6 weeks. The exact pathophysiologic mechanisms responsible for the condition may vary from patient to patient. Severe thrombocytopenia and bleeding typically occur at the platelet nadir. Oral contraceptive medications, androgens, azathioprine, and thrombopoietic growth factors have been used successfully in the management of cyclic thrombocytopenia.

INCREASED PLATELET DESTRUCTION

1. Immune Thrombocytopenia

ESSENTIALS OF DIAGNOSIS

▸ Isolated thrombocytopenia.
▸ Assess for any new causative medications and HIV and hepatitis C infections.
▸ ITP is a diagnosis of exclusion.

▶ General Considerations

ITP is an autoimmune condition in which pathogenic antibodies bind platelets, accelerating their clearance from the circulation. Many patients with ITP also lack appropriate compensatory platelet production, thought, at least in part, to reflect the antibody's effect on megakaryocytopoiesis and thrombopoiesis. The disorder is primary and idiopathic in most adult patients, although it can be associated with connective tissue disease (such as systemic lupus erythematosus), lymphoproliferative disease (such as lymphoma), medications, and infections (such as hepatitis C virus and HIV infections). Targets of antiplatelet antibodies include glycoproteins IIb/IIIa and Ib/IX on the platelet membrane, although antibodies are demonstrable in only two-thirds of patients. In addition to production of antiplatelet antibodies, HIV and hepatitis C virus may lead to thrombocytopenia through additional mechanisms (for instance, by direct suppression of platelet production [HIV] and cirrhosis-related splenomegaly [hepatitis C virus]).

▶ **Clinical Findings**

A. Symptoms and Signs

Mucocutaneous bleeding may be present, depending on the platelet count. Clinically relevant spontaneous bruising, nosebleeds, gingival bleeding, or other types of hemorrhage generally do not occur until the platelet count has fallen below 20,000–30,000/mcL. Individuals with secondary ITP (such as due to collagen vascular disease, HIV or HCV infection, or lymphoproliferative malignancy) may have additional disease-specific findings.

B. Laboratory Findings

Typically, patients have isolated thrombocytopenia. If bleeding has occurred, anemia may also be present.

Hepatitis B and C viruses and HIV infections should be excluded by serologic testing. Bone marrow should be examined in patients with unexplained cytopenias, in patients older than 60 years, or in those who did not respond to primary ITP-specific therapy. A bone marrow biopsy is not necessary in all cases to make a diagnosis in younger patients. Megakaryocyte abnormalities and hypocellularity or hypercellularity are not characteristic of ITP. If there are clinical findings suggestive of a lymphoproliferative malignancy, a CT scan should be performed. In the absence of such findings, otherwise asymptomatic patients with unexplained isolated thrombocytopenia of recent onset may be considered to have ITP.

▶ **Treatment**

Individuals with platelet counts less than 20,000–30,000/mcL or those with significant bleeding should be treated; the remainder may be monitored serially for progression, but that is a patient-specific decision. The mainstay of initial treatment of new-onset primary ITP is a short course of corticosteroids with or without intravenous immunoglobulin (IVIG) or anti-D (WinRho) (Figure 14–1). Responses are generally seen within 3–5 days of initiating treatment, with responses to IVIG typically seen in 24–36 hours. Platelet transfusions may be given concomitantly if active bleeding is present. The addition of the monoclonal anti-B cell antibody rituximab to corticosteroids as

▲ **Figure 14–1.** Management of immune thrombocytopenia (ITP).

first-line treatment may improve the initial response rate, but it is associated with increased toxicity and is not regarded as standard first-line therapy in most centers.

Although over two-thirds of patients with ITP respond to initial treatment, most relapse following reduction of the corticosteroid dose. Patients with a persistent platelet count less than 30,000/mcL or clinically significant bleeding are appropriate candidates for second-line treatments (Figure 14–1). These treatments are chosen empirically, bearing in mind potential toxicities and the patient's preference. Anti-D (WinRho) or IVIG temporarily increases platelet counts (duration, up to 3 weeks or longer), although serial anti-D treatment (platelet counts less than 30,000/mcL) may allow adult patients to delay or avoid splenectomy. Rituximab leads to clinical responses in about 50% of adults with corticosteroid-refractory chronic ITP, which decrease to about 20% at 5 years. Romiplostim (administered subcutaneously weekly) and eltrombopag (taken orally daily) are approved for use in adult patients with chronic ITP who have not responded durably to corticosteroids, IVIG, or splenectomy and are typically taken indefinitely to maintain the platelet response. Splenectomy has a durable response rate of over 60% and may be considered for cases of severe thrombocytopenia that fail to respond durably to initial treatment or are refractory to second-line agents; patients should receive pneumococcal, *Haemophilus influenzae* type b, and meningococcal vaccination at least 2 weeks before therapeutic splenectomy. If available, laparoscopic splenectomy is preferred. Additional treatments for ITP are found in Figure 14–1.

The goals of management of pregnancy-associated ITP are a platelet count of 10,000–30,000/mcL in the first trimester, greater than 30,000/mcL during the second or third trimester, and greater than 50,000/mcL prior to cesarean section or vaginal delivery. Moderate-dose oral prednisone or intermittent infusions of IVIG are standard. Splenectomy is reserved for failure to respond to these therapies and may be performed in the first or second trimester.

For thrombocytopenia associated with HIV or hepatitis C virus, effective treatment of either infection leads to an amelioration of thrombocytopenia in most cases; refractory thrombocytopenia may be treated with infusion of IVIG or anti-D (HIV and hepatitis C virus), splenectomy (HIV), or interferon-alpha or eltrombopag (hepatitis C virus, including eradication). Treatment with corticosteroids is not recommended in hepatitis C virus infection. Occasionally, ITP treatment response is impaired due to *Helicobacter pylori* infection, so that should be ruled out in the appropriate situation.

▶ When to Refer

Chronic thrombocytopenia will develop in most adult patients with newly diagnosed ITP. All patients with ITP should be referred to a subspecialist for evaluation at the time of diagnosis.

▶ When to Admit

Patients with major hemorrhage or very severe thrombocytopenia associated with bleeding should be admitted and monitored in-hospital until the platelet count has risen to more than 20,000–30,000/mcL and hemodynamic stability has been achieved.

Afdhal NH et al; ELEVATE Study Group. Eltrombopag before procedures in patients with cirrhosis and thrombocytopenia. N Engl J Med. 2012 Aug 23;367(8):716–24. [PMID: 22913681]

Gudbrandsdottir S et al. Rituximab and dexamethasone vs dexamethasone monotherapy in newly diagnosed patients with primary immune thrombocytopenia. Blood. 2013 Mar 14; 121(11):1976–81. [PMID: 23293082]

Kuter DJ et al. TPO concentrations and response to romiplostim. Am J Hematol. 2014 Dec;89(12):1155–6. [PMID: 25132329]

Liebman HA et al. Diagnosis and management of immune thrombocytopenia in the era of thrombopoietin mimetics. Hematology Am Soc Hematol Educ Program. 2011;2011: 384–90. [PMID: 22160062]

Neunert C et al. Severe bleeding events in adults and children with primary immune thrombocytopenia: a systematic review. J Thromb Haemost. 2015 Mar;13(3):457–64. [PMID: 25495497]

2. Thrombotic Microangiopathy

ESSENTIALS OF DIAGNOSIS

▶ Microangiopathic hemolytic anemia and thrombocytopenia, in the absence of another plausible explanation, are sufficient for the diagnosis of thrombotic microangiopathy (TMA).

▶ Fever, neurologic abnormalities, and kidney disease may occur concurrently but are not required for diagnosis.

▶ Kidney dysfunction is more common and more severe in hemolytic-uremic syndrome (HUS).

▶ General Considerations

The TMAs include, but are not limited to, thrombotic thrombocytopenic purpura (TTP) and HUS. These disorders are characterized by thrombocytopenia due to the incorporation of platelets into thrombi in the microvasculature, and microangiopathic hemolytic anemia, which results from shearing of erythrocytes in fibrin networks in the microcirculation.

In idiopathic TTP, autoantibodies against ADAMTS-13 (a disintegrin and metalloproteinase with thrombospondin type 1 repeat, member 13), also known as the von Willebrand factor cleaving protease (vWFCP), lead to accumulation of ultra-large von Willebrand factor (vWF) multimers. These multimers bridge and aggregate platelets in the absence of hemostatic triggers, which in turn leads to the vessel obstruction and various organ manifestations seen in TTP. Classic HUS, also called Shiga-toxin–mediated HUS, is thought to be secondary to toxin-mediated endothelial damage and is often contracted through the ingestion of undercooked ground beef contaminated with *Escherichia coli* (especially types O157:H7 or O145).

Atypical HUS is not related to Shiga toxin. It is a chronic disorder that typically leads to acute kidney injury and often kidney failure. Patients with atypical HUS often have genetic defects in proteins that regulate complement activity. Damage to endothelial cells—such as the damage that occurs in endemic HUS due to presence of toxins from *E coli* (especially type O157:H7 or O145) or in the setting of cancer, hematopoietic stem cell transplantation, or HIV infection—may also lead to TMA. Certain drugs (eg, cyclosporine, quinine, ticlopidine, clopidogrel, mitomycin C, and bleomycin) have been associated with the development of TMA, possibly by promoting injury to endothelial cells, although inhibitory antibodies to ADAMTS-13 have been demonstrated in some cases.

▶ Clinical Findings

A. Symptoms and Signs

Microangiopathic hemolytic anemia and thrombocytopenia are presenting signs in all patients with TTP and most patients with HUS; in a subset of patients with HUS, the platelet count remains in the normal range. Only approximately 25% of patients with TMA manifest all components of the original pentad of findings (microangiopathic hemolytic anemia, thrombocytopenia, fever, kidney disease, and neurologic system abnormalities) (Table 14–4). Most patients (especially children) with HUS have a recent or current diarrheal illness. Neurologic manifestations, including headache, somnolence, delirium, seizures, paresis, and coma, may result from deposition of microthrombi in the cerebral vasculature.

B. Laboratory Findings

Laboratory features of TMA include those associated with microangiopathic hemolytic anemia (anemia, elevated lactate dehydrogenase [LD], elevated indirect bilirubin, decreased haptoglobin, reticulocytosis, schistocytes on the blood smear, and a negative direct antiglobulin test); thrombocytopenia; elevated creatinine; positive stool culture for *E coli* O157:H7 or stool assays for Shiga-toxin producing *E coli* to detect non-O157:H7 such as *E coli* O145 (HUS only); reductions in ADAMTS-13 activity (idiopathic TTP); and mutations of genes encoding complement proteins (atypical HUS; specialized laboratory assessment). Routine coagulation studies are within the normal range in most patients with TMA.

▶ Treatment

Immediate administration of plasma exchange is essential in most cases because the mortality rate is more than 95% without treatment. With the exception of children or adults with endemic diarrhea-associated HUS, who generally recover with supportive care only, plasma exchange must be initiated as soon as the diagnosis of TMA is suspected and in all cases of TTP. Plasma exchange usually is administered once daily until the platelet count and LD have returned to normal for at least 2 days, after which the frequency of treatments may be tapered slowly while the platelet count and LD are monitored for relapse. In cases of insufficient response to once-daily plasma exchange, twice-daily treatments can be given. Fresh frozen plasma (FFP) may be administered if immediate access to plasma exchange is not

Table 14–4. Presentation and management of thrombotic microangiopathies.

	TTP	Atypical HUS	Endemic HUS
Patient population	Adult patients	Children (occasionally adults)	Usually children, often following bloody diarrhea
Pathogenesis	Acquired auto-antibody to ADAMTS-13	Some cases: heritable deficiency in function of complement regulatory proteins	Bacterial (such as enterotoxigenic *Escherichia coli*; Shiga toxin)
Thrombocytopenia	Typically severe, except in very early clinical course	Variable	May be mild/absent in a minority of patients
Fever	Typical	Variable	Atypical
Kidney disease	Typical, but may be mild	Typical	Typical
Neurologic impairment	Variable	Less than half of cases	Less than half of cases
Laboratory investigation	Decreased activity of ADAMTS-13; inhibitor usually identified	Defects in complement regulatory proteins	Typically normal ADAMTS-13 activity Positive stool culture for *E coli* 0157:H7 or detectable antibody to Shiga toxin
Management	TPE Hemodialysis for severe renal impairment Platelet transfusions contraindicated unless TPE underway	Immediate TPE in most cases Supportive care Hemodialysis for severe renal impairment Eculizumab (selected cases)	Hemodialysis for severe renal impairment Supportive care TPE rarely beneficial (exception: selected cases in adults)

ADAMTS-13, a disintegrin and metalloproteinase with a thrombospondin type 1 motif, member 13; HUS, hemolytic-uremic syndrome; TPE, therapeutic plasma exchange; TTP, thrombotic thrombocytopenic purpura.

available or in cases of familial TMA. *Platelet transfusions are contraindicated* in the treatment of TMAs due to reports of worsening TMA, possibly due to propagation of platelet-rich microthrombi. In cases of documented life-threatening bleeding, however, platelet transfusions may be given slowly and after plasma exchange is underway. Red blood cell transfusions may be administered in cases of clinically significant anemia. Hemodialysis should be considered for patients with significant kidney disease.

In cases of TTP relapse following initial treatment, plasma exchange should be reinstituted. If ineffective, or in cases of primary refractoriness, second-line treatments should be considered including rituximab (which has shown efficacy when administered preemptively in selected cases of relapsing TTP), corticosteroids, IVIG, vincristine, cyclophosphamide, and splenectomy.

Cases of atypical HUS may respond to plasma infusion initially, and serial infusions of the anti-complement C5 antibody eculizumab have produced sustained remissions in some patients. If irreversible kidney disease has occurred, hemodialysis or kidney transplantation may be necessary.

▶ When to Refer

Consultation by a hematologist or transfusion medicine specialist familiar with plasma exchange is required at the time of presentation. Patients with refractory or relapsing TMA require ongoing care by a hematologist.

▶ When to Admit

All patients with newly suspected or diagnosed TMA should be hospitalized initially.

Deford CC et al. Multiple major morbidities and increased mortality during long-term follow-up after recovery from thrombotic thrombocytopenic purpura. Blood. 2013 Sep 19;122(12):2023–9. [PMID: 23838348]

George JN et al. Syndromes of thrombotic microangiopathy associated with pregnancy. Hematology Am Soc Hematol Educ Program. 2015 Dec 5;2015(1):644–8. [PMID: 26637783]

Hie M et al; French Thrombotic Microangiopathies Reference Centre. Preemptive rituximab infusions after remission efficiently prevent relapses in acquired thrombotic thrombocytopenic purpura. Blood. 2014 Jul 10;124(2):204–10. [PMID: 24869941]

Legendre CM et al. Terminal complement inhibitor eculizumab in atypical hemolytic-uremic syndrome. N Engl J Med. 2013 Jun 6;368(23):2169–81. [PMID: 23738544]

Sayani FA et al. How I treat refractory thrombotic thrombocytopenic purpura. Blood. 2015 Jun 18;125(25):3860–7. [PMID: 25784681]

3. Heparin-Induced Thrombocytopenia

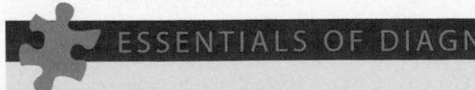

ESSENTIALS OF DIAGNOSIS

▶ Thrombocytopenia within 5–14 days of exposure to heparin.

▶ Decline in baseline platelet count of 50% or greater.

▶ Thrombosis occurs in up to 50% of cases; bleeding is uncommon.

▶ General Considerations

Heparin-induced thrombocytopenia (HIT) is an acquired disorder that affects approximately 3% of patients exposed to unfractionated heparin and 0.6% of patients exposed to low-molecular-weight heparin (LMWH). The condition results from formation of IgG antibodies to heparin-platelet factor 4 (PF4) complexes; the antibody:heparin-PF2 complex binds to and activates platelets independent of physiologic hemostasis, which leads to thrombocytopenia and a pro-thrombotic state.

▶ Clinical Findings

A. Symptoms and Signs

Patients are usually asymptomatic, and due to the pro-thrombotic nature of HIT, bleeding usually does not occur. Thrombosis (at any venous or arterial site), however, may be detected in up to 50% of patients, up to 30 days post-diagnosis.

B. Laboratory Findings

A presumptive diagnosis of HIT is made when new-onset thrombocytopenia is detected in a patient (frequently a hospitalized patient) within 5–14 days of exposure to heparin; other presentations (eg, rapid-onset HIT) are less common. A decline of 50% or more from the baseline platelet count is typical. The 4T score (http://www.qxmd.com/calculate-online/hematology/hit-heparin-induced-thrombocytopenia-probability) is a clinical prediction rule that may assist in assessment of pretest probability for HIT, although low scores have been shown to be more predictive of excluding HIT, than are intermediate or high scores of predicting its presence. Once HIT is clinically suspected, the clinician must establish the diagnosis by performing a screening PF4-heparin antibody enzyme-linked immunosorbent assay (ELISA). If the PF4-heparin antibody ELISA is positive, the diagnosis must be confirmed using a functional assay (such as serotonin release assay). The magnitude of a positive ELISA result correlates with the clinical probability of HIT.

▶ Treatment

Treatment should be initiated as soon as the diagnosis of HIT is suspected, before results of laboratory testing are available.

Management of HIT (Table 14–5) involves the immediate discontinuation of all forms of heparin.

If thrombosis has not already been detected, duplex Doppler ultrasound of the lower extremities should be performed to rule out subclinical deep venous thrombosis (DVT). Despite thrombocytopenia, platelet transfusions are rarely necessary and should be avoided. Due to the substantial frequency of thrombosis among HIT patients, an alternative anticoagulant, typically a direct thrombin inhibitor (DTI) such as argatroban or bivalirudin should be administered immediately. The DTI should be continued until the platelet count has recovered to at least 100,000/mcL, at which point treatment with a vitamin K antagonist (warfarin) may be initiated. The DTI should be continued

Table 14–5. Management of suspected or proven HIT.

I. Discontinue all forms of heparin. Send PF4-heparin ELISA (if indicated).

II. Begin treatment with direct thrombin inhibitor.

Agent	Indication	Dosing
Argatroban	Prophylaxis or treatment of HIT	Continuous intravenous infusion of 0.5–1.2 mcg/kg/min, titrate to aPTT = 1.5 to 3 × the baseline value.[1] Max infusion rate ≤ 10 mcg/kg/min.
Bivalirudin	Percutaneous coronary intervention[2]	Bolus of 0.75 mg/kg intravenously followed by initial continuous intravenous infusion of 1.75 mg/kg/h. Manufacturer indicates monitoring should be by ACT.

III. Perform Doppler ultrasound of lower extremities to rule out subclinical thrombosis (if indicated).

IV. Follow platelet counts daily until recovery occurs.

V. When platelet count has recovered, transition anticoagulation to warfarin; treat for 30 days (HIT) or 3–6 months (HITT).

VI. Document heparin allergy in medical record (confirmed cases).

[1]Hepatic insufficiency: initial infusion rate = 0.5 mcg/kg/min.
[2]Not approved for HIT/HITT.
ACT, activated clotting time; aPTT, activated partial thromboplastin time; ELISA, enzyme-linked immunosorbent assay; HIT, heparin-induced thrombocytopenia; HITT, heparin-induced thrombocytopenia and thrombosis; PF4, platelet factor 4.

until therapeutic anticoagulation with the vitamin K antagonist has been achieved (international normalized ratio [INR] of 2.0–3.0) due to the warfarin effect; the infusion of argatroban must be temporarily discontinued for 2 hours before the INR is obtained so that it reflects the anticoagulant effect of warfarin alone. There is growing use of the subcutaneous indirect anti-Xa inhibitor fondaparinux for initial treatment of HIT. In all patients with HIT, some form of anticoagulation (warfarin or other) subsequently should be continued for at least 30 days, due to a persistent risk of thrombosis even after the platelet count has recovered, but in patients in whom thrombosis has been documented, anticoagulation should continue for 3–6 months.

Subsequent exposure to heparin should be avoided in all patients with a prior history of HIT, if possible. If its use is regarded as necessary for a procedure, it should be withheld until PF4-heparin antibodies are no longer detectable by ELISA (usually as of 100 days following an episode of HIT), and exposure should be limited to the shortest time period possible.

When to Refer

Due to the tremendous thrombotic potential of the disorder and the complexity of use of the DTI, all patients with HIT should be evaluated by a hematologist.

When to Admit

Most patients with HIT are hospitalized at the time of detection of thrombocytopenia. Any outpatient in whom HIT is suspected should be admitted because the DTIs must be administered by continuous intravenous infusion.

Chaudhary RK et al. Emerging therapy options in heparin-induced thrombocytopenia. Cardiovasc Hematol Agents Med Chem. 2014;12(1):50–8. [PMID: 25374012]
Cuker A et al. Predictive value of the 4Ts scoring system for heparin-induced thrombocytopenia: a systematic review and meta-analysis. Blood. 2012 Nov 15;120(20):4160–7. [PMID: 22990018]
McKenzie SE et al. Advances in the pathophysiology and treatment of heparin-induced thrombocytopenia. Curr Opin Hematol. 2014 Sep;21(5):380–7. [PMID: 24992313]
Warkentin TE et al. Serological investigation of patients with a previous history of heparin-induced thrombocytopenia who are reexposed to heparin. Blood. 2014 Apr 17;123(16):2485–93. [PMID: 24516044]

4. Disseminated Intravascular Coagulation

ESSENTIALS OF DIAGNOSIS

► A frequent cause of thrombocytopenia in hospitalized patients.
► Prolonged activated partial thromboplastin time and prothrombin time.
► Thrombocytopenia and decreased fibrinogen levels.

General Considerations

Disseminated intravascular coagulation (DIC) results from uncontrolled local or systemic activation of coagulation, which leads to depletion of coagulation factors and fibrinogen as well as to thrombocytopenia as platelets are activated and consumed.

The numerous disorders that are associated with DIC include sepsis (in which coagulation is activated by presence of lipopolysaccharide), cancer, trauma, burns, and pregnancy-associated complications (in which tissue factor is released). Aortic aneurysm and cavernous hemangiomas may promote localized intravascular coagulation, and snake bites may result in DIC due to the introduction of exogenous toxins.

Clinical Findings

A. Symptoms and Signs

Bleeding in DIC usually occurs at multiple sites, such as intravenous catheters or incisions, and may be widespread (purpura fulminans). Malignancy-related DIC may manifest principally as thrombosis (Trousseau syndrome).

B. Laboratory Findings

In early DIC, the platelet count and fibrinogen levels may remain within the normal range, albeit reduced from baseline levels. There is progressive thrombocytopenia (rarely severe), prolongation of the prothrombin time (PT), decrease in fibrinogen levels, and eventually elevation in the activated partial thromboplastin time (aPTT). D-dimer levels typically are elevated due to the activation of coagulation and diffuse cross-linking of fibrin. Schistocytes on the blood smear, due to shearing of red cells through the microvasculature, are present in 10–20% of patients. Laboratory abnormalities in the HELLP syndrome (hemolysis, elevated liver enzymes, low platelets), a severe form of DIC with a particularly high mortality rate that occurs in peripartum women, include elevated liver transaminases and (many cases) kidney injury due to gross hemoglobinuria and pigment nephropathy. Malignancy-related DIC may feature normal platelet counts and coagulation studies, but clinicians often see a dropping platelet count and fibrinogen, with a rising INR.

Treatment

The underlying causative disorder must be treated (eg, antimicrobials, chemotherapy, surgery, or delivery of conceptus). If clinically significant bleeding is present, hemostasis must be achieved (Table 14–6).

Blood products should be administered only if clinically significant hemorrhage has occurred or is thought likely to occur without intervention (Table 14–6). The goal of platelet therapy for most cases is greater than 20,000/mcL or greater than 50,000/mcL for serious bleeding, such as

Table 14–6. Management of DIC.

I. Assess for underlying cause of DIC and treat.
II. Establish baseline platelet count, PT, aPTT, D-dimer, fibrinogen.

III. Transfuse blood products only if ongoing bleeding or high risk of bleeding:	Platelets: goal > 20,000/mcL (most patients) or > 50,000/mcL (severe bleeding, eg, intracranial hemorrhage)
	Cryoprecipitate: goal fibrinogen level > 80–100 mg/dL
	Fresh frozen plasma: goal PT and aPTT < 1.5 × normal
	Packed red blood cells: goal hemoglobin > 8 g/dL or Improvement in symptomatic anemia

IV. Follow platelets, aPTT/PT, fibrinogen every 4–6 hours or as clinically indicated.
V. If persistent bleeding, consider use of heparin[1] (initial infusion, 5–10 units/kg/h); do not administer bolus.
VI. Follow laboratory parameters every 4–6 hours until DIC resolved and underlying condition successfully treated

[1]Contraindicated if platelets cannot be maintained at > 50,000/mcL, in cases of gastrointestinal or central nervous system bleeding, in conditions that may require surgical management, or placental abruption.

aPTT, activated partial thromboplastin time; DIC, disseminated intravascular coagulation; PT, prothrombin time.

intracranial bleeding. FFP should be given only to patients with a prolonged aPTT and PT and significant bleeding. Cryoprecipitate may be given for bleeding or for fibrinogen levels less than 80–100 mg/dL. The clinician should correct the fibrinogen level with cryoprecipitate prior to giving FFP for prolonged PT and aPTT, to see if the fibrinogen replacement alone corrects the PT and aPTT. The PT, aPTT, fibrinogen, and platelet count should be monitored at least every 6–8 hours in acutely ill patients with DIC.

In some cases of refractory bleeding despite replacement of blood products, administration of low doses of heparin can be considered. The clinician must remember that DIC is primarily excessive clotting with secondary fibrinolysis, and heparin can interfere with thrombin generation, which could then lead to a lessened consumption of coagulation proteins and platelets. An infusion of 5–10 units/kg/h (no bolus) may be used with appropriate clinical judgement. *Heparin, however, is contraindicated if the platelet count cannot be maintained at 50,000/mcL or more and in cases of central nervous system hemorrhage, gastrointestinal bleeding, placental abruption, and any other condition that is likely to require imminent surgery.* Fibrinolysis inhibitors may be considered in some patients with refractory DIC, but this can promote dangerous clotting and should not be undertaken without consulting a hematologist.

The treatment of **HELLP syndrome** must include evacuation of the uterus (eg, delivery of a term or near-term infant or removal of retained placental or fetal fragments). Patients with **Trousseau syndrome** require treatment of the underlying malignancy or administration of unfractionated heparin or subcutaneous therapeutic-dose LMWH as treatment of thrombosis, since warfarin typically is ineffective at secondary prevention of thromboembolism in the disorder. Typically, the fibrinogen rises, platelets rise, and PT (INR) and aPTT normalize, but it can take days. Immediate initiation of chemotherapy (usually within 24 hours of diagnosis) is required for patients with **acute promyelocytic leukemia (APL)–associated DIC,** along with administration of blood products as clinically indicated.

When to Refer

- Diffuse bleeding that is unresponsive to administration of blood products should be evaluated by a hematologist.
- All patients with DIC starting treatment with heparin or LMWH.

When to Admit

Most patients with DIC are hospitalized when DIC is detected.

Feinstein DI. Disseminated intravascular coagulation in patients with solid tumors. Oncology (Williston Park). 2015 Feb;29(2):96–102. [PMID: 25683828]

Iba T et al. Anticoagulant therapy for sepsis-associated disseminated intravascular coagulation: the view from Japan. J Thromb Haemost. 2014 Jul;12(7):1010–9. [PMID: 24801203]

Levi M. Diagnosis and treatment of disseminated intravascular coagulation. Int J Lab Hematol. 2014 Jun;36(3):228–36. [PMID: 24750668]

McMahon CM et al. Hospital-acquired thrombocytopenia. Hosp Pract (1995). 2014 Oct;42(4):142–52. [PMID: 25502138]

Wada H et al. Disseminated intravascular coagulation: testing and diagnosis. Clin Chim Acta. 2014 Sep 25;436:130–4. [PMID: 24792730]

OTHER CONDITIONS CAUSING THROMBOCYTOPENIA

1. Drug-Induced Thrombocytopenia

The mechanisms underlying drug-induced thrombocytopenia are thought in most cases to be immune, although exceptions exist (such as chemotherapy). Table 14–7 lists medications associated with thrombocytopenia. The typical presentation of **drug-induced** (or **drug-related**) **thrombocytopenia** is severe thrombocytopenia and mucocutaneous bleeding 7–14 days after exposure to a new drug, although a range of presentations is possible. Discontinuation of the offending agent leads to resolution of thrombocytopenia within 7–10 days in most cases, but recovery kinetics depends on rate of drug clearance, which can be affected by liver and kidney function. Patients with severe thrombocytopenia should be given platelet transfusions with (immune cases only) or without IVIG.

2. Posttransfusion Purpura

Posttransfusion purpura (PTP) is a rare disorder that features sudden-onset thrombocytopenia in an individual who recently has received transfusion of red cells, platelets, or plasma within 1 week prior to detection of thrombocytopenia. Antibodies against the human platelet antigen PlA1 are detected in most individuals with PTP. Patients with PTP almost universally are either multiparous women or persons who have received transfusions previously. Severe thrombocytopenia and bleeding are typical. Initial treatment consists of administration of IVIG (1 g/kg/day for 2 days), which should be administered as soon as the diagnosis is suspected. Platelets are not indicated unless severe bleeding is present, but if they are to be administered, HLA-matched platelets are preferred. A second course or IVIG, plasma exchange, corticosteroids, or splenectomy may be used in case of refractoriness. PlA1-negative or washed blood products are preferred for subsequent transfusions.

3. von Willebrand Disease Type 2B

von Willebrand disease (vWD) type 2B leads to chronic, characteristically mild to moderate thrombocytopenia via an abnormal vWF molecule that binds platelets with increased affinity, resulting in aggregation and clearance.

4. Platelet Sequestration

At any given time, one-third of the platelet mass is sequestered in the spleen. Splenomegaly, due to a variety of conditions, may lead to thrombocytopenia of variable severity. Whenever possible, treatment of the underlying disorder

Table 14–7. Selected medications causing drug-associated thrombocytopenia.

Class	Examples
Chemotherapy	Most agents
Antiplatelet agents	Anagrelide Abciximab Eptifibatide Tirofiban Ticlopidine
Antimicrobial agents	Penicillins Isoniazid Rifampin Sulfa drugs Vancomycin Adefovir Indinavir Ritonavir Fluconazole Linezolid
Cardiovascular agents	Digoxin Amiodarone Captopril Hydrochlorothiazide Procainamide Atorvastatin Simvastatin
Gastrointestinal agents	Cimetidine Ranitidine Famotidine
Neuropsychiatric agents	Haloperidol Carbamazepine Methyldopa Phenytoin
Analgesic agents	Acetaminophen Ibuprofen Sulindac Diclofenac Naproxen
Anticoagulant agents	Heparin Low-molecular-weight heparin
Immunomodulator agents	Interferon-alpha Rituximab
Immunosuppressant agents	Mycophenolate mofetil Tacrolimus
Other agents	Iodinated contrast dye Immunizations

should be pursued, but splenectomy, splenic embolization, or splenic irradiation may be considered in selected cases.

5. Pregnancy

Gestational thrombocytopenia is thought to result from progressive expansion of the blood volume that typically occurs during pregnancy, leading to hemodilution. Cytopenias result, although production of blood cells is normal or increased. Platelet counts less than 100,000/mcL, however, are observed in less than 10% of pregnant women in the third trimester; decreases to less than 70,000/mcL should prompt consideration of pregnancy-related ITP as well as preeclampsia or a pregnancy-related thrombotic microangiopathy.

6. Infection or Sepsis

Both immune- and platelet production–mediated defects are possible, and there may be significant overlap with concomitant DIC. In either case, the platelet count typically improves with effective antimicrobial treatment or after the infection has resolved. In some critically ill patients, a defect in immunomodulation may lead to bone marrow macrophages (histiocytes) engulfing cellular components of the marrow in a process also called hemophagocytosis. The phenomenon typically resolves with resolution of the infection, but with certain infections (Epstein-Barr virus) immunosuppression may be required. Hemophagocytosis also may arise in the setting of malignancy, in which case the disorder is usually unresponsive to treatment with immunosuppression. Sepsis-related thrombocytopenia may be due to increased hepatic clearance of platelets caused by loss of asialoglycoprotein moieties on the platelet surface.

7. Pseudothrombocytopenia

Pseudothrombocytopenia results from EDTA anticoagulant-induced platelet clumping; the phenomenon typically disappears when blood is collected in a tube containing citrate anticoagulant.

Grewal PK et al. Inducing host protection in pneumococcal sepsis by preactivation of the Ashwell-Morell receptor. Proc Natl Acad Sci U S A. 2013 Dec 10;110(50):20218–23. [PMID: 24284176]

Grozovsky R et al. The Ashwell-Morell receptor regulates hepatic thrombopoietin production via JAK2-STAT3 signaling. Nat Med. 2015 Jan;21(1):47–54. [PMID: 25485912]

Kasai J et al. Clinical features of gestational thrombocytopenia difficult to differentiate from immune thrombocytopenia diagnosed during pregnancy. J Obstet Gynaecol Res. 2015 Jan;41(1):44–9. [PMID: 25163390]

Perdomo J et al. Quinine-induced thrombocytopenia: drug-dependent GPIb/IX antibodies inhibit megakaryocyte and proplatelet production in vitro. Blood. 2011 Jun 2;117(22): 5975–86. [PMID: 21487107]

QUALITATIVE PLATELET DISORDERS

CONGENITAL DISORDERS OF PLATELET FUNCTION

ESSENTIALS OF DIAGNOSIS

► Usually diagnosed in childhood.

► Family history usually is positive.

► May be diagnosed in adulthood when there is excessive bleeding.

► General Considerations

Heritable qualitative platelet disorders are far less common than acquired disorders of platelet function and lead to variably severe bleeding, often beginning in childhood. Occasionally, however, disorders of platelet function may go undetected until later in life when excessive bleeding occurs following a sufficient hemostatic insult. Thus, the true incidence of hereditary qualitative platelet disorders is unknown.

Bernard-Soulier syndrome (BSS) is a rare, autosomal recessive bleeding disorder due to reduced or abnormal platelet membrane expression of glycoprotein Ib/IX (vWF receptor).

Glanzmann thrombasthenia results from a qualitative or quantitative abnormality in glycoprotein IIb/IIIa receptors on the platelet membrane, which are required to bind fibrinogen and vWF, both of which bridge platelets during aggregation. Inheritance is autosomal recessive.

Under normal circumstances, activated platelets release the contents of platelet granules to reinforce the aggregatory response. **Storage pool disease** is caused by defects in release of alpha or dense (delta) platelet granules, or both (alpha-delta storage pool disease).

► Clinical Findings

A. Symptoms and Signs

In patients with **Glanzmann thrombasthenia,** the onset of bleeding is usually in infancy or childhood. The degree of deficiency in IIb/IIIa may not correlate well with bleeding symptoms. Patients with **storage pool disease** are affected by variable bleeding, ranging from mild and trauma-related to spontaneous.

B. Laboratory Findings

In **Bernard-Soulier syndrome,** there are abnormally large platelets (approaching the size of red cells), moderate thrombocytopenia, and a prolonged bleeding time. Platelet aggregation studies show a marked defect in response to ristocetin, whereas aggregation in response to other agonists is normal; the addition of normal platelets corrects the abnormal aggregation. The diagnosis can be confirmed by platelet flow cytometry.

In **Glanzmann thrombasthenia,** platelet aggregation studies show marked impairment of aggregation in response to stimulation with typical agonists.

Storage pool disease describes defects in the number or content of platelet alpha or dense granules, or both. The **gray platelet syndrome** comprises abnormalities of platelet alpha granules, thrombocytopenia, and marrow fibrosis. The blood smear shows agranular platelets, and the diagnosis is confirmed with electron microscopy.

Albinism-associated storage pool disease involves defective dense granules in disorders of oculocutaneous albinism, such as the Hermansky-Pudlak and Chediak-Higashi syndromes. Electron microscopy confirms the diagnosis.

Non–albinism-associated storage pool disease results from quantitative or qualitative defects in dense granules and is seen in Ehlers-Danlos and Wiskott-Aldrich syndromes, among others.

The **Quebec platelet disorder** comprises mild thrombocytopenia, an abnormal platelet factor V molecule, and a prolonged bleeding time. Patients typically experience moderate bleeding. Interestingly, platelet transfusion does not ameliorate the bleeding.

Patients have a prolonged bleeding time. Platelet aggregation studies characteristically show platelet dissociation following an initial aggregatory response, and electron microscopy confirms the diagnosis.

► Treatment

The mainstay of treatment (including periprocedural prophylaxis) is transfusion of normal platelets, although desmopressin acetate (DDAVP), antifibrinolytic agents, and recombinant human activated factor VII also have been used successfully.

Andrews RK et al. Bernard-Soulier syndrome: an update. Semin Thromb Hemost. 2013 Sep;39(6):656–62. [PMID: 23929303]
Lambert MP. What to do when you suspect an inherited platelet disorder. Hematology Am Soc Hematol Educ Program. 2011;2011:377–83. [PMID: 22160061]

ACQUIRED DISORDERS OF PLATELET FUNCTION

Platelet dysfunction is more commonly acquired than inherited; the widespread use of platelet-altering medications accounts for most of the cases of qualitative defects (Table 14–8). In cases where platelet function is irreversibly altered, platelet inhibition typically recovers within 5–10 days following discontinuation of the drug. In cases where platelet function is non-irreversibly affected, platelet inhibition recovers with clearance of the drug from the system. Transfusion of platelets may be required if clinically significant bleeding is present.

DISORDERS OF COAGULATION

CONGENITAL DISORDERS OF COAGULATION

1. Hemophilia A & B

ESSENTIALS OF DIAGNOSIS

► **Hemophilia A:** congenital deficiency of coagulation factor VIII.

► **Hemophilia B:** congenital deficiency of coagulation factor IX.

► Recurrent hemarthroses and arthropathy.

► Risk of development of inhibitory antibodies to factor VIII or factor IX.

► In many older patients, infection with HIV or hepatitis C virus from receipt of contaminated blood products.

► General Considerations

The frequency of hemophilia A is 1 per 5000 live male births, whereas hemophilia B occurs in approximately 1 in 25,000 live male births. Inheritance is X-linked recessive, leading to affected males and carrier females. There is no race predilection. Testing is indicated for male infants with a hemophilic pedigree who are asymptomatic or who experience excessive bleeding, or for an otherwise asymptomatic adolescent or adult who experiences unexpected excessive bleeding with trauma or invasive procedures.

Inhibitors to factor VIII will develop in approximately 30% of patients with severe hemophilia A, and inhibitors to factor IX will develop in less than 5% of patients with severe hemophilia B.

A substantial proportion of older patients with hemophilia acquired infection with HIV or HCV or both in the 1980s due to exposure to contaminated factor concentrates and blood products.

► Clinical Findings

A. Symptoms and Signs

Severe hemophilia (factor VIII activity less than 1%) presents in infant males or in early childhood with spontaneous bleeding into joints, soft tissues, or other locations. Spontaneous bleeding is rare in patients with mild hemophilia (factor VIII activity greater than 5%), but bleeding may occur with a significant hemostatic challenge (eg, surgery, trauma). Intermediate clinical symptoms are seen in patients with moderate hemophilia (factor VIII activity 1–5%). Female carriers of hemophilia are usually asymptomatic.

Significant hemophilic arthropathy is usually avoided in patients who have received long-term prophylaxis with factor concentrate starting in childhood, whereas joint disease is common in adults who have experienced recurrent hemarthroses.

Inhibitor development to factor VIII or factor IX is characterized by bleeding episodes that are resistant to treatment with clotting factor VIII or IX concentrate, and by new or atypical bleeding.

B. Laboratory Findings

Hemophilia is diagnosed by demonstration of an isolated reproducibly low factor VIII or factor IX activity level, in the absence of other conditions. If the aPTT is prolonged, it typically corrects upon mixing with normal plasma. A variety of mutations, including inversions, large and small deletions, insertions, missense mutations, and nonsense mutations may be causative. Depending on the level of residual factor VIII or factor IX activity and the sensitivity of the thromboplastin used in the aPTT coagulation reaction, the aPTT may or may not be prolonged (although it typically is markedly prolonged in severe hemophilia). Hemophilia is classified according to the level of factor activity in the plasma. **Severe hemophilia** is characterized by less than 1% factor activity, **mild hemophilia** features greater than 5% factor activity, and **moderate hemophilia** features 1–5% factor activity. Female carriers may become

Table 14–8. Causes of acquired platelet dysfunction.

Cause	Mechanism(s)	Treatment of Bleeding
Drug-induced		
Salicylates (eg, aspirin)	Irreversible inhibition of platelet cyclooxygenase	Discontinuation of drug; platelet transfusion
NSAIDs (eg, ibuprofen)	Reversible inhibition of cyclooxygenase	
Glycoprotein IIb/IIIa inhibitors (eg, abciximab, tirofiban, eptifibatide)	↓ Binding of fibrinogen to PM IIb/IIIa receptor	
Thienopyridines (eg, clopidogrel, ticlopidine)	↓ ADP binding to PM receptor	
Dipyridamole	↓ Intracellular cAMP metabolism	
SSRIs (eg, paroxetine, fluoxetine)	↓ Serotonin in dense granules	
Omega-3 fatty acids (eg, DHA, EHA)	Disruption of PM phospholipid	
Antibiotics, (eg, high-dose penicillin, nafcillin, ticarcillin, cephalothin, moxalactam)	Not fully elucidated; PM binding may interfere with receptor-ligand interactions	
Alcohol	↓ TXA2 release	
Disease-related		
Uremia	↑ Nitric oxide; ↓ release of granules	DDAVP, high-dose estrogens; platelet transfusion, dialysis
Myeloproliferative disorder/myelodysplastic syndrome	Abnormal PM receptors, signal transduction, and/or granule release	Platelet transfusion; myelosuppressive treatment (myeloproliferative disorder)
Surgical procedure–related		
Cardiac bypass	Platelet activation in bypass circuit	Platelet transfusion

ADP, adenosine diphosphate; cAMP, cyclic adenosine monophosphate; DDAVP, desmopressin acetate; DHA, docosahexaenoic acid; EHA, eicosahexaenoic acid; NSAIDs, nonsteroidal anti-inflammatory drugs; PM, platelet membrane; SSRIs, selective serotonin release inhibitors; TXA2, thromboxane A2.

symptomatic if significant lyonization has occurred favoring the defective factor VIII or factor IX gene, leading to factor VIII or factor IX activity level markedly less than 50%. Typically, a clinical bleeding diathesis occurs once the factor activity is less than 20%.

In the presence of an inhibitor to factor VIII or factor IX, there is accelerated clearance of and suboptimal or absent rise in measured activity of infused factor, and the aPTT does not correct on mixing. The Bethesda assay measures the potency of the inhibitor.

▶ **Treatment**

Plasma-derived or recombinant factor VIII or IX products are the mainstay of treatment. The standard of care for most individuals with severe hemophilia is primary prophylaxis: by the age of 4 years, most children with severe hemophilia have begun twice- or thrice-weekly infusions of factor to prevent the recurrent joint bleeding that otherwise would characterize the disorder and lead to severe musculoskeletal morbidity. In selected cases of nonsevere hemophilia, or as an adjunct to prophylaxis in severe hemophilia, treatment with factor products may also be given periprocedurally, prior to high-risk activities (such as sports), or as needed for bleeding episodes (Table 14–9). Recombinant FVIII and FIX molecules that are

bioengineered to have an extended half-life have been approved for clinical use and may allow for extended dosing intervals in patients who are treated prophylactically. The decision to switch to a long-acting product is patient specific. The long-acting factor IX products have clear added value in reducing frequency of factor injections. This is not so clear with the newly approved long-acting factor VIII products. Patients with mild hemophilia A may respond to as-needed intravenous or intranasal treatment with DDAVP. Antifibrinolytic agents may be useful in cases of mucosal bleeding and are commonly used adjunctively, such as following dental procedures. Delivery of a functional factor IX gene using modified viral vectors continues to be explored in clinical trials, with early results among patients with severe hemophilia B showing improvement in the baseline factor IX level so as to reduce or eliminate the need for prophylactic infusions of factor IX protein.

It may be possible to overcome low-titer inhibitors (less than 5 Bethesda units [BU]) by giving larger doses of factor, whereas treatment of bleeding in the presence of a high-titer inhibitor (more than 5 BU) requires infusion of an activated prothrombin complex concentrate (such as FEIBA [factor eight inhibitor bypassing activity]) or recombinant activated factor VII. Inhibitor tolerance induction, achieved by giving large doses (50–300 units/kg intravenously of factor VIII daily) for 6–18 months,

Table 14–9. Treatment of bleeding in selected inherited disorders of hemostasis.

Disorder	Subtype	Treatment for Minor Bleeding	Treatment for Major Bleeding	Comment
Hemophilia A	Mild	DDAVP[1]	DDAVP[1] or factor VIII product	Treat for 3–10 days for major bleeding or following surgery, keeping factor activity level 50–80% initially. Adjunctive aminocaproic acid (EACA) may be useful for mucosal bleeding or procedures
	Moderate or severe	Factor VIII product	Factor VIII product	
Hemophilia B	Mild, moderate, or severe	Factor IX product	Factor IX product	
von Willebrand disease	Type 1	DDAVP	DDAVP, vWF product	
	Type 2	DDAVP,[1] vWF product	vWF product	
	Type 3	vWF product	vWF product	
Factor XI deficiency	—	FFP or aminocaproic acid	FFP	Adjunctive aminocaproic acid should be used for mucosal bleeding or procedures

[1]Mild hemophilia A and type 2A or 2B vWD patients: therapeutic trial must have previously confirmed an adequate response (ie, elevation of factor VIII or vWF activity level into the normal range) and (for type 2B) no exacerbation of thrombocytopenia. DDAVP is not typically effective for type 2M vWD. A vWF-containing factor VIII concentrate is preferred for treatment of type 2N vWD.

Notes:

DDAVP dose is 0.3 mcg/kg intravenously in 50 mL saline over 20 minutes, or nasal spray 300 mcg for weight > 50 kg or 150 mcg for < 50 kg, every 12–24 hours, maximum of three doses in a 48-hour period. If more than two doses are used in a 12- to 24-hour period, free water restriction and monitoring for hyponatremia is essential.

EACA dose is 50 mg/kg orally four times daily for 3–5 days; maximum 24 g/day, useful for mucosal bleeding/dental procedures.

Factor VIII product dose is 50 units/kg intravenously initially followed by 25 units/kg every 8 hours followed by lesser doses at longer intervals once hemostasis has been established.

Factor IX product dose is 100 units/kg (120 units/kg if using Benefix) intravenously initially followed by 50 units/kg (60 units/kg if using Benefix) every 8 hours followed by lesser doses at longer intervals once hemostasis has been established.

vWF-containing factor VIII product dose is 60–80 RCoF units/kg intravenously every 12 hours initially followed by lesser doses at longer intervals once hemostasis has been established.

FFP is typically administered in 4-unit boluses and may not need to be re-bolused after the initial administration due to the long half-life of factor XI.

DDAVP, desmopressin acetate; FFP, fresh frozen plasma; vWF, von Willebrand factor.

succeeds in eradicating the inhibitor in 70% of patients with hemophilia A and in 30% of patients with hemophilia B. Patients with hemophilia B who receive inhibitor tolerance induction, however, are at risk for development of nephrotic syndrome and anaphylactic reactions, making eradication of their inhibitors less feasible. Additional immunomodulation may allow for eradication in selected inhibitor tolerance induction–refractory patients.

Antiretroviral treatment is almost universally administered to individuals with HIV infection. Patients with hepatitis C infection should be referred for treatment to eradicate the virus.

▶ **When to Refer**

All patients with hemophilia should be seen regularly in a comprehensive hemophilia treatment center.

▶ **When to Admit**

- Major invasive procedures because of the need for serial infusions of clotting factor concentrate.
- Bleeding that is unresponsive to outpatient treatment.

Aledort L et al. Factor VIII therapy for hemophilia A: current and future issues. Expert Rev Hematol. 2014 Jun;7(3):373–85. [PMID: 24717090]

Astermark J. FVIII inhibitors: pathogenesis and avoidance. Blood. 2015 Mar 26;125(13):2045–51. [PMID: 25712994]

Baghaipour MR et al. Strategies for inhibitor treatment and costs in the short and long term: a critical evaluation of recent clinical studies. Eur J Haematol. 2015 Feb;94(Suppl 77):30–7. [PMID: 25560792]

Coppola A et al. Treatment for preventing bleeding in people with haemophilia or other congenital bleeding disorders undergoing surgery. Cochrane Database Syst Rev. 2015 Feb 9; 2:CD009961. [PMID: 25922858]

Franchini M. Current management of hemophilia B: recommendations, complications and emerging issues. Expert Rev Hematol. 2014 Oct;7(5):573–81. [PMID: 25112898]

Nathwani AC et al. Long-term safety and efficacy of factor IX gene therapy in hemophilia B. N Engl J Med. 2014 Nov 20;371(21):1994–2004. [PMID: 25409372]

Oldenburg J. Optimal treatment strategies for hemophilia: achievements and limitations of current prophylactic regimens. Blood. 2015 Mar 26;125(13):2038–44. [PMID: 25712992]

Srivastava A et al; Treatment Guidelines Working Group of Behalf of The World Federation Of Hemophilia. Guidelines for the management of hemophilia. Haemophilia. 2013 Jan;19(1):e1–47. [PMID: 22776238]

2. von Willebrand Disease

ESSENTIALS OF DIAGNOSIS

▶ The most common inherited bleeding disorder.

▶ von Willebrand factor binds platelets to subendo-thelial surfaces, aggregates platelets, and prolongs the half-life of factor VIII.

General Considerations

vWF is an unusually large multimeric glycoprotein that binds to its receptor, platelet glycoprotein Ib, bridging platelets together and tethering them to the subendothelial matrix at the site of vascular injury. vWF also has a binding site for factor VIII, prolonging its half-life in the circulation.

Between 75% and 80% of patients with vWD have type 1, a quantitative abnormality of the vWF molecule that usually does not feature an identifiable causal mutation in the vWF gene.

Type 2 vWD is seen in 15–20% of patients with vWD. In type 2A or 2B vWD, a qualitative defect in the vWF molecule is causative. Type 2N and 2M vWD are due to defects in vWF that decrease binding to factor VIII or to platelets, respectively. Importantly, type 2N vWD clinically resembles hemophilia A, with the exception of a family history that shows affected females. Factor VIII activity levels are markedly decreased, and vWF activity and antigen (Ag) are normal. Type 2M vWD features a normal multimer pattern. Type 3 vWD is rare, and like type 1, is a quantitative defect, but mutational homozygosity or double heterozygosity leads to undetectable levels of vWF and severe bleeding in infancy or childhood.

Clinical Findings

A. Symptoms and Signs

Patients with type 1 vWD usually have mild or moderate platelet-type bleeding (especially involving the integument and mucous membranes). Patients with type 2 vWD usually have moderate to severe bleeding that presents in childhood or adolescence. Patient with type 3 vWD demonstrate a severe bleeding phenotype.

B. Laboratory Findings

In type 1 vWD, the vWF activity (by ristocetin co-factor assay) and Ag are mildly depressed, whereas the vWF multimer pattern is normal (Table 14–10). Laboratory testing of type 2A or 2B vWD typically shows a ratio of vWF Ag:vWF activity of approximately 2:1 and a multimer pattern that lacks the highest molecular weight multimers. Thrombocytopenia is common in type 2B vWD due to a gain-of-function mutation of the vWF molecule, which leads to increased binding to its receptor on platelets, resulting in clearance; a ristocetin-induced platelet aggregation (RIPA) study shows an increase in platelet aggregation in response to low concentrations of ristocetin. Except in the more severe forms of vWD that feature a significantly decreased factor VIII activity, the aPTT and PT in vWD are usually normal.

Treatment

The treatment of vWD is summarized in Table 14–9. DDAVP is useful in the treatment of mild bleeding in most cases of type 1 and some cases of type 2 vWD. DDAVP causes release of vWF and factor VIII from storage sites, leading to increases in vWF and factor VIII twofold to sevenfold that of baseline levels. Cryoprecipitate should not be given due to lack of viral inactivation. Antifibrinolytic agents (eg, aminocaproic acid) may be used adjunctively for mucosal bleeding or procedures. Pregnant patients with vWD usually do not require treatment at the time of delivery because of the natural physiologic increase in vWF levels (up to threefold that of baseline) that are observed by parturition; however, if excessive bleeding is encountered, vWF products may be given. Moreover, patients are at risk for significant bleeding for a few days postpartum when vWF levels fall secondary to the fall in estrogen levels.

Abshire TC et al. Prophylaxis in severe forms of von Willebrand's disease: results from the von Willebrand Disease Prophylaxis Network (VWD PN). Haemophilia. 2013 Jan;19(1):76–81. [PMID: 22823000]

Castaman G et al. Laboratory aspects of von Willebrand disease: test repertoire and options for activity assays and genetic analysis. Haemophilia. 2014 May;20(Suppl 4):65–70. [PMID: 24762278]

Lenting PJ et al. von Willebrand factor biosynthesis, secretion, and clearance: connecting the far ends. Blood. 2015 Mar 26; 125(13):2019–28. [PMID: 25712991]

Neff AT. Current controversies in the diagnosis and management of von Willebrand disease. Ther Adv Hematol. 2015 Aug; 6(4):209–16. [PMID: 26288715]

Stone ME et al. Current management of von Willebrand disease and von Willebrand syndrome. Curr Opin Anaesthesiol. 2014 Jun;27(3):353–8. [PMID: 24709665]

3. Factor XI Deficiency

Factor XI deficiency (sometimes referred to as **hemophilia C**) is inherited in an autosomal recessive manner, leading to heterozygous or homozygous defects. It is most prevalent among individuals of Ashkenazi Jewish descent. Levels of factor XI, while variably reduced, do not correlate well with bleeding symptoms. Mild bleeding is most common, and surgery or trauma may expose or worsen the bleeding tendency. FFP is the mainstay of treatment in locales where the plasma-derived factor XI concentrate is not available. Administration of adjunctive aminocaproic acid is regarded as mandatory for procedures or bleeding episodes involving the mucosa (Table 14–9).

James P et al. Rare bleeding disorders—bleeding assessment tools, laboratory aspects and phenotype and therapy of FXI deficiency. Haemophilia. 2014 May;20(Suppl 4):71–5. [PMID: 24762279]

4. Less Common Heritable Disorders of Coagulation

Congenital deficiencies of clotting factors II, V, VII, and X are rare and typically are inherited in an autosomal recessive pattern. A prolongation in the PT (and aPTT for

Table 14–10. Laboratory diagnosis of von Willebrand disease.

Type		vWF Activity	vWF Antigen	FVIII	RIPA	Multimer Analysis
1		↓	↓	NI or ↓	↓	Normal pattern; uniform ↓ intensity of bands
2	A	↓↓	↓	↓	↓	Large and intermediate multimers decreased or absent
	B	↓↓	↓	↓	↑	Large multimers decreased or absent
	M	↓	↓	↓	↓	Normal pattern; uniform ↓ intensity of bands
	N	NI	NI	↓↓	NI	NI
3		↓↓↓	↓↓↓	↓↓↓	↓↓↓	Multimers absent

NI, normal; RIPA, ristocetin-induced platelet aggregation; vWF, von Willebrand factor.

factor X, factor V, and factor II deficiency) that corrects upon mixing with normal plasma is typical. The treatment of factor II deficiency is with a prothrombin complex concentrate; factor V deficiency is treated with infusions of FFP or platelets (which contain factor V in alpha granules); factor VII deficiency is treated with recombinant human activated factor VII at 15–30 mcg/kg every 4–6 hours. In the past, factor X deficiency was treated with FFP, but a new FDA-approved plasma-derived factor X product (Coagadex) is now available.

Deficiency of factor XIII, a transglutamase that cross-links fibrin, characteristically leads to delayed bleeding that occurs hours to days after a hemostatic challenge (such as surgery or trauma). The condition is usually life-long, and spontaneous intracranial hemorrhages as well as recurrent pregnancy loss appear to occur with increased frequency in these patients compared with other congenital deficiencies. Cryoprecipitate or infusion of a plasma-derived factor XIII concentrate (appropriate for patients with A-subunit deficiency only) is the treatment of choice for bleeding or surgical prophylaxis.

Acharya SS. Rare bleeding disorders in children: identification and primary care management. Pediatrics. 2013 Nov;132(5):882–92. [PMID: 24127475]
Peyvandi F et al. Rare bleeding disorders: worldwide efforts for classification, diagnosis, and management. Semin Thromb Hemost. 2013 Sep;39(6):579–84. [PMID: 23888434]

ACQUIRED DISORDERS OF COAGULATION

1. Acquired Antibodies to Factor VIII

Spontaneous antibodies to factor VIII occasionally occur in adults without a prior history of hemophilia; the elderly and patients with lymphoproliferative malignancy or connective tissue disease and those who are postpartum, or postsurgical are at highest risk. The clinical presentation typically includes extensive soft-tissue ecchymoses, hematomas, and mucosal bleeding, as opposed to hemarthrosis in congenital hemophilia A. The aPTT is typically prolonged and does not correct upon mixing; factor VIII activity is found to be low and a Bethesda assay reveals the titer of the inhibitor. Inhibitors of low titer (less than 5 BU) may often be overcome by infusion of high doses of factor VIII concentrates, whereas high-titer inhibitors (greater

than 5 BU) must be treated with serial infusions of activated prothrombin complex concentrates, recombinant human activated factor VII, or recombinant porcine FVIII (hemophilia A patients only). Along with establishment of hemostasis by one of these measures, immunosuppressive treatment with corticosteroids and oral cyclophosphamide should be instituted; treatment with IVIG, rituximab, or plasmapheresis can be considered in refractory cases. Unlike in congenital factor VIII deficiency, the patient's bleeding does not correlate well with the factor VIII activity level, so the clinician must be concerned with any elevation of aPTT secondary to acquired factor VIII inhibitor. All such patients require referral to a hematologist.

Astermark J. FVIII inhibitors: pathogenesis and avoidance. Blood. 2015 Mar 26;125(13):2045–51. [PMID: 25712994]
Tiede A et al. Prognostic factors for remission and survival in acquired hemophilia A (AHA): results from the GTH-AH 01/2010 study. Blood. 2015 Feb 12;125(7):1091–7. [PMID: 25525118]
Zeng Y et al. Interventions for treating acute bleeding episodes in people with acquired hemophilia A. Cochrane Database Syst Rev. 2014 Aug 28;8:CD010761. [PMID: 25165992]

2. Acquired Antibodies to Factor II

Patients with antiphospholipid antibodies occasionally manifest specificity to coagulation factor II (prothrombin), leading typically to a severe hypoprothrombinemia and bleeding. Mixing studies may or may not reveal presence of an inhibitor, as the antibody typically binds a non-enzymatically active portion of the molecule that leads to accelerated clearance, but characteristically the PT is prolonged and levels of factor II are low. FFP should be administered for treatment of bleeding. Treatment is immunosuppressive.

3. Acquired Antibodies to Factor V

Products containing bovine factor V (such as topical thrombin or fibrin glue, frequently used in surgical procedures) can lead to formation of an anti-factor V antibody that cross-reacts with human factor V. Clinicopathologic manifestations range from a prolonged PT in an otherwise asymptomatic individual to severe bleeding. Mixing studies suggest the presence of an inhibitor, and the factor V activity level is low. In cases of serious or life-threatening bleeding, IVIG or platelet transfusions, or both, should be administered, and immunosuppression (as for acquired inhibitors to factor VIII) may be offered.

4. Vitamin K Deficiency

Vitamin K deficiency may occur as a result of deficient dietary intake of vitamin K (from green leafy vegetables, soybeans, and other sources), malabsorption, or decreased production by intestinal bacteria (due to treatment with chemotherapy or antibiotics). Vitamin K is required for normal function of vitamin K epoxide reductase that assists in posttranslational gamma-carboxylation of the coagulation factors II, VII, IX, and X, which is necessary for their activity. Thus, vitamin K deficiency typically features a prolonged PT (in which the activity of the vitamin K–dependent factors is more reflected than in the aPTT) that corrects upon mixing; activity levels of individual clotting factors II, VII, IX, and X typically are low. Importantly, a concomitantly low factor V activity level is not indicative of isolated vitamin K deficiency, and may indicate an underlying defect in liver synthetic function.

For treatment, vitamin K_1 (phytonadione) may be administered via intravenous or oral routes; the subcutaneous route is not recommended due to erratic absorption. The oral dose is 5–10 mg/day and absorption is typically excellent; at least partial improvement in the PT should be observed within 1 day of administration. Intravenous administration (1–5 mg/day) results in even faster normalization of a prolonged PT than oral administration; due to descriptions of anaphylaxis, parenteral doses should be administered at lower doses and slowly (eg, over 30 minutes) with concomitant monitoring.

5. Coagulopathy of Liver Disease

Impaired hepatic function due to cirrhosis or other causes leads to decreased synthesis of clotting factors, including factors II, V, VII, and IX, and fibrinogen, whereas factor VIII levels may be elevated in spite of depressed levels of other coagulation factors. The PT (and with advanced disease, the aPTT) is typically prolonged and usually corrects on mixing with normal plasma. A normal factor V level, in spite of decreases in the activity of factors II, VII, IX, and X, however, suggests vitamin K deficiency rather than liver disease. Qualitative and quantitative deficiencies of fibrinogen also are prevalent among patients with advanced liver disease, typically leading to a prolonged PT, thrombin time, and reptilase time.

The coagulopathy of liver disease usually does not require hemostatic treatment until bleeding complications occur. Infusion of FFP may be considered if active bleeding is present and the aPTT and PT are markedly prolonged; however, the effect is transient and concern for volume overload may limit infusions. Patients with bleeding and a fibrinogen level consistently below 80–100 mg/dL should receive cryoprecipitate. Liver transplantation, if feasible, results in production of coagulation factors at normal levels. The use of recombinant human activated factor VII in patients with bleeding varices is controversial, although some patient subgroups may experience benefit.

Bianchini M et al. Coagulopathy in liver diseases: complication or therapy? Dig Dis. 2014;32(5):609–14. [PMID: 25034295]

Franchini M et al. Acquired factor V inhibitors: a systematic review. J Thromb Thrombolysis. 2011 May;31(4):449–57. [PMID: 21052780]

Saja MF et al. The coagulopathy of liver disease: does vitamin K help? Blood Coagul Fibrinolysis. 2013 Jan;24(1):10–7. [PMID: 23080365]

Tripodi A et al. The coagulopathy of chronic liver disease. N Engl J Med. 2011 Jul 14;365(2):147–56. [PMID: 21751907]

6. Warfarin Ingestion

See **Antithrombotic Therapy** section, below.

7. Disseminated Intravascular Coagulation

The consumptive coagulopathy of DIC is typically initiated by excessive tissue factor exposure or release and results in decreases in the activity of clotting factors. The result can be bleeding or thrombosis in any given patient. The aPTT and PT are characteristically prolonged, and platelets and fibrinogen levels are reduced from baseline.

8. Heparin/Fondaparinux/Direct-Acting Oral Anticoagulant Use

The thrombin time is dramatically prolonged in the presence of heparin. Patients who are receiving heparin and who have bleeding should be managed by discontinuation of the heparin and, in some cases, administration of protamine sulfate; 1 mg of protamine neutralizes approximately 100 units of heparin sulfate, and the maximum dose is 50 mg intravenously. LMWHs typically do not prolong clotting times and are incompletely reversible with protamine. There is no reversal agent for fondaparinux, although some experts have suggested using recombinant human activated factor VIIa for cases of life-threatening bleeding. The direct-acting oral anticoagulants (DOACs) include DTIs (eg, dabigatran) and factor Xa inhibitors (eg, rivaroxaban, apixaban, and edoxaban). Dabigatran has a reversal agent, a monoclonal antibody called idarucizumab. Reversal agents for the factor Xa inhibitors are still in development or awaiting FDA approval (eg, andexanet alfa, a recombinant modified human factor Xa decoy protein).

Das A et al. Novel antidotes for target specific oral anticoagulants. Exp Hematol Oncol. 2015 Sep 15;4:25. [PMID: 26380149]

Pollack CV Jr et al. Idarucizumab for dabigatran reversal. N Engl J Med. 2015 Aug 6;373(6):511–20. [PMID: 26095746]

Siegal DM et al. Acute management of bleeding in patients on novel oral anticoagulants. Eur Heart J. 2013 Feb;34(7): 489–498b. [PMID: 23220847]

Siegal DM et al. Andexanet alfa for the reversal of factor Xa inhibitor activity. N Engl J Med. 2015 Dec 17;373(25):2413–24. [PMID: 26559317]

9. Lupus Anticoagulants

Lupus anticoagulants prolong clotting times (aPTT) by binding proteins associated with phospholipid, which is a necessary component of coagulation reactions, but they do not lead to bleeding. In fact, they predispose to thrombosis. Lupus anticoagulants were so named because of their early identification in patients with connective tissue disease, although they also occur with increased frequency in individuals with underlying infection, inflammation, or malignancy, and they also can occur in asymptomatic individuals in the general population. A prolongation in the aPTT is observed that does not correct completely on mixing but that normalizes with excessive phospholipid. Specialized testing such as the hexagonal phase phospholipid neutralization assay, the dilute Russell viper venom time, and platelet neutralization assays can confirm the presence of a lupus anticoagulant.

Adams M. Measurement of lupus anticoagulants: an update on quality in laboratory testing. Semin Thromb Hemost. 2013 Apr;39(3):267–71. [PMID: 23424052]

OTHER CAUSES OF BLEEDING

Occasionally, abnormalities of the vasculature and integument may lead to bleeding despite normal hemostasis; congenital or acquired disorders may be causative. These abnormalities include Ehlers-Danlos syndrome, osteogenesis imperfecta, Osler-Weber-Rendu disease, and Marfan syndrome (heritable defects) and integumentary thinning due to prolonged corticosteroid administration or normal aging, amyloidosis, vasculitis, and scurvy (acquired defects). The bleeding time often is prolonged. If possible, treatment of the underlying condition should be pursued, but if this is not possible or feasible (ie, congenital syndromes), globally hemostatic agents such as DDAVP can be considered for treatment of bleeding. Topical bevacizumab has been effective in some patients with refractory nosebleeds.

Gaillard S et al; ATERO Study Group. Tranexamic acid for epistaxis in hereditary hemorrhagic telangiectasia patients: a European cross-over controlled trial in a rare disease. J Thromb Haemost. 2014 Sep;12(9):1494–502. [PMID: 25040799]
Kanellopoulou T et al. Bevacizumab in the treatment of hereditary hemorrhagic telangiectasia. Expert Opin Biol Ther. 2013 Sep;13(9):1315–23. [PMID: 23815519]
McDonald J et al. Hereditary hemorrhagic telangiectasia: an overview of diagnosis, management, and pathogenesis. Genet Med. 2011 Jul;13(7):607–16. [PMID: 21546842]

ANTITHROMBOTIC THERAPY

The currently available anticoagulants include unfractionated heparin, LMWHs, fondaparinux, vitamin K antagonist (ie, warfarin), and DOACs (ie, dabigatran, rivaroxaban, apixaban, edoxaban). (For a discussion of the injectable DTIs, see section on **Heparin-Induced Thrombocytopenia**.)

▶ Classes of Anticoagulants

A. Unfractionated Heparin and LMWHs

Unfractionated heparin is a repeating polymer of sulfated glycosaminoglycans that is most commonly derived from porcine intestinal tissue, which is rich in heparin-bearing mast cells. A biologic product, it is extremely heterogeneous with respect to sulfation and polymer length; individual molecules may range from 3000 to 30,000.

In addition, only about one-third of the molecules in a given preparation of unfractionated heparin contain the crucial pentasaccharide sequence that is necessary for binding of antithrombin and, through conversion of thrombin from a slow inhibitor of coagulation factor activity to a rapid inhibitor, exertion of its anticoagulant effect. Heparin is highly negatively charged, and upon intravenous infusion, it binds to a large array of blood components, such as endothelial cells, platelets, mast cells, and plasma proteins. The pharmacokinetics of unfractionated heparin are poorly predictable, and the degree of anticoagulation is typically monitored (by aPTT or anti-Xa level) in patients who are receiving the drug in therapeutic doses. Only a fraction of an infused dose of heparin is metabolized by the kidneys, however, making it safe to use in most patients with significant kidney disease.

The LMWHs are produced from chemical depolymerization of unfractionated heparin, resulting in products of lower molecular weight (mean molecular weight, 4500–6500D, depending on the LMWH). Due to less protein and cellular binding, the pharmacokinetics of the LMWHs are much more predictable than those of unfractionated heparin, allowing for fixed weight-based dosing. All LMWHs are principally renally cleared and must be avoided or used with extreme caution in individuals with creatinine clearance less than 30 mL/min. A longer half-life permits once- or twice-daily subcutaneous dosing, allowing for greater convenience and outpatient therapy in selected cases. Most patients do not require monitoring, although monitoring using the anti-Xa activity level is appropriate for patients with moderate kidney disease, those with elevated body mass index or low weight, and selected pregnant patients. About 30% of the molecules in a dose of LMWH are long enough (ie, sufficiently negatively charged) to bind protamine sulfate, allowing for some neutralization of anticoagulant effect. LMWHs are associated with a lower frequency of HIT (approximately 0.6%) than unfractionated heparin.

B. Fondaparinux

Fondaparinux, which is chemically related to LMWHs, is a synthetic molecule consisting of the highly active pentasaccharide sequence. As such, it exerts almost no thrombin inhibition and works to indirectly inhibit factor Xa through binding to antithrombin. Fondaparinux, like the LMWHs, is almost exclusively metabolized by the kidneys, and should be avoided in patients with creatinine clearance less than 30 mL/min. Predictable pharmacokinetics allow for weight-based dosing. A particularly long half-life (17–21 hours) allows for once-daily subcutaneous dosing, but the absence of necessary charge characteristics leads to a lack of binding to protamine sulfate; therefore, unlike heparin, no effective neutralizing agent exists.

C. Vitamin K Antagonist (Warfarin)

The vitamin K antagonist **warfarin** inhibits the activity of the vitamin K–dependent carboxylase that is important for the posttranslational modification of coagulation factors II, VII, IX, and X. Although warfarin may be taken orally, leading to a significant advantage over the heparins and heparin derivatives, which must be given parenterally or subcutaneously, inter-individual differences in response to the agent related to nutritional status, comorbid diseases, concomitant medications, and genetic polymorphisms lead to a poorly predictable anticoagulant response. Individuals taking warfarin must undergo periodic monitoring to verify the intensity of the anticoagulant effect. The intensity of anticoagulant effect is reported as the INR, which corrects for differences in potency of commercially available thromboplastin used to perform the PT.[1]

D. Direct-Acting Oral Anticoagulants (Table 14–11)

Dabigatran etexilate is an oral DOAC that is approved for use in the United States for the following indications: (1) preventing stroke and systemic embolism in nonvalvular atrial fibrillation, (2) treating DVT and pulmonary embolism (PE) in patients who have been received a parenteral anticoagulant for 5–10 days, and (3) reducing the risk of recurrence of DVT and PE in patients who have been previously treated. It prevents thrombus formation by inhibiting both clotbound and free thrombin and thrombin-induced platelet aggregation. It is a prodrug that is converted to dabigatran with peak effect within 2 hours. Steady state is reached within 3 days. As renal excretion accounts for about 80% of clearance, dose adjustment is required for creatinine clearance 15–30 mL/min; this agent cannot be recommended for patients with creatinine clearances less than 15–30 mL/min depending on indication (Table 14–11). As a substrate of the p-glycoprotein (P-gp) transport system, concomitant use of strong inducers, eg, rifampin, should be avoided and caution is advised with concomitant use of strong P-gp inhibitors (eg, ketoconazole and dronedarone) in patients with normal kidney function while drug dose reduction or avoidance is recommended for concomitant use in those with creatinine clearances less than 30–50 mL/min or less depending on indication (Table 14–11). The half-life of the dabigatran etexilate is 12–17 hours. Non–life-threatening bleeding may be treated by holding dabigatran, maintaining diuresis, providing supportive measures, and administering charcoal (if a dose was recently ingested). Idarucizumab is an antibody fragment that binds to dabigatran to neutralize its activity, reversing the anticoagulant effect in minutes. Its intended use is to reverse the anticoagulant effect in patients taking dabigatran when emergency surgery or urgent procedures are needed or when life-threatening or uncontrolled bleeding is present.

Rivaroxaban is an oral direct factor Xa inhibitor that is approved in the United States for the following indications: (1) preventing venous thrombosis following hip or knee replacement, (2) preventing nonvalvular atrial fibrillation–associated stroke, (3) treating acute venous thrombosis, and (4) reducing the risk of recurrence of VTE. Its half-life ranges from 5 hours to 13 hours (longer in the elderly). As renal excretion accounts for about 35% of clearance, dose adjustment is required for creatinine clearances 30–50 mL/min

in patients with atrial fibrillation. This agent cannot be recommended for patients with creatinine clearances less than 15–30 mL/min (Table 14–11). Concomitant use of agents that are strong inducers or inhibitors of P-gp should be avoided and caution is recommended with the concomitant administration of combined P-gp inhibitors and/or weak or moderate inhibitors of CYP3A4 (eg, amiodarone, azithromycin, diltiazem, dronedarone, erythromycin, felodipine, quinidine, ranolazine, verapamil) particularly in patients with impaired renal function. As it has no antidote, rivaroxaban-associated bleeding may be treated by withholding the drug while the anticoagulant effect dissipates and by administration of activated charcoal (if a dose was recently ingested). For patients with life-threatening bleeding, use of prothrombin complex concentrate, 4-component prothrombin complex concentrate, rFVIIa may be considered. Protamine and vitamin K are not expected to affect the anticoagulant activity of the DOACs.

Apixaban is an oral direct factor Xa inhibitor approved in the United States for the following indications: (1) preventing stroke in nonvalvular atrial fibrillation, (2) prophylaxis of DVT following hip and knee surgery, (3) treating acute VTE, and (4) preventing recurrent VTE. It has a half-life of about 12 hours in patients with normal kidney function. Simultaneous use of strong inducers of CYP3A4 and P-gp reduces blood levels of apixaban, and concomitant use should be avoided. Strong dual inhibitors of CYP3A4 and P-gp increase blood levels of apixaban, and concomitant use should be avoided but if necessary dose reduction is recommended. While all four of the currently approved DOACs are renally cleared, apixaban, relies least on the kidneys; only 25% is renally excreted. However, dose reduction is still recommended in patients with two of three of the following: older than 80 years and less than 60 kg or serum creatinine greater than 1.5 mg/dL. This agent cannot be recommended for patients with creatinine clearances less than 15 mL/min (Table 14–11.) The approach to life-threatening bleeding is the same as outlined for rivaroxaban.

Edoxaban is an oral direct factor Xa inhibitor approved in the United States for the following indications: (1) reducing the risk of stroke and systemic embolism in patients with nonvalvular atrial fibrillation, and (2) treating DVT and PE after 5–10 days of initial therapy with a parenteral anticoagulant. Its onset of action is 1–2 hours and half-life is 10–14 hours. Edoxaban should not be used in patients with creatinine clearance greater than 95 mL/min as therapy for nonvalvular atrial fibrillation because of an increased risk of ischemic stroke compared to warfarin. As renal excretion accounts for about 50% of clearance, dose adjustment is required for patients with creatinine clearances less than 15–50 mL/min, and it cannot be recommended in those with creatinine clearances less than 15 mL/min (Table 14–11). Dose reduction is also recommended if the patient's weight is less than 60 kg and if used concomitantly with certain p-Gp inhibitors. The approach to life-threatening bleeding is the same as rivaroxaban.

Routine monitoring is not recommended for patients taking DOACs. However, there are clinical scenarios where assessing anticoagulant activity would be helpful, including active bleeding, pending urgent surgery, suspected

---

[1] Importantly, because the INR is not standardized for abnormalities of factor V and fibrinogen, the INR should be used only in reference to anticoagulation in patients who are receiving warfarin.

Table 14–11. Direct-acting oral anticoagulants (DOACs).[1]

	Dabigatran	Rivaroxaban	Apixaban	Edoxaban
Mechanism	Oral direct thrombin inhibitor	Oral direct factor Xa inhibitor	Oral direct factor Xa inhibitor	Oral direct factor Xa inhibitor
Approved uses	Atrial fibrillation VTE treatment and secondary prevention VTE replacement prophylaxis following hip replacement	Atrial fibrillation VTE treatment and secondary prevention VTE prophylaxis post-hip or knee replacement	Atrial fibrillation VTE treatment and secondary prevention VTE prophylaxis post-hip or knee replacement	Atrial fibrillation VTE treatment and secondary prevention
Frequency of dosing	Twice daily for most indications Once daily following hip replacement	Daily for atrial fibrillation Twice daily for first 21 days of acute VTE, then daily	Twice daily	Once daily
Dosing	**Atrial Fibrillation** CrCl > 30 mL/min: 150 mg orally twice daily CrCl 15–30 mL/min: 75 mg orally twice daily CrCl ≤ 15 mL/min or on dialysis: dosing recommendations cannot be provided CrCl 30–50 mL/min and coadministered with dronedarone or ketoconazole: 75 mg orally twice daily. Avoid if CrCl < 30 mL/min with concomitant use of P-gp inhibitors **VTE Treatment** Following 5 to 10 days of initial therapy with a parenteral anticoagulant: CrCl > 30 mL/min: 150 mg orally twice daily CrCl ≤ 30 mL/min or on dialysis: dosing recommendations cannot be provided based on studies Avoid if CrCl < 50 mL/min with concomitant use of P-gp inhibitors **VTE Prevention Following Hip Replacement** CrCl > 30 mL/min: 110 mg 1–4 h post-surgery, then 220 mg daily for 28–35 days CrCl ≤ 30 mL/min or on dialysis: dosing recommendations cannot be provided based on studies	**Atrial Fibrillation** CrCl > 50 mL/min: 20 mg orally once a day CrCl 30–50 mL/min: 15 mg orally once a day CrCl ≤ 15mL/min or on dialysis: dosing recommendations cannot be provided based on studies **VTE Treatment and Secondary Prevention** CrCl ≥ 30 mL/min: 15 mg orally twice daily for 21 days, then 20 mg daily CrCl ≤ 30 mL/min or on dialysis **VTE Prevention Following Hip or Knee Replacement** 10 mg orally once daily with or without food for 35 days (hip) or 12 days (knee), starting 6–10 hours postoperatively, after hemostasis achieved CrCl 30–50 mL/min: observe carefully and evaluate for symptoms or signs of bleeding CrCl ≤ 30 mL/min or on dialysis: avoid use	**Atrial Fibrillation** 5 mg orally twice daily 2.5 mg orally twice daily if two or more of the following: ≥ 80 years old, ≤ 60 kg, SCr ≥ 1.5 mg/dL 2.5 mg orally twice daily if coadministered with strong 3A4/P-gp dual inhibitors **VTE Treatment and Secondary Prevention** 10 mg taken orally twice daily for the first 7 days. After 7 days, then reduce dose to 5 mg taken orally twice daily. CrCl < 15 mL/min not on dialysis: no dosing change recommended by manufacturer but recommendation is not based on studies **VTE Prevention Following Hip or Knee Replacement** 2.5 mg taken orally twice daily for 35 days post-hip replacement and for 12 days post-knee replacement. The initial dose should be taken 12 to 24 hours after surgery. CrCl < 15 mL/min not on dialysis: no dosing change recommended by manufacturer but recommendation is not based on studies	**Atrial Fibrillation** 60 mg orally once daily Assess CrCl before initiating therapy Do not use in patients with CrCl > 95 mL/min Reduce dose to 30 mg once daily if CrCl 15–50 mL/min **VTE Treatment** 60 mg orally once daily following 5–10 days of initial therapy with a parenteral anticoagulant, reduce dose to 30 mg once daily in patients with CrCl 15–50 mL/min weight ≤ 60 kg, or if taking certain concomitant P-gp inhibitor medications CrCl < 15 mL/min or on dialysis: dosing recommendations cannot be provided based on studies
Food	With or without food	With food (for 15 and 20 mg tablets)	With or without food	With or without food
Crushable?	No	Can crush; do not administer via J tube	Can crush and administer orally or via NG tube	No data
Renal clearance	80%	30–60%	25%	50%
Kinetics	t ½ = 12–17 hours; tmax = 2 hours	t ½ = 5–9 hours; tmax = 3 hours	t ½ = 12 hours; tmax = 3 hours	t ½ = 10–14 hours; tmax = 2 hours

(continued)

Table 14–11. Direct-acting oral anticoagulants (DOACs).[1] (continued)

	Dabigatran	Rivaroxaban	Apixaban	Edoxaban
Influences INR?	↑ (or →)	↑↑ (or → at low concentrations)	↑ (or →)	↑
Influences aPTT?	↑↑	↑	↑	↑
Drug interactions (list not comprehensive)	**Avoid** rifampin, St John's wort, and possibly carbamazepine **Caution** with amiodarone, clarithromycin, dronedarone, ketoconazole, quinidine, verapamil. No dosage adjustment of dabigatran is recommended if CrCl > 50 mL/min **Reduce dose** to 75 mg orally twice daily if CrCl 30–50 mL/min and coadministered with dronedarone or ketoconazole	**Avoid** carbamazepine, conivaptan, indinavir/ritonavir, itraconazole, ketoconazole, lopinavir/ritonavir, phenytoin, rifampin, ritonavir, St John's wort **Caution** with the concomitant administration of combined P-gp inhibitors and/or weak or moderate inhibitors of CYP3A4 (eg, amiodarone, azithromycin, diltiazem, dronedarone, erythromycin, felodipine, quinidine, ranolazine, verapamil) with rivaroxaban, particularly in patients with impaired renal function	**Avoid** carbamazepine, phenytoin, rifampin, St John's wort **Avoid** clarithromycin, itraconazole, ketoconazole, and ritonavir in patients already taking apixaban at a reduced dose of 2.5 mg twice daily **Caution** with clarithromycin, itraconazole, ketoconazole, and ritonavir	**Avoid** rifampin Reduce dose with certain P-gp inhibitors. Use has not been studied with many other P-gp inhibitors and inducers Some recommend avoiding concomitant use altogether
Switching from DOAC to warfarin	Consider discontinuing dabigatran and bridging with parenteral anticoagulant (Initiate parenteral anticoagulant 12 h [CrCl ≥ 30 mL/min] or 24 h [CrCl < 30 mL/min] after the last dose of dabigatran)	Consider discontinuing rivaroxaban and bridging with parenteral anticoagulant (Initiate parenteral anticoagulant at the time the next dose of rivaroxaban would have been taken)	Consider discontinuing apixaban and bridging with parenteral anticoagulant (Initiate parenteral anticoagulant at the time the next dose of apixaban would have been taken)	Consider discontinuing edoxaban and bridging with parenteral anticoagulant (Initiate parenteral anticoagulant at the time the next dose of edoxaban would have been taken) Alternatively, could cut dose of edoxaban in half and start warfarin. Measure INR frequently and just prior to edoxaban dose and stop edoxaban when INR reaches 2.0
Warfarin to DOAC	INR < 2.0	INR < 3.0	INR < 2.0	INR < 2.5
Special considerations	Dyspepsia is common and starts within first 10 days GI bleeding risk higher with dabigatran vs warfarin	GI bleeding risk higher with rivaroxaban vs warfarin		Do not use if CrCl ≥ 95 mL/min
Management of life-threatening bleeding	Idarucizumab 2 doses of 2.5 g intravenously no more than 15 min apart	Activated charcoal, supportive care, consider 4-component PCC	Activated charcoal, supportive care, consider 4-component PCC	Activated charcoal, supportive care, consider 4-component PCC

[1]Previously called new (novel) oral anticoagulants and target-specific oral anticoagulants.

[2]If surgery has a high risk of bleeding, hold dose for max number of days.

aPTT, activated partial thromboplastin time; CrCl, creatinine clearance; GI, gastrointestinal; INR, international normalized ratio; NG, nasogastric; PCC, prothrombin complex concentrate; P-gp, p-glycoprotein; SCr, serum creatinine; VTE, venous thromboembolism.

therapeutic failure, or concern for accumulation. There is no standardized laboratory assay to measure anticoagulant effect of the DOACs. They have varying effects on the PT and aPTT. A normal thrombin time excludes the presence of clinically relevant dabigatran levels; a normal aPTT likely excludes excess drug levels of dabigatran. A negative anti-Xa level likely excludes clinically relevant levels of rivaroxaban, apixaban, or edoxaban; a normal PT likely excludes excess drug levels of rivaroxaban but not apixaban or edoxaban. The INR is completely unreliable for the evaluation of factor Xa activity.

Ageno W et al. Oral anticoagulant therapy: Antithrombotic Therapy and Prevention of Thrombosis, 9th ed: American College of Chest Physicians Evidence-Based Clinical Practice Guidelines. Chest. 2012 Feb;141(2 Suppl):e44S–88S. [PMID: 22315269]

Cuker A et al. Laboratory measurement of the anticoagulant activity of the non-vitamin K oral anticoagulants. J Am Coll Cardiol. 2014 Sep 16;64(11):1128–39. [PMID: 25212648]

Dale BJ et al. Laboratory measurement of the direct oral anticoagulants. Br J Haematol. 2016 Feb;172(3):315–36. [PMID: 26492202]

Garcia DA et al. Parenteral anticoagulants: Antithrombotic Therapy and Prevention of Thrombosis, 9th ed: American College of Chest Physicians Evidence-Based Clinical Practice Guidelines. Chest. 2012 Feb;141(2 Suppl):e24S–43S. Erratum in: Chest. 2012 May;141(5):1369. Dosage error in article text. [PMID: 22315264]

Heidbuchel H et al. Updated European Heart Rhythm Association Practical Guide on the use of non-vitamin K antagonist anticoagulants in patients with non-valvular atrial fibrillation. Europace. 2015 Oct;17(10):1467–507. [PMID: 26324838]

The Hokusai-VTE Investigators. Edoxaban versus warfarin for the treatment of symptomatic venous thromboembolism. N Engl J Med. 2013 Oct 10;369(15):1406–15. [PMID: 23991658]

Holbrook A et al. Evidence-based management of anticoagulant therapy: Antithrombotic Therapy and Prevention of Thrombosis, 9th ed: American College of Chest Physicians Evidence-Based Clinical Practice Guidelines. Chest. 2012 Feb;141(2 Suppl):e152S–84S. [PMID: 22315259]Pollack CV Jr et al. Idarucizumab for dabigatran reversal. N Engl J Med. 2015 Aug 6;373(6):511–20. [PMID: 26095746]

Robertson L et al. Oral direct thrombin inhibitors or oral factor Xa inhibitors for the treatment of deep vein thrombosis. Cochrane Database Syst Rev. 2015 Jun 30;6:CD010956. [PMID: 26123214]

Robertson L et al. Oral direct thrombin inhibitors or oral factor Xa inhibitors for the treatment of pulmonary embolism. Cochrane Database Syst Rev. 2015 Dec 4;12:CD010957. [PMID: 26636644]

Siegal DM et al. Andexanet alfa for the reversal of factor Xa inhibitor activity. N Engl J Med. 2015 Dec 17;373(25):2413–24. [PMID: 26559317]

Sugerman DT. JAMA patient page. Blood thinners. JAMA. 2013 Dec 18;310(23):2579. [PMID: 24347004]

▶ Prevention of Venous Thromboembolic Disease

The frequency of venous thromboembolic disease (VTE) among hospitalized patients ranges widely; up to 20% of medical patients and 80% of critical care patients and high-risk surgical patients have been reported to experience this complication, which includes DVT and PE.

Avoidance of fatal PE, which occurs in up to 5% of high-risk inpatients as a consequence of hospitalization or

Table 14–12. Risk stratification for DVT/VTE among surgical inpatients.

High risk
- Recent major orthopedic surgery/arthroplasty/fracture
- Abdominal/pelvic cancer undergoing surgery
- Recent spinal cord injury or major trauma within 90 days
- More than three of the intermediate risk factors (see below)

Intermediate risk
- Not ambulating independently outside of room at least twice daily
- Active infectious or inflammatory process
- Active malignancy
- Major surgery (nonorthopedic)
- History of VTE
- Stroke
- Central venous access or PICC line
- Inflammatory bowel disease
- Prior immobilization (> 72 hours) preoperatively
- Obesity (BMI > 30)
- Patient age > 50 years
- Hormone replacement or oral contraceptive therapy
- Hypercoagulable state
- Nephrotic syndrome
- Burns
- Cellulitis
- Varicose veins
- Paresis
- HF (systolic dysfunction)
- COPD exacerbation

Low risk
- Minor procedure and age < 40 years with no additional risk factors
- Ambulatory with expected length of stay of < 24 hours or minor surgery

surgery is a major goal of pharmacologic prophylaxis. Tables 14–12 and 14–13 provide risk stratification for DVT/VTE among hospitalized surgical and medical inpatients. Standard prophylactic regimens are listed in Table 14–14. Prophylactic strategies should be guided by individual risk stratification, with all moderate- and high-risk patients receiving pharmacologic prophylaxis, unless

Table 14–13. Padua Risk Assessment Model for VTE prophylaxis in hospitalized medical patients.

Condition	Points[1]
Active cancer, history of VTE, immobility, laboratory thrombophilia	3 points each
Recent (≤ 1 mo) trauma and/or surgery	2 points each
Age ≥ 70, acute MI or CVA, acute infection, rheumatologic disorder, BMI ≥ 30, hormonal therapy	1 point each

[1]A score ≥ 4 connotes high risk of VTE in the noncritically ill medical patients and pharmacologic prophylaxis is indicated, absent absolute contraindications.
BMI, body mass index; CVA, cerebrovascular accident; MI, myocardial infarction; VTE, venous thromboembolism.

Table 14–14. Pharmacologic prophylaxis of VTE in selected clinical scenarios.[1]

Anticoagulant	Dose	Frequency	Clinical Scenario	Comment
Enoxaparin	40 mg subcutaneously	Once daily	Most medical inpatients and critical care patients	—
			Surgical patients (moderate risk for VTE)	
			Abdominal/pelvic cancer surgery	Consider continuing for 4 weeks, total duration for abdomino-pelvic cancer surgery
		Twice daily	Bariatric surgery	Higher doses may be required
	30 mg subcutaneously	Twice daily	Orthopedic surgery[2]	Give for at least 10 days. For THR, TKA, or HFS, consider continuing up to 1 month after surgery in high-risk patients
			Major trauma	Not applicable to patients with isolated lower extremity trauma
			Acute spinal cord injury	—
Dalteparin	2500 units subcutaneously	Once daily	Most medical inpatients	—
			Abdominal surgery (moderate risk for VTE)	Give for 5–10 days
	5000 units subcutaneously	Once daily	Orthopedic surgery[2]	First dose = 2500 units. Give for at least 10 days. For THR, TKA, or HFS, consider continuing up to 1 month after surgery in high-risk patients
			Abdominal surgery (higher-risk for VTE)	Give for 5–10 days
			Medical inpatients	—
Fondaparinux	2.5 mg subcutaneously	Once daily	Orthopedic surgery[2]	Give for at least 10 days. For THR, TKA, or HFS, consider continuing up to 1 month after surgery in high-risk patients
Rivaroxaban	10 mg orally	Once daily	Orthopedic surgery: total hip and total knee replacement	Give for 12 days following total knee replacement; give for 35 days following total hip replacement
Apixaban	2.5 mg orally	Twice daily	Following hip or knee replacement surgery	Give for 12 days following total knee replacement; give for 35 days following total hip replacement
Edoxaban	60 mg orally	Once daily	For nonvalvular atrial fibrillation	—
Unfractionated heparin	5000 units subcutaneously	Three times daily	Higher VTE risk with low bleeding risk	Includes gynecologic surgery for malignancy and urologic surgery, medical patients with multiple risk factors for VTE
	5000 units subcutaneously	Twice daily	Hospitalized patients at intermediate risk for VTE	Includes gynecologic surgery (moderate risk)
			Patients with epidural catheters	LMWHs usually avoided due to risk of spinal hematoma
			Patients with severe kidney disease[3]	LMWHs contraindicated
Warfarin	(variable) oral	Once daily	Orthopedic surgery[2]	Titrate to goal INR = 2.5. Give for at least 10 days. For high-risk patients undergoing THR, TKA, or HFS, consider continuing up to 1 month after surgery

[1]All regimens administered subcutaneously, except for warfarin.
[2]Includes TKA, THR, and HFS.
[3]Defined as creatinine clearance < 30 mL/min.
HFS, hip fracture surgery; LMWH, low-molecular-weight heparin; THR, total hip replacement; TKA, total knee arthroplasty; VTE, venous thromboembolic disease.

Table 14–15. Contraindications to VTE prophylaxis for medical or surgical hospital inpatients at high risk for VTE.

Absolute contraindications
  Acute hemorrhage from wounds or drains or lesions
  Intracranial hemorrhage within prior 24 hours
  Heparin-induced thrombocytopenia (HIT): consider using fondaparinux
  Severe trauma to head or spinal cord or extremities
  Epidural anesthesia/spinal block within 12 hours of initiation of anticoagulation (concurrent use of an epidural catheter and anticoagulation other than low prophylactic doses of unfractionated heparin should require review and approval by service who performed the epidural or spinal procedure, eg, anesthesia/pain service and in many cases should be avoided entirely)
  Currently receiving warfarin or heparin or LMWH or direct thrombin inhibitor for other indications
Relative contraindications
  Coagulopathy (INR > 1.5)
  Intracranial lesion or neoplasm
  Severe thrombocytopenia (platelet count < 50,000/mcL)
  Intracranial hemorrhage within past 6 months
  Gastrointestinal or genitourinary hemorrhage within past 6 months

INR, international normalized ratio; LMWH, low-molecular-weight heparin; VTE, venous thromboembolic disease.
Adapted from Guidelines used at the VA Medical Center, San Francisco, CA.

contraindicated. Contraindications to VTE prophylaxis for hospital inpatients at high risk for VTE are listed in Table 14–15.

It is recommended that VTE prophylaxis be used judiciously in hospitalized medical patients who are not critically ill since a comprehensive review of evidence suggested harm from bleeding in low-risk patients given low-dose heparin and skin necrosis in stroke patients given compression stockings. The Padua Risk Score provides clinicians with a simple approach to risk stratification in medical patients (Table 14–13). Certain high-risk surgical patients should be considered for extended-duration prophylaxis of approximately 1 month, including those undergoing total hip replacement, hip fracture repair, and abdominal and pelvic cancer surgery. If bleeding is present, if the risk of bleeding is high, or if the risk of VTE is high for the inpatient (Table 14–12) and therefore combined prophylactic strategies are needed, some measure of thromboprophylaxis may be provided through use of mechanical devices, including intermittent pneumatic compression devices, venous foot pumps, or graduated compression stockings.

Buesing KL et al. Deep venous thrombosis and venous thromboembolism prophylaxis. Surg Clin North Am. 2015 Apr;95(2):285–300. [PMID: 25814107]
Di Nisio M et al. Primary prophylaxis for venous thromboembolism in ambulatory cancer patients receiving chemotherapy. Cochrane Database Syst Rev. 2014 Aug 29;8:CD008500. [PMID: 25171736]

Falck-Ytter Y et al. Prevention of VTE in orthopedic surgery patients: Antithrombotic Therapy and Prevention of Thrombosis, 9th ed: American College of Chest Physicians Evidence-Based Clinical Practice Guidelines. Chest. 2012 Feb;141(2 Suppl):e278S–325S. [PMID: 22315265]
Gould MK et al. Prevention of VTE in nonorthopedic surgical patients: Antithrombotic Therapy and Prevention of Thrombosis, 9th ed: American College of Chest Physicians Evidence-Based Clinical Practice Guidelines. Chest. 2012 Feb;141(2 Suppl):e227S–77S. Erratum in: Chest. 2012 May;141(5):1369. [PMID: 22315263]
Kahn SR et al. Prevention of VTE in nonsurgical patients: Antithrombotic Therapy and Prevention of Thrombosis, 9th ed: American College of Chest Physicians Evidence-Based Clinical Practice Guidelines. Chest. 2012 Feb;141(2 Suppl):e195S–226S. [PMID: 2231526]
Mandernach MW et al. Apixaban for the prophylaxis and treatment of deep vein thrombosis and pulmonary embolism: an evidence-based review. Ther Clin Risk Manag. 2015 Aug 26;11:1273–82. [PMID: 26345156]
Sachdeva A et al. Graduated compression stockings for prevention of deep vein thrombosis. Cochrane Database Syst Rev. 2014 Dec 17;12:CD001484. [PMID: 25517473]
Zalpour A et al. Update on edoxaban for the prevention and treatment of thromboembolism: clinical applications based on current evidence. Adv Hematol. 2015;2015:920361. [PMID: 26351456]

► Treatment of Venous Thromboembolic Disease

A. Anticoagulant Therapy

Treatment for VTE should be offered to patients with objectively confirmed DVT or PE, or to those in whom the clinical suspicion is high for the disorder but who have not yet undergone diagnostic testing (see Chapter 9). The management of VTE primarily involves administration of anticoagulants; the goal is to prevent recurrence, extension and embolization of thrombosis and to reduce the risk of postthrombotic syndrome. Suggested anticoagulation regimens are found in Table 14–16.

B. Selecting Appropriate Anticoagulant Therapy

Most patients with DVT alone may be treated as outpatients, provided that their risk of bleeding is low, and they have good follow-up. Table 14–17 outlines proposed selection criteria for outpatient treatment of DVT.

Among patients with PE, risk stratification should be done at time of diagnosis to direct treatment and triage. Patients with persistent hemodynamic instability are classified as high-risk patients (previously referred to as having "massive PE") and have an early PE-related mortality of more than 15%. These patients should be admitted to an intensive care unit and generally receive thrombolysis in addition to anticoagulation. Intermediate-risk patients (previously, "submassive PE") have a mortality rate of up to 15% and should be admitted to a higher level of inpatient care, with consideration of thrombolysis on a case-by-case basis. Low-risk patients have a mortality rate less than 3% and are candidates for expedited discharge or outpatient therapy.

Because both intermediate- and low-risk patients are hemodynamically stable, additional assessment is

Table 14–16. Initial anticoagulation for VTE.[1]

Anticoagulant	Dose/Frequency	DVT, Lower Extremity	DVT, Upper Extremity	PE	VTE, with Concomitant Severe Renal Impairment[2]	VTE, Cancer-Related	Comment
					Clinical Scenario		
Unfractionated Heparin							
Unfractionated heparin	80 units/kg intravenous bolus, then continuous intravenous infusion of 18 units/kg/h	×	×	×	×		Bolus may be omitted if risk of bleeding is perceived to be elevated. Maximum bolus, 10,000 units. Requires aPTT monitoring. Most patients: begin warfarin at time of initiation of heparin.
	330 units/kg subcutaneously × 1, then 250 units/kg subcutaneously every 12 hours	×					Fixed-dose; no aPTT monitoring required
LMWH and Fondaparinux							
Enoxaparin[3]	1 mg/kg subcutaneously every 12 hours	×	×	×			Most patients: begin warfarin at time of initiation of LMWH
Dalteparin[3]	200 units/kg subcutaneously once daily for first month, then 150 units/kg/day	×	×	×		×	Cancer: administer LMWH for ≥ 3–6 months; reduce dose to 150 units/kg after first month of treatment
Fondaparinux	5–10 mg subcutaneously once daily (see Comment)	×	×	×			Use 7.5 mg for body weight 50–100 kg; 10 mg for body weight > 100 kg
Direct-Acting Oral Anticoagulants (DOACs)							
Rivaroxaban	15 mg orally twice daily with food for 21 days then 20 mg orally daily with food	×	×	×			Contraindicated if CrCl < 30 mL/min
Apixaban	10 mg orally twice daily for first 7 days then 5 mg twice daily	×	×	×			Contraindicated if CrCl < 25 mL/min
Dabigatran	5–10 days of parenteral anticoagulation, then 150 mg twice daily	×	×	×			Contraindicated if CrCl < 15 mL/min
Edoxaban	5–10 days of parenteral anticoagulation, then 60 mg once daily; 30 mg once daily recommended if CrCl is between 15 and 50 mL/min, if weight ≤ 60 kg, or if certain P-gp inhibitors are present	×	×	×			Contraindicated if CrCl < 15 mL/min or > 95 mL/min

Note: An "×" denotes appropriate use of the anticoagulant.
[1]Obtain baseline hemoglobin, platelet count, aPTT, PT/INR, creatinine, prior to initiation of anticoagulation.
Anticoagulation is contraindicated in the setting of active bleeding.
[2]Defined as creatinine clearance < 30 mL/min.
[3]Body weight < 50 kg: reduce dose and monitor anti-Xa levels.
CrCl, creatinine clearance; DVT, deep venous thrombosis; PE, pulmonary embolism; VTE, venous thromboembolic disease (includes DVT and PE).

Table 14–17. Patient selection for outpatient treatment of DVT.

Patients considered appropriate for outpatient treatment
No clinical signs or symptoms of PE and pain controlled
Motivated and capable of self-administration of injections
Confirmed prescription insurance that covers injectable medication or patient can pay out-of-pocket for injectable agents
Capable and willing to comply with frequent follow-up
Initially, patients may need to be seen daily to weekly
Potential contraindications for outpatient treatment
DVT involving inferior vena cava, iliac, common femoral, or upper extremity vein (these patients might benefit from vascular intervention)
Comorbid conditions
Active peptic ulcer disease, GI bleeding in past 14 days, liver synthetic dysfunction
Brain metastases, current or recent CNS or spinal cord injury/surgery in the last 10 days, CVA ≤ 4–6 weeks
Familial bleeding diathesis
Active bleeding from source other than GI
Thrombocytopenia
Creatinine clearance < 30 mL/min
Patient weighs < 55 kg (male) or < 45 kg (female)
Recent surgery, spinal or epidural anesthesia in the past 3 days
History of heparin-induced thrombocytopenia
Inability to inject medication at home, reliably follow medication schedule, recognize changes in health status, understand or follow directions

Table 14–18. Simplified Pulmonary Embolism Severity Index (PESI).

	Points	
Age > 80	1	
Cancer	1	
Chronic cardiopulmonary disease	1	
Systolic blood pressure < 100 mm Hg	1	
Oxygen saturation ≤ 90%	1	
Severity Class	**Points**	**30-day Mortality**
Low risk	0	1%
High risk	≥ 1	10%

Adapted, with permission, from Jiménez D et al; RIETE Investigators. Simplification of the pulmonary embolism severity index for prognostication in patients with acute symptomatic pulmonary embolism. Arch Intern Med. 2010 Aug 9;170(15):1383–9. [PMID: 20696966]

necessary to differentiate the two. Echocardiography can be used to identify patients with right ventricular dysfunction, which connotes intermediate risk. An RV/LV ratio less than 1.0 on chest CT angiogram has been shown to have good negative predictive value for adverse outcome but suffers from inter-observer variability. Serum biomarkers such as B-type natriuretic peptide and troponin have been studied and are most useful for their negative predictive value, and mainly in combination with other predictors. The PE severity index (PESI) and simplified PESI clinical risk scores, which do not require additional testing, accurately identify patients at low risk for 30-day PE-related mortality (Table 14–18) and thus potential candidates for expedited discharge or outpatient treatment. The PESI48 and sPESI48 scores identify a subgroup of patients hospitalized with intermediate-risk PE who are reclassified as low risk by 48 hours and may be appropriate for early discharge.

1. Heparin—Selection of a parenteral anticoagulant should be determined by patient characteristics (kidney function, immediate bleeding risk, weight) and the clinical scenario (eg, whether thrombolysis is being considered). LMWHs are more effective than unfractionated heparin in the immediate treatment of DVT and PE and are preferred as initial treatment because of predictable pharmacokinetics, which allow for subcutaneous, once- or twice-daily dosing with no

requirement for monitoring in most patients. Monitoring of the therapeutic effect of LMWH may be indicated in pregnancy, compromised kidney function, and extremes of weight. Accumulation of LMWH and increased rates of bleeding have been observed among patients with severe chronic kidney disease (creatinine clearance less than 30 mL/min), leading to a recommendation to use intravenous unfractionated heparin preferentially in these patients. *If concomitant thrombolysis is being considered, unfractionated heparin is indicated.* Patients with VTE and a perceived higher risk of bleeding (ie, post-surgery) may be better candidates for treatment with unfractionated heparin than LMWH given its shorter half-life and reversibility. Unfractionated heparin can be effectively neutralized with the positively charged protamine sulfate while protamine may only have partial reversal effect at best on LMWH. Use of unfractionated heparin leads to HIT in approximately 3% of patients, so most individuals require serial platelet count determinations during the initial 10–14 days of exposure.

Weight-based, fixed-dose daily subcutaneous fondaparinux (a synthetic factor Xa inhibitor) may also be used for the initial treatment of DVT and PE, with no increase in bleeding over that observed with LMWH. Its lack of reversibility, long half-life, and renal clearance limit its use in patients with an increased risk of bleeding or kidney disease.

2. Warfarin—Patients with DVT with or without PE require a minimum of 3 months of anticoagulation in order to reduce the risk of recurrence of thrombosis. An oral vitamin K antagonist, such as warfarin, is usually initiated along with the parenteral anticoagulant, although patients with cancer-related thrombosis may benefit from ongoing treatment with LMWH alone. Most patients require 5 mg of warfarin daily for initial treatment, but lower doses (2.5 mg daily) should be considered for patients of Asian descent, the elderly, and those with hyperthyroidism, heart failure, liver disease, recent major surgery, malnutrition, certain polymorphisms for the *CYP2C9* or the *VKORC1* genes or who are receiving concurrent medications that increase sensitivity to warfarin. Conversely, individuals of African descent, those with larger body mass index or hypothyroidism, and those who are receiving medications that increase warfarin metabolism may require higher initial doses (7.5 mg daily). Daily INR results should guide dosing adjustments in the hospitalized patient while at least biweekly INR results guide dosing in the outpatient. (Table 14–19). Web-based warfarin dosing calculators that consider these clinical and genetic factors are available to help clinicians choose the appropriate starting dose (eg, see www.warfarindosing.org).

Because an average of 5 days is required to achieve a steady-state reduction in the activity of vitamin K–dependent coagulation factors, the parenteral anticoagulant should be continued for at least 5 days and until the INR is more than 2.0 on 2 consecutive days. Meticulous follow-up should be arranged for all patients taking warfarin because of the bleeding risk that is associated with initiation of therapy. Once stabilized, the INR should be checked at an interval no longer than every 6 weeks and warfarin dosing should be adjusted by guidelines (Table 14–20) since this strategy has been shown to improve the time patients spend in the therapeutic range and their clinical outcomes. Supratherapeutic

Table 14–19. Warfarin adjustment guidelines.

Measurement Day	INR	Action
For hospitalized patients newly starting therapy		
Day 1		5 mg (2.5 or 7.5 mg in select populations[1])
Day 2	< 1.5	Continue dose
	≥ 1.5	Decrease or hold dose[2]
Day 3	≤ 1.2	Increase dose[2]
	> 1.2 and < 1.7	Continue dose
	≥ 1.7	Decrease dose[2]
Day 4 until therapeutic	Daily increase < 0.2 units	Increase dose[2]
	Daily increase 0.2–0.3 units	Continue dose
	Daily increase 0.4–0.6 units	Decrease dose[2]
	Daily increase ≥ 0.7 units	Hold dose
For outpatients newly starting therapy		
Measure PT/INR on Day 1	Baseline	Start treatment with 2–7.5 mg
Measure PT/INR on Day 3–4	< 1.5	Increase weekly dose by 5–25%
	1.5–1.9	No dosage change
	2.0–2.5	Decrease weekly dose by 25–50%
	> 2.5	Decrease weekly dose by 50% or HOLD dose
Measure PT/INR on Day 5–7	< 1.5	Increase weekly dose by 10–25%
	1.5–1.9	Increase weekly dose by 0–20%
	2.0–3.0	No dosage change
	> 3.0	Decrease weekly dose by 10–25% or HOLD dose
Measure PT/INR on Day 8–10	< 1.5	Increase weekly dose by 15–35%
	1.5–1.9	Increase weekly dose by 5–20%
	2.0–3.0	No dosage change
	> 3.0	Decrease weekly dose by 10–25% or HOLD dose
Measure PT/INR on Day 11–14	< 1.6	Increase weekly dose by 15–35%
	1.6–1.9	Increase weekly dose by 5–20%
	2.0–3.0	No dosage change
	> 3.0	Decrease weekly dose by 5–20% or HOLD dose

[1] See text
[2] In general, dosage adjustments should not exceed 2.5 mg or 50%.
Data from Kim YK et al. *J Thromb Haemost* 2010;8:101–6. From Center for Health Quality, Outcomes, and Economic Research VA Medical Center Bedford MA.

Table 14–20. Warfarin-dosing adjustment guidelines for patients receiving long-term therapy, with target INR 2–3.

| Patient INR | Weekly Dosing Change | |
	Dose change	Follow-up INR
≤ 1.5	Increase by 10–15%	Within 1 week
1.51–1.79	If falling or low on two or more occasions, increase weekly dose by 5–10%.	7–14 days
1.80–2.29	Consider not changing the dose unless a consistent pattern has been observed.	7–14 days
2.3–3.0 (in range)	No change in dosage.	28 days (42 days if INR in range three times consecutively)
3.01–3.20	Consider not changing the dose unless a consistent pattern has been observed.	7–14 days
3.21–3.69	Do not hold warfarin. If rising or high on two or more occasions, decrease weekly dose by 5–10%.	7–14 days
3.70–4.99	Hold warfarin for 1 day and decrease weekly dose by 5–10%.	Within 1 week, sooner if clinically indicated
5.0–8.99	Hold warfarin. Clinical evaluation for bleeding. When INR is therapeutic, restart at lower dose (decrease weekly dose by 10–15%). Check INR at least weekly until stable.	Within 1 week, sooner if clinically indicated, then weekly until stabilized
≥ 9	See Table 14–21	

From Center for Health Quality, Outcomes, and Economic Research VA Medical Center Bedford, MA. Data from Kim YK et al. *J Thromb Haemost* 2010;8:101–6. See also Van Spall HE et al. Variation in warfarin dose adjustment practice is responsible for differences in the quality of anticoagulation control between centers and countries: an analysis of patients receiving warfarin in the randomized evaluation of long-term anticoagulation therapy (RE-LY) trial. Circulation. 2012 Nov 6;126(19):2309–16. [PMID: 23027801]

INRs should be managed according to evidence-based guidelines (Table 14–21).

3. Direct-acting oral anticoagulants—DOACs have a predictable dose effect, few drug-drug interactions, rapid onset of action, and freedom from laboratory monitoring (Table 14–11). Dabigatran, rivaroxaban, apixaban, and edoxaban are approved for treatment of acute DVT and PE. While rivaroxaban and apixaban can be used as monotherapy eliminating the need for parenteral therapy, patients who will be treated with dabigatran or edoxaban must first receive 5–10 days of parenteral anticoagulation and then be transitioned to the oral agent. Compared to warfarin and LMWH, the DOACs are all "noninferior" with respect to prevention of recurrent VTE; both rivaroxaban and apixaban boast a lower bleeding risk than warfarin and LMWH. Agent selection for acute treatment of VTE should be individualized and consider renal function, concomitant medications, ability to use LMWH bridge therapy, cost, and adherence.

There are limited data available regarding the use of DOACs in cancer patients. LMWH is still the preferred agent for treatment of cancer-related VTE.

4. Duration of anticoagulation therapy—The clinical scenario in which the thrombosis occurred is the strongest predictor of recurrence and, in most cases, guides duration of anticoagulation (Table 14–22). In the first year after discontinuation of anticoagulation therapy, the frequency of recurrent VTE among individuals whose thrombosis occurred in the setting of a transient, major, reversible risk factor (such as surgery) is approximately 3% after completing 3 months of anticoagulation, compared with at least 8% for individuals whose thrombosis was unprovoked, and greater than 20% in patients with cancer. Patients with provoked VTE are generally treated with a minimum of 3 months of anticoagulation, whereas unprovoked VTE should prompt consideration of indefinite anticoagulation. Merely extending duration of anticoagulation beyond 3 months will not reduce risk of recurrence once anticoagulation is stopped; if anticoagulants are stopped after 6, 12, or 18 months, the risk of recurrence can be expected to be similar to that after 3 months. Individual risk stratification may help identify patients most likely to suffer recurrent disease and thus most likely to benefit from ongoing anticoagulation therapy. Normal D-dimer levels 1 month after cessation of anticoagulation are associated with lower recurrence risk, although some would argue not low enough to consider stopping anticoagulant therapy, particularly in men. One risk scoring system uses body mass index, age, D-dimer, and post-phlebitic symptoms to identify women at lower risk for recurrence after unprovoked VTE. The Vienna Prediction Model, a simple scoring system based on age, sex, D-dimer, and location of thrombosis, can help estimate an individual's recurrence risk to guide duration of therapy decisions. The following facts are important to consider when determining duration of therapy: (1) men have a greater than twofold higher risk of recurrent VTE compared to women, (2) recurrent PE is more likely to develop in patients with clinically apparent PE than in those with DVT alone and has a case fatality rate of 10%, and (3) proximal DVT has a higher recurrence risk than distal DVT. Laboratory work-up for thrombophilia is not recommended routinely for determining duration of therapy because clinical presentation is a much stronger predictor of recurrence risk. The work-up may be pursued in patients younger than 50 years, with a strong family history, with a clot in unusual locations, or with recurrent thromboses (Table 14–23). In addition, a work-up for thrombophilia should be considered in women of

Table 14–21. American College of Chest Physicians Evidence-based Clinical Practice Guidelines for the Management of Nontherapeutic INR.

Clinical Situation	INR	Recommendations
No significant bleed	Above therapeutic range but < 5.0	• Lower dose or omit dose • Monitor more frequently and resume at lower dose when INR falls within therapeutic range (if INR only slightly above range, may not be necessary to decrease dose)
	≥ 5.0 but < 9.0	• Hold next 1–2 doses • Monitor more frequently and resume therapy at lower dose when INR falls within therapeutic range • *Patients at high risk for bleeding*[1]: Hold warfarin and consider giving vitamin K$_1$ 1–2.5 mg orally; check INR in 24–48 h to ensure response to therapy
	≥ 9.0	• Hold warfarin • Vitamin K$_1$ 2.5–5 mg orally • Monitor frequently and resume therapy at lower dose when INR within therapeutic range
Serious/life-threatening bleed		• Hold warfarin and give 10 mg vitamin K by slow intravenous infusion supplemented by FFP, PCC, or recombinant factor VIIa (PCC preferred)

[1]Patients at higher risk for bleeding include the elderly; conditions that increase the risk of bleeding include kidney disease, hypertension, falls, liver disease, and history of gastrointestinal or genitourinary bleeding.
FFP, fresh frozen plasma; INR, international normalized ratio; PCC, prothrombin complex concentrate.

childbearing age in whom results may influence fertility and pregnancy outcomes and management or in those patients in whom results will influence duration of therapy. The most important hypercoagulable state to identify is antiphospholipid syndrome [APS] because these patients have a marked increase in recurrence rates, are at risk for both arterial and venous disease, and in general receive bridge therapy during any interruption of anticoagulation. Due to effects of anticoagulants and acute thrombosis on many of the tests, the thrombophilia work-up should be delayed in most cases until at least 3 months after the acute event, if it is indicated at all (Table 14–24). The benefit of anticoagulation must be weighed against the bleeding risks posed, and the benefit-risk ratio should be assessed at the initiation of therapy, at 3 months, and then at least annually in any patient receiving prolonged anticoagulant therapy.

While bleeding risk scores have been developed to estimate risk of these complications, their performance may not offer any advantage over a clinician's subjective assessment, particularly in the elderly. Compared with placebo, aspirin has been shown to reduce risk of recurrent VTE by 30% in patients with idiopathic VTE. Low-dose aspirin therapy (81 mg/day) should be considered in patients with unprovoked VTE who are not candidates for ongoing anticoagulation.

Brighton TA et al; ASPIRE Investigators. Low-dose aspirin for preventing recurrent venous thromboembolism. N Engl J Med. 2012 Nov 22;367(21):1979–87. [PMID: 23121403]
Castellucci LA et al. Clinical and safety outcomes associated with treatment of acute venous thromboembolism: a systematic review and meta-analysis. JAMA. 2014 Sep 17;312(11): 1122–35. [PMID: 25226478]

Table 14–22. Duration of treatment of VTE.

Scenario	Suggested Duration of Therapy	Comments
Major transient risk factor (eg, major surgery, major trauma, major hospitalization)	3 months	VTE prophylaxis upon future exposure to transient risk factors
Cancer-related	≥ 3–6 months or as long as cancer active, whichever is longer	LMWH recommended for initial treatment (see Table 14–16)
Unprovoked	At least 3 months; consider indefinite if bleeding risk allows	May individually risk-stratify for recurrence with D-dimer, clinical risk scores and clinical presentation
Recurrent unprovoked	Indefinite	
Underlying significant thrombophilia (eg, antiphospholipid antibody syndrome, antithrombin deficiency, protein C deficiency, protein S deficiency, ≥ two concomitant thrombophilic conditions)	Indefinite	To avoid false positives, consider delaying investigation for laboratory thrombophilia until 3 months after event

LMWH, low-molecular-weight heparin; VTE, venous thromboembolic disease.

Table 14–23. Candidates for thrombophilia work-up if results will influence management.

Patients younger than 50 years
Strong family history of VTE
Clot in unusual locations
Recurrent thromboses
Women of childbearing age
Suspicion for APS

APS, antiphospholipid syndrome; VTE, venous thromboembolism.

Couturaud F et al; PADIS-PE Investigators. Six months vs extended oral anticoagulation after a first episode of pulmonary embolism: the PADIS-PE randomized clinical trial. JAMA. 2015 Jul 7;314(1):31–40. [PMID: 26151264]

Erkens PM et al. Does the Pulmonary Embolism Severity Index accurately identify low risk patients eligible for outpatient treatment? Thromb Res. 2012 Jun;129(6):710–4. [PMID: 21906787]

Heidbuchel H et al. European Heart Rhythm Association Practical Guide on the use of new oral anticoagulants in patients with non-valvular atrial fibrillation. Europace. 2013 May; 15(5):625–51. [PMID: 23625942]

Jiménez D et al. Simplification of the Pulmonary Embolism Severity Index for prognostication in patients with acute symptomatic pulmonary embolism. Arch Intern Med. 2010;170(15):1383–9. [PMID: 20696966]

Kaatz S et al. Reversal of target-specific oral anticoagulants. J Thromb Thrombolysis. 2013 Aug;36(2):195–202. [PMID: 23657589]

Kearon C et al. Antithrombotic therapy for VTE disease: Antithrombotic Therapy and Prevention of Thrombosis, 9th ed: American College of Chest Physicians Evidence-Based Clinical Practice Guidelines. Chest. 2012 Feb;141(2 Suppl): e419S–94S. [PMID: 22315268]

Kearon C et al. Duration of anticoagulant therapy for deep vein thrombosis and pulmonary embolism. Blood. 2014 Mar 20;123(12):1794–801. [PMID: 24497538]

Kearon C et al; D-dimer Optimal Duration Study Investigators. D-dimer testing to select patients with a first unprovoked venous thromboembolism who can stop anticoagulant therapy: a cohort study. Ann Intern Med. 2015 Jan 6;162(1): 27–34. [PMID: 25560712]

Konstantinides SV et al; Task Force for the Diagnosis and Management of Acute Pulmonary Embolism of the European Society of Cardiology (ESC). 2014 ESC guidelines on the diagnosis and management of acute pulmonary embolism. Eur Heart J. 2014 Nov 14;35(43):3033–69, 3069a-3069k. Erratum in: Eur Heart J. 2015 Oct 14;36(39):2666. Eur Heart J. 2015 Oct 14;36(39):2642. [PMID: 25173341]

Moll S. Thrombophilia: clinical-practical aspects. J Thromb Thrombolysis. 2015 Apr;39(3):367–78. [PMID: 25724822]

Moores L et al; Instituto Ramón y Cajal de Investigación Sanitaria Pulmonary Embolism Study Group. Changes in PESI scores predict mortality in intermediate-risk patients with acute pulmonary embolism. Eur Respir J. 2013 Feb;41(2): 354–9. [PMID: 22743671]

Palareti G et al; DULCIS (D-dimer and ULtrasonography in Combination Italian Study) Investigators. D-dimer to guide the duration of anticoagulation in patients with venous thromboembolism: a management study. Blood. 2014 Jul 10; 124(2):196–203. [PMID: 24879813]

Table 14–24. Laboratory evaluation of thrombophilia.

Hypercoagulable State	When to Suspect	Laboratory Work-Up	Influence of Anticoagulation and Acute Thrombosis
Antiphospholipid antibody syndrome	Unexplained DVT/PE CVA/TIA age < 50 Recurrent thrombosis (despite anticoagulation) Thrombosis at an unusual site Arterial and venous thrombosis Livedo reticularis, Raynaud phenomenon, thrombocytopenia, recurrent early pregnancy loss	Anti-cardiolipin IgG and/or IgM medium or high titer (ie, > 40 GPL or MPL, or > the 99th percentile)[1] Anti-beta-2 glycoprotein I IgG and/or IgM medium or high titer (> the 99th percentile)[1] Lupus anticoagulant[1]	Lupus anticoagulant can be falsely positive or falsely negative on anticoagulation
Protein C, S, antithrombin deficiencies	Thrombosis < 50 years of age with family history of VTE	Screen with protein C activity, free protein S, protein S activity, antithrombin activity	Acute thrombosis can result in decreased protein C, S and antithrombin activity. Warfarin can decrease protein C and S activity, heparin can cause decrease antithrombin activity. DOACs can increase protein C, S, and antithrombin activity
Factor V Leiden, prothrombin gene mutation	Thrombosis on OCPs, cerebral vein thrombosis, DVT/PE in white population	PCR for factor V Leiden or prothrombin gene mutation	No influence
Hyperhomocysteinemia		Fasting homocysteine	No influence

[1]Detected on two occasions not less than 12 weeks apart.
CVA/TIA, cerebrovascular accident/transient ischemic attack; DOACs, direct-acting oral anticoagulants; DVT/PE, deep venous thrombosis/pulmonary embolism; OCPs, oral contraceptives; PCR, polymerase chain reaction; VTE, venous thromboembolism.

C. Thrombolytic Therapy

Anticoagulation alone is appropriate treatment for most patients with PE; however, those with high-risk, massive PE, defined as PE with persistent hemodynamic instability, have an in-hospital mortality rate that approaches 30% and require immediate thrombolysis in combination with anti-coagulation (Table 14–25). Thrombolytic therapy has been used in selected patients with intermediate-risk, submassive PE, defined as PE without hemodynamic instability but with evidence of right ventricular compromise and myocardial injury. Thrombolysis in this cohort decreases risk of hemodynamic compromise but increases the risk of major hemorrhage and stroke. A "safe dose" of tPA (50% or less of the standard dose [100 mg] commonly used for the treatment of PE) has been evaluated in small trials of both massive and submassive PE showing similar efficacy and a better safety profile. The use of thrombolysis in hemodynamically stable intermediate risk PE patients should be considered on a case-by-case basis.

Limited data suggest that patients with large proximal iliofemoral DVT may also benefit from catheter-directed thrombolysis in addition to treatment with anticoagulation. However, standardized guidelines are lacking, and use of the intervention may be limited by institutional availability and provider experience. Importantly, thrombolytics should be considered only in patients who have a low risk of bleeding, as rates of bleeding are increased in patients who receive these products compared with rates of hemorrhage in those who are treated with anticoagulation alone.

Chatterjee S et al. Thrombolysis for pulmonary embolism and risk of all-cause mortality, major bleeding, and intracranial hemorrhage: a meta-analysis. JAMA. 2014 Jun 18;311(23):2414–21. [PMID: 24938564]

Howard LS. Thrombolytic therapy for submassive pulmonary embolus? PRO viewpoint. Thorax. 2014 Feb;69(2):103–5. [PMID: 23624534]

Jaff MR et al. Management of massive and submassive pulmonary embolism, iliofemoral deep vein thrombosis, and chronic thromboembolic pulmonary hypertension: a scientific statement from the American Heart Association. Circulation. 2011 Apr 26;123(16):1788–830. Erratum in: Circulation. 2012 Aug 14;126(7):e104. Circulation. 2012 Mar 20;125(11):e495. [PMID: 21422387]

Kearon C et al; American College of Chest Physicians. Antithrombotic therapy for VTE disease: Antithrombotic Therapy and Prevention of Thrombosis, 9th ed: American College of Chest Physicians Evidence-Based Clinical Practice Guidelines. Chest. 2012 Feb;141(2 Suppl):e419S–94S. [PMID: 22315268]

Meyer G et al; PEITHO Investigators. Fibrinolysis for patients with intermediate-risk pulmonary embolism. N Engl J Med. 2014 Apr 10;370(15):1402–11. [PMID: 24716681]

Sharifi M et al. Moderate pulmonary embolism treated with thrombolysis (from the "MOPETT" Trial). Am J Cardiol. 2013 Jan 15;111(2):273–7. [PMID: 23102885]

Simpson AJ. Thrombolysis for acute submassive pulmonary embolism: CON viewpoint. Thorax. 2014 Feb;69(2):105–7. [PMID: 24046127]

Watson L et al. Thrombolysis for acute deep vein thrombosis. Cochrane Database Syst Rev. 2014 Jan 23;1:CD002783. [PMID: 24452314]

D. Nonpharmacologic Therapy

1. Graduated compression stockings—Although use of graduated compression stockings with 30–40 mm Hg pressure at the ankle in patients with DVT on the affected lower extremity had been advocated for 1–2 years after diagnosis, a randomized placebo-controlled trial failed to show a reduction in the postthrombotic syndrome at 6 months. Stockings may provide symptomatic relief to selected patients with ongoing swelling or pain; however, they are contraindicated in patients with peripheral vascular disease.

2. Inferior vena caval (IVC) filters—There is a paucity of data to support the use of IVC filters for the prevention of

Table 14–25. Thrombolytic therapies for pulmonary embolism.

Thrombolytic Agent	Dose	Frequency	Comment
High Risk (Massive Pulmonary Embolism)			
Alteplase	100 mg	Continuous intravenous infusion over 2 hours	Follow with continuous intravenous infusion of unfractionated heparin (see Table 14–16 for dosage)
	100 mg	Intravenous bolus × 1	Appropriate for acute management of cardiac arrest and suspected pulmonary embolism
Urokinase	4400 international units/kg	Intravenous bolus × 1 followed by 4400 international units/kg continuous intravenous infusion for 12 hours	Unfractionated heparin should be administered concurrently (see Table 14–16 for dosage)
Intermediate Risk (Submassive Pulmonary Embolism)			
rt-PA	50 mg/2 hours	Continuous infusion over 2 hours	
Tenecteplase	30–50 mg	Intravenous bolus × 1	
Alteplase	100 mg	(10-mg intravenous bolus, followed by a 90-mg intravenous infusion 2 hours)	

(rtPA, recombinant tissue plasminogen activator).

PE in any clinical scenario. There are two randomized, controlled trials of IVC filters for prevention of PE. In the first study, patients with documented DVT received full intensity, time-limited anticoagulation with or without placement of a permanent IVC filter. Patients with IVC filters had a lower rate of nonfatal asymptomatic PE at 12 days but an increased rate of DVT at 2 years. In the second study, patients with symptomatic PE and residual DVT plus at least one additional risk factor for severity received anticoagulation with or without a retrievable IVC filter. IVC filter use did not reduce the risk of symptomatic recurrent PE at 3 months. Most experts agree with placement of an IVC filter in patients with acute proximal DVT and an absolute contraindication to anticoagulation despite lack of evidence to support this practice. While IVC filters were once commonly used to prevent VTE recurrence in the setting of anticoagulation failure, many experts now recommend switching to an alternative agent or increasing the intensity of the current anticoagulant regimen instead. The remainder of the indications (submassive/intermediate-risk PE, free-floating iliofemoral DVT, perioperative risk reduction) are controversial. If the contraindication to anticoagulation is temporary (active bleeding with subsequent resolution), placement of a retrievable IVC filter should be considered so that the device can be removed once anticoagulation has been started and has been shown to be tolerated. Rates of IVC filter retrieval are very low, often due to a failure to arrange for its removal. Thus, if a device is placed, removal should be arranged at the time of device placement.

Complications of IVC filters include local thrombosis, tilting, migration, fracture, and inability to retrieve the device. When considering placement of an IVC filter, it is best to consider both short- and long-term complications, since devices intended for removal may become permanent. To improve patient safety, institutions should develop systems that guide appropriate patient selection for IVC filter placement, tracking, and removal.

Kahn SR et al. Graduated compression stockings to treat acute leg pain associated with proximal DVT. A randomised controlled trial. Thromb Haemost. 2014 Dec 1;112(6):1137–41. [PMID: 25183442]

Milovanovic L et al. Procedural and indwelling complications with inferior vena cava filters: frequency, etiology, and management. Semin Intervent Radiol. 2015 Mar;32(1):34–41. [PMID: 25762846]
Mismetti P et al; PREPIC2 Study Group. Effect of a retrievable inferior vena cava filter plus anticoagulation vs anticoagulation alone on risk of recurrent pulmonary embolism: a randomized clinical trial. JAMA. 2015 Apr 28;313(16):1627–35. [PMID: 25919526]
PREPIC Study Group. Eight-year follow-up of patients with permanent vena cava filters in the prevention of pulmonary embolism: the PREPIC (Prévention du Risque d'Embolie Pulmonaire par Interruption Cave) randomized study. Circulation. 2005 Jul 19;112(3):416–22. [PMID: 16009794]
Sarosiek S et al. Indications, complications, and management of inferior vena cava filters: the experience in 952 patients at an academic hospital with a level I trauma center. JAMA Intern Med. 2013 Apr 8;173(7):513–7. [PMID: 23552968]

► **When to Refer**

- Presence of large iliofemoral VTE, IVC thrombosis, portal vein thrombosis, or Budd-Chiari syndrome for consideration of catheter-directed thrombolysis.
- Massive PE for urgent embolectomy.
- History of HIT or prolonged PTT plus renal failure for alternative anticoagulation regimens.
- Consideration of IVC filter placement.
- Presence of clots in unusual locations (eg, renal vein, hepatic vein, cerebral vein), or simultaneous arterial and venous thrombosis, to assess possibility of a hypercoagulable state.

► **When to Admit**

- Documented or suspected PE (some patients with low-risk PE may not require admission).
- DVT with poorly controlled pain, high bleeding risk, concerns about follow-up.
- Large iliofemoral DVT for consideration of thrombolysis.
- Acute DVT and absolute contraindication to anticoagulation for IVC filter placement.
- Venous thrombosis despite therapeutic anticoagulation.

Gastrointestinal Disorders

15

Kenneth R. McQuaid, MD

DYSPEPSIA

ESSENTIALS OF DIAGNOSIS

► Epigastric pain or burning, early satiety, or post-prandial fullness.

► Endoscopy is warranted in patients with alarm features or in those older than 55 years.

► All other patients should first undergo testing for *Helicobacter pylori* or a trial of empiric proton pump inhibitor.

► General Considerations

Dyspepsia refers to acute, chronic, or recurrent pain or discomfort centered in the upper abdomen. An international committee of clinical investigators (Rome III Committee) has defined dyspepsia as epigastric pain or burning, early satiety, or postprandial fullness. Heartburn (retrosternal burning) should be distinguished from dyspepsia. When heartburn is the dominant complaint, gastroesophageal reflux is nearly always present. Dyspepsia occurs in 15% of the adult population and accounts for 3% of general medical office visits.

► Etiology

A. Food or Drug Intolerance

Acute, self-limited "indigestion" may be caused by overeating, eating too quickly, eating high-fat foods, eating during stressful situations, or drinking too much alcohol or coffee. Many medications cause dyspepsia, including aspirin, nonsteroidal anti-inflammatory drugs (NSAIDs), antibiotics (metronidazole, macrolides), dabigatran, diabetes drugs (metformin, alpha-glucosidase inhibitors, amylin analogs, GLP-1 receptor antagonists), antihypertensive medications (angiotensin-converting enzyme [ACE] inhibitors, angiotensin-receptor blockers), cholesterol-lowering agents (niacin, fibrates), neuropsychiatric medications (cholinesterase inhibitors [donepezil, rivastigmine]), SSRIs (fluoxetine, sertraline), serotonin-norepinephrine-reuptake inhibitors (venlafaxine, duloxetine), Parkinson drugs (dopamine agonists, monoamine oxidase [MAO]-B inhibitors), corticosteroids, estrogens, digoxin, iron, and opioids.

B. Functional Dyspepsia

This is the most common cause of *chronic* dyspepsia. Up to three-fourths of patients have no obvious organic cause for their symptoms after evaluation. Symptoms may arise from a complex interaction of increased visceral afferent sensitivity, gastric delayed emptying or impaired accommodation to food, or psychosocial stressors. Although benign, these symptoms may be chronic and difficult to treat.

C. Luminal Gastrointestinal Tract Dysfunction

Peptic ulcer disease is present in 5–15% of patients with dyspepsia. Gastroesophageal reflux disease (GERD) is present in up to 20% of patients with dyspepsia, even without significant heartburn. Gastric or esophageal cancer is identified in less than 1% but is extremely rare in persons under age 50 years with uncomplicated dyspepsia. Other causes include gastroparesis (especially in diabetes mellitus), lactose intolerance or malabsorptive conditions, and parasitic infection (*Giardia, Strongyloides, Anisakis*).

D. *Helicobacter pylori* Infection

Although chronic gastric infection with *H pylori* is an important cause of peptic ulcer disease, it is an uncommon cause of dyspepsia in the absence of peptic ulcer disease. The prevalence of *H pylori*–associated chronic gastritis in patients with dyspepsia without peptic ulcer disease is the same as in the general population.

E. Pancreatic Disease

Pancreatic carcinoma and chronic pancreatitis may initially be mistaken for dyspepsia but usually are associated with more severe pain, anorexia and rapid weight loss, steatorrhea, or jaundice.

F. Biliary Tract Disease

The abrupt onset of epigastric or right upper quadrant pain due to cholelithiasis or choledocholithiasis should be readily distinguished from dyspepsia.

G. Other Conditions

Diabetes mellitus, thyroid disease, chronic kidney disease, myocardial ischemia, intra-abdominal malignancy, gastric volvulus or paraesophageal hernia, chronic gastric or intestinal ischemia, and pregnancy are sometimes accompanied by dyspepsia.

▶ Clinical Findings

A. Symptoms and Signs

Given the nonspecific nature of dyspeptic symptoms, the history has limited diagnostic utility. It should clarify the chronicity, location, and quality of the discomfort, and its relationship to meals. The discomfort may be characterized by one or more upper abdominal symptoms including epigastric pain or burning, early satiety, postprandial fullness, bloating, nausea, or vomiting. Concomitant weight loss, persistent vomiting, constant or severe pain, dysphagia, hematemesis, or melena warrants endoscopy or abdominal imaging. Potentially offending medications and excessive alcohol use should be identified and discontinued if possible. The patient's reason for seeking care should be determined. Recent changes in employment, marital discord, physical and sexual abuse, anxiety, depression, and fear of serious disease may all contribute to the development and reporting of symptoms. Patients with functional dyspepsia often are younger, report a variety of abdominal and extragastrointestinal complaints, show signs of anxiety or depression, or have a history of use of psychotropic medications.

The symptom profile alone does not differentiate between functional dyspepsia and organic gastrointestinal disorders. Based on the clinical history alone, primary care clinicians misdiagnose nearly half of patients with peptic ulcers or gastroesophageal reflux and have less than 25% accuracy in diagnosing functional dyspepsia.

The physical examination is rarely helpful. Signs of serious organic disease such as weight loss, organomegaly, abdominal mass, or fecal occult blood are to be further evaluated.

B. Laboratory Findings

In patients older than age of 50 years, initial laboratory work should include a blood count, electrolytes, liver enzymes, calcium, and thyroid function tests. In patients younger than 50 years with uncomplicated dyspepsia (in whom gastric cancer is rare), initial noninvasive strategies should be pursued. The cost-effectiveness of routine laboratory studies is uncertain. In most clinical settings, a noninvasive test for H pylori (urea breath test, fecal antigen test, or IgG serology) should be performed first. Although serologic tests are inexpensive, performance characteristics are poor in low-prevalence populations, whereas breath

and fecal antigen tests have 95% accuracy. If H pylori breath test or fecal antigen test results are negative in a patient not taking NSAIDs, peptic ulcer disease is virtually excluded.

C. Upper Endoscopy

Upper endoscopy is indicated to look for gastric cancer or other serious organic disease in all patients over age 50 years with new-onset dyspepsia and in all patients with "alarm" features, such as weight loss, dysphagia, recurrent vomiting, evidence of bleeding, or anemia. Upper endoscopy is the study of choice to diagnose gastroduodenal ulcers, erosive esophagitis, and upper gastrointestinal malignancy. It is also helpful for patients who are concerned about serious underlying disease. For patients born in regions in which there is a higher incidence of gastric cancer, such as Central or South America, China and Southeast Asia, or Africa, an age threshold of 45 years may be appropriate.

Endoscopic evaluation is also warranted when symptoms fail to respond to initial empiric management strategies within 4–8 weeks or when frequent symptom relapse occurs after discontinuation of antisecretory therapy.

D. Other Tests

In patients with refractory symptoms or progressive weight loss, antibodies for celiac disease or stool testing for ova and parasites or Giardia antigen, fat, or elastase may be considered. Abdominal imaging (ultrasonography or CT scanning) is performed only when pancreatic, biliary tract, vascular disease, or volvulus is suspected. Gastric emptying studies are valuable only in patients with recurrent vomiting. Ambulatory esophageal pH-impedance testing may be of value when atypical gastroesophageal reflux is suspected.

▶ Treatment

Initial empiric treatment is warranted for patients who are younger than 50 years and who have no alarm features (defined above). All other patients as well as patients whose symptoms fail to respond or relapse after empiric treatment should undergo upper endoscopy with subsequent treatment directed at the specific disorder (eg, peptic ulcer, gastroesophageal reflux, cancer). Most patients will have no significant findings on endoscopy and will be given a diagnosis of functional dyspepsia.

A. Empiric Therapy

Young patients with uncomplicated dyspepsia may be treated empirically with either a proton pump inhibitor or evaluated with a noninvasive test for H pylori, followed if positive by treatment. The prevalence of H pylori in the population influences recommendations for the timing of these empiric therapies. In clinical settings in which the prevalence of H pylori infection in the population is low (less than 10%), it may be more cost-effective to initially treat patients with a 4-week trial of a proton pump inhibitor. Patients who have symptom relapse after discontinuation of the proton pump inhibitor should be tested for H pylori and treated if results are positive. In clinical settings in which *H pylori* prevalence is greater than 10%, it may be more cost-effective to initially test patients for *H pylori* infection. *H pylori*–negative patients most likely have functional dyspepsia or atypical GERD and can be treated with an antisecretory agent (proton pump inhibitor) for 4 weeks. For patients who have symptom relapse after discontinuation of the proton pump inhibitor, intermittent or long-term proton pump inhibitor therapy may be considered. For patients in whom test results are positive for *H pylori*, antibiotic therapy proves definitive for patients with underlying peptic ulcers and may improve symptoms in a small subset (less than 10%) of infected patients with functional dyspepsia. Patients with persistent dyspepsia after *H pylori* eradication can be given a trial of proton pump inhibitor therapy.

B. Treatment of Functional Dyspepsia

1. General measures—Most patients have mild, intermittent symptoms that respond to reassurance and lifestyle changes. Alcohol and caffeine should be reduced or discontinued. Patients with postprandial symptoms should be instructed to consume small, low-fat meals. A food diary, in which patients record their food intake, symptoms, and daily events, may reveal dietary or psychosocial precipitants of pain.

2. Pharmacologic agents—Drugs have demonstrated limited efficacy in the treatment of functional dyspepsia. One-third of patients derive relief from placebo. Antisecretory therapy for 4–8 weeks with oral proton pump inhibitors (omeprazole, esomeprazole, or rabeprazole 20 mg, dexlansoprazole or lansoprazole 30 mg, or pantoprazole 40 mg) may benefit 10–15% of patients, particularly those with dyspepsia characterized as epigastric pain ("ulcer-like dyspepsia") or dyspepsia and heartburn ("reflux-like dyspepsia"). Low doses of antidepressants (eg, desipramine or nortriptyline, 25–50 mg orally at bedtime) benefit some patients, possibly by moderating visceral afferent sensitivity. A 2015 multicenter controlled trial reported adequate symptom improvement in 53% of patients treated with amitriptyline (50 mg/day) at 10 weeks compared with placebo (40%) and escitalopram (38%), particularly those with upper abdominal pain (ulcer-like dyspepsia). Doses should be increased slowly to minimize side effects. Metoclopramide (5–10 mg three times daily) may improve symptoms, but improvement does not correlate with the presence or absence of gastric emptying delay. In 2009, the FDA issued a black box warning that metoclopramide use for more than 3 months is associated with a high incidence of tardive dyskinesia and should be avoided. The elderly, particularly elderly women, are most at risk.

3. Anti-*H pylori* treatment—Meta-analyses have suggested that a small number of patients with functional dyspepsia (less than 10%) derive benefit from *H pylori* eradication therapy. Therefore, patients with functional dyspepsia should be tested and treated for *H pylori* as recommended above.

4. Alternative therapies—Psychotherapy and hypnotherapy may be of benefit in selected motivated patients with functional dyspepsia. Herbal therapies (peppermint, caraway) may offer benefit with little risk of adverse effects.

Shaukat A et al; ASGE Standards of Practice Committee. The role of endoscopy in dyspepsia. Gastrointest Endosc. 2015 Aug; 82(2):227–32. [PMID: 26032200]
Talley NJ et al. Effect of amitriptyline and escitalopram on functional dyspepsia: a multicenter, randomized controlled study. Gastroenterology. 2015 Aug;149(2):340–9.e2. [PMID: 25921377]
Talley NJ et al. Functional dyspepsia. N Engl J Med. 2015 Nov 5; 373(19):1853–63. [PMID: 26535514]

NAUSEA & VOMITING

Nausea is a vague, intensely disagreeable sensation of sickness or "queasiness" and is distinguished from anorexia. Vomiting often follows, as does retching (spasmodic respiratory and abdominal movements). Vomiting should be distinguished from regurgitation, the effortless reflux of liquid or food stomach contents; and from rumination, the chewing and swallowing of food that is regurgitated volitionally after meals.

The brainstem vomiting center is composed of a group of neuronal areas (area postrema, nucleus tractus solitarius, and central pattern generator) within the medulla that coordinate emesis. It may be stimulated by four different sources of afferent input: (1) Afferent vagal fibers from the gastrointestinal viscera are rich in serotonin 5-HT$_3$ receptors; these may be stimulated by biliary or gastrointestinal distention, mucosal or peritoneal irritation, or infections. (2) Fibers of the vestibular system, which have high concentrations of histamine H$_1$ and muscarinic cholinergic receptors. (3) Higher central nervous system centers (amygdala); here, certain sights, smells, or emotional experiences may induce vomiting. For example, patients receiving chemotherapy may start vomiting in anticipation of its administration. (4) The chemoreceptor trigger zone, located outside the blood-brain barrier in the area postrema of the medulla, which is rich in opioid, serotonin 5-HT$_3$, neurokinin 1 (NK$_1$) and dopamine D$_2$ receptors. This region may be stimulated by drugs and chemotherapeutic agents, toxins, hypoxia, uremia, acidosis, and radiation therapy. Although the causes of nausea and vomiting are many, a simplified list is provided in Table 15–1.

▶ Clinical Findings

A. Symptoms and Signs

Acute symptoms without abdominal pain are typically caused by food poisoning, infectious gastroenteritis, drugs, or systemic illness. Inquiry should be made into recent changes in medications, diet, other intestinal symptoms, or similar illnesses in family members. The acute onset of severe pain and vomiting suggests peritoneal irritation, acute gastric or intestinal obstruction, or pancreaticobiliary disease. Persistent vomiting suggests pregnancy, gastric outlet obstruction, gastroparesis, intestinal dysmotility, psychogenic disorders, and central nervous system or systemic disorders. Vomiting that occurs in the morning before breakfast is common with pregnancy, uremia, alcohol intake, and increased intracranial pressure. Vomiting

Table 15–1. Causes of nausea and vomiting.

Visceral afferent stimulation	**Infections**
	Mechanical obstruction
	    Gastric outlet obstruction: peptic ulcer disease, malignancy, gastric volvulus
	    Small intestinal obstruction: adhesions, hernias, volvulus, Crohn disease, carcinomatosis
	Dysmotility
	    Gastroparesis: diabetic, postviral, postvagotomy
	    Small intestine: scleroderma, amyloidosis, chronic intestinal pseudo-obstruction, familial myoneuropathies
	Peritoneal irritation
	    Peritonitis: perforated viscus, appendicitis, spontaneous bacterial peritonitis
	    Viral gastroenteritis: Norwalk agent, rotavirus
	    "Food poisoning": toxins from *Bacillus cereus, Staphylococcus aureus, Clostridium perfringens*
	    Hepatitis A or B
	    Acute systemic infections
	Hepatobiliary or pancreatic disorders
	    Acute pancreatitis
	    Cholecystitis or choledocholithiasis
	Topical gastrointestinal irritants
	    Alcohol, NSAIDs, oral antibiotics
	Postoperative
	Other
	    Cardiac disease: acute myocardial infarction, heart failure
	    Urologic disease: stones, pyelonephritis

Vestibular disorders	**Vestibular disorders** Labyrinthitis, Meniere syndrome, motion sickness

CNS disorders	**Increased intracranial pressure**
	    CNS tumors, subdural or subarachnoid hemorrhage
	Migraine
	Infections
	    Meningitis, encephalitis
	Psychogenic
	    Anticipatory vomiting, anorexia nervosa and bulimia, psychiatric disorders

Irritation of chemoreceptor trigger zone	**Antitumor chemotherapy**
	Medications and drugs
	    Opioids
	    Anticonvulsants
	    Antiparkinsonism drugs
	    Beta-blockers, antiarrhythmics, digoxin
	    Nicotine
	    Oral contraceptives
	    Cholinesterase inhibitors
	    Diabetes medications (metformin, acarbose, pramlintide, exenatide)
	Radiation therapy
	Systemic disorders
	    Diabetic ketoacidosis
	    Uremia
	    Adrenocortical crisis
	    Parathyroid disease
	    Hypothyroidism
	    Pregnancy
	    Paraneoplastic syndrome

CNS, central nervous system; NSAIDs, nonsteroidal anti-inflammatory drugs.

immediately after meals strongly suggests bulimia or psychogenic causes. Vomiting of undigested food one to several hours after meals is characteristic of gastroparesis or a gastric outlet obstruction; physical examination may reveal a succussion splash. Patients with acute or chronic symptoms should be asked about neurologic symptoms (eg, headache, stiff neck, vertigo, and focal paresthesias or weakness) that suggest a central nervous system cause.

B. Special Examinations

With vomiting that is severe or protracted, serum electrolytes should be obtained to look for hypokalemia, azotemia, or metabolic alkalosis resulting from loss of gastric contents. Flat and upright abdominal radiographs or abdominal CT are obtained in patients with severe pain or suspicion of mechanical obstruction to look for free intraperitoneal air or dilated loops of small bowel. The cause of gastric outlet obstruction is best demonstrated by upper endoscopy, and the cause of small intestinal obstruction is best demonstrated with abdominal CT imaging. Gastroparesis is confirmed by nuclear scintigraphic studies or ^{13}C-octanoic acid breath tests, which show delayed gastric emptying and either upper endoscopy or barium upper gastrointestinal series showing no evidence of mechanical gastric outlet obstruction. Abnormal liver biochemical tests or elevated amylase or lipase suggest pancreaticobiliary disease, which may be investigated with an abdominal sonogram or CT scan. Central nervous system causes are best evaluated with either head CT or MRI.

► Complications

Complications include dehydration, hypokalemia, metabolic alkalosis, aspiration, rupture of the esophagus (Boerhaave syndrome), and bleeding secondary to a mucosal tear at the gastroesophageal junction (Mallory-Weiss syndrome).

► Treatment

A. General Measures

Most causes of acute vomiting are mild, self-limited, and require no specific treatment. Patients should ingest clear liquids (broths, tea, soups, carbonated beverages) and small quantities of dry foods (soda crackers). Ginger may be an effective nonpharmacologic treatment. For more severe acute vomiting, hospitalization may be required. Patients unable to eat and losing gastric fluids may become dehydrated, resulting in hypokalemia with metabolic alkalosis. Intravenous 0.45% saline solution with 20 mEq/L of potassium chloride is given in most cases to maintain hydration. A nasogastric suction tube for gastric or mechanical small bowel obstruction improves patient comfort and permits monitoring of fluid loss.

B. Antiemetic Medications

Medications may be given either to prevent or to control vomiting. Combinations of drugs from different classes may provide better control of symptoms with less toxicity in some patients. Table 15–2 outlines common antiemetic dosing regimens.

1. Serotonin 5-HT3-receptor antagonists—Ondansetron, granisetron, dolasetron, and palonosetron are effective in preventing chemotherapy- and radiation-induced emesis when initiated prior to treatment. Although 5-HT$_3$-receptor antagonists are effective as single agents for the prevention of chemotherapy-induced nausea and vomiting, their efficacy is enhanced by combination therapy with a corticosteroid (dexamethasone) and NK$_1$-receptor antagonist. Serotonin antagonists increasingly are used for the prevention of postoperative nausea and vomiting because of increased restrictions on the use of other antiemetic agents (such as droperidol).

2. Corticosteroids—Corticosteroids (eg, dexamethasone) have antiemetic properties, but the basis for these effects is

Table 15–2. Common antiemetic dosing regimens.

	Dosage	Route
Serotonin 5-HT$_3$ Antagonists		
Ondansetron	Doses vary: 4–8 mg twice daily for postoperative nausea and vomiting	Intravenously, orally
	8 mg twice daily for moderately or highly emetogenic chemotherapy	Intravenously, orally
Granisetron	1 mg once daily	Intravenously
	1–2 mg once daily	Orally
Dolasetron	12.5 mg postoperatively	Intravenously
	100 mg once daily	Orally
Palonosetron	0.25 mg once as a single dose 30 min before start of chemotherapy	Intravenously
	0.5 mg once as single dose	Orally
Corticosteroids		
Dexamethasone	4 mg once pre-induction for prevention of postoperative nausea and vomiting	Intravenously, orally
	8 mg once daily for chemotherapy	Intravenously, orally
Methylprednisolone	40–100 mg once daily	Intravenously, intramuscularly, orally
Dopamine Receptor Antagonists		
Metoclopramide	10–20 mg or 0.5 mg/kg every 6–8 hours	Intravenously
	10–20 mg every 6–8 hours	Orally
Prochlorperazine	5–10 mg every 4–6 hours	Intravenously, intramuscularly, orally
	25 mg suppository every 6 hours	Per rectum
Promethazine	12.5–25 mg every 6–8 hours	Intravenously, orally
	25 mg every 6–8 hours	Per rectum
Trimethobenzamide	200 mg every 6–8 hours	Orally
	250–300 mg every 6–8 hours	Intravenously, orally
Neurokinin Receptor Antagonists[1]		
Aprepitant	125 mg once before chemotherapy; then 80 mg on days 1 and 2 after chemotherapy	Orally
Rolapitant	180 mg once before chemotherapy	Orally
Fosaprepitant	115 mg once 30 minutes before chemotherapy	Intravenously

[1]Neurokinin receptor antagonists are used solely for highly emetogenic chemotherapy regimens in combination with 5-HT$_3$ antagonists or dexamethasone or both.

unknown. These agents enhance the efficacy of serotonin receptor antagonists for preventing acute and delayed nausea and vomiting in patients receiving moderately to highly emetogenic chemotherapy regimens.

3. Neurokinin receptor antagonists—Aprepitant, fosaprepitant, and rolapitant are highly selective antagonists for NK_1-receptors in the area postrema. They are used in combination with corticosteroids and serotonin antagonists for the prevention of acute and delayed nausea and vomiting with highly emetogenic chemotherapy regimens. Combined therapy with a neurokinin-1 receptor antagonist prevents acute emesis in 80–90% and delayed emesis in more than 70% of patients treated with highly emetogenic regimens.

4. Dopamine antagonists—The phenothiazines, butyrophenones, and substituted benzamides (eg, prochlorperazine, promethazine) have antiemetic properties that are due to dopaminergic blockade as well as to their sedative effects. High doses of these agents are associated with antidopaminergic side effects, including extrapyramidal reactions and depression. With the advent of more effective and safer antiemetics, these agents are infrequently used, mainly in outpatients with minor, self-limited symptoms.

5. Antihistamines and anticholinergics—These drugs (eg, meclizine, dimenhydrinate, transdermal scopolamine) may be valuable in the prevention of vomiting arising from stimulation of the labyrinth, ie, motion sickness, vertigo, and migraines. They may induce drowsiness. A combination of oral vitamin B_6 and doxylamine is recommended by the American College of Obstetricians and Gynecologists as first-line therapy for nausea and vomiting during pregnancy.

6. Cannabinoids—Marijuana has been used widely as an appetite stimulant and antiemetic. Pure Delta[9]-tetrahydrocannabinol (THC) is the major active ingredient in marijuana and the most psychoactive and is available by prescription as dronabinol. In doses of 5–15 mg/m², oral dronabinol is effective in treating nausea associated with chemotherapy, but it is associated with central nervous system side effects in most patients. Some states allow the use of medical marijuana with a clinician's certification. Strains of medical marijuana with different proportions of various naturally occurring cannabinoids (primarily THC and Cannabidiol [CBD]) can be chosen to minimize its psychoactive effects.

Matthews A et al. Interventions for nausea and vomiting in early pregnancy. Cochrane Database Syst Rev. 2014 Mar 21;3: CD007575. [PMID: 24659261]

Navari RM. Management of chemotherapy-induced nausea and vomiting: focus on newer agents and new uses for older agents. Drugs. 2013 Mar;73(3):249–62. [PMID: 23404093]

Tageja N et al. Chemotherapy-induced nausea and vomiting: an overview and comparison of three consensus guidelines. Postgrad Med J. 2016 Jan;92(1083):34–40. [PMID: 26561590]

Thomson M et al. Effects of ginger for nausea and vomiting in early pregnancy: a meta-analysis. J Am Board Fam Med. 2014 Jan–Feb;27(1):115–22. [PMID: 24390893]

HICCUPS (Singultus)

Though usually a benign and self-limited annoyance, hiccups may be persistent and a sign of serious underlying illness. In patients on mechanical ventilation, hiccups can trigger a full respiratory cycle and result in respiratory alkalosis.

Causes of benign, self-limited hiccups include gastric distention (carbonated beverages, air swallowing, overeating), sudden temperature changes (hot then cold liquids, hot then cold shower), alcohol ingestion, and states of heightened emotion (excitement, stress, laughing). There are over 100 causes of recurrent or persistent hiccups due to gastrointestinal, central nervous system, cardiovascular, and thoracic disorders.

► Clinical Findings

Evaluation of the patient with persistent hiccups should include a detailed neurologic examination, serum creatinine, liver chemistry tests, and a chest radiograph. When the cause remains unclear, CT or MRI of the head, chest, and abdomen, echocardiography, and upper endoscopy may help.

► Treatment

A number of simple remedies may be helpful in patients with acute benign hiccups. (1) Irritation of the nasopharynx by tongue traction, lifting the uvula with a spoon, catheter stimulation of the nasopharynx, or eating 1 teaspoon (tsp) (7 g) of dry granulated sugar. (2) Interruption of the respiratory cycle by breath holding, Valsalva maneuver, sneezing, gasping (fright stimulus), or rebreathing into a bag. (3) Stimulation of the vagus by carotid massage. (4) Irritation of the diaphragm by holding knees to chest or by continuous positive airway pressure during mechanical ventilation. (5) Relief of gastric distention by belching or insertion of a nasogastric tube.

A number of drugs have been promoted as being useful in the treatment of hiccups. Chlorpromazine, 25–50 mg orally or intramuscularly, is most commonly used. Other agents reported to be effective include anticonvulsants (phenytoin, carbamazepine), benzodiazepines (lorazepam, diazepam), metoclopramide, baclofen, gabapentin, and occasionally general anesthesia.

Bredenoord AJ. Management of belching, hiccups, and aerophagia. Clin Gastroenterol Hepatol. 2013 Jan;11(1):6–12. [PMID: 22982101]

Moretto EN et al. Interventions for treating persistent and intractable hiccups in adults. Cochrane Database Syst Rev. 2013 Jan 31;1:CD008768. [PMID: 23440833]

CONSTIPATION

Constipation occurs in 15% of adults and up to one-third of elderly adults and is a common reason for seeking medical attention. It is more common in women. The elderly are predisposed due to comorbid medical conditions, medications, poor eating habits, decreased mobility and, in some cases, inability to sit on a toilet (bed-bound patients).

Table 15–3. Causes of constipation in adults.

Most common
Inadequate fiber or fluid intake
Poor bowel habits
Systemic disease
Endocrine: hypothyroidism, hyperparathyroidism, diabetes mellitus
Metabolic: hypokalemia, hypercalcemia, uremia, porphyria
Neurologic: Parkinson disease, multiple sclerosis, sacral nerve damage (prior pelvic surgery, tumor), paraplegia, autonomic neuropathy
Medications
Opioids
Diuretics
Calcium channel blockers
Anticholinergics
Psychotropics
Calcium and iron supplements
NSAIDs
Clonidine
Cholestyramine
Structural abnormalities
Anorectal: rectal prolapse, rectocele, rectal intussusception, anorectal stricture, anal fissure, solitary rectal ulcer syndrome
Perineal descent
Colonic mass with obstruction: adenocarcinoma
Colonic stricture: radiation, ischemia, diverticulosis
Hirschsprung disease
Idiopathic megarectum
Slow colonic transit
Idiopathic: isolated to colon
Psychogenic
Eating disorders
Chronic intestinal pseudo-obstruction
Pelvic floor dyssynergia
Irritable bowel syndrome

NSAIDs, nonsteroidal anti-inflammatory drugs.

The first step in evaluating the patient is to determine what is meant by "constipation." Patients may define constipation as infrequent stools (fewer than three in a week), hard stools, excessive straining, or a sense of incomplete evacuation. Table 15–3 summarizes the many causes of constipation, which are discussed below.

► **Etiology**

A. Primary Constipation

Most patients have constipation that cannot be attributed to any structural abnormalities or systemic disease. Some of these patients have normal colonic transit time; however, a subset have slow colonic transit or defecatory disorders. Normal colonic transit time is approximately 35 hours; more than 72 hours is significantly abnormal. Slow colonic transit is commonly idiopathic but may be part of a generalized gastrointestinal dysmotility syndrome. Patients may complain of infrequent bowel movements and abdominal bloating. Slow transit is more common in women, some of whom have a history of psychosocial problems (depression, anxiety, eating disorder, childhood trauma) or sexual abuse. Normal defecation requires coordination between relaxation of the anal sphincter and pelvic floor musculature while abdominal pressure is increased. Patients with defecatory disorders (also known dyssynergic defecation)—women more often than men—have impaired relaxation or paradoxical contraction of the anal sphincter and/or pelvic floor muscles during attempted defecation that impedes the bowel movement. This problem may be acquired during childhood or adulthood. Patients may complain of excessive straining, sense of incomplete evacuation, or need for digital manipulation. Patients with primary complaints of abdominal pain or bloating with alterations in bowel habits (constipation, or alternating constipation and diarrhea) may have irritable bowel syndrome.

B. Secondary Constipation

Constipation may be caused by systemic disorders, medications, or obstructing colonic lesions. Systemic disorders can cause constipation because of neurologic gut dysfunction, myopathies, endocrine disorders, or electrolyte abnormalities (eg, hypercalcemia or hypokalemia); medication side effects are often responsible (eg, anticholinergics or opioids). Colonic lesions that obstruct fecal passage, such as neoplasms and strictures, are an uncommon cause but important in new-onset constipation. Such lesions should be excluded in patients older than 50 years, in patients with "alarm" symptoms or signs (hematochezia, weight loss, anemia, or positive fecal occult blood tests [FOBT] or fecal immunochemical tests [FIT]), and in patients with a family history of colon cancer or inflammatory bowel disease. Defecatory difficulties also can be due to a variety of anorectal problems that impede or obstruct flow (perineal descent, rectal prolapse, rectocele), some of which may require surgery, and Hirschsprung disease (usually suggested by lifelong constipation).

► **Clinical Findings**

A. Symptoms and Signs

All patients should undergo a history and physical examination to distinguish primary from secondary causes of constipation. Physical examination should include digital rectal examination with assessment for anatomic abnormalities, such as anal stricture, rectocele, rectal prolapse, or perineal descent during straining as well as assessment of pelvic floor motion during simulated defecation (ie, the patient's ability to "expel the examiner's finger"). Further diagnostic tests should be performed in patients with any of the following: age 50 years or older, severe constipation, signs of an organic disorders, alarm symptoms (hematochezia, weight loss, positive FOBT or FIT), or a family history of colon cancer or inflammatory bowel disease. These tests should include laboratory studies (complete blood count; serum electrolytes, calcium, glucose, and thyroid-stimulating hormone) and a colonoscopy or flexible sigmoidoscopy.

B. Special Examinations

Patients with refractory constipation not responding to routine medical management warrant further diagnostic studies. Anorectal manometry including a balloon expulsion test should be performed first to evaluate for defecatory disorders. Inability to expel a balloon (attached to a 16F Foley catheter) filled with 50 mL of warm water within 2 minutes while sitting on a toilet is strongly suggestive of pelvic floor dyssenergia. Defecography to further assess pelvic floor function may be considered in selected patients. Subsequent colon transit studies are recommended only after defecatory disorders have been excluded. Colon transit time may be assessed by radiopaque markers, scintigraphy, or wireless motility capsule.

▶ **Treatment**

A. Chronic Constipation

1. Dietary and lifestyle measures—Adverse psychosocial issues should be identified and addressed. Patients should be instructed on normal defecatory function and optimal toileting habits, including regular timing, proper positioning, and abdominal pressure. Adequate dietary fluid and fiber intake should be emphasized. A trial of fiber supplements is recommended (Table 15–4). Increased dietary fiber may cause distention or flatulence,

Table 15–4. Pharmacologic management of constipation.

Agent	Dosage	Onset of Action	Comments
Fiber laxatives			
Bran powder	1–4 tbsp orally twice daily	Days	Inexpensive; may cause gas, flatulence
Psyllium	1 tsp once or twice daily	Days	(Metamucil; Perdiem)
Methylcellulose	1 tsp once or twice daily	Days	(Citrucel) Less gas, flatulence
Calcium polycarbophil	1 or 2 tablets once or twice daily	12–24 hours	(FiberCon) Does not cause gas; pill form
Guargum	1 tbsp once or twice daily	Days	(Benefiber) Non-gritty, tasteless, less gas
Stool surfactants			
Docusate sodium	100 mg once or twice daily	12–72 hours	(Colace) Marginal benefit
Mineral oil	15–45 mL once or twice daily	6–8 hours	May cause lipoid pneumonia if aspirated
Osmotic laxatives			
Magnesium hydroxide	15–30 mL orally once or twice daily	6–24 hours	(Milk of magnesia; Epsom salts)
Lactulose or 70% sorbitol	15–60 mL orally once daily to three times daily	6–48 hours	Cramps, bloating, flatulence
Polyethylene glycol (PEG 3350)	17 g in 8 oz liquid once or twice daily	6–24 hours	(Miralax) Less bloating than lactulose, sorbitol
Stimulant laxatives			
Bisacodyl	5–20 mg orally as needed	6–8 hours	May cause cramps; avoid daily use if possible
Bisacodyl suppository	10 mg per rectum as needed	1 hour	
Cascara	4–8 mL or 2 tablets as needed	8–12 hours	(Nature's Remedy) May cause cramps; avoid daily use if possible
Senna	8.6–17.2 mg orally as needed	8–12 hours	(ExLax; Senekot) May cause cramps; avoid daily use if possible
Lubiprostone	24 mcg orally twice daily	12–48 hours	Expensive; may cause nausea. Contraindicated in pregnancy
Linaclotide	145 mcg orally once daily		Expensive; contraindicated in pediatric patients
Enemas			
Tap water	500 mL per rectum	5–15 minutes	
Sodium phosphate enema	120 mL per rectum	5–15 minutes	Commonly used for acute constipation or to induce movement prior to medical procedures
Mineral oil enema	100–250 mL per rectum	5–15 minutes	To soften and lubricate fecal impaction
Agents used for acute purgative or to clean bowel prior to medical procedures			
Polyethylene glycol (PEG 3350)	4 L orally administered over 2–4 hours	< 4 hours	(GoLYTELY; CoLYTE; NuLYTE, MoviPrep) Used to cleanse bowel before colonoscopy
Magnesium citrate	10 oz orally	3–6 hours	Lemon-flavored

which often diminishes over several days. Response to fiber therapy is not immediate, and increases in dosage should be made gradually over 7–10 days. Fiber is most likely to benefit patients with normal colonic transit, but it may not benefit patients with colonic inertia, defecatory disorders, opioid-induced constipation, or irritable bowel syndrome; it may even exacerbate symptoms in these patients. Regular exercise is associated with a decreased risk of constipation. When possible, discontinue medications that may be causing or contributing to constipation. Probiotics are widely promoted to patients in direct advertising for treatment of constipation. A 2014 meta-analysis of randomized controlled trials suggests probiotics improve stool frequency and consistency; however, more study is needed.

2. Laxatives—Laxatives may be given on an intermittent or chronic basis for constipation that does not respond to dietary and lifestyle changes (Table 15–4). There is no evidence that long-term use of these agents is harmful.

A. Osmotic laxatives—Treatment usually is initiated with regular (daily) use of an osmotic laxative. Nonabsorbable osmotic agents increase secretion of water into the intestinal lumen, thereby softening stools and promoting defecation. Magnesium hydroxide, nondigestible carbohydrates (sorbitol, lactulose), and polyethylene glycol are all efficacious and safe for treating acute and chronic cases. The dosages are adjusted to achieve soft to semi-liquid movements. Magnesium-containing saline laxatives should not be given to patients with chronic renal insufficiency. Nondigestible carbohydrates may induce bloating, cramps, and flatulence. Polyethylene glycol 3350 (Miralax) is a component of solutions traditionally used for colonic lavage prior to colonoscopy and does not cause flatulence. When used in conventional doses, the onset of action of these osmotic agents is generally within 24 hours. For more rapid treatment of acute constipation, purgative laxatives may be used, such as magnesium citrate. Magnesium citrate may cause hypermagnesemia.

B. Stimulant laxatives—For patients with incomplete response to osmotic agents, stimulant laxatives may be prescribed as needed as a "rescue" agent or on a regular basis three or four times a week. These agents stimulate fluid secretion and colonic contraction, resulting in a bowel movement within 6–12 hours after oral ingestion or 15–60 minutes after rectal administration. Oral agents are usually administered once daily at bedtime. Common preparations include bisacodyl, senna, and cascara (Table 15–4).

C. Chloride secretory agents—Lubiprostone and linaclotide stimulate intestinal chloride secretion through activation of chloride channels or guanylcyclase C, respectively, resulting in increased intestinal fluid and accelerated colonic transit. In multicenter controlled trials, patients treated with lubiprostone 24 mcg orally twice daily or linaclotide 145 mcg once daily increased the number of bowel movements compared with patients treated with placebo. Because these agents are expensive, they should be reserved for patients who have suboptimal response or side effects with less expensive agents.

D. Opioid-receptor antagonists—Long-term use of opioids can cause constipation by inhibiting peristalsis and increasing intestinal fluid absorption. Methylnaltrexone is a mu-opioid receptor antagonist that blocks peripheral opioid receptors (including the gastrointestinal tract) without affecting central analgesia. It is approved for the treatment of opioid-induced constipation in patients receiving palliative care for advanced illness who have not responded to conventional laxative regimens. In controlled trials, methylnaltrexone subcutaneously (8 mg [38–62 kg], 12 mg [62–114 kg], or 0.15 mg/kg [less 38 kg] every other day) achieves laxation in 50% of patients compared with 15% of patients who received placebo.

B. Fecal Impaction

Severe impaction of stool in the rectal vault may result in obstruction to further fecal flow, leading to partial or complete large bowel obstruction. Predisposing factors include medications (eg, opioids), severe psychiatric disease, prolonged bed rest, neurogenic disorders of the colon, and spinal cord disorders. Clinical presentation includes decreased appetite, nausea and vomiting, and abdominal pain and distention. There may be paradoxical "diarrhea" as liquid stool leaks around the impacted feces. Firm feces are palpable on digital examination of the rectal vault. Initial treatment is directed at relieving the impaction with enemas (saline, mineral oil, or diatrizoate) or digital disruption of the impacted fecal material. Long-term care is directed at maintaining soft stools and regular bowel movements (as above).

▶ When to Refer

- Patients with refractory constipation for anorectal testing.
- Patients with defecatory disorders may benefit from biofeedback therapy.
- Patients with alarm symptoms or who are over age 50 should be referred for colonoscopy.
- Rarely, surgery (subtotal colectomy) is required for patients with severe colonic inertia.

American Gastroenterological Association medical position statement on constipation. Gastroenterology. 2013 Jan;144(1): 211–7. [PMID: 23261064]

ASGE Standards of Practice Committee; Cash BD et al. The role of endoscopy in the management of constipation. Gastrointest Endosc. 2014 Oct;80(4):563–5. [PMID: 25150599]

Bader S et al. Methylnaltrexone for the treatment of opioid-induced constipation. Expert Rev Gastroenterol Hepatol. 2013 Jan;7(1):13–26. [PMID: 23265145]

Chiarioni G et al. Validation of the balloon evacuation test: reproducibility and agreement with findings from anorectal manometry and electromyography. Clin Gastroenterol Hepatol. 2014 Dec;12(12):2049–54. [PMID: 24674941]

Dimidi E et al. The effect of probiotics on functional constipation in adults: a systematic review and meta-analysis of randomized controlled trials. Am J Clin Nutr. 2014 Oct;100(4): 1075–84. [PMID: 25099542]

Jamal MM et al. A randomized, placebo-controlled trial of lubiprostone for opioid-induced constipation in chronic noncancer pain. Am J Gastroenterol. 2015 May;110(5):725–32. [PMID: 25916220]

Jin J. JAMA patient page. Over-the-counter laxatives. JAMA. 2014 Sep 17;312(11):1167. [PMID: 25226492]

Shah BJ et al. In the clinic. Constipation. Ann Intern Med. 2015 Apr 7;162(7):ITC1. [PMID: 25845017]

Sugerman DT. JAMA patient page. Constipation. JAMA. 2013 Oct 2;310(13):1416. [PMID: 24084936]

GASTROINTESTINAL GAS

▶ Belching

Belching (eructation) is the involuntary or voluntary release of gas from the stomach or esophagus. It occurs most frequently after meals, when gastric distention results in transient lower esophageal sphincter (LES) relaxation. Belching is a normal reflex and does not itself denote gastrointestinal dysfunction. Virtually all stomach gas comes from swallowed air. With each swallow, 2–5 mL of air is ingested, and excessive amounts may result in distention, flatulence, and abdominal pain. This may occur with rapid eating, gum chewing, smoking, and the ingestion of carbonated beverages. Evaluation should be restricted to patients with other complaints such as dysphagia, heartburn, early satiety, or vomiting.

Chronic excessive belching is almost always caused by supragastric belching (voluntary diaphragmatic contraction, followed by upper esophageal relaxation with air inflow to the esophagus) or true air swallowing (aerophagia), both of which are behavioral disorders that are more common in patients with anxiety or psychiatric disorders. These patients may benefit from referral to a behavioral or speech therapist.

Kessing BF et al. The pathophysiology, diagnosis and treatment of excessive belching symptoms. Am J Gastroenterol. 2014 Aug;109(8):1196–203. [PMID: 25001253]

▶ Flatus

The rate and volume of expulsion of flatus is highly variable. Healthy adults pass flatus up to 20 times daily and excrete up to 750 mL. Flatus is derived from two sources: swallowed air (primarily nitrogen) and bacterial fermentation of undigested carbohydrate (which produces H_2, CO_2, and methane). A number of short-chain carbohydrates (fermentable oligosaccharides, disaccharides, monosaccharides, and polypols or "FODMAPS") are incompletely absorbed in the small intestine and pass into the colon. These include lactose (dairy products); fructose (fruits, corn syrups, and some sweeteners); polypols (stone-fruits, mushrooms, and some sweeteners); and fructans (legumes, cruciferous vegetables, pasta, and whole grains). Abnormal gas production may be caused by increased ingestion of these carbohydrates or, less commonly, by disorders of malabsorption. Foul odor may be caused by garlic, onion, eggplant, mushrooms, and certain herbs and spices.

Determining abnormal from normal amounts of flatus is difficult. Patients with a long-standing history of flatulence and no other symptoms or signs of malabsorption disorders can be treated conservatively. Gum chewing and carbonated beverages should be avoided to reduce air swallowing. Lactose intolerance may be assessed by a 2-week trial of a lactose-free diet or by a hydrogen breath test. A list of foods containing FODMAPS should be provided. Multiple low-FODMAP dietary guides are available; however, referral to a knowledgeable dietician may be helpful.

The nonprescription agent Beano (alpha-d-galactosidase enzyme) reduces gas caused by foods containing galacto-oligosaccharides (legumes, chickpeas, lentils) but not other FODMAPS. Activated charcoal may afford relief. Simethicone is of no proved benefit.

Complaints of chronic abdominal distention or bloating are common. Some of these patients may produce excess gas. However, many patients have impaired small bowel gas propulsion or enhanced visceral sensitivity to gas distention. Many of these patients have an underlying functional gastrointestinal disorder such as irritable bowel syndrome or functional dyspepsia. Reduction of dietary fat, which delays intestinal gas clearance, may be helpful. Rifaximin, 400 mg twice daily, a nonabsorbable oral antibiotic with high activity against enteric bacteria, has been shown to reduce abdominal bloating and flatulence in approximately 40% of treated patients compared with 20% of controls. Symptom improvement may be attributable to suppression of gas-producing colonic bacteria; however, relapse commonly occurs within days after stopping the antibiotic. Further trials are needed to clarify the role of nonabsorbable antibiotics in symptom management. Many patients report reduced flatus production with use of probiotics, although there has been limited controlled study of these agents for this purpose. Patients interested in complementary medical therapies may be offered a trial of 4–8 ounces daily of Kefir, a commercially available fermented milk drink containing multiple probiotics.

Manichanh C et al. Anal gas evacuation and colonic microbiota in patients with flatulence: effect of diet. Gut. 2014 Mar;63(3):401–8. [PMID: 23766444]

Shepherd SJ et al. Short-chain carbohydrates and functional gastrointestinal disorders. Am J Gastroenterol. 2013 May;108(5):707–17. [PMID: 23588241]

Sugerman DT. JAMA patient page. Abdominal bloating. JAMA. 2013 Oct 16;310(15):1637. [PMID: 24129477]

DIARRHEA

Diarrhea can range in severity from an acute self-limited episode to a severe, life-threatening illness. To properly evaluate the complaint, the clinician must determine the patient's normal bowel pattern and the nature of the current symptoms.

Approximately 10 L of fluid enter the duodenum daily, of which all but 1.5 L are absorbed by the small intestine. The colon absorbs most of the remaining fluid, with less than 200 mL lost in the stool. Although diarrhea sometimes is defined as a stool weight of more than 200–300 g/24 h, quantification of stool weight is necessary only in some patients with chronic diarrhea. In most cases, the physician's working definition of diarrhea is increased stool frequency (more than three bowel movements per day) or liquidity of feces.

The causes of diarrhea are myriad. In clinical practice, it is helpful to distinguish acute from chronic diarrhea, as the evaluation and treatment are entirely different (Tables 15–5 and 15–6).

Table 15–5. Causes of acute infectious diarrhea.

Noninflammatory Diarrhea	Inflammatory Diarrhea
Viral	**Viral**
Noroviruses	Cytomegalovirus
Rotavirus	
Protozoal	**Protozoal**
Giardia lamblia	Entamoeba histolytica
Cryptosporidium	
Cyclospora	
Bacterial	**Bacterial**
1. Preformed enterotoxin production	1. Cytotoxin production
Staphylococcus aureus	Enterohemorrhagic E coli O157:H5 (EHEC)
Bacillus cereus	Vibrio parahaemolyticus
Clostridium perfringens	Clostridium difficile
2. Enterotoxin production	2. Mucosal invasion
Enterotoxigenic E coli (ETEC)	Shigella
Vibrio cholerae	Campylobacter jejuni
	Salmonella
	Enteroinvasive E coli (EIEC)
	Aeromonas
	Plesiomonas
	Yersinia enterocolitica
	Chlamydia
	Neisseria gonorrhoeae
	Listeria monocytogenes

1. Acute Diarrhea

ESSENTIALS OF DIAGNOSIS

▶ Diarrhea of less than 2 weeks' duration is most commonly caused by invasive or noninvasive pathogens and their enterotoxins.

Acute noninflammatory diarrhea

▶ Watery, nonbloody.

▶ Usually mild, self-limited.

▶ Caused by a virus or noninvasive bacteria.

▶ Diagnostic evaluation is limited to patients with diarrhea that is severe or persists beyond 7 days.

Acute inflammatory diarrhea

▶ Blood or pus, fever.

▶ Usually caused by an invasive or toxin-producing bacterium.

▶ Diagnostic evaluation requires routine stool bacterial cultures (including E coli O157:H7) in all and testing as clinically indicated for Clostridium difficile toxin, and ova and parasites.

Table 15–6. Causes of chronic diarrhea.

Osmotic diarrhea
  CLUES: Stool volume decreases with fasting; increased stool osmotic gap
    1. Medications: antacids, lactulose, sorbitol
    2. Disaccharidase deficiency: lactose intolerance
    3. Factitious diarrhea: magnesium (antacids, laxatives)
Secretory diarrhea
  CLUES: Large volume (> 1 L/day); little change with fasting; normal stool osmotic gap
    1. Hormonally mediated: VIPoma, carcinoid, medullary carcinoma of thyroid (calcitonin), Zollinger-Ellison syndrome (gastrin)
    2. Factitious diarrhea (laxative abuse); phenolphthalein, cascara, senna
    3. Villous adenoma
    4. Bile salt malabsorption (idiopathic, ileal resection; Crohn ileitis; postcholecystectomy)
    5. Medications
Inflammatory conditions
  CLUES: Fever, hematochezia, abdominal pain
    1. Ulcerative colitis
    2. Crohn disease
    3. Microscopic colitis
    4. Malignancy: lymphoma, adenocarcinoma (with obstruction and pseudodiarrhea)
    5. Radiation enteritis
Medications
  Common offenders: SSRIs, cholinesterase inhibitors, NSAIDs, proton pump inhibitors, angiotensin II receptor blockers, metformin, allopurinol

Malabsorption syndromes
  CLUES: Weight loss, abnormal laboratory values; fecal fat > 10 g/24h
    1. Small bowel mucosal disorders: celiac sprue, tropical sprue, Whipple disease, eosinophilic gastroenteritis, small bowel resection (short bowel syndrome), Crohn disease
    2. Lymphatic obstruction: lymphoma, carcinoid, infectious (tuberculosis, MAI), Kaposi sarcoma, sarcoidosis, retroperitoneal fibrosis
    3. Pancreatic disease: chronic pancreatitis, pancreatic carcinoma
    4. Bacterial overgrowth: motility disorders (diabetes, vagotomy), scleroderma, fistulas, small intestinal diverticula
Motility disorders
  CLUES: Systemic disease or prior abdominal surgery
    1. Postsurgical: vagotomy, partial gastrectomy, blind loop with bacterial overgrowth
    2. Systemic disorders: scleroderma, diabetes mellitus, hyperthyroidism
    3. Irritable bowel syndrome
Chronic infections
    1. Parasites: Giardia lamblia, Entamoeba histolytica, Strongyloidiasis stercoralis, Capillaria philippinensis
    2. AIDS-related:
      Viral: Cytomegalovirus, HIV infection (?)
      Bacterial: Clostridium difficile, Mycobacterium avium complex
      Protozoal: Microsporida (Enterocytozoon bieneusi), Cryptosporidium, Isospora belli
Factitious
  See Osmotic and Secretory diarrhea above

MAI, Mycobacterium avium-intracellulare; NSAIDs, nonsteroidal anti-inflammatory drugs; SSRIs, selective serotonin reuptake inhibitors.

► Etiology & Clinical Findings

Diarrhea acute in onset and persisting for less than 2 weeks is most commonly caused by infectious agents, bacterial toxins (either preformed or produced in the gut), or medications. Community outbreaks (including nursing homes, schools, cruise ships) suggest a viral etiology or a common food source. Similar recent illnesses in family members suggest an infectious origin. Ingestion of improperly stored or prepared food implicates food poisoning. Pregnant women have an increased risk of developing listeriosis. Day care attendance or exposure to unpurified water (camping, swimming) may result in infection with *Giardia* or *Cryptosporidium*. Large *Cyclospora* outbreaks have been traced to contaminated produce. Recent travel abroad suggests "traveler's diarrhea" (see Chapter 30). Antibiotic administration within the preceding several weeks increases the likelihood of *C difficile* colitis. Finally, risk factors for HIV infection or sexually transmitted diseases should be determined. (AIDS-associated diarrhea is discussed in Chapter 31; infectious proctitis is discussed in this chapter under Anorectal Disorders.) Persons engaging in anal intercourse or oral-anal sexual activities are at risk for a variety of infections that cause proctitis, including gonorrhea, syphilis, lymphogranuloma venereum, and herpes simplex.

The nature of the diarrhea helps distinguish among different infectious causes (Table 15–5).

A. Noninflammatory Diarrhea

Watery, nonbloody diarrhea associated with periumbilical cramps, bloating, nausea, or vomiting suggests a small bowel source caused by either a toxin-producing bacterium (enterotoxigenic *E coli* [ETEC], *Staphylococcus aureus, Bacillus cereus, Clostridium perfringens*) or other agents (viruses, *Giardia*) that disrupt normal absorption and secretory process in the small intestine. Prominent vomiting suggests viral enteritis or *S aureus* food poisoning. Although typically mild, the diarrhea (which originates in the small intestine) can be voluminous and result in dehydration with hypokalemia and metabolic acidosis (eg, cholera). Because tissue invasion does not occur, fecal leukocytes are not present.

B. Inflammatory Diarrhea

The presence of fever and bloody diarrhea (dysentery) indicates colonic tissue damage caused by invasion (shigellosis, salmonellosis, *Campylobacter* or *Yersinia* infection, amebiasis) or a toxin (*C difficile*, Shiga-toxin–producing *E coli* [STEC; also known as enterohemorrhagic *E coli*]). Because these organisms predominantly involve the colon, the diarrhea is small in volume (less than 1 L/day) and associated with left lower quadrant cramps, urgency, and tenesmus. Fecal leukocytes or lactoferrin usually are present in infections with invasive organisms. *E coli* O157:H7 is a Shiga-toxin–producing noninvasive organism most commonly acquired from contaminated meat that has resulted in several outbreaks of an acute, often severe hemorrhagic colitis. In 2011, an outbreak of severe gastroenteritis in Germany,

caused by an unusual Shiga-toxin–producing strain, *E coli* O104:H4, was traced to contaminated sprouts. A major complication of STEC is hemolytic-uremic syndrome, which develops in 6–22% of cases. In immunocompromised and HIV-infected patients, cytomegalovirus (CMV) can cause intestinal ulceration with watery or bloody diarrhea.

Infectious dysentery must be distinguished from acute ulcerative colitis, which may also present acutely with fever, abdominal pain, and bloody diarrhea. Diarrhea that persists for more than 14 days is not attributable to bacterial pathogens (except for *C difficile*) and should be evaluated as chronic diarrhea.

► Evaluation

In over 90% of patients with acute noninflammatory diarrhea, the illness is mild and self-limited, responding within 5 days to simple rehydration therapy or antidiarrheal agents; diagnostic investigation is unnecessary.

The isolation rate of bacterial pathogens from stool cultures in patients with acute noninflammatory diarrhea is under 3%. Thus, the goal of initial evaluation is to distinguish patients with mild disease from those with more serious illness. If diarrhea worsens or persists for more than 7 days, stool should be sent for fecal leukocyte or lactoferrin determination, ovum and parasite evaluation, and bacterial culture.

Prompt medical evaluation is indicated in the following situations (Figure 15–1): (1) Signs of inflammatory diarrhea manifested by any of the following: fever (higher than 38.5°C), WBC 15,000/mcL or more, bloody diarrhea, or severe abdominal pain. (2) The passage of six or more unformed stools in 24 hours. (3) Profuse watery diarrhea and dehydration. (4) Frail older patients or nursing home residents. (5) Immunocompromised patients (AIDS, post-transplantation). (6) Exposure to antibiotics. (7) Hospital-acquired diarrhea (onset following at least 3 days of hospitalization). (8) Systemic illness.

Physical examination pays note to the patient's level of hydration, mental status, and the presence of abdominal tenderness or peritonitis. Peritoneal findings may be present in infection with *C difficile* or STEC. Hospitalization is required in patients with severe dehydration, organ failure, marked abdominal pain, or altered mental status. Stool specimens should be sent for examination for routine bacterial cultures.

The rate of positive bacterial cultures in such patients is 60–75%. For bloody stools, the laboratory should be directed to perform serotyping for Shiga-toxin–producing *E coli*. Special culture media are required for *Yersinia, Vibrio*, and *Aeromonas*. In patients who are hospitalized or who have a history of antibiotic exposure, a stool sample should be tested for *C difficile* toxin.

In patients with diarrhea that persists for more than 10 days, who have a history of travel to areas where amebiasis is endemic, or who engage in oral-anal sexual practices, three stool examinations for ova and parasites should also be performed. The stool antigen detection tests for both *Giardia* and *Entamoeba histolytica* are more sensitive than stool microscopy for detection of these organisms. A serum

Acute diarrhea (≤ 7 days)

Are the following present?
1. Severe illness: T > 38.5°C, abdominal pain,
   bloody diarrhea, > 6 stools/24 h, dehydration
2. Immunocompromised patient: AIDS, posttransplantation
3. Elderly patient (> 70 yrs)

No ◄──────────────────► Yes

Symptomatic therapy
Antidiarrheal agents: loperamide,
bismuth subsalicylate

Illness resolves

Illness persists for 7–10
days or worsens

Send stool for following:
1. Fecal leukocytes
2. Routine stool culture
3. *C difficile* assay, if recent hospitalization or antibiotics
4. Ova and parasite testing, if:
   a. Diarrhea > 10 days
   b. Travel to endemic region
   c. Community water-borne outbreak
   d. HIV infection or men who have sex with men

&

Consider empiric antibiotic therapy while awaiting
culture, if:
1. Fecal leukocyte positive
2. Bloody diarrhea, fever, abdominal pain
3. Dehydration or > 8 stools/24 h
4. Immunocompromised
5. Hospitalization required

▲ **Figure 15–1.** Evaluation of acute diarrhea.

antigen detection test for *E histolytica* is also available. *Cyclospora* and *Cryptosporidium* are detected by fecal acid-fast staining.

▶ Treatment

A. Diet

Most mild diarrhea will not lead to dehydration provided the patient takes adequate oral fluids containing carbohydrates and electrolytes. Patients find it more comfortable to rest the bowel by avoiding high-fiber foods, fats, milk products, caffeine, and alcohol. Frequent feedings of tea, "flat" carbonated beverages, and soft, easily digested foods (eg, soups, crackers, bananas, apple sauce, rice, toast) are encouraged.

B. Rehydration

In more severe diarrhea, dehydration can occur quickly, especially in children, the frail, and the elderly. Oral rehydration with fluids containing glucose, Na⁺, K⁺, Cl⁻, and bicarbonate or citrate is preferred when feasible. A convenient mixture is ½ tsp salt (3.5 g), 1 tsp baking soda (2.5 g $NaHCO_3$), 8 tsp sugar (40 g), and 8 oz orange juice (1.5 g KCl), diluted to 1 L with water. Alternatively, oral electrolyte solutions (eg, Pedialyte, Gatorade) are readily available.

Fluids should be given at rates of 50–200 mL/kg/24 h depending on the hydration status. Intravenous fluids (lactated Ringer injection) are preferred in patients with severe dehydration.

C. Antidiarrheal Agents

Antidiarrheal agents may be used safely in patients with mild to moderate diarrheal illnesses to improve patient comfort. Opioid agents help decrease the stool number and liquidity and control fecal urgency. However, they should not be used in patients with bloody diarrhea, high fever, or systemic toxicity and should be discontinued in patients whose diarrhea is worsening despite therapy. With these provisos, such drugs provide excellent symptomatic relief. Loperamide is preferred, in a dosage of 4 mg orally initially, followed by 2 mg after each loose stool (maximum: 16 mg/24 h).

Bismuth subsalicylate (Pepto-Bismol), two tablets or 30 mL orally four times daily, reduces symptoms in patients with traveler's diarrhea by virtue of its anti-inflammatory and antibacterial properties. It also reduces vomiting associated with viral enteritis. Anticholinergic agents (eg, diphenoxylate with atropine) are contraindicated in acute diarrhea because of the rare precipitation of toxic megacolon.

D. Antibiotic Therapy

1. Empiric treatment—Empiric antibiotic treatment of all patients with acute diarrhea is not indicated. Even patients with inflammatory diarrhea caused by invasive pathogens usually have symptoms that will resolve within several days without antimicrobials. Empiric treatment may be considered in patients with non–hospital-acquired diarrhea with moderate to severe fever, tenesmus, or bloody stools or the presence of fecal lactoferrin while the stool bacterial culture is incubating, provided that infection with STEC is not suspected. It should also be considered in patients who are immunocompromised or who have significant dehydration. The oral drugs of choice for empiric treatment are the fluoroquinolones (eg, ciprofloxacin 500 mg, ofloxacin 400 mg, or norfloxacin 400 mg, twice daily, or levofloxacin 500 mg once daily) for 5–7 days. Alternatives include trimethoprim-sulfamethoxazole, 160/800 mg twice daily; or doxycycline, 100 mg twice daily. Macrolides and penicillins are no longer recommended because of widespread microbial resistance to these agents. Rifaximin, a nonabsorbed oral antibiotic, 200 mg three times daily for 3 days, is approved for empiric treatment of noninflammatory traveler's diarrhea (see Chapter 30).

2. Specific antimicrobial treatment—Antibiotics are not recommended in patients with nontyphoid *Salmonella*, *Campylobacter*, Shiga-toxin–producing *E coli*, *Aeromonas*, or *Yersinia*, except in severe disease, because they do not hasten recovery or reduce the period of fecal bacterial excretion. The infectious diarrheas for which treatment is recommended are shigellosis, cholera, extraintestinal salmonellosis, listeriosis, traveler's diarrhea, *C difficile* infection, giardiasis, and amebiasis. Therapy for traveler's diarrhea, infectious (sexually transmitted) proctitis, and AIDS-related diarrhea is presented in other chapters of this book.

► When to Admit

- Severe dehydration for intravenous fluids, especially if vomiting or unable to maintain sufficient oral fluid intake.
- Bloody diarrhea that is severe or worsening in order to distinguish infectious versus noninfectious cause.
- Severe abdominal pain, worrisome for toxic colitis, inflammatory bowel disease, intestinal ischemia, or surgical abdomen.
- Signs of severe infection or sepsis (temperature higher than 39.5°C, leukocytosis, rash).
- Severe or worsening diarrhea in patients who are older than 70 years or immunocompromised.
- Signs of hemolytic-uremic syndrome (acute kidney injury, thrombocytopenia, hemolytic anemia).

DuPont HL. Acute infectious diarrhea in immunocompetent adults. N Engl J Med. 2014 Apr 17;370(16):1532–40. [PMID: 24738670]

2. Chronic Diarrhea

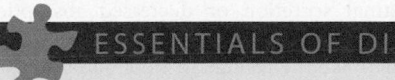

ESSENTIALS OF DIAGNOSIS

► Diarrhea present for longer than 4 weeks.
► Before embarking on extensive work-up, common causes should be excluded, including medications, chronic infections, and irritable bowel syndrome.

► Etiology

The causes of chronic diarrhea may be grouped into the following major pathophysiologic categories: medications, osmotic diarrheas, secretory conditions, inflammatory conditions, malabsorptive conditions, motility disorders, chronic infections, and systemic disorders (Table 15–6).

A. Medications

Numerous medications can cause diarrhea. Common offenders include cholinesterase inhibitors, SSRIs, angiotensin II-receptor blockers, proton pump inhibitors, NSAIDs, metformin, allopurinol, and orlistat. All medications should be carefully reviewed, and discontinuation of potential culprits should be considered.

B. Osmotic Diarrheas

As stool leaves the colon, fecal osmolality is equal to the serum osmolality, ie, approximately 290 mOsm/kg. Under normal circumstances, the major osmoles are Na^+, K^+, Cl^-, and HCO_3^-. The stool osmolality may be estimated by multiplying the stool $(Na^+ + K^+) \times 2$. The **osmotic gap** is the difference between the *measured* osmolality of the stool (or serum) and the *estimated* stool osmolality and is normally less than 50 mOsm/kg. An increased osmotic gap (greater than 75 mOsm/kg) implies that the diarrhea is caused by ingestion or malabsorption of an osmotically active substance. The most common causes are carbohydrate malabsorption (lactose, fructose, sorbitol), laxative abuse, and malabsorption syndromes. Osmotic diarrheas resolve during fasting. Those caused by malabsorbed carbohydrates are characterized by abdominal distention, bloating, and flatulence due to increased colonic gas production.

Carbohydrate malabsorption is common and should be considered in all patients with chronic, postprandial diarrhea. Patients should be asked about their intake of dairy products (lactose), fruits and artificial sweeteners (fructose and sorbitol), and alcohol. The diagnosis of carbohydrate malabsorption may be established by an elimination trial for 2–3 weeks or by hydrogen breath tests.

Ingestion of magnesium- or phosphate-containing compounds (laxatives, antacids) should be considered in enigmatic chronic diarrhea. The fat substitute olestra also causes diarrhea and cramps in occasional patients.

C. Secretory Conditions

Increased intestinal secretion or decreased absorption results in a high-volume watery diarrhea with a normal osmotic gap. There is little change in stool output during the fasting state, and dehydration and electrolyte imbalance may develop. Causes include endocrine tumors (stimulating intestinal or pancreatic secretion) and bile salt malabsorption (stimulating colonic secretion).

D. Inflammatory Conditions

Diarrhea is present in most patients with inflammatory bowel disease (ulcerative colitis, Crohn disease). A variety of other symptoms may be present, including abdominal pain, fever, weight loss, and hematochezia. Microscopic colitis is a common cause of chronic watery diarrhea in the elderly (see Inflammatory Bowel Disease, below).

E. Malabsorptive Conditions

The major causes of malabsorption are small mucosal intestinal diseases, intestinal resections, lymphatic obstruction, small intestinal bacterial overgrowth, and pancreatic insufficiency. Its characteristics are weight loss, osmotic diarrhea, steatorrhea, and nutritional deficiencies. Significant diarrhea in the absence of weight loss is not likely to be due to malabsorption. The physical and laboratory abnormalities related to deficiencies of vitamins or minerals are discussed in Chapter 29.

F. Motility Disorders (Including Irritable Bowel Syndrome)

Irritable bowel syndrome is the most common cause of chronic diarrhea in young adults (see Irritable Bowel Syndrome). It should be considered in patients with lower abdominal pain and altered bowel habits who have no other evidence of serious organic disease (weight loss, nocturnal diarrhea, anemia, or gastrointestinal bleeding). Abnormal intestinal motility secondary to systemic disorders or surgery may result in diarrhea due to rapid transit or to stasis of intestinal contents with bacterial overgrowth, resulting in malabsorption.

G. Chronic Infections

Chronic parasitic infections may cause diarrhea through a number of mechanisms. Pathogens most commonly associated with diarrhea include the protozoans *Giardia, E histolytica*, and *Cyclospora* as well as the intestinal nematodes. Strongyloidiasis and capillariasis should be excluded in patients from endemic regions, especially in the presence of eosinophilia. Bacterial infections with *C difficile* and, uncommonly, *Aeromonas* and *Plesiomonas* may cause chronic diarrhea.

Immunocompromised patients are susceptible to infectious organisms that can cause acute or chronic diarrhea (see Chapter 31), including Microsporida, *Cryptosporidium*, CMV, *Isospora belli, Cyclospora*, and *Mycobacterium avium* complex.

H. Systemic Conditions

Chronic systemic conditions, such as thyroid disease, diabetes, and collagen vascular disorders, may cause diarrhea through alterations in motility or intestinal absorption.

▶ Clinical Findings

The history and physical examination commonly suggest the underlying pathophysiology that guides the subsequent diagnostic work-up (Figure 15–2). The clinician should establish whether the diarrhea is continuous or intermittent, its relationship to meals, and whether it occurs at night or during fasting. The stool appearance may suggest a malabsorption disorder (greasy or malodorous), inflammatory disorder (containing blood or pus), or a secretory process (watery). The presence of abdominal pain suggests irritable bowel syndrome or inflammatory bowel disease. Medications, diet, and recent psychosocial stressors should be reviewed. Physical examination should assess for signs of malnutrition, dehydration, and inflammatory bowel disease.

Because chronic diarrhea is caused by so many conditions, the subsequent diagnostic approach is guided by the relative suspicion for the underlying cause, and no specific algorithm can be followed in all patients. Prior to embarking on an extensive evaluation, the most common causes of chronic diarrhea should be considered, including medications, irritable bowel syndrome, and lactose intolerance. The presence of nocturnal diarrhea, weight loss, anemia, or positive results on FOBT are inconsistent with these disorders and warrant further evaluation. AIDS-associated diarrhea is discussed in Chapter 31.

A. Initial Diagnostic Tests

1. Routine laboratory tests—Complete blood count, serum electrolytes, liver function tests, calcium, phosphorus, albumin, thyroid-stimulating hormone, vitamin A and D levels, INR, erythrocyte sedimentation rate, and C-reactive protein should be obtained in most patients. Serologic testing for celiac disease with an IgA tissue transglutaminase (tTG) test may be recommended in the evaluation of most patients with chronic diarrhea and all patients with signs of malabsorption. Anemia occurs in malabsorption syndromes (folate, iron deficiency, or vitamin B_{12}) as well as inflammatory conditions. Hypoalbuminemia is present in malabsorption, protein-losing enteropathies, and inflammatory diseases. Hyponatremia and nonanion gap metabolic acidosis occur in secretory diarrheas. Increased erythrocyte sedimentation rate or C-reactive protein suggests inflammatory bowel disease.

2. Routine stool studies—Stool sample should be analyzed for ova and parasites, electrolytes (to calculate osmotic gap), qualitative staining for fat (Sudan stain), occult blood, and leukocytes or lactoferrin. The presence of *Giardia* and *E histolytica* may be detected in wet mounts. However, fecal antigen detection tests for *Giardia* and *E histolytica* are a more sensitive and specific method of detection. *Cryptosporidium* and *Cyclospora* are found with modified acid-fast staining. As discussed previously,

▲ Figure 15–2. Decision diagram for diagnosis of causes of chronic diarrhea.

an increased osmotic gap suggests an osmotic diarrhea or disorder of malabsorption. A positive fecal fat stain suggests a disorder of malabsorption. The presence of fecal leukocytes or lactoferrin may suggest inflammatory bowel disease.

3. Endoscopic examination and mucosal biopsy—Most patients with chronic persistent diarrhea undergo colonoscopy with mucosal biopsy to exclude inflammatory bowel disease (including Crohn disease and ulcerative colitis), microscopic colitis, and colonic neoplasia. Upper endoscopy with small bowel biopsy is performed when a small intestinal malabsorptive disorder is suspected (celiac disease, Whipple disease) from abnormal laboratory studies or a positive fecal fat stain. It may also be done in patients with advanced AIDS to document *Cryptosporidium*, Microsporida, and *M avium-intracellulare* infection.

B. Further Studies

If the cause of diarrhea is still not apparent, further studies may be warranted.

1. 24-hour stool collection quantification of total weight and fat—A stool weight of less than 200–300 g/24 h excludes diarrhea and suggests a functional disorder such as irritable bowel syndrome. A weight greater than 1000–1500 g suggests a significant secretory process, including neuroendocrine tumors. A fecal fat determination in excess of 10 g/24 h confirms a malabsorptive disorder. Fecal elastase less than 100 mcg/g may be caused by pancreatic insufficiency. (See Celiac Disease and specific tests for malabsorption, below.)

2. Other imaging studies—Calcification on a plain abdominal radiograph confirms a diagnosis of chronic pancreatitis, although abdominal CT and endoscopic ultrasonography are more sensitive for the diagnosis of chronic pancreatitis as well as pancreatic cancer. Small intestinal imaging with barium, CT, or MRI is helpful in the diagnosis of Crohn disease, small bowel lymphoma, carcinoid, and jejunal diverticula. Neuroendocrine tumors may be localized using somatostatin receptor scintigraphy. Retention of less than 11% at 7 days of intravenous 75Se-homotaurocholate on scintigraphy suggests bile salt malabsorption.

3. Laboratory tests—

A. SEROLOGIC TESTS FOR NEUROENDOCRINE TUMORS— Secretory diarrheas due to neuroendocrine tumors are rare but should be considered in patients with chronic, high-volume watery diarrhea (greater than 1 L/day) with a normal osmotic gap that persists during fasting. Measurements of the secretagogues of various neuroendocrine tumors may be assayed, including serum chromogranin A, vasoactive intestinal peptide (VIP) (VIPoma), calcitonin (medullary thyroid carcinoma), gastrin (Zollinger-Ellison syndrome), and urinary 5-hydroxyindoleacetic acid (5-HIAA) (carcinoid).

B. BREATH TEST—The diagnosis of small bowel bacterial overgrowth is confirmed with noninvasive breath tests (glucose or lactulose) or by obtaining an aspirate of small intestinal contents for quantitative aerobic and anaerobic bacterial culture.

▶ Treatment

A number of antidiarrheal agents may be used in certain patients with chronic diarrheal conditions and are listed below. Opioids are safe in most patients with chronic, stable symptoms.

Loperamide: 4 mg orally initially, then 2 mg after each loose stool (maximum: 16 mg/day).

Diphenoxylate with atropine: One tablet orally three or four times daily as needed.

Codeine and deodorized tincture of opium: Because of potential habituation, these drugs are avoided except in cases of chronic, intractable diarrhea. Codeine may be given in a dosage of 15–60 mg orally every 4 hours; tincture of opium, 0.3–1.2 mL orally every 6 hours as needed.

Clonidine: Alpha-2-adrenergic agonists inhibit intestinal electrolyte secretion. Clonidine, 0.1–0.3 mg orally twice daily, or a clonidine patch, 0.1–0.2 mg/day, may help in some patients with secretory diarrheas, diabetic diarrhea, or cryptosporidiosis.

Octreotide: This somatostatin analog stimulates intestinal fluid and electrolyte absorption and inhibits intestinal fluid secretion and the release of gastrointestinal peptides. It is given for secretory diarrheas due to neuroendocrine tumors (VIPomas, carcinoid). Effective doses range from 50 mcg to 250 mcg subcutaneously three times daily.

Bile salt binders: Cholestyramine or colestipol (2–4 g once to three times daily) or colesevelam (625 mg, 1–3 tablets once or twice daily) may be useful in patients with bile salt-induced diarrhea, which may be idiopathic or secondary to intestinal resection or ileal disease.

Li Z et al. Treatment of chronic diarrhea. Best Pract Res Clin Gastroenterol. 2012 Oct;26(5):677–87. [PMID: 23384811]

Money ME et al. Review: management of postprandial diarrhea syndrome. Am J Med. 2012 Jun;125(6):538–44. [PMID: 22624684]

Schiller LR. Definitions, pathophysiology, and evaluation of chronic diarrhoea. Best Pract Res Clin Gastroenterol. 2012 Oct; 26(5):551–62. [PMID: 23384801]

GASTROINTESTINAL BLEEDING

1. Acute Upper Gastrointestinal Bleeding

ESSENTIALS OF DIAGNOSIS

▶ Hematemesis (bright red blood or "coffee grounds").

▶ Melena in most cases; hematochezia in massive upper gastrointestinal bleeds.

▶ Volume status to determine severity of blood loss; hematocrit is a poor early indicator of blood loss.

▶ Endoscopy diagnostic and may be therapeutic.

▶ General Considerations

There are over 250,000 hospitalizations a year in the United States for acute upper gastrointestinal bleeding. In the United States, the mortality rate for nonvariceal upper gastrointestinal bleeding has declined steadily over the past 20 years to 2.1% in 2009. Mortality is higher in patients who are older than 60 years and in patients in whom bleeding develops during hospitalization. Patients seldom die of exsanguination but rather of complications from an underlying disease.

The most common presentation of upper gastrointestinal bleeding is hematemesis or melena. Hematemesis may be either bright red blood or brown "coffee grounds" material. Melena develops after as little as 50–100 mL of blood loss in the upper gastrointestinal tract, whereas hematochezia requires a loss of more than 1000 mL. Although hematochezia generally suggests a lower bleeding source (eg, colonic), severe upper gastrointestinal bleeding may present with hematochezia in 10% of cases.

Upper gastrointestinal bleeding is self-limited in 80% of patients; urgent medical therapy and endoscopic evaluation are obligatory in the rest. Patients with bleeding more than 48 hours prior to presentation have a low risk of recurrent bleeding.

▶ Etiology

Acute upper gastrointestinal bleeding may originate from a number of sources. These are listed in order of their frequency and discussed in detail below.

A. Peptic Ulcer Disease

Peptic ulcers account for 40% of major upper gastrointestinal bleeding with an overall mortality rate of less than 5%. In North America, the incidence of bleeding from ulcers is declining due to eradication of *H pylori* and prophylaxis with proton pump inhibitors in high-risk patients.

B. Portal Hypertension

Portal hypertension accounts for 10–20% of upper gastrointestinal bleeding. Bleeding usually arises from esophageal varices and less commonly gastric or duodenal varices or portal hypertensive gastropathy. Approximately 25% of patients with cirrhosis have medium to large esophageal varices, of whom 30% experience acute variceal bleeding within a 2-year period. Due to improved care, the hospital mortality rate has declined over the past 20 years from 40% to 15%. Nevertheless, a mortality rate of 60–80% is expected at 1–4 years due to recurrent bleeding or other complications of chronic liver disease.

C. Mallory-Weiss Tears

Lacerations of the gastroesophageal junction cause 5–10% of cases of upper gastrointestinal bleeding. Many patients report a history of heavy alcohol use or retching. Less than 10% have continued or recurrent bleeding.

D. Vascular Anomalies

Vascular anomalies are found throughout the gastrointestinal tract and may be the source of chronic or acute gastrointestinal bleeding. They account for 7% of cases of acute upper tract bleeding. The most common are **angioectasias** (angiodysplasias) which are 1–10 mm distorted, aberrant submucosal vessels caused by chronic, intermittent obstruction of submucosal veins. They have a bright red stellate appearance and occur throughout the gastrointestinal tract but most commonly in the right colon. **Telangiectasias** are small, cherry red lesions caused by dilation of venules that may be part of systemic conditions (hereditary hemorrhagic telangiectasia, CREST syndrome) or occur sporadically. The **Dieulafoy lesion** is an aberrant, large-caliber submucosal artery, most commonly in the proximal stomach that causes recurrent, intermittent bleeding.

E. Gastric Neoplasms

Gastric neoplasms result in 1% of upper gastrointestinal hemorrhages.

F. Erosive Gastritis

Because this process is superficial, it is a relatively unusual cause of severe gastrointestinal bleeding (less than 5% of cases) and more commonly results in chronic blood loss. Gastric mucosal erosions are due to NSAIDs, alcohol, or severe medical or surgical illness (stress-related mucosal disease).

G. Erosive Esophagitis

Severe erosive esophagitis due to chronic gastroesophageal reflux may rarely cause significant upper gastrointestinal bleeding, especially in patients who are bed bound long-term.

H. Others

An aortoenteric fistula complicates 2% of abdominal aortic grafts or, rarely, can occur as the initial presentation of a previously untreated aneurysm. Unusual causes of upper gastrointestinal bleeding include hemobilia (from hepatic tumor, angioma, penetrating trauma), pancreatic malignancy, and pseudoaneurysm (hemosuccus pancreaticus).

▶ Initial Evaluation & Treatment

A. Stabilization

The initial step is assessment of the hemodynamic status. A systolic blood pressure lower than 100 mm Hg identifies a high-risk patient with severe acute bleeding. A heart rate over 100 beats/min with a systolic blood pressure over 100 mm Hg signifies moderate acute blood loss. A normal systolic blood pressure and heart rate suggest relatively minor hemorrhage. Postural hypotension and tachycardia are useful when present but may be due to causes other than blood loss. Because the hematocrit may take 24–72 hours to equilibrate with the extravascular fluid, it is not a reliable indicator of the severity of acute bleeding.

In patients with significant bleeding, two 18-gauge or larger intravenous lines should be started prior to further diagnostic tests. Blood is sent for complete blood count, prothrombin time with international normalized ratio (INR), serum creatinine, liver enzymes, and blood typing and screening (in anticipation of the possible need for transfusion). In patients without hemodynamic compromise or overt active bleeding, aggressive fluid repletion can be delayed until the extent of the bleeding is further clarified. Patients with evidence of hemodynamic compromise are given 0.9% saline or lactated Ringer injection and cross-matched for 2–4 units of packed red blood cells. It is rarely necessary to administer type-specific or O-negative blood. Central venous pressure monitoring is desirable in some cases, but line placement should not interfere with rapid volume resuscitation.

Placement of a nasogastric tube is not routinely needed but may be helpful in the initial assessment and triage of selected patients with suspected active upper tract bleeding. The aspiration of red blood or "coffee grounds" confirms an upper gastrointestinal source of bleeding, though up to 18% of patients with confirmed upper tract sources of bleeding have nonbloody aspirates—especially when bleeding originates in the duodenum. An aspirate of bright red blood indicates active bleeding and is associated with the highest risk of further bleeding and complications, while a clear aspirate identifies patients at lower initial risk. Erythromycin (250 mg) administered intravenously 30 minutes prior to upper endoscopy promotes gastric emptying and may improve the quality of endoscopic evaluation when substantial amounts of blood or clot in the stomach is suspected. Efforts to stop or slow bleeding by gastric lavage with large volumes of fluid are of no benefit and expose the patient to an increased risk of aspiration.

B. Blood Replacement

The amount of fluid and blood products required is based on assessment of vital signs, evidence of active bleeding from nasogastric aspirate, and laboratory tests. Sufficient packed red blood cells should be given to maintain a hemoglobin of 7–9 g/dL, based on the patient's hemodynamic status, comorbidities (especially cardiovascular disease), and presence of continued bleeding. In the absence of continued bleeding, the hemoglobin should rise approximately 1 g/dL for each unit of transfused packed red cells. Transfusion of blood should not be withheld from patients with massive active bleeding regardless of the hemoglobin value. It is desirable to transfuse blood in anticipation of the nadir hematocrit. In actively bleeding patients, platelets are transfused if the platelet count is under 50,000/mcL and considered if there is impaired platelet function due to aspirin or clopidogrel use (regardless of the platelet count). Uremic patients (who also have dysfunctional platelets) with active bleeding are given three doses of desmopressin (DDAVP), 0.3 mcg/kg intravenously, at 12-hour intervals. Fresh frozen plasma is administered for actively bleeding patients with a coagulopathy and an INR greater than 1.8; however, endoscopy may be performed safely if the INR is less than 2.5. In the face of massive bleeding, administration of four factor prothrombin complex concentrates is preferred (rather than fresh frozen plasma) because it is more rapid and effective at correcting the INR and requires a smaller volume.

C. Initial Triage

A preliminary assessment of risk based on several clinical factors aids in the resuscitation as well as the rational triage of the patient. Clinical predictors of increased risk of rebleeding and death include age over 60 years, comorbid illnesses, systolic blood pressure less than 100 mm Hg, pulse greater than 100 beats/min, and bright red blood in the nasogastric aspirate or on rectal examination.

1. High risk—Patients with active bleeding manifested by hematemesis or bright red blood on nasogastric aspirate, shock, persistent hemodynamic derangement despite fluid resuscitation, serious comorbid medical illness, or evidence of advanced liver disease require admission to an intensive care unit (ICU). After adequate resuscitation, endoscopy should be performed within 2–24 hours in most patients but may be delayed in selected patients with serious comorbidities (eg, acute coronary syndrome) who do not have signs of continued bleeding.

2. Low to moderate risk—All other patients are admitted to a step-down unit or medical ward after appropriate stabilization for further evaluation and treatment. Patients without evidence of active bleeding undergo nonemergent endoscopy usually within 24 hours.

▶ Subsequent Evaluation & Treatment

Specific treatment of the various causes of upper gastrointestinal bleeding is discussed elsewhere in this chapter. The following general comments apply to most patients with bleeding.

The clinician's impression of the bleeding source is correct in only 40% of cases. Signs of chronic liver disease implicate bleeding due to portal hypertension, but a different lesion is identified in 25% of patients with cirrhosis. A history of dyspepsia, NSAID use, or peptic ulcer disease suggests peptic ulcer. Acute bleeding preceded by heavy alcohol ingestion or retching suggests a Mallory-Weiss tear, though most of these patients have neither.

A. Upper Endoscopy

Virtually all patients with upper tract bleeding should undergo upper endoscopy within 24 hours of arriving in

the emergency department. The benefits of endoscopy in this setting are threefold.

1. To identify the source of bleeding—The appropriate acute and long-term medical therapy is determined by the cause of bleeding. Patients with portal hypertension will be treated differently from those with ulcer disease. If surgery or radiologic interventional therapy is required for uncontrolled bleeding, the source of bleeding as determined at endoscopy will determine the approach.

2. To determine the risk of rebleeding and guide triage—Patients with a nonbleeding Mallory-Weiss tear, esophagitis, gastritis, and ulcers that have a clean, white base have a very low risk (less than 5%) of rebleeding. Patients with one of these findings who are younger than 60 years, without hemodynamic instability or transfusion requirement, without serious coexisting illness, and who have stable social support may be discharged from the emergency department or medical ward after endoscopy with outpatient follow-up. All others with one of these low-risk lesions should be observed on a medical ward for 24–48 hours. Patients with ulcers that are actively bleeding or have a visible vessel or adherent clot, or who have variceal bleeding usually require at least a 3-day hospitalization with closer initial observation in an ICU or step down unit.

3. To render endoscopic therapy—Hemostasis can be achieved in actively bleeding lesions with endoscopic modalities such as cautery, injection, or endoclips. About 90% of bleeding or nonbleeding varices can be effectively treated immediately with injection of a sclerosant or application of rubber bands to the varices. Similarly, 90% of bleeding ulcers, angiomas, or Mallory-Weiss tears can be controlled with either injection of epinephrine, direct cauterization of the vessel by a heater probe or multipolar electrocautery probe, or application of an endoclip. Certain nonbleeding lesions such as ulcers with visible blood vessels, and angioectasias are also treated with these therapies. Specific endoscopic therapy of varices, peptic ulcers, and Mallory-Weiss tears is dealt with elsewhere in this chapter.

B. Acute Pharmacologic Therapies

1. Acid inhibitory therapy—Intravenous proton pump inhibitors (esomeprazole or pantoprazole, 80 mg bolus, followed by 8 mg/h continuous infusion for 72 hours) reduce the risk of rebleeding in patients with peptic ulcers with high-risk features (active bleeding, visible vessel, or adherent clot) after endoscopic treatment. **Oral proton pump inhibitors** (omeprazole, esomeprazole, or pantoprazole 40 mg; lansoprazole or dexlansoprazole 30–60 mg) once or twice daily are sufficient for lesions at low-risk for rebleeding (eg, esophagitis, gastritis, clean-based ulcers, and Mallory-Weiss tears).

Administration of continuous intravenous proton pump inhibitor *before* endoscopy results in a decreased number of ulcers with lesions that require endoscopic therapy. It therefore is standard clinical practice at many institutions to administer either an intravenous or a high-dose oral proton pump inhibitor prior to endoscopy in patients with significant upper gastrointestinal bleeding.

Based on the findings during endoscopy, the intravenous proton pump inhibitor may be continued or discontinued.

2. Octreotide—Continuous intravenous infusion of octreotide (100 mcg bolus, followed by 50–100 mcg/h) reduces splanchnic blood flow and portal blood pressures and is effective in the initial control of bleeding related to portal hypertension. It is administered promptly to all patients with active upper gastrointestinal bleeding and evidence of liver disease or portal hypertension until the source of bleeding can be determined by endoscopy. In countries where it is available, terlipressin may be preferred to octreotide for the treatment of bleeding related to portal hypertension because of its sustained reduction of portal and variceal pressures and its proven reduction in mortality.

C. Other Treatment

1. Intra-arterial embolization—Angiographic treatment is used in patients with persistent bleeding from ulcers, angiomas, or Mallory-Weiss tears who have failed endoscopic therapy and are poor operative risks.

2. Transvenous intrahepatic portosystemic shunts (TIPS)—Placement of a wire stent from the hepatic vein through the liver to the portal vein provides effective decompression of the portal venous system and control of acute variceal bleeding. It is indicated in patients in whom endoscopic modalities have failed to control acute variceal bleeding.

Abougergi MS et al. The in-hospital mortality rate for upper GI hemorrhage has decreased over 2 decades in the United States: a nationwide analysis. Gastrointest Endosc. 2015 Apr;81(4):882–8.e1. [PMID: 25484324]

Greenspoon J et al; International Consensus Upper Gastrointestinal Bleeding Conference Group. Management of patients with nonvariceal upper gastrointestinal bleeding. Clin Gastroenterol Hepatol. 2012 Mar;10(3):234–9. [PMID: 21820395]

Jairath V et al. Restrictive versus liberal blood transfusion for acute upper gastrointestinal bleeding (TRIGGER): a pragmatic, open-label, cluster randomized feasibility trial. Lancet. 2015 Jul 11;386(9989):137–44. [PMID: 25956718]

Lau JY et al. Challenges in the management of acute peptic ulcer bleeding. Lancet. 2013 Jun 8;381(9882):2033–43. [PMID: 23746903]

Villanueva C et al. Transfusion for acute upper gastrointestinal bleeding. N Engl J Med. 2013 Apr 4;368(1):11–21. [PMID: 23550677]

2. Acute Lower Gastrointestinal Bleeding

ESSENTIALS OF DIAGNOSIS

▶ Hematochezia usually present.

▶ Ten percent of cases of hematochezia due to upper gastrointestinal source.

▶ Evaluation with colonoscopy in stable patients.

▶ Massive active bleeding calls for evaluation with sigmoidoscopy, upper endoscopy, angiography, or nuclear bleeding scan.

▶ General Considerations

Lower gastrointestinal bleeding is defined as that arising below the ligament of Treitz, ie, the small intestine or colon; however, up to 95% of cases arise from the colon. The severity of lower gastrointestinal bleeding ranges from mild anorectal bleeding to massive, large-volume hematochezia. Bright red blood that drips into the bowl after a bowel movement or is mixed with solid brown stool signifies mild bleeding, usually from an anorectosigmoid source, and can be evaluated in the outpatient setting. In patients hospitalized with gastrointestinal bleeding, lower tract bleeding is one-third as common as upper gastrointestinal hemorrhage and tends to have a more benign course. Patients hospitalized with lower gastrointestinal tract bleeding are less likely to present with shock or orthostasis (less than 20%) or to require transfusions (less than 40%). Spontaneous cessation of bleeding occurs in over 75% of cases, and hospital mortality is less than 4%.

▶ Etiology

The cause of these lesions depends on both the age of the patient and the severity of the bleeding. In patients under 50 years of age, the most common causes are infectious colitis, anorectal disease, and inflammatory bowel disease. In older patients, significant hematochezia is most often seen with diverticulosis, angiectasias, malignancy, or ischemia. In 20% of acute bleeding episodes, no source of bleeding can be identified. There is an increased risk of lower gastrointestinal bleeding in patients taking aspirin, nonaspirin antiplatelet agents, and NSAIDs.

A. Diverticulosis

Hemorrhage occurs in 3–5% of all patients with diverticulosis and is the most common cause of major lower tract bleeding, accounting for 50% of cases. Diverticular bleeding usually presents as acute, painless, large-volume maroon or bright red hematochezia in patients over age 50 years. More than 95% of cases require less than 4 units of blood transfusion. Bleeding subsides spontaneously in 80% but may recur in up to 25% of patients.

B. Angioectasias

Angioectasias (angiodysplasias) occur throughout the upper and lower intestinal tracts and cause painless bleeding ranging from melena or hematochezia to occult blood loss. They are responsible for 4% of cases of lower gastrointestinal bleeding, where they are most often seen in the cecum and ascending colon. They are flat, red lesions (2–10 mm) with ectatic peripheral vessels radiating from a central vessel, and are most common in patients over 70 years and in those with chronic renal failure. Bleeding in younger patients more commonly arises from the small intestine.

Ectasias can be identified in up to 6% of persons over age 60 years, so the mere presence of ectasias does not prove that the lesion is the source of bleeding, since active bleeding is seldom seen.

C. Neoplasms

Benign polyps and carcinoma are associated with chronic occult blood loss or intermittent anorectal hematochezia. Furthermore, they may cause up to 7% of acute lower gastrointestinal hemorrhage. After endoscopic removal of colonic polyps, important bleeding may occur up to 2 weeks later in 0.3% of patients. In general, prompt colonoscopy is recommended to treat postpolypectomy hemorrhage and minimize the need for transfusions.

D. Inflammatory Bowel Disease

Patients with inflammatory bowel disease (especially ulcerative colitis) often have diarrhea with variable amounts of hematochezia. Bleeding varies from occult blood loss to recurrent hematochezia usually mixed with stool. Symptoms of abdominal pain, tenesmus, and urgency are often present.

E. Anorectal Disease

Anorectal disease (hemorrhoids, fissures) usually results in small amounts of bright red blood noted on the toilet paper, streaking of the stool, or dripping into the toilet bowl; clinically significant blood loss can sometimes occur. Hemorrhoids are the source in 10% of patients admitted with lower bleeding. Rectal ulcers may account for up to 8% of lower bleeding, usually in elderly or debilitated patients with constipation.

F. Ischemic Colitis

This condition is seen commonly in older patients, most of whom have atherosclerotic disease. Most cases occur spontaneously due to transient episodes of nonocclusive ischemia. Ischemic colitis may also occur in 5% of patients after surgery for ileoaortic or abdominal aortic aneurysm. In young patients, colonic ischemia may develop due to vasculitis, coagulation disorders, estrogen therapy, and long distance running. Ischemic colitis results in hematochezia or bloody diarrhea associated with mild cramps. In most patients, the bleeding is mild and self-limited.

G. Others

Radiation-induced proctitis causes anorectal bleeding that may develop months to years after pelvic radiation. Endoscopy reveals multiple rectal telangiectasias. Acute infectious colitis (see Acute Diarrhea) commonly causes bloody diarrhea. Rare causes of lower tract bleeding include vasculitic ischemia, solitary rectal ulcer, NSAID-induced ulcers in the small bowel or right colon, small bowel diverticula, and colonic varices.

▶ Clinical Findings

A. Symptoms and Signs

The color of the stool helps distinguish upper from lower gastrointestinal bleeding, especially when observed by the clinician. Brown stools mixed or streaked with blood predict a source in the rectosigmoid or anus. Large volumes of bright red blood suggest a colonic source; maroon stools imply a lesion in the right colon or small intestine; and black stools (melena) predict a source proximal to the ligament of Treitz. Although 10% of patients admitted with self-reported hematochezia have an upper gastrointestinal source of bleeding (eg, peptic ulcer), this almost always occurs in the setting of massive hemorrhage with hemodynamic instability. Painless large-volume bleeding usually suggests diverticular bleeding. Bloody diarrhea associated with cramping abdominal pain, urgency, or tenesmus is characteristic of inflammatory bowel disease, infectious colitis, or ischemic colitis.

B. Diagnostic Tests

Important considerations in management include exclusion of an upper tract source, anoscopy and sigmoidoscopy, colonoscopy, nuclear bleeding scans and angiography, and small intestine push enteroscopy or capsule imaging.

1. Exclusion of an upper tract source—A nasogastric tube with aspiration should be considered, especially in patients with hemodynamic compromise. Aspiration of red blood or dark brown ("coffee grounds") guaiac-positive material strongly implicates an upper gastrointestinal source of bleeding. Upper endoscopy should be performed in most patients presenting with hematochezia and hemodynamic instability to exclude an upper gastrointestinal source before proceeding with evaluation of the lower gastrointestinal tract.

2. Anoscopy and sigmoidoscopy—In otherwise healthy patients without anemia under age 45 years with small-volume bleeding, anoscopy and sigmoidoscopy are performed to look for evidence of anorectal disease, inflammatory bowel disease, or infectious colitis. If a lesion is found, no further evaluation is needed immediately unless the bleeding persists or is recurrent. In patients over age 45 years with small-volume hematochezia, the entire colon must be evaluated with colonoscopy to exclude tumor.

3. Colonoscopy—In patients with acute, large-volume bleeding requiring hospitalization, colonoscopy is the preferred initial study in most cases. The bowel first is purged rapidly by administration of a high-volume colonic lavage solution, given until the effluent is clear of blood and clots (4–8 L of GoLYTELY, CoLYTE, NuLYTE given orally or 1 L every 30 minutes over 2–5 hours by nasogastric tube). For patients with stable vital signs and whose lower gastrointestinal bleeding appears to have stopped (more than 75% of patients), colonoscopy can be performed electively within 24 hours of admission. For patients with signs of hemodynamically significant bleeding (unstable vital signs) or who have signs of continued active bleeding during bowel preparation (less than 25% of patients), urgent colonoscopy should be performed within 1–2 hours of completing the bowel purgative, when the bowel discharge is without clots. The probable site of bleeding can be identified in 70–85% of patients, and a high-risk lesion can be identified and treated in up to 20%.

4. Nuclear bleeding scans and angiography—Technetium-labeled red blood cell scanning can detect significant active bleeding and, in some cases, can localize the source to the small intestine, right colon, or left colon. Because most bleeding is slow or intermittent, less than half of nuclear studies are diagnostic and the accuracy of localization is poor. Thus, the main utility of scintigraphy is to determine whether bleeding is ongoing in order to determine whether angiography should be pursued. Less than half of patients with a positive nuclear study have positive angiography. Accordingly, angiograms are performed only in patients with positive technetium scans believed to have significant, ongoing bleeding.

In patients with massive lower gastrointestinal bleeding manifested by continued hemodynamic instability and hematochezia, urgent angiography should be performed without attempt at colonoscopy or scintigraphy.

5. Small intestine push enteroscopy or capsule imaging—Up to 5% of acute episodes of lower gastrointestinal bleeding arise from the small intestine, eluding diagnostic evaluation with upper endoscopy and colonoscopy. Because of the difficulty of examining the small intestine and its relative rarity as a source of acute bleeding, evaluation of the small bowel is not usually pursued in patients during the initial episode of acute lower gastrointestinal bleeding. However, the small intestine is investigated in patients with unexplained recurrent hemorrhage of obscure origin.

Treatment

Initial stabilization, blood replacement, and triage are managed in the same manner as described above for Acute Upper Gastrointestinal Bleeding.

A. Therapeutic Colonoscopy

High-risk lesions (eg, angioectasia or diverticulum, rectal ulcer with active bleeding, or a visible vessel) may be treated endoscopically with epinephrine injection, cautery (bipolar or heater probe), or application of metallic endoclips or bands. In diverticular hemorrhage with high-risk lesions identified at colonoscopy, rebleeding occurs in half of untreated patients compared with virtually no rebleeding in patients treated endoscopically. Radiation proctitis is effectively treated with applications of cautery therapy to the rectal telangiectasias, preferably with an argon plasma coagulator.

B. Intra-arterial Embolization

When a bleeding lesion is identified, angiography with selective embolization achieves immediate hemostasis in more than 95% of patients. Major complications occur in 5% (mainly ischemic colitis) and rebleeding occurs in up to 25%.

C. Surgical Treatment

Emergency surgery is required in less than 5% of patients with acute lower gastrointestinal bleeding due to the efficacy of colonoscopic and angiographic therapies. It is indicated in patients with ongoing bleeding that requires more than 6 units of blood within 24 hours or more than 10 total units in whom attempts at endoscopic or angiographic therapy failed. Most such hemorrhages are caused by a bleeding diverticulum or angioectasia.

Surgery may also be indicated in patients with two or more hospitalizations for diverticular hemorrhage depending on the severity of bleeding and the patient's other comorbid conditions.

Aoki T et al. Recurrence and mortality among patients hospitalized for acute lower gastrointestinal bleeding. Clin Gastroenterol Hepatol. 2015 Mar;13(3):488–94.e1. [PMID: 24997327]
ASGE Standards of Practice Committee; Pasha SF et al. The role of endoscopy in the patient with lower GI bleeding. Gastrointest Endosc. 2014 Jun;79(6):875–85. [PMID: 24703084]
Navaneethan U et al. Timing of colonoscopy and outcomes in patients with lower GI bleeding: a nationwide population-based study. Gastrointest Endosc. 2014 Feb;79(2):297–306. [PMID: 24060518]

3. Small Bowel Bleeding

Bleeding from the small intestine can be overt or occult. *Overt* small bowel bleeding manifests as melena, maroon stools, or bright red blood per rectum. Up to 5–10% of patients admitted to hospitals with clinically overt gastrointestinal bleeding do not have a cause identified on upper endoscopy or colonoscopy and are presumed to have a small bowel source. In up to one-third of cases, however, a source of bleeding has been overlooked in the upper or lower tract on prior endoscopic studies. *Occult* small bowel bleeding refers to bleeding that is manifested by recurrent positive FOBTs or FITs or recurrent iron deficiency anemia, or both in the absence of visible blood loss.

The likely etiology of small bowel bleeding depends on the age of the patient. The most common causes of small intestinal bleeding in patients younger than 40 years are neoplasms (stromal tumors, lymphomas, adenocarcinomas, carcinoids), Crohn disease, celiac disease, and Meckel diverticulum. These disorders also occur in patients over age 40; however, angioectasias and NSAID-induced ulcers are far more common.

Evaluation of Small Bowel Bleeding

The evaluation of small bowel bleeding depends on the age and overall health status of the patient, associated symptoms, and severity of the bleeding. In an older patient with significant comorbid illnesses, no gastrointestinal symptoms, and occult bleeding in whom the suspected source of bleeding is angioectasias, it may be reasonable to limit diagnostic evaluations, provided the anemia can be managed with long-term iron therapy or occasional transfusions. On the other hand, aggressive diagnostic evaluation is warranted in younger patients with obscure bleeding (in whom small bowel tumors are the most common cause) and symptomatic older patients with overt bleeding. Upper endoscopy and colonoscopy should be repeated to ascertain that a lesion in these regions has not been overlooked. If these studies are unrevealing, capsule endoscopy should be performed to evaluate the small intestine. Capsule endoscopy is superior to radiographic studies and standard push enteroscopy for the detection of small bowel abnormalities, demonstrating possible sources of occult bleeding in 50% of patients, most commonly vascular abnormalities (25%), ulcers (10–25%), and neoplasms (less than 1–10%).

Further management depends on the capsule endoscopic findings. Abdominal CT may be considered to exclude a hepatic or pancreatic source of bleeding. CT enterography may be performed if video capsule and abdominal CT are unrevealing. Laparotomy is warranted if a small bowel tumor is identified by capsule endoscopy or radiographic studies. Most other lesions identified by capsule imaging can be further evaluated with enteroscopes that use over-tubes with balloons to advance the scope through most of the small intestine in a forward and retrograde direction. Neoplasms can be biopsied or resected, and angioectasias may be cauterized. For massive or hemodynamically significant acute bleeding, angiography may be superior to enteroscopy for localization and embolization of a bleeding vascular abnormality. For hemodynamically stable overt bleeding, CT angiography may be useful to localize bleeding and guide other interventions (enteroscopy or angiography with embolization). A nuclear scan for Meckel diverticulum should be obtained in patients under age 30. With the advent of capsule imaging and advanced endoscopic technologies for evaluating and treating bleeding lesions in the small intestine, intraoperative enteroscopy of the small bowel is seldom required.

4. Occult Gastrointestinal Bleeding

Occult gastrointestinal bleeding refers to bleeding that is not apparent to the patient. Chronic gastrointestinal blood loss of less than 100 mL/day may cause no appreciable change in stool appearance. Thus, occult bleeding in an adult is identified by a positive FOBT, FIT, or by iron deficiency anemia in the absence of visible blood loss. FOBT or FIT may be performed in patients with gastrointestinal symptoms or as a screening test for colorectal neoplasia (see Chapter 39). From 2% to 6% of patients in screening programs have a positive FOBT or FIT.

In the United States, 2% of men and 5% of women have iron deficiency anemia (serum ferritin less than 30–45 mcg/L). In premenopausal women, iron deficiency anemia is most commonly attributable to menstrual and pregnancy-associated iron loss; however, a gastrointestinal source of chronic blood loss is present in 10%. Occult blood loss may arise from anywhere in the gastrointestinal tract. Among men and postmenopausal women, a potential gastrointestinal cause of blood loss can be identified in the colon in 15–30% and in the upper gastrointestinal tract in 35–55%; a malignancy is present in 10%. Iron deficiency on rare occasions is caused by malabsorption (especially celiac disease) or malnutrition. The most common causes of occult bleeding with iron deficiency are (1) neoplasms; (2) vascular abnormalities (angioectasias); (3) acid-peptic lesions (esophagitis, peptic ulcer disease, erosions in hiatal hernia); (4) infections (nematodes, especially hookworm; tuberculosis); (5) medications (especially NSAIDs or aspirin); and (6) other causes such as inflammatory bowel disease.

Evaluation of Occult Bleeding

Asymptomatic adults with positive FOBTs or FITs that are performed for routine colorectal cancer screening should undergo colonoscopy (see Chapter 39). All symptomatic adults with positive FOBTs or FITs or iron deficiency anemia should undergo evaluation of the lower and upper gastrointestinal tract with colonoscopy and upper endoscopy, unless the anemia can be definitively ascribed to a nongastrointestinal source (eg, menstruation, blood donation, or recent surgery). Patients with iron deficiency anemia should be evaluated for possible celiac disease with either IgA anti-tissue transglutaminase or duodenal biopsy. After evaluation of the upper and lower gastrointestinal tract with upper endoscopy and colonoscopy, the origin of occult bleeding remains unexplained in 30–50% of patients.

In patients younger than 60 years with unexplained occult bleeding or iron deficiency, it is recommended to pursue further evaluation of the small intestine for a source of obscure-occult bleeding (as described above) in order to exclude a small intestinal neoplasm or inflammatory bowel disease. Patients over age 60 with occult bleeding who have a normal initial endoscopic evaluation and no other worrisome symptoms or signs (eg, abdominal pain, weight loss) most commonly have blood loss from angioectasias, which may be clinically unimportant. Therefore, it is reasonable to give an empiric trial of iron supplementation and observe the patient for evidence of clinically significant bleeding. For anemia that responds poorly to iron supplementation or recurrent or persistent chronic occult gastrointestinal blood loss, further evaluation is pursued for a source of obscure-occult bleeding (as described above). When possible, antiplatelet agents (aspirin, NSAIDs, clopidogrel) should be discontinued.

ASGE Technology Committee; Chauhan SS et al. Enteroscopy. Gastrointest Endosc. 2015 Dec;82(6):975–90. [PMID: 26388546]
Camaschella C. Iron-deficiency anemia. N Engl J Med. 2015 May 7;372(19):1832–43. [PMID: 25946282]
Gerson LB et al. ACG clinical guideline: diagnosis and management of small bowel bleeding. Am J Gastroenterol. 2015 Sep;110(9):1265–87. [PMID: 26303132]

DISEASES OF THE PERITONEUM

ASSESSMENT OF THE PATIENT WITH ASCITES

Etiology of Ascites

The term "ascites" denotes the pathologic accumulation of fluid in the peritoneal cavity. Healthy men have little or no intraperitoneal fluid, but women normally may have up to 20 mL depending on the phase of the menstrual cycle. The causes of ascites may be classified into two broad pathophysiologic categories: that which is associated with a normal peritoneum and that which occurs due to a diseased peritoneum (Table 15–7). The most common cause of ascites is portal hypertension secondary to chronic liver disease, which accounts for over 80% of patients with ascites. The management of portal hypertensive ascites is discussed in Chapter 16. The most common causes of nonportal hypertensive ascites include infections (tuberculous peritonitis), intra-abdominal malignancy, inflammatory disorders of the peritoneum, and ductal disruptions (chylous, pancreatic, biliary).

Table 15–7. Causes of ascites.

Normal Peritoneum
Portal hypertension (SAAG ≥ 1.1 g/dL)
1. Hepatic congestion[1]
Heart failure
Constrictive pericarditis
Tricuspid insufficiency
Budd-Chiari syndrome
Veno-occlusive disease
2. Liver disease[2]
Cirrhosis
Alcoholic hepatitis
Fulminant hepatic failure
Massive hepatic metastases
Hepatic fibrosis
Acute fatty liver of pregnancy
3. Portal vein occlusion
Hypoalbuminemia (SAAG < 1.1 g/dL)
Nephrotic syndrome
Protein-losing enteropathy
Severe malnutrition with anasarca
Miscellaneous conditions (SAAG < 1.1 g/dL)
Chylous ascites
Pancreatic ascites
Bile ascites
Nephrogenic ascites
Urine ascites
Myxedema (SAAG ≥ 1.1 g/dL)
Ovarian disease
Diseased Peritoneum (SAAG < 1.1 g/dL)[2]
Infections
Bacterial peritonitis
Tuberculous peritonitis
Fungal peritonitis
HIV-associated peritonitis
Malignant conditions
Peritoneal carcinomatosis
Primary mesothelioma
Pseudomyxoma peritonei
Massive hepatic metastases
Hepatocellular carcinoma
Other conditions
Familial Mediterranean fever
Vasculitis
Granulomatous peritonitis
Eosinophilic peritonitis

[1]Hepatic congestion usually associated with SAAG ≥ 1.1 g/dL and ascitic fluid total protein > 2.5 g/dL.

[2]There may be cases of "mixed ascites" in which portal hypertensive ascites is complicated by a secondary process such as infection. In these cases, the SAAG is ≥ 1.1 g/dL.

SAAG, serum-ascites albumin gradient = serum albumin minus ascitic fluid albumin.

► **Clinical Findings**

A. Symptoms and Signs

The history usually is one of increasing abdominal girth, with the presence of abdominal pain depending on the cause. Because most ascites is secondary to chronic liver disease with portal hypertension, patients should be asked about risk factors for liver disease, especially alcohol consumption, transfusions, tattoos, injection drug use, a history of viral hepatitis or jaundice, and birth in an area endemic for hepatitis. A history of cancer or marked weight loss arouses suspicion of malignant ascites. Fevers may suggest infected peritoneal fluid, including bacterial peritonitis (spontaneous or secondary). Patients with chronic liver disease and ascites are at greatest risk for developing spontaneous bacterial peritonitis. In immigrants, immunocompromised hosts, or severely malnourished alcoholics, tuberculous peritonitis should be considered.

Physical examination should emphasize signs of portal hypertension and chronic liver disease. Elevated jugular venous pressure may suggest right-sided heart failure or constrictive pericarditis. A large tender liver is characteristic of acute alcoholic hepatitis or Budd-Chiari syndrome (thrombosis of the hepatic veins). The presence of large abdominal wall veins with cephalad flow also suggests portal hypertension; inferiorly directed flow implies hepatic vein obstruction. Signs of chronic liver disease include palmar erythema, cutaneous spider angiomas, gynecomastia, and muscle wasting. Asterixis secondary to hepatic encephalopathy may be present. Anasarca results from cardiac failure or nephrotic syndrome with hypoalbuminemia. Finally, firm lymph nodes in the left supraclavicular region or umbilicus may suggest intra-abdominal malignancy.

The physical examination is relatively insensitive for detecting ascitic fluid. In general, patients must have at least 1500 mL of fluid to be detected reliably by this method. Even the experienced clinician may find it difficult to distinguish between obesity and small-volume ascites. Abdominal ultrasound establishes the presence of fluid.

B. Laboratory Testing

1. Abdominal paracentesis—Abdominal paracentesis is performed as part of the diagnostic evaluation in all patients with new onset of ascites to help determine the cause. It also is recommended for patients admitted to the hospital with cirrhosis and ascites (in whom the prevalence of bacterial peritonitis is 10–20%) and when patients with known ascites deteriorate clinically (development of fever, abdominal pain, rapid worsening of renal function, or worsened hepatic encephalopathy) to exclude bacterial peritonitis.

A. INSPECTION—Cloudy fluid suggests infection. Milky fluid is seen with chylous ascites due to high triglyceride levels. Bloody fluid is most commonly attributable to a traumatic paracentesis, but up to 20% of cases of malignant ascites are bloody.

B. ROUTINE STUDIES

(1) Cell count—A white blood cell count with differential is the most important test. Normal ascitic fluid contains less than 500 leukocytes/mcL and less than 250 polymorphonuclear neutrophils (PMNs)/mcL. Any inflammatory condition can cause an elevated ascitic white blood cell count. A PMN count of greater than 250/mcL (neutrocytic ascites) with a percentage of more than 75% of

all white cells is highly suggestive of bacterial peritonitis, either spontaneous primary peritonitis or secondary peritonitis (ie, caused by an intra-abdominal source of infection, such as a perforated viscus or appendicitis). An elevated white count with a predominance of lymphocytes arouses suspicion of tuberculosis or peritoneal carcinomatosis.

(2) Albumin and total protein—The serum-ascites albumin gradient (SAAG) is the best single test for the classification of ascites into portal hypertensive and nonportal hypertensive causes (Table 15–7). Calculated by subtracting the ascitic fluid albumin from the serum albumin, the gradient correlates directly with the portal pressure. An SAAG of 1.1 g/dL or more suggests underlying portal hypertension, while gradients less than 1.1 g/dL implicate nonportal hypertensive causes.

The accuracy of the SAAG exceeds 95% in classifying ascites. It should be recognized, however, that approximately 4% of patients have "mixed ascites," ie, underlying cirrhosis with portal hypertension complicated by a second cause for ascites formation (such as malignancy or tuberculosis). Thus, a high SAAG is indicative of portal hypertension but does not exclude concomitant malignancy.

The ascitic fluid total protein provides some additional clues to the cause. An elevated SAAG and a high protein level (greater than 2.5 g/dL) are seen in most cases of hepatic congestion secondary to cardiac disease or Budd-Chiari syndrome. However, an increased ascitic fluid protein is also found in up to 20% of cases of uncomplicated cirrhosis. Two-thirds of patients with malignant ascites have a total protein level more than 2.5 g/dL.

(3) Culture and Gram stain—The best technique consists of the inoculation of aerobic and anaerobic blood culture bottles with 5–10 mL of ascitic fluid at the patient's bedside, which increases the sensitivity for detecting bacterial peritonitis to over 85% in patients with neutrocytic ascites (greater than 250 PMNs/mcL), compared with approximately 50% sensitivity by conventional agar plate or broth cultures.

c. Optional studies—Other laboratory tests are of utility in some specific clinical situations. Glucose and lactate dehydrogenase (LD) may be helpful in distinguishing spontaneous from secondary bacterial peritonitis. An elevated amylase may suggest pancreatic ascites or a perforation of the gastrointestinal tract with leakage of pancreatic secretions into the ascitic fluid. Perforation of the biliary tree is suspected with an ascitic bilirubin concentration that is greater than the serum bilirubin. An elevated ascitic creatinine suggests leakage of urine from the bladder or ureters. Ascitic fluid cytologic examination is ordered if peritoneal carcinomatosis is suspected. Adenosine deaminase may be useful for the diagnosis of tuberculous peritonitis.

C. Imaging

Abdominal ultrasound is useful in confirming the presence of ascites and in the guidance of paracentesis. Both ultrasound and CT imaging are useful in distinguishing between causes of portal and nonportal

hypertensive ascites. Doppler ultrasound and CT can detect Budd-Chiari syndrome. In patients with nonportal hypertensive ascites, these studies are useful in detecting lymphadenopathy and masses of the mesentery and of solid organs such as the liver, ovaries, and pancreas. Furthermore, they permit directed percutaneous needle biopsies of these lesions. Ultrasound and CT are poor procedures for the detection of peritoneal carcinomatosis; the role of positron emission tomography (PET) imaging is unclear.

D. Laparoscopy

Laparoscopy is an important test in the evaluation of some patients with nonportal hypertensive ascites (low SAAG) or mixed ascites. It permits direct visualization and biopsy of the peritoneum, liver, and some intra-abdominal lymph nodes. Cases of suspected peritoneal tuberculosis or suspected malignancy with nondiagnostic CT imaging and ascitic fluid cytology are best evaluated by this method.

Gordon FD. Ascites. Clin Liver Dis. 2012 May;16(2):285–99. [PMID: 22541699]
Rahimi RS et al. End-stage liver disease complications. Curr Opin Gastroenterol. 2013 May;29(3):257–63. [PMID: 23429468]

SPONTANEOUS BACTERIAL PERITONITIS

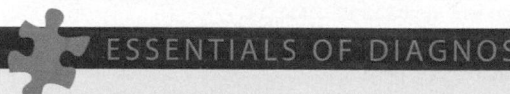

ESSENTIALS OF DIAGNOSIS

► A history of chronic liver disease and ascites.
► Fever and abdominal pain.
► Peritoneal signs uncommonly encountered on examination.
► Ascitic fluid neutrophil count greater than 250 white blood cells/mcL.

► General Considerations

"Spontaneous" bacterial infection of ascitic fluid occurs in the absence of an apparent intra-abdominal source of infection. It is seen with few exceptions in patients with ascites caused by chronic liver disease. Translocation of enteric bacteria across the gut wall or mesenteric lymphatics leads to seeding of the ascitic fluid, as may bacteremia from other sites. Approximately 20–30% of cirrhotic patients with ascites develop spontaneous peritonitis; however, the incidence is greater than 40% in patients with ascitic fluid total protein less than 1 g/dL, probably due to decreased ascitic fluid opsonic activity.

Virtually all cases of spontaneous bacterial peritonitis are caused by a monomicrobial infection. The most common pathogens are enteric gram-negative bacteria (*E coli, Klebsiella pneumoniae*) or gram-positive bacteria (*Streptococcus pneumoniae*, viridans streptococci, *Enterococcus* species). Anaerobic bacteria are not associated with spontaneous bacterial peritonitis.

Clinical Findings

A. Symptoms and Signs

Eighty to ninety percent of patients with spontaneous bacterial peritonitis are symptomatic; in many cases the presentation is subtle. Spontaneous bacterial peritonitis may be present in 10–20% of patients hospitalized with chronic liver disease, sometimes in the absence of any suggestive symptoms or signs.

The most common symptoms are fever and abdominal pain, present in two-thirds of patients. Spontaneous bacterial peritonitis may also present with a change in mental status due to exacerbation or precipitation of hepatic encephalopathy, or sudden worsening of renal function. Physical examination typically demonstrates signs of chronic liver disease with ascites. Abdominal tenderness is present in less than 50% of patients, and its presence suggests other processes.

B. Laboratory Findings

The most important diagnostic test is abdominal paracentesis. Ascitic fluid should be sent for cell count with differential, and blood culture bottles should be inoculated at the bedside; Gram stain and reagent strips are insensitive.

In the proper clinical setting, an ascitic fluid PMN count of greater than 250 cells/mcL (neutrocytic ascites) is presumptive evidence of bacterial peritonitis. The percentage of PMNs is greater than 50–70% of the ascitic fluid white blood cells and commonly approximates 100%. Patients with neutrocytic ascites are presumed to be infected and should be started—regardless of symptoms—on antibiotics. Although 10–30% of patients with neutrocytic ascites have negative ascitic bacterial cultures ("culture-negative neutrocytic ascites"), it is presumed that these patients have bacterial peritonitis and should be treated empirically. Occasionally, a positive blood culture identifies the organism when ascitic fluid is sterile.

Differential Diagnosis

Spontaneous bacterial peritonitis must be distinguished from secondary bacterial peritonitis, in which ascitic fluid has become secondarily infected by an intra-abdominal infection. Even in the presence of perforation, clinical symptoms and signs of peritonitis may be lacking owing to the separation of the visceral and parietal peritoneum by the ascitic fluid. Causes of secondary bacterial peritonitis include appendicitis, diverticulitis, perforated peptic ulcer, and perforated gallbladder. Secondary bacterial infection accounts for 3% of cases of infected ascitic fluid.

Ascitic fluid total protein, LD, and glucose are useful in distinguishing spontaneous bacterial peritonitis from secondary infection. Up to two-thirds of patients with secondary bacterial peritonitis have at least two of the following: decreased glucose level (less than 50 mg/dL), an elevated LD level (greater than serum), and total protein greater than 1 g/dL. Ascitic neutrophil counts greater than 10,000/mcL also are suspicious; however, most patients with secondary peritonitis have neutrophil counts within the range of spontaneous peritonitis. The presence of multiple organisms on ascitic fluid Gram stain or culture is diagnostic of secondary peritonitis.

If secondary bacterial peritonitis is suspected, abdominal CT imaging of the upper and lower gastrointestinal tracts should be obtained to look for evidence of an intra-abdominal source of infection. If these studies are negative and secondary peritonitis still is suspected, repeat paracentesis should be performed after 48 hours of antibiotic therapy to confirm that the PMN count is decreasing. Secondary bacterial peritonitis should be suspected in patients in whom the PMN count is not below the pretreatment value at 48 hours.

Neutrocytic ascites may also be seen in some patients with peritoneal carcinomatosis, pancreatic ascites, or tuberculous ascites. In these circumstances, however, PMNs account for less than 50% of the ascitic white blood cells.

Prevention

Up to 70% of patients who survive an episode of spontaneous bacterial peritonitis will have another episode within 1 year. Oral once-daily prophylactic therapy—with norfloxacin, 400 mg, ciprofloxacin, 250–500 mg, or trimethoprim-sulfamethoxazole, one double-strength tablet—has been shown to reduce the rate of recurrent infections to less than 20% and is recommended. Prophylaxis should be considered also in patients who have not had prior bacterial peritonitis but are at increased risk of infection due to low-protein ascites (total ascitic protein less than 1 g/dL). Although improvement in survival in cirrhotic patients with ascites treated with prophylactic antibiotics has not been shown, decision analytic modeling suggests that in patients with prior bacterial peritonitis or low ascitic fluid protein, the use of prophylactic antibiotics is a cost-effective strategy.

Treatment

Empiric therapy for spontaneous bacterial peritonitis should be initiated with a third-generation cephalosporin (such as cefotaxime, 2 g intravenously every 8–12 hours, or ceftriaxone, 1–2 g intravenously every 24 hours) or a combination beta-lactam/beta-lactamase agent (such as ampicillin/sulbactam, 2 g/1 g intravenously every 6 hours). Because of a high risk of nephrotoxicity in patients with chronic liver disease, aminoglycosides should not be used. A repeat paracentesis is recommended after 48 hours of treatment in patients without clinical improvement. If the ascitic neutrophil count has not decreased by 25%, antibiotic coverage should be adjusted (guided by culture and sensitivity results, if available) and secondary causes of peritonitis excluded. Although the optimal duration of therapy is unknown, a course of 5–10 days is sufficient in most patients, or until the ascites fluid PMN count decreases to less than 250 cells/mcL.

Kidney injury develops in up to 40% of patients and is a major cause of death. Intravenous albumin increases effective arterial circulating volume and renal perfusion, decreasing the incidence of kidney injury and mortality. Intravenous albumin, 1.5 g/kg on day 1 and 1 g/kg on day 3, should be administered to patients at high risk for hepatorenal failure (ie, patients with baseline creatinine greater than 1 mg/dL, blood urea nitrogen [BUN] more than 30 mg/dL, or bilirubin more than 4 mg/dL). Nonselective beta-blockers increase the risk of hepatorenal syndrome in patients with bacterial peritonitis and should be discontinued permanently due to their adverse impact on cardiac output and renal perfusion in advanced cirrhosis which is associated with decreased long-term survival. Patients with suspected secondary bacterial peritonitis should be given broad-spectrum coverage for enteric aerobic and anaerobic flora with a third-generation cephalosporin and metronidazole pending identification and definitive (usually surgical) treatment of the cause.

▶ **Prognosis**

The mortality rate of spontaneous bacterial peritonitis exceeds 30%. However, if the disease is recognized and treated early, the rate is less than 10%. As the majority of patients have underlying severe liver disease, many may die of liver failure, hepatorenal syndrome, or bleeding complications from portal hypertension. The most effective treatment for recurrent spontaneous bacterial peritonitis is liver transplant.

Mandorfer M et al. Nonselective β blockers increase risk for hepatorenal syndrome and death in patients with cirrhosis and spontaneous bacterial peritonitis. Gastroenterology. 2014 Jun; 146(7):1680–90. [PMID: 24631577]
Orman ES et al. Paracentesis is associated with reduced mortality in patients hospitalized with cirrhosis and ascites. Clin Gastroenterol Hepatol. 2014 Mar;12(3):496–503. [PMID: 23978348]
Salerno F et al. Albumin infusion improves outcomes of patients with spontaneous bacterial peritonitis: a meta-analysis of randomized trials. Clin Gastroenterol Hepatol. 2013 Feb; 11(2):123–30. [PMID: 23178229]
Tandon P et al. Renal dysfunction is the most important independent predictor of mortality in cirrhotic patients with spontaneous bacterial peritonitis. Clin Gastroenterol Hepatol. 2011 Mar;9(3):260–5. [PMID: 21145427]

MALIGNANT ASCITES

Two-thirds of cases of malignant ascites are caused by peritoneal carcinomatosis. The most common tumors causing carcinomatosis are primary adenocarcinomas of the ovary, uterus, pancreas, stomach, colon, lung, or breast. The remaining one-third is due to lymphatic obstruction or portal hypertension due to hepatocellular carcinoma or diffuse hepatic metastases. Patients present with nonspecific abdominal discomfort and weight loss associated with increased abdominal girth. Nausea or vomiting may be caused by partial or complete intestinal obstruction. Abdominal CT may be useful to demonstrate the primary malignancy or hepatic metastases but seldom confirms the diagnosis of peritoneal carcinomatosis. In patients with carcinomatosis, paracentesis demonstrates a low serum ascites-albumin gradient (less than 1.1 mg/dL), an increased total protein (greater than 2.5 g/dL), and an

elevated white cell count (often both neutrophils and mononuclear cells) but with a lymphocyte predominance. Cytology is positive in over 95%, but laparoscopy may be required in patients with negative cytology to confirm the diagnosis and to exclude tuberculous peritonitis, with which it may be confused. Malignant ascites attributable to portal hypertension usually is associated with an increased serum ascites-albumin gradient (greater than 1.1 g/dL), a variable total protein, and negative ascitic cytology. Ascites caused by peritoneal carcinomatosis does not respond to diuretics.

Patients may be treated with periodic large-volume paracentesis for symptomatic relief. Indwelling catheters can be left in place for patients approaching the end of life who require periodic paracentesis for symptomatic relief. Intraperitoneal chemotherapy is sometimes used to shrink the tumor, but the overall prognosis is extremely poor, with only 10% survival at 6 months. Ovarian cancers represent an exception to this rule. With newer treatments consisting of surgical debulking and intraperitoneal chemotherapy, long-term survival from ovarian cancer is possible.

Cavazzoni E et al. Malignant ascites: pathophysiology and treatment. Int J Clin Oncol. 2013 Feb;18(1):1–9. [PMID: 22460778]

FAMILIAL MEDITERRANEAN FEVER

This is a rare autosomal recessive disorder of unknown pathogenesis that almost exclusively affects people of Mediterranean ancestry, especially Sephardic Jews, Armenians, Turks, and Arabs. Patients lack a protease in serosal fluids that normally inactivates interleukin-8 and the chemotactic complement factor 5A. Symptoms present in most patients before the age of 20 years. It is characterized by episodic bouts of acute peritonitis that may be associated with serositis involving the joints and pleura. Peritoneal attacks are marked by the sudden onset of fever, severe abdominal pain, and abdominal tenderness with guarding or rebound tenderness. If left untreated, attacks resolve within 24–48 hours. Because symptoms resemble those of surgical peritonitis, patients may undergo unnecessary exploratory laparotomy. Colchicine, 0.6 mg orally two or three times daily, has been shown to decrease the frequency and severity of attacks.

MESOTHELIOMA

(See Chapter 39.)

▼ DISEASES OF THE ESOPHAGUS

(See Chapter 39 for Esophageal Cancer.)

▶ **Symptoms**

Heartburn, dysphagia, and odynophagia almost always indicate a primary esophageal disorder.

A. Heartburn

Heartburn (pyrosis) is the feeling of substernal burning, often radiating to the neck. Caused by the reflux of acidic (or, rarely, alkaline) material into the esophagus, it is highly specific for GERD.

B. Dysphagia

Difficulties in swallowing may arise from problems in transferring the food bolus from the oropharynx to the upper esophagus (oropharyngeal dysphagia) or from impaired transport of the bolus through the body of the esophagus (esophageal dysphagia). The history usually leads to the correct diagnosis.

1. Oropharyngeal dysphagia—The oropharyngeal phase of swallowing is a complex process requiring elevation of the tongue, closure of the nasopharynx, relaxation of the upper esophageal sphincter, closure of the airway, and pharyngeal peristalsis. A variety of mechanical and neuromuscular conditions can disrupt this process (Table 15–8). Problems with the oral phase of swallowing cause drooling or spillage of food from the mouth, inability to chew or initiate swallowing, or dry mouth. Pharyngeal dysphagia is characterized by an immediate sense of the bolus catching in the neck, the need to swallow repeatedly to clear food from the pharynx, or coughing or choking during meals. There may be associated dysphonia, dysarthria, or other neurologic symptoms.

2. Esophageal dysphagia—Esophageal dysphagia may be caused by **mechanical obstructions** of the esophagus or by

Table 15–8. Causes of oropharyngeal dysphagia.

Neurologic disorders
Brainstem cerebrovascular accident, mass lesion
Amyotrophic lateral sclerosis, multiple sclerosis, pseudobulbar palsy, post-polio syndrome, Guillain-Barré syndrome
Parkinson disease, Huntington disease, dementia
Tardive dyskinesia
Muscular and rheumatologic disorders
Myopathies, polymyositis
Oculopharyngeal dystrophy
Sjögren syndrome
Metabolic disorders
Thyrotoxicosis, amyloidosis, Cushing disease, Wilson disease
Medication side effects: anticholinergics, phenothiazines
Infectious disease
Polio, diphtheria, botulism, Lyme disease, syphilis, mucositis (*Candida*, herpes)
Structural disorders
Zenker diverticulum
Cervical osteophytes, cricopharyngeal bar, proximal esophageal webs
Oropharyngeal tumors
Postsurgical or radiation changes
Pill-induced injury
Motility disorders
Upper esophageal sphincter dysfunction

Table 15–9. Causes of esophageal dysphagia.

Cause	Clues
Mechanical obstruction	**Solid foods worse than liquids**
Schatzki ring	Intermittent dysphagia; not progressive
Peptic stricture	Chronic heartburn; progressive dysphagia
Esophageal cancer	Progressive dysphagia; age over 50 years
Eosinophilic esophagitis	Young adults; small-caliber lumen, proximal stricture, corrugated rings, or white papules
Motility disorder	**Solid and liquid foods**
Achalasia	Progressive dysphagia
Diffuse esophageal spasm	Intermittent; not progressive; may have chest pain
Scleroderma	Chronic heartburn; Raynaud phenomenon
Ineffective esophageal motility	Intermittent; not progressive; commonly associated with GERD

motility disorders (Table 15–9). Patients with mechanical obstruction experience dysphagia, primarily for solids. This is recurrent, predictable, and, if the lesion progresses, will worsen as the lumen narrows. Patients with **motility disorders** have dysphagia for both solids and liquids. It is episodic, unpredictable, and can be progressive.

C. Odynophagia

Odynophagia is sharp substernal pain on swallowing that may limit oral intake. It usually reflects severe erosive disease. It is most commonly associated with infectious esophagitis due to *Candida*, herpesviruses, or CMV, especially in immunocompromised patients. It may also be caused by corrosive injury due to caustic ingestions and by pill-induced ulcers.

▶ Diagnostic Studies

A. Upper Endoscopy

Endoscopy is the study of choice for evaluating persistent heartburn, dysphagia, odynophagia, and structural abnormalities detected on barium esophagography. In addition to direct visualization, it allows biopsy of mucosal abnormalities and of normal mucosa (to evaluate for eosinophilic esophagitis) as well as dilation of strictures.

B. Videoesophagography

Oropharyngeal dysphagia is best evaluated with rapid-sequence videoesophagography.

C. Barium Esophagography

Patients with esophageal dysphagia often are evaluated first with a radiographic barium study to differentiate between mechanical lesions and motility disorders, providing important information about the latter in particular. In patients with esophageal dysphagia and a suspected motility disorder, barium esophagoscopy should be obtained first. In patients in whom there is a high suspicion of a mechanical lesion, many clinicians will proceed first to endoscopic evaluation because it better identifies mucosa lesions (eg, erosions) and permits mucosal biopsy and dilation. However, barium study is more sensitive for detecting subtle esophageal narrowing due to rings, achalasia, and proximal esophageal lesions.

D. Esophageal Manometry

Esophageal motility may be assessed using manometric techniques. They are indicated: (1) to determine the location of the LES to allow precise placement of a conventional electrode pH probe; (2) to establish the etiology of dysphagia in patients in whom a mechanical obstruction cannot be found, especially if a diagnosis of achalasia is suspected by endoscopy or barium study; (3) for the preoperative assessment of patients being considered for antireflux surgery to exclude an alternative diagnosis (eg, achalasia) or possibly to assess peristaltic function in the esophageal body. High-resolution manometry may be superior to conventional manometry for distinguishing motility disorders.

E. Esophageal pH Recording and Impedance Testing

The pH within the esophageal lumen may be monitored continuously for 24–48 hours. There are two kinds of systems in use: catheter-based and wireless. Traditional systems use a long transnasal catheter that is connected directly to the recording device. Wireless systems are increasingly used; in these systems, a capsule is attached directly to the esophageal mucosa under endoscopic visualization and data are transmitted by radiotelemetry to the recording device. The recording provides information about the amount of esophageal acid reflux and the temporal correlations between symptoms and reflux.

Esophageal pH monitoring devices provide information about the amount of esophageal acid reflux but not nonacid reflux. Techniques using combined pH and multichannel intraluminal impedance allow assessment of acid and nonacid liquid reflux. They may be useful in evaluation of patients with atypical reflux symptoms or persistent symptoms despite therapy with proton pump inhibitors to diagnose hypersensitivity, functional symptoms, and symptoms caused by nonacid reflux.

Pugliese D et al. pH impedance vs. traditional pH monitoring in clinical practice: an outcome study. J Gastroenterol. 2016 Feb; 51(2):130–7. [PMID: 26033511]

Xiao Y et al. Tailored therapy for the refractory GERD patients by combined multichannel intraluminal impedance-pH monitoring. J Gastroenterol Hepatol. 2016 Feb;31(2):350–4. [PMID: 26202002]

GASTROESOPHAGEAL REFLUX DISEASE

► Heartburn; may be exacerbated by meals, bending, or recumbency.

► Typical uncomplicated cases do not require diagnostic studies.

► Endoscopy demonstrates abnormalities in one-third of patients.

► General Considerations

GERD is a condition that develops when the reflux of stomach contents causes troublesome symptoms or complications. GERD affects 20% of adults, who report at least weekly episodes of heartburn, and up to 10% complain of daily symptoms. Although most patients have mild disease, esophageal mucosal damage (reflux esophagitis) develops in up to one-third and more serious complications develop in a few others. Several factors may contribute to GERD.

A. Dysfunction of the Gastroesophageal Junction

The antireflux barrier at the gastroesophageal junction depends on LES pressure, the intra-abdominal location of the sphincter (resulting in a "flap valve" caused by angulation of the esophageal-gastric junction), and the extrinsic compression of the sphincter by the crural diaphragm. In most patients with GERD, baseline LES pressures are normal (10–35 mm Hg). Most reflux episodes occur during transient relaxations of the LES that are triggered by gastric distention by a vagovagal reflex. A subset of patients with GERD have an incompetent (less than 10 mm Hg) LES that results in increased acid reflux, especially when supine or when intra-abdominal pressures are increased by lifting or bending. A hypotensive sphincter is present in up to 50% of patients with severe erosive GERD.

Hiatal hernias are found in one-fourth of patients with nonerosive GERD, three-fourths of patients with severe erosive esophagitis, and over 90% of patients with Barrett esophagus. They are caused by movement of the LES above the diaphragm, resulting in dysfunction of the gastroesophageal junction reflux barrier. Hiatal hernias are common and may cause no symptoms; however, in patients with gastroesophageal reflux, they are associated with higher amounts of acid reflux and delayed esophageal acid clearance, leading to more severe esophagitis and Barrett esophagus. Increased reflux episodes occur during normal swallowing-induced relaxation, transient LES relaxations, and straining due to reflux of acid from the hiatal hernia sac into the esophagus.

Truncal obesity may contribute to GERD, presumably due to an increased intra-abdominal pressure, which contributes to dysfunction of the gastroesophageal junction and increased likelihood of hiatal hernia.

B. Irritant Effects of Refluxate

Esophageal mucosal damage is related to the potency of the refluxate and the amount of time it is in contact with the mucosa. Acidic gastric fluid (pH less than 4.0) is extremely caustic to the esophageal mucosa and is the major injurious agent in the majority of cases. In some patients, reflux of bile or alkaline pancreatic secretions may be contributory.

Most acid reflux episodes occur after meals, despite the buffering effect of food that raises intragastric pH. In fact, meal-stimulated acid secretion from the proximal stomach mixes poorly with gastric contents, forming an unbuffered "acid pocket" that floats on top of the meal contents. In patients with GERD, this acid pocket is located near the gastroesophageal junction and may extend into the LES or hiatal hernia.

C. Abnormal Esophageal Clearance

Acid refluxate normally is cleared and neutralized by esophageal peristalsis and salivary bicarbonate. One-half of patients with severe GERD have diminished clearance due to hypotensive peristaltic contractions (less than 30 mm Hg) or intermittent failed peristalsis after swallowing. Certain medical conditions such as scleroderma are associated with diminished peristalsis. Sjögren syndrome, anticholinergic medications, and oral radiation therapy may exacerbate GERD due to impaired salivation.

D. Delayed Gastric Emptying

Impaired gastric emptying due to gastroparesis or partial gastric outlet obstruction potentiates GERD.

▶ Clinical Findings

A. Symptoms and Signs

The typical symptom is heartburn. This most often occurs 30–60 minutes after meals and upon reclining. Patients often report relief from taking antacids or baking soda. When this symptom is dominant, the diagnosis is established with a high degree of reliability. Many patients, however, have less specific dyspeptic symptoms with or without heartburn. Overall, a clinical diagnosis of gastroesophageal reflux has a sensitivity and specificity of only 65%. Severity is not correlated with the degree of tissue damage. In fact, some patients with severe esophagitis are only mildly symptomatic. Patients may complain of regurgitation—the spontaneous reflux of sour or bitter gastric contents into the mouth. Dysphagia occurs in one-third of patients and may be due to erosive esophagitis, abnormal esophageal peristalsis, or the development of an esophageal stricture.

"Atypical" or "extraesophageal" manifestations of gastroesophageal disease may occur, including asthma, chronic cough, chronic laryngitis, sore throat, noncardiac chest pain, and sleep disturbances. Gastroesophageal reflux, especially unrecognized nocturnal reflux, may be either a causative or an exacerbating factor in a subset of these patients. In the absence of heartburn or regurgitation, atypical symptoms are unlikely to be related to gastroesophageal reflux.

Physical examination and laboratory data are normal in uncomplicated disease.

B. Special Examinations

Initial diagnostic studies are not warranted for patients with typical GERD symptoms suggesting uncomplicated reflux disease. Patients with typical symptoms of heartburn and regurgitation should be treated empirically with a once daily proton pump inhibitor for 4–8 weeks. Symptomatic response to empiric treatment (while clinically desirable) only has a 78% sensitivity and 54% specificity for GERD. Therefore, further investigation is required in patients with symptoms that persist despite empiric proton pump inhibitor therapy to identify complications of reflux disease and to diagnose other conditions, particularly in patients with "alarm features" (troublesome dysphagia, odynophagia, weight loss, iron deficiency anemia).

1. Upper endoscopy—Upper endoscopy is excellent for documenting the type and extent of tissue damage in gastroesophageal reflux; for detecting other gastroesophageal lesions that may mimic GERD; and for detecting GERD complications, including esophageal stricture, Barrett metaplasia, and esophageal adenocarcinoma. In the absence of prior antisecretory therapy, up to one-third of patients with GERD have visible mucosal damage (known as reflux esophagitis), characterized by single or multiple erosions or ulcers in the distal esophagus at the squamocolumnar junction. In patients treated with a proton pump inhibitor prior to endoscopy, preexisting reflux esophagitis may be partially or completely healed. The Los Angeles (LA) classification grades reflux esophagitis on a scale of A (one or more isolated mucosal breaks 5 mm or less that do not extend between the tops of two mucosal folds) to D (one or more mucosal breaks that involve at least 75% of the esophageal circumference).

2. Barium esophagography—This study should not be performed to diagnose GERD. In patients with severe dysphagia, it is sometimes obtained prior to endoscopy to identify a stricture.

3. Esophageal pH or combined esophageal pH-impedance testing—Esophageal pH monitoring is unnecessary in most patients but may be indicated to document abnormal esophageal acid exposure in patients who have atypical or extraesophageal symptoms or who are being considered for antireflux surgery. Combined impedance-pH monitoring is indicated in patients with persistent symptoms despite proton pump inhibitor therapy to determine whether symptoms are caused by acid or nonacid reflux (40%) or are unrelated to reflux and indicative of a functional disorder.

▶ Differential Diagnosis

Symptoms of GERD may be similar to those of other diseases such as esophageal motility disorders, peptic ulcer, angina pectoris, or functional disorders. Reflux erosive esophagitis may be confused with pill-induced damage, eosinophilic esophagitis, or infections (CMV, herpes, *Candida*).

▶ Complications

A. Barrett Esophagus

This is a condition in which the squamous epithelium of the esophagus is replaced by metaplastic columnar epithelium containing goblet and columnar cells (specialized intestinal metaplasia). Present in up to 10% of patients with chronic reflux, Barrett esophagus is believed to arise from chronic reflux-induced injury to the esophageal squamous epithelium; however, it is also increased in patients with truncal obesity independent of GERD. Barrett esophagus is suspected at endoscopy from the presence of orange, gastric type epithelium that extends upward from the stomach into the distal tubular esophagus in a tongue-like or circumferential fashion. Biopsies obtained at endoscopy confirm the diagnosis. Three types of columnar epithelium may be identified: gastric cardiac, gastric fundic, and specialized intestinal metaplasia. There is agreement that the latter carries an increased risk of dysplasia; however, some authorities believe that gastric cardiac mucosa also raises risk.

Barrett esophagus does not provoke specific symptoms but gastroesophageal reflux does. Most patients have a long history of reflux symptoms, such as heartburn and regurgitation. Barrett esophagus should be treated with long-term proton pump inhibitors once or twice daily to control reflux symptoms. Although these medications do not appear to cause regression of Barrett esophagus, they may reduce the risk of cancer. Paradoxically, one-third of patients report minimal or no symptoms of GERD, suggesting decreased acid sensitivity of Barrett epithelium. Indeed, over 90% of individuals with Barrett esophagus in the general population do not seek medical attention.

The most serious complication of Barrett esophagus is esophageal adenocarcinoma. It is believed that most adenocarcinomas of the esophagus and many such tumors of the gastric cardia arise from dysplastic epithelium in Barrett esophagus. In recent studies, the incidence of adenocarcinoma in patients with Barrett esophagus has been estimated at 0.12–0.33%/year. Although this still is an 11-fold increased risk compared with patients without Barrett esophagus, adenocarcinoma of the esophagus remains a relatively uncommon malignancy in the United States (7000 cases/year). Given the large number of adults with chronic GERD relative to the small number in whom adenocarcinoma develops, 2011 clinical guidelines recommend against endoscopic screening for Barrett esophagus in adults with GERD except in those with multiple risk factors for adenocarcinoma (chronic GERD, hiatal hernia, obesity, white race, male gender, and age 50 years of older).

In patients known to have Barrett esophagus, surveillance endoscopy every 3–5 years is recommended to look for low- or high-grade dysplasia or adenocarcinoma. The risk of progression to adenocarcinoma is a 0.8% risk per year for patients with low-grade dysplasia and a 6% risk per year for high-grade dysplasia. Patients with low-grade dysplasia require repeat endoscopic surveillance in 6 months to exclude coexisting high-grade dysplasia or cancer and, if low-grade dysplasia persists, endoscopic surveillance should be repeated yearly.

Approximately 13% of patient with high-grade dysplasia may harbor an unrecognized invasive esophageal cancer. Therefore, patients with high-grade dysplasia should undergo repeat staging endoscopy with resection of visible mucosal nodules and random mucosal biopsies in order to exclude invasive cancer. The subsequent management of patients with intramucosal cancer or high-grade dysplasia has rapidly evolved. Until recently, esophagectomy was recommended for patients deemed to have a low operative risk; however, this procedure is associated with high morbidity and mortality rates (40% and 1–5%, respectively). Therefore, it is now recommended that endoscopic therapy be performed for most patients with high-grade dysplasia or intramucosal adenocarcinoma. Endoscopic therapies can remove or ablate dysplastic Barrett epithelium, using mucosal snare resection and radiofrequency wave ablation electrocautery. Snare resection is performed of visible neoplastic mucosal nodules to exclude submucosal invasion (which favors surgical resection). Of the patients who have cancer confined to the mucosa, less than 2% have recurrence of cancer or high-grade dysplasia after snare resection. Radiofrequency wave ablation electrocautery is used to ablate Barrett epithelium with flat (non-nodular) dysplasia and to ablate Barrett epithelium that remains after snare resection of dysplastic mucosal nodules. The efficacy of endoscopic ablation therapies in patients with Barrett dysplasia is supported by several studies. When high-dose proton pump inhibitors are administered to normalize intraesophageal pH, radiofrequency wave ablation electrocautery eradication of Barrett columnar epithelium is followed by complete healing with normal squamous epithelium in greater than 90% of patients. In a 2011 randomized, sham-controlled trial in 127 patients with Barrett dysplasia with 3-year follow up, eradication of high-grade dysplasia occurred in 98% after radiofrequency ablation (HALO) and progression to cancer was only 0.55%/year. After initial ablation, Barrett esophagus recurs (with or without dysplasia) in up to 33% within 2 years, justifying periodic surveillance endoscopy.

Endoscopic ablation techniques have a risk of complications (bleeding, perforation, strictures). Therefore, endoscopic eradication therapy currently is not recommended for patients with nondysplastic Barrett esophagus for whom the risk of developing esophageal cancer is low and treatment does not appear to be cost-effective.

B. Peptic Stricture

Stricture formation occurs in about 5% of patients with esophagitis. It is manifested by the gradual development of solid food dysphagia progressive over months to years. Often there is a reduction in heartburn because the stricture acts as a barrier to reflux. Most strictures are located at the gastroesophageal junction. Endoscopy with biopsy is mandatory in all cases to differentiate peptic stricture from stricture by esophageal carcinoma. Active erosive esophagitis is often present. Up to 90% of symptomatic patients are effectively treated with dilation with graduated polyvinyl catheters passed over a wire placed at the time of endoscopy or fluoroscopically, or balloons passed fluoroscopically or through an endoscope. Dilation is continued over one to several sessions. A luminal diameter of 13–17 mm is usually sufficient to relieve dysphagia. Long-term therapy with a proton pump inhibitor is required to decrease the likelihood of stricture recurrence. Some patients require intermittent dilation to maintain luminal patency, but operative management for strictures that do not respond to dilation is seldom required. Refractory strictures may benefit from endoscopic injection of triamcinolone into the stricture.

► **Treatment**

A. Medical Treatment

The goal of treatment is to provide symptomatic relief, to heal esophagitis (if present), and to prevent complications. In the majority of patients with uncomplicated disease, empiric treatment is initiated based on a compatible history without the need for further confirmatory studies. Patients not responding and those with suspected complications undergo further evaluation with upper endoscopy or esophageal manometry and pH recording.

1. Mild, intermittent symptoms—Patients with mild or intermittent symptoms that do not impact adversely on quality of life may benefit from lifestyle modifications with medical interventions taken as needed. Patients may find that eating smaller meals and elimination of acidic foods (citrus, tomatoes, coffee, spicy foods), foods that precipitate reflux (fatty foods, chocolate, peppermint, alcohol), and cigarettes may reduce symptoms. Weight loss should be recommended for patients who are overweight or have had recent weight gain. All patients should be advised to avoid lying down within 3 hours after meals (the period of greatest reflux). Patients with nocturnal symptoms should also elevate the head of the bed on 6-inch blocks or a foam wedge to reduce reflux and enhance esophageal clearance.

Patients with infrequent heartburn (less than once weekly) may be treated on demand with antacids or oral H_2-receptor antagonists. Antacids provide rapid relief of heartburn; however, their duration of action is less than 2 hours. Many are available over the counter. Those containing magnesium should not be used for patients with kidney disease, and patients with acute or chronic kidney disease should be cautioned appropriately.

All oral H_2-receptor antagonists are available in over-the-counter formulations: cimetidine 200 mg, ranitidine and nizatidine 75 mg, famotidine 10 mg—all of which are half of the typical prescription strength. When taken for active heartburn, these agents have a delay in onset of at least 30 minutes. However, once these agents take effect, they provide heartburn relief for up to 8 hours. When taken before meals known to provoke heartburn, these agents reduce the symptom.

2. Troublesome symptoms

A. Initial therapy—Patients with troublesome reflux symptoms and patients with known complications of GERD should be treated with a once-daily oral proton pump inhibitor (omeprazole or rabeprazole, 20 mg; omeprazole, 40 mg with sodium bicarbonate; lansoprazole, 30 mg; dexlansoprazole, 60 mg; esomeprazole or

pantoprazole, 40 mg) taken 30 minutes before breakfast for 4–8 weeks. Because there appears to be little difference between these agents in efficacy or side effect profiles, the choice of agent is determined by cost. Oral omeprazole, 20 mg, and lansoprazole, 15 mg, are available as over-the-counter formulations. Once-daily proton pump inhibitors achieve adequate control of heartburn in 80–90% of patients, complete heartburn resolution in over 50%, and healing of erosive esophagitis (when present) in over 80%. Because of their superior efficacy and ease of use, proton pump inhibitors are preferred to H_2-receptor antagonists for the treatment of acute and chronic GERD. Approximately 10–20% of patients do not achieve symptom relief with a once-daily dose within 2–4 weeks and require a twice-daily proton pump inhibitor (taken 30 minutes before breakfast and dinner). Patients with inadequate symptom relief with empiric twice-daily proton pump inhibitor therapy should undergo evaluation with upper endoscopy. Many providers prefer to prescribe initial twice-daily proton pump inhibitor therapy for patients who have documented severe erosive esophagitis (Los Angeles Grade C or D), Barrett esophagus, or peptic stricture.

B. Long-term therapy—In those who achieve good symptomatic relief with a course of empiric once-daily proton pump inhibitor, therapy may be discontinued after 8–12 weeks. Most patients (over 80%) will experience relapse of GERD symptoms, usually within 3 months. Patients whose symptoms relapse may be treated with either continuous proton pump inhibitor therapy, intermittent 2–4 week courses, or "on demand" therapy (ie, drug taken until symptoms abate) depending on symptom frequency and patient preference. Alternatively, twice daily H_2-receptor antagonists may be used to control symptoms in patients without erosive esophagitis. Patients who require twice-daily proton pump inhibitor therapy for initial symptom control and patients with complications of GERD, including severe erosive esophagitis, Barrett esophagus, or peptic stricture, should be maintained on long-term therapy with a once- or twice-daily proton pump inhibitor titrated to the lowest effective dose to achieve satisfactory symptom control.

Side effects of proton pump inhibitors are uncommon. Headache, diarrhea, and abdominal pain may occur with any of the agents but generally resolve when another formulation is tried. Potential risks of long-term use of proton pump inhibitors include an increased risk of infectious gastroenteritis (including *C difficile*), iron and vitamin B_{12} deficiency, hypomagnesemia, pneumonia, hip fractures (possibly due to impaired calcium absorption), and fundic gland polyps (which appear to be of no clinical significance).

3. Extraesophageal reflux manifestations—Establishing a causal relationship between gastroesophageal reflux and extraesophageal symptoms (eg, asthma, hoarseness, cough, sleep disturbances) is difficult. Gastroesophageal reflux seldom is the sole cause of extraesophageal disorders but may be a contributory factor. Although ambulatory esophageal pH testing can document the presence of increased acid esophageal reflux, it does not prove a causative connection. Current guidelines recommend that a trial of a twice-daily proton pump inhibitor be administered for 2–3 months in patients with suspected extraesophageal GERD syndromes who also have typical GERD symptoms. Improvement of extraesophageal symptoms suggests but does not prove that acid reflux is the causative factor. Esophageal impedance-pH testing may be performed in patients whose extraesophageal symptoms persist after 3 months of twice-daily proton pump inhibitor therapy and may be considered before proton pump inhibitor therapy in patients without typical GERD symptoms in whom other causes of extraesophageal symptoms have been excluded.

4. Unresponsive disease—Approximately 5% do not respond to twice-daily proton pump inhibitors or a change to a different proton pump inhibitor. These patients should undergo endoscopy for detection of severe, inadequately treated reflux esophagitis and for other gastroesophageal lesions (including eosinophilic esophagitis) that may mimic GERD. The presence of active erosive esophagitis usually is indicative of inadequate acid suppression and can almost always be treated successfully with higher proton pump inhibitor doses (eg, esomeprazole, 40 mg twice daily). Alginate is a naturally occurring polymer that forms a viscous raft that floats on the gastric acid pocket and significantly reduces postprandial reflux episodes in patients with GERD and large hiatal hernias. A proprietary antacid-alginate formulation (Gaviscon Double Action Liquid) is available in Europe but not the United States. Truly refractory esophagitis may be caused by gastrinoma with gastric acid hypersecretion (Zollinger-Ellison syndrome), pill-induced esophagitis, resistance to proton pump inhibitors, and medical noncompliance. Patients without endoscopically visible esophagitis should undergo ambulatory impedance-pH monitoring while taking a twice-daily proton pump inhibitor to determine whether the symptoms are correlated with acid or nonacid reflux episodes. The pH study is performed on therapy if the suspicion for GERD is high (to determine whether therapy has adequately suppressed acid esophageal reflux) and off therapy if the suspicion for GERD is low (to determine whether the patient has reflux disease). Combined esophageal pH monitoring with impedance monitoring is preferred over pH testing alone because of its ability to detect both acid and nonacid reflux events. Approximately 60% of patients with unresponsive symptoms do not have increased reflux and may be presumed to have a functional disorder. Treatment with a low-dose tricyclic antidepressant (eg, imipramine or nortriptyline 25 mg at bedtime) may be beneficial.

B. Surgical Treatment

Surgical fundoplication affords good to excellent relief of symptoms and healing of esophagitis in over 85% of properly selected patients and can be performed laparoscopically with low complication rates in most instances. Although patient satisfaction is high, typical reflux symptoms recur in 10–30% of patients. Furthermore, new symptoms of dysphagia, bloating, increased flatulence, dyspepsia, or diarrhea develop in over 30% of patients. In 2011, results from a randomized trial comparing laparoscopic fundoplication with prolonged medical therapy (esomeprazole 40 mg/day) for chronic GERD were reported. After 5 years, adequate GERD symptom control (symptom remission) was similar, occurring in 85–92% of patients; however, patients who had undergone fundoplication had increased dysphagia, bloating, and flatulence. In 2012, the FDA approved a novel, minimally invasive magnetic artificial sphincter for the treatment of GERD. The device is made up of a flexible, elastic string of titanium beads (wrapped around a magnetic core) that is placed laparoscopically below the diaphragm at the gastroesophageal junction. A 2013 prospective study of 100 patients reported that 64% of patients had significant reductions in esophageal acid reflux. Further experience with this device is needed before widespread adoption can be recommended.

Surgical treatment is not recommended for patients who are well controlled with medical therapies but should be considered for: (1) otherwise healthy, carefully selected patients with extraesophageal manifestations of reflux, as these symptoms often require high doses of proton pump inhibitors and may be more effectively controlled with antireflux surgery; (2) those with severe reflux disease who are unwilling to accept lifelong medical therapy due to its expense, inconvenience, or theoretical risks; and (3) patients with large hiatal hernias and persistent regurgitation despite proton pump inhibitor therapy. Gastric bypass (rather than fundoplication) should be considered for obese patients with GERD.

▶ When to Refer

- Patients with typical GERD whose symptoms do not resolve with empiric management with a twice-daily proton pump inhibitor.

- Patients with suspected extraesophageal GERD symptoms that do not resolve with 3 months of twice-daily proton pump inhibitor therapy.

- Patients with significant dysphagia or other alarm symptoms for upper endoscopy.

- Patients with Barrett esophagus for endoscopic surveillance.

- Patients who have Barrett esophagus with dysplasia or early mucosal cancer.

- Surgical fundoplication is considered.

Bennett C et al. Consensus statements for management of Barrett's dysplasia and early-stage esophageal adenocarcinoma, based on a Delphi process. Gastroenterology. 2012 Aug;143(2):336–46. [PMID: 22537613]

Di Pietro M et al. Screening for Barrett's esophagus. Gastroenterology. 2015 May;148(5):912–23. [PMID: 25701083]

Galmiche JP et al; LOTUS Trial Collaborators. Laparoscopic antireflux surgery vs esomeprazole treatment for chronic GERD. JAMA. 2011 May 18;305(19):1969–77. [PMID: 21586712]

Ganz RA et al. Esophageal sphincter device for gastroesophageal reflux disease. N Engl J Med. 2013 May 23;368(21):2039–40. [PMID: 23697523]

Gupta M et al. Recurrence of esophageal intestinal metaplasia after endoscopic mucosal resection and radiofrequency ablation of Barrett's esophagus: results from a US Multicenter Consortium. Gastroenterology. 2013 Jul;145(1):79–86. [PMID: 23499759]

Harnik IG. In the Clinic. Gastroesophageal reflux disease. Ann Intern Med. 2015 Jul 7;163(1):ITC1. [PMID: 26148292]

Johnson DA et al. Reported side effects and complications of long-term proton pump inhibitor use: dissecting the evidence. Clin Gastroenterol Hepatol. 2013 May;11(5):458–64. Erratum in: Clin Gastroenterol Hepatol. 2013 Jul;11(7):880. [PMID: 23247326]

Katz PO et al. Guidelines for the diagnosis and management of gastroesophageal reflux disease. Am J Gastroenterol. 2013 Mar; 108(3):308–28. Erratum in: Am J Gastroenterol. 2013 Oct; 108(10):1672. [PMID: 23419381]

Phoa KN et al. Radiofrequency ablation vs endoscopic surveillance for patients with Barrett esophagus and low-grade dysplasia: a randomized clinical trial. JAMA. 2014 Mar 26; 311(12):1209–17. [PMID: 24668102]

Richter JE. Gastroesophageal reflux disease treatment: side effects and complications of fundoplication. Clin Gastroenterol Hepatol. 2013 May;11(5):465–71. [PMID: 23267868]

Rohof WO et al. An alginate-antacid formulation localizes to the acid pocket to reduce acid reflux in patients with gastroesophageal reflux disease. Clin Gastroenterol Hepatol. 2013 Dec;11(12):1585–91. [PMID: 23669304]

Small AJ et al. Radiofrequency ablation is associated with decreased neoplastic progression in patients with Barrett's esophagus and confirmed low-grade dysplasia. Gastroenterology. 2015 Sep;149(3):567–76. [PMID: 25917785]

Spechler SJ. Barrett esophagus and risk of esophageal cancer: a clinical review. JAMA. 2013 Aug 14;310(6):627–36. [PMID: 23942681]

Sugerman DT. JAMA patient page. Gastroesophageal reflux disease. JAMA. 2014 Jun 18;311(23):2452. [PMID: 24938579]

Vaezi MF. Ambulatory monitoring for gastroesophageal reflux disease: where do we stand? Clin Gastroenterol Hepatol. 2015 May;13(5):892–4. [PMID: 25451884]

Weijenborg PW et al. Effects of antidepressants in patients with functional esophageal disorders or gastroesophageal reflux disease: a systematic review. Clin Gastroenterol Hepatol. 2015 Feb;13(2):251–9.e1. [PMID: 24997325]

INFECTIOUS ESOPHAGITIS

ESSENTIALS OF DIAGNOSIS

▶ Immunosuppressed patient.

▶ Odynophagia, dysphagia, and chest pain.

▶ Endoscopy with biopsy establishes diagnosis.

▶ General Considerations

Infectious esophagitis occurs most commonly in immunosuppressed patients. Patients with AIDS, solid organ transplants, leukemia, lymphoma, and those receiving immunosuppressive drugs are at particular risk for opportunistic infections. *Candida albicans*, herpes simplex, and CMV are the most common pathogens. *Candida* infection may occur also in patients who have uncontrolled diabetes

and those being treated with systemic corticosteroids, radiation therapy, or systemic antibiotic therapy. Herpes simplex can affect normal hosts, in which case the infection is generally self-limited.

▶ Clinical Findings

A. Symptoms and Signs

The most common symptoms are odynophagia and dysphagia. Substernal chest pain occurs in some patients. Patients with candidal esophagitis are sometimes asymptomatic. Oral thrush is present in only 75% of patients with candidal esophagitis and 25–50% of patients with viral esophagitis and is therefore an unreliable indicator of the cause of esophageal infection. Patients with esophageal CMV infection may have infection at other sites such as the colon and retina. Oral ulcers (herpes labialis) are often associated with herpes simplex esophagitis.

B. Special Examinations

Treatment may be empiric. For diagnostic certainty, endoscopy with biopsy and brushings (for microbiologic and histopathologic analysis) is preferred because of its high diagnostic accuracy. The endoscopic signs of candidal esophagitis are diffuse, linear, yellow-white plaques adherent to the mucosa. CMV esophagitis is characterized by one to several large, shallow, superficial ulcerations. Herpes esophagitis results in multiple small, deep ulcerations.

▶ Treatment

A. Candidal Esophagitis

Systemic therapy is required for esophageal candidiasis. An empiric trial of antifungal therapy is often administered without performing diagnostic endoscopy. Initial therapy is generally with fluconazole, 400 mg on day 1, then 200–400 mg/day orally for 14–21 days. Patients not responding to empiric therapy within 3–5 days should undergo endoscopy with brushings, biopsy, and culture to distinguish resistant fungal infection from other infections (eg, CMV, herpes). Esophageal candidiasis not responding to fluconazole therapy may be treated with itraconazole suspension (not capsules), 200 mg/day orally, or voriconazole, 200 mg orally twice daily. Refractory infection may be treated intravenously with caspofungin, 50 mg daily.

B. Cytomegalovirus Esophagitis

In patients with HIV infection, immune restoration with antiretroviral therapy is the most effective means of controlling CMV disease. Initial therapy is with ganciclovir, 5 mg/kg intravenously every 12 hours for 3–6 weeks. Neutropenia is a frequent dose-limiting side effect. Once resolution of symptoms occurs, it may be possible to complete the course of therapy with oral valganciclovir, 900 mg once daily. Patients who either do not respond to or cannot tolerate ganciclovir are treated acutely with foscarnet, 90 mg/kg intravenously every 12 hours for 3–6 weeks.

The principal toxicity is acute renal injury, hypocalcemia, and hypomagnesemia.

C. Herpetic Esophagitis

Immunocompetent patients may be treated symptomatically and generally do not require specific antiviral therapy. Immunosuppressed patients may be treated with oral acyclovir, 400 mg orally five times daily, or 250 mg/m² intravenously every 8–12 hours, usually for 14–21 days. Oral famciclovir, 500 mg orally three times daily, or valacyclovir, 1 g twice daily, are also effective but more expensive than generic acyclovir. Nonresponders require therapy with foscarnet, 40 mg/kg intravenously every 8 hours for 21 days.

▶ Prognosis

Most patients with infectious esophagitis can be effectively treated with complete symptom resolution. Depending on the patient's underlying immunodeficiency, relapse of symptoms off therapy can raise difficulties. Long-term suppressive therapy is sometimes required.

Almashat SJ et al. Non-reflux esophagitis: a review of inflammatory diseases of the esophagus exclusive of reflux esophagitis. Semin Diagn Pathol. 2014 Mar;31(2):89–99. [PMID: 24815935]
Kim KY et al. Acid suppression therapy as a risk factor for *Candida* esophagitis. Dig Dis Sci. 2013 May;58(5):1282–6. [PMID: 23306845]

PILL-INDUCED ESOPHAGITIS

A number of different medications may injure the esophagus, presumably through direct, prolonged mucosal contact or mechanisms that disrupt mucosal integrity. The most commonly implicated are the NSAIDs, potassium chloride pills, quinidine, zalcitabine, zidovudine, alendronate and risedronate, emepronium bromide, iron, vitamin C, and antibiotics (doxycycline, tetracycline, clindamycin, trimethoprim-sulfamethoxazole). Because injury is most likely to occur if pills are swallowed without water or while supine, hospitalized or bed-bound patients are at greater risk. Symptoms include severe retrosternal chest pain, odynophagia, and dysphagia, often beginning several hours after taking a pill. These may occur suddenly and persist for days. Some patients (especially the elderly) have relatively little pain, presenting with dysphagia. Endoscopy may reveal one to several discrete ulcers that may be shallow or deep. Chronic injury may result in severe esophagitis with stricture, hemorrhage, or perforation. Healing occurs rapidly when the offending agent is eliminated. To prevent pill-induced damage, patients should take pills with 4 oz of water and remain upright for 30 minutes after ingestion. Known offending agents should not be given to patients with esophageal dysmotility, dysphagia, or strictures.

Kim SH et al. Clinical and endoscopic characteristics of drug-induced esophagitis. World J Gastroenterol. 2014 Aug 21; 20(31):10994–9. [PMID: 25152603]

BENIGN ESOPHAGEAL LESIONS

1. Mallory-Weiss Syndrome (Mucosal Laceration of Gastroesophageal Junction)

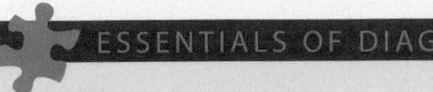

ESSENTIALS OF DIAGNOSIS

▶ Hematemesis; usually self-limited.
▶ Prior history of vomiting, retching in 50%.
▶ Endoscopy establishes diagnosis.

▶ General Considerations

Mallory-Weiss syndrome is characterized by a nonpenetrating mucosal tear at the gastroesophageal junction that is hypothesized to arise from events that suddenly raise transabdominal pressure, such as lifting, retching, or vomiting. Alcoholism is a strong predisposing factor. Mallory-Weiss tears are responsible for approximately 5% of cases of upper gastrointestinal bleeding.

▶ Clinical Findings

A. Symptoms and Signs

Patients usually present with hematemesis with or without melena. A history of retching, vomiting, or straining is obtained in about 50% of cases.

B. Special Examinations

As with other causes of upper gastrointestinal hemorrhage, upper endoscopy should be performed after the patient has been appropriately resuscitated. The diagnosis is established by identification of a 0.5- to 4-cm linear mucosal tear usually located either at the gastroesophageal junction or, more commonly, just below the junction in the gastric mucosa.

▶ Differential Diagnosis

At endoscopy, other potential causes of upper gastrointestinal hemorrhage are found in over 35% of patients with Mallory-Weiss tears, including peptic ulcer disease, erosive gastritis, arteriovenous malformations, and esophageal varices. Patients with underlying portal hypertension are at higher risk for continued or recurrent bleeding.

▶ Treatment

Patients are initially treated as needed with fluid resuscitation and blood transfusions. Most patients stop bleeding spontaneously and require no therapy. Endoscopic hemostatic therapy is employed in patients who have continuing active bleeding. Injection with epinephrine (1:10,000), cautery with a bipolar or heater probe coagulation device, or mechanical compression of the artery by application of an endoclip or band is effective in 90–95% of cases. Angiographic arterial embolization or operative intervention is required in patients who fail endoscopic therapy.

Brown JD. Hiccups: an unappreciated cause of the Mallory-Weiss syndrome. Am J Med. 2015 Dec;128(12):e19–20. [PMID: 26232752]

Nojkov B et al. Distinctive aspects of peptic ulcer disease, Dieulafoy's lesion, and Mallory-Weiss syndrome in patients with advanced alcoholic liver disease or cirrhosis. World J Gastroenterol. 2016 Jan 7;22(1):446–66. [PMID: 26755890]

2. Eosinophilic Esophagitis

General Considerations

Eosinophilia of the esophagus may be caused by several conditions, most commonly eosinophilic esophagitis; GERD; proton pump inhibitor–responsive eosinophilia; and celiac disease, Crohn disease, and pemphigus (although rarely).

Eosinophilic esophagitis is a disorder in which food or environmental antigens are thought to stimulate an inflammatory response. Initially recognized in children, it is increasingly identified in young or middle-aged adults (estimated 57/100,000), predominantly men (75%). A history of allergies or atopic conditions (asthma, eczema, hay fever) is present in over half of patients.

Clinical Findings

Most adults have a long history of dysphagia for solid-foods or an episode of food impaction. Heartburn may be present. Children may have abdominal pain, vomiting, chest pain, or failure to thrive. On laboratory tests, a few have eosinophilia or elevated IgE levels. Barium swallow studies may demonstrate a small-caliber esophagus; focal or long, tapered strictures; or multiple concentric rings. However, endoscopy with esophageal biopsy and histologic evaluation is required to establish the diagnosis. Endoscopic appearances include white exudates or papules, red furrows, corrugated concentric rings, and strictures; however, the esophagus is grossly normal in up to 10% of patients. Multiple biopsies (at least 2–4) from the proximal and distal esophagus should be obtained to demonstrate multiple (greater than 15/high-powered field) eosinophils in the mucosa. Most children have other coexisting atopic disorders. Skin testing for food allergies may be helpful to identify causative factors, especially in children.

Treatment

Before making a diagnosis of eosinophilic esophagitis, all patients should be given an empiric trial of a proton pump inhibitor orally twice daily for 2 months followed by repeat endoscopy and mucosal biopsy to exclude GERD and so-called proton pump inhibitor–responsive eosinophilia, a distinct entity that is not necessarily related to GERD. Up to 50% of symptomatic patients with increased esophageal eosinophils have clinical and histologic improvement with proton pump inhibitor treatment.

Eosinophilic esophagitis is diagnosed in patients with persistent symptoms and eosinophilia; the optimal treatment of this condition is uncertain. Referral to an allergist for evaluation of coexisting atopic disorders and for testing for food and environmental allergens may be considered.

Elimination of suspected dietary allergens leads to clinical, endoscopic and histologic improvement in 50–70% of adults. The most common allergenic foods are dairy, eggs, wheat, soy, peanuts, and shellfish. Reintroduction of the trigger food results in prompt recurrence of symptoms. Topical corticosteroids lead to symptom resolution in 70% of adults. Either budesonide suspension (1 mg orally) may be administered twice daily or one to two puffs of fluticasone (440 mcg/puff inhaler without a spacer twice daily after meals) may be swallowed after activation instead of inhaled. Symptomatic relapse is common after discontinuation of therapy and may require maintenance therapy. Graduated dilation of strictures should be conducted in patients with dysphagia and strictures or narrow-caliber esophagus but should be performed cautiously because there is an increased risk of perforation and postprocedural chest pain.

Dellon ES et al. ACG Clinical Guideline: evidence based approach to the diagnosis and management of esophageal eosinophilia and eosinophilic esophagitis. Am J Gastroenterol. 2013 May;108(5):679–92. [PMID: 23567357]

Furuta GT et al. Eosinophilic esophagitis. N Engl J Med. 2015 Oct 22;373(17):1640–8. [PMID: 26488694]

Wolf WA et al. Dietary elimination therapy is an effective option for adults with eosinophilic esophagitis. Clin Gastroenterol Hepatol. 2014 Aug;12(8):1272–9. [PMID: 24440337]

3. Esophageal Webs & Rings

Esophageal webs are thin, diaphragm-like membranes of squamous mucosa that typically occur in the mid or upper esophagus and may be multiple. They may be congenital but also occur with eosinophilic esophagitis, graft-versus-host disease, pemphigoid, epidermolysis bullosa, pemphigus vulgaris, and, rarely, in association with iron deficiency anemia (Plummer-Vinson syndrome). Esophageal "Schatzki" rings are smooth, circumferential, thin (less than 4 mm in thickness) mucosal structures located in the distal esophagus at the squamocolumnar junction. Their pathogenesis is controversial. They are associated in nearly all cases with a hiatal hernia, and reflux symptoms are common, suggesting that acid gastroesophageal reflux may be contributory in many cases. Most webs and rings are over 20 mm in diameter and are asymptomatic. Solid food dysphagia most often occurs with rings less than 13 mm in diameter. Characteristically, dysphagia is intermittent and not progressive. Large poorly chewed food boluses such as beefsteak are most likely to cause symptoms. Obstructing boluses may pass by drinking extra liquids or after regurgitation. In some cases, an impacted bolus must be extracted endoscopically. Esophageal webs and rings are best visualized using a barium esophagogram with full esophageal distention. Endoscopy is less sensitive than barium esophagography.

The majority of symptomatic patients with a single ring or web can be effectively treated with the passage of bougie dilators to disrupt the lesion or endoscopic electrosurgical incision of the ring. A single dilation may suffice, but repeat dilations are required in many patients. Patients who have heartburn or who require repeated dilation should receive long-term acid suppressive therapy with a proton pump inhibitor.

Jouhourian C et al. Abdominal compression during endoscopy (the Bolster technique) demonstrates hidden Schatzki rings (with videos). Gastrointest Endosc. 2015 Nov 10. [Epub ahead of print] [PMID: 26548850]

Novak SH et al. Effective treatment of symptomatic lower esophageal (Schatzki) rings with acid suppression therapy: confirmed on barium esophagography. AJR Am J Roentgenol. 2015 Dec;205(6):1182–7. [PMID: 26587923]

4. Zenker Diverticulum

Zenker diverticulum is a protrusion of pharyngeal mucosa that develops at the pharyngoesophageal junction between the inferior pharyngeal constrictor and the cricopharyngeus. The cause is believed to be loss of elasticity of the upper esophageal sphincter, resulting in restricted opening during swallowing. Symptoms of dysphagia and regurgitation tend to develop insidiously over years in older, predominantly male patients. Initial symptoms include vague oropharyngeal dysphagia with coughing or throat discomfort. As the diverticulum enlarges and retains food, patients may note halitosis, spontaneous regurgitation of undigested food, nocturnal choking, gurgling in the throat, or a protrusion in the neck. Complications include aspiration pneumonia, bronchiectasis, and lung abscess. The diagnosis is best established by a video esophagography.

Symptomatic patients require upper esophageal myotomy and, in most cases, surgical diverticulectomy. Minimally invasive intraluminal approaches have been developed in which the septum between the esophagus and diverticulum is incised using a rigid or flexible endoscope or a diverticuloscope. Significant improvement occurs in over 90% of patients treated surgically. Small asymptomatic diverticula may be observed.

Bonavina L et al. Long-term outcome and quality of life after transoral stapling for Zenker diverticulum. World J Gastroenterol. 2015 Jan 28;21(4):1167–72. [PMID: 25632189]

Huberty V et al. Endoscopic treatment for Zenker's diverticulum: long-term results (with video). Gastrointest Endosc. 2013 May;77(5):701–7. [PMID: 23394840]

Law R et al. Zenker's diverticulum. Clin Gastroenterol Hepatol. 2014 Nov;12(11):1773–82. [PMID: 24055983]

5. Esophageal Varices

ESSENTIALS OF DIAGNOSIS

► Develop secondary to portal hypertension.
► Found in 50% of patients with cirrhosis.
► One-third of patients with varices develop upper gastrointestinal bleeding.
► Diagnosis established by upper endoscopy.

► General Considerations

Esophageal varices are dilated submucosal veins that develop in patients with underlying portal hypertension and may result in serious upper gastrointestinal bleeding.

The causes of portal hypertension are discussed in Chapter 16. Under normal circumstances, there is a 2–6 mm Hg pressure gradient between the portal vein and the inferior vena cava. When the gradient exceeds 10–12 mm Hg, significant portal hypertension exists. Esophageal varices are the most common cause of important gastrointestinal bleeding due to portal hypertension, though gastric varices and, rarely, intestinal varices may also bleed. Bleeding from esophageal varices most commonly occurs in the distal 5 cm of the esophagus.

The most common cause of portal hypertension is cirrhosis. Approximately 50% of patients with cirrhosis have esophageal varices. Bleeding from varices occurs in 30% of patients with esophageal varices. In the absence of any treatment, variceal bleeding spontaneously stops in about 50% of patients. Patients surviving this bleeding episode have a 60% chance of recurrent variceal bleeding, usually within the first 6 weeks. With current therapies, the in-hospital mortality rate associated with bleeding esophageal varices is 15%.

A number of factors have been identified that may portend an increased risk of bleeding from esophageal varices. The most important are: (1) the size of the varices; (2) the presence at endoscopy of red wale markings (longitudinal dilated venules on the varix surface); (3) the severity of liver disease (as assessed by Child scoring); and (4) active alcohol abuse—patients with cirrhosis who continue to drink have an extremely high risk of bleeding.

► Clinical Findings

A. Symptoms and Signs

Patients with bleeding esophageal varices present with symptoms and signs of acute gastrointestinal hemorrhage. (See Acute Upper Gastrointestinal Bleeding, above.) In some cases, there may be preceding retching or dyspepsia attributable to alcoholic gastritis or withdrawal. Varices per se do not cause symptoms of dyspepsia, dysphagia, or retching. Variceal bleeding usually is severe, resulting in hypovolemia manifested by postural vital signs or shock. Twenty percent of patients with chronic liver disease in whom bleeding develops have a nonvariceal source of bleeding.

B. Laboratory Findings

These are identical to those listed above in the section on acute upper gastrointestinal tract bleeding.

► Initial Management

A. Acute Resuscitation

The initial management of patients with acute upper gastrointestinal bleeding is also discussed in the section on acute upper gastrointestinal bleeding. Variceal hemorrhage is life-threatening; rapid assessment and resuscitation with fluids or blood products are essential. Overtransfusion should be avoided as it leads to increased central and portal venous pressures, increasing the risk of rebleeding. Many patients with bleeding esophageal varices have coagulopathy due to underlying cirrhosis; fresh frozen plasma

(20 mL/kg loading dose, then 10 mg/kg every 6 hours) or platelets should be administered to patients with INRs greater than 1.8–2.0 or with platelet counts less than 50,000/mcL in the presence of active bleeding. Recombinant factor VIIa has not demonstrated efficacy in controlled studies and is not recommended. The role of prothrombin complex concentrates requires further study. Patients with advanced liver disease are at high risk for poor outcome regardless of the bleeding source and should be transferred to an ICU.

B. Pharmacologic Therapy

1. Antibiotic prophylaxis—Cirrhotic patients admitted with upper gastrointestinal bleeding have a greater than 50% chance of developing a severe bacterial infection during hospitalization—such as bacterial peritonitis, pneumonia, or urinary tract infection. Most infections are caused by gram-negative organisms of gut origin. Prophylactic administration of oral or intravenous fluoroquinolones (eg, norfloxacin, 400 mg orally twice daily) or intravenous third-generation cephalosporins (eg, ceftriaxone, 1 g/day) for 5–7 days reduces the risk of serious infection to 10–20% as well as hospital mortality, especially in patients with Child-Pugh class C cirrhosis. Because of a rising incidence of infections caused by gram-positive organisms as well as fluoroquinolone-resistant organisms, intravenous third-generation cephalosporins may be preferred.

2. Vasoactive drugs—Somatostatin and octreotide infusions reduce portal pressures in ways that are poorly understood. Somatostatin (250 mcg/h)—not available in the United States—or octreotide (50 mcg intravenous bolus followed by 50 mcg/h) reduces splanchnic and hepatic blood flow and portal pressures in cirrhotic patients. Both agents appear to provide acute control of variceal bleeding in up to 80% of patients although neither has been shown to reduce mortality. Data about the absolute efficacy of both are conflicting, but they may be comparable in efficacy to endoscopic therapy. Combined treatment with octreotide or somatostatin infusion and endoscopic therapy (band ligation or sclerotherapy) is superior to either modality alone in controlling acute bleeding and early rebleeding, and it may improve survival. In patients with advanced liver disease and upper gastrointestinal hemorrhage, it is reasonable to initiate therapy with octreotide or somatostatin on admission and continue for 3–5 days if varices are confirmed by endoscopy. If bleeding is determined by endoscopy not to be secondary to portal hypertension, the infusion can be discontinued.

Terlipressin, 1–2 mg intravenous every 4 hours, (not available in the United States) is a synthetic vasopressin analog that causes a significant and sustained reduction in portal and variceal pressures while preserving renal perfusion. Where available, terlipressin may be preferred to somatostatin or octreotide. Terlipressin is contraindicated in patients with significant coronary, cerebral, or peripheral vascular disease.

3. Vitamin K—In cirrhotic patients with an abnormal prothrombin time, vitamin K (10 mg) should be administered intravenously.

4. Lactulose—Encephalopathy may complicate an episode of gastrointestinal bleeding in patients with severe liver disease. In patients with encephalopathy, lactulose should be administered in a dosage of 30 mL orally every 1–2 hours until evacuation occurs then reduced to 15–45 mL/h every 8–12 hours as needed to promote two or three bowel movements daily. (See Chapter 16.)

C. Emergent Endoscopy

Emergent endoscopy is performed after the patient's hemodynamic status has been appropriately stabilized (usually within 2–12 hours). In patients with active bleeding, endotracheal intubation is commonly performed to protect against aspiration during endoscopy. An endoscopic examination is performed to exclude other or associated causes of upper gastrointestinal bleeding such as Mallory-Weiss tears, peptic ulcer disease, and portal hypertensive gastropathy. In many patients, variceal bleeding has stopped spontaneously by the time of endoscopy, and the diagnosis of variceal bleeding is made presumptively. Immediate endoscopic treatment of the varices generally is performed with banding. In clinical practice, sclerotherapy seldom is used. These techniques arrest active bleeding in 80–90% of patients and reduce the chance of in-hospital recurrent bleeding to about 20%.

If banding is chosen, repeat sessions are scheduled at intervals of 2–4 weeks until the varices are obliterated or reduced to a small size. Banding achieves lower rates of rebleeding, complications, and death than sclerotherapy and should be considered the endoscopic treatment of choice.

D. Balloon Tube Tamponade

Mechanical tamponade with specially designed nasogastric tubes containing large gastric and esophageal balloons (Minnesota or Sengstaken-Blakemore tubes) provides initial control of active variceal hemorrhage in 60–90% of patients; rebleeding occurs in 50%. Given its high rate of complications, mechanical tamponade is used as a temporizing measure only in patients with bleeding that cannot be controlled with pharmacologic or endoscopic techniques until more definitive decompressive therapy (eg, TIPS) can be provided.

E. Portal Decompressive Procedures

In the 10–20% of patients with variceal bleeding that cannot be controlled with pharmacologic or endoscopic therapy, emergency portal decompression may be considered.

1. Transvenous intrahepatic portosystemic shunts (TIPS)—Over a wire that is passed through a catheter inserted in the jugular vein, an expandable wire mesh stent (8–12 mm in diameter) is passed through the liver parenchyma, creating a portosystemic shunt from the portal vein to the hepatic vein. TIPS can control acute hemorrhage in over 90% of patients actively bleeding from gastric or esophageal varices. However, when TIPS is performed in the actively bleeding patient, the mortality approaches 40%, especially in patients requiring ventilatory support or blood pressure support and patients with renal insufficiency, bilirubin greater than 3 mg/dL, or encephalopathy. Therefore, TIPS should be considered in the 10–20% of patients with acute variceal bleeding that cannot be controlled with pharmacologic and endoscopic therapy, but it may not be warranted in patients with a particularly poor prognosis.

2. Emergency portosystemic shunt surgery—Emergency portosystemic shunt surgery is associated with a 40–60% mortality rate. At centers where TIPS is available, that procedure has become the preferred means of providing emergency portal decompression.

⏵ Prevention of Rebleeding

Once the initial bleeding episode has been controlled, therapy is warranted to reduce the high risk (60%) of rebleeding.

A. Combination Beta-Blockers and Variceal Band Ligation

Nonselective beta-adrenergic blockers (propranolol, nadolol) reduce the risk of rebleeding from esophageal varices to about 40%. Likewise, long-term treatment with band ligation reduces the incidence of rebleeding to about 30%. In most patients, two to six treatment sessions (performed at 2- to 4-week intervals) are needed to eradicate the varices.

Meta-analyses of randomized controlled trials suggest that a *combination* of band ligation plus beta-blockers is superior to either variceal band ligation alone (RR 0.68) or beta-blockers alone (RR 0.71). Therefore, combination therapy is recommended for patients without contraindications to beta-blockers. Recommended starting doses of beta-blockers are propranolol (20 mg orally twice daily), long-acting propranolol (60 mg orally once daily), or nadolol (20–40 mg orally once daily), with gradual increases in the dosage every 1–2 weeks until the heart rate falls by 25% or reaches 55–60 beats/min, provided the systolic blood pressure remains above 90 mm Hg and the patient has no side effects. The average dosage of long-acting propranolol is 120 mg once daily and for nadolol, 80 mg once daily. One-third of patients with cirrhosis are intolerant of beta-blockers, experiencing fatigue or hypotension. Drug administration at bedtime may reduce the frequency and severity of side effects.

B. Transvenous Intrahepatic Portosystemic Shunt

TIPS has resulted in a significant reduction in recurrent bleeding compared with endoscopic sclerotherapy or band ligation—either alone or in combination with beta-blocker therapy. At 1 year, rebleeding rates in patients treated with TIPS versus various endoscopic therapies average 20% and 40%, respectively. However, TIPS was also associated with a higher incidence of encephalopathy (35% vs 15%) and did not result in a decrease in mortality. Another limitation of TIPS is that stenosis and thrombosis of the stents occur in the majority of patients over time with a consequent risk of rebleeding. Therefore, periodic monitoring with Doppler ultrasonography or hepatic venography is required.

Stent patency usually can be maintained by balloon angioplasty or additional stent placement. Given these problems, TIPS should be reserved for patients who have recurrent (two or more) episodes of variceal bleeding that have failed endoscopic or pharmacologic therapies. TIPS is also useful in patients with recurrent bleeding from gastric varices or portal hypertensive gastropathy (for which endoscopic therapies cannot be used). TIPS is likewise considered in patients who are noncompliant with other therapies or who live in remote locations (without access to emergency care).

C. Surgical Portosystemic Shunts

Shunt surgery has a significantly lower rate of rebleeding compared with endoscopic therapy but also a higher incidence of encephalopathy. With the advent and widespread adoption of TIPS, surgical shunts are seldom performed.

D. Liver Transplantation

Candidacy for orthotopic liver transplantation should be assessed in all patients with chronic liver disease and bleeding due to portal hypertension. Transplant candidates should be treated with band ligation or TIPS to control bleeding pretransplant.

⏵ Prevention of First Episodes of Variceal Bleeding

Among patients with varices that have not previously bled, bleeding occurs in 12% of patients each year, with a lifetime risk of 30%. Because of the high mortality rate associated with variceal hemorrhage, prevention of the initial bleeding episode is desirable. Therefore, patients with cirrhosis should undergo diagnostic endoscopy or capsule endoscopy to determine whether varices are present. Varices are present in 40% of patients with Child-Turcotte-Pugh class A cirrhosis and in 85% with Child-Turcotte-Pugh class C cirrhosis. In patients without varices on screening endoscopy, a repeat endoscopy is recommended in 3 years, since varices develop in 8% of patients per year. Patients with varices have a higher risk of bleeding if they have varices larger than 5 mm, varices with red wale markings, or Child-Turcotte-Pugh class B or C cirrhosis. The risk of bleeding in patients with varices smaller than 5 mm is 5% per year and with large varices is 15–20% per year. Patients with small varices without red wale marks and compensated (Child-Turcotte-Pugh class A) cirrhosis have a low-risk of bleeding; hence, prophylaxis is unnecessary, but endoscopy should be repeated in 1–2 years to reassess size.

Nonselective beta-adrenergic blockers are recommended to reduce the risk of first variceal hemorrhage in patients with medium/large varices and patients with small varices who either have variceal red wale marks or advanced cirrhosis (Child-Turcotte-Pugh class B or C). (See Combination Beta-Blockers and Variceal Band Ligation, above.) Band ligation is not recommended for small varices due to technical difficulties in band application. Prophylactic band ligation may be preferred over beta-blockers for patients at higher risk for bleeding, especially patients with medium/large varices with red wale markings or with advanced cirrhosis (Child-Turcotte-Pugh class B or C) as well as patients with contraindications to or intolerance of beta-blockers.

When to Refer

- All patients with upper gastrointestinal bleeding and suspected varices should be evaluated by a physician skilled in therapeutic endoscopy.
- Patients being considered for TIPS procedures or liver transplantation.
- Patients with cirrhosis for endoscopic evaluation for varices.

When to Admit

All patients with acute upper gastrointestinal bleeding and suspected cirrhosis should be admitted to an ICU.

ASGE Standards of Practice Committee; Hwang JH et al. The role of endoscopy in the management of variceal hemorrhage. Gastrointest Endosc. 2014 Aug;80(2):221–7. [PMID: 25034836]

Cárdenas A et al. Endoscopic hemostasis in acute esophageal variceal bleeding. Gastroenterol Clin North Am. 2014 Dec; 43(4):795–806. [PMID: 25440926]

Sauerbruch T et al; German Study Group for Prophylaxis of Variceal Rebleeding. Prevention of rebleeding from esophageal varices in patients with cirrhosis receiving small-diameter stents versus hemodynamically controlled medical therapy. Gastroenterology. 2015 Sep;149(3):660–8.e1. [PMID: 25989386]

Tandon P et al. Risk of bacterial infection in patients with cirrhosis and acute variceal hemorrhage, based on Child-Pugh class and effects of antibiotics. Clin Gastroenterol Hepatol. 2015 Jun;13(6):1189–96.e2. [PMID: 25460564]

ESOPHAGEAL MOTILITY DISORDERS

1. Achalasia

ESSENTIALS OF DIAGNOSIS

- Gradual, progressive dysphagia for solids and liquids.
- Regurgitation of undigested food.
- Barium esophagogram with "bird's beak" distal esophagus.
- Esophageal manometry confirms diagnosis.

General Considerations

Achalasia is an idiopathic motility disorder characterized by loss of peristalsis in the distal two-thirds (smooth muscle) of the esophagus and impaired relaxation of the LES. There appears to be denervation of the esophagus resulting primarily from loss of nitric oxide-producing inhibitory neurons in the myenteric plexus. The cause of the neuronal degeneration is unknown.

Clinical Findings

A. Symptoms and Signs

There is a steady increase in the incidence of achalasia with age; however, it can be seen in individuals as young as 25 years. Patients complain of the gradual onset of dysphagia for solid foods and, in the majority, of liquids also. Symptoms at presentation may have persisted for months to years. Substernal discomfort or fullness may be noted after eating. Many patients eat more slowly and adopt specific maneuvers such as lifting the neck or throwing the shoulders back to enhance esophageal emptying. Regurgitation of undigested food is common and may occur during meals or up to several hours later. Nocturnal regurgitation can provoke coughing or aspiration. Up to 50% of patients report substernal chest pain that is unrelated to meals or exercise and may last up to hours. Weight loss is common. Physical examination is unhelpful.

B. Imaging

Chest radiographs may show an air-fluid level in the enlarged, fluid-filled esophagus. Barium esophagography discloses characteristic findings, including esophageal dilation, loss of esophageal peristalsis, poor esophageal emptying, and a smooth, symmetric "bird's beak" tapering of the distal esophagus. Without treatment, the esophagus may become markedly dilated ("sigmoid esophagus").

C. Special Examinations

After esophagography, endoscopy is always performed to evaluate the distal esophagus and gastroesophageal junction to exclude a distal stricture or a submucosal infiltrating carcinoma. The diagnosis is confirmed by esophageal manometry. The manometric features are complete absence of normal peristalsis and incomplete lower esophageal sphincteric relaxation with swallowing. Using high-resolution esophageal topographic tracings, three achalasia subtypes are recognized. Type III is a spastic variant with less favorable treatment outcomes (66%) than types I (81%) or II (96%).

Differential Diagnosis

Chagas disease is associated with esophageal dysfunction that is indistinguishable from idiopathic achalasia and should be considered in patients from endemic regions (Central and South America); it is becoming more common in the southern United States. Primary or metastatic tumors can invade the gastroesophageal junction, resulting in a picture resembling that of achalasia, called "pseudo-achalasia." Endoscopic ultrasonography and chest CT may be required to examine the distal esophagus in suspicious cases.

Treatment

A. Botulinum Toxin Injection

Endoscopically guided injection of botulinum toxin directly into the LES results in a marked reduction in LES pressure with initial improvement in symptoms in 65–85%

of patients. However, symptom relapse occurs in over 50% of patients within 6–9 months and in all patients within 2 years. Three-fourths of initial responders who relapse have improvement with repeated injections. Because it is inferior to pneumatic dilation therapy and surgery in producing sustained symptomatic relief, this therapy is most appropriate for patients with comorbidities who are poor candidates for more invasive procedures.

B. Pneumatic Dilation

Up to 90% of patients derive good to excellent relief of dysphagia after one to three sessions of pneumatic dilation of the LES. Dilation is less effective in patients who are younger than age 45, have the type III variant, or have a dilated esophagus. Symptoms recur following pneumatic dilation in up to 35% within 10 years but usually respond to repeated dilation. Perforations occur in less than 3% of dilations and may require operative repair. The success of laparoscopic myotomy is not compromised by prior pneumatic dilation.

C. Surgery

A modified Heller cardiomyotomy of the LES and cardia results in good to excellent symptomatic improvement in over 90% of patients. Because gastroesophageal reflux develops in up to 20% of patients after myotomy, most surgeons also perform an antireflux procedure (fundoplication), and all patients are prescribed a once-daily proton pump inhibitor. Myotomy is performed with a laparoscopic approach and is preferred to the open surgical approach. Symptoms recur following cardiomyotomy in greater than 25% of cases within 10 years but usually respond to pneumatic dilation. A 2015 systematic review of nine randomized controlled trials reported treatment efficacy in 70–90% of patients treated with pneumatic dilation and 88–95% with laparoscopic myotomy. Thus, in experienced hands, the initial efficacies of pneumatic dilation and laparoscopic myotomy are nearly equivalent. Pneumatic dilation may be less effective in men younger than 45 years, so surgical myotomy may be preferred for them. Surgical myotomy may also be preferred for patients with the type III variant. Complete esophagectomy or percutaneous gastrostomy is required in 2–5% of patients in whom massive dilation of the esophagus (megaesophagus) develops despite dilation or myotomy. In megaesophagus, dysphagia, food retention, and regurgitation may decrease nutrition and quality of life and increase risk of aspiration.

D. Per Oral Endoscopic Myotomy (POEM)

Since 2011, selected, highly experienced centers in Southeast Asia and in the United States, have reported excellent results with a less invasive, endoscopic procedure in which an endoscope is inserted into the patient's mouth and passed into the upper esophagus. After a small incision is made in the esophageal mucosa, the endoscope dissects through the submucosal space to the lower esophageal sphincter, where the circular muscle fibers are incised. In uncontrolled studies, success rates of 80–90% have been reported.

Boeckxstaens GE et al. Achalasia. Lancet. 2014 Jan 4;383(9911): 83–93. [PMID: 23871090]

NOSCAR POEM White Paper Committee; Stavropoulos SN et al. Per-oral endoscopic myotomy white paper summary. Gastrointest Endosc. 2014 Jul;80(1):1–15. [PMID: 24950639]

Pandolfino JE et al. Achalasia: a systematic review. JAMA. 2015 May 12;313(18):1841–52. [PMID: 25965233]

Tirresan F et al. Treatment of achalasia in the era of high-resolution manometry. Am J Gastroenterol. 2015 Jul–Sep;28(3):301–8. [PMID: 26130022]

2. Other Primary Esophageal Motility Disorders

▶ Clinical Findings

A. Symptoms and Signs

Abnormalities in esophageal motility may cause dysphagia or chest pain. Dysphagia for liquids as well as solids tends to be intermittent and nonprogressive. Periods of normal swallowing may alternate with periods of dysphagia, which usually is mild though bothersome—rarely severe enough to result in significant alterations in lifestyle or weight loss. Dysphagia may be provoked by stress, large boluses of food, or hot or cold liquids. Some patients may experience anterior chest pain that may be confused with angina pectoris but usually is nonexertional. The pain generally is unrelated to eating. (See Chest Pain of Undetermined Origin, below.)

B. Diagnostic Tests

The evaluation of suspected esophageal motility disorders includes barium esophagography, upper endoscopy, and, in some cases, esophageal manometry. Barium esophagography is useful to exclude mechanical obstruction and to evaluate esophageal motility. The presence of simultaneous contractions (spasm), disordered peristalsis, or failed peristalsis supports a diagnosis of esophageal dysmotility. Upper endoscopy also is performed to exclude a mechanical obstruction (as a cause of dysphagia) and to look for evidence of erosive reflux esophagitis (a common cause of chest pain) or eosinophilic esophagitis (confirmed by esophageal biopsy). Manometry is not routinely used for mild to moderate symptoms because the findings seldom influence further medical management, but it may be useful in patients with persistent, disabling dysphagia to exclude achalasia and to look for other disorders of esophageal motility. These include diffuse esophageal spasm, hypercontractile esophagus, esophagogastric junction outflow obstruction, and findings of ineffective esophageal peristalsis (failed or weak esophageal peristalsis). The further evaluation of noncardiac chest pain is discussed in a subsequent section.

▶ Treatment

For patients with mild symptoms of dysphagia, therapy is directed at symptom reduction and reassurance. Patients should be instructed to eat more slowly and take smaller bites of food. In some cases, a warm liquid at the start of a meal may facilitate swallowing. Because unrecognized gastroesophageal reflux may cause dysphagia, a trial of a proton pump inhibitor (esomeprazole 40 mg, lansoprazole 30 mg) orally twice daily should be administered for 4–8 weeks. Treatment of patients with severe dysphagia is empiric. Suspected spastic disorders may be treated with isosorbide (10–20 mg four times daily) or nitroglycerin (0.4 mg sublingually as needed) and nifedipine (10 mg) or diltiazem (60–90 mg) 30–45 minutes before meals may be tried; their efficacy is unproved. Phosphodiesterase type 5 inhibitors (eg, sildenafil) promote smooth muscle relaxation and improve esophageal motility in small numbers of patients with spastic disorders but require further clinical study before they can be recommended. Injection of botulinum toxin into the lower esophagus may improve chest pain and dysphagia in some patients for a limited time. For unclear reasons, esophageal dilation provides symptomatic relief in some cases.

Carlson DA et al. Diagnosis of esophageal motility disorders: esophageal pressure topography vs. conventional line tracing. Am J Gastroenterol. 2015 Jul;110(7):967–77. [PMID: 26032151]
Roman S et al. The Chicago Classification of motility disorders: an update. Gastrointest Endosc Clin N Am. 2014 Oct;24(4): 545–61. [PMID: 25216902]

CHEST PAIN OF UNDETERMINED ORIGIN

One-third of patients with chest pain undergo negative cardiac evaluation. Patients with recurrent noncardiac chest pain thus pose a difficult clinical problem. Because coronary artery disease is common and can present atypically, it must be excluded prior to evaluation for other causes.

Causes of noncardiac chest pain may include the following.

A. Chest Wall and Thoracic Spine Disease

These are easily diagnosed by history and physical examination.

B. Gastroesophageal Reflux

Up to 50% of patients have increased amounts of gastroesophageal acid reflux or a correlation between acid reflux episodes and chest pain demonstrated on esophageal pH testing. An empiric 4-week trial of acid-suppressive therapy with a high-dose proton pump inhibitor is recommended (eg, omeprazole or rabeprazole, 40 mg orally twice daily; lansoprazole, 30–60 mg orally twice daily; or esomeprazole or pantoprazole, 40 mg orally twice daily), especially in patients with reflux symptoms. In patients with persistent symptoms, ambulatory esophageal pH or impedance and pH study may be useful to exclude definitively a relationship between acid and nonacid reflux episodes and chest pain events.

C. Esophageal Dysmotility

Esophageal motility abnormalities such as diffuse esophageal spasm or hypertensive peristalsis (nutcracker esophagus) are uncommon causes of noncardiac chest pain. In patients with chest pain and dysphagia, a barium swallow radiograph should be obtained to look for evidence of achalasia or diffuse esophageal spasm. Esophageal manometry is not routinely performed because of low specificity and the unlikelihood of finding a clinically significant disorder, but it may be recommended in patients with frequent symptoms.

D. Heightened Visceral Sensitivity

Some patients with noncardiac chest pain report pain in response to a variety of minor noxious stimuli such as physiologically normal amounts of acid reflux, inflation of balloons within the esophageal lumen, injection of intravenous edrophonium (a cholinergic stimulus), or intracardiac catheter manipulation. Low doses of oral antidepressants such as trazodone 50 mg or imipramine 10–50 mg reduce chest pain symptoms and are thought to reduce visceral afferent awareness. In a 2010 controlled crossover trial, over 50% of patients treated with venlafaxine, 75 mg once daily at bedtime, achieved symptomatic improvement compared with only 4% treated with placebo.

E. Psychological Disorders

A significant number of patients have underlying depression, anxiety, and panic disorder. Patients reporting dyspnea, sweating, tachycardia, suffocation, or fear of dying should be evaluated for panic disorder.

Bowers SP. Esophageal motility disorders. Surg Clin North Am. 2015 Jun;95(3):467–82. [PMID: 25965124]
Coss-Adame E et al. Treatment of esophageal (noncardiac) chest pain: an expert review. Clin Gastroenterol Hepatol. 2014 Aug; 12(8):1224–45. [PMID: 23994670]
Flook NW et al. Acid-suppressive therapy with esomeprazole for relief of unexplained chest pain in primary care: a randomized, double-blind, placebo-controlled trial. Am J Gastroenterol. 2013 Jan;108(1):56–64. [PMID: 23147520]
Hershcovici T et al. Systematic review: the treatment of noncardiac chest pain. Aliment Pharmacol Ther. 2012 Jan;35(1):5–14. [PMID: 22077344]

DISEASES OF THE STOMACH & DUODENUM

(See Chapter 39 for Gastric Cancers.)

GASTRITIS & GASTROPATHY

The term "gastropathy" should be used to denote conditions in which there is epithelial or endothelial damage without inflammation, and "gastritis" should be used to denote conditions in which there is histologic evidence of inflammation. In clinical practice, the term "gastritis" is commonly applied to three categories: (1) erosive and hemorrhagic "gastritis" (gastropathy); (2) nonerosive, nonspecific (histologic) gastritis; and (3) specific types of gastritis, characterized by distinctive histologic and endoscopic features diagnostic of specific disorders.

1. Erosive & Hemorrhagic "Gastritis" (Gastropathy)

- ▶ Most commonly seen in alcoholic or critically ill patients, or patients taking NSAIDs.
- ▶ Often asymptomatic; may cause epigastric pain, nausea, and vomiting.
- ▶ May cause hematemesis; usually insignificant bleeding.

General Considerations

The most common causes of erosive gastropathy are medications (especially NSAIDs), alcohol, stress due to severe medical or surgical illness, and portal hypertension ("portal gastropathy"). Major risk factors for stress gastritis include mechanical ventilation, coagulopathy, trauma, burns, shock, sepsis, central nervous system injury, liver failure, kidney disease, and multiorgan failure. The use of enteral nutrition reduces the risk of stress-related bleeding. Uncommon causes of erosive gastropathy include ischemia, caustic ingestion, and radiation. Erosive and hemorrhagic gastropathy typically are diagnosed at endoscopy, often being performed because of dyspepsia or upper gastrointestinal bleeding. Endoscopic findings include subepithelial hemorrhages, petechiae, and erosions. These lesions are superficial, vary in size and number, and may be focal or diffuse. There usually is no significant inflammation on histologic examination.

Clinical Findings

A. Symptoms and Signs

Erosive gastropathy is usually asymptomatic. Symptoms, when they occur, include anorexia, epigastric pain, nausea, and vomiting. There is poor correlation between symptoms and the number or severity of endoscopic abnormalities. The most common clinical manifestation of erosive gastritis is upper gastrointestinal bleeding, which presents as hematemesis, "coffee grounds" emesis, or bloody aspirate in a patient receiving nasogastric suction, or as melena. Because erosive gastritis is superficial, hemodynamically significant bleeding is rare.

B. Laboratory Findings

The laboratory findings are nonspecific. The hematocrit is low if significant bleeding has occurred; iron deficiency may be found.

C. Special Examinations

Upper endoscopy is the most sensitive method of diagnosis. Although bleeding from gastritis is usually insignificant, it cannot be distinguished on clinical grounds from more serious lesions such as peptic ulcers or esophageal varices. Hence, endoscopy is generally performed within 24 hours in patients with upper gastrointestinal bleeding to identify the source. An upper gastrointestinal series is sometimes obtained in lieu of endoscopy in patients with hemodynamically insignificant upper gastrointestinal bleeds to exclude serious lesions but is insensitive for the detection of gastritis.

Differential Diagnosis

Epigastric pain may be due to peptic ulcer, gastroesophageal reflux, gastric cancer, biliary tract disease, food poisoning, viral gastroenteritis, and functional dyspepsia. With severe pain, one should consider a perforated or penetrating ulcer, pancreatic disease, esophageal rupture, ruptured aortic aneurysm, gastric volvulus, gastrointestinal ischemia, and myocardial ischemia. Causes of upper gastrointestinal bleeding include peptic ulcer disease, esophageal varices, Mallory-Weiss tear, and angioectasias.

Specific Causes & Treatment

A. Stress Gastritis

1. Prophylaxis—Stress-related mucosal erosions and subepithelial hemorrhages may develop within 72 hours in critically ill patients. Clinically overt bleeding occurs in 6% of ICU patients, but clinically important bleeding in less than 1.5%. Bleeding is associated with a higher mortality rate but is seldom the cause of death. Two of the most important risk factors for bleeding are coagulopathy (platelets less than 50,000/mcL or INR greater than 1.5) and respiratory failure with the need for mechanical ventilation for over 48 hours. When these two risk factors are absent, the risk of significant bleeding is only 0.1%. Other risk factors include traumatic brain injury, severe burns, sepsis, vasopressor therapy, corticosteroid therapy, and prior history of peptic ulcer disease and gastrointestinal bleeding. Early enteral tube feeding may decrease the risk of significant bleeding.

Prophylaxis should be routinely administered to critically ill patients with risk factors for significant bleeding upon admission. Prophylactic suppression of gastric acid with intravenous H_2-receptor antagonists or proton pump inhibitors (oral or intravenous) has been shown to reduce the incidence of clinically overt and significant bleeding but may increase the risk of nosocomial pneumonia. A 2012 meta-analysis of 13 randomized trials found that oral and intravenous proton pump inhibitors significantly decreased the incidence of clinically significant bleeding compared with intravenous H_2-receptor antagonists (1.3% vs 6.6%, OR 0.30).

The optimal, cost-effective prophylactic regimen remains uncertain, hence clinical practices vary. For patients with nasoenteric tubes, immediate-release omeprazole (40 mg at 1 and 6 hours on day 1; then 40 mg once daily beginning on day 2) may be preferred because of lower cost and ease of administration. For patients requiring intravenous administration, continuous intravenous infusions of H_2-receptor antagonists provide adequate control of intragastric pH in most patients in the following doses over 24 hours: cimetidine (900–1200 mg), ranitidine (150 mg), or famotidine (20 mg). Alternatively, intravenous proton pump inhibitors, although more expensive, may be preferred due to superior efficacy. The optimal dosing of intravenous proton pump inhibitors is uncertain; however, in clinical trials pantoprazole doses ranging from 40 mg to 80 mg and administered every 8–24 hours appear equally effective.

2. Treatment—Once bleeding occurs, patients should receive continuous infusions of a proton pump inhibitor (esomeprazole or pantoprazole, 80 mg intravenous bolus, followed by 8 mg/h continuous infusion) as well as sucralfate suspension, 1 g orally every 4 to 6 hours. Endoscopy should be performed in patients with clinically significant bleeding to look for treatable causes, especially stress-related peptic ulcers with active bleeding or visible vessels. When bleeding arises from diffuse gastritis, endoscopic hemostasis techniques are not helpful.

B. NSAID Gastritis

Of patients receiving NSAIDs in clinical trials, 25–50% have gastritis and 10–20% have ulcers at endoscopy; however, symptoms of significant dyspepsia develop in about 5%. NSAIDs that are more selective for the cyclooxygenase (COX)-2 enzyme ("coxibs"), such as celecoxib, etodolac, and meloxicam, decrease the incidence of endoscopically visible ulcers by approximately 75% and significant ulcer complications by up to 50% compared with nonselective NSAIDs (nsNSAIDs). However, a twofold increase in the incidence in cardiovascular complications (myocardial infarction, cerebrovascular infarction, and death) in patients taking coxibs compared with placebo led to the withdrawal of two highly selective coxibs (rofecoxib and valdecoxib) from the market by the manufacturers. Celecoxib and all currently available nsNSAIDs (with notable exception of aspirin and possibly naproxen) are associated with increased risk of cardiovascular complications and therefore should be used with caution in patients with cardiovascular risk factors.

In population surveys, the rate of dyspepsia is increased 1.5- to 2-fold with nsNSAID and coxib use. However, dyspeptic symptoms correlate poorly with significant mucosal abnormalities or the development of adverse clinical events (ulcer bleeding or perforation). Given the frequency of dyspeptic symptoms in patients taking NSAIDs, it is neither feasible nor desirable to investigate all such cases. Patients with alarm symptoms or signs, such as severe pain, weight loss, vomiting, gastrointestinal bleeding, or anemia, should undergo diagnostic upper endoscopy. For other patients, symptoms may improve with discontinuation of the agent, reduction to the lowest effective dose, or administration with meals. Proton pump inhibitors have demonstrated efficacy in controlled trials for the treatment of NSAID-related dyspepsia and superiority to H_2-receptor antagonists for healing of NSAID-related ulcers even in the setting of continued NSAID use. Therefore, an empiric 2–4 week trial of an oral proton pump inhibitor (omeprazole, rabeprazole, or esomeprazole 20–40 mg/day; lansoprazole or dexlansoprazole, 30 mg/day; pantoprazole, 40 mg/day) is recommended for patients with NSAID-related dyspepsia, especially those in whom continued NSAID treatment is required. If symptoms do not improve, diagnostic upper endoscopy should be conducted.

C. Alcoholic Gastritis

Excessive alcohol consumption may lead to dyspepsia, nausea, emesis, and minor hematemesis—a condition sometimes labeled "alcoholic gastritis." However, it is not proven that alcohol alone actually causes significant erosive gastritis. Therapy with H_2-receptor antagonists, proton pump inhibitors, or sucralfate for 2–4 weeks often is empirically prescribed.

D. Portal Hypertensive Gastropathy

Portal hypertension commonly results in gastric mucosal and submucosal congestion of capillaries and venules, which is correlated with the severity of the portal hypertension and underlying liver disease. Usually asymptomatic, it may cause chronic gastrointestinal bleeding in 10% of patients and, less commonly, clinically significant bleeding with hematemesis. Treatment with propranolol or nadolol reduces the incidence of recurrent acute bleeding by lowering portal pressures. Patients who fail propranolol therapy may be successfully treated with portal decompressive procedures (see section above on treatment of esophageal varices).

Bardou M et al. Stress-related mucosal disease in the critically ill patient. Nat Rev Gastroenterol Hepatol. 2015 Feb;12(2): 98–107. [PMID: 25560847]
Barkun AN et al. Proton pump inhibitors vs. histamine 2 receptor antagonists for stress-related mucosal bleeding prophylaxis in critically ill patients: a meta-analysis. Am J Gastroenterol. 2012 Apr;107(4):507–20. [PMID: 22290403]

2. Nonerosive, Nonspecific Gastritis

The diagnosis of nonerosive gastritis is based on histologic assessment of mucosal biopsies. Endoscopic findings are normal in many cases and do not reliably predict the presence of histologic inflammation. The main types of nonerosive gastritis are those due to *H pylori* infection, those associated with pernicious anemia, and eosinophilic gastritis. (See Specific Types of Gastritis below.)

A. *Helicobacter pylori* Gastritis

H pylori is a spiral gram-negative rod that resides beneath the gastric mucous layer adjacent to gastric epithelial cells. Although not invasive, it causes gastric mucosal inflammation with PMNs and lymphocytes. The mechanisms of injury and inflammation may in part be related to the products of two genes, *vacA* and *cagA*.

In developed countries the prevalence of *H pylori* is rapidly declining. In the United States, the prevalence rises from less than 10% in non-immigrants under age 30 years to over 50% in those over age 60 years. The prevalence is higher in non-whites and immigrants from developing countries and is correlated inversely with socioeconomic status. Transmission is from person to person, mainly during infancy and childhood; however, the mode of transmission is unknown.

Acute infection with *H pylori* may cause a transient clinical illness characterized by nausea and abdominal pain that may last for several days and is associated with acute histologic gastritis with PMNs. After these symptoms resolve, the majority progress to chronic infection with chronic, diffuse mucosal inflammation (gastritis) characterized by PMNs and lymphocytes. Although chronic *H pylori* infection with gastritis is present in 30–50% of the population, most persons are asymptomatic and suffer no sequelae. Three gastritis phenotypes occur which determine clinical outcomes. Most infected people have a mild, diffuse gastritis that does not disrupt acid secretion and seldom causes clinically important outcomes. About 15% of infected people have inflammation that predominates in the gastric antrum but spares the gastric body (where acid is secreted). People with this phenotype tend to have increased gastrin; increased acid production; and increased risk of developing peptic ulcers, especially duodenal ulcers. An even smaller subset of infected adults have inflammation that predominates in the gastric body. Over time, this may lead to destruction of acid-secreting glands with resultant mucosal atrophy, decreased acid secretion, and intestinal metaplasia. This phenotype is associated with an increased risk of gastric ulcers and gastric cancer. Long-term treatment with proton pump inhibitors can potentiate the development of *H pylori*–associated atrophic gastritis. Chronic *H pylori* gastritis leads to the development of duodenal or gastric ulcers in up to 10%, gastric cancer in 0.1–3%, and low-grade B cell gastric lymphoma (mucosa-associated lymphoid tissue lymphoma; MALToma) in less than 0.01%.

Eradication of *H pylori* may be achieved with antibiotics in over 85% of patients and leads to resolution of the chronic gastritis (see section on Peptic Ulcer Disease). Testing for *H pylori* is indicated for patients with either active or a past history of documented peptic ulcer disease or gastric MALToma and for patients with a family history of gastric carcinoma. Testing and empiric treatment is cost-effective in young patients (less than 55 years of age) with uncomplicated dyspepsia prior to further medical evaluation. The role of testing and treating *H pylori* in patients with functional dyspepsia remains controversial but is generally recommended (see Dyspepsia, above). *H pylori* eradication decreases the risk of gastric cancer in patients with peptic ulcer disease. Some groups recommend population-based screening of all asymptomatic persons in regions in which there is a high prevalence of *H pylori* and gastric cancer (such as Japan, Korea, and China) to reduce the incidence of gastric cancer. Population-based screening of asymptomatic individuals is not recommended in western countries, in which the incidence of gastric cancer is low, but should be considered in immigrants from high-prevalence regions.

1. Noninvasive testing for *H pylori*—Although serologic tests are easily obtained and widely available, most clinical guidelines no longer endorse their use for testing for *H pylori* infection because they are less accurate than other noninvasive tests that measure active infection. Laboratory-based quantitative serologic ELISA tests have an overall accuracy of only 80%. In comparison, the fecal antigen immunoassay and [^{13}C] urea breath test have excellent sensitivity and specificity (greater than 95%) at a cost of less than $60. Although more expensive and cumbersome to perform, these tests of active infection are more cost-effective in most clinical settings because they reduce unnecessary treatment for patients without active infection.

Recent proton pump inhibitors or antibiotics significantly reduce the sensitivity of urea breath tests and fecal antigen assays (but not serologic tests). Prior to testing, proton pump inhibitors should be discontinued for 7–14 days and antibiotics for at least 28 days.

2. Endoscopic testing for *H pylori*—Endoscopy is not indicated to diagnose *H pylori* infection in most circumstances. However, when it is performed for another reason, gastric biopsy specimens can be obtained for detection of *H pylori* and tested for active infection by urease production. This simple, inexpensive ($10) test has excellent sensitivity (90%) and specificity (95%). In patients with active upper gastrointestinal bleeding or patients recently taking proton pump inhibitors or antibiotics, histologic assessment for *H pylori* is preferred. Histologic assessment of biopsies from the gastric antrum and body is more definitive but more expensive ($150–$250) than a rapid urease test. Histologic assessment is also indicated in patients with suspected MALTomas and, possibly, in patients with suspected infection whose rapid urease test is negative. However, serologic testing is the most cost-effective means of confirming *H pylori* infection in patients with a negative rapid urease test.

Malfertheiner P et al; European Helicobacter Study Group. Management of *Helicobacter pylori* infection—the Maastricht IV/Florence Consensus Report. Gut. 2012 May;61(5):646–64. [PMID: 22491499]

McColl KE. Clinical practice. *Helicobacter pylori* infection. N Engl J Med. 2010 Apr 29;362(17):1597–1604. [PMID: 20427808]

Yazbek PB et al. Challenges to the treatment and new perspectives for the eradication of *Helicobacter pylori*. Dig Dis Sci. 2015 Oct;60(10):2901–12. [PMID: 25999247]

B. Pernicious Anemia Gastritis

Pernicious anemia gastritis is a rare autoimmune disorder involving the fundic glands with resultant achlorhydria, decreased intrinsic factor secretion, and vitamin B_{12} malabsorption. Of patients with B_{12} deficiency, a small number have pernicious anemia. Most patients have malabsorption secondary to chronic *H pylori* infection that results in atrophic gastritis, small intestine bacterial overgrowth, or dietary insufficiency. Fundic histology in pernicious anemia is characterized by severe gland atrophy and intestinal metaplasia caused by autoimmune destruction of the gastric fundic mucosa. Anti-intrinsic factor antibodies are present in 70% of patients. Achlorhydria leads to pronounced hypergastrinemia (greater than 1000 pg/mL) due to loss of acid inhibition of gastrin G cells. Hypergastrinemia may induce hyperplasia of gastric enterochromaffin-like cells that may lead to the development of small, multicentric carcinoid tumors in 5% of patients. Metastatic spread is uncommon in lesions smaller than 2 cm. The risk of gastric adenocarcinoma is increased threefold, with a prevalence of 1–3%. Endoscopy with biopsy is indicated in patients with pernicious anemia at the time of diagnosis. Patients with extensive atrophy and metaplasia involving the antrum and body, dysplasia or small carcinoids require periodic endoscopic surveillance. Pernicious anemia is discussed in detail in Chapter 13.

Bizzaro N et al. Diagnosis and classification of pernicious anemia. Autoimmun Rev. 2014 Apr–May;13(4–5):565–8. [PMID: 24424200]
Murphy G et al. Cancer risk after pernicious anemia in the US elderly population. Clin Gastroenterol Hepatol. 2015 Dec; 13(13):2282–9.e4. [PMID: 26079040]

3. Specific Types of Gastritis

A number of disorders are associated with specific mucosal histologic features.

Infections

Acute bacterial infection of the gastric submucosa and muscularis with a variety of aerobic or anaerobic organisms produces a rare, rapidly progressive, life-threatening condition known as phlegmonous or necrotizing gastritis, which requires broad-spectrum antibiotic therapy and, in many cases, emergency gastric resection. Viral infection with CMV is seen in patients with AIDS and after bone marrow or solid organ transplantation. Endoscopic findings include thickened gastric folds and ulcerations. Fungal infection with mucormycosis and *Candida* may occur in immunocompromised and diabetic patients. Larvae of *Anisakis marina* ingested in raw fish or sushi may become embedded in the gastric mucosa, producing severe abdominal pain. Pain persists for several days until the larvae die. Endoscopic removal of the larvae provides rapid symptomatic relief.

Okano K et al. Acute abdomen with epigastric pain and vomiting in an adult healthy patient. Gastroenterology. 2010 Nov; 139(5):1465. [PMID: 20875783]

PEPTIC ULCER DISEASE

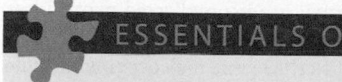
ESSENTIALS OF DIAGNOSIS

- ▶ History of dyspepsia present in 80–90% of patients with variable relationship to meals.
- ▶ Ulcer symptoms characterized by rhythmicity and periodicity.
- ▶ Ulcer complications present without antecedent symptoms in 10–20% of patients.
- ▶ Most NSAID-induced ulcers are asymptomatic.
- ▶ Upper endoscopy with gastric biopsy for *H pylori* is the diagnostic procedure of choice in most patients.
- ▶ Gastric ulcer biopsy or documentation of complete healing necessary to exclude gastric malignancy.

General Considerations

Peptic ulcer is a break in the gastric or duodenal mucosa that arises when the normal mucosal defensive factors are impaired or are overwhelmed by aggressive luminal factors such as acid and pepsin. By definition, ulcers extend through the muscularis mucosae and are usually over 5 mm in diameter. In the United States, there are about 500,000 new cases per year of peptic ulcer and 4 million ulcer recurrences; the lifetime prevalence of ulcers in the adult population is approximately 10%. Ulcers occur either in the duodenum, where over 95% are in the bulb or pyloric channel, or in the stomach, where benign ulcers are located most commonly in the antrum (60%) or at the junction of the antrum and body on the lesser curvature (25%).

Although ulcers can occur in any age group, duodenal ulcers most commonly occur in patients between the ages of 30 and 55 years, whereas gastric ulcers are more common in patients between the ages of 55 and 70 years. The incidence of duodenal ulcer disease has been declining dramatically for the past 30 years (due to the eradication of *H pylori*), but the incidence of gastric ulcers has not been declining (due to the widespread use of NSAIDs and low-dose aspirin).

Etiology

There are two major causes of peptic ulcer disease: NSAIDs and chronic *H pylori* infection. Evidence of *H pylori* infection or NSAID ingestion should be sought in all patients with peptic ulcer. Alcohol, dietary factors, and stress do not appear to cause ulcer disease. Less than 5–10% of ulcers are caused by other conditions, including acid hypersecretory states (such as Zollinger-Ellison syndrome or systemic mastocytosis), CMV (especially in transplant recipients), Crohn disease, lymphoma, medications (eg, alendronate), chronic medical illness (cirrhosis or chronic kidney disease), or are idiopathic. NSAID and *H pylori*-associated ulcers will be presented in this section; Zollinger-Ellison syndrome will be discussed subsequently.

A. H pylori–Associated Ulcers

H pylori infection with associated gastritis and, in some cases, duodenitis appears to be a necessary cofactor for the majority of duodenal and gastric ulcers not associated with NSAIDs. Ulcer disease will develop in an estimated 10% of infected patients. The prevalence of *H pylori* infection in duodenal ulcer patients is 70–90%. The association with gastric ulcers is lower, but *H pylori* is found in most patients in whom NSAIDs cannot be implicated.

The natural history of *H pylori*–associated peptic ulcer disease is well defined. In the absence of specific antibiotic treatment to eradicate the organism, 85% of patients will have an endoscopically visible recurrence within 1 year. Half of these will be symptomatic. After successful eradication of *H pylori* with antibiotics, ulcer recurrence rates are reduced dramatically to 5–20% at 1 year. Most of these ulcer recurrences are due to NSAID use or, rarely, reinfection with *H pylori*.

B. NSAID-Induced Ulcers

There is a 10–20% prevalence of gastric ulcers and a 2–5% prevalence of duodenal ulcers in long-term NSAID users. Approximately 2–5%/year of long-term NSAID users will have an ulcer that causes clinically significant dyspepsia or a serious complication. The incidence of serious gastrointestinal complications (hospitalization, bleeding, perforation) is 0.2–1.9%/year. Meta-analyses of clinical trials detected an increased risk of upper gastrointestinal bleeding in patients taking low-dose aspirin (1 of 1000), coxibs (2 of 1000), and nsNSAIDs (4–6 of 1000). The risk of NSAID complications is greater within the first 3 months of therapy and in patients who are older than 60 years; who have a prior history of ulcer disease; or who take NSAIDs in combination with aspirin, corticosteroids, or anticoagulants.

Traditional nsNSAIDs inhibit prostaglandins through reversible inhibition of both COX-1 and COX-2 enzymes. Aspirin causes irreversible inhibition of COX-1 and COX-2 as well as of platelet aggregation. Coxibs (or selective NSAIDs) preferentially inhibit COX-2—the principal enzyme involved in prostaglandin production at sites of inflammation—while providing relative sparing of COX-1, the principal enzyme involved with mucosal cytoprotection in the stomach and duodenum. Celecoxib is the only coxib currently available in the United States, although other older NSAIDs (etodolac, meloxicam) may have similar COX-2/COX-1 selectivity.

Coxibs decrease the incidence of endoscopically visible ulcers by approximately 75% compared with nsNSAIDs. Of greater clinical importance, the risk of significant clinical events (obstruction, perforation, bleeding) is reduced by up to 50% in patients taking coxibs versus nsNSAIDs. However, a twofold increase in the incidence in cardiovascular complications (myocardial infarction, cerebrovascular infarction, and death) has been detected in patients taking coxibs compared with placebo, prompting the voluntary withdrawal of two highly selective coxibs (rofecoxib and valdecoxib) from the market by the manufacturers. A review by an FDA panel suggested that all NSAIDs (other than aspirin and, possibly, naproxen) may be associated with an increased risk of cardiovascular complications, but concluded that celecoxib, which has less COX-2 selectivity than rofecoxib and valdecoxib, does not have higher risk than other nsNSAIDs when used in currently recommended doses (200 mg/day).

Use of even low-dose aspirin (81–325 mg/day) leads to a twofold increased risk of gastrointestinal bleeding complications. In randomized controlled trials, the absolute annual increase of gastrointestinal bleeding attributable to low-dose aspirin is only 0.12% higher than with placebo therapy. However, in population studies, gastrointestinal bleeding occurs in 1.2% of patients each year. Patients with a prior history of peptic ulcers or gastrointestinal bleeding have a markedly increased risk of complications on low-dose aspirin. It should be noted that low-dose aspirin in combination with NSAIDs or coxibs increases the risk of ulcer complications by up to tenfold compared with NSAIDs or low-dose aspirin alone. Dual antiplatelet therapy with aspirin and a thienopyridine (eg, clopidogrel) incurs a twofold to threefold increased risk of bleeding compared with aspirin alone.

H pylori infection increases the risk of ulcer disease and complications over threefold in patients taking NSAIDs or low-dose aspirin. It is hypothesized that NSAID initiation may potentiate or aggravate ulcer disease in susceptible infected individuals.

▶ Clinical Findings

A. Symptoms and Signs

Epigastric pain (dyspepsia), the hallmark of peptic ulcer disease, is present in 80–90% of patients. However, this complaint is not sensitive or specific enough to serve as a reliable diagnostic criterion for peptic ulcer disease. The clinical history cannot accurately distinguish duodenal from gastric ulcers. Less than 25% of patients with dyspepsia have ulcer disease at endoscopy. Twenty percent of patients with ulcer complications such as bleeding have no antecedent symptoms ("silent ulcers"). Nearly 60% of patients with NSAID-related ulcer complications do not have prior symptoms.

Pain is typically well localized to the epigastrium and not severe. It is described as gnawing, dull, aching, or "hunger-like." Approximately 50% of patients report relief of pain with food or antacids (especially duodenal ulcers) and a recurrence of pain 2–4 hours later. However, many patients deny any relationship to meals or report worsening of pain. Two-thirds of duodenal ulcers and one-third of gastric ulcers cause nocturnal pain that awakens the patient. A change from a patient's typical rhythmic discomfort to constant or radiating pain may reflect ulcer penetration or perforation. Most patients have symptomatic periods lasting up to several weeks with intervals of months to years in which they are pain free (periodicity).

Nausea and anorexia may occur with gastric ulcers. Significant vomiting and weight loss are unusual with uncomplicated ulcer disease and suggest gastric outlet obstruction or gastric malignancy.

The physical examination is often normal in uncomplicated peptic ulcer disease. Mild, localized epigastric tenderness to deep palpation may be present. FOBT or FIT is positive in one-third of patients.

B. Laboratory Findings

Laboratory tests are normal in uncomplicated peptic ulcer disease but are ordered to exclude ulcer complications or confounding disease entities. Anemia may occur with acute blood loss from a bleeding ulcer or less commonly from chronic blood loss. Leukocytosis suggests ulcer penetration or perforation. An elevated serum amylase in a patient with severe epigastric pain suggests ulcer penetration into the pancreas. A fasting serum gastrin level to screen for Zollinger-Ellison syndrome is obtained in some patients.

C. Endoscopy

Upper endoscopy is the procedure of choice for the diagnosis of duodenal and gastric ulcers. Duodenal ulcers are virtually never malignant and do not require biopsy. Three to 5 percent of benign-appearing gastric ulcers prove to be malignant. Hence, biopsies of the ulcer margin are almost always performed. Provided that the gastric ulcer appears benign to the endoscopist and adequate biopsy specimens reveal no evidence of cancer, dysplasia, or atypia, the patient may be monitored without further endoscopy. If these conditions are not fulfilled, follow-up endoscopy should be performed 12 weeks after the start of therapy to document complete healing; nonhealing ulcers are suspicious for malignancy.

D. Imaging

Because barium upper gastrointestinal series is less sensitive for detection of ulcers and less accurate for distinguishing benign from malignant ulcers, it has been supplanted by upper endoscopy in most settings. Abdominal CT imaging is obtained in patients with suspected complications of peptic ulcer disease (perforation, penetration, or obstruction).

E. Testing for *H pylori*

In patients in whom an ulcer is diagnosed by endoscopy, gastric mucosal biopsies should be obtained both for a rapid urease test and for histologic examination. The specimens for histology are discarded if the urease test is positive.

In patients with a history of peptic ulcer or when an ulcer is diagnosed by upper gastrointestinal series, noninvasive assessment for *H pylori* with fecal antigen assay or urea breath testing should be done, which both have a sensitivity and specificity of 95%. Proton pump inhibitors may cause false-negative urea breath tests and fecal antigen tests and should be withheld for at least 14 days before testing. Because of its lower sensitivity (85%) and specificity (79%), serologic testing should not be performed unless fecal antigen testing or urea breath testing is unavailable.

▶ Differential Diagnosis

Peptic ulcer disease must be distinguished from other causes of epigastric distress (dyspepsia). Over 50% of patients with dyspepsia have no obvious organic explanation for their symptoms and are classified as having functional dyspepsia (see sections above on Dyspepsia and Functional Dyspepsia). Atypical gastroesophageal reflux may be manifested by epigastric symptoms. Biliary tract disease is characterized by discrete, intermittent episodes of pain that should not be confused with other causes of dyspepsia. Severe epigastric pain is atypical for peptic ulcer disease unless complicated by a perforation or penetration. Other causes include acute pancreatitis, acute cholecystitis or choledocholithiasis, esophageal rupture, gastric volvulus, gastric or intestinal ischemia, and ruptured aortic aneurysm.

▶ Pharmacologic Agents

The pharmacology and use of several agents that enhance the healing of peptic ulcers is briefly discussed here. They may be divided into three categories: (1) acid-antisecretory agents, (2) mucosal protective agents, and (3) agents that promote healing through eradication of *H pylori*.

A. Acid-Antisecretory Agents

1. Proton pump inhibitors—Proton pump inhibitors covalently bind the acid-secreting enzyme H^+-K^+-ATPase, or "proton pump," permanently inactivating it. Restoration of acid secretion requires synthesis of new pumps, which have a half-life of 18 hours. Thus, although these agents have a serum half-life of less than 60 minutes, their duration of action exceeds 24 hours.

There are six oral proton pump inhibitors currently available: omeprazole, rabeprazole, esomeprazole, lansoprazole, dexlansoprazole, and pantoprazole. The available oral agents inhibit over 90% of 24-hour acid secretion, compared with under 65% for H_2-receptor antagonists in standard dosages. Despite minor differences in their pharmacology, they are equally efficacious in the treatment of peptic ulcer disease. Treatment with oral proton pump inhibitors results in over 90% healing of duodenal ulcers after 4 weeks and 90% of gastric ulcers after 8 weeks when given once daily (30 minutes before breakfast) at the following recommended doses: omeprazole, 20–40 mg; esomeprazole, 40 mg; rabeprazole, 20 mg; lansoprazole, 30 mg; dexlansoprazole, 30–60 mg; pantoprazole, 40 mg. Compared with H_2-receptor antagonists, proton pump inhibitors provide faster pain relief and more rapid ulcer healing.

The proton pump inhibitors are remarkably safe for short-term therapy. Long-term use may lead to mild decreases in vitamin B_{12}, iron, and calcium absorption. Observational studies suggest an increased risk of enteric infections, including *C difficile* and bacterial gastroenteritis, a modest (1.4-fold) increased risk of hip fracture, and pneumonia. Serum gastrin levels rise significantly in 3% of patients receiving long-term therapy but return to normal limits within 2 weeks after discontinuation.

2. H_2-receptor antagonists—Although H_2-receptor antagonists are effective in the treatment of peptic ulcer disease, proton pump inhibitors are now the preferred agents because of their ease of use and superior efficacy. Four H_2-receptor antagonists are available: cimetidine, ranitidine, famotidine, and nizatidine. For uncomplicated peptic ulcers, H_2-receptor antagonists may be administered once daily at bedtime as follows: ranitidine and nizatidine 300 mg, famotidine 40 mg, and cimetidine 800 mg. Duodenal and gastric ulcer healing rates of 85–90% are obtained within 6 weeks and 8 weeks, respectively.

B. Agents Enhancing Mucosal Defenses

Bismuth sucralfate, misoprostol, and antacids all have been shown to promote ulcer healing through the enhancement of mucosal defensive mechanisms. Given the greater efficacy and safety of antisecretory agents and better compliance of patients, these agents are no longer used as first-line therapy for active ulcers in most clinical settings.

C. *H pylori* Eradication Therapy

Eradication of *H pylori* has proved difficult. Combination regimens that use two or three antibiotics with a proton pump inhibitor or bismuth are required to achieve adequate rates of eradication and to reduce the number of failures due to antibiotic resistance. In the United States, up to 50% of strains are resistant to metronidazole and 10–20% are resistant to clarithromycin. Recommended regimens are listed in Table 15–10. At present, experts disagree on the optimal regimen; however, updated Maastricht consensus guidelines were published in 2012. Ideally, the optimal regimen would be determined by antibiotic susceptibility testing. However, this requires endoscopic biopsy, and few laboratories are equipped for *H pylori* cultures. Thus, in most clinical settings, therapy is chosen empirically. In areas of low clarithromycin resistance, including the United States, a 14-day course of "triple therapy," with an oral proton pump inhibitor, clarithromycin 500 mg, and amoxicillin 1 g (or, if penicillin allergic,

metronidazole 500 mg), all given twice daily for 14 days, is still recommended for first-line therapy. In the United States, this regimen achieves rates of eradication approaching 90%. "Quadruple therapy," with a proton pump inhibitor, bismuth, tetracycline, and metronidazole or tinidazole for 14 days (Table 15–10) is a more complicated regimen that achieves greater than 90% eradication, even in strains with metronidazole resistance. A 2013 large multicenter European controlled trial conducted in regions of high clarithromycin resistance reported 92% eradication with a 14-day quadruple therapy consisting of a proton pump inhibitor, amoxicillin, clarithromycin, and nitroimidazole (the latter drug not available in the United States). Bismuth-based quadruple therapy is recommended as first-line therapy for patients in areas with high clarithromycin resistance

Table 15–10. Treatment options for peptic ulcer disease.

Active *Helicobacter pylori*–associated ulcer

1. Treat with anti-*H pylori* regimen for 14 days. Treatment options:

   Standard Triple Therapy
   - Proton pump inhibitor orally twice daily[1]
   - Clarithromycin 500 mg orally twice daily[2]
   - Amoxicillin 1 g orally twice daily (OR metronidazole 500 mg orally twice daily, if penicillin allergic[3])

   Standard Quadruple Therapy
   - Proton pump inhibitor orally twice daily[1,4]
   - Bismuth subsalicylate two tablets orally four times daily
   - Tetracycline 500 mg orally four times daily
   - Metronidazole 500 mg three times daily
     (OR bismuth subcitrate potassium 140 mg/metronidazole 125 mg/tetracycline 125 mg [Pylera] three capsules orally four times daily)[5]

2. After completion of course of *H pylori* eradication therapy, continue treatment with proton pump inhibitor[1] once daily for 4–6 weeks if ulcer is large (> 1 cm) or complicated.

3. Confirm successful eradication of *H pylori* with urea breath test, fecal antigen test, or endoscopy with biopsy at least 4 weeks after completion of antibiotic treatment and 1–2 weeks after proton pump inhibitor treatment.

Active ulcer not attributable to *H pylori*

1. Consider other causes: NSAIDs, Zollinger-Ellison syndrome, gastric malignancy. Treatment options:
   - Proton pump inhibitors[1]:
     Uncomplicated duodenal ulcer: treat for 4 weeks
     Uncomplicated gastric ulcer: treat for 8 weeks
   - H₂-receptor antagonists:
     Uncomplicated duodenal ulcer: cimetidine 800 mg, ranitidine or nizatidine 300 mg, famotidine 40 mg, orally once daily at bedtime for 6 weeks
     Uncomplicated gastric ulcer: cimetidine 400 mg, ranitidine or nizatidine 150 mg, famotidine 20 mg, orally twice daily for 8 weeks
     Complicated ulcers: proton pump inhibitors are the preferred drugs

Prevention of ulcer relapse

1. NSAID-induced ulcer: prophylactic therapy for high-risk patients (prior ulcer disease or ulcer complications, use of corticosteroids or anticoagulants, age > 60 years, serious comorbid illnesses). Treatment options:
   - Proton pump inhibitor once daily[1]
   - Celecoxib (contraindicated in patients with increased risk of cardiovascular disease)
   - Misoprostol 200 mcg orally 4 times daily

2. Long-term "maintenance" therapy indicated in patients with recurrent ulcers who either are *H pylori*–negative or who have failed attempts at eradication therapy: once-daily oral proton pump inhibitor[1]

---

[1]Oral proton pump inhibitors: omeprazole 40 mg, rabeprazole 20 mg, lansoprazole 30 mg, dexlansoprazole 30–60 mg, pantoprazole 40 mg, esomeprazole 40 mg. Proton pump inhibitors are administered 30 minutes before meals.
[2]If region with high clarithromycin resistance or if patient has previously been treated with macrolide antibiotic, choose another regimen.
[3]Avoid in areas of known high metronidazole resistance or in patients who have failed a course of treatment that included metronidazole.
[4]Preferred regimen in regions with high clarithromycin resistance or in patients who have previously received a macrolide antibiotic or are penicillin allergic. Effective against metronidazole-resistant organisms.
[5]Pylera is an FDA-approved formulation containing bismuth subcitrate 140 mg/tetracycline 125 mg/metronidazole 125 mg per capsule.
NSAIDs, nonsteroidal anti-inflammatory drugs.

(greater than 20%), in patients who have previously been treated with a macrolide antibiotic, or as second-line therapy for patients whose infection persists after an initial course of triple therapy. Previous studies reported eradication rates of more than 90% using a 10-day sequential regimen consisting of four drugs: a proton pump inhibitor and amoxicillin for 5 days, followed by a proton pump inhibitor, clarithromycin, and tinidazole for 5 days. However, a 2013 meta-analysis did not detect superiority compared with 14-day triple therapy or bismuth-based therapy, except in patients with organisms exhibiting clarithromycin resistance.

▶ Medical Treatment

Patients should be encouraged to eat balanced meals at regular intervals. There is no justification for bland or restrictive diets. Moderate alcohol intake is not harmful. Smoking retards the rate of ulcer healing and increases the frequency of recurrences and should be prohibited.

A. Treatment of *H pylori*–Associated Ulcers

1. Treatment of active ulcer—The goals of treatment of active *H pylori*–associated ulcers are to relieve dyspeptic symptoms, to promote ulcer healing, and to eradicate *H pylori* infection. Uncomplicated *H pylori*–associated ulcers should be treated for 14 days with one of the proton pump inhibitor-based *H pylori* eradication regimens listed in Table 15–10. At that point, no further antisecretory therapy is needed, provided the ulcer was small (less than 1 cm) and dyspeptic symptoms have resolved. For patients with large or complicated ulcers, an antisecretory agent should be continued for an additional 2–4 weeks (duodenal ulcer) or 4–6 weeks (gastric ulcer) after completion of the antibiotic regimen to ensure complete ulcer healing. A once-daily oral proton pump inhibitor (as listed in Table 15–10) is recommended. Confirmation of *H pylori* eradication is recommended for all patients more than 4 weeks after completion of antibiotic therapy and more than 2 weeks after discontinuation of the proton pump inhibitor either with noninvasive tests (urea breath test, fecal antigen test) or endoscopy with biopsy for histology.

2. Therapy to prevent recurrence—Successful eradication reduces ulcer recurrences to less than 20% after 1–2 years. The most common cause of recurrence after antibiotic therapy is failure to achieve successful eradication. Once cure has been achieved, reinfection rates are less than 0.5% per year. Although *H pylori* eradication has reduced the need for long-term maintenance antisecretory therapy to prevent ulcer recurrences, there remains a subset of patients who require long-term therapy with a proton pump inhibitor once daily. This subset includes patients with *H pylori*–positive ulcers who have not responded to repeated attempts at eradication therapy, patients with a history of *H pylori*–positive ulcers who have recurrent ulcers despite successful eradication, and patients with idiopathic ulcers (ie, *H pylori*–negative and not taking NSAIDs). In all patients with recurrent ulcers, NSAID usage (unintentional or surreptitious) and hypersecretory states (including gastrinoma) should be excluded.

B. Treatment of NSAID-Associated Ulcers

1. Treatment of active ulcers—In patients with NSAID-induced ulcers, the offending agent should be discontinued whenever possible. Both gastric and duodenal ulcers respond rapidly to therapy with H_2-receptor antagonists or proton pump inhibitors (Table 15–10) once NSAIDs are eliminated. In some patients with severe inflammatory diseases, it may not be feasible to discontinue NSAIDs. These patients should be treated with concomitant proton pump inhibitors once daily, which results in ulcer healing rates of approximately 80% at 8 weeks in patients continuing to take NSAIDs. All patients with NSAID-associated ulcers should undergo testing for *H pylori* infection. Antibiotic eradication therapy should be given if *H pylori* tests are positive.

2. Prevention of NSAID-induced ulcers—Clinicians should carefully weigh the benefits of NSAID therapy with the risks of cardiovascular and gastrointestinal complications. Both coxibs and nsNSAIDs with the possible exception of naproxen increase the risk of cardiovascular complications. Ulcer complications occur in up to 2% of all nsNSAID-treated patients per year but in up to 10–20% per year of patients with multiple risk factors. These include age over 60 years, history of ulcer disease or complications, concurrent use of antiplatelet therapy (low-dose aspirin or clopidogrel, or both), concurrent therapy with anticoagulants or corticosteroids, and serious underlying medical illness. After considering the patient's risk of cardiovascular and gastrointestinal complications due to NSAID use, the clinician can decide what type of NSAID (nsNSAID vs coxib) is appropriate and what strategies should be used to reduce the risk of such complications. To minimize cardiovascular and gastrointestinal risks, all NSAIDs should be used at the lowest effective dose and for the shortest time necessary.

A. TEST FOR AND TREAT *H PYLORI* INFECTION—All patients with a known history of peptic ulcer disease who are treated with NSAIDs or antiplatelet agents (aspirin, clopidogrel) should be tested for *H pylori* infection and treated, if positive. Although *H pylori* eradication may decrease the risk of NSAID-related complications, co-therapy with a proton pump inhibitor is still required in high-risk patients.

B. PROTON PUMP INHIBITOR—Treatment with an oral proton pump inhibitor given once daily (rabeprazole 20 mg, omeprazole 20–40 mg, lansoprazole 30 mg, dexlansoprazole 30–60 mg, or pantoprazole or esomeprazole 40 mg) is effective in the prevention of NSAID-induced gastric and duodenal ulcers and is approved by the FDA for this indication. Among high-risk patients taking nsNSAIDs or coxibs, the incidence of endoscopically visible gastric and duodenal ulcers after 6 months of therapy in patients treated with esomeprazole 20–40 mg/day was 5%, compared with 17% who were given placebo. Nonetheless, proton pump inhibitors are not fully protective in high-risk patients in preventing NSAID-related complications. In prospective, controlled trials of patients with a prior history of NSAID-related ulcer complications, the incidence of recurrent bleeding was almost 5% after 6 months in patients taking nsNSAIDs and a proton pump inhibitor. In prospective, controlled trials of patients with a prior history of ulcer complications related to low-dose aspirin, the incidence of recurrent ulcer bleeding in patients taking low-dose aspirin alone was approximately 15% per year compared with 0–2% per year in patients taking low-dose aspirin and proton pump inhibitor and 9–14% per year in patients taking clopidogrel. Thus, proton pump inhibitors are highly effective in preventing complications related to low-dose aspirin, even in high-risk patients. Enteric coating of aspirin may reduce direct topical damage to the stomach but does not reduce complications.

C. Recommendations to reduce risk of ulcer complications from nsNSAIDs and coxibs—For patients with a low-risk of cardiovascular disease who have no risk factors for gastrointestinal complications, an nsNSAID alone may be given. For patients with one or two gastrointestinal risk factors, a coxib alone or an nsNSAID with a proton pump inhibitor once daily should be given to reduce the risk of gastrointestinal complications. NSAIDs should be avoided if possible in patients with multiple risk factors; if required, however, combination therapy with a coxib or a partially COX-2 selective nsNSAID (etodolac, meloxicam) and a proton pump inhibitor once daily is recommended.

For patients with an increased risk of cardiovascular complications, it is preferable to avoid NSAIDs, if possible. If an NSAID is required, naproxen is preferred because it appears to have reduced risk of cardiovascular complications compared with other nsNSAIDs. Coxibs should not be prescribed in patients with increased cardiovascular risk. Almost all patients with increased cardiovascular risk also will be taking antiplatelet therapy with low-dose aspirin or clopidogrel, or both. Because combination therapy with an nsNSAID and antiplatelet therapy increases the risks of gastrointestinal complications, these patients should all receive cotherapy with a proton pump inhibitor once daily or misoprostol.

D. Recommendations to reduce risk of ulcer complications with use of antiplatelet agents—The risk of significant gastrointestinal complications in persons taking low-dose aspirin (81–325 mg/day) or clopidogrel, or both, for cardiovascular prophylaxis is 0.5%/year. Aspirin, 81 mg/day, is recommended in most patients because it has a lower risk of gastrointestinal complications but equivalent cardiovascular protection compared with higher aspirin doses. Complications are increased with combinations of aspirin and clopidogrel or aspirin and anticoagulants. Clopidogrel does not cause gastrointestinal ulcers or erosions. However, its antiplatelet activity may promote bleeding from erosions or ulcers caused by low-dose aspirin or *H pylori*. Patients with dyspepsia or prior ulcer disease should be tested for *H pylori* infection and treated, if positive. Patients younger than 60–70 years who have no other risk factors for gastrointestinal complications may be treated with low-dose aspirin or dual antiplatelet therapy without a proton pump inhibitor. Virtually all other patients who require low-dose aspirin or aspirin plus anticoagulant therapy should receive a proton pump inhibitor once daily.

At the present time, the optimal management of patients who require dual antiplatelet therapy with clopidogrel and aspirin is uncertain. Clopidogrel is a prodrug that is activated by the cytochrome P450 CYP2C19 enzyme. All proton pump inhibitors inhibit CYP2C19 to varying degrees, with omeprazole having the highest and pantoprazole the least level of inhibition. In vitro and in vivo platelet aggregation studies demonstrate that proton pump inhibitors (especially omeprazole) may attenuate the antiplatelet effects of clopidogrel, although the clinical importance of this interaction is uncertain. In 2009 the FDA issued a warning that patients should avoid using clopidogrel with omeprazole, stating further that the safety of other proton pump inhibitors also was uncertain. Faced with this warning, the optimal strategy to reduce the risk of upper gastrointestinal bleeding in patients taking clopidogrel (with or without aspirin) is uncertain. A 2010 expert consensus panel concluded that once daily treatment with an oral proton pump inhibitor (pantoprazole 40 mg; rabeprazole 20 mg; lansoprazole or dexlansoprazole 30 mg) may still be recommended for patients who have an increased risk of upper gastrointestinal bleeding (prior history of peptic ulcer disease or gastrointestinal bleeding; concomitant NSAIDs). In keeping with the FDA warning and product labeling, omeprazole and esomeprazole should not be used. For patients with a lower risk of gastrointestinal bleeding, the risks and benefits of proton pump inhibitors must be weighed. Pending further recommendations, an acceptable alternative is to treat with an oral H_2-receptor antagonist (famotidine 20 mg, ranitidine 150 mg, nizatidine 150 mg) twice daily; however, proton pump inhibitors are more effective in preventing upper gastrointestinal bleeding. Cimetidine is a CYP2C19 inhibitor and should not be used. An alternative strategy is ticagrelor, an antiplatelet agent approved for use with low-dose aspirin in the treatment of acute coronary syndrome. Like clopidogrel, ticagrelor blocks the platelet ADP p2y12 receptor; however, it does not require hepatic activation, it does not interact with the CYP2C19 enzyme, and its efficacy is not diminished by proton pump inhibitors.

C. Refractory Ulcers

Ulcers that are truly refractory to medical therapy are now uncommon. Less than 5% of ulcers are unhealed after 8 weeks of once daily therapy with proton pump inhibitors, and almost all benign ulcers heal with twice daily therapy. Thus, noncompliance is the most common cause of ulcer nonhealing. NSAID and aspirin use, sometimes surreptitious, are commonly implicated in refractory ulcers and must be stopped. *H pylori* infection should be sought and the infection treated, if present, in all refractory ulcer patients. Single or multiple linear gastric ulcers may occur in large hiatal hernias where the stomach slides back and forth through the diaphragmatic hiatus ("Cameron lesions"), which may be a cause of iron deficiency anemia. Other causes of nonhealing ulcers include acid hypersecretion (Zollinger-Ellison syndrome), unrecognized malignancy (adenocarcinoma or lymphoma), medications causing gastrointestinal ulceration (eg, iron or bisphosphonates), Crohn disease, and unusual infections (*H heilmanii*, CMV, mucormycosis). Fasting serum gastrin levels should be obtained to exclude gastrinoma with acid hypersecretion (Zollinger-Ellison syndrome). Repeat ulcer biopsies are mandatory after 2–3 months of therapy in all nonhealed ulcers to look for malignancy or infection. Patients with persistent nonhealing ulcers are referred for surgical therapy after exclusion of NSAID use and persistent *H pylori* infection.

Abraham NS et al. ACCF/ACG/AHA 2010 expert consensus document on the concomitant use of proton pump inhibitors and thienopyridines: a focused update of the ASSG/ACG/AHA 2008 expert consensus document on reducing the gastrointestinal risks of antiplatelet therapy and NSAID use. Am J Gastroenterol. 2010 Dec;105(12):2533–49. [PMID: 21131924]

Chan FK et al. Effects of *Helicobacter pylori* infection on long-term risk of peptic ulcer bleeding in low-dose aspirin users. Gastroenterology. 2013 Mar;144(3):528–35. [PMID: 23333655]

Gatta L et al. Global eradication rates for *Helicobacter pylori* infection: systematic review and meta-analysis of sequential therapy. BMJ. 2013 Aug 7;347:f4587. [PMID: 23926315]

Graham DY. *Helicobacter pylori* update: gastric cancer, reliable therapy, and possible benefits. Gastroenterology. 2015 Apr; 148(4):719–31.e3. [PMID: 25655557]

Graham DY et al. Rational *Helicobacter pylori* therapy: evidence-based medicine rather than medicine-based evidence. Clin Gastroenterol Hepatol. 2014 Feb;12(2):177–86. [PMID: 23751282]

Laine L. NSAID-associated gastrointestinal bleeding: assessing the role of concomitant medications. Gastroenterology. 2014 Oct; 147(4):730–3. [PMID: 25167988]

Malfertheiner P et al; European Helicobacter Study Group. Management of *Helicobacter pylori* infection—the Maastricht IV/ Florence Consensus Report. Gut. 2012 May;61(5):646–64. [PMID: 22491499]

Molina-Infante J et al. Optimized nonbismuth quadruple therapies cure most patients with *Helicobacter pylori* infection in populations with high rates of antibiotic resistance. Gastroenterology. 2013 Jul;145(1):121–8. [PMID: 23562754]

Park CS et al. Pretreatment antimicrobial susceptibility-guided vs. clarithromycin-based triple therapy for *Helicobacter pylori* eradication in a region with high rates of multiple drug resistance. Am J Gastroenterol. 2014 Oct;109(10):1595–602. [PMID: 25091062]

Scheiman JM. The use of proton pump inhibitors in treating and preventing NSAID-induced mucosal damage. Arthritis Res Ther. 2013;15 (Suppl 3):S5. [PMID: 24267413]

COMPLICATIONS OF PEPTIC ULCER DISEASE

1. Gastrointestinal Hemorrhage

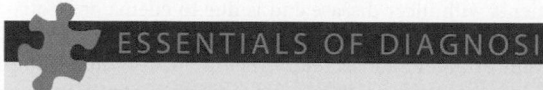
ESSENTIALS OF DIAGNOSIS

- ▶ "Coffee grounds" emesis, hematemesis, melena, or hematochezia.

- ▶ Emergent upper endoscopy is diagnostic and therapeutic.

▶ General Considerations

Approximately 50% of all episodes of upper gastrointestinal bleeding are due to peptic ulcer. Clinically significant bleeding occurs in 10% of ulcer patients. About 80% of patients stop bleeding spontaneously and generally have an uneventful recovery; the remaining 20% have more severe bleeding. The overall mortality rate for ulcer bleeding is 7%, but it is higher in the elderly, in patients with comorbid medical problems, and in patients with hospital-associated bleeding. Mortality is also higher in patients who present with persistent hypotension or shock, bright red blood in the vomitus or nasogastric lavage fluid, or severe coagulopathy.

▶ Clinical Findings

A. Symptoms and Signs

Up to 20% of patients have no antecedent symptoms of pain; this is particularly true of patients receiving NSAIDs. Common presenting signs include melena and hematemesis. Massive upper gastrointestinal bleeding or rapid gastrointestinal transit may result in hematochezia rather than melena; this may be misinterpreted as signifying a lower tract bleeding source. Nasogastric lavage that demonstrates "coffee grounds" or bright red blood confirms an upper tract source. Recovered nasogastric lavage fluid that is negative for blood does not exclude active bleeding from a duodenal ulcer.

B. Laboratory Findings

The hematocrit may fall as a result of bleeding or expansion of the intravascular volume with intravenous fluids. The BUN may rise as a result of absorption of blood nitrogen from the small intestine and prerenal azotemia.

▶ Treatment

The assessment and initial management of upper gastrointestinal tract bleeding are discussed above. Specific issues pertaining to peptic ulcer bleeding are described below.

A. Medical Therapy

1. Antisecretory agents—Intravenous proton pump inhibitors should be administered for 3 days in patients with ulcers whose endoscopic appearance suggests a high risk of rebleeding after endoscopic therapy. Intravenous proton pump inhibitors have been associated with a reduction in rebleeding, transfusions, the need for further endoscopic therapy, and surgery in the subset of patients with high-risk ulcers, ie, an ulcer with active bleeding, visible vessel, or adherent clot. After initial successful endoscopic treatment of ulcer hemorrhage, intravenous esomeprazole, pantoprazole, or omeprazole (80 mg bolus injection, followed by 8 mg/h continuous infusion for 72 hours) reduces the rebleeding rate from approximately 20% to less than 10%; however, intravenous omeprazole is not available in the United States.

High-dose oral proton pump inhibitors (omeprazole 40 mg twice daily) also appear to be effective in reducing rebleeding but have not been compared with the intravenous regimen. Intravenous H$_2$-receptor antagonists have not been demonstrated to be of any benefit in the treatment of acute ulcer bleeding.

2. Long-term prevention of rebleeding—Recurrent ulcer bleeding develops within 3 years in one-third of patients if no specific therapy is given. In patients with bleeding ulcers who are *H pylori*-positive, successful eradication effectively prevents recurrent ulcer bleeding in almost all cases. It is therefore recommended that all patients with bleeding ulcers be tested for *H pylori* infection and treated if positive. Four to 8 weeks after completion of antibiotic therapy, a urea breath or fecal antigen test for *H pylori* should be administered or endoscopy performed with biopsy for histologic confirmation of successful eradication. In patients in whom *H pylori* persists or the small subset of patients whose ulcers are not associated with NSAIDs or *H pylori*, long-term acid suppression with a once-daily proton pump inhibitor should be prescribed to reduce the likelihood of recurrence of bleeding.

B. Endoscopy

Endoscopy is the preferred diagnostic procedure in almost all cases of upper gastrointestinal bleeding because of its high diagnostic accuracy, its ability to predict the likelihood of recurrent bleeding, and its availability for therapeutic intervention in high-risk lesions. Endoscopy should be performed within 24 hours in most cases. In cases of severe active bleeding, endoscopy is performed as soon as patients have been appropriately resuscitated and are hemodynamically stable.

On the basis of clinical and endoscopic criteria, it is possible to predict which patients are at a higher risk of rebleeding and therefore to make more rational use of hospital resources. Nonbleeding ulcers under 2 cm in size with a base that is clean have a less than 5% chance of rebleeding. Most young (under age 60 years), otherwise healthy patients with clean-based ulcers may be safely discharged from the emergency department or hospital after endoscopy. Ulcers that have a flat red or black spot have a less than 10% chance of significant rebleeding. Patients who are hemodynamically stable with these findings should be admitted to a hospital ward for 24–72 hours and may begin immediate oral feedings and antiulcer (or anti-*H pylori*) medication.

By contrast, the risk of rebleeding or continued bleeding in ulcers with a nonbleeding visible vessel is 50%, and with active bleeding it is 80–90%. Endoscopic therapy with thermocoagulation (bipolar or heater probes) or application of endoscopic clips (akin to a staple) is the standard of care for such lesions because it reduces the risk of rebleeding, the number of transfusions, and the need for subsequent surgery. The optimal treatment of ulcers with a dense clot that adheres despite vigorous washing is controversial; removal of the clot followed by endoscopic treatment of an underlying vessel may be considered in selected high-risk patients. For actively bleeding ulcers, a combination of epinephrine injection followed by

thermocoagulation or clip application commonly is used. These techniques achieve successful hemostasis of actively bleeding lesions in 90% of patients. After endoscopic therapy followed by an intravenous proton pump inhibitor, significant rebleeding occurs in less than 10%, of which over 70% can be managed successfully with repeat endoscopic treatment. After endoscopic treatment, patients should remain hospitalized for at least 72 hours, when the risk of rebleeding falls to below 3%.

C. Surgical Treatment

Patients with recurrent bleeding or bleeding that cannot be controlled by endoscopic techniques should be evaluated by a surgeon. However, less than 5% of patients treated with hemostatic therapy require surgery for continued or recurrent bleeding. Overall surgical mortality for emergency ulcer bleeding is less than 6%. The prognosis is poorer for patients over age 60 years, those with serious underlying medical illnesses or chronic kidney disease, and those who require more than 10 units of blood transfusion. Percutaneous arterial embolization is an alternative to surgery for patients in whom endoscopic therapy has failed.

2. Ulcer Perforation

Perforations develop in less than 5% of ulcer patients, usually from ulcers on the anterior wall of the stomach or duodenum. Perforation results in a chemical peritonitis that causes sudden, severe generalized abdominal pain that prompts most patients to seek immediate attention. Elderly or debilitated patients and those receiving long-term corticosteroid therapy may experience minimal initial symptoms, presenting late with bacterial peritonitis, sepsis, and shock. On physical examination, patients appear ill, with a rigid, quiet abdomen and rebound tenderness. Hypotension develops later after bacterial peritonitis has developed. If hypotension is present early with the onset of pain, other abdominal emergencies should be considered such as a ruptured aortic aneurysm, mesenteric infarction, or acute pancreatitis. Leukocytosis is almost always present. A mildly elevated serum amylase (less than twice normal) is sometimes seen. Abdominal CT usually establishes the diagnosis without need for further studies. The absence of free air may lead to a misdiagnosis of pancreatitis, cholecystitis, or appendicitis.

Laparoscopic perforation closure can be performed in many centers, significantly reducing operative morbidity compared with open laparotomy.

3. Gastric Outlet Obstruction

Gastric outlet obstruction occurs in less than 2% of patients with ulcer disease and is due to edema or cicatricial narrowing of the pylorus or duodenal bulb. With the advent of potent antisecretory therapy with proton pump inhibitors and the eradication of *H pylori*, obstruction now is less commonly caused by peptic ulcers than by gastric neoplasms or extrinsic duodenal obstruction by intraabdominal neoplasms. The most common symptoms are early satiety, vomiting, and weight loss. Later, vomiting may develop that typically occurs one to several hours after eating and consists of partially digested food contents. Patients may develop dehydration, metabolic alkalosis, and hypokalemia. On physical examination, a succussion splash may be heard in the epigastrium. In most cases, nasogastric aspiration will result in evacuation of a large amount (greater than 200 mL) of foul-smelling fluid, which establishes the diagnosis. Patients are treated initially with intravenous isotonic saline and KCl to correct fluid and electrolyte disorders, an intravenous proton pump inhibitor, and nasogastric decompression of the stomach. Upper endoscopy is performed after 24–72 hours to define the nature of the obstruction and to exclude gastric neoplasm.

Chiu PW et al. What if endoscopic hemostasis fails? Alternative treatment strategies: surgery. Gastroenterol Clin North Am. 2014 Dec;43(4):753–63. [PMID: 25440923]

Laine L et al. Management of patients with ulcer bleeding. Am J Gastroenterol. 2012 Mar;107(3):345–60. [PMID: 22310222]

Lau JY et al. Challenges in the management of acute peptic ulcer bleeding. Lancet. 2013 Jun 8;381(9882):2033–43. [PMID: 23746903]

Lu Y et al. Multidisciplinary management strategies for acute non-variceal upper gastrointestinal bleeding. Br J Surg. 2014 Jan; 101(1):e34–50. [PMID: 24277160]

Sanabria A et al. Laparoscopic repair for perforated peptic ulcer disease. Cochrane Database Syst Rev. 2013 Feb 28;2:CD004778. [PMID: 23450555]

ZOLLINGER-ELLISON SYNDROME (Gastrinoma)

ESSENTIALS OF DIAGNOSIS

▶ Peptic ulcer disease; may be severe and atypical.

▶ Gastric acid hypersecretion.

▶ Diarrhea common, relieved by nasogastric suction.

▶ Most cases are sporadic; 25% with multiple endocrine neoplasia type 1 (MEN 1).

▶ General Considerations

Zollinger-Ellison syndrome is caused by gastrin-secreting gut neuroendocrine tumors (gastrinomas), which result in hypergastrinemia and acid hypersecretion. Less than 1% of peptic ulcer disease is caused by gastrinomas. Primary gastrinomas may arise in the pancreas (25%), duodenal wall (45%), or lymph nodes (5–15%), and in other locations or of unknown primary (20%). Approximately 80% arise within the "gastrinoma triangle" bounded by the porta hepatis, the neck of the pancreas, and the third portion of the duodenum. Most gastrinomas are solitary or multifocal nodules that are potentially resectable. Approximately 25% of patients have small multicentric gastrinomas associated with MEN 1 that are more difficult to resect. Over two-thirds of gastrinomas are malignant, and one-third have already metastasized to the liver at initial presentation.

▶ Clinical Findings

A. Symptoms and Signs

Over 90% of patients with Zollinger-Ellison syndrome develop peptic ulcers. In most cases, the symptoms are indistinguishable from other causes of peptic ulcer disease and therefore the syndrome may go undetected for years. Ulcers usually are solitary and located in the duodenal bulb, but they may be multiple or occur more distally in the duodenum. Isolated gastric ulcers do not occur. Gastroesophageal reflux symptoms occur often. Diarrhea occurs in one-third of patients, in some cases in the absence of peptic symptoms. Gastric acid hypersecretion can cause direct intestinal mucosal injury and pancreatic enzyme inactivation, resulting in diarrhea, steatorrhea, and weight loss; nasogastric aspiration of stomach acid stops the diarrhea. Screening for Zollinger-Ellison syndrome with fasting gastrin levels should be obtained in patients with ulcers that are refractory to standard therapies, giant ulcers (larger than 2 cm), ulcers located distal to the duodenal bulb, multiple duodenal ulcers, frequent ulcer recurrences, ulcers associated with diarrhea, ulcers occurring after ulcer surgery, and patients with ulcer complications. Ulcer patients with hypercalcemia or family histories of ulcers (suggesting MEN 1) should also be screened. Finally, patients with peptic ulcers who are *H pylori* negative and who are not taking NSAIDs should be screened.

B. Laboratory Findings

The most sensitive and specific method for identifying Zollinger-Ellison syndrome is demonstration of an increased fasting serum gastrin concentration (greater than 150 pg/mL [150 ng/L]). If possible, levels should be obtained with patients not taking H_2-receptor antagonists for 24 hours or proton pump inhibitors for 6 days; however, withdrawal of the proton pump inhibitor may be accompanied by massive gastric hypersecretion with serious consequences and should be closely monitored. The median gastrin level is 500–700 pg/mL (500–700 ng/L), and 60% of patients have levels less than 1000 pg/mL (1000 ng/L). Hypochlorhydria with increased gastric pH is a much more common cause of hypergastrinemia than is gastrinoma. Therefore, a measurement of gastric pH (and, where available, gastric secretory studies) is performed in patients with fasting hypergastrinemia. Most patients have a basal acid output of over 15 mEq/h. A gastric pH of greater than 3.0 implies hypochlorhydria and excludes gastrinoma. In a patient with a serum gastrin level of greater than 1000 pg/mL (1000 ng/L) and acid hypersecretion, the diagnosis of Zollinger-Ellison syndrome is established. With lower gastrin levels (150–1000 pg/mL [150–1000 ng/L]) and acid secretion, a secretin stimulation test may be performed to distinguish Zollinger-Ellison syndrome from other causes of hypergastrinemia. Intravenous secretin (2 units/kg) produces a rise in serum gastrin of over 200 pg/mL (200 ng/L) within 2–30 minutes in 85% of patients with gastrinoma. An elevated serum calcium suggests hyperparathyroidism and MEN 1 syndrome. In all patients with Zollinger-Ellison syndrome, a serum parathyroid hormone (PTH), prolactin, luteinizing hormone-follicle-stimulating hormone (LH-FSH), and growth hormone (GH) level should be obtained to exclude MEN 1.

C. Imaging

Imaging studies are obtained in an attempt to determine whether there is metastatic disease and, if not, to identify the site of the primary tumor. CT and MRI scans are commonly obtained first to look for large hepatic metastases and primary lesions, but they have low sensitivity for small lesions. Gastrinomas express somatostatin receptors that bind radiolabeled octreotide. Somatostatin receptor scintigraphy (SRS) with single photon emission computed tomography (SPECT) allows total body imaging for detection of primary gastrinomas in the pancreas and lymph nodes, primary gastrinomas in unusual locations, and metastatic gastrinomas (liver and bone). The 80% sensitivity for tumor detection of SRS exceeds all other imaging studies combined. If SRS is positive for tumor localization, further imaging studies are not necessary. In patients with negative SRS, endoscopic ultrasonography (EUS) may be useful to detect small gastrinomas in the duodenal wall, pancreas, or peripancreatic lymph nodes. With a combination of SRS and EUS, more than 90% of primary gastrinomas can be localized preoperatively.

▶ Differential Diagnosis

Gastrinomas are one of several gut neuroendocrine tumors that have similar histopathologic features and arise either from the gut or pancreas. These include carcinoid, insulinoma, VIPoma, glucagonoma, and somatostatinoma. These tumors usually are differentiated by the gut peptides that they secrete; however, poorly differentiated neuroendocrine tumors may not secrete any hormones. Patients may present with symptoms caused by tumor metastases (jaundice, hepatomegaly) rather than functional symptoms. Once a diagnosis of a neuroendocrine tumor is established from the liver biopsy, the specific type of tumor can subsequently be determined. Both carcinoid and gastrinoma tumors may be detected incidentally during endoscopy after biopsy of a submucosal nodule and must be distinguished by subsequent studies.

Hypergastrinemia due to gastrinoma must be distinguished from other causes of hypergastrinemia. Atrophic gastritis with decreased acid secretion is detected by gastric secretory analysis. Other conditions associated with hypergastrinemia (eg, gastric outlet obstruction, vagotomy, chronic kidney disease) are associated with a negative secretin stimulation test.

▶ Treatment

A. Metastatic Disease

The most important predictor of survival is the presence of hepatic metastases. In patients with multiple hepatic metastases, initial therapy should be directed at controlling hypersecretion. Oral proton pump inhibitors (omeprazole, esomeprazole, rabeprazole, pantoprazole, or lansoprazole)

are given at a dose of 40–120 mg/day, titrated to achieve a basal acid output of less than 10 mEq/h. At this level, there is complete symptomatic relief and ulcer healing. Owing to the slow growth of these tumors, 30% of patients with hepatic metastases have a survival of 10 years.

B. Localized Disease

Cure can be achieved only if the gastrinoma can be resected before hepatic metastatic spread has occurred. Lymph node metastases do not adversely affect prognosis. Laparotomy should be considered in all patients in whom preoperative studies fail to demonstrate hepatic or other distant metastases. A combination of preoperative studies, duodenotomy with careful duodenal inspection, and intraoperative palpation and sonography allows successful localization and resection in the majority of cases. The 15-year survival of patients who do not have liver metastases at initial presentation is over 95%. Surgery usually is not recommended in patients with MEN 1 due to the presence of multifocal tumors and long-term survival in the absence of surgery in most patients.

Epelboym I et al. Zollinger-Ellison syndrome: classical considerations and current controversies. Oncologist. 2014 Jan; 19(1):44–50. [PMID: 24319020]

� DISEASES OF THE SMALL INTESTINE

MALABSORPTION

The term "malabsorption" denotes disorders in which there is a disruption of digestion and nutrient absorption. The clinical and laboratory manifestations of malabsorption are summarized in Table 15–11.

1. Celiac Disease

ESSENTIALS OF DIAGNOSIS

▶ *Typical symptoms*: weight loss, chronic diarrhea, abdominal distention, growth retardation.

▶ *Atypical symptoms*: dermatitis herpetiformis, iron deficiency anemia, osteoporosis.

▶ Abnormal serologic test results.

▶ Abnormal small bowel biopsy.

▶ Clinical improvement on gluten-free diet.

▶ General Considerations

Celiac disease (also called sprue, celiac sprue, and gluten enteropathy) is a permanent dietary disorder caused by an immunologic response to gluten, a storage protein found in certain grains, that results in diffuse damage to the proximal small intestinal mucosa with malabsorption of nutrients. Although symptoms may manifest between 6 months and 24 months of age after the introduction of weaning

Table 15–11. Clinical manifestations and laboratory findings in malabsorption of various nutrients.

Manifestations	Laboratory Findings	Malabsorbed Nutrients
Steatorrhea (bulky, light-colored stools)	Increased fecal fat; decreased serum cholesterol; decreased serum carotene, vitamin A, vitamin D	Triglycerides, fatty acids, phospholipids, cholesterol. Fat soluble vitamins: A, D, E, K
Diarrhea (increased fecal water)	Increased stool volume and weight; increased fecal fat; increased stool osmolality gap	Fats, carbohydrates
Weight loss; muscle wasting	Increased fecal fat; decreased carbohydrate (D-xylose) absorption	Fat, protein, carbohydrates
Microcytic anemia	Low serum iron	Iron
Macrocytic anemia	Decreased serum vitamin B_{12} or red blood cell folate	Vitamin B_{12} or folic acid
Paresthesia; tetany; positive Trousseau and Chvostek signs	Decreased serum calcium or magnesium	Calcium, vitamin D, magnesium
Bone pain; pathologic fractures; skeletal deformities	Osteopenia on radiograph; osteoporosis (adults); osteomalacia (children)	Calcium, vitamin D
Bleeding tendency (ecchymoses, epistaxis)	Prolonged prothrombin time or INR	Vitamin K
Edema	Decreased serum total protein and albumin; increased fecal loss of alpha-1-antitrypsin	Protein
Milk intolerance (cramps, bloating, diarrhea)	Abnormal lactose tolerance test	Lactose

INR, international normalized ratio.

foods, the majority of cases present in childhood or adulthood. Population screening with serologic tests suggests that the disease is present in 1:100 whites of Northern European ancestry, in whom a clinical diagnosis of celiac disease is made in only 10%, suggesting that most cases are undiagnosed or asymptomatic. Celiac disease only develops in people with the HLA-DQ2 (95%) or -DQ8 (5%) class II molecules, which are present in 40% of the population. Although the precise pathogenesis is unclear, celiac disease arises in a small subset of genetically susceptible (-DQ2 or -DQ8) individuals when dietary gluten stimulates an inappropriate immunologic response.

▶ Clinical Findings

The most important step in diagnosing celiac disease is to consider the diagnosis. Symptoms are present for more than 10 years in most adults before the correct diagnosis is established. Because of its protean manifestations, celiac disease is grossly underdiagnosed in the adult population.

A. Symptoms and Signs

The gastrointestinal symptoms and signs of celiac disease depend on the length of small intestine involved and the patient's age when the disease presents. "Classic" symptoms of malabsorption, including diarrhea, steatorrhea, weight loss, abdominal distention, weakness, muscle wasting, or growth retardation, more commonly present in infants (younger than 2 years). Older children and adults are less likely to manifest signs of serious malabsorption. They may report chronic diarrhea, dyspepsia, or flatulence due to colonic bacterial digestion of malabsorbed nutrients, but

the severity of weight loss is variable. Many adults have minimal or no gastrointestinal symptoms but present with extraintestinal "atypical" manifestations, including fatigue, depression, iron deficiency anemia, osteoporosis, short stature, delayed puberty, amenorrhea, or reduced fertility. Approximately 40% of patients with positive serologic tests consistent with disease have no symptoms of disease; the natural history of these patients with "silent" disease is unclear.

Physical examination may be normal in mild cases or may reveal signs of malabsorption such as loss of muscle mass or subcutaneous fat, pallor due to anemia, easy bruising due to vitamin K deficiency, hyperkeratosis due to vitamin A deficiency, bone pain due to osteomalacia, or neurologic signs (peripheral neuropathy, ataxia) due to vitamin B_{12} or vitamin E deficiency (Table 15–11). Abdominal examination may reveal distention with hyperactive bowel sounds.

Dermatitis herpetiformis is regarded as a cutaneous variant of celiac disease. It is a characteristic skin rash consisting of pruritic papulovesicles over the extensor surfaces of the extremities and over the trunk, scalp, and neck. Dermatitis herpetiformis occurs in less than 10% of patients with celiac disease; however, almost all patients who present with dermatitis herpetiformis have evidence of celiac disease on intestinal mucosal biopsy, though it may not be clinically evident.

B. Laboratory Findings

1. Routine laboratory tests—Depending on the severity of illness and the extent of intestinal involvement, nonspecific laboratory abnormalities may be present that may raise the suspicion of malabsorption and celiac disease (Table 15–11). Limited proximal involvement may result only in microcytic anemia due to iron deficiency. Up to 5% of adults with iron deficiency not due to gastrointestinal blood loss have undiagnosed celiac disease. More extensive involvement results in a megaloblastic anemia due to folate or vitamin B$_{12}$ deficiency. Low serum calcium or elevated alkaline phosphatase may reflect impaired calcium or vitamin D absorption with osteomalacia or osteoporosis. Dual-energy x-ray densitometry scanning is recommended for all patients with sprue to screen for osteoporosis. Elevations of prothrombin time, or decreased vitamin A or D levels reflect impaired fat-soluble vitamin absorption. A low serum albumin may reflect small intestine protein loss or poor nutrition. Other deficiencies may include zinc and vitamin B$_6$. Mild elevations of aminotransferases are found in up to 40%.

2. Serologic tests—Serologic tests should be performed in all patients in whom there is a suspicion of celiac disease. The recommended test is the IgA tissue transglutaminase (IgA tTG) antibody, which has a 95% sensitivity and 95% specificity for the diagnosis of celiac disease. Antigliadin antibodies are not recommended because of their lower sensitivity and specificity. IgA antiendomysial antibodies are no longer recommended due to the lack of standardization among laboratories. An IgA level should be obtained in patients with a negative IgA tTG antibody when celiac disease is strongly suspected because up to 3% of patients with celiac disease have IgA deficiency. A test that measures IgG antibodies to deamidated gliadin peptides (anti-DGP) has excellent sensitivity and specificity and is useful in patients with IgA deficiency and young children. Levels of all antibodies become undetectable after 3–12 months of dietary gluten withdrawal and may be used to monitor dietary compliance, especially in patients whose symptoms fail to resolve after institution of a gluten-free diet.

C. Mucosal Biopsy

Endoscopic mucosal biopsy of the proximal duodenum (bulb) and distal duodenum is the standard method for confirmation of the diagnosis in patients with a positive serologic test for celiac disease. Mucosal biopsy should also be pursued in patients with negative serologies when symptoms and laboratory studies are strongly suggestive of celiac disease. At endoscopy, atrophy or scalloping of the duodenal folds may be observed. Histology reveals abnormalities ranging from intraepithelial lymphocytosis alone to extensive infiltration of the lamina propria with lymphocytes and plasma cells with hypertrophy of the intestinal crypts and blunting or complete loss of intestinal villi. An adequate normal biopsy excludes the diagnosis. Partial or complete reversion of these abnormalities occurs within 3–24 months after a patient is placed on a gluten-free diet, but symptom resolution remains incomplete in 30% of patients. If a patient with a compatible biopsy demonstrates prompt clinical improvement on a gluten-free diet and a decrease in serologic markers, a repeat biopsy is unnecessary.

Differential Diagnosis

Many patients with chronic diarrhea or flatulence are erroneously diagnosed as having irritable bowel syndrome. Celiac sprue must be distinguished from other causes of malabsorption, as outlined above. Severe panmalabsorption of multiple nutrients is almost always caused by mucosal disease. The histologic appearance of celiac sprue may resemble other mucosal diseases such as tropical sprue, bacterial overgrowth, cow's milk intolerance, viral gastroenteritis, eosinophilic gastroenteritis, and mucosal damage caused by acid hypersecretion associated with gastrinoma. Documentation of clinical response to gluten withdrawal therefore is essential to the diagnosis.

Some patients complain of symptoms after gluten ingestion but do not have serologic or histologic evidence of celiac disease. The frequency and cause of this entity is debated. A large 2013 study found that symptoms improved in gluten-sensitive patients when placed on a FODMAP-restricted diet and worsened to similar degrees when challenged in a double-blind crossover trial with gluten or whey proteins. These data suggest that nonceliac gluten sensitivity may not be a true entity and that the symptom improvement reported by patients with gluten restriction may be due to broader FODMAP elimination.

Treatment

Removal of all gluten from the diet is essential to therapy—all wheat, rye, and barley must be eliminated. Although oats appear to be safe for many patients, commercial products may be contaminated with wheat or barley during processing. Because of the pervasive use of gluten products in manufactured foods and additives, in medications, and by restaurants, it is imperative that patients and their families confer with a knowledgeable dietitian to comply satisfactorily with this lifelong diet. Several excellent dietary guides and patient support groups are available. Most patients with celiac disease also have lactose intolerance either temporarily or permanently and should avoid dairy products until the intestinal symptoms have improved on the gluten-free diet. Dietary supplements (folate, iron, zinc, calcium, and vitamins A, B$_6$, B$_{12}$, D, and E) should be provided in the initial stages of therapy but usually are not required long-term with a gluten-free diet. Patients with confirmed osteoporosis may require long-term calcium, vitamin D, and bisphosphonate therapy.

Improvement in symptoms should be evident within a few weeks on the gluten-free diet. The most common reason for treatment failure is incomplete removal of gluten. Intentional or unintentional rechallenge with gluten may trigger acute severe diarrhea with dehydration, electrolyte imbalance, and may require TPN and intravenous or oral corticosteroids (prednisone 40 mg or budesonide 9 mg) for 2 or more weeks as a gluten-free diet is re-initiated.

Prognosis & Complications

If appropriately diagnosed and treated, patients with celiac disease have an excellent prognosis. Celiac disease may be associated with other autoimmune disorders, including

Addison disease, Graves disease, type 1 diabetes mellitus, myasthenia gravis, scleroderma, Sjögren syndrome, atrophic gastritis, and pancreatic insufficiency. In some patients, celiac disease may evolve and become refractory to the gluten-free diet. The most common cause is intentional or unintentional dietary noncompliance, which may be suggested by positive serologic tests. Celiac disease that is truly refractory to gluten withdrawal occurs in less than 5% and generally carries a poor prognosis. There are two types of refractory disease, which are distinguished by their intraepithelial lymphocyte phenotype. This diagnosis should be considered in patients previously responsive to the gluten-free diet in whom new weight loss, abdominal pain, and malabsorption develop.

Biesiekierski JR et al. No effects of gluten in patients with self-reported non-celiac gluten sensitivity after dietary reduction of fermentable, poorly absorbed, short-chain carbohydrates. Gastroenterology. 2013 Aug;145(2):320–8. [PMID: 23648697]
Celiac Disease Foundation, 13251 Ventura Blvd, Suite #1, Studio City, CA 91604-1838. http://www.celiac.org
Fasano A et al. Nonceliac gluten sensitivity. Gastroenterology. 2015 May;148(6):1195–204. [PMID: 25583468]
Kelly CP et al. Advances in diagnosis and management of celiac disease. Gastroenterology. 2015 May;148(6):1175–86. [PMID: 25662623]

2. Whipple Disease

ESSENTIALS OF DIAGNOSIS

▸ Multisystem disease.

▸ Fever, lymphadenopathy, arthralgias.

▸ Weight loss, malabsorption, chronic diarrhea.

▸ Duodenal biopsy with periodic acid-Schiff (PAS)-positive macrophages with characteristic bacillus.

▸ General Considerations

Whipple disease is a rare multisystem illness caused by infection with the bacillus *Tropheryma whipplei*. It may occur at any age but most commonly affects white men in the fourth to sixth decades. The source of infection is unknown, but no cases of human-to-human spread have been documented.

▸ Clinical Findings

A. Symptoms and Signs

The clinical manifestations are protean; however, the most common are arthralgias, diarrhea, abdominal pain, and weight loss. Arthralgias or a migratory, nondeforming arthritis occurs in 80% and is typically the first symptom experienced. Gastrointestinal symptoms occur in approximately 75% of cases. They include abdominal pain, diarrhea, and some degree of malabsorption with distention, flatulence, and steatorrhea. Weight loss is the most common presenting symptom—seen in almost all patients. Loss of protein due to intestinal or lymphatic involvement

may result in protein-losing enteropathy with hypoalbuminemia and edema. In the absence of gastrointestinal symptoms, the diagnosis often is delayed for several years. Intermittent low-grade fever occurs in over 50% of cases.

Physical examination may reveal hypotension (a late finding), low-grade fever, and evidence of malabsorption (see Table 15–11). Lymphadenopathy is present in 50%. Heart murmurs due to valvular involvement may be evident. Peripheral joints may be enlarged or warm, and peripheral edema may be present. Neurologic findings are cited above. Hyperpigmentation on sun-exposed areas is evident in up to 40%.

B. Laboratory Findings

If significant malabsorption is present, patients may have laboratory abnormalities as outlined in Table 15–11. There may be steatorrhea.

C. Histologic Evaluation

The diagnosis of Whipple disease is established in 90% of cases by endoscopic biopsy of the duodenum with histologic evaluation, which demonstrates infiltration of the lamina propria with PAS-positive macrophages that contain gram-positive bacilli (which are not acid-fast) and dilation of the lacteals. The remainder of cases are diagnosed by *T whipplei*–specific polymerase chain reaction (PCR) or immunohistochemistry of duodenal biopsies or extraintestinal fluids (cerebrospinal, synovial) or tissue (lymph nodes, synovium, endocardium). The sensitivity of PCR is 97% and the specificity 100%. Because asymptomatic central nervous system infection occurs in 40% of patients, examination of the cerebrospinal fluid by PCR for *T whipplei* should be performed routinely.

▸ Differential Diagnosis

Whipple disease should be considered in patients who present with signs of malabsorption, fever of unknown origin, lymphadenopathy, seronegative arthritis, culture-negative endocarditis, or multisystem disease. Small bowel biopsy readily distinguishes Whipple disease from other mucosal malabsorptive disorders, such as celiac sprue.

▸ Treatment

Antibiotic therapy results in a dramatic clinical improvement within several weeks, even in some patients with neurologic involvement. The optimal regimen is unknown. Complete clinical response usually is evident within 1–3 months; however, relapse may occur in up to one-third of patients after discontinuation of treatment. Therefore, prolonged treatment for at least 1 year is required. Drugs that cross the blood-brain barrier are preferred. A randomized controlled trial in 40 patients with 3–10 years' follow-up demonstrated 100% remission with either ceftriaxone 1 g intravenously twice daily or meropenem 1 g intravenously three times daily for 2 weeks, followed by trimethoprim-sulfamethoxazole 160/800 mg twice daily for 12 months. After treatment, repeat duodenal biopsies for histologic analysis and cerebrospinal fluid PCR should be obtained every 6 months for at least 1 year. The absence of PAS-positive material predicts a low likelihood of clinical relapse.

▶ Prognosis

If untreated, the disease is fatal. Because some neurologic signs may be permanent, the goal of treatment is to prevent this progression. Patients must be followed closely after treatment for signs of symptom recurrence.

Günther U et al. Gastrointestinal diagnosis of classical Whipple disease: clinical, endoscopic, and histopathologic features in 191 patients. Medicine (Baltimore). 2015 Apr;94(15):e714. [PMID: 25881849]

Puéchal X. Whipple's disease. Postgrad Med J. 2013 Nov; 89(1057):659–65. [PMID: 24129033]

Schwartzman S et al. Whipple's disease. Rheum Dis Clin North Am. 2013 May;39(2):313–21. [PMID: 23597966]

3. Bacterial Overgrowth

ESSENTIALS OF DIAGNOSIS

▶ Symptoms of distention, flatulence, diarrhea, and weight loss.

▶ Increased qualitative or quantitative fecal fat.

▶ Advanced cases associated with deficiencies of iron or vitamins A, D, and B_{12}.

▶ Diagnosis suggested by breath tests using glucose, lactulose, or ^{14}C-xylose as substrates.

▶ Diagnosis confirmed by jejunal aspiration with quantitative bacterial cultures.

▶ General Considerations

The small intestine normally contains a small number of bacteria. Bacterial overgrowth in the small intestine of whatever cause may result in malabsorption via a number of mechanisms. Bacterial deconjugation of bile salts may lead to inadequate micelle formation, resulting in decreased fat absorption with steatorrhea and malabsorption of fat-soluble vitamins (A, D). Microbial uptake of specific nutrients reduces absorption of vitamin B_{12} and carbohydrates. Bacterial proliferation also causes direct damage to intestinal epithelial cells and the brush border, further impairing absorption of proteins, carbohydrates, and minerals. Passage of the malabsorbed bile acids and carbohydrates into the colon leads to an osmotic and secretory diarrhea and increased flatulence.

Causes of bacterial overgrowth include: (1) gastric achlorhydria (including proton pump inhibitor therapy); (2) anatomic abnormalities of the small intestine with stagnation (afferent limb of Billroth II gastrojejunostomy, resection of ileocecal valve, small intestine diverticula, obstruction, blind loop); (3) small intestine motility disorders (vagotomy, scleroderma, diabetic enteropathy, chronic intestinal pseudo-obstruction); (4) gastrocolic or coloenteric fistula

(Crohn disease, malignancy, surgical resection); and (5) miscellaneous disorders. Bacterial overgrowth is an important cause of malabsorption in the elderly, perhaps because of decreased gastric acidity or impaired intestinal motility. It may also be present in a subset of patients with irritable bowel syndrome.

▶ Clinical Findings

Many patients with bacterial overgrowth are asymptomatic. Symptoms are nonspecific and include flatulence, weight loss, abdominal pain, diarrhea, and sometimes steatorrhea. Severe cases may result in clinically significant vitamin and mineral deficiencies, including fat-soluble vitamins A or D, vitamin B_{12}, and iron (Table 15–11). Qualitative or quantitative fecal fat assessment typically is abnormal. Bacterial overgrowth should be considered in any patient with diarrhea, flatulence, weight loss, or macrocytic anemia, especially if the patient has a predisposing cause (such as prior gastrointestinal surgery). A stool collection should be obtained to corroborate the presence of steatorrhea. Vitamins A, D, B_{12}, and serum iron should be measured. A specific diagnosis can be established firmly only by an aspirate and culture of proximal jejunal secretion that demonstrates over 10^5 organisms/mL. However, this is an invasive and laborious test that requires careful collection and culturing techniques and therefore is not available in many clinical settings. Noninvasive breath tests are easier to perform and have a sensitivity of 60–90% and a specificity of 85% compared with jejunal cultures. Breath hydrogen and methane tests with glucose or lactulose as substrates are commonly done because of their ease of use. A small bowel study (CT or MR enterography, barium radiography) may be obtained to look for mechanical factors predisposing to intestinal stasis.

Owing to the lack of an optimal test for bacterial overgrowth, many clinicians use an empiric antibiotic trial as a diagnostic and therapeutic maneuver in patients with predisposing conditions for bacterial overgrowth in whom unexplained diarrhea or steatorrhea develops.

▶ Treatment

Where possible, the anatomic defect that has potentiated bacterial overgrowth should be corrected. Otherwise, treatment as follows for 1–2 weeks with oral broad-spectrum antibiotics effective against enteric aerobes and anaerobes usually leads to dramatic improvement: twice-daily ciprofloxacin 500 mg, norfloxacin 400 mg, or amoxicillin clavulanate 875 mg, or a combination of metronidazole 250 mg three times daily plus either trimethoprim-sulfamethoxazole (one double-strength tablet) twice daily or cephalexin 250 mg four times daily. Rifaximin 400 mg three times daily is a nonabsorbable antibiotic that also appears to be effective but has fewer side effects than the other systemically absorbed antibiotics.

In patients in whom symptoms recur off antibiotics, cyclic therapy (eg, 1 week out of 4) may be sufficient. Continuous antibiotics should be avoided, if possible, to avoid development of bacterial antibiotic resistance.

Grace E et al. Review article: small intestinal bacterial over-growth—prevalence, clinical features, current and developing diagnostic tests, and treatment. Aliment Pharmacol Ther. 2013 Oct;38(7):674–88. [PMID: 23957651]

Saad RJ et al. Breath testing for small intestinal bacterial over-growth: maximizing test accuracy. Clin Gastroenterol Hepatol. 2014 Dec;12(12):1964–72. [PMID: 24095975]

4. Short Bowel Syndrome

Short bowel syndrome is the malabsorptive condition that arises secondary to removal of significant segments of the small intestine. The most common causes in adults are Crohn disease, mesenteric infarction, radiation enteritis, volvulus, tumor resection, and trauma. The type and degree of malabsorption depend on the length and site of the resection and the degree of adaptation of the remaining bowel.

▶ Terminal Ileal Resection

Resection of the terminal ileum results in malabsorption of bile salts and vitamin B_{12}, which are normally absorbed in this region. Patients with low serum vitamin B_{12} levels or resection of over 50 cm of ileum require monthly subcutaneous or intramuscular vitamin B_{12} injections. In patients with less than 100 cm of ileal resection, bile salt malabsorption stimulates fluid secretion from the colon, resulting in watery diarrhea. This may be treated with bile salt-binding resins (colestipol or cholestyramine, 2–4 g orally three times daily with meals or colesevelam, 625 mg, 1–3 tablets twice daily). Resection of over 100 cm of ileum leads to a reduction in the bile salt pool that results in steatorrhea and malabsorption of fat-soluble vitamins. Treatment is with a low-fat diet and vitamins supplemented with medium-chain triglycerides, which do not require micellar solubilization. Unabsorbed fatty acids bind with calcium, reducing its absorption and enhancing the absorption of oxalate. Oxalate kidney stones may develop. Calcium supplements should be administered to bind oxalate and increase serum calcium. Cholesterol gallstones due to decreased bile salts are common also. In patients with resection of the ileocolonic valve, bacterial overgrowth may occur in the small intestine, further complicating malabsorption (as outlined above).

▶ Extensive Small Bowel Resection

Resection of up to 40–50% of the total length of small intestine usually is well tolerated. A more massive resection may result in "short-bowel syndrome," characterized by weight loss and diarrhea due to nutrient, water, and electrolyte malabsorption. If the colon is preserved, 100 cm of proximal jejunum may be sufficient to maintain adequate oral nutrition with a low-fat, high complex-carbohydrate diet, though fluid and electrolyte losses may still be significant. In patients in whom the colon has been removed, at least 200 cm of proximal jejunum is typically required to maintain oral nutrition. Antidiarrheal agents (loperamide, 2–4 mg orally three times daily) slow transit and reduce

diarrheal volume. Octreotide reduces intestinal transit time and fluid and electrolyte secretion. Gastric hypersecretion initially complicates intestinal resection and should be treated with proton pump inhibitors.

Patients with less than 100–200 cm of proximal jejunum remaining almost always require parenteral nutrition. Teduglutide is a glucagon-like peptide-2 analogue that stimulates small bowel growth and absorption and is FDA approved for the treatment of short-bowel syndrome. In clinical trials, it resulted in a reduced need for parenteral nutrition. Small intestine transplantation has reported 5-year graft survival rates of 40%. Currently, it is performed chiefly in patients in whom serious problems develop due to parenteral nutrition.

Jeppesen PB et al. Teduglutide reduces need for parenteral support among patients with short bowel syndrome with intestinal failure. Gastroenterology. 2012 Dec;143(6):1473–1481.e3. [PMID: 22982184]

Wall EA. An overview of short bowel syndrome management: adherence, adaptation, and practical recommendations. J Acad Nutr Diet. 2013 Sep;113(9):1200–8. [PMID: 23830324]

5. Lactase Deficiency

ESSENTIALS OF DIAGNOSIS

- ▶ Diarrhea, bloating, flatulence, and abdominal pain after ingestion of milk-containing products.
- ▶ Diagnosis supported by symptomatic improvement on lactose-free diet.
- ▶ Diagnosis confirmed by hydrogen breath test.

▶ General Considerations

Lactase is a brush border enzyme that hydrolyzes the disaccharide lactose into glucose and galactose. The concentration of lactase enzyme levels is high at birth but declines steadily in most people of non-European ancestry during childhood and adolescence and into adulthood. As many as 90% of Asian Americans, 70% of African Americans, 95% of Native Americans, 50% of Mexican Americans, and 60% of Jewish Americans are lactose intolerant compared with less than 25% of white adults. Lactase deficiency may also arise secondary to other gastrointestinal disorders that affect the proximal small intestinal mucosa. These include Crohn disease, celiac disease, viral gastroenteritis, giardiasis, short bowel syndrome, and malnutrition. Malabsorbed lactose is fermented by intestinal bacteria, producing gas and organic acids. The nonmetabolized lactose and organic acids result in an increased stool osmotic load with an obligatory fluid loss.

▶ Clinical Findings

A. Symptoms and Signs

Patients have great variability in clinical symptoms, depending both on the severity of lactase deficiency and the amount of lactose ingested. Because of the nonspecific nature of these symptoms, there is a tendency for both lactose-intolerant and lactose-tolerant individuals to mistakenly attribute a variety of abdominal symptoms to lactose intolerance. Most patients with lactose intolerance can drink one or two 8 oz glasses of milk daily without symptoms if taken with food at wide intervals, though rare patients have almost complete intolerance. With mild to moderate amounts of lactose malabsorption, patients may experience bloating, abdominal cramps, and flatulence. With higher lactose ingestions, an osmotic diarrhea will result. Isolated lactase deficiency does not result in other signs of malabsorption or weight loss. If these findings are present, other gastrointestinal disorders should be pursued. Diarrheal specimens reveal an increased osmotic gap and a pH of less than 6.0.

B. Laboratory Findings

The most widely available test for the diagnosis of lactase deficiency is the hydrogen breath test. After ingestion of 50 g of lactose, a rise in breath hydrogen of more than 20 ppm within 90 minutes is a positive test, indicative of bacterial carbohydrate metabolism. In clinical practice, many clinicians prescribe an empiric trial of a lactose-free diet for 2 weeks. Resolution of symptoms (bloating, flatulence, diarrhea) is suggestive of lactase deficiency (though a placebo response cannot be excluded) and may be confirmed, if necessary, with a breath hydrogen study.

▶ Differential Diagnosis

The symptoms of late-onset lactose intolerance are nonspecific and may mimic a number of gastrointestinal disorders, such as inflammatory bowel disease, mucosal malabsorptive disorders, irritable bowel syndrome, and pancreatic insufficiency. Furthermore, lactase deficiency frequently develops secondary to other gastrointestinal disorders (as listed above). Concomitant lactase deficiency should always be considered in these gastrointestinal disorders.

▶ Treatment

The goal of treatment in patients with isolated lactase deficiency is achieving patient comfort. Patients usually find their "threshold" of intake at which symptoms will occur. Foods that are high in lactose include milk (12 g/cup), ice cream (9 g/cup), and cottage cheese (8 g/cup). Aged cheeses have a lower lactose content (0.5 g/oz). Unpasteurized yogurt contains bacteria that produce lactase and is generally well tolerated.

By spreading dairy product intake throughout the day in quantities of less than 12 g of lactose (one cup of milk), most patients can take dairy products without symptoms and do not require lactase supplements. Most food markets provide milk that has been pretreated with lactase, rendering it 70–100% lactose free. Lactase enzyme replacement is commercially available as nonprescription formulations (Lactaid, Lactrase, Dairy Ease). Caplets or drops of lactase

may be taken with milk products, improving lactose absorption and eliminating symptoms. The number of caplets ingested depends on the degree of lactose intolerance. Patients who choose to restrict or eliminate milk products may have increased risk of osteoporosis. Calcium supplementation (calcium carbonate 500 mg orally two to three times daily) is recommended for susceptible patients.

Carter SL et al. The diagnosis and management of patients with lactose intolerance. Nurse Pract. 2013 Jul 10;38(7):23–8. [PMID: 23778177]

Suchy FJ et al. National Institutes of Health Consensus Development Conference: lactose intolerance and health. Ann Intern Med. 2010 Jun 15;152(12):792–6. [PMID: 20404261]

INTESTINAL MOTILITY DISORDERS

1. Acute Paralytic Ileus

ESSENTIALS OF DIAGNOSIS

▶ Precipitating factors: surgery, peritonitis, electrolyte abnormalities, medications, severe medical illness.

▶ Nausea, vomiting, obstipation, distention.

▶ Minimal abdominal tenderness; decreased bowel sounds.

▶ Plain abdominal radiography with gas and fluid distention in small and large bowel.

▶ General Considerations

Ileus is a condition in which there is neurogenic failure or loss of peristalsis in the intestine in the absence of any mechanical obstruction. It is commonly seen in hospitalized patients as a result of: (1) intra-abdominal processes such as recent gastrointestinal or abdominal surgery or peritoneal irritation (peritonitis, pancreatitis, ruptured viscus, hemorrhage); (2) severe medical illness such as pneumonia, respiratory failure requiring intubation, sepsis or severe infections, uremia, diabetic ketoacidosis, and electrolyte abnormalities (hypokalemia, hypercalcemia, hypomagnesemia, hypophosphatemia); and (3) medications that affect intestinal motility (opioids, anticholinergics, phenothiazines). Following surgery, small intestinal motility usually normalizes first (often within hours), followed by the stomach (24–48 hours), and the colon (48–72 hours). Postoperative ileus is reduced by the use of patient-controlled or epidural analgesia and avoidance of intravenous opioids as well as early ambulation, gum chewing, and initiation of a clear liquid diet.

▶ Clinical Findings

A. Symptoms and Signs

Patients who are conscious report mild diffuse, continuous abdominal discomfort with nausea and vomiting.

Generalized abdominal distention is present with minimal abdominal tenderness but no signs of peritoneal irritation (unless due to the primary disease). Bowel sounds are diminished to absent.

B. Laboratory Findings

The laboratory abnormalities are attributable to the underlying condition. Serum electrolytes, including potassium, magnesium, phosphorus, and calcium, should be obtained to exclude abnormalities as contributing factors.

C. Imaging

Plain film radiography of the abdomen demonstrates distended gas-filled loops of the small and large intestine. Air-fluid levels may be seen. Under some circumstances, it may be difficult to distinguish ileus from partial small bowel obstruction. A CT scan may be useful in such instances to exclude mechanical obstruction, especially in postoperative patients.

► Differential Diagnosis

Ileus must be distinguished from mechanical obstruction of the small bowel or proximal colon. Pain from small bowel mechanical obstruction is usually intermittent, cramping, and associated initially with profuse vomiting. Acute gastroenteritis, acute appendicitis, and acute pancreatitis may all present with ileus.

► Treatment

The primary medical or surgical illness that has precipitated adynamic ileus should be treated. Most cases of ileus respond to restriction of oral intake with gradual liberalization of diet as bowel function returns. Severe or prolonged ileus requires nasogastric suction and parenteral administration of fluids and electrolytes. Alvimopan is a peripherally acting mu-opioid receptor antagonist with limited absorption or systemic activity that reverses opioid-induced inhibition of intestinal motility. In five randomized controlled trials, it reduced the time to first flatus, bowel movement, solid meal, and hospital discharge compared with placebo in postoperative patients. Alvimopan, 12 mg orally twice daily (available only through a restricted program for short-term use—no more than 15 doses), may be considered in patients undergoing partial large or small bowel resection when postoperative opioid therapy is anticipated.

Delaney CP et al. Evaluation of clinical outcomes with alvimopan in clinical practice: a national matched-cohort study in patients undergoing bowel resection. Ann Surg. 2012 Apr; 255(4):731–8. [PMID: 22388106]

Doorly MG et al. Pathogenesis and clinical and economic consequences of paralytic ileus. Surg Clin North Am. 2012 Apr; 92(2):259–72. [PMID: 22414412]

2. Acute Colonic Pseudo-obstruction (Ogilvie Syndrome)

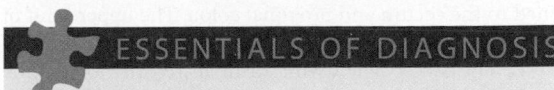

ESSENTIALS OF DIAGNOSIS

► Severe abdominal distention.

► Arises in postoperative state or with severe medical illness.

► May be precipitated by electrolyte imbalances, medications.

► Absent to mild abdominal pain; minimal tenderness.

► Massive dilation of cecum or right colon.

► General Considerations

Spontaneous massive dilation of the cecum and proximal colon may occur in a number of different settings in hospitalized patients. Progressive cecal dilation may lead to spontaneous perforation with dire consequences. The risk of perforation correlates poorly with absolute cecal size and duration of colonic distention. Early detection and management are important to reduce morbidity and mortality. Colonic pseudo-obstruction is most commonly detected in postsurgical patients (mean 3–5 days), after trauma, and in medical patients with respiratory failure, metabolic imbalance, malignancy, myocardial infarction, heart failure, pancreatitis, or a recent neurologic event (stroke, subarachnoid hemorrhage, trauma). Liberal use of opioids or anticholinergic agents may precipitate colonic pseudo-obstruction in susceptible patients. It may also occur as a manifestation of colonic ischemia.

► Clinical Findings

A. Symptoms and Signs

Many patients are on ventilatory support or are unable to report symptoms due to altered mental status. Abdominal distention is frequently noted by the clinician as the first sign, often leading to a plain film radiograph that demonstrates colonic dilation. Some patients are asymptomatic, although most report constant but mild abdominal pain. Nausea and vomiting may be present. Bowel movements may be absent, but up to 40% of patients continue to pass flatus or stool. Abdominal tenderness with some degree of guarding or rebound tenderness may be detected; however, signs of peritonitis are absent unless perforation has occurred. Bowel sounds may be normal or decreased.

B. Laboratory Findings

Laboratory findings reflect the underlying medical or surgical problems. Serum sodium, potassium, magnesium, phosphorus, and calcium should be obtained to exclude abnormalities as contributing factors. Significant fever or leukocytosis raises concern for colonic ischemia or perforation.

C. Imaging

Radiographs demonstrate colonic dilation, usually confined to the cecum and proximal colon. The upper limit of normal for cecal size is 9 cm. A cecal diameter greater than 10–12 cm is associated with an increased risk of colonic perforation. Varying amounts of small intestinal dilation and air-fluid levels due to adynamic ileus may be seen. Because the dilated appearance of the colon may raise concern that there is a distal colonic mechanical obstruction due to malignancy, volvulus, or fecal impaction, a CT scan or water-soluble (diatrizoate meglumine) enema may sometimes be performed.

► Differential Diagnosis

Colonic pseudo-obstruction should be distinguished from distal colonic mechanical obstruction (as above) and toxic megacolon, which is acute dilation of the colon due to inflammation (inflammatory bowel disease) or infection (*C difficile*–associated colitis, CMV). Patients with toxic megacolon manifest fever; dehydration; significant abdominal pain; leukocytosis; and diarrhea, which is often bloody.

► Treatment

Conservative treatment is the appropriate first step for patients with no or minimal abdominal tenderness, no fever, no leukocytosis, and a cecal diameter smaller than 12 cm. The underlying illness is treated appropriately. A nasogastric tube and a rectal tube should be placed. Patients should be ambulated or periodically rolled from side to side and to the knee-chest position in an effort to promote expulsion of colonic gas. All drugs that reduce intestinal motility, such as opioids, anticholinergics, and calcium channel blockers, should be discontinued if possible. Enemas may be administered judiciously if large amounts of stool are evident on radiography. Oral laxatives are not helpful and may cause perforation, pain, or electrolyte abnormalities.

Conservative treatment is successful in over 80% of cases within 1–2 days. Patients must be watched for signs of worsening distention or abdominal tenderness. Cecal size should be assessed by abdominal radiographs every 12 hours. Intervention should be considered in patients with any of the following: (1) no improvement or clinical deterioration after 24–48 hours of conservative therapy; (2) cecal dilation greater than 10 cm for a prolonged period (more than 3–4 days); (3) patients with cecal dilation greater than 12 cm. Neostigmine injection should be given unless contraindicated. A single dose (2 mg intravenously) results in rapid (within 30 minutes) colonic decompression in 75–90% of patients. Cardiac monitoring during neostigmine infusion is indicated for possible bradycardia that may require atropine administration. Colonoscopic decompression is indicated in patients who fail to respond to neostigmine. Colonic decompression with aspiration of air or placement of a decompression tube is successful in 70% of patients. However, the procedure is technically difficult in an unprepared bowel and has been associated with perforations in the distended colon. Dilation recurs in up to 50% of patients. In patients in whom colonoscopy is unsuccessful, a tube cecostomy can be created through a small laparotomy or with percutaneous radiologically guided placement.

► Prognosis

In most cases, the prognosis is related to the underlying illness. The risk of perforation or ischemia is increased with cecal diameter more than 12 cm and when distention has been present for more than 6 days. With aggressive therapy, the development of perforation is unusual.

Elsner JL et al. Intravenous neostigmine for postoperative acute colonic pseudo-obstruction. Ann Pharmacother. 2012 Mar; 46(3):430–5. [PMID: 22388328]

Harrison ME et al; ASGE Standards of Practice Committee. The role of endoscopy in the management of patients with known and suspected colonic obstruction and pseudo-obstruction. Gastrointest Endosc. 2010 Apr;71(4):669–79. [PMID: 20363408]

3. Chronic Intestinal Pseudo-obstruction & Gastroparesis

Gastroparesis and chronic intestinal pseudo-obstruction are chronic conditions characterized by intermittent, waxing and waning symptoms and signs of gastric or intestinal obstruction in the absence of any mechanical lesions to account for the findings. They are caused by a heterogeneous group of endocrine disorders (diabetes mellitus, hypothyroidism, cortisol deficiency), postsurgical conditions (vagotomy, partial gastric resection, fundoplication, gastric bypass, Whipple procedure), neurologic conditions (Parkinson disease, muscular and myotonic dystrophy, autonomic dysfunction, multiple sclerosis, postpolio syndrome, porphyria), rheumatologic syndromes (progressive systemic sclerosis), infections (postviral, Chagas disease), amyloidosis, paraneoplastic syndromes, medications, and eating disorders (anorexia); a cause may not always be identified.

► Clinical Findings

A. Symptoms and Signs

Gastric involvement leads to chronic or intermittent symptoms of gastroparesis with postprandial fullness (early satiety), nausea, and vomiting (1–3 hours after meals). Patients with predominantly small bowel involvement may have abdominal distention, vomiting, diarrhea, and varying degrees of malnutrition. Abdominal pain is not common and should prompt investigation for structural causes of obstruction. Bacterial overgrowth in the stagnant intestine may result in malabsorption. Colonic involvement may result in constipation or alternating diarrhea and constipation.

B. Imaging

Plain film radiography may demonstrate dilation of the esophagus, stomach, small intestine, or colon resembling ileus or mechanical obstruction. Mechanical obstruction of the stomach, small intestine, or colon is much more common than gastroparesis or intestinal pseudo-obstruction and must be excluded with endoscopy or CT or barium enterography, especially in patients with prior surgery, recent onset of symptoms, or abdominal pain. In cases of unclear origin, studies based on the clinical picture are obtained to exclude underlying systemic disease. Gastric scintigraphy with a low-fat solid meal is the optimal means for assessing gastric emptying. Gastric retention of 60% after 2 hours or more than 10% after 4 hours is abnormal. Small bowel manometry is useful for distinguishing visceral from myopathic disorders and for excluding cases of mechanical obstruction that are otherwise difficult to diagnose by endoscopy or radiographic studies.

▶ Treatment

There is no specific therapy for gastroparesis or pseudo-obstruction. Acute exacerbations are treated with nasogastric suction and intravenous fluids. Long-term treatment is directed at maintaining nutrition. Patients should eat small, frequent meals that are low in fiber, milk, gas-forming foods, and fat. Some patients may require liquid enteral supplements. Agents that reduce gastrointestinal motility (opioids, anticholinergics) should be avoided. In diabetic patients, glucose levels should be maintained below 200 mg/dL, as hyperglycemia may slow gastric emptying even in the absence of diabetic neuropathy, and amylin and GLP-1 analogs (exenatide or pramlintide) should be discontinued. Metoclopramide (5–20 mg orally or 5–10 mg intravenously or subcutaneously four times daily) and erythromycin (50–125 mg orally three times daily) before meals are each of benefit in treatment of gastroparesis but not small bowel dysmotility. Since the use of metoclopramide for more than 3 months is associated with a less than 1% risk of tardive dyskinesia, patients are advised to discontinue the medication if neuromuscular side effects, particularly involuntary movements, develop. The elderly are at greatest risk. Gastric electrical stimulation with internally implanted neurostimulators has shown reduction in nausea and vomiting in small studies and one controlled trial in some patients with severe gastroparesis (especially those with diabetes mellitus); however, the mechanism of action is uncertain as improvement is not correlated with changes in gastric emptying. Bacterial overgrowth should be treated with intermittent antibiotics. Patients with predominant small bowel distention may require a venting gastrostomy to relieve distress. Some patients may require placement of a jejunostomy for long-term enteral nutrition. Patients unable to maintain adequate enteral nutrition require TPN or small bowel transplantation. Difficult cases should be referred to centers with expertise in this area.

Bharucha AE et al. Relationship between glycemic control and gastric emptying in poorly controlled type 2 diabetes. Clin Gastroenterol Hepatol. 2015 Mar;13(3):466–476.e1. [PMID: 25041866]

Camilleri M et al. Clinical guideline: management of gastroparesis. Am J Gastroenterol. 2013 Jan;108(1):18–37. [PMID: 23147521]

De Giorgio R et al. Chronic intestinal pseudo-obstruction: clinical features, diagnosis, and therapy. Gastroenterol Clin North Am. 2011 Dec;40(4):787–807. [PMID: 22100118]

APPENDICITIS

ESSENTIALS OF DIAGNOSIS

▶ *Early:* periumbilical pain; *later:* right lower quadrant pain and tenderness.

▶ Anorexia, nausea and vomiting, obstipation.

▶ Tenderness or localized rigidity at McBurney point.

▶ Low-grade fever and leukocytosis.

▶ General Considerations

Appendicitis is the most common abdominal surgical emergency, affecting approximately 10% of the population. It occurs most commonly between the ages of 10 and 30 years. It is initiated by obstruction of the appendix by a fecalith, inflammation, foreign body, or neoplasm. Obstruction leads to increased intraluminal pressure, venous congestion, infection, and thrombosis of intramural vessels. If untreated, gangrene and perforation develop within 36 hours.

▶ Clinical Findings

A. Symptoms and Signs

Appendicitis usually begins with vague, often colicky periumbilical or epigastric pain. Within 12 hours the pain shifts to the right lower quadrant, manifested as a steady ache that is worsened by walking or coughing. Almost all patients have nausea with one or two episodes of vomiting. Protracted vomiting or vomiting that begins before the onset of pain suggests another diagnosis. A sense of constipation is typical, and some patients administer cathartics in an effort to relieve their symptoms—though some report diarrhea. Low-grade fever (below 38°C) is typical; high fever or rigors suggest another diagnosis or appendiceal perforation.

On physical examination, localized tenderness with guarding in the right lower quadrant can be elicited with gentle palpation with one finger. When asked to cough, patients may be able to precisely localize the painful area, a sign of peritoneal irritation. Light percussion may also elicit pain. Although rebound tenderness is also present, it is unnecessary to elicit this finding if the above signs are present. The psoas sign (pain on passive extension of the right hip) and the obturator sign (pain with passive flexion and internal rotation of the right hip) are indicative of adjacent inflammation and strongly suggestive of appendicitis.

B. Atypical Presentations of Appendicitis

Owing to the variable location of the appendix, there are a number of "atypical" presentations. Because the retrocecal appendix does not touch the anterior abdominal wall, the pain remains less intense and poorly localized; abdominal tenderness is minimal and may be elicited in the right flank. The psoas sign may be positive. With pelvic appendicitis, there is pain in the lower abdomen, often on the left, with an urge to urinate or defecate. Abdominal tenderness is absent, but tenderness is evident on pelvic or rectal examination; the obturator sign may be present. In the elderly, the diagnosis of appendicitis is often delayed because patients present with minimal, vague symptoms and mild abdominal tenderness. Appendicitis in pregnancy may present with pain in the right lower quadrant, periumbilical area, or right subcostal area owing to displacement of the appendix by the uterus.

C. Laboratory Findings

Moderate leukocytosis (10,000–20,000/mcL) with neutrophilia is common. Microscopic hematuria and pyuria are present in 25% of patients.

D. Imaging

Both abdominal ultrasound and CT scanning are useful in diagnosing appendicitis as well as excluding other diseases presenting with similar symptoms, including adnexal disease in younger women. However, CT scanning appears to be more accurate (sensitivity 94%, specificity 95%, positive likelihood ratio 13.3, negative likelihood ratio 0.09). Abdominal CT scanning is also useful in cases of suspected appendiceal perforation to diagnose a periappendiceal abscess. In patients in whom there is a clinically high suspicion of appendicitis, some surgeons feel that preoperative diagnostic imaging is unnecessary. However, studies suggest that even in this group, imaging studies suggest an alternative diagnosis in up to 15%.

Differential Diagnosis

Given its frequency and myriad presentations, appendicitis should be considered in the differential diagnosis of all patients with abdominal pain. It is difficult to reliably diagnose the disease in some cases. A several-hour period of close observation with reassessment usually clarifies the diagnosis. Absence of the classic migration of pain (from the epigastrium to the right lower abdomen), right lower quadrant pain, fever, or guarding makes appendicitis less likely. Ten to twenty percent of patients with suspected appendicitis have either a negative examination at laparotomy or an alternative surgical diagnosis. The widespread use of ultrasonography and CT has reduced the number of incorrect diagnoses to less than 2%. Still, in some cases diagnostic laparotomy or laparoscopy is required. The most common causes of diagnostic confusion are gastroenteritis and gynecologic disorders. Viral gastroenteritis presents with nausea, vomiting, low-grade fever, and diarrhea and can be difficult to distinguish from appendicitis. The onset of vomiting before pain makes appendicitis less likely. As a rule, the pain of gastroenteritis is more generalized and the tenderness less well localized. Acute salpingitis or tubo-ovarian abscess should be considered in young, sexually active women with fever and bilateral abdominal

or pelvic tenderness. A twisted ovarian cyst may also cause sudden severe pain. The sudden onset of lower abdominal pain in the middle of the menstrual cycle suggests mittelschmerz. Sudden severe abdominal pain with diffuse pelvic tenderness and shock suggests a ruptured ectopic pregnancy. A positive pregnancy test and pelvic ultrasonography are diagnostic. Retrocecal or retroileal appendicitis (often associated with pyuria or hematuria) may be confused with ureteral colic or pyelonephritis. Other conditions that may resemble appendicitis are diverticulitis, Meckel diverticulitis, carcinoid of the appendix, perforated colonic cancer, Crohn ileitis, perforated peptic ulcer, cholecystitis, and mesenteric adenitis. It is virtually impossible to distinguish appendicitis from Meckel diverticulitis, but both require surgical treatment.

Complications

Perforation occurs in 20% of patients and should be suspected in patients with pain persisting for over 36 hours, high fever, diffuse abdominal tenderness or peritoneal findings, a palpable abdominal mass, or marked leukocytosis. Localized perforation results in a contained abscess, usually in the pelvis. A free perforation leads to suppurative peritonitis with toxicity. Septic thrombophlebitis (pylephlebitis) of the portal venous system is rare and suggested by high fever, chills, bacteremia, and jaundice.

Treatment

The treatment of early, uncomplicated appendicitis is surgical appendectomy in most patients. When possible, a laparoscopic approach is preferred to open laparotomy. Prior to surgery, patients should be given broad-spectrum antibiotics with gram-negative and anaerobic coverage to reduce the incidence of postoperative infections. Recommended preoperative intravenous regimens include cefoxitin or cefotetan 1–2 g every 8 hours; ampicillin-sulbactam 3 g every 6 hours; or ertapenem 1 g as a single dose. Up to 80% of patients with uncomplicated appendicitis treated with antibiotics alone for 7 days have resolution of symptoms and signs. Conservative management may be considered in patients with surgical contraindications or with a strong preference to avoid surgery; however, appendectomy generally still is recommended in most patients to prevent recurrent appendicitis (20–35% within 1 year).

Emergency appendectomy is required in patients with perforated appendicitis with generalized peritonitis. Likewise, the optimal treatment of stable patients with perforated appendicitis and a contained abscess is controversial. Surgery in this setting can be difficult. Many recommend percutaneous CT-guided drainage of the abscess with intravenous fluids and antibiotics to allow the inflammation to subside. An interval appendectomy may be performed after 6 weeks to prevent recurrent appendicitis.

Prognosis

The mortality rate from uncomplicated appendicitis is extremely low. Even with perforated appendicitis, the mortality rate in most groups is only 0.2%, though it approaches 15% in the elderly.

Flum DR. Clinical practice. Acute appendicitis—appendectomy or the "antibiotics first" strategy. N Engl J Med. 2015 May 14; 372(20):1937–43. Erratum in: N Engl J Med. 2015 Jun 4; 372(23):2274. [PMID: 25970051]

Markar SR et al. Systematic review and meta-analysis of single-incision versus conventional multiport appendectomy. Br J Surg. 2013 Dec;100(13):1709–18. [PMID: 24227355]

Salminen P et al. Antibiotic therapy vs appendectomy for treatment of uncomplicated acute appendicitis: the APPAC randomized controlled trial. JAMA. 2015;313(23):2340–8. [PMID: 26080338]

INTESTINAL TUBERCULOSIS

Intestinal tuberculosis is common in underdeveloped countries but rare in the United States except in immigrant groups or in patients with untreated AIDS. It is caused by both *Mycobacterium tuberculosis* and *M bovis*. Active pulmonary disease is present in less than 50% of patients. The most frequent site of involvement is the ileocecal region; however, any region of the gastrointestinal tract may be involved. Patients may be without symptoms or complain of chronic abdominal pain, obstructive symptoms, weight loss, and diarrhea. An abdominal mass may be palpable. Complications include intestinal obstruction, hemorrhage, and fistula formation. The purified protein derivative (PPD) skin test may be negative, especially in patients with weight loss or AIDS. Abdominal CT may show thickening of the cecum and ileocecal valve and massive lymphadenopathy. Colonoscopy may demonstrate an ulcerated mass, multiple ulcers with steep edges and adjacent small sessile polyps, small ulcers or erosions, or small diverticula, most commonly in the ileocecal region. The differential diagnosis includes Crohn disease, carcinoma, and intestinal amebiasis. The diagnosis is established by either endoscopic or surgical biopsy revealing acid-fast bacilli, caseating granuloma, or positive cultures from the organism. Detection of tubercle bacilli in biopsy specimens by PCR is now the most sensitive means of diagnosis.

Treatment with standard antituberculous regimens is effective.

Yu H et al. Clinical, endoscopic and histological differentiations between Crohn's disease and intestinal tuberculosis. Digestion. 2012;85(3):202–9. [PMID: 22354097]

PROTEIN-LOSING ENTEROPATHY

Protein-losing enteropathy comprises a number of conditions that result in excessive loss of serum proteins into the gastrointestinal tract.

Hypoalbuminemia is the sine qua non of protein-losing enteropathy. However, a number of other serum proteins such as alpha-1-antitrypsin also are lost from the gut epithelium. In protein-losing enteropathy caused by lymphatic obstruction, loss of lymphatic fluid commonly results in lymphocytopenia (less than 1000/mcL), hypoglobulinemia, and hypocholesterolemia.

In most cases, protein-losing enteropathy is recognized as a sequela of a known gastrointestinal disorder. In patients in whom the cause is unclear, evaluation is indicated and is guided by the clinical suspicion. Protein-losing enteropathy must be distinguished from other causes of hypoalbuminemia, which include liver disease and nephrotic syndrome, and from heart failure. Protein-losing enteropathy is confirmed by determining the gut alpha-1-antitrypsin clearance (24-hour volume of feces × stool concentration of alpha-1-antitrypsin ÷ serum alpha-1-antitrypsin concentration). A clearance of more than 27 mL/24 h is abnormal.

Laboratory evaluation of protein-losing enteropathy includes serum protein electrophoresis, lymphocyte count, and serum cholesterol to look for evidence of lymphatic obstruction. Serum ANA and C3 levels are useful to screen for autoimmune disorders. Stool samples should be examined for ova and parasites. Evidence of malabsorption is evaluated by means of a stool qualitative fecal fat determination. Intestinal imaging is performed with small bowel enteroscopy biopsy, CT enterography, or wireless capsule endoscopy of the small intestine. Colonic diseases are excluded with colonoscopy. A CT scan of the abdomen is performed to look for evidence of neoplasms or lymphatic obstruction. Rarely, lymphangiography is helpful. In some situations, laparotomy with full-thickness intestinal biopsy is required to establish a diagnosis.

Treatment is directed at the underlying cause.

DISEASES OF THE COLON & RECTUM

(See Chapter 39 for Colorectal Cancer.)

IRRITABLE BOWEL SYNDROME

ESSENTIALS OF DIAGNOSIS

► Chronic functional disorder characterized by abdominal pain or discomfort with alterations in bowel habits.

► Symptoms usually begin in late teens to early twenties.

► Limited evaluation to exclude organic causes of symptoms.

► General Considerations

The functional gastrointestinal disorders are characterized by a variable combination of chronic or recurrent gastrointestinal symptoms *not explicable by the presence of structural or biochemical abnormalities*. Several clinical entities are included under this broad rubric, including chest pain of unclear origin (noncardiac chest pain), functional dyspepsia, and biliary dyskinesia (sphincter of Oddi dysfunction). There is a large overlap among these entities. For example, over 50% of patients with noncardiac chest pain and over one-third with functional dyspepsia also have symptoms compatible with irritable bowel syndrome. In none of these disorders is there a definitive diagnostic study. Rather, the diagnosis is a subjective one based on the presence of a compatible profile and the exclusion of similar disorders.

Irritable bowel syndrome can be defined, therefore, as an idiopathic clinical entity characterized by chronic (more than 6 months) abdominal pain or discomfort that occurs in association with altered bowel habits. These symptoms may be continuous or intermittent. Consensus definition of irritable bowel syndrome is abdominal discomfort or pain that has two of the following three features: (1) relieved with defecation, (2) onset associated with a change in frequency of stool, or (3) onset associated with a change in form (appearance) of stool. Other symptoms supporting the diagnosis include abnormal stool frequency; abnormal stool form (lumpy or hard; loose or watery); abnormal stool passage (straining, urgency, or feeling of incomplete evacuation); passage of mucus; and bloating or a feeling of abdominal distention.

Patients may have other somatic or psychological complaints such as dyspepsia, heartburn, chest pain, headaches, fatigue, myalgias, urologic dysfunction, gynecologic symptoms, anxiety, or depression.

The disorder is a common problem presenting to both gastroenterologists and primary care physicians. Up to 10% of the adult population have symptoms compatible with the diagnosis, but most never seek medical attention. Approximately two-thirds of patients with irritable bowel syndrome are women.

▶ Pathogenesis

A number of pathophysiologic mechanisms have been identified and may have varying importance in different individuals.

A. Abnormal Motility

A variety of abnormal myoelectrical and motor abnormalities have been identified in the colon and small intestine. In some cases, these are temporally correlated with episodes of abdominal pain or emotional stress. Whether they represent a primary motility disorder or are secondary to psychosocial stress is debated. Differences between patients with constipation-predominant and diarrhea-predominant syndromes are reported.

B. Visceral Hypersensitivity

Patients often have a lower visceral pain threshold, reporting abdominal pain at lower volumes of colonic gas insufflation or colonic balloon inflation than controls. Many patients complain of bloating and distention, which may be due to a number of different factors including increased visceral sensitivity, increased gas production (due to small bowel bacterial overgrowth or carbohydrate malabsorption), impaired gas transit through the intestine, or impaired rectal expulsion. Many patients report rectal urgency despite small rectal volumes of stool.

C. Enteric Infection

Symptoms compatible with irritable bowel syndrome develop within 1 year in up to 10% of patients after an episode of bacterial gastroenteritis compared with less than 2% of controls. Women and patients with increased life stressors at the onset of gastroenteritis appear to be at increased risk for developing "postinfectious" irritable bowel syndrome. Increased inflammatory cells have been found in the mucosa, submucosa, and muscularis of some patients with irritable bowel syndrome, but their importance is unclear. Chronic inflammation is postulated by some investigators to contribute to alterations in motility or visceral hypersensitivity.

Some investigators suggest that alterations in the numbers and distribution of bacterial species (estimated 30,000 different species) may affect bowel transit time, gas production, and sensitivity. An increase in breath hydrogen or methane excretion after lactulose ingestion has been reported in 65% of patients with irritable bowel syndrome, believed by some investigators to indicate small intestinal bacterial overgrowth. However, many investigators dispute these findings because overgrowth was confirmed in only 4% of patients using jejunal aspiration and bacterial culture. Small bowel bacterial overgrowth may be more likely in patients with bloating, postprandial discomfort, and loose stools. It is hypothesized that bacterial overgrowth may lead to immune alterations that affect motility or visceral sensitivity or to degradation of carbohydrates in the small intestine that may cause increased postprandial gas, bloating, and distention.

D. Psychosocial Abnormalities

More than 50% of patients with irritable bowel who seek medical attention have underlying depression, anxiety, or somatization. By contrast, those who do not seek medical attention are similar psychologically to normal individuals. Psychological abnormalities may influence how the patient perceives or reacts to illness and minor visceral sensations. Chronic stress may alter intestinal motility or modulate pathways that affect central and spinal processing of visceral afferent sensation.

▶ Clinical Findings

A. Symptoms and Signs

Irritable bowel is a chronic condition. Symptoms usually begin in the late teens to twenties. Symptoms should be present for at least 3 months before the diagnosis can be considered. The diagnosis is established in the presence of compatible symptoms and the judicious use of tests to exclude organic disease.

Abdominal pain usually is intermittent, crampy, and in the lower abdominal region. As previously stated, the onset of pain typically is associated with a change in stool frequency or form and commonly is relieved by defecation. It does not usually occur at night or interfere with sleep. Patients with irritable bowel syndrome may be classified into one of three categories based on the predominant bowel habit: irritable bowel syndrome with diarrhea; irritable bowel syndrome with constipation; or irritable bowel syndrome with mixed constipation and diarrhea. It is important to clarify what the patient means by these complaints. Patients with irritable bowel and constipation report infrequent bowel movements (less than three per week), hard or lumpy stools, or straining. Patients with irritable bowel syndrome with diarrhea refer to loose or watery stools, frequent stools (more than three per day), urgency, or fecal incontinence. Many patients report that they have a firm stool in the morning followed by progressively looser movements. Complaints of visible distention and bloating are common, though these are not always clinically evident.

The patient should be asked about "alarm symptoms" that suggest a diagnosis other than irritable bowel syndrome and warrant further investigation. The acute onset of symptoms raises the likelihood of organic disease, especially in patients older than 40–50 years. Nocturnal diarrhea, severe constipation or diarrhea, hematochezia, weight loss, and fever are incompatible with a diagnosis of irritable bowel syndrome and warrant investigation for underlying disease. Patients who have a family history of cancer, inflammatory bowel disease, or celiac disease should undergo additional evaluation.

A physical examination should be performed to look for evidence of organic disease and to allay the patient's anxieties. The physical examination usually is normal. Abdominal tenderness, especially in the lower abdomen, is common but not pronounced. A new onset of symptoms in a patient over age 40 years warrants further examination.

B. Laboratory Findings and Special Examinations

In patients whose symptoms fulfill the diagnostic criteria for irritable bowel syndrome and who have no other alarm symptoms, evidence-based consensus guidelines do not support further diagnostic testing, as the likelihood of serious organic diseases does not appear to be increased. Although the vague nature of symptoms and patient anxiety may prompt clinicians to consider a variety of diagnostic studies, overtesting should be avoided. A 2013 study of primary care patients aged 30–50 years with suspected irritable bowel found that patients randomized to a strategy of extensive testing prior to diagnosis had higher health care costs but similar symptoms and satisfaction at 1 year as patients randomized to a strategy of minimal testing but a positive clinical diagnosis. The use of routine blood tests (complete blood count, chemistry panel, serum albumin, thyroid function tests, erythrocyte sedimentation rate) is unnecessary in most patients. Stool specimen examinations for ova and parasites should be obtained only in patients with increased likelihood of infection (eg, day care workers, campers, foreign travelers). Routine sigmoidoscopy or colonoscopy is not recommended in young patients with symptoms of irritable bowel syndrome without alarm symptoms but should be considered in patients who do not improve with conservative management. In all patients age 50 years or older who have not had a previous evaluation, colonoscopy should be obtained to exclude malignancy. When colonoscopy is performed, random mucosal biopsies should be obtained to look for evidence of microscopic colitis (which may have similar symptoms). In patients with irritable bowel syndrome with diarrhea, serologic tests for celiac disease should be performed. Routine testing for bacterial overgrowth with hydrogen breath tests are not recommended.

Differential Diagnosis

A number of disorders may present with similar symptoms. Examples include colonic neoplasia, inflammatory bowel disease (ulcerative colitis, Crohn disease, microscopic colitis), hyperthyroidism or hypothyroidism, parasites, malabsorption (especially celiac disease, bacterial overgrowth, lactase deficiency), causes of chronic secretory diarrhea (carcinoid), and endometriosis. Psychiatric disorders such as depression, panic disorder, and anxiety must be considered as well. Women with refractory symptoms have an increased incidence of prior sexual and physical abuse. These diagnoses should be excluded in patients with presumed irritable bowel syndrome who do not improve within 2–4 weeks of empiric treatment or in whom subsequent alarm symptoms develop.

Treatment

A. General Measures

As with other functional disorders, the most important interventions the clinician can offer are reassurance, education, and support. This includes identifying and responding to the patient's concerns, careful explanation of the pathophysiology and natural history of the disorder, setting realistic treatment goals, and involving the patient in the treatment process. Because irritable bowel symptoms are chronic, the patient's reasons for seeking consultation at this time should be determined. These may include major life events or recent psychosocial stressors, dietary or medication changes, concerns about serious underlying disease, or reduced quality of life and impairment of daily activities. In discussing with the patient the importance of the mind-gut interaction, it may be helpful to explain that alterations in visceral motility and sensitivity may be exacerbated by environmental, social, or psychological factors such as foods, medications, hormones, and stress. Symptoms such as pain, bloating, and altered bowel habits may lead to anxiety and distress, which in turn may further exacerbate bowel disturbances due to disordered communication between the gut and the central nervous system. Fears that the symptoms will progress, require surgery, or degenerate into serious illness should be allayed. The patient should understand that irritable bowel syndrome is a chronic disorder characterized by periods of exacerbation and quiescence. The emphasis should be shifted from finding the cause of the symptoms to finding a way to cope with them. Moderate exercise is beneficial. Clinicians must resist the temptation to chase chronic complaints with new or repeated diagnostic studies.

B. Dietary Therapy

Patients commonly report dietary intolerances. Proposed mechanisms for dietary intolerance include food allergy, hypersensitivity, effects of gut hormones, changes in bacterial flora, increased bacterial gas production (arising in the small or large intestine), and direct chemical irritation. Fatty foods and caffeine are poorly tolerated by many patients with irritable bowel syndrome. In patients with diarrhea, bloating, and flatulence, lactose intolerance should be excluded with a hydrogen breath test or a trial of a lactose-free diet. A host of poorly absorbed, fermentable, monosaccharides and short-chain carbohydrates ("FODMAPS") may exacerbate bloating, flatulence, and diarrhea in some patients. These include fructose (corn syrups, apples, pears, honey, watermelon, raisins), lactose, fructans (garlic, onions, leeks, asparagus, artichokes), wheat-based products (breads, pasta, cereals, cakes), sorbitol (stone fruits), and raffinose (legumes, lentils, brussel sprouts, soybeans, cabbage). Dietary restriction of these fermentable carbohydrates may improve symptoms. A 2014 crossover trial showed that patients experienced a marked reduction in overall symptoms, including bloating, pain, and flatus, while on the low FODMAP diet.

A high-fiber diet and fiber supplements appears to be of little value in patients with irritable bowel syndrome. Many patients report little change in bowel frequency but increased gas and distention.

C. Pharmacologic Measures

More than two-thirds of patients with irritable bowel syndrome have mild symptoms that respond readily to education, reassurance, and dietary interventions. Drug therapy should be reserved for patients with moderate to severe symptoms that do not respond to conservative measures. These agents should be viewed as being adjunctive rather than curative. Given the wide spectrum of symptoms, no single agent is expected to provide relief in all or even most patients. Nevertheless, therapy targeted at the specific dominant symptom (pain, constipation, or diarrhea) may be beneficial.

1. Antispasmodic agents—Anticholinergic agents are used by some practitioners for treatment of acute episodes of pain or bloating despite a lack of well-designed trials demonstrating efficacy. Available agents include hyoscyamine, 0.125 mg orally (or sublingually as needed) or sustained-release, 0.037 mg or 0.75 mg orally twice daily; dicyclomine, 10–20 mg orally; or methscopolamine 2.5–5 mg orally before meals and at bedtime. Anticholinergic side effects are common, including urinary retention, constipation, tachycardia, and dry mouth. Hence, these agents should be used with caution in the elderly and in patients with constipation. Peppermint oil formulations (which relax smooth muscle) may be helpful.

2. Antidiarrheal agents—Loperamide (2 mg orally three or four times daily) is effective for the treatment of patients with diarrhea, reducing stool frequency, liquidity, and urgency. It may best be used "prophylactically" in situations in which diarrhea is anticipated (such as stressful situations) or would be inconvenient (social engagements). Increased intracolonic bile acids due to alterations in enterohepatic circulation may contribute to diarrhea in a subset of patients with diarrhea. An empiric trial of bile salt-binding agents (cholestyramine 2–4 g with meals; colesevelam, 625 mg, 1–3 tablets twice daily) may be considered.

3. Anticonstipation agents—Treatment with oral osmotic laxatives polyethylene glycol 3350 (Miralax, 17–34 g/day)

may increase stool frequency, improve stool consistency, and reduce straining. Lactulose or sorbitol produces increased flatus and distention, which are poorly tolerated in patients with irritable bowel syndrome and should be avoided. Lubiprostone (8 mcg orally twice daily) and linaclotide (290 mcg orally once daily) are newer agents approved for treatment of irritable bowel syndrome with constipation. Through different mechanisms, both stimulate increased intestinal chloride and fluid secretion, resulting in accelerated colonic transit. In clinical trials, lubiprostone led to global symptom improvement in 18% of patients compared with 10% of patients who received placebo. Trials of linaclotide included similar patient populations but measured different primary end points. Higher combined response rates (defined as greater than 30% reduction in abdominal pain and more than three spontaneous bowel movements per week, including an increase of one or more from baseline) were found in 12.5% of linaclotide-treated patients compared with 4% of placebo-treated patients. Patients with intractable constipation should undergo further assessment for slow colonic transit and pelvic floor dysfunction (see Constipation, above).

4. Psychotropic agents—Patients with predominant symptoms of pain or bloating may benefit from low doses of tricyclic antidepressants, which are believed to have effects on motility, visceral sensitivity, and central pain perception that are independent of their psychotropic effects. Because of their anticholinergic effects, these agents may be more useful in patients with diarrhea-predominant than constipation-predominant symptoms. Oral nortriptyline, desipramine, or imipramine, may be started at a low dosage of 10 mg at bedtime and increased gradually to 50–150 mg as tolerated. Response rates do not correlate with dosage, and many patients respond to doses of 50 mg or less daily. Side effects are common, and lack of efficacy with one agent does not preclude benefit from another. Improvement should be evident within 4 weeks. The oral serotonin reuptake inhibitors (sertraline, 25–100 mg daily; citalopram 10–20 mg; paroxetine 20–50 mg daily; or fluoxetine, 10–40 mg daily) may lead to improvement in overall sense of well-being but have little impact on abdominal pain or bowel symptoms. Anxiolytics should not be used chronically in irritable bowel syndrome because of their habituation potential. Patients with major depression or anxiety disorders should be identified and treated with therapeutic doses of appropriate agents.

5. Serotonin receptor agonists and antagonists—Serotonin is an important mediator of gastrointestinal motility and sensation. In patients with irritable bowel syndrome with diarrhea, 5-HT$_3$ antagonists may reduce diarrhea and improve overall symptoms through central and peripheral mechanisms. Alosetron is a 5-HT$_3$ antagonist that is FDA-approved for the treatment of women with severe irritable bowel syndrome with predominant diarrhea. Unfortunately, due to cases of severe constipation and a small (1:1000) but significant risk of ischemic colitis, alosetron is restricted to women with severe irritable bowel syndrome with diarrhea who have not responded to conventional therapies and who have been educated about the relative risks and benefits of the agent. It should not be used in patients with constipation. A randomized crossover trial of another 5-HT$_3$ antagonist, ondansetron 4–8 mg three times daily, showed overall superior symptom improvement, including stool frequency, consistency, and urgency. At this time, 5-HT$_3$ antagonists may be considered after careful discussion of the risks and benefits in carefully selected patients with severe diarrhea-predominant irritable bowel syndrome.

6. Nonabsorbable antibiotics—Rifaximin is not approved for the treatment of irritable bowel syndrome but may be considered in patients with refractory symptoms, especially bloating. A 2012 meta-analysis identified a 9.9% greater improvement in bloating compared with placebo, a modest gain that is similar to other less expensive therapies. Symptom improvement may be attributable to suppression of bacteria in either the small intestine or colon, resulting in decreased bacterial carbohydrate fermentation, diarrhea, and bloating.

7. Probiotics—Meta-analyses of small controlled clinical trials report improved symptoms in some patients treated with one probiotic, *Bifidobacterium infantis*, but not with another probiotic, *Lactobacillus salivarius*, or placebo. It is hypothesized that alterations in gut flora may reduce symptoms through suppression of inflammation or reduction of bacterial gas production, resulting in reduced distention, flatus, and visceral sensitivity. Such therapy is attractive because it is safe, well tolerated, and inexpensive. Although promising, further study is needed to define the efficacy and optimal formulations of probiotic therapy. The probiotics VSL#3 (1 packet twice daily) or *Bifidobacterium infantis* (1 tablet twice daily) have shown modest benefit in small studies.

D. Psychological Therapies

Cognitive-behavioral therapies, relaxation techniques, and hypnotherapy appear to be beneficial in some patients. Patients with underlying psychological abnormalities may benefit from evaluation by a psychiatrist or psychologist. Patients with severe disability should be referred to a pain treatment center.

► Prognosis

The majority of patients with irritable bowel syndrome learn to cope with their symptoms and lead productive lives.

Begtrup LM et al. A positive diagnostic strategy is noninferior to a strategy of exclusion for patients with irritable bowel syndrome. Clin Gastroenterol Hepatol. 2013 Aug;11(8):956–62. [PMID: 23357491]

Böhn L et al. Diet low in FODMAPs reduces symptoms of irritable bowel syndrome as well as traditional dietary advice: a randomized controlled trial. Gastroenterology. 2015 Nov; 149(6):1399–407.e2. [PMID: 26255043]

Chey WD et al. JAMA patient page. Irritable bowel syndrome. JAMA. 2015 Mar 3;313(9):982. [PMID: 25734751]

Ford AC et al. Effect of antidepressants and psychological therapies, including hypnotherapy, in irritable bowel syndrome: systematic review and meta-analysis. Am J Gastroenterol. 2014 Sep;109(9):1350–65. [PMID: 24935275]

Ford AC et al; Task Force on the Management of Functional Bowel Disorders. American College of Gastroenterology monograph on the management of irritable bowel syndrome and chronic idiopathic constipation. Am J Gastroenterol. 2014 Aug;109(Suppl 1):S2–26. [PMID: 25091148]

Garsed K et al. A randomised trial of ondansetron for the treatment of irritable bowel syndrome with diarrhoea. Gut. 2014 Oct; 63(10):1617–25. [PMID: 24334242]

Halmos EP et al. A diet low in FODMAPs reduces symptoms of irritable bowel syndrome. Gastroenterology. 2014 Jan; 146(1):67–75. [PMID: 24076059]

Lacy BE. The science, evidence, and practice of dietary interventions in irritable bowel syndrome. Clin Gastroenterol Hepatol. 2015 Nov;13(11):1899–906. [PMID: 25769411]

Sugerman DT. JAMA patient page. Abdominal bloating. JAMA. 2013 Oct 16;310(15):1637. [PMID: 24129477]

Videlock EJ et al. Effects of linaclotide in patients with irritable bowel syndrome with constipation or chronic constipation: a meta-analysis. Clin Gastroenterol Hepatol. 2013 Sep;11(9): 1084–92. [PMID: 23644388]

Weinberg DS et al. American Gastroenterological Association Institute guideline on the pharmacological management of irritable bowel syndrome. Gastroenterology. 2014 Nov; 147(5):1146–8. [PMID: 25224526]

ANTIBIOTIC-ASSOCIATED COLITIS

ESSENTIALS OF DIAGNOSIS

► Most cases of antibiotic-associated diarrhea are not attributable to *C difficile* and are usually mild and self-limited.

► Symptoms of antibiotic-associated colitis vary from mild to fulminant; almost all colitis is attributable to *C difficile*.

► Diagnosis in most cases established by stool assay.

► General Considerations

Antibiotic-associated diarrhea is a common clinical occurrence. Characteristically, the diarrhea occurs during the period of antibiotic exposure, is dose related, and resolves spontaneously after discontinuation of the antibiotic. In most cases, this diarrhea is mild, self-limited, and does not require any specific laboratory evaluation or treatment. Stool examination usually reveals no fecal leukocytes, and stool cultures reveal no pathogens. Although *C difficile* is identified in the stool of 15–25% of cases of antibiotic-associated diarrhea, it is also identified in 5–10% of patients treated with antibiotics who do not have diarrhea. Most cases of antibiotic-associated diarrhea are due to changes in colonic bacterial fermentation of carbohydrates and are not due to *C difficile*.

Antibiotic-associated colitis is a significant clinical problem almost always caused by *C difficile* infection that colonizes the colon and releases two toxins: TcdA and TcdB. This anaerobic bacterium is acquired by fecal-oral transmission of spores that colonize the colon of 3% of healthy adults and 8% of hospitalized patients. *C difficile* colitis is the major cause of diarrhea in patients hospitalized for more than 3 days, affecting up to 15 of every 1000 patients and increasing mean hospital stay costs as much as $30,000. In the United States, there are an estimated 453,000 cases per year with 29,000 associated deaths. Found throughout hospitals in patient rooms and bathrooms, *C difficile* is readily transmitted from patient to patient by hospital personnel. Fastidious hand washing and use of disposable gloves are helpful in minimizing transmission and reducing infections in hospitalized patients. In hospitalized patients, *C difficile* colitis occurs in approximately 20% of those who are colonized at admission and 3.5% of those not colonized. In both hospital-associated and community infections, most episodes of colitis occur in people who have received antibiotics that disrupt the normal bowel flora and thus allow the spores to germinate and the bacterium to flourish. Although almost all antibiotics have been implicated, colitis most commonly develops after use of ampicillin, clindamycin, third-generation cephalosporins, and fluoroquinolones. In clinical trials, prophylactic administration of the probiotics "DanActiv" and "Bio-K+," containing *Lactobacillus casei, Lactobacillus bulgaricus*, and *Streptococcus thermophilus*, to hospitalized patients who are receiving antibiotics reduced the incidence of *C difficile*–associated diarrhea. Symptoms usually begin during or shortly after antibiotic therapy but may be delayed for up to 8 weeks. All patients with acute diarrhea should be asked about recent antibiotic exposure. Patients who are elderly; debilitated; immunocompromised; receiving multiple antibiotics or prolonged (more than 10 days) antibiotic therapy; receiving enteral tube feedings, proton pump inhibitors, or chemotherapy; or who have inflammatory bowel disease have a higher risk of acquiring *C difficile* and developing *C difficile*–associated diarrhea.

A more virulent strain of *C difficile* (NAP1) has emerged that contains an 18-base pair deletion of the TcdC inhibitory gene, resulting in higher toxin A and B production. This hypervirulent strain is more prevalent among hospital-associated infections (31%) than community-acquired infections (19%) and has been associated with outbreaks of severe disease with up to 7% mortality.

► Clinical Findings

A. Symptoms and Signs

Most patients report mild to moderate greenish, foul-smelling watery diarrhea 5–15 times per day with lower abdominal cramps. Physical examination is normal or reveals mild left lower quadrant tenderness. The stools may have mucus but seldom gross blood. In most patients, colitis is most severe in the distal colon and rectum. Over half of hospitalized patients diagnosed with *C difficile* colitis have a white blood count greater than 15,000/mcL, and *C difficile* should be considered in all hospitalized patients with unexplained leukocytosis.

Severe or fulminant disease occurs in 10–15% of patients. It is characterized by fever; hemodynamic instability; and abdominal distention, pain, and tenderness. Most patients have profuse diarrhea (up to 30 stools/day); however, diarrhea may be absent or appear to be improving in patients with fulminant disease or ileus. Laboratory data

suggestive of severe disease include a white blood count greater than 30,000/mcL, albumin less than 2.5 g/dL (due to protein-losing enteropathy), elevated serum lactate, or rising creatinine.

B. Special Examinations

1. Stool studies—Pathogenic strains of *C difficile* produce two toxins: toxin TcdA is an enterotoxin and toxin TcdB is a cytotoxin. Rapid enzyme immunoassays (EIAs) for toxins TcdA and TcdB have a 75–90% sensitivity with a single stool specimen; sensitivity increases to 90–95% with two specimens; however, these have now been supplanted in many laboratories by nucleic acid amplification tests (eg, PCR assays) that amplify the toxin TcdB gene. PCR assays are superior to EIA tests due to their high sensitivity (97%) as well as their ability to detect the NAP1 hypervirulent strain. Some laboratories first perform an assay for glutamate dehydrogenase (a common *C difficile* antigen), which has a high sensitivity and negative predictive value (greater than 95%). A negative glutamate dehydrogenase assay effectively excludes infection, while a positive assay requires confirmation with PCR or EIA to determine whether the strain that is present is toxin producing.

2. Flexible sigmoidoscopy—Flexible sigmoidoscopy is not needed in patients who have typical symptoms and a positive stool toxin assay. It may clarify the diagnosis in patients with positive *C difficile* toxin assays who have atypical symptoms or who have persistent diarrhea despite appropriate therapy. In patients with mild to moderate symptoms, there may be no abnormalities or only patchy or diffuse, nonspecific colitis indistinguishable from other causes. In patients with severe illness, true **pseudomembranous colitis** is seen.

3. Imaging studies—Abdominal radiographs or noncontrast abdominal CT scans are obtained in patients with severe or fulminant symptoms to look for evidence of colonic dilation and wall thickening. Abdominal CT also is useful in the evaluation of hospitalized patients with abdominal pain or ileus without significant diarrhea, in whom the presence of colonic wall thickening suggests unsuspected *C difficile* colitis. CT scanning is also useful in the detection of possible perforation.

► Differential Diagnosis

In the hospitalized patient in whom acute diarrhea develops after admission, the differential diagnosis includes simple antibiotic-associated diarrhea (not related to *C difficile*), enteral feedings, medications, and ischemic colitis. Other infectious causes are unusual in hospitalized patients in whom diarrhea develops more than 72 hours after admission, and it is not cost-effective to obtain stool cultures unless tests for *C difficile* are negative. Rarely, other organisms (staphylococci, *Clostridium perfringens*) have been associated with pseudomembranous colitis. *Klebsiella oxytoca* may cause a distinct form of antibiotic-associated hemorrhagic colitis that is segmental (usually in the right or transverse colon); spares the rectum; and is more common in younger, healthier outpatients.

▶ Complications

Severe colitis may progress quickly to fulminant disease, resulting in hemodynamic instability, respiratory failure, metabolic acidosis, megacolon (more than 7 cm diameter), perforation, and death. Chronic untreated colitis may result in weight loss and protein-losing enteropathy.

▶ Treatment

A. Immediate Treatment

If possible, antibiotic therapy should be discontinued and therapy with metronidazole, vancomycin, or fidaxomicin (a poorly absorbable macrolide antibiotic) should be initiated. For patients with mild disease, oral metronidazole (500 mg orally three times daily), vancomycin (125 mg orally four times daily), or fidaxomicin, (200 mg orally two times daily) are equally effective for initial treatment. Vancomycin and fidaxomicin are significantly more expensive than metronidazole. At present, metronidazole remains the preferred first-line therapy in patients with mild disease, except in patients who are intolerant of metronidazole, pregnant women, and children, although vancomycin is increasingly used due to its superior efficacy against the NAP1 strain and the decreased cost of its generic version. The duration of initial therapy is usually 10–14 days. Symptomatic improvement occurs in most patients within 72 hours.

For patients with severe disease, characterized by a white blood cell count greater than 15,000/mcL, serum albumin less than 3 g/dL, or a rise in serum creatinine to more than 1.5 times baseline, vancomycin, 125 mg orally four times daily, is the preferred agent because it achieves significantly higher response rates (97%) than metronidazole (76%). In patients with severe, complicated disease, characterized by fever higher than 38.5°C, hypotension, mental status changes, ileus, megacolon, or WBC greater than 30,000/mcL, intravenous metronidazole, 500 mg every 6 hours, should be given—supplemented by vancomycin (500 mg four times daily administered by nasoenteric tube) and, in some cases, vancomycin enemas (500 mg in 100 mL every 6 hours). Intravenous vancomycin does not penetrate the bowel and should not be used. The efficacy of fidaxomicin for severe or fulminant disease requires further investigation. Early surgical consultation is recommended for all patients with severe or fulminant disease. Total abdominal colectomy or loop ileostomy with colonic lavage may be required in patients with toxic megacolon, perforation, sepsis, or hemorrhage.

B. Treatment of Relapse

Up to 25% of patients have a relapse of diarrhea from *C difficile* within 1 or 2 weeks after stopping initial therapy. This may be due to reinfection or failure to eradicate the organism. The optimal treatment regimen for recurrent relapses is evolving. The first episode of recurrent infection usually responds promptly to a second course of the same regimen used for the initial episode. Some patients, however, have further relapses that can be difficult to treat. For patients with two relapses, a 7-week tapering regimen of vancomycin is recommended: 125 mg orally four times daily for 14 days; twice daily for 7 days; once daily for 7 days; every other day for 7 days; and every third day for 2–8 weeks. Fidaxomicin may be appropriate for patients with recurrent *C difficile* infection or as initial therapy in patients believed to be at higher risk for recurrent disease. Patients treated with fidaxomicin have lower recurrence rates (15%) of non-NAP1 *C difficile* strains than patients treated with vancomycin (25%). For patients with three or more relapses, updated 2013 guidelines recommend consideration of an installation of a suspension of fecal bacteria from a healthy donor ("fecal microbiota transplant"). In uncontrolled case reports and case series involving several hundred patients, such "fecal transplantation" into the terminal ileum or proximal colon (by colonoscopy) or into the duodenum and jejunum (by nasoenteric tube) results in disease remission after a single treatment in over 90% of patients with recurrent *C difficile* infection. In a 2013 randomized study, duodenal infusion of donor feces led to resolution of *C difficile* diarrhea in 94%, which was dramatically higher than vancomycin treatment (31%), prompting early study termination. Despite uncertainties, fecal transplantation should be considered in patients with refractory infection. A 2014 open label study demonstrated resolution of diarrhea in 18/20 (90%) patients with recurrent *C difficile* infection after oral treatment with capsules containing frozen feces from healthy volunteers.

Bagdasarian N et al. Diagnosis and treatment of *Clostridium difficile* in adults: a systematic review. JAMA. 2015 Jan 27; 313(4):398–408. [PMID: 25626036]

Brandt LJ. American Journal of Gastroenterology Lecture: intestinal microbiota and the role of fecal microbiota transplant (FMT) in treatment of *C. difficile* infection. Am J Gastroenterol. 2013 Feb;108(2):177–85. [PMID: 23318479]

Brandt LJ et al. Long-term follow-up of colonoscopic fecal microbiota transplant for recurrent *Clostridium difficile* infection. Am J Gastroenterol. 2012 Jul;107(7):1079–87. [PMID: 22450732]

Kelly CR et al. Update on fecal microbiota transplantation 2015: indications, methodologies, mechanisms, and outlook. Gastroenterology. 2015 Jul;149(1):223–37. [PMID: 25982290]

Leffler DA et al. *Clostridium difficile* infection. N Engl J Med. 2015 Apr 16;372(16):1539–48. [PMID: 25875259]

Lessa FC et al. Burden of *Clostridium difficile* infection in the United States. N Engl J Med. 2015 Feb 26;372(9):825–34. [PMID: 25714160]

Surawicz CM et al. Guidelines for diagnosis, treatment, and prevention of *Clostridium difficile* infections. Am J Gastroenterol. 2013 Apr;108(4):478–98. [PMID: 23439232]

van Nood E et al. Duodenal infusion of donor feces for recurrent *Clostridium difficile*. N Engl J Med. 2013 Jan 31;368(5):407–15. [PMID: 23323867]

Youngster I et al. Oral, capsulized, frozen fecal microbiota transplantation for relapsing *Clostridium difficile* infection. JAMA. 2014 Nov 5;312(17):1772–8. [PMID: 25322359]

Zacharioudakis IM et al. Colonization with toxinogenic *C. difficile* upon hospital admission, and risk of infection: a systematic review and meta-analysis. Am J Gastroenterol. 2015 Mar; 110(3):381–90. [PMID: 25732416]

INFLAMMATORY BOWEL DISEASE

The term "inflammatory bowel disease" includes ulcerative colitis and Crohn disease. Ulcerative colitis is a chronic, recurrent disease characterized by diffuse mucosal inflammation involving only the colon. Ulcerative colitis invariably involves the rectum and may extend proximally in a continuous fashion to involve part or all of the colon. Crohn disease is a chronic, recurrent disease characterized by patchy transmural inflammation involving any segment of the gastrointestinal tract from the mouth to the anus.

Crohn disease and ulcerative colitis may be associated in 50% of patients with a number of extraintestinal manifestations, including oral ulcers, oligoarticular or polyarticular nondeforming peripheral arthritis, spondylitis or sacroiliitis, episcleritis or uveitis, erythema nodosum, pyoderma gangrenosum, hepatitis and sclerosing cholangitis, and thromboembolic events.

▶ Pharmacologic Therapy

Although ulcerative colitis and Crohn disease appear to be distinct entities, the same pharmacologic agents are used to treat both. Despite extensive research, there are still no specific therapies for these diseases. The mainstays of therapy are 5-aminosalicylic acid derivatives, corticosteroids, immunomodulating agents (such as mercaptopurine or azathioprine and methotrexate), and biologic agents.

A. 5-Aminosalicylic Acid (5-ASA)

5-ASA is a topically active agent that has a variety of anti-inflammatory effects. It is used in the active treatment of ulcerative colitis and Crohn disease and during disease inactivity to maintain remission. It is readily absorbed from the small intestine but demonstrates minimal colonic absorption. A number of oral and topical compounds have been designed to target delivery of 5-ASA to the colon or small intestine while minimizing absorption. Commonly used formulations of 5-ASA are sulfasalazine, mesalamine, and azo compounds. Side effects of these compounds are uncommon but include nausea, rash, diarrhea, pancreatitis, and acute interstitial nephritis.

1. Oral mesalamine agents—These 5-ASA agents are coated in various pH-sensitive resins (Asacol, Apriso, and Lialda) or packaged in timed-release capsules (Pentasa). Pentasa releases 5-ASA slowly throughout the small intestine and colon. Asacol, Apriso, and Lialda tablets dissolve at pH 6.0–7.0, releasing 5-ASA in the terminal small bowel and proximal colon. Lialda has a multi-matrix system that gradually releases 5-ASA throughout the colon.

2. Azo compounds—Sulfasalazine, balsalazide and olsalazine contain 5-ASA linked by an azo bond that requires cleavage by colonic bacterial azoreductases to release 5-ASA. Absorption of these drugs from the small intestine is negligible. After release within the colon, the 5-ASA works topically and is largely unabsorbed.

Sulfasalazine contains 5-ASA linked to a sulfapyridine moiety. It is unclear whether the sulfapyridine group has any anti-inflammatory effects. One gram of sulfasalazine contains 400 mg of 5-ASA. The sulfapyridine group, however, is absorbed and may cause side effects in 15–30% of patients—much higher than with other 5-ASA compounds. Dose-related side effects include nausea, headaches,

leukopenia, oligospermia, and impaired folate metabolism. Allergic and idiosyncratic side effects are fever, rash, hemolytic anemia, neutropenia, worsened colitis, hepatitis, pancreatitis, and pneumonitis. Because of its side effects, sulfasalazine is less frequently used than other 5-ASA agents. It should always be administered in conjunction with folate. Eighty percent of patients intolerant of sulfasalazine can tolerate mesalamine.

3. Topical mesalamine—5-ASA is provided in the form of suppositories (Canasa; 1000 mg) and enemas (Rowasa; 4 g/60 mL). These formulations can deliver much higher concentrations of 5-ASA to the distal colon than oral compounds. Side effects are uncommon.

B. Corticosteroids

A variety of intravenous, oral, and topical corticosteroid formulations have been used in inflammatory bowel disease. They have utility in the short-term treatment of moderate to severe disease. However, long-term use is associated with serious, potentially irreversible side effects and is to be avoided. The agents, route of administration, duration of use, and tapering regimens used are based more on personal bias and experience than on data from rigorous clinical trials. The most commonly used intravenous formulations have been hydrocortisone or methylprednisolone, which are given by continuous infusion or every 6 hours. Oral formulations are prednisone or methylprednisolone. Adverse events commonly occur during short-term systemic corticosteroid therapy, including mood changes, insomnia, dyspepsia, weight gain, edema, elevated serum glucose levels, acne, and moon facies. Side effects of long-term use include osteoporosis, osteonecrosis of the femoral head, myopathy, cataracts, and susceptibility to infections. Calcium and vitamin D supplementation should be administered to all patients receiving long-term corticosteroid therapy. Bone densitometry should be considered in patients with inflammatory bowel disease with other risk factors for osteoporosis and in all patients with a lifetime use of corticosteroids for 3 months or more. Budesonide is an oral corticosteroid with high topical anti-inflammatory activity but low systemic activity due to high first-pass hepatic metabolism. A controlled-release formulation is available (Entocort) that targets delivery to the terminal ileum and proximal colon. An enteric coated, multi-matrix, delayed-release formulation is available (Uceris) that releases budesonide throughout the colon. Budesonide produces less suppression of the hypothalamic-pituitary-adrenal axis and fewer steroid-related side effects than hydrocortisone or prednisone. Topical preparations are provided as hydrocortisone suppositories (100 mg), foam (90 mg), enemas (100 mg), and as budesonide foam (2 mg).

C. Immunomodulating Drugs: Mercaptopurine, Azathioprine, or Methotrexate

Mercaptopurine and azathioprine are thiopurine drugs that are used in many patients with moderate to severe Crohn disease and ulcerative colitis either in combination with anti-TNF agents or in patients who are corticosteroid-dependent in an attempt to reduce or withdraw the corticosteroids and to maintain patients in remission. Azathioprine is converted in vivo to mercaptopurine. It is believed that the active metabolite of mercaptopurine is 6-thioguanine. Monitoring of 6-thioguanine levels is performed in some clinical settings but is of unproven value in the management of most patients. Side effects of mercaptopurine and azathioprine, including allergic reactions (fever, rash, or arthralgias) and nonallergic reactions (nausea, vomiting, pancreatitis, hepatotoxicity, bone marrow suppression, infections), occur in 15% of patients. Thiopurines are associated with up to a fivefold increased risk of non-Hodgkin lymphomas (1/1000 patient-years). The risk rises after 1–2 years of exposure and is higher in men younger than 30 years and patients older than 50 years. Thiopurines also are associated with a risk of human papillomavirus (HPV)–related cervical dysplasia; and with an increased risk of non-melanoma skin cancer. Younger patients also are at risk for severe primary Epstein-Barr virus (EBV) infection, if not previously exposed.

Three competing enzymes are involved in the metabolism of mercaptopurine to its active (6-thioguanine) and inactive metabolites. About 1 person in 300 has a homozygous mutation of one of the enzymes that metabolizes thiopurine methyltransferase (TPMT), placing them at risk for profound immunosuppression; 1 person in 9 is heterozygous for TPMT, resulting in intermediate enzyme activity. Measurement of TPMT functional activity is recommended prior to initiation of therapy. Treatment should be withheld in patients with absent TPMT activity. The most effective dose of mercaptopurine is 1–1.5 mg/kg. For azathioprine, it is 2–3 mg/kg daily. For patients with normal TPMT activity, both drugs may be initiated at the weight-calculated dose. A complete blood count should be obtained weekly for 4 weeks, biweekly for 4 weeks, and then every 1–3 months for the duration of therapy. Liver biochemical tests should be measured periodically. Some clinicians prefer gradual dose-escalation, especially for patients with intermediate TPMT activity or in whom TPMT measurement is not available; both drugs may be started at 25 mg/day and increased by 25 mg every 1–2 weeks while monitoring for myelosuppression until the target dose is reached. If the white blood count falls below 3000–4000/mcL or the platelet count falls below 100,000/mcL, the medication should be held for at least 1 week before reducing the daily dose by 25–50 mg.

Methotrexate is used in the treatment of patients with inflammatory bowel disease, especially patients with Crohn disease who are intolerant of mercaptopurine. Methotrexate is an analog of dihydrofolic acid. Although at high doses it interferes with cell proliferation through inhibition of nucleic acid metabolism, at low doses it has anti-inflammatory properties, including inhibition of expression of tumor necrosis factor (TNF) in monocytes and macrophages. Methotrexate may be given intramuscularly, subcutaneously, or orally. Side effects of methotrexate include nausea, vomiting, stomatitis, infections, bone marrow suppression, hepatic fibrosis, and life-threatening pneumonitis. A complete blood count and liver function tests should be monitored every 1–3 months. Folate supplementation (1 mg/day) should be administered.

D. Biologic Therapies

Although the etiology of inflammatory bowel disorders is uncertain, it appears that an abnormal response of the mucosal innate immune system to luminal bacteria may trigger inflammation, which is perpetuated by dysregulation of cellular immunity. A number of biologic therapies are available or in clinical testing that more narrowly target various components of the immune system. Biologic agents are highly effective for patients with corticosteroid-dependent or refractory disease and potentially may improve the natural history of disease. The potential benefits of these agents, however, must be carefully weighed with their high cost and risk of serious and potentially life-threatening side effects.

1. Anti-TNF therapies—TNF is one of the key proinflammatory cytokines in the T_H1 response. TNF exists in two biologically active forms: a soluble form (sTNF), which is enzymatically cleaved from its cell surface, and a membrane-bound precursor (tmTNF). When either form binds to the TNF-receptors on effector cells, they initiate a variety of signaling pathways that lead to inflammatory gene activation. Four monoclonal antibodies to TNF currently are available for the treatment of inflammatory bowel disease: infliximab, adalimumab, golimumab, and certolizumab. All four agents bind and neutralize soluble as well as membrane-bound TNF on macrophages and activated T lymphocytes, thereby preventing TNF stimulation of effector cells.

Infliximab is a chimeric (75% human/25% mouse) IgG_1 antibody that is administered by intravenous infusion. A three-dose regimen of 5 mg/kg administered at 0, 2, and 6 weeks is recommended for acute induction, followed by infusions every 8 weeks for maintenance therapy. Acute infusion reactions occur in 5–10% of infusions but occur less commonly in patients receiving regularly scheduled infusions or concomitant immunomodulators (ie, azathioprine or methotrexate). Most reactions are mild or moderate (nausea; headache; dizziness; urticaria; diaphoresis; or mild cardiopulmonary symptoms that include chest tightness, dyspnea, or palpitations) and can be treated by slowing the infusion rate and administering acetaminophen and diphenhydramine. Severe reactions (hypotension, severe shortness of breath, rigors, severe chest discomfort) occur in less than 1% and may require oxygen, diphenhydramine, hydrocortisone, and epinephrine. Delayed serum sickness-like reactions occur in 1%. With repeated, intermittent intravenous injections, antibodies to infliximab develop in up to 40% of patients, which are associated with a shortened duration or loss of response and increased risk of acute or delayed infusion reactions. Giving infliximab in a regularly scheduled maintenance therapy (eg, every 8 weeks), concomitant use of infliximab with other immunomodulating agents (azathioprine, mercaptopurine, or methotrexate), or preinfusion treatment with corticosteroids (intravenous hydrocortisone 200 mg) significantly reduces the development of antibodies to approximately 10%.

Adalimumab and golimumab are fully human IgG_1 antibodies that are administered by subcutaneous injection. For adalimumab, a dose of 160 mg at week 0 and 80 mg at week 2 is recommended for acute induction, followed by maintenance therapy with 40 mg subcutaneously every other week. For golimumab, a dose of 200 mg at week 0 and 100 mg at week 2 is recommended for acute induction, followed by maintenance therapy with 100 mg subcutaneously every 4 weeks.

Certolizumab is a fusion compound in which the Fab1 portion of a chimeric (95% human/5% mouse) TNF-antibody is bound to polyethylene glycol in order to prolong the drug half-life. A dose of 400 mg at weeks 0, 2, and 4 is recommended for acute induction, followed by maintenance therapy with 400 mg subcutaneously every 4 weeks. Injection site reactions (burning, pain, redness, itching) are relatively common but are usually minor and self-limited.

Acute and delayed hypersensitivity reactions are rare with subcutaneous anti-TNF therapies. Antibodies to adalimumab or golimumab develop in 5% of patients and to certolizumab in 10%, which may lead to shortened duration or loss of response to the drug.

Serious infections with anti-TNF therapies may occur in 2–5% of patients, including sepsis, pneumonia, abscess, and cellulitis; however, controlled studies suggest the increased risk may be attributable to increased severity of disease and concomitant use of corticosteroids. Patients treated with anti-TNF therapies are at increased risk for the development of opportunistic infections with intracellular bacterial pathogens including tuberculosis, mycoses (candidiasis, histoplasmosis, coccidioidomycosis, nocardiosis), and listeriosis, and with reactivation of viral infections, including hepatitis B, herpes simplex, varicella zoster, and EBV. Prior to use of these agents, patients should be screened for latent tuberculosis with PPD testing and a chest radiograph. Antinuclear and anti-DNA antibodies occur in a large percentage of patients; however, the development of drug-induced lupus is rare. All agents may cause severe hepatic reactions leading to acute hepatic failure; liver biochemical tests should be monitored routinely during therapy. Anti-TNF therapies increase the risk of non-melanoma skin cancer and, possibly, non-Hodgkin lymphoma. Most lymphomas, however, are associated with a combination of an anti-TNF agent and a thiopurine, and it appears that the risk of anti-TNF monotherapy is very low. Rare cases of optic neuritis and demyelinating diseases, including multiple sclerosis have been reported. Anti-TNF therapies may worsen heart failure in patients with cardiac disease.

2. Anti-integrins—Two monoclonal antibodies are available that target integrins, decreasing the trafficking of circulating leukocytes through the vasculature and reducing chronic inflammation. Natalizumab is a humanized monoclonal antibody targeted against alpha-4-integrins that blocks leukocytes trafficking to the gut and brain. Although natalizumab is efficacious for the induction and maintenance of response and remission in patients with Crohn disease, there is an increased incidence of progressive multifocal leukoencephalopathy (PML) caused by reactivation of the JC virus, in approximately 1:250 patients with a positive JC virus antibody test result receiving therapy for longer than 18 months.

Vedolizumab is a new anti-integrin that blocks the $alpha_4 beta_7$ heterodimer, selectively blocking gut, but not brain, lymphocyte trafficking. The greater selectivity may prevent JC virus reactivation. Thus far, it appears to have a negligible incidence of any serious side effects.

Beaugerie L. Lymphoma: the bête noire of the long-term use of thiopurines in adult and elderly patients with inflammatory bowel disease. Gastroenterology. 2013 Nov;145(5):927–30. [PMID: 24070724]

Bernstein CN. Treatment of IBD: where we are and where we are going. Am J Gastroenterol. 2015 Jan;110(1):114–26. [PMID: 25488896]

Coskun M et al. Tumor necrosis factor inhibitors for inflammatory bowel disease. N Engl J Med. 2013 Dec 26;369(26):2561–2. [PMID: 24369082]

Jin J. JAMA patient page. Inflammatory bowel disease. JAMA. 2014 May 21;311(19):2034. [PMID: 24846049]

Kotlyar DS et al. Risk of lymphoma in patients with inflammatory bowel disease treated with azathioprine and 6-mercaptopurine: a meta-analysis. Clin Gastroenterol Hepatol. 2015 May; 13(5):847–58.e4. [PMID: 24879926]

Targownik LE et al. Infectious and malignant complications of TNF inhibitor therapy in IBD. Am J Gastroenterol. 2013 Dec; 108(12):1835–42. [PMID: 24042192]

► Social Support for Patients

Inflammatory bowel disease is a lifelong illness that can have profound emotional and social impacts on the individual. Patients should be encouraged to become involved in the Crohn's and Colitis Foundation of America (CCFA). National headquarters may be contacted at 733 Third Avenue, Suite 510, New York, NY 10017; phone 800-932-2423. Internet address: http://www.ccfa.org.

1. Crohn Disease

ESSENTIALS OF DIAGNOSIS

► Insidious onset.

► Intermittent bouts of low-grade fever, diarrhea, and right lower quadrant pain.

► Right lower quadrant mass and tenderness.

► Perianal disease with abscess, fistulas.

► Radiographic or endoscopic evidence of ulceration, stricturing, or fistulas of the small intestine or colon.

► General Considerations

One-third of cases of Crohn disease involve the small bowel only, most commonly the terminal ileum (ileitis). Half of all cases involve the small bowel and colon, most often the terminal ileum and adjacent proximal ascending colon (ileocolitis). In 20% of cases, the colon alone is affected. One-third of patients have associated perianal disease (fistulas, fissures, abscesses). Less than 5% patients have symptomatic involvement of the upper intestinal tract. Unlike ulcerative colitis, Crohn disease is a transmural process that can result in mucosal inflammation and ulceration, stricturing, fistula development, and abscess formation. Cigarette smoking is strongly associated with the development of Crohn disease, resistance to medical therapy, and early disease relapse.

▶ Clinical Findings

A. Symptoms and Signs

Because of the variable location of involvement and severity of inflammation, Crohn disease may present with a variety of symptoms and signs. In eliciting the history, the clinician should take particular note of fevers, the patient's general sense of well-being, weight loss, the presence of abdominal pain, the number of liquid bowel movements per day, and prior surgical resections. Physical examination should focus on the patient's temperature, weight, and nutritional status, the presence of abdominal tenderness or an abdominal mass, rectal examination, and extraintestinal manifestations (described below). Most commonly, there is one or a combination of the following clinical constellations.

1. Chronic inflammatory disease—This is the most common presentation and is often seen in patients with ileitis or ileocolitis. Patients report malaise, weight loss, and loss of energy. In patients with ileitis or ileocolitis, there may be diarrhea, which is usually nonbloody and often intermittent. In patients with colitis involving the rectum or left colon, there may be bloody diarrhea and fecal urgency, which may mimic the symptoms of ulcerative colitis. Cramping or steady right lower quadrant or periumbilical pain is common. Physical examination reveals focal tenderness, usually in the right lower quadrant. A palpable, tender mass that represents thickened or matted loops of inflamed intestine may be present in the lower abdomen.

2. Intestinal obstruction—Narrowing of the small bowel may occur as a result of inflammation, spasm, or fibrotic stenosis. Patients report postprandial bloating, cramping pains, and loud borborygmi. This may occur in patients with active inflammatory symptoms (as above) or later in the disease from chronic fibrosis without other systemic symptoms or signs of inflammation.

3. Penetrating disease and fistulae—Sinus tracts that penetrate through the bowel, where they may be contained or form fistulas to adjacent structures, develop in a subset of patients. Penetration through the bowel can result in an intra-abdominal or retroperitoneal phlegmon or abscess manifested by fevers, chills, a tender abdominal mass, and leukocytosis. Fistulas between the small intestine and colon commonly are asymptomatic but can result in diarrhea, weight loss, bacterial overgrowth, and malnutrition. Fistulas to the bladder produce recurrent infections. Fistulas to the vagina result in malodorous drainage and problems with personal hygiene. Fistulas to the skin usually occur at the site of surgical scars.

4. Perianal disease—One-third of patients with either large or small bowel involvement develop perianal disease manifested by large painful skin tags, anal fissures, perianal abscesses, and fistulas.

5. Extraintestinal manifestations—Extraintestinal manifestations may be seen with both Crohn disease and ulcerative colitis. These include arthralgias, arthritis, iritis or uveitis, pyoderma gangrenosum, or erythema nodosum. Oral aphthous lesions are common. There is an increased prevalence of gallstones due to malabsorption of bile salts from the terminal ileum. Nephrolithiasis with urate or calcium oxalate stones may occur.

B. Laboratory Findings

There is a poor correlation between laboratory studies and the patient's clinical picture. Laboratory values may reflect inflammatory activity or nutritional complications of disease. A complete blood count and serum albumin should be obtained in all patients. Anemia may reflect chronic inflammation, mucosal blood loss, iron deficiency, or vitamin B_{12} malabsorption secondary to terminal ileal inflammation or resection. Leukocytosis may reflect inflammation or abscess formation or may be secondary to corticosteroid therapy. Hypoalbuminemia may be due to intestinal protein loss (protein-losing enteropathy), malabsorption, bacterial overgrowth, or chronic inflammation. The sedimentation rate or C-reactive protein level is elevated in many patients during active inflammation. Fecal calprotectin levels also are increased in patients with intestinal inflammation. Stool specimens are sent for examination for routine pathogens, ova and parasites, leukocytes, fat, and *C difficile* toxin.

C. Special Diagnostic Studies

In most patients, the initial diagnosis of Crohn disease is based on a compatible clinical picture with supporting endoscopic, pathologic, and radiographic findings. Colonoscopy usually is performed first to evaluate the colon and terminal ileum and to obtain mucosal biopsies. Typical endoscopic findings include aphthoid, linear or stellate ulcers, strictures, and segmental involvement with areas of normal-appearing mucosa adjacent to inflamed mucosa. In 10% of cases, it may be difficult to distinguish ulcerative colitis from Crohn disease. Granulomas on biopsy are present in less than 25% of patients but are highly suggestive of Crohn disease. CT or MR enterography or a barium upper gastrointestinal series with small bowel follow-through often is obtained in patients with suspected small bowel involvement. Suggestive findings include ulcerations, strictures, and fistulas; in addition, CT or MR enterography may identify bowel wall thickening and vascularity, mucosal enhancement, and fat stranding. Capsule imaging may help establish a diagnosis when clinical suspicion for small bowel involvement is high but radiographs are normal or nondiagnostic.

▶ Complications

A. Abscess

The presence of a tender abdominal mass with fever and leukocytosis suggests an abscess. Emergent CT of the abdomen is necessary to confirm the diagnosis. Patients should be given broad-spectrum antibiotics. Percutaneous drainage or surgery is usually required.

B. Obstruction

Small bowel obstruction may develop secondary to active inflammation or chronic fibrotic stricturing and is often acutely precipitated by dietary indiscretion. Patients should be given intravenous fluids with nasogastric suction. Systemic corticosteroids are indicated in patients with symptoms or signs of active inflammation but are unhelpful in patients with inactive, fixed disease. Patients unimproved on medical management require surgical resection of the stenotic area or stricturoplasty.

C. Abdominal and Rectovaginal Fistulas

Many fistulas are asymptomatic and require no specific therapy. Most symptomatic fistulas eventually require surgical therapy; however, medical therapy is effective in a subset of patients and is usually tried first in outpatients who otherwise are stable. Large abscesses associated with fistulas require percutaneous or surgical drainage. After percutaneous drainage, long-term antibiotics are administered in order to reduce recurrent infections until the fistula is closed or surgically resected. Fistulas may close temporarily in response to TPN or oral elemental diets but recur when oral feedings are resumed. Anti-TNF agents may promote closure in up to 60% within 10 weeks; however, relapse occurs in over one-half of patients within 1 year despite continued therapy. Surgical therapy is required for symptomatic fistulas that do not respond to medical therapy. Fistulas that arise above (proximal to) areas of intestinal stricturing commonly require surgical treatment.

D. Perianal Disease

Patients with fissures, fistulas, and skin tags commonly have perianal discomfort. Successful treatment of active intestinal disease also may improve perianal disease. Specific treatment of perianal disease can be difficult and is best approached jointly with a surgeon with an expertise in colorectal disorders. Pelvic MRI is the best noninvasive study for evaluating perianal fistulas. Patients should be instructed on proper perianal skin care, including gentle wiping with a premoistened pad (baby wipes) followed by drying with a cool hair dryer, daily cleansing with sitz baths or a water wash, and use of perianal cotton balls or pads to absorb drainage. Oral antibiotics (metronidazole, 250 mg three times daily, or ciprofloxacin, 500 mg twice daily) may promote symptom improvement or healing in patients with fissures or uncomplicated fistulas; however, recurrent symptoms are common. Refractory fissures may benefit from mesalamine suppositories or topical 0.1% tacrolimus ointment. Immunomodulators or anti-TNF agents or both promote short-term symptomatic improvement from anal fistulas in two-thirds of patients and complete closure in up to one-half of patients; however, less than one-third maintain symptomatic remission during long-term maintenance treatment.

Anorectal abscesses should be suspected in patients with severe, constant perianal pain, or perianal pain in association with fever. Superficial abscesses are evident on perianal examination, but deep perirectal abscesses may be detected by digital examination or pelvic CT scan. Depending on the abscess location, surgical drainage may be achieved by incision, or catheter or seton placement. Surgery should be considered for patients with severe, refractory symptoms but is best approached after medical therapy of the Crohn disease has been optimized.

E. Carcinoma

Patients with colonic Crohn disease are at increased risk for developing colon carcinoma; hence, annual screening colonoscopy to detect dysplasia or cancer is recommended for patients with a history of 8 or more years of Crohn colitis. Patients with Crohn disease have an increased risk of lymphoma and of small bowel adenocarcinoma; however, both are rare.

F. Hemorrhage

Unlike ulcerative colitis, severe hemorrhage is unusual in Crohn disease.

G. Malabsorption

Malabsorption may arise after extensive surgical resections of the small intestine and from bacterial overgrowth in patients with enterocolonic fistulas, strictures, and stasis resulting in bacterial overgrowth.

▶ Differential Diagnosis

Chronic cramping abdominal pain and diarrhea are typical of both irritable bowel syndrome and Crohn disease, but radiographic examinations are normal in the former. Celiac disease may cause diarrhea with malabsorption. Acute fever and right lower quadrant pain may resemble appendicitis or *Yersinia enterocolitica* enteritis. Intestinal lymphoma causes fever, pain, weight loss, and abnormal small bowel radiographs that may mimic Crohn disease. Patients with undiagnosed AIDS may present with fever and diarrhea. Segmental colitis may be caused by tuberculosis, *E histolytica*, *Chlamydia*, or ischemic colitis. *C difficile* or CMV infection may develop in patients with inflammatory bowel disease, mimicking disease recurrence. Diverticulitis or appendicitis with abscess formation may be difficult to distinguish acutely from Crohn disease. NSAIDs may exacerbate inflammatory bowel disease and may also cause NSAID-induced colitis characterized by small bowel or colonic ulcers, erosion, or strictures that tend to be most severe in the terminal ileum and right colon.

▶ Treatment of Active Disease

Crohn disease is a chronic lifelong illness characterized by exacerbations and periods of remission. As no specific therapy exists, current treatment is directed toward symptomatic improvement and control of the disease process, in order to improve quality of life and reduce disease progression and complications. Although sustained clinical remission should be the therapeutic goal, this cannot be achieved in all patients. Choice of therapies depends on the disease location and severity, patient age and comorbidities, and patient preference. Early introduction of biologic therapy should be considered strongly in patients with risk factors for aggressive disease, including young age, perianal disease, stricturing disease, or need for corticosteroids. All patients with Crohn disease should be counseled to discontinue cigarettes.

A. Nutrition

1. Diet—Patients should eat a well-balanced diet with as few restrictions as possible. Eating smaller but more frequent meals may be helpful. Patients with diarrhea should be encouraged to drink fluids to avoid dehydration. Many patients report that certain foods worsen symptoms, especially fried or greasy foods. Because lactose intolerance is common, a trial off dairy products is warranted if flatulence or diarrhea is a prominent complaint. Patients with obstructive symptoms should be placed on a low-roughage diet, ie, no raw fruits or vegetables, popcorn, nuts, etc. Resection of more than 100 cm of terminal ileum results in fat malabsorption for which a low-fat diet is recommended. Parenteral vitamin B_{12} (1000 mcg subcutaneously per month) commonly is needed for patients with previous ileal resection or extensive terminal ileal disease.

2. Enteral therapy—Supplemental enteral therapy via nasogastric tube may be required for children and adolescents with poor intake and growth retardation.

3. Total parenteral nutrition—TPN is used short term in patients with active disease and progressive weight loss or those awaiting surgery who have malnutrition but cannot tolerate enteral feedings because of high-grade obstruction, high-output fistulas, severe diarrhea, or abdominal pain. It is required long term in a small subset of patients with extensive intestinal resections resulting in short bowel syndrome with malnutrition.

B. Symptomatic Medications

There are several potential mechanisms by which diarrhea may occur in Crohn disease in addition to active Crohn disease. A rational empiric treatment approach often yields therapeutic improvement that may obviate the need for corticosteroids or immunosuppressive agents. Involvement of the terminal ileum with Crohn disease or prior ileal resection may lead to reduced absorption of bile acids that may induce secretory diarrhea from the colon. This diarrhea commonly responds to cholestyramine 2–4 g, colestipol 5 g, or colesevelam 625 mg one to two times daily before meals to bind the malabsorbed bile salts. Patients with extensive ileal disease (requiring more than 100 cm of ileal resection) have such severe bile salt malabsorption that steatorrhea may arise. Such patients may benefit from a low-fat diet; bile salt-binding agents will exacerbate the diarrhea and should not be given. Patients with Crohn disease are at risk for the development of small intestinal bacterial overgrowth due to enteral fistulas, ileal resection, and impaired motility and may benefit from a course of broad-spectrum antibiotics (see Bacterial Overgrowth, above). Other causes of diarrhea include lactase deficiency and short bowel syndrome (described in other sections).

Use of oral antidiarrheal agents may provide benefit in some patients. Loperamide (2–4 mg), diphenoxylate with atropine (one tablet), or tincture of opium (5–15 drops) may be given as needed up to four times daily. Because of the risk of toxic megacolon, these drugs should not be used in patients with active severe colitis.

C. Specific Drug Therapy

1. 5-Aminosalicylic acid agents—Mesalamine has long been used as initial therapy for the treatment of mild to moderately active colonic and ileocolonic Crohn disease. However, meta-analyses of published and unpublished trial data suggest that mesalamine is of no value in either the treatment of active Crohn disease or the maintenance of remission. Current treatment guidelines recommend against its use for Crohn disease.

2. Antibiotics—Antibiotics also are widely used by clinicians for the treatment of active luminal Crohn disease, although meta-analyses of controlled trials suggest that they have little or no efficacy. It is hypothesized that antibiotics may reduce inflammation through alteration of gut flora, reduction of bacterial overgrowth, or treatment of microperforations. Oral metronidazole (10 mg/kg/day) or ciprofloxacin (500 mg twice daily), or rifaximin (800 mg twice daily) are commonly administered for 6–12 weeks.

3. Corticosteroids—Approximately one-half of patients with Crohn disease require corticosteroids at some time in their illness. Corticosteroids dramatically suppress the acute clinical symptoms or signs in most patients with both small and large bowel disease; however, they do not alter the underlying disease. An ileal-release budesonide preparation (Entocort), 9 mg once daily for 8–16 weeks, induces remission in 50–70% of patients with mild to moderate Crohn disease involving the terminal ileum or ascending colon. After initial treatment, budesonide is tapered over 2–4 weeks in 3 mg increments. In some patients, low-dose budesonide (6 mg/day) may be used for up to 1 year to maintain remission. Budesonide is superior to mesalamine but somewhat less effective than prednisone. However, because budesonide has markedly reduced acute and chronic steroid-related adverse effects, including smaller reductions of bone mineral density, it is preferred to other systemic corticosteroids for the treatment of mild to moderate Crohn disease involving the terminal ileum or ascending colon.

Prednisone or methylprednisolone, 40–60 mg/day, is generally administered to patients with Crohn disease that is severe, that involves the distal colon or proximal small intestine, or that has failed treatment with budesonide. Remission or significant improvement occurs in greater than 80% of patients after 8–16 weeks of therapy. After improvement at 2 weeks, tapering proceeds at 5 mg/wk until a dosage of 20 mg/day is being given. Thereafter, slow tapering by 2.5 mg/wk is recommended. Approximately 20% of patients cannot be completely withdrawn from corticosteroids without experiencing a symptomatic flare-up. Furthermore, more than 50% of patients who achieve initial remission on corticosteroids will experience a relapse within 1 year. Use of long-term low corticosteroid doses (2.5–10 mg/day) should be avoided because of associated complications. Patients requiring long-term corticosteroid treatment should be given immunomodulatory drugs (as described below) in an effort to wean them from corticosteroids.

Patients with persisting symptoms despite oral corticosteroids or those with high fever, persistent vomiting, evidence of intestinal obstruction, severe weight loss, severe abdominal tenderness, or suspicion of an abscess should be hospitalized. In patients with a tender, palpable inflammatory abdominal mass, CT scan of the abdomen should be obtained prior to administering corticosteroids to rule out an abscess. If no abscess is identified, parenteral corticosteroids should be administered (as described for ulcerative colitis below).

4. Immunomodulating drugs: Azathioprine, mercaptopurine, or methotrexate—The two main indications for immunomodulators in Crohn disease are (1) for maintenance of remission after induction with corticosteroids; and (2) for the induction of remission, in combination with anti-TNF therapy, in patients with moderate to severe active Crohn disease (discussed in next section). In the United States, mercaptopurine or azathioprine are more commonly used than methotrexate. Immunomodulators are used in up to 60% of patients with Crohn disease for maintenance after induction of remission with corticosteroids. Although the magnitude of benefit is debated, meta-analysis of controlled trials suggest that patients treated with thiopurines are 2.3 times as likely to maintain remission as patients treated with placebo, reducing the 3-year relapse rate from more than 60% to less than 25%. Methotrexate (25 mg subcutaneously weekly for 12 weeks, followed by 12.5–15 mg once weekly) is used in patients who are unresponsive to, or intolerant of, mercaptopurine or azathioprine. Because oral absorption may be erratic, parenteral administration of methotrexate is preferred. Immunomodulators do not appear to be effective at inducing remission. Two 2013 randomized controlled trials in patients with newly diagnosed Crohn disease (treated with or without corticosteroids) found equivalent corticosteroid-free remissions rates in patients treated with thiopurines or placebo. A 2013 AGA guideline has recommended against the use of thiopurine monotherapy to induce remission.

5. Anti-TNF therapies—Infliximab, adalimumab, and certolizumab are used to induce and maintain remission in patients with moderate to severe Crohn disease, including fistulizing disease. These agents are also used to treat extraintestinal manifestations of Crohn disease (except optic neuritis).

A. ACUTE INDUCTION THERAPY—Anti-TNF therapies are recommended as the preferred first-line agents to induce remission in patients with moderate to severe Crohn disease, either as monotherapy or in combination with thiopurines. Currently, there are two major controversies about the use of anti-TNF agents: (1) whether anti-TNF agents should be reserved as second-line therapy in patients with moderate to severe Crohn disease who have not responded to prior therapy with corticosteroids and immunomodulators ("step-up" therapy) or whether it should be used early in

the course of illness with the goal of inducing early remission and altering the natural history of the disease; (2) whether anti-TNF therapy should be used alone or in combination with an immunomodulator to enhance remission and reduce the development of antibodies to the anti-TNF agent. The best data support the use of anti-TNF agents early in the course of disease and suggest that "step-up therapy" (corticosteroids, followed by azathioprine, followed by infliximab) is obsolete. Furthermore, for most patients, anti-TNF therapy should be used in combination with an immunomodulator—at least during the first year of treatment. Data in support of use of early combination therapy come from a large 2010 trial (SONIC) that compared three treatment arms: combination therapy with infliximab and azathioprine versus infliximab alone or azathioprine alone in patients with moderate to severe Crohn disease who had not previously been treated with immunomodulators or anti-TNF agents. After 6 months, clinical remission (57%) and mucosal healing (44%) was significantly higher with combination therapy than with either agent alone. Combination therapy with anti-TNF and azathioprine beyond 1 year may not be appropriate in men younger than 30 years of age in whom there is a higher risk of hepatosplenic T-cell lymphoma and in adults older than 50–60 years in whom there is a higher risk of lymphoma and infectious complications. Anti-TNF serum trough levels should be obtained after induction therapy to optimize drug dosing. Low trough levels are associated with a decreased likelihood of remission and increased risk of developing anti-drug antibodies.

The doses for acute induction therapy are described above. Up to two-thirds of patients have significant clinical improvement during acute induction therapy.

B. MAINTENANCE THERAPY—After initial clinical response, symptom relapse occurs in more than 80% of patients within 1 year in the absence of further maintenance therapy. Therefore, scheduled maintenance therapy is usually recommended (infliximab, 5 mg/kg infusion every 8 weeks; adalimumab, 40 mg subcutaneous injection every 2 weeks; certolizumab, 400 mg subcutaneous injection every 4 weeks). With long-term maintenance therapy, approximately two-thirds have continued clinical response and up to one-half have complete symptom remission. Loss of efficacy is due to low anti-TNF levels, the development of antibodies to the anti-TNF agent, or inflammation that is unresponsive to anti-TNF therapy. Serum anti-TNF trough levels and drug antibody levels may guide subsequent therapy in patients who have lost response. Patients with antibodies to the anti-TNF agent should be switched to another anti-TNF agent. Patients with low serum anti-TNF trough levels and absent drug antibodies should receive increased anti-TNF dosing (infliximab 10 mg/kg; adalimumab 80 mg) or decreased dosing intervals (infliximab every 6 weeks; adalimumab every week). Patients with inadequate response despite adequate anti-TNF trough levels should be changed to an alternative agent, such as vedolizumab. Concomitant therapy with anti-TNF agents and immunomodulating agents (azathioprine, mercaptopurine, or methotrexate) reduces the risk of development of antibodies to the anti-TNF agent but may increase the risk of complications (non-Hodgkin lymphoma and opportunistic infections). At this time, there is uncertainty about whether combination therapy with anti-TNF agents and immunomodulators should be continued indefinitely or converted after 1–2 years to anti-TNF monotherapy.

6. Anti-integrins—Anti-integrins may offer a therapeutic option for patients who do not respond to, or who lose response to, anti-TNF agents.

Vedolizumab, a monoclonal antibody directed against the $alpha_4beta_7$ heterodimer, is FDA-approved for the treatment of moderate to severe Crohn disease. Its purported specificity for gut leukocyte trafficking may mitigate the risk of PML. Pending further clinical studies, vedolizumab is used primarily in patients with moderate to severe Crohn disease in whom anti-TNF therapy has failed or is not tolerated. A 2014 phase III trial studying patients with Crohn disease showed that when response was lost or side effects developed to one anti-TNF therapy, switching to vedolizumab (300 mg intravenously at weeks 0 and 2) resulted in clinical remission in 26.6% of patients at week 10 compared to 12.1% of patients treated with placebo. In another phase III trial, among patients demonstrating initial clinical improvement with vedolizumab induction therapy, 39% of patients treated with long-term vedolizumab (300 mg every 8 weeks) were in remission at 1 year compared with 21.6% of patients given placebo.

Indications for Surgery

Over 50% of patients will require at least one surgical procedure. The main indications for surgery are intractability to medical therapy, intra-abdominal abscess, massive bleeding, symptomatic refractory internal or perianal fistulas, and intestinal obstruction. Patients with chronic obstructive symptoms due to a short segment of ileal stenosis are best treated with resection or stricturoplasty (rather than long-term medical therapy), which promotes rapid return of well-being and elimination of corticosteroids. After surgery, endoscopic evidence of recurrence occurs in 60% within 1 year. Endoscopic recurrence precedes clinical recurrence by months to years; clinical recurrence occurs in 20% of patients within 1 year and 80% within 10–15 years. Therapy with metronidazole, 250 mg three times daily for 3 months, or long-term therapy with immunomodulators (mercaptopurine or azathioprine) has only been modestly effective in preventing clinical and endoscopic recurrence after ileocolic resection; however, small uncontrolled studies suggest that anti-TNF therapies may prevent endoscopic recurrence in up to 90% of patients. Clinicians may choose to perform endoscopy in high-risk patients 6–12 months after surgery in order to identify patients with early endoscopic recurrence who may benefit from anti-TNF therapy.

Prognosis

With proper medical and surgical treatment, the majority of patients are able to cope with this chronic disease and its complications and lead productive lives. Few patients die as a direct consequence of the disease.

When to Refer

- For expertise in endoscopic procedures or capsule endoscopy.
- For follow-up of any patient requiring hospitalization.
- Patients with moderate to severe disease for whom therapy with immunomodulators or biologic agents is being considered.
- When surgery may be necessary.

When to Admit

- An intestinal obstruction is suspected.
- An intra-abdominal or perirectal abscess is suspected.
- A serious infectious complication is suspected, especially in patients who are immunocompromised due to concomitant use of corticosteroids, immunomodulators, or anti-TNF agents.
- Patients with severe symptoms of diarrhea, dehydration, weight loss, or abdominal pain.
- Patients with severe or persisting symptoms despite treatment with corticosteroids.

Cheifetz A. JAMA patient page. Crohn disease. JAMA. 2014 Oct 22–29;312(16):1708. [PMID: 25335164]

Jones JL et al. Effects of concomitant immunomodulator therapy on efficacy and safety of anti-tumor necrosis factor therapy for Crohn's disease: a meta-analysis of placebo-controlled trials. Clin Gastroenterol Hepatol. 2015 Dec;13(13):2233–40.e2. [PMID: 26142167]

Lee D et al. Diet in the pathogenesis and treatment of inflammatory bowel diseases. Gastroenterology. 2015 May;148(6):1087–106. [PMID: 25597840]

Panés J et al; AZTEC Study Group. Early azathioprine therapy is no more effective than placebo for newly diagnosed Crohn's disease. Gastroenterology. 2013 Oct;145(4):766–74.e1. [PMID: 23770132]

Sandborn WJ et al; GEMINI 2 Study Group. Vedolizumab as induction and maintenance therapy for Crohn's disease. N Engl J Med. 2013 Aug 22;369(8):711–21. [PMID: 23964933]

Sands BE et al. Effects of vedolizumab induction therapy for patients with Crohn's disease in whom tumor necrosis factor antagonist treatment failed. Gastroenterology. 2014 Sep;147(3):618–627.e3. [PMID: 24859203]

Savarino E et al. Adalimumab is more effective than azathioprine and mesalamine at preventing postoperative recurrence of Crohn's disease: a randomized controlled trial. Am J Gastroenterol. 2013 Nov;108(11):1731–42. [PMID: 24019080]

Schwartz DA et al. Guidelines for medical treatment of Crohn's perianal fistulas: critical evaluation of therapeutic trials. Inflamm Bowel Dis. 2015 Apr;21(4):737–52. [PMID: 25751068]

Terdiman JP et al. American Gastroenterological Association Institute guide on the use of thiopurines, methotrexate, and anti-TNF-alpha biologic drugs for the induction and maintenance of remission in inflammatory Crohn's disease. Gastroenterology. 2013 Dec;145(6):1459–63. [PMID: 24267474]

Vande Casteele N et al. Trough concentrations of infliximab guide dosing for patients with inflammatory bowel disease. Gastroenterology. 2015 Jun;148(7):1320–9.e3. [PMID: 25724455]

Yanai H et al. Levels of drug and antidrug antibodies are associated with outcome of interventions after loss of response to infliximab or adalimumab. Clin Gastroenterol Hepatol. 2015 Mar;13(3):522–30.e2. [PMID: 25066837]

2. Ulcerative Colitis

▶ Bloody diarrhea.

▶ Lower abdominal cramps and fecal urgency.

▶ Anemia, low serum albumin.

▶ Negative stool cultures.

▶ Sigmoidoscopy is the key to diagnosis.

General Considerations

Ulcerative colitis is an idiopathic inflammatory condition that involves the mucosal surface of the colon, resulting in diffuse friability and erosions with bleeding. Approximately one-third of patients have disease confined to the rectosigmoid region (proctosigmoiditis); one-third have disease that extends to the splenic flexure (left-sided colitis); and one-third have disease that extends more proximally (extensive colitis). In patients with distal colitis, the disease progresses with time to more extensive involvement in 25–50%. There is some correlation between disease extent and symptom severity. In most patients, the disease is characterized by periods of symptomatic flare-ups and remissions. Ulcerative colitis is more common in nonsmokers and former smokers. Disease severity may be lower in active smokers and may worsen in patients who stop smoking. Appendectomy before the age of 20 years for acute appendicitis is associated with a reduced risk of developing ulcerative colitis.

Clinical Findings

A. Symptoms and Signs

The clinical profile in ulcerative colitis is highly variable. Bloody diarrhea is the hallmark. On the basis of several clinical and laboratory parameters, it is clinically useful to classify patients as having mild, moderate, or severe disease (Table 15–12). Patients should be asked about stool frequency, the presence and amount of rectal bleeding, cramps, abdominal pain, fecal urgency, and tenesmus. Physical examination should focus on the patient's volume status as determined by orthostatic blood pressure and pulse measurements and by nutritional status. On abdominal examination, the clinician should look for tenderness and evidence of peritoneal inflammation. Red blood may be present on digital rectal examination.

1. Mild to moderate disease—Patients with mild disease have a gradual onset of infrequent diarrhea (less than four movements per day) with intermittent rectal bleeding and mucus. Stools may be formed or loose in consistency. Because of rectal inflammation, there is fecal urgency and tenesmus. Left lower quadrant cramps relieved by defecation are common, but there is no significant abdominal tenderness. Patients with moderate disease have more severe diarrhea with frequent bleeding. Abdominal pain and tenderness may be present but are not severe. There may be mild fever, anemia, and hypoalbuminemia.

2. Severe disease—Patients with severe disease have more than six bloody bowel movements per day, resulting in severe anemia, hypovolemia, and impaired nutrition with hypoalbuminemia. Abdominal pain and tenderness are present. "Fulminant colitis" is a subset of severe disease characterized by rapidly worsening symptoms with signs of toxicity.

B. Laboratory Findings

The degree of abnormality of the hematocrit, sedimentation rate, and serum albumin reflects disease severity.

C. Endoscopy

In acute colitis, the diagnosis is readily established by sigmoidoscopy. The mucosal appearance is characterized by edema, friability, mucopus, and erosions. Colonoscopy should not be performed in patients with fulminant disease because of the risk of perforation. After patients have demonstrated improvement on therapy, colonoscopy is performed to determine the extent of disease.

D. Imaging

Plain abdominal radiographs are obtained in patients with severe colitis to look for significant colonic dilation. Barium enemas are of little utility in the evaluation of acute ulcerative colitis and may precipitate toxic megacolon in patients with severe disease.

Differential Diagnosis

The initial presentation of ulcerative colitis is indistinguishable from other causes of colitis, clinically as well as endoscopically. Thus, the diagnosis of idiopathic ulcerative colitis is reached after excluding other known causes of colitis. Infectious colitis should be excluded by sending stool specimens for routine bacterial cultures (to exclude *Salmonella*, *Shigella*, and *Campylobacter*, as well as specific assays for *E coli* O157), ova and parasites (to exclude amebiasis), and stool toxin assay for *C difficile*. Mucosal biopsy

Table 15–12. Ulcerative colitis: Assessment of disease activity.

	Mild	Moderate	Severe
Stool frequency (per day)	< 4	4–6	> 6 (mostly bloody)
Pulse (beats/min)	< 90	90–100	> 100
Hematocrit (%)	Normal	30–40	< 30
Weight loss (%)	None	1–10	> 10
Temperature (°F)	Normal	99–100	> 100
ESR (mm/h)	< 20	20–30	> 30
Albumin (g/dL)	Normal	3–3.5	< 3

ESR, erythrocyte sedimentation rate.

can distinguish amebic colitis from ulcerative colitis. CMV colitis occurs in immunocompromised patients, including patients receiving prolonged corticosteroid therapy, and is diagnosed on mucosal biopsy. Gonorrhea, chlamydial infection, herpes, and syphilis are considerations in sexually active patients with proctitis. In elderly patients with cardiovascular disease, ischemic colitis may involve the rectosigmoid. A history of radiation to the pelvic region can result in proctitis months to years later. Crohn disease involving the colon but not the small intestine may be confused with ulcerative colitis. In 10% of patients, a distinction between Crohn disease and ulcerative colitis may not be possible.

► **Treatment**

There are two main treatment objectives: (1) to terminate the acute, symptomatic attack and (2) to prevent recurrence of attacks. The treatment of acute ulcerative colitis depends on the extent of colonic involvement and the severity of illness.

Patients with mild to moderate disease should eat a regular diet but limit their intake of caffeine and gas-producing vegetables. Antidiarrheal agents should not be given in the acute phase of illness but are safe and helpful in patients with mild chronic symptoms. Oral loperamide (2 mg) or diphenoxylate with atropine (one tablet) may be given up to four times daily. Such remedies are particularly useful at nighttime and when taken prophylactically for occasions when patients may not have reliable access to toilet facilities.

A. Mild to Moderate Distal Colitis

Patients with disease confined to the rectum or rectosigmoid region generally have mild to moderate but distressing symptoms. Patients may be treated with topical mesalamine, topical corticosteroids, or oral aminosalicylates (5-ASA) according to patient preference and cost considerations. Topical mesalamine is the drug of choice and is superior to topical corticosteroids and 5-ASA. Mesalamine is administered as a suppository, 1000 mg once daily at bedtime for proctitis, and as an enema, 4 g at bedtime for proctosigmoiditis, for 4–8 weeks, with 75% of patients improving. Patients who either decline or are unable to manage topical therapy may be treated with oral 5-ASA, as discussed below. Topical corticosteroids are a less expensive alternative to mesalamine but are also less effective. Hydrocortisone enema or foam (80–100 mg) or budesonide foam are prescribed for proctitis or proctosigmoiditis. Systemic effects from short-term use are very slight. For patients with distal disease who do not improve with topical or oral mesalamine therapy, the following options may be considered: (1) a combination of a topical agent with an oral 5-ASA agent is more effective than either drug alone; (2) combination topical therapy with a 5-ASA suppository or enema at bedtime and a corticosteroid enema or foam in the morning; or (3) a combination of oral 5-ASA agent, topical 5-ASA agent, and a topical corticosteroid. Patients with distal colitis who are refractory to all of these therapies or who have severe disease may require treatment with oral prednisone 40–60 mg/day or infliximab, as described below.

Most patients with proctitis or proctosigmoiditis who achieve complete remission with oral or rectal 5-ASA should continue indefinitely on the same therapy to reduce the likelihood of symptomatic relapse. Maintenance treatment with 5-ASA reduces the 12-month relapse rate from 75% to less than 40%. Some patients, however, may prefer intermittent therapy for symptomatic relapse. Topical corticosteroids are ineffective for maintaining remission of distal colitis.

B. Mild to Moderate Colitis

1. 5-ASA Agents—Disease extending above the sigmoid colon is best treated with oral 5-ASA agents (mesalamine, balsalazide, or sulfasalazine), which result in symptomatic improvement in 50–75% of patients. The optimal dose for induction of remission of mild disease is 2.4 g once daily and for moderate disease is 2.4–4.8 g once daily. Most patients improve within 4–8 weeks. These agents achieve clinical improvement in 50–70% of patients and remission in 20–30%. Oral sulfasalazine is comparable in efficacy to mesalamine and because of its low cost is still commonly used as a first-line agent by many providers, though it is associated with greater side effects. To minimize side effects, sulfasalazine is begun at a dosage of 500 mg twice daily and increased gradually over 1–2 weeks to 2 g twice daily. Total doses of 5–6 g/day may have greater efficacy but are poorly tolerated. Folic acid, 1 mg/day orally, should be administered to all patients taking sulfasalazine.

2. Corticosteroids—Patients with mild to moderate disease who do not improve within 4–8 weeks of 5-ASA therapy should have corticosteroid therapy added. Prednisone and methylprednisolone are most commonly used. Depending on the severity of illness, the initial oral dose of prednisone is 40–60 mg daily. Rapid improvement is observed in most cases within 2 weeks. Thereafter, tapering of prednisone should proceed by 5–10 mg/wk. After tapering to 20 mg/day, slower tapering (2.5 mg/week) is sometimes required. Complete tapering without symptomatic flare-ups is possible in the majority of patients. Delayed-release budesonide (Uceris) 9 mg ER orally once daily has shown modest benefit in mild to moderate colitis, achieving remission in 17.5% of patients after 8 weeks compared with 12.5% with placebo. In view of its low incidence of corticosteroid-associated side-effects, it may be considered in patients with mild colitis for whom other systemic corticosteroids are deemed high risk.

3. Immunomodulating agents—Approximately 30% of patients either do not respond to corticosteroids or have symptomatic flares during attempts at corticosteroid tapering and develop steroid dependency. Patients with steroid dependency may be treated with thiopurines (mercaptopurine or azathioprine), although rigorous controlled trials are lacking and their absolute benefit appears to be modest compared with other alternatives (anti-TNF or vedolizumab). Methotrexate does not appear to be effective.

The anti-TNF agents infliximab, adalimumab, and golimumab are approved in the United States for the treatment of patients with moderate to severe ulcerative colitis who have had an inadequate response to conventional therapies (oral corticosteroids, mercaptopurine or azathioprine, and mesalamine). Following a three-dose induction regimen of infliximab 5 mg/kg administered at 0, 2, and 6 weeks, clinical response occurs in 65%. In two, large, controlled studies of patients with active moderate to severe colitis, initial induction therapy was followed by infliximab maintenance infusions (5 mg/kg) administered every 8 weeks for 30–54 weeks. At the end of the study (30 or 54 weeks), 35% were in clinical remission (and 21% were in corticosteroid-free remission), a modest but impressive response in patients with more refractory disease. By comparison, phase III trials of adalimumab and golimumab reported clinical response rates of 50–59% and remission rates of 16–21% after 8 weeks. Although the response and remission rates appear lower with adalimumab and golimumab than infliximab, differences in study design and patient populations limit comparisons. Importantly, 40% of patients in the adalimumab trials were previously treated with other anti-TNF agents, in whom lower response rates were noted. When initiating anti-TNF therapy, it should be combined in most patients with an immunomodulator (azathioprine, mercaptopurine, or methotrexate) for at least the first year. Combination therapy increases the likelihood of disease remission and reduces the development of antibodies that may result in secondary loss of response to anti-TNF therapies. After initiating anti-TNF therapy, serum trough levels and anti-drug antibody titers should be obtained at least once in order to optimize drug dosing.

4. Anti-integrin therapy—Vedolizumab, a monoclonal antibody directed against the alpha$_4$beta$_7$ heterodimer, is FDA-approved for the treatment of moderate to severe ulcerative colitis in patients who have not responded to, lost response to, or been intolerant of other therapies. In a phase III clinical trial of patients with moderate to severe ulcerative colitis, vedolizumab induction (300 mg intravenously at 0, 2, and 6 weeks) led to clinical improvement in 47.1% of patients compared with 25.5% who were given placebo. Among patients who demonstrated initial clinical improvement, 41.8% of those given long-term maintenance treatment with vedolizumab (300 mg intravenous every 8 weeks) were in clinical remission at 1 year compared with 15.9% of those given placebo. At present, vedolizumab is recommended for treatment of acute cases and maintenance therapy in patients with moderate to severe ulcerative colitis who have not responded to or have lost response to anti-TNF therapy or immunomodulator therapy, or both.

5. Probiotics—VSL#3 (two packets twice daily), a probiotic compound containing eight different nonpathogenic strains of lactobacilli, bifidobacteria, and streptococci, has demonstrated significant benefit versus placebo in the treatment of mild to moderate ulcerative colitis in two randomized, controlled multicenter trials. Although its efficacy relative to other agents is unclear, it may be considered as an adjunctive therapy for mild to moderate disease.

C. Severe and Fulminant Colitis

About 15% of patients with ulcerative colitis have a more severe course. Of these, a small subset has a fulminant course with rapid progression of symptoms over 1–2 weeks and signs of severe toxicity. These patients appear quite ill, with fever, prominent hypovolemia, hemorrhage requiring transfusion, and abdominal distention with tenderness. Toxic megacolon develops in less than 2% of cases of ulcerative colitis. It is characterized by colonic dilation of more than 6 cm on plain films with signs of toxicity.

1. General measures—Discontinue all oral intake for 24–48 hours or until the patient demonstrates clinical improvement. TPN is indicated only in patients with poor nutritional status or if feedings cannot be reinstituted within 7–10 days. All opioid or anticholinergic agents should be discontinued. Restore circulating volume with fluids, correct electrolyte abnormalities, and consider transfusion for significant anemia (hematocrit less than 25–28%). A plain abdominal radiograph should be ordered on admission to look for evidence of colonic dilation. Send stools for bacterial culture, *C difficile* toxin assay, and examination for ova and parasites. CMV superinfection should be considered in patients receiving long-term immunosuppressive therapy who are unresponsive to corticosteroid therapy. Due to a high risk of venous thromboembolic disease, prophylaxis should be administered to all hospitalized patients with inflammatory bowel disease. Surgical consultation should be sought for all patients with severe disease.

Patients with fulminant disease are at higher risk for perforation or toxic megacolon and must be monitored closely. Abdominal examinations should be repeated to look for evidence of worsening distention or pain. Broad-spectrum antibiotics should be administered to cover anaerobes and gram-negative bacteria. In addition to the therapies outlined above, nasogastric suction should be initiated. Patients should be instructed to roll from side to side and onto the abdomen in an effort to decompress the distended colon. Serial abdominal plain films should be obtained to look for worsening dilation or signs of ischemia. Patients with fulminant disease or toxic megacolon who worsen or do not improve within 48–72 hours should undergo surgery to prevent perforation. If the operation is performed before perforation, the mortality rate should be low.

2. Corticosteroid therapy—Methylprednisolone, 48–64 mg, or hydrocortisone, 300 mg, is administered intravenously in four divided doses or by continuous infusion over 24 hours. Higher or "pulse" doses are of no benefit. Hydrocortisone enemas (100 mg) may also be administered twice daily for treatment of urgency or tenesmus. Approximately 50–75% of patients achieve remission with systemic corticosteroids within 7–10 days. Once symptomatic improvement has occurred, oral fluids are reinstituted. If fluids are well tolerated, intravenous corticosteroids are discontinued and the patient is started on oral prednisone (as described for moderate disease). Patients without significant improvement within 3–5 days of intravenous corticosteroid therapy should be referred for surgery or considered for anti-TNF therapies or cyclosporine.

3. Anti-TNF therapies—Infusion of infliximab, 5 mg/kg, has been shown in controlled and uncontrolled studies to be effective in treating severe colitis in patients who did not improve within 4–7 days of intravenous corticosteroid therapy. In a controlled study of patients hospitalized for ulcerative colitis, colectomy was required within 3 months in 69% who received placebo therapy, compared with 47% who received infliximab. Thus, infliximab therapy should be considered in patients with severe ulcerative colitis who have not improved with intravenous corticosteroid therapy. Recent studies have demonstrated more rapid clearance of infliximab in patients with severe ulcerative colitis. Uncontrolled trials have found lower colectomy rates in patients administered higher doses of infliximab (three infusions of 5–10 mg/kg within 2–3 weeks) than with conventional dosing (5 mg/kg at 0, 2, and 6 weeks). (See Crohn Disease.)

4. Cyclosporine—Intravenous cyclosporine (2–4 mg/kg/day as a continuous infusion) benefits 60–75% of patients with severe colitis who have not improved after 7–10 days of corticosteroids, but it is associated with significant toxicity (nephrotoxicity, seizures, infection, hypertension). Up to two-thirds of responders may be maintained in remission with a combination of oral cyclosporine for 3 months and long-term therapy with mercaptopurine or azathioprine. A 2011 randomized study of patients with severe colitis refractory to intravenous corticosteroids found similar response rates (85%) with cyclosporine and infliximab therapy.

5. Surgical therapy—Patients with severe disease who do not improve after corticosteroid, infliximab, or cyclosporine therapy are unlikely to respond to further medical therapy, and surgery is recommended.

Risk of Colon Cancer

In patients with ulcerative colitis with disease proximal to the rectum and in patients with Crohn colitis, there is an increased risk of developing colon carcinoma. Although older meta-analyses from referral centers reported a high risk (8% after 20 years), more recent systematic reviews of population-based studies report a 2.4-fold increased risk (1.4% after a mean of 14 years follow up). Retrospective studies suggest that the risk of colon cancer may be reduced in patients treated with long-term 5-ASA therapy. Ingestion of folic acid, 1 mg/day, also is associated with a decreased risk of cancer development. Colonoscopies are recommended every 1–2 years in patients with colitis, beginning 8 years after diagnosis. Several prospective studies demonstrate that dye spraying with methylene blue or indigo carmine ("chromoendoscopy") enhances the detection of subtle mucosal lesions, thereby significantly increasing the detection of dysplasia compared with standard colonoscopy. At colonoscopy, all adenoma-like polyps should be resected, when possible, and biopsies obtained of non-endoscopically resectable mass lesions.

Surgery in Ulcerative Colitis

Surgery is required in 25% of patients. Severe hemorrhage, perforation, and documented carcinoma are absolute indications for surgery. Surgery is indicated also in patients with fulminant colitis or toxic megacolon that does not improve within 48–72 hours, in patients with invisible flat dysplasia or non-endoscopically resectable dysplastic lesions on surveillance colonoscopy, and in patients with refractory disease requiring long-term corticosteroids to control symptoms.

Although total proctocolectomy (with placement of an ileostomy) provides complete cure of the disease, most patients seek to avoid it out of concern for the impact it may have on their bowel function, their self-image, and their social interactions. After complete colectomy, patients may have a standard ileostomy with an external appliance, a continent ileostomy, or an internal ileal pouch that is anastomosed to the anal canal (ileal pouch-anal anastomosis). The latter maintains intestinal continuity, thereby obviating an ostomy. Under optimal circumstances, patients have five to seven loose bowel movements per day without incontinence. Endoscopic or histologic inflammation in the ileal pouch ("pouchitis") develops in over 40% of patients, resulting in increased stool frequency, fecal urgency, cramping, and bleeding, but usually resolves with a 2-week course of oral metronidazole (250–500 mg three times daily) or ciprofloxacin (500 mg twice daily). Patients with frequently relapsing pouchitis may need continuous antibiotics. Probiotics containing nonpathogenic strains of lactobacilli, bifidobacteria, and streptococci (VSL#3) are effective in the maintenance of remission in patients with recurrent pouchitis.

Prognosis

Ulcerative colitis is a lifelong disease characterized by exacerbations and remissions. For most patients, the disease is readily controlled by medical therapy without need for surgery. The majority never require hospitalization. A subset of patients with more severe disease will require surgery, which results in complete cure of the disease. Properly managed, most patients with ulcerative colitis lead close to normal productive lives.

When to Refer

- Colonoscopy: for evaluation of activity and extent of active disease and for surveillance for neoplasia in patients with quiescent disease for more than 8–10 years.
- For follow-up of any patient requiring hospitalization.
- When surgical colectomy is indicated.

When to Admit

- Patients with severe disease manifested by frequent bloody stools, anemia, weight loss, and fever.
- Patients with fulminant disease manifested by rapid progression of symptoms, worsening abdominal pain, distention, high fever, tachycardia.
- Patients with moderate to severe symptoms that do not respond to oral corticosteroids and require a trial of bowel rest and intravenous corticosteroids.

Autenrieth DM et al. Toxic megacolon. Inflamm Bowel Dis. 2012 Mar;18(3):584–91. [PMID: 22009735]

Beaugerie L et al. Cancers complicating inflammatory bowel disease. N Engl J Med. 2015 Apr 9;372(15):1441–52. [PMID: 25853748]

Bitton A et al; Canadian Association of Gastroenterology Severe Ulcerative Colitis Consensus Group. Treatment of hospitalized adult patients with severe ulcerative colitis: Toronto consensus statements. Am J Gastroenterol. 2012 Feb; 107(2):179–94. [PMID: 22108451]

Bressler B et al. Clinical practice guidelines for the medical management of nonhospitalized ulcerative colitis: the Toronto consensus. Gastroenterology. 2015 May;148(5):1035–58.e3. [PMID: 25747596]

Danese S et al. Biological agents for moderately to severely active ulcerative colitis: a systematic review and network meta-analysis. Ann Intern Med. 2014 May 20;160(10):704–11. [PMID: 24842416]

Feagan BG et al; GEMINI 1 Study Group. Vedolizumab as induction and maintenance therapy for ulcerative colitis. N Engl J Med. 2013 Aug 22;369(8):699–710. [PMID: 23964932]

Gibson DJ et al. An accelerated infliximab induction regimen reduces the need for early colectomy in patients with acute severe ulcerative colitis. Clin Gastroenterol Hepatol. 2015 Feb; 13(2):330–5.e1. [PMID: 25086187]

Laine L et al. SCENIC international consensus statement on surveillance and management of dysplasia in inflammatory bowel disease. Gastrointest Endosc. 2015 Mar;81(3):489–501. e26. [PMID: 25708752]

Nguyen GC et al. Consensus statements on the risk, prevention, and treatment of venous thromboembolism in inflammatory bowel disease: Canadian Association of Gastroenterology. Gastroenterology. 2014 Mar;146(3):835–48.e6. [PMID: 24462530]

Ordás I et al. Ulcerative colitis. Lancet. 2012 Nov 3; 380(9853):1606–19. [PMID: 22914296]

Sandborn WJ et al. Budesonide foam induces remission in patients with mild to moderate ulcerative proctitis and ulcerative proctosigmoiditis. Gastroenterology. 2015 Apr; 148(4):740–50.e2. [PMID: 25644096]

Sandborn WJ et al. Subcutaneous golimumab induces clinical response and remission in patients with moderate-to-severe ulcerative colitis. Gastroenterology. 2014 Jan;146(1):85–95. [PMID: 23735746]

Soetikno R et al. The detection of nonpolypoid (flat and depressed) colorectal neoplasms in patients with inflammatory bowel disease. Gastroenterology. 2013 Jun;144(7): 1349–52.e1–6. [PMID: 23583483]

3. Microscopic Colitis

Microscopic colitis is an idiopathic condition that is found in up to 15% of patients who have chronic or intermittent watery diarrhea with normal-appearing mucosa at endoscopy. There are two major subtypes—lymphocytic colitis and collagenous colitis. In both, histologic evaluation of mucosal biopsies reveals chronic inflammation (lymphocytes, plasma cells) in the lamina propria and increased intraepithelial lymphocytes. Collagenous colitis is further characterized by the presence of a thickened band (greater than 10 mcm) of subepithelial collagen. Both forms occur more commonly in women, especially in the fifth to sixth decades. Symptoms tend to be chronic or recurrent but may remit in most patients after several years. A more severe illness characterized by abdominal pain, fatigue, dehydration, and weight loss may develop in a subset of patients. The cause of microscopic colitis usually is unknown. Several medications have been implicated as etiologic agents, including NSAIDs, proton pump inhibitors, low-dose aspirin, selective serotonin reuptake inhibitors, ACE inhibitors, and beta-blockers. Diarrhea usually abates within 30 days of stopping the offending medication. Celiac disease may be present in up to 20% of patients and should be excluded with serologic testing (antitissue transglutaminase IgA). Treatment is largely empiric since there are few well-designed, controlled treatment trials. Antidiarrheal therapy with loperamide is the first-line treatment, providing symptom improvement in up to 70%. For patients who do not respond to loperamide, the next option is delayed-release budesonide (Entocort), 9 mg/day for 6–8 weeks. Budesonide has been shown in three prospective controlled studies to induce clinical remission in greater than 80% of patients; however, relapse occurs in most patients after stopping therapy. In two prospective studies, remission was maintained in 75% of patients treated with budesonide 6 mg/day compared with 25% of persons given placebo. In clinical practice, budesonide is tapered to the lowest effective dose for suppressing symptoms. For patients who do not respond to budesonide, uncontrolled studies report that treatment with bile-salt binding agents (cholestyramine, colestipol) or 5-ASAs (sulfasalazine, mesalamine) may be effective in some patients. A small unpublished controlled trial demonstrated efficacy for bismuth subsalicylate (two tablets three times daily) for 2 months; however, clinical experience with it has shown only modest benefit. Less than 3% of patients have refractory or severe symptoms, which may be treated with immunosuppressive agents (azathioprine or methotrexate) or anti-TNF agents (infliximab, adaliumumab).

Masclee GM et al. Increased risk of microscopic colitis with use of proton pump inhibitors and non-steroidal anti-inflammatory drugs. Am J Gastroenterol. 2015 May;110(5):749–59. [PMID: 25916221]

Münch A et al. Microscopic colitis: clinical and pathologic perspectives. Clin Gastroenterol Hepatol. 2015 Feb;13(2):228–36. [PMID: 24407107]

Tong J et al. Incidence, prevalence, and temporal trends of microscopic colitis: a systematic review and meta-analysis. Am J Gastroenterol. 2015 Feb;110(2):265–76. [PMID: 25623658]

DIVERTICULAR DISEASE OF THE COLON

Colonic diverticulosis increases with age, ranging from 5% in those under age 40, to 30% at age 60, to more than 50% over age 80 years in Western societies. Most are asymptomatic, discovered incidentally at endoscopy or on barium enema. Complications occur in less than 5%, including gastrointestinal bleeding and diverticulitis.

Colonic diverticula may vary in size from a few millimeters to several centimeters and in number from one to several dozen. Almost all patients with diverticulosis have involvement in the sigmoid and descending colon; however, only 15% have proximal colonic disease.

For over 40 years, it has been believed that diverticulosis arises after many years of a diet deficient in fiber. Recent epidemiologic studies challenge this theory, finding no association between the prevalence of asymptomatic diverticulosis and low dietary fiber intake or constipation. Thus, the etiology of diverticulosis is uncertain. The extent to which abnormal motility and hereditary factors contribute to diverticular disease is unknown. Patients with abnormal connective tissue are also disposed to development of diverticulosis, including Ehlers-Danlos syndrome, Marfan syndrome, and scleroderma.

1. Uncomplicated Diverticulosis

More than 90% of patients with diverticulosis have uncomplicated disease and no specific symptoms. In most, diverticulosis is an incidental finding detected during colonoscopic examination or barium enema examination. Some patients have nonspecific complaints of chronic constipation, abdominal pain, or fluctuating bowel habits. It is unclear whether these symptoms are due to alterations in the colonic motility, visceral hypersensitivity, gut microbiota, or low-grade inflammation. Physical examination is usually normal but may reveal mild left lower quadrant tenderness with a thickened, palpable sigmoid and descending colon. Screening laboratory studies should be normal in uncomplicated diverticulosis.

There is no reason to perform imaging studies for the purpose of diagnosing asymptomatic, uncomplicated disease. Diverticula are well seen on barium enema, colonoscopy and CT imaging. Involved segments of colon may also be narrowed and deformed.

Patients in whom diverticulosis is discovered, especially patients with symptoms or a history of complicated disease should be treated with a high-fiber diet or fiber supplements (bran powder, 1–2 tbsp twice daily; psyllium or methylcellulose) (see section on constipation). Retrospective studies suggest that such treatment may decrease the likelihood of subsequent complications.

Almerie MQ et al. Diagnosing and treating diverticular disease. Practitioner. 2015 Sep;259(1785):29–33. [PMID: 26591654]
Elisei W et al. Recent advances in the treatment of colonic diverticular disease and prevention of acute diverticulitis. Ann Gastroenterol. 2016 Jan–Mar;29(1):24–32. [PMID: 26752946]

2. Diverticulitis

ESSENTIALS OF DIAGNOSIS

▶ Acute abdominal pain and fever.
▶ Left lower abdominal tenderness and mass.
▶ Leukocytosis.

▶ Clinical Findings

A. Symptoms and Signs

Diverticulitis is defined as macroscopic inflammation of a diverticulum that may reflect a spectrum from inflammation alone, to microperforation with localized paracolic

inflammation, to macroperforation with either abscess or generalized peritonitis. Thus, there is a range from mild to severe disease. Most patients with localized inflammation or infection report mild to moderate aching abdominal pain, usually in the left lower quadrant. Constipation or loose stools may be present. Nausea and vomiting are frequent. In many cases, symptoms are so mild that the patient may not seek medical attention until several days after onset. Physical findings include a low-grade fever, left lower quadrant tenderness, and a palpable mass. Stool occult blood is common, but hematochezia is rare. Leukocytosis is mild to moderate. Patients with free perforation present with a more dramatic picture of generalized abdominal pain and peritoneal signs.

B. Imaging

In patients with mild symptoms and a presumptive diagnosis of diverticulitis, empiric medical therapy is started without further imaging in the acute phase. Patients who respond to acute medical management should undergo complete colonic evaluation with colonoscopy or radiologic imaging (CT colonography or barium enema) after resolution of clinical symptoms to corroborate the diagnosis or exclude other disorders such as colonic neoplasms. In patients who do not improve rapidly after 2–4 days of empiric therapy and in those with severe disease, CT scan of the abdomen is obtained to look for evidence of diverticulitis and determine its severity, and to exclude other disorders that may cause lower abdominal pain. The presence of colonic diverticula and wall thickening, pericolic fat infiltration, abscess formation, or extraluminal air or contrast suggests diverticulitis. Endoscopy and colonography are contraindicated during the initial stages of an acute attack because of the risk of free perforation.

▶ Differential Diagnosis

Diverticulitis must be distinguished from other causes of lower abdominal pain, including perforated colonic carcinoma, Crohn disease, appendicitis, ischemic colitis, *C difficile*-associated colitis, and gynecologic disorders (ectopic pregnancy, ovarian cyst or torsion) by abdominal CT scan, pelvic ultrasonography, or radiographic studies of the distal colon that use water-soluble contrast enemas.

▶ Complications

Chronic inflammation or an untreated abscess may lead to fistula formation that may involve the bladder, ureter, vagina, uterus, bowel, and abdominal wall. Acute or chronic inflammation may result in stricturing of the colon with partial or complete obstruction.

▶ Treatment

A. Medical Management

Most patients can be managed with conservative measures. Patients with mild symptoms and no peritoneal signs may be managed initially as outpatients on a clear liquid diet.

Although broad-spectrum oral antibiotics with anaerobic activity commonly are prescribed, large clinical trials confirm that antibiotics are not beneficial in uncomplicated disease. A 2015 American Gastroenterological Association guideline suggests that antibiotics should be used selectively for uncomplicated disease. Reasonable regimens include amoxicillin and clavulanate potassium (875 mg/125 mg) twice daily; or metronidazole, 500 mg three times daily; plus either ciprofloxacin, 500 mg twice daily, or trimethoprim-sulfamethoxazole, 160/800 mg twice daily orally, for 7–10 days or until the patient is afebrile for 3–5 days. Symptomatic improvement usually occurs within 3 days, at which time the diet may be advanced. Once the acute episode has resolved, a high-fiber diet is often recommended. Patients with increasing pain, fever, or inability to tolerate oral fluids require hospitalization. Patients with severe diverticulitis (high fevers, leukocytosis, or peritoneal signs) and patients who are elderly or immunosuppressed or who have serious comorbid disease require hospitalization acutely. Patients should be given nothing by mouth and should receive intravenous fluids. If ileus is present, a nasogastric tube should be placed. Intravenous antibiotics should be given to cover anaerobic and gram-negative bacteria. Single-agent therapy with either a second-generation cephalosporin (eg, cefoxitin), piperacillin-tazobactam, or ticarcillin clavulanate appears to be as effective as combination therapy (eg, metronidazole or clindamycin plus an aminoglycoside or third-generation cephalosporin [eg, ceftazidime, cefotaxime]). Symptomatic improvement should be evident within 2–3 days. Intravenous antibiotics should be continued for 5–7 days, before changing to oral antibiotics.

B. Surgical Management

Surgical consultation and repeat abdominal CT imaging should be obtained on all patients with severe disease or those who do not improve after 72 hours of medical management. Patients with a localized abdominal abscess 4 cm in size or larger are usually treated urgently with a percutaneous catheter drain placed by an interventional radiologist. This permits control of the infection and resolution of the immediate infectious inflammatory process. In this manner, a subsequent elective one-stage surgical operation can be performed (if deemed necessary) in which the diseased segment of colon is removed and primary colonic anastomosis performed. After recovery, the decision to perform elective surgery depends on the patient's age, comorbid disease, and frequency and severity of attacks. Patients with chronic disease resulting in fistulas or colonic obstruction will require elective surgical resection.

Indications for emergent surgical management include generalized peritonitis, large undrainable abscesses, and clinical deterioration despite medical management and percutaneous drainage. Surgery may be performed in one- or two-stage operations depending on the patient's nutritional status, severity of illness, and extent of intra-abdominal peritonitis and abscess formation.

Prognosis

Diverticulitis recurs in 10–30% of patients treated with medical management over 10–20 years. However, less than 5% have more than two recurrences. Recurrent attacks may warrant elective surgical resection in selected patients. Diverticulosis is not associated with an increased risk of colorectal cancer. Nonetheless, colorectal cancer may cause symptoms that may be confused with diverticulitis. Therefore, colonoscopy is recommended in patients over age 50 who have not undergone appropriate screening and should be considered in other high-risk patients, especially those with suspicious radiologic imaging, diverticulitis with complications or protracted symptoms, or family history of colorectal cancer.

When to Refer

- Failure to improve within 72 hours of medical management.
- Presence of significant peridiverticular abscesses (4 cm or larger) requiring possible percutaneous or surgical drainage.
- Generalized peritonitis or sepsis.
- Recurrent attacks.
- Chronic complications including colonic strictures or fistulas.

When to Admit

- Severe pain or inability to tolerate oral intake.
- Signs of sepsis or peritonitis.
- CT scan showing signs of complicated disease (abscess, perforation).
- Failure to improve with outpatient management.
- Immunocompromised or frail, elderly patient.

Bharucha AE et al. Temporal trends in the incidence and natural history of diverticulitis: a population-based study. Am J Gastroenterol. 2015 Nov;110(11):1589–96. [PMID: 26416187]

Daniels L et al. Routine colonoscopy after left-sided acute uncomplicated diverticulitis: a systematic review. Gastrointest Endosc. 2014 Mar;79(3):378–89. [PMID: 24434085]

Huang WY et al. Association between colonic diverticular disease and colorectal cancer: a nationwide population-based study. Clin Gastroenterol Hepatol. 2014 Aug;12(8):1288–94. [PMID: 24361412]

Peery AF et al. Diverticular disease: reconsidering conventional wisdom. Clin Gastroenterol Hepatol. 2013 Dec;11(12):1532–7. [PMID: 23669306]

Stollman N et al. American Gastroenterological Association Institute Guideline on the management of acute diverticulitis. Gastroenterology. 2015 Dec;149(7):1944–9. [PMID: 26453777]

3. Diverticular Bleeding

Half of all cases of acute lower gastrointestinal bleeding are attributable to diverticulosis. For a full discussion, see the section on Acute Lower Gastrointestinal Bleeding, above.

POLYPS OF THE COLON

Polyps are discrete mass lesions that protrude into the intestinal lumen. Although most commonly sporadic, they may be inherited as part of a familial polyposis syndrome. Polyps may be divided into four major pathologic groups: mucosal adenomatous polyps (tubular, tubulovillous, and villous), mucosal serrated polyps (hyperplastic, sessile serrated polyps, and traditional serrated adenoma), mucosal nonneoplastic polyps (juvenile polyps, hamartomas, inflammatory polyps), and submucosal lesions (lipomas, lymphoid aggregates, carcinoids, pneumatosis cystoides intestinalis). Of polyps removed at colonoscopy, over 70% are adenomatous; most of the remainder are serrated. Adenomatous polyps and serrated polyps have significant clinical implications and will be considered further below.

NONFAMILIAL ADENOMATOUS & SERRATED POLYPS

Adenomas and serrated polyps may be non-polypoid (flat, slightly elevated, or depressed), sessile, or pedunculated (containing a stalk). They are present in 30% of adults over 50 years of age. Their significance is that over 95% of cases of adenocarcinoma of the colon are believed to arise from these lesions. It is proposed that there is a polyp → carcinoma sequence whereby nonfamilial colorectal cancer develops through a continuous process from normal mucosa to adenoma or serrated polyps to carcinoma. The majority of cancers arise in adenomas after inactivation of the *APC* gene leads to chromosomal instability and inactivation or loss of other tumor suppressor genes. By contrast, cancers arising in the serrated pathway appear to have either *Kras* (traditional serrated adenomas) mutations or *BRAF* oncogene activation (sessile serrated adenomas) with methylation of CpG-rich promoter regions that leads to inactivation of tumor suppressor genes or mismatch repair genes (*MLH1*) with microsatellite instability.

Most adenomas are smaller than 1 cm and have a low risk of becoming malignant; less than 5% of these enlarge with time. Adenomas and serrated polyps are classified as "advanced" if they are 1 cm or larger, or contain villous features or high-grade dysplasia. Advanced lesions are believed to have a higher risk of harboring or progressing to malignancy. It has been estimated from longitudinal studies that it takes an average of 5 years for a medium-sized polyp to develop from normal-appearing mucosa and 10 years for a gross cancer to arise. The prevalence of advanced adenomas is 6% and colorectal cancer 0.3%.

Most sessile serrated polyps and traditional serrated adenomas are believed to arise from hyperplastic polyps. It is believed that sessile serrated polyps and traditional serrated adenomas harbor an increased risk of colorectal cancer similar or greater to that of adenomas. Many pathologists cannot reliably distinguish between hyperplastic polyps and sessile serrated polyps. Hyperplastic polyps smaller than 5 mm located in the rectosigmoid region are of no consequence, except that they cannot reliably be distinguished from adenomatous lesions other than

by biopsy. Hyperplastic polyps located in the proximal colon (ie, proximal to the splenic flexure) may be associated with an increased prevalence of advanced neoplasia, particularly those larger than 1 cm.

► Clinical Findings

A. Symptoms and Signs

Most patients with adenomatous and serrated polyps are completely asymptomatic. Chronic occult blood loss may lead to iron deficiency anemia. Large polyps may ulcerate, resulting in intermittent hematochezia.

B. Fecal Occult Blood or Multitarget DNA Tests

FOBT, FIT, and fecal DNA tests are available as part of colorectal cancer screening programs (see Chapter 39). FIT is a fecal immunochemical test for hemoglobin that is more sensitive than guaiac-based tests for the detection of colorectal cancer and advanced adenomas. In 2014, a test combining a fecal DNA test with a fecal immunochemical test for stool hemoglobin (under the proprietary name "Cologuard") was approved by the FDA. In a prospective comparative trial conducted in persons at average risk for colorectal cancer undergoing colonoscopy, the sensitivity for colorectal cancer for "Cologuard" was 92.3% compared to 73.8% for FIT and the sensitivity for large (greater than 1 cm) adenomas or serrated polyps for "Cologuard" was 42.4% compared to 23.8% for FIT.

C. Radiologic Tests

Polyps are identified by means of barium enema examinations or CT colonography. Both studies require bowel cleansing with laxatives before the study and insertion of a rectal catheter for air insufflation during the study. CT colonography ("virtual colonoscopy") uses data from helical CT imaging with computer-enabled luminal image reconstruction to generate two-dimensional and three-dimensional images of the colon. Using optimal imaging software with multidetector helical CT scanners, several studies report a sensitivity of 90% or more for the detection of polyps larger than 10 mm in size. However, the accuracy for detection of polyps 5–9 mm in size is significantly lower (sensitivity 50%). A small proportion of these small polyps harbor advanced histology (up to 1.2%) or carcinoma (less than 1%). Abdominal CT imaging results in a radiation exposure that may lead to a small risk of cancer. CT colonography is endorsed by the US Multisociety Task Force as an acceptable option for screening for colorectal adenomatous polyps and cancer in average-risk asymptomatic adults. Barium enema is no longer recommended due to its poor diagnostic accuracy.

D. Endoscopic Tests

Colonoscopy allows evaluation of the entire colon and is the best means of detecting and removing adenomatous and serrated polyps. It should be performed in all patients who have positive FOBT, FIT, fecal, or DNA tests or iron deficiency anemia (see Occult Gastrointestinal

Bleeding above), as the prevalence of colonic neoplasms is increased in these patients. Colonoscopy should also be performed in patients with polyps detected on radiologic imaging studies (barium enema or CT colonography) or adenomas detected on flexible sigmoidoscopy to remove these polyps and to fully evaluate the entire colon. The newest generation of capsule endoscopy of the colon has an 88% sensitivity and 82% specificity for detection of adenomas greater than 6 mm compared with colonoscopy but only 29% sensitivity and 33% specificity for sessile serrated polyps. The bowel preparation required for the colon capsule study is more extensive than for colonoscopy and 10–30% of studies may be inadequate due to poor bowel preparation or failure to excrete the capsule. At this time, colonoscopy remains the best test in most patients to detect colorectal polyps. However, capsule endoscopy may be considered in patients with an incomplete colonoscopy or those who are unsuitable or unwilling to undergo colonoscopy.

▶ Treatment

A. Colonoscopic Polypectomy

Most adenomatous and serrated polyps are amenable to colonoscopic removal with biopsy forceps or snare cautery. Sessile polyps larger than 2–3 cm may be removed by snare cautery using a variety of techniques (eg, piecemeal or saline-lift assisted mucosal resection) or may require surgical resection. Patients with large sessile polyps removed in piecemeal fashion should undergo repeated colonoscopy in 2–6 months to verify complete polyp removal. Complications after colonoscopic polypectomy include perforation in 0.2% and clinically significant bleeding in 0.3–1% of patients.

B. Postpolypectomy Surveillance

Adenomas and serrated polyps can be found in 30–40% of patients when another colonoscopy is performed within 3–5 years after the initial examination and polyp removal. Periodic colonoscopic surveillance is therefore recommended to detect these "metachronous" lesions, which either may be new or may have been overlooked during the initial examination. Most of these polyps are small, without high-risk features and of little immediate clinical significance. The probability of detecting advanced neoplasms at surveillance colonoscopy depends on the number, size, and histologic features of the polyps removed on initial (index) colonoscopy. Patients with 1–2 tubular adenomas smaller than 1 cm (without villous features or high-grade dysplasia) should have their next colonoscopy in 5–10 years. Patients with 3–10 adenomas, an adenoma larger than 1 cm, or an adenoma with villous features or high-grade dysplasia should have their next colonoscopy at 3 years. Patients with more than 10 adenomas should have a repeat colonoscopy at 1–2 years and may be considered for evaluation for a familial polyposis syndrome. Surveillance colonoscopy at 5 years is appropriate for patients with small (less than 1 cm) serrated polyps without cytologic dysplasia; surveillance colonoscopy at 3 years should be considered for serrated polyps larger than 1 cm and those with cytologic atypia. No surveillance is recommended for

patients with small, typical hyperplastic polyps located in the distal colon and rectum.

Adrián-de-Ganzo Z et al. Uptake of colon capsule endoscopy vs colonoscopy for screening relatives of patients with colorectal cancer. Clin Gastroenterol Hepatol. 2015 Dec;13(13):2293–301. e1. [PMID: 26133904]

Imperiale TF et al. Multitarget stool DNA testing for colorectal-cancer screening. N Engl J Med. 2014 Apr 3;370(14):1287–97. [PMID: 24645800]

Lieberman D et al. Management of diminutive colon polyps based on endoluminal imaging. Clin Gastroenterol Hepatol. 2015 Nov;13(11):1860–6. [PMID: 26192139]

Lieberman DA et al. Guidelines for colonoscopy surveillance after screening and polypectomy: a consensus update by the US Multi-Society Task Force on Colorectal Cancer. Gastroenterology. 2012 Sep;143(3):844–57. [PMID: 22763141]

Naini BV et al. Advanced precancerous lesions (APL) in the colonic mucosa. Best Pract Res Clin Gastroenterol. 2013 Apr; 27(2):235–56. [PMID: 23809243]

Payne SR et al. Endoscopic detection of proximal serrated lesions and pathologic identification of sessile serrated adenomas/polyps vary on the basis of center. Clin Gastroenterol Hepatol. 2014 Jul;12(7):1119–26. [PMID: 24333512]

Rex DK et al. Accuracy of capsule colonoscopy in detecting colorectal polyps in a screening population. Gastroenterology. 2015 May;148(5):948–57.e2. [PMID: 25620668]

Rosty C et al. Serrated polyps of the large intestine: current understanding of diagnosis, pathogenesis, and clinical management. J Gastroenterol. 2013 Mar;48(3):287–302. [PMID: 23208018]

Zauber AG et al. Colonoscopic polypectomy and long-term prevention of colorectal-cancer deaths. N Engl J Med. 2012 Feb 23;366(8):687–96. [PMID: 22356322]

HEREDITARY COLORECTAL CANCER & POLYPOSIS SYNDROMES

Up to 4% of all colorectal cancers are caused by germline genetic mutations that impose on carriers a high lifetime risk of developing colorectal cancer (see Chapter 39). Because the diagnosis of these disorders has important implications for treatment of affected members and for screening of family members, it is important to consider these disorders in patients with a family history of colorectal cancer that has affected more than one family member, those with a personal or family history of colorectal cancer developing at an early age (50 years or younger), those with a personal or family history of multiple polyps (more than 20), and those with a personal or family history of multiple extracolonic malignancies.

1. Familial Adenomatous Polyposis

 ESSENTIALS OF DIAGNOSIS

- ▶ Inherited condition characterized by early development of hundreds to thousands of colonic adenomatous polyps and adenocarcinoma.

- ▶ Variety of extracolonic manifestations, including duodenal adenomas, desmoid tumors, and osteomas.

- Attenuated variant with fewer than 500 (average 25) colonic adenomas.
- Genetic testing confirms mutation of *APC* gene (90%) or *MUTYH* gene (8%).
- Prophylactic colectomy recommended to prevent otherwise inevitable colon cancer.

General Considerations

Familial adenomatous polyposis (FAP) is a syndrome affecting 1:10,000 people and accounts for approximately 0.5% of colorectal cancer. The classic form of FAP is characterized by the development of hundreds to thousands of colonic adenomatous polyps and a variety of extracolonic manifestations. Of patients with classic FAP, approximately 90% have a mutation in the *APC* gene that is inherited in an autosomal dominant fashion and 8% have mutations in the *MUTYH* gene that are inherited in an autosomal recessive fashion. FAP arises de novo in 15% of patients in the absence of genetic mutations in the parents. An attenuated variant of FAP also has been recognized in which an average of only 25 polyps (range of 1–500) develop.

Clinical Findings

A. Symptoms and Signs

Colorectal polyps develop by a mean age of 15 years and cancer at 40 years. Unless prophylactic colectomy is performed, colorectal cancer is inevitable by age 50 years. In attenuated FAP, the mean age for development of cancer is about 56 years.

Adenomatous polyps of the duodenum and periampullary area develop in over 90% of patients, resulting in a 5–8% lifetime risk of adenocarcinoma. Adenomas occur less frequently in the gastric antrum and small bowel and in those locations have a lower risk of malignant transformation. Gastric fundus gland polyps occur in over 50% but have an extremely low (0.6%) malignant potential.

A variety of other benign extraintestinal manifestations, including soft tissue tumors of the skin, desmoid tumors, osteomas, and congenital hypertrophy of the retinal pigment, develop in some patients with FAP. These extraintestinal manifestations vary among families, depending in part on the type or site of mutation in the *APC* gene. Desmoid tumors are locally invasive fibromas, most commonly intra-abdominal, that may cause bowel obstruction, ischemia, or hemorrhage. They occur in 15% of patients and are the second leading cause of death in FAP. Malignancies of the central nervous system (Turcot syndrome) and tumors of the thyroid and liver (hepatoblastomas) may also develop in patients with FAP.

B. Genetic Testing

Genetic counseling and testing should be offered to patients found to have multiple adenomatous polyps at endoscopy and to first-degree family members of patients with FAP. Genetic testing is best performed by sequencing the *APC* gene to identify disease-associated mutations followed by

MUTYH mutational assessment in patients with no detachable *APC* mutations. *APC* gene mutations are identified in 80% of patients with more than 1000, and 56% with 100–1000 polyps (ie, the classic phenotype of FAP). Recent guidelines also recommend that genetic testing be considered in individuals with as few as 10 adenomas to exclude a diagnosis of attenuated disease. *APC* or *MUTYH* mutations are found in10% and 7%, respectively, of patients with 20–100 adenomas and 5% and 4%, respectively, of those with 10–19 adenomas.

Treatment

Once the diagnosis has been established, complete proctocolectomy with ileoanal anastomosis or colectomy with ileorectal anastomosis is recommended, usually before age 20 years. Ileorectal anastomosis affords superior bowel function but has a 5% risk of development of rectal cancer, and for that reason frequent sigmoidoscopy with fulguration of polyps is required. Upper endoscopic evaluation of the stomach, duodenum, and periampullary area should be performed every 1–3 years to look for adenomas or carcinoma. Periampullary adenomas larger than 2 cm require surgical resection. Sulindac and celecoxib have been shown to decrease the number and size of polyps in the rectal stump but not the duodenum.

Grover S et al. Prevalence and phenotypes of *APC* and *MUTYH* mutations in patients with multiple colorectal adenomas. JAMA. 2012 Aug 1;308(5):485–92. [PMID: 22851115]

Kerr SE et al. *APC* germline mutations in individuals being evaluated for familial adenomatous polyposis: a review of the Mayo Clinic experience with 1591 consecutive tests. J Mol Diagn. 2013 Jan;15(1):31–43. [PMID: 23159591]

Stoffel EM et al. Familial colorectal cancer, beyond Lynch syndrome. Clin Gastroenterol Hepatol. 2014 Jul;12(7):1059–68. [PMID: 23962553]

2. Hamartomatous Polyposis Syndromes

Hamartomatous polyposis syndromes are rare and account for less than 0.1% of colorectal cancers.

Peutz-Jeghers syndrome is an autosomal dominant condition characterized by hamartomatous polyps throughout the gastrointestinal tract (most notably in the small intestine) as well as mucocutaneous pigmented macules on the lips, buccal mucosa, and skin. The hamartomas may become large, leading to bleeding, intussusception, or obstruction. Although hamartomas are not malignant, gastrointestinal malignancies (stomach, small bowel, and colon) develop in 40–60%, breast cancer in 30–50%, as well as a host of other malignancies of nonintestinal organs (gonads, pancreas). The defect has been localized to the serine threonine kinase 11 gene, and genetic testing is available.

Familial juvenile polyposis is also autosomal dominant and is characterized by several (more than ten) juvenile hamartomatous polyps located most commonly in the colon. There is an increased risk (up to 50%) of adenocarcinoma due to synchronous adenomatous polyps or mixed hamartomatous-adenomatous polyps. Genetic defects have been identified to loci on 18q and 10q (*MADH4* and *BMPR1A*). Genetic testing is available.

PTEN multiple hamartoma syndrome (Cowden disease) is characterized by hamartomatous polyps and lipomas throughout the gastrointestinal tract, trichilemmomas, and cerebellar lesions. An increased rate of malignancy is demonstrated in the thyroid, breast, and urogenital tract.

Stoffel EM et al. Familial colorectal cancer, beyond Lynch syndrome. Clin Gastroenterol Hepatol. 2014 Jul;12(7):1059–68. [PMID: 23962553]

3. Lynch Syndrome

ESSENTIALS OF DIAGNOSIS

- ▶ Autosomally dominant inherited condition.
- ▶ Caused by mutations in a gene that detects and repairs DNA base-pair mismatches, resulting in DNA microsatellite instability and inactivation of tumor suppressor genes.
- ▶ Increased lifetime risk of colorectal cancer (22–75%), endometrial cancer (30–60%), and other cancers that may develop at young age.
- ▶ Evaluation warranted in patients with personal history of early-onset colorectal cancer or family history of colorectal, endometrial, or other Lynch syndrome–related cancers at young age or in multiple members.
- ▶ Diagnosis suspected by tumor tissue immunohistochemical staining for mismatch repair proteins or testing for microsatellite instability.
- ▶ Diagnosis confirmed by genetic testing.

General Considerations

Lynch syndrome (also known as hereditary nonpolyposis colon cancer [HNPCC]) is an autosomal dominant condition in which there is a markedly increased risk of developing colorectal cancer as well as a host of other cancers, including endometrial, ovarian, renal or bladder, hepatobiliary, gastric, and small intestinal cancers. It is estimated to account for up to 3% of all colorectal cancers. Affected individuals have a 22–75% lifetime risk of developing colorectal carcinoma and a 30–60% lifetime risk of endometrial cancer, depending on the affected gene. Unlike individuals with familial adenomatous polyposis, patients with Lynch syndrome develop only a few adenomas, which may be flat and more often contain villous features or high-grade dysplasia. In contrast to the traditional polyp → cancer progression (which may take over 10 years), these polyps are believed to undergo rapid transformation over 1–2 years from normal tissue → adenoma → cancer. Colon and endometrial cancer tend to develop at an earlier age than sporadic, nonhereditary cancers (mean age 45–50 years). Compared with patients with sporadic tumors of similar pathologic stage, those with Lynch syndrome tumors have improved survival. Synchronous or metachronous cancers occur within 10 years in up to 45% of patients.

Lynch syndrome is caused by a defect in one of several genes that are important in the detection and repair of DNA base-pair mismatches: *MLH1, MSH2, MSH6,* and *PMS2.* Germline mutations in *MLH1* and *MSH2* account for almost 90% of the known mutations in families with Lynch syndrome. Mutations in any of these mismatch repair genes result in a characteristic phenotypic DNA abnormality known as microsatellite instability.

▶ Clinical Findings

A thorough family cancer history is essential to identify families that may be affected with Lynch syndrome so that appropriate genetic and colonoscopic screening can be offered. Owing to the limitations of genetic testing and the medical, psychological, and social implications that such testing may have, families should be evaluated first by a genetic counselor and give informed consent before genetic testing is performed.

Patients whose families meet any of the revised "Bethesda criteria" have an increased likelihood of harboring a germline mutation in one of the mismatch repair genes and should be considered for genetic testing. The "Bethesda criteria" are (1) colorectal cancer under age 50; (2) synchronous or metachronous colorectal or Lynch syndrome–associated tumor regardless of age (endometrial, stomach, ovary, pancreas, ureter and renal pelvis, biliary tract, brain); (3) colorectal cancer with one or more first-degree relatives with colorectal or Lynch syndrome–related cancer, with one of the cancers occurring before age 50; (4) colorectal cancer with two or more second-degree relatives with colorectal or Lynch syndrome–related cancer, regardless of age; (5) tumors with infiltrating lymphocytes, mucinous/signet ring differentiation, or medullary growth pattern in patients younger than 60 years.

The Bethesda criteria identify approximately 70% of mutation-positive Lynch syndrome families but overlook 30%. For this reason, 2014 consensus, multisociety guidelines recommend that *all* colorectal cancers should undergo testing for Lynch syndrome with either immunohistochemistry or microsatellite instability. Universal testing has the greatest sensitivity for the diagnosis of Lynch syndrome and is cost-effective. Individuals whose tumors have normal immunohistochemical staining or do not have microsatellite instability are unlikely to have germline mutations in mismatch repair genes, do not require further genetic testing, and do not require intensive cancer surveillance. Up to 15% of sporadic (noninherited) tumors have microsatellite instability or absent *MLH1* staining due to somatic (noninherited) methylation of the *MLH1* gene promoter and somatic *BRAF* mutations, which must be excluded before further genetic testing is considered. Germline testing for gene mutations is positive in more than 90% of individuals whose tumors show absent histochemical staining of one of the mismatch repair genes or high level of microsatellite instability without a *BRAF* mutation. Germline testing is also warranted in families with a strong history consistent with Lynch syndrome when tumors from affected members are unavailable for assessment. If a mutation is detected in a patient with cancer in one of the known mismatch genes, genetic testing of other first-degree family members is indicated.

Screening & Treatment

If genetic testing documents a Lynch syndrome gene mutation, affected relatives should be screened with colonoscopy every 1–2 years beginning at age 25 (or at age 5 years younger than the age at diagnosis of the youngest affected family member). If cancer is found, subtotal colectomy with ileorectal anastomosis (followed by annual surveillance of the rectal stump) should be performed. Women should undergo screening for endometrial and ovarian cancer beginning at age 30–35 years with pelvic examination, transvaginal ultrasound, and endometrial sampling. Prophylactic hysterectomy and oophorectomy is recommended to women at age 40 or once they have finished childbearing. Screening for gastric cancer with upper endoscopy should be considered every 2–3 years beginning at age 30–35 years.

Giardiello FM et al. Guidelines on genetic evaluation and management of Lynch syndrome: a consensus statement by the US Multi-Society Task Force on colorectal cancer. Gastroenterology. 2014 Aug;147(2):502–26. [PMID: 25043945]

Rubenstein JH et al. American Gastroenterological Association Institute Guideline on the diagnosis and management of Lynch syndrome. Gastroenterology. 2015 Sep;149(3):777–82. [PMID: 26226577]

Syngal S et al. ACG clinical guideline: genetic testing and management of hereditary gastrointestinal cancer syndromes. Am J Gastroenterol. 2015 Feb;110(2):223–62. [PMID: 25645574]

ANORECTAL DISEASES

(See Chapter 39 for Carcinoma of the Anus.)

HEMORRHOIDS

ESSENTIALS OF DIAGNOSIS

▶ Bright red blood per rectum.

▶ Protrusion, discomfort.

▶ Characteristic findings on external anal inspection and anoscopic examination.

General Considerations

Internal hemorrhoids are subepithelial vascular cushions consisting of connective tissue, smooth muscle fibers, and arteriovenous communications between terminal branches of the superior rectal artery and rectal veins. They are a normal anatomic entity, occurring in all adults, that contribute to normal anal pressures and ensure a water-tight closure of the anal canal. They commonly occur in three primary locations—right anterior, right posterior, and left lateral. External hemorrhoids arise from the inferior hemorrhoidal veins located below the dentate line and are covered with squamous epithelium of the anal canal or perianal region.

Hemorrhoids may become symptomatic as a result of activities that increase venous pressure, resulting in distention and engorgement. Straining at stool, constipation, prolonged sitting, pregnancy, obesity, and low-fiber diets all may contribute. With time, redundancy and enlargement of the venous cushions may develop and result in bleeding or protrusion.

Clinical Findings

A. Symptoms and Signs

Patients often attribute a variety of perianal complaints to "hemorrhoids." However, the principal problems attributable to internal hemorrhoids are bleeding, prolapse, and mucoid discharge. Bleeding is manifested by bright red blood that may range from streaks of blood visible on toilet paper or stool to bright red blood that drips into the toilet bowl after a bowel movement. Uncommonly, bleeding is severe and prolonged enough to result in anemia. Initially, internal hemorrhoids are confined to the anal canal (stage I). Over time, the internal hemorrhoids may gradually enlarge and protrude from the anal opening. At first, this mucosal prolapse occurs during straining and reduces spontaneously (stage II). With progression over time, the prolapsed hemorrhoids may require manual reduction after bowel movements (stage III) or may remain chronically protruding (stage IV). Chronically prolapsed hemorrhoids may result in a sense of fullness or discomfort and mucoid perianal discharge, resulting in irritation and soiling of underclothes. Pain is unusual with internal hemorrhoids, occurring only when there is extensive inflammation and thrombosis of irreducible tissue or with thrombosis of an external hemorrhoid.

B. Examination

External hemorrhoids are readily visible on perianal inspection. Nonprolapsed internal hemorrhoids are not visible but may protrude through the anus with gentle straining while the clinician spreads the buttocks. Prolapsed hemorrhoids are visible as protuberant purple nodules covered by mucosa. The perianal region should also be examined for other signs of disease such as fistulas, fissures, skin tags, condyloma, anal cancer, or dermatitis. On digital examination, uncomplicated internal hemorrhoids are neither palpable nor painful. Anoscopic evaluation, best performed in the prone jackknife position, provides optimal visualization of internal hemorrhoids.

Differential Diagnosis

Small volume rectal bleeding may be caused by anal fissure or fistula, neoplasms of the distal colon or rectum, ulcerative colitis or Crohn colitis, infectious proctitis, or rectal ulcers. Rectal prolapse, in which a full thickness of rectum protrudes concentrically from the anus, is readily distinguished from mucosal hemorrhoidal prolapse. Proctosigmoidoscopy or colonoscopy should be performed in all patients with hematochezia to exclude disease in the rectum or sigmoid colon that could be misinterpreted in the presence of hemorrhoidal bleeding.

Treatment

A. Conservative Measures

Most patients with early (stage I and stage II) disease can be managed with conservative treatment. To decrease straining with defecation, patients should be given instructions for a high-fiber diet and told to increase fluid intake with meals. Dietary fiber may be supplemented with bran powder (1–2 tbsp twice daily added to food or in 8 oz of liquid) or with commercial bulk laxatives (eg, Benefiber, Metamucil, Citrucel). Suppositories and rectal ointments have no demonstrated utility in the management of mild disease. Mucoid discharge may be treated effectively by the local application of a cotton ball tucked next to the anal opening after bowel movements.

B. Medical Treatment

Patients with stage I, stage II, and stage III hemorrhoids and recurrent bleeding despite conservative measures may be treated without anesthesia with injection sclerotherapy, rubber band ligation, or application of electrocoagulation (bipolar cautery or infrared photocoagulation). The choice of therapy is dictated by operator preference, but rubber band ligation is preferred due to its ease of use and high rate of efficacy. Major complications occur in less than 2%, including pelvic sepsis, pelvic abscess, urinary retention, and bleeding. Recurrence is common unless patients alter their dietary habits. Edematous, prolapsed (stage IV) internal hemorrhoids, may be treated acutely with topical creams, foams, or suppositories containing various combinations of emollients, topical anesthetics, (eg, pramoxine, dibucaine), vasoconstrictors (eg, phenylephrine), astringents (witch hazel) and corticosteroids. Common preparations include Preparation H (several formulations), Anusol HC, Proctofoam, Nupercainal, Tucks, and Doloproct (not available in the United States).

C. Surgical Treatment

Surgical excision (hemorrhoidectomy) is reserved for less than 5–10% of patients with chronic severe bleeding due to stage III or stage IV hemorrhoids or patients with acute thrombosed stage IV hemorrhoids with necrosis. Complications of surgical hemorrhoidectomy include postoperative pain (which may persist for 2–4 weeks) and impaired continence.

Thrombosed External Hemorrhoid

Thrombosis of the external hemorrhoidal plexus results in a perianal hematoma. It most commonly occurs in otherwise healthy young adults and may be precipitated by coughing, heavy lifting, or straining at stool. The condition is characterized by the relatively acute onset of an exquisitely painful, tense and bluish perianal nodule covered with skin that may be up to several centimeters in size. Pain is most severe within the first few hours but gradually eases over 2–3 days as edema subsides. Symptoms may be relieved with warm sitz baths, analgesics, and ointments. If the patient is evaluated in the first 24–48 hours, removal of the clot may hasten symptomatic relief. With the patient in

the lateral position, the skin around and over the lump is injected subcutaneously with 1% lidocaine using a tuberculin syringe with a 30-gauge needle. An ellipse of skin is then excised and the clot evacuated. A dry gauze dressing is applied for 12–24 hours, and daily sitz baths are then begun.

When to Refer

- Stage I, II, or III: When conservative measures fail and expertise in medical procedures is needed (injection, banding, thermocoagulation).
- Stage IV: When surgical excision is required.

Jacobs D. Clinical practice. Hemorrhoids. N Engl J Med. 2014 Sep 4;371(10):944–51. [PMID: 25184866]
Sugerman DT. JAMA patient page. Hemorrhoids. JAMA. 2014 Dec 24–31;312(24):2698. [PMID: 25536271]

ANORECTAL INFECTIONS

A number of organisms can cause inflammation of the anal and rectal mucosa. Proctitis is characterized by anorectal discomfort, tenesmus, constipation, and mucus or bloody discharge. Most cases of proctitis are sexually transmitted, especially by anal-receptive intercourse. Infectious proctitis must be distinguished from noninfectious causes of anorectal symptoms, including anal fissures or fistulae, perirectal abscesses, anorectal carcinomas, and inflammatory bowel disease (ulcerative colitis or Crohn disease).

Etiology & Management

Several organisms may cause infectious proctitis.

A. Neisseria gonorrhoeae

Gonorrhea may cause itching, burning, tenesmus, and a mucopurulent discharge, although many anorectal infections are asymptomatic. Rectal swab specimens should be taken during anoscopy for culture; Gram staining is unreliable. Cultures should also be taken from the pharynx and urethra in men and from the pharynx and cervix in women. Complications of untreated infections include strictures, fissures, fistulas, and perirectal abscesses. (For treatment, see Chapter 33.)

B. Treponema pallidum

Anal syphilis may be asymptomatic or may lead to perianal pain and discharge. With primary syphilis, the chancre may be at the anal margin or within the anal canal and may mimic a fissure, fistula, or ulcer. Proctitis or inguinal lymphadenopathy may be present. With secondary syphilis, condylomata lata (pale-brown, flat verrucous lesions) may be seen, with secretion of foul-smelling mucus. Although the diagnosis may be established with dark-field microscopy or fluorescent antibody testing of scrapings from the chancre or condylomas, this requires proper equipment and trained personnel. The VDRL or RPR test is positive in 75% of primary cases and in 99% of secondary cases. (For treatment, see Chapter 34.)

C. Chlamydia trachomatis

Chlamydial infection may cause proctitis similar to gonorrheal proctitis; however, some infections are asymptomatic. It also may cause lymphogranuloma venereum, characterized by proctocolitis with fever and bloody diarrhea, painful perianal ulcerations, anorectal strictures and fistulas, and inguinal adenopathy (buboes). Previously rare in developed countries, an increasing number of cases have been identified among men who have sex with men. The diagnosis is established by serology, culture, or PCR-based testing of rectal discharge or rectal biopsy. Recommended treatment is doxycycline 100 mg orally twice daily for 21 days.

D. Herpes Simplex Type 2

Herpes simplex virus is a common cause of anorectal infection. Symptoms occur 4–21 days after exposure and include severe pain, itching, constipation, tenesmus, urinary retention, and radicular pain from involvement of lumbar or sacral nerve roots. Small vesicles or ulcers may be seen in the perianal area or anal canal. Sigmoidoscopy is not usually necessary but may reveal vesicular or ulcerative lesions in the distal rectum. Diagnosis is established by viral culture, PCR, or antigen detection assays of vesicular fluid. Symptoms resolve within 2 weeks, but viral shedding may continue for several weeks. Patients may remain asymptomatic with or without viral shedding or may have recurrent mild relapses. Treatment of acute infection for 7–10 days with acyclovir, 400 mg, or famciclovir, 250 mg orally three times daily, or valacyclovir, 1 g twice daily, has been shown to reduce the duration of symptoms and viral shedding. Patients with AIDS and recurrent relapses may benefit from long-term suppressive therapy (see Chapter 31).

E. Condylomata Acuminata

Condylomata acuminata (warts) are a significant cause of anorectal symptoms. Caused by the HPV, they may occur in the perianal area, the anal canal, or the genitals. Perianal or anal warts are seen in up to 25% of men who have sex with men. HIV-positive individuals with condylomas have a higher relapse rate after therapy and a higher rate of progression to high-grade dysplasia or anal cancer. The warts are located on the perianal skin and extend within the anal canal up to 2 cm above the dentate line. Patients may have no symptoms or may report itching, bleeding, and pain. The warts may be small and flat or verrucous, or may form a confluent mass that may obscure the anal opening. Warts must be distinguished from condyloma lata (secondary syphilis) or anal cancer. Biopsies should be obtained from large or suspicious lesions. Treatment can be difficult. Sexual partners should also be examined and treated. The treatment of anogenital warts is discussed in Chapter 30. HPV vaccines have demonstrated efficacy in preventing anogenital warts and routine vaccination is now recommended for all children and adults 9–26 years old (see Chapters 1 and 30). Vaccination also should be considered in men who have sex with men. HIV-positive individuals with condylomas who have detectable serum HIV RNA levels should have anoscopic surveillance every 3–6 months.

Hoentjen F et al. Infectious proctitis: when to suspect it is not inflammatory bowel disease. Dig Dis Sci. 2012 Feb;57(2):269–73. [PMID: 21994137]

Palefsky JM et al. HPV vaccine against anal HPV infection and anal intraepithelial neoplasia. N Engl J Med. 2011 Oct 27; 365(17):1576–85. [PMID: 22029979]

Workowski KA et al; Centers for Disease Control and Prevention (CDC). Sexually transmitted diseases treatment guidelines, 2015. MMWR Recomm Rep. 2015 Jun 5;64(RR-03):1–137. Erratum in: MMWR Recomm Rep. 2015 Aug 28;64(33):924. [PMID: 26042815]

FECAL INCONTINENCE

There are five general requirements for bowel continence: (1) solid or semisolid stool (even healthy young adults have difficulty maintaining continence with liquid rectal contents); (2) a distensible rectal reservoir (as sigmoid contents empty into the rectum, the vault must expand to accommodate); (3) a sensation of rectal fullness (if the patient cannot sense this, overflow may occur before the patient can take appropriate action); (4) intact pelvic nerves and muscles; and (5) the ability to reach a toilet in a timely fashion.

► Minor Incontinence

Many patients complain of inability to control flatus or slight soilage of undergarments that tends to occur after bowel movements or with straining or coughing. This may be due to local anal problems such as prolapsed hemorrhoids that make it difficult to form a tight anal seal or isolated weakness of the internal anal sphincter, especially if stools are somewhat loose. Patients should be treated with fiber supplements to provide greater stool bulk. Coffee and other caffeinated beverages should be eliminated. The perianal skin should be cleansed with moist, lanolin-coated tissue (baby wipes) to reduce excoriation and infection. After wiping, loose application of a cotton ball near the anal opening may absorb small amounts of fecal leakage. Prolapsing hemorrhoids may be treated with band ligation or surgical hemorrhoidectomy. Control of flatus and seepage may be improved by Kegel perineal exercises. Conditions such as ulcerative proctitis that cause tenesmus and urgency, chronic diarrheal conditions, and irritable bowel syndrome may result in difficulty in maintaining complete continence, especially if a toilet is not readily available. Loperamide may be helpful to reduce urge incontinence in patients with loose stools and may be taken in anticipation of situations in which a toilet may not be readily available. The elderly may require more time or assistance to reach a toilet, which may lead to incontinence. Scheduled toileting and the availability of a bedside commode are helpful. Elderly patients with chronic constipation may develop stool impaction leading to "overflow" incontinence.

► Major Incontinence

Complete uncontrolled loss of stool reflects a significant problem with central perception or neuromuscular function. Incontinence that occurs without awareness suggests a loss of central awareness (eg, dementia, cerebrovascular accident, multiple sclerosis) or peripheral nerve injury (eg, spinal cord injury, cauda equina syndrome, pudendal nerve damage due to obstetric trauma or pelvic floor prolapse, aging, or diabetes mellitus). Incontinence that occurs despite awareness and active efforts to retain stool suggests sphincteric damage, which may be caused by traumatic childbirth (especially forceps delivery), episiotomy, prolapse, prior anal surgery, and physical trauma.

Physical examination should include careful inspection of the perianal area for hemorrhoids, rectal prolapse, fissures, fistulas, and either gaping or a keyhole defect of the anal sphincter (indicating severe sphincteric injury or neurologic disorder). The perianal skin should be stimulated to confirm an intact anocutaneous reflex. Digital examination during relaxation gives valuable information about resting tone (due mainly to the internal sphincter) and contraction of the external sphincter and pelvic floor during squeezing. It also excludes fecal impaction. Anoscopy is required to evaluate for hemorrhoids, fissures, and fistulas. Proctosigmoidoscopy is useful to exclude rectal carcinoma or proctitis. Anal ultrasonography or pelvic MRI is the most reliable test for definition of anatomic defects in the external and internal anal sphincters. Anal manometry may also be useful to define the severity of weakness, to assess sensation, and to predict response to biofeedback training. In special circumstances, surface electromyography is useful to document sphincteric denervation and proctography to document perineal descent or rectal intussusception.

Patients who are incontinent only of loose or liquid stools are treated with bulking agents and antidiarrheal drugs (eg, loperamide, 2 mg before meals and prophylactically before social engagements, shopping trips, etc). Patients with incontinence of solid stool benefit from scheduled toilet use after glycerin suppositories or tap water enemas. Biofeedback training with anal sphincteric strengthening (Kegel) exercises (alternating 5-second squeeze and 10-second rest for 10 minutes twice daily) may be helpful in motivated patients to lower the threshold for awareness of rectal filling—or to improve anal sphincter squeeze function—or both. In 2012, the FDA approved two interventions for fecal incontinence. The first is a sterile gel (containing dextranomer and sodium hyaluronate) for submucosal injection into the proximal anal canal for the treatment of anal incontinence for patients who have not responded to conservative therapies, such as fiber supplements and antidiarrheal agents. This treatment is hypothesized to reduce incontinence episodes by bulking and narrowing the anal canal. In clinical trials, more than one-half of treated patients reported a greater than 50% reduction in the number of fecal incontinence episodes. The second is a sacral nerve stimulation device. In uncontrolled trials in selected patients, 83% of patients were improved with sacral stimulation. Further study is needed to determine optimal candidates and the true efficacy of these treatments. Operative management is seldom needed but should be considered in patients with major incontinence due to prior injury to the anal sphincter who have not responded to medical therapy.

When to Refer

- Conservative measures fail.
- Anorectal tests are deemed necessary (manometry, ultrasonography, electromyography).
- A surgically correctable lesion is suspected.

Bharucha AE et al. Epidemiology, pathophysiology, and classification of fecal incontinence: state of the science summary for the National Institute of Diabetes and Digestive and Kidney Diseases (NIDDK) workshop. Am J Gastroenterol. 2015 Jan; 110(1):127–36. [PMID: 25533002]

Brown SR et al. Surgery for faecal incontinence in adults. Cochrane Database Syst Rev. 2013 Jul 2;7:CD001757. [PMID: 23821339]

Kunduru L et al. Factors that affect consultation and screening for fecal incontinence. Clin Gastroenterol Hepatol. 2015 Apr; 13(4):709–16. [PMID: 25148761]

Soh JS et al. The diagnostic value of a digital rectal examination compared with high-resolution anorectal manometry in patients with chronic constipation and fecal incontinence. Am J Gastroenterol. 2015 Aug;110(8):1197–204. [PMID: 26032152]

Whitehead WE et al. Treatment of fecal incontinence: state of the science summary for the National Institute of Diabetes and Digestive and Kidney Diseases workshop. Am J Gastroenterol. 2015 Jan;110(1):138–46. [PMID: 25331348]

OTHER ANAL CONDITIONS

Anal Fissures

Anal fissures are linear or rocket-shaped ulcers that are usually less than 5 mm in length. Most fissures are believed to arise from trauma to the anal canal during defecation, perhaps caused by straining, constipation, or high internal sphincter tone. They occur most commonly in the posterior midline, but 10% occur anteriorly. Fissures that occur off the midline should raise suspicion for Crohn disease, HIV/AIDS, tuberculosis, syphilis, or anal carcinoma. Patients complain of severe, tearing pain during defecation followed by throbbing discomfort that may lead to constipation due to fear of recurrent pain. There may be mild associated hematochezia, with blood on the stool or toilet paper. Anal fissures are confirmed by visual inspection of the anal verge while gently separating the buttocks. Acute fissures look like cracks in the epithelium. Chronic fissures result in fibrosis and the development of a skin tag at the outermost edge (sentinel pile). Digital and anoscopic examinations may cause severe pain and may not be possible. Medical management is directed at promoting effortless, painless bowel movements. Fiber supplements and sitz baths should be prescribed. Topical anesthetics (5% lidocaine; 2.5% lidocaine plus 2.5% prilocaine) may provide temporary relief. Healing occurs within 2 months in up to 45% of patients with conservative management. Chronic fissures may be treated with topical 0.2–0.4% nitroglycerin or diltiazem 2% ointment (1 cm of ointment) applied twice daily just inside the anus with the tip of a finger for 4–8 weeks or injection of botulinum toxin (20 units) into the internal anal sphincter. All of these treatments result in healing in 50–80% of patients with chronic anal fissure, but headaches occur in up to 40% of patients treated with nitroglycerin. Fissures recur in up to 40% of patients after treatment. Chronic or recurrent fissures benefit from lateral internal sphincterotomy; however, minor incontinence may complicate this procedure.

Barnes TG et al. Fissurectomy combined with high-dose botulinum toxin is a safe and effective treatment for chronic anal fissure and a promising alternative to surgical sphincterotomy. Dis Colon Rectum. 2015 Oct;58(10):967–73. [PMID: 26347969]

Dat A et al. Botulinum toxin therapy for chronic anal fissures: where are we at currently? ANZ J Surg. 2015 Sep 30. [Epub ahead of print] [PMID: 26423046]

Liang J et al. Lateral internal sphincterotomy for surgically recurrent chronic anal fissure. Am J Surg. 2015 Oct; 210(4):715–9. [PMID: 26231724]

Malaty HM et al. Time trends, clinical characteristics, and risk factors of chronic anal fissure among a national cohort of patients with inflammatory bowel disease. Dig Dis Sci. 2016 Mar; 61(3):861–4. [PMID: 26514675]

Sugerman DT. JAMA patient page. Anal fissure. JAMA. 2014 Mar 19;311(11):1171. [PMID: 24643618]

Perianal Abscess & Fistula

The anal glands located at the base of the anal crypts at the dentate line may become infected, leading to abscess formation. Other causes of abscess include anal fissure and Crohn disease. Abscesses may extend upward or downward through the intersphincteric plane. Symptoms of perianal abscess are throbbing, continuous perianal pain. Erythema, fluctuance, and swelling may be found in the perianal region on external examination or in the ischiorectal fossa on digital rectal examination. Perianal abscesses are treated with local incision and drainage, while ischiorectal abscesses require drainage in the operating room. After drainage of an abscess, most patients are found to have a fistula in ano.

Fistula in ano most often arises in an anal crypt and is usually preceded by an anal abscess. In patients with fistulas that connect to the rectum, other disorders such as Crohn disease, lymphogranuloma venereum, rectal tuberculosis, and cancer should be considered. Fistulas are associated with purulent discharge that may lead to itching, tenderness, and pain. The treatment of Crohn-related fistula is discussed elsewhere in this chapter. Treatment of simple idiopathic fistula in ano is by surgical incision or excision under anesthesia. Care must be taken to preserve the anal sphincters. Surgical fistulotomy for treatment of complex (high, transphincteric) anal fissures carries a high risk of incontinence. Techniques for healing the fistula while preserving the sphincter include an endoanal advancement flap over the internal opening and insertion of a bioprosthetic plug into the fistula opening.

Lange EO et al. Ligation of intersphincteric fistula tract: a sphincter-sparing option for complex fistula-in-ano. J Gastrointest Surg. 2016 Feb;20(2):439–44. [PMID: 26394877]

Ratto C et al. Fistulotomy or fistulectomy and primary sphincteroplasty for anal fistula (FIPS): a systematic review. Tech Coloproctol. 2015 Jul;19(7):391–400. [PMID: 26062740]

Perianal Pruritus

Perianal pruritus is characterized by perianal itching and discomfort. It may be caused by poor anal hygiene associated with fistulas, fissures, prolapsed hemorrhoids, skin tags, and minor incontinence. Conversely, overzealous cleansing with soaps may contribute to local irritation or contact dermatitis. Contact dermatitis, atopic dermatitis, bacterial infections (*Staphylococcus* or *Streptococcus*), parasites (pinworms, scabies), candidal infection (especially in diabetics), sexually transmitted disease (condylomata acuminata, herpes, syphilis, molluscum contagiosum), and other skin conditions (psoriasis, Paget, lichen sclerosis) must be excluded. In patients with idiopathic perianal pruritus, examination may reveal erythema, excoriations, or lichenified, eczematous skin. Education is vital to successful therapy. Spicy foods, coffee, chocolate, and tomatoes may cause irritation and should be eliminated. After bowel movements, the perianal area should be cleansed with nonscented wipes premoistened with lanolin followed by gentle drying. A piece of cotton ball should be tucked next to the anal opening to absorb perspiration or fecal seepage. Anal ointments and lotions may exacerbate the condition and should be avoided. A short course of high-potency topical corticosteroid may be tried, although efficacy has not been demonstrated. Diluted capsaicin cream (0.006%) led to symptomatic relief in 75% of patients in a double-blind crossover study.

Foxx-Orenstein AE et al. Common anorectal disorders. Gastroenterol Hepatol (N Y). 2014 May;10(5):294–301. [PMID: 24987313]

Nasseri YY et al. Pruritus ani: diagnosis and treatment. Gastroenterol Clin North Am. 2013 Dec;42(4):801–13. [PMID: 24280401]

Liver, Biliary Tract, & Pancreas Disorders

Lawrence S. Friedman, MD

JAUNDICE & EVALUATION OF ABNORMAL LIVER BIOCHEMICAL TESTS

ESSENTIALS OF DIAGNOSIS

▶ Jaundice results from accumulation of bilirubin in body tissues; the cause may be hepatic or nonhepatic.

▶ Hyperbilirubinemia may be due to abnormalities in the formation, transport, metabolism, or excretion of bilirubin.

▶ Persistent mild elevations of the aminotransferase levels are common in clinical practice and caused most often by nonalcoholic fatty liver disease.

▶ Evaluation of obstructive jaundice begins with ultrasonography and is usually followed by cholangiography.

General Considerations

Jaundice (icterus) results from the accumulation of bilirubin—a product of heme metabolism—in body tissues. Hyperbilirubinemia may be due to abnormalities in the formation, transport, metabolism, or excretion of bilirubin. Total serum bilirubin is normally 0.2–1.2 mg/dL (3.42–20.52 mcmol/L). Mean levels are higher in men than women, higher in whites and Hispanics than blacks, and correlate with an increased risk of symptomatic gallstone disease and inversely with the risk of stroke, respiratory disease, cardiovascular disease, and mortality, presumably because of an antioxidant effect. Jaundice may not be recognizable until serum bilirubin levels are about 3 mg/dL (51.3 mcmol/L).

Jaundice is caused by predominantly unconjugated or conjugated bilirubin in the serum (Table 16–1). Unconjugated hyperbilirubinemia may result from overproduction of bilirubin because of hemolysis; impaired hepatic uptake of bilirubin due to certain drugs; or impaired conjugation of bilirubin by glucuronide, as in Gilbert syndrome, due to mild decreases in uridine diphosphate (UDP) glucuronyl transferase, or Crigler-Najjar syndrome,

caused by moderate decreases or absence of UDP glucuronyl transferase. Hemolysis alone rarely elevates the serum bilirubin level to more than 7 mg/dL (119.7 mcmol/L). Predominantly conjugated hyperbilirubinemia may result from impaired excretion of bilirubin from the liver due to hepatocellular disease, drugs, sepsis, or hereditary hepatocanalicular transport defects (such as Dubin-Johnson syndrome, progressive familial intrahepatic cholestasis syndromes, and intrahepatic cholestasis of pregnancy) or from extrahepatic biliary obstruction. Features of some hyperbilirubinemic syndromes are summarized in Table 16–2. The term "cholestasis" denotes retention of bile in the liver, and the term "cholestatic jaundice" is often used when conjugated hyperbilirubinemia results from impaired bile flow. Mediators of pruritus due to cholestasis have been identified to be lysophosphatidic acid and autotaxin, the enzyme that forms lysophosphatidic acid.

Clinical Findings

A. Unconjugated Hyperbilirubinemia

Stool and urine color are normal, and there is mild jaundice and indirect (unconjugated) hyperbilirubinemia with no bilirubin in the urine. Splenomegaly occurs in all hemolytic disorders except in sickle cell disease.

B. Conjugated Hyperbilirubinemia

1. Hereditary cholestatic syndromes or intrahepatic cholestasis—The patient may be asymptomatic; cholestasis is often accompanied by pruritus, light colored stools, and jaundice.

2. Hepatocellular disease—Malaise, anorexia, low-grade fever, and right upper quadrant discomfort are frequent. Dark urine, jaundice, and, in women, amenorrhea occur. An enlarged tender liver, spider telangiectasias, palmar erythema, ascites, gynecomastia, sparse body hair, fetor hepaticus, and asterixis may be present, depending on the cause, severity, and chronicity of liver dysfunction.

C. Biliary Obstruction

There may be right upper quadrant pain, weight loss (suggesting carcinoma), jaundice, pruritus, dark urine, and

Table 16–1. Classification of jaundice.

Type of Hyperbilirubinemia	Location and Cause
Unconjugated hyperbilirubinemia (predominantly indirect bilirubin)	Increased bilirubin production (eg, hemolytic anemias, hemolytic reactions, hematoma, pulmonary infarction) Impaired bilirubin uptake and storage (eg, posthepatitis hyperbilirubinemia, Gilbert syndrome, Crigler-Najjar syndrome, drug reactions)
Conjugated hyperbilirubinemia (predominantly direct bilirubin)	**Hereditary Cholestatic Syndromes** (see also Table 16–2)
	Faulty excretion of bilirubin conjugates (eg, Dubin-Johnson syndrome, Rotor syndrome) or mutation in genes coding for bile salt transport proteins (eg, progressive familial intrahepatic cholestasis syndromes, benign recurrent intrahepatic cholestasis, and some cases of intrahepatic cholestasis of pregnancy)
	Hepatocellular Dysfunction
	Biliary epithelial and hepatocyte damage (eg, hepatitis, hepatic cirrhosis) Intrahepatic cholestasis (eg, certain drugs, biliary cirrhosis, sepsis, postoperative jaundice) Hepatocellular damage or intrahepatic cholestasis resulting from miscellaneous causes (eg, spirochetal infections, infectious mononucleosis, cholangitis, sarcoidosis, lymphomas, industrial toxins)
	Biliary Obstruction
	Choledocholithiasis, biliary atresia, carcinoma of biliary duct, sclerosing cholangitis, choledochal cyst, external pressure on bile duct, pancreatitis, pancreatic neoplasms

Table 16–2. Hyperbilirubinemic disorders.

	Nature of Defect	Type of Hyperbilirubinemia	Clinical and Pathologic Characteristics
Gilbert syndrome[1]	Reduced activity of uridine diphosphate glucuronyl transferase	Unconjugated (indirect) bilirubin	Benign, asymptomatic hereditary jaundice. Hyperbilirubinemia increased by 24- to 36-hour fast. No treatment required. Associated with reduced mortality from cardiovascular disease.
Dubin-Johnson syndrome[2]	Reduced excretory function of hepatocytes	Conjugated (direct) bilirubin	Benign, asymptomatic hereditary jaundice. Gallbladder does not visualize on oral cholecystography. Liver darkly pigmented on gross examination. Biopsy shows centrilobular brown pigment. Prognosis excellent.
Rotor syndrome[3]	Reduced hepatic reuptake of bilirubin conjugates	Conjugated (direct) bilirubin	Similar to Dubin-Johnson syndrome, but liver is not pigmented and the gallbladder is visualized on oral cholecystography. Prognosis excellent.
Recurrent intrahepatic cholestasis[4]	Cholestasis, often on a familial basis	Predominantly conjugated (direct) bilirubin	Episodic attacks of jaundice, itching, and malaise. Onset in early life and may persist for a lifetime. Alkaline phosphatase increased. Cholestasis found on liver biopsy. (Biopsy may be normal during remission.) Prognosis is generally excellent for "benign" recurrent intrahepatic cholestasis but may not be for familial forms.
Intrahepatic cholestasis of pregnancy[5]	Cholestasis	Predominantly conjugated (direct) bilirubin	Benign cholestatic jaundice, usually occurring in the third trimester of pregnancy. Itching, gastrointestinal symptoms, and abnormal liver excretory function tests. Cholestasis noted on liver biopsy. Prognosis excellent, but recurrence with subsequent pregnancies or use of oral contraceptives is characteristic.

[1]Gilbert syndrome generally results from the addition of extra dinucleotide(s) TA sequences to the TATA promoter of the conjugating enzyme *UGT1A1*.

[2]Dubin-Johnson syndrome is caused by a mutation in the *ABCC2* gene coding for organic anion transporter multidrug resistance protein 2 in bile canaliculi on chromosome 10q24.

[3]Rotor syndrome is caused by mutations in the genes coding for organic anion transporting polypeptides OATP1B1 and OATP1B3 on chromosome 12p.

[4]Mutations in genes that control hepatocellular transport systems that are involved in the formation of bile and inherited as autosomal recessive traits are on chromosomes 18q21–22, 2q24, and 7q21 in families with progressive familial intrahepatic cholestasis. Gene mutations on chromosome 18q21–22 alter a P-type ATPase expressed in the small intestine and liver and other tissues on chromosome 2q24 alter the bile acid export pump and also cause benign recurrent intrahepatic cholestasis.

[5]Mutations in genes (especially *ABCB4* and *ABCB11*) that encode biliary canalicular transporters account for many cases of intrahepatic cholestasis of pregnancy.

light-colored stools. Symptoms and signs may be intermittent if caused by a stone, carcinoma of the ampulla, or cholangiocarcinoma. Pain may be absent early in pancreatic cancer. Occult blood in the stools suggests cancer of the ampulla. Hepatomegaly and a palpable gallbladder (Courvoisier sign) are characteristic, but neither specific nor sensitive, of a pancreatic head tumor. Fever and chills are more common in benign obstruction with associated cholangitis.

► Diagnostic Studies (Tables 16–3, 16–4)

A. Laboratory Findings

Elevated serum alanine and aspartate aminotransferase (ALT and AST) levels reflect hepatocellular injury. Normal reference values for ALT and AST are lower than generally reported when persons with risk factors for fatty liver are excluded. Levels decrease with age and correlate with body mass index and mortality from liver disease and inversely with caffeine consumption and possibly serum vitamin D levels. There is controversy about whether an elevated ALT level is associated with mortality from coronary artery disease, cancer, diabetes mellitus, and all causes. Truncal fat and early-onset paternal obesity are risk factors for increased ALT levels. Levels are mildly elevated in more than 25% of persons with untreated celiac disease and in type 1 diabetic patients with so-called glycogenic hepatopathy and often rise transiently in healthy persons who begin taking 4 g of acetaminophen per day or experience rapid weight gain on a fast-food diet. Levels may rise strikingly but transiently in patients with acute biliary obstruction from choledocholithiasis. Nonalcoholic fatty liver disease is by far the most common cause of mildly to moderately elevated aminotransferase levels. Elevated ALT and AST levels, often greater than 1000 units/L (20 mckat/L), are the hallmark of hepatocellular necrosis or inflammation. Elevated alkaline phosphatase levels are seen in cholestasis or infiltrative liver disease (such as tumor, granulomas, or amyloidosis). Isolated alkaline phosphatase

Table 16–4. Causes of serum aminotransferase elevations.[1]

Mild Elevations (5 × normal)	Severe Elevations (> 15 × normal)
Hepatic: ALT-predominant	Acute viral hepatitis
Chronic hepatitis B, C, and D	(A–E, herpes)
Acute viral hepatitis (A-E, EBV, CMV)	Medications/toxins
Steatosis/steatohepatitis	Ischemic hepatitis
Hemochromatosis	Autoimmune hepatitis
Medications/toxins	Wilson disease
Autoimmune hepatitis	Acute bile duct
Alpha-1-antitrypsin	obstruction
(alpha-1-antiprotease) deficiency	Acute Budd-Chiari
Wilson disease	syndrome
Celiac disease	Hepatic artery ligation
Glycogenic hepatopathy	
Hepatic: AST–predominant	
Alcohol-related liver injury	
(AST:ALT > 2:1)	
Cirrhosis	
Nonhepatic	
Strenuous exercise	
Hemolysis	
Myopathy	
Thyroid disease	
Macro-AST	

[1]Almost any liver disease can cause moderate aminotransferase elevations (5–15 × normal).
ALT, alanine aminotransferase; AST, aspartate aminotransferase; CMV, cytomegalovirus; EBV, Epstein-Barr virus.
Adapted with permission from Green RM et al. AGA technical review on the evaluation of liver chemistry tests. Gastroenterology. 2002 Oct;123(4):1367–84.

elevations of hepatic rather than bone, intestinal, or placental origin are confirmed by concomitant elevation of gamma-glutamyl transpeptidase or 5′-nucleotidase levels. Serum gamma-glutamyl transpeptidase levels appear to correlate with the risk of mortality and disability in the

Table 16–3. Liver biochemical tests: Normal values and changes in hepatocellular and obstructive jaundice.

Tests	Normal Values	Hepatocellular Jaundice	Obstructive Jaundice
Bilirubin[1]			
Direct	0.1–0.3 mg/dL (1.71–5.13 mcmol/L)	Increased	Increased
Indirect	0.2–0.7 mg/dL (3.42–11.97 mcmol/L)	Increased	Increased
Urine bilirubin	None	Increased	Increased
Serum albumin	3.5–5.5 g/dL (35–55 g/L)	Decreased	Generally unchanged
Alkaline phosphatase	30–115 units/L (0.6–2.3 mkat/L)	Mildly increased (+)	Markedly increased (++++)
Prothrombin time	INR of 1.0–1.4. After vitamin K, 10% decrease in 24 hours	Prolonged if damage is severe; does not respond to parenteral vitamin K	Prolonged if obstruction is marked; generally responds to parenteral vitamin K
ALT, AST	ALT, ≤ 30 units/L (0.6 mkat/L) (men), ≤ 19 units/L (0.38 mkat/L) (women); AST, 5–40 units/L (0.1–0.8 mkat/L)	Increased, as in viral hepatitis	Minimally increased

[1]Measured by the van den Bergh reaction, which overestimates direct bilirubin in normal persons.
ALT, alanine aminotransferase; AST, aspartate aminotransferase; INR, international normalized ratio.

general population. The differential diagnosis of any liver test elevation includes toxicity caused by drugs, herbal remedies, and toxins.

B. Imaging

Demonstration of dilated bile ducts by ultrasonography or CT indicates biliary obstruction (90–95% sensitivity). Ultrasonography, CT, and MRI may also demonstrate hepatomegaly, intrahepatic tumors, and portal hypertension. Use of color Doppler ultrasonography or contrast agents that produce microbubbles increases the sensitivity of transcutaneous ultrasonography for detecting small neoplasms. MRI is the most accurate technique for identifying isolated liver lesions such as hemangiomas, focal nodular hyperplasia, or focal fatty infiltration and for detecting hepatic iron overload. The most sensitive techniques for detection of individual small hepatic metastases in patients eligible for resection are multiphasic helical or multislice CT; CT arterial portography, in which imaging follows intravenous contrast infusion via a catheter placed in the superior mesenteric artery; MRI with use of gadolinium or ferumoxides as contrast agents; and intraoperative ultrasonography. Dynamic gadolinium-enhanced MRI and MRI following administration of superparamagnetic iron oxide show promise in visualizing hepatic fibrosis. Because of its much lower cost, ultrasonography is preferable to CT (~six times more expensive) or MRI (~seven times more expensive) as a screening test. Positron emission tomography (PET) can be used to detect small pancreatic tumors and metastases. Ultrasonography can detect gallstones with a sensitivity of 95%.

Magnetic resonance cholangiopancreatography (MRCP) is a sensitive, noninvasive method of detecting bile duct stones, strictures, and dilatation; however, it is less reliable than endoscopic retrograde cholangiopancreatography (ERCP) for distinguishing malignant from benign strictures. ERCP requires a skilled endoscopist and may be used to demonstrate pancreatic or ampullary causes of jaundice, carry out sphincterotomy and stone extraction, insert a stent through an obstructing lesion, or facilitate direct cholangiopancreatoscopy. Complications of ERCP include pancreatitis (5% or less) and, less commonly, cholangitis, bleeding, or duodenal perforation after sphincterotomy. Risk factors for post-ERCP pancreatitis include female sex, prior post-ERCP pancreatitis, suspected sphincter of Oddi dysfunction, and a difficult or failed cannulation. Percutaneous transhepatic cholangiography (PTC) is an alternative approach to evaluating the anatomy of the biliary tract. Serious complications of PTC occur in 3% and include fever, bacteremia, bile peritonitis, and intraperitoneal hemorrhage. Endoscopic ultrasonography (EUS) is the most sensitive test for detecting small lesions of the ampulla or pancreatic head and for detecting portal vein invasion by pancreatic cancer. It is also accurate in detecting or excluding bile duct stones.

C. Liver Biopsy

Percutaneous liver biopsy is the definitive study for determining the cause and histologic severity of hepatocellular dysfunction or infiltrative liver disease. In patients with suspected metastatic disease or a hepatic mass, it is performed under ultrasound or CT guidance. A transjugular route can be used in patients with coagulopathy or ascites. The risk of bleeding after a percutaneous liver biopsy is approximately 0.5% and is increased in persons with a platelet count of 60,000/mcL (60×10^9/mcL) or less. Panels of blood tests (eg, FibroSure) and ultrasound (transient or acoustic radiation force impulse) elastography or magnetic resonance elastography to measure liver stiffness are used increasingly for estimating the stage of liver fibrosis and degree of portal hypertension without the need for liver biopsy.

► When to Refer

Patients with jaundice should be referred for diagnostic procedures.

► When to Admit

Patients with liver failure should be hospitalized.

Castillo NE et al. Prevalence of abnormal liver function tests in celiac disease and the effect of a gluten-free diet in the US population. Am J Gastroenterol. 2015 Aug;110(8):1216–22. [PMID: 26150087]

European Association for Study of Liver; Asociacion Latino-americana para el Estudio del Higado. EASL-ALEH Clinical Practice Guidelines: non-invasive tests for evaluation of liver disease severity and prognosis. J Hepatol. 2015 Jul;63(1):237–64. [PMID: 25911335]

Singh S et al. Diagnostic performance of magnetic resonance elastography in staging liver fibrosis: a systematic review and meta-analysis of individual participant data. Clin Gastroenterol Hepatol. 2015 Mar;13(3):440–51. [PMID: 25305349]

Van Beers BE et al. New imaging techniques for liver diseases. J Hepatol. 2015 Mar;62(3):690–700. [PMID: 25457198]

DISEASES OF THE LIVER

See Chapter 39 for Hepatocellular Carcinoma.

ACUTE HEPATITIS A

ESSENTIALS OF DIAGNOSIS

► Prodrome of anorexia, nausea, vomiting, malaise, aversion to smoking.

► Fever, enlarged and tender liver, jaundice.

► Normal to low white cell count; markedly elevated aminotransferases.

► General Considerations

Hepatitis can be caused by viruses, including the five hepatotropic viruses—A, B, C, D, and E—and many drugs and toxic agents; the clinical manifestations may be similar regardless of cause. Hepatitis A virus (HAV) is a 27-nm RNA hepatovirus (in the picornavirus family) that causes epidemics or sporadic cases of hepatitis. The virus is transmitted by the fecal-oral route, and its spread is favored by crowding and poor sanitation. Since introduction of the HAV vaccine in the United States in 1995, the incidence rate of HAV infection has declined from as much as 14 to 0.4 per 100,000 population, with a corresponding decline in the mortality rate from 0.1 to 0.02 deaths per 100,000 population and an increase in the mean age of death. International travel has emerged as the leading risk factor, accounting for over 40% of cases, with another 18% of cases attributable to exposure to an international traveler. Common source outbreaks may still result from contaminated water or food, including inadequately cooked shellfish. In 2013, an outbreak in the United States resulted from frozen pomegranate arils imported from Turkey, and HAV has been described as a reemerging foodborne public health threat in Europe. Outbreaks among people who inject drugs or who are unvaccinated residents in institutions and cases among international adoptees and their contacts also have been reported.

The incubation period averages 30 days. HAV is excreted in feces for up to 2 weeks before clinical illness but rarely after the first week of illness. The mortality rate for hepatitis A is low, and fulminant hepatitis A is uncommon except for rare instances in which it occurs in a patient with concomitant chronic hepatitis C. There is no chronic carrier state. In the United States, about 30% of the population have serologic evidence of previous HAV infection.

► Clinical Findings

A. Symptoms and Signs

Figure 16–1 shows the typical course of acute hepatitis A. Clinical illness is more severe in adults than in children, in whom it is usually asymptomatic. The onset may be abrupt or insidious, with malaise, myalgia, arthralgia, easy

▲ **Figure 16–1.** The typical course of acute type A hepatitis. (HAV, hepatitis A virus; anti-HAV, antibody to hepatitis A virus; ALT, alanine aminotransferase.) (Reprinted, with permission, from Koff RS. Acute viral hepatitis. In: Friedman LS, Keeffe EB [editors]. *Handbook of Liver Disease*, 3rd ed. Philadelphia: Saunders Elsevier, 2012.)

fatigability, upper respiratory symptoms, and anorexia. A distaste for smoking, paralleling anorexia, may occur early. Nausea and vomiting are frequent, and diarrhea or constipation may occur. Fever is generally present but is low-grade except in occasional cases in which systemic toxicity may occur. Defervescence and a fall in pulse rate often coincide with the onset of jaundice.

Abdominal pain is usually mild and constant in the right upper quadrant or epigastrium, often aggravated by jarring or exertion, and rarely may be severe enough to simulate cholecystitis.

Jaundice occurs after 5–10 days but may appear at the same time as the initial symptoms. In many patients, jaundice never develops. With the onset of jaundice, prodromal symptoms often worsen, followed by progressive clinical improvement. Stools may be acholic during this phase.

The acute illness usually subsides over 2–3 weeks with complete clinical and laboratory recovery by 9 weeks. In some cases, clinical, biochemical, and serologic recovery may be followed by one or two relapses, but recovery is the rule. Acute cholecystitis occasionally complicates the course of acute hepatitis A.

Hepatomegaly—rarely marked—is present in over half of cases. Liver tenderness is usually present. Splenomegaly is reported in 15% of patients, and soft, enlarged lymph nodes—especially in the cervical or epitrochlear areas—may occur.

B. Laboratory Findings

The white blood cell count is normal to low, especially in the preicteric phase. Large atypical lymphocytes may occasionally be seen. Mild proteinuria is common, and bilirubinuria often precedes the appearance of jaundice. Strikingly elevated ALT or AST levels occur early, followed by elevations of bilirubin and alkaline phosphatase; in a minority of patients, the latter persist after aminotransferase levels have normalized. Cholestasis is occasionally marked. Antibody to hepatitis A (anti-HAV) appears early in the course of the illness (Figure 16–1). Both IgM and IgG anti-HAV are detectable in serum soon after the onset. Peak titers of IgM anti-HAV occur during the first week of clinical disease and disappear within 3–6 months. Detection of IgM anti-HAV is an excellent test for diagnosing acute hepatitis A but is not recommended for the evaluation of asymptomatic persons with persistently elevated serum aminotransferase levels because false-positive results occur. False-negative results have been described in a patient receiving rituximab for rheumatoid arthritis. Titers of IgG anti-HAV rise after 1 month of the disease and may persist for years. IgG anti-HAV (in the absence of IgM anti-HAV) indicates previous exposure to HAV, noninfectivity, and immunity.

► Differential Diagnosis

The differential diagnosis includes other viruses that cause hepatitis, particularly hepatitis B and C, and diseases such as infectious mononucleosis, cytomegalovirus infection, herpes simplex virus infection, Middle East respiratory syndrome, and infections caused by many other viruses, including influenza and Ebola virus; spirochetal diseases such as leptospirosis and secondary syphilis; brucellosis; rickettsial diseases such as Q fever; drug-induced liver injury; and ischemic hepatitis (shock liver). Occasionally, autoimmune hepatitis may have an acute onset mimicking acute viral hepatitis. Rarely, metastatic cancer of the liver, lymphoma, or leukemia may present as a hepatitis-like picture.

The prodromal phase of viral hepatitis must be distinguished from other infectious disease such as influenza, upper respiratory infections, and the prodromal stages of the exanthematous diseases. Cholestasis may mimic obstructive jaundice.

▶ Prevention

Strict isolation of patients is not necessary, but hand washing after bowel movements is required. Unvaccinated persons who are exposed to HAV are advised to receive postexposure prophylaxis with a single dose of HAV vaccine or immune globulin (0.02 mL/kg) as soon as possible. The vaccine is preferred in healthy persons ages 1 year to 40 years, whereas immune globulin is preferred in those who are younger than 1 year or older than 40 years, are immunocompromised, or have chronic liver disease.

Two effective inactivated hepatitis A vaccines are available in the United States and recommended for persons living in or traveling to endemic areas (including military personnel), patients with chronic liver disease upon diagnosis after prescreening for immunity (although the cost-effectiveness of vaccinating all patients with concomitant chronic hepatitis C has been questioned), persons with clotting-factor disorders who are treated with concentrates, men who have sex with men, animal handlers, illicit drug users, sewage workers, food handlers, close personal contacts of international adoptees, and children and caregivers in day-care centers and institutions. For healthy travelers, a single dose of vaccine at any time before departure can provide adequate protection. Routine vaccination is advised for all children in states with an incidence of hepatitis A at least twice the national average and has been approved by the Advisory Committee on Immunization Practices of the Centers for Disease Control and Prevention (CDC) for use in all children between ages 1 and 2 in the United States. HAV vaccine is also effective in the prevention of secondary spread to household contacts of primary cases. The recommended dose for adults is 1 mL (1440 ELISA units) of Havrix (GlaxoSmithKline) or 1 mL (50 units) of Vaqta (Merck) intramuscularly, followed by a booster dose at 6–18 months. A combined hepatitis A and B vaccine (Twinrix, GlaxoSmithKline) is available. HIV infection impairs the response to the HAV vaccine, especially in persons with a CD4 count less than 200/mcL.

▶ Treatment

Bed rest is recommended only if symptoms are marked. If nausea and vomiting are pronounced or if oral intake is substantially decreased, intravenous 10% glucose is indicated.

Dietary management consists of palatable meals as tolerated, without overfeeding; breakfast is usually tolerated best. Strenuous physical exertion, alcohol, and hepatotoxic agents should be avoided. Small doses of oxazepam are safe because metabolism is not hepatic; morphine sulfate should be avoided.

Corticosteroids have no benefit in patients with viral hepatitis, including those with fulminant disease.

▶ Prognosis

In most patients, clinical recovery is generally complete within 3 months. Laboratory evidence of liver dysfunction may persist for a longer period, but most patients recover completely. Hepatitis A does not cause chronic liver disease, although it may persist for up to 1 year, and clinical and biochemical relapses may occur before full recovery. The mortality rate is less than 1.0%, with a higher rate in older adults than in younger persons.

▶ When to Admit

- Encephalopathy is present.
- INR greater than 1.6.
- The patient is unable to maintain hydration.

Collier MG et al. Hepatitis A hospitalizations in the United States, 2002–2011. Hepatology. 2015 Feb;61(2):481–5. [PMID: 25266085]

Ly KN et al. Trends in disease and complications of hepatitis A virus infection in the United States, 1999–2011: a new concern for adults. J Infect Dis. 2015 Jul 15;212(2):176–82. [PMID: 25637352]

Wenzel JJ et al. Hepatitis A as a foodborne infection. Lancet Infect Dis. 2014 Oct;14(10):907–8. [PMID: 25195177]

ACUTE HEPATITIS B

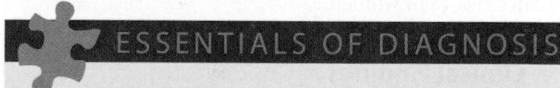

ESSENTIALS OF DIAGNOSIS

- ▶ Prodrome of anorexia, nausea, vomiting, malaise, aversion to smoking.
- ▶ Fever, enlarged and tender liver, jaundice.
- ▶ Normal to low white blood cell count; markedly elevated aminotransferases early in the course.
- ▶ Liver biopsy shows hepatocellular necrosis and mononuclear infiltrate but is rarely indicated.

▶ General Considerations

Hepatitis B virus (HBV) is a 42-nm hepadnavirus with a partially double-stranded DNA genome, inner core protein (hepatitis B core antigen, HBcAg), and outer surface coat (hepatitis B surface antigen, HBsAg). There are eight different genotypes (A–H), which may influence the course of infection and responsiveness to antiviral therapy. HBV is usually transmitted by inoculation of infected blood or blood products or by sexual contact and is present in saliva, semen, and vaginal secretions. HBsAg-positive mothers may transmit HBV at delivery; the risk of chronic infection in the infant is as high as 90%.

Since 1990, the incidence of HBV infection in the United States has decreased from 8.5 to 1.5 cases per 100,000 population. The prevalence is 0.27% in persons aged 6 or over. Because of universal vaccination since 1992, exposure to HBV is now very low among persons aged 18 or younger. HBV is prevalent in men who have sex with men and in people who inject drugs (about 7% of HIV-infected persons are coinfected with HBV), but the greatest number of cases result from heterosexual transmission. Other groups at risk include patients and staff at hemodialysis centers, physicians, dentists, nurses, and personnel working in clinical and pathology laboratories and blood banks. Half of all patients with acute hepatitis B in the United States have previously been incarcerated or treated for a sexually transmitted disease. The risk of HBV infection from a blood transfusion in the United States is no higher than 1 in 350,000 units transfused. Screening for HBV infection is recommended for high-risk groups by the US Preventive Services Task Force.

The incubation period of hepatitis B is 6 weeks to 6 months (average 12–14 weeks). The onset of hepatitis B is more insidious and the aminotransferase levels are higher on average than in HAV infection. Fulminant hepatitis occurs in less than 1%, with a mortality rate of up to 60%. Following acute hepatitis B, HBV infection persists in 1–2% of immunocompetent adults but in a higher percentage of children and immunocompromised adults. There are as many as 2.2 million persons (including an estimated 1.32 million foreign-born persons from endemic areas) with chronic hepatitis B in the United States and 248 million worldwide. Persons with chronic hepatitis B, particularly when HBV infection is acquired early in life and viral replication persists, are at substantial risk for cirrhosis and hepatocellular carcinoma (up to 25–40%); men are at greater risk than women.

▶ Clinical Findings

A. Symptoms and Signs

The clinical picture of viral hepatitis is extremely variable, ranging from asymptomatic infection without jaundice to a fulminating disease and death in a few days. Figure 16–2 shows the typical course of acute HBV infection. The onset may be abrupt or insidious, and the clinical features are similar to those for acute hepatitis A. Serum sickness may be seen early in acute hepatitis B. Fever is generally present and is low-grade. Defervescence and a fall in pulse rate often coincide with the onset of jaundice. Infection caused by HBV may be associated with glomerulonephritis and polyarteritis nodosa.

The acute illness usually subsides over 2–3 weeks with complete clinical and laboratory recovery by 16 weeks. In 5–10% of cases, the course may be more protracted, but less than 1% will have a fulminant course. Hepatitis B may become chronic.

▲ **Figure 16–2.** The typical course of acute type B hepatitis. (anti-HBs, antibody to HBsAg; HBeAg, hepatitis Be antigen; HBsAg, hepatitis B surface antigen; anti-HBe, antibody to HBeAg; anti-HBc, antibody to hepatitis B core antigen; ALT, alanine aminotransferase.) (Reprinted, with permission, from Koff RS. Acute viral hepatitis. In: Friedman LS, Keeffe EB [editors]. *Handbook of Liver Disease*, 3rd ed. Philadelphia: Saunders Elsevier, 2012.)

B. Laboratory Findings

The laboratory features are similar to those for acute hepatitis A, although serum aminotransferase levels are higher on average in acute hepatitis B, and marked cholestasis is not a feature. Marked prolongation of the prothrombin time in severe hepatitis correlates with increased mortality.

There are several antigens and antibodies as well as HBV DNA that relate to HBV infection and that are useful in diagnosis. Interpretation of common serologic patterns is shown in Table 16–5.

1. HBsAg—The appearance of HBsAg in serum is the first evidence of infection, appearing before biochemical evidence of liver disease, and persisting throughout the clinical illness. Persistence of HBsAg more than 6 months after the acute illness signifies chronic hepatitis B.

2. Anti-HBs—Specific antibody to HBsAg (anti-HBs) appears in most individuals after clearance of HBsAg and after successful vaccination against hepatitis B. Disappearance of HBsAg and the appearance of anti-HBs signal recovery from HBV infection, noninfectivity, and immunity.

3. Anti-HBc—IgM anti-HBc appears shortly after HBsAg is detected. (HBcAg alone does not appear in serum.) In the setting of acute hepatitis, IgM anti-HBc indicates a diagnosis of acute hepatitis B, and it fills the serologic gap in rare patients who have cleared HBsAg but do not yet have detectable anti-HBs. IgM anti-HBc can persist for 3–6 months, and sometimes longer. IgM anti-HBc may also reappear during flares of previously inactive chronic hepatitis B. IgG anti-HBc also appears during acute hepatitis B

Table 16–5. Common serologic patterns in hepatitis B virus infection and their interpretation.

HBsAg	Anti-HBs	Anti-HBc	HBeAg	Anti-HBe	Interpretation
+	–	IgM	+	–	Acute hepatitis B
+	–	IgG[1]	+	–	Chronic hepatitis B with active viral replication
+	–	IgG	–	+	Inactive HBV carrier state (low HBV DNA level) or HBeAg-negative chronic hepatitis B with active viral replication (high HBV DNA level)
+	+	IgG	+ or –	+ or –	Chronic hepatitis B with heterotypic anti-HBs (about 10% of cases)
–	–	IgM	+ or –	–	Acute hepatitis B
–	+	IgG	–	+ or –	Recovery from hepatitis B (immunity)
–	+	–	–	–	Vaccination (immunity)
–	–	IgG	–	–	False-positive; less commonly, infection in remote past

[1]Low levels of IgM anti-HBc may also be detected.

but persists indefinitely, whether the patient recovers (with the appearance of anti-HBs in serum) or chronic hepatitis B develops (with persistence of HBsAg). In asymptomatic blood donors, an isolated anti-HBc with no other positive HBV serologic results may represent a falsely positive result or latent infection in which HBV DNA is detectable in serum only by polymerase chain reaction (PCR) testing.

4. HBeAg—HBeAg is a secretory form of HBcAg that appears in serum during the incubation period shortly after the detection of HBsAg. HBeAg indicates viral replication and infectivity. Persistence of HBeAg beyond 3 months indicates an increased likelihood of chronic hepatitis B. Its disappearance is often followed by the appearance of anti-HBe, generally signifying diminished viral replication and decreased infectivity.

5. HBV DNA—The presence of HBV DNA in serum generally parallels the presence of HBeAg, although HBV DNA is a more sensitive and precise marker of viral replication and infectivity. Very low levels of HBV DNA, detectable only by PCR testing, may persist in serum and liver long after a patient has recovered from acute hepatitis B, but the HBV DNA in serum is bound to IgG and is rarely infectious. In some patients with chronic hepatitis B, HBV DNA is present at high levels without HBeAg in serum because of development of a mutation in the core promoter or precore region of the gene that codes HBcAg; these mutations prevent synthesis of HBeAg in infected hepatocytes. When additional mutations in the core gene are present, the precore mutant enhances the severity of HBV infection and increases the risk of cirrhosis.

▶ **Differential Diagnosis**

The differential diagnosis includes hepatitis A and the same disorders listed for the differential diagnosis of acute hepatitis A. In addition, coinfection with HDV must be considered.

▶ **Prevention**

Strict isolation of patients is not necessary. Thorough hand washing by medical staff who may contact contaminated utensils, bedding, or clothing is essential. Medical staff should handle disposable needles carefully and not recap them. Screening of donated blood for HBsAg, anti-HBc, and anti-HCV has reduced the risk of transfusion-associated hepatitis markedly. All pregnant women should undergo testing for HBsAg. HBV-infected persons should practice safer sex. Although cesarean section, in combination with immunoprophylaxis of the neonate, reduces the risk of perinatal transmission of HBV infection when the mother's serum HBV DNA level is 200,000 international units/mL or higher, it is preferable to initiate antiviral therapy of the mother in the third trimester (see Chronic Hepatitis B & Chronic Hepatitis D). HBV-infected health care workers are not precluded from practicing medicine or dentistry if they follow CDC guidelines.

Hepatitis B immune globulin (HBIG) may be protective—or may attenuate the severity of illness—if given within 7 days after exposure (adult dose is 0.06 mL/kg body weight) followed by initiation of the HBV vaccine series. This approach is currently recommended for persons exposed to HBsAg-contaminated material via mucous membranes or through breaks in the skin and for individuals who have had sexual contact with a person with HBV infection (irrespective of the presence or absence of HBeAg in the source). HBIG is also indicated for newborn infants of HBsAg-positive mothers followed by initiation of the vaccine series.

The CDC recommends HBV vaccination of all infants and children in the United States and all adults who are at risk for hepatitis B (including persons under age 60 with diabetes mellitus) or who request vaccination. Over 90% of recipients of the vaccine mount protective antibody to hepatitis B; immunocompromised persons, including patients receiving dialysis (especially those with diabetes mellitus), respond poorly (see Table 30–7). Reduced response to the vaccine may have a genetic basis in some cases and has also been associated with age over 40 years and celiac disease. The standard regimen for adults is 10–20 mcg (depending on the formulation) repeated again at 1 and 6 months, but alternative schedules have been approved, including accelerated schedules of 0, 1, 2, and 12 months and of 0, 7, and 21 days plus 12 months. For greatest reliability of absorption, the deltoid muscle is the preferred site of innoculation. Vaccine formulations free of the mercury-containing preservative thimerosal are given to infants under 6 months of age. When documentation of seroconversion is considered desirable, postimmunization anti-HBs titers may be checked. Protection appears to be excellent even if the titer wanes—at least for 20 years—and booster reimmunization is not routinely recommended but is advised for immunocompromised persons in whom anti-HBs titers fall below 10 milli-international units/mL. For vaccine nonresponders, three additional vaccine doses may elicit seroprotective anti-HBs levels in 30–50% of persons. Doubling of the standard dose may also be effective. Universal vaccination of neonates in countries endemic for HBV has reduced the incidence of hepatocellular carcinoma. Incomplete immunization is the most important predictor of liver disease among vaccinees.

Treatment

Treatment of acute hepatitis B is the same as that for acute hepatitis A. Encephalopathy or severe coagulopathy indicates acute liver failure, and hospitalization at a liver transplant center is mandatory. Antiviral therapy is generally unnecessary in patients with acute hepatitis B but is usually prescribed in cases of fulminant hepatitis B as well as in spontaneous reactivation of chronic hepatitis B presenting as acute-on-chronic liver failure.

Prognosis

In most patients, clinical recovery is complete in 3–6 months. Laboratory evidence of liver dysfunction may persist for a longer period, but most patients recover completely. The mortality rate for acute hepatitis B is 0.1–1% but is higher with superimposed hepatitis D.

Chronic hepatitis, characterized by elevated aminotransferase levels for more than 3–6 months, develops in 1–2% of immunocompetent adults with acute hepatitis B but in as many as 90% of infected neonates and infants and a substantial proportion of immunocompromised adults. Ultimately, cirrhosis develops in up to 40% of those with chronic hepatitis B; the risk of cirrhosis is even higher in HBV-infected patients coinfected with hepatitis C or HIV. Patients with cirrhosis are at risk for hepatocellular carcinoma at a rate of 3–5% per year. Even in the absence of cirrhosis, patients with chronic hepatitis B—particularly those with active viral replication—are at increased risk for hepatocellular carcinoma.

When to Refer

Refer patients with acute hepatitis who require liver biopsy for diagnosis.

When to Admit

- Encephalopathy is present.
- INR greater than 1.6.
- The patient is unable to maintain hydration.

Chen HL et al. Efficacy of maternal tenofovir disoproxil fumarate in interrupting mother-to-infant transmission of hepatitis B virus. Hepatology. 2015 Aug;62(2):375–86. [PMID: 25851052]

LeFevre ML et al. Screening for hepatitis B virus infection in nonpregnant adolescents and adults: U.S. Preventive Services Task Force recommendation statement. Ann Intern Med. 2014 Jul 1;161(1):58–66. [PMID: 24863637]

Rajbhandari R et al. HBV infection is associated with greater mortality in hospitalised patients compared to HCV infection or alcoholic liver disease. Aliment Pharmacol Ther. 2015 May;41(10):928–38. [PMID: 25786514]

Trépo C et al. Hepatitis B virus infection. Lancet. 2014 Dec 6; 384(9959):2053–63. [PMID: 24954675]

Wu Q et al. Telbivudine prevents vertical transmission of hepatitis B virus from women with high viral loads: a prospective long-term study. Clin Gastroenterol Hepatol. 2015 Jun;13(6):1170–6. [PMID: 25251571]

Zeisel MB et al. Towards an HBV cure: state-of-the-art and unresolved questions—report of the ANRS workshop on HBV cure. Gut. 2015 Aug;64(8):1314–26. [PMID: 25670809]

ACUTE HEPATITIS C & OTHER CAUSES OF ACUTE VIRAL HEPATITIS

Viruses other than HAV and HBV that can cause hepatitis are hepatitis C virus (HCV), hepatitis D virus (HDV) (delta agent), and hepatitis E virus (HEV) (an enterically transmitted hepatitis seen in epidemic form in Asia, the Middle East, and North Africa). Human pegivirus (formerly hepatitis G virus [HGV]) rarely, if ever, causes frank hepatitis. A related virus has been named human hepegivirus-1. A DNA virus designated the TT virus (TTV) has been identified in up to 7.5% of blood donors and found to be transmitted readily by blood transfusions, but an association between this virus and liver disease has not been established. A related virus known as SEN-V has been found in 2% of US blood donors, is transmitted by transfusion, and may account for some cases of transfusion-associated non-ABCDE hepatitis. In immunocompromised and rare immunocompetent persons, cytomegalovirus, Epstein-Barr virus, and herpes simplex virus should be considered in the differential diagnosis of hepatitis. Middle East respiratory syndrome (MERS), severe acute respiratory syndrome (SARS), Ebola virus infection, and influenza may be associated with marked serum aminotransferase elevations. Unidentified pathogens account for a small percentage of cases of acute viral hepatitis.

1. Hepatitis C

HCV is a single-stranded RNA virus (hepacivirus) with properties similar to those of flaviviruses. Seven major genotypes of HCV have been identified. In the past, HCV was responsible for over 90% of cases of posttransfusion hepatitis, yet only 4% of cases of hepatitis C were attributable to blood transfusions. Over 50% of cases are transmitted by injection drug use, and both reinfection and superinfection of HCV are common in people who actively inject drugs. Body piercing, tattoos, and hemodialysis are risk factors. The risk of sexual and maternal–neonatal transmission is low and may be greatest in a subset of patients with high circulating levels of HCV RNA. Having multiple sexual partners may increase the risk of HCV infection, and HIV coinfection, unprotected receptive anal intercourse with ejaculation, and sex while high on meth-amphetamine increase the risk of HCV transmission in men who have sex with men. Transmission via breastfeeding has not been documented. An outbreak of hepatitis C in patients with immune deficiencies has occurred in some recipients of intravenous immune globulin. Hospital- and outpatient facility–acquired transmission has occurred via multidose vials of saline used to flush Portacaths; through reuse of disposable syringes; through drug "diversion" and tampering with injectable opioids by an infected health care worker; through contamination of shared saline, radiopharmaceutical, and sclerosant vials; via inadequately disinfected endoscopy equipment; and between hospital-ized patients on a liver unit. In the developing world, unsafe medical practices lead to a substantial number of cases of HCV infection. Covert transmission during bloody fisticuffs has even been reported, and incarceration in prison is a risk factor, with a frequency of 26% in the United States. In many patients, the source of infection is unknown. Coinfection with HCV is found in at least 30% of HIV-infected persons. HIV infection leads to an increased risk of acute liver failure and more rapid progres-sion of chronic hepatitis C to cirrhosis; in addition, HCV increases the hepatotoxicity of highly active antiretroviral therapy. The number of cases of chronic HCV infections in the United States is reported to have decreased from 3.2 million in 2001 to 2.3 million in 2013, although estimates of at least 4.6 million exposed and 3.5 million currently infected have also been reported. The incidence of new cases of acute, symptomatic hepatitis C declined from 1992 to 2005, but an increase was observed in persons aged 15 to 24 after 2002, as a result of injection drug use.

► **Clinical Findings**

A. Symptoms and Signs

Figure 16–3 shows the typical course of HCV infection. The incubation period for hepatitis C averages 6–7 weeks, and clinical illness is often mild, usually asymptomatic, and characterized by waxing and waning aminotransferase ele-vations and a high rate (greater than 80%) of chronic hepa-titis. Spontaneous clearance of HCV following acute infection is more common (64%) in persons with the CC genotype of the *IFNL3* (*IL28B*) gene than in those with the CT or TT genotype (24% and 6%, respectively). In persons with the CC genotype, jaundice is more likely to develop during the course of acute hepatitis C. Patients with the CC genotype and chronic hepatitis C are more likely to respond to therapy with pegylated interferon (see Chronic Viral Hepatitis). In pregnant patients with chronic hepatitis C, serum aminotransferase levels frequently normalize despite persistence of viremia, only to increase again after delivery.

▲ **Figure 16–3.** The typical course of acute and chronic hepatitis C. (ALT, alanine aminotransferase; Anti-HCV, antibody to hepatitis C virus by enzyme immunoas-say; HCV RNA [PCR], hepatitis C viral RNA by polymerase chain reaction.)

B. Laboratory Findings

Diagnosis of hepatitis C is based on an enzyme immunoas-say (EIA) that detects antibodies to HCV. Anti-HCV is not protective, and in patients with acute or chronic hepatitis, its presence in serum generally signifies that HCV is the cause. Limitations of the EIA include moderate sensitivity (false-negatives) for the diagnosis of acute hepatitis C early in the course and low specificity (false-positives) in some persons with elevated gamma-globulin levels. In these situ-ations, a diagnosis of hepatitis C may be confirmed by using an assay for HCV RNA. Occasional persons are found to have anti-HCV in serum, without HCV RNA in serum, suggesting recovery from HCV infection in the past.

► **Complications**

HCV is a pathogenic factor in mixed cryoglobulinemia and membranoproliferative glomerulonephritis and may be related to lichen planus, autoimmune thyroiditis, lympho-cytic sialadenitis, idiopathic pulmonary fibrosis, sporadic porphyria cutanea tarda, and monoclonal gammopathies. HCV infection confers a 20–30% increased risk of non-Hodgkin lymphoma. Hepatic steatosis is a particular fea-ture of infection with HCV genotype 3 and may also occur in patients infected with other HCV genotypes who have risk factors for fatty liver. On the other hand, chronic HCV infection is associated with a decrease in serum cholesterol and low-density lipoprotein levels.

► **Prevention**

Testing donated blood for HCV has helped reduce the risk of transfusion-associated hepatitis C from 10% in 1990 to about 1 case per 2 million units in 2011. Birth cohort screening of persons born between 1945 and 1965 ("baby boomers") for HCV infection has been recommended by the CDC and the US Preventive Services Task Force and could identify over 900,000 new cases. HCV-infected persons should practice safe sex, but there is little evidence that HCV is spread easily by sexual contact or perinatally, and no specific preventive measures are recommended for persons in a monogamous relationship or for pregnant women. Vaccination against HAV (after prescreening for prior immunity) and HBV is recommended for patients with chronic hepatitis C, and vaccination against HAV is also recommended for patients with chronic hepatitis B.

▶ **Treatment**

In the past, treatment of patients with acute hepatitis C with peginterferon for 6–24 weeks was shown to appreciably decrease the risk of chronic hepatitis. Because 20% of patients with acute hepatitis C, particularly those who are symptomatic, clear the virus without such treatment, reserving treatment for patients in whom serum HCV RNA levels failed to clear after 3 months was advised. Ribavirin was added if HCV RNA failed to clear after 3 months of peginterferon, but some authorities recommended using ribavirin with peginterferon from the start of therapy. New oral direct-acting agents are now supplanting interferon-based therapy (see Chronic Viral Hepatitis).

▶ **Prognosis**

In most patients, clinical recovery is complete in 3–6 months. Laboratory evidence of liver dysfunction may persist for a longer period. The overall mortality rate is less than 1%, but the rate is reportedly higher in older people. Fulminant hepatitis C is rare in the United States.

Chronic hepatitis, which progresses very slowly in many cases, develops in as many as 85% of all persons with acute hepatitis C. Ultimately, cirrhosis develops in up to 30% of those with chronic hepatitis C; the risk of cirrhosis and hepatic decompensation is higher in patients coinfected with both HCV and HBV or HIV. Patients with cirrhosis are at risk for hepatocellular carcinoma at a rate of 3–5% per year. Long-term morbidity and mortality in patients with chronic hepatitis C is lower in black than in white patients and lowest in those infected with HCV genotype 2 and highest in those with HCV genotype 3.

2. Hepatitis D (Delta Agent)

HDV is a defective RNA virus that causes hepatitis only in association with HBV infection and specifically only in the presence of HBsAg; it is cleared when the latter is cleared.

HDV may coinfect with HBV or may superinfect a person with chronic hepatitis B, usually by percutaneous exposure. When acute hepatitis D is coincident with acute HBV infection, the infection is generally similar in severity to acute hepatitis B alone. In chronic hepatitis B, superinfection by HDV appears to carry a worse short-term prognosis, often resulting in fulminant hepatitis or severe chronic hepatitis that progresses rapidly to cirrhosis.

New cases of hepatitis D are now infrequent in the United States primarily because of the control of HBV infection (although rates of testing HBV carriers for HDV are inappropriately low), and cases seen today are usually from cohorts infected years ago who survived the initial impact of hepatitis D and now have cirrhosis. These patients are at risk for decompensation and have a threefold increased risk of hepatocellular carcinoma. New cases are seen primarily in immigrants from endemic areas, including Africa, central Asia, Eastern Europe, and the Amazon region of Brazil. More than 15 million people are infected worldwide. The diagnosis of hepatitis D is made by detection of antibody to hepatitis D antigen (anti-HDV) and, where available, hepatitis D antigen (HDAg) or HDV RNA in serum.

3. Hepatitis E

HEV is a 29- to 32-nm RNA hepevirus (in the Hepeviridae family) that is a major cause of acute hepatitis throughout Central and Southeast Asia, the Middle East, and North Africa, where it is responsible for waterborne hepatitis outbreaks. It is uncommon in the United States but should be considered in patients with acute hepatitis after a trip to an endemic area. In rare cases, hepatitis E can be mistaken for drug-induced liver injury. In industrialized countries, it may be spread by swine, and having a pet in the home and consuming undercooked organ meats are risk factors. Illness generally is self-limited (no carrier state), but instances of chronic hepatitis with rapid progression to cirrhosis attributed to HEV have been reported in transplant recipients (particularly when tacrolimus rather than cyclosporine is used as the main immunosuppressant) and, rarely, in persons with HIV infection, preexisting liver disease, or cancer undergoing chemotherapy. The diagnosis of acute hepatitis E is made most readily by testing for IgM anti-HEV in serum, although available tests may not be reliable. Reported extrahepatic manifestations include arthritis; pancreatitis; monoclonal gammopathy; thrombocytopenia; and a variety of neurologic complications, including Guillain-Barré syndrome and peripheral neuropathy. In endemic regions, the mortality rate is high (10–20%) in pregnant women and correlates with high levels of HEV RNA in serum and gene mutations that lead to reduced expression of progesterone receptors. The risk of hepatic decompensation is increased in patients with underlying chronic liver disease. A 3-month course of treatment with oral ribavirin has been reported to induce sustained clearance of HEV RNA from the serum in 78% of patients. Improved public hygiene reduces the risk of HEV infection in endemic areas. Recombinant vaccines against HEV have shown promise in clinical trials, and one (Hecolin) is approved in China.

Hatia RI et al. Nosocomial hepatitis C virus transmission from tampering with injectable anesthetic opioids. Hepatology. 2015 Jul;62(1):101–10. [PMID: 25808284]

Sugerman DT. JAMA patient page. Hepatitis C. JAMA. 2014 Aug 13; 312(6):664. [PMID: 25117147]

Webster DP et al. Hepatitis C. Lancet. 2015 Mar 21; 385(9973):1124–35. [PMID: 25687730]

Zhang J et al. Long-term efficacy of a hepatitis E vaccine. N Engl J Med. 2015 Mar 5;372(10):914–22. [PMID: 25738667]

ACUTE LIVER FAILURE

ESSENTIALS OF DIAGNOSIS

▸ May be fulminant or subfulminant; both forms carry a poor prognosis.

▸ Acetaminophen and idiosyncratic drug reactions are the most common causes.

▸ General Considerations

Acute liver failure may be fulminant or subfulminant. Fulminant hepatic failure is characterized by the development of hepatic encephalopathy within 8 weeks after the onset of acute liver disease. Coagulopathy (international normalized ratio [INR] 1.5 or higher) is invariably present. Subfulminant hepatic failure occurs when these findings appear between 8 weeks and 6 months after the onset of acute liver disease and carries an equally poor prognosis. Acute-on-chronic liver failure refers to acute deterioration in liver function in a person with preexisting chronic liver disease.

An estimated 1600 cases of acute liver failure occur each year in the United States. Acetaminophen toxicity is the most common cause, accounting for at least 45% of cases. Suicide attempts account for 44% of cases of acetaminophen-induced hepatic failure, and unintentional overdoses ("therapeutic misadventures"), which are often a result of a decrease in the threshold toxic dose because of chronic alcohol use or fasting and have been reported after weight loss surgery, account for at least 48%. Other causes include idiosyncratic drug reactions (the second most common cause, with antituberculosis drugs, antiepileptics, and antibiotics implicated most commonly), viral hepatitis, poisonous mushrooms (*Amanita phalloides*), shock, hyperthermia or hypothermia, Budd-Chiari syndrome, malignancy (most commonly lymphomas), Wilson disease, Reye syndrome, fatty liver of pregnancy and other disorders of fatty acid oxidation, autoimmune hepatitis, parvovirus B19 infection and, rarely, grand mal seizures. The risk of acute liver failure is increased in patients with diabetes mellitus, and outcome is worsened by obesity. Herbal and dietary supplements are thought to be contributory to acute liver failure in a substantial portion of cases, regardless of cause. Acute-on-chronic liver failure is often precipitated by infection or an alcohol binge and alcoholic hepatitis.

Viral hepatitis now accounts for only 12% of all cases of acute liver failure. The decline of viral hepatitis as the principal cause of acute liver failure is due to universal vaccination of infants and children against hepatitis B and the availability of the hepatitis A vaccine. In endemic areas, hepatitis E is an important cause of acute liver failure. Hepatitis C is a rare cause of acute liver failure in the United States, but acute hepatitis A or B superimposed on chronic hepatitis C may cause fulminant hepatitis.

▸ Clinical Findings

Gastrointestinal symptoms, systemic inflammatory response, renal dysfunction, and hemorrhagic phenomena are common. Adrenal insufficiency and subclinical myocardial injury manifesting as an elevated serum troponin I level often complicate acute liver failure. Jaundice may be absent or minimal early, but laboratory tests show severe hepatocellular damage. In acetaminophen toxicity, serum aminotransferase elevations are often towering (greater than 5000 units/L). In acute liver failure due to microvesicular steatosis (eg, fatty liver of pregnancy), serum aminotransferase elevations may be modest (less than 300 units/L). Over 10% of patients have an elevated serum amylase level at least three times the upper limit of normal, often as a result of renal dysfunction. The blood ammonia level is typically elevated and correlates (along with the Model for End-Stage Liver Disease [MELD] score) with the development of encephalopathy and intracranial hypertension. Intracranial hypertension rarely develops when the blood ammonia level is less than 75 mcmol/L and is invariable when it is greater than 200 mcmol/L. The severity of extrahepatic organ dysfunction (as assessed by the Sequential Organ Failure Assessment [SOFA]) also correlates with the likelihood of intracranial hypertension. Acute kidney injury frequently complicates acute-on-chronic liver failure.

▸ Treatment

The treatment of acute liver failure is directed toward achieving metabolic and hemodynamic stability. Intravascular volume should be preserved, but large-volume infusions of hypotonic fluids should be avoided. Hypoglycemia should be prevented. Intermittent renal replacement therapy may be required. To preserve muscle mass and immune function, enteral administration of protein, 1–1.5 g/kg/day, is advised, with careful monitoring of the ammonia level. Cerebral edema and sepsis are the leading causes of death. Prophylactic antibiotic therapy decreases the risk of infection, observed in up to 90%, but has no effect on survival and is not routinely recommended. For suspected sepsis, broad coverage is indicated. Despite a high rate of adrenal insufficiency, corticosteroids are of uncertain value and may lower overall survival in patients with a high MELD score. Stress gastropathy prophylaxis with an H_2-receptor blocker or proton pump inhibitor is recommended. Administration of acetylcysteine (140 mg/kg orally followed by 70 mg/kg orally every 4 hours for an additional 17 doses or 150 mg/kg in 5% dextrose intravenously over 15 minutes followed by 50 mg/kg over 4 hours and then 100 mg/kg over 16 hours) is indicated for acetaminophen toxicity up to 72 hours after ingestion. For massive acetaminophen overdoses, treatment with intravenous acetylcysteine may need to be extended in duration until the serum aminotransferase levels are declining and serum acetaminophen levels are undetectable. Treatment with acetylcysteine improves cerebral blood flow and oxygenation as well as transplant-free survival in patients with stage 1 or 2 encephalopathy due to fulminant hepatic failure of any cause. (Acetylcysteine treatment can prolong the prothrombin time, leading to the erroneous assumption that liver failure is worsening; it can also cause nausea, vomiting, and an anaphylactoid reaction [especially in persons with a history of asthma].) Penicillin G (300,000 to 1 million units/kg/day) or silibinin (silymarin or milk thistle), which is not licensed in the United States, is administered to patients with mushroom poisoning. Nucleoside analogs are recommended for patients with fulminant hepatitis B (see Chronic Viral Hepatitis), and intravenous acyclovir has shown benefit in those with herpes simplex virus hepatitis. Plasmapheresis combined with D-penicillamine has been used in fulminant Wilson disease. Subclinical seizure activity is common in patients with acute liver failure, but the value of prophylactic phenytoin is uncertain.

Early transfer to a liver transplantation center is essential. The head of the patient's bed should be elevated to 30 degrees, and patients with stage 3 or 4 encephalopathy should be intubated. Extradural sensors may be placed to monitor intracranial pressure for impending cerebral edema with the goal of maintaining the intracranial pressure below 20 mm Hg and the cerebral perfusion pressure above 70 mm Hg. Recombinant activated factor VIIa may be administered to reduce the risk of bleeding associated with intracranial pressure monitoring. Lactulose is generally avoided. Mannitol, 0.5 g/kg, or 100–200 mL of a 20% solution by intravenous infusion over 10 minutes, may decrease cerebral edema but should be used with caution in patients with advanced chronic kidney disease. Intravenously administered hypertonic saline to induce hypernatremia (serum sodium concentration of 145–155 mEq/L [145–155 mmol/L]) also may reduce intracranial hypertension. Hypothermia to a temperature of 32–34°C may reduce intracranial pressure when other measures have failed and may improve survival long enough to permit liver transplantation, although a controlled trial showed no benefit and some authorities recommend a target core temperature of 35–36°C. The value of hyperventilation and intravenous prostaglandin E_1 is uncertain. A short-acting barbiturate, propofol, or intravenous boluses of indomethacin, 25 mg, is considered for refractory intracranial hypertension.

Prognosis

With earlier recognition of acute liver failure, the frequency of cerebral edema has declined, and overall survival has improved steadily since the 1970s and is now as high as 75%. The survival rate in fulminant hepatic failure with severe encephalopathy is as low as 20%, except for acetaminophen hepatotoxicity, in which the transplant-free survival is 65% and no more than 8% of patients undergo liver transplantation. For patients with fulminant hepatic failure of other causes, the outlook is poor in patients younger than 10 and older than 40 years of age and in those with an idiosyncratic drug reaction but appears to be improved when acetylcysteine is administered to patients with stage 1 or 2 encephalopathy. Spontaneous recovery is less likely for hepatitis B than for hepatitis A. Other adverse prognostic factors are a serum bilirubin level greater than 18 mg/dL (307.8 mcmol/L), INR higher than 6.5, onset of encephalopathy more than 7 days after the onset of jaundice, and a low factor V level (less than 20% of normal). For acetaminophen-induced fulminant hepatic failure, indicators of a poor outcome are acidosis (pH < 7.3), INR greater than 6.5, and azotemia (serum creatinine 3.4 mg/dL [283.22 mcmol/L] or higher), whereas a rising serum

alpha-fetoprotein level predicts a favorable outcome. An elevated blood lactate level (greater than 3.5 mEq/L [3.5 mmol/L]), elevated blood ammonia level (greater than 211 mcg/dL [124 mcmol/L]), and possibly hyperphosphatemia (greater than 3.7 mg/dL [1.2 mmol/L]) also predict poor survival. One study has shown that patients with persistent elevation of the arterial ammonia level (211 mcg/dL [122 mcmol/L] or higher) for 3 days have greater rates of complications and mortality than those with decreasing ammonia levels. A number of prognostic indices have been proposed: the "BiLE" score, based on the serum bilirubin, serum lactate, and etiology; the Acute Liver Failure Early Dynamic (ALFED) model, based on the arterial ammonia level, serum bilirubin, INR, and hepatic encephalopathy; and the Acute Liver Failure Study Group (ALFSG) index, based on coma grade, INR, serum bilirubin and phosphorous levels, and serum levels of M30, a cleavage product of cytokeratin-18 caspase. Emergency liver transplantation is considered for patients with stage 2 to stage 3 encephalopathy (see Cirrhosis) and is associated with a 70% survival rate at 5 years. For mushroom poisoning, liver transplantation should be considered when the interval between ingestion and the onset of diarrhea is less than 8 hours or the INR is 6.0 or higher, even in the absence of encephalopathy. Acute liver failure superimposed on chronic liver disease (acute-on-chronic liver failure) is often precipitated by a bacterial infection or active alcoholism and has a poor prognosis when associated with renal dysfunction.

When to Admit

All patients with acute liver failure should be hospitalized.

Manka P et al. Hepatitis E virus infection as a possible cause of acute liver failure in Europe. Clin Gastroenterol Hepatol. 2015 Oct;13(10):1836–42. [PMID: 25912835]

Moreau R et al. Acute-on-chronic liver failure: a new clinical entity. Clin Gastroenterol Hepatol. 2015 May;13(5):836–41 [PMID: 24583872]

Rich NE et al. Malignant infiltration of the liver presenting as acute liver failure. Clin Gastroenterol Hepatol. 2015 May; 13(5):1025–8. [PMID: 25277846]

Tujios SR et al. Risk factors and outcomes of acute kidney injury in patients with acute liver failure. Clin Gastroenterol Hepatol. 2015 Feb;13(2):352–9. [PMID: 25019700]

CHRONIC VIRAL HEPATITIS

ESSENTIALS OF DIAGNOSIS

▶ Defined by chronic infection (HBV, HCV, HDV) for longer than 3–6 months.

▶ Diagnosis is usually made by antibody tests and viral nucleic acid in serum.

General Considerations

Chronic hepatitis is defined as chronic necroinflammation of the liver of more than 3–6 months' duration, demonstrated by persistently elevated serum aminotransferase levels or characteristic histologic findings. In many cases, the diagnosis of chronic hepatitis may be made on initial presentation. The causes of chronic hepatitis include HBV, HCV, and HDV as well as autoimmune hepatitis; alcoholic and nonalcoholic steatohepatitis; certain medications, such as isoniazid and nitrofurantoin; Wilson disease; alpha-1-antiprotease deficiency; and, rarely, celiac disease. Mortality from chronic HBV and HCV infection has been rising in the United States, and HCV has surpassed HIV as a cause of death. Chronic hepatitis is categorized on the basis of etiology; the grade of portal, periportal, and lobular inflammation (minimal, mild, moderate, or severe); and the stage of fibrosis (none, mild, moderate, severe, cirrhosis). In the absence of advanced cirrhosis, patients are often asymptomatic or have mild nonspecific symptoms.

1. Chronic Hepatitis B & Chronic Hepatitis D

► Clinical Findings & Diagnosis

Chronic hepatitis B afflicts 248 million people worldwide (2 billion overall have been infected; endemic areas include Asia and sub-Saharan Africa) and up to 2.2 million (predominantly males) in the United States. It may be noted as a continuum of acute hepatitis B or diagnosed because of repeated detection of HBsAg in serum, often with elevated aminotransferase levels.

Four phases of HBV infection are recognized: immune tolerant phase, immune clearance phase, inactive HBsAg carrier state, and reactivated chronic hepatitis B phase. In the **immune tolerant phase,** HBeAg and HBV DNA are present in serum, which is indicative of active viral replication, and serum aminotransferase levels are normal, with little necroinflammation in the liver. This phase is common in infants and young children whose immature immune system fails to mount an immune response to HBV. Persons in the immune tolerant phase and those who acquire HBV infection later in life may enter an **immune clearance phase,** in which aminotransferase levels are elevated and necroinflammation is present in the liver, with a risk of progression to cirrhosis (at a rate of 2–5.5% per year) and of hepatocellular carcinoma (at a rate of more than 2% per year in those with cirrhosis); low-level IgM anti-HBc is present in serum in about 70%.

Patients enter the **inactive HBsAg carrier state** when biochemical improvement follows immune clearance. This improvement coincides with disappearance of HBeAg and reduced HBV DNA levels (less than 10^5 copies/mL, or less than 20,000 international units/mL) in serum, appearance of anti-HBe, and integration of the HBV genome into the host genome in infected hepatocytes. Patients in this phase are at a low risk for cirrhosis (if it has not already developed) and hepatocellular carcinoma, and those with persistently normal serum aminotransferase levels infrequently have histologically significant liver disease, especially if the HBsAg level is low.

The **reactivated chronic hepatitis B phase** may result from infection by a pre-core mutant of HBV or spontaneous mutation of the pre-core or core promoter region of the HBV genome during the course of chronic hepatitis

caused by wild-type HBV. So-called HBeAg-negative chronic hepatitis B accounts for less than 10% of cases of chronic hepatitis B in the United States, up to 50% in southeast Asia, and up to 90% in Mediterranean countries, reflecting in part differences in the frequencies of HBV genotypes. In reactivated chronic hepatitis B, there is a rise in serum HBV DNA levels and possible progression to cirrhosis (at a rate of 8–10% per year), particularly when additional mutations in the core gene of HBV are present. Risk factors for reactivation include male sex and HBV genotype C. In patients with either HBeAg-positive or HBeAg-negative chronic hepatitis B, the risk of cirrhosis and of hepatocellular carcinoma correlates with the serum HBV DNA level. Other risk factors include advanced age, male sex, alcohol use, cigarette smoking, HBV genotype C, and coinfection with HCV or HDV. HIV coinfection is also associated with an increased frequency of cirrhosis when the CD4 count is low.

Acute **hepatitis D** infection superimposed on chronic HBV infection may result in severe chronic hepatitis, which may progress rapidly to cirrhosis and may be fatal. Patients with long-standing chronic hepatitis D and B often have inactive cirrhosis and are at risk for decompensation and hepatocellular carcinoma. The diagnosis is confirmed by detection of anti-HDV or HDAg (or HDV RNA) in serum.

► Treatment

Patients with active viral replication (HBeAg and HBV DNA [10^5 copies/mL or more, or 20,000 international units/mL or more] in serum and elevated aminotransferase levels) may be treated with a nucleoside or nucleotide analog or with pegylated interferon. Nucleoside and nucleotide analogs are preferred because they are better tolerated and can be taken orally. For patients who are HBeAg-negative, the threshold for treatment is a serum HBV DNA level of 10^4 copies/mL or more, or 2000 international units/mL or more. If the threshold HBV DNA level for treatment is met but the serum ALT level is normal, treatment may still be considered in patients over age 35–40 if liver biopsy demonstrates a fibrosis stage of 2 of 4 (moderate) or higher. Therapy is aimed at reducing and maintaining the serum HBV DNA level to the lowest possible levels, thereby leading to normalization of the ALT level and histologic improvement. An additional goal in HBeAg-positive patients is seroconversion to anti-HBe, and some responders eventually clear HBsAg. Although nucleoside and nucleotide analogs generally have been discontinued 6–12 months after HBeAg-to-anti-HBe seroconversion, some patients (especially Asian patients) serorevert to HBeAg after discontinuation, have a rise in HBV DNA levels and recurrence of hepatitis activity, and require long-term therapy, which also is required when seroconversion does not occur. HBeAg-negative patients with chronic hepatitis B also generally require long-term therapy because relapse is frequent when therapy is stopped.

The available nucleoside and nucleotide analogs—entecavir, tenofovir, lamivudine, adefovir, and telbivudine—differ in efficacy and rates of resistance; however, in HBeAg-positive patients, they all achieve an HBeAg-to-anti-HBe seroconversion rate of about 20% at 1 year, with higher rates after more prolonged therapy. The preferred first-line oral agents are entecavir and tenofovir. Entecavir is rarely associated with resistance unless a patient is already resistant to lamivudine. The daily dose is 0.5 mg orally for patients not resistant to lamivudine and 1 mg for patients who previously became resistant to lamivudine. Suppression of HBV DNA in serum occurs in nearly all treated patients, and histologic improvement is observed in 70% of patients. Entecavir has been reported to cause lactic acidosis when used in patients with decompensated cirrhosis. Tenofovir, 300 mg orally daily, is equally effective and is used as a first-line agent or when resistance to a nucleoside analog has developed. Like entecavir, tenofovir has a low rate of resistance when used as initial therapy. Long-term use may lead to an elevated serum creatinine level and reduced serum phosphate level (Fanconi-like syndrome) that is reversible with discontinuation of the drug.

The first available nucleoside analog was lamivudine, 100 mg orally daily. By the end of 1 year of therapy with lamivudine, however, 15–30% of responders experience a relapse (and occasionally frank decompensation). The rate of resistance reaches 70% by 5 years of therapy, and the drug is no longer considered first-line therapy in the United States but may be used in countries in which cost is a deciding factor. Adefovir dipivoxil has activity against wild-type and lamivudine-resistant HBV but is the least potent of the oral antiviral agents for HBV. The standard dose is 10 mg orally once a day for at least 1 year. As with lamivudine, only a small number of patients achieve sustained suppression of HBV replication with adefovir, and long-term suppressive therapy is often required. Resistance to adefovir occurs in up to 29% of patients treated for 5 years. Patients with underlying kidney dysfunction are at risk for nephrotoxicity from adefovir. Telbivudine, given in a daily dose of 600 mg orally, is more potent than either lamivudine or adefovir. Resistance to this drug may develop, however, particularly in patients who are resistant to lamivudine, and elevated creatine kinase levels are common in patients treated with telbivudine. Strategies using multiple drugs have not proved advantageous. Other antiviral agents are under study.

The development of resistance occasionally results in hepatic decompensation. Resistance is most likely to develop to lamivudine and may develop to adefovir and telbivudine, but these drugs are no longer used as first-line agents in the United States. Sequential addition of a second antiviral agent is usually effective after resistance to the first agent has developed. Combined use of peginterferon and a nucleoside or nucleotide analog has not been shown convincingly to have a substantial advantage over the use of either type of drug alone. Nucleoside and nucleotide analogs are well tolerated even in patients with decompensated cirrhosis (for whom the treatment threshold may be an HBV DNA level less than 10^4 copies/mL) and may be effective in patients with rapidly progressive hepatitis B ("fibrosing cholestatic hepatitis") following organ transplantation.

Nucleoside analogs are also recommended for inactive HBV carriers (and those positive only for anti-HBc) prior to the initiation of immunosuppressive therapy (including rituximab or anti-tumor necrosis factor antibody therapy) or cancer chemotherapy to prevent reactivation; entecavir has been shown to be more effective than lamivudine. In patients infected with both HBV and HIV, antiretroviral therapy, including two drugs active against both viruses (eg, tenofovir plus lamivudine or emtricitabine), has been recommended when treatment of HIV infection is indicated. Telbivudine and tenofovir are classified as pregnancy category B drugs, and lamivudine, a category C drug, has been shown to be safe in pregnant women with HIV infection. Antiviral therapy has been recommended, beginning in the third trimester, when the mother's serum HBV DNA level is 200,000 international units/mL or higher to reduce levels at the time of delivery.

Peginterferon alfa-2a is still an alternative to the oral agents in selected cases. A dose of 180 mcg subcutaneously once weekly for 48 weeks leads to sustained normalization of aminotransferase levels, disappearance of HBeAg and HBV DNA from serum, appearance of anti-HBe, and improved survival in up to 40% of treated patients. A response is most likely in patients with a low baseline HBV DNA level and high aminotransferase levels and is more likely in those who are infected with HBV genotype A than with other genotypes (especially genotype D). Moreover, most complete responders eventually clear HBsAg and develop anti-HBs in serum, and are thus cured. Relapses are uncommon in complete responders who seroconvert from HBeAg to anti-HBe. Peginterferon may be considered in order to avoid long-term therapy with an oral agent, as in young women who may want to become pregnant in the future. Patients with HBeAg-negative chronic hepatitis B have a response rate of 60% after 48 weeks of therapy with peginterferon, but the response may not be durable once peginterferon is stopped. A rapid decline in serum HBsAg titers predicts a sustained response and ultimate clearance of HBsAg. The response to peginterferon is poor in patients with HIV coinfection.

In **chronic hepatitis D**, peginterferon alfa-2b (1.5 mcg/kg/wk for 48 weeks) may lead to normalization of serum aminotransferase levels, histologic improvement, and elimination of HDV RNA from serum in 20–50% of patients, but relapse may occur and tolerance is poor. Nucleoside and nucleotide analogs are generally not effective in treating chronic hepatitis D; prenylation inhibitors are under study.

► Prognosis

The course of chronic hepatitis B is variable. The sequelae of chronic hepatitis secondary to hepatitis B include cirrhosis, liver failure, and hepatocellular carcinoma. The 5-year mortality rate is 0–2% in those without cirrhosis, 14–20% in those with compensated cirrhosis, and 70–86% following decompensation. The risk of cirrhosis and hepatocellular carcinoma correlates with serum HBV DNA levels, and a focus of therapy is to suppress HBV DNA levels below 300 copies/mL (60 international units/mL). HBV genotype C is associated with a higher risk of cirrhosis and hepatocellular carcinoma than other genotypes. Antiviral treatment improves the prognosis in responders, prevents (or leads to regression of) cirrhosis, and decreases the frequency of liver-related complications (although the risk of hepatocellular carcinoma does not become as low as that in inactive HBV carriers).

2. Chronic Hepatitis C

▶ Clinical Findings & Diagnosis

Chronic hepatitis C develops in up to 85% of patients with acute hepatitis C. It is clinically indistinguishable from chronic hepatitis due to other causes and may be the most common. Worldwide, 170 million people are infected with HCV, with 1.8% of the US population infected. Peak prevalence in the United States (about 4%) is in persons born between 1945 and 1964. In approximately 40% of cases, serum aminotransferase levels are persistently normal. The diagnosis is confirmed by detection of anti-HCV by EIA. In rare cases of suspected chronic hepatitis C but a negative EIA, HCV RNA is detected by PCR testing. Progression to cirrhosis occurs in 20% of affected patients after 20 years, with an increased risk in men, those who drink more than 50 g of alcohol daily, and those who acquire HCV infection after age 40 years. The rate of fibrosis progression accelerates after age 50. African Americans have a higher rate of chronic hepatitis C but lower rates of fibrosis progression and response to therapy than whites. Immunosuppressed persons—including patients with hypogammaglobulinemia or HIV infection with a low CD4 count or those receiving immunosuppressants—appear to progress more rapidly to cirrhosis than immunocompetent persons with chronic hepatitis C. Tobacco and cannabis smoking and hepatic steatosis also appear to promote progression of fibrosis, but coffee consumption appears to slow progression. Persons with chronic hepatitis C and persistently normal serum aminotransferase levels usually have mild chronic hepatitis with slow or absent progression to cirrhosis; however, cirrhosis is present in 10% of these patients. Serum FibroSure testing or ultrasound elastography may be used to identify the absence of fibrosis or presence of cirrhosis.

▶ Treatment

The introduction of direct-acting and host-targeting antiviral agents is rapidly expanding the therapeutic armamentarium against HCV (Table 16–6). Standard therapy for HCV infection from the late 1990s to the early 2010s was a combination of peginterferon plus ribavirin, and ribavirin continues to be used in some all-oral regimens. Sustained virologic response rates (negative HCV RNA in serum at 24 weeks after completion of therapy) to peginterferon plus ribavirin were 45% in patients with HCV genotype 1 infection and 70–80% in those with genotype 2 or 3 infection. Response of genotype 1 infection to peginterferon plus ribavirin was associated most strongly with the CC genotype of the *IFNL3* (*IL28B*) gene, with sustained response rates as high as 80%, compared to 40% for the CT genotype and 30% for the TT genotype.

Higher rates of response were achieved in persons infected with HCV genotype 1 when a direct-acting antiviral agent—boceprevir (or telaprevir, an agent no longer

available in the United States), a nonstructural (NS) 3/4A serine protease inhibitor—was added to peginterferon plus ribavirin. Sustained response rates were as high as 75% for HCV genotype 1 with a standard three-drug regimen. With the addition of the protease inhibitor, the treatment duration for HCV genotype 1 infection could be shortened to 24 weeks, depending on the rapidity of clearance of HCV RNA from serum—so-called response-guided therapy.

The definition of clearance of HCV RNA requires use of a sensitive real-time reverse transcriptase-PCR assay to monitor HCV RNA during treatment (the lower limit of quantification should be 25 international units/mL or less, and the limit of detection should be 10–15 international units/mL). With newer regimens, the criterion for a sustained virologic response has been shortened from 24 to 12 weeks after the completion of treatment.

Treatment with peginterferon-based therapy is associated with frequent, often distressing, side effects, and discontinuation rates have been as high as 15–30%. Peginterferon alfa is contraindicated in pregnant or breastfeeding women and those with decompensated cirrhosis, profound cytopenias, severe psychiatric disorders, autoimmune diseases, or an inability to self-administer or comply with treatment. Men and women taking ribavirin must practice strict contraception until 6 months after the conclusion of therapy because of its teratogenic effects in animals. Ribavirin should be used with caution in persons over 65 years of age and in others in whom hemolysis could pose a risk of angina or stroke.

Several types of direct-acting antiviral agents have been developed. HCV protease inhibitors ("…previrs") generally have high antiviral potency but differ with respect to the development of resistance (although resistance-associated variants of HCV tend not to persist after therapy is stopped). Most of the compounds show better response rates in HCV genotype 1b than in genotype 1a infection. The HCV protease inhibitors currently approved by the FDA are boceprevir and simeprevir (Table 16–6). Both of these drugs were used initially in combination with peginterferon and ribavirin for HCV genotype 1 infection, although simeprevir was less effective in patients with genotype 1a and a nonstructural protein Q80K mutation than in those without the mutation.

NS5A inhibitors ("…asvirs") are characterized by high antiviral potency at picomolar doses. The cross-genotype efficacy of these agents varies. Ledipasvir was the first NS5A inhibitor approved by the FDA in 2014 (Table 16–6). Ledipasvir has potent activity against genotypes 1, 4, 5, and 6 HCV and has been formulated in combination with sofosbuvir. The combination is highly effective in both treatment-naive and treatment-experienced patients, even those with cirrhosis. The combination is given in a fixed dose of ledipasvir 90 mg and sofosbuvir 400 mg once daily for 12 weeks in HCV genotype 1–infected treatment-naive patients and treatment-experienced patients without cirrhosis and for 24 weeks in treatment-experienced patients with cirrhosis. In treatment-naive patients without cirrhosis, the duration of treatment can be shortened to 8 weeks if the baseline HCV RNA level is less than 6 million international units/mL. Sustained virologic response rates are well

Table 16–6. Direct-acting antiviral agents for HCV infection.

Agent	Genotype(s)	Dose[1]	Comment
NS3/4A Protease Inhibitors			
Boceprevir	1	800 mg orally three times daily	Used in combination with pegylated interferon and ribavirin; no longer recommended
Telaprevir	1	1125 mg orally twice daily	Used in combination with pegylated interferon and ribavirin; no longer recommended Drug discontinued in the United States
Simeprevir	1 and 4	150 mg orally once daily	Used in combination with pegylated interferon and ribavirin or with sofosbuvir
Paritaprevir	1 and 4	150 mg orally once daily	Used in combination with ombitasvir and dasabuvir; ritonavir (100 mg) boosted[2]; for genotype 1b with cirrhosis and genotype 1a, used with ribavirin. Used in combination with ombitasvir, ritonavir boosting, and ribavirin for genotype 4[3]
Asunaprevir[4]	1 and 4	200 mg orally twice daily	Used in combination with daclatasvir or with daclatasvir and beclabuvir
Grazoprevir	1, 4–6	100 mg orally once daily	Used in combination with elbasvir[5]
NS5A Inhibitors			
Daclatasvir[6]	1–6	60 mg orally once daily	Used in combination with sofosbuvir (genotypes 1–6) or with pegylated interferon and ribavirin (genotype 4) or with asunaprevir (with or without beclabuvir; under study)
Ledipasvir	1, 4–6	90 mg orally once daily	Used in combination with sofosbuvir[7]
Ombitasvir	1 and 4	25 mg orally once daily	Used in combination with paritaprevir (ritonavir boosted) with or without dasabuvir and with or without ribavirin as per paritaprevir above
Elbasvir	1–6	50 mg orally once daily	Used in combination with grazoprevir
Velpatasvir[4]	1–6	100 mg orally once daily	Used in combination with sofosbuvir
NS5B Nucleos(t)ide Polymerase Inhibitor			
Sofosbuvir	1–6	400 mg orally once daily	Used in combination with pegylated interferon and ribavirin (all genotypes) or with ribavirin alone (genotypes 2 and 3) or with simeprevir (genotypes 1 and 4) or with daclatasvir (all genotypes) or with ledipasvir (genotypes 1, 3, and 4) or with velpatasvir
NS5B Non-nucleos(t)ide Polymerase Inhibitors			
Dasabuvir	1 and 4	250 mg orally twice daily	Used in combination with paritaprevir (ritonavir boosted) and ombitasvir with or without ribavirin as per paritaprevir above
Beclabuvir[4]	1	75 mg orally twice daily	Used in combination with daclatasvir and asunaprevir

[1]The preferred regimen and duration of treatment may vary depending on HCV genotype, presence or absence of cirrhosis, or nonresponse to prior therapy for HCV infection.
[2]Marketed as Viekira Pak (AbbVie).
[3]Marketed as Technivie (AbbVie).
[4]Agent has not been approved by the FDA as of early 2016; additional drugs are under study.
[5]Marketed as Zepatier (Merck).
[6]Approved by the FDA for use with sofosbuvir in HCV genotype 3 infection.
[7]Marketed as Harvoni (Gilead Sciences).

above 90%, including patients coinfected with HIV, and this regimen has emerged as a first-line therapy for HCV genotype 1. The combination of ledipasvir, sofosbuvir, and ribavirin achieves high rates of sustained virologic response in patients with HCV genotype 3. Side effects are mild and include fatigue and headache. The optimal retreatment of occasional nonresponders or relapsers with resistance-associated variants is under study. FDA approval of the highly effective combination of the NS3/4A protease inhibitor grazoprevir 100 mg and the NS5A inhibitor elbasvir 50 mg daily for HCV genotypes 1, 4, and 6 is expected in 2016.

HCV polymerase inhibitors ("...buvirs") are categorized as nucleoside or nucleotide analog and non-nucleoside polymerase inhibitors. Nucleoside analogs are active against all HCV genotypes and have a high barrier to resistance. Non-nucleoside polymerase inhibitors are the weakest class of compounds against HCV because of a low barrier to resistance. Most drugs in this class are more active against HCV genotype 1b than HCV genotype 1a. They are being developed to be used only in combination with the other direct-acting antiviral agents, mainly protease inhibitors and NS5A inhibitors. The first approved

HCV NS5B nucleotide polymerase inhibitor was sofosbuvir in 2013.

Sofosbuvir was initially approved for use in combination with peginterferon and ribavirin in patients with HCV genotype 1 infection and with ribavirin alone in patients with HCV genotype 2 or 3 infection (Table 16–6). Most patients with HCV genotypes 2 or 3 infection, including those with HIV coinfection, are cured with 12 or 24 weeks of therapy, respectively. HCV genotype 2 responds much better to interferon-free sofosbuvir-based therapy than HCV genotype 3, but the sustained virologic response is 20–30% lower in patients with cirrhosis. Importantly, no sofosbuvir-resistant variants have been selected during therapy. The combination of sofosbuvir and simeprevir has been found to be effective in HCV genotype 1 infection and was approved by the FDA in 2014; the approval was extended to HCV genotypes 4, 5, and 6 in 2015.

The combination of paritaprevir (an NS3/4A protease inhibitor), boosted by ritonavir, plus ombitasvir (an NS5A inhibitor) and dasabuvir (an NS5B non-nucleoside polymerase inhibitor) is effective in HCV genotype-1 treatment-naive and prior nonresponders to interferon-based therapy, with or without cirrhosis, and was approved by the FDA in late 2014. The same combination without dasabuvir was FDA approved in 2015 for HCV genotype 4 infection. Instances of hepatotoxicity have been reported with these regimens in patients with advanced cirrhosis. Daclatasvir in combination with sofosbuvir has proven effective in genotypes 1-, 2-, and 3-infected patients, including those coinfected with HIV, and was FDA approved in 2015 for HCV genotype 3 infection. The combination of velpatasvir, an NS5A inhibitor, and sofosbuvir is effective for all HCV genotypes. The combination of daclatasvir and asunaprevir is highly effective in genotype 1b-, 4-, 5-, and 6-infected patients but less effective in genotype 1a-infected patients. The combination of daclatasvir, asunaprevir, and beclabuvir (a non-nucleoside NS5B inhibitor) is effective in genotype 1a- and 1b-infected patients. As of early 2016, asunaprevir, beclabuvir, and velpatasvir were not available in the United States.

Numerous other antiviral agents with various, often novel, mechanisms of action are under study, and several regimens have become commercially available, although not all are approved by the US FDA (Table 16–6). However, despite the efficacy of the new regimens, their cost is high and insurance coverage is often a barrier to their use. Other agents that have been studied include NS3/4A protease inhibitors (eg, danoprevir, faldaprevir); polymerase inhibitors (eg, mericitabine); virus entry, assembly, and secretion inhibitors; microRNA-122 antisense oligonucleotides (eg, miravirsen); cyclophilin A inhibitors (eg, alisporivir); interferon lambda-3; and therapeutic vaccines. HCV genotype 1 has become easy to cure with oral direct-acting agents, with expected sustained virologic response rates above 90%, and virtually all HCV genotype 2 infection is curable with all-oral regimens. HCV genotype 3 infection, particularly in association with cirrhosis, remains the most challenging to treat. Nonetheless, interferon is now rarely required, and the need for ribavirin will likely decline.

Antiviral therapy has been shown to be beneficial in the treatment of cryoglobulinemia associated with chronic hepatitis C; an acute flare of cryoglobulinemia may first require treatment with rituximab, cyclophosphamide plus methylprednisolone, or plasma exchange. As noted above, patients with HCV and HIV coinfection have been shown to benefit from treatment of HCV infection. Moreover, in persons coinfected with HCV and HIV, long-term liver disease–related mortality increases as HIV infection–related mortality is reduced by current antiretroviral therapy.

▶ **Prognosis**

Chronic hepatitis C is an indolent, often subclinical disease that may lead to cirrhosis and hepatocellular carcinoma after decades. The overall mortality rate in patients with transfusion-associated hepatitis C may be no different from that of an age-matched control population. Nevertheless, mortality or transplantation rates clearly rise to 5% per year once cirrhosis develops, and mortality from cirrhosis and hepatocellular carcinoma due to hepatitis C is rising. A risk score combining age, sex, platelet count, and AST-to-ALT ratio has been proposed. There is some evidence that HCV genotype 1b is associated with a higher risk of hepatocellular carcinoma than other genotypes. Antiviral therapy has a beneficial effect on mortality and quality of life, is cost-effective, appears to retard and even reverse fibrosis, and reduces (but does not eliminate) the risk of decompensated cirrhosis and hepatocellular carcinoma in responders. Even patients who achieve a sustained virologic response remain at an increased risk for mortality compared with the general population. The risk of mortality from drug addiction is higher than that for liver disease in patients with chronic hepatitis C. Statin use has been reported to be associated with improved virologic response to antiviral therapy and decreased progression of liver fibrosis and frequency of hepatocellular carcinoma.

▶ **When to Refer**

- For liver biopsy.
- For antiviral therapy.

▶ **When to Admit**

For complications of decompensated cirrhosis.

Butt AA et al. Effect of addition of statins to antiviral therapy in hepatitis C virus-infected persons: results from ERCHIVES. Hepatology. 2015 Aug;62(2):365–74. [PMID: 25847403]

Hézode C et al. Ombitasvir plus paritaprevir plus ritonavir with or without ribavirin in treatment-naive and treatment-experienced patients with genotype 4 chronic hepatitis C virus infection (PEARL-I): a randomised, open-label trial. Lancet. 2015 Jun 20;385(9986):2502–9. [PMID: 25837829]

Lawitz E et al. Efficacy and safety of ombitasvir, paritaprevir, and ritonavir in an open-label study of patients with genotype 1b chronic hepatitis C virus infection with and without cirrhosis. Gastroenterology. 2015 Oct;149(4):971–80. [PMID: 26170136]

Naggie S et al; ION-4 Investigators. Ledipasvir and sofosbuvir for HCV in patients coinfected with HIV-1. N Engl J Med. 2015 Aug 20;373(8):705–13. [PMID: 26196665]

Nelson DR et al. All-oral 12-week treatment with daclatasvir plus sofosbuvir in patients with hepatitis C virus genotype 3 infection: ALLY-3 phase III study. Hepatology. 2015 Apr;61(4):1127–35. [PMID: 25614962]

AUTOIMMUNE HEPATITIS

ESSENTIALS OF DIAGNOSIS

▶ Usually young to middle-aged women.

▶ Chronic hepatitis with high serum globulins and characteristic liver histology.

▶ Positive antinuclear antibody (ANA) and/or smooth muscle antibody in most common type.

▶ Responds to corticosteroids.

General Considerations

Although autoimmune hepatitis is usually seen in young women, it can occur in either sex at any age. The incidence, which has been rising, and prevalence are estimated to be 8.5 and 107 per million population, respectively.

Clinical Findings

A. Symptoms and Signs

The onset is usually insidious, but about 20% of cases present with acute (occasionally fulminant) hepatitis and some cases follow a viral illness (such as hepatitis A, Epstein-Barr infection, or measles) or exposure to a drug or toxin (such as nitrofurantoin, minocycline, or infliximab). Exacerbations may occur postpartum. Amenorrhea may be a presenting feature, and the frequency of depression appears to be increased. Thirty-four percent of patients, and particularly elderly patients, are asymptomatic. Typically, examination reveals a healthy-appearing young woman with multiple spider telangiectasias, cutaneous striae, acne, hirsutism, and hepatomegaly. Extrahepatic features include arthritis, Sjögren syndrome, thyroiditis, nephritis, ulcerative colitis, and Coombs-positive hemolytic anemia. Patients, especially elderly patients, with autoimmune hepatitis are at increased risk for cirrhosis, which, in turn, increases the risk of hepatocellular carcinoma (at a rate of about 1% per year).

B. Laboratory Findings

Serum aminotransferase levels may be greater than 1000 units/L, and the total bilirubin is usually increased. In type I (classic) autoimmune hepatitis, ANA or smooth muscle antibodies (either or both) are usually detected in serum. Serum gamma-globulin levels are typically elevated (up to 5–6 g/dL [0.05–0.06 g/L]); in such patients, the EIA for antibody to HCV may be falsely positive. Other antibodies, including atypical perinuclear antineutrophil cytoplasmic antibodies (pANCA) and antibodies to histones, F-actin, and alpha-actinin may be found. Antibodies to soluble liver antigen (anti-SLA) characterize a variant of type I that is marked by severe disease, a high relapse rate after treatment, and absence of the usual antibodies (ANA and smooth muscle antibodies). Type II, seen more often in girls under age 14 in Europe, is characterized by circulating antibodies to liver-kidney microsome type 1 (anti-LKM1)

without smooth muscle antibodies or ANA. In some cases, antibodies to liver cytosol type 1, are detected. Type II autoimmune hepatitis can be seen in patients with autoimmune polyglandular syndrome type 1. Concurrent primary biliary cholangitis (PBC; formerly primary biliary cirrhosis) or primary sclerosing cholangitis ("overlap syndrome") has been recognized in 7–13% and 6–11% of patients with autoimmune hepatitis, respectively. Liver biopsy is indicated to help establish the diagnosis (interface hepatitis is the hallmark), evaluate disease severity, and determine the need for treatment.

Simplified diagnostic criteria based on the detection of autoantibodies (1 point for a titer of > 1:40 or 2 points for a titer of > 1:80), elevated IgG levels (1 point for IgG level ≥ upper limit of normal or 2 points for level ≥ 1.1 times upper limit of normal), and characteristic histologic features (1 or 2 points depending on how typical the features are) and exclusion of viral hepatitis (2 points) can be useful for diagnosis; a score of 6 indicates probable and a score of 7 indicates definite autoimmune hepatitis with a high degree of specificity but moderate sensitivity. Diagnostic criteria for an overlap of autoimmune hepatitis and PBC ("Paris criteria") have been proposed.

Treatment

Prednisone with or without azathioprine improves symptoms; decreases the serum bilirubin, aminotransferase, and gamma-globulin levels; and reduces hepatic inflammation. Symptomatic patients with aminotransferase levels elevated tenfold (or fivefold if the serum globulins are elevated at least twofold) are optimal candidates for therapy, and asymptomatic patients with modest enzyme elevations may be considered for therapy depending on the clinical circumstances and histologic severity; however, asymptomatic patients usually remain asymptomatic, have either mild hepatitis or inactive cirrhosis on liver biopsy specimens, and have a good long-term prognosis without therapy.

Prednisone is given initially in a dose of 30 mg orally daily with azathioprine, 50 mg orally daily, which is generally well tolerated and permits the use of lower corticosteroid doses than a regimen beginning with prednisone 60 mg orally daily alone. Intravenous corticosteroids or prednisone, 60 mg orally daily, is recommended for patients with acute severe autoimmune hepatitis. Budesonide, 3 mg orally two or three daily, may be at least as effective as prednisone in noncirrhotic autoimmune hepatitis and associated with fewer side effects. Whether patients should undergo testing for the genotype or level of thiopurine methyltransferase prior to treatment with azathioprine to predict toxicity is debated. Blood counts are monitored weekly for the first 2 months of therapy and monthly thereafter because of the small risk of bone marrow suppression. The dose of prednisone is lowered from 30 mg/day after 1 week to 20 mg/day and again after 2 or 3 weeks to 15 mg/day. Treatment is response guided, and ultimately, a maintenance dose of 10 mg/day should be achieved. While symptomatic improvement is often prompt, biochemical improvement is more gradual, with normalization of serum aminotransferase levels after an average of 22 months.

Histologic resolution of inflammation lags biochemical remission by 3–6 months, and repeat liver biopsy is recommended at least 3 months after the aminotransferase levels have normalized. Failure of aminotransferase levels to return to normal invariably predicts lack of histologic resolution.

The response rate to therapy with prednisone and azathioprine is 80% with remission in 65% by 3 years. Older patients and those with HLA genotype *DRB1*04* are more likely to respond than younger patients and those with HLA *DRB1*03*, hyperbilirubinemia, or a high MELD score (12 or higher, see Cirrhosis). Fibrosis may reverse with therapy and rarely progresses after apparent biochemical and histologic remission. Once complete remission is achieved, therapy may be withdrawn, but the subsequent relapse rate is 90% by 3 years. Relapses may again be treated in the same manner as the initial episode, with the same remission rate. After successful treatment of a relapse, the patient may continue taking azathioprine (up to 2 mg/kg) or the lowest dose of prednisone with or without azathioprine (50 mg/day) needed to maintain aminotransferase levels as close to normal as possible; another attempt at withdrawing therapy may be considered in patients remaining in remission long term (eg, 4 years or longer). During pregnancy, flares can be treated with prednisone, and maintenance azathioprine does not have to be discontinued.

Nonresponders to corticosteroids and azathioprine (failure of serum aminotransferase levels to decrease by 50% after 6 months) may be considered for a trial of cyclosporine, tacrolimus, sirolimus, everolimus, methotrexate, rituximab, or infliximab. Mycophenolate mofetil, 1 g twice daily, is an effective alternative to azathioprine in patients who cannot tolerate it but is less effective in nonresponders to azathioprine. Bone density should be monitored—particularly in patients receiving maintenance corticosteroid therapy—and measures undertaken to prevent or treat osteoporosis (see Chapter 26). Liver transplantation may be required for treatment failures and patients with a fulminant presentation, but the outcome may be worse than that for PBC because of an increased rate of infectious complications. As immunosuppression is reduced, the disease has been recognized to recur in up to 70% of transplanted livers at 5 years (and rarely to develop de novo); sirolimus can be effective in such cases. Overall long-term mortality of patients with autoimmune hepatitis appears to be twofold higher than that of the general population despite response to immunosuppressive therapy. Factors that predict the need for liver transplantation or that predict liver-related death include the following: (1) age 20 years or younger or older than 60 years at presentation, (2) low serum albumin level at diagnosis, (3) cirrhosis at diagnosis, (4) the presence of anti-SLA, and (5) incomplete normalization of the serum ALT level after 6 months of treatment.

▶ When to Refer

- For liver biopsy.
- For immunosuppressive therapy.

▶ When to Admit

- Hepatic encephalopathy.
- INR greater than 1.6.

Dhaliwal HK et al. Long-term prognostic significance of persisting histological activity despite biochemical remission in autoimmune hepatitis. Am J Gastroenterol. 2015 Jul; 110(7):993–9. [PMID: 26010310]

European Association for the Study of the Liver. EASL Clinical Practice Guidelines: Autoimmune hepatitis. J Hepatol. 2015 Oct; 63(4):971–1004. [PMID: 26341719]

Hartl J et al. Patient selection based on treatment duration and liver biochemistry increases success rates after treatment withdrawal in autoimmune hepatitis. J Hepatol. 2015 Mar; 62(3):642–6. [PMID: 25457202]

Muratori P et al. Type 1 and type 2 autoimmune hepatitis in adults share the same clinical phenotype. Aliment Pharmacol Ther. 2015 Jun;41(12):1281–7. [PMID: 25898847]

ALCOHOLIC LIVER DISEASE

ESSENTIALS OF DIAGNOSIS

- ▶ Chronic alcohol intake usually exceeds 80 g/day in men and 30–40 g/day in women with alcoholic hepatitis or cirrhosis.

- ▶ Fatty liver is often asymptomatic.

- ▶ Fever, right upper quadrant pain, tender hepatomegaly, and jaundice characterize alcoholic hepatitis, but the patient may be asymptomatic.

- ▶ AST is usually elevated but usually not above 300 units/L (6 mckat/L); AST is greater than ALT, usually by a factor of 2 or more.

- ▶ Alcoholic hepatitis is often reversible but it is the most common precursor of cirrhosis in the United States.

▶ General Considerations

Excessive alcohol intake can lead to fatty liver, hepatitis, and cirrhosis. Alcoholic hepatitis is characterized by acute or chronic inflammation and parenchymal necrosis of the liver induced by alcohol. Alcoholic hepatitis is often a reversible disease but the most common precursor of cirrhosis in the United States. It is associated with four to five times the number of hospitalizations and deaths as hepatitis C, which is the second most common cause of cirrhosis.

The frequency of alcoholic cirrhosis is estimated to be 10–15% among persons who consume over 50 g of alcohol (4 oz of 100-proof whiskey, 15 oz of wine, or four 12-oz cans of beer) daily for over 10 years (although the risk of cirrhosis may be lower for wine than for a comparable intake of beer or spirits). The risk of cirrhosis is lower (5%) in the absence of other cofactors such as chronic viral hepatitis and obesity. Genetic factors may also account for differences in susceptibility to and severity of liver disease.

Women appear to be more susceptible than men, in part because of lower gastric mucosal alcohol dehydrogenase levels.

Clinical Findings

A. Symptoms and Signs

The clinical presentation of alcoholic liver disease can vary from asymptomatic hepatomegaly to a rapidly fatal acute illness or end-stage cirrhosis. A recent period of heavy drinking, complaints of anorexia and nausea, and the demonstration of hepatomegaly and jaundice strongly suggest the diagnosis. Abdominal pain and tenderness, splenomegaly, ascites, fever, and encephalopathy may be present. Infection, including invasive aspergillosis, is common in patients with severe alcoholic hepatitis.

B. Laboratory Findings

In patients with steatosis, mild liver enzyme elevations may be the only laboratory abnormality. Anemia (usually macrocytic) may be present. Leukocytosis with a shift to the left is common in patients with severe alcoholic hepatitis. Leukopenia is occasionally seen and resolves after cessation of drinking. About 10% of patients have thrombocytopenia related to a direct toxic effect of alcohol on megakaryocyte production or to hypersplenism.

AST is usually elevated but infrequently above 300 units/L (6 mckat/L). AST is greater than ALT, usually by a factor of 2 or more. Serum alkaline phosphatase is generally elevated, but seldom more than three times the normal value. Serum bilirubin is increased in 60–90% of patients with alcoholic hepatitis.

Serum bilirubin levels greater than 10 mg/dL (171 mcmol/L) and marked prolongation of the prothrombin time (6 seconds or more above control) indicate severe alcoholic hepatitis with a mortality rate as high as 50%. The serum albumin is depressed, and the gamma-globulin level is elevated in 50–75% of individuals, even in the absence of cirrhosis. Increased transferrin saturation, hepatic iron stores, and sideroblastic anemia are found in many alcoholic patients. Folic acid deficiency may coexist.

C. Imaging

Imaging studies can detect moderate to severe hepatic steatosis reliably but not inflammation or fibrosis. Ultrasonography helps exclude biliary obstruction and identifies subclinical ascites. CT with intravenous contrast or MRI may be indicated in selected cases to evaluate patients for collateral vessels, space-occupying lesions of the liver, or concomitant disease of the pancreas.

D. Liver Biopsy

Liver biopsy, if done, demonstrates macrovesicular fat and, in patients with alcoholic hepatitis, polymorphonuclear infiltration with hepatic necrosis, Mallory (or Mallory-Denk) bodies (alcoholic hyaline), and perivenular and perisinusoidal fibrosis. Micronodular cirrhosis may be present as well. The findings are identical to those of non-alcoholic steatohepatitis.

Differential Diagnosis

Alcoholic hepatitis may be closely mimicked by cholecystitis and cholelithiasis and by drug toxicity. Other causes of hepatitis or chronic liver disease may be excluded by serologic or biochemical testing, imaging studies, or liver biopsy. A formula based on the AST/ALT ratio, body mass index, mean corpuscular volume, and sex has been reported to reliably distinguish alcoholic liver disease from nonalcoholic fatty liver disease (NAFLD).

Treatment

A. General Measures

Abstinence from alcohol is essential. Naltrexone, acamprosate, or baclofen may be considered in combination with counseling to reduce the likelihood of recidivism. Fatty liver is quickly reversible with abstinence. Every effort should be made to provide sufficient amounts of carbohydrates and calories in anorectic patients to reduce endogenous protein catabolism, promote gluconeogenesis, and prevent hypoglycemia. Nutritional support (40 kcal/kg with 1.5–2 g/kg as protein) improves liver disease, but not necessarily survival, in patients with malnutrition. Use of liquid formulas rich in branched-chain amino acids does not improve survival beyond that achieved with less expensive caloric supplementation. The administration of micronutrients, particularly folic acid, thiamine, and zinc, is indicated, especially when deficiencies are noted; glucose administration increases the thiamine requirement and can precipitate Wernicke-Korsakoff syndrome if thiamine is not coadministered.

B. Pharmacologic Measures

Methylprednisolone, 32 mg/day orally, or the equivalent, for 1 month, may reduce short-term mortality in patients with alcoholic hepatitis and encephalopathy or a Maddrey discriminant function index (defined by the patient's prothrombin time minus the control prothrombin time times 4.6 plus the total bilirubin in mg/dL) of 32 or more, or a MELD score of 18 or more (see Cirrhosis). Concomitant gastrointestinal bleeding or infection may not preclude treatment with corticosteroids if otherwise indicated. The combination of corticosteroids and N-acetylcysteine has been reported to improve 1-month but not 6-month survival and reduce the risk of hepatorenal syndrome and infections; the combination may be superior to corticosteroids alone, but more data are needed.

Pentoxifylline, 400 mg orally three times daily for 4 weeks, may reduce 1-month mortality rates in patients with severe alcoholic hepatitis, primarily by decreasing the risk of hepatorenal syndrome. It may be less effective in reducing short-term mortality than corticosteroids and is often used when corticosteroids are contraindicated. Whether the addition of pentoxifylline to prednisolone improves survival or reduces the frequency of hepatorenal syndrome compared with prednisolone alone is uncertain.

Prognosis

A. Short-Term

The overall mortality rate is 34% (20% within 1 month) without corticosteroid therapy. Individuals in whom the prothrombin time prohibits liver biopsy have a 42% mortality rate at 1 year. Other unfavorable prognostic factors are older age, a serum bilirubin greater than 10 mg/dL (171 mcmol/L), hepatic encephalopathy, coagulopathy, azotemia, leukocytosis, sepsis and other infections, lack of response to corticosteroid therapy, and possibly a paucity of steatosis on a liver biopsy specimen and reversal of portal blood flow by Doppler ultrasonography. Concomitant gastrointestinal bleeding does not appear to worsen survival. Failure of the serum bilirubin level to decline after 7 days of treatment with corticosteroids predicts nonresponse and poor long-term survival, as does the Lille model (which includes age, serum creatinine, serum albumin, prothrombin time [or INR], serum bilirubin on admission, and serum bilirubin on day 7). The MELD score used for cirrhosis and the Glasgow alcoholic hepatitis score (based on age, white blood cell count, blood urea nitrogen, prothrombin time ratio, and bilirubin level) also correlate with mortality from alcoholic hepatitis and have higher specificities than the discriminant function and Lille score. A scoring system based on age, serum bilirubin, INR, and serum creatinine (ABIC) has been proposed, and one study has shown that the development of acute kidney injury is the most accurate predictor of 90-day mortality. The combination of the MELD score and Lille model has also been reported to be the best predictor of short-term mortality among the scoring systems. Histologic features associated with 90-day mortality include the degree of fibrosis and neutrophil infiltration, presence of metamitochondria, and bilirubinostasis.

B. Long-Term

Overall mortality from alcoholic liver disease has declined slightly in the United States since 1980. Nevertheless, the 3-year mortality rate of persons who recover from acute alcoholic hepatitis is ten times greater than that of control individuals of comparable age; the 5-year mortality rate is as high as 85%. Histologically severe disease is associated with continued excessive mortality rates after 3 years, whereas the death rate is not increased after the same period in those whose liver biopsies show only mild alcoholic hepatitis. Complications of portal hypertension (ascites, variceal bleeding, hepatorenal syndrome), coagulopathy, and severe jaundice following recovery from acute alcoholic hepatitis also suggest a poor long-term prognosis. Alcoholic cirrhosis is a risk factor for hepatocellular carcinoma, and the risk is highest in carriers of the *C282Y* mutation for hemochromatosis or those with increased hepatic iron.

The most important prognostic consideration is continued excessive drinking. A 6-month period of abstinence is generally required before liver transplantation is considered, although this requirement has been questioned and early liver transplantation has been performed in selected patients with alcoholic hepatitis, with good outcomes. Optimal candidates have adequate social support, do not smoke, have no psychosis or personality disorder, are adherent to therapy, and have regular appointments with a psychiatrist or psychologist who specializes in addiction treatment. Patients with alcoholic liver disease are at higher risk for posttransplant malignancy than those with other types of liver disease because of alcohol and tobacco use.

When to Refer

Refer patients with alcoholic hepatitis who require liver biopsy for diagnosis.

When to Admit

- Hepatic encephalopathy.
- INR greater than 1.6.
- Total bilirubin 10 mg/dL or more.
- Inability to maintain hydration.

Askgaard G et al. Alcohol drinking pattern and risk of alcoholic liver cirrhosis: a prospective cohort study. J Hepatol. 2015 May; 62(5):1061–7. [PMID: 25634330]

Louvet A et al. Combining data from liver disease scoring systems better predicts outcomes of patients with alcoholic hepatitis. Gastroenterology. 2015 Aug;149(2):398–406.e8. [PMID: 25935634]

Rudler M et al. Prognosis of treated severe alcoholic hepatitis in patients with gastrointestinal bleeding. J Hepatol. 2015 Apr; 62(4):816–21. [PMID: 25450199]

Singh S et al. Comparative effectiveness of pharmacological interventions for severe alcoholic hepatitis: a systematic review and network meta-analysis. Gastroenterology. 2015 Oct; 149(4):958–70. [PMID: 26091937]

Thursz MR et al; STOPAH Trial. Prednisolone or pentoxifylline for alcoholic hepatitis. N Engl J Med. 2015 Apr 23;372 (17):1619–28. [PMID: 25901427]

DRUG- & TOXIN-INDUCED LIVER INJURY

ESSENTIALS OF DIAGNOSIS

▶ Drug-induced liver injury can mimic viral hepatitis, biliary tract obstruction, or other types of liver disease.

▶ Clinicians must inquire about the use of many widely used therapeutic agents, including over-the-counter "natural" and herbal products, in any patient with liver disease.

General Considerations

Many therapeutic agents may cause drug-induced liver injury, and up to 10% of patients with drug-induced liver injury die or undergo liver transplantation within

6 months of onset. The medications most commonly implicated are nonsteroidal anti-inflammatory drugs and antibiotics because of their widespread use. In any patient with liver disease, the clinician must inquire carefully about the use of potentially hepatotoxic drugs or exposure to hepatotoxins, including over-the-counter "natural" and herbal products. In some cases, coadministration of a second agent may increase the toxicity of the first (eg, isoniazid and rifampin, acetaminophen and alcohol). A relationship between increased serum ALT levels in premarketing clinical trials and postmarketing reports of hepatotoxicity has been identified. Except for drugs used to treat tuberculosis and HIV infection and possibly azithromycin, the risk of hepatotoxicity is not increased in patients with preexisting cirrhosis, but hepatotoxicity may be more severe and the outcome worse when it does occur. Older persons may be at higher risk for hepatotoxicity from certain agents, such as amoxicillin-clavulanic acid, isoniazid, and nitrofurantoin, and more likely to have persistent and cholestatic, rather than hepatocellular, injury compared with younger persons. Drug toxicity may be categorized on the basis of pathogenesis or predominant histologic appearance. Drug-induced liver injury can mimic viral hepatitis, biliary tract obstruction, or other types of liver disease. The development of jaundice predicts a mortality rate of at least 10%. A useful resource is the website www.livertox.nih.gov/.

Categorization by Pathogenesis

A. Direct Hepatotoxicity

Liver toxicity caused by this group of drugs is characterized by: (1) dose-related severity, (2) a latent period following exposure, and (3) susceptibility in all individuals. Examples include acetaminophen (toxicity is enhanced by fasting and chronic alcohol use because of depletion of glutathione and induction of cytochrome P450 2E1 and possibly reduced by statins, fibrates, and nonsteroidal anti-inflammatory drugs), alcohol, carbon tetrachloride, chloroform, heavy metals, mercaptopurine, niacin, plant alkaloids, phosphorus, pyrazinamide, tetracyclines, tipranavir, valproic acid, and vitamin A.

B. Idiosyncratic Reactions

Except for acetaminophen, most severe hepatotoxicity is idiosyncratic. Reactions of this type are (1) sporadic, (2) not related to dose above a general threshold of 100 mg/day, and (3) occasionally associated with features suggesting an allergic reaction, such as fever and eosinophilia, which may be associated with a favorable outcome. In many instances, the drug is lipophilic, and toxicity results directly from a metabolite that is produced only in certain individuals on a genetic basis. Drug-induced liver injury may be observed only during post-marketing surveillance and not during preclinical trials. Examples include abacavir, amiodarone, aspirin, carbamazepine, chloramphenicol, diclofenac, disulfiram, duloxetine, ezetimibe, flavocoxid (a "medical food"), fluoroquinolones

(levofloxacin and moxifloxacin, in particular), flutamide, halothane, isoniazid, ketoconazole, lamotrigine, methyldopa, natalizumab, nevirapine, oxacillin, phenytoin, pyrazinamide, quinidine, rivaroxaban, streptomycin, thiazolidinediones, tolvaptan, and perhaps tacrine. Statins, like all cholesterol-lowering agents, may cause serum aminotransferase elevations but rarely cause true hepatitis, and even more rarely cause acute liver failure, and are no longer considered contraindicated in patients with liver disease.

Categorization by Histopathology

A. Cholestasis

1. Noninflammatory—Drug-induced cholestasis results from inhibition or genetic deficiency of various hepatobiliary transporter systems. The following drugs cause cholestasis: anabolic steroids containing an alkyl or ethinyl group at carbon 17, azathioprine, cetirizine, cyclosporine, diclofenac, estrogens, indinavir (increased risk of indirect hyperbilirubinemia in patients with Gilbert syndrome), mercaptopurine, methyltestosterone, tamoxifen, temozolomide, and ticlopidine.

2. Inflammatory—The following drugs cause inflammation of portal areas with bile duct injury (cholangitis), often with allergic features such as eosinophilia: amoxicillin-clavulanic acid (among the most common causes of drug-induced liver injury), azathioprine, azithromycin, captopril, celecoxib, cephalosporins, chlorothiazide, chlorpromazine, chlorpropamide, erythromycin, mercaptopurine, penicillamine, prochlorperazine, semisynthetic penicillins (eg, cloxacillin), and sulfadiazine. Ketamine abuse may cause secondary biliary cirrhosis. Cholestatic and mixed cholestatic hepatocellular toxicity is more likely than pure hepatocellular toxicity to lead to chronic liver disease.

B. Acute or Chronic Hepatitis

Medications that may result in acute or chronic hepatitis that is histologically and in some cases clinically similar to autoimmune hepatitis include minocycline and nitrofurantoin, most commonly, as well as aspirin, isoniazid (increased risk in HBV and HCV carriers), methyldopa, nonsteroidal anti-inflammatory drugs, propylthiouracil, terbinafine, tumor necrosis factor inhibitors, and varenicline. Histologic features that favor a drug cause include portal tract neutrophils and hepatocellular cholestasis. Hepatitis also can occur in patients taking cocaine, diclofenac, methylenedioxymethamphetamine (MDMA; Ecstasy), efavirenz, imatinib mesylate, ipilimumab, nafazodone (has a black box warning for a potential to cause liver failure), nevirapine (like other protease inhibitors, increased risk in HBV and HCV carriers), pioglitazone, ritonavir (greater rate than other protease inhibitors), rosiglitazone, saquinavir, sulfonamides, telithromycin, and zafirlukast, as well as a variety of alternative remedies (eg, chaparral, germander, green tea extracts, Herbalife products, Hydroxycut, jin bu huan, kava, saw palmetto, skullcap, possibly black cohosh, and other traditional Chinese herbal preparations), as well as dietary supplements (eg, 1, 3-dimethylamylamine in OxyELITE Pro, a weight loss supplement withdrawn from the US market). In patients with jaundice due to drug-induced hepatitis, the mortality rate without liver transplantation is at least 10%.

C. Other Reactions

1. Fatty liver

A. MACROVESICULAR—This type of liver injury may be produced by alcohol, amiodarone, corticosteroids, irinotecan, methotrexate, tamoxifen, vinyl chloride (in exposed workers), zalcitabine, and possibly oxaliplatin.

B. MICROVESICULAR—Often resulting from mitochondrial injury, this condition is associated with didanosine, stavudine, tetracyclines, valproic acid, and zidovudine.

2. Granulomas—Allopurinol, phenytoin, pyrazinamide, quinidine, and quinine can lead to granulomas.

3. Fibrosis and cirrhosis—Methotrexate and vitamin A are associated with fibrosis and cirrhosis.

4. Sinusoidal obstruction syndrome (veno-occlusive disease)—This disorder may result from treatment with antineoplastic agents (eg, pre-bone marrow transplant, oxaliplatin), and pyrrolizidine alkaloids (eg, Comfrey).

5. Peliosis hepatis (blood-filled cavities)—Peliosis hepatis may be caused by anabolic steroids and oral contraceptive steroids as well as azathioprine and mercaptopurine, which may also cause nodular regenerative hyperplasia.

6. Neoplasms—Neoplasms may result from therapy with oral contraceptive steroids, including estrogens (hepatic adenoma but not focal nodular hyperplasia), and vinyl chloride (angiosarcoma).

▶ When to Refer

Refer patients with drug- and toxin-induced hepatitis who require liver biopsy for diagnosis.

▶ When to Admit

Patients with liver failure should be hospitalized.

Alqahtani SA et al. Identification and characterization of cefazolin-induced liver injury. Clin Gastroenterol Hepatol. 2015 Jul; 13(7):1328–36. [PMID: 25528012]

Chalasani N et al. Features and outcomes of 899 patients with drug-induced liver injury: the DILIN Prospective Study. Gastroenterology. 2015 Jun;148(7):1340–52. [PMID: 25754159]

Chalasani NP et al. ACG Clinical Guideline: the diagnosis and management of idiosyncratic drug-induced liver injury. Am J Gastroenterol. 2014 Jul;109(7):950–66. [PMID: 24935270]

Martinez MA et al. Clinical and histologic features of azithromycin-induced liver injury. Clin Gastroenterol Hepatol. 2015 Feb; 13(2):369–76. [PMID: 25111234]

Seeff LB et al. Herbal products and the liver: a review of adverse effects and mechanisms. Gastroenterology. 2015 Mar;148 (3):517–32. [PMID: 25500423]

NONALCOHOLIC FATTY LIVER DISEASE

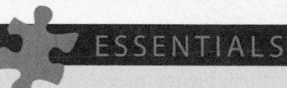

ESSENTIALS OF DIAGNOSIS

▶ Often asymptomatic.

▶ Elevated aminotransferase levels and/or hepatomegaly.

▶ Predominantly macrovesicular steatosis with or without inflammation and fibrosis on liver biopsy.

▶ General Considerations

Nonalcoholic fatty liver disease (NAFLD) is estimated to affect 20–45% of the US population. The principal causes of NAFLD are obesity (present in 40% or more of affected patients), diabetes mellitus (in 20% or more), and hypertriglyceridemia (in 20% or more) in association with insulin resistance as part of the metabolic syndrome. The risk of NAFLD in persons with metabolic syndrome is 4 to 11 times higher than that of persons without insulin resistance. Other causes of fatty liver include corticosteroids, amiodarone, diltiazem, tamoxifen, irinotecan, oxaliplatin, highly active antiretroviral therapy, toxins (vinyl chloride, carbon tetrachloride, yellow phosphorus), endocrinopathies such as Cushing syndrome and hypopituitarism, polycystic ovary syndrome, hypothyroidism, hypobetalipoproteinemia and other metabolic disorders, obstructive sleep apnea (with chronic intermittent hypoxia), excessive dietary fructose consumption, starvation and refeeding syndrome, and total parenteral nutrition. Genetic factors play a role, and may account in part for an increased risk in Hispanics. The risk of NAFLD is increased in persons with psoriasis and appears to correlate with the activity of psoriasis. Soft drink consumption and cholecystectomy have been reported to be associated with NAFLD. Physical activity protects against the development of NAFLD.

In addition to macrovesicular steatosis, histologic features may include focal infiltration by polymorphonuclear neutrophils and Mallory hyalin, a picture indistinguishable from that of alcoholic hepatitis and referred to as nonalcoholic steatohepatitis (NASH), which affects 3–5% of the US population. In patients with NAFLD, older age, obesity, and diabetes mellitus are risk factors for advanced hepatic fibrosis and cirrhosis, whereas coffee consumption appears to reduce the risk. Cirrhosis caused by NASH appears to be uncommon in African Americans. Persons with NAFLD appear to be at increased risk for cardiovascular disease, chronic kidney disease, and colorectal cancer.

Microvesicular steatosis is seen with Reye syndrome, didanosine or stavudine toxicity, valproic acid toxicity, high-dose tetracycline, or acute fatty liver of pregnancy and may result in fulminant hepatic failure. Women in whom fatty liver of pregnancy develops often have a defect in fatty acid oxidation due to reduced long-chain 3-hydroxyacyl-CoA dehydrogenase activity.

► Clinical Findings

A. Symptoms and Signs

Most patients with NAFLD are asymptomatic or have mild right upper quadrant discomfort. Hepatomegaly is present in up to 75% of patients, but stigmata of chronic liver disease are uncommon. Rare instances of subacute liver failure caused by previously unrecognized NASH have been described. Signs of portal hypertension generally signify advanced liver fibrosis or cirrhosis but occasionally occur in patients with mild and no fibrosis and severe steatosis.

B. Laboratory Findings

Laboratory studies may show mildly elevated aminotransferase and alkaline phosphatase levels; however, laboratory values may be normal in up to 80% of persons with hepatic steatosis. In contrast to alcoholic liver disease, the ratio of ALT to AST is almost always greater than 1 in NAFLD, but it decreases to less than 1 as advanced fibrosis and cirrhosis develop. Antinuclear or smooth muscle antibodies and an elevated serum ferritin level may each be detected in one-fourth of patients with NASH. Elevated serum ferritin levels may signify so-called dysmetabolic iron overload syndrome and mildly increased body iron stores, which may play a causal role in insulin resistance and oxidative stress in hepatocytes and correlate with advanced fibrosis; the frequency of mutations in the *HFE* gene for hemochromatosis is not increased in patients with NAFLD. Iron deficiency is also common and associated with female sex, obesity, increased waist circumference, diabetes mellitus, and black or Native American race.

C. Imaging

Macrovascular steatosis may be demonstrated on ultrasonography, CT, or MRI. However, imaging does not distinguish steatosis from steatohepatitis or detect fibrosis.

D. Liver Biopsy

Percutaneous liver biopsy is diagnostic and is the standard approach to assessing the degree of inflammation and fibrosis. The risks of the procedure must be balanced against the impact of the added information on management decisions and assessment of prognosis. Liver biopsy is generally not recommended in asymptomatic persons with unsuspected hepatic steatosis detected on imaging but normal liver biochemistry test results. The histologic spectrum of NAFLD includes fatty liver, isolated portal fibrosis, steatohepatitis, and cirrhosis. A risk score for predicting advanced fibrosis, known as BARD, is based on body mass index more than 28, AST/ALT ratio 0.8 or more, and diabetes mellitus; it has a 96% negative predictive value (ie, a low score reliably excludes advanced fibrosis). Another risk score for advanced fibrosis, the NAFLD Fibrosis Score (http://nafldscore.com) based on age, hyperglycemia, body mass index, platelet count, albumin, and AST/ALT ratio, has a positive predictive value of over 80% and identifies patients at increased risk for liver-related complications and death. A clinical scoring system to predict the

likelihood of NASH in morbidly obese persons includes six predictive factors: hypertension, type 2 diabetes mellitus, sleep apnea, AST greater than 27 units/L (0.54 mckat/L), ALT greater than 27 units/L (0.54 mckat/L), and non-black race.

► Treatment

Treatment consists of lifestyle changes to remove or modify the offending factors. Weight loss, dietary fat restriction, and exercise (through reduction of abdominal obesity) often lead to improvement in liver biochemical tests and steatosis in obese patients with NAFLD. Loss of 3–5% of body weight appears necessary to improve steatosis, but loss of at least 10% may be needed to improve necroinflammation and fibrosis. Exercise may reduce liver fat with minimal or no weight loss and no reduction in ALT levels. Resistance training and aerobic exercise are equally effective in reducing hepatic fat content in patients with NAFLD and type 2 diabetes mellitus. Various drugs are under study. Vitamin E 800 international units/day (to reduce oxidative stress) appears to be of benefit in patients with NASH who do not have diabetes mellitus. Thiazolidinediones reverse insulin resistance and, in most relevant studies, have improved both serum aminotransferase levels and histologic features of steatohepatitis but lead to weight gain. Metformin, which reduces insulin resistance, improves abnormal liver chemistries but may not reliably improve liver histology. Pentoxifylline improves liver biochemical test levels but is associated with a high rate of side effects, particularly nausea. Ursodeoxycholic acid, 12–15 mg/kg/day, has not consistently resulted in biochemical and histologic improvement in patients with NASH but may be effective when given in combination with vitamin E. Hepatic steatosis due to total parenteral nutrition may be ameliorated—and perhaps prevented—with supplemental choline. Other approaches under study include obeticholic acid, a semisynthetic bile acid analog. Statins are not contraindicated in persons with NAFLD and may protect against histologic progression in some patients. Gastric bypass may be considered in patients with a body mass index greater than 35 and leads to histologic regression of NASH in most patients. Liver transplantation is indicated in appropriate candidates with advanced cirrhosis caused by NASH, now the third most common (and most rapidly increasing) indication for liver transplantation in the United States. Liver transplantation for NASH with advanced cirrhosis may be associated with increased mortality from cardiovascular disease and sepsis compared with liver transplantation for other indications.

► Prognosis

Fatty liver often has a benign course and is readily reversible with discontinuation of alcohol (or no more than one glass of wine per day, which may actually reduce the frequency of NASH in persons with NAFLD), or treatment of other underlying conditions; if untreated, fibrosis progresses at an average rate of 1 stage every 14 years, with a subset progressing more rapidly. In patients with NAFLD, the likelihood of NASH is increased by the following factors:

obesity, older age, non–African American ethnicity, female sex, diabetes mellitus, hypertension, higher ALT or AST level, higher AST/ALT ratio, low platelet count, elevated fasting C-peptide level, and a high ultrasound steatosis score. NASH may be associated with hepatic fibrosis in 40% of cases with progression at a rate of 1 stage every 7 years; cirrhosis develops in 9–25%; and decompensated cirrhosis occurs in 30–50% of cirrhotic patients over 10 years. The course may be more aggressive in diabetic persons than in nondiabetic persons. Mortality is increased in patients with NAFLD, correlates with fibrosis stage, and is more likely to be the result of malignancy and ischemic heart disease than liver disease. Risk factors for mortality are older age, male sex, white race, smoking, higher body mass index, hypertension, diabetes mellitus, and cirrhosis. Steatosis is a cofactor for the progression of fibrosis in patients with other causes of chronic liver disease, such as hepatitis C. Hepatocellular carcinoma is a complication of cirrhosis caused by NASH, as it is for other causes of cirrhosis, and has been reported even in the absence of cirrhosis. NASH accounts for a substantial percentage of cases labeled as cryptogenic cirrhosis and can recur following liver transplantation. Central obesity is an independent risk factor for death from cirrhosis of any cause.

► When to Refer

Refer patients with NAFLD who require liver biopsy for diagnosis.

Angulo P et al. Liver fibrosis, but no other histologic features, is associated with long-term outcomes of patients with nonalcoholic fatty liver disease. Gastroenterology. 2015 Aug;149(2):389–97. [PMID: 25935633]

Ekstedt M et al. Fibrosis stage is the strongest predictor for disease-specific mortality in NAFLD after up to 33 years of follow-up. Hepatology. 2015 May;61(5):1547–54. [PMID: 25125077]

Rinella ME. Nonalcoholic fatty liver disease: a systematic review. JAMA. 2015 Jun 9;313(22):2263–73. [PMID: 26057287]

Singh S et al. Fibrosis progression in nonalcoholic fatty liver vs nonalcoholic steatohepatitis: a systematic review and meta-analysis of paired-biopsy studies. Clin Gastroenterol Hepatol. 2015 Apr;13(4):643–54. [PMID: 24768810]

Vilar-Gomez E et al. Weight loss through lifestyle modification significantly reduces features of nonalcoholic steatohepatitis. Gastroenterology. 2015 Aug;149(2):367–78.e5 [PMID: 25865049]

CIRRHOSIS

ESSENTIALS OF DIAGNOSIS

► End result of injury that leads to both fibrosis and regenerative nodules.

► May be reversible if cause is removed.

► The clinical features result from hepatic cell dysfunction, portosystemic shunting, and portal hypertension.

► General Considerations

Cirrhosis, the twelfth leading cause of death in the United States with a prevalence rate of 0.27%, is the end result of hepatocellular injury that leads to both fibrosis and regenerative nodules throughout the liver. Hospitalization rates for cirrhosis and portal hypertension are rising in the United States. Causes include chronic viral hepatitis, alcohol, drug toxicity, autoimmune and metabolic liver diseases, and miscellaneous disorders. Celiac disease appears to be associated with an increased risk of cirrhosis. Many patients have more than one risk factor (eg, chronic hepatitis and alcohol use). Mexican Americans and African Americans have a higher frequency of cirrhosis than whites because of a higher rate of risk factors. In persons at increased risk for liver injury (eg, heavy alcohol use, obesity, iron overload), higher coffee and tea consumption has been reported to reduce the risk of cirrhosis. The risk of hospitalization or death due to cirrhosis has been reported to correlate with protein and cholesterol consumption and with hyperuricemia and inversely with carbohydrate consumption.

Clinically, cirrhosis is considered to progress through three stages that correlate with the thickness of fibrous septa: compensated, compensated with varices, and decompensated (ascites, variceal bleeding, encephalopathy, or jaundice).

► Clinical Findings

A. Symptoms and Signs

The clinical features of cirrhosis result from hepatocyte dysfunction, portosystemic shunting, and portal hypertension. Patients may have no symptoms for long periods. The onset of symptoms may be insidious or, less often, abrupt. Fatigue, disturbed sleep, muscle cramps, and weight loss are common. In advanced cirrhosis, anorexia is usually present and may be extreme, with associated nausea and occasional vomiting, as well as reduced muscle strength and exercise capacity. Abdominal pain may be present and is related either to hepatic enlargement and stretching of Glisson capsule or to the presence of ascites. Menstrual abnormalities (usually amenorrhea), erectile dysfunction, loss of libido, sterility, and gynecomastia may occur. Hematemesis is the presenting symptom in 15–25%. The risk of falls is increased in hospitalized patients with cirrhosis who are taking psychoactive medications.

Skin manifestations consist of spider telangiectasias (invariably on the upper half of the body), palmar erythema (mottled redness of the thenar and hypothenar eminences), and Dupuytren contractures. Evidence of vitamin deficiencies (glossitis and cheilosis) is common. Weight loss, wasting (due to sarcopenia), and the appearance of chronic illness are present. Jaundice—usually not an initial sign—is mild at first, increasing in severity during the later stages of the disease. In 70% of cases, the liver is enlarged, palpable, and firm if not hard and has a sharp or nodular edge; the left lobe may predominate. Splenomegaly is present in 35–50% of cases and is associated with an increased risk of complications of portal hypertension. The superficial veins of the abdomen and thorax are dilated, reflecting the intrahepatic obstruction to portal blood flow, as do rectal varices. The abdominal wall veins fill from below when compressed. Ascites, pleural effusions, peripheral edema, and ecchymoses are late findings. Encephalopathy, characterized by day-night reversal, asterixis, tremor, dysarthria, delirium, drowsiness and, ultimately coma also occurs late in the course except when precipitated by an acute hepatocellular insult or an episode of gastrointestinal bleeding or infection. Fever is present in up to 35% of patients and usually reflects associated alcoholic hepatitis, spontaneous bacterial peritonitis, or intercurrent infection.

B. Laboratory Findings

Laboratory abnormalities are either absent or minimal in early or compensated cirrhosis. Anemia, a frequent finding, is often macrocytic; causes include suppression of erythropoiesis by alcohol as well as folate deficiency, hemolysis, hypersplenism, and occult or overt blood loss from the gastrointestinal tract. The white blood cell count may be low, reflecting hypersplenism, or high, suggesting infection. Thrombocytopenia, the most common cytopenia in cirrhotic patients, is secondary to alcoholic marrow suppression, sepsis, folate deficiency, or splenic sequestration. Prolongation of the prothrombin time may result from reduced levels of clotting factors (except factor VIII). However, bleeding risk correlates poorly with the prothrombin time because of concomitant abnormalities of fibrinolysis, and among hospitalized patients under age 45, cirrhosis is associated with an increased risk of venous thromboembolism.

Blood chemistries reflect hepatocellular injury and dysfunction, manifested by modest elevations of AST and alkaline phosphatase and progressive elevation of the bilirubin. Serum albumin decreases as the disease progresses; gamma-globulin levels are increased and may be as high as in autoimmune hepatitis. The risk of diabetes mellitus is increased in patients with cirrhosis, particularly when associated with HCV infection, alcoholism, hemochromatosis, or NAFLD. Vitamin D deficiency has been reported in as many as 91% of patients with cirrhosis. Patients with alcoholic cirrhosis may have elevated serum cardiac troponin I and B-type natriuretic peptide (BNP) levels. Blunted cardiac inotropic and chronotropic responses to exercise, stress, and drugs, as well as systolic and diastolic ventricular dysfunction in the absence of other known causes of cardiac disease ("cirrhotic cardiomyopathy"), and prolongation of the QT interval in the setting of a hyperkinetic circulation, are common in cirrhosis of all causes, but overt heart failure is rare in the absence of alcoholism. Relative adrenal insufficiency appears to be common in patients with advanced cirrhosis, even in the absence of sepsis, and may relate in part to reduced synthesis of cholesterol and increased levels of proinflammatory cytokines.

C. Imaging

Ultrasonography is helpful for assessing liver size and detecting ascites or hepatic nodules, including small

hepatocellular carcinomas. Together with a Doppler study, it may establish patency of the splenic, portal, and hepatic veins. Hepatic nodules are characterized further by contrast-enhanced CT or MRI. Nodules suspicious for malignancy may be biopsied under ultrasound or CT guidance.

D. Liver Biopsy

Liver biopsy may show inactive cirrhosis (fibrosis with regenerative nodules) with no specific features to suggest the underlying cause. Alternatively, there may be additional features of alcoholic liver disease, chronic hepatitis, NASH, or other specific causes of cirrhosis. Liver biopsy may be performed by laparoscopy or, in patients with coagulopathy and ascites, by a transjugular approach. Combinations of routine blood tests (eg, AST, platelet count), including the FibroSure test, serum markers of hepatic fibrosis (eg, hyaluronic acid, amino-terminal propeptide of type III collagen, tissue inhibitor of matrix metalloproteinase 1), and ultrasound or magnetic resonance elastography are potential alternatives to liver biopsy for the diagnosis or exclusion of cirrhosis. In persons with chronic hepatitis C, for example, a low FibroSure or elastography score reliably excludes advanced fibrosis, a high score reliably predicts advanced fibrosis, and intermediate scores are inconclusive.

E. Other Tests

Esophagogastroduodenoscopy confirms the presence of varices and detects specific causes of bleeding in the esophagus, stomach, and proximal duodenum. In selected cases, wedged hepatic vein pressure measurement may establish the presence and cause of portal hypertension.

▶ Differential Diagnosis

The most common causes of cirrhosis are alcohol, chronic hepatitis C infection, NAFLD, and hepatitis B infection. Hemochromatosis is the most commonly identified genetic disorder that causes cirrhosis. Other diseases associated with cirrhosis include Wilson disease, alpha-1-antitrypsin (alpha-1-antiprotease) deficiency, and celiac disease. PBC occurs more frequently in women than men. Secondary biliary cirrhosis may result from chronic biliary obstruction due to a stone, stricture, or neoplasm. Heart failure and constrictive pericarditis may lead to hepatic fibrosis ("cardiac cirrhosis") complicated by ascites. Hereditary hemorrhagic telangiectasia can lead to portal hypertension because of portosystemic shunting and nodular transformation of the liver as well as high-output heart failure. Many cases of cirrhosis are "cryptogenic," in which unrecognized NAFLD may play a role.

▶ Complications

Upper gastrointestinal tract bleeding may occur from varices, portal hypertensive gastropathy, or gastroduodenal ulcer (see Chapter 15). Varices may also result from portal vein thrombosis, which may complicate cirrhosis. Liver failure may be precipitated by alcoholism, surgery, and infection. Hepatic Kupffer cell (reticuloendothelial) dysfunction and decreased opsonic activity lead to an increased risk of systemic infection (which may be increased further by the use of proton pump inhibitors), and which increase mortality fourfold. These infections include nosocomial infections, which may be classified as spontaneous bloodstream infections, urinary tract infections, pulmonary infections, spontaneous bacterial peritonitis, *Clostridium difficile* infection, and intervention-related infections. These nosocomial infections are increasingly caused by multidrug-resistant bacteria. Osteoporosis occurs in 12–55% of patients with cirrhosis. The risk of hepatocellular carcinoma is increased greatly in persons with cirrhosis (see Chapter 39).

▶ **Treatment**

A. General Measures

Most important is abstinence from alcohol. The diet should be palatable, with adequate calories (25–35 kcal/kg body weight per day in those with compensated cirrhosis and 35–45 kcal/kg/day in those with malnutrition) and protein (1–1.5 g/kg/day in those with compensated cirrhosis and 1.5 g/kg/day in those with malnutrition) and, if there is fluid retention, sodium restriction. In the presence of hepatic encephalopathy, protein intake should be reduced to no less than 60–80 g/day. Specialized supplements containing branched-chain amino acids to prevent or treat hepatic encephalopathy or delay progressive liver failure are generally unnecessary. Vitamin supplementation is desirable. Muscle cramps may be helped by L-carnitine, 300 mg orally four times a day. Patients with cirrhosis should receive the HAV, HBV, and pneumococcal vaccines and a yearly influenza vaccine. Liver transplantation in appropriate candidates is curative.

B. Treatment of Complications

1. Ascites and edema—Diagnostic paracentesis is indicated for patients who have new ascites or who have been hospitalized for a complication of cirrhosis; it reduces mortality, especially if performed within 12 hours of admission. Serious complications of paracentesis, including bleeding, infection, or bowel perforation, occur in 1.6% of procedures and are associated with therapeutic (vs diagnostic) paracentesis and possibly with Child-Pugh class C, a platelet count less than 50,000/mcL (50 × 10⁹/L), and alcoholic cirrhosis. In patients with coagulopathy, however, pre-paracentesis prophylactic transfusions do not appear to be necessary. In addition to a cell count and culture, the ascitic albumin level should be determined: a serum-ascites albumin gradient (serum albumin minus ascitic fluid albumin) greater than or equal to 1.1 suggests portal hypertension. An elevated ascitic adenosine deaminase level is suggestive of tuberculous peritonitis. Occasionally, cirrhotic ascites is chylous (rich in triglycerides); other causes of chylous ascites are malignancy, tuberculosis, and recent abdominal surgery or trauma.

In individuals with ascites, the urinary sodium concentration is often less than 10 mEq/L (10 mmol/L). Free water excretion is also impaired in cirrhosis, and hyponatremia may develop.

In all patients with cirrhotic ascites, dietary sodium intake may initially be restricted to 2000 mg/day; the intake of sodium may be liberalized slightly after diuresis ensues. Nonsteroidal anti-inflammatory drugs are contraindicated, and angiotensin-converting enzyme inhibitors and angiotensin II antagonists should be avoided. In some patients, ascites diminishes promptly with bed rest and dietary sodium restriction alone. Fluid intake (800–1000 mL/day) is often restricted in patients with hyponatremia. Treatment of severe hyponatremia (serum sodium less than 125 mEq/L [125 mmol/L]) with vasopressin receptor antagonists (eg, intravenous conivaptan, 20 mg daily) can be considered but such treatment is expensive, causes thirst, and does not improve survival; oral tolvaptan is contraindicated in patients with liver disease because of potential hepatotoxicity.

A. Diuretics—Spironolactone, generally in combination with furosemide, should be used in patients who do not respond to salt restriction alone. An initial trial of furosemide 80 mg intravenously demonstrating a rise in urine sodium to 750 mmol in 8 hours may predict response to diuretic therapy. The dose of spironolactone is initially 100 mg orally daily and may be increased by 100 mg every 3–5 days (up to a maximal conventional daily dose of 400 mg/day, although higher doses have been used) until diuresis is achieved, typically preceded by a rise in the urinary sodium concentration. A "spot" urine sodium concentration that exceeds the potassium concentration correlates with a 24-hour sodium excretion greater than 78 mmol/day, which predicts diuresis in patients adherent to a salt-restricted diet. Monitoring for hyperkalemia is important. In patients who cannot tolerate spironolactone because of side effects, such as painful gynecomastia, amiloride (another potassium-sparing diuretic) may be used in a starting dose of 5–10 mg orally daily. Diuresis is augmented by the addition of a loop diuretic such as furosemide. This potent diuretic, however, will maintain its effect even with a falling glomerular filtration rate, with resulting prerenal azotemia. The dose of oral furosemide ranges from 40 mg/day to 160 mg/day, and the drug should be administered while blood pressure, urinary output, mental status, and serum electrolytes (especially potassium) are monitored. The goal of weight loss in the ascitic patient without associated peripheral edema should be no more than 1–1.5 lb/day (0.5–0.7 kg/day).

B. Large-volume paracentesis—In patients with massive ascites and respiratory compromise, ascites refractory to diuretics ("diuretic resistant"), or intolerable diuretic side effects ("diuretic intractable"), large-volume paracentesis (more than 5 L) is effective. Intravenous albumin concomitantly at a dosage of 6–8 g/L of ascites fluid removed protects the intravascular volume and may prevent postparacentesis circulatory dysfunction, although the usefulness of this practice is debated and the use of albumin is expensive. Large-volume paracentesis can be repeated daily until ascites is largely resolved and may decrease the need for hospitalization. If possible, diuretics should be continued in the hope of preventing recurrent ascites.

c. Transjugular intrahepatic portosystemic shunt (TIPS)—TIPS is an effective treatment of variceal bleeding refractory to standard therapy (eg, endoscopic band ligation) and has shown benefit in the treatment of severe refractory ascites. The technique involves insertion of an expandable metal stent between a branch of the hepatic vein and the portal vein over a catheter inserted via the internal jugular vein. Increased renal sodium excretion and control of ascites refractory to diuretics can be achieved in about 75% of selected cases. The success rate is lower in patients with underlying chronic kidney disease. TIPS appears to be the treatment of choice for refractory hepatic hydrothorax (translocation of ascites across the diaphragm to the pleural space); video-assisted thoracoscopy with pleurodesis using talc may be effective when TIPS is contraindicated. Complications of TIPS include hepatic encephalopathy in 20–30% of cases, infection, shunt stenosis in up to 60% of cases, and shunt occlusion in up to 30% of cases when bare stents are used; polytetrafluoroethylene-covered stents are associated with long-term patency rates of 80–90%. Long-term patency often requires periodic shunt revisions. In most cases, patency can be maintained by balloon dilation, local thrombolysis, or placement of an additional stent. TIPS is particularly useful in patients who require short-term control of variceal bleeding or ascites until liver transplantation can be performed. In patients with refractory ascites, TIPS results in lower rates of ascites recurrence and hepatorenal syndrome but a higher rate of hepatic encephalopathy than occurs with repeated large-volume paracentesis; a benefit in survival has been demonstrated in one study and a meta-analysis. Chronic kidney disease, diastolic cardiac dysfunction, refractory encephalopathy, and hyperbilirubinemia (greater than 5 mg/dL [85.5 mcmol/L]) are associated with mortality after TIPS.

2. Spontaneous bacterial peritonitis—Spontaneous bacterial peritonitis is heralded by abdominal pain, increasing ascites, fever, and progressive encephalopathy in a patient with cirrhotic ascites; symptoms are typically mild. (Analogously, spontaneous bacterial empyema may complicate hepatic hydrothorax and is managed similarly.) Risk factors in cirrhotic patients with ascites include gastroesophageal variceal bleeding and possibly use of a proton pump inhibitor. Paracentesis reveals an ascitic fluid with, most commonly, a total white cell count of up to 500 cells/mcL with a high polymorphonuclear (PMN) cell count (250/mcL or more) and a protein concentration of 1 g/dL (10 g/L) or less, corresponding to decreased ascitic opsonic activity. Rapid diagnosis of bacterial peritonitis can be made with a high degree of specificity with rapid reagent strips ("dipsticks") that detect leukocyte esterase in ascitic fluid, but the sensitivity is too low for routine use. Cultures of ascites give the highest yield—80–90% positive—using specialized culture bottles inoculated at the bedside. Common isolates are *Escherichia coli* and *Streptococcus* spp. Gram-positive cocci are the most common isolates in patients who have undergone an invasive procedure such as central venous line placement, and the frequency of enterococcal isolates is increasing. Anaerobes are uncommon. Pending culture results, if there are 250 or more

PMNs/mcL or symptoms or signs of infection, intravenous antibiotic therapy should be initiated with cefotaxime, 2 g every 8–12 hours for at least 5 days. Alternative choices include ceftriaxone, amoxicillin-clavulanic acid, and levofloxacin (in patients not receiving fluoroquinolone prophylaxis). Oral ofloxacin, 400 mg twice daily for 7 days, or, in a patient not already taking a fluoroquinolone for prophylaxis against bacterial peritonitis, a 2-day course of intravenous ciprofloxacin, 200 mg twice daily, followed by oral ciprofloxacin, 500 mg twice daily for 5 days, may be effective alternative regimens in selected patients. A carbapenem has been recommended for patients with hospital-acquired spontaneous bacterial peritonitis. Supplemental administration of intravenous albumin (which may have anti-inflammatory effects in addition to expanding plasma volume) prevents further renal impairment and reduces mortality, particularly in patients with a serum creatinine greater than 1 mg/dL (83.3 mcmol/L), blood urea nitrogen greater than 30 mg/dL (10.8 mmol/L), or total bilirubin greater than 4 mg/dL (68.4 mcmol/L). Response to therapy can be documented, if necessary, by a decrease in the PMN count of at least 50% on repeat paracentesis 48 hours after initiation of therapy. The overall mortality rate is high—up to 30% during hospitalization and up to 70% by 1 year. Mortality may be predicted by the 22/11 model: MELD score greater than 22 and peripheral white blood cell count higher than 11,000/mcL (11×10^9/L). Patients with cirrhosis and septic shock have a high frequency of relative adrenal insufficiency, which if present requires administration of hydrocortisone.

In survivors of bacterial peritonitis, the risk of recurrent peritonitis may be decreased by long-term norfloxacin, 400 mg orally daily; ciprofloxacin (eg, 500 mg orally once or twice a day), although with recurrence the causative organism is often resistant to fluoroquinolones; or trimethoprim-sulfamethoxazole (eg, one double-strength tablet five times a week). In high-risk cirrhotic patients without prior peritonitis (eg, those with an ascitic protein less than 1.5 g/dL and serum bilirubin greater than 3 mg/dL (51.3 mcmol/L), serum creatinine greater than 1.2 mg/dL (99.96 mcmol/L), blood urea nitrogen 25 mg/dL or more (9 mmol/L or more), or sodium 130 mEq/L or less [130 mmol/L or less]), the risk of peritonitis, hepatorenal syndrome, and mortality for at least 1 year may be reduced by prophylactic norfloxacin, 400 mg orally once a day. In patients hospitalized for acute variceal bleeding, oral norfloxacin (400 mg orally twice a day) or intravenous ceftriaxone (1 g per day), which may be preferable, for 7 days reduces the risk of bacterial peritonitis.

3. Hepatorenal syndrome—Hepatorenal syndrome occurs in up to 10% of patients with advanced cirrhosis and ascites. It is characterized by (1) azotemia (increase in serum creatinine level of greater than 0.3 mg/dL [26.5 mcmol/L]) within 48 hours or increase by 50% or more from baseline within the previous 7 days in the absence of current or recent nephrotoxic drug use, (2) macroscopic signs of structural kidney injury, (3) shock, and (4) failure of kidney function to improve following 2 days of diuretic withdrawal and volume expansion with albumin, 1 g/kg up to a maximum of 100 g/day. Oliguria, hyponatremia, and a low urinary sodium concentration are typical features. Hepatorenal syndrome is diagnosed only when other causes of acute kidney injury (including prerenal azotemia and acute tubular necrosis) have been excluded. Urinary neutrophil gelatinase-associated lipocalin levels (normal, 20 ng/mL) and other biomarkers may help distinguish hepatorenal syndrome (105 ng/mL) from chronic kidney disease (50 ng/mL) and acute kidney injury (325 ng/mL). Type I hepatorenal syndrome is characterized by doubling of the serum creatinine to a level greater than 2.5 mg/dL (208.25 mcmol/L) or by halving of the creatinine clearance to less than 20 mL/min (0.34 mL/s/1.73 m² BSA) in less than 2 weeks. Type II hepatorenal syndrome is more slowly progressive and chronic. An acute decrease in cardiac output is often the precipitating event. In addition to discontinuation of diuretics, clinical improvement and an increase in short-term survival may follow intravenous infusion of albumin in combination with one of the following vasoconstrictor regimens for 7–14 days: oral midodrine plus octreotide, subcutaneously or intravenously; intravenous terlipressin (not yet available in the United States but perhaps the preferred agent where available); or intravenous norepinephrine. Oral midodrine, 7.5 mg three times daily, added to diuretics, to increase blood pressure has also been reported to convert refractory ascites to diuretic-sensitive ascites. Prolongation of survival has been associated with use of MARS, a modified dialysis method that selectively removes albumin-bound substances. Improvement and sometimes normalization of kidney function may also follow placement of a TIPS; survival after 1 year is reported to be predicted by the combination of a serum bilirubin level less than 3 mg/dL (50 mcmol/L) and a platelet count greater than 75,000/mcL (75 ×10⁹/L). Continuous venovenous hemofiltration and hemodialysis are of uncertain value in hepatorenal syndrome. Liver transplantation is the treatment of choice, but many patients die before a donor liver can be obtained. Mortality correlates with the MELD score and presence of a systemic inflammatory response. Type 1 hepatorenal syndrome is often irreversible in patients with a systemic infection. The 3-month probability of survival in cirrhotic patients with hepatorenal syndrome (15%) is lower than that for renal failure associated with infections (31%), hypovolemia (46%), and parenchymal kidney disease (73%).

4. Hepatic encephalopathy—Hepatic encephalopathy is a state of disordered central nervous system function resulting from failure of the liver to detoxify noxious agents of gut origin because of hepatocellular dysfunction and portosystemic shunting. The clinical spectrum ranges from day-night reversal and mild intellectual impairment to coma. Patients with covert (formerly minimal) hepatic encephalopathy have no recognizable clinical symptoms but demonstrate mild cognitive, psychomotor, and attention deficits on standardized psychometric tests and an increased rate of traffic accidents. The stages of overt encephalopathy are: (1) mild confusion, (2) drowsiness, (3) stupor, and (4) coma. A revised staging system known as SONIC (spectrum of neurocognitive impairment in cirrhosis) encompasses absent, covert, and stages 2 to 4

encephalopathy. Ammonia is the most readily identified and measurable toxin but is not solely responsible for the disturbed mental status. Bleeding into the intestinal tract may significantly increase the amount of protein in the bowel and precipitate encephalopathy. Other precipitants include constipation, alkalosis, and potassium deficiency induced by diuretics, opioids, hypnotics, and sedatives; medications containing ammonium or amino compounds; paracentesis with consequent hypovolemia; hepatic or systemic infection; and portosystemic shunts (including TIPS). The diagnosis is based primarily on detection of characteristic symptoms and signs, including asterixis. A smartphone app called EncephalApp using the "Stroop test" (asking the patient to name the color of a written word rather than the word itself, even when the word is the name of a different color) has proved useful for detecting covert hepatic encephalopathy. The role of neuroimaging studies (eg, cerebral PET, magnetic resonance spectroscopy) in the diagnosis of hepatic encephalopathy is evolving.

Protein is withheld during acute episodes if the patient cannot eat. When the patient resumes oral intake, protein intake should be 60–80 g/day as tolerated; vegetable protein is better tolerated than meat protein. Gastrointestinal bleeding should be controlled and blood purged from the gastrointestinal tract. This can be accomplished with 120 mL of magnesium citrate by mouth or nasogastric tube every 3–4 hours until the stool is free of gross blood or by administration of lactulose. The value of treating patients with covert hepatic encephalopathy is uncertain; probiotic agents may have some benefit.

Lactulose, a nonabsorbable synthetic disaccharide syrup, is digested by bacteria in the colon to short-chain fatty acids, resulting in acidification of colon contents. This acidification favors the formation of ammonium ion in the $NH_4^+ \leftrightarrow NH_3 + H^+$ equation; NH_4^+ is not absorbable, whereas NH_3 is absorbable and thought to be neurotoxic. Lactulose also leads to a change in bowel flora so that fewer ammonia-forming organisms are present. When given orally, the initial dose of lactulose for acute hepatic encephalopathy is 30 mL three or four times daily. The dose should then be titrated so that the patient produces 2–3 soft stools per day. When given rectally because the patient is unable to take medicines orally, the dose is 300 mL of lactulose in 700 mL of saline or sorbitol as a retention enema for 30–60 minutes; it may be repeated every 4–6 hours. Bowel cleansing with a polyethylene glycol colonoscopy preparation is also effective in patients with acute overt hepatic encephalopathy. Continued use of lactulose after an episode of acute encephalopathy reduces the frequency of recurrences.

The ammonia-producing intestinal flora may also be controlled with an oral antibiotic. The nonabsorbable agent rifaximin, 550 mg orally twice daily, is preferred and has been shown as well to maintain remission of and reduce the risk of rehospitalization for hepatic encephalopathy over a 24-month period, with or without the concomitant use of lactulose. Metronidazole, 250 mg orally three times daily, has also shown benefit. Patients who do not respond to lactulose alone may improve with a course of an antibiotic added to treatment with lactulose.

Opioids and sedatives metabolized or excreted by the liver should be avoided. If agitation is marked, oxazepam, 10–30 mg, which is not metabolized by the liver, may be given cautiously by mouth or by nasogastric tube. Zinc deficiency should be corrected, if present, with oral zinc sulfate, 600 mg/day in divided doses. Sodium benzoate, 5 g orally twice daily, ornithine aspartate, 9 g orally three times daily, and L-acyl-carnitine (an essential factor in the mitochrondrial transport of long-chain fatty acids), 4 g orally daily, may lower blood ammonia levels, but there is less experience with these drugs than with lactulose. Flumazenil is effective in about 30% of patients with severe hepatic encephalopathy, but the drug is short-acting and intravenous administration is required. Use of special dietary supplements enriched with branched-chain amino acids is usually unnecessary except in occasional patients who are intolerant of standard protein supplements.

5. Coagulopathy—Hypoprothrombinemia caused by malnutrition and vitamin K deficiency may be treated with vitamin K (eg, phytonadione, 5 mg orally or intravenously daily); however, this treatment is ineffective when synthesis of coagulation factors is impaired because of hepatic disease. In such cases, correcting the prolonged prothrombin time requires large volumes of fresh frozen plasma (see Chapter 14). Because the effect is transient, plasma infusions are not indicated except for active bleeding or before an invasive procedure, and even then, their value has been questioned because of concomitant alterations in antihemostatic factors and because bleeding risk does not correlate with the INR. Recombinant activated factor VIIa may be an alternative but is expensive and poses a 1–2% risk of thrombotic complications. Eltrombopag reduces the need for platelet transfusions in patients with cirrhosis and a platelet count less than 50,000/mcL (50×10^9/L) who undergo invasive procedures, but eltrombopag is associated with an increased risk of portal vein thrombosis and arterial thromboembolism.

6. Hemorrhage from esophageal varices—See Chapter 15.

7. Hepatopulmonary syndrome and portopulmonary hypertension—Shortness of breath in patients with cirrhosis may result from pulmonary restriction and atelectasis caused by massive ascites or hepatic hydrothorax. The hepatopulmonary syndrome—the triad of chronic liver disease, an increased alveolar-arterial gradient while the patient is breathing room air, and intrapulmonary vascular dilatations or arteriovenous communications that result in a right-to-left intrapulmonary shunt—occurs in 5–32% of patients with cirrhosis. Patients often have greater dyspnea (platypnea) and arterial deoxygenation (orthodeoxia) in the upright than in the recumbent position. The diagnosis should be suspected in a cirrhotic patient with a pulse oximetry level of 96% or less.

Contrast-enhanced echocardiography is a sensitive screening test for detecting pulmonary vascular dilatations, whereas macroaggregated albumin lung perfusion scanning is more specific and may be used to confirm the diagnosis. High-resolution CT may be useful for detecting dilated pulmonary vessels that may be amenable to embolization in patients with severe hypoxemia (PO_2 less than

60 mm Hg [7.8 kPa]) who respond poorly to supplemental oxygen.

Medical therapy has been disappointing; experimentally, intravenous methylene blue, oral garlic powder, oral norfloxacin, and mycophenolate mofetil may improve oxygenation by inhibiting nitric oxide-induced vasodilatation and angiogenesis, and pentoxifylline may prevent hepatopulmonary syndrome by inhibiting production of tumor necrosis factor. Long-term oxygen therapy is recommended for severely hypoxemic patients. The syndrome may reverse with liver transplantation, although postoperative mortality is increased in patients with a preoperative arterial PO_2 less than 44 mm Hg (5.9 kPa) or with substantial intrapulmonary shunting. TIPS may provide palliation in patients with hepatopulmonary syndrome awaiting transplantation.

Portopulmonary hypertension occurs in 0.7% of patients with cirrhosis. Female sex and autoimmune hepatitis have been reported to be risk factors, and large spontaneous portosystemic shunts are present in many affected patients and are associated with a lack of response to treatment. In cases confirmed by right-sided heart catheterization, treatment with the prostaglandin epoprostenol, the endothelin-receptor antagonists bosentan or ambrisentan, or the phosphodiesterase-5 inhibitors sildenafil or tadalafil may reduce pulmonary hypertension and thereby facilitate liver transplantation; beta-blockers worsen exercise capacity and are contraindicated, and calcium channel blockers should be used with caution because they may worsen portal hypertension. Liver transplantation is contraindicated in patients with moderate to severe pulmonary hypertension (mean pulmonary pressure greater than 35 mm Hg).

C. Liver Transplantation

Liver transplantation is indicated in selected cases of irreversible, progressive chronic liver disease, acute liver failure, and certain metabolic diseases in which the metabolic defect is in the liver. Absolute contraindications include malignancy (except relatively small hepatocellular carcinomas in a cirrhotic liver—see Chapter 39), advanced cardiopulmonary disease (except hepatopulmonary syndrome), and sepsis. Relative contraindications include age over 70 years, morbid obesity, portal and mesenteric vein thrombosis, active alcohol or drug abuse, severe malnutrition, and lack of patient understanding. With the emergence of effective antiretroviral therapy for HIV disease, a major cause of mortality in these patients has shifted to liver disease caused by HCV and HBV infection; experience to date suggests that the outcome of liver transplantation is comparable to that for non–HIV-infected liver transplant recipients. Patients with alcoholism should be abstinent for 6 months. Liver transplantation should be considered in patients with worsening functional status, rising bilirubin, decreasing albumin, worsening coagulopathy, refractory ascites, recurrent variceal bleeding, or worsening encephalopathy; prioritization is based on the MELD score. Combined liver-kidney transplantation is indicated in patients with associated kidney failure presumed to be irreversible. The major impediment to more widespread use of liver transplantation is a shortage of donor organs. Adult living donor liver transplantation is an option for some patients, and extended-criteria donors are being used. Five-year survival rates over 80% are now reported. Hepatocellular carcinoma, hepatitis B and C, and some cases of Budd-Chiari syndrome and autoimmune liver disease may recur in the transplanted liver. The incidence of recurrence of hepatitis B can be reduced by preoperative and postoperative treatment with a nucleoside or nucleotide analog and perioperative administration of HBIG, and hepatitis C can be treated with direct-acting antiviral agents. Immunosuppression is achieved with combinations of cyclosporine, tacrolimus or sirolimus, corticosteroids, azathioprine, and mycophenolate mofetil and may be complicated by infections, advanced chronic kidney disease, neurologic disorders, and drug toxicity, as well as graft rejection, vascular occlusion, or bile leaks. Patients taking these drugs are at risk for obesity, diabetes mellitus, and hyperlipidemia.

▶ Prognosis

Prognostic scoring systems for cirrhosis include the Child-Pugh score and MELD score (Table 16–7). The MELD score, which incorporates the serum bilirubin and creatinine levels and the INR, is also a measure of mortality risk in patients with end-stage liver disease and is particularly useful for predicting short- and intermediate-term survival and complications of cirrhosis (eg, bacterial peritonitis) as

well as determining allocation priorities for donor livers. Additional (MELD-exception) points are given for patients with conditions such as hepatopulmonary syndrome and hepatocellular carcinoma that may benefit from liver transplantation. A MELD score of greater than 14 is required for liver transplant listing. In patients with a relatively low MELD score (less than 21) and a low priority for liver transplantation, a low serum sodium concentration (below 130 mEq/L [130 mmol/L]), an elevated hepatic venous pressure gradient, persistent ascites, and a low health-related quality of life appear to be additional independent predictors of mortality, and modifications of the MELD score, including one that incorporates the serum sodium (MELDNa), are under consideration. Only 50% of patients with severe hepatic dysfunction (serum albumin less than 3 g/dL [30 g/L], bilirubin greater than 3 mg/dL [51.3 mcmol/L]), ascites, encephalopathy, cachexia, and upper gastrointestinal bleeding) survive 6 months without transplantation. The risk of death in this subgroup of patients with advanced cirrhosis is associated with muscle wasting, age 65 years or older, mean arterial pressure 82 mm Hg or less, renal failure, cognitive dysfunction, ventilatory insufficiency, prothrombin time 16 seconds or longer, delayed and suboptimal treatment of sepsis, and second infections. For cirrhotic patients admitted to an intensive care unit, the Royal Free Hospital score, consisting of the serum bilirubin, INR, serum lactate, alveolar-arterial oxygen gradient, and blood urea nitrogen, has been reported to predict mortality. Renal failure increases mortality up to sevenfold in patients with cirrhosis. Obesity and diabetes mellitus appear to be risk factors for clinical deterioration and cirrhosis-related mortality, as is continued alcohol use in patients with alcoholic cirrhosis. The use of beta-blockers for portal hypertension is beneficial early in the course but is associated with reduced survival in patients with refractory ascites or spontaneous bacterial peritonitis because of their negative effect on cardiac compensatory reserve. Patients with cirrhosis are at risk for the development of hepatocellular carcinoma, with rates of 3–5% per year for alcoholic and viral hepatitis-related cirrhosis. Liver transplantation has markedly improved the outlook for patients with cirrhosis who are candidates and are referred for evaluation early in the course. Patients with compensated cirrhosis are given additional priority for liver transplantation if they are found to have a lesion larger than 2 cm in diameter consistent with hepatocellular carcinoma. In-hospital mortality from cirrhosis declined from 9.1% in 2002 to 5.4% in 2010 and that from variceal bleeding in patients with cirrhosis declined from over 40% in 1980 to 15% in 2000. Patients hospitalized with cirrhosis and an infection are at high risk for subsequent infections, particularly if they are older, taking a proton pump inhibitor, or receiving antibiotic prophylaxis for spontaneous bacterial peritonitis.

Table 16–7. Child-Pugh and Model for End-Stage Liver Disease (MELD) scoring systems for staging cirrhosis.

Child-Pugh scoring system			
Parameter	Numerical Score		
	1	2	3
Ascites	None	Slight	Moderate to severe
Encephalopathy	None	Slight to moderate	Moderate to severe
Bilirubin, mg/dL (mcmol/L)	< 2.0 (34.2)	2–3 (34.2–51.3)	> 3.0 (51.3)
Albumin, g/dL (g/L)	> 3.5 (35)	2.8–3.5 (28–35)	< 2.8 (28)
Prothrombin time (seconds increased)	1–3	4–6	> 6.0

Total Numerical Score and Corresponding Child-Pugh Class	
Score	Class
5–6	A
7–9	B
10–15	C

MELD scoring system
MELD = 11.2 $\log_e$ (INR) + 3.78 $\log_e$ (bilirubin [mg/dL]) + 9.57 $\log_e$ (creatinine [mg/dL]) + 6.43. (Range 6–40).

INR, international normalized ratio.

▶ When to Refer

- For liver biopsy.
- When the MELD score is 14 or higher.
- For upper endoscopy to screen for gastroesophageal varices.

When to Admit

- Gastrointestinal bleeding.
- Stage 3–4 hepatic encephalopathy.
- Worsening kidney function.
- Severe hyponatremia.
- Serious infection.
- Profound hypoxia.

Angeli P et al. Diagnosis and management of acute kidney injury in patients with cirrhosis: revised consensus recommendations of the International Club of Ascites. Gut. 2015 Apr; 64(4):531–7. [PMID: 25631669]

Bajaj JS et al. Validation of EncephalApp, smartphone-based Stroop test, for the diagnosis of covert hepatic encephalopathy. Clin Gastroenterol Hepatol. 2015 Oct;13(10):1828–35. [PMID: 24846278]

Dever JB et al. Review article: spontaneous bacterial peritonitis—bacteriology, diagnosis, treatment, risk factors and prevention. Aliment Pharmacol Ther. 2015 Jun;41(11):1116–31. [PMID: 25819304]

O'Leary JG et al; North American Consortium for the Study of End-Stage Liver Disease. Long-term use of antibiotics and proton pump inhibitors predict development of infections in patients with cirrhosis. Clin Gastroenterol Hepatol. 2015 Apr; 13(4):753–9. [PMID: 25130937]

Tsochatzis EA et al. Liver cirrhosis. Lancet. 2014 May 17; 383(9930):1749–61. [PMID: 24480518]

PRIMARY BILIARY CHOLANGITIS (Primary Biliary Cirrhosis)

ESSENTIALS OF DIAGNOSIS

- ► Occurs in middle-aged women.
- ► Often asymptomatic.
- ► Elevation of alkaline phosphatase, positive antimitochondrial antibodies, elevated IgM, increased cholesterol.
- ► Characteristic liver biopsy.
- ► In later stages, can present with fatigue, jaundice, features of cirrhosis, xanthelasma, xanthoma, steatorrhea.

General Considerations

Primary biliary cholangitis (PBC) is a chronic disease of the liver characterized by autoimmune destruction of small intrahepatic bile ducts and cholestasis. The designation "primary biliary cholangitis" has been proposed instead of primary biliary cirrhosis because many patients do not have cirrhosis. The disease is insidious in onset, occurs usually in women aged 40–60 years, and is often detected by the chance finding of elevated alkaline phosphatase levels. Estimated incidence and prevalence rates in the United States are 4.5 and 65.4 per 100,000, respectively, in women, and 0.7 and 12.1 per 100,000, respectively, in men. These rates may be increasing. The frequency of the disease among first-degree relatives of affected persons is

1.3–6%, and the concordance rate in identical twins is high. PBC is associated with HLA *DRB1*08* and *DQB1*. The disease may be associated with Sjögren syndrome, autoimmune thyroid disease, Raynaud syndrome, scleroderma, hypothyroidism, and celiac disease. Infection with *Novosphingobium aromaticivorans* or *Chlamydophila pneumoniae* may trigger or cause PBC. A history of urinary tract infections (caused by *E coli* or *Lactobacillus delbrueckii*) and smoking, and possibly use of hormone replacement therapy and hair dye, are risk factors, and clustering of cases in time and space argues for a causative role of environmental agents.

Clinical Findings

A. Symptoms and Signs

Many patients are asymptomatic for years. The onset of clinical illness is insidious and is heralded by fatigue (excessive daytime somnolence) and pruritus. With progression, physical examination reveals hepatosplenomegaly. Xanthomatous lesions may occur in the skin and tendons and around the eyelids. Jaundice, steatorrhea, and signs of portal hypertension are late findings, although occasional patients have esophageal varices despite an early histologic stage. Autonomic dysfunction, including orthostatic hypotension and associated with fatigue, and cognitive dysfunction appear to be common. The risk of low bone density, osteoporosis, and fractures is increased in patients with PBC (who tend to be older women) possibly due in part to polymorphisms of the vitamin D receptor.

B. Laboratory Findings

Blood counts are normal early in the disease. Liver biochemical tests reflect cholestasis with elevation of alkaline phosphatase, cholesterol (especially high-density lipoproteins), and, in later stages, bilirubin. Antimitochondrial antibodies are present in 95% of patients, and serum IgM levels are elevated.

Diagnosis

The diagnosis of PBC is based on the detection of cholestatic liver chemistries (often initially an isolated elevation of the alkaline phosphatase) and antimitochondrial antibodies in serum. Liver biopsy is not essential for diagnosis but permits histologic staging: I, portal inflammation with granulomas; II, bile duct proliferation, periportal inflammation; III, interlobular fibrous septa; and IV, cirrhosis. Estimation of histologic stage by an "enhanced liver fibrosis assay" that incorporates serum levels of hyaluronic acid, tissue inhibitor of metalloproteinase-1, and procollagen III aminopeptide has shown promise.

Differential Diagnosis

The disease must be differentiated from chronic biliary tract obstruction (stone or stricture), carcinoma of the bile ducts, primary sclerosing cholangitis, sarcoidosis, cholestatic drug toxicity (eg, chlorpromazine), and in some cases chronic hepatitis. Patients with a clinical and histologic picture of PBC but no antimitochondrial antibodies are said to have antimitochondrial antibody-negative PBC ("autoimmune cholangitis"), which has been associated with lower serum IgM levels and a greater frequency of smooth muscle antibodies and ANA. Many such patients are found to have antimitochondrial antibodies by immunoblot against recombinant proteins (rather than standard immunofluorescence). Some patients have overlapping features of PBC and autoimmune hepatitis.

Treatment

Cholestyramine (4 g) in water or juice three times daily may be beneficial for pruritus; colestipol and colesevelam have not been shown to reduce pruritus. Rifampin, 150–300 mg orally twice daily, is inconsistently beneficial. Opioid antagonists (eg, naloxone, 0.2 mcg/kg/min by intravenous infusion, or naltrexone, starting at 12.5 mg/day by mouth) show promise in the treatment of pruritus but may cause opioid withdrawal symptoms. The 5-hydroxytryptamine (5-HT$_3$) serotonin receptor antagonist ondansetron, 4 mg orally three times a day as needed, and the selective serotonin reuptake inhibitor sertraline, 75–100 mg/day orally, may also provide some benefit. For refractory pruritus, plasmapheresis or extracorporeal albumin dialysis may be needed. Modafinil, 100–200 mg/day orally, may improve daytime somnolence but is poorly tolerated. Deficiencies of vitamins A, D, and K may occur if steatorrhea is present and are aggravated when cholestyramine is administered.

Because of its lack of toxicity, ursodeoxycholic acid (13–15 mg/kg/day in one or two doses) is the preferred (and only FDA approved) medical treatment for PBC. It has been shown to slow the progression of disease (particularly in early-stage disease), stabilize histology, improve long-term survival, reduce the risk of developing esophageal varices, and delay (and possibly prevent) the need for liver transplantation. Complete normalization of liver biochemical tests occurs in 20% of treated patients within 2 years and 40% within 5 years, and survival is similar to that of healthy controls when the drug is given to patients with stage 1 or 2 PBC. Response rates have been reported to be lower in men than women (72% vs 80%) and higher in women diagnosed after age 70 than before age 30 (90% vs 50%). Ursodeoxycholic acid has also been reported to reduce the risk of recurrent colorectal adenomas in patients with PBC. Side effects include weight gain and rarely loose stools.

Colchicine (0.6 mg orally twice daily) and methotrexate (15 mg/wk orally) have had some reported benefit in improving symptoms and serum levels of alkaline phosphatase and bilirubin. Methotrexate may also improve liver histology in some patients, but overall response rates have been disappointing. Penicillamine, prednisone, and azathioprine have proved to be of no benefit. Budesonide may improve liver histology but worsens bone density. For patients with advanced disease, liver transplantation is the treatment of choice.

Prognosis

Without liver transplantation, survival averages 7–10 years once symptoms develop but has improved for younger women since the introduction of ursodeoxycholic acid.

Progression to liver failure and portal hypertension may be accelerated by smoking. Patients with early-stage disease in whom the alkaline phosphatase and AST are less than 1.5 times normal and bilirubin is 1 mg/dL (17.1 mcmol/L) or less after 1 year of therapy with ursodeoxycholic acid (Paris II criteria) are at low long-term risk for cirrhosis and have a life expectancy similar to that of the healthy population. Pregnancy is well tolerated in younger patients. In advanced disease, an adverse prognosis is indicated by a high Mayo risk score that includes older age, high serum bilirubin, edema, low serum albumin, and prolonged prothrombin time as well as by variceal hemorrhage. Other prognostic models include the Globe index, which is based on age, serum bilirubin, serum albumin, serum alkaline phosphatase, and platelet count. A prediction tool for varices has been proposed based on the serum albumin, serum alkaline phosphatase, platelet count, and splenomegaly. Fatigue is associated with an increased risk of cardiac mortality and may not be reversed by liver transplantation. Among asymptomatic patients, at least one-third will become symptomatic within 15 years. The risk of hepatocellular carcinoma appears to be increased in patients with PBC; risk factors include older age, male sex, prior blood transfusions, advanced histologic stage, and signs of cirrhosis or portal hypertension. Liver transplantation for advanced PBC is associated with a 1-year survival rate of 85–90%. The disease recurs in the graft in 20% of patients by 3 years, but this does not seem to affect survival.

When to Refer

- For liver biopsy.
- For liver transplant evaluation.

When to Admit

- Gastrointestinal bleeding.
- Stage 3–4 hepatic encephalopathy.
- Worsening kidney function.
- Severe hyponatremia.
- Profound hypoxia.

Beuers U et al. Changing nomenclature for PBC: From 'cirrhosis' to 'cholangitis'. Hepatology. 2015 Nov;62(5):1620–2. [PMID: 26372460]

Carey EJ et al. Primary biliary cirrhosis. Lancet. 2015 Oct 17; 386(10003):1565–75. [PMID: 26364546]

Hirschfield GM et al. Efficacy of obeticholic acid in patients with primary biliary cirrhosis and inadequate response to ursodeoxycholic acid. Gastroenterology. 2015 Apr;148(4):751–61. [PMID: 25500425]

Hosonuma K et al. A prospective randomized controlled study of long-term combination therapy using ursodeoxycholic acid and bezafibrate in patients with primary biliary cirrhosis and dyslipidemia. Am J Gastroenterol. 2015 Mar;110(3):423–31. [PMID: 25732417]

Karlsen TH et al. Review article: controversies in the management of primary biliary cirrhosis and primary sclerosing cholangitis. Aliment Pharmacol Ther. 2014 Feb;39(3):282–301. [PMID: 24372568]

HEMOCHROMATOSIS

General Considerations

Hemochromatosis is an autosomal recessive disease caused in most cases by a mutation in the *HFE* gene on chromosome 6. The HFE protein is thought to play an important role in the process by which duodenal crypt cells sense body iron stores, leading in turn to increased iron absorption from the duodenum. A decrease in the synthesis or expression of hepcidin, the principal iron regulatory hormone, is thought to be a key pathogenic factor in all forms of hemochromatosis. About 85% of persons with well-established hemochromatosis are homozygous for the *C282Y* mutation. The frequency of the gene mutation averages 7% in Northern European and North American white populations, resulting in a 0.5% frequency of homozygotes (of whom 38–50% will develop biochemical evidence of iron overload but only 28% of men and 1% of women will develop clinical symptoms). Polymorphisms in modifier genes have been shown to lead to a high iron phenotype. The *HFE* gene mutation and hemochromatosis are uncommon in blacks and Asian-American populations. A second genetic mutation (*H63D*) may contribute to the development of iron overload in a small percentage (1.5%) of persons who are compound heterozygotes for *C282Y* and *H63D*; iron overload-related disease develops in few patients (particularly those who have a comorbidity such as diabetes mellitus and fatty liver). Rare instances of hemochromatosis result from mutations in the genes that encode transferrin receptor 2 (*TFR2*) and ferroportin (*FPN1*). A juvenile-onset variant that is characterized by severe iron overload, cardiac dysfunction, hypogonadotropic hypogonadism, and a high mortality rate is usually linked to a mutation of a gene on chromosome 1q designated *HJV* that produces a protein called hemojuvelin or, rarely, to a mutation in the *HAMP* gene on chromosome 19 that encodes hepcidin, but not to the *C282Y* mutation.

Hemochromatosis is characterized by increased accumulation of iron as hemosiderin in the liver, pancreas, heart, adrenals, testes, pituitary, and kidneys. Cirrhosis is more likely to develop in affected persons who drink alcohol excessively or have obesity-related hepatic steatosis than in those who do not. Eventually, hepatic and pancreatic insufficiency, heart failure, and hypogonadism may develop; overall mortality is increased slightly. Heterozygotes do not develop cirrhosis in the absence of associated disorders such as viral hepatitis or NAFLD.

▶ Clinical Findings

A. Symptoms and Signs

The onset of clinical disease is usually after age 50 years—earlier in men than in women; however, because of widespread liver biochemical testing and iron screening, the diagnosis is usually made long before symptoms develop. Early symptoms are nonspecific (eg, fatigue, arthralgia). Later clinical manifestations include arthropathy (and ultimately the need for joint replacement surgery in some cases), hepatomegaly and evidence of hepatic dysfunction, skin pigmentation (combination of slate-gray due to iron and brown due to melanin, sometimes resulting in a bronze color), cardiac enlargement with or without heart failure or conduction defects, diabetes mellitus with its complications, and erectile dysfunction in men. Interestingly, population studies have shown an increased prevalence of liver disease but not of diabetes mellitus, arthritis, or heart disease in *C282Y* homozygotes. In patients in whom cirrhosis develops, bleeding from esophageal varices may occur, and there is a 15–20% frequency of hepatocellular carcinoma. Affected patients are at increased risk of infection with *Vibrio vulnificus*, *Listeria monocytogenes*, *Yersinia enterocolitica*, and other siderophilic organisms. The risk of porphyria cutanea tarda is increased in persons with the *C282Y* or *H63D* mutation, and *C282Y* homozygotes have twice the risk of colorectal and breast cancer than persons without the *C282Y* variant.

B. Laboratory Findings

Laboratory findings include mildly abnormal liver tests (AST, alkaline phosphatase), an elevated plasma iron with greater than 45% transferrin saturation, and an elevated serum ferritin (although a normal iron saturation or a normal ferritin does not exclude the diagnosis). Affected men are more likely than affected women to have an elevated ferritin level. Testing for *HFE* mutations is indicated in any patient with evidence of iron overload. Interestingly, in persons with an elevated serum ferritin, the likelihood of detecting *C282Y* homozygosity decreases with increasing ALT and AST levels, which are likely to reflect hepatic inflammation and secondary iron overload.

C. Imaging

MRI and CT may show changes consistent with iron overload of the liver, and MRI can quantitate hepatic iron stores and help assess the degree of hepatic fibrosis.

D. Liver Biopsy

In patients who are homozygous for *C282Y*, liver biopsy is often indicated to determine whether cirrhosis is present. Biopsy can be deferred, however, in patients in whom the serum ferritin level is less than 1000 mcg/L, serum AST level is normal, and hepatomegaly is absent; the likelihood of cirrhosis is low in these persons. The combination of a serum ferritin level of 1000 mcg/L or more and a serum hyaluronic acid level of 46.5 mcg/L or more has been reported to identify all patients with cirrhosis, with a high specificity. Risk factors for advanced fibrosis include male sex, excess alcohol consumption, and diabetes mellitus. Liver biopsy is also indicated when iron overload is suspected even though the patient is neither homozygous for *C282Y* nor a *C282Y/H63D* compound heterozygote. In patients with hemochromatosis, the liver biopsy characteristically shows extensive iron deposition in hepatocytes and in bile ducts, and the hepatic iron index—hepatic iron content per gram of liver converted to micromoles and divided by the patient's age—is generally higher than 1.9. Only 5% of patients with hereditary hemochromatosis identified by screening in a primary care setting have cirrhosis.

▶ Screening

Iron studies and *HFE* testing are recommended for all first-degree family members of a proband; children of an affected person (*C282Y* homozygote) need to be screened only if the patient's spouse carries the *C282Y* or *H63D* mutation. Average-risk population screening for hemochromatosis is not recommended because the clinical penetrance of *C282Y* homozygosity and morbidity and mortality from hemochromatosis are low. Patients with otherwise unexplained chronic liver disease, chondrocalcinosis, erectile dysfunction, and type 1 diabetes mellitus (especially late-onset) should be screened for iron overload.

▶ Treatment

Affected patients should avoid foods rich in iron (such as red meat), alcohol, vitamin C, raw shellfish, and supplemental iron. Weekly phlebotomies of 1 or 2 units (250–500 mL) of blood (each containing about 250 mg of iron) is indicated in all symptomatic patients, those with a serum ferritin level of at least 1000 mcg/L, and those with an increased fasting iron saturation and should be continued for up to 2–3 years to achieve depletion of iron stores. The hematocrit and serum iron values should be monitored. When iron store depletion is achieved (iron saturation less than 50% and serum ferritin level 50–100 mcg/L), phlebotomies (every 2–4 months) to maintain serum ferritin levels between 50 mcg/L and 100 mcg/L are continued, although compliance has been reported to decrease with time; administration of a proton pump inhibitor, which reduces intestinal iron absorption, appears to decrease the maintenance phlebotomy blood volume requirement. In *C282Y* homozygous women, a body mass index greater than 28 is associated with a lower phlebotomy requirement, possibly because hepcidin levels are increased by overweight. Complications of hemochromatosis—arthropathy, diabetes mellitus, heart disease, portal hypertension, and hypopituitarism—also require treatment.

The chelating agent deferoxamine is indicated for patients with hemochromatosis and anemia or in those with secondary iron overload due to thalassemia who cannot tolerate phlebotomies. The drug is administered intravenously or subcutaneously in a dose of 20–40 mg/kg/day infused over 24 hours and can mobilize 30 mg of iron per day; however, treatment is painful and time-consuming. Two oral chelators, deferasirox, 20 mg/kg once daily, and deferiprone, 25 mg/kg three times daily, have been approved for treatment of iron overload due to blood transfusions and may be appropriate in persons with hemochromatosis who cannot tolerate phlebotomy; however, these agents have a number of side effects and drug-drug interactions.

The course of hemochromatosis is favorably altered by phlebotomy therapy. Hepatic fibrosis may regress, and in precirrhotic patients, cirrhosis may be prevented. Cardiac conduction defects and insulin requirements improve with treatment. In patients with cirrhosis, varices may reverse, and the risk of variceal bleeding declines, although the risk of hepatocellular carcinoma persists. In those with an initial serum ferritin level greater than 1000 mcg/L (2247 pmol/L), the risk of death is fivefold greater than in those with a serum ferritin 1000 mcg/L (2247 pmol/L) or less. In treated patients, only those with a serum ferritin greater than 2000 mcg/L (4494 pmol/L) have increased mortality, mainly related to liver disease. Since 1997, posttransplant survival rates have been excellent. Following liver transplantation, serum iron studies and hepcidin levels are normal, and phlebotomy is not required.

▶ When to Refer

- For liver biopsy.
- For initiation of therapy.

Bardou-Jacquet E et al. Decreased cardiovascular and extrahepatic cancer-related mortality in treated patients with mild HFE hemochromatosis. J Hepatol. 2015 Mar;62(3):682–9. [PMID: 25450707]

McLaren CE et al. Exome sequencing in *HFE* C282Y homozygous men with extreme phenotypes identifies a *GNPAT* variant associated with severe iron overload. Hepatology. 2015 Aug; 62(2):429–39. [PMID: 25605615]

WILSON DISEASE (Hepatolenticular Degeneration)

ESSENTIALS OF DIAGNOSIS

- ▶ Rare autosomal recessive disorder that usually occurs in persons under age 40.
- ▶ Excessive deposition of copper in the liver and brain.
- ▶ Serum ceruloplasmin, the plasma copper-carrying protein, is low.
- ▶ Urinary excretion of copper and hepatic copper concentration are high.

General Considerations

Wilson disease (hepatolenticular degeneration) is a rare autosomal recessive disorder that usually occurs in persons under age 40. The worldwide prevalence is about 30 per million population. The condition is characterized by excessive deposition of copper in the liver and brain. The genetic defect, localized to chromosome 13, has been shown to affect a copper-transporting adenosine triphosphatase (*ATP7B*) in the liver and leads to copper accumulation in the liver and oxidative damage of hepatic mitochondria. Most patients are compound heterozygotes (ie, carry two different mutations). Over 500 mutations in the Wilson disease gene have been identified. The *H1069Q* mutation accounts for 37–63% of disease alleles in populations of Northern European descent. The major physiologic aberration in Wilson disease is excessive absorption of copper from the small intestine and decreased excretion of copper by the liver, resulting in increased tissue deposition, especially in the liver, brain, cornea, and kidney.

▲ **Figure 16–4.** Brownish Kayser-Fleischer ring at the rim of the cornea in a patient with Wilson disease. (From Marc Solioz, University of Berne; used, with permission, from Usatine RP, Smith MA, Mayeaux EJ Jr, Chumley H, Tysinger J. *The Color Atlas of Family Medicine.* McGraw-Hill, 2009.)

Clinical Findings

Wilson disease tends to present as liver disease in adolescents and neuropsychiatric disease in young adults, but there is great variability, and onset of symptoms after age 40 is more common than previously thought. The diagnosis should always be considered in any child or young adult with hepatitis, splenomegaly with hypersplenism, Coombs-negative hemolytic anemia, portal hypertension, and neurologic or psychiatric abnormalities. Wilson disease should also be considered in persons under 40 years of age with chronic or fulminant hepatitis.

Hepatic involvement may range from elevated liver biochemical tests (although the alkaline phosphatase may be low) to cirrhosis and portal hypertension. In patients with acute liver failure (seen much more often in females than males), the diagnosis of Wilson disease is suggested by an alkaline phosphatase (in units/L)-to-total bilirubin (in mg/dL) ratio less than 4 and an AST-to-ALT ratio greater than 2.2. The neurologic manifestations of Wilson disease are related to basal ganglia dysfunction and include an akinetic-rigid syndrome similar to parkinsonism, pseudosclerosis with tremor, ataxia, and a dystonic syndrome. Dysarthria, dysphagia, incoordination, and spasticity are common. Migraines, insomnia, and seizures have been reported. Psychiatric features include behavioral and personality changes and emotional lability and may precede characteristic neurologic features. The pathognomonic sign of the condition is the brownish or gray-green Kayser-Fleischer ring, which represents fine pigmented granular deposits in Descemet membrane in the cornea (Figure 16–4). The ring is usually most marked at the superior and inferior poles of the cornea. It is sometimes seen with the naked eye and is readily detected by slit-lamp examination. It may be absent in patients with hepatic manifestations only but is usually present in those with neuropsychiatric disease. Renal calculi, aminoaciduria, renal tubular acidosis, hypoparathyroidism, infertility, hemolytic anemia, and subcutaneous lipomas may occur.

Diagnosis

The diagnosis can be challenging, even with the use of scoring systems (eg, the Leipzig criteria), and is generally based on demonstration of increased urinary copper excretion (greater than 40 mcg/24 h and usually greater than 100 mcg/24 h) or low serum ceruloplasmin levels (less than 20 mg/dL [200 mg/L]; less than 5 mg/dL [50 mg/L] is diagnostic), and elevated hepatic copper concentration (greater than 210–250 mcg/g of dry liver), as well as Kayser-Fleischer rings, neurologic symptoms, and Coombs-negative hemolytic anemia. However, increased urinary copper and a low serum ceruloplasmin level (by a standard immunologic assay) are neither completely sensitive nor specific for Wilson disease, although an enzymatic assay for ceruloplasmin appears to be more accurate. The ratio of exchangeable copper to total copper in serum has been reported to improve diagnostic accuracy. In equivocal cases (when the serum ceruloplasmin level is normal), the diagnosis may require demonstration of a rise in urinary copper after a penicillamine challenge, although the test has been validated only in children. Liver biopsy may show acute or chronic hepatitis or cirrhosis. MRI of the brain may show evidence of increased basal ganglia, brainstem, and cerebellar copper even early in the course of the disease. If available, molecular analysis of *ATP7B* mutations can be diagnostic.

Treatment

Early treatment to remove excess copper before it can produce hepatic or neurologic damage is essential. Early in treatment, restriction of dietary copper (shellfish, organ foods, nuts, mushrooms, and chocolate) may be of value. Oral penicillamine (0.75–2 g/day in divided doses taken 1 h before or 2 h after food) has been the drug of choice and enhances urinary excretion of chelated copper. Oral pyridoxine, 50 mg per week, is added because penicillamine is an antimetabolite of this vitamin. If penicillamine treatment cannot be tolerated because of gastrointestinal intolerance, hypersensitivity, autoimmune reactions, nephrotoxicity, or bone marrow toxicity, consider the use of trientine, 250–500 mg three times a day, a chelating agent as effective as penicillamine but with a lower rate of adverse effects. However, the cost of trientine has become exorbitant. Oral zinc acetate or zinc gluconate, 50 mg three times a day, interferes with intestinal absorption of copper, promotes fecal copper excretion, and has been used as first-line therapy in presymptomatic or pregnant patients and those with neurologic disease and as maintenance therapy after decoppering with a chelating agent, but adverse gastrointestinal effects often lead to discontinuation and its long-term efficacy and safety (including a risk of hepatotoxicity) have been questioned. Ammonium tetrathiomolybdate, which complexes copper in the intestinal tract, has shown promise as initial therapy for neurologic Wilson disease.

Treatment should continue indefinitely. The doses of penicillamine and trientine should be reduced during pregnancy. Supplemental vitamin E, an antioxidant, has been recommended but not rigorously studied. Once the serum nonceruloplasmin copper level is within the normal range (50–150 mcg/L), the dose of chelating agent can be reduced to the minimum necessary for maintaining that level. The prognosis is good in patients who are effectively treated before liver or brain damage has occurred, but long-term survival is reduced in patients with cirrhosis at diagnosis (84% after 20 years). Liver transplantation is indicated for fulminant hepatitis (often after plasma exchange or dialysis with MARS as a stabilizing measure), end-stage cirrhosis (with excellent outcomes), and, in selected cases, intractable neurologic disease, although survival is lower when liver transplantation is undertaken for neurologic disease than for liver disease. Family members, especially siblings, require screening with serum ceruloplasmin, liver biochemical tests, and slit-lamp examination or, if the causative mutation is known, with mutation analysis.

When to Refer

All patients with Wilson disease should be referred for diagnosis and treatment.

When to Admit

- Acute liver failure.
- Gastrointestinal bleeding.
- Stage 3–4 hepatic encephalopathy.
- Worsening kidney function.
- Severe hyponatremia.
- Profound hypoxia.

Beinhardt S et al. Long-term outcomes of patients with Wilson disease in a large Austrian cohort. Clin Gastroenterol Hepatol. 2014 Apr;12(4):683–9. [PMID: 24076416]

Hunt DP et al. Case records of the Massachusetts General Hospital. Case 30-2014. A 29-year-old man with diarrhea, nausea, and weight loss. N Engl J Med. 2014 Sep 25;371(13):1238–47. [PMID: 25251619]

Yang X et al. Prospective evaluation of the diagnostic accuracy of hepatic copper content, as determined using the entire core of a liver biopsy sample. Hepatology. 2015 Dec;62(6):1731–41. [PMID: 26095812]

HEPATIC VEIN OBSTRUCTION (Budd-Chiari Syndrome)

ESSENTIALS OF DIAGNOSIS

- ▶ Right upper quadrant pain and tenderness.
- ▶ Ascites.
- ▶ Imaging studies show occlusion/absence of flow in the hepatic vein(s) or inferior vena cava.
- ▶ Clinical picture is similar in sinusoidal obstruction syndrome but major hepatic veins are patent.

▶ General Considerations

Factors that predispose patients to hepatic vein obstruction, or Budd-Chiari syndrome, including hereditary and acquired hypercoagulable states, can be identified in 75% of affected patients; multiple disorders are found in up to 45%. Up to 50% of cases are associated with polycythemia vera or other myeloproliferative neoplasms (which has a risk of Budd-Chiari syndrome of 1%). These cases (37% of patients with Budd-Chiari syndrome) are often associated with a specific mutation (V617F) in the gene that codes for JAK2 tyrosine kinase and may otherwise be subclinical. In some cases, somatic mutations in the gene coding for calreticulin have been found. Other predispositions to thrombosis (eg, activated protein C resistance [factor V Leiden mutation] [25% of cases], protein C or S or antithrombin deficiency, hyperprothrombinemia [factor II G20210A mutation] [rarely], the methylenetetrahydrofolate reductase TT677 mutation, antiphospholipid antibodies) may be identified in other cases. Hepatic vein obstruction may be associated with caval webs, right-sided heart failure or constrictive pericarditis, neoplasms that cause hepatic vein occlusion, paroxysmal nocturnal hemoglobinuria, Behçet syndrome, blunt abdominal trauma, use of oral contraceptives, and pregnancy. Some cytotoxic agents and pyrrolizidine alkaloids (Comfrey or "bush teas") may cause sinusoidal obstruction syndrome (previously known as veno-occlusive disease because the terminal venules are often occluded), which mimics Budd-Chiari syndrome clinically. Sinusoidal obstruction syndrome is common in patients who have undergone hematopoietic stem cell transplantation, particularly those with pretransplant serum aminotransferase elevations or fever during cytoreductive therapy with cyclophosphamide, azathioprine, carmustine, busulfan, or etoposide or those receiving high-dose cytoreductive therapy or high-dose total body irradiation. In India, China, and South Africa, Budd-Chiari syndrome is associated with a poor standard of living and often the result of occlusion of the hepatic portion of the inferior vena cava, presumably due to prior thrombosis. The clinical presentation is mild but the course is frequently complicated by hepatocellular carcinoma.

▶ Clinical Findings

A. Symptoms and Signs

The presentation may be fulminant, acute, subacute, or chronic. An insidious (subacute) onset is most common. Clinical manifestations generally include tender, painful hepatic enlargement, jaundice, splenomegaly, and ascites. With chronic disease, bleeding varices and hepatic encephalopathy may be evident; hepatopulmonary syndrome may occur.

B. Imaging

Hepatic imaging studies may show a prominent caudate lobe, since its venous drainage may be occluded. The screening test of choice is contrast-enhanced, color, or pulsed-Doppler ultrasonography, which has a sensitivity of 85% for detecting evidence of hepatic venous or inferior vena caval thrombosis. MRI with spin-echo and gradient-echo sequences and intravenous gadolinium injection allows visualization of the obstructed veins and collateral vessels. Direct venography can delineate caval webs and occluded hepatic veins ("spider-web" pattern) most precisely.

C. Liver Biopsy

Percutaneous or transjugular liver biopsy in Budd-Chiari syndrome may be considered when the results of noninvasive imaging are inconclusive and frequently shows characteristic centrilobular congestion and fibrosis and often multiple large regenerative nodules. Liver biopsy is often contraindicated in sinusoidal obstruction syndrome because of thrombocytopenia, and the diagnosis is based on clinical findings.

▶ Treatment

Ascites should be treated with salt and fluid restriction and diuretics. Treatable causes of Budd-Chiari syndrome should be sought. Prompt recognition and treatment of an underlying hematologic disorder may avoid the need for surgery; however, the optimal anticoagulation regimen is uncertain, and anticoagulation is associated with a high risk of bleeding, particularly in patients with portal hypertension and those undergoing invasive procedures. Low-molecular-weight heparins are preferred over unfractionated heparin because of a high rate of heparin-induced thrombocytopenia with the latter. Infusion of a thrombolytic agent into recently occluded veins has been attempted with success. Defibrotide, an adenosine receptor agonist that increases endogenous tissue plasminogen activator levels, has shown promise in the prevention and treatment of sinusoidal obstruction syndrome. TIPS placement may be attempted in patients with Budd-Chiari syndrome and persistent hepatic congestion or failed thrombolytic therapy and possibly in those with sinusoidal obstruction syndrome. Late TIPS dysfunction is less frequent with the use of polytetra-fluoroethylene-covered stents than uncovered stents. TIPS is now preferred over surgical decompression (side-to-side

portacaval, mesocaval, or mesoatrial shunt), which, in contrast to TIPS, has generally not been proven to improve long-term survival. Older age, a higher serum bilirubin level, and a greater INR predict a poor outcome with TIPS. Balloon angioplasty, in some cases with placement of an intravascular metallic stent, is preferred in patients with an inferior vena caval web and is being performed increasingly in patients with a short segment of thrombosis in the hepatic vein. Liver transplantation can be considered in patients with fulminant hepatic failure, cirrhosis with hepatocellular dysfunction, and failure of a portosystemic shunt, and outcomes have improved with the advent of patient selection based on the MELD score. Patients with Budd-Chiari syndrome often require lifelong anticoagulation and treatment of the underlying myeloproliferative disease; antiplatelet therapy with aspirin and hydroxyurea has been suggested as an alternative to warfarin in patients with a myeloproliferative disorder.

▶ Prognosis

The overall 5-year survival rate is 50–90% with treatment (but less than 10% without intervention). Adverse prognostic factors in patients with Budd-Chiari syndrome are older age, high Child-Pugh score, ascites, encephalopathy, elevated total bilirubin, prolonged prothrombin time, elevated serum creatinine, concomitant portal vein thrombosis, and histologic features of acute liver disease superimposed on chronic liver injury; 3-month mortality may be predicted by the Rotterdam score, which is based on encephalopathy, ascites, prothrombin time, and bilirubin. A serum ALT level at least fivefold above the upper limit of normal on presentation indicates hepatic ischemia and also predicts a poor outcome, particularly when the ALT level decreases slowly. The risk of hepatocellular carcinoma is increased; risk factors include cirrhosis, combined hepatic vein and inferior vena cava obstruction, and a long-segment interior vena cava block.

▶ When to Admit

All patients with hepatic vein obstruction should be hospitalized.

European Association for the Study of the Liver. EASL Clinical Practice Guidelines: vascular diseases of the liver. J Hepatol. 2016 Jan;64(1):179–202. [PMID: 26516032]

Paul SB et al. Incidence and risk factors of hepatocellular carcinoma in patients with hepatic venous outflow tract obstruction. Aliment Pharmacol Ther. 2015 May;41(10):961–71. [PMID: 25809735]

Pavri TM et al. Budd-Chiari syndrome: a single-center experience. World J Gastroenterol. 2014 Nov 21;20(43):16236–44. [PMID: 25473178]

THE LIVER IN HEART FAILURE

Ischemic hepatitis, also called **ischemic hepatopathy, hypoxic hepatitis, shock liver**, or **acute cardiogenic liver injury** may affect 2.5 of every 100 patients admitted to an intensive care unit and results from an acute fall in cardiac output due to acute myocardial infarction, arrhythmia, or septic or hemorrhagic shock, usually in a patient with passive congestion of the liver. Clinical hypotension may be absent (or unwitnessed). In some cases, the precipitating event is arterial hypoxemia due to respiratory failure, sleep apnea, severe anemia, heat stroke, carbon monoxide poisoning, cocaine use, or bacterial endocarditis. More than one precipitant is common. Statin therapy prior to admission may protect against ischemic hepatitis. The hallmark is a rapid and striking elevation of serum aminotransferase levels (often greater than 5000 units/L); an early rapid rise in the serum lactate dehydrogenase (LD) level (with an ALT-to-LD ratio less than 1.5) is also typical. Elevations of serum alkaline phosphatase and bilirubin are usually mild, but jaundice is associated with worse outcomes. The prothrombin time may be prolonged, and encephalopathy or hepatopulmonary syndrome may develop. The mortality rate due to the underlying disease is high (particularly in patients receiving vasopressor therapy or with septic shock, acute kidney disease, or coagulopathy), but in patients who recover, the aminotransferase levels return to normal quickly, usually within 1 week—in contrast to viral hepatitis.

In patients with **passive congestion of the liver** ("nutmeg liver") due to right-sided heart failure, the serum bilirubin level may be elevated, occasionally as high as 40 mg/dL (684 mcmol/L), due in part to hypoxia of perivenular hepatocytes, and the level is a predictor of mortality and morbidity. Serum alkaline phosphatase levels are normal or slightly elevated, and aminotransferase levels are only mildly elevated in the absence of superimposed ischemia. Hepatojugular reflux is present, and with tricuspid regurgitation the liver may be pulsatile. Ascites may be out of proportion to peripheral edema, with a high serum ascites-albumin gradient (greater than or equal to 1.1) and a protein content of more than 2.5 g/dL (25 g/L). A markedly elevated serum N-terminal-proBNP or BNP (greater than 364 pg/mL [364 ng/L]) level has been reported to distinguish ascites due to heart failure from ascites due to cirrhosis in the absence of renal insufficiency. In severe cases, signs of encephalopathy may develop.

Drolz A et al. Statin therapy is associated with reduced incidence of hypoxic hepatitis in critically ill patients. J Hepatol. 2014 Jun;60(6):1187–93. [PMID: 24509409]

Farias AQ et al. Serum B-type natriuretic peptide in the initial workup of patients with new onset ascites: a diagnostic accuracy study. Hepatology. 2014 Mar;59(3):1043–51. [PMID: 23907731]

Tapper EB et al. The incidence and outcomes of ischemic hepatitis: a systematic review with meta-analysis. Am J Med. 2015 Dec;128(12):1314–21. [PMID: 26299319]

NONCIRRHOTIC PORTAL HYPERTENSION

ESSENTIALS OF DIAGNOSIS

▸ Splenomegaly or upper gastrointestinal bleeding from esophageal or gastric varices in patients without liver disease.

▸ Portal vein thrombosis complicating cirrhosis.

▶ General Considerations

Causes of noncirrhotic portal hypertension include extrahepatic portal vein obstruction (portal vein thrombosis often with cavernous transformation [portal cavernoma]), splenic vein obstruction (presenting as gastric varices without esophageal varices), schistosomiasis, nodular regenerative hyperplasia, and arterial-portal vein fistula. Idiopathic noncirrhotic portal hypertension is common in India and has been attributed to chronic infections, exposure to medications or toxins, prothrombotic disorders, immunologic disorders, and genetic disorders that result in obliterative vascular lesions in the liver. It is rare in Western countries, where increased mortality is attributable to associated disorders and older age. Portal vein thrombosis may occur in 10–25% of patients with cirrhosis, is associated with the severity of the liver disease, and may be associated with hepatocellular carcinoma but not with increased mortality. Other risk factors are oral contraceptive use, pregnancy, chronic inflammatory diseases (including pancreatitis), injury to the portal venous system (including surgery), other malignancies, and treatment of thrombocytopenia with eltrombopag. Splenic vein thrombosis may complicate pancreatitis or pancreatic cancer. Pylephlebitis (septic thrombophlebitis of the portal vein) may complicate intra-abdominal inflammatory disorders such as appendicitis or diverticulitis, particularly when anaerobic organisms (especially *Bacteroides* species) are involved. Nodular regenerative hyperplasia results from altered hepatic perfusion and can be associated with collagen vascular diseases; myeloproliferative disorders; and drugs, including azathioprine, 5-fluorouracil, and oxaliplatin. In patients infected with HIV, long-term use of didanosine and use of a combination of didanosine and stavudine have been reported to account for some cases of noncirrhotic portal hypertension often due to nodular regenerative hyperplasia, and genetic factors may play a role. The term "obliterative portal venopathy" is used to describe primary occlusion of intrahepatic portal veins in the absence of cirrhosis, inflammation, or hepatic neoplasia.

▶ Clinical Findings

A. Symptoms and Signs

Acute portal vein thrombosis usually causes abdominal pain. Aside from splenomegaly, the physical findings are not remarkable, although hepatic decompensation can follow severe gastrointestinal bleeding or a concurrent hepatic disorder, and intestinal infarction may occur when portal vein thrombosis is associated with mesenteric venous thrombosis. Ascites may occur in 25% of persons with noncirrhotic portal hypertension. Minimal hepatic encephalopathy is reported to be common in patients with noncirrhotic portal vein thrombosis.

B. Laboratory Findings

Liver biochemical test levels are usually normal, but there may be findings of hypersplenism. An underlying hypercoagulable state is found in many patients with portal vein thrombosis; this includes myeloproliferative neoplasms (often associated with a specific mutation [V617F] in the gene coding for JAK2 tyrosine kinase, which is found in 24% of cases of portal vein thrombosis, or occasionally with a mutation in the gene coding for calreticulin), mutation G20210A of prothrombin, factor V Leiden mutation, protein C and S deficiency, antiphospholipid syndrome, mutation TT677 of methylenetetrahydrofolate reductase, elevated factor VIII levels, hyperhomocysteinemia, and a mutation in the gene that codes for thrombin-activatable fibrinolysis inhibitor. It is possible, however, that in many cases evidence of hypercoagulability is a secondary phenomenon due to portosystemic shunting and reduced hepatic blood flow.

C. Imaging

Color Doppler ultrasonography and contrast-enhanced CT are usually the initial diagnostic tests for portal vein thrombosis. Magnetic resonance angiography (MRA) of the portal system is generally confirmatory. EUS may be helpful in some cases. In patients with jaundice, magnetic resonance cholangiography may demonstrate compression of the bile duct by a large portal cavernoma (portal biliopathy), a finding that may be more common in patients with an underlying hypercoagulable state than in those without one. In patients with pylephlebitis, CT may demonstrate an intra-abdominal source of infection, thrombosis or gas in the portal venous system, and a hepatic abscess.

D. Other Studies

Endoscopy shows esophageal or gastric varices. Needle biopsy of the liver may be indicated to diagnose schistosomiasis, nodular regenerative hyperplasia, and noncirrhotic portal fibrosis and may demonstrate sinusoidal dilatation.

▶ Treatment

If splenic vein thrombosis is the cause of variceal bleeding, splenectomy is curative. For other causes of noncirrhotic portal hypertension, band ligation (or, less commonly, sclerotherapy) followed by beta-blockers to reduce portal pressure is initiated for variceal bleeding, and portosystemic shunting (including TIPS) is reserved for failures of endoscopic therapy; rarely progressive liver dysfunction requires liver transplantation. Anticoagulation particularly with low-molecular-weight heparin or thrombolytic therapy may be indicated for isolated acute portal vein thrombosis (and leads to at least partial recanalization in up to 75% of cases) and possibly for acute splenic vein thrombosis; an oral anticoagulant is continued long-term if a hypercoagulable disorder is identified or if an acute portal vein thrombosis extends into the mesenteric veins. The use of enoxaparin to prevent portal vein thrombosis and hepatic decompensation in patients with cirrhosis has shown promise.

▶ When to Refer

All patients with noncirrhotic portal hypertension should be referred.

Berry K et al. Portal vein thrombosis is not associated with increased mortality among patients with cirrhosis. Clin Gastroenterol Hepatol. 2015 Mar;13(3):585–93. [PMID: 25459555]

Kumar A et al. Review article: portal vein obstruction—epidemiology, pathogenesis, natural history, prognosis and treatment. Aliment Pharmacol Ther. 2015 Feb;41(3):276–92. [PMID: 25475582]

Nery F et al. Causes and consequences of portal vein thrombosis in 1,243 patients with cirrhosis: results of a longitudinal study. Hepatology. 2015 Feb;61(2):660–7. [PMID: 25284616]

PYOGENIC HEPATIC ABSCESS

ESSENTIALS OF DIAGNOSIS

▶ Fever, right upper quadrant pain, jaundice.

▶ Often in setting of biliary disease, but up to 40% are "cryptogenic" in origin.

▶ Detected by imaging studies.

▶ General Considerations

The incidence of liver abscess is 3.6 per 100,000 population in the United States and has increased since the 1990s. The liver can be invaded by bacteria via (1) the bile duct (ascending cholangitis); (2) the portal vein (pylephlebitis); (3) the hepatic artery, secondary to bacteremia; (4) direct extension from an infectious process; and (5) traumatic implantation of bacteria through the abdominal wall. Risk factors for liver abscess include older age and male sex. Predisposing conditions and factors include presence of malignancy, diabetes mellitus, inflammatory bowel disease, and cirrhosis; necessity for liver transplantation; and use of proton pump inhibitors. Pyogenic liver abscess has been observed to be associated with a subsequent increased risk of gastrointestinal malignancy.

Ascending cholangitis resulting from biliary obstruction due to a stone, stricture, or neoplasm is the most common identifiable cause of hepatic abscess in the United States. In 10% of cases, liver abscess is secondary to appendicitis or diverticulitis. At least 40% of abscesses have no demonstrable cause and are classified as cryptogenic; a dental source is identified in some cases. The most frequently encountered organisms are *E coli*, *Klebsiella pneumoniae*, *Proteus vulgaris*, *Enterobacter aerogenes*, and multiple microaerophilic and anaerobic species (eg, *Streptococcus anginosus* [also known as *S milleri*]). Liver abscess caused by virulent strains of *K pneumoniae* may be associated with thrombophlebitis of the portal or hepatic veins and hematogenously spread septic ocular or central nervous system complications. *Staphylococcus aureus* is usually the causative organism in patients with chronic granulomatous disease. Uncommon causative organisms include *Salmonella*, *Haemophilus*, *Yersinia*, and *Listeria*. Hepatic candidiasis, tuberculosis, and actinomycosis are seen in immunocompromised patients and those with hematologic malignancies. Rarely, hepatocellular carcinoma can present as a pyogenic abscess because of tumor necrosis, biliary obstruction, and superimposed bacterial infection (see Chapter 39). The possibility of an amebic liver abscess must always be considered (see Chapter 35).

▶ Clinical Findings

A. Symptoms and Signs

The presentation is often insidious. Fever is almost always present and may antedate other symptoms or signs. Pain may be a prominent complaint and is localized to the right upper quadrant or epigastric area. Jaundice, tenderness in the right upper abdomen, and either steady or spiking fever are the chief physical findings.

B. Laboratory Findings

Laboratory examination reveals leukocytosis with a shift to the left. Liver biochemical tests are nonspecifically abnormal. Blood cultures are positive in 50–100% of cases.

C. Imaging

Chest radiographs usually reveal elevation of the diaphragm if the abscess is in the right lobe of the liver. Ultrasonography, CT, or MRI may reveal the presence of intrahepatic lesions. On MRI, characteristic findings include high signal intensity on T2-weighted images and rim enhancement. The characteristic CT appearance of hepatic candidiasis, usually seen in the setting of systemic candidiasis, is that of multiple "bull's-eyes," but imaging studies may be negative in neutropenic patients.

▶ Treatment

Treatment should consist of antimicrobial agents (generally a third-generation cephalosporin such as cefoperazone 1–2 g intravenously every 12 hours and metronidazole 500 mg intravenously every 6 hours) that are effective against coliform organisms and anaerobes. Antibiotics are administered for 2–3 weeks, and sometimes up to 6 weeks. If the abscess is at least 5 cm in diameter or the response to antibiotic therapy is not rapid, intermittent needle aspiration, percutaneous or endoscopic ultrasound-guided catheter drainage or stent placement or, if necessary, surgical (eg, laparoscopic) drainage should be done. Other suggested indications for abscess drainage are patient age of at least 55 years, symptom duration of at least 7 days, and involvement of two lobes of the liver. The underlying source (eg, biliary disease, dental infection) should be identified and treated. The mortality rate is still substantial (at least 5% in most studies) and is highest in patients with underlying biliary malignancy or severe multiorgan dysfunction. Other risk factors for mortality include older age, cirrhosis, chronic kidney disease, and other cancers. Hepatic candidiasis often responds to intravenous amphotericin B (total dose of 2–9 g). Fungal abscesses are associated with mortality rates of up to 50% and are treated with intravenous amphotericin B and drainage.

▶ When to Admit

Nearly all patients with pyogenic hepatic abscess should be hospitalized.

Tonozuka R et al. EUS-guided drainage of hepatic abscess and infected biloma using short and long metal stents (with videos). Gastrointest Endosc. 2015 Jun;81(6):1463–9. [PMID: 25843615]

Wang YP et al. Proton pump inhibitor use significantly increases the risk of cryptogenic liver abscess: a population-based study. Aliment Pharmacol Ther. 2015 Jun;41(11):1175–81. [PMID: 25871643]

BENIGN LIVER NEOPLASMS

Benign neoplasms of the liver must be distinguished from hepatocellular carcinoma, intrahepatic cholangiocarcinoma, and metastases (see Chapter 39). The most common benign neoplasm of the liver is the **cavernous hemangioma,** often an incidental finding on ultrasonography or CT. This lesion may enlarge in women who take hormonal therapy and must be differentiated from other space-occupying intrahepatic lesions, usually by contrast-enhanced MRI, CT, or ultrasonography. Rarely, fine-needle biopsy is necessary to differentiate these lesions and does not appear to carry an increased risk of bleeding. Surgical resection of cavernous hemangiomas is rarely necessary but may be required for abdominal pain or rapid enlargement, to exclude malignancy, or to treat Kasabach-Merritt syndrome (consumptive coagulopathy complicating a hemangioma).

In addition to rare instances of sinusoidal dilatation and peliosis hepatis, two distinct benign lesions with characteristic clinical, radiologic, and histopathologic features have been described in women taking oral contraceptives— focal nodular hyperplasia and hepatocellular adenoma. **Focal nodular hyperplasia** occurs at all ages and in both sexes and is probably not caused by the oral contraceptives. It is often asymptomatic and appears as a hypervascular mass, often with a central hypodense "stellate" scar on CT or MRI. Microscopically, focal nodular hyperplasia consists of hyperplastic units of hepatocytes that stain positively for glutamine synthetase with a central stellate scar containing proliferating bile ducts. It is not a true neoplasm but a proliferation of hepatocytes in response to altered blood flow. Focal nodular hyperplasia is associated with an elevated angiopoietin 1/angiopoietin 2 mRNA ratio that is thought to promote angiogenesis and may also occur in patients with cirrhosis, with exposure to certain drugs such as azathioprine, and in antiphospholipid syndrome. The prevalence of hepatic hemangiomas is increased in patients with focal nodular hyperplasia.

Hepatocellular adenoma occurs most commonly in women in the third and fourth decades of life and is usually caused by oral contraceptives; acute abdominal pain may occur if the tumor undergoes necrosis or hemorrhage. The tumor may be associated with mutations in: (1) the gene coding for hepatocyte nuclear factor 1 alpha (*HNF1alpha*) in 30–40% of cases (characterized by steatosis and a low risk of malignant transformation, although in men concomitant metabolic syndrome appears to increase the risk of malignant transformation); (2) the gene coding for beta-catenin (characterized by a high rate of malignant transformation) in 10–15% of cases; or (3) neither gene with the designation of inflammatory adenoma (previously termed "telangiectatic focal nodular hyperplasia"), which is associated with a high body mass index and serum biomarkers of inflammation (such as C-reactive protein) in 40–50% of cases. Unclassified adenomas account for 10% of tumors. Rare instances of multiple hepatocellular adenomas in association with maturity-onset diabetes of the young occur in families with a germline mutation in *HNF1alpha*. Hepatocellular adenomas also occur in patients with glycogen storage disease (inflammatory or unclassified adenomas) and familial adenomatous polyposis. The tumor is hypovascular. Grossly, the cut surface appears structureless. As seen microscopically, the hepatocellular adenoma consists of sheets of hepatocytes without portal tracts or central veins.

Cystic neoplasms of the liver, such as cystadenoma and cystadenocarcinoma, must be distinguished from simple and echinococcal cysts, von Meyenburg complexes (hamartomas), and polycystic liver disease.

► Clinical Findings

The only physical finding in focal nodular hyperplasia or hepatocellular adenoma is a palpable abdominal mass in a minority of cases. Liver function is usually normal. Arterial phase helical CT and multiphase dynamic MRI with contrast can distinguish an adenoma from focal nodular hyperplasia in 80–90% of cases and may suggest a specific subtype of adenoma (eg, homogeneous fat pattern in *HNF1alpha*-mutated adenomas and marked and persistent arterial enhancement in inflammatory adenomas).

► Treatment

While oral contraceptives should not necessarily be discontinued in women who have focal nodular hyperplasia, affected women who continue taking oral contraceptives should undergo annual ultrasonography for 2–3 years to ensure the lesion is not enlarging. The prognosis is excellent. Hepatocellular adenoma may undergo bleeding, necrosis, and rupture, often after hormone therapy, in the third trimester of pregnancy, or in men in whom the rate of malignant transformation is high. Resection is advised in all affected men and in women in whom the tumor causes symptoms or is 5 cm or greater in diameter, even in the absence of symptoms. If an adenoma is less than 5 cm in size, resection is also recommended if a beta-catenin gene mutation is present in a biopsy sample. In selected cases, laparoscopic resection or percutaneous radiofrequency ablation may be feasible. Rarely, liver transplantation is required. Regression of benign hepatic tumors may follow cessation of oral contraceptives. Transarterial embolization is the initial treatment for adenomas complicated by hemorrhage.

► When to Refer

- Diagnostic uncertainty.
- For surgery.

► When to Admit

- Severe pain.
- Rupture.

Agrawal S et al. Management of hepatocellular adenoma: recent advances. Clin Gastroenterol Hepatol. 2015 Jul;13(7):1221–30. [PMID: 24909909]

Alagusundaramoorthy SS et al. Role of transplantation in the treatment of benign solid tumors of the liver: a review of the United Network of Organ Sharing data set. JAMA Surg. 2015 Apr;150(4):337–42. [PMID: 25714928]

Margonis GA et al. Benign solid tumors of the liver: management in the modern era. J Gastrointest Surg. 2015 Jun;19(6):1157–68. [PMID: 25560181]

Marrero JA et al. ACG clinical guideline: the diagnosis and management of focal liver lesions. Am J Gastroenterol. 2014 Sep; 109(9):1328–47. [PMID: 25135008]

DISEASES OF THE BILIARY TRACT

See Chapter 39 for Carcinoma of the Biliary Tract.

CHOLELITHIASIS (Gallstones)

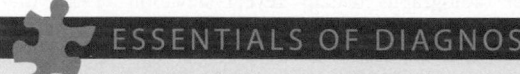

ESSENTIALS OF DIAGNOSIS

- ► Often asymptomatic.
- ► Classic biliary pain ("episodic gallbladder pain") characterized by infrequent episodes of steady severe pain in epigastrium or right upper quadrant with radiation to right scapula.
- ► Detected on ultrasonography.

► General Considerations

Gallstones are more common in women than in men and increase in incidence in both sexes and all races with age. In the United States, the prevalence of gallstones is 8.6% in women and 5.5% in men, with the highest rates in persons over age 60 and higher rates in Mexican-Americans than in non-Hispanic whites and African Americans, and gallstone disease is associated with increased overall, cardiovascular, and cancer mortality. Although cholesterol gallstones are less common in black people, cholelithiasis attributable to hemolysis occurs in over a third of individuals with sickle cell disease. Native Americans of both the Northern and Southern hemispheres have a high rate of cholesterol cholelithiasis, probably because of a predisposition resulting from "thrifty" (*LITH*) genes that promote efficient calorie utilization and fat storage. As many as 75% of Pima and other American Indian women over the age of 25 years have cholelithiasis. Other genetic mutations that predispose persons to gallstones have been identified. Obesity is a risk factor for gallstones, especially in women. Rapid weight loss, as occurs after bariatric surgery, also increases the risk of symptomatic gallstone formation. Diabetes mellitus, glucose intolerance, and insulin resistance are risk factors for gallstones, and a high intake of carbohydrate and high dietary glycemic load increase the risk of cholecystectomy in women. Hypertriglyceridemia may promote gallstone formation by impairing gallbladder motility. The prevalence of gallbladder disease is increased in men (but not women) with cirrhosis and hepatitis C virus infection. Moreover, cholecystectomy has been reported to be associated with an increased risk of NAFLD and cirrhosis, possibly because gallstones and liver disease have some risk factors in common. A low-carbohydrate diet, physical activity, and cardiorespiratory fitness may help prevent gallstones. Consumption of caffeinated coffee appears to protect against gallstones in women, and a high intake of magnesium and of polyunsaturated and monounsaturated fats reduces the risk of gallstones in men. A diet high in fiber, a diet rich in fruits and vegetables, and statin use reduce the risk of cholecystectomy, particularly in women. The incidence of gallstones is high in individuals with Crohn disease; approximately one-third of those with inflammatory involvement of the terminal ileum have gallstones due to disruption of bile salt resorption that results in decreased solubility of the bile. Drugs such as clofibrate, octreotide, and ceftriaxone can cause gallstones. In contrast, aspirin and other nonsteroidal anti-inflammatory drugs may protect against gallstones. Prolonged fasting (over 5–10 days) can lead to formation of biliary "sludge" (microlithiasis), which usually resolves with refeeding but can lead to gallstones or biliary symptoms. Pregnancy, particularly in obese women and those with insulin resistance, is associated with an increased risk of gallstones and of symptomatic gallbladder disease. Hormone replacement therapy appears to increase the risk of gallbladder disease and need for cholecystectomy; the risk is lower with transdermal than oral therapy.

Gallstones are classified according to their predominant chemical composition as cholesterol or calcium bilirubinate stones. The latter comprise less than 20% of the gallstones found in patients in the United States or Europe but 30–40% of gallstones found in patients in Japan.

▶ Clinical Findings

Table 16–8 lists the clinical and laboratory features of several diseases of the biliary tract as well as their treatment. Cholelithiasis is frequently asymptomatic and is discovered in the course of routine radiographic study, operation, or autopsy. Symptoms (biliary [or "episodic gallbladder"] pain) develop in 10–25% of patients (1–4% annually), and acute cholecystitis develops in 20% of these symptomatic persons over time. Occasionally, small intestinal obstruction due to "gallstone ileus" (or Bouveret syndrome when the obstructing stone is in pylorus or duodenum) presents as the initial manifestation of cholelithiasis.

Table 16–8. Diseases of the biliary tract.

	Clinical Features	Laboratory Features	Diagnosis	Treatment
Asymptomatic gallstones	Asymptomatic	Normal	Ultrasonography	None
Symptomatic gallstones	Biliary pain	Normal	Ultrasonography	Laparoscopic cholecystectomy
Cholesterolosis of gallbladder	Usually asymptomatic	Normal	Oral cholecystography	None
Adenomyomatosis	May cause biliary pain	Normal	Oral cholecystography	Laparoscopic cholecystectomy if symptomatic
Porcelain gallbladder	Usually asymptomatic, high risk of gallbladder cancer	Normal	Radiograph or CT	Laparoscopic cholecystectomy
Acute cholecystitis	Epigastric or right upper quadrant pain, nausea, vomiting, fever, Murphy sign	Leukocytosis	Ultrasonography, HIDA scan	Antibiotics, laparoscopic cholecystectomy
Chronic cholecystitis	Biliary pain, constant epigastric or right upper quadrant pain, nausea	Normal	Ultrasonography (stones), oral cholecystography (nonfunctioning gallbladder)	Laparoscopic cholecystectomy
Choledocholithiasis	Asymptomatic or biliary pain, jaundice, fever; gallstone pancreatitis	Cholestatic liver biochemical tests; leukocytosis and positive blood cultures in cholangitis; elevated amylase and lipase in pancreatitis	Ultrasonography (dilated ducts), EUS, MRCP, ERCP	Endoscopic sphincterotomy and stone extraction; antibiotics for cholangitis

ERCP, endoscopic retrograde cholangiopancreatography; EUS, endoscopic ultrasonography; HIDA, hepatic iminodiacetic acid; MRCP, magnetic resonance cholangiopancreatography.

Treatment

Nonsteroidal anti-inflammatory drugs (eg, diclofenac 50–75 mg intramuscularly) can be used to relieve biliary pain. Laparoscopic cholecystectomy is the treatment of choice for symptomatic gallbladder disease. Pain relief after cholecystectomy is most likely in patients with episodic pain (generally once a month or less), pain lasting 30 minutes to 24 hours, pain in the evening or at night, and the onset of symptoms 1 year or less before presentation. Patients may go home within 1 day of the procedure and return to work within days (instead of weeks for those undergoing open cholecystectomy). The procedure is often performed on an outpatient basis and is suitable for most patients, including those with acute cholecystitis. Conversion to a conventional open cholecystectomy may be necessary in 2–8% of cases (higher for acute cholecystitis than for uncomplicated cholelithiasis). Bile duct injuries occur in 0.1% of cases done by experienced surgeons. There is generally no need for prophylactic cholecystectomy in an asymptomatic person unless the gallbladder is calcified, gallstones are 3 cm or greater in diameter, or the patient is a Native American or a candidate for bariatric surgery or cardiac transplantation. Cholecystectomy may increase the risk of esophageal, proximal small intestinal, and colonic adenocarcinomas because of increased duodenogastric reflux and changes in intestinal exposure to bile. In pregnant patients a conservative approach to biliary pain is advised, but for patients with repeated attacks of biliary pain or acute cholecystitis, cholecystectomy can be performed—even by the laparoscopic route—preferably in the second trimester. Enterolithotomy alone is considered adequate treatment in most patients with gallstone ileus. Cholecystectomy via natural orifice translumenal endoscopic surgery (NOTES) has been performed and is under study.

Ursodeoxycholic acid is a bile salt that when given orally for up to 2 years dissolves some cholesterol stones and may be considered in occasional, selected patients who refuse cholecystectomy. The dose is 8–13 mg/kg in divided doses daily. It is most effective in patients with a functioning gallbladder, as determined by gallbladder visualization on oral cholecystography, and multiple small "floating" gallstones (representing not more than 15% of patients with gallstones). In half of patients, gallstones recur within 5 years after treatment is stopped. Ursodeoxycholic acid, 500–600 mg daily, and diets higher in fat reduce the risk of gallstone formation with rapid weight loss. Lithotripsy in combination with bile salt therapy for single radiolucent stones smaller than 20 mm in diameter was an option in the past but is no longer generally used in the United States.

When to Refer

Patients should be referred when they require surgery.

Gurusamy KS et al. Gallstones. BMJ. 2014 Apr 22;348:g2669. [PMID: 24755732]

Nordenvall C et al. Inverse association between coffee consumption and risk of cholecystectomy in women but not in men. Clin Gastroenterol Hepatol. 2015 Jun;13(6):1096–102. [PMID: 25245628]

Zhang YP et al. Systematic review with meta-analysis: coffee consumption and the risk of gallstone disease. Aliment Pharmacol Ther. 2015 Sep;42(6):637–48. [PMID: 26198295]

ACUTE CHOLECYSTITIS

ESSENTIALS OF DIAGNOSIS

▶ Steady, severe pain and tenderness in the right hypochondrium or epigastrium.

▶ Nausea and vomiting.

▶ Fever and leukocytosis.

General Considerations

Cholecystitis is associated with gallstones in over 90% of cases. It occurs when a stone becomes impacted in the cystic duct and inflammation develops behind the obstruction. Acalculous cholecystitis should be considered when unexplained fever or right upper quadrant pain occurs within 2–4 weeks of major surgery or in a critically ill patient who has had no oral intake for a prolonged period; multiorgan failure is often present. Acute cholecystitis may be caused by infectious agents (eg, cytomegalovirus, cryptosporidiosis, or microsporidiosis) in patients with AIDS or by vasculitis (eg, polyarteritis nodosa, Henoch-Schönlein purpura).

Clinical Findings

A. Symptoms and Signs

The acute attack is often precipitated by a large or fatty meal and is characterized by the sudden appearance of steady pain localized to the epigastrium or right hypochondrium, which may gradually subside over a period of 12–18 hours. Vomiting occurs in about 75% of patients and in half of instances affords variable relief. Fever is typical. Right upper quadrant abdominal tenderness (often with a Murphy sign, or inhibition of inspiration by pain on palpation of the right upper quadrant) is almost always present and is usually associated with muscle guarding and rebound tenderness (Table 16–8). A palpable gallbladder is present in about 15% of cases. Jaundice is present in about 25% of cases and, when persistent or severe, suggests the possibility of choledocholithiasis.

B. Laboratory Findings

The white blood cell count is usually high (12,000–15,000/mcL [12–15 ×10⁹/L]). Total serum bilirubin values of 1–4 mg/dL (17.1–68.4 mcmol/L) may be seen even in the absence of bile duct obstruction. Serum aminotransferase and alkaline phosphatase levels are often elevated—the former as high as 300 units/mL, and even higher when associated with acute (ascending) cholangitis. Serum amylase may also be moderately elevated.

C. Imaging

Plain films of the abdomen may show radiopaque gallstones in 15% of cases. ^{99m}Tc hepatobiliary imaging (using iminodiacetic acid compounds), also known as the hepatic iminodiacetic acid (HIDA) scan, is useful in demonstrating an obstructed cystic duct, which is the cause of acute cholecystitis in most patients. This test is reliable if the bilirubin is under 5 mg/dL (85.5 mcmol/L) (98% sensitivity and 81% specificity for acute cholecystitis). False-positive results can occur with prolonged fasting, liver disease, and chronic cholecystitis, and the specificity can be improved by intravenous administration of morphine, which induces spasm of the sphincter of Oddi. Right upper quadrant abdominal ultrasonography, which is often performed first, may show gallstones but is not as sensitive for acute cholecystitis (67% sensitivity, 82% specificity); findings suggestive of acute cholecystitis are gallbladder wall thickening, pericholecystic fluid, and a sonographic Murphy sign. CT may show complications of acute cholecystitis, such as perforation or gangrene.

Differential Diagnosis

The disorders most likely to be confused with acute cholecystitis are perforated peptic ulcer, acute pancreatitis, appendicitis in a high-lying appendix, perforated colonic carcinoma or diverticulum of the hepatic flexure, liver abscess, hepatitis, pneumonia with pleurisy on the right side, and even myocardial ischemia. Definite localization of pain and tenderness in the right upper quadrant, with radiation around to the infrascapular area, strongly favors the diagnosis of acute cholecystitis. True cholecystitis without stones suggests acalculous cholecystitis.

Complications

A. Gangrene of the Gallbladder

Continuation or progression of right upper quadrant abdominal pain, tenderness, muscle guarding, fever, and leukocytosis after 24–48 hours suggests severe inflammation and possible gangrene of the gallbladder, resulting from ischemia due to splanchnic vasoconstriction and intravascular coagulation. Necrosis may occasionally develop without specific signs in the obese, diabetic, elderly, or immunosuppressed patient. Gangrene may lead to gallbladder perforation, usually with formation of a pericholecystic abscess, and rarely to generalized peritonitis. Other serious acute complications include emphysematous cholecystitis (secondary infection with a gas-forming organism) and empyema.

B. Chronic Cholecystitis and Other Complications

Chronic cholecystitis results from repeated episodes of acute cholecystitis or chronic irritation of the gallbladder wall by stones and is characterized pathologically by varying degrees of chronic inflammation of the gallbladder. Calculi are usually present. In about 4–5% of cases, the villi of the gallbladder undergo polypoid enlargement due to deposition of cholesterol that may be visible to the naked eye ("strawberry gallbladder," cholesterolosis). In other instances, hyperplasia of all or part of the gallbladder wall may be so marked as to give the appearance of a myoma (adenomyomatosis). Hydrops of the gallbladder results when acute cholecystitis subsides but cystic duct obstruction persists, producing distention of the gallbladder with a clear mucoid fluid. Occasionally, a stone in the neck of the gallbladder may compress the common hepatic duct and cause jaundice (Mirizzi syndrome). Xanthogranulomatous cholecystitis is a rare, aggressive variant of chronic cholecystitis characterized by grayish-yellow nodules or streaks, representing lipid-laden macrophages, in the wall of the gallbladder and often presents with acute jaundice.

Cholelithiasis with chronic cholecystitis may be associated with acute exacerbations of gallbladder inflammation, bile duct stone, fistulization to the bowel, pancreatitis and, rarely, carcinoma of the gallbladder. Calcified (porcelain) gallbladder is associated with gallbladder carcinoma and is generally an indication for cholecystectomy; the risk of gallbladder cancer may be higher when calcification is mucosal rather than intramural.

Treatment

Acute cholecystitis will usually subside on a conservative regimen (withholding of oral feedings, intravenous alimentation, analgesics, and intravenous antibiotics—generally a second- or third-generation cephalosporin such as cefoperazone, 1–2 g intravenously every 12 hours, with the addition of metronidazole, 500 mg intravenously every 6 hours; in severe cases, a fluoroquinolone such as ciprofloxacin, 250 mg intravenously every 12 hours, plus metronidazole may be given). Morphine or meperidine may be administered for pain. Because of the high risk of recurrent attacks (up to 10% by 1 month and over 30% by 1 year), cholecystectomy—generally laparoscopically—should generally be performed within 24 hours of admission to the hospital for acute cholecystitis. Compared with delayed surgery, surgery within 24 hours is associated with a shorter length of stay, lower costs, and greater patient satisfaction. If nonsurgical treatment has been elected, the patient (especially if diabetic or elderly) should be watched carefully for recurrent symptoms, evidence of gangrene of the gallbladder, or cholangitis. In high-risk patients, ultrasound-guided aspiration of the gallbladder, if feasible, percutaneous cholecystostomy, or endoscopic insertion of a stent or nasobiliary drain into the gallbladder may postpone or even avoid the need for surgery. Immediate cholecystectomy is mandatory when there is evidence of gangrene or perforation.

Surgical treatment of chronic cholecystitis is the same as for acute cholecystitis. If indicated, cholangiography can be performed during laparoscopic cholecystectomy. Choledocholithiasis can also be excluded by either preoperative or postoperative MRCP or ERCP.

Prognosis

The overall mortality rate of cholecystectomy is less than 0.2%, but hepatobiliary tract surgery is a more formidable procedure in the elderly, in whom mortality rates are higher; mortality rates are also higher in persons with diabetes mellitus and cirrhosis. A technically successful surgical procedure in an appropriately selected patient is generally followed by complete resolution of symptoms.

▶ When to Admit

All patients with acute cholecystitis should be hospitalized.

Baron TH et al. Interventional approaches to gallbladder disease. N Engl J Med. 2015 Jul 23;373(4):357–65. [PMID: 26200981]
Cao AM et al. Early cholecystectomy is superior to delayed cholecystectomy for acute cholecystitis: a meta-analysis. J Gastrointest Surg. 2015 May;19(5):848–57. [PMID: 25749854]

PRE- & POSTCHOLECYSTECTOMY SYNDROMES

1. Precholecystectomy

In a small group of patients (mostly women) with biliary pain, conventional radiographic studies of the upper gastrointestinal tract and gallbladder—including cholangiography—are unremarkable. Emptying of the gallbladder may be markedly reduced on gallbladder scintigraphy following injection of cholecystokinin; cholecystectomy may be curative in such cases. Histologic examination of the resected gallbladder may show chronic cholecystitis or microlithiasis. An additional diagnostic consideration is sphincter of Oddi dysfunction.

2. Postcholecystectomy

Following cholecystectomy, some patients complain of continuing symptoms, ie, right upper quadrant pain, flatulence, and fatty food intolerance. The persistence of symptoms in this group of patients suggests the possibility of an incorrect diagnosis prior to cholecystectomy, eg, esophagitis, pancreatitis, radiculopathy, or functional bowel disease. Choledocholithiasis or bile duct stricture should be ruled out. Pain may also be associated with dilatation of the cystic duct remnant, neuroma formation in the ductal wall, foreign body granuloma, or traction on the bile duct by a long cystic duct.

The clinical presentation of right upper quadrant pain, chills, fever, or jaundice suggests biliary tract disease. EUS or retrograde cholangiography may be necessary to demonstrate a stone or stricture. Biliary pain associated with elevated liver biochemical tests or a dilated bile duct in the absence of an obstructing lesion suggests sphincter of Oddi dysfunction. Biliary manometry may be useful for documenting elevated baseline sphincter of Oddi pressures typical of sphincter dysfunction when biliary pain is associated with elevated liver biochemical tests (twofold) or a dilated bile duct (greater than 12 mm) ("sphincter disorder," formerly type II sphincter of Oddi dysfunction) but is not necessary when both are present ("sphincter stenosis," formerly type I sphincter of Oddi dysfunction) and is associated with a high risk of pancreatitis. In the absence of either elevated liver biochemical tests or a dilated bile duct ("functional pain," formerly type III sphincter of Oddi dysfunction), a nonbiliary source of symptoms should be

suspected, and biliary sphincterotomy does not benefit this group. (Analogous criteria have been developed for pancreatic sphincter dysfunction.) Biliary scintigraphy after intravenous administration of morphine and MRCP following intravenous administration of secretin are under study as screening tests for sphincter dysfunction. Endoscopic sphincterotomy is most likely to relieve symptoms in patients with a sphincter disorder or stenosis, although many patients continue to have some pain. In some cases, treatment with a calcium channel blocker, long-acting nitrate, or phosphodiesterase inhibitor (eg, vardenafil) or possibly injection of the sphincter with botulinum toxin may be beneficial. The rate of psychosocial comorbidity with sphincter of Oddi dysfunction does not appear to differ from that of the general population. In refractory cases, surgical sphincteroplasty or removal of the cystic duct remnant may be considered.

▶ When to Refer

Patients with sphincter of Oddi dysfunction should be referred for diagnostic procedures.

Sugawa C et al. The role of endoscopic biliary sphincterotomy for the treatment of type 1 biliary dysfunction (papillary stenosis) with or without biliary stones. Am J Surg. 2014 Jan; 207(1):65–9. [PMID: 24070665]
Wilcox CM. Sphincter of Oddi dysfunction type III: new studies suggest new approaches are needed. World J Gastroenterol. 2015 May 21;21(19):5755–61. [PMID: 26019439]
Yaghoobi M et al. Sphincter of Oddi dysfunction: updates from the recent literature. Curr Gastroenterol Rep. 2015 Aug; 17(8):31. [PMID: 26143628]

CHOLEDOCHOLITHIASIS & CHOLANGITIS

ESSENTIALS OF DIAGNOSIS

▶ Often a history of biliary pain, which may be accompanied by jaundice.

▶ Occasional patients present with painless jaundice.

▶ Nausea and vomiting.

▶ Cholangitis should be suspected with fever followed by hypothermia and gram-negative shock, jaundice, and leukocytosis.

▶ Stones in bile duct most reliably detected by ERCP or EUS.

▶ General Considerations

About 15% of patients with gallstones have choledocholithiasis (bile duct stones). The percentage rises with age, and the frequency in elderly people with gallstones may be as high as 50%. Bile duct stones usually originate in the gallbladder but may also form spontaneously in the bile duct after cholecystectomy. The risk is increased twofold in persons with a juxtapapillary duodenal diverticulum. Symptoms, including cholangitis, result if there is obstruction.

▶ Clinical Findings

A. Symptoms and Signs

A history of biliary pain or jaundice may be obtained. Biliary pain results from rapid increases in bile duct pressure due to obstructed bile flow. The features that suggest the presence of a bile duct stone are: (1) frequently recurring attacks of right upper abdominal pain that is severe and persists for hours; (2) chills and fever associated with severe pain; and (3) a history of jaundice associated with episodes of abdominal pain (Table 16–8). The combination of pain, fever (and chills), and jaundice represents **Charcot triad** and denotes the classic picture of acute cholangitis. The addition of altered mental status and hypotension (**Reynolds pentad**) signifies acute suppurative cholangitis and is an endoscopic emergency. According to the Tokyo guidelines (2006), the diagnosis of acute cholangitis is established by the presence of either (1) the Charcot triad or (2) two elements of the Charcot triad plus laboratory evidence of an inflammatory response (eg, elevated white blood cell count, C-reactive protein), elevated liver biochemical test levels, and imaging evidence of biliary dilatation or a cause of obstruction.

Hepatomegaly may be present in calculous biliary obstruction, and tenderness is usually present in the right upper quadrant and epigastrium. Bile duct obstruction lasting more than 30 days results in liver damage leading to cirrhosis. Hepatic failure with portal hypertension occurs in untreated cases. In a population-based study from Denmark, acute cholangitis was reported to be a marker of occult gastrointestinal cancer.

B. Laboratory Findings

Acute obstruction of the bile duct typically produces a transient albeit striking increase in serum aminotransferase levels (often greater than 1000 units/L [20 mckat/L]). Bilirubinuria and elevation of the serum bilirubin are present if the bile duct remains obstructed; levels commonly fluctuate. Serum alkaline phosphatase levels rise more slowly. Not uncommonly, serum amylase elevations are present because of secondary pancreatitis. When extrahepatic obstruction persists for more than a few weeks, differentiation of obstruction from chronic cholestatic liver disease becomes more difficult. Leukocytosis is present in patients with acute cholangitis. Prolongation of the prothrombin time can result from the obstructed flow of bile to the intestine. In contrast to hepatocellular dysfunction, hypoprothrombinemia due to obstructive jaundice will respond to intravenous vitamin K, 10 mg, or water-soluble oral vitamin K (phytonadione, 5 mg) within 24–36 hours.

C. Imaging

Ultrasonography and CT may demonstrate dilated bile ducts, and radionuclide imaging may show impaired bile flow. EUS, helical CT, and magnetic resonance cholangiography are accurate in demonstrating bile duct stones and may be used in patients thought to be at intermediate risk for choledocholithiasis (age older than 55 years,

cholecystitis, bile duct diameter greater than 6 mm on ultrasonography, serum bilirubin 1.8–4 mg/dL [30.78–68.4 mcmol/L], elevated serum liver enzymes, pancreatitis). ERCP (occasionally with intraductal ultrasonography) or percutaneous transhepatic cholangiography provides the most direct and accurate means of determining the cause, location, and extent of obstruction, but in patients at intermediate risk of choledocholithiasis, initial cholecystectomy and intraoperative cholangiography result in a shorter length of hospital stay, fewer bile duct investigations, and no increase in morbidity. If the likelihood that obstruction is caused by a stone is high (bile duct diameter greater than 6 mm, bile duct stone seen on ultrasonography, serum bilirubin greater than 4 mg/dL [68.4 mcmol/L]) or acute cholangitis is present, ERCP with sphincterotomy and stone extraction or stent placement is the procedure of choice; meticulous technique is required to avoid causing acute cholangitis. Because the sensitivity of these criteria for choledocholithiasis is only 80%, it is not unreasonable for magnetic resonance cholangiography or EUS to be done before ERCP.

▶ Differential Diagnosis

The most common cause of obstructive jaundice is a bile duct stone. Next in frequency are neoplasms of the pancreas, ampulla of Vater, or bile duct or an obstructed stent placed previously for decompression of an obstructing tumor. Extrinsic compression of the bile duct may result from metastatic carcinoma (usually from the gastrointestinal tract or breast) involving porta hepatis lymph nodes or, rarely, from a large duodenal diverticulum. Gallbladder cancer extending into the bile duct often presents as obstructive jaundice. Chronic cholestatic liver diseases (PBC, sclerosing cholangitis, drug-induced) must be considered. Hepatocellular jaundice can usually be differentiated by the history, clinical findings, and liver biochemical tests, but liver biopsy is necessary on occasion. Recurrent pyogenic cholangitis should be considered in persons from Asia (and occasionally elsewhere) with intrahepatic biliary stones (particularly in the left ductal system) and recurrent cholangitis.

▶ Treatment

In general, bile duct stones, even small ones, should be removed, even in an asymptomatic patient. A bile duct stone in a patient with cholelithiasis or cholecystitis is usually treated by endoscopic sphincterotomy and stone extraction followed by laparoscopic cholecystectomy within 72 hours in patients with cholecystitis and within 2 weeks in those without cholecystitis. An alternative approach, which is associated with a shorter duration of hospitalization in patients at intermediate risk for choledocholithiasis, is laparoscopic cholecystectomy and bile duct exploration. For patients older than 70 years or poor-risk patients with cholelithiasis and choledocholithiasis, cholecystectomy may be deferred after endoscopic sphincterotomy because the risk of subsequent cholecystitis is low. ERCP with sphincterotomy, generally within 48 hours, should be performed before cholecystectomy in patients with gallstones and cholangitis, jaundice (serum total bilirubin greater than 4 mg/dL [68.4 mcmol/L]), a dilated bile duct (greater than 6 mm), or stones in the bile duct seen on ultrasonography or CT. (Stones may ultimately recur in up to 12% of patients, particularly in the elderly, when the bile duct diameter is 15 mm or greater, or when brown pigment stones are found at the time of the initial sphincterotomy.) Endoscopic balloon dilation of the sphincter of Oddi may be associated with a higher rate of pancreatitis than endoscopic sphincterotomy unless adequate dilation for more than 1 min is carried out but may also be associated with a lower rate of stone recurrence. This procedure is generally reserved for patients with coagulopathy because the risk of bleeding is lower with balloon dilation than with sphincterotomy. Endoscopic ultrasound-guided biliary drainage and PTC with drainage are second-line approaches if ERCP fails or is not possible. In patients with biliary pancreatitis that resolves rapidly, the stone usually passes into the intestine, and ERCP prior to cholecystectomy is not necessary if an intraoperative cholangiogram is planned.

Choledocholithiasis discovered at laparoscopic cholecystectomy may be managed via laparoscopic or, if necessary, open bile duct exploration or by postoperative endoscopic sphincterotomy. Operative findings of choledocholithiasis are palpable stones in the bile duct, dilatation or thickening of the wall of the bile duct, or stones in the gallbladder small enough to pass through the cystic duct. Laparoscopic intraoperative cholangiography (or intraoperative ultrasonography) should be done at the time of cholecystectomy in patients with liver enzyme elevations but a bile duct diameter of less than 5 mm; if a ductal stone is found, the duct should be explored. In the post-cholecystectomy patient with choledocholithiasis, endoscopic sphincterotomy with stone extraction is preferable to transabdominal surgery. Lithotripsy (endoscopic or external), peroral cholangioscopy (choledoscopy), or biliary stenting may be a therapeutic consideration for large stones. For the patient with a T tube and bile duct stone, the stone may be extracted via the T tube.

Postoperative antibiotics are not administered routinely after biliary tract surgery. Cultures of the bile are always taken at operation. If biliary tract infection was present preoperatively or is apparent at operation, ampicillin (500 mg every 6 hours intravenously) with gentamicin (1.5 mg/kg intravenously every 8 hours) and metronidazole (500 mg intravenously every 6 hours) or ciprofloxacin (250 mg intravenously every 12 hours) or a third-generation cephalosporin (eg, cefoperazone, 1–2 g intravenous every 12 hours) is administered postoperatively until the results of sensitivity tests on culture specimens are available. A T-tube cholangiogram should be done before the tube is removed, usually about 3 weeks after surgery. A small amount of bile frequently leaks from the tube site for a few days.

Urgent ERCP with sphincterotomy and stone extraction is generally indicated for choledocholithiasis complicated by acute cholangitis and is preferred to surgery. Before ERCP, liver function should be evaluated thoroughly. The prothrombin time should be restored to normal by intravenous administration of vitamin K. For mild-to-moderately severe community-acquired acute cholangitis, ciprofloxacin, 500 mg intravenously every 12 hours, penetrates well into bile and is effective treatment, with the possible addition of metronidazole, 500 mg every 6–8 hours. Alternative regimens include intravenous cefoxitin, 1–2 g every 6 hours, ampicillin, 2 g every 6 hours, plus gentamicin, 1.7 mg/kg every 8 hours, or ceftriaxone 1–2 g daily, among others. Regimens for severe or hospital-acquired acute cholangitis include intravenous piperacillin and tazobactam, 3.375 g every 6 hours; ticarcillin and clavulanate, 3.1 g every 6 hours; ceftriaxone, 1–2 g daily, plus metronidazole, 500 mg every 6–8 hours; or, in patients at high risk for harboring antibiotic-resistant pathogens, meropenem, 1 g every 8 hours. Aminoglycosides should not be given for more than a few days because the risk of aminoglycoside nephrotoxicity is increased in patients with cholestasis. Regimens that include drugs active against anaerobes are required when a biliary-enteric communication is present. Emergent decompression of the bile duct, generally by ERCP, is required for patients who are septic or fail to improve on antibiotics within 12–24 hours. Medical therapy alone is most likely to fail in patients with tachycardia, serum albumin less than 3 g/dL (30 g/L), marked hyperbilirubinemia, high serum ALT level, high white blood cell count, and prothrombin time greater than 14 seconds on admission. If sphincterotomy cannot be performed, the bile duct can be decompressed by a biliary stent or nasobiliary catheter. Once decompression is achieved, antibiotics are generally continued for at least another 3 days. Elective cholecystectomy can be undertaken after resolution of cholangitis, unless the patient remains unfit for surgery. Mortality from acute cholangitis has been reported to correlate with a high total bilirubin level, prolonged partial thromboplastin time, presence of a liver abscess, and unsuccessful ERCP.

▶ When to Refer

All symptomatic patients with choledocholithiasis should be referred.

▶ When to Admit

All patients with acute cholangitis should be hospitalized.

Iranmanesh P et al. Initial cholecystectomy vs sequential common duct endoscopic assessment and subsequent cholecystectomy for suspected gallstone migration: a randomized clinical trial. JAMA. 2014 Jul;312(2):137–44. [PMID: 25005650]

James PD et al. Decreasing mortality from acute biliary diseases that require endoscopic retrograde cholangiopancreatography: a nationwide cohort study. Clin Gastroenterol Hepatol. 2014 Jul;12(7):1151–9. [PMID: 24095977]

Lee F et al. Delayed endoscopic retrograde cholangiopancreatography is associated with persistent organ failure in hospitalised patients with acute cholangitis. Aliment Pharmacol Ther. 2015 Jul;42(2):212–20. [PMID: 25997554]

BILIARY STRICTURE

Benign biliary strictures are the result of surgical (including liver transplantation) anastomosis or injury in about 95% of cases. The remainder of cases are caused by blunt external injury to the abdomen, pancreatitis, erosion of the duct by a gallstone, or prior endoscopic sphincterotomy.

Signs of injury to the duct may or may not be recognized in the immediate postoperative period. If complete occlusion has occurred, jaundice will develop rapidly; more often, however, a tear has been made accidentally in the duct, and the earliest manifestation of injury may be excessive or prolonged loss of bile from the surgical drains. Bile leakage resulting in a bile collection (biloma) may predispose to localized infection, which in turn accentuates scar formation and the ultimate development of a fibrous stricture.

Cholangitis is the most common complication of stricture. Typically, the patient experiences episodes of pain, fever, chills, and jaundice within a few weeks to months after cholecystectomy. Physical findings may include jaundice during an acute attack of cholangitis and right upper quadrant abdominal tenderness. Serum alkaline phosphatase is usually elevated. Hyperbilirubinemia is variable, fluctuating during exacerbations and usually remaining in the range of 5–10 mg/dL (85.5–171 mcmol/L). Blood cultures may be positive during an acute episode of cholangitis. Secondary biliary cirrhosis will inevitably develop if a stricture is not treated.

MRCP can be valuable in demonstrating the stricture, whereas ERCP permits biopsy and cytologic specimens to exclude malignancy (in conjunction with EUS-guided fine-needle aspiration, an even more sensitive test for distal bile duct malignancy), sphincterotomy to allow closure of a bile leak, and dilation (often repeated) and stent placement, thereby avoiding surgical repair in some cases; when ERCP is unsuccessful, dilation of a stricture may be accomplished by PTC. Placement of multiple plastic stents appears to be more effective than placement of a single stent. The use of covered metal stents, which are more easily removed endoscopically than uncovered metal stents, as well as bioabsorbable stents, is an alternative to use of plastic stents. Uncovered metal stents, which often cannot be removed endoscopically, are generally avoided in benign strictures unless life expectancy is less than 2 years. Strictures related to chronic pancreatitis are more difficult than postsurgical strictures to treat endoscopically and may be best managed with a temporary covered metal stent. Following liver transplantation, endoscopic management is more successful for anastomotic than for nonanastomotic strictures, although results for nonanastomotic strictures may be improved with repeated dilation or the use of multiple plastic stents. Biliary strictures after live liver donor liver transplantation, particularly in patients with a late-onset (after 24 weeks) stricture or with intrahepatic biliary dilatation, are also challenging and require aggressive endoscopic therapy; in addition, the risk of post-ERCP pancreatitis appears to be increased. When malignancy cannot be excluded with certainty, additional endoscopic diagnostic approaches may be considered—if available—including EUS, intraductal ultrasonography, peroral cholangioscopy, and confocal laser endomicroscopy. Differentiation from cholangiocarcinoma may ultimately require surgical exploration. Operative treatment of a stricture frequently necessitates performance of an end-to-end ductal repair, choledochojejunostomy, or hepaticojejunostomy to reestablish bile flow into the intestine.

► When to Refer

All patients with biliary stricture should be referred.

► When to Admit

Patients with acute cholangitis should be hospitalized.

ASGE Standards of Practice Committee; Chathadi KV et al. The role of ERCP in benign diseases of the biliary tract. Gastrointest Endosc. 2015 Apr;81(4):795–803. [PMID: 25665931]

Devière J et al; Benign Biliary Stenoses Working Group. Successful management of benign biliary strictures with fully covered self-expanding metal stents. Gastroenterology. 2014 Aug;147(2):385–95. [PMID: 24801350]

Navaneethan U et al. Single-operator cholangioscopy and targeted biopsies in the diagnosis of indeterminate biliary strictures: a systematic review. Gastrointest Endosc. 2015 Oct;82(4):608–14. [PMID: 26071061]

PRIMARY SCLEROSING CHOLANGITIS

ESSENTIALS OF DIAGNOSIS

- ► Most common in men aged 20–50 years.
- ► Often associated with ulcerative colitis.
- ► Progressive jaundice, itching, and other features of cholestasis.
- ► Diagnosis based on characteristic cholangiographic findings.
- ► At least 10% risk of cholangiocarcinoma.

► General Considerations

Primary sclerosing cholangitis is an uncommon disease thought to result from an increased immune response to intestinal endotoxins and characterized by diffuse inflammation of the biliary tract leading to fibrosis and strictures of the biliary system. The disease is most common in men aged 20–50 years, with an incidence of nearly 3.3 per 100,000 in Asian Americans, 2.8 per 100,000 in Hispanic Americans, and 2.1 per 100,000 in African Americans, and an intermediate incidence in whites (possibly increasing) and a prevalence of 21 per 100,000 men and 6 per 100,000 women in the United States. Primary sclerosing cholangitis is closely associated with inflammatory bowel disease (more commonly ulcerative colitis than Crohn colitis), which is present in approximately two-thirds of patients with primary sclerosing cholangitis; however, clinically significant sclerosing cholangitis develops in only 1–4% of patients with ulcerative colitis. Smoking is associated with a decreased risk of primary sclerosing cholangitis in patients who also have inflammatory bowel disease. Coffee consumption is also associated with a decreased risk of primary sclerosing cholangitis. Women with primary sclerosing cholangitis may be more likely to have recurrent urinary tract infections and less likely to use hormone replacement therapy than healthy controls. Associations with cardiovascular disease and diabetes mellitus have been reported. Primary sclerosing cholangitis is associated with the histocompatibility antigens HLA-B8 and -DR3 or -DR4, and first-degree relatives of patients with primary sclerosing cholangitis have a fourfold increased risk of primary sclerosing cholangitis and a threefold increased risk of ulcerative colitis. A subset of patients with primary sclerosing cholangitis have increased serum IgG_4 levels and distinct HLA associations but do not meet criteria for IgG_4-associated cholangitis. The diagnosis of primary sclerosing cholangitis may be difficult to make after biliary surgery.

Clinical Findings

A. Symptoms and Signs

Primary sclerosing cholangitis presents as progressive obstructive jaundice, frequently associated with fatigue, pruritus, anorexia, and indigestion. Patients may be diagnosed in the presymptomatic phase because of an elevated alkaline phosphatase level. Complications of chronic cholestasis, such as osteoporosis and malabsorption of fat-soluble vitamins, may occur late in the course. Risk factors for osteoporosis include older age, lower body mass index, and longer duration of inflammatory bowel disease. Esophageal varices on initial endoscopy are most likely in patients with a higher Mayo risk score based on age, bilirubin, albumin, and AST and a higher AST/ALT ratio, and new varices are likely to develop in those with a lower platelet count and higher bilirubin at 2 years. In patients with primary sclerosing cholangitis, ulcerative colitis is frequently characterized by rectal sparing and backwash ileitis.

B. Diagnostic Findings

The diagnosis of primary sclerosing cholangitis is increasingly made by MRCP, the sensitivity of which approaches that of ERCP. Characteristic cholangiographic findings are segmental fibrosis of bile ducts with saccular dilatations between strictures. Biliary obstruction by a stone or tumor should be excluded. Liver biopsy is not necessary for diagnosis when cholangiographic findings are characteristic. The disease may be confined to small intrahepatic bile ducts in about 15% of cases, in which case MRCP and ERCP are normal and the diagnosis is suggested by liver biopsy findings. These patients have a longer survival than patients with involvement of the large ducts and do not appear to be at increased risk for cholangiocarcinoma unless large-duct sclerosing cholangitis develops (which occurs in about 20% over 7–10 years). Liver biopsy may show characteristic periductal fibrosis ("onion-skinning") and allows staging, which is based on the degree of fibrosis and which correlates with liver stiffness as measured by ultrasound elastography. Perinuclear ANCA (directed

against myeloid-specific tubulin-beta isotype 5) as well as antinuclear, anticardiolipin, antithyroperoxidase, and anti-Saccharomyces cerevisiae antibodies and rheumatoid factor are frequently detected in serum. Occasional patients have clinical and histologic features of both sclerosing cholangitis and autoimmune hepatitis. An association with autoimmune pancreatitis is also seen, and this entity (IgG_4-associated cholangitis) is often responsive to corticosteroids, although it may be difficult to distinguish from primary sclerosing cholangitis and even cholangiocarcinoma. Primary sclerosing cholangitis must be distinguished from idiopathic adulthood ductopenia (a rare disorder that affects young to middle-aged adults who manifest cholestasis resulting from loss of interlobular and septal bile ducts yet who have a normal cholangiogram and that is caused in some cases by a mutation in the canalicular phospholipid transporter gene ABCB4) and from other cholangiopathies (including PBC; cystic fibrosis; eosinophilic cholangitis; AIDS cholangiopathy; histiocytosis X, allograft rejection; graft-versus-host disease; ischemic cholangiopathy [often with biliary "casts," a rapid progression to cirrhosis, and a poor outcome] caused by hepatic artery thrombosis, shock, respiratory failure, or drugs; intra-arterial chemotherapy; and sarcoidosis).

Complications

Cholangiocarcinoma may complicate the course of primary sclerosing cholangitis in up to 20% of cases (1.2% per year) and may be difficult to diagnose by cytologic examination or biopsy because of false-negative results. A serum CA 19-9 level above 100 units/mL is suggestive but not diagnostic of cholangiocarcinoma. Annual right-upper-quadrant ultrasonography or MRI with MRCP and serum CA 19-9 testing (a level of 20 is the threshold for further investigation) are recommended for surveillance, with ERCP and biliary cytology if the results are suggestive of malignancy. PET and peroral cholangioscopy may play roles in the early detection of cholangiocarcinoma. Patients with ulcerative colitis and primary sclerosing cholangitis are at high risk (tenfold higher than ulcerative colitis patients without primary sclerosing cholangitis) for colorectal neoplasia. The risks of gallstones, cholecystitis, gallbladder polyps, and gallbladder carcinoma appear to be increased in patients with primary sclerosing cholangitis.

Treatment

Episodes of acute bacterial cholangitis may be treated with ciprofloxacin (750 mg twice daily orally or intravenously). Ursodeoxycholic acid in standard doses (10–15 mg/kg/day orally) may improve liver biochemical test results but does not appear to alter the natural history. However, withdrawal of ursodeoxycholic acid may result in worsening of liver biochemical test levels and increased pruritus, and ursodeoxycholic acid in intermediate doses (17–23 mg/kg/day) has been reported to be beneficial. High-dose ursodeoxycholic acid (25–30 mg/kg/day) has been shown not to reduce cholangiographic progression and liver fibrosis, nor to improve survival or prevent cholangiocarcinoma, and has been shown to increase the risk of death and need for liver transplantation in patients with a normal serum bilirubin level and an early histologic stage. Other drugs such as antibiotics (vancomycin, metronidazole, minocycline, azithromycin), obeticholic acid (a farsenoid-X receptor agonist), 24-norursodeoxycholic acid, budesonide, antitumor necrosis factor antibodies, cyclosporine, tacrolimus, and antifibrotic agents are under study. Careful endoscopic evaluation of the biliary tract may permit balloon dilation of localized strictures, and repeated dilation of a dominant stricture may improve survival, although such patients have reduced survival compared with patients who do not have a dominant stricture. Short-term (2–3 weeks) placement of a stent in a major stricture also may relieve symptoms and improve biochemical abnormalities, with sustained improvement after the stent is removed; however, long-term stenting may increase the rate of complications such as cholangitis and is not recommended. Cholecystectomy is indicated in patients with primary sclerosing cholangitis and a gallbladder polyp greater than 8 mm in diameter. In patients without cirrhosis, surgical resection of a dominant bile duct stricture may lead to longer survival than endoscopic therapy by decreasing the subsequent risk of cholangiocarcinoma. When feasible, extensive surgical resection of cholangiocarcinoma complicating primary sclerosing cholangitis may result in 5-year survival rates of greater than 50%. In patients with ulcerative colitis, primary sclerosing cholangitis is an independent risk factor for the development of colorectal dysplasia and cancer (especially in the right colon), and strict adherence to a colonoscopic surveillance program (yearly for those with ulcerative colitis and every 5 years for those without ulcerative colitis) is recommended. Whether treatment with ursodeoxycholic acid reduces the risk of colorectal dysplasia and carcinoma in patients with ulcerative colitis and primary sclerosing cholangitis is still uncertain. For patients with cirrhosis and clinical decompensation, liver transplantation is the procedure of choice; primary sclerosing cholangitis recurs in the graft in 30% of cases, with a possible reduction in the risk of recurrence when colectomy has been performed for ulcerative colitis before transplantation.

▶ Prognosis

Survival of patients with primary sclerosing cholangitis averages 9–17 years, and up to 21 years in population-based studies. Adverse prognostic markers are older age, hepatosplenomegaly, higher serum bilirubin and AST levels, lower albumin levels, a history of variceal bleeding, a dominant bile duct stricture, and extrahepatic duct changes. Variceal bleeding is also a risk factor for cholangiocarcinoma. Patients in whom serum alkaline phosphatase levels decline by 40% or more (spontaneously, with ursodeoxycholic acid therapy, or after treatment of a dominant stricture) have longer transplant-free survival times than those in whom the alkaline phosphatase does not decline. Moreover, improvement in the serum alkaline phosphatase to less than 1.5 times the upper limit of normal is associated with a reduced risk of cholangiocarcinoma. Transplant-free survival can also be predicted by serum levels of markers of liver fibrosis—hyaluronic acid,

tissue inhibitor of metalloproteinase-1, and propeptide of type III procollagen. Reduced quality of life is associated with older age, large-duct disease, and systemic symptoms. Although maternal primary sclerosing cholangitis is associated with preterm birth and cesarean section delivery, the risk of congenital malformations is not increased. Interestingly, patients with milder ulcerative colitis tend to have more severe primary cholangitis and a higher rate of liver transplantation. Actuarial survival rates with liver transplantation are as high as 85% at 3 years, but rates are much lower once cholangiocarcinoma has developed. Following transplantation, patients have an increased risk of nonanastomotic biliary strictures and—in those with ulcerative colitis—colon cancer. The retransplantation rate is higher than that for PBC. Those patients who are unable to undergo liver transplantation will ultimately require high-quality palliative care (see Chapter 5).

Eaton JE et al. A comprehensive assessment of environmental exposures among 1000 North American patients with primary sclerosing cholangitis, with and without inflammatory bowel disease. Aliment Pharmacol Ther. 2015 May;41(10):980–90. [PMID: 25783671]

Joshi D et al. Immunoglobulin G4-related sclerosing cholangitis. Hepatology. 2015 Apr;61(4):1432–4. [PMID: 25179687]

Lazaridis KN et al. The cholangiopathies. Mayo Clin Proc. 2015 Jun;90(6):791–800. [PMID: 25957621]

Lindor KD et al. ACG clinical guideline: primary sclerosing cholangitis. Am J Gastroenterol. 2015 May;110(5):646–59. [PMID: 25869391]

DISEASES OF THE PANCREAS

See Chapter 39 for Carcinoma of the Pancreas and Periampullary Area.

ACUTE PANCREATITIS

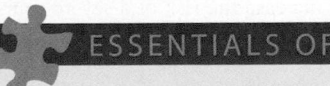

ESSENTIALS OF DIAGNOSIS

► Abrupt onset of deep epigastric pain, often with radiation to the back.

► History of previous episodes, often related to alcohol intake.

► Nausea, vomiting, sweating, weakness.

► Abdominal tenderness and distention and fever.

► Leukocytosis, elevated serum amylase, elevated serum lipase.

▶ General Considerations

The annual incidence of acute pancreatitis ranges from 13 to 45 per 100,000 population and has increased since 1990. Most cases of acute pancreatitis are related to biliary tract disease (a passed gallstone, usually 5 mm or less in diameter) or heavy alcohol intake. The exact pathogenesis is not known but may include edema or obstruction of the ampulla of Vater, reflux of bile into pancreatic ducts, and direct injury of pancreatic acinar cells by prematurely activated pancreatic enzymes. Among the numerous other causes or associations are hypercalcemia, hyperlipidemias (chylomicronemia, hypertriglyceridemia, or both), abdominal trauma (including surgery), drugs (including azathioprine, mercaptopurine, asparaginase, pentamidine, didanosine, valproic acid, tetracyclines, dapsone, isoniazid, metronidazole, estrogen and tamoxifen [by raising serum triglycerides], sulfonamides, mesalamine, celecoxib, sulindac, leflunomide, thiazides, simvastatin, fenofibrate, enalapril, methyldopa, procainamide, sitagliptin, exenatide, possibly corticosteroids, and others), vasculitis, infections (eg, mumps, cytomegalovirus, *M avium intracellulare* complex), peritoneal dialysis, cardiopulmonary bypass, single- or double-balloon enteroscopy, and ERCP. In patients with pancreas divisum, a congenital anomaly in which the dorsal and ventral pancreatic ducts fail to fuse, acute pancreatitis may result from stenosis of the minor papilla with obstruction to flow from the accessory pancreatic duct, although concomitant genetic mutations, particularly in the cystic fibrosis transmembrane conductance regulator (*CFTR*) gene, have also been reported to account for acute pancreatitis in some patients with pancreas divisum. Genetic mutations also predispose to chronic pancreatitis, particularly in persons younger than 30 years of age if no other cause is evident and a family history of pancreatic disease is present. Acute pancreatitis may also result from the anomalous union of the pancreaticobiliary duct. Rarely, acute pancreatitis may be the presenting manifestation of a pancreatic or ampullary neoplasm. Celiac disease appears to be associated with an increased risk of acute and chronic pancreatitis. Apparently "idiopathic" acute pancreatitis is often caused by occult biliary microlithiasis and may be caused by sphincter of Oddi dysfunction involving the pancreatic duct. Between 15% and 25% of cases are truly idiopathic. Smoking, high dietary glycemic load, and abdominal adiposity increase the risk of pancreatitis, and older age and obesity increase the risk of a severe course; vegetable consumption and use of statins may reduce the risk of pancreatitis.

► Clinical Findings

A. Symptoms and Signs

Epigastric abdominal pain, generally abrupt in onset, is steady, boring, and severe and often made worse by walking and lying supine and better by sitting and leaning forward. The pain usually radiates into the back but may radiate to the right or left. Nausea and vomiting are usually present. Weakness, sweating, and anxiety are noted in severe attacks. There may be a history of alcohol intake or a heavy meal immediately preceding the attack or a history of milder similar episodes or biliary pain in the past.

The abdomen is tender mainly in the upper part, most often without guarding, rigidity, or rebound. The abdomen may be distended, and bowel sounds may be absent with associated ileus. Fever of 38.4–39°C, tachycardia, hypotension (even shock), pallor, and cool clammy skin are present in severe cases. Mild jaundice may be seen. Occasionally, an upper abdominal mass due to the inflamed pancreas or a pseudocyst may be palpated.

Acute kidney injury (usually prerenal) may occur early in the course of acute pancreatitis.

B. Laboratory Findings

Serum amylase and lipase are elevated—usually more than three times the upper limit of normal—within 24 hours in 90% of cases; their return to normal is variable depending on the severity of disease. Lipase remains elevated longer than amylase and is slightly more accurate for the diagnosis of acute pancreatitis. Leukocytosis (10,000–30,000/mcL), proteinuria, granular casts, glycosuria (10–20% of cases), hyperglycemia, and elevated serum bilirubin may be present. Blood urea nitrogen and serum alkaline phosphatase may be elevated and coagulation tests abnormal. An elevated serum creatinine level (greater than 1.8 mg/dL [149.94 mcmol/L]) at 48 hours is associated with the development of pancreatic necrosis. In patients with clear evidence of acute pancreatitis, a serum ALT level of more than 150 units/L (3 mkat/L) suggests biliary pancreatitis. A decrease in serum calcium may reflect saponification and correlates with severity of the disease. Levels lower than 7 mg/dL (1.75 mmol/L) (when serum albumin is normal) are associated with tetany and an unfavorable prognosis. Patients with acute pancreatitis caused by hypertriglyceridemia generally have fasting triglyceride levels above 1000 mg/dL (10 mmol/L); in some cases, the serum amylase is not elevated substantially because of an inhibitor in the serum of patients with marked hypertriglyceridemia that interferes with measurement of serum amylase. An early rise in the hematocrit value above 44% suggests hemoconcentration and predicts pancreatic necrosis. An elevated C-reactive protein concentration (greater than 150 mg/L [1500 mg/L]) at 48 hours suggests severe disease.

Other diagnostic tests that offer the possibility of simplicity, rapidity, ease of use, and low cost—including urinary trypsinogen-2, trypsinogen activation peptide, and carboxypeptidase B—are not widely available. In patients in whom ascites or a left pleural effusion develops, fluid amylase content is high. Electrocardiography may show ST–T wave changes.

C. Assessment of Severity

In addition to the individual laboratory parameters noted above, the severity of acute alcoholic pancreatitis can be assessed using several scoring systems, including the **Ranson criteria** (Table 16–9). The **Sequential Organ Failure Assessment (SOFA)** score or **modified Marshall scoring system** can be used to assess injury to other organs, and the **Acute Physiology and Chronic Health Evaluation (APACHE II)** score is another tool for assessing severity. A simple 5-point clinical scoring system (the **Bedside Index for Severity in Acute Pancreatitis,** or **BISAP**) based on blood urea nitrogen above 25 mg/dL (9 mmol/L), impaired mental status, systemic inflammatory response syndrome, age older than 60 years, and pleural effusion during the first 24 hours (before the onset of organ failure) identifies patients at increased risk for mortality. More simply, the presence of a systemic inflammatory response alone and an elevated blood urea nitrogen level on admission as well as

Table 16–9. Ranson criteria for assessing the severity of acute pancreatitis.

Three or more of the following predict a severe course complicated by pancreatic necrosis with a sensitivity of 60–80%	
Age over 55 years	
White blood cell count > 16 × 10³/mcL (> 16 × 10⁹/L)	
Blood glucose > 200 mg/dL (> 11 mmol/L)	
Serum lactic dehydrogenase > 350 units/L (> 7 mkat/L)	
Aspartate aminotransferase > 250 units/L (> 5 mkat/L)	
Development of the following in the first 48 hours indicates a worsening prognosis	
Hematocrit drop of more than 10 percentage points	
Blood urea nitrogen rise > 5 mg/dL (> 1.8 mmol/L)	
Arterial Po₂ of < 60 mm Hg (< 7.8 kPa)	
Serum calcium of < 8 mg/dL (< 0.2 mmol/L)	
Base deficit over 4 mEq/L	
Estimated fluid sequestration of > 6 L	

Mortality rates correlate with the number of criteria present[1]

Number of Criteria	Mortality Rate
0–2	1%
3–4	16%
5–6	40%
7–8	100%

[1]An APACHE II score ≥ 8 also correlates with mortality.

a rise in blood urea nitrogen within the first 24 hours of hospitalization are independently associated with increased mortality; the greater the rise in blood urea nitrogen after admission, the greater the mortality rate. A model based on the change in serum amylase in the first 2 days after admission and the body mass index has been proposed. An early rise in serum levels of neutrophil gelatinase-associated lipocalin has also been proposed as a marker of severe acute pancreatitis. The absence of rebound abdominal tenderness or guarding, a normal hematocrit value, and a normal serum creatinine level (the "**harmless acute**

pancreatitis score," or **HAPS**) predicts a nonsevere course with 98% accuracy. The **revised Atlanta classification** of the severity of acute pancreatitis uses the following three categories: (1) **mild** disease is the absence of organ failure and local ([peri]pancreatic necrosis or fluid collections) or systemic complications; (2) **moderate** disease is the presence of transient (under 48 hours) organ failure or local or systemic complications, or both; and (3) **severe** disease is the presence of persistent (48 hours or more) organ failure. A similar "determinant-based" classification includes a category of critical acute pancreatitis characterized by both persistent organ failure and infected peripancreatic necrosis.

D. Imaging

Plain radiographs of the abdomen may show gallstones (if calcified), a "sentinel loop" (a segment of air-filled small intestine most commonly in the left upper quadrant), the "colon cutoff sign"—a gas-filled segment of transverse colon abruptly ending at the area of pancreatic inflammation—or focal linear atelectasis of the lower lobe of the lungs with or without pleural effusion. Ultrasonography is often not helpful in diagnosing acute pancreatitis because of intervening bowel gas but may identify gallstones in the gallbladder. Unenhanced CT is useful for demonstrating an enlarged pancreas when the diagnosis of pancreatitis is uncertain, differentiating pancreatitis from other possible intra-abdominal catastrophes, and providing an initial assessment of prognosis but is often unnecessary early in the course (Table 16–10). Rapid-bolus intravenous contrast-enhanced CT following aggressive volume resuscitation is of particular value after the first 3 days of severe acute pancreatitis for identifying areas of necrotizing pancreatitis and assessing the degree of necrosis, although the use of intravenous contrast may increase the risk of complications of pancreatitis and of acute kidney injury and should be avoided when the serum creatinine level is above 1.5 mg/dL (124.95 mcmol/L). MRI appears to be a suitable alternative to CT. Perfusion CT on day 3 demonstrating areas of ischemia in the pancreas has been reported to predict the development of pancreatic necrosis. The

Table 16–10. Severity index for acute pancreatitis.

CT Grade	Points	Pancreatic Necrosis	Additional Points	Severity Index[1]	Mortality Rate[2]
A Normal pancreas	0	0%	0	0	0%
B Pancreatic enlargement	1	0%	0	1	0%
C Pancreatic inflammation and/or peripancreatic fat	2	< 30%	2	4	< 3%
D Single acute peripancreatic fluid collection	3	30–50%	4	7	6%
E Two or more acute peripancreatic fluid collections or retroperitoneal air	4	> 50%	6	10	> 17%

[1]Severity Index = CT Grade *Points* + Pancreatic Necrosis *Additional Points*.
[2]Based on the Severity Index.
Adapted with permission from Balthazar EJ. Acute pancreatitis: assessment of severity with clinical and CT evaluation. Radiology. 2002 Jun;223(3):603–13.

presence of a fluid collection in the pancreas correlates with an increased mortality rate. CT-guided needle aspiration of areas of necrotizing pancreatitis after the third day may disclose infection, usually by enteric organisms, which typically requires debridement. The presence of gas bubbles on CT implies infection by gas-forming organisms. EUS is useful in identifying occult biliary disease (eg, small stones, sludge, microlithiasis), which is present in a majority of patients with apparently idiopathic acute pancreatitis, and is indicated in persons over age 40 to exclude malignancy. ERCP is generally not indicated after a first attack of acute pancreatitis unless there is associated cholangitis or jaundice or a bile duct stone is known to be present, but EUS or MRCP should be considered, especially after repeated attacks of idiopathic acute pancreatitis. In selected cases, aspiration of bile for crystal analysis may confirm the suspicion of microlithiasis, and manometry of the pancreatic duct sphincter may detect sphincter of Oddi dysfunction as a cause of recurrent pancreatitis.

▶ Differential Diagnosis

Acute pancreatitis must be differentiated from an acutely perforated duodenal ulcer, acute cholecystitis, acute intestinal obstruction, leaking aortic aneurysm, renal colic, and acute mesenteric ischemia. Serum amylase may also be elevated in high intestinal obstruction, in gastroenteritis, in mumps not involving the pancreas (salivary amylase), in ectopic pregnancy, after administration of opioids, and after abdominal surgery. Serum lipase may also be elevated in many of these conditions.

▶ Complications

Intravascular volume depletion secondary to leakage of fluids in the pancreatic bed and ileus with fluid-filled loops of bowel may result in prerenal azotemia and even acute tubular necrosis without overt shock. This sequence usually occurs within 24 hours of the onset of acute pancreatitis and lasts 8–9 days. Some patients require renal replacement therapy.

According to the revised Atlanta classification, fluid collections and necrosis may be acute (within the first 4 weeks) or chronic (after 4 weeks) and sterile or infected. Chronic collections, including pseudocysts and walled-off necrosis, are characterized by encapsulation. Sterile or infected necrotizing pancreatitis may complicate the course of 5–10% of cases and accounts for most of the deaths. The risk of infection does not correlate with the extent of necrosis. Pancreatic necrosis is often associated with fever, leukocytosis, and, in some cases, shock and is associated with organ failure (eg, gastrointestinal bleeding, respiratory failure, acute kidney injury) in 50% of cases. Because infected pancreatic necrosis is often an indication for debridement, fine-needle aspiration of necrotic tissue under CT guidance should be performed (if necessary, repeatedly) for Gram stain and culture.

A serious complication of acute pancreatitis is acute respiratory distress syndrome (ARDS); cardiac dysfunction may be superimposed. It usually occurs 3–7 days after the onset of pancreatitis in patients who have required large volumes of fluid and colloid to maintain blood pressure and urinary output. Most patients with ARDS require intubation, mechanical ventilation, and supplemental oxygen.

Pancreatic abscess (also referred to as infected or suppurative pseudocyst) is a suppurative process characterized by rising fever, leukocytosis, and localized tenderness and an epigastric mass usually 6 or more weeks into the course of acute pancreatitis. The abscess may be associated with a left-sided pleural effusion or an enlarging spleen secondary to splenic vein thrombosis. In contrast to infected necrosis, the mortality rate is low following drainage.

Pseudocysts, encapsulated fluid collections with high amylase content, commonly appear in pancreatitis when CT is used to monitor the evolution of an acute attack. Pseudocysts that are smaller than 6 cm in diameter often resolve spontaneously. They most commonly are within or adjacent to the pancreas but can present almost anywhere (eg, mediastinal, retrorectal) by extension along anatomic planes. Multiple pseudocysts are seen in 14% of cases. Pseudocysts may become secondarily infected, necessitating drainage as for an abscess. Pancreatic ascites may present after recovery from acute pancreatitis as a gradual increase in abdominal girth and persistent elevation of the serum amylase level in the absence of frank abdominal pain. Marked elevations in ascitic protein (greater than 3 g/dL) and amylase (greater than 1000 units/L [20 mkat/L]) concentrations are typical. The condition results from disruption of the pancreatic duct or drainage of a pseudocyst into the peritoneal cavity.

Rare complications of acute pancreatitis include hemorrhage caused by erosion of a blood vessel to form a pseudoaneurysm and colonic necrosis. Portosplenomesenteric venous thrombosis frequently develops in patients with necrotizing acute pancreatitis but rarely leads to complications. Chronic pancreatitis develops in about 10% of cases. Permanent diabetes mellitus and exocrine pancreatic insufficiency occur uncommonly after a single acute episode.

▶ Treatment

A. Treatment of Acute Disease

1. Mild disease—In most patients, acute pancreatitis is a mild disease ("nonsevere acute pancreatitis") that subsides spontaneously within several days. The pancreas is "rested" by a regimen of withholding food and liquids by mouth, bed rest, and, in patients with moderately severe pain or ileus and abdominal distention or vomiting, nasogastric suction. Early fluid resuscitation (one-third of the total 72-hour fluid volume administered within 24 hours of presentation, 250–500 mL/h initially) may reduce the frequency of systemic inflammatory response syndrome and organ failure in this group of patients, and lactated Ringer solution may be preferable to normal saline; however, overly aggressive fluid resuscitation may lead to morbidity as well. Pain is controlled with meperidine, up to 100–150 mg intramuscularly every 3–4 hours as necessary. In those with severe liver or kidney dysfunction, the dose may need to be reduced. Morphine had been thought to cause sphincter of Oddi spasm but is now considered an acceptable alternative and, given the potential side effects of meperidine, may even be preferable. Oral intake of fluid and foods can be resumed when the patient is largely free of pain and has bowel sounds (even if the serum amylase is still elevated). Clear liquids are given first (this step may be skipped in patients with mild acute pancreatitis), followed by gradual advancement to a low-fat diet, guided by the patient's tolerance and by the absence of pain. Pain may recur on refeeding in 20% of patients. Following recovery from acute biliary pancreatitis, laparoscopic cholecystectomy is generally performed, preferably during the same hospital admission, and is associated with a reduced rate of recurrent gallstone-related complications compared with delayed cholecystectomy. In selected cases endoscopic sphincterotomy alone may be done. In patients with recurrent pancreatitis associated with pancreas divisum, insertion of a stent in the minor papilla (or minor papilla sphincterotomy) may reduce the frequency of subsequent attacks, although complications of such therapy are frequent. In patients with recurrent acute pancreatitis attributed to pancreatic sphincter of Oddi dysfunction, biliary sphincterotomy alone is as effective as combined biliary and pancreatic sphincterotomy in reducing the frequency of recurrent acute pancreatitis, but chronic pancreatitis may still develop in treated patients. Hypertriglyceridemia with acute pancreatitis has been treated with insulin, heparin, or apheresis, but the benefit of these approaches has not been proven.

2. Severe disease—In more severe pancreatitis—particularly necrotizing pancreatitis—there may be considerable leakage of fluids, necessitating large amounts of intravenous fluids (eg, 500–1000 mL/h for several hours, then 250–300 mL/h) to maintain intravascular volume. Risk factors for high levels of fluid sequestration include younger age, alcohol etiology, higher hematocrit value, higher serum glucose, and systemic inflammatory response syndrome in the first 48 hours of hospital admission. Hemodynamic monitoring in an intensive care unit is required, and the importance of aggressive intravenous hydration targeted to result in adequate urinary output, stabilization of blood pressure and heart rate, restoration of central venous pressure, and a modest decrease in hematocrit value cannot be overemphasized. Calcium gluconate must be given intravenously if there is evidence of hypocalcemia with tetany. Infusions of fresh frozen plasma or serum albumin may be necessary in patients with coagulopathy or hypoalbuminemia. With colloid solutions, the risk of ARDS may be increased. If shock persists after adequate volume replacement (including packed red cells), pressors may be required. For the patient requiring a large volume of parenteral fluids, central venous pressure and blood gases should be monitored at regular intervals. Enteral nutrition via a nasojejunal or possibly nasogastric feeding tube is preferable to parenteral nutrition in patients who will otherwise be without oral nutrition for at least 7–10 days and reduces the risk of multiorgan failure and mortality when started within 48 hours of admission, but may not be tolerated in some patients with an ileus and does not reduce the rates of infection and death compared with the introduction of an oral diet after 72 hours. Parenteral nutrition (including lipids) should be considered in patients who have severe pancreatitis and ileus; glutamine supplementation appears to reduce the risk of infectious complications and mortality. The routine use of antibiotics to prevent conversion of sterile pancreatic necrosis to infected necrosis is still controversial and generally is not indicated in those with less than 30% pancreatic necrosis. Imipenem (500 mg every 8 hours intravenously) and possibly cefuroxime (1.5 g intravenously three times daily, then 250 mg orally twice daily) administered for no more than 14 days to patients with sterile pancreatic necrosis has been reported in some studies to reduce the risk of pancreatic infection and mortality; meropenem and the combination of ciprofloxacin and metronidazole do not appear to reduce the frequency of infected necrosis, multiorgan failure, or mortality. When infected necrosis is confirmed, imipenem or meropenem should be continued. In occasional cases, a fungal infection is found, and appropriate antifungal therapy should be prescribed. The role of intravenous somatostatin in severe acute pancreatitis is uncertain, and octreotide is thought to have no benefit. A small study has suggested benefit from pentoxifylline. To date, probiotic agents have not been shown to reduce infectious complications of severe pancreatitis and may increase mortality. Nonsteroidal anti-inflammatory drugs (eg, indomethacin administered rectally) and aggressive hydration with lactated Ringer solution have been reported to reduce the frequency and severity of post-ERCP pancreatitis in persons at high risk, and rectal indomethacin has become standard practice. There is some evidence that the risk of pancreatitis after ERCP can be reduced by the administration of somatostatin, octreotide, nafamostat and other protease inhibitors, ulinastatin, and nitroglycerin, but further studies are needed. Placement of a stent across the pancreatic duct or orifice has been shown to reduce the risk of post-ERCP pancreatitis and is a common practice but has not been compared directly with rectal indomethacin.

B. Treatment of Complications and Follow-Up

A surgeon should be consulted in all cases of severe acute pancreatitis. If the diagnosis is in doubt and investigation indicates a strong possibility of a serious surgically correctable lesion (eg, perforated peptic ulcer), exploratory laparotomy is indicated. When acute pancreatitis is found unexpectedly, it is usually wise to close without intervention. If the pancreatitis appears mild and cholelithiasis or microlithiasis is present, cholecystectomy or cholecystostomy may be justified. When severe pancreatitis results from choledocholithiasis and jaundice (serum total bilirubin above 5 mg/dL [85.5 mcmol/L]) or cholangitis is present, ERCP with endoscopic sphincterotomy and stone extraction is indicated. MRCP may be useful in selecting patients for therapeutic ERCP. Endoscopic sphincterotomy does not appear to improve the outcome of severe pancreatitis in the absence of cholangitis or jaundice.

Necrosectomy may improve survival in patients with necrotizing pancreatitis and clinical deterioration with multiorgan failure or lack of resolution by 4 weeks and is often indicated for infected necrosis, although a select group of relatively stable patients with infected pancreatic necrosis may be managed with antibiotics alone. The goal is to debride necrotic pancreas and surrounding tissue and establish adequate drainage. Outcomes are best if necrosectomy is delayed until the necrosis has organized, usually about 4 weeks after disease onset. A "step-up" approach in which nonsurgical drainage of walled-off pancreatic necrosis under radiologic guidance with subsequent open surgical necrosectomy if necessary has been shown to reduce mortality and resource utilization in selected patients with necrotizing pancreatitis and confirmed or suspected secondary infection. Endoscopic (transgastric or transduodenal) drainage combined with percutaneous drainage and, in some cases, laparoscopic guidance are additional options, depending on local expertise. Treatment is labor intensive, and multiple procedures are often required. Peritoneal lavage has not been shown to improve survival in severe acute pancreatitis, in part because the risk of late septic complications is not reduced.

The development of a pancreatic abscess is an indication for prompt percutaneous or surgical drainage. Chronic pseudocysts require endoscopic, percutaneous catheter, or surgical drainage when infected or associated with persisting pain, pancreatitis, or bile duct obstruction. For pancreatic infections, imipenem, 500 mg every 8 hours intravenously, is a good choice of antibiotic because it achieves bactericidal levels in pancreatic tissue for most causative organisms. Pancreatic duct leaks and fistulas may require endoscopic or surgical therapy.

▶ Prognosis

Mortality rates for acute pancreatitis have declined from at least 10% to around 5% since the 1980s, but the mortality rate for severe acute pancreatitis (more than three Ranson criteria; Table 16–9) remains at least 20%, with rates of 10% and 25% in those with sterile and infected necrosis, respectively. Severe acute pancreatitis is predicted by features of the systemic inflammatory response on admission; a persistent systemic inflammatory response is associated with a mortality rate of 25% and a transient response with a mortality rate of 8%. Half of the deaths occur within the first 2 weeks, usually from multiorgan failure. Multiorgan failure is associated with a mortality rate of at least 30%, and if it persists beyond the first 48 hours, the mortality rate is over 50%. Later deaths occur because of complications of infected necrosis. The risk of death doubles when both organ failure and infected necrosis are present. Moreover, hospital-acquired infections increase the mortality of acute pancreatitis, independent of severity. Readmission to the hospital for acute pancreatitis within 30 days may be predicted by a scoring system based on five factors during the index admission: eating less than a solid diet at discharge; nausea, vomiting, or diarrhea at discharge; pancreatic necrosis; use of antibiotics at discharge; and pain at discharge. Male sex, an alcohol etiology, and severe acute disease are risk factors. Recurrences are common in alcoholic pancreatitis but can be reduced by repeated, regularly scheduled interventions to eliminate alcohol consumption

after discharge from the hospital. A severe initial attack and smoking also increase the risk of recurrence. The risk of chronic pancreatitis following an episode of acute alcoholic pancreatitis is 13% in 10 years and 16% in 20 years, and the risk of diabetes mellitus is increased more than twofold over 5 years. Overall, chronic pancreatitis develops in 36% of patients with recurrent acute pancreatitis; alcohol use and smoking are principal risk factors.

▶ When to Admit

Nearly all patients with acute pancreatitis should be hospitalized.

Bertilsson S et al. Factors that affect disease progression after first attack of acute pancreatitis. Clin Gastroenterol Hepatol. 2015 Sep;13(9):1662–9.e3. [PMID: 25911118]

Choksi NS et al; United States Cooperative for Outcomes Research in Endoscopy. The risk of post-ERCP pancreatitis and the protective effect of rectal indomethacin in cases of attempted but unsuccessful prophylactic pancreatic stent placement. Gastrointest Endosc. 2015 Jan;81(1):150–5. [PMID: 25527053]

da Costa DW et al; Dutch Pancreatitis Study Group. Same-admission versus interval cholecystectomy for mild gallstone pancreatitis (PONCHO): a multicentre randomised controlled trial. Lancet. 2015 Sep 26;386(10000):1261–8. [PMID: 26460661]

Kubiliun NM et al; United States Cooperative for Outcomes Research in Endoscopy (USCORE). Evaluation of pharmacologic prevention of pancreatitis after endoscopic retrograde cholangiopancreatography: a systematic review. Clin Gastroenterol Hepatol. 2015 Jul;13(7):1231–9. [PMID: 25579870]

Kumaravel A et al. A model to predict the severity of acute pancreatitis based on serum level of amylase and body mass index. Clin Gastroenterol Hepatol. 2015 Aug;13(8):1496–501. [PMID: 25818080]

Lankisch PG et al. Acute pancreatitis. Lancet. 2015 Jul 4; 386(9988):85–96. [PMID: 25616312]

CHRONIC PANCREATITIS

 ESSENTIALS OF DIAGNOSIS

- ▶ Chronic or intermittent epigastric pain, steatorrhea, weight loss, abnormal pancreatic imaging.

- ▶ A mnemonic for the predisposing factors of chronic pancreatitis is TIGAR-O: toxic-metabolic, idiopathic, genetic, autoimmune, recurrent and severe acute pancreatitis, or obstructive.

▶ General Considerations

Chronic pancreatitis occurs most often in patients with alcoholism (45–80% of all cases). The risk of chronic pancreatitis increases with the duration and amount of alcohol consumed, but pancreatitis develops in only 5–10% of heavy drinkers. Tobacco smoking is a risk factor for idiopathic chronic pancreatitis and has been reported to accelerate progression of alcoholic chronic pancreatitis. About 2% of patients with hyperparathyroidism develop pancreatitis. In tropical Africa and Asia, tropical pancreatitis, related in part to malnutrition, is the most common cause of chronic pancreatitis. A stricture, stone, or tumor obstructing the pancreas can lead to obstructive chronic pancreatitis. Autoimmune pancreatitis is associated with hypergammaglobulinemia (IgG_4 in particular), often with autoantibodies and other autoimmune diseases, and is responsive to corticosteroids. Affected persons are at increased risk for various cancers. Type 1 autoimmune pancreatitis (or simply "autoimmune pancreatitis") is a multisystem disease characterized by lymphoplasmacytic sclerosing pancreatitis on biopsy, associated bile duct strictures, retroperitoneal fibrosis, renal and salivary gland lesions, and a high rate of relapse after treatment. It is the pancreatic manifestation of IgG_4-related disease. Type 2 ("idiopathic duct-centric chronic pancreatitis") affects the pancreas alone and is characterized by duct-centric pancreatitis on biopsy, lack of systemic IgG_4 involvement, an association with inflammatory bowel disease in 25% of cases, often a tumor-like mass, and a low rate of relapse after treatment. Between 10% and 30% of cases of chronic pancreatitis are idiopathic, with either early onset (median age 23) or late onset (median age 62). Genetic factors may predispose to chronic pancreatitis in some of these cases and include mutations of the cystic fibrosis transmembrane conductance regulator (*CFTR*) gene, the pancreatic secretory trypsin inhibitory gene (*PSTI*, serine protease inhibitor, *SPINK1*), and possibly the gene for uridine 5′-diphosphate glucuronosyltransferase. Mutation of the cationic trypsinogen gene on chromosome 7 (serine protease 1, *PRSS1*) is associated with hereditary pancreatitis, transmitted as an autosomal dominant trait with variable penetrance. A useful mnemonic for the predisposing factors to chronic pancreatitis is TIGAR-O: toxic-metabolic, idiopathic, genetic, autoimmune, recurrent and severe acute pancreatitis, or obstructive.

The pathogenesis of chronic pancreatitis may be explained by the SAPE (sentinel *a*cute *p*ancreatitis *e*vent) hypothesis by which the first (sentinel) acute pancreatitis event initiates an inflammatory process that results in injury and later fibrosis ("necrosis-fibrosis"). In many cases, chronic pancreatitis is a self-perpetuating disease characterized by chronic pain or recurrent episodes of acute pancreatitis and ultimately by pancreatic exocrine or endocrine insufficiency (sooner in alcoholic pancreatitis than in other types). After many years, chronic pain may resolve spontaneously or as a result of surgery tailored to the cause of pain. Over 80% of adults develop diabetes mellitus within 25 years after the clinical onset of chronic pancreatitis.

▶ Clinical Findings

A. Symptoms and Signs

Persistent or recurrent episodes of epigastric and left upper quadrant pain are typical. The pain results in part from impaired inhibitory pain modulation by the central nervous system. Anorexia, nausea, vomiting, constipation, flatulence, and weight loss are common. During attacks, tenderness over the pancreas, mild muscle guarding, and

ileus may be noted. Attacks may last only a few hours or as long as 2 weeks; pain may eventually be almost continuous. Steatorrhea (as indicated by bulky, foul, fatty stools) may occur late in the course.

B. Laboratory Findings

Serum amylase and lipase may be elevated during acute attacks; however, normal values do not exclude the diagnosis. Serum alkaline phosphatase and bilirubin may be elevated owing to compression of the bile duct. Glycosuria may be present. Excess fecal fat may be demonstrated on chemical analysis of the stool. Pancreatic insufficiency generally is confirmed by response to therapy with pancreatic enzyme supplements; the secretin stimulation test can be used if available (and has a high negative predictive factor for ruling out early acute chronic pancreatitis), as can detection of decreased fecal chymotrypsin or elastase levels, although the latter tests lack sensitivity and specificity. Vitamin B_{12} malabsorption is detectable in about 40% of patients, but clinical deficiency of vitamin B_{12} and fat-soluble vitamins is rare. Accurate diagnostic tests are available for the major trypsinogen gene mutations, but because of uncertainty about the mechanisms linking heterozygous *CFTR* and *PSTI* mutations with pancreatitis, genetic testing for mutations in these two genes is not currently recommended. Elevated IgG_4 levels, ANA, and antibodies to lactoferrin and carbonic anhydrase II are often found in patients with autoimmune pancreatitis (especially type 1). Pancreatic biopsy, if necessary, shows a lymphoplasmacytic inflammatory infiltrate with characteristic IgG_4 immunostaining, which is also found in biopsy specimens of the major papilla, bile duct, and salivary glands, in type 1 autoimmune pancreatitis.

C. Imaging

Plain films show calcifications due to pancreaticolithiasis in 30% of affected patients. CT may show calcifications not seen on plain films as well as ductal dilatation and heterogeneity or atrophy of the gland. Occasionally, the findings raise suspicion of pancreatic cancer ("tumefactive chronic pancreatitis"). ERCP is the most sensitive imaging study for chronic pancreatitis and may show dilated ducts, intraductal stones, strictures, or pseudocyst but is infrequently used for diagnosis alone; moreover, the results may be normal in patients with so-called minimal change pancreatitis. MRCP (including secretin-enhanced MRCP) and EUS (with pancreatic tissue sampling) are less invasive alternatives to ERCP. Endoscopic ultrasonographic ("Rosemont") criteria for the diagnosis of chronic pancreatitis include hyperechoic foci with shadowing indicative of calculi in the main pancreatic duct and lobularity with honeycombing of the pancreatic parenchyma. Characteristic imaging features of autoimmune pancreatitis include diffuse enlargement of the pancreas, a peripheral rim of hypoattenuation, and irregular narrowing of the main pancreatic duct. In the United States, the diagnosis of autoimmune pancreatitis is based on the HISORt criteria: *his*tology, *i*maging, *s*erology, *o*ther *o*rgan involvement, and *r*esponse to corticosteroid *t*herapy.

Complications

Opioid addiction is common. Other frequent complications include often brittle diabetes mellitus, pancreatic pseudocyst or abscess, cholestatic liver enzymes with or without jaundice, bile duct stricture, steatorrhea, malnutrition, osteoporosis, and peptic ulcer. Pancreatic cancer develops in 4% of patients after 20 years; the risk may relate to tobacco and alcohol use. In patients with hereditary pancreatitis, the risk of pancreatic cancer rises after age 50 years and reaches 19% by age 70 years (see Chapter 39).

Treatment

Correctable coexistent biliary tract disease should be treated surgically.

A. Medical Measures

A low-fat diet should be prescribed. Alcohol is forbidden because it frequently precipitates attacks. Opioids should be avoided if possible. Preferred agents for pain are acetaminophen, nonsteroidal anti-inflammatory drugs, and tramadol, along with pain-modifying agents such as tricyclic antidepressants, selective serotonin reuptake inhibitors, and gabapentin or pregabalin. Steatorrhea is treated with pancreatic supplements that are selected on the basis of their high lipase activity (Table 16–11). A total dose of at least 40,000 units of lipase in capsules is given with each meal (during and after the meal). Doses of 90,000 units or more of lipase per meal may be required in some cases. The tablets should be taken at the start of, during, and at the end of a meal. Concurrent administration of a H_2-receptor antagonist (eg, ranitidine, 150 mg orally twice daily), a proton pump inhibitor (eg, omeprazole, 20–60 mg orally daily), or sodium bicarbonate, 650 mg orally before and after meals, decreases the inactivation of lipase by acid and may thereby further decrease steatorrhea. In selected cases of alcoholic pancreatitis and in cystic fibrosis, enteric-coated microencapsulated preparations may offer an advantage. However, in patients with cystic fibrosis, high-dose pancreatic enzyme therapy has been associated with strictures of the ascending colon. Pain secondary to idiopathic chronic pancreatitis may be alleviated in some cases by the use of pancreatic enzymes (not enteric-coated) or octreotide, 200 mcg subcutaneously three times daily. Associated diabetes mellitus should be treated (see Chapter 27). Autoimmune pancreatitis is treated with prednisone 40 mg/day orally for 1–2 months, followed by a taper of 5 mg every 2–4 weeks. Nonresponse or relapse occurs in 45% of type 1 cases (particularly in those with concomitant IgG_4-associated cholangitis); rituximab is an effective induction and maintenance agent, and azathioprine appears to reduce the risk of relapse.

B. Endoscopic and Surgical Treatment

Endoscopic therapy or surgery may be indicated in chronic pancreatitis to treat underlying biliary tract disease, ensure free flow of bile into the duodenum, drain persistent pseudocysts, treat other complications, eliminate obstruction of the pancreatic duct, attempt to relieve pain, or exclude

Table 16–11. FDA-approved pancreatic enzyme (pancrelipase) preparations.

Product	Enzyme Content/Unit Dose, USP Units		
	Lipase	Amylase	Protease
Immediate-Release Capsule			
Nonenteric-coated			
Viokace 10,440	10,440	39,150	39,150
Viokace 20,880	20,880	78,300	78,300
Delayed-Release Capsules			
Enteric-coated minimicrospheres			
Creon 3000	3000	15,000	9500
Creon 6000	6000	30,000	19,000
Creon 12,000	12,000	60,000	38,000
Creon 24,000	24,000	120,000	76,000
Creon 36,000	36,000	180,000	114,000
Enteric-coated minitablets			
Ultresa 13,800	13,800	27,600	27,600
Ultresa 20,700	20,700	46,000	41,400
Ultresa 23,000	23,000	46,000	41,400
Enteric-coated beads			
Zenpep 3000	3000	16,000	10,000
Zenpep 5000	5000	27,000	17,000
Zenpep 10,000	10,000	55,000	34,000
Zenpep 15,000	15,000	82,000	51,000
Zenpep 20,000	20,000	109,000	68,000
Zenpep 25,000	25,000	136,000	85,000
Enteric-coated microtablets			
Pancreaze 4200	4200	17,500	10,000
Pancreaze 10,500	10,500	43,750	25,000
Pancreaze 16,800	16,800	70,000	40,000
Pancreaze 21,000	21,000	61,000	37,000
Bicarbonate-buffered enteric-coated microspheres			
Peptyze 8000	8000	30,250	28,750
Peptyze 16,000	16,000	60,500	57,500

FDA, US Food and Drug Administration; USP, US Pharmacopeia.

pancreatic cancer. Liver fibrosis may regress after biliary drainage. Distal bile duct obstruction may be relieved by endoscopic placement of multiple bile duct stents. When obstruction of the duodenal end of the pancreatic duct can be demonstrated by ERCP, dilation of or placement of a stent in the duct and pancreatic duct stone lithotripsy or surgical resection of the tail of the pancreas with implantation of the distal end of the duct by pancreaticojejunostomy may be performed. Endoscopic therapy is successful in about 50% of cases. In patients who do not respond to endoscopic therapy, surgery is successful in about 50%.

When the pancreatic duct is diffusely dilated, anastomosis between the duct after it is split longitudinally and a defunctionalized limb of jejunum (modified Puestow procedure), in some cases combined with resection of the head of the pancreas (Beger or Frey procedure), is associated with relief of pain in 80% of cases. In advanced cases, subtotal or total pancreatectomy may be considered as a last resort but has variable efficacy and causes pancreatic insufficiency and diabetes mellitus. Perioperative administration of somatostatin or octreotide may reduce the risk of postoperative pancreatic fistulas. Endoscopic or surgical (including laparoscopic) drainage is indicated for symptomatic pseudocysts and, in many cases, those over 6 cm in diameter. EUS may facilitate selection of an optimal site for endoscopic drainage. Pancreatic ascites or pancreaticopleural fistulas due to a disrupted pancreatic duct can be managed by endoscopic placement of a stent across the disrupted duct. Pancreatic sphincterotomy or fragmentation of stones in the pancreatic duct by lithotripsy and endoscopic removal of stones from the duct may relieve pain in selected patients. For patients with chronic pain and nondilated ducts, a percutaneous celiac plexus nerve block may be considered under either CT or endoscopic ultrasound guidance, with pain relief (albeit often short-lived) in approximately 50% of patients. A single session of radiation therapy to the pancreas has been reported to relieve otherwise refractory pain.

Prognosis

Chronic pancreatitis often leads to disability and reduced life expectancy; pancreatic cancer is the main cause of death. The prognosis is best in patients with recurrent acute pancreatitis caused by a remediable condition, such as cholelithiasis, choledocholithiasis, stenosis of the sphincter of Oddi, or hyperparathyroidism, and in those with autoimmune pancreatitis. Medical management of hyperlipidemia, if present, may also prevent recurrent attacks of pancreatitis. In alcoholic pancreatitis, pain relief is most likely when a dilated pancreatic duct can be decompressed. In patients with disease not amenable to decompressive surgery, addiction to opioids is a frequent outcome of treatment. The quality of life is poorer in patients with constant pain than in those with intermittent pain.

When to Refer

All patients with chronic pancreatitis should be referred for diagnostic and therapeutic procedures.

When to Admit

- Severe pain.
- New jaundice.
- New fever.

Bang UC et al. Mortality, cancer, and comorbidities associated with chronic pancreatitis: a Danish nationwide matched-cohort study. Gastroenterology. 2014 Apr;146(4):989–94. [PMID: 24389306]

Hart PA et al. Recent advances in autoimmune pancreatitis. Gastroenterology. 2015 Jul;149(1):39–51. [PMID: 25770706]

Kamisawa T et al. IgG$_4$-related disease. Lancet. 2015 Apr 11; 385(9976):1460–71. [PMID: 25481618]

Wilcox CM et al. Chronic pancreatitis pain pattern and severity are independent of abdominal imaging findings. Clin Gastroenterol Hepatol. 2015 Mar;13(3):552–60. [PMID: 25424572]

Breast Disorders

Armando E. Giuliano, MD

Sara A. Hurvitz, MD

FIBROCYSTIC CONDITION

ESSENTIALS OF DIAGNOSIS

- ► Painful, often multiple, usually bilateral masses in the breast.
- ► Rapid fluctuation in the size of the masses is common.
- ► Frequently, pain occurs or worsens and size increases during premenstrual phase of cycle.
- ► Most common age is 30–50. Rare in postmenopausal women not receiving hormonal replacement.

► General Considerations

Fibrocystic condition is the most frequent lesion of the breast. Although commonly referred to as "fibrocystic disease," it does not, in fact, represent a pathologic or anatomic disorder. It is common in women 30–50 years of age but rare in postmenopausal women who are not taking hormonal replacement. Estrogen is considered a causative factor. There may be an increased risk in women who drink alcohol, especially women between 18 and 22 years of age.

The microscopic findings of fibrocystic condition include cysts (gross and microscopic), papillomatosis, adenosis, fibrosis, and ductal epithelial hyperplasia. Although fibrocystic condition has generally been considered to increase the risk of subsequent breast cancer, only the variants with a component of epithelial proliferation (especially with atypia), papillomatosis, or increased breast density on mammogram represent true risk factors.

► Clinical Findings

A. Symptoms and Signs

Fibrocystic condition may produce an asymptomatic mass in the breast that is discovered by accident, but pain or tenderness often calls attention to it. Discomfort often occurs or worsens during the premenstrual phase of the cycle, at which time the cysts tend to enlarge. Fluctuations in size and rapid appearance or disappearance of a breast mass are common with this condition as are multiple or bilateral masses and serous nipple discharge. Patients will give a history of a transient lump in the breast or cyclic breast pain.

B. Diagnostic Tests

Mammography and ultrasonography should be used to evaluate a mass in a patient with fibrocystic condition. Ultrasonography alone may be used in women under 30 years of age. Because a mass due to fibrocystic condition is difficult to distinguish from carcinoma on the basis of clinical findings, suspicious lesions should be biopsied. Core needle biopsy, rather than fine-needle aspiration (FNA), is the preferable technique. Excisional biopsy is rarely necessary but should be done for lesions with atypia or where imaging and biopsy results are discordant. Surgery should be conservative, since the primary objective is to exclude cancer. Occasionally, FNA cytology will suffice. Simple mastectomy or extensive removal of breast tissue is rarely, if ever, indicated for fibrocystic condition.

► Differential Diagnosis

Pain, fluctuation in size, and multiplicity of lesions are the features most helpful in differentiating fibrocystic condition from carcinoma. If a dominant mass is present, the diagnosis of cancer should be assumed until disproven by biopsy. Mammography may be helpful, but the breast tissue in these young women is usually too radiodense to permit a worthwhile study. Sonography is useful in differentiating a cystic mass from a solid mass, especially in women with dense breasts. Final diagnosis, however, depends on analysis of a biopsy specimen.

► Treatment

When the diagnosis of fibrocystic condition has been established by previous biopsy or is likely because the history is classic, aspiration of a discrete mass suggestive of a cyst is indicated to alleviate pain and, more importantly, to confirm the cystic nature of the mass. The patient is reexamined at intervals thereafter. If no fluid is obtained by aspiration, if fluid is bloody, if a mass persists after aspiration, or if at any time during follow-up a persistent or recurrent mass is noted, biopsy should be performed.

Breast pain associated with generalized fibrocystic condition is best treated by avoiding trauma and by wearing a good supportive brassiere during the night and day. Hormone therapy is not advisable, because it does not cure the condition and has undesirable side effects. Danazol (100–200 mg orally twice daily), a synthetic androgen, is the only treatment approved by the US Food and Drug Administration (FDA) for patients with severe pain. This treatment suppresses pituitary gonadotropins, but androgenic effects (acne, edema, hirsutism) usually make this treatment intolerable; in practice, it is rarely used. Similarly, tamoxifen reduces some symptoms of fibrocystic condition, but because of its side effects, it is not useful for young women unless it is given to reduce the risk of cancer. Postmenopausal women receiving hormone replacement therapy may stop or change doses of hormones to reduce pain. Oil of evening primrose, a natural form of gamolenic acid, has been shown to decrease pain in 44–58% of users. The dosage of gamolenic acid is six capsules of 500 mg orally twice daily. Studies have also demonstrated a low-fat diet or decreasing dietary fat intake may reduce the painful symptoms associated with fibrocystic condition. Topical treatments such as nonsteroidal anti-inflammatory drugs or anti-hormonal drugs such as tamoxifen are rarely of value.

The role of caffeine consumption in the development and treatment of fibrocystic condition is controversial. Some studies suggest that eliminating caffeine from the diet is associated with improvement while other studies refute the benefit entirely. Many patients are aware of these studies and report relief of symptoms after giving up coffee, tea, and chocolate. Similarly, many women find vitamin E (400 international units daily) helpful; however, these observations remain anecdotal.

▶ Prognosis

Exacerbations of pain, tenderness, and cyst formation may occur at any time until menopause, when symptoms usually subside, except in patients receiving hormonal replacement. The patient should be advised to examine her own breasts regularly just after menstruation and to inform her clinician if a mass appears. The risk of breast cancer developing in women with fibrocystic condition with a proliferative or atypical epithelial hyperplasia or papillomatosis is higher than that of the general population. These women should be monitored carefully with physical examinations and imaging studies.

Liu Y et al. Intakes of alcohol and folate during adolescence and risk of proliferative benign breast disease. Pediatrics. 2012 May;129(5):e1192–8. [PMID: 22492774]

Onstad M et al. Benign breast disorders. Obstet Gynecol Clin North Am. 2013 Sep;40(3):459–73. [PMID: 24021252]

FIBROADENOMA OF THE BREAST

This common benign neoplasm occurs most frequently in young women, usually within 20 years after puberty. It is somewhat more frequent and tends to occur at an earlier age in black women. Multiple tumors are found in 10–15% of patients.

The typical **fibroadenoma** is a round or ovoid, rubbery, discrete, relatively movable, nontender mass 1–5 cm in diameter. It is usually discovered accidentally. Clinical diagnosis in young patients is generally not difficult. In women over 30 years, fibrocystic condition of the breast and carcinoma of the breast must be considered. Cysts can be identified by aspiration or ultrasonography. Fibroadenoma does not normally occur after menopause but may occasionally develop after administration of hormones.

No treatment is usually necessary if the diagnosis can be made by core needle biopsy. Excision with pathologic examination of the specimen is performed if the diagnosis is uncertain or the lesion grows significantly. Cryoablation, or freezing of the fibroadenoma, appears to be a safe procedure if the lesion is a biopsy-proven fibroadenoma prior to ablation. Cryoablation is not appropriate for all fibroadenomas because some are too large to freeze or the diagnosis may not be certain. There is no obvious advantage to cryoablation of a histologically proven fibroadenoma except that some patients may feel relief that a mass is gone. However, at times a mass of scar or fat necrosis replaces the mass of the fibroadenoma. Reassurance seems preferable. It is usually not possible to distinguish a large fibroadenoma from a phyllodes tumor on the basis of needle biopsy results or imaging alone and histology is usually required. Presumed fibroadenomas larger than 3–4 cm should be excised to rule out phyllodes tumors.

Phyllodes tumor is a fibroadenoma-like tumor with cellular stroma that grows rapidly. It may reach a large size and, if inadequately excised, will recur locally. The lesion can be benign or malignant. If benign, phyllodes tumor is treated by local excision. The treatment of malignant phyllodes tumor is more controversial, but complete removal of the tumor with a margin of normal tissue avoids recurrence. Because these tumors may be large, total mastectomy is sometimes necessary. Lymph node dissection is not performed, since the sarcomatous portion of the tumor metastasizes to the lungs and not the lymph nodes.

Hubbard JL et al. Criteria for excision of suspected fibroadenomas of the breast. Am J Surg. 2015 Feb;209(2):297–301. [PMID: 25682095]

Sala MA et al. Indications for diagnostic open biopsy of mammographic screen-detected lesions preoperatively diagnosed as fibroadenomas by needle biopsy and their outcomes. Clin Radiol. 2015 May;70(5):507–14. [PMID: 25656661]

NIPPLE DISCHARGE

In order of decreasing frequency, the following are the most common causes of nipple discharge in the nonlactating breast: duct ectasia, intraductal papilloma, and carcinoma. The important characteristics of the discharge and

Table 17–1. Characteristics of nipple discharge in the nonpregnant, nonlactating woman.

Finding	Significance
Serous	Most likely benign FCC, ie, duct ectasia
Bloody	More likely neoplastic–papilloma, carcinoma
Associated mass	More likely neoplastic
Unilateral	Either neoplastic or non-neoplastic
Bilateral	Most likely non-neoplastic
Single duct	More likely neoplastic
Multiple ducts	More likely FCC
Milky	Endocrine disorders, medications
Spontaneous	Either neoplastic or non-neoplastic
Produced by pressure at single site	Either neoplastic or non-neoplastic
Persistent	Either neoplastic or non-neoplastic
Intermittent	Either neoplastic or non-neoplastic
Related to menses	More likely FCC
Premenopausal	More likely FCC
Taking hormones	More likely FCC

FCC, fibrocystic condition.

some other factors to be evaluated by history and physical examination are listed in Table 17–1.

Spontaneous, unilateral, serous or serosanguineous discharge from a single duct is usually caused by an ectatic duct or an intraductal papilloma or, rarely, by an intraductal cancer. A mass may not be palpable. The involved duct may be identified by pressure at different sites around the nipple at the margin of the areola. Bloody discharge is suggestive of cancer but is more often caused by a benign papilloma in the duct. Cytologic examination may identify malignant cells, but negative findings do not rule out cancer, which is more likely in women over age 50 years. In any case, the involved bloody duct—and a mass if present—should be excised. A ductogram (a mammogram of a duct after radiopaque dye has been injected), like cytology, is of limited value since excision of the suspicious ductal system is indicated regardless of findings. Ductoscopy, evaluation of the ductal system with a small scope inserted through the nipple, has been attempted but is not effective management.

In premenopausal women, spontaneous multiple duct discharge, unilateral or bilateral, most noticeable just before menstruation, is often due to fibrocystic condition. Discharge may be green or brownish. Papillomatosis and ductal ectasia are usually detected only by biopsy. If a mass is present, it should be removed.

A milky discharge from multiple ducts in the nonlactating breast may occur from hyperprolactinemia. Serum prolactin levels should be obtained to search for a pituitary tumor. Thyroid-stimulating hormone (TSH) helps exclude causative hypothyroidism. Numerous antipsychotic drugs and other drugs may also cause a milky discharge that ceases on discontinuance of the medication.

Oral contraceptive agents or estrogen replacement therapy may cause clear, serous, or milky discharge from a single duct, but multiple duct discharge is more common. In the premenopausal woman, the discharge is more evident just before menstruation and disappears on stopping the medication. If it does not stop, is from a single duct, and is copious, exploration should be performed since this may be a sign of cancer.

A purulent discharge may originate in a subareolar abscess and require removal of the abscess and the related lactiferous sinus.

When localization is not possible, no mass is palpable, and the discharge is nonbloody, the patient should be reexamined every 3 or 4 months for a year, and a mammogram and an ultrasound should be performed. Although most discharge is from a benign process, patients may find it annoying or disconcerting. To eliminate the discharge, proximal duct excision can be performed both for treatment and diagnosis.

Ashfaq A et al. Validation study of a modern treatment algorithm for nipple discharge. Am J Surg. 2014 Aug;208(2):222–7. [PMID: 24767970]

Morgan HS. Primary care management of the female patient presenting with nipple discharge. Nurse Pract. 2015 Mar 12; 40(3):1–6. [PMID: 25679138]

Patel BK et al. Management of nipple discharge and the associated imaging findings. Am J Med. 2015 Apr;128(4):353–60. [PMID: 25447625]

FAT NECROSIS

Fat necrosis is a rare lesion of the breast but is of clinical importance because it produces a mass (often accompanied by skin or nipple retraction) that is usually indistinguishable from carcinoma even with imaging studies. Trauma is presumed to be the cause, though only about 50% of patients give a history of injury. Ecchymosis is occasionally present. If untreated, the mass gradually disappears. The safest course is to obtain a biopsy. Core needle biopsy is often adequate, but frequently the entire mass must be excised to exclude carcinoma. Fat necrosis is common after segmental resection, radiation therapy, or flap reconstruction after mastectomy.

Kerridge WD et al. Fat necrosis of the breast: a pictorial review of the mammographic, ultrasound, CT, and MRI findings with histopathologic correlation. Radiol Res Pract. 2015;2015: 613139. [PMID: 25861475]

BREAST ABSCESS

During nursing, an area of redness, tenderness, and induration may develop in the breast. The organism most commonly found in these abscesses is *Staphylococcus aureus* (see Puerperal Mastitis, Chapter 19).

Infection in the nonlactating breast is rare. A subareolar abscess may develop in young or middle-aged women who

▲ **Figure 17–1.** Breast abscess and cellulitis. (Reproduced, with permission, from Richard P. Usatine, MD.)

are not lactating (Figure 17–1). These infections tend to recur after incision and drainage unless the area is explored during a quiescent interval, with excision of the involved lactiferous duct or ducts at the base of the nipple. In the nonlactating breast, inflammatory carcinoma must always be considered. Thus, incision and biopsy of any indurated tissue with a small piece of erythematous skin is indicated when suspected abscess or cellulitis in the nonlactating breast does not resolve promptly with antibiotics. Often needle or catheter drainage is adequate to treat an abscess, but surgical incision and drainage may be necessary.

Dixon JM. Breast infection. BMJ. 2013 Dec 16;347:f3291. [PMID: 24344239]
Trop I et al. Breast abscesses: evidence-based algorithms for diagnosis, management, and follow-up. Radiographics. 2011 Oct;31(6):1683–99. [PMID: 21997989]

DISORDERS OF THE AUGMENTED BREAST

At least 4 million American women have had breast implants. Breast augmentation is performed by placing implants under the pectoralis muscle or, less desirably, in the subcutaneous tissue of the breast. Most implants are made of an outer silicone shell filled with a silicone gel, saline, or some combination of the two. Capsule contraction or scarring around the implant develops in about 15–25% of patients, leading to a firmness and distortion of the breast that can be painful. Some require removal of the implant and surrounding capsule.

Implant rupture may occur in as many as 5–10% of women, and bleeding of gel through the capsule is noted even more commonly. Although silicone gel may be an immunologic stimulant, there is no increase in autoimmune disorders in patients with such implants. The FDA has advised symptomatic women with ruptured silicone implants to discuss possible surgical removal with their clinicians. However, women who are asymptomatic and have no evidence of rupture of a silicone gel prosthesis should probably not undergo removal of the implant.

Women with symptoms of autoimmune illnesses often undergo removal, but no benefit has been shown.

Studies have failed to show any association between implants and an increased incidence of breast cancer. However, breast cancer may develop in a patient with an augmentation prosthesis, as it does in women without them. Detection in patients with implants may be more difficult because mammography is less able to detect early lesions. Mammography is better if the implant is subpectoral rather than subcutaneous. Prostheses should be placed retropectorally after mastectomy to facilitate detection of a local recurrence of cancer, which is usually cutaneous or subcutaneous and is easily detected by palpation. Rarely lymphoma of the breast with silicone implants has been reported.

If a cancer develops in a patient with implants, it should be treated in the same manner as in women without implants. Such women should be offered the option of mastectomy or breast-conserving therapy, which may require removal or replacement of the implant. Radiotherapy of the augmented breast often results in marked capsular contracture. Adjuvant treatments should be given for the same indications as for women who have no implants.

Gidengil CA et al. Breast implant-associated anaplastic large cell lymphoma: a systematic review. Plast Reconstr Surg. 2015 Mar; 135(3):713–20. [PMID: 25490539]
Jewell ML. Silicone gel breast implants at 50: the state of the science. Aesthet Surg J. 2012 Nov;32(8):1031–4. [PMID: 23012658]
Lavigne E et al. Breast cancer detection and survival among women with cosmetic breast implants: systematic review and meta-analysis of observational studies. BMJ. 2013 Apr 29;346: f2399. [PMID: 23637132]

CARCINOMA OF THE FEMALE BREAST

 ESSENTIALS OF DIAGNOSIS

▶ Risk factors include age, delayed childbearing, positive family history of breast cancer or genetic mutations (*BRCA1*, *BRCA2*), and personal history of breast cancer or some types of proliferative conditions.

▶ **Early findings:** Single, nontender, firm to hard mass with ill-defined margins; mammographic abnormalities and no palpable mass.

▶ **Later findings:** Skin or nipple retraction; axillary lymphadenopathy; breast enlargement, erythema, edema, pain; fixation of mass to skin or chest wall.

▶ Incidence & Risk Factors

Breast cancer will develop in one of eight American women. Next to skin cancer, breast cancer is the most common cancer in women; it is second only to lung cancer as a cause of death. In 2015, there were approximately 234,190 new cases and 40,730 deaths from breast cancer in the

United States. In addition, an estimated 60,290 cases of breast carcinoma in situ were diagnosed in women in the United States, principally by screening mammography. Worldwide, breast cancer is diagnosed in approximately 1.38 million women, and about 458,000 die of breast cancer each year, with the highest rates of diagnosis in Western and Northern Europe, Australia, New Zealand, and North America and lowest rates in Sub-Saharan Africa and Asia. These regional differences in incidence are likely due to the variable availability of screening mammography as well as differences in reproductive and hormonal factors. In western countries, incidence rates decreased with a reduced use of postmenopausal hormone therapy and mortality declined with increased use of screening and improved treatments. In contrast, incidence and mortality from breast cancer in many African and Asian countries have increased as reproductive factors have changed (such as delayed childbearing) and as the incidence of obesity has risen.

The most significant risk factor for the development of breast cancer is age. A woman's risk of breast cancer rises rapidly until her early 60s, peaks in her 70s, and then declines. A significant family history of breast or ovarian cancer may also indicate a high risk of developing breast cancer. Germline mutations in the BRCA family of tumor suppressor genes accounts for approximately 5–10% of breast cancer diagnoses and tend to cluster in certain ethnic groups, including women of Ashkenazi Jewish descent. Women with a mutation in the BRCA1 gene, located on chromosome 17, have an estimated 85% chance of developing breast cancer in their lifetime. Other genes associated with an increased risk of breast and other cancers include BRCA2 (associated with a gene on chromosome 13); ataxia-telangiectasia mutation; and mutation of the tumor suppressor gene p53. If a woman has a compelling family history (such as breast cancer diagnosed in two first-degree relatives, especially if diagnosed younger than age 50; ovarian cancer; male breast cancer; or a first-degree relative with bilateral breast cancer), genetic testing may be appropriate. In general, it is best for a woman who has a strong family history to meet with a genetics counselor to undergo a risk assessment and decide whether genetic testing is indicated.

Even when genetic testing fails to reveal a predisposing genetic mutation, women with a strong family history of breast cancer are at higher risk for development of breast cancer. Compared with a woman with no affected family members, a woman who has one first-degree relative with breast cancer has double the risk of developing breast cancer and a woman with two first-degree relatives with breast cancer has triple the risk of developing breast cancer. The risk is further increased for a woman whose affected family member was premenopausal at the time of diagnosis or had bilateral breast cancer. Lifestyle and reproductive factors also contribute to risk of breast cancer. Nulliparous women and women whose first full-term pregnancy occurred after the age of 30 have an elevated risk. Late menarche and artificial menopause are associated with a lower incidence, whereas early menarche (under age 12) and late natural menopause (after age 55) are associated

with an increase in risk, especially for hormone receptor positive breast cancer. Combined oral contraceptive pills may increase the risk of breast cancer. Several studies show that concomitant administration of progesterone and estrogen to postmenopausal women may markedly increase the incidence of breast cancer, compared with the use of estrogen alone or with no hormone replacement treatment. The Women's Health Initiative prospective randomized study of hormone replacement therapy stopped treatment with estrogen and progesterone early because of an increased risk of breast cancer compared with untreated women or women treated with estrogen alone. Alcohol consumption, high dietary intake of fat, and lack of exercise may also increase the risk of breast cancer. Fibrocystic breast condition, when accompanied by proliferative changes, papillomatosis, or atypical epithelial hyperplasia, and increased breast density on mammogram are also associated with an increased incidence. A woman who had cancer in one breast is at increased risk for cancer developing in the other breast. In these women, a contralateral cancer develops at rate of 1% or 2% per year. Women with cancer of the uterine corpus have a risk of breast cancer significantly higher than that of the general population, and women with breast cancer have a comparably increased risk of endometrial cancer. Socioeconomic and racial factors have also been associated with breast cancer risk. Breast cancer tends to be diagnosed more frequently in women of higher socioeconomic status. In the past, breast cancer was noted to be more frequent in white women than in black women; however, in 2012 the rates converged.

Women at greater than average risk for developing breast cancer (Table 17–2) should be identified by their clinicians and monitored carefully. Several risk assessment models have been validated (most extensively the Gail 2 model) to evaluate a woman's risk of developing cancer. Those with an exceptional family history should be counseled about the option of genetic testing. Some of these high-risk women may consider prophylactic mastectomy, oophorectomy, tamoxifen, or an aromatase inhibitor.

Women with genetic mutations in whom breast cancer develops may be treated in the same way as women who do

Table 17–2. Factors associated with increased risk of breast cancer.

Race	White
Age	Older
Family history	Breast cancer in parent, sibling, or child (especially bilateral or premenopausal)
Genetics	BRCA1 or BRCA2 mutation
Previous medical history	Endometrial cancer Proliferative forms of fibrocystic disease Cancer in other breast
Menstrual history	Early menarche (under age 12) Late menopause (after age 50)
Reproductive history	Nulliparous or late first pregnancy

not have mutations (ie, lumpectomy), though there is an increased risk of ipsilateral and contralateral breast cancer after lumpectomy for these women. One study showed that of patients with a diagnosis of breast cancer who were found to be carriers of a *BRCA* mutation, approximately 50% chose to undergo bilateral mastectomy.

Anderson KN et al. Reproductive risk factors and breast cancer subtypes: a review of the literature. Breast Cancer Res Treat. 2014 Feb;144(1):1–10. [PMID: 24477977]
DeSantis CE et al. Breast cancer statistics, 2015: convergence of incidence rates between black and white women. CA Cancer J Clin. 2016 Jan;66(1):31–42. [PMID: 26513636]
Siegel RL et al. Cancer statistics, 2015. CA Cancer J Clin. 2015 Jan–Feb;65(1):5–29. [PMID: 25559415]
Vineis P et al. Global cancer patterns: causes and prevention. Lancet. 2014 Feb 8;383(9916):549–57. [PMID: 24351322]

Prevention

Several clinical trials have evaluated the use of selective estrogen receptor modulators (SERMs), including tamoxifen and raloxifene, for prevention of breast cancer in women with no personal history of breast cancer but at high risk for developing the disease. A meta-analysis of nine of these studies including 83,399 women with a median follow-up of 65 months demonstrated a 38% reduction in breast cancer incidence (hazard ratio [HR], 0.62; 95% CI, 0.56, 0.69) with a 10-year cumulative incidence of 6.3% in control groups and 4.2% in SERM-treated groups. An increased risk of endometrial cancer, cataracts and venous thromboembolic events but a reduced risk of vertebral fractures was seen in SERM groups. While SERMs have been shown to be effective at reducing the risk of breast cancer, the uptake of this intervention by women has been relatively low, possibly due to the perceived risks and side effects of therapy. A cost-effectiveness study based on a meta-analysis of four randomized prevention trials showed that tamoxifen saves costs and improves life expectancy when higher risk (Gail 5-year risk at least 1.66%) women under the age of 55 years were treated.

Similar to SERMs, aromatase inhibitors (AIs), such as exemestane and anastrozole, have shown success in preventing breast cancer with a lower risk of uterine cancer and thromboembolic events, although bone loss is a significant side effect of this treatment.

Cuzick J et al; IBIS-II investigators. Anastrozole for prevention of breast cancer in high-risk postmenopausal women (IBIS-II): an international, double-blind, randomised placebo-controlled trial. Lancet. 2014 Mar 22;383(9922):1041–8. [PMID: 24333009]
Cuzick J et al; SERM Chemoprevention of Breast Cancer Overview Group. Selective oestrogen receptor modulators in prevention of breast cancer: an updated meta-analysis of individual participant data. Lancet. 2013 May 25;381(9880):1827–34. [PMID: 23639488]
Nelson HD et al. Use of medications to reduce risk for primary breast cancer: a systematic review for the U.S. Preventive Services Task Force. Ann Intern Med. 2013 Apr 16;158(8):604–14. [PMID: 23588749]

Early Detection of Breast Cancer

A. Screening Programs

A number of large screening programs, consisting of physical and mammographic examination of asymptomatic women, have been conducted over the years. On average, these programs identify 10 cancers per 1000 women over the age of 50 and 2 cancers per 1000 women under the age of 50. Screening detects cancer before it has spread to the lymph nodes in about 80% of the women evaluated. This increases the chance of survival to about 85% at 5 years.

The American Cancer Society no longer recommends the use of clinical breast examination for cancer screening in average risk women. Similarly, the US Preventive Services Task Force concludes that current evidence is insufficient to infer that clinical breast examination adds any benefit over routine screening mammography. Substantial evidence supports the use of routine screening mammography; however, recommendations relating to timing and frequency vary by different agencies and countries. About one-third of the abnormalities detected on screening mammograms will be found to be malignant when biopsy is performed. The probability of cancer on a screening mammogram is directly related to the Breast Imaging Reporting and Data System (BIRADS) assessment, and work-up should be performed based on this classification. The sensitivity of mammography varies from approximately 60% to 90%. This sensitivity depends on several factors, including patient age, breast density, tumor size, tumor histology (lobular versus ductal), location, and mammographic appearance. In young women with dense breasts, mammography is less sensitive than in older women with fatty breasts, in whom mammography can detect at least 90% of malignancies. Smaller tumors, particularly those without calcifications, are more difficult to detect, especially in dense breasts. The lack of sensitivity and the low incidence of breast cancer in young women have led to questions concerning the value of mammography for screening in women 40–50 years of age. The specificity of mammography in women under 50 years varies from about 30% to 40% for nonpalpable mammographic abnormalities to 85% to 90% for clinically evident malignancies. In 2009, the US Preventive Services Task Force recommended against routine screening mammography in this age range, and also recommended mammography be performed every 2 years for women between the ages of 50 and 74. The change in recommendation for screening women aged 40–50 was particularly controversial in light of several meta-analyses that included women in this age group and showed a 15–20% reduction in the relative risk of death from breast cancer with screening mammography. To add to the controversy, an analysis of the Surveillance, Epidemiology and End Results (SEER) database from 1976 to 2008 suggests that screening mammography has led to substantial increases in the number of breast cancer cases diagnosed but has only had a minor impact on the rate of women presenting with advanced disease. Currently, the American College of Radiology recommends annual mammography screening for women aged 40 and older and the American Cancer Society recommends screening average-risk women annually starting at the age of 45 and offering mammography to women who choose to do so starting at the age of 40. Thus, clinicians should have an informed discussion with patients about screening mammography regarding its potential risks (eg, false positives, overdiagnosis) and benefits (eg, early diagnosis), taking into consideration a patient's individual risk factors.

B. Clinical Breast Examination and Self-Examination

Breast self-examination has not been shown to improve survival. Because of the lack of strong evidence demonstrating value, the American Cancer Society no longer recommends monthly breast self-examination. While breast self-examination is not a recommended practice, patients should recognize and report any breast changes to their clinicians as it remains an important facet of proactive care.

C. Imaging

Mammography is the most reliable means of detecting breast cancer before a mass can be palpated. Most slowly growing cancers can be identified by mammography at least 2 years before reaching a size detectable by palpation. Film screen mammography delivers less than 0.4 cGy to the mid breast per view. Although full-field digital mammography provides an easier method to maintain and review mammograms and may improve image quality, it has not been proven to improve overall cancer detection and is less economical. It may offer screening benefits to women younger than age 50 years and to women with dense breasts. While computer-assisted detection may increase the sensitivity of mammography, it has not been shown to improve mortality rates. Tomosynthesis creates tomographic "slices" of the breast volume with a single acquisition. This technique may improve the sensitivity of mammogram especially in patients with dense breast tissue but has not yet been shown in prospective studies to improve patient outcomes.

Calcifications are the most easily recognized mammographic abnormality. The most common findings associated with carcinoma of the breast are clustered pleomorphic microcalcifications. Such calcifications are usually at least five to eight in number, aggregated in one part of the breast and differing from each other in size and shape, often including branched or V- or Y-shaped configurations. There may be an associated mammographic mass density or, at times, only a mass density with no calcifications. Such a density usually has irregular or ill-defined borders and may lead to architectural distortion within the breast but may be subtle and difficult to detect.

Indications for mammography are as follows: (1) to screen at regular intervals asymptomatic women at risk for developing breast cancer; (2) to evaluate each breast when a diagnosis of potentially curable breast cancer has been made, and at regular intervals thereafter; (3) to evaluate a questionable or ill-defined breast mass or other suspicious change in the breast; (4) to search for an occult breast cancer in a woman with metastatic disease in axillary nodes or elsewhere from an unknown primary; (5) to screen women

prior to cosmetic operations or prior to biopsy of a mass, to examine for an unsuspected cancer; (6) to monitor those women with breast cancer who have been treated with breast-conserving surgery and radiation; and (7) to monitor the contralateral breast in those women with breast cancer treated with mastectomy.

Patients with a dominant or suspicious mass on examination must undergo biopsy despite mammographic findings. The mammogram should be obtained prior to biopsy so that other suspicious areas can be noted and the contralateral breast can be evaluated. Mammography is never a substitute for biopsy because it may not reveal clinical cancer, especially in a very dense breast.

Communication and documentation among the patient, the referring clinician, and the interpreting physician are critical for high-quality screening and diagnostic mammography. The patient should be told about *how* she will receive timely results of her mammogram; that mammography does not "rule out" cancer; and that she may receive a correlative examination such as ultrasound at the mammography facility if referred for a suspicious lesion. She should also be aware of the technique and need for breast compression and that this may be uncomfortable. The mammography facility should be informed in writing by the clinician of abnormal physical examination findings. The Agency for Health Care Policy and Research (AHCPR) Clinical Practice Guidelines strongly recommend that all mammography reports be communicated in writing to the patient and referring clinician. Legislation has been passed in a number of US states that requires imaging facilities to report to patients the density of their breasts. This may prompt women with dense breasts to discuss with their clinician whether or not additional screening options would be appropriate in addition to mammogram.

MRI and ultrasound may be useful screening modalities in women who are at high risk for breast cancer but not for the general population. The sensitivity of MRI is much higher than mammography; however, the specificity is significantly lower and this results in multiple unnecessary biopsies. The increased sensitivity despite decreased specificity may be considered a reasonable trade-off for those at increased risk for developing breast cancer but not for normal-risk population. Starting in 2009, the National Comprehensive Cancer Network (NCCN) guidelines recommended MRI in addition to screening mammography for high-risk women, including those with *BRCA1/2* mutations, those who have a lifetime risk of breast cancer of greater than 20%, and those with a personal history of LCIS. Women who received radiation therapy to the chest in their teens or twenties are also known to be at high risk for developing breast cancer and screening MRI may be considered in addition to mammography. MRI is useful in women with breast implants to determine the character of a lesion present in the breast and to search for implant rupture and at times is helpful in patients with prior lumpectomy and radiation.

Hendrick RE et al. United States Preventive Services Task Force screening mammography recommendations: science ignored. AJR Am J Roentgenol. 2011 Feb;196(2):W112–6. [PMID: 21257850]

Independent UK Panel on Breast Cancer Screening. The benefits and harms of breast cancer screening: an independent review. Lancet. 2012 Nov 17;380(9855):1778–86. [PMID: 23117178]

Miller AB et al. Twenty five year follow-up for breast cancer incidence and mortality of the Canadian National Breast Screening Study: randomised screening trial. BMJ. 2014 Feb 11; 348:g366. [PMID: 24519768]

Myers ER et al. Benefits and harms of breast cancer screening: a systematic review. JAMA. 2015 Oct 20;314(15):1615–34. [PMID: 26501537]

Oeffinger KC et al. Breast cancer screening for women at average risk: 2015 guideline update from the American Cancer Society. JAMA. 2015 Oct 20;314(15):1599–614. [PMID: 26501536]

Onega T et al. Breast cancer screening in an era of personalized regimens: a conceptual model and National Cancer Institute initiative for risk-based and preference-based approaches at a population level. Cancer. 2014 Oct 1;120(19):2955–64. [PMID: 24830599]

Pace LE et al. A systematic assessment of benefits and risks to guide breast cancer screening decisions. JAMA. 2014 Apr 2; 311(13):1327–35. [PMID: 24691608]

► Clinical Findings Associated with Early Detection of Breast Cancer

A. Symptoms and Signs

The presenting complaint in about 70% of patients with breast cancer is a lump (usually painless) in the breast. About 90% of these breast masses are discovered by the patient. Less frequent symptoms are breast pain; nipple discharge; erosion, retraction, enlargement, or itching of the nipple; and redness, generalized hardness, enlargement, or shrinking of the breast. Rarely, an axillary mass or swelling of the arm may be the first symptom. Back or bone pain, jaundice, or weight loss may be the result of systemic metastases, but these symptoms are rarely seen on initial presentation.

The relative frequency of carcinoma in various anatomic sites in the breast is shown in Figure 17–2.

▲ **Figure 17–3.** Peau d'orange sign (resemblance to the skin of an orange due to lymphedema) in advanced breast cancer. (Reproduced, with permission, from Richard P. Usatine, MD.)

Inspection of the breast is the first step in physical examination and should be carried out with the patient sitting, arms at her sides and then overhead. Abnormal variations in breast size and contour, minimal nipple retraction, and slight edema, redness, or retraction of the skin can be identified (Figure 17–3). Asymmetry of the breasts and retraction or dimpling of the skin can often be accentuated by having the patient raise her arms overhead or press her hands on her hips to contract the pectoralis muscles. Axillary and supraclavicular areas should be thoroughly palpated for enlarged nodes with the patient sitting (Figure 17–4). Palpation of the breast for masses or other changes should be performed with the patient both seated

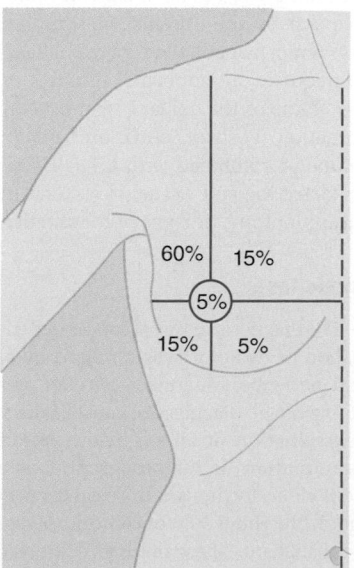

▲ **Figure 17–2.** Frequency of breast carcinoma at various anatomic sites.

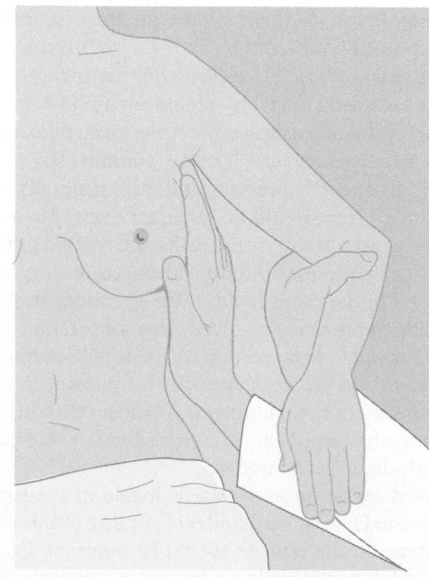

▲ **Figure 17–4.** Palpation of axillary region for enlarged lymph nodes.

▲ **Figure 17–5.** Palpation of breasts. Palpation is performed with the patient supine and arm abducted.

and supine with the arm abducted (Figure 17–5). Palpation with a rotary motion of the examiner's fingers as well as a horizontal stripping motion has been recommended.

Breast cancer usually consists of a nontender, firm or hard mass with poorly delineated margins (caused by local infiltration). Very small (1–2 mm) erosions of the nipple epithelium may be the only manifestation of Paget disease of the breast. Watery, serous, or bloody discharge from the nipple is an occasional early sign but is more often associated with benign disease.

A lesion smaller than 1 cm in diameter may be difficult or impossible for the examiner to feel but may be discovered by the patient. She should always be asked to demonstrate the location of the mass; if the clinician fails to confirm the patient's suspicions and imaging studies are normal, the examination should be repeated in 2–3 months, preferably 1–2 weeks after the onset of menses. During the premenstrual phase of the cycle, increased innocuous nodularity may suggest neoplasm or may obscure an underlying lesion. If there is any question regarding the nature of an abnormality under these circumstances, the patient should be asked to return after her menses.

Metastases tend to involve regional lymph nodes, which may be palpable. One or two movable, nontender, not particularly firm axillary lymph nodes 5 mm or less in diameter are frequently present and are generally of no significance. Firm or hard nodes larger than 1 cm are typical of metastases. Axillary nodes that are matted or fixed to skin or deep structures indicate advanced disease (at least stage III). On the other hand, if the examiner thinks that the axillary nodes are involved, that impression will be borne out by histologic section in about 85% of cases. The incidence of positive axillary nodes increases with the size of the primary tumor. Noninvasive cancers (in situ) do not metastasize. Metastases are present in about 30% of patients with clinically negative nodes.

In most cases, no nodes are palpable in the supraclavicular fossa. Firm or hard nodes of any size in this location or just beneath the clavicle should be biopsied. Ipsilateral supraclavicular or infraclavicular nodes containing cancer indicate that the tumor is in an advanced stage (stage III or IV). Edema of the ipsilateral arm, commonly caused by metastatic infiltration of regional lymphatics, is also a sign of advanced cancer.

B. Laboratory Findings

Liver or bone metastases may be associated with elevation of serum alkaline phosphatase. Hypercalcemia is an occasional important finding in advanced cancer of the breast. Serum tumor markers such as carcinoembryonic antigen (CEA) and CA 15-3 or CA 27-29 are not recommended for diagnosis of early lesions or for routine surveillance for recurrence after a breast cancer diagnosis.

C. Imaging

1. For lesions felt only by the patient—Ultrasound is often valuable and mammography essential when an area is felt by the patient to be abnormal but the clinician feels no mass. MRI may be considered, but the lack of specificity should be discussed by the clinician and the patient. MRI should not be used to rule out cancer because MRI has a false-negative rate of about 3–5%. Although lower than mammography, this false-negative rate cannot permit safe elimination of the possibility of cancer. False-negative results are more likely seen in infiltrating lobular carcinomas and DCIS than invasive ductal carcinoma.

2. For metastatic lesions—For patients with suspicious symptoms or signs (bone pain, abdominal symptoms, elevated liver biochemical tests) or locally advanced disease (clinically abnormal lymph nodes or large primary tumors), staging scans are indicated prior to surgery or systemic therapy. Chest imaging with CT or radiographs may be done to evaluate for pulmonary metastases. Abdominal imaging with CT or ultrasound may be obtained to evaluate for liver metastases. Bone scans using ^{99m}Tc-labeled phosphates or phosphonates are more sensitive than skeletal radiographs in detecting metastatic breast cancer. Bone scanning has not proved to be of clinical value as a routine preoperative test in the absence of symptoms, physical findings, or abnormal alkaline phosphatase or calcium levels. The frequency of abnormal findings on bone scan parallels the status of the axillary lymph nodes on pathologic examination. Positron emission tomography (PET) scanning alone or combined with CT (PET-CT) may also be used for detecting soft tissue or visceral metastases in patients with symptoms or signs of metastatic disease.

D. Diagnostic Tests

1. Biopsy—The diagnosis of breast cancer depends ultimately on examination of tissue or cells removed by biopsy. Treatment should never be undertaken without an unequivocal histologic or cytologic diagnosis of cancer. **The safest course is biopsy examination of all suspicious lesions found on physical examination or mammography, or both.** About 60% of lesions clinically thought to be cancer prove on biopsy to be benign, while about 30% of clinically benign lesions are found to be malignant. These findings demonstrate the fallibility of clinical judgment and the necessity for biopsy.

All breast masses require a histologic diagnosis with one probable exception: a nonsuspicious, presumably

▲ **Figure 17–6.** Evaluation of breast masses in premenopausal women. (Adapted, with permission, from Chang S, Haigh PI, Giuliano AE. Breast disease. In: Berek JS, Hacker NF [editors], *Practical Gynecologic Oncology,* 4th edition, LWW, 2004.)

fibrocystic mass, in a premenopausal woman. Rather, these masses can be observed through one or two menstrual cycles. However, if the mass is not cystic and does not completely resolve during this time, it must be biopsied. Figures 17–6 and 17–7 present algorithms for management of breast masses in premenopausal and postmenopausal patients.

The simplest biopsy method is needle biopsy, either by aspiration of tumor cells (FNA cytology) or by obtaining a small core of tissue with a hollow needle (core biopsy).

Large-needle (core needle) biopsy removes a core of tissue with a large cutting needle and is **the diagnostic procedure of choice** for both palpable and image-detected abnormalities. Hand-held biopsy devices make large-core needle biopsy of a palpable mass easy and cost effective in the office with local anesthesia. As in the case of any needle

biopsy, the main problem is sampling error due to improper positioning of the needle, giving rise to a false-negative test result. This is extremely unusual with image-guided biopsies. Core biopsy allows the tumor to be tested for the expression of biological markers, such as estrogen receptor (ER), progesterone receptor (PR) and *HER2*.

FNA cytology is a technique whereby cells are aspirated with a small needle and examined cytologically. This technique can be performed easily with virtually no morbidity and is much less expensive than excisional or open biopsy. The main disadvantages are that it requires a pathologist skilled in the cytologic diagnosis of breast cancer and it is subject to sampling problems, particularly because deep lesions may be missed. Furthermore, noninvasive cancers usually cannot be distinguished from invasive cancers and immunohistochemical tests to determine expression of

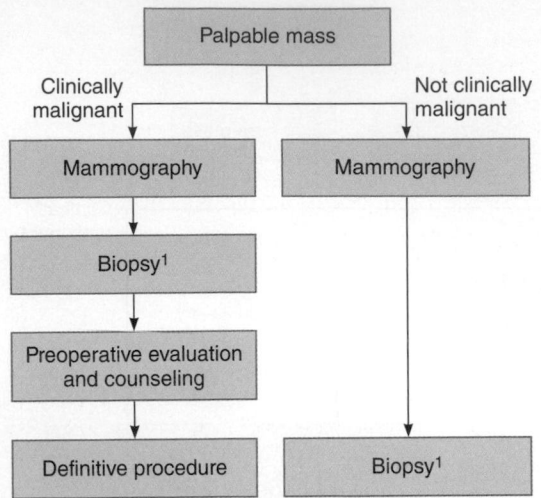

```
              ┌─────────────────┐
              │  Palpable mass  │
              └─────────────────┘
        Clinically          Not clinically
        malignant           malignant
         ┌──────────────┐   ┌──────────────┐
         │ Mammography  │   │ Mammography  │
         └──────────────┘   └──────────────┘
         ┌──────────────┐
         │   Biopsy¹    │
         └──────────────┘
    ┌──────────────────────┐
    │ Preoperative evaluation │
    │    and counseling    │
    └──────────────────────┘
    ┌──────────────────────┐   ┌──────────────┐
    │ Definitive procedure │   │   Biopsy¹    │
    └──────────────────────┘   └──────────────┘
```

¹Biopsy may be excisional or by needle cytology, but if cytology appears benign and the mass persists, it should be excised.

▲ **Figure 17–7.** Evaluation of breast masses in post-menopausal women. (Adapted, with permission, from Chang S, Haigh PI, Giuliano AE. Breast disease. In: Berek JS, Hacker NF [editors], *Practical Gynecologic Oncology,* 4th edition, LWW, 2004.)

hormone receptors and the amplification of the *HER2* oncogene cannot be reliably performed on FNA biopsies. The incidence of false-positive diagnoses is extremely low, perhaps 1–2%. The false-negative rate is as high as 10%. Most experienced clinicians would not leave a suspicious dominant mass in the breast even when FNA cytology is negative unless the clinical diagnosis, breast imaging studies, and cytologic studies were all in agreement, such as a fibrocystic lesion or fibroadenoma. Given the stated limitations, FNA is not the modality of choice for sampling an abnormal breast mass.

Open biopsy under local anesthesia as a separate procedure prior to deciding upon definitive treatment is becoming less common with the increasing use of core needle biopsy. Needle biopsy, when positive, offers a more rapid approach with less expense and morbidity, but when nondiagnostic it must be followed by open biopsy. It generally consists of an excisional biopsy, which is done through an incision with the intent to remove the entire abnormality, not simply a sample. Additional evaluation for metastatic disease and therapeutic options can be discussed with the patient after the histologic or cytologic diagnosis of cancer has been established. As an alternative in highly suspicious circumstances, the diagnosis may be made on a frozen section of tissue obtained by open biopsy under general anesthesia. If the frozen section is positive, the surgeon can proceed immediately with the definitive operation. This one-step method is rarely used today except when a cytologic study has suggested cancer but is not diagnostic and there is a high clinical suspicion of malignancy in a patient well prepared for the diagnosis of cancer and its treatment options.

In general, the two-step approach—outpatient large-needle biopsy followed by definitive operation at a later date—is preferred in the diagnosis and treatment of breast cancer, because patients can be given time to adjust to the diagnosis of cancer, can consider alternative forms of therapy, and can seek a second opinion if they wish. **There is no adverse effect from the few week delay of the two-step procedure.**

2. Biopsy with ultrasound guidance—Ultrasonography is performed primarily to differentiate cystic from solid lesions but may show signs suggestive of carcinoma. Ultrasonography may show an irregular mass within a cyst in the rare case of intracystic carcinoma. If a tumor is palpable and feels like a cyst, an 18-gauge needle can be used to aspirate the fluid and make the diagnosis of cyst. If a cyst is aspirated and the fluid is nonbloody, it does not have to be examined cytologically. If the mass does not recur, no further diagnostic test is necessary. Nonpalpable mammographic densities that appear benign should be investigated with ultrasound to determine whether the lesion is cystic or solid. These may even be needle biopsied with ultrasound guidance.

3. Biopsy with mammographic guidance ("stereotactic biopsy")—When a suspicious abnormality is identified by mammography alone and cannot be palpated by the clinician, the lesion should be biopsied under mammographic guidance. In the **computerized stereotactic guided core needle** technique, a biopsy needle is inserted into the lesion with mammographic guidance, and a core of tissue for histologic examination can then be examined. Vacuum assistance increases the amount of tissue obtained and improves diagnosis.

Mammographic localization biopsy is performed by obtaining a mammogram in two perpendicular views and placing a needle or hook-wire near the abnormality so that the surgeon can use the metal needle or wire as a guide during operation to locate the lesion. After mammography confirms the position of the needle in relation to the lesion, an incision is made and the subcutaneous tissue is dissected until the needle is identified. Often, the abnormality cannot even be palpated through the incision—as is the case with microcalcifications—and thus it is essential to obtain a mammogram of the specimen to document that the lesion was excised. At that time, a second marker needle can further localize the lesion for the pathologist. Stereotactic core needle biopsies have proved equivalent to mammographic localization biopsies. Core biopsy is preferable to mammographic localization for accessible lesions since an operation can be avoided. A metal clip should be placed after any image-guided core biopsy to facilitate finding the site of the lesion if subsequent treatment is necessary.

4. Other imaging modalities—Other modalities of breast imaging have been investigated for diagnostic purposes. Automated breast ultrasonography is useful in distinguishing cystic from solid lesions but should be used only as a supplement to physical examination and mammography. Ductography may be useful to define the site of a lesion causing a bloody discharge, but since biopsy is almost always indicated, ductography may be omitted and the blood-filled nipple system excised. Ductoscopy has shown some promise in identifying intraductal lesions, especially in the case of pathologic nipple discharge, but in practice, this technique is rarely used. MRI is highly sensitive but not specific and should not be used for screening except in highly selective cases. For example, MRI is useful in differentiating scar from recurrence postlumpectomy and may be valuable to screen high-risk women (eg, women with *BRCA* mutations). It may also be of value to examine for multicentricity when there is a known primary cancer; to examine the contralateral breast in women with cancer; to examine the extent of cancer, especially lobular carcinomas; or to determine the response to neoadjuvant chemotherapy. Moreover, MRI-detected suspicious findings that are not seen on mammogram or ultrasound may be biopsied under MRI-guidance. PET scanning does not appear useful in evaluating the breast itself but is useful to examine for distant metastases.

5. Cytology—Cytologic examination of nipple discharge or cyst fluid may be helpful on rare occasions. As a rule, mammography (or ductography) and breast biopsy are required when nipple discharge or cyst fluid is bloody or cytologically questionable.

▶ Differential Diagnosis

The lesions to be considered most often in the differential diagnosis of breast cancer are the following, in descending order of frequency: fibrocystic condition of the breast, fibroadenoma, intraductal papilloma, lipoma, and fat necrosis.

▶ Staging

The American Joint Committee on Cancer and the International Union Against Cancer have agreed on a TNM (tumor, regional lymph nodes, distant metastases) staging system for breast cancer. Using the TNM staging system enhances communication between researchers and clinicians. Table 17–3 outlines the TNM classification.

▶ Pathologic Types

Numerous pathologic subtypes of breast cancer can be identified histologically (Table 17–4).

Except for the in situ cancers, the histologic subtypes have only a slight bearing on prognosis when outcomes are compared after accurate staging. The noninvasive cancers by definition are confined by the basement membrane of the ducts and lack the ability to spread. Histologic parameters for invasive cancers, including lymphovascular invasion and tumor grade, have been shown to be of prognostic value. Immunohistochemical analysis for expression of hormone receptors and for overexpression of *HER2* in the primary tumor offers prognostic and therapeutic information.

▶ Special Clinical Forms of Breast Cancer

A. Paget Carcinoma

Paget carcinoma is not common (about 1% of all breast cancers). Over 85% of cases are associated with an underlying invasive or noninvasive cancer, usually a well differentiated infiltrating ductal carcinoma or a DCIS. The ducts of the nipple epithelium are infiltrated, but gross nipple changes are often minimal, and a tumor mass may not be palpable.

Because the nipple changes appear innocuous, the diagnosis is frequently missed. The first symptom is often itching or burning of the nipple, with superficial erosion or ulceration. These are often diagnosed and treated as dermatitis or bacterial infection, leading to delay or failure in detection. The diagnosis is established by biopsy of the area of erosion. When the lesion consists of nipple changes only, the incidence of axillary metastases is less than 5%, and the prognosis is excellent. When a breast mass is also present, the incidence of axillary metastases rises, with an associated marked decrease in prospects for cure by surgical or other treatment.

B. Inflammatory Carcinoma

This is the most malignant form of breast cancer and constitutes less than 3% of all cases. The clinical findings consist of a rapidly growing, sometimes painful mass that enlarges the breast. The overlying skin becomes erythematous, edematous, and warm. Often there is no distinct mass, since the tumor infiltrates the involved breast diffusely. The inflammatory changes, often mistaken for an infection, are caused by carcinomatous invasion of the subdermal lymphatics, with resulting edema and hyperemia. If the clinician suspects infection but the lesion does not respond rapidly (1–2 weeks) to antibiotics, biopsy should be performed. The diagnosis should be made when the redness involves more than one-third of the skin over the breast and biopsy shows infiltrating carcinoma with invasion of the subdermal lymphatics. Metastases tend to occur early and widely, and for this reason inflammatory carcinoma is rarely curable. Radiation, hormone therapy (if hormone receptor positive), anti-*HER2* therapy (if *HER2* overexpressing or amplified), and chemotherapy are the measures most likely to be of value initially rather than operation. Mastectomy is indicated when chemotherapy and radiation have resulted in clinical remission with no evidence of distant metastases. In these cases, residual disease in the breast may be eradicated.

▶ Breast Cancer Occurring during Pregnancy or Lactation

Breast cancer complicates up to one in 3000 pregnancies. The diagnosis is frequently delayed, because physiologic changes in the breast may obscure the lesion and screening mammography is not done in young or pregnant women. Data are insufficient to determine whether interruption of pregnancy improves the prognosis of patients who are identified to have potentially curable breast cancer and who receive definitive treatment during pregnancy. Theoretically, the high levels of estrogen produced by the placenta as the pregnancy progresses could be detrimental to the patient with occult metastases of hormone-sensitive breast cancer. However, retrospective studies have *not* shown a worse prognosis for women with gestational breast cancer. The decision whether or not to terminate the

Table 17–3. TNM staging for breast cancer.

Primary Tumor (T)	
	Definitions for classifying the primary tumor (T) are the same for clinical and for pathologic classification. If the measurement is made by physical examination, the examiner will use the major headings (T1, T2, or T3). If other measurements, such as mammographic or pathologic measurements, are used, the subsets of T1 can be used. Tumors should be measured to the nearest 0.1 cm increment.
TX	Primary tumor cannot be assessed
T0	No evidence of primary tumor
Tis	Carcinoma in situ
Tis (DCIS)	Ductal carcinoma in situ
Tis (LCIS)	Lobular carcinoma in situ
Tis (Paget)	Paget disease of the nipple with no tumor

Note: Paget disease associated with a tumor is classified according to the size of the tumor.

T1	Tumor 2 cm or less in greatest dimension
T1mic	Microinvasion 0.1 cm or less in greatest dimension
T1a	Tumor more than 0.1 cm but not more than 0.5 cm in greatest dimension
T1b	Tumor more than 0.5 cm but not more than 1 cm in greatest dimension
T1c	Tumor more than 1 cm but not more than 2 cm in greatest dimension
T2	Tumor more than 2 cm but not more than 5 cm in greatest dimension
T3	Tumor more than 5 cm in greatest dimension
T4	Tumor of any size with direct extension to (a) chest wall or (b) skin, only as described below
T4a	Extension to chest wall, not including pectoralis muscle
T4b	Edema (including peau d'orange [see Figure 17–3]) or ulceration of the skin of the breast, or satellite skin nodules confined to the same breast
T4c	Both T4a and T4b
T4d	Inflammatory carcinoma

Regional Lymph Nodes (N)	
Clinical	
NX	Regional lymph nodes cannot be assessed (eg, previously removed)
N0	No regional lymph node metastasis
N1	Metastasis in movable ipsilateral axillary lymph node(s)
N2	Metastases in ipsilateral axillary lymph nodes fixed or matted, or in clinically apparent[1] ipsilateral internal mammary nodes in the *absence* of clinically evident axillary lymph node metastasis
N2a	Metastasis in ipsilateral axillary lymph nodes fixed to one another (matted) or to other structures

N2b	Metastasis only in clinically apparent[1] ipsilateral internal mammary nodes and in the *absence* of clinically evident axillary lymph node metastasis
N3	Metastasis in ipsilateral infraclavicular lymph node(s) with or without axillary lymph node involvement, or in clinically apparent[1] ipsilateral internal mammary lymph node(s) and in the *presence* of clinically evident axillary lymph node metastasis; or metastasis in ipsilateral supraclavicular lymph node(s) with or without axillary or internal mammary lymph node involvement
N3a	Metastasis in ipsilateral infraclavicular lymph node(s)
N3b	Metastasis in ipsilateral internal mammary lymph node(s) and axillary lymph node(s)
N3c	Metastasis in ipsilateral supraclavicular lymph node(s)

Regional Lymph Nodes (pN)[2]

pNX	Regional lymph nodes cannot be assessed (eg, previously removed, or not removed for pathologic study)
pN0	No regional lymph node metastasis histologically, no additional examination for isolated tumor cells

Note: Isolated tumor cells (ITC) are defined as single tumor cells or small cell clusters not > 0.2 mm, usually detected only by immunohistochemical (IHC) or molecular methods but which may be verified on hematoxylin and eosin stains. ITCs do not usually show evidence of malignant activity, eg, proliferation or stromal reaction.

pN0(i−)	No regional lymph node metastasis histologically, negative IHC
pN0(i+)	No regional lymph node metastasis histologically, positive IHC, no IHC cluster > 0.2 mm
pN0(mol−)	No regional lymph node metastasis histologically, negative molecular findings (RT-PCR)[3]
pN0(mol+)	No regional lymph node metastasis histologically, positive molecular findings (RT-PCR)[3]
pN1	Metastasis in one to three axillary lymph nodes, and/or in internal mammary nodes with microscopic disease detected by sentinel lymph node dissection but not clinically apparent[4]
pN1mi	Micrometastasis (> 0.2 mm, none > 2.0 mm)
pN1a	Metastasis in one to three axillary lymph nodes
pN1b	Metastasis in internal mammary nodes with microscopic disease detected by sentinel lymph node dissection but not clinically apparent[4]
pN1c	Metastasis in one to three axillary lymph nodes and in internal mammary lymph nodes with microscopic disease detected by sentinel lymph node dissection but not clinically apparent.[4] (If associated with greater than three positive axillary lymph nodes, the internal mammary nodes are classified as pN3b to reflect increased tumor burden)

(continued)

Table 17–3. TNM staging for breast cancer. (continued)

		Distant Metastasis (M)		
pN2	Metastasis in four to nine axillary lymph nodes, or in clinically apparent[1] internal mammary lymph nodes in the absence of axillary lymph node metastasis	MX	Distant metastasis cannot be assessed	
		M0	No distant metastasis	
pN2a	Metastasis in four to nine axillary lymph nodes (at least one tumor deposit > 2.0 mm)	M1	Distant metastasis	
pN2b	Metastasis in clinically apparent[1] internal mammary lymph nodes in the absence of axillary lymph node metastasis	**Stage Grouping**		
		Stage 0	Tis	N0	M0

		Stage Grouping		
pN2b	Metastasis in clinically apparent[1] internal mammary lymph nodes in the absence of axillary lymph node metastasis	Stage 0	Tis N0 M0	
pN3	Metastasis in 10 or more axillary lymph nodes, or in infraclavicular lymph nodes, or in clinically apparent[1] ipsilateral internal mammary lymph nodes in the presence of one or more positive axillary lymph nodes; or in more than three axillary lymph nodes with clinically negative microscopic metastasis in internal mammary lymph nodes; or in ipsilateral supraclavicular lymph nodes	Stage 1	T1[5] N0 M0	
		Stage IIA	T0 N1 M0 / T1[5] N1 M0 / T2 N0 M0	
		Stage IIB	T2 N1 M0 / T3 N0 M0	
pN3a	Metastasis in 10 or more axillary lymph nodes (at least one tumor deposit > 2.0 mm), or metastasis to the infraclavicular lymph nodes	Stage IIIA	T0 N2 M0 / T1[5] N2 M0 / T2 N2 M0 / T3 N1 M0 / T3 N2 M0	
pN3b	Metastasis in clinically apparent[1] ipsilateral internal mammary lymph nodes in the presence of one or more positive axillary lymph nodes; or in more than three axillary lymph nodes and in internal mammary lymph nodes with microscopic disease detected by sentinel lymph node dissection but not clinically apparent[4]	Stage IIIB	T4 N0 M0 / T4 N1 M0 / T4 N2 M0	
		Stage IIIC	Any T N3 M0	
pN3c	Metastasis in ipsilateral supraclavicular lymph nodes	Stage IV	Any T Any N M1	

Note: Stage designation may be changed if postsurgical imaging studies reveal the presence of distant metastases, provided that the studies are carried out within 4 months of diagnosis in the absence of disease progression and provided that the patient has not received neoadjuvant therapy.

[1]*Clinically apparent* is defined as detected by imaging studies (excluding lymphoscintigraphy) or by clinical examination or grossly visible pathologically.

[2]Classification is based on axillary lymph node dissection with or without sentinel lymph node dissection. Classification based solely on sentinel lymph node dissection without subsequent axillary lymph node dissection is designated (sn) for "sentinel node," eg, pN0(i+)(sn).

[3]RT-PCR, reverse transcriptase/polymerase chain reaction.

[4]*Not clinically apparent* is defined as not detected by imaging studies (excluding lymphoscintigraphy) or by clinical examination.

[5]T1 includes T1mic.

Reproduced, with permission, of the American Joint Committee on Cancer (AJCC), Chicago, Illinois, *AJCC Cancer Staging Manual,* 7th edition, Springer-Science and Business Media LLC, New York, 2010, www.springer.com.

pregnancy must be made on an individual basis, taking into account the patient's clinical stage of the cancer and overall prognosis, the gestational age of the fetus, the potential for premature ovarian failure in the future with systemic therapy, and the patient's wishes.

A retrospective analysis of women who were younger than 36 years when breast cancer was diagnosed showed that while women with pregnancy-associated breast cancer were more frequently diagnosed with later stage breast cancer, they had similar rates of local regional recurrence, distant metastases, and overall survival as women with nonpregnancy-associated breast cancer. It is thus important for primary care and reproductive specialists to aggressively work up any breast abnormality discovered in a pregnant woman. Pregnancy (or lactation) is not a contraindication to operation or treatment, and therapy should be based on the stage of the disease as in the nonpregnant (or nonlactating) woman. Women with early-stage gestational breast cancer who choose to continue their pregnancy should undergo surgery to remove the tumor and systemic therapy if indicated. Retrospective reviews of patients treated with anthracycline-containing regimens for gestational cancers (including leukemia and lymphomas) have established the relative safety of these regimens during pregnancy for both the patient and the fetus. Taxane-based and trastuzumab-based regimens have not been evaluated extensively, however. Radiation therapy should be delayed until after delivery. Overall survival rates have improved, since cancers are now diagnosed in pregnant women earlier than in the past and treatment has improved.

Table 17–4. Histologic types of breast cancer.

Type	Frequency of Occurrence
Infiltrating ductal (not otherwise specified)	80–90%
Medullary	5–8%
Colloid (mucinous)	2–4%
Tubular	1–2%
Papillary	1–2%
Invasive lobular	6–8%
Noninvasive	4–6%
Intraductal	2–3%
Lobular in situ	2–3%
Rare cancers	< 1%
Juvenile (secretory)	
Adenoid cystic	
Epidermoid	
Sudoriferous	

Bilateral Breast Cancer

Bilateral breast cancer occurs in less than 5% of cases, but there is as high as a 20–25% incidence of later occurrence of cancer in the second breast. Bilaterality occurs more often in familial breast cancer, in women under age 50 years, and when the tumor in the primary breast is lobular. The incidence of second breast cancers increases directly with the length of time the patient is alive after her first cancer—about 1–2% per year.

In patients with breast cancer, mammography should be performed before primary treatment and at regular intervals thereafter, to search for occult cancer in the opposite breast or conserved ipsilateral breast. MRI may be useful in this high-risk group.

Noninvasive Cancer

Noninvasive cancer can occur within the ducts (DCIS) or lobules (LCIS). DCIS tends to be unilateral and **most often progresses to invasive cancer if untreated.** In approximately 40–60% of women who have DCIS treated with biopsy alone, invasive cancer develops within the same breast. LCIS is generally agreed to be a marker of an increased risk of breast cancer rather than a direct precursor of breast cancer itself. The probability of breast cancer (DCIS or invasive in either breast) in a woman in whom LCIS has been diagnosed is estimated to be 1% per year. If LCIS is detected on core needle biopsy, an excisional biopsy without lymph node sampling should be performed to rule out DCIS or invasive cancer since these are found in 10–20% of patients. The incidence of LCIS is rising, likely due to increased use of screening mammography. In addition, the rate of mastectomy after the diagnosis of LCIS is increasing in spite of the fact that mastectomy is only recommended in those patients who otherwise have an increased risk of breast cancer through family history, genetic mutation, or past exposure to thoracic radiation. Pleomorphic LCIS may behave more like DCIS and may be associated with invasive carcinoma. For this reason, pleomorphic LCIS should be surgically removed with clear margins.

The treatment of intraductal lesions is controversial. DCIS can be treated by wide excision with or without radiation therapy or with total mastectomy. Conservative management is advised in patients with small lesions amenable to lumpectomy. Patients in whom LCIS is diagnosed or who have received lumpectomy for DCIS may discuss chemoprevention (with hormonal therapy) with their clinician, which is effective in preventing invasive breast cancer in both LCIS and DCIS that has been completely excised by breast-conserving surgery. Axillary metastases from in situ cancers should not occur unless there is an occult invasive cancer. Because one cannot perform a sentinel lymph node biopsy after mastectomy, one might consider performing a sentinel node biopsy in a patient undergoing mastectomy for DCIS in case an invasive component is discovered.

Genin AS et al. Association with pregnancy increases the risk of local recurrence but does not impact overall survival in breast cancer: a case-control study of 87 cases. Breast. 2015 Oct 8. [Epub ahead of print] [PMID: 26456897]

Portschy PR et al. Trends in incidence and management of lobular carcinoma in situ: a population-based analysis. Ann Surg Oncol. 2013 Oct;20(10):3240–6. [PMID: 23846782]

Biomarkers & Gene Expression Profiling

Determining the ER, PR, and *HER2* status of the tumor at the time of diagnosis of early breast cancer and, if possible, at the time of recurrence is critical, both to gauge a patient's prognosis and to determine the best treatment regimen. In addition to ER status and PR status, the rate at which tumor divides (assessed by an immunohistochemical stain for Ki-67) and the grade and differentiation of the cells are also important prognostic factors. These markers may be obtained on core biopsy or surgical specimens, but not reliably on FNA cytology. Patients whose tumors are hormone receptor-positive tend to have a more indolent disease course than those whose tumors are receptor-negative. Moreover, treatment with an anti-hormonal agent is an essential component of therapy for hormone-receptor positive breast cancer at any stage. While up to 60% of patients with metastatic breast cancer will respond to hormonal manipulation if their tumors are ER-positive, less than 5% of patients with metastatic, ER-negative tumors will respond.

Another key element in determining treatment and prognosis is the amount of the *HER2* oncogene present in the cancer. *HER2* overexpression is measured by an immunohistochemical assay that is scored using a numerical system: 0 and 1+ are considered negative for overexpression, 2+ is borderline/indeterminate, and 3+ is overexpression. In the case of 2+ expression, fluorescence in situ hybridization (FISH) is recommended to more accurately assess *HER2* amplification. Guidelines for the interpretation of *HER2* results by IHC and FISH have been published by the College of American Pathologists. Occasionally, a tumor has an indeterminate *HER2* result by both immuno-histochemistry and FISH testing. The College of American Pathologists guidelines provide direction for further analysis in this situation.

Individually these biomarkers are predictive and thus provide insight to guide appropriate therapy. Moreover, when combined they provide useful information regarding risk of recurrence and prognosis. In general, tumors that lack expression of *HER2*, ER, and PR ("triple negative") have a higher risk of recurrence and metastases and are associated with a worse survival compared with other types. Neither endocrine therapy nor *HER2*-targeted agents are useful for this type of breast cancer, leaving chemotherapy as the only treatment option. In contrast, patients with early stage, hormone receptor–positive breast cancer may not benefit from the addition of chemotherapy to hormonally targeted treatments. Several molecular tests have been developed to assess risk of recurrence and to predict which patients are most likely to benefit from chemotherapy.

Cuzick J et al. Prognostic value of a combined estrogen receptor, progesterone receptor, Ki-67, and human epidermal growth factor receptor 2 immunohistochemical score and comparison with the Genomic Health recurrence score in early breast cancer. J Clin Oncol. 2011 Nov 10;29(32):4273–8. [PMID: 21990413]

Galanina N et al. Molecular predictors of response to therapy for breast cancer. Cancer J. 2011 Mar–Apr;17(2):96–103. [PMID: 21427553]

Gangi A et al. Breast-conserving therapy for triple-negative breast cancer. JAMA Surg. 2014 Mar;149(3):252–8. [PMID: 24382582]

Lang JE et al. Molecular markers for breast cancer diagnosis, prognosis and targeted therapy. J Surg Oncol. 2015 Jan; 111(1): 81–90. [PMID: 25091830]

Sparano JA et al. Prospective validation of a 21-gene expression assay in breast cancer. N Engl J Med. 2015 Nov 19;373(21): 2005–14. [PMID: 26412349]

Stefansson OA et al. Epigenetic modifications in breast cancer and their role in personalized medicine. Am J Pathol. 2013 Oct;183(4):1052–63. [PMID: 23899662]

Wolff AC et al. Recommendations for human epidermal growth factor receptor 2 testing in breast cancer: American Society of Clinical Oncology/College of American Pathologists clinical practice guideline update. J Clin Oncol. 2013 Nov 1;31(31): 3997–4013. [PMID: 24101045]

▶ **Curative Treatment**

Clearly, not all breast cancer is systemic at the time of diagnosis. For this reason, a pessimistic attitude concerning the management of breast cancer is unwarranted. Most patients with early breast cancer can be cured. Treatment with a curative intent is advised for clinical stage I, II, and III disease (see Tables 17–3, 39–3). Patients with locally advanced (T3, T4) and even inflammatory tumors may be cured with multimodality therapy, but metastatic disease will be diagnosed in most patients and at that point, palliation becomes the goal of therapy. Treatment with palliative intent is appropriate for all patients with stage IV disease and for patients with unresectable local cancers.

A. Choice and Timing of Primary Therapy

The extent of disease and its biologic aggressiveness are the principal determinants of the outcome of primary therapy. Clinical and pathologic staging help in assessing extent of disease (see Table 17–3), but each is to some extent imprecise. Other factors such as tumor grade, hormone receptor assays, and *HER2* oncogene amplification are of prognostic value and are key to determining systemic therapy, but are not as relevant in determining the type of local therapy.

Controversy has surrounded the choice of primary therapy of stage I, II, and III breast carcinoma. Currently, the standard of care for stage I, stage II, and most stage III cancer is surgical resection followed by adjuvant radiation or systemic therapy, or both, when indicated. Neoadjuvant therapy is becoming more popular since large tumors may be shrunk by chemotherapy prior to surgery, making some patients who require mastectomy candidates for lumpectomy. It is important for patients to understand all of the surgical options, including reconstructive options, prior to having surgery. Patients with large primary tumors, inflammatory cancer, or palpably enlarged lymph nodes should have staging scans performed to rule out distant metastatic disease prior to definitive surgery. In general, adjuvant systemic therapy is started when the breast has adequately healed, usually within 4–8 weeks after surgery. While no prospective studies have defined the appropriate timing of adjuvant chemotherapy, a single institution study of over 6800 patients suggests that systemic therapy should be started within 60 days of surgery, especially in women with stage II or III breast cancer, triple-negative breast cancer or *HER2*-positive disease.

B. Surgical Resection

1. Breast-conserving therapy—Multiple, large, randomized studies including the Milan and NSABP trials show that disease-free and overall survival rates are similar for patients with stage I and stage II breast cancer treated with partial mastectomy (breast-conserving lumpectomy or "breast conservation") plus axillary dissection followed by radiation therapy and for those treated by modified radical mastectomy (total mastectomy plus axillary dissection).

Tumor size is a major consideration in determining the feasibility of breast conservation. The NSABP lumpectomy trial randomized patients with tumors as large as 4 cm. To achieve an acceptable cosmetic result, the patient must have a breast of sufficient size to enable excision of a 4-cm tumor without considerable deformity. Therefore, large tumor size is only a relative contraindication. Subareolar tumors, also difficult to excise without deformity, are not contraindications to breast conservation. Clinically detectable multifocality is a relative contraindication to breast-conserving surgery, as is fixation to the chest wall or skin or involvement of the nipple or overlying skin. The patient—not the surgeon—should be the judge of what is cosmetically acceptable. Given the relatively high risk of poor outcome after radiation, concomitant scleroderma is a contraindication to breast-conserving surgery. A history of prior therapeutic radiation to the ipsilateral breast or chest wall (or both) is also generally a contraindication for breast conservation.

▲ **Figure 17–8.** Sentinel node. (Used, with permission, from Armando E. Giuliano, MD.)

Axillary dissection is primarily used to properly stage cancer and plan radiation and systemic therapy. Intraoperative lymphatic mapping and sentinel node biopsy identify lymph nodes most likely to harbor metastases if present (Figure 17–8). Sentinel node biopsy is a reasonable alternative to axillary dissection in patients without clinical evidence of axillary lymph node metastases. If sentinel node biopsy reveals no evidence of axillary metastases, it is highly likely that the remaining lymph nodes are free of disease and axillary dissection may be omitted. An important study from the American College of Surgeons Oncology group randomized women with sentinel node metastases to undergo completion of axillary dissection or to receive no further axillary treatment after lumpectomy; no difference in survival was found, showing that axillary dissection is not necessary for selected patients with node involvement who are treated with lumpectomy, whole breast irradiation, and adjuvant systemic therapy. Omission of axillary dissection is accepted at many major cancer institutions.

Breast-conserving surgery with radiation is the preferred form of treatment for patients with early-stage breast cancer. Despite the numerous randomized trials showing no survival benefit of mastectomy over breast-conserving partial mastectomy and irradiation, breast-conserving surgery still appears to be underutilized.

2. Mastectomy—Modified radical mastectomy was the standard therapy for most patients with early-stage breast cancer. This operation removes the entire breast, overlying skin, nipple, and areolar complex usually with underlying pectoralis fascia with the axillary lymph nodes in continuity. The major advantage of modified radical mastectomy is that radiation therapy may not be necessary, although radiation may be used when lymph nodes are involved with cancer or when the primary tumor is 5 cm or larger. The disadvantage of mastectomy is the cosmetic and psychological impact associated with breast loss. Radical mastectomy, which removes the underlying pectoralis muscle, should be performed rarely, if at all. Axillary node dissection is not indicated for noninvasive cancers because nodal metastases are rarely present. Skin-sparing and nipple-sparing mastectomy is currently gaining favor but is not appropriate for all patients. Breast reconstruction, immediate or delayed, should be discussed with patients who choose or require mastectomy. Patients should have an interview with a reconstructive plastic surgeon to discuss options prior to making a decision regarding reconstruction. Time is well spent preoperatively in educating the patient and family about these matters.

C. Radiotherapy

Radiotherapy after partial mastectomy consists of 5–7 weeks of five daily fractions to a total dose of 5000–6000 cGy. Most radiation oncologists use a boost dose to the cancer location. Shorter fractionation schedules may be reasonable for women over the age of 50 with early stage, lymph node–negative breast cancer. Accelerated partial breast irradiation, in which only the portion of the breast from which the tumor was resected is irradiated for 1–2 weeks, appears effective in achieving local control for selected patients; however, the results of prospective randomized trials, such as the NSABP B-39/RTOG 0413, are awaited. In women over the age of 70 with small (less than 2 cm), lymph node–negative, hormone receptor–positive cancers, radiation therapy may be avoided. The recurrence rates after intraoperative radiation, while low, appear significantly higher than postoperative whole breast radiation therapy. However, in all of these situations, a balanced discussion with a radiation oncologist to weigh the risks and benefits of each approach is warranted.

Current studies suggest that radiotherapy after mastectomy may improve recurrence rates and survival in younger patients and those with tumors 5 cm or larger or positive lymph nodes. The AMAROS study randomized women with sentinel node metastases to ALND or nodal irradiation and found no significant difference in survival but lower lymphedema rates after radiation. An ACOSOG study (Z0010) and large NSABP trial (B-32) showed no adverse impact of micrometastases on survival and support no alteration in treatment when found. A Canadian trial (MA20) of postoperative nodal irradiation after lumpectomy and axillary dissection showed improved disease-free survival but not overall survival with nodal irradiation.

D. Adjuvant Systemic Therapy

The goal of systemic therapy, including hormone-modulating drugs (endocrine therapy), cytotoxic chemotherapy, and *HER2*-targeted agents such as trastuzumab, is to kill cancer cells that have escaped the breast and axillary lymph nodes as micrometastases before they become macrometastases (ie, stage IV cancer). Systemic therapy improves survival and is advocated for most patients with curable breast cancer. In practice, most medical oncologists are currently using adjuvant chemotherapy for patients with either node-positive or higher-risk (eg, hormone receptor-negative or *HER2*-positive) node-negative breast cancer and using endocrine therapy for all hormone receptor–positive invasive breast cancer unless contraindicated. Prognostic factors other than nodal status that are used to determine the patient's risks of recurrence are tumor size, ER and PR status, nuclear grade,

Table 17–5. Prognostic factors in node-negative breast cancer.

Prognostic Factors	Increased Recurrence	Decreased Recurrence
Size[1]	T3, T2	T1, T0
Hormone receptors	Negative	Positive
DNA flow cytometry	Aneuploid	Diploid
Histologic grade	High	Low
Tumor labeling index	< 3%	> 3%
S phase fraction	> 5%	< 5%
Lymphatic or vascular invasion	Present	Absent
Cathepsin D	High	Low
HER2 oncogene	High	Low
Epidermal growth factor receptor	High	Low

[1]See Table 17–3 for TNM staging for breast cancer.

histologic type, proliferative rate, oncogene expression (Table 17–5), and patient's age and menopausal status. In general, systemic chemotherapy decreases the chance of recurrence by about 30%, hormonal modulation decreases the relative risk of recurrence by 40–50% (for hormone receptor–positive cancer), and HER2-targeted therapy decreases the relative risk of recurrence by up to 40% (for HER2-positive cancer). Systemic chemotherapy is usually given sequentially, rather than concurrently with radiation. In terms of sequencing, typically chemotherapy is given before radiation and endocrine therapy is started concurrent with or after radiation therapy.

The long-term advantage of systemic therapy has been well established. All patients with invasive hormone receptor–positive tumors should consider the use of hormone-modulating therapy. Most patients with HER2-positive tumors should receive trastuzumab-containing chemotherapy regimens. In general, adjuvant systemic chemotherapy should not be given to women who have small node-negative breast cancers with favorable histologic findings and tumor markers. The ability to predict more accurately which patients with HER2-negative, hormone receptor–positive, lymph node–negative tumors should receive chemotherapy is improving with the advent of prognostic tools, such as Oncotype DX and Mamma-print. These tests are undergoing prospective evaluation in two clinical trials (TAILORx and MINDACT).

1. Chemotherapy—The Early Breast Cancer Trialists' Collaborative Group (EBCTCG) meta-analysis involving over 28,000 women enrolled in 60 trials of adjuvant polychemotherapy versus no chemotherapy demonstrated a significant beneficial impact of chemotherapy on clinical outcome in non–stage IV breast cancer. This study showed that adjuvant chemotherapy reduces the risk of recurrence and breast cancer–specific mortality in all women and also

showed that women under the age of 50 derive the greatest benefit. On the basis of the superiority of anthracycline-containing regimens in metastatic breast cancer, both doxorubicin and epirubicin have been studied extensively in the adjuvant setting. Studies comparing Adriamycin (doxorubicin) and cyclophosphamide (AC) or epirubicin and cyclophosphamide (EC) to cyclophosphamide-methotrexate-5-fluorouracil (CMF) have shown that treatments with anthracycline-containing regimens are at least as effective as treatment with CMF. The EBCTCG analysis including over 14,000 patients enrolled in trials comparing anthracycline-based regimens to CMF, showed a small but statistically significant improved disease-free and overall survival with the use of anthracycline-based regimens. It should be noted, however, that most of these studies included a mixed population of patients with HER2-positive and HER2-negative breast cancer and were performed before the introduction of trastuzumab. Retrospective analyses of a number of these studies suggest that anthracyclines may be primarily effective in tumors with HER2 overexpression or alteration in the expression of topoisomerase IIa (the target of anthracyclines and close to the HER2 gene). Given this, for HER2-negative, node-negative breast cancer, four cycles of AC or six cycles of CMF are probably equally effective.

When taxanes (paclitaxel and docetaxel) emerged in the 1990s, multiple trials were conducted to evaluate their use in combination with anthracycline-based regimens. The majority of these trials showed an improvement in disease-free survival and at least one showed an improvement in overall survival with the taxane-based regimen. A meta-analysis of taxane versus non-taxane anthracycline-based regimen trials showed an improvement in disease-free and overall survival for the taxane-based regimens. Several regimens have been reported including AC followed by paclitaxel (AC-P) or docetaxel (Taxotere) (AC-T), docetaxel concurrent with AC (TAC), 5-fluorouracil-epirubicine-cyclophosphamide (FEC)-docetaxel and FEC-paclitaxel.

The US Oncology trial 9735 compared four cycles of AC with four cycles of docetaxel (Taxotere) and cyclophosphamide (TC). With a median of 7 years follow-up, this study showed a statistically significantly improved disease-free survival and overall survival in the patients who received TC.

An important ongoing study (US Oncology 06090) is prospectively evaluating whether anthracyclines add any incremental benefit to a taxane-based regimen by comparing six cycles of TAC to six cycles of TC in patients with HER2-negative breast cancer. A third arm was added to evaluate the benefit of adding bevacizumab, a monoclonal antibody directed against vascular endothelial growth factor (VEGF), to TC. While awaiting the results of this trial, oncologists are faced with choosing from among the above treatment regimens for HER2-negative breast cancer. Given the benefits described above, taxanes are now used for most patients receiving chemotherapy for early breast cancer.

The overall duration of adjuvant chemotherapy still remains uncertain. However, based on the meta-analysis performed in the Oxford Overview (EBCTCG), the current recommendation is for 3–6 months of the commonly used regimens. Although it is clear that dose intensity to a specific threshold is essential, there is no evidence to support the long-term survival benefit of high-dose chemotherapy with stem cell support.

Chemotherapy side effects are now generally well controlled. Nausea and vomiting are abated with drugs that directly affect the central nervous system, such as ondansetron and granisetron. Infertility and premature ovarian failure are common side effects of chemotherapy and should be discussed with patients prior to starting treatment. The risk of life-threatening neutropenia associated with chemotherapy can be reduced by use of growth factors such as pegfilgrastim and filgrastim (G-CSF), which stimulate proliferation and differentiation of hematopoietic cells. Long-term toxicities from chemotherapy, including cardiomyopathy (anthracyclines), peripheral neuropathy (taxanes), and leukemia/myelodysplasia (anthracyclines and alkylating agents), remain a small but significant risk.

2. Targeted therapy—Targeted therapy refers to agents that are directed specifically against a protein or molecule expressed uniquely on tumor cells or in the tumor microenvironment.

A. HER2 OVEREXPRESSION—Approximately 20% of breast cancers are characterized by amplification of the *HER2* oncogene leading to overexpression of the *HER2* oncoprotein. The poor prognosis associated with *HER2* overexpression has been drastically improved with the development of *HER2*-targeted therapy. Trastuzumab (Herceptin [H]), a monoclonal antibody that binds to *HER2*, has proved effective in combination with chemotherapy in patients with *HER2*-overexpressing metastatic and early breast cancer. In the adjuvant setting, the first and most commonly studied chemotherapy backbone used with trastuzumab is AC-T. Subsequently, the BCIRG006 study showed similar efficacy for AC-TH and a nonanthracycline-containing regimen, TCH (docetaxel, carboplatin, trastuzumab). Both were significantly better than AC-T in terms of disease-free and overall survival and TCH had a lower risk of cardiac toxicity. Both AC-TH and TCH are FDA-approved for nonmetastatic, *HER2*-positive breast cancer. In these regimens, trastuzumab is given with chemotherapy and then continues beyond the course of chemotherapy to complete a full year. At least one study (N9831) suggests that concurrent, rather than sequential, delivery of trastuzumab with chemotherapy may be more beneficial. Neoadjuvant chemotherapy plus dual *HER2*-targeted therapy with trastuzumab and pertuzumab (also a *HER2*-targeted monoclonal antibody that prevents dimerization of *HER2* with *HER3* and has been shown to be synergistic in combination with trastuzumab) was FDA approved in 2013 and is now a standard of care option available to patients with nonmetastatic *HER2*. Another question being addressed in trials is whether to treat small (less than 1 cm), node-negative tumors with trastuzumab plus chemotherapy. Retrospective studies have shown that even small (stage T1a,b) *HER2*-positive tumors have a worse prognosis compared with same-sized *HER2*-negative tumors and may thus be appropriate for trastuzumab-based regimens. The NSABP B43 study is also ongoing to evaluate whether the addition of trastuzumab to radiation therapy is warranted for DCIS.

Cardiomyopathy develops in a small but significant percent (0.4–4%) of patients who receive trastuzumab-based regimens. For this reason, anthracyclines and trastuzumab are rarely given concurrently and cardiac function is monitored periodically throughout therapy.

B. ENDOCRINE THERAPY—Adjuvant hormone modulation therapy is highly effective in decreasing relative risk of recurrence by 40–50% and mortality by 25% in women with hormone receptor–positive tumors regardless of menopausal status. The traditional regimen had been 5 years of the estrogen-receptor antagonist/agonist tamoxifen until the 2012 reporting of the Adjuvant Tamoxifen Longer Against Shorter (ATLAS) trial in which 5 versus 10 years of adjuvant tamoxifen were compared. In this study, disease-free and overall survival were significantly improved in women who received 10 years of tamoxifen, particularly after year 10. The Adjuvant Tamoxifen—To offer more? (aTTom) study confirmed these results. Though these results are impressive, the clinical application of long-term tamoxifen use must be discussed with patients individually, taking into consideration risks of tamoxifen (such as secondary uterine cancers, venous thromboembolic events, and side effects that impact quality of life). The addition of ovarian suppression to tamoxifen has not been shown to significantly improve recurrence rates or survival compared to tamoxifen alone in randomized clinical trials (Zoladex in Premenopausal Patients [ZIPP] and Suppression of Ovarian Function Trial [SOFT] studies). AIs, including anastrozole, letrozole, and exemestane, reduce estrogen production and are also effective in the adjuvant setting for postmenopausal women. Approximately seven large randomized trials enrolling more than 24,000 patients have compared the use of AIs with tamoxifen or placebo as adjuvant therapy. All of these studies have shown small but statistically significant improvements in disease-free survival (absolute benefits of 2–6%) with the use of AIs. In addition, AIs have been shown to reduce the risk of contralateral breast cancers and to have fewer associated serious side effects (such as endometrial cancers and thromboembolic events) than tamoxifen. However, they are associated with accelerated bone loss and an increased risk of fractures as well as a musculoskeletal syndrome characterized by arthralgias or myalgias (or both) in up to 50% of patients. The American Society of Clinical Oncology and the NCCN have recommended that postmenopausal women with hormone receptor–positive breast cancer be offered an AI either initially or after tamoxifen therapy. *HER2* status should not affect the use or choice of hormone therapy. Until recently, the use of AIs was restricted to postmenopausal women whose ovaries were not producing estrogen. A combined analysis of the SOFT and Tamoxifen and Exemestane Trial (TEXT) studies showed for the first time that exemestane plus ovarian suppression was associated with a reduced risk of relapse compared to tamoxifen plus ovarian suppression, making this a viable adjuvant therapy option for young women with high-risk ER-positive breast cancers.

3. Bisphosphonates—Multiple randomized studies have evaluated the use of adjuvant bisphosphonates in addition to standard local and systemic therapy for early-stage breast cancer and have shown, in addition to improvement in bone density, a consistent reduction in the risk of metastatic recurrence in postmenopausal patients. A meta-analysis evaluating more than 18,000 women with early-stage breast cancer treated with bisphosphonates or placebo showed that bisphosphonates reduce the risk of cancer recurrence (especially in bone) and improve breast cancer-specific survival primarily in postmenopausal women. Side effects associated with bisphosphonate therapy include bone pain, fever, osteonecrosis of the jaw (rare, less than 1%), esophagitis or ulcers (for oral bisphosphonates), and renal failure. Although the FDA has not yet approved the adjuvant use of bisphosphonates to reduce the risk of breast cancer recurrence, the use of these agents in women with breast cancer is becoming more common, especially in the setting of a patient who has concomitant osteopenia or osteoporosis. In addition, denosumab (another bone stabilizing drug), which is an antibody directed against receptor activator of nuclear factor kappa B ligand (RANK-B), is being investigated for its impact on breast cancer recurrence rates.

4. Adjuvant therapy in older women—Data relating to the optimal use of adjuvant systemic treatment for women over the age of 65 are limited. Results from the EBCTCG overview indicate that while adjuvant chemotherapy yields a smaller benefit for older women compared with younger women, it still improves clinical outcomes. Moreover, individual studies do show that older women with higher risk disease derive benefits from chemotherapy. One study compared the use of oral chemotherapy (capecitabine) to standard chemotherapy in older women and concluded that standard chemotherapy is preferred. Another study (USO TC vs AC) showed that women over the age of 65 derive similar benefits from the taxane-based regimen as women who are younger. The benefits of endocrine therapy for hormone receptor-positive disease appear to be independent of age. In general, decisions relating to the use of systemic therapy should take into account a patient's comorbidities and physiological age, more so than chronologic age.

E. Neoadjuvant Therapy

The use of chemotherapy or endocrine therapy prior to resection of the primary tumor (neoadjuvant) is gaining popularity. This enables the assessment of in vivo chemo-sensitivity. Patients with hormone receptor–negative, triple negative, or HER2-positive breast cancer are more likely to have a pathologic complete response to neoadjuvant chemotherapy than those with hormone receptor–positive breast cancer. A complete pathologic response at the time of surgery is associated with improvement in event-free and overall survival. Neoadjuvant chemotherapy also increases the chance of breast conservation by shrinking the primary tumor in women who would otherwise need mastectomy for local control. Survival after neoadjuvant chemotherapy is similar to that seen with postoperative adjuvant chemotherapy.

1. HER2-positive breast cancer—Dual targeting of HER2 with two monoclonal antibodies, trastuzumab and pertuzumab, showed positive results in two clinical trials in the neoadjuvant setting, the TRYPHAENA and the NEO-SPHERE studies.

Based on these clinical trials, three regimens have received FDA approval in the HER2-positive neoadjuvant setting: docetaxel [T], cyclophosphamide [C], trastuzumab [H], and pertuzumab [P] (TCHP) for six cycles; 5-fluorouracil, epirubicin, cyclophosphamide [FEC] for 3 cycles followed by THP for 3 cycles; or THP for 4 cycles (followed by three cycles of postoperative FEC). Pertuzumab is not FDA-approved for the adjuvant setting, though the National Comprehensive Cancer Network guidelines list pertuzumab plus trastuzumab as an appropriate adjuvant therapy if pertuzumab was not given in the neoadjuvant setting. Postoperatively, all patients should continue to receive trastuzumab to complete a full year.

2. Hormone receptor–positive, HER2-negative breast cancer—Patients with hormone receptor-positive breast cancer have a lower chance of achieving a pathologic complete response with neoadjuvant therapy than those patients with triple negative or HER2-positive breast cancers. Studies are ongoing to evaluate hormonally targeted regimens in the neoadjuvant setting. Outside of the clinical trial setting, the use of neoadjuvant hormonal therapy is generally restricted to postmenopausal patients who are unwilling or unable to tolerate chemotherapy.

3. Triple negative breast cancer—No targeted therapy has been identified for patients with breast cancer that is lacking in HER2 amplification or hormone receptor expression. Neoadjuvant chemotherapy leads to pathologic complete response in up to 40–50% of patients with triple negative breast cancer. Patients who achieve a pathologic complete response seem to have a similar prognosis to other breast cancer subtypes with pathologic complete response. However, those patients with residual disease at the time of surgery have a poor prognosis. Based on the theory that triple negative breast cancers may be more vulnerable to DNA-damaging agents, several studies are evaluating whether the addition of platinum salts to a neoadjuvant chemotherapy regimen is beneficial in this disease subtype. A randomized phase II trial (GeparSixto) randomly assigned 595 patients with triple negative or HER2-positive breast cancer to weekly paclitaxel plus weekly liposomal doxorubicin (18 weeks) alone or with weekly carboplatin. Patients with triple negative disease also received bevacizumab. Those patients with triple negative disease who received carboplatin had a pathologic complete response rate of 53.2% compared to those who did not receive carboplatin (36.9%; $P = 0.005$). The 3-year disease-free survival (DFS) data were presented in 2015; the addition of carboplatin improved disease-free survival from 76.1% to 85.8% (HR 0.56, 95% CI (0.33, 0.96), $P = 0.0350$) Similarly designed studies are ongoing to evaluate the pathologic complete response rates and long-term outcomes associated with incorporating platinums into standard chemotherapy regimens.

4. Timing of sentinel lymph node biopsy in neoadjuvant setting—There is considerable concern about the timing of sentinel lymph node biopsy, since the chemotherapy may affect cancer present in the lymph nodes. Several studies have shown that sentinel node biopsy can be done after neoadjuvant therapy. However, a large multicenter study, ACOSOG 1071, demonstrated a false-negative rate of 10.7%, well above the false-negative rate outside the neoadjuvant setting (less than 1–5%). Some physicians recommend performing sentinel lymph node biopsy before administering the chemotherapy in order to avoid a false-negative result and to aid in planning subsequent radiation therapy. Others prefer to perform sentinel lymph node biopsy after neoadjuvant therapy to avoid a second operation and assess post-chemotherapy nodal status. If a complete dissection is desired, this can be performed at the time of the definitive breast surgery. The SENTINA trial showed similarly poor results for sentinel node biopsy after neoadjuvant therapy. No study has evaluated the impact of no axillary treatment for node-positive patients who become node-negative after neoadjuvant therapy.

Important questions remaining to be answered are the timing and duration of adjuvant and neoadjuvant chemotherapy, which chemotherapeutic agents should be applied for which subgroups of patients, the use of combinations of hormonal therapy and chemotherapy as well as possibly targeted therapy, and the value of prognostic factors other than hormone receptors in predicting response to therapy.

▶ Palliative Treatment

Palliative treatments are those to manage symptoms, improve quality of life, and even prolong survival, without the expectation of achieving cure. In the United States, it is uncommon to have distant metastases at the time of diagnosis (de novo metastases). However, most patients who have a breast cancer recurrence after initial local and adjuvant therapy have a metastatic rather than local (in breast) disease. Breast cancer most commonly metastasizes to the liver, lungs and bone, causing symptoms such as fatigue, change in appetite, abdominal pain, cough, dyspnea, or bone pain. Headaches, imbalance, vision changes, vertigo, and other neurologic symptoms may be signs of brain metastases. Triple negative (ER-, PR-, *HER2*-negative) and *HER2*-positive tumors have a higher rate of brain metastases than hormone-receptor positive, *HER2*-negative tumors.

A. Radiotherapy and Bisphosphonates

Palliative radiotherapy may be advised for primary treatment of locally advanced cancers with distant metastases to control ulceration, pain, and other manifestations in the breast and regional nodes. Irradiation of the breast and chest wall and the axillary, internal mammary, and supraclavicular nodes should be undertaken in an attempt to cure locally advanced and inoperable lesions when there is no evidence of distant metastases. A small number of patients in this group are cured in spite of extensive breast and regional node involvement.

Palliative irradiation is of value also in the treatment of certain bone or soft-tissue metastases to control pain or avoid fracture. Radiotherapy is especially useful in the treatment of isolated bony metastases, chest wall recurrences, brain metastases and sometimes, in lieu of the preferred option of orthopedic surgery for acute spinal cord compression.

In addition to radiotherapy, bisphosphonate therapy has shown excellent results in delaying and reducing skeletal events in women with bony metastases. Pamidronate and zoledronic acid are FDA-approved intravenous bisphosphonates given for bone metastases or hypercalcemia of malignancy from breast cancer. Denosumab, a fully human monoclonal antibody that targets RANK-ligand, is approved by the FDA for the treatment of bone metastases from breast cancer, with data showing that it reduced the time to first skeletal-related event (eg, pathologic fracture) compared to zoledronic acid.

Caution should be exercised when combining radiation therapy with chemotherapy because toxicity of either or both may be augmented by their concurrent administration. In general, only one type of therapy should be given at a time unless it is necessary to irradiate a destructive lesion of weight-bearing bone while the patient is receiving chemotherapy. Systemic therapy should be changed only if the disease is clearly progressing. This is especially difficult to determine for patients with destructive bone metastases, since changes in the status of these lesions are difficult to determine radiographically.

B. Targeted Therapy

1. Endocrine therapy for metastatic disease—The first targeted therapy for cancer was the use of antiestrogen therapy in hormone receptor–positive breast cancer. The following therapies have all been shown to be effective in hormone receptor–positive metastatic breast cancer: administration of drugs that block or downregulate hormone receptors (such as tamoxifen or fulvestrant, respectively) or drugs that block the synthesis of hormones (such as AIs); ablation of the ovaries, adrenals, or pituitary; and the administration of hormones (eg, estrogens, androgens, progestins); see Table 17–6. Palliative treatment of metastatic cancer should be based on the ER status of the primary tumor or the metastases. Because only 5–10% of women with ER-negative tumors respond, they should not receive endocrine therapy. The rate of response is nearly equal in premenopausal and postmenopausal women with ER-positive tumors. A favorable response to hormonal manipulation occurs in about one-third of patients with metastatic breast cancer. Of those whose tumors contain ER, the response is about 60% and perhaps as high as 80% for patients whose tumors contain PR as well. The choice of endocrine therapy depends on the menopausal status of the patient. Women within 1 year of their last menstrual period are arbitrarily considered to be premenopausal and should receive tamoxifen therapy or ovarian ablation (surgical or hormonal) plus an AI, whereas women whose menses ceased more than a year before are postmenopausal and may receive tamoxifen, fulvestrant, or an AI. Women with ER-positive tumors who do not respond to first-line endocrine therapy or experience progression should be given a different form of hormonal manipulation. Because the quality of life during endocrine manipulation is usually superior to that during cytotoxic chemotherapy, it is best to try endocrine manipulation

Table 17–6. Agents commonly used for hormonal management of metastatic breast cancer.

Drug	Action	Dose, Route, Frequency	Major Side Effects
Tamoxifen citrate (Nolvadex)	SERM	20 mg orally daily	Hot flushes, uterine bleeding, thrombophlebitis, rash
Fulvestrant (Faslodex)	Steroidal estrogen receptor antagonist	500 mg intramuscularly days 1, 15, 29 and then monthly	Gastrointestinal upset, headache, back pain, hot flushes, pharyngitis
Toremifene citrate (Fareston)	SERM	40 mg orally daily	Hot flushes, sweating, nausea, vaginal discharge, dry eyes, dizziness
Diethylstilbestrol (DES)	Estrogen	5 mg orally three times daily	Fluid retention, uterine bleeding, thrombophlebitis, nausea
Goserelin (Zoladex)	Synthetic luteinizing hormone releasing analog	3.6 mg subcutaneously monthly	Arthralgias, blood pressure changes, hot flushes, headaches, vaginal dryness
Megestrol acetate (Megace)	Progestin	40 mg orally four times daily	Fluid retention
Letrozole (Femara)	AI	2.5 mg orally daily	Hot flushes, arthralgia/arthritis, myalgia, bone loss
Anastrozole (Arimidex)	AI	1 mg orally daily	Hot flushes, skin rashes, nausea and vomiting, bone loss
Exemestane (Aromasin)	AI	25 mg orally daily	Hot flushes, increased arthralgia/arthritis, myalgia, bone loss

AI, aromatase inhibitor; SERM, selective estrogen receptor modulator.

whenever possible. However, when receptor status is unknown, disease is progressing rapidly or is threatening visceral organs, chemotherapy may be used as first-line treatment.

A. THE PREMENOPAUSAL PATIENT

(1) Primary hormonal therapy—The most extensively studied method of endocrine therapy in premenopausal patients is tamoxifen, in large part because it can be given with less morbidity and fewer side effects than cytotoxic chemotherapy and does not require oophorectomy. Tamoxifen is given orally in a dose of 20 mg daily. The average clinical benefit associated with tamoxifen lasts about 12 months.

There is no significant difference in survival or response between tamoxifen therapy and bilateral oophorectomy. Bilateral oophorectomy is less desirable than tamoxifen in premenopausal women because tamoxifen is so well tolerated. However, oophorectomy can be achieved rapidly and safely either by surgery, by irradiation of the ovaries if the patient is a poor surgical candidate, or by chemical ovarian ablation using a gonadotropin-releasing hormone (GnRH) analog. Oophorectomy presumably works by eliminating estrogens, progestins, and androgens, which stimulate growth of the tumor. AIs should not be used in a patient with functioning ovaries since they do not block ovarian production of estrogen.

(2) Secondary or tertiary hormonal therapy—Patients who do not respond to tamoxifen or ovarian ablation may be treated with chemotherapy or may try a second endocrine regimen, such as GnRH analog plus AI or fulvestrant. Whether to opt for chemotherapy or another endocrine measure depends largely on the sites of metastatic disease (visceral being more serious than bone-only, thus sometimes

warranting the use of chemotherapy), the disease burden, the rate of growth of disease, and patient preference. Patients who take chemotherapy and then later have progressive disease may subsequently respond to another form of endocrine treatment (Table 17–6). The optimal choice for secondary endocrine manipulation has not been clearly defined for the premenopausal patient.

Patients who improve after oophorectomy but subsequently relapse should receive fulvestrant, tamoxifen or an AI; if one fails, the other may be tried. Megestrol acetate, a progesterone agent, may also be considered.

B. THE POSTMENOPAUSAL PATIENT

(1) Primary hormonal therapy—For postmenopausal women with metastatic breast cancer amenable to endocrine manipulation, fulvestrant, tamoxifen or an AI is the initial therapy of choice. AIs may be more effective. The side effect profile of AIs differs from tamoxifen. The main side effects of tamoxifen are nausea, skin rash, and hot flushes. Rarely, tamoxifen induces hypercalcemia in patients with bony metastases. Tamoxifen also increases the risk of venous thromboembolic events and uterine hyperplasia and cancer. The main side effects of AIs include hot flushes, vaginal dryness, and joint stiffness; however, osteoporosis and bone fractures are significantly higher than with tamoxifen. Phase II data from the randomized Fulvestrant fIRst line Study comparing endocrine Treatments (FIRST) suggest that the pure estrogen antagonist fulvestrant may be even more effective than front-line anastrozole in terms of time to progression and overall survival. Results from the phase III FALCON study are awaited to confirm these data. The combination of fulvestrant plus anastrozole may also be more effective than anastrozole alone, although two studies evaluating this question have yielded conflicting results.

(2) Secondary or tertiary hormonal therapy—AIs are also used for the treatment of advanced breast cancer in postmenopausal women after tamoxifen or fulvestrant treatment. In the event that the patient responds to an AI but then has progression of disease, fulvestrant has shown efficacy with about 20–30% of women benefiting from use. Postmenopausal women who respond initially to a SERM or AI but later manifest progressive disease may be crossed over to another hormonal therapy. Until recently, patients who experienced disease progression during or after treatment with a SERM or AI were routinely offered chemotherapy. This standard practice changed in 2012 with the approval of **everolimus** (Afinitor), an oral inhibitor of the mammalian target of rapamycin (MTOR)—a protein whose activation has been associated with the development of endocrine resistance. A phase III, placebo-controlled trial (BOLERO-2) evaluated exemestane with or without everolimus in 724 patients with AI-resistant, hormone receptor–positive metastatic breast cancer and found that patients treated with everolimus had a significantly improved progression-free survival (7.8 months vs 3.2 months; HR, 0.45; 95% CI, 0.38–0.54; $P < 0.0001$) but no significant difference in overall survival.

(3) Cyclin dependent kinase inhibition—The preclinical observation that hormonally driven breast cancer may be particularly sensitive to inhibition of cell cycle regulatory proteins, called cyclin dependent kinases (CDK), led to a randomized study evaluating letrozole with or without an oral CDK 4/6 inhibitor (palbociclib) for the first-line treatment of postmenopausal women with hormone receptor–positive advanced breast cancer. This phase II trial demonstrated a striking and highly significant doubling of progression-free survival with palbociclib compared to the control arm. These results led to the accelerated FDA approval in 2015 of palbociclib in combination with letrozole for patients with previously untreated ER-positive *HER2*-negative metastatic breast cancer. Results from the phase III confirmatory study (PALOMA-2) in the first-line setting are awaited. Shortly after the regulatory approval of palbociclib, results from the phase III PALOMA-3 study were published that showed the addition of palbociclib to fulvestrant in *pretreated* patients with ER-positive metastatic breast cancer more than doubled progression free survival. In general, palbociclib is well tolerated; however, it is associated with grade 3/4 leukopenia and neutropenia, thus monitoring patients closely is required. Several other CDK4/6 inhibitors (abemaciclib and ribociclib) are being evaluated in clinical trials.

2. *HER2*-targeted agents—For patients with *HER2*-overexpressing or amplified tumors, trastuzumab plus chemotherapy has been shown to significantly improve clinical outcomes, including survival compared to chemotherapy alone. Trastuzumab plus chemotherapy was therefore the standard first-line treatment for *HER2*-positive metastatic breast cancer until 2012 when pertuzumab was granted FDA approval. **Pertuzumab** is a monoclonal antibody that targets the extracellular domain of *HER2* at a different epitope than targeted by trastuzumab and inhibits receptor dimerization. A phase III placebo-controlled randomized study (CLEOPATRA) showed that patients treated with the combination of pertuzumab, trastuzumab, and docetaxel had a significantly longer progression-free survival (18.5 months vs 12.4 months; HR, 0.62; 95% CI, 0.51–0.75; $P < 0.001$) compared with those treated with docetaxel and trastuzumab. Longer follow-up revealed a significant overall survival benefit associated with pertuzumab as well.

Lapatinib, an oral targeted drug that inhibits the intracellular tyrosine kinases of the epidermal growth factor and *HER2* receptors, is FDA-approved for the treatment of trastuzumab-resistant *HER2*-positive metastatic breast cancer in combination with capecitabine, thus, a completely oral regimen. The combination of trastuzumab plus lapatinib has been shown to be more effective than lapatinib alone for trastuzumab-resistant metastatic breast cancer. Moreover, several trials have shown a significant clinical benefit for continuing *HER2*-targeted agents beyond progression. **T-DM1 (trastuzumab emtansine)** is a novel antibody drug conjugate in which trastuzumab is stably linked to a derivative of maytansine, enabling targeted delivery of the cytotoxic chemotherapy to *HER2*-overexpressing cells. The phase III trial (EMILIA) that evaluated T-DM1 in patients with *HER2*-positive, trastuzumab-pretreated advanced disease showed that T-DM1 is associated with improved progression-free and overall survival compared to lapatinib plus capecitabine (EMILIA). Regulatory approval of T-DM1 (Kadcyla [ado-trastuzumab emtansine]) was received in February 2013. Ado-trastuzumab emtansine (Kadcyla) with or without pertuzumab was compared to trastuzumab plus a taxane for the first-line treatment of *HER2*-positive advanced breast cancer in the phase III MARIANNE study. This study showed that the two ado-trastuzumab containing arms were noninferior (but not superior) to the trastuzumab plus taxane arm. Thus, for the time being, ado-trastuzumab is primarily used in the second-line setting and beyond. Several other drugs targeting *HER2* and its associated signaling pathways are in development, including everolimus, neratinib, and *HER2*-targeted vaccines.

3. Targeting "triple-negative" breast cancer—Breast cancers lacking expression of the hormone receptors ER, PR, and *HER2* have only been amenable to therapy with cytotoxic chemotherapy. This type of "triple-negative" breast cancer, while heterogeneous, generally behaves aggressively and is associated with a poor prognosis. Newer classes of targeted agents are being evaluated specifically for triple-negative breast cancer, although none have been shown to improve outcomes to date. Early phase clinical trials show promise for immune checkpoint inhibitors (such as monoclonal antibodies that target PDL-1 or PD-1) and androgen receptor inhibitors. Research in this area is rapidly expanding with multiple clinical trials of molecularly targeted agents ongoing.

C. Palliative Chemotherapy

Cytotoxic drugs should be considered for the treatment of metastatic breast cancer (1) if visceral metastases are present (especially brain, liver, or lymphangitic pulmonary), (2) if hormonal treatment is unsuccessful or the disease has progressed after an initial response to hormonal manipulation, or (3) if the tumor is ER-negative or *HER2*-positive. Prior adjuvant chemotherapy does not seem to alter response rates in patients who relapse. A number of chemotherapy drugs (including vinorelbine, paclitaxel, docetaxel, gemcitabine, ixabepilone, carboplatin, cisplatin, capecitabine, albumin-bound paclitaxel, eribulin, and liposomal doxorubicin) may be used as single agents with first-line objective response rates ranging from 30% to 50%.

Combination chemotherapy yields statistically significantly higher response rates and progression-free survival rates, but has not been conclusively shown to improve overall survival rates compared with sequential single-agent therapy. Combinations that have been tested in phase III studies and have proven efficacy compared with single-agent therapy include capecitabine/docetaxel, gemcitabine/paclitaxel, and capecitabine/ixabepilone (see Tables 39–11 and 39–12). Various other combinations of drugs have been tested in phase II studies, and a number of clinical trials are ongoing to identify effective combinations. Patients should be encouraged to participate in clinical trials given the number of promising targeted therapies in development. It is generally appropriate to treat willing patients with multiple sequential lines of therapy as long as they tolerate the treatment and as long as their performance status is good (eg, at least ambulatory and able to care for self, up out of bed more than 50% of waking hours).

Amiri-Kordestani L et al. First FDA approval of neoadjuvant therapy for breast cancer: pertuzumab for the treatment of patients with *HER2*-positive breast cancer. Clin Cancer Res. 2014 Nov 1;20(21):5359–64. [PMID: 25204553]

Baselga J et al; CLEOPATRA Study Group. Pertuzumab plus trastuzumab plus docetaxel for metastatic breast cancer. N Engl J Med. 2012 Jan 12;366(2):109–19. [PMID: 22149875]

Dengel LT et al. Axillary dissection can be avoided in the majority of clinically node-negative patients undergoing breast-conserving therapy. Ann Surg Oncol. 2014 Jan;21(1):22–7. [PMID: 23975314]

Donker M et al. Radiotherapy or surgery of the axilla after a positive sentinel node in breast cancer (EORTC 10981-22023 AMAROS): a randomized, multi-centre, open-label, phase 3 non-inferiority trial. Lancet Oncol. 2014 Nov;15(12):1303–10. [PMID: 25439688]

Early Breast Cancer Trialists' Collaborative Group. Adjuvant bisphosphonate treatment in early breast cancer: meta-analyses of individual patient data from randomized trials. Lancet. 2015 Oct 3;386(10001):1353–61. [PMID: 26211824]

Ellis MJ et al. Fulvestrant 500 mg versus anastrozole 1 mg for the first-line treatment of advanced breast cancer: overall survival analysis from the Phase II FIRST Study. J Clin Oncol. 2015 Nov 10;33(32):3781–7. [PMID: 26371134]

Ellis PA et al. Phase III, randomized study of trastuzumab emtansine (T-DM1) ± pertuzumab (P) vs trastuzumab + taxane (HT) for first-line treatment of HER2-positive MBC: primary results from the MARIANNE study. J Clin Oncol. 2015;33(Suppl; abstr 507).

Finn RS et al. The cyclin-dependent kinase 4/6 inhibitor palbociclib in combination with letrozole versus letrozole alone as first-line treatment of oestrogen receptor-positive, HER2-negative, advanced breast cancer (PALOMA-1/TRIO-18): a randomised phase 2 study. Lancet Oncol. 2015 Jan;16(1):25–35. [PMID: 25524798]

Giuliano AE et al. Axillary dissection vs no axillary dissection in women with invasive breast cancer and sentinel node metastasis: a randomized clinical trial. JAMA. 2011 Feb 9;305(6):569–75. [PMID: 21304082]

Goldhirsch A et al; Herceptin Adjuvant (HERA) Trial Study Team. 2 years versus 1 year of adjuvant trastuzumab for *HER2*-positive breast cancer (HERA): an open-label, randomised controlled trial. Lancet. 2013 Sep 21;382(9897):1021–8. [PMID: 23871490]

Haviland JS et al. The UK Standardisation of Breast Radiotherapy (START) trials of radiotherapy hypofractionation for treatment of early breast cancer: 10-year follow-up results of two randomised controlled trials. Lancet Oncol. 2013 Oct;14(11):1086–94. [PMID: 24055415]

Jagsi R et al. Progress and controversies: radiation therapy for invasive breast cancer. CA Cancer J Clin. 2014 Mar–Apr;64(2):135–52. [PMID: 24357525]

Kümmel S et al. Surgical treatment of primary breast cancer in the neoadjuvant setting. Br J Surg. 2014 Jul;101(8):912–24. [PMID: 24838656]

Moore HC et al; POEMS/S0230 Investigators. Goserelin for ovarian protection during breast cancer adjuvant chemotherapy. N Engl J Med. 2015 Mar 5;372(10):923–32. [PMID: 25738668]

National Comprehensive Cancer Network. NCCN Guidelines: Breast Cancer. http://www.nccn.org/professionals/physician_gls/f_guidelines.asp

Pagani O et al; TEXT and SOFT Investigators; International Breast Cancer Study Group. Adjuvant exemestane with ovarian suppression in premenopausal breast cancer. N Engl J Med. 2014 Jul 10;371(2):107–18. [PMID: 24881463]

Perez EA et al. Trastuzumab plus adjuvant chemotherapy for human epidermal growth factor receptor 2-positive breast cancer: planned joint analysis of overall survival from NSABP B-31 and NCCTG N9831. J Clin Oncol. 2014 Nov 20;32(33):3744–52. [PMID: 25332249]

Piccart M et al. Everolimus plus exemestane for hormone-receptor-positive, human epidermal growth factor receptor-2-negative advanced breast cancer: overall survival results from BOLERO-2†. Ann Oncol. 2014 Dec;25(12):2357–62. [PMID: 25231953]

Poortmans PM et al; EORTC Radiation Oncology and Breast Cancer Groups. Internal mammary and medial supraclavicular irradiation in breast cancer. N Engl J Med. 2015 Jul 23;373(4):317–27. [PMID: 26200978]

Slamon D et al; Breast Cancer International Research Group. Adjuvant trastuzumab in *HER2*-positive breast cancer. N Engl J Med. 2011 Oct 6;365(14):1273–83. [PMID: 21991949]

Tolaney SM et al. Adjuvant paclitaxel and trastuzumab for node-negative, HER2-positive breast cancer. N Engl J Med. 2015 Jan 8;372(2):134–41. Erratum in: N Engl J Med. 2015 Nov 12;373(20):1989. [PMID: 25564897]

Turner NC et al; PALOMA3 Study Group. Palbociclib in hormone-receptor-positive advanced breast cancer. N Engl J Med. 2015 Jul 16;373(3):209–19. [PMID: 26030518]

Verma S et al; EMILIA Study Group. Trastuzumab emtansine for *HER2*-positive advanced breast cancer. N Engl J Med. 2012 Nov 8;367(19):1783–91. [PMID: 23020162]

von Minckwitz G et al. Neoadjuvant carboplatin in patients with triple-negative and *HER2*-positive early breast cancer (GeparSixto; GBG 66): a randomised phase 2 trial. Lancet Oncol. 2014 Jun;15(7):747–56. [PMID: 2479424]

von Minckwitz G et al. Early survival analysis of the randomized phase II trial investigating the addition of carboplatin to neoadjuvant therapy for triple-negative and HER2-positive early breast cancer (GeparSixto). SABCS 2015, Abstract S02-04.

Whelan TJ et al; MA.20 Study Investigators. Regional nodal irradiation in early-stage breast cancer. N Engl J Med. 2015 Jul 23;373(4):307–16. [PMID: 26200977]

Prognosis

Stage of breast cancer is the most reliable indicator of prognosis (Table 17–7). Axillary lymph node status is the best-analyzed prognostic factor and correlates with survival at all tumor sizes. When cancer is localized to the breast with no evidence of regional spread after pathologic examination, the clinical cure rate with most accepted methods of therapy is 75% to more than 90%. In fact, patients with small mammographically detected biologically favorable tumors and no evidence of axillary spread have a 5-year survival rate greater than 95%. When the axillary lymph nodes are involved with tumor, the survival rate drops to 50–70% at 5 years and probably around 25–40% at 10 years. Increasingly, the use of biologic markers, such as ER, PR, grade, and *HER2*, is helping to identify high-risk tumor types as well as direct treatment used (see Biomarkers & Gene Expression Profiling). Tumors with marked aneuploidy have a poor prognosis (see Table 17–5). Gene analysis studies, such as Oncotype Dx, can predict disease-free survival for some subsets of patients.

Five-year statistics do not accurately reflect the final outcome of therapy. The mortality rate of breast cancer patients exceeds that of age-matched normal controls for nearly 20 years. Thereafter, the mortality rates are equal, though deaths that occur among breast cancer patients are often directly the result of tumor.

In general, breast cancer appears to be somewhat more aggressive and associated with worse outcomes in younger than in older women, and this may be related to the fact that fewer younger women have ER-positive tumors. Disparities in treatment outcome for different racial and ethnic backgrounds have been reported by several studies. These differences appear to be not only due to different socioeconomic factors (and a resulting difference in access to healthcare) but also due to differences in the subtype of breast cancer diagnosed.

For those patients whose disease progresses despite treatment, studies suggest supportive group therapy may improve survival. As they approach the end of life, such patients will require meticulous palliative care (see Chapter 5).

Iqbal J et al. Differences in breast cancer stage at diagnosis and cancer-specific survival by race and ethnicity in the United States. JAMA. 2015 Jan 13;313(2):165–73. Erratum in: JAMA. 2015 Jun 9;313(22):2287. [PMID: 25585328]

Rakha EA. Pitfalls in outcome prediction of breast cancer. J Clin Pathol. 2013 Jun;66(6):458–64. [PMID: 23618694]

Warner ET al. Racial and ethnic differences in breast cancer survival: mediating effect of tumor characteristics and sociodemographic and treatment factors. J Clin Oncol. 2015 Jul 10;33(20):2254–61. [PMID: 25964252]

Follow-up Care

After primary therapy, patients with breast cancer should be monitored long-term in order to detect recurrences and to observe the opposite breast for a second primary carcinoma. Local and distant recurrences occur most frequently within the first 2–5 years. During the first 2 years, most patients should be examined every 6 months then annually thereafter. Special attention is paid to the contralateral breast because a new primary breast malignancy will develop in 20–25% of patients. In some cases, metastases are dormant for long periods and may appear 10–15 years or longer after removal of the primary tumor. Although studies have failed to show an adverse effect of hormonal replacement in disease-free patients, it is rarely used after breast cancer treatment, particularly if the tumor was hormone receptor–positive. Even pregnancy has not been associated with shortened survival of patients rendered disease free—yet many oncologists are reluctant to advise a young patient with breast cancer that it is safe to become pregnant. The use of estrogen replacement for conditions such as osteoporosis, vaginal dryness and hot flushes may be considered for a woman with a history of breast cancer after discussion of the benefits and risks; however, it is not routinely recommended, especially given the availability of nonhormonal agents for these conditions (such as bisphosphonates and denosumab for osteoporosis). Vaginal estrogen is frequently used to treat vaginal atrophy with no obvious ill effects.

A. Local Recurrence

The incidence of local recurrence correlates with tumor size, the presence and number of involved axillary nodes, the histologic type of tumor, the presence of skin edema or skin and fascia fixation with the primary tumor, and the type of definitive surgery and local irradiation. Local recurrence on the chest wall after total mastectomy and axillary dissection develops in as many as 8% of patients. When the axillary nodes are not involved, the local recurrence rate is less than 5%, but the rate is as high as 25% when they are heavily involved. A similar difference in local recurrence rate was noted between small and large tumors. Factors such as multifocal cancer, in situ tumors, positive resection margins, chemotherapy, and radiotherapy have an effect on local recurrence in patients treated with breast-conserving surgery. Adjuvant systemic therapy greatly decreases the rate of local recurrence.

Chest wall recurrences usually appear within the first several years but may occur as late as 15 or more years after

Table 17–7. Approximate survival of patients with breast cancer by TNM stage.

TNM Stage	5 Years	10 Years
0	95%	90%
I	85%	70%
IIA	70%	50%
IIB	60%	40%
IIIA	55%	30%
IIIB	30%	20%
IV	5–10%	2%
All	65%	30%

mastectomy. All suspicious nodules and skin lesions should be biopsied. Local excision or localized radiotherapy may be feasible if an isolated nodule is present. If lesions are multiple or accompanied by evidence of regional involvement in the internal mammary or supraclavicular nodes, the disease is best managed by radiation treatment of the entire chest wall including the parasternal, supraclavicular, and axillary areas and usually by systemic therapy.

Local recurrence after mastectomy usually signals the presence of widespread disease and is an indication for studies to search for evidence of metastases. Distant metastases will develop within a few years in most patients with locally recurrent tumor after mastectomy. When there is no evidence of metastases beyond the chest wall and regional nodes, irradiation for cure after complete local excision should be attempted. After partial mastectomy, local recurrence does not have as serious a prognostic significance as after mastectomy. However, those patients in whom a recurrence develops have a worse prognosis than those who do not. It is speculated that the ability of a cancer to recur locally after radiotherapy is a sign of aggressiveness and resistance to therapy. Completion of the mastectomy should be done for local recurrence after partial mastectomy; some of these patients will survive for prolonged periods, especially if the breast recurrence is DCIS or occurs more than 5 years after initial treatment. Systemic chemotherapy or hormonal treatment should be used for women in whom disseminated disease develops or those in whom local recurrence occurs.

B. Breast Cancer Survivorship Issues

Given that most women with non-metastatic breast cancer will be cured, a significant number of women face survivorship issues stemming from either the diagnosis or the treatment of the breast cancer. These challenges include psychological struggles, upper extremity lymphedema, cognitive decline (also called "chemo brain"), weight management problems, cardiovascular issues, bone loss, postmenopausal side effects, and fatigue. One randomized study reported that survivors who received psychological intervention from the time of diagnosis had a lower risk of recurrence and breast cancer–related mortality. A randomized study in older, overweight cancer survivors showed that diet and exercise reduced the rate of self-reported functional decline compared with no intervention. Cognitive dysfunction is a commonly reported symptom experienced by women who have undergone systemic treatment for early breast cancer. Studies are ongoing to understand the pathophysiology leading to this syndrome. An interesting study reported that 200 mg of modafinil daily improved speed and quality of memory as well as attention for breast cancer survivors dealing with cognitive dysfunction. This promising study requires validation in a larger clinical trial.

1. Edema of the arm—Significant edema of the arm occurs in about 10–30% of patients after axillary dissection with or without mastectomy. It occurs more commonly if radiotherapy has been given or if there was postoperative infection. Partial mastectomy with radiation to the axillary lymph nodes is followed by chronic edema of the arm in 10–20% of patients. Sentinel lymph node dissection has proved to be a more accurate form of axillary staging without the side effects of edema or infection. Judicious use of radiotherapy, with treatment fields carefully planned to spare the axilla as much as possible, can greatly diminish the incidence of edema, which will occur in only 5% of patients if no radiotherapy is given to the axilla after a partial mastectomy and lymph node dissection.

Late or secondary edema of the arm may develop years after treatment, as a result of axillary recurrence or infection in the hand or arm, with obliteration of lymphatic channels. When edema develops, a careful examination of the axilla for recurrence or infection is performed. Infection in the arm or hand on the dissected side should be treated with antibiotics, rest, and elevation. If there is no sign of recurrence or infection, the swollen extremity should be treated with rest and elevation. A mild diuretic may be helpful. If there is no improvement, a compressor pump or manual compression decreases the swelling, and the patient is then fitted with an elastic glove or sleeve. Most patients are not bothered enough by mild edema to wear an uncomfortable glove or sleeve and will treat themselves with elevation or manual compression alone. Benzopyrones have been reported to decrease lymphedema but are not approved for this use in the United States. Rarely, edema may be severe enough to interfere with use of the limb. A prospective randomized study has shown that twice weekly progressive weight lifting improves lymphedema symptoms and exacerbations and improves extremity strength.

2. Breast reconstruction—Breast reconstruction is usually feasible after total or modified radical mastectomy. Reconstruction should be discussed with patients prior to mastectomy, because it offers an important psychological focal point for recovery. Reconstruction is not an obstacle to the diagnosis of recurrent cancer. The most common breast reconstruction has been implantation of a silicone gel or saline prosthesis in the subpectoral plane between the pectoralis minor and pectoralis major muscles. Alternatively, autologous tissue can be used for reconstruction.

Autologous tissue flaps have the advantage of not feeling like a foreign body to the patient. The most popular autologous technique currently is reconstruction using abdominal tissue flaps. This includes the deep inferior epigastric perforator (DIEP) flap and the more traditional transrectus abdominis muscle (TRAM) flap. A latissimus dorsi flap can be swung from the back but offers less volume than the TRAM flap and thus often requires supplementation with an implant. Reconstruction may be performed immediately (at the time of initial mastectomy) or may be delayed until later, usually when the patient has completed adjuvant therapy. When considering reconstructive options, concomitant illnesses should be considered, since the ability of an autologous flap to survive depends on medical comorbidities. In addition, the need for radiotherapy may affect the choice of reconstruction as radiation may increase fibrosis around an implant or decrease the volume of a flap.

3. Risks of pregnancy—Clinicians are often asked to advise patients regarding the potential risk of future pregnancy after definitive treatment for early-stage breast cancer. To date, no adverse effect of pregnancy on survival of women who have had breast cancer has been demonstrated. When counseling patients, oncologists must take into consideration the patients' overall prognosis, age, comorbidities, and life goals.

In patients with inoperable or metastatic cancer (stage IV disease), induced abortion may be advisable because of the possible adverse effects of hormonal treatment, radiotherapy, or chemotherapy upon the fetus in addition to the expectant mother's poor prognosis.

Berger AM et al. Cancer-related fatigue: implications for breast cancer survivors. Cancer. 2012 Apr 15;118(8 Suppl):2261–9. [PMID: 22488700]

DeSantis CE et al. Cancer treatment and survivorship statistics, 2014. CA Cancer J Clin. 2014 Jul–Aug;64(4):252–71. [PMID: 24890451]

Hermelink K. Acute and late onset cognitive dysfunction associated with chemotherapy in women with breast cancer. Cancer. 2011 Mar 1;117(5):1103. [PMID: 20960507]

Lee ES et al. Health-related quality of life in survivors with breast cancer 1 year after diagnosis compared with the general population: a prospective cohort study. Ann Surg. 2011 Jan; 253(1):101–8. [PMID: 21294288]

Thong MS et al. Population-based cancer registries for quality-of-life research: a work-in-progress resource for survivorship studies? Cancer. 2013 Jun 1;119(Suppl 11):2109–23. [PMID: 23695923]

CARCINOMA OF THE MALE BREAST

ESSENTIALS OF DIAGNOSIS

▶ A painless lump beneath the areola in a man usually over 50 years of age.

▶ Nipple discharge, retraction, or ulceration may be present.

▶ Generally poorer prognosis than in women.

General Considerations

Breast cancer in men is a rare disease; the incidence is only about 1% of all breast cancer diagnoses. The average age at occurrence is about 70 years and there may be an increased incidence of breast cancer in men with prostate cancer. As in women, hormonal influences are probably related to the development of male breast cancer. There is a high incidence of both breast cancer and gynecomastia in Bantu men, theoretically owing to failure of estrogen inactivation by associated liver disease. It is important to note that first-degree relatives of men with breast cancer are considered to be at high risk. This risk should be taken into account when discussing options with the patient and family. In addition, *BRCA2* mutations are common in men with breast cancer. Men with breast cancer, especially with a history of prostate cancer, should receive genetic counseling. The prognosis, even in stage I cases, is worse in men than in women.

Clinical Findings

A painless lump, occasionally associated with nipple discharge, retraction, erosion, or ulceration, is the primary complaint. Examination usually shows a hard, ill-defined, nontender mass beneath the nipple or areola. Gynecomastia not uncommonly precedes or accompanies breast cancer in men. Nipple discharge is an uncommon presentation for breast cancer in men but is an ominous finding associated with carcinoma in nearly 75% of cases.

Breast cancer staging is the same in men as in women. Gynecomastia and metastatic cancer from another site (eg, prostate) must be considered in the differential diagnosis. Benign tumors are rare, and biopsy should be performed on all males with a defined breast mass.

Treatment

Treatment consists of modified radical mastectomy in operable patients, who should be chosen by the same criteria as women with the disease. Breast conserving therapy is rarely performed. Irradiation is the first step in treating localized metastases in the skin, lymph nodes, or skeleton that are causing symptoms. Examination of the cancer for hormone receptors and *HER2* overexpression is of value in determining adjuvant therapy. Over 95% of men have ER-positive tumors and less than 10% have overexpression of *HER2*. Androgen receptor is also commonly overexpressed in male breast cancer. Adjuvant systemic therapy and radiation are used for the same indications as in breast cancer in women.

Because breast cancer in men is frequently a disseminated disease, endocrine therapy is of considerable importance in its management. Tamoxifen is the main drug for management of advanced breast cancer in men. Tamoxifen (20 mg orally daily) should be the initial treatment. There is little data regarding the use of AIs in men. Castration in advanced breast cancer is a successful measure and more beneficial than the same procedure in women but is rarely used. Objective evidence of regression may be seen in 60–70% of men with endocrine therapy for metastatic disease—approximately twice the proportion in women. Bone is the most frequent site of metastases from breast cancer in men (as in women), and endocrine therapy relieves bone pain in most patients so treated. The longer the interval between mastectomy and recurrence, the longer the remission following treatment is likely. Corticosteroid therapy alone has been considered to be efficacious but probably has no value when compared with major endocrine ablation.

Chemotherapy should be administered for the same indications and using the same dosage schedules as for women with metastatic disease or for adjuvant treatment.

Prognosis

Men with breast cancer *seem* to have a worse prognosis than women with breast cancer because breast cancer is diagnosed in men at a later stage. However, a large population based, international study reported that after adjustment for prognostic features (age, stage, treatment), men had a significantly improved relative survival from breast cancer compared to women. For node-positive disease, 5-year survival is approximately 69%, and for node-negative disease, it is 88%. A practice-patterns database study reported that based on NCCN guidelines, only 59% of patients received the recommended chemotherapy, 82% received the recommended hormonal therapy, and 71% received the recommended post-mastectomy radiation, indicating a relatively low adherence to NCCN guidelines for men.

For those patients whose disease progresses despite treatment, meticulous efforts at palliative care are essential (see Chapter 5).

Bird ST et al. Male breast cancer and 5 alpha-reductase inhibitors finasteride and dutasteride. J Urol. 2013 Nov; 190(5):1811–4. [PMID: 23665270]

Colfry AJ 3rd. Miscellaneous syndromes and their management: occult breast cancer, breast cancer in pregnancy, male breast cancer, surgery in stage IV disease. Surg Clin North Am. 2013 Apr;93(2):519–31. [PMID: 23464700]

Ruddy KJ et al. Male breast cancer: risk factors, biology, diagnosis, treatment, and survivorship. Ann Oncol. 2013 Jun;24(6): 1434–43. [PMID: 23425944]

Sousa B et al. An update on male breast cancer and future directions for research and treatment. Eur J Pharmacol. 2013 Oct 5; 717(1–3):71–83. [PMID: 23545364]

Gynecologic Disorders

Jason Woo, MD, MPH, FACOG

Alicia Y. Armstrong, MD, MHSCR

PREMENOPAUSAL ABNORMAL UTERINE BLEEDING

ESSENTIALS OF DIAGNOSIS

► Accurate diagnosis of abnormal uterine bleeding (AUB) depends on appropriate categorization and diagnostic tests.

► Pregnancy should always be ruled out as a cause of AUB in reproductive age women.

► The evaluation of AUB depends on the age and risk factors of the patient.

► General Considerations

Normal menstrual bleeding lasts an average of 5 days (range, 2–7 days), with a mean blood loss of 40 mL per cycle. **Menorrhagia** is defined as blood loss of over 80 mL per cycle and frequently produces anemia. **Metrorrhagia** is defined as bleeding between periods. **Polymenorrhea** is defined as bleeding that occurs more often than every 21 days, and **oligomenorrhea** is defined as bleeding that occurs less frequently than every 35 days.

A classification system, known by the acronym PALM-COEIN, is used by the International Federation of Gynecology and Obstetrics (FIGO) and does not use the term "dysfunctional uterine bleeding." Instead, **abnormal uterine bleeding (AUB)** is the overarching term paired with descriptive terms denoting the bleeding pattern (ie, heavy, light and menstrual, intermenstrual) and by etiology (**P**olyp, **A**denomyosis, **L**eiomyoma, **M**alignancy and hyperplasia, **C**oagulopathy, **O**vulatory dysfunction, **E**ndometrial, **I**atrogenic, and **N**ot yet classified). In adolescents, AUB often occurs as a result of persistent anovulation due to the immaturity of the hypothalamic-pituitary-ovarian axis and represents normal physiology. Once regular menses has been established during adolescence, **ovulatory** AUB (AUB-O) accounts for most cases. AUB in women aged 19–39 years is often a result of pregnancy, structural lesions, anovulatory cycles, use of hormonal contraception, or endometrial hyperplasia.

► Clinical Findings

A. Symptoms and Signs

The diagnosis usually depends on the following: (1) A careful description of the duration and amount of flow, related pain, and relationship to the last menstrual period (LMP), with the presence of blood clots or the degree of inconvenience caused by the bleeding serving as useful indicators; (2) A history of pertinent illnesses, such as recent systemic infections or hospitalizations, or weight change; (3) A history of medications or herbal remedies that might cause AUB (such as black cohosh, chamomile, feverfew, fish oil, garlic, ginger, ginkgo, and ginseng); (4) A history of coagulation disorders in the patient or family members; (5) A physical examination to look for general findings of excessive weight, signs of polycystic ovary syndrome (PCOS), thyroid disease or insulin resistance; and (6) A pelvic examination for vulvar, vaginal or cervical lesions, pregnancy, uterine myomas, adnexal masses, adenomyosis, or infection.

B. Laboratory Studies

A complete blood count and a pregnancy test should be done as well as thyroid function studies. For adolescents with heavy menstrual bleeding and adults with a positive screening history, coagulation studies should be considered, since up to 18% of women with severe menorrhagia may have a coagulopathy. Cervical samples should be obtained for cytology and culture.

C. Imaging

Ultrasound may be useful to evaluate endometrial thickness or to diagnose intrauterine or ectopic pregnancy or adnexal masses. Sonohysterography or hysteroscopy may be used to diagnose endometrial polyps or subserous myomas. MRI is not a primary imaging modality for AUB but can definitively diagnose submucous myomas and adenomyosis.

D. Cervical Biopsy and Endometrial Sampling

The primary role of endometrial sampling is to determine whether carcinoma or premalignant lesions are present, even though other pathology related to bleeding may be found. Sampling methods and other gynecologic

Table 18–1. Common gynecologic diagnostic procedures.

Colposcopy
Visualization of cervical, vaginal, or vulvar epithelium under 5–50 × magnification with and without dilute acetic acid to identify abnormal areas requiring biopsy. An office procedure.

Dilation & curettage (D&C)
Dilation of the cervix and curettage of the entire endometrial cavity, using a metal curette or suction cannula and often using forceps for the removal of endometrial polyps. Can usually be done in the office under local anesthesia.

Endometrial biopsy
Removal of one or more areas of the endometrium by means of a curette or small aspiration device without cervical dilation. Diagnostic accuracy similar to D&C. An office procedure performed under local anesthesia.

Endocervical curettage
Removal of endocervical epithelium with a small curette for diagnosis of cervical dysplasia and cancer. An office procedure performed under local anesthesia.

Hysteroscopy
Visual examination of the uterine cavity with a small fiberoptic endoscope passed through the cervix. Biopsies and excision of myomas can be performed. Can be done in the office under local anesthesia or in the operating room under general anesthesia.

Saline infusion sonohysterography
Introduction of saline solution into endometrial cavity with a catheter to visualize submucous myomas or endometrial polyps by transvaginal ultrasound. May be performed in the office with oral analgesia.

Hysterosalpingography
Injection of radiopaque dye through the cervix to visualize the uterine cavity and oviducts. Mainly used in investigation of infertility.

Laparoscopy
Visualization of the abdominal and pelvic cavity through a small fiberoptic endoscope passed through a subumbilical incision. Permits diagnosis, tubal sterilization, and treatment of many conditions previously requiring laparotomy. General anesthesia is usually used.

diagnostic procedures are described in Table 18–1. Polyps, endometrial hyperplasia, and submucous myomas are commonly identified in this way. **Endometrial sampling should be performed in patients with AUB who are older than 45 years, or in younger patients with a history of unopposed estrogen exposure or failed medical management and persistent AUB.** If the Papanicolaou smear abnormality requires it, or a gross cervical lesion is seen, colposcopic-directed biopsies and endocervical curettage are usually indicated.

► **Treatment**

Premenopausal patients with AUB include those with submucosal myomas, infection, early abortion, thrombophilias, or pelvic neoplasms. The history, physical examination, laboratory findings, imaging, and endometrial sampling should identify such patients, who require definitive therapy. A large group of patients remain, most of whom have AUB-O.

AUB-O can usually be treated hormonally. Progestins, which limit and stabilize endometrial growth, are generally effective. For patients with irregular or light bleeding, medroxyprogesterone acetate, 10 mg/day orally, or norethindrone acetate, 5 mg/day orally, should be given for 10 days, following which withdrawal bleeding (so-called *medical curettage*) will occur. If successful, the treatment can be repeated for several cycles, starting medication on day 15 of subsequent cycles, or it can be reinstituted if amenorrhea or dysfunctional bleeding recurs. In women who are experiencing heavier bleeding, any of the combination oral contraceptives (with 30–35 mcg of estrogen estradiol) can be given four times daily for 1 or 2 days followed by two pills daily through day 5 and then one pill daily through day 20; after withdrawal bleeding occurs, pills are taken in the usual dosage for three cycles. In cases of intractable heavy bleeding, a gonadotropin-releasing hormone (GnRH) agonist such as depot leuprolide, 3.75 mg intramuscularly monthly, or nafarelin, 0.2–0.4 mg intranasally twice daily, can be used for up to 6 months to create a temporary cessation of menstruation by ovarian suppression. These therapies require 2–4 weeks to downregulate the pituitary and stop bleeding and will not stop bleeding acutely. In cases of heavy bleeding requiring hospitalization, intravenous conjugated estrogens, 25 mg every 4 hours for three or four doses, can be used, followed by oral conjugated estrogens, 2.5 mg daily, or ethinyl estradiol, 20 mcg orally daily, for 3 weeks, with the addition of medroxyprogesterone acetate, 10 mg orally daily for the last 10 days of treatment, or a combination oral contraceptive daily for 3 weeks. This will thicken the endometrium and control the bleeding. Nonsteroidal anti-inflammatory drugs (NSAIDs), such as naproxen or mefenamic acid, in the usual anti-inflammatory doses, will often reduce blood loss in menorrhagia—even that associated with a copper intrauterine device (IUD).

If the abnormal bleeding is not controlled by hormonal treatment, hysteroscopy with tissue sampling or saline infusion sonohysterography is used to evaluate for structural lesions (such as polyps, submucous myomas) or neoplasms (such as endometrial cancer). In the absence of specific pathology, bleeding unresponsive to medical therapy may be treated with endometrial ablation, levonorgestrel-releasing IUD, or hysterectomy. While hysterectomy was used commonly in the past for bleeding unresponsive to medical therapy, the low risk of complications and the good short-term results of both endometrial ablation and levonorgestrel-releasing IUD make them attractive alternatives to hysterectomy. Endometrial ablation may be performed through the hysteroscope with laser photocoagulation or electrocautery. Nonhysteroscopic techniques include balloon thermal ablation, cryoablation, free-fluid thermal ablation, impedence bipolar radiofrequency ablation, and microwave ablation. The latter methods are well-adapted to outpatient therapy under local anesthesia.

The levonorgestrel-releasing IUD markedly reduces menstrual blood loss and may be a good alternative to other therapies. However, while short-term results with endometrial ablation and levonorgestrel-releasing IUD are satisfactory, at 5 years after either the endometrial ablation procedure or placement of the levonorgestrel IUD, up to 40% of women will have had either repeat ablation procedures or a hysterectomy.

When to Refer

- If bleeding is not controlled with first-line therapy.
- If expertise is needed for a surgical procedure.

When to Admit

If bleeding is uncontrollable with first-line therapy or the patient is not hemodynamically stable.

American College of Obstetricians and Gynecologists. ACOG Committee Opinion No. 557: Management of acute abnormal uterine bleeding in nonpregnant reproductive-aged women. Obstet Gynecol. 2013 Apr;121(4):891–6. [PMID: 23635706]

American College of Obstetricians and Gynecologists. Practice Bulletin No. 128: Diagnosis of abnormal uterine bleeding in reproductive-aged women. Obstet Gynecol. 2012 Jul;120 (1):197–206. [PMID: 22914421]

Committee on Practice Bulletins—Gynecology. Practice Bulletin No. 136: Management of abnormal uterine bleeding associated with ovulatory dysfunction. Obstet Gynecol. 2013 Jul; 122(1):176–85. [PMID: 23787936]

POSTMENOPAUSAL VAGINAL BLEEDING

 ESSENTIALS OF DIAGNOSIS

- ▶ Vaginal bleeding that occurs 6 months or more following cessation of menstrual function.
- ▶ Postmenopausal bleeding of any amount always should be investigated. Transvaginal ultrasound measurement of the endometrium is a very helpful tool in evaluating postmenopausal bleeding.

General Considerations

Vaginal bleeding that occurs 6 months or more following cessation of menstrual function should be investigated. The most common causes are atrophic endometrium, endometrial proliferation or hyperplasia, endometrial or cervical cancer, and administration of estrogens with or without added progestin. Other causes include atrophic vaginitis, trauma, endometrial polyps, friction ulcers of the cervix associated with prolapse of the uterus, and blood dyscrasias. **Bleeding of any amount in a postmenopausal woman should always be investigated.**

Diagnosis

The vulva and vagina should be inspected for areas of bleeding, ulcers, or neoplasms. A cytologic smear of the cervix and vaginal pool should be taken. If available, transvaginal sonography should be used to measure endometrial thickness. A measurement of 4 mm or less indicates a low likelihood of hyperplasia or endometrial cancer. If the thickness is greater than 4 mm or there is a heterogeneous

appearance to the endometrium, it should be determined if the thickening is global or focal. Sonohysterography may assist in making this distinction. If the thickening is global, endometrial biopsy or D&C is appropriate. If focal, guided sampling with hysteroscopy should be done.

Treatment

Simple endometrial hyperplasia calls for cyclic or continuous progestin therapy (medroxyprogesterone acetate, 10 mg/day orally, or norethindrone acetate, 5 mg/day orally) for 21 or 30 days of each month for 3 months. The use of a levonorgestrel intrauterine system is also a treatment option. Repeat sampling should be performed if symptoms recur. If endometrial hyperplasia with atypia or if carcinoma of the endometrium is found, hysterectomy is necessary.

When to Refer

- Expertise in performing ultrasonography is required.
- Complex endometrial hyperplasia with atypia is present.
- Hysteroscopy is indicated.

Morelli M et al. Efficacy of the levonorgestrel intrauterine system (LNG-IUS) in the prevention of the atypical endometrial hyperplasia and endometrial cancer: retrospective data from selected obese menopausal symptomatic women. Gynecol Endocrinol. 2013 Feb;29(2):156–9. [PMID: 23134558]

Null DB et al. Postmenopausal bleeding-first steps in the workup. J Fam Pract. 2012 Oct;61(10):597–604. [PMID: 23106061]

PREMENSTRUAL SYNDROME (Premenstrual Tension)

The premenstrual syndrome (PMS) is a recurrent, variable cluster of troublesome physical and emotional symptoms that develop during the 5 days before the onset of menses and subside within 4 days after menstruation occurs. PMS intermittently affects about 40% of all premenopausal women, primarily those 25–40 years of age. In about 5–8% of affected women, the syndrome may be severe. Although not every woman experiences all the symptoms or signs at one time, many describe bloating, breast pain, ankle swelling, a sense of increased weight, skin disorders, irritability, aggressiveness, depression, inability to concentrate, libido change, lethargy, and food cravings. When emotional or mood symptoms predominate, along with physical symptoms, and there is a clear functional impairment with work or personal relationships, the term "premenstrual dysphoric disorder" (PMDD) may be applied. The pathogenesis of PMS/PMDD is still uncertain, and current treatment methods are mainly empiric. The clinician should provide support for both the patient's emotional and physical distress. This includes the following:

1. Careful evaluation of the patient, with understanding, explanation, and reassurance.
2. Advise the patient to keep a daily diary of all symptoms for 2–3 months, such as the Daily Record of Severity of Problems, to evaluate the timing and characteristics of her symptoms. If her symptoms occur throughout the month rather than in the 2 weeks before menses, she

may have depression or other mental health problems instead of or in addition to PMS.

3. For mild to moderate symptoms, a program of aerobic exercise; reduction of caffeine, salt, and alcohol intake; the use of alternative therapies, such as an increase in dietary calcium (to 1200 mg/day), vitamin D, or magnesium, and complex carbohydrates in the diet, acupuncture, and herbal treatments may be helpful, although these interventions remain unproven.

4. Medications that prevent ovulation, such as hormonal contraceptives, may lessen physical symptoms. A combined oral contraceptive containing the progestin drospirenone with a 4-day pill-free interval has been approved by the US Food and Drug Administration (FDA) for the treatment of PMDD. NSAIDs, such as mefenamic acid, 500 mg orally three times a day, will reduce a number of symptoms but not breast pain. When the above regimens are not effective, ovarian function can be suppressed with continuous high-dose progestin (20–30 mg/day of oral medroxyprogesterone acetate or 150 mg of depot medroxyprogesterone acetate [DMPA] orally every 3 months or GnRH agonist with add-back therapy, such as conjugated equine estrogen, 0.625 mg orally daily with medroxyprogesterone acetate, 2.5–5 mg orally daily).

5. When mood disorders predominate, several serotonin reuptake inhibitors (such as fluoxetine, 20 mg orally, either daily or only on symptom days) have been shown to be effective in relieving tension, irritability, and dysphoria with few side effects. First-line medication therapy includes serotonergic antidepressants (citalopram, escitalopram, fluoxetine, sertraline, venlafaxine). There is little data to support the use of calcium, vitamin D, and vitamin B_6 supplementation. There is insufficient evidence to support cognitive behavioral therapy.

Kelderhouse K et al. A review of treatment and management modalities for premenstrual dysphoric disorder. Nurs Womens Health. 2013 Aug–Sep;17(4):294–305. [PMID: 23957795]
Panay N. Treatment of premenstrual syndrome: a decision-making algorithm. Menopause Int. 2012 Jun;18(2):90–2. [PMID: 22611230]

PELVIC PAIN

1. Primary Dysmenorrhea

Primary dysmenorrhea is menstrual pain associated with menstrual cycles in the absence of pathologic findings. The pain usually begins within 1–2 years after the menarche and may become more severe with time. The frequency of cases increases up to age 20 and then decreases with age and markedly with parity. Fifty to 75 percent of women are affected at some time and 5–6% have incapacitating pain.

Clinical Findings

Primary dysmenorrhea is low, midline, wave-like, cramping pelvic pain often radiating to the back or inner thighs. Cramps may last for 1 or more days and may be associated with nausea, diarrhea, headache, and flushing. The pain is produced by uterine vasoconstriction, anoxia, and sustained contractions mediated by prostaglandins. The pelvic examination is normal between menses; examination during menses may produce discomfort, but there are no pathologic findings.

Treatment

NSAIDs (ibuprofen, ketoprofen, mefenamic acid, naproxen) and the cyclooxygenase (COX)-2 inhibitor celecoxib are generally helpful. The medication should be started 1–2 days before expected menses. Symptoms can be suppressed with use of oral contraceptives, DMPA, or the levonorgestrel-releasing IUD. Continuous use of oral contraceptives can be used to suppress menstruation completely and prevent dysmenorrhea. For women who do not wish to use hormonal contraception, other therapies that have shown at least some benefit include local heat; thiamine, 100 mg/day orally; vitamin E, 200 units/day orally from 2 days prior to and for the first 3 days of menses; and high-frequency transcutaneous electrical nerve stimulation.

2. Other Categories of Pelvic Pain

Unlike primary dysmenorrhea, other causes of pelvic pain may or may not be associated with the menstrual cycle but are more likely to be associated with pelvic pathology. Conditions such as endometriosis, fibroids, pelvic inflammatory disease (PID), or other anatomic abnormalities of the pelvic organs, including the bowels or bladder, may present with symptoms during the menstrual cycle or with a more chronic nature.

Clinical Findings

The history and physical examination may suggest endometriosis or fibroids. Other causes may be PID, submucous myoma(s), adenomyosis, IUD use, cervical stenosis with obstruction, or blind uterine horn (rare). Careful review of associated bowel or bladder symptoms should be considered to rule out other pelvic organ origination.

Diagnosis

Pelvic imaging is useful for detecting the presence of uterine fibroids or other anomalies. Adenomyosis, the presence of islands of endometrial tissue in the myometrium, may be diagnosed with ultrasound or, preferably, with MRI. Cervical stenosis may result from induced abortion, creating crampy pain at the time of expected menses with obstruction of blood flow; this is easily cured by passing a sound into the uterine cavity after administering a paracervical block. Laparoscopy may be used to diagnose endometriosis or other pelvic abnormalities not visualized by imaging.

Treatment

A. Specific Measures

The combined oral contraceptive pill alleviates the symptoms of dysmenorrhea. Periodic use of analgesics, including the NSAIDs given for primary dysmenorrhea, may be beneficial, and oral contraceptives may give relief, particularly in endometriosis. GnRH agonists are effective in the treatment of endometriosis, although their long-term use may be limited by cost or side effects. Adenomyosis may respond to the levonorgestrel-releasing intrauterine system, uterine artery embolization, or hormonal approaches used to treat endometriosis, but hysterectomy remains the definitive treatment of choice for women for whom childbearing is not a consideration.

B. Surgical Measures

If disability is marked or prolonged, laparoscopy or exploratory laparotomy is usually warranted. Definitive surgery depends on the degree of disability and the findings at operation. Uterine fibroids may be removed or treated by uterine artery embolization. Hysterectomy may be done if other treatments have not worked but is usually a last resort.

▶ When to Refer

- Standard therapy fails to relieve pain.
- Suspicion of pelvic pathology, such as endometriosis, leiomyomas, or adenomyosis.

American College of Obstetricians and Gynecologists. FAQ099 gynecologic problems: chronic pelvic pain. 2011 Aug. http://www.acog.org/-/media/For-Patients/faq099.pdf

European Society of Human Reproduction and Embryology. Study finds convincing evidence that the combined oral contraceptive pill helps painful periods. 2012 Jan 18. http://www.eshre.eu/Press-Room/Press-releases/Press-releases-2012/Combined-oral-contraceptive-pill.aspx

Harel Z. Dysmenorrhea in adolescents and young adults: an update on pharmacological treatments and management strategies. Expert Opin Pharmacother. 2012 Oct; 13(15):2157–70. [PMID: 22984937]

Osayande AS et al. Diagnosis and initial management of dysmenorrhea. Am Fam Physician. 2014 Mar 1;89(5):341–6. [PMID: 24695505]

Royal College of Obstetricians and Gynecologists. Green-top Guideline No. 41: The initial management of chronic pelvic pain. 2012 May. https://www.rcog.org.uk/globalassets/documents/guidelines/gtg_41.pdf

VAGINITIS

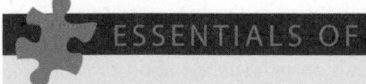

ESSENTIALS OF DIAGNOSIS

- ▶ Vaginal irritation.
- ▶ Pruritus.
- ▶ Unusual or malodorous discharge.

▶ General Considerations

Inflammation and infection of the vagina are common gynecologic problems, resulting from a variety of pathogens, allergic reactions to vaginal contraceptives or other products, vaginal atrophy, or the friction of coitus. The normal vaginal pH is 4.5 or less, and *Lactobacillus* is the predominant

organism. Normal secretions during the middle of the cycle, or during pregnancy, can be confused with vaginitis by concerned women.

▶ Clinical Findings

When the patient complains of vaginal irritation, pain, or unusual or malodorous discharge, a history should be taken, noting the onset of the LMP; recent sexual activity; use of contraceptives, tampons, or douches; recent changes in medications or use of antibiotics; and the presence of vaginal burning, pain, pruritus, or unusually profuse or malodorous discharge. The physical examination should include careful inspection of the vulva and speculum examination of the vagina and cervix. The cervix is sampled for gonococcus and *Chlamydia* if appropriate. A specimen of vaginal discharge is examined under the microscope in a drop of 0.9% saline solution to look for trichomonads or clue cells and in a drop of 10% potassium hydroxide to search for *Candida*. The vaginal pH should be tested; it is frequently greater than 4.5 in infections due to trichomonads and bacterial vaginosis. A bimanual examination to look for evidence of pelvic infection should follow. Point-of-care testing is available for all three organisms that cause vaginitis. It can be used if microscopy is not available or for confirmatory testing of microscopy.

A. Vulvovaginal Candidiasis

Pregnancy, diabetes, and use of broad-spectrum antibiotics or corticosteroids predispose patients to *Candida* infections. Heat, moisture, and occlusive clothing also contribute to the risk. Pruritus, vulvovaginal erythema, and a white curd-like discharge that is not malodorous are found (Figure 18–1). Microscopic examination with 10% potassium hydroxide reveals hyphae and spores. Cultures with Nickerson medium may be used if *Candida* is suspected but not demonstrated.

B. *Trichomonas vaginalis* Vaginitis

This protozoal flagellate infects the vagina, Skene ducts, and lower urinary tract in women and the lower genitourinary tract in men. It is sexually transmitted. Pruritus and a

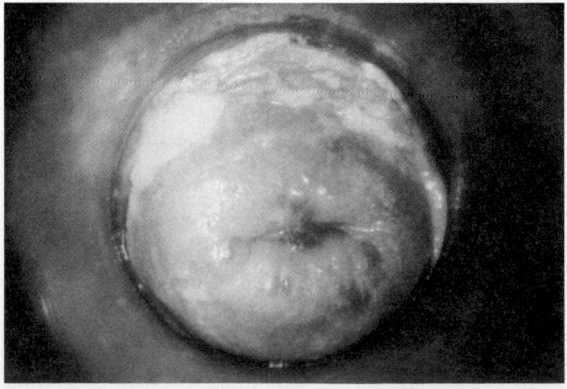

▲ **Figure 18–1.** Cervical candidiasis. (Public Health Image Library, CDC.)

▲ **Figure 18–3.** Clue cells seen in bacterial vaginosis due to *Gardnerella vaginalis.* (Reproduced, with permission, from Richard P. Usatine, MD.)

▲ **Figure 18–2.** Strawberry cervix in *Trichomonas vaginalis* infection, with inflammation and punctate hemorrhages. (Used, with permission, from Richard P. Usatine, MD.)

malodorous frothy, yellow-green discharge occur, along with diffuse vaginal erythema and red macular lesions on the cervix in severe cases ("strawberry cervix," Figure 18–2). Motile organisms with flagella are seen by microscopic examination of a wet mount with saline solution.

C. Bacterial Vaginosis

This condition is considered to be a polymicrobial disease that is not sexually transmitted. An overgrowth of *Gardnerella* and other anaerobes is often associated with increased malodorous discharge without obvious vulvitis or vaginitis. The discharge is grayish and sometimes frothy, with a pH of 5.0–5.5. An amine-like ("fishy") odor is present if a drop of discharge is alkalinized with 10% potassium hydroxide. On wet mount in saline, epithelial cells are covered with bacteria to such an extent that cell borders are obscured (*clue cells,* Figure 18–3). Vaginal cultures are generally not useful in diagnosis.

► Treatment

A. Vulvovaginal Candidiasis

A variety of regimens are available to treat vulvovaginal candidiasis. Women with uncomplicated vulvovaginal candidiasis will usually respond to a 1- to 3-day regimen of a topical azole. Women with complicated infection (including four or more episodes in 1 year [*recurrent* vulvovaginal candidiasis], severe signs and symptoms, non-albicans

species, uncontrolled diabetes, HIV infection, corticosteroid treatment, or pregnancy) should receive 7–14 days of a topical regimen or two doses of oral fluconazole 3 days apart. Pregnant women should use only topical azoles. In recurrent non-albicans infections, 600 mg of boric acid in a gelatin capsule intravaginally once daily for 2 weeks is approximately 70% effective. If recurrence occurs, referral to an infectious disease specialist is indicated.

1. Single-dose regimens—Effective single-dose regimens include miconazole (1200-mg vaginal suppository), tioconazole (6.5% cream, 5 g vaginally), sustained-release butoconazole (2% cream, 5 g vaginally), or fluconazole (150 mg oral tablet).

2. Three-day regimens—Effective 3-day regimens include butoconazole (2% cream, 5 g vaginally once daily), clotrimazole (2% cream, 5 g vaginally once daily), terconazole (0.8% cream, 5 g, or 80 mg vaginal suppository once daily), or miconazole (200 mg vaginal suppository once daily).

3. Seven-day regimens—The following regimens are given once daily: clotrimazole (1% cream), miconazole (2% cream, 5 g, or 100 mg vaginal suppository), or terconazole (0.4% cream, 5 g).

4. Fourteen-day regimen—An effective 14-day regimen is nystatin (100,000-unit vaginal tablet once daily).

5. Recurrent vulvovaginal candidiasis (maintenance therapy)—Clotrimazole (500 mg vaginal suppository once weekly or 200 mg cream twice weekly) or fluconazole (100, 150, or 200 mg orally once weekly) are effective regimens for maintenance therapy for up to 6 months.

B. *Trichomonas vaginalis* Vaginitis

Treatment of both partners simultaneously is recommended; metronidazole or tinidazole, 2 g orally as a single dose or 500 mg orally twice a day for 7 days, is usually used.

In the case of treatment failure with metronidazole in the absence of reexposure, the patient should be re-treated with metronidazole, 500 mg orally twice a day for 7 days, or tinidazole, 2 g orally as a single dose. If treatment failure occurs again, give metronidazole or tinidazole, 2 g orally once daily for 5 days. If this is not effective in eradicating the organisms, metronidazole and tinidazole susceptibility testing can be arranged with the Centers for Disease Control and Prevention (CDC) at 404-718-4141 or at http://www.cdc.gov/std. Women infected with *T vaginalis* are at increased risk for concurrent infection with other sexually transmitted diseases.

C. Bacterial Vaginosis

The recommended regimens are metronidazole (500 mg orally, twice daily for 7 days), clindamycin vaginal cream (2%, 5 g, once daily for 7 days), or metronidazole gel (0.75%, 5 g, twice daily for 5 days). Alternative regimens include clindamycin (300 mg orally twice daily for 7 days), clindamycin ovules (100 g intravaginally at bedtime for 3 days), tinidazole (2 g orally once daily for 3 days), or tinidazole (1 g orally once daily for 7 days).

The CDC offers a helpful training module to clinicians to review current recommendations for treatment of vaginitis (http://www2a.cdc.gov/stdtraining/self-study/vaginitis/default.htm).

CONDYLOMA ACUMINATA

Warty growths on the vulva, perianal area, vaginal walls, or cervix are caused by various types of the human papillomavirus (HPV). Pregnancy and immunosuppression favor growth. Ninety percent of genital warts are caused by HPV 6 and 11. Despite the relatively low uptake in use of a quadrivalent HPV vaccine in the United States, the prevalence of HPV types 6, 11, 16 and 18 decreased from 11.5% in 2003–2006 to 5.1% in 2007–2010. Vulvar lesions may be obviously wart-like or may be diagnosed only after application of 4% acetic acid (vinegar) and colposcopy, when they appear whitish, with prominent papillae. Vaginal lesions may show diffuse hypertrophy or a cobblestone appearance. Recommended treatments for vulvar warts include podophyllum resin 10–25% in tincture of benzoin (do not use during pregnancy or on bleeding lesions) or 80–90% trichloroacetic or bichloroacetic acid, carefully applied to avoid the surrounding skin. Surgical removal may be accomplished with tangential scissor excision, tangential shave excision, curettage, or electrotherapy. The pain of bichloroacetic or trichloroacetic acid application can be lessened by a sodium bicarbonate paste applied immediately after treatment. Podophyllum resin must be washed off after 2–4 hours. Freezing with liquid nitrogen or a cryoprobe and electrocautery are also effective. Patient-applied regimens, useful when the entire lesion is accessible to the patient, include podofilox 0.5% solution or gel, imiquimod 5% cream, or sinecatechins 15% ointment. Vaginal warts may be treated with cryotherapy with liquid nitrogen or trichloroacetic acid. Extensive warts may require treatment with CO_2 laser under local or general anesthesia.

Dunne EF et al. Reduction in human papillomavirus vaccine type prevalence among young women screened for cervical cancer in an integrated US healthcare delivery system in 2007 and 2012–2013. J Infect Dis. 2015 Dec 15;212(12):1970–5. [PMID: 26123561]

Workowski KA et al; Centers for Disease Control and Prevention. Sexually transmitted diseases treatment guidelines, 2015. MMWR Recomm Rep. 2015 Jun 5;64(RR-03):1–137. [PMID: 26042815] http://www.cdc.gov/mmwr/preview/mmwrhtml/rr6403a1.htm

CERVICAL POLYPS

Cervical polyps commonly occur after menarche and are occasionally noted in postmenopausal women. The cause is not known, but inflammation may play an etiologic role. The principal symptoms are discharge and abnormal vaginal bleeding. However, abnormal bleeding should not be ascribed to a cervical polyp without sampling the endocervix and endometrium. The polyps are visible in the cervical os on speculum examination.

Cervical polyps must be differentiated from polypoid neoplastic disease of the endometrium, small submucous pedunculated myomas, large nabothian cysts, and endometrial polyps. Cervical polyps rarely contain dysplasia (0.5%) or malignant (0.5%) foci. Asymptomatic polyps in women under age 45 may be left untreated.

► Treatment

Cervical polyps can generally be removed in the office by avulsion with uterine packing forceps or ring forceps.

BARTHOLIN DUCT CYSTS & ABSCESSES

Trauma or infection may involve the Bartholin duct, causing obstruction of the gland. Drainage of secretions is prevented, leading to pain, swelling, and abscess formation (Figure 18–4). The infection usually resolves and pain disappears, but stenosis of the duct outlet with distention often persists. Reinfection causes recurrent tenderness and further enlargement of the duct.

▲ **Figure 18–4.** Right-sided Bartholin cyst (abscess). The Bartholin gland is located in the lower two-thirds of the introitus. (Used, with permission, from Susan Lindsley, Public Health Image Library, CDC.)

The principal symptoms are periodic painful swelling on either side of the introitus and dyspareunia. A fluctuant swelling 1–4 cm in diameter lateral to either labium minus is a sign of occlusion of Bartholin duct. Tenderness is evidence of active infection.

Pus or secretions from the gland should be cultured for *Chlamydia* and other pathogens and treated accordingly (see Chapter 33); frequent warm soaks may be helpful. If an abscess develops, aspiration or incision and drainage are the simplest forms of therapy, but the problem may recur. Marsupialization (in the absence of an abscess), incision, and drainage with the insertion of an indwelling Word catheter, or laser treatment will establish a new duct opening. Antibiotics are unnecessary unless cellulitis is present. An asymptomatic cyst does not require therapy.

▶ When to Refer

Surgical therapy (marsupialization) is indicated.

CERVICAL INTRAEPITHELIAL NEOPLASIA (CIN) (Dysplasia of the Cervix)

ESSENTIALS OF DIAGNOSIS

▶ The presumptive diagnosis is made by an abnormal Papanicolaou smear of an asymptomatic woman with no grossly visible cervical changes.

▶ Diagnose by colposcopically directed biopsy.

▶ General Considerations

The squamocolumnar junction of the cervix is an area of active squamous cell proliferation. In childhood, this junction is located on the exposed vaginal portion of the cervix. At puberty, because of hormonal influence and possibly because of changes in the vaginal pH, the squamous margin begins to encroach on the single-layered, mucus-secreting epithelium, creating an area of metaplasia (transformation zone). Factors associated with infection with HPV (see Prevention, below) may lead to cellular abnormalities, which over a period of time can result in the development of squamous cell dysplasia or cancer. There are varying degrees of dysplasia (Table 18–2), defined by the degree of cellular atypia; all types must be observed and treated if they persist or become more severe.

▶ Clinical Findings

There are no specific symptoms or signs of CIN. The presumptive diagnosis is made by cytologic screening of an asymptomatic population with no grossly visible cervical changes. All visibly abnormal cervical lesions should be biopsied (Figure 18–5).

Table 18–2. Classification systems for Papanicolaou smears.

Numerical	Dysplasia	CIN	Bethesda System
1	Benign	Benign	Normal
2	Benign with inflammation	Benign with inflammation	Normal, ASC-US
3	Mild dysplasia	CIN I	Low-grade SIL
3	Moderate dysplasia	CIN II	High-grade SIL
3	Severe dysplasia	CIN III	
4	Carcinoma in situ		
5	Invasive cancer	Invasive cancer	Invasive cancer

ASC-US, atypical squamous cells of undetermined significance; CIN, cervical intraepithelial neoplasia; SIL, squamous intraepithelial lesion.

▶ Screening & Diagnosis

A. Cytologic Examination (Papanicolaou Smear)

Screening should begin at age 21. The recommendation to start screening at age 21 years regardless of the age of onset of sexual intercourse is based in part on the very low incidence of cancer in younger women. In contrast to the high rate of infection with HPV in sexually active adolescents, invasive cervical cancer is very rare in women younger than age 21 years. The recommendation is also based on the potential for adverse effects associated with follow-up of young women with abnormal cytology screening results. **The US Preventive Services Task Force (USPSTF) recommends screening for cervical cancer in women age 21 to 65 years with cytology (Papanicolaou smear) every 3 years or, for women age 30 to 65 years who want to lengthen the screening interval, screening with a**

▲ **Figure 18–5.** Erosion of the cervix due to cervical intraepithelial neoplasia (CIN), a precursor lesion to cervical cancer. (Public Health Image Library, CDC.)

combination of cytology and HPV testing every 5 years. Screening may be done with either liquid-based or conventional cytology. Women with risk factors that place them at higher risk for CIN may require more frequent screening. These risk factors include HIV infection, immunosuppression, exposure to diethylstilbesterol in utero, and previous treatment for CIN 2, CIN 3, or cervical cancer. The USPSTF recommends against screening for cervical cancer with HPV testing, alone or in combination with cytology, in women younger than age 30 years. The USPSTF recommends against screening for cervical cancer in women older than age 65 years who have had adequate prior screening and are not otherwise at high risk for cervical cancer. Online guidelines are available for the management of abnormal Papanicolaou smears (http://www.imedicalapps. com/2013/04/cervical-cancer-screening-medical-app-asccp-obgyn-physicians/ and http://www.uspreventiveservicestask-force.org/Page/Document/RecommendationStatementFinal/ cervical-cancer-screening).

Exfoliated cells are collected from the transformation zone of the cervix and may be transferred to a vial of liquid preservative that is processed in the laboratory to produce a slide for interpretation—the liquid-based technique—or may be transferred directly to the slide and fixed using the conventional technique. Performance of conventional cervical cytology requires avoidance of contaminating blood, discharge, and lubricant.

Cytologic reports from the laboratory may describe findings in one of several ways (see Table 18–2). The Bethesda System uses the terminology "atypical squamous cells of unknown significance" (ASC-US) and "squamous intraepithelial lesions," either low-grade (LSIL) or high-grade (HSIL). Cytopathologists consider a Papanicolaou smear to be a medical consultation and will recommend further diagnostic procedures, treatment for infection, and comments on factors preventing adequate evaluation of the specimen.

Testing for HPV DNA is used as an adjunct in cervical cancer screening as a triage test to stratify risk to women aged 21 years and older with a cytologic diagnosis of ASC-US and postmenopausal women with a cytologic diagnosis of LSIL. In April 2014 the FDA approved the first HPV DNA test that can be used alone to screen women aged 25 years or older who should undergo additional diagnostic testing for cervical cancer. This approval did not change current medical practice guidelines for cervical cancer screening, though, which are developed by groups other than the FDA. This test may continue to be used as an adjunct to cytology for primary screening in women older than 30 years. It also may be used as a follow-up test after CIN 1 or negative findings on colposcopy in women whose prior cytologic diagnosis is ASC-US, atypical squamous cells, cannot rule out a high-grade lesion (ASC-H), LSIL, or atypical glandular cells, and in follow-up after treatment for CIN 2 and CIN 3. **HPV testing should not be used in females younger than 21 years** and if inadvertently performed, a positive result should not influence management.

B. Colposcopy

Women with ASC-US and a negative HPV screening may be followed-up in 1 year. If the HPV screen is positive, colposcopy should be performed. If HPV screening is unavailable, repeat cytology may be done at 4- to 6-month intervals until two consecutive normal results, or the patient may be referred directly for colposcopy. **All patients with SIL or atypical glandular cells should undergo colposcopy.** Viewing the cervix with 10–20 × magnification allows for assessment of the size and margins of an abnormal transformation zone and determination of extension into the endocervical canal. The application of 3–5% acetic acid (vinegar) dissolves mucus, and the acid's desiccating action sharpens the contrast between normal and actively proliferating squamous epithelium. Abnormal changes include white patches and vascular atypia, which indicate areas of greatest cellular activity.

C. Biopsy

Colposcopically directed punch biopsy and endocervical curettage are office procedures. If colposcopy is not available, the normal-appearing cervix shedding atypical cells can be evaluated by endocervical curettage and multiple punch biopsies of nonstaining squamous epithelium or biopsies from each quadrant of the cervix. Data from both cervical biopsy and endocervical curettage are important in deciding on treatment.

▶ Prevention

Cervical infection with the HPV is associated with a high percentage of all cervical dysplasias and cancers. There are over 70 recognized HPV subtypes, of which types 6 and 11 tend to cause genital warts and mild dysplasia, while types 16, 18, 31, and others cause higher-grade cellular changes. Vaccination can prevent cervical cancer and vaginal and vulvar pre-cancers caused by HPV types 16 and 18 and to protect against low-grade and pre-cancerous lesions caused by HPV types 16 and 18. The bivalent vaccine (known as Cervarix) provides protection against HPV types 16 and 18. The quadrivalent HPV 6/11/16/18 L1 virus-like-particle vaccine (known as Gardasil) also provides protection against genital warts caused by HPV types 6 and 11. **Gardasil is recommended for all girls and women aged 9 to 26.** Both vaccines provide partial protection against several other HPV types that cause approximately 30% of cervical cancers. Gardisil-9 was approved by FDA in December 2014 and expanded protection to HPV types 31, 33, 45, 52, and 58 to cover the strains causing up to 90% of cervical cancers; in addition, it has been proven to protect against anal cancer and anal intraepithelial neoplasia caused by these strains. The use of HPV vaccination in the United States continues to increase but varies by state. In 2014, more than 60% of girls and 40% of boys ages 13–17 received one or more doses of the HPV vaccine; however, these percentages are still below the target goal of 80% adherence by 2020 set by the CDC. Because complete coverage of all carcinogenic HPV types is not provided by either vaccine, all women need to have regular cytologic screening as outlined above. In addition to vaccination, preventive measures include limiting the number of sexual partners, using a diaphragm or condom for coitus, and stopping smoking or exposure to second-hand smoke.

► Treatment

Treatment varies depending on the degree and extent of CIN. Biopsies should always precede treatment.

A. Cryosurgery

The use of freezing (cryosurgery) is effective for noninvasive small lesions visible on the cervix without endocervical extension.

B. CO_2 Laser

This well-controlled method minimizes tissue destruction. It is colposcopically directed and requires special training. It may be used with large visible lesions. In current practice, it involves the vaporization of the transformation zone on the cervix and the distal 5–7 mm of endocervical canal.

C. Loop Excision

When the CIN is clearly visible in its entirety, a wire loop can be used for excisional biopsy. This office procedure, called LEEP (loop electrosurgical excision procedure), with local anesthesia is quick and uncomplicated. Cutting and hemostasis are achieved with a low-voltage electrosurgical machine.

D. Conization of the Cervix

Conization is surgical removal of the entire transformation zone and endocervical canal. It should be reserved for cases of severe dysplasia (CIN III) or cancer in situ, particularly those with endocervical extension. The procedure can be performed with the scalpel, the CO_2 laser, the needle electrode, or by large-loop excision.

E. Follow-Up

Because recurrence is possible—especially in the first 2 years after treatment—and because the false-negative rate of a single cervical cytologic test is 20%, close follow-up after colposcopy and biopsy is imperative. For CIN II or III, cytologic examination or cytology and colposcopy should be repeated at 4- to 6-month intervals for up to 2 years. For CIN I, cytology should be performed at 6 and 12 months or HPV DNA testing can be done at 12 months. If testing is normal, routine cytologic screening can be resumed.

The American Society for Colposcopy and Cervical Pathology Guidelines for cervical cancer screening and management of abnormal Papanicolaou smears are available for purchase in an online application (http://www.imedicalapps.com/2013/04/cervical-cancer-screening-medical-app-asccp-obgyn-physicians/).

► When to Refer

- Patients with CIN II/III should be referred to an experienced colposcopist.
- Patients requiring conization biopsy should be referred to a gynecologist.

Erickson BK et al. Human papillomavirus: what every provider should know. Am J Obstet Gynecol. 2013 Mar;208(3):169–75. [PMID: 23021131]

Joura EA et al. A 9-valent HPV vaccine against infection and intraepithelial neoplasia in women. N Engl J Med. 2015 Feb 19; 372(8):711–23. [PMID: 25693011]
Markowitz LE et al. Reduction in human papillomavirus (HPV) prevalence among young women following HPV vaccine introduction in the United States, National Health and Nutrition Examination Surveys, 2003–2010. J Infect Dis. 2013 Aug 1; 208(3):385–93. [PMID: 23785124]
Moyer VA. Screening for cervical cancer: U.S. Preventive Services Task Force recommendation statement. Ann Intern Med. 2012 Jun 19;156(12):880–91. [PMID: 22711081]

CARCINOMA OF THE CERVIX

ESSENTIALS OF DIAGNOSIS

► Increased risk in women who smoke and those with HIV or high-risk HPV types.

► Gross lesions should be evaluated by colposcopically directed biopsies and not cytology alone. Cervical lesion may be visible on inspection as a tumor or ulceration but a diagnosis of cervical cancer requires a tissue diagnosis.

► General Considerations

Cervical cancer is the third most common cancer in the world and the leading cause of cancer death among women in developing countries. It can be considered a sexually transmitted disease. Both squamous cell and adenocarcinoma of the cervix are etiologically related to infection with HPV, primarily types 16 and 18. Women infected with HIV are at an increased risk for high-risk HPV infection and CIN. Smoking and possibly dietary factors such as decreased circulating vitamin A appear to be cofactors. Squamous cell carcinoma (SCC) accounts for approximately 80% of cervical cancers, while adenocarcinoma accounts for 15% and adenosquamous carcinoma for 3–5%; neuroendocrine or small cell carcinomas are rare.

SCC appears first in the intraepithelial layers (the preinvasive stage, or carcinoma in situ). Preinvasive cancer (CIN III) is a common diagnosis in women 25–40 years of age. Two to 10 years are required for carcinoma to penetrate the basement membrane and invade the tissues. While cervical cancer mortality has declined steadily in the United States due to high rates of screening and improved treatment, the rate of decline has slowed in recent years. In general, black women experienced much higher incidence and mortality than white women. The 5-year survival rate ranges from 63% for stage II cervical cancer to less than 20% for stage IV.

► Clinical Findings

A. Symptoms and Signs

The most common signs are metrorrhagia, postcoital spotting, and cervical ulceration. Bladder and rectal dysfunction or fistulas and pain are late symptoms.

B. Cervical Biopsy and Endocervical Curettage or Conization

These procedures are necessary steps after a positive Papanicolaou smear to determine the extent and depth of invasion of the cancer. Even if the smear is positive, treatment is never justified until definitive diagnosis has been established through biopsy.

C. "Staging" or Estimate of Gross Spread of Cancer of the Cervix

Staging of invasive cervical cancer is achieved by clinical evaluation, usually conducted under anesthesia. Further examinations, such as ultrasonography, CT, MRI, lymphangiography, laparoscopy, and fine-needle aspiration, are valuable for treatment planning.

▶ Complications

Metastases to regional lymph nodes occur with increasing frequency from stage I to stage IV. Paracervical extension occurs in all directions from the cervix. The ureters may become obstructed lateral to the cervix, causing hydroureter and hydronephrosis and consequently impaired kidney function. Almost two-thirds of patients with untreated carcinoma of the cervix die of uremia when ureteral obstruction is bilateral. Pain in the back, in the distribution of the lumbosacral plexus, is often indicative of neurologic involvement. Gross edema of the legs may be indicative of vascular and lymphatic stasis due to tumor.

Vaginal fistulas to the rectum and urinary tract are severe late complications. Hemorrhage is the cause of death in 10–20% of patients with extensive invasive carcinoma.

▶ Prevention

Vaccination with Gardasil and/or Cervarix can prevent cervical cancer caused by HPV types 16 and 18, and protect against low-grade and precancerous lesions caused by these types (see Cervical Intraepithelial Neoplasia).

▶ Treatment

A. Emergency Measures

Vaginal hemorrhage originates from gross ulceration and cavitation in stage II–IV cervical carcinoma. Ligation and suturing of the cervix are usually not feasible, but ligation of the uterine or hypogastric arteries may be lifesaving when other measures fail. Styptics such as Monsel solution or acetone are effective, although delayed sloughing may result in further bleeding. Wet vaginal packing is helpful. Emergency irradiation usually controls bleeding.

B. Specific Measures

1. Carcinoma in situ (stage 0)—In women for whom childbearing is not a consideration, total hysterectomy is the treatment of choice. In women who wish to retain the uterus, acceptable alternatives include cervical conization or ablation of the lesion with cryotherapy or laser.

Close follow-up with Papanicolaou smears every 3 months for 1 year and every 6 months for another year is necessary after cryotherapy or laser.

2. Invasive carcinoma—Microinvasive carcinoma (stage IA1) is treated with simple, extrafascial hysterectomy. Stages IA2, IB1, and IIA cancers may be treated with either radical hysterectomy with concomitant radiation and chemotherapy or with radiation plus chemotherapy alone. Women with stage IB1 may be candidates for fertility-sparing surgery that includes radical trachelectomy and lymph node dissection with preservation of the uterus and ovaries. Stages IB2, IIB, III, and IV cancers are treated with radiation therapy plus concurrent chemotherapy.

▶ Prognosis

The overall 5-year relative survival rate for carcinoma of the cervix is 68% in white women and 55% in black women in the United States. Survival rates are inversely proportionate to the stage of cancer: stage 0, 99–100%; stage IA, more than 95%; stage IB–IIA, 80–90%; stage IIB, 65%; stage III, 40%; and stage IV, less than 20%.

▶ When to Refer

All patients with invasive cervical carcinoma (stage 1A or higher) should be referred to a gynecologic oncologist.

American Cancer Society. Survival rates for cervical cancer by stage. http://www.cancer.org/cancer/cervicalcancer/detailedguide/cervical-cancer-survival

Apgar BS et al. Gynecologic procedures: colposcopy, treatments for cervical intraepithelial neoplasia and endometrial assessment. Am Fam Physician. 2013 Jun 15;87(12):836–43. [PMID: 23939565]

Berger JL et al. Surgical management of cervical carcinoma. Hematol Oncol Clin North Am. 2012 Feb;26(1):63–78. [PMID: 22244662]

Dickinson JA et al. Reduced cervical cancer incidence and mortality in Canada: national data from 1932 to 2006. BMC Public Health. 2012 Nov 16;12:992. [PMID: 23158654]

LEIOMYOMA OF THE UTERUS (Fibroid Tumor)

ESSENTIALS OF DIAGNOSIS

▶ Irregular enlargement of the uterus (may be asymptomatic).

▶ Heavy or irregular vaginal bleeding, dysmenorrhea.

▶ Pelvic pain and pressure.

▶ General Considerations

Uterine leiomyoma is the most common benign neoplasm of the female genital tract. It is a discrete, round, firm, often multiple uterine tumor composed of smooth muscle and connective tissue. The most convenient classification is by anatomic location: (1) intramural, (2) submucous, (3) subserous, (4) intraligamentous, (5) parasitic (ie, deriving its blood supply from an organ to which it becomes attached), and (6) cervical. A submucous myoma may become pedunculated and descend through the cervix into the vagina.

Clinical Findings

A. Symptoms and Signs

In nonpregnant women, myomas are frequently asymptomatic. The two most common symptoms of uterine leiomyomas for which women seek treatment are AUB and pelvic pain or pressure. Occasionally, degeneration occurs, causing intense pain. The risk of miscarriage is increased if the myoma significantly distorts the uterine cavity. Fibroids rarely cause infertility by causing bilateral tubal blockage; they more commonly cause miscarriage and pregnancy complications such as preterm labor and preterm delivery as well as malpresentation.

B. Laboratory Findings

Iron deficiency anemia may result from blood loss; in rare cases, polycythemia is present, presumably as a result of the production of erythropoietin by the myomas.

C. Imaging

Ultrasonography will confirm the presence of uterine myomas and can be used sequentially to monitor growth. When multiple subserous or pedunculated myomas are being followed, ultrasonography is important to exclude ovarian masses. MRI can delineate intramural and submucous myomas accurately. Hysterography or hysteroscopy can also confirm cervical or submucous myomas.

Differential Diagnosis

Irregular myomatous enlargement of the uterus must be differentiated from the similar but symmetric enlargement that may occur with pregnancy or adenomyosis. Subserous myomas must be distinguished from ovarian tumors. Leiomyosarcoma is an unusual tumor occurring in 0.5% of women operated on for symptomatic myoma. It is very rare under the age of 40 and increases in incidence thereafter.

Treatment

A. Emergency Measures

Emergency surgery may be required for acute torsion of a pedunculated myoma. If the patient is markedly anemic as a result of long, heavy menstrual periods, preoperative treatment with DMPA, 150 mg intramuscularly every 28 days, or use of a GnRH agonist, such as depot leuprolide, 3.75 mg intramuscularly monthly, or nafarelin, 0.2–0.4 mg intranasally twice daily, will slow or stop bleeding, and medical treatment of anemia can be given prior to surgery. Levonorgestrel-containing IUDs have also been used to decrease the bleeding associated with fibroids, but IUD placement is more technically challenging in these patients. The only emergency indication for myomectomy during pregnancy is torsion. This surgery is not likely to cause abortion.

B. Specific Measures

Women who have small asymptomatic myomas should be examined annually. Surgical intervention is based on the patient's symptoms and desire for future fertility. Uterine size alone is no longer considered an indication for surgery. Cervical myomas larger than 3–4 cm in diameter or pedunculated myomas that protrude through the cervix must be removed because they often cause bleeding, infection, degeneration, pain, and urinary retention. Submucous myomas can be removed using a hysteroscope and laser or resection instruments.

Because the risk of surgical complications increases with the increasing size of the myoma, preoperative reduction of myoma size is desirable. GnRH analogs such as depot leuprolide, 3.75 mg intramuscularly monthly, or nafarelin, 0.2–0.4 mg intranasally twice a day, are used preoperatively for 3- to 4-month periods to induce reversible hypogonadism, which temporarily reduces the size of myomas, suppresses their further growth, and reduces surrounding vascularity. Low-dose (5–10 mg/day) mifepristone and other selective progesterone-receptor modulators have shown some promise for long-term medical treatment of myomas. Ulipristal acetate, a selective progesterone receptor modulator, has been approved in Europe and Canada for the preoperative treatment of fibroids in daily doses of 5 mg for up to 3 months.

C. Surgical Measures

Surgical measures available for the treatment of myoma are laparoscopic or abdominal myomectomy and total or subtotal abdominal, vaginal, or laparoscopy-assisted vaginal hysterectomy. Myomectomy is the treatment of choice for women who wish to preserve fertility. Uterine artery embolization is a minimally invasive treatment for some uterine fibroids. In uterine artery embolization the goal is to block the blood vessels supplying the fibroids, causing them to shrink. Magnetic resonance–guided high-intensity focused ultrasound, myolysis/radiofrequency ablation, and laparoscopic or vaginal occlusion of uterine vessels are newer interventions, with a smaller body of evidence.

Prognosis

Surgical therapy is curative. In women desiring future fertility, myomectomy can be offered, but patients should be counseled that recurrence is common, postoperative pelvic adhesions may impact fertility, and cesarean delivery may be necessary.

When to Refer

Refer to a gynecologist for treatment of symptomatic leiomyomata.

When to Admit

For acute abdomen associated with an infarcted leiomyoma or hemorrhage not controlled by outpatient measures.

Guo XC et al. The impact and management of fibroids for fertility: an evidence-based approach. Obstet Gynecol Clin North Am. 2012 Dec;39(4):521–33. [PMID: 23182558]

Islam MS et al. Uterine leiomyoma: available medical treatments and new possible therapeutic options. J Clin Endocrinol Metab. 2013 Mar;98(3):921–34. [PMID: 23393173]

van der Kooij SM et al. Review of nonsurgical/minimally invasive treatments for uterine fibroids. Curr Opin Obstet Gynecol. 2012 Dec;24(6):368–75. [PMID: 23014141]

Zimmermann A et al. Prevalence, symptoms and management of uterine fibroids: an international internet-based survey of 21,746 women. BMC Womens Health. 2012 Mar 26;12:6. [PMID: 22448610]

CARCINOMA OF THE ENDOMETRIUM

ESSENTIALS OF DIAGNOSIS

▸ Abnormal bleeding is the presenting sign in 90% of cases.

▸ Papanicolaou smear is frequently negative.

▸ After a negative pregnancy test, endometrial tissue is required to confirm the diagnosis.

General Considerations

Adenocarcinoma of the endometrium is the second most common cancer of the female genital tract. It occurs most often in women 50–70 years of age. Obesity, nulliparity, diabetes, and polycystic ovaries with prolonged anovulation, unopposed estrogen therapy, and the extended use of tamoxifen for the treatment of breast cancer are also risk factors. Women with a family history of colon cancer (hereditary nonpolyposis colorectal cancer, Lynch syndrome) are at significantly increased risk, with a lifetime incidence as high as 30%.

Abnormal bleeding is the presenting sign in 90% of cases. Any postmenopausal bleeding requires investigation. Pain generally occurs late in the disease, with metastases or infection.

Papanicolaou smears of the cervix occasionally show atypical endometrial cells but are an insensitive diagnostic tool. **Endocervical and endometrial sampling is the only reliable means of diagnosis.** Simultaneous hysteroscopy can be a valuable addition in order to localize polyps or other lesions within the uterine cavity. Vaginal ultrasonography may be used to determine the thickness of the endometrium as an indication of hypertrophy and possible neoplastic change. The finding of a thin endometrial lining on ultrasound is helpful in cases where very little tissue is obtainable through endometrial biopsy.

Pathologic assessment is important in differentiating hyperplasias, which often can be treated with cyclic oral progestins.

Prevention

Prompt endometrial sampling for patients who report abnormal menstrual bleeding or postmenopausal uterine bleeding will reveal many incipient as well as clinical cases of endometrial cancer. Younger women with chronic anovulation are at risk for endometrial hyperplasia and subsequent endometrial cancer. They can reduce the risk of hyperplasia almost completely with the use of oral contraceptives or cyclic progestin therapy.

Staging

Staging and prognosis are based on surgical and pathologic evaluation only. Examination under anesthesia, endometrial and endocervical sampling, chest radiography, intravenous urography, cystoscopy, sigmoidoscopy, transvaginal sonography, and MRI will help determine the extent of the disease and its appropriate treatment.

Treatment

Treatment consists of total hysterectomy and bilateral salpingo-oophorectomy. Peritoneal material for cytologic examination is routinely taken and lymph node sampling may be done. If invasion deep into the myometrium has occurred or if sampled lymph nodes are positive for tumor, postoperative irradiation is indicated. Patients with stage III endometrial cancer are generally treated with surgery followed by chemotherapy or radiation therapy or both. A review by the Society of Gynecologic Oncology Clinical Practice Committee concluded "the use of adjuvant chemotherapy to treat stage I or II endometrial carcinoma is not supported by the available evidence." Palliation of advanced or metastatic endometrial adenocarcinoma may be accomplished with large doses of progestins, eg, medroxyprogesterone, 400 mg weekly intramuscularly, or megestrol acetate, 80–160 mg daily orally.

Prognosis

With early diagnosis and treatment, the overall 5-year survival is 80–85%. With stage I disease, the depth of myometrial invasion is the strongest predictor of survival, with a 98% 5-year survival with less than 66% depth of invasion and 78% survival with 66% or more invasion.

When to Refer

All patients with endometrial carcinoma should be referred to a gynecologic oncologist.

Freeman SJ et al. The revised FIGO staging system for uterine malignancies: implications for MR imaging. Radiographics. 2012 Oct;32(6):1805–27. [PMID: 23065170]

Landrum LM et al. Phase II trial of vaginal cuff brachytherapy followed by chemotherapy in early stage endometrial cancer patients with high-intermediate risk factors. Gynecol Oncol. 2014 Jan;132(1):50–4. [PMID: 24219982]

SGO Clinical Practice Endometrial Cancer Working Group; Burke WM et al; Society of Gynecologic Oncology Clinical Practice Committee. Endometrial cancer: a review and current management strategies: part II. Gynecol Oncol. 2014 Aug; 134(2):393–402. [PMID: 24929052]

Trimble CL et al; Society of Gynecologic Oncology Clinical Practice Committee. Management of endometrial precancers. Obstet Gynecol. 2012 Nov;120(5):1160–75. [PMID: 23090535]

CARCINOMA OF THE VULVA

> ## ESSENTIALS OF DIAGNOSIS
>
> ▶ History of genital warts.
> ▶ History of prolonged vulvar irritation, with pruritus, local discomfort, or slight bloody discharge.
> ▶ Early lesions may suggest or include non-neoplastic epithelial disorders.
> ▶ Late lesions appear as a mass, an exophytic growth, or a firm, ulcerated area in the vulva.
> ▶ Biopsy is necessary for diagnosis.

General Considerations

The majority of cancers of the vulva are squamous lesions that classically have occurred in women over 50 years of age. Several subtypes (particularly 16, 18, and 31) of HPV have been identified in some but not all vulvar cancers. About 70–90% of vulvar intraepithelial neoplasia (VIN) and 40–60% of vulvar cancers are HPV associated. As with squamous cell lesions of the cervix, a grading system of VIN from mild dysplasia to carcinoma in situ is used.

Differential Diagnosis

Benign vulvar disorders that must be excluded in the diagnosis of carcinoma of the vulva include chronic granulomatous lesions (eg, lymphogranuloma venereum, syphilis), condylomas, hidradenoma, or neurofibroma. Lichen sclerosus and other associated leukoplakic changes in the skin should be biopsied. The likelihood that a superimposed vulvar cancer will develop in a woman with a nonneoplastic epithelial disorder (vulvar dystrophy) is 1–5%.

Diagnosis

Biopsy is essential for the diagnosis of VIN and vulvar cancer and should be performed with any localized atypical vulvar lesion, including white patches. Multiple skin-punch specimens can be taken in the office under local anesthesia, with care to include tissue from the edges of each lesion sampled. Colposcopy of vulva, vagina, and cervix can help in identifying areas for biopsy and in planning further treatment.

Staging

Vulvar cancer generally spreads by direct extension into the vagina, urethra, perineum, and anus, with discontinuous spread into the inguinal and femoral lymph nodes. CT or MRI of the pelvis or abdomen is generally not required except in advanced cases for planning therapeutic options.

Treatment

A. General Measures

Early diagnosis and treatment of irritative or other predisposing causes, such as lichen sclerosis and VIN, should be pursued. A 7:3 combination of betamethasone and crotamiton is particularly effective for itching. After an initial response, fluorinated steroids should be replaced with hydrocortisone because of their skin atrophying effect. For lichen sclerosus, recommended treatment is clobetasol propionate cream 0.05% twice daily for 2–3 weeks, then once daily until symptoms resolve. Application one to three times a week can be used for long-term maintenance therapy.

B. Surgical Measures

High-grade VIN may be treated with a variety of approaches including topical chemotherapy, laser ablation, wide local excision, skinning vulvectomy, and simple vulvectomy. Small, invasive basal cell carcinoma of the vulva should be excised with a wide margin. If the VIN is extensive or multicentric, laser therapy or superficial surgical removal of vulvar skin may be required. In this way, the clitoris and uninvolved portions of the vulva may be spared.

Invasive carcinoma confined to the vulva without evidence of spread to adjacent organs or to the regional lymph nodes is treated with wide local excision and inguinal lymphadenectomy or wide local excision alone if invasion is less than 1 mm. To avoid the morbidity of inguinal lymphadenectomy, some guidelines recommend sentinel lymph node sampling for women with early-stage vulvar cancer. Patients with more advanced disease may receive preoperative radiation, chemotherapy, or both.

Prognosis

Basal cell vulvar carcinomas very seldom metastasize, and carcinoma in situ by definition has not metastasized. With adequate excision, the prognosis for both lesions is excellent. Patients with invasive vulvar SCC 2 cm in diameter or less, without inguinal lymph node metastases, have an 85–90% 5-year survival rate. If the lesion is larger than 2 cm and lymph node involvement is present, the likelihood of 5-year survival is approximately 40%.

When to Refer

All patients with invasive vulvar carcinoma should be referred to a gynecologic oncologist.

Carter JS et al. Vulvar and vaginal cancer. Obstet Gynecol Clin North Am. 2012 Jun;39(2):213–31. [PMID: 22640712]
de Gregorio N et al. The role of preoperative ultrasound evaluation of inguinal lymph nodes in patients with vulvar malignancy. Gynecol Oncol. 2013 Oct;131(1):113–7. [PMID: 23932893]
Dittmer C et al. Diagnosis and treatment options of vulvar cancer: a review. Arch Gynecol Obstet. 2012 Jan;285(1):183–93. [PMID: 21909752]

ENDOMETRIOSIS

ESSENTIALS OF DIAGNOSIS

▶ Dysmenorrhea.

▶ Dyspareunia.

▶ Increased frequency among infertile women.

▶ Abnormal uterine bleeding.

▶ General Considerations

Endometriosis is an aberrant growth of endometrium outside the uterus, particularly in the dependent parts of the pelvis and in the ovaries, whose principal manifestations are chronic pain and infertility. While retrograde menstruation is the most widely accepted cause, its pathogenesis and natural course are not fully understood. The overall prevalence in the United States is 6–10% and is fourfold to fivefold greater among infertile women.

▶ Clinical Findings

The clinical manifestations of endometriosis are variable and unpredictable in both presentation and course. Dysmenorrhea, chronic pelvic pain, and dyspareunia, are among the well-recognized manifestations. A significant number of women with endometriosis, however, remain asymptomatic and most women with endometriosis have a normal pelvic examination. However, in some women, pelvic examination can disclose tender nodules in the cul-de-sac or rectovaginal septum, uterine retroversion with decreased uterine mobility, cervical motion tenderness, or an adnexal mass or tenderness.

Endometriosis must be distinguished from PID, ovarian neoplasms, and uterine myomas. Bowel invasion by endometrial tissue may produce blood in the stool that must be distinguished from bowel neoplasm.

Imaging is of limited value and is only useful in the presence of a pelvic or adnexal mass. Transvaginal ultrasonography is the imaging modality of choice to detect the presence of deeply penetrating endometriosis of the rectum or rectovaginal septum, while MRI should be reserved for equivocal cases of rectovaginal or bladder endometriosis. Ultimately, a definitive diagnosis of endometriosis is made only by histology of lesions removed at surgery.

▶ Treatment

A. Medical Treatment

Although there is no conclusive evidence that NSAIDs improve pain associated with endometriosis, these agents are reasonable options in appropriately selected patients. Medical treatment, using a variety of hormonal therapies, is effective in the amelioration of pain associated with endometriosis. However, there is no evidence that any of these agents increase the likelihood of pregnancy. Their preoperative use is of questionable value in reducing the difficulty of surgery. Most of these regimens are designed

to inhibit ovulation over 4–9 months and lower hormone levels, thus preventing cyclic stimulation of endometriotic implants and inducing atrophy. The optimum duration of therapy is not clear, and the relative merits in terms of side effects and long-term risks and benefits show insignificant differences when compared with each other and, in mild cases, with placebo. Commonly used medical regimens include the following:

1. Low-dose **oral contraceptives** can also be given cyclically; prolonged suppression of ovulation often inhibits further stimulation of residual endometriosis, especially if taken after one of the therapies mentioned here. Any of the combination oral contraceptives, the contraceptive patch, or vaginal ring may be used continuously for 6–12 months. Breakthrough bleeding can be treated with conjugated estrogens, 1.25 mg orally daily for 1 week, or estradiol, 2 mg daily orally for 1 week.

2. **Progestins,** specifically oral norethindrone acetate and subcutaneous DMPA, have been approved by the FDA for treatment of endometriosis-associated pain.

3. **GnRH agonists** are highly effective in reducing the pain syndromes associated with endometriosis. However, they are not superior to other methods such as combined oral contraceptives as first-line therapy. The GnRH analogs (such as nafarelin nasal spray, 0.2–0.4 mg twice daily, or long-acting injectable leuprolide acetate, 3.75 mg intramuscularly monthly, used for 6 months) suppress ovulation. Side effects of vasomotor symptoms and bone demineralization may be relieved by "add-back" therapy, such as conjugated equine estrogen, 0.625 mg, or norethindrone, 5 mg orally daily.

4. **Danazol** is an androgenic drug that has been used for the treatment of endometriosis-associated pain. It should be used for 4–6 months in the lowest dose necessary to suppress menstruation, usually 200–400 mg orally twice daily. However, danazol has a high incidence of androgenic side effects that are more severe than other medications available, including decreased breast size, weight gain, acne, and hirsutism.

5. Intrauterine progestin use with the **levonorgestrel intrauterine system** also has been shown to be effective in reducing endometriosis-associated pelvic pain and should be tried before radical surgery.

6. The use of **aromatase inhibitors** (such as anastrozole or letrozole) has been evaluated in women with chronic pain resistant to other forms of medical management or surgical management. Although promising, there are insufficient data to recommend their routine use.

B. Surgical Measures

Surgical treatment of endometriosis—particularly extensive disease—is effective both in reducing pain and in promoting fertility. Laparoscopic ablation of endometrial implants significantly reduces pain. Ablation of implants and, if necessary, removal of ovarian endometriomas enhance fertility, although subsequent pregnancy rates are inversely related to the severity of disease. Women with disabling pain for whom childbearing is not a consideration can be treated definitively with total abdominal hysterectomy and bilateral salpingo-oophorectomy. In premenopausal women, hormone replacement then may be used to relieve vasomotor symptoms. However, hormone replacement may lead to a recurrence of endometriosis and associated pain.

▶ Prognosis

There is little systematic research regarding either the progression of the disease or the prediction of clinical outcomes. The prognosis for reproductive function in early or moderately advanced endometriosis appears to be good with conservative therapy. Hysterectomy, with bilateral salpingo-oophorectomy, often is regarded as definitive therapy for the treatment of endometriosis associated with intractable pelvic pain, adnexal masses, or multiple previous ineffective conservative surgical procedures. However, symptoms may recur in women even after hysterectomy and oophorectomy.

▶ When to Refer

Refer to a gynecologist for laparoscopic diagnosis or treatment.

▶ When to Admit

Rarely necessary except for acute abdomen associated with ruptured or bleeding endometrioma.

Abu Hashim H. Potential role of aromatase inhibitors in the treatment of endometriosis. Int J Womens Health. 2014 Jul 21; 6:671–80. [PMID: 25092998]
American College of Obstetricians and Gynecologists. ACOG Practice Bulletin No. 114: Management of endometriosis. Obstet Gynecol. 2010 July:116(1):223–36. [Reaffirmed 2014] [PMID: 20567196]
Burney RO et al. Pathogenesis and pathophysiology of endometriosis. Fertil Steril. 2012 Sep;98(3):511–9. [PMID: 22819144]
Johnson NP et al; World Endometriosis Society Montpellier Consortium. Consensus on current management of endometriosis. Hum Reprod. 2013 Jun;28(6):1552–68. [PMID: 23528916]
Schrager S et al. Evaluation and treatment of endometriosis. Am Fam Physician. 2013 Jan 15;87(2):107–13. [PMID: 23317074]
Tafi E et al. Advances in pharmacotherapy for treating endometriosis. Expert Opin Pharmacother. 2015 Nov;16(16):2465–83. [PMID: 26569155]

PELVIC ORGAN PROLAPSE

▶ General Considerations

Cystocele, rectocele, and enterocele are vaginal hernias commonly seen in multiparous women. **Cystocele** is a hernia of the bladder wall into the vagina, causing a soft anterior fullness. Cystocele may be accompanied by **urethrocele,** which is not a hernia but a sagging of the urethra following its detachment from the pubic symphysis during childbirth. **Rectocele** is a herniation of the terminal rectum into the posterior vagina, causing a collapsible pouch-like fullness. **Enterocele** is a vaginal vault hernia containing small intestine, usually in the posterior vagina and resulting from a deepening of the pouch of Douglas. Two or all

three types of hernia may occur in combination. Risk factors may include vaginal birth, genetic predisposition, advancing age, prior pelvic surgery, connective tissue disorders, and increased intra-abdominal pressure associated with obesity or straining associated with chronic constipation or coughing.

▶ Clinical Findings

Symptoms of pelvic organ prolapse may include sensation of a bulge or protrusion in the vagina, urinary or fecal incontinence, constipation, a sense of incomplete bladder emptying, and dyspareunia. The cause of pelvic organ prolapse, including prolapse of the uterus, vaginal apex, and anterior or posterior vaginal walls, is likely multifactorial.

▶ Treatment

The type of therapy depends on the extent of prolapse and the patient's age and her desire for menstruation, pregnancy, and coitus.

A. General Measures

Supportive measures include a high-fiber diet and laxatives to improve constipation. Weight reduction in obese patients and limitation of straining and lifting are helpful. Pelvic muscle training (Kegel exercises) is a simple, noninvasive intervention that may improve pelvic function that has clearly demonstrated benefit for women with urinary or fecal symptoms, especially incontinence. Pessaries may reduce cystocele, rectocele, or enterocele and are helpful in women who do not wish to undergo surgery or are poor surgical candidates.

B. Surgical Measures

The most common surgical procedure is vaginal or abdominal hysterectomy with additional attention to restoring apical support after the uterus is removed, including suspension by either uterosacral or sacrospinous fixation vaginally or abdominal sacral colpopexy. Since stress incontinence is common after vault suspension procedures, an anti-incontinence procedure should be considered. While the use of various surgical mesh materials with these procedures increased substantially since 2000, several safety advisories recommend a more cautious use of mesh materials. If the patient desires pregnancy, the same procedures for vaginal suspension can be performed without hysterectomy, though limited data on pregnancy outcomes or prolapse outcomes are available. For elderly women who do not desire coitus, colpocleisis, the partial obliteration of the vagina, is surgically simple and effective. Uterine suspension with sacrospinous cervicocolpopexy may be an effective approach in older women who wish to avoid hysterectomy but preserve coital function.

▶ When to Refer

• Refer to urogynecologist or gynecologist for incontinence evaluation.

• Refer if nonsurgical therapy is ineffective.

Committee on Gynecologic Practice. Vaginal placement of synthetic mesh for pelvic organ prolapse. Female Pelvic Med Reconstr Surg. 2012 Jan–Feb;18(1):5–9. [PMID: 22453257]

Kenton K et al; Pelvic Floor Disorders Network. Pelvic floor symptoms improve similarly after pessary and behavioral treatment for stress incontinence. Female Pelvic Med Reconstr Surg. 2012 Mar–Apr;18(2):118–21. [PMID: 22453323]

Wei JT et al; Pelvic Floor Disorders Network. A midurethral sling to reduce incontinence after vaginal prolapse repair. N Engl J Med. 2012 Jun 21;366(25):2358–67. [PMID: 22716974]

PELVIC INFLAMMATORY DISEASE
(Salpingitis, Endometritis)

 ESSENTIALS OF DIAGNOSIS

- ▶ Uterine, adnexal, or cervical motion tenderness.
- ▶ Abnormal discharge from the vagina or cervix.
- ▶ Absence of a competing diagnosis.

▶ General Considerations

Pelvic inflammatory disease (PID) is a polymicrobial infection of the upper genital tract associated with the sexually transmitted organisms *N gonorrhoeae* and *Chlamydia trachomatis* as well as endogenous organisms, including anaerobes, *Haemophilus influenzae*, enteric gram-negative rods, and streptococci. It is most common in young, nulliparous, sexually active women with multiple partners and is a leading cause of infertility and ectopic pregnancy. The use of barrier methods of contraception may provide significant protection.

Tuberculous salpingitis is rare in the United States but more common in developing countries; it is characterized by pelvic pain and irregular pelvic masses not responsive to antibiotic therapy. It is not sexually transmitted.

▶ Clinical Findings

A. Symptoms and Signs

Patients with PID may have lower abdominal pain, chills and fever, menstrual disturbances, purulent cervical discharge, and cervical and adnexal tenderness. Right upper quadrant pain (Fitz-Hugh and Curtis syndrome) may indicate an associated perihepatitis. However, diagnosis of PID is complicated by the fact that many women may have subtle or mild symptoms that are not readily recognized as PID, such as postcoital bleeding, urinary frequency, or low back pain.

B. Minimum Diagnostic Criteria

Women with uterine, adnexal, or cervical motion tenderness should be considered to have PID and be treated with antibiotics unless there is a competing diagnosis such as ectopic pregnancy or appendicitis.

C. Additional Criteria

No single historical, physical or laboratory finding is definitive for acute PID. The following criteria may be used to enhance the specificity of the diagnosis: (1) oral temperature higher than 38.3°C, (2) abnormal cervical or vaginal discharge with white cells on saline microscopy (greater than 1 leukocyte per epithelial cell), (3) elevated erythrocyte sedimentation rate, (4) elevated C-reactive protein, and (5) laboratory documentation of cervical infection with *N gonorrhoeae* or *C trachomatis*. Endocervical culture should be performed routinely, but treatment should not be delayed while awaiting results.

▶ Differential Diagnosis

Appendicitis, ectopic pregnancy, septic abortion, hemorrhagic or ruptured ovarian cysts or tumors, twisted ovarian cyst, degeneration of a myoma, and acute enteritis must be considered. PID is more likely to occur when there is a history of PID, recent sexual contact, recent onset of menses, recent insertion of an IUD, or if the partner has a sexually transmitted disease. **Acute PID is highly unlikely when recent (within 60 days) intercourse has not taken place.** A sensitive serum pregnancy test should be obtained to rule out ectopic pregnancy. Pelvic and vaginal ultrasonography is helpful in the differential diagnosis of ectopic pregnancy of over 6 weeks. Laparoscopy is often used to diagnose PID, and it is imperative if the diagnosis is not certain or if the patient has not responded to antibiotic therapy after 48 hours. The appendix should be visualized at laparoscopy to rule out appendicitis. Cultures obtained at the time of laparoscopy are often specific and helpful.

▶ Treatment

A. Antibiotics

Early treatment with appropriate antibiotics effective against *N gonorrhoeae*, *C trachomatis*, and the endogenous organisms listed above is essential to prevent long-term sequelae. The sexual partner should be examined and treated appropriately. Most women with mild to moderate disease can be treated successfully as an outpatient. The recommended outpatient regimen is a single dose of cefoxitin, 2 g intramuscularly, with probenecid, 1 g orally, plus doxycycline 100 mg orally twice a day for 14 days, or ceftriaxone 250 mg intramuscularly plus doxycycline, 100 mg orally twice daily, for 14 days. Metronidazole 500 mg orally twice daily for 14 days may also be added to either of these two regimens to treat bacterial vaginosis that is frequently associated with PID. For patients with severe disease or those who meet the other criteria for hospitalization, there are two recommended regimens. One regimen includes either cefotetan, 2 g intravenously every 12 hours, or cefoxitin, 2 g intravenously every 6 hours, plus doxycycline 100 mg orally or intravenously every 12 hours. The other recommended regimen is clindamycin, 900 mg intravenously every 8 hours, plus gentamicin, a loading dose of 2 mg/kg intravenously or intramuscularly followed by a maintenance dose of 1.5 mg/kg every 8 hours (or as a single daily dose, 3–5 mg/kg). These regimens should be continued for a minimum of 24 hours after the patient shows significant clinical improvement. Then, an oral regimen should be given for a total course of antibiotics of 14 days with either doxycycline, 100 mg orally twice a day, or clindamycin, 450 mg orally four times a day. If a tuboovarian abscess is present, clindamycin should be given because of the better anaerobic coverage it provides.

B. Surgical Measures

Tubo-ovarian abscesses may require surgical excision or transcutaneous or transvaginal aspiration. Unless rupture is suspected, institute high-dose antibiotic therapy in the hospital, and monitor therapy with ultrasound. In 70% of cases, antibiotics are effective; in 30%, there is inadequate response in 48–72 hours, and surgical intervention is required. Unilateral adnexectomy is acceptable for unilateral abscess. Hysterectomy and bilateral salpingo-oophorectomy may be necessary for overwhelming infection or in cases of chronic disease with intractable pelvic pain.

▶ Prognosis

In spite of treatment, long-term sequelae, including repeated episodes of infection, chronic pelvic pain, dyspareunia, ectopic pregnancy, or infertility, develop in onefourth of women with acute disease. The risk of infertility increases with repeated episodes of salpingitis: it is estimated at 10% after the first episode, 25% after a second episode, and 50% after a third episode.

▶ When to Admit

The following patients with acute PID should be admitted for intravenous antibiotic therapy:

- The patient has a tubo-ovarian abscess (direct inpatient observation for at least 24 hours before switching to outpatient parenteral therapy).
- The patient is pregnant.
- The patient is unable to follow or tolerate an outpatient regimen.
- The patient has not responded clinically to outpatient therapy within 72 hours.
- The patient has severe illness, nausea and vomiting, or high fever.
- Another surgical emergency, such as appendicitis, cannot be ruled out.

Liu B et al. Improving adherence to guidelines for the diagnosis and management of pelvic inflammatory disease: a systematic review. Infect Dis Obstet Gynecol. 2012;2012:325108. [PMID: 22973085]
Markle W et al. Sexually transmitted diseases. Prim Care. 2013 Sep; 40(3):557–87. [PMID: 23958358]
Sweet RL. Treatment of acute pelvic inflammatory disease. Infect Dis Obstet Gynecol. 2011;2011:561909. [PMID: 22228985]

OVARIAN CANCER & OVARIAN TUMORS

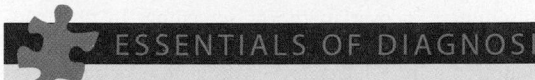

ESSENTIALS OF DIAGNOSIS

▶ Vague gastrointestinal discomfort, pelvic pressure, or pain.

▶ Many cases of early-stage cancer are asymptomatic.

▶ Pelvic examination and ultrasound are mainstays of diagnosis.

▶ General Considerations

Ovarian tumors are common. Most are benign, but malignant ovarian tumors are the leading cause of death from reproductive tract cancer. The wide range of types and patterns of ovarian tumors is due to the complexity of ovarian embryology and differences in tissues of origin.

In women with no family history of ovarian cancer, the lifetime risk is 1.6%, whereas a woman with one affected first-degree relative has a 5% lifetime risk. **Ultrasound or tumor marker screening for women with one or no affected first-degree relatives have not been shown to reduce mortality from ovarian cancer,** and the risks associated with unnecessary prophylactic surgical procedures outweigh the benefits in low-risk women. With two or more affected first-degree relatives, the risk is 7%. Approximately 3% of women with two or more affected first-degree relatives will have a hereditary ovarian cancer syndrome with a lifetime risk of 40%. Women with a *BRCA1* gene mutation have a 45% lifetime risk of ovarian cancer and those with a *BRCA2* mutation a 25% risk. Consideration should be given to screening these women every 6 months with transvaginal sonography and serum CA 125 testing, starting at age 35 or 5–10 years earlier than the earliest age that ovarian cancer was first diagnosed in a family member. Because this screening regimen has not been shown to reduce mortality, oophorectomy is recommended by age 35 or whenever childbearing is not a consideration because of the high risk of disease.

▶ Clinical Findings

A. Symptoms and Signs

Unfortunately, **most women with both benign and malignant ovarian neoplasms are either asymptomatic or experience only mild nonspecific gastrointestinal symptoms or pelvic pressure.** Women with early disease are typically detected on routine pelvic examination. Women with advanced malignant disease may experience abdominal pain and bloating, and a palpable abdominal mass with ascites is often present.

B. Laboratory Findings

CA 125 is elevated in 80% of women with epithelial ovarian cancer overall but in only 50% of women with early disease.

Serum CA 125 may be elevated in premenopausal women with benign disease (such as endometriosis), minimizing its usefulness in ovarian cancer screening. In premenopausal women, other markers (such as human chorionic gonadotropin [hCG], lactate dehydrogenase, or alpha fetoprotein) may be indicators of the type of tumor present.

C. Imaging Studies

Transvaginal sonography is useful for screening high-risk women but has inadequate sensitivity for screening low-risk women. Ultrasound is helpful in differentiating ovarian masses that are benign and likely to resolve spontaneously from those with malignant potential. Color Doppler imaging may further enhance the specificity of ultrasound diagnosis.

Differential Diagnosis

Once an ovarian mass has been detected, it must be categorized as functional, benign neoplastic, or potentially malignant. Predictive factors include age, size of the mass, ultrasound configuration, CA 125 levels, the presence of symptoms, and whether the mass is unilateral or bilateral. Simple cysts up to 10 cm in diameter are almost universally benign in both premenopausal and postmenopausal patients. Most will resolve spontaneously and may be monitored without intervention. If the mass is larger or unchanged on repeat pelvic examination and transvaginal sonography, surgical evaluation is warranted.

Laparoscopy may be used when an ovarian mass is small enough to be removed with a laparoscopic approach. If malignancy is suspected, because of findings on transvaginal ultrasound with morphologic scoring, color Doppler assessment of vascular quality, and serum CA 125 level, then laparotomy is preferable.

Treatment

If a malignant ovarian mass is suspected, surgical evaluation should be performed by a gynecologic oncologist. For benign neoplasms, tumor removal or unilateral oophorectomy is usually performed. For ovarian cancer in an early stage, the standard therapy is complete surgical staging followed by abdominal hysterectomy and bilateral salpingo-oophorectomy with omentectomy and selective lymphadenectomy. With more advanced disease, aggressive removal of all visible tumor improves survival. Except for women with low-grade ovarian cancer in an early stage, postoperative chemotherapy is indicated (see Table 39–11). Several chemotherapy regimens are effective, such as the combination of cisplatin or carboplatin with paclitaxel, with clinical response rates of up to 60–70% (see Table 39–12).

Prognosis

Unfortunately, **advanced disease is diagnosed in approximately 75% of women with ovarian cancer.** The overall 5-year survival is approximately 17% with distant metastases, 36% with local spread, and 89% with early disease.

When to Refer

If a malignant mass is suspected, surgical evaluation should be performed by a gynecologic oncologist.

Arie S. Routine testing for women with ovarian cancer. BMJ. 2014 Feb 26;348:g1200. [PMID: 24574473]

Banerjee S et al. Recent advances in systemic treatments for ovarian cancer. Cancer Imaging. 2012 Sep 28;12:305–9. [PMID: 23022887]

Centers for Disease Control and Prevention. Ovarian cancer screening. 2013 Aug 29. http://www.cdc.gov/cancer/ovarian/basic_info/screening.htm

Committee opinion no. 634: Hereditary cancer syndromes and risk assessment. Obstet Gynecol. 2015 Jun;125(6):1538–43. [PMID: 26000542]

Girolimetti G et al. *BRCA*-associated ovarian cancer: from molecular genetics to risk management. Biomed Res Int. 2014;2014:787143. [PMID: 25136623]

Rooth C. Ovarian cancer: risk factors, treatment and management. Br J Nurs. 2013 Sep 12-25;22(17):S23–30. [PMID: 24067270]

POLYCYSTIC OVARY SYNDROME

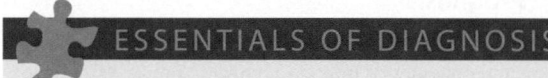

ESSENTIALS OF DIAGNOSIS

▶ Clinical or biochemical evidence of hyperandrogenism.

▶ Oligoovulation or anovulation.

▶ Polycystic ovaries on ultrasonography.

General Considerations

Polycystic ovary syndrome (PCOS) is a common endocrine disorder of unknown etiology affecting 5–10% of women of reproductive age. It is characterized by chronic anovulation, polycystic ovaries, and hyperandrogenism. It is associated with hirsutism and obesity as well as an increased risk of diabetes mellitus, cardiovascular disease, and metabolic syndrome. Unrecognized or untreated PCOS is an important risk factor for cardiovascular disease. The Rotterdam Criteria identify **androgen production, ovulatory dysfunction,** and **polycystic ovaries** as the key diagnostic features of the disorder in adult women. The classification system has been endorsed by the National Institutes of Health.

Clinical Findings

PCOS often presents as a menstrual disorder (from amenorrhea to menorrhagia) and infertility. Skin disorders due to peripheral androgen excess, including hirsutism and acne, are common. Patients may also show signs of insulin resistance and hyperinsulinemia, and these women are at increased risk for early-onset type 2 diabetes and metabolic syndrome. Patients who do become pregnant are at increased risk for perinatal complications. In addition, they have an increased long-term risk of cancer of the endometrium because of unopposed estrogen secretion.

Differential Diagnosis

Anovulation in the reproductive years may also be due to: (1) premature ovarian failure (high FSH and LH levels); (2) rapid weight loss, extreme physical exertion (normal FSH and LH levels for age), or obesity; (3) discontinuation of hormonal contraceptives (anovulation for 6 months or more occasionally occurs); (4) pituitary adenoma with elevated prolactin (galactorrhea may or may not be present); and (5) hyperthyroidism or hypothyroidism. To rule out other etiologies in women with suspected PCOS, serum FSH, LH, prolactin, and TSH should be checked. **Because of the high risk of insulin resistance and dyslipidemia, all women with suspected PCOS should have a hemoglobin A_{1C} and fasting glucose along with a lipid and lipoprotein profile.** Women with clinical evidence of androgen excess should have total testosterone and sex hormone-binding globulin or free (bioavailable) testosterone, and 17-hydroxyprogesterone measured. Women with stigmata of Cushing syndrome should have a 24-hour urinary free-cortisol or a low-dose dexamethasone suppression test. Congenital adrenal hyperplasia and androgen-secreting adrenal tumors also tend to have high circulating androgen levels and anovulation with polycystic ovaries; these disorders must also be ruled out in women with presumed PCOS.

Treatment

In obese patients with PCOS, weight reduction and exercise are often effective in reversing the metabolic effects and in inducing ovulation. For those women who do not respond to weight loss and exercise, metformin therapy may be helpful and may be offered along with contraceptive counseling to prevent unplanned pregnancy in case of a return of ovulatory cycles. Metformin is beneficial for metabolic or glucose abnormalities, and it can improve menstrual function. Metformin has little or no benefit in the treatment of hirsutism, acne, or infertility. For women who are seeking pregnancy and remain anovulatory, clomiphene or other medications can be used for ovulatory stimulation (see section on Infertility below). Clomiphene is the first-line therapy for infertility. If induction of ovulation fails with the above regimens, treatment with gonadotropins, but at low dose to lower the risk of ovarian hyperstimulation syndrome, may be successful. Second-line therapies such as use of aromatase inhibitors or laparoscopic "ovarian drilling" may be considered but are of unproved benefit. Women with PCOS are at greater risk than normal women for twin gestation with ovulation induction.

If the patient does not desire pregnancy, medroxyprogesterone acetate, 10 mg/day orally for the first 10 days of each month, should be given to ensure regular shedding of the endometrium and avoid hyperplasia. If contraception is desired, a low-dose combination oral contraceptive can be used; this is also useful in controlling hirsutism, for which treatment must be continued for 6–12 months before results are seen.

Spironolactone is useful for hirsutism in doses of 25 mg three or four times daily. Flutamide, 125–250 mg orally daily, and finasteride, 5 mg orally daily, are also effective for treating hirsutism. Because these three agents are potentially teratogenic, they should be used only in conjunction with secure contraception. Topical eflornithine cream applied to affected facial areas twice daily for 6 months may be helpful in the majority of women. Hirsutism may also be managed with depilatory creams, electrolysis, and laser therapy. The combination of laser therapy and topical eflornithine may be particularly effective.

Weight loss, exercise, and treatment of unresolved metabolic derangements are important in preventing cardiovascular disease. Women with PCOS should be managed aggressively and should have regular monitoring of lipid profiles and glucose. In adolescent patients with PCOS hormonal contraceptives and metformin are treatment options.

When to Refer

- If expertise in diagnosis is needed.
- If patient is infertile.

Bates GW et al. Longterm management of Polycystic Ovarian Syndrome (PCOS). Mol Cell Endocrinol. 2013 Jul 5;373(1–2): 91–7. [PMID: 23261983]

Blume-Peytavi U. How to diagnose and treat medically women with excessive hair. Dermatol Clin. 2013 Jan;31(1):57–65. [PMID: 23159176]

Legro RS et al. Diagnosis and treatment of polycystic ovary syndrome: an endocrine society clinical practice guideline. J Clin Endocrinol Metab. 2013 Dec;98(12):4565–92. [PMID: 24151290]

Legro RS. Obesity and PCOS: implications for diagnosis and treatment. Semin Reprod Med. 2012 Dec;30(6):496–506. [PMID: 23074008]

FEMALE SEXUAL DYSFUNCTION

General Considerations

Female sexual dysfunction is a common problem. Depending on the questions asked, surveys have shown that from **35% to 98% of women report sexual concerns.** Questions related to sexual functioning should be asked as part of the routine medical history. Three helpful questions are: "Are you currently involved in a sexual relationship?", "With men, women, or both?", and "Are there any sexual concerns or pain with sex?" If the woman is not involved in a sexual relationship, she should be asked about any concerns that are contributing to a lack of sexual behavior. If a history of sexual dysfunction is elicited, a complete history of factors that may affect sexual function should be taken. These factors include her reproductive history (including pregnancies and mode of delivery) as well as history of infertility, sexually transmitted diseases, rape or sexual abuse, gynecologic or urologic disorders, endocrine abnormalities (such as diabetes mellitus or thyroid disease), neurologic problems, cardiovascular disease, psychiatric disease, and current prescription and over-the-counter medication use. A detailed history of the specific sexual dysfunction should be elicited, and a gynecologic examination should focus on findings that may contribute to sexual complaints.

▶ **Etiology**

A. Disorders of Sexual Desire

Sexual desire in women is a complex and poorly understood phenomenon. Emotion is a key factor in sexual desire. Anger toward a partner, fear or anxiety related to previous sexual encounters, or history of sexual abuse may contribute. Physical factors, such as chronic illness, fatigue, depression, and specific medical disorders (such as diabetes mellitus, thyroid disease, or adrenal insufficiency) may contribute to a lack of desire. Attitudes toward aging and menopause may play a role. In addition, sexual desire may be influenced by other sexual dysfunctions, such as arousal disorders, dyspareunia, or anorgasmia.

B. Sexual Arousal Disorders

Sexual arousal disorders may be both subjective and objective. Sexual stimulation normally leads to genital vasocongestion and lubrication. Some women may have a physiologic response to sexual stimuli but may not subjectively feel aroused because of factors such as distractions; negative expectations; anxiety; fatigue; depression; or medications, such as selective serotonin reuptake inhibitors (SSRIs) or oral contraceptives. Other women may lack both a subjective and physiologic response to sexual stimuli related to vaginal atrophy.

C. Orgasmic Disorders

In spite of subjective and physiologic arousal, women may experience a marked delay in orgasm, diminished sensation of an orgasm, or anorgasmia. The etiology is complex and typically multifactorial, but the disorder is usually amenable to treatment.

D. Sexual Pain Disorders

Dyspareunia and vaginismus are two subcategories of sexual pain disorders. **Dyspareunia** is defined as recurrent or persistent genital pain associated with sexual intercourse that is not caused exclusively by lack of lubrication or by vaginismus and causes marked distress or interpersonal difficulty. **Vaginismus** is defined as recurrent or persistent involuntary spasm of the musculature of the outer third of the vagina that interferes with sexual intercourse, resulting from fear, pain, sexual trauma, or a negative attitude toward sex, often learned in childhood, and causing marked distress or interpersonal difficulty. Other medical causes of sexual pain may include vulvovaginitis; vulvar disease, including lichen planus, lichen sclerosus, and lichen simplex chronicus; pelvic disease, such as endometriosis or chronic PID; vulvodynia; or vaginal atrophy. Vulvodynia is the most frequent cause of dyspareunia in premenopausal women. It is characterized by a sensation of burning along with other symptoms, including pain, itching, stinging, irritation, and rawness. The discomfort may be constant or intermittent, focal or diffuse, and experienced as either deep or superficial. There are generally no physical findings except minimal erythema that may be associated in a subset of patients with vulvodynia, those with vulvar vestibulitis. Vulvar vestibulitis is normally asymptomatic, but pain is associated with touching or pressure on the vestibule, such as with vaginal entry or insertion of a tampon. Pain occurring with deep thrusting during coitus is usually due to acute or chronic infection of the cervix, uterus, or adnexa; endometriosis; adnexal tumors; or adhesions resulting from prior pelvic disease or operation.

▶ **Treatment**

A. Disorders of Sexual Desire

In the absence of specific medical disorders, arousal or orgasmic disorders or dyspareunia, the focus of therapy is psychological. Cognitive behavioral therapy, sexual therapy, and couples therapy may all play a role. Success with pharmacologic therapy, particularly the use of dopamine agonists or testosterone with estrogen has been reported, but data from large long-term clinical trials are lacking.

B. Sexual Arousal Disorders

As with disorders of sexual desire, arousal disorders may respond to psychological therapy. The use of the phosphodiesterase inhibitors used in men does not appear to benefit the majority of women with sexual arousal disorders. However, there is some evidence to suggest a role for sildenafil in women with sexual dysfunction due to multiple sclerosis, type 1 diabetes mellitus, spinal cord injury, and antidepressant medications, if other, better established, approaches fail. Flibanserin (Addyi), an antidepressant, was approved by FDA in August 2015 as an effective treatment of hypoactive sexual desire disorder in premenopausal women; however, it must be used long-term to be effective and has significant risks that require specific certifications of providers and pharmacies for dispensation to patients in the United States.

C. Orgasmic Disorders

For many women, brief sexual counseling along with the use of educational books (such as *For Yourself*, by Lonnie Barbach) may be adequate therapy. Also, there is an FDA-approved vacuum device that increases clitoral blood flow and may improve the likelihood of orgasm.

D. Sexual Pain Disorders

Specific medical disorders, such as endometriosis, vulvovaginitis, or vaginal atrophy, should be treated as outlined in other sections of this chapter. Lichen planus and lichen simplex chronicus are addressed in Chapter 6. Lichen sclerosus, a thinning and whitening of the vulvar epithelium is treated with clobetasol propionate 0.05% ointment, applied twice daily for 2–3 months.

Vaginismus may be treated initially with sexual counseling and education on anatomy and sexual functioning. The patient can be instructed in self-dilation, using a lubricated finger or test tubes of graduated sizes. Before coitus (with adequate lubrication) is attempted, the patient—and then her partner—should be able to easily and painlessly introduce two fingers into the vagina. Penetration should never be forced, and the woman should always be the one to control the depth of insertion during dilation or intercourse. Injection of botulinum toxin has been used successfully in refractory cases.

Since the cause of vulvodynia is unknown, management is difficult. Few treatment approaches have been subjected to methodologically rigorous trials. A variety of topical agents have been tried, although only topical anesthetics (eg, estrogen cream and a compounded mixture of topical amitriptyline 2% and baclofen 2% in a water washable base) have been useful in relieving vulvodynia. Useful oral medications include tricyclic antidepressants, such as amitriptyline in gradually increasing doses from 10 mg/day to 75–100 mg/day; various SSRIs; and anticonvulsants, such as gabapentin, starting at 300 mg three times daily and increasing to 1200 mg three times daily. Biofeedback and physical therapy, with a physical therapist experienced with the treatment of vulvar pain, have been shown to be helpful. Surgery—usually consisting of vestibulectomy—has been useful for women with introital dyspareunia.

▶ When to Refer

- When symptoms or concerns persist despite first-line therapy.
- For expertise in surgical procedures.

American College of Obstetricians and Gynecologists. ACOG Practice Bulletin No. 119: Female sexual dysfunction. Obstet Gynecol. 2011 Apr;117(4):96–1007. [Reaffirmed 2013] [PMID: 21422879]

Buster JE. Managing female sexual dysfunction. Fertil Steril. 2013 Oct;100(4):905–15. [PMID: 24074537]

Fooladi E et al. An update on the pharmacological management of female sexual dysfunction. Expert Opin Pharmacother. 2012 Oct;13(15):2131–42. [PMID: 22984935]

Management of symptomatic vulvovaginal atrophy: 2013 position statement of The North American Menopause Society. Menopause. 2013 Sep;20(9):888–902. [PMID: 23985562]

Nappi RE et al. Advances in pharmacotherapy for treating female sexual dysfunction. Expert Opin Pharmacother. 2015 Apr;16(6):875–87. [PMID: 25732267]

Nastri CO et al. Hormone therapy for sexual function in perimenopausal and postmenopausal women. Cochrane Database Syst Rev. 2013 Jun 5;6:CD009672. [PMID: 23737033]

INFERTILITY

A couple is said to be infertile if pregnancy does not result after 1 year of normal sexual activity without contraceptives. About 25% of couples experience infertility at some point in their reproductive lives; the incidence of infertility increases with age, with a decline in fertility beginning in the early 30s and accelerating in the late 30s. **The male partner contributes to about 40% of cases of infertility**, and a combination of factors is common. The most recent data from the CDC National Survey of Family Growth noted that 6.0% of married women in the United States aged 15–44 received a diagnosis of infertility.

A. Initial Testing

During the initial interview, the clinician can present an overview of infertility and discuss a plan of study. Private consultations with each partner separately are then conducted, allowing appraisal of psychosexual adjustment without embarrassment or criticism. Pertinent details (eg, sexually transmitted disease or prior pregnancies) must be obtained. The ill effects of cigarettes, alcohol, and other recreational drugs on male fertility should be discussed. Prescription medications that impair male potency and factors that may lead to scrotal hyperthermia, such as tight underwear or frequent use of saunas or hot tubs, should be discussed. The gynecologic history should include the menstrual pattern, the use and types of contraceptives, douching, libido, sex techniques, frequency and success of coitus, and correlation of intercourse with time of ovulation. Family history includes repeated spontaneous abortions. The American Society for Reproductive Medicine provides patient information on the infertility evaluation and treatment (http://www.asrm.org/FactSheetsandBooklets/).

General physical and genital examinations are performed on the female partner. Basic laboratory studies include complete blood count, urinalysis, cervical culture for *Chlamydia,* rubella antibody determination, and thyroid function tests. If the woman has regular menses, the likelihood of ovulatory cycles is very high. A luteal phase serum progesterone above 3 ng/mL establishes ovulation. Couples should be advised that coitus resulting in conception occurs during the 6-day window around the day of ovulation. Ovulation predictor kits have in many cases replaced basal body temperatures for predicting ovulation, but temperature charting is a natural and inexpensive way to identify most fertile days. Basal body temperature charts cannot predict ovulation; they can only retrospectively confirm ovulation occurred.

A semen analysis to rule out a male factor for infertility should be completed. Men must abstain from sexual activity for at least 3 days before the semen is obtained. A clean, dry, wide-mouthed bottle for collection is preferred. Semen should be examined within 1–2 hours after collection. Semen is considered normal with the following minimum values: volume, 2.0 mL; concentration, 20 million sperm per milliliter; motility, 50% or more forward progression, 25% or more rapid progression; and normal forms, 30%. If the sperm count is abnormal, further evaluation includes physical examination of the male partner and a search for exposure to environmental and workplace toxins, alcohol or drug abuse.

B. Further Testing

1. Gross deficiencies of sperm (number, motility, or appearance) require repeat analysis. Intracytoplasmic sperm injection (ICSI) is the treatment option available for sperm deficiencies except for azoospermia (absence of sperm). ICSI requires the female partner to undergo in vitro fertilization (IVF).

2. A screening pelvic ultrasound and hysterosalpingography to identify uterine cavity or tubal anomalies should be performed. Hysterosalpingography using an oil dye is performed within 3 days following the menstrual period if structural abnormalities are suspected. This radiographic study will demonstrate uterine abnormalities (septa, polyps, submucous myomas) and tubal obstruction.

Oil-based (versus water-soluble) contrast media may improve pregnancy rates but reports of complications using oil-based media resulted in a decrease in its usage. Women who have had prior pelvic inflammation should receive doxycycline, 100 mg orally twice daily, beginning immediately before and for 7 days after the radiographic study. IVF is recommended as the primary treatment option for tubal disease, but surgery can be considered in young women with mild tubal disease.

3. Absent or infrequent ovulation requires additional laboratory evaluation. Elevated FSH and LH levels and low estradiol levels indicate ovarian insufficiency. Elevated LH levels in the presence of normal FSH levels may indicate the presence of polycystic ovaries. Elevation of blood prolactin (PRL) levels suggests a pituitary adenoma. In women over age 35, ovarian reserve should be assessed. A markedly elevated FSH (greater than 15–20 international units/L) on day 3 of the menstrual cycle suggests inadequate ovarian reserve. Although less widely used clinically, a Clomiphene Citrate Challenge Test, with measurement of FSH on day 10 after administration of clomiphene from day 5–9, can help confirm a diagnosis of diminished ovarian reserve. The number of antral follicles during the early follicular phase of the cycle can provide useful information about ovarian reserve and can confirm serum testing. Antimullerian hormone can be used as part of the assessment of ovarian reserve. Unlike FSH, it can be measured at any time during the menstrual cycle and is less likely to be affected by hormones.

4. If all the above testing is normal, **unexplained infertility** is diagnosed. In approximately 25% of women whose basic evaluation is normal, the first-line therapy is usually controlled ovarian hyperstimulation (usually clomiphene citrate) and intrauterine insemination. IVF may be recommended as second-line therapy.

► Treatment

A. Medical Measures

Fertility may be restored by treatment of endocrine abnormalities, particularly hypothyroidism or hyperthyroidism. Women who are anovulatory as a result of low body weight or exercise may become ovulatory when they gain weight or decrease their exercise levels.

B. Surgical Measures

Excision of ovarian tumors or ovarian foci of endometriosis can improve fertility. Microsurgical relief of tubal obstruction due to salpingitis or tubal ligation will reestablish fertility in a significant number of cases, although with severe disease or proximal obstruction, IVF is preferable. Peritubal adhesions or endometriotic implants often can be treated via laparoscopy.

In a male with a varicocele, sperm characteristics may be improved following surgical treatment. For men who have sperm production but obstructive azoospermia, trans-epidermal sperm aspiration or microsurgical epidermal sperm aspiration has been successful.

C. Induction of Ovulation

1. Clomiphene citrate—Clomiphene citrate stimulates gonadotropin release, especially FSH. It acts as a selective estrogen receptor modulator, similar to tamoxifen and raloxifene, and binds to the estrogen receptor. The body perceives a low level of estrogen, decreasing the negative feedback on the hypothalamus, and there is an increased release of FSH and LH. When FSH and LH are present in the appropriate amounts and timing, ovulation occurs.

After a normal menstrual period or induction of withdrawal bleeding with progestin, 50 mg of clomiphene orally daily for 5 days, typically on days 3–7 of the cycle, should be given. If ovulation does not occur, the dosage is increased to 100 mg daily for 5 days. If ovulation still does not occur, the course is repeated with 150 mg daily and then 200 mg daily for 5 days. The maximum dosage is 200 mg. Ovulation and appropriate timing of intercourse can be facilitated with the addition of chorionic gonadotropin, 10,000 units intramuscularly. Monitoring of the follicles by transvaginal ultrasound usually is necessary to appropriately time the hCG injection. The rate of ovulation following this treatment is 90% in the absence of other infertility factors. The pregnancy rate is high. Twinning occurs in 5% of these patients, and three or more fetuses are found in rare instances (less than 0.5% of cases). Pregnancy is most likely to occur within the first three ovulatory cycles, and unlikely to occur after cycle six. In addition, several studies have suggested a twofold to threefold increased risk of ovarian cancer with the use of clomiphene for more than 1 year, so treatment with clomiphene is usually limited to a maximum of six cycles.

In the presence of increased androgen production (DHEA-S greater than 200 mcg/dL), the addition of dexamethasone, 0.5 mg orally, or prednisone, 5 mg orally, at bedtime, improves the response to clomiphene in selected patients. Dexamethasone should be discontinued after pregnancy is confirmed.

2. Letrozole—The aromatase inhibitor, letrozole, appears to be at least as effective as clomiphene for ovulation induction in women with PCOS. There is a reduced risk of multiple pregnancy, a lack of antiestrogenic effects, and a reduced need for ultrasound monitoring. The dose is 5–7.5 mg daily, starting on day 3 of the menstrual cycle. In women who have a history of estrogen dependent tumors, such as breast cancer, letrozole is preferred as the estrogen levels with this medication are much lower.

3. Carbergoline or bromocriptine—Carbergoline or bromocriptine is used only if PRL levels are elevated and there is no withdrawal bleeding following progesterone administration (otherwise, clomiphene is used). The initial dosage is 2.5 mg orally once daily, increased to two or three times daily in increments of 1.25 mg. The medication is discontinued once pregnancy has occurred. Carbergoline causes fewer adverse effects than bromocriptine. However, it is much more expensive. Carbergoline is often used in patients who cannot tolerate the adverse effects of bromocriptine or in those who do not respond to bromocriptine.

4. Human menopausal gonadotropins (hMG) or recombinant FSH—hMG or recombinant FSH is indicated in cases of hypogonadotropism and most other types of anovulation resistant to clomiphene treatment. Because of the complexities, laboratory tests, and expense associated with this treatment, these patients should be referred to an infertility specialist.

D. Treatment of Endometriosis

See above.

E. Artificial Insemination in Azoospermia

If azoospermia is present, artificial insemination by a donor usually results in pregnancy, assuming female function is normal. The use of frozen sperm is the only option because it provides the opportunity for screening for sexually transmitted diseases, including HIV infection.

F. Assisted Reproductive Technologies (ART)

Couples who have not responded to traditional infertility treatments, including those with tubal disease, severe endometriosis, oligospermia, and immunologic or unexplained infertility, may benefit from IVF. Gamete intrafallopian transfer and zygote intrafallopian transfer are rarely performed, although it may be an option in a few selected patients. These techniques are complex and require a highly organized team of specialists. All of the procedures involve ovarian stimulation to produce multiple oocytes, oocyte retrieval by transvaginal sonography–guided needle aspiration, and handling of the oocytes outside the body. With IVF, the eggs are fertilized in vitro and the embryos transferred to the uterus. ICSI allows fertilization with a single sperm. While originally intended for couples with male factor infertility, it is now used in two-thirds of all IVF procedures in the United States.

The chance of a multiple gestation pregnancy (ie, twins, triplets) is increased in all assisted reproductive procedures, increasing the risk of preterm delivery and other pregnancy complications. To minimize this risk, most infertility specialists recommend only transferring one embryo in appropriately selected patients with a favorable prognosis. In women with prior failed IVF cycles who are over the age of 40 who have poor embryo quality, up to 4 embryos may be transferred. In the event of a multiple gestation pregnancy, a couple may consider selective reduction to avoid the medical issues generally related to multiple births. This issue should be discussed with the couple before embryo transfer.

Prognosis

The prognosis for conception and normal pregnancy is good if minor (even multiple) disorders can be identified and treated; it is poor if the causes of infertility are severe, untreatable, or of prolonged duration (over 3 years).

It is important to remember that **in the absence of identifiable causes of infertility, 60% of couples will achieve a pregnancy within 3 years.** Couples with unexplained infertility who do not achieve pregnancy within 3 years may be offered ovulation induction or assisted reproductive technology. Women over the age of

35 should be offered a more aggressive approach, with consideration of ART within 3–6 months of not achieving pregnancy with more conservative approaches. Also, offering appropriately timed information about adoption is considered part of a complete infertility regimen.

When to Refer

Refer to reproductive endocrinologist if ART are indicated, or surgery is required.

Beall SA et al. History and challenges surrounding ovarian stimulation in the treatment of infertility. Fertil Steril. 2012 Apr; 97(4):795–801. [PMID: 22463773]
Legro RS et al; Eunice Kennedy Shriver NICHD Reproductive Medicine Network. Letrozole or clomiphene for infertility in the polycystic ovary syndrome. N Engl J Med. 2014 Oct 9; 371(15):1463–4. [PMID: 25295506]

CONTRACEPTION

Unintended pregnancies are a worldwide problem but disproportionately impact developing countries. Studies estimate that 40% of the 213 million pregnancies that occurred in 2012 were unintended. Globally, 50% ended in abortion, 13% ended in miscarriage, and 38% resulted in an unplanned birth. **It is important for primary care providers to educate their patients about the benefits of contraception** and to provide options that are appropriate and desirable for the patient.

1. Oral Contraceptives

A. Combined Oral Contraceptives

1. Efficacy and methods of use—Combined oral contraceptives have a perfect use failure rate of 0.3% and a typical use failure rate of 8%. Their primary mode of action is suppression of ovulation. The pills can be initially started on the first day of the menstrual cycle, the first Sunday after the onset of the cycle or on any day of the cycle. If started on any day other than the first day of the cycle, a backup method should be used. If an active pill is missed at any time, and no intercourse occurred in the past 5 days, two pills should be taken immediately and a backup method should be used for 7 days. If intercourse occurred in the previous 5 days, emergency contraception should be used immediately, and the pills restarted the following day. A backup method should be used for 5 days.

2. Benefits of oral contraceptives—Noncontraceptive benefits of oral contraceptives include lighter menses, reducing the likelihood of anemia, and improvement of dysmenorrhea symptoms. Functional ovarian cysts are less likely with oral contraceptive use. The risk of ovarian and endometrial cancer is decreased. Acne is usually improved. The frequency of developing myomas is lower in patients who have taken oral contraceptives for longer than 4 years. There is also a beneficial effect on bone mass.

3. Selection of an oral contraceptive—Any of the combination oral contraceptives containing 35 mcg or less of ethinyl estradiol or 3 mg of estradiol valerate are suitable for most women. There is some variation in potency of the various progestins in the pills, but **there are essentially no clinically significant differences for most women among the progestins in the low-dose pills.** The available evidence is insufficient to determine whether triphasic oral contraceptives differ from monophasic oral contraceptives in effectiveness, bleeding patterns or discontinuation rates. **Therefore, monophasic pills are recommended as a first choice for women starting oral contraceptive use.** Women who have acne or hirsutism may benefit from treatment with desogestrel, drospirenone, or norgestimate, since they are the least androgenic. A combination regimen with 84 active and 7 inert pills that results in only four menses per year is available. There is also a combination regimen that is taken continuously with no regular menses. At the end of one years' use, 58% of the women had amenorrhea, and nearly 80% reported no bleeding requiring sanitary protection. **Studies have not shown any significant risk from long-term amenorrhea in patients taking continuous oral contraceptives.** The low-dose oral contraceptives commonly used in the United States are listed in Table 18–3.

4. Drug interactions—Several medications interact with oral contraceptives to decrease their efficacy by causing induction of microsomal enzymes in the liver, or by other mechanisms. Some commonly prescribed medications in this category are phenytoin, phenobarbital (and other barbiturates), primidone, topiramate, carbamazepine, and rifampin and St. John's Wort. Women taking these medications should use another means of contraception for maximum safety.

Antiretroviral medications, specifically ritonavir-boosted protease inhibitors, may significantly decrease the efficacy of combined oral contraceptives, and the concomitant use of oral contraceptives may increase the toxicity of these antiretroviral agents. Non-nucleoside reverse transcriptase inhibitors have smaller effects on oral contraceptive efficacy, while nucleoside reverse transcriptase inhibitors appear to have no effect.

5. Contraindications and adverse effects—Oral contraceptives have been associated with many adverse effects; they are contraindicated in some situations and should be used with caution in others (Table 18–4).

A. MYOCARDIAL INFARCTION—The risk of heart attack is higher with use of oral contraceptives, particularly with pills containing 50 mcg of estrogen or more. Cigarette smoking, obesity, hypertension, diabetes, or hypercholesterolemia increases the risk. Young nonsmoking women have minimal increased risk. Smokers over age 35 and women with other cardiovascular risk factors should use other methods of birth control.

B. THROMBOEMBOLIC DISEASE—An increased rate of venous thromboembolism is found in oral contraceptive users, especially if the dose of estrogen is 50 mcg or more. While the overall risk is very low (5–6 per 100,000 woman-years compared to 50–300 per 100,000 pregnancies), several studies have reported a twofold increased risk in women using oral contraceptives containing the progestins

gestodene (not available in the United States), drosperinone, or desogestrel compared with women using oral contraceptives with levonorgestrel and norethindrone. Women in whom thrombophlebitis develops should stop using this method, as should those at increased risk for thrombophlebitis because of surgery, fracture, serious injury, hypercoagulable condition, or immobilization. Women with a known thrombophilia should not use oral contraceptives.

C. CEREBROVASCULAR DISEASE—Overall, a small increased risk of hemorrhagic stroke and subarachnoid hemorrhage and a somewhat greater increased risk of thrombotic stroke have been found; smoking, hypertension, and age over 35 years are associated with increased risk. Women should stop using contraceptives if such warning symptoms as severe headache, blurred or lost vision, or other transient neurologic disorders develop.

D. CARCINOMA—There is no increased risk of breast cancer in women aged 35–64 who are current or former users of oral contraceptives. Women with a family history of breast cancer or women who started oral contraceptive use at a young age are not at increased risk. Combination oral contraceptives reduce the risk of endometrial carcinoma by 40% after 2 years of use and 60% after 4 or more years of use. The risk of ovarian cancer is reduced by 30% with pill use for less than 4 years, by 60% with use for 5–11 years, and by 80% after 12 or more years. Rarely, oral contraceptives have been associated with the development of benign or malignant hepatic tumors; this may lead to rupture of the liver, hemorrhage, and death. The risk increases with higher dosage, longer duration of use, and older age.

E. HYPERTENSION—Oral contraceptives may cause hypertension in some women; the risk is increased with longer duration of use and older age. Women in whom hypertension develops while using oral contraceptives should use other contraceptive methods. However, with regular blood pressure monitoring, nonsmoking women with well-controlled mild hypertension may use oral contraceptives.

F. HEADACHE—Migraine or other vascular headaches may occur or worsen with pill use. If severe or frequent headaches develop while using this method, it should be discontinued. Women with migraine headaches *with an aura* should not use oral contraceptives.

G. LACTATION—Combined oral contraceptives can impair the quantity and quality of breast milk. While it is preferable to avoid the use of combination oral contraceptives during lactation, the effects on milk quality are small and are not associated with developmental abnormalities in infants. Combination oral contraceptives should be started no earlier than 6 weeks postpartum to allow for establishment of lactation. Progestin-only pills, levonorgestrel implants, and DMPA are alternatives with no adverse effects on milk quality.

H. OTHER DISORDERS—Depression may occur or be worsened with oral contraceptive use. Fluid retention may occur. Patients who had cholestatic jaundice during pregnancy may develop it while taking birth control pills.

Table 18–3. Commonly used low-dose oral contraceptives.

Name	Progestin	Estrogen (Ethinyl Estradiol)	Cost per Month[1]
Combination			
Alesse[2,3]	0.1 mg levonorgestrel	20 mcg	$35.16
Loestrin 1/20[2]	1 mg norethindrone acetate	20 mcg	$28.66
Mircette[2]	0.15 mg desogestrel	20 mcg	$59.92
Yaz	3 mg drospirenone	20 mcg	$70.81
Loestrin 1.5/30[2]	1.5 mg norethindrone acetate	30 mcg	$25.79
Lo-Ovral[2]	0.3 mg norgestrel	30 mcg	$30.52
Levlen[2]	0.15 mg levonorgestrel	30 mcg	$30.93
Ortho-Cept[2] Desogen[2]	0.15 mg desogestrel	30 mcg	$39.34
Yasmin	3 mg drospirenone	30 mcg	$76.68
Brevicon[2] Modicon[2]	0.5 mg norethindrone	35 mcg	$32.14
Demulen 1/35[2]	1 mg ethynodiol diacetate	35 mcg	$29.88
Ortho-Novum 1/35[2]	1 mg norethindrone	35 mcg	$29.50
Ortho-Cyclen[2]	0.25 mg norgestimate	35 mcg	$32.23
Ovcon 35[2]	0.4 mg norethindrone	35 mcg	$44.84
Combination: Extended-Cycle			
Seasonale (91 day cycle)	0.15 mg levonorgestrel	30 mcg	$52.98
Seasonique (91 day cycle)	0.15 mg levonorgestrel (days 1–84)/0 mg levonorgestrel (days 85–91)	30 mcg (84 days)/10 mcg (7 days)	$112.94
LoSeasonique (91 day cycle)	0.10 mg levonorgestrel (days 1–84)/0 mg levonorgestrel (days 85–91)	20 mcg (84 days)/10 mcg (7 days)	$112.94
Amethyst (28 day pack)	90 mcg levonorgestrel	20 mcg	$59.40
Triphasic			
Estrostep	1 mg norethindrone acetate (days 1–5) 1 mg norethindrone acetate (days 6–12) 1 mg norethindrone acetate (days 13–21)	20 mcg 30 mcg 35 mcg	$57.15
Cyclessa[2]	0.1 mg desogestrel (days 1–7) 0.125 mg desogestrel (days 8–14) 0.15 mg desogestrel (days 15–21)	25 mcg	$33.33
Ortho-Tri-Cyclen Lo	0.18 norgestimate (days 1–7) 0.21 norgestimate (days 8–14) 0.25 norgestimate (days 15–21)	25 mcg	$39.32
Triphasil[2,3]	0.05 mg levonorgestrel (days 1–6) 0.075 mg levonorgestrel (days 7–11) 0.125 mg levonorgestrel (days 12–21)	30 mcg 40 mcg 30 mcg	$27.50
Ortho-Novum 7/7/7[2,3]	0.5 mg norethindrone (days 1–7) 0.75 mg norethindrone (days 8–14) 1 mg norethindrone (days 15–21)	35 mcg	$32.23
Ortho-Tri-Cyclen[2,3]	0.18 mg norgestimate (days 1–7) 0.215 mg norgestimate (days 8–14) 0.25 mg norgestimate (days 15–21)	35 mcg	$39.32
Tri-Norinyl[2,3]	0.5 mg norethindrone (days 1–7) 1 mg norethindrone (days 8–16) 0.5 mg norethindrone (days 17–21)	35 mcg	$39.35
Progestin-Only Minipill			
Ortho Micronor[2,3]	0.35 mg norethindrone to be taken continuously	None	$36.92

[1]Average wholesale price (AWP, for AB-rated generic when available) for quantity listed. Source: *Red Book Online, 2015, Truven Health Analytics, Inc.* AWP may not accurately represent the actual pharmacy cost because wide contractual variations exist among institutions.
[2]Generic equivalent available.
[3]Multiple other brands available.

Table 18–4. Contraindications to use of oral contraceptives.

Absolute contraindications
Pregnancy
Thrombophlebitis or thromboembolic disorders (past or present)
Stroke or coronary artery disease (past or present)
Cancer of the breast (known or suspected)
Undiagnosed abnormal vaginal bleeding
Estrogen-dependent cancer (known or suspected)
Benign or malignant tumor of the liver (past or present)
Uncontrolled hypertension
Diabetes mellitus with vascular disease
Age over 35 and smoking > 15 cigarettes daily
Known thrombophilia
Migraine with aura
Active hepatitis
Surgery or orthopedic injury requiring prolonged immobilization
Relative contraindications
Migraine without aura
Hypertension
Heart or kidney disease
Diabetes mellitus
Gallbladder disease
Cholestasis during pregnancy
Sickle cell disease (S/S or S/C type)
Lactation

I. OBESITY—Some studies have suggested that oral contraceptives are less effective in overweight women. In addition, obesity is a risk factor for thromboembolic complications. It is important that obese women are not denied effective contraception as a result of concerns about complications or efficacy of oral contraceptives. Alternatives, including progestin only injections, implants, or intrauterine devices, should be considered as first options instead of oral contraceptives.

6. Minor side effects—Nausea and dizziness may occur in the first few months of pill use. A weight gain of 2–5 lb (0.9–2.25 kg) commonly occurs. Spotting or breakthrough bleeding between menstrual periods may occur, especially if a pill is skipped or taken late; this may be helped by switching to a pill of slightly greater potency (see section 3, above). Missed menstrual periods may occur, especially with low-dose pills. A pregnancy test should be performed if pills have been skipped or if two or more expected menstrual periods are missed. Fatigue and decreased libido can occur. Chloasma may occur, as in pregnancy, and is increased by exposure to sunlight.

B. Progestin Minipill

1. Efficacy and methods of use—A formulation containing 0.35 mg of norethindrone is available in the United States. The efficacy is similar to that of combined oral contraceptives. The minipill is believed to prevent conception by causing thickening of the cervical mucus to make it hostile to sperm, alteration of ovum transport (which may

account for the slightly higher rate of ectopic pregnancy with these pills), and inhibition of implantation. Ovulation is inhibited inconsistently with this method. The minipill is begun on the first day of a menstrual cycle and then taken continuously for as long as contraception is desired.

2. Advantages—The low dose of progestin and absence of estrogen make the minipill safe during lactation; it may increase the flow of milk. It is often tried by women who want minimal doses of hormones and by patients who are over age 35. They lack the cardiovascular side effects of combination pills. The minipill can be safely used by women with sickle cell disease (S/S or S/C).

3. Complications and contraindications—Minipill users often have bleeding irregularities (eg, prolonged flow, spotting, or amenorrhea); such patients may need regular pregnancy tests. Ectopic pregnancies are more frequent, and complaints of abdominal pain should be investigated with this in mind. Many of the absolute contraindications and relative contraindications listed in Table 18–4 apply to the minipill; however, the contraceptive benefit of the minipill may outweigh the risks for patients who smoke, who are over age 35, or who have such conditions as superficial deep venous thrombosis or known thromboembolic disorders or diabetes with vascular disease. Minor side effects of combination oral contraceptives such as weight gain and mild headache may also occur with the minipill.

Centers for Disease Control and Prevention (CDC). Update to CDC's U.S. Medical Eligibility Criteria for Contraceptive Use, 2010: revised recommendations for the use of hormonal contraception among women at high risk for HIV infection or infected with HIV. MMWR Morb Mortal Wkly Rep. 2012 Jun 22;61(24):449–52. [PMID: 22717514]
Edelman A et al. Continuous or extended cycle vs. cyclic use of combined hormonal contraceptives for contraception. Cochrane Database Syst Rev. 2014 Jul 29;7:CD004695. [PMID: 25072731]
Jin J. JAMA patient page. Oral contraceptives. JAMA. 2014 Jan 15; 311(3):321. [PMID: 24430333]
Shaw KA et al. Obesity and oral contraceptives: a clinician's guide. Best Pract Res Clin Endocrinol Metab. 2013 Feb; 27(1):55–65. [PMID: 23384746]

2. Contraceptive Injections & Implants (Long-Acting Progestins)

The injectable progestin DMPA is approved for contraceptive use in the United States. There has been extensive worldwide experience with this method over the past 3 decades. The medication is given as a deep intramuscular injection of 150 mg every 3 months and has a contraceptive efficacy of 99.7%. A subcutaneous preparation, containing 104 mg of DMPA is available in the United States. Common side effects include irregular bleeding, amenorrhea, weight gain, and headache. It is associated with bone mineral loss that is usually reversible after discontinuation of the method. Users commonly have irregular bleeding initially and subsequently develop amenorrhea. Ovulation may be delayed after the last injection. Contraindications are similar to those for the minipill.

A single-rod, subdermal progestin implant, Nexplanon, is approved for use in the United States. Nexplanon is a 40-mm by 2-mm rod containing 68 mg of the progestin etonogestrel that is inserted in the inner aspect of the non-dominant arm and remains effective for 3 years. Hormone levels drop rapidly after removal, and there is no delay in the return of fertility. In clinical trials, the pregnancy rate was 0.0% with 3 years of use. The side effect profile is similar to minipills, and DMPA. Irregular bleeding has been the most common reason for discontinuation. Implanon, a predecessor to Nexplanon, is not marketed in the United States but is still widely used in many developing countries. A list of countries that offer Implanon may be found at http://www.implanon.md/. Both the American College of Obstetricians and Gynecologists and the American Academy of Pediatrics have recommended that adolescents should be encouraged to consider long-acting reversible contraception methods. In a large prospective study, a 75% reduction in unintended pregnancy was demonstrated with the use of long-acting reversible contraception.

Mommers E et al. Nexplanon, a radiopaque etonogestrel implant in combination with a next-generation applicator: 3-year results of a noncomparative multicenter trial. Am J Obstet Gynecol. 2012 Nov;207(5):388.e1–6. [PMID: 22939402]

Secura GM et al. Provision of no-cost, long-acting contraception and teenage pregnancy. N Engl J Med. 2014 Oct 2;371(14): 1316–23. [PMID: 25271604]

3. Other Hormonal Methods

A transdermal contraceptive patch containing 150 mcg norelgestromin and 20 mcg ethinyl estradiol and measuring 20 cm^2 is available. The patch is applied to the lower abdomen, upper torso, or buttock once a week for 3 consecutive weeks, followed by 1 week without the patch. It appears that the average steady-state concentration of ethinyl estradiol with the patch is approximately 60% higher than with a 35 mcg pill. However, there is currently no evidence for an increased incidence of estrogen-related side effects. The mechanism of action, side effects, and efficacy are similar to those associated with oral contraceptives, although compliance may be better. However, discontinuation for side effects is more frequent.

A contraceptive vaginal ring that releases 120 mcg of etonogestrel and 15 mcg of ethinyl estradiol daily is available. The ring is soft and flexible and is placed in the upper vagina for 3 weeks, removed, and replaced 1 week later. The efficacy, mechanism of action, and systemic side effects are similar to those associated with oral contraceptives. Ring users may experience an increased incidence of vaginal discharge.

Lopez LM et al. Skin patch and vaginal ring versus combined oral contraceptives for contraception. Cochrane Database Syst Rev. 2013 Apr 30;4:CD003552. [PMID: 23633314]

4. Intrauterine Devices

In the United States, the following devices are available: the **Mirena** and the **Skyla** IUDs (both of which release levonorgestrel) and the copper-bearing **TCu380A.** The mechanism of action of IUDs is thought to involve either spermicidal or inhibitory effects on sperm capacitation and transport. IUDs are not abortifacients.

Skyla is effective for 3 years, Mirena for 5 years, and the TCu380A for 10 years. The hormone-containing IUDs have the advantage of reducing cramping and menstrual flow.

The IUD is an excellent contraceptive method for most women. The devices are highly effective, with failure rates similar to those achieved with surgical sterilization. Nulliparity is not a contraindication to IUD use. Adolescents are also candidates for IUD use. Women who are not in mutually monogamous relationships should use condoms for protection from sexually transmitted diseases. Levonorgestrel-containing IUDs may have a protective effect against upper tract infection similar to that of the oral contraceptives.

A. Insertion

Insertion can be performed during or after the menses, at midcycle to prevent implantation, or later in the cycle if the patient has not become pregnant. There is growing evidence to suggest that IUDs can be safely inserted in the immediate postabortal and postpartum periods.

Both types of IUDs (levonorgestrel-releasing and copper bearing) may be inserted up to 48 hours after vaginal delivery, or prior to closure of the uterus at the time of cesarean section. Insertion immediately following abortion is acceptable if there is no sepsis and if follow-up insertion a month later will not be possible; otherwise, it is wise to wait until 4 weeks post abortion. Misoprostol (200 mcg the night before) and NSAIDs given as premedications may help insertions in nulliparous patients or when insertion is not performed during menses.

B. Contraindications & Complications

Contraindications to use of IUDs are outlined in Table 18–5.

1. Pregnancy—A copper-containing IUD can be inserted within 5 days following a single episode of unprotected mid-cycle coitus as a postcoital contraceptive. An IUD should not be inserted into a pregnant uterus. If pregnancy occurs as an IUD failure, there is a greater chance of spontaneous abortion if the IUD is left in situ (50%) than if it is removed (25%). Spontaneous abortion with an IUD in

Table 18–5. Contraindications to IUD use.

Absolute contraindications
Pregnancy
Acute or subacute pelvic inflammatory disease or purulent cervicitis
Significant anatomic abnormality of uterus
Unexplained uterine bleeding
Active liver disease (Mirena only)
Relative contraindications
History of pelvic inflammatory disease since the last pregnancy
Lack of available follow-up care
Menorrhagia or severe dysmenorrhea (copper IUD)
Cervical or uterine neoplasia

place is associated with a high risk of severe sepsis, and death can occur rapidly. Women using an IUD who become pregnant should have the IUD removed if the string is visible. It can be removed at the time of abortion if this is desired. If the string is not visible and the patient wants to continue the pregnancy, she should be informed of the serious risk of sepsis and, occasionally, death with such pregnancies. She should be informed that any flu-like symptoms such as fever, myalgia, headache, or nausea warrant immediate medical attention for possible septic abortion.

Since the ratio of ectopic to intrauterine pregnancies is increased among IUD wearers, clinicians should search for adnexal masses in early pregnancy and should always check the products of conception for placental tissue following abortion.

2. Pelvic infection—There is an increased risk of pelvic infection during the first month following insertion; however, prophylactic antibiotics given at the time of insertion do not appear to decrease this risk. The subsequent risk of pelvic infection appears to be primarily related to the risk of acquiring sexually transmitted infections. Infertility rates do not appear to be increased among women who have previously used the currently available IUDs. At the time of insertion, women with an increased risk of sexually transmitted diseases should be screened for gonorrhea and *Chlamydia*. Women with a history of recent or recurrent pelvic infection are not good candidates for IUD use.

3. Menorrhagia or severe dysmenorrhea—The copper IUD can cause heavier menstrual periods, bleeding between periods, and more cramping, so it is generally not suitable for women who already suffer from these problems. Alternatively, the hormone-releasing IUD Mirena has been approved by the FDA to treat heavy menstrual bleeding. NSAIDs are also helpful in decreasing bleeding and pain in IUD users.

4. Complete or partial expulsion—Spontaneous expulsion of the IUD occurs in 10–20% of cases during the first year of use. Any IUD should be removed if the body of the device can be seen or felt in the cervical os.

5. Missing IUD strings—If the transcervical tail cannot be seen, this may signify unnoticed expulsion, perforation of the uterus with abdominal migration of the IUD, or simply retraction of the string into the cervical canal or uterus owing to movement of the IUD or uterine growth with pregnancy. Once pregnancy is ruled out, a cervical speculum may be used to visualize the IUD string in the cervical canal. If not visualized, one should probe for the IUD with a sterile sound or forceps designed for IUD removal after administering a paracervical block. If the IUD cannot be detected, pelvic ultrasound will demonstrate the IUD if it is in the uterus. Alternatively, obtain anteroposterior and lateral radiographs of the pelvis with another IUD or a sound in the uterus as a marker to confirm an extrauterine IUD. If the IUD is in the abdominal cavity, it should generally be removed by laparoscopy or laparotomy. Perforations of the uterus are less likely if insertion is performed slowly, with meticulous care taken to follow directions applicable to each type of IUD.

Lopez LM et al. Immediate postpartum insertion of intrauterine device for contraception. Cochrane Database Syst Rev. 2015 Jun 26;6:CD003036. [PMID: 26115018]
Okusanya BO et al. Immediate postabortal insertion of intrauterine devices. Cochrane Database Syst Rev. 2014 Jul 28; 7:CD001777. [PMID: 25101364]

5. Diaphragm & Cervical Cap

The diaphragm (with contraceptive jelly) is a safe and effective contraceptive method with features that make it acceptable to some women and not others. Failure rates range from 6% to 16%, depending on the motivation of the woman and the care with which the diaphragm is used. The advantages of this method are that it has no systemic side effects and gives significant protection against pelvic infection and cervical dysplasia as well as pregnancy. The disadvantages are that it must be inserted near the time of coitus and that pressure from the rim predisposes some women to cystitis after intercourse.

The cervical cap (with contraceptive jelly) is similar to the diaphragm but fits snugly over the cervix only (the diaphragm stretches from behind the cervix to behind the pubic symphysis). The cervical cap is more difficult to insert and remove than the diaphragm. The main advantages are that it can be used by women who cannot be fitted for a diaphragm because of a relaxed anterior vaginal wall or by women who have discomfort or develop repeated bladder infections with the diaphragm. However, failure rates are 9% (perfect use) and 16% (typical use) in nulliparous women and 26% (perfect use) and 32% (typical use) in parous women.

Because of the small risk of toxic shock syndrome, a cervical cap or diaphragm should not be left in the vagina for over 12–18 hours, nor should these devices be used during the menstrual period.

6. Contraceptive Foam, Cream, Film, Sponge, Jelly, & Suppository

These products are available without prescription, are easy to use, and are fairly effective, with typical failure rates of 10–22%. All contain the spermicide nonoxynol-9, which also has some virucidal and bactericidal activity. Nonoxynol-9 does not appear to adversely affect the vaginal colonization of hydrogen peroxide-producing lactobacilli. The FDA requires products containing nonoxynol-9 to include a warning that the products do not protect against HIV or other sexually transmitted diseases and that use of these products can irritate the vagina and rectum and may increase the risk of getting the AIDS virus from an infected partner. Low-risk women using a nonoxynol-9 product, with coital activity two to three times per week, are not at increased risk for epithelial disruption, compared with couples using condoms alone.

7. Condom

The male condom of latex or animal membrane affords good protection against pregnancy—equivalent to that of a diaphragm and spermicidal jelly; latex (but not animal membrane) condoms also offer protection against many sexually transmitted diseases, including HIV. When a spermicide, such as vaginal foam, is used with the condom, the failure rate (approximately 2% with perfect use and 15% with typical use) approaches that of oral contraceptives. The disadvantages of condoms are dulling of sensation and spillage of semen due to tearing, slipping, or leakage with detumescence of the penis.

Two female condoms, one made of polyurethane and the other of synthetic nitrile, are available in the United States. The reported failure rates range from 5% to 21%; the efficacy is comparable to that of the diaphragm. These are the only female-controlled method that offers significant protection from both pregnancy and sexually transmitted diseases.

8. Contraception Based on Awareness of Fertile Periods

These methods are most effective when the couple restricts intercourse to the post-ovular phase of the cycle or uses a barrier method at other times. Well-instructed, motivated couples may be able to achieve low pregnancy rates with fertility awareness methods. However, properly done randomized clinical trials comparing the efficacy of most of these methods with other contraceptive methods do not exist.

9. Emergency Contraception

If unprotected intercourse occurs in midcycle and if the woman is certain she has not inadvertently become pregnant earlier in the cycle, the following regimens are effective in preventing implantation. These methods should be started as soon as possible and **within 120 hours after unprotected coitus.** (1) Levonorgestrel, 1.5 mg orally as a single dose (available in the United States prepackaged as Plan B and available over-the-counter for women aged 17 years and older), has a 1% failure rate when taken within 72 hours. It remains efficacious up to 120 hours after intercourse, though less so compared with earlier use. (2) If the levonorgestrel regimen is not available, a combination oral contraceptive containing ethinyl estradiol and levonorgestrel given twice in 12 hours may be used. At least 20 brands of pills may be used in this way. For specific dosages and instructions for each pill brand, consult www.not-2-late.com. Used within 72 hours, the failure rate of these regimens is approximately 3%, but antinausea medication is often necessary. (3) Ulipristal, 30 mg orally as a single dose, has been shown to be more effective than levonorgestrel, particularly when used between 72 and 120 hours, particularly among overweight women. It is available by prescription in the United States and Western Europe. (4) IUD insertion within 5 days after one episode of unprotected midcycle coitus will also prevent pregnancy; copper-bearing IUDs have been tested and used for many years for this purpose. All victims of sexual assault should be offered emergency contraception.

Information on clinics or individual clinicians providing emergency contraception in the United States may be obtained by calling 1-888-668-2528.

Brache V et al. Ulipristal acetate prevents ovulation more effectively than levonorgestrel: analysis of pooled data from three randomized trials of emergency contraception regimens. Contraception. 2013 Nov;88(5):611–8. [PMID: 23809278]
Cleland K et al. The efficacy of intrauterine devices for emergency contraception: a systematic review of 35 years of experience. Hum Reprod. 2012 Jul;27(7):1994–2000. [PMID: 22570193]

10. Abortion

Since the legalization of abortion in the United States in 1973, the related maternal mortality rate has fallen markedly, because illegal and self-induced abortions have been replaced by safer medical procedures. Abortions in the first trimester of pregnancy are performed by vacuum aspiration under local anesthesia or with medical regimens. Dilation and evacuation, a variation of vacuum aspiration is generally used in the second trimester. Techniques utilizing intra-amniotic instillation of hypertonic saline solution or various prostaglandins regimens, along with medical or osmotic dilators are occasionally used after 18 weeks. Several medical abortion regimens utilizing mifepristone and multiple doses of misoprostol have been reported as being effective in the second trimester. Overall, legal abortion in the United States has a mortality rate of less than 1:100,000. Rates of morbidity and mortality rise with length of gestation. In the United States, more than 60% of abortions are performed before 9 weeks, and more than 90% are performed before 13 weeks' gestation; only 1.2% are performed after 20 weeks. **If abortion is chosen, every effort should be made to encourage the patient to seek an early procedure.** In the United States, while numerous state laws limiting access to abortion and a federal law banning a rarely used variation of dilation and evacuation have been enacted, abortion remains legal and available until fetal viability, between 24 and 28 weeks gestation, under Roe v. Wade.

Complications resulting from abortion include retained products of conception (often associated with infection and heavy bleeding) and unrecognized ectopic pregnancy. Immediate analysis of the removed tissue for placenta can exclude or corroborate the diagnosis of ectopic pregnancy. Women who have fever, bleeding, or abdominal pain after abortion should be examined; use of broad-spectrum antibiotics and reaspiration of the uterus are frequently necessary. Hospitalization is advisable if acute salpingitis requires intravenous administration of antibiotics. Complications following illegal abortion often need emergency care for hemorrhage, septic shock, or uterine perforation.

Rh immune globulin should be given to all Rh-negative women following abortion. Contraception should be thoroughly discussed and contraceptive supplies or pills provided at the time of abortion. There is growing evidence to support the safety and efficacy of immediate postabortal insertion of IUDs. Prophylactic antibiotics are indicated for surgical abortion; for example a one-dose regimen of doxycycline, 200 mg orally 1 hour before the procedure. Many clinics prescribe tetracycline, 500 mg orally four times daily for 5 days after the procedure, as presumptive treatment for *Chlamydia*.

Mifepristone (RU 486) is approved by the FDA as an oral abortifacient at a dose of 600 mg on day 1, followed by 400 mcg orally of misoprostol on day 3. This combination is 95% successful in terminating pregnancies of up to 9 weeks' duration with minimum complications. A more commonly used, evidence-based regimen is mifepristone, 200 mg orally on day 1, followed by misoprostol, 800 mcg vaginally either immediately or within 6–8 hours. Although not approved by the FDA for this indication, a combination of intramuscular methotrexate, 50 mg/m² of body surface area, followed 3–7 days later by vaginal misoprostol, 800 mcg, is 98% successful in terminating pregnancy at 8 weeks or less. Minor side effects, such as nausea, vomiting, and diarrhea, are common with these regimens. There is a 5–10% incidence of hemorrhage or incomplete abortion requiring curettage. **Medical abortion is generally considered as safe as surgical abortion in the first trimester but is associated with more pain and a lower success rate** (requiring surgical abortion). Overall, the risk of uterine infection is lower with medical than with surgical abortion.

Grimes DA et al. Immediate postabortal insertion of intrauterine devices. Cochrane Database Syst Rev. 2010 Jun 16;(6): CD001777. Update in: Cochrane Database Syst Rev. 2014; 7:CD001777. [PMID: 20556754]
Guiahi M et al. First-trimester abortion in women with medical conditions: release date October 2012 SFP guideline #20122. Contraception. 2012 Dec;86(6):622–30. [PMID: 23039921]

11. Sterilization

In the United States, sterilization is the most popular method of birth control for couples who want no more children. Although sterilization is reversible in some instances, reversal surgery in both men and women is costly, complicated, and not always successful. Therefore, patients should be counseled carefully before sterilization and should view the procedure as permanent.

Vasectomy is a safe, simple procedure in which the vas deferens is severed and sealed through a scrotal incision under local anesthesia. Long-term follow-up studies on vasectomized men show no excess risk of cardiovascular disease. Several studies have shown a possible association with prostate cancer, but the evidence is weak and inconsistent.

Female sterilization procedures include laparoscopic bipolar electrocoagulation, or plastic ring application on the uterine tubes, or minilaparotomy with Pomeroy tubal resection. The advantages of laparoscopy are minimal postoperative pain, small incisions, and rapid recovery. The advantages of minilaparotomy are that it can be performed with standard surgical instruments under local or general anesthesia. However, there is more postoperative pain and a longer recovery period. The cumulative 10-year failure rate for all methods combined is 1.85%, varying from 0.75% for postpartum partial salpingectomy and laparoscopic unipolar coagulation to 3.65% for spring clips; this fact should be discussed with women preoperatively. Some studies have found an increased risk of menstrual irregularities as a long-term complication of tubal

ligation, but findings in different studies have been inconsistent. Two methods of transcervical sterilization, Essure and Adiana, can be performed as outpatient procedures. Essure involves the placement of an expanding microcoil of titanium into the proximal uterine tube under hysteroscopic guidance. The efficacy rate at 1 year is 99.8%. Adiana involves hysteroscopically guided superficial radiofrequency damage to the tubal lumen and immediate placement of a nonabsorbable silicone elastomer matrix in the tube to allow tissue in-growth. The efficacy rate at 1 year is 98.9%. Both procedures should have tubal occlusion confirmed at 3 months with a hysterosalpingogram.

▶ When to Refer

Refer to experienced clinicians for Implanon or Nexplanon or other subcutaneous insertion, IUD insertion, tubal occlusion or ligation, vasectomy, or therapeutic abortion.

Dhruva SS et al. Revisiting Essure—toward safe and effective sterilization. N Engl J Med. 2015 Oct 8;373(15):e17. [PMID: 26397951]
Division of Reproductive Health, National Center for Chronic Disease Prevention and Health Promotion, Centers for Disease Control and Prevention (CDC). U.S. Selected Practice Recommendations for Contraceptive Use, 2013: adapted from the World Health Organization selected practice recommendations for contraceptive use, 2nd edition. MMWR Recomm Rep. 2013 Jun 21;62(RR-05):1–60. [PMID: 23784109]

SEXUAL VIOLENCE

ESSENTIALS OF DIAGNOSIS

▶ The legal definition of rape varies by state and geographic location. The term "sexual violence" is used by the CDC and will be used in this discussion. It can be committed by a stranger, but more commonly by an assailant known to the victim, including a current or former partner or spouse (a form of intimate partner violence [IPV]).

▶ All victims of sexual violence should be offered emergency contraception, and counseled that this method does not induce abortion.

▶ The large number of individuals affected, the enormous health care costs, and the need for a multidisciplinary approach make rape and IPV important health care issues.

▶ Knowledge of state laws and collection of evidence requirements are essential for clinicians evaluating possible victims of sexual violence, including IPV.

▶ General Considerations

Rape, or sexual assault, is legally defined in different ways in various jurisdictions. Clinicians and emergency department personnel who deal with victims of sexual violence should be familiar with the laws pertaining to sexual assault in their own state. From a medical and psychological viewpoint, **it is essential that persons treating victims of sexual violence recognize the nonconsensual and violent nature of the crime**. About 95% of reported victims of sexual violence are women. Each year in the United States, 4.8 million incidents of physical or sexual assault are reported by women. Penetration may be vaginal, anal, or oral and may be by the penis, hand, or a foreign object. The absence of genital injury does not imply consent by the victim. The assailant may be unknown to the victim or, more frequently, may be an acquaintance or even the spouse.

"Unlawful sexual intercourse," or statutory rape, is intercourse with a female before the age of majority even with her consent.

Health care providers can have a significant impact in increasing the reporting of sexual assault and in identifying resources for the victims. The International Rescue Committee has developed a multimedia training tool to encourage competent, compassionate, and confidential clinical care for sexual assault survivors in low-resource settings. They studied this intervention in over a 100 healthcare providers, and found knowledge and confidence in clinical care for sexual assault survivors increased from 49% to 62% ($P < 0.001$) and 58% to 73% ($P < 0.001$), respectively following training. There was also a documented increase in eligible survivors receiving emergency contraception from 50% to 82% ($P < 0.01$), HIV postexposure prophylaxis from 42% to 92% ($P < 0.001$), and sexually transmitted infection prophylaxis and treatment from 45% to 96% ($P < 0.01$). This training will encourage providers to offer care in the areas of pregnancy and sexually transmitted infection prevention as well as assistance for psychological trauma.

Because sexual violence is a personal crisis, each patient will react differently, but anxiety disorders and posttraumatic stress disorder (PTSD) are common sequelae. The rape trauma syndrome comprises two principal phases. (1) Immediate or acute: Shaking, sobbing, and restless activity may last from a few days to a few weeks. The patient may experience anger, guilt, or shame or may repress these emotions. Reactions vary depending on the victim's personality and the circumstances of the attack. (2) Late or chronic: Problems related to the attack may develop weeks or months later. The lifestyle and work patterns of the individual may change. Sleep disorders or phobias often develop. Loss of self-esteem can lead to suicide albeit rarely.

Clinicians and emergency department personnel who deal with victims of sexual violence should work with community rape crisis centers or other sources of ongoing psychological support and counseling.

▶ General Office Procedures

The clinician who first sees the alleged victim of sexual violence should be empathetic and prepared with appropriate evidence collection and treatment materials. Standardized information and training, such as the program created by the International Rescue Committee, can be a helpful resource to the providers caring for these patients.

Many emergency departments have a protocol for sexual assault victims and personnel who are trained in interviewing and examining victims of sexual violence.

1. Secure written consent from the patient, guardian, or next of kin for gynecologic examination and for photographs if they are likely to be useful as evidence. Although there are differences in state requirements, most states require health care providers to report sexual assault and physical abuse.

2. Obtain and record the history in the patient's own words. The sequence of events, ie, the time, place, and circumstances, must be included. Note the date of the LMP, whether or not the woman is pregnant, and the time of the most recent coitus prior to the sexual assault. Note the details of the assault such as body cavities penetrated, use of foreign objects, and number of assailants. Note whether the victim is calm, agitated, or confused (drugs or alcohol may be involved). Record whether the patient came directly to the hospital or whether she bathed or changed her clothing. Record findings but do not issue even a tentative diagnosis lest it be erroneous or incomplete.

3. Have the patient disrobe while standing on a white sheet. Hair, dirt, leaves, underclothing, and any torn or stained clothing should be kept as evidence. Scrape material from beneath fingernails and comb pubic hair for evidence. Place all evidence in separate clean paper bags or envelopes and label carefully.

4. Examine the patient, noting any traumatized areas that should be photographed. Examine the body and genitals with a Wood light to identify semen, which fluoresces; positive areas should be swabbed with a premoistened swab and air-dried in order to identify acid phosphatase. Colposcopy can be used to identify small areas of trauma from forced entry especially at the posterior fourchette.

5. Perform a pelvic examination, explaining all procedures and obtaining the patient's consent before proceeding gently with the examination. Use a narrow speculum lubricated with water only. Collect material with sterile cotton swabs from the vaginal walls and cervix and make two air-dried smears on clean glass slides. Wet and dry swabs of vaginal secretions should be collected and refrigerated for subsequent acid phosphatase and DNA evaluation. Swab the mouth (around molars and cheeks) and anus in the same way, if appropriate. Label all slides carefully. Collect secretions from the vagina, anus, or mouth with a premoistened cotton swab, place at once on a slide with a drop of saline, and cover with a coverslip. Look for motile or nonmotile sperm under high, dry magnification, and record the percentage of motile forms.

6. Perform appropriate laboratory tests as follows. Culture the vagina, anus, or mouth (as appropriate) for *N gonorrhoeae* and *Chlamydia*. Perform a Papanicolaou smear of the cervix, a wet mount for *T vaginalis*, a baseline pregnancy test, and VDRL test. A confidential test for HIV viral load or antibody can be obtained if desired by the patient. Antibody testing can be repeated in

2–4 months if initially negative. Repeat the pregnancy test if the next menses is missed, and repeat the VDRL test in 6 weeks. Obtain blood (10 mL without anticoagulant) and urine (100 mL) specimens if there is a history of forced ingestion or injection of drugs or alcohol.

7. Transfer clearly labeled evidence, eg, laboratory specimens, directly to the clinical pathologist in charge or to the responsible laboratory technician, in the presence of witnesses (never via messenger), so that the rules of evidence will not be breached.

▶ Treatment

Give analgesics or sedatives if indicated. Administer tetanus toxoid if deep lacerations contain soil or dirt particles.

Give ceftriaxone, 125 mg intramuscularly, to prevent gonorrhea. In addition, give metronidazole, 2 g as a single dose, and azithromycin 1 g orally or doxycycline, 100 mg orally twice daily for 7 days to treat chlamydial infection. Incubating syphilis will probably be prevented by these medications, but the VDRL test should be repeated 6 weeks after the assault.

Prevent pregnancy by using one of the methods discussed under Emergency Contraception.

Vaccinate against hepatitis B. Consider HIV prophylaxis (see Chapter 31).

Because women who are sexually assaulted are at increased risk for long-term psychological sequelae, such as PTSD and anxiety disorders, it is critical that the patient and her family and friends have a source of ongoing counseling and psychological support.

▶ When to Refer

All women who seek care for sexual assault should be referred to a facility that has expertise in the management of victims of sexual assault and is capable of performing expert forensic examination, if requested.

Newton M. The forensic aspects of sexual violence. Best Pract Res Clin Obstet Gynaecol. 2013 Feb;27(1):77–90. [PMID: 23062592]
Smith JR et al. Clinical care for sexual assault survivors multimedia training: a mixed-methods study of effect on healthcare providers' attitudes, knowledge, confidence, and practice in humanitarian settings. Confl Health. 2013 Jul 3;7(1):14. [PMID: 23819561]

MENOPAUSAL SYNDROME

ESSENTIALS OF DIAGNOSIS

- ▶ Menopause is a retrospective diagnosis after 12 months of amenorrhea.

- ▶ Approximately 80% of women will experience hot flushes and night sweats.

- ▶ Elevated follicle-stimulating hormone (FSH) and low estradiol can help confirm the diagnosis.

▶ General Considerations

The term "menopause" denotes the final cessation of menstruation, either as a normal part of aging or as the result of surgical removal of both ovaries. In a broader sense, as the term is commonly used, it denotes a 1- to 3-year period during which a woman adjusts to a diminishing and then absent menstrual flow and the physiologic changes that may be associated with lowered estrogen levels—hot flushes, night sweats, and vaginal dryness.

The average age at menopause in Western societies today is 51 years. Premature menopause is defined as ovarian failure and menstrual cessation before age 40; this often has a genetic or autoimmune basis. Surgical menopause due to bilateral oophorectomy is common and can cause more severe symptoms owing to the sudden rapid drop in sex hormone levels.

There is no objective evidence that cessation of ovarian function is associated with severe emotional disturbance or personality changes. However, mood changes toward depression and anxiety can occur at this time. Disruption of sleep patterns associated with the menopause can affect mood and concentration and cause fatigue. Furthermore, the time of menopause often coincides with other major life changes, such as departure of children from the home, a midlife identity crisis, or divorce.

▶ Clinical Findings

A. Symptoms and Signs

1. Cessation of menstruation—Menstrual cycles generally become irregular as menopause approaches. Anovular cycles occur more often, with irregular cycle length and occasional menorrhagia. Menstrual flow usually diminishes in amount owing to decreased estrogen secretion, resulting in less abundant endometrial growth. Finally, cycles become longer, with missed periods or episodes of spotting only. When no bleeding has occurred for 1 year, the menopausal transition can be said to have occurred. **Any bleeding after 6 months of the cessation of menses warrants investigation by endometrial curettage or aspiration to rule out endometrial cancer.**

2. Hot flushes—Hot flushes (feelings of intense heat over the trunk and face, with flushing of the skin and sweating) occur in over 80% of women as a result of the decrease in ovarian hormones. Hot flushes can begin before the cessation of menses. Menopausal vasomotor symptoms last longer than previously thought, and there are ethnic differences in the duration of symptoms. Vasomotor symptoms were found to last more than 7 years in more than 50% of the women. African American women reported the longest duration of vasomotor symptoms. The etiology of hot flushes is unknown. Occurring at night, they often cause sweating and insomnia and result in fatigue on the following day.

3. Vaginal atrophy—With decreased estrogen secretion, thinning of the vaginal mucosa and decreased vaginal lubrication occur and may lead to dyspareunia. The introitus decreases in diameter. Pelvic examination reveals pale, smooth vaginal mucosa and a small cervix and uterus. The ovaries are not normally palpable after the menopause. Continued sexual activity will help prevent vaginal atrophy.

4. Osteoporosis—Osteoporosis may occur as a late sequela of menopause. The US Preventive Services Task Force recommends screening for osteoporosis at age 65. A complete summary can be found at http://www.uspreventiveservicestaskforce.org/uspstf/uspsoste.htm.

B. Laboratory Findings

Serum FSH, LH, and estradiol levels are of little diagnostic value because of unpredictable variability during the menopausal transition but can provide confirmation if the FSH is elevated and the estradiol is low. Vaginal cytologic examination will show a low estrogen effect with predominantly parabasal cells, indicating lack of epithelial maturation due to hypoestrogenism.

▶ Treatment

A. Natural Menopause

Education and support from health providers, midlife discussion groups, and reading material will help most women having difficulty adjusting to the menopause. Physiologic symptoms can be treated as follows.

1. Vasomotor symptoms—For women with moderate to severe vasomotor symptoms, estrogen or estrogen/progestin regimens are the most effective approach to symptom relief. Conjugated estrogens, 0.3 mg, 0.45 mg, or 0.625 mg; 17-beta-estradiol, 0.5 or 1 mg; or estrone sulfate, 0.625 mg can be given once daily orally; or estradiol can be given transdermally as skin patches that are changed once or twice weekly and secrete 0.05–0.1 mg of hormone daily. Unless the patient has undergone hysterectomy, a combination regimen of an estrogen with a progestin such as medroxyprogesterone, 1.5 or 2.5 mg, or norethindrone, 0.1, 0.25, or 0.5 mg, should be used to prevent endometrial hyperplasia or cancer. There is also a patch available containing estradiol and the progestin levonorgestrel. The oral hormones can be given in several differing regimens. Give estrogen on days 1–25 of each calendar month, with 5–10 mg of oral medroxyprogesterone acetate added on days 14–25. Withhold hormones from day 26 until the end of the month, when the endometrium will be shed, producing a light, generally painless monthly period. Alternatively, give the estrogen along with a progestin daily, without stopping. This regimen causes some initial bleeding or spotting, but within a few months it produces an atrophic endometrium that will not bleed. If the patient has had a hysterectomy, a progestin need not be used.

Postmenopausal women generally should not use combination progestin-estrogen therapy for more than 3 or 4 years (see discussion below). Women who cannot find relief with alternative approaches may wish to consider continuing use of combination therapy after a thorough discussion of the risks and benefits. Alternatives to hormone therapy for vasomotor symptoms include SSRIs such

as paroxetine, 12.5 mg or 25 mg/day orally, or venlafaxine, 75 mg/day orally. Gabapentin, an antiseizure medication, is also effective at 900 mg/day orally. Clonidine given orally or transdermally, 100–150 mcg daily, may also reduce the frequency of hot flushes, but its use is limited by side effects, including dry mouth, drowsiness, and hypotension. There is some evidence that soy isoflavones may be effective in treating menopausal symptoms. Other compounds including red clover and black cohosh have not been shown to be effective. Because little is known about adverse effects, particularly with long-term use, dietary supplements should be used with caution.

2. Vaginal atrophy—A vaginal ring containing 2 mg of estradiol can be left in place for 3 months and is suitable for long-term use. Short-term use of estrogen vaginal cream will relieve symptoms of atrophy, but because of variable absorption, therapy with either the vaginal ring or systemic hormone replacement is preferable. A low-dose estradiol tablet (10 mcg) is available and is inserted in the vagina daily for 2 weeks and then twice a week for long-term use. Testosterone propionate 1–2%, 0.5–1 g, in a vanishing cream base used in the same manner is also effective if estrogen is contraindicated. A bland lubricant such as unscented cold cream or water-soluble gel can be helpful at the time of coitus. Although serum estrogen level increases associated with vaginal rings are lower than other routes of administration, it is recommended that the ring be used with caution.

3. Osteoporosis—(See also discussion in Chapter 26.) Women should ingest at least 800 mg of calcium daily throughout life. Nonfat or low-fat milk products, calcium-fortified orange juice, green leafy vegetables, corn tortillas, and canned sardines or salmon consumed with the bones are good dietary sources. Vitamin D, at least 800 international units/day from food, sunlight, or supplements, is necessary to enhance calcium absorption and maintain bone mass. A daily program of energetic walking and exercise to strengthen the arms and upper body helps maintain bone mass. Screening bone densitometry is recommended for women beginning at age 65 (see Chapter 1). Women most at risk for osteoporotic fractures should consider bisphosphonates, raloxifene, or hormone replacement therapy. This includes white and Asian women, especially if they have a family history of osteoporosis, are thin, short, cigarette smokers, have a history of hyperthyroidism, use corticosteroid medications long-term, or are physically inactive.

B. Risks of Hormone Therapy

Double-blind, randomized, controlled trials have shown no overall cardiovascular benefit with estrogen-progestin replacement therapy in a group of postmenopausal women with or without established coronary disease. Both in the Women's Health Initiative (WHI) trial and the Heart and Estrogen/Progestin Replacement Study (HERS), the overall health risks (increased risk of coronary heart events; strokes; thromboembolic disease; gallstones; and breast cancer, including an increased risk of mortality from breast cancer) exceeded the benefits from the long-term use of combination estrogen and progesterone. An ancillary study of the WHI study showed that not only did estrogen-progestin hormone replacement therapy not benefit cognitive function but there was a small increased risk of cognitive decline in that group compared with women in the placebo group. The unopposed estrogen arm of the WHI trial demonstrated a decrease in the risk of hip fracture, a small but not significant decrease in breast cancer, but an increased risk of stroke and no evidence of protection from coronary heart disease. The study also showed a small increase in the combined risk of mild cognitive impairment and dementia with estrogen use compared with placebo, similar to the estrogen-progestin arm. **Women who have been receiving long-term estrogen-progestin hormone replacement therapy, even in the absence of complications, should be encouraged to stop, especially if they do not have menopausal symptoms.** However, the risks appear to be lower in women starting therapy at the time of menopause and higher in previously untreated women starting therapy long after menopause. Therapy should be individualized as the risk-benefit profile varies with age and individual risk factors. (See also discussions of estrogen and progestin replacement therapy in Chapter 26.)

C. Surgical Menopause

The abrupt hormonal decrease resulting from oophorectomy generally results in severe vasomotor symptoms and rapid onset of dyspareunia and osteoporosis unless treated. If not contraindicated, estrogen replacement is generally started immediately after surgery. Conjugated estrogens 1.25 mg orally, estrone sulfate 1.25 mg orally, or estradiol 2 mg orally is given for 25 days of each month. After age 45–50 years, this dose can be tapered to 0.625 mg of conjugated estrogens or equivalent.

Avis NE et al; Study of Women's Health Across the Nation. Duration of menopausal vasomotor symptoms over the menopause transition. JAMA Intern Med. 2015 Apr;175(4):531–9. [PMID: 25686030]

Hodis HN et al. The timing hypothesis for coronary heart disease prevention with hormone therapy: past, present and future in perspective. Climacteric. 2012 Jun;15(3):217–28. [PMID: 22612607]

LeFevre ML. Screening for vitamin D deficiency in adults: U.S. Preventive Services Task Force Recommendation Statement. Ann Intern Med. 2015 Jan 20;162(2):133–40. [PMID: 25419853]

Wills S et al. Effects of vaginal estrogens on serum estradiol levels in postmenopausal breast cancer survivors and women at risk of breast cancer taking an aromatase inhibitor or a selective estrogen receptor modulator. J Oncol Pract. 2012 May;8(3):144–8. [PMID: 22942807]

Obstetrics & Obstetric Disorders

Vanessa L. Rogers, MD

Kevin C. Worley, MD

DIAGNOSIS OF PREGNANCY

It is advantageous to diagnose pregnancy as promptly as possible when a sexually active woman misses a menstrual period or has symptoms suggestive of pregnancy. In the event of a desired pregnancy, prenatal care can begin early, and potentially harmful medications and activities such as drug and alcohol use, smoking, and occupational chemical exposure can be halted. In the event of an unwanted pregnancy, counseling about adoption or termination of the pregnancy can be provided at an early stage.

▶ Pregnancy Tests

All urine or blood pregnancy tests rely on the detection of human chorionic gonadotropin (hCG) produced by the placenta. Levels increase shortly after implantation, approximately double every 48 hours (this rise can range from 30% to 100% in normal pregnancies), reach a peak at 50–75 days, and fall to lower levels in the second and third trimesters. Pregnancy tests are performed on serum or urine and are accurate at the time of the missed period or shortly after it.

Compared with intrauterine pregnancies, **ectopic pregnancies** may show lower levels of hCG that plateau or fall in serial determinations. Quantitative assays of hCG repeated at 48-hour intervals are used in the diagnosis of ectopic pregnancy as well as in cases of molar pregnancy, threatened abortion, and missed abortion. Comparison of hCG levels between laboratories may be misleading in a given patient because different international standards may produce results that vary by as much as twofold. hCG levels can also be problematic because they require a series of measurements. Progesterone levels, however, remain relatively stable in the first trimester. A single measurement of progesterone is the best indicator of whether a pregnancy is viable, although there is a broad indeterminate zone. A value less than 5 ng/mL (16 nmol/L) predicts pregnancy failure while a value greater than 25 ng/mL (80 nmoL/L) indicates a pregnancy will be successful. There is uncertainty when the value is between these two points. Combining several serum biomarkers (beta hCG and progesterone) may provide a better prediction of pregnancy viability. **Pregnancy of unknown location** is a term used to describe a situation where a woman has a positive pregnancy test but the location and viability of the pregnancy is not known because it is not seen on transvaginal ultrasound.

Senapati S et al. Biomarkers for ectopic pregnancy and pregnancy of unknown location. Fertil Steril. 2013 Mar 15;99(4): 1107–16. [PMID: 23290746]

▶ Manifestations of Pregnancy

The following symptoms and signs are usually due to pregnancy, but none are diagnostic. A record of the time and frequency of coitus is helpful for diagnosing and dating a pregnancy.

A. Symptoms

Amenorrhea, nausea and vomiting, breast tenderness and tingling, urinary frequency and urgency, "quickening" (perception of first movement noted at about the 18th week), weight gain.

B. Signs (in Weeks from Last Menstrual Period)

Breast changes (enlargement, vascular engorgement, colostrum) start to occur very early in pregnancy and continue until the postpartum period. Cyanosis of the vagina and cervical portio and softening of the cervix occur in about the seventh week. Softening of the cervicouterine junction takes place in the eighth week, and generalized enlargement and diffuse softening of the corpus occurs after the eighth week. When a woman's abdomen will start to enlarge depends on her body habitus but typically starts in the sixteenth week.

The uterine fundus is palpable above the pubic symphysis by 12–15 weeks from the last menstrual period and reaches the umbilicus by 20–22 weeks. Fetal heart tones can be heard by Doppler at 10–12 weeks of gestation.

▶ Differential Diagnosis

The nonpregnant uterus enlarged by myomas can be confused with the gravid uterus, but it is usually very firm and irregular. An ovarian tumor may be found midline, displacing the nonpregnant uterus to the side or posteriorly. Ultrasonography and a pregnancy test will provide accurate diagnosis in these circumstances.

ESSENTIALS OF PRENATAL CARE

The first prenatal visit should occur as early as possible after the diagnosis of pregnancy and should include the following: history, physical examination, advice to the patient, and appropriate tests and procedures.

▶ History

The patient's age, ethnic background, and occupation should be obtained. The onset of the last menstrual period and its normality, possible conception dates, bleeding after the last menstruation, medical history, all prior pregnancies (duration, outcome, and complications), and symptoms of present pregnancy should be documented. The patient's nutritional habits should be discussed with her, as well as any use of caffeine, tobacco, alcohol, or drugs (Tables 19–1 and 19–2). Whether there is any family history of congenital anomalies and heritable diseases, a personal history of childhood varicella, prior sexually transmitted diseases (STDs), or risk factors for HIV infection should be determined. The woman should also be asked about domestic violence.

▶ Physical Examination

Height, weight, and blood pressure should be measured, and a general physical examination should be done, including a breast examination. Abdominal and pelvic examination should include the following: (1) estimate of uterine size or measure of fundal height; (2) evaluation of bony pelvis for symmetry and adequacy; (3) evaluation of cervix for structural anatomy, infection, effacement, dilation; (4) detection of fetal heart tones by Doppler device after 10 weeks.

Table 19–1. Common drugs that are teratogenic or fetotoxic.[1]

ACE inhibitors	Lithium
Alcohol	Methotrexate
Androgens	Misoprostol
Angiotensin-II receptor blockers	NSAIDs (third trimester)
	Opioids (prolonged use)
Antiepileptics (phenytoin, valproic acid, carbamazepine)	Radioiodine (antithyroid)
	Reserpine
Benzodiazepines	Ribavirin
Carbarsone (amebicide)	SSRIs
Chloramphenicol (third trimester)	Sulfonamides (third trimester)
	Tetracycline (third trimester)
Cyclophosphamide	Thalidomide
Diazoxide	Tobacco smoking
Diethylstilbestrol	Trimethoprim (third trimester)
Disulfiram	Warfarin and other coumarin anticoagulants
Ergotamine	
Estrogens	
Griseofulvin	
Isotretinoin	

[1]Many other drugs are also contraindicated during pregnancy. Evaluate any drug for its need versus its potential adverse effects. Further information can be obtained from the manufacturer or from any of several teratogenic registries around the country.
ACE, angiotensin-converting enzyme; NSAIDs, nonsteroidal anti-inflammatory drugs; SSRIs, selective serotonin reuptake inhibitors.

Table 19–2. Drugs and substances that require a careful assessment of risk before they are prescribed for breast-feeding women.[1]

Category of Drug	Specific Drug	Concern
ACE inhibitors	Lisinopril	Unknown effects. Captopril or enalapril is preferred if an agent from this category is needed.
Alkylating agents	Cyclophosphamide	Neonatal neutropenia. No breastfeeding.
Analgesic	Codeine, oxycodone	Cause CNS depression. Unpredictable metabolism.
Antibiotics	Ciprofloxacin	Association with adverse effects on fetal cartilage and bone. Must weigh risks versus benefits.
	Doxycycline	Concern for bone growth and dental staining.
Antiepileptics	Valproic acid	Long-term effects are unknown. Although levels in milk are low, it is teratogenic, so it should be avoided if possible.
Antidepressants	Fluoxetine	Present in breast milk in higher levels than other SSRIs. Watch for adverse effects like an infant's fussiness and crying.
Antihistamine	Diphenhydramine	Present in very small quantities in milk; sources are conflicting with regard to its safety.
Beta-blockers	Atenolol	Has been associated with hypotension and bradycardia in the infant. Metoprolol and propranolol are preferred.
Mood stabilizer	Lithium	Circulating levels in the neonate are variable. Follow infant's serum creatinine and blood urea nitrogen levels and thyroid function tests.

[1]The above list is not all-inclusive. For additional information, see the below reference from which this information is adapted or the online drug and lactation database, Lactmed, at http://toxnet.nlm.nih.gov/newtoxnet/lactmed.htm.
ACE, angiotensin-converting enzyme; CNS, central nervous system; SSRIs, selective serotonin reuptake inhibitors.
Data from Rowe H et al. Maternal medication, drug use, and breastfeeding. Pediatr Clin North Am. 2013 Feb;60(1):275–94. [PMID: 23178070]

Laboratory Tests

See Tests & Procedures, below.

Advice to Patients

A. Prenatal Visits

Prenatal care should begin early and maintain a schedule of regular prenatal visits: 4–28 weeks, every 4 weeks; 28–36 weeks, every 2 weeks; 36 weeks on, weekly.

B. Diet

The patient should be counseled to eat a balanced diet containing the major food groups. See Nutrition in Pregnancy, below.

1. Prenatal vitamins with iron and folic acid should be prescribed. Supplements that are not specified for pregnant women should be avoided as they may contain dangerous amounts of certain vitamins.
2. Caffeine intake should be decreased to 0–1 cup of coffee, tea, or caffeinated cola daily.
3. The patient should be advised to avoid eating raw or rare meat as well as fish known to contain elevated levels of mercury.
4. Patients should be encouraged to eat fresh fruits and vegetables (washed before eating).

C. Medications

Only medications prescribed or authorized by the obstetric provider should be taken.

D. Alcohol and Other Drugs

Patients should be encouraged to abstain from alcohol, tobacco, and all recreational ("street") drugs. No safe level of alcohol intake has been established for pregnancy. Fetal effects are manifest in the **fetal alcohol syndrome,** which includes growth restriction; facial, skeletal, and cardiac abnormalities; and serious central nervous system dysfunction. These effects are thought to result from direct toxicity of ethanol as well as of its metabolites such as acetaldehyde.

Cigarette smoking results in fetal exposure to carbon monoxide and nicotine, and this is thought to eventuate in a number of adverse pregnancy outcomes. An increased risk of placental abruption (abruptio placentae), placenta previa, and premature rupture of the membranes is documented among women who smoke. Preterm delivery, low birth weight, and ectopic pregnancy are also more likely among smokers. Women who smoke should quit smoking or at least reduce the number of cigarettes smoked per day to as few as possible. Clinicians should ask all pregnant women about their smoking history and offer smoking cessation counseling during pregnancy, since women are more motivated to change at this time. Pregnant women should also avoid exposure to environmental smoke ("passive smoking"), smokeless tobacco, and e-cigarettes (Tables 1–4, 1–5). Pharmacotherapy for smoking cessation has been used with mixed results. Studies of buproprion

and nicotine replacement systems have not demonstrated any definitive drawbacks, but prolonged cessation from smoking has not been proven either.

Sometimes compounding the above effects on pregnancy outcome are the independent adverse effects of illicit drugs. Cocaine use in pregnancy is associated with an increased risk of premature rupture of membranes, preterm delivery, placental abruption, intrauterine growth restriction, neurobehavioral deficits, and sudden infant death syndrome. Similar adverse pregnancy effects are associated with amphetamine use, perhaps reflecting the vasoconstrictive potential of both amphetamines and cocaine. Adverse effects associated with opioid use include intrauterine growth restriction, prematurity, and fetal death.

E. Radiographs and Noxious Exposures

Radiographs should be avoided unless essential and approved by a clinician. Abdominal shielding should be used whenever possible. The patient should be told to inform her other health care providers that she is pregnant. Chemical or radiation hazards should be avoided as should excessive heat in hot tubs or saunas. Patients should be told to avoid handling cat feces or cat litter and to wear gloves when gardening to avoid infection with toxoplasmosis.

F. Rest and Activity

The patient should be encouraged to obtain adequate rest each day. She should abstain from strenuous physical work or activities, particularly when heavy lifting or weight bearing is required. Regular exercise can be continued at a mild to moderate level; however, exhausting or hazardous exercises or new athletic training programs should be avoided during pregnancy. Exercises that require a great deal of balance should also be done with caution.

G. Birth Classes

The patient should be encouraged to enroll in a childbirth preparation class with her partner well before her due date.

Tests & Procedures

A. Each Visit

Weight, blood pressure, fundal height, and fetal heart rate are measured, and a urine specimen is obtained and tested for protein and glucose. Any concerns the patient may have about pregnancy, health, and nutrition should be addressed.

B. 6–12 Weeks

Confirm uterine size and growth by pelvic examination. Document fetal heart tones (audible at 10–12 weeks of gestation by Doppler). Urinalysis; culture of a clean-voided midstream urine sample; random blood glucose; complete blood count (CBC) with red cell indices; serologic test for syphilis, rubella antibody titer; varicella immunity; blood group; Rh type; antibody screening for anti-Rh$_o$(D), hepatitis B surface antigen (HBsAg), and HIV should be performed. Cervical cultures are usually obtained for *Chlamydia trachomatis* and possibly *Neisseria gonorrhoeae*, along with a Papanicolaou smear of the cervix. All black women should have sickle cell screening. Women of African, Asian, or Mediterranean ancestry with anemia or low mean corpuscular volume (MCV) values should have hemoglobin electrophoresis performed to identify abnormal hemoglobins (Hb S, C, F, alpha-thalassemia, beta-thalassemia). Tuberculosis testing is indicated for high-risk populations. Blood screening for Tay-Sachs, Canavan disease, and familial dysautonomia is offered to couples who are of Eastern European Jewish (Ashkenazi) descent. Couples of French-Canadian or Cajun ancestry should also be screened as possible Tay-Sachs carriers. Screening for cystic fibrosis is offered to all pregnant women. Hepatitis C antibody screening should be offered to pregnant women who are at high risk for infection. Fetal aneuploidy screening is available in the first and second trimester and should be offered to all women, ideally before 20 weeks gestation. Noninvasive first trimester screening for Down syndrome includes ultrasonographic nuchal translucency and serum levels of PAPP-A (pregnancy-associated plasma protein A) and the free beta subunit of hCG. For pregnancies at high risk for aneuploidy, noninvasive testing with cell free fetal DNA from maternal plasma can be performed. It screens only for trisomy 13, 18, and 21. If indicated and requested by the patient, chorionic villus sampling can be performed during this period (11–13 weeks).

C. 16–20 Weeks

The "quad screen" and amniocentesis are performed as indicated and requested by the patient during this time. First and second trimester tests have similar detection rates. When first and second trimester screening for Down syndrome are combined (integrated screening), the detection rates are even higher. Fetal ultrasound examination to determine pregnancy dating and evaluate fetal anatomy is also done. An earlier examination provides the most accurate dating, and a later examination demonstrates fetal anatomy in greatest detail. The best compromise is at 18–20 weeks of gestation. Cervical length measurement (greater than 2.5 cm is normal) is not performed universally in all practices, but is used by some clinicians to identify women at risk for preterm birth.

D. 24 Weeks to Delivery

The patient should be instructed about the symptoms and signs of preterm labor and rupture of membranes. Ultrasound examination is performed as indicated. Typically, fetal size and growth are evaluated when fundal height is 3 cm less than or more than expected for gestational age. In multi-fetal pregnancies, ultrasound should be performed every 2–6 weeks to evaluate for discordant growth.

E. 24–28 Weeks

Screening for gestational diabetes is performed using a 50-g glucose load (Glucola) and a 1-hour post-Glucola blood glucose determination. Abnormal values (greater than or equal to 140 mg/dL or 7.8 mmol/L) should be followed up with a 3-hour glucose tolerance test (see Table 19–4).

F. 28 Weeks

If initial antibody screen for anti-Rh$_o$(D) is negative, repeat antibody testing for Rh-negative patients is performed, but the result is not required before Rh$_o$(D) immune globulin is administered.

G. 28–32 Weeks

A CBC is done to evaluate for anemia of pregnancy. Screening for syphilis and HIV is also performed at this time. Providers should familiarize themselves with the laws in their state since testing requirements vary.

H. 28 Weeks to Delivery

Fetal position and presentation are determined. The patient is asked about symptoms or signs of preterm labor or rupture of membranes at each visit. Maternal perception of fetal movement should be assessed at each visit. Antepartum fetal testing in the form of nonstress tests and biophysical profiles can be performed as medically indicated.

I. 36 Weeks to Delivery

Repeat syphilis and HIV testing (depending on state laws) and cervical cultures for *N gonorrhoeae* and *C trachomatis* should be performed in at-risk patients. The indicators of onset of labor, admission to the hospital, management of labor and delivery, and options for analgesia and anesthesia should be discussed with the patient. Weekly cervical examinations are not necessary unless indicated to assess a specific clinical situation. Elective delivery (whether by induction or cesarean section) prior to 39 weeks of gestation requires confirmation of fetal lung maturity.

The CDC recommends universal prenatal culture-based screening for group B streptococcal colonization in pregnancy. A single standard culture of the distal vagina and anorectum is collected at 35–37 weeks. No prophylaxis is needed if the screening culture is negative. Patients whose cultures are positive receive intrapartum penicillin prophylaxis during labor. Except when group B streptococci are found in urine, asymptomatic colonization is not to be treated before labor. Patients who have had a previous infant with invasive group B streptococcal disease or who have group B streptococcal bacteriuria during this pregnancy should receive intrapartum prophylaxis regardless, so rectovaginal cultures are not needed. Patients whose cultures at 35–37 weeks were not done or whose results are not known should receive prophylaxis if they have a risk factor for early-onset neonatal disease, including intrapartum temperature 38°C or higher, membrane rupture more than 18 hours, or delivery before 37 weeks gestation.

The routine recommended regimen for prophylaxis is penicillin G, 5 million units intravenously as a loading dose and then 2.5 million units intravenously every 4 hours until delivery. In penicillin-allergic patients not at high risk for anaphylaxis, 2 g of cefazolin can be given intravenously as an initial dose and then 1 g intravenously every 8 hours until delivery. In patients at high risk for anaphylaxis, vancomycin 1 g intravenously every 12 hours until delivery is used or, after confirmed susceptibility testing of group B streptococcal isolate, clindamycin 900 mg intravenously every 8 hours or erythromycin 500 mg intravenously every 6 hours until delivery.

J. 41 Weeks

The patient should have a cervical examination to determine the probability of successful induction of labor. Induction is undertaken if the cervix is favorable (generally, cervix 2 cm or more dilated, 50% or more effaced, vertex at –1 station, soft cervix, and midposition); if unfavorable, antepartum fetal testing is begun. Induction is performed at 42 weeks gestation regardless of the cervical examination findings; some providers elect induction at 41 weeks regardless of the cervical examination findings.

ACOG Committee on Genetics. Committee Opinion No. 442: Preconception and prenatal carrier screening for genetic diseases in individuals of Eastern European Jewish descent. Obstet Gynecol. 2009 Oct;114(4):950–3. [Reaffirmed 2014] [PMID: 19888064]
Dooley EK et al. Prenatal care: touching the future. Prim Care. 2012 Mar;39(1):17–37. [PMID: 22309579]
O'Neill M et al. Ambulatory obstetric care. Clin Obstet Gynecol. 2012 Sep;55(3):714–21. [PMID: 22828104]

NUTRITION IN PREGNANCY

Nutrition in pregnancy can affect maternal health and infant size and well-being. Pregnant women should have nutrition counseling early in prenatal care and access to supplementary food programs if necessary. Counseling should stress abstention from alcohol, smoking, and recreational drugs. Caffeine and artificial sweeteners should be used only in small amounts.

Recommendations regarding weight gain in pregnancy should be based on maternal body mass index (BMI) preconceptionally or at the first prenatal visit. According to the Institute of Medicine guidelines, total weight gain should be 25–35 lbs (11.3–15.9 kg) for normal weight women (BMI of 18.5–24.9) and 15–25 lbs (6.8–11.3 kg) for overweight women. For obese women (BMI of 30 or greater), weight gain should be limited to 11–20 lbs (5.0–9.1 kg). Excessive maternal weight gain has been associated with increased birth weight as well as postpartum retention of weight. Not gaining weight in pregnancy, conversely, has been associated with low birth weight. Nutrition counseling must be tailored to the individual patient.

The increased calcium needs of pregnancy (1200 mg/day) can be met with milk, milk products, green vegetables, soybean products, corn tortillas, and calcium carbonate supplements.

The increased need for iron and folic acid should be met with foods as well as vitamin and mineral supplements. (See Anemia section.) Megavitamins should not be taken in pregnancy, as they may result in fetal malformation or disturbed metabolism. However, a balanced prenatal supplement containing 30–60 mg of elemental iron, 0.5–0.8 mg of folate, and the recommended daily allowances of various vitamins and minerals is widely used in the United States

and is probably beneficial to many women with marginal diets. There is evidence that periconceptional folic acid supplements can decrease the risk of neural tube defects in the fetus. For this reason, the United States Public Health Service recommends the consumption of 0.4 mg of folic acid per day for all pregnant and reproductive age women. Women with a prior pregnancy complicated by neural tube defect may require higher supplemental doses as determined by their providers.

American College of Obstetricians and Gynecologists. ACOG Committee Opinion No. 548: Weight gain during pregnancy. Obstet Gynecol. 2013 Jan;121(1):210–2. [PMID: 23262962]
Blumfield ML et al. A systematic review and meta-analysis of micronutrient intakes during pregnancy in developed countries. Nutr Rev. 2013 Feb;71(2):118–32. [PMID: 23356639]
Lassi ZS et al. Folic acid supplementation during pregnancy for maternal health and pregnancy outcomes. Cochrane Database Syst Rev. 2013 Mar 28;3:CD006896. [PMID: 23543547]

PREVENTION OF RHESUS ALLOIMMUNIZATION

The antibody anti-Rh_o(D) causes severe hemolytic disease of the newborn. About 15% of whites and much lower proportions of blacks and Asians are Rh_o(D)–negative. If an Rh_o(D)–negative woman carries an Rh_o(D)–positive fetus, antibodies against Rh_o(D) may develop in the mother when fetal red cells enter her circulation during small fetomaternal bleeding episodes in the early third trimester or during delivery, abortion, ectopic pregnancy, placental abruption, or other instances of antepartum bleeding. This antibody, once produced, remains in the woman's circulation and poses the threat of hemolytic disease for subsequent Rh-positive fetuses.

Passive immunization against hemolytic disease of the newborn is achieved with Rh_o(D) immune globulin, a purified concentrate of antibodies against Rh_o(D) antigen. The Rh_o(D) immune globulin (one vial of 300 mcg intramuscularly) is given to the mother within 72 hours after delivery (or spontaneous or induced abortion or ectopic pregnancy). The antibodies in the immune globulin destroy fetal Rh-positive cells so that the mother will not produce anti-Rh_o(D). During her next Rh-positive gestation, erythroblastosis will be prevented. An additional safety measure is the routine administration of the immune globulin at the 28th week of pregnancy. The passive antibody titer that results is too low to significantly affect an Rh-positive fetus. The maternal clearance of the globulin is slow enough that protection will continue for 12 weeks. Once a woman is alloimmunized, Rh_o(D) immune globulin is no longer helpful and should not be given.

Karanth L et al. Anti-D administration after spontaneous miscarriage for preventing Rhesus alloimmunisation. Cochrane Database Syst Rev. 2013 Mar 28;3:CD009617. [PMID: 23543581]
Okwundu CI et al. Intramuscular versus intravenous anti-D for preventing Rhesus alloimmunization during pregnancy. Cochrane Database Syst Rev. 2013 Jan 31;1:CD007885. [PMID: 23440818]

LACTATION

Breastfeeding should be encouraged by education throughout pregnancy and the puerperium. Mothers should be told the benefits of breastfeeding, including infant immunity, emotional satisfaction, mother-infant bonding, and economic savings. The period of amenorrhea associated with frequent and consistent breastfeeding provides some (although not reliable) birth control until menstruation begins at 6–12 months postpartum or the intensity of breastfeeding diminishes. If the mother must return to work, even a brief period of nursing is beneficial. Transfer of immunoglobulins, macrophages, and lymphocytes in colostrum and breast milk immunoprotects the infant against many systemic and enteric infections. The intestinal flora of breastfed infants inhibits the growth of pathogens. Breastfed infants have fewer bacterial and viral infections, fewer gastrointestinal tract infections, and fewer allergy problems than bottle-fed infants. Furthermore, they are less apt to be obese as children and adults.

Frequent breastfeeding on an infant-demand schedule enhances milk flow and successful breastfeeding. Mothers breastfeeding for the first time need help and encouragement from providers, nurses, and other nursing mothers. Milk supply can be increased by increased suckling and increased rest.

Nursing mothers should have a fluid intake of over 3 L/day. The United States RDA calls for 21 g of extra protein (over the 44 g/day baseline for an adult woman) and 550 extra kcal/day in the first 6 months of nursing. Calcium intake should be 1200 mg/day. Continuation of a prenatal vitamin and mineral supplement is wise. Strict vegetarians who eschew both milk and eggs should always take vitamin B_{12} supplements during pregnancy and lactation.

1. Effects of Drugs in a Nursing Mother

Drugs taken by a nursing mother may accumulate in milk and be transmitted to the infant (Table 19–2). The amount of drug entering the milk depends on the drug's lipid solubility, mechanism of transport, and degree of ionization.

2. Suppression of Lactation

The simplest and safest method of suppressing lactation after it has started is to gradually transfer the baby to a bottle or a cup over a 3-week period. Milk supply will decrease with decreased demand, and minimal discomfort ensues. If nursing must be stopped abruptly, the mother should avoid nipple stimulation, refrain from expressing milk, and use a snug brassiere. Ice packs and analgesics can be helpful. This same technique can be used in cases where suppression is desired before nursing has begun. Engorgement will gradually recede over a 2- to 3-day period. Hormonal suppression of lactation is no longer practiced.

Denne SC. Neonatal nutrition. Pediatr Clin North Am. 2015 Apr; 62(2):427–38. [PMID: 25836706]

Oladapo OT et al. Treatments for suppression of lactation. Cochrane Database Syst Rev. 2012 Sep 12;9:CD005937. [PMID: 22972088]

TRAVEL & IMMUNIZATIONS DURING PREGNANCY

During an otherwise normal low-risk pregnancy, travel can be planned most safely up to the 32nd week. Commercial flying in pressurized cabins does not pose a threat to the fetus. An aisle seat will allow frequent walks. Adequate fluids should be taken during the flight. It is not advisable to travel to endemic areas of yellow fever in Africa or Latin America; similarly, it is inadvisable to travel to areas of Africa or Asia where chloroquine-resistant falciparum malaria is a hazard, since complications of malaria are more common in pregnancy.

Ideally, all immunizations should precede pregnancy. Live virus products are contraindicated during pregnancy (measles, rubella, yellow fever, and smallpox.) Inactivated polio vaccine (IPV) should be given subcutaneously instead of the oral live-attenuated vaccine. The varicella vaccine should be given 1–3 months before becoming pregnant. Vaccines against pneumococcal pneumonia, meningococcal meningitis, and hepatitis A can be used as indicated. Pregnant women who are considered to be at high-risk for hepatitis B and who have not been previously vaccinated should be vaccinated during pregnancy.

The CDC lists pregnant women as a high-risk group for influenza. Annual influenza vaccination is indicated in all women who are pregnant or will be pregnant during the "flu season." It can be given in the first trimester. The CDC also recommends that every pregnant woman receive a dose of Tdap during each pregnancy irrespective of her prior vaccination history. The optimal timing for such Tdap administration is between 27 and 36 weeks of gestation, in order to maximize the antibody response of the pregnant woman and the passive antibody transfer to the infant. For any woman who was not previously vaccinated with Tdap and for whom the vaccine was not given during her pregnancy, Tdap should be administered immediately postpartum. Further, any teenagers or adults not previously vaccinated who will have close contact with the infant should also receive it, ideally 2 weeks before exposure to the child. This vaccination strategy is referred to as "cocooning," and its purpose is to protect the infant aged younger than 12 months who is at particularly high risk for lethal pertussis.

Hepatitis A vaccine contains formalin-inactivated virus and can be given in pregnancy when needed. Pooled immune globulin to prevent hepatitis A is safe and does not carry risk of HIV transmission. Chloroquine can be used for malaria prophylaxis in pregnancy, and proguanil is also safe.

Water should be purified by boiling, since iodine purification may provide more iodine than is safe during pregnancy.

Prophylactic antibiotics or bismuth subsalicylate should not be used during pregnancy to prevent diarrhea. Oral rehydration and treatment of bacterial diarrhea with erythromycin or ampicillin if necessary is preferred.

Centers for Disease Control and Prevention (CDC). Updated recommendations for use of tetanus toxoid, reduced diphtheria toxoid and acellular pertussis vaccine (Tdap) in pregnant women—Advisory Committee on Immunization Practices (ACIP), 2012. MMWR Morb Mortal Wkly Rep. 2013 Feb 22; 62(7):131–5. [PMID: 23425962]

OBSTETRIC COMPLICATIONS OF THE FIRST & SECOND TRIMESTERS

VOMITING OF PREGNANCY (Morning Sickness) & HYPEREMESIS GRAVIDARUM

ESSENTIALS OF DIAGNOSIS

▶ Morning or evening nausea and vomiting.

▶ Persistent vomiting severe enough to result in weight loss, dehydration, starvation ketosis, hypochloremic alkalosis, hypokalemia.

▶ May have transient elevation of liver enzymes.

▶ Appears related to high or rising serum hCG.

▶ More common with multi-fetal pregnancies or hydatidiform mole.

General Considerations

Nausea and vomiting begin soon after the first missed period and cease by the fifth month of gestation. Up to three-fourths of women complain of nausea and vomiting during early pregnancy, with the vast majority noting nausea throughout the day. This problem exerts no adverse effects on the pregnancy and does not presage other complications.

Persistent, severe vomiting during pregnancy—hyperemesis gravidarum—can be disabling and require hospitalization. Thyroid dysfunction can be associated with hyperemesis gravidarum, so it is advisable to determine thyroid-stimulating hormone (TSH) and free thyroxine (FT_4) values in these patients. Of note, these patients will not have a goiter.

Treatment

A. Mild Nausea and Vomiting of Pregnancy

In most instances, only reassurance and dietary advice are required. Because of possible teratogenicity, drugs used during the first half of pregnancy should be restricted to those of major importance to life and health. Antiemetics, antihistamines, and antispasmodics are generally unnecessary to treat nausea of pregnancy. Vitamin B_6 (pyridoxine), 50–100 mg/day orally, is nontoxic and may be helpful in some patients. Pyridoxine alone or in combination with doxylamine is first-line pharmacotherapy.

B. Hyperemesis Gravidarum

With more severe nausea and vomiting, it may become necessary to hospitalize the patient. In this case, a private room with limited activity is preferred. It is recommended to give nothing by mouth until the patient is improving, and maintain hydration and electrolyte balance by giving appropriate parenteral fluids and vitamin supplements as indicated. Antiemetics such as promethazine (25 mg orally, rectally, or intravenously every 4–6 hours), metoclopramide (10 mg orally or intravenously every 6 hours), or ondansetron (4–8 mg orally or intravenously every 8 hours) should be started. Ondansetron has been associated in some studies with congenital anomalies. Data are limited, but the risks and benefits of treatment should be addressed with the patient. Antiemetics will likely need to be given intravenously initially. Rarely, total parenteral nutrition may become necessary but only if enteral feedings cannot be done. As soon as possible, the patient should be placed on a dry diet consisting of six small feedings daily. Antiemetics may be continued orally as needed. After in-patient stabilization, the patient can be maintained at home even if she requires intravenous fluids in addition to her oral intake. There are conflicting studies regarding the use of corticosteroids for the control of hyperemesis gravidarum, and it has also been associated with fetal anomalies. Therefore, this treatment should be withheld before 10 weeks gestation and until more accepted treatments have been exhausted.

▶ When to Refer

• Patient does not respond to first-line outpatient management.

• There is concern for other pathology (ie, hydatidiform mole).

▶ When to Admit

• Patient is unable to tolerate any food or water.

• Condition precludes the patient from ingesting necessary medications.

• Weight loss.

• Presence of a hydatidiform mole.

American College of Obstetricians and Gynecologists. ACOG Practice Bulletin No. 153: Nausea and vomiting of pregnancy. Obstet Gynecol. 2015 Sep;126(3):e12–24. [PMID: 26287788]

SPONTANEOUS ABORTION

ESSENTIALS OF DIAGNOSIS

▶ Intrauterine pregnancy at less than 20 weeks.

▶ Low or falling levels of hCG.

▶ Bleeding, midline cramping pain.

▶ Open cervical os.

▶ Complete or partial expulsion of products of conception.

General Considerations

About three-fourths of spontaneous abortions occur before the 16th week; of these, three-fourths occur before the eighth week. Almost 20% of all clinically recognized pregnancies terminate in spontaneous abortion.

More than 60% of spontaneous abortions result from chromosomal defects due to maternal or paternal factors; about 15% appear to be associated with maternal trauma, infections, dietary deficiencies, diabetes mellitus, hypothyroidism, the lupus anticoagulant-anticardiolipin-antiphospholipid antibody syndrome, or anatomic malformations. There is no reliable evidence that abortion may be induced by psychic stimuli such as severe fright, grief, anger, or anxiety. In about one-fourth of cases, the cause of abortion cannot be determined. There is no evidence that video display terminals or associated electromagnetic fields are related to an increased risk of spontaneous abortion.

It is important to distinguish women with a history of incompetent cervix from those with more typical early abortion. Characteristically, incompetent cervix presents as "silent" cervical dilation (ie, with minimal uterine contractions) in the second trimester. Women with incompetent cervix often present with significant cervical dilation (2 cm or more) and minimal symptoms. When the cervix reaches 4 cm or more, active uterine contractions or rupture of the membranes may occur secondary to the degree of cervical dilation. This does not change the primary diagnosis. Factors that predispose to incompetent cervix are a history of incompetent cervix with a previous pregnancy, cervical conization or surgery, cervical injury, diethylstilbestrol (DES) exposure, and anatomic abnormalities of the cervix. Prior to pregnancy or during the first trimester, there are no methods for determining whether the cervix will eventually be incompetent. After 14–16 weeks, ultrasound may be used to evaluate the internal anatomy of the lower uterine segment and cervix for the funneling and shortening abnormalities consistent with cervical incompetence.

Clinical Findings

A. Symptoms and Signs

1. Threatened abortion—Bleeding or cramping occurs, but the pregnancy continues. The cervix is not dilated.

2. Inevitable abortion—The cervix is dilated and the membranes may be ruptured, but passage of the products of conception has not yet occurred. Bleeding and cramping persist, and passage of the products of conception is considered inevitable.

3. Complete abortion—Products of conception are completely expelled. Pain ceases, but spotting may persist. Cervical os is closed.

4. Incomplete abortion—The cervix is dilated. Some portion of the products of conception (usually placental) remains in the uterus. Only mild cramps are reported, but bleeding is persistent and often excessive.

5. Missed abortion—The pregnancy has ceased to develop, but the conceptus has not been expelled. Symptoms of pregnancy disappear. There may be a brownish vaginal discharge but no active bleeding. Pain does not develop. The cervix is semifirm and slightly patulous; the uterus becomes smaller and irregularly softened; the adnexa are normal.

B. Laboratory Findings

Pregnancy tests show low or falling levels of hCG. A CBC should be obtained if bleeding is heavy. Determine Rh type, and give $Rh_o(D)$ immune globulin if Rh-negative. All tissue recovered should be assessed by a pathologist and may be sent for genetic analysis in selected cases.

C. Ultrasonographic Findings

The gestational sac can be identified at 5–6 weeks from the last menstruation, a fetal pole at 6 weeks, and fetal cardiac activity at 6–7 weeks by transvaginal ultrasound. Serial observations are often required to evaluate changes in size of the embryo. Diagnostic criteria of early pregnancy loss are a crown-rump length of 7 mm or more and no heartbeat, a mean sac diameter of 25 mm or more and no embryo, no heartbeat 2 weeks after an ultrasound that demonstrated a gestational sac without a yolk sac, and no heartbeat 11 days or more after an ultrasound demonstrating a gestational sac with a yolk sac.

Differential Diagnosis

The bleeding that occurs in abortion of a uterine pregnancy must be differentiated from the abnormal bleeding of an ectopic pregnancy and anovulatory bleeding in a nonpregnant woman. The passage of hydropic villi in the bloody discharge is diagnostic of hydatidiform mole.

Treatment

A. General Measures

1. Threatened abortion—Bed rest for 24–48 hours followed by gradual resumption of usual activities has been offered in the past. Studies do not support that this strategy is beneficial. Abstinence from sexual activity has also been suggested without proven benefit. Data are lacking to support the administration of progestins to all women with a threatened abortion. If during the patient's evaluation, an infection is diagnosed (ie, urinary tract infection), it should be treated.

2. Missed abortion—This calls for counseling regarding the fate of the pregnancy and planning for its elective termination at a time chosen by the patient and clinician. Management can be medical or surgical. Each has risk and benefits. Medically induced first-trimester termination with prostaglandins (ie, misoprostol given vaginally or orally in a dose of 200–800 mcg) is safe, effective, less invasive, and more private than surgical intervention; however, if it is unsuccessful or if there is excessive bleeding, a surgical procedure (dilation and curettage) may still be needed. Patients must be counseled about the different therapeutic options.

B. Surgical Measures

1. Incomplete or inevitable abortion—Prompt removal of any products of conception remaining within the uterus is required to stop bleeding and prevent infection. Analgesia and a paracervical block are useful, followed by uterine exploration with ovum forceps or uterine aspiration. Regional anesthesia may be required.

2. Cerclage and restriction of activities—A cerclage is the treatment of choice for incompetent cervix, but a viable intrauterine pregnancy should be confirmed prior to placement of the cerclage.

A variety of suture materials including a 5-mm Mersilene tape or No. 2 nonabsorbable monofilament suture can be used to create a purse-string type of stitch around the cervix, using either the McDonald or Shirodkar method. Cerclage should be undertaken with caution when there is advanced cervical dilation or when the membranes are prolapsed into the vagina. Rupture of the membranes and infection are specific contraindications to cerclage. Cervical cultures for *N gonorrhoeae*, *C trachomatis*, and group B streptococci should be obtained before elective placement of a cerclage. *N gonorrhoeae* and *C trachomatis* should be treated before placement.

▶ **When to Refer**

- Patient with history of two second-trimester losses.
- Vaginal bleeding in a pregnant patient that resembles menstruation in a nonpregnant woman.
- Patient with an open cervical os.
- No signs of uterine growth in serial examinations of a pregnant patient.
- Leakage of amniotic fluid.

▶ **When to Admit**

- Open cervical os.
- Heavy vaginal bleeding.
- Leakage of amniotic fluid.

American College of Obstetricians and Gynecologists. ACOG Practice Bulletin No. 150: Early pregnancy loss. Obstet Gynecol. 2015 May;125(5):1258–67. [PMID: 25932865]

Brix N et al; CERVO group. Randomised trial of cervical cerclage, with and without occlusion, for the prevention of preterm birth in women suspected for cervical insufficiency. BJOG. 2013 Apr;120(5):613–20. [PMID: 23331924]

RECURRENT (Habitual) ABORTION

Recurrent abortion has been defined as the loss of three or more previable (less than 20 weeks gestation or 500 g) pregnancies in succession. Recurrent abortion affects about 1% of couples. Abnormalities related to recurrent abortion can be identified in approximately 50% of these couples. If a woman has lost three previous pregnancies without identifiable cause, she still has at least a 65% chance of carrying a fetus to viability.

Recurrent abortion is a clinical rather than pathologic diagnosis. The clinical findings are similar to those observed in other types of abortion. It is appropriate to begin a medical evaluation in a woman who has had two first-trimester losses.

▶ **Treatment**

A. Preconception Therapy

Preconception therapy is aimed at detection of maternal or paternal defects that may contribute to abortion. A thorough history and examination is essential. A random blood glucose test and thyroid function studies (including thyroid antibodies) can be done if history indicates a possible predisposition to diabetes mellitus or thyroid disease. Detection of lupus anticoagulant and other hemostatic abnormalities (proteins S and C and antithrombin deficiency, hyperhomocysteinemia, anticardiolipin antibody, factor V Leiden mutations) and an antinuclear antibody test may be indicated. Hysteroscopy, saline infusion sonogram, or hysterography can be used to exclude submucosal myomas and congenital anomalies of the uterus. In women with recurrent losses, resection of a uterine septum, if present, has been recommended. Chromosomal (karyotype) analysis of both partners can be done to rule out balanced translocations (found in 3–4% of infertile couples), but karyotyping is expensive and may not be helpful.

Many therapies have been tried to prevent recurrent pregnancy loss from immunologic causes. Low-molecular-weight heparin (LMWH), aspirin, intravenous immunoglobulin, and corticosteroids have all been used but the definitive treatment has not yet been determined. Prophylactic dose heparin and low-dose aspirin have been recommended for women with antiphospholipid antibodies and recurrent pregnancy loss.

B. Postconception Therapy

The patient should be provided early prenatal care and scheduled frequent office visits. Empiric sex steroid hormone therapy is complicated and should be done by an expert if undertaken.

▶ **Prognosis**

The prognosis is excellent if the cause of abortion can be corrected or treated.

Shahine L et al. Recurrent pregnancy loss: evaluation and treatment. Obstet Gynecol Clin North Am. 2015 Mar;42(1):117–34. [PMID: 25681844]

ECTOPIC PREGNANCY

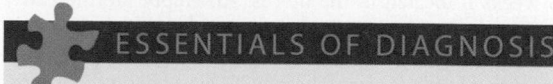

ESSENTIALS OF DIAGNOSIS

- ▶ Amenorrhea or irregular bleeding and spotting.
- ▶ Pelvic pain, usually adnexal.
- ▶ Adnexal mass by clinical examination or ultrasound.
- ▶ Failure of serum level of beta-hCG to double *every 48 hours*.
- ▶ No intrauterine pregnancy on transvaginal ultrasound with serum beta-hCG greater than 2000 milli-units/mL.

General Considerations

Ectopic implantation occurs in about one out of 150 live births. About 98% of ectopic pregnancies are tubal. Other sites of ectopic implantation are the peritoneum or abdominal viscera, the ovary, and the cervix. Any condition that prevents or retards migration of the fertilized ovum to the uterus can predispose to an ectopic pregnancy, including a history of infertility, pelvic inflammatory disease, ruptured appendix, and prior tubal surgery. Combined intrauterine and extrauterine pregnancy (heterotopic) may occur rarely. In the United States, undiagnosed or undetected ectopic pregnancy is one of the most common causes of maternal death during the first trimester.

Clinical Findings

A. Symptoms and Signs

Severe lower quadrant pain occurs in almost every case. It is sudden in onset, stabbing, intermittent, and does not radiate. Backache may be present during attacks. Shock occurs in about 10%, often after pelvic examination. At least two-thirds of patients give a history of abnormal menstruation; many have been infertile.

Blood may leak from the tubal ampulla over a period of days, and considerable blood may accumulate in the peritoneum. Slight but persistent vaginal spotting is usually reported, and a pelvic mass may be palpated. Abdominal distention and mild paralytic ileus are often present.

B. Laboratory Findings

The CBC may show anemia and slight leukocytosis. Quantitative serum pregnancy tests will show levels generally lower than expected for normal pregnancies of the same duration. If beta-hCG levels are followed over a few days, there may be a slow rise or a plateau rather than the near doubling every 2 days associated with normal early intrauterine pregnancy or the falling levels that occur with spontaneous abortion. A progesterone level can also be measured to assess the viability of the pregnancy.

C. Imaging

Ultrasonography can reliably demonstrate a gestational sac 5–6 weeks from the last menstruation and a fetal pole at 6 weeks if located in the uterus. An empty uterine cavity raises a strong suspicion of extrauterine pregnancy, which can occasionally be revealed by transvaginal ultrasound. Specified levels of serum beta-hCG have been reliably correlated with ultrasound findings of an intrauterine pregnancy. For example, a beta-hCG level of 6500 milli-units/mL with an empty uterine cavity by transabdominal ultrasound is highly suspicious for an ectopic pregnancy. Similarly, a beta-hCG value of 2000 milli-units/mL or more can be indicative of an ectopic pregnancy if no products of conception are detected within the uterine cavity by transvaginal ultrasound. Serum beta-hCG values can vary by laboratory.

D. Special Examinations

With the advent of high-resolution transvaginal ultrasound, culdocentesis is rarely used in evaluation of possible ectopic pregnancy. Laparoscopy is the surgical procedure of choice both to confirm an ectopic pregnancy and in most cases to permit removal of the ectopic pregnancy without the need for exploratory laparotomy.

Differential Diagnosis

Clinical and laboratory findings suggestive or diagnostic of pregnancy will distinguish ectopic pregnancy from many acute abdominal illnesses such as acute appendicitis, acute pelvic inflammatory disease, ruptured corpus luteum cyst or ovarian follicle, and urinary calculi. Uterine enlargement with clinical findings similar to those found in ectopic pregnancy is also characteristic of an aborting uterine pregnancy or hydatidiform mole. Ectopic pregnancy should be suspected when postabortal tissue examination fails to reveal chorionic villi. Steps must be taken for immediate diagnosis, including prompt microscopic tissue examination, ultrasonography, and serial beta-hCG titers every 48 hours.

Treatment

Patients must be warned about the complications of an ectopic pregnancy and monitored closely. In a stable patient with normal liver and renal function tests, methotrexate (50 mg/m^2) intramuscularly—given as single or multiple doses—is acceptable medical therapy for early ectopic pregnancy. Favorable criteria are that the pregnancy should be < 3.5 cm in largest dimension and unruptured, with no active bleeding and no fetal heart tones.

When a patient with an ectopic pregnancy is unstable or when surgical therapy is planned, the patient is hospitalized. Blood is typed and cross-matched. The goal is to diagnose and operate before there is frank rupture of the tube and intra-abdominal hemorrhage. The use of methotrexate in an unstable patient is absolutely contraindicated.

Surgical treatment is definitive. In most patients, diagnostic laparoscopy is the initial surgical procedure performed. Depending on the size of the ectopic pregnancy and whether or not it has ruptured, salpingostomy with removal of the ectopic pregnancy or a partial or complete salpingectomy can usually be performed. Clinical conditions permitting, patency of the contralateral tube can be established by injection of indigo carmine into the uterine cavity and flow through the contralateral tube confirmed visually by the surgeon; iron therapy for anemia may be necessary during convalescence. Rh$_o$(D) immune globulin (300 mcg) should be given to Rh-negative patients.

Prognosis

Repeat tubal pregnancy occurs in about 10% of cases. This should not be regarded as a contraindication to future pregnancy, but the patient requires careful observation and early ultrasound confirmation of an intrauterine pregnancy.

When to Refer

- Severe abdominal pain.
- Palpation of an adnexal mass on pelvic examination.
- Abdominal pain and vaginal bleeding in a pregnant patient.

When to Admit

Presence of symptoms or signs of a ruptured ectopic pregnancy.

Capmas P et al. Treatment of ectopic pregnancies in 2014: new answers to some old questions. Fertil Steril. 2014 Mar;101(3): 615–20. [PMID: 24559615]
Crochet JR et al. Does this woman have an ectopic pregnancy? The rational clinical examination systematic review. JAMA. 2013 Apr 24;309(16):1722–9. [PMID: 23613077]

GESTATIONAL TROPHOBLASTIC DISEASE (Hydatidiform Mole & Choriocarcinoma)

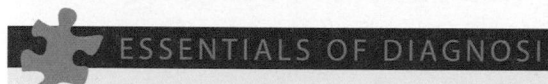

ESSENTIALS OF DIAGNOSIS

Hydatidiform Mole

- ► Amenorrhea.
- ► Irregular uterine bleeding.
- ► Serum beta-hCG greater than 40,000 milli-units/mL.
- ► Passage of grapelike clusters of enlarged edematous villi per vagina.
- ► Ultrasound of uterus shows characteristic heterogeneous echogenic image and no fetus or placenta.
- ► Cytogenetic composition is 46, XX (85%), of paternal origin.

Choriocarcinoma

- ► Persistence of detectable beta-hCG after mole evacuation.

General Considerations

Gestational trophoblastic disease is a spectrum of disorders that includes hydatidiform mole (partial and complete), invasive mole (local extension into the uterus or vagina), choriocarcinoma (malignancy often complicated by distant metastases), and placental site trophoblastic tumor. Complete moles show no evidence of a fetus on ultrasonography. The majority are 46, XX, with all chromosomes of paternal origin. Partial moles generally show evidence of an embryo or gestational sac; are triploid, slower-growing, and less symptomatic; and often present clinically as a missed abortion. Partial moles tend to follow a benign course, while complete moles have a greater tendency to become choriocarcinoma.

In the United States, the frequency of gestational trophoblastic disease is 1:1500 pregnancies. The highest rates occur in Asians. Risk factors include prior spontaneous abortion, a history of mole, and age younger than 21 or older than 35. Approximately 10% of women require further treatment after evacuation of the mole; choriocarcinoma develops in 2–3% of women.

Clinical Findings

A. Symptoms and Signs

Uterine bleeding, beginning at 6–16 weeks, is observed in most instances. In some cases, the uterus is larger than would be expected in a normal pregnancy of the same duration. Excessive nausea and vomiting may occur. Bilaterally enlarged cystic ovaries are sometimes palpable. They are the result of ovarian hyperstimulation due to excess beta-hCG.

Preeclampsia-eclampsia may develop during the second trimester of an untreated molar pregnancy, but this is unusual because most are diagnosed early.

Choriocarcinoma may be manifested by continued or recurrent uterine bleeding after evacuation of a mole or following delivery, abortion, or ectopic pregnancy. The presence of an ulcerative vaginal tumor, pelvic mass, or distant metastases may be the presenting manifestation.

B. Laboratory Findings

Hydatidiform moles are generally characterized by high serum beta-hCG values, which can range from high normal to the millions. Levels are higher with complete moles than with partial moles. Serum beta-hCG values, if extremely high, can assist in making the diagnosis, but they are more helpful in managing response to treatment. Hematocrit, creatinine, blood type, liver function tests, and thyroid function tests should also be measured. High beta-hCG levels can cause the release of thyroid hormone, and rarely, symptoms of hyperthyroidism. Patients with hyperthyroidism may require beta-blocker therapy until the mole has been evacuated.

C. Imaging

Ultrasound has virtually replaced all other means of preoperative diagnosis of hydatidiform mole. Placental vesicles can be easily seen on transvaginal ultrasound. A preoperative chest film is indicated to rule out pulmonary metastases of the trophoblast.

Treatment

A. Specific (Surgical) Measures

The uterus should be emptied as soon as the diagnosis of hydatidiform mole is established, preferably by suction curettage. Ovarian cysts should not be resected nor ovaries removed; spontaneous regression of theca lutein cysts will occur with elimination of the mole. The products of conception removed from the uterus should be sent to a pathologist for review. In patients who have completed their childbearing, hysterectomy is an acceptable alternative. Hysterectomy does not preclude the need for follow-up of beta-hCG levels.

B. Follow-Up Measures

Weekly quantitative beta-hCG level measurements are initially required. Following successful surgical evacuation, moles show a progressive decline in beta-hCG. After three negative weekly tests (less than 5 milli-units/mL), the interval may be increased to every 1–3 months for an additional 6 months. The purpose of this follow-up is to identify persistent nonmetastatic and metastatic disease, including choriocarcinoma, which is more likely to occur if the initial beta-hCG is high and the uterus is large. If levels plateau or begin to rise, the patient should be evaluated by repeat laboratory tests, chest film, and dilatation and curettage (D&C) before the initiation of chemotherapy. Effective contraception (preferably birth control pills) should be prescribed to avoid the hazard and confusion of elevated beta-hCG from a new pregnancy. The beta-hCG levels should be negative for 6 months before pregnancy is attempted again. Because the risk of recurrence of a molar pregnancy is 1%, an ultrasound should be performed in the first trimester of the pregnancy following a mole to ensure that the pregnancy is normal. In addition, a beta-hCG level should then be checked 6 weeks postpartum (after the subsequent normal pregnancy) to ensure there is no persistent trophoblastic tissue, and the placenta should be examined by a pathologist.

C. Antitumor Chemotherapy

If malignant tissue is discovered at surgery or during the follow-up examination, chemotherapy is indicated. For low-risk patients with a good prognosis, methotrexate is considered first-line therapy followed by dactinomycin (see Table 39–11). Patients with a poor prognosis should be referred to a cancer center, where multiple-agent chemotherapy probably will be given.

▶ Prognosis

Five-year survival after courses of chemotherapy, even when metastases have been demonstrated, can be expected in at least 85% of cases of choriocarcinoma.

▶ When to Refer

- Uterine size exceeds that anticipated for gestational age.
- Vaginal bleeding similar to menstruation.
- Pregnant patient with a history of a molar pregnancy.

▶ When to Admit

- Confirmed molar pregnancy by ultrasound and laboratory studies.
- Heavy vaginal bleeding in a pregnant patient under evaluation.

Berkowitz RS et al. Current advances in the management of gestational trophoblastic disease. Gynecol Oncol. 2013 Jan; 128(1):3–5. [PMID: 22846466]

Deng L et al. Combination chemotherapy for primary treatment of high-risk gestational trophoblastic tumour. Cochrane Database Syst Rev. 2013 Jan 31;1:CD005196. [PMID: 23440800]

PDQ Adult Treatment Editorial Board. Gestational trophoblastic disease treatment (PDQ®): health professional version. 2015 Feb 25. [Internet] [PMID: 26389414] http://www.ncbi.nlm.nih.gov/books/NBK65977/

OBSTETRIC COMPLICATIONS OF THE SECOND & THIRD TRIMESTERS

PREECLAMPSIA-ECLAMPSIA

 ESSENTIALS OF DIAGNOSIS

Preeclampsia

▶ Blood pressure of 140 mm Hg or higher systolic or 90 mm Hg or higher diastolic after 20 weeks of gestation.

▶ Proteinuria of 0.3 g or more in 24 hours.

Severe Preeclampsia (one or more of below)

▶ Blood pressure of 160 mm Hg or higher systolic or 110 mm Hg or higher diastolic.

▶ Progressive kidney injury.

▶ Thrombocytopenia.

▶ Hemolysis, elevated liver enzymes, low platelets (HELLP).

▶ Pulmonary edema.

▶ Vision changes or headache.

Eclampsia

▶ Seizures in a patient with evidence of preeclampsia.

▶ General Considerations

Preeclampsia is defined as the presence of newly elevated blood pressure and proteinuria during pregnancy. Eclampsia is diagnosed when seizures develop in a patient with evidence of preeclampsia. Historically, the presence of three elements was required for the diagnosis of preeclampsia: hypertension, proteinuria, and edema. Edema was difficult to objectively quantify and is no longer a required element.

Preeclampsia-eclampsia can occur any time after 20 weeks of gestation and up to 6 weeks postpartum. It is a disease unique to pregnancy, with the only cure being delivery of the fetus and placenta. Preeclampsia develops in approximately 7% of pregnant women in the United States; of those, eclampsia will develop in 5% (0.04% of pregnant women). Primiparas are most frequently affected; however, the incidence of preeclampsia-eclampsia is increased with multi-fetal pregnancies, chronic hypertension, diabetes mellitus, kidney disease, collagen-vascular and autoimmune disorders, and gestational trophoblastic disease. Uncontrolled eclampsia is a significant cause of maternal death.

Clinical Findings

Clinically, the severity of preeclampsia-eclampsia can be measured with reference to the six major sites in which it exerts its effects: the central nervous system, the kidneys, the liver, the hematologic system, the vascular system, and the fetal-placental unit. By evaluating each of these areas for the presence of mild to severe preeclampsia, the degree of involvement can be assessed, and an appropriate management plan can be formulated that balances the severity of disease and gestational age (Table 19–3).

A. Preeclampsia

1. Mild—Patients usually have few complaints, and the diastolic blood pressure is less than 110 mm Hg. Edema may be present. The platelet count is over 100,000/mcL, antepartum fetal testing is reassuring (see Tests & Procedures, above), central nervous system irritability is minimal, epigastric pain is not present, and liver enzymes are not elevated.

2. Severe—Symptoms are more dramatic and persistent. Patients may complain of headache and changes in vision. The blood pressure is often above 160/110 mm Hg. Thrombocytopenia (platelet count less than 100,000/mcL) may be present and progress to disseminated intravascular coagulation. Severe epigastric pain may be present from hepatic subcapsular hemorrhage with significant stretch or rupture of the liver capsule. HELLP syndrome (hemolysis, elevated liver enzymes, low platelets) is an advanced form of severe preeclampsia.

B. Eclampsia

The occurrence of seizures defines eclampsia. It is a manifestation of severe central nervous system involvement. Other findings of preeclampsia are observed.

Differential Diagnosis

Preeclampsia-eclampsia can mimic and be confused with many other diseases, including chronic hypertension, chronic kidney disease, primary seizure disorders, gallbladder and pancreatic disease, immune thrombocytopenia, thrombotic thrombocytopenic purpura, and hemolytic-uremic syndrome. It must always be considered in any pregnant woman beyond 20 weeks of gestation with consistent signs and symptoms. Although it is most common in the third trimester, it can occur earlier, especially in women with comorbid conditions like hypertension, kidney disease, and systemic lupus erythematosus. It is particularly difficult to diagnose when a preexisting disease such as hypertension is present.

Treatment

In clinical studies, diuretics, dietary restriction or enhancement, sodium restriction, and vitamin-mineral supplements (eg, calcium or vitamin C and E) have not been

Table 19–3. Indicators of mild to moderate versus severe preeclampsia-eclampsia.

Site	Indicator	Mild to Moderate	Severe
Central nervous system	Symptoms and signs	Hyperreflexia	Seizures
			Blurred vision
			Scotomas
			Headache
			Clonus
			Irritability
Kidney	Proteinuria	0.3–5 g/24 h	> 5 g/24 h or catheterized urine with 4+ protein
	Urinary output	> 30 mL/h	< 30 mL/h
Liver	AST, ALT, LD	Normal liver enzymes	Elevated liver enzymes
			Epigastric pain
			Ruptured liver
Hematologic	Platelets		< 100,000/mcL
	Hemoglobin	Normal	Low, normal, or elevated
Vascular	Blood pressure	< 160/110 mm Hg	> 160/110 mm Hg
	Retina	Arteriolar spasm	Retinal hemorrhages
Fetal-placental unit	Growth restriction	Absent	Present
	Oligohydramnios	Absent	Present
	Fetal distress	Absent	Present

ALT, alanine aminotransferase; AST, aspartate aminotransferase; LD, lactate dehydrogenase.

confirmed to be useful. The only cure is delivery of the fetus at a time as favorable as possible for its survival.

A. Preeclampsia

Early recognition is the key to treatment. This requires careful attention to the details of prenatal care—especially subtle changes in blood pressure and weight. The objectives are to prolong pregnancy if possible to allow fetal lung maturity while preventing progression to severe disease and eclampsia. The critical factors are the gestational age of the fetus, fetal pulmonary maturity, and the severity of maternal disease. Preeclampsia-eclampsia at term is managed by delivery. Prior to term, severe preeclampsia-eclampsia requires delivery with very few exceptions. Epigastric pain, seizures, severe range blood pressures, thrombocytopenia, and visual disturbances are strong indications for delivery of the fetus. Marked proteinuria alone can be managed more conservatively.

1. Home management—Home management may be attempted for patients with mild preeclampsia and a stable home situation. This requires assistance at home, rapid access to the hospital, a reliable patient, and the ability to obtain frequent blood pressure readings. A home health nurse can often provide frequent home visits and assessments.

2. Hospital care—Hospitalization is required for women with severe preeclampsia or those with unreliable home situations. Regular assessments of blood pressure, urine protein, and fetal heart tones and activity are required. A CBC with platelet count, electrolyte panel, and liver enzymes should be checked regularly, with frequency dependent on severity. A 24-hour urine collection for total protein and creatinine clearance should be obtained on admission and repeated as indicated. Magnesium sulfate is not used until the diagnosis of severe preeclampsia is made and delivery planned (see Eclampsia, below).

Fetal evaluation should be obtained as part of the workup. If the patient is being admitted to the hospital, fetal testing should be performed on the same day to assess fetal wellbeing. This may be done by fetal heart rate testing with nonstress testing or by biophysical profile. A regular schedule of fetal surveillance must then be followed. Daily fetal kick counts can be recorded by the patient herself. If the fetus is less than 34 weeks gestation, corticosteroids (betamethasone 12 mg intramuscularly every 24 h for two doses, or dexamethasone 6 mg intramuscularly every 12 h for four doses) can be administered to the mother. *However, when a woman is clearly suffering from unstable severe preeclampsia, delivery should not be delayed for fetal lung maturation or administration of corticosteroids.*

The method of delivery is determined by the maternal and fetal status. A vaginal delivery is preferred because it has less blood loss than a cesarean section and requires less coagulation factors. Cesarean section is reserved for the usual fetal indications. For mild preeclampsia, delivery should take place at term.

B. Eclampsia

1. Emergency care—If the patient is convulsing, she is turned on her side to prevent aspiration and to improve

blood flow to the placenta. The seizure may be stopped by giving an intravenous bolus of either magnesium sulfate, 4–6 g, or lorazepam, 2–4 mg over 4 minutes or until the seizure stops. Magnesium sulfate is the preferred agent, and alternatives should only be used if magnesium sulfate is unavailable. A continuous intravenous infusion of magnesium sulfate is then started at a rate of 2–3 g/h unless the patient is known to have significantly reduced kidney function. Magnesium blood levels are then checked every 4–6 hours and the infusion rate adjusted to maintain a therapeutic blood level (4–6 mEq/L). Urinary output is checked hourly and the patient assessed for signs of possible magnesium toxicity such as loss of deep tendon reflexes or decrease in respiratory rate and depth, which can be reversed with calcium gluconate, 1 g intravenously over 2 minutes.

2. General care—In patients with severe preeclampsia, magnesium sulfate should be given intravenously, 4- to 6-g load over 15–20 minutes followed by 2–3 g/h maintenance, for seizure prophylaxis. The occurrence of eclampsia necessitates delivery once the patient is stabilized. It is important, however, that assessment of the status of the patient and fetus take place first. Continuous fetal monitoring must be performed and maternal blood typed and cross-matched quickly. A urinary catheter is inserted to monitor urinary output, and a CBC with platelets, electrolytes, creatinine, and liver enzymes are obtained. If hypertension is present with systolic values of 160 mm Hg or higher or diastolic values 110 mm Hg or higher, antihypertensive medications should be administered to reduce the blood pressure to 140–150/90–100 mm Hg. Lower blood pressures than this may induce placental insufficiency through reduced perfusion. Hydralazine given in 5- to 10-mg increments intravenously every 20 minutes is frequently used to lower blood pressure. Labetalol, 10–20 mg intravenously, every 20 minutes as needed, can also be used.

3. Delivery—Delivery is mandated once eclampsia has occurred. Vaginal delivery is preferred. The rapidity with which delivery must be achieved depends on the fetal and maternal status following the seizure and the availability of laboratory data on the patient. Oxytocin, given intravenously and titrated to a dose that results in adequate contractions, may be used to induce or augment labor. Oxytocin should only be administered by a clinician specifically trained in its use. Regional analgesia or general anesthesia is acceptable. Cesarean section is used for the usual obstetric indications.

4. Postpartum—Magnesium sulfate infusion (2–3 g/h) should be continued for 24 hours postpartum. Late-onset preeclampsia-eclampsia can occur during the postpartum period. It is usually manifested by either hypertension or seizures. Treatment is the same as prior to delivery—ie, with hydralazine and magnesium sulfate.

▶ When to Refer

- New onset of hypertension and proteinuria in a pregnant patient more than 20 weeks' gestation.
- New onset of seizure activity in a pregnant patient.

When to Admit

- Symptoms of severe preeclampsia in a pregnant patient with elevated blood pressure above baseline.
- Evaluation for preeclampsia when severe disease is suspected.
- Evaluation for preeclampsia in a patient with an unstable home environment.
- Evidence of eclampsia.

Abildgaard U et al. Pathogenesis of the syndrome of hemolysis, elevated liver enzymes, and low platelet count (HELLP): a review. Eur J Obstet Gynecol Reprod Biol. 2013 Feb;166(2): 117–23. [PMID: 23107053]

American College of Obstetricians and Gynecologists et al. Hypertension in pregnancy. Report of the American College of Obstetricians and Gynecologists' Task Force on Hypertension in Pregnancy. Obstet Gynecol. 2013 Nov;122(5): 1122–31. [PMID: 24150027]

Repke JT. What is new in preeclampsia? Best articles from the past year. Obstet Gynecol. 2013 Mar;121(3):682–3. [PMID: 23635633]

PRETERM LABOR

ESSENTIALS OF DIAGNOSIS

- ▶ Preterm regular uterine contractions approximately 5 minutes apart.
- ▶ Cervical dilatation, effacement, or both.

General Considerations

Preterm birth is defined as delivery prior to 37 weeks gestation, and spontaneous preterm labor with or without premature rupture of the fetal membranes is responsible for at least two-thirds of all preterm births. Prematurity is the largest single contributor to infant mortality, and survivors are at risk for a myriad of short- and long-term complications. Rates of infant death and long-term neurologic impairment are inversely related to gestational age at birth. The cusp of viability in contemporary practice is 23–25 weeks gestation, and infants born prior to 23 weeks rarely survive. About two-thirds of the preterm births occur between 34 weeks and 36 weeks and 6 days (termed **late preterm birth**), and good outcomes are expected at these gestational ages. Importantly, however, even these late preterm infants are at significantly increased risk for both morbidity and mortality when compared to those infants born at term.

Major risk factors for spontaneous preterm labor include a **past history of preterm birth** and a **short cervical length** as measured by transvaginal ultrasound. Patients with one or both of these risk factors have largely been the focus of recent intervention trials aiming to prevent preterm birth. Other known risk factors are many but include black race, multi-fetal pregnancies, intrauterine infection, substance abuse, smoking, periodontal disease, and socioeconomic deprivation.

Clinical Findings

In women with regular uterine contractions and cervical change, the diagnosis of preterm labor is straightforward. However, symptoms such as pelvic pressure, cramping, or vaginal discharge may be the first complaints in high-risk patients who later develop preterm labor. Because these complaints may be vague and irregular uterine contractions are common, distinguishing which patients merit further evaluation can be problematic. In some cases, this distinction can be facilitated by the use of fetal fibronectin measurement in cervicovaginal specimens. This test is most useful when it is negative (less than 50 ng/mL), since the negative predictive value for delivery within 7–14 days is 93–97%. A negative test, therefore, usually means the patient can be reassured and discharged home. Because of its low sensitivity, however, fetal fibronectin is not recommended as a screening test in asymptomatic women.

Treatment

A. General Measures

Patients must be educated to identify symptoms associated with preterm labor to avoid unnecessary delay in their evaluation. In patients who are believed to be at increased risk for preterm delivery, conventional recommendations are for limited activity and bed rest. Randomized trials, however, have failed to demonstrate improved outcomes in women placed on activity restriction. Paradoxically, such recommendations may place a woman at an *increased* risk to deliver preterm. Women with preterm labor at the threshold of viability present unique ethical and obstetric challenges and are best managed in consultation with maternal-fetal medicine and neonatology specialists. The families in such situations should be actively and continually engaged about decisions regarding the aggressiveness of resuscitative efforts.

B. Corticosteroids

In pregnancies between 24 and 34 weeks gestation where preterm birth is anticipated, a single short course of corticosteroids should be administered to promote fetal lung maturity. Such therapy has been demonstrated to reduce the frequency of respiratory distress syndrome, intracranial hemorrhage, and even death in preterm infants. Betamethasone, 12 mg intramuscularly repeated once 24 hours later, or dexamethasone, 6 mg intramuscularly repeated every 12 hours for four doses, both cross the placenta and are the preferred treatments in this setting. Repeat courses are not recommended. Although antibiotics have not been proven to forestall delivery, women in preterm labor should receive antimicrobial prophylaxis against group B streptococcus.

C. Tocolytic Agents

Numerous pharmacologic agents—tocolytics—have been given in an attempt to forestall preterm birth, although none are completely effective, and there is no evidence that such therapy directly improves neonatal outcomes. Administering tocolytic agents, however, remains a reasonable approach to the initial management of preterm labor and may provide sufficient prolongation of pregnancy to administer a course of corticosteroids and (if appropriate) transport the patient to a facility better equipped to care for premature infants. Maintenance therapy (continuation of treatment beyond 48 hours) is not effective at preventing preterm birth and is not recommended. Likewise, despite the finding that preterm labor is associated with intrauterine infection in certain cases, there is no evidence that antibiotics forestall delivery in women with preterm labor and intact membranes.

Magnesium sulfate is commonly used, and there is evidence that it may also be protective against cerebral palsy in infants whose mothers were receiving magnesium infusions at time of birth. Magnesium sulfate is given intravenously as a 4- to 6-g bolus followed by a continuous infusion of 2 g/h. Magnesium levels are not typically checked but should be monitored if there is any concern for toxicity. Magnesium sulfate is entirely cleared by the kidney and must, therefore, be used with caution in women with any degree of kidney disease.

Beta-adrenergic drugs such as **terbutaline** can be given as an intravenous infusion starting at 2.5 mcg/min or as a subcutaneous injection starting at 250 mcg given every 30 minutes. Oral terbutaline is not recommended because of the lack of proven efficacy and concerns about maternal safety. Serious maternal side effects have been reported with the use of terbutaline and include tachycardia, pulmonary edema, arrhythmias, metabolic derangements (such as hyperglycemia and hypokalemia), and even death. Pulmonary edema occurs with increased frequency with concomitant administration of corticosteroids, large volume intravenous fluid infusion, maternal sepsis, or prolonged tocolysis. Because of these safety concerns, the US Food and Drug Administration warns that terbutaline be administered exclusively in a hospital setting and discontinued after 48–72 hours of treatment.

Nifedipine, 20 mg orally every 6 hours, and **indomethacin,** 50 mg orally once then 25 mg orally every 6 hours up to 48 hours, have also been used with limited success. Nifedipine should not be given in conjunction with magnesium sulfate.

Before attempts are made to prevent preterm delivery with tocolytic agents, the patient should be assessed for conditions in which delivery would be indicated. Severe preeclampsia, lethal fetal anomalies, placental abruption, and intrauterine infection are all examples of indications for preterm delivery. In such cases, attempts to forestall delivery would be inappropriate.

▶ **Preterm Birth Prevention**

Strategies aimed at preventing preterm birth in high-risk women—principally those with a history of preterm birth or a shortened cervix (or both)—have focused on the administration of progesterone or progesterone compounds and the use of cervical cerclage. Prospective randomized controlled trials have demonstrated reductions in rates of preterm birth in high-risk women with singleton pregnancies who received progesterone supplementation,

although the optimal preparation, dose, and route of administration (intramuscular injection versus vaginal suppository) are unclear. Although the issue has not been adequately studied, there is also some evidence that progesterone therapy may decrease rates of preterm birth in nulliparous women who are found to have a shortened cervix as measured by transvaginal ultrasound. Universal screening of cervical length, however, is controversial and has not been proven to be cost effective.

There is also evidence that women with a previous spontaneous preterm birth and a shortened cervix (less than 25 mm before 24 weeks gestation) may benefit from placement of a cervical cerclage. The use of cervical cerclage in conjunction with progesterone supplementation has not been adequately studied. In twin and triplet gestations, however, neither progesterone administration nor cervical cerclage placement has been effective at prolonging pregnancy, and these therapies are not recommended in women with multi-fetal pregnancies.

▶ **When to Refer**

- Symptoms of increased pelvic pressure or cramping in high-risk patients.
- Regular uterine contractions.
- Rupture of membranes.
- Vaginal bleeding.

▶ **When to Admit**

- Cervical dilation of 2 cm or more prior to 34 weeks gestation.
- Contractions that cause cervical change.
- Rupture of membranes.

American College of Obstetricians and Gynecologists. ACOG Practice Bulletin No. 127: Management of preterm labor. Obstet Gynecol. 2012 Jun;119(6):1308–17. [Reaffirmed 2014] [PMID: 22617615]

American College of Obstetricians and Gynecologists. ACOG Practice Bulletin No. 130: Prediction and prevention of preterm birth. Obstet Gynecol. 2012 Oct;120(4):964–73. [Reaffirmed 2014] [PMID: 22996126]

Grobman WA et al. Activity restriction among women with a short cervix. Obstet Gynecol. 2013 Jun;121(6):1181–6. [PMID: 23812450]

Grobman WA et al. 17 alpha-hydroxyprogesterone caproate to prevent prematurity in nulliparas with cervical length less than 30 mm. Am J Obstet Gynecol. 2012 Nov;207(5):390.e1–8. [PMID: 23010094]

Iams JD. Clinical practice. Prevention of preterm parturition. N Engl J Med. 2014 Jan 16;370(3):254–61. [PMID: 24428470]

Obstetric Care Consensus No. 3: Periviable birth. Obstet Gynecol. 2015 Nov;126(5):e82–94. [PMID: 26488525]

THIRD-TRIMESTER BLEEDING

Five to 10 percent of women have vaginal bleeding in late pregnancy. The clinician must distinguish between placental causes (placenta previa, placental abruption, vasa previa) and nonplacental causes (labor, infection, disorders of the lower genital tract, systemic disease). The approach to bleeding in late pregnancy depends on the underlying cause, the gestational age at presentation, the degree of blood loss, and the overall status of the mother and her fetus.

▶ Treatment

A. General Measures

The patient should initially be observed closely with continuous fetal monitoring to assess for fetal distress. A complete blood count with platelets and a prothrombin time (INR) should be obtained and repeated serially if the bleeding continues. If hemorrhage is significant or if there is evidence of acute hypovolemia, the need for transfusion should be anticipated and an appropriate volume of red cells prepared with cross matching. Ultrasound examination should be performed to determine placental location. Digital pelvic examinations are done only after ultrasound examination has ruled out placenta previa. Administration of anti-D immune globulin may be required for women who are Rh negative.

B. Placenta Previa

Placenta previa occurs when the placenta implants over the internal cervical os. Risk factors for this condition include previous cesarean delivery, increasing maternal age, multiparity, and smoking. If the diagnosis is initially made in the first or second trimester, the ultrasound should be repeated in the third trimester. Persistence of placenta previa at this point is an indication for cesarean as the route of delivery. Painless vaginal bleeding is the characteristic symptom in placenta previa and can range from light spotting to profuse hemorrhage. Hospitalization for extended evaluation is the appropriate initial management approach. For pregnancies that have reached 37 weeks gestation or beyond with continued bleeding, delivery is generally indicated. Pregnancies at 36 weeks or earlier are candidates for expectant management provided the bleeding is not prodigious, and a subset of these women can be discharged if the bleeding and contractions completely subside.

C. Morbidly Adherent Placenta

Morbidly adherent placenta is a general term describing an abnormally adherent placenta that has invaded into the uterus. The condition can be further classified depending on whether the depth of invasion is limited to the endometrium (*accreta*), extends into the myometrium (*increta*), or invades beyond the uterine serosa (*percreta*). The most important risk factor for a morbidly adherent placenta is a prior uterine scar—typically from one or more prior cesarean deliveries. The focus of invasion usually involves the scar itself, and *placenta previa* is commonly associated with morbid adherence. Of serious concern for the field of obstetrics, the incidence of these syndromes has increased dramatically over the last 50 years commensurate with the increasing cesarean delivery rate.

After delivery of the infant, the morbidly adherent placenta does not separate normally, and the bleeding that results can be torrential. Emergency hysterectomy is usually required to stop the hemorrhage, and transfusion requirements are often massive. Because of the considerable increase in both maternal morbidity and mortality associated with this condition, careful preoperative planning is imperative when the diagnosis is suspected antenatally. Ultrasound findings such as intraplacental lacunae, bridging vessels into the bladder, and loss of the retroplacental clear space suggest placental invasion in women who have placenta previa. *Importantly, however, even if ultrasound findings are subtle, an abnormally adherent placenta should be suspected in any patient with one or more prior cesarean deliveries and an anterior placenta previa.* Ideally, delivery planning should involve a multidisciplinary team, and the surgery should take place at an institution with appropriate personnel and a blood bank equipped to handle patients requiring massive transfusion. It has been demonstrated that a systematic approach to management with a multidisciplinary team improves patient outcomes. Evidence-based recommendations regarding delivery timing are lacking, but the goal is to have a planned, late-preterm cesarean delivery. As such, delivery at 34–36 weeks in a stable patient seems a reasonable approach.

D. Placental Abruption

Placental abruption is the premature separation of the placenta from its implantation site before delivery. Hypertension is a known risk factor for abruption. Other risk factors include multiparity, cocaine use, smoking, previous abruption, and thrombophilias. Classic symptoms are vaginal bleeding, uterine tenderness, and frequent contractions, but the clinical presentation is highly variable. Profound coagulopathy and acute hypovolemia from blood loss can occur and are more likely with an abruption severe enough to kill the fetus. Ultrasound may be helpful to exclude placenta previa, but failure to identify a retroplacental clot does not exclude abruption. In most cases, abruption is an indication for immediate delivery because of the high risk of fetal death.

American College of Obstetricians and Gynecologists. Committee Opinion No. 529: Placenta accreta. Obstet Gynecol. 2012 Jul;120(1):207–11. [Reaffirmed 2014] [PMID: 22914422]

Shamshirsaz AA et al. Maternal morbidity in patients with morbidly adherent placenta treated with and without a standardized multidisciplinary approach. Am J Obstet Gynecol. 2015 Feb;212(2):218.e1-9. [PMID: 25173187]

Silver RM. Abnormal placentation: placenta previa, vasa previa, and placenta accreta. Obstet Gynecol. 2015 Sep;126(3): 654–68. [PMID: 26244528]

▼ OBSTETRIC COMPLICATIONS OF THE PERIPARTUM PERIOD

PUERPERAL MASTITIS (See also Chapter 17)

Postpartum mastitis occurs sporadically in nursing mothers, usually with symptom onset after discharge from the hospital. *Staphylococcus aureus* is usually the causative agent. Women nursing for the first time and those with difficulty breastfeeding appear to be at greatest risk. Rarely, inflammatory carcinoma of the breast can be mistaken for puerperal mastitis. Unfortunately, strategies aimed at preventing mastitis in breastfeeding women have been unsuccessful.

Mastitis frequently begins within 3 months after delivery and may start with an engorged breast and a sore or fissured nipple. Cellulitis is typically unilateral with the affected area of breast being red, tender, and warm. Fever and chills are common complaints as well. Treatment consists of antibiotics effective against penicillin-resistant staphylococci (dicloxacillin 500 mg orally every 6 hours or a cephalosporin for 10–14 days) and regular emptying of the breast by nursing or by using a mechanical suction device. Although nursing of the infected breast is safe for the infant, local inflammation of the nipple may complicate latching. Failure to respond to usual antibiotics within 3 days may represent an organizing abscess or infection with a resistant organism. When the causative organism is methicillin-resistant *S aureus* (MRSA), the risk for abscess formation is increased when compared with infection caused by nonresistant staphylococcal species. If an abscess is suspected, ultrasound of the breast can help confirm the diagnosis. In these cases, aspiration or surgical evacuation is usually required.

Crepinsek MA et al. Interventions for preventing mastitis after childbirth. Cochrane Database Syst Rev. 2012 Oct 17;10: CD007239. [PMID: 23076933]
Dixon JM et al. Treatment of breast infection. BMJ. 2011 Feb 11; 342:d396. [PMID: 21317199]

CHORIOAMNIONITIS & METRITIS

ESSENTIALS OF DIAGNOSIS

▶ Fever not attributable to another source.

▶ Uterine tenderness.

▶ Tachycardia in the mother, fetus, or both.

▶ General Considerations

Pelvic infections are relatively common problems encountered during the peripartum period. Uterine infections diagnosed during pregnancy are referred to as chorioamnionitis—a generalized infection of all of the contents of the gravid uterus. Uterine infection after delivery is often called endometritis or endomyometritis, but the term "metritis" is probably most accurate to emphasize that the infection extends throughout the uterine tissue. These infections are polymicrobial and are most commonly attributed to urogenital pathogens. The single most important risk factor for puerperal infection is cesarean delivery, which increases the risk from 5- to 20-fold. Other recognized risk factors include prolonged labor, use of internal monitors, nulliparity, multiple pelvic examinations, prolonged rupture of membranes, and lower genital tract infections. Although maternal complications such as dysfunctional labor and

postpartum hemorrhage are increased with clinical chorioamnionitis, the principal reason to initiate treatment is to prevent morbidity in the offspring. Neonatal complications such as sepsis, pneumonia, intraventricular hemorrhage, and cerebral palsy are increased in the setting of chorioamnionitis. Intrapartum initiation of antibiotics, however, significantly reduces neonatal morbidity.

▶ Clinical Findings

Puerperal infections are diagnosed principally by the presence of **fever** (38°C or higher) in the absence of any other source and one or more of the following signs: maternal or fetal tachycardia (or both), and uterine tenderness. Foul-smelling lochia may be present but is an insensitive marker of infection as many women without infection also experience an unpleasant odor. Likewise, some life-threatening infections such as necrotizing fasciitis are typically odorless. Cultures are typically not done because of the polymicrobial nature of the infection.

▶ Treatment

Treatment is empiric with broad-spectrum antibiotics that will cover gram-positive and gram-negative organisms if still pregnant and gram-negative organisms and anaerobes if postpartum. A common regimen for chorioamnionitis is ampicillin, 2 g intravenously every 6 hours, and gentamicin, 2 mg/kg intravenous load then 1.5 mg/kg intravenously every 8 hours. A common regimen for metritis is gentamicin, 2 mg/kg intravenous load then 1.5 mg/kg intravenously every 8 hours, and clindamycin, 900 mg intravenously every 8 hours. Antibiotics are stopped in the mother when she has been afebrile for 24 hours. No oral antibiotics are subsequently needed. Patients with metritis who do not respond in the first 24–48 hours may have enterococcus and require additional gram-positive coverage (such as ampicillin) to the regimen.

Conroy K et al. Infectious morbidity after cesarean delivery: 10 strategies to reduce risk. Rev Obstet Gynecol. 2012;5(2):69–77. [PMID: 22866185]
Martinelli P et al. Chorioamnionitis and prematurity: a critical review. J Matern Fetal Neonatal Med. 2012 Oct;25(Suppl 4): 29–31. [PMID: 22958008]

MEDICAL CONDITIONS COMPLICATING PREGNANCY

ANEMIA

Normal pregnancy is characterized by an increase in maternal plasma volume of about 50% and an increase in red cell volume of about 25%. Because of these changes, the mean hemoglobin and hematocrit values are lower than in the nonpregnant state. Anemia in pregnancy is considered when the hemoglobin measurement is below 11 g/dL. By far, the most common causes are iron deficiency and acute blood loss anemia, the latter usually occurring in the peripartum period. Symptoms such as fatigue and dyspnea that would otherwise suggest the presence of anemia in nonpregnant women are common in pregnant women; therefore, periodic measurement of CBCs in pregnancy is essential so that anemia can be identified and treated. In addition to its impact on maternal health, untoward pregnancy outcomes such as low birthweight and preterm delivery have been associated with second- and third-trimester anemia.

A. Iron Deficiency Anemia

The increased requirement for iron over the course of pregnancy is appreciable in order to support fetal growth and expansion of maternal blood volume. Dietary intake of iron is generally insufficient to meet this demand, and it is recommended that all pregnant women receive about 30 mg of elemental iron per day in the second and third trimesters. Oral iron therapy is commonly associated with gastrointestinal side effects, such as nausea and constipation, and these symptoms often contribute to noncompliance. If supplementation is inadequate, however, anemia often becomes evident by the third trimester of pregnancy. Because iron deficiency is by far the most common cause of anemia in pregnancy, treatment is usually empiric and consists of 60–100 mg of elemental iron per day and a diet containing iron-rich foods. Iron studies can confirm the diagnosis if necessary (see Chapter 13), and further evaluation should be considered in patients who do not respond to oral iron. Intermittent iron supplementation (eg, every other day) has been associated with fewer side effects and may be reasonable for women who cannot tolerate daily therapy.

B. Folic Acid Deficiency Anemia

Megaloblastic anemia in pregnancy is almost always caused by folic acid deficiency, since vitamin B_{12} deficiency is extremely uncommon in the childbearing years. Folate deficiency is usually caused by inadequate dietary intake of fresh leafy vegetables, legumes, and animal proteins.

The diagnosis is made by finding macrocytic red cells and hypersegmented neutrophils on a blood smear (see Chapter 13). However, blood smears in pregnancy may be difficult to interpret, since they frequently show iron deficiency changes as well. With established folate deficiency, a supplemental dose of 1 mg/day and a diet with increased folic acid is generally sufficient to correct the anemia.

C. Sickle Cell Anemia

Women with sickle cell anemia are subject to serious complications in pregnancy. The anemia becomes more severe, and acute pain crises often occur more frequently. When compared with women who do not have hemoglobinopathies, women with hemoglobin SS are at increased risk for infections (especially pulmonary and urinary tract), thromboembolic events, pregnancy-related hypertension, transfusion, cesarean delivery, preterm birth, and fetal growth restriction. There also continues to be an increased rate of maternal mortality, despite an increased recognition of the high-risk nature of these pregnancies. Intensive medical treatment may improve the outcomes for both mother and fetus. Prophylactically transfusing packed red

cells to lower the level of hemoglobin S and elevate the level of hemoglobin A is a controversial practice without clear benefit. Most women with sickle cell disease will not require iron supplementation, but folate requirements can be appreciable due to red cell turnover from hemolysis.

D. Other Anemias

Although many of the inherited or acquired causes of anemia are relatively rare in women of childbearing age, they can be encountered in pregnancy. The implications for the mother and her offspring vary widely depending on the etiology of anemia. For example, mild microcytic anemia may be caused by iron deficiency, but it could also represent anemia of chronic disease as a result of previously undiagnosed malignancy. As such, women who have anemia caused by a disorder besides a nutritional deficiency are best managed in conjunction with a maternal fetal medicine specialist and a hematologist. Additionally, women who have an inherited form of anemia (hemoglobinopathies and thalassemia syndromes, for example) should be offered genetic counseling; prenatal diagnosis, if available, should be discussed if the parents wish to know whether the fetus is affected.

American College of Obstetricians and Gynecologists. ACOG Practice Bulletin No. 95: Anemia in pregnancy. Obstet Gynecol. 2008 Jul;112(1):201–7. [Reaffirmed 2015] [PMID: 18591330]

Boulet SL et al. Sickle cell disease in pregnancy: maternal complications in a Medicaid-enrolled population. Matern Child Health J. 2013 Feb;17(2):200–7. [PMID: 23315242]

Kumar KJ et al. Maternal anemia in various trimesters and its effect on newborn weight and maturity: an observational study. Int J Prev Med. 2013 Feb;4(2):193–9. [PMID: 23543625]

ANTIPHOSPHOLIPID SYNDROME

(See also Chapter 20.)

The antiphospholipid syndrome (APS) is characterized by the presence of specific autoantibodies in association with certain clinical conditions, most notably arterial and venous thrombosis and adverse pregnancy outcomes. Clinically, the diagnosis can be suspected after any of the following outcomes: an episode of thrombosis, three or more unexplained consecutive spontaneous abortions prior to 10 weeks gestation, one or more unexplained deaths of a morphologically normal fetus after 10 weeks gestation, or a preterm delivery at less than 34 weeks due to preeclampsia or placental insufficiency. In addition to these clinical features, laboratory criteria include the identification of at least one of the following antiphospholipid antibodies: the lupus anticoagulant, anticardiolipin antibodies, or anti-beta-2-glycoprotein I antibodies. The lupus anticoagulant cannot be directly assayed, but it is tested for in several different phospholipid-dependent clotting tests and is interpreted as either present or absent. Anticardiolipin antibodies may be detected with enzyme-linked immunosorbent assay (ELISA) testing but should be considered diagnostic only when the IgG or IgM isotypes are present in medium to high titer (40 GPL or MPL, respectively). Likewise, anti-beta-2-glycoprotein I antibodies are detected with ELISA but should only be considered positive when they are present in a titer that is greater than 99th percentile for a normal population. The diagnosis of APS requires two positive antiphospholipid antibody test results at least 12 weeks apart since transient positive results can occur.

The optimal treatment for APS in pregnancy is unclear but generally involves administration of a heparin compound and low-dose aspirin (81 mg). Although anticoagulation is particularly prudent in women with a history of thrombosis, there is also evidence that this management reduces the risk for spontaneous abortion in women with recurrent pregnancy loss from APS. It is not clear whether continuation of therapy beyond the first trimester decreases the risk for stillbirth or placental dysfunction; however, treatment is typically continued through pregnancy and the early postpartum period for thromboprophylaxis. LMWH is also commonly used for this indication; however, it is not clear that LMWH has the same effect on reducing the risk of recurrent abortion as unfractionated heparin. Either prophylactic or therapeutic dosing strategies may be appropriate depending on the patient's history and clinical risk factors. The use of corticosteroids and intravenous immunoglobulin is of unclear benefit in these patients, and neither treatment is recommended.

ACOG Committee on Practice Bulletins—Obstetrics. ACOG Practice Bulletin No. 132: Antiphospholipid syndrome. Obstet Gynecol. 2012 Dec;120(6):1514–21. [Reaffirmed 2015] [PMID: 23168789]
de Jesus GR et al. 14th International Congress on Antiphospholipid Antibodies Task Force report on obstetric antiphospholipid syndrome. Autoimmun Rev. 2014 Aug;13(8):795–813. [PMID: 24650941]

THYROID DISEASE

Thyroid disease is relatively common in pregnancy, and in their overt states, both hypothyroidism and hyperthyroidism have been consistently associated with adverse pregnancy outcomes. Fortunately, these risks are mitigated by adequate treatment. It is essential to understand the gestational age-specific effects that pregnancy has on thyroid function tests, since these biochemical markers are required to make the diagnosis of thyroid dysfunction. Failure to recognize these physiologic alterations can result in misclassification or misdiagnosis. Women who have a history of a thyroid disorder or symptoms that suggest thyroid dysfunction should be screened with thyroid function tests. Screening asymptomatic pregnant women, however, is of unproven benefit and is not currently recommended.

Overt hypothyroidism is defined by an elevated serum TSH level with a depressed FT_4 level. The condition in pregnancy has consistently been associated with an increase in complications such as spontaneous abortion, preterm birth, preeclampsia, placental abruption, and impaired neuropsychological development in the offspring. The most common etiology is Hashimoto (autoimmune) thyroiditis. Many of the symptoms of hypothyroidism mimic those of normal pregnancy, making its clinical identification difficult. Initial treatment is empiric with oral

levothyroxine started at 75–100 mcg/day. Thyroid function tests can be repeated at 4–6 weeks and the dose adjusted as necessary with the goal of normalizing the TSH level (preferably to a trimester-specific gestational reference range). An increase in the dose of levothyroxine may be required in the second and third trimesters.

Subclinical hypothyroidism is defined as an increased serum TSH with a normal FT_4 level. Although some studies have found associations with untoward pregnancy outcomes such as miscarriage, preterm birth, and preeclampsia, others have failed to confirm these findings. There is currently no evidence, however, that identification and treatment of subclinical hypothyroidism will prevent any of these outcomes. Early observational studies also suggested that cognitive function was impaired in offspring of women with untreated subclinical hypothyroidism. Data from a more recent randomized, controlled trial, however, demonstrated no improvement in cognitive function of 3-year-olds born to women screened and treated for subclinical hypothyroidism. For these reasons, the American College of Obstetricians and Gynecologists and the American Association of Clinical Endocrinologists recommend against universal screening for thyroid disease in pregnancy.

Overt hyperthyroidism, defined as excessive production of thyroxine with a depressed (usually undetectable) serum TSH level, is also associated with increased risks in pregnancy. Spontaneous abortion, preterm birth, preeclampsia, and maternal heart failure occur with increased frequency with untreated thyrotoxicosis. Thyroid storm, although rare, can be a life-threatening complication. Medical treatment of thyrotoxicosis is usually accomplished with the antithyroid drugs propylthiouracil or methimazole. Although teratogenicity has not been clearly established, in utero exposure to methimazole has been associated with aplasia cutis and choanal and esophageal atresia in the offspring of pregnancies so treated. Propylthiouracil is not believed to be teratogenic, but it has been associated with the rare complications of hepatotoxicity and agranulocytosis. Recommendations by the American Thyroid Association are to treat with propylthiouracil in the first trimester and convert to methimazole for the remainder of the pregnancy. The therapeutic target for the FT_4 level is the upper limit of the normal reference range. The TSH levels generally stay suppressed even with adequate treatment. A beta-blocker can be used for such symptoms as palpitations or tremors. Fetal hypothyroidism or hyperthyroidism is uncommon but can occur with maternal Graves disease, which is the most common cause of hyperthyroidism in pregnancy. Radioiodine ablation is absolutely contraindicated in pregnancy because it may destroy the fetal thyroid as well.

Transient autoimmune thyroiditis can occur in the postpartum period and is evident within the first year after delivery. The first phase, occurring up to 4 months postpartum, is a hyperthyroid state. Over the next few months, there is a transition to a hypothyroid state, which may require treatment with levothyroxine. Spontaneous resolution to a euthyroid state within the first year is the expected course; however, some women remain hypothyroid beyond this time (see Chapter 26).

American College of Obstetricians and Gynecologists. Practice Bulletin No. 148: Thyroid disease in pregnancy. Obstet Gynecol. 2015 Apr;125(4):996–1005. [PMID: 25798985]

De Groot L et al. Management of thyroid dysfunction during pregnancy and postpartum: an Endocrine Society clinical practice guideline. J Clin Endocrinol Metab. 2012 Aug;97(8): 2543–65. [PMID: 22869843]

Lazarus JH et al. Antenatal thyroid screening and childhood cognitive function. N Engl J Med. 2012 Feb 9;366(6):493–501. [PMID: 22316443]

DIABETES MELLITUS

Normal pregnancy can be characterized as a state of increased insulin resistance that helps ensure a steady stream of glucose delivery to the developing fetus. Thus, both mild fasting hypoglycemia and postprandial hyperglycemia are physiologic. These metabolic changes are felt to be hormonally mediated with likely contributions from human placental lactogen, estrogen, and progesterone.

A. Gestational Diabetes Mellitus

Gestational diabetes mellitus is abnormal glucose tolerance in pregnancy and is generally believed to be an exaggeration of the pregnancy-induced physiologic changes in carbohydrate metabolism. Alternatively, pregnancy may unmask an underlying propensity for glucose intolerance, which will be evident in the nonpregnant state at some future time if not in the immediate postpartum period. Indeed, at least 50% of women with gestational diabetes are diagnosed with overt diabetes at some point in their lifetime. During the pregnancy, the principal concern in women identified to have gestational diabetes is excessive fetal growth, which can result in increased maternal and perinatal morbidity. Shoulder dystocia occurs more frequently in infants of diabetic mothers because of fetal overgrowth and increased fat deposition on the shoulders. Cesarean delivery and preeclampsia are also significantly increased in women with diabetes, both gestational and overt.

All asymptomatic pregnant women should undergo laboratory screening for gestational diabetes after 24 weeks gestation. The diagnostic thresholds for glucose tolerance tests in pregnancy are not universally agreed upon, and importantly, adverse pregnancy outcomes appear to occur along a continuum of glucose intolerance even if the diagnosis of gestational diabetes is not formally assigned. A two-stage testing strategy is recommended by the American College of Obstetricians and Gynecologists, starting with a 50-g screening test offered to all pregnant women at 24–28 weeks gestation. If this test is abnormal, the diagnostic test is a 100-g oral glucose tolerance test (Table 19–4).

Women in whom gestational diabetes is diagnosed should undergo nutrition counseling, and medications are typically initiated for those with persistent fasting hyperglycemia. Insulin has historically been considered the standard medication used to achieve glycemic control; however, oral medications appear to be equivalent in efficacy, and either are appropriate first-line therapy. Insulin regimens commonly include multiple daily injections of a split dose mix of intermediate-acting and short-acting

Table 19–4. Screening and diagnostic criteria for gestational diabetes mellitus.

Screening for gestational diabetes mellitus
1. 50-g oral glucose load, administered between 24 and 28 weeks, without regard to time of day or time of last meal. Universal blood glucose screening is indicated for all women.
2. Venous plasma glucose measured 1 hour later.
3. Value of 140 mg/dL (7.8 mmol/L) or above in venous plasma indicates the need for a diagnostic glucose tolerance test.

Diagnosis of gestational diabetes mellitus
1. 100-g oral glucose load, administered in the morning after overnight fast lasting at least 8 hours but not more than 14 hours, and following at least 3 days of unrestricted diet (> 150 g carbohydrate) and physical activity.
2. Venous plasma glucose is measured fasting and at 1, 2, and 3 hours. Subject should remain seated and should not smoke throughout the test.
3. The diagnosis of gestational diabetes is made when two or more of the following venous plasma concentrations are met or exceeded: fasting, 95 mg/dL (5.3 mmol/L); 1 hour, 180 mg/dL (10 mmol/L); 2 hours, 155 mg/dL (8.6 mmol/L); 3 hours, 140 mg/dL (7.8 mmol/L).

agents. Although regular and NPH insulins have been used most commonly, newer analogs—including insulin lispro and aspart—have been used in pregnancy and do not cross the placenta. Oral hypoglycemic agents, principally glyburide and metformin, have been evaluated in clinical trials and appear to achieve similar degrees of glycemic control without increasing maternal or neonatal outcomes. These medications, however, have not been approved by the US Food and Drug Administration for this indication, and the long-term safety of oral agents has not been adequately studied in the women so treated or in their offspring. Once therapy is initiated, blood glucose surveillance is important to assess for adequacy of glycemic control. Capillary blood glucose levels should be checked four times per day, once fasting and three times after meals. Euglycemia is considered to be 60–90 mg/dL (3.3–5.0 mmol/L) while fasting and less than 120 mg/dL (6.7 mmol/L) 2 hours postprandially. Intensive therapy with dietary modifications or insulin therapy, or both, has been demonstrated to decrease rates of macrosomia, shoulder dystocia, and preeclampsia. Because of the increased prevalence of overt diabetes in women identified to have gestational diabetes, they should be screened at 6–12 weeks postpartum with a fasting plasma glucose test or a 2-hour oral glucose tolerance test (75-g glucose load).

B. Overt Diabetes Mellitus

Overt diabetes is diabetes mellitus that antedates the pregnancy. As in gestational diabetes, fetal overgrowth from inadequately controlled hyperglycemia remains a significant concern because of the increased maternal and perinatal morbidity that accompany macrosomia. Women with overt diabetes are subject to a number of other complications as well. Spontaneous abortions and third trimester stillbirths occur with increased frequency in these women. There is also at least a twofold to threefold increased risk for fetal malformations, as hyperglycemia during organogenesis is teratogenic. The most common malformations in offspring of diabetic women are cardiac, skeletal, and neural tube defects. For the mother, the likelihood of infections and pregnancy-related hypertension is increased.

Preconception counseling and evaluation in a diabetic woman is ideal to maximize the pregnancy outcomes. This provides an opportunity to optimize glycemic control and evaluate for evidence of end-organ damage. The initial evaluation of diabetic women should include a complete chemistry panel, HbA$_{1c}$ determination, 24-hour urine collection for total protein and creatinine clearance, funduscopic examination, and an ECG. Hypertension is common and may require treatment. Optimally, euglycemia should be established before conception and maintained during pregnancy with daily home glucose monitoring by the patient. There is an inverse relationship between glycemic control and the occurrence of fetal malformations, and women whose periconceptional glycosylated hemoglobin levels are at or near normal levels have rates of malformations that approach baseline. A well-planned dietary program is a key component, with an intake of 1800–2200 kcal/day divided into three meals and three snacks. Insulin is given subcutaneously in a split-dose regimen as described above for women with gestational diabetes. The use of continuous insulin pump therapy may be helpful for some patients.

Throughout the pregnancy, diabetic women should be seen every 2–3 weeks and more frequently depending on the clinical condition. Adjustments in the insulin regimen may be necessary as the pregnancy progresses to maintain optimal glycemic control. A specialized ultrasound is often performed around 20 weeks to screen for fetal malformations. Symptoms and signs of infections should be evaluated and promptly treated. In the third trimester, fetal surveillance is indicated, and women with diabetes should receive serial antenatal testing (usually in the form of a nonstress test or biophysical profile). The timing of delivery is dictated by the quality of diabetic control, the presence or absence of medical complications, and fetal status. The goal is to reach 39 weeks (38 completed weeks) and then proceed with delivery. Confirmation of lung maturity may be appropriate if preterm delivery is contemplated.

ACOG Committee on Practice Bulletins—Obstetrics. Practice Bulletin No. 137: Gestational diabetes mellitus. Obstet Gynecol. 2013 Aug;122(2 Pt 1):406–16. [PMID: 23969827]

Moyer VA et al. Screening for gestational diabetes mellitus: U.S. Preventive Services Task Force recommendation statement. Ann Intern Med. 2014 Mar 18;160(6):414–20. [PMID: 24424622]

Wahabi HA et al. Pre-pregnancy care for women with pregestational diabetes mellitus: a systematic review and meta-analysis. BMC Public Health. 2012 Sep 17;12:792. [PMID: 22978747]

CHRONIC HYPERTENSION

Chronic hypertension is estimated to complicate up to 5% of pregnancies. To establish this diagnosis, hypertension should antedate the pregnancy or be evident before 20 weeks gestation to differentiate it from pregnancy-related hypertension. This distinction can be problematic when the initial presentation is after 20 weeks, but chronic hypertension is confirmed if the blood pressure remains elevated beyond 12 weeks postpartum. Risk factors for chronic hypertension include older maternal age, African American race, and obesity. While essential hypertension is by far the most common cause, secondary causes should be sought when clinically indicated.

Women with chronic hypertension are at increased risk for adverse maternal and perinatal outcomes. Superimposed preeclampsia develops in up to 20% of women with mild hypertension, but the risk increases up to 50% when there is severe baseline hypertension (160/110 mm Hg or higher) and may be even higher when there is evidence of end-organ damage. When preeclampsia is superimposed on chronic hypertension, there is a tendency for it to occur at an earlier gestational age, be more severe, and impair fetal growth. Women with chronic hypertension are also at increased risk for placental abruption, cesarean delivery, preterm birth, and perinatal mortality.

Ideally, women with chronic hypertension should undergo a preconceptional evaluation to detect end-organ damage, assess the need for antihypertensive therapy, and discontinue teratogenic medications. The specific tests ordered may vary depending on the severity of the hypertensive disorder, but an evaluation of renal and cardiac function is appropriate.

If the woman is not known to have chronic hypertension, then initiation of antihypertensive therapy in pregnant women is indicated only if the blood pressure is sustained at or above 160/105 mm Hg or if there is evidence of end-organ damage. Treatment of hypertension has not been demonstrated to improve pregnancy outcomes, but it is indicated in women with significant hypertension for long-term maternal cardiovascular health. Although methyldopa has the longest record of safety in pregnancy, nifedipine and labetalol are also acceptable, and these three agents are recommended above all others when initiating therapy in pregnancy. Care must be taken not to excessively reduce the blood pressure, as this may decrease uteroplacental perfusion. The goal is a modest reduction in blood pressure and avoidance of severe hypertension.

If a woman with mild chronic hypertension is stable on a medical regimen when she becomes pregnant, it is usually appropriate to continue this therapy, although the benefits of doing so are not well established. Angiotensin-converting enzyme (ACE) inhibitors and angiotensin receptor blockers, however, are contraindicated in all trimesters of pregnancy. These medications are teratogenic in the first trimester and cause fetal hypocalvaria and acute kidney injury in the second and third trimesters.

When there is sustained severe hypertension despite multiple medications or significant end-organ damage from hypertensive disease, pregnancy is not likely to be tolerated well. In these situations, therapeutic abortion may be appropriate. If the pregnancy is continued, the woman must be counseled that the maternal and perinatal risks are appreciable, and complications such as superimposed preeclampsia and fetal growth restriction should be anticipated.

Abalos E et al. Antihypertensive drug therapy for mild to moderate hypertension during pregnancy. Cochrane Database Syst Rev. 2014 Feb 6;2:CD002252. [PMID: 24504933]

American College of Obstetricians and Gynecologists; Task Force on Hypertension in Pregnancy. Hypertension in pregnancy. Obstet Gynecol. 2013 Nov;122(5):1122–31. [PMID: 24150027]

Bramham K et al. Chronic hypertension and pregnancy outcomes: systematic review and meta-analysis. BMJ. 2014 Apr 15; 348:g2301. [PMID: 24735917]

HEART DISEASE

Normal pregnancy physiology is characterized by cardiovascular adaptations in the mother. Cardiac output increases markedly as a result of both augmented stroke volume and an increase in the resting heart rate, and the maternal blood volume expands by up to 50%. These changes may not be tolerated well in women with functional or structural abnormalities of the heart. Thus, although only a small number of pregnancies are complicated by cardiac disease, these contribute disproportionately to overall rates of maternal morbidity and mortality. Most cardiac disease in women of childbearing age in the United States is caused by congenital heart disease. Ischemic heart disease, however, is being seen more commonly in pregnant women due to increasing rates of comorbid conditions, such as diabetes mellitus, hypertension, and obesity.

For practical purposes, the best single measurement of cardiopulmonary status is defined by the New York Heart Association Functional Classification. Most pregnant women with cardiac disease have class I or II functional disability, and although good outcomes are generally anticipated in this group, complications such as preeclampsia, preterm birth, and low birth weight appear to occur with increased frequency. Women with more severe disability (class III or IV) are rare in contemporary obstetrics; however, the maternal mortality is markedly increased in this setting and is usually the result of heart failure. Because of these risks, therapeutic abortion for maternal health should be considered in women who are severely disabled from cardiac disease. Specific conditions that have been associated with a particularly high risk for maternal death include Eisenmenger syndrome, primary pulmonary hypertension, Marfan syndrome with aortic root dilatation, and severe aortic or mitral stenosis. In general, these conditions should be considered contraindications to pregnancy.

The importance of preconceptional counseling for women with heart disease cannot be overstated. A thorough evaluation prior to pregnancy provides an opportunity for comprehensive risk assessment and detailed planning. Once pregnant, women with cardiac disease are best treated by a team of practitioners with experience in caring for such patients. Heart failure is the most common cardiovascular complication associated with heart disease in pregnancy, and adverse maternal and fetal outcomes are increased when heart failure occurs. Symptoms of volume overload should therefore be evaluated and treated promptly. Labor management depends on the underlying cardiac lesion and the degree of disability. Cesarean delivery is generally reserved for obstetric indications but may be appropriate for women in whom Valsalva maneuvers are contraindicated. The early postpartum period is a critical time for fluid management. Patients who are predisposed to heart failure should be monitored closely during the puerperium.

Infective endocarditis prophylaxis is not recommended for a vaginal or cesarean delivery in the absence of infection, except in the very small subset of patients at highest risk for adverse outcomes from endocarditis. The women at highest risk include those with cyanotic heart disease, prosthetic valves, or both. If infection is present, such as chorioamnionitis, the underlying infection should be treated with the usual regimen and additional agents are not needed specifically for endocarditis prophylaxis. Prophylaxis, if required, should be given intravenously (see Table 33–6).

Brickner ME. Cardiovascular management in pregnancy: congenital heart disease. Circulation. 2014 Jul 15;130(3):273–82. [PMID: 25024123]

Ruys TP et al. Heart failure in pregnant women with cardiac disease: data from the ROPAC. Heart. 2014 Feb;100(3):231–8. [PMID: 24293523]

ASTHMA

(See also Chapter 9.)

Asthma is one of the most common medical conditions encountered in pregnancy. Women with mild to moderate asthma can generally expect excellent pregnancy outcomes, but severe or poorly controlled asthma has been associated with a number of pregnancy complications, including preterm birth, small-for-gestational-age infants, and preeclampsia. The effects of pregnancy on asthma are likely minimal as asthma severity in the pregnancy has been reported to be similar to its severity during the year preceding the pregnancy. Strategies for treatment are similar to those in nonpregnant women. Patients should be educated about symptom management and avoidance of asthma triggers. Baseline pulmonary function tests can provide an objective assessment of lung function and may help the patient with self-monitoring of her asthma severity using a peak flow meter. As in nonpregnant women, treatment algorithms generally follow a step-wise approach, and commonly used medications, particularly those for mild to moderate asthma symptoms, are generally considered safe in pregnancy. Concerns about teratogenicity and medication effects on the fetus should be thoroughly discussed with the patient to decrease noncompliance rates. Inhaled beta-2-agonists are indicated for all asthma patients, and low to moderate dose inhaled corticosteroids are added for persistent symptoms when a rescue inhaler alone is inadequate. Systemic corticosteroid administration is reserved for severe exacerbations but should not be withheld, if indicated, irrespective of gestational age. The primary goals of management in pregnancy include minimizing symptoms and avoiding hypoxic episodes to the fetus. Prostaglandin F2a and ergonovine—medications frequently used to treat postpartum uterine atony—should be avoided because they can precipitate bronchospasm in women with asthma.

Gregersen TL et al. Safety of bronchodilators and corticosteroids for asthma during pregnancy: what we know and what we need to do better. J Asthma Allergy. 2013 Nov 15;6:117–25. [PMID: 24259987]

McCallister JW. Asthma in pregnancy: management strategies. Curr Opin Pulm Med. 2013 Jan;19(1):13–7. [PMID: 23154712]

SEIZURE DISORDERS

Epilepsy is one of the most common serious neurologic disorders in pregnant women. Many of the commonly used antiepileptic drugs are known human teratogens. Therefore, the principal objectives in managing pregnancy in epileptic women are achieving adequate control of seizures while minimizing exposure to medications that can cause congenital malformations. Certain women who are contemplating pregnancy and have been seizure-free for 2–5 years may be considered candidates for discontinuation of antiseizure medication prior to pregnancy. For those who continue to require treatment, however, therapy with one medication is preferred. Selecting a regimen should be based on the type of seizure disorder and the risks associated with each medication. Valproic acid should not be considered first-line therapy because it has consistently been associated with higher rates of fetal malformations than most other commonly used antiepileptic drugs. Additionally, evidence is accumulating that in utero exposure to valproate may be associated with impaired neurocognitive development in the offspring. Phenytoin and carbamazepine are also older medications that are still used, and both have established patterns of associated fetal malformations. Concerns about teratogenicity have prompted increasing use of the newer antiepileptic drugs such as lamotrigine, topiramate, oxcarbazepine, and levetiracetam. Although the safety of these medications in pregnancy continues to be evaluated, experiences from ongoing registries and large, population-based studies suggest that in utero exposure to the newer antiepileptic drugs in the first trimester of pregnancy carries a lower risk of major malformations than older medications. Although it is recommended that pregnant women with epilepsy be given supplemental folic acid, it is unclear if supplemental folate decreases rates of fetal malformations in women taking anticonvulsant therapy.

Hernández-Díaz S et al; North American AED Pregnancy Registry. Comparative safety of antiepileptic drugs during pregnancy. Neurology. 2012 May 22;78(21):1692–9. [PMID: 22551726]

Meador KJ et al. Developmental effects of antiepileptic drugs and the need for improved regulations. Neurology. 2015 Oct 30. [Epub ahead of print] [PMID: 26519545]

Shallcross R et al; Liverpool and Manchester Neurodevelopment Group; UK Epilepsy and Pregnancy Register. In utero exposure to levetiracetam vs valproate: development and language at 3 years of age. Neurology. 2014 Jan 21;82(3):213–21. [PMID: 24401687]

▼ INFECTIOUS CONDITIONS COMPLICATING PREGNANCY

URINARY TRACT INFECTION

The urinary tract is especially vulnerable to infections during pregnancy because the altered secretions of steroid sex hormones and the pressure exerted by the gravid uterus on the ureters and bladder cause hypotonia and congestion and predispose to urinary stasis. Labor and delivery and urinary retention postpartum also may initiate or aggravate infection. *Escherichia coli* is the offending organism in over two-thirds of cases.

From 2% to 8% of pregnant women have asymptomatic bacteriuria, which some believe to be associated with an increased risk of preterm birth. It is estimated that pyelonephritis will develop in 20–40% of these women if untreated.

An evaluation for asymptomatic bacteriuria at the first prenatal visit is recommended for all pregnant women. If a urine culture is positive, treatment should be initiated. Nitrofurantoin (100 mg orally twice daily), ampicillin (250 mg orally four times daily), and cephalexin (250 mg orally four times daily) are acceptable medications for 4–7 days. Sulfonamides should be avoided in the third trimester because they may interfere with bilirubin binding and thus impose a risk of neonatal hyperbilirubinemia and kernicterus. Fluoroquinolones are also contraindicated because of their potential teratogenic effects on fetal cartilage and bone. Patients with recurrent bacteriuria should receive suppressive medication (once daily dosing of an appropriate antibiotic) for the remainder of the pregnancy. Acute pyelonephritis requires hospitalization for intravenous administration of antibiotics and crystalloids until the patient is afebrile; this is followed by a full course of oral antibiotics.

Glaser AP et al. Urinary tract infection and bacteriuria in pregnancy. Urol Clin North Am. 2015 Nov;42(4):547–60. [PMID: 26475951]

GROUP B STREPTOCOCCAL INFECTION

Group B streptococci frequently colonize the lower female genital tract, with an asymptomatic carriage rate in pregnancy of 10–30%. This rate depends on maternal age, gravidity, and geographic variation. Vaginal carriage is asymptomatic and intermittent, with spontaneous clearing in approximately 30% and recolonization in about 10% of women. Adverse perinatal outcomes associated with group B streptococcal colonization include urinary tract infection, intrauterine infection, premature rupture of membranes, preterm delivery, and postpartum metritis.

Women with postpartum metritis due to infection with group B streptococci, especially after cesarean section, develop fever, tachycardia, and abdominal pain, usually within 24 hours after delivery. Approximately 35% of these women are bacteremic.

Group B streptococcal infection is a common cause of neonatal sepsis. Transmission rates are high, yet the rate of neonatal sepsis is surprisingly low at less than 1:1000 live births. Unfortunately, the mortality rate associated with early-onset disease can be as high as 20–30% in premature infants. In contrast, it is approximately 2–3% in those at term. Moreover, these infections can contribute markedly to chronic morbidity, including mental retardation and neurologic disabilities. Late-onset disease develops through contact with hospital nursery personnel. Up to 45% of these health care workers can carry the bacteria on their skin and transmit the infection to newborns.

CDC recommendations for screening and prophylaxis for group B streptococcal colonization are set forth above (see Essentials of Prenatal Care: Tests and Procedures).

Clifford V et al. Prevention of neonatal group B streptococcus disease in the 21st century. J Paediatr Child Health. 2012 Sep; 48(9):808–15. [PMID: 22151082]
Ohlsson A et al. Intrapartum antibiotics for known maternal Group B streptococcal colonization. Cochrane Database Syst Rev. 2014 Jun 10;6:CD007467. [PMID: 24915629]

VARICELLA

Commonly known as chickenpox, varicella-zoster virus (VZV) infection has a fairly benign course when incurred during childhood but may result in serious illness in adults, particularly during pregnancy. Infection results in lifelong immunity. Approximately 95% of women born in the United States have VZV antibodies by the time they reach reproductive age. The incidence of VZV infection during pregnancy has been reported as up to 7:10,000.

▶ **Clinical Findings**

A. Symptoms and Signs

The incubation period for this infection is 10–20 days. A primary infection follows and is characterized by a flu-like syndrome with malaise, fever, and development of a pruritic maculopapular rash on the trunk, which becomes vesicular and then crusts. Pregnant women are prone to the development of VZV pneumonia, often a fulminant infection sometimes requiring respiratory support. After primary infection, the virus becomes latent, ascending to dorsal root ganglia. Subsequent reactivation can occur as zoster, often under circumstances of immunocompromise, although this is rare during pregnancy.

Two types of fetal infection have been documented. The first is congenital VZV syndrome, which typically occurs in 0.4–2% of fetuses exposed to primary VZV infection during the first trimester. Anomalies include limb and digit abnormalities, microphthalmos, and microcephaly.

Infection during the second and third trimesters is less threatening. Maternal IgG crosses the placenta, protecting the fetus. The only infants at risk for severe infection are those born after maternal viremia but before development of maternal protective antibody. Maternal infection manifesting 5 days before or up to 2 days after delivery is the time period believed to be most hazardous for transmission to the fetus.

B. Laboratory Findings

Diagnosis is commonly made on clinical grounds. Laboratory verification is made by ELISA, fluorescent antibody, and hemagglutination inhibition antibody techniques. Serum obtained by cordocentesis may be tested for VZV IgM to document fetal infection.

▶ **Treatment**

Varicella-zoster immune globulin (VZIG) has been shown to prevent or modify the symptoms of infection in exposed persons. Treatment success depends on identification of susceptible women at or just following exposure. Exposed women with a questionable or negative history of chickenpox should be checked for antibody, since the overwhelming majority will have been previously exposed. If the antibody is negative, VZIG (625 units intramuscularly) should ideally be given within 96 hours of exposure for greatest efficacy, but the CDC reports it can be given for up to 10 days. There are no known adverse effects of VZIG administration during pregnancy, although the incubation period for disease can be lengthened. Infants born to women in whom symptoms develop in the period from 5 days before delivery to 2 days after delivery should also receive VZIG (125 units).

Pregnant women with varicella may benefit from treatment with oral acyclovir if started within 24 hours of rash onset. Treatment has been shown to improve maternal symptoms but does not prevent congenital varicella. Infected pregnant women should be closely observed and hospitalized at the earliest signs of pulmonary involvement. Intravenous acyclovir (10 mg/kg intravenously every 8 hours) is recommended in the treatment of VZV pneumonia.

American College of Obstetricians and Gynecologists. ACOG Practice Bulletin No. 151: Cytomegalovirus, parvovirus B19, varicella zoster, and toxoplasmosis in pregnancy. Obstet Gynecol. 2015 Jun;125(6):1510–25. [PMID: 26000539]
Centers for Disease Control and Prevention (CDC). Updated recommendations for use of VariZIG—United States, 2013. MMWR Morb Mortal Wkly Rep. 2013 July 19;62(28):574–6. [PMID: 23863705]

TUBERCULOSIS

The diagnosis of tuberculosis in pregnancy is made by history taking, physical examination, and testing, with special attention to women in high-risk groups. Women at high risk include those who are from endemic areas, those infected with HIV, drug users, health care workers, and close contacts of people with tuberculosis. Chest radiographs should not be obtained as a routine screening measure in pregnancy but should be used only in patients with a positive test or with suggestive findings in the history and physical examination. Abdominal shielding must be used if a chest radiograph is obtained. Both tuberculin skin testing and interferon gamma release assays are acceptable tests in pregnancy.

Decisions on treatment depend on whether the patient has active disease or is at high risk for progression to active disease. Pregnant women with latent disease not at high risk for disease progression can receive treatment postpartum, which does not preclude breastfeeding. The concentration of medication in breast milk is neither toxic nor adequate for treatment of the newborn. Treatment is with isoniazid and ethambutol or isoniazid and rifampin (see Chapters 9 and 33). Because isoniazid therapy may result in vitamin B_6 deficiency, a supplement of 50 mg/day of vitamin B_6 should be given simultaneously. There is concern that isoniazid, particularly in pregnant women, can cause hepatitis. Liver function tests should be performed regularly in pregnant women who receive treatment. Streptomycin, ethionamide, and most other antituberculous drugs should be avoided in pregnancy. If adequately treated, tuberculosis in pregnancy has an excellent prognosis.

Mathad JS et al. Tuberculosis in pregnant and postpartum women: epidemiology, management, and research gaps. Clin Infect Dis. 2012 Dec;55(11):1532–49. [PMID: 22942202]

Taylor AW et al. Pregnancy outcomes in HIV-infected women receiving long-term isoniazid prophylaxis for tuberculosis and antiretroviral therapy. Infect Dis Obstet Gynecol. 2013;2013:195637. [PMID: 23533318]

HIV/AIDS DURING PREGNANCY

Heterosexual acquisition and injection drug use are the principal identified modes of HIV infection in women. Asymptomatic infection is associated with a normal pregnancy rate and no increased risk of adverse pregnancy outcomes. There is no evidence that pregnancy causes AIDS progression.

Previously, two-thirds of HIV-positive neonates acquired their infection close to, or during, the time of delivery. Routine HIV screening in pregnancy, including the use of rapid HIV tests in Labor and Delivery units, and the use of antiretroviral drugs has markedly reduced this transmission risk to approximately 2%. In an HIV-positive pregnant woman, a CD4 count, plasma RNA level, and resistance testing (if virus is detectable, and the patient has not already had this) should be obtained at the first prenatal visit. Treatment should not be delayed while waiting for the results of resistance testing. Prior or current antiretroviral use should be reviewed. A woman already taking and tolerating an acceptable antiretroviral regimen does not have to discontinue it in the first trimester. Patients should also be tested for hepatitis C, tuberculosis, toxoplasmosis, and cytomegalovirus.

Women not taking medication should be offered combination antiretroviral therapy (commonly a dual nucleoside reverse transcriptase inhibitor combination and a ritonavir-boosted protease inhibitor) after counseling regarding the potential impact of therapy on both mother and fetus. Antiretroviral therapy should be offered regardless of viral load and CD4 count. Whether to start in the first or second trimester should be determined on a case-by-case basis. It can be started in the first trimester after explanation of risks and benefits, provided the mother is not experiencing nausea and vomiting. The majority of drugs used to treat HIV/AIDS have thus far proven to be safe in pregnancy with an acceptable risk/benefit ratio. Efavirenz has been clearly linked with anomalies (myelomeningocele) and should not be used in the first trimester of pregnancy. However, efavirenz does not need to be discontinued if a pregnant patient presents for obstetrical care already taking the drug. Standard of care also includes administration of intravenous zidovudine prior to cesarean delivery and during labor in women whose viral load near delivery is greater than or equal to 1000 copies/mL or unknown. Antiretroviral therapy on the patient's usual schedule should also be continued in labor.

The use of prophylactic elective cesarean section at 38 weeks (before the onset of labor or rupture of the membranes) to prevent vertical transmission of HIV infection from mother to fetus has been shown to further reduce the transmission rate. In patients with a viral load of less than 1000 copies/mL, there may be no additional benefit of cesarean delivery, and those women can be offered a vaginal delivery. Amniotomy should not be performed, and internal monitors, particularly the fetal scalp electrode, should be avoided. Methergine (used for postpartum hemorrhage) should be avoided in patients receiving certain regimens. HIV-infected women should be advised not to breastfeed their infants.

The Public Health Task Force provides guidelines for the management of HIV/AIDS in pregnancy that are regularly updated and available at http://www.aidsinfo.nih.gov/. In addition, there is the National Perinatal HIV Hotline, which provides free consultation regarding perinatal HIV care (1-888-448-8765).

U.S. Department of Health & Human Services Panel on Treatment of HIV-Infected Pregnant Women and Prevention of Perinatal Transmission. Recommendations for use of antiretroviral drugs in pregnant HIV-1 infected women for maternal health and interventions to reduce perinatal HIV transmission in the United States. 2015 Aug 6:1–264. http://aidsinfo.nih.gov/ContentFiles/lvguidelines/PerinatalGL.pdf

MATERNAL HEPATITIS B & C CARRIER STATE (See also Chapter 1)

There are an estimated 350 million chronic carriers of **hepatitis B virus** worldwide. Among these people, there is an increased incidence of chronic active hepatitis, cirrhosis, and hepatocellular carcinoma. In the United States, 1.4 million people are infected, with the highest rate among Asian Americans. All pregnant women should be screened for HBsAg. Transmission of the virus to the baby after delivery is likely if both surface antigen and e antigen are positive. Vertical transmission can be blocked by the immediate postdelivery administration to the newborn of hepatitis B immunoglobulin and hepatitis B vaccine intramuscularly. The vaccine dose is repeated at 1 and 6 months of age. Third trimester administration of lamivudine, telbivudine, or tenofovir to women with a viral load of greater than 10^8 copies/mL has been shown to reduce vertical transmission particularly if the viral load is less than 10^6 copies/mL at delivery. This therapy is safe in pregnancy although long-term follow-up data are lacking. Pregnant women with chronic hepatitis B should have liver function tests and viral load testing during the pregnancy. Hepatitis B infection is not a contraindication to breastfeeding, and antiviral therapy if given does not need to be continued postpartum.

Hepatitis C virus infection is the most common chronic blood-borne infection in the United States. Risk factors for transmission include blood transfusion, injection drug use, employment in patient care or clinical laboratory work, exposure to a sex partner or household member who has had a history of hepatitis, exposure to multiple sex partners, and low socioeconomic level. The average rate of hepatitis C virus (HCV) infection among infants born to HCV-positive, HIV-negative women is

5–6%. However, the average infection rate increases to 15–25% when mothers are coinfected with HCV and HIV. The principal factor associated with transmission is the presence of HCV RNA in the mother at the time of birth. Treatment is not recommended in pregnancy. Interferon and ribavirin have been considered contraindicated. Ledipasvir/sofosbuvir (Harvoni) has been shown to be safe in animal studies, but there are no human studies on safety or efficacy at reducing vertical transmission.

Rac MW et al. Prevention and management of viral hepatitis in pregnancy. Obstet Gynecol Clin North Am. 2014 Dec;41(4):573–92. [PMID: 25454991]
Sarkar M et al. Ending vertical transmission of hepatitis B: the third trimester intervention. Hepatology. 2014 Aug;60(2):448–51. [PMID: 24668789]

HERPES GENITALIS

Infection of the lower genital tract by herpes simplex virus type 2 (HSV-2) (see also Chapter 6) is a common STD with potentially serious consequences to pregnant women and their newborn infants. Although up to 20% of women in an obstetric practice may have antibodies to HSV-2, a history of the infection is unreliable and the incidence of neonatal infection is low (10–60/100,000 live births). Most infected neonates are born to women with no history, symptoms, or signs of infection.

Women who have had *primary* herpes infection late in pregnancy are at high risk for shedding virus at delivery. Some authors suggest use of prophylactic acyclovir, 400 mg orally three times daily, to decrease the likelihood of active lesions at the time of labor and delivery.

Women with a history of *recurrent* genital herpes have a lower neonatal attack rate than women infected during the pregnancy, but they should still be monitored with clinical observation and culture of any suspicious lesions. Since asymptomatic viral shedding is not predictable by antepartum cultures, current recommendations do not include routine cultures in individuals with a history of herpes without active disease. However, when labor begins, vulvar and cervical inspection should be performed. Cesarean delivery is indicated at the time of labor if there are prodromal symptoms or active genital lesions.

For treatment, see Chapter 32. The use of acyclovir in pregnancy is acceptable, and prophylaxis starting at 36 weeks gestation has been shown to decrease the number of cesarean sections performed for active disease.

Pinninti SG et al. Maternal and neonatal herpes simplex virus infections. Am J Perinatol. 2013 Feb;30(2):113–9. [PMID: 23303485]
Stephenson-Famy A et al. Herpes simplex virus infection during pregnancy. Obstet Gynecol Clin North Am. 2014 Dec;41(4):601–14. [PMID: 25454993]

SYPHILIS, GONORRHEA, & C TRACHOMATIS INFECTION (See also Chapters 33 & 34)

These STDs have significant consequences for mother and child. Untreated syphilis in pregnancy can cause late abortion, stillbirth, transplacental infection, and congenital syphilis. Gonorrhea can produce large-joint arthritis by hematogenous spread as well as ophthalmia neonatorum. Maternal chlamydial infections are largely asymptomatic but are manifested in the newborn by inclusion conjunctivitis and, at age 2–4 months, by pneumonia. The diagnosis of each can be reliably made by appropriate laboratory tests. All women should be tested for syphilis and *C trachomatis* as part of their routine prenatal care. Repeat testing is dependent on risk factors, prevalence, and state laws. Women at risk should be tested for gonorrhea. The sexual partners of women with STDs should be identified and treated also if possible; the local health department can assist with this process.

Hawkes SJ et al. Early antenatal care: does it make a difference to outcomes of pregnancy associated with syphilis? A systematic review and meta-analysis. PLoS One. 2013;8(2):e56713. [PMID: 23468875]
Workowski KA et al; Centers for Disease Control and Prevention (CDC). Sexually transmitted diseases treatment guidelines, 2015. MMWR Recomm Rep. 2015 Jun 5;64(RR-03):1–137. [PMID: 26042815]

GASTROINTESTINAL, HEPATIC, & BILIARY DISORDERS OF PREGNANCY

Complications involving the gastrointestinal tract, liver, and gallbladder are common in pregnancy. Nausea and vomiting in the first trimester affect the majority of pregnant women to some degree (see Obstetric Complications of the First & Second Trimesters). Nausea and vomiting in the last half of pregnancy, however, are never normal; a thorough evaluation of such complaints is mandatory. Some of these conditions are incidental to pregnancy (eg, appendicitis), while others are related to the gravid state and tend to resolve with delivery (eg, acute fatty liver of pregnancy). Importantly, the myriad anatomic and physiologic changes associated with normal pregnancy must be considered when assessing for a disease state. Likewise, interpretation of laboratory studies must take into account the pregnancy-associated changes in hepatic protein production.

For conditions in which surgery is clinically indicated, operative intervention should never be withheld based soley on the fact that a woman is pregnant. While purely elective surgery is avoided during pregnancy, women who undergo surgical procedures for an urgent or emergent indication during pregnancy do not appear to be at increased risk for adverse outcomes. Obstetric complications, when they occur, are more likely to be associated with the underlying maternal illness. Recommendations have held that the optimal time for semi-elective surgery is the second trimester to avoid exposure to anesthesia in the first trimester and the enlarged uterus in the third. Importantly, however, there is no convincing evidence that general anesthesia induces malformations or increases the risk for abortion.

CHOLELITHIASIS & CHOLECYSTITIS

Cholelithiasis is common in pregnancy as physiologic changes such as increased cholesterol production and incomplete gallbladder emptying predispose to gallstone formation. The diagnosis is usually suspected based on classic symptoms of nausea, vomiting, and right upper quadrant pain, usually after meals, and is confirmed with right upper quadrant ultrasound. Symptomatic cholelithiasis without cholecystitis is usually managed conservatively, but recurrent symptoms are common. Cholecystitis results from obstruction of the cystic duct and often is accompanied by bacterial infection. Medical management with antibiotics is reasonable in selected cases, but definitive treatment with cholecystectomy will help prevent complications such as gallbladder perforation and pancreatitis. Cholecystectomy has successfully been performed in all trimesters of pregnancy and should not be withheld based on the stage of pregnancy if clinically indicated. Laparoscopy is preferred in the first half of pregnancy but becomes more technically challenging in the last trimester due to the enlarged uterus and cephalad displacement of abdominal contents.

Obstruction of the common bile duct, which can lead to cholangitis, is an indication for surgical removal of gallstones and establishment of biliary drainage. Increasingly, endoscopic retrograde cholangiopancreatography (ERCP) with or without sphincterotomy is being performed in this situation. Pregnant women can safely undergo ERCP provided that precautions are taken to minimize fetal exposure to radiation. There does, however, appear to be a slightly higher rate of post-procedure pancreatitis in pregnant women who undergo ERCP. Magnetic resonance cholangiopancreatography (MRCP) can also be of use in patients with suspected common bile duct obstruction. This study is particularly useful for those women in whom the etiology of common duct dilatation is unclear on ultrasound. MRCP can provide detailed evaluation of the entire biliary system and the pancreas while avoiding ionizing radiation.

Fine S et al. Continued evidence for safety of endoscopic retrograde cholangiopancreatography during pregnancy. World J Gastrointest Endosc. 2014 Aug 16;6(8):352–8. [PMID: 25132918]

ACUTE FATTY LIVER OF PREGNANCY

Acute fatty liver of pregnancy, a disorder limited to the gravid state, occurs in the third trimester of pregnancy and causes acute hepatic failure. With improved recognition and immediate delivery, the maternal mortality rate in contemporary reports is about 4%. The disorder is usually seen after the 35th week of gestation and is more common in primigravidas and those with twins. The incidence is about 1:10,000 deliveries.

The etiology of acute fatty liver of pregnancy is likely poor placental mitochondrial function. Many cases may be due to a homozygous fetal deficiency of long-chain acyl coenzyme A dehydrogenase (LCHAD).

▶ Clinical Findings

Pathologic findings are unique to the disorder, with fatty engorgement of hepatocytes. Clinical onset is gradual, with nausea and vomiting being the most common presenting symptoms. Varying degrees of flu-like symptoms are also typical. Eventually, symptoms progress to those of fulminant hepatic failure: jaundice, encephalopathy, disseminated intravascular coagulation, and death. On examination, the patient shows signs of hepatic failure.

Laboratory findings include marked elevation of alkaline phosphatase but only moderate elevations of alanine aminotransferase (ALT) and aspartate aminotransferase (AST). Hypocholesterolemia and hypofibrinogenemia are typical, and hypoglycemia can be extreme. Coagulopathy is also frequently seen with depressed procoagulant protein production. Renal function should be assessed as well, since hepatorenal syndrome commonly causes acute kidney injury. The white blood cell count is elevated, and the platelet count is depressed.

▶ Differential Diagnosis

The differential diagnosis is that of fulminant hepatitis. Liver aminotransferases for fulminant hepatitis are higher (greater than 1000 units/mL) than those for acute fatty liver of pregnancy (usually 500–1000 units/mL). Preeclampsia may involve the liver but typically does not cause jaundice; the elevations in liver function tests in patients with preeclampsia usually do not reach the levels seen in patients with acute fatty liver of pregnancy.

▶ Treatment

Diagnosis of acute fatty liver of pregnancy mandates immediate delivery. Intensive supportive care with ICU-level observation is essential and typically includes administration of blood products and glucose as well as correction of acidemia. Vaginal delivery is preferred. Resolution of encephalopathy and laboratory derangements occurs over days with supportive care, and recovery is usually complete. Rare cases of liver transplantation have been reported.

Nelson DB et al. Acute fatty liver of pregnancy: clinical outcomes and expected duration of recovery. Am J Obstet Gynecol. 2013 Nov;209(5):456.e1–7. [PMID: 23860212]

INTRAHEPATIC CHOLESTASIS OF PREGNANCY

Intrahepatic cholestasis of pregnancy is characterized by incomplete clearance of bile acids in genetically susceptible women. The principal symptom is pruritus, which can be generalized but tends to have a predilection for the palms and soles. Presentation is typically in the third trimester, and women with multi-fetal pregnancies are at increased risk. The finding of an elevated serum bile acid level, ideally performed in the fasting state, confirms the diagnosis. Associated laboratory derangements include modest elevations in hepatic transaminase levels and mild hyperbilirubinemia. Although rare, the bilirubin level may be sufficiently elevated to result in clinical jaundice. The symptoms and laboratory abnormalities resolve quickly after delivery but can recur in subsequent pregnancies or with exposure to combination oral contraceptives.

Ursodeoxycholic acid (8–10 mg/kg/day) is the treatment of choice and results in decreased pruritus in most women.

Adverse fetal outcomes, particularly preterm birth, nonreassuring fetal status, meconium-stained amniotic fluid, and stillbirth, have consistently been reported in women with cholestasis of pregnancy. The risk for adverse perinatal outcomes appears to correlate with disease severity as measured by the degree of bile acid elevation, and women with fasting bile acids greater than 40 mcmol/L have been reported to be at greatest risk. Because of the risks associated with cholestasis of pregnancy, many clinicians recommend antenatal testing in the third trimester and elective early delivery in attempt to avoid stillbirth. Evidence-based recommendations regarding such management practices, however, are not currently available.

Geenes V et al. Association of severe intrahepatic cholestasis of pregnancy with adverse pregnancy outcomes: a prospective population-based case-control study. Hepatology. 2014 Apr; 59(4):1482–91. [PMID: 23857305]

Williamson C et al. Intrahepatic cholestasis of pregnancy. Obstet Gynecol. 2014 Jul;124(1):120–33. [PMID: 24901263]

APPENDICITIS

Appendicitis occurs in about 1 of 1500 pregnancies. The diagnosis is more difficult to make clinically in pregnant women where the appendix is displaced cephalad from McBurney point. Furthermore, nausea, vomiting, and mild leukocytosis occur in normal pregnancy, so with or without these findings, any complaint of right-sided pain should raise suspicion. Imaging can help confirm the diagnosis if clinical findings are equivocal. Abdominal sonography is a reasonable initial imaging choice, but nonvisualization of the appendix is common in pregnancy. CT scanning is more sensitive than ultrasound, and with proper shielding, the radiation exposure to the fetus is minimized. MRI is also being increasingly used to evaluate for appendicitis in pregnant women and is a reasonable alternative to CT scanning. Unfortunately, the diagnosis of appendicitis is not made until the appendix has ruptured in at least 20% of obstetric patients. Peritonitis in these cases can lead to preterm labor or abortion. With early diagnosis and appendectomy, the prognosis is good for mother and baby.

Cheng HT et al. Laparoscopic appendectomy versus open appendectomy in pregnancy: a population-based analysis of maternal outcome. Surg Endosc. 2015 Jun;29(6):1394–9. [PMID: 25171885]

Dewhurst C et al. MRI evaluation of acute appendicitis in pregnancy. J Magn Reson Imaging. 2013 Mar;37(3):566–75. [PMID: 23423797]

Rheumatologic, Immunologic, & Allergic Disorders

David B. Hellmann, MD, MACP

John B. Imboden Jr., MD

RHEUMATOLOGIC DISORDERS

▶ Diagnosis & Evaluation

A. Examination of the Patient

Two helpful clinical clues for diagnosing arthritis are the **joint pattern and the presence or absence of extra-articular manifestations.** The joint pattern is defined by the answers to three questions: (1) Is inflammation present? (2) How many joints are involved? and (3) What joints are affected? Joint inflammation manifests as warmth, swelling, and morning stiffness of at least 30 minutes' duration. Overlying erythema occurs with the intense inflammation of crystal-induced and septic arthritis. Both the number of affected joints and the specific sites of involvement affect the differential diagnosis (Table 20–1). Some diseases—gout, for example—are characteristically monarticular, whereas other diseases, such as rheumatoid arthritis, are usually polyarticular. The location of joint involvement can also be distinctive. Only two diseases frequently cause prominent involvement of the distal interphalangeal (DIP) joint: osteoarthritis and psoriatic arthritis. Extra-articular manifestations such as fever (eg, gout, Still disease, endocarditis), rash (eg, systemic lupus erythematosus [SLE], psoriatic arthritis, Still disease), nodules (eg, rheumatoid arthritis, gout), or neuropathy (eg, polyarteritis nodosa, granulomatosis with polyangiitis [formerly Wegener granulomatosis]) narrow the differential diagnosis further.

B. Arthrocentesis and Examination of Joint Fluid

If the diagnosis is uncertain, synovial fluid should be examined whenever possible (Table 20–2). Most large joints are easily aspirated, and contraindications to arthrocentesis are few. The aspirating needle should never be passed through an overlying cellulitis or psoriatic plaque because of the risk of introducing infection. For patients who are receiving long-term anticoagulation therapy with warfarin, joints can be aspirated with a small-gauge needle (eg, 22F) if the international normalized ratio (INR) is less than 3.0.

1. Types of studies

A. GROSS EXAMINATION—Clarity is an approximate guide to the degree of inflammation. Noninflammatory fluid is transparent, mild inflammation produces translucent fluid, and purulent effusions are opaque. Bleeding disorders, trauma, and traumatic taps are the most common causes of bloody effusions.

B. CELL COUNT—The synovial fluid white cell count discriminates between **noninflammatory** (less than 2000 white cells/mcL [2.0×10^9/L]), **inflammatory** (2000–75,000 white cells/mcL [2.0×10^9/L–75.0×10^9/L]), and **purulent** (greater than 100,000 white cells/mcL [100×10^9/L]) joint effusions. Synovial fluid glucose and protein levels add little information and should not be ordered.

C. MICROSCOPIC EXAMINATION—Compensated polarized light microscopy identifies and distinguishes monosodium urate (gout, negatively birefringent) and calcium pyrophosphate (pseudogout, positive birefringent) crystals. Gram stain has specificity but limited sensitivity (50%) for septic arthritis.

D. CULTURE—Bacterial cultures as well as special studies for gonococci, tubercle bacilli, or fungi are ordered as appropriate.

2. Interpretation—Synovial fluid analysis is diagnostic in infectious or microcrystalline arthritis. Although the severity of inflammation in synovial fluid can overlap among various conditions, the synovial fluid white cell count is a helpful guide to diagnosis (Table 20–3).

DEGENERATIVE & CRYSTAL-INDUCED ARTHRITIS

DEGENERATIVE JOINT DISEASE (Osteoarthritis)

- ▶ A degenerative disorder with minimal articular inflammation.
- ▶ No systemic symptoms.
- ▶ Pain relieved by rest; morning stiffness brief.
- ▶ Radiographic findings: narrowed joint space, osteophytes, increased density of subchondral bone, bony cysts.

Table 20–1. Diagnostic value of the joint pattern.

Characteristic	Status	Representative Disease
Inflammation	Present	Rheumatoid arthritis, systemic lupus erythematosus, gout
	Absent	Osteoarthritis
Number of involved joints	Monarticular	Gout, trauma, septic arthritis, Lyme disease, osteoarthritis
	Oligoarticular (2–4 joints)	Reactive arthritis, psoriatic arthritis, inflammatory bowel disease
	Polyarticular (≥ 5 joints)	Rheumatoid arthritis, systemic lupus erythematosus
Site of joint involvement	Distal interphalangeal	Osteoarthritis, psoriatic arthritis (not rheumatoid arthritis)
	Metacarpophalangeal, wrists	Rheumatoid arthritis, systemic lupus erythematosus, calcium pyrophosphate deposition disease (not osteoarthritis)
	First metatarsal phalangeal	Gout, osteoarthritis

General Considerations

Osteoarthritis, the most common form of joint disease, is chiefly a disease of aging. Ninety percent of all people have radiographic features of osteoarthritis in weight-bearing joints by age 40. Symptomatic disease also increases with age. Sex is also a risk factor; osteoarthritis develops in women more frequently than in men.

This arthropathy is characterized by degeneration of cartilage and by hypertrophy of bone at the articular margins. Inflammation is usually minimal. Hereditary and mechanical factors may be involved in the pathogenesis.

Obesity is a risk factor for osteoarthritis of the knee, hand, and probably of the hip. Recreational running does not increase the incidence of osteoarthritis, but participation in competitive contact sports does. Jobs requiring frequent bending and carrying increase the risk of knee osteoarthritis (see Chapter 41).

Clinical Findings

A. Symptoms and Signs

Degenerative joint disease is divided into two types: (1) primary, which most commonly affects some or all of the following: the DIP and the proximal interphalangeal (PIP) joints of the fingers, the carpometacarpal joint of the thumb, the hip, the knee, the metatarsophalangeal (MTP) joint of the big toe, and the cervical and lumbar spine; and (2) secondary, which may occur in any joint as a sequela to articular injury resulting from either intra-articular (including rheumatoid arthritis) or extra-articular causes. The injury may be acute, as in a fracture; or chronic, as that due to occupational overuse of a joint, metabolic disease (eg, hyperparathyroidism, hemochromatosis, ochronosis), or neurologic disorders (syringomyelia; see below).

The onset is insidious. Initially, there is articular stiffness, seldom lasting more than 15 minutes; this develops later into pain on motion of the affected joint and is made worse by activity or weight bearing and relieved by rest. Flexion contracture or varus deformity of the knee is not unusual, and bony enlargements of the DIP (Heberden nodes) and PIP (Bouchard nodes) are occasionally prominent (Figure 20–1). There is no ankylosis, but limitation of motion of the affected joint or joints is common. Crepitus may often be felt over the knee. Joint effusion and other articular signs of inflammation are mild. There are no systemic manifestations.

B. Laboratory Findings

Osteoarthritis does not cause elevation of the erythrocyte sedimentation rate (ESR) or other laboratory signs of inflammation. Synovial fluid is noninflammatory.

Table 20–2. Examination of joint fluid.

Measure	(Normal)	Group I (Noninflammatory)	Group II (Inflammatory)	Group III (Purulent)
Volume (mL) (knee)	< 3.5	Often > 3.5	Often > 3.5	Often > 3.5
Clarity	Transparent	Transparent	Translucent to opaque	Opaque
Color	Clear	Yellow	Yellow to opalescent	Yellow to green
WBC (per mcL)	< 200	< 2000	2000–75,000[1]	> 100,000[2]
Polymorphonuclear leukocytes	< 25%	< 25%	50% or more	75% or more
Culture	Negative	Negative	Negative	Usually positive[2]

[1]Gout, rheumatoid arthritis, and other inflammatory conditions occasionally have synovial fluid WBC counts > 75,000/mcL but rarely > 100,000/mcL.
[2]Most purulent effusions are due to septic arthritis. Septic arthritis, however, can present with group II synovial fluid, particularly if infection is caused by organisms of low virulence (eg, *Neisseria gonorrhoeae*) or if antibiotic therapy has been started.
WBC, white blood cell count.

Table 20–3. Differential diagnosis by joint fluid groups.

Group I (Noninflammatory) (< 2000 white cells/mcL)	Group II (Inflammatory) (2000–75,000 white cells/mcL)	Group III (Purulent) (> 100,000 white cells/mcL)	Hemorrhagic
Degenerative joint disease Trauma[1] Osteochondritis dissecans Osteochondromatosis Neuropathic arthropathy[1] Subsiding or early inflammation Hypertrophic osteoarthropathy[2] Pigmented villonodular synovitis[1]	Rheumatoid arthritis Acute crystal-induced synovitis (gout and pseudogout) Reactive arthritis Ankylosing spondylitis Rheumatic fever[2] Tuberculosis	Pyogenic bacterial infections	Hemophilia or other hemorrhagic diathesis Trauma with or without fracture Neuropathic arthropathy Pigmented villonodular synovitis Synovioma Hemangioma and other benign neoplasms

[1]May be hemorrhagic.
[2]Noninflammatory or inflammatory group.
Reproduced, with permission, from Rodnan GP (editor). Primer on the rheumatic diseases, 7th ed. JAMA. 1973;224(Suppl):662. Copyright © 1973 American Medical Association. All rights reserved.

C. Imaging

Radiographs may reveal narrowing of the joint space; osteophyte formation and lipping of marginal bone; and thickened, dense subchondral bone. Bone cysts may also be present.

▶ Differential Diagnosis

Because articular inflammation is minimal and systemic manifestations are absent, degenerative joint disease should seldom be confused with other arthritides. The distribution of joint involvement in the hands also helps distinguish osteoarthritis from rheumatoid arthritis. Osteoarthritis chiefly affects the DIP and PIP joints and spares the wrist and metacarpophalangeal (MCP) joints; rheumatoid arthritis involves the wrists and MCP joints and spares the DIP joints. Furthermore, the joint enlargement is bony-hard and cool in osteoarthritis but spongy and warm in rheumatoid arthritis. Skeletal symptoms due to degenerative changes in joints—especially in the spine—may cause coexistent metastatic neoplasia, osteoporosis, multiple myeloma, or other bone disease to be overlooked.

▲ **Figure 20–1.** Osteoarthritis with bony enlargement of the distal interphalangeal (DIP) joints (Heberden nodes) and proximal interphalangeal (PIP) joints (Bouchard nodes). (Reproduced, with permission, from Richard P. Usatine, MD.)

▶ Prevention

Weight reduction reduces the risk of developing symptomatic knee osteoarthritis. Correcting leg length discrepancy of greater than 1 cm with shoe modification may prevent knee osteoarthritis from developing in the shorter leg. Maintaining normal vitamin D levels may reduce the occurrence and progression of osteoarthritis, in addition to being important for bone health.

▶ Treatment

A. General Measures

Patients with osteoarthritis of the hand may benefit from assistive devices and instruction on techniques for joint protection; splinting is beneficial for those with symptomatic osteoarthritis of the first carpometacarpal joint. Patients with mild to moderate osteoarthritis of the knee or hip should participate in a regular exercise program (eg, a supervised walking program, hydrotherapy classes) and, if overweight, should lose weight. The use of assistive devices (eg, a cane on the contralateral side) can improve functional status.

B. Medical Management

1. Acetaminophen—First-line therapy for patients with mild osteoarthritis is acetaminophen (2.6–4 g/day orally).

2. Nonsteroidal anti-inflammatory—NSAIDs (see Table 5–2) are more effective than acetaminophen for osteoarthritis but have greater toxicity. NSAIDs inhibit cyclooxygenase (COX), the enzyme that converts arachidonic acid to prostaglandins. Although prostaglandins play important roles in promoting inflammation and pain, they also help maintain homeostasis in several organs—especially the stomach, where prostaglandin E serves as a local hormone responsible for gastric mucosal cytoprotection. COX exists in two isomers—COX-1, which is expressed continuously in many cells and is responsible for the homeostatic effects of prostaglandins, and COX-2, which is induced by cytokines and expressed in inflammatory tissues. Most NSAIDs inhibit both isomers. Celecoxib is the only selective COX-2 inhibitor currently available in the United States.

Gastrointestinal toxicity, such as gastric ulceration, perforation, and gastrointestinal hemorrhage, are the most common serious side effects of NSAIDs. NSAIDs can also affect the lower intestinal tract, causing perforation or aggravating inflammatory bowel disease. The overall rate of bleeding with NSAID use in the general population is low (1:6000 users or less) but is increased by the risk factors of long-term use, higher NSAID dose, concomitant corticosteroids or anticoagulants, the presence of rheumatoid arthritis, history of peptic ulcer disease or alcoholism, and age over 70. Proton pump inhibitors (eg, omeprazole 20 mg orally daily) reduce the incidence of serious gastrointestinal toxicity and should be used for patients with risk factors for NSAID-induced gastrointestinal toxicity. Patients who have recently recovered from an NSAID-induced bleeding gastric ulcer appear to be at high risk for rebleeding (about 5% in 6 months) when an NSAID is reintroduced, even if prophylactic measures (such as proton pump inhibitors) are used. Compared with nonselective NSAIDs, celecoxib may be less likely in some circumstances to cause upper gastrointestinal tract adverse events. However, long-term use of COX-2 inhibitors, particularly in the absence of concomitant aspirin use, has been associated with an increased risk of cardiovascular events.

All of the NSAIDs, including aspirin and celecoxib, can produce renal toxicity, including interstitial nephritis, nephrotic syndrome, prerenal azotemia, and aggravation of hypertension. Hyperkalemia due to hyporeninemic hypoaldosteronism is seen rarely. The risk of renal toxicity is low but is increased by the following risk factors: age older than 60 years; history of kidney disease; heart failure; ascites; and diuretic use.

The FDA has warned that all NSAIDs can increase the risk of myocardial infarction and stroke in patients with or without risk factors for heart disease or known heart disease. While the cardiovascular risk is related to the dose and duration of treatment, stroke and myocardial infarction can occur within the first week of treatment. Cardiovascular risks may be lower with naproxen than with other NSAIDs.

All NSAIDs, except the nonacetylated salicylates and the COX-2 inhibitor celecoxib, interfere with platelet function and prolong bleeding time. Aspirin irreversibly inhibits platelet function, so the bleeding time effect resolves only as new platelets are made. In contrast, the effect of nonselective NSAIDs on platelet function is reversible and resolves as the drug is cleared. Concomitant administration of a nonselective NSAID can interfere with the ability of aspirin to acetylate platelets and thus may interfere with the cardioprotective effects of low-dose aspirin.

Topical NSAIDs (eg, 4 g of diclofenac gel 1% applied to the affected joint four times daily) appear more effective than placebo for knee and hand osteoarthritis and have lower rates of systemic side effects than with oral NSAIDs. Few studies have compared the efficacy of oral and topical NSAIDs.

Topical capsaicin may be of benefit for osteoarthritis of the hand but is not recommended for osteoarthritis of the knee or hip.

Chondroitin sulfate and glucosamine, alone or in combination, are no better than placebo in reducing pain in patients with knee or hip osteoarthritis.

3. Intra-articular injections—Intra-articular injections of triamcinolone (20–40 mg) for patients with osteoarthritis of the knee or hip may reduce the need for analgesics or NSAIDs and can be repeated up to four times a year. The American College of Rheumatology does not recommend corticosteroid injections for osteoarthritis of the hand.

Intra-articular injections of sodium hyaluronate produce moderate reduction in symptoms in some patients with osteoarthritis of the knee.

C. Surgical Measures

Total hip and knee replacements provide excellent symptomatic and functional improvement when involvement of that joint severely restricts walking or causes pain at rest, particularly at night. Arthroscopic surgery for knee osteoarthritis is ineffective.

▶ Prognosis

Symptoms may be quite severe and limit activity considerably (especially with involvement of the hips, knees, and cervical spine).

▶ When to Refer

Refer patients to an orthopedic surgeon when recalcitrant symptoms or functional impairment, or both, warrant consideration of joint replacement surgery of the hip or knee.

Bannuru RR et al. Comparative effectiveness of pharmacologic interventions for knee osteoarthritis: a systematic review and network meta-analysis. Ann Intern Med. 2015 Jan 6; 162(1):46–54. [PMID: 25560713]

Bennell KL et al. Effect of physical therapy on pain and function in patients with hip osteoarthritis: a randomized clinical trial. JAMA. 2014 May 21;311(19):1987–97. [PMID: 24846036]

Glyn-Jones S et al. Osteoarthritis. Lancet. 2015 Jul 25; 386(9991):376–87. [PMID: 25748615]

Skou ST et al. A randomized, controlled trial of total knee replacement. N Engl J Med. 2015 Oct 22;373(17):1597–606. [PMID: 26488691]

CRYSTAL DEPOSITION ARTHRITIS

1. Gouty Arthritis

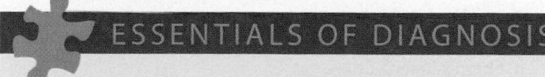

ESSENTIALS OF DIAGNOSIS

▶ Acute onset, usually monarticular, recurring attacks, often involving the first MTP joint.

▶ Polyarticular involvement more common in patients with long-standing disease.

▶ Identification of urate crystals in joint fluid or tophi is diagnostic.

▶ Dramatic therapeutic response to NSAIDs.

▶ With chronicity, urate deposits in subcutaneous tissue, bone, cartilage, joints, and other tissues.

► General Considerations

Gout is a metabolic disease of a heterogeneous nature, often familial, associated with abnormal deposits of urate in tissues and characterized initially by a recurring acute arthritis, usually monarticular, and later by chronic deforming arthritis. Urate deposition occurs when serum uric acid is supersaturated (ie, at levels greater than 6.8 mg/dL [404.5 mcmol/L]). Hyperuricemia is due to overproduction or underexcretion of uric acid—sometimes both. The disease is especially common in Pacific islanders, eg, Filipinos and Samoans. Primary gout has a heritable component, and genome-wide surveys have linked risk of gout to several genes whose products regulate urate handling by the kidney. Secondary gout, which may have a heritable component, is related to acquired causes of hyperuricemia, eg, medication use (especially diuretics, low-dose aspirin, cyclosporine, and niacin), myeloproliferative disorders, multiple myeloma, hemoglobinopathies, chronic kidney disease, hypothyroidism, psoriasis, sarcoidosis, and lead poisoning (Table 20–4). Alcohol ingestion promotes hyperuricemia by increasing urate production and decreasing the renal excretion of uric acid. Finally, hospitalized patients frequently suffer attacks of gout because of changes in diet, fluid intake, or medications that lead either to rapid reductions or increases in the serum urate level.

About 90% of patients with primary gout are men, usually over 30 years of age. In women, the onset is typically postmenopausal. The characteristic lesion is the tophus, a nodular deposit of monosodium urate monohydrate crystals with an associated foreign body reaction. Tophi are found in cartilage, subcutaneous and periarticular tissues, tendon, bone, the kidneys, and elsewhere. Urates have been demonstrated in the synovial tissues (and fluid) during acute arthritis; indeed, the acute inflammation of gout is believed to be initiated by the ingestion of uncoated urate crystals by monocytes and synoviocytes. Once inside the cells, the gout crystals are processed through Toll-like receptors and activate NALP-3 inflammasomes that in turn release a variety of chemotactic agents and cytokines capable of mediating inflammation. The precise relationship of hyperuricemia to gouty arthritis is still obscure, since chronic hyperuricemia is found in people who never develop gout or uric acid stones. Rapid fluctuations in serum urate levels, either increasing or decreasing, are important factors in precipitating acute gout. The mechanism of the late, chronic stage of gouty arthritis is better understood. This is characterized pathologically by tophaceous invasion of the articular and periarticular tissues, with structural derangement and secondary degeneration (osteoarthritis).

Uric acid kidney stones are present in 5–10% of patients with gouty arthritis. Hyperuricemia correlates highly with the likelihood of developing stones, with the risk of stone formation reaching 50% in patients with a serum urate level greater than 13 mg/dL. Chronic urate nephropathy is caused by the deposition of monosodium urate crystals in the renal medulla and pyramids. Although progressive chronic kidney disease occurs in a substantial percentage of patients with chronic gout, the role of hyperuricemia in causing this outcome is controversial, because many patients with gout have numerous confounding risk factors for chronic kidney disease (eg, hypertension, alcohol use, lead exposure, and other risk factors for vascular disease).

► Clinical Findings

A. Symptoms and Signs

Acute gouty arthritis is sudden in onset and frequently nocturnal. It may develop without apparent precipitating cause or may follow rapid increases or decreases in serum urate levels. Common precipitants are alcohol excess (particularly beer), changes in medications that affect urate metabolism, and, in the hospitalized patient, fasting before medical procedures. The MTP joint of the great toe is the most susceptible joint ("podagra"), although others, especially those of the feet, ankles, and knees, are commonly affected. Gouty attacks may develop in periarticular soft tissues such as the arch of the foot. Hips and shoulders are rarely affected. More than one joint may occasionally be affected during the same attack; in such cases, the distribution of the arthritis is usually asymmetric. As the attack progresses, the pain becomes intense. The involved joints are swollen and exquisitely tender and the overlying skin tense, warm, and dusky red. Fever is common and may reach 39°C. Local desquamation and pruritus during recovery from the acute arthritis are characteristic of gout but are not always present. Tophi may be found in the external ears, feet, olecranon and prepatellar bursae, and hands (Figure 20–2). They usually develop years after the initial attack of gout.

Asymptomatic periods of months or years commonly follow the initial acute attack. After years of recurrent

Table 20–4. Origin of hyperuricemia.

Primary hyperuricemia
A. Increased production of purine
1. Idiopathic
2. Specific enzyme defects (eg, Lesch-Nyhan syndrome, glycogen storage diseases)
B. Decreased renal clearance of uric acid (idiopathic)
Secondary hyperuricemia
A. Increased catabolism and turnover of purine
1. Myeloproliferative disorders
2. Lymphoproliferative disorders
3. Carcinoma and sarcoma (disseminated)
4. Chronic hemolytic anemias
5. Cytotoxic drugs
6. Psoriasis
B. Decreased renal clearance of uric acid
1. Intrinsic kidney disease
2. Functional impairment of tubular transport
a. Drug-induced (eg, thiazides, low-dose aspirin)
b. Hyperlacticacidemia (eg, lactic acidosis, alcoholism)
c. Hyperketoacidemia (eg, diabetic ketoacidosis, starvation)
d. Diabetes insipidus (vasopressin-resistant)
e. Bartter syndrome

Modified, with permission, from Rodnan GP. Gout and other crystalline forms of arthritis. Postgrad Med. 1975 Oct;58(5):6–14.

▲ **Figure 20–2.** Acute gouty arthritis superimposed on tophaceous gout. (Reproduced, with permission, from Geiderman JM. An elderly woman with a warm, painful finger. West J Med. 2000 Jan;172 (1):51–52.)

severe monoarthritis attacks of the lower extremities and untreated hyperuricemia, gout can evolve into a chronic, deforming polyarthritis of upper and lower extremities that mimics rheumatoid arthritis.

B. Laboratory Findings

Although serial measurements of the serum uric acid detect hyperuricemia in 95% of patients, a single uric acid determination during an acute flare of gout is normal in up to 25% of cases. A normal serum uric acid level, therefore, does not exclude gout, especially in patients taking urate-lowering drugs. During an acute attack, the peripheral blood white cell count is frequently elevated. Identification of sodium urate crystals in joint fluid or material aspirated from a tophus establishes the diagnosis. The crystals, which may be extracellular or found within neutrophils, are needle-like and negatively birefringent when examined by polarized light microscopy.

C. Imaging

Early in the disease, radiographs show no changes. Later, punched-out erosions with an overhanging rim of cortical bone ("rat bite") develop. When these are adjacent to a soft tissue tophus, they are diagnostic of gout.

▶ Differential Diagnosis

Acute gout is often confused with cellulitis. Bacteriologic studies usually exclude acute pyogenic arthritis. Pseudogout is distinguished by the identification of calcium pyrophosphate crystals (positive birefringence) in the joint fluid, usually normal serum uric acid, and the radiographic appearance of chondrocalcinosis.

Chronic tophaceous arthritis may resemble chronic rheumatoid arthritis; gout is suggested by an earlier history of monoarthritis and is established by the demonstration of urate crystals in a suspected tophus. Likewise, hips and shoulders are generally spared in tophaceous gout. Biopsy may be necessary to distinguish tophi from rheumatoid nodules. A radiographic appearance similar to that of gout may be found in rheumatoid arthritis, sarcoidosis, multiple myeloma, hyperparathyroidism, or Hand-Schüller-Christian disease. Chronic lead intoxication may result in attacks of gouty arthritis (saturnine gout).

▶ Treatment

A. Asymptomatic Hyperuricemia

Asymptomatic hyperuricemia should not be treated; uric acid–lowering drugs should not be instituted until arthritis, renal calculi, or tophi become apparent.

B. Acute Attack

Treatment of the acute attack focuses on reducing inflammation, not lowering serum uric acid. Indeed, sudden reduction of serum uric acid often precipitates further episodes of gouty arthritis.

1. NSAIDs—Oral NSAIDs in full dose (eg, naproxen 500 mg twice daily or indomethacin 25–50 mg every 8 hours; see Table 5–2) are effective treatment for acute gout and should be continued until the symptoms have resolved (usually 5–10 days). Contraindications include active peptic ulcer disease, impaired kidney function, and a history of allergic reaction to NSAIDs.

2. Colchicine—Oral colchicine is an appropriate treatment option for acute gout, provided the duration of the attack is less than 36 hours. For acute gout, colchicine should be administered orally as follows: a loading dose of 1.2 mg followed by a dose of 0.6 mg 1 hour later and then dosing for prophylaxis (0.6 mg once or twice daily) beginning 12 hours later. Patients who are already taking prophylactic doses of colchicine and have an acute flare of gout may receive the full loading dose (1.2 mg) followed by 0.6 mg 1 hour later (before resuming the usual 0.6 mg once or twice daily) provided they have not received this regimen within the preceding 14 days (in which case, NSAIDs or corticosteroids should be used). The use of oral colchicine during the intercritical period to prevent gout attacks is discussed below.

3. Corticosteroids—Corticosteroids often give dramatic symptomatic relief in acute episodes of gout and will control most attacks. They are most useful in patients with contraindications to the use of NSAIDs. Corticosteroids may be given intravenously (eg, methylprednisolone, 40 mg/day) or orally (eg, prednisone, 40–60 mg/day). These corticosteroids can be given at the suggested dose for 5–10 days and then simply discontinued or given at the suggested initial dose for 2–5 days and then tapered over

7–10 days. If the patient's gout is monarticular or oligoarticular, intra-articular administration of the corticosteroid (eg, triamcinolone, 10–40 mg depending on the size of the joint) is very effective. Because gouty and septic arthritis can coexist, albeit rarely, joint aspiration and Gram stain with culture of synovial fluid should be performed when intra-articular corticosteroids are given.

4. Interleukin-1 inhibitors—Anakinra (an interleukin-1 receptor antagonist), canakinumab (a monoclonal antibody against interleukin-1 beta), and rilonacept (a chimera composed of IgG constant domains and the extracellular components of the interleukin-1 receptor) have efficacy for the management of acute gout but these drugs have not been approved by the US Food and Drug Administration (FDA) for this indication.

C. Management between Attacks

Treatment during symptom-free periods is intended to minimize urate deposition in tissues, which causes chronic tophaceous arthritis, and to reduce the frequency and severity of recurrences. Potentially reversible causes of hyperuricemia are a high-purine diet, obesity, alcohol consumption, and use of certain medications (see below). Patients with a single episode of gout who are willing to lose weight and stop drinking alcohol are at low risk for another attack and may not require long-term medical therapy. In contrast, individuals with mild chronic kidney disease or with a history of multiple attacks of gout are likely to benefit from pharmacologic treatment. In general, the higher the uric acid level and the more frequent the attacks, the more likely that long-term medical therapy will be beneficial. All patients with tophaceous gout should receive urate-lowering therapy.

1. Diet—Excessive alcohol consumption can precipitate attacks and should be avoided. Beer consumption appears to confer a higher risk of gout than does whiskey or wine. Although dietary purines usually contribute only 1 mg/dL to the serum uric acid level, moderation in eating foods with high purine content is advisable (Table 20–5). Patients should avoid organ meats and beverages sweetened with high fructose corn syrup. A high liquid intake and, more importantly, a daily urinary output of 2 L or more will aid urate excretion and minimize urate precipitation in the urinary tract.

2. Avoidance of hyperuricemic medications—Thiazide and loop diuretics inhibit renal excretion of uric acid and, if possible, should be avoided in patients with gout. Similarly, niacin can raise serum uric acid levels and should be discontinued if there are therapeutic alternatives. Low doses of aspirin also aggravate hyperuricemia but, in general, should be continued due to their overriding benefits in cardiovascular prophylaxis.

3. Colchicine prophylaxis—There are two indications for daily colchicine administration. First, colchicine can be used to prevent future attacks for the individual who has mild hyperuricemia and only occasional attacks of gouty arthritis. Second, colchicine can be used when urate-lowering therapy (see below) is started, to suppress attacks

Table 20–5. The purine content of foods.[1]

Low-purine foods
Refined cereals and cereal products, cornflakes, white bread, pasta, flour, arrowroot, sago, tapioca, cakes
Milk, milk products, and eggs
Sugar, sweets, and gelatin
Butter, polyunsaturated margarine, and all other fats
Fruit, nuts, and peanut butter
Lettuce, tomatoes, and green vegetables (except those listed below)
Cream soups made with low-purine vegetables but without meat or meat stock
Water, fruit juice, cordials, and carbonated drinks
High-purine foods
All meats, including organ meats, and seafood
Meat extracts and gravies
Yeast and yeast extracts, beer, and other alcoholic beverages
Beans, peas, lentils, oatmeal, spinach, asparagus, cauliflower, and mushrooms

[1]The purine content of a food reflects its nucleoprotein content and turnover. Foods containing many nuclei (eg, liver) have many purines, as do rapidly growing foods such as asparagus. The consumption of large amounts of a food containing a small concentration of purines may provide a greater purine load than consumption of a small amount of a food containing a large concentration of purines.
Reproduced, with permission, from Emmerson BT. The management of gout. N Engl J Med. 1996 Feb 15;334(7):445–51.

precipitated by abrupt changes in the serum uric acid level. For either indication, the usual dose is 0.6 mg either once or twice a day. Colchicine is renally cleared. Patients who have coexisting moderate chronic kidney disease should take colchicine only once a day or once every other day in order to avoid peripheral neuromyopathy and other complications of colchicine toxicity.

4. Reduction of serum uric acid—Indications for a urate-lowering therapy in a person with gout include frequent acute arthritis (two or more episodes per year), tophaceous deposits, or chronic kidney disease (stage 2 or worse). If instituted, the minimum goal of urate-lowering therapy is to maintain the serum uric acid at or below 6 mg/dL or 357 mcmol/L (ie, below the level at which serum is supersaturated with uric acid, thereby allowing urate crystals to solubilize); in some cases, control of gout may require lowering serum uric acid to less than 5 mg/dL or 297.4 mcmol/L. Lowering serum uric acid levels is not of benefit for the treatment of an acute gout flare.

Three classes of agents may be used to lower the serum uric acid—xanthine oxidase inhibitors (allopurinol or febuxostat), uricosuric agents, and uricase (pegloticase). Xanthine oxidase inhibitors are the preferred first-line agents for urate lowering. The uricosuric agent, probenecid, is an acceptable alternative, provided the serum creatinine clearance is greater than 50 mL/minute and there is no history of nephrolithiasis. The uricase, pegloticase, requires intravenous administration and is indicated only in patients with chronic gout refractory to other treatments.

A. Xanthine oxidase inhibitors—The xanthine oxidase inhibitors, allopurinol and febuxostat, lower plasma uric acid levels by blocking the final enzymatic steps in the production of uric acid. Allopurinol and febuxostat should not be used together but they can be tried sequentially if the initial agent fails to lower serum uric acid to the target level or if it is not tolerated. The most frequent adverse effect with either medication is the precipitation of an acute gouty attack; thus, patients generally should be receiving prophylactic doses of colchicine.

Hypersensitivity to allopurinol occurs in 2% of cases, usually within the first few months of therapy, and it can be life-threatening. The most common sign of hypersensitivity is a pruritic rash that may progress to toxic epidermal necrolysis, particularly if allopurinol is continued; vasculitis and hepatitis are other manifestations. Patients should be instructed to stop allopurinol immediately if a rash develops. Chronic kidney disease and concomitant thiazide therapy are risk factors. In certain ethnic groups, there is a strong association between HLA-B*5801 and allopurinol hypersensitivity. Current recommendations are to screen for HLA-B*5801 prior to initiating allopurinol in Han Chinese, those of Thai descent, and Koreans with stage 3 or worse chronic kidney disease.

The initial daily dose of allopurinol is 100 mg/day orally (50 mg/day for those with stage 4 or worse chronic kidney disease); the dose of allopurinol should be titrated upward every 2–5 weeks to achieve the target serum uric acid level (either less than or equal to 6.0 mg/dL [357 mcmol/L] for men or less than or equal to 5.0 mg/dL [297.4 mcmol/L] for women). Successful treatment usually requires a dose of at least 300 mg of allopurinol daily. The maximum daily dose is 800 mg.

Allopurinol interacts with other drugs. The combined use of allopurinol and ampicillin causes a drug rash in 20% of patients. Allopurinol can increase the half-life of probenecid, while probenecid increases the excretion of allopurinol. Thus, a patient taking both drugs may need to use slightly higher than usual doses of allopurinol and lower doses of probenecid.

Febuxostat does not cause the hypersensitivity reactions seen with allopurinol and can be given without dose adjustment to patients with mild to moderate kidney disease. However, abnormal liver tests may develop in 2–3% of patients taking febuxostat. In addition, one clinical study showed that febuxostat was associated with a slightly higher rate of fatal and nonfatal cardiovascular events than allopurinol (0.97 vs 0.58 per 100 patient-years). The initial dose of febuxostat is 40 mg/day orally. If the target serum uric acid is not reached, the dose of febuxostat can be increased to 80 mg/day and then to the maximum dose of 120 mg/day.

B. Uricosuric drugs—Uricosuric drugs lower serum uric acid levels by blocking the tubular reabsorption of filtered urate, thereby increasing uric acid excretion by the kidney. Probenecid (0.5 g/day orally) is the uricosuric of choice in the United States. It is an acceptable alternative when xanthine oxidase inhibitors cannot be used and can be added when monotherapy with a xanthine oxidase inhibitor fails to reach the target serum uric acid. Probenecid should not be used in patients with a creatinine clearance of less than 50 mL/min due to limited efficacy; contraindications include a history of nephrolithiasis (uric acid or calcium stones) and evidence of overproduction of uric acid (ie, greater than 800 mg of uric acid in a 24-hour urine collection). To reduce the development of uric acid stones (which occur in up to 11%), patients should be advised to increase their fluid intake and clinicians should consider prescribing an alkalinizing agent (eg, potassium citrate, 30–80 mEq/day orally) to maintain a urine pH > 6.0.

C. Uricase—Pegloticase, a recombinant uricase that must be administered intravenously (8 mg every 2 weeks), is indicated for the rare patient with refractory chronic tophaceous gout. Pegloticase carries a "Black Box Warning," which advises administering the drug only in health care settings and by health care professionals prepared to manage anaphylactic and other serious infusion reactions.

D. Chronic Tophaceous Arthritis

With rigorous medical compliance, allopurinol or febuxostat or pegloticase shrinks tophi and in time can lead to their disappearance. Resorption of extensive tophi requires maintaining a serum uric acid below 6 mg/dL. Surgical excision of large tophi offers mechanical improvement in selected deformities.

E. Gout in the Transplant Patient

Hyperuricemia and gout commonly develop in many transplant patients because they have decreased kidney function and require drugs that inhibit uric acid excretion (especially cyclosporine and diuretics). Treating acute gout in these patients is challenging. Often the best approach for monarticular gout—after excluding infection—is injecting corticosteroids into the joint (see above). For polyarticular gout, increasing the dose of systemic corticosteroid may be the only alternative. Since transplant patients often have multiple attacks of gout, long-term relief requires lowering the serum uric acid with allopurinol or febuxostat. (Kidney dysfunction seen in many transplant patients makes uricosuric agents ineffective.) Both allopurinol and febuxostat inhibit the metabolism of azathioprine and should be avoided in patients who must take azathioprine.

▶ Prognosis

Without treatment, the acute attack may last from a few days to several weeks. The intervals between acute attacks vary up to years, but the asymptomatic periods often become shorter if the disease progresses. Chronic gouty arthritis occurs after repeated attacks of acute gout, but only after inadequate treatment. The younger the patient at the onset of disease, the greater the tendency to a progressive course. Destructive arthropathy is rarely seen in patients whose first attack is after age 50.

Patients with gout are anecdotally thought to have an increased incidence of hypertension, kidney disease (eg, nephrosclerosis, interstitial nephritis, pyelonephritis), diabetes mellitus, hypertriglyceridemia, and atherosclerosis.

Khanna D et al. 2012 American College of Rheumatology guidelines for management of gout. Part 1: systemic nonpharmacologic and pharmacologic therapeutic approaches to hyperuricemia. Arthritis Care Res (Hoboken). 2012 Oct; 64(10):1431–46. [PMID: 23024028]

Khanna D et al. 2012 American College of Rheumatology guidelines for management of gout. Part 2: therapy and antiinflammatory prophylaxis of acute gouty arthritis. Arthritis Care Res (Hoboken). 2012 Oct;64(10):1447–61. [PMID: 23024029]

van Durme CM et al. Nonsteroidal anti-inflammatory drugs for treatment of acute gout. JAMA. 2015 Jun 9;313(22):2276–7. [PMID: 26057289]

2. Calcium Pyrophosphate Deposition

Calcium pyrophosphate deposition (CPPD) in fibrocartilage and hyaline cartilage (chondrocalcinosis) can cause an acute crystal-induced arthritis ("pseudogout"), a degenerative arthropathy, and a chronic inflammatory polyarthritis ("pseudorheumatoid arthritis"). CPPD also can be an asymptomatic condition detected as incidental chondrocalcinosis on radiographs. The prevalence of CPPD increases with age. Hyperparathyroidism, hemochromatosis, and hypomagnesemia confer risk of CPPD, but most cases have no associated condition.

Pseudogout is most often seen in persons age 60 or older, is characterized by acute, recurrent and rarely chronic arthritis involving large joints (most commonly the knees and the wrists) and is almost always accompanied by radiographic chondrocalcinosis of the affected joints. The crowned dens syndrome, caused by pseudogout of the atlantoaxial junction associated with "crown-like" calcifications around the dens, manifests with severe neck pain, rigidity, and high fever that can mimic meningitis or polymyalgia rheumatica. Pseudogout, like gout, frequently develops 24–48 hours after major surgery. Identification of calcium pyrophosphate crystals in joint aspirates is diagnostic. NSAIDs are helpful in the treatment of acute episodes. Colchicine, 0.6 mg orally once or twice daily, is more effective for prophylaxis than for acute attacks. Aspiration of the inflamed joint and intra-articular injection of triamcinolone, 10–40 mg, depending on the size of the joint, are also of value in resistant cases.

The degenerative arthropathy associated with CPPD can involve joints not usually affected by osteoarthritis (eg, glenohumeral joint, wrist, patellofemoral compartment of the knee). The "pseudorheumatoid arthritis" of CPPD affects the metacarpophalangeal joints and wrists. In both conditions, radiographs demonstrate chondrocalcinosis and degenerative changes such as asymmetric joint space narrowing and osteophyte formation.

Filippucci E et al. Tips and tricks to recognize microcrystalline arthritis. Rheumatology (Oxford). 2012 Dec;51(Suppl 7): vii18–21. [PMID: 23230088]

Oka A et al. Crowned dens syndrome: report of three cases and a review of the literature. Emerg Med. 2015 Jul;49(1):e9–13. [PMID: 25910825]

AUTOIMMUNE DISEASES

RHEUMATOID ARTHRITIS

ESSENTIALS OF DIAGNOSIS

► Usually insidious onset with morning stiffness and pain in affected joints.

► Symmetric polyarthritis with predilection for small joints of the hands and feet; deformities common with progressive disease.

► Radiographic findings: juxta-articular osteoporosis, joint erosions, and joint space narrowing.

► Rheumatoid factor and antibodies to cyclic citrullinated peptides (anti-CCP) are present in 70–80%.

► Extra-articular manifestations: subcutaneous nodules, interstitial lung disease, pleural effusion, pericarditis, splenomegaly with leukopenia, and vasculitis.

► General Considerations

Rheumatoid arthritis is a chronic systemic inflammatory disease whose major manifestation is synovitis of multiple joints. It has a prevalence of 1% and is more common in women than men (female:male ratio of 3:1). Rheumatoid arthritis can begin at any age, but the peak onset is in the fourth or fifth decade for women and the sixth to eighth decades for men. The cause is not known. Susceptibility to rheumatoid arthritis is genetically determined with multiple genes contributing. Inheritance of HLA DRB1 alleles encoding a distinctive five-amino-acid sequence known as the "shared epitope" is the best characterized genetic risk factor. Untreated, rheumatoid arthritis causes joint destruction with consequent disability and shortens life expectancy. Early, aggressive treatment is the standard of care.

The pathologic findings in the joint include chronic synovitis with formation of a pannus, which erodes cartilage, bone, ligaments, and tendons. In the acute phase, effusion and other manifestations of inflammation are common. In the late stage, organization may result in fibrous ankylosis; true bony ankylosis is rare.

► Clinical Findings

A. Symptoms and Signs

1. Joint symptoms—The clinical manifestations of rheumatoid disease are highly variable, but joint symptoms usually predominate. Although acute presentations may occur, the onset of articular signs of inflammation is usually insidious, with prodromal symptoms of vague periarticular pain or stiffness. Symmetric swelling of multiple joints with tenderness and pain is characteristic. Monarticular disease is occasionally seen initially. Stiffness persisting for longer than 30 minutes (and usually many hours) is prominent in the morning. Stiffness may recur after daytime inactivity and be much more severe after

▲ **Figure 20–3.** Rheumatoid arthritis with ulnar deviation at the metacarpophalangeal (MCP) joints. (Reproduced, with permission, from Richard P. Usatine, MD.)

▲ **Figure 20–4.** Rheumatoid nodules over the extensor surface of the forearm. (Reproduced, with permission, from Richard P. Usatine, MD.)

strenuous activity. Although any diarthrodial joint may be affected, PIP joints of the fingers, MCP joints (Figure 20–3), wrists, knees, ankles, and MTP joints are most often involved. Synovial cysts and rupture of tendons may occur. Entrapment syndromes are common—particularly of the median nerve at the carpal tunnel of the wrist. Rheumatoid arthritis can affect the neck but spares the other components of the spine and does not involve the sacroiliac joints. In advanced disease, atlantoaxial (C1–C2) subluxation can lead to myelopathy.

2. Rheumatoid nodules—Twenty percent of patients have subcutaneous rheumatoid nodules, most commonly situated over bony prominences but also observed in the bursae and tendon sheaths (Figure 20–4). Nodules are occasionally seen in the lungs, the sclerae, and other tissues. Nodules correlate with the presence of rheumatoid factor in serum ("seropositivity"), as do most other extra-articular manifestations.

3. Ocular symptoms—Dryness of the eyes, mouth, and other mucous membranes is found especially in advanced disease (see Sjögren syndrome). Other ocular manifestations include episcleritis, scleritis, and scleromalacia due to scleral nodules.

4. Other symptoms—Interstitial lung disease is not uncommon (estimates of prevalence vary widely according to method of detection) and manifests clinically as cough and progressive dyspnea. Pericarditis and pleural disease, when present, are usually silent clinically. Patients with active joint disease often have palmar erythema. Occasionally, a small vessel vasculitis develops and manifests as tiny hemorrhagic infarcts in the nail folds or finger pulps. Necrotizing arteritis is well reported but rare. A small subset of patients with rheumatoid arthritis have Felty syndrome, the

occurrence of splenomegaly and neutropenia, usually in the setting of severe, destructive arthritis. Felty syndrome must be distinguished from the large granular lymphoproliferative disorder, with which it shares many features.

Aortitis is a rare late complication that can result in aortic regurgitation or rupture and is usually associated with evidence of rheumatoid vasculitis elsewhere in the body.

B. Laboratory Findings

Anti-CCP antibodies and rheumatoid factor, an IgM antibody directed against the Fc fragment of IgG, are present in 70–80% of patients with established rheumatoid arthritis. Rheumatoid factor has a sensitivity of only 50% in early disease. Anti-CCP antibodies are the most specific blood test for rheumatoid arthritis (specificity ~95%). Rheumatoid factor can occur in other autoimmune disease and in chronic infections, including hepatitis C, syphilis, subacute bacterial endocarditis, and tuberculosis. The prevalence of rheumatoid factor positivity also rises with age in healthy individuals. Approximately 20% of rheumatoid patients have antinuclear antibodies.

The ESR and levels of C-reactive protein are typically elevated in proportion to disease activity. A moderate hypochromic normocytic anemia is common. The white cell count is normal or slightly elevated, but leukopenia may occur, often in the presence of splenomegaly (eg, Felty syndrome). The platelet count is often elevated, roughly in proportion to the severity of overall joint inflammation. Initial joint fluid examination confirms the inflammatory nature of the arthritis (see Table 20–2). Arthrocentesis is needed to diagnose superimposed septic arthritis, which is a common complication of rheumatoid arthritis and should be considered whenever a patient with rheumatoid arthritis has one joint inflamed out of proportion to the rest.

C. Imaging

Of all the laboratory tests, radiographic changes are the most specific for rheumatoid arthritis. Radiographs obtained during the first 6 months of symptoms, however, are usually normal. The earliest changes occur in the hands or feet and consist of soft tissue swelling and juxta-articular demineralization. Later, diagnostic changes of uniform joint space narrowing and erosions develop. The erosions are often first evident at the ulnar styloid and at the juxta-articular margin, where the bony surface is not protected by cartilage. Characteristic changes also occur in the cervical spine, with C1–2 subluxation, but these changes usually take many years to develop. Although both MRI and ultrasonography are more sensitive than radiographs in detecting bony and soft tissue changes in rheumatoid arthritis, their value in early diagnosis relative to that of plain radiographs has not been established.

▶ Differential Diagnosis

The differentiation of rheumatoid arthritis from other joint conditions and immune-mediated disorders can be difficult. In 2010, the American College of Rheumatology updated their classification criteria for rheumatoid arthritis. In contrast to rheumatoid arthritis, osteoarthritis spares the wrist and the MCP joints. Osteoarthritis is not associated with constitutional manifestations, and the joint pain is characteristically relieved by rest, unlike the morning stiffness of rheumatoid arthritis. Signs of articular inflammation, prominent in rheumatoid arthritis, are usually minimal in degenerative joint disease. CPPD disease can cause a degenerative arthropathy of the MCPs and wrists; radiographs are usually diagnostic. Although gouty arthritis is almost always intermittent and monarticular in the early years, it may evolve with time into a chronic polyarticular process that mimics rheumatoid arthritis. Gouty tophi can resemble rheumatoid nodules but are not associated with rheumatoid factor, whose sensitivity for rheumatoid nodules approaches 100%. The early history of intermittent monoarthritis and the presence of synovial urate crystals are distinctive features of gout. Spondyloarthropathies, particularly earlier in their course, can be a source of diagnostic uncertainty; predilection for lower extremities and involvement of the spine and sacroiliac joints point to the correct diagnosis. Chronic Lyme arthritis typically involves only one joint, most commonly the knee, and is associated with positive serologic tests (see Chapter 34). Human parvovirus B19 infection in adults can mimic early rheumatoid arthritis. However, arthralgias are more prominent than arthritis, fever is common, IgM antibodies to parvovirus B19 are present, and the arthritis usually resolves within weeks. Infection with hepatitis C can cause a chronic nonerosive polyarthritis associated with rheumatoid factor; tests for anti-CCP antibodies are negative.

Malar rash, photosensitivity, discoid skin lesions, alopecia, high titer antibodies to double-stranded DNA, glomerulonephritis, and central nervous system abnormalities point to the diagnosis of SLE. Polymyalgia rheumatica occasionally causes polyarthralgias in patients over age 50, but these patients remain rheumatoid factor–negative and

have chiefly proximal muscle pain and stiffness, centered on the shoulder and hip girdles. Joint pain that can be confused with rheumatoid arthritis presents in a substantial minority of patients with granulomatosis with polyangiitis (formerly Wegener granulomatosis). This diagnostic error can be avoided by recognizing that, in contrast to rheumatoid arthritis, the arthritis of granulomatosis with polyangiitis preferentially involves large joints (eg, hips, ankles, wrists) and usually spares the small joints of the hand. Rheumatic fever is characterized by the migratory nature of the arthritis, an elevated antistreptolysin titer, and a more dramatic and prompt response to aspirin; carditis and erythema marginatum may occur in adults, but chorea and subcutaneous nodules virtually never do. Finally, a variety of cancers produce paraneoplastic syndromes, including polyarthritis. One form is hypertrophic pulmonary osteoarthropathy most often produced by lung and gastrointestinal carcinomas, characterized by a rheumatoid-like arthritis associated with clubbing, periosteal new bone formation, and a negative rheumatoid factor. Diffuse swelling of the hands with palmar fasciitis occurs in a variety of cancers, especially ovarian carcinoma.

▶ Treatment

The primary objectives in treating rheumatoid arthritis are reduction of inflammation and pain, preservation of function, and prevention of deformity. Success requires early, effective pharmacologic intervention. Disease-modifying antirheumatic drugs (DMARDs) should be started as soon as the diagnosis of rheumatoid disease is certain and then adjusted with the aim of suppressing disease activity. NSAIDs provide some symptomatic relief in rheumatoid arthritis but do not prevent erosions or alter disease progression. They are not appropriate for monotherapy and should only be used in conjunction with DMARDs, if at all. The American College of Rheumatology recommends using standardized assessments, such as the Disease Activity Score 28 Joints (DAS28), to gauge therapeutic responses, with the target of mild disease activity or remission by these measures. In advanced disease, surgical intervention may help improve function of damaged joints and to relieve pain.

A. Corticosteroids

Low-dose corticosteroids (eg, oral prednisone 5–10 mg daily) produce a prompt anti-inflammatory effect in rheumatoid arthritis and slow the rate of articular erosion. These often are used as a "bridge" to reduce disease activity until the slower acting DMARDs take effect or as adjunctive therapy for active disease that persists despite treatment with DMARDs. No more than 10 mg of prednisone or equivalent per day is appropriate for articular disease. Many patients do reasonably well on 5–7.5 mg daily. (The use of 1 mg tablets, to facilitate doses of less than 5 mg/day, is encouraged.) Higher doses are used to manage serious extra-articular manifestations (eg, pericarditis, necrotizing scleritis). When the corticosteroids are to be discontinued, they should be tapered gradually on a planned schedule appropriate to the duration of treatment. All patients receiving long-term corticosteroid therapy should take measures to prevent osteoporosis.

Intra-articular corticosteroids may be helpful if one or two joints are the chief source of difficulty. Intra-articular triamcinolone, 10–40 mg depending on the size of the joint to be injected, may be given for symptomatic relief but not more than four times a year.

B. Synthetic DMARDs

1. Methotrexate—Methotrexate is usually the initial synthetic DMARD of choice for patients with rheumatoid arthritis. It is generally well tolerated and often produces a beneficial effect in 2–6 weeks. The usual initial dose is 7.5 mg of methotrexate orally once weekly. If the patient has tolerated methotrexate but has not responded in 1 month, the dose can be increased to 15 mg orally once per week. The maximal dose is usually 20–25 mg/wk. The most frequent side effects are gastric irritation and stomatitis. Cytopenia, most commonly leukopenia or thrombocytopenia but rarely pancytopenia, due to bone marrow suppression is another important potential problem. The risk of developing pancytopenia is much higher in patients with elevation of the serum creatinine (greater than 2 mg/dL [176.8 mcmol/L]). Hepatotoxicity with fibrosis and cirrhosis is an important toxic effect that correlates with cumulative dose and is uncommon with appropriate monitoring of liver function tests. Methotrexate is contraindicated in a patient with any form of chronic hepatitis. Heavy alcohol use increases the hepatotoxicity, so patients should be advised to drink alcohol in extreme moderation, if at all. Diabetes mellitus, obesity, and kidney disease also increase the risk of hepatotoxicity. Liver function tests should be monitored at least every 12 weeks, along with a complete blood count. The dose of methotrexate should be reduced if aminotransferase levels are elevated, and the drug should be discontinued if abnormalities persist despite dosage reduction. Gastric irritation, stomatitis, cytopenias, and hepatotoxicity are reduced by prescribing either daily folate (1 mg orally) or weekly leucovorin calcium (2.5–5 mg taken orally 24 hours after the dose of methotrexate). Hypersensitivity to methotrexate can cause an acute or subacute interstitial pneumonitis that can be life-threatening but which usually responds to cessation of the drug and institution of corticosteroids. Because methotrexate is teratogenic, women of childbearing age as well as men must use effective contraception while taking the medication. Methotrexate is associated with an increased risk of B-cell lymphomas, some of which resolve following the discontinuation of the medication. The combination of methotrexate and other folate antagonists, such as trimethoprim-sulfamethoxazole, should be used cautiously since pancytopenia can result. Amoxicillin can decrease renal clearance of methotrexate, leading to toxicity. Probenecid also increases methotrexate drug levels and toxicity and should be avoided.

2. Sulfasalazine—This drug is a second-line agent for rheumatoid arthritis. It is usually introduced at a dosage of 0.5 g orally twice daily and then increased each week by 0.5 g until the patient improves or the daily dose reaches 3 g. Side effects, particularly neutropenia and thrombocytopenia, occur in 10–25% and are serious in 2–5%. Sulfasalazine also causes hemolysis in patients with glucose-6-phosphate dehydrogenase (G6PD) deficiency, so a G6PD level should be checked before initiating sulfasalazine. Patients with aspirin sensitivity should not be given sulfasalazine. Patients taking sulfasalazine should have complete blood counts monitored every 2–4 weeks for the first 3 months, then every 3 months.

3. Leflunomide—Leflunomide, a pyrimidine synthesis inhibitor, is also FDA-approved for treatment of rheumatoid arthritis and is administered as a single oral daily dose of 20 mg. The most frequent side effects are diarrhea, rash, reversible alopecia, and hepatotoxicity. Some patients experience dramatic unexplained weight loss. The drug is carcinogenic, teratogenic, and has a half-life of 2 weeks. Thus, it is contraindicated in premenopausal women or in men who wish to father children.

4. Antimalarials—Hydroxychloroquine sulfate is the antimalarial agent most often used against rheumatoid arthritis. Monotherapy with hydroxychloroquine should be reserved for patients with mild disease because only a small percentage will respond and in some of those cases only after 3–6 months of therapy. Hydroxychloroquine is often used in combination with other conventional DMARDs, particularly methotrexate and sulfasalazine. The advantage of hydroxychloroquine is its comparatively low toxicity, especially at a dosage of 200–400 mg/day orally (not to exceed 5 mg/kg/day). The prevalence of the most important reaction, pigmentary retinitis causing visual loss, is a function of duration of therapy, occurring in less than 2% of patients (dosed properly) during the first 10 years of use, but rising to 20% after 20 years of treatment. Ophthalmologic examinations every 12 months are required. Other reactions include neuropathies and myopathies of both skeletal and cardiac muscle, which usually improve when the drug is withdrawn.

5. Tofacitinib—Tofacitinib, an inhibitor of Janus kinase 3, is used to manage severe rheumatoid arthritis that is refractory to methotrexate. While it appears to be superior to methotrexate as initial monotherapy for rheumatoid arthritis, it has greater toxicity. Tofacitinib can be used either as monotherapy or in combination with methotrexate. It is administered orally in a dose of 5 mg or 10 mg twice daily. Patients should be screened and treated for latent tuberculosis prior to receiving the drug.

C. Biologic DMARDs

1. Tumor necrosis factor inhibitors—Inhibitors of tumor necrosis factor (TNF)—a pro-inflammatory cytokine—are frequently added to the treatment of patients who have not responded adequately to methotrexate and are increasingly used as initial therapy in combination with methotrexate for patients with poor prognostic factors.

Five inhibitors are in use: etanercept, infliximab, adalimumab, golimumab, and certolizumab pegol. Etanercept, a soluble recombinant TNF receptor:Fc fusion protein, is usually administered at a dosage of 50 mg subcutaneously once per week. Infliximab, a chimeric monoclonal antibody, is administered at a dosage of 3–10 mg/kg intravenously; infusions are repeated after 2, 6, 10, and 14 weeks and then are administered every 8 weeks. Adalimumab, a human monoclonal antibody that binds to TNF, is given at a dosage of 40 mg subcutaneously every other week. The dose for golimumab, a human anti-TNF monoclonal antibody, is 50 mg subcutaneously once monthly. Certolizumab pegol is a PEGylated monoclonal antibody TNF inhibitor; the dose is 200–400 mg subcutaneously every 2 to 4 weeks. Each drug produces substantial improvement in more than 60% of patients. Each is usually very well tolerated. Minor irritation at injection sites is the most common side effect of etanercept and adalimumab. Rarely, nonrecurrent leukopenia develops in patients. TNF plays a physiologic role in combating many types of infection; TNF inhibitors have been associated with a several-fold increased risk of serious bacterial infections and a striking increase in granulomatous infections, particularly reactivation of tuberculosis. Screening for latent tuberculosis (see Chapter 9) is mandatory before the initiation of TNF blockers. It is prudent to suspend TNF blockers when a fever or other manifestations of a clinically important infection develops in a patient. Demyelinating neurologic complications that resemble multiple sclerosis have been reported rarely in patients taking etanercept, but the true magnitude of this risk—likely quite small—has not been determined with precision. While there are conflicting data with respect to increased risk of malignancy, in 2009, the FDA issued a safety alert about case reports of malignancies, including leukemias, in patients treated with TNF inhibitors. Contrary to expectation, TNF inhibitors were not effective in the treatment of heart failure. The use of infliximab, in fact, was associated with increased morbidity in a heart failure trial. Consequently, TNF inhibitors should be used with extreme caution in patients with heart failure. Infliximab can rarely cause anaphylaxis and induce anti-DNA antibodies (but rarely clinically evident SLE).

2. Abatacept—Abatacept, a recombinant protein made by fusing a fragment of the Fc domain of human IgG with the extracellular domain of a T-cell inhibitory receptor (CTLA4), blocks T-cell costimulation and produces clinically meaningful responses in approximately 50% of individuals whose disease is active despite the combination of methotrexate and a TNF inhibitor.

3. Rituximab—Rituximab, a humanized mouse monoclonal antibody that depletes B cells, can be used in combination with methotrexate for patients whose disease has been refractory to treatment with a TNF inhibitor.

4. Tocilizumab—Tocilizumab is a monoclonal antibody that blocks the receptor for IL-6, an inflammatory cytokine involved in the pathogenesis of rheumatoid arthritis. It is used most often in combination with methotrexate for patients whose disease has been refractory to treatment with a TNF inhibitor.

D. DMARD Combinations

As a general rule, DMARDs have greater efficacy when administered in combination than when used individually.

Currently, the most commonly used combination is that of methotrexate with one of the TNF inhibitors, which clearly is superior to methotrexate alone. The combination of methotrexate, sulfasalazine, and hydroxychloroquine is also effective and is not inferior to the combination of methotrexate plus etanercept for those who have not responded to methotrexate monotherapy.

► **Course & Prognosis**

After months or years, deformities may occur; the most common are ulnar deviation of the fingers, boutonnière deformity (hyperextension of the DIP joint with flexion of the PIP joint), "swan-neck" deformity (flexion of the DIP joint with extension of the PIP joint), valgus deformity of the knee, and volar subluxation of the MTP joints. The excess mortality associated with rheumatoid arthritis is largely due to cardiovascular disease that is unexplained by traditional risk factors and that appears to be a result of deleterious effects of chronic systemic inflammation on the vascular system.

► **When to Refer**

Early referral to a rheumatologist is essential for appropriate diagnosis and the timely introduction of effective therapy.

Lee EB et al; ORAL Start Investigators. Tofacitinib versus methotrexate in rheumatoid arthritis. N Engl J Med. 2014 Jun 19; 370(25):2377–86. [PMID: 24941177]

Melles RB et al. The risk of toxic retinopathy in patients on long-term hydroxychloroquine therapy. JAMA Ophthalmol. 2014 Dec; 132(12):1453–60. [PMID: 25275721]

Sethi MK et al. Combination conventional DMARDs compared to biologicals: what is the evidence? Curr Opin Rheumatol. 2015 Mar;27(2):183–8. [PMID: 25603037]

Singh JA et al. Risk of serious infection in biological treatment of patients with rheumatoid arthritis: a systematic review and meta-analysis. Lancet. 2015 Jul 18;386(9990):258–65. [PMID: 25975452]

ADULT STILL DISEASE

Still disease is a systemic form of juvenile chronic arthritis in which high spiking fevers are much more prominent, especially at the outset, than arthritis. This syndrome also occurs in adults. Most adults are in their 20s or 30s; onset after age 60 is rare. The fever is dramatic, often with daily spikes to 40°C, associated with sweats and chills, and then plunging to normal or several degrees below normal in the absence of antipyretics. Many patients initially complain of sore throat. An evanescent salmon-colored nonpruritic rash, chiefly on the chest and abdomen, is a characteristic feature. The rash can easily be missed since it often appears only with the fever spike. Many patients also have lymphadenopathy and pericardial effusions. Joint symptoms are mild or absent in the beginning, but a destructive arthritis, especially of the wrists, may develop months later. Anemia and leukocytosis, with white blood counts sometimes exceeding 40,000/mcL, are the rule. The diagnosis of adult Still disease is strongly suggested by the quotidian fever pattern, sore throat, and the classic rash but requires exclusion of other causes of fever. About half of the patients respond to NSAIDs, and half require prednisone, sometimes in doses greater than 60 mg/day orally. Targeting IL-1 with anakinra or canakinumab or IL-6 with tocilizumab can be effective for patients with refractory disease. The course of adult Still disease can be monophasic, intermittent, or chronic. Macrophage activation syndrome is a life-threatening complication of adult Still disease and manifests as fever; splenomegaly; cytopenias; hypertriglyceridemia; hypofibrinogenemia; marked elevation of serum ferritin; and hemophagocytosis in bone marrow, spleen, and lymph nodes.

Kadavath S et al. Adult-onset Still's disease-pathogenesis, clinical manifestations, and new treatment options. Ann Med. 2015 Feb; 47(1):6–14. [PMID: 25613167]

SYSTEMIC LUPUS ERYTHEMATOSUS

ESSENTIALS OF DIAGNOSIS

▶ Occurs mainly in young women.

▶ Rash over areas exposed to sunlight.

▶ Joint symptoms in 90% of patients. Multiple system involvement.

▶ Anemia, leukopenia, thrombocytopenia.

▶ Glomerulonephritis, central nervous system disease, and complications of antiphospholipid antibodies are major sources of disease morbidity.

▶ Serologic findings: antinuclear antibodies (100%), anti–double-stranded DNA antibodies (approximately two-thirds), and low serum complement levels (particularly during disease flares).

General Considerations

SLE is an inflammatory autoimmune disorder characterized by autoantibodies to nuclear antigens. It can affect multiple organ systems. Many of its clinical manifestations are secondary to the trapping of antigen-antibody complexes in capillaries of visceral structures or to autoantibody-mediated destruction of host cells (eg, thrombocytopenia). The clinical course is marked by spontaneous remission and relapses. The severity may vary from a mild episodic disorder to a rapidly fulminant, life-threatening illness.

The incidence of SLE is influenced by many factors, including sex, race, and genetic inheritance. About 85% of patients are women. Sex hormones appear to play some role; most cases develop after menarche and before menopause. Among older individuals, the sex distribution is more equal. Race is also a factor, as SLE occurs in 1:1000 white women but in 1:250 black women. Familial occurrence of SLE has been repeatedly documented, and the

disorder is concordant in 25–70% of identical twins. If a mother has SLE, her daughters' risks of developing the disease are 1:40 and her sons' risks are 1:250. Aggregation of serologic abnormalities (positive antinuclear antibody) is seen in asymptomatic family members, and the prevalence of other rheumatic diseases is increased among close relatives of patients. The importance of specific genes in SLE is emphasized by the high frequency of certain HLA haplotypes, especially DR2 and DR3, and null complement alleles.

The diagnosis of SLE should be suspected in patients having a multisystem disease with a positive test for antinuclear antibodies. It is imperative to ascertain that the condition has not been induced by a drug (see Drug-Induced Lupus below). Differential diagnosis also includes rheumatoid arthritis, systemic vasculitis, scleroderma, inflammatory myopathies, viral hepatitis, sarcoidosis, and acute drug reactions.

The diagnosis of SLE can be made with reasonable probability if 4 of the 11 criteria set forth in Table 20–6 are met. These criteria, developed as guidelines for the inclusion of patients in research studies, do not supplant clinical judgment in the diagnosis of SLE.

Table 20–6. Criteria for the classification of SLE. (A patient is classified as having SLE if any 4 or more of 11 criteria are met.)

1. Malar rash
2. Discoid rash
3. Photosensitivity
4. Oral ulcers
5. Arthritis
6. Serositis
7. Kidney disease
a. > 0.5 g/day proteinuria, or
b. ≥ 3+ dipstick proteinuria, or
c. Cellular casts
8. Neurologic disease
a. Seizures, or
b. Psychosis (without other cause)
9. Hematologic disorders
a. Hemolytic anemia, or
b. Leukopenia (< 4000/mcL), or
c. Lymphopenia (< 1500/mcL), or
d. Thrombocytopenia (< 100,000/mcL)
10. Immunologic abnormalities
a. Antibody to native DNA, or
b. Antibody to Sm, or
c. Antibodies to antiphospholipid antibodies based on (1) IgG or IgM anticardiolipin antibodies, (2) lupus anticoagulant, or (3) false-positive serologic test for syphilis
11. Positive ANA

ANA, antinuclear antibody; SLE, systemic lupus erythematosus. Modified and reproduced, with permission, from Tan EM et al. The 1982 revised criteria for the classification of systemic lupus erythematosus. Arthritis Rheum. 1982 Nov;25(11):1271–7, and Hochberg MC. Updating the American College of Rheumatology revised criteria for the classification of systemic lupus erythematosus. Arthritis Rheum. 1997 Sep;40(9):1725.

Clinical Findings

A. Symptoms and Signs

The systemic features include fever, anorexia, malaise, and weight loss. Most patients have skin lesions at some time; the characteristic "butterfly" (malar) rash affects less than half of patients. Other cutaneous manifestations are panniculitis (lupus profundus), discoid lupus, typical fingertip lesions, periungual erythema, nail fold infarcts, and splinter hemorrhages. Alopecia is common. Mucous membrane lesions tend to occur during periods of exacerbation. Raynaud phenomenon, present in about 20% of patients, often antedates other features of the disease.

Joint symptoms, with or without active synovitis, occur in over 90% of patients and are often the earliest manifestation. The arthritis can lead to reversible swan-neck deformities, but erosive changes are almost never noted on radiographs. Subcutaneous nodules are rare.

Ocular manifestations include conjunctivitis, photophobia, transient or permanent monocular blindness, and blurring of vision. Cotton-wool spots on the retina (cytoid bodies) represent degeneration of nerve fibers due to occlusion of retinal blood vessels.

Pleurisy, pleural effusion, bronchopneumonia, and pneumonitis are frequent. Restrictive lung disease can develop. Alveolar hemorrhage is uncommon but life-threatening. Interstitial lung disease is rare.

The pericardium is affected in the majority of patients. Heart failure may result from myocarditis and hypertension. Cardiac arrhythmias are common. Atypical verrucous endocarditis of Libman-Sacks is usually clinically silent but occasionally can produce acute or chronic valvular regurgitation—most commonly mitral regurgitation.

Mesenteric vasculitis occasionally occurs in SLE and may closely resemble polyarteritis nodosa, including the presence of aneurysms in medium-sized blood vessels. Abdominal pain (particularly postprandial), ileus, peritonitis, and perforation may result.

Neurologic complications of SLE include psychosis, cognitive impairment, seizures, peripheral and cranial neuropathies, transverse myelitis, and strokes. Severe depression and psychosis are sometimes exacerbated by the administration of large doses of corticosteroids.

Several forms of glomerulonephritis may occur, including mesangial, focal proliferative, diffuse proliferative, and membranous (see Chapter 22). Some patients may also have interstitial nephritis. With appropriate therapy, the survival rate even for patients with serious chronic kidney disease (proliferative glomerulonephritis) is favorable, albeit a substantial portion of patients with severe lupus nephritis still eventually require renal replacement therapy.

B. Laboratory Findings

(Tables 20–7 and 20–8.) SLE is characterized by the production of many different autoantibodies. Antinuclear antibody tests based on immunofluorescence assays using HEp-2 cells (a human cell line) as a source of nuclei are nearly 100% sensitive for SLE but not specific—ie, they are positive in low titer in up to 20% of healthy adults and also in many patients with nonlupus conditions such as rheumatoid arthritis, autoimmune thyroid disease, scleroderma, and Sjögren syndrome. False-negative results can

Table 20–7. Frequency (%) of autoantibodies in rheumatic diseases.[1]

	ANA	Anti-Native DNA	Rheumatoid Factor	Anti-Sm	Anti-SS-A	Anti-SS-B	Anti-SCL-70	Anti-Centromere	Anti-Jo-1	ANCA
Rheumatoid arthritis	30–60	0–5	70	0	0–5	0–2	0	0	0	0
Systemic lupus erythematosus	95–100	60	20	10–25	15–20	5–20	0	0	0	0–1
Sjögren syndrome	95	0	75	0	65	65	0	0	0	0
Diffuse scleroderma	>95	0	30	0	0	0	33	1	0	0
Limited scleroderma (CREST syndrome)	>95	0	30	0	0	0	20	50	0	0
Polymyositis/ dermatomyositis	80	0	33	0	0	0	0	0	20–30	0
Granulomatosis with polyangiitis (formerly Wegener granulomatosis)	0–15	0	50	0	0	0	0	0	0	93–96[1]

[1]Frequency for generalized, active disease.

ANA, antinuclear antibodies; Anti-Sm, anti-Smith antibody; anti-SCL-70, anti-scleroderma antibody; ANCA, antineutrophil cytoplasmic antibody; CREST, calcinosis cutis, Raynaud phenomenon, esophageal motility disorder, sclerodactyly, and telangiectasia.

Table 20–8. Frequency (%) of laboratory abnormalities in systemic lupus erythematosus.

Anemia	60%
Leukopenia	45%
Thrombocytopenia	30%
Antiphospholipid antibodies	
Biologic false-positive test for syphilis	25%
Lupus anticoagulant	7%
Anti-cardiolipin antibody	25%
Direct Coombs-positive	30%
Proteinuria	30%
Hematuria	30%
Hypocomplementemia	60%
ANA	95–100%
Anti-native DNA	50%
Anti-Sm	20%

ANA, antinuclear antibody; Anti-Sm, anti-Smith antibody.
Modified and reproduced, with permission, from Hochberg MC et al. Systemic lupus erythematosus: a review of clinicolaboratory features and immunologic matches in 150 patients with emphasis on demographic subsets. Medicine (Baltimore). 1985 Sep;64(5): 285–95.

occur with tests for antinuclear antibodies based on multiplex assays that use specific nuclear antigens rather than cell lines. Therefore, SLE should not be excluded on the basis of a negative multiplex assay for antinuclear antibodies. Antibodies to double-stranded DNA and to Sm are specific for SLE but not sensitive, since they are present in only 60% and 30% of patients, respectively. Depressed serum complement—a finding suggestive of disease activity—often returns toward normal in remission. Anti-double-stranded DNA antibody levels also correlate with disease activity in some patients; anti-Sm levels do not.

Three types of antiphospholipid antibodies occur (Table 20–8). The first causes the biologic false-positive tests for syphilis; the second is the lupus anticoagulant, which despite its name is a risk factor for venous and arterial thrombosis and for miscarriage. The lupus anticoagulant often causes prolongation of the activated partial thromboplastin time, and its presence is confirmed by an abnormal Russell viper venom time (RVVT) that corrects with the addition of phospholipid but not normal plasma. Anti-cardiolipin antibodies are the third type of antiphospholipid antibodies. In many cases, the "antiphospholipid antibody" appears to be directed at a serum cofactor (beta-2-glycoprotein-I) rather than at phospholipid itself. Abnormality of urinary sediment is almost always found in association with renal lesions. Showers of red blood cells, with or without casts, and proteinuria (varying from mild to nephrotic range) are frequent during exacerbation of the disease.

▶ **Treatment**

Since the various manifestations of SLE affect prognosis differently and since SLE activity often waxes and wanes,

drug therapy—both the choice of agents and the intensity of their use—must be tailored to match disease severity. Patients should be cautioned against sun exposure and should apply a protective lotion to the skin while out of doors. Skin lesions often respond to the local administration of corticosteroids. Minor joint symptoms can usually be alleviated by rest and NSAIDs.

Antimalarials (hydroxychloroquine) may be helpful in treating lupus rashes or joint symptoms and appear to reduce the incidence of severe disease flares. The dose of hydroxychloroquine is 200 or 400 mg/day orally and should not exceed 5 mg/kg/day; annual monitoring for retinal changes is recommended. Drug-induced neuropathy and myopathy may be erroneously ascribed to the underlying disease.

Corticosteroids are required for the control of certain complications. (Systemic corticosteroids are not usually given for minor arthritis, skin rash, leukopenia, or the anemia associated with chronic disease.) Glomerulonephritis, hemolytic anemia, pericarditis or myocarditis, alveolar hemorrhage, central nervous system involvement, and thrombotic thrombocytopenic purpura all require corticosteroid treatment and often other interventions as well. Forty to 60 mg of oral prednisone is often needed initially; however, the lowest dose of corticosteroid that controls the condition should be used. Central nervous system lupus may require higher doses of corticosteroids than are usually given; however, corticosteroid psychosis may mimic lupus cerebritis, in which case reduced doses are appropriate. Immunosuppressive agents such as cyclophosphamide, mycophenolate mofetil, and azathioprine are used in cases resistant to corticosteroids. Treatment of severe lupus nephritis includes an induction phase and a maintenance phase. Cyclophosphamide, which improves renal survival but not patient survival, has been used for many years as the standard treatment for both phases of lupus nephritis. Cyclophosphamide can be administered according to the National Institutes of Health regimen (3–6 monthly intravenous pulses [0.5–1 g/m^2] for induction followed by maintenance infusions every 3 months) or the Euro-Lupus regimen (500 mg intravenously every 2 weeks for 6 doses followed by maintenance with azathioprine). Mycophenolate mofetil appears to be an equally effective alternative treatment to cyclophosphamide for many patients with lupus nephritis. Very close follow-up is needed to watch for potential side effects when immunosuppressants are given; these agents should be administered by clinicians experienced in their use. When cyclophosphamide is required, gonadotropin-releasing hormone analogs can be given to protect a woman against the risk of premature ovarian failure. Belimumab, a monoclonal antibody that inhibits the activity of a B-cell growth factor, has received FDA approval for treating antibody-positive SLE patients with active disease who have not responded to standard therapies (eg, NSAIDs, antimalarials, or immunosuppressive therapies). However, the precise indications for its use have not been defined, and its efficacy in severe disease activity is unknown. Belimumab appears less effective in blacks. While observational studies suggested that rituximab was effective in SLE, one large randomized-controlled trial demonstrated it was no more effective than placebo. For patients with the **antiphospholipid syndrome**—the presence of antiphospholipid antibodies and compatible clinical events—anticoagulation is the treatment of choice (see Antiphospholipid Syndrome, below). Moderately intensive anticoagulation with warfarin to achieve an INR of 2.0–3.0 is as effective as more intensive regimens. Pregnant patients with recurrent fetal loss associated with antiphospholipid antibodies should be treated with low-molecular-weight heparin plus aspirin. Sulfa-containing antibiotics should be used cautiously in SLE; these agents can provoke flares in some patients, and 30% of SLE patients are allergic to sulfonamides.

► Course & Prognosis

Ten-year survival rates exceeding 85% are routine. In most patients, the illness pursues a relapsing and remitting course. Prednisone, often needed in doses of 40 mg/day orally or more during severe flares, can usually be tapered to low doses (5–10 mg/day) when the disease is inactive. However, there are some in whom the disease pursues a virulent course, leading to serious impairment of vital structures such as lungs, heart, brain, or kidneys, and the disease may lead to death. With improved control of lupus activity and with increasing use of corticosteroids and immunosuppressive drugs, the mortality and morbidity patterns in lupus have changed. Mortality in SLE shows a bimodal pattern. In the early years after diagnosis, infections—especially with opportunistic organisms—are the leading cause of death, followed by active SLE, chiefly due to kidney or central nervous system disease. In later years, accelerated atherosclerosis, linked to chronic inflammation, becomes a major cause of death. Indeed, the incidence of myocardial infarction is five times higher in persons with SLE than in the general population. Therefore, it is especially important for SLE patients to avoid smoking and to minimize other conventional risk factors for atherosclerosis (eg, hypercholesterolemia, hypertension, obesity, and inactivity). Patients with SLE should receive influenza vaccination every year and pneumococcal vaccination every 5 years. Since SLE patients have a higher risk of developing malignancy (especially lymphoma, lung cancer, and cervical cancer), preventive cancer screening recommendations should be followed assiduously. With more patients living longer, it has become evident that avascular necrosis of bone, affecting most commonly the hips and knees, is responsible for substantial morbidity. Nonetheless, the outlook for most patients with SLE has become increasingly favorable.

► When to Refer

- Appropriate diagnosis and management of SLE requires the active participation of a rheumatologist.
- The severity of organ involvement dictates referral to other subspecialists, such as nephrologists and pulmonologists.

► When to Admit

- Rapidly progressive glomerulonephritis, pulmonary hemorrhage, transverse myelitis, and other severe organ-threatening manifestations of lupus usually require inpatient assessment and management.

- Severe infections, particularly in the setting of immunosuppressant therapy, should prompt admission.

Buyon JP et al. Predictors of pregnancy outcomes in patients with lupus: a cohort study. Ann Intern Med. 2015 Aug 4; 163(3):153–63. [PMID: 26098843]

Murphy et al. Systemic lupus erythematosus and other autoimmune rheumatic diseases: challenges to treatment. Lancet. 2013 Aug 31;382(9894):809–18. [PMID: 23972423]

Walsh M et al. Mycophenolate mofetil or intravenous cyclophosphamide for lupus nephritis with poor kidney function: a subgroup analysis of the Aspreva Lupus Management Study. Am J Kidney Dis. 2013 May;61(5):710–5. [PMID: 23375819]

DRUG-INDUCED LUPUS

Drug-induced lupus shares several clinical and serologic features with SLE but is due to ongoing exposure to a drug and resolves when the offending drug is discontinued. In contrast to SLE, the sex ratio is nearly equal. As a general rule, drug-induced lupus presents with fever, arthralgia, myalgia, and serositis but not renal involvement, neurologic symptoms, or other features of SLE. Serologic testing reveals elevated titers of antinuclear antibodies in all patients, but antibodies to DNA, Sm, RNP, SS-A, and SS-B are rare. Antibodies to histones are common but also are seen in SLE and thus do not distinguish drug-induced lupus from SLE. Complement levels are usually normal. There are definite associations between the development of drug-induced lupus and the use of hydralazine, isoniazid, and minocycline as well as several medications no longer commonly prescribed (procainamide, quinidine, methyldopa, chlorpromazine). The list of drugs implicated as possible causes of drug-induced lupus in observational studies and case reports is extensive. The incidence of drug-induced lupus in patients taking hydralazine for a year or longer is as high as 5–8%; for most other medications, the risk is considerably lower (less than 1%). TNF inhibitors can induce antibodies to DNA, but the incidence of lupus-like syndromes on these medications is low (0.5–1%).

Rubin RL. Drug-induced lupus. Expert Opin Drug Saf. 2015 Mar; 14(3):361–78. [PMID: 25554102]

ANTIPHOSPHOLIPID SYNDROME

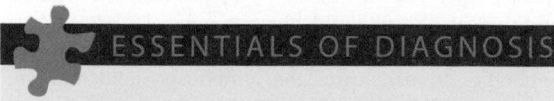
ESSENTIALS OF DIAGNOSIS

- ► Hypercoagulability, with recurrent thromboses in either the venous or arterial circulation.
- ► Thrombocytopenia is common.
- ► Pregnancy complications, specifically pregnancy losses after the first trimester.
- ► Lifelong anticoagulation with warfarin is recommended currently for patients with serious complications of this syndrome because recurrent events are common.

General Considerations

Primary **antiphospholipid syndrome** (APS) is diagnosed in patients who have venous or arterial occlusions or recurrent fetal loss in the presence of persistent (12 weeks or longer), high-titer, diagnostic antiphospholipid antibodies but no other features of SLE. Diagnostic antiphospholipid antibodies are IgG or IgM anticardiolipin, or IgG or IgM antibodies to beta-2-glycoprotein I, and lupus anticoagulant. In less than 1% of patients with antiphospholipid antibodies, a potentially devastating syndrome known as the "catastrophic antiphospholipid syndrome" occurs, leading to diffuse thromboses, thrombotic microangiopathy, and multiorgan system failure.

Clinical Findings

A. Symptoms and Signs

Patients are often asymptomatic until suffering a thrombotic complication of this syndrome or a pregnancy loss. Thrombotic events may occur in either the arterial or venous circulations. Thus, deep venous thromboses, pulmonary emboli, and cerebrovascular accidents are typical clinical events among patients with the APS. In case-control studies, 3.1% of patients in the general population who experienced a venous thrombotic event (in the absence of cancer) tested positive for the lupus anticoagulant (versus 0.9% of controls, yielding an odds ratio of 3.6). For women younger than 50 years in whom stroke developed, the odds ratio for having the lupus anticoagulant is 43.1. Budd-Chiari syndrome, cerebral sinus vein thrombosis, myocardial or digital infarctions, and other thrombotic events also occur. A variety of other symptoms and signs are often attributed to the APS, including thrombocytopenia, mental status changes, livedo reticularis, skin ulcers, microangiopathic nephropathy, adrenal insufficiency, and cardiac valvular dysfunction—typically mitral regurgitation due to Libman-Sacks endocarditis. Livedo reticularis is strongly associated with the subset of patients with APS in whom arterial ischemic events develop. Pregnancy losses that are associated with APS include unexplained fetal death after the first trimester, one or more premature births before 34 weeks because of eclampsia or preeclampsia, or three or more unexplained miscarriages during the first trimester.

B. Laboratory Findings

As noted in the discussion of SLE, three types of antiphospholipid antibody are associated with this syndrome: (1) anticardiolipin antibodies; (2) antibodies to beta-2 glycoprotein; and (3) a "lupus anticoagulant" that prolongs certain phospholipid-dependent coagulation tests (see below). Antibodies to cardiolipin and to beta-2 glycoprotein are typically measured with enzyme immunoassays. Anti-cardiolipin antibodies can produce a biologic false-positive test for syphilis (ie, a positive rapid plasma reagin but negative specific anti-treponemal assay). In general, IgG anti-cardiolipin antibodies are believed to be more pathologic than IgM. Presence of the lupus anticoagulant is a stronger risk factor for thrombosis or pregnancy loss than is the presence of antibodies to either beta-2-glycoprotein I or anticardiolipin.

A clue to the presence of a lupus anticoagulant, which may occur in individuals who do not have SLE, may be detected by a prolongation of the partial thromboplastin time (which, paradoxically, is associated with a thrombotic tendency rather than a bleeding risk). Testing for the lupus anticoagulant involves phospholipid-dependent functional assays of coagulation, such as the Russell viper venom time (RVVT). In the presence of a lupus anticoagulant, the RVVT is prolonged and does not correct with mixing studies but does with the addition of excess phospholipid.

Differential Diagnosis

The exclusion of other autoimmune disorders, particularly those in the SLE spectrum, is essential because such disorders may be associated with additional complications requiring alternative treatments. Other genetic or acquired conditions associated with hypercoagulability such as protein C, protein S, or antithrombin deficiency and factor V Leiden should be excluded. Catastrophic APS has a broad differential, including sepsis, pulmonary-renal syndromes, systemic vasculitis, disseminated intravascular coagulation, and thrombotic thrombocytopenic purpura.

Treatment

Present recommendations for anticoagulation are to treat patients with warfarin to maintain an INR of 2.0–3.0. Patients who have recurrent thrombotic events on this level of anticoagulation may require higher INRs (greater than 3.0), but the bleeding risk increases substantially with this degree of anticoagulation. Guidelines indicate that patients with APS should be treated with anticoagulation for life. Because of the teratogenic effects of warfarin, subcutaneous heparin and low-dose aspirin (81 mg) is the usual approach to prevent pregnancy complications in women with APS. In patients with catastrophic APS, a three-pronged approach is taken in the acute setting: intravenous heparin, high doses of corticosteroids, and either intravenous immune globulin or plasmapheresis.

Cervera R et al; Euro-Phospholipid Project Group. Morbidity and mortality in the antiphospholipid syndrome during a 10-year period: a multicentre prospective study of 1000 patients. Ann Rheum Dis. 2015 Jun;74(6):1011–8. [PMID: 24464962]

Giannakopoulos B et al. The pathogenesis of the antiphospholipid syndrome. N Engl J Med. 2013 Mar 14;368(11):1033–44. [PMID: 23484830]

Pons-Estel GJ et al. Renal involvement in antiphospholipid syndrome. Curr Rheumatol Rep. 2014 Feb;16(2):397. [PMID: 24357443]

RAYNAUD PHENOMENON

ESSENTIALS OF DIAGNOSIS

▶ Paroxysmal bilateral digital pallor and cyanosis followed by rubor.

▶ Precipitated by cold or emotional stress; relieved by warmth.

▶ Primary form of Raynaud phenomenon is benign and usually affects young women.

▶ Secondary form can cause digital ulceration or gangrene.

General Considerations

Raynaud phenomenon (RP) is a syndrome of paroxysmal digital ischemia, most commonly caused by an exaggerated response of digital arterioles to cold or emotional stress. The initial phase of RP, mediated by excessive vasoconstriction, consists of well-demarcated digital pallor or cyanosis; the subsequent (recovery) phase of RP, caused by vasodilation, leads to intense hyperemia and rubor. Although RP chiefly affects fingers, it can also affect toes and other acral areas such as the nose and ears. RP is classified as primary (idiopathic or Raynaud disease) or secondary. Nearly one-third of the population reports being "sensitive to the cold" but does not experience the paroxysms of digital pallor, cyanosis, and erythema characteristic of RP. Primary RP occurs in 2–6% of adults, is especially common in young women, and poses more of a nuisance than a threat to good health. In contrast, secondary RP is less common, is chiefly associated with rheumatic diseases (especially scleroderma), and is frequently severe enough to cause digital ulceration or gangrene.

Clinical Findings

In early attacks of RP, only one or two fingertips may be affected; as it progresses, all fingers down to the distal palm may be involved. The thumbs are rarely affected. During recovery there may be intense rubor, throbbing, paresthesia, pain, and slight swelling. Attacks usually terminate spontaneously or upon returning to a warm room or putting the extremity in warm water. The patient is usually asymptomatic between attacks. Sensory changes that often accompany vasomotor manifestations include numbness, stiffness, diminished sensation, and aching pain.

Primary RP appears first between ages 15 and 30, almost always in women. It tends to be mildly progressive and, unlike secondary RP (which may be unilateral and may involve only one or two fingers), symmetric involvement of the fingers of both hands is the rule. Spasm becomes more frequent and prolonged. Unlike secondary RP, primary RP does not cause digital pitting, ulceration, or gangrene.

Nailfold capillary abnormalities are among the earliest clues that a person has secondary rather than primary RP. The nailfold capillary pattern can be visualized by placing a drop of grade B immersion oil at the patient's cuticle and then viewing the area with an ophthalmoscope set to 20–40 diopters. Dilation or dropout of the capillary loops indicates the patient has a secondary form of RP, most commonly scleroderma (Table 20–9). While highly specific for secondary RP, nailfold capillary changes have a low sensitivity. Digital pitting or ulceration or other abnormal physical findings (eg, skin tightening, loss of extremity pulse, rash, swollen joints) can also provide evidence of secondary RP.

Table 20–9. Causes of secondary Raynaud phenomenon.

Rheumatic diseases
Scleroderma
Systemic lupus erythematosus
Dermatomyositis/polymyositis
Sjögren syndrome
Vasculitis (polyarteritis nodosa, Takayasu disease, Buerger disease)
Neurovascular compression and occupational
Carpal tunnel syndrome
Thoracic outlet obstruction
Vibration injury
Medications
Serotonin agonists (sumatriptan)
Sympathomimetic drugs (decongestants)
Chemotherapy (bleomycin, vinblastine)
Ergotamine
Caffeine
Nicotine
Hematologic disorders
Cryoglobulinemia
Polycythemia vera
Paraproteinemia
Cold agglutinins
Endocrine disorders
Hypothyroidism
Pheochromocytoma
Miscellaneous
Atherosclerosis
Embolic disease
Migraine
Exposure to epoxy resins
Sequela of frostbite

Primary RP must be differentiated from the numerous causes of secondary RP (Table 20–9). The history and examination may suggest the diagnosis of scleroderma, SLE, and mixed connective tissue disease; RP is often the first manifestation of limited scleroderma (CREST syndrome). The diagnosis of many of these rheumatic diseases can be confirmed with specific serologic tests (see Table 20–7).

RP may occur in patients with the thoracic outlet syndromes. In these disorders, involvement is generally unilateral, and symptoms referable to brachial plexus compression tend to dominate the clinical picture. Carpal tunnel syndrome should also be considered, and nerve conduction tests are appropriate in selected cases.

Differential Diagnosis

The differentiation from Buerger disease (thromboangiitis obliterans) is usually not difficult, since thromboangiitis obliterans is generally a disease of men, particularly smokers; peripheral pulses are often diminished or absent; and, when RP occurs in association with thromboangiitis obliterans, it is usually in only one or two digits.

In acrocyanosis, cyanosis of the hands is permanent and diffuse; the sharp and paroxysmal line of demarcation with pallor does not occur with acrocyanosis. Frostbite may lead to chronic RP.

RP may be mimicked by type I cryoglobulinemia, in which a monoclonal antibody cryoprecipitates in the cooler distal circulation. Type I cryoglobulinemia is usually associated with multiple myeloma or with lymphoproliferative disorders.

Erythromelalgia can mimic the rubor phase of RP; exacerbation by heat and relief with cold readily distinguish erythromelalgia from RP.

Treatment

A. General Measures

Patients should wear gloves or mittens whenever outside in temperatures that precipitate attacks. Keeping the body warm is also a cornerstone of initial therapy. Wearing warm shirts, coats, and hats will help prevent the exaggerated vasospasm that causes RP and that is not prevented by warming only the hands. The hands should be protected from injury at all times; wounds heal slowly, and infections are consequently hard to control. Softening and lubricating lotion to control the fissured dry skin should be applied to the hands frequently. Smoking should be stopped and sympathomimetic drugs (eg, decongestants, diet pills, and amphetamines) should be avoided. For most patients with primary RP, general measures alone are sufficient to control symptoms. Medical or surgical therapy should be considered in patients who have severe symptoms or are experiencing tissue injury from digital ischemia.

B. Medications

Calcium channel blockers are first-line therapy for RP. Calcium channel blockers produce a modest benefit and are more effective in primary RP than secondary RP. Slow release nifedipine (30–180 mg/day orally), amlodipine (5–20 mg/day orally), felodipine, isradipine, or nisoldipine are popular and more effective than verapamil, nicardipine, and diltiazem. Other medications that are sometimes effective in treating RP include angiotensin-converting enzyme inhibitors, sympatholytic agents (eg, prazosin), topical nitrates, phosphodiesterase inhibitors (eg, sildenafil, tadalafil, and vardenafil), selective serotonin reuptake inhibitors (fluoxetine), endothelin-receptor inhibitors (ie, bosentan), statins, parenteral prostaglandins (prostaglandin E_1), and oral prostaglandins (misoprostol).

C. Surgical Measures

Sympathectomy may be indicated when attacks have become frequent and severe, when they interfere with work and well-being, and particularly when trophic changes have developed and medical measures have failed. Cervical sympathectomy is modestly effective for primary but not secondary RP. Digital sympathectomy may improve secondary RP.

Prognosis

Primary RP is benign and largely a nuisance for affected individuals who are exposed to cold winters or excessive air conditioning. The prognosis of secondary RP depends on

the severity of the underlying disease. Unfortunately, severe pain from ulceration and gangrene is not rare with scleroderma, especially the CREST variant.

When to Refer

Appropriate management of patients with secondary RP often requires consultation with a rheumatologist.

When to Admit

Patients with severe digital ischemia as evidenced by demarcation should be admitted for intensive therapy.

Hughes M et al. Prediction and impact of attacks of Raynaud's phenomenon, as judged by patient perception. Rheumatology (Oxford). 2015 Aug;54(8):1443–7. [PMID: 25752312]

Landry GJ. Current medical and surgical management of Raynaud's syndrome. J Vasc Surg. 2013 Jun;57(6):1710–6. [PMID: 23618525]

Pavlov-Dolijanovic S et al. Late appearance and exacerbation of primary Raynaud's phenomenon attacks can predict future development of connective tissue disease: a retrospective chart review of 3,035 patients. Rheumatol Int. 2013 Apr; 33(4):921–6. [PMID: 22821334]

SCLERODERMA (Systemic Sclerosis)

ESSENTIALS OF DIAGNOSIS

▶ Limited disease (80% of patients): thickening of skin confined to the face, neck, and distal extremities.

▶ Diffuse disease (20%): widespread thickening of skin, including truncal involvement, with areas of increased pigmentation and depigmentation.

▶ Raynaud phenomenon and antinuclear antibodies are present in virtually all patients.

▶ Systemic features of gastroesophageal reflux, hypomotility of gastrointestinal tract, pulmonary fibrosis, pulmonary hypertension, and renal involvement.

General Considerations

Scleroderma (systemic sclerosis) is a rare chronic disorder characterized by diffuse fibrosis of the skin and internal organs. Symptoms usually appear in the third to fifth decades, and women are affected two to three times as frequently as men.

Two forms of scleroderma are generally recognized: limited (80% of patients) and diffuse (20%). In limited scleroderma, which is also known as the CREST syndrome (representing calcinosis cutis, Raynaud phenomenon, esophageal motility disorder, sclerodactyly, and telangiectasia), the hardening of the skin (scleroderma) is limited to the face and hands. In contrast, in diffuse scleroderma, the skin changes also involve the trunk and proximal extremities. Tendon friction rubs over the forearms and shins occur uniquely (but not universally) in diffuse scleroderma. In general, patients with limited scleroderma have better outcomes than those with diffuse disease, largely because kidney disease or interstitial lung disease rarely develops in patients with limited disease. Cardiac disease is also more characteristic of diffuse scleroderma. Patients with limited disease, however, are more susceptible to digital ischemia, leading to finger loss, and to life-threatening pulmonary hypertension. Small and large bowel hypomotility, which may occur in either form of scleroderma, can cause constipation alternating with diarrhea, malabsorption due to bacterial overgrowth, pseudoobstruction, and severe bowel distension with rupture.

Clinical Findings

A. Symptoms and Signs

Raynaud phenomenon is usually the initial manifestation and can precede other signs and symptoms by years in cases of limited scleroderma. Polyarthralgia, weight loss, and malaise are common early features of diffuse scleroderma but are infrequent in limited scleroderma. Cutaneous disease usually, but not always, develops before visceral involvement and can manifest initially as non-pitting subcutaneous edema associated with pruritus. With time the skin becomes thickened and hidebound, with loss of normal folds. Telangiectasia, pigmentation, and depigmentation are characteristic. Ulceration about the fingertips and subcutaneous calcification are seen. Dysphagia and symptoms of reflux due to esophageal dysfunction are common and result from abnormalities in motility and later from fibrosis. Fibrosis and atrophy of the gastrointestinal tract cause hypomotility. Large-mouthed diverticuli occur in the jejunum, ileum, and colon. Diffuse pulmonary fibrosis and pulmonary vascular disease are reflected in restrictive lung physiology and low diffusing capacities. Cardiac abnormalities include pericarditis, heart block, myocardial fibrosis, and right heart failure secondary to pulmonary hypertension. Scleroderma renal crisis, resulting from intimal proliferation of smaller renal arteries and usually associated with hypertension, is a marker for a poor outcome even though many cases can be treated effectively with angiotensin-converting enzyme inhibitors.

B. Laboratory Findings

Mild anemia is often present. In scleroderma renal crisis, the peripheral blood smear shows findings consistent with a microangiopathic hemolytic anemia (due to mechanical damage to red cells from diseased small vessels). Elevation of the ESR is unusual. Proteinuria appears in association with renal involvement. Antinuclear antibody tests are nearly always positive, frequently in high titers (Table 20–7). The scleroderma antibody (anti-SCL-70), directed against topoisomerase III, is found in one-third of patients with diffuse systemic sclerosis and in 20% of those with CREST syndrome. Although present in only a small number of patients with diffuse scleroderma, anti-SCL-70 antibodies may portend a poor prognosis, with a high likelihood of serious internal organ involvement (eg, interstitial lung disease). Anticentromere antibodies are seen in 50% of

those with CREST syndrome and in 1% of individuals with diffuse scleroderma (Table 20–7). Anticentromere antibodies are highly specific for limited scleroderma, but they also occur occasionally in overlap syndromes. Anti-RNA polymerase III antibodies develop in 10–20% of scleroderma patients overall and correlate with the development of diffuse skin disease and renal hypertensive crisis.

Differential Diagnosis

Early in its course, scleroderma can cause diagnostic confusion with other causes of Raynaud phenomenon, particularly SLE, mixed connective tissue disease, and the inflammatory myopathies. Scleroderma can be mistaken for other disorders characterized by skin hardening. Eosinophilic fasciitis is a rare disorder presenting with skin changes that resemble diffuse scleroderma. The inflammatory abnormalities, however, are limited to the fascia rather than the dermis and epidermis. Moreover, patients with eosinophilic fasciitis are distinguished from those with scleroderma by the presence of peripheral blood eosinophilia, the absence of Raynaud phenomenon, the good response to prednisone, and an association (in some cases) with paraproteinemias. Diffuse skin thickening and visceral involvement are features of scleromyxedema; the presence of a paraprotein, the absence of Raynaud phenomenon, and distinct skin histology point to scleromyxedema. Diabetic cheiropathy typically develops in long-standing, poorly controlled diabetes and can mimic sclerodactyly. Nephrogenic fibrosing dermopathy produces thickening and hardening of the skin of the trunk and extremities in patients with chronic kidney disease; exposure to gadolinium may play a pathogenic role. Morphea and linear scleroderma cause sclerodermatous changes limited to circumscribed areas of the skin and usually have excellent outcomes.

Treatment

Treatment of scleroderma is symptomatic and supportive and focuses on the organ systems involved. There is no effective therapy for the underlying disease process. However, interventions for management of specific organ manifestations of this disease have improved substantially. Severe Raynaud syndrome may respond to calcium channel blockers, eg, long-acting nifedipine, 30–120 mg/day orally, or to losartan, 50 mg/day orally, or to sildenafil 50 mg orally twice daily. Patients with esophageal disease should take medications in liquid or crushed form. Esophageal reflux can be reduced and the risk of scarring diminished by avoidance of late-night meals and by the use of proton pump inhibitors (eg, omeprazole, 20–40 mg/day orally), which achieve near-complete inhibition of gastric acid production and are remarkably effective for refractory esophagitis. Patients with delayed gastric emptying maintain their weight better if they eat small, frequent meals and remain upright for at least 2 hours after eating. Malabsorption due to bacterial overgrowth also responds to antibiotics, eg, tetracycline, 500 mg four times orally daily, often prescribed cyclically. The hypertensive crises associated with systemic sclerosis renal crisis must be treated early and aggressively (in the hospital) with angiotensin-converting enzyme inhibitors, eg, captopril, initiated at 25 mg orally every 6 hours and titrated up as tolerated to a maximum of 100 mg every 6 hours. Apart from the patient with myositis, prednisone has little or no role in the treatment of scleroderma; doses higher than 15 mg/day have been associated with scleroderma renal crisis. Cyclophosphamide improves dyspnea and pulmonary function tests modestly in patients with severe interstitial lung disease; this highly toxic drug should only be administered by physicians familiar with its use. Methotrexate has been used in the treatment of skin disease, arthritis, and myositis. Mycophenolate mofetil, 1 g twice daily, stabilized lung function in small, uncontrolled studies of patients with interstitial lung disease. Bosentan, an endothelin receptor antagonist, improves exercise capacity and cardiopulmonary hemodynamics in patients with pulmonary hypertension and helps prevent digital ulceration. Sildenafil or prostaglandins (delivered by continuous intravenous infusion or intermittent inhalation) may also be useful in treating pulmonary hypertension. At an experimental level, immunoablative therapy with or without stem cell rescue has achieved promising results for some patients with severe, rapidly progressive diffuse scleroderma.

The 9-year survival rate in scleroderma averages approximately 40%. The prognosis tends to be worse in those with diffuse scleroderma, in blacks, in males, and in older patients. Lung disease—in the form of pulmonary fibrosis or pulmonary arterial hypertension—is now the number one cause of mortality. Death from advanced heart failure or chronic kidney disease is also common. Those persons in whom severe internal organ involvement does not develop in the first 3 years have a substantially better prognosis, with 72% surviving at least 9 years. Breast and lung cancer may be more common in patients with scleroderma. Studies conducted in a small number of patients with simultaneous onset of cancer and scleroderma have demonstrated that the scleroderma developed as a consequence of an immune response directed at the cancer.

▶ When to Refer

- Appropriate management of scleroderma requires frequent consultations with a rheumatologist.
- Severity of organ involvement dictates referral to other subspecialists, such as pulmonologists or gastroenterologists.

Alhajeri H et al. 2013 American College of Rheumatology/European League against Rheumatism classification criteria for systemic sclerosis outperform the 1980 criteria: data from the Canadian Scleroderma Research Group. Arthritis Care Res (Hoboken). 2015 Apr;67(4):582–7. [PMID: 25233870]

Gelber AC et al. Race and association with disease manifestations and mortality in scleroderma: a 20-year experience at the Johns Hopkins Scleroderma Center and review of the literature. Medicine (Baltimore). 2013 Jul;92(4):191–205. [PMID: 23793108]

Joseph CG et al. Association of the autoimmune disease scleroderma with an immunologic response to cancer. Science. 2014 Jan 10;343(6167):152–7. [PMID: 24310608]

McMahan ZH et al. Novel investigational agents for the treatment of scleroderma. Expert Opin Investig Drugs. 2014 Feb;23(2):183–98. [PMID: 24261610]

IDIOPATHIC INFLAMMATORY MYOPATHIES (Polymyositis & Dermatomyositis)

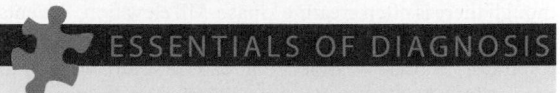

ESSENTIALS OF DIAGNOSIS

- ▶ Bilateral proximal muscle weakness.
- ▶ Characteristic cutaneous manifestations in dermatomyositis (Gottron papules, heliotrope rash).
- ▶ Diagnostic tests: elevated creatine kinase, muscle biopsy, electromyography, MRI.
- ▶ Increased risk of malignancy, particularly in dermatomyositis.
- ▶ Inclusion body myositis can mimic polymyositis but is less responsive to treatment.

▶ General Considerations

Polymyositis and dermatomyositis are systemic disorders of unknown cause whose principal manifestation is muscle weakness. Although their clinical presentations (aside from the presence of certain skin findings in dermatomyositis, some of which are pathognomonic) and treatments are similar, the two diseases are pathologically quite distinct. They affect persons of any age group, but the peak incidence is in the fifth and sixth decades of life. Women are affected twice as commonly as men, and the diseases (particularly polymyositis) also occur more often among blacks than whites. There is an increased risk of malignancy in adult patients with dermatomyositis. Indeed, up to one patient in four with dermatomyositis has an occult malignancy. Malignancies may be evident at the time of presentation with the muscle disease but may not be detected until months afterward in some cases. Patients may have skin disease without overt muscle involvement, a condition termed "dermatomyositis sine myositis." Myositis may also be associated with other connective tissue diseases, especially scleroderma, lupus, mixed connective tissue disease, and Sjögren syndrome.

▶ Clinical Findings

A. Symptoms and Signs

Polymyositis may begin abruptly, but the usual presentation is one of progressive muscle weakness over weeks to months. The weakness chiefly involves proximal muscle groups of the upper and lower extremities as well as the neck. Leg weakness (eg, difficulty in rising from a chair or climbing stairs) typically precedes arm symptoms. In contrast to myasthenia gravis, polymyositis and dermatomyositis do not cause facial or ocular muscle weakness. Pain and tenderness of affected muscles occur in one-fourth of cases, but these are rarely the chief complaints. About one-fourth of patients have dysphagia. In contrast to scleroderma, which affects the smooth muscle of the lower esophagus and can cause a "sticking" sensation below the sternum, polymyositis or dermatomyositis involves the striated muscles of the upper pharynx and can make initiation of swallowing difficult. Muscle atrophy and contractures occur as late complications of advanced disease. Clinically significant myocarditis is uncommon even though there is often creatine kinase-MB elevation. Patients who are bed-bound from myositis should be screened for respiratory muscle weakness that can be severe enough to cause CO_2 retention and can progress to require mechanical ventilation.

The characteristic rash of **dermatomyositis** is dusky red and may appear in a malar distribution mimicking the classic rash of SLE. Facial erythema beyond the malar distribution is also characteristic of dermatomyositis. Erythema also occurs over other areas of the face, neck, shoulders, and upper chest and back ("shawl sign"). Periorbital edema and a purplish (heliotrope) suffusion over the eyelids are typical signs (Figure 20–5). Coloration of the heliotrope and other rashes of dermatomyositis can be affected by skin tone. In blacks, the rashes may appear more hyperpigmented than erythematous or violaceous. Periungual erythema, dilations of nailfold capillaries, Gottron papules (raised violaceous lesions overlying the dorsa of DIP, PIP, and MCP joints) and Gottron sign (erythematous rash on the extensors surfaces of the fingers, elbows, and knees) are highly suggestive. Scalp involvement by dermatomyositis may mimic psoriasis. Infrequently, the cutaneous findings of this disease precede the muscle inflammation by weeks or months. Diagnosing polymyositis in patients over age 70 years can be difficult because weakness may be overlooked or attributed erroneously to idiopathic frailty. Polymyositis can remain undiagnosed or will be misdiagnosed as hepatitis because of elevations in alanine aminotransferase (ALT) and aspartate aminotransferase (AST) levels. A subset of patients with polymyositis and dermatomyositis develop the **"antisynthetase syndrome,"** a group of findings including inflammatory arthritis, fever, Raynaud phenomenon, "mechanic's hands" (hyperkeratosis along the radial and palmar aspects of the fingers), interstitial lung disease, and often severe muscle disease associated with certain autoantibodies (eg, anti-Jo-1 antibodies).

B. Laboratory Findings

Measurement of serum levels of muscle enzymes, especially creatine kinase and aldolase, is most useful in diagnosis and in assessment of disease activity. Anemia is uncommon. The ESR and C-reactive protein are often normal and are not reliable indicators of disease activity. Rheumatoid factor is found in a minority of patients. Antinuclear antibodies are present in many patients, especially those who have an associated connective tissue disease. A number of autoantibodies are seen exclusively in patients with myositis and are associated with distinctive clinical features (Table 20–10). The most common myositis-specific antibody, anti-Jo-1 antibody, is seen in the subset of patients who have associated interstitial lung disease, nonerosive polyarthritis, fever, and "mechanic's hands." The other myositis-specific autoantibodies are anti-Mi-2, associated with dermatomyositis; anti-SRP (anti-signal recognition particle), associated with rapidly progressive, severe polymyositis, and dysphagia; and anti-155/140, strongly associated with dermatomyositis with malignancy (malignancy in 71% with versus 11% without this antibody). In the absence of the anti-synthetase syndrome, chest radiographs are usually normal. Electromyographic abnormalities can point toward a myopathic, rather than a neurogenic, cause of weakness. MRI can detect early and patchy muscle involvement, can guide biopsies, and often is more useful than electromyography. The malignancies most commonly associated with dermatomyositis in descending order of frequency are ovarian, lung, pancreatic, stomach,

Table 20–10. Myositis-specific antibodies.

Antibody	Clinical Association
Anti-Jo-1 and other antisynthetase antibodies	Polymyositis or dermatomyositis with interstitial lung disease, arthritis, mechanic's hands
Anti-Mi-2	Dermatomyositis with rash more than myositis
Anti-MDA5 (anti-CADM 140)	Dermatomyositis with rapidly progressive lung disease, cutaneous ulcers
Anti-155/140	Cancer-associated myositis
Anti-140	Juvenile dermatomyositis
Anti-SAE	Cancer-associated dermatomyositis, dermatomyositis with rapidly progressive lung disease
Anti-signal recognition particle	Severe, acute necrotizing myopathy
Anti-HMG CoA reductase	Necrotizing myopathy related to statin use

Adapted, with permission, from Imboden JB, Hellmann DB, Stone JH (editors): *Current Diagnosis & Treatment Rheumatology*, 3rd ed. McGraw-Hill, 2013.

▲ **Figure 20–5.** Heliotrope (violaceous) rash around the eyes in a patient with dermatomyositis. (Reproduced, with permission, from Richard P. Usatine, MD.)

colorectal, and non-Hodgkin lymphoma. The search for an occult malignancy should begin with a history and physical examination, supplemented with a complete blood count, comprehensive biochemical panel, serum protein electrophoresis, and urinalysis, and should include age- and risk-appropriate cancer screening tests. Given the especially strong association of ovarian carcinoma and dermatomyositis, transvaginal ultrasonography, CT scanning, and CA-125 levels may be useful in women. No matter how extensive the initial screening, some malignancies will not become evident for months after the initial presentation.

C. Muscle Biopsy

Biopsy of clinically involved muscle is the only specific diagnostic test. The pathology findings in polymyositis and dermatomyositis are distinct. Although both include lymphoid inflammatory infiltrates, the findings in dermatomyositis are localized to perivascular regions and there is evidence of humoral and complement-mediated destruction of microvasculature associated with the muscle. In addition to its vascular orientation, the inflammatory infiltrate in dermatomyositis centers on the interfascicular septa and is located around, rather than in, muscle fascicles. A pathologic hallmark of dermatomyositis is perifascicular atrophy. In contrast, the pathology of polymyositis characteristically includes endomysial infiltration of the inflammatory infiltrate. However, false-negative biopsies sometimes occur in both disorders because of the sometimes patchy distribution of pathologic abnormalities.

► Differential Diagnosis

Muscle inflammation may occur as a component of SLE, scleroderma, Sjögren syndrome, and overlap syndromes. In those cases, associated findings usually permit the precise diagnosis of the primary condition.

Inclusion body myositis, because of its tendency to mimic polymyositis, is a common cause of "treatment-resistant polymyositis." In contrast to the epidemiologic features of polymyositis, however, the typical inclusion body myositis patient is white, male, and over the age of 50. The onset of inclusion body myositis is more insidious than that of polymyositis or dermatomyositis (eg, occurring over years rather than months), and asymmetric distal motor weakness is common in inclusion body myositis. Creatine kinase levels in inclusion body myositis are often minimally elevated and are normal in 25%. Electromyography may show a mixed picture of myopathic and neurogenic abnormalities. Muscle biopsy shows characteristic intracellular vacuoles by light microscopy and either tubular or filamentous inclusions in the nucleus or cytoplasm by electron microscopy. Inclusion body myositis is less likely to respond to therapy.

Hypothyroidism is a common cause of proximal muscle weakness associated with elevations of serum creatine kinase. Hyperthyroidism and Cushing disease may both be associated with proximal muscle weakness with normal levels of creatine kinase. Patients with polymyalgia rheumatica are over the age of 50 and—in contrast to patients with polymyositis—have pain but no objective weakness;

creatine kinase levels are normal. Disorders of the peripheral and central nervous systems (eg, chronic inflammatory polyneuropathy, multiple sclerosis, myasthenia gravis, Lambert-Eaton disease, and amyotrophic lateral sclerosis) can produce weakness but are distinguished by characteristic symptoms and neurologic signs and often by distinctive electromyographic abnormalities. A number of systemic vasculitides (polyarteritis nodosa, microscopic polyangiitis, the Churg-Strauss syndrome, granulomatosis with polyangiitis, and mixed cryoglobulinemia) can produce profound weakness through vasculitic neuropathy. The muscle weakness associated with these disorders, however, is typically distal and asymmetric, at least in the early stages.

Limb-girdle muscular dystrophy can present in early adulthood with a clinical picture that mimics polymyositis: proximal muscle weakness, elevations in serum levels of creatine kinase, and inflammatory changes on muscle biopsy. Failure to respond to treatment for polymyositis or the presence of atypical clinical features such as scapular winging or weakness of ankle plantar flexors should prompt genetic testing for limb-girdle muscular dystrophy.

Many drugs, including corticosteroids, alcohol, clofibrate, penicillamine, tryptophan, and hydroxychloroquine, can produce proximal muscle weakness. Long-term use of colchicine at doses as low as 0.6 mg twice a day in patients with moderate chronic kidney disease can produce a mixed neuropathy-myopathy that mimics polymyositis. The weakness and muscle enzyme elevation reverse with cessation of the drug. Polymyositis can occur as a complication of HIV or HTLV-1 infection and with zidovudine therapy as well.

HMG-CoA reductase inhibitors can cause myopathy and rhabdomyolysis. Although only about 0.1% of patients taking a statin drug alone develop myopathy, concomitant administration of other drugs (especially gemfibrozil, cyclosporine, niacin, macrolide antibiotics, azole antifungals, and protease inhibitors) increases the risk. Statin use has also been linked to the development of an autoimmune-mediated necrotizing myositis, which persists after the statin has been discontinued and is associated with autoantibodies to HMG-CoA reductase.

► Treatment

Most patients respond to corticosteroids. Often a daily dose of 40–60 mg or more of oral prednisone is required initially. The dose is then adjusted downward while monitoring muscle strength and serum levels of muscle enzymes. Long-term use of corticosteroids is often needed, and the disease may recur or reemerge when they are withdrawn. Patients with an associated neoplasm have a poor prognosis, although remission may follow treatment of the tumor; corticosteroids may or may not be effective in these patients. In patients resistant or intolerant to corticosteroids, therapy with methotrexate or azathioprine may be helpful. Intravenous immune globulin is effective for dermatomyositis resistant to prednisone. Mycophenolate mofetil (1–1.5 g orally twice daily) may be useful as a steroid-sparing agent. Rituximab has achieved encouraging results in some patients with inflammatory myositis unresponsive to prednisone. Since the rash of dermatomyositis is often photosensitive, patients should limit sun exposure. Hydroxychloroquine (200–400 mg/day orally not to exceed 5 mg/kg) can also help ameliorate the skin disease.

▶ When to Refer

- Appropriate management of myositis usually requires frequent consultations with a rheumatologist or neurologist.
- Severe lung disease may require consultation with a pulmonologist.

▶ When to Admit

- Signs of rhabdomyolysis.
- New onset of dysphagia.
- Respiratory insufficiency with hypoxia or carbon dioxide retention.

Cavagna L et al; AENEAS (American, European Network of Antisynthetase Syndrome) Collaborative Group. Clinical spectrum time course in anti Jo-1 positive antisynthetase syndrome: results from an international retrospective multi-center study. Medicine (Baltimore). 2015 Aug;94(32):e1144. [PMID: 26266346]
Dalakas MC. Inflammatory muscle diseases. N Engl J Med. 2015 Jul 23;373(4):393–4. [PMID: 26200989]
Venalis P et al. Immune mechanisms in polymyositis and dermatomyositis and potential targets for therapy. Rheumatology (Oxford). 2014 Mar;53(3):397–405. [PMID: 23970542]

SJÖGREN SYNDROME

ESSENTIALS OF DIAGNOSIS

- ▶ Women are 90% of patients; the average age is 50 years.
- ▶ Dryness of eyes and dry mouth (sicca components) are the most common features; they occur alone or in association with rheumatoid arthritis or other connective tissue disease.
- ▶ Rheumatoid factor and antinuclear antibodies are common.
- ▶ Increased incidence of lymphoma.

▶ General Considerations

Sjögren syndrome is a systemic autoimmune disorder whose clinical presentation is usually dominated by dryness of the eyes and mouth due to immune-mediated dysfunction of the lacrimal and salivary glands. The disorder is predominantly seen in women, with a ratio of 9:1; most cases develop between the ages of 40 and 60 years. Sjögren syndrome can occur in isolation ("primary" Sjögren syndrome) or in association with another rheumatic disease.

Sjögren syndrome is most frequently associated with rheumatoid arthritis but also occurs with SLE, primary biliary cholangitis, scleroderma, polymyositis, Hashimoto thyroiditis, polyarteritis, and interstitial pulmonary fibrosis.

▶ Clinical Findings

A. Symptoms and Signs

Keratoconjunctivitis sicca results from inadequate tear production caused by lymphocyte and plasma cell infiltration of the lacrimal glands. Ocular symptoms are usually mild. Burning, itching, and the sensation of having a foreign body or a grain of sand in the eye occur commonly. For some patients, the initial manifestation is the inability to tolerate wearing contact lenses. Many patients with more severe ocular dryness notice ropy secretions across their eyes, especially in the morning. Photophobia may signal corneal ulceration resulting from severe dryness. For most patients, symptoms of dryness of the mouth (xerostomia) dominate those of dry eyes. Patients frequently complain of a "cotton mouth" sensation and difficulty swallowing foods, especially dry foods like crackers, unless they are washed down with liquids. The persistent oral dryness causes most patients to carry water bottles or other liquid dispensers from which they sip constantly. A few patients have such severe xerostomia that they have difficulty speaking. Persistent xerostomia results often in rampant dental caries; caries at the gum line strongly suggest Sjögren syndrome. Some patients are most troubled by loss of taste and smell. Parotid enlargement, which may be chronic or relapsing, develops in one-third of patients. Desiccation may involve the nose, throat, larynx, bronchi, vagina, and skin.

Systemic manifestations include dysphagia, small vessel vasculitis, pleuritis, obstructive airways disease and interstitial lung disease (in the absence of smoking), neuropsychiatric dysfunction (most commonly peripheral neuropathies), and pancreatitis; they may be related to the associated diseases noted above. Renal tubular acidosis (type I, distal) occurs in 20% of patients. Chronic interstitial nephritis, which may result in impaired kidney function, may be seen.

B. Laboratory Findings

Laboratory findings include mild anemia, leukopenia, and eosinophilia. Polyclonal hypergammaglobulinemia, rheumatoid factor positivity (70%), and antinuclear antibodies (95%) are all common findings. Antibodies against SS-A and SS-B (also called Ro and La, respectively) are often present in primary Sjögren syndrome and tend to correlate with the presence of extra-glandular manifestations (Table 20–7). Thyroid-associated autoimmunity is a common finding among patients with Sjögren syndrome.

Useful ocular diagnostic tests include the Schirmer test, which measures the quantity of tears secreted. Lip biopsy, a simple procedure, reveals characteristic lymphoid foci in accessory salivary glands. Biopsy of the parotid gland should be reserved for patients with atypical presentations such as unilateral gland enlargement that suggest a neoplastic process.

Differential Diagnosis

Isolated complaints of dry mouth are most commonly due to medication side effects. Chronic hepatitis C can cause sicca symptoms and rheumatoid factor positivity. Minor salivary gland biopsies reveal lymphocytic infiltrates but not to the extent of Sjögren syndrome, and tests for anti-SS-A and anti-SS-B are negative. Involvement of the lacrimal or salivary glands, or both in sarcoidosis can mimic Sjögren syndrome; biopsies reveal noncaseating granulomas. Rarely, amyloid deposits in the lacrimal and salivary glands produce sicca symptoms. IgG$_4$-related systemic disease (characterized by high serum IgG$_4$ levels and infiltration of tissues with IgG$_4^+$ plasma cells) can result in lacrimal and salivary gland enlargement that mimics Sjögren syndrome.

Treatment & Prognosis

Treatment of sicca symptoms is symptomatic and supportive. Artificial tears applied frequently will relieve ocular symptoms and avert further desiccation. Topical ocular 0.05% cyclosporine also improves ocular symptoms and signs of dryness. The mouth should be kept well lubricated. Sipping water frequently or using sugar-free gums and hard candies usually relieves dry mouth symptoms. Pilocarpine (5 mg orally four times daily) and the acetylcholine derivative cevimeline (30 mg orally three times daily) may improve xerostomia symptoms. Atropinic drugs and decongestants decrease salivary secretions and should be avoided. A program of oral hygiene, including fluoride treatment, is essential in order to preserve dentition. If there is an associated rheumatic disease, its systemic treatment is not altered by the presence of Sjögren syndrome.

Although Sjögren syndrome may compromise patients' quality of life significantly, the disease is usually consistent with a normal life span. Poor prognoses are influenced mainly by the presence of systemic features associated with underlying disorders, the development in some patients of lymphocytic vasculitis, the occurrence of a painful peripheral neuropathy, and the complication (in a minority of patients) of lymphoma. Severe systemic inflammatory manifestations are treated with prednisone or various immunosuppressive medications. The patients (3–10% of the total Sjögren population) at greatest risk for developing lymphoma are those with severe exocrine dysfunction, marked parotid gland enlargement, splenomegaly, vasculitis, peripheral neuropathy, anemia, and mixed monoclonal cryoglobulinemia.

When to Refer

- Presence of systemic symptoms or signs.
- Symptoms or signs of ocular dryness not responsive to artificial tears.

When to Admit

Presence of severe systemic signs such as vasculitis unresponsive to outpatient management.

Colafrancesco S et al. Myositis in primary Sjögren's syndrome: data from a multicentre cohort. Clin Exp Rheumatol. 2015 Jul–Aug;33(4):457–64. [PMID: 26088683]

Quartuccio L et al. Clinical and biological differences between cryoglobulinaemic and hypergammaglobulinaemic purpura in primary Sjögren's syndrome: results of a large multicentre study. Scand J Rheumatol. 2015;44(1):36–41. [PMID: 25268749]

St Clair EW et al; Autoimmunity Centers of Excellence. Rituximab therapy for primary Sjögren's syndrome: an open-label clinical trial and mechanistic analysis. Arthritis Rheum. 2013 Apr; 65(4):1097–106. [PMID: 23334994]

IgG$_4$-RELATED DISEASE

 ESSENTIALS OF DIAGNOSIS

- ▶ Predominantly affects men (75% of patients); average age older than 50 years.
- ▶ Protean manifestations caused by lymphoplasmacytic infiltrates in any organ or tissue, especially the pancreas, lacrimal glands, biliary tract, and retroperitoneum.
- ▶ Subacute onset; fever, constitutional symptoms rare.
- ▶ Diagnosis rests on specific histopathological findings that include presence of IgG$_4$-bearing plasma cells.

General Considerations

IgG$_4$-related disease is a systemic disorder of unknown cause marked by highly characteristic fibroinflammatory changes that can affect virtually any organ. Elevations of serum IgG$_4$ levels occur often but are not diagnostic. The disorder chiefly affects men over the age of 50 years.

Clinical Findings

A. Symptoms and Signs

IgG$_4$-related disease has been compared with sarcoidosis: both disorders can affect any organ of the body, can be localized or generalized, demonstrate the same distinctive histopathology at all sites of involvement, produce protean manifestations depending on location and extent of involvement, and cause disease that ranges in severity from asymptomatic to organ- or life-threatening. The inflammatory infiltration in IgG$_4$-related disease frequently produces tumefactive masses that can be seen on physical examination or on imaging. Some of the common presenting manifestations include enlargement of submandibular glands, proptosis from periorbital infiltration, retroperitoneal fibrosis, mediastinal fibrosis, inflammatory aortic aneurysm, and pancreatic mass with autoimmune pancreatitis. IgG$_4$-related disease can also affect the thyroid, kidney, meninges, sinuses, lung, prostate, breast, and bone. Most symptomatic patients with IgG$_4$-related disease present subacutely; fever and constitutional symptoms are usually absent. Nearly half of the patients with IgG$_4$-related disease also have allergic disorders such as sinusitis or asthma.

B. Laboratory Findings

The infiltrating lesions in IgG$_4$-related disease often produce tumors or fibrotic changes that are evident on CT or MRI imaging. However, the cornerstone of diagnosis is the histopathology. The key pathological findings are a dense lymphoplasmacytic infiltrate rich in IgG$_4$ plasma cells, storiform (matted and irregularly whorled) fibrosis, and obliterative phlebitis. Serum IgG$_4$ levels are usually, but not invariably, elevated so this finding cannot be used as the sole diagnostic criterion.

Differential Diagnosis

IgG$_4$-related disease can mimic many disorders including Sjögren syndrome (lacrimal gland enlargement), pancreatic cancer (pancreatic mass), and granulomatosis with polyangiitis (proptosis). It is now recognized that some cases of retroperitoneal fibrosis and mediastinal fibrosis are caused by IgG$_4$-related disease. Lymphoma can mimic some of the histopathologic features of IgG$_4$-related disease.

Treatment & Prognosis

Patients who are asymptomatic and have no organ-threatening disease can be monitored carefully. Spontaneous resolution can occur. The optimal therapy for symptomatic patients has not been defined, but initial therapy is usually oral prednisone 0.6 mg/kg/day, tapered over weeks or months depending on response. Patients who do not respond to prednisone or respond only to sustained high doses of prednisone can be treated with rituximab, mycophenolate mofetil, or azathioprine. The degree of fibrosis in affected organs determines the patient's responsiveness to treatment.

When to Refer

- Presence of systemic symptoms or signs.
- Symptoms or signs not responsive to prednisone.

When to Admit

Presence of severe systemic signs unresponsive to outpatient management.

Kamisawa et al. IgG$_4$-related disease. Lancet. 2015 Apr 11;385 (9976):1460–71. [PMID: 25481618]

RHABDOMYOLYSIS

ESSENTIALS OF DIAGNOSIS

- ▶ Associated with crush injuries to muscle, prolonged immobility, drug toxicities, hypothermia, and other causes.
- ▶ Massive acute elevations of muscle enzymes that peak quickly and usually resolve within days once the inciting injury has been identified and removed.

General Considerations

Rhabdomyolysis is a syndrome of acute necrosis of skeletal muscle associated with myoglobinuria and markedly elevated creatine kinase levels. Acute tubular necrosis is a common complication of rhabdomyolysis and is due to the toxic effects of filtering excessive quantities of myoglobin in the setting of hypovolemia (See Acute Tubular Necrosis in Chapter 22). Many patients in whom rhabdomyolysis develops are volume-contracted and, therefore, oliguric renal failure is encountered routinely.

Cocaine use and alcohol intoxication, particularly in the setting of prolonged immobility and exposure hypothermia, are leading causes of admissions due to rhabdomyolysis on the medical services of inner-city hospitals. Use of statins is another important cause of rhabdomyolysis. The presence of compromised kidney and liver function, diabetes mellitus, and hypothyroidism as well as concomitant use of other medications increase the risk of rhabdomyolysis in patients taking statins. The cytochrome P450 liver enzymes metabolize all statins except for pravastatin and rosuvastatin. Drugs that block the action of cytochrome P450 include protease inhibitors, erythromycin, itraconazole, clarithromycin, diltiazem, and verapamil. Use of these drugs concomitantly with the statins (but not pravastatin or rosuvastatin) can increase the risk of development of rhabdomyolysis. The likelihood of rhabdomyolysis also increases when statins are used with niacin and fibric acids (gemfibrozil, clofibrate, and fenofibrate). Rhabdomyolysis is an uncommon complication of polymyositis, dermatomyositis, and the myopathy of hypothyroidism, despite the high levels of creatine kinase often seen in these conditions.

Often there is little evidence for muscle injury on clinical assessment of the patients with rhabdomyolysis—specifically, myalgias and weakness are usually absent. The first clue to muscle necrosis in such individuals may be a urinary dipstick testing positive for "blood" (actually myoglobin) in the absence of red cells in the sediment. This myoglobinuria results in a false-positive reading for hemoglobin. Urine tests for myoglobin are insensitive, however, positive in only 25% of patients with rhabdomyolysis. Such an abnormality should prompt determination of the serum creatine kinase level, which invariably is elevated (usually markedly so). Other commonly encountered laboratory abnormalities in rhabdomyolysis include elevated serum levels of AST, ALT, and lactate dehydrogenase due to release of these enzymes from skeletal muscle.

Treatment

Vigorous fluid resuscitation (4–6 L/day, with careful monitoring for volume overload) is indicated. Infusion of mannitol (100 mg/day) and urine alkalinization (to minimize precipitation of myoglobin within tubules) have been recommended as measures to reduce kidney injury, but definitive evidence for the efficacy of these measures is lacking. Myopathic complications of statins usually resolve within several weeks of discontinuing the drug.

Panzio N et al. Molecular mechanisms and novel therapeutic approaches to rhabdomyolysis-induced acute kidney injury. Kidney Blood Press Res. 2015;40(5):520–32. [PMID: 26512883]

VASCULITIS SYNDROMES

"Vasculitis" is a heterogeneous group of disorders characterized by inflammation within the walls of affected blood vessels. The major forms of primary systemic vasculitis are listed in Table 20–11. The first consideration in classifying cases of vasculitis is the size of the major vessels involved: large, medium, or small. The presence of the clinical signs and symptoms shown in Table 20–12 helps distinguish among these three groups. After determining the size of the major vessels involved, other issues that contribute to the classification include the following:

- Does the process involve arteries, veins, or both?
- What are the patient's demographic characteristics (age, sex, ethnicity, smoking status)?
- Which organs are involved?
- Is there hypocomplementemia or other evidence of immune complex deposition?
- Is there granulomatous inflammation on tissue biopsy?
- Are antineutrophil cytoplasmic antibodies (ANCA) present?

In addition to the disorders considered to be primary vasculitides, there are also multiple forms of vasculitis that are associated with other known underlying conditions. These "secondary" forms of vasculitis occur in the setting of chronic infections (eg, hepatitis B or C, subacute bacterial endocarditis), connective tissue disorders, inflammatory bowel disease, malignancies, and reactions to medications. Only the major primary forms of vasculitis are discussed here.

Gwathmey KG et al. Vasculitic neuropathies. Lancet Neurol. 2014 Jan;13(1):67–82. [PMID: 24331794]

Table 20–11. Classification scheme of primary vasculitides according to size of predominant blood vessels involved.

Predominantly large-vessel vasculitides
Takayasu arteritis
Giant cell arteritis (temporal arteritis)
Behçet disease[1]
Predominantly medium-vessel vasculitides
Polyarteritis nodosa
Buerger disease
Primary angiitis of the central nervous system
Predominantly small-vessel vasculitides
Immune-complex mediated
Cutaneous leukocytoclastic angiitis ("hypersensitivity vasculitis")
Henoch-Schönlein purpura
Essential cryoglobulinemia[2]
"ANCA-associated" disorders[3]
Granulomatosis with polyangiitis (formerly Wegener granulomatosis)[2]
Microscopic polyangiitis[2]
Eosinophilic granulomatosis with polyangiitis (formerly Churg-Strauss syndrome)[2]

[1]May involve small-, medium-, and large-sized blood vessels.
[2]Frequent overlap of small and medium-sized blood vessel involvement.
[3]Not all forms of these disorders are always associated with ANCA.
ANCA, antineutrophil cytoplasmic antibodies.

Table 20–12. Typical clinical manifestations of large-, medium-, and small-vessel involvement by vasculitis.

Large	Medium	Small
Constitutional symptoms: fever, weight loss, malaise, arthralgias/arthritis		
Limb claudication	Cutaneous nodules	Purpura
Asymmetric blood pressures	Ulcers	Vesiculobullous lesions
Absence of pulses	Livedo reticularis	Urticaria
Bruits	Digital gangrene	Glomerulonephritis
Aortic dilation	Mononeuritis multiplex	Alveolar hemorrhage
	Microaneurysms	Cutaneous extravascular necrotizing granulomas
		Splinter hemorrhages
		Uveitis
		Episcleritis
		Scleritis

POLYMYALGIA RHEUMATICA & GIANT CELL ARTERITIS

ESSENTIALS OF DIAGNOSIS

- ▶ Age over 50 years.
- ▶ Giant cell (temporal) arteritis is characterized by headache, jaw claudication, polymyalgia rheumatica, visual abnormalities, and a markedly elevated ESR.
- ▶ The hallmark of polymyalgia rheumatica is pain and stiffness in shoulders and hips lasting for several weeks without other explanation.

General Considerations

Polymyalgia rheumatica and giant cell arteritis probably represent a spectrum of one disease: Both affect the same population (patients over the age of 50), show preference for the same HLA haplotypes, and show similar patterns of cytokines in blood and arteries. Polymyalgia rheumatica and giant cell arteritis also frequently coexist. The important differences between the two conditions are that polymyalgia rheumatica alone does not cause blindness and responds to low-dose (10–20 mg/day orally) prednisone therapy, whereas giant cell arteritis can cause blindness and large artery complications and requires high-dose (40–60 mg/day) prednisone.

► Clinical Findings

A. Polymyalgia Rheumatica

Polymyalgia rheumatica is a clinical diagnosis based on pain and stiffness of the shoulder and pelvic girdle areas, frequently in association with fever, malaise, and weight loss. In approximately two-thirds of cases, polymyalgia occurs in the absence of giant cell arteritis. Because of the stiffness and pain in the shoulders, hips, and lower back, patients have trouble combing their hair, putting on a coat, or rising from a chair. In contrast to polymyositis and poly-arteritis nodosa, polymyalgia rheumatica does not cause muscular weakness either through primary muscle inflam-mation or secondary to nerve infarction. A few patients have joint swelling, particularly of the knees, wrists, and sternoclavicular joints.

B. Giant Cell Arteritis

Giant cell arteritis is a systemic panarteritis affecting medium-sized and large vessels in patients over the age of 50. The incidence of this disease increases with each decade of life. The mean age at onset is approximately 79 years. Giant cell arteritis is also called temporal arteritis because that artery is frequently involved, as are other extracranial branches of the carotid artery. About 50% of patients with giant cell arteritis also have polymyalgia rheumatica. The classic symptoms suggesting that a patient has arteritis are headache, scalp tenderness, visual symptoms (particularly amaurosis fugax or diplopia), jaw claudication, or throat pain. Of these symptoms, jaw claudication has the highest positive predictive value. The temporal artery is usually normal on physical examination but may be nodular, enlarged, tender, or pulseless. Blindness usually results from the syndrome of anterior ischemic optic neuropathy, caused by occlusive arteritis of the posterior ciliary branch of the ophthalmic artery. The ischemic optic neuropathy of giant cell arteritis may produce no funduscopic findings for the first 24–48 hours after the onset of blindness.

Asymmetry of pulses in the arms, a murmur of aortic regurgitation, or bruits heard near the clavicle resulting from subclavian artery stenoses identify patients in whom giant cell arteritis has affected the aorta or its major branches. Clinically evident large vessel involvement—characterized chiefly by aneurysm of the thoracic aorta or stenosis of the subclavian, vertebral, carotid, and basilar arteries—occurs in approximately 25% of patients with giant cell arteritis, sometimes years after the diagnosis. Subclinical large artery disease is the rule: positron emis-sion tomography scans reveal inflammation in the aorta and its major branches in nearly 85% of untreated patients. Forty percent of patients with giant cell arteritis have non-classic symptoms at presentation, chiefly respiratory tract problems (most frequently dry cough), mononeuritis mul-tiplex (most frequently with painful paralysis of a shoul-der), or fever of unknown origin. Giant cell arteritis accounts for 15% of all cases of fever of unknown origin in patients over the age of 65. The fever can be as high as 40°C and is frequently associated with rigors and sweats. In con-trast to patients with infection, patients with giant cell arteritis and fever usually have normal white blood cell counts (before prednisone is started). Thus, in an older patient with fever of unknown origin, marked elevations of acute phase reactants, and a normal white blood count, giant cell arteritis must be considered even in the absence of specific features such as headache or jaw claudication. In some cases, instead of having the well-known symptom of jaw claudication, patients complain of vague pain affecting other locations, including the tongue, nose, or ears. Indeed, unexplained head or neck pain in an older patient may signal the presence of giant cell arteritis.

C. Laboratory Findings

1. Polymyalgia rheumatica—Anemia and elevated acute phase reactants (often markedly elevated ESRs, for exam-ple) are present in the most cases, but cases of polymyalgia rheumatica occurring with normal acute phase reactants are well documented.

2. Giant cell arteritis—Nearly 90% of patients with giant cell arteritis have ESRs higher than 50 mm/h. The ESR in this disorder is often more than 100 mm/h, but cases in which the ESR is lower or even normal do occur. In one series, 5% of patients with biopsy-proven giant cell arteritis had ESRs below 40 mm/h. Although the C-reactive protein is slightly more sensitive, patients with biopsy-proven giant cell arteritis with normal C-reactive proteins have also been described. Most patients also have a mild normochro-mic, normocytic anemia and thrombocytosis. The alkaline phosphatase (liver source) is elevated in 20% of patients with giant cell arteritis.

► Differential Diagnosis

The differential diagnosis of malaise, anemia, and striking acute phase reactant elevations includes rheumatic diseases (such as rheumatoid arthritis, other systemic vasculitides, multiple myeloma, and other malignant disorders) and chronic infections (such as bacterial endocarditis and osteomyelitis).

► Treatment

A. Polymyalgia Rheumatica

Patients with isolated polymyalgia rheumatica (ie, those not having "above the neck" symptoms of headache, jaw claudication, scalp tenderness, or visual symptoms) are treated with prednisone, 10–20 mg/day orally. If the patient does not experience a dramatic improvement within 72 hours, the diagnosis should be revisited. Usually after 2–4 weeks of treatment, slow tapering of the prednisone can be attempted. Most patients require some dose of pred-nisone for a minimum of approximately 1 year; 6 months is too short in most cases. Disease flares are common (50% or more) as prednisone is tapered. The addition of weekly methotrexate may increase the chance of successfully tapering prednisone in some patients.

B. Giant Cell Arteritis

The urgency of early diagnosis and treatment in giant cell arteritis relates to the prevention of blindness. Once blindness develops, it is usually permanent. Therefore, when a patient has symptoms and findings suggestive of temporal arteritis, therapy with prednisone (60 mg/day orally) should be initiated immediately and a temporal artery biopsy performed promptly. For patients who seek medical attention for visual loss, intravenous pulse methylprednisolone (eg, 1 g daily for 3 days) has been advocated; unfortunately, few patients recover vision no matter what the initial treatment. One study—too small and too preliminary to change the standard therapy recommendations mentioned above—suggested that initiating treatment with intravenous pulse methylprednisolone may increase the chance that a patient with giant cell arteritis will achieve remission and be able to taper off of prednisone. Retrospective studies suggest that low-dose aspirin (~81 mg/day orally) may reduce the chance of visual loss or stroke in patients with giant cell arteritis and should be added to prednisone in the initial treatment. Although it is prudent to obtain a temporal artery biopsy as soon as possible after instituting treatment, diagnostic findings of giant cell arteritis may still be present 2 weeks (or even considerably longer) after starting corticosteroids. Typically, a positive biopsy shows inflammatory infiltrate in the media and adventitia with lymphocytes, histiocytes, plasma cells, and giant cells. An adequate biopsy specimen is essential (at least 2 cm in length is ideal), because the disease may be segmental. Unilateral temporal artery biopsies are positive in approximately 80–85% of patients, but bilateral biopsies add incrementally to the yield (10–15% in some studies, less in others). Temporal artery biopsy is abnormal in only 50% of patients with large artery disease (eg, arm claudication and unequal upper extremity blood pressures). In these patients, magnetic resonance angiography or CT angiography will establish the diagnosis by demonstrating long stretches of narrowing of the subclavian and axillary arteries. Prednisone should be continued in a dosage of 60 mg/day orally for about 1 month before tapering. When only the symptoms of polymyalgia rheumatica are present, temporal artery biopsy is not necessary.

After 1 month of high-dose prednisone, almost all patients will have a normal ESR. When tapering and adjusting the dosage of prednisone, the ESR (or C-reactive protein) is a useful but not absolute guide to disease activity. A common error is treating the ESR rather than the patient. The ESR often rises slightly as the prednisone is tapered, even as the disease remains quiescent. Because elderly individuals often have baseline ESRs that are above the normal range, mild ESR elevations should not be an occasion for renewed treatment with prednisone in patients who are asymptomatic. Unfortunately, no highly effective prednisone-sparing therapy has been identified. Methotrexate was modestly effective in one double-blind, placebo-controlled treatment trial but ineffective in another. Anti-TNF therapies do not work in giant cell arteritis, but there may be a role for the anti-interleukin-6 receptor monoclonal antibody tocilizumab. Thoracic aortic aneurysms occur 17 times more frequently in patients with giant cell arteritis than in normal individuals and can result in aortic regurgitation, dissection, or rupture. The aneurysms can develop at any time but typically occur 7 years after the diagnosis of giant cell arteritis is made.

González-Gay MA et al. Giant cell arteritis and polymyalgia rheumatica: an update. Curr Rheumatol Rep. 2015 Feb;17(2):6. [PMID: 25618572]

Weyand CM et al. Clinical practice. Giant-cell arteritis and polymyalgia rheumatica. N Engl J Med. 2014 Jul 3;371(1):50–7. [PMID: 24988557]

TAKAYASU ARTERITIS

Takayasu arteritis is a granulomatous vasculitis of the aorta and its major branches. Rare in North America but more prevalent in the Far East, it primarily affects women and typically has its onset in early adulthood. Takayasu arteritis can present with nonspecific constitutional symptoms of malaise, fever, and weight loss or with manifestations of vascular damage (diminished pulses, unequal blood pressures in the arms, bruits over carotids and subclavian arteries, limb claudication, and hypertension). There are no specific laboratory abnormalities; the ESR and the C-reactive protein level are elevated in most cases. The diagnosis is established by imaging studies, usually MRI, which can detect inflammatory thickening of the walls of affected vessels, or CT angiography, which can provide images of the stenoses, occlusions, and dilations characteristic of arteritis. Corticosteroids (eg, oral prednisone, 1 mg/kg for 1 month, followed by a taper over several months to 10 mg daily) are the mainstays of treatment. The addition of methotrexate or mycophenolate mofetil to the prednisone may be more effective than the prednisone alone. Takayasu arteritis has a chronic relapsing and remitting course that requires ongoing monitoring and adjustment of therapy.

Clifford A et al. Recent advances in the medical management of Takayasu arteritis: an update on use of biological therapies. Curr Opin Rheumatol. 2014 Jan;26(1):7–15. [PMID: 24225487]

POLYARTERITIS NODOSA

 ESSENTIALS OF DIAGNOSIS

▶ Medium-sized arteries are always affected; smaller arterioles are sometimes involved; lung is spared but kidney often affected, causing renin-mediated hypertension.

▶ Clinical findings depend on the arteries involved.

▶ Common features include fever, abdominal pain, extremity pain, livedo reticularis, mononeuritis multiplex, anemia, and elevated acute phase reactants (ESR or C-reactive protein or both).

▶ Associated with hepatitis B (10% of cases).

General Considerations

Polyarteritis nodosa, described in 1866, is acknowledged widely as the first form of vasculitis reported in the medical literature. For many years, all forms of inflammatory vascular disease were termed "polyarteritis nodosa." In recent decades, numerous subtypes of vasculitis have been recognized, greatly narrowing the spectrum of vasculitis called polyarteritis nodosa. Currently, the term is reserved for necrotizing arteritis of medium-sized vessels that has a predilection for involving the skin, peripheral nerves, mesenteric vessels (including renal arteries), heart, and brain, but polyarteritis nodosa can actually involve almost any organ. Polyarteritis nodosa is relatively rare, with a prevalence of about 30 per 1 million people. Approximately 10% of cases of polyarteritis nodosa are caused by hepatitis B. Most cases of hepatitis B–associated disease occur within 6 months of hepatitis B infection. A mutation in the gene for adenosine deaminase 2 has been identified in the rare cases of familial polyarteritis.

Clinical Findings

A. Symptoms and Signs

The clinical onset is usually insidious, with fever, malaise, weight loss, and other symptoms developing over weeks to months. Pain in the extremities is often a prominent early feature caused by arthralgia, myalgia (particularly affecting the calves), or neuropathy. The combination of mononeuritis multiplex (with the most common finding being foot-drop) and features of a systemic illness is one of the earliest specific clues to the presence of an underlying vasculitis. Polyarteritis nodosa is among the forms of vasculitis most commonly associated with vasculitic neuropathy.

In polyarteritis nodosa, the typical skin findings—livedo reticularis, subcutaneous nodules, and skin ulcers—reflect the involvement of deeper, medium-sized blood vessels. Digital gangrene is not an unusual occurrence. The most common cutaneous presentation is lower extremity ulcerations, usually occurring near the malleoli. Involvement of the renal arteries leads to a renin-mediated hypertension (much less characteristic of vasculitides involving smaller blood vessels). For unclear reasons, classic polyarteritis nodosa seldom (if ever) involves the lung, with the occasional exception of the bronchial arteries.

Abdominal pain—particularly diffuse periumbilical pain precipitated by eating—is common but often difficult to attribute to mesenteric vasculitis in the early stages. Nausea and vomiting are common symptoms. Infarction compromises the function of major viscera and may lead to acalculous cholecystitis or appendicitis. Some patients present dramatically with an acute abdomen caused by mesenteric vasculitis and gut perforation or with hypotension resulting from rupture of a microaneurysm in the liver, kidney, or bowel.

Subclinical cardiac involvement is common in polyarteritis nodosa, and overt cardiac dysfunction occasionally occurs (eg, myocardial infarction secondary to coronary vasculitis, or myocarditis).

B. Laboratory Findings

Most patients with polyarteritis nodosa have a slight anemia, and leukocytosis is common. Acute-phase reactants are often (but not always) strikingly elevated. A major challenge in making the diagnosis of polyarteritis nodosa, however, is the absence of a disease-specific serologic test (eg, an autoantibody). Patients with classic polyarteritis nodosa are ANCA-negative and may have low titers of rheumatoid factor or antinuclear antibodies, both of which are nonspecific findings. In patients with polyarteritis nodosa, appropriate serologic tests for active hepatitis B infection (HBsAg, HBeAg) must be performed.

C. Biopsy and Angiography

The diagnosis of polyarteritis nodosa requires confirmation with either a tissue biopsy or an angiogram. Biopsies of symptomatic sites such as skin (from the edge of an ulcer or the center of a nodule), nerve, or muscle have sensitivities of approximately 70%. The least invasive tests should usually be obtained first, but biopsy of an involved organ is essential. If performed by experienced clinicians, tissue biopsies normally have high benefit-risk ratios because of the importance of establishing the diagnosis. Patients in whom polyarteritis nodosa is suspected—eg, on the basis of mesenteric ischemia or new-onset hypertension occurring in the setting of a systemic illness—may be diagnosed by the angiographic finding of aneurysmal dilations in the renal, mesenteric, or hepatic arteries. Angiography must be performed cautiously in patients with baseline renal dysfunction.

Treatment

For polyarteritis nodosa, corticosteroids in high doses (up to 60 mg of oral prednisone daily) may control fever and constitutional symptoms and heal vascular lesions. Pulse methylprednisolone (eg, 1 g intravenously daily for 3 days) may be necessary for patients who are critically ill at presentation. Immunosuppressive agents, especially cyclophosphamide, lower the risk of disease-related death and morbidity among patients who have severe disease. For patients with polyarteritis nodosa associated with hepatitis B, the preferred treatment regimen is a short course of prednisone accompanied by anti-HBV therapy and plasmapheresis (three times a week for up to 6 weeks).

Prognosis

Without treatment, the 5-year survival rate in this disorder is poor—on the order of 10%. With appropriate therapy, remissions are possible in many cases and the 5-year survival rate has improved to 60–90%. Poor prognostic factors are chronic kidney disease with serum creatinine greater than 1.6 mg/dL (141 mcmol/L), proteinuria greater than 1 g/day, gastrointestinal ischemia, central nervous system disease, and cardiac involvement. In the absence of any of these five factors, 5-year survival is nearly 90%. Survival at 5 years drops to 75% with one poor prognostic factor present and to about 50% with two or more factors. Substantial morbidity and even death may result from adverse effects of cyclophosphamide and corticosteroids. Consequently, these therapies require careful monitoring and expert management. In contrast to many other forms of systemic vasculitis, disease relapses in polyarteritis following the successful induction of remission are the exception rather than the rule, occurring in only about 20% of cases.

Diamantopoulos AP et al. Polyarteritis nodosa. J Rheumatol. 2013 Jan;40(1):87–8. [PMID: 23280163]

Forbess L et al. Polyarteritis nodosa. Rheum Dis Clin North Am. 2015;41(1):33–46. [PMID: 25399938]

Navon Elkan P et al. Mutant adenosine deaminase 2 in a polyarteritis nodosa vasculopathy. N Engl J Med. 2014 Mar 6;370(10): 921–31. [PMID: 24552285]

GRANULOMATOSIS WITH POLYANGIITIS (Formerly Wegener Granulomatosis)

ESSENTIALS OF DIAGNOSIS

- ▶ Classic triad of upper and lower respiratory tract disease and glomerulonephritis.
- ▶ Suspect if mild respiratory symptoms (eg, nasal congestion, sinusitis) are refractory to usual treatment.
- ▶ Pathology defined by the triad of small-vessel vasculitis, granulomatous inflammation, and necrosis.
- ▶ ANCAs (90% of patients), usually directed against proteinase-3 (less commonly against myeloperoxidase present in severe, active disease).
- ▶ Kidney disease often rapidly progressive without treatment.

▶ General Considerations

Granulomatosis with polyangiitis, which has an estimated incidence of approximately 12 cases per million individuals per year, is the prototype of diseases associated with antineutrophil cytoplasmic antibodies (ANCA). (Other "ANCA-associated vasculitides" include microscopic polyangiitis and the Churg-Strauss syndrome.) Granulomatosis with polyangiitis is characterized in its full expression by vasculitis of small arteries, arterioles, and capillaries, necrotizing granulomatous lesions of both upper and lower respiratory tract, glomerulonephritis, and other organ manifestations. Without treatment, generalized disease is invariably fatal, with most patients surviving less than 1 year after diagnosis. It occurs most commonly in the fourth and fifth decades of life and affects men and women with equal frequency.

▶ Clinical Findings

A. Symptoms and Signs

The disorder usually develops over 4–12 months. Upper respiratory tract symptoms develop in 90% of patients and lower respiratory tract symptoms develop in 60% of

patients; some patients may have both upper and lower respiratory tract symptoms. Upper respiratory tract symptoms can include nasal congestion, sinusitis, otitis media, mastoiditis, inflammation of the gums, or stridor due to subglottic stenosis. Since many of these symptoms are common, the underlying disease is not often suspected until the patient develops systemic symptoms or the original problem is refractory to treatment. The lungs are affected initially in 40% and eventually in 80%, with symptoms including cough, dyspnea, and hemoptysis. Other early symptoms can include a migratory oligoarthritis with a predilection for large joints; a variety of symptoms related to ocular disease (unilateral proptosis from orbital pseudotumor; red eye from scleritis [Figure 20–6], episcleritis, anterior uveitis, or peripheral ulcerative keratitis); purpura or other skin lesions; and dysesthesia due to neuropathy. Renal involvement, which develops in three-fourths of the cases, may be subclinical until kidney disease is advanced. Fever, malaise, and weight loss are common.

Physical examination can be remarkable for congestion, crusting, ulceration, bleeding, and even perforation of the nasal septum. Destruction of the nasal cartilage with "saddle nose" deformity occurs late. Otitis media, proptosis, scleritis, episcleritis, and conjunctivitis are other common findings. Newly acquired hypertension, a frequent feature of polyarteritis nodosa, is rare in granulomatosis with polyangiitis. Venous thrombotic events (eg, deep venous thrombosis and pulmonary embolism) are a common occurrence in granulomatosis with polyangiitis, at least in part because of the tendency of the disease to involve veins as well as arteries. Although limited forms of granulomatosis with polyangiitis have been described in which the kidney is spared initially, kidney disease will develop in the majority of untreated patients.

▲ **Figure 20–6.** Scleritis in a patient with granulomatosis with polyangiitis (formerly Wegener granulomatosis). (From Everett Allen, MD; reproduced, with permission, from Usatine RP, Smith MA, Mayeaux EJ Jr, Chumley H, Tysinger J. *The Color Atlas of Family Medicine*. McGraw-Hill, 2009.)

B. Laboratory Findings

1. Serum tests and urinalysis—Most patients have slight anemia, mild leukocytosis, and elevated acute-phase reactants. If there is renal involvement, there is proteinuria and the urinary sediment contains red cells, with or without white cells, and often has red cell casts.

Serum tests for ANCA help in the diagnosis of granulomatosis with polyangiitis and related forms of vasculitis (Table 20–7). Several different types of ANCA are recognized, but the two subtypes relevant to systemic vasculitis are those directed against proteinase-3 (PR3) and myeloperoxidase (MPO). Antibodies to these two antigens are termed "PR3-ANCA" and "MPO-ANCA," respectively. The cytoplasmic pattern of immunofluorescence (c-ANCA) caused by PR3-ANCA has a high specificity (more than 90%) for either granulomatosis with polyangiitis or a closely related disease, microscopic polyangiitis (or, less commonly, the Churg-Strauss syndrome). In the setting of active disease, particularly cases in which the disease is severe and generalized to multiple organ systems, the sensitivity of PR3-ANCA is greater than 95%. A substantial percentage of patients with "limited" granulomatosis with polyangiitis—disease that does not pose an immediate threat to life and is often confined to the respiratory tract—are ANCA-negative. Although ANCA testing may be very helpful when used properly, it does not eliminate the need in most cases for confirmation of the diagnosis by tissue biopsy. Furthermore, ANCA levels correlate erratically with disease activity, and changes in titer should not dictate changes in therapy in the absence of supporting clinical data. The perinuclear (p-ANCA) pattern, caused by MPO-ANCA, is more likely to occur in microscopic polyangiitis or Churg-Strauss but may also be found in granulomatosis with polyangiitis. Approximately 10–25% of patients with classic granulomatosis with polyangiitis have MPO-ANCA. All positive immunofluorescence assays for ANCA should be confirmed by enzyme immunoassays for the specific autoantibodies directed against PR3 or MPO.

2. Histologic findings—Histologic features of granulomatosis with polyangiitis include vasculitis, granulomatous inflammation, geographic necrosis, and acute and chronic inflammation. The full range of pathologic changes is usually evident only on thoracoscopic lung biopsy. Granulomas, observed only rarely in renal biopsy specimens, are found much more commonly on lung biopsy specimens. Nasal biopsies often do not show vasculitis but may show chronic inflammation and other changes which, interpreted by an experienced pathologist, can serve as convincing evidence of the diagnosis. Renal biopsy discloses a segmental necrotizing glomerulonephritis with multiple crescents; this is characteristic but not diagnostic. Pathologists characterize the renal lesion of granulomatosis with polyangiitis (and other forms of "ANCA-associated vasculitis") as a pauci-immune glomerulonephritis because of the relative absence (compared with immune complex–mediated disorders) of immunoreactants—IgG, IgM, IgA, and complement proteins—within glomeruli.

C. Imaging

Chest CT is more sensitive than chest radiography; lesions include infiltrates, nodules, masses, and cavities. Pleural effusions are uncommon. Often the radiographs prompt concern about lung cancer. Hilar adenopathy large enough to be evident on chest film is unusual in granulomatosis with polyangiitis; if present, sarcoidosis, tumor, or infection is more likely. Other common radiographic abnormalities include extensive sinusitis and even bony sinus erosions.

▶ Differential Diagnosis

In most patients with granulomatosis with polyangiitis, refractory sinusitis or otitis media is initially suspected. When upper respiratory tract inflammation persists and is accompanied by additional systemic inflammatory signs (eg, red eye from scleritis, joint pain, and swelling), the diagnosis of granulomatosis with polyangiitis should be considered. Rheumatoid arthritis will wrongly be suspected in a substantial minority of patients who chiefly complain of joint pain. Arriving at the correct diagnosis is aided by awareness that rheumatoid arthritis typically involves small joints of the hand, whereas granulomatosis with polyangiitis favors large joints, such as the hip, knee, elbow, and shoulder. Lung cancer may be the first diagnostic consideration for some middle-aged patients in whom cough, hemoptysis, and lung masses are presenting symptoms and signs; typically, evidence of glomerulonephritis, a positive ANCA or, ultimately, the lung biopsy findings will point to the proper diagnosis. Granulomatosis with polyangiitis shares with SLE, anti–glomerular basement membrane disease, and microscopic polyangiitis the ability to cause an acute pulmonary-renal syndrome. Approximately 10–25% of patients with classic granulomatosis with polyangiitis have MPO-ANCA. Owing to involvement of the same types of blood vessels, similar patterns of organ involvement, and the possibility of failing to identify granulomatous pathology on tissue biopsies because of sampling error, granulomatosis with polyangiitis is often difficult to differentiate from microscopic polyangiitis. The crucial distinctions between the two disorders are the tendencies for granulomatosis with polyangiitis to involve the upper respiratory tract (including the ears) and to cause granulomatous inflammation. Cocaine use can cause destruction of midline tissues—the nose and palate—that mimics granulomatosis with polyangiitis. Indeed, distinguishing between the two conditions can be challenging because patients with cocaine-mediated midline destructive disease frequently have positive tests for PR-3-ANCA and lesional biopsies that demonstrate vasculitis. In contrast to granulomatosis with polyangiitis, cocaine-mediated midline destructive disease does not cause pulmonary or renal disease.

▶ Treatment

Early treatment is crucial in preventing the devastating end-organ complications of this disease, and often in preserving life. While granulomatosis with polyangiitis may involve the sinuses or lung for months, once proteinuria or hematuria develops, progression to advanced chronic kidney disease can be rapid (over several weeks). Current practice divides treatment into 2 phases: induction of remission and maintenance of remission. Choice of induction therapy is dictated by whether the patient has mild disease (ie, no significant renal dysfunction or immediately life-threatening disease) or severe disease (ie, life- or organ-threatening disease such as rapidly progressive glomerulonephritis or pulmonary hemorrhage).

For patients with severe disease, there are now two treatment options for inducing remission: cyclophosphamide plus corticosteroids or rituximab plus corticosteroids. For several decades, the combination of cyclophosphamide and prednisone had been the standard of care for patients with severe disease. Remissions can be induced in more than 90% of patients treated with prednisone (1 mg/kg daily) plus cyclophosphamide (2 mg/kg/day orally with adjustments required for acute or chronic kidney disease and patients over age 70). Cyclophosphamide is best given daily by mouth; intermittent high-dose intravenous cyclophosphamide is less effective. Whenever cyclophosphamide is used, *Pneumocystis jirovecii* prophylaxis with either single-strength oral trimethoprim-sulfamethoxazole daily or dapsone 100 mg/day is essential. To minimize toxicity, patients are treated with cyclophosphamide for only 3–6 months; once remission is achieved, the patient is switched to a maintenance regimen more likely to be tolerated well. There are three options for maintaining remission in patients with normal or near normal renal function after cyclophosphamide induction: azathioprine (up to 2 mg/kg/day orally), methotrexate (20–25 mg/wk administered either orally or intramuscularly), or rituximab (500 mg administered intravenously when remission is achieved, repeated in 14 days, then repeated every 6 months three more times). Methotrexate should not be used in patients with renal dysfunction. One randomized, controlled trial comparing azathioprine and rituximab for maintenance of remission showed that the risk of relapse over 28 months was 5% with rituximab and 29% with azathioprine. Before the institution of azathioprine, patients should be tested (through a commercially available blood test) for deficiencies in the level of thiopurine methyltransferase, an enzyme essential to the metabolism of azathioprine.

The other option for induction therapy of severe granulomatosis with polyangiitis is rituximab, a B-cell depleting antibody. The FDA has approved rituximab in combination with corticosteroids for the treatment of granulomatosis with polyangiitis and microscopic polyangiitis. Studies demonstrate that rituximab is not less effective for remission-induction in these conditions. Indeed, post-hoc analysis of one clinical trial demonstrated that rituximab is more effective than cyclophosphamide for treating relapses of granulomatosis with polyangiitis and microscopic polyangiitis. Both rituximab and cyclophosphamide increase the risk of developing life-threatening opportunistic infections (including progressive multifocal leukoencephalopathy [PML]).

Because of its superior side-effect profile, methotrexate is viewed as an appropriate substitute for cyclophosphamide or rituximab for initial and maintenance treatment in patients who have mild disease and normal renal function.

Hilhorst M et al; Limburg Renal Registry. Proteinase 3-ANCA vasculitis versus myeloperoxidase-ANCA vasculitis. J Am Soc Nephrol. 2015 Oct;26(10):2314–27. [PMID: 25956510]

Lyons PA et al. Genetically distinct subsets within ANCA-associated vasculitis. N Engl J Med. 2012 Jul 19;367(3):214–23. [PMID: 22808956]

Stone JH et al. Rituximab versus cyclophosphamide for ANCA-associated vasculitis. N Engl J Med. 2010 Jul 15;363(3):221–32. [PMID: 20647199]

Unizony S et al; RAVE-ITN Research Group. Clinical outcomes of treatment of anti-neutrophil cytoplasmic antibody (ANCA)-associated vasculitis based on ANCA type. Ann Rheum Dis. 2015 Nov 30. [Epub ahead of print] [PMID: 26621483]

MICROSCOPIC POLYANGIITIS

ESSENTIALS OF DIAGNOSIS

▶ Necrotizing vasculitis of small- and medium-sized arteries and veins.

▶ Most common cause of pulmonary-renal syndrome: diffuse alveolar hemorrhage and glomerulonephritis.

▶ Associated with ANCA in 75% of cases, usually anti-myeloperoxidase antibodies (MPO-ANCA) that cause a p-ANCA pattern on immunofluorescence testing. ANCA directed against proteinase-3 (PR3-ANCA) can also be observed.

▶ General Considerations

Microscopic polyangiitis is a pauci-immune nongranulomatous necrotizing vasculitis that (1) affects small blood vessels (capillaries, venules, or arterioles), (2) often causes glomerulonephritis and pulmonary capillaritis, and (3) is often associated with ANCA on immunofluorescence testing (directed against MPO, a constituent of neutrophil granules). Because microscopic polyangiitis may involve medium-sized as well as small blood vessels and because it tends to affect capillaries within the lungs and kidneys, its spectrum overlaps those of both polyarteritis nodosa and granulomatosis with polyangiitis.

In rare instances, medications, particularly propylthiouracil, hydralazine, allopurinol, penicillamine, minocycline, and sulfasalazine, induce a systemic vasculitis associated with high titers of MPO-ANCA and features of microscopic polyangiitis.

▶ Clinical Findings

A. Symptoms and Signs

A wide variety of findings suggesting vasculitis of small blood vessels may develop in microscopic polyangiitis. These include "palpable" (or "raised") purpura and other signs of cutaneous vasculitis (ulcers, splinter hemorrhages, vesiculobullous lesions).

Microscopic polyangiitis is the most common cause of pulmonary-renal syndromes, being several times more common than anti–glomerular basement membrane disease. Interstitial lung fibrosis that mimics usual interstitial pneumonitis is the presenting condition. Pulmonary hemorrhage may occur. The pathologic findings in the lung are typically those of capillaritis.

Vasculitic neuropathy (mononeuritis multiplex) is also common in microscopic polyangiitis.

B. Laboratory Findings

As noted, three-fourths of patients with microscopic polyangiitis are ANCA-positive. Elevated acute-phase reactants are also typical of active disease. Microscopic hematuria, proteinuria, and red blood cell casts in the urine may occur. The renal lesion is a segmental, necrotizing glomerulonephritis, often with localized intravascular coagulation and the observation of intraglomerular thrombi upon renal biopsy.

▶ Differential Diagnosis

Distinguishing this disease from granulomatosis with polyangiitis may be challenging in some cases. Microscopic polyangiitis is not associated with the chronic destructive upper respiratory tract disease often found in granulomatosis with polyangiitis. Moreover, as noted, a critical difference between the two diseases is the absence of granulomatous inflammation in microscopic polyangiitis. Because their treatments may differ, microscopic polyangiitis must also be differentiated from polyarteritis nodosa.

▶ Treatment

Microscopic polyangiitis is usually treated in the same way as granulomatosis with polyangiitis: patients with severe disease, typically involving pulmonary hemorrhage and glomerulonephritis, require urgent induction treatment with corticosteroids and either cyclophosphamide or rituximab. If cyclophosphamide is chosen, it may be administered either in an oral daily regimen or via intermittent (usually monthly) intravenous pulses; following induction of remission, cyclophosphamide may be replaced with azathioprine, rituximab, or methotrexate (provided the patient has normal renal function). In cases of drug-induced MPO-ANCA–associated vasculitis, the offending medication should be discontinued; significant organ involvement (eg, pulmonary hemorrhage, glomerulonephritis) requires immunosuppressive therapy.

▶ Prognosis

The key to effecting good outcomes is early diagnosis. Compared with patients who have granulomatosis with polyangiitis, those who have microscopic polyangiitis are more likely to have significant fibrosis on renal biopsy because of later diagnosis. The likelihood of disease recurrence following remission in microscopic polyangiitis is about 33%.

Cartin-Ceba R et al. Diffuse alveolar hemorrhage secondary to ANCA-associated vasculitis: predictors of respiratory failure and clinical outcomes. Arthritis Rheumatol. 2015 Dec 29. [Epub ahead of print] [PMID: 26713723]
Schönermarck U et al. Treatment of ANCA-associated vasculitis. Nat Rev Nephrol. 2014 Jan;10(1):25–36. [PMID: 24189648]

LEVAMISOLE-ASSOCIATED PURPURA

Exposure to levamisole, a prevalent adulterant of illicit cocaine in North America, can induce a distinctive clinical syndrome of retiform purpura and cutaneous necrosis affecting the extremities, ears, and skin overlying the zygomatic arch. Biopsies reveal widespread thrombosis of small cutaneous vessels with varying degrees of vasculitis. The syndrome is associated with the lupus anticoagulant, IgM antibodies to cardiolipin, and very high titers of p-ANCAs (due to autoantibodies to elastase, lactoferrin, cathepsin-G, and other neutrophil components rather than to myeloperoxidase alone). There is no consensus on treatment of levamisole-induced purpura, but early lesions can resolve with abstinence. Use of levamisole-adulterated cocaine also has been linked to neutropenia, agranulocytosis, and pauci-immune glomerulonephritis.

Graf J et al. Purpura, cutaneous necrosis, and anti-neutrophil cytoplasmic antibodies associated with levamisole-adulterated cocaine. Arthritis Rheum. 2011 Dec;63(12):3998–4001. [PMID: 22127712]

CRYOGLOBULINEMIA

Cryoglobulinemia can be associated with an immune-complex mediated, small-vessel vasculitis. Chronic infection with hepatitis C is the most common underlying condition; cryoglobulinemic vasculitis also can occur with other chronic infections (such as subacute bacterial endocarditis, osteomyelitis, HIV, and hepatitis B), with connective tissues diseases (especially Sjögren syndrome), and with lymphoproliferative disorders. The cryoglobulins associated with vasculitis are cold-precipitable immune complexes consisting of rheumatoid factor and IgG (rheumatoid factor is an autoantibody to the constant region of IgG). The rheumatoid factor component can be monoclonal (type II cryoglobulins) or polyclonal (type III cryoglobulins). (Type I cryoglobulins are cryoprecipitable monoclonal proteins that lack rheumatoid factor activity; these cause cold-induced hyperviscosity syndromes, not vasculitis, and are associated with lymphoproliferative disease.)

▶ Clinical Findings

Cryoglobulinemic vasculitis typically manifests as recurrent palpable purpura and peripheral neuropathy. A proliferative glomerulonephritis can develop and can manifest as rapidly progressive glomerulonephritis. Abnormal liver function tests, abdominal pain, digital gangrene, and pulmonary disease may also occur. The diagnosis is based on a compatible clinical picture and a positive serum test for cryoglobulins. The presence of a disproportionately low C4 level can be a diagnostic clue to the presence of cryoglobulinemia.

▶ Treatment

Treatment depends on the cause and the severity of the vasculitis. Asymptomatic cryoglobulinemia is common in hepatitis C–infected individuals and does not in itself warrant treatment. Patients with severe vasculitis (eg, extensive digital gangrene, extensive neuropathy, and rapidly progressive glomerulonephritis) and hepatitis C are first given immunosuppressive therapy with corticosteroids and either rituximab or cyclophosphamide for 2–4 months. Once improved, patients with severe vasculitis from hepatitis C can then be given antiviral therapy.

Cacoub P et al. Hepatitis C virus–induced vasculitis: therapeutic options. Ann Rheum Dis. 2014 Jan;73(1):24–30. [PMID: 23921995]

Sise ME et al. Treatment of hepatitis C virus-associated mixed cryoglobulinemia with direct-acting antiviral agents. Hepatology. 2016 Feb;63(2):408–17. [PMID: 26474537]

HENOCH-SCHÖNLEIN PURPURA

Henoch-Schönlein purpura, the most common systemic vasculitis in children, occurs in adults as well. Typical features are palpable purpura (see Figure 22–6), arthritis, and hematuria. Abdominal pain occurs less frequently in adults than in children. Pathologic features include leukocytoclastic vasculitis with IgA deposition. The cause is not known.

The purpuric skin lesions are typically located on the lower extremities but may also be seen on the hands, arms, trunk, and buttocks. Joint symptoms are present in the majority of patients, the knees and ankles being most commonly involved. Abdominal pain secondary to vasculitis of the intestinal tract is often associated with gastrointestinal bleeding. Hematuria signals the presence of a renal lesion that is usually reversible, although it occasionally may progress to chronic kidney disease. Children tend to have more frequent and more serious gastrointestinal vasculitis, whereas adults more often suffer from chronic kidney disease. Biopsy of the kidney reveals segmental glomerulonephritis with crescents and mesangial deposition of IgA.

Chronic courses with persistent or intermittent skin disease are more likely to occur in adults than in children. The value of corticosteroids has been controversial. In children, prednisone (1–2 mg/kg/day orally) does not decrease the frequency of proteinuria 1 year after onset of disease. The incremental efficacy of steroid-sparing drugs such as azathioprine and mycophenolate mofetil—often used in the setting of kidney disease—is not known.

Komatsu H et al. Clinical manifestations of Henoch-Schönlein purpura nephritis and IgA nephropathy: comparative analysis of data from the Japan Renal Biopsy Registry (J-RBR). Clin Exp Nephrol. 2015 Oct 11. [Epub ahead of print] [PMID: 26456327]

RELAPSING POLYCHONDRITIS

This disease is characterized by inflammatory destructive lesions of cartilaginous structures, principally the ears, nose, trachea, and larynx. Nearly 40% of cases are associated with another disease, especially either other immunologic disorders (such as SLE, rheumatoid arthritis, or Hashimoto thyroiditis) or cancers (such as multiple myeloma) or hematologic disorders (such as myelodysplastic syndrome). The disease, which is usually episodic, affects males and females equally. The cartilage is painful, swollen, and tender during an attack and subsequently

becomes atrophic, resulting in permanent deformity. Biopsy of the involved cartilage shows inflammation and chondrolysis. Noncartilaginous manifestations of the disease include fever, episcleritis, uveitis, deafness, aortic regurgitation, and rarely glomerulonephritis. In 85% of patients, a migratory, asymmetric, and seronegative arthropathy occurs, affecting both large and small joints and the costochondral junctions. Diagnosing this uncommon disease is especially difficult since the signs of cartilage inflammation (such as red ears or nasal pain) may be more subtle than the fever, arthritis, rash, or other systemic manifestations.

Prednisone, 0.5–1 mg/kg/day orally, is often effective. Dapsone (100–200 mg/day orally) or methotrexate (7.5–20 mg orally per week) may also have efficacy, sparing the need for long-term high-dose corticosteroid treatment. Involvement of the tracheobronchial tree, leading to tracheomalacia, may lead to difficult management issues.

Vitale A et al. Relapsing polychondritis: an update on pathogenesis, clinical features, diagnostic tools, and therapeutic perspectives. Curr Rheumatol Rep. 2016 Jan;18(1):3. [PMID: 26711694]

BEHÇET SYNDROME

ESSENTIALS OF DIAGNOSIS

▶ Most commonly occurs among persons of Asian, Turkish, or Middle Eastern background, but may affect persons of any demographic profile.

▶ Recurrent, painful aphthous ulcers of the mouth and genitals.

▶ Erythema nodosum–like lesions; a follicular rash; and the pathergy phenomenon (formation of a sterile pustule at the site of a needle stick).

▶ Either anterior or posterior uveitis. Posterior uveitis may be asymptomatic until significant damage to the retina has occurred.

▶ Variety of neurologic lesions that can mimic multiple sclerosis, particularly through involvement of the white matter of the brainstem.

▶ General Considerations

Named after the Turkish dermatologist who first described it, this disease is of unknown cause. Its protean manifestations are believed to result from vasculitis that may involve all types of blood vessels: small, medium, and large, on both the arterial and venous side of the circulation.

▶ Clinical Findings

A. Symptoms and Signs

The hallmark of Behçet disease is painful aphthous ulcerations in the mouth (see Figure 8–7). These lesions, which usually occur multiply, may be found on the tongue, gums, and inner surfaces of the oral cavity. Genital lesions, similar in appearance, are also common but do not occur in all patients. Other cutaneous lesions of Behçet disease include tender, erythematous, papular lesions that resemble erythema nodosum. (On biopsy, however, many of these lesions are shown to be secondary to vasculitis rather than septal panniculitis.) These erythema nodosum–like lesions have a tendency to ulcerate, a major difference between the lesions of Behçet disease and the erythema nodosum seen in cases of sarcoidosis and inflammatory bowel disease. An erythematous follicular rash that occurs frequently on the upper extremities may be a subtle feature of the disease. The pathergy phenomenon is frequently underappreciated (unless the patient is asked); in this phenomenon, sterile pustules develop at sites where needles have been inserted into the skin (eg, for phlebotomy) in some patients.

A nonerosive arthritis occurs in about two-thirds of patients, most commonly affecting the knees and ankles. Eye involvement may be one of the most devastating complications of Behçet disease. Posterior uveitis, in essence a retinal venulitis, may lead to the insidious destruction of large areas of the retina before the patient becomes aware of visual problems. Anterior uveitis, associated with photophobia and a red eye, is intensely symptomatic. This complication may lead to a hypopyon, the accumulation of pus in the anterior chamber. If not treated properly with mydriatic agents to dilate the pupil and corticosteroid eyedrops to diminish inflammation, the anterior uveitis may lead to synechial formation between the iris and lens, resulting in permanent pupillary distortion.

Central nervous system involvement is another cause of major potential morbidity. The central nervous system lesions that may mimic multiple sclerosis radiologically often result in serious disability or death. Findings include sterile meningitis (recurrent meningeal headaches associated with a lymphocytic pleocytosis), cranial nerve palsies, seizures, encephalitis, mental disturbances, and spinal cord lesions. Aphthous ulcerations of the ileum and cecum and other forms of gastrointestinal involvement develop in approximately a quarter of patients. Large vessel vasculitis can lead to pulmonary artery aneurysms and life-threatening pulmonary hemorrhage. Finally, patients have a hypercoagulable tendency that may lead to complicated venous thrombotic events, particularly multiple deep venous thrombosis, pulmonary emboli, cerebral sinus thrombosis, and other problems associated with clotting.

The clinical course may be chronic but is often characterized by remissions and exacerbations.

B. Laboratory Findings

There are no pathognomonic laboratory features of Behçet disease. Although acute-phase reactants are often elevated, there is no autoantibody or other assay that is distinctive. No markers of hypercoagulability specific to Behçet have been identified.

▶ Treatment

Both colchicine (0.6 mg once to three times daily orally) and thalidomide (100 mg/day orally) help ameliorate the mucocutaneous findings. Apremilast, a selective phosphodiesterase-4 inhibitor, is effective for the treatment of the oral ulcers. Corticosteroids (1 mg/kg/day of oral prednisone) are a mainstay of initial therapy for severe disease manifestations. Azathioprine (2 mg/kg/day orally) may be an effective steroid-sparing agent. Infliximab, cyclosporine, or cyclophosphamide is indicated for severe ocular and central nervous system complications of Behçet disease.

Hatemi G et al. Apremilast for Behçet's syndrome—a phase 2, placebo-controlled study. N Engl J Med. 2015 Apr 16;372(16): 1510–8. [PMID: 25875256]

PRIMARY ANGIITIS OF THE CENTRAL NERVOUS SYSTEM

Primary angiitis of the central nervous system is a syndrome with several possible causes that produces small- and medium-sized vasculitis limited to the brain and spinal cord. Biopsy-proved cases have predominated in men who have a history of weeks to months of headaches, encephalopathy, and multifocal strokes. Systemic symptoms and signs are absent, and routine laboratory tests are usually normal. MRI of the brain is almost always abnormal, and the spinal fluid often reveals a mild lymphocytosis and a modest increase in protein level. Angiograms classically reveal a "string of beads" pattern produced by alternating segments of arterial narrowing and dilation. However, neither the MRI nor the angiogram appearance is specific for vasculitis. Indeed, in one study, none of the patients who had biopsy-proved central nervous system vasculitis had an angiogram showing "the string of beads," and none of the patients with the classic angiographic findings had a positive brain biopsy for vasculitis. Review of many studies suggests that the sensitivity of angiography varies greatly (from 40% to 90%) and the specificity is only approximately 30%. Many conditions, including vasospasm, can produce the same angiographic pattern as vasculitis. Definitive diagnosis requires a compatible clinical picture; exclusion of infection, neoplasm, or metabolic disorder or drug exposure (eg, cocaine) that can mimic primary angiitis of the central nervous system; and a positive brain biopsy. In contrast to biopsy-proved cases, patients with angiographically defined central nervous system vasculopathy are chiefly women who have had an abrupt onset of headaches and stroke (often in the absence of encephalopathy) with normal spinal fluid findings. Many patients who fit this clinical profile may have reversible cerebral vasoconstriction rather than true vasculitis. Such cases may best be treated with calcium channel blockers (such as nimodipine or verapamil) and possibly a short course of corticosteroids. Biopsy-proved cases usually improve with prednisone therapy and often require cyclophosphamide. In recent years, cases of central nervous system vasculitis associated with cerebral amyloid angiopathy have been reported. These cases often respond well to corticosteroids, albeit the long-term natural history remains poorly defined.

de Boysson H et al; French Vasculitis Study Group and the French NeuroVascular Society. Primary angiitis of the central nervous system: description of the first fifty-two adults enrolled in the French cohort of patients with primary vasculitis of the central nervous system. Arthritis Rheumatol. 2014 May;66(5):1315–26. [PMID: 24782189]

John S et al. CNS vasculitis. Semin Neurol. 2014 Sep;34(4):405–12. [PMID: 25369436]

LIVEDO RETICULARIS & LIVEDO RACEMOSA

Livedo reticularis produces a mottled, purplish discoloration of the skin with reticulated cyanotic areas surrounding paler central cores. This distinctive "fishnet" pattern is caused by spasm or obstruction of perpendicular arterioles, combined with pooling of blood in surrounding venous plexuses. Idiopathic livedo reticularis is a benign condition that worsens with cold exposure, improves with warming, and primarily affects the extremities. Apart from cosmetic concerns, it is usually asymptomatic. Systemic symptoms or the development of cutaneous ulcerations point to the presence of an underlying disease.

Secondary livedo reticularis, now more properly known as livedo racemosa, occurs in association with a variety of diseases that cause vascular obstruction or inflammation. Livedo racemosa resembles idiopathic livedo reticularis but has a wider distribution (often found on trunk and buttocks as well as extremities) and its lesions are more irregular, broken, and circular. Of particular importance is the link with antiphospholipid antibody syndrome. Livedo racemosa is the presenting manifestation of 25% of patients with antiphospholipid antibody syndrome and is strongly associated with the subgroup that has arterial thromboses, including those with Sneddon syndrome (livedo reticularis and cerebrovascular events). Other underlying causes of livedo racemosa include the vasculitides (particularly polyarteritis nodosa), cholesterol emboli syndrome, thrombocythemia, cryoglobulinemia, cold agglutinin disease, primary hyperoxaluria (due to vascular deposits of calcium oxalate), and disseminated intravascular coagulation.

Sajjan VV et al. Livedo reticularis: a review of the literature. Indian Dermatol Online J. 2015 Sep–Oct;6(5):315–21. [PMID: 26500860]

SERONEGATIVE SPONDYLOARTHROPATHIES

The seronegative spondyloarthropathies are ankylosing spondylitis, psoriatic arthritis, reactive arthritis, the arthritis associated with inflammatory bowel disease, and undifferentiated spondyloarthropathy. These disorders are noted for male predominance, onset usually before age 40, inflammatory arthritis of the spine and sacroiliac joints, asymmetric oligoarthritis of large peripheral joints, enthesopathy (inflammation of where ligaments, tendons, and joint capsule insert into bone), uveitis in a significant minority, the absence of autoantibodies in the serum, and a striking association with HLA-B27. HLA-B27 is positive in up to 90% of patients with ankylosing spondylitis and 75% with reactive arthritis. HLA-B27 also occurs in 50% of the psoriatic and inflammatory bowel disease patients who have sacroiliitis. Patients with only peripheral arthritis in these latter two syndromes do not show an increase in HLA-B27.

ANKYLOSING SPONDYLITIS

ESSENTIALS OF DIAGNOSIS

▶ Chronic low backache in young adults, generally worst in the morning.

▶ Progressive limitation of back motion and of chest expansion.

▶ Transient (50%) or persistent (25%) peripheral arthritis.

▶ Anterior uveitis in 20–25%.

▶ Diagnostic radiographic changes in sacroiliac joints.

▶ Negative serologic tests for rheumatoid factor and anti-CCP antibodies.

▶ HLA-B27 testing is most helpful when there is an intermediate probability of disease.

▶ General Considerations

Ankylosing spondylitis is a chronic inflammatory disease of the joints of the axial skeleton, manifested clinically by pain and progressive stiffening of the spine. The age at onset is usually in the late teens or early 20s. The incidence is greater in males than in females, and symptoms are more prominent in men, with ascending involvement of the spine more likely to occur.

▶ Clinical Findings

A. Symptoms and Signs

The onset is usually gradual, with intermittent bouts of back pain that may radiate into the buttocks. The back pain is worse in the morning and usually associated with stiffness that lasts hours. The pain and stiffness improve with activity, in contrast to back pain due to mechanical causes and degenerative disease, which improves with rest and worsens with activity. As the disease advances, symptoms progress in a cephalad direction, and back motion becomes limited, with the normal lumbar curve flattened and the thoracic curvature exaggerated. Chest expansion is often limited as a consequence of costovertebral joint involvement. In advanced cases, the entire spine becomes fused, allowing no motion in any direction. Transient acute arthritis of the peripheral joints occurs in about 50% of cases, and permanent changes in the peripheral joints—most commonly the hips, shoulders, and knees—are seen in about 25%. Enthesopathy, a hallmark of the spondyloarthropathies, can manifest as swelling of the Achilles tendon at its insertion, plantar fasciitis (producing heel pain), or "sausage" swelling of a finger or toe (less common in ankylosing spondylitis than in psoriatic arthritis).

Anterior uveitis is associated in as many as 25% of cases and may be a presenting feature. Spondylitic heart disease, characterized chiefly by atrioventricular conduction defects and aortic regurgitation occurs in 3–5% of patients with long-standing severe disease. Constitutional symptoms similar to those of rheumatoid arthritis are absent in most patients.

B. Laboratory Findings

The ESR is elevated in 85% of cases, but serologic tests for rheumatoid factor and anti-CCP antibodies are negative. Anemia may be present but is often mild. HLA-B27 is found in 90% of white patients and 50% of black patients with ankylosing spondylitis. Because this antigen occurs in 8% of the healthy white population (and 2% of healthy blacks), it is not a specific diagnostic test.

C. Imaging

The earliest radiographic changes are usually in the sacroiliac joints. In the first 2 years of the disease process, the sacroiliac changes may be detectable only by MRI. Later, erosion and sclerosis of these joints are evident on plain radiographs; the sacroiliitis of ankylosing spondylitis is bilateral and symmetric. Inflammation where the annulus fibrosus attaches to the vertebral bodies initially causes sclerosis ("the shiny corner sign") and then characteristic squaring of the vertebral bodies. The term "bamboo spine" describes the late radiographic appearance of the spinal column in which the vertebral bodies are fused by vertically oriented, bridging syndesmophytes formed by the ossification of the annulus fibrosus and calcification of the anterior and lateral spinal ligaments. Fusion of the posterior facet joints of the spine is also common.

Additional radiographic findings include periosteal new bone formation on the iliac crest, ischial tuberosities and calcanei, and alterations of the pubic symphysis and sternomanubrial joint similar to those of the sacroiliacs. Radiologic changes in peripheral joints, when present, tend to be asymmetric and lack the demineralization and erosions seen in rheumatoid arthritis.

Differential Diagnosis

Low back pain due to mechanical causes, disk disease, and degenerative arthritis is very common. Onset of back pain prior to age 30 and an "inflammatory" quality of the back pain (ie, morning stiffness and pain that improve with activity) should raise the possibility of ankylosing spondylitis. In contrast to ankylosing spondylitis, rheumatoid arthritis predominantly affects multiple, small, peripheral joints of the hands and feet. Rheumatoid arthritis spares the sacroiliac joints and only affects the cervical component of the spine. Bilateral sacroiliitis indistinguishable from ankylosing spondylitis is seen with the spondylitis associated with inflammatory bowel disease. Sacroiliitis associated with reactive arthritis and psoriasis, on the other hand, is often asymmetric or even unilateral. Osteitis condensans ilii (sclerosis on the iliac side of the sacroiliac joint) is an asymptomatic, postpartum radiographic finding that is occasionally mistaken for sacroiliitis. **Diffuse idiopathic skeletal hyperostosis (DISH)** causes exuberant osteophytes ("enthesophytes") of the spine that occasionally are difficult to distinguish from the syndesmophytes of ankylosing spondylitis. The enthesophytes of DISH are thicker and more anterior than the syndesmophytes of ankylosing spondylitis, and the sacroiliac joints are normal in DISH.

Treatment

NSAIDs remain first-line treatment of ankylosing spondylitis and may slow radiographic progression of spinal disease. TNF inhibitors have established efficacy for NSAID-resistant axial disease; responses are often substantial and durable. Etanercept (50 mg subcutaneously once a week), adalimumab (40 mg subcutaneously every other week), infliximab (5 mg/kg every other month by intravenous infusion), or golimumab (50 mg subcutaneously once a month) is reasonable for patients whose symptoms are refractory to NSAIDs. Initial results with secukinumab, an inhibitor of the proinflammatory cytokine IL-17, suggest that targeting the IL-17 pathway will prove highly effective in the treatment of ankylosing spondylitis. Sulfasalazine (1000 mg orally twice daily) is sometimes useful for peripheral arthritis but lacks effectiveness for spinal and sacroiliac joint disease. Corticosteroids have minimal impact on the arthritis—particularly the spondylitis—of ankylosing spondylitis and can worsen osteopenia. All patients should be referred to a physical therapist for instruction in postural exercises.

Prognosis

Almost all patients have persistent symptoms over decades; rare individuals experience long-term remissions. The severity of disease varies greatly, with about 10% of patients having work disability after 10 years. Developing hip disease within the first 2 years of disease onset presages a worse prognosis. The availability of TNF inhibitors has provided symptomatic relief and improved quality of life for many patients with ankylosing spondylitis.

Baeten D et al; MEASURE 1 Study Group; MEASURE 2 Study Group. Secukinumab, an interleukin-17A inhibitor, in ankylosing spondylitis. N Engl J Med. 2015 Dec 24;373(26):2534–48. [PMID: 26699169]
Dougados M et al. Symptomatic efficacy of etanercept and its effects on objective signs of inflammation in early nonradiographic axial spondyloarthritis: a multicenter, randomized, double-blind, placebo-controlled trial. Arthritis Rheumatol. 2014 Aug;66(8):2091–102. [PMID: 24891317]

PSORIATIC ARTHRITIS

ESSENTIALS OF DIAGNOSIS

► Psoriasis precedes onset of arthritis in 80% of cases.
► Arthritis usually asymmetric, with "sausage" appearance of fingers and toes but a polyarthritis that resembles rheumatoid arthritis also occurs.
► Sacroiliac joint involvement common; ankylosis of the sacroiliac joints may occur.
► Radiographic findings: osteolysis; pencil-in-cup deformity; relative lack of osteoporosis; bony ankylosis; asymmetric sacroiliitis and atypical syndesmophytes.

General Considerations

Although psoriasis usually precedes the onset of arthritis, arthritis precedes (by up to 2 years) or occurs simultaneously with the skin disease in approximately 20% of cases.

Clinical Findings

A. Symptoms and Signs

The patterns or subsets of psoriatic arthritis include the following:

1. A symmetric polyarthritis that resembles rheumatoid arthritis. Usually, fewer joints are involved than in rheumatoid arthritis.
2. An oligoarticular form that may lead to considerable destruction of the affected joints.
3. A pattern of disease in which the DIP joints are primarily affected. Early, this may be monarticular, and often the joint involvement is asymmetric. Pitting of the nails and onycholysis frequently accompany DIP involvement.
4. A severe deforming arthritis (arthritis mutilans) in which osteolysis is marked.
5. A spondylitic form in which sacroiliitis and spinal involvement predominate; 50% of these patients are HLA-B27-positive.

Arthritis is at least five times more common in patients with severe skin disease than in those with only mild skin findings. Occasionally, however, patients may have a single patch of psoriasis (typically hidden in the scalp, gluteal cleft, or umbilicus) and are unaware of its presence. Thus, a detailed search for cutaneous lesions is essential in patients with arthritis of new onset. Also, the psoriatic lesions may have cleared when arthritis appears—in such cases, the history is most useful in diagnosing previously unexplained cases of mono- or oligoarthritis. Nail pitting is sometimes a clue. "Sausage" swelling of one or more digits is a common manifestation of enthesopathy in psoriatic arthritis.

B. Laboratory Findings

Laboratory studies show an elevation of the ESR, but rheumatoid factor is not present. Uric acid levels may be high, reflecting the active turnover of skin affected by psoriasis. There is a correlation between the extent of psoriatic involvement and the level of uric acid, but gout is no more common than in patients without psoriasis. Desquamation of the skin may also reduce iron stores.

C. Imaging

Radiographic findings are most helpful in distinguishing the disease from other forms of arthritis. There are marginal erosions of bone and irregular destruction of joint and bone, which, in the phalanx, may give the appearance of a sharpened pencil. Fluffy periosteal new bone may be marked, especially at the insertion of muscles and ligaments into bone. Such changes will also be seen along the shafts of metacarpals, metatarsals, and phalanges. Psoriatic spondylitis causes asymmetric sacroiliitis and syndesmophytes, which are coarser than those seen in ankylosing spondylitis.

Treatment

NSAIDs are usually sufficient for mild cases. Methotrexate (7.5–20 mg orally once a week) is generally considered the drug of choice for patients who have not responded to NSAIDs; methotrexate can improve both the cutaneous and arthritic manifestations. For cases with disease that is refractory to methotrexate, the addition of TNF inhibitors (at doses similar to the treatment of ankylosing spondylitis) is usually effective for both arthritis and psoriatic skin disease. Patients who do not respond to TNF inhibitors can be treated with ustekinumab, a monoclonal antibody that inhibits IL-12 and IL-23, or secukinumab, which inhibits IL-17. Apremilast, a novel oral phosphodiesterase-4 inhibitor, is an option for patients who cannot use, or choose not to use, biologic agents. Corticosteroids are less effective in psoriatic arthritis than in other forms of inflammatory arthritis and may precipitate pustular psoriasis during tapers. Successful treatment directed at the skin lesions alone (eg, by PUVA therapy) occasionally is accompanied by an improvement in peripheral articular symptoms.

Gossec L et al. European League Against Rheumatism (EULAR) recommendations for the management of psoriatic arthritis with pharmacological therapies: 2015 update. Ann Rheum Dis. 2016 Mar;75(3):499–510. [PMID: 26644232]
Olivieri I et al. Advances in the management of psoriatic arthritis. Nat Rev Rheumatol. 2014 Sep;10(9):531–42. [PMID: 25003762]

REACTIVE ARTHRITIS (Formerly Reiter Syndrome)

ESSENTIALS OF DIAGNOSIS

▶ Fifty to eighty percent of patients are HLA-B27-positive.

▶ Oligoarthritis, conjunctivitis, urethritis, and mouth ulcers most common features.

▶ Usually follows dysentery or a sexually transmitted infection.

General Considerations

Reactive arthritis is precipitated by antecedent gastrointestinal and genitourinary infections and manifests as an asymmetric sterile oligoarthritis, typically of the lower extremities. It is frequently associated with enthesitis. Extra-articular manifestations are common and include urethritis, conjunctivitis, uveitis, and mucocutaneous lesions. Reactive arthritis occurs most commonly in young men and is associated with HLA-B27 in 80% of white patients and 50–60% of blacks.

► Clinical Findings

A. Symptoms and Signs

Most cases of reactive arthritis develop within 1–4 weeks after either a gastrointestinal infection (with *Shigella*, *Salmonella*, *Yersinia*, *Campylobacter*) or a sexually transmitted infection (with *Chlamydia trachomatis* or perhaps *Ureaplasma urealyticum*). Whether the inciting infection is sexually transmitted or dysenteric does not affect the subsequent manifestations but does influence the gender ratio: The ratio is 1:1 after enteric infections but 9:1 with male predominance after sexually transmitted infections. Synovial fluid from affected joints is culture-negative. A clinically indistinguishable syndrome can occur without an apparent antecedent infection, suggesting that subclinical infection can precipitate reactive arthritis or that there are other, as yet unrecognized, triggers.

The arthritis is most commonly asymmetric and frequently involves the large weight-bearing joints (chiefly the knee and ankle); sacroiliitis or ankylosing spondylitis is observed in at least 20% of patients, especially after frequent recurrences. Systemic symptoms including fever and weight loss are common at the onset of disease. The mucocutaneous lesions may include balanitis (Figure 20–7), stomatitis, and keratoderma blennorrhagicum (Figure 20–8), indistinguishable from pustular psoriasis. Involvement of the fingernails in reactive arthritis also mimics psoriatic changes. When present, conjunctivitis is mild and occurs early in the disease course. Anterior uveitis, which can develop at any time in HLA-B27-positive patients, is a more clinically significant ocular complication. Carditis and aortic regurgitation may occur. While most signs of the disease disappear within days or weeks, the arthritis may persist for several months or become chronic. Recurrences involving any combination of the clinical manifestations are common and are sometimes followed by permanent sequelae, especially in the joints (eg, articular destruction).

▲ **Figure 20–8.** Keratoderma blennorrhagica of the soles due to reactive arthritis (Reiter syndrome). (From Susan Lindsley, Public Health Image Library, CDC.)

B. Imaging

Radiographic signs of permanent or progressive joint disease may be seen in the sacroiliac as well as the peripheral joints.

► Differential Diagnosis

Gonococcal arthritis can initially mimic reactive arthritis, but the marked improvement after 24–48 hours of antibiotic administration and the culture results distinguish the two disorders. Rheumatoid arthritis, ankylosing spondylitis, and psoriatic arthritis must also be considered. By causing similar oral, ocular, and joint lesions, Behçet disease may also mimic reactive arthritis. The oral lesions of reactive arthritis, however, are typically painless, in contrast to those of Behçet disease.

The association of reactive arthritis and HIV has been debated, but evidence now indicates that it is equally common in sexually active men regardless of HIV status.

► Treatment

NSAIDs have been the mainstay of therapy. Antibiotics given at the time of a nongonococcal sexually transmitted infection reduce the chance that the individual will develop this disorder. For chronic reactive arthritis associated with chlamydial infection, combination antibiotics taken for 6 months are more effective than placebo. Patients who do not respond to NSAIDs may respond to sulfasalazine, 1000 mg orally twice daily, or to methotrexate, 7.5–20 mg orally per week. For those patients with recent-onset disease that is refractory to NSAIDs and these DMARDs, anti-TNF agents, which are effective in the other spondyloarthropathies, may be effective.

▲ **Figure 20–7.** Circinate balanitis due to reactive arthritis (Reiter syndrome). (From Susan Lindsley, Dr. M. F. Rein, Public Health Image Library, CDC.)

Selmi C et al. Diagnosis and classification of reactive arthritis. Autoimmun Rev. 2014 Apr–May;13(4–5):546–9. [PMID: 24418301]

ARTHRITIS & INFLAMMATORY INTESTINAL DISEASES

One-fifth of patients with **inflammatory bowel disease** have arthritis, which complicates **Crohn disease** somewhat more frequently than it does **ulcerative colitis.** In both diseases, two distinct forms of arthritis occur. The first is peripheral arthritis—usually a nondeforming asymmetric oligoarthritis of large joints—in which the activity of the joint disease parallels that of the bowel disease. The arthritis usually begins months to years after the bowel disease, but occasionally the joint symptoms develop earlier and may be prominent enough to cause the patient to overlook intestinal symptoms. The second form of arthritis is a spondylitis that is indistinguishable by symptoms or radiographs from ankylosing spondylitis and follows a course independent of the bowel disease. About 50% of these patients are HLA-B27-positive.

Controlling the intestinal inflammation usually eliminates the peripheral arthritis. The spondylitis often requires NSAIDs, which need to be used cautiously since these agents may activate the bowel disease in a few patients. Range-of-motion exercises as prescribed for ankylosing spondylitis can be helpful.

About two-thirds of patients with **Whipple disease** experience arthralgia or arthritis, most often an episodic, large-joint polyarthritis. The arthritis usually precedes the gastrointestinal manifestations by years and often resolves as the diarrhea develops. Thus, Whipple disease should be considered in the differential diagnosis of unexplained episodic arthritis.

Perez-Alamino R et al. Rheumatic manifestations in inflammatory bowel diseases: a link between GI and rheumatology. Clin Rheumatol. 2016 Feb;35(2):291–6. [PMID: 26573206]

INFECTIOUS ARTHRITIS[1]

NONGONOCOCCAL ACUTE BACTERIAL (Septic) ARTHRITIS

ESSENTIALS OF DIAGNOSIS

▶ Acute onset of inflammatory monarticular arthritis, most often in large weight-bearing joints and wrists.

▶ Common risk factors include previous joint damage and injection drug use.

▶ Infection with causative organisms commonly found elsewhere in body.

▶ Joint effusions are usually large, with white blood counts commonly over 50,000/mcL.

[1]Lyme disease is discussed in Chapter 34.

▶ General Considerations

Nongonococcal acute bacterial arthritis is most often due to hematogenous seeding of the joint; direct inoculation from penetrating trauma is rare. The key risk factors are bacteremia (eg, injection drug use, endocarditis, infection at other sites), damaged joints (eg, rheumatoid arthritis), prosthetic joints, compromised immunity (eg, diabetes mellitus, advanced chronic kidney disease, alcoholism, cirrhosis, and immunosuppressive therapy), and loss of skin integrity (eg, cutaneous ulcer or psoriasis). *Staphylococcus aureus* is the most common cause of nongonococcal septic arthritis, accounting for about 50% of all cases. Methicillin-resistant *S aureus* (MRSA) and group B streptococcus have become increasing frequent and important causes of septic arthritis. Gram-negative septic arthritis causes about 10% of cases and is especially common in injection drug users and in immunocompromised persons. *Escherichia coli* and *Pseudomonas aeruginosa* are the most common gram-negative isolates in adults. Pathologic changes include varying degrees of acute inflammation, with synovitis, effusion, abscess formation in synovial or subchondral tissues, and, if treatment is not adequate, articular destruction.

▶ Clinical Findings

A. Symptoms and Signs

The onset is usually acute, with pain, swelling, and heat of the affected joint worsening over hours. The knee is most frequently involved; other commonly affected sites are the hip, wrist, shoulder, and ankle. Unusual sites, such as the sternoclavicular or sacroiliac joint, can be involved in injection drug users. Chills and fever are common but are absent in up to 20% of patients. Infection of the hip usually does not produce apparent swelling but results in groin pain greatly aggravated by walking. More than one joint is involved in 15% of cases of septic arthritis; risk factors for multiple joint involvement include rheumatoid arthritis, associated endocarditis, and infection with group B streptococci.

B. Laboratory Findings

Synovial fluid analysis is critical for diagnosis. The leukocyte count of the synovial fluid is always inflammatory (greater than 2000/mcL), usually exceeds 50,000/mcL, and often is more than 100,000/mcL, with 90% or more polymorphonuclear cells (Table 20–2). Gram stain of the synovial fluid is positive in 75% of staphylococcal infections and in 50% of gram-negative infections. Synovial fluid cultures are positive in 70–90% of cases; administration of antibiotics prior to arthrocentesis reduces the likelihood of a positive culture result. Blood cultures are positive in approximately 50% of patients.

C. Imaging

Imaging tests generally add little to the diagnosis of septic arthritis. Indeed, other than demonstrating joint effusion, radiographs are usually normal early in the disease;

however, evidence of demineralization may develop within days of onset. MRI and CT are more sensitive in detecting fluid in joints that are not accessible to physical examination (eg, the hip). Bony erosions and narrowing of the joint space followed by osteomyelitis and periostitis may be seen within 2 weeks.

► Differential Diagnosis

Gout and pseudogout can cause acute, very inflammatory monarticular arthritis and high-grade fever; the failure to find crystals on synovial fluid analysis excludes these diagnoses. A well-recognized but uncommon initial presentation of rheumatoid arthritis is an acute inflammatory monoarthritis ("pseudoseptic"). The most common articular manifestation of chronic Lyme disease is inflammatory monoarthritis of the knee, which yields synovial fluid that is Gram stain and culture negative. Acute rheumatic fever commonly involves several joints; Still disease may mimic septic arthritis, but laboratory evidence of infection is absent. Pyogenic arthritis may be superimposed on other types of joint disease, notably rheumatoid arthritis. Indeed, septic arthritis must be excluded (by joint fluid examination) in any patient with rheumatoid arthritis who has a joint strikingly more inflamed than the other joints.

► Prevention

There is no evidence that patients with prosthetic joints undergoing procedures should receive antibiotic prophylaxis to prevent joint infection unless the patient has a prosthetic heart valve or the procedure requires antibiotics to prevent a surgical site infection. However, the topic remains controversial. The American Academy of Orthopedic Surgeons advocates prescribing antibiotic prophylaxis for any patient with a prosthetic joint replacement undergoing a procedure that can cause bacteremia.

► Treatment

The effective treatment of septic arthritis requires appropriate antibiotic therapy together with drainage of the infected joint. Hospitalization is always necessary. If the likely causative organism cannot be determined clinically or from the synovial fluid Gram stain, treatment should be started with broad-spectrum antibiotic coverage effective against staphylococci, streptococci, and gram-negative organisms. The recommendation for initial treatment is to give vancomycin (1 g intravenously every 12 hours, adjusted for age, weight, and renal function) plus a third-generation cephalosporin: ceftriaxone, 1–2 g intravenously daily (or every 12 hours if concomitant meningitis or endocarditis is suspected); or cefotaxime, 1–2 g intravenously every 8 hours; or ceftazidime, 1–2 g intravenously every 8 hours. Antibiotic therapy should be adjusted when culture results become available; the duration of antibiotic therapy is usually 4–6 weeks.

Early orthopedic consultation is essential. Effective drainage is usually achieved through early arthroscopic lavage and debridement together with drain placement.

Open surgical drainage should be performed when conservative treatment fails, when there is concomitant osteomyelitis requiring debridement, or when the involved joint (eg, hip, shoulder, sacroiliac joint) cannot be drained by more conservative means. Immobilization with a splint and elevation are used at the onset of treatment. Early active motion exercises within the limits of tolerance will hasten recovery.

► Prognosis

The outcome of septic arthritis depends largely on the antecedent health of the patient, the causative organism (eg, *S aureus* bacterial arthritis is associated with a poor functional outcome in about 40% of cases), and the promptness of treatment. Five to 10 percent of patients with an infected joint die of respiratory complications of sepsis. The mortality rate is 30% for patients with polyarticular sepsis. Bony ankylosis and articular destruction commonly also occur if treatment is delayed or inadequate.

Kennedy N et al. Native joint septic arthritis: epidemiology, clinical features, and microbiological causes in a New Zealand population. J Rheumatol. 2015 Dec;42(12):2392–7. [PMID: 26523022]

Salar O et al. Septic arthritis in the era of immunosuppressive treatments. Ann R Coll Surg Engl. 2014 Mar;96(2):e11–2. [PMID: 24780657]

Zmistowski B et al. Diagnosis of periprosthetic joint infection. J Orthop Res. 2014 Jan;32(Suppl 1):S98–107. [PMID: 24464903]

GONOCOCCAL ARTHRITIS

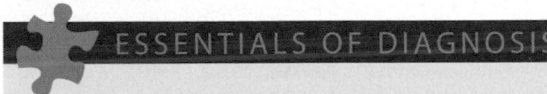

► Prodromal migratory polyarthralgias.
► Tenosynovitis is the most common sign.
► Purulent monoarthritis in 50%.
► Characteristic skin lesions.
► Most common in young women during menses or pregnancy.
► Symptoms of urethritis frequently absent.
► Dramatic response to antibiotics.

► General Considerations

In contrast to nongonococcal bacterial arthritis, gonococcal arthritis usually occurs in otherwise healthy individuals. Host factors, however, influence the expression of the disease: gonococcal arthritis is two to three times more common in women than in men, is especially common during menses and pregnancy, and is rare after age 40. Gonococcal arthritis is also common in men who have sex with men, whose high incidence of asymptomatic gonococcal pharyngitis and proctitis predisposes them to disseminated gonococcal infection. Recurrent disseminated gonococcal infection should prompt testing of the patient's CH50 level to evaluate for a congenital deficiency of a terminal complement component (C5, C6, C7, or C8).

Clinical Findings

A. Symptoms and Signs

One to 4 days of migratory polyarthralgias involving the wrist, knee, ankle, or elbow are common at the outset. Thereafter, two patterns emerge. The first pattern is characterized by tenosynovitis that most often affects wrists, fingers, ankles, or toes and is seen in 60% of patients. The second pattern is purulent monoarthritis that most frequently involves the knee, wrist, ankle, or elbow and is seen in 40% of patients. Less than half of patients have fever, and less than one-fourth have any genitourinary symptoms. Most patients will have asymptomatic but highly characteristic skin lesions that usually consist of two to ten small necrotic pustules distributed over the extremities, especially the palms and soles.

B. Laboratory Findings

The peripheral blood leukocyte count averages about 10,000 cells/mcL and is elevated in less than one-third of patients. The synovial fluid white blood cell count usually ranges from 30,000 to 60,000 cells/mcL. The synovial fluid Gram stain is positive in one-fourth of cases and culture in less than half. Positive blood cultures are uncommon. Urethral, throat, cervical, and rectal cultures should be done in all patients, since they are often positive in the absence of local symptoms. Urinary nucleic acid amplification tests have excellent sensitivity and specificity for the detection of Neisseria gonorrhoeae in genitourinary sites.

C. Imaging

Radiographs are usually normal or show only soft tissue swelling.

Differential Diagnosis

Reactive arthritis can produce acute monoarthritis, urethritis, and fever in a young person but is distinguished by negative cultures and failure to respond to antibiotics. Lyme disease involving the knee is less acute, does not show positive cultures, and may be preceded by known tick exposure and characteristic rash. The synovial fluid analysis will exclude gout, pseudogout, and nongonococcal bacterial arthritis. Rheumatic fever and sarcoidosis can produce migratory tenosynovitis but have other distinguishing features. Infective endocarditis with septic arthritis can mimic disseminated gonococcal infection. Meningococcemia occasionally presents with a clinical picture that resembles disseminated gonococcal infection; blood cultures establish the correct diagnosis. Early hepatitis B infection is associated with circulating immune complexes that can cause a rash and polyarthralgias. In contrast to disseminated gonococcal infection, the rash in hepatitis B is urticarial.

Treatment

In most cases, patients in whom gonococcal arthritis is suspected should be admitted to the hospital to confirm the diagnosis, to exclude endocarditis, and to start treatment. The recommendation for initial treatment is to give azithromycin (1 g orally as a single dose) and a third-generation cephalosporin: ceftriaxone, 1 g intravenously daily (or every 12 hours if concomitant meningitis or endocarditis is suspected); or cefotaxime, 1 g intravenously every 8 hours; or ceftizoxime, 1 g intravenously every 8 hours. Azithromycin enhances eradication of gonorrhea and covers potential coinfection with Chlamydia. Because of the increasing prevalence of resistant strains of gonococci, step-down treatment from parenteral to oral antibiotics is no longer recommended. Indeed, once improvement has been achieved for 24–48 hours, patients must receive ceftriaxone 250 mg intramuscularly every 24 hours to complete a 7–14 day course.

Prognosis

Generally, gonococcal arthritis responds dramatically in 24–48 hours after initiation of antibiotics, and drainage of the infected joint(s) is required infrequently. Complete recovery is the rule.

RHEUMATIC MANIFESTATIONS OF HIV INFECTION

Infection with HIV has been associated with various rheumatic disorders, most commonly arthralgias and arthritis. HIV painful articular syndrome causes severe arthralgias in an oligoarticular, asymmetric pattern that resolve within 24 hours; the joint examination is normal. HIV-associated arthritis is an asymmetric oligoarticular process with objective findings of arthritis and a self-limited course that ranges from weeks to months. Psoriatic arthritis and reactive arthritis occur in HIV-infected individuals and can be severe; it remains uncertain whether the incidence of these disorders is increased in HIV-infected populations. These spondyloarthropathies can respond to NSAIDs, though many cases are unresponsive. Along with antiretroviral therapies, immunosuppressive medications can be used if necessary in HIV-infected patients, though with caution. Muscle weakness associated with an elevated creatine kinase can be due to nucleoside reverse transcriptase inhibitor-associated myopathy or HIV-associated myopathy; the clinical presentations of each resemble idiopathic polymyositis but the muscle biopsies show minimal inflammation. Less commonly, an inflammatory myositis indistinguishable from idiopathic polymyositis occurs. Other rheumatic manifestations of HIV include diffuse infiltrative lymphocytosis syndrome (with parotid gland enlargement) and various forms of vasculitis. The introduction of HAART has been associated with a marked decreased frequency of painful articular syndromes, psoriatic arthritis, spondyloarthropathy, and diffuse infiltrative lymphocytosis syndrome, and an increased frequency of the immune reconstitution inflammatory syndrome (IRIS) and osteoporosis.

Lawson E et al. The changing spectrum of rheumatic disease in HIV infection. Br Med Bull. 2012 Sep;103(1):203–21. [PMID: 22879627]

VIRAL ARTHRITIS

Arthralgias occur frequently in the course of acute infections with many viruses, but frank arthritis is uncommon with the notable exceptions of acute parvovirus B19 infection and Chikungunya fever. Parvovirus B19 causes an acute polyarthritis in 50–60% of adult cases (infected children develop the febrile exanthem known as "slapped cheek fever"). The arthritis can mimic rheumatoid arthritis but is almost always self-limited and resolves within several weeks. The diagnosis is established by the presence of IgM antibodies specific for parvovirus B19. Chikungunya fever is an arthropod-borne viral infection that is endemic to West Africa but has spread to multiple locations including the Indian Ocean islands, the Caribbean and Central and Latin America. Clinical manifestations include high fever, rash, and incapacitating bone pain. Acute polyarthralgia and polyarthritis are common and can persist for months or years.

Self-limited polyarthritis is common in acute hepatitis B infection and typically occurs before the onset of jaundice. Urticaria or other types of skin rash may be present. Indeed, the clinical picture resembles that of serum sickness. Serum transaminase levels are elevated, and tests for hepatitis B surface antigen are positive. Serum complement levels are often low during active arthritis and become normal after remission of arthritis. The incidence of hepatitis B–associated polyarthritis has fallen substantially with the introduction of hepatitis B vaccination. Effective vaccination programs in the United States have eliminated acute rubella infections, formerly a common cause of virally induced polyarthritis. Changes in the rubella vaccine (an attenuated live vaccine) have greatly reduced the incidence of rubella vaccine–induced polyarthritis as well.

Chronic infection with hepatitis C is associated with chronic polyarthralgia in up to 20% of cases and with chronic polyarthritis in 3–5%. Both can mimic rheumatoid arthritis, and the presence of rheumatoid factor in most hepatitis C–infected individuals leads to further diagnostic confusion. Indeed, hepatitis C–associated arthritis is frequently misdiagnosed as rheumatoid arthritis. Distinguishing hepatitis C–associated arthritis/arthralgias from the co-occurrence of hepatitis C and rheumatoid arthritis can be difficult. Rheumatoid arthritis always causes objective arthritis (not just arthralgias) and can be erosive (hepatitis C–associated arthritis is nonerosive). The presence of anti-CCP antibodies points to the diagnosis of rheumatoid arthritis.

Miner JJ et al. Chikungunya viral arthritis in the United States: a mimic of seronegative rheumatoid arthritis. Arthritis Rheumatol. 2015 May;67(5):1214–20. [PMID: 25605621]

INFECTIONS OF BONES

ACUTE PYOGENIC OSTEOMYELITIS

 ESSENTIALS OF DIAGNOSIS

► Fever and chills associated with pain and tenderness of involved bone.

► Diagnosis usually requires culture of bone biopsy.

► ESR often extremely high (eg, greater than 100 mm/h).

► Radiographs early in the course are typically negative.

► General Considerations

Osteomyelitis is a serious infection that is often difficult to diagnose and treat. Infection of bone occurs as a consequence of (1) hematogenous dissemination of bacteria, (2) invasion from a contiguous focus of infection, and (3) skin breakdown in the setting of vascular insufficiency.

► Clinical Findings

A. Symptoms and Signs

1. Hematogenous osteomyelitis—Osteomyelitis resulting from bacteremia is a disease associated with sickle cell disease, injection drug users, diabetes mellitus, or the elderly. Patients with this form of osteomyelitis often present with sudden onset of high fever, chills, and pain and tenderness of the involved bone. The site of osteomyelitis and the causative organism depend on the host. Among patients with hemoglobinopathies such as sickle cell anemia, osteomyelitis is caused most often by salmonellae; *S aureus* is the second most common cause. Osteomyelitis in injection drug users develops most commonly in the spine. Although in this setting *S aureus* is most common, gram-negative infections, especially *P aeruginosa* and *Serratia* species, are also frequent pathogens. Rapid progression to epidural abscess causing fever, pain, and sensory and motor loss is not uncommon. In older patients with hematogenous osteomyelitis, the most common sites are the thoracic and lumbar vertebral bodies. Risk factors for these patients include diabetes, intravenous catheters, and indwelling urinary catheters. These patients often have more subtle presentations, with low-grade fever and gradually increasing bone pain.

2. Osteomyelitis from a contiguous focus of infection—Prosthetic joint replacement, pressure ulcer, neurosurgery, and trauma most frequently cause soft tissue infections that can spread to bone. *S aureus* and *Staphylococcus epidermidis* are the most common organisms. Polymicrobial infections, rare in hematogenously spread osteomyelitis, are more common in osteomyelitis due to contiguous spread. Localized signs of inflammation are usually evident, but high fever and other signs of toxicity are usually absent. Septic arthritis and cellulitis can also spread to contiguous bone.

3. Osteomyelitis associated with vascular insufficiency—
Patients with diabetes mellitus and vascular insufficiency are susceptible to developing a very challenging form of osteomyelitis. The foot and ankle are the most commonly affected sites. Infection originates from an ulcer or other break in the skin that is usually still present when the patient presents but may appear disarmingly unimpressive. Bone pain is often absent or muted by the associated neuropathy. Fever is also commonly absent. Two of the best bedside clues that the patient has osteomyelitis are the ability to easily advance a sterile probe through a skin ulcer to bone and an ulcer area larger than 2 cm^2.

B. Imaging and Laboratory Findings

The ESR and serum C-reactive protein are almost always elevated and can be useful parameters to follow during the course of therapy.

The plain film is the most readily available imaging procedure to establish the diagnosis of osteomyelitis, but it can be falsely negative early. Early radiographic findings may include soft tissue swelling, loss of tissue planes, and periarticular demineralization of bone. About 2 weeks after onset of symptoms, erosion of bone and alteration of cancellous bone appear, followed by periostitis.

MRI, CT, and nuclear medicine bone scanning are more sensitive than conventional radiography. MRI is the most sensitive and is particularly helpful in demonstrating the extent of soft tissue involvement. Radionuclide bone scanning is most valuable when osteomyelitis is suspected but no site is obvious. Nuclear medicine studies may also detect multifocal sites of infection. Ultrasound is useful in diagnosing the presence of effusions within joints and extra-articular soft tissue fluid collections but not in detecting bone infections.

Identifying the offending organism is a crucial step in selection of antibiotic therapy. Bone biopsy for culture is required except in those with hematogenous osteomyelitis, who have positive blood cultures. Cultures from overlying ulcers, wounds, or fistulas are unreliable.

▶ Differential Diagnosis

Acute hematogenous osteomyelitis should be distinguished from suppurative arthritis, rheumatic fever, and cellulitis. More subacute forms must be differentiated from tuberculosis or mycotic infections of bone and Ewing sarcoma or, in the case of vertebral osteomyelitis, from metastatic cancer. When osteomyelitis involves the vertebrae, it commonly traverses the disk—a finding not observed in cancer. Charcot arthropathy of the foot or ankle can mimic osteomyelitis, particularly in patients with diabetes; elevated ESR and serum C-reactive protein point to the presence of osteomyelitis in such cases.

▶ Complications

Inadequate treatment of bone infections results in chronicity of infection, and this possibility is increased by delaying diagnosis and treatment. Extension to adjacent bone or joints may complicate acute osteomyelitis. Recurrence of bone infections often results in anemia, a markedly elevated ESR, weight loss, weakness and, rarely, amyloidosis or nephrotic syndrome. Pseudoepitheliomatous hyperplasia, squamous cell carcinoma, or fibrosarcoma may occasionally arise in persistently infected tissues.

▶ Treatment

Most patients require both debridement of necrotic bone and prolonged administration of antibiotics. Patients with vertebral body osteomyelitis and epidural abscess may require urgent neurosurgical decompression. Depending on the site and extent of debridement, surgical procedures to stabilize, fill in, cover, or revascularize may be needed. Oral therapy with quinolones (eg, ciprofloxacin, 750 mg twice daily) for 6–8 weeks has been shown to be as effective as standard parenteral antibiotic therapy for chronic osteomyelitis with susceptible organisms. When treating osteomyelitis caused by *S aureus*, quinolones are usually combined with rifampin, 300 mg orally twice daily.

▶ Prognosis

If sterility of the lesion is achieved within 2–4 days, a good result can be expected in most cases if there is no compromise of the patient's immune system. However, progression of the disease to a chronic form may occur. It is especially common in the lower extremities and in patients in whom circulation is impaired (eg, diabetics).

Berbari EF et al. Executive Summary: 2015 Infectious Diseases Society of America (IDSA) clinical practice guidelines for the diagnosis and treatment of native vertebral osteomyelitis in adults. Clin Infect Dis. 2015 Sep 15;61(6):859–63. [PMID: 26316526]

TUBERCULOSIS OF BONES & JOINTS

SPINAL TUBERCULOSIS (Pott Disease)

ESSENTIALS OF DIAGNOSIS

▶ Seen primarily in immigrants from developing countries or immunocompromised patients.

▶ Back pain and gibbus deformity.

▶ Radiographic evidence of vertebral involvement.

▶ Evidence of *Mycobacterium tuberculosis* in aspirate or biopsies of spinal lesions.

▶ General Considerations

In the developing world, children primarily bear the burden of musculoskeletal tuberculosis. In the United States, however, musculoskeletal infection is more often seen in adult immigrants from countries where tuberculosis is prevalent, or it develops in the setting of immunosuppression (eg, HIV infection, therapy with TNF inhibitors). Spinal tuberculosis (Pott disease) accounts for about 50% of musculoskeletal infection due to *M tuberculosis* (see Chapter 9). Seeding of the vertebrae may occur through hematogenous spread from the respiratory tract at the time of primary infection, with clinical disease developing years later as a consequence of reactivation. The thoracic and lumbar vertebrae are the most common sites of spinal involvement; vertebral infection is associated with paravertebral cold abscesses in 75% of cases.

▶ **Clinical Findings**

A. Symptoms and Signs

Patients complain of back pain, often present for months and sometimes associated with radicular pain and lower extremity weakness. Constitutional symptoms are usually absent, and less than 20% have active pulmonary disease. Destruction of the anterior aspect of the vertebral body can produce the characteristic gibbus deformity.

B. Laboratory Findings

Most patients have a positive reaction to purified protein derivative (PPD) or a positive interferon-gamma release assay. Cultures of paravertebral abscesses and biopsies of vertebral lesions are positive in up to 70–90%. Biopsies reveal characteristic caseating granulomas in most cases. Isolation of *M tuberculosis* from an extraspinal site is sufficient to establish the diagnosis in the proper clinical setting.

C. Imaging

Radiographs can reveal lytic and sclerotic lesions and bony destruction of vertebrae but are normal early in the disease course. CT scanning can demonstrate paraspinal soft tissue extensions of the infection; MRI is the imaging technique of choice to detect compression of the spinal cord or cauda equina.

▶ **Differential Diagnosis**

Spinal tuberculosis must be differentiated from subacute and chronic spinal infections due to pyogenic organisms, *Brucella*, and fungi as well as from malignancy.

▶ **Complications**

Paraplegia due to compression of the spinal cord or cauda equina is the most serious complication of spinal tuberculosis.

▶ **Treatment**

Antimicrobial therapy should be administered for 6–9 months, usually in the form of isoniazid, rifampin, pyrazinamide, and ethambutol for 2 months followed by isoniazid and rifampin for an additional 4–7 months (see also Chapter 9). Medical management alone is often sufficient. Surgical intervention, however, may be indicated when there is neurologic compromise or severe spinal instability.

Batirel A et al. The course of spinal tuberculosis (Pott disease): results of the multinational, multicentre Backbone-2 study. Clin Microbiol Infect. 2015 Nov;21(11):1008.e9–18. [PMID: 26232534]

Varatharajah S et al. Update on the surgical management of Pott's disease. Orthop Traumatol Surg Res. 2014 Apr;100(2):229–35. [PMID: 24613439]

TUBERCULOUS ARTHRITIS

Infection of peripheral joints by *M tuberculosis* usually presents as a monoarticular arthritis lasting for weeks to months (or longer), but less often, it can have an acute presentation that mimics septic arthritis. Any joint can be involved; the hip and knee are most commonly affected. Constitutional symptoms and fever are present in only a small number of cases. Tuberculosis also can cause a chronic tenosynovitis of the hand and wrist. Joint destruction occurs far more slowly than in septic arthritis due to pyogenic organisms. Synovial fluid is inflammatory but not to the degree seen in pyogenic infections, with synovial white cell counts in the range of 10,000–20,000 cells/mcL. Smears of synovial fluid are positive for acid-fast bacilli in a minority of cases; synovial fluid cultures, however, are positive in 80% of cases. Because culture results may take weeks, the diagnostic procedure of choice usually is synovial biopsy, which yields characteristic pathologic findings and positive cultures in greater than 90%. Antimicrobial therapy is the mainstay of treatment. Rarely, a reactive, sterile polyarthritis associated with erythema nodosum (Poncet disease) develops in patients with active pulmonary tuberculosis.

Zeng M et al. Cementless total hip arthroplasty in advanced tuberculosis of the hip. Int Orthop. 2015 Nov;39(11):2103–7. [PMID: 26395010]

Zeng M et al. Total knee arthroplasty in advanced tuberculous arthritis of the knee. Int Orthop. 2015 Nov 18. [Epub ahead of print] [PMID: 26578080]

ARTHRITIS IN SARCOIDOSIS

The frequency of arthritis among patients with sarcoidosis is variously reported between 10% and 35%. It is usually acute in onset, but articular symptoms may appear insidiously and often antedate other manifestations of the disease. Knees and ankles are most commonly involved, but any joint may be affected. Distribution of joint involvement is usually polyarticular and symmetric. The arthritis is commonly self-limited, resolving after several weeks or months and rarely resulting in chronic arthritis, joint destruction, or significant deformity. Sarcoid arthropathy is often associated with erythema nodosum, but the diagnosis is contingent on the demonstration of other extra-articular manifestations of sarcoidosis and, notably, biopsy evidence of noncaseating granulomas. Despite the clinical appearance of an inflammatory arthritis, synovial fluid often is noninflammatory (ie, less than 2000 leukocytes/mcL). In chronic arthritis, radiographs show typical changes in the bones of the extremities with intact cortex and cystic changes.

Treatment of arthritis in sarcoidosis is usually symptomatic and supportive. Colchicine may be of value. A short course of corticosteroids may be effective in patients with severe and progressive joint disease.

Ungprasert P et al. Clinical characteristics of sarcoid arthropathy: a population-based study. Arthritis Care Res (Hoboken). 2015 Sep 28. [Epub ahead of print] [PMID: 26415117]

MISCELLANEOUS RHEUMATOLOGIC DISORDERS

THORACIC OUTLET SYNDROMES

Thoracic outlet syndromes result from compression of the neurovascular structures supplying the upper extremity. Symptoms and signs arise from intermittent or continuous pressure on elements of the brachial plexus (more than 90% of cases) or the subclavian or axillary vessels (veins or arteries) by a variety of anatomic structures of the shoulder girdle region. The neurovascular bundle can be compressed between the anterior or middle scalene muscles and a normal first thoracic rib or a cervical rib. Most commonly thoracic outlet syndromes are caused by scarred scalene neck muscle secondary to neck trauma or sagging of the shoulder girdle resulting from aging, obesity, or pendulous breasts. Faulty posture, occupation, or thoracic muscle hypertrophy from physical activity (eg, weight-lifting, baseball pitching) may be other predisposing factors.

Thoracic outlet syndromes present in most patients with some combination of four symptoms involving the upper extremity, namely pain, numbness, weakness, and swelling. The predominant symptoms depend on whether the compression chiefly affects neural or vascular structures. The onset of symptoms is usually gradual but can be sudden. Some patients spontaneously notice aggravation of symptoms with specific positioning of the arm. Pain radiates from the point of compression to the base of the neck, the axilla, the shoulder girdle region, arm, forearm, and hand. Paresthesias are common and distributed to the volar aspect of the fourth and fifth digits. Sensory symptoms may be aggravated at night or by prolonged use of the extremities. Weakness and muscle atrophy are the principal motor abnormalities. Vascular symptoms consist of arterial ischemia characterized by pallor of the fingers on elevation of the extremity, sensitivity to cold and, rarely, gangrene of the digits or venous obstruction marked by edema, cyanosis, and engorgement.

The symptoms of thoracic outlet syndromes can be provoked within 60 seconds over 90% of the time by having a patient elevate the arms in a "stick-em-up" position (ie, abducted 90 degrees in external rotation). Reflexes are usually not altered. Obliteration of the radial pulse with certain maneuvers of the arm or neck, once considered a highly sensitive sign of thoracic outlet obstruction, does not occur in most cases.

Chest radiography will identify patients with cervical rib (although most patients with cervical ribs are asymptomatic). MRI with the arms held in different positions is useful in identifying sites of impaired blood flow.

Intra-arterial or venous obstruction is confirmed by angiography. Determination of conduction velocities of the ulnar and other peripheral nerves of the upper extremity may help localize the site of their compression.

Thoracic outlet syndrome must be differentiated from osteoarthritis of the cervical spine, tumors of the superior pulmonary sulcus, cervical spinal cord, or nerve roots, and periarthritis of the shoulder.

Treatment is directed toward relief of compression of the neurovascular bundle. Greater than 95% of patients can be treated successfully with conservative therapy consisting of physical therapy and avoiding postures or activities that compress the neurovascular bundle. Some women will benefit from a support bra. Operative treatment, required by less than 5% of patients, is more likely to relieve the neurologic rather than the vascular component that causes symptoms.

Buller LT et al. Thoracic outlet syndrome: current concepts, imaging features, and therapeutic strategies. Am J Orthop (Belle Mead NJ). 2015 Aug;44(8):376–82. [PMID: 26251937]
Kuhn JE et al. Thoracic outlet syndrome. J Am Acad Orthop Surg. 2015 Apr;23(4):222–32. [PMID: 25808686]
Povlsen B et al. Treatment for thoracic outlet syndrome. Cochrane Database Syst Rev. 2014 Nov 26;11:CD007218. [PMID: 25427003]

FIBROMYALGIA

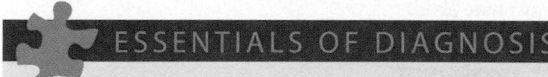 ESSENTIALS OF DIAGNOSIS

► Most frequent in women aged 20–50.
► Chronic widespread musculoskeletal pain syndrome with multiple tender points.
► Fatigue, headaches, numbness common.
► Objective signs of inflammation absent; laboratory studies normal.

General Considerations

Fibromyalgia is a common syndrome, affecting 3–10% of the general population. It shares many features with the chronic fatigue syndrome, namely, an increased frequency among women aged 20–50, absence of objective findings, and absence of diagnostic laboratory test results. While many of the clinical features of the two conditions overlap, musculoskeletal pain predominates in fibromyalgia whereas lassitude dominates the chronic fatigue syndrome.

The cause is unknown, but aberrant perception of painful stimuli, sleep disorders, depression, and viral infections have all been proposed. Fibromyalgia can be a rare complication of hypothyroidism, rheumatoid arthritis or, in men, sleep apnea.

Clinical Findings

The patient complains of chronic aching pain and stiffness, frequently involving the entire body but with prominence of pain around the neck, shoulders, low back, and hips.

Fatigue, sleep disorders, subjective numbness, chronic headaches, and irritable bowel symptoms are common. Even minor exertion aggravates pain and increases fatigue. Physical examination is normal except for "trigger points" of pain produced by palpation of various areas such as the trapezius, the medial fat pad of the knee, and the lateral epicondyle of the elbow.

▶ Differential Diagnosis

Fibromyalgia is a diagnosis of exclusion. A detailed history and repeated physical examination can obviate the need for extensive laboratory testing. Rheumatoid arthritis and SLE present with objective physical findings or abnormalities on routine testing. Thyroid function tests are useful, since hypothyroidism can produce a secondary fibromyalgia syndrome. Polymyositis produces weakness rather than pain. The diagnosis of fibromyalgia probably should be made hesitantly in a patient over age 50 and should never be invoked to explain fever, weight loss, or any other objective signs. Polymyalgia rheumatica produces shoulder and pelvic girdle pain, is associated with anemia and an elevated ESR, and occurs after age 50. Hypophosphatemic states, such as oncogenic osteomalacia, should also be included in the differential diagnosis of musculoskeletal pain unassociated with physical findings. In contrast to fibromyalgia, oncogenic osteomalacia usually produces pain in only a few areas and is associated with a low serum phosphate level.

▶ Treatment

A multidisciplinary approach is most effective. Patient education is essential. Patients can be comforted that they have a diagnosable syndrome treatable by specific though imperfect therapies and that the course is not progressive. Cognitive behavioral therapy, including programs that emphasize mindfulness meditation, is often helpful. There is modest efficacy of amitriptyline, fluoxetine, duloxetine, milnacipran, chlorpromazine, cyclobenzaprine, pregabalin, or gabapentin. Amitriptyline is initiated at a dosage of 10 mg orally at bedtime and gradually increased to 40–50 mg depending on efficacy and toxicity. Less than 50% of the patients experience a sustained improvement. Exercise programs are also beneficial. NSAIDs are generally ineffective. Tramadol and acetaminophen combinations have ameliorated symptoms modestly in short-term trials. Opioids and corticosteroids are ineffective and should not be used to treat fibromyalgia. Acupuncture is also ineffective.

▶ Prognosis

All patients have chronic symptoms. With treatment, however, many do eventually resume increased activities. Progressive or objective findings do not develop.

Clauw DJ. Fibromyalgia and related conditions. Mayo Clin Proc. 2015 May;90(5):680–92. [PMID: 25939940]
Sugerman DT. JAMA patient page. Fibromyalgia. JAMA. 2014 Apr 16;311(15):1577. [PMID: 24737379]

COMPLEX REGIONAL PAIN SYNDROME

Complex regional pain syndrome (formerly called reflex sympathetic dystrophy) is a rare disorder of the extremities characterized by autonomic and vasomotor instability. The cardinal symptoms and signs are pain localized to an arm or leg, swelling of the involved extremity, disturbances of color and temperature in the affected limb, dystrophic changes in the overlying skin and nails, and limited range of motion. Strikingly, the findings are not limited to the distribution of a single peripheral nerve. Most cases are preceded by direct physical trauma, often of a relatively minor nature, to the soft tissues, bone, or nerve. Early mobilization after injury or surgery reduces the likelihood of developing the syndrome. Any extremity can be involved, but the syndrome most commonly occurs in the hand and is associated with ipsilateral restriction of shoulder motion ("shoulder-hand" syndrome). This syndrome proceeds through phases: pain, swelling, and skin color and temperature changes develop early and, if untreated, lead to atrophy and dystrophy. The swelling in complex regional pain syndrome is diffuse ("catcher's mitt hand") and not restricted to joints. Pain is often burning in quality, intense, and often greatly worsened by minimal stimuli such as light touch. The shoulder-hand variant of this disorder sometimes complicates myocardial infarction or injuries to the neck or shoulder. Complex regional pain syndrome may occur after a knee injury or after arthroscopic knee surgery. There are no systemic symptoms. In the early phases of the syndrome, bone scans are sensitive, showing diffuse increased uptake in the affected extremity. Radiographs eventually reveal severe generalized osteopenia. In the posttraumatic variant, this is known as Sudeck atrophy. Symptoms and findings are bilateral in some. This syndrome should be differentiated from other cervicobrachial pain syndromes, rheumatoid arthritis, thoracic outlet obstruction, and scleroderma, among others.

Early treatment offers the best prognosis for recovery. For mild cases, NSAIDs (eg, naproxen 250–500 mg twice daily orally) can be effective. For more severe cases associated with edema, prednisone, 30–60 mg/day orally for 2 weeks and then tapered over 2 weeks, can be effective. Pain management is important and facilitates physical therapy, which plays a critical role in efforts to restore function. Some patients will also benefit from antidepressant agents (eg, nortriptyline initiated at a dosage of 10 mg orally at bedtime and gradually increased to 40–75 mg at bedtime) or from anticonvulsants (eg, gabapentin 300 mg three times daily orally). Bisphosphonates, calcitonin, intravenous immunoglobulin, regional nerve blocks, and dorsal-column stimulation have also been demonstrated to be helpful. Patients who have restricted shoulder motion may benefit from the treatment described for scapulohumeral periarthritis. The prognosis partly depends on the stage in which the lesions are encountered and the extent and severity of associated organic disease.

Birklein F et al. Complex regional pain syndrome: an optimistic perspective. Neurology. 2015 Jan 6;84(1):89–96. [PMID: 25471395]

Borchers AT et al. Complex regional pain syndrome: a comprehensive and critical review. Autoimmun Rev. 2014 Mar; 13(3):242–65. [PMID: 24161450]

Freedman M et al. Complex regional pain syndrome: diagnosis and treatment. Phys Med Rehabil Clin N Am. 2014 May; 25(2):291–303. [PMID: 24787334]

Rockett M. Diagnosis, mechanisms and treatment of complex regional pain syndrome. Curr Opin Anaesthesiol. 2014 Oct; 27(5):494–500. [PMID: 25111604]

RHEUMATOLOGIC MANIFESTATIONS OF CANCER

Rheumatologic syndromes may be the presenting manifestations for a variety of cancers. Dermatomyositis in adults, for example, is often associated with cancer. Hypertrophic pulmonary osteoarthropathy, which is characterized by the triad of polyarthritis, new onset of clubbing, and periosteal new bone formation, is associated with both malignant diseases (eg, lung and intrathoracic cancers) and nonmalignant ones (eg, cyanotic heart disease, cirrhosis, and lung abscess). Cancer-associated polyarthritis is rare, has both oligoarticular and polyarticular forms, and should be considered when "seronegative rheumatoid arthritis" develops abruptly in an elderly patient. Palmar fasciitis manifests as bilateral palmar swelling with finger contractures and may be the first indication of cancer, particularly ovarian carcinoma. Remitting seronegative synovitis with non-pitting edema ("RS3PE") presents with a symmetric small-joint polyarthritis associated with non-pitting edema of the hands; it can be idiopathic or associated with malignancy. Palpable purpura due to leukocytoclastic vasculitis may be the presenting complaint in myeloproliferative disorders. Hairy cell leukemia can be associated with medium-sized vessel vasculitis such as polyarteritis nodosa. Acute leukemia can produce joint pains that are disproportionately severe in comparison to the minimal swelling and heat that are present. Leukemic arthritis complicates approximately 5% of cases. Rheumatic manifestations of myelodysplastic syndromes include cutaneous vasculitis, lupus-like syndromes, neuropathy, and episodic intense arthritis. Erythromelalgia, a painful warmth and redness of the extremities that (unlike Raynaud) improves with cold exposure or with elevation of the extremity, is often associated with myeloproliferative diseases, particularly essential thrombocythemia.

Kisacik B et al. Diagnostic dilemma of paraneoplastic arthritis: case series. Int J Rheum Dis. 2014 Jul;17(6):640–5. [PMID: 24433553]

Mekinian A et al; Société Nationale Française de Médecine Interne (SNFMI). Inflammatory arthritis in patients with myelodysplastic syndromes: a multicenter retrospective study and literature review of 68 cases. Medicine (Baltimore). 2014 Jan;93(1):1–10. [PMID: 24378738]

NEUROGENIC ARTHROPATHY (Charcot Joint)

Neurogenic arthropathy is joint destruction resulting from loss or diminution of proprioception, pain, and temperature perception. Although initially described in the knees

of patients with tabes dorsalis, it is more frequently seen in association with diabetic neuropathy (foot and ankle) or syringomyelia (shoulder). As normal muscle tone and protective reflexes are lost, secondary degenerative joint disease ensues, resulting in an enlarged, boggy, relatively painless joint with extensive cartilage erosion, osteophyte formation, and multiple loose joint bodies. Radiographs can reveal striking osteolysis that mimics osteomyelitis or dramatic destruction of the joint with subluxation, fragmentation of bone, and bony sclerosis.

Treatment is directed toward the primary disease; mechanical devices are used to assist in weight bearing and prevention of further trauma. In some instances, amputation becomes unavoidable.

Bariteau JT et al. Charcot arthropathy of the foot and ankle in patients with idiopathic neuropathy. Foot Ankle Int. 2014 Oct; 35(10):996–1001. [PMID: 25104748]

Blume PA et al. Charcot neuroarthropathy of the foot and ankle: diagnosis and management strategies. Clin Podiatr Med Surg. 2014 Jan;31(1):151–72. [PMID: 24296023]

DiPreta JA. Outpatient assessment and management of the diabetic foot. Med Clin North Am. 2014 Mar;98(2):353–73. [PMID: 24559880]

PALINDROMIC RHEUMATISM

Palindromic rheumatism is a disease of unknown cause characterized by frequent recurring attacks (at irregular intervals) of acutely inflamed joints. Periarticular pain with swelling and transient subcutaneous nodules may also occur. The attacks cease within several hours to several days. The knee and finger joints are most commonly affected, but any peripheral joint may be involved. Systemic manifestations other than fever do not occur. Although hundreds of attacks may take place over a period of years, there is no permanent articular damage. Laboratory findings are usually normal. Palindromic rheumatism must be distinguished from acute gouty arthritis and an atypical acute onset of rheumatoid arthritis. In some patients, palindromic rheumatism is a prodrome of rheumatoid arthritis.

Symptomatic treatment with NSAIDs is usually all that is required during the attacks. Hydroxychloroquine may be of value in preventing recurrences.

OSTEONECROSIS (Avascular Necrosis of Bone)

Osteonecrosis is a complication of corticosteroid use, alcoholism, trauma, SLE, pancreatitis, gout, sickle cell disease, dysbaric syndromes (eg, "the bends"), knee menisectomy, and infiltrative diseases (eg, Gaucher disease). The most commonly affected sites are the proximal and distal femoral heads, leading to hip or knee pain. Other commonly affected sites include the ankle, shoulder, and elbow. Osteonecrosis of the jaw has been rarely associated with use of bisphosphonate therapy, almost always when the bisphosphonate is used for treating metastatic cancer or multiple myeloma rather than osteoporosis. Initially, radiographs are often normal; MRI, CT scan, and bone scan are all more sensitive techniques. Treatment involves avoidance of weight bearing on the affected joint for at least several weeks. The value of surgical core decompression is controversial. For osteonecrosis of the hip, a variety of procedures designed to preserve the femoral head have been developed for early disease, including vascularized and nonvascularized bone grafting procedures. These procedures are most effective in avoiding or forestalling the need for total hip arthroplasty in young patients who do not have advanced disease. Without a successful intervention of this nature, the natural history of avascular necrosis is usually progression of the bony infarction to cortical collapse, resulting in significant joint dysfunction. Total hip replacement is the usual outcome for all patients who are candidates for that procedure.

Moya-Angeler J et al. Current concepts on osteonecrosis of the femoral head. World J Orthop. 2015 Sep 18;6(8):590–601. [PMID: 26396935]

Ruggiero SL. Diagnosis and staging of medication-related osteonecrosis of the jaw. Oral Maxillofac Surg Clin North Am. 2015 Nov;27(4):479–87. [PMID: 26293329]

▼ ALLERGIC & IMMUNOLOGIC DISORDERS

R. Anthony Orden, MD & N. Franklin Adkinson, Jr., MD

Allergy is an immunologically mediated hypersensitivity reaction to a foreign antigen manifested by tissue inflammation and organ dysfunction. The clinical expression of allergic disease depends on prior immunologic responsiveness, antigen exposure, and genetically influenced host factors such as atopy. Atopic patients have a genetically aggregated predisposition to a limited number of disorders: allergic rhinitis (Chapter 8), allergic asthma (Chapter 9), atopic dermatitis (Chapter 6), and IgE-mediated food allergies. Although these disorders tend to aggregate in families designated as "atopic," each of these disorders can occur in individuals without personal or familial history of an atopic diathesis. In addition, many mast cell and IgE-dependent disorders (eg, many drug and chemical sensitivities, eosinophilic disorders, mast cell stability syndromes, chronic urticaria) occur equally frequently in atopic and nonatopic persons.

The timing of the onset of clinical allergic syndromes after exposure to a suspected allergen serves as a useful clinical marker on which to base diagnosis and treatment. Reactions will usually be either *immediate* (generally occurring within 60 minutes after initial exposure), or *delayed*, appearing after many hours to days or weeks of antigen exposure.

IMMEDIATE HYPERSENSITIVITY

IgE antibodies occupy receptor sites on mast cells. Within minutes after exposure to the allergen, a multivalent antigen links adjacent IgE molecules, activating and degranulating mast cells. Clinical manifestations can be explained by the effects of released mediators on target end organs. Both preformed and newly generated mediators cause vasodilation and permeability changes, visceral smooth muscle contraction, mucous secretory gland stimulation, vascular permeability, and tissue inflammation. Arachidonic acid metabolites, cytokines, and other mediators (such as chemoattractants) induce a late-phase inflammatory response that appears several hours later in affected tissues when antigen exposure is continuous (eg, pollen) or chronic.

1. Anaphylaxis

▶ General Considerations

Anaphylaxis is the most serious and potentially life-threatening clinical manifestation of mast cell and basophil mediator release. Anaphylaxis is defined clinically under the following circumstances: (1) an allergen exposure followed by the acute onset of illness involving skin or mucosal tissue and either respiratory compromise or hypotension (systolic blood pressure less than 90 mm Hg or 30% less than known baseline); (2) a likely allergen exposure followed by the acute onset of two or more of the following conditions: skin or mucosal tissue involvement, respiratory compromise, hypotension, and persistent gastrointestinal symptoms; or (3) a known allergen exposure followed by hypotension.

IgE-dependent anaphylaxis is usually an acute syndrome initiated by a new allergen exposure after a prior silent exposure has sensitized the patient with IgE antibodies. Thus, anaphylaxis (or systemic allergic reactions which do not meet the definition of anaphylaxis) cannot occur on first-time exposure to allergens like drugs, insect venoms, latex, and foods. In contrast, **idiopathic anaphylaxis** (sometimes called "anaphylactoid"), such as reactions to radiocontrast media and most NSAID and opioid reactions, is pseudoallergic without known immunologic mechanisms and can occur with first-time exposure.

▶ Clinical Findings

A. Symptoms and Signs

Symptoms and signs typically occur within 30 minutes of initial exposure but may appear up to several hours later. These include (in order of frequency): (1) skin manifestations, typically urticaria but also flushing, blotchy rashes, and pruritus; (2) respiratory distress, including wheezing, stridor, bronchospasm, and airway angioedema; (3) gastrointestinal symptoms, including cramping, emesis, and diarrhea (especially in food allergy); and (4) hypotension, often manifested as lightheadedness, dizziness, or syncope. The condition is potentially fatal, especially if untreated, and can affect both nonatopic and atopic persons.

B. Laboratory Findings

Identification of anaphylaxis is clinical as the need for treatment is urgent. Elevated serum levels of mast cell mediators, such as tryptase and histamine, may be detected shortly after a reaction providing support to the diagnosis. Referral to an allergy specialist is standard because of concern for a future reaction and need for appropriate interventions and education. Specific IgE serum or skin testing may be performed to suspected allergens. Skin testing, which is usually more sensitive, optimally occurs 4–6 weeks after a severe reaction to avoid falsely negative testing during a post-reaction "refractory" period. The positive predictive value of these tests is highly dependent on a suggestive temporal relationship to putative allergen exposure.

▶ **Treatment**

Early administration of intramuscular epinephrine at the onset of a suspected anaphylactic response is the cornerstone of therapy. Supportive measures, such as oxygen, intravenous fluids and, if required, airway management are also appropriate. Adjunctive pharmacologic therapies include antihistamines, bronchodilators, and corticosteroids. Self-administered epinephrine at the earliest signs of recurrence can be life-sparing, whereas antihistamines and corticosteroids have limited value in reversing anaphylactic syndromes.

▶ **When to Refer**

Patients with new or unexplained onset of anaphylaxis should be evaluated by an allergist.

Lieberman P et al. Anaphylaxis—a practice parameter update 2015. Ann Allergy Asthma Immunol. 2015 Nov;115(5): 341–84. [PMID: 26505932]

2. Food Allergy

Immediate allergic reactions within 2 hours of ingestion of foods are much less common among adults than children. Most acute systemic food allergy is caused by proteins in milk, egg, wheat, soy, fish, shellfish, peanuts, and tree nuts. Milk and egg allergies in atopic children are often outgrown by adulthood. Shellfish, peanuts, and tree nuts are the most common causes of food anaphylaxis in adults. Diagnosis of food allergy relies on a combination of history, skin tests, and specific IgE tests. There is no role for specific IgG testing for evaluating food hypersensitivity. Because of frequent false-positive IgE tests, especially among atopic patients, oral food challenge remains the gold standard for diagnosis. However, this procedure should only be conducted by an experienced provider in a well-equipped setting. Management involves strict avoidance of the culprit food and guaranteed access to self-administered epinephrine.

Other IgE-mediated food reactions include oral allergy syndrome and hypersensitivity to alpha-gal (galactose-alpha-1,3-galactose). Oral allergy syndrome, also known as pollen-associated food allergy syndrome, is the result of cross-reactivity between food and pollen proteins. Affected individuals have known seasonal pollen allergies (most commonly tree pollens) and experience itching of the oral mucosa upon ingestion of certain raw fruits and vegetables. In contrast to systemic food allergy, symptoms are limited to the oropharynx and usually do not involve other organ systems or progress to anaphylaxis.

Alpha-gal (galactose-alpha-1,3-galactose) is a carbohydrate found in red mammalian meats, including beef, pork and lamb but not in human tissues. Sensitization to this epitope has been linked to tick bites, so nonatopic individuals are at risk. In contrast to conventional systemic food allergy, the reaction to red meat typically occurs 4–6 hours after ingestion.

Ho MH et al. Clinical spectrum of food allergies: a comprehensive review. Clin Rev Allergy Immunol. 2014 Jun;46(3):225–40. [PMID: 23229594]
Kattan JD et al. Optimizing the diagnosis of food allergy. Immunol Allergy Clin North Am. 2015 Feb;35(1):61–76. [PMID: 25459577]
Muraro A et al. EAACI food allergy and anaphylaxis guidelines: diagnosis and management of food allergy. Allergy. 2014 Aug; 69(8):1008–25. [PMID: 24909706]
Muraro A et al. EAACI food allergy and anaphylaxis guidelines: managing patients with food allergy in the community. Allergy. 2014 Aug;69(8):1046–57. [PMID: 24905609]
Savage J et al. Food allergy: epidemiology and natural history. Immunol Allergy Clin North Am. 2015 Feb;35(1):45–59. [PMID: 25459576]
Turnbull JL et al. Review article: the diagnosis and management of food allergy and food intolerances. Aliment Pharmacol Ther. 2015 Jan;41(1):3–25. [PMID: 25316115]
Valenta R et al. Food allergies: the basics. Gastroenterology. 2015 May;148(6):1120–31.e4. [PMID: 25680669]

3. Drug Allergy

Skin testing for immediate allergy to drugs is reliable for high molecular weight proteins (eg, cytokines, antisera, enzymes) but often not as reliable for low-molecular-weight compounds (eg, most drugs), which must bind to larger proteins (as haptens) to become immunogenic. With the exception of beta-lactam antibiotics like penicillins and some intraoperative drugs, in vivo skin testing for low-molecular-weight drugs is largely unvalidated, and interpretable only if the test is positive at a nonirritating concentration. Testing for IgE-mediated allergy to penicillin is available because the immunochemistry has been delineated and appropriate skin testing reagents are available. Skin testing with the major and minor metabolic determinants of penicillin has a very high (more than 98%) negative predictive value. Referral of individuals who relate histories of acute penicillin reactions to an allergist for skin testing is worthwhile because more than 90% have negative testing, indicating loss of allergic sensitization. Such patients may safely receive penicillins and related antibiotics.

Chiriac AM et al. Drug allergy diagnosis. Immunol Allergy Clin North Am. 2014 Aug;34(3):461–7. [PMID: 25017672]
Kelso JM. Drug and vaccine allergy. Immunol Allergy Clin North Am. 2015 Feb;35(1):221–30. [PMID: 25459586]
Mirakian R et al; Standards of Care Committee of the British Society for Allergy and Clinical Immunology. Management of allergy to penicillins and other beta-lactams. Clin Exp Allergy. 2015 Feb;45(2):300–27. [PMID: 25623506]
Romano A et al. Antibiotic allergy. Immunol Allergy Clin North Am. 2014 Aug;34(3):489–506. [PMID: 25017674]
Sicherer SH et al. Advances in allergic skin disease, anaphylaxis, and hypersensitivity reactions to foods, drugs, and insects in 2014. J Allergy Clin Immunol. 2015 Feb;135(2):357–67. [PMID: 25662305]
Vultaggio A et al. Hypersensitivity reactions to biologic agents. Immunol Allergy Clin North Am. 2014 Aug;34(3):615–32. [PMID: 25017680]

4. Venom Allergy

The most common insects causing systemic allergic reactions include honeybees, vespids (yellow jackets, hornets, wasps), and fire ants. Systemic reactions often occur after several unremarkable stinging events and can develop at any age. Patients at highest risk for a severe reaction are those who have had a history of recent and severe reactions. The risk of a systemic reaction appears to decline over time since the last sting. If a systemic allergy is suspected, referral to an allergist for testing and, if appropriate, initiation of venom immunotherapy, is recommended. In the interim, making self-administered epinephrine available is indicated for those with continuing exposure.

Antolín-Amérigo D et al. Venom immunotherapy: an updated review. Curr Allergy Asthma Rep. 2014 Jul;14(7):449. [PMID: 24934908]
Golden DB. New directions in diagnostic evaluation of insect allergy. Curr Opin Allergy Clin Immunol. 2014 Aug;14(4):334–9. [PMID: 24915545]
Pesek RD et al. Treatment of *Hymenoptera* venom allergy: an update. Curr Opin Allergy Clin Immunol. 2014 Aug; 14(4):340–6. [PMID: 24887986]
Sicherer SH et al. Advances in allergic skin disease, anaphylaxis, and hypersensitivity reactions to foods, drugs, and insects in 2014. J Allergy Clin Immunol. 2015 Feb;135(2):357–67. [PMID: 25662305]

5. Pseudoallergic Reactions

Pseudoallergic reactions (Table 20–13) resemble immediate hypersensitivity reactions but are not mediated by allergen-IgE interaction. Examples include radiocontrast reactions, opioid reactions (direct mast cell activation), and "red man syndrome" from rapid infusion of vancomycin. Patients with mast cell disorders may be more prone to these reactions due to more easily triggered mast cell degranulation. In contrast to IgE-mediated reactions, these can often be prevented by prophylactic medical regimens.

▶ Radiocontrast Media Reactions

Reactions to radiocontrast media are not IgE antibody–mediated, yet they are clinically similar to anaphylaxis and can be life-threatening. If a patient has had an anaphylactoid reaction to conventional radiocontrast media, the risk for a second reaction upon reexposure may be as high as 30%. Patients with a history of atopy are at increased risk.

Management includes use of the low-osmolality contrast preparations and prophylactic administration of prednisone (50 mg orally every 6 hours beginning 13 hours before the procedure) and diphenhydramine (25–50 mg orally, intramuscularly or intravenously 60 minutes before the procedure). The use of the lower-osmolality radiocontrast media in combination with the pretreatment regimen decreases the incidence of recurrent reactions to less than 1%.

Brockow K et al. Hypersensitivity to contrast media and dyes. Immunol Allergy Clin North Am. 2014 Aug;34(3):547–64. [PMID: 25017677]
Davis PL. Anaphylactoid reactions to the nonvascular administration of water-soluble iodinated contrast media. AJR Am J Roentgenol. 2015 Jun;204(6):1140–5. [PMID: 26001221]
Egbert RE et al. Delayed adverse reactions to the parenteral administration of iodinated contrast media. AJR Am J Roentgenol. 2014 Dec;203(6):1163–70. [PMID: 25415693]

6. Aspirin (NSAID) Exacerbated Respiratory Disease

Although aspirin (NSAID) hypersensitivity is a feature of this condition, the reaction is a result of aberrant arachidonic acid metabolism, rather than a product of an IgE activated process. The inhibition of cyclooxygenase-1 (COX-1) by these anti-inflammatory drugs results in the overproduction of cysteinyl leukotrienes and increased expression of leukotriene receptors, leading to increased airway responsiveness, bronchospasm, rhinorrhea, and nasal congestion. Reactions outside of the respiratory system can also occur, including ocular, cutaneous, and gastric symptoms.

In addition to aspirin or NSAID sensitivity, patients with aspirin exacerbated respiratory disease typically have a chronic rhinosinusitis with nasal polyps and asthma, a syndrome referred to as "Samter triad" or "triad asthma." Diagnosis is largely based on history and clinical findings. If required, a positive aspirin challenge can demonstrate the NSAID hypersensitivity, the presence of which may suggest increased responsiveness to treatments such as nasal polypectomy and aspirin desensitization. Patients who require daily aspirin or NSAID treatment for cardiovascular or rheumatologic disorders can be desensitized to permit such treatment. Desensitization and long-term aspirin therapy have also been shown to reduce the need for nasal polypectomy and asthma therapy. Referral to an allergy specialist is appropriate for consideration of such desensitization.

Morales DR et al. Safety risks for patients with aspirin-exacerbated respiratory disease after acute exposure to selective nonsteroidal anti-inflammatory drugs and COX-2 inhibitors: meta-analysis of controlled clinical trials. J Allergy Clin Immunol. 2014 Jul;134(1):40–5. [PMID: 24388008]
Saff RR et al. Management of patients with nonaspirin-exacerbated respiratory disease aspirin hypersensitivity reactions. Allergy Asthma Proc. 2015 Jan–Feb;36(1):34–9. [PMID: 25562554]
Simon RA et al. Update on aspirin desensitization for chronic rhinosinusitis with polyps in aspirin-exacerbated respiratory disease (AERD). Curr Allergy Asthma Rep. 2015 Mar;15(3):508. [PMID: 25663486]

DELAYED HYPERSENSITIVITY

According to the Gell and Coombs classification, type IV delayed hypersensitivity is mediated by activated T cells, which accumulate in areas of antigen deposition. A common example is allergic contact dermatitis, which develops when a low-molecular-weight sensitizing substance serves as a hapten for dermal proteins, becoming a complete antigen. Sensitized T cells release cytokines, activating macrophages and promoting subsequent dermal inflammation;

Table 20–13. Uncommon allergic and pseudoallergic conditions.

Disease	Pathogenesis	Symptoms and Signs	Diagnostic Findings[1]	Treatment
Allergic bronchopulmonary aspergillosis	Immunologic response to pulmonary fungal colonization	Often underlying moderate to severe allergic asthma and/or cystic fibrosis, with wheezing, cough productive of thick brown sputum, fever, weight loss, fatigue	**Elevated serum total IgE (> 1000 ng/mL); SPT positive to *Aspergillus*; positive *Aspergillus* precipitins,** eosinophilia (off corticosteroids) (total eosinophils > 1000 cells/mcL), pulmonary infiltrates, central bronchiectasis	Oral corticosteroids, antifungal (azole) agent
Hereditary angioedema	Quantitative or functional C1 esterase inhibitor deficiency, resulting in increased serum bradykinin levels	Unpredictable swelling of face, lips, tongue, hands, feet; no urticaria; gastrointestinal tract swelling causing severe abdominal pain	**Decreased C1 esterase inhibitor serum level and/or function,** decreased serum C4 level	Prophylactic treatment: Danazol, tranexamic acid Acute treatment: C1 esterase inhibitor product, kallikrein inhibitor, bradykinin B_2-receptor antagonist
Hypereosinophilic syndromes	Leukoproliferative disorder characterized by overproduction of eosinophils	Symptoms related to eosinophilic infiltration of organs: angioedema, urticaria, pruritic papules, chronic cough, splenomegaly, heart failure	**Eosinophilia (eosinophils > 1500 cells/mcL),** elevated serum vitamin B_{12} level, elevated serum tryptase level, anemia, PDGFRA gene mutation	Corticosteroids, tyrosine kinase inhibitors
Mastocytosis	Mast cell hyperplasia	Pruritus, flushing, nausea, vomiting, diarrhea, abdominal pain, hypotension	**Dense bone marrow mast cell infiltrate (≥ 15/hpf) on biopsy, elevated serum tryptase level (> 20 ng/mL),** atypical mast cell morphology, *cKIT* mutation	Antihistamine, cromolyn, epinephrine, chemotherapy directed at underlying mast cell hyperplasia
"Red man syndrome" (acute infusion reaction)	Direct activation of mast cells by vancomycin (opioids and other drugs)	Flushing, pruritus, and erythema, especially of the upper body, during intravenous infusion of drug	Clinical history and physical examination, no role for laboratory testing	Antihistamine pretreatment 1 hour prior to subsequent vancomycin (or opioid and other causative drug) infusions, decreased rate of infusion
Serum sickness (and serum sickness-like syndromes)	Mediated by circulating immune complexes	Fever, pruritic urticarial or maculopapular rash, lymphadenopathy, arthralgias, arthritis, nephritis	**Increased ESR, leukocytosis,** possible low serum C3 and C4 levels	Self-limited illness: NSAIDs, antihistamines Severe illness: Corticosteroids, plasma exchange

[1]Key diagnostic findings in bold.

cKIT, stem cell factor receptor or CD117; ESR, erythrocyte sedimentation rate; NSAID, nonsteroidal anti-inflammatory drug; PDGFRA, platelet-derived growth factor receptor alpha; SPT, skin prick test.

this typically occurs 48–72 hours after contact. Another common expression of delayed hypersensitivity is drug allergy that occurs after a similar process and that often results in maculopapular or morbilliform exanthems. T cell–mediated hypersensitivity is now understood to involve both Th1 and Th2 cells. In addition, subsequent inflammation and tissue damage occurs via various effector cell types, including monocytes, eosinophils, and neutrophils.

1. Drug Exanthems

The clinical manifestation of these reactions is vast (Chapter 6), ranging from the commonly observed morbilliform drug rash to the skin sloughing observed in Stevens-Johnson syndrome and toxic epidermal necrolysis. Given the range of cutaneous findings, the differential diagnosis is broad and includes miliaria, lichen planus, folliculitis, pityriasis rosea, tinea corporis, and mycosis fungoides. Physical examination of rash characteristics, dermatologic consultation, and biopsy findings can help narrow the differential. While a whole spectrum of drugs can result in exanthems, there are no commercially available laboratory or other diagnostic tests to reliably identify the culprit drug.

Management consists mainly of immediate cessation of suspected medications and monitoring for symptom resolution. Systemic corticosteroids may be indicated for extensive dermatitis or other organ involvement.

Martin SF. New concepts in cutaneous allergy. Contact Dermatitis. 2015 Jan;72(1):2–10. [PMID: 25348820]

Naisbitt DJ et al. In vitro diagnosis of delayed-type drug hypersensitivity: mechanistic aspects and unmet needs. Immunol Allergy Clin North Am. 2014 Aug;34(3):691–705. [PMID: 25017686]

Pavlos R et al. T cell-mediated hypersensitivity reactions to drugs. Annu Rev Med. 2015;66:439–54. [PMID: 25386935]

2. Drug-Induced Hypersensitivity Syndrome (Drug Reaction with Eosinophilia & Systemic Symptoms)

▶ General Considerations

Potentially life-threatening, systemic drug-induced hypersensitivity reactions most commonly occur with exposure to anticonvulsants and sulfonamides, although many other classes of drugs, including other antimicrobials and antidepressants, have been implicated. The onset of symptoms typically occurs 2–6 weeks after drug initiation. As suggested by its alternative name, drug reaction with eosinophilia and systemic symptoms (DRESS), it typically involves the development of eosinophilia and/or lymphocytosis and systemic symptoms such as fever and lymph node enlargement, along with the rash. The exact pathogenesis of DRESS is not well-elucidated but may include deficient drug metabolism due to genetic mutations in specific detoxification enzymes; reactivation of herpesviruses including HHV-6, HHV-7, cytomegalovirus, and Epstein-Barr virus; and a genetic predisposition based on the presence of specific HLA haplotypes.

▶ HLA Haplotypes & Risk of Delayed-Onset Drug Hypersensitivity Syndromes

Activated cytotoxic CD8 T lymphocytes play a key role in the pathogenesis of serious, drug-induced adverse cutaneous reactions, such as toxic epidermal necrolysis. There are striking, medication-specific associations between inheritance of particular HLA-B alleles and risk of these hypersensitivity reactions in defined populations. Most notably, B*57:01 confers risk for reactions to abacavir; B*15:02, for carbamazepine; B*58:01, for allopurinol; and B*13:01, for dapsone. The most likely mechanism is a direct interaction between the drug and the antigen-binding cleft of the HLA-B molecule, such that many "self" antigens subsequently bound by the HLA-B molecule are perceived as "foreign," eliciting massive CD8 T-cell activation. Current FDA recommendations call for testing for the relevant HLA-B allele prior to initiating therapy with abacavir in all patients and with carbamazepine in Asian patients. The American College of Rheumatology recommends such testing before starting allopurinol therapy in patients of Korean descent, especially those with kidney disease, and Han Chinese and individuals of Thai extraction. Pretreatment HLA testing for other drugs or in other populations may not be useful at the present time due to low prevalence of the implicated isotypes.

▶ Clinical Findings

A. Symptoms and Signs

DRESS often begins with pruritus and fever, but cutaneous manifestations generally follow soon thereafter. The most common cutaneous manifestation is an erythematous morbilliform rash. Although the entire skin surface can be involved, the face, trunk, and upper and lower extremities are the commonly affected areas. The most common systemic findings involve the lymphatic (lymphadenopathy), hematologic and hepatic systems, although renal, pulmonary and cardiac involvement is also documented.

B. Laboratory Findings

Laboratory abnormalities include leukocytosis with eosinophilia (greater than 1.5×10^9/L) and atypical lymphocytosis; elevated hepatic transaminases (more than 2 times upper limits of normal) and alkaline phosphatase, and increased serum creatinine, pyuria, and proteinuria, which may indicate the development of interstitial nephritis. The most common skin biopsy findings are a dense, perivascular lymphocytic infiltrate in the papillary dermis with eosinophils and dermal edema.

▶ Treatment

Management consists of cessation of the causative medication and initiation of systemic corticosteroids. A dose of 1.0 mg/kg of oral prednisone is recommended as a starting dose, followed by a gradual taper occurring over 3–6 months after laboratory normalization and stabilization. Additional supportive therapies may include antipyretics for

Table 20–14. Selected immunodeficiency syndromes.

Disease	Clinical Presentation	Diagnosis[1]	Treatment
Common variable immunodeficiency	Recurrent sinopulmonary infections, parasitic (especially *Giardia lamblia*) and microbial gastrointestinal infections, autoimmune diseases and increased risk of malignancy	**Poor humoral response to immunizations,** low serum quantitative immunoglobulin levels, T-cell dysfunction	Antibiotics, intravenous immunoglobulin G (IVIG) every 3–4 weeks, subcutaneous IVIG weekly
Selective IgA deficiency	Most prevalent primary immunodeficiency (1 in 600 individuals); most cases asymptomatic; recurrent sinopulmonary infections; atopic disorders, rheumatoid arthritis and systemic lupus erythematosus common; rarely, anaphylaxis to transfusion of blood or blood products	**Low to absent serum IgA levels (< 15 mcg/dL),** normal serum IgG and IgM levels	Early use of antibiotics; monitor for development of common variable immunodeficiency
Adult T-cell deficiencies	Opportunistic infections (similar to HIV)	**Exclude HIV infection; obtain T-cell profiles.** A subtype, the Wiskott-Aldrich syndrome, is associated with thrombocytopenia, small platelets, and eczema	Antimicrobials, bone marrow transplantation for Wiskott-Aldrich syndrome
Complement disorders	"Early" complement component deficiencies: Autoimmune diseases "Late" complement component (C5–C8) deficiencies: Recurrent meningococcal or gonococcal infections	**Serum complement levels**	Prompt administration of antibiotics

[1]**Key diagnostic findings in bold.**
Modified, with permission, from Ashar B, Miller R, Sisson S (editors): Johns Hopkins Internal Medicine Board Review Certification and Recertification, 5th ed. © Elsevier, 2015.

fever, topical steroids for skin lesions, or fluid and electrolyte replacement in the case of more severe exfoliative dermatitis.

Cheng CY et al. HLA associations and clinical implications in T-cell mediated drug hypersensitivity reactions: an updated review. J Immunol Res. 2014;2014:565320. [PMID: 24901010]
Husain Z et al. DRESS syndrome: Part I. Clinical perspectives. J Am Acad Dermatol. 2013 May;68(5):693.e1–14. [PMID: 23602182]
Husain Z et al. DRESS syndrome: Part II. Management and therapeutics. J Am Acad Dermatol. 2013 May;68(5):709.e1–9. [PMID: 23602183]
Radonjic-Hoesli S et al. Novel targeted therapies for eosinophil-associated diseases and allergy. Annu Rev Pharmacol Toxicol. 2015;55:633–56. [PMID: 25340931]
Schwartz RA et al. Toxic epidermal necrolysis. Part I. Introduction, history, classification, clinical diagnosis, systemic manifestations, etiology, and immunopathogenesis. J Am Acad Dermatol. 2013 Aug;69(2):173.e1-13. [PMID: 23866878]

PRIMARY IMMUNODEFICIENCY DISORDERS IN ADULTS

Most primary immunologic deficiency diseases are rare and, because they are genetically determined, usually present in childhood. Nonetheless, several important immunodeficiency disorders can present in adulthood, most notably selective IgA deficiency, common variable immunodeficiency, and deficiencies in the terminal components of the complement pathway, which confer susceptibility to *Neisseria* infections (Table 20–14). Specific antibody deficiency may predispose patients to common conditions such as refractory chronic rhinosinusitis or chronic obstructive pulmonary disease with frequent exacerbations, and thus additional immunologic evaluation may be warranted. Autoantibodies that neutralize cytokines are a recognized mechanism of acquired immunodeficiency in adulthood. For example, neutralizing autoantibodies against interferon-gamma can lead to severe opportunistic infections with nontuberculous mycobacteria, and antibodies to granulocyte macrophage-colony stimulating factor are associated with cryptococcal meningitis in otherwise immunocompetent individuals.

Bonilla FA et al. Practice parameter for the diagnosis and management of primary immunodeficiency. J Allergy Clin Immunol. 2015 Nov;136(5):1186–205. [PMID: 26371839]
Browne SK. Anticytokine autoantibody-associated immunodeficiency. Annu Rev Immunol. 2014;32:635–57. [PMID: 24499273]
Wall LA et al. Specific antibody deficiencies. Immunol Allergy Clin North Am. 2015 Nov;35(4):659–70. [PMID: 26454312]

1. Selective Immunoglobulin A Deficiency

Selective IgA deficiency is the most common primary immunodeficiency disorder and is characterized by serum

IgA levels lower than 15 mg/dL (0.15 g/L) with normal levels of IgG and IgM; its prevalence is about 1 in 500 individuals. Most affected individuals are asymptomatic because of compensatory increases in secreted IgG and IgM. Some affected patients have frequent and recurrent infections, such as sinusitis, otitis, and bronchitis. Some cases of IgA deficiency spontaneously remit. When IgG$_2$ subclass deficiency occurs in combination with IgA deficiency, affected patients are more susceptible to infections with encapsulated bacteria (ie, *Haemophilus influenzae*, *Streptococcus pneumoniae*, *Neisseria meningitidis*, Group B streptococcus, *Klebsiella pneumoniae*, and *Salmonella typhi*), and the degree of immune impairment is more severe. Selective IgA deficiency can be associated with atopic diseases and autoimmune disorders, including Graves disease, SLE, juvenile rheumatoid arthritis, type 1 diabetes mellitus, and celiac disease. Treatment with commercial immune globulin is ineffective, since IgA and IgM are present only in trace quantities in these preparations.

Some individuals with undetectable levels of serum IgA may have high titers of anti-IgA antibodies and are at risk for anaphylactic reactions to IgA following exposure to it through infusions of plasma (or blood transfusions).

When to Refer

- Refer patients with anaphylaxis following infusions of plasma (or blood transfusions) to an immunologist for further evaluation of possible IgA deficiency.
- Refer patients with low serum IgA and recurrent sinopulmonary infections, celiac disease, giardiasis or a family history of immunodeficiency to an immunologist for further evaluation of possible IgA deficiency.

Singh K et al. IgA deficiency and autoimmunity. Autoimmun Rev. 2014 Feb;13(2):163–77. [PMID: 24157629]
Wang N et al. IgA deficiency: what is new? Curr Opin Allergy Clin Immunol. 2012 Dec;12(6):602–8. [PMID: 23026772]

2. Common Variable Immunodeficiency

ESSENTIALS OF DIAGNOSIS

- Defect in terminal differentiation of B cells, with absent plasma cells and deficient synthesis of secreted antibody; primary defect may be with B cells or T cells.
- Frequent sinopulmonary infections secondary to humoral immune deficiency.
- Confirmation by evaluation of serum immunoglobulin levels and deficient functional antibody responses.

General Considerations

The most common cause of panhypogammaglobulinemia in adults is common variable immunodeficiency, a heterogeneous immunodeficiency disorder clinically characterized by an increased incidence of recurrent infections, autoimmune phenomena, and neoplastic diseases. The onset is generally during adolescence or early adulthood but it can occur at any age. The prevalence of common variable immunodeficiency is about 1 in 80,000 in the United States. Most cases are sporadic; 10–20% are familial.

Clinical Findings

A. Symptoms and Signs

Increased susceptibility to pyogenic infections is the hallmark of the disease. Virtually all patients suffer from recurrent sinusitis, with bronchitis, otitis, pharyngitis, and pneumonia also being common infections. Infections may be prolonged or associated with unusual complications such as meningitis or sepsis.

Gastrointestinal infections and dysfunction are commonly associated with common variable immunodeficiency, and a sprue-like syndrome, with diarrhea, steatorrhea, malabsorption, protein-losing enteropathy, and hepatosplenomegaly, may develop in patients. Paradoxically, there is an increased incidence of autoimmune disease (20%), although patients may not display the usual serologic markers. Autoimmune cytopenias are most common, but autoimmune endocrinopathies, seronegative rheumatic disease, and gastrointestinal disorders are also commonly seen. Lymph nodes may be enlarged in these patients, yet biopsies show marked reduction in plasma cells. Noncaseating granulomas are frequently found in the spleen, liver, lungs, or skin. There is an increased propensity for the development of B-cell neoplasms (50- to 400-fold increased risk of lymphoma), gastric carcinomas, and skin cancers.

B. Laboratory Findings

The pattern of immunoglobulin isotype deficiency is variable. Most patients present with significantly depressed IgG levels, but over time all antibody classes (IgG, IgA, and IgM) may be affected. Diagnosis is confirmed in patients with recurrent infections by demonstration of functional or quantitative defects in antibody production. Decreased or absent functional antibody responses to common vaccines establish the diagnosis. Secondary causes of decreased antibody production should be carefully considered and ruled out and may include immunosuppression from drugs, most commonly corticosteroids but also other immunosuppressive agents used to treat cancer or transplant patients, and protein-losing states (eg, protein-losing gastroenteropathy, nephrotic syndrome, peritoneal dialysis).

The causes of the hypogammaglobulinemia in patients with common variable immunodeficiency include intrinsic B-cell defects that prevent terminal maturation into antibody-secreting plasma cells. The absolute B-cell count in the peripheral blood in most patients, despite the underlying cellular defect, is normal. A subset of these patients have concomitant T-cell immunodeficiency with increased numbers of activated CD8 cells, splenomegaly, and decreased delayed-type hypersensitivity.

► Treatment

Patients with common variable immunodeficiency should be treated aggressively with antibiotics at the first sign of infection. Since antibody deficiency predisposes patients to high-risk pyogenic infections, antibiotic coverage should be sure to cover encapsulated bacteria (listed above). Only after the development of bronchiectasis or after sinus surgery do patients become significantly affected by more virulent organisms such as *S aureus* or *P aeruginosa*. Maintenance intravenous immune globulin therapy is indicated, with infusions of 300–500 mg/kg of intravenous immune globulin given at about monthly intervals. An alternative is weekly subcutaneous injections of IgG that can be self-administered at home. Adjustment of dosage or of the infusion interval is made on the basis of clinical responses and steady-state trough serum IgG levels. Such therapy is effective in decreasing the incidence of potentially life-threatening infections and increasing quality of life.

Gathmann B et al; European Society for Immunodeficiencies Registry Working Party. Clinical picture and treatment of 2212 patients with common variable immunodeficiency. J Allergy Clin Immunol. 2014 Jul;134(1):116–26. [PMID: 24582312]

Jolles S. The variable in common variable immunodeficiency: a disease of complex phenotypes. J Allergy Clin Immunol Pract. 2013 Nov–Dec;1(6):545–56. [PMID: 24565700]

Paquin-Proulx D et al. Persistent immune activation in CVID and the role of IVIg in its suppression. Front Immunol. 2014 Dec 16;5:637. [PMID: 25566250]

Wehr C et al; Inborn Errors Working Party of the European Society for Blood and Marrow Transplantation and the European Society for Immunodeficiency. Multicenter experience in hematopoietic stem cell transplantation for serious complications of common variable immunodeficiency. J Allergy Clin Immunol. 2015 Apr;135(4):988–97.e6. [PMID: 25595268]

Electrolyte & Acid-Base Disorders

Kerry C. Cho, MD

ASSESSMENT OF THE PATIENT

The diagnosis and treatment of fluid and electrolyte disorders are based on (1) careful history, (2) physical examination and assessment of total body water and its distribution, (3) serum electrolyte concentrations, (4) urine electrolyte concentrations, and (5) serum osmolality. The pathophysiology of electrolyte disorders is rooted in basic principles of total body water and its distribution across fluid compartments.

A. Body Water and Fluid Distribution

Total body water is different in men than in women, and it decreases with aging (Table 21–1). Approximately 50–60% of total body weight is water; two-thirds (40% of body weight) is intracellular, while one-third (20% of body weight) is extracellular. One-fourth of extracellular fluid (5% of body weight) is intravascular. Water may be lost from either or both compartments (intracellular and extracellular). Changes in total body water content are best evaluated by documenting changes in body weight. Effective circulating volume may be assessed by physical examination (eg, blood pressure, pulse, jugular venous distention). Quantitative measurements of effective circulating volume and intravascular volume may be invasive (ie, central venous pressure or pulmonary wedge pressure) or noninvasive (ie, inferior vena cava diameter and right atrial pressure by echocardiography) but still require careful interpretation.

B. Serum Electrolytes

The cause of electrolyte disorders may be determined by reviewing the history, underlying diseases, and medications.

C. Evaluation of Urine

The urine concentration of an electrolyte indicates renal handling of the electrolyte and whether the kidney is appropriately excreting or retaining the electrolyte. A 24-hour urine collection for daily electrolyte excretion is the gold standard for renal electrolyte handling, but it is slow and onerous. A more convenient method is the

fractional excretion (F_E) of an electrolyte X (F_{E_x}) calculated from a spot urine sample:

$$F_{E_x}(\%) = \frac{\text{Urine X/Serum X}}{\text{Urine Cr/Serum Cr}} \times 100$$

A low fractional excretion indicates renal reabsorption (high avidity or electrolyte retention), while a high fractional excretion indicates renal wasting (low avidity or electrolyte excretion). Thus, the fractional excretion helps the clinician determine whether the kidney's response is appropriate for a specific electrolyte disorder.

D. Serum Osmolality

Solute concentration is measured by osmolality in millimoles per kilogram. Osmolarity is measured in millimoles of solute per liter of solution. At physiologic solute concentrations (normally 285–295 mmol/kg), the two measurements are clinically interchangeable. Tonicity refers to osmolytes that are impermeable to cell membranes. Differences in osmolyte concentration across cell membranes lead to osmosis and fluid shifts, stimulation of thirst, and secretion of antidiuretic hormone (ADH). Substances that easily permeate cell membranes (eg, urea, ethanol) are ineffective osmoles that do not cause fluid shifts across fluid compartments.

Serum osmolality can be estimated using the following formula:

$$\text{Osmolality} = 2(Na^+ \text{ mEq/L}) + \frac{\text{Glucose mg/dL}}{18} + \frac{\text{BUN mg/dL}}{2.8}$$

(1 mOsm/L of glucose equals 180 mg/L or 18 mg/dL and 1 mOsm/L of urea nitrogen equals 28 mg/L or 2.8 mg/dL). Sodium is the major extracellular cation; doubling the serum sodium in the formula for estimated osmolality accounts for counterbalancing anions. A discrepancy between measured and estimated osmolality of greater than 10 mmol/kg suggests an osmolal gap, which is the presence of unmeasured osmoles such as ethanol, methanol, isopropanol, and ethylene glycol (see Table 38–5).

Table 21–1. Total body water (as percentage of body weight) in relation to age and sex.

Age	Male	Female
18–40	60%	50%
41–60	60–50%	50–40%
Over 60	50%	40%

DISORDERS OF SODIUM CONCENTRATION

HYPONATREMIA

ESSENTIALS OF DIAGNOSIS

▶ Volume status and serum osmolality are essential to determine etiology.

▶ Hyponatremia usually reflects excess water retention relative to sodium rather than sodium deficiency. The sodium concentration is not a measure of total body sodium.

▶ Hypotonic fluids commonly cause hyponatremia in hospitalized patients.

▶ General Considerations

Defined as a serum sodium concentration less than 135 mEq/L (135 mmol/L), hyponatremia is the most common electrolyte abnormality in hospitalized patients. The clinician should be wary about hyponatremia since mismanagement can result in neurologic catastrophes from cerebral osmotic demyelination. Indeed, iatrogenic complications from aggressive or inappropriate therapy can be more harmful than hyponatremia itself.

A common misconception is that the sodium concentration is a reflection of total body sodium or total body water. In fact, total body water and sodium can be low, normal, or high in hyponatremia since the kidney independently regulates sodium and water homeostasis. Most cases of hyponatremia reflect water imbalance and abnormal water handling, not sodium imbalance, indicating the primary role of ADH in the pathophysiology of hyponatremia. A diagnostic algorithm using serum osmolality and volume status separates the causes of hyponatremia into therapeutically useful categories (Figure 21–1).

▶ Etiology

A. Isotonic & Hypertonic Hyponatremia

Serum osmolality identifies isotonic and hypertonic hyponatremia, although these cases can often be identified by careful history or previous laboratory tests.

▲ **Figure 21–1.** Evaluation of hyponatremia using serum osmolality and extracellular fluid volume status. ACE, angiotensin-converting enzyme; SIADH, syndrome of inappropriate antidiuretic hormone. (Adapted, with permission, from Narins RG et al. Diagnostic strategies in disorders of fluid, electrolyte and acid-base homeostasis. Am J Med. 1982 Mar;72(3):496–520.)

Pseudohyponatremia does not occur with newer sodium assays because they use a direct assay method for sodium. With older assays, lipemia (including chylomicrons, triglycerides, and cholesterol) and hyperproteinemia (greater than 10 g/dL [100 g/L], eg, paraproteinemias and intravenous immunoglobulin therapy) cause pseudohyponatremia when the serum osmolality is isotonic because lipids and proteins do not affect osmolality measurement.

Hypertonic hyponatremia occurs with hyperglycemia and mannitol administration for increased intracranial pressure. Glucose and mannitol osmotically pull intracellular water into the extracellular space. The translocation of water lowers the serum sodium concentration. Translocational hyponatremia is not pseudohyponatremia or an artifact of sodium measurement. The sodium concentration falls 2 mEq/L (or 2 mmol/L) for every 100 mg/dL (or 5.56 mmol/L) rise in glucose when the glucose concentration is between 200 mg/dL and 400 mg/dL (11.1 mmol/L and 22.2 mmol/L). If the glucose concentration is more than 400 mg/dL, the sodium concentration falls 4 mEq/L for every 100 mg/dL rise in glucose. There is some controversy about the correction factor for the serum sodium in the presence of hyperglycemia. Many guidelines recommend a correction factor, whereby the serum sodium concentration decreases by 1.6 mEq/L (or 1.6 mmol/L) for every 100 mg/dL (5.56 mmol/L) rise in plasma glucose above normal, but there is evidence that the decrease may be greater when patients have more severe hyperglycemia (greater than 400 mg/dL or 22.2 mmol/L) or volume depletion, or both. One group has suggested (based on short-term exposure of normal volunteers to markedly elevated glucose levels) that when the serum glucose is more than 200 mg/dL, the serum sodium concentration decreases by at least 2.4 mEq/L (or 2.4 mmol/L).

B. Hypotonic Hyponatremia

Most cases of hyponatremia are hypotonic, highlighting sodium's role as the predominant extracellular osmole. The next step is classifying hypotonic cases by the patient's volume status.

1. Hypovolemic hypotonic hyponatremia—Hypovolemic hyponatremia occurs with renal or extrarenal volume loss and hypotonic fluid replacement (Figure 21–1). Total body sodium and total body water are decreased. To maintain intravascular volume, the pituitary increases ADH secretion, causing free water retention from hypotonic fluid replacement. The body sacrifices serum osmolality to preserve intravascular volume. In short, losses of water and salt are replaced by water alone. Without ongoing hypotonic fluid intake, the renal or extrarenal volume loss would produce hypovolemic hypernatremia.

Cerebral salt wasting is a distinct and rare subset of hypovolemic hyponatremia seen in patients with intracranial disease (eg, infections, cerebrovascular accidents, tumors, and neurosurgery). Clinical features include refractory hypovolemia and hypotension, often requiring continuous infusion of isotonic or hypertonic saline and ICU monitoring. The exact pathophysiology is unclear but includes renal sodium wasting possibly through B-type

natriuretic peptide, ADH release, and decreased aldosterone secretion.

2. Euvolemic hypotonic hyponatremia—Euvolemic hyponatremia has the broadest differential diagnosis. Most causes are mediated directly or indirectly through ADH, including hypothyroidism, adrenal insufficiency, medications, and the syndrome of inappropriate ADH (SIADH). The exceptions are primary polydipsia, beer potomania, and reset osmostat.

A. HORMONAL ABNORMALITIES—Hypothyroidism and adrenal insufficiency can cause hyponatremia. Exactly how hypothyroidism induces hyponatremia is unclear but may be related to ADH. Adrenal insufficiency may be associated with the hyperkalemia and metabolic acidosis of hypoaldosteronism. Cortisol provides feedback inhibition for ADH release.

B. THIAZIDE DIURETICS AND OTHER MEDICATIONS—Thiazides induce hyponatremia typically in older female patients within days of initiating therapy. The mechanism appears to be a combination of mild diuretic-induced volume contraction, ADH effect, and intact urinary concentrating ability resulting in water retention and hyponatremia. Loop diuretics do not cause hyponatremia as frequently because of disrupted medullary concentrating gradient and impaired urine concentration.

Nonsteroidal anti-inflammatory drugs (NSAIDs) increase ADH by inhibiting prostaglandin formation. Prostaglandins and selective serotonin reuptake inhibitors (eg, fluoxetine, paroxetine, and citalopram) can cause hyponatremia, especially in geriatric patients. Enhanced secretion or action of ADH may result from increased serotonergic tone. Angiotensin-converting enzyme (ACE) inhibitors do not block the conversion of angiotensin I to angiotensin II in the brain. Angiotensin II stimulates thirst and ADH secretion. Hyponatremia during amiodarone loading has been reported; it usually improves with dose reduction.

Abuse of 3,4-methylenedioxymethamphetamine (MDMA, also known as Ecstasy) can lead to hyponatremia and severe neurologic symptoms, including seizures, cerebral edema, and brainstem herniation. MDMA and its metabolites increase ADH release from the hypothalamus. Primary polydipsia may contribute to hyponatremia since MDMA users typically increase fluid intake to prevent hyperthermia.

C. NAUSEA, PAIN, SURGERY, AND MEDICAL PROCEDURES—Nausea and pain are potent stimulators of ADH release. Severe hyponatremia can develop after elective surgery in healthy patients, especially premenopausal women. Hypotonic fluids in the setting of elevated ADH levels can produce severe, life-threatening hyponatremia. Medical procedures such as colonoscopy have also been associated with hyponatremia.

D. HIV INFECTION—Hyponatremia is seen in up to 50% of hospitalized HIV-infected patients and 20% of ambulatory HIV-infected patients. The differential diagnosis is broad: medication effect, adrenal insufficiency, hypoaldosteronism, central nervous system or pulmonary disease, SIADH, malignancy, and volume depletion.

E. **Exercise-associated hyponatremia**—Hyponatremia after exercise, especially endurance events such as triathlons and marathons, may be caused by a combination of excessive hypotonic fluid intake and continued ADH secretion. Reperfusion of the exercise-induced ischemic splanchnic bed causes delayed absorption of excessive quantities of hypotonic fluid ingested during exercise. Sustained elevation of ADH prevents water excretion in this setting. Current guidelines suggest that endurance athletes drink water according to thirst rather than according to specified hourly rates of fluid intake. Specific universal recommendations for fluid replacement rates are not possible given the variability of sweat production, renal water excretion, and environmental conditions. Electrolyte-containing sport drinks do not protect against hyponatremia since they are markedly hypotonic relative to serum.

F. **Syndrome of inappropriate antidiuretic hormone secretion**—Under normal circumstances, hypovolemia and hyperosmolality stimulate ADH secretion. ADH release is inappropriate without these physiologic cues. Normal regulation of ADH release occurs from both the central nervous system and the chest via baroreceptors and neural input. The major causes of SIADH (Table 21–2) are disorders affecting the central nervous system (structural, metabolic, psychiatric, or pharmacologic processes) or the lungs (infectious, mechanical, oncologic). Medications commonly cause SIADH by increasing ADH or its action. Some carcinomas, especially small cell lung carcinoma, can autonomously secrete ADH.

G. **Psychogenic polydipsia and beer potomania**—Marked free water intake (generally greater than 10 L/day) may produce hyponatremia. Euvolemia is maintained through renal excretion of sodium. Urine sodium is therefore generally elevated (greater than 20 mEq/L), and ADH levels are appropriately suppressed. As the increased free water is excreted, the urine osmolality approaches the minimum of 50 mOsm/kg (or 50 mmol/kg). Polydipsia occurs in psychiatric patients. Psychiatric medications may interfere with water excretion or increase thirst through anticholinergic side effects, further increasing water intake. The hyponatremia of beer potomania occurs in patients who consume large amounts of beer. Free water excretion is decreased because of decreased solute consumption and production; muscle wasting and malnutrition are contributing factors. Without enough solute, these patients have decreased free water excretory capacity even if they maximally dilute the urine.

H. **Reset osmostat**—Reset osmostat is a rare cause of hyponatremia characterized by appropriate ADH regulation in response to water deprivation and fluid challenges. Patients with reset osmostat regulate serum sodium and serum osmolality around a lower set point, concentrating or diluting urine in response to hyperosmolality and hypoosmolality. The mild hypo-osmolality of pregnancy is a form of reset osmostat.

3. Hypervolemic hypotonic hyponatremia—Hypervolemic hyponatremia occurs in the edematous states of cirrhosis, heart failure, nephrotic syndrome, and advanced kidney disease (Figure 21–1). In cirrhosis and heart failure, effective circulating volume is decreased due to peripheral vasodilation

Table 21–2. Causes of syndrome of inappropriate ADH secretion (SIADH).

Central nervous system disorders
Head trauma
Stroke
Subarachnoid hemorrhage
Hydrocephalus
Brain tumor
Encephalitis
Guillain-Barré syndrome
Meningitis
Acute psychosis
Acute intermittent porphyria
Pulmonary lesions
Tuberculosis
Bacterial pneumonia
Aspergillosis
Bronchiectasis
Neoplasms
Positive pressure ventilation
Malignancies
Bronchogenic carcinoma
Pancreatic carcinoma
Prostatic carcinoma
Renal cell carcinoma
Adenocarcinoma of colon
Thymoma
Osteosarcoma
Lymphoma
Leukemia
Drugs
Increased ADH production
Antidepressants: tricyclics, monoamine oxidase inhibitors, SSRIs
Antineoplastics: cyclophosphamide, vincristine
Carbamazepine
Methylenedioxymethamphetamine (MDMA; Ecstasy)
Clofibrate
Neuroleptics: thiothixene, thioridazine, fluphenazine, haloperidol, trifluoperazine
Potentiated ADH action
Carbamazepine
Chlorpropamide, tolbutamide
Cyclophosphamide
NSAIDs
Somatostatin and analogs
Amiodarone
Others
Postoperative
Pain
Stress
AIDS
Pregnancy (physiologic)
Hypokalemia

ADH, antidiuretic hormone; NSAIDs, nonsteroidal anti-inflammatory drugs; SSRIs, selective serotonin reuptake inhibitors.

or decreased cardiac output. Increased renin-angiotensin-aldosterone system activity and ADH secretion result in water retention. Note the pathophysiologic similarity to hypovolemic hyponatremia—the body sacrifices osmolality in an attempt to restore effective circulating volume.

The pathophysiology of hyponatremia in nephrotic syndrome is not completely understood, but the primary disturbance may be renal sodium retention, resulting in overfilling of the intravascular space and secondary edema formation as fluid enters the interstitial space. Previously, it was thought that the decreased oncotic pressure of hypoalbuminemia caused fluid shifts from the intravascular space to the interstitial compartment. Intravascular underfilling led to secondary renal sodium retention. However, patients receiving therapy for glomerular disease and nephrotic syndrome often have edema resolution prior to normalization of the serum albumin.

Patients with advanced kidney disease typically have sodium retention and decreased free water excretory capacity, resulting in hypervolemic hyponatremia.

Clinical Findings

A. Symptoms and Signs

Whether hyponatremia is symptomatic depends on its severity and acuity. Chronic disease can be severe (sodium concentration less than 110 mEq/L), yet remarkably asymptomatic because the brain has adapted by decreasing its tonicity over weeks to months. Acute disease that has developed over hours to days can be severely symptomatic with relatively modest hyponatremia. Mild hyponatremia (sodium concentrations of 130–135 mEq/L) is usually asymptomatic.

Mild symptoms of nausea and malaise progress to headache, lethargy, and disorientation as the sodium concentration drops. The most serious symptoms are respiratory arrest, seizure, coma, permanent brain damage, brainstem herniation, and death. Premenopausal women are much more likely than menopausal women to die or suffer permanent brain injury from hyponatremic encephalopathy, suggesting a hormonal role in the pathophysiology.

Evaluation starts with a careful history for new medications, changes in fluid intake (polydipsia, anorexia, intravenous fluid rates and composition), fluid output (nausea and vomiting, diarrhea, ostomy output, polyuria, oliguria, insensible losses). The physical examination should help categorize the patient's volume status into hypovolemia, euvolemia, or hypervolemia.

B. Laboratory Findings

Laboratory assessment should include serum electrolytes, creatinine, and osmolality as well as urine sodium. The etiology of most cases of hyponatremia will be apparent from the history, physical, and basic laboratory tests. Additional tests of thyroid and adrenal function will occasionally be necessary.

SIADH is a clinical diagnosis characterized by (1) hyponatremia; (2) decreased osmolality (less than 280 mOsm/kg [280 mmol/kg]); (3) absence of heart, kidney, or liver disease; (4) normal thyroid and adrenal function (see Chapter 26); and (5) urine sodium usually over 20 mEq/L. In clinical practice, ADH levels are not measured. Patients with SIADH may have low blood urea nitrogen (BUN) (less than 10 mg/dL [3.6 mmol/L]) and hypouricemia (less than 4 mg/dL [238 mcmol/L]), which are not only dilutional but result from increased urea and uric acid clearances

in response to the volume-expanded state. Azotemia may reflect volume contraction, ruling out SIADH, which is seen in euvolemic patients.

Complications

The most serious complication of hyponatremia is iatrogenic cerebral osmotic demyelination from overly rapid sodium correction. Also called central pontine myelinolysis, cerebral osmotic demyelination may occur outside the brainstem. Demyelination may occur days after sodium correction or initial neurologic recovery from hyponatremia. Hypoxic episodes during hyponatremia may contribute to demyelination. The neurologic effects are generally catastrophic and irreversible.

Treatment

Regardless of the etiology of hyponatremia and the patient's volume status, restriction of free water and hypotonic fluid intake is the initial step in hyponatremia management since excessive free water intake will exacerbate hyponatremia. Free water clearance by the kidneys must exceed free water intake for the serum sodium concentration to rise. Free water intake should generally be less than 1–1.5 L/day, although more severe free water restriction may be necessary in patients with minimal free water clearance, and hypertonic saline may be necessary in patients with negative free water clearance.

Hypovolemic patients require adequate fluid resuscitation from isotonic fluids (either normal saline or lactated Ringer solution) to suppress the hypovolemic stimulus for ADH release. Patients with **cerebral salt wasting** may require hypertonic saline to prevent circulatory collapse; some may respond to fludrocortisone. **Hypervolemic** patients may require loop diuretics or dialysis, or both, to correct increased total body water and sodium. **Euvolemic** patients may respond to free water restriction alone.

Pseudohyponatremia from hypertriglyceridemia or hyperproteinemia requires no therapy except confirmation with the clinical laboratory. **Translocational hyponatremia** from glucose or mannitol can be managed with glucose correction or mannitol discontinuation (if possible). No specific therapy is necessary in patients with **reset osmostat** since they successfully regulate their serum sodium with fluid challenges and water deprivation.

Symptomatic and severe hyponatremia generally require hospitalization for careful monitoring of fluid balance and weights, treatment, and frequent sodium checks. Inciting medications should be discontinued if possible.

Guidelines established in 2014 provide consensus recommendations for the optimal rate of sodium correction in symptomatic hyponatremic patients. First, a relatively small increase of 4–6 mEq/L in the serum sodium may be all that is necessary to reverse the neurologic manifestations of symptomatic hyponatremia. Second, acute hyponatremia (eg, exercise-associated hyponatremia) with severe neurologic manifestations can be reversed rapidly with 100 mL of 3% hypertonic saline infused over 10 minutes (repeated twice as necessary). Third, correction rates for chronic hyponatremia are low (4–8 mEq/L per 24 hours in patients at high risk for demyelination). Fourth, chronic hyponatremic patients at high risk for demyelination who are corrected too rapidly are candidates for treatment with a combination of DDAVP and intravenous dextrose 5% to relower the serum sodium. In severely symptomatic patients, the clinician should calculate the sodium deficit and deliver 3% **hypertonic saline.** The sodium deficit can be calculated by the following formula:

Sodium deficit = Total body water (TBW)
× (Desired serum Na–Actual serum Na)

where TBW is typically 50% of total mass in women and 55% of total mass in men. For example, a nonedematous, severely symptomatic 70 kg woman with a serum sodium of 124 mEq/L should have her serum sodium corrected to approximately 130 mEq/L in the first 24 hours. Her sodium deficit is calculated as:

Sodium deficit = 70 kg × 0.5 × (130 mEq/L – 124 mEq/L)
= 210 mEq

3% hypertonic saline has a sodium concentration of 513 mEq/1000 mL. The delivery rate for hypertonic saline can be calculated as:

Delivery rate = Sodium deficit/(513 mEq/1000 mL)/
24 hours
= 210 mEq / (513 mEq/1000 mL)/24 hours
= 17 mL/hour

In general, the 3% hypertonic saline infusion rate should be approximately 0.25 mL/kg body weight/h and should not exceed 0.5 mL/kg body weight/h; higher rates may represent a mathematical error or overly aggressive sodium correction. Hypertonic saline in hypervolemic patients can be hazardous, resulting in worsening volume overload, pulmonary edema, and ascites.

For patients who cannot adequately restrict free water or have an inadequate response to conservative measures, demeclocycline (300–600 mg orally twice daily) inhibits the effect of ADH on the distal tubule. Onset of action may require 1 week, and urinary concentrating ability may be permanently impaired, resulting in nephrogenic diabetes insipidus (DI) and even hypernatremia. Cirrhosis may increase the nephrotoxicity of demeclocycline.

Vasopressin antagonists have transformed the treatment of euvolemic and hypervolemic hyponatremia, especially in heart failure. Tolvaptan, lixivaptan, and satavaptan are oral selective vasopressin-2 receptor antagonists; conivaptan is an intravenous agent. Tolvaptan and conivaptan are available in the United States, but lixivaptan and satavaptan are not approved by the US Food and Drug Administration (FDA).

V_2 receptors mediate the diuretic effect of ADH, and V_2 receptor antagonists are recommended for use in hospitalized patients with euvolemic SIADH or hyponatremic patients with heart failure. V_2 receptor antagonists (eg, tolvaptan) can be considered for patients who are unable to maintain a serum sodium above 120 mEq/L despite adequate resuscitation for hypovolemia, hypertonic saline therapy, or both. The starting dose of **tolvaptan** is 15 mg orally daily; it can be increased to 30 mg daily and 60 mg daily at 24 hour intervals if hyponatremia persists or if the increase in sodium concentration is less than 4–6 mEq/L over the preceding 24 hours. Tolvaptan is contraindicated in patients with liver disease, including cirrhosis, and should not be used for longer than 30 days due to the potential for liver toxicity. Conivaptan is given as an intravenous loading dose of 20 mg delivered over 30 minutes, then as 20 mg continuously over 24 hours. Subsequent infusions may be administered every 1–3 days at 20–40 mg/day by continuous infusion. The standard free water restriction for hyponatremic patients should be lifted for patients receiving vasopressin antagonists since the aquaresis can result in excessive sodium correction in a fluid-restricted patient. Frequent monitoring of the serum sodium is necessary.

► When to Refer

- Nephrology or endocrinology consultation should be considered in severe, symptomatic, refractory, or complicated cases of hyponatremia.
- Aggressive therapies with hypertonic saline, demeclocycline, vasopressin antagonists, or dialysis mandate specialist consultation.
- Consultation may be necessary with end-stage liver or heart disease.

► When to Admit

Hospital admission is necessary for symptomatic patients or those requiring aggressive therapies for close monitoring and frequent laboratory testing.

Berl T. Vasopressin antagonists. N Engl J Med. 2015 Jun 4; 372(23):2207–16. [PMID: 26039601]

Gharaibeh KA et al. Risk factors, complication and measures to prevent or reverse catastrophic sodium overcorrection in chronic hyponatremia. Am J Med Sci. 2015 Feb;349(2):170–5. [PMID: 25163018]

Henry DA. In the clinic: hyponatremia. Ann Intern Med. 2015 Aug 4;163(3):ITC1–19. [PMID: 26237763]

Spasovski G et al; Hyponatraemia Guideline Development Group. Clinical practice guideline on diagnosis and treatment of hyponatraemia. Eur J Endocrinol. 2014 Feb 25;170(3): G1–47. Erratum in: Eur J Endocrinol. 2014 Jul;171(1):X1. [PMID: 24569125]

Sterns RH. Disorders of plasma sodium—causes, consequences, and correction. N Engl J Med. 2015 Jan 1;372(1):55–65. [PMID: 25551526]

HYPERNATREMIA

 ESSENTIALS OF DIAGNOSIS

- ► Increased thirst and water intake is the first defense against hypernatremia.
- ► Urine osmolality helps differentiate renal from nonrenal water loss.

General Considerations

Hypernatremia is defined as a sodium concentration greater than 145 mEq/L. All patients with hypernatremia have hyperosmolality, unlike hyponatremic patients who can have a low, normal, or high serum osmolality. The hypernatremic patient is typically hypovolemic due to free water losses, although hypervolemia is frequently seen, often as an iatrogenic complication in hospitalized patients with impaired access to free water. Rarely, excessive sodium intake may cause hypernatremia. Hypernatremia in primary aldosteronism is mild and usually does not cause symptoms.

An intact thirst mechanism and access to water are the primary defense against hypernatremia. The hypothalamus can sense minimal changes in serum osmolality, triggering the thirst mechanism and increased water intake. Thus, whatever the underlying disorder (eg, dehydration, encephalopathy, lactulose or mannitol therapy, central and nephrogenic DI), excess water loss can cause hypernatremia only when adequate water intake is not possible.

Clinical Findings

A. Symptoms and Signs

When the patient is dehydrated, orthostatic hypotension and oliguria are typical findings. Because water shifts from the cells to the intravascular space to protect volume status, these symptoms may be delayed. Lethargy, irritability, and weakness are early signs. Hyperthermia, delirium, seizures, and coma may be seen with severe hypernatremia (ie, sodium greater than 158 mEq/L). Symptoms in the elderly may not be specific; a recent change in consciousness is associated with a poor prognosis. Osmotic cerebral demyelination is an uncommon but reported consequence of severe hypernatremia.

B. Laboratory Findings

1. Urine osmolality greater than 400 mOsm/kg—Renal water-conserving ability is functioning.

A. Nonrenal losses—Hypernatremia will develop if water intake falls behind hypotonic fluid losses from excessive sweating, the respiratory tract, or bowel movements. Lactulose causes an osmotic diarrhea with loss of free water.

B. Renal losses—While severe hyperglycemia can cause translocational hyponatremia, progressive volume depletion from glucosuria can result in hypernatremia. Osmotic diuresis can occur with the use of mannitol or urea.

2. Urine osmolality less than 250 mOsm/kg—Hypernatremia with a dilute urine (osmolality less than 250 mOsm/kg) is characteristic of DI. Central DI results from inadequate ADH release. Nephrogenic DI results from renal insensitivity to ADH; common causes include lithium, demeclocycline, relief of urinary obstruction, interstitial nephritis, hypercalcemia, and hypokalemia.

Treatment

Treatment of hypernatremia includes correcting the cause of the fluid loss, replacing water, and replacing electrolytes (as needed). In response to increases in plasma osmolality,

brain cells synthesize solutes called idiogenic osmoles, which cause intracellular fluid shifts. Osmole production begins 4–6 hours after dehydration and takes several days to reach steady state. If hypernatremia is rapidly corrected, the osmotic imbalance may cause cerebral edema and potentially severe neurologic impairment. Fluids should be administered over a 48-hour period, aiming for serum sodium correction of approximately 1 mEq/L/h (1 mmol/L/h). There is no consensus about the optimal rates of sodium correction in hypernatremia.

A. Choice of Type of Fluid for Replacement

1. Hypernatremia with hypovolemia—Hypovolemic patients should receive isotonic 0.9% normal saline to restore euvolemia and to treat hyperosmolality because normal saline (308 mOsm/kg or 308 mmol/kg) is hypoosmolar compared with plasma. After adequate volume resuscitation with normal saline, 0.45% saline or 5% dextrose (or both) can be used to replace any remaining free water deficit. Milder volume deficits may be treated with 0.45% saline and 5% dextrose.

2. Hypernatremia with euvolemia—Water ingestion or intravenous 5% dextrose will result in the excretion of excess sodium in the urine. If the glomerular filtration rate (GFR) is decreased, diuretics will increase urinary sodium excretion but may impair renal concentrating ability, increasing the quantity of water that needs to be replaced.

3. Hypernatremia with hypervolemia—Treatment includes 5% dextrose solution to reduce hyperosmolality. Loop diuretics may be necessary to promote natriuresis and lower total body sodium. In severe rare cases with kidney disease, hemodialysis may be necessary to correct the excess total body sodium and water.

B. Calculation of Water Deficit

Fluid replacement should include the free water deficit and additional maintenance fluid to replace ongoing and anticipated fluid losses.

1. Acute hypernatremia—In acute dehydration without much solute loss, free water loss is similar to the weight loss. Initially, a 5% dextrose solution may be used. As correction of water deficit progresses, therapy should continue with 0.45% saline with dextrose.

2. Chronic hypernatremia—The water deficit is calculated to restore normal sodium concentration, typically 140 mEq/L. Total body water (TBW) (Table 21–1) correlates with muscle mass and therefore decreases with advancing age, cachexia, and dehydration and is lower in women than in men. Current TBW equals 40–60% current body weight. (See Table 21–1.)

$$\text{Volume (in L) to be replaced} = \text{Current TBW} \times \frac{[Na^+] - 140}{140}$$

When to Refer

Patients with refractory or unexplained hypernatremia should be referred for subspecialist consultation.

When to Admit

- Patients with symptomatic hypernatremia require hospitalization for evaluation and treatment.
- Significant comorbidities or concomitant acute illnesses, especially if contributing to hypernatremia, may necessitate hospitalization.

Al-Absi A et al. A clinical approach to the treatment of chronic hypernatremia. Am J Kidney Dis. 2012 Dec;60(6):1032–8. [PMID: 22959761]

Lindner G et al. Hypernatremia in critically ill patients. J Crit Care. 2013 Apr;28(2):216.e11–20. [PMID: 22762930]

Ryu JH et al. Induced and sustained hypernatremia for the prevention and treatment of cerebral edema following brain injury. Neurocrit Care. 2013 Oct;19(2):222–31. [PMID: 23468135]

Sam R et al. Understanding hypernatremia. Am J Nephrol. 2012;36(1):97–104. [PMID: 22739333]

Shah MK et al. Hypernatremia in the geriatric population. Clin Interv Aging. 2014 Nov 19;9:1987–92. [PMID: 25429210]

HYPEROSMOLAR DISORDERS & OSMOLAR GAPS

HYPEROSMOLALITY WITH TRANSIENT OR NO SIGNIFICANT SHIFT IN WATER

Urea and alcohol readily cross cell membranes and can produce hyperosmolality. Urea is an ineffective osmole with little effect on osmotic water movement across cell membranes. Alcohol quickly equilibrates between the intracellular and extracellular compartments, adding 22 mOsm/L for every 100 mg/dL (or 21.7 mmol/L) of ethanol. Ethanol ingestion should be considered in any case of stupor or coma with an elevated osmol gap (measured osmolality – calculated osmolality greater than 10 mOsm/kg [10 mmol/kg]). Other toxic alcohols such as methanol and ethylene glycol cause an osmol gap and a metabolic acidosis with an increased anion gap (see Chapter 38). The combination of an increased anion gap metabolic acidosis and an osmol gap exceeding 10 mOsm/kg (or 10 mmol/kg) is not specific for toxic alcohol ingestion and may occur with alcoholic ketoacidosis or lactic acidosis (see Metabolic Acidosis).

Al-Jaghbeer M et al. Acid-base disturbances in intensive care patients: etiology, pathophysiology and treatment. Nephrol Dial Transplant. 2015 Jul;30(7):1104–11. [PMID: 25213433]

Kruse JA. Methanol and ethylene glycol intoxication. Crit Care Clin. 2012 Oct;28(4):661–711. [PMID: 22998995]

Roberts DM et al; EXTRIP Work Group. Recommendations for the role of extracorporeal treatments in the management of acute methanol poisoning: a systematic review and consensus statement. Crit Care Med. 2015 Feb;43(2):461–72. [PMID: 25493973]

HYPEROSMOLALITY ASSOCIATED WITH SIGNIFICANT SHIFTS IN WATER

Increased concentrations of solutes that do not readily enter cells cause a shift of water from intracellular to extracellular. Hyperosmolality of effective osmoles such as sodium and glucose causes symptoms, primarily neurologic. The severity of symptoms depends on the degree of hyperosmolality and rapidity of development. In acute hyperosmolality, somnolence and confusion can appear when the osmolality exceeds 320–330 mOsm/kg (320–330 mmol/kg); coma, respiratory arrest, and death can result when osmolality exceeds 340–350 mOsm/kg (340–350 mmol/kg).

Kraut JA et al. Approach to the evaluation of a patient with an increased serum osmolal gap and high-anion-gap metabolic acidosis. Am J Kidney Dis. 2011 Sep;58(3):480–4. [PMID: 21794966]

Wiener SW. Toxicologic acid-base disorders. Emerg Med Clin North Am. 2014 Feb;32(1):149–65. [PMID: 24275173]

DISORDERS OF POTASSIUM CONCENTRATION

HYPOKALEMIA

 ESSENTIALS OF DIAGNOSIS

- ▶ Serum potassium level less than 3.5 mEq/L (3.5 mmol/L)
- ▶ Severe hypokalemia may induce dangerous arrhythmias and rhabdomyolysis.
- ▶ Transtubular potassium concentration gradient (TTKG) can distinguish renal from nonrenal loss of potassium.

General Considerations

Hypokalemia can result from insufficient dietary potassium intake, intracellular shifting of potassium from the extracellular space, extrarenal potassium loss, or renal potassium loss (Table 21–3). Cellular uptake of potassium is increased by insulin and beta-adrenergic stimulation and blocked by alpha-adrenergic stimulation. Aldosterone is an important regulator of total body potassium, increasing potassium secretion in the distal renal tubule. The most common cause of hypokalemia, especially in developing countries, is gastrointestinal loss from infectious diarrhea. The potassium concentration in intestinal secretion is ten times higher (80 mEq/L) than in gastric secretions. Hypokalemia in the presence of acidosis suggests profound potassium depletion and requires urgent treatment. Self-limited hypokalemia occurs in 50–60% of trauma patients, perhaps related to enhanced release of epinephrine.

Hypokalemia increases the likelihood of digitalis toxicity. In patients with heart disease, hypokalemia induced by beta-2-adrenergic agonists and diuretics may substantially increase the risk of arrhythmias. Numerous genetic mutations affect fluid and electrolyte metabolism, including disorders of potassium metabolism (Table 21–4).

Magnesium is an important cofactor for potassium uptake and maintenance of intracellular potassium levels.

Table 21–3. Causes of hypokalemia.

Decreased potassium intake
Potassium shift into the cell
Increased postprandial secretion of insulin
Alkalosis
Trauma (via beta-adrenergic stimulation?)
Periodic paralysis (hypokalemic)
Barium intoxication
Renal potassium loss
Increased aldosterone (mineralocorticoid) effects
Primary hyperaldosteronism
Secondary aldosteronism (dehydration, heart failure)
Renovascular hypertension
Malignant hypertension
Ectopic ACTH-producing tumor
Gitelman syndrome
Bartter syndrome
Cushing syndrome
Licorice (European)
Renin-producing tumor
Congenital abnormality of steroid metabolism
(eg, adrenogenital syndrome, 17-alpha-hydroxylase
defect, apparent mineralocorticoid excess,
11-beta-hydroxylase deficiency)
Increased flow to distal nephron
Diuretics (furosemide, thiazides)
Salt-losing nephropathy
Hypomagnesemia
Unreabsorbable anion
Carbenicillin, penicillin
Renal tubular acidosis (type I or II)
Metabolic alkalosis (bicarbonaturia)
Congenital defect of distal nephron
Liddle syndrome
Extrarenal potassium loss
Vomiting, diarrhea, laxative abuse
Villous adenoma, Zollinger-Ellison syndrome

Loop diuretics (eg, furosemide) cause substantial renal potassium and magnesium losses. Magnesium depletion should be considered in refractory hypokalemia.

▶ Clinical Findings

A. Symptoms and Signs

Muscular weakness, fatigue, and muscle cramps are frequent complaints in mild to moderate hypokalemia. Gastrointestinal smooth muscle involvement may result in constipation or ileus. Flaccid paralysis, hyporeflexia, hypercapnia, tetany, and rhabdomyolysis may be seen with severe hypokalemia (less than 2.5 mEq/L). The presence of hypertension may be a clue to the diagnosis of hypokalemia from aldosterone or mineralocorticoid excess (Table 21–4). Renal manifestations include nephrogenic DI and interstitial nephritis.

B. Laboratory Findings

Urinary potassium concentration is low (less than 20 mEq/L) as a result of extrarenal loss (eg, diarrhea, vomiting) and

Table 21–4. Genetic disorders associated with electrolyte metabolism disturbances.

Disease	Site of Mutation
Potassium	
Hypokalemia	
Hypokalemic periodic paralysis	Dihydropyridine-sensitive skeletal muscle voltage-gated calcium channel
Bartter syndrome	Na⁺-K⁺-2Cl⁻ cotransporter, K⁺ channel (ROMK), or Cl⁻ channel of thick ascending limb of Henle (hypofunction), barttin
Gitelman syndrome	Thiazide-sensitive Na⁺-Cl⁻ cotransporter
Liddle syndrome	Beta or gamma subunit of amiloride-sensitive Na⁺ channel (hyperfunction)
Apparent mineralocorticoid excess	11-beta-hydroxysteroid dehydrogenase (failure to inactivate cortisol)
Glucocorticoid-remediable hyperaldosteronism	Regulatory sequence of 11-beta-hydroxysteroid controls aldosterone synthase inappropriately
Hyperkalemia	
Hyperkalemic periodic paralysis	Alpha subunit of calcium channel
Pseudohypo-aldosteronism type I	Beta or gamma subunit of amiloride-sensitive Na⁺ channel (hypofunction)
Pseudohypo-aldosteronism type II (Gordon syndrome)	WNK2, WNK4
Calcium	
Familial hypocalciuric hypercalcemia	Ca²⁺-sensing protein (hypofunction)
Familial hypocalcemia	Ca²⁺-sensing protein (hyperfunction)
Phosphate	
Hypophosphatemic rickets	*PEX* gene, FGF23
Magnesium	
Hypomagnesemia-hypercalciuria syndrome	Paracellin-1
Water	
Nephrogenic diabetes insipidus	Vasopressin receptor-2 (Type 1), aquaporin-2
Acid-base	
Proximal RTA	Na⁺ HCO₃⁻ cotransporter
Distal RTA	Cl⁻ HCO₃⁻ exchanger, H⁺-ATPase
Proximal and distal RTA	Carbonic anhydrase II

FGF23, fibroblast growth factor 23; RTA, renal tubular acidosis.

inappropriately high (greater than 40 mEq/L) with renal loss (eg, mineralocorticoid excess, Bartter syndrome, Liddle syndrome) (Table 21–3).

The transtubular [K^+] gradient (TTKG) is a simple and rapid evaluation of net potassium secretion. TTKG is calculated as follows:

$$TTKG = \frac{Urine\ K^+/Plasma\ K^+}{Urine\ Osm/Plasma\ Osm}$$

Hypokalemia with a TTKG more than 4 suggests renal potassium loss with increased distal K^+ secretion. In such cases, plasma renin and aldosterone levels are helpful in differential diagnosis. The presence of nonabsorbed anions, such as bicarbonate, increases the TTKG.

C. Electrocardiogram

The electrocardiogram (ECG) may show decreased amplitude and broadening of T waves, prominent U waves, premature ventricular contractions, and depressed ST segments.

▶ Treatment

Oral potassium supplementation is the safest and easiest treatment for mild to moderate deficiency. Dietary potassium is almost entirely coupled to phosphate—rather than chloride—and is therefore not effective in correcting potassium loss associated with chloride depletion from diuretics or vomiting. In the setting of abnormal kidney function and mild to moderate diuretic dosage, 20 mEq/day of oral potassium is generally sufficient to prevent hypokalemia, but 40–100 mEq/day over a period of days to weeks is needed to treat hypokalemia and fully replete potassium stores.

Intravenous potassium is indicated for patients with severe hypokalemia and for those who cannot take oral supplementation. For severe deficiency, potassium may be given through a peripheral intravenous line in a concentration up to 40 mEq/L and at rates up to 10 mEq/h. Concentrations of up to 20 mEq/h may be given through a central venous catheter. Continuous ECG monitoring is indicated, and the serum potassium level should be checked every 3–6 hours. Avoid glucose-containing fluid to prevent further shifts of potassium into the cells. Magnesium deficiency should be corrected, particularly in refractory hypokalemia.

▶ When to Refer

Patients with unexplained hypokalemia, refractory hypokalemia, or clinical features suggesting alternative diagnoses (eg, aldosteronism or hypokalemic periodic paralysis) should be referred for endocrinology or nephrology consultation.

▶ When to Admit

Patients with symptomatic or severe hypokalemia, especially with cardiac manifestations, require cardiac monitoring, potassium supplementation, and frequent laboratory testing.

Gumz ML et al. An integrated view of potassium homeostasis. N Engl J Med. 2015 Jul 2;373(1):60–72. Erratum in: N Engl J Med. 2015 Sep 24;373(13):1281. [PMID: 26132942]

Jensen HK et al. Hypokalemia in acute medical patients: risk factors and prognosis. Am J Med. 2015 Jan;128(1):60–7.e1. [PMID: 25107385]

Marti G et al. Etiology and symptoms of severe hypokalemia in emergency department patients. Eur J Emerg Med. 2014 Feb; 21(1):46–51. [PMID: 23839104]

Pepin J et al. Advances in diagnosis and management of hypokalemic and hyperkalemic emergencies. Emerg Med Pract. 2012 Feb;14(2):1–18. [PMID: 22413702]

HYPERKALEMIA

ESSENTIALS OF DIAGNOSIS

▶ Serum potassium level greater than 5.0 mEq/L (5.0 mmol/L).

▶ Hyperkalemia may develop in patients taking ACE inhibitors, angiotensin-receptor blockers, potassium-sparing diuretics, or their combination, even with no or only mild kidney dysfunction.

▶ The ECG may show peaked T waves, widened QRS and biphasic QRS–T complexes, or may be normal despite life-threatening hyperkalemia.

▶ Measurement of plasma potassium level differentiates potassium leak from blood cells in cases of clotting, leukocytosis, and thrombocytosis from truly elevated serum potassium.

▶ Rule out extracellular potassium shift from the cells in acidosis and assess renal potassium excretion.

▶ General Considerations

Hyperkalemia usually occurs in patients with advanced kidney disease but can also develop with normal kidney function (Table 21–5). Acidosis causes intracellular potassium to shift extracellularly. Serum potassium concentration rises about 0.7 mEq/L for every decrease of 0.1 pH unit during acidosis. Fist clenching during venipuncture may raise the potassium concentration by 1–2 mEq/L by causing acidosis and potassium shift from cells. In the absence of acidosis, serum potassium concentration rises about 1 mEq/L when there is a total body potassium excess of 1–4 mEq/kg. However, the higher the serum potassium concentration, the smaller the excess necessary to raise the potassium levels further.

Mineralocorticoid deficiency from Addison disease or chronic kidney disease (CKD) is another cause of hyperkalemia with decreased renal excretion of potassium. Mineralocorticoid resistance due to genetic disorders, interstitial kidney disease, or urinary tract obstruction also leads to hyperkalemia.

ACE inhibitors or angiotensin-receptor blockers (ARBs), commonly used in patients with heart failure or CKD, may cause hyperkalemia. The concomitant use of spironolactone, eplerenone, or beta-blockers further

Table 21–5. Causes of hyperkalemia.

Spurious/Pseudohyperkalemia
Leakage from erythrocytes when separation of serum from clot is delayed (plasma K^+ normal)
Marked thrombocytosis or leukocytosis with release of intracellular K^+ (plasma K^+ normal)
Repeated fist clenching during phlebotomy, with release of K^+ from forearm muscles
Specimen drawn from arm with intravenous K^+ infusion
Decreased K^+ excretion
Kidney disease, acute and chronic
Renal secretory defects (may or may not have reduced kidney function): kidney transplant, interstitial nephritis, systemic lupus erythematosus, sickle cell disease, amyloidosis, obstructive nephropathy
Hyporeninemic hypoaldosteronism (often in diabetic patients with mild to moderate diabetic nephropathy) or selective hypoaldosteronism (eg, AIDS patients)
Drugs that inhibit potassium excretion: spironolactone, eplerenone, drospirenone, NSAIDs, ACE inhibitors, angiotensin II receptor blockers, triamterene, amiloride, trimethoprim, pentamidine, cyclosporine, tacrolimus
Shift of K^+ from within the cell
Massive release of intracellular K^+ in burns, rhabdomyolysis, hemolysis, severe infection, internal bleeding, vigorous exercise
Metabolic acidosis (in the case of organic acid accumulation— eg, lactic acidosis—a shift of K^+ does not occur since organic acid can easily move across the cell membrane)
Hypertonicity (solvent drag)
Insulin deficiency (metabolic acidosis may not be apparent)
Hyperkalemic periodic paralysis
Drugs: succinylcholine, arginine, digitalis toxicity, beta- adrenergic antagonists
Alpha-adrenergic stimulation?
Excessive intake of K^+
Especially in patients taking medications that decrease potassium secretion (see above)

ACE, angiotensin-converting enzyme; NSAIDs, nonsteroidal anti-inflammatory drugs.

increases the risk of hyperkalemia. Thiazide or loop diuretics and sodium bicarbonate may minimize hyperkalemia. Persistent mild hyperkalemia in the absence of ACE inhibitor or ARB therapy is usually due to type IV renal tubular acidosis (RTA). Heparin inhibits aldosterone production in the adrenal glands, causing hyperkalemia.

Trimethoprim is structurally similar to amiloride and triamterene, and all three drugs inhibit renal potassium excretion through suppression of sodium channels in the distal nephron.

Cyclosporine and tacrolimus can induce hyperkalemia in organ transplant recipients, especially kidney transplant patients, partly due to suppression of the basolateral Na^+–K^+-ATPase in principal cells. Hyperkalemia is commonly seen in HIV patients and has been attributed to impaired renal excretion of potassium due to pentamidine or trimethoprim-sulfamethoxazole or to hyporeninemic hypoaldosteronism.

Clinical Findings

Hyperkalemia impairs neuromuscular transmission, causing muscle weakness, flaccid paralysis, and ileus. Electrocardiography is not a sensitive method for detecting hyperkalemia, since nearly half of patients with a serum potassium level greater than 6.5 mEq/L will not manifest ECG changes. ECG changes in hyperkalemia include bradycardia, PR interval prolongation, peaked T waves, QRS widening, and biphasic QRS–T complexes. Conduction disturbances, such as bundle branch block and atrioventricular block, may occur. Ventricular fibrillation and cardiac arrest are terminal events.

Prevention

Inhibitors of the renin-angiotensin-aldosterone axis (ie, ACE inhibitors, ARBs, and spironolactone) and potassium-sparing diuretics (eplerenone, triamterene) should be used cautiously in patients with heart failure, liver failure, and kidney disease. Laboratory monitoring should be performed within 1 week of drug initiation or dosage increase.

Treatment

The diagnosis should be confirmed by repeat laboratory testing to rule out spurious hyperkalemia, especially in the absence of medications that cause hyperkalemia or in patients without kidney disease or a previous history of hyperkalemia. Plasma potassium concentration can be measured to avoid spurious hyperkalemia due to potassium leakage out of red cells, white cells, and platelets. Kidney dysfunction should be ruled out at the initial assessment.

Treatment consists of withholding exogenous potassium, identifying the cause, reviewing the patient's medications and dietary potassium intake, and correcting the hyperkalemia. Emergent treatment is indicated when cardiac toxicity, muscle paralysis, or severe hyperkalemia (potassium greater than 6.5 mEq/L) is present, even in the absence of ECG changes. Insulin, bicarbonate, and beta-agonists shift potassium intracellularly within minutes of administration (Table 21–6). Intravenous calcium may be given to antagonize the cell membrane effects of potassium, but its use should be restricted to life-threatening hyperkalemia in patients taking digitalis because hypercalcemia may cause digitalis toxicity. Hemodialysis may be required to remove potassium in patients with acute or chronic kidney injury. Patiromer binds potassium in the intestine and is approved by the FDA for the treatment of chronic hyperkalemia in patients with CKD who take at least one drug that inhibits the renin-angiotensin-aldosterone system. Patiromer may decrease the absorption of orally administered drugs. Another potassium binder zirconium cyclosilicate has been studied for chronic hyperkalemia treatment but has not received FDA approval. Neither agent has been studied in acute hyperkalemia or in patients with end-stage renal disease. Sodium polystyrene has been widely used for decades although its efficacy and safety have been questioned. It may not increase potassium excretion above laxatives alone and has been associated with colonic necrosis, both with and without sorbitol coadministration. In 2009, the FDA recommended that sodium polystyrene should not be administered in

Table 21–6. Treatment of hyperkalemia.

IMMEDIATE					
Modality	Mechanism of Action	Onset	Duration	Prescription	K+ Removed from Body
Calcium	Antagonizes cardiac conduction abnormalities	0–5 minutes	1 hour	Calcium gluconate 10%, 5–30 mL intravenously; or calcium chloride 5%, 5–30 mL intravenously	None
Bicarbonate	Distributes K+ into cells	15–30 minutes	1–2 hours	NaHCO$_3$, 50–100 mEq intravenously **Note:** Sodium bicarbonate may not be effective in end-stage renal disease patients; dialysis is more expedient and effective. Some patients may not tolerate the additional sodium load of bicarbonate therapy.	None
Insulin	Distributes K+ into cells	15–60 minutes	4–6 hours	Regular insulin, 5–10 units intravenously, plus glucose 50%, 25 g intravenously	None
Albuterol	Distributes K+ into cells	15–30 minutes	2–4 hours	Nebulized albuterol, 10–20 mg in 4 mL normal saline, inhaled over 10 minutes **Note:** Much higher doses are necessary for hyperkalemia therapy (10–20 mg) than for airway disease (2.5 mg).	None

URGENT				
Modality	Mechanism of Action	Onset of Action	Prescription	K+ Removed from Body
Loop diuretic	Renal K+ excretion	0.5–2 hours	Furosemide, 40–160 mg intravenously **Note:** Diuretics may not be effective in patients with acute and chronic kidney diseases.	Variable
Sodium polystyrene sulfonate (eg, Kayexalate)	Ion-exchange resin binds K+	1–3 hours	Oral: 15–60 g in 20% sorbitol (60–240 mL) Rectal: 30–60 g in 20% sorbitol **Note:** Resins with sorbitol may cause bowel necrosis and intestinal perforation, especially in patients with abnormal bowel function.	0.5–1 mEq/g resin
Hemodialysis[1]	Extracorporeal K+ removal	1–8 hours	Dialysate [K+] 0–1 mEq/L **Note:** A fast and effective therapy for hyperkalemia, hemodialysis can be delayed by vascular access placement and equipment and/or staffing availability. Serum K can be rapidly corrected within minutes, but post-dialysis rebound can occur.	25–50 mEq/h **Note:** Serum K can be rapidly and effectively corrected within minutes; post-dialysis rebound can occur. Hemo-dialysis can be delayed by vascular access placement and equipment and/or staffing availability.
Peritoneal dialysis	Peritoneal K+ removal	1–4 hours	Frequent exchanges	200–300 mEq

[1]Can be both acute immediate and urgent treatment of hyperkalemia.
Modified and reproduced, with permission, from Cogan MG. *Fluid and Electrolytes: Physiology and Pathophysiology.* McGraw-Hill, 1991.

sorbitol, but the mixture remains commonly available. Its use should be restricted to patients with life-threatening hyperkalemia when dialysis is not available and other therapies (eg, diuretics) have failed. Sodium polystyrene is contraindicated in patients with risk factors for colonic necrosis, such as bowel obstruction, ileus, and postoperative state.

► When to Refer

- Patients with hyperkalemia from kidney disease and reduced renal potassium excretion should see a nephrologist.
- Transplant patients may need adjustment of their immunosuppression regimen by transplant specialists.

► When to Admit

Patients with severe hyperkalemia greater than 6 mEq/L, any degree of hyperkalemia associated with ECG changes, or concomitant illness (eg, tumor lysis, rhabdomyolysis, metabolic acidosis) should be sent to the emergency department for immediate treatment.

Medford-Davis L et al. Derangements of potassium. Emerg Med Clin North Am. 2014 May;32(2):329–47. [PMID: 24766936]

Packham DK et al. Sodium zirconium cyclosilicate in hyperkalemia. N Engl J Med. 2015 Jan 15;372(3):222–31. [PMID: 25415807]

Pitt B et al. New potassium binders for the treatment of hyperkalemia: current data and opportunities for the future. Hypertension. 2015 Oct;66(4):731–8. [PMID: 26303290]

Weir MR et al; the OPAL-HK Investigators. Patiromer in patients with kidney disease and hyperkalemia receiving RAAS inhibitors. N Engl J Med. 2015 Jan 15;372(3):211–21. [PMID: 25415805]

DISORDERS OF CALCIUM CONCENTRATION

The normal total plasma (or serum) calcium concentration is 8.5–10.5 mg/dL (or 2.1–2.6 mmol/L). Ionized calcium (normal: 4.6–5.3 mg/dL [or 1.15–1.32 mmol/L]) is physiologically active and necessary for muscle contraction and nerve function.

The calcium-sensing receptor, a transmembrane protein that detects the extracellular calcium concentration, has been identified in the parathyroid gland and the kidney. Functional defects in this protein are associated with diseases of abnormal calcium metabolism such as familial hypocalcemia and familial hypocalciuric hypercalcemia (Table 21–4).

HYPOCALCEMIA

ESSENTIALS OF DIAGNOSIS

- ► Often mistaken as a neurologic disorder.
- ► Check for decreased serum parathyroid hormone (PTH), vitamin D, or magnesium levels.
- ► If the ionized calcium level is normal despite a low total serum calcium, calcium metabolism is usually normal.

Table 21–7. Causes of hypocalcemia.

Decreased intake or absorption
Malabsorption
Small bowel bypass, short bowel
Vitamin D deficit (decreased absorption, decreased production of 25-hydroxyvitamin D or 1,25-dihydroxyvitamin D)
Increased loss
Alcoholism
Chronic kidney disease
Diuretic therapy
Endocrine disease
Hypoparathyroidism (genetic, acquired; including hypomagnesemia and hypermagnesemia)
Post-parathyroidectomy (hungry bone syndrome)
Pseudohypoparathyroidism
Calcitonin secretion with medullary carcinoma of the thyroid
Familial hypocalcemia
Associated diseases
Pancreatitis
Rhabdomyolysis
Septic shock
Physiologic causes
Associated with decreased serum albumin[1]
Decreased end-organ response to vitamin D
Hyperphosphatemia
Induced by aminoglycoside antibiotics, plicamycin, loop diuretics, foscarnet

[1]Ionized calcium concentration is normal.

► General Considerations

The most common cause of low total serum calcium is hypoalbuminemia. When serum albumin concentration is lower than 4 g/dL (40 g/L), serum Ca^{2+} concentration is reduced by 0.8–1 mg/dL (0.20–0.25 mmol/L) for every 1 g/dL (10 g/L) of albumin.

The most accurate measurement of serum calcium is the ionized calcium concentration. True hypocalcemia (decreased ionized calcium) implies insufficient action of PTH or active vitamin D. Important causes of hypocalcemia are listed in Table 21–7.

The most common cause of hypocalcemia is advanced CKD, in which decreased production of active vitamin D_3 (1,25 dihydroxyvitamin D_3) and hyperphosphatemia both play a role (see Chapter 22). Some cases of primary hypoparathyroidism are due to mutations of the calcium-sensing receptor in which inappropriate suppression of PTH release leads to hypocalcemia (see Chapter 26). Magnesium depletion reduces both PTH release and tissue responsiveness to PTH, causing hypocalcemia. Hypocalcemia in pancreatitis is a marker of severe disease. Elderly hospitalized patients with hypocalcemia and hypophosphatemia, with or without an elevated PTH level, are likely vitamin D deficient.

► Clinical Findings

A. Symptoms and Signs

Hypocalcemia increases excitation of nerve and muscle cells, primarily affecting the neuromuscular and cardiovascular systems. Spasm of skeletal muscle causes cramps and tetany. Laryngospasm with stridor can obstruct the airway. Convulsions, perioral and peripheral paresthesias, and abdominal pain can develop. Classic physical findings include Chvostek sign (contraction of the facial muscle in response to tapping the facial nerve) and Trousseau sign (carpal spasm occurring with occlusion of the brachial artery by a blood pressure cuff). QT prolongation predisposes to ventricular arrhythmias. In chronic hypoparathyroidism, cataracts and calcification of basal ganglia may appear (see Chapter 26).

B. Laboratory Findings

Serum calcium concentration is low (less than 8.5 mg/dL [2.1 mmol/L]). In true hypocalcemia, the ionized serum calcium concentration is also low (less than 4.6 mg/dL [1.15 mmol/L]). Serum phosphate is usually elevated in hypoparathyroidism or in advanced CKD, whereas it is suppressed in early CKD or vitamin D deficiency.

Serum magnesium concentration is commonly low. In respiratory alkalosis, total serum calcium is normal but ionized calcium is low. The ECG shows a prolonged QT interval.

▶ Treatment[1]

A. Severe, Symptomatic Hypocalcemia

In the presence of tetany, arrhythmias, or seizures, intravenous calcium gluconate is indicated.[1] Because of the short duration of action, continuous calcium infusion is usually required. Ten to 15 milligrams of calcium per kilogram body weight, or six to eight 10-mL vials of 10% calcium gluconate (558–744 mg of calcium), is added to 1 L of D_5W and infused over 4–6 hours. By monitoring the serum calcium level frequently (every 4–6 hours), the infusion rate is adjusted to maintain the serum calcium level at 7–8.5 mg/dL.

B. Asymptomatic Hypocalcemia

Oral calcium (1–2 g) and vitamin D preparations, including active vitamin D sterols, are used. Calcium carbonate is well tolerated and less expensive than many other calcium tablets. A check of urinary calcium excretion is recommended after the initiation of therapy because hypercalciuria (urine calcium excretion greater than 300 mg or 7.5 mmol per day) or urine calcium:creatinine ratio greater than 0.3 may impair kidney function in these patients. The low serum calcium associated with hypoalbuminemia does not require replacement therapy. If serum Mg^{2+} is low, therapy must include magnesium replacement, which by itself will usually correct hypocalcemia.

▶ When to Refer

Patients with complicated hypocalcemia from hypoparathyroidism, familial hypocalcemia, or CKD require referral to an endocrinologist or nephrologist.

***

[1] See also Chapter 26 for discussion of the treatment of hypoparathyroidism.

▶ When to Admit

Patients with tetany, arrhythmias, seizures, or other symptoms of hypocalcemia require immediate evaluation and therapy.

Al-Azem H et al. Hypoparathyroidism. Best Pract Res Clin Endocrinol Metab. 2012 Aug;26(4):517–22. [PMID: 22863393]

Fong J et al. Hypocalcemia: updates in diagnosis and management for primary care. Can Fam Physician. 2012 Feb;58(2):158–62. [PMID: 22439169]

Kelly A et al. Hypocalcemia in the critically ill patient. J Intensive Care Med. 2013 May–Jun;28(3):166–77. [PMID: 21841146]

HYPERCALCEMIA

ESSENTIALS OF DIAGNOSIS

▶ Primary hyperparathyroidism and malignancy-associated hypercalcemia are the most common causes.

▶ Hypercalciuria usually precedes hypercalcemia.

▶ Most often, asymptomatic, mild hypercalcemia (greater than or equal to 10.5 mg/dL [2.6 mmol/L]) is due to primary hyperparathyroidism; symptomatic, severe hypercalcemia (greater than or equal to 14 mg/dL [3.5 mmol/L]) is usually due to hypercalcemia of malignancy.

▶ General Considerations

Important causes of hypercalcemia are listed in Table 21–8. Primary hyperparathyroidism and malignancy account for 90% of cases. Primary hyperparathyroidism is the most common cause of hypercalcemia (usually mild) in ambulatory patients. Chronic hypercalcemia (over 6 months) or some manifestation such as nephrolithiasis also suggests a benign cause. Tumor production of PTH-related proteins (PTHrP) is the most common paraneoplastic endocrine syndrome, accounting for most cases of hypercalcemia in inpatients. The neoplasm is clinically apparent in nearly all cases when the hypercalcemia is detected, and the prognosis is poor. Granulomatous diseases, such as sarcoidosis and tuberculosis, cause hypercalcemia via overproduction of active vitamin D_3 (1,25 dihydroxyvitamin D_3).

Milk-alkali syndrome has had a resurgence due to calcium ingestion for prevention of osteoporosis. Heavy calcium carbonate intake causes hypercalcemic acute kidney injury, likely from renal vasoconstriction. The decreased GFR impairs bicarbonate excretion, while hypercalcemia stimulates proton secretion and bicarbonate reabsorption. Metabolic alkalosis decreases calcium excretion, maintaining hypercalcemia.

Hypercalcemia causes nephrogenic DI through activation of calcium-sensing receptors in collecting ducts, which reduces ADH-induced water permeability. Volume depletion further worsens hypercalcemia.

Table 21–8. Causes of hypercalcemia.

Increased intake or absorption
Milk-alkali syndrome
Vitamin D or vitamin A excess
Endocrine disorders
Primary hyperparathyroidism
Secondary or tertiary hyperparathyroidism (usually associated with hypocalcemia)
Acromegaly
Adrenal insufficiency
Pheochromocytoma
Thyrotoxicosis
Neoplastic diseases
Tumors producing PTH-related proteins (ovary, kidney, lung)
Multiple myeloma (elaboration of osteoclast-activating factor)
Lymphoma (occasionally from production of calcitriol)
Miscellaneous causes
Thiazide diuretic use
Granulomatous diseases (production of calcitriol)
Paget disease of bone
Hypophosphatasia
Immobilization
Familial hypocalciuric hypercalcemia
Complications of kidney transplantation
Lithium intake

PTH, parathyroid hormone.

▶ Clinical Findings

A. Symptoms and Signs

The history and physical examination should focus on the duration of hypercalcemia and evidence for a neoplasm. Hypercalcemia may affect gastrointestinal, kidney, and neurologic function. Mild hypercalcemia is often asymptomatic. Symptoms usually occur if the serum calcium is higher than 12 mg/dL (3 mmol/L) and tend to be more severe if hypercalcemia develops acutely. Symptoms include constipation and polyuria, except in hypocalciuric hypercalcemia, in which polyuria is absent. Other symptoms include nausea, vomiting, anorexia, peptic ulcer disease, renal colic, and hematuria from nephrolithiasis. Polyuria from hypercalciuria-induced nephrogenic DI can result in volume depletion and acute kidney injury. Neurologic manifestations range from mild drowsiness to weakness, depression, lethargy, stupor, and coma in severe hypercalcemia. Ventricular ectopy and idioventricular rhythm occur and can be accentuated by digitalis.

B. Laboratory Findings

The ionized calcium exceeds 1.32 mmol/L. A high serum chloride concentration and a low serum phosphate concentration in a ratio greater than 33:1 (or greater than 102 if SI units are utilized) suggests primary hyperparathyroidism where PTH decreases proximal tubular phosphate reabsorption. A low serum chloride concentration with a high serum bicarbonate concentration, along with elevated BUN and creatinine, suggests milk-alkali syndrome. Severe

hypercalcemia (greater than 15 mg/dL [3.75 mmol/L]) generally occurs in malignancy. More than 300 mg (7.5 mmol) per day of urinary calcium excretion suggests hypercalciuria; less than 100 mg (2.5 mmol) per day suggests hypocalciuria. Hypercalciuric patients—such as those with malignancy or those receiving oral active vitamin D therapy—may easily develop hypercalcemia in case of volume depletion. Serum phosphate may or may not be low, depending on the cause. Hypocalciuric hypercalcemia occurs in milk-alkali syndrome, thiazide diuretic use, and familial hypocalciuric hypercalcemia.

The chest radiograph may reveal malignancy or granulomatous disease. The ECG shows a shortened QT interval. Measurements of PTH and PTHrP help distinguish between hyperparathyroidism (elevated PTH) and malignancy-associated hypercalcemia (suppressed PTH, elevated PTHrP).

▶ Treatment

Until the primary cause can be identified and treated, renal excretion of calcium is promoted through aggressive hydration and forced calciuresis. The tendency in hypercalcemia is hypovolemia from nephrogenic DI. In dehydrated patients with normal cardiac and kidney function, 0.45% saline or 0.9% saline can be given rapidly (250–500 mL/h). A meta-analysis questioned the efficacy and safety profile of intravenous furosemide for hypercalcemia. Thiazides can worsen hypercalcemia.

Bisphosphonates are the treatment of choice for hypercalcemia of malignancy. Although they are safe, effective, and normalize calcium in more than 70% of patients, bisphosphonates may require up to 48–72 hours before reaching full therapeutic effect. Calcitonin may be helpful in the short-term until bisphosphonates reach therapeutic levels. In emergency cases, dialysis with low calcium dialysate may be needed. The calcimimetic agent cinacalcet suppresses PTH secretion and decreases serum calcium concentration; it has been recommended for use in patients with symptomatic or severe primary hyperparathyroidism who are unable to undergo parathyroidectomy and patients with inoperable parathyroid carcinoma. (See Chapters 26 and 39.)

Typically, if dialysis patients do not receive proper supplementation of calcium and active vitamin D, hypocalcemia and hyperphosphatemia develop. On the other hand, hypercalcemia can sometimes develop, particularly in the setting of severe secondary hyperparathyroidism, characterized by high PTH levels and subsequent release of calcium from bone. Therapy may include intravenous vitamin D, which further increases the serum calcium concentration. Another type of hypercalcemia occurs when PTH levels are low. Bone turnover is decreased, which results in a low buffering capacity for calcium. When calcium is administered in calcium-containing phosphate binders or dialysate, or when vitamin D is administered, hypercalcemia results. Hypercalcemia in dialysis patients usually occurs in the presence of hyperphosphatemia, and metastatic calcification may occur. Malignancy should be considered as a cause of the hypercalcemia.

When to Refer

- Patients may require referral to an oncologist or endocrinologist depending on the underlying cause of hypercalcemia.
- Patients with granulomatous diseases (eg, tuberculosis and other chronic infections, granulomatosis with polyangiitis [formerly Wegener granulomatosis], sarcoidosis) may require assistance from infectious disease specialists, rheumatologists, or pulmonologists.

When to Admit

- Patients with symptomatic or severe hypercalcemia require immediate treatment.
- Unexplained hypercalcemia with associated conditions, such as acute kidney injury or suspected malignancy, may require urgent treatment and expedited evaluation.

Crowley R et al. How to approach hypercalcaemia. Clin Med. 2013 Jun;13(3):287–90. [PMID: 23760705]
Cusano NE et al. Parathyroid hormone in the evaluation of hypercalcemia. JAMA. 2014 Dec 24–31;312(24):2680–1. [PMID: 25536261]
Donovan PJ et al. PTHrP-mediated hypercalcemia: causes and survival in 138 patients. J Clin Endocrinol Metab. 2015 May;100(5):2024–9. [PMID: 25719931]
Powe NR et al. Case records of the Massachusetts General Hospital. Case 27-2015. A 78-year-old man with hypercalcemia and renal failure. N Engl J Med. 2015 Aug 27;373(9):864–73. [PMID: 26308688]

DISORDERS OF PHOSPHORUS CONCENTRATION

Plasma phosphorus is mainly inorganic phosphate and represents a small fraction (less than 0.2%) of total body phosphate. Important determinants of plasma inorganic phosphate are renal excretion, intestinal absorption, and shift between the intracellular and extracellular spaces. The kidney is the most important regulator of the serum phosphate level. PTH decreases reabsorption of phosphate in the proximal tubule while 1,25-dihydroxyvitamin D_3 increases reabsorption. Renal proximal tubular reabsorption of phosphate is decreased by volume expansion, corticosteroids, and proximal tubular dysfunction (as in Fanconi syndrome). Fibroblast growth factor 23 (FGF23) is a potent phosphaturic hormone. Intestinal absorption of phosphate is facilitated by active vitamin D. PTH stimulates phosphate release from bone and renal phosphate excretion; primary hyperparathyroidism can lead to hypophosphatemia and depletion of bone phosphate stores. By contrast, growth hormone augments proximal tubular reabsorption of phosphate. Cellular phosphate uptake is stimulated by various factors and conditions, including alkalemia, insulin, epinephrine, feeding, hungry bone syndrome, and accelerated cell proliferation.

Phosphorus metabolism and homeostasis are intimately related to calcium metabolism. See sections on metabolic bone disease in Chapter 26.

HYPOPHOSPHATEMIA

ESSENTIALS OF DIAGNOSIS

- ▶ Severe hypophosphatemia may cause tissue hypoxia and rhabdomyolysis.
- ▶ Renal loss of phosphate can be diagnosed by measuring urinary phosphate excretion and by calculating maximal tubular phosphate reabsorption rate (TmP/GFR).
- ▶ PTH and FGF23 are the major factors that decrease TmP/GFR, leading to renal loss of phosphate.

General Considerations

The leading causes of hypophosphatemia are listed in Table 21–9. Hypophosphatemia may occur in the presence

Table 21–9. Causes of hypophosphatemia.

Diminished supply or absorption
Starvation
Parenteral alimentation with inadequate phosphate content
Malabsorption syndrome, small bowel bypass
Absorption blocked by oral antacids with aluminum or magnesium
Vitamin D–deficient and vitamin D–resistant osteomalacia
Increased loss
Phosphaturic drugs: theophylline, diuretics, bronchodilators, corticosteroids
Hyperparathyroidism (primary or secondary)
Hyperthyroidism
Renal tubular defects with excessive phosphaturia (congenital, Fanconi syndrome induced by monoclonal gammopathy, heavy metal poisoning), alcoholism
Hypokalemic nephropathy
Inadequately controlled diabetes mellitus
Hypophosphatemic rickets
Phosphatonins of oncogenic osteomalacia (eg, FGF23 production)
Intracellular shift of phosphorus
Administration of glucose
Anabolic steroids, estrogen, oral contraceptives, beta-adrenergic agonists, xanthine derivatives
Hungry bone syndrome
Respiratory alkalosis
Salicylate poisoning
Electrolyte abnormalities
Hypercalcemia
Hypomagnesemia
Metabolic alkalosis
Abnormal losses followed by inadequate repletion
Diabetes mellitus with acidosis, particularly during aggressive therapy
Recovery from starvation or prolonged catabolic state
Chronic alcoholism, particularly during restoration of nutrition; associated with hypomagnesemia
Recovery from severe burns

FGF23, fibroblast growth factor 23.

of normal phosphate stores. Serious depletion of body phosphate stores may exist with low, normal, or high serum phosphate concentrations.

Serum phosphate levels decrease transiently after food intake, thus fasting samples are recommended for accuracy. **Moderate hypophosphatemia** (1.0–2.4 mg/dL [0.32–0.79 mmol/L]) occurs commonly in hospitalized patients and may not reflect decreased phosphate stores.

In **severe hypophosphatemia** (less than 1 mg/dL [0.32 mmol/L]), the affinity of hemoglobin for oxygen increases through a decrease in the erythrocyte 2,3-biphosphoglycerate concentration, impairing tissue oxygenation and cell metabolism and resulting in muscle weakness or even rhabdomyolysis. Severe hypophosphatemia is common and multifactorial in alcoholic patients. In acute alcohol withdrawal, increased plasma insulin and epinephrine along with respiratory alkalosis promote intracellular shift of phosphate. Vomiting, diarrhea, and poor dietary intake contribute to hypophosphatemia. Chronic alcohol use results in a decrease in the renal threshold of phosphate excretion. This renal tubular dysfunction reverses after a month of abstinence. Patients with chronic obstructive pulmonary disease and asthma commonly have hypophosphatemia, attributed to xanthine derivatives causing shifts of phosphate intracellularly and the phosphaturic effects of beta-adrenergic agonists, loop diuretics, xanthine derivatives, and corticosteroids. Refeeding or glucose administration to phosphate-depleted patients may cause fatal hypophosphatemia.

▶ Clinical Findings

A. Symptoms and Signs

Acute, severe hypophosphatemia (less than 1.0 mg/dL [0.32 mmol/L]) can lead to rhabdomyolysis, paresthesias, and encephalopathy (irritability, confusion, dysarthria, seizures, and coma). Respiratory failure or failure to wean from mechanical ventilation may occur as a result of diaphragmatic weakness. Arrhythmias and heart failure are uncommon but serious manifestations. Hematologic manifestations include acute hemolytic anemia from erythrocyte fragility, platelet dysfunction with petechial hemorrhages, and impaired chemotaxis of leukocytes (leading to increased susceptibility to gram-negative sepsis).

Chronic severe depletion may cause anorexia, pain in muscles and bones, and fractures.

B. Laboratory Findings

Urine phosphate excretion is a useful clue in the evaluation of hypophosphatemia. The normal renal response to hypophosphatemia is decreased urinary phosphate excretion to less than 100 mg/day. The fractional excretion of phosphate (F_EPO_4) should be less than 5%. The main factors regulating F_EPO_4 are PTH and phosphate intake. Increased PTH or phosphate intake decreases F_EPO_4 (ie, more phosphate is excreted into the urine).

Measurement of plasma PTH or PTHrP levels may be helpful. The clinical utility of serum FGF levels is undetermined except in uncommon diseases.

Other clinical features may be suggestive of hypophosphatemia, such as hemolytic anemia and rhabdomyolysis. Fanconi syndrome may present with any combination of uricosuria, aminoaciduria, normoglycemic glucosuria, normal anion gap metabolic acidosis, and phosphaturia. In chronic hypophosphatemia, radiographs and bone biopsies show changes resembling osteomalacia.

▶ Treatment

Hypophosphatemia can be prevented by including phosphate in repletion and maintenance fluids. A rapid decline in calcium levels can occur with parenteral administration of phosphate; oral replacement of phosphate is preferable. Moderate hypophosphatemia (1.0–2.5 mg/dL [or 0.32–0.79 mmol/L]) is usually asymptomatic and does not require treatment. The hypophosphatemia in patients with diabetic ketoacidosis (DKA) will usually correct with normal dietary intake. Chronic hypophosphatemia can be treated with oral phosphate repletion. Mixtures of sodium and potassium phosphate salts may be given to provide 0.5–1 g (16–32 mmol) of phosphate per day. For severe, symptomatic hypophosphatemia (less than 1 mg/dL [0.32 mmol/L]), an infusion should provide 279–310 mg/12 h (or 9–10 mmol/12 h) until the serum phosphorus exceeds 1 mg/dL and the patient can be switched to oral therapy. The infusion rate should be decreased if hypotension occurs. Monitoring of plasma phosphate, calcium, and potassium every 6 hours is necessary because the response to phosphate supplementation is not predictable. Magnesium deficiency often coexists and should be treated.

Contraindications to phosphate replacement include hypoparathyroidism, advanced CKD, tissue damage and necrosis, and hypercalcemia. When an associated hyperglycemia is treated, phosphate accompanies glucose into cells, and hypophosphatemia may ensue.

▶ When to Refer

- Patients with refractory hypophosphatemia with increased urinary phosphate excretion may require evaluation by an endocrinologist (for such conditions as hyperparathyroidism and vitamin D disorders) or a nephrologist (for such conditions as renal tubular defects).

- Patients with decreased gastrointestinal absorption may require referral to a gastroenterologist.

▶ When to Admit

Patients with severe or refractory hypophosphatemia will require intravenous phosphate.

Felsenfeld AJ et al. Approach to treatment of hypophosphatemia. Am J Kidney Dis. 2012 Oct;60(4):655–61. [PMID: 22863286]

Hall AM et al. J. Drug-induced renal Fanconi syndrome. QJM. 2014 Apr;107(4):261–9. [PMID: 24368854]

Suzuki S et al. Hypophosphatemia in critically ill patients. J Crit Care. 2013 Aug;28(4):536.e9–19. [PMID: 23265292]

HYPERPHOSPHATEMIA

ESSENTIALS OF DIAGNOSIS

► Advanced CKD is the most common cause.
► Hyperphosphatemia in the presence of hypercalcemia imposes a high risk of metastatic calcification.

General Considerations

Advanced CKD with decreased urinary excretion of phosphate is the most common cause of hyperphosphatemia. Other causes are listed in Table 21–10.

Clinical Findings

A. Symptoms and Signs

The clinical manifestations are those of the underlying disorder or associated condition.

B. Laboratory Findings

In addition to elevated phosphate, blood chemistry abnormalities are those of the underlying disease.

Treatment

Treatment is directed at the underlying cause. Exogenous sources of phosphate, including enteral or parenteral nutrition and medications, should be reduced or eliminated. Dietary phosphate absorption can be reduced by oral phosphate binders, such as calcium carbonate, calcium acetate,

Table 21–10. Causes of hyperphosphatemia.

Massive load of phosphate into the extracellular fluid
Exogenous sources
Hypervitaminosis D
Laxatives or enemas containing phosphate
Intravenous phosphate supplement
Endogenous sources
Rhabdomyolysis (especially if chronic kidney disease coexists)
Cell lysis by chemotherapy of malignancy, particularly lymphoproliferative diseases
Metabolic acidosis (lactic acidosis, ketoacidosis)
Respiratory acidosis (phosphate incorporation into cells is disturbed)
Decreased excretion into urine
Chronic kidney disease
Acute kidney injury
Hypoparathyroidism
Pseudohypoparathyroidism
Acromegaly
Pseudohyperphosphatemia
Multiple myeloma
Hyperbilirubinemia
Hypertriglyceridemia
Hemolysis in vitro

sevelamer carbonate, lanthanum carbonate, and aluminum hydroxide. Sevelamer, lanthanum, and aluminum may be used in patients with hypercalcemia, although aluminum use should be limited to a few days because of the risk of aluminum accumulation and neurotoxicity. In acute kidney injury and advanced CKD, dialysis will reduce serum phosphate.

When to Admit

Patients with acute severe hyperphosphatemia require hospitalization for emergent therapy, possibly including dialysis. Concomitant illnesses, such as acute kidney injury or cell lysis, may necessitate admission.

Leaf DE et al. A physiologic-based approach to the evaluation of a patient with hyperphosphatemia. Am J Kidney Dis. 2013 Feb;61(2):330–6. [PMID: 22938849]
Malberti F. Hyperphosphataemia: treatment options. Drugs. 2013 May;73(7):673–88. [PMID: 23625273]
Wilson FP et al. Tumor lysis syndrome: new challenges and recent advances. Adv Chronic Kidney Dis. 2014 Jan;21(1):18–26. [PMID: 24359983]

DISORDERS OF MAGNESIUM CONCENTRATION

Normal plasma magnesium concentration is 1.8–3.0 mg/dL (or 0.75–1.25 mmol/L), with about one-third bound to protein and two-thirds existing as free cation. Magnesium excretion is via the kidney. Magnesium's physiologic effects on the nervous system resemble those of calcium.

Altered magnesium concentration usually provokes an associated alteration of Ca^{2+}. Both hypomagnesemia and hypermagnesemia can decrease PTH secretion or action. Severe hypermagnesemia (greater than 5 mg/dL [2.1 mmol/L]) suppresses PTH secretion with consequent hypocalcemia; this disorder is typically seen only in patients receiving magnesium therapy for preeclampsia. Severe hypomagnesemia causes PTH resistance in end-organs and eventually decreased PTH secretion in severe cases.

HYPOMAGNESEMIA

ESSENTIALS OF DIAGNOSIS

► Serum concentration of magnesium may not be decreased even in the presence of magnesium depletion. Check urinary magnesium excretion if renal magnesium wasting is suspected.
► Causes neurologic symptoms and arrhythmias.
► Impairs release of PTH.

General Considerations

Causes of hypomagnesemia are listed in Table 21–11. Normomagnesemia does not exclude magnesium depletion

Table 21–11. Causes of hypomagnesemia.

Diminished absorption or intake
Malabsorption, chronic diarrhea, laxative abuse
Proton pump inhibitors
Prolonged gastrointestinal suction
Small bowel bypass
Malnutrition
Alcoholism
Total parenteral alimentation with inadequate Mg^{2+} content
Increased renal loss
Diuretic therapy (loop diuretics, thiazide diuretics)
Hyperaldosteronism, Gitelman syndrome (a variant of Bartter syndrome)
Hyperparathyroidism, hyperthyroidism
Hypercalcemia
Volume expansion
Tubulointerstitial diseases
Transplant kidney
Drugs (aminoglycoside, cetuximab, cisplatin, amphotericin B, pentamidine)
Others
Diabetes mellitus
Post-parathyroidectomy (hungry bone syndrome)
Respiratory alkalosis
Pregnancy

because only 1% of total body magnesium is in the extracellular fluid (ECF). Hypomagnesemia and hypokalemia share many etiologies, including diuretics, diarrhea, alcoholism, aminoglycosides, and amphotericin. Renal potassium wasting also occurs from hypomagnesemia, and is refractory to potassium replacement until magnesium is repleted. Hypomagnesemia also suppresses PTH release and causes end-organ resistance to PTH and low 1,25-dihydroxyvitamin D_3 levels. The resultant hypocalcemia is refractory to calcium replacement until the magnesium is normalized. Molecular mechanisms of magnesium wasting have been revealed in some hereditary disorders. The FDA has issued a warning about hypomagnesemia for patients taking proton pump inhibitors. The presumed mechanism is decreased intestinal magnesium absorption, but it is not clear why this complication develops in only a small fraction of patients taking these medications.

▶ Clinical Findings

A. Symptoms and Signs

Common symptoms are those of hypokalemia and hypocalcemia, with weakness and muscle cramps. Marked neuromuscular and central nervous system hyperirritability may produce tremors, athetoid movements, jerking, nystagmus, Babinski response, confusion, and disorientation. Cardiovascular manifestations include hypertension, tachycardia, and ventricular arrhythmias.

B. Laboratory Findings

Urinary excretion of magnesium exceeding 10–30 mg/day or a fractional excretion greater than 2% indicates renal magnesium wasting. Hypocalcemia and hypokalemia are

often present. The ECG shows a prolonged QT interval, due to lengthening of the ST segment. PTH secretion is often suppressed (see Hypocalcemia).

▶ Treatment

Magnesium oxide, 250–500 mg orally once or twice daily, is useful for treating chronic hypomagnesemia. Symptomatic hypomagnesemia requires intravenous magnesium sulfate 1–2 g over 5–60 minutes mixed in either dextrose 5% or 0.9% normal saline. Torsades de pointes in the setting of hypomagnesemia can be treated with 1–2 g of magnesium sulfate in 10 mL of dextrose 5% solution pushed intravenously over 15 minutes. Severe, non–life-threatening deficiency can be treated at a rate to 1–2 g/h over 3–6 hours. Magnesium sulfate may also be given intramuscularly in a dosage of 200–800 mg/day (8–33 mmol/day) in four divided doses. Serum levels must be monitored daily and dosage adjusted to keep the concentration from rising above 3 mg/dL (1.23 mmol/L). Tendon reflexes may be checked for hyporeflexia of hypermagnesemia. K^+ and Ca^{2+} replacement may be required, but patients with hypokalemia and hypocalcemia of hypomagnesemia do not recover without magnesium supplementation.

Patients with normal kidney function can excrete excess magnesium; hypermagnesemia should not develop with replacement dosages. In patients with CKD, magnesium replacement should be done cautiously to avoid hypermagnesemia. Reduced doses (50–75% dose reduction) and more frequent monitoring (at least twice daily) are indicated.

Alhosaini M et al. Magnesium and dialysis: the neglected cation. Am J Kidney Dis. 2015 Sep;66(3):523–31. [PMID: 25864370]

Ayuk J et al. Treatment of hypomagnesemia. Am J Kidney Dis. 2014 Apr;63(4):691–5. [PMID: 24100128]

Cheungpasitporn W et al. Dysmagnesemia in hospitalized patients: prevalence and prognostic importance. Mayo Clin Proc. 2015 Aug;90(8):1001–10. [PMID: 26250725]

Danziger J et al. Proton-pump inhibitor use is associated with low serum magnesium concentrations. Kidney Int. 2013 Apr;83(4):692–9. [PMID: 23325090]

Konrad M et al. Inherited disorders of renal hypomagnesaemia. Nephrol Dial Transplant. 2014 Sep;29(Suppl 4):iv63–71. [PMID: 25165187]

HYPERMAGNESEMIA

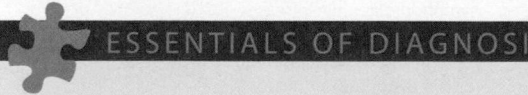
ESSENTIALS OF DIAGNOSIS

▶ Often associated with advanced CKD and chronic intake of magnesium-containing drugs.

▶ General Considerations

Hypermagnesemia is almost always the result of advanced CKD and impaired magnesium excretion. Antacids and laxatives are underrecognized sources of magnesium. Pregnant patients may have severe hypermagnesemia from intravenous magnesium for preeclampsia and eclampsia. Magnesium replacement should be done cautiously in patients with CKD; dose reductions up to 75% may be necessary to avoid hypermagnesemia.

▶ Clinical Findings

A. Symptoms and Signs

Muscle weakness, decreased deep tendon reflexes, mental obtundation, and confusion are characteristic manifestations. Weakness, flaccid paralysis, ileus, urinary retention, and hypotension are noted. Serious findings include respiratory muscle paralysis and cardiac arrest.

B. Laboratory Findings

Serum Mg^{2+} is elevated. In the common setting of CKD, BUN, creatinine, potassium, phosphate, and uric acid may all be elevated. Serum Ca^{2+} is often low. The ECG shows increased PR interval, broadened QRS complexes, and peaked T waves, probably related to associated hyperkalemia.

▶ Treatment

Exogenous sources of magnesium should be discontinued. Calcium antagonizes Mg^{2+} and may be given intravenously as calcium chloride, 500 mg or more at a rate of 100 mg (4.1 mmol) per minute. Hemodialysis or peritoneal dialysis may be necessary to remove magnesium, particularly with severe kidney disease.

Long-term use of magnesium hydroxide and magnesium sulfate should be avoided in patients with advanced stages of CKD.

Chang WT et al. Calcium, magnesium, and phosphate abnormalities in the emergency department. Emerg Med Clin North Am. 2014 May;32(2):349–66. [PMID: 24766937]
Volpe SL. Magnesium in disease prevention and overall health. Adv Nutr. 2013 May 1;4(3):378S–83S. [PMID: 23674807]

▼ ACID–BASE DISORDERS

Assessment of a patient's acid–base status requires measurement of arterial pH, P_{CO_2}, and plasma bicarbonate (HCO_3^-). Blood gas analyzers directly measure pH and P_{CO_2}. The HCO_3^- value is calculated from the Henderson–Hasselbalch equation:

$$pH = 6.1 + \log \frac{HCO_3^-}{0.03 \times PCO_2}$$

The total venous CO_2 measurement is a more direct determination of HCO_3^-. Because of the dissociation characteristics of carbonic acid (H_2CO_3) at body pH, dissolved CO_2 is almost exclusively in the form of HCO_3^-, and for clinical purposes the total carbon dioxide content is equivalent (± 3 mEq/L) to the HCO_3^- concentration:

$$H^+ + HCO_3^- \leftrightarrow H_2CO_3 \leftrightarrow CO_2 + H_2O$$

Venous blood gases can provide useful information for acid–base assessment since the arteriovenous differences in pH and P_{CO_2} are small and relatively constant. Venous blood pH is usually 0.03–0.04 units lower than arterial blood pH, and venous blood P_{CO_2} is 7 or 8 mm Hg higher than arterial blood P_{CO_2}. Calculated HCO_3^- concentration in venous blood is at most 2 mEq/L higher than arterial blood HCO_3^-. Arterial and venous blood gases will not be equivalent during a cardiopulmonary arrest; arterial samples should be obtained for the most accurate measurements of pH and P_{CO_2}.

TYPES OF ACID–BASE DISORDERS

There are two types of acid–base disorders: acidosis and alkalosis. These disorders can be either metabolic (decreased or increased HCO_3^-) or respiratory (decreased or increased P_{CO_2}). Primary respiratory disorders affect blood acidity by changes in P_{CO_2}, and primary metabolic disorders are disturbances in HCO_3^- concentration. A primary disturbance is usually accompanied by a compensatory response, but the compensation does not fully correct the pH disturbance of the primary disorder. If the pH is < 7.40, the primary process is acidosis, either respiratory (P_{CO_2} greater than 40 mm Hg) or metabolic (HCO_3^- less than 24 mEq/L). If the pH is > 7.40, the primary process is alkalosis, either respiratory (P_{CO_2} less than 40 mm Hg) or metabolic (HCO_3^- greater than 24 mEq/L). One respiratory or metabolic disorder with its appropriate compensatory response is a simple acid-base disorder.

MIXED ACID–BASE DISORDERS

Two or three simultaneous disorders can be present in a mixed acid-base disorder, but there can never be two primary respiratory disorders. Uncovering a mixed acid-base disorder is clinically important, but requires a methodical approach to acid-base analysis (see box, Step-by-Step Analysis of Acid-Base Status). Once the primary disturbance has been determined, the clinician should assess whether the compensatory response is appropriate (Table 21–12). An inadequate or an exaggerated response indicates the presence of another primary acid-base disturbance.

STEP-BY-STEP ANALYSIS OF ACID-BASE STATUS

Step 1: Determine the primary (or main) disorder—whether it is metabolic or respiratory—from blood pH, HCO_3^-, and P_{CO_2} values.
Step 2: Determine the presence of mixed acid-base disorders by calculating the range of compensatory responses (see Table 21–12).
Step 3: Calculate the anion gap (see Table 21–13).
Step 4: Calculate the corrected HCO_3^- concentration if the anion gap is increased (see above).
Step 5: Examine the patient to determine whether the clinical signs are compatible with the acid-base analysis.

Table 21–12. Primary acid-base disorders and expected compensation.

Disorder	Primary Defect	Compensatory Response	Magnitude of Compensation
Respiratory acidosis			
Acute	$\uparrow PCO_2$	$\uparrow HCO_3^-$	$\uparrow HCO_3^-$ 1 mEq/L per 10 mm Hg $\uparrow PCO_2$
Chronic	$\uparrow PCO_2$	$\uparrow HCO_3^-$	$\uparrow HCO_3^-$ 3.5 mEq/L per 10 mm Hg $\uparrow PCO_2$
Respiratory alkalosis			
Acute	$\downarrow PCO_2$	$\downarrow HCO_3^-$	$\downarrow HCO_3^-$ 2 mEq/L per 10 mm Hg $\downarrow PCO_2$
Chronic	$\downarrow PCO_2$	$\downarrow HCO_3^-$	$\downarrow HCO_3^-$ 5 mEq/L per 10 mm Hg $\downarrow PCO_2$
Metabolic acidosis	$\downarrow HCO_3^-$	$\downarrow PCO_2$	$\downarrow PCO_2$ 1.3 mm Hg per 1 mEq/L $\downarrow HCO_3^-$
Metabolic alkalosis	$\uparrow HCO_3^-$	$\uparrow PCO_2$	$\uparrow PCO_2$ 0.7 mm Hg per 1 mEq/L $\uparrow HCO_3^-$

The anion gap should always be calculated for two reasons. First, it is possible to have an abnormal anion gap even if the sodium, chloride, and bicarbonate concentrations are normal. Second, an anion gap larger than 20 mEq/L suggests a primary metabolic acid-base disturbance regardless of the pH or serum bicarbonate level because a markedly abnormal anion gap is never a compensatory response to a respiratory disorder. In patients with an increased anion gap metabolic acidosis, clinicians should calculate the corrected bicarbonate. In increased anion gap acidoses, there should be a mole for mole decrease in HCO_3^- as the anion gap increases. A corrected HCO_3^- value higher or lower than normal (24 mEq/L) indicates the concomitant presence of metabolic alkalosis or normal anion gap metabolic acidosis, respectively.

Berend K et al. Physiological approach to assessment of acid-base disturbances. N Engl J Med. 2014 Oct 9;371(15): 1434–45. Erratum in: N Engl J Med. 2014 Nov 13;371(20):1948. [PMID: 25295502]
Seifter JL. Integration of acid-base and electrolyte disorders. N Engl J Med. 2014 Nov 6;371(19):1821–31. [PMID: 25372090]
Wiener SW. Toxicologic acid-base disorders. Emerg Med Clin North Am. 2014 Feb;32(1):149–65. [PMID: 24275173]

METABOLIC ACIDOSIS

ESSENTIALS OF DIAGNOSIS

▶ Decreased HCO_3^- with acidemia.

▶ Classified into increased anion gap acidosis and normal anion gap acidosis.

▶ Lactic acidosis, ketoacidosis, and toxins produce metabolic acidoses with the largest anion gaps.

▶ Normal anion gap acidosis is mainly caused by gastrointestinal HCO_3^- loss or RTA. Urinary anion gap may help distinguish between these causes.

▶ General Considerations

The hallmark of metabolic acidosis is decreased HCO_3^-. Metabolic acidoses are classified by the anion gap, usually normal or increased (Table 21–13). The anion gap is the difference between readily measured anions and cations.

In plasma,

$$Na^+ + \frac{Unmeasured}{cations} = (HCO_3^- + Cl^-) + \frac{Unmeasured}{anions}$$

$$Anion\ gap = Na^+ - (HCO_3^- + Cl^-)$$

Table 21–13. Anion gap in metabolic acidosis.[1]

Decreased (< 6 mEq)
Hypoalbuminemia (decreased unmeasured anion)
Plasma cell dyscrasias
Monoclonal protein (cationic paraprotein) (accompanied by chloride and bicarbonate)
Bromide intoxication
Increased (> 12 mEq)
Metabolic anion
Diabetic ketoacidosis
Alcoholic ketoacidosis
Lactic acidosis
Chronic kidney disease (advanced stages) (PO_4^{3-}, SO_4^{2-})
Starvation
Metabolic alkalosis (increased number of negative charges on protein)
5-oxoproline acidosis from acetaminophen toxicity
Drug or chemical anion
Salicylate intoxication
Sodium carbenicillin therapy
Methanol (formic acid)
Ethylene glycol (oxalic acid)
Normal (6–12 mEq)
Loss of HCO_3
Diarrhea
Recovery from diabetic ketoacidosis
Pancreatic fluid loss, ileostomy (unadapted)
Carbonic anhydrase inhibitors
Chloride retention
Renal tubular acidosis
Ileal loop bladder
Administration of HCl equivalent or NH_4Cl
Arginine and lysine in parenteral nutrition

[1]Reference ranges for anion gap may vary based on differing laboratory methods.

Major unmeasured cations are calcium (2 mEq/L), magnesium (2 mEq/L), gamma-globulins, and potassium (4 mEq/L). Major unmeasured anions are albumin (2 mEq/L per g/dL), phosphate (2 mEq/L), sulfate (1 mEq/L), lactate (1–2 mEq/L), and other organic anions (3–4 mEq/L). Traditionally, the normal anion gap has been 12 ± 4 mEq/L. With current auto-analyzers, the reference range may be lower (6 ± 1 mEq/L), primarily from an increase in Cl^- values. Despite its usefulness, the anion gap can be misleading. Non–acid-base disorders may cause errors in anion gap interpretation; these disorders include hypoalbuminemia, hypernatremia, or hyponatremia; antibiotics (eg, carbenicillin is an unmeasured anion; polymyxin is an unmeasured cation) may also cause errors in anion gap interpretation. Although not usually associated with metabolic acidosis, a decreased anion gap can occur because of a reduction in unmeasured anions or an increase in unmeasured cations. In hypoalbuminemia, a 2 mEq/L decrease in anion gap will occur for every 1 g/dL decline in serum albumin.

INCREASED ANION GAP ACIDOSIS (Increased Unmeasured Anions)

Normochloremic metabolic acidosis generally results from addition of organic acids such as lactate, acetoacetate, beta-hydroxybutyrate, and exogenous toxins. Other anions such as isocitrate, alpha-ketoglutarate, malate and d-lactate, may contribute to the anion gap of lactic acidosis, DKA, and acidosis of unknown etiology. Uremia causes an increased anion gap metabolic acidosis from unexcreted organic acids and anions.

A. Lactic Acidosis

Lactic acid is formed from pyruvate in anaerobic glycolysis, typically in tissues with high rates of glycolysis, such as gut (responsible for over 50% of lactate production), skeletal muscle, brain, skin, and erythrocytes. Normally, lactate levels remain low (1 mEq/L) because of metabolism of lactate principally by the liver through gluconeogenesis or oxidation via the Krebs cycle. The kidneys metabolize about 30% of lactate.

In lactic acidosis, lactate levels are at least 4–5 mEq/L but commonly 10–30 mEq/L. There are two basic types of lactic acidosis.

Type A (hypoxic) lactic acidosis is more common, resulting from decreased tissue perfusion; cardiogenic, septic, or hemorrhagic shock; and carbon monoxide or cyanide poisoning. These conditions increase peripheral lactic acid production and decrease hepatic metabolism of lactate as liver perfusion declines.

Type B lactic acidosis may be due to metabolic causes (eg, diabetes, ketoacidosis, liver disease, kidney disease, infection, leukemia, or lymphoma) or toxins (eg, ethanol, methanol, salicylates, isoniazid, or metformin). Propylene glycol can cause lactic acidosis from decreased liver metabolism; it is used as a vehicle for intravenous drugs, such as nitroglycerin, etomidate, and diazepam. Parenteral nutrition without thiamine causes severe refractory lactic acidosis from deranged pyruvate metabolism. Patients with short bowel syndrome may develop d-lactic acidosis with encephalopathy due to carbohydrate malabsorption and subsequent fermentation by colonic bacteria. Nucleoside analog reverse transcriptase inhibitors can cause type B lactic acidosis due to mitochondrial toxicity.

Idiopathic lactic acidosis, usually in debilitated patients, has an extremely high mortality rate. (For treatment of lactic acidosis, see below and Chapter 27.)

B. Diabetic Ketoacidosis (DKA)

DKA is characterized by hyperglycemia and metabolic acidosis with an increased anion gap:

$$H^+ + B^- + NaHCO_3 \leftrightarrow CO_2 + NaB + H_2O$$

where B^- is beta-hydroxybutyrate or acetoacetate, the ketones responsible for the increased anion gap. The anion gap should be calculated from the measured serum electrolytes; correction of the serum sodium for the dilutional effect of hyperglycemia will exaggerate the anion gap. Diabetics with ketoacidosis may have lactic acidosis from tissue hypoperfusion and increased anaerobic metabolism.

During the recovery phase of DKA, a hyperchloremic non-anion gap acidosis can develop because saline resuscitation results in chloride retention, restoration of GFR, and ketoaciduria. Ketone salts (NaB) are formed as bicarbonate is consumed:

$$HB + NaHCO_3 \rightarrow NaB + H_2CO_3$$

The kidney reabsorbs ketone anions poorly but can compensate for the loss of anions by increasing the reabsorption of Cl^-.

Patients with DKA and normal kidney function may have marked ketonuria and severe metabolic acidosis but only a mildly increased anion gap. Thus, the size of the anion gap correlates poorly with the severity of the DKA; the urinary loss of Na^+ or K^+ salts of beta-hydroxybutyrate will lower the anion gap without altering the H^+ excretion or the severity of the acidosis. Urine dipsticks for ketones test primarily for acetoacetate and, to a lesser degree, acetone but not the predominant ketoacid, beta-hydroxybutyrate. Dipstick tests for ketones may become more positive even as the patient improves due to the metabolism of beta-hydroxybutyrate. Thus, the patient's clinical status and pH are better markers of improvement than the anion gap or ketone levels.

C. Alcoholic Ketoacidosis

Chronically malnourished patients who consume large quantities of alcohol daily may develop alcoholic ketoacidosis. Most of these patients have mixed acid–base disorders (10% have a triple acid–base disorder). Although decreased HCO_3^- is usual, 50% of the patients may have normal or alkalemic pH. Three types of metabolic acidosis are seen in alcoholic ketoacidosis: (1) Ketoacidosis is due to beta-hydroxybutyrate and acetoacetate excess. (2) Lactic acidosis: Alcohol metabolism increases the NADH:NAD ratio, causing increased production and decreased utilization of lactate. Accompanying thiamine deficiency, which inhibits pyruvate carboxylase, further enhances lactic acid production in many cases. Moderate to severe elevations of lactate (greater than 6 mmol/L) are seen with concomitant disorders such as sepsis, pancreatitis, or hypoglycemia. (3) Hyperchloremic acidosis from bicarbonate loss in the urine is associated with ketonuria (see above). Metabolic alkalosis occurs from volume contraction and vomiting. Respiratory alkalosis results from alcohol withdrawal, pain, or associated disorders such as sepsis or liver disease. Half of the patients have hypoglycemia or hyperglycemia. When serum glucose levels are greater than 250 mg/dL (13.88 mmol/L), the distinction from DKA is difficult. The absence of a diabetic history and normoglycemia after initial therapy support the diagnosis of alcoholic ketoacidosis.

D. Toxins

(See also Chapter 38.) Multiple toxins and drugs increase the anion gap by increasing endogenous acid production. Common examples include methanol (metabolized to formic acid), ethylene glycol (glycolic and oxalic acid), and salicylates (salicylic acid and lactic acid). The latter can cause a mixed disorder of metabolic acidosis with respiratory alkalosis. In toluene poisoning, the metabolite hippurate is rapidly excreted by the kidney and may present as a normal anion gap acidosis. Isopropanol, which is metabolized to acetone, increases the osmolar gap, but not the anion gap.

E. Uremic Acidosis

As the GFR drops below 15–30 mL/min, the kidneys are increasingly unable to synthesize NH_3. The reduced excretion of H^+ and organic acids (eg, phosphate and sulfate) as NH_4Cl results in an increased anion gap metabolic acidosis.

NORMAL ANION GAP ACIDOSIS

The two major causes are gastrointestinal HCO_3^- loss and defects in renal acidification (renal tubular acidosis) (Table 21–14). The urinary anion gap can differentiate between these causes.

A. Gastrointestinal HCO_3^- Loss

The gastrointestinal tract secretes bicarbonate at multiple sites. Small bowel and pancreatic secretions contain large amounts of HCO_3^-; massive diarrhea or pancreatic drainage can result in HCO_3^- loss. Hyperchloremia occurs because the ileum and colon secrete HCO_3^- in exchange for Cl^- by countertransport. The resultant volume contraction causes increased Cl^- retention by the kidney in the setting of decreased HCO_3^-. Patients with ureterosigmoidostomies can develop hyperchloremic metabolic acidosis because the colon secretes HCO_3^- in the urine in exchange for Cl^-.

B. Renal Tubular Acidosis (RTA)

Hyperchloremic acidosis with a normal anion gap and normal (or near normal) GFR, and in the absence of diarrhea, defines RTA. The defect is either inability to excrete H^+ (inadequate generation of new HCO_3^-) or inappropriate reabsorption of HCO_3^-. Three major types can be differentiated by the clinical setting, urinary pH, urinary anion gap, and serum K^+ level. The pathophysiologic mechanisms of RTA have been elucidated by identifying the responsible molecules and gene mutations.

1. Classic distal RTA (type I)—This disorder is characterized by selective deficiency in H^+ secretion in alpha intercalated cells in the collecting tubule. Despite acidosis, urinary pH cannot be acidified and is above 5.5, which retards the binding of H^+ to phosphate ($H^+ + HPO_4^{2-} \rightarrow H_2PO_4$) and inhibits titratable acid excretion. Furthermore, urinary excretion of $NH_4^+Cl^-$ is decreased, and the urinary anion gap is positive. Enhanced K^+ excretion occurs probably because there is less competition from H^+ in the distal nephron transport system. Furthermore, hyperaldosteronism occurs in response to renal salt wasting, which will increase potassium excretion. Nephrocalcinosis and nephrolithiasis are often seen in patients with distal RTA since chronic acidosis decreases tubular calcium reabsorption. Hypercalciuria, alkaline urine, and lowered level of urinary

Table 21–14. Hyperchloremic, normal anion gap metabolic acidoses.

	Renal Defect	Serum [K+]	Distal H+ Secretion			Treatment
			Urinary NH₄⁺ Plus Minimal Urine pH	Titratable Acid	Urinary Anion Gap	
Gastrointestinal HCO_3^- loss	None	↓	< 5.5	↑↑	Negative	Na⁺, K⁺, and HCO_3^- as required
Renal tubular acidosis						
I. Classic distal	Distal H⁺ secretion	↓	> 5.5	↓	Positive	$NaHCO_3$ (1–3 mEq/kg/day)
II. Proximal secretion	Proximal H⁺	↓	< 5.5	Normal	Positive	$NaHCO_3$ or $KHCO_3$ (10–15 mEq/kg/day), thiazide
IV. Hyporeninemic hypoaldosteronism	Distal Na⁺ reabsorption, K⁺ secretion, and H⁺ secretion	↑	< 5.5	↓	Positive	Fludrocortisone (0.1–0.5 mg/day), dietary K⁺ restriction, furosemide (40–160 mg/day), $NaHCO_3$ (1–3 mEq/kg/day)

Modified and reproduced, with permission, from Cogan MG. *Fluid and Electrolytes: Physiology and Pathophysiology.* McGraw-Hill, 1991.

citrate cause calcium phosphate stones and nephrocalcinosis. Distal RTA develops as a consequence of paraproteinemias, autoimmune disease, and drugs and toxins such as amphotericin.

2. Proximal RTA (type II)—Proximal RTA is due to a selective defect in the proximal tubule's ability to reabsorb filtered HCO_3^-. Carbonic anhydrase inhibitors (acetazolamide) can cause proximal RTA. About 90% of filtered HCO_3^- is absorbed by the proximal tubule. A proximal defect in HCO_3^- reabsorption will overwhelm the distal tubule's limited capacity to reabsorb HCO_3^-, resulting in bicarbonaturia and metabolic acidosis. Distal delivery of HCO_3^- declines as the plasma HCO_3^- level decreases. When the plasma HCO_3^- level drops to 15–18 mEq/L, the distal nephron can reabsorb the diminished filtered load of HCO_3^-. Bicarbonaturia resolves, and the urinary pH can be acidic. Thiazide-induced volume contraction can be used to enhance proximal HCO_3^- reabsorption, leading to the decrease in distal HCO_3^- delivery and improvement of bicarbonaturia and renal acidification. The increased delivery of HCO_3^- to the distal nephron increases K^+ secretion, and hypokalemia results if a patient is loaded with excess HCO_3^- and K^+ is not adequately supplemented. Proximal RTA can exist with other proximal reabsorption defects, such as Fanconi syndrome, resulting in glucosuria, aminoaciduria, phosphaturia, and uricosuria. Causes include multiple myeloma and nephrotoxic drugs.

3. Hyporeninemic hypoaldosteronemic RTA (type IV)—Type IV is the most common RTA in clinical practice. The defect is aldosterone deficiency or antagonism, which impairs distal nephron Na^+ reabsorption and K^+ and H^+ excretion. Renal salt wasting and hyperkalemia are frequently present. Common causes are diabetic nephropathy, tubulointerstitial renal diseases, hypertensive nephrosclerosis, and AIDS. In patients with these disorders, drugs, such as ACE inhibitors, spironolactone, and NSAIDs, can exacerbate the hyperkalemia.

C. Dilutional Acidosis

Rapid dilution of plasma volume by 0.9% NaCl may cause hyperchloremic acidosis.

D. Recovery from DKA

See Increased Anion Gap Acidosis (Increased Unmeasured Anions).

E. Posthypocapnia

In prolonged respiratory alkalosis, HCO_3^- decreases and Cl^- increases from decreased renal $NH_4^+Cl^-$ excretion. If the respiratory alkalosis is corrected quickly, HCO_3^- will remain low until the kidneys can generate new HCO_3^-, which generally takes several days. In the meantime, the increased PCO_2 with low HCO_3^- causes metabolic acidosis.

F. Hyperalimentation

Hyperalimentation fluids may contain amino acid solutions that acidify when metabolized, such as arginine hydrochloride and lysine hydrochloride.

Assessment of Hyperchloremic Metabolic Acidosis by Urinary Anion Gap

Increased renal $NH_4^+Cl^-$ excretion to enhance H^+ removal is the normal physiologic response to metabolic acidosis. The daily urinary excretion of NH_4Cl can be increased from 30 mEq to 200 mEq in response to acidosis.

The urinary anion gap ($Na^+ + K^+ - Cl^-$) reflects the ability of the kidney to excrete NH_4Cl. The urinary anion gap differentiates between gastrointestinal and renal causes of hyperchloremic acidosis. If the cause is gastrointestinal HCO_3^- loss (diarrhea), renal acidification remains normal and NH_4Cl excretion increases, and the urinary anion gap is negative. If the cause is distal RTA, the urinary anion gap is positive, since the basic lesion in the disorder is the inability of the kidney to excrete H^+ as NH_4Cl. In proximal (type II) RTA, the kidney has defective HCO_3^- reabsorption, leading to increased HCO_3^- excretion rather than decreased NH_4Cl excretion; the urinary anion gap is often negative.

Urinary pH may not readily differentiate between the two causes. Despite acidosis, if volume depletion from diarrhea causes inadequate Na^+ delivery to the distal nephron and therefore decreased exchange with H^+, urinary pH may not be lower than 5.3. In the presence of this relatively high urinary pH, however, H^+ excretion continues due to buffering of NH_3 to NH_4^+, since the pK of this reaction is as high as 9.1. Potassium depletion, which can accompany diarrhea (and surreptitious laxative abuse), may also impair renal acidification. Thus, when volume depletion is present, the urinary anion gap is a better measure of ability to acidify the urine than urinary pH.

When large amounts of other anions are present in the urine, the urinary anion gap may not be reliable. In such a situation, NH_4^+ excretion can be estimated using the urinary osmolar gap.

$$NH_4^+ \text{ excretion (mmol/L)} = 0.5 \times \text{Urinary osmolar gap}$$
$$= 0.5 \text{ [U Osm} - 2(\text{U Na}^+ + \text{U K}^+) + \text{U urea} + \text{U glucose]}$$

where urine concentrations and osmolality are in mmol/L.

Clinical Findings

A. Symptoms and Signs

Symptoms of metabolic acidosis are mainly those of the underlying disorder. Compensatory hyperventilation is an important clinical sign and may be misinterpreted as a primary respiratory disorder; Kussmaul breathing (deep, regular, sighing respirations) may be seen with severe metabolic acidosis.

B. Laboratory Findings

Blood pH, serum HCO_3^-, and PCO_2 are decreased. Anion gap may be normal (hyperchloremic) or increased (normochloremic). Hyperkalemia may be seen.

Treatment

A. Increased Anion Gap Acidosis

Treatment is aimed at the underlying disorder, such as insulin and fluid therapy for diabetes and appropriate volume resuscitation to restore tissue perfusion. The metabolism of lactate will produce HCO_3^- and increase pH. Supplemental HCO_3^- is indicated for treatment of hyperkalemia (see Table 21–6) and some forms of normal anion gap acidosis but has been controversial for treatment of increased anion gap metabolic acidosis with respect to efficacy and safety. Large amounts of HCO_3^- may have deleterious effects, including hypernatremia, hyperosmolality, volume overload, and worsening of intracellular acidosis.

In addition, alkali administration stimulates phosphofructokinase activity, thus exacerbating lactic acidosis via enhanced lactate production. Ketogenesis is also augmented by alkali therapy.

In salicylate intoxication, alkali therapy must be started to decrease central nervous system damage unless blood pH is already alkalinized by respiratory alkalosis, since an increased pH converts salicylate to more impermeable salicylic acid. In alcoholic ketoacidosis, thiamine should be given with glucose to avoid Wernicke encephalopathy. The bicarbonate deficit can be calculated as follows:

$$HCO_3^- \text{ deficit} = 0.5 \times \text{body weight in kg} \times (24 - HCO_3^-)$$

Half of the calculated deficit should be administered within the first 3–4 hours to avoid overcorrection and volume overload. In methanol intoxication, inhibition of alcohol dehydrogenase by fomepizole is standard care. Ethanol had previously been used as a competitive substrate for alcohol dehydrogenase, which metabolizes to formaldehyde.

B. Normal Anion Gap Acidosis

Treatment of RTA is mainly achieved by administration of alkali (either as bicarbonate or citrate) to correct metabolic abnormalities and prevent nephrocalcinosis and CKD.

Large amounts of oral alkali (10–15 mEq/kg/day) (Table 21–14) may be required to treat proximal RTA because most of the alkali is excreted into the urine, which exacerbates hypokalemia. Thus, a mixture of sodium and potassium salts is preferred. Thiazides may reduce the amount of alkali required, but hypokalemia may develop. Treatment of type 1 distal RTA requires less alkali (1–3 mEq/kg/day) than proximal RTA. Potassium supplementation may be necessary.

For type IV RTA, dietary potassium restriction may be necessary and potassium-retaining drugs should be withdrawn. Fludrocortisone may be effective in cases with hypoaldosteronism, but should be used with care, preferably in combination with loop diuretics. In some cases, oral alkali supplementation (1–3 mEq/kg/day) may be required.

▶ When to Refer

Most clinicians will refer patients with renal tubular acidoses to a nephrologist for evaluation and possible alkali therapy.

▶ When to Admit

Patients will require emergency department evaluation or hospital admission depending on the severity of the acidosis and underlying conditions.

Emmett M. Acetaminophen toxicity and 5-oxoproline (pyroglutamic acid): a tale of two cycles, one an ATP-depleting futile cycle and the other a useful cycle. Clin J Am Soc Nephrol. 2014 Jan;9(1):191–200. [PMID: 24235282]

Kamel KS et al. Acid-base problems in diabetic ketoacidosis. N Engl J Med. 2015 Feb 5;372(6):546–54. [PMID: 25651248]

Kraut JA et al. Lactic acidosis. N Engl J Med. 2014 Dec 11; 371(24):2309–19. [PMID: 25494270]

Kraut JA et al. The serum anion gap in the evaluation of acid-base disorders: what are its limitations and can its effectiveness be improved? Clin J Am Soc Nephrol. 2013 Nov;8(11): 2018–24. [PMID: 23833313]

Palmer BF et al. Electrolyte and acid-base disturbances in patients with diabetes mellitus. N Engl J Med. 2015 Aug 6; 373(6):548–59. [PMID: 26244308]

Rice M et al. Approach to metabolic acidosis in the emergency department. Emerg Med Clin North Am. 2014 May;32(2): 403–20. [PMID: 24766940]

Vichot AA et al. Use of anion gap in the evaluation of a patient with metabolic acidosis. Am J Kidney Dis. 2014 Oct;64(4): 653–7. [PMID: 25132207]

METABOLIC ALKALOSIS

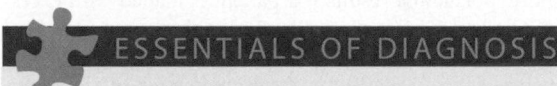 ESSENTIALS OF DIAGNOSIS

▶ High HCO_3^- with alkalemia.

▶ Evaluate effective circulating volume by physical examination.

▶ Check urinary chloride concentration to differentiate saline-responsive alkalosis from saline-unresponsive alkalosis.

▶ Classification

Metabolic alkalosis is characterized by high HCO_3^-. Abnormalities that generate HCO_3^- are called "initiation factors," whereas abnormalities that promote renal conservation of HCO_3^- are called "maintenance factors." Thus, metabolic alkalosis may remain even after the initiation factors have resolved.

The causes of metabolic alkalosis are classified into two groups based on "saline responsiveness" using the urine Cl^- as a marker for volume status (Table 21–15). Saline-responsive metabolic alkalosis is a sign of extracellular volume contraction, and saline-unresponsive alkalosis implies excessive total body bicarbonate with either euvolemia or hypervolemia. The compensatory increase in PCO_2 rarely exceeds 55 mm Hg; higher PCO_2 values imply a superimposed primary respiratory acidosis.

A. Saline-Responsive Metabolic Alkalosis

Much more common than saline-unresponsive alkalosis, saline-responsive alkalosis is characterized by normotensive extracellular volume contraction and hypokalemia. Hypotension and orthostasis may be seen. In vomiting or nasogastric suction, loss of acid (HCl) initiates the

Table 21–15. Metabolic alkalosis.

Saline-Responsive (U_{Cl} < 25 mEq/L)	Saline-Unresponsive (U_{Cl} > 40 mEq/L)

Excessive body bicarbonate content
Renal alkalosis
  Diuretic therapy
  Poorly reabsorbable anion therapy: carbenicillin,
    penicillin, sulfate, phosphate
  Posthypercapnia
Gastrointestinal alkalosis
  Loss of HCl from vomiting or nasogastric suction
  Intestinal alkalosis: chloride diarrhea
  NaHCO$_3$ (baking soda)
  Sodium citrate, lactate, gluconate, acetate
  Transfusions
  Antacids
Normal body bicarbonate content
  "Contraction alkalosis"
	Excessive body bicarbonate content
	Renal alkalosis
	  Normotensive
	    Bartter syndrome (renal salt wasting and secondary
	      hyperaldosteronism)
	    Severe potassium depletion
	    Refeeding alkalosis
	    Hypercalcemia and hypoparathyroidism
	Hypertensive
	  Endogenous mineralocorticoids
	    Primary aldosteronism
	    Hyperreninism
	    Adrenal enzyme (11-beta-hydroxylase and 17-alpha-hydroxylase)
	      deficiency
	    Liddle syndrome
	  Exogenous alkali
	  Exogenous mineralocorticoids
	  Licorice

Modified and reproduced, with permission, from Narins RG et al. Diagnostic strategies in disorders of fluid, electrolyte and acid-base homeostasis. Am J Med. 1982 Mar;72(3):496–520.

alkalosis, but volume contraction from Cl⁻ loss maintains the alkalosis because the kidney avidly reabsorbs Na⁺ to restore the ECF. Increased sodium reabsorption necessitates increased HCO$_3$⁻ reabsorption proximally, and the urinary pH remains acidic despite alkalemia (paradoxical aciduria). Renal Cl⁻ reabsorption is high, and urine Cl⁻ is low (less than 10–20 mEq/L). In alkalosis, bicarbonaturia may force Na⁺ excretion as the accompanying cation even if volume depletion is present. Therefore, urine Cl⁻ is preferred to urine Na⁺ as a measure of extracellular volume. Diuretics may limit the utility of urine chloride by increasing urine chloride and sodium excretion, even in the setting of volume contraction.

Metabolic alkalosis is generally associated with hypokalemia due to the direct effect of alkalosis on renal potassium excretion and secondary hyperaldosteronism from volume depletion. Hypokalemia exacerbates the metabolic alkalosis by increasing bicarbonate reabsorption in the proximal tubule and hydrogen ion secretion in the distal tubule. Administration of KCl will correct the disorder.

1. Contraction alkalosis—Diuretics decrease extracellular volume from urinary loss of NaCl and water. The plasma HCO$_3$⁻ concentration increases because the extracellular fluid volume contracts around a stable total body bicarbonate. Contraction alkalosis is the opposite of dilutional acidosis.

2. Posthypercapnia alkalosis—In chronic respiratory acidosis, the kidney decreases bicarbonate excretion, increasing plasma HCO$_3$ concentration (see Table 21–12). Hypercapnia directly affects the proximal tubule to decrease NaCl reabsorption, which can cause extracellular volume depletion. If PCO_2 is rapidly corrected, metabolic alkalosis will exist until the kidney excretes the retained bicarbonate. Many patients with chronic respiratory acidosis

receive diuretics, which further exacerbates the metabolic alkalosis.

B. Saline-Unresponsive Alkalosis

1. Hyperaldosteronism—Primary hyperaldosteronism causes extracellular volume expansion and hypertension by increasing distal sodium reabsorption. Aldosterone increases H⁺ and K⁺ excretion, producing metabolic alkalosis and hypokalemia. In an attempt to decrease extracellular volume, high levels of NaCl are excreted resulting in a high urine Cl⁻ (greater than 20 mEq/L). Therapy with NaCl will only increase volume expansion and hypertension and will not treat the underlying problem of mineralocorticoid excess.

2. Alkali administration with decreased GFR—The normal kidney has a substantial capacity for bicarbonate excretion, protecting against metabolic alkalosis even with large HCO$_3$⁻ intake. However, urinary excretion of bicarbonate is inadequate in CKD. If large amounts of HCO$_3$⁻ are consumed, as with intensive antacid therapy, metabolic alkalosis will occur. Lactate, citrate, and gluconate can also cause metabolic alkalosis because they are metabolized to bicarbonate. In milk-alkali syndrome, sustained heavy ingestion of absorbable antacids and milk causes hypercalcemic kidney injury and metabolic alkalosis. Volume contraction from renal hypercalcemic effects exacerbates the alkalosis.

▶ Clinical Findings

A. Symptoms and Signs

There are no characteristic symptoms or signs. Orthostatic hypotension may be encountered. Concomitant hypokalemia may cause weakness and hyporeflexia. Tetany and neuromuscular irritability occur rarely.

B. Laboratory Findings

The arterial blood pH and bicarbonate are elevated. With respiratory compensation, the arterial P_{CO_2} is increased. Serum potassium and chloride are decreased. There may be an increased anion gap. The urine chloride can differentiate between saline-responsive (less than 25 mEq/L) and unresponsive (greater than 40 mEq/L) causes.

▶ Treatment

Mild alkalosis is generally well tolerated. Severe or symptomatic alkalosis (pH > 7.60) requires urgent treatment.

A. Saline-Responsive Metabolic Alkalosis

Therapy for saline-responsive metabolic alkalosis is correction of the extracellular volume deficit with isotonic saline. Diuretics should be discontinued. H_2-blockers or proton pump inhibitors may be helpful in patients with alkalosis from nasogastric suctioning. If pulmonary or cardiovascular disease prohibits adequate resuscitation, acetazolamide will increase renal bicarbonate excretion. Hypokalemia may develop because bicarbonate excretion may induce kaliuresis. Severe cases, especially those with reduced kidney function, may require dialysis with low-bicarbonate dialysate.

B. Saline-Unresponsive Metabolic Alkalosis

Therapy for saline-unresponsive metabolic alkalosis includes surgical removal of a mineralocorticoid-producing tumor and blockage of aldosterone effect with an ACE inhibitor or with spironolactone (see Chapter 26). Metabolic alkalosis in primary aldosteronism can be treated only with potassium repletion.

Feldman M et al. Respiratory compensation to a primary metabolic alkalosis in humans. Clin Nephrol. 2012 Nov;78(5):365–9. [PMID: 22854166]
Peixoto AJ et al. Treatment of severe metabolic alkalosis in a patient with congestive heart failure. Am J Kidney Dis. 2013 May;61(5):822–7. [PMID: 23481366]
Soifer JT et al. Approach to metabolic alkalosis. Emerg Med Clin North Am. 2014 May;32(2):453–63. [PMID: 24766943]
Yi JH et al. Metabolic alkalosis from unsuspected ingestion: use of urine pH and anion gap. Am J Kidney Dis. 2012 Apr;59(4):577–81. [PMID: 22265393]

RESPIRATORY ACIDOSIS (HYPERCAPNIA)

Respiratory acidosis results from hypoventilation and subsequent hypercapnia. Pulmonary and extrapulmonary disorders can cause hypoventilation.

Acute respiratory failure is associated with severe acidosis and only a small increase in the plasma bicarbonate. After 6–12 hours, the primary increase in P_{CO_2} evokes a renal compensation to excrete more acid and to generate more HCO_3^-; complete metabolic compensation by the kidney takes several days.

Chronic respiratory acidosis is generally seen in patients with underlying lung disease, such as chronic obstructive pulmonary disease. Renal excretion of acid as NH_4Cl results in hypochloremia. When chronic respiratory acidosis is corrected suddenly, posthypercapnic metabolic alkalosis ensues until the kidneys excrete the excess bicarbonate over 2–3 days.

▶ Clinical Findings

A. Symptoms and Signs

With acute onset, somnolence, confusion, mental status changes, asterixis, and myoclonus may develop. Severe hypercapnia increases cerebral blood flow, cerebrospinal fluid pressure, and intracranial pressure; papilledema and pseudotumor cerebri may be seen.

B. Laboratory Findings

Arterial pH is low and P_{CO_2} is increased. Serum HCO_3^- is elevated but does not fully correct the pH. If the disorder is chronic, hypochloremia is seen. Respiratory etiologies of respiratory acidosis usually have a wide A-a gradient; a relatively normal A-a gradient suggests a nonpulmonary (eg, central) etiology.

▶ Treatment

If opioid overdose is a possible diagnosis or there is no other obvious cause for hypoventilation, the clinician should consider a diagnostic and therapeutic trial of intravenous naloxone (see Chapter 38). In all forms of respiratory acidosis, treatment is directed at the underlying disorder to improve ventilation.

Adrogué HJ. Diagnosis and management of severe respiratory acidosis. Am J Kidney Dis. 2010 Nov;56(5):994–1000. [PMID: 20673604]
Bruno CM et al. Acid-base disorders in patients with chronic obstructive pulmonary disease: a pathophysiological review. J Biomed Biotechnol. 2012;2012:915150. [PMID: 22500110]
Chebbo A et al. Hypoventilation syndromes. Med Clin North Am. 2011 Nov;95(6):1189–202. [PMID: 22032434]
Schwartzstein RM et al. Rising PaCO2 in the ICU: using a physiologic approach to avoid cognitive biases. Chest. 2011 Dec;140(6):1638–42. [PMID: 22147823]

RESPIRATORY ALKALOSIS (HYPOCAPNIA)

Respiratory alkalosis occurs when hyperventilation reduces the P_{CO_2}, increasing serum pH. The most common cause of respiratory alkalosis is hyperventilation syndrome (Table 21–16), but bacterial septicemia and cirrhosis are other common causes. In pregnancy, progesterone stimulates the respiratory center, producing an average P_{CO_2} of 30 mm Hg and respiratory alkalosis. Symptoms of acute respiratory alkalosis are related to decreased cerebral blood flow induced by the disorder.

Determination of appropriate metabolic compensation may reveal an associated metabolic disorder (see Mixed Acid-Base Disorders).

As in respiratory acidosis, the metabolic compensation is greater if the respiratory alkalosis is chronic (see Table 21–12). Although serum HCO_3^- is frequently less than 15 mEq/L in metabolic acidosis, such a low level in respiratory alkalosis is unusual and may represent a concomitant primary metabolic acidosis.

Table 21–16. Causes of respiratory alkalosis.

Hypoxia
Decreased inspired oxygen tension
High altitude
Ventilation/perfusion inequality
Hypotension
Severe anemia
CNS-mediated disorders
Voluntary hyperventilation
Anxiety-hyperventilation syndrome
Neurologic disease
Cerebrovascular accident (infarction, hemorrhage)
Infection
Trauma
Tumor
Pharmacologic and hormonal stimulation
Salicylates
Nicotine
Xanthines
Pregnancy (progesterone)
Hepatic failure
Gram-negative septicemia
Recovery from metabolic acidosis
Heat exposure
Pulmonary disease
Interstitial lung disease
Pneumonia
Pulmonary embolism
Pulmonary edema
Mechanical overventilation

Adapted, with permission, from Gennari FJ. Respiratory acidosis and alkalosis. In: *Maxwell and Kleeman's Clinical Disorders of Fluid and Electrolyte Metabolism,* 5th ed. Narins RG (editor). McGraw-Hill, 1994.

► Clinical Findings

A. Symptoms and Signs

In acute cases (hyperventilation), there is light-headedness, anxiety, perioral numbness, and paresthesias. Tetany occurs from a low ionized calcium, since severe alkalosis increases calcium binding to albumin.

B. Laboratory Findings

Arterial blood pH is elevated, and P_{CO_2} is low. Serum bicarbonate is decreased in chronic respiratory alkalosis.

► Treatment

Treatment is directed toward the underlying cause. In acute hyperventilation syndrome from anxiety, the traditional treatment of breathing into a paper bag should be discouraged because it does not correct P_{CO_2} and may decrease P_{O_2}. Reassurance may be sufficient for the anxious patient, but sedation may be necessary if the process persists. Hyperventilation is usually self-limited since muscle weakness caused by the respiratory alkalemia will suppress ventilation. Rapid correction of chronic respiratory alkalosis may result in metabolic acidosis as P_{CO_2} is increased with a previous compensatory decrease in HCO_3^-. The severity of hypocapnia in critically ill patients has been associated with adverse outcomes.

Palmer BF. Evaluation and treatment of respiratory alkalosis. Am J Kidney Dis. 2012 Nov;60(5):834–8. [PMID: 22871240]

▼ FLUID MANAGEMENT

Daily parenteral maintenance fluids and electrolytes for an average adult of 70 kg would include at least 2 L of water in the form of 0.45% saline with 20 mEq/L of potassium chloride. Patients with hypoglycemia, starvation ketosis, or ketoacidosis being treated with insulin may require 5% dextrose-containing solutions. Guidelines for gastrointestinal fluid losses are shown in Table 21–17.

Weight loss or gain is the best indication of water balance. Insensible water loss should be considered in febrile patients. Water loss increases by 100–150 mL/day for each degree of body temperature over 37°C.

In patients requiring maintenance and possibly replacement of fluid and electrolytes by parenteral infusion, the

Table 21–17. Replacement guidelines for sweat and gastrointestinal fluid losses.

	Average Electrolyte Composition					Replacement Guidelines per Liter Lost			
	Na+ (mEq/L)	K+ (mEq/L)	Cl− (mEq/L)	HCO3− (mEq/L)	0.9% Saline (mL)	0.45% Saline (mL)	D5W (mL)	KCl (mEq/L)	7.5% NaHCO3 (45 mEq HCO3−/amp)
Sweat	30–50	5	50			500	500	5	
Gastric secretions	20	10	10			300	700	20	
Pancreatic juice	130	5	35	115		400	600	5	2 amps
Bile	145	5	100	25	600		400	5	0.5 amp
Duodenal fluid	60	15	100	10		1000		15	0.25 amp
Ileal fluid	100	10	60	60		600	400	10	1 amp
Colonic diarrhea	140[1]	10	85	60		1000		10	1 amp

[1]In the absence of diarrhea, colonic fluid Na+ levels are low (40 mEq/L).

total daily ration should be administered continuously over 24 hours to ensure optimal utilization.

If intravenous fluids are the only source of water, electrolytes, and calories for longer than a week, parenteral nutrition containing amino acids, lipids, trace metals, and vitamins may be indicated. (See Chapter 29.)

The ideal resuscitation fluid composition and dose are not established; and there is little evidence that one type of fluid (crystalloid, colloid, or semisynthetic colloid) is superior to or safer than another. Excessive fluid resuscitation and maintenance are complications in hospitalized patients, especially those with critical illness or acute kidney injury, and have been associated with worsened outcomes such as

prolonged mechanical ventilation, dependence on dialysis, and longer hospitalization with increased mortality.

Moritz ML et al. Maintenance intravenous fluids in acutely ill patients. N Engl J Med. 2015 Oct;373(14):1350–60. [PMID: 26422725]

Myburgh JA et al. Resuscitation fluids. N Engl J Med. 2013 Sep 26; 369(13):1243–51. [PMID: 24066745]

Raghunathan K et al. What is the ideal crystalloid? Curr Opin Crit Care. 2015 Aug;21(4):309–14. [PMID: 26103144]

Seymour CW et al. Septic shock: advances in diagnosis and treatment. JAMA. 2015 Aug 18;314(7):708–17. Erratum in: JAMA. 2015 Oct 6;314(13):1404. [PMID: 26284722]

Kidney Disease

22

Suzanne Watnick, MD

Tonja C. Dirkx, MD

Kidney disease can be discovered incidentally during a routine medical evaluation or with evidence of kidney dysfunction, such as hypertension, edema, nausea, or hematuria. The initial approach in both situations should be to assess the cause and severity of renal abnormalities. In all cases, this evaluation includes (1) an estimation of disease duration, (2) a careful urinalysis, and (3) an assessment of the glomerular filtration rate (GFR). The history and physical examinations, though equally important, are variable among renal syndromes—thus, specific symptoms and signs are discussed under each disease entity.

ASSESSMENT OF KIDNEY DISEASE

▶ Disease Duration

Kidney disease may be acute or chronic. Acute kidney injury is worsening of kidney function over hours to days, resulting in the retention of nitrogenous wastes (such as urea nitrogen) and creatinine in the blood. Retention of these substances is called azotemia. Chronic kidney disease (CKD) results from an abnormal loss of kidney function over months to years. Differentiating between the two is important for diagnosis, treatment, and outcome. Oliguria is unusual in CKD. Anemia (from low kidney erythropoietin production) is rare in the initial period of acute kidney injury. Small kidneys are most consistent with CKD, whereas normal to large-size kidneys can be seen with both chronic and acute disease.

▶ Urinalysis

A urinalysis can provide information similar to a kidney biopsy in a way that is cost-effective and noninvasive. The urine is collected in midstream or, if that is not feasible, by bladder catheterization. The urine should be examined within 1 hour after collection to avoid destruction of formed elements. Urinalysis includes a dipstick examination followed by microscopic assessment if the dipstick has positive findings. The dipstick examination measures urinary pH, protein, hemoglobin, glucose, ketones, bilirubin, nitrites, and leukocyte esterase. Urinary specific gravity is often reported. Microscopy provides examination of formed elements—crystals, cells, casts, and infecting organisms.

Various findings on the urinalysis are indicative of certain patterns of kidney disease. A bland (normal) urinary sediment is common, especially in CKD and acute disorders that are not intrinsic to the kidney, such as limited effective blood flow to the kidney or obstruction of the urinary outflow tract. Casts are composed of Tamm-Horsfall urinary mucoprotein in the shape of the nephron segment where they were formed. Heavy proteinuria and lipiduria are consistent with the nephrotic syndrome. The presence of hematuria with dysmorphic red blood cells, red blood cell casts, and proteinuria is indicative of glomerulonephritis. Dysmorphic red blood cells are misshapen during abnormal passage from the capillary through the glomerular basement membrane (GBM) into the urinary space of the Bowman capsule. Pigmented granular casts (also termed "muddy brown casts") and renal tubular epithelial cells alone or in casts suggest acute tubular necrosis. White blood cells, including neutrophils and eosinophils, white blood cell casts (Table 22–1), red blood cells, and small amounts of protein can be found in interstitial nephritis and pyelonephritis; Wright and Hansel stains can detect eosinophiluria. Pyuria alone can indicate a urinary tract infection. Hematuria and proteinuria are discussed more thoroughly below.

A. Proteinuria

Proteinuria is defined as excessive protein excretion in the urine, generally greater than 150–160 mg/24 h in adults. Significant proteinuria is a sign of an underlying kidney abnormality, usually glomerular in origin when more than 1–2 g/day. Less than 1 g/day can be due to multiple causes along the nephron segment, as listed below. Proteinuria can be accompanied by other clinical abnormalities—elevated blood urea nitrogen (BUN) and serum creatinine levels, abnormal urinary sediment, or evidence of systemic illness (eg, fever, rash, vasculitis).

There are several reasons for development of proteinuria: (1) **Functional proteinuria** is a benign process stemming from stressors such as acute illness, exercise, and "orthostatic proteinuria." The latter condition, generally found in people under age 30 years, usually results in urinary protein excretion of less than 1 g/day. The orthostatic nature of the proteinuria is confirmed by measuring an

Table 22–1. Significance of specific urinary casts.

Type	Significance
Hyaline casts	Concentrated urine, febrile disease, after strenuous exercise, in the course of diuretic therapy (not indicative of renal disease)
Red cell casts	Glomerulonephritis
White cell casts	Pyelonephritis, interstitial nephritis (indicative of infection or inflammation)
Renal tubular cell casts	Acute tubular necrosis, interstitial nephritis
Coarse, granular casts	Nonspecific; can represent acute tubular necrosis
Broad, waxy casts	Chronic kidney disease (indicative of stasis in enlarged collecting tubules)

8-hour overnight supine urinary protein excretion, which should be less than 50 mg. (2) **Overload proteinuria** can result from overproduction of circulating, filterable plasma proteins (monoclonal gammopathies), such as Bence Jones proteins associated with multiple myeloma. Urinary protein electrophoresis will exhibit a discrete protein peak. Other examples of overload proteinuria include myoglobinuria in rhabdomyolysis and hemoglobinuria in hemolysis. (3) **Glomerular proteinuria** results from effacement of epithelial cell foot processes and altered glomerular permeability with an increased filtration fraction of normal plasma proteins, as in diabetic nephropathy. Glomerular diseases exhibit some degree of proteinuria. The urinary protein electrophoresis will have a pattern exhibiting a large albumin spike indicative of increased permeability of albumin across a damaged GBM. (4) **Tubular proteinuria** occurs as a result of faulty reabsorption of normally filtered proteins in the proximal tubule, such as beta-2-microglobulin and immunoglobulin light chains. Causes include acute tubular necrosis, toxic injury (lead, aminoglycosides), drug-induced interstitial nephritis, and hereditary metabolic disorders (Wilson disease and Fanconi syndrome).

Evaluation of proteinuria by urinary dipstick primarily detects albumin, while overlooking positively charged light chains of immunoglobulins. These proteins can be detected by the addition of sulfosalicylic acid to the urine specimen. Precipitation without dipstick detection of albumin indicates the presence of paraproteins.

The next step is an estimation of daily urinary protein excretion. The simplest method is to collect a random urine sample. The ratio of urinary protein concentration to urinary creatinine concentration ($[U_{protein}]/[U_{creatinine}]$) correlates with a 24-hour urine protein collection (less than 0.2 is normal and corresponds to excretion of less than 200 mg/24 h). The benefit of a urine protein-to-creatinine ratio is the ease of collection and the lack of error from overcollection or undercollection of urine. In a 24-hour urine collection, a finding of greater than 150–160 mg is abnormal, and greater than 3.5 g is consistent with nephrotic-range proteinuria. If a patient has proteinuria with or without

loss of kidney function, kidney biopsy may be indicated, particularly if the kidney disease is acute in onset. The clinical sequelae of proteinuria are discussed in the section Nephrotic Spectrum Glomerular Diseases below.

B. Hematuria

Hematuria is significant if there are more than three red cells per high-power field on at least two occasions. It is usually detected incidentally by the urine dipstick examination or clinically following an episode of macroscopic hematuria. The diagnosis must be confirmed via microscopic examination, as false-positive dipstick tests can be caused by myoglobin, oxidizing agents, beets and rhubarb, hydrochloric acid, and bacteria. Transient hematuria is common, but in patients younger than 40 years, it is less often of clinical significance due to lower concern for malignancy.

Hematuria may be due to renal or extrarenal causes. Extrarenal causes are addressed in Chapters 23 and 39; most worrisome are urologic malignancies. Renal causes account for approximately 10% of cases and are best considered anatomically as glomerular or extraglomerular. The most common extraglomerular sources include cysts, calculi, interstitial nephritis, and renal neoplasia. Glomerular causes include immunoglobulin A (IgA) nephropathy, thin GBM disease, membranoproliferative glomerulonephritis (MPGN), other hereditary glomerular diseases (eg, Alport syndrome), and systemic nephritic syndromes. Currently, due to insufficient evidence, the United States Preventive Services Task Force gives no recommendation to screen for hematuria to test for bladder cancer in asymptomatic adults. See Chapter 23 for evaluation of hematuria.

▶ **Estimation of GFR**

The GFR provides a useful index of kidney function at the level of the glomerulus. Patients with kidney disease can have a decreased GFR from any process that causes loss of nephron (and thus glomerular) mass. However, they can also have a normal or increased GFR, either from hyperfiltration at the glomerulus or disease at a different segment of the nephron, interstitium, or vascular supply. The GFR measures the amount of plasma ultrafiltered across the glomerular capillaries and correlates with the ability of the kidneys to filter fluids and various substances. Daily GFR in normal individuals is variable, with a range of 150–250 L/24 h or 100–120 mL/min/1.73 m² of body surface area. GFR can be measured indirectly by determining the renal clearance of plasma substances that are not bound to plasma proteins, are freely filterable across the glomerulus, and are neither secreted nor reabsorbed along the renal tubules. The formula used to determine the renal clearance of a substance is

$$C = \frac{U \times \dot{V}}{P}$$

where C is the clearance, U and P are the urine and plasma concentrations of the substance (mg/dL), and $\dot{V}$ is the urine flow rate (mL/min). In clinical practice, the clearance rate of endogenous creatinine, the creatinine clearance, is one way of estimating GFR. Creatinine is a product of muscle metabolism produced at a relatively constant rate and cleared by renal excretion. It is freely filterable by the glomerulus and not reabsorbed by the renal tubules. With stable kidney function, creatinine production and excretion are equal; thus, plasma creatinine concentrations remain constant. However, it is not a perfect indicator of GFR for the following reasons: (1) A small amount is normally eliminated by tubular secretion, and the fraction secreted progressively increases as GFR declines (overestimating GFR); (2) with severe kidney failure, gut microorganisms degrade creatinine; (3) an individual's meat intake and muscle mass affect baseline plasma creatinine levels; (4) commonly used drugs such as aspirin, cimetidine, probenecid, and trimethoprim reduce tubular secretion of creatinine, increasing the plasma creatinine concentration and falsely indicating kidney dysfunction; and (5) the accuracy of the measurement necessitates a stable plasma creatinine concentration over a 24-hour period, so that during the development of and recovery from acute kidney injury, when the serum creatinine is changing, the creatinine clearance is unhelpful. Of note, the creatinine clearance is the traditional estimation equation used for consideration of drug dosing in patients with kidney disease.

One way to measure creatinine clearance is to collect a timed urine sample and determine the plasma creatinine level midway through the collection. An incomplete or prolonged urine collection is a common source of error. A method of estimating the completeness of the collection is to calculate a 24-hour creatinine excretion; the amount should be constant:

$$U_{cr} \times \dot{V} = 15\text{--}20 \text{ mg/kg for healthy young women}$$

$$U_{cr} \times \dot{V} = 20\text{--}25 \text{ mg/kg for healthy young men}$$

The creatinine clearance (C_{cr}) is approximately 100 mL/min/1.73 m^2 in healthy young women and 120 mL/min/1.73 m^2 in healthy young men. The creatinine clearance declines by an average of 0.8 mL/min/yr after age 40 years as part of the aging process, but this is variable, with 35% of subjects in one study having no decline in kidney function over 10 years.

The Kidney Disease Improving Global Outcomes workgroup recommends that estimated glomerular filtration rate (eGFR) in adults be reported when serum creatinine is measured. They recommend using the 2009 CKD-Epidemiology (EPI) Collaboration creatinine equation. An alternative creatinine-based GFR estimating equation is acceptable if it improves accuracy over the CKD-EPI equation. Several web-based calculators will calculate the eGFR (eg, www.nephron.com).

Creatinine clearance (C_{cr}) can also be estimated using the Cockcroft and Gault formula, which incorporates age, sex, and weight to estimate creatinine clearance from plasma creatinine levels without any urinary measurements:

$$C_{cr} = \frac{(140 - \text{Age}) \times \text{Weight (kg)}}{P_{cr} \times 72}$$

Table 22–2. Conditions affecting BUN independently of GFR.

Increased BUN
Reduced effective circulating blood volume (prerenal azotemia)
Catabolic states (gastrointestinal bleeding, corticosteroid use)
High-protein diets
Tetracycline
Decreased BUN
Liver disease
Malnutrition
Sickle cell anemia
SIADH

BUN, blood urea nitrogen; GFR, glomerular filtration rate; SIADH, syndrome of inappropriate antidiuretic hormone.

For women, the creatinine clearance is multiplied by 0.85 because muscle mass is less. This formula overestimates GFR in patients who are obese or edematous and is most accurate when normalized for a body surface area of 1.73 m^2. Dosing of many medications is still based on values of creatinine clearance from the Cockcroft-Gault equation.

BUN is another index used in assessing kidney function. It is synthesized mainly in the liver and is the end product of protein catabolism. Urea is freely filtered by the glomerulus, and about 30–70% is reabsorbed in the renal tubules. Unlike creatinine clearance, which overestimates GFR, urea clearance underestimates GFR. Urea reabsorption may be decreased in volume replete patients, whereas volume depletion causes increased urea reabsorption, in conjunction with increased sodium reabsorption, from the kidney, increasing BUN. A normal BUN:creatinine ratio is 10:1, although this can vary between individuals. With volume depletion, the ratio can increase to 20:1 or higher. Other causes of increased BUN include increased catabolism (gastrointestinal [GI] bleeding, cell lysis, and corticosteroid usage), increased dietary protein, and decreased renal perfusion (heart failure, renal artery stenosis) (Table 22–2). Reduced BUN levels are seen in liver disease and in the syndrome of inappropriate antidiuretic hormone (SIADH).

As patients approach ESRD, a more accurate measure of GFR than creatinine clearance is the average of the creatinine and urea clearances. The creatinine clearance overestimates GFR, as mentioned above, while the urea clearance underestimates GFR. Therefore, an average of the two more accurately approximates the true GFR.

KIDNEY BIOPSY

Indications for percutaneous needle biopsy include (1) unexplained acute kidney injury or CKD; (2) acute nephritic syndromes; (3) unexplained proteinuria and hematuria; (4) previously identified and treated lesions to plan future therapy; (5) systemic diseases associated with kidney dysfunction, such as systemic lupus erythematosus (SLE), Goodpasture syndrome, and granulomatosis with polyangiitis (formerly Wegener granulomatosis), to confirm the extent of renal involvement and to guide management; (6) suspected transplant rejection, to differentiate it from other causes of acute kidney injury; and (7) to guide treatment. If a patient is unwilling to accept therapy based on biopsy findings, the risk of biopsy may outweigh its benefit. Relative contraindications include a solitary or ectopic kidney (exception: transplant allografts), horseshoe kidney, ESRD, congenital anomalies, and multiple cysts. Absolute contraindications include an uncorrected bleeding disorder, severe uncontrolled hypertension, renal infection, renal neoplasm, hydronephrosis, or an uncooperative patient.

Prior to biopsy, patients should not use medications that prolong clotting times and should have well-controlled blood pressure. Blood work should include a hemoglobin, platelet count, prothrombin time, and partial thromboplastin time. After biopsy, hematuria occurs in nearly all patients. Less than 10% will have macroscopic hematuria. Patients should remain supine for 4–6 hours postbiopsy. Patients should be closely monitored when the hematocrit is lower than baseline by more than 3% at 6 hours postbiopsy.

Percutaneous kidney biopsies are generally safe. Approximately 1% of patients will experience significant bleeding requiring blood transfusions. More than half of patients will have at least a small hematoma. Risk of major bleeding persists up to 72 hours after the biopsy. Any type of anticoagulation therapy should be held for 5–7 days postbiopsy if possible. The risks of nephrectomy and mortality are about 0.06–0.08%. When a percutaneous needle biopsy is technically not feasible and kidney tissue is deemed clinically essential, a closed biopsy via interventional radiologic techniques or open biopsy under general anesthesia can be done.

Levey AS et al. GFR estimation: from physiology to public health. Am J Kidney Dis. 2014 May;63(5):820–34. [PMID: 24485147]

Shlipak MG et al; CKD Prognosis Consortium. Cystatin C versus creatinine in determining risk based on kidney function. N Engl J Med. 2013 Sep 5;369(10):932–43. [PMID: 24004120]

Vivante A et al. Hematuria and risk for end-stage kidney disease. Curr Opin Nephrol Hypertens. 2013 May;22(3):325–30. [PMID: 23449218]

ACUTE KIDNEY INJURY

 ESSENTIALS OF DIAGNOSIS

► Rapid increase in serum creatinine.
► Oliguria may be present.
► Symptoms and signs depend on cause.

General Considerations

Acute kidney injury is defined as a rapid decrease in kidney function, resulting in an inability to maintain acid-base, fluid, and electrolyte balance and to excrete nitrogenous wastes. The 2012 Kidney Disease Improving Global Outcomes Clinical Practice Guidelines for Acute Kidney Injury describes three progressive levels of acute kidney injury (Stage 1, 2, or 3) based on the elevation in serum creatinine or decline in urinary output, which correlates with prognosis. **Stage 1** is defined as a 1.0- to 1.5-fold increase in serum creatinine or a decline in urinary output to 0.5 mL/kg/h over 6–12 hours; **stage 2** as a 2.0- to 2.9-fold increase in serum creatinine or decline in urinary output to 0.5 mL/kg/h over 12 hours or longer; **stage 3** as a 3-fold or greater increase in serum creatinine or decline in urinary output to less than 0.3 mL/kg/h for 24 hours or longer or anuria for 12 hours or longer. In the absence of functioning kidneys, serum creatinine concentration will typically increase by 1–1.5 mg/dL daily, although with certain conditions, such as rhabdomyolysis, serum creatinine can increase more rapidly. On average, 5% of hospital admissions and 30% of intensive care unit (ICU) admissions carry a diagnosis of acute kidney injury, and it will develop in 25% of hospitalized patients. Patients with acute kidney injury of any type are at higher risk for all-cause mortality according to prospective cohorts, whether or not there is substantial renal recovery. The rates of acute kidney injury in the hospital setting have increased steadily since the 1980s and are continuing to rise.

► Clinical Findings

A. Symptoms and Signs

The uremic milieu of acute kidney injury can cause nonspecific symptoms. When present, symptoms are often due to uremia or its underlying cause. Uremia can cause nausea, vomiting, malaise, and altered sensorium. Hypertension can occur, and fluid homeostasis is often altered. Hypovolemia can cause states of low blood flow to the kidneys, sometimes termed "prerenal" states, whereas hypervolemia can result from intrinsic or "postrenal" disease. Pericardial effusions can occur with uremia, and a pericardial friction rub can be present. Effusions may result in cardiac tamponade. Arrhythmias occur, especially with hyperkalemia. The lung examination may show rales in the presence of hypervolemia. Acute kidney failure can cause nonspecific diffuse abdominal pain and ileus as well as platelet dysfunction; thus, bleeding and clotting disorders are more common in these patients. The neurologic examination reveals encephalopathic changes with asterixis and confusion; seizures may ensue.

B. Laboratory Findings

Elevated BUN and serum creatinine levels are present, though these elevations do not distinguish acute kidney disease from CKD. Hyperkalemia can occur from impaired renal potassium excretion. With hyperkalemia, the ECG can reveal peaked T waves, PR prolongation, and QRS widening. A long QT segment can occur with hypocalcemia. Anion gap and non-gap metabolic acidosis (due to decreased organic and nonorganic acid clearance) are often noted. Hyperphosphatemia occurs when phosphorus cannot be secreted by damaged tubules either with or without increased cell catabolism. Anemia can occur as a result of decreased erythropoietin production over weeks, and associated platelet dysfunction is typical.

Table 22–3. Classification and differential diagnosis of acute kidney injury.

			Intrinsic Renal Disease		
	Prerenal Azotemia	Postrenal Azotemia	Acute Tubular Necrosis (Oliguric or Polyuric)	Acute Glomerulonephritis	Acute Interstitial Nephritis
Etiology	Poor renal perfusion	Obstruction of the urinary tract	Ischemia, nephrotoxins	Immune complex-mediated, pauci-immune, anti-GBM related	Allergic reaction; drug reaction; infection, collagen vascular disease
Serum BUN:Cr ratio	> 20:1	> 20:1	< 20:1	> 20:1	< 20:1
Urinary indices					
U_{Na} (mEq/L)	< 20	Variable	> 20	< 20	Variable
FE_{Na} (%)	< 1	Variable	> 1 (when oliguric)	< 1	< 1; > 1
Urine osmolality (mOsm/kg)	> 500	< 400	250–300	Variable	Variable
Urinary sediment	Benign or hyaline casts	Normal or red cells, white cells, or crystals	Granular (muddy brown) casts, renal tubular casts	Red cells, dysmorphic red cells and red cell casts	White cells, white cell casts, with or without eosinophils

BUN:Cr, blood urea nitrogen:creatinine ratio; FE_{Na}, fractional excretion of sodium; GBM, glomerular basement membrane; U_{Na}, urinary concentration of sodium.

► Classification & Etiology

Acute kidney injury can be divided into three categories: prerenal causes (kidney hypoperfusion leading to lower GFR), intrinsic kidney disease, and postrenal causes (obstructive uropathy or other obstruction to outflow). Identifying the cause is the first step toward treating the patient (Table 22–3).

A. Prerenal Causes

Prerenal causes are the most common etiology of acute kidney insults and injury, accounting for 40–80% of cases, depending on the population studied. Prerenal azotemia is due to renal hypoperfusion, which is an appropriate physiologic change. If reversed quickly with restoration of renal blood flow, renal parenchymal damage often does not occur. If hypoperfusion persists, ischemia can result, causing intrinsic kidney injury.

Decreased renal perfusion can occur in several ways, such as a decrease in intravascular volume, a change in vascular resistance, or low cardiac output. Causes of volume depletion include hemorrhage, GI losses, dehydration, excessive diuresis, extravascular space sequestration, pancreatitis, burns, trauma, and peritonitis.

Changes in vascular resistance can occur systemically with sepsis, anaphylaxis, anesthesia, and afterload-reducing drugs. Blockers of the renin-angiotensin-aldosterone system, such as angiotensin-converting enzyme (ACE) inhibitors, limit efferent renal arteriolar constriction out of proportion to the afferent arteriolar constriction; thus, GFR will decrease with these medications. Nonsteroidal anti-inflammatory drugs (NSAIDs) minimize afferent arteriolar vasodilation by inhibiting prostaglandin-mediated signals.

Thus, in cirrhosis and heart failure, when prostaglandins are recruited to increase renal blood flow, NSAIDs will have particularly deleterious effects. Epinephrine, norepinephrine, high-dose dopamine, anesthetic agents, and cyclosporine also can cause renal vasoconstriction. Renal artery stenosis causes increased resistance and decreased renal perfusion.

Low cardiac output is a state of low effective renal arterial blood flow. This occurs in states of cardiogenic shock, heart failure, pulmonary embolism, and pericardial tamponade. Arrhythmias and valvular disorders can also reduce cardiac output. In the ICU setting, positive pressure ventilation will decrease venous return, also decreasing cardiac output.

When GFR falls acutely, it is important to determine whether acute kidney injury is due to prerenal or intrinsic renal causes. The history and physical examination are important, and urinalysis can be helpful. The BUN:creatinine ratio will typically exceed 20:1 due to increased urea reabsorption. In an oliguric patient, another useful index is the fractional excretion of sodium (FE_{Na}). With decreased GFR, the kidney will reabsorb salt and water avidly if there is no intrinsic tubular dysfunction. Thus, patients with prerenal causes should have a low fractional excretion percent of sodium (less than 1%). Oliguric patients with intrinsic kidney dysfunction typically have a high fractional excretion of sodium (greater than 1–2%). The FE_{Na} is calculated as follows: FE_{Na} = clearance of Na^+/GFR = clearance of Na^+/C_{cr}:

$$FE_{Na} = \frac{Urine_{Na} \, / \, Serum_{Na}}{Urine_{cr} \, / \, Serum_{cr}} \times 100\%$$

Renal sodium handling is more accurately assessed by the FE_{Na} in oliguric states than in nonoliguric states because the FE_{Na} could be relatively low in nonoliguric acute tubular necrosis if sodium intake and excretion are relatively low. (Oliguria is defined as urinary output less than 400–500 mL/day, or less than 20 mL/h.) The equation was created and validated to assess the difference between oliguric acute tubular necrosis and prerenal states. Diuretics can cause increased sodium excretion. Thus, if the FE_{Na} is high within 12–24 hours after diuretic administration, the cause of acute kidney injury may not be accurately predicted. Acute kidney injury due to glomerulonephritis can have a low FE_{Na} because sodium reabsorption and tubular function may not be compromised.

Treatment of prerenal insults depends entirely on the causes, but maintenance of euvolemia, attention to serum electrolytes, and avoidance of nephrotoxic drugs are benchmarks of therapy. This involves careful assessment of volume status, cardiac function, diet, and drug usage.

B. Postrenal Causes

Postrenal causes are the least common reason for acute kidney injury, accounting for approximately 5–10% of cases, but important to detect because of their reversibility. Postrenal azotemia occurs when urinary flow from both kidneys, or a single functioning kidney, is obstructed. Occasionally, postrenal uropathies can occur when a single kidney is obstructed if the contralateral kidney cannot adjust for the loss in function, (eg, in a patient with advanced CKD). Obstruction leads to elevated intraluminal pressure, causing kidney parenchymal damage, with marked effects on renal blood flow and tubular function, and a decrease in GFR.

Postrenal causes include urethral obstruction, bladder dysfunction or obstruction, and obstruction of both ureters or renal pelvises. In men, benign prostatic hyperplasia is the most common cause. Patients taking anticholinergic drugs are particularly at risk. Obstruction can also be caused by bladder, prostate, and cervical cancers; retroperitoneal fibrosis; and neurogenic bladder. Less common causes are blood clots, bilateral ureteral stones, urethral stones or strictures, and bilateral papillary necrosis.

Patients may be anuric or polyuric and may complain of lower abdominal pain. Polyuria can occur in the setting of partial obstruction with resultant tubular dysfunction and an inability to appropriately reabsorb salt and water loads. Obstruction can be constant or intermittent and partial or complete. On examination, the patient may have an enlarged prostate, distended bladder, or mass detected on pelvic examination.

Laboratory examination may initially reveal high urine osmolality, low urine sodium, high BUN:creatinine ratio, and low FE_{Na} (as tubular function may not be compromised initially). These indices are similar to a prerenal picture because extensive intrinsic renal damage has not occurred. After several days, the urine sodium increases as the kidneys fail and are unable to concentrate the urine—thus, isosthenuria is present. The urine sediment is generally benign.

Patients with acute kidney injury and suspected postrenal insults should undergo bladder catheterization and ultrasonography to assess for hydroureter and hydronephrosis. After reversal of the underlying process, these patients often undergo a postobstructive diuresis, and care should be taken to avoid volume depletion. Rarely, obstruction is not diagnosed by ultrasonography. For example, patients with retroperitoneal fibrosis from tumor or radiation may not show dilation of the urinary tract. If suspicion does exist, a CT scan or MRI can establish the diagnosis. Prompt treatment of obstruction within days by catheters, stents, or other surgical procedures can result in partial or complete reversal of the acute process.

C. Intrinsic Acute Kidney Injury

Intrinsic renal disorders account for up to 50% of all cases of acute kidney injury referred to a nephrologist. Intrinsic dysfunction is considered after prerenal and postrenal causes have been excluded. The sites of injury are the tubules, interstitium, vasculature, and glomeruli.

▶ When to Refer

- If a patient has signs of acute kidney injury that have not reversed over 1–2 weeks, but no signs of acute uremia, the patient can usually be referred to a nephrologist rather than admitted.
- If a patient has signs of persistent urinary tract obstruction, the patient should be referred to a urologist.

▶ When to Admit

The patient should be admitted if there is sudden loss of kidney function resulting in abnormalities that cannot be handled expeditiously in an outpatient setting (eg, hyperkalemia, volume overload, uremia) or other requirements for acute intervention, such as emergent urologic intervention or dialysis.

Okusa MD et al. Reading between the (guide)lines—the KDIGO practice guideline on acute kidney injury in the individual patient. Kidney Int. 2014 Jan;85(1):39–48. [PMID: 24067436]
Walther CP et al. Summary of clinical practice guidelines for acute kidney injury. Hosp Pract (1995). 2014 Feb;42(1):7–14. [PMID: 24566591]

ACUTE TUBULAR NECROSIS

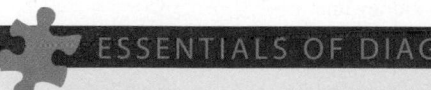

ESSENTIALS OF DIAGNOSIS

▶ Acute kidney injury.
▶ Ischemic or toxic insult or underlying sepsis.
▶ Urine sediment with pigmented granular casts and renal tubular epithelial cells is pathognomonic but not essential.

▶ General Considerations

Acute kidney injury due to tubular damage is termed "acute tubular necrosis" and accounts for approximately 85% of intrinsic acute kidney injury. The two major causes of acute tubular necrosis are ischemia and nephrotoxin exposure. Ischemic acute kidney injury is characterized not only by inadequate GFR but also by renal blood flow inadequate to maintain parenchymal cellular perfusion. Renal tubular damage with low effective arterial blood flow to the kidney can result in tubular necrosis and apoptosis. This occurs in the setting of prolonged hypotension or hypoxemia, such as volume depletion or shock. Underlying sepsis can also be an independent risk factor for acute tubular necrosis. Major surgical procedures can involve prolonged periods of hypoperfusion, which are exacerbated by vasodilating anesthetic agents.

A. Exogenous Nephrotoxins

Aminoglycosides cause some degree of acute tubular necrosis in up to 25% of hospitalized patients receiving therapeutic levels of the drugs. Nonoliguric kidney injury typically starts to occur after 5–10 days of exposure. Predisposing factors include underlying kidney damage, volume depletion, and advanced age. Aminoglycosides can remain in renal tissues for up to a month, so kidney function may not recover for some time after stopping the medication. Monitoring of peak and trough levels is important, but trough levels are more helpful in predicting renal toxicity. Gentamicin and tobramycin are equally nephrotoxic; streptomycin is the least nephrotoxic of the aminoglycosides, likely due to the number of cationic amino side chains present on each molecule.

Amphotericin B is typically nephrotoxic after a dose of 2–3 g. This causes a type I renal tubular acidosis with severe vasoconstriction and distal tubular damage, which can lead to hypokalemia and nephrogenic diabetes insipidus. **Vancomycin,** intravenous **acyclovir,** and several **cephalosporins** have been known to cause acute tubular necrosis.

Radiographic contrast media may be directly nephrotoxic. Contrast nephropathy is the third leading cause of new-onset acute kidney injury in hospitalized patients. It probably results from the synergistic combination of direct renal tubular epithelial cell toxicity and renal medullary ischemia. Predisposing factors include advanced age, preexisting kidney disease (serum creatinine greater than 2 mg/dL), volume depletion, diabetic nephropathy, heart failure, multiple myeloma, repeated doses of contrast, and recent exposure to other nephrotoxic agents, including NSAIDs and ACE inhibitors. The combination of preexisting diabetes mellitus and kidney dysfunction poses the greatest risk (15–50%) for contrast nephropathy. Lower volumes of contrast with lower osmolality are recommended in high-risk patients. Toxicity usually occurs within 24–48 hours after the radiocontrast study. Nonionic contrast media may be less toxic, but this has not been well proven. Prevention should be the goal when using these agents. The mainstay of therapy is a liter of intravenous 0.9% saline over 10–12 hours both before and after the contrast administration—cautiously in patients with preexisting cardiac dysfunction. Isotonic intravenous volume repletion is superior to hypotonic intravenous solutions which are both superior to oral solutions in small studies. Neither mannitol nor furosemide offers benefit over 0.9%

(normal) saline administration. In fact, furosemide may lead to increased rates of renal dysfunction in this setting. It is unclear whether N-acetylcysteine can prevent kidney injury. In some small studies, N-acetylcysteine given before and after contrast decreases the incidence of dye-induced nephrotoxicity. However, a large prospective randomized controlled trial showed no benefit of N-acetylcysteine in over 2300 patients, some of whom had CKD, randomized to either 1200 mg orally twice versus placebo before and after angiographic procedures. Acetylcysteine is a thiol-containing antioxidant with little toxicity whose mechanism of action is unclear. With little harm and possible benefit, administering acetylcysteine 600 mg orally every 12 hours twice, before and after a dye load, for patients with preexisting risk factors at risk for acute kidney injury, is a reasonable strategy. Intravenous N-acetylcysteine, 1200 mg prior to an emergent procedure, has shown benefit compared with placebo and may be a good option if a patient needs contrast dye urgently. Some investigators have shown a benefit using sodium bicarbonate (154 mEq/L, intravenously at 3 mL/kg/h for 1 hour before the procedure, then 1 mL/kg/h for 6 hours after the procedure) over a more conventional regimen of normal saline as the isotonic volume expander. However, others have shown sodium bicarbonate was not superior to sodium chloride when using similar administration regimens. Other nephrotoxic agents should be avoided during the day before and after dye administration. The largest ongoing randomized trial to date is investigating intravenous normal saline versus bicarbonate and N-acetylcysteine versus placebo to prevent contrast-induced nephropathy in a 2×2 design, with a result expected for 2019.

Cyclosporine toxicity is usually dose dependent. It causes distal tubular dysfunction (a type 4 renal tubular acidosis) and severe vasoconstriction. Regular blood level monitoring is important to prevent both acute and chronic nephrotoxicity. With patients who are taking cyclosporine to prevent kidney allograft rejection, kidney biopsy is often necessary to distinguish transplant rejection from cyclosporine toxicity. Renal function usually improves after reducing the dose or stopping the drug.

Other exogenous nephrotoxins include antineoplastics, such as cisplatin and organic solvents, and heavy metals such as mercury, cadmium, and arsenic. Exogenous nephrotoxins more commonly cause damage than endogenous nephrotoxins.

B. Endogenous Nephrotoxins

Endogenous nephrotoxins include heme-containing products, uric acid, and paraproteins. **Myoglobinuria** as a consequence of rhabdomyolysis leads to acute tubular necrosis. Necrotic muscle releases large amounts of myoglobin, which is freely filtered across the glomerulus. The myoglobin is reabsorbed by the renal tubules, and direct damage can occur. Distal tubular obstruction from pigmented casts and intrarenal vasoconstriction can also cause damage. This type of kidney injury occurs in the setting of crush injury, or muscle necrosis from prolonged unconsciousness, seizures, cocaine, and alcohol abuse. Dehydration and acidosis predispose to the development of myoglobinuric acute kidney injury. Patients may complain of muscular pain and often have signs of muscle injury. Rhabdomyolysis of clinical importance commonly occurs with a serum creatine kinase (CK) greater than 20,000–50,000 international units/L. One study showed that 58% of patients with acute kidney injury from rhabdomyolysis had CK levels greater than 16,000 international units/L. Only 11% of patients without kidney injury had CK values greater than 16,000 international units/L. The globin moiety of myoglobin will cause the urine dipstick to read falsely positive for hemoglobin: the urine appears dark brown, but no red cells are present. With lysis of muscle cells, patients also become hyperkalemic, hyperphosphatemic, and hyperuricemic. Hypocalcemia may ensue due to phosphorus and calcium precipitation. The mainstay of treatment is volume repletion. Adjunctive treatments with mannitol and alkalinization of the urine have not been proved to change outcomes in human trials. As the patient recovers, calcium can move back from tissues to plasma, so early exogenous calcium administration for hypocalcemia is not recommended unless the patient is symptomatic or the level becomes exceedingly low in an unconscious patient. Such repletion could result in hypercalcemia later in the course of the illness.

Hemoglobin can cause a similar form of acute tubular necrosis. Massive intravascular hemolysis is seen in transfusion reactions and in certain hemolytic anemias. Reversal of the underlying disorder and hydration are the mainstays of treatment.

Hyperuricemia can occur in the setting of rapid cell turnover and lysis. Chemotherapy for germ cell neoplasms and leukemia and lymphoma are the primary causes. Spontaneous tumor lysis syndrome is a less common cause. Acute kidney injury occurs with intratubular deposition of uric acid crystals; serum uric acid levels are often greater than 15–20 mg/dL and urine uric acid levels greater than 600 mg/24 h. A urine uric acid to urine creatinine ratio greater than 1.0 indicates risk of acute kidney injury. Allopurinol or rasburicase can be used prophylactically, and rasburicase with or without dialysis is often used for treatment in diagnosed cases.

Bence Jones protein seen in conjunction with multiple myeloma can cause direct tubular toxicity and tubular obstruction. Other renal complications from multiple myeloma include hypercalcemia and renal tubular dysfunction, including proximal renal tubular acidosis (see Multiple Myeloma, below).

▶ Clinical Findings

A. Symptoms and Signs

See Acute Kidney Injury.

B. Laboratory Findings

Hyperkalemia and hyperphosphatemia are commonly encountered. BUN:creatinine ratio is usually less than 20:1 because tubular function is not intact, per the mechanisms described in the general section on acute kidney injury (Table 22–3). Urinary output can be either oliguric or nonoliguric, with oliguria portending a worse prognosis. Urine sodium concentration and the FE_{Na} are typically elevated, indicative of tubular dysfunction, as discussed above. Urinalysis may show evidence of acute tubular damage; the presence of two or more muddy brown casts or renal tubular epithelial cells are strongly predictive of acute tubular necrosis and have a low negative predictive value (see Table 22–1).

▶ Treatment

Treatment is aimed at hastening recovery and avoiding complications. Preventive measures should be taken to avoid volume overload and hyperkalemia. A prospective randomized controlled trial did not show a benefit from loop diuretics in large doses on either recovery from acute kidney injury or death. Widespread use of diuretics in critically ill patients with acute kidney injury should be encouraged only in states of volume overload when appropriate. Disabling side effects of supranormal dosing include hearing loss and cerebellar dysfunction. This is mainly due to peak furosemide levels; this risk can be minimized by the use of a furosemide drip. A starting dose of 0.1–0.3 mg/kg/h is appropriate, increasing to a maximum of 0.5–1 mg/kg/h. A bolus of 1–1.5 mg/kg should be administered at the beginning of each dose escalation. Intravenous thiazide diuretics can be used to augment urinary output; chlorothiazide, 250–500 mg intravenously every 8–12 hours, is a reasonable choice. Another good choice to augment diuresis is metolazone at doses of 2.5–5 mg given orally once to twice daily, 30 minutes prior to loop diuretics. It is less expensive than intravenous chlorothiazide and has reasonable bioavailability. Short-term effects of loop diuretics include activation of the renin–angiotensin system. A 2012 prospective randomized trial did not show a benefit on mortality from plasma ultrafiltration over the use of intravenous diuretics in patients with decompensated heart failure. This intervention can be considered in ICU patients with acute kidney injury in need of volume removal who are nonresponsive to diuretics with the caveat that the intervention has not ultimately improved population-based survival. Nutritional support should maintain adequate intake while preventing excessive catabolism. Dietary protein restriction of 0.6 g/kg/day helps prevent metabolic acidosis. Hypocalcemia and hyperphosphatemia can be improved with diet and phosphate-binding agents taken with meals three times daily; examples include aluminum hydroxide (500 mg orally) over the short term, and calcium carbonate (500–1500 mg orally), calcium acetate (667 mg, two or three tablets), sevelamer carbonate (800–1600 mg orally), and lanthanum carbonate (1000 mg orally) over longer periods. Hypocalcemia should not be treated in patients with rhabdomyolysis unless they are symptomatic. Hypermagnesemia can occur because of reduced magnesium excretion by the renal tubules, so magnesium-containing antacids and laxatives should be avoided in these patients. Dosages of all medications must be adjusted according to the estimated degree of renal impairment for drugs eliminated by the kidney.

Indications for dialysis in acute kidney injury from acute tubular necrosis or other intrinsic disorders include life-threatening electrolyte disturbances (such as hyperkalemia), volume overload unresponsive to diuresis, worsening acidosis, and uremic complications (eg, encephalopathy, pericarditis, and seizures). In gravely ill patients, less severe but worsening abnormalities may also be indications for dialytic support. Two large prospective randomized control trials showed that an intensive dialysis dose was not superior to a more conventional dose.

▶ Course & Prognosis

The clinical course of acute tubular necrosis is often divided into three phases: initial injury, maintenance, and recovery. The maintenance phase is expressed as either oliguric (urinary output less than 500 mL/day) or nonoliguric. Nonoliguric acute tubular necrosis has a better outcome. Conversion from oliguric to nonoliguric states with the use of diuretics has not been shown to change the prognosis. While dopamine has sometimes been used for this purpose, numerous studies have shown that its use in this setting has not been beneficial. Average duration of the maintenance phase is 1–3 weeks but may be several months. Cellular repair and removal of tubular debris occur during this period. The recovery phase can be heralded by diuresis. This can be due to inability of recovering renal tubules to reabsorb salt and water appropriately, and a solute diuresis from elevated BUN levels. GFR begins to rise; BUN and serum creatinine fall.

The mortality rate associated with acute kidney injury is 20–50% in hospitalized settings, and up to 70% for those in the ICU requiring dialysis with additional comorbid illnesses. Increased mortality is associated with advanced age, severe underlying disease, and multisystem organ failure. Leading causes of death are infections, fluid and electrolyte disturbances, and worsening of underlying disease. Mortality rates have started to improve slightly according to two retrospective cohort studies conducted within the last 10 years.

▶ When to Refer

- Studies have shown that nephrology referral improves outcome in acute kidney injury.
- For fluid, electrolyte, and acid-base abnormalities that are recalcitrant to interventions.

▶ When to Admit

A patient with symptoms or signs of acute kidney injury that require immediate intervention, such as administration of intravenous fluids, dialytic therapy, or that requires a team approach that cannot be coordinated as an outpatient.

Perazella MA. The urine sediment as a biomarker of kidney disease. Am J Kidney Dis. 2015 Nov;66(5):748–55. [PMID: 25943719]

INTERSTITIAL NEPHRITIS

ESSENTIALS OF DIAGNOSIS

▶ Fever.

▶ Transient maculopapular rash.

▶ Acute or chronic kidney injury.

▶ Pyuria (including eosinophiluria), white blood cell casts, and hematuria.

▶ General Considerations

Acute interstitial nephritis accounts for 10–15% of cases of intrinsic renal failure. An interstitial inflammatory response with edema and possible tubular cell damage is the typical pathologic finding.

Although drugs account for over 70% of cases, acute interstitial nephritis also occurs in infectious diseases, immunologic disorders, or as an idiopathic condition. The most common drugs are penicillins and cephalosporins, sulfonamides and sulfonamide-containing diuretics, NSAIDs, rifampin, phenytoin, and allopurinol. Proton pump inhibitors can also cause acute interstitial nephritis. Infectious causes include streptococcal infections, leptospirosis, cytomegalovirus, histoplasmosis, and Rocky Mountain spotted fever. Immunologic entities are more commonly associated with glomerulonephritis, but SLE, Sjögren syndrome, sarcoidosis, and cryoglobulinemia can cause interstitial nephritis.

▶ Clinical Findings

Clinical features can include fever (more than 80% of cases), rash (25–50%), arthralgias, and peripheral blood eosinophilia (80%). The classic triad of fever, rash, and arthralgias is present in only 10–15% of cases. The urine often contains white cells (95%), red cells, and white cell casts. Proteinuria can be a feature, particularly in NSAID-induced interstitial nephritis, but is usually modest (less than 2 g/24 h). Eosinophiluria is neither very sensitive nor specific but can be detected by Wright or Hansel stain.

▶ Treatment & Prognosis

Acute interstitial nephritis often carries a good prognosis. Recovery occurs over weeks to months. Urgent dialytic therapy may be necessary in up to one-third of all referred patients before resolution but patients rarely progress to ESRD. Those with prolonged courses of oliguric failure and advanced age have a worse prognosis. Treatment consists of supportive measures and removal of the inciting agent. If kidney injury persists after these steps, a short course of corticosteroids can be given, although the data to support use of corticosteroids are not substantial. Short-term, high-dose methylprednisolone (0.5–1 g/day intravenously for 1–4 days) or prednisone (60 mg/day orally for 1–2 weeks) followed by a prednisone taper can be used in these more severe cases of drug-induced interstitial nephritis.

GLOMERULONEPHRITIS

ESSENTIALS OF DIAGNOSIS

▶ Hematuria, mild proteinuria.

▶ Non-dysmorphic or dysmorphic red cells.

▶ Red cell casts pathognomonic but not required for diagnosis.

▶ Dependent edema and hypertension.

▶ Acute kidney injury.

▶ General Considerations

Acute glomerulonephritis is a relatively uncommon cause of acute kidney injury, accounting for about 5% of cases. Pathologically, inflammatory glomerular lesions are seen. These include mesangioproliferative, focal and diffuse proliferative, and crescentic lesions. The larger the percentage of glomeruli involved and the more severe the lesion, the more likely it is that the patient will have a poor clinical outcome.

Categorization of acute glomerulonephritis can be done by serologic analysis. Markers include anti-GBM antibodies, antineutrophil cytoplasmic antibodies (ANCAs), and other immune markers of disease.

Immune complex deposition usually occurs when moderate antigen excess over antibody production occurs. Complexes formed with marked antigen excess tend to remain in the circulation. Antibody excess with large antigen–antibody aggregates usually results in phagocytosis and clearance of the precipitates by the mononuclear phagocytic system in the liver and spleen. Causes include IgA nephropathy (Berger disease), peri-infectious or post-infectious glomerulonephritis, endocarditis, lupus nephritis, cryoglobulinemic glomerulonephritis (often associated with hepatitis C virus [HCV]), and MPGN.

Anti-GBM–associated acute glomerulonephritis is either confined to the kidney or associated with pulmonary hemorrhage. The latter is termed "Goodpasture syndrome." Injury is related to autoantibodies aimed against type IV collagen in the GBM rather than to immune complex deposition.

Pauci-immune acute glomerulonephritis is a form of small-vessel vasculitis associated with ANCAs, causing primary and secondary kidney diseases that do not have direct immune complex deposition or antibody binding. Tissue injury is believed to be due to cell-mediated immune processes. An example is granulomatosis with polyangiitis, a systemic necrotizing vasculitis of small arteries and veins associated with intravascular and extravascular granuloma formation. In addition to glomerulonephritis, these patients can have upper airway, pulmonary, and skin manifestations of disease. Cytoplasmic ANCA (c-ANCA) is the common pattern. Microscopic polyangiitis is another pauci-immune vasculitis causing acute glomerulonephritis. Perinuclear staining (p-ANCA) is the common pattern in this scenario. ANCA-associated and anti-GBM-associated acute glomerulonephritis can evolve to crescentic glomerulonephritis and often have poor outcomes unless treatment is started early. Both are described more fully below.

Other vascular causes of acute glomerulonephritis include hypertensive emergencies and the thrombotic microangiopathies such as hemolytic-uremic syndrome and thrombotic thrombocytopenic purpura (see Chapter 14).

▶ Clinical Findings

A. Symptoms and Signs

Patients with acute glomerulonephritis are often hypertensive and edematous, and have an abnormal urinary sediment. The edema is found first in body parts with low tissue tension, such as the periorbital and scrotal regions.

B. Laboratory Findings

Serum creatinine can rise over days to months, depending on the rapidity of the underlying process. The BUN:creatinine ratio is not a reliable marker of kidney function and is more reflective of the underlying volume status of the patient. Dipstick and microscopic evaluation will reveal evidence of hematuria and mild proteinuria (usually less than 3 g/day); there may be cellular elements such as dysmorphic red cells, red cell casts, and white cells, or only normomorphic red cells. Red cell casts are specific for glomerulonephritis, and a detailed search is warranted. Either spot urinary protein-creatinine ratios or 24-hour urine collections can quantify protein excretion; the latter can quantify creatinine clearance when renal function is stable. However, in cases of rapidly changing serum creatinine values, the urinary creatinine clearance is an unreliable marker of GFR. The FE_{Na} is usually low unless the renal tubulo-interstitial space is affected, and renal dysfunction is marked (see Table 22–3).

Further tests include complement levels (C3, C4, CH50) that are low in immune complex glomerulonephritis aside from IgA nephropathy and normal in pauci immune and anti-GBM related glomerulonephritis. Other tests include ASO titers, anti-GBM antibody levels, ANCAs, antinuclear antibody titers, cryoglobulins, hepatitis serologies, blood cultures, renal ultrasound, and kidney biopsy in the appropriate setting.

▶ Treatment

Depending on the nature and severity of disease, treatment can consist of high-dose corticosteroids and cytotoxic agents such as cyclophosphamide. Plasma exchange can be used in Goodpasture syndrome and pauci-immune glomerulonephritis as a temporizing measure until chemotherapy can take effect. Treatment and prognosis for specific diseases are discussed more fully below.

Ad-hoc working group of ERBP; Fliser D et al. A European Renal Best Practice (ERBP) position statement on the Kidney Disease Improving Global Outcomes (KDIGO) clinical practice guidelines on acute kidney injury: part 1: definitions, conservative management and contrast-induced nephropathy. Nephrol Dial Transplant. 2012 Dec;27(12):4263–72. [PMID: 23045432]

Hebert LA et al. Differential diagnosis of glomerular disease: a systematic and inclusive approach. Am J Nephrol. 2013;38(3):253–66. [PMID: 24052039]

Perazella MA. Diagnosing drug-induced AIN in the hospitalized patient: a challenge for the clinician. Clin Nephrol. 2014 Jun;81(6):381–8. [PMID: 24691017]

CARDIORENAL SYNDROME

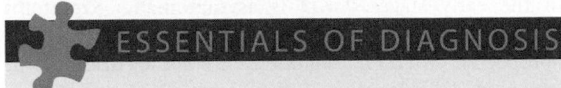

ESSENTIALS OF DIAGNOSIS

► Cardiac dysfunction: acute or chronic symptoms or signs of heart failure, ischemic injury or arrhythmias.

► Kidney disease: acute or chronic, depending on type of cardiorenal syndrome.

General Considerations

Cardiorenal syndrome is a pathophysiologic disorder of the heart and kidneys wherein the acute or chronic deterioration of one organ results in the acute or chronic deterioration of the other. This syndrome has been classified into five types.

Type 1 consists of acute kidney injury stemming from acute cardiac disease. Type 2 is CKD due to chronic cardiac disease. Type 3 is acute cardiac disease as a result of acute kidney injury. Type 4 is chronic cardiac decompensation from CKD. Type 5 consists of heart and kidney dysfunction due to other acute or chronic systemic disorders (such as sepsis). Identifying and defining this common syndrome may assist in the future with treatments to improve its morbidity and mortality. Although novel agents are being examined for future therapies, the mainstay of treatment is to address the primary underlying cardiac or renal dysfunction.

Braam B et al. Cardiorenal syndrome—current understanding and future perspectives. Nat Rev Nephrol. 2014 Jan;10(1):48–55. [PMID: 24247284]

CHRONIC KIDNEY DISEASE

ESSENTIALS OF DIAGNOSIS

► Decline in the GFR over months to years.

► Persistent proteinuria or abnormal renal morphology may be present.

► Hypertension in most cases.

► Symptoms and signs of uremia when nearing end-stage disease.

► Bilateral small or echogenic kidneys on ultrasound in advanced disease.

General Considerations

CKD affects approximately 13% of Americans. Most are unaware of the condition because they remain asymptomatic until the disease is near end-stage. The National Kidney Foundation's staging system helps clinicians formulate practice plans (Table 22–4). Over 70% of cases of late-stage CKD (stage 5 CKD and ESRD) in the United States are due to diabetes mellitus or hypertension/vascular disease. Glomerulonephritis, cystic diseases, chronic tubulointerstitial

Table 22–4. Stages of chronic kidney disease: A clinical action plan.[1,2]

Stage[3]	Description	GFR (mL/min/1.73 m^2)	Action
1	Kidney damage with normal or ↑↑ GFR	≥ 90	Diagnosis and treatment of underlying etiology if possible. Treatment of comorbid conditions. Estimate progression, work to slow progression. Cardiovascular disease risk reduction.
2	Kidney damage with mildly ↓ GFR	60–89	
3a	Mildly-moderately ↓ GFR	45–59	As above, and evaluating and treating complications.
3b	Moderately-severely ↓ GFR	30–44	
4	Severely ↓ GFR	15–29	Preparation for End-stage renal disease (ESRD).
5	End-stage renal disease (ESRD)	< 15 (or dialysis)	Dialysis, transplant, or palliative care.

[1]Based on National Kidney Foundation, KDOQI, and KDIGO Chronic Kidney Disease Guidelines.
[2]Chronic kidney disease is defined as either kidney damage or GFR < 60 mL/min/1.73 m^2 for 3 or more months. Kidney damage is defined as pathologic abnormalities or markers of damage, including abnormalities in blood or urine tests or imaging studies.
[3]At all stages, persistent albuminuria confers added risk for CKD progression and cardiovascular disease in the following gradations: < 30 mg/day = lowest added risk, 30–300 mg/day = mildly increased risk, > 300–1000 mg/day moderately increased risk, > 1000 mg/day = severely increased risk.
GFR, glomerular filtration rate.
(Modified and reproduced, with permission, from Kidney Disease: Improving Global Outcomes (KDIGO) CKD Work Group. KDIGO 2012 Clinical Practice Guideline for the Evaluation and Management of Chronic Kidney Disease. Kidney Int. 2013 Jan;3(1) (Suppl):1–150.)

Table 22–5. Major causes of chronic kidney disease.

Glomerular diseases
Primary glomerular diseases
Focal segmental glomerulosclerosis
Membranoproliferative glomerulonephritis
IgA nephropathy
Membranous nephropathy
Alport syndrome (hereditary nephritis)
Secondary glomerular diseases
Diabetic nephropathy
Renal amyloidosis
Postinfectious glomerulonephritis
HIV-associated nephropathy
Collagen-vascular diseases (eg, SLE)
HCV-associated membranoproliferative glomerulonephritis
Tubulointerstitial nephritis
Drug hypersensitivity
Heavy metals
Analgesic nephropathy
Reflux/chronic pyelonephritis
Sickle cell nephropathy
Idiopathic
Cystic diseases
Polycystic kidney disease
Medullary cystic disease
Obstructive nephropathies
Prostatic disease
Nephrolithiasis
Retroperitoneal fibrosis/tumor
Congenital
Vascular diseases
Hypertensive nephrosclerosis
Renal artery stenosis

HCV, hepatitis C virus; SLE, systemic lupus erythematosus.

diseases, and other urologic diseases account for the remainder (Table 22–5). Genetic polymorphisms of the *APOL-1* gene have been shown to be associated with an increased risk of the development of CKD in African Americans.

CKD usually leads to a progressive decline in kidney function even if the inciting cause can be identified and treated or removed. Destruction of nephrons leads to compensatory hypertrophy and supranormal GFR of the remaining nephrons in order to maintain overall homeostasis. As a result, the serum creatinine may remain relatively normal even in the face of significant loss of renal mass and is, therefore, a relatively insensitive marker for renal damage and scarring. In addition, compensatory hyperfiltration leads to overwork injury in the remaining nephrons, which in turn causes progressive glomerular sclerosis and interstitial fibrosis. Angiotensin receptor blockers (ARBs) and ACE inhibitors can help reduce hyperfiltration injury and are particularly helpful in slowing the progression of proteinuric CKD.

While CKD is an independent risk factor for cardiovascular disease (CVD); proteinuric CKD confers the highest risk. Most patients with stage 3 CKD die of underlying CVD prior to progression to ESRD.

▶ Clinical Findings

A. Symptoms and Signs

In the early stages, CKD is asymptomatic. Symptoms develop slowly with the progressive decline in GFR, are nonspecific, and do not manifest until kidney disease is far advanced (GFR less than 5–10 mL/min/1.73 m²). At this point, the accumulation of metabolic waste products, or uremic toxins, results in the uremic syndrome (Table 22–6). General symptoms of uremia may include fatigue and weakness; anorexia, nausea, vomiting, and a metallic taste in the mouth are also common. Patients or family members may report irritability, memory impairment, insomnia, restless legs, paresthesias, and twitching. Generalized pruritus without rash may occur. Decreased libido and menstrual irregularities are common. Pericarditis, a rare complication of CKD, may present with pleuritic chest pain. Drug toxicity can develop as renal clearance worsens; in particular, since insulin is renally cleared, hypoglycemia may develop and can be life-threatening in patients with diabetes.

Table 22–6. Symptoms and signs of uremia.

Organ System	Symptoms	Signs
General	Fatigue, weakness	Sallow-appearing, chronically ill
Skin	Pruritus, easy bruisability	Pallor, ecchymoses, excoriations, edema, xerosis
ENT	Metallic taste in mouth, epistaxis	Urinous breath
Eye		Pale conjunctiva
Pulmonary	Shortness of breath	Rales, pleural effusion
Cardiovascular	Dyspnea on exertion, retrosternal pain on inspiration (pericarditis)	Hypertension, cardiomegaly, friction rub
Gastrointestinal	Anorexia, nausea, vomiting, hiccups	
Genitourinary	Nocturia, erectile dysfunction	Isosthenuria
Neuromuscular	Restless legs, numbness and cramps in legs	
Neurologic	Generalized irritability and inability to concentrate, decreased libido	Stupor, asterixis, myoclonus, peripheral neuropathy

Table 22–7. Reversible causes of kidney injury.

Reversible Factors	Diagnostic Clues
Infection	Urine culture and sensitivity tests
Obstruction	Bladder catheterization, then renal ultrasound
Extracellular fluid volume depletion or significant hypotension relative to baseline	Blood pressure and pulse, including orthostatic pulse
Hypokalemia, hypercalcemia, and hyperuricemia (usually >15 mg/dL)	Serum electrolytes, calcium, phosphate, uric acid
Nephrotoxic agents	Drug history
Severe/urgent hypertension	Blood pressure, chest radiograph
Heart failure	Physical examination, chest radiograph

[1] Value of serum creatinine level = 1.0 mg/dL
[2] Value of serum creatinine level = 2.0 mg/dL
[3] Value of serum creatinine level = 5.0 mg/dL

▲ **Figure 22–1.** Decline in kidney function (expressed as the reciprocal of serum creatinine as shown here, or as estimated glomerular filtration rate [eGFR]) plotted against time to end-stage renal disease (ESRD). The solid line indicates the linear decline in kidney function over time. The dotted line indicates the approximate time to ESRD.

The most common physical finding in CKD is hypertension—due in part to impaired sodium excretion. It is often present in early stages of CKD and tends to worsen with CKD progression. In later stages of CKD, sodium retention may lead to typical physical signs of volume overload. Uremic signs are seen with a profound decrease in GFR (less than 5–10 mL/min/1.73 m²) and may include a generally sallow and ill appearance, halitosis (uremic fetor), and the uremic encepholopathic signs of decreased mental status, asterixis, myoclonus, and possibly seizures.

Symptoms and signs of uremia warrant immediate hospital admission and nephrology consultation for initiation of dialysis. The uremic syndrome improves or resolves with dialytic therapy.

In any patient with kidney disease, it is important to identify and correct all possibly reversible insults or exacerbating factors (Table 22–7). Urinary tract infections, obstruction, hypovolemia, hypotension, nephrotoxins (such as NSAIDs, aminoglycosides, or proton pump inhibitors), severe or emergent hypertension, and heart failure should be excluded.

B. Laboratory Findings

CKD is usually defined by an abnormal GFR persisting for at least 3 months. Persistent proteinuria or abnormalities on renal imaging (eg, polycystic kidneys) are also diagnostic of CKD, even when eGFR is normal. It is helpful to plot the inverse of serum creatinine ($1/S_{Cr}$) versus time or eGFR (if reported by the laboratory) versus time. If three or more prior measurements are available, the time to ESRD can be roughly estimated (Figure 22–1). If the slope of the line acutely declines, new and potentially reversible renal insults should be excluded as outlined above. Anemia, hyperphosphatemia, hypocalcemia, hyperkalemia, and metabolic acidosis are common complications of advanced CKD. The urinary sediment may show broad waxy casts as a result of dilated, hypertrophic nephrons. Proteinuria may be present. If so, it should be quantified as described above.

Quantification of urinary protein is important for several reasons. First, it helps narrow the differential diagnosis of the etiology of the CKD (Table 22–5); for example, glomerular diseases tend to present with protein excretion of more than 1 g/day. Second, the presence of proteinuria is associated with more rapid progression of CKD and with increased risk of cardiovascular mortality.

C. Imaging

The finding of small, echogenic kidneys bilaterally (less than 9–10 cm) by ultrasonography supports a diagnosis of CKD, although normal or even large kidneys can be seen with adult polycystic kidney disease, diabetic nephropathy, HIV-associated nephropathy, multiple myeloma, amyloidosis, and obstructive uropathy.

► Complications

The complications of CKD tend to occur at relatively predictable stages of disease as noted in Figure 22–2.

A. Cardiovascular Complications

Patients with CKD experience greater morbidity and mortality from CVD in comparison to the general population. Roughly 80% of patients with CKD die, primarily of CVD, before reaching the need for dialysis. Of those undergoing dialysis, 45% will die of a cardiovascular cause. The precise biologic mechanisms for this enhanced mortality are

▲ **Figure 22–2.** Complications of chronic kidney disease (CKD) by stage and glomerular filtration rate (GFR). Complications arising from CKD tend to occur at the stages depicted, although there is considerable variability noted in clinical practice. HTN, hypertension; PTH, parathyroid hormone. (Adapted, with permission, from William Bennett, MD.)

unclear but may have to do with the uremic milieu including abnormal phosphorus and calcium homeostasis, increased burden of oxidative stress, increased vascular reactivity, increased left ventricular hypertrophy, and underlying coexistent comorbidities such as hypertension and diabetes mellitus.

1. Hypertension—Hypertension is the most common complication of CKD; it tends to be progressive and salt-sensitive. Hyperreninemic states and exogenous erythropoietin administration can also exacerbate hypertension.

As with other patient populations, control of hypertension should focus on both nonpharmacologic therapy (eg, diet, exercise, weight loss, treatment of obstructive sleep apnea) and pharmacologic therapy. CKD results in disturbed sodium homeostasis such that the ability of the kidney to adjust to variations in sodium and water intake becomes limited as GFR declines. A low salt diet (2 g/day) is often essential to control blood pressure and help avoid overt volume overload. Diuretics are nearly always needed to help control hypertension (see Table 11–5); thiazides work well in early CKD, but in those with a GFR less than 30 mL/min/1.73 m², loop diuretics are more effective. However, volume contraction as a result of very low sodium intake (especially with intercurrent illness) or over-diuresis in the presence of impaired sodium homeostasis can result in acute kidney injury. Initial drug therapy for proteinuric patients should include ACE inhibitors or ARBs (see Table 11–7). When an ACE inhibitor or an ARB is initiated or uptitrated, patients must have serum creatinine and potassium checked within 7–14 days. Hyperkalemia or a rise in serum creatinine greater than 30% from baseline mandates reduction or cessation of the drug. An ACE inhibitor and ARB should not be used in combination. Hypertension in CKD can be difficult to control and additional agents from other classes are often needed. Current guidelines from the Joint National Commission suggest a blood pressure goal of less than 140/90 mm Hg for patients with CKD. However, the SPRINT trial, which enrolled over 2800 nondiabetic patients with CKD, showed substantial cardiovascular and mortality benefit with systolic blood pressure goal of less than 120 mm Hg, including in those aged 75 years and older. Further analysis of this data will help direct therapy goals for future guidelines.

2. Coronary artery disease—Patients with CKD are at higher risk for death from CVD than the general population. Traditional modifiable risk factors for CVD, such as hypertension, tobacco use, and hyperlipidemia, should be aggressively treated in patients with CKD. Uremic vascular calcification involving disordered phosphorus homeostasis and other mediators may also be a cardiovascular risk factor in these patients.

3. Heart failure—The complications of CKD result in increased cardiac workload via hypertensive disease, volume overload, and anemia. Patients with CKD may also have accelerated rates of atherosclerosis and vascular calcification resulting in vessel stiffness. All of these factors contribute to left ventricular hypertrophy and heart failure with preserved ejection fraction, which are present in most patients starting dialysis. Over time, heart failure with decreased ejection fraction may also develop. Diuretic therapy, in addition to prudent fluid and salt restriction, is usually necessary. Thiazides may be adequate therapy for most patients through CKD stage 3, but loop diuretics are usually needed when the GFR is less than 30 mL/min/1.73 m²; higher doses may be needed as kidney function declines. Digoxin is excreted by the kidney, and its toxicity is exacerbated in the presence of electrolyte disturbances, which are common in CKD. ACE inhibitors and ARBs can be used for patients with advanced CKD with close monitoring of blood pressure as well as close monitoring for hyperkalemia and worsening kidney function.

4. Pericarditis—Pericarditis rarely develops in uremic patients; typical findings include pleuritic chest pain and a friction rub. Development of a significant effusion may result in pulsus paradoxus, an enlarged cardiac silhouette on chest radiograph, and low QRS voltage and electrical alternans on ECG. The effusion is generally hemorrhagic, and anticoagulants should be avoided if this diagnosis is suspected. Cardiac tamponade can occur; therefore, uremic pericarditis is a mandatory indication for hospitalization and initiation of hemodialysis.

B. Disorders of Mineral Metabolism

The metabolic bone disease of CKD refers to the complex disturbances of calcium and phosphorus metabolism, parathyroid hormone (PTH), active vitamin D, and fibroblast growth factor-23 (FGF-23) homeostasis (see Chapter 21 and Figure 22–3). A typical pattern seen as early as CKD stage 3 is hyperphosphatemia, hypocalcemia, and hypovitaminosis D, resulting in secondary hyperparathyroidism. These abnormalities can cause vascular calcification, which may be partly responsible for the accelerated CVD and excess mortality seen in the CKD population. Epidemiologic studies in humans show an association between elevated phosphorus levels and increased risk of cardiovascular mortality in early CKD through ESRD. As yet, there are no intervention trials suggesting the best course of treatment in these patients; control of mineral and PTH levels per current guidelines is discussed below.

Bone disease, or **renal osteodystrophy,** in advanced CKD is common and there are several types of lesions. Renal osteodystrophy can be diagnosed only by bone biopsy, which is rarely done. The most common bone disease, **osteitis fibrosa cystica,** is a result of secondary hyperparathyroidism and the osteoclast-stimulating effects of PTH. This is a high-turnover disease with bone resorption and subperiosteal lesions; it can result in bone pain and proximal muscle weakness. **Adynamic bone disease,** or low-bone turnover, is becoming more common; it may result iatrogenically from suppression of PTH or via spontaneously low PTH production. **Osteomalacia** is characterized by lack of bone mineralization. In the past, osteomalacia was associated with aluminum toxicity—either as a result of chronic ingestion of prescribed aluminum-containing phosphorus binders or from high levels of aluminum in impure dialysate water. Currently, osteomalacia is more likely to result from hypovitaminosis D; there is

also theoretical risk of osteomalacia associated with use of bisphosphonates in advanced CKD.

All of the above entities increase the risk of fractures. Aluminum exposure should be avoided. In addition, treatment may involve correction of calcium, phosphorus, and 25-OH vitamin D levels toward normal values, and mitigation of hyperparathyroidism. Understanding the interplay between these abnormalities can help target therapy (Figure 22–3). Declining GFR leads to phosphorus retention. This results in hypocalcemia as phosphorus complexes with calcium, deposits in soft tissues, and stimulates PTH. Loss of renal mass and low 25-OH vitamin D levels often seen in CKD patients result in low 1,25(OH) vitamin D production by the kidney. Because 1,25(OH) vitamin D is a suppressor of PTH production, hypovitaminosis D also leads to secondary hyperparathyroidism.

The first step in treatment of metabolic bone disease is control of hyperphosphatemia (defined as a serum phosphorus of less than or equal to 4.5 mg/dL in pre-ESRD CKD, or less than or equal to 5.5 mg/dL in ESRD patients). This involves dietary phosphorus restriction initially (see section on dietary management), followed by the administration of oral phosphorus binders if targets are not achieved (see below). Oral phosphorus binders, such as calcium carbonate (650 mg/tablet) or calcium acetate (667 mg/capsule), block absorption of dietary phosphorus in the gut and are given thrice daily with meals. These should be titrated to a serum phosphorus of less than 4.6 mg/dL in stage 3–4 CKD and less than 4.6–5.5 mg/dL in ESRD. Maximal recommended elemental calcium doses are 1500 mg/day (eg, nine tablets of calcium acetate); doses should be decreased if serum calcium rises above 10 mg/dL. Phosphorus-binding agents that do not contain calcium are sevelamer and lanthanum. Sevelamer, 800–3200 mg, and lanthanum carbonate, 500–1000 mg, are given orally at the beginning of meals and may be combined with calcium-containing binders. Aluminum hydroxide is a highly effective phosphorus binder but can cause osteomalacia and neurologic complications when used long-term. It can be used in the acute setting for serum phosphorus greater than 7 mg/dL or for short periods (eg, 3 weeks) in CKD patients.

Once serum phosphorus levels are controlled, active vitamin D (1,25[OH] vitamin D, or calcitriol) or active vitamin D analogs are recommended to treat secondary hyperparathyroidism in stage 3–5 CKD. Serum 25-OH vitamin D levels should be measured and brought to normal (see Chapter 26) prior to considering administration of active vitamin D. Active vitamin D (calcitriol) increases serum calcium and phosphorus levels; both need to be monitored closely during calcitriol therapy, and its dose should be decreased if hypercalcemia or hyperphosphatemia occurs. Typical calcitriol dosing is 0.25 or 0.5 mcg orally daily or every other day. Cinacalcet targets the calcium-sensing receptors of the parathyroid gland and suppresses PTH production. Cinacalcet, 30–90 mg orally once a day, can be used if elevated serum phosphorus or calcium levels prohibit the use of vitamin D analogs; cinacalcet can cause serious hypocalcemia, and patients should be closely monitored for this complication. Optimal PTH levels in

▲ **Figure 22–3.** Mineral abnormalities of chronic kidney disease (CKD). Decline in glomerular filtration rate (GFR) and loss of renal mass lead directly to increased serum phosphorus and hypovitaminosis D. Both of these abnormalities result in hypocalcemia and hyperparathyroidism. Many CKD patients also have nutritional 25(OH) vitamin D deficiency. PTH, parathyroid hormone.

CKD are not known, but because skeletal resistance to PTH develops with uremia, relatively high levels are targeted in advanced CKD to avoid adynamic bone disease. Expert guidelines generally suggest goal PTH levels near or just above the upper limit of normal for moderate CKD, and at least twofold and up to ninefold the upper limit of normal for ESRD.

C. Hematologic Complications

1. Anemia—The anemia of CKD is primarily due to decreased erythropoietin production, which often becomes clinically significant during stage 3 CKD. Many patients are iron deficient as well due to impaired GI iron absorption.

Erythropoiesis-stimulating agents (ESAs, eg, recombinant erythropoietin [epoetin] and darbepoetin) are used to treat the anemia of CKD if other treatable causes are excluded. There is likely no benefit of starting an ESA before Hgb values are less than 9 g/dL. The starting dose of epoetin is 50 units/kg (3000–4000 units/dose) once or twice a week, and darbepoetin is started at 0.45 mcg/kg and can be administered every 2–4 weeks. These agents can be given intravenously (eg, to the hemodialysis patient) or subcutaneously (to both the predialysis or dialysis patient); subcutaneous dosing of erythropoietin is roughly 30% more effective than intravenous dosing. ESAs should be titrated to an Hgb of 10–11 g/dL for optimal safety; studies show that targeting a higher Hgb increases the risk of stroke and possibly other cardiovascular events. When titrating doses, Hgb levels should rise no more than 1 g/dL every 3–4 weeks. Hypertension is a complication of treatment with ESAs in about 20% of patients. The dosage may require adjustment, or antihypertensive drugs may need to be given.

Iron stores must be adequate to ensure response to ESAs. Hepcidin, a molecule that blocks GI iron absorption and mobilization of iron from body stores, tends to be high in CKD. Therefore, traditional measures of iron stores are measured in CKD patients but are targeted to higher goals; in CKD, a serum ferritin below 100–200 ng/mL or iron saturation less than 20% is suggestive of iron deficiency. Iron stores should be repleted with oral or parenteral iron prior to the initiation of an ESA. Iron therapy should probably be withheld if the serum ferritin is greater than 500–800 ng/mL, even if the iron saturation is less than 20%. Oral therapy with ferrous sulfate, gluconate, or fumarate, 325 mg once to three times daily, is the initial therapy in pre-ESRD CKD. For those who do not respond due to poor GI absorption or lack of tolerance, intravenous iron may be necessary.

The preliminary investigation of anemia in any CKD patient should also include assessment of thyroid function tests, and serum vitamin B_{12} testing prior to initiating therapy with an ESA.

2. Coagulopathy—The bleeding diathesis that may occur in advanced stage CKD is mainly due to platelet dysfunction, but severe anemia may also contribute.

Treatment is required only in patients who are symptomatic. Raising the Hgb to 9–10 g/dL in anemic patients can reduce risk of bleeding via improved clot formation.

Desmopressin (25 mcg intravenously every 8–12 hours for two doses) is a short-lived but effective treatment for platelet dysfunction and it is often used in preparation for surgery. Conjugated estrogens, 2.5–5 mg orally for 5–7 days, may have an effect for several weeks but are seldom used. Dialysis improves the bleeding time. Cryoprecipitate (10–15 bags) is rarely used and lasts less than 24 hours.

D. Hyperkalemia

Potassium balance generally remains intact in CKD until stages 4–5. However, hyperkalemia may occur at earlier stages when certain conditions are present, such as type 4 renal tubular acidosis (seen in patients with diabetes mellitus), high potassium diets, or medications that decrease renal potassium secretion (amiloride, triamterene, spironolactone, eplerenone, NSAIDs, ACE inhibitors, ARBs) or block cellular potassium uptake (beta-blockers). Other causes include acidemic states and any type of cellular destruction causing release of intracellular contents, such as hemolysis and rhabdomyolysis.

Treatment of acute hyperkalemia is discussed in Chapter 21 (see Table 21–6). Cardiac monitoring is indicated for any ECG changes seen with hyperkalemia or a serum potassium level greater than 6.0–6.5 mEq/L. Chronic hyperkalemia is best treated with dietary potassium restriction (2 g/day) and minimization or elimination of any medications that may impair renal potassium excretion, as noted above. Loop diuretics may also be administered for their kaliuretic effect as long as the patient is not volume-depleted.

E. Acid–Base Disorders

Damaged kidneys are unable to excrete the 1 mEq/kg/day of acid generated by metabolism of dietary animal proteins in the typical Western diet. The resultant metabolic acidosis is primarily due to decreased GFR; proximal or distal tubular defects may contribute to or worsen the acidosis. Excess hydrogen ions are buffered by bone; the consequent leaching of calcium and phosphorus from the bone contributes to the metabolic bone disease described above and to growth retardation in children with CKD. Chronic acidosis can also result in muscle protein catabolism, and may accelerate progression of CKD. The serum bicarbonate level should be maintained at greater than 21 mEq/L. Reduction in the intake of dietary animal protein and the administration of oral sodium bicarbonate (in doses of 0.5–1.0 mEq/kg/day divided twice daily and titrated as needed) may achieve this goal. Citrate salts increase the absorption of dietary aluminum and should be avoided in CKD.

F. Neurologic Complications

Uremic encephalopathy, resulting from the aggregation of uremic toxins, does not occur until GFR falls below 5–10 mL/min/1.73 m^2. Symptoms begin with difficulty in concentrating and can progress to lethargy, confusion, seizure, and coma. Physical findings may include altered mental status, weakness, and asterixis. These findings improve with dialysis.

Other neurologic complications, which can manifest with advanced CKD include peripheral neuropathies (stocking-glove or isolated mononeuropathies), erectile dysfunction, autonomic dysfunction, and restless leg syndrome. These may not improve with dialysis therapy.

G. Endocrine Disorders

There is risk of hypoglycemia in treated diabetic patients with advanced CKD due to decreased renal elimination of insulin. Doses of oral hypoglycemics and insulin may need reduction. Metformin is associated with risk of lactic acidosis when the GFR is less than 50 mL/min/1.73 m^2 and should be discontinued at this point.

Decreased libido and erectile dysfunction are common in advanced CKD. Men have decreased testosterone levels; women are often anovulatory. Women with serum creatinine less than 1.4 mg/dL are not at increased risk for poor outcomes in pregnancy; however, those with serum creatinine greater than 1.4 mg/dL may experience faster progression of CKD with pregnancy. Fetal survival is not compromised, however, unless CKD is advanced. Despite a high degree of infertility in patients with ESRD, pregnancy can occur in this setting; however, fetal mortality approaches 50%, and babies who survive are often premature. In female patients with ESRD, renal transplantation with a well-functioning allograft affords the best chances for a successful pregnancy.

▶ Treatment

A. Slowing Progression

Treatment of the underlying cause of CKD is vital. Control of diabetes should be aggressive in early CKD; risk of hypoglycemia increases in advanced CKD, and glycemic targets may need to be relaxed to avoid this dangerous complication. Blood pressure control is vital to slow progression of all forms of CKD; agents that block the renin-angiotensin-aldosterone system are particularly important in proteinuric disease (see section on hypertension regarding blood pressure goals). Several small studies suggest a possible benefit of oral bicarbonate therapy in slowing CKD progression when acidemia is present; there is also theoretic value in lowering uric acid levels in those with concomitant hyperuricemia, but clinical data are lacking. Obese patients should be encouraged to lose weight. Management of traditional cardiovascular risk factors should also be emphasized.

B. Dietary Management

Patients with CKD should be evaluated by a renal nutritionist. Patient-specific recommendations should be made concerning protein, salt, water, potassium, and phosphorus intake to help manage CKD progression and complications.

1. Protein restriction—Reduced intake of animal protein to 0.6-0.8 g/kg/day may retard CKD progression and is likely not harmful in the otherwise well-nourished patient; it is not advisable in those with cachexia or low serum albumin in the absence of the nephrotic syndrome.

2. Salt and water restriction—In advanced CKD, the kidney is unable to adapt to large changes in sodium intake. Intake of greater than 3–4 g/day can lead to hypertension and hypervolemia, whereas intake of less than 1 g/day can lead to volume depletion and hypotension. A goal of 2 g/day of sodium is reasonable for most patients. Daily fluid restriction to 2 L may be needed if volume overload is present.

3. Potassium restriction—Restriction is needed once the GFR has fallen below 10–20 mL/min/1.73 m^2, or earlier if the patient is hyperkalemic. Patients should receive detailed lists describing potassium content of foods and should limit their intake to less than 50–60 mEq/day (2 g/day). An aggressive bowel regimen should be instituted for patients with hyperkalemia (more than two bowel movements daily), since a higher percentage of potassium is excreted through the gastrointestinal tract as GFR declines.

4. Phosphorus restriction—The phosphorus level should be kept in the "normal" range (less than 4.5 mg/dL) predialysis, and between 3.5 and 5.5 mg/dL in ESRD, with a dietary restriction of 800–1000 mg/day. Foods rich in phosphorus such as cola beverages, eggs, dairy products, nuts, beans, and meat should be limited, although care must be taken to avoid protein malnutrition. Processed foods are often preserved with highly bioavailable phosphorus and should be avoided. When GFR is less than 20–30 mL/min/1.73 m^2, dietary restriction is rarely sufficient to reach target levels, and phosphorus binders are usually required (see above).

C. Medication Management

Many drugs are excreted by the kidney; dosages should be adjusted for GFR. Insulin doses may need to be decreased as noted above. Magnesium-containing medications, such as laxatives or antacids, and phosphorus-containing medicines, (eg, cathartics) should be avoided. Active morphine metabolites can accumulate in advanced CKD; this problem is not encountered with other opioid agents. Drugs with potential nephrotoxicity (NSAIDs, intravenous contrast, as well as others noted in the Acute Kidney Injury section) should be avoided.

D. Treatment of End-Stage Renal Disease

When GFR declines to 5–10 mL/min/1.73 m^2, renal replacement therapy (hemodialysis, peritoneal dialysis, or kidney transplantation) is required to sustain life. Patient education is important in understanding which mode of therapy is most suitable, as is timely preparation for treatment; therefore, referral to a nephrologist should take place in late stage 3 CKD, or when the GFR is declining rapidly. Such referral has been shown to improve mortality. Preparation for ESRD treatment requires a team approach with the involvement of dieticians, social workers, primary care clinicians, and nephrologists. For very elderly patients, or those with multiple debilitating or life-limiting comorbidities, dialysis therapy may not meaningfully prolong life, and the option of palliative care should be discussed with the patient and family. Conversely, for patients who are otherwise relatively healthy, evaluation for possible kidney transplantation should be considered prior to initiation of dialysis.

1. Dialysis—Dialysis initiation should be considered when GFR is 10 mL/min/1.73 m². Studies suggest that the well-selected patient without overt uremic symptoms may wait to initiate dialysis until GFR is closer to 7 mL/min/1.73 m². Other indications for dialysis, which may occur when GFR is 10–15 mL/min/1.73 m² include (1) uremic symptoms, (2) fluid overload unresponsive to diuresis, and (3) refractory hyperkalemia.

A. Hemodialysis—Vascular access for hemodialysis can be accomplished by an arteriovenous fistula (the preferred method) or prosthetic graft; creation of dialysis access should be considered well before dialysis initiation. An indwelling catheter is used when there is no useable vascular access. Because catheters confer a high risk of bloodstream infection, they should be considered a temporary measure. Native fistulas typically last longer than prosthetic grafts but require a longer time after surgical construction for maturation (6–8 weeks for a fistula versus 2 weeks for a graft). Infection, thrombosis, and aneurysm formation are complications seen more often in grafts than fistulas. *Staphylococcus* species are the most common cause of soft-tissue infections and bacteremia.

Treatment at a hemodialysis center occurs three times a week. Sessions last 3–5 hours depending on patient size and type of dialysis access. Home hemodialysis is often performed more frequently (3–6 days per week for shorter sessions) and requires a trained helper. Results of trials comparing quotidian modalities (nocturnal and frequent home hemodialysis) to conventional in-center dialysis have not thus far shown significant mortality differences, but there may be improvements in blood pressure control, mineral metabolism, and quality of life.

B. Peritoneal dialysis—With peritoneal dialysis, the peritoneal membrane is the "dialyzer." Dialysate is instilled into the peritoneal cavity through an indwelling catheter; water and solutes move across the capillary bed that lies between the visceral and parietal layers of the membrane into the dialysate during a "dwell." After equilibration, the dialysate is drained, and fresh dialysate is instilled—this is an "exchange."

The most common complication of peritoneal dialysis is peritonitis. Peritonitis may present with nausea and vomiting, abdominal pain, diarrhea or constipation, and fever. The normally clear dialysate becomes cloudy; and a diagnostic peritoneal fluid cell count greater than 100 white blood cells/mcL with a differential of greater than 50% polymorphonuclear neutrophils is present. *Staphylococcus aureus* is the most common infecting organism, but streptococci and gram-negative species are also common.

2. Kidney transplantation—Up to 50% of all patients with ESRD are otherwise healthy enough to be suitable for transplantation, although standard criteria for recipient selection are lacking between transplant centers. Older age

is becoming less of a barrier, as long as reasonable life expectancy is anticipated. Two-thirds of kidney allografts come from deceased donors, with the remainder from living related or unrelated donors. Over 100,000 patients are on the waiting list for a deceased donor transplant in the United States; the average wait is 2–6 years, depending on geographic location and recipient blood type.

The 1- and 5-year kidney graft survival rates are approximately 95% and 80%, respectively, for living donor transplants and 89% and 66%, respectively, for deceased donor transplants.

3. Medical management of ESRD—As noted above, some patients are not candidates for kidney transplantation and may not benefit from dialysis. Very elderly persons may die soon after dialysis initiation; those who do not may nonetheless rapidly lose functional status in the first year of treatment. The decision to initiate dialysis in patients with limited life expectancy should be weighed against possible deterioration in quality of life. For patients with ESRD who elect not to undergo dialysis or who withdraw from dialysis, progressive uremia with gradual suppression of sensorium results in a painless death within days to months. Hyperkalemia may intervene with a fatal cardiac dysrythmia. Diuretics, volume restriction, and opioids, as described in Chapter 5, may help decrease the symptoms of volume overload. Involvement of a palliative care team is essential.

▶ **Prognosis in ESRD**

Compared with kidney transplant recipients and age-matched controls, mortality is higher for patients undergoing dialysis. There is likely little difference in survival for well-matched peritoneal versus hemodialysis patients.

Survival rates on dialysis depend on the underlying disease process. Five-year Kaplan-Meier survival rates vary from 37% for patients with diabetes to 54% for patients with glomerulonephritis. Overall 5-year survival is currently estimated at 40%. Patients undergoing dialysis have an average life-expectancy of 3–5 years, but survival for as long as 25 years may be achieved depending on comorbidities. The most common cause of death is cardiac disease (more than 50%). Other causes include infection, cerebrovascular disease, and malignancy. Diabetes, advanced age, a low serum albumin, lower socioeconomic status, and inadequate dialysis are all significant predictors of mortality; high fibroblast growth factor (FGF)-23 levels are a novel marker for mortality in ESRD.

▶ **When to Refer**

- A patient with stage 3–5 CKD should be referred to a nephrologist for management in conjunction with the primary care provider.
- A patient with other forms of CKD such as those with proteinuria greater than 1 g/day or polycystic kidney disease should be referred to a nephrologist at earlier stages.

When to Admit

- Admission should be considered for patients with decompensation of problems related to CKD, such as worsening of acid-base status, electrolyte abnormalities, and volume status that cannot be appropriately treated in the outpatient setting.

- Admission is appropriate when a patient needs to start dialysis and is not stable for outpatient initiation.

Gansevoort RT et al. Chronic kidney disease and cardiovascular risk: epidemiology, mechanisms, and prevention. Lancet. 2013 Jul 27;382(9889):339–52. [PMID: 23727170]

Malindretos P et al. Phosphate binders, past—present—future. A critical appraisal. Expert Opin Pharmacother. 2016 Feb;17(3):297–300. [PMID: 26679256]

Mendu ML et al. Clinical predictors of diagnostic testing utility in the initial evaluation of chronic kidney disease. Nephrology (Carlton). 2015 Nov 26. [Epub ahead of print] [PMID: 26610178]

Ponticelli C et al. Drug management in the elderly adult with chronic kidney disease: a review for the primary care physician. Mayo Clin Proc. 2015 May;90(5):633–45. [PMID: 25771152]

Sinnakirouchenan R et al. Role of sodium restriction and diuretic therapy for "resistant" hypertension in chronic kidney disease. Semin Nephrol. 2014;34(5):514–9. [PMID: 25416660]

SPRINT Research Group, Wright JT Jr et al. A randomized trial of intensive versus standard blood-pressure control. N Engl J Med. 2015 Nov 26;373(22):2103–16. [PMID: 26551272]

Vassalotti JA et al; National Kidney Foundation Kidney Disease Outcomes Quality Initiative. Practical approach to detection and management of chronic kidney disease for the primary care clinician. Am J Med. 2016 Feb;129(2):153–162.e7. [PMID: 26391748]

RENAL ARTERY STENOSIS

 ESSENTIALS OF DIAGNOSIS

- Produced by atherosclerotic occlusive disease (80–90% of patients) or fibromuscular dysplasia (10–15%).

- Hypertension.

- Acute kidney injury in patients starting ACE inhibitor therapy.

General Considerations

Atherosclerotic ischemic renal disease accounts for most cases of renal artery stenosis. Fibromuscular dysplasia is a less common cause of renal artery stenosis. Approximately 5% of Americans with hypertension suffer from renal artery stenosis. It occurs most commonly in those over 45 years of age with a history of atherosclerotic disease. Other risk factors include CKD, diabetes mellitus, tobacco use, and hypertension.

Clinical Findings

A. Symptoms and Signs

Patients with atherosclerotic ischemic renal disease may have refractory hypertension, new-onset hypertension (in an older patient), pulmonary edema with poorly controlled blood pressure, and acute kidney injury upon starting an ACE inhibitor. In addition to hypertension, physical examination may reveal an audible abdominal bruit on the affected side. Fibromuscular dysplasia primarily affects young women. Unexplained hypertension in a woman younger than 40 years is reason to screen for this disorder.

B. Laboratory Findings

Laboratory values can show elevated BUN and serum creatinine levels in the setting of significant renal ischemia.

C. Imaging

Abdominal ultrasound can reveal asymmetric kidney size when one renal artery is affected out of proportion to the other or small hyperechoic kidneys if both are affected.

Three prevailing methods used for screening are Doppler ultrasonography, CT angiography, and magnetic resonance angiography (MRA). According to the American College of Cardiology/American Heart Association guidelines, one of these should be undertaken if a corrective procedure would be performed when a positive test result is found. **Doppler ultrasonography** is highly sensitive and specific (85% and 92% respectively in a meta-analysis of 88 studies) and relatively inexpensive. However, this method is extremely operator and patient dependent.

CT angiography consists of intravenous digital subtraction angiography with arteriography and is a noninvasive procedure. The procedure uses a spiral (helical) CT scan with intravenous contrast injection. The sensitivities from various studies range from 77% to 98%, with less varying specificities in a range of 90–94%.

MRA is an excellent but expensive way to screen for renal artery stenosis, particularly in those with atherosclerotic disease. Sensitivity is 77–100%, although one study with particular flaws showed a sensitivity of only 62%. Specificity ranges from 71% to 96%. Turbulent blood flow can cause false-positive results. The imaging agent for MRA (gadolinium) has been associated with nephrogenic systemic fibrosis, which occurs primarily in patients with a GFR of less than 15 mL/min/1.73 m², and rarely in patients with a GFR of 15–30 mL/min/1.73 m². It has also been seen in those with acute kidney injury and kidney transplants.

Renal angiography is the gold standard for diagnosis but more invasive than the screening tests above. Thus, this is performed after a positive screening test. CO_2 subtraction angiography can be used in place of dye when the risk of dye nephropathy exists—eg, in diabetic patients with kidney injury. Lesions are most commonly found in the proximal third or ostial region of the renal artery. The risk of atheroembolic phenomena after angiography ranges from 5% to 10%. Fibromuscular dysplasia has a characteristic "beads-on-a-string" appearance on angiography.

► Treatment

Treatment of atherosclerotic ischemic renal disease is controversial. Options include medical management, angioplasty with or without stenting, and surgical bypass. Two large randomized trials have shown that vascular intervention is no better than optimal medical management in typical patients with renal artery stenosis. Angioplasty might reduce the number of antihypertensive medications but does not significantly change the progression of kidney dysfunction in comparison to patients medically managed. Stenting produces significantly better angioplastic results. However, blood pressure and serum creatinines are similar at 6 months of observation compared with both angioplasty and stents. Angioplasty is equally as effective as, and safer than, surgical revision.

Treatment of **fibromuscular dysplasia** with percutaneous transluminal angioplasty is often curative, which is in stark contrast to treatment for atherosclerotic causes.

Boateng FK et al. Renal artery stenosis: prevalence of, risk factors for, and management of in-stent stenosis. Am J Kidney Dis. 2013 Jan;61(1):147–60. [PMID: 23122491]

Cooper CJ et al; CORAL Investigators. Stenting and medical therapy for atherosclerotic renal-artery stenosis. N Engl J Med. 2014 Jan 2;370(1):13–22. [PMID: 24245566]

Sattur S et al. Renal artery stenosis—an update. Postgrad Med. 2013 Sep;125(5):43–50. [PMID: 24113662]

▼ GLOMERULAR DISEASES

Abnormalities of glomerular function can be caused by damage to the major components of the glomerulus: the epithelium (podocytes), basement membrane, capillary endothelium, or mesangium. The damage may be caused by overwork injury, as in CKD; by an inflammatory process, such as SLE; by a podocyte protein mutation, as in hereditary focal segmental glomerulosclerosis (FSGS); or a deposition disease, as in diabetes or amyloidosis. A specific histologic pattern of glomerular injury results from this damage and can be seen on kidney biopsy.

► Classification

Clinically, a glomerular disease can be classified as being in one of two spectra—either in the nephritic spectrum or the nephrotic spectrum (Figure 22–4). In the "least severe" end of the **nephritic spectrum,** the findings of glomerular hematuria (ie, dysmorphic red blood cells with some degree of proteinuria) are characteristic. The nephritic *syndrome,* comprising glomerular hematuria, subnephrotic proteinuria (less than 3 g/day), edema, and elevated creatinine, falls in the mid-portion of the spectrum. The rapidly progressive glomerulonephridities (RPGNs) are at the "most severe" and clinically urgent end of the nephritic spectrum. The **nephrotic spectrum** comprises diseases

▲ **Figure 22–4.** Glomerular diseases present within one of the clinical spectra shown, the exact presentation is determined by the severity of the underlying disease and the pattern of injury. Nephritic diseases are characterized by the presence of an active urine sediment with glomerular hematuria and often with proteinuria. Nephrotic spectrum diseases are proteinuric with bland urine sediments (no cells or cellular casts). All glomerular diseases may progress to a chronic, scarred state. (Adapted, with permission, from Megan Troxell, MD, PhD.)

that present primarily with proteinuria of at least 0.5–1 g/day and a bland urine sediment (no cells or cellular casts). The more severe end of the nephrotic spectrum comprises the nephrotic *syndrome*, which is characterized by the constellation of nephrotic-range proteinuria of greater than 3 g/day, hypoalbuminuria, edema, and hyperlipidemia. Differentiating between a clinical presentation within the *nephritic* spectrum versus the *nephrotic* spectrum is important because it helps narrow the differential diagnosis of the underlying glomerular disease (Tables 22–8 and 22–9).

Glomerular diseases can also be classified according to whether they cause only renal abnormalities (primary renal disease) or whether the renal abnormalities result from a systemic disease (secondary renal disease).

Further evaluation prior to kidney biopsy may include serologic testing for systemic diseases that can result in glomerular damage (Figure 22–5).

Table 22–8. Classification and findings in glomerulonephritis: Nephritic spectrum presentations.

	Typical Presentation	Association/Notes	Serology
Postinfectious glomerulonephritis	Children: abrupt onset of nephritic syndrome and acute kidney injury but can present anywhere in nephritic spectrum	Streptococci, other bacterial infections (eg, staphylococci, endocarditis, shunt infections)	Rising ASO titers, low complement levels
IgA nephropathy (Berger disease) and Henoch-Schönlein purpura, systemic IgA vasculitis	Classically: gross hematuria with respiratory tract infection; can present anywhere in nephritic spectrum; Henoch-Schönlein purpura with vasculitic rash and gastrointestinal hemorrhage	Abnormal IgA glycosylation in both primary (familial predisposition) and secondary disease (associated with cirrhosis, HIV, celiac disease) Henoch-Schönlein purpura in children after an inciting infection	No serologic tests helpful; complement levels are normal
Pauci-immune (granulomatosis with polyangiitis, eosinophilic granulomatosis with polyangiitis [formerly Churg-Strauss], polyarteritis, idiopathic crescentic glomerulonephritis)	Classically as crescentic or RPGN, but can present anywhere in nephritic spectrum; may have respiratory tract/sinus symptoms in granulomatosis with polyangiitis	See Figure 22–5	ANCAs: MPO or PR3 titers high; complement levels normal
Anti-GBM glomerulonephritis; Goodpasture syndrome	Classically as crescentic or RPGN, but can present anywhere in nephritic spectrum; with pulmonary hemorrhage in Goodpasture syndrome	May develop as a result of respiratory irritant exposure (chemicals or tobacco use)	Anti-GBM antibody titers high; complement levels normal
Cryoglobulin-associated glomerulonephritis	Often acute nephritic syndrome; often with systemic vasculitis including rash and arthritis	Most commonly associated with chronic hepatitis C; may occur with other chronic infections or some connective tissue diseases	Cryoglobulins positive; rheumatoid factor may be elevated; complement levels low
Idiopathic MPGN	Classically presents with acute nephritic syndrome, but can see nephrotic syndrome features in addition	Most patients are < 30 years old Type I most common Type II (dense deposit disease) associated with C3 nephritic factor	Low complement levels
Hepatitis C infection	Anywhere in nephritic spectrum	Can cause MPGN pattern of injury or cryoglobulinemic glomerulonephritis; membranous nephropathy pattern of injury uncommon	Low complement levels; positive hepatitis C serology; rheumatoid factor may be elevated
Systemic lupus erythematosus	Anywhere in nephritic spectrum, depending on pattern/severity of injury	Treatment depends on clinical course and International Society of Nephrology and Renal Pathology Society (ISN/RPS) classification on biopsy	High ANA and anti-double-stranded DNA titers; low complement levels

ANA, antinuclear antibodies; ANCAs: antineutrophil cytoplasmic antibodies; GBM, glomerular basement membrane; MPGN, membranoproliferative glomerulonephritis; MPO, myeloperoxidase; PR3, proteinase 3; RPGN, rapidly progressive glomerulonephritis.

Table 22–9. Classification and findings in glomerulonephritis: Nephrotic spectrum presentations.

Disease	Typical Presentation	Association/Notes
Minimal change disease (nil disease; lipoid nephrosis)	Child with sudden onset of full nephrotic syndrome	Children: associated with allergy or viral infection Adults: associated with Hodgkin disease, NSAIDs
Membranous nephropathy	Anywhere in nephrotic spectrum, but nephrotic syndrome not uncommon; particular predisposition to hypercoagulable state	Primary (idiopathic) may be associated with antibodies to PLA₂R Secondary may be associated with non-Hodgkin lymphoma, carcinoma (gastrointestinal, renal, bronchogenic, thyroid), gold therapy, penicillamine, SLE, chronic hepatitis B or C infection
Focal and segmental glomerulosclerosis	Anywhere in nephrotic spectrum; children with congenital disease have nephrotic syndrome	Children: congenital disease with podocyte gene mutation, or in spectrum of disease with minimal change disease Adults: Associated with heroin abuse, HIV infection, reflux nephropathy, obesity, pamidronate, podocyte protein mutations, *APOL1* mutations in blacks
Amyloidosis	Anywhere in nephrotic spectrum	AL: plasma cell dyscrasia with Ig light chain over-production and deposition; check SPEP and UPEP AA: serum amyloid protein A over-production and deposition in response to chronic inflammatory disease (rheumatoid arthritis, inflammatory bowel disease, chronic infection)
Diabetic nephropathy	High GFR (hyperfiltration) → microalbuminuria → frank proteinuria → decline in GFR	Diabetes diagnosis precedes diagnosis of nephropathy by years
HIV-associated nephropathy	Heavy proteinuria, often nephrotic syndrome, progresses to ESRD relatively quickly	Usually seen in antiviral treatment-naïve patients (rare in HAART era), predilection for those of African descent (*APOL1* mutations)
Membranoproliferative glomerulonephropathy	Can present with nephrotic syndrome, but usually with nephritic features as well (glomerular hematuria)	See Table 22–8

ESRD, end-stage renal disease; GFR, glomerular filtration rate; HAART, highly active antiretroviral therapy; NSAIDs, nonsteroidal anti-inflammatory drugs; PLA₂R, phospholipase A₂ receptor; SLE, systemic lupus erythematosus; SPEP/UPEP: serum and urine protein electrophoresis.

Caliskan Y et al. Novel biomarkers in glomerular disease. Adv Chronic Kidney Dis. 2014 Mar;21(2):205–16. [PMID: 24602470]

Cattran D. KDIGO clinical practice guideline for glomerulonephritis. Chapter 2: General principles in the management of glomerular disease. 2012 Dec;(Suppl 2):156–62. http://kdigo.org/home/glomerulonephritis-gn

Couser WG et al. The etiology of glomerulonephritis: roles of infection and autoimmunity. Kidney Int. 2014 Nov;86 (5):905–14. [PMID: 24621918]

Hogan J et al. Diagnostic tests and treatment options in glomerular disease: 2014 update. Am J Kidney Dis. 2014 Apr;63(4):656–66. [PMID: 24239051]

NEPHRITIC SPECTRUM GLOMERULAR DISEASES

ESSENTIALS OF DIAGNOSIS

► Glomerular hematuria (dysmorphic red blood cells) and modest proteinuria (usually 0.3–3 g/day).

► Red blood cell casts may be present if glomerular bleeding is heavy.

► Nephritic syndrome in more severe/inflammatory cases:

–Glomerular hematuria and proteinuria.

–Hypertension.

–Edema.

–Rising creatinine over days to months.

► Rapidly progressive glomerulonephritis in most severe cases:

–Glomerular hematuria and proteinuria.

–Hypertension and edema uncommon.

–Rising creatinine over days to months.

► General Considerations

Glomerulonephritis is a term given to those diseases that present in the nephritic spectrum and usually signifies an inflammatory process causing renal dysfunction. It can be acute, developing over days to weeks, with or without resolution, or may be more chronic and indolent with progressive scarring. As noted above, diseases that cause a nephritic

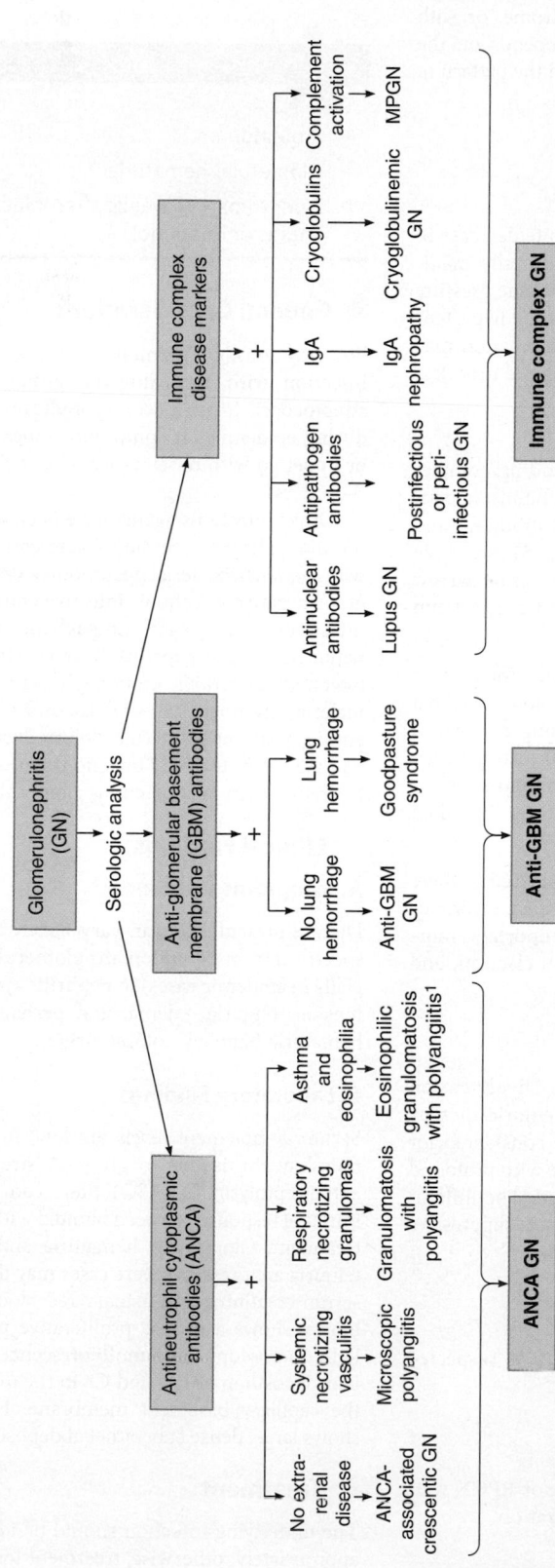

▲ **Figure 22–5.** Serologic analysis of patients with glomerulonephritis. MPGN, membranoproliferative glomerulonephritis. (Modified, with permission, from Greenberg A et al. *Primer on Kidney Diseases.* Academic Press, 1994 and Jennette JC, Falk RJ. Diagnosis and management of glomerulonephritis and vasculitis presenting as acute renal failure. Med Clin North Am. 1990;74(4):893–908. © Elsevier.)

¹Formerly Churg-Strauss syndrome.

spectrum presentation may present with glomerular hematuria and proteinuria, with nephritic syndrome, or with RPGN (Figure 22–4). The presentation depends on the severity of the underlying inflammation and the pattern of injury caused by the disease process.

▶ Clinical Findings

A. Symptoms and Signs

If the nephritic syndrome is present, the acute decrease in GFR leads to sodium retention. This is clinically manifested by edema, first seen in regions of low tissue pressure such as the periorbital and scrotal areas, and by hypertension. Heavy glomerular bleeding from inflammation may result in gross hematuria (smoky or cola-colored urine).

B. Laboratory Findings

1. Serologic testing—Serologic tests, including complement levels, antinuclear antibodies, cryoglobulins, hepatitis serologies, ANCAs, anti-GBM antibodies, and antistreptolysin O (ASO) titers (Figure 22–5), are done based on the history and physical examination to narrow the differential diagnosis of the nephritic spectrum disorder.

2. Urinalysis—The urine dipstick is positive for protein and blood. Urinary microscopy reveals red blood cells that are misshapen or dysmorphic from traversing a damaged glomerular filtration barrier. Red blood cell casts are seen with heavy glomerular bleeding and tubular stasis. When quantified, proteinuria is usually subnephrotic (less than 3 g/day).

3. Biopsy—Kidney biopsy should be considered if there are no contraindications (eg, bleeding disorders, thrombocytopenia, uncontrolled hypertension). Important morphologic information is gleaned from light, electron, and immunofluorescent microscopy.

▶ Treatment

General measures for all include treatment of hypertension and of fluid overload if present. Antiproteinuric therapy with an ACE inhibitor or ARB should be considered for those without acute kidney injury. For those with profound acute kidney injury, dialysis may be needed. The inflammatory glomerular injury may require immunosuppressive agents (see specific diseases discussed below).

▶ When to Refer

Any patient in whom a glomerulonephritis is suspected should be referred to a nephrologist.

▶ When to Admit

Any suspicion of acute nephritic syndrome or RPGN warrants consideration of immediate hospitalization.

Kazi SN et al. Work-up of hematuria. Prim Care. 2014 Dec;41(4):737–48. [PMID: 25439531]

1. Postinfectious Glomerulonephritis

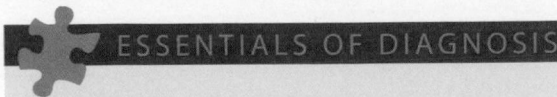

ESSENTIALS OF DIAGNOSIS

► Proteinuria.
► Glomerular hematuria.
► Symptoms 1–3 weeks after infection (often pharyngitis or impetigo).

▶ General Considerations

Postinfectious glomerulonephritis is most often due to infection with nephritogenic group A beta-hemolytic streptococci. It can occur sporadically or in clusters and during epidemics. It commonly appears after pharyngitis or impetigo with onset 1–3 weeks after infection (average 7–10 days).

Other infectious agents have been associated with glomerulonephritis including bacteremic states (especially with *S aureus*), bacterial pneumonias, deep-seated abscesses, gram-negative infections, infective endocarditis, and shunt infections; viral, fungal, and parasitic causes of glomerulonephritis include hepatitis B or C, HIV, cytomegalovirus infection, infectious mononucleosis, coccidioidomycosis, malaria, mycobacteria, syphilis, and toxoplasmosis. These entities result in glomerular injury during active infection, and are better termed "infection-related glomerulonephritis" rather than postinfectious glomerulonephritis.

▶ Clinical Findings

A. Symptoms and Signs

Disease presentation can vary widely across the nephritic spectrum from asymptomatic glomerular hematuria (especially in epidemic cases) to nephritic syndrome with hypertension, oliguria, edema, and perhaps gross glomerular hematuria (smokey-colored urine).

B. Laboratory Findings

Serum complement levels are low; in postinfectious glomerulonephritis due to group A streptococcal infection, anti-streptolysin O (ASO) titers can be high unless the immune response has been blunted with previous antibiotic treatment. Glomerular hematuria and subnephrotic proteinuria are present; severe cases may demonstrate elevated serum creatinine and urinary red blood cell casts. Kidney biopsy shows a diffuse proliferative pattern of injury on light microscopy. Immunofluorescence demonstrates granular deposition of IgG and C3 in the mesangium and along the capillary basement membrane. Electron microscopy shows large, dense subepithelial deposits or "humps."

▶ Treatment

The underlying infection should be identified and treated appropriately; otherwise, treatment for postinfectious glomerulonephritis is supportive. Antihypertensives, salt restriction, and diuretics should be used if needed.

Corticosteroids have not been shown to improve outcomes but have been tried in severe cases. Prognosis depends on the severity of the glomerular injury and age of the patient. Children are more likely to fully recover; adults are more prone to the development of severe disease (RPGN with crescent formation) and CKD.

Cattran D et al. KDIGO clinical practice guideline for glomerulonephritis. Chapter 9: infection-related glomerulonephritis. Kidney Int. 2012 Dec;(Suppl 2):200–8. http://www.kdigo.org/clinical_practice_guidelines/GN.php

Glassock RJ et al. *Staphylococcus*-related glomerulonephritis and poststreptococcal glomerulonephritis: why defining "post" is important in understanding and treating infection-related glomerulonephritis. Am J Kidney Dis. 2015 Jun;65(6):826–32. [PMID: 25890425]

Pinto SW et al. Ten-year follow-up of patients with epidemic post infectious glomerulonephritis. PLoS One. 2015 May 11;10(5):e0125313. [PMID: 25962068]

2. IgA Nephropathy

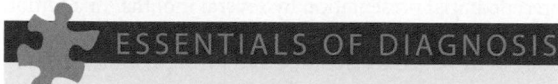

ESSENTIALS OF DIAGNOSIS

▶ Proteinuria: minimal to nephrotic range.

▶ Glomerular hematuria: microscopic is common; macroscopic (gross) after infection.

▶ Positive IgA staining on kidney biopsy.

▶ General Considerations

IgA nephropathy (Berger disease) is a primary renal disease of IgA deposition in the glomerular mesangium. The inciting cause is unknown but is likely due to deficient O-linked glycosylation of IgA subclass 1 molecules. IgA nephropathy can be a primary (renal-limited) disease, or it can be secondary to hepatic cirrhosis, celiac disease, and infections such as HIV and cytomegalovirus. Susceptibility to IgA nephropathy seems to be inheritable.

IgA nephropathy is the most common primary glomerular disease worldwide, particularly in Asia. It is most commonly seen in children and young adults, with males affected two to three times more commonly than females.

▶ Clinical Findings

An episode of gross hematuria is the most common presenting symptom. Frequently, this is associated with a mucosal viral infection such as an upper respiratory infection. The urine becomes red or smokey-colored 1–2 days after illness onset—a so-called "synpharyngitic" presentation in contradistinction to the latent period seen in postinfectious glomerulonephritis. IgA nephropathy can present anywhere along the nephritic spectrum from asymptomatic microscopic hematuria to RPGN. Rarely, nephrotic syndrome can be present as well.

There are no serologic tests that aid in this diagnosis; serum IgA subclass 1 testing may be a possibility in the future. Serum complements are normal. The typical pattern of injury seen on kidney biopsy is a focal glomerulonephritis with mesangial proliferation; immunofluorescence demonstrates diffuse mesangial IgA and C3 deposits.

▶ Treatment

The disease course of primary IgA nephropathy varies widely among patients; treatment approach needs to be tailored to risk for progression. Patients with low risk for progression (no hypertension, normal GFR, minimal proteinuria) can be monitored annually. Patients at higher risk (proteinuria greater than 1.0 g/day, decreased GFR, or hypertension or any combination of these three conditions) should be treated with an ACE inhibitor or ARB. Therapy should be titrated to reduce proteinuria to less than 1 g/day and to control blood pressure in the range of 125/75 mm Hg to 130/80 mm Hg. Addition of corticosteroids may be beneficial in patients with GFR greater than 50 mL/min/1.73 m² and persistent proteinuria greater than 1 g/day; the most commonly used regimen is methylprednisolone, 1 g/day intravenously for 3 days during months 1, 3, and 5, plus prednisone in a dosage of 0.5 mg/kg orally every other day for 6 months. Azathioprine and mycophenolate mofetil have also been used in patients at high risk for progression, but studies with these agents are small. For the rare patient with IgA neuropathy and a rapidly progressive clinical course with crescent formation on biopsy, cyclophosphamide and corticosteroid therapy should be considered (see section on ANCA-associated vasculitis below). Kidney transplantation is an excellent option for patients with ESRD, but recurrent disease has been documented in 30% of patients 5–10 years posttransplant. Fortunately, recurrent disease rarely leads to failure of the allograft.

▶ Prognosis

Approximately one-third of patients experience spontaneous clinical remission. Progression to ESRD occurs in 20–40% of patients. The remaining patients have chronic microscopic hematuria and a stable serum creatinine. The most unfavorable prognostic indicator is proteinuria greater than 1 g/day; other unfavorable prognostic indicators include hypertension, tubulointerstitial fibrosis, glomerulosclerosis, or glomerular crescents on biopsy, and abnormal GFR on presentation.

Rauen T et al; STOP-IgAN Investigators. Intensive supportive care plus immunosuppression in IgA nephropathy. N Engl J Med. 2015 Dec 3;373(23):2225–36. [PMID: 26630142]

Vecchio M et al. Immunosuppressive agents for treating IgA nephropathy. Cochrane Database Syst Rev. 2015 Aug 3;8:CD003965. [PMID: 26235292]

3. Henoch-Schönlein Purpura

Henoch-Schönlein purpura is a systemic small-vessel leukocytoclastic vasculitis associated with IgA subclass 1 deposition in vessel walls. It is most common in children and is often associated with an inciting infection, such as group A streptococcus or other exposure. There is a male predominance. It classically presents with palpable purpura in the lower extremities (Figure 22–6) and buttock

▲ **Figure 22–6.** Henoch-Schönlein purpura, with palpable purpura over both lower extremities. (Used, with permission, from Dean SM, Satiani B, Abraham WT. *Color Atlas and Synopsis of Vascular Diseases.* McGraw-Hill, 2014.)

area; arthralgias; and abdominal symptoms, such as nausea, colic, and melena. A decrease in GFR is common with a nephritic presentation. The renal lesions can be identical to those found in IgA nephropathy, and the underlying pathophysiology appears to be similar. Most patients with microscopic hematuria and minimal proteinuria recover fully over several weeks. Progressive CKD and possibly ESRD are more likely to develop in those with the nephrotic syndrome and the presence of both nephritic and nephrotic syndrome poses the worst renal prognosis. Histologic classification of the lesions in children may also provide prognostic information. To date, although several treatment regimens of various immunosuppressive agents have been clinically tested, none have been definitively proven to alter the course of severe Henoch-Schönlein purpura nephritis. Rituximab treatment and plasma exchange have been successful for severe disease according to several case reports, but clinical trials are lacking. Rapidly progressive disease with crescent formation on biopsy may be treated as in ANCA-associated vasculitis (see section below).

Further details about Henoch-Schönlein purpura are provided in Chapter 20.

Audemard-Verger A et al. IgA vasculitis (Henoch-Shönlein purpura) in adults: diagnostic and therapeutic aspects. Autoimmun Rev. 2015 Jul;14(7):579–85. [PMID: 25688001]

4. Pauci-Immune Glomerulonephritis (Anca-Associated)

Pauci-immune necrotizing glomerulonephritis is caused by the following systemic ANCA-associated small-vessel vasculitides: granulomatosis with polyangiitis (formerly known as Wegener granulomatosis), microscopic polyangiitis, and eosinophilic granulomatosis with polyangiitis (formerly Churg-Strauss disease; see Chapter 20). ANCA-associated glomerulonephritis can also present as a primary renal lesion without systemic involvement; this is termed "idiopathic crescentic glomerulonephritis." The pathogenesis of these entities appears to involve cytokine-primed neutrophils presenting cytoplasmic antigens on their surfaces (proteinase 3 and myeloperoxidase). Circulating ANCAs then bind to these antigens and activate a neutrophil respiratory burst with consequent vascular damage; primed neutrophils also appear to activate the alternative complement pathway. Putative environmental exposures that may encite the initial response include *S aureus* and silica. Immunofluorescence of kidney biopsy specimens do not reveal any evidence of immunoglobulin or complement deposition, hence the term "pauci-immune." Renal involvement classically presents as an RPGN, but more indolent presentations can be seen as well.

▶ Clinical Findings

A. Symptoms and Signs

Symptoms of a systemic inflammatory disease, including fever, malaise, and weight loss may be present and usually precede initial presentation by several months. In addition to hematuria and proteinuria from glomerular inflammation, some patients exhibit purpura from dermal capillary involvement and mononeuritis multiplex from nerve arteriolar involvement. Ninety percent of patients with granulomatosis with polyangiitis have upper (especially sinus) or lower respiratory tract symptoms with nodular lesions that can cavitate and bleed. Hemoptysis is a concerning sign and usually warrants hospitalization and aggressive immunosuppression.

B. Laboratory Findings

Serologically, ANCA subtype analysis is done to determine whether antiproteinase-3 antibodies (PR3-ANCA) or antimyeloperoxidase antibodies (MPO-ANCA) are present. Most patients with granulomatosis with polyangiitis are PR3 positive; the remainder are MPO positive or, more rarely, do not demonstrate circulating ANCA. Microscopic angiitis is generally associated with MPO ANCA. Renal biopsy demonstrates necrotizing lesions and crescents on light microscopy; immunofluorescence is negative for immune complex deposition.

▶ Treatment

Treatment should be instituted early if aggressive disease is present. Induction therapy of high-dose corticosteroids (methylprednisolone, 1–2 g/day intravenously for 3 days, followed by prednisone, 1 mg/kg orally for 1 month, with a slow taper over the next 6 months) and cytotoxic agents (cyclophosphamide, 0.5–1 g/m² intravenously per month or 1.5–2 mg/kg orally for 3–6 months) is followed by long-term azathioprine or mycophenolate mofetil. Rituximab has been shown to be noninferior to cyclophosphamide for induction and is also used in refractory or relapsing cases and as an alternative to azathioprine for maintenance of remission. Plasma exchange has been used in conjunction with induction therapy in particularly severe cases; however, its efficacy is controversial. Patients receiving cyclophosphamide should receive prophylaxis for

Pneumocystis jirovecii, such as trimethoprim-sulfamethoxazole double-strength orally 3 days per week.

▶ Prognosis

Without treatment, prognosis is extremely poor. However, with aggressive treatment, complete remission can be achieved in about 75% of patients. Prognosis depends on the extent of renal involvement before treatment is started and may be worse in those with PR3-associated disease. ANCA titers may be monitored to follow treatment efficacy; rising titers may herald relapse.

Beck L et al. KDOQI US commentary on the 2012 KDIGO clinical practice guideline for glomerulonephritis. Am J Kidney Dis. 2013 Sep;62(3):429–33. [PMID: 23871408]

Guillevin L et al; French Vasculitis Study Group. Rituximab versus azathioprine for maintenance in ANCA-associated vasculitis. N Engl J Med. 2014 Nov 6;371(19):1771–80. [PMID: 25372085]

Walters G et al. Interventions for renal vasculitis in adults. Cochrane Database Syst Rev. 2015 Sep 24;9:CD003232. [PMID: 26400765]

5. Anti-Glomerular Basement Membrane Glomerulonephritis & Goodpasture Syndrome

Goodpasture syndrome is defined by the clinical constellation of glomerulonephritis and pulmonary hemorrhage; injury to both the kidneys and the lungs is mediated by antibodies to epitopes in the GBM (Figure 22–5). Up to one-third of patients with anti-GBM glomerulonephritis have no evidence of concomitant lung injury (anti-GBM disease). Anti-GBM–associated glomerulonephritis accounts for 10–20% of patients with acute RPGN. The incidence peaks in the second and third decades of life during which time males are predominantly affected and lung involvement is more common, and again in the sixth and seventh decades with less male sex predominance. Lung involvement has been associated with pulmonary infection, tobacco use, and hydrocarbon solvent exposure; HLA-DR2 and -B7 antigens may predispose as well.

▶ Clinical Findings

A. Symptoms and Signs

The onset of disease may be preceded by an upper respiratory tract infection; hemoptysis, dyspnea, and possible respiratory failure may ensue. Other findings are consistent with an RPGN, although some cases may present with much milder forms of the nephritic spectrum of disease (eg, glomerular hematuria and proteinuria with minimal renal dysfunction).

B. Laboratory Findings

Chest radiographs may demonstrate pulmonary infiltrates if pulmonary hemorrhage is present. Serum complement levels are normal. Circulating anti-GBM antibodies are present in over 90% of patients. A small percentage of patients also have elevated ANCA titers; these patients should be treated with plasma exchange as for anti-GBM

disease. Kidney biopsy typically shows crescent formation on light microscopy, with linear IgG staining along the GBM on immunofluorescence.

▶ Treatment

Treatment is a combination of plasma exchange therapy daily for up to 2 weeks to remove circulating antibodies, and administration of corticosteroids and cyclophosphamide to prevent formation of new antibodies and control the inflammatory response. Rituximab has been used in a small number of patients with refractory disease. Patients with oliguria and a serum creatinine greater than 6–7 mg/dL, or who require dialysis upon presentation have a poor prognosis. Anti-GBM antibody titers should decrease as the clinical course improves.

Beck L et al. KDOQI US commentary on the 2012 KDIGO clinical practice guideline for glomerulonephritis. Am J Kidney Dis. 2013 Sep;62(3):433–34. [PMID: 23871408]

Greco A et al. Goodpasture's syndrome: a clinical update. Autoimmun Rev. 2015 Mar;14(3):246–53. [PMID: 25462583]

6. Cryoglobulin-Associated Glomerulonephritis

Essential (mixed) cryoglobulinemia is a vasculitis associated with cold-precipitable immunoglobulins (cryoglobulins). The most common underlying etiology is HCV infection; in these cases, there is clonal expansion of B lymphocytes, which produce IgM rheumatoid factor. Rheumatoid factor, HCV antigen and polyclonal anti-HCV IgG form complexes that deposit in vessels and incite inflammation. Other overt or occult infections (eg, viral, bacterial, and fungal) as well as some connective tissue diseases can also be causative.

Patients exhibit purpuric and necrotizing skin lesions in dependent areas, arthralgias, fever, and hepatosplenomegaly. Serum complement levels are depressed. Rheumatoid factor is often elevated when cryoglobulins are present. Kidney biopsy may show several different patterns of injury; there may be crescent formation, glomerular capillary thrombi, or MPGN (see below). Treatment consists of aggressively targeting the causative infection. Pulse corticosteroids, plasma exchange, rituximab and cytotoxic agents have been used when risk of exacerbating the underlying infection is resolved, or when no infection is present. See also section on Hepatitis C Virus–Associated Renal Disease.

Cacoub P et al. Cryoglobulinemia vasculitis. Am J Med. 2015 Sep;128(9):950–5. [PMID: 25837517]

De Vita S et al. A randomized controlled trial of rituximab for the treatment of severe cryoglobulinemic vasculitis. Arthritis Rheum. 2012 Mar;64(3):843–53. [PMID: 22147661]

7. Membranoproliferative Glomerulonephritis & C3 Glomerulopathies

MPGN is a relatively rare pattern of glomerular injury that can be caused by a wide range of known etiologies or can be idiopathic. Clinically, it can present anywhere along the nephritic spectrum from asymptomatic glomerular hematuria to acute nephritic syndrome with bouts of gross hematuria to RPGN; nephrotic syndrome can also be seen. Traditionally, MPGN has been classified into several histologic subtypes; this classification is now in evolution. Type I is relatively more common and can be idiopathic (especially in children and young adults) or secondary to chronic infection (most commonly HCV), a paraproteinemia, or an underlying autoimmune disease such as lupus. The pathogenesis is likely a chronic antigenemia leading to classical complement pathway activation with immune complex deposition; however, it is now recognized that some cases may result from alternative complement pathway dysregulation. Type II MPGN is caused by several inherited or acquired abnormalities in the alternative complement pathway. Both types result in low circulating C3 complement; immune complex type I also has low C4. Light microscopy of both types shows varying degrees of mesangial hypercellularity, endocapillary proliferation and capillary wall remodeling resulting in double contours of the GBM ("tram track" appearance). Immunofluorescence and electron microscopy provide distinguishing information. Type II MPGN reveals C3 deposition without immunoglobulin staining on immunofluorescence, and electron microscopy demonstrates thick ribbon-like electron dense deposits along the GBM; thus, type II disease is also known as "dense deposit disease." Conversely, type I MPGN has scattered subendothelial and subepithelial deposits on electron microscopy. When there is immunoglobulin and C3 staining on immunofluorescence in type I MPGN, it is also called immune complex MPGN (more common type); when a type I case demonstrates only C3 staining on immunofluorescence, it is now termed C3 glomerulonephritis (C3 GN). Together, dense deposit disease (type II) and C3 GN are now termed "C3 glomerulopathies"; both result from inherited or acquired alternative complement dysregulation/activation.

Treatment of type I immune complex MPGN should be directed at the underlying cause, if such is found. Treatment of idiopathic immune complex disease is controversial and controlled trial data are lacking. For those with nephrotic syndrome and declining GFR, a combination of oral cyclophosphamide or mycophenolate mofetil plus corticosteroids could be considered; patients with RPGN and crescents on biopsy may be treated the same as those with ANCA-associated disease provided secondary causes have been ruled out. Despite therapy, most will progress to ESRD. Treatment for the C3 glomerulopathies is in evolution as novel therapies to target the dysregulated alternative complement cascade are being explored; small, uncontrolled series suggest a possible benefit of eculizumab. Less favorable prognostic findings include type II/dense deposit disease, early decline in GFR, hypertension, and persistent nephrotic syndrome. All types of MPGN recur with high frequency after renal transplantation; however, type II recurs more commonly. Plasma exchange has been used with mixed results to treat post-transplant recurrence of MPGN.

Beck L et al. KDOQI US commentary on the 2012 KDIGO clinical practice guideline for glomerulonephritis. Am J Kidney Dis. 2013 Sep;62(3):417–19. [PMID: 23871408]

Noris M et al. Glomerular diseases dependent on complement activation, including atypical hemolytic uremic syndrome, membranoproliferative glomerulonephritis, and C3 glomerulopathy: core curriculum 2015. Am J Kidney Dis. 2015 Aug;66(2):359–75. [PMID: 26032627]

8. Hepatitis C Virus–Associated Renal Disease

Renal disease can occur in the setting of HCV infection. The three patterns of renal injury associated with HCV are secondary MPGN (type I disease), cryoglobulinemic glomerulonephritis, and membranous nephropathy—the former is the most common lesion seen. The clinical presentation is dictated by the underlying pattern of injury. Many patients have elevated serum transaminases and an elevated rheumatoid factor. Hypocomplementemia is very common, with C4 typically more reduced than C3; complement levels and rheumatoid factor tend to be normal if there is a membranous pattern of injury.

► **Treatment**

Viral suppression or eradication is the cornerstone of treatment of HCV–associated renal disease; the main indications for therapy are poor kidney function, nephrotic syndrome, new or worsening hypertension, tubulointerstitial disease on biopsy, and progressive disease. IFN-alpha may result in suppression of viremia and improvement in hepatic function. Renal function rarely improves unless viral suppression occurs, and renal function often worsens when therapy is stopped. Ribavirin may cause hemolysis in those with significant kidney impairment and is relatively contraindicated in that population. Despite this, some case series have shown benefit with combined IFN-alpha and ribavirin in closely monitored settings. Rituximab may be considered in addition to antiviral therapy, although controlled trials are lacking. Small, uncontrolled studies suggest an emerging role for sofosbuvir in the treatment of cryoglobulinemic vasculitis with or without kidney involvement. There are several small, uncontrolled series suggesting safety of sofosbuvir use in those with markedly impaired GFR or ESRD; however, there are several case reports of new kidney injury associated with the use of teleprevir, and point to a need for greater clinical experience with these agents.

Cacoub P et al. Cryoglobulinemia vasculitis. Am J Med. 2015 Sep;128(9):950–5. [PMID: 25837517]
Gupta A et al. Glomerular diseases associated with hepatitis B and C. Adv Chronic Kidney Dis. 2015 Sep;22(5):343–51. [PMID: 26311595]

9. Systemic Lupus Erythematosus

Renal involvement in SLE is very common, with estimates ranging from 35% to 90%—the higher estimates encompassing subclinical disease. Rates of lupus nephritis are highest in non-whites. The pathogenesis may be dysregulated cellular apoptosis resulting in autoantibodies against nucleosomes; antibody/nucleosome complexes then bind to components of the glomerulus to form immune complex glomerular disease. See Chapter 20 for further discussion of SLE.

The term "lupus nephritis" encompasses many possible patterns of renal injury—most cases present within the nephritic spectrum (class I–IV). Nonglomerular syndromes include tubulointerstitial nephritis and vasculitis. All patients with SLE should have routine urinalyses to monitor for the appearance of hematuria or proteinuria. If urinary abnormalities are detected, kidney biopsy is often performed. The 2003 International Society of Nephrology and Renal Pathology Society (ISN/RPS) classification of renal glomerular lesions is class I, minimal mesangial nephritis; class II, mesangial proliferative nephritis; class III, focal (less than 50% of glomeruli affected with capillary involvement) proliferative nephritis; class IV, diffuse (greater than 50% of glomeruli affected with capillary involvement) proliferative nephritis; class V, membranous nephropathy; and class VI, advanced sclerosis without residual disease activity. Classes III and IV, the most severe forms of lupus nephritis, are further classified as active or chronic, and global or segmental, which confers additional prognostic value.

Treatment

Individuals with **class I** and **class II lesions** generally require no treatment; corticosteroids or calcineurin inhibitors should be considered for those with class II lesions with nephrotic-range proteinuria. Transformation of these types to a more active lesion may occur and is usually accompanied by an increase in lupus serologic activity (eg, rising titers of anti-double-stranded DNA antibodies and falling C3 and C4 levels) and increasing proteinuria or falling GFR. Repeat biopsy in such patients is recommended. Some experts recommend hydroxychloroquine treatment in all patients with lupus nephritis, regardless of histological class. Patients with extensive **class III lesions** and all **class IV lesions** should receive aggressive immunosuppressive therapy. The features signifying the poorest prognosis in patients with class III or IV lesions include elevated serum creatinine, lower complement levels, male sex, presence of antiphospholipid antibodies, nephrotic-range proteinuria, black race (possibly in association with *APOL1* risk alleles), and poor response to therapy. Immunosuppressive therapy for class V lupus nephritis is indicated if superimposed proliferative lesions exist. Class VI lesions should not be treated.

Treatment of **class III** or **IV lupus nephritis** consists of induction therapy, followed by maintenance treatment. All induction therapy includes corticosteroids (eg, methylprednisolone 1 g intravenously daily for 3 days followed by prednisone, 1 mg/kg orally daily with subsequent taper over 6–12 months) in combination with either cyclophosphamide or mycophenolate mofetil. Data suggest that blacks and Hispanics respond more favorably to mycophenolate mofetil rather than cyclophosphamide; in addition, mycophenolate mofetil has a more favorable side-effect profile than cyclophosphamide and should be favored when preservation of fertility is a consideration. Mycophenolate mofetil induction is typically given at 2–3 g/day, then tapered to 1–2 g/day for maintenance. Cyclophosphamide induction regimens vary but usually involve monthly

intravenous pulse doses (500–1000 mg/m²) for 6 months. Induction is followed by daily oral mycophenolate mofetil or azathioprine maintenance therapy; mycophenolate mofetil may be superior to azathioprine maintenance and causes few adverse effects. Maintenance with calcineurin inhibitors may also be considered, but the relapse rate is high upon discontinuation of these agents. With standard therapy, remission rates with induction vary from 80% for partial remission to 50–60% for full remission; it may take more than 6 months to see these effects. Relapse is common and rates of disease flare are higher in those who do not experience complete remission; similarly, progression to ESRD is more common in those who relapse more frequently, or in whom no remission has been achieved. Studies to assess safety and efficacy of newer biologic immunomodulatory drugs for lupus nephritis are ongoing.

The normalization of various laboratory tests (double-stranded DNA antibodies, serum C3, C4, CH₅₀ levels) can be useful in monitoring treatment. Urinary protein levels and sediment activity are also helpful markers. Patients with SLE who undergo dialysis have a favorable prospect for long-term survival; interestingly, systemic lupus symptoms may become quiescent with the development of ESRD. Patients with SLE undergoing kidney transplants can have recurrent renal disease, although rates are relatively low.

Bose B et al. Ten common mistakes in the management of lupus nephritis. Am J Kidney Dis. 2014 Apr;63(4):667–76. [PMID: 24332767]
Furie R et al. Lessons learned from the clinical trials of novel biologics and small molecules in lupus nephritis. Semin Nephrol. 2015 Sep;35(5):509–20. [PMID: 26573553]
Schwartz N et al. The pathogenesis, diagnosis and treatment of lupus nephritis. Curr Opin Rheumatol. 2014 Sep;26(5):502–9. [PMID: 25014039]
Wilhelmus S et al. Lupus nephritis management guidelines compared. Nephrol Dial Transplant. 2015 Apr 28. [Epub ahead of print] [PMID: 25920920]

NEPHROTIC SPECTRUM GLOMERULAR DISEASES

 ESSENTIALS OF DIAGNOSIS

► Bland urine sediment (few if any cells or cellular casts).
► Nephrotic syndrome is characterized by the following:
  – Heavy proteinuria (urine protein excretion greater than 3 g per 24 hours).
  – Hypoalbuminemia (albumin less than 3 g/dL).
  – Peripheral edema.
  – Hyperlipidemia.
  – Oval fat bodies may be seen in the urine.

General Considerations

In American adults, the most common cause of nephrotic spectrum glomerular disease is diabetes mellitus. Other causes of this presentation include minimal change disease, FSGS, membranous nephropathy, and amyloidosis. Any of these entities can present on the less severe end of the spectrum with a bland urinalysis and proteinuria, or with the most severe presentation of the nephrotic syndrome. Serum creatinine may or may not be abnormal at the time of presentation, depending on the severity, acuity and chronicity of the disease.

Clinical Findings

A. Symptoms and Signs

Patients with subnephrotic range proteinuria do not manifest symptoms of the renal disease. In those with the nephrotic syndrome, peripheral edema is present and is most likely due to sodium retention and, at albumin levels less than 2 g/dL (20 g/L), arterial underfilling from low plasma oncotic pressure. Edema may present in dependent regions, such as the lower extremities, or it may become generalized and include periorbital edema. Dyspnea due to pulmonary edema, pleural effusions, and diaphragmatic compromise with ascites can occur.

B. Laboratory Findings

1. Urinalysis—Proteinuria occurs as a result of effacement of podocytes (foot processes) and an alteration of the negative charge of the GBM. The urinary dipstick is a good screening test for proteinuria; however, it only detects albumin. The addition of sulfosalicylic acid to the urine causes total protein to precipitate, allowing for the possible discovery of paraproteins (and albumin). A spot urine protein to urine creatinine ratio gives a reasonable approximation of grams of protein excreted per day; a 24-hour urine sample for protein excretion is rarely needed.

Microscopically, the urinary sediment has relatively few cellular elements or casts. However, if marked hyperlipidemia is present, urinary oval fat bodies may be seen. They appear as "grape clusters" under light microscopy and "Maltese crosses" under polarized light.

2. Blood chemistries—The nephrotic syndrome results in hypoalbuminemia (less than 3 g/dL [30 g/L]) and hypoproteinemia (less than 6 g/dL [60 g/L]). Hyperlipidemia occurs in over 50% of patients with early nephrotic syndrome, and becomes more frequent and worsens in degree as the severity of the nephrotic syndrome increases. A fall in oncotic pressure triggers increased hepatic production of lipids (cholesterol and apolipoprotein B). There is also decreased clearance of very low-density lipoproteins, causing hypertriglyceridemia. Patients may also have an elevated erythrocyte sedimentation rate as a result of alterations in some plasma components such as increased levels of fibrinogen. Patients may become deficient in vitamin D, zinc, and copper from loss of binding proteins in the urine.

Laboratory testing to determine the underlying cause may include complement levels, serum and urine protein electrophoresis, antinuclear antibodies, and serologic tests for viral hepatitides.

3. Kidney biopsy—Kidney biopsy is often performed in adults with new-onset idiopathic nephrotic syndrome if a primary renal disease that may require immunosuppressive therapy is suspected. Chronically and significantly decreased GFR indicates irreversible kidney disease mitigating the usefulness of kidney biopsy. In the setting of long-standing diabetes mellitus type 1 or 2, proteinuric renal disease is rarely biopsied unless atypical features (such as significant glomerular hematuria or cellular casts) are also present, or if there is other reason to suspect an additional renal lesion.

Treatment

A. Protein Loss

In those with subnephrotic proteinuria or mild nephrotic syndrome, dietary protein restriction may be helpful in slowing progression of renal disease (see CKD section). In those with proteinuria greater than 10 g/day, protein malnutrition may occur and daily protein intake should replace daily urinary protein losses.

In both diabetic and nondiabetic patients, therapy that is aimed at reducing proteinuria may also reduce progression of renal disease. ACE inhibitors and ARBs lower urine protein excretion by reducing glomerular capillary pressure; they also have antifibrotic effects. These agents can be used in patients with reduced GFR as long as significant hyperkalemia (potassium greater than 5.2–5.5 mEq/L) does not occur and serum creatinine rises less than 30%; patients should be monitored closely to avoid acute kidney injury and hyperkalemia. Combination therapy of an ARB and an ACE inhibitor is not recommended because of the risk of acute kidney injury and hyperkalemia.

B. Edema

Dietary salt restriction is essential for managing edema; most patients also require diuretic therapy. Both thiazide and loop diuretics are highly protein bound; therefore, with hypoalbuminemia and decreased GFR, diuretic delivery to the kidney is reduced, and patients often require larger doses. A combination of loop and thiazide diuretics can potentiate the diuretic effect and may be needed for patients with refractory fluid retention.

C. Hyperlipidemia

Hypercholesterolemia and hypertriglyceridemia occur as noted above. Dietary modification and exercise should be advocated; however, effective lipid-lowering usually also requires pharmacologic treatment (see Chapter 28). Rhabdomyolysis, however, is more common in patients with CKD who take gemfibrozil in combination with statins; combining fenofibrate or niacin with a statin poses less risk.

D. Hypercoagulable State

Patients with serum albumin less than 2 g/dL can become hypercoagulable. Nephrotic patients have urinary losses of antithrombin, protein C, and protein S and increased platelet activation. Patients are prone to renal vein thrombosis, pulmonary embolus, and other venous thromboemboli, particularly with membranous nephropathy. Anticoagulation therapy with warfarin is warranted for at least 3–6 months in patients with evidence of thrombosis in any location. Patients with renal vein thrombosis, pulmonary embolus, or recurrent thromboemboli require indefinite anticoagulation. After an initial clotting event, ongoing nephrotic syndrome poses a risk of thrombosis recurrence, and continued anticoagulation should be considered until resolution of the nephrotic syndrome.

► When to Refer

Any patient noted to have nephrotic syndrome should be referred immediately to a nephrologist for consideration of volume and blood pressure management, assessment for kidney biopsy, and treatment of the underlying disease. Proteinuria of more than 1 g/day without the nephrotic syndrome also merits nephrology referral, though with less urgency.

► When to Admit

Patients with edema refractory to outpatient therapy or rapidly worsening kidney function that may require inpatient interventions should be admitted.

Fried LF et al; VA NEPHRON-D Investigators. Combined angiotensin inhibition for the treatment of diabetic nephropathy. N Engl J Med. 2013 Nov 14;369(20):892–903. [PMID: 24206457]

Gbadegesin RA et al. Genetic testing in nephrotic syndrome—challenges and opportunities. Nat Rev Nephrol. 2013 Mar;9(3):179–84. [PMID: 23321566]

Snyder S et al. Workup for proteinuria. Prim Care. 2014 Dec;41(4):719–35. [PMID: 25439530]

NEPHROTIC SPECTRUM DISEASE IN PRIMARY RENAL DISORDERS

MINIMAL CHANGE DISEASE

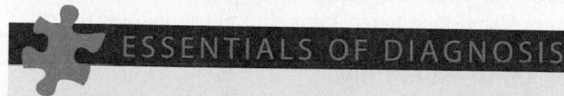

ESSENTIALS OF DIAGNOSIS

▸ Nephrotic-range proteinuria.

▸ Kidney biopsy shows no changes on light microscopy.

▸ Characteristic foot-process effacement on electron microscopy.

► General Considerations

Minimal change disease is the most common cause of proteinuric renal disease in children, accounting for about 80% of cases. It often remits upon treatment with a course of corticosteroids. Indeed, children with nephrotic

syndrome are often treated for minimal change disease empirically without a biopsy diagnosis. Biopsy should be considered for children with nephrotic syndrome who exhibit unusual features (such as signs of other systemic illness), who are steroid-resistant (see below), or who relapse frequently upon withdrawal of corticosteroid therapy. Minimal change disease is less common in adults, accounting for 20–25% of cases of primary nephrotic syndrome in those over age 40 years. This entity can be idiopathic but also occurs following viral upper respiratory infections (especially in children), in association with neoplasms such as Hodgkin disease, with drugs (lithium), and with hypersensitivity reactions (especially to NSAIDs and bee stings).

► Clinical Findings

A. Symptoms and Signs

Patients often exhibit the manifestations of full-blown nephrotic syndrome. They are more susceptible to infection, have a tendency toward thromboembolic events, develop severe hyperlipidemia, and may experience protein malnutrition. Minimal change disease can rarely cause acute kidney injury due to tubular changes and interstitial edema.

B. Laboratory and Histologic Findings

There is no helpful serologic testing. Glomeruli show no changes on light microscopy or immunofluorescence. On electron microscopy, there is a characteristic effacement of podocyte foot processes. Mesangial cell proliferation may be seen in a subgroup of patients; this finding is associated with more hematuria and hypertension and poor response to standard corticosteroid treatment.

► Treatment

Treatment is with prednisone, 60 mg/m^2/day orally; remission in steroid-responsive minimal change disease generally occurs within 4–8 weeks. Adults often require longer courses of therapy than children, requiring up to 16 weeks to achieve a response. Treatment should be continued for several weeks after complete remission of proteinuria, and dosing tapers should be individualized. A significant number of patients will relapse and require repeated corticosteroid treatment. Patients with frequent relapses or corticosteroid resistance may require cyclophosphamide, a calcineurin inhibitor (tacrolimus, cyclosporine), or rituximab to induce subsequent remissions. Progression to ESRD is rare. Complications most often arise from prolonged corticosteroid use.

Iijima K et al; Rituximab for Childhood-onset Refractory Nephrotic Syndrome (RCRNS) Study Group. Rituximab for childhood-onset, complicated, frequently relapsing nephrotic syndrome or steroid-dependent nephrotic syndrome: a multicentre, double-blind, randomised, placebo-controlled trial. Lancet. 2014 Oct 4;384(9950):1273–81. [PMID: 24965823]

Zhao L et al. Enhanced steroid therapy in adult minimal change nephrotic syndrome: a systematic review and meta-analysis. Intern Med. 2015;54(17):2101–8. [PMID: 26328632]

FOCAL SEGMENTAL GLOMERULOSCLEROSIS

General Considerations

This relatively common renal pattern of injury results from damage to podocytes. Possible causes of podocyte injury include both primary and secondary renal diseases. Primary causes fall into three categories: (1) heritable abnormalities in any one of several podocyte proteins, or to underlying type 4 collagen mutations, (2) polymorphisms in the *APOL1* gene in those of African descent, or (3) increased levels of a circulating permeability factor. Secondary causes include renal overwork injury, obesity, hypertension, chronic urinary reflux, HIV infection, or analgesic or bisphosphonate exposure. Genetic testing in primary cases is becoming more common, especially in the pediatric population.

Clinical Findings

Proteinuria is present in patients with FSGS. In FSGS caused by a primary renal disease, 80% of children and 50% of adults have overt nephrotic syndrome; however, when it develops due to a secondary cause, frank nephrotic syndrome is uncommon. Decreased GFR is present in 25–50% of those with FSGS at time of diagnosis. ESRD typically develops in patients with FSGS and nephrotic syndrome in 6–8 years.

Diagnosis requires kidney biopsy; there is no helpful serologic test. Light microscopy shows sclerosis of portions (segments) of some, but not all, glomeruli (thus, focal, not diffuse, disease). On immunofluorescence, IgM and C3 are seen in the sclerotic lesions, although it is presumed that these immune components are simply trapped in the sclerotic glomeruli and not pathogenetic. As in minimal change disease, electron microscopy shows fusion of epithelial foot processes.

Treatment

Treatment for all forms of FSGS should include diuretics for edema, ACE inhibitors or ARBs for proteinuria and hypertension, and statins or niacin for hyperlipidemia. Immunosuppression therapy (oral prednisone, 1 mg/kg/day for 4–16 weeks followed by a slow taper) is reserved for nephrotic primary FSGS cases presumed to be due to a circulating permeability factor; in those with steroid-resistance or intolerance, calcineurin inhibitors and mycophenolate mofetil can be considered. Kidney transplantation in this subgroup of FSGS patients is complicated by a relatively high relapse rate and risk of graft loss. Plasma exchange therapy, and possibly rituximab, just prior to the transplant surgery and with early signs of relapse, appear to be beneficial. Those with *APOL1*-associated and nonhereditary primary renal disease may not benefit from immunosuppression, although robust clinical trials are lacking. Patients with secondary FSGS do not benefit from immunosuppressive therapy; treatment should be directed at the inciting cause.

Beck L et al. KDOQI US commentary on the 2012 KDIGO clinical practice guideline for glomerulonephritis. Am J Kidney Dis. 2013 Sep;62(3):410–13. [PMID: 23871408]

Fogo AB. Causes and pathogenesis of focal segmental glomerulosclerosis. Nat Rev Nephrol. 2015 Feb;11(2):76–87. [PMID: 25447132]

Sethi S et al. Focal and segmental glomerulosclerosis: towards a better understanding for the practicing nephrologist. Nephrol Dial Transplant. 2015 Mar;30(3):375–84. [PMID: 24589721]

MEMBRANOUS NEPHROPATHY

ESSENTIALS OF DIAGNOSIS

▶ Varying degrees of proteinuria, may have nephrotic syndrome.

▶ Associated with coagulopathy, eg, renal vein thrombosis, if nephrotic syndrome present.

▶ "Spike and dome" pattern on kidney biopsy from subepithelial deposits.

▶ Secondary causes notably include hepatitis B virus and carcinomas.

General Considerations

Membranous nephropathy is the most common cause of primary nephrotic syndrome in adults and often presents in the fifth and sixth decades. It is an immune-mediated disease characterized by immune complex deposition in the subepithelial portion of glomerular capillary walls. The antigen in the primary form of the disease appears to be a phospholipase A_2 receptor (PLA_2R) on the podocyte in 70–80% of patients. Secondary disease is associated with underlying carcinomas; infections, such as hepatitis B and C, endocarditis, and syphilis; autoimmune disease, such as SLE, mixed connective tissue disease, and thyroiditis; and certain drugs, such as NSAIDs and captopril. The course of disease is variable, with about 50% of patients progressing to ESRD over 3–10 years. Poorer outcome is associated with concomitant tubulointerstitial fibrosis, male sex, elevated serum creatinine, hypertension, and proteinuria greater than 10 g/day.

Patients with membranous nephropathy and nephrotic syndrome have a higher risk of hypercoagulable state than those with nephrosis from other etiologies; there is a particular predisposition to renal vein thrombosis in these patients.

Clinical Findings

A. Symptoms and Signs

Patients may be asymptomatic or may have edema or frothy urine. Venous thrombosis, such as an unprovoked deep venous thrombosis may be an initial sign. There may be symptoms or signs of an underlying infection or neoplasm (especially lung, stomach, breast, and colon cancers) in secondary membranous nephropathy.

B. Laboratory Findings

See above for laboratory findings in the nephrotic syndrome. Evaluation for secondary causes including serologic testing for SLE, syphilis, viral hepatitides, and age- and risk-appropriate cancer screening should be performed. Serum evaluation for circulating PLA$_2$R antibodies to assess for idiopathic membranous nephropathy may be available in the future. By light microscopy, capillary wall thickness is increased without inflammatory changes or cellular proliferation; when stained with silver methenamine, a "spike and dome" pattern results from projections of excess GBM between the subepithelial deposits. Immunofluorescence shows IgG and C3 staining along capillary loops. Electron microscopy shows a discontinuous pattern of dense deposits along the subepithelial surface of the basement membrane.

► Treatment

Underlying causes must be excluded prior to consideration of treatment. Idiopathic/primary disease treatment depends on the risk of renal disease progression. Roughly 30% of patients present with subnephrotic proteinuria (less than 3 g/day) and most have a good prognosis with conservative management, including antiproteinuric therapy with ACE inhibitor or ARB if blood pressure is greater than 125/75 mm Hg. Spontaneous remission may develop even in those with heavy proteinuria (about 30% of cases). Thus, use of immunosuppressive agents should be limited to those at highest risk for progression and with salvageable renal function. Patients with nephrotic syndrome despite 6 months of conservative management and serum creatinine less than 3.0 may elect therapy with corticosteroids and chlorambucil or cyclophosphamide for 6 months. Calcineurin inhibitors with or without corticosteroids may be considered as well. Uncontrolled trials with rituximab have shown benefit. Remission may take up to 6 months. Patients with primary membranous nephropathy are excellent candidates for transplant.

Beck L et al. KDOQI US commentary on the 2012 KDIGO clinical practice guideline for glomerulonephritis. Am J Kidney Dis. 2013 Sep;62(3):413–17. [PMID: 23871408]
Chen Y et al. Immunosuppressive treatment for idiopathic membranous nephropathy in adults with nephrotic syndrome. Cochrane Database Syst Rev. 2014 Oct 16;10:CD004293. [PMID: 25318831]

NEPHROTIC SPECTRUM DISEASE FROM SYSTEMIC DISORDERS

DIABETIC NEPHROPATHY

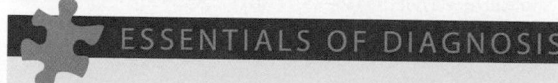

ESSENTIALS OF DIAGNOSIS

► Prior evidence of diabetes mellitus, typically over 10 years.

► Albuminuria usually precedes decline in GFR.

► Other end-organ damage, such as retinopathy, is common.

► General Considerations

Diabetic nephropathy is the most common cause of ESRD in the United States. Type 1 diabetes mellitus carries a 30–40% risk of nephropathy after 20 years, whereas type 2 has a 15–20% risk after 20 years. ESRD is much more likely to develop in persons with type 1 diabetes mellitus, in part due to fewer comorbidities and deaths before ESRD ensues. With the current epidemic of obesity and type 2 diabetes mellitus, rates of diabetic nephropathy are projected to continue to increase. Patients at higher risk include males, African Americans, Native Americans, and those with a positive family history. Mortality rates are higher for diabetics with kidney disease compared to those without CKD.

► Clinical Findings

Diabetic nephropathy develops about 10 years after the onset of diabetes mellitus. It may be present at the time type 2 diabetes mellitus is diagnosed. The first stage of classic diabetic nephropathy is hyperfiltration with an increase in GFR, followed by the development of microalbuminuria (30–300 mg/day). With progression, albuminuria increases to greater than 300 mg/day and can be detected on a urine dipstick as overt proteinuria; the GFR subsequently declines over time. Yearly screening for microalbuminuria is recommended for all diabetic patients to detect disease at its earliest stage; however, diabetic nephropathy can, less commonly result in nonproteinuric CKD.

The most common lesion in diabetic nephropathy is diffuse glomerulosclerosis, but nodular glomerulosclerosis (Kimmelstiel-Wilson nodules) is pathognomonic. The kidneys are usually enlarged as a result of cellular hypertrophy and proliferation. Kidney biopsy is not required in most patients, though, unless atypical findings are present, such as sudden onset of proteinuria, nephritic spectrum features (see above), massive proteinuria (greater than 10 g/day), urinary cellular casts, or rapid decline in GFR.

Patients with diabetes are prone to other renal diseases. These include papillary necrosis, chronic interstitial nephritis, and type 4 (hyporeninemic hypoaldosteronemic) renal tubular acidosis. Patients are more susceptible to acute kidney injury from many insults, including intravenous contrast material and concomitant use of an ACE inhibitor or ARB with NSAID.

► Treatment

With the onset of microalbuminuria, aggressive treatment is necessary. Strict glycemic control should be emphasized early in diabetic nephropathy, with recognition of risk of hypoglycemia as CKD becomes advanced (see CKD section). Recommended blood pressure goals should be tailored to the individual patient: based on the ACCORD trial, those with microalbuminuria (30–300 mg/day) and preserved GFR and those with significant CVD likely derive little benefit from blood pressure lowering much below 140/90 mm Hg. Those with overt proteinuria (especially when more than 1 g/day) benefit from a goal of less than 130/80 mm Hg. ACE inhibitors and ARBs in those with microalbuminuria lower the rate of progression to overt proteinuria and slow progression to ESRD by reducing intraglomerular pressure and via antifibrotic effects; these agents are not absolutely indicated in diabetics with normal blood pressure and no microalbuminuria. In patients with markedly diminished GFR, ACE inhibitors and ARBs may provide benefit; close monitoring for hyperkalemia or a decline in GFR more than 30% with the initiation or uptitration of this therapy is required. Combination ARB and ACE inhibitor therapy is not recommended due to lack of efficacy and increased adverse events of hyperkalemia and acute kidney injury. Non-dihydropyridine calcium channel blockers are the recommended anti-proteinuric agents for patients taking ACE inhibitors or ARBs in whom hyperkalemia develops. Treatment of other cardiovascular risk factors and obesity is crucial. Many with diabetes have multiple comorbid conditions; therefore, in patients undergoing dialysis who progress to ESRD, mortality over the first 5 years is high. Patients who are relatively healthy, however, benefit from renal transplantation.

Agrawal V et al. The effects of glucose-lowering therapies on diabetic kidney disease. Curr Diabetes Rev. 2015;11(3):191–200. [PMID: 25824237]

Bilo H et al. Clinical practice guideline on management of patients with diabetes and chronic kidney disease stage 3b or higher (eGFR < 45 mL/min). Nephrol Dial Transplant. 2015 May;30(Suppl 2):ii1–142. [PMID: 25940656]

Gilbert MP. Screening and treatment by the primary care provider of common diabetes complications. Med Clin North Am. 2015 Jan;99(1):201–19. [PMID: 25456651]

Palmer SC et al. Comparative efficacy and safety of blood pressure-lowering agents in adults with diabetes and kidney disease: a network meta-analysis. Lancet. 2015 May 23;385(9982): 2047–56. [PMID: 26009228]

HIV-ASSOCIATED NEPHROPATHY

HIV-associated nephropathy usually presents as the nephrotic syndrome and declining GFR in patients with active HIV infection. Most patients are of African descent, likely due to the association of *APOL1* polymorphisms with increased risk for HIV-associated nephropathy. Often, patients have low CD4 counts and have AIDS, but HIV-associated nephropathy can also be the initial presentation of HIV disease. Patients with HIV are at risk for kidney disease other than HIV-associated nephropathy (eg, toxicity from antiretroviral medications such as tenofovir, vascular disease, and diabetes, or an immune complex–mediated glomerular disease); such diseases tend to be nonnephrotic.

Kidney biopsy shows an FSGS pattern of injury (described above) with glomerular collapse; severe tubulointerstitial damage may also be present.

HIV-associated nephropathy is becoming less common in the era of HIV screening and more effective antiretroviral therapy. Small, uncontrolled studies have shown that HAART slows progression of disease. ACE inhibitors or ARBs can be used to control blood pressure and slow disease progression. Corticosteroid treatment has been used with variable success at a dosage of 1 mg/kg/day, along with cyclosporine. Patients who progress to ESRD and are otherwise healthy are good candidates for renal transplantation.

Lucas GM et al. Clinical practice guideline for the management of chronic kidney disease in patients infected with HIV: 2014 update by the HIV Medicine Association of the Infectious Diseases Society of America. Clin Infect Dis. 2014 Nov 1;59(9):e96–138. [PMID: 25234519]

Rosenberg AZ et al. HIV-associated nephropathies: epidemiology, pathology, mechanisms and treatment. Nat Rev Nephrol. 2015 Mar;11(3):150–60. [PMID: 25686569]

Yombi JC et al. Monitoring of kidney function in HIV-positive patients. HIV Med. 2015 Sep;16(8):457–67. [PMID: 25944246]

RENAL AMYLOIDOSIS

Amyloidosis is caused by extracellular deposition of an abnormally folded protein (amyloid). Several different proteins can form amyloid fibrils. Primary amyloidosis, the most common form, is due to a plasma cell dyscrasia. In this so-called "AL amyloidosis," the protein is a monoclonal Ig light chain (see Chapter 13). Secondary amyloidosis results from a chronic inflammatory disease such as rheumatoid arthritis, inflammatory bowel disease, or chronic infection. In this so-called "AA amyloid disease," there is deposition of an acute phase reactant, serum amyloid A protein.

Proteinuria, decreased GFR, and nephrotic syndrome are presenting symptoms and signs of renal involvement in amyloidosis; evidence of other organ involvement is common. Serum and urine protein electrophoresis should be done as screening tests; if a monoclonal spike is found on either, serum free light chains should be quantified by immunoelectrophoresis. Amyloid-affected kidneys are often larger than 10 cm. Pathologically, glomeruli are filled with amorphous deposits that show green birefringence with Congo red staining.

AL amyloidosis progresses to ESRD in an average of 2–3 years. Five-year overall survival is less than 20%, with death occurring from ESRD and heart disease. Treatment options are few. The use of alkylating agents and corticosteroids—eg, melphalan and prednisone—can reduce proteinuria and improve renal function in a small percentage of patients. New therapies, including the proteosome inhibitor bortezomib, may hold promise but data from controlled trials are lacking. A greater than 90% reduction in the level of serum free light chain has been shown to correlate with improved renal outcomes. Melphalan and stem cell transplantation are associated with a high (45%) mortality rate, but can induce remission in 80% of survivors; however, few patients are eligible for this treatment. In AA amyloidosis, remissions can occur if the underlying disease is treated. Renal transplantation is an option.

Gertz MA. Immunoglobulin light chain amyloidosis: 2013 update on diagnosis, prognosis, and treatment. Am J Hematol. 2013 May;88(5):416–25. [PMID: 23605846]

Gillmore JD et al. Pathophysiology and treatment of systemic amyloidosis. Nat Rev Nephrol. 2013 Oct;9(10):574–86. [PMID: 23979488]

▼ TUBULOINTERSTITIAL DISEASES

Tubulointerstitial disease may be acute or chronic. Acute disease is most commonly associated with medications, infectious agents, and systemic rheumatologic disorders. Interstitial edema, infiltration with polymorphonuclear neutrophils, and tubular cell necrosis can be seen. (See Acute Kidney Injury, above, and Table 22–10.) Chronic disease is associated with insults from an acute factor or progressive insults without any obvious acute cause.

Table 22–10. Causes of acute tubulointerstitial nephritis (abbreviated list).

Drug reactions
Antibiotics
Beta-lactam antibiotics: methicillin, penicillin, ampicillin, cephalosporins
Ciprofloxacin
Erythromycin
Sulfonamides
Tetracycline
Vancomycin
Trimethoprim-sulfamethoxazole
Ethambutol
Rifampin
Nonsteroidal anti-inflammatory drugs
Diuretics
Thiazides
Furosemide
Miscellaneous
Allopurinol
Cimetidine
Phenytoin
Systemic infections
Bacteria
Streptococcus
Corynebacterium diphtheriae
Legionella
Viruses
Epstein-Barr
Others
Mycoplasma
Rickettsia rickettsii
Leptospira icterohaemorrhagiae
Toxoplasma
Idiopathic
Tubulointerstitial nephritis-uveitis (TIN–U)

Interstitial fibrosis and tubular atrophy are present, with a mononuclear cell predominance. The chronic disorders are described below.

CHRONIC TUBULOINTERSTITIAL DISEASES

ESSENTIALS OF DIAGNOSIS

- ► Kidney size is small and contracted.
- ► Decreased urinary concentrating ability.
- ► Hyperchloremic metabolic acidosis.
- ► Reduced GFR.

► General Considerations

The primary causes of chronic tubulointerstitial disease are discussed below. Other causes include multiple myeloma and gout, which are discussed in the section on multisystem disease with variable kidney involvement.

The most common cause of chronic tubulointerstitial disease is **obstructive uropathy** from prolonged obstruction of the urinary tract. The major causes are prostatic disease in men; ureteral calculus in a single functioning kidney; bilateral ureteral calculi; carcinoma of the cervix, colon, or bladder; and retroperitoneal tumors or fibrosis.

Reflux nephropathy from **vesicoureteral reflux** is primarily a disorder of childhood and occurs when urine passes retrograde from the bladder to the kidneys during voiding. It is the second most common cause of chronic tubulointerstitial disease. It occurs as a result of an incompetent vesicoureteral sphincter. Urine can extravasate into the interstitium; an inflammatory response develops, and fibrosis occurs. The inflammatory response is due to either bacteria or normal urinary components.

Analgesic nephropathy is most commonly seen in patients who ingest large quantities of analgesic combinations. The drugs of concern are phenacetin, paracetamol, aspirin, and NSAIDs, with acetaminophen a possible but less certain culprit. Ingestion of at least 1 g/day for 3 years of these analgesics is considered necessary for kidney dysfunction to develop. This disorder occurs most frequently in individuals who are using analgesics for chronic headaches, muscular pains, and arthritis. Most patients grossly underestimate their analgesic use.

Tubulointerstitial inflammation and papillary necrosis are seen on pathologic examination. Papillary tip and inner medullary concentrations of some analgesics are tenfold higher than in the renal cortex. Phenacetin—once a common cause of this disorder and now rarely available—is metabolized in the papillae by the prostaglandin hydroperoxidase pathway to reactive intermediates that bind covalently to interstitial cell macromolecules, causing necrosis. Aspirin and other NSAIDs can cause damage by their metabolism to active intermediates which can result in cell necrosis. These drugs also decrease medullary blood flow (via inhibition of prostaglandin synthesis) and decrease glutathione levels, which are necessary for detoxification.

Environmental exposure to **heavy metals**—such as lead, cadmium, mercury, and bismuth—is seen infrequently now in the United States but can cause tubulointerstitial disease. Individuals at risk for lead-induced tubulointerstitial disease are those with occupational exposure (eg, welders who work with lead-based paint) and drinkers of alcohol distilled in automobile radiators ("moonshine" whiskey users). Lead is filtered by the glomerulus and is transported across the proximal convoluted tubules, where it accumulates and causes cell damage. Fibrosed arterioles and cortical scarring also lead to damaged kidneys. The proximal tubular dysfunction from cadmium exposure can cause hypercalciuria and nephrolithiasis.

► Clinical Findings

A. General Findings

Polyuria is common because tubular damage leads to inability to concentrate the urine. Volume depletion can also occur as a result of a salt-wasting defect in some individuals.

Patients can become hyperkalemic both because the GFR is lower and the distal tubules become aldosterone resistant. A hyperchloremic renal tubular acidosis is characteristic from a component of type 4 or type 1 renal tubular acidosis. Less commonly, a proximal renal tubular acidosis is seen due to direct proximal tubular damage. The cause of the renal tubular acidosis is threefold: (1) reduced ammonia production, (2) inability to acidify the distal tubules, and (3) proximal tubular bicarbonate wasting. The urinalysis is nonspecific, as opposed to that seen in acute interstitial nephritis. Proteinuria is typically less than 2 g/day (owing to inability of the proximal tubule to reabsorb freely filterable proteins); a few cells may be seen; and broad waxy casts are often present.

B. Specific Findings

1. Obstructive uropathy—In partial obstruction, patients can exhibit polyuria (possibly due to vasopressin insensitivity and poor ability to concentrate the urine) or oliguria (due to decreased GFR). Azotemia and hypertension (due to increased renin-angiotensin production) are usually present. Abdominal, rectal, and genitourinary examinations are helpful. Urinalysis can show hematuria, pyuria, and bacteriuria but is often benign. Abdominal ultrasound may detect mass lesions, hydroureter, and hydronephrosis. CT scanning and MRI provide more detailed information.

2. Vesicoureteral reflux—Typically vesicoureteral reflux is diagnosed in young children with a history of recurrent urinary tract infections. This entity can be detected before birth via screening fetal ultrasonography. After birth, a voiding cystourethrogram can be done. Less commonly, this entity is not diagnosed until adolescence or young adulthood when patients present with hypertension and substantial proteinuria, unusual in most tubular diseases. At this point, renal ultrasound or IVP can show renal scarring and hydronephrosis. IVP is relatively contraindicated in patients with kidney dysfunction who are at higher risk for contrast nephropathy. On kidney biopsy, FSGS can be seen in those with kidney damage. Although most damage occurs before age 5 years, progressive renal deterioration to ESRD continues as a result of the early insults.

3. Analgesics—Patients can exhibit hematuria, mild proteinuria, polyuria (from tubular damage), anemia (from GI bleeding or erythropoietin deficiency), and sterile pyuria. As a result of papillary necrosis, sloughed papillae can be found in the urine. An IVP may be helpful for detecting these—contrast will fill the area of the sloughed papillae, leaving a "ring shadow" sign at the papillary tip. However, IVP is rarely used in patients with significant kidney dysfunction, given the need for dye and associated acute kidney injury.

4. Heavy metals—Proximal tubular damage from lead exposure can cause decreased secretion of uric acid, resulting in hyperuricemia and saturnine gout. Patients commonly are hypertensive. Diagnosis is most reliably performed with a calcium disodium edetate (EDTA) chelation test. Urinary excretion of greater than 600 mg of lead in 24 hours following 1 g of EDTA indicates excessive lead exposure. The proximal tubular dysfunction from cadmium can cause hypercalciuria and nephrolithiasis.

▶ Treatment

Treatment depends first on identifying the disorder responsible for kidney dysfunction. The degree of interstitial fibrosis that has developed can help predict recovery of renal function. Once there is evidence for loss of parenchyma (small shrunken kidneys or interstitial fibrosis on biopsy), little can prevent the progression toward ESRD. Treatment is then directed at medical management. Tubular dysfunction may require potassium and phosphorus restriction and sodium, calcium, or bicarbonate supplements.

If hydronephrosis is present, relief of obstruction should be accomplished promptly. Prolonged obstruction leads to further tubular damage—particularly in the distal nephron—which may be irreversible despite relief of obstruction. Neither surgical correction of reflux nor medical therapy with antibiotics can prevent deterioration toward ESRD once renal scarring has occurred.

Patients in whom lead nephropathy is suspected should continue chelation therapy with EDTA if there is no evidence of irreversible renal damage (eg, renal scarring or small kidneys). Continued exposure should be avoided.

Treatment of analgesic nephropathy requires withdrawal of all analgesics. Stabilization or improvement of renal function may occur if significant interstitial fibrosis is not present. Ensuring volume repletion during exposure to analgesics may also have some beneficial effects.

▶ When to Refer

- Patients with stage 3–5 CKD should be referred to a nephrologist when tubulointerstitial diseases are suspected. Other select cases of stage 1–2 CKD should also be referred.

- Patients with urologic abnormalities should be referred to a urologist.

Gratzke C et al. EAU guidelines on the assessment of non-neurogenic male lower urinary tract symptoms including benign prostatic obstruction. Eur Urol. 2015 Jun;67(6):1099–109. [PMID: 25613154]
Nderitu P et al. Non-steroidal anti-inflammatory drugs and chronic kidney disease progression: a systematic review. Fam Pract. 2013 Jun;30(3):247–55. [PMID: 23302818]

▼ CYSTIC DISEASES OF THE KIDNEY

Renal cysts are epithelium-lined cavities filled with fluid or semisolid material. They develop primarily from renal tubular elements. One or more simple cysts are found in 50% of individuals over the age of 50 years. They are rarely symptomatic and have little clinical significance. In contrast, generalized cystic diseases are associated with cysts scattered throughout the cortex and medulla of both kidneys and can progress to ESRD (Table 22–11).

Table 22–11. Clinical features of renal cystic disease.

	Simple Renal Cysts	Acquired Renal Cysts	Autosomal Dominant Polycystic Kidney Disease	Medullary Sponge Kidney	Medullary Cystic Kidney
Prevalence	Common	Dialysis patients	1:1000	1:5000	Rare
Inheritance	None	None	Autosomal dominant	None	Autosomal dominant
Age at onset	...	...	20–40	40–60	Adulthood
Kidney size	Normal	Small	Large	Normal	Small
Cyst location	Cortex and medulla	Cortex and medulla	Cortex and medulla	Collecting ducts	Corticomedullary junction
Hematuria	Occasional	Occasional	Common	Rare	Rare
Hypertension	None	Variable	Common	None	None
Associated complications	None	Adenocarcinoma in cysts	Urinary tract infections, renal calculi, cerebral aneurysms 10–15%, hepatic cysts 40–60%	Renal calculi, urinary tract infections	Polyuria, salt wasting
Kidney failure	Never	Always	Frequently	Never	Always

SIMPLE OR SOLITARY CYSTS

Simple cysts account for 65–70% of all renal masses. They are generally found at the outer cortex and contain fluid that is consistent with an ultrafiltrate of plasma. Most are found incidentally on ultrasonographic examination. Simple cysts are typically asymptomatic but can become infected.

The main concern with simple cysts is to differentiate them from malignancy, abscess, or polycystic kidney disease. Renal cystic disease can develop in dialysis patients. These cysts have a potential for progression to malignancy. Ultrasound and CT scanning are the recommended procedures for evaluating these masses. Simple cysts must meet three sonographic criteria to be considered benign: (1) echo free, (2) sharply demarcated mass with smooth walls, and (3) an enhanced back wall (indicating good transmission through the cyst). Complex cysts can have thick walls, calcifications, solid components, and mixed echogenicity. On CT scan, the simple cyst should have a smooth thin wall that is sharply demarcated. It should not enhance with contrast media. A renal cell carcinoma will enhance but typically is of lower density than the rest of the parenchyma. Arteriography can also be used to evaluate a mass preoperatively. A renal cell carcinoma is hypervascular in 80%, hypovascular in 15%, and avascular in 5% of cases.

If a cyst meets the criteria for being benign, periodic reevaluation is the standard of care. If the lesion is not consistent with a simple cyst, follow-up with a urologic consultant and possible surgical exploration is recommended.

Skolarikos A et al. Conservative and radiological management of simple cysts: a comprehensive review. BJU Int. 2012 Jul;110(2):170–8. [PMID: 22414207]

AUTOSOMAL DOMINANT POLYCYSTIC KIDNEY DISEASE

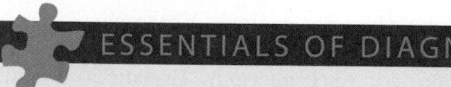 ESSENTIALS OF DIAGNOSIS

► Multiple cysts in both kidneys; total number of cysts depends on patient age.
► Combination of hypertension and abdominal mass suggestive of disease.
► Autosomal dominant inheritance pattern chromosomal abnormalities present in some patients.
► Family history and large, palpable kidneys are compelling but not necessary.

► General Considerations

Polycystic kidney disease is among the most common hereditary diseases in the United States, affecting 500,000 individuals, or 1 in 800 live births. Fifty percent of patients will have ESRD by age 60 years. The disease has variable penetrance but accounts for 10% of dialysis patients in the United States. At least two genes account for this disorder: *ADPKD1* on the short arm of chromosome 16 (85–90% of patients) and *ADPKD2* on chromosome 4 (10–15%). Patients with the *PKD2* mutation have slower progression of disease and longer life expectancy than those with *PKD1*. Other sporadic cases without these mutations have also been recognized.

► Clinical Findings

Abdominal or flank pain and microscopic or gross hematuria are present in most patients. A history of urinary tract infections and nephrolithiasis is common. A family history is positive in 75% of cases, and more than 50% of patients have hypertension (see below) that may antedate the clinical manifestations of the disease. Patients have large kidneys that may be palpable on abdominal examination. The combination of hypertension and an abdominal mass should suggest the disease. Forty to 50 percent have concurrent hepatic cysts. Pancreatic and splenic cysts occur also. Hemoglobin and hematocrit tend to be maintained as a result of erythropoietin production by the cysts. The urinalysis may show hematuria and mild proteinuria. In patients with *PKD1*, ultrasonography confirms the diagnosis—two or more cysts in patients under age 30 years (sensitivity of 88.5%), two or more cysts in each kidney in patients aged 30–59 years (sensitivity of 100%), and four or more cysts in each kidney in patients age 60 years or older are diagnostic for autosomal dominant polycystic kidney disease. If sonographic results are unclear, CT scan is recommended and highly sensitive.

▶ Complications & Treatment

A. Pain

Abdominal or flank pain is caused by infection, bleeding into cysts, and nephrolithiasis. Bed rest and analgesics are recommended. Cyst decompression can help with chronic pain.

B. Hematuria

Gross hematuria is most commonly due to rupture of a cyst into the renal pelvis, but it can also be caused by a kidney stone or urinary tract infection. Hematuria typically resolves within 7 days with bed rest and hydration. Recurrent bleeding should suggest the possibility of underlying renal cell carcinoma, particularly in men over age 50 years.

C. Renal Infection

An infected renal cyst should be suspected in patients who have flank pain, fever, and leukocytosis. Blood cultures may be positive, and urinalysis may be normal because the cyst does not communicate directly with the urinary tract. CT scans can be helpful because an infected cyst may have an increased wall thickness. Bacterial cyst infections are difficult to treat. Antibiotics with cystic penetration should be used, eg, fluoroquinolones or trimethoprim-sulfamethoxazole and chloramphenicol. Treatment may require 2 weeks of parenteral therapy followed by long-term oral therapy.

D. Nephrolithiasis

Up to 20% of patients have kidney stones, primarily calcium oxalate. Hydration (2–3 L/day) is recommended.

E. Hypertension

Fifty percent of patients have hypertension at time of presentation, and it will develop in most patients during the course of the disease. Cyst-induced ischemia appears to cause activation of the renin–angiotensin system, and cyst decompression can lower blood pressure temporarily. Hypertension should be treated, trying to prolong the time to ESRD. However, a randomized controlled trial showed that aggressive blood pressure control (blood pressures 95–110/60–75 mm Hg), when compared to usual care (blood pressures 120–130/70–80 mm Hg), slowed the increase of kidney volume, but not the decline in GFR.

F. Cerebral Aneurysms

About 10–15% of these patients have arterial aneurysms in the circle of Willis. Screening arteriography is not recommended unless the patient has a family history of aneurysms, is employed in a high risk profession (such as airline pilot), or is undergoing elective surgery with a high risk of developing moderate to severe perioperative hypertension.

G. Other Complications

Vascular problems include mitral valve prolapse in up to 25% of patients, aortic aneurysms, and aortic valve abnormalities. Colonic diverticula are more common in patients with polycystic kidneys.

▶ Prognosis

Vasopressin receptor antagonists have been shown to slow down the rate of change in total kidney volume and to lower the rate of worsening kidney function. Other agents, octreotide and sirolimus, have shown a decreased rate of cyst growth but no decrease in the rate of decline in kidney function. Avoidance of caffeine may prevent cyst formation due to effects on G-coupled proteins. Treatment of hypertension and a low-protein diet may slow the progression of disease, although this is not well proven.

Ong AC et al; ERA-EDTA Working Group for Inherited Kidney Diseases. Autosomal dominant polycystic kidney disease: the changing face of clinical management. Lancet. 2015 May 16;385(9981):1993–2002. Erratum in: Lancet. 2015 Jun 27;385(9987):2576. [PMID: 26090645]

Schrier RW et al; HALT-PKD Trial Investigators. Blood pressure in early autosomal dominant polycystic kidney disease. N Engl J Med. 2014 Dec 11;371(24):2255–66. [PMID: 25399733]

Torres VE et al; TEMPO 3:4 Trial Investigators. Tolvaptan in patients with autosomal dominant polycystic kidney disease. N Engl J Med. 2012 Dec 20;367(25):2407–18. [PMID: 23121377]

MEDULLARY SPONGE KIDNEY

This disease is a relatively common and benign disorder that is present at birth and not usually diagnosed until the fourth or fifth decade. It can be caused by autosomal dominant mutations in the *MCKD1* or *MCKD2* genes on chromosomes 1 and 16, respectively. Kidneys have a marked irregular enlargement of the medullary and interpapillary collecting ducts. This is associated with medullary cysts that are diffuse, giving a "Swiss cheese" appearance in these regions.

▶ Clinical Findings

Medullary sponge kidney presents with gross or microscopic hematuria, recurrent urinary tract infections, or nephrolithiasis. Common abnormalities are a decreased urinary concentrating ability and nephrocalcinosis; less common is incomplete type I distal renal tubular acidosis. The diagnosis can be made by CT, which shows cystic dilatation of the distal collecting tubules, a striated appearance in this area, and calcifications in the renal collecting system.

▶ Treatment

There is no known therapy. Adequate fluid intake (2 L/day) helps prevent stone formation. If hypercalciuria is present, thiazide diuretics are recommended because they decrease calcium excretion. Alkali therapy is recommended if renal tubular acidosis is present.

▶ Prognosis

Renal function is well maintained unless there are complications from recurrent urinary tract infections and nephrolithiasis.

JUVENILE NEPHRONOPHTHISIS-MEDULLARY CYSTIC DISEASE

This is a disorder previously believed to be rare but is now recognized as more common and as the cause of ESRD in younger individuals. It is associated with almost universal progression to ESRD. The childhood type—juvenile nephronophthisis—is an autosomal recessive disorder caused by mutations in the *NPH1*, *NPH2*, and *NPH3* genes; the type appearing in adulthood—medullary cystic disease—is autosomal dominant. Both types are manifested by multiple small renal cysts at the corticomedullary junction and medulla. The cortex becomes fibrotic, and as the disease progresses, interstitial inflammation and glomerular sclerosis appear.

▶ Clinical Findings

Patients with both forms exhibit polyuria, pallor, and lethargy. Hypertension occurs at the later stages of disease. The juvenile form causes growth retardation and ESRD before age 20 years. Patients require large amounts of salt and water as a result of renal salt wasting. Ultrasound and CT scan show small, scarred kidneys, and an open kidney biopsy may be necessary to recover tissue from the corticomedullary junction.

▶ Treatment & Prognosis

There is no current medical therapy that will prevent progression to renal failure. Adequate salt and water intake are essential to replenish renal losses.

MULTISYSTEM DISEASES WITH VARIABLE KIDNEY INVOLVEMENT[1]

MULTIPLE MYELOMA

Multiple myeloma is a malignancy of plasma cells (see Chapter 13).[1] Renal involvement occurs in about 25% of all patients. "Myeloma kidney" is the presence of light chain immunoglobulins (Bence Jones protein) in the urine

---

[1]Other diseases with variable involvement described elsewhere in this chapter include systemic lupus erythematosus, diabetes mellitus, and the vasculitides such as granulomatosis with polyangiitis and Goodpasture syndrome.

causing renal toxicity. Bence Jones protein causes direct renal tubular toxicity and results in tubular obstruction by precipitating in the tubules. The earliest tubular damage results in Fanconi syndrome (a type II proximal renal tubular acidosis). The proteinuria seen with multiple myeloma is primarily due to light chains that are not detected on urine dipstick, which mainly detects albumin. Hypercalcemia and hyperuricemia are frequently seen. Glomerular amyloidosis can develop in patients with multiple myeloma; in these patients, dipstick protein determinations are positive due to glomerular epithelial cell foot process effacement and albumin "spilling" into the Bowman capsule with resultant albuminuria. Other conditions resulting in renal dysfunction include plasma cell infiltration of the renal parenchyma and a hyperviscosity syndrome compromising renal blood flow. Therapy for acute kidney injury attributed to multiple myeloma includes correction of hypercalcemia, volume repletion, and chemotherapy for the underlying malignancy. Plasmapheresis had been considered appropriate to decrease the burden of existing monoclonal proteins while awaiting chemotherapeutic regimens to take effect. However, in the largest randomized prospective trial to date, plasmapheresis did not provide any renal benefit to these patients. Pheresis therapy still remains controversial.

Haynes R et al. Myeloma kidney: improving clinical outcomes? Adv Chronic Kidney Dis. 2012 Sep;19(5):342–51. [PMID: 22920645]
Leung N et al. Myeloma-related kidney disease. Adv Chronic Kidney Dis. 2014 Jan;21(1):36–47. [PMID: 24359985]

SICKLE CELL DISEASE

Kidney dysfunction associated with sickle cell disease is most commonly due to sickling of red blood cells in the renal medulla because of low oxygen tension and hypertonicity. Congestion and stasis lead to hemorrhage, interstitial inflammation, and papillary infarcts. Clinically, hematuria is common. Damage to renal capillaries also leads to diminished concentrating ability. Isosthenuria (urine osmolality equal to that of serum) is routine, and patients can easily become dehydrated. Papillary necrosis occurs as well. These abnormalities are also encountered in patients with sickle cell trait. Sickle cell glomerulopathy is less common but will inexorably progress to ESRD. Its primary clinical manifestation is proteinuria. Optimal treatment requires adequate hydration and control of the sickle cell disease.

Ataga KI et al. The glomerulopathy of sickle cell disease. Am J Hematol. 2014 Sep;89(9):907–14. [PMID: 24840607]
Gosmanova EO et al. Prevalence and progression of chronic kidney disease in adult patients with sickle cell disease. J Investig Med. 2014 Jun;62(5):804–7. [PMID: 24781553]
Nath KA et al. Vasculature and kidney complications in sickle cell disease. J Am Soc Nephrol. 2012 May;23(5):781–4. [PMID: 22440903]

TUBERCULOSIS

The classic renal manifestation of tuberculosis is the presence of microscopic pyuria with a sterile urine culture—or "sterile pyuria." More often, other bacteria are also present.

Microscopic hematuria is often present with pyuria. Urine cultures are the gold standard for diagnosis. Three to six first morning midstream specimens should be performed to improve sensitivity. Papillary necrosis and cavitation of the renal parenchyma occur less frequently, as do ureteral strictures and calcifications. Adequate drug therapy can result in resolution of renal involvement.

Chapagain A et al. Presentation, diagnosis, and treatment outcome of tuberculous-mediated tubulointerstitial nephritis. Kidney Int. 2011 Mar;79(6):671–7. [PMID: 21160461]
Latus J et al. Tubulointerstitial nephritis in active tuberculosis—a single center experience. Clin Nephrol. 2012 Oct;78(4):297–302. [PMID: 22704252]

GOUT & THE KIDNEY

The kidney is the primary organ for excretion of uric acid. Patients with proximal tubular dysfunction have decreased excretion of uric acid and are more prone to gouty arthritis attacks. Depending on the pH and uric acid concentration, deposition can occur in the tubules, the interstitium, or the urinary tract. The more alkaline pH of the interstitium causes urate salt deposition, whereas the acidic environment of the tubules and urinary tract causes uric acid crystal deposition at high concentrations.

Three disorders are commonly seen: (1) uric acid nephrolithiasis, (2) acute uric acid nephropathy, and (3) chronic urate nephropathy. Kidney dysfunction with uric acid nephrolithiasis stems from obstructive physiology. Acute uric acid nephropathy presents similarly to acute tubulointerstitial nephritis with direct toxicity from uric acid crystals. Chronic urate nephropathy is caused by deposition of urate crystals in the alkaline medium of the interstitium; this can lead to fibrosis and atrophy. Epidemiologically, hyperuricemia and gout have been associated with worsening cardiovascular outcomes.

Treatment between gouty attacks involves avoidance of food and drugs causing hyperuricemia (see Chapter 20), aggressive hydration, and pharmacotherapy aimed at reducing serum uric acid levels (such as with allopurinol and febuxostat). The three disorders mentioned above are seen in both "overproducers" and "underexcretors" of uric acid. The latter situation may seem counterintuitive; however, these patients have hyperacidic urine, which explains the deposition of relatively insoluble uric acid crystals. For those with uric acid nephrolithiasis, fluid intake should exceed 3 L/day, and use of a urinary alkalinizing agent can be considered.

Gibson T. Hyperuricemia, gout and the kidney. Curr Opin Rheumatol. 2012 Mar;24(2):127–31. [PMID: 22157498]
Johnson RJ et al. Uric acid and chronic kidney disease: which is chasing which? Nephrol Dial Transplant. 2013 Sep;28(9):2221–8. [PMID: 23543594]

NEPHROGENIC SYSTEMIC FIBROSIS

Nephrogenic systemic fibrosis is a multisystem disorder seen only in patients with CKD (primarily with an eGFR less than 15 mL/min/1.73 m^2, but rarely with a GFR of 15–29 mL/min/1.73 m^2), acute kidney injury, and after kidney transplantation. Histopathologically, there is an increase in dermal spindle cells positive for CD34 and procollagen I. Collagen bundles with mucin and elastic fibers are also noted.

Nephrogenic systemic fibrosis was first recognized in hemodialysis patients in 1997 and has been strongly linked to use of contrast agents containing gadolinium. Incidence is projected to be 1–4% in the highest risk (ESRD) population that has received gadolinium, and lower in patients with less severe kidney dysfunction. There is an FDA warning regarding avoidance of exposure to this agent for patients with an eGFR less than 30 mL/min/1.73 m^2.

▶ Clinical Findings

Nephrogenic systemic fibrosis affects several organ systems, including the skin, muscles, lungs, and cardiovascular system. The most common manifestation is a debilitating fibrosing skin disorder that can range from skin-colored to erythematous papules, which coalesce to brawny patches. The skin can be thick and woody in areas and is painful out-of-proportion to findings on examination.

▶ Treatment

Several case reports and series have described benefit for patients after treatment with corticosteroids, photopheresis, plasmapheresis, and sodium thiosulfate. The true effectiveness of these interventions is still unclear. Alternative or no imaging agents should be used for patients requiring MR with contrast at risk for nephrogenic systemic fibrosis.

Daftari Besheli L et al. Current status of nephrogenic systemic fibrosis. Clin Radiol. 2014 Jul;69(7):661–8. [PMID: 24582176]

Urologic Disorders

Maxwell V. Meng, MD, FACS

Thomas J. Walsh, MD, MS

Thomas D. Chi, MD

HEMATURIA

ESSENTIALS OF DIAGNOSIS

▶ Both gross and microscopic hematuria require evaluation.

▶ The upper urinary tract should be imaged, and cystoscopy should be performed if there is hematuria in the absence of infection.

General Considerations

An **upper tract source** (kidneys and ureters) can be identified in 10% of patients with gross or microscopic hematuria. For upper tract sources, stone disease accounts for 40%, medical kidney disease (medullary sponge kidney, glomerulonephritis, papillary necrosis) for 20%, renal cell carcinoma for 10%, and urothelial cell carcinoma of the ureter or renal pelvis for 5%. Drug ingestion and associated medical problems may provide diagnostic clues. Analgesic use (papillary necrosis), cyclophosphamide (chemical cystitis), antibiotics (interstitial nephritis), diabetes mellitus, sickle cell trait or disease (papillary necrosis), a history of stone disease, or malignancy should all be investigated. The **lower tract source** of gross hematuria (in the absence of infection) is most commonly from urothelial cell carcinoma of the bladder. Microscopic hematuria in the male is most commonly from benign prostatic hyperplasia. **The presence of hematuria in patients receiving anticoagulation therapy cannot be presumed to be due the anticoagulation;** a complete evaluation is warranted consisting of upper tract imaging, cystoscopy, and urine cytology (see Chapter 39 for Bladder Cancer, Cancers of the Ureter & Renal Pelvis, Renal Cell Carcinoma, and Other Primary Tumors of the Kidney).

Clinical Findings

A. Symptoms and Signs

If gross hematuria occurs, a description of the timing (initial, terminal, total) may provide a clue to the localization of disease. Associated symptoms (ie, renal colic, irritative voiding symptoms, constitutional symptoms) should be investigated. Physical examination should emphasize signs of systemic disease (fever, rash, lymphadenopathy, abdominal or pelvic masses) as well as signs of medical kidney disease (hypertension, volume overload). Urologic evaluation may demonstrate an enlarged prostate, flank mass, or urethral disease.

B. Laboratory Findings

Initial laboratory investigations include a urinalysis and urine culture. Proteinuria and casts suggest renal origin. Irritative voiding symptoms, bacteriuria, and a positive urine culture in the female suggest urinary tract infection, but follow-up urinalysis is important after treatment to ensure resolution of the hematuria. An estimate of the kidney function should be obtained, since intrinsic kidney disease has implications for further evaluation and management of patients with hematuria.

Urinary cytology should be performed to evaluate for urothelial neoplasm either prior to or at the time of cystoscopy.

C. Imaging

The upper tract should be imaged using abdominal and pelvic CT scanning without and with contrast to identify neoplasms of the kidney or ureter as well as benign conditions such as urolithiasis, obstructive uropathy, papillary necrosis, medullary sponge kidney, or polycystic kidney disease. The role of ultrasonographic evaluation of the urinary tract for hematuria is unclear. Although it may provide adequate information for the kidney, its sensitivity in detecting ureteral disease is lower.

D. Cystoscopy

Cystoscopy can be used to assess for bladder or urethral neoplasm, benign prostatic enlargement, and radiation or chemical cystitis. For gross hematuria, cystoscopy is ideally performed while the patient is actively bleeding to allow better localization (ie, lateralize to one side of the upper tracts, bladder, or urethra).

Follow-up

In patients with negative evaluations, repeat evaluations may be warranted to avoid a missed malignancy; however, the ideal frequency of such evaluations is not defined. Urinary cytology can be obtained after initial negative evaluation, and cystoscopy and upper tract imaging after a year.

When to Refer

In the absence of infection or other benign etiology, hematuria (either gross or microscopic) requires evaluation.

Daher Ede F et al. Renal tuberculosis in the modern era. Am J Trop Med Hyg. 2013 Jan;88(1):54–64. [PMID: 23303798]

Davis R et al. Diagnosis, evaluation and follow-up of asymptomatic microhematuria (AMH) in adults: AUA guideline. J Urol. 2012 Dec;188(6 Suppl):2473–81. [PMID: 23098784]

Dick-Biascoechea MA et al. Asymptomatic microscopic hematuria. Curr Opin Obstet Gynecol. 2012 Oct;24(5):324–30. [PMID: 22954764]

GENITOURINARY TRACT INFECTIONS

1. Acute Cystitis

ESSENTIALS OF DIAGNOSIS

- ▶ Irritative voiding symptoms.
- ▶ Patient usually afebrile.
- ▶ Positive urine culture; blood cultures may also be positive.

General Considerations

Acute cystitis is an infection of the bladder most commonly due to the coliform bacteria (especially *Escherichia coli*) and occasionally gram-positive bacteria (enterococci). The route of infection is typically ascending from the urethra. Viral cystitis due to adenovirus is sometimes seen in children but is rare in adults. Uncomplicated cystitis in men is rare and implies a pathologic process such as infected stones, prostatitis, or chronic urinary retention requiring further investigation.

Clinical Findings

A. Symptoms and Signs

Irritative voiding symptoms (frequency, urgency, dysuria) and suprapubic discomfort are common. Women may experience gross hematuria, and symptoms may often appear following sexual intercourse. Physical examination may elicit suprapubic tenderness, but examination is often unremarkable. Systemic toxicity is absent.

B. Laboratory Findings

Urinalysis shows pyuria, bacteriuria, and varying degrees of hematuria. The degree of pyuria and bacteriuria does not necessarily correlate with the severity of symptoms. **Urine culture is positive for the offending organism, but colony counts exceeding 10^5/mL are not essential for the diagnosis.**

C. Imaging

Because uncomplicated cystitis is rare in men, elucidation of the underlying problem with appropriate investigations, such as abdominal ultrasonography or cystoscopy (or both), is warranted. Follow-up imaging using CT scanning is warranted if pyelonephritis, recurrent infections, or anatomic abnormalities are suspected.

Differential Diagnosis

In women, infectious processes such as vulvovaginitis and pelvic inflammatory disease can usually be distinguished by pelvic examination and urinalysis. In men, urethritis and prostatitis may be distinguished by physical examination (urethral discharge or prostatic tenderness).

Noninfectious causes of cystitis-like symptoms include pelvic irradiation, chemotherapy (cyclophosphamide), bladder carcinoma, interstitial cystitis, voiding dysfunction disorders, and psychosomatic disorders.

Prevention

Women who have more than three episodes of cystitis per year are considered candidates for prophylactic antibiotic therapy to prevent recurrence after treatment of urinary tract infection. Prior to institution of therapy, a thorough urologic evaluation is warranted to exclude any anatomic abnormality (eg, stones, reflux, fistula). The three most commonly used oral agents for prophylaxis are trimethoprim-sulfamethoxazole (40 mg/200 mg), nitrofurantoin (100 mg), and cephalexin (250 mg). Single dosing at bedtime or at the time of intercourse is the recommended schedule.

The risk of acquiring a catheter-associated urinary tract infection in hospitalized patients can be minimized by using indwelling catheters only when necessary, implementing systems to ensure removal of catheters when no longer needed, using antimicrobial catheters in high-risk patients, using external collection devices in select men, identifying significant postvoid residuals by ultrasound, maintaining proper insertion techniques, and utilizing alternatives such as intermittent catheterization.

Treatment

Uncomplicated cystitis in women can be treated with short-term antimicrobial therapy, which consists of single-dose therapy or 1–9 days of therapy. Cephalexin, nitrofurantoin, trimethoprim-sulfamethoxazole, and fluoroquinolones are the medications of choice for uncomplicated cystitis (Table 23–1). Local patterns of bacterial resistance should be consulted to identify best treatment options. Some antibiotics may be ineffective because of the emergence of resistant organisms. A review of the literature proposed that acute uncomplicated cystitis in women can be diagnosed without office evaluation or urine culture, and that appropriate

Table 23–1. Empiric therapy for urinary tract infections.

Diagnosis	Antibiotic	Route	Duration	Cost per Duration Noted[1]
Acute pyelonephritis	Ampicillin, 1 g every 6 hours, and gentamicin, 1 mg/kg every 8 hours	Intravenous	14 days	$540.00 not including intravenous supplies
	Ciprofloxacin, 750 mg every 12 hours[2]	Oral	7–14 days	$79.00–158.00
	Levofloxacin, 750 mg daily	Oral	5 days	$181.00
	Trimethoprim-sulfamethoxazole, 160/800 mg every 12 hours[3]	Oral	10–14 days	$18.00-25.00
Chronic pyelonephritis	Same as for acute pyelonephritis		3–6 months	
Acute cystitis	Cephalexin, 250–500 mg every 6 hours	Oral	1–3 days	$16.60/3 days (500 mg)
	Nitrofurantoin (macrocrystals), 100 mg every 12 hours	Oral	7 days	$47.00
	Ciprofloxacin, 250–500 mg every 12 hours	Oral	1–3 days	$32.00/3 days (500 mg)
	Norfloxacin, 400 mg every 12 hours	Oral	1–3 days	Not available in the United States
	Levofloxacin, 750 mg daily	Oral	5 days	$181.00
	Trimethoprim-sulfamethoxazole, 160/800 mg, two tablets[2]	Oral	Single dose	$1.80
Acute bacterial prostatitis	Same as for acute pyelonephritis		21 days	
Chronic bacterial prostatitis	Ciprofloxacin, 250–500 mg every 12 hours	Oral	1–3 months	$322.00/1 month (500 mg)
	Levofloxacin, 750 mg daily	Oral	5 days	$181.00
	Trimethoprim-sulfamethoxazole, 160/800 mg every 12 hours[2]	Oral	1–3 months	$54.00/1 month
Acute epididymitis				
Sexually transmitted	Ceftriaxone, 250 mg as single dose, **plus** Doxycycline, 100 mg every 12 hours	Intramuscular Oral	Once 10 days	$1.00/250 mg $95.00
Non-sexually transmitted	Same as for chronic bacterial prostatitis	Oral	3 weeks	

[1]Average wholesale price, (AWP, for AB-rated generic when available) for quantity listed. Source: *Red Book* (electronic version), Truven Health Analytics Information, http://www.micromedexsolutions.com, accessed April 8, 2016. AWP may not accurately represent the actual pharmacy cost because wide contractual variations exist among institutions.
[2]Increasing resistance noted.
[3]Increasing resistance noted (up to 20%).

first-line therapies include trimethoprim-sulfamethoxazole (100 mg twice daily for 3 days), nitrofurantoin (100 mg twice daily for 5–7 days), and fosfomycin trometamol (3 g single dose). In men, uncomplicated urinary tract infection is rare, and thus, the duration of antibiotic therapy depends on the underlying etiology. Hot sitz baths or urinary analgesics (phenazopyridine, 200 mg orally three times daily) may provide symptomatic relief.

▶ **Prognosis**

Infections typically respond rapidly to therapy, and failure to respond suggests resistance to the selected medication or anatomic abnormalities requiring further investigation.

▶ **When to Refer**

- Suspicion or radiographic evidence of anatomic abnormality.

- Evidence of urolithiasis.

- Recurrent cystitis due to bacterial persistence.

Grigoryan L et al. Diagnosis and management of urinary tract infection in the outpatient setting: a review. JAMA. 2014 Oct 22–29;312(16):1677–84. [PMID: 25335150]

Marschall J et al. Antibiotic prophylaxis for urinary tract infections after removal of urinary catheter: meta-analysis. BMJ. 2013 Jun 11;346:f3147. Erratum in: BMJ. 2013;347:f5325. [PMID: 23757735]

Mody L et al. JAMA patient page. Urinary tract infections in older women. JAMA. 2014 Feb 26;311(8):874. [PMID: 24570259]

Shepherd AK et al. Management of urinary tract infections in the era of increasing antimicrobial resistance. Med Clin North Am. 2013 Jul;97(4):737–57. [PMID: 23809723]

Tambyah PA et al. Catheter-associated urinary tract infection. Curr Opin Infect Dis. 2012 Aug;25(4):365–70. [PMID: 22691687]

Torpy JM et al. JAMA patient page. Urinary tract infection. JAMA. 2012 May 2;307(17):1877. [PMID: 22550203]

2. Acute Pyelonephritis

ESSENTIALS OF DIAGNOSIS

▸ Fever.

▸ Flank pain.

▸ Irritative voiding symptoms.

▸ Positive urine culture.

▶ General Considerations

Acute pyelonephritis is an infectious inflammatory disease involving the kidney parenchyma and renal pelvis. Gram-negative bacteria are the most common causative agents including *E coli*, *Proteus*, *Klebsiella*, *Enterobacter*, and *Pseudomonas*. Gram-positive bacteria are less commonly seen but include *Enterococcus faecalis* and *Staphylococcus aureus*. The infection usually ascends from the lower urinary tract—with the exception of *S aureus*, which usually is spread by a hematogenous route.

▶ Clinical Findings

A. Symptoms and Signs

Symptoms include fever, flank pain, shaking chills, and irritative voiding symptoms (urgency, frequency, dysuria). Associated nausea and vomiting, and diarrhea are common. Signs include fever and tachycardia. Costovertebral angle tenderness is usually pronounced.

B. Laboratory Findings

Complete blood count shows leukocytosis and a left shift. Urinalysis shows pyuria, bacteriuria, and varying degrees of hematuria. White cell casts may be seen. Urine culture demonstrates heavy growth of the offending organism, and blood culture may also be positive.

C. Imaging

In complicated pyelonephritis, renal ultrasound may show hydronephrosis from a stone or other source of obstruction.

▶ Differential Diagnosis

The differential diagnosis includes acute cystitis or a lower urinary source. Acute intra-abdominal disease such as appendicitis, cholecystitis, pancreatitis, or diverticulitis must be distinguished from pyelonephritis. A normal urinalysis is usually seen in gastrointestinal disorders; however, on occasion, inflammation from adjacent bowel (appendicitis or diverticulitis) may result in hematuria or sterile pyuria. Abnormal liver biochemical tests or elevated amylase levels may assist in the differentiation. Lower-lobe pneumonia is distinguishable by the abnormal chest radiograph.

In males, the main differential diagnosis for acute pyelonephritis also includes acute epididymitis and acute prostatitis. Physical examination and the location of the pain should permit this distinction.

▶ Complications

Sepsis with shock can occur with acute pyelonephritis. In diabetic patients, emphysematous pyelonephritis resulting from gas-producing organisms may be life threatening if not adequately treated. Healthy adults usually recover complete kidney function, yet if coexistent kidney disease is present, scarring or chronic pyelonephritis may result. Inadequate therapy could result in abscess formation.

▶ Treatment

Urine and blood cultures are obtained to identify the causative agent and to determine antimicrobial sensitivity. In the inpatient setting, intravenous ampicillin and an aminoglycoside are initiated prior to obtaining sensitivity results (Table 23–1). In the outpatient setting, a quinolone may be initiated (Table 23–1). Antibiotics are adjusted according to sensitivities. Fevers may persist for up to 72 hours even with appropriate antibiotics; failure to respond within 48 hours warrants imaging (CT or ultrasound) to exclude complicating factors that may require intervention. Catheter drainage may be necessary in the face of urinary retention and nephrostomy drainage if there is ureteral obstruction. In inpatients, intravenous antibiotics are continued for 24 hours after the fever resolves, and oral antibiotics are then given to complete a 14-day course of therapy. However, a shorter 7-day course may be just as effective with fewer side effects, such as mucosal candidiasis. Follow-up urine cultures are mandatory following the completion of treatment. Randomized trial data suggest that ceftolozane-tazobactam may yield better response rates compared to high-dose levofloxacin in the treatment of complicated lower urinary tract infection and pyelonephritis.

▶ Prognosis

With prompt diagnosis and appropriate treatment, acute pyelonephritis carries a good prognosis. Complicating factors, underlying kidney disease, and increasing patient age may lead to a less favorable outcome.

▶ When to Refer

• Evidence of complicating factors (urolithiasis, obstruction).

• Absence of clinical improvement in 48 hours.

▶ When to Admit

• Severe infections or complicating factors, evidence of sepsis or need for parenteral antibiotics.

• Need for radiographic imaging or drainage of urinary tract obstruction.

Meng MV. Infection of the upper urinary tract. In: Wessells H (editor). *Urological Emergencies: A Practical Guide*. New York: Humana Press, 2012.

Sandberg T et al. Ciprofloxacin for 7 days versus 14 days in women with acute pyelonephritis: a randomised, open-label and double-blind, placebo-controlled, non-inferiority trial. Lancet. 2012 Aug 4;380(9840):484–90. [PMID: 22726802]

Wagenlehner FM et al. Ceftolozane-tazobactam compared with levofloxacin in the treatment of complicated urinary-tract infections, including pyelonephritis: a randomised, double-blind, phase 3 trial (ASPECT-cUTI). Lancet. 2015 May 16; 385(9981):1949–56. [PMID: 25931244]

3. Acute Bacterial Prostatitis

ESSENTIALS OF DIAGNOSIS

► Fever.

► Irritative voiding symptoms.

► Perineal or suprapubic pain; exquisite tenderness common on rectal examination.

► Positive urine culture.

► General Considerations

Acute bacterial prostatitis is usually caused by gram-negative rods, especially *E coli* and *Pseudomonas* species and less commonly by gram-positive organisms (eg, enterococci). The most likely routes of infection include ascent up the urethra and reflux of infected urine into the prostatic ducts. Lymphatic and hematogenous routes are probably rare.

► Clinical Findings

A. Symptoms and Signs

Perineal, sacral, or suprapubic pain, fever, and irritative voiding complaints are common. Varying degrees of obstructive symptoms may occur as the acutely inflamed prostate swells, which may lead to urinary retention. High fevers and a warm and often exquisitely tender prostate are detected on examination. Care should be taken to perform a gentle rectal examination, since vigorous manipulations may result in septicemia. **Prostatic massage is contraindicated.**

B. Laboratory Findings

Complete blood count shows leukocytosis and a left shift. Urinalysis shows pyuria, bacteriuria, and varying degrees of hematuria. Urine cultures will demonstrate the offending pathogen (Table 23–2).

► Differential Diagnosis

Acute pyelonephritis or acute epididymitis should be distinguishable by the location of pain as well as by physical examination. Acute diverticulitis is occasionally confused with acute prostatitis; however, the history and urinalysis should permit clear distinction. Urinary retention from benign or malignant prostatic enlargement is distinguishable by initial or follow-up rectal examination.

► Treatment

Hospitalization may be required, and parenteral antibiotics (ampicillin and aminoglycoside) should be initiated until organism sensitivities are available (Table 23–1). After the patient is afebrile for 24–48 hours, oral antibiotics (eg, quinolones) are used to complete 4–6 weeks of therapy. If urinary retention develops, a percutaneous suprapubic tube is required as urethral catheterization is contraindicated. Follow-up urine culture and examination of prostatic secretions should be performed after the completion of therapy to ensure eradication.

► Prognosis

With effective treatment, chronic bacterial prostatitis is rare.

► When to Refer

• Evidence of urinary retention.

• Evidence of chronic prostatitis.

► When to Admit

• Signs of sepsis.

• Need for surgical drainage of bladder or prostatic abscess.

Campeggi A et al. Acute bacterial prostatitis after transrectal ultrasound-guided prostate biopsy: epidemiological, bacteria and treatment patterns from a 4-year prospective study. Int J Urol. 2014 Feb;21(2):152–5. [PMID: 23906113]

Dickson G. Prostatitis—diagnosis and treatment. Aust Fam Physician. 2013 Apr;42(4):216–9. [PMID: 23550248]

Nagy V et al. Acute bacterial prostatitis in humans: current microbiological spectrum, sensitivity to antibiotics and clinical findings. Urol Int. 2012;89(4):445–50. [PMID: 23095643]

Wagenlehner FM et al. Bacterial prostatitis. World J Urol. 2013 Aug;31(4):711–6. [PMID: 23519458]

Yoon BI et al. Clinical courses following acute bacterial prostatitis. Prostate Int. 2013;1(2):89–93. [PMID: 24223408]

Table 23–2. Clinical characteristics of prostatitis and prostatodynia syndromes.

Findings	Acute Bacterial Prostatitis	Chronic Bacterial Prostatitis	Nonbacterial Prostatitis	Prostatodynia
Fever	+	–	–	–
Urinalysis	+	–	–	–
Expressed prostate secretions	Contraindicated	+	+	–
Bacterial culture	+	+	–	–

4. Chronic Bacterial Prostatitis

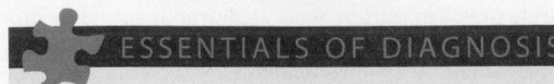

> ► Irritative voiding symptoms.
> ► Perineal or suprapubic discomfort, often dull and poorly localized.
> ► Positive expressed prostatic secretions and culture.

General Considerations

Although chronic bacterial prostatitis may evolve from acute bacterial prostatitis, many men have no history of acute infection. Gram-negative rods are the most common etiologic agents, but only one gram-positive organism (*Enterococcus*) is associated with chronic infection. Routes of infection are the same as discussed for acute infection.

Clinical Findings

A. Symptoms and Signs

Clinical manifestations are variable. Some patients are asymptomatic, but most have varying degrees of irritative voiding symptoms. Low back and perineal pain are not uncommon. Many patients report a history of urinary tract infections. Physical examination is often unremarkable, although the prostate may feel normal, boggy, or indurated.

B. Laboratory Findings

Urinalysis is normal unless a secondary cystitis is present. Expressed prostatic secretions demonstrate increased numbers of leukocytes (greater than 10 per high-power field), especially lipid-laden macrophages. However, this finding is consistent with inflammation and is not diagnostic of bacterial prostatitis (Table 23–2). Leukocyte and bacterial counts from expressed prostatic secretions do not correlate with severity of symptoms. **Culture of the secretions or the postprostatic massage urine specimen is necessary to make the diagnosis.**

C. Imaging

Imaging tests are not necessary, although pelvic radiographs or transrectal ultrasound may demonstrate prostatic calculi.

Differential Diagnosis

Chronic urethritis may mimic chronic prostatitis, though cultures of the fractionated urine may localize the source of infection to the initial specimen, which would come from the urethra. Cystitis may be secondary to prostatitis, but urine samples after prostatic massage may localize the infection to the prostate. Anal disease may share some of the symptoms of prostatitis, but physical examination should distinguish between the two.

Treatment

Few antimicrobial agents attain therapeutic intraprostatic levels in the absence of acute inflammation. Trimethoprim does diffuse into the prostate, and trimethoprim-sulfamethoxazole is associated with the best cure rates (Table 23–1). However, increasing resistance to this antibiotic up to 20% has been noted. Other effective agents include quinolones, cephalexin, erythromycin, and carbenicillin. The optimal duration of therapy remains controversial, ranging from 6 to 12 weeks. Symptomatic relief may be provided by anti-inflammatory agents (indomethacin, ibuprofen) and hot sitz baths.

Prognosis

Chronic bacterial prostatitis is difficult to cure, but its symptoms and tendency to cause recurrent urinary tract infections can be controlled by suppressive antibiotic therapy.

When to Refer

- Persistent symptoms.
- Consideration of enrollment in clinical trials.

Perletti G et al. Antimicrobial therapy for chronic bacterial prostatitis. Cochrane Database Syst Rev. 2013 Aug 12;8:CD009071. [PMID: 23934982]

5. Nonbacterial Prostatitis

> ► Irritative voiding symptoms.
> ► Perineal or suprapubic discomfort, similar to that of chronic bacterial prostatitis.
> ► Positive expressed prostatic secretions, but negative culture.

General Considerations

Nonbacterial prostatitis is the most common of the prostatitis syndromes, and its cause is unknown. Speculation implicates chlamydiae, mycoplasmas, ureaplasmas, and viruses, but no substantial proof exists. In some cases, nonbacterial prostatitis may represent a noninfectious inflammatory or autoimmune disorder. Because the cause of nonbacterial prostatitis remains unknown, the diagnosis is usually one of exclusion.

Clinical Findings

A. Symptoms and Signs

The clinical presentation is identical to that of chronic bacterial prostatitis; however, no history of urinary tract infections is present. The National Institutes of Health Chronic Prostatitis Symptom Index (NIH-CPSI) (www.prostatitisclinic.com/graphics/questionnaire2.pdf) has been validated to quantify symptoms of chronic nonbacterial prostatitis or chronic pelvic pain syndrome.

B. Laboratory Findings

Increased numbers of leukocytes are seen on expressed prostatic secretions, but all cultures are negative.

▶ Differential Diagnosis

The major distinction is from chronic bacterial prostatitis. The absence of a history of urinary tract infection and of positive cultures makes the distinction (Table 23–2). In older men with irritative voiding symptoms and negative cultures, bladder cancer must be excluded. Urinary cytologic examination and cystoscopy are warranted.

▶ Treatment

Because of the uncertainty regarding the etiology of nonbacterial prostatitis, a trial of antimicrobial therapy directed against *Ureaplasma, Mycoplasma,* or *Chlamydia* is warranted. Erythromycin (250 mg orally four times daily) can be initiated for 14 days, yet should be continued for 3–6 weeks only if a favorable clinical response ensues. Some symptomatic relief may be obtained with nonsteroidal anti-inflammatory agents or sitz baths. Dietary restrictions are not necessary unless the patient relates a history of symptom exacerbation by certain substances such as alcohol, caffeine, or particular foods.

▶ Prognosis

Annoying, recurrent symptoms are common, but serious sequelae have not been identified.

Chung SD et al. Association between chronic prostatitis/chronic pelvic pain syndrome and anxiety disorder: a population-based study. PLoS One. 2013 May 15;8(5):e64630. [PMID: 23691256]
Ismail M et al. Contemporary treatment options for chronic prostatitis/chronic pelvic pain syndrome. Drugs Today (Barc). 2013 Jul;49(7):457–62. [PMID: 23914354]
Nickel JC. Understanding chronic prostatitis/chronic pelvic pain syndrome (CP/CPPS). World J Urol. 2013 Aug;31(4):709–10. [PMID: 23812415]
Pontari M et al. New developments in the diagnosis and treatment of chronic prostatitis/chronic pelvic pain syndrome. Curr Opin Urol. 2013 Nov;23(6):565–9. [PMID: 24080807]

6. Prostatodynia

Prostatodynia is a noninflammatory disorder that affects young and middle-aged men and has variable causes, including voiding dysfunction and pelvic floor musculature dysfunction. The term "prostatodynia" is a misnomer, since the prostate is actually normal.

▶ Clinical Findings

A. Symptoms and Signs

Symptoms are the same as those seen with chronic prostatitis, yet there is no history of urinary tract infection. Additional symptoms may include hesitancy and interruption of flow. Patients may relate a lifelong history of voiding difficulty. Physical examination is unremarkable, but increased anal sphincter tone and periprostatic tenderness may be observed.

B. Laboratory Findings

Urinalysis is normal. Expressed prostatic secretions show normal numbers of leukocytes (Table 23–2). Urodynamic testing may show signs of dysfunctional voiding (detrusor contraction without urethral relaxation, high urethral pressures, spasms of the urinary sphincter) and is indicated in patients who do not respond to empiric treatment.

▶ Differential Diagnosis

Normal urinalysis will distinguish it from acute infectious processes. Examination of expressed prostatic secretions will distinguish nonbacterial prostatitis from other etiologies of prostadynia (Table 23–2).

▶ Treatment

Bladder neck and urethral spasms can be treated by alpha-blocking agents (terazosin, 1–10 mg orally once a day, or doxazosin, 1–8 mg orally once a day). Pelvic floor muscle dysfunction may respond to diazepam and biofeedback techniques. Sitz baths may contribute to symptomatic relief.

▶ Prognosis

Prognosis is variable depending on the specific cause.

Chung SD et al. Association between chronic prostatitis/chronic pelvic pain syndrome and anxiety disorder: a population-based study. PLoS One. 2013 May 15;8(5):e64630. [PMID: 23691256]
Ismail M et al. Contemporary treatment options for chronic prostatitis/chronic pelvic pain syndrome. Drugs Today (Barc). 2013 Jul;49(7):457–62. [PMID: 23914354]
Nickel JC. Understanding chronic prostatitis/chronic pelvic pain syndrome (CP/CPPS). World J Urol. 2013 Aug;31(4):709–10. [PMID: 23812415]
Pontari M et al. New developments in the diagnosis and treatment of chronic prostatitis/chronic pelvic pain syndrome. Curr Opin Urol. 2013 Nov;23(6):565–9. [PMID: 24080807]

7. Acute Epididymitis

ESSENTIALS OF DIAGNOSIS

- ▶ Fever.
- ▶ Irritative voiding symptoms.
- ▶ Painful enlargement of epididymis.

▶ General Considerations

Most cases of acute epididymitis are infectious and can be divided into one of two categories that have different age distributions and etiologic agents. **Sexually transmitted** forms typically occur in men under age 40 years, are associated with urethritis, and result from *Chlamydia trachomatis* or *Neisseria gonorrhoeae*. **Non-sexually transmitted forms** typically occur in older men, are associated with urinary tract infections and prostatitis, and are caused by gram-negative rods. The route of infection is probably via the urethra to the ejaculatory duct and then down the vas deferens to the epididymis. Amiodarone has been associated with self-limited epididymitis, which is a dose-dependent phenomenon.

▶ Clinical Findings

A. Symptoms and Signs

Symptoms may follow acute physical strain (heavy lifting), trauma, or sexual activity. Associated symptoms of urethritis (pain at the tip of the penis and urethral discharge) or cystitis (irritative voiding symptoms) may occur. Pain develops in the scrotum and may radiate along the spermatic cord or to the flank. Fever and scrotal swelling are usually apparent. Early in the course, the epididymis may be distinguishable from the testis; however, later the two may appear as one enlarged, tender mass. The prostate may be tender on rectal examination.

B. Laboratory Findings

Complete blood count shows leukocytosis and a left shift. In the sexually transmitted variety, Gram staining of a smear of urethral discharge may be diagnostic of gram-negative intracellular diplococci *(N gonorrhoeae)*. White cells without visible organisms on urethral smear represent nongonococcal urethritis, and *C trachomatis* is the most likely pathogen. In the non-sexually transmitted variety, urinalysis shows pyuria, bacteriuria, and varying degrees of hematuria. Urine cultures will demonstrate the offending pathogen.

C. Imaging

Scrotal ultrasound may aid in the diagnosis if examination is difficult because of the presence of a large hydrocele or because questions exist regarding the diagnosis.

▶ Differential Diagnosis

Tumors generally cause painless enlargement of the testis. Urinalysis is negative, and examination reveals a normal epididymis. Scrotal ultrasound is helpful to define the pathology. Testicular torsion usually occurs in prepubertal males but is occasionally seen in young adults. Acute onset of symptoms and a negative urinalysis favor testicular torsion or torsion of one of the testicular or epididymal appendages. Prehn sign (elevation of the scrotum above the pubic symphysis improves pain from epididymitis) may be helpful but is not reliable.

▶ Treatment

Bed rest with scrotal elevation is important in the acute phase. Treatment is directed toward the identified pathogen (Table 23–1). The sexually transmitted variety is

treated with 10–21 days of antibiotics, and **the sexual partner must be treated as well.** Non-sexually transmitted forms are treated for 21–28 days with appropriate antibiotics, at which time evaluation of the urinary tract is warranted to identify underlying disease.

▶ Prognosis

Prompt treatment usually results in a favorable outcome. Delayed or inadequate treatment may result in epididymo-orchitis, decreased fertility, or abscess formation.

▶ When to Refer

- Persistent symptoms and infection despite antibiotic therapy.
- Signs of sepsis or abscess formation.

Pilatz A et al. Acute epididymitis in ultrasound: results of a prospective study with baseline and follow-up investigations in 134 patients. Eur J Radiol. 2013 Dec;82(12):e762–8. [PMID: 24094645]
Srinath H. Acute scrotal pain. Aust Fam Physician. 2013 Nov; 42(11):790–2. [PMID: 24217099]

INTERSTITIAL CYSTITIS

 ESSENTIALS OF DIAGNOSIS

- ▶ Pain with a full bladder or urinary urgency.
- ▶ Submucosal petechiae or ulcers on cystoscopic examination.
- ▶ Diagnosis of exclusion.

▶ General Considerations

Interstitial cystitis (painful bladder syndrome) is characterized by pain with bladder filling that is relieved by emptying and is often associated with urgency and frequency. This is a diagnosis of exclusion, and patients must have a negative urine culture and cytology and no other obvious cause such as radiation cystitis, chemical cystitis (cyclophosphamide), vaginitis, urethral diverticulum, or genital herpes. Up to 40% of patients referred to urologists for interstitial cystitis may actually be found to have a different diagnosis after careful evaluation.

Population-based studies have demonstrated a prevalence of between 18 and 40 per 100,000 people. Both sexes are involved, but most patients are women, with a mean age of 40 years at onset. Patients with interstitial cystitis are more likely to report bladder problems in childhood, and there appears to be a higher prevalence of these in women. Up to 50% of patients may experience spontaneous remission of symptoms, with a mean duration of 8 months without treatment.

The etiology of interstitial cystitis is unknown, and it is most likely not a single disease but rather several diseases with similar symptoms. Associated diseases include severe allergies, irritable bowel syndrome, or inflammatory bowel disease. Theories regarding the cause of interstitial cystitis include increased epithelial permeability, neurogenic causes (sensory nervous system abnormalities), and autoimmunity.

► Clinical Findings

A. Symptoms and Signs

Pain with bladder filling that is relieved with urination or urgency, frequency, and nocturia are the most common symptoms. Patients should be asked about exposure to pelvic radiation or treatment with cyclophosphamide. Examination should exclude genital herpes, vaginitis, or a urethral diverticulum.

B. Laboratory Findings

Urinalysis, urine culture, and urinary cytologies are obtained to examine for infectious causes and bladder malignancy. Urodynamic testing assesses bladder sensation and compliance and excludes detrusor instability.

C. Cystoscopy

The bladder is distended with fluid (hydrodistention) to detect glomerulations (submucosal hemorrhage), which may or may not be present. Biopsy should be performed to exclude other causes such as carcinoma, eosinophilic cystitis, and tuberculous cystitis. The presence of submucosal mast cells is not needed to make the diagnosis of interstitial cystitis.

► Differential Diagnosis

Exposures to radiation or cyclophosphamide are obtained by the history. Bacterial cystitis, genital herpes, or vaginitis can be excluded by urinalysis, culture, and physical examination. A urethral diverticulum may be suspected if palpation of the urethra demonstrates an indurated mass that results in the expression of pus from the urethral meatus. Urethral carcinoma presents as a firm mass on palpation.

► Treatment

There is no cure for interstitial cystitis, but most patients achieve symptomatic relief from one of several approaches, including hydrodistention, which is usually done as part of the diagnostic evaluation. Approximately 20–30% of patients notice symptomatic improvement following this maneuver. Also of importance is the measurement of bladder capacity during hydrodistention, since patients with very small bladder capacities (less than 200 mL) are unlikely to respond to medical therapy.

Amitriptyline (10–75 mg/day orally) is often used as first-line medical therapy in patients with interstitial cystitis. Both central and peripheral mechanisms may contribute to its activity. Nifedipine (30–60 mg/day orally) and other calcium channel blockers have also demonstrated some activity in patients with interstitial cystitis. Pentosan polysulfate sodium (Elmiron) is an oral synthetic sulfated polysaccharide that helps restore integrity to the epithelium of the bladder in a subset of patients and has been

evaluated in a placebo-controlled trial. Other options include intravesical instillation of dimethyl sulfoxide (DMSO) and heparin. Intravesical bacillus Calmette-Guérin (BCG) is not beneficial.

Further treatment modalities include transcutaneous electric nerve stimulation (TENS) and acupuncture. Surgical therapy for interstitial cystitis should be considered only as a last resort and may require cystourethrectomy with urinary diversion.

► When to Refer

Persistent and bothersome symptoms in the absence of identifiable cause.

Matsuoka PK et al. Intravesical treatment of painful bladder syndrome: a systematic review and meta-analysis. Int Urogynecol J. 2012 Sep;23(9):1147–53. [PMID: 22569686]

Quillin RB et al. Management of interstitial cystitis/bladder pain syndrome: a urology perspective. Urol Clin North Am. 2012 Aug;39(3):389–96. [PMID: 22877722]

Quillin RB et al. Practical use of the new American Urological Association interstitial cystitis guidelines. Curr Urol Rep. 2012 Oct;13(5):394–401. [PMID: 22828913]

Torpy JM et al. JAMA patient page. Interstitial cystitis. JAMA. 2012 May 23;307(20):2211. [PMID: 22618932]

URINARY STONE DISEASE

ESSENTIALS OF DIAGNOSIS

► Severe flank pain.

► Nausea and vomiting.

► Identification on noncontrast CT or ultrasonography.

► General Considerations

Urinary stone disease is exceeded in frequency as a urinary tract disorder only by infections and prostatic disease and is estimated to afflict 240,000–720,000 Americans per year. While men are more frequently affected by urolithiasis than women, with a ratio of 2.5:1, the incidence in women appears to be rising over time. Initial presentation predominates between the third and fifth decade.

Urinary calculi are polycrystalline aggregates composed of varying amounts of crystalloid and a small amount of organic matrix. Stone formation requires saturated urine that is dependent on pH, ionic strength, solute concentration, and complexation. There are five major types of urinary stones: **calcium oxalate, calcium phosphate, struvite** (magnesium ammonium phosphate), **uric acid,** and **cystine.** The most common types are composed of calcium, and for that reason most urinary stones (85%) are radiopaque on plain abdominal radiographs. Uric acid stones frequently are composed of a combination of uric acid and calcium oxalate and thus are frequently radiopaque, though pure uric acid stones are radiolucent. Cystine stones frequently have a smooth-edged ground-glass appearance and are radiolucent.

Geographic factors contribute to the development of stones. Areas of high humidity and elevated temperatures appear to be contributing factors, and the incidence of symptomatic ureteral stones is greatest during hot summer months. Persons with sedentary lifestyles have a higher incidence of stones, which have also been associated with higher rates of hypertension, carotid calcification, and cardiovascular disease.

High protein and salt intake as well as inadequate hydration appear to be the most important factors in the development of urinary stones.

Genetic factors may contribute to urinary stone formation. While approximately 50% of calcium-based stones are thought to have a heritable component, other stone types are better characterized genetically. For example, cystinuria is an autosomal recessive disorder. Homozygous individuals have markedly increased excretion of cystine and frequently have numerous recurrent episodes of urinary stones. Distal renal tubular acidosis may be transmitted as a hereditary trait, and urolithiasis occurs in up to 75% of affected patients.

▶ Clinical Findings

A. Symptoms and Signs

Obstructing urinary stones usually present with acute and severe colic. Pain usually occurs suddenly and may awaken patients from sleep. It is localized to the flank, is usually severe, unremitting, and may be associated with nausea and vomiting. Patients are constantly moving trying to find a comfortable position—in sharp contrast to those with an acute abdomen. The pain may occur episodically and may radiate anteriorly over the abdomen. As the stone progresses down the ureter, the pain may be referred into the ipsilateral groin. If the stone becomes lodged at the uretero-vesicular junction, patients will complain of marked urinary urgency and frequency and in men, pain may radiate to the tip of the penis. After the stone passes into the bladder, there typically is minimal pain with passage through the urethra. Stone size does not correlate with the severity of the symptoms.

B. Laboratory Findings

In patients with either symptomatic or asymptomatic kidney stones, urinalysis usually reveals microscopic or gross hematuria (~90%). However, the absence of microhematuria does not exclude urinary stones. Urinary pH is a valuable clue to the cause of the possible stone. Normal urine pH is 5.8–6.2. Numerous dipstick measurements are valuable in the complete work-up of a patient in whom urinary stones are suspected. Persistent urinary pH < 5.5 is suggestive of uric acid or cystine stones. In contrast, a persistent urinary pH > 7.2 is suggestive of a struvite infection stone or calcium phosphate stone (when above 7.5). Patients with calcium oxalate–based stones typically have a urinary pH between 5.5 and 6.8.

C. Metabolic Evaluation

Patients should strain their urine through cheesecloth or a urine strainer during a symptomatic episode to facilitate stone analysis on recovered stones. Patients with uncomplicated first-time stones should undergo dietary counseling as outlined below and can be offered an optional complete metabolic evaluation.

General dietary counseling includes encouraging patients to change their diet to reduce sodium intake, reduce their animal protein intake during individual meals, and to ingest adequate fluid to achieve a voided volume of 1.5–2.0 L/day of urine. **Complete metabolic evaluation is recommended for patients who have recurrent stones or those with a family history of nephrolithiasis.** This includes a 24-hour urine collection to ascertain urinary volume, pH, calcium, uric acid, oxalate, phosphate, sodium, and citrate excretion. Serum parathyroid hormone (PTH), calcium, uric acid, electrolytes (including bicarbonate), creatinine, and BUN should also be obtained. Table 23–3 demonstrates the diagnostic criteria for the hypercalciuric states.

Table 23–3. Diagnostic criteria of different types of hypercalciuria.

	Absorptive Type I	Absorptive Type II	Absorptive Type III	Resorptive	Renal
Serum					
Calcium	N	N	N	↑	N
Phosphorus	N	N	↓	↓	N
PTH	N	N	N	↑	↑
Vitamin D	N	N	↑	↑	↑
Urinary calcium					
Fasting	N	N	↑	↑	↑
Restricted calcium intake	↑	N	↑	↑	↑
After calcium load	↑	↑	↑	↑	↑

N, normal; PTH, parathyroid hormone; ↑, elevated; ↓, low.

D. Imaging

A plain abdominal radiograph (kidneys-ureters-bladder [KUB]) and renal ultrasound examination will diagnose most stones. More than 60% of patients with acute renal colic will have a stone in the distal 4 cm of the ureter; attention should be directed to that region when examining plain radiographs and abdominal ultrasonographic studies. **Spiral CT is the most accurate imaging tool in evaluating flank pain** given its increased sensitivity and specificity over other tests; however, ultrasound (which is devoid of ionizing radiation) is a safe and effective alternative for evaluating renal colic that can be used in the emergency department with good accuracy. If CT scan is used, it should be obtained in the prone position to help differentiate distal ureterovesicular stones from those that have already passed into the urinary bladder. Repeated CT scans should be avoided due to the substantial radiation exposure to these patients with recurrent stones. Stone density can be estimated with Hounsfield units (HU) on CT scans to help determine stone type. Stones with low HU (less than 450) are more likely composed of uric acid, while those with high HU (greater than 1200) are more likely composed of calcium oxalate monohydrate. All stones whether radiopaque or radiolucent on plain abdominal radiographs will be visible on noncontrast CT except the rare calculi due to protease inhibitors (classically indinavir).

▶ Medical Treatment & Prevention

To reduce the recurrence rate of urinary stones, dietary modification is important. Additional metabolic evaluation often identifies a modifiable risk factor that can further reduce stone recurrence rates. If no medical treatment is provided after surgical stone removal, stones will generally recur in 50% of patients within 5 years. Some stone types (eg, uric acid, cystine) are more prone to rapid recurrence than others. **Of greatest importance in reducing stone recurrence is an increased fluid intake.** Absolute volumes are not established, but increasing fluid intake to ensure a voided volume of 1.5–2.0 L/day is recommended (normal average voided volume is 1.6 L/day). Patients are encouraged to ingest fluids during meals, 2 hours after each meal (when the body is most dehydrated), and prior to going to sleep in the evening—enough to awaken the patient to void—and to ingest additional fluids during the night. Increasing fluids only during daylight hours may not dilute a supersaturated urine overnight and thus initiate a new stone.

A. Diet

Sodium intake should be restricted to keep urinary sodium levels less than 150 mEq/day. Increased sodium intake will increase renal sodium and calcium excretion, increase urinary monosodium urates (that can act as a nidus for stone growth), increase the relative saturation of calcium phosphate, and decrease urinary citrate excretion. All of these factors encourage stone growth. Animal protein intake should be spread out through the day, not all consumed during any individual meal, and is best limited to 1 g/kg/day. An increased protein load during an individual meal can also increase calcium, oxalate, and uric acid excretion and decrease urinary citrate excretion.

Excessive intake of oxalate and purines can increase the incidence of stones in predisposed individuals. Dietary calcium or calcium supplements should not be routinely decreased. In fact, decreased calcium consumption has been found to increase stone recurrence. Only type II absorptive hypercalciuric patients (Table 23–3) benefit from a low-calcium diet.

B. Calcium Nephrolithiasis

1. Hypercalciuric—Hypercalciuric calcium nephrolithiasis (greater than 250 mg/24 h; greater than 4 mg/kg/24 h) can be caused by absorptive, resorptive, and renal disorders.

Absorptive hypercalciuria is secondary to increased absorption of calcium at the level of the small bowel, predominantly in the jejunum, and can be further subdivided into types I, II, and III. **Type I** absorptive hypercalciuria is independent of calcium intake. There is increased urinary calcium on a regular or even a calcium-restricted diet. Thiazide diuretics decrease renal calcium and result in increased bone density of approximately 1% per year. Thiazides have limited long-term utility (less than 5 years) since they may lose their hypocalciuric effect with continued therapy. Decreasing bowel absorption of calcium with a chelating agent, such as cellulose phosphate (10–15 g in three divided doses), is another treatment modality. It binds to the calcium and impedes small bowel absorption due to its increased bulk. Cellulose phosphate does not change the intestinal transport mechanism. It should be given with meals so it will be available to bind to the dietary calcium. Taking this chelating agent prior to bedtime is ineffective. Postmenopausal women should be treated with caution. Inappropriate use may result in a negative calcium balance and a secondary parathyroid stimulation and consequent bone reabsorption. However, there is generally no enhanced decline in bone density with long-term use. Long-term use without follow-up metabolic surveillance may result in hypomagnesuria and secondary hyperoxaluria and recurrent calculi. Routine follow-up every 6–8 months will help encourage medical compliance and permit adjustments in medical therapy based on repeat metabolic studies.

Type II absorptive hypercalciuria is diet-dependent and fortunately rare. Decreasing calcium intake by 50% (approximately 400 mg/day) will decrease the hypercalciuria to normal values (150–200 mg/24 h). There is no specific medical therapy.

Type III absorptive hypercalciuria is secondary to a renal phosphate leak. This results in increased vitamin D synthesis and secondarily increased small bowel absorption of calcium. This can be readily reversed by orthophosphates (250 mg orally three to four times per day), presently available without need for a prescription. Orthophosphates do not change intestinal absorption but rather inhibit vitamin D synthesis.

Resorptive hypercalciuria is secondary to hyperparathyroidism. Hypercalcemia, hypophosphatemia, hypercalciuria, and an elevated serum PTH value are found. Appropriate surgical resection of the parathyroid adenoma cures the disease, although recurrent urinary stones can still occur in 10% of patients after parathyroidectomy. Medical management invariably fails.

Renal hypercalciuria occurs when the renal tubules are unable to efficiently reabsorb filtered calcium, and hypercalciuria results. Spilling calcium in the urine results in secondary hyperparathyroidism. Serum calcium typically is normal. Thiazides are an effective long-term therapy in patients with this disorder.

2. Hyperuricosuric—Hyperuricosuric calcium nephrolithiasis is secondary to dietary purine excess or endogenous uric acid metabolic defects. Most cases (85%) can be treated with purine dietary restrictions; those that are not reversed with dietary modification are successfully treated with allopurinol. In contrast to uric acid nephrolithiasis, patients with hyperuricosuric calcium stones typically maintain a urinary pH > 5.5. Monosodium urates absorb and adsorb inhibitors and promote heterogeneous nucleation. Hyperuricosuric calcium nephrolithiasis is initiated with epitaxy, or heterogeneous nucleation. In such situations, similar crystal structures (ie, uric acid and calcium oxalate) can grow together with the aid of a protein matrix infrastructure.

3. Hyperoxaluric—Hyperoxaluric calcium nephrolithiasis (greater than 40 mg oxalate/24 h urine) is usually due to primary intestinal disorders. Patients often have a history of chronic diarrhea frequently associated with inflammatory bowel disease. In these situations, increased bowel fat or bile (or both) combine with intraluminal calcium to form a soap-like product. Calcium is therefore unavailable to bind to oxalate in the gut, which is then freely and rapidly absorbed. A small increase in oxalate absorption will significantly increase stone formation. If the diarrhea or steatorrhea cannot be effectively curtailed, oral calcium should be taken with meals, either by ingesting milk products or taking calcium carbonate supplements (250–500 mg). This helps to bind dietary oxalate in the gut and oxalate movement into the kidneys. Excess ascorbic acid (greater than 2 g/day) will substantially increase urinary oxalate levels. Rare enzymatic liver defects can lead to primary hyperoxaluria that is routinely fatal without a combined liver and kidney transplantation.

4. Hypocitraturic—Hypocitraturic calcium nephrolithiasis may be secondary to chronic diarrhea, type I (distal) renal tubular acidosis, chronic hydrochlorothiazide treatment, or in any condition that results in a metabolic acidosis. The metabolic acidosis enhances citrate transport into the proximal tubular cells where it is consumed by the citric acid cycle in their mitochondria, resulting in hypocitraturia (less than 450 mg/24h). Hypocitraturia is frequently associated with calcium stone formation. Urinary citrate binds to calcium in solution, thereby decreasing available calcium for precipitation and subsequent stone formation. Potassium citrate supplements are usually effective treatment in these situations. Urinary citrate is decreased in acidosis and is increased during alkalosis. The potassium will supplement the frequently associated hypokalemic states, and citrate will help correct the acidosis. A typical dose is 60 mEq total daily intake, divided either into three times daily as tablets or twice daily as the crystal

formulations dissolved in water (it is also available as a solution). Alternatively, oral lemonade has been shown to increase urinary citrate by about 150 mg/24h.

C. Uric Acid Calculi

The average normal urinary pH is 5.8–5.9. Urinary pH is consistently less than 5.5 in persons who form uric acid stones. Increasing the urinary pH to > 6.2 dramatically increases uric acid solubility, can effectively dissolve large calculi at a rate of 1 cm per month, and effectively prevents future uric acid stone formation. Urinary alkalinization with potassium citrate or an equivalent agent is the key to stone dissolution and prophylaxis. The target should be a urinary pH > 6.2 and < 6.5 (to avoid calcium phosphate precipitation). Other precipitating factors include hyperuricemia, myeloproliferative disorders, malignancy with increased uric acid production, abrupt and dramatic weight loss, and uricosuric medications. If hyperuricemia is present in addition to hyperuricosuria, allopurinol (300 mg/day orally) may be given for stone prevention. Although pure uric acid stones are relatively radiolucent, most have some calcium components and can be visualized on plain abdominal radiographs.

D. Struvite Calculi

Struvite stones are radiodense magnesium-ammonium-phosphate stones. They are most common in women with recurrent urinary tract infections with urease-producing organisms, including *Proteus, Pseudomonas, Providencia* and, less commonly, *Klebsiella, Staphylococcus*, and *Mycoplasma* (but not *E coli*). They rarely present as ureteral stones with colic without prior upper tract endourologic intervention. Frequently, a struvite stone is discovered as a large staghorn calculus forming a cast of the renal collecting system. Urinary pH is high, routinely above 7.2. Struvite stones are relatively soft and amenable to percutaneous removal. Appropriate perioperative antibiotics are required. They can recur rapidly, and efforts should be taken to render the patient stone-free. Acetohydroxamic acid is an effective urease inhibitor that can dissolve and prevent struvite stones, but it is poorly tolerated by most patients because of gastrointestinal side effects.

E. Cystine Calculi

Cystine stones are a result of abnormal excretion of cystine. These stones are particularly difficult to manage medically. Prevention is centered around marked increased fluid intake during the day and evening to achieve a urinary volume of 3–4 L/day, urinary alkalinization with a urinary pH > 7.0 (monitored with Nitrazine pH paper), and disulfide inhibitors such as tiopronin (alpha-mercaptoproprionylglycine) or penicillamine. There are no known inhibitors of cystine calculi.

▶ Surgical Treatment

In the acute setting, forced intravenous fluids will not push stones down the ureter. Forced diuresis can be counterproductive and exacerbate the pain; instead, a euvolemic state should be achieved. Signs of infection, including associated fever, tachycardia, or elevated white blood cell count may indicate a urinary tract infection behind the obstructing stone. **Any obstructing stone with associated infection is a medical emergency requiring urology consultation and prompt drainage by a ureteral catheter or a percutaneous nephrostomy tube.** Antibiotics alone are inadequate unless the obstruction is drained.

A. Ureteral Stones

Impediment to urine flow by ureteral stones usually occurs at three sites: the ureteropelvic junction, the crossing of the ureter over the iliac artery, or the ureterovesicular junction. Prediction of spontaneous stone passage is difficult. Stones smaller than 5–6 mm in diameter on a plain abdominal radiograph usually pass spontaneously. Medical expulsive therapy with alpha-blockers (such as tamsulosin, 0.4 mg orally once daily) in combination with a nonsteroidal anti-inflammatory agent (such as ibuprofen 600 mg orally three times per day with a full stomach), with or without a short course of a low-dose oral corticosteroid (such as prednisone 10 mg orally daily for 3–5 days) dramatically increases the rate of spontaneous stone passage though it is less effective for larger or more proximal stones. Medical expulsive therapy with appropriate pain medications is appropriate for the first few weeks. If the stone fails to pass within 4 weeks, the patient has fever, intolerable pain or persistent nausea or vomiting, or the patient must return to work or anticipates travel, then therapeutic intervention is indicated.

Ureteral stones are best managed with ureteroscopic stone extraction or in situ extracorporeal shock wave lithotripsy (SWL). Ureteroscopic stone extraction involves placement of a small endoscope through the urethra and into the ureter. Under direct vision, basket extraction or stone laser fragmentation followed by extraction is performed. Complications during endoscopic retrieval increase if medical expulsive therapy has been attempted for more than 6 weeks.

In situ SWL utilizes an external energy source focused on the stone with the aid of fluoroscopy or ultrasonography. SWL can be performed under anesthesia as an outpatient procedure and results in a high rate of stone fragmentation. Most stone fragments then pass uneventfully within 2 weeks, but those that have not passed within 6 weeks are unlikely to do so without intervention. Decreased SWL success rates are associated with lower pole and distal stone location, as well as larger stone burden. Women of childbearing age with a stone in the lower ureter are best not treated with SWL because its impact on the ovary is unknown.

Proximal and midureteral stones—those above the inferior margin of the sacroiliac joint—as well as intrarenal stones can be treated with SWL or ureteroscopy. SWL is delivered directly to the stone in situ. Occasionally, stone fragments will obstruct the ureter after SWL. Conservative management will usually result in spontaneous resolution with eventual passage of the stone fragments. In rare instances, ureteroscopic extraction will be required.

B. Renal Calculi

Patients with renal calculi but without pain, urinary tract infection, or obstruction may not warrant surgical treatment. If surveillance is elected, they should be monitored with serial abdominal radiographs or renal ultrasonographic examinations every 6–12 months. If calculi are growing or become symptomatic, intervention should be undertaken. Renal calculi smaller than 1.5 cm in diameter are best treated with SWL or ureteroscopic extraction. Calculi of larger diameter, located in the inferior calices, and staghorn stones (large branched stones occupying at least two renal calices) are best treated via percutaneous nephrolithotomy. Percutaneous nephrolithotomy is performed by inserting a needle into the appropriate renal calyx and dilating a tract large enough to allow a nephroscope to pass directly into the kidney. In this fashion, larger and more complex renal stones can be inspected, fragmented, and removed. Perioperative antibiotic coverage for any stone procedure should be given, ideally based on preoperative urine culture.

▶ When to Refer

- Evidence of urinary obstruction.
- Urinary stone with associated flank pain.
- Anatomic abnormalities or solitary kidney.
- Concomitant pyelonephritis or recurrent infection.

▶ When to Admit

- Intractable nausea and vomiting or pain.
- Obstructing stone with signs of infection.

Fink HA et al. Medical management to prevent recurrent nephrolithiasis in adults: a systematic review for an American College of Physicians Clinical Guideline. Ann Intern Med. 2013 Apr 2;158(7):535–43. [PMID: 23546565]

Goldfarb DS et al. Metabolic evaluation of first-time and recurrent stone formers. Urol Clin North Am. 2013 Feb;40(1):13–20. [PMID: 23177631]

Matlaga BR et al. Treatment of ureteral and renal stones: a systematic review and meta-analysis of randomized, controlled trials. J Urol. 2012 Jul;188(1):130–7. [PMID: 22591962]

Pickard R et al. Medical expulsive therapy in adults with ureteric colic: a multicentre, randomised, placebo-controlled trial. Lancet. 2015 Jul 25;386(9991):341–9. [PMID: 25998582]

Smith-Bindman R et al. Ultrasonography versus computed tomography for suspected nephrolithiasis. N Engl J Med. 2014 Sep 18;371(12):1100–10. [PMID: 25229916]

MALE ERECTILE DYSFUNCTION & SEXUAL DYSFUNCTION

 ESSENTIALS OF DIAGNOSIS

- ▶ Erectile dysfunction can have organic and psychogenic etiologies, and the two frequently overlap.
- ▶ Organic erectile dysfunction may be an early sign of cardiovascular disease and requires evaluation.
- ▶ Peyronie disease is a common, benign fibrotic disorder of the penis that causes pain, penile deformity, and sexual dysfunction.

General Considerations

Erectile dysfunction is the consistent inability to attain or maintain a sufficiently rigid penile erection for sexual performance. More than half of men aged 40–70 years experience erectile dysfunction and its incidence is age-related. Normal male erection is a neurovascular event relying on an intact autonomic and somatic nerve supply to the penis, smooth and striated musculature of the corpora cavernosa and pelvic floor, and arterial blood flow supplied by the paired cavernosal arteries. Erection is caused and maintained by an increase in arterial flow, active relaxation of the smooth muscle within the sinusoids of the paired corpora cavernosa, and an increase in venous resistance. Contraction of the bulbocavernosus and ischiocavernosus muscles results in further rigidity of the penis with intracavernosal pressures exceeding systolic blood pressure. Nitric oxide is a key neurotransmitter that initiates and sustains erections; however, other molecules contribute, including acetylcholine, prostaglandins, and vasoactive intestinal peptide.

Male sexual dysfunction may be manifested in a variety of ways, and patient history is critical to the proper classification and treatment. A **loss of libido** may indicate androgen deficiency. **Loss of erections** may result from arterial, venous, neurogenic, hormonal, or psychogenic causes. Concurrent medical problems may damage one or more of the mechanisms. Endothelial dysfunction results from the decreased bioavailability of nitric oxide with subsequent impairment of arterial vasodilation. Erectile dysfunction may be an early manifestation of endothelial dysfunction, which precedes more severe atherosclerotic cardiovascular disease. Many medications, especially antihypertensive, antidepressant, and opioid agents, are associated with erectile dysfunction.

Peyronie disease is a fibrotic disorder of the tunica albuginea of the penis resulting in varying degrees of penile pain, curvature, or deformity. Peyronie disease develops in approximately 5–10% of men and is more common with increased age. While 10% of men improve spontaneously, 50% will stabilize and the remainder will progress if left untreated. Penile deformity can impair normal sexual function and impact self-esteem.

Priapism is the occurrence of penile erection lasting longer than 4 hours resulting in ischemic injury of the corpora cavernosa from venous congestion and cessation of arterial inflow (low flow or "ischemic" priapism). Ischemic priapism may be caused by red blood cell dyscrasias, drug use, and any of the treatments for erectile dysfunction. **Ischemic priapism is a medical emergency requiring immediate medical or surgical intervention to avoid irreversible penile damage.**

Anejaculation is the **loss of seminal emission** and may result from androgen deficiency by decreasing prostate and seminal vesicle secretions, or by sympathetic denervation as a result of diabetes mellitus or pelvic or retroperitoneal surgery or radiation. **Retrograde ejaculation** may occur as a result of mechanical disruption of the bladder neck, due to transurethral resection of the prostate, pelvic radiation,

sympathetic denervation, or treatment with alpha-blockers. **Premature ejaculation** is the persistent or recurrent ejaculation with minimal stimulation before a person desires (associated with distress). It may be primary or secondary to erectile dysfunction. The former is common and may be treated with behavioral modification, sexual health counseling, local anesthetic agents, and systemic medications. The latter will often correct with treatment of erectile dysfunction.

Clinical Findings

A. Symptoms and Signs

Erectile dysfunction should be distinguished from problems of penile deformity, ejaculation, libido, and orgasm. The severity of erectile dysfunction (maintaining vs attaining; chronic, occasional, or situational) and its timing should be noted. The history should include inquiries about dyslipidemia, hypertension, depression, neurologic disease, diabetes mellitus, chronic kidney disease, endocrine disorders, and cardiac or peripheral vascular disease. Pelvic trauma, surgery, or irradiation increases a man's likelihood of erectile dysfunction. A history of penile deformity or curvature that prevents normal intercourse indicates Peyronie disease. The history should clarify the severity of curvature, loss of penile length, and other problems that may prevent normal sexual intercourse. The ability to attain but not maintain an erection may be the first sign of endothelial dysfunction and further cardiovascular risk stratification is warranted. The gradual loss of erections over time is more suggestive of an organic cause. Medication use should be reviewed. Alcohol, tobacco, and recreational drug use are associated with an increased risk of sexual dysfunction.

During the physical examination, vital signs, body habitus (obesity), and secondary sexual characteristics should be assessed. Thorough cardiovascular examination should be performed with auscultation of the heart as well as palpation and quantification of lower extremity arterial pulsations. Motor and sensory examination should be performed. The genitalia should be examined, noting the stretched length of the penis, the presence of penile scarring or plaque formation (Peyronie disease) and any abnormalities in size or consistency of either testicle.

B. Laboratory Findings

Laboratory evaluation should be performed in select cases based on patient history and examination. Possible testing includes a lipid profile and glucose, testosterone, and prolactin. Patients with abnormalities of testosterone or prolactin require further evaluation with measurement of free testosterone and luteinizing hormone (LH) to distinguish hypothalamic-pituitary dysfunction from primary testicular failure.

C. Special Tests

Further testing is based on the patient's history and is performed when etiology is unclear. Organic and psychogenic erectile dysfunction most frequently occur in tandem, given that erectile dysfunction can cause emotional stress and decreased quality of life. Psychogenic erectile dysfunction typically occurs in young men and can generally be differentiated by patient history, whereby men will describe normal nocturnal or morning erections, situational erectile dysfunction, or erectile dysfunction that is solely partner related.

Treatment of patients with oral medications (sildenafil, vardenafil, tadalafil, and avanafil) provides insight into the etiology and severity of erectile dysfunction. Patients with inadequate response to oral medications may undergo further evaluation with direct injection of vasoactive medications into the penis. These medications (prostaglandin E_1, papaverine, phentolamine or a combination) induce erections in men with intact vascular systems. Patients who respond with a rigid erection require no further vascular evaluation. Such testing also allows for visualization and quantification of penile curvature and deformity.

Additional vascular testing is indicated in select patients who do not achieve an erection after penile injection and who are candidates for vascular reconstructive surgery. Duplex ultrasound, penile cavernosography, and pudendal arteriography can distinguish arterial from venous erectile dysfunction and help predict which patients may benefit from vascular surgery.

▶ **Treatment**

Treatment of men suffering from sexual dysfunction should be patient centered and goal oriented. Men who have a significant psychogenic component to their erectile dysfunction will benefit from behaviorally oriented sex therapy or counseling. Lifestyle modification and reduction of cardiovascular risk factors are important components to any treatment plan. This should potentially include smoking cessation; reduction of alcohol intake; diet; exercise; and close monitoring and treatment of diabetes, dyslipidemia, and hypertension.

A. Hormonal Replacement

Testosterone replacement therapy may be offered to men with hypogonadism who have undergone complete endocrinologic evaluation and in whom there is no evidence of prostate cancer or other contraindication to treatment (eg, erythrocytosis). (See also the Male Hypogonadism section in Chapter 26.)

B. Vasoactive Therapy

1. Oral agents—Sildenafil, vardenafil, tadalafil, and avanafil inhibit phosphodiesterase-5 (PDE-5), preventing the degradation of cGMP, thereby enhancing inflow of blood into the erect penis. **These medications are similarly effective, but patients who do not respond to one PDE-5 inhibitor may respond to one of the other agents.** Because of differences in receptor binding affinity and pharmacokinetics, the medications have variable durations of activity and side effects. Each medication should be initiated at the lowest dose and titrated to effect. There is no

effect on libido, and priapism is exceedingly rare. When taken with nitrate medications, there may be exaggerated cardiac preload reduction and hypotension; therefore, these medications are contraindicated in patients taking nitroglycerin or nitrates. All patients being evaluated for acute chest pain should be asked if they are taking a PDE-5 inhibitor before administering nitroglycerin and close monitoring of blood pressure is warranted if there is concern regarding medication overlap.

The combination of PDE-5 inhibitors and alpha-receptor blockers (which may be prescribed for lower urinary tract symptoms) may cause a larger reduction in systemic blood pressure than when PDE-5 inhibitors are used alone. However, these two classes of medication may be safely used in combination if they are started in a stepwise fashion, with escalation of dose when there is no evidence of hypotension or syncope.

2. Injectable medications—Injection of prostaglandin E_2 into the penis is an acceptable form of treatment for many men with erectile dysfunction. Injections are performed using a tuberculin-type syringe or a metered-dose injection device. The base and lateral aspect of the penis is used as the injection site to avoid injury to the superficial blood and nerve supply located anteriorly. Complications are rare and include priapism, penile pain, bruising, dizziness, fibrosis, and infection. Prostaglandin E_2 (alprostadil) can also be delivered via a urethral suppository albeit with less effectiveness. Prostaglandin E_2 is often compounded with papaverine, phentolamine, or atropine in order to increase effectiveness. Patients using compounded agents should be cautioned about the increased risk of priapism.

Priapism requires immediate medical attention to prevent ischemia and fibrosis of the cavernosal tissues. Initial treatment is aspiration of blood from the penis and the injection of sympathomimetic drugs (epinephrine or phenylephrine); if these maneuvers are not successful, surgical arteriovenous shunts should be performed to allow detumescence.

C. Vacuum Erection Device

The vacuum erection device creates a vacuum chamber around the penis and draws blood into the corpora cavernosa. Once adequate tumescence is achieved, an elastic constriction band is placed around the penile base to prevent loss of erection, and the vacuum cylinder is removed. Such devices are effective in many cases; however, the devices are cumbersome and may cause penile discomfort leading to a high rate of disuse. Serious complications are rare.

D. Penile Prosthetic Surgery

Penile prostheses are implanted directly into the paired corporal bodies. Penile prostheses may be semi-rigid (malleable) or inflatable. Each is manufactured in a variety of sizes and is custom-fit to the individual. Inflatable devices result in a more natural appearance and function in most cases, since they emulate the tumescence and detumescence of the native erection. Complications of surgery are rare but include mechanical failure, infection, and injury to adjacent anatomic structures. For men who elect this treatment, personal and partner satisfaction rates are very high due to enhanced spontaneity and reliability of erections.

E. Vascular Reconstruction

Patients with disorders of the arterial system are candidates for various forms of arterial reconstruction, including end-arterectomy and balloon dilation for proximal arterial occlusion and arterial bypass procedures utilizing arterial (epigastric) or venous (deep dorsal vein) segments for distal occlusion. Patients with venous disorders may be managed with ligation of certain veins (deep dorsal or emissary veins) or the crura of the corpora cavernosa. Experience with vascular reconstructive procedures is limited, and many patients so treated still fail to achieve a rigid erection.

F. Medical and Surgical Therapy for Peyronie Disease

A wide range of medical and surgical treatments have been used. Clostridial collagenase is the only FDA-approved medication for the treatment of Peyronie disease. Collagenase is administered to the central portion of the penile plaque by needle injection; it causes enzymatic digestion of the lesion with subsequent correction of penile curvature. The intraplaque injection of verapamil or interferon improves penile deformity in some patients. No oral therapies for Peyronie disease are approved by the FDA; however, off-label use of multiple vasodilatory, anti-inflammatory, and antioxidant medications is common. Surgical treatment is an alternative for men with compromised sexual function due to severe curvature or lesions causing penile instability. The choice of corrective procedure should be tailored to each patient after a detailed evaluation of disease severity and sexual function.

▶ When to Refer

- Patients with inadequate response to oral medications, who are unable to tolerate side effects or who are dissatisfied with their current treatment.
- Patients with Peyronie disease or other penile deformity.
- Patients with a history of pelvic or perineal trauma, surgery, or radiation.
- Ischemic priapism is a medical emergency and requires immediate referral to a urologist or the emergency department for intervention to allow restoration of penile blood perfusion.

Gandaglia G et al. A systematic review of the association between erectile dysfunction and cardiovascular disease. Eur Urol. 2014 May;65(5):968–78. [PMID: 24011423]

Levine LA et al. Clinical safety and effectiveness of collagenase *Clostridium histolyticum* injection in patients with Peyronie's disease: a phase 3 open-label study. J Sex Med. 2015 Jan; 12(1):248–58. [PMID: 25388099]

McCabe MP et al. A systematic review of the psychosocial outcomes associated with erectile dysfunction: does the impact of erectile dysfunction extend beyond a man's inability to have sex? J Sex Med. 2014 Feb;11(2):347–63. [PMID: 24251371]

MALE INFERTILITY

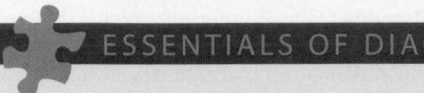

ESSENTIALS OF DIAGNOSIS

► The male partner contributes to 50% of infertility cases.

► Causes include decreased or absent sperm production or function, or obstruction of the male genital tract.

► Detailed history, physical examination, and repeated semen analysis are important for diagnosis and treatment.

► Abnormal semen quality may indicate poor health or increased risk of certain health conditions.

▶ General Considerations

Infertility, the inability of a couple to conceive a child after 1 year of sexual intercourse without contraceptive use, affects 15–20% of US couples. Approximately one-half of cases result from male factors; therefore, evaluation of both partners is critical. Following a detailed history and physical examination, a semen analysis should be performed at least twice, on two separate occasions (Figure 23–1). Because spermatogenesis requires approximately 74 days, it is important to review health events and gonadotoxic exposures from the preceding 3 months. Male infertility is associated with a higher risk for the later development of testicular germ cell cancer and with a higher rate of medical comorbidity; thus, these men should be counseled and screened appropriately and taught testicular self-examination.

▶ Clinical Findings

A. Symptoms and Signs

The history should include prior testicular insults (torsion, cryptorchidism, trauma), infections (mumps orchitis, epididymitis, sexually transmitted infections), environmental factors (excessive heat, radiation, chemotherapy, prolonged pesticide exposure), medications (testosterone, finasteride, cimetidine, selective serotonin reuptake inhibitors, and spironolactone may affect spermatogenesis; phenytoin may lower FSH; sulfasalazine and nitrofurantoin affect sperm motility; tamsulosin causes retrograde ejaculation), and other drugs (alcohol, tobacco, marijuana). Sexual function, frequency and timing of intercourse, use of lubricants, and each partner's previous fertility are important. Loss of libido, headaches, visual disturbances, or galactorrhea may indicate a pituitary tumor. The past medical or surgical history may reveal chronic disease, including, obesity, cardiovascular, thyroid, or liver disease (decreased spermatogenesis); diabetes mellitus (decreased spermatogenesis, retrograde or anejaculation); or radical pelvic or retroperitoneal surgery (absent seminal emission secondary to sympathetic nerve injury).

▲ **Figure 23–1.** Couple-based approach to evaluation and treatment of male factor infertility. FNA, fine-needle aspiration.

Physical examination should pay particular attention to features of hypogonadism: underdeveloped sexual characteristics, diminished male pattern hair distribution (axillary, body, facial, pubic), body habitus, gynecomastia, and obesity. The scrotal contents should be carefully evaluated. Testicular size should be noted (normal size approximately 4.5 × 2.5 cm, volume 18 mL). **Varicoceles** are abnormally dilated and refluxing veins of the pampiniform plexus that can be identified in the standing position by gentle palpation of the spermatic cord and, on occasion, may only be appreciated with the Valsalva maneuver. The vas deferens, epididymis, and prostate should be palpated (absence of all or part of the vas deferens may indicate the presence of a cystic fibrosis variant, congenital bilateral or unilateral absence of the vas deferens).

B. Laboratory Findings

Semen analysis should be performed after 2 to 3 days of ejaculatory abstinence. The specimen should be analyzed within 1 hour after collection. Abnormal sperm concentrations are less than 15 million/mL (**oligozoospermia** is the

presence of less than 15 million sperm/mL in the ejaculate; **azoospermia** is the complete absence of sperm). Normal semen volumes range between 1.5 mL and 5 mL (volumes less than 1.5 mL may result in inadequate buffering of the vaginal acidity and may be due to retrograde ejaculation, ejaculatory duct obstruction, congenital bilateral absence of the vasa deferentia, or androgen insufficiency). Normal sperm motility and morphology demonstrate greater than 45% motile cells and greater than 3% normal morphology (World Health Organization). Abnormal motility may result from varicocele, antisperm antibodies, infection, abnormalities of the sperm flagella, or partial ejaculatory duct obstruction. Abnormal morphology may result from a varicocele, infection, or exposure to gonadotoxins (eg, tobacco smoke).

Endocrine evaluation is warranted if sperm concentration is below normal or if the history and physical examination suggest an endocrinologic origin. Initial testing should include serum testosterone and FSH. Specific abnormalities in these hormones should prompt additional testing, including serum LH, prolactin, and estradiol levels. Elevated FSH and LH levels and low testosterone levels (hypergonadotropic hypogonadism) are associated with primary testicular failure. Low FSH and LH associated with low testosterone occur in secondary testicular failure (hypogonadotropic hypogonadism) and may be of hypothalamic or pituitary origin. Elevation of serum prolactin may indicate the presence of prolactinoma. Elevation of estradiol may impair normal gonadotropin production and impact normal spermatogenesis.

C. Genetic Testing

Men with sperm concentrations less than 10 million/mL should consider testing for Y chromosome microdeletions and karyotypic abnormalities. Gene deletions from the long arm of the Y chromosome may cause azoospermia or oligozoospermia with age-related decline in spermatogenesis that is transmissible to male offspring. Karyotyping may reveal Klinefelter syndrome. Partial or complete absence of the vas deferens should prompt testing for cystic fibrosis mutations.

D. Imaging

Scrotal ultrasound can aid in characterizing the testes and may detect a subclinical varicocele. Men with low ejaculate volume and no evidence of retrograde ejaculation should undergo transrectal ultrasound to evaluate the prostate and seminal vesicles. MRI of the sella turcica should be performed in men with markedly elevated prolactin or hypogonadotropic hypogonadism to evaluate the anterior pituitary gland. MRI of the pelvis and scrotum should be considered in men for whom the testes cannot be identified in the scrotum by physical examination or ultrasound. Men with unilateral absence of the vas deferens should have abdominal ultrasound or CT to exclude absence of the ipsilateral kidney, given the association of these two conditions.

E. Special Tests

Patients with low volume ejaculate should have post-ejaculation urine samples centrifuged and analyzed for sperm to evaluate for retrograde ejaculation. In cases of disproportionately low motility, sperm vitality and the presence of autoantibodies should be assessed. Round cells in concentrations greater than 1 million/mL should prompt leukocyte esterase or peroxidase staining (immature germ cells are found normally, but inflammatory cells may require treatment).

▶ Treatment

A. General Measures

Education about the proper timing for intercourse in relation to the woman's ovulatory cycle as well as the avoidance of spermicidal lubricants should be discussed. In cases of gonadotoxic exposure or medication-related factors, the offending agent should be removed whenever feasible. Patients with active genitourinary tract infections should be treated with appropriate antibiotics. Healthy lifestyle habits, including healthy diet, moderate exercise, and avoidance of gonadotoxins (such as tobacco smoke, excessive alcohol, and marijuana) should be reinforced.

B. Varicocele

Varicocelectomy is performed by stopping retrograde blood flow in spermatic cord veins. Surgical ligation may be accomplished via subinguinal, inguinal, retroperitoneal, or laparoscopic approaches; however, a microsurgical subinguinal approach should be considered the gold-standard given its highest success and lowest complication rates. Percutaneous venographic embolization of varicoceles is feasible but may have a higher recurrence rate.

C. Endocrine Therapy

Hypogonadotropic hypogonadism may be treated with chorionic gonadotropin once primary pituitary disease has been excluded or treated. Dosage is usually 2000 international units intramuscularly three times a week. If sperm concentration fails to rise after 12 months, FSH therapy should be initiated.

D. Ejaculatory Dysfunction Therapy

Patients with retrograde ejaculation may benefit from alpha-adrenergic agonists (pseudoephedrine, 60 mg orally three times a day) or imipramine (25 mg orally three times a day). Medical failures may require the collection of post-ejaculation urine for intrauterine insemination. Anejaculation can be treated with vibratory stimulation or electroejaculation in select cases.

E. Ductal Obstruction

Obstruction of the ejaculatory ducts may be corrected by transurethral resection of the ducts in the prostatic urethra. If obstruction of the vas deferens or epididymis is suspected, the level of obstruction must be determined via vasography or direct surgical inspection prior to surgical reconstruction, with the exception of prior vasectomy. Obstruction of the vas deferens is best managed by microsurgical vasovasostomy or vasoepididymostomy.

F. Assisted Reproductive Techniques

Intrauterine insemination, in vitro fertilization, and intracytoplasmic sperm injection are alternatives for patients in whom other means of treating reduced sperm concentration, motility, or functionality have failed. Intrauterine insemination should be performed only when adequate numbers of motile sperm are noted on an ejaculate sample. With the use of intracytoplasmic sperm injection, some men with azoospermia can father their genetic progeny by surgical retrieval of sperm from the testicle, epididymis, or vas deferens.

▶ When to Refer

- Couples with clinical infertility or who are concerned about their fertility potential.
- Men with known genital insults, genetic diagnoses, or syndromes that preclude natural fertility.
- Reproductive-aged men with newly diagnosed cancer or other disease that may require cytotoxic therapies with interest in fertility preservation.

Eisenberg ML et al. Relationship between semen production and medical comorbidity. Fertil Steril. 2015 Jan;103(1):66–71. [PMID: 25497466]

Lopushnyan NA et al. Surgical techniques for the management of male infertility. Asian J Androl. 2012 Jan;14(1):94–102. [PMID: 22120932]

Ostrowski KA et al. Infertility with testicular cancer. Urol Clin North Am. 2015 Aug;42(3):409–20. [PMID: 26216827]

Winters BR et al. The epidemiology of male infertility. Urol Clin North Am. 2014 Feb;41(1):195–204. [PMID: 24286777]

BENIGN PROSTATIC HYPERPLASIA

 ESSENTIALS OF DIAGNOSIS

- ▸ Obstructive or irritative voiding symptoms.
- ▸ May have enlarged prostate on rectal examination.
- ▸ Absence of urinary tract infection, neurologic disorder, stricture disease, prostatic or bladder malignancy.

General Considerations

Benign prostatic hyperplasia is the most common benign tumor in men, and its incidence is age related. The prevalence of histologic benign prostatic hyperplasia in autopsy studies rises from approximately 20% in men aged 41–50 years, to 50% in men aged 51–60, and to over 90% in men over 80 years of age. Although clinical evidence of disease occurs less commonly, symptoms of prostatic obstruction are also age related. At age 55 years, approximately 25% of men report obstructive voiding symptoms. At age 75 years, 50% of men report a decrease in the force and caliber of the urinary stream.

Risk factors for the development of benign prostatic hyperplasia are poorly understood. Some studies have suggested a genetic predisposition and some have noted racial differences. Approximately 50% of men under age 60 years who undergo surgery for benign prostatic hyperplasia may have a heritable form of the disease. This form is most likely an autosomal dominant trait, and first-degree male relatives of such patients carry an increased relative risk of approximately fourfold.

Clinical Findings

A. Symptoms

The symptoms of benign prostatic hyperplasia can be divided into obstructive and irritative complaints. **Obstructive symptoms** include hesitancy, decreased force and caliber of the stream, sensation of incomplete bladder emptying, double voiding (urinating a second time within 2 hours), straining to urinate, and postvoid dribbling. **Irritative symptoms** include urgency, frequency, and nocturia.

The **American Urological Association (AUA) symptom index** (Table 23–4) is perhaps the single most important tool used in the evaluation of patients with this disorder and should be calculated for all patients before

Table 23–4. American Urological Association symptom index for benign prostatic hyperplasia.[1]

Questions to Be Answered	Not at All	Less Than One Time in Five	Less Than Half the Time	About Half the Time	More Than Half the Time	Almost Always
1. Over the past month, how often have you had a sensation of not emptying your bladder completely after you finish urinating?	0	1	2	3	4	5
2. Over the past month, how often have you had to urinate again less than 2 hours after you finished urinating?	0	1	2	3	4	5
3. Over the past month, how often have you found you stopped and started again several times when you urinated?	0	1	2	3	4	5
4. Over the past month, how often have you found it difficult to postpone urination?	0	1	2	3	4	5
5. Over the past month, how often have you had a weak urinary stream?	0	1	2	3	4	5
6. Over the past month, how often have you had to push or strain to begin urination?	0	1	2	3	4	5
7. Over the past month, how many times did you most typically get up to urinate from the time you went to bed at night until the time you got up in the morning?	0	1	2	3	4	5

[1]Sum of seven circled numbers equals the symptom score. See text for explanation.
Reproduced, with permission, from Barry MJ et al. The American Urological Association symptom index for benign prostatic hyperplasia. J Urol. 1992 Nov;148(5):1549–57.

starting therapy. The answers to seven questions quantitate the severity of obstructive or irritative complaints on a scale of 0–5. Thus, the score can range from 0 to 35, in increasing severity of symptoms.

A detailed history focusing on the urinary tract should be obtained to exclude other possible causes of symptoms such as prostate cancer or disorders unrelated to the prostate such as urinary tract infection, neurogenic bladder, or urethral stricture.

B. Signs

A physical examination, digital rectal examination (DRE), and a focused neurologic examination should be performed on all patients. The size and consistency of the prostate should be noted, but prostate size does not correlate with the severity of symptoms or the degree of obstruction. Benign prostatic hyperplasia usually results in a smooth, firm, elastic enlargement of the prostate. Induration, if detected, must alert the clinician to the possibility of cancer, and further evaluation is needed (ie, prostate-specific antigen [PSA] testing, transrectal ultrasound, and biopsy). Examination of the lower abdomen should be performed to assess for a distended bladder.

C. Laboratory Findings

Urinalysis should be performed to exclude infection or hematuria. A serum PSA is considered optional, yet most clinicians will include it in the initial evaluation, particularly if life expectancy is longer than 10 years. PSA certainly increases the ability to detect prostate cancer over DRE alone; however, because there is much overlap between levels seen in benign prostatic hyperplasia and prostate cancer, its use remains controversial (see Chapter 39).

D. Imaging

Upper tract imaging (CT or renal ultrasound) is recommended only in the presence of concomitant urinary tract disease or complications from benign prostatic hyperplasia (ie, hematuria, urinary tract infection, chronic kidney disease, history of stone disease). As included in the Choosing Wisely (ABIM Foundation) initiative, neither creatinine nor imaging should be routinely ordered for patients with benign prostatic hyperplasia.

E. Cystoscopy

Cystoscopy is not recommended to determine the need for treatment but may assist in determining the surgical approach in patients opting for invasive therapy.

F. Additional Tests

Cystometrograms and urodynamic profiles should be reserved for patients with suspected neurologic disease or those who have failed prostate surgery. Flow rates, postvoid residual urine determination, and pressure-flow studies are considered optional.

▶ Differential Diagnosis

A history of prior urethral instrumentation, urethritis, or trauma should be elucidated to exclude urethral stricture or bladder neck contracture. Hematuria and pain are commonly associated with bladder stones. Carcinoma of the prostate may be detected by abnormalities on the DRE or an elevated PSA (see Chapter 39). A urinary tract infection can mimic the irritative symptoms of benign prostatic hyperplasia and can be readily identified by urinalysis and culture; however, a urinary tract infection can also be a complication of benign prostatic hyperplasia. Carcinoma of the bladder, especially carcinoma in situ, may also present with irritative voiding complaints; however, urinalysis usually shows evidence of hematuria (see Chapter 39). Patients with a neurogenic bladder may also have many of the same symptoms and signs as those with benign prostatic hyperplasia; however, a history of neurologic disease, stroke, diabetes mellitus, or back injury may be obtained, and diminished perineal or lower extremity sensation or alterations in rectal sphincter tone or the bulbocavernosus reflex might be observed on examination. Simultaneous alterations in bowel function (constipation) might also suggest the possibility of a neurologic disorder.

▶ Treatment

Clinical practice guidelines exist for the evaluation and treatment of patients with benign prostatic hyperplasia (Figure 23–2). Following evaluation as outlined above, patients should be offered various forms of therapy for benign prostatic hyperplasia. Patients are advised to consult with their primary care clinicians and make an educated decision on the basis of the relative efficacy and side effects of the treatment options (Table 23–5).

Patients with mild symptoms (AUA scores 0–7) should be managed by watchful waiting only. Absolute surgical indications include refractory urinary retention (failing at least one attempt at catheter removal), large bladder diverticula, or any of the following sequelae of benign prostatic hyperplasia: recurrent urinary tract infection, recurrent gross hematuria, bladder stones, or chronic kidney disease.

A. Watchful Waiting

The risk of progression or complications is uncertain. However, in men with symptomatic disease, it is clear that progression is not inevitable and that some men undergo spontaneous improvement or resolution of their symptoms.

Retrospective studies on the natural history of benign prostatic hyperplasia are inherently subject to bias, relating in part to patient selection and also to the type and extent of follow-up. Very few prospective studies addressing the natural history have been reported. One small series demonstrated that approximately 10% of symptomatic men may progress to urinary retention while 50% of patients demonstrate marked improvement or resolution of symptoms. A large randomized study compared finasteride with placebo in men with moderate to severely symptomatic disease and enlarged prostates on DRE. Patients in the placebo arm demonstrated a 7% risk of developing urinary retention over 4 years.

Men with moderate or severe symptoms can also be observed if they so choose. The optimal interval for follow-up is not defined, nor are the specific end points for intervention.

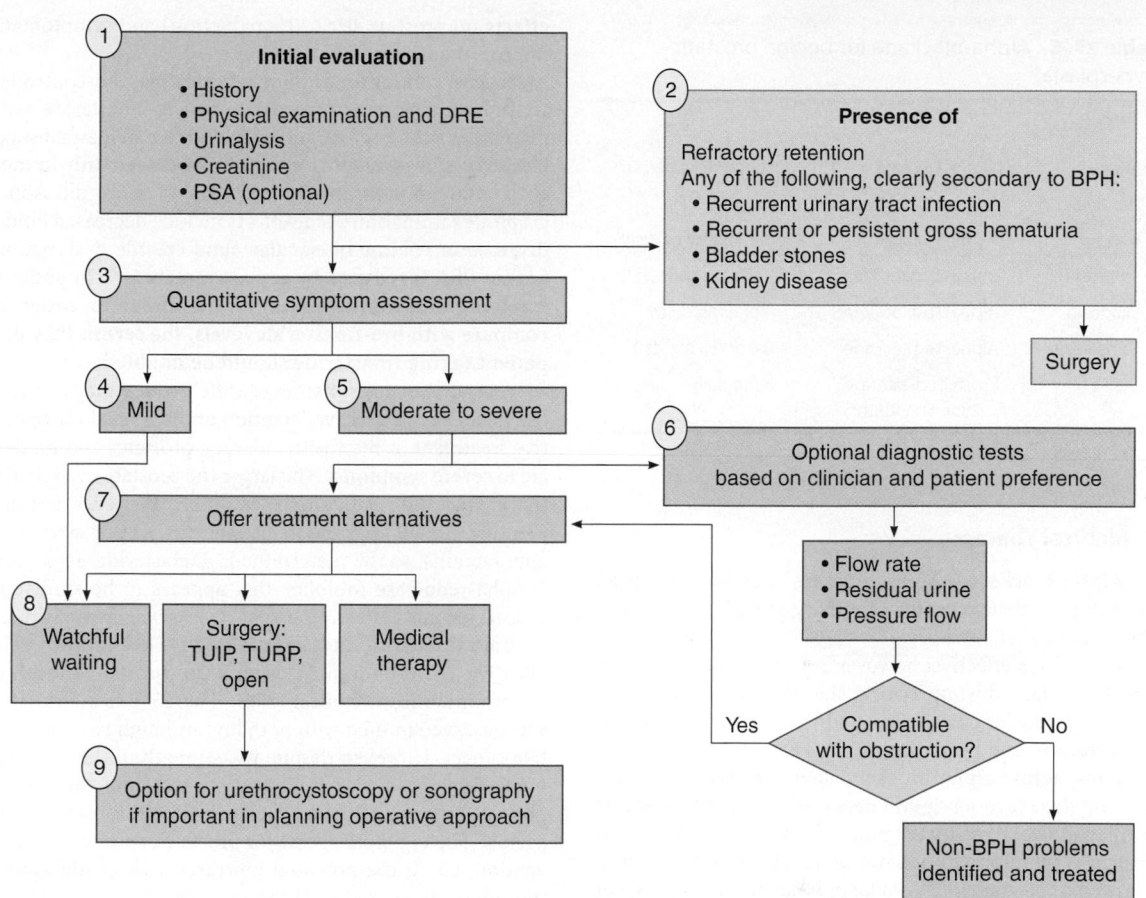

▲ **Figure 23–2.** Benign prostatic hyperplasia decision diagram. BPH, benign prostatic hyperplasia; DRE, digital rectal examination; PSA, prostate-specific antigen; TUIP, transurethral incision of the prostate; TURP, transurethral resection of the prostate.

Table 23–5. Summary of benign prostatic hyperplasia treatment outcomes.[1]

Outcome	TUIP	Open Surgery	TURP	Watchful Waiting	Alpha-Blockers	Finasteride[2]
Chance for improvement[1]	78–83%	94–99.8%	75–96%	31–55%	59–86%	54–78%
Degree of symptom improvement (% reduction in symptom score)	73%	79%	85%	Unknown	51%	31%
Morbidity and complications[1]	2.2–33.3%	7–42.7%	5.2–30.7%	1–5%	2.9–43.3%	13.6–8.8%
Death within 30–90 days[1]	0.2–1.5%	1–4.6%	0.5–3.3%	0.8%	0.8%	0.8%
Total incontinence[1]	0.1–1.1%	0.3–0.7%	0.7–1.4%	2%	2%	2%
Need for operative treatment for surgical complications[1]	1.3–2.7%	0.6–14.1%	0.7–10.1%	0	0	0
Erectile dysfunction[1]	3.9–24.5%	4.7–39.2%	3.3–34.8%	3%	3%	2.5–5.3%
Retrograde ejaculation	6–55%	36–95%	25–99%	0	4–11%	0
Loss of work in days	7–21	21–28	7–21	1	3.5	1.5
Hospital stay in days	1–3	5–10	3–5	0	0	0

[1]90% confidence interval.
[2]Most of the data reviewed for finasteride are derived from three trials that have required an enlarged prostate for entry. The chance of improvement in men with symptoms yet minimally enlarged prostates may be much less, as noted from the VA Cooperative Trial.
TUIP, transurethral incision of the prostate; TURP, transurethral resection of the prostate.

Table 23–6. Alpha-blockade for benign prostatic hyperplasia.

Agent	Action	Oral Dose
Alfuzosin	Alpha-1a-blockade	10 mg daily
Doxazosin	Alpha-1-blockade	1–8 mg daily
Prazosin	Alpha-1-blockade	1–5 mg twice daily
Terazosin	Alpha-1-blockade	1–10 mg daily
Silodosin	Alpha-1a-blockade	4 or 8 mg daily
Tamsulosin	Alpha-1a-blockade	0.4 or 0.8 mg daily
Tadalafil	Phosphodiesterase type 5 inhibitor	5 mg daily

B. Medical Therapy

1. Alpha-blockers—Alpha-blockers can be classified according to their receptor selectivity as well as their half-life (Table 23–6).

Prazosin is effective; however, it requires dose titration and twice daily dosing. Typical side effects include orthostatic hypotension, dizziness, tiredness, retrograde ejaculation, rhinitis, and headache.

Long-acting alpha-blockers allow for once-a-day dosing, but dose titration is still necessary because side effects similar to those seen with prazosin may occur. Terazosin improves symptoms and in numerous studies is superior to placebo or finasteride. Terazosin is started at a dosage of 1 mg orally daily for 3 days, increased to 2 mg orally daily for 11 days, then 5 mg orally daily. Additional dose escalation to 10 mg orally daily can be performed if necessary. Doxazosin is started at a dosage of 1 mg orally daily for 7 days, increased to 2 mg orally daily for 7 days, then 4 mg orally daily. Additional dose escalation to 8 mg orally daily can be performed if necessary.

Alpha-1a-receptors are localized to the prostate and bladder neck. Selective blockade of these receptors results in fewer systemic side effects than alpha-blocker therapy (orthostatic hypotension, dizziness, tiredness, rhinitis, and headache), thus obviating the need for dose titration. The typical dose of tamsulosin is 0.4 mg orally daily taken 30 minutes after a meal. Alfuzosin is a long-acting alpha-1a-blocker; its dose is 10 mg orally once daily with food and does not require titration. Several randomized, double-blind, placebo-controlled trials have been performed comparing terazosin, doxazosin, tamsulosin, and alfuzosin with placebo. All agents have demonstrated safety and efficacy. However, floppy eye syndrome, a complication of cataract surgery, can occur in patients taking alpha-blockers and alpha-1a-blockers.

2. 5-alpha-reductase inhibitors—Finasteride is a 5-alpha-reductase inhibitor that blocks the conversion of testosterone to dihydrotestosterone. This medication impacts upon the epithelial component of the prostate, resulting in reduction in size of the gland and improvement in symptoms. **Six months of therapy is required for maximum effects** on prostate size (20% reduction) and symptomatic improvement.

Several randomized, double-blind, placebo-controlled trials have been performed comparing finasteride with placebo. Efficacy, safety, and durability are well established. However, **symptomatic improvement is seen only in men with enlarged prostates** (greater than 40 mL by ultrasonographic examination). Side effects include decreased libido, decrease in volume of ejaculate, and erectile dysfunction. **Serum PSA is reduced by approximately 50% in patients receiving finasteride therapy. Therefore, in order to compare with pre-finasteride levels, the serum PSA of a patient taking finasteride should be doubled.**

A report suggests that finasteride therapy may decrease the incidence of urinary retention and the need for operative treatment in men with enlarged prostates and moderate to severe symptoms. The larger the prostate over 40 mL, the greater the relative-risk reduction. However, optimal identification of appropriate patients for prophylactic therapy remains to be determined. Dutasteride is a dual 5-alpha-reductase inhibitor that appears to be similar to finasteride in its effectiveness; its dose is 0.5 mg orally daily.

Both finasteride and dutasteride have been shown to be effective chemopreventive agents for prostate cancer in large, randomized clinical trials. The 25% risk reduction was observed in men with both low and high risk for prostate cancer. However, despite the strength of the evidence for 5-alpha-reductase inhibitors in reducing the risk of prostate cancer, an FDA advisory committee recommended against labeling these agents for prostate cancer chemoprevention, citing the potential increased risk of high-grade tumors in these studies (1.8% vs 1.0% for finasteride and 1% vs 0.5% for dutasteride), isolated risk reduction in low-grade tumors, and inability to apply the findings to the general population. Moreover, the FDA has included the increased risk of being diagnosed with high-grade prostate cancer in the labels of all 5-alpha-reductase inhibitors.

3. Phosphodiesterase-5 inhibitor—Tadalafil is approved by the FDA to treat the signs and symptoms of benign prostatic hyperplasia; it is also approved for use in men with both urinary symptoms and erectile dysfunction. The data from two randomized, double-blind, placebo-controlled trials demonstrated significant improvements in standardized measurements of urinary function between 2 and 4 weeks after initiating treatment at 5 mg, with minimal adverse effects.

4. Combination therapy—The four-arm Veterans Administration Cooperative Trial compared placebo, finasteride alone, terazosin alone, and combination of finasteride and terazosin. Over 1200 patients participated, and significant decreases in symptom scores and increases in urinary flow rates were seen only in the arms containing terazosin. However, enlarged prostates were not an entry criterion; in fact, prostate size in this study was much smaller than in previous controlled trials using finasteride (32 versus 52 mL). The Medical Therapy of Prostatic Symptoms (MTOPS) trial was a large, randomized, placebo-controlled trial comparing finasteride, doxazosin, the combination of the two, and placebo in 3047 men observed for a mean of 4.5 years. Long-term combination therapy with doxazosin and finasteride was safe and reduced the risk of overall clinical progression of benign prostatic hyperplasia significantly more than did treatment with either medication alone. Combination therapy and finasteride alone reduced the long-term risk of acute urinary retention and the need for invasive therapy. Combination therapy had the risks of additional side effects and the cost of two medications.

5. Phytotherapy—Phytotherapy is the use of plants or plant extracts for medicinal purposes. Several plant extracts have been popularized, including the saw palmetto berry, the bark of *Pygeum africanum*, the roots of *Echinacea purpurea* and *Hypoxis rooperi*, pollen extract, and the leaves of the trembling poplar. The mechanisms of action of these agents are unknown. A 2006 prospective, randomized, double-blind, placebo-controlled trial revealed no improvement in symptoms, urinary flow rate, or quality of life for men with benign prostatic hyperplasia with saw palmetto treatment compared with placebo.

C. Conventional Surgical Therapy

1. Transurethral resection of the prostate (TURP)—Ninety-five percent of simple prostatectomies can be performed endoscopically (TURP). Most of these procedures are performed under a spinal anesthetic and require a 1- to 2-day hospital stay. Symptom scores and flow rate improvement are superior following TURP relative to any minimally invasive therapy; however, the length of the hospital stay is greater. Much controversy revolves around possible higher rates of morbidity and mortality associated with TURP in comparison with open surgery, but the higher rates observed in one study probably related to more significant comorbidities in the TURP patients compared with the patients who received open surgical treatment. Several other studies could not confirm the difference in mortality when controlling for age and comorbidities. The risks of TURP include retrograde ejaculation (75%), erectile dysfunction (5–10%), and urinary incontinence (less than 1%). Potential complications include (1) bleeding; (2) urethral stricture or bladder neck contracture; (3) perforation of the prostate capsule with extravasation; and (4) **transurethral resection syndrome,** a hypervolemic, hyponatremic state resulting from absorption of the hypotonic irrigating solution. Clinical manifestations of the syndrome include nausea, vomiting, confusion, hypertension, bradycardia, and visual disturbances. The risk of transurethral resection syndrome increases with resection times over 90 minutes. Treatment includes diuresis and, in severe cases, hypertonic saline administration (see Hyponatremia, Chapter 21).

2. Transurethral incision of the prostate (TUIP)—Men with moderate to severe symptoms and small prostates often have posterior commissure hyperplasia or an "elevated bladder neck." These patients will often benefit from incision of the prostate. The procedure is more rapid and less morbid than TURP. Outcomes in well-selected patients

are comparable, though a lower rate of retrograde ejaculation has been reported (25%).

3. Open simple prostatectomy—When the prostate is too large to remove endoscopically, open enucleation is necessary. What size is "too large" depends upon the surgeon's experience with TURP. Glands over 100 g are usually considered for open enucleation. In addition to size, other relative indications for open prostatectomy include concomitant bladder diverticulum or bladder stone and whether dorsal lithotomy positioning is or is not possible.

Open prostatectomies can be performed with either a suprapubic or retropubic approach. Simple suprapubic prostatectomy is performed transvesically and is the operation of choice if there is concomitant bladder pathology. After the prostatic adenoma is removed, both a urethral and a suprapubic catheter are inserted prior to closure.

In simple retropubic prostatectomy, the bladder is not entered but rather a transverse incision is made in the surgical capsule of the prostate and the adenoma is enucleated as described above; only a urethral catheter is needed at the end of the case.

D. Minimally Invasive Therapy

1. Laser therapy—Several coagulation necrosis techniques have been utilized. Transurethral laser-induced prostatectomy (TULIP) is performed under transrectal ultrasound guidance. The instrument is placed in the urethra and transrectal ultrasound is used to direct the device as it is slowly pulled from the bladder neck to the apex. The depth of treatment is monitored with ultrasound.

Most urologists prefer to use visually directed laser techniques. Visual coagulative necrosis is performed under cystoscopic control, and the laser fiber is pulled through the prostate at several designated areas depending on the size and configuration of the gland. Coagulative techniques do not create an immediate visual defect in the prostatic urethra—tissue is sloughed over the course of several weeks up to 3 months following the procedure.

Visual contact ablative techniques take longer in the operating room because the laser fiber is placed in direct contact with the prostate tissue, which is vaporized. Photovaporization of the prostate (PVP), an alternative laser technique, uses a high-power KTP laser. An immediate defect is obtained in the prostatic urethra, similar to that seen during TURP.

Interstitial laser therapy places laser fibers directly into the prostate, usually under cystoscopic control. Irritative voiding symptoms may be less in these patients as the urethral mucosa is spared and prostate tissue is resorbed by the body rather than sloughed.

Advantages to laser surgery include minimal blood loss, rarity of transurethral resection syndrome, ability to treat patients during anticoagulant therapy, and outpatient surgery. Disadvantages are the lack of tissue for pathologic examination, longer postoperative catheterization time, more frequent irritative voiding complaints, and expense of laser fibers and generators.

Large multicenter, randomized studies with long-term follow-up are needed to compare laser prostate surgery with TURP and other forms of minimally invasive surgery.

2. Transurethral needle ablation of the prostate (TUNA)—
This procedure uses a specially designed urethral catheter
that is passed into the urethra. Interstitial radiofrequency
needles are then deployed from the tip of the catheter,
piercing the mucosa of the prostatic urethra. Radiofre-
quencies are then used to heat the tissue, resulting in
coagulative necrosis. Subjective and objective improvement in voiding occurs. In randomized trials comparing
TUNA to TURP, similar improvement was seen when
comparing life scores, peak urinary flow rates, and postvoid residual urine. Bladder neck and median lobe enlargement are not well treated by TUNA.

3. Transurethral electrovaporization of the prostate—
This technique uses the standard resectoscope. High current densities result in heat vaporization of tissue, creating
a cavity in the prostatic urethra. This procedure usually
takes longer than a standard TURP. Long-term comparative data are needed.

4. Hyperthermia—Microwave hyperthermia is most commonly delivered with a transurethral catheter. Some
devices cool the urethral mucosa to decrease the risk of
injury. However, if temperatures do not go above 45°C,
cooling is unnecessary. Symptom score and flow rate
improvement are obtained, but (as with laser surgery) large
randomized studies with long-term follow-up are needed
to assess durability and cost-effectiveness.

5. Implant to open prostatic urethra—A minimally invasive, FDA-approved implant can be used to retract the
enlarged lobes of the prostate in symptomatic men 50 years
and older with an enlarged prostate. Data from trials suggest that the technique improved symptoms and voiding
flow while having minimal impact on ejaculation.

▶ **When to Refer**

- Progression to urinary retention.
- Patient dissatisfaction with medical therapy.
- Need for surgical intervention or further evaluation
  (cystoscopy).

Juliao AA et al. American Urological Association and European
Association of Urology guidelines in the management of
benign prostatic hypertrophy: revisited. Curr Opin Urol. 2012
Jan;22(1):34–9. [PMID: 22123290]

McNicholas TA et al. Minimally invasive prostatic urethral lift:
surgical technique and multinational experience. Eur Urol.
2013 Aug;64(2):292–9. [PMID: 23357348]

McVary KT et al. Update on AUA guideline on the management
of benign prostatic hyperplasia. J Urol. 2011 May;185(5):
1793–803. [PMID: 21420124]

Toren P et al. Effect of dutasteride on clinical progression of
benign prostatic hyperplasia in asymptomatic men with
enlarged prostate: a post hoc analysis of the REDUCE study.
BMJ. 2013 Apr 15;346:f2109. [PMID: 23587564]

Nervous System Disorders

Michael J. Aminoff, MD, DSc, FRCP

Vanja C. Douglas, MD

HEADACHE

Headache is such a common complaint and can occur for so many different reasons that its proper evaluation may be difficult. New, severe, or acute headaches are more likely than chronic headaches to relate to an intracranial disorder; the approach to such headaches is discussed in Chapter 2. **Chronic headaches** may be primary or secondary to another disorder. Common primary headache syndromes include migraine, tension-type headache, and cluster headache. Important secondary causes to consider include intracranial lesions, head injury, cervical spondylosis, dental or ocular disease, temporomandibular joint dysfunction, sinusitis, hypertension, depression, and a wide variety of general medical disorders. Although underlying structural lesions are not present in most patients presenting with headache, it is nevertheless important to bear this possibility in mind. About one-third of patients with brain tumors, for example, present with a primary complaint of headache.

1. Migraine

ESSENTIALS OF DIAGNOSIS

- ► Headache, usually pulsatile, lasting 4–72 hours.
- ► Pain is typically, but not always, unilateral.
- ► Nausea, vomiting, photophobia, and phonophobia are common accompaniments.
- ► Pain is aggravated with routine physical activity.
- ► An aura of transient neurologic symptoms (commonly visual) may precede head pain.
- ► Commonly, head pain occurs with no aura.

► General Considerations

The pathophysiology of migraine probably relates to neuronal dysfunction in the trigeminal system resulting in release of vasoactive neuropeptides such as calcitonin gene-related peptide leading to neurogenic inflammation, sensitization, and headache. Migraine aura is hypothesized

to result from cortical spreading depression, a wave of neuronal and glial depolarization that moves slowly across the cerebral cortex corresponding to the clinical symptoms (ie, occipital cortex and visual aura). Migraine often exhibits a complex, polygenic pattern of inheritance. Sometimes, an autosomal dominant inheritance pattern is apparent, as in **familial hemiplegic migraine** (FHM), in which attacks of lateralized weakness represent the aura. Mutations in three associated genes—*ATP1A2*, *CACNA1A*, and *SCN1A*—account for about three-quarters of cases.

► Clinical Findings

Typical migrainous headache is a lateralized throbbing headache that occurs episodically following its onset in adolescence or early adult life. In many cases, however, the headaches do not conform to this pattern, although their associated features and response to antimigrainous preparations nevertheless suggest a similar basis. In this broader sense, migrainous headaches may be lateralized or generalized, may be dull or throbbing, and are sometimes associated with anorexia, nausea, vomiting, photophobia, phonophobia, osmophobia, cognitive impairment, and blurring of vision. They usually build up gradually and last several hours or longer. Focal disturbances of neurologic function (migraine aura) may precede or accompany the headaches and have been attributed to cortical spreading depression. Visual disturbances occur commonly and may consist of field defects; of luminous visual hallucinations such as stars, sparks, unformed light flashes (photopsia), geometric patterns, or zigzags of light; or of some combination of field defects and luminous hallucinations (scintillating scotomas). Other focal disturbances such as aphasia or numbness, paresthesias, clumsiness, dysarthria, dysequilibrium, or weakness in a circumscribed distribution may also occur.

In rare instances, the neurologic or somatic disturbance accompanying typical migrainous headaches becomes the sole manifestation of an attack ("migraine equivalent"). Very rarely, the patient may be left with a permanent neurologic deficit following a migrainous attack, and migraine with aura may be a risk factor for stroke.

Patients often give a family history of migraine. Attacks may be triggered by emotional or physical stress, lack or excess of sleep, missed meals, specific foods (eg, chocolate), alcoholic beverages, bright lights, loud noise, menstruation, or use of oral contraceptives.

An uncommon variant is **basilar artery migraine,** in which blindness or visual disturbances throughout both visual fields are initially accompanied or followed by dysarthria, dysequilibrium, tinnitus, and perioral and distal paresthesias and are sometimes followed by transient loss or impairment of consciousness or by a confusional state. This, in turn, is followed by a throbbing (usually occipital) headache, often with nausea and vomiting.

In **ophthalmoplegic migraine,** lateralized pain—often about the eye—is accompanied by nausea, vomiting, and diplopia due to transient external ophthalmoplegia. The ophthalmoplegia is due to third nerve palsy, sometimes with accompanying sixth nerve involvement, and may outlast the orbital pain by several days or even weeks. The ophthalmic division of the fifth nerve has also been affected in some patients. Ophthalmoplegic migraine is rare and a diagnosis of exclusion; more common causes of a painful ophthalmoplegia are internal carotid artery aneurysms and diabetes.

▶ Treatment

Management of migraine consists of avoidance of any precipitating factors, together with prophylactic or symptomatic pharmacologic treatment if necessary.

A. Symptomatic Therapy

During acute attacks, rest in a quiet, darkened room may be helpful until symptoms subside. A simple analgesic (eg, aspirin, acetaminophen, ibuprofen, or naproxen) taken right away often provides relief, but treatment with prescription therapy is sometimes necessary. *To prevent medication overuse, use of simple analgesics should be limited to 15 days or less per month, and combination analgesics should be limited to no more than 10 days per month.*

1. Ergotamines—Cafergot, a combination of ergotamine tartrate (1 mg) and caffeine (100 mg), is often particularly helpful; one or two tablets are taken at the onset of headache or warning symptoms, followed by one tablet every 30 minutes, if necessary, up to six tablets per attack and no more than 10 days per month. Because of vomiting during acute attacks, oral medication sometimes fails to help. Cafergot given rectally as suppositories (one-half to one suppository containing 2 mg of ergotamine) or dihydroergotamine mesylate (0.5–1 mg intravenously or 1–2 mg subcutaneously or intramuscularly) may be useful in such cases. Ergotamine-containing preparations should be avoided in pregnancy and when cardiovascular disease or risk factors are present.

2. Triptans—Sumatriptan, which has a high affinity for 5-HT$_1$ receptors, is a rapidly effective agent for aborting attacks when given subcutaneously by an autoinjection device (4–6 mg once subcutaneously, may repeat once after 2 hours if needed; maximum dose 12 mg/24 h). Nasal and oral preparations are available but may be less effective due to slower absorption. Zolmitriptan, another selective

5-HT$_1$ receptor agonist, has high bioavailability after oral administration and is also effective for the immediate treatment of migraine. The optimal initial oral dose is 5 mg, and relief usually occurs within 1 hour; may repeat once after 2 hours. It is also available in a nasal formulation, which has a rapid onset of action; the dose is 5 mg in one nostril once and it may be repeated once after 2 hours. The maximum dose for both formulations is 10 mg/24 h. Other triptans are available, including rizatriptan (5–10 mg orally at onset, may repeat every 2 hours twice [maximum dose 30 mg/24 h]); naratriptan (1–2.5 mg orally at onset, may repeat once after 4 hours [maximum dose 5 mg/24 h]); almotriptan (6.25–12.5 mg orally at onset, may repeat dose once after 2 hours [maximum dose 25 mg/24 h]); frovatriptan (2.5 mg orally at onset, may repeat after 2 hours once [maximum dose 7.5 mg/24]); and eletriptan (20–40 mg orally at onset; may repeat after 2 hours once [maximum dose 80 mg/24 h]). Eletriptan is useful for immediate therapy and frovatriptan, which has a longer half-life, may be worthwhile for patients with prolonged attacks or attacks provoked by menstrual periods.

Triptans may cause nausea and vomiting. They should probably be avoided in women who are pregnant, in patients with hemiplegic or basilar migraine, and in patients with risk factors for stroke (such as uncontrolled hypertension, prior stroke or transient ischemic attack (TIA), diabetes mellitus, hypercholesterolemia, obesity). In patients whose hypertension is controlled, triptans are commonly used safely although caution is advised. Triptans are contraindicated in patients with coronary or peripheral vascular disease. Patients often experience greater benefit when the triptan is combined with naproxen (500 mg orally).

3. Other agents—Prochlorperazine is effective and may be administered rectally (25 mg suppository), intravenously or intramuscularly (5–10 mg), or orally (5–10 mg). Intravenous metoclopramide (10–20 mg) or chlorpromazine (25–50 mg) is also particularly useful in the emergency department setting. Various butalbital-containing combination oral analgesics risk overuse and dependence and should only be used as a last resort. Opioid analgesics should be avoided because of high rates of rebound headache and the tendency to develop medication overuse headache.

B. Preventive Therapy

Preventive treatment may be necessary if migraine headaches occur more frequently than two or three times a month or significant disability is associated with attacks. Avoidance of triggers and maintenance of homeostasis with regular sleep, meals, and hydration should not be neglected; a headache diary may be useful to identify triggers. Some of the more common drugs used for prophylaxis are listed in Table 24–1. Their mode of action is unclear but may involve alteration of central neurotransmission. Several drugs may have to be tried in turn before headaches are brought under control. Once a drug has been found to help, it should be continued for several months. If the patient remains headache-free, the dose may

Table 24–1. Pharmacologic prophylaxis of migraine.

Drug	Usual Adult Oral Daily Dose	Common Side Effects
Antiepileptic[1]		
Topiramate	100 mg (divided twice daily)	Somnolence, nausea, dyspepsia, irritability, dizziness, ataxia, nystagmus, diplopia, glaucoma, renal calculi, weight loss, hypohidrosis, hyperthermia.
Valproic acid[2,3]	500–1000 mg (divided twice daily)	Nausea, vomiting, diarrhea, drowsiness, alopecia, weight gain, hepatotoxicity, thrombocytopenia, tremor, pancreatitis.
Cardiovascular		
Candesartan[3]	8–32 mg	Dizziness, cough, diarrhea, fatigue.
Guanfacine	1 mg	Dry mouth, somnolence, dizziness, constipation, erectile dysfunction.
Propranolol[4]	80–240 mg (divided twice to four times daily)	Fatigue, dizziness, hypotension, bradycardia, depression, insomnia, nausea, vomiting, constipation.
Verapamil[5]	80–240 mg (divided three times daily)	Headache, hypotension, flushing, edema, constipation. May aggravate atrioventricular nodal heart block and heart failure.
Antidepressant[6]		
Amitriptyline[7]	10–150 mg	Sedation, dry mouth, constipation, weight gain, blurred vision, edema, hypotension, urinary retention.
Venlafaxine	37.5–150 mg extended release	Nausea, somnolence, dry mouth, dizziness, diaphoresis, sexual dysfunction, anxiety, weight loss.
Other		
Botulinum toxin A	Intramuscular injection	Injection site reaction, hypersensitivity, muscle weakness.
Riboflavin	400 mg	Yellow-orange discoloration of urine
Butterbur	100–150 mg (divided twice daily)	Belching, headache, itchy eyes, gastrointestinal issues, asthma, fatigue, drowsiness, allergic reaction. **Do not use unprocessed butterbur, which contains hepatotoxic pyrrolizidine alkaloids.**

[1]Gabapentin and possibly other antiepileptics have also been used successfully.
[2]Avoid during pregnancy.
[3]Not FDA-approved for this indication.
[4]Other beta-adrenergic antagonists, such as atenolol, metoprolol, nadolol, and timolol are similarly effective.
[5]Other calcium channel antagonists (eg, nimodipine, nicardipine, and diltiazem) may also help.
[6]Depression is commonly comorbid with migraine disorder and may warrant separate treatment.
[7]Other tricyclic antidepressants (eg, nortriptyline and imipramine) may similarly help.

be tapered and the drug eventually withdrawn. Botulinum toxin type A, injected into specific head and neck muscles, reduces headache frequency in patients with chronic migraine (at least 15 days per month with headaches lasting 4 hours per day or longer). A 2009 Cochrane review suggested acupuncture as effective as prophylactic drug treatment, but comparison with sham acupuncture showed no benefit. Some neurostimulation techniques look promising, including occipital nerve stimulation, but critical appraisal is necessary. Blockade of calcitonin gene-related peptide signaling by a receptor antagonist or monoclonal antibody looks promising, but no therapy is yet approved.

2. Tension-type Headache

This is the most common type of primary headache disorder. Patients frequently complain of pericranial tenderness, poor concentration, and other nonspecific symptoms, in addition to constant daily headaches that are often vise-like or tight in quality but not pulsatile. Headaches may be exacerbated by emotional stress, fatigue, noise, or glare.

The headaches are usually generalized, may be most intense about the neck or back of the head, and are not associated with focal neurologic symptoms. There is diagnostic overlap with migraine.

The therapeutic approach is similar to that in migraine, except that triptan drugs are not indicated. Treatment of comorbid anxiety or depression is important. Behavioral therapies that may be effective include biofeedback and relaxation training.

3. Cluster Headache

Cluster headache affects predominantly middle-aged men. The pathophysiology is unclear but may relate to activation of cells in the ipsilateral hypothalamus, triggering the trigeminal autonomic vascular system. There is often no family history of headache or migraine. Episodes of severe unilateral periorbital pain occur daily for several weeks and are often accompanied by one or more of the following: ipsilateral nasal congestion, rhinorrhea, lacrimation, redness of the eye, and Horner syndrome (ptosis of the eyelid, meiosis or constriction of the pupil, and anhidrosis or reduced sweat secretion). During attacks, patients are often restless and agitated. Episodes typically occur at night, awaken the patient, and last between 15 minutes and 3 hours. Spontaneous remission then occurs, and the patient remains well for weeks or months before another bout of closely spaced attacks. Bouts may last for 4 to 8 weeks and may occur up to several times per year. During a bout, many patients report alcohol triggers an attack; others report that stress, glare, or ingestion of specific foods occasionally precipitates attacks. In occasional patients, remission does not occur. This variant has been referred to as chronic cluster headache. In longstanding cases, Horner syndrome may persist between attacks.

Cluster headache is one of the trigeminal autonomic cephalgias, which include hemicrania continua, paroxysmal hemicranias, and short-lasting neuralgiform headache attacks with conjunctival injection and tearing. Similar to cluster headache, the other trigeminal autonomic cephalgias consist of unilateral periorbital pain associated with ipsilateral autonomic symptoms; they are distinguished from cluster headache by different attack duration and frequency and their exquisite responsiveness to indomethacin.

Treatment of an individual attack with oral drugs is generally unsatisfactory, but subcutaneous (6 mg dose) or intranasal (20 mg/spray) sumatriptan or inhalation of 100% oxygen (12–15 L/min for 15 minutes via a nonrebreather mask) may be effective. Zolmitriptan (5- and 10-mg nasal spray) is also effective. Dihydroergotamine (0.5–1 mg intramuscularly or intravenously) or viscous lidocaine (1 mg of 4–6% solution intranasally) is sometimes effective.

Various prophylactic agents include oral medications such as lithium carbonate (start at 300 mg daily, titrating according to serum levels and treatment response up to a typical total daily dose of 900–1200 mg, divided three or four times), verapamil (start at 240 mg daily, increase by 80 mg every 2 weeks to 960 mg daily, with routine ECG to monitor the PR interval), topiramate (100–400 mg daily), and civamide (not available in the United States). As there is often a delay before these medications are effective, transitional therapy is often used. Prednisone (60 mg daily for 5 days followed by gradual withdrawal) is effective in 70–80% of patients, and suboccipital corticosteroid injection about the greater occipital nerve is effective in 75%. Ergotamine tartrate can be given as rectal suppositories (0.5–1 mg at night or twice daily), by mouth (2 mg daily), or by subcutaneous injection (0.25 mg three times daily for 5 days per week). As in migraine, limited evidence suggests that electrical stimulation of the occipital nerve by an implantable device may be helpful.

4. Posttraumatic Headache

A variety of nonspecific symptoms may follow closed head injury, regardless of whether consciousness is lost (see Head Injury). Headache is often a conspicuous feature. It usually appears within a day or so following injury, may worsen over the ensuing weeks, and then gradually subsides. It is usually a constant dull ache, with superimposed throbbing that may be localized, lateralized, or generalized. Headaches are sometimes accompanied by nausea, vomiting, or scintillating scotomas and often respond to simple analgesics; severe headaches may necessitate preventive treatment as outlined for migraine. Headaches occurring more than 1–2 weeks after the inciting event are probably not directly attributable to the head injury.

5. Primary Cough Headache

Severe head pain may be produced by coughing (and by straining, sneezing, and laughing) but, fortunately, usually lasts for only a few minutes or less. The pathophysiologic basis of the complaint is not known, and often there is no underlying structural lesion. However, intracranial lesions, usually in the posterior fossa (eg, Arnold-Chiari malformation), are present in about 10% of cases, and brain tumors or other space-occupying lesions may present in this way. Accordingly, CT scanning or MRI should be undertaken in all patients and repeated annually for several years, since a small structural lesion may not show up initially.

The disorder is usually self-limited, although it may persist for several years. For unknown reasons, symptoms sometimes clear completely after lumbar puncture. Indomethacin (75–150 mg daily orally) may provide relief. Similar activity-triggered headache syndromes include primary exertional headache and primary headache associated with sexual activity.

6. Headache Due to Giant Cell (Temporal or Cranial) Arteritis

This topic is discussed in Chapter 20.

7. Headache Due to Intracranial Mass Lesions

Intracranial mass lesions of all types may cause headache owing to displacement of vascular structures and other pain-sensitive tissues. While pain and location are nonspecific, headache may be worse upon lying down, awaken the patient at night, or peak in the morning after overnight recumbency. The key feature prompting brain imaging is a new or worsening headache in middle or later life. Other features suggesting an intracranial lesion include signs or symptoms of infection or malignancy such as fever, night sweats, and weight loss; immunocompromise; or history of malignancy. Signs of focal or diffuse cerebral dysfunction or of increased intracranial pressure (eg, papilledema) also necessitate investigation.

8. Medication Overuse (Analgesic Rebound) Headache

In approximately half of all patients with chronic daily headaches, medication overuse is responsible. Patients have chronic pain or severe headache unresponsive to medication. Early initiation of a migraine preventive therapy permits withdrawal of analgesics and eventual relief of headache.

9. Headache Due to Other Neurologic Causes

Cerebrovascular disease may be associated with headache, but the mechanism is unclear. Headache may occur with internal carotid artery occlusion or carotid dissection and after carotid endarterectomy. Acute severe headache accompanies subarachnoid hemorrhage and meningeal infections; accompanying signs of impairment of consciousness and sign of meningeal irritation indicate the need for further investigations. Headaches are also a feature of pseudotumor cerebri (idiopathic intracranial hypertension).

Dull or throbbing headache is a frequent sequela of lumbar puncture and may last for several days. It is aggravated by the erect posture and alleviated by recumbency. The mechanism is unclear, but the headache is commonly attributed to leakage of cerebrospinal fluid through the dural puncture site. Its incidence may be reduced if an atraumatic needle (instead of a beveled, cutting needle) is used for the lumbar puncture.

▶ When to Refer

- Thunderclap onset.
- Increasing headache unresponsive to simple measures.
- History of trauma, hypertension, fever, visual changes.
- Presence of neurologic signs or of scalp tenderness.

▶ When to Admit

Suspected subarachnoid hemorrhage or structural intracranial lesion.

Bigal ME et al. Safety and tolerability of TEV-48125 for preventive treatment of high-frequency episodic migraine: a multicenter, randomized, double-blind, placebo-controlled, phase 2b study. Lancet Neurol. 2015 Nov;14(11):1081–90. [PMID: 26432182]

Chiang CC et al. Treatment of medication-overuse headache: a systematic review. Cephalalgia. 2015 Jun 29. [Epub ahead of print] [PMID: 26122645]

Diener HC et al. New therapeutic approaches for the prevention and treatment of migraine. Lancet Neurol. 2015 Oct; 14(10):1010–22. [PMID: 26376968]

Holland S et al. Evidence-based guideline update: NSAIDs and other complementary treatments for episodic migraine prevention in adults: report of the Quality Standards Subcommittee of the American Academy of Neurology and the American Headache Society. Neurology. 2012 Apr 24;78(17):1346–53. [PMID: 22529203]

Minen MT et al. Evaluation and treatment of migraine in the emergency department: a review. Headache. 2014 Jul–Aug; 54(7):1131–45. [PMID: 24898930]

Nierenburg Hdel C et al. Systematic review of preventive and acute treatment of menstrual migraine. Headache. 2015 Sep; 55(8):1052–71. [PMID: 26264117]

Silberstein SD et al. Evidence-based guideline update: pharmacologic treatment for episodic migraine prevention in adults: report of the Quality Standards Subcommittee of the American Academy of Neurology and the American Headache Society. Neurology. 2012 Apr 24;78(17):1337–45. [PMID: 22529202]

FACIAL PAIN

1. Trigeminal Neuralgia

◆ ESSENTIALS OF DIAGNOSIS

- ▶ Brief episodes of stabbing facial pain.
- ▶ Pain is in the territory of the second and third division of the trigeminal nerve.
- ▶ Pain exacerbated by touch.

▶ General Considerations

Trigeminal neuralgia ("tic douloureux") is most common in middle and later life. It affects women more frequently than men. Pain may be due to an anomalous artery or vein impinging on the trigeminal nerve.

▶ Clinical Findings

Momentary episodes of sudden lancinating facial pain commonly arise near one side of the mouth and shoot toward the ear, eye, or nostril on that side. The pain may be triggered or precipitated by such factors as touch, movement, drafts, and eating. Indeed, in order to lessen the likelihood of triggering further attacks, many patients try to hold the face still while talking. Spontaneous remissions for several months or longer may occur. As the disorder progresses, however, the episodes of pain become more frequent, remissions become shorter and less common, and a dull ache may persist between the episodes of stabbing pain. Symptoms remain confined to the distribution of the trigeminal nerve (usually the second or third division) on one side only.

▶ Differential Diagnosis

The characteristic features of the pain in trigeminal neuralgia usually distinguish it from other causes of facial pain. Neurologic examination shows no abnormality except in a few patients in whom trigeminal neuralgia is symptomatic of some underlying lesion, such as multiple sclerosis or a brainstem neoplasm, in which case the finding will depend on the nature and site of the lesion. Multiple sclerosis must be suspected in a patient younger than 40 years in whom trigeminal neuralgia is the presenting symptom, even if there are no other neurologic signs. Bilateral symptoms should also prompt further investigation. Brain MRI need only be obtained when a secondary cause is suspected; it is usually normal in classic trigeminal neuralgia. If MRI is not readily available, trigeminal reflexes, measured in an electrophysiology laboratory, can distinguish between symptomatic and idiopathic trigeminal neuralgia but are rarely performed.

▶ Treatment

The drugs most helpful for treatment are oxcarbazepine (although not approved by the FDA for this indication) or carbamazepine, with monitoring by serial blood counts and liver function tests. If these medications are ineffective or cannot be tolerated, phenytoin should be tried. (Doses and side effects of these drugs are shown in Table 24–3). Baclofen (10–20 mg orally three or four times daily), topiramate (50 mg orally twice daily), or lamotrigine (400 mg orally daily) may also be helpful, either alone or in combination with one of these other agents. Gabapentin may also relieve pain, especially in patients who do not respond to conventional medical therapy and those with multiple sclerosis. Depending on response and tolerance, up to 3600 mg daily orally is given in divided doses.

For neuralgia due to vascular impingement on the trigeminal nerve (despite normal findings on CT scans, MRI, or arteriograms), microvascular surgical decompression and separation of the anomalous vessel from the nerve root produce lasting relief of symptoms. In elderly patients with a limited life expectancy, radiofrequency rhizotomy is sometimes preferred because it is easy to perform, has few complications, and provides symptomatic relief for a period of time. Gamma radiosurgery to the trigeminal root is another noninvasive approach that appears to be successful in most patients, with essentially no side effects other than facial paresthesias in a few instances; up to one-third of patients achieved a pain-free state without need for medication after the procedure. Surgical exploration is inappropriate in patients with trigeminal neuralgia due to multiple sclerosis.

Cheng JS et al. A review of percutaneous treatments for trigeminal neuralgia. Neurosurgery. 2014 Mar;10(Suppl 1):25–33. [PMID: 24509496]
Torpy JM et al. JAMA patient page: Trigeminal neuralgia. JAMA. 2013 Mar 13;309(10):1058. [PMID: 23483182]

2. Atypical Facial Pain

Facial pain without the typical features of trigeminal neuralgia is generally a constant, often burning pain that may have a restricted distribution at its onset but soon spreads to the rest of the face on the affected side and sometimes involves the other side, the neck, or the back of the head as well. The disorder is especially common in middle-aged women, many of them depressed, but it is not clear whether depression is the cause of or a reaction to the pain. Simple analgesics should be given a trial, as should tricyclic antidepressants, carbamazepine, oxcarbazepine, and phenytoin; the response is often disappointing. Opioid analgesics pose a danger of addiction in patients with this disorder. Attempts at surgical treatment are not indicated.

3. Glossopharyngeal Neuralgia

Glossopharyngeal neuralgia is an uncommon disorder in which pain similar in quality to that in trigeminal neuralgia occurs in the throat, about the tonsillar fossa, and sometimes deep in the ear and at the back of the tongue. The pain may be precipitated by swallowing, chewing, talking, or yawning and is sometimes accompanied by syncope. In most instances, no underlying structural abnormality is present; multiple sclerosis is sometimes responsible. Oxcarbazepine and carbamazepine are the treatments of choice

and should be tried before any surgical procedures are considered. Microvascular decompression is often effective and is generally preferred over destructive surgical procedures such as partial rhizotomy in medically refractory cases.

Reddy GD et al. Trigeminal and glossopharyngeal neuralgia. Neurol Clin. 2014 May;32(2):539–52. [PMID: 24703544]

4. Postherpetic Neuralgia

Postherpetic neuralgia develops in about 15% of patients who have herpes zoster (shingles). This complication seems especially likely to occur in elderly or immunocompromised persons, when the rash is severe, and when the first division of the trigeminal nerve is affected. It also relates to the duration of the rash before medical consultation. A history of shingles and the presence of cutaneous scarring resulting from shingles aid in the diagnosis. Severe pain with shingles correlates with the intensity of postherpetic symptoms.

Acyclovir (800 mg five times daily) or valacyclovir (1000 mg three times daily), when given within 72 hours of rash onset, reduces the incidence of postherpetic neuralgia by almost half; systemic corticosteroids do not help (see Chapter 6). Management of the established complication is essentially medical. If simple analgesics fail to help, a trial of a tricyclic antidepressant (eg, amitriptyline or nortriptyline, up to 100–150 mg daily orally) is often effective. Other patients respond to carbamazepine (up to 1200 mg daily orally), phenytoin (300 mg daily orally), gabapentin (up to 3600 mg daily orally), or pregabalin (up to 600 mg/daily orally). A combination of gabapentin and morphine taken orally may provide better analgesia at lower doses of each agent than either taken alone. Topical application of capsaicin cream (eg, Zostrix, 0.025%) may be helpful, but a transdermal patch (8%) had no effect. Topical lidocaine (5%) is also worthy of trial. The administration of live-attenuated zoster vaccine to patients over the age of 60 years is important in reducing the likelihood of herpes zoster and reducing the severity of postherpetic neuralgia should a reactivation occur.

Johnson RW et al. Clinical practice. Postherpetic neuralgia. N Engl J Med. 2014 Oct 16;371(16):1526–33. [PMID: 25317872]

5. Facial Pain Due to Other Causes

Facial pain may be caused by temporomandibular joint dysfunction in patients with malocclusion, abnormal bite, or faulty dentures. There may be tenderness of the masticatory muscles, and sometimes pain begins at the onset of chewing. This pattern differs from that of jaw (masticatory) claudication, a symptom of giant cell arteritis, in which pain develops progressively with mastication. Treatment of the underlying joint dysfunction relieves symptoms.

A relationship of facial pain to chewing or temperature changes may suggest a dental disturbance. The cause is sometimes not obvious, and diagnosis requires careful dental examination and radiographs. Sinusitis and ear infections causing facial pain are usually recognized by a history of respiratory tract infection, fever and, in some instances, nasal or aural discharge. There may be localized tenderness. Radiologic evidence of sinus infection or mastoiditis is confirmatory.

Glaucoma is an important ocular cause of facial pain, usually localized to the periorbital region.

On occasion, pain in the jaw may be the principal manifestation of angina pectoris. Precipitation by exertion and radiation to more typical areas suggests a cardiac origin.

▶ When to Refer

- Worsening pain unresponsive to simple measures.
- Continuing pain of uncertain cause.
- For consideration of surgical treatment (trigeminal or glossopharyngeal neuralgia).

EPILEPSY

ESSENTIALS OF DIAGNOSIS

- ▶ Recurrent seizures.
- ▶ Characteristic electroencephalographic changes accompany seizures.
- ▶ Mental status abnormalities or focal neurologic symptoms may persist for hours postictally.

▶ General Considerations

The term "epilepsy" denotes any disorder characterized by recurrent unprovoked seizures. A seizure is a transient disturbance of cerebral function due to an abnormal paroxysmal neuronal discharge in the brain. Epilepsy is common, affecting approximately 0.5% of the population in the United States.

Patients with recurrent seizures provoked by a readily reversible cause, such as withdrawal from alcohol or drugs, hypoglycemia, hyperglycemia, or uremia, are not considered to have epilepsy.

▶ Etiology

According to the International League Against Epilepsy classification system, the many etiologies of recurrent seizures can be grouped into three categories.

A. Genetic Epilepsy

This category encompasses a broad range of disorders, for which the age at onset ranges from the neonatal period to adolescence or even later in life. Monogenic disorders tend to exhibit an autosomal dominant pattern of inheritance, and where the mutation is known, the responsible gene often encodes a neuronal ion channel.

B. Structural/Metabolic Epilepsy

1. Pediatric age groups—Congenital abnormalities and perinatal injuries may result in seizures presenting in infancy or childhood.

2. Metabolic disorders—Inborn errors of metabolism and other inherited conditions may cause epilepsy as one of their manifestations (eg, pyridoxine deficiency, mitochondrial disease); these disorders typically present during childhood. Autoimmune diseases such as systemic lupus erythematosus and autoimmune limbic encephalitis may also cause epilepsy.

3. Mesial temporal sclerosis—Hippocampal sclerosis is a recognized cause of focal and secondarily generalized seizures of uncertain etiology.

4. Trauma—Trauma is an important cause of seizures at any age, but especially in young adults. Posttraumatic epilepsy is more likely to develop if the dura mater was penetrated and generally becomes manifest within 2 years following the injury. However, seizures developing in the first week after head injury do not necessarily imply that future attacks will occur. There is no evidence that prophylactic anticonvulsant drug treatment reduces the incidence of posttraumatic epilepsy.

5. Tumors and other space-occupying lesions—Neoplasms may lead to seizures at any age, but they are an especially important cause of seizures in middle and later life, when the incidence of neoplastic disease increases. Seizures are commonly the initial symptoms of the tumor and often are focal in character. They are most likely to occur with structural lesions involving the frontal, parietal, or temporal regions. Tumors must be excluded by imaging studies (MRI preferred over CT) in all patients with onset of seizures after 20 years of age, focal seizures or signs, or a progressive seizure disorder.

6. Vascular diseases—Stroke and other vascular diseases become increasingly frequent causes of seizures with advancing age and are the most common cause of seizures with onset at age 60 years or older.

7. Degenerative disorders—Alzheimer disease and other degenerative disorders are a cause of seizures in later life.

8. Infectious diseases—Infectious diseases must be considered in all age groups as potentially reversible causes of seizures. Seizures may occur with an acute infective or inflammatory illness, such as bacterial meningitis or herpes encephalitis, or in patients with more longstanding or chronic disorders, such as neurosyphilis or cerebral cysticercosis. In patients with AIDS, seizures may result from central nervous system toxoplasmosis, cryptococcal meningitis, secondary viral encephalitis, or other infective complications. Seizures are a common sequela of supratentorial brain abscess, developing most frequently in the first year after treatment.

C. Unknown

In many cases, the cause of epilepsy cannot be determined.

▶ Classification of Seizures

The International League Against Epilepsy distinguishes seizures affecting only part of the brain (focal seizures) from those that are generalized (Table 24–2).

Table 24–2. Seizure classification.

Seizure Type	Key Features	Other Associated Features
Focal seizures	Involvement of only a restricted part of brain; may evolve to a bilateral, convulsive seizure	
Without impairment of consciousness		Observable focal motor or autonomic symptoms, or subjective sensory or psychic symptoms may occur
With impairment of consciousness		Above symptoms may precede, accompany, or follow the period of altered responsiveness
Generalized seizures	Diffuse involvement of brain at onset	
Absence (petit mal)	Consciousness impaired briefly; patient often unaware of attacks	May have clonic, tonic, or atonic (ie, loss of postural tone) components; autonomic components (eg, enuresis); or accompanying automatisms. Almost always begin in childhood and frequently cease by age 20
Atypical absenc	May be more gradual in onset and termination than typical absence	More marked changes in tone may occur
Myoclonic	Single or multiple myoclonic jerks	
Tonic	Bilaterally increased tone and stiffening of limbs with associated loss of consciousness	Onset may be accompanied by expiratory grunt
Clonic	Bilateral rhythmic jerking with associated loss of consciousness	
Tonic-clonic (grand mal)	Tonic phase: Sudden loss of consciousness, with rigidity and arrest of respiration, lasting < 1 minute. Clonic phase: Jerking, usually for < 2–3 minutes. Flaccid coma: Variable duration	May be accompanied by tongue biting, incontinence, or aspiration; commonly followed by postictal confusion variable in duration
Atonic	Sudden loss of tone, very brief (< 2 seconds)	Often result in recurrent falls
Status epilepticus	Repeated seizures without intervening recovery of consciousness; a fixed and enduring epileptic condition lasting ≥ 30 minutes	

A. Focal Seizures

The initial clinical and electroencephalographic manifestations of partial seizures indicate that only a restricted part of one cerebral hemisphere has been activated. The ictal manifestations depend on the area of the brain involved. Focal seizures sometimes involve impairment of consciousness and may evolve to convulsive seizures, in a process previously called secondary generalization.

1. Without impairment of consciousness—Seizures may be manifested by focal motor symptoms (convulsive jerking) or somatosensory symptoms (eg, paresthesias or tingling) that spread (or "march") to different parts of the limb or body depending on their cortical representation; such seizures were previously described as "simple partial" seizures. In other instances, special sensory symptoms (eg, light flashes or buzzing) indicate involvement of visual, auditory, olfactory, or gustatory regions of the brain, or there may be autonomic symptoms or signs (eg, abnormal epigastric sensations, sweating, flushing, pupillary dilation). The sole manifestations of some seizures are phenomena such as dysphasia, dysmnesic symptoms (eg, déjà

vu, jamais vu), affective disturbances, illusions, or structured hallucinations, but such symptoms are usually accompanied by impairment of consciousness.

2. With impairment of consciousness—Impaired consciousness or responsiveness may be preceded, accompanied, or followed by the various symptoms mentioned above, and automatisms may occur. Such dyscognitive seizures were previously called "complex partial" seizures.

B. Generalized Seizures

There are several different varieties of generalized seizures, as outlined below. In some circumstances, seizures cannot be classified because of incomplete information or because they do not fit into any category.

1. Absence seizures—These are characterized by impairment of consciousness, sometimes with mild clonic, tonic, or atonic components (ie, reduction or loss of postural tone), autonomic components (eg, enuresis), or accompanying automatisms. Onset and termination of attacks are abrupt. If attacks occur during conversation, the patient may miss a few words or may break off in midsentence for a few seconds. The impairment of external awareness is so brief that the patient is unaware of it. Absence ("petit mal") seizures almost always begin in childhood and frequently cease by the age of 20 years or are then replaced by other forms of generalized seizure. Electroencephalographically, such attacks are associated with bursts of bilaterally synchronous and symmetric 3-Hz spike-and-wave activity. A normal background in the electroencephalogram and normal or above-normal intelligence imply a good prognosis for the ultimate cessation of these seizures.

2. Atypical absence seizures—There may be more marked changes in tone, or attacks may have a more gradual onset and termination than in typical absence seizures. They commonly occur in patients with multiple seizure types, may be accompanied by developmental delay or mental retardation, and are associated with slower spike-wave discharges than those in typical absence attacks.

3. Myoclonic seizures—Myoclonic seizures consist of single or multiple myoclonic jerks.

4. Tonic-clonic ("grand mal") seizures—In these seizures, which are characterized by sudden loss of consciousness, the patient becomes rigid and falls to the ground, and respiration is arrested. This tonic phase, which usually lasts for under 1 minute, is followed by a clonic phase in which there is jerking of the body musculature that may last for 2 or 3 minutes and is then followed by a stage of flaccid coma. During the seizure, the tongue or lips may be bitten, urinary or fecal incontinence may occur, and the patient may be injured. Immediately after the seizure, the patient may recover consciousness, drift into sleep, have a further convulsion without recovery of consciousness between the attacks (**status epilepticus**), or after recovering consciousness have a further convulsion (**serial seizures**). In other cases, patients will behave in an abnormal fashion in the immediate postictal period, without subsequent awareness or memory of events (**postepileptic automatism**). Headache, disorientation, confusion, drowsiness, nausea, soreness of the muscles, or some combination of these symptoms commonly occurs postictally.

5. Tonic, clonic, or atonic seizures—Loss of consciousness may occur with either the tonic or clonic accompaniments described above, especially in children. Atonic seizures consist of very brief (less than 2 seconds) loss of muscle tone and often result in falls (**epileptic drop attacks**).

▶ Clinical Findings

A. Symptoms and Signs

Nonspecific changes such as headache, mood alterations, lethargy, and myoclonic jerking alert some patients to an impending seizure hours before it occurs. These prodromal symptoms are distinct from the aura; the aura that may precede a generalized seizure by a few seconds or minutes is itself a part of the seizure indicating focal onset from a restricted part of the brain.

In most patients, seizures occur unpredictably at any time and without any relationship to posture or ongoing activities. Occasionally, however, they occur at a particular time (eg, during sleep) or in relation to external precipitants such as lack of sleep, missed meals, emotional stress, menstruation, alcohol ingestion (or alcohol withdrawal), or use of certain drugs. Fever and nonspecific infections may also precipitate seizures in epileptic patients. In a few patients, seizures are provoked by specific stimuli such as flashing lights or a flickering television set (**photosensitive epilepsy**), music, or reading.

Clinical examination between seizures shows no abnormality in patients with idiopathic epilepsy, but in the immediate postictal period, extensor plantar responses may be seen. The presence of lateralized or focal signs postictally suggests that seizures may have a focal origin. In patients with symptomatic epilepsy, the findings on examination will reflect the underlying cause.

B. Imaging

Some clinicians routinely order MRI for all patients with new-onset seizure disorders, but this may be unnecessary. MRI is indicated for patients with focal neurologic symptoms or signs, focal seizures, or electroencephalographic findings of a focal disturbance. It should also be performed in patients with clinical evidence of a progressive disorder and in those with new onset of seizures after the age of 20 years because of the possibility of an underlying neoplasm. CT is generally less sensitive than MRI in detecting small structural brain abnormalities but may be used when MRI is contraindicated or unavailable.

C. Laboratory and Other Studies

Initial investigations after a first seizure should include complete blood count, serum glucose, electrolytes, creatinine, calcium, magnesium, and liver function tests to exclude various causes of provoked seizures and to provide a baseline for subsequent monitoring of long-term effects of treatment. Routine laboratory investigations are not usually necessary after recurrent seizures in patients with known epilepsy. A lumbar puncture may be necessary when any sign of infection is present or in the evaluation of new-onset seizures in the acute setting.

Electroencephalography may support the clinical diagnosis of epilepsy (by demonstrating paroxysmal abnormalities containing spikes or sharp waves), provide a guide to prognosis, and help classify the seizure disorder. Classification of the disorder is important for determining the most appropriate anticonvulsant drug with which to start treatment. For example, absence and focal seizures with impairment of consciousness may be difficult to distinguish clinically, but the electroencephalographic findings and treatment of choice differ in these two conditions. Finally, by localizing the epileptogenic source, the electroencephalographic findings are important in evaluating candidates for surgical treatment.

▶ Differential Diagnosis

The distinction between the various disorders likely to be confused with generalized seizures is usually made on the basis of the history. The importance of obtaining an eyewitness account of the attacks cannot be overemphasized.

A. Differential Diagnosis of Focal Seizures

1. TIAs—These are distinguished from seizures by their longer duration, lack of spread, and negative (eg, weakness or numbness) rather than positive (eg, convulsive jerking or paresthesias) symptoms. Level of consciousness, which is unaltered, does not distinguish them.

2. Rage attacks—Rage attacks are usually situational and lead to goal-directed aggressive behavior.

3. Panic attacks—These may be hard to distinguish from focal seizures unless there is evidence of an anxiety disorder between attacks and the attacks have a clear relationship to external circumstances.

B. Differential Diagnosis of Generalized Seizures

1. Syncope—Syncopal episodes usually occur in relation to postural change, emotional stress, instrumentation, pain, or straining. They are typically preceded by pallor, sweating, nausea, and malaise and lead to loss of consciousness accompanied by flaccidity; recovery occurs rapidly with recumbency, and there is no postictal headache or confusion. In some instances, however, motor accompaniments and urinary incontinence may simulate a seizure.

2. Cardiac disease—Cerebral hypoperfusion due to a disturbance of cardiac rhythm should be suspected in patients with known cardiac or vascular disease or in elderly patients who present with episodic loss of consciousness. Prodromal symptoms are typically absent. Repeated Holter monitoring may be necessary to establish the diagnosis; external event recorders or implantable loop recorders may be valuable if the disturbances of consciousness are rare. A relationship of attacks to physical activity and the finding of a systolic murmur are suggestive of aortic stenosis.

3. Brainstem ischemia—Loss of consciousness is preceded or accompanied by other brainstem signs. Basilar artery migraine and vertebrobasilar vascular disease are discussed elsewhere in this chapter.

4. Psychogenic nonepileptic seizure (PNES)—Simulating an epileptic seizure, a PNES may occur due to a conversion disorder or malingering. Many patients also have true seizures or a family history of epilepsy. A history of childhood physical or sexual abuse is common. Although a PNES tends to occur at times of emotional stress, this may also be the case with true seizures.

Clinically, the attacks superficially resemble tonic-clonic seizures, but there may be obvious preparation before a PNES. Moreover, there is usually no tonic phase; instead, there may be an asynchronous thrashing of the limbs and the attack rarely leads to injury. Eyes are often forcibly closed during PNES, unlike epileptic seizures, in which they are typically open. Consciousness may be normal or "lost," but in the latter context the occurrence of goal-directed behavior or of shouting, swearing, etc, indicates that it is feigned. Postictally, there are no changes in behavior or neurologic findings.

Often, clinical observation is insufficient to discriminate epileptic from nonepileptic seizures and video electroencephalographic monitoring is required. Elevation of serum prolactin level to at least twice the upper limit of normal can be seen between 10 and 20 minutes after a seizure or syncopal event but not after a PNES. However, the test has limited clinical utility because levels are normal after an epileptic seizure in roughly half of patients and a baseline prolactin must be drawn 6 hours after the attack.

► Treatment

A. General Measures

For patients with epilepsy, drug treatment is prescribed with the goal of preventing further attacks and is usually continued until there have been no seizures for at least 2 years. Epileptic patients should be advised to avoid situations that could be dangerous or life-threatening if further seizures should occur. Legislation may require clinicians to report to the state authorities any patients with seizures or other episodic disturbances of consciousness; driving cessation for 6 months or as legislated is appropriate following an unprovoked seizure.

1. Choice of medication—Drug selection depends on seizure type (Table 24–3). The dose of the selected drug is gradually increased until seizures are controlled or side effects prevent further increases. If seizures continue despite treatment at the maximal tolerated dose, a second drug is added and the dose increased depending on tolerance; the first drug is then gradually withdrawn. In most patients with seizures of a single type, satisfactory control can be achieved with a single anticonvulsant drug. Treatment with two drugs may further reduce seizure frequency or severity but usually only at the cost of greater toxicity. Treatment with more than two drugs is almost always unhelpful unless the patient is having seizures of different types. Other factors to consider in selecting an anticonvulsant drug include likely side effects, teratogenicity, interactions with other drugs and oral contraceptives, and route of metabolism.

All antiepileptics are potentially teratogenic, although the teratogenicity of the newer antiseizure medications is less clear. Nevertheless, antiepileptic medication must be given to pregnant women with epilepsy to prevent seizures, which can pose serious risk to the fetus from trauma, hypoxia, or other factors.

2. Monitoring—Individual differences in drug metabolism cause a given dose of a drug to produce different blood concentrations in different patients, and this will affect the therapeutic response. In general, the dose of an antiepileptic agent is increased depending on the clinical response regardless of the serum drug level. When a dose is achieved that either controls seizures or is the maximum tolerated, then a steady-state trough drug level may be obtained for future reference; rechecking this level may be appropriate during pregnancy, if a breakthrough seizure occurs, a dose change occurs, or another (potentially interacting) drug is added to the regimen. A laboratory's therapeutic range for a drug is only a guide; many patients achieve good seizure control with no adverse effect at serum levels that exceed the stipulated range, and in these

Table 24–3. Drug treatment for seizures in adults.

Drug	Usual Adult Daily Oral Dose	Minimum No. of Daily Doses	Time to Steady-State Drug Levels	Optimal Drug Level and Laboratory Monitoring[1]	Selected Side Effects and Idiosyncratic Reactions
Generalized or focal seizures					
Phenytoin	200–400 mg	1	5–10 days	10–20 mcg/mL CBC, LFTs, folate	Nystagmus, ataxia, dysarthria, sedation, confusion, gingival hyperplasia, hirsutism, megaloblastic anemia, blood dyscrasias, skin rashes, fever, systemic lupus erythematosus, lymphadenopathy, peripheral neuropathy, dyskinesias.
Carbamazepine	400–1600 mg (immediate or extended release)	2	3–4 days	4–8 mcg/mL CBC, LFTs, BUN/Cr	Nystagmus, dysarthria, diplopia, ataxia, drowsiness, nausea, blood dyscrasias, hepatotoxicity, hyponatremia, Stevens-Johnson syndrome.[2] **May exacerbate myoclonic seizures.**
Valproic acid	1500–2000 mg	2–3	2–4 days	50–100 mcg/mL CBC, LFTs	Nausea, vomiting, diarrhea, drowsiness, alopecia, weight gain, hepatotoxicity, thrombocytopenia, tremor, pancreatitis. **Teratogenic; avoid in women of childbearing age.**
Phenobarbital	100–200 mg	1	14–21 days	10–40 mcg/mL CBC, LFTs, BUN/Cr	Drowsiness, nystagmus, ataxia, skin rashes, learning difficulties, hyperactivity.
Primidone	750–1500 mg	3	4–7 days	5–15 mcg/mL CBC	Sedation, nystagmus, ataxia, vertigo, nausea, skin rashes, megaloblastic anemia, irritability.
Lamotrigine[3–5]	100–500 mg	2	4–5 days		Sedation, skin rash, visual disturbances, dyspepsia, ataxia.
Topiramate[3,4,6,7]	200–400 mg	2	4 days	Serum bicarbonate; BUN/Cr in elderly patients	Somnolence, nausea, dyspepsia, irritability, dizziness, ataxia, nystagmus, diplopia, glaucoma, renal calculi, weight loss, hypohidrosis, hyperthermia.
Oxcarbazepine[3,6]	900–1800 mg	2	2–3 days	Serum sodium	As for carbamazepine.
Levetiracetam[3,4]	1000–3000 mg	2	2 days		Somnolence, ataxia, headache, behavioral changes.
Zonisamide[3]	200–600 mg	1	14 days	BUN/Cr, serum bicarbonate	Somnolence, ataxia, anorexia, nausea, vomiting, rash, confusion, renal calculi. Do not use in patients with sulfonamide allergy.
Tiagabine[3]	32–56 mg	2	2 days		Somnolence, anxiety, dizziness, poor concentration, tremor, diarrhea.
Pregabalin[3]	150–300 mg	2	2–4 days		Somnolence, dizziness, poor concentration, weight gain, thrombocytopenia, skin rashes, anaphylactoid reactions.
Gabapentin[3]	900–3600 mg	3	1 day		Sedation, fatigue, ataxia, nystagmus, weight loss.
Felbamate[3,6,8]	1200–3600 mg	3	4–5 days	CBC and reticulocytes, LFTs	Anorexia, nausea, vomiting, headache, insomnia, weight loss, dizziness, hepatotoxicity, fatal aplastic anemia; reserved for refractory epilepsy.
Lacosamide[3]	100–400 mg	2	3 days	ECG if known cardiac conduction problems or severe cardiac disease	Vertigo, diplopia, nausea, headache, fatigue, ataxia, tremor, anaphylactoid reactions, PR prolongation, cardiac dysrhythmia, suicidality.
Ezogabine[3]	300–1200 mg	3	2–3 days	ECG to assess QT interval	Dizziness, somnolence, confusion, vertigo, nausea, ataxia, psychiatric disturbances, prolonged QT interval, retinal abnormalities.[9]
Perampanel	4–12 mg	1	3 weeks		Dizziness, somnolence, irritability, weight gain, falls, ataxia, dysarthria, blurred vision.

(continued)

Table 24–3. Drug treatment for seizures in adults. (continued)

Drug	Usual Adult Daily Oral Dose	Minimum No. of Daily Doses	Time to Steady-State Drug Levels	Optimal Drug Level and Laboratory Monitoring[1]	Selected Side Effects and Idiosyncratic Reactions
Clorazepate[3]	22.5–90 mg	2	10 days		Sedation, dizziness, confusion, ataxia, depression, dependency/abuse.
Eslicarbazepine[3]	400–1200 mg daily	1	4 days	Serum sodium and chloride; LFTs	As for carbamazepine.
Vigabatrin[3,4]	3000 mg	2	2 days		Somnolence, anorexia, nausea, vomiting, agitation, hostility, confusion, suicidality, neutropenia, Stevens-Johnson syndrome, permanent visual field loss.[9]
Clobazam[10]	10–40 mg	2	7–10 days		Lethargy and somnolence, ataxia, insomnia, dysarthria, aggression, constipation, fever, Stevens-Johnson syndrome
Rufinamide[10]	800–3200 mg daily	2	2 days		Somnolence, headache, dizziness, suicidality, Stevens-Johnson syndrome, leukopenia, shortened QT interval, nausea, vomiting
Absence seizures					
Ethosuximide	100–1500 mg	2	5–10 days	40–100 mcg/mL CBC; LFTs; urinalysis	Nausea, vomiting, anorexia, headache, lethargy, unsteadiness, blood dyscrasias, systemic lupus erythematosus, urticaria, pruritus.
Valproic acid	1500–2000 mg	3	2–4 days	See above	Nausea, vomiting, diarrhea, drowsiness, alopecia, weight gain, hepatotoxicity, thrombocytopenia, tremor, pancreatitis.
Clonazepam	0.04–0.2 mg/kg	2	?	20–80 ng/mL CBC; LFTs	Drowsiness, ataxia, irritability, behavioral changes, exacerbation of tonic-clonic seizures.
Myoclonic seizures					
Valproic acid	1500–2000 mg	3	2–4 days	See above	Nausea, vomiting, diarrhea, drowsiness, alopecia, weight gain, hepatotoxicity, thrombocytopenia, tremor, pancreatitis.
Clonazepam	0.04–0.2 mg/kg	2	?	See above	Drowsiness, ataxia, irritability, behavioral changes, exacerbation of tonic-clonic seizures.

BUN, blood urea nitrogen; CBC, complete blood count; Cr, creatinine; ECG, electrocardiogram; LFTs, liver function tests.

[1]Patients starting treatment with any antiepileptic drug should be monitored for new or worsening depression or suicidal thoughts, especially during the first weeks of therapy. Baseline measurement of creatinine clearance is advisable in renally metabolized drugs.

[2]Carriers of the HLA-B*1502 allele are at higher risk for Stevens-Johnson syndrome.

[3]Approved as adjunctive therapy for focal-onset seizures.

[4]Approved as adjunctive therapy for primary generalized tonic-clonic seizures.

[5]Approved as monotherapy (after conversion from another drug) in focal-onset seizures.

[6]Approved as initial monotherapy for focal-onset seizures.

[7]Approved as initial monotherapy for primary generalized tonic-clonic seizures.

[8]Not to be used as a first-line drug; when used, blood counts should be performed regularly (every 2–4 weeks). Should be used only in selected patients because of risk of aplastic anemia and hepatic failure. It is advisable to obtain written informed consent before use.

[9] Regular ophthalmologic examination is recommended.

[10]Approved as adjunctive therapy for Lennox-Gastaut syndrome.

cases no dose adjustment is needed. The most common cause of a lower concentration of drug than expected for the prescribed dose is suboptimal patient adherence. Adherence can be improved by limiting to a minimum the number of daily doses. Recurrent seizures or status epilepticus may result if drugs are taken erratically, and in some circumstances nonadherent patients may be better off

without any medication. All anticonvulsant drugs have side effects, and many require baseline and regular laboratory monitoring (Table 24–3).

3. Discontinuance of medication—Only when adult patients have been seizure-free for 2 years should withdrawal of medication be considered. Unfortunately, there is no way of predicting which patients can be managed successfully without treatment, although seizure recurrence is more likely in patients who initially did not respond to therapy, those with seizures having focal features or of multiple types, and those with continuing electroencephalographic abnormalities. Dose reduction should be gradual (over weeks or months), and drugs should be withdrawn one at a time. If seizures recur, treatment is reinstituted with the previously effective drug regimen.

4. Surgical treatment—Patients with seizures refractory to pharmacologic management may be candidates for operative treatment. Surgical resection is most efficacious when there is a single well-defined seizure focus, particularly in the temporal lobe. Among well-chosen patients, up to 70% remain seizure-free after extended follow-up. Bilateral deep brain stimulation of the anterior thalamus for medically refractory focal-onset seizures may be of benefit, and there is an evolving role for electrical stimulation of other cortical and subcortical targets.

5. Vagal nerve stimulation—Treatment by chronic vagal nerve stimulation for adults and adolescents with medically refractory focal seizures is approved in the United States and provides an alternative approach for patients who are not optimal candidates for surgical treatment. The mechanism of therapeutic action is unknown. Adverse effects consist mainly of transient hoarseness during stimulus delivery.

B. Special Circumstances

1. Solitary seizures—In patients who have had only one seizure or a flurry of seizures over a brief period of several hours, investigation as outlined earlier should exclude an underlying cause requiring specific treatment. An electroencephalogram should be obtained, preferably within 24 hours after the seizure. Prophylactic anticonvulsant drug treatment is generally not required unless further attacks occur or investigations reveal underlying pathology. The risk of seizure recurrence varies in different series between about 30% and 70%, with higher risk of recurrence in patients with structural brain lesions or abnormalities on electroencephalogram. Epilepsy should not be diagnosed on the basis of a solitary seizure. If seizures occur in the context of transient, nonrecurrent systemic disorders such as hyponatremia or hypoglycemia, the diagnosis of epilepsy is inaccurate, and long-term prophylactic anticonvulsant drug treatment is unnecessary.

2. Alcohol withdrawal seizures—The characteristic alcohol withdrawal seizure pattern is one or more generalized tonic-clonic seizures that may occur within 48 hours or so of withdrawal from alcohol after a period of high or prolonged intake. If the seizures have consistently focal features, the possibility of an associated structural abnormality, often traumatic in origin, must be considered. Head CT scan or MRI should be performed in patients with new onset of generalized seizures and whenever there are focal features. Treatment with anticonvulsant drugs is generally not required for alcohol withdrawal seizures, since they are self-limited. Benzodiazepines (diazepam or lorazepam,

dosed as needed to reduce withdrawal symptoms and to avoid oversedation) are effective and safe for preventing further seizures (see Chapter 25). Status epilepticus may complicate alcohol withdrawal and is managed along conventional lines. Further attacks will not occur if the patient abstains from alcohol.

3. Tonic-clonic status epilepticus—Poor adherence to the anticonvulsant drug regimen is the most common cause; other causes include alcohol withdrawal, intracranial infection or neoplasms, metabolic disorders, and drug overdose. The mortality rate may be as high as 20%, and among survivors the incidence of neurologic and cognitive sequelae is high. The prognosis relates to the underlying cause as well as the length of time between onset of status epilepticus and the start of effective treatment.

Status epilepticus is a medical emergency. Initial management includes maintenance of the airway and 50% dextrose (25–50 mL) intravenously in case hypoglycemia is responsible. If seizures continue, an intravenous bolus of lorazepam, 4 mg, is given at a rate of 2 mg/min and repeated once after 10 minutes if necessary; alternatively, 10 mg of midazolam is given intramuscularly, and again after 10 minutes if necessary. Diazepam can also be given rectally as a gel (0.2 mg/kg). These measures are usually effective in halting seizures for a brief period. Respiratory depression and hypotension may complicate the treatment and are treated as in other circumstances; this treatment may include intubation and mechanical ventilation and admission to an intensive care unit.

Regardless of the response to lorazepam or midazolam, fosphenytoin or phenytoin should be administered intravenously to initiate long-term seizure control. Fosphenytoin (18–20 mg phenytoin equivalents [PE]/kg) is rapidly and completely converted to phenytoin following intravenous administration and is preferred because it is less likely to cause reactions at the infusion site, can be given with all common intravenous solutions, and may be administered at a faster rate (150 mg PE/min). When fosphenytoin is not available, phenytoin (18–20 mg/kg) is given intravenously at a rate of 50 mg/min. Phenytoin is best injected directly but can also be given in saline; it precipitates, however, if injected into glucose-containing solutions. Because arrhythmias may develop during rapid administration of phenytoin or fosphenytoin, electrocardiographic monitoring is prudent. Hypotension may occur, especially if diazepam has also been given.

If seizures continue, phenobarbital is then given in a loading dose of 10–20 mg/kg intravenously by slow or intermittent injection (50 mg/min). Respiratory depression and hypotension are especially common with this therapy. Alternatively or additionally, intravenous valproate is used for status epilepticus (loading dose 25–30 mg/kg over 15 min; then 100 mg/h); although valproate is not approved by the FDA for this indication, it has been used with success.

If these measures fail, general anesthesia with ventilatory assistance may be required; some experts recommend proceeding directly to general anesthesia if convulsions do not cease after the initial 18–20 PE/kg fosphenytoin load. Intravenous midazolam may provide control of refractory status epilepticus; the suggested loading dose is 0.2 mg/kg, followed by 0.05–0.2 mg/kg/h. Propofol (1–2 mg/kg as an intravenous bolus, followed by infusion at 2–15 mg/kg/h depending on response) may also be used, as may pentobarbital (15 mg/kg intravenously, followed by 0.5–4 mg/kg/h).

After status epilepticus is controlled, an oral drug program for the long-term management of seizures is started, and investigations into the cause of the disorder are pursued.

4. Nonconvulsive status epilepticus—In some cases, status epilepticus presents not with convulsions, but with a fluctuating abnormal mental status, confusion, impaired responsiveness, and automatism. Electroencephalography is helpful in establishing the diagnosis. The treatment approach outlined above applies to any type of status epilepticus, although intravenous anesthesia is usually not necessary. The prognosis is a reflection of the underlying cause rather than of continuing seizures.

▶ When to Refer

- Behavioral episodes of uncertain nature.
- Seizures are difficult to control with monotherapy.
- There is a progressive neurologic disorder.
- For inpatient monitoring when PNES is suspected.

▶ When to Admit

- Status epilepticus.
- Frequent seizures requiring rapid medication titration and electroencephalographic monitoring.

Angus-Leppan H. First seizures in adults. BMJ. 2014 Apr 15; 348:g2470. [PMID: 24736280]

Betjemann JP et al. Status epilepticus in adults. Lancet Neurol. 2015 Jun;14(6):615–24. [PMID: 25908090]

Glauser T et al. Updated ILAE evidence review of antiepileptic drug efficacy and effectiveness as initial monotherapy for epileptic seizures and syndromes. Epilepsia. 2013 Mar;54(3):551–63. [PMID: 23350722]

Moshé SL et al. Epilepsy: new advances. Lancet. 2015 Mar 7; 385(9971):884–98. [PMID: 25260236]

Ryvlin P et al. Epilepsy surgery in children and adults. Lancet Neurol. 2014 Nov;13(11):1114–26. [PMID: 25316018]

DYSAUTONOMIA

ESSENTIALS OF DIAGNOSIS

▶ Postural hypotension or abnormal heart rate regulation.

▶ Abnormalities of sweating, intestinal motility, sexual function, or sphincter control.

▶ Syncope may occur.

▶ Symptoms occur in isolation or any combination.

▶ General Considerations

Dysautonomia may occur as a result of central or peripheral pathologic processes. It is manifested by a variety of symptoms that may occur in isolation or in various combinations and relates to abnormalities of blood pressure regulation, thermoregulatory sweating, gastrointestinal function, sphincter control, sexual function, respiration, and ocular function. Syncope, a symptom of dysautonomia, is characterized by a transient loss of consciousness, usually accompanied by hypotension and bradycardia. It may occur in response to emotional stress, postural hypotension, vigorous exercise in a hot environment, obstructed venous return to the heart, acute pain or its anticipation, fluid loss, and a variety of other circumstances.

A. Central Neurologic Causes

Disease at certain sites in the central nervous system, regardless of its nature, may lead to dysautonomic symptoms. Postural hypotension, which is usually the most troublesome and disabling symptom, may result from spinal cord transection and other myelopathies (eg, due to tumor or syringomyelia) above the T6 level or from brainstem lesions such as syringobulbia and posterior fossa tumors. Sphincter or sexual disturbances may result from cord lesions below T6. Certain primary degenerative disorders are responsible for dysautonomia occurring in isolation (**pure autonomic failure**) or in association with more widespread abnormalities (**multisystem atrophy**) that may include parkinsonian, pyramidal symptoms, and cerebellar deficits.

B. Peripheral Neurologic Causes

A pure autonomic neuropathy may occur acutely or subacutely after a viral infection or as a paraneoplastic disorder related usually to small cell lung cancer, particularly in association with certain antibodies, such as anti-Hu or those directed at neuronal nicotinic ganglionic acetylcholine receptors. Dysautonomia is often conspicuous in patients with Guillain-Barré syndrome, manifesting with marked hypotension or hypertension or cardiac arrhythmias that may have a fatal outcome. It may also occur with diabetic, uremic, amyloidotic, and various other metabolic or toxic neuropathies; in association with leprosy or Chagas disease; and as a feature of certain hereditary neuropathies with autosomal dominant or recessive inheritance or an X-linked pattern. Autonomic symptoms are prominent in the crises of hepatic porphyria. Patients with botulism or the Lambert-Eaton myasthenic syndrome may have constipation, urinary retention, and a sicca syndrome as a result of impaired cholinergic function.

▶ Clinical Findings

A. Symptoms and Signs

Dysautonomic symptoms include syncope, postural hypotension, paroxysmal hypertension, persistent tachycardia without other cause, facial flushing, hypohidrosis or hyperhidrosis, vomiting, constipation, diarrhea, dysphagia, abdominal distention, disturbances of micturition or defecation, erectile dysfunction, apneic episodes, and declining night vision. In syncope, prodromal malaise, nausea, headache, diaphoresis, pallor, visual disturbance, loss of postural tone, and a sense of weakness and impending loss of consciousness are followed by actual loss of consciousness. Although the patient is usually flaccid, some motor activity is not uncommon, and urinary (and rarely fecal) incontinence may also occur, thereby simulating a seizure. Recovery is rapid once the patient becomes recumbent, but headache, nausea, and fatigue are common postictally.

B. Evaluation of the Patient

Testing of autonomic function includes evaluating the cardiovascular response to the Valsalva maneuver, startle, mental stress, postural change, and deep respiration, and the sudomotor (sweating) responses to warming or a deep inspiratory gasp. Tilt-table testing may reproduce syncopal or presyncopal symptoms. Pharmacologic studies to evaluate the pupillary responses, radiologic studies of the bladder or gastrointestinal tract, uroflowmetry and urethral pressure profiles, and recording of nocturnal penile tumescence may also be necessary in selected cases. Further investigation depends on the presence of other associated neurologic abnormalities. In patients with a peripheral cause, work-up for peripheral neuropathy may be required and should include testing for ganglionic acetylcholine receptor antibody. For those with evidence of a central lesion, imaging studies will exclude a treatable structural cause. Reversible, nonneurologic causes of symptoms must be considered. Postural hypotension and syncope may relate to a reduced cardiac output, paroxysmal cardiac dysrhythmias, volume depletion, various medications, and endocrine and metabolic disorders such as Addison disease, hypothyroidism or hyperthyroidism, pheochromocytoma, and carcinoid syndrome.

▶ Treatment

The most disabling symptoms are usually postural hypotension and syncope. Abrupt postural change, prolonged recumbency, and other precipitants should be avoided. Medications associated with postural hypotension should be discontinued or reduced in dose. Treatment may include wearing waist-high elastic hosiery, salt supplementation, sleeping in a semierect position (which minimizes the natriuresis and diuresis that occur during recumbency), and fludrocortisone (0.1–0.5 mg orally daily). Vasoconstrictor agents may be helpful and include midodrine (2.5–10 mg orally three times daily) and ephedrine (15–30 mg orally three times daily). Other agents that have been used occasionally or experimentally are dihydroergotamine, yohimbine, pyridostigmine, and clonidine; refractory cases may respond to erythropoietin (epoetin alfa) or desmopressin. Patients must be monitored for recumbent hypertension. Postprandial hypotension is helped by caffeine. There is no satisfactory treatment for disturbances of sweating, but an air-conditioned environment is helpful in avoiding extreme swings in body temperature.

▶ When to Refer

- When the diagnosis is uncertain.
- When symptoms persist despite conventional treatment.

Benarroch EE. The clinical approach to autonomic failure in neurological disorders. Nat Rev Neurol. 2014 Jul;10(7):396–407. [PMID: 24866874]
Iodice V et al. Autonomic neuropathies. Continuum (Minneap Minn). 2014 Oct;20(5):1373–97. [PMID: 25299288]

TRANSIENT ISCHEMIC ATTACKS

ESSENTIALS OF DIAGNOSIS

▸ Focal neurologic deficit of acute onset.

▸ Clinical deficit resolves completely within 24 hours.

▸ Risk factors for vascular disease often present.

▶ General Considerations

Transient ischemic attacks (TIAs) are characterized by focal ischemic cerebral neurologic deficits that last for less than 24 hours (usually less than 1–2 hours). About 30% of patients with stroke have a history of TIAs and 5–10% of patients with TIAs will have a stroke within 90 days. Urgent intervention in TIA patients reduces rates of subsequent stroke, and the condition should be treated with a similar sense of urgency as unstable angina.

▶ Etiology

An important cause of transient cerebral ischemia is embolization. In many patients with these attacks, a source is readily apparent in the heart or a major extracranial artery to the head, and emboli sometimes are visible in the retinal arteries. An embolic phenomenon explains why separate attacks may affect different parts of the territory supplied by the same major vessel. Cardiac causes of embolic ischemic attacks include atrial fibrillation, severe heart failure, infective and noninfective endocarditis, atrial myxoma, and mural thrombi complicating myocardial infarction. Atrial septal defects and patent foramen ovale may permit venous thromboemboli to reach the brain (paradoxical emboli). An ulcerated plaque on a major artery to the brain may serve as a source of emboli. In the anterior circulation, atherosclerotic changes occur most commonly in the region of the carotid bifurcation extracranially; these changes may cause a bruit. Atherosclerosis also affects the vertebrobasilar system and the major intracranial vessels including the middle and anterior cerebral arteries.

Less common abnormalities of blood vessels that may cause TIAs include fibromuscular dysplasia, which affects particularly the cervical internal carotid artery; atherosclerosis of the aortic arch; inflammatory arterial disorders such as giant cell arteritis, polyarteritis, and granulomatous angiitis; and meningovascular syphilis. Critical stenosis of a major extracranial or intracranial artery may cause TIA, especially in the setting of hypotension.

Hematologic causes of TIA include polycythemia, sickle cell disease, hyperviscosity syndromes, and the antiphospholipid antibody syndrome. Severe anemia may also lead to transient focal neurologic deficits in patients with preexisting cerebral arterial disease.

The **subclavian steal syndrome** may lead to transient vertebrobasilar ischemia. Symptoms develop when there is localized stenosis or occlusion of one subclavian artery proximal to the source of the vertebral artery, so that blood is "stolen" from this artery. A bruit in the supraclavicular fossa, unequal radial pulses, and a difference of 20 mm Hg or more between the systolic blood pressures in the arms should suggest the diagnosis in patients with vertebrobasilar TIAs.

▶ Clinical Findings

A. Symptoms and Signs

The symptoms of TIAs vary markedly among patients; however, the symptoms in a given individual tend to be constant in type. Onset is abrupt and without warning, and recovery usually occurs rapidly, often within a few minutes. The specific symptoms depend on the arterial distribution affected, as outlined in the subsequent section on stroke. Of note, TIA is a rare cause of loss of consciousness or acute confusion but is often erroneously blamed for such symptoms.

The natural history of attacks is variable. Some patients will have a major stroke after only a few attacks, whereas others may have frequent attacks for weeks or months without having a stroke. The risk of stroke is high in the first 3 months after an attack, particularly in the first month and especially within the first 48 hours. Attacks may occur intermittently over a long period of time, or they may stop spontaneously. In general, carotid ischemic attacks are more liable than vertebrobasilar ischemic attacks to be followed by stroke. The stroke risk is greater in patients older than 60 years, in patients with diabetes, or after TIAs that last longer than 10 minutes and with symptoms or signs of weakness, speech impairment, or gait disturbance.

B. Imaging

CT or MRI scan is indicated within 24 hours of symptom onset, in part to exclude the possibility of a small cerebral hemorrhage or a cerebral tumor masquerading as a TIA. MRI with diffusion-weighted sequences is particularly sensitive for revealing acute or subacute infarction, which is seen in up to one-third of cases despite resolution of clinical symptoms. Noninvasive imaging of the cervical vasculature should also be performed; carotid duplex ultrasonography is useful for detecting significant stenosis of the internal carotid artery, and MR or CT angiography permits broader visualization of cervical and intracranial vasculature.

C. Laboratory and Other Studies

Clinical and laboratory evaluation must include assessment for hypertension, heart disease, hematologic disorders, diabetes mellitus, hyperlipidemia, and peripheral vascular disease. It should include complete blood count, fasting blood glucose and serum cholesterol determinations, and an ECG and may include serologic tests for syphilis and HIV infection depending on the circumstances. Echocardiography with agitated saline contrast is performed if a cardiac source is likely, and blood cultures are obtained if endocarditis is suspected. Holter monitoring is indicated to detect paroxysmal atrial fibrillation and, if the cause of the TIA remains elusive, for extended cardiac event monitoring.

▶ Differential Diagnosis

Focal seizures usually cause abnormal motor or sensory phenomena such as clonic limb movements, paresthesias, or tingling, rather than weakness or loss of feeling. Symptoms generally spread ("march") up the limb and may lead to a generalized tonic-clonic seizure.

Classic migraine is easily recognized by the visual premonitory symptoms, followed by nausea, headache, and photophobia, but less typical cases may be hard to distinguish. The patient's age and medical history (including family history) may be helpful in this regard. Patients with migraine commonly have a history of episodes since adolescence and report that other family members have a similar disorder.

Focal neurologic deficits may occur during periods of hypoglycemia in diabetic patients receiving insulin or oral hypoglycemic agent therapy.

▶ Treatment

A. Medical Measures

Hospitalization should be considered for patients seen within a week of the attack, when they are at increased risk for early recurrence. One commonly used method to assess recurrence risk is the ABCD2 score; points are assigned for each of the following criteria: age 60 years or older (1 point), blood pressure 140/90 mm Hg or higher (1 point), clinical symptoms of focal weakness (2 points) or speech impairment without weakness (1 point), duration 60 minutes or longer (2 points) or 10–59 minutes (1 point), or diabetes mellitus (1 point). An ABCD2 score of 4 or more points has been suggested as a threshold for hospital admission. The ABCD2I (with an additional 3 points for any abnormal diffusion-weighted MRI finding or any infarct [new or old] on noncontrast CT) has been proposed as a better predictor of subsequent stroke risk. Admission is also advisable for patients with crescendo attacks, symptomatic carotid stenosis, or a known cardiac source of emboli or hypercoagulable state; such hospitalization facilitates early intervention for any recurrence and rapid institution of secondary prevention measures.

Medical treatment is aimed at preventing further attacks and stroke. Treat diabetes mellitus; hematologic disorders; and hypertension, preferably with an angiotensin-converting enzyme inhibitor or angiotensin receptor blocker. A statin should be started regardless of the current low-density lipoprotein level (LDL), although this practice is only supported by randomized trial data in patients with an LDL greater than 100 mg/dL. Cigarette smoking should be stopped, and cardiac sources of embolization should be treated appropriately. Weight reduction and regular physical activity should be encouraged when appropriate.

1. Anticoagulation—The chief indication for anticoagulation after TIA is atrial fibrillation. Patients with metal heart valves, left ventricular thrombus, and the antiphospholipid antibody syndrome should also receive anticoagulation therapy. A randomized trial of patients with heart failure and an ejection fraction under 35% failed to show a benefit of warfarin over aspirin. If anticoagulants are indicated, they should be started immediately, provided that their use is not contraindicated and that if an acute cerebral infarct has occurred, it is small. Treatment is with warfarin (target INR 2.0–3.0); bridging warfarin with heparin is not necessary, but some experts advocate treatment with aspirin until the INR becomes therapeutic. For long-term anticoagulation in the setting of atrial fibrillation, dabigatran (150 mg orally twice daily), rivaroxaban (20 mg orally daily), apixaban (2.5–5 mg orally twice daily) are options; these are usually not started in the acute setting due to limited experience and lack of reversal agents for the latter two. Combination antiplatelet-anticoagulation therapy is only indicated in patients with mechanical heart valves or those with a separate indication for antiplatelet therapy such as a cardiac stent.

2. Antiplatelet therapy—All patients in whom anticoagulation is not indicated should be treated with antiplatelet therapy to reduce the frequency of TIAs and the incidence of stroke. Aspirin (81 mg daily orally), aspirin combined with extended-release dipyridamole (200 mg twice daily orally), or clopidogrel (75 mg daily orally) all have similar efficacy. Cilostazol (100 mg twice daily) had similar efficacy as aspirin at stroke prevention in an Asian population with less risk of hemorrhage. Combining clopidogrel with aspirin for the long term increases the risk of hemorrhagic complications and is not recommended. However, short-term combination antiplatelet therapy may be beneficial. A large Chinese trial showed that when treatment was initiated within 24 hours after the TIA, a single loading dose of clopidogrel (300 mg) followed by 75 mg/day for 90 days plus aspirin (75 mg daily for the first 21 days) was more effective at reducing 90-day stroke risk than aspirin alone. An international trial using a similar protocol is ongoing.

B. Surgical or Endovascular Measures

When arteriography reveals a surgically accessible high-grade stenosis (70–99% in luminal diameter) on the side appropriate to carotid ischemic attacks, operative treatment (carotid endarterectomy) or endovascular intervention reduces the risk of ipsilateral carotid stroke, especially when TIAs are of recent onset (less than 1 month) and when the perioperative morbidity and mortality risk is estimated to be less than 6%. Endovascular therapy carries a slightly higher procedural stroke risk than endarterectomy in patients older than 70 years and is generally reserved for younger patients whose neck anatomy is unfavorable for surgery. Patients with a symptomatic carotid stenosis of 50–69% derive moderate benefit from intervention, but surgery is not indicated for mild stenosis (less than 50%).

▶ When to Refer

All patients should be referred for urgent investigation and treatment to prevent stroke.

▶ When to Admit

If seen within a week of a TIA, patients should be considered for admission when they have an ABCD2 score of 4 points or more, when outpatient evaluation is impractical, or when there are multiple attacks, carotid stenosis of greater than 70%, or other concern for early recurrence or stroke.

Kernan WN et al. Guidelines for the prevention of stroke in patients with stroke and transient ischemic attack: a guideline for healthcare professionals from the American Heart Association/American Stroke Association. Stroke. 2014 Jul;45(7):2160–236. [PMID: 24788967]

Sposato LA et al. Diagnosis of atrial fibrillation after stroke and transient ischaemic attack: a systematic review and meta-analysis. Lancet Neurol. 2015 Apr;14(4):377–87. [PMID: 25748102]

Wang Y et al; CHANCE Investigators. Clopidogrel with aspirin in acute minor stroke or transient ischemic attack. N Engl J Med. 2013 Jul 4;369(1):11–9. [PMID: 23803136]

STROKE

ESSENTIALS OF DIAGNOSIS

▶ Sudden onset of neurologic deficit of cerebrovascular origin.

▶ Patient often has history of hypertension, diabetes mellitus, tobacco use, atrial fibrillation, or atherosclerosis.

▶ Distinctive neurologic signs reflect the region of the brain involved.

▶ General Considerations

In the United States, stroke is the fifth leading cause of death and a leading cause of disability, despite a general decline in the incidence of stroke in the last 30 years. The precise reasons for this decline are uncertain, but increased awareness of risk factors (hypertension, diabetes mellitus, hyperlipidemia, cigarette smoking, cardiac disease, HIV infection, recreational drug abuse, heavy alcohol consumption, family history of stroke) and improved prophylactic measures and surveillance of those at increased risk have been contributory.

Strokes are subdivided pathologically into infarcts and hemorrhages. The distinction may be difficult clinically, but CT scanning usually clarifies the pathologic basis (Table 24–4).

1. Lacunar Infarction

Lacunar infarcts are small lesions (usually less than 5 mm in diameter) that occur in the distribution of short penetrating arterioles in the basal ganglia, pons, cerebellum,

Table 24–4. Features of the major stroke subtypes.

Stroke Type and Subtype	Clinical Features	Diagnosis	Treatment
Ischemic stroke			
Lacunar infarct	Small (< 5 mm) lesions in the basal ganglia, pons, cerebellum, or internal capsule; less often in deep cerebral white matter; prognosis generally good; clinical features depend on location, but may worsen over first 24–36 hours.	MRI with diffusion-weighted sequences usually defines the area of infarction; CT is insensitive acutely but can be used to exclude hemorrhage.	Antiplatelet; control risk factors (hypertension, tobacco use, hypercholesterolemia, and diabetes mellitus).
Carotid circulation obstruction	See text—signs vary depending on occluded vessel.	Noncontrast CT to exclude hemorrhage but findings may be normal during first 6–24 hours of an ischemic stroke; diffusion-weighted MRI is gold standard for identifying acute stroke; electrocardiography, carotid duplex studies, echocardiography, blood glucose, complete blood count, and tests for hyperlipidemia are indicated; Holter and extended monitoring in selected instances; CTA, MRA, or conventional angiography in selected cases; tests for hypercoagulable states in selected cases.	0–3 hours in United States: intravenous thrombolytics (approved in Europe for up to 4.5 hours) 0–6 hours: endovascular mechanical embolectomy Secondary prevention: Antiplatelet agent is first-line therapy; anticoagulation without heparin bridge for cardioembolic strokes due to atrial fibrillation and other select cases when no contraindications exist; control risk factors as above.
Vertebrobasilar occlusion	See text—signs vary based on location of occluded vessel.	As for carotid circulation obstruction.	As for carotid circulation obstruction.
Hemorrhagic stroke			
Spontaneous intracerebral hemorrhage	Commonly associated with hypertension; also with bleeding disorders, amyloid angiopathy. Hypertensive hemorrhage is located commonly in the basal ganglia, pons, thalamus, cerebellum, and less commonly the cerebral white matter.	Noncontrast CT is superior to MRI for detecting bleeds of < 48 hours duration; laboratory tests to identify bleeding disorder: angiography may be indicated to exclude aneurysm or AVM in younger patients without hypertension. Do not perform lumbar puncture.	Lower systolic blood pressure to < 140 mm Hg; cerebellar bleeds or hematomas with gross mass effect may require urgent surgical evacuation. AVM: surgical resection indicated to prevent further bleeding; other modalities to treat nonoperable AVMs available at specialized centers.
Subarachnoid hemorrhage	Present with sudden onset of worst headache of life, may lead rapidly to loss of consciousness; signs of meningeal irritation often present; etiology usually aneurysm or AVM, but 20% have no source identified.	CT to confirm diagnosis, but may be normal in rare instances; if CT negative and suspicion high, perform lumbar puncture to look for red blood cells or xanthochromia; angiography to determine source of bleed in candidates for treatment.	Lower systolic blood pressure to < 140 mm Hg immediately. Aneurysm: prevent further bleeding by clipping aneurysm or coil embolization; nimodipine helps prevent vasospasm; once aneurysm has been obliterated intravenous fluids and induced hypertension to prevent vasospasm; angioplasty may also reverse symptomatic vasospasm. AVM: as above.

AVMs, arteriovenous malformations; CTA, computed tomography angiography; MRA, magnetic resonance angiography.

internal capsule, thalamus and, less commonly, the deep cerebral white matter (Table 24–4). Lacunar infarcts are associated with poorly controlled hypertension or diabetes and have been found in several clinical syndromes, including contralateral pure motor or pure sensory deficit, ipsilateral ataxia with crural paresis, and dysarthria with clumsiness of the hand. The neurologic deficit may progress over 24–36 hours before stabilizing.

Early mortality and risk of stroke recurrence is higher for patients with nonlacunar than lacunar infarcts. The prognosis for recovery from the deficit produced by a lacunar infarct is usually good, with partial or complete resolution occurring over the following 4–6 weeks in many instances. Treatment is as described for TIA and cerebral infarction.

2. Cerebral Infarction

Thrombotic or embolic occlusion of a major vessel leads to cerebral infarction. Causes include the disorders predisposing to TIAs and atherosclerosis of cerebral arteries. The resulting deficit depends on the particular vessel involved and the extent of any collateral circulation. Cerebral ischemia leads to release of excitatory and other neuropeptides that may augment calcium flux into neurons, thereby leading to cell death and increasing the neurologic deficit.

▶ Clinical Findings

A. Symptoms and Signs

Onset is usually abrupt, and there may then be very little progression except that due to brain swelling. Clinical evaluation should always include examination of the heart and auscultation over the subclavian and carotid vessels to determine whether there are any bruits.

1. Obstruction of carotid circulation—Occlusion of the **ophthalmic or central retinal artery** is probably symptomless in most cases because of the rich orbital collaterals, but its transient embolic obstruction can lead to amaurosis fugax—sudden and brief loss of vision in one eye.

Occlusion of the **anterior cerebral artery** distal to its junction with the anterior communicating artery causes weakness and cortical sensory loss in the contralateral leg and sometimes mild weakness of the arm, especially proximally. There may be a contralateral grasp reflex, paratonic rigidity, and abulia (lack of initiative) or frank confusion. Urinary incontinence is not uncommon, particularly if behavioral disturbances are conspicuous. Bilateral anterior cerebral infarction is especially likely to cause marked behavioral changes and memory disturbances. Unilateral anterior cerebral artery occlusion proximal to the junction with the anterior communicating artery is generally well tolerated because of the collateral supply from the other side.

Middle cerebral artery occlusion leads to contralateral hemiplegia, hemisensory loss, and homonymous hemianopia (ie, bilaterally symmetric loss of vision in half of the visual fields), with the eyes deviated to the side of the lesion. If the dominant hemisphere is involved, global aphasia is also present. It may be impossible to distinguish this clinically from occlusion of the internal carotid artery. With occlusion of either of these arteries, there may also be considerable swelling of the hemisphere during the first 72 hours. For example, an infarct involving one cerebral hemisphere may lead to such swelling that the function of the other hemisphere or the rostral brainstem is disturbed and coma results. Occlusions of different branches of the middle cerebral artery cause more limited findings. For example, involvement of the superior division in the dominant hemisphere leads to a predominantly expressive aphasia and to contralateral paralysis and loss of sensations in the arm, the face and, to a lesser extent, the leg. Inferior branch occlusion in the dominant hemisphere produces a receptive (Wernicke) aphasia and a homonymous visual field defect. With involvement of the nondominant hemisphere, speech and comprehension are preserved, but there may be a left hemispatial neglect syndrome or constructional and visuospatial deficits.

2. Obstruction of vertebrobasilar circulation—Occlusion of the **posterior cerebral artery** may lead to a thalamic syndrome in which contralateral hemisensory disturbance occurs, followed by the development of spontaneous pain and hyperpathia. There is often a macular-sparing homonymous hemianopia and sometimes a mild, usually temporary, hemiparesis. Depending on the site of the lesion and the collateral circulation, the severity of these deficits varies and other deficits may also occur, including involuntary movements and alexia. Occlusion of the main artery beyond the origin of its penetrating branches may lead solely to a macular-sparing hemianopia.

Vertebral artery occlusion below the origin of the anterior spinal and posterior inferior cerebellar arteries may be clinically silent because the circulation is maintained by the other vertebral artery. If the remaining vertebral artery is congenitally small or severely atherosclerotic, however, a deficit similar to that of basilar artery occlusion is seen unless there is good collateral circulation from the anterior circulation through the circle of Willis. An obstruction of the **posterior inferior cerebellar artery** or an obstruction of the vertebral artery just before it branches to this vessel leads to ipsilateral spinothalamic sensory loss involving the face, ninth and tenth cranial nerve lesions, limb ataxia and numbness, and Horner syndrome, combined with contralateral spinothalamic sensory loss involving the limbs.

Occlusion of both **vertebral arteries** or the **basilar artery** leads to coma with pinpoint pupils, flaccid quadriplegia and sensory loss, and variable cranial nerve abnormalities. With partial basilar artery occlusion, there may be diplopia, visual loss, vertigo, dysarthria, ataxia, weakness or sensory disturbances in some or all of the limbs, and discrete cranial nerve palsies. In patients with hemiplegia of pontine origin, the eyes are often deviated to the paralyzed side, whereas in patients with a hemispheric lesion, the eyes commonly deviate from the hemiplegic side. When the small paramedian arteries arising from the basilar artery are occluded, contralateral hemiplegia and sensory deficit occur in association with an ipsilateral cranial nerve palsy at the level of the lesion.

Occlusion of any of the major **cerebellar arteries** produces vertigo, nausea, vomiting, nystagmus, ipsilateral limb ataxia, and contralateral spinothalamic sensory loss in the limbs. If the superior cerebellar artery is involved, the contralateral spinothalamic loss also involves the face; with occlusion of the anterior inferior cerebellar artery, there is ipsilateral spinothalamic sensory loss involving the face, usually in conjunction with ipsilateral facial weakness and deafness (due to cochlear infarction). Massive cerebellar infarction may lead to coma, tonsillar herniation, and death.

B. Imaging

A CT scan of the head (without contrast) should be performed immediately, before the administration of aspirin or other antithrombotic agents, to exclude cerebral hemorrhage (Table 24–4). CT is relatively insensitive to acute ischemic stroke, and subsequent MRI with diffusion-weighted sequences helps define the distribution and extent of infarction as well as to exclude tumor or other differential considerations. If patients present within 6 hours of stroke onset, CT angiography of the head and neck should be performed to identify large vessel occlusions potentially amenable to endovascular therapy. Regardless of timing of presentation, imaging of the cervical vasculature, by CT angiography, MR angiography, carotid duplex ultrasonography, or conventional catheter angiography, is indicated as part of a search to identify the source of the stroke.

C. Laboratory and Other Studies

Investigations should include a complete blood count, blood glucose determination, and fasting lipid panel. It may include serologic tests for syphilis and HIV infection depending on the circumstances. Screening for antiphospholipid antibodies (lupus anticoagulants and anticardiolipin antibodies); the factor V Leiden mutation; abnormalities of protein C, protein S, or antithrombin; or a prothrombin gene mutation is indicated only if a hypercoagulable disorder is suspected (eg, a young patient without apparent risk factors for stroke). While elevated serum homocysteine is a risk factor for stroke, lowering homocysteine levels with vitamin supplementation has not been shown to decrease stroke risk, and therefore, routinely checking homocysteine is not recommended. Electrocardiography or continuous cardiac monitoring for at least 24 hours will help exclude a recent myocardial infarction or a cardiac arrhythmia that might be serving as a source of embolization. While atrial fibrillation will be discovered in approximately 10% of patients with ischemic stroke during their hospitalization, it is estimated that an arrhythmia will be found in an additional 10% with continuous cardiac event monitoring after discharge; this testing is indicated in cases where atrial fibrillation is suspected (eg, nonlacunar stroke and left atrial enlargement on echocardiography or lack of intracranial or carotid atherosclerosis) but has not been demonstrated. Echocardiography (with agitated saline contrast) should be performed in cases of nonlacunar stroke to exclude valvular disease, left-to-right shunting, and cardiac thrombus. Blood cultures should be performed if endocarditis is suspected but are not required routinely. Examination of the cerebrospinal fluid is not always necessary but may be helpful if cerebral vasculitis or another inflammatory or infectious cause of stroke is suspected, but it should be delayed until after CT or MRI to exclude any risk for herniation due to mass effect.

▶ Treatment

Management is divided into acute and chronic phases, the first aimed at minimizing disability and the second aimed at preventing recurrent stroke. The most important initial determination is the time at which the patient was last normal; this is considered the time of stroke onset. If patients receive medical attention within 6 hours of stroke onset, a CT and CT angiogram should be performed to rule out hemorrhage and to identify large vessel occlusions.

Intravenous thrombolytic therapy with recombinant tissue plasminogen activator (rtPA; 0.9 mg/kg to a maximum of 90 mg, with 10% given as a bolus over 1 minute and the remainder over 1 hour) improves the chance of recovery without significant disability at 90 days from 26% to 39% if given within 3 hours from stroke onset; it is still effective up to 4.5 hours from stroke onset. Treatment should be initiated as soon as possible; outcome is directly related to the time from stroke onset to treatment. Intravenous thrombolysis is approved in Europe for use up to 4.5 hours from stroke onset but only for up to 3 hours in the United States although off-label use during the 3- to 4.5-hour window is standard.

The risk of rtPA is hemorrhage; when given beyond 4.5 hours, the risk of intracerebral hemorrhage outweighs any benefit. Contraindications to rtPA include the following: (1) significant head trauma or prior stroke in the previous 3 months, (2) symptoms suggestive of subarachnoid hemorrhage, (3) recent arterial puncture at a noncompressible site, (4) previous intracranial hemorrhage, (5) intracranial neoplasm or arteriovenous malformation, (6) recent intracranial or intraspinal surgery, (7) active internal bleeding or bleeding diathesis (eg, platelets less than 100,000/mcL, recent use of heparin with an elevated aPTT, INR greater than 1.7, current use of direct thrombin or factor Xa inhibitors), (8) glucose less than 50 mg/dL (2.7 mmol/L), (9) large cerebral infarction on CT, and (10) systolic pressure greater than 185 mm Hg or diastolic pressure greater than 110 mm Hg. The blood pressure should be lowered immediately to less than 185/110 mm Hg to enable rtPA administration. Additional relative contraindications include minor stroke, seizure at stroke onset, pregnancy, major surgery within previous 14 days, gastrointestinal or urinary tract hemorrhage within previous 21 days, and myocardial infarction within previous 3 months.

Several randomized trials have demonstrated an increased likelihood of achieving functional independence with the use of endovascular mechanical embolectomy by stent retrievers as an adjunct to intravenous rtPA. Only patients with large vessel occlusion (about 20% of patients with acute ischemic stroke) are eligible for embolectomy, which must be performed within 6 hours of stroke onset.

Early management of a completed stroke otherwise requires general supportive measures. Management in a stroke care unit has been shown to improve outcomes, likely due to early rehabilitation and prevention of medical complications. During the acute stage, there may be marked brain swelling and edema, with symptoms and signs of increasing intracranial pressure, an increasing neurologic deficit, or herniation syndrome. Elevated intracranial pressure is managed by head elevation and osmotic agents such as mannitol. Maintenance of an adequate cerebral perfusion pressure helps prevent further ischemia. Early decompressive hemicraniectomy (within 48 hours of stroke onset) for malignant middle cerebral artery infarctions reduces mortality and improves functional outcome. Attempts to lower the blood pressure of hypertensive patients during the acute phase (ie, within 72 hours) of a stroke should generally be avoided unless the purpose is to enable the safe administration of rtPA, as there is loss of cerebral autoregulation, and lowering the blood pressure may further compromise ischemic areas. However, if the systolic pressure exceeds 220 mm Hg, it can be lowered using intravenous labetalol or nicardipine with continuous monitoring to 170–200 mm Hg and then, after 72 hours, it can be reduced further to less than 140/90 mm Hg. Blood pressure augmentation is usually not necessary in patients with relative hypotension but maintenance of intravenous hydration is important.

Prophylactic and medical measures were discussed earlier in the section on TIAs and should guide management. In patients not eligible for thrombolytic therapy and in whom hemorrhage has been excluded by CT, the immediate administration of aspirin 325 mg orally daily is indicated. Anticoagulant drugs are started when indicated, as discussed earlier in the section on TIAs. There is generally no advantage in delay, and the common fear of causing hemorrhage into a previously infarcted area is misplaced, since there is a far greater risk of further embolism to the cerebral circulation if treatment is withheld.

Physical therapy has an important role in the management of patients with impaired motor function. Passive movements at an early stage will help prevent contractures. As cooperation increases and some recovery begins, active movements will improve strength and coordination. In all cases, early mobilization and active rehabilitation are important. Occupational therapy may improve morale and motor skills, while speech therapy may help expressive dysphasia or dysarthria. Because of the risk for dysphagia following stroke, access to food and drink is typically restricted until an appropriate swallowing evaluation; the head of the bed should be kept elevated to prevent aspiration. Urinary catheters should not be placed and, if placed, removed within 24–48 hours.

▶ **Prognosis**

The prognosis for survival after cerebral infarction is better than after cerebral or subarachnoid hemorrhage. Patients receiving treatment with rtPA are at least 30% more likely to have minimal or no disability at 3 months than those not treated by this means. Those treated with mechanical embolectomy are also at least 30% more likely to achieve functional independence. Loss of consciousness after a cerebral infarct implies a poorer prognosis than otherwise. The extent of the infarct governs the potential for rehabilitation. Patients who have had a cerebral infarct are at risk for additional strokes and for myocardial infarcts. The prophylactic measures discussed earlier reduce this risk. Antiplatelet therapy (same treatment guidelines as for TIA) reduces the recurrence rate by 30% among patients without a cardiac cause for the stroke who are not candidates for carotid endarterectomy. Nevertheless, the cumulative risk of recurrence of noncardioembolic stroke is still 3–7% annually.

Patients with massive strokes from which meaningful recovery is unlikely should receive palliative care (see Chapter 5).

▶ **When to Refer**

All patients should be referred.

▶ **When to Admit**

All patients should be hospitalized, preferably in a stroke care unit.

Jauch EC et al. Guidelines for the early management of patients with acute ischemic stroke: a guideline for healthcare professionals from the American Heart Association/American Stroke Association. Stroke. 2013 Mar;44(3):870–947. [PMID: 23370205]
Jüttler E et al; DESTINY II Investigators. Hemicraniectomy in older patients with extensive middle-cerebral-artery stroke. N Engl J Med. 2014 Mar 20;370(12):1091–100. [PMID: 24645942]
Mackey J. Evaluation and management of stroke in young adults. Continuum (Minneap Minn). 2014 Apr;20(2 Cerebrovascular Disease):352–69. [PMID: 24699486]
Powers WJ et al. 2015 American Heart Association/American Stroke Association focused update of the 2013 guidelines for the early management of patients with acute ischemic stroke regarding endovascular treatment: a guideline for healthcare professionals from the American Heart Association/American Stroke Association. Stroke. 2015 Oct;46(10):3020–35. [PMID: 26123479]
Prabhakaran S et al. Acute stroke intervention: a systematic review. JAMA. 2015 Apr 14;313(14):1451–62. [PMID: 25871671]

3. Intracerebral Hemorrhage

Spontaneous, nontraumatic intracerebral hemorrhage in patients with no angiographic evidence of an associated vascular anomaly (eg, aneurysm or angioma) is usually due to hypertension. The pathologic basis for hemorrhage is probably the presence of microaneurysms that develop on perforating vessels in hypertensive patients. Hypertensive intracerebral hemorrhage occurs most frequently in the basal ganglia, pons, thalamus, cerebellum and less commonly in the cerebral white matter. Hemorrhage may extend into the ventricular system or subarachnoid space, and signs of meningeal irritation are then found. Hemorrhages usually occur suddenly and without warning, often during activity. In the elderly, cerebral amyloid angiopathy is another important and frequent cause of hemorrhage, which is usually lobar in distribution, sometimes recurrent, and associated with a better prognosis than hypertensive hemorrhage. Arteriovenous malformations are an important cause of intracerebral hemorrhage in younger patients.

Other causes of nontraumatic intracerebral hemorrhage include hematologic and bleeding disorders (eg, leukemia, thrombocytopenia, hemophilia, or disseminated intravascular coagulation), anticoagulant therapy, liver disease, high alcohol intake, and primary or secondary brain tumors. There is also an association with advancing age and male sex. Bleeding is primarily into the subarachnoid space when it occurs from an intracranial aneurysm, but it may be partly intraparenchymal as well. In some cases, no specific cause for cerebral hemorrhage can be identified.

▶ **Clinical Findings**

A. Symptoms and Signs

With hemorrhage into the cerebral hemisphere, consciousness is initially lost or impaired in about one-half of patients. Vomiting occurs very frequently at the onset of bleeding, and headache is sometimes present. Focal symptoms and signs then develop, depending on the site of the hemorrhage. With hypertensive hemorrhage, there is generally a rapidly evolving neurologic deficit with hemiplegia or hemiparesis. A hemisensory disturbance is also present with more deeply placed lesions. With lesions of the putamen, loss of conjugate lateral gaze may be conspicuous. With thalamic hemorrhage, there may be a loss of upward gaze, downward or skew deviation of the eyes, lateral gaze palsies, and pupillary inequalities.

Cerebellar hemorrhage may present with sudden onset of nausea and vomiting, dysequilibrium, headache, and loss of consciousness that may terminate fatally within 48 hours. Less commonly, the onset is gradual and the course episodic or slowly progressive—clinical features suggesting an expanding cerebellar lesion. In yet other cases, however, the onset and course are intermediate, and examination shows lateral conjugate gaze palsies to the side of the lesion; small reactive pupils; contralateral hemiplegia; peripheral facial weakness; ataxia of gait, limbs, or trunk; periodic respiration; or some combination of these findings.

B. Imaging

CT scanning (without contrast) is important not only in confirming that hemorrhage has occurred but also in determining the size and site of the hematoma. MRI is equally sensitive when magnetic susceptibility weighted sequences (eg, gradient echo) are used. If the patient's condition permits further intervention, CT angiography, MR angiography, or cerebral angiography may be undertaken thereafter to determine whether an aneurysm or arteriovenous malformation is present. In patients under age 55 with lobar hemorrhage and no history of hypertension, a contrast-enhanced MRI may indicate a nonhypertensive cause such as an underlying neoplasm.

C. Laboratory and Other Studies

A complete blood count, platelet count, prothrombin and partial thromboplastin times, and liver and kidney function tests may reveal a predisposing cause for the hemorrhage. Lumbar puncture is contraindicated because it may precipitate a herniation syndrome in patients with a large hematoma, and CT scanning is superior in detecting intracerebral hemorrhage.

▶ Treatment

Patients should be admitted to an intensive care unit for observation and supportive care. The systolic blood pressure should be lowered to 140 mm Hg. Thrombocytopenia should be treated with platelet transfusion; the specific threshold for treatment and the goal platelet count after transfusion vary with patient characteristics and provider experience. Coagulopathies should be reversed using fresh frozen plasma, prothrombin complex concentrates, vitamin K, or specific reversal agents (eg, protamine for heparin, idarucizumab for dabigatran). Hemostatic therapy with recombinant activated factor VII in patients without underlying coagulopathy has not improved survival or

functional outcome. Intracranial pressure may require monitoring and osmotic therapy. Ventricular drainage may be required in patients with intraventricular hemorrhage and acute hydrocephalus. Decompression may be helpful when a superficial hematoma in cerebral white matter is exerting a mass effect and causing incipient herniation. In patients with cerebellar hemorrhage, prompt surgical evacuation of the hematoma is appropriate, because spontaneous unpredictable deterioration may otherwise lead to a fatal outcome and because operative treatment may lead to complete resolution of the clinical deficit. The treatment of underlying structural lesions or bleeding disorders depends on their nature. There is no specific treatment for cerebral amyloid angiopathy.

▶ When to Refer

All patients should be referred.

▶ When to Admit

All patients should be hospitalized.

Hemphill JC 3rd et al. Guidelines for the management of spontaneous intracerebral hemorrhage: a guideline for healthcare professionals from the American Heart Association/American Stroke Association. Stroke. 2015 Jul;46(7):2032–60. [PMID: 26022637]

4. Spontaneous Subarachnoid Hemorrhage

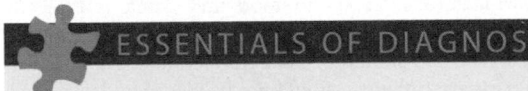 ESSENTIALS OF DIAGNOSIS

- ▶ Sudden severe headache.
- ▶ Signs of meningeal irritation usually present.
- ▶ Obtundation is common.
- ▶ Focal deficits frequently absent.

▶ General Considerations

Between 5% and 10% of strokes are due to subarachnoid hemorrhage. Trauma is the most common cause of subarachnoid hemorrhage, the prognosis of which depends on the severity of the head injury. Spontaneous (nontraumatic) subarachnoid hemorrhage frequently results from the rupture of an arterial saccular ("berry") aneurysm or from an arteriovenous malformation. Occasional patients with aneurysms have headaches, sometimes accompanied by nausea and neck stiffness, a few hours or days before massive subarachnoid hemorrhage occurs. This has been attributed to "warning leaks" of a small amount of blood from the aneurysm.

▶ Clinical Findings

A. Symptoms and Signs

Subarachnoid hemorrhage has a characteristic clinical picture. Its onset is with sudden headache of a severity never experienced previously by the patient. This may be followed by nausea and vomiting and by a loss or impairment of consciousness that can either be transient or progress inexorably to deepening coma and death. If consciousness is regained, the patient is often confused and irritable and may show other symptoms of an altered mental status. Neurologic examination generally reveals nuchal rigidity and other signs of meningeal irritation, except in deeply comatose patients.

Aneurysms may cause a focal neurologic deficit by compressing adjacent structures. However, most are asymptomatic or produce only nonspecific symptoms until they rupture, at which time subarachnoid hemorrhage results. A higher risk of subarachnoid hemorrhage is associated with older age, female sex, "nonwhite" ethnicity, hypertension, tobacco smoking, high alcohol consumption (exceeding 150 g per week), previous symptoms, posterior circulation aneurysms, and larger aneurysms. Focal neurologic signs are usually absent but, when present, may relate either to a focal intracerebral hematoma (from arteriovenous malformations) or to ischemia in the territory of the vessel with a ruptured aneurysm.

B. Imaging

A CT scan (preferably with CT angiography) should be performed immediately to confirm that hemorrhage has occurred and to search for clues regarding its source. It is preferable to MRI because it is faster and more sensitive in detecting hemorrhage in the first 24 hours. CT findings sometimes are normal in patients with suspected hemorrhage, and the cerebrospinal fluid must then be examined for the presence of blood or xanthochromia before the possibility of subarachnoid hemorrhage is discounted.

Cerebral arteriography is undertaken to determine the source of bleeding. In general, bilateral carotid and vertebral arteriography are necessary because aneurysms are often multiple, while arteriovenous malformations may be supplied from several sources. The procedure allows an interventional radiologist to treat an underlying aneurysm or arteriovenous malformation by various techniques. If arteriograms show no abnormality, the examination should be repeated after 2 weeks because vasospasm or thrombus may have prevented detection of an aneurysm or other vascular anomaly during the initial study. CT or MR angiography may also be revealing but is less sensitive than conventional arteriography.

C. Laboratory and Other Studies

The cerebrospinal fluid is bloodstained. Electro-cardiographic evidence of arrhythmias or myocardial ischemia has been well described and probably relates to excessive sympathetic activity. Peripheral leukocytosis and transient glycosuria are also common findings.

▶ Treatment

All patients should be hospitalized and seen by a neurologist. The measures outlined below in the section on stupor and coma are applied to comatose patients. Conscious patients are confined to bed, advised against any exertion or straining, treated symptomatically for headache and anxiety, and given laxatives or stool softeners. The systolic blood pressure should be lowered to 140 mm Hg until the aneurysm is secured. Phenytoin is sometimes prescribed to prevent seizures, but the evidence of benefit is conflicting (see Table 24–3). Patients are generally hospitalized for at least 14 days to monitor, prevent, and treat vasospasm.

The major aim of treatment is to prevent further hemorrhage. The risk of further hemorrhage from a ruptured aneurysm is greatest within a few days of the first hemorrhage; approximately 20% of patients will have further bleeding within 2 weeks and 40% within 6 months. Definitive treatment, ideally within 2 days of the hemorrhage, requires surgical clipping of the aneurysm or endovascular treatment by interventional radiologists; the latter is sometimes feasible even for inoperable aneurysms and has a lower morbidity than surgery.

▶ Complications

Spontaneous subarachnoid hemorrhage may result in severe complications, so monitoring is necessary, usually in an intensive care unit. Hemiplegia or other focal deficit sometimes may follow aneurysmal bleeding after a delay of 2–14 days due to focal arterial spasm. The etiology of vasospasm is uncertain and likely multifactorial, and it sometimes leads to significant cerebral ischemia or infarction and may further aggravate any existing increase in intracranial pressure. Transcranial Doppler ultrasound may be used to screen noninvasively for vasospasm, but conventional arteriography is required to document and treat vasospasm when the clinical suspicion is high. Nimodipine has been shown to reduce the incidence of ischemic deficits from arterial spasm. The dose of nimodipine is 60 mg every 4 hours orally for 21 days. After surgical obliteration of all aneurysms, symptomatic vasospasm may also be treated by intravascular volume expansion and induced hypertension; transluminal balloon angioplasty of involved intracranial vessels is also helpful. Aspirin provides no benefit. Prophylactic administration of intravenous magnesium sulfate does not change overall clinical outcomes.

Acute hydrocephalus, which sometimes occurs due to cerebrospinal fluid outflow disruption by the subarachnoid blood, should be suspected if the patient deteriorates clinically; a repeat CT scan should be obtained. Acute hydrocephalus frequently causes intracranial hypertension severe enough to require temporary, and less commonly prolonged or permanent, intraventricular cerebrospinal fluid shunting. Renal salt-wasting is another complication of subarachnoid hemorrhage that may develop abruptly during the first several days of hospitalization. The resulting hyponatremia and cerebral edema may exacerbate intracranial hypertension and may require carefully titrated treatment with oral sodium chloride or intravenous hyperosmotic sodium solution. Daily measurement of the serum sodium level allows for the early detection of this complication. Hypopituitarism may occur as a late complication of subarachnoid hemorrhage.

Blok KM et al. CT within 6 hours of headache onset to rule out subarachnoid hemorrhage in nonacademic hospitals. Neurology. 2015 May 12;84(19):1927–32. [PMID: 25862794]

Perry JJ et al. Differentiation between traumatic tap and aneurysmal subarachnoid hemorrhage: prospective cohort study. BMJ. 2015 Feb 18;350:h568. [PMID: 25694274]

Raya AK et al. Treatment of subarachnoid hemorrhage. Crit Care Clin. 2014 Oct;30(4):719–33. [PMID: 25257737]

5. Intracranial Aneurysm

ESSENTIALS OF DIAGNOSIS

▶ Subarachnoid hemorrhage or focal deficit.

▶ Abnormal imaging studies.

General Considerations

Saccular aneurysms ("berry" aneurysms) tend to occur at arterial bifurcations, are frequently multiple (20% of cases), and are usually asymptomatic. They may be associated with polycystic kidney disease and coarctation of the aorta. Risk factors for aneurysm formation include smoking, hypertension, and hypercholesterolemia. Most aneurysms are located on the anterior part of the circle of Willis—particularly on the anterior or posterior communicating arteries, at the bifurcation of the middle cerebral artery, and at the bifurcation of the internal carotid artery. Mycotic aneurysms resulting from septic embolism occur in more distal vessels and often at the cortical surface. The most significant complication of intracranial aneurysms is a subarachnoid hemorrhage, which is discussed in the preceding section. A higher risk of subarachnoid hemorrhage is associated with older age, female sex, "non-white" ethnicity, hypertension, tobacco smoking, high alcohol consumption (exceeding 150 g per week), previous symptoms, posterior circulation aneurysms, and larger aneurysms.

Clinical Findings

A. Symptoms and Signs

Aneurysms may cause a focal neurologic deficit by compressing adjacent structures. However, most are asymptomatic or produce only nonspecific symptoms until they rupture, at which time subarachnoid hemorrhage results. Its manifestations, complications, and management were outlined in the preceding section.

B. Imaging

Definitive evaluation is by angiography (bilateral carotid and vertebral studies), which generally indicates the size and site of the lesion, sometimes reveals multiple aneurysms, and may show arterial spasm if rupture has occurred. Visualization by CT or MR angiography is not usually adequate if operative treatment is under consideration because lesions may be multiple and small lesions are sometimes missed.

Treatment

The major aim of treatment is to prevent hemorrhage. Management of ruptured aneurysms was described in the section on subarachnoid hemorrhage. Symptomatic but unruptured aneurysms merit prompt treatment, either surgically or by endovascular techniques, whereas small asymptomatic ones discovered incidentally are often monitored arteriographically and corrected only if they increase in size to over 10 mm.

When to Refer

All patients should be referred.

When to Admit

• All patients with a subarachnoid hemorrhage.

• All patients for detailed imaging.

• All patients undergoing surgical or endovascular treatment.

Brown RD Jr et al. Unruptured intracranial aneurysms: epidemiology, natural history, management options, and familial screening. Lancet Neurol. 2014 Apr;13(4):393–404. [PMID: 24646873]

Greving JP et al. Development of the PHASES score for prediction of risk of rupture of intracranial aneurysms: a pooled analysis of six prospective cohort studies. Lancet Neurol. 2014 Jan;13(1):59–66. [PMID: 24290159]

6. Arteriovenous Malformations

ESSENTIALS OF DIAGNOSIS

▶ Sudden onset of subarachnoid and intracerebral hemorrhage.

▶ Distinctive neurologic signs reflect the region of the brain involved.

▶ Signs of meningeal irritation in patients presenting with subarachnoid hemorrhage.

▶ Seizures or focal deficits may occur.

General Considerations

Arteriovenous malformations are congenital vascular malformations that result from a localized maldevelopment of part of the primitive vascular plexus and consist of abnormal arteriovenous communications without intervening capillaries. They vary in size, ranging from massive lesions that are fed by multiple vessels and involve a large part of the brain to lesions so small that they are hard to identify at arteriography, surgery, or autopsy. In approximately 10% of cases, there is an associated arterial aneurysm, while 1–2% of patients presenting with aneurysms have associated arteriovenous malformations. Clinical presentation may relate to hemorrhage from the malformation or an associated aneurysm or may relate to cerebral ischemia due to diversion of blood by the anomalous arteriovenous shunt or due to venous stagnation. Regional maldevelopment of the brain, compression or distortion of adjacent cerebral tissue by enlarged anomalous vessels, and progressive gliosis due to mechanical and ischemic factors may also be contributory. In addition, communicating or obstructive hydrocephalus may occur and lead to symptoms.

► Clinical Findings

A. Symptoms and Signs

1. Supratentorial lesions—Most cerebral arteriovenous malformations are supratentorial, usually lying in the territory of the middle cerebral artery. Initial symptoms consist of hemorrhage in 30–60% of cases, recurrent seizures in 20–40%, headache in 5–25%, and miscellaneous complaints (including focal deficits) in 10–15%. Up to 70% of arteriovenous malformations bleed at some point in their natural history, most commonly before the patient reaches the age of 40 years. This tendency to bleed is unrelated to the lesion site or to the patient's sex, but small arteriovenous malformations are more likely to bleed than large ones. Arteriovenous malformations that have bled once are more likely to bleed again. Hemorrhage is commonly intracerebral as well as into the subarachnoid space, and it has a fatal outcome in about 10% of cases. Focal or generalized seizures may accompany or follow hemorrhage, or they may be the initial presentation, especially with frontal or parietal arteriovenous malformations. Headaches are especially likely when the external carotid arteries are involved in the malformation. These sometimes simulate migraine but more commonly are nonspecific in character, with nothing about them to suggest an underlying structural lesion.

In patients presenting with subarachnoid hemorrhage, examination may reveal an abnormal mental status and signs of meningeal irritation. Additional findings may help localize the lesion and sometimes indicate that intracranial pressure is increased. A cranial bruit always suggests the possibility of a cerebral arteriovenous malformation, but bruits may also be found with aneurysms, meningiomas, acquired arteriovenous fistulas, and arteriovenous malformations involving the scalp, calvarium, or orbit. Bruits are best heard over the ipsilateral eye or mastoid region and are of some help in lateralization but of no help in localization. Absence of a bruit does not exclude the possibility of arteriovenous malformation.

2. Infratentorial lesions—Brainstem arteriovenous malformations are often clinically silent, but they may hemorrhage, cause obstructive hydrocephalus, or lead to progressive or relapsing brainstem deficits. Cerebellar arteriovenous malformations may also be clinically inconspicuous but sometimes lead to cerebellar hemorrhage.

B. Imaging

In patients presenting with suspected hemorrhage, CT scanning indicates whether subarachnoid or intracerebral bleeding has recently occurred, helps localize its source, and may reveal the arteriovenous malformation. If the CT scan shows no evidence of bleeding but subarachnoid hemorrhage is diagnosed clinically, a lumbar puncture should be performed to examine the cerebrospinal fluid for blood.

When intracranial hemorrhage is confirmed but the source of hemorrhage is not evident on the CT scan, arteriography is necessary to exclude aneurysm or arteriovenous malformation. MR and CT angiography are not sensitive enough for this purpose. Even if the findings on CT scan suggest arteriovenous malformation, arteriography is required to establish the nature of the lesion with certainty and to determine its anatomic features so that treatment can be planned. The examination must generally include bilateral opacification of the internal and external carotid arteries and the vertebral arteries. Arteriovenous malformations typically appear as a tangled vascular mass with distended tortuous afferent and efferent vessels, a rapid circulation time, and arteriovenous shunting.

In patients presenting without hemorrhage, CT scan or MRI usually reveals the underlying abnormality, and MRI frequently also shows evidence of old or recent hemorrhage that may have been asymptomatic. The nature and detailed anatomy of any focal lesion identified by these means are delineated by angiography, especially if operative treatment is under consideration.

C. Laboratory and Other Studies

Electroencephalography is usually indicated in patients presenting with seizures and may show consistently focal or lateralized abnormalities resulting from the underlying cerebral arteriovenous malformation. This should be followed by CT scanning.

► Treatment

Surgical treatment to prevent further hemorrhage is justified in patients with arteriovenous malformations that have bled, provided that the lesion is accessible and the patient has a reasonable life expectancy. Surgical treatment is also appropriate if intracranial pressure is increased and to prevent further progression of a focal neurologic deficit. In patients presenting solely with seizures, anticonvulsant drug treatment is usually sufficient, and operative treatment is unnecessary unless seizures cannot be controlled medically.

Definitive operative treatment consists of excision of the arteriovenous malformation if it is surgically accessible. Arteriovenous malformations that are inoperable because of their location are sometimes treated solely by embolization; although the risk of hemorrhage is not reduced, neurologic deficits may be stabilized or even reversed by this procedure. Two other techniques for the treatment of intracerebral arteriovenous malformations are injection of a vascular occlusive polymer through a flow-guided microcatheter and permanent occlusion of feeding vessels by positioning detachable balloon catheters in the desired sites and then inflating them with quickly solidifying contrast material. Stereotactic radiosurgery is also useful in the management of inoperable cerebral arteriovenous malformations.

▶ When to Refer

All patients should be referred.

▶ When to Admit

- All patients with a subarachnoid or cerebral hemorrhage.
- All patients for detailed imaging.
- All patients undergoing surgical or endovascular treatment.

Asif K et al. Cerebral arteriovenous malformation diagnosis and management. Semin Neurol. 2013 Nov;33(5):468–75. [PMID: 24504610]

Mohr JP et al; international ARUBA investigators. Medical management with or without interventional therapy for unruptured brain arteriovenous malformations (ARUBA): a multicentre, non-blinded, randomised trial. Lancet. 2014 Feb 15;383(9917):614–21. [PMID: 24268105]

7. Intracranial Venous Thrombosis

Intracranial venous thrombosis may occur in association with intracranial or maxillofacial infections, hypercoagulable states, polycythemia, sickle cell disease, and cyanotic congenital heart disease and in pregnancy or during the puerperium. Genetic factors are also important. The disorder is characterized by headache, focal or generalized convulsions, drowsiness, confusion, increased intracranial pressure, and focal neurologic deficits—and sometimes by evidence of meningeal irritation. The diagnosis is confirmed by CT or MR venography or angiography.

Treatment includes anticonvulsant drugs if seizures have occurred and—if necessary— measures to reduce intracranial pressure. Anticoagulation with dose-adjusted intravenous heparin or weight-adjusted subcutaneous low-molecular-weight heparin, followed by oral warfarin anticoagulation for 6 months reduces morbidity and mortality of venous sinus thrombosis. Concomitant intracranial hemorrhage related to the venous thrombosis does not contraindicate heparin therapy. In cases refractory to heparin, endovascular techniques including catheter-directed thrombolytic therapy (urokinase) and thrombectomy, are sometimes helpful but may increase the risk for major hemorrhage.

▶ When to Refer

All patients should be referred.

▶ When to Admit

All patients should be hospitalized.

Bushnell C et al. Evaluation and management of cerebral venous thrombosis. Continuum (Minneap Minn). 2014 Apr;20 (2 Cerebrovascular Disease):335–51. [PMID: 24699485]

8. Spinal Cord Vascular Diseases

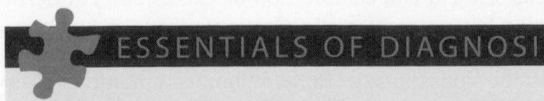

▶ Sudden onset of back or limb pain and neurologic deficit in limbs.

▶ Motor, sensory, or reflex changes in limbs depending on level of lesion.

▶ Imaging studies distinguish between infarct and hematoma.

▶ Infarction of the Spinal Cord

Infarction of the spinal cord is rare. It typically occurs in the territory of the anterior spinal artery because this vessel, which supplies the anterior two-thirds of the cord, is itself supplied by only a limited number of feeders. Infarction usually results from interrupted flow in one or more of these feeders, eg, with aortic dissection, aortography, polyarteritis, or severe hypotension, or after surgical resection of the thoracic aorta. The paired posterior spinal arteries, by contrast, are supplied by numerous arteries at different levels of the cord. Spinal cord hypoperfusion may lead to a central cord syndrome with distal weakness of lower motor neuron type and loss of pain and temperature appreciation, with preserved posterior column function.

Since the anterior spinal artery receives numerous feeders in the cervical region, infarcts almost always occur caudally. Clinical presentation is characterized by acute onset of flaccid, areflexive paraplegia that evolves after a few days or weeks into a spastic paraplegia with extensor plantar responses. There is an accompanying dissociated sensory loss, with impairment of appreciation of pain and temperature but preservation of sensations of vibration and position.

The risk of spinal cord infarction in the setting of abdominal aortic surgery and thoracic endovascular repair may be reduced by intraoperative cerebrospinal fluid drainage through a catheter placed in the lumbar subarachnoid space to reduce intraspinal pressure. If signs of infarction are noted after surgery, blood pressure augmentation for 24–48 hours in addition to lumbar drainage has been noted anecdotally to improve outcomes. Treatment is otherwise symptomatic.

▶ Epidural or Subdural Hemorrhage

Epidural or subdural hemorrhage may lead to sudden severe back pain followed by an acute compressive myelopathy necessitating urgent spinal MRI or myelography and surgical evacuation. It may occur in patients with bleeding disorders or those who are taking anticoagulant drugs, sometimes following trauma or lumbar puncture. Epidural hemorrhage may also be related to a vascular malformation or tumor deposit.

▶ Spinal Dural Arteriovenous Fistulae

Spinal dural arteriovenous fistulae are congenital lesions that present with spinal subarachnoid hemorrhage or myeloradiculopathy. Since most of these malformations are located in the thoracolumbar region, they lead to motor and sensory disturbances in the legs and to sphincter disorders. Pain in the legs or back is often severe. Examination reveals an upper, lower, or mixed motor deficit in the legs; sensory deficits are also present and are usually extensive, although occasionally they are confined to a radicular distribution. Cervical spinal dural arteriovenous fistulae lead also to symptoms and signs in the arms. Spinal MRI may not detect the spinal dural arteriovenous fistula although most cases show either T2 hyperintensity in the cord or perimedullary flow voids. Myelography (performed with the patient prone and supine) may detect serpiginous filling defects due to enlarged vessels. Selective spinal arteriography is required to confirm the diagnosis and plan treatment. Most lesions are extramedullary, are posterior to the cord (lying either intradurally or extradurally), and can easily be treated by ligation of feeding vessels and excision of the fistulous anomaly or by embolization procedures. Delay in treatment may lead to increased and irreversible disability or to death from recurrent subarachnoid hemorrhage.

► When to Refer

All patients should be referred.

► When to Admit

All patients should be hospitalized.

Rabinstein AA. Vascular myelopathies. Continuum (Minneap Minn). 2015 Feb;21(1 Spinal Cord Disorders):67–83. [PMID: 25651218]

INTRACRANIAL & SPINAL MASS LESIONS

1. Primary Intracranial Tumors

ESSENTIALS OF DIAGNOSIS

- ► Generalized or focal disturbance of cerebral function, or both.
- ► Increased intracranial pressure in some patients.
- ► Neuroradiologic evidence of space-occupying lesion.

► General Considerations

Half of all primary intracranial neoplasms (Table 24–5) are gliomas, and the remainder are meningiomas, pituitary adenomas (see Chapter 26), neurofibromas, and other tumors. Certain tumors, especially neurofibromas, hemangioblastomas, and retinoblastomas, may have a familial basis, and congenital factors bear on the development of craniopharyngiomas. Tumors may occur at any age, but certain gliomas show particular age predilections.

► Clinical Findings

A. Symptoms and Signs

Intracranial tumors may lead to a generalized disturbance of cerebral function and to symptoms and signs of increased intracranial pressure. In consequence, there may be personality changes, intellectual decline, emotional lability, seizures, headaches, nausea, and malaise. If the pressure is increased in a particular cranial compartment, brain tissue may herniate into a compartment with lower pressure. The most familiar syndrome is herniation of the temporal lobe uncus through the tentorial hiatus, which causes compression of the third cranial nerve, midbrain, and posterior cerebral artery. The earliest sign of this is ipsilateral pupillary dilation, followed by stupor, coma, decerebrate posturing, and respiratory arrest. Another important herniation syndrome consists of displacement of the cerebellar tonsils through the foramen magnum, which causes medullary compression leading to apnea, circulatory collapse, and death. Other herniation syndromes are less common and of less clear clinical importance.

Intracranial tumors also lead to focal deficits depending on their location.

1. Frontal lobe lesions—Tumors of the frontal lobe often lead to progressive intellectual decline, slowing of mental activity, personality changes, and contralateral grasp reflexes. They may lead to expressive aphasia if the posterior part of the left inferior frontal gyrus is involved. Anosmia may also occur as a consequence of pressure on the olfactory nerve. Precentral lesions may cause focal motor seizures or contralateral pyramidal deficits.

2. Temporal lobe lesions—Tumors of the uncinate region may be manifested by seizures with olfactory or gustatory hallucinations, motor phenomena such as licking or smacking of the lips, and some impairment of external awareness without actual loss of consciousness. Temporal lobe lesions also lead to depersonalization, emotional changes, behavioral disturbances, sensations of déjà vu or jamais vu, micropsia or macropsia (objects appear smaller or larger than they are), visual field defects (crossed upper quadrantanopia), and auditory illusions or hallucinations. Left-sided lesions may lead to dysnomia and receptive aphasia, while right-sided involvement sometimes disturbs the perception of musical notes and melodies.

3. Parietal lobe lesions—Tumors in this location characteristically cause contralateral disturbances of sensation and may cause sensory seizures, sensory loss or inattention, or some combination of these symptoms. The sensory loss is cortical in type and involves postural sensibility and tactile discrimination, so that the appreciation of shape, size, weight, and texture is impaired. Objects placed in the hand may not be recognized (astereognosis). Extensive parietal lobe lesions may produce contralateral hyperpathia and spontaneous pain (thalamic syndrome). Involvement of the optic radiation leads to a contralateral homonymous field defect that sometimes consists solely of lower quadrantanopia. Lesions of the left angular gyrus cause Gerstmann syndrome (a combination of alexia, agraphia, acalculia, right-left confusion, and finger agnosia), whereas involvement of the left submarginal gyrus

Table 24–5. Primary intracranial tumors.

Tumor	Clinical Features	Treatment and Prognosis
Glioblastoma multiforme	Presents commonly with nonspecific complaints and increased intracranial pressure. As it grows, focal deficits develop.	Course is rapidly progressive, with poor prognosis. Total surgical removal is usually not possible. Radiation therapy and chemotherapy may prolong survival.
Astrocytoma	Presentation similar to glioblastoma multiforme but course more protracted, often over several years. Cerebellar astrocytoma may have a more benign course.	Prognosis is variable. By the time of diagnosis, total excision is usually impossible; tumor may be radiosensitive and chemotherapy may also be helpful. In cerebellar astrocytoma, total surgical removal is often possible.
Medulloblastoma	Seen most frequently in children. Generally arises from roof of fourth ventricle and leads to increased intracranial pressure accompanied by brainstem and cerebellar signs. May seed subarachnoid space.	Treatment consists of surgery combined with radiation therapy and chemotherapy.
Ependymoma	Glioma arising from the ependyma of a ventricle, especially the fourth ventricle; leads to early signs of increased intracranial pressure. Arises also from central canal of cord.	Tumor is best treated surgically if possible. Radiation therapy may be used for residual tumor.
Oligodendroglioma	Slow-growing. Usually arises in cerebral hemisphere in adults. Calcification may be visible on skull radiograph.	Treatment is surgical and usually successful. Radiation and chemotherapy may be used if tumor has malignant features.
Brainstem glioma	Presents during childhood with cranial nerve palsies and then with long tract signs in the limbs. Signs of increased intracranial pressure occur late.	Tumor is inoperable; treatment is by irradiation and shunt for increased intracranial pressure.
Cerebellar hemangioblastoma	Presents with dysequilibrium, ataxia of trunk or limbs, and signs of increased intracranial pressure. Sometimes familial. May be associated with retinal and spinal vascular lesions, polycythemia, and renal cell carcinoma.	Treatment is surgical. Radiation is used for residual tumor.
Pineal tumor	Presents with increased intracranial pressure, sometimes associated with impaired upward gaze (Parinaud syndrome) and other deficits indicative of midbrain lesion.	Ventricular decompression by shunting is followed by surgical approach to tumor; irradiation is indicated if tumor is malignant. Prognosis depends on histopathologic findings and extent of tumor.
Craniopharyngioma	Originates from remnants of Rathke pouch above the sella, depressing the optic chiasm. May present at any age but usually in childhood, with endocrine dysfunction and bitemporal visual field defects.	Treatment is surgical, but total removal may not be possible. Radiation may be used for residual tumor.
Acoustic neurinoma	Ipsilateral hearing loss is most common initial symptom. Subsequent symptoms may include tinnitus, headache, vertigo, facial weakness or numbness, and long tract signs. (May be familial and bilateral when related to neurofibromatosis.) Most sensitive screening tests are MRI and brainstem auditory evoked potential.	Treatment is excision by translabyrinthine surgery, craniectomy, or a combined approach. Outcome is usually good.
Meningioma	Originates from the dura mater or arachnoid; compresses rather than invades adjacent neural structures. Increasingly common with advancing age. Tumor size varies greatly. Symptoms vary with tumor site—eg, unilateral proptosis (sphenoidal ridge); anosmia and optic nerve compression (olfactory groove). Tumor is usually benign and readily detected by CT scanning; may lead to calcification and bone erosion visible on plain radiographs of skull.	Treatment is surgical. Tumor may recur if removal is incomplete.
Primary cerebral lymphoma	Associated with AIDS and other immunodeficient states. Presentation may be with focal deficits or with disturbances of cognition and consciousness. May be indistinguishable from cerebral toxoplasmosis.	Treatment is high-dose methotrexate and corticosteroids followed by radiation therapy. Prognosis depends on CD4 count at diagnosis.

causes ideational apraxia. Anosognosia (the denial, neglect, or rejection of a paralyzed limb) is seen in patients with lesions of the nondominant (right) hemisphere. Constructional apraxia and dressing apraxia may also occur with right-sided lesions.

4. Occipital lobe lesions—Tumors of the occipital lobe characteristically produce crossed homonymous hemianopia or a partial field defect. With left-sided or bilateral lesions, there may be visual agnosia both for objects and for colors, while irritative lesions on either side can cause unformed visual hallucinations. Bilateral occipital lobe involvement causes cortical blindness in which there is preservation of pupillary responses to light and lack of awareness of the defect by the patient. There may also be loss of color perception, prosopagnosia (inability to identify a familiar face), simultagnosia (inability to integrate and interpret a composite scene as opposed to its individual elements), and Balint syndrome (failure to turn the eyes to a particular point in space, despite preservation of spontaneous and reflex eye movements). The denial of blindness or a field defect constitutes Anton syndrome.

5. Brainstem and cerebellar lesions—Brainstem lesions lead to cranial nerve palsies, ataxia, incoordination, nystagmus, and pyramidal and sensory deficits in the limbs on one or both sides. Intrinsic brainstem tumors, such as gliomas, tend to produce an increase in intracranial pressure only late in their course. Cerebellar tumors produce marked ataxia of the trunk if the vermis cerebelli is involved and ipsilateral appendicular deficits (ataxia, incoordination and hypotonia of the limbs) if the cerebellar hemispheres are affected.

6. False localizing signs—Tumors may lead to neurologic signs other than by direct compression or infiltration, thereby leading to errors of clinical localization. These false localizing signs include third or sixth nerve palsy and bilateral extensor plantar responses produced by herniation syndromes, and an extensor plantar response occurring ipsilateral to a hemispheric tumor as a result of compression of the opposite cerebral peduncle against the tentorium.

B. Imaging

MRI with gadolinium enhancement is the preferred method to detect the lesion and to define its location, shape, and size; the extent to which normal anatomy is distorted; and the degree of any associated cerebral edema or mass effect. CT scanning with radiocontrast enhancement could be performed; however, it is less helpful than MRI for small lesions or tumors in the posterior fossa. Newer neuroimaging techniques may help identify brain tumors by increased blood perfusion (perfusion-weighted MRI, single photon-emission computed tomography, positron-emission tomography) and high metabolism or cell turnover (magnetic resonance spectroscopy, positron-emission tomography), but non-neoplastic diseases, such as stroke and inflammatory or infectious diseases, are sometimes associated with hyperperfusion and hypermetabolism. Diffusion-weighted MRI may also be helpful. Arteriography is largely reserved for presurgical embolization of highly vascular tumors. In patients with normal hormone levels and an intrasellar mass, angiography is sometimes necessary to distinguish with confidence between a pituitary adenoma and an arterial aneurysm.

C. Laboratory and Other Studies

The electroencephalogram provides supporting information concerning cerebral function and may show either a focal disturbance due to the neoplasm or a more diffuse change reflecting altered mental status. Lumbar puncture is rarely necessary; the findings are seldom diagnostic, and the procedure carries the risk of causing a herniation syndrome.

▶ Treatment

Treatment depends on the type and site of the tumor (Table 24–5) and the condition of the patient. Some benign tumors, especially meningiomas discovered incidentally during brain imaging for another purpose, may be monitored with serial annual imaging. For symptomatic tumors, complete surgical removal may be possible if the tumor is extra-axial (eg, meningioma, acoustic neuroma) or is not in a critical or inaccessible region of the brain (eg, cerebellar hemangioblastoma). Surgery also permits the diagnosis to be verified and may be beneficial in reducing intracranial pressure and relieving symptoms even if the neoplasm cannot be completely removed. Clinical deficits are sometimes due in part to obstructive hydrocephalus, in which case simple surgical shunting procedures often produce dramatic benefit. In patients with malignant gliomas, survival correlates to the extent of initial resection. Radiation therapy increases median survival rates regardless of any preceding surgery, and its combination with chemotherapy provides additional benefit. Indications for irradiation in the treatment of patients with other primary intracranial neoplasms depend on tumor type and accessibility and the feasibility of complete surgical removal. Temozolomide is a commonly used oral and intravenous chemotherapeutic for gliomas, and the use of monoclonal antibodies like bevacizumab as a component of therapy may be helpful (see Table 39–4). Corticosteroids help reduce cerebral edema and are usually started before surgery. Herniation is treated with intravenous dexamethasone (10–20 mg as a bolus, followed by 4 mg every 6 hours) and intravenous mannitol (20% solution given in a dose of 1.5 g/kg over about 30 minutes). Anticonvulsants are also commonly administered in standard doses (see Table 24–3) but are not indicated for prophylaxis in patients who have no history of seizures. Long-term neurocognitive deficits may complicate radiation therapy. For those patients whose disease deteriorates despite treatment, palliative care is important (see Chapter 5).

▶ When to Refer

All patients should be referred.

▶ When to Admit

- All patients with increased intracranial pressure.
- All patients requiring biopsy, surgical treatment, or shunting procedures.

Hoang-Xuan K et al. Diagnosis and treatment of primary CNS lymphoma in immunocompetent patients: guidelines from the European Association for Neuro-Oncology. Lancet Oncol. 2015 Jul;16(7):e322–32. [PMID: 26149884]

Olson JJ et al; AANS/CNS Joint Guidelines Committee. The role of targeted therapies in the management of progressive glioblastoma: a systematic review and evidence-based clinical practice guideline. J Neurooncol. 2014 Jul;118(3):557–99. [PMID: 24740195]

2. Metastatic Intracranial Tumors

A. Cerebral Metastases

Metastatic brain tumors present in the same way as other cerebral neoplasms, ie, with increased intracranial pressure, with focal or diffuse disturbance of cerebral function, or with both of these manifestations. Indeed, in patients with a single cerebral lesion, the metastatic nature of the lesion may become evident only on histopathologic examination. In other patients, there is evidence of widespread metastatic disease, or an isolated cerebral metastasis develops during treatment of the primary neoplasm.

The most common source of intracranial metastasis is carcinoma of the lung; other primary sites are the breast, kidney, skin (melanoma), and gastrointestinal tract. Most cerebral metastases are located supratentorially. Laboratory and radiologic studies used to evaluate patients with metastases are those described for primary neoplasms. They include MRI and CT scanning performed both with and without contrast material. Lumbar puncture is necessary only in patients with suspected carcinomatous meningitis. In patients with verified cerebral metastasis from an unknown primary, investigation is guided by symptoms and signs. In women, mammography is indicated; in men under 50, germ cell origin is sought since both have therapeutic implications.

In patients with only a single, surgically accessible cerebral metastasis who are otherwise well (ie, a high level of functioning and little or no evidence of extracranial disease), it may be possible to remove the lesion and then treat with irradiation; the latter may also be selected as the sole treatment. In patients with multiple metastases or widespread systemic disease, the prognosis is poor; stereotactic radiosurgery, whole-brain radiotherapy, or both, may help in some instances, but in others treatment is palliative only.

Ba JL et al. Current and emerging treatments for brain metastases. Oncology (Williston Park). 2015 Apr;29(4):250–7. [PMID: 25952487]

B. Leptomeningeal Metastases (Carcinomatous Meningitis)

The neoplasms metastasizing most commonly to the leptomeninges are carcinoma of the breast, lymphomas, and leukemia (see Chapter 39). Leptomeningeal metastases lead to multifocal neurologic deficits, which may be associated with infiltration of cranial and spinal nerve roots, direct invasion of the brain or spinal cord, obstructive or communicating hydrocephalus, or some combination of these factors.

The diagnosis is confirmed by examination of the cerebrospinal fluid. Findings may include elevated cerebrospinal fluid pressure, pleocytosis, increased protein concentration, and decreased glucose concentration. Cytologic studies may indicate that malignant cells are present; if not, lumbar puncture should be repeated at least twice to obtain further samples for analysis.

CT scans showing contrast enhancement in the basal cisterns or showing hydrocephalus without any evidence of a mass lesion support the diagnosis. Gadolinium-enhanced MRI frequently shows enhancing foci in the leptomeninges. Myelography may show deposits on multiple nerve roots.

Treatment is by irradiation to symptomatic areas, combined with intrathecal chemotherapy in select patients. The long-term prognosis is poor—only about 10% of patients survive for 1 year—and palliative care is therefore important (see Chapter 5).

Passarin MG et al. Leptomeningeal metastasis from solid tumors: a diagnostic and therapeutic challenge. Neurol Sci. 2015 Jan; 36(1):117–23. [PMID: 25022241]

3. Intracranial Mass Lesions in AIDS Patients

Primary cerebral lymphoma is a common complication in patients with AIDS. This leads to disturbances in cognition or consciousness, focal motor or sensory deficits, aphasia, seizures, and cranial neuropathies. Similar clinical disturbances may result from **cerebral toxoplasmosis,** which is also a common complication in patients with AIDS (see Chapters 31 and 35). Neither CT nor MRI findings distinguish these two disorders, and serologic tests for toxoplasmosis are unreliable in AIDS patients. Accordingly, for neurologically stable patients, a trial of treatment for toxoplasmosis with pyrimethamine and sulfadiazine is recommended for 3 weeks (see Table 31–5); the imaging studies are then repeated, and if any lesion has improved, the regimen is continued indefinitely. If any lesion does not improve, cerebral biopsy is necessary. Primary cerebral lymphoma in AIDS patients is treated with corticosteroids, high-dose methotrexate, and antiretroviral therapy. Whole-brain irradiation may not be necessary.

Cryptococcal meningitis is a common opportunistic infection in AIDS patients. Clinically, it may resemble cerebral toxoplasmosis or lymphoma, but cranial CT scans are usually normal (see Chapter 36).

Uldrick TS et al. Factors associated with survival among patients with AIDS-related primary central nervous system lymphoma. AIDS. 2014 Jan 28;28(3):397–405. [PMID: 24076659]

4. Primary & Metastatic Spinal Tumors

Approximately 10% of spinal tumors are intramedullary. Ependymoma is the most common type of intramedullary tumor; the remainder are other types of glioma. Extramedullary tumors may be extradural or intradural in location. Among the primary extramedullary tumors, neurofibromas and meningiomas are relatively common, benign, and may be intradural or extradural. Carcinomatous metastases, lymphomatous or leukemic deposits, and myeloma are usually extradural; in the case of metastases, the prostate, breast, lung, and kidney are common primary sites.

Tumors may lead to spinal cord dysfunction by direct compression, by ischemia secondary to arterial or venous obstruction and, in the case of intramedullary lesions, by invasive infiltration.

► Clinical Findings

A. Symptoms and Signs

Symptoms usually develop insidiously. Pain is often conspicuous with extradural lesions; is characteristically aggravated by coughing or straining; may be radicular, localized to the back, or felt diffusely in an extremity; and may be accompanied by motor deficits, paresthesias, or numbness, especially in the legs. Bladder, bowel, and sexual dysfunction may occur. When sphincter disturbances occur, they are usually particularly disabling. Pain, however, often precedes specific neurologic symptoms from epidural metastases.

Examination may reveal localized spinal tenderness. A segmental lower motor neuron deficit or dermatomal sensory changes (or both) are sometimes found at the level of the lesion, while an upper motor neuron deficit and sensory disturbance are found below it.

B. Imaging

MRI with contrast or CT myelography is used to identify and localize the lesion. The combination of known tumor elsewhere in the body, back pain, and either abnormal plain films of the spine or neurologic signs of cord compression is an indication to perform this on an urgent basis.

C. Laboratory Findings

The cerebrospinal fluid is often xanthochromic and contains a greatly increased protein concentration with normal cell content and glucose concentration.

► Treatment

Intramedullary tumors are treated by decompression and surgical excision (when feasible) and by irradiation. The prognosis depends on the cause and severity of cord compression before it is relieved.

Treatment of epidural spinal metastases consists of irradiation, irrespective of cell type. Dexamethasone is also given in a high dosage (eg, 10–96 mg once intravenously, followed by 4–25 mg four times daily for 3 days orally or intravenously, followed by rapid tapering of the dosage, depending on initial dose and response) to reduce cord swelling and relieve pain. Surgical decompression is reserved for patients with tumors that are unresponsive to irradiation or who have previously been irradiated, for those with spinal instability, and for patients in whom there is some uncertainty about the diagnosis. The long-term outlook is poor, but radiation treatment may at least delay the onset of major disability.

Chamberlain MC. Neoplastic myelopathies. Continuum (Minneap Minn). 2015 Feb;21(1 Spinal Cord Disorders):132–45. [PMID: 25651222]

5. Brain Abscess

ESSENTIALS OF DIAGNOSIS

► Symptoms and signs of expanding intracranial mass.
► Signs of primary infection or congenital heart disease are sometimes present.
► Fever may be absent.

► General Considerations

Brain abscess presents as an intracranial space-occupying lesion and arises as a sequela of disease of the ear or nose, may be a complication of infection elsewhere in the body, or may result from infection introduced intracranially by trauma or surgical procedures. The most common infective organisms are streptococci, staphylococci, and anaerobes; mixed infections are not uncommon.

► Clinical Findings

A. Symptoms and Signs

Headache, drowsiness, inattention, confusion, and seizures are early symptoms, followed by signs of increasing intracranial pressure and then a focal neurologic deficit. There may be little or no systemic evidence of infection.

B. Imaging and Other Investigations

A CT scan of the head characteristically shows an area of contrast enhancement surrounding a low-density core. Similar abnormalities may be found in patients with metastatic neoplasms. MRI findings often permit earlier recognition of focal cerebritis or an abscess. Stereotactic needle aspiration may enable a specific etiologic organism to be identified. Examination of the cerebrospinal fluid does not help in diagnosis and may precipitate a herniation syndrome. Peripheral leukocytosis is sometimes present.

► Treatment

Treatment consists of intravenous antibiotics, combined with surgical drainage (aspiration or excision) if necessary to reduce the mass effect, or sometimes to establish the diagnosis. Abscesses smaller than 2 cm can often be cured medically. Broad-spectrum antibiotics, selected based on risk factors and likely organisms, are used if the infecting organism is unknown (see Chapter 33). An initial empiric multi-antibiotic regimen typically includes ceftriaxone (2 g intravenously every 12 hours), metronidazole (15 mg/kg intravenous loading dose, followed by 7.5 mg/kg intravenously every 6 hours), and vancomycin (1 g intravenously every 12 hours). The regimen is altered once culture and sensitivity data are available.

Antimicrobial treatment is usually continued parenterally for 6–8 weeks, followed by orally for 2–3 months. The patient should be monitored by serial CT scans or MRI every 2 weeks and at deterioration. Dexamethasone (4–25 mg four times daily intravenously or orally, depending on severity, followed by tapering of dose, depending on response) may reduce any associated edema, but intravenous mannitol is sometimes required.

Brouwer MC et al. Brain abscess. N Engl J Med. 2014 Jul 31; 371(5):447–56. [PMID: 25075836]

NONMETASTATIC NEUROLOGIC COMPLICATIONS OF MALIGNANT DISEASE

A variety of nonmetastatic neurologic complications of malignant disease can be recognized. Metabolic encephalopathy due to electrolyte abnormalities, infections, drug overdose, or the failure of some vital organ may be reflected by drowsiness, lethargy, restlessness, insomnia, agitation, confusion, stupor, or coma. The mental changes are usually associated with tremor, asterixis, and multifocal myoclonus. The electroencephalogram is generally diffusely slowed. Laboratory studies are necessary to detect the cause of the encephalopathy, which must then be treated appropriately.

Immune suppression resulting from either the malignant disease or its treatment (eg, by chemotherapy) predisposes patients to brain abscess, progressive multifocal leukoencephalopathy, meningitis, herpes zoster infection, and other opportunistic infectious diseases. Moreover, an overt or occult cerebrospinal fluid fistula, as occurs with some tumors, may also increase the risk of infection. MRI or CT scanning aids in the early recognition of a brain abscess, but metastatic brain tumors may have a similar appearance. Examination of the cerebrospinal fluid is essential in the evaluation of patients with meningitis and encephalitis but is of no help in the diagnosis of brain abscess.

Cerebrovascular disorders that cause neurologic complications in patients with systemic cancer include nonbacterial thrombotic endocarditis and septic embolization. Cerebral, subarachnoid, or subdural hemorrhages may occur in patients with myelogenous leukemia and may be found in association with metastatic tumors, especially melanoma. Spinal subdural hemorrhage sometimes occurs after lumbar puncture in patients with marked thrombocytopenia.

Disseminated intravascular coagulation occurs most commonly in patients with acute promyelocytic leukemia or with some adenocarcinomas and is characterized by a fluctuating encephalopathy, often with associated seizures, that frequently progresses to coma or death. There may be few accompanying neurologic signs. Venous sinus thrombosis, which usually presents with convulsions and headaches, may also occur in patients with leukemia or lymphoma. Examination commonly reveals papilledema and focal or diffuse neurologic signs. Anticonvulsants, anticoagulants, and drugs to lower the intracranial pressure may be of value.

Autoimmune paraneoplastic disorders occur when the immune system reacts against neuronal antigens expressed by tumor cells. The clinical manifestations depend on the autoantibody. Symptoms may precede those due to the neoplasm itself. Several distinct syndromes are common, including paraneoplastic cerebellar degeneration, limbic encephalitis, encephalomyelitis, anti-NMDA receptor-associated encephalitis, opsoclonus/myoclonus, sensory neuronopathy, and dermatomyositis.

Paraneoplastic cerebellar degeneration occurs most commonly in association with carcinoma of the lung, but also in breast and gynecologic cancers and Hodgkin lymphoma. Typically, there is a pancerebellar syndrome causing dysarthria, nystagmus, and ataxia of the trunk and limbs. The disorder is associated with anti-Yo, -Tr, -voltage-gated calcium channel (VGCC), and -Zic antibodies. Treatment is of the underlying malignant disease. **Limbic encephalitis,** characterized by impaired recent memory, disturbed affect, hallucinations, and seizures, occurs in some patients with tumors of the lungs, breast, thymus, and germ cells. Associated antibodies include anti-Hu, -Ma2, -CV2/CRMP5, -voltage-gated potassium channel (VGKC), -leucine rich glioma inactivated 1 (LGI1), -contactin associated protein-like 2 (Caspr2), dipeptidyl-peptidase-like protein-6 (DPPX), -AMPA receptor, -GABA$_A$ receptor, and -GABA$_B$ receptor. Anti-DPPX encephalitis is typically preceded by a severe and prolonged diarrheal prodrome. A more generalized **encephalomyelitis** occurs with anti-Hu, -CV2/CRMP5, -Ma2, and -amphiphysin antibodies in the context of a similar spectrum of tumors. **Anti-NMDA receptor-associated encephalitis** causes a characteristic syndrome of severe psychiatric symptoms, dyskinesias, dysautonomia, and hypoventilation, and is frequently associated with ovarian teratoma. **Opsoclonus/myoclonus,** a syndrome of involuntary, erratic, and conjugate saccadic eye movements and myoclonic movements of the limbs, occurs in patients with lung, breast, and gynecologic tumors, often without an identifiable antibody. **Sensory neuronopathy,** typically caused by anti-Hu antibodies in small cell lung cancer or other carcinomas, manifests itself with asymmetric, multifocal sensory nerve root deficits leading to pain, numbness, sensory ataxia, and sometimes hearing loss. **Dermatomyositis** (see Chapter 20) or the **Lambert-Eaton myasthenic syndrome** (discussed below) may be seen in patients with underlying carcinoma. Identification of an antibody is not always possible in a suspected autoimmune paraneoplastic condition, and a search for an underlying neoplasm should not be deterred. Treatment of the neoplasm takes priority and offers the best hope for stabilization or improvement of the neurologic symptoms, which often are not completely reversible. Specific treatment of the antibody-mediated symptoms by intravenous immunoglobulin (IVIG) administration, plasmapheresis, corticosteroids, or other immunosuppressive regimens is frequently attempted despite limited evidence of efficacy. Encephalitides involving antibodies directed against neuronal cell surface antigens, such as VGKC, LGI1, Caspr2, AMPA, NMDA, GABA$_{B \text{ and } A}$ receptors, and DPPX can occur either as paraneoplastic phenomena or in isolation, and typically respond well to immunotherapy.

Didelot A et al. Paraneoplastic disorders of the central and peripheral nervous systems. Handb Clin Neurol. 2014;121:1159–79. [PMID: 24365410]

McKeon A. Paraneoplastic and other autoimmune disorders of the central nervous system. Neurohospitalist. 2013 Apr; 3(2):53–64. [PMID: 23983888]

PSEUDOTUMOR CEREBRI (Idiopathic Intracranial Hypertension)

 ESSENTIALS OF DIAGNOSIS

► Headache, worse on straining.

► Visual obscurations or diplopia may occur.

► Examination reveals papilledema.

► Abducens palsy is commonly present.

General Considerations

There are many causes of pseudotumor cerebri. Thrombosis of the transverse venous sinus as a noninfectious complication of otitis media or chronic mastoiditis is one cause, and sagittal sinus thrombosis may lead to a clinically similar picture. Other causes include chronic pulmonary disease, systemic lupus erythematosus, uremia, endocrine disturbances such as hypoparathyroidism, hypothyroidism, or Addison disease, vitamin A toxicity, and the use of tetracycline or oral contraceptives. Cases have also followed withdrawal of corticosteroids after long-term use. In most instances, however, no specific cause can be found, and the disorder remits spontaneously after several months. This idiopathic variety—known as idiopathic intracranial hypertension—occurs most commonly among overweight women aged 20–44. In all cases, screening for a space-occupying lesion of the brain is important.

Clinical Findings

A. Symptoms and Signs

Symptoms consist of headache, diplopia, and other visual disturbances due to papilledema and abducens nerve dysfunction. Pulse-synchronous tinnitus may also occur. Examination reveals papilledema and some enlargement of the blind spots, but patients otherwise look well.

B. Imaging

Investigations reveal no evidence of a space-occupying lesion. CT scan shows small or normal ventricles. MR venography is important in screening for thrombosis of the intracranial venous sinuses.

C. Laboratory Findings

Lumbar puncture confirms the presence of intracranial hypertension, but the cerebrospinal fluid is normal. Laboratory studies help exclude some of the other causes mentioned earlier.

Treatment

Untreated intracranial hypertension sometimes leads to secondary optic atrophy and permanent visual loss. Acetazolamide (250–500 mg orally three times daily, increasing slowly to a maintenance dose of 1000–2000 mg daily, divided two to four times daily) reduces formation of cerebrospinal fluid. Like acetazolamide, the antiepileptic drug topiramate (Table 24–3) is a carbonic anhydrase inhibitor and was shown to be similarly effective in an open label study; topiramate has the added benefit of causing weight loss. Furosemide (20–40 mg daily) may be helpful as adjunct therapy. Corticosteroids (eg, prednisone 60–80 mg daily) are sometimes prescribed but side effects and the risk of relapse on withdrawal have discouraged their use. Obese patients should be advised to lose weight. Repeated lumbar puncture to lower the intracranial pressure by removal of cerebrospinal fluid is effective as a temporizing measure, but pharmacologic approaches to treatment provide better long-term relief. Treatment is monitored by checking visual acuity and visual fields, funduscopic appearance, and pressure of the cerebrospinal fluid. The disorder may worsen after a period of stability, indicating the need for long-term follow-up.

If medical treatment fails to control the intracranial pressure, surgical placement of a lumboperitoneal or ventriculoperitoneal shunt or optic nerve sheath fenestration should be undertaken to preserve vision.

In addition to the above measures, any specific cause of intracranial hypertension requires appropriate treatment. Thus, hormone therapy should be initiated if there is an underlying endocrine disturbance. Discontinuing the use of tetracycline, oral contraceptives, or vitamin A will allow for resolution of intracranial hypertension due to these agents. If corticosteroid withdrawal is responsible, the medication should be reintroduced and then tapered more gradually.

When to Refer

All patients should be referred.

When to Admit

All patients with worsening vision requiring shunt placement or optic nerve sheath fenestration should be hospitalized.

NORDIC Idiopathic Intracranial Hypertension Study Group Writing Committee et al. Effect of acetazolamide on visual function in patients with idiopathic intracranial hypertension and mild visual loss: the idiopathic intracranial hypertension treatment trial. JAMA. 2014 Apr 23–30;311(16):1641–51. [PMID: 24756514]

SELECTED NEUROCUTANEOUS DISEASES

Because the nervous system develops from the epithelial layer of the embryo, a number of congenital diseases include both neurologic and cutaneous manifestations. Among these disorders, three are discussed below, and von Hippel-Lindau disease is discussed in Chapter 26.

1. Tuberous Sclerosis

Tuberous sclerosis may occur sporadically or on a familial basis with autosomal dominant inheritance. Neurologic presentation is with seizures and progressive psychomotor retardation beginning in early childhood. The cutaneous abnormality, adenoma sebaceum, becomes manifest usually between 5 and 10 years of age and typically consists of reddened nodules on the face (cheeks, nasolabial folds, sides of the nose, and chin) and sometimes on the forehead and neck. Other typical cutaneous lesions include subungual fibromas, shagreen patches (leathery plaques of subepidermal fibrosis, situated usually on the trunk), and leaf-shaped hypopigmented spots. Associated abnormalities include retinal lesions and tumors, benign rhabdomyomas of the heart, lung cysts, benign tumors in the viscera, and bone cysts.

The disease is slowly progressive and leads to increasing mental deterioration. There is no specific treatment, but anticonvulsant drugs may help in controlling seizures.

Curatolo P et al. Neurological and neuropsychiatric aspects of tuberous sclerosis complex. Lancet Neurol. 2015 Jul;14(7):733–45. [PMID: 26067126]

2. Neurofibromatosis

Neurofibromatosis may occur either sporadically or on a familial basis with autosomal dominant inheritance. Two distinct forms are recognized: **Type 1 (Recklinghausen disease)** is characterized by multiple hyperpigmented macules and neurofibromas, and results from mutations in the *NF1* gene on chromosome 17. **Type 2** is characterized by bilateral eighth nerve tumors, often accompanied by other intracranial or intraspinal tumors, and is associated with mutations in the *NF2* (merlin) gene on chromosome 22.

Neurologic presentation is usually with symptoms and signs of tumor. Multiple neurofibromas characteristically are present and may involve spinal or cranial nerves, especially the eighth nerve (Figure 24–1). Examination of the superficial cutaneous nerves usually reveals palpable mobile nodules. In some cases, there is an associated marked overgrowth of subcutaneous tissues (plexiform neuromas), sometimes with an underlying bony abnormality. Associated cutaneous lesions include axillary freckling and patches of cutaneous pigmentation (café au lait spots). Malignant degeneration of neurofibromas occasionally occurs and may lead to peripheral sarcomas. Meningiomas, gliomas (especially optic nerve gliomas), bone cysts, pheochromocytomas, scoliosis, and obstructive hydrocephalus may also occur.

Hirbe AC et al. Neurofibromatosis type 1: a multidisciplinary approach to care. Lancet Neurol. 2014 Aug;13(8):834–43. [PMID: 25030515]
Karajannis MA et al. Neurofibromatosis-related tumors: emerging biology and therapies. Curr Opin Pediatr. 2015 Feb;27(1):26–33. [PMID: 25490687]

3. Sturge-Weber Syndrome

Sturge-Weber syndrome consists of a congenital, usually unilateral, cutaneous capillary angioma involving the upper face, leptomeningeal angiomatosis and, in many patients, choroidal angioma. It has no sex predilection and usually occurs sporadically. The cutaneous angioma sometimes has a more extensive distribution over the head and neck and is often quite disfiguring, especially if there is associated overgrowth of connective tissue. Focal or generalized seizures are the usual neurologic presentation and may commence at any age. There may be contralateral homonymous hemianopia, hemiparesis and hemisensory disturbance, ipsilateral glaucoma, and mental subnormality. Skull radiographs taken after the first 2 years of life usually reveal gyriform ("tramline") intracranial calcification, especially in the parieto-occipital region, due to mineral deposition in the cortex beneath the intracranial angioma.

Treatment is aimed at controlling seizures pharmacologically, but surgical treatment may be necessary. Ophthalmologic advice should be sought concerning the management of choroidal angioma and of increased intraocular pressure.

Sudarsanam A et al. Sturge-Weber syndrome: from the past to the present. Eur J Paediatr Neurol. 2014 May;18(3):257–66. [PMID: 24275166]

MOVEMENT DISORDERS

1. Benign Essential (Familial) Tremor

ESSENTIALS OF DIAGNOSIS

► Postural tremor of hands, head, or voice.
► Family history common.
► May improve temporarily with alcohol.
► No abnormal findings other than tremor.

▲ **Figure 24–1. Neurofibromatosis.** (From Jack Resnick, Sr, MD; reproduced with permission from Usatine RP, Smith MA, Mayeaux EJ, Jr, Chumley H, Tysinger J. *The Color Atlas of Family Medicine.* McGraw-Hill, 2009.)

General Considerations

The cause of benign essential tremor is uncertain, but it is sometimes inherited in an autosomal dominant manner. Responsible genes have been identified at 3q13, 2p22-p25, and 6p23.

Clinical Findings

Tremor may begin at any age and is enhanced by emotional stress. The tremor usually involves one or both hands, the head, or the hands and head, while the legs tend to be spared. Examination reveals no other abnormalities. Ingestion of a small quantity of alcohol commonly provides remarkable but short-lived relief by an unknown mechanism.

Although the tremor may become more conspicuous with time, it generally leads to little disability. Occasionally, it interferes with manual skills and leads to impairment of handwriting. Speech may also be affected if the laryngeal muscles are involved.

Treatment

Treatment is often unnecessary. When it is required because of disability, propranolol (60–240 mg daily orally) may be helpful. Long-term therapy is typical; however, intermittent therapy is sometimes useful in patients whose tremor becomes exacerbated in specific predictable situations. Primidone may be helpful when propranolol is ineffective, but patients with essential tremor are often very sensitive to it. Therefore, the starting dose is 50 mg daily orally, and the daily dose is increased by 50 mg every 2 weeks depending on the patient's response; a maintenance dose of 125 mg three times daily orally is commonly effective. Occasional patients do not respond to these measures but are helped by alprazolam (up to 3 mg daily orally in divided doses), topiramate (titrated up to a dose of 400 mg daily orally in divided doses over about 8 weeks), or gabapentin (1800 mg daily orally in divided doses). Botulinum toxin A may reduce tremor, but adverse effects include dose-dependent weakness of the injected muscles. Levetiracetam, flunarizine, and 3,4-diaminopyridine are probably ineffective, and there is insufficient evidence to support the use of pregabalin, zonisamide, and clozapine.

Disabling tremor unresponsive to medical treatment may be helped by high-frequency thalamic stimulation on one or both sides, according to the laterality of symptoms. Subdural motor cortex stimulation has also been effective in a small trial.

When to Refer

- When refractory to first-line treatment with propranolol or primidone.
- When additional neurologic signs are present (ie, parkinsonism).

When to Admit

Patients requiring surgical treatment (deep brain stimulator placement) should be hospitalized.

Schneider SA et al. Medical and surgical treatment of tremors. Neurol Clin. 2015 Feb;33(1):57–75. [PMID: 25432723]

2. Parkinsonism

ESSENTIALS OF DIAGNOSIS

- ▶ Any combination of tremor, rigidity, bradykinesia, and progressive postural instability.
- ▶ Cognitive impairment is sometimes prominent.

General Considerations

Parkinsonism is a relatively common disorder that occurs in all ethnic groups, with an approximately equal sex distribution. The most common variety, idiopathic Parkinson disease, begins most often between 45 and 65 years of age and is a progressive disease.

Etiology

Parkinsonism may rarely occur on a familial basis, and the parkinsonian phenotype may result from mutations of several different genes (alpha-synuclein, parkin, *LRRK2*, *DJ1*, and *PINK1*). Mutations in *LRRK2* also account for some cases of apparently sporadic Parkinson disease. Postencephalitic parkinsonism is becoming increasingly rare. Exposure to certain toxins (eg, manganese dust, carbon disulfide) and severe carbon monoxide poisoning may lead to parkinsonism. Reversible parkinsonism may develop in patients receiving neuroleptic drugs (see Chapter 25), reserpine, or metoclopramide. Only rarely is hemiparkinsonism the presenting feature of a progressive space-occupying lesion.

In idiopathic Parkinson disease, dopamine depletion due to degeneration of the dopaminergic nigrostriatal system leads to an imbalance of dopamine and acetylcholine, which are neurotransmitters normally present in the corpus striatum. Treatment of the motor disturbance is directed at redressing this imbalance by blocking the effect of acetylcholine with anticholinergic drugs or by the administration of levodopa, the precursor of dopamine. Prior use of ibuprofen is associated with a decreased risk of developing Parkinson disease; age, family history, male sex, ongoing herbicide/pesticide exposure, and significant prior head trauma are risk factors.

Clinical Findings

Tremor, rigidity, bradykinesia, and postural instability are the cardinal motor features of parkinsonism and may be present in any combination. There may also be a mild decline in intellectual function. Depression, anxiety, anosmia, constipation, and sleep disturbances are common. The tremor of about four to six cycles per second is most conspicuous at rest, is enhanced by emotional stress, and is often less severe during voluntary activity. Although it may ultimately be present in all limbs, the tremor is commonly confined to one limb or to the limbs on one side for months or years before it becomes more generalized. In some patients, tremor is absent.

Rigidity (an increase in resistance to passive movement) is responsible for the characteristically flexed posture seen in many patients, but the most disabling symptoms of parkinsonism are due to bradykinesia, manifested as a slowness of voluntary movement and a reduction in automatic movements such as swinging of the arms while walking. Curiously, however, effective voluntary activity may briefly be regained during an emergency (eg, the patient is able to leap aside to avoid an oncoming motor vehicle).

Clinical diagnosis of the well-developed syndrome is usually simple. The patient has a relatively immobile face with widened palpebral fissures, infrequent blinking, and a fixity of facial expression. Seborrhea of the scalp and face is common. There is often mild blepharoclonus, and a tremor may be present about the mouth and lips. Repetitive tapping (about twice per second) over the bridge of the nose produces a sustained blink response (Myerson sign). Other findings may include saliva drooling from the mouth, perhaps due to impairment of swallowing; soft and poorly modulated voice; a variable rest tremor and rigidity in some or all of the limbs; slowness of voluntary movements; impairment of fine or rapidly alternating movements; and micrographia. There is typically no muscle weakness (provided that sufficient time is allowed for power to be developed) and no alteration in the tendon reflexes or plantar responses. It is difficult for the patient to arise from a sitting position and begin walking. The gait itself is characterized by small shuffling steps and a loss of the normal automatic arm swing; there may be unsteadiness on turning, difficulty in stopping, and a tendency to fall. The serum urate level may be a prognostic indicator—the rate of progression declines as the urate level increases.

Differential Diagnosis

Diagnostic problems may occur in mild cases, especially if tremor is minimal or absent. For example, mild hypokinesia or slight tremor is commonly attributed to old age. Depression, with its associated expressionless face, poorly modulated voice, and reduction in voluntary activity, can be difficult to distinguish from mild parkinsonism, especially since the two disorders may coexist; in some cases, a trial of antidepressant drug therapy is necessary. The family history, the character of the tremor, and lack of other neurologic signs should distinguish essential tremor from parkinsonism. **Wilson disease** can be distinguished by its early age at onset, the presence of other abnormal movements, Kayser-Fleischer rings, and chronic hepatitis, and by increased concentrations of copper in the tissues. **Huntington disease** presenting with rigidity and bradykinesia may be mistaken for parkinsonism unless the family history and accompanying dementia are recognized. In **multisystem atrophy** (previously called the **Shy-Drager syndrome**), autonomic insufficiency (leading to postural hypotension, anhidrosis, disturbances of sphincter control, erectile dysfunction, etc) may be accompanied by parkinsonism, pyramidal deficits, lower motor neuron signs, or cerebellar dysfunction. In **progressive supranuclear palsy,** bradykinesia and rigidity are accompanied by a supranuclear disorder of eye movements, pseudobulbar palsy,

pseudo-emotional lability (pseudobulbar affect), and axial dystonia. **Creutzfeldt-Jakob disease** may be accompanied by features of parkinsonism, but progression is rapid, dementia is usual, myoclonic jerking is common, ataxia and pyramidal signs may be conspicuous, and the MRI and electroencephalographic findings are usually characteristic. In **corticobasal degeneration,** asymmetric parkinsonism is accompanied by conspicuous signs of cortical dysfunction (eg, apraxia, sensory inattention, dementia, aphasia).

▶ Treatment

Treatment is symptomatic. There is great interest in developing disease-modifying therapies, but trials of several putative neuroprotective agents have shown no benefit. Trials of various gene therapies have shown limited or no benefit.

A. Medical Measures

Drug treatment is not required early in the course of Parkinson disease, but the nature of the disorder and the availability of medical treatment for use when necessary should be discussed with the patient.

1. Amantadine—Patients with mild symptoms but no disability may be helped by amantadine. This drug improves all of the clinical features of parkinsonism, but its mode of action is unclear. Side effects include restlessness, confusion, depression, skin rashes, edema, nausea, constipation, anorexia, postural hypotension, and disturbances of cardiac rhythm. However, these are relatively uncommon with the usual dose (100 mg twice daily orally). It also ameliorates dyskinesias resulting from chronic levodopa therapy.

2. Levodopa—Levodopa, which is converted in the body to dopamine, improves all of the major features of parkinsonism, including bradykinesia, but does not stop progression of the disorder. The most common early side effects of levodopa are nausea, vomiting, and hypotension, but cardiac arrhythmias may also occur. Dyskinesias, restlessness, confusion, and other behavioral changes tend to occur somewhat later and become more common with time. Levodopa-induced dyskinesias may take any conceivable form, including chorea, athetosis, dystonia, tremor, tics, and myoclonus. An even later complication is the "wearing off effect" or the "on-off phenomenon," in which abrupt but transient fluctuations in the severity of parkinsonism occur unpredictably but frequently during the day. The "off" period of marked bradykinesia has been shown to relate in some instances to falling plasma levels of levodopa. During the "on" phase, dyskinesias are often conspicuous but mobility is increased. However, such response fluctuations may relate to advancing disease rather than to levodopa therapy itself.

Carbidopa, which inhibits the enzyme responsible for the breakdown of levodopa to dopamine, does not cross the blood-brain barrier. When levodopa is given in combination with carbidopa, the extracerebral breakdown of levodopa is diminished. This reduces the amount of levodopa required daily for beneficial effects, and it lowers the incidence of nausea, vomiting, hypotension, and cardiac irregularities. Such a combination does not prevent the development of response fluctuations and the incidence of other side effects (dyskinesias or psychiatric complications) may actually be increased.

Sinemet, a commercially available preparation that contains carbidopa and levodopa in a fixed ratio (1:10 or 1:4), is generally used. Treatment is started with a small dose—eg, one tablet of Sinemet 25/100 (containing 25 mg of carbidopa and 100 mg of levodopa) three times daily—and gradually increased depending on the response. Sinemet CR is a controlled-release formulation (containing 25 or 50 mg of carbidopa and 100 or 200 mg of levodopa). It is sometimes helpful in reducing fluctuations in clinical response to treatment and in reducing the frequency with which medication must be taken. A novel formulation of carbidopa/levodopa (Rytary) that contains both immediate- and delayed-release beads is also available and provides a smoother response in patients with fluctuations. The commercially available combination of levodopa with both carbidopa and entacapone (Stalevo) may also be helpful in this context and is discussed in the following section on COMT inhibitors. Response fluctuations are also reduced by keeping the daily intake of protein at the recommended minimum and taking the main protein meal as the last meal of the day.

The dyskinesias and behavioral side effects of levodopa are dose-related, but reduction in dose may eliminate any therapeutic benefit. Levodopa-induced dyskinesias may also respond to amantadine or possibly levetiracetam.

Levodopa therapy is contraindicated in patients with psychotic illness or narrow-angle glaucoma. It should not be given to patients taking monoamine oxidase A inhibitors or within 2 weeks of their withdrawal, because hypertensive crises may result. Levodopa should be used with care in patients with suspected melanomas or with active peptic ulcers because of concerns that it may exacerbate these disorders.

3. Dopamine agonists—Dopamine agonists, such as pramipexole and ropinirole, act directly on dopamine receptors, and their use in parkinsonism is associated with a lower incidence of the response fluctuations and dyskinesias that occur with long-term levodopa therapy. They are effective in both early and advanced stages of Parkinson disease. They are often given either before the introduction of levodopa or with a low dose of Sinemet 25/100 (carbidopa 25 mg and levodopa 100 mg, one tablet three times daily) when dopaminergic therapy is first introduced; the dose of Sinemet is kept constant, while the dose of the agonist is gradually increased.

Pramipexole is started at a dosage of 0.125 mg three times daily orally, and the dose is doubled after 1 week and again after another week; the daily dose is then increased by 0.75 mg at weekly intervals depending on response and tolerance. Most patients require between 0.5 and 1.5 mg three times daily orally. Ropinirole is begun in a dosage of 0.25 mg three times daily orally, and the total daily dose is increased at weekly intervals by 0.75 mg until the fourth week and by 1.5 mg thereafter. Most patients require between 2 and 8 mg three times daily for benefit. Extended-release, once-daily formulations of pramipexole and ropinirole are available with similar efficacy and tolerability as the immediate release

versions. Rotigotine is a dopamine agonist absorbed transdermally from a skin patch; it is started at 2 mg once daily and increasing weekly by 2 mg daily until achieving an optimal response, up to a maximum of 8 mg daily. Adverse effects of these various agonists include fatigue, somnolence, nausea, peripheral edema, dyskinesias, confusion, and postural hypotension. Less commonly, an irresistible urge to sleep may occur, sometimes in inappropriate and hazardous circumstances. Impulse control disorders involving gambling, shopping, or sexual activity have also been related to use of dopamine agonists. Local skin reactions may occur with the rotigotine patch.

4. Selective monoamine oxidase inhibitors—Rasagiline, a selective monoamine oxidase B inhibitor, has a clear symptomatic benefit in a daily oral dose of 1 mg, taken in the morning; it may also be used for adjunctive therapy in patients with response fluctuations to levodopa. Selegiline (5 mg orally with breakfast and lunch) is another monoamine oxidase B inhibitor that is sometimes used as adjunctive treatment for parkinsonism. By inhibiting the metabolic breakdown of dopamine, these drugs may improve fluctuations or declining response to levodopa. Although it is sometimes advised that tyramine-rich foods be avoided when either rasagiline or selegiline is taken because of the theoretical possibility of a hypertensive ("cheese") effect, there is no clinical evidence to support the need for such dietary precautions when they are taken at the recommended dosage.

Studies have suggested (but failed to show conclusively) that rasagiline may slow the progression of Parkinson disease, and it appears to delay the need for other symptomatic therapies. For these reasons, rasagiline is often started early, particularly for patients who are young or have mild disease. However, the FDA has rejected an expansion of rasagiline's indication to include disease modification.

5. COMT inhibitors—Catecholamine-O-methyltransferase (COMT) inhibitors reduce the metabolism of levodopa to 3-O-methyldopa and thereby alter the plasma pharmacokinetics of levodopa, leading to more sustained plasma levels and more constant dopaminergic stimulation of the brain. Two such agents, tolcapone and entacapone, are currently available and may be used as an adjunct to levodopa-carbidopa in patients with response fluctuations or an otherwise inadequate response. Treatment results in reduced response fluctuations, with a greater period of responsiveness to administered levodopa; however, the use of these agents does not delay the eventual development of levodopa-induced dyskinesias. Tolcapone is given in a dosage of 100 mg or 200 mg three times daily orally, and entacapone is given as 200 mg with each dose of Sinemet. With either preparation, the dose of Sinemet taken concurrently may have to be reduced by up to one-third to avoid side effects such as dyskinesias, confusion, hypotension, and syncope. Diarrhea is sometimes troublesome. Because rare cases of fulminant hepatic failure have followed its use, tolcapone should be avoided in patients with preexisting liver disease. Serial liver function tests should be performed at 2-week intervals for the first year and at longer intervals thereafter in patients receiving the drug—as recommended by the manufacturer. Hepatotoxicity has not been reported with entacapone, which is therefore the preferred agent, and serial liver function tests are not required.

Stalevo is the commercial preparation of levodopa combined with both carbidopa and entacapone. It is best used in patients already stabilized on equivalent doses of carbidopa/levodopa and entacapone. It is priced at or below the price of the individual ingredients (ie, carbidopa/levodopa and entacapone) and has the added convenience of requiring fewer tablets to be taken daily. It is available in three strengths: Stalevo 50 (12.5 mg of carbidopa, 50 mg of levodopa, and 200 mg of entacapone), Stalevo 100 (25 mg of carbidopa, 100 mg of levodopa, and 200 mg of entacapone), and Stalevo 150 (37.5 mg of carbidopa, 150 mg of levodopa, and 200 mg of entacapone).

6. Anticholinergic drugs—Anticholinergics are more helpful in alleviating tremor and rigidity than bradykinesia. Treatment is started with a small dose and gradually increased until benefit occurs or side effects limit further increments. If treatment is ineffective, the drug is gradually withdrawn and another preparation then tried.

Side effects limit the routine use of these drugs, and include dryness of the mouth, nausea, constipation, palpitations, cardiac arrhythmias, urinary retention, confusion, agitation, restlessness, drowsiness, mydriasis, increased intraocular pressure, and defective accommodation. Anticholinergic drugs are contraindicated in patients with prostatic hyperplasia, narrow-angle glaucoma, or obstructive gastrointestinal disease and are often tolerated poorly by the elderly. They are best avoided whenever cognitive impairment or a predisposition to delirium exists.

7. Atypical antipsychotics—Confusion and psychotic symptoms may occur as a side effect of dopaminergic therapy or as a part of the underlying illness. They often respond to atypical antipsychotic agents, which have few extrapyramidal side effects and do not block the effects of dopaminergic medication. The most effective of these agents is clozapine, a dibenzodiazepine derivative; olanzapine, quetiapine, and risperidone may be tried. Clozapine may rarely cause marrow suppression, and weekly blood counts are therefore necessary for patients taking it. The patient is started on 6.25 mg at bedtime and the dosage increased to 25–100 mg/day as needed. In low doses, it may also improve iatrogenic dyskinesias.

B. General Measures

Physical therapy or speech therapy helps many patients. Cognitive impairment and psychiatric symptoms may be helped by a cholinesterase inhibitor, such as rivastigmine (3–12 mg orally daily or 4.6 or 9.5 mg/24 hours transdermally daily). The quality of life can often be improved by the provision of simple aids to daily living, eg, rails or banisters placed strategically about the home, special table cutlery with large handles, nonslip rubber table mats, and devices to amplify the voice.

C. Brain Stimulation

High-frequency stimulation of the subthalamic nuclei or globus pallidus internus may benefit all the major features

of the disease but does not affect its natural history. Electrical stimulation of the brain has the advantage over ablative procedures of being reversible and of causing minimal or no damage to the brain, and is therefore the preferred surgical approach to treatment. Deep brain stimulation is reserved for patients without cognitive impairment or psychiatric disorder who have a good response to levodopa but in whom dyskinesias or response fluctuations are problematic. It frequently takes 3–6 months after surgery to adjust stimulator programming and to achieve optimal results. Side effects include depression, apathy, impulsivity, executive dysfunction, and decreased verbal fluency in a subset of patients. Because of the nondestructive nature of brain stimulation, it has supplanted thalamotomy and pallidotomy, older ablative procedures aimed at achieving the same result.

D. Gene Therapy

Injections of adeno-associated viruses encoding various human genes have been made into the subthalamic nucleus or putamen in various clinical trials. The procedure appears to be safe, but results have been disappointing except that transfer of the gene for glutamic acid decarboxylase (the enzyme that produces the inhibitory neurotransmitter gamma-aminobutyric acid [GABA]) into the subthalamic nucleus seems to improve motor function in patients with Parkinson disease. It is unclear whether this provides any greater benefit than subthalamic deep brain stimulation.

▶ When to Refer

All patients should be referred.

▶ When to Admit

Patients requiring surgical treatment should be admitted.

Connolly BS et al. Pharmacological treatment of Parkinson disease: a review. JAMA. 2014 Apr 23–30;311(16):1670–83. [PMID: 24756517]
Kalia SK et al. Deep brain stimulation for Parkinson's disease and other movement disorders. Curr Opin Neurol. 2013 Aug; 26(4):374–80. [PMID: 23817213]
Stamelou M et al. Atypical parkinsonism: diagnosis and treatment. Neurol Clin. 2015 Feb;33(1):39–56. [PMID: 25432722]

3. Huntington Disease

ESSENTIALS OF DIAGNOSIS

▶ Gradual onset and progression of chorea and dementia or behavioral change.
▶ Family history of the disorder.
▶ Responsible gene identified on chromosome 4.

▶ General Considerations

Huntington disease is characterized by chorea and dementia. It is inherited in an autosomal dominant manner and occurs throughout the world, in all ethnic groups, with a prevalence rate of about 5 per 100,000. There is an expanded and unstable CAG trinucleotide repeat in the huntingtin gene at 4p16.3; longer repeat lengths correspond to an earlier age of onset and faster disease progression.

Clinical Findings

A. Symptoms and Signs

Clinical onset is usually between 30 and 50 years of age. The disease is progressive and usually leads to a fatal outcome within 15–20 years. The initial symptoms may consist of either abnormal movements or intellectual changes, but ultimately both occur. The earliest mental changes are often behavioral, with irritability, moodiness, antisocial behavior, or a psychiatric disturbance, but a more obvious dementia subsequently develops. The dyskinesia may initially be no more than an apparent fidgetiness or restlessness, but eventually choreiform movements and some dystonic posturing occur. Progressive rigidity and akinesia (rather than chorea) sometimes occur in association with dementia, especially in cases with childhood onset.

B. Imaging

CT scanning or MRI usually demonstrates cerebral atrophy and atrophy of the caudate nucleus in established cases. Positron emission tomography (PET) has shown reduced striatal metabolic rate.

Differential Diagnosis

The diagnosis is established with a widely available genetic test, although such testing should be pursued under the guidance of a licensed genetic counselor. Chorea developing with no family history of choreoathetosis should not be attributed to Huntington disease, at least not until other causes of chorea have been excluded clinically and by appropriate laboratory studies. Nongenetic causes of chorea include stroke, systemic lupus erythematosus and antiphospholipid antibody syndrome, paraneoplastic syndromes, infection with HIV, and various medications. In younger patients, self-limiting Sydenham chorea develops after group A streptococcal infections on rare occasions. If a patient presents solely with progressive intellectual failure, it may not be possible to distinguish Huntington disease from other causes of dementia unless there is a characteristic family history or a dyskinesia develops.

Huntington disease–like (HDL) disorders resemble Huntington disease but the CAG trinucleotide repeat number of the huntingtin gene is normal. There are autosomal dominant (HDL1, a familial prion disease involving a mutation in the *PRNP* gene on chromosome 20; and HDL2, a triplet repeat disease involving the gene for junctophilin-3 on chromosome 16) and recessive forms (HDL3, 4p15.3).

A clinically similar autosomal dominant disorder (**dentatorubral-pallidoluysian atrophy**), manifested by chorea, dementia, ataxia, and myoclonic epilepsy, is uncommon except in persons of Japanese ancestry. It is due to a mutation in the *ATN1* gene mapping to 12p13.31. Treatment is as for Huntington disease.

Treatment

There is no cure for Huntington disease; progression cannot be halted; and treatment is purely symptomatic. The reported biochemical changes suggest a relative underactivity of neurons containing GABA and acetylcholine or a relative overactivity of dopaminergic neurons. Tetrabenazine, a drug that interferes with the vesicular storage of biogenic amines, is widely used to treat the dyskinesia. The starting dose is 12.5 mg twice or three times daily orally, increasing by 12.5 mg every 5 days depending on response and tolerance; the usual maintenance dose is 25 mg three times daily. Side effects include depression, postural hypotension, drowsiness, and parkinsonian features; tetrabenazine should not be given within 14 days of taking monoamine oxidase inhibitors and is not indicated for the treatment of levodopa-induced dyskinesias. Reserpine is similar in depleting central monoamines but has more peripheral effects and a worse side-effect profile, making its use problematic in Huntington disease; if utilized, the dose is built up gradually to between 2 mg and 5 mg orally daily, depending on the response. Treatment with drugs blocking dopamine receptors, such as phenothiazines or haloperidol, may control the dyskinesia and any behavioral disturbances. Haloperidol treatment is usually begun with a dose of 1 mg once or twice daily orally, which is then increased every 3 or 4 days depending on the response; alternatively, atypical antipsychotic agents such as quetiapine (increasing from 25 mg daily orally up to 100 mg twice daily orally as tolerated) may be tried. Amantadine in a dose of 200 mg to 400 mg daily orally is sometimes helpful for chorea. Behavioral disturbances may respond to clozapine. Attempts to compensate for the relative GABA deficiency by enhancing central GABA activity or to compensate for the relative cholinergic underactivity by giving choline chloride have not been therapeutically helpful. Neuroprotective strategies are being explored.

Offspring should be offered genetic counseling. Genetic testing permits presymptomatic detection and definitive diagnosis of the disease.

When to Refer

All patients should be referred.

Dayalu P et al. Huntington disease: pathogenesis and treatment. Neurol Clin. 2015 Feb;33(1):101–14. [PMID: 25432725]

4. Idiopathic Torsion Dystonia

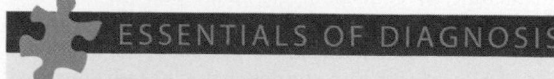
ESSENTIALS OF DIAGNOSIS

» Dystonic movements and postures.
» Normal birth and developmental history. No other neurologic signs.
» Investigations (including CT scan or MRI) reveal no cause of dystonia.

General Considerations

Idiopathic torsion dystonia may occur sporadically or on a hereditary basis, with autosomal dominant, autosomal recessive, and X-linked recessive modes of transmission. Symptoms may begin in childhood or later and persist throughout life.

Clinical Findings

The disorder is characterized by the onset of abnormal movements and postures in a patient with a normal birth and developmental history, no relevant past medical illness, and no other neurologic signs. Investigations (including CT scan) reveal no cause for the abnormal movements. Dystonic movements of the head and neck may take the form of torticollis, blepharospasm, facial grimacing, or forced opening or closing of the mouth. The limbs may also adopt abnormal but characteristic postures. The age at onset influences both the clinical findings and the prognosis. With onset in childhood, there is usually a family history of the disorder, symptoms commonly commence in the legs, and progression is likely until there is severe disability from generalized dystonia. In contrast, when onset is later, a positive family history is unlikely, initial symptoms are often in the arms or axial structures, and severe disability does not usually occur, although generalized dystonia may ultimately develop in some patients. If all cases are considered together, about one-third of patients eventually become so severely disabled that they are confined to chair or bed, while another one-third are affected only mildly.

Differential Diagnosis

Perinatal anoxia, birth trauma, and kernicterus are common causes of dystonia, but abnormal movements usually then develop before the age of 5, the early development of the patient is usually abnormal, and a history of seizures is not unusual. Moreover, examination may reveal signs of mental retardation or pyramidal deficit in addition to the movement disorder. Dystonic posturing may also occur in Wilson disease, Huntington disease, or parkinsonism; as a sequela of encephalitis lethargica or previous neuroleptic drug therapy; and in certain other disorders. In these cases, diagnosis is based on the history and accompanying clinical manifestations.

Treatment

Idiopathic torsion dystonia usually responds poorly to drugs. Levodopa, diazepam, baclofen, carbamazepine, amantadine, or anticholinergic medication (in high dosage) is occasionally helpful; if not, a trial of treatment with tetrabenazine, phenothiazines, or haloperidol may be worthwhile. In each case, the dose has to be individualized, depending on response and tolerance. However, the doses of these latter drugs that are required for benefit lead usually to mild parkinsonism. Pallidal deep brain stimulation is helpful for medically refractory dystonia and has a lower morbidity than stereotactic thalamotomy, which is sometimes helpful in patients with predominantly unilateral limb dystonia. Potential adverse events of deep brain stimulation include cerebral infection or hemorrhage, broken leads, affective changes, and dysarthria.

A distinct variety of dominantly inherited dystonia, caused by a mutation in the gene for GTP cyclohydrolase I on chromosome 14q, is remarkably responsive to levodopa; therefore, a levodopa trial is warranted in all patients.

When to Refer

All patients should be referred.

When to Admit

Patients requiring surgical treatment should be admitted.

Balint B et al. Dystonia: an update on phenomenology, classification, pathogenesis and treatment. Curr Opin Neurol. 2014 Aug; 27(4):468–76. [PMID: 24978640]

5. Focal Torsion Dystonia

A number of the dystonic manifestations that occur in idiopathic torsion dystonia may also occur as isolated phenomena. They are best regarded as focal dystonias that either occur as formes frustes of idiopathic torsion dystonia in patients with a positive family history or represent a focal manifestation of the adult-onset form of that disorder when there is no family history. Mapping of responsible genes to chromosome 8 (*DYT6*) and chromosome 18 (*DYT7*) has been reported in some instances of cervical or cranial dystonia. Medical treatment is generally unsatisfactory. A trial of the drugs used in idiopathic torsion dystonia is worthwhile, however, since a few patients do show some response. In addition, with restricted dystonias such as blepharospasm or torticollis, local injection of botulinum A toxin into the overactive muscles may produce worthwhile benefit for several weeks or months and can be repeated as needed.

Both blepharospasm and oromandibular dystonia may occur as an isolated focal dystonia. The former is characterized by spontaneous involuntary forced closure of the eyelids for a variable interval. Oromandibular dystonia is manifested by involuntary contraction of the muscles about the mouth causing, for example, involuntary opening or closing of the mouth, roving or protruding tongue movements, and retraction of the platysma.

Spasmodic torticollis, usually with onset between 25 and 50 years of age, is characterized by a tendency for the neck to twist to one side. This initially occurs episodically, but eventually the neck is held to the side. Some patients have a sensory trick ("geste antagoniste") that lessens the dystonic posture, eg, touching the side of the face. Spontaneous resolution may occur in the first year or so. The disorder is otherwise usually lifelong. Selective section of the spinal accessory nerve and the upper cervical nerve roots is sometimes helpful if medical treatment is unsuccessful. Local injection of botulinum A toxin provides benefit in most cases.

Writer's cramp is characterized by dystonic posturing of the hand and forearm when the hand is used for writing and sometimes when it is used for other tasks, eg, playing the piano or using a screwdriver or eating utensils. Drug treatment is usually unrewarding, and patients are often best advised to learn to use the other hand for activities requiring manual dexterity. Injections of botulinum A toxin are helpful in some instances.

Fox MD et al. Brain stimulation for torsion dystonia. JAMA Neurol. 2015 Jun;72(6):713–9. [PMID: 25894231]

6. Myoclonus

Occasional myoclonic jerks may occur in anyone, especially when drifting into sleep. General or multifocal myoclonus is common in patients with idiopathic epilepsy and is especially prominent in certain hereditary disorders characterized by seizures and progressive intellectual decline, such as the lipid storage diseases. It is also a feature of subacute sclerosing panencephalitis and Creutzfeldt-Jakob disease. Generalized myoclonic jerking may accompany uremic and other metabolic encephalopathies, result from therapy with levodopa or tricyclic antidepressants, occur in alcohol or drug withdrawal states, or follow anoxic brain damage. It also occurs on a hereditary or sporadic basis as an isolated phenomenon in otherwise healthy subjects.

Segmental myoclonus is a rare manifestation of a focal spinal cord lesion. It may also be the clinical expression of **epilepsia partialis continua,** a disorder in which a repetitive focal epileptic discharge arises in the contralateral sensorimotor cortex, sometimes from an underlying structural lesion. An electroencephalogram is often helpful in clarifying the epileptic nature of the disorder, and CT or MRI scan may reveal the causal lesion.

Myoclonus may respond to certain anticonvulsant drugs, especially valproic acid or levetiracetam, or to one of the benzodiazepines, particularly clonazepam (see Table 24–3). It may also respond to piracetam (up to 16.8 g daily; not available in the United States). Myoclonus following anoxic brain damage is often responsive to oxitriptan (5-hydroxy-tryptophan), the precursor of serotonin, and sometimes to clonazepam. Oxitriptan is given in gradually increasing doses up to 1–1.5 mg daily. In patients with segmental myoclonus, a localized lesion should be searched for and treated appropriately.

Mills K et al. An update and review of the treatment of myoclonus. Curr Neurol Neurosci Rep. 2015 Jan;15(1):512. [PMID: 25398378]

7. Wilson Disease

In this metabolic disorder, abnormal movement and posture may occur with or without coexisting signs of liver involvement. Psychiatric and neuropsychological manifestations are common. Wilson disease is discussed in Chapter 16.

8. Drug-Induced Abnormal Movements

Phenothiazines, butyrophenones, and metoclopramide may produce a wide variety of abnormal movements, including parkinsonism, akathisia (ie, motor restlessness),

acute dystonia, chorea, and tardive dyskinesias or dystonia; several of these are also produced by aripiprazole. These complications are discussed in Chapter 25. Chorea may also develop in patients receiving levodopa, bromocriptine, anticholinergic drugs, phenytoin, carbamazepine, lithium, amphetamines, or oral contraceptives, and it resolves with withdrawal of the offending substance. Similarly, dystonia may be produced by levodopa, bromocriptine, lithium, or carbamazepine; and parkinsonism by reserpine and tetrabenazine. Postural tremor may occur with a variety of drugs, including epinephrine, isoproterenol, theophylline, caffeine, lithium, thyroid hormone, tricyclic antidepressants, and valproic acid.

Mehta SH et al. Drug-induced movement disorders. Neurol Clin. 2015 Feb;33(1):153–74. [PMID: 25432728]

9. Restless Legs Syndrome

This disorder may occur as a primary (idiopathic) disorder or in relation to Parkinson disease, pregnancy, iron deficiency anemia, peripheral neuropathy (especially uremic or diabetic), or periodic leg movements of sleep. It may have a hereditary basis, and several genetic loci have been associated with the disorder (12q12-q21, 14q13-q21, 9p24-p22, 2q33, 20p13, 6p21, and 2p14-p13). Restlessness and curious sensory disturbances lead to an irresistible urge to move the limbs, especially during periods of relaxation. Disturbed nocturnal sleep and excessive daytime somnolence may result. Therapy is with nonergot dopamine agonists, such as pramipexole (0.125–0.5 mg orally once daily), ropinirole (0.25–4 mg orally once daily 2 to 3 hours before bedtime), or rotigotine (1–3 mg/24h transdermal patch once daily) or with benzodiazepines, such as clonazepam (0.5–2 mg orally once daily). Gabapentin (starting with 300 mg orally daily, increasing to approximately 1800 mg daily depending on response and tolerance), pregabalin (150–300 mg orally divided twice to three times daily), or gabapentin enacarbil (600 mg extended release daily) are related drugs that improve symptoms. Levodopa is helpful but may lead to an augmentation of symptoms, so that its use is generally reserved for those who do not respond to other measures. In some instances, opioids are required to control symptoms.

Garcia-Borreguero D et al. An update on restless legs syndrome (Willis-Ekbom disease): clinical features, pathogenesis and treatment. Curr Opin Neurol. 2014 Aug;27(4):493–501. [PMID: 24978636]

10. Gilles de la Tourette Syndrome

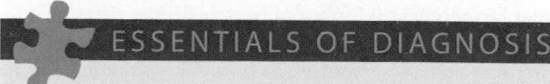
ESSENTIALS OF DIAGNOSIS

▶ Multiple motor and phonic tics.

▶ Symptoms begin before age 18 years.

▶ Tics occur frequently for at least 1 year.

▶ Tics vary in number, frequency, and nature over time.

Clinical Findings

Simple tics occur transiently in up to 25% of children, remit within weeks to months, and do not require treatment. Tourette syndrome is a more complex disorder, with diagnostic criteria as defined above. Motor tics are the initial manifestation in 80% of cases and most commonly involve the face, whereas in the remaining 20%, the initial symptoms are phonic tics; ultimately a combination of different motor and phonic tics develop in all patients. Tics are preceded by an urge that is relieved upon performance of the movement or vocalization; they can be temporarily suppressed but eventually the urge becomes overwhelming. These are noted first in childhood, generally between the ages of 2 and 15. Motor tics occur especially about the face, head, and shoulders (eg, sniffing, blinking, frowning, shoulder shrugging, head thrusting, etc). Phonic tics commonly consist of grunts, barks, hisses, throat-clearing, coughs, etc, but sometimes also of verbal utterances including coprolalia (obscene speech). There may also be echolalia (repetition of the speech of others), echopraxia (imitation of others' movements), and palilalia (repetition of words or phrases). Some tics may be self-mutilating in nature, such as nail-biting, hair-pulling, or biting of the lips or tongue. The disorder is chronic, but the course may be punctuated by relapses and remissions. Obsessive-compulsive behaviors are commonly associated and may be more disabling than the tics themselves. A family history is sometimes obtained.

Examination usually reveals no abnormalities other than the tics. In addition to obsessive-compulsive behavior disorders, psychiatric disturbances may occur because of the associated cosmetic and social embarrassment. The diagnosis of the disorder is often delayed for years, the tics being interpreted as psychiatric illness or some other form of abnormal movement. Patients are thus often subjected to unnecessary treatment before the disorder is recognized. The tic-like character of the abnormal movements and the absence of other neurologic signs should differentiate this disorder from other movement disorders presenting in childhood. Wilson disease, however, can simulate the condition and should be excluded.

Treatment

Treatment is symptomatic and may need to be continued indefinitely. Habit reversal training or other forms of behavioral therapy can be effective alone or in combination with pharmacotherapy. Alpha-adrenergic agonists, such as clonidine (start 0.05 mg orally at bedtime, titrating to 0.3–0.4 mg orally daily, divided three to four times per day) or guanfacine (start 0.5 mg orally at bedtime, titrating to a maximum of 3–4 mg orally daily, divided twice daily) are first-line therapies because of a favorable side-effect profile compared with typical antipsychotics, which are the only FDA-approved therapies for the disorder. Many specialists favor the use of tetrabenazine. Topiramate has yielded mixed results in several studies. Atypical antipsychotics, including risperidone and aripiprazole, have shown possible efficacy and may be tried before the typical antipsychotic agents. When a typical antipsychotic is required in cases of severe tics, haloperidol is generally regarded as the drug of choice. It is started in a low dose (0.25 mg daily orally) that is gradually increased (by 0.25 mg every 4 or 5 days) until there is maximum benefit with a minimum of side effects or until side effects limit further increments. A total daily oral dose of between 2 mg and 8 mg is usually optimal, but higher doses are sometimes necessary. Fluphenazine (1–15 mg orally daily) or pimozide (1–10 mg orally daily) are alternatives. Typical antipsychotics can cause significant weight gain and carry a risk of tardive dyskinesias and other long-term, potentially irreversible motor side effects.

Injection of botulinum toxin type A at the site of the most distressing tics is sometimes worthwhile and has fewer side effects than systemic antipsychotic therapy. Bilateral high-frequency deep brain stimulation at various sites has been helpful in some, otherwise intractable, cases.

When to Refer

All patients with Gilles de la Tourette syndrome should be referred.

When to Admit

Patients undergoing surgical (deep brain stimulation) treatment should be admitted.

Schrock LE et al; Tourette Syndrome Association International Deep Brain Stimulation (DBS) Database and Registry Study Group. Tourette syndrome deep brain stimulation: a review and updated recommendations. Mov Disord. 2015 Apr; 30(4):448–71. [PMID: 25476818]

Serajee FJ et al. Advances in Tourette syndrome: diagnoses and treatment. Pediatr Clin North Am. 2015 Jun;62(3):687–701. [PMID: 26022170]

Wile DJ et al. Behavior therapy for Tourette syndrome: a systematic review and meta-analysis. Curr Treat Options Neurol. 2013 Aug; 15(4):385–95. [PMID: 23645295]

DEMENTIA

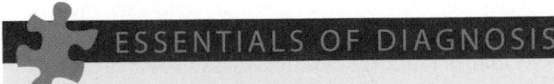

ESSENTIALS OF DIAGNOSIS

▶ Progressive intellectual decline.

▶ Not due to delirium or psychiatric disease.

▶ Age is the main risk factor, followed by family history and vascular disease risk factors.

General Considerations

Dementia is a progressive decline in intellectual function that is severe enough to compromise social or occupational functioning. "Mild cognitive impairment" describes a decline that has not resulted in a change in the level of function. Although a few patients identify a precipitating event, most experience an insidious onset and gradual progression of symptoms.

Dementia typically begins after age 60, and the prevalence doubles approximately every 5 years thereafter; in persons aged 85 and older, around half have dementia. In most, the cause of dementia is acquired, either as a sporadic primary neurodegenerative disease or as the result of another disorder, such as stroke (Table 24–6). Other risk factors for dementia include family history, diabetes mellitus and other vascular disease risk factors, and a history of significant head injury. Vitamin D deficiency and chronic sleep deprivation may also increase the risk of dementia. Dementia is more prevalent among women, but this may be accounted for by their longer life expectancy. Education and ongoing intellectual stimulation may be protective, perhaps by promoting a "cognitive reserve," an improved capacity to compensate for insidious neurodegeneration.

Dementia is distinct from delirium and psychiatric disease. **Delirium** is an acute confusional state that often occurs in response to an identifiable trigger, such as drug or alcohol intoxication or withdrawal (eg, Wernicke encephalopathy, described below), medication side effects (especially drugs with anticholinergic properties, antihistamines, benzodiazepines, sleeping aids, opioids, neuroleptics, corticosteroids, and other sedative or psychotropic agents),

infection (consider occult urinary tract infection or pneumonia in elderly patients), metabolic disturbance (including an electrolyte abnormality; hypoglycemia or hyperglycemia; or a nutritional, endocrine, renal, or hepatic disorder), sleep deprivation, or other neurologic disease (seizure, including a postictal state, or stroke). Delirium typically involves fluctuating levels of arousal, including drowsiness or agitation, and it improves after removal or treatment of the precipitating factor. Patients with dementia are especially susceptible to episodes of delirium, but recognition of dementia is not possible until delirium lifts. For this reason, dementia is typically diagnosed in outpatients who are otherwise medically stable, rather than in acutely ill patients in the hospital.

Psychiatric disease sometimes leads to complaints of impaired cognition. Impaired attention is usually to blame, and in some patients with depression or anxiety, poor focus and concentration may even be a primary complaint. The symptoms should improve with appropriate psychiatric treatment. Mood disorders are commonly seen in patients with neurodegenerative disease and in some cases are an

Table 24–6. Common causes of age-related dementia.

Disorder	Pathology	Clinical Features
Alzheimer disease	Plaques containing beta-amyloid peptide, and neurofibrillary tangles containing tau protein, occur throughout the neocortex	• Most common age-related neurodegenerative disease; incidence doubles every 5 years after age 60 • Short-term memory impairment is early and prominent in most cases • Variable deficits of executive function, visuospatial function, and language
Vascular dementia	Multifocal ischemic change	• Stepwise or progressive accumulation of cognitive deficits in association with repeated strokes • Symptoms depend on localization of strokes
Dementia with Lewy bodies	Histologically indistinguishable from Parkinson disease: alpha-synuclein-containing Lewy bodies occur in the brainstem, midbrain, olfactory bulb, and neocortex. Alzheimer pathology may coexist.	• Cognitive dysfunction, with prominent visuospatial and executive deficits • Psychiatric disturbance, with anxiety, visual hallucinations, and fluctuating delirium • Parkinsonian motor deficits with or after other features • Cholinesterase inhibitors lessen delirium; poor tolerance of neuroleptics and dopaminergics
Frontotemporal dementia (FTD)	Neuropathology is variable and defined by the protein found in intraneuronal aggregates. Tau protein, TAR DNA-binding protein 43 (TDP-43), or fused-in-sarcoma (FUS) protein account for most cases.	• Peak incidence in the sixth decade; approximately equal to Alzheimer disease as a cause of dementia in patients under 60 years old • Familial cases result from mutations in genes for tau, progranulin, or others **Behavioral variant FTD** • Deficits in empathy, social comportment, insight, abstract thought, and executive function • Behavior is disinhibited, impulsive, and ritualistic, with prominent apathy and increased interest in sex or sweet/fatty foods • Relative preservation of memory • Focal right frontal atrophy • Association with amyotrophic lateral sclerosis **Semantic variant primary progressive aphasia** • Deficits in word-finding, single-word comprehension, object and category knowledge, and face recognition • Behaviors may be similar to behavioral variant FTD • Focal, asymmetric temporal pole atrophy **Nonfluent/agrammatic variant primary progressive aphasia** • Speech is effortful with dysarthria, phonemic errors, sound distortions, and poor grammar • Focal extrapyramidal signs and apraxia of the right arm and leg are common; overlaps with corticobasal degeneration • Focal left frontal atrophy

early symptom. There is some evidence that a persistent, untreated mood disorder may predispose to the development of an age-related dementia, and psychiatric symptoms can clearly exacerbate cognitive impairment in patients who already have dementia; therefore, suspicion of dementia should not distract from appropriate screening for and treatment of depression or anxiety.

► Clinical Findings

A. Symptoms and Signs

Symptoms and signs of the common causes of dementia are detailed in Table 24–6. Clinicians should be aware that a patient's insight into a cognitive change may be vague or absent, and collateral history is essential to a proper evaluation. As patients age, primary care clinicians should inquire periodically about the presence of any cognitive symptoms.

Symptoms depend on the area of the brain affected. **Short-term memory loss**, involving the repeating of questions or stories and a diminished ability to recall the details of recent conversations or events, frequently results from pathologic changes in the hippocampus. **Word-finding difficulty** often involves difficulty recalling the names of people, places, or objects, with low-frequency words affected first, eventually resulting in speech laden with pronouns and circumlocutions. This problem is thought to arise from pathology at the temporoparietal junction of the left hemisphere. Problems with articulation, fluency, comprehension, or word meaning are anatomically distinct and less common. **Visuospatial dysfunction** may result in poor navigation and getting lost in familiar places, impaired recognition of previously familiar faces and buildings, or trouble discerning an object against a background. The right parietal lobe is one of the brain areas implicated in such symptoms. **Executive dysfunction** may manifest by easy distractibility, impulsivity, mental inflexibility, concrete thought, slowed processing speed, poor planning and organization, or impaired judgment. Localization may vary and could include the frontal lobes or subcortical areas like the basal ganglia or cerebral white matter. **Apathy** or indifference, separate from depression, is common and may have a similar anatomy as executive dysfunction. **Apraxia**, or the loss of learned motor behaviors, may result from dysfunction of the frontal or parietal lobes, especially the left parietal lobe.

The time of symptom onset must be established, but subtle, early symptoms are often apparent only in retrospect. Another event, such as an illness or hospitalization, may lead to a new recognition of existing symptoms. Symptoms often accumulate over time, and the nature of the earliest symptom is most helpful in forming the differential diagnosis. The history should establish risk factors for dementia, including family history, other chronic illnesses, and vascular disease risk factors. Finally, it is important to document the patient's current capacity to perform basic and instrumental activities of daily living (see Chapter 4) and to note the extent of decline from the premorbid level of function. Indeed, it is this functional assessment that defines the presence and severity of a dementia.

The physical examination is important to identify any occult medical illness. In addition, eye movement abnormalities, parkinsonism, or other motor abnormalities may help identify an underlying neurologic condition. The workup should prioritize the exclusion of conditions that are reversible or require separate therapy. Screening for depression is necessary, along with imaging and laboratory workup, as indicated below.

B. Neuropsychological Assessment

Brief quantification of cognitive impairment is indicated in a patient complaining of cognitive symptoms. The Folstein Mini Mental State Exam (MMSE), Montreal Cognitive Assessment (MoCA), Mini-Cog, and other similar tests are brief, objective, and widely used but have important limitations: they are insensitive to mild cognitive impairment, they may be biased negatively by the presence of language or attention problems, and they do not correlate with functional capacity.

An evaluation by a trained neuropsychologist or psychometrician may be appropriate. The goal of such testing is to enhance localization by defining the cognitive domains that are impaired as well as to quantify the degree of impairment. There is no standard battery of tests, but a variety of metrics is commonly used to assess all of the symptom types highlighted above. Assessments are most accurate when a patient is well-rested, comfortable, and otherwise medically stable.

C. Imaging

Brain imaging with MRI or CT without contrast is indicated in any patient with a new, progressive cognitive complaint. The goal is to exclude occult cerebrovascular disease, tumor, or other identifiable structural abnormality, rather than to provide positive evidence of a neurodegenerative disease. Global or focal brain atrophy may be worse than expected for age and could suggest a particular neurodegenerative process, but such findings are rarely specific.

Positron-emission tomography (PET) with fluorodeoxyglucose (FDG) does not confirm or exclude any specific cause of dementia but may be useful as an element of the workup in specific clinical circumstances, such as discriminating between Alzheimer disease and frontotemporal dementia in a patient with some symptoms of each. PET imaging with a radiolabeled ligand for beta-amyloid, one of the pathologic proteins in Alzheimer disease, is highly sensitive to amyloid pathology and may help provide positive evidence for Alzheimer disease in a patient with cognitive decline. However, after age 60 or 70, amyloid plaques can accumulate in the absence of cognitive impairment; thus, the specificity of a positive amyloid scan diminishes with age. Single photon-emission computed tomography offers similar information as FDG-PET but is less sensitive. PET imaging with radiolabeled ligands for tau, a pathogenic protein in Alzheimer disease, progressive supranuclear palsy, and some forms of frontotemporal dementia, has entered clinical trials and may help refine premortem diagnostic accuracy.

D. Laboratory Findings

Serum levels of vitamin B_{12}, free T_4, and thyroid-stimulating hormone should be measured for any patient with cognitive symptoms. A serum rapid plasma reagin (RPR) and testing for HIV should be considered. Other testing should be driven by clinical suspicion, and often includes a complete blood count, serum electrolytes, glucose, and lipid profile.

Although the presence of one or two ApoE epsilon-4 alleles indicates an increased risk of Alzheimer disease and ApoE genotyping is clinically available, it is of limited clinical utility. Finding an ApoE epsilon-4 allele in a young patient with dementia might raise the index of suspicion for Alzheimer disease, but obtaining a genotype in an elderly patient is unlikely to be helpful, and doing so in an asymptomatic patient as a marker of risk for Alzheimer disease is inappropriate until a preventive therapy becomes available. Spinal fluid protein measurements are also available; levels of beta-amyloid decrease and tau protein increase in Alzheimer disease, but this testing shares some of the same concerns as amyloid PET imaging. Serum tests for Alzheimer disease are in the early stages of development.

▶ Differential Diagnosis

In elderly patients with gradually progressive cognitive symptoms and no other complaint or sign, a neurodegenerative disease is likely (Table 24–6). Decline beginning before age 60, rapid progression, fluctuating course, unintended weight loss, systemic complaints, or other unexplained symptoms or signs raise suspicion for another process. In this case, the differential is broad and includes infection or inflammatory disease (consider a lumbar puncture to screen for cells or antibodies in the spinal fluid), neoplasm or a paraneoplastic condition, endocrine or metabolic disease, drugs or toxins, or other conditions. **Normal pressure hydrocephalus** is a difficult diagnosis to establish. Symptoms include gait apraxia (sometimes described as a "magnetic" gait, as if the feet are stuck to the floor), urinary incontinence, and dementia. CT scanning or MRI of the brain reveals ventricles that are enlarged in obvious disproportion to sulcal widening and overall brain atrophy.

▶ Treatment

A. Nonpharmacologic Approaches

Aerobic exercise (45 minutes most days of the week) and frequent mental stimulation may reduce the rate of functional decline and decrease the demented patient's caregiving needs, and these interventions may reduce the risk of dementia in normal individuals. The most efficacious manner of mental stimulation is a matter of debate: maintaining as active a role in the family and community as practically possible is most likely to be of benefit, emphasizing activities at which the patient feels confident. Patients with neurodegenerative diseases have a limited capacity to regain lost skills; for instance, memory drills in a patient with Alzheimer disease are more likely to lead to frustration than benefit and studies show that computerized cognitive training does not improve cognition or function in demented patients.

B. Cognitive Symptoms

Cholinesterase inhibitors are first-line therapy for Alzheimer disease and dementia with Lewy bodies (Table 24–6). They provide modest, symptomatic treatment for cognitive dysfunction and may prolong the capacity for independence but do not prevent disease progression. Commonly used medications include donepezil (start at 5 mg orally daily for 4 weeks, then increase to 10 mg daily; a 23 mg daily dose is approved for moderate to severe Alzheimer disease, although its very modest additional efficacy over the 10 mg dose is overshadowed by an increased risk of side effects); rivastigmine (start at 1.5 mg orally twice daily, then increasing every 2 weeks by 1.5 mg twice daily to a goal of 3–6 mg twice daily; or 4.6, 9.5, or 13.3 mg/24 hours transdermally daily); and galantamine (start at 4 mg orally twice daily, then increasing every 4 weeks by 4 mg twice daily to a goal of 8–12 mg twice daily; a once-daily extended-release formulation is also available). Cholinesterase inhibitors are not given for frontotemporal dementia because they may worsen behavioral symptoms. Nausea and diarrhea are common side effects; syncope and cardiac dysrhythmia are uncommon but more serious. An ECG is often obtained before and after starting therapy, particularly in a patient with cardiac disease or a history of syncope.

Memantine (start at 5 mg orally daily, then increase by 5 mg per week up to a target of 10 mg twice daily) is approved for the treatment of moderate to severe Alzheimer disease. In frontotemporal dementia, memantine is ineffective and may worsen cognition. There is some evidence that memantine may improve cognition and behavior among patients with dementia with Lewy bodies.

Disease-modifying drugs are not yet available for Alzheimer disease. Immunotherapy directed against beta-amyloid has not shown promise in phase III trials.

C. Mood and Behavioral Disturbances

Selective serotonin reuptake inhibitors are generally safe and well-tolerated in elderly, cognitively impaired patients, and they may be efficacious for the treatment of depression, anxiety, or agitation. There is evidence to support the use of citalopram for agitation; however, side effects also occur, including QTc prolongation. Paroxetine should be avoided because it has anticholinergic effects; avoid all tricyclic antidepressants for the same reason. Other antidepressant agents, such as buproprion or venlafaxine, may also be tried.

Insomnia is common, and trazodone (25–50 mg orally at bedtime as needed) can be safe and effective. Over-the-counter antihistamine hypnotics must be avoided, along with benzodiazepines, because of their tendency to worsen cognition and precipitate delirium. Other prescription hypnotics such as zolpidem may result in similar adverse reactions.

For agitation, impulsivity, and other behaviors that interfere with safe caregiving, causes of delirium (detailed above) should first be considered. When no reversible trigger is identified, treatment should be approached in a staged manner. Behavioral interventions, such as reorientation and distraction from anxiety-provoking stimuli, are first-line. Ensure that the patient is kept active during the day with both physical exercise and mentally stimulating activities, and that there is adequate sleep at night. Reassess the level of caregiving, and consider increasing the time spent directly with an attendant. Next, ensure that appropriate pharmacologic treatment of cognition and mood is optimized. Finally, as a last resort, when other measures prove insufficient and the patient's behaviors raise safety concerns, consider low doses of an atypical antipsychotic medication, such as quetiapine (start 25 mg orally daily as needed, increasing to two to three times daily as needed); even though atypical agents cause extrapyramidal side effects less frequently than typical antipsychotics, they should be used with particular caution in a patient at risk for falls, especially if parkinsonian signs are already present. Regularly scheduled dosing is not recommended, and if implemented should be reassessed on a frequent basis (eg, weekly), with attempts to taper off as tolerated. There is an FDA black box warning against the use of all antipsychotic medications in demented patients because of an increased risk of death. The combination of dextromethorphan and quinidine (up to 30/10 mg orally twice daily) has shown promise in early clinical trials.

Finally, psychostimulants like methylphenidate have been studied as a means to treat apathy in dementia. While such treatment may be of benefit to selected patients, the possibility of causing agitation or cardiovascular strain limits routine use.

▶ Special Circumstances

A. Rapidly Progressive Dementia

When dementia develops quickly, with obvious decline over a few weeks to a few months, the syndrome may be classified as a rapidly progressive dementia. The differential diagnosis for typical dementias is still relevant, but additional etiologies must be considered, including prion disease; infections; toxins; neoplasms; and autoimmune and inflammatory diseases, including corticosteroid-responsive (Hashimoto) encephalopathy and antibody-mediated paraneoplastic syndromes. Workup should begin with brain MRI with contrast and diffusion-weighted imaging, routine laboratory studies (serum vitamin B_{12}, free T_4, and thyroid-stimulating hormone levels), serum RPR, HIV antibody, Lyme serology, rheumatologic tests (erythrocyte sedimentation rate, C-reactive protein, and antinuclear antibody), anti-thyroglobulin and anti-thyroperoxidase antibody levels, paraneoplastic autoimmune antibodies, and cerebrospinal fluid studies (cell count and differential; protein and glucose levels; protein electrophoresis for oligoclonal bands; IgG index [spinal-fluid-to-serum gamma-globulin level] ratio; and VDRL). Depending on the clinical context, it may be necessary to exclude Wilson disease (24-hour urine copper level), heavy metal intoxication (24-hour urine heavy metal panel), and infectious encephalitis (cerebrospinal fluid polymerase chain reaction for Whipple disease, herpes simplex virus, cytomegalovirus, varicella-zoster virus, and other viruses).

Creutzfeldt-Jakob disease is a relatively common cause of rapidly progressive dementia (see Chapter 32). Family history is important since mutations in *PRNP*, the gene for the prion protein, account for around 15% of cases. Diffusion-weighted MRI is the most helpful diagnostic tool, classically revealing cortical ribboning (a gyral pattern of hyperintensity) as well as restricted diffusion in the caudate and anterior putamen. Reflecting the high rate of neuronal death, cerebrospinal fluid levels of the intraneuronal proteins tau, 14-3-3, and neuron-specific enolase are often elevated, although this finding is neither sensitive nor specific. An electroencephalogram often shows periodic complexes.

B. Driving and Dementia

It is recommended that any patient with mild dementia or worse should discontinue driving. Most states have laws regulating driving among cognitively impaired individuals, and many require the clinician to report the patient's diagnosis to the public health department or department of motor vehicles. There is no evidence that driving classes help patients with neurodegenerative diseases.

▶ When to Refer

All patients with new, unexplained cognitive decline should be referred.

▶ When to Admit

Dementia alone is not an indication for admission, but admission is sometimes necessary when a superimposed delirium poses safety risks at home.

Cooper C et al. Modifiable predictors of dementia in mild cognitive impairment: a systematic review and meta-analysis. Am J Psychiatry. 2015 Apr;172(4):323–34. [PMID: 25698435]

Galasko D. The diagnostic evaluation of a patient with dementia. Continuum (Minneap Minn). 2013 Apr;19(2):397–410. [PMID: 23558485]

Mitchell SL. Clinical Practice. Advanced dementia. N Engl J Med. 2015 Jun 25;372(26):2533–40. [PMID: 26107053]

Paterson RW et al. Diagnosis and treatment of rapidly progressive dementias. Neurol Clin Pract. 2012 Sep;2(3):187–200. [PMID: 23634367]

Reitz C et al. Alzheimer disease: epidemiology, diagnostic criteria, risk factors and biomarkers. Biochem Pharmacol. 2014 Apr 15;88(4):640–51. [PMID: 24398425]

MULTIPLE SCLEROSIS

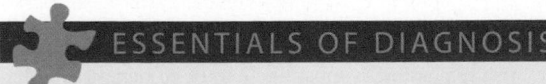

ESSENTIALS OF DIAGNOSIS

▶ Episodic neurologic symptoms.

▶ Patient usually under 55 years of age at onset.

▶ Single pathologic lesion cannot explain clinical findings.

▶ Multiple foci best visualized by MRI.

General Considerations

This common neurologic disorder, which probably has an autoimmune basis, has its greatest incidence in young adults. Epidemiologic studies indicate that multiple sclerosis is much more common in persons of western European lineage who live in temperate zones. No population with a high risk for multiple sclerosis exists between latitudes 40° N and 40° S. A genetic susceptibility to the disease is present, based on twin studies, familial cases, and an association with specific HLA antigens (HLA-DR2) and alleles of *IL2RA* (the interleukin-2 receptor alpha gene) and *IL7RA* (the interleukin-7 receptor alpha gene). Pathologically, focal—often perivenular—areas of demyelination with reactive gliosis are found scattered in the white matter of the brain and spinal cord and in the optic nerves. Axonal damage also occurs.

Clinical Findings

A. Symptoms and Signs

The common initial presentation is weakness, numbness, tingling, or unsteadiness in a limb; spastic paraparesis; retrobulbar optic neuritis; diplopia; dysequilibrium; or a sphincter disturbance such as urinary urgency or hesitancy. Symptoms may disappear after a few days or weeks, although examination often reveals a residual deficit.

Several forms of the disease are recognized. In most patients, there is an interval of months or years after the initial episode before new symptoms develop or the original ones recur (**relapsing-remitting disease**). Eventually, however, relapses and usually incomplete remissions lead to increasing disability, with weakness, spasticity, and ataxia of the limbs, impaired vision, and urinary incontinence. The findings on examination at this stage commonly include optic atrophy; nystagmus; dysarthria; and pyramidal, sensory, or cerebellar deficits in some or all of the limbs. In some of these patients, the clinical course changes so that a steady deterioration occurs, unrelated to acute relapses (**secondary progressive disease**). Less commonly, symptoms are steadily progressive from their onset, and disability develops at a relatively early stage (**primary progressive disease**). The diagnosis cannot be made with confidence unless the total clinical picture indicates involvement of different parts of the central nervous system at different times. Fatigue is common in all forms of the disease.

A number of factors (eg, infection) may precipitate or trigger exacerbations. Relapses are reduced in pregnancy but are more likely during the 2 or 3 months following pregnancy, possibly because of the increased demands and stresses that occur in the postpartum period.

B. Imaging

MRI of the brain and cervical cord has a major role in excluding other causes of neurologic dysfunction and in demonstrating the presence of multiple lesions. In T1-weighted images, hypointense "black holes" probably represent areas of permanent axonal damage. Gadolinium-enhanced T1-weighted images may highlight areas of active inflammation with breakdown of the blood-brain barrier, which helps identify newer lesions. T2-weighted images provide information about disease burden or total number of lesions, which typically appear as areas of high signal intensity. CT scans are less helpful than MRI.

In patients with myelopathy alone and no clinical or laboratory evidence of more widespread disease, MRI or myelography is necessary to exclude a congenital or acquired surgically treatable lesion. In patients with mixed pyramidal and cerebellar deficits in the limbs, the foramen magnum region must be visualized to exclude the possibility of Arnold-Chiari malformation, in which parts of the cerebellum and lower brainstem are displaced into the cervical canal.

C. Laboratory and Other Studies

A definitive diagnosis can never be based solely on the laboratory findings. If there is clinical evidence of only a single lesion in the central nervous system, multiple sclerosis cannot properly be diagnosed unless it can be shown that other regions are affected subclinically. Visual, brainstem auditory, and somatosensory evoked potentials are helpful in this regard, but other disorders may also be characterized by multifocal electrophysiologic abnormalities reflecting disease of central white matter. Certain infections (eg, HIV, Lyme disease, syphilis), connective tissue diseases, sarcoidosis, metabolic disorders (eg, vitamin B_{12} deficiency), and lymphoma may therefore require exclusion.

There may be mild lymphocytosis or a slightly increased protein concentration in the cerebrospinal fluid, especially soon after an acute relapse. Elevated IgG in cerebrospinal fluid and discrete bands of IgG (oligoclonal bands) are present in many patients. The presence of such bands is not specific, however, since they have been found in a variety of inflammatory neurologic disorders and occasionally in patients with vascular or neoplastic disorders of the nervous system.

Vitamin D deficiency may be associated with an increased risk of developing multiple sclerosis; whether supplementation prevents the disease or disease progression is under study.

D. Diagnosis

Multiple sclerosis should not be diagnosed unless there is evidence that two or more different regions of the central white matter (dissemination in space) have been affected at different times (dissemination in time). The diagnosis may be made in a patient with two or more typical attacks and two or more MRI lesions. To fulfill the criterion of dissemination in space in a patient with only one lesion, repeat imaging in a few months should demonstrate at least one lesion in at least two of four typical sites (periventricular, juxtacortical, infratentorial, or spinal); alternatively, an additional attack localized to a different site suffices. To fulfill the criterion of dissemination in time in a patient with only one attack, the simultaneous presence of asymptomatic gadolinium-enhancing and nonenhancing lesions at any time (including at initial examination) suffices;

alternatively, await a new lesion on follow-up MRI or a second attack. Primary progressive disease requires at least a year of progressive disease, plus two of three of the following: at least one typical brain lesion, at least two spinal lesions, or oligoclonal banding in the cerebrospinal fluid.

In patients with a single clinical event who do not satisfy criteria for multiple sclerosis, a diagnosis of a **clinically isolated syndrome (CIS)** is made. Such patients are at risk for developing multiple sclerosis and are sometimes offered beta-interferon or glatiramer acetate therapy, which may delay progression to clinically definite disease. Follow-up MRI should be considered 6–12 months later to assess for the presence of any new lesion.

▶ Treatment

At least partial recovery from acute exacerbations can reasonably be expected, but further relapses may occur without warning. Some disability is likely to result eventually, but about half of all patients are without significant disability even 10 years after onset of symptoms. Current treatments are chiefly aimed at preventing relapses, thereby reducing the accumulation of disability.

Recovery from acute relapses may be hastened by treatment with corticosteroids, but the extent of recovery is unchanged. Intravenous therapy is given first—typically methylprednisolone 1 g daily for 3 days—followed by oral prednisone at 60–80 mg daily for 1 week with a taper over the ensuing 2–3 weeks. Long-term treatment with corticosteroids provides no benefit and does not prevent further relapses. Transient exacerbations of symptoms relating to intercurrent infection requires no added treatment.

In patients with relapsing disease, numerous medications have well-established efficacy at reducing the frequency of attacks (Table 24–7). Natalizumab is highly effective but increases the risk of developing progressive multifocal leukoencephalopathy; its use is therefore generally restricted to patients in whom testing for JC virus antibodies is negative and it is stopped if seroconversion occurs during the course of therapy. Progressive multifocal

Table 24–7. Treatment of multiple sclerosis.

Medication	Dose
Acute episode, including relapse[1]	
Methylprednisolone	1 g intravenously daily for 3–5 days
Prednisone	1000 mg orally daily for 3–5 days
Dexamethasone	160 mg orally daily for 3–5 days
Relapse prevention, first-line treatment[2]	
Interferon β-1a (Rebif)	44 mcg subcutaneously three times per week
Interferon β-1a (Aconex)	30 mcg intramuscularly once per week
Interferon β-1b (Betaseron, Extavia)	0.25 mg subcutaneously on alternate days
Glatiramer acetate (Copaxone)	20 mg subcutaneously daily
Fingolimod (Gilenya)[3]	0.5 mg orally daily
Teriflunomide (Aubagio)[4]	14 mg orally daily
Dimethyl fumarate (Techfidera)	240 mg orally twice daily
Relapse prevention for disease activity despite use of first-line treatment	
Natalizumab (Tysabri)[5]	300 mg intravenously monthly
Fingolimod (Gilenya)[3]	0.5 mg orally daily
Teriflunomide (Aubagio)[4]	14 mg orally daily
Dimethyl fumarate (Techfidera)	240 mg orally twice daily
Alemtuzumab (Lemtrada)	12 mg intravenously daily for 5 days; 3-day course given 1 year later
Mitoxantrone	12 mg/m^2 intravenously every 3 months; maximum lifetime dose, 140 mg/m^2
High disease activity (typically with multiple gadolinium-enhancing lesions on MRI)	
Natalizumab (Tysabri)[5]	300 mg intravenously monthly
Alemtuzumab (Lemtrada)	12 mg intravenously daily for 5 days; 3-day course given 1 year later

Reproduced, with permission from Aminoff MJ et al. *Clinical Neurology*, 9th ed, McGraw-Hill Education, 2015.
[1]For corticosteroid-refractory relapses, plasmapheresis may be used.
[2]High-dose high-frequency interferons, fingolimod, and glatiramer acetate are more efficacious than once weekly interferon.
[3]Heart rate should be monitored for 6 hours after the first dose of fingolimod or if restarted after an interval of ≥ 2 weeks.
[4]Pregnancy category X; if patient becomes pregnant, need to wash out drug; monitor for hepatotoxicity.
[5]Need to monitor JC antibody status every 6 months.

leukoencephalopathy has developed in several patients taking dimethyl fumarate. Fingolimod is associated with fatal disseminated varicella zoster infection, and immunity must be demonstrated prior to treatment initiation. Alemtuzumab is also associated with disseminated zoster as well as development of autoimmune disease and malignancy.

For patients with severe or progressive disease, limited evidence supports immunosuppressive therapy with rituximab, cyclophosphamide, azathioprine, methotrexate, or mitoxantrone. Plasmapheresis is sometimes helpful in patients with severe relapses unresponsive to corticosteroids.

Symptomatic therapy for spasticity, neurogenic bladder, or fatigue may be required. Fatigue is especially common in multiple sclerosis, and modafinil (200 mg orally every morning) is an effective and FDA-approved therapy for this indication. Dalfampridine (an extended-release formulation of 4-aminopyridine administered as 10 mg orally twice daily) is efficacious at improving timed gait in multiple sclerosis. Depression and even suicidality can occur in multiple sclerosis and may worsen with interferon beta-1a therapy; screening and conventional treatment of such symptoms are appropriate.

▶ When to Refer

All patients, but especially those with progressive disease despite standard therapy, should be referred.

▶ When to Admit

- Patients requiring plasma exchange for severe relapses unresponsive to corticosteroids.
- During severe relapses.
- Patients unable to manage at home.

Carrithers MD. Update on disease-modifying treatments for multiple sclerosis. Clin Ther. 2014 Dec 1;36(12):1938–45. [PMID: 25218310]

Feinstein A et al. Treatment of progressive multiple sclerosis: what works, what does not, and what is needed. Lancet Neurol. 2015 Feb;14(2):194–207. [PMID: 25772898]

Filippini G et al. Immunomodulators and immunosuppressants for multiple sclerosis: a network meta-analysis. Cochrane Database Syst Rev. 2013 Jun 6;6:CD008933. [PMID: 23744561]

Gelfand JM. Multiple sclerosis: diagnosis, differential diagnosis, and clinical presentation. Handb Clin Neurol. 2014;122:269–90. [PMID: 24507522]

NEUROMYELITIS OPTICA

This disorder is characterized by optic neuritis and acute myelitis with MRI changes that extend over at least three segments of the spinal cord. An isolated myelitis or optic neuritis may also occur. Previously known as Devic disease and once regarded as a variant of multiple sclerosis, neuromyelitis optica is associated with a specific antibody marker (NMO-IgG) targeting the water channel aquaporin-4. MRI of the brain typically does not show widespread white matter involvement, but such changes do not exclude the diagnosis. Treatment is by long-term immunosuppression. First-line therapy is with rituximab (two 1 g

intravenous infusions spaced by 2 weeks, or four weekly infusions of 375 mg/m^2; re-dosing may occur every 6 months or when CD19/20-positive or CD27-positive lymphocytes become detectable), mycophenolate mofetil (500–1500 mg orally twice daily, titrated until the absolute lymphocyte count falls below 1500/mcL), or with azathioprine (2.5–3 mg/kg orally). Acute relapses are treated with corticosteroids at doses similar to those outlined for multiple sclerosis, with plasma exchange for severe relapses unresponsive to corticosteroids.

Trebst C et al. Update on the diagnosis and treatment of neuromyelitis optica: Recommendations of the Neuromyelitis Optica Study Group (NEMOS). J Neurol. 2014 Jan;261(1):1–16. [PMID: 24272588]

Wingerchuk DM et al; International Panel for NMO Diagnosis. International consensus diagnostic criteria for neuromyelitis optica spectrum disorders. Neurology. 2015 Jul 14;85(2):177–89. [PMID: 26092914]

VITAMIN E DEFICIENCY

Vitamin E deficiency may produce a disorder somewhat similar to Friedreich ataxia. There is spinocerebellar degeneration involving particularly the posterior columns of the spinal cord and leading to limb ataxia, sensory loss, absent tendon reflexes, slurring of speech and, in some cases, pigmentary retinal degeneration. The disorder may occur as a consequence of malabsorption or on a hereditary basis (eg, abetalipoproteinemia).

Pfeiffer RF. Neurologic manifestations of malabsorption syndromes. Handb Clin Neurol. 2014;120:621–32. [PMID: 24365342]

SPASTICITY

The term "spasticity" is commonly used for an upper motor neuron deficit, but it properly refers to a velocity-dependent increase in resistance to passive movement that affects different muscles to a different extent, is not uniform in degree throughout the range of a particular movement, and is commonly associated with other features of pyramidal deficit. It is often a major complication of stroke, cerebral or spinal injury, static perinatal encephalopathy, and multiple sclerosis.

Physical therapy with appropriate stretching programs is important during rehabilitation after the development of an upper motor neuron lesion and in subsequent management of the patient. The aim is to prevent joint and muscle contractures and perhaps to modulate spasticity.

Drug management is important also, but treatment may increase functional disability when increased extensor tone is providing additional support for patients with weak legs. Dantrolene weakens muscle contraction by interfering with the role of calcium. It is best avoided in patients with poor respiratory function or severe myocardial disease. Treatment is begun with 25 mg once daily, increased by 25 mg every 3 days, depending on tolerance, to a maximum of 100 mg four times daily. Side effects include diarrhea, nausea, weakness, hepatic dysfunction (that may rarely be fatal, especially in women older than 35), drowsiness, light-headedness, and hallucinations.

Baclofen is an effective drug for treating spasticity of spinal origin and painful flexor (or extensor) spasms. The maximum recommended daily oral dose is 80 mg; treatment is started with a dose of 5 or 10 mg twice daily orally and then built up gradually. Side effects include gastrointestinal disturbances, lassitude, fatigue, sedation, unsteadiness, confusion, and hallucinations. Diazepam may modify spasticity by its action on spinal interneurons and perhaps also by influencing supraspinal centers, but effective doses often cause intolerable drowsiness and vary with different patients. Tizanidine, a centrally acting alpha-2-adrenergic agonist, is as effective as these other agents and is probably better tolerated. The daily dose is built up gradually, usually to 8 mg taken three times daily. Side effects include sedation, lassitude, hypotension, and dryness of the mouth.

Intramuscular injection of botulinum toxin has been used to relax targeted muscles.

In patients with severe spasticity that is unresponsive to other therapies and is associated with marked disability, intrathecal injection of phenol or alcohol may be helpful. Surgical options include implantation of an intrathecal baclofen pump, rhizotomy, or neurectomy. Severe contractures may be treated by surgical tendon release.

Spasticity may be exacerbated by decubitus ulcers, urinary or other infections, and nociceptive stimuli.

Nair KP et al. The management of spasticity in adults. BMJ. 2014 Aug 5;349:g4737. [PMID: 25096594]

MYELOPATHIES IN AIDS

A variety of myelopathies may occur in patients with AIDS. These are discussed in Chapter 31.

MYELOPATHY OF HUMAN T-CELL LEUKEMIA VIRUS INFECTION

Human T-cell leukemia virus (HTLV-1), a human retrovirus, is transmitted by breast-feeding, sexual contact, blood transfusion, and contaminated needles. Most patients are asymptomatic, but after a variable latent period (which may be as long as several years) a myelopathy develops in some instances. The MRI, electrophysiologic, and cerebrospinal fluid findings are similar to those of multiple sclerosis, but HTLV-1 antibodies are present in serum and spinal fluid. There is no specific treatment, but intravenous or oral corticosteroids may help in the initial inflammatory phase of the disease. Prophylactic measures are important. Needles or syringes should not be shared; infected patients should not breastfeed their infants or donate blood, semen, or other tissue. Infected patients should use condoms to prevent sexual transmission.

Dhasmana D et al. Human T-lymphotropic virus/HIV co-infection: a clinical review. Curr Opin Infect Dis. 2014 Feb;27(1):16–28. [PMID: 24305042]

SUBACUTE COMBINED DEGENERATION OF THE SPINAL CORD

Subacute combined degeneration of the spinal cord is due to vitamin B_{12} deficiency, such as occurs in pernicious anemia. It is characterized by myelopathy with spasticity, weakness, proprioceptive loss, and numbness, sometimes in association with polyneuropathy, mental changes, or optic neuropathy. Megaloblastic anemia may also occur, but this does not parallel the neurologic disorder, and the former may be obscured if folic acid supplements have been taken. Treatment is with vitamin B_{12}. For pernicious anemia, a convenient therapeutic regimen is 1000 mcg cyanocobalamin intramuscularly daily for 1 week, then weekly for 1 month, and then monthly for the remainder of the patient's life. Oral cyanocobalamin replacement is not advised for pernicious anemia when neurologic symptoms are present. A similar syndrome is caused by recreational abuse of inhaled nitrous oxide due to its interference with vitamin B_{12} metabolism.

WERNICKE ENCEPHALOPATHY & KORSAKOFF SYNDROME

Wernicke encephalopathy is characterized by confusion, ataxia, and nystagmus leading to ophthalmoplegia (lateral rectus muscle weakness, conjugate gaze palsies); peripheral neuropathy may also be present. It is due to thiamine deficiency and in the United States occurs most commonly in patients with alcoholism. It may also occur in patients with AIDS or hyperemesis gravidarum, and after bariatric surgery. In suspected cases, thiamine (100 mg) is given intravenously immediately and then intramuscularly on a daily basis until a satisfactory diet can be ensured. Intravenous glucose given before thiamine may precipitate the syndrome or worsen the symptoms. The diagnosis is confirmed by the response in 1 or 2 days to treatment, which must not be delayed while awaiting laboratory confirmation of thiamine deficiency from a blood sample obtained prior to thiamine administration. **Korsakoff syndrome** occurs in more severe cases; it includes anterograde and retrograde amnesia and sometimes confabulation, and may not be recognized until after the initial delirium has lifted.

Latt N et al. Thiamine in the treatment of Wernicke encephalopathy in patients with alcohol use disorders. Intern Med J. 2014 Sep;44(9):911–5. [PMID: 25201422]

STUPOR & COMA

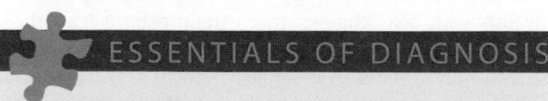

ESSENTIALS OF DIAGNOSIS

► Level of consciousness is depressed.

► Stuporous patients respond only to repeated vigorous stimuli.

► Comatose patients are unarousable and unresponsive.

General Considerations

The patient who is stuporous is unresponsive except when subjected to repeated vigorous stimuli, while the comatose patient is unarousable and unable to respond to external events or inner needs, although reflex movements and posturing may be present.

Coma is a major complication of serious central nervous system disorders. It can result from seizures, hypothermia, metabolic disturbances, or structural lesions causing bilateral cerebral hemispheric dysfunction or a disturbance of the brainstem reticular activating system. A mass lesion involving one cerebral hemisphere may cause coma by compression of the brainstem.

Assessment & Emergency Measures

The diagnostic workup of the comatose patient must proceed concomitantly with management. Supportive therapy for respiration or blood pressure is initiated; in hypothermia, all vital signs may be absent and all such patients should be rewarmed before the prognosis is assessed.

The patient can be positioned on one side with the neck partly extended, dentures removed, and secretions cleared by suction; if necessary, the patency of the airways is maintained with an oropharyngeal airway. Blood is drawn for serum glucose, electrolyte, and calcium levels; arterial blood gases; liver and kidney function tests; and toxicologic studies as indicated. Dextrose 50% (25 g), naloxone (0.4–1.2 mg), and thiamine (100 mg) are given intravenously without delay.

Further details are then obtained from attendants of the patient's medical history, the circumstances surrounding the onset of coma, and the time course of subsequent events. Abrupt onset of coma suggests subarachnoid hemorrhage, brainstem stroke, or intracerebral hemorrhage, whereas a slower onset and progression occur with other structural or mass lesions. Urgent noncontrast CT scanning of the head is appropriate if it can be obtained directly from the emergency department, in order to identify intracranial hemorrhage, brain herniation, or other structural lesion that may require immediate neurosurgical intervention. A metabolic cause is likely with a preceding intoxicated state or agitated delirium. On examination, attention is paid to the behavioral response to painful stimuli, the pupils and their response to light, the position of the eyes and their movement in response to passive movement of the head and ice-water caloric stimulation, and the respiratory pattern.

A. Response to Painful Stimuli

Purposeful limb withdrawal from painful stimuli implies that sensory pathways from and motor pathways to the stimulated limb are functionally intact. Unilateral absence of responses despite application of stimuli to both sides of the body in turn implies a corticospinal lesion; bilateral absence of responsiveness suggests brainstem involvement, bilateral pyramidal tract lesions, or psychogenic unresponsiveness. Inappropriate responses may also occur. Decorticate (flexor) posturing may occur with lesions of the internal capsule and rostral cerebral peduncle, decerebrate (extensor) posturing with dysfunction or destruction of the midbrain and rostral pons, and decerebrate posturing in the arms accompanied by flaccidity or slight flexor responses in the legs in patients with extensive brainstem damage extending down to the pons at the trigeminal level.

B. Ocular Findings

1. Pupils—Hypothalamic disease processes may lead to unilateral Horner syndrome, while bilateral diencephalic involvement or destructive pontine lesions may lead to small but reactive pupils. Ipsilateral pupillary dilation with no direct or consensual response to light occurs with compression of the third cranial nerve, eg, with uncal herniation. The pupils are slightly smaller than normal but responsive to light in many metabolic encephalopathies; however, they may be fixed and dilated following overdosage with atropine or scopolamine, and pinpoint (but responsive) with opioids.

2. Eye movements—Conjugate deviation of the eyes to the side suggests the presence of an ipsilateral hemispheric lesion, a contralateral pontine lesion, or ongoing seizures from the contralateral hemisphere. A mesencephalic lesion leads to downward conjugate deviation. Dysconjugate ocular deviation in coma implies a structural brainstem lesion unless there was preexisting strabismus.

The oculomotor responses to passive head turning and to caloric stimulation relate to each other and provide complementary information. In response to brisk rotation of the head from side to side and to flexion and extension of the head, normally conscious patients with open eyes do not exhibit contraversive conjugate eye deviation (oculocephalic reflex) unless there is voluntary visual fixation or bilateral frontal pathology. With cortical depression in lightly comatose patients, a brisk oculocephalic reflex is seen. With brainstem lesions, this oculocephalic reflex becomes impaired or lost, depending on the site of the lesion.

The oculovestibular reflex is tested by caloric stimulation using irrigation with ice water. In normal subjects, jerk nystagmus is elicited for about 2 or 3 minutes, with the slow component toward the irrigated ear. In unconscious patients with an intact brainstem, the fast component of the nystagmus disappears, so that the eyes tonically deviate toward the irrigated side for 2–3 minutes before returning to their original position. With impairment of brainstem function, the response becomes perverted and finally disappears. In metabolic coma, oculocephalic and oculovestibular reflex responses are preserved, at least initially.

C. Respiratory Patterns

Diseases causing coma may lead to respiratory abnormalities. Cheyne-Stokes respiration (in which episodes of deep breathing alternate with periods of apnea) may occur with bihemispheric or diencephalic disease or in metabolic disorders. Central neurogenic hyperventilation occurs with lesions of the brainstem tegmentum; apneustic breathing (in which there are prominent end-inspiratory pauses) suggests damage at the pontine level (eg, due to basilar artery occlusion); and atactic breathing (a completely irregular pattern of breathing with deep and shallow breaths occurring randomly) is associated with lesions of the lower pontine tegmentum and medulla.

1. Stupor & Coma Due to Structural Lesions

Supratentorial mass lesions tend to affect brain function in an orderly way. There may initially be signs of hemispheric dysfunction, such as hemiparesis. As coma develops and deepens, cerebral function becomes progressively disturbed, producing a predictable progression of neurologic signs that suggest rostrocaudal deterioration.

Thus, as a supratentorial mass lesion begins to impair the diencephalon, the patient becomes drowsy, then stuporous, and finally comatose. There may be Cheyne-Stokes respiration; small but reactive pupils; normal oculocephalic responses with side-to-side head movements but sometimes an impairment of reflex upward gaze with brisk flexion of the head; tonic ipsilateral deviation of the eyes in response to vestibular stimulation with cold water; and initially a positive response to pain but subsequently only decorticate posturing. With further progression, midbrain failure occurs. Motor dysfunction progresses from decorticate to bilateral decerebrate posturing in response to painful stimuli; Cheyne-Stokes respiration is gradually replaced by sustained central hyperventilation; the pupils become middle-sized and fixed; and the oculocephalic and oculovestibular reflex responses become impaired, perverted, or lost. As the pons and then the medulla fail, the pupils remain unresponsive; oculovestibular responses are unobtainable; respiration is rapid and shallow; and painful stimuli may lead only to flexor responses in the legs. Finally, respiration becomes irregular and stops, the pupils often then dilating widely.

In contrast, a subtentorial (ie, brainstem) lesion may lead to an early, sometimes abrupt disturbance of consciousness without any orderly rostrocaudal progression of neurologic signs. Compressive lesions of the brainstem, especially cerebellar hemorrhage, may be clinically indistinguishable from intraparenchymal processes.

A structural lesion is suspected if the findings suggest focality. In such circumstances, a CT scan should be performed before, or instead of, a lumbar puncture in order to avoid any risk of cerebral herniation. Further management is of the causal lesion and is considered separately under the individual disorders.

2. Stupor & Coma Due to Metabolic Disturbances

Patients with a metabolic cause of coma generally have signs of patchy, diffuse, and symmetric neurologic involvement that cannot be explained by loss of function at any single level or in a sequential manner, although focal or lateralized deficits may occur in hypoglycemia. Pupillary reactivity is usually preserved. Comatose patients with meningitis, encephalitis, or subarachnoid hemorrhage may also exhibit little in the way of focal neurologic signs, however, and clinical evidence of meningeal irritation is sometimes very subtle in comatose patients. Examination of the

cerebrospinal fluid in such patients is essential to establish the correct diagnosis.

In patients with coma due to cerebral ischemia and hypoxia, the absence of pupillary light reflexes 24 hours after return of spontaneous circulation indicates that there is little chance of regaining independence; absent corneal reflexes or absent or extensor motor responses at 72 hours also indicate a grim prognosis. Physical findings are less reliable predictors of outcome among those treated with therapeutic hypothermia, although absent corneal or pupillary light reflexes at 72 hours likely indicate a poor prognosis.

Treatment of metabolic encephalopathy is of the underlying disturbance and is considered in other chapters. If the cause of the encephalopathy is obscure, all drugs except essential ones may have to be withdrawn in case they are responsible for the altered mental status.

3. Brain Death

The definition of brain death is controversial, and diagnostic criteria have been published by many different professional organizations. In order to establish brain death, the irreversibly comatose patient must be shown to have lost all brainstem reflex responses, including the pupillary, corneal, oculovestibular, oculocephalic, oropharyngeal, and respiratory reflexes, and should have been in this condition for at least 6 hours, with adequate time allowed for all sedating medications to be metabolized. Spinal reflex movements do not exclude the diagnosis, but ongoing seizure activity or decerebrate or decorticate posturing is not consistent with brain death. The apnea test (presence or absence of spontaneous respiratory activity at a $Paco_2$ of at least 60 mm Hg or after a rise of 20 mm Hg from baseline) serves to determine whether the patient is capable of respiratory activity.

Reversible coma simulating brain death may be seen with hypothermia (temperature lower than 32°C) and overdosage with central nervous system depressant drugs, and these conditions must be excluded. Certain ancillary tests may assist the determination of brain death but are not essential. An isoelectric electroencephalogram, when the recording is made according to the recommendations of the American Electroencephalographic Society, may help in confirming the diagnosis. Alternatively, the demonstration of an absent cerebral circulation by intravenous radioisotope cerebral angiography or by four-vessel contrast cerebral angiography is confirmatory.

4. Persistent Vegetative State

Patients with severe bilateral hemispheric disease may show some improvement from an initially comatose state, so that, after a variable interval, they appear to be awake but lie motionless and without evidence of awareness or higher mental activity. This persistent vegetative state has been variously referred to as akinetic mutism, apallic state, or coma vigil. Most patients in this persistent vegetative state will die in months or years, but partial recovery has occasionally occurred and in rare instances has been sufficient to permit communication or even independent living.

5. Minimally Conscious State

In this state, patients exhibit inconsistent evidence of consciousness. There is some degree of functional recovery of behaviors suggesting self- or environmental awareness, such as basic verbalization or context-appropriate gestures, emotional responses (eg, smiling) to emotional but not neutral stimuli, or purposive responses to environmental stimuli (eg, a finger movement or eye blink apparently to command). Further improvement is manifest by the restoration of communication with the patient. The minimally conscious state may be temporary or permanent. Little information is available about its natural history or long-term outlook, which reflects the underlying cause. The likelihood of useful functional recovery diminishes with time; after 12 months, patients are likely to remain severely disabled and without a reliable means of communication. Prognostication is difficult.

6. Locked-In Syndrome (De-efferented State)

Acute destructive lesions (eg, infarction, hemorrhage, demyelination, encephalitis) involving the ventral pons and sparing the tegmentum may lead to a mute, quadriparetic but conscious state in which the patient is capable of blinking and voluntary eye movement in the vertical plane, with preserved pupillary responses to light. Such a patient can mistakenly be regarded as comatose. Clinicians should recognize that "locked-in" individuals are fully aware of their surroundings. The prognosis is usually poor, but recovery has occasionally been reported in some cases, including resumption of independent daily life. A similar condition may occur with severe Guillain-Barré syndrome and has a better prognosis.

Barbic D et al. Locked-in syndrome: a critical and time-dependent diagnosis. CJEM. 2012 Sep;14(5):317–20. [PMID: 22967701]

Bouwes A et al. Prognosis of coma after therapeutic hypothermia: a prospective cohort study. Ann Neurol. 2012 Feb;71(2):206–12. [PMID: 22367993]

Edlow JA et al. Diagnosis of reversible causes of coma. Lancet. 2014 Dec 6;384(9959):2064–76. [PMID: 24767707]

Giacino JT et al. Disorders of consciousness after acquired brain injury: the state of the science. Nat Rev Neurol. 2014 Feb; 10(2):99–114. [PMID: 24468878]

Grandhi R et al. Surgical management of traumatic brain injury: a review of guidelines, pathophysiology, neurophysiology, outcomes, and controversies. J Neurosurg Sci. 2014 Dec; 58(4):249–59. [PMID: 25418276]

Wijdicks EF. Brain death. Handb Clin Neurol. 2013;118:191–203. [PMID: 24182378]

HEAD INJURY

Trauma is the most common cause of death in young people, and head injury accounts for almost half of these trauma-related deaths. Head injury severity ranges from concussion to severe traumatic brain injury (TBI). Concussion is broadly defined as an alteration in mental status caused by trauma with or without loss of consciousness. The term concussion is often used synonymously with mild TBI. Grades of TBI are traditionally defined by the

Table 24–8. Glasgow Coma Scale.[1]

Points	Eye Opening	Verbal Response	Motor Response
1	None	None	None
2	To pain	Vocal but not verbal	Extension
3	To voice	Verbal but not conversational	Flexion
4	Spontaneous	Conversational but disoriented	Withdraws from pain
5	--	Oriented	Localizes pain
6	--	--	Obeys commands

[1]GSC score indicating severity of traumatic brain injury (TBI): **mild,** 13–15; **moderate,** 9–12; **severe,** ≤ 8.
From Aminoff MJ et al. *Clinical Neurology*, 9th ed, McGraw-Hill Education, 2015; Reproduced, with permission from Teasdale G, Jennett B. Assessment of coma and impaired consciousness. A practical scale. *Lancet.* 1974;2:81–84.

Glasgow Coma Scale (GCS) measured 30 minutes after injury (Table 24–8).

Head trauma may cause cerebral injury through a variety of mechanisms (Table 24–9). Central to management is determination of which patients need head imaging and observation. Of particular concern is identification of patients with epidural and subdural hematoma, who may present with normal neurologic findings shortly after injury (lucid interval) but rapidly deteriorate thereafter, and in whom surgical intervention is life-saving.

▶ Clinical Findings

A. Symptoms and Signs

Common symptoms of concussion that develop acutely include headache, nausea, vomiting, confusion, disorientation, dizziness, and imbalance. A period of amnesia encompassing the traumatic event and a variable period of time leading up to the trauma is typical. Loss of consciousness may occur. Additional symptoms of photophobia, phonophobia, difficulty concentrating, irritability, and sleep and mood disturbances may develop over the following hours to days. Examination is usually normal, although orientation and attention, short-term memory, and reaction time may be impaired. Persistent or progressive decline in the level of consciousness after the initial injury, or focal neurologic findings, suggests the need for urgent imaging and neurosurgical consultation.

Patients should also be examined for signs of scalp lacerations, facial and skull fracture, and neck injury. The clinical signs of basilar skull fracture include bruising about the orbit (raccoon sign), blood in the external auditory meatus (Battle sign), and leakage of cerebrospinal fluid (which can be identified by its glucose or beta-2-transferrin content) from the ear or nose. Cranial nerve palsies (involving especially the first, second, third, fourth, fifth, seventh, and eighth nerves in any combination) may

Table 24–9. Acute cerebral sequelae of head injury.

Sequelae	Clinical Features	Pathology
Concussion	A transient, trauma-induced alteration in mental status that may or may not involve loss of consciousness. Symptoms and signs include headache, nausea, disorientation, irritability, amnesia, clumsiness, visual disturbances, and focal neurologic deficit.	Unknown; likely mild diffuse axonal injury and excitotoxic neuronal injury. Cerebral contusion may occur.
Cerebral contusion or laceration	Loss of consciousness longer than with concussion. Focal neurologic deficits are often present. May lead to death or severe residual neurologic deficit.	Bruising on side of impact (coup injury) or contralaterally (contrecoup injury). Vasogenic edema, multiple petechial hemorrhages, and mass effect. May have subarachnoid bleeding. Herniation may occur in severe cases. Cerebral laceration specifically involves tearing of the cerebral tissue and pia-arachnoid overlying a contusion.
Acute epidural hemorrhage	Headache, confusion, somnolence, seizures, and focal deficits occur several hours after injury (lucid interval) and lead to coma, respiratory depression, and death unless treated by surgical evacuation.	Tear in meningeal artery, vein, or dural sinus, leading to hematoma visible on CT scan.
Acute subdural hemorrhage	Similar to epidural hemorrhage, but interval before onset of symptoms is longer. Neurosurgical consultation for consideration of evacuation.	Hematoma from tear in veins from cortex to superior sagittal sinus or from cerebral laceration, visible on CT scan.
Cerebral hemorrhage	Generally develops immediately after injury. Clinically resembles hypertensive hemorrhage. Surgery to relieve mass effect is sometimes necessary.	Hematoma, visible on CT scan.
Diffuse axonal injury	Persistent loss of consciousness, coma, or persistent vegetative state resulting from severe rotational shearing forces or deceleration.	Imaging may be normal or may show tiny, scattered white matter hemorrhages. Histology reveals torn axons.

also occur. The head should be immobilized until imaging can be performed.

B. Imaging and Other Investigations

Current recommendations are that head CT be performed in patients with concussion and any of the following: GCS score less than 15; focal neurologic deficit; seizure; coagulopathy; age 65 or older; skull fracture; persistent headache or vomiting; retrograde amnesia exceeding 30 minutes; intoxication; or soft tissue injury of the head or neck. Otherwise, patients can be sent home as long as a responsible caregiver can check the patient at hourly intervals for the next 24 hours. Patients requiring imaging should be admitted unless the head CT is normal, the GCS score is 15, there have been no seizures, there is no predisposition to bleeding, and they can be monitored by a caregiver at home.

Because injury to the spine may have accompanied head trauma, cervical spine radiographs (three views) or CT should always be obtained in comatose patients and in patients with severe neck pain or a deficit possibly related to cord compression.

▶ Treatment

Head injury can often be prevented by helmets, seatbelts, and other protective equipment.

After intracranial bleeding has been excluded clinically or by head CT, treatment of mild TBI is aimed at promoting resolution of postconcussive symptoms and preventing recurrent injury, which increases the risk of chronic neurobehavioral impairment and delays recovery. Rarely, a recurrent concussion while a patient is still symptomatic from their first concussion may lead to fatal cerebral edema (second impact syndrome). These observations form the basis of the recommendation that patients at risk for recurrent concussion (eg, athletes) be held out of the risky activity until their concussive symptoms have fully resolved.

In patients hospitalized with moderate or severe TBI, management often requires a multidisciplinary approach due to multiple concomitant injuries. Elevated intracranial pressure can result from diffuse axonal injury or a hematoma requiring surgical evacuation, or from a variety of medical causes. Decompressive craniectomy may reduce otherwise refractory intracranial hypertension but does not improve neurologic outcome. Hypothermia is associated with worsened functional outcomes.

Because bridging veins between the brain and venous sinuses become more vulnerable to shear injury as the brain atrophies, a subdural hematoma may develop days or weeks following head injury in elderly patients or even occur spontaneously. Clinical presentation can be subtle, often with mental changes such as slowness, drowsiness, headache, confusion, or memory disturbance. Focal neurologic deficits such as hemiparesis or hemisensory disturbance are less common. Surgical intervention is indicated if the hematoma is 10 mm or more in thickness or there is a midline shift of 5 mm ore more; if there is a decline in GCS score of 2 or more from injury to hospital admission; or if one or both pupils are fixed and dilated.

Scalp lacerations and depressed skull fractures should be treated surgically as appropriate. Simple skull fractures require no specific treatment. If there is any leakage of cerebrospinal fluid, conservative treatment, with elevation of the head, restriction of fluids, and administration of acetazolamide (250 mg orally four times daily), is often helpful; if the leak continues for more than a few days, lumbar subarachnoid drainage may be necessary. Antibiotics are given if infection occurs, based on culture and sensitivity studies. Only very occasional patients require intracranial repair of the dural defect because of persistence of the leak or recurrent meningitis.

Prognosis

Moderate and severe TBI may result in permanent cognitive and motor impairment depending on the severity and location of the initial injury. Initial GCS and head CT findings have prognostic value. Among patients with a GCS score of 8 or less at presentation, mortality approaches 30% and only one-third of survivors regain functional independence. Cognitive impairment tends to affect frontal and temporal lobe function, causing deficits in attention, memory, judgment, and executive function. Behavioral dysregulation, depression, and disinhibition can impair social functioning. Anosmia, presumably due to shearing of fibers from the nasal epithelium, is common.

Epilepsy can develop after TBI, especially with more severe injury. Among patients with severe TBI (typically loss of consciousness for at least 12–24 hours, intracranial hematoma, depressed skull fracture, or cerebral contusion), phenytoin is typically given for 7 days to reduce the incidence of early posttraumatic seizures; this is done exclusively to minimize acute complications resulting from such seizures and does not prevent the development of posttraumatic epilepsy.

Among patients with mild TBI, symptoms of concussion resolve in most patients by 1 month and in the vast majority by 3 months. Prolonged postconcussive symptoms are rare, persisting at 1 year in only 10–15% of patients. Risk factors for prolonged postconcussive symptoms included active litigation regarding the injury; repeated concussions; and GCS score of 13 at presentation. Headaches often have migrainous features and may respond to tricyclic antidepressants or beta-blockers (Table 24–1). Opioids should be avoided to minimize the risk of medication overuse headache. Mood symptoms may respond to antidepressants, anxiolytics, and cognitive behavioral therapy.

There appears to be an association between head trauma and the later development of neurodegenerative disease, such as Alzheimer disease, Parkinson disease, or amyotrophic lateral sclerosis. **Chronic traumatic encephalopathy** may represent a distinct pathologic entity and is characterized by mood and cognitive changes after repetitive, mild head injury, as has been observed in athletes or military personnel, and is due to the abnormal aggregation

of tau or other proteins either focally or globally in the cerebral cortex. Whether a specific number of concussions is required to increase an individual's risk of future neurodegenerative disease is not known. Normal pressure hydrocephalus may also occur.

When to Refer

• Patients with focal neurologic deficits, altered consciousness, or skull fracture.

• Patients with late complications of head injury, eg, posttraumatic seizure disorder or normal pressure hydrocephalus.

When to Admit

• Patients with concussion and GCS score less than 15, predisposition to bleeding, seizure, or no responsible caregiver at home.

• Patients with abnormal head CT.

Levin HS et al. Diagnosis, prognosis, and clinical management of mild traumatic brain injury. Lancet Neurol. 2015 May; 14(5):506–17. [PMID: 25801547]
McKee AC et al. The spectrum of disease in chronic traumatic encephalopathy. Brain. 2013 Jan;136(Pt 1):43–64. [PMID: 23208308]
Pasquina P et al. Moderate-to-severe traumatic brain injury. Semin Neurol. 2014 Nov;34(5):572–83. [PMID: 25520028]
Vos PE et al; European Federation of Neurological Societies. Mild traumatic brain injury. Eur J Neurol. 2012 Feb;19(2):191–8. [PMID: 22260187]

SPINAL TRAUMA

ESSENTIALS OF DIAGNOSIS

▶ History of preceding trauma.
▶ Development of acute neurologic deficit.
▶ Signs of myelopathy on examination.

General Considerations

While spinal cord damage may result from whiplash injury, severe injury usually relates to fracture-dislocation causing compression or angular deformity of the cord either cervically or in the lower thoracic and upper lumbar regions. Extreme hypotension following injury may also lead to cord infarction.

Clinical Findings

Total cord transection results in immediate flaccid paralysis and loss of sensation below the level of the lesion. Reflex activity is lost for a variable period, and there is urinary and fecal retention. As reflex function returns over the following days and weeks, spastic paraplegia or quadriplegia develops, with hyperreflexia and extensor plantar responses, but a flaccid atrophic (lower motor neuron) paralysis may be found depending on the segments of the cord that are affected. The bladder and bowels also regain some reflex function, permitting urine and feces to be expelled at intervals. As spasticity increases, flexor or extensor spasms (or both) of the legs become troublesome, especially if the patient develops bed sores or a urinary tract infection. Paraplegia with the legs in flexion or extension may eventually result.

With lesser degrees of injury, patients may be left with mild limb weakness, distal sensory disturbance, or both. Sphincter function may also be impaired, urinary urgency and urge incontinence being especially common. More particularly, a unilateral cord lesion leads to an ipsilateral motor disturbance with accompanying impairment of proprioception and contralateral loss of pain and temperature appreciation below the lesion (Brown-Séquard syndrome). A central cord syndrome may lead to a lower motor neuron deficit and loss of pain and temperature appreciation, with sparing of posterior column functions. A radicular deficit may occur at the level of the injury—or, if the cauda equina is involved, there may be evidence of disturbed function in several lumbosacral roots.

▶ Treatment

Treatment of the injury consists of immobilization and—if there is cord compression—early decompressive laminectomy and fusion (within 24 hours). Early treatment with high doses of corticosteroids (eg, methylprednisolone, 30 mg/kg by intravenous bolus, followed by 5.4 mg/kg/h for 23 hours) may improve neurologic recovery if commenced within 8 hours after injury, although the evidence is limited and some neurosurgical guidelines do not recommend their use. Anatomic realignment of the spinal cord by traction and other orthopedic procedures is important. Subsequent care of the residual neurologic deficit—paraplegia or quadriplegia—requires treatment of spasticity and care of the skin, bladder, and bowels.

▶ When to Refer

All patients with focal neurologic deficits should be referred.

▶ When to Admit

- Patients with neurologic deficits.
- Patients with spinal cord injury, compression, or acute epidural or subdural hematoma.
- Patients with vertebral fracture-dislocation likely to compress the cord.

Bracken MB. Steroids for acute spinal cord injury. Cochrane Database Syst Rev. 2012 Jan 18;1:CD001046. [PMID: 22258943]
Stein DM et al. Management of acute spinal cord injury. Continuum (Minneap Minn). 2015 Feb;21(1 Spinal Cord Disorders):159–87. [PMID: 25651224]

Zhang S et al. Spine and spinal cord trauma: diagnosis and management. Neurol Clin. 2013 Feb;31(1):183–206. [PMID: 23186900]

SYRINGOMYELIA

Destruction or degeneration of gray and white matter adjacent to the central canal of the cervical spinal cord leads to cavitation and accumulation of fluid within the spinal cord. The precise pathogenesis is unclear, but many cases are associated with Arnold-Chiari malformation, in which there is displacement of the cerebellar tonsils, medulla, and fourth ventricle into the spinal canal, sometimes with accompanying meningomyelocele. In such circumstances, the cord cavity connects with and may merely represent a dilated central canal. In other cases, the cause of cavitation is less clear. There is a characteristic clinical picture, with segmental atrophy, areflexia and loss of pain and temperature appreciation in a "cape" distribution, owing to the destruction of fibers crossing in front of the central canal in the mid-cervical spinal cord. Thoracic kyphoscoliosis is usually present. With progression, involvement of the long motor and sensory tracts occurs as well, so that a pyramidal and sensory deficit develops in the legs. Upward extension of the cavitation (syringobulbia) leads to dysfunction of the lower brainstem and thus to bulbar palsy, nystagmus, and sensory impairment over one or both sides of the face.

Syringomyelia, ie, cord cavitation, may also occur in association with an intramedullary tumor or following severe cord injury, and the cavity then does not communicate with the central canal.

In patients with Arnold-Chiari malformation, CT scans reveal a small posterior fossa and enlargement of the foramen magnum, along with other associated skeletal abnormalities at the base of the skull and upper cervical spine. MRI reveals the syrinx as well as the characteristic findings of the Arnold-Chiari malformation, including the caudal displacement of the fourth ventricle and herniation of the cerebellar tonsils through the foramen magnum. Focal cord enlargement is found at myelography or by MRI in patients with cavitation related to past injury or intramedullary neoplasms.

Treatment of Arnold-Chiari malformation with associated syringomyelia is by suboccipital craniectomy and upper cervical laminectomy, with the aim of decompressing the malformation at the foramen magnum. The cord cavity should be drained, and if necessary an outlet for the fourth ventricle can be made. In cavitation associated with intramedullary tumor, treatment is surgical, but radiation therapy may be necessary if complete removal is not possible. Posttraumatic syringomyelia is also treated surgically if it leads to increasing neurologic deficits or to intolerable pain.

Vandertop WP. Syringomyelia. Neuropediatrics. 2014 Feb; 45(1):3–9. [PMID: 24272770]

DEGENERATIVE MOTOR NEURON DISEASES

ESSENTIALS OF DIAGNOSIS

- ► Weakness.
- ► No sensory loss or sphincter disturbance.
- ► Progressive course.
- ► No identifiable underlying cause other than genetic basis in familial cases.

General Considerations

This group of degenerative disorders is characterized clinically by weakness and variable wasting of affected muscles, without accompanying sensory changes.

Motor neuron disease in adults generally commences between 30 and 60 years of age. There is degeneration of the anterior horn cells in the spinal cord, the motor nuclei of the lower cranial nerves, and the corticospinal and corticobulbar pathways. The disorder is usually sporadic, but familial cases may occur and several genetic mutations or loci have been identified. Cigarette smoking may be one risk factor.

Classification

Five varieties have been distinguished on clinical grounds.

A. Progressive Bulbar Palsy

Bulbar involvement predominates owing to disease processes affecting primarily the motor nuclei of the cranial nerves.

B. Pseudobulbar Palsy

Bulbar involvement predominates in this variety also, but it is due to bilateral corticobulbar disease and thus reflects upper motor neuron dysfunction. There may be a "pseudobulbar affect," with uncontrollable episodes of laughing or crying to stimuli that would not normally have elicited such marked reactions.

C. Progressive Spinal Muscular Atrophy

This is characterized primarily by a lower motor neuron deficit in the limbs due to degeneration of the anterior horn cells in the spinal cord.

D. Primary Lateral Sclerosis

There is a purely upper motor neuron deficit in the limbs.

E. Amyotrophic Lateral Sclerosis

A mixed upper and lower motor neuron deficit is found in the limbs. This disorder is sometimes associated with cognitive decline (in a pattern consistent with frontotemporal dementia), a pseudobulbar affect, or parkinsonism.

Approximately 10% of cases of amyotrophic lateral sclerosis are familial and have been associated with mutations at several different genetic loci, including a hexanucleotide repeat on chromosome 9 that also associates with frontotemporal dementia.

Differential Diagnosis

The spinal muscular atrophies (SMAs) are inherited syndromes caused most often by mutations of the survival motor neuron (*SMN*) gene on chromosome 5.

Pure motor syndromes resembling motor neuron disease may also occur in association with monoclonal gammopathy or multifocal motor neuropathies with conduction block. A motor neuronopathy may also develop in Hodgkin disease and has a relatively benign prognosis. Infective anterior horn cell diseases (polio virus or West Nile virus infection) can generally be distinguished by the acute onset and monophasic course of the illness, as discussed in Chapter 32.

Clinical Findings

A. Symptoms and Signs

Difficulty in swallowing, chewing, coughing, breathing, and talking (dysarthria) occur with bulbar involvement. In progressive bulbar palsy, there is drooping of the palate; a depressed gag reflex; pooling of saliva in the pharynx; a weak cough; and a wasted, fasciculating tongue. In pseudobulbar palsy, the tongue is contracted and spastic and cannot be moved rapidly from side to side. Limb involvement is characterized by motor disturbances (weakness, stiffness, wasting, fasciculations) reflecting lower or upper motor neuron dysfunction; there are no objective changes on sensory examination, although there may be vague sensory complaints. The sphincters are generally spared. Cognitive changes or pseudobulbar affect may be present. The disorder is progressive, and amyotrophic lateral sclerosis is usually fatal within 3–5 years; death usually results from pulmonary infections. Patients with bulbar involvement generally have the poorest prognosis, while patients with primary lateral sclerosis often have a longer survival despite profound quadriparesis and spasticity.

B. Laboratory and Other Studies

Electromyography may show changes of chronic partial denervation, with abnormal spontaneous activity in the resting muscle and a reduction in the number of motor units under voluntary control. In patients with suspected SMA or amyotrophic lateral sclerosis, the diagnosis should not be made with confidence unless such changes are found in at least three spinal regions (cervical, thoracic, lumbosacral) or two spinal regions and the bulbar musculature. Motor conduction velocity is usually normal but may be slightly reduced, and sensory conduction studies are also normal. Biopsy of a wasted muscle shows the histologic changes of denervation. The serum creatine kinase may be slightly elevated but never reaches the extremely high values seen in some of the muscular dystrophies. The cerebrospinal fluid is normal. There are abnormal findings on rectal biopsy and reduced hexosaminidase A in serum and leukocytes in patients with juvenile SMA due to hexosaminidase deficiency.

▶ Treatment

Riluzole, 50 mg orally twice daily, which reduces the presynaptic release of glutamate, is the only medication shown to increase short-term survival in amyotrophic lateral sclerosis in randomized trials. Noninvasive ventilation at least 4 hours per day in patients with a maximal inspiratory pressure less than 60 cm H_2O may prolong survival. There is otherwise no specific treatment except in patients with gammopathy, in whom plasmapheresis and immunosuppression may lead to improvement. Symptomatic and supportive measures may include trials of anticholinergic drugs (such as trihexyphenidyl, amitriptyline, or atropine) or use of a portable suction machine if drooling is troublesome, braces or a walker to improve mobility, and physical therapy to prevent contractures. Combination dextromethorphan/quinidine (20 mg/10 mg, one tablet orally once or twice daily) may relieve symptoms of pseudobulbar affect. Behavioral modification (eg, exercising facial muscles and encouraging frequent swallowing) or over-the-counter decongestants may also help mild drooling. Spasticity may be helped by baclofen or diazepam. A semi-liquid diet or gastrostomy tube feeding may be needed if dysphagia is severe; it is advisable to perform the procedure before the forced vital capacity falls below 50% of predicted to minimize the risk of complications. Tracheostomy is sometimes performed if respiratory muscles are severely affected; however, in the terminal stages of these disorders, the focus of treatment should be on quality of life and realistic expectations should be discussed well in advance. Information on palliative care is provided in Chapter 5.

▶ When to Refer

All patients (to exclude other treatable causes of symptoms and signs) should be referred.

▶ When to Admit

Patients may need to be admitted for initiation or titration of noninvasive ventilation, or for periods of increased requirement of noninvasive ventilator support during pulmonary infections.

Connolly S et al. End-of-life management in patients with amyotrophic lateral sclerosis. Lancet Neurol. 2015 Apr;14(4):435–42. [PMID: 25728958]
Malik R et al. Amyotrophic lateral sclerosis. Semin Neurol. 2014 Nov;34(5):534–41. [PMID: 25520025]

PERIPHERAL NEUROPATHIES

Peripheral neuropathies can be categorized on the basis of the structure primarily affected. The predominant pathologic feature may be axonal degeneration (axonal or neuronal neuropathies) or paranodal or segmental demyelination. The distinction may be possible on the basis of

neurophysiologic findings. Motor and sensory conduction velocity can be measured in accessible segments of peripheral nerves. In axonal neuropathies, conduction velocity is normal or reduced only mildly and needle electromyography provides evidence of denervation in affected muscles. In demyelinating neuropathies, conduction may be slowed considerably in affected fibers, and in more severe cases, conduction is blocked completely, without accompanying electromyographic signs of denervation.

POLYNEUROPATHIES & MONONEURITIS MULTIPLEX

ESSENTIALS OF DIAGNOSIS

▶ Weakness, sensory disturbances, or both in the extremities.

▶ Pain is common.

▶ Depressed or absent tendon reflexes.

▶ May be family history of neuropathy.

▶ May be history of systemic illness or toxic exposure.

▶ General Considerations

Diffuse **polyneuropathies** lead to a symmetric sensory, motor, or mixed deficit, often most marked distally. They include the hereditary, metabolic, and toxic disorders; idiopathic inflammatory polyneuropathy (Guillain-Barré syndrome); and the peripheral neuropathies that may occur as a nonmetastatic complication of malignant diseases. Involvement of motor fibers leads to flaccid weakness that is most marked distally; dysfunction of sensory fibers causes impaired sensory perception. Tendon reflexes are depressed or absent. Paresthesias, pain, and muscle tenderness may also occur. Multiple **mononeuropathies** suggest a patchy multifocal disease process such as vasculopathy (eg, diabetes, arteritis), an infiltrative process (eg, leprosy, sarcoidosis), radiation damage, or an immunologic disorder (eg, brachial plexopathy).

▶ Clinical Findings

The cause of polyneuropathy or mononeuritis multiplex is suggested by the history, mode of onset, and predominant clinical manifestations. Laboratory workup includes a complete blood count and erythrocyte sedimentation rate, serum protein electrophoresis and immunofixation, determination of plasma urea and electrolytes, liver and thyroid function tests, tests for rheumatoid factor and antinuclear antibody, HBsAg determination, a serologic test for syphilis, fasting blood glucose level, urinary heavy metal levels, cerebrospinal fluid examination, and chest radiography. These tests should be ordered selectively, as guided by symptoms and signs. Measurement of nerve conduction velocity is important in confirming the peripheral nerve origin of symptoms and providing a means of following clinical changes, as well as indicating the likely disease process (ie, axonal or demyelinating neuropathy). Cutaneous nerve biopsy may help establish a precise diagnosis (eg, polyarteritis, amyloidosis). In about half of cases, no specific cause can be established; of these, slightly less than half are subsequently found to be familial.

▶ Treatment

Treatment is of the underlying cause, when feasible, and is discussed below under the individual disorders. Physical therapy helps prevent contractures, and splints can maintain a weak extremity in a position of useful function. Anesthetic extremities must be protected from injury. To guard against burns, patients should check the temperature of water and hot surfaces with a portion of skin having normal sensation, measure water temperature with a thermometer, and use cold water for washing or lower the temperature setting of their hot-water heaters. Shoes should be examined frequently during the day for grit or foreign objects in order to prevent pressure lesions.

Patients with polyneuropathies or mononeuritis multiplex are subject to additional nerve injury at pressure points and should therefore avoid such behavior as leaning on elbows or sitting with crossed legs for lengthy periods.

Neuropathic, burning pain may respond to simple analgesics, such as aspirin or nonsteroidal anti-inflammatory agents, and to gabapentin (300 mg orally three times daily, titrated up to a maximum of 1200 mg orally three times daily as necessary). Duloxetine (60 mg orally daily) or venlafaxine (start 37.5 mg orally twice daily, and titrate up to 75 mg orally two to three times daily) may be helpful, especially in painful diabetic neuropathy. Opioids may be necessary for severe hyperpathia or pain induced by minimal stimuli, but their use should be avoided as much as possible. The use of a frame or cradle to reduce contact with bedclothes may be helpful. Many patients experience episodic stabbing pains, which may respond to gabapentin, pregabalin (100 mg orally three times daily), carbamazepine (start 100 mg orally twice daily, and titrate up to 400 mg orally twice daily), or tricyclic antidepressants (eg, amitriptyline 10–150 mg orally at bedtime daily).

Symptoms of autonomic dysfunction are occasionally troublesome. Postural hypotension is often helped by wearing waist-high elastic stockings and sleeping in a semierect position at night. Fludrocortisone reduces postural hypotension, but doses as high as 1 mg/day are sometimes necessary for patients with diabetes and may lead to recumbent hypertension. Midodrine, an alpha-agonist, is sometimes helpful in a dose of 2.5–10 mg three times daily. Erectile dysfunction and diarrhea are difficult to treat; a flaccid neuropathic bladder may respond to parasympathomimetic drugs such as bethanechol chloride, 10–50 mg three or four times daily.

Callaghan BC et al. Distal symmetric polyneuropathy: a review. JAMA. 2015 Nov 24;314(20):2172–81. [PMID: 26599185]

Chaparro LE et al. Combination pharmacotherapy for the treatment of neuropathic pain in adults. Cochrane Database Syst Rev. 2012 Jul 11;7:CD008943. [PMID: 22786518]

Watson JC et al. Peripheral neuropathy: a practical approach to diagnosis and symptom management. Mayo Clin Proc. 2015 Jul;90(7):940–51. [PMID: 26141332]

1. Inherited Neuropathies

A. Charcot-Marie-Tooth Disease (HMSN Type I, II)

Several distinct varieties of Charcot-Marie-Tooth disease can be recognized. There is usually an autosomal dominant mode of inheritance, but occasional cases occur on a sporadic, recessive, or X-linked basis. Clinical presentation may be with foot deformities or gait disturbances in childhood or early adult life. Slow progression leads to the typical features of polyneuropathy, with distal weakness and wasting that begin in the legs, a variable amount of distal sensory loss, and depressed or absent tendon reflexes. Tremor is a conspicuous feature in some instances. Hereditary motor and sensory neuropathy (HMSN) type I is characterized by demyelination on electrodiagnostic studies and is usually caused by mutations in the peripheral myelin protein 22 or myelin protein zero gene. In HMSN type II, electrodiagnostic studies show axonal loss rather than demyelination; one-third of cases are due to mutations in the gene mitofusin 2.

A similar disorder may occur in patients with progressive distal SMA, but there is no sensory loss; electrophysiologic investigation reveals that motor conduction velocity is normal or only slightly reduced, and nerve action potentials are normal.

Saporta MA. Charcot-Marie-Tooth disease and other inherited neuropathies. Continuum (Minneap Minn). 2014 Oct; 20(5):1208–25. [PMID: 25299278]

B. Dejerine-Sottas Disease (HMSN Type III)

The disorder may occur on a sporadic, autosomal dominant or, less commonly, autosomal recessive basis. Onset in infancy or childhood leads to a progressive motor and sensory polyneuropathy with weakness, ataxia, sensory loss, and depressed or absent tendon reflexes. The peripheral nerves may be palpably enlarged and are characterized pathologically by segmental demyelination, Schwann cell hyperplasia, and thin myelin sheaths. Electrophysiologically, there is a slowing of conduction, and sensory action potentials may be unrecordable.

C. Friedreich Ataxia

This disorder, the only known autosomal recessive trinucleotide repeat disease, is caused by expansion of a poly-GAA locus in the gene for frataxin on chromosome 9, leading to symptoms in childhood or early adult life. The gait becomes ataxic, the hands become clumsy, and other signs of cerebellar dysfunction develop accompanied by weakness of the legs and extensor plantar responses. Involvement of peripheral sensory fibers leads to sensory disturbances in the limbs and depressed tendon reflexes.

There is bilateral pes cavus. Pathologically, there is a marked loss of cells in the posterior root ganglia and degeneration of peripheral sensory fibers. In the central nervous system, changes are conspicuous in the posterior and lateral columns of the cord. Electrophysiologically, conduction velocity in motor fibers is normal or only mildly reduced, but sensory action potentials are small or absent. Cardiac disease is the most common cause of death.

In the differential diagnosis for Friedreich ataxia are other spinocerebellar ataxias, a growing group of at least 30 inherited disorders, each involving a different identified gene. These heterogeneous disorders, which frequently (but not exclusively) exhibit an autosomal dominant inheritance pattern and poly-CAG expansion of the affected gene, typically cause cerebellar ataxia and varying combinations of other symptoms (such as peripheral neuropathy, ophthalmoparesis, dysarthria, and pyramidal and extrapyramidal signs).

Parkinson MH et al. Clinical features of Friedreich's ataxia: classical and atypical phenotypes. J Neurochem. 2013 Aug;126(Suppl 1): 103–17. [PMID: 23859346]

D. Refsum Disease (HMSN Type IV)

This autosomal recessive disorder is due to a disturbance in phytanic acid metabolism. Clinically, pigmentary retinal degeneration is accompanied by progressive sensorimotor polyneuropathy and cerebellar signs. Auditory dysfunction, cardiomyopathy, and cutaneous manifestations may also occur. Motor and sensory conduction velocities are reduced, often markedly, and there may be electromyographic evidence of denervation in affected muscles. Dietary restriction of phytanic acid and its precursors may be helpful therapeutically. Plasmapheresis to reduce stored phytanic acid may help at the initiation of treatment.

Zolotov D et al. Long-term strategies for the treatment of Refsum's disease using therapeutic apheresis. J Clin Apher. 2012;27(2):99–105. [PMID: 22267052]

E. Porphyria

Peripheral nerve involvement may occur during acute attacks in both variegate porphyria and acute intermittent porphyria. Motor symptoms usually occur first, and weakness is often most marked proximally and in the upper limbs rather than the lower. Sensory symptoms and signs may be proximal or distal in distribution. Autonomic involvement is sometimes pronounced. The electrophysiologic findings are in keeping with the results of neuropathologic studies suggesting that the neuropathy is axonal in type. Hematin (4 mg/kg intravenously over 15 minutes once or twice daily) may lead to rapid improvement. A high-carbohydrate diet and, in severe cases, intravenous glucose or levulose may also be helpful. Propranolol (up to 100 mg orally every 4 hours) may control tachycardia and hypertension in acute attacks.

2. Neuropathies Associated with Systemic & Metabolic Disorders

A. Diabetes Mellitus

In this disorder, involvement of the peripheral nervous system may lead to symmetric sensory or mixed polyneuropathy, asymmetric motor radiculoneuropathy or plexopathy (diabetic amyotrophy), thoracoabdominal radiculopathy, autonomic neuropathy, or isolated lesions of individual nerves. These may occur singly or in any combination and are discussed in Chapter 27.

Snedecor SJ et al. Systematic review and meta-analysis of pharmacological therapies for painful diabetic peripheral neuropathy. Pain Pract. 2014 Feb;14(2):167–84. [PMID: 23534696]

B. Uremia

Uremia may lead to a symmetric sensorimotor polyneuropathy that tends to affect the lower limbs more than the upper limbs and is more marked distally than proximally (see Chapter 22). The diagnosis can be confirmed electrophysiologically, for motor and sensory conduction velocity is moderately reduced. The neuropathy improves both clinically and electrophysiologically with kidney transplantation and to a lesser extent with chronic dialysis.

C. Alcoholism and Nutritional Deficiency

Many patients with alcoholism have an axonal distal sensorimotor polyneuropathy that is frequently accompanied by painful cramps, muscle tenderness, and painful paresthesias and is often more marked in the legs than in the arms. Symptoms of autonomic dysfunction may also be conspicuous. Motor and sensory conduction velocity may be slightly reduced, even in subclinical cases, but gross slowing of conduction is uncommon. A similar distal sensorimotor polyneuropathy is a well-recognized feature of beriberi (thiamine deficiency). In vitamin B_{12} deficiency, distal sensory polyneuropathy may develop but is usually overshadowed by central nervous system manifestations (eg, myelopathy, optic neuropathy, or intellectual changes).

D. Paraproteinemias

A symmetric sensorimotor polyneuropathy that is gradual in onset, progressive in course, and often accompanied by pain and dysesthesias in the limbs may occur in patients (especially men) with multiple myeloma. The neuropathy is of the axonal type in classic lytic myeloma, but segmental demyelination (primary or secondary) and axonal loss may occur in sclerotic myeloma and lead to predominantly motor clinical manifestations. Both demyelinating and axonal neuropathies are also observed in patients with paraproteinemias without myeloma. A small fraction will develop myeloma if serially followed. The demyelinating neuropathy in these patients may be due to the monoclonal proteins reacting to a component of the nerve myelin. The neuropathy of classic multiple myeloma is poorly responsive to therapy. The polyneuropathy of benign monoclonal gammopathy may respond to immunosuppressant drugs and plasmapheresis.

Polyneuropathy may also occur in association with monoclonal gammopathy of unknown significance, macroglobulinemia, and cryoglobulinemia and sometimes responds to plasmapheresis. Many patients with an IgM M-protein will have antibodies to myelin-associated glycoprotein (MAG); these patients may respond to treatment with rituximab. Entrapment neuropathy, such as carpal tunnel syndrome, is more common than polyneuropathy in patients with (nonhereditary) generalized amyloidosis. With polyneuropathy due to amyloidosis, sensory and autonomic symptoms are especially conspicuous, whereas distal wasting and weakness occur later; there is no specific treatment.

3. Neuropathies Associated with Infectious & Inflammatory Diseases

A. Leprosy

Leprosy is an important cause of peripheral neuropathy in certain parts of the world. Sensory disturbances are mainly due to involvement of intracutaneous nerves. In tuberculoid leprosy, they develop at the same time and in the same distribution as the skin lesion but may be more extensive if nerve trunks lying beneath the lesion are also involved. In lepromatous leprosy, there is more extensive sensory loss, and this develops earlier and to a greater extent in the coolest regions of the body, such as the dorsal surfaces of the hands and feet, where the bacilli proliferate most actively. Motor deficits result from involvement of superficial nerves where their temperature is lowest, eg, the ulnar nerve in the region proximal to the olecranon groove, the median nerve as it emerges from beneath the forearm flexor muscle to run toward the carpal tunnel, the peroneal nerve at the head of the fibula, and the posterior tibial nerve in the lower part of the leg; patchy facial muscular weakness may also occur owing to involvement of the superficial branches of the seventh cranial nerve.

Motor disturbances in leprosy are suggestive of multiple mononeuropathy, whereas sensory changes resemble those of distal polyneuropathy. Examination, however, relates the distribution of sensory deficits to the temperature of the tissues; in the legs, for example, sparing frequently occurs between the toes and in the popliteal fossae, where the temperature is higher. Treatment is with antileprotic agents (see Chapter 33).

B. AIDS

A variety of neuropathies occur in HIV-infected patients (see Chapter 31).

C. Lyme Borreliosis

The neurologic manifestations of Lyme disease include meningitis, meningoencephalitis, polyradiculoneuropathy, mononeuropathy multiplex, and cranial neuropathy. Serologic tests establish the underlying disorder. Lyme disease and its treatment are discussed in depth in Chapter 34.

D. Sarcoidosis

Cranial nerve palsies (especially facial palsy), multiple mononeuropathy and, less commonly, symmetric

polyneuropathy may all occur, the latter sometimes preferentially affecting either motor or sensory fibers. Improvement may occur with use of corticosteroids.

E. Polyarteritis

Involvement of the vasa nervorum by the vasculitic process may result in infarction of the nerve. Clinically, one encounters an asymmetric sensorimotor polyneuropathy (mononeuritis multiplex) that pursues a waxing and waning course. Corticosteroids and cytotoxic agents—especially cyclophosphamide—may be of benefit in severe cases (Chapter 20).

F. Rheumatoid Arthritis

Compressive or entrapment neuropathies, ischemic neuropathies, mild distal sensory polyneuropathy, and severe progressive sensorimotor polyneuropathy can occur in rheumatoid arthritis.

4. Neuropathy Associated with Critical Illness

Patients in intensive care units with sepsis and multiorgan failure sometimes develop polyneuropathies. This may be manifested initially by unexpected difficulty in weaning patients from a mechanical ventilator and in more advanced cases by wasting and weakness of the extremities and loss of tendon reflexes. Sensory abnormalities are relatively inconspicuous. The neuropathy is axonal in type. Its pathogenesis is obscure, and treatment is supportive. The prognosis is good provided patients recover from the underlying critical illness.

5. Toxic Neuropathies

Axonal polyneuropathy may follow exposure to industrial agents or pesticides such as acrylamide, organophosphorus compounds, hexacarbon solvents, methyl bromide, and carbon disulfide; metals such as arsenic, thallium, mercury, and lead; and drugs such as phenytoin, perhexiline, isoniazid, nitrofurantoin, vincristine, and pyridoxine in high doses. Detailed occupational, environmental, and medical histories and recognition of clusters of cases are important in suggesting the diagnosis. Treatment is by preventing further exposure to the causal agent. Isoniazid neuropathy is prevented by pyridoxine supplementation.

Diphtheritic neuropathy results from a neurotoxin released by the causative organism and is common in many areas. Palatal weakness may develop 2–4 weeks after infection of the throat, and infection of the skin may similarly be followed by focal weakness of neighboring muscles. Disturbances of accommodation may occur about 4–5 weeks after infection and distal sensorimotor demyelinating polyneuropathy after 1–3 months.

6. Neuropathies Associated with Malignant Diseases

Both a sensorimotor and a purely sensory polyneuropathy may occur as a nonmetastatic complication of malignant diseases, and have been associated with circulating anti-MAG or anti-Hu antibodies that can be detected by a paraneoplastic antibody panel that is available commercially. The sensorimotor polyneuropathy may be mild and occur in the course of known malignant disease, or it may have an acute or subacute onset, lead to severe disability, and occur before there is any clinical evidence of the cancer, occasionally following a remitting course. An autonomic neuropathy may also occur as a paraneoplastic disorder related to the presence of anti-Hu antibodies or to an antibody against ganglionic acetylcholine receptors (anti-nAChR).

7. Acute Idiopathic Polyneuropathy (Guillain-Barré Syndrome)

ESSENTIALS OF DIAGNOSIS

- ► Acute or subacute progressive polyradiculoneuropathy.
- ► Weakness is more severe than sensory disturbances.
- ► Acute dysautonomia may be life-threatening.

▶ General Considerations

This acute or subacute polyradiculoneuropathy sometimes follows infective illness, inoculations, or surgical procedures. There is an association with preceding *Campylobacter jejuni* enteritis. The disorder probably has an immunologic basis, but the precise mechanism is unclear.

▶ Clinical Findings

A. Symptoms and Signs

The main complaint is of weakness that varies widely in severity in different patients and often has a proximal emphasis and symmetric distribution. It usually begins in the legs, spreading to a variable extent but frequently involving the arms and often one or both sides of the face. The muscles of respiration or deglutition may also be affected. Sensory symptoms are usually less conspicuous than motor ones, but distal paresthesias and dysesthesias are common, and neuropathic or radicular pain is present in many patients. Autonomic disturbances are also common, may be severe, and are sometimes life-threatening; they include tachycardia, cardiac irregularities, hypotension or hypertension, facial flushing, abnormalities of sweating, pulmonary dysfunction, and impaired sphincter control. The axonal subtypes of the syndrome (acute motor axonal neuropathy [AMAN] and acute motor and sensory axonal neuropathy [AMSAN]) are caused by antibodies to gangliosides on the axon membrane, including anti-GM1, anti-GM1b, anti-GD1a, anti-GD1b, and (in AMAN) anti-GalNAC-GD1a antibodies. The Miller Fisher syndrome, another subtype, is characterized by the clinical triad of ophthalmoplegia, ataxia, and areflexia, and is associated with anti-GQ1b antibodies.

B. Laboratory Findings

The cerebrospinal fluid characteristically contains a high protein concentration with a normal cell count, but these changes may take up to 2 weeks to develop.

Electrophysiologic studies may reveal marked abnormalities, which do not necessarily parallel the clinical disorder in their temporal course. Pathologic examination shows primary demyelination or, less commonly, axonal degeneration.

▶ Differential Diagnosis

When the diagnosis is made, the history and appropriate laboratory studies should exclude the possibility of porphyric, diphtheritic, or toxic (heavy metal, hexacarbon, organophosphate) neuropathies, and of HIV infection. The temporal course excludes other peripheral neuropathies. Poliomyelitis, botulism, and tick paralysis must also be considered as they cause weakness of acute onset. The presence of pyramidal signs, a markedly asymmetric motor deficit, a sharp sensory level, or early sphincter involvement should suggest a focal cord lesion.

▶ Treatment

Treatment with prednisone is ineffective and may prolong recovery time. Plasmapheresis is of value; it is best performed within the first few days of illness and is particularly useful for clinically severe or rapidly progressive cases or those with ventilatory impairment. IVIG (400 mg/kg/day for 5 days) is equally helpful. Patients should be admitted to intensive care units if their forced vital capacity is declining, and intubation is considered if the forced vital capacity reaches 15 mL/kg, the maximum inspiratory pressure reaches –30 mm Hg, or dyspnea becomes evident. Declining oxygen saturation is a late indicator of neuromuscular respiratory failure. Respiratory toilet and chest physical therapy help prevent atelectasis. Marked hypotension may respond to volume replacement or pressor agents. Thromboprophylaxis is important.

▶ Prognosis

Most patients eventually make a good recovery, but this may take many months, and about 20% of patients are left with persisting disability. Approximately 3% of patients with acute idiopathic polyneuropathy have one or more clinically similar relapses, sometimes several years after the initial illness.

▶ When to Refer

All patients should be referred.

▶ When to Admit

All patients should be hospitalized until their condition is stable and there is no respiratory compromise.

Hughes RA et al. Corticosteroids for Guillain-Barré syndrome. Cochrane Database Syst Rev. 2012 Aug 15;8:CD001446. [PMID: 22895921]

Hughes RA et al. Intravenous immunoglobulin for Guillain-Barré syndrome. Cochrane Database Syst Rev. 2014 Sep 19;9: CD002063. [PMID: 25238327]

Raphaël JC et al. Plasma exchange for Guillain-Barré syndrome. Cochrane Database Syst Rev. 2012 Jul 11;7:CD001798. [PMID: 22786475] van den Berg B et al. Guillain-Barré syndrome: pathogenesis, diagnosis, treatment and prognosis. Nat Rev Neurol. 2014 Aug;10(8):469–82. [PMID: 25023340]

8. Chronic Inflammatory Polyneuropathy

Chronic inflammatory demyelinating polyneuropathy, an acquired immunologically mediated disorder, is clinically similar to Guillain-Barré syndrome except that it has a relapsing or steadily progressive course over months or years and that autonomic dysfunction is generally less common. It may present as an exclusively motor disorder or with a mixed sensorimotor disturbance. In the relapsing form, partial recovery may occur after some relapses, but in other instances there is no recovery between exacerbations. Although remission may occur spontaneously with time, the disorder frequently follows a progressive downhill course leading to severe functional disability.

Electrodiagnostic studies show marked slowing of motor and sensory conduction, and focal conduction block. Signs of partial denervation may also be present owing to secondary axonal degeneration. Nerve biopsy may show chronic perivascular inflammatory infiltrates in the endoneurium and epineurium, without accompanying evidence of vasculitis. However, a normal nerve biopsy result or the presence of nonspecific abnormalities does not exclude the diagnosis.

Corticosteroids may arrest or reverse the downhill course. Treatment is usually begun with prednisone, 60–80 mg orally daily, continued for 2–3 months or until a definite response has occurred. If no response has occurred despite 3 months of treatment, a higher dose may be tried. In responsive cases, the dose is gradually tapered, but most patients become corticosteroid-dependent, often requiring prednisone, 20 mg daily on alternate days, on a long-term basis. IVIG can be used in place of, or in addition to corticosteroids and is best used as the initial treatment in pure motor syndromes. When both IVIG and corticosteroids are ineffective, plasma exchange may be worthwhile. Consistent with the notion that the condition is antibody mediated, rituximab has shown promise. Immunosuppressant or immunomodulatory drugs (such as azathioprine) may be added when the response to other measures is unsatisfactory or to enable maintenance doses of corticosteroids to be lowered. Symptomatic treatment is also important.

Latov N. Diagnosis and treatment of chronic acquired demyelinating polyneuropathies. Nat Rev Neurol. 2014 Aug;10(8):435–46. [PMID: 24980070]

MONONEUROPATHIES

ESSENTIALS OF DIAGNOSIS

▶ Focal motor or sensory deficit.

▶ Deficit is in territory of an individual peripheral nerve.

An individual nerve may be injured along its course or may be compressed, angulated, or stretched by neighboring anatomic structures, especially at a point where it passes through a narrow space (entrapment neuropathy). The relative contributions of mechanical factors and ischemia to the local damage are not clear. With involvement of a sensory or mixed nerve, pain is commonly felt distal to the lesion. Symptoms never develop with some entrapment neuropathies, resolve rapidly and spontaneously in others, and become progressively more disabling and distressing in yet other cases. The precise neurologic deficit depends on the nerve involved. Percussion of the nerve at the site of the lesion may lead to paresthesias in its distal distribution.

Entrapment neuropathy may be the sole manifestation of subclinical polyneuropathy, and this must be borne in mind and excluded by nerve conduction studies. Such studies are also indispensable for the localization of the focal lesion.

In patients with acute compression neuropathy such as may occur in intoxicated individuals ("Saturday night palsy"), no treatment is necessary. Complete recovery generally occurs, usually within 2 months, presumably because the underlying pathology is demyelination. However, axonal degeneration can occur in severe cases, and recovery then takes longer and may never be complete.

In chronic compressive or entrapment neuropathies, avoidance of aggravating factors and correction of any underlying systemic conditions are important. Local infiltration of the region about the nerve with corticosteroids may be of value; in addition, surgical decompression may help if there is a progressively increasing neurologic deficit or if electrodiagnostic studies show evidence of partial denervation in weak muscles.

Peripheral nerve tumors are uncommon, except in neurofibromatosis type 1, but also give rise to mononeuropathy. This may be distinguishable from entrapment neuropathy only by noting the presence of a mass along the course of the nerve and by demonstrating the precise site of the lesion with appropriate electrophysiologic studies. Treatment of symptomatic lesions is by surgical removal if possible.

1. Carpal Tunnel Syndrome

See Chapter 41.

2. Pronator Teres or Anterior Interosseous Syndrome

The median nerve gives off its motor branch, the anterior interosseous nerve, below the elbow as it descends between the two heads of the pronator teres muscle. A lesion of either nerve may occur in this region, sometimes after trauma or owing to compression from, for example, a fibrous band. With anterior interosseous nerve involvement, there is no sensory loss, and weakness is confined to the pronator quadratus, flexor pollicis longus, and the flexor digitorum profundus to the second and third digits. Weakness is more widespread and sensory changes occur in an appropriate distribution when the median nerve itself is affected. The prognosis is variable. If improvement does not occur spontaneously, decompressive surgery may be helpful.

3. Ulnar Nerve Lesions

Ulnar nerve lesions are likely to occur in the elbow region as the nerve runs behind the medial epicondyle and descends into the cubital tunnel. In the condylar groove, the ulnar nerve is exposed to pressure or trauma. Moreover, any increase in the carrying angle of the elbow, whether congenital, degenerative, or traumatic, may cause excessive stretching of the nerve when the elbow is flexed. Ulnar nerve lesions may also result from thickening or distortion of the anatomic structures forming the cubital tunnel, and the resulting symptoms may also be aggravated by flexion of the elbow, because the tunnel is then narrowed by tightening of its roof or inward bulging of its floor. A severe lesion at either site causes sensory changes in the fifth and medial half of the fourth digits and along the medial border of the hand. There is weakness of the ulnar-innervated muscles in the forearm and hand. With a cubital tunnel lesion, however, there may be relative sparing of the flexor carpi ulnaris muscle. Electrophysiologic evaluation using nerve stimulation techniques allows more precise localization of the lesion.

If conservative measures are unsuccessful in relieving symptoms and preventing further progression, surgical treatment may be necessary. This consists of nerve transposition if the lesion is in the condylar groove, or a release procedure if it is in the cubital tunnel.

Ulnar nerve lesions may also develop at the wrist or in the palm of the hand, usually owing to repetitive trauma or to compression from ganglia or benign tumors. They can be subdivided depending on their presumed site. Compressive lesions are treated surgically. If repetitive mechanical trauma is responsible, this is avoided by occupational adjustment or job retraining.

4. Radial Nerve Lesions

The radial nerve is particularly liable to compression or injury in the axilla (eg, by crutches or by pressure when the arm hangs over the back of a chair). This leads to weakness or paralysis of all the muscles supplied by the nerve, including the triceps. Sensory changes may also occur but are often surprisingly inconspicuous, being marked only in a small area on the back of the hand between the thumb and index finger. Injuries to the radial nerve in the spiral groove occur characteristically during deep sleep, as in intoxicated individuals (Saturday night palsy), and there is then sparing of the triceps muscle, which is supplied more proximally. The nerve may also be injured at or above the elbow; its purely motor posterior interosseous branch, supplying the extensors of the wrist and fingers, may be involved immediately below the elbow, but then there is sparing of the extensor carpi radialis longus, so that the wrist can still be extended. The superficial radial nerve may be compressed by handcuffs or a tight watch strap.

5. Femoral Neuropathy

The clinical features of femoral nerve palsy consist of weakness and wasting of the quadriceps muscle, with

sensory impairment over the anteromedian aspect of the thigh and sometimes also of the leg to the medial malleolus, and a depressed or absent knee jerk. Isolated femoral neuropathy may occur in patients with diabetes or from compression by retroperitoneal neoplasms or hematomas (eg, expanding aortic aneurysm). Femoral neuropathy may also result from pressure from the inguinal ligament when the thighs are markedly flexed and abducted, as in the lithotomy position.

6. Meralgia Paresthetica

The lateral femoral cutaneous nerve, a sensory nerve arising from the L2 and L3 roots, may be compressed or stretched in obese or diabetic patients and during pregnancy. The nerve usually runs under the outer portion of the inguinal ligament to reach the thigh, but the ligament sometimes splits to enclose it. Hyperextension of the hip or increased lumbar lordosis—such as occurs during pregnancy—leads to nerve compression by the posterior fascicle of the ligament. However, entrapment of the nerve at any point along its course may cause similar symptoms, and several other anatomic variations predispose the nerve to damage when it is stretched. Pain, paresthesia, or numbness occurs about the outer aspect of the thigh, usually unilaterally, and is sometimes relieved by sitting. The pain stops at the knee, unlike the pain from lower lumbar sciatica that radiates to the foot. Examination shows no abnormalities except in severe cases when cutaneous sensation is impaired in the affected area. Symptoms are usually mild and commonly settle spontaneously. Hydrocortisone injections medial to the anterosuperior iliac spine often relieve symptoms temporarily, while nerve decompression by transposition may provide more lasting relief.

7. Sciatic & Common Peroneal (Fibular) Nerve Palsies

Misplaced deep intramuscular injections are probably still the most common cause of sciatic nerve palsy. Trauma to the buttock, hip, or thigh may also be responsible. The resulting clinical deficit depends on whether the whole nerve has been affected or only certain fibers. In general, the peroneal (fibular) fibers of the sciatic nerve are more susceptible to damage than those destined for the tibial nerve. A sciatic nerve lesion may therefore be difficult to distinguish from peroneal (fibular) neuropathy unless there is electromyographic evidence of involvement of the short head of the biceps femoris muscle. The common peroneal (fibular) nerve itself may be compressed or injured in the region of the head and neck of the fibula, eg, by sitting with crossed legs or wearing high boots. There is weakness of dorsiflexion and eversion of the foot, accompanied by numbness or blunted sensation of the anterolateral aspect of the calf and dorsum of the foot.

8. Tarsal Tunnel Syndrome

The tibial nerve, the other branch of the sciatic, supplies several muscles in the lower extremity, gives origin to the sural nerve, and then continues as the posterior tibial nerve to supply the plantar flexors of the foot and toes. It passes through the tarsal tunnel behind and below the medial malleolus, giving off calcaneal branches and the medial and lateral plantar nerves that supply small muscles of the foot and the skin on the plantar aspect of the foot and toes. Compression of the posterior tibial nerve or its branches between the bony floor and ligamentous roof of the tarsal tunnel leads to pain, paresthesias, and numbness over the bottom of the foot, especially at night, with sparing of the heel. Muscle weakness may be hard to recognize clinically. Compressive lesions of the individual plantar nerves may also occur more distally, with clinical features similar to those of the tarsal tunnel syndrome. Treatment is surgical decompression.

9. Facial Neuropathy

An isolated facial palsy is most often idiopathic (Bell palsy, see later) but may occur in patients with HIV seropositivity, sarcoidosis, Lyme disease (Figure 24–2; also see Chapter 34) or with any process causing an inflammatory reaction in the subarachnoid space, such as meningitis. Whenever facial palsies occur bilaterally, or a facial palsy occurs in conjunction with other neurologic deficits, MRI brain imaging should be undertaken and other investigations considered.

▶ When to Refer

- If there is uncertainty about the diagnosis.
- Symptoms or signs are progressing despite treatment.

▲ **Figure 24–2.** Facial palsy caused by an infection with *Borrelia burgdorferi* (**Lyme disease**). (Public Health Image Library, CDC.)

BELL PALSY

ESSENTIALS OF DIAGNOSIS

- ▶ Sudden onset of lower motor neuron facial palsy.
- ▶ Hyperacusis or impaired taste may occur.
- ▶ No other neurologic abnormalities.

▶ General Considerations

Bell palsy is an idiopathic facial paresis of lower motor neuron type that has been attributed to an inflammatory reaction involving the facial nerve near the stylomastoid foramen or in the bony facial canal. Increasing evidence incriminates reactivation of herpes simplex or varicella zoster virus infection in the geniculate ganglion at least in some instances. The disorder is more common in pregnant women and in persons with diabetes mellitus.

▶ Clinical Findings

The facial paresis (Figure 24–2) generally comes on abruptly, but it may worsen over the following day or so. Pain about the ear precedes or accompanies the weakness in many cases but usually lasts for only a few days. The face itself feels stiff and pulled to one side. There may be ipsilateral restriction of eye closure and difficulty with eating and fine facial movements. A disturbance of taste is common, owing to involvement of chorda tympani fibers, and hyperacusis due to involvement of fibers to the stapedius occurs occasionally.

▶ Treatment

Other disorders that can produce a facial palsy and require specific treatment, such as tumors, Lyme disease, AIDS, sarcoidosis, and herpes zoster infection of the geniculate ganglion, must be excluded. Approximately 60% of cases of Bell palsy recover completely without treatment, presumably because the lesion is so mild that it leads merely to conduction block. Treatment with corticosteroids (prednisone 60 mg orally daily for 5 days followed by a 5-day taper, or prednisolone 25 mg orally twice daily for 10 days) increases the chance of a complete recovery at 9–12 months by 12–15%. Treatment with acyclovir or valacyclovir is only indicated when there is evidence of herpetic vesicles in the external ear canal. It is helpful to protect the eye with lubricating drops (or lubricating ointment at night) and a patch if eye closure is not possible. There is no evidence that surgical procedures to decompress the facial nerve are of benefit. Physical therapy may improve facial function.

Schwartz SR et al. Reconciling the clinical practice guidelines on Bell's palsy from the AAO-HNSF and the AAN. Neurology. 2014 May 27;82(21):1927–9. [PMID: 24793182]

DISCOGENIC NECK PAIN

▶ General Considerations

A variety of congenital abnormalities may involve the cervical spine and lead to neck pain; these include hemivertebrae, fused vertebrae, basilar impression, and instability of the atlantoaxial joint. Traumatic, degenerative, infective, and neoplastic disorders may also lead to pain in the neck. When rheumatoid arthritis involves the spine, it tends to affect especially the cervical region, leading to pain, stiffness, and reduced mobility; displacement of vertebrae or atlantoaxial subluxation may lead to cord compression that can be life-threatening if not treated by fixation. Further details are given in Chapter 41 (including a discussion on low back pain), and discussion here is restricted to disk disease.

1. Acute Cervical Disk Protrusion

Acute cervical disk protrusion leads to pain in the neck and radicular pain in the arm, exacerbated by head movement. With lateral herniation of the disk, motor, sensory, or reflex changes may be found in a radicular (usually C6 or C7) distribution on the affected side (Figure 24–3); with more centrally directed herniations, the spinal cord may also be involved, leading to spastic paraparesis and sensory disturbances in the legs, sometimes accompanied by impaired sphincter function. The diagnosis is confirmed by MRI or CT myelography. In mild cases, bed rest or intermittent neck traction may help, followed by immobilization of the neck in a collar for several weeks. If these measures are unsuccessful or the patient has a significant neurologic deficit, surgical removal of the protruding disk may be necessary.

2. Cervical Spondylosis

Cervical spondylosis results from chronic cervical disk degeneration, with herniation of disk material, secondary calcification, and associated osteophytic outgrowths. One or more of the cervical nerve roots may be compressed, stretched, or angulated; and myelopathy may also develop as a result of compression, vascular insufficiency, or recurrent minor trauma to the cord. Patients present with neck pain and restricted head movement, occipital headaches, radicular pain and other sensory disturbances in the arms, weakness of the arms or legs, or some combination of these symptoms. Examination generally reveals that lateral

flexion and rotation of the neck are limited. A segmental pattern of weakness or dermatomal sensory loss (or both) may be found unilaterally or bilaterally in the upper limbs, and tendon reflexes mediated by the affected root or roots are depressed. The C5 and C6 nerve roots are most commonly involved, and examination frequently then reveals weakness of muscles supplied by these roots (eg, deltoids, supraspinatus and infraspinatus, biceps, brachioradialis), pain or sensory loss about the shoulder and outer border of the arm and forearm, and depressed biceps and brachioradialis reflexes. Spastic paraparesis may also be present if there is an associated myelopathy, sometimes accompanied by posterior column or spinothalamic sensory deficits in the legs.

Plain radiographs of the cervical spine show osteophyte formation, narrowing of disk spaces, and encroachment on the intervertebral foramina, but such changes are common in middle-aged persons and may be unrelated to the presenting complaint. CT or MRI helps confirm the diagnosis and exclude other structural causes of the myelopathy.

Restriction of neck movements by a cervical collar may relieve pain. Local injection of anesthetics or corticosteroids, for instance by a pain management specialist, may be of benefit. Operative treatment may be necessary to prevent further progression if there is a significant neurologic deficit or if root pain is severe, persistent, and unresponsive to conservative measures.

▶ When to Refer

- Pain unresponsive to simple measures.
- Patients with neurologic deficits.
- Patients in whom surgical treatment is under consideration.

▶ When to Admit

- Patients with progressive or significant neurologic deficit.
- Patients with sphincter involvement (from cord compression).
- Patients requiring surgical treatment.

Corey DL et al. Cervical radiculopathy. Med Clin North Am. 2014 Jul;98(4):791–9. [PMID: 24994052]

BRACHIAL & LUMBAR PLEXUS LESIONS

1. Brachial Plexus Neuropathy

Brachial plexus neuropathy may be idiopathic, sometimes occurring in relationship to a number of different nonspecific illnesses or factors. In other instances, brachial plexus lesions follow trauma or result from congenital anomalies, neoplastic involvement, or injury by various physical agents. In rare instances, the disorder occurs on a familial basis.

Peripheral nerve

- Trigeminal
  - Ophthalmic branch
  - Maxillary branch
  - Mandibular branch
- Anterior cutaneous nerve of neck
- Supraclavicular nerves
- Axillary nerve
- Medial cutaneous nerve of arm
- Lateral cutaneous nerve of arm (branch of radial nerve)
- Medial cutaneous nerve of forearm
- Lateral cutaneous nerve of forearm
- Radial
- Median
- Ulnar
- Lateral femoral cutaneous
- Obturator
- Anterior femoral cutaneous
- Lateral cutaneous nerve of calf
- Saphenous
- Superficial peroneal
- Sural
- Lateral and medial plantar
- Deep peroneal

Nerve root

C3, C4, C5, T2, T3, T4, T5, T6, T7, T8, T9, T10, T11, T12, T2, T1, C6, C6, C8, C7, L1, L1, L2, L3, L4, L5, S1

Post. Mid. Ant.

Lateral thoracic rami
Anterior thoracic rami

x = Iliohypogastric
† = Ilioinguinal
★ = Genitofemoral
■ Dorsal nerve of penis
■ Perineal nerve of penis

▲ **Figure 24–3.** Cutaneous innervation. The segmental or radicular (root) distribution is shown on the left side of the body and the peripheral nerve distribution on the right side. Above: anterior view; next page: posterior view. (Reproduced, with permission, from Aminoff MJ, Greenberg DA, Simon RP. Clinical Neurology, 9th ed. McGraw-Hill Education, 2015.)

Idiopathic brachial plexus neuropathy (neuralgic amyotrophy) characteristically begins with severe pain about the shoulder, followed within a few days by weakness, reflex changes, and sensory disturbances involving especially the C5 and C6 segments but affecting any nerve in the brachial plexus. Symptoms and signs are usually unilateral but may be bilateral. Wasting of affected muscles is sometimes profound. The disorder relates to disturbed function of cervical roots or part of the brachial plexus, but its precise cause is unknown. Recovery occurs over the ensuing months but may be incomplete. Treatment is purely symptomatic.

Nerve root **Peripheral nerve**

Great occipital

Lesser occipital
Great auricular

Posterior rami of cervical nerves

Supraclavicular

Axillary

Lateral cutaneous nerve of arm
Posterior cutaneous nerve of arm
Medial cutaneous nerve of arm

Lateral cutaneous nerve of forearm
Posterior cutaneous nerve of forearm
Medial cutaneous nerve of forearm

Posterior lumbar rami

Posterior sacral rami

Radial

Median

Ulnar

Lateral femoral cutaneous
Obturator
Anterior femoral cutaneous

Posterior femoral cutaneous
Lateral cutaneous nerve of calf

Superficial peroneal

Saphenous

Sural

Calcaneal

Lateral plantar
Medial plantar

x = Iliohypogastric

▲ **Figure 24–3** (continued)

2. Cervical Rib Syndrome

Compression of the C8 and T1 roots or the lower trunk of the brachial plexus by a cervical rib or band arising from the seventh cervical vertebra leads to weakness and wasting of intrinsic hand muscles, especially those in the thenar eminence, accompanied by pain and numbness in the medial two fingers and the ulnar border of the hand and forearm. The subclavian artery may also be compressed, and this forms the basis of the Adson test for diagnosing the disorder; the radial pulse is diminished or obliterated on the affected side when the seated patient inhales deeply and turns the head to one side or the other. Electromyography, nerve conduction studies, and somatosensory evoked potential studies may help confirm the diagnosis. MRI may be especially helpful in revealing the underlying compressive structure. Plain radiographs or CT scanning sometimes shows the cervical rib or a large transverse process of the seventh cervical vertebra, but normal findings do not exclude the possibility of a cervical band. Treatment of the disorder is by surgical excision of the rib or band.

3. Lumbosacral Plexus Lesions

A lumbosacral plexus lesion may develop in association with diseases such as diabetes, cancer, or bleeding disorders or in relation to injury. It occasionally occurs as an isolated phenomenon similar to idiopathic brachial plexopathy, and pain and weakness then tend to be more conspicuous than sensory symptoms. The distribution of symptoms and signs depends on the level and pattern of neurologic involvement.

Van Alfen N et al. Diagnosis of brachial and lumbosacral plexus lesions. Handb Clin Neurol. 2013;115:293–310. [PMID: 23931788]

DISORDERS OF NEUROMUSCULAR TRANSMISSION

1. Myasthenia Gravis

ESSENTIALS OF DIAGNOSIS

▶ Fluctuating weakness of commonly used voluntary muscles, producing symptoms such as diplopia, ptosis, and difficulty in swallowing.

▶ Activity increases weakness of affected muscles.

▶ Short-acting anticholinesterases transiently improve the weakness.

▶ General Considerations

Myasthenia gravis occurs at all ages, sometimes in association with a thymic tumor or thyrotoxicosis, as well as in rheumatoid arthritis and lupus erythematosus. It is most common in young women with HLA-DR3; if thymoma is associated, older men are more commonly affected. Onset is usually insidious, but the disorder is sometimes unmasked by a coincidental infection that leads to exacerbation of symptoms. Exacerbations may also occur before the menstrual period and during or shortly after pregnancy. Symptoms are due to a variable degree of block of neuromuscular transmission caused by autoantibodies binding to acetylcholine receptors; these are found in most patients with the disease and have a primary role in reducing the number of functioning acetylcholine receptors. Additionally, cellular immune activity against the receptor is found.

▶ Clinical Findings

A. Symptoms and Signs

Patients present with ptosis, diplopia, difficulty in chewing or swallowing, respiratory difficulties, limb weakness, or some combination of these problems. Weakness may remain localized to a few muscle groups or may become generalized. The external ocular muscles and certain other cranial muscles, including the masticatory, facial, and pharyngeal muscles, are especially likely to be affected, and the respiratory and limb muscles may also be involved. Symptoms often fluctuate in intensity during the day, and this diurnal variation is superimposed on a tendency to longer-term spontaneous relapses and remissions that may last for weeks. Nevertheless, the disorder follows a slowly progressive course and may have a fatal outcome owing to respiratory complications such as aspiration pneumonia.

Clinical examination confirms the weakness and fatigability of affected muscles. In most cases, the extraocular muscles are involved, and this leads to ocular palsies and ptosis, which are commonly asymmetric. Pupillary responses are normal. The bulbar and limb muscles are often weak, but the pattern of involvement is variable. Sustained activity of affected muscles increases the weakness, which improves after a brief rest. Sensation is normal, and there are usually no reflex changes.

Life-threatening exacerbations of myasthenia (so-called **myasthenic crisis**) may lead to respiratory weakness requiring immediate admission to the intensive care unit, where respiratory function can be monitored and ventilator support is readily available.

B. Imaging

A CT scan of the chest with and without contrast should be obtained to demonstrate a coexisting thymoma, but a normal study does not exclude this possibility.

C. Laboratory and Other Studies

Electrophysiologic demonstration of a decrementing muscle response to repetitive 2- or 3-Hz stimulation of motor nerves indicates a disturbance of neuromuscular transmission. Such an abnormality may even be detected in clinically strong muscles with certain provocative procedures. Needle electromyography of affected muscles shows a marked variation in configuration and size of individual motor unit potentials, and single-fiber electromyography reveals an increased jitter, or variability, in the time interval between two muscle fiber action potentials from the same motor unit.

Assay of serum for elevated levels of circulating acetylcholine receptor antibodies is useful because it has a sensitivity of 80–90% for the diagnosis of myasthenia gravis. Certain patients without antibodies to acetylcholine receptors have serum antibodies to muscle-specific tyrosine kinase (MuSK), which should therefore be determined; these patients are more likely to have facial, respiratory, and proximal muscle weakness than those with antibodies to acetylcholine receptors. Other antibodies associated with myasthenia gravis include low-density lipoprotein receptor-related protein 4 (LRP4) and agrin, but tests for these antibodies are not widely commercially available.

▶ Treatment

Anticholinesterase drugs provide symptomatic benefit without influencing the course of the disease. Neostigmine, pyridostigmine, or both can be used, the dose being determined on an individual basis. The usual dose of neostigmine is 7.5–30 mg (average, 15 mg) orally taken four times daily; of pyridostigmine, 30–180 mg (average, 60 mg) orally four times daily. Overmedication may temporarily increase weakness. A wide range of medications (eg, aminoglycosides) may exacerbate myasthenia gravis and should be avoided.

Thymectomy should be performed when a thymoma is present. Even in the absence of a radiologically identifiable thymoma, thymectomy may lead to symptomatic benefit or remission and should be considered in all patients younger than age 60, unless weakness is restricted to the extraocular muscles, despite an absence of randomized controlled trial data supporting this approach. If the disease is of recent onset and only slowly progressive, operation is sometimes delayed for a year or so, in the hope that spontaneous remission will occur.

Treatment with corticosteroids is indicated for patients who have responded poorly to anticholinesterase drugs and have already undergone thymectomy. It is often introduced with the patient in the hospital, since weakness may initially be aggravated. Once weakness has stabilized after 2–3 weeks or any improvement is sustained, further management can be on an outpatient basis. Alternate-day treatment is usually well tolerated, but if weakness is enhanced on the nontreatment day it may be necessary for medication to be taken daily. The dose of corticosteroids is determined on an individual basis, but an initial high daily dose (eg, prednisone, 60–100 mg orally daily) can gradually be tapered to a relatively low maintenance level (eg, 10 mg orally daily) as improvement occurs; total withdrawal is difficult, however. Treatment with azathioprine may be effective in allowing a lower dose of corticosteroids. The usual dose is 2–3 mg/kg orally daily after a lower initial dose. Mycophenolate mofetil or cyclosporine is typically reserved for more refractory cases or as a strategy to reduce the corticosteroid dose.

In patients with major disability, plasmapheresis or IVIG therapy may be beneficial and have similar efficacy. It is also useful for stabilizing patients before thymectomy and for managing acute crisis.

▶ When to Refer

All patients should be referred.

▶ When to Admit

- Patients with acute exacerbation or respiratory involvement.
- Patients requiring plasmapheresis.
- Patients who are starting corticosteroid therapy.
- For thymectomy.

Diaz A et al. Is thymectomy in non-thymomatous myasthenia gravis of any benefit? Interact Cardiovasc Thorac Surg. 2014 Mar;18(3):381–9. [PMID: 24351507]

Sieb JP. Myasthenia gravis: an update for the clinician. Clin Exp Immunol. 2014 Mar;175(3):408–18. [PMID: 24117026]

2. Myasthenic Syndrome (Lambert-Eaton Syndrome)

ESSENTIALS OF DIAGNOSIS

▶ Variable weakness, typically improving with activity.

▶ Dysautonomic symptoms may also be present.

▶ A history of malignant disease may be obtained.

▶ General Considerations

Myasthenic syndrome may be associated with small-cell carcinoma, sometimes developing before the tumor is diagnosed, and occasionally occurs with certain autoimmune diseases. There is defective release of acetylcholine in response to a nerve impulse, caused by P/Q-type voltage-gated calcium-channel antibodies, and this leads to weakness, especially of the proximal muscles of the limbs. Unlike myasthenia gravis, however, power steadily increases with sustained contraction. The diagnosis can be confirmed electrophysiologically, because the muscle response to stimulation of its motor nerve increases remarkably after exercise or if the nerve is stimulated repetitively at high rates (50 Hz), even in muscles that are not clinically weak.

Treatment with plasmapheresis and immunosuppressive drug therapy (prednisone and azathioprine) may lead to clinical and electrophysiologic improvement, in addition to therapy aimed at tumor when present. Prednisone is usually initiated in a daily dose of 60–80 mg orally and azathioprine in a daily dose of 2 mg/kg orally. Symptomatic therapy includes the use of potassium channel antagonists; of these, 3,4-diaminopyridine (60–80 mg/day orally in three divided doses) has been best studied and appears efficacious. Guanidine hydrochloride (25–50 mg/kg/day orally in divided doses) is an alternative and is occasionally helpful in seriously disabled patients, but adverse effects of the drug include marrow suppression. The response to treatment with anticholinesterase drugs such as pyridostigmine or neostigmine is usually disappointing.

Hülsbrink R et al. Lambert-Eaton myasthenic syndrome—diagnosis, pathogenesis and therapy. Clin Neurophysiol. 2014 Dec;125(12):2328–36. [PMID: 25065299]

3. Botulism

The toxin of *Clostridium botulinum* prevents the release of acetylcholine at neuromuscular junctions and autonomic synapses. Botulism occurs most commonly following the ingestion of contaminated home-canned food; outbreaks have also occurred among drug abusers due to wound infection after injection of contaminated heroin. The diagnosis should be suggested by the development of sudden, fluctuating, severe weakness in a previously healthy person. Symptoms begin within 72 hours following ingestion of the toxin and may progress for several days. Typically, there is diplopia, ptosis, facial weakness, dysphagia, and nasal speech, followed by respiratory difficulty and finally by weakness that appears last in the limbs. Blurring of vision (with unreactive dilated pupils) is characteristic, and there may be dryness of the mouth, constipation (paralytic ileus), and postural hypotension. Sensation is preserved, and the tendon reflexes are not affected unless the involved muscles are very weak. If the diagnosis is suspected, the local health authority should be notified and a sample of serum and contaminated food (if available) sent to be assayed for toxin. Support for the diagnosis may be obtained by electrophysiologic studies; with repetitive stimulation of motor nerves at fast rates, the muscle response increases in size progressively.

Patients should be hospitalized in case respiratory assistance becomes necessary. Treatment is with trivalent antitoxin, once it is established that the patient is not allergic to horse serum. Potassium channel antagonists may provide symptomatic relief as they do in Lambert-Eaton myasthenic syndrome. Anticholinesterase drugs are of no value. Respiratory assistance and other supportive measures should be provided as necessary. Further details are provided in Chapter 33.

Chalk C et al. Medical treatment for botulism. Cochrane Database Syst Rev. 2011 Mar 16;(3):CD008123. [PMID: 21412916]

4. Disorders Associated with Use of Aminoglycosides

Aminoglycoside antibiotics, eg, gentamicin, may produce a clinical disturbance similar to botulism by preventing the release of acetylcholine from nerve endings, but symptoms subside rapidly as the responsible drug is eliminated from the body. These antibiotics are particularly dangerous in patients with preexisting disturbances of neuromuscular transmission and are therefore best avoided in patients with myasthenia gravis.

MYOPATHIC DISORDERS

1. Muscular Dystrophies

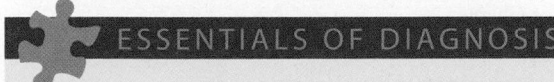

ESSENTIALS OF DIAGNOSIS

▶ Muscle weakness, often in a characteristic distribution.

▶ Age at onset and inheritance pattern depend on the specific dystrophy.

▶ General Considerations

These inherited myopathic disorders are characterized by progressive muscle weakness and wasting. They are subdivided by mode of inheritance, age at onset, and clinical features, as shown in Table 24–10. In the Duchenne type,

pseudohypertrophy of muscles frequently occurs at some stage; intellectual retardation is common; and there may be skeletal deformities, muscle contractures, and cardiac involvement. The serum creatine kinase level is increased, especially in the Duchenne and Becker varieties, and mildly increased also in limb-girdle dystrophy. Electromyography may help confirm that weakness is myopathic rather than neurogenic. Similarly, histopathologic examination of a muscle biopsy specimen may help confirm that weakness is due to a primary disorder of muscle and to distinguish between various muscle diseases.

A genetic defect on the short arm of the X chromosome has been identified in Duchenne dystrophy. The affected gene codes for the protein dystrophin, which is markedly reduced or absent from the muscle of patients with the disease. Dystrophin levels are generally normal in the Becker variety, but the protein is qualitatively altered. The diagnosis is usually made with genetic testing; muscle biopsy is needed occasionally. Duchenne muscular dystrophy can be recognized early in pregnancy in about 95% of women by genetic studies; in late pregnancy, DNA probes can be used on fetal tissue obtained for this purpose by amniocentesis. The genes causing some of the other muscular dystrophies are listed in Table 24–10.

There is no specific treatment for the muscular dystrophies, but it is important to encourage patients to lead as normal lives as possible. Prednisone (0.75 mg/kg orally daily) improves muscle strength and function in boys with Duchenne dystrophy, but side effects need to be monitored. Prolonged bed rest must be avoided, as inactivity often leads to worsening of the underlying muscle disease. Physical therapy and orthopedic procedures may help counteract deformities or contractures.

Kang PB et al. Advances in muscular dystrophies. JAMA Neurol. 2015 Jul;72(7):741–2. [PMID: 25985443]
Wein N et al. Genetics and emerging treatments for Duchenne and Becker muscular dystrophy. Pediatr Clin North Am. 2015 Jun;62(3):723–42. [PMID: 26022172]

2. Myotonic Dystrophy

Myotonic dystrophy, a slowly progressive, dominantly inherited disorder, usually manifests itself in the third or fourth decade but occasionally appears early in childhood. Two types, with a different genetic basis, have been recognized. Myotonia leads to complaints of muscle stiffness and is evidenced by the marked delay that occurs before affected muscles can relax after a contraction. This can often be demonstrated clinically by delayed relaxation of the hand after sustained grip or by percussion of the belly of a muscle. In addition, there is weakness and wasting of the facial, sternocleidomastoid, and distal limb muscles. Associated clinical features include cataracts, frontal baldness, testicular atrophy, diabetes mellitus, cardiac abnormalities, and intellectual changes. Electromyographic sampling of affected muscles reveals myotonic discharges in addition to changes suggestive of myopathy.

It is difficult to determine whether drug therapy for myotonia is safe or effective. When myotonia is disabling, treatment with a sodium channel blocker—such as

Table 24–10. The muscular dystrophies.[1]

Disorder	Inheritance	Age at Onset (years)	Distribution	Prognosis	Genetic Association
Duchenne type	X-linked recessive	1–5	Pelvic, then shoulder girdle; later, limb and respiratory muscles.	Rapid progression. Death within about 15 years after onset.	Xp21; Dystrophin (loss of functional expression)
Becker	X-linked recessive	5–25	Pelvic, then shoulder girdle.	Slow progression. May have normal life span.	Xp21; Dystrophin (reduced functional expression)
Limb-girdle (Erb)	Autosomal recessive, dominant, or sporadic	10–30	Pelvic or shoulder girdle initially, with later spread to the other.	Variable severity and rate of progression. Possible severe disability in middle life.	Multiple
Facioscapulo-humeral	Autosomal dominant	Any age	Face and shoulder girdle initially; later, pelvic girdle and legs.	Slow progression. Minor disability. Usually normal life span.	4q35.2; Double homeobox protein 4 18p11.32; Structural maintenance of chromosome's flexible hinge domain-containing protein 1
Emery-Dreifuss	X-linked recessive or autosomal dominant	5–10	Humeroperoneal or scapuloperoneal.	Variable.	Multiple
Distal	Autosomal dominant or recessive	40–60	Onset distally in extremities; proximal involvement later.	Slow progression.	Multiple
Oculopharyngeal	Autosomal dominant	Any age	As in the ocular form but with dysphagia.		14q11.2–q13; Poly (A)-binding protein-2
Myotonic dystrophy	Autosomal dominant	Any age (usually 20–40)	Face, neck, distal limbs.	Slow progression.	19q13.32; Myotonin-protein kinase 3q21.3; Cellular nucleic acid-binding protein

[1]Not all possible genetic loci are shown.

phenytoin (100 mg orally three times daily), procainamide (0.5–1 g orally four times daily), or mexiletine (150–200 mg orally three times daily)—may be helpful, but the associated side effects, particularly for antiarrhythmic drugs, are often limiting. Neither the weakness nor the course of the disorder is influenced by treatment. Cardiac function should be monitored, and pacemaker placement may be considered if there is evidence of heart block.

Turner C et al. Myotonic dystrophy: diagnosis, management and new therapies. Curr Opin Neurol. 2014 Oct;27(5):599–606. [PMID: 25121518]

3. Myotonia Congenita

Myotonia congenita is commonly inherited as a dominant trait. The responsible gene on chromosome 7 encodes a voltage-gated chloride channel. Generalized myotonia without weakness is usually present from birth, but symptoms may not appear until early childhood. Patients complain of muscle stiffness that is enhanced by cold and inactivity and relieved by exercise. Muscle hypertrophy, at

times pronounced, is also a feature. A recessive form with later onset is associated with slight weakness and atrophy of distal muscles. Treatment with procainamide, tocainide, mexiletine, or phenytoin may help the myotonia, as in myotonic dystrophy.

4. Polymyositis & Dermatomyositis

See Chapter 20.

5. Inclusion Body Myositis

This disorder, of unknown cause, begins insidiously, usually after middle age, with progressive proximal weakness of first the lower and then the upper extremities, and affecting facial and pharyngeal muscles. Weakness often begins in the quadriceps femoris in the lower limbs and the forearm flexors in the upper limbs. Distal weakness is usually mild. Serum creatine kinase levels may be normal or increased. The diagnosis is confirmed by muscle biopsy. Corticosteroid and immunosuppressive therapy is sometimes offered but is usually ineffective, and IVIG therapy is not recommended.

Dimachkie MM et al. Inclusion body myositis. Neurol Clin. 2014 Aug;32(3):629–46. [PMID: 25037082]

6. Mitochondrial Myopathies

The mitochondrial myopathies are a clinically diverse group of disorders that on pathologic examination of skeletal muscle with the modified Gomori stain show characteristic "ragged red fibers" containing accumulations of abnormal mitochondria. Patients may present with progressive external ophthalmoplegia or with limb weakness that is exacerbated or induced by activity. Other patients present with central neurologic dysfunction, eg, myoclonic epilepsy (myoclonic epilepsy, ragged red fiber syndrome, or MERRF), or the combination of myopathy, encephalopathy, lactic acidosis, and stroke-like episodes (MELAS). These disorders result from separate abnormalities of mitochondrial DNA. Treatment is symptomatic and palliative, but various experimental approaches are being explored.

A mitochondrial myopathy may develop in patients receiving zidovudine for treatment of AIDS, and patients receiving combined antiretroviral therapy for HIV infection may develop a lipodystrophy, with fat accumulating in muscle.

Sharp LJ et al. Metabolic and mitochondrial myopathies. Neurol Clin. 2014 Aug;32(3):777–99. [PMID: 25037090]

7. Myopathies Associated with Other Disorders

Myopathy may occur in association with chronic hypokalemia, any endocrinopathy, and in patients taking corticosteroids, chloroquine, colchicine, clofibrate, emetine, aminocaproic acid, statin drugs, or bretylium tosylate. Weakness is mainly proximal, and serum creatine kinase is typically normal, except in hypothyroidism and some of the toxic myopathies. Treatment is of the underlying cause. Myopathy also occurs with chronic alcoholism, whereas acute reversible muscle necrosis may occur shortly after acute alcohol intoxication. Inflammatory myopathy may occur in patients taking penicillamine; myotonia may be induced by clofibrate, and preexisting myotonia may be exacerbated or unmasked by depolarizing muscle relaxants (eg, suxamethonium), beta-blockers (eg, propranolol), fenoterol, ritodrine and, possibly, certain diuretics.

▶ When to Refer

All patients should be referred to establish the diagnosis and underlying cause.

▶ When to Admit

- For respiratory assistance.
- For rhabdomyolysis.

PERIODIC PARALYSIS SYNDROMES

Periodic paralysis may have a familial (dominant inheritance) basis. The syndromes to be described are channelopathies that manifest as abnormal, often potassium-sensitive, muscle-membrane excitability and lead clinically to episodes of flaccid weakness or paralysis, sometimes in association with abnormalities of the plasma potassium level. Strength is normal between attacks. Mutations in genes encoding three ion channels (*CACNA1S [1q32], SCN4A [17q23.1-q25.3],* and *KCNJ2 [17q23.1-q24.2]*) account for most cases. **Hypokalemic periodic paralysis** has been related to mutations in the *CACNL1A3, SCN4A,* or *KCNE3 (11q13-q14)* gene and is characterized by attacks that tend to occur on awakening, after exercise, or after a heavy meal and may last for several days. Patients should avoid excessive exertion. A low-carbohydrate and low-salt diet may help prevent attacks, as may acetazolamide, 250–750 mg orally daily. Nonselective beta-adrenergic blockers may also prevent recurrent paralytic attacks. An ongoing attack may be aborted by potassium chloride given orally or by intravenous drip, provided the ECG can be monitored and kidney function is satisfactory. In young Asian men, it is commonly associated with hyperthyroidism and has been related to polymorphism in the *CACNA1S* gene; treatment of the endocrine disorder prevents recurrences. In **hyperkalemic periodic paralysis,** which is mostly associated with mutations in the *SCN4A* gene, attacks also tend to occur after exercise but usually last for less than 1 hour. They may be terminated by intravenous calcium gluconate (1–2 g) or by intravenous diuretics (furosemide, 20–40 mg), glucose, or glucose and insulin; daily acetazolamide or chlorothiazide may prevent recurrences. **Normokalemic periodic paralysis** is similar clinically to the hyperkalemic variety, but the plasma potassium level remains normal during attacks; treatment is with acetazolamide.

▶ When to Refer

All patients should be referred.

Cope TE et al. Thyrotoxic periodic paralysis: correct hypokalemia with caution. J Emerg Med. 2013 Sep;45(3):338–40. [PMID: 23849367]

Suetterlin K et al. Muscle channelopathies: recent advances in genetics, pathophysiology and therapy. Curr Opin Neurol. 2014 Oct;27(5):583–90. [PMID: 25188014]

25

Psychiatric Disorders

Nolan Williams, MD

Charles DeBattista, DMH, MD

The fifth edition of the American Psychiatric Association's *Diagnostic and Statistical Manual (DSM-5)* utilizes specific criteria with which to objectively assess symptoms, rather than purely discrete diagnostic categories. For example, personality dimensions are more prominent than they were in *DSM-IV*. Nonetheless, the diagnosis is still based on a solid history and examination.

COMMON PSYCHIATRIC DISORDERS

STRESS & ADJUSTMENT DISORDERS (Situational Disorders)

ESSENTIALS OF DIAGNOSIS

► Anxiety or depression in reaction to an identifiable stress.

► Subsequent symptoms of anxiety or depression commonly elicited by similar stress of lesser magnitude.

► Alcohol and other drugs are commonly used in self-treatment.

► General Considerations

An individual experiences stress when the adaptive capacity of the individual is overwhelmed by events. The event may be an insignificant one when objectively considered, and even favorable changes (eg, promotion and transfer) requiring adaptive behavior can produce stress. For each individual, stress is subjectively defined, and the response to stress is a function of each person's personality and physiologic endowment.

Opinion differs about what events are most apt to produce stress reactions. The causes of stress are different at different ages—eg, in young adulthood, the sources of stress are found in the marriage or parent-child relationship, the employment relationship, and the struggle to achieve financial stability; in the middle years, the focus shifts to changing spousal relationships, problems with

aging parents, and problems associated with having young adult offspring who themselves are encountering stressful situations; in old age, the principal concerns are apt to be retirement, loss of physical and mental capacity, major personal losses, and thoughts of death.

► Clinical Findings

An individual may react to stress by becoming anxious or depressed, by developing a physical symptom, by running away, drinking alcohol, overeating, starting an affair, or in limitless other ways. Common subjective responses are anxiety, sadness, fear, rage, guilt, and shame. Acute and reactivated stress may be manifested by restlessness, irritability, fatigue, increased startle reaction, and a feeling of tension. Inability to concentrate, sleep disturbances (insomnia, bad dreams), and somatic preoccupations often lead to self-medication, most commonly with alcohol or other central nervous system depressants. Maladaptive behavior in response to stress is called **adjustment disorder**, with the major symptom specified (eg, "adjustment disorder with depressed mood"). Even with an identifiable stressor, if the patient meets syndromal criteria for another disorder such as major depression, then the convention would be to diagnose a major depression and not an adjustment disorder with depressed mood.

► Differential Diagnosis

Adjustment disorders are distinguished from anxiety disorders, mood disorders, bereavement, other stress disorders such as posttraumatic stress disorder (PTSD), and personality disorders exacerbated by stress and from somatic disorders with psychic overlay. Unlike many other psychiatric disorders, such as bipolar disorder or schizophrenia, adjustment disorders are wholly situational and usually resolve when the stressor resolves or the individual effectively adapts to the situation. Adjustment disorders may have symptoms that overlap with other disorders, such as anxiety symptoms, but they occur in reaction to an identifiable life stressor such as a difficult work situation or romantic breakup. An adjustment disorder that persists and worsens can potentially evolve into another psychiatric disorder such as major depression or generalized anxiety disorder (GAD). However, that is not the case for most patients. Patients with adjustment disorders have marked distress after a stressor and significant impairment in social or occupational functioning but not to the degree experienced by patients with a more severe disorder such as major depressive disorder or PTSD. By definition, an adjustment disorder occurs within 3 months of an identifiable stressor.

▶ Treatment

A. Behavioral

Stress reduction techniques include immediate symptom reduction (eg, rebreathing in a bag for hyperventilation) or early recognition and removal from a stress source before full-blown symptoms appear. It is often helpful for the patient to keep a daily log of stress precipitators, responses, and alleviators. Relaxation, mindfulness-based stress reduction, and exercise techniques are also helpful in reducing the reaction to stressful events.

B. Social

The stress reactions of life crisis problems are a function of psychosocial upheaval, and patients frequently present with somatic symptoms. While it is not easy for the patient to make necessary changes (or they would have been made long ago), it is important for the clinician to establish the framework of the problem, since the patient's denial system may obscure the issues. Clarifying the problem allows the patient to begin viewing it within the proper context and facilitates the difficult decisions the patient eventually must make (eg, change of job).

C. Psychological

Prolonged in-depth psychotherapy is seldom necessary in cases of isolated stress response or adjustment disorder. Supportive psychotherapy (see above) with an emphasis on the here and now and strengthening of existing coping mechanisms is a helpful approach so that time and the patient's own resiliency can restore the previous level of function. In addition, cognitive behavioral therapy has long been established to treat acute stress and facilitate recovery in patients with an adjustment disorder.

D. Medical

Judicious use of sedatives (eg, lorazepam, 0.5–1 mg two or three times daily orally) for a limited time and as part of an overall treatment plan can provide relief from acute anxiety symptoms. Problems arise when the situation becomes chronic through inappropriate treatment or when the treatment approach supports the development of chronicity. There are occasions where the short-term use of selective serotonin reuptake inhibitors (SSRIs) targeting dysphoria and anxiety may be useful.

▶ Prognosis

Return to satisfactory function after a short period is part of the clinical picture of this syndrome. Resolution may be delayed if others' responses to the patient's difficulties are thoughtlessly harmful or if the secondary gains outweigh the advantages of recovery. The longer the symptoms persist, the worse the prognosis.

Birnie K et al. Psychological benefits for cancer patients and their partners participating in mindfulness-based stress reduction (MBSR). Psychooncology. 2010 Sep;19(9):1004–9. [PMID: 19918956]

TRAUMA & STRESSOR-RELATED DISORDERS

ESSENTIALS OF DIAGNOSIS

▶ Exposure to a traumatic or life-threatening event.

▶ Symptoms, such as flashbacks, intrusive images, and nightmares, often represent reexperiencing the event.

▶ Avoidance symptoms, including numbing, social withdrawal, and avoidance of stimuli associated with the event.

▶ Increased vigilance, such as startle reactions and difficulty falling asleep.

▶ Symptoms impair functioning.

▶ General Considerations

Posttraumatic stress disorder (PTSD) has been reclassified from an anxiety disorder to a trauma and stressor-related disorder in the *DSM-5*. PTSD is a syndrome characterized by "reexperiencing" a traumatic event (eg, sexual assault, severe burns, military combat) and decreased responsiveness and avoidance of current events when associated with the trauma. Data indicate that 13% of veterans who served in Iraq and 6% of those who served in Afghanistan have experienced PTSD. The 2005 National Comorbidity Survey Report estimated the lifetime prevalence of PTSD among adult Americans at 6.8% with a point prevalence of 3.6% and with women having rates twice as high as men. PTSD is more common when the event is associated with physical injury than when it is not. Many individuals with PTSD (20–40%) have experienced other associated problems, including divorce, parenting problems, difficulties with the law, and substance abuse. Since the terrorist attacks in the United States on September 11, 2001, estimates of PTSD have ranged from 4.7% to 10.2% in those witnessing the live attacks and have been associated with functional impairment as well as increased rates of substance use.

▶ Clinical Findings

The key to establishing the diagnosis of PTSD lies in the history of exposure to a *life-threatening event* followed by intrusive (eg, flashbacks, nightmares) or avoidance (eg, withdrawal) symptoms. Patients with PTSD experience physiologic hyperarousal, including startle reactions, intrusive thoughts, illusions, overgeneralized associations, sleep problems, nightmares, dreams about the precipitating event, impulsivity, difficulties in concentration, and hyperalertness. The symptoms may be precipitated or exacerbated by events that are a reminder of the original traumatic event. Symptoms frequently arise after a long latency period (eg, child abuse can result in later-onset PTSD). *DSM-5* includes the requirement that the symptoms persist for at least 1 month. In some individuals, the symptoms fade over months or years, and in others it may persist for a lifetime.

▶ Differential Diagnosis

In 75% of cases, PTSD occurs with comorbid depression or panic disorder, and there is considerable overlap in the symptom complexes of all three conditions. Acute stress disorder occurs during or shortly after a traumatic event and has many of the same symptoms as PTSD but lasts between 2 and 28 days. Some individuals with dissociative features, such as borderline personality disorders, may mimic some of the symptoms of PTSD, but those disorders are typically more related to chronic childhood maltreatment not a specific traumatic event. The other major comorbidity is alcohol and substance abuse.

▶ Treatment

A. Psychotherapy

Psychotherapy should be initiated as soon as possible after the traumatic event, and it should be brief (typically 8–12 sessions), once the individual is in a safe environment. Cognitive behavior therapy, exposure therapy, and eye-movement desensitization reprocessing have been effective in significantly reducing the duration of symptoms. In all of these approaches, the individual confronts the traumatic situation and learns to view it with less reactivity. Psychological debriefing in a single session, once a mainstay in prevention of PTSD, is now considered to be ineffective and possibly harmful. Posttraumatic stress syndromes respond to interventions that help patients integrate the event in an adaptive way with some sense of mastery in having survived the trauma. Partner relationship problems are a major area of concern, and it is important that the clinician have available a dependable referral source when marriage counseling is indicated.

Treatment initiated later, when symptoms have crystallized, includes programs for cessation of alcohol and other drug use, group and individual psychotherapy, and improved social support systems. The therapeutic approach is to facilitate the normal recovery that was blocked at the time of the trauma.

Treatment of any comorbid substance abuse is an essential part of the recovery process for patients with PTSD. Support groups and 12-step programs such as Alcoholic Anonymous are often very helpful.

B. Medication

SSRIs in full dosage are helpful in ameliorating depression, panic attacks, sleep disruption, and startle responses in chronic PTSD. Sertraline and paroxetine are approved by the US Food and Drug Administration (FDA) for this

purpose, and the SSRIs are the only class of medications approved for the treatment of PTSD. They are, therefore, considered the pharmacotherapy of choice for PTSD. Early treatment of anxious arousal with beta-blockers (eg, propranolol, 80–160 mg orally daily) may lessen the peripheral symptoms of anxiety (eg, tremors, palpitations) but has not been shown to help prevent PTSD. Similarly, noradrenergic agents such as clonidine (titrated from 0.1 mg orally at bedtime to 0.2 mg three times a day) have been shown to help with the hyperarousal symptoms of PTSD. The alpha-adrenergic blocking agent prazosin (2–10 mg orally at bedtime) decreases nightmares and improves quality of sleep in PTSD. Antiseizure medications such as carbamazepine (400–800 mg orally daily) will often mitigate impulsivity and difficulty with anger management. Benzodiazepines, such as clonazepam (1–4 mg orally daily, divided into one or two doses), will reduce anxiety and panic attacks when used in adequate dosage, but dependency problems are a concern, particularly when the patient has had such problems in the past. Trazodone (25–100 mg orally at bedtime) is commonly prescribed as a non–habit forming hypnotic agent. Second-generation antipsychotics have not demonstrated significant utility in the the treatment of PTSD but agents such as quetiapine 50–300 mg/day may have a limited role in treating agitation and sleep disturbance in PTSD patients.

▶ Prognosis

The sooner therapy is initiated after the trauma, the better the prognosis. Approximately half of patients experience chronic symptoms. Prognosis is best in those with good premorbid psychiatric functioning. Individuals experiencing an acute stress disorder typically do better than those experiencing a delayed posttraumatic disorder. Individuals who experience trauma resulting from a natural disaster (eg, earthquake or hurricane) tend to do better than those who experience a traumatic interpersonal encounter (eg, rape or combat).

Hoskins M et al. Pharmacotherapy for post-traumatic stress disorder: systematic review and meta-analysis. Br J Psychiatry. 2015 Feb;206(2):93–100. [PMID: 25644881]

Spoont M. JAMA patient page. Posttraumatic stress disorder (PTSD). JAMA. 2015 Aug 4;314(5):532. [PMID: 26241611]

ANXIETY DISORDERS

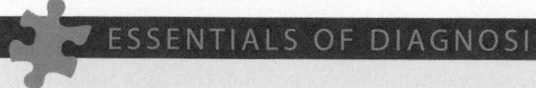

ESSENTIALS OF DIAGNOSIS

▶ Overt anxiety or an overt manifestation of a coping mechanism (such as a phobia), or both.

▶ Not limited to an adjustment disorder.

▶ Somatic symptoms referable to the autonomic nervous system or to a specific organ system (eg, dyspnea, palpitations, paresthesias).

▶ Not a result of physical disorders, psychiatric conditions (eg, schizophrenia), or drug abuse (eg, cocaine).

General Considerations

Stress, fear, and anxiety all tend to be interactive. The principal components of anxiety are **psychological** (tension, fears, difficulty in concentration, apprehension) and **somatic** (tachycardia, hyperventilation, shortness of breath, palpitations, tremor, sweating). Sympathomimetic symptoms of anxiety are both a response to a central nervous system state and a reinforcement of further anxiety. Anxiety can become self-generating, since the symptoms reinforce the reaction, causing it to spiral. This is often the case when the anxiety is an epiphenomenon of other medical or psychiatric disorders.

Anxiety may be free-floating, resulting in acute anxiety attacks, occasionally becoming chronic. When coping mechanisms for stress management are not functioning, the consequences are problems such as phobias, conversion reactions, and dissociative states. Lack of structure is frequently a contributing factor, as noted in those people who have "Sunday neuroses." They do well during the week with a planned work schedule but cannot tolerate the unstructured weekend. Planned-time activities tend to bind anxiety, and many people have increased difficulties when this is lost, as in retirement.

Some believe that various manifestations of anxiety are not a result of unconscious conflicts but are "habits"—persistent patterns of nonadaptive behavior acquired by learning. The "habits," being nonadaptive, are unsatisfactory ways of dealing with life's problems—hence the resultant anxiety. Help is sought only when the anxiety becomes too painful. Exogenous factors such as stimulants (eg, caffeine, cocaine) must be considered as a contributing factor.

Clinical Findings

A. Generalized Anxiety Disorder

This is among the most common of the clinically significant anxiety disorders. Initial manifestations appear at age 20–35 years, and the rate appears to increase with age. GAD becomes chronic in many patients with over half of patients having the disorder for longer than 2 years. About 7% of women and 4% of men will meet criteria for GAD over a lifetime. The anxiety symptoms of apprehension, worry, irritability, difficulty in concentrating, insomnia, and somatic complaints are present more days than not for at least 6 months. Manifestations can include cardiac (eg, tachycardia, increased blood pressure), gastrointestinal (eg, increased acidity, nausea, epigastric pain), and neurologic (eg, headache, near-syncope) systems. The focus of the anxiety may be a number of everyday activities.

B. Panic Disorder

This is characterized by recurrent, unpredictable episodes of intense anxiety accompanied by marked physiologic manifestations. **Agoraphobia**, fear of being in places where escape is difficult, such as open spaces or public places where one cannot easily hide, may be present and may lead the individual to confine his or her life to the home environment. Distressing symptoms and signs such as dyspnea, tachycardia, palpitations, headaches, dizziness, paresthesias, choking, smothering feelings, nausea, and bloating are associated with feelings of impending doom (alarm response). Although these symptoms may lead to overlap with some of the same bodily complaints found in the somatic symptom disorders, the key to the diagnosis of panic disorder is the psychic pain and suffering the individual expresses. Recurrent **sleep panic attacks** (not nightmares) occur in about 30% of panic disorders. Anticipatory anxiety develops in all these patients and further constricts their daily lives. Panic disorder tends to be familial, with onset usually under age 25; it affects 3–5% of the population, and the female-to-male ratio is 2:1. The premenstrual period is one of heightened vulnerability. Patients frequently undergo emergency medical evaluations (eg, for "heart attacks" or "hypoglycemia") before the correct diagnosis is made. Gastrointestinal symptoms (eg, stomach pain, heartburn, diarrhea, constipation, nausea and vomiting) are especially common, occurring in about one-third of cases. Myocardial infarction, pheochromocytoma, hyperthyroidism, and various recreational drug reactions can mimic panic disorder. Mitral valve prolapse may be present but is not usually a significant factor. Patients who have recurrent panic disorder often become demoralized, hypochondriacal, agoraphobic, and depressed. These individuals are at increased risk for major depression and the suicide attempts associated with that disorder. Alcohol abuse (in about 20%) results from self-treatment and is frequently combined with dependence on sedatives. Some patients have atypical panic attacks associated with seizure-like symptoms that often include psychosensory phenomena (a history of stimulant abuse often emerges). About 25% of panic disorder patients also have obsessive-compulsive disorder (OCD).

C. Phobic Disorders

Phobias are fears of a specific object or situation (eg, spiders, height) that are out of proportion to the danger posed and they tend to be chronic. Social phobias are global or specific; in the former, all social situations are poorly tolerated, while the latter group includes performance anxiety (eg, fear of public speaking). Agoraphobia is frequently associated with severe panic attacks, and it often develops in early adult life, making a normal lifestyle difficult. Patients with agoraphobia experience intense fear about common situations, such as being in open spaces (eg, marketplaces), enclosed spaces (eg, theaters), standing in line, or being alone outside of their homes. While patients with simple phobias such as fear of heights may function as long as they do not have to be in tall buildings or airplanes, a patient with agoraphobia may not be able to function vocationally or interpersonally. Thus, patients with agoraphobia are much more likely to seek treatment than those with simple or even social phobia.

Treatment

In all cases, underlying medical disorders must be ruled out (eg, cardiovascular, endocrine, respiratory, and neurologic disorders and substance-related syndromes, both intoxication and withdrawal states). These and other disorders can coexist with panic disorder.

A. Medical

1. Generalized anxiety—Antidepressants including the SSRIs and serotonin norepinephrine reuptake inhibitors (SNRIs) are safe and effective in the long-term management of GAD. The antidepressants appear to be as effective as the benzodiazepines without the risks of tolerance or dependence. However, **benzodiazepines are the anxiolytics of choice in the acute management of generalized anxiety** (Table 25–1). They are almost immediately effective.

All of the benzodiazepines may be given orally, and several are available in parenteral formulations. Benzodiazepines such as lorazepam are absorbed rapidly when given intramuscularly. In psychiatric disorders, the benzodiazepines are usually given orally; in controlled medical environments (eg, the ICU), where the rapid onset of respiratory depression can be assessed, they are often given intravenously. Diazepam and clorazepate are the most rapidly absorbed oral benzodiazepines, which may explain the popularity of diazepam. In the average case of anxiety, diazepam, 5–10 mg orally twice daily as needed, is a reasonable starting regimen.

Benzodiazepines such as lorazepam do not produce active metabolites and have intermediate half-lives of

Table 25–1. Commonly used antianxiety and hypnotic agents.

Drug	Usual Daily Oral Doses	Usual Daily Maximum Doses	Cost for 30 Days Treatment Based on Maximum Dosage[1]
Benzodiazepines (used for anxiety)			
Alprazolam (Xanax)[2]	0.5 mg	4 mg	$223.80
Chlordiazepoxide (Librium)[3]	10–20 mg	100 mg	$37.20
Clonazepam (Klonopin)[3]	1–2 mg	10 mg	$122.40
Clorazepate (Tranxene)[3]	15–30 mg	60 mg	$260.40
Diazepam (Valium)[3]	5–15 mg	30 mg	$30.60
Lorazepam (Ativan)[2]	2–4 mg	4 mg	$69.00
Oxazepam (Serax)[2]	10–30 mg	60 mg	$95.40
Benzodiazepines (used for sleep)			
Estazolam (Prosom)[2]	1 mg	2 mg	$29.70
Flurazepam (Dalmane)[3]	15 mg	30 mg	$11.40
Midazolam (Versed)[4]	5 mg		$1.00/dose
Quazepam (Doral)[3]	7.5 mg	15 mg	$138.00
Temazepam (Restoril)[2]	15 mg	30 mg	$26.40
Triazolam (Halcion)[5]	0.125 mg	0.25 mg	$82.20
Miscellaneous (used for anxiety)			
Buspirone (Buspar)[2]	10–30 mg	60 mg	$217.80
Phenobarbital[3]	15–30 mg	90 mg	$37.80
Miscellaneous (used for sleep)			
Eszopiclone (Lunesta)[5]	2–3 mg	3 mg	$349.80
Hydroxyzine (Vistaril)[2]	50 mg	100 mg	$62.40
Suvorexant (Belsomra)	5–10 mg	20 mg	$341.10
Ramelteon (Rozerem)	8 mg	8 mg	$367.04
Zaleplon (Sonata)[6]	5–10 mg	10 mg	$108.30
Zolpidem (Ambien)[5]	5–10 mg	10 mg	$138.60

[1]Average wholesale price (AWP, for AB-rated generic when available) for quantity listed. Source: *Red Book (electronic version)*, Truven Health Analytic Information, http://www.micormedexsolutions.com, accessed April 8, 2016. AWP may not accurately represent the actual pharmacy cost because wide contractual variations exist among institutions.
[2]Intermediate physical half-life (10–20 hours).
[3]Long physical half-life (> 20 hours).
[4]Intravenously for procedures.
[5]Short physical half-life (1–6 hours).
[6]Short physical half-life (about 1 hour).

10–20 hours, characteristics useful in treating elderly patients. Ultra-short-acting agents such as triazolam have half-lives of 1–3 hours and may lead to rebound withdrawal anxiety. Longer-acting benzodiazepines such as flurazepam and diazepam produce active metabolites, have half-lives of 20–120 hours, and should be avoided in the elderly. Since people vary widely in their response and since the medications are long lasting, the dosage must be individualized. Once this is established, an adequate dose early in the course of symptom development will obviate the need for "pill popping," which contributes to dependency problems.

Antidepressants are the first-line medications for sustained treatment of GAD, having the advantage of not causing physiologic dependency problems. Antidepressants can themselves be anxiogenic—thus, at the initiation of treatment, concomitant short-term treatment with a benzodiazepine is often indicated. Venlafaxine and duloxetine are FDA-approved for the treatment of GAD in usual antidepressant doses. Initial daily dosing should start low (37.5–75 mg for venlafaxine and 30 mg for duloxetine) and be titrated upward as needed. SSRIs, such as paroxetine, are also used. While most antidepressants including tricyclic antidepressants (TCAs) and monoamine oxidase (MAO) inhibitors are often effective in the treatment of anxiety disorders, their side effects and drug interactions make them second- or third-line agents. Bupropion may be the most anxiogenic antidepressant and has no clear usefulness in treatment of anxiety disorders. Buspirone, sometimes used as an augmenting agent in the treatment of depression and compulsive behaviors, is also effective for generalized anxiety. Buspirone is usually given in a total dose of 15–60 mg/day in three divided doses. Higher doses tend to be counterproductive and produce gastrointestinal symptoms and dizziness. There is a 2- to 4-week delay before antidepressants and buspirone take effect, and patients require education regarding this lag. Sleep is sometimes negatively affected. Gabapentin (titrated to doses of 900–1800 mg orally daily) appears effective and lacks the habit-forming potential of the benzodiazepines. Unfortunately, like buspirone, many patients find gabapentin less effective than benzodiazepines in the management of acute anxiety. Beta-blockers, such as propranolol, may help reduce peripheral somatic symptoms. Alcohol is the most frequently self-administered drug and should be interdicted.

2. Panic disorder—Antidepressants are the first-line pharmacotherapy for panic disorder. Several SSRIs, including fluoxetine, paroxetine, and sertraline, are approved for the treatment of panic disorder. The SNRI venlafaxine is FDA approved for treatment of panic disorder. As with GAD, panic disorder is often a chronic condition; the long-term use of high-dose benzodiazepines can result in benzodiazepine dependence. While, panic disorder often responds to high-potency benzodiazepines such as clonazepam and alprazolam, the best use of these agents is generally early in the course of treatment concurrently with an antidepressant. Once the antidepressant has begun working after 4 or more weeks, the benzodiazepine may be tapered. Thus, those benzodiazepines and the antidepressants are the most commonly used agents for panic disorder.

Whether the indications for benzodiazepines are **anxiety** or **insomnia**, the medications should be used judiciously. The longer-acting benzodiazepines are used for the treatment of alcohol withdrawal and anxiety symptoms; the intermediate medications are useful as sedatives for insomnia (eg, lorazepam), while short-acting agents (eg, midazolam) are used for medical procedures such as endoscopy.

The side effects of all the benzodiazepine antianxiety agents are patient and dose dependent. As the dosage exceeds the levels necessary for sedation, the side effects include disinhibition, ataxia, dysarthria, nystagmus, and delirium. (The patient should be told not to operate machinery and drive with caution until he or she is well stabilized without side effects.)

Paradoxical agitation, anxiety, psychosis, confusion, mood lability, and anterograde amnesia have been reported, particularly with the shorter-acting benzodiazepines. These agents produce cumulative clinical effects with repeated dosage (especially if the patient has not had time to metabolize the previous dose), additive effects when given with other classes of sedatives or alcohol (many apparently "accidental" deaths are the result of concomitant use of sedatives and alcohol), and residual effects after termination of treatment (particularly in the case of medications that undergo slow biotransformation).

Overdosage results in respiratory depression, hypotension, shock syndrome, coma, and death. Flumazenil, a benzodiazepine antagonist, is effective in overdosage. Overdosage (see Chapter 38) and withdrawal states are medical emergencies. Serious side effects of chronic excessive dosage are development of tolerance, resulting in increasing dose requirements, and physiologic dependence, resulting in withdrawal symptoms similar in appearance to alcohol and barbiturate withdrawal (withdrawal effects must be distinguished from reemergent anxiety). Abrupt withdrawal of sedative medications may cause serious and even fatal convulsive seizures. Psychosis, delirium, and autonomic dysfunction have also been described. Both duration of action and duration of exposure are major factors related to likelihood of withdrawal.

Common withdrawal symptoms after low to moderate daily use of benzodiazepines are classified as somatic (disturbed sleep, tremor, nausea, muscle aches), psychological (anxiety, poor concentration, irritability, mild depression), or perceptual (poor coordination, mild paranoia, mild confusion). The presentation of symptoms will vary depending on the half-life of the drug. There are no significant side effects on organ systems other than the brain, and the medications are safe in most medical conditions. Benzodiazepine interactions with other medications are listed in Table 25–2.

Panic attacks may be treated in several ways. A sublingual dose of alprazolam (0.5–1 mg) or clonazepam (0.5–1 mg) is often effective for urgent treatment. For sustained treatment, SSRIs are the initial medications of choice (adequate blood levels will require dosages similar to those used in the treatment of depression). For example, sertraline starting at 25 mg/day and increased after 1 week to 50 mg/day may be effective. Because of initial agitation in response to

Table 25–2. Benzodiazepine interactions with other medications.

Drug	Effects
Antacids	Decreased absorption of benzodiazepines
Cimetidine	Increased half-life of diazepam and triazolam
Contraceptives	Increased levels of diazepam and triazolam
Digoxin	Alprazolam and diazepam raise digoxin level
Disulfiram	Increased duration of action of sedatives
Isoniazid	Increased plasma diazepam
Levodopa	Inhibition of antiparkinsonism effect
Propoxyphene	Impaired clearance of diazepam
Rifampin	Decreased plasma diazepam
Warfarin	Decreased prothrombin time

antidepressants, doses should start low and be very gradually increased. High-potency benzodiazepines may be used for symptomatic treatment as the antidepressant dose is titrated upward. Clonazepam (1–6 mg/day orally) and alprazolam (0.5–6 mg/day orally) are effective alternatives to antidepressants. Both medications may produce marked withdrawal if stopped abruptly and should always be tapered. Because of chronicity of the disorders and the problem of dependency with benzodiazepine medications, it is generally desirable to use antidepressant medications as the principal pharmacologic approach. Antidepressants have been used in conjunction with beta-blockers in resistant cases. Propranolol (40–160 mg/day orally) can mute the peripheral symptoms of anxiety without significantly affecting motor and cognitive performance. They block symptoms mediated by sympathetic stimulation (eg, palpitations, tremulousness) but not nonadrenergic symptoms (eg, diarrhea, muscle tension). Contrary to common belief, they usually do not cause depression as a side effect and can be used cautiously in patients with depression. The most effective long-term pharmacotherapy for panic disorder is treatment with an antidepressant. While not as rapidly acting as the benzodiazepines, the antidepressants are not habit forming. The SSRIs are known to be effective in the management of panic disorder and several are FDA approved for the treatment of panic disorder including sertraline, paroxetine, and fluoxetine. In addition, the SNRI venlafaxine is approved by the FDA for the treatment of panic disorder. Other antidepressants, including the TCAs and MAO inhibitors, are often effective when safer and easier to use medications prove ineffective.

3. Phobic disorders—A phobic disorder may be part of the panic disorder or may occur independently. Social phobias and agoraphobia may be treated with SSRIs, such as paroxetine, sertraline, and fluvoxamine. In addition, phobic disorders often respond to SNRIs such as venlafaxine. Gabapentin, an antiseizure medication with anxiolytic properties, is an alternative to antidepressants in the treatment of social phobia in a dosage of 300–3600 mg/day,

depending on response versus sedation. Specific phobias such as performance or test anxiety may respond to moderate doses of beta-blockers, such as propranolol, 20–40 mg 1 hour prior to exposure. Specific phobias tend to respond to behavioral therapies such as systematic desensitization, which is when the patient is gradually exposed to the feared object or situation in a controlled setting. A meta-analysis has demonstrated that the antituberculous drug D-cycloserine (DCS) enhances extinction of fear responses with exposures. Importantly, such medications must be used in combination with cognitive behavioral exposure strategies.

B. Behavioral

Behavioral approaches are widely used in various anxiety disorders, often in conjunction with medication. Any of the behavioral techniques can be used beneficially in altering the contingencies (precipitating factors or rewards) supporting any anxiety-provoking behavior. Relaxation techniques can sometimes be helpful in reducing anxiety. Desensitization, by exposing the patient to graded doses of a phobic object or situation, is an effective technique and one that the patient can practice outside the therapy session. Emotive imagery, wherein the patient imagines the anxiety-provoking situation while at the same time learning to relax, helps decrease the anxiety when the patient faces the real-life situation. Physiologic symptoms in panic attacks respond well to relaxation training. Both GAD and panic disorder appear to respond as well to cognitive behavioral therapy as they do to medications.

C. Psychological

Cognitive behavioral approaches have been effective in treatment of panic disorder, GAD, and phobias when erroneous beliefs need correction. These approaches share a common behavioral technique of exposing the individual to the feared object or situation. The combination of medical and cognitive behavioral therapy is more effective than either alone. Group therapy is the treatment of choice when the anxiety is clearly a function of the patient's difficulties in dealing with social settings. Acceptance and commitment therapy has been used with some success in anxiety disorders. It encourages individuals to keep focused on life goals while they "accept" the presence of anxiety in their lives.

D. Social

Peer support groups for panic disorder and agoraphobia have been particularly helpful. Social modification may require measures such as family counseling to aid acceptance of the patient's symptoms and avoid counterproductive behavior in behavioral training. Any help in maintaining the social structure is anxiety-alleviating, and work, school, and social activities should be maintained. School and vocational counseling may be provided by professionals, who often need help from the clinician in defining the patient's limitations.

Prognosis

Anxiety disorders are usually long-standing and may be difficult to treat. All can be relieved to varying degrees with medications and behavioral techniques. The prognosis is better if the commonly observed anxiety-panic-phobia-depression cycle can be broken with a combination of the therapeutic interventions discussed above.

Buoli M et al. New approaches to the pharmacological management of generalized anxiety disorder. Expert Opin Pharmacother. 2013 Feb;14(2):175–84. [PMID: 23282069]

Katzman MA et al; Canadian Anxiety Guidelines Initiative Group on behalf of the Anxiety Disorders Association of Canada and McGill University. Canadian clinical practice guidelines for the management of anxiety, posttraumatic stress and obsessive-compulsive disorders. BMC Psychiatry. 2014;14(Suppl 1):S1. [PMID: 25081580]

Porter E et al. A systematic review of predictors and moderators of improvement in cognitive-behavioral therapy for panic disorder and agoraphobia. Clin Psychol Rev. 2015 Dec;42:179–92. [PMID: 26443228]

OBSESSIVE-COMPULSIVE DISORDER & RELATED DISORDERS

ESSENTIALS OF DIAGNOSIS

▶ Anxiety is alleviated only by ritualistic performance of the action or by deliberate contemplation of the intruding idea or emotion.

▶ Other behaviors may overlap with OCD resulting in "OCD spectrum."

▶ Neurologic abnormalities of fine motor coordination and involuntary movements are common.

General Considerations

Obsessive compulsive disorder (OCD), classified as an anxiety disorder in the *DSM-IV,* now is part of a separate category of Obsessive-Compulsive Disorder and Related Disorders in *DSM-5.* The new category includes such disorders as trichotillomania and compulsive gambling in addition to OCD. In OCD, the irrational idea or the impulse persistently intrudes into awareness. Obsessions (recurring anxiety provoking thoughts such as fears of exposure to germs) and compulsions (repetitive actions such as washing the hands many times or cognitions such as counting rituals) are recognized by the individual as absurd and are resisted, but anxiety is alleviated only by ritualistic performance of the action or by deliberate contemplation of the intruding idea or emotion. Many patients do not mention the symptoms and must be asked about them. These patients are often predictable, orderly, conscientious, and intelligent—traits that are seen in many compulsive behaviors such as food binging and purging and compulsive exercise. There is an overlapping of OCD and other behaviors ("OCD spectrum"), including tics, trichotillomania (hair pulling),

excoriation disorder (skin picking), hoarding, onychophagia (nail biting), Tourette syndrome, and eating disorders (see Chapter 29). The incidence of OCD in the general population is 2–3% and there is a high comorbidity with major depression: major depression will develop in two-thirds of OCD patients during their lifetime. Male to female ratios are similar, with the highest rates occurring in the young, divorced, separated, and unemployed (all high-stress categories). Neurologic abnormalities of fine motor coordination and involuntary movements are common. Under extreme stress, these patients sometimes exhibit paranoid and delusional behaviors, often associated with depression, and can mimic schizophrenia.

Treatment

A. Medical

OCD responds to serotonergic antidepressants including the SSRIs and clomipramine in about 60% of cases and usually requires a longer response time than for depression (up to 12 weeks). Clomipramine has proved effective in doses equivalent to those used for depression. Fluoxetine has been widely used in this disorder but in doses higher than those used in depression (up to 60–80 mg orally daily). The other SSRI medications, such as sertraline, paroxetine, and fluvoxamine, are used with comparable efficacy each with its own side-effect profile. Buspirone in doses of 15–60 mg orally daily appears to be effective primarily as an anti-obsessional augmenting agent for the SSRI medications. There is some evidence that antipsychotics may be helpful as adjuncts to the SSRIs in treatment-resistant cases. Alternatively, low-dose clomipramine may be an effective adjunct to an SSRI in some patients. Psychosurgery has a limited place in selected cases of severe unremitting OCD. Experimental work has suggested a role for deep brain stimulation in OCD and it is FDA approved on a compassionate basis for refractory OCD patients.

B. Behavioral

OCD may respond to a variety of behavioral techniques. One common strategy is systematic desensitization. As in the treatment of simple phobias, systematic desensitization involves gradually exposing the OCD spectrum patient to situations that the patient fears, such as perceived germs or situations that a hoarder must part with things they are hoarding. By gradually exposing the patient to increasingly stressful situations and helping them manage their anxiety, OCD spectrum patients are often able to develop some mastery over the compulsions.

A technique used to help quell obsessive thoughts is "thought stopping." In this technique, the patient is taught to identify an obsessive thought and then to derail it. For example, the patient may be taught to say STOP any time an obsessive thought is present. In time, thought stopping can mitigate some of the obsessive thoughts.

C. Psychological

In addition to behavioral techniques, OCD may respond to psychological therapies including cognitive behavioral therapy in which the patient learns to identify maladaptive cognitions associated with obsessive thoughts and challenge those cognitions. For example, an OCD patient may fear that if he does not wash his hands 50 times after shaking hands he or someone close to him might develop a serious disease. These cognitions can be identified and gradually replaced with more rational thoughts.

D. Social

OCD can have devastating effects on the ability of a patient to lead a normal life. Educating both the patient and family about the course of illness and treatment options is extremely useful in setting appropriate expectations. Severe OCD is commonly associated with vocational disability, and the clinician may sometimes need to facilitate a leave of absence from work or encourage vocational rehabilitation to get the patient back to work.

▶ Prognosis

OCD is usually a chronic disorder with a waxing and waning course. As many as 40% of patients in whom OCD problems develop in childhood will experience remission as adults. However, it is less common for OCD to remit without treatment when it develops during adulthood.

SOMATIC SYMPTOM DISORDERS
(Abnormal Illness Behaviors)

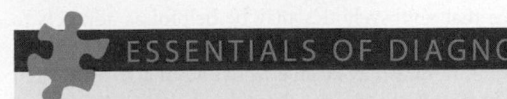

ESSENTIALS OF DIAGNOSIS

▶ Physical symptoms may involve one or more organ systems and are not intentional.

▶ Subjective complaints exceed objective findings.

▶ Correlations of symptom development and psychosocial stresses.

▶ Combination of biogenetic and developmental patterns.

▶ General Considerations

Any organ system can be affected in somatic symptom disorders. In *DSM-5*, somatic symptom disorders encompass disorders that were listed under somatic disorders in *DSM-IV*, including conversion disorder, hypochondriasis, somatization disorder, and pain disorder secondary to psychological factors. Vulnerability in one or more organ systems and exposure to family members with somatization problems plays a major role in the development of particular symptoms, and the "functional" versus "organic" dichotomy is a hindrance to good treatment. Clinicians should suspect psychiatric disorders in a number of conditions. For example, 45% of patients complaining of palpitations had lifetime psychiatric diagnoses including generalized anxiety, depression, panic, and somatization disorders. Similarly, 33–44% of patients who undergo

coronary angiography for chest pain but have negative results have been found to have panic disorder.

In any patient presenting with a condition judged to be somatic symptom disorder, depression must be considered in the diagnosis.

▶ Clinical Findings

A. Conversion Disorder

"Conversion" of psychic conflict into physical symptoms in parts of the body innervated by the sensorimotor system (eg, paralysis, aphonic) is a disorder that is more common in individuals from lower socioeconomic classes and certain cultures. The somatic manifestation that takes the place of anxiety is often paralysis, and in some instances the organ dysfunction may have symbolic meaning (eg, arm paralysis in marked anger so the individual cannot use the arm to strike someone). Pseudoepileptic ("hysterical") seizures are often difficult to differentiate from intoxication states or panic attacks and commonly occur in patients who also have seizures of organic etiology. Retention of consciousness, random flailing with asynchronous movements of the right and left sides, and resistance to having the nose and mouth pinched closed during the attack, all point toward a pseudoepileptic event. Electroencephalography, particularly in a video-electroencephalography assessment unit, during the attack is the most helpful diagnostic aid in excluding genuine seizure states. Serum prolactin levels rise abruptly in the postictal state only in true epilepsy. La belle indifférence (an unconcerned affect) is not a significant identifying characteristic, as commonly believed, since individuals even with genuine medical illness may exhibit a high level of denial. Important conversion disorder criteria include a history of conversion or somatization disorder, modeling the symptom after someone else who had a similar presentation, a serious precipitating emotional event, associated psychopathology (eg, depression, schizophrenia, personality disorders), a temporal correlation between the precipitating event and the symptom, and a temporary "solving of the problem" by the conversion. It is important to identify physical disorders with unusual presentations (eg, multiple sclerosis, systemic lupus erythematosus).

B. Somatic Symptom Disorder

Somatic symptom disorder is characterized by one or more somatic symptoms that are associated with significant distress or disability. The somatic symptoms may be associated with persistent thoughts about the seriousness of the symptoms, a high level of anxiety about health, or excessive time and energy devoted to these symptoms. The patient's focus on somatic symptoms is usually chronic. Panic, anxiety, and depression are often present, and **major depression** is an important consideration in the differential diagnosis. There is a significant relationship (20%) to a lifetime history of panic-agoraphobia-depression. It usually occurs before age 30 and is ten times more common in women. Polysurgery is often a feature of the history. Preoccupation with medical and surgical therapy becomes a lifestyle that may exclude other activities. The symptoms indicate maladaptive coping techniques and there is often evidence of longstanding somatic complaints, including multiple pain and gastrointestinal symptoms (such as dyspareunia, dysmenorrhea, headache, backache, abdominal pain, vomiting, bloating) and pseudoneurologic symptoms (such as amnesia or pseudoepileptic seizures), often with a history of similar organ system involvement in other family members. Multiple symptoms that constantly change and the inability of more than three doctors to make a diagnosis are strong clues to the problem.

C. Somatic Symptom Disorder with Predominant Pain

This involves a long history of complaints of severe pain out of proportion to biomedical findings that are present. This diagnosis must be one of exclusion and should be made only after extended evaluation has established a clear correlation of psychogenic factors with exacerbations and remissions of complaints.

D. Factitious Disorders

These disorders, in which symptom production is intentional, are not somatic symptom conditions in that symptoms are produced consciously, in contrast to the unconscious process of the other somatic symptom disorders. They are characterized by self-induced symptoms or false physical and laboratory findings for the purpose of deceiving clinicians or other health care personnel. The deceptions may involve self-mutilation, fever, hemorrhage, hypoglycemia, seizures, and an almost endless variety of manifestations—often presented in an exaggerated and dramatic fashion (**Munchausen syndrome**). "Munchausen by proxy" is the term used when a parent creates an illness in a child so the adult (usually the mother) can maintain a relationship with clinicians. The duplicity may be either simple or extremely complex and difficult to recognize. The patients are frequently connected in some way with the health professions and there is no apparent external motivation other than achieving the patient role. A poor clinician-patient relationship and "doctor shopping" tend to exacerbate the problem. The only secondary gain of inducing symptoms in Munchausen syndrome is being the focus of medical attention rather than obtaining disability benefits or being excused from work or school in malingering situations.

▶ Complications

Sedative and analgesic dependency is the most common iatrogenic complication. Patients may pursue medical or surgical treatments that induce iatrogenic problems. Thus, identifying patients with a potential somatic symptom disorder and attempting to limit tests, procedures, and medications that may lead to harm is quite important.

▶ Treatment

A. Medical

Medical support with careful attention to building a therapeutic clinician-patient relationship is the mainstay of treatment. It must be accepted that the patient's distress is real. Every problem not found to have an organic basis is not necessarily a mental disease. Diligent attempts should be made to relate symptoms to adverse developments in the patient's life. It may be useful to have the patient keep a meticulous diary, paying particular attention to various pertinent factors evident in the history. Regular, frequent, short appointments that are not symptom-contingent may be helpful. Medications (frequently abused) should not be prescribed to replace appointments. One person should be the primary clinician, and consultants should be used mainly for evaluation. An empathic, realistic, optimistic approach must be maintained in the face of the expected ups and downs. Ongoing reevaluation is necessary, since somatization can coexist with a concurrent physical illness.

B. Psychological

The primary clinician can use psychological approaches when it is clear that the patient is ready to make some changes in lifestyle in order to achieve symptomatic relief. This is often best approached on a here-and-now basis and oriented toward pragmatic changes rather than an exploration of early experiences that the patient frequently fails to relate to current distress. Group therapy with other individuals who have similar problems is sometimes of value to improve coping, allow ventilation, and focus on interpersonal adjustment. Hypnosis or lorazepam interviews used early are helpful in resolving conversion disorders. If the primary clinician has been working with the patient on psychological problems related to the physical illness, the groundwork is often laid for successful psychiatric referral.

For patients who have been identified as having a factitious disorder, early psychiatric consultation is indicated. There are two main treatment strategies for these patients. One consists of a conjoint confrontation of the patient by both the primary clinician and the psychiatrist. The patient's disorder is portrayed as a cry for help, and psychiatric treatment is recommended. The second approach avoids direct confrontation and attempts to provide a face-saving way to relinquish the symptom without overt disclosure of the disorder's origin. Techniques such as biofeedback and self-hypnosis may foster recovery using this strategy. Another face-saving approach is to use a double bind with the patient. For example, the patient is told there are two possible diagnoses: (1) an organic disease that should respond to the next medical intervention (usually modest and noninvasive), or (2) factitious disorder for which the patient will need psychiatric treatment. Given these options, many patients will choose to recover and not have to admit the origin of their problem.

C. Behavioral

Behavioral therapy is probably best exemplified by biofeedback techniques. In biofeedback, the particular abnormality (eg, increased peristalsis) must be recognized and monitored by the patient and therapist (eg, by an electronic stethoscope to amplify the sounds). This is immediate feedback, and after learning to recognize it, the patient can then learn to identify any change thus produced (eg, a decrease in bowel sounds) and so become a conscious originator of the feedback instead of a passive recipient. Relief of the symptom operantly conditions the patient to utilize the maneuver that relieves symptoms (eg, relaxation causing a decrease in bowel sounds). With emphasis on this type of learning, the patient is able to identify symptoms early and initiate the countermaneuvers, thus decreasing the symptomatic problem. Migraine and tension headaches have been particularly responsive to biofeedback methods.

D. Social

Social endeavors include family, work, and other interpersonal activity. Family members should come for some appointments with the patient so they can learn how best to live with the patient. This is particularly important in treatment of somatization and pain disorders. Peer support groups provide a climate for encouraging the patient to accept and live with the problem. Ongoing communication with the employer may be necessary to encourage long-term continued interest in the employee. Employers can become just as discouraged as clinicians in dealing with employees who have chronic problems.

▶ Prognosis

The prognosis is better if the primary clinician is able to intervene early before the situation has deteriorated. After the problem has crystallized into chronicity, it is difficult to effect change.

> Gordon-Elliott JS et al. An approach to the patient with multiple physical symptoms or chronic disease. Med Clin North Am. 2010 Nov;94(6):1207–16. [PMID: 20951278]
> Katz J et al. Chronic pain, psychopathology, and DSM-5 somatic symptom disorder. Can J Psychiatry. 2015 Apr;60(4):160–7. [PMID: 26174215]
> Tavel ME. Somatic symptom disorders without known physical causes: one disease with many names? Am J Med. 2015 Oct;128(10):1054–8. [PMID: 26031885]

CHRONIC PAIN DISORDERS

ESSENTIALS OF DIAGNOSIS

- ▶ Chronic complaints of pain.
- ▶ Symptoms frequently exceed signs.
- ▶ Minimal relief with standard treatment.
- ▶ History of having seen many clinicians.
- ▶ Frequent use of several nonspecific medications.

▶ General Considerations

A problem in the management of pain is the lack of distinction between acute and chronic pain syndromes. Most clinicians are adept at dealing with acute pain problems but have difficulty treating the patient with a chronic pain disorder. This type of patient frequently takes too many medications, stays in bed a great deal, has seen many clinicians, has lost skills, and experiences little joy in either work or play. All relationships suffer (including those with clinicians), and life becomes a constant search for relief. The search results in complex clinician-patient relationships that usually include many drug trials, particularly sedatives, with adverse consequences (eg, irritability, depressed mood) related to long-term use. Treatment failures provoke angry responses and depression from both the patient and the clinician, and the pain syndrome is exacerbated. When frustration becomes too great, a new clinician is found, and the cycle is repeated. The longer the existence of the pain disorder, the more important become the psychological factors of anxiety and depression. As with all other conditions, it is counterproductive to speculate about whether the pain is "real." It is real to the patient, and acceptance of the problem must precede a mutual endeavor to alleviate the disturbance.

▶ Clinical Findings

Components of the chronic pain syndrome consist of anatomic changes, chronic anxiety and depression, anger, and changed lifestyle. Usually, the anatomic problem is irreversible, since it has already been subjected to many interventions with increasingly unsatisfactory results. An algorithm for assessing chronic pain and differentiating it from other psychiatric conditions is illustrated in Figure 25–1.

Chronic anxiety and depression produce heightened irritability and overreaction to stimuli. A marked decrease in pain threshold is apparent. This pattern develops into a hypochondriacal preoccupation with the body and a constant need for reassurance. The pressure on the clinician becomes wearing and often leads to covert rejection of the patient, such as not being available or making referrals to other clinicians.

This is perceived by the patient, who then intensifies the effort to find help, and the typical cycle is repeated. Anxiety and depression are seldom discussed, almost as if there is a tacit agreement not to deal with these issues.

Changes in lifestyle involve some of the pain behaviors. These usually take the form of a family script in which the patient accepts the role of being sick, and this role then becomes the focus of most family interactions and may become important in maintaining the family, so that neither the patient nor the family wants the patient's role to change. Demands for attention and efforts to control the behavior of others revolve around the central issue of control of other people (including clinicians). Cultural factors frequently play a role in the behavior of the patient and how the significant people around the patient cope with the problem. Some cultures encourage demonstrative behavior, while others value the stoic role.

Another secondary gain that frequently maintains the patient in the sick role is financial compensation or other benefits. Frequently, such systems are structured so that they reinforce the maintenance of sickness and discourage any attempts to give up the role. Clinicians unwittingly

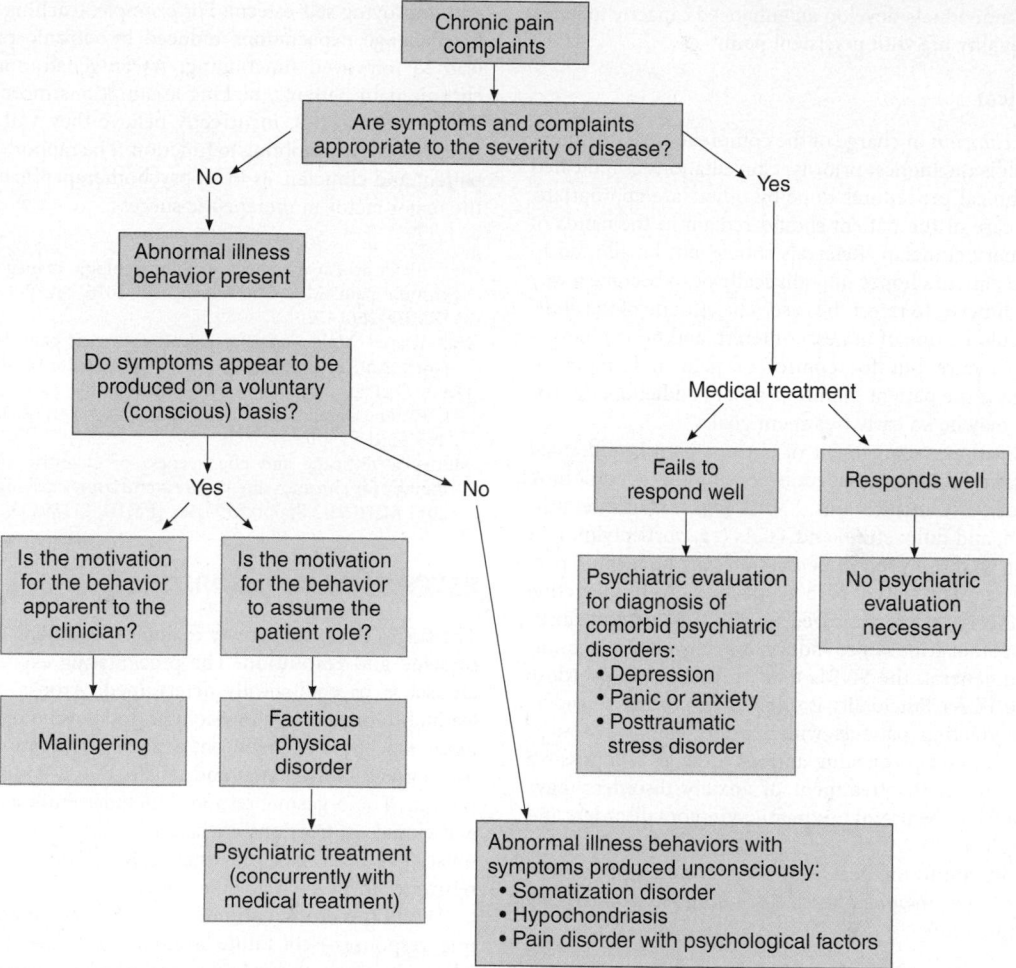

▲ **Figure 25–1.** Algorithm for assessing psychiatric component of chronic pain. (Adapted and reproduced, with permission, from Eisendrath SJ. Psychiatric aspects of chronic pain. Neurology. 1995 Dec;45(12 Suppl 9):S26–34.)

reinforce this role because of the very nature of the practice of medicine, which is to respond to complaints of illness. Helpful suggestions from the clinician are often met with responses like, "Yes, but…." Medications then become the principal approach, and drug dependency problems may develop.

▶ Treatment

A. Behavioral

The cornerstone of a unified approach to chronic pain syndromes is a comprehensive behavioral program. This is necessary to identify and eliminate pain reinforcers, to decrease drug use, and to use effectively those positive reinforcers that shift the focus from the pain. It is critical that the patient be made a partner in the effort to manage and function better in the setting of ongoing pain symptoms. The clinician must shift from the idea of biomedical cure to ongoing care of the patient. The patient should agree to discuss the pain only with the clinician and not with family members; this tends to stabilize the patient's personal life, since the family is usually tired of the subject.

At the beginning of treatment, the patient should be assigned self-help tasks graded up to maximal activity as a means of positive reinforcement. The tasks should not exceed capability. The patient can also be asked to keep a self-rating chart to log accomplishments, so that progress can be measured and remembered. Instruct the patient to record degrees of pain on a self-rating scale in relation to various situations and mental attitudes so that similar circumstances can be avoided or modified.

Avoid positive reinforcers for pain such as marked sympathy and attention to pain. Emphasize a positive response to productive activities, which remove the focus of attention from the pain. Activity is also desensitizing, since the patient learns to tolerate increasing activity levels.

Biofeedback techniques (see Somatic Symptom Disorders, above) and hypnosis have been successful in ameliorating some pain syndromes. Hypnosis tends to be most effective in patients with a high level of denial, who are more responsive to suggestion. Hypnosis can be used to lessen anxiety, alter perception of the length of time that pain is experienced, and encourage relaxation. Mindfulness-based stress reduction programs have been useful in helping individuals develop an enhanced capacity to live a higher quality life with persistent pain.

B. Medical

A *single clinician* in charge of the comprehensive treatment approach is the highest priority. Consultations as indicated and technical procedures done by others are appropriate, but the care of the patient should remain in the hands of the primary clinician. Referrals should not be allowed to raise the patient's hopes unrealistically or to become a way for the clinician to reject the case. The attitude of the clinician should be one of honesty, interest, and hopefulness—not for a cure but for control of pain and improved function. If the patient manifests opioid addiction, detoxification may be an early treatment goal.

Medication management of chronic pain is addressed in Chapter 5. A fixed schedule lessens the conditioning effects of these medications. SNRIs (eg, venlafaxine, milnacipran, and duloxetine) and TCAs (eg, nortriptyline), in doses up to those used in depression may be helpful, particularly in neuropathic pain syndromes. Both duloxetine and milnacipran are approved for the treatment of fibromyalgia; duloxetine is also indicated in chronic pain conditions. In general, the SNRIs tend to be safer in overdose than the TCAs. Suicidality is often an important consideration in treating patients with chronic pain syndromes. Gabapentin and pregabalin, anticonvulsants with possible applications in the treatment of anxiety disorders, have been shown to be useful in somatic symptom disorders and fibromyalgia.

In addition to medications, a variety of nonpharmacologic strategies may be offered, including physical therapy and acupuncture.

C. Social

Involvement of family members and other significant persons in the patient's life should be an early priority. The best efforts of both patient and therapists can be unwittingly sabotaged by other persons who may feel that they are "helping" the patient. They frequently tend to reinforce the negative aspects of the chronic pain disorder. The patient becomes more dependent and less active, and the pain syndrome becomes an immutable way of life. The more destructive pain behaviors described by many experts in chronic pain disorders are the results of well-meaning but misguided efforts of family members. Ongoing therapy with the family can be helpful in the early identification and elimination of these behavior patterns.

D. Psychological

In addition to group therapy with family members and others, groups of patients can be helpful if properly led. The major goal, whether of individual or group therapy, is to gain patient involvement. A group can be a powerful instrument for achieving this goal, with the development of group loyalties and cooperation. People will frequently make efforts with group encouragement that they would never make alone. Individual therapy should be directed toward strengthening existing coping mechanisms

and improving self-esteem. For example, teaching patients to challenge expectations induced by chronic pain may lead to improved functioning. As an illustration, many chronic pain patients, making assumptions more derived from acute injuries, incorrectly believe they will damage themselves by attempting to function. The rapport between patient and clinician, as in all psychotherapeutic efforts, is the major factor in therapeutic success.

Beal BR et al. An overview of pharmacologic management of chronic pain. Med Clin North Am. 2016 Jan;100(1):65–79. [PMID: 26614720]

Dale R et al. Multimodal treatment of chronic pain. Med Clin North Am. 2016 Jan;100(1):55–64. [PMID: 26614719]

Derry S et al. Nortriptyline for neuropathic pain in adults. Cochrane Database Syst Rev. 2015 Jan 8;1:CD011209. [PMID: 25569864]

Morley S. Efficacy and effectiveness of cognitive behaviour therapy for chronic pain: progress and some challenges. Pain. 2011 Mar;152(3 Suppl):S99–106. [PMID: 21159433]

PSYCHOSEXUAL DISORDERS

The stages of sexual activity include **excitement** (arousal), **orgasm**, and **resolution**. The precipitating excitement or arousal is psychologically determined. Arousal response leading to orgasm is a physiologic and psychological phenomenon of vasocongestion, a parasympathetic reaction causing erection in men and labial-clitoral congestion in women. The orgasmic response includes emission in men and clonic contractions of the analogous striated perineal muscles of both men and women. Resolution is a gradual return to normal physiologic status.

While the arousal stimuli—vasocongestive and orgasmic responses—constitute a single response in a well-adjusted person, they can be considered as separate stages that can produce different syndromes responding to different treatment procedures.

▶ Clinical Findings

There are three major groups of sexual disorders.

A. Paraphilias (Sexual Arousal Disorders)

In these conditions, formerly called "deviations" or "variations," the excitement stage of sexual activity is associated with sexual objects or orientations different from those usually associated with adult sexual stimulation. The stimulus may be a woman's shoe, a child, animals, instruments of torture, or incidents of aggression. The pattern of sexual stimulation is usually one that has early psychological roots. Poor experiences with sexual activity frequently reinforce this pattern over time. Paraphilias include exhibitionism, transvestism, voyeurism, pedophilia, incest, sexual sadism, and sexual masochism.

B. Gender Identity Disorder

Core gender identity reflects a biologic self-image—the conviction that "I am a boy" or "I am a girl" that is usually well developed by age 3 or 4. Gender dysphoria refers to the development of a sexual identity that is the opposite of the biologic one.

Transsexualism is an attempt to deny and reverse biologic sex by maintaining sexual identity with the opposite gender. Transsexuals do not alternate between gender roles; rather, they assume a fixed role of attitudes, feelings, fantasies, and choices consonant with those of the opposite sex, all of which clearly date back to early development. For example, male to female transsexuals in early childhood behave, talk, and fantasize as if they were girls. They do not grow out of feminine patterns; they do not work in professions traditionally considered to be masculine; and they have no interest in their own penises either as evidence of maleness or as organs for erotic behavior. The desire for sex change starts early and may culminate in assumption of a feminine lifestyle, hormonal treatment, and use of surgical procedures, eg, castration and vaginoplasty.

C. Psychosexual Dysfunction

This category includes a large group of vasocongestive and orgasmic disorders. Often, they involve problems of sexual adaptation, education, and technique that are often initially discussed with, diagnosed by, and treated by the primary care provider.

There are two conditions common in men: erectile dysfunction and ejaculation disturbances.

Erectile dysfunction is inability to achieve or maintain an erection firm enough for satisfactory intercourse; patients sometimes use the term to mean premature ejaculation. Decreased nocturnal penile tumescence occurs in some depressed patients. **Psychological erectile dysfunction** is caused by interpersonal or intrapsychic factors (eg, partner disharmony, depression). **Organic factors** are discussed in Chapter 23.

Ejaculation disturbances include premature ejaculation, inability to ejaculate, and retrograde ejaculation. (Ejaculation is possible in patients with erectile dysfunction.) Ejaculation is usually connected with orgasm, and ejaculatory control is an acquired behavior that is minimal in adolescence and increases with experience. Pathogenic factors are those that interfere with learning control, most frequently sexual ignorance. Intrapsychic factors (anxiety, guilt, depression) and interpersonal maladaptation (partner problems, unresponsiveness of mate, power struggles) are also common. Organic causes include interference with sympathetic nerve distribution (often due to surgery or radiation) and the effects of pharmacologic agents (eg, SSRIs or sympatholytics).

In women, the most common forms of sexual dysfunction are orgasmic disorder and hyposexual desire disorder (see Chapter 18).

Orgasmic disorder is a complex condition in which there is a general lack of sexual responsiveness. The woman has difficulty in experiencing erotic sensation and does not have the vasocongestive response. Sexual activity varies from active avoidance of sex to an occasional orgasm. Orgasmic dysfunction—in which a woman has a vasocongestive response but varying degrees of difficulty in reaching orgasm—is sometimes differentiated from anorgasmia. Causes for the dysfunctions include poor sexual techniques,

early traumatic sexual experiences, interpersonal disharmony (partner struggles, use of sex as a means of control), and intrapsychic problems (anxiety, fear, guilt). Organic causes include any conditions that might cause pain in intercourse, pelvic pathology, mechanical obstruction, and neurologic deficits.

Hyposexual desire disorder consists of diminished or absent libido in either sex and may be a function of organic or psychological difficulties (eg, anxiety, phobic avoidance). Any chronic illness can reduce desire as can aging. Hormonal disorders, including hypogonadism or use of antiandrogen compounds such as cyproterone acetate, and chronic kidney disease contribute to deterioration in sexual desire. Although menopause may lead to diminution of sexual desire in some women, the relationship between menopause and libido is complicated and may be influenced by sociocultural factors. Alcohol, sedatives, opioids, marijuana, and some medications may affect sexual drive and performance.

► Treatment

A. Paraphilias and Gender Identity Disorders

1. Psychological—Sexual arousal disorders involving variant sexual activity (paraphilia), particularly those of a more superficial nature (eg, voyeurism) and those of recent onset, are responsive to psychotherapy in some cases. The prognosis is much better if the motivation comes from the individual rather than the legal system; unfortunately, judicial intervention is frequently the only stimulus to treatment because the condition persists and is reinforced until conflict with the law occurs. Therapies frequently focus on barriers to normal arousal response; the expectation is that the variant behavior will decrease as normal behavior increases.

2. Behavioral—Aversive and operant conditioning techniques have been tried frequently in gender role disorders but have only occasionally been successful. In some cases, the sexual arousal disorders improve with modeling, role-playing, and conditioning procedures. Emotive imagery is occasionally helpful in lessening anxiety in fetish problems.

3. Social—Although they do not produce a change in sexual arousal patterns or gender role, self-help groups have facilitated adjustment to an often hostile society. Attention to the family is particularly important in helping persons in such groups to accept their situation and alleviate their guilt about the role they think they had in creating the problem.

4. Medical—Medroxyprogesterone acetate, a suppressor of libidinal drive, is used to mute disruptive sexual behavior in men of all ages. Onset of action is usually within 3 weeks, and the effects are generally reversible. Fluoxetine or other SSRIs at depression doses may reduce some of the compulsive sexual behaviors including the paraphilias. A focus of study in the treatment of severe paraphilia has been agonists of luteinizing hormone–releasing hormone (LHRH). Case reports and open label studies suggest that LHRH-agonists may play a role in preventing relapse in some patients with paraphilia. While some transsexuals are treated with genital reconstructive surgery, many others are screened out by trial periods of living as the other sex prior to operation.

B. Psychosexual Dysfunction

1. Medical—Even if the condition is not reversible, identification of the specific cause helps the patient to accept the condition. Partner disharmony, with its exacerbating effects, may thus be avoided. Of all the sexual dysfunctions, erectile dysfunction is the condition most likely to have an organic basis. Sildenafil, tadalafil, and vardenafil are phosphodiesterase type 5 inhibitors that are effective oral agents for the treatment of penile erectile dysfunction (eg, sildenafil 25–100 mg orally 1 hour prior to intercourse). These agents are effective for SSRI-induced erectile dysfunction in men and in some cases for SSRI-associated sexual dysfunction in women. Use of the medications in conjunction with any nitrates can have significant hypotensive effects leading to death in rare cases. Because of their common effect in delaying ejaculation, the SSRIs have been effective in premature ejaculation.

Flibanserin is a 5-HT$_{1A}$-agonist/5-HT$_2$-antagonist that is FDA approved for the treatment of female hyposexual desire disorder. This is the first drug marketed to improve sexual desire in women. The data suggest that compared to placebo, women treated flibanserin have somewhat higher number of sexual events. The drug interacts with alcohol, causing hypotensive events, so patients need to be educated about this risk. Flibanserin is taken 100 mg orally at bedtime to circumvent the side effects of dizzinesss, sleepiness, and nausea.

2. Behavioral—Syndromes resulting from conditioned responses have been treated by conditioning techniques, with excellent results. Masters and Johnson have used behavioral approaches in all of the sexual dysfunctions, with concomitant supportive psychotherapy and with improvement of the communication patterns of the couple.

3. Psychological—The use of psychotherapy by itself is best suited for those cases in which interpersonal difficulties or intrapsychic problems predominate. Anxiety and guilt about parental injunctions against sex may contribute to sexual dysfunction. Even in these cases, however, a combined behavioral-psychological approach usually produces results most quickly.

4. Social—The proximity of other people (eg, a mother-in-law) in a household is frequently an inhibiting factor in sexual relationships. In such cases, some social engineering may alleviate the problem.

Jin J. JAMA patient page. Flibanserin for treating low sexual desire in women. JAMA. 2015 Sep 22–29;314(12):1312. [PMID: 26393863]

Nehra A et al. The Princeton III Consensus recommendations for the management of erectile dysfunction and cardiovascular disease. Mayo Clin Proc. 2012 Aug;87(8):766–78. [PMID: 22862865]

Robinson K et al. First pharmacological therapy for hypoactive sexual desire disorder in premenopausal women: flibanserin. Ann Pharmacother. 2016 Feb;50(2):125–32. [PMID: 26692273]

Simopoulos EF et al. Male erectile dysfunction: integrating psychopharmacology and psychotherapy. Gen Hosp Psychiatry. 2013 Jan;35(1):33–8. [PMID: 23044247]

PERSONALITY DISORDERS

ESSENTIALS OF DIAGNOSIS

▶ Long history dating back to childhood.

▶ Recurrent maladaptive behavior.

▶ Low self-esteem.

▶ Minimal introspective ability with a tendency to blame others for all problems.

▶ Major difficulties with interpersonal relationships or society.

▶ Depression with anxiety when maladaptive behavior fails.

▶ General Considerations

An individual's personality structure, or character, is an integral part of self-image. It reflects genetics, interpersonal influences, and recurring patterns of behavior adopted in order to cope with the environment. The classification of subtypes of personality disorders depends on the predominant symptoms and their severity. The most severe disorders—those that bring the patient into greatest conflict with society—tend to be classified as antisocial (psychopathic) or borderline.

Personality disorders can be considered a matrix for some of the more severe psychiatric problems (eg, schizotypal, relating to schizophrenia, and avoidance types, relating to some anxiety disorders).

▶ Classification & Clinical Findings

See Table 25–3.

▶ Differential Diagnosis

Patients with personality disorders tend to show anxiety and depression when pathologic coping mechanisms fail, and their symptoms can be similar to those disorders. Occasionally, the more severe cases may decompensate into psychosis under stress and mimic other psychotic disorders.

▶ Treatment

A. Social

Social and therapeutic environments such as day hospitals, halfway houses, and self-help communities utilize peer pressure to modify the self-destructive behavior. The patient with a personality disorder often has failed to profit from experience, and difficulties with authority impair the learning experience. The use of peer relationships and the

Table 25–3. Personality disorders: Classification and clinical findings.

Personality Disorder	Clinical Findings
Antisocial	Selfish, callous, promiscuous, impulsive, unable to learn from experience, often has legal problems.
Avoidant	Fears rejection, hyperreacts to rejection and failure, with poor social endeavors and low self-esteem.
Borderline	Impulsive; has unstable and intense interpersonal relationships; is suffused with anger, fear, and guilt; lacks self-control and self-fulfillment; has identity problems and affective instability; is suicidal (a serious problem—up to 80% of hospitalized borderline patients make an attempt at some time during treatment, and the incidence of completed suicide is as high as 5%); aggressive behavior, feelings of emptiness, and occasional psychotic decompensation. This group has a high drug abuse rate, which plays a role in symptoms. There is extensive overlap with other diagnostic categories, particularly mood disorders and posttraumatic stress disorder.
Dependent	Passive, overaccepting, unable to make decisions, lacks confidence, with poor self-esteem.
Histrionic (hysterical)	Dependent, immature, seductive, egocentric, vain, emotionally labile.
Narcissistic	Exhibitionist, grandiose, preoccupied with power, lacks interest in others, with excessive demands for attention.
Obsessive compulsive	Perfectionist, egocentric, indecisive, with rigid thought patterns and need for control.
Paranoid	Defensive, oversensitive, secretive, suspicious, hyperalert, with limited emotional response.
Schizoid	Shy, introverted, withdrawn, avoids close relationships.
Schizotypal	Superstitious, socially isolated, suspicious, with limited interpersonal ability, eccentric behaviors, and odd speech.

repetition possible in a structured setting of a helpful community enhance the behavioral treatment opportunities and increase learning. When problems are detected early, both the school and the home can serve as foci of intensified social pressure to change the behavior, particularly with the use of behavioral techniques.

B. Behavioral

The behavioral techniques used are principally operant conditioning and aversive conditioning. The former simply emphasizes the recognition of acceptable behavior and its reinforcement with praise or other tangible rewards. Aversive responses usually mean punishment, although this can range from a mild rebuke to some specific punitive responses such as deprivation of privileges. Extinction plays a role in that an attempt is made not to respond to inappropriate behavior, and the lack of response eventually causes the person to abandon that type of behavior. Pouting and tantrums, for example, diminish quickly when such behavior elicits no reaction. Dialectical behavioral therapy is a program of individual and group therapy specifically designed for patients with chronic suicidality and borderline personality disorder. It blends mindfulness and a cognitive-behavioral model to address self-awareness, interpersonal functioning, affective lability, and reactions to stress.

C. Psychological

Psychological interventions can be conducted in group and individual settings. Group therapy is helpful when specific interpersonal behavior needs to be improved. This mode of treatment also has a place with so-called "acting-out" patients, ie, those who frequently act in an impulsive and inappropriate way. The peer pressure in the group tends to impose restraints on rash behavior. The group also quickly identifies the patient's types of behavior and helps improve the validity of the patient's self-assessment, so that the antecedents of the unacceptable behavior can be effectively handled, thus decreasing its frequency. Individual therapy should initially be supportive, ie, helping the patient to restabilize and mobilize coping mechanisms. If the individual has the ability to observe his or her own behavior, a longer-term and more introspective therapy may be warranted. The therapist must be able to handle countertransference feelings (which are frequently negative), maintain appropriate boundaries in the relationship (no physical contact, however well-meaning), and refrain from premature confrontations and interpretations.

D. Medical

Hospitalization is indicated in the case of serious suicidal or homicidal danger. In most cases, treatment can be accomplished in the day treatment center or self-help community. Pharmacotherapy should be directed to specific symptom clusters. Antidepressants have improved anxiety, depression, and sensitivity to rejection in some patients with borderline personality disorder. SSRIs also have a role in reducing aggressive behavior in impulsive aggressive patients (eg, fluoxetine 20–60 mg orally daily or sertraline 50–200 mg orally daily). Antipsychotics may be helpful in targeting hostility, agitation, and as adjuncts to antidepressant therapy (eg, olanzapine [2.5–10 mg/day orally], risperidone [0.5–2 mg/day orally], or haloperidol [0.5–2 mg/day orally, split into two doses]). In some cases, these medications are required only for several days and can be discontinued after the patient has regained a previously established level of adjustment; they can also provide ongoing support. Anticonvulsants including, carbamazepine, 400–800 mg orally daily in divided doses, lamotrigine, 50–200 mg/day and valproate 500–2000 mg/day have been shown to decrease the severity of behavioral dyscontrol in some personality disorder patients.

▶ Prognosis

Antisocial and borderline categories generally have a guarded prognosis. Those patients with a history of parental abuse and a family history of mood disorder tend to have the most challenging treatments. Patients with a schizotypal personality often improve with antipsychotics, while those with avoidant personality may benefit from strategies that reduce anxiety, including the use of SSRIs and benzodiazepines.

Ingenhoven T et al. Effectiveness of pharmacotherapy for severe personality disorders: meta-analyses of randomized controlled trials. J Clin Psychiatry. 2010 Jan;71(1):14–25. [PMID: 19778496]

Stoffers JM et al. Pharmacotherapy for borderline personality disorder—current evidence and recent trends. Curr Psychiatry Rep. 2015 Jan;17(1):534. [PMID: 25413640]

Stoffers JM et al. Psychological therapies for people with borderline personality disorder. Cochrane Database Syst Rev. 2012 Aug 15;8:CD005652. [PMID: 22895952]

SCHIZOPHRENIA SPECTRUM DISORDERS

ESSENTIALS OF DIAGNOSIS

▶ Social withdrawal, usually slowly progressive; deterioration in personal care.

▶ Loose thought associations; often slowed thinking and rapid shifting from topic to topic.

▶ Autistic absorption in inner thoughts; frequent sexual or religious preoccupations.

▶ Auditory hallucinations, often of a derogatory nature.

▶ Delusions, frequently of a persecutory nature.

▶ Symptoms of at least 6 months' duration.

▶ General Considerations

Schizophrenia is manifested by a massive disruption of thinking, mood, and overall behavior as well as poor filtering of stimuli. The characterization and nomenclature of the disorders are quite arbitrary and are influenced by sociocultural factors and schools of psychiatric thought.

The cause of schizophrenia is believed to be multifactorial, with genetic, environmental, and neurotransmitter pathophysiologic components. Studies have demonstrated that schizophrenia is at least eight distinct disorders. At present, there is no laboratory method for confirming the diagnosis of schizophrenia. There may or may not be a

history of a major disruption in the individual's life (failure, loss, physical illness) before gross psychotic deterioration is evident.

"Other psychotic disorders" are conditions that are similar to schizophrenic disorders in their acute symptoms but have a less pervasive influence over the long term. The patient usually attains higher levels of functioning. The acute psychotic episodes tend to be less disruptive of the person's lifestyle, with a fairly quick return to previous levels of functioning.

▶ Classification

A. Schizophrenic Disorders

Schizophrenia is the most common of the psychotic disorders that are all characterized by a loss of contact with reality. While about 1% if the population suffers from schizophrenia, those with the diagnosis account for up to 50% of all long-term psychiatric hospitalizations. Schizophrenia is a chronic disorder that is characterized by increasing social and vocational disability that begins in late adolescence or early adulthood and tends to continue through life. Schizophrenic symptoms have been classified into positive and negative categories. Positive symptoms include hallucinations, delusions, disorganized speech and behavior; these symptoms appear to be related to increased dopaminergic (D_2) activity in the mesolimbic region. Negative symptoms include diminished sociability, restricted affect, and poverty of speech; these symptoms appear to be related to decreased D_2 activity in the mesocortical system.

B. Delusional Disorder

Delusional disorders are psychoses in which the predominant symptoms are persistent delusions with minimal impairment of daily functioning. (The schizophrenic disorders show significant impairment.) Intellectual and occupational activities are little affected, whereas social and partner functioning tends to be markedly involved. Hallucinations are not usually present. Common delusional themes include paranoid delusions of persecution, delusions of being related to or loved by a well-known person, and delusions that one's partner is unfaithful.

C. Schizoaffective Disorder

Schizoaffective disorders are those cases that fail to fit comfortably either in the schizophrenic or in the affective categories. They are usually cases with affective symptoms (either a major depressive episode, manic episode, or hypomanic episode) that precede or develop concurrently with psychotic manifestations and the psychotic symptoms occur in the absence of any mood symptoms. There has been increasing interest in studying prodromal schizophrenia with a goal of prevention or early treatment.

D. Schizophreniform Disorders

Schizophreniform disorders are similar in their symptoms to schizophrenic disorders except that the duration of prodromal, acute, and residual symptoms is longer than 1 week but less than 6 months.

E. Brief Psychotic Disorders

These disorders last less than 1 week. They are the result of psychological stress. The shorter duration is significant and correlates with a more acute onset and resolution as well as a much better prognosis.

▶ Clinical Findings

A. Symptoms and Signs

The symptoms and signs of schizophrenia vary markedly among individuals as well as in the same person at different times. The patient's **appearance** may be bizarre, although the usual finding is a mild to moderate unkempt blandness. **Motor activity** is generally reduced, although extremes ranging from catatonic stupor to frenzied excitement occur. **Social behavior** is characterized by marked withdrawal coupled with disturbed interpersonal relationships and a reduced ability to experience pleasure. Dependency and a poor self-image are common. **Verbal utterances** are variable, the language being concrete yet symbolic, with unassociated rambling statements (at times interspersed with mutism) during an acute episode. Neologisms (made-up words or phrases), echolalia (repetition of words spoken by others), and verbigeration (repetition of senseless words or phrases) are occasionally present. **Affect** is usually flattened, with occasional inappropriateness. **Depression** is present in almost all cases but may be less apparent during the acute psychotic episode and more obvious during recovery. Depression is sometimes confused with akinetic side effects of antipsychotic medications. It is also related to boredom, which increases symptoms and decreases the response to treatment. Work is generally unavailable and time unfilled, providing opportunities for counterproductive activities such as drug abuse, withdrawal, and increased psychotic symptoms.

Thought content may vary from a paucity of ideas to a rich complex of delusional fantasy with archaic thinking. One frequently notes after a period of conversation that little if any information has actually been conveyed. Incoming stimuli produce varied responses. In some cases a simple question may trigger explosive outbursts, whereas at other times there may be no overt response whatsoever (catatonia). When paranoid ideation is present, the patient is often irritable and less cooperative. **Delusions** (false beliefs) are characteristic of paranoid thinking, and they usually take the form of a preoccupation with the supposedly threatening behavior exhibited by other individuals. This ideation may cause the patient to adopt active countermeasures such as locking doors and windows, taking up weapons, covering the ceiling with aluminum foil to counteract radar waves, and other bizarre efforts. Somatic delusions revolve around issues of bodily decay or infestation. **Perceptual distortions** usually include auditory hallucinations—visual hallucinations are more commonly associated with organic mental states—and may include illusions (distortions of reality) such as figures changing in size or lights varying in intensity. Cenesthetic hallucinations

(eg, a burning sensation in the brain, feeling blood flowing in blood vessels) occasionally occur. Lack of humor, feelings of dread, depersonalization (a feeling of being apart from the self), and fears of annihilation may be present. Any of the above symptoms generate higher anxiety levels, with heightened arousal and occasional panic and suicidal ideation, as the individual fails to cope.

The development of the acute episode in schizophrenia frequently is the end product of a gradual decompensation. Frustration and anxiety appear early, followed by depression and alienation, along with progressive ineffectiveness in day-to-day coping. This often leads to feelings of panic and increasing disorganization, with loss of the ability to test and evaluate the reality of perceptions. The stage of so-called psychotic resolution includes delusions, autistic preoccupations, and psychotic insight, with acceptance of the decompensated state. The process is frequently complicated by the use of caffeine, alcohol, and other recreational drugs. Life expectancy of schizophrenic patients is as much as 20% shorter than that of cohorts in the general population and is often associated with comorbid conditions such as the metabolic syndrome, which may be induced or exacerbated by the atypical antipsychotic agents.

Polydipsia may produce water intoxication with hyponatremia—characterized by symptoms of confusion, lethargy, psychosis, seizures, and occasionally death—in any psychiatric disorder, but most commonly in schizophrenia. These problems exacerbate the schizophrenic symptoms and can be confused with them. Possible pathogenetic factors in polydipsia include a hypothalamic defect, inappropriate antidiuretic hormone (ADH) secretion, antipsychotic medications (anticholinergic effects, stimulation of hypothalamic thirst center, effect on ADH), smoking (nicotine and syndrome of inappropriate antidiuretic hormone [SIADH]), psychotic thought processes (delusions), and other medications (eg, diuretics, antidepressants, lithium, alcohol) (see Chapter 21).

B. Imaging

Ventricular enlargement and cortical atrophy, as seen on CT scan, have been correlated with chronic course, severe cognitive impairment, and nonresponsiveness to antipsychotic medications. Decreased frontal lobe activity seen on PET scan has been associated with negative symptoms.

▶ Differential Diagnosis

The diagnosis of schizophrenia is best made over time because repeated observations increase the reliability of the diagnosis. One should not hesitate to reconsider the diagnosis of schizophrenia in any person who has received that diagnosis in the past, particularly when the clinical course has been atypical. A number of these patients have been found to actually have bipolar disorder, which has responded well to lithium. Manic episodes often mimic schizophrenia. However, schizophrenia is less likely to be associated with the decreased need for sleep, increase in goal directed activity, and overconfidence, symptoms that are typical of mania. However, thought disorder, auditory hallucinations, and delusions are commonly seen in manic psychosis.

Psychotic depressions, brief reactive psychosis, delusional disorder, and any illness with psychotic ideation tend to be confused with schizophrenia, partly because of the regrettable tendency to use the terms interchangeably.

Medical disorders such as thyroid dysfunction, adrenal and pituitary disorders, reactions to toxic materials (eg, mercury, PCBs), and almost all of the organic mental states in the early stages must be ruled out. Postpartum psychosis is discussed under Mood Disorders. **Complex partial seizures**, especially when psychosensory phenomena are present, are an important differential consideration. **Toxic drug states** arising from prescription, over-the-counter, herbal and street drugs may mimic all of the psychotic disorders. The chronic use of amphetamines, cocaine, and other stimulants frequently produces a psychosis that is almost identical to the acute paranoid schizophrenic episode. Drug-induced psychoses can have all the positive symptoms of schizophrenia but less commonly have the negative symptoms. The presence of formication (sensation of insects crawling on or under the skin) and stereotypy suggests the possibility of stimulant abuse. Phencyclidine, a common street drug, may cause a reaction that is difficult to distinguish from other psychotic disorders. Cerebellar signs, excessive salivation, dilated pupils, and increased deep tendon reflexes should alert the clinician to the possibility of a toxic psychosis. Industrial chemical toxicity (both organic and metallic), degenerative disorders, and metabolic deficiencies must be considered in the differential diagnosis.

Catatonia, frequently assumed to exist solely as a component of schizophrenic disorders, is actually the end product of a number of illnesses, including a number of organic conditions as well as other psychiatric disorders such as bipolar disorder. Neoplasms, viral and bacterial encephalopathies, central nervous system hemorrhage, metabolic derangements such as diabetic ketoacidosis, sedative withdrawal, and liver and kidney malfunction have all been implicated. It is particularly important to realize that drug toxicity (eg, overdoses of antipsychotic medications such as fluphenazine or haloperidol) can cause catatonic syndrome, which may be misdiagnosed as a catatonic schizophrenic disorder and inappropriately treated with more antipsychotic medication. Catatonia is also seen in other major psychiatric disorders, including bipolar disorder and major depression.

▶ Treatment

A. Medical (see Side Effects, below)

Hospitalization is often necessary, particularly when the patient's behavior shows gross disorganization. The presence of competent family members lessens the need for hospitalization, and each case should be judged individually. The major considerations are to prevent self-inflicted harm or harm to others and to provide the patient's basic needs. A full medical evaluation and CT scan or MRI of the brain should be considered in first episodes of schizophreniform disorder and other psychotic episodes of unknown cause.

Antipsychotic medications are the treatment of choice. The relapse rate can be reduced by 50% with proper maintenance antipsychotic therapy. Long-acting, injectable depot antipsychotics are used in nonadherant patients or nonresponders to oral medication.

Antipsychotic medications include the **"typical or first-generation"** antipsychotics (phenothiazines, thioxanthenes, butyrophenones, dihydroindolones, dibenzoxazepines, and benzisoxazoles) and the newer **"atypical or second-generation"** antipsychotics (clozapine, risperidone, olanzapine, quetiapine, aripiprazole, ziprasidone, paliperidone, asenapine, iloperidone, lurasidone, and cariprazine) (Tables 25–4 and 25–5). Generally, increasing milligram potency of the typical antipsychotics is associated with decreasing anticholinergic and adrenergic side effects and increasing extrapyramidal symptoms. Data suggest similar antipsychotic efficacy for both classes and a tendency for the second-generation antipsychotics being better tolerated leading to enhanced compliance.

The phenothiazines comprise the bulk of the currently used "typical" antipsychotic medications. The only butyrophenone commonly used in psychiatry is haloperidol, which is different in structure but similar in action and side effects to the piperazine phenothiazines such as fluphenazine, perphenazine, and trifluoperazine. These medications and haloperidol (dopamine [D_2] receptor blockers) have high potency and a paucity of autonomic side effects and act to markedly lower arousal levels.

Clozapine, the first "atypical" (novel) antipsychotic drug developed, has dopamine (D_4) receptor-blocking activity as well as central serotonergic, histaminergic, and alpha-noradrenergic receptor-blocking activity. It is effective in the treatment of about 30% of psychoses resistant to other antipsychotic medications, and it may have specific efficacy in decreasing suicidality in patients with schizophrenia. Risperidone is an antipsychotic that blocks some serotonin receptors (5-HT_2) and dopamine receptors (D_2). Risperidone causes fewer extrapyramidal side effects than the typical antipsychotics at doses less than 6 mg. It appears to be as effective as haloperidol and possibly as effective as clozapine in treatment-resistant patients without necessitating weekly white cell counts, as required with clozapine therapy. Risperidone is available in a long-acting injectable preparation.

Olanzapine is a potent blocker of 5-HT_2 and dopamine D_1, D_2, and D_4 receptors. High doses of olanzapine (10–20 mg daily) appear to be more effective than lower doses. The drug is somewhat more effective than haloperidol in the treatment of negative symptoms, such as withdrawal, psychomotor retardation, and poor interpersonal relationships. It is available in an orally disintegrating form for patients who are unable to tolerate standard oral dosing and in an injectable form for the management of acute agitation associated with schizophrenia and bipolar disorder. Olanzapine is available in a long-term injectable preparation but this formulation tends to be used less commonly than other depot formulations because some patients experience severe sedation and delirium.

Quetiapine is an antipsychotic with greater 5-HT_2 relative to D_2 receptor blockade as well as a relatively high affinity for alpha-1- and alpha-2-adrenergic receptors. It appears to be as efficacious as haloperidol in treating

Table 25–4. Commonly used antipsychotics and medications.

Drug	Usual Daily Oral Dose	Usual Daily Maximum Dose[1]	Cost per Unit	Cost for 30 Days Treatment Based on Maximum Dosage[2]
Aripiprazole (Abilify)	10–15 mg	30 mg	$45.41/30 mg	$1362.30
Asenapine (Saphris)	10–20 mg	20 mg	$13.79/10 mg	$827.40
Cariprazine (Vraylar)	1.5–6 mg	6 mg	$40.24/6 mg	$1207.30
Chlorpromazine (Thorazine; others)	100–400 mg	1 g	$13.74/200 mg	$2061.00
Clozapine (Clozaril)	300–450 mg	900 mg	$8.17/100 mg	$2205.90
Fluphenazine (Permitil, Prolixin)[3]	2–10 mg	60 mg	$1.15/10 mg	$207.00
Haloperidol (Haldol)	2–5 mg	60 mg	$2.76/20 mg	$248.40
Iloperidone (Fanapt)	12–24 mg	24 mg	$36.49/12 mg	$2189.40
Loxapine (Loxitane)	20–60 mg	200 mg	$2.57/50 mg	$308.40
Lurasidone (Latuda)	40–80 mg	80 mg	$36.88/80 mg	$1106.40
Olanzapine (Zyprexa)	5–10 mg	20 mg	$39.83/20 mg	$1194.90
Paliperidone (Invega)	6–12 mg	12 mg	$30.53/6 mg	$1831.80
Perphenazine (Trilafon)[3]	16–32 mg	64 mg	$3.90/16 mg	$468.00
Quetiapine (Seroquel)	200–400 mg	800 mg	$19.93/400 mg	$1195.80
Risperidone (Risperdal)[4]	2–6 mg	10 mg	$7.59/2 mg	$946.16
Thiothixene (Navane)[3]	5–10 mg	80 mg	$0.65/10 mg	$156.00
Trifluoperazine (Stelazine)	5–15 mg	60 mg	$2.45/10 mg	$441.00
Ziprasidone (Geodon)	40–160 mg	160 mg	$10.76/80 mg	$645.60

[1]Can be higher in some cases.
[2]Average wholesale price (AWP, for AB-rated generic when available) for quantity listed. Source: *Red Book* (electronic version), Truven Health Analytics Information, http://www.micormedexsolutions.com, accessed April 8, 2016. AWP may not accurately represent the actual pharmacy cost because wide contractual variations exist among institutions.
[3]Indicates piperazine structure.
[4]For risperidone, daily doses above 6 mg increase the risk of extrapyramidal syndrome. Risperidone 6 mg is approximately equivalent to haloperidol 20 mg.

Table 25–5. Relative potency and side effects of antipsychotic medications.

Drug	Chlorpromazine: Drug Potency Ratio	Anticholinergic Effects[1]	Extrapyramidal Effect[1]
Aripiprazole	1:20	1	1
Chlorpromazine	1:1	4	1
Clozapine	1:1	4	—
Fluphenazine	1:50	1	4
Haloperidol	1:50	1	4
Iloperidone	1:25	1	1
Loxapine	1:10	2	3
Lurasidone	1:5	1	2
Olanzapine	1:20	1	1
Perphenazine	1:10	2	3
Quetiapine	1:1	1	1
Risperidone	1:50	1	3
Thiothixene	1:20	1	4
Trifluoperazine	1:20	1	4
Ziprasidone	1:1	1	1

[1]1, weak effect; 4, strong effect.

positive and negative symptoms of schizophrenia, with fewer extrapyramidal side effects even at high doses.

Ziprasidone has both anti-dopamine receptor and anti-serotonin receptor effects, with good efficacy for both positive and negative symptoms of schizophrenia. Aripiprazole is a partial agonist at the dopamine D_2 and serotonin 5-HT_1 receptors and an antagonist at 5-HT_2 receptors, it is effective against positive and negative symptoms of schizophrenia. It functions as an antagonist or agonist, depending on the dopaminergic activity at the dopamine receptors. This may help decrease side effects. Aripiprazole is approved as an augmentation agent for treatment-resistant depression, even when psychosis is not present, and as a maintenance treatment for bipolar disorder. Aripiprazole is available as an acute injectable preparation as well as a long-term injectable preparation that is given once monthly in patients who are not able to adhere to daily oral dosing. Asenapine, approved for the treatment of schizophrenia and bipolar disorder (mixed or manic state), appears to be particularly helpful in treating negative symptoms of schizophrenia. Paliperidone, the active metabolite of risperidone, is available as a capsule and a monthly injection. Lurasidone is FDA-approved and has been shown to be effective in treating acute decompensation in patients with chronic schizophrenia. Cariprazine is a partial agonist of the D_2 and D_3 receptor and is approved by the FDA for the treatment of schizophrenia and bipolar disorder. Akithisia, weight gain, and insomnia are among the more commonly reported side effects with cariprazine. Because cariprazine is not a potent D_2-antagonist, it is less likely to increase prolactin levels than most antipsychotics. Despite higher costs, atypical antipsychotics are often considered preferable to traditional antipsychotics because they are thought to be associated with reduced extrapyramidal symptoms and a lesser risk of tardive dyskinesia.

Clinical Indications

The antipsychotics are used to treat all forms of the schizophrenias as well as psychotic ideation in delirium, drug-induced psychoses, psychotic depression, augmentation of unipolar depression, acute mania, and the prevention of mood cycles in bipolar disorder. They are also effective in Tourette syndrome and behavioral dyscontrol in autistic patients. While frequently used to treat agitation in dementia patients, no antipsychotic has been shown to be reliably effective in this population and may increase the risk of early mortality in elderly dementia patients. Antipsychotics quickly lower the arousal (activity) level and, perhaps indirectly, gradually improve socialization and thinking. The improvement rate for treating positive symptoms is about 80%. Patients whose behavioral symptoms worsen with use of antipsychotic medications may have an undiagnosed organic condition such as anticholinergic toxicity.

Symptoms that are ameliorated by these medications include hyperactivity, hostility, aggression, delusions, hallucinations, irritability, and poor sleep. Individuals with acute psychosis and good premorbid function respond quite well. The most common cause of failure in the treatment of acute psychosis is inadequate dosage, and the most common cause of relapse is noncompliance.

Although first-generation antipsychotics are efficacious in the treatment of positive symptoms of schizophrenia, such as hallucinations and delusions, second-generation antipsychotics are thought to have efficacy in reducing positive symptoms and some efficacy in treating negative symptoms. Antidepressant medications may be used in conjunction with antipsychotics if significant depression is present. Resistant cases may require concomitant use of lithium, carbamazepine, or valproic acid. The addition of a benzodiazepine drug to the antipsychotic regimen may prove helpful in treating the agitated or catatonic psychotic patient who has not responded to antipsychotics alone—lorazepam, 1–2 mg orally, can produce a rapid resolution of catatonic symptoms and may allow maintenance with a lower antipsychotic dose. Electroconvulsive therapy (ECT) has also been effective in treating catatonia.

Dosage Forms & Patterns

The dosage range is quite broad (Table 25–4). For example, risperidone, 0.25–1 mg orally at bedtime, may be sufficient for the elderly person with mild dementia with psychosis (especially in view of the increased risk of stroke and death in the elderly), whereas up to 6 mg/day may be used in a young patient with acute schizophrenia. For quick response, an atypical antipsychotic may be started in combination with a benzodiazepine (eg, risperidone oral solution, 2 mg, or olanzapine, 10 mg orally, and lorazepam, 2 mg orally, every 2–4 hours as needed). In an acutely distressed, psychotic patient one might use haloperidol, 10 mg intramuscularly, which is absorbed rapidly and achieves an initial tenfold plasma level advantage over equal oral doses. Psychomotor agitation, racing thoughts, and general arousal are quickly reduced. The dose can be repeated every 3–4 hours; when the patient is less symptomatic, oral doses can replace parenteral administration in most cases. In the elderly, both atypical (eg, risperidone 0.25 mg–0.5 mg daily or olanzapine 1.25 mg daily) and typical (eg, haloperidol 0.5 mg daily or perphenazine 2 mg daily) antipsychotics, often used effectively in small doses for behavioral control, have been linked to premature death in some cases.

Absorption of oral medications may be increased or decreased by concomitant administration of other medications (eg, antacids tend to decrease the absorption of antidepressants). Previous gastrointestinal surgery may alter pH, motility, and surface areas available for drug absorption. There are racial differences in metabolizing the antipsychotic medications—eg, many Asians require only about half the usual dosage. Bioavailability is influenced by other factors such as smoking or hepatic microsomal enzyme stimulation with alcohol or barbiturates and enzyme-altering medications such as carbamazepine or methylphenidate. Antipsychotic plasma drug level determinations are not currently of major clinical assistance.

Divided daily doses are not necessary after a maintenance dose has been established, and most patients can then be maintained on a single daily dose, usually taken at bedtime. This is particularly appropriate in a case where the sedative effect of the drug is desired for nighttime sleep, and undesirable sedative effects can be avoided during the day. Risperidone is an exception, being given twice daily.

First-episode patients especially should be tapered off medications after about 6 months of stability and carefully monitored; their rate of relapse is lower than that of multiple-episode patients.

Psychiatric patients—particularly paranoid individuals—often neglect to take their medication. In these cases and in nonresponders to oral medication, the enanthate and decanoate (the latter is slightly longer-lasting and has fewer extrapyramidal side effects) forms of fluphenazine or the decanoate form of haloperidol may be given by deep subcutaneous injection or intramuscularly to achieve an effect that will usually last 7–28 days. A patient who cannot be depended on to take oral medication (or who overdoses on minimal provocation) will generally agree to come to the clinician's office for a "shot." The usual dose of the fluphenazine long-acting preparations is 25 mg every 2 weeks. Dosage and frequency of administration vary from about 100 mg weekly to 12.5 mg monthly. Use the smallest effective amount as infrequently as possible. A monthly injection of 25 mg of fluphenazine decanoate is equivalent to about 15–20 mg of oral fluphenazine daily. Risperidone was the first atypical antipsychotic available in a long-acting injectable form (25–50 mg intramuscularly every 2 weeks). Concomitant use of a benzodiazepine (eg, lorazepam, 2 mg orally twice daily) may permit reduction of the required dosage of oral or parenteral antipsychotic drug. Long-acting injectables are now available for risperidone, paliperidone, aripiprazole, and olanzapine.

Intravenous haloperidol, the antipsychotic most commonly used by this route, is often used in critical care units in the management of agitated, delirious patients. Intravenous haloperidol should be given no faster than 1 mg/min to reduce cardiovascular side effects, such as torsades de pointes. Current practice indicates that ECG monitoring should be used whenever haloperidol is being administered intravenously.

Some antipsychotic agents are available for intranasal administration. The intranasal form of loxapine has a more rapid onset of action for the treatment of agitation (about 10 minutes) than either intramuscular or oral antipsychotic agents. Also, intranasal administration tends to be less traumatic to patients than getting an injection. However, intranasal loxapine requires the cooperation of the patient and is more expensive than generic antipsychotic injectable preparations.

Side Effects

For both typical and atypical antipsychotic agents, a range of side effects has been reported. The most common anticholinergic side effects include **dry mouth** (which can lead to ingestion of caloric liquids and weight gain or hyponatremia), **blurred near vision, urinary retention** (particularly in elderly men with enlarged prostates), **delayed gastric emptying, esophageal reflux, ileus, delirium,** and precipitation of **acute glaucoma** in patients with narrow anterior chamber angles. Other autonomic effects include **orthostatic hypotension** and **sexual dysfunction**—problems in achieving erection, ejaculation (including retrograde ejaculation), and orgasm in men (approximately 50% of cases) and women (approximately 30%). Delay in achieving orgasm is often a factor in medication noncompliance. **Electrocardiographic changes** occur frequently, but clinically significant arrhythmias are much less common. Elderly patients and those with preexisting cardiac disease are at greater risk. The most frequently seen electrocardiographic changes include diminution of the T wave amplitude, appearance of prominent U waves, depression of the ST segment, and prolongation of the QT interval (Table 25–6). Ziprasidone can produce QTc prolongation. A pretreatment ECG is indicated for patients at risk for cardiac sequelae (including patients taking other medications that might prolong the QTc interval). In some critical care patients, torsades de pointes has been associated with the use of high-dose intravenous haloperidol (usually greater than 30 mg/24 h).

Associations have been suggested between the atypical antipsychotics and **new-onset diabetes, hyperlipidemia,** and **weight gain** (Table 25–6). The FDA has particularly noted the risk of hyperglycemia and new-onset diabetes in this class of medication that is not related to weight gain. The risk of diabetes mellitus is increased in patients taking

Table 25–6. Adverse factors associated with atypical antipsychotic medications.

	Weight Gain	Hyperlipidemia	New-Onset Diabetes Mellitus	QTc Prolongation[1]
Asenapine	+/–	+/–	+/–	+++
Aripiprazole	+/–	–	–	++
Clozapine	+++	+++	+++	+/–
Lurasidone	–	–	–	–
Olanzapine	+++	+++	+++	+/–
Paliperidone	+	+/—	+/–	+++
Quetiapine	++	++	++	+++
Risperidone	++	++	++	+
Ziprasidone	+/–	—	–	+++

[1]QTc prolongation is a side effect of many medications and suggests a possible risk for arrhythmia. Prescriber's Letter 2011;18(12):271207.

clozapine and olanzapine. Monitoring of weight, fasting blood sugar and lipids prior to initiation of treatment and at regular intervals thereafter is an important part of medication monitoring. The addition of metformin to olanzapine may improve drug-induced weight gain in patients with drug-naïve, first-episode schizophrenia. Antipsychotic medications in general may have **metabolic and endocrine effects,** including weight gain, hyperglycemia, impaired temperature regulation in hot weather, and water intoxication, that may be due to inappropriate ADH secretion. Lactation and menstrual irregularities are common (antipsychotic medications should be avoided, if possible, in breast cancer patients because of potential trophic effects of elevated prolactin levels on the breast). Both antipsychotic and antidepressant medications inhibit sperm motility. **Bone marrow depression** and **cholestatic jaundice** occur rarely; these are hypersensitivity reactions, and they usually appear in the first 2 months of treatment. They subside on discontinuance of the drug. There is cross-sensitivity among all of the phenothiazines, and a drug from a different group should be used when allergic reactions occur.

Clozapine is associated with a 1.6% risk of agranulocytosis (higher in persons of Ashkenazi Jewish ancestry), and its use must be strictly monitored with weekly blood counts during the first 6 months of treatment, with monitoring every other week thereafter. The risk of developing agranulocytosis is approximately 2.5 times higher in patients with a polymorphism for *HLADQB1* gene. Thus, this genetic test may be worthwhile to perform before initiating clozapine. Discontinuation of the medication requires weekly monitoring of the white blood cell count for 1 month. Clozapine has been associated with fatal myocarditis and is contraindicated in patients with severe heart disease. In addition, clozapine lowers the seizure threshold and has many side effects, including sedation, hypotension, increased liver enzyme levels, hypersalivation, respiratory arrest, weight gain, and changes in both the ECG and the electroencephalogram. Notably, adynamic ileus is a rare side effect of clozapine that can be fatal.

Photosensitivity, retinopathy, and **hyperpigmentation** are associated with use of fairly high dosages of chlorpromazine. The appearance of particulate melanin deposits in the lens of the eye is related to the total dose given, and patients on long-term medication should have periodic eye examinations. Teratogenicity has not been causally related to these medications, but prudence is indicated particularly in the first trimester of pregnancy. The seizure threshold is lowered, but it is safe to use these medications in epileptics who take anticonvulsants.

The **neuroleptic malignant syndrome (NMS)** is a catatonia-like state manifested by extrapyramidal signs, blood pressure changes, altered consciousness, and hyperpyrexia; it is an uncommon but serious complication of antipsychotic treatment. Muscle rigidity, involuntary movements, confusion, dysarthria, and dysphagia are accompanied by pallor, cardiovascular instability, fever, pulmonary congestion, and diaphoresis and may result in stupor, coma, and death. The cause may be related to a number of factors, including poor dosage control of antipsychotic medication, affective illness, decreased serum iron, dehydration, and increased sensitivity of dopamine receptor sites. Lithium in combination with an antipsychotic drug may increase vulnerability, which is already increased in patients with an affective disorder. In most cases, the symptoms develop within the first 2 weeks of antipsychotic drug treatment. The syndrome may occur with small doses of the medications. Intramuscular administration is a risk factor. Elevated creatine kinase and leukocytosis with a shift to the left are present early in about half of cases. Treatment includes controlling fever and providing fluid support. Dopamine agonists such as bromocriptine, 2.5–10 mg orally three times a day, and amantadine, 100–200 mg orally twice a day, have also been useful. Dantrolene, 50 mg intravenously as needed, is used to alleviate rigidity (do not exceed 10 mg/kg/day due to hepatotoxicity risk). There is ongoing controversy about the efficacy of these three agents as well as the use of calcium channel blockers and benzodiazepines. ECT has been used effectively in resistant cases. Clozapine has been used with relative safety and fair success as an antipsychotic drug for patients who have had NMS.

Akathisia is the most common (about 20%) extrapyramidal symptom. It usually occurs early in treatment (but may persist after antipsychotics are discontinued) and is frequently mistaken for anxiety or exacerbation of psychosis. It is characterized by a subjective desire to be in constant motion followed by an inability to sit or stand still and consequent pacing. It may induce suicidality or feelings of fright, rage, terror, or sexual torment. Insomnia is often present. It is crucial to educate patients in advance about these potential side effects so that the patients do not misinterpret them as signs of increased illness. In all cases, reevaluate the dosage requirement or the type of antipsychotic drug. One should inquire also about cigarette smoking, which in women has been associated with an increased incidence of akathisia. Antiparkinsonism medications (such as trihexyphenidyl, 2–5 mg orally three times daily) may be helpful, but first-line treatment often includes a benzodiazepine (such as clonazepam 0.5–1 mg orally three times daily). In resistant cases, symptoms may be alleviated by propranolol, 30–80 mg/day orally, diazepam, 5 mg orally three times daily, or amantadine, 100 mg orally three times daily.

Acute dystonias usually occur early, although a late (tardive) occurrence is reported in patients (mostly men after several years of therapy) who previously had early severe dystonic reactions and a mood disorder. Younger patients are at higher risk for acute dystonias. The most common signs are bizarre muscle spasms of the head, neck, and tongue. Frequently present are torticollis, oculogyric crises, swallowing or chewing difficulties, and masseter spasms. Laryngospasm is particularly dangerous. Back, arm, or leg muscle spasms are occasionally reported. Diphenhydramine, 50 mg intramuscularly, is effective for the acute crisis; one should then give benztropine mesylate, 2 mg orally twice daily, for several weeks, and then discontinue gradually, since few of the extrapyramidal symptoms require long-term use of the antiparkinsonism medications (all of which are about equally efficacious—though trihexyphenidyl tends to be mildly stimulating and benztropine mildly sedating).

Drug-induced parkinsonism is indistinguishable from idiopathic parkinsonism, but it is reversible, occurs later in treatment than the preceding extrapyramidal symptoms, and in some cases appears after antipsychotic withdrawal. The condition includes the typical signs of apathy and reduction of facial and arm movements (akinesia, which can mimic depression), festinating gait, rigidity, loss of postural reflexes, and pill-rolling tremor. AIDS patients seem particularly vulnerable to extrapyramidal side effects. High-potency antipsychotics often require antiparkinsonism medications (see Table 24–6). The antipsychotic dosage should be reduced, and immediate relief can be achieved with antiparkinsonism medications in the same dosages as above. After 4–6 weeks, these antiparkinsonism medications can often be discontinued with no recurrent symptoms. In any of the extrapyramidal symptoms, amantadine, 100–400 mg orally daily, may be used instead of the antiparkinsonism medications. Antipsychotic-induced catatonia is similar to catatonic stupor with rigidity, drooling, urinary incontinence, and cogwheeling. It usually responds slowly to withdrawal of the offending medication and use of antiparkinsonism agents.

Tardive dyskinesia is a syndrome of abnormal involuntary stereotyped movements of the face, mouth, tongue, trunk, and limbs that may occur after months or (usually) years of treatment with antipsychotic agents. The syndrome affects 20–35% of patients who have undergone long-term antipsychotic therapy. Predisposing factors include older age, many years of treatment, cigarette smoking, and diabetes mellitus. Pineal calcification is higher in this condition by a margin of 3:1. There are no clearcut differences among the antipsychotic medications in the development of tardive dyskinesia. (Although the atypical antipsychotics appear to offer a lower risk of tardive dyskinesia, long-term effects have not been investigated.) Early manifestations of tardive dyskinesia include fine worm-like movements of the tongue at rest, difficulty in sticking out the tongue, facial tics, increased blink frequency, or jaw movements of recent onset. Later manifestations may include bucco-linguo-masticatory movements, lip smacking, chewing motions, mouth opening and closing, disturbed gag reflex, puffing of the cheeks, disrupted speech, respiratory distress, or choreoathetoid movements of the extremities (the last being more prevalent in younger patients). The symptoms do not necessarily worsen and in rare cases may lessen even though antipsychotic medications are continued. The dyskinesias do not occur during sleep and can be voluntarily suppressed for short periods. Stress and movements in other parts of the body will often aggravate the condition.

Early signs of dyskinesia must be differentiated from those reversible signs produced by ill-fitting dentures or nonantipsychotic medications such as levodopa, TCAs, antiparkinsonism agents, anticonvulsants, and antihistamines. Other neurologic conditions such as Huntington chorea can be differentiated by history and examination.

The emphasis should be on prevention of side effects. Use the least amount of antipsychotic drug necessary to mute the psychotic symptoms, and use atypical antipsychotics as first-line agents. Detect early manifestations of dyskinesias. When these occur, stop anticholinergic medications and gradually discontinue antipsychotic medications, if clinically feasible. Weight loss and cachexia sometimes appear on withdrawal of antipsychotics. In an indeterminate number of cases, the dyskinesias will remit. Keep the patient off the medications until reemergent psychotic symptoms dictate their resumption, at which point they are restarted in low doses and gradually increased until there is clinical improvement. If antipsychotic medications are restarted, clozapine and olanzapine appear to offer less risk of recurrence. The use of adjunctive agents such as benzodiazepines or lithium may help directly or indirectly by allowing control of psychotic symptoms with a low dosage of antipsychotics. If the dyskinesic syndrome recurs and it is necessary to continue antipsychotic medications to control psychotic symptoms, informed consent should be obtained. Benzodiazepines, buspirone (in doses of 15–60 mg/day orally), phosphatidylcholine, clonidine, calcium channel blockers, vitamin E, omega-3 fatty acids, and propranolol all have had limited usefulness in treating the dyskinetic side effects.

B. Social

Environmental considerations are most important in the individual with a chronic illness, who usually has a history of repeated hospitalizations, a continued low level of functioning, and symptoms that never completely remit. Family rejection and work failure are common. In these cases, board and care homes staffed by personnel experienced in caring for psychiatric patients are most important. There is frequently an inverse relationship between stability of the living situation and the amounts of required antipsychotic medications, since the most salutary environment is one that reduces stimuli. Nonresidential self-help groups such as Recovery, Inc., should be utilized whenever possible. They provide a setting for sharing, learning, and mutual support and are frequently the only social involvement with which this type of patient is comfortable. Vocational rehabilitation and work agencies (eg, Goodwill Industries, Inc.) provide assessment, training, and job opportunities at a level commensurate with the person's clinical condition.

C. Psychological

The need for psychotherapy varies markedly depending on the patient's current status and history. In a person with a single psychotic episode and a previously good level of adjustment, supportive psychotherapy may help the patient reintegrate the experience, gain some insight into antecedent problems, and become a more self-observant individual who can recognize early signs of stress. Insight-oriented psychotherapy is often counterproductive in this type of disorder. Research suggests that cognitive behavioral therapy—in conjunction with medication management—may have some efficacy in the treatment of symptoms of schizophrenia. Cognitive behavioral therapy for schizophrenia involves helping the individual challenge psychotic thinking and alters response to hallucinations. Similarly, a form of psychotherapy called acceptance and commitment therapy has shown value in helping prevent hospitalizations in schizophrenia. Cognitive remediation therapy is another approach to treatment that may help patients with schizophrenia become better able to focus their disorganized thinking. Family therapy may also help alleviate the patient's stress and to assist relatives in coping with the patient.

D. Behavioral

Behavioral techniques (see above) are most frequently used in therapeutic settings such as day treatment centers, but they can also be incorporated into family situations or any therapeutic setting. Many behavioral techniques (eg, positive reinforcement—whether it be a word of praise or an approving nod—after some positive behavior), can be a powerful instrument for helping a person learn behaviors that will facilitate social acceptance. Music from portable digital players with earphones is one of many ways to divert the patient's attention from auditory hallucinations.

▶ Prognosis

For most patients with any psychosis, the prognosis is good for alleviation of positive symptoms such as hallucinations or delusions treated with medication. Negative symptoms such as diminished affect and sociability are much more difficult to treat but appear mildly responsive to atypical antipsychotics. Cognitive deficits, such as the executive dysfunction that is common to schizophrenia, also do not appear as responsive to antipsychotics as do positive symptoms. Unfortunately, both negative symptoms and cognitive deficits appear to contribute more to long-term disability in schizophrenic patients than do positive symptoms. Unavailability of structured work situations and lack of family therapy are two other reasons why the prognosis is so guarded in such a large percentage of schizophrenic patients. Psychosis connected with a history of serious drug abuse has a guarded prognosis because of the central nervous system damage, usually from the medications themselves and associated medical illnesses.

Arnedo J et al; Molecular Genetics of Schizophrenia Consortium. Uncovering the hidden risk architecture of the schizophrenias: confirmation in three independent genome-wide association studies. Am J Psychiatry. 2015 Feb 1;172(2):139–53. [PMID: 25219520]

Buckley PF et al. Schizophrenia research: a progress report. Psychiatr Clin North Am. 2015 Sep;38(3):373–7. [PMID: 26300028]

Hasnain M et al. Metabolic syndrome associated with schizophrenia and atypical antipsychotics. Curr Diab Rep. 2010 Jun;10(3):209–16. [PMID: 20425584]

Stahl SM et al. "Meta-guidelines" for the management of patients with schizophrenia. CNS Spectr. 2013 Jun;18(3):150–62. [PMID: 23591126]

MOOD DISORDERS (Depression & Mania)

ESSENTIALS OF DIAGNOSIS

Present in most depressions

▶ Mood varies from mild sadness to intense despondency and feelings of guilt, worthlessness, and hopelessness.

▶ Difficulty in thinking, including inability to concentrate, ruminations, and lack of decisiveness.

▶ Loss of interest, with diminished involvement in work and recreation.

▶ Somatic complaints such as headache; disrupted, lessened, or excessive sleep; loss of energy; change in appetite; decreased sexual drive.

▶ Anxiety.

Present in some severe depressions

▶ Psychomotor retardation or agitation.

▶ Delusions of a somatic or persecutory nature.

▶ Withdrawal from activities.

▶ Physical symptoms of major severity, eg, anorexia, insomnia, reduced sexual drive, weight loss, and various somatic complaints.

▶ Suicidal ideation.

Present in mania

▶ Mood ranging from euphoria to irritability.

▶ Sleep disruption.

▶ Hyperactivity.

▶ Racing thoughts.

▶ Grandiosity or extreme overconfidence.

▶ Variable psychotic symptoms.

▶ General Considerations

Depression is extremely common, with up to 30% of primary care patients having depressive symptoms. Depression may be the final expression of (1) genetic factors (neurotransmitter dysfunction), (2) developmental problems (personality problems, childhood events), or (3) psychosocial stresses (divorce, unemployment). It frequently presents in the form of somatic complaints with negative medical workups. Although sadness and grief are normal responses to loss, depression is not. Patients experiencing normal grief tend to produce sympathy and sadness in the clinician caregiver; depression often produces frustration and irritation in the clinician. Grief is usually accompanied by intact self-esteem, whereas depression is marked by a sense of guilt and worthlessness.

Mania is often combined with depression and may occur alone, together with depression in a mixed episode, or in cyclic fashion with depression.

▶ Clinical Findings

In general, there are four major types of depression, with similar symptoms in each group.

A. Adjustment Disorder with Depressed Mood

Depression may occur in reaction to some identifiable stressor or adverse life situation, usually loss of a person by death (grief reaction), divorce, etc; financial reversal (crisis); or loss of an established role, such as being needed. Anger is frequently associated with the loss, and this in turn often produces a feeling of guilt. The disorder occurs within 3 months of the stressor and causes significant impairment in social or occupational functioning. The symptoms range from mild sadness, anxiety, irritability, worry, and lack of concentration, discouragement, and somatic complaints to the more severe symptoms of frank depression. When the full criteria for major depressive disorder are present, then that diagnosis should be made and treatment instituted even when there is a known stressor. The presence of a stressor is not the determining diagnostic driver, it is the resultant syndromal complex. One should not neglect treatment for major depression simply because it may appear to be an understandable reaction to a particular stress or difficulty.

B. Depressive Disorders

The subclassifications include major depressive disorder and dysthymia.

1. Major depressive disorder—A major depressive disorder consists of a syndrome of mood, physical and cognitive symptoms that occurs at any time of life. Many consider a physiologic or metabolic aberration to be causative. Complaints vary widely but most frequently include a loss of interest and pleasure (anhedonia), withdrawal from activities, and feelings of guilt. Also included are inability to concentrate, some cognitive dysfunction, anxiety, chronic fatigue, feelings of worthlessness, somatic complaints (unexplained somatic complaints frequently indicate depression), loss of sexual drive, and thoughts of death. Unemployment has been associated with increase in depression risk. Diurnal variation with improvement as the day progresses is common. Vegetative signs that frequently occur are insomnia, anorexia with weight loss, and constipation. Occasionally, severe agitation and psychotic ideation are present. Psychotic major depression occurs up to 14% of all patients with major depression and 25% of patients who are hospitalized with depression. Psychotic symptoms (delusions, paranoia) are more common in depressed persons who are older than 50 years. Paranoid symptoms may range from general suspiciousness to ideas of reference with delusions. The somatic delusions frequently revolve around feelings of impending annihilation or somatic concerns (eg, that the body is rotting away with cancer). Hallucinations are less common than unusual beliefs and tend not to occur independent of delusions.

In addition to psychotic major depression, other subcategories include **major depression with atypical features** that is characterized by hypersomnia, overeating, lethargy,

and mood reactivity in which the mood brightens in response to positive events or news. Melancholic major depression is characterized by a lack of mood reactivity seen in atypical depression, the presence of a prominent anhedonia and more severe vegetative symptoms. **Major depression with a seasonal onset (seasonal affective disorder)** is a dysfunction of circadian rhythms that occurs more commonly in the fall and winter months and is believed to be due to decreased exposure to full-spectrum light. Common symptoms include carbohydrate craving, lethargy, hyperphagia, and hypersomnia. **Major depression with postpartum onset** usually occurs 2 weeks to 6 months postpartum.

Most women (up to 80%) experience some mild letdown of mood in the postpartum period. For some of these (10–15%), the symptoms are more severe and similar to those usually seen in serious depression, with an increased emphasis on concerns related to the baby (obsessive thoughts about harming it or inability to care for it). When psychotic symptoms occur, there is frequently associated sleep deprivation, volatility of behavior, and manic-like symptoms. Postpartum psychosis is much less common (less than 2%), often occurs within the first 2 weeks, and requires early and aggressive management. Biologic vulnerability with hormonal changes and psychosocial stressors all play a role. The chances of a second episode are about 25% and may be reduced with prophylactic treatment.

2. Dysthymia—Dysthymia is a chronic depressive disturbance. Sadness, loss of interest, and withdrawal from activities over a period of 2 or more years with a relatively persistent course is necessary for this diagnosis. Generally, the symptoms are milder but longer-lasting than those in a major depressive episode.

3. Premenstrual dysphoric disorder—Depressive symptoms occur during the late luteal phase (last 2 weeks) of the menstrual cycle. (See also Chapter 18.)

C. Bipolar Disorder

Bipolar disorder consists of episodic mood shifts into mania, major depression, hypomania, and mixed mood states. The ability of bipolar disorder to mimic aspects of many other coincident major mental health disorders and a high comorbidity with substance abuse can make the initial diagnosis of bipolar disorder difficult. Bipolar I is diagnosed when an individual has both depressive and manic episodes. For individuals who experience depressive and hypomanic episodes without frank mania, the diagnosis is Bipolar II.

1. Mania—A manic episode is a mood state characterized by elation with hyperactivity, overinvolvement in life activities, increased irritability, flight of ideas, easy distractibility, and little need for sleep. The overenthusiastic quality of the mood and the expansive behavior initially attract others, but the irritability, mood lability with swings into depression, aggressive behavior, and grandiosity usually lead to marked interpersonal difficulties. Activities may occur that are later regretted, eg, excessive spending, resignation from a job, a hasty marriage, sexual acting out, and exhibitionistic behavior, with alienation of friends and family. Atypical manic episodes can include gross delusions, paranoid ideation of severe proportions, and auditory hallucinations usually related to some grandiose perception. The episodes begin abruptly (sometimes precipitated by life stresses) and may last from several days to months. Spring and summer tend to be the peak periods. Generally, the manic episodes are of shorter duration than the depressive episodes. In almost all cases, the manic episode is part of a broader bipolar (manic-depressive) disorder. Patients with four or more discrete episodes of a mood disturbance in 1 year are called "rapid cyclers." (Substance abuse, particularly cocaine, can mimic rapid cycling.) These patients have a higher incidence of hypothyroidism. Manic patients differ from patients with schizophrenia in that the former use more effective interpersonal maneuvers, are more sensitive to the social maneuvers of others, and are more able to utilize weakness and vulnerability in others to their own advantage. Creativity has been positively correlated with mood disorders, but the best work done is between episodes of mania and depression.

2. Cyclothymic disorders—These are chronic mood disturbances with episodes of subsyndromal depression and hypomania. The symptoms must have at least a 2-year duration and are milder than those that occur in depressive or manic episodes. Occasionally, the symptoms will escalate into a full-blown manic or depressive episode, in which case reclassification as bipolar I or II would be warranted.

D. Mood Disorders Secondary to Illness and Medications

Any illness, severe or mild, can cause significant depression. Conditions such as rheumatoid arthritis, multiple sclerosis, stroke, and chronic heart disease are particularly likely to be associated with depression, as are other chronic illnesses. Depression is common in cancer, as well, with a particularly high degree of comorbidity in pancreatic cancer. Hormonal variations clearly play a role in some depressions. Varying degrees of depression occur at various times in schizophrenic disorders, central nervous system disease, and organic mental states. **Alcohol dependency** frequently coexists with serious depression.

The classic model of **drug-induced depression** occurred with the use of reserpine, both in clinical settings and as a pharmacologic probe in research settings. Corticosteroids and oral contraceptives are commonly associated with mood changes such as depression and hypomania. Antihypertensive medications such as methyldopa, guanethidine, and clonidine have been associated with the development of depressive syndromes, as have digitalis and antiparkinsonism medications (eg, levodopa). Interferon is strongly associated with depressed mood and fatigue as a side effect; consultation with a psychiatrist prior to prescribing these agents is indicated in cases where there is a history of depression. It is unusual for beta-blockers to produce depression when given for short periods, such as in the treatment of performance anxiety. Sustained use of beta-blockers for medical conditions such as hypertension

may be associated with depression in some patients, although most individuals do not suffer this adverse effect. One study associated the use of beta-blockers with a significant reduction in risk of depressive symptoms 1 year after a percutaneous coronary intervention. Infrequently, disulfiram and anticholinesterase medications may be associated with symptoms of depression. All stimulant use results in a depressive syndrome when the drug is withdrawn. Alcohol, sedatives, opioids, and most of the psychedelic drugs are depressants and, paradoxically, are often used in self-treatment of depression. Corticosteroids may be associated with hypomania.

▶ Differential Diagnosis

Since depression may be a part of any illness—either reactively or as a secondary symptom—careful attention must be given to personal life adjustment problems and the role of medications (eg, reserpine, corticosteroids, levodopa). Schizophrenia, partial complex seizures, organic brain syndromes, panic disorders, and anxiety disorders must be differentiated. Thyroid dysfunction and other endocrinopathies should be ruled out. Malignancies, including central and gastrointestinal tumors are sometimes associated with depressive symptoms and may antecede the diagnosis of tumor. Strokes, particularly dominant hemisphere lesions, can occasionally present with a syndrome that looks like major depression. Medication-induced depressive symptoms are also quite common.

▶ Complications

The most important complication is **suicide**, which often includes some elements of aggression. Suicide rates in the general population vary from 9 per 100,000 in Spain to 20 per 100,000 in the United States to 58 per 100,000 in Hungary. In individuals hospitalized for depression, the lifetime risk rises to 10–15%. In patients with bipolar I disorder, the risk is higher, with up to 20% of individuals dying of suicide. Men over the age of 50 are more likely to complete a suicide because of their tendency to attempt suicide with more violent means, particularly guns. On the other hand, women make more attempts but are less likely to complete a suicide. An increased suicide rate is being observed in the younger population, aged 15–35. Patients with cancer, respiratory illnesses, AIDS, and those being maintained on hemodialysis have higher suicide rates. Alcohol use is a significant factor in many suicide attempts.

There are several groups of people who make suicide attempts. One group includes those individuals with acute situational problems. These individuals may be acutely distressed by a recent breakup in a relationship or another type of disappointment. This group also includes those who may not be diagnosed as having depression but who are overwhelmed by a stressful situation often with an aspect of public humiliation (eg, victims of cyber-bullying). A suicide attempt in such cases may be an impulsive or aggressive act not associated with significant depression. In such cases, a suicide attempt is clearly a stratagem for controlling or hurting others or an attempted escape.

Another high-risk group includes individuals with severe depression. Severe depression may be due to conditions such as medical illness (eg, AIDS, whose victims have a suicide rate over 20 times that of the general population) or comorbid psychiatric disorders (eg, panic disorders). Anxiety, panic, and fear are major findings in suicidal behavior. A patient may seem to make a dramatic improvement, but the lifting of depression may be due to the patient's decision to commit suicide. Another high-risk group are individuals with psychotic illness who tend not to verbalize their concerns, are unpredictable, and are often successful in their suicide attempt, although they make up only a small percentage of the total.

Finally, suicide is 10 times more prevalent in patients with schizophrenia than in the general population, and jumping from bridges is a more common means of attempted suicide by patients with schizophrenia than by others. In one study of 100 "jumpers," 47% had schizophrenia.

The immediate goal of psychiatric evaluation is to assess the current suicidal risk and the need for hospitalization versus outpatient management. Perhaps the one most useful question is to ask the person how many hours per day he or she thinks about suicide. If it is more than 1 hour, the individual is at high risk. Further assessing the risk by inquiring about intent, plans, means, and suicide-inhibiting factors (eg, strong ties to children or the church) is essential. The intent is less likely to be truly suicidal, for example, if small amounts of poison or medication were ingested or scratching of wrists was superficial, if the act was performed in the vicinity of others or with early notification of others, or if the attempt was arranged so that early detection would be anticipated. Alcohol, hopelessness, delusional thoughts, and complete or nearly complete loss of interest in life or ability to experience pleasure are all positively correlated with suicide attempts. Other risk factors are previous attempts, a family history of suicide, medical or psychiatric illness (eg, anxiety, depression, psychosis), male sex, older age, contemplation of violent methods, a humiliating social stressor, and drug use (including long-term sedative or alcohol use), which contributes to impulsiveness or mood swings. Successful treatment of the patient at risk for suicide cannot be achieved if the patient continues to abuse drugs.

The patient's current mood status is best evaluated by direct evaluation of plans and concerns about the future, personal reactions to the attempt, and thoughts about the reactions of others. Measurement of mood is often facilitated by using a standardized instrument such as the Hamilton or Montgomery-Asberg clinician-administered rating scales or the self-administered Patient Health Questionnaire-9. Blood tests are being developed to diagnose depression and predict antidepressant response. However, more testing is needed to determine the usefulness in routine clinical practice. Common antidepressant scales such as the PHQ-9 allow for initial assessment as well as ongoing treatment tracking. The patient's immediate resources should also be assessed—people who can be significantly involved (most important), family support, job situation, financial resources, etc. Suicide risk can be specifically assessed using an instrument such as the Columbia-Suicide Severity Risk Scale.

If hospitalization is not indicated (eg, gestures, impulsive attempts; see above), the clinician must formulate and institute a treatment plan or make an adequate referral. (National Suicide Prevention Lifeline, 1-800-273-8255, may be of assistance.) Medication should be dispensed in small amounts to at-risk patients. Although TCAs and SSRIs are associated with an equal incidence of suicide attempts, the risk of a completed suicide is much higher with TCA overdose. Guns and medications should be removed from the patient's household. Driving should be interdicted until the patient improves. The problem is often worsened by the long-term complications of the suicide attempt, eg, brain damage due to hypoxia, peripheral neuropathies caused by staying for long periods in one position causing nerve compressions, and medical or surgical problems such as esophageal strictures and tendon dysfunctions.

Sleep disturbances in the depressions are discussed below.

▶ Treatment of Depression

A. Medical

Milder forms of depression usually do not require drug therapy and can be managed by psychotherapy and the passage of time. In severe cases—particularly when vegetative signs are significant and symptoms have persisted for more than a few weeks—antidepressant drug therapy is often effective. Drug therapy is also suggested by a family history of major depression in first-degree relatives or a past history of prior episodes.

The antidepressant medications may be classified into four groups: (1) the newer antidepressants, including the SSRIs, SNRIs, and bupropion, vilazodone, vortioxetine, and mirtazapine, (2) the TCAs and clinically similar medications, (3) the MAO inhibitors (Table 25–7), and (4) stimulants. ECT and repetitive transcranial magnetic stimulation are procedural treatments for depression. These modalities are described in greater detail below.

Hospitalization is necessary if suicide is a major consideration or if complex treatment modalities are required.

Medication selection is influenced by the history of previous response or lack thereof if that information is available. A positive family history of response to a particular drug suggests that the patient may respond similarly. If no background information is available, a drug such as sertraline, 25 mg orally daily and increasing gradually up to 200 mg, or venlafaxine at 37.5 mg/day and titrated gradually to a maximum dose of 225 mg/day can be selected and a *full trial* instituted. The medication trial should be monitored for worsening mood or suicidal ideation with patient assessments every 1–2 weeks until week 6. In patients under 25 years of age, there is an association between antidepressant use and increased suicidality. Younger patients, therefore, should be monitored closely during the first 6–8 weeks of treatment. The STAR*D trial suggests that if the response to the first medication is inadequate, the best alternatives are to switch to a second agent that may be

Table 25–7. Commonly used antidepressants.

Drug	Usual Daily Oral Dose (mg)	Usual Daily Maximum Dose (mg)	Sedative Effects[1]	Anticholinergic Effects[1]	Cost per Unit	Cost for 30 Days Treatment Based on Maximum Dosage[2]
SSRIs						
Citalopram (Celexa)	20	40	< 1	1	$2.53/40 mg	$75.90
Escitalopram (Lexapro)	10	20	< 1	1	$4.51/20 mg	$135.30
Fluoxetine (Prozac, Sarafem)	5–40	80	< 1	< 1	$2.67/20 mg	$320.40
Fluvoxamine (Luvox)	100–300	300	1	< 1	$2.64/100 mg	$237.60
Paroxetine (Paxil)	20–30	50	1	1	$2.64/20 mg	$161.10
Sertraline (Zoloft)	50–150	200	< 1	< 1	$2.85/100 mg	$171.00
SNRIs						
Desvenlafaxine (Pristiq)	50	100	1	< 1	$11.84/100 mg	$355.20
Duloxetine (Cymbalta)	40	60	2	3	$5.93/60 mg	$177.90
Levomilnacipran (Fetzima)	40	120	1	1	$11.97/80 mg	$359.10
Milnacipran (Savella)	100	200	1	1	$5.36/100 mg	$321.60
Venlafaxine XR (Effexor)	150–225	225	1	< 1	$4.67/75 mg	$420.30
Tricyclic and clinically similar compounds						
Amitriptyline (Elavil)	150–250	300	4	4	$2.14/150 mg	$128.40
Amoxapine (Asendin)	150–200	400	2	2	$1.67/100 mg	$200.40
Clomipramine (Anafranil)	100	250	3	3	$11.24/75 mg	$1348.80
Desipramine (Norpramin)	100–250	300	1	1	$5.74/100 mg	$498.60
Doxepin (Sinequan)	150–200	300	4	3	$1.79/100 mg	$161.10
Imipramine (Tofranil)	150–200	300	3	3	$0.64/50 mg	$115.20
Maprotiline (Ludiomil)	100–200	300	4	2	$2.34/75 mg	$280.80
Nortriptyline (Aventyl, Pamelor)	100–150	150	2	2	$4.00/75 mg	$240.00
Protriptyline (Vivactil)	15–40	60	1	3	$3.30/10 mg	$594.00
Trimipramine (Surmontil)	75–200	200	4	4	$11.43/100 mg	$685.80
Monoamine oxidase inhibitors						
Phenelzine (Nardil)	45–60	90	...	...	$0.84/15 mg	$151.20
Selegiline transdermal (Emsam)	6 (skin patch)	12	...	...	$60.54/6 mg patch	$1816.20
Tranylcypromine (Parnate)	20–30	50	...	...	$7.07/10 mg	$1060.50
Other compounds						
Bupropion SR (Wellbutrin SR)	300	400[3]	< 1	< 1	$3.59/200 mg	$215.40
Bupropion XL (Wellbutrin XL)	300[4]	450[4]	< 1	< 1	$4.77/300 mg	$286.20
Mirtazapine (Remeron)	15–45	45	4	2	$2.80/30 mg	$85.53
Nefazodone (Serzone)	150-600	600	3	1	$3.99/200 mg	$239.40
Trazodone (Desyrel)	100–300	400	4	< 1	$0.73/100 mg	$87.60
Vilazodone (Viibryd)	10-40	40	1	1	$8.33/40 mg	$249.90
Vortioxetine (Brintellix)	10	20	<1	< 1	$11.58/20 mg	$347.40

[1]1, weak effect; 4, strong effect.
[2]Average wholesale price (AWP, for AB-rated generic when available) for quantity listed. Source: *Red Book* (electronic version), Truven Health Analytics, Information, http://www.micormedxsolutions.com, accessed April 8, 2016. AWP may not accurately represent the actual pharmacy cost because wide contractual variations exist among institutions.
[3]200 mg twice daily.
[4]Wellbutrin XL is a once-daily form of bupropion. Bupropion is still available as immediate release, and, if used, no single dose should exceed 150 mg.
SSRIs, selective serotonin reuptake inhibitors.

from the same or different class of antidepressant; another option is to try augmenting the first agent with bupropion (150–450 mg/day), lithium (eg, 300–900 mg/day orally), thyroid medication (eg, liothyronine, 25–50 mcg/day orally) or a second-generation antipsychotic (eg, aripiprazole [5–15 mg/day] or olanzapine [5–15 mg/day]). The latter course is often taken when there has been at least a partial response to the initial drug. The Agency for Health Care Policy and Research has produced clinical practice guidelines that outline one algorithm of treatment decisions (Figure 25–2).

Psychotic depression should be treated with a combination of an antipsychotic such as olanzapine and an antidepressant such as an SSRI at their usual doses. Mifepristone may have specific and early activity against psychotic depression. ECT is generally regarded as the single most effective treatment for psychotic depression.

Major depression with atypical features or seasonal onset can be treated with bupropion or an SSRI with good results. MAO inhibitors appear more effective than TCAs and an MAO inhibitor may be used if more benign antidepressant strategies prove unsuccessful.

Melancholic depression may respond to ECT, TCAs, and SNRIs, which are preferable to SSRIs. However, SSRIs are often used in the treatment of melancholic depression and are effective in many cases.

Caution: Depressed patients often have suicidal thoughts, and the amount of drug dispensed should be appropriately controlled particularly if prescribing an MAO inhibitor, TCA, and to a lesser extent, venlafaxine. At the same time, adults with untreated depression are at higher risk for suicide than those who are treated sufficiently to reduce symptoms. It has been thought that in children and adolescent populations, antidepressants may be associated with some slightly increased risk of suicidality. One meta-analysis indicates that suicidality persists even after symptoms of depression are treated suggesting other causes, such as increased impulsivity among younger patients. After age 25, antidepressants may have neutral or possibly protective effects until age 65 years or older. The older TCAs have a narrow therapeutic index. One advantage of the newer medications is their wider margin of safety. Nonetheless, even with newer agents, because of the possibility of suicidality early in antidepressant treatment, close follow-up is indicated. In all cases of pharmacologic management of depressed states, caution is indicated until the risk of suicide is considered minimal.

1. SSRIs, SNRIs, and atypical antidepressants—The SSRIs include fluoxetine, sertraline, paroxetine, fluvoxamine, citalopram and its enantiomer escitalopram (Table 25–7). The chief advantages of these agents are that they are generally well tolerated, the starting dose is typically a therapeutic dose for most patients, and they have much lower lethality in overdose compared to TCAs or MAO inhibitors. (Notably, citalopram carries a warning regarding QT prolongation in doses above 40 mg, and caution should be used in prescribing in patients at risk for arrhythmia. There is no similar FDA warning for escitalopram as of this writing.) The SNRIs include venlafaxine, desvenlafaxine, duloxetine,

milnacipran, and levomilnacipran. In addition to possessing the strong serotonin reuptake blocking properties of the SSRIs, the SNRIs are also norepinephrine reuptake blockers. The combined serotonergic-noradrenergic properties of these drugs may provide benefits in pain conditions such as neuropathy and fibromyalgia as well as conditions such as stress incontinence. The atypical antidepressants are bupropion, nefazodone, trazodone, vilazodone, vortioxetine, and mirtazapine (Table 25–7). All of these antidepressants are effective in the treatment of depression, both typical and atypical. The SSRI medications have been effective in the treatment of panic disorder, bulimia, GAD, OCD, and PTSD.

Most of the medications in this group tend to be activating and are given in the morning so as not to interfere with sleep. Some patients, however, may have sedation, requiring that the drug be given at bedtime. This reaction occurs most commonly with paroxetine, fluvoxamine, and mirtazapine. The SSRIs can be given in once-daily dosage. Nefazodone and trazodone are usually given twice daily. Bupropion and venlafaxine are available in extended-release formulations and can be given once daily. There is usually some delay in response; fluoxetine, for example, requires 2–6 weeks to act in depression, 4–8 weeks to be effective in panic disorder, and 6–12 weeks in treatment of OCD. The starting dose (10 mg) is given for 1 week before increasing to the average daily oral dose of 20 mg for depression, while OCD may require up to 80 mg daily. Some patients, particularly the elderly, may tolerate and benefit from as little as 10 mg/day or every other day. The other SSRIs have shorter half-lives and a lesser effect on hepatic enzymes, which reduces their impact on the metabolism of other medications (thus not increasing significantly the serum concentrations of other medications as much as fluoxetine). The shorter half-lives also allow for more rapid clearing if adverse side effects appear. Venlafaxine appears to be more effective with doses greater than 200 mg/day orally, although some individuals respond to doses as low as 75 mg/day.

The **side effects** common to all of these medications are headache, nausea, tinnitus, insomnia, and nervousness. Akathisia has been common with the SSRIs; other extrapyramidal symptoms (eg, dystonias) have occurred infrequently but particularly in withdrawal states. Because SSRIs affect platelet serotonin levels, abnormal bleeding can occur. Sertraline and citalopram appear to be the safest agents in this class when used with warfarin. Sexual side effects of erectile dysfunction, retrograde ejaculation, and dysorgasmia are very common with the SSRIs. Oral phosphodiesterase-5 inhibitors (such as sildenafil, 25–50 mg; tadalafil, 5-20 mg; or vardenafil, 10–20 mg taken 1 hour prior to sexual activity) can improve erectile dysfunction in some patients and have been shown to improve other SSRI-induced sexual dysfunction in both men and women. Adjunctive bupropion (75–150 mg orally daily) may also enhance sexual arousal. Cyproheptadine, 4 mg orally prior to sexual activity, may be helpful in countering drug-induced anorgasmia but also is quite sedating and may counter the therapeutic benefits of SSRIs as well. The SSRIs are strong serotonin uptake blockers and may in high

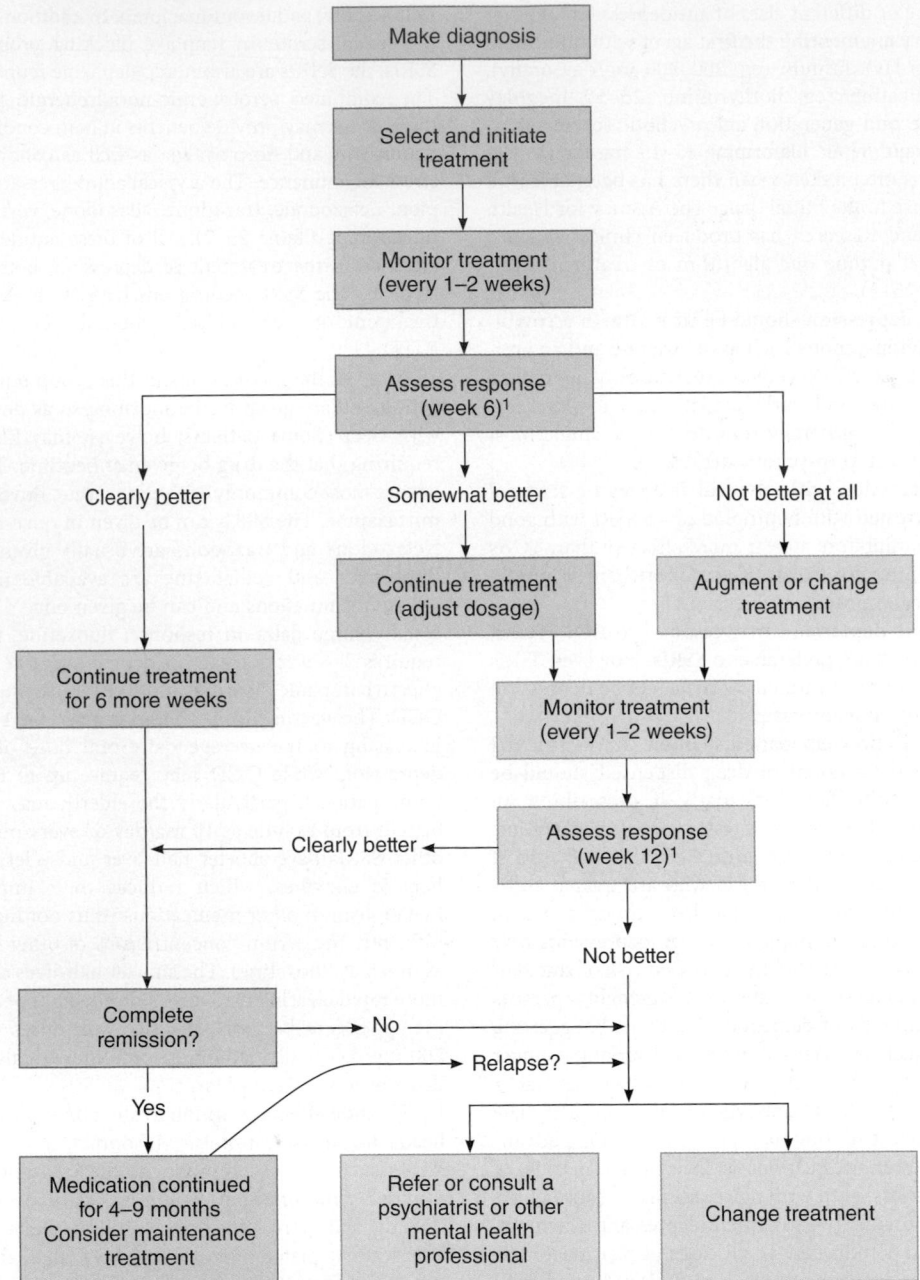

▲ Figure 25-2. Overview of treatment for depression. (Reproduced from Agency for Health Care Policy and Research: Depression in Primary Care. Vol. 2: Treatment of Major Depression. United States Department of Health and Human Services, 1993.)

dosage or in combination with MAO inhibitors, including the antiparkinsonian drug selegiline, cause a **"serotonin syndrome."** This syndrome is manifested by rigidity, hyperthermia, autonomic instability, myoclonus, confusion, delirium, and coma. This syndrome can be a particularly troublesome problem in the elderly. Research indicates that SSRIs are safer agents to use than TCAs in patients

with cardiac disease; the SSRI sertraline is a safe and effective antidepressant treatment in patients with acute myocardial infarction or unstable angina.

Withdrawal symptoms, including dizziness, paresthesias, dysphoric mood, agitation, and a flu-like state, have been reported for the shorter-acting SSRIs and SNRIs but may occur with other classes including the TCAs and

MAO inhibitors. These medications should be discontinued gradually over a period of weeks or months to reduce the risk of withdrawal phenomena.

Fluoxetine, fluvoxamine, sertraline, venlafaxine, and citalopram in customary antidepressant doses may increase the risk of major fetal malformation when used during pregnancy; however, the absolute risk of congenital defects is considered low. Maternal major mood disorder in pregnancy by itself carries its own risks to the mother and fetus and has been linked to low birth weight and preterm delivery. Postpartum effects of prenatal depression have not been studied. The decision to use SSRIs and other psychotropic agents during pregnancy and postpartum must be a collaborative decision based on a thorough risk-benefit analysis for each individual.

Venlafaxine lacks significant anticholinergic side effects. Nausea, nervousness, and profuse sweating appear to be the major side effects. Venlafaxine appears to have few drug-drug interactions. It does require monitoring of blood pressure because dose-related hypertension may develop in some individuals. Venlafaxine prescribing in the United Kingdom has been restricted to psychiatrists. Venlafaxine appears to carry a greater risk of lethal arrhythmias in instances of overdose relative to the SSRIs, but less risk than with the TCAs. Desvenlafaxine, a newer form of the drug, is started at its target dose of 50 mg/day orally and does not require upward titration although higher doses have been well studied and some patients benefit from 100 mg/day. Duloxetine may also result in small increases in blood pressure. Common side effects include dry mouth, dizziness, and fatigue. Inhibitors of 1A2 and 2D6 may increase duloxetine levels with a risk of toxicity. Milnacipran, approved for the treatment of fibromyalgia, and levomilnacipran, approved for the treatment of major depression, carry many of the side effects common to other SNRIs including a mild tachycardia, hypertension, sexual side effects, mydriasis, urinary constriction, and occasional abnormal bleeding. Levomilnacipran is started at 20 mg/day orally then increased to 40 mg/day after 2-3 days. The target dose is 40-120 mg given once daily. Milnacipran is typically started at 12.5 mg/day orally, titrated to 12.5 mg twice daily after 2 days, and then to 25 mg twice daily after 7 days. The target dose is typically 100-200 mg/day given in in two divided doses. While not approved for the treatment of major depression, the evidence suggests that milnacipran, like levomilnacipran, is an effective antidepressant agent.

Nefazodone appears to lack the anticholinergic effects of the TCAs and the agitation sometimes induced by SSRIs. Nefazodone should not be given with terfenadine, astemizole, or cisapride, which are not commercially available in the United States. Because nefazodone inhibits the liver's cytochrome P450 3A4 isoenzymes, concurrent use of these medications can lead to serious QT prolongation, ventricular tachycardia, or death. Through the same mechanism of enzyme inhibition, nefazodone can elevate cyclosporine levels sixfold to tenfold. Nefazodone carries an FDA warning given its association with liver failure in rare cases. Pretreatment and ongoing monitoring of liver enzymes are indicated.

Mirtazapine is thought to enhance central noradrenergic and serotonergic activity with minimal sexual side effects compared with the SSRIs. Its action as a potent antagonist of histaminergic receptors may make it a useful agent for patients with depression and insomnia. It is also an effective antiemetic due to its antagonism of the 5-HT$_3$ receptor. Its most common adverse side effects include somnolence, increased appetite, weight gain, lipid abnormalities, and dizziness. The labeling for mirtazapine indicated that agranulocytosis was seen in 2 of 2796 patients in premarketing studies. Since 2004, a few case reports have linked mirtazapine to neutropenia. However, given the widespread use of mirtazapine over the past 10 years, the association of agranulocytosis or a clinically significant neutropenia with the drug appears to be modest. Although it is metabolized by P450 isoenzymes, it is not an inhibitor of this system. It is given in a single oral dose at bedtime starting at 15 mg and increasing in 15-mg increments every week or every other week up to 45 mg.

Vortioxetine is a newer antidepressant that blocks serotonin reuptake, is a partial agonist of the 5-HT$_{1A}$ receptor, and effects a variety of other serotonin receptor sites. The side effects attributed to its serotonergic effects include gastrointestinal upset and sexual dysfunction. Vortioxetine has demonstrated efficacy in improving cognitive symptoms of depression and received regulatory approval for this indication in Europe. Vortioxetine is typically dosed at 10 mg/day orally and may be increased to 20 mg/day.

2. Tricyclic antidepressants (TCAs) and clinically similar medications—TCAs were the mainstay of drug therapy for depression for many years. They have also been effective in panic disorder, pain syndromes, and anxiety states. Specific ones have been effective in OCD (clomipramine), enuresis (imipramine), psychotic depression (amoxapine), and reduction of craving in cocaine withdrawal (desipramine).

TCAs are characterized more by their similarities than by their differences. They tend to affect both serotonin and norepinephrine reuptake; some medications act mainly on the former and others principally on the latter neurotransmitter system. Individuals receiving the same dosages vary markedly in therapeutic drug levels achieved (elderly patients require smaller doses), and determination of plasma drug levels is helpful when clinical response has been disappointing. Nortriptyline is usually effective when plasma levels are between 50 and 150 ng/mL; imipramine at plasma levels of 200-250 ng/mL; and desipramine at plasma levels of 100-250 ng/mL. High blood levels are not more effective than moderate levels and may be counterproductive (eg, delirium, seizures). Patients with gastrointestinal side effects benefit from plasma level monitoring to assess absorption of the drug. Most TCAs can be given in a single dose at bedtime, starting at fairly low doses (eg, nortriptyline 25 mg orally) and increasing by 25 mg every several days as tolerated until the therapeutic response is achieved (eg, nortriptyline, 100-150 mg) or to maximum dose if necessary (eg, nortriptyline, 150 mg). The most common cause of treatment failure is an inadequate trial. A full trial consists of giving a therapeutic daily dosage for at least 6 weeks. Because of marked anticholinergic and sedating side effects, clomipramine is started at a low dose (25 mg/day orally) and increased slowly in divided doses up to 100 mg/day, held at that level for several days, and then gradually increased as necessary up to 250 mg/day. Any of the TCA-like medications should be started at very low doses (eg, 10–25 mg/day) and increased slowly in the treatment of panic disorder.

The TCAs have anticholinergic side effects to varying degrees (amitriptyline 100 mg is equivalent to atropine 5 mg). One must be particularly wary of the effect in elderly men with prostatic hyperplasia. The anticholinergic effects also predispose to other medical problems such as constipation, confusion, heat stroke, or dental problems from xerostomia. Orthostatic hypotension is fairly common, is not dose-dependent and may not remit with time on medication; this may predispose to falls and hip fractures in the elderly. Cardiac effects of the TCAs are functions of the anticholinergic effect, direct myocardial depression, quinidine-like effect, and interference with adrenergic neurons. These factors may produce altered rate, rhythm, and contractility, particularly in patients with preexisting cardiac disease, such as bundle-branch or bifascicular block. Even relatively small overdoses (eg, 1500 mg of imipramine) have resulted in lethal arrhythmias. Electrocardiographic changes range from benign ST segment and T wave changes and sinus tachycardia to a variety of complex and serious arrhythmias, the latter requiring a change in medication. Because TCAs have class I antiarrhythmic effects, they should be used with caution in patients with ischemic heart disease, arrhythmias, or conduction disturbances. SSRIs or the atypical antidepressants are better initial choices for this population. TCAs lower the seizure threshold so this is of particular concern in patients with a propensity for seizures. Loss of libido and erectile, ejaculatory, and orgasmic dysfunction are fairly common and can compromise compliance. Trazodone rarely causes priapism (1 in 9000), but when it occurs, it requires treatment within 12 hours (epinephrine 1:1000 injected into the corpus cavernosum). Delirium, agitation, and mania are infrequent complications of the TCAs but can occur. Sudden discontinuation of some of these medications can produce "cholinergic rebound," manifested by headaches and nausea with abdominal cramps. Overdoses of TCAs are often serious because of the narrow therapeutic index and quinidine-like effects (see Chapter 38).

3. Monoamine oxidase inhibitors—The MAO inhibitors are generally used as third-line medications for depression (after a failure of SSRIs, SNRIs, TCAs, or the atypical antidepressants) because of the dietary and other restrictions required (Table 25–8). They should be considered third-line medications for refractory panic disorder as well as depression; however, this hierarchy has become more flexible since MAO inhibitor skin patches (selegiline) have become available. They deliver the MAO inhibitor to the bloodstream bypassing the gastrointestinal tract so that dietary restrictions are not necessary in the lowest dosage strength (6 mg/24 h).

The MAO inhibitors commonly cause symptoms of orthostatic hypotension (which may persist) and

Table 25–8. Principal dietary restrictions in MAOI use.

1. Cheese, except cream cheese and cottage cheese and fresh yogurt
2. Fermented or aged meats such as bologna, salami
3. Broad bean pods such as Chinese bean pods
4. Liver of all types
5. Meat and yeast extracts
6. Red wine, sherry, vermouth, cognac, beer, ale
7. Soy sauce, shrimp paste, sauerkraut

MAOI, monoamine oxidase inhibitor.

sympathomimetic effects of tachycardia, sweating, and tremor. Nausea, insomnia (often associated with intense afternoon drowsiness), and sexual dysfunction are common. Zolpidem 5–10 mg orally at bedtime can ameliorate MAO-induced insomnia. Central nervous system effects include agitation and toxic psychoses. Dietary limitations (see Table 25–8) and abstinence from drug products containing phenylpropanolamine, phenylephrine, meperidine, dextromethorphan, and pseudoephedrine are mandatory for MAO-A type inhibitors (those marketed for treatment of depression), since the reduction of available MAO leaves the patient vulnerable to exogenous amines (eg, tyramine in foodstuffs).

4. Stimulants—Dextroamphetamine (5–30 mg/day orally) and methylphenidate (10–45 mg/day orally) may be effective for the short-term treatment of some depressive symptoms in medically ill and geriatric patients. The stimulants are notable for rapid onset of action (hours) and a paucity of side effects (tachycardia, agitation) in most patients. They are usually given in two divided doses early in the day (eg, 7 am and noon) so as to avoid interfering with sleep. These agents may also be useful as adjunctive agents in refractory depression. Ketamine infusion has been shown to lead to a rapid improvement in depressive symptoms in some patients; however, effects of a single treatment are short-lived (about 3–7 days). Ketamine and other NMDA antagonists continue to be evaluated in the treatment of resistant depression.

5. Switching and combination therapy—If the therapeutic response has been poor after an adequate trial with the chosen drug, the diagnosis should be reassessed. Assuming that the trial has been adequate and the diagnosis is correct, a trial with a second drug is appropriate. In switching from one group to another, an adequate "washout time" must be allowed. This is critical in certain situations—eg, in switching from an MAO inhibitor to a TCA, allow 2–3 weeks between stopping one drug and starting another; in switching from an SSRI to an MAO inhibitor, allow 4–5 weeks for fluoxetine and at least 2 weeks for other SSRIs. In switching within groups—eg, from one TCA to another (amitriptyline to desipramine, etc)—no washout time is needed, and one can rapidly decrease the dosage of one drug while increasing the other. In clinical practice, adjunctive treatment with lithium, buspirone, or thyroid hormone may be helpful in depression. The adjunctive use of low-dose atypical antipsychotics such as aripiprazole, olanzapine, and quetiapine in the treatment of patients with refractory depression is supported by research. The side effect risk is the same as when treating psychosis. Monotherapy with aripiprazole or quetiapine is FDA approved for this purpose as well as the combination of fluoxetine and olanzapine. Adding an atypical agent requires monitoring body mass index, lipids, and glucose. Combining two antidepressants, or adding an antipsychotic to an antidepressant, requires caution and is usually reserved for clinicians who feel comfortable managing this or after psychiatric consultation.

6. Maintenance and tapering—When clinical relief of symptoms is obtained, medication is continued for 12 months in the effective maintenance dosage, which is the dosage required in the acute stage. The full dosage should be continued indefinitely when the individual has a first episode before age 20 or after age 50, is over age 40 with two episodes, at least one episode after age 50, or has had three episodes at any age. Major depression should often be considered a chronic disease. If the medication is being tapered, it should be done gradually over several months, monitoring closely for relapse.

7. Drug interactions—Interactions with other medications are listed in Table 25–9.

8. Electroconvulsive therapy—ECT causes a generalized central nervous system seizure (peripheral convulsion is not necessary) by means of electric current. The key objective is to exceed the seizure threshold, which can be accomplished by a variety of means. The mechanism of action is not known, but it is thought to involve major neurotransmitter responses at the cell membrane. Electrical current insufficient to cause a seizure produces no therapeutic benefit.

ECT is the most effective (about 70–85%) treatment of severe depression—particularly the delusions and agitation commonly seen with depression in the elderly. It is indicated when medical conditions preclude the use of antidepressants, nonresponsiveness to these medications, and extreme suicidality. Comparative controlled studies of ECT in severe depression show that it is more effective than pharmacotherapy. It is also effective in the treatment of mania and psychoses during pregnancy (when medications may be contraindicated). It has not been shown to be helpful in chronic schizophrenic disorders, and it is generally not used in acute schizophrenic episodes unless medications are not effective and it is urgent that the psychosis be controlled (eg, a catatonic stupor complicating an acute medical condition).

The most common side effects are memory disturbance and headache. Memory loss or confusion is usually related to the number and frequency of ECT treatments and proper oxygenation during treatment. Unilateral ECT is associated with less memory loss than bilateral ECT. Both anterograde and retrograde memory loss may occur, but short term-retrograde memory loss is more common. While some memory deficits may persist, memory loss tends to improve in a few weeks after the last

Table 25–9. Antidepressant drug interactions with other medications.

Drug	Effects
Tricyclic and other non-MAOI antidepressants	
Antacids	Decreased absorption of antidepressants
Anticoagulants	Increased hypoprothrombinemic effect
Cimetidine	Increased antidepressant blood levels and psychosis
Clonidine	Decreased antihypertensive effect
Digitalis	Increased incidence of heart block
Disulfiram	Increased antidepressant blood levels
Haloperidol	Increased antidepressant levels
Insulin	Decreased blood sugar
Lithium	Increased lithium levels with fluoxetine
Methyldopa	Decreased antihypertensive effect
Other anticholinergic medications	Marked anticholinergic responses
Phenytoin	Increased blood levels
Procainamide	Decreased ventricular conduction
Procarbazine	Hypertensive crisis
Propranolol	Increased hypotension
Quinidine	Decreased ventricular conduction
Rauwolfia derivatives	Increased stimulation
Sedatives	Increased sedation
Sympathomimetic medications	Increased vasopressor effect
Terfenadine,[1] astemizole,[1] cisapride[1]	Torsades de pointes
MAOIs	
Antihistamines	Increased sedation
Belladonna-like medications	Increased blood pressure
Dextromethorphan	Same as meperidine
Guanethidine	Decreased blood pressure
Insulin	Decreased blood sugar
Levodopa	Increased blood pressure
Meperidine	Increased agitation, serotonin syndrome, death
Methyldopa	Decreased blood pressure
Pseudoephedrine	Hypertensive crisis (increased blood pressure)
Reserpine	Increased blood pressure and temperature
Succinylcholine	Increased neuromuscular blockade
Sulfonylureas	Decreased blood sugar
Sympathomimetic medications	Increased blood pressure/hypertensive crisis
SSRIs, SNRIs, triptans	Serotonin syndrome, death

[1]Terfenadine, astemizole, and cisapride are not commercially available in the United States.
MAOIs, monoamine oxidase inhibitors; SNRIs, serotonin norepinephrine reuptake inhibitors; SSRIs, selective serotonin reuptake inhibitors.

ECT treatment. There have been reports that lithium administration concurrent with ECT resulted in greater memory loss.

Increased intracranial pressure is a relative contraindication. Other problems such as cardiac disorders, aortic aneurysms, bronchopulmonary disease, and venous thrombosis must be evaluated in light of the severity of the medical problem versus the need for ECT. Serious complications arising from ECT occur in less than 1 in 1000 cases. Most of these problems are cardiovascular or respiratory in nature (eg, aspiration of gastric contents, arrhythmias, myocardial infarction). Poor patient understanding and lack of acceptance of the technique by the public are the biggest obstacles to the use of ECT.

9. Phototherapy—Phototherapy is used in major depression with seasonal onset. It consists of exposure to a light source of greater than 2500 lux for 2 hours daily to increase the photoperiod of the day. Light visors are an adaptation that provides greater mobility and an adjustable light intensity but may not be as effective. The dosage varies, with some patients requiring morning and night exposure. One effect is alteration of biorhythm through melatonin mechanisms.

10. Other treatments—Transcranial magnetic stimulation appears to be effective in nonpsychotic depression and involves the application of electromagnetic pulses to the dorsolateral prefrontal cortex. Its use in depression is approved by the FDA for individuals who have not tolerated or responded to standard medications. It is usually delivered in a course of 20–30 sessions over 4–6 weeks. While not as effective as ECT, transcranial magnetic stimulation neither requires general anesthesia nor is it associated with cognitive side effects. Vagus nerve stimulation has shown promise in about one-third of extremely refractory cases and is approved by the FDA but has not been approved by many insurers. Deep brain stimulation continues to be explored for the treatment of refractory depression but controlled studies have not shown success to date.

B. Psychological

It is seldom possible to engage an individual in penetrating psychotherapeutic endeavors during the acute stage of a severe depression. While medications may be taking effect, a supportive approach to strengthen existing coping mechanisms and appropriate consideration of the patient's continuing need to function at work, to engage in recreational activities, etc, are necessary as the severity of the depression lessens. If the patient is not seriously depressed, it is often appropriate to initiate intensive psychotherapeutic efforts, since flux periods are a good time to effect change. A catharsis of repressed anger and guilt may be beneficial. Therapy during or just after the acute stage may focus on coping techniques, with some practice of alternative choices. Depression-specific psychotherapies help improve self-esteem, increase assertiveness, and lessen dependency. Interpersonal psychotherapy for depression has shown efficacy in the treatment of acute depression, helping patients master interpersonal stresses and develop new coping strategies. Cognitive behavioral therapy for depression addresses patients' patterns of negative thoughts, called cognitive distortions, which lead to feelings of depression and anxiety. Treatment usually includes homework assignments such as keeping a journal of cognitive distortions and of positive responses to them. The combination of drug therapy plus interpersonal psychotherapy or cognitive behavioral therapy is generally more effective than either modality alone. It is usually helpful to involve the spouse or other significant family members early in treatment. Mindfulness-based cognitive therapy has reduced relapse rates in several randomized controlled trials. In two studies, it was as effective as maintenance medication in preventing relapse. This therapy incorporates meditation and teaches patients to distance themselves from depressive thinking. It may be a preferable alternative for individuals who wish to have an alternative to long-term medications to stay free of depressive episodes.

C. Social

Flexible use of appropriate social services can be of major importance in the treatment of depression. Since alcohol abuse is often associated with depression, early involvement in alcohol treatment programs such as Alcoholics Anonymous can be important to future success (see Alcohol Use Disorder [Alcoholism]). The structuring of daily activities during severe depression is often quite difficult for the patient, and loneliness is often a major factor. The help of family, employer, or friends is often necessary to mobilize the patient who experiences no joy in daily activities and tends to remain uninvolved and to deteriorate. Insistence on sharing activities will help involve the patient in simple but important daily functions. In some severe cases, the use of day treatment centers or support groups of a specific type (eg, mastectomy groups) is indicated. It is not unusual for a patient to have multiple legal, financial, and vocational problems requiring legal and vocational assistance.

D. Behavioral

When depression is a function of self-defeating coping techniques such as passivity, the role-playing approach can be useful. Behavioral techniques, including desensitization, may be used in problems such as phobias where depression is a by-product. When depression is a regularly used interpersonal style, behavioral counseling to family members or others can help in extinguishing the behavior in the patient. Behavioral activation, a technique of motivating depressed patients to begin engaging in pleasurable activities, has been shown to be a useful depression-specific psychotherapy.

▶ Treatment of Mania

Acute manic or hypomanic symptoms will respond to lithium or valproic acid after several days of treatment, but it is increasingly common to use second-generation antipsychotics as first-line agents. The antipsychotics act more rapidly than agents such as lithium or valproate and do not require serum level monitoring. High-potency benzodiazepines (eg, clonazepam) may also be useful adjuncts in managing the agitation and sleep disturbance that are features of manic and hypomanic episodes. Some schizoaffective disorders and some cases of so-called schizophrenia are probably atypical bipolar affective disorder, for which lithium treatment may be effective.

A. Antipsychotics

Acute manic symptoms may be treated initially with a second-generation antipsychotic such as olanzapine, (eg, 5–20 mg orally), risperidone (2–3 mg orally), or aripiprazole (15–30 mg) in conjunction with a benzodiazepine if indicated. All of the available oral second-generation antipsychotics and many of the first-generation agents appear to be more rapidly effective in the management of acute mania than are mood stabilizers such as lithium or valproate. Alternatively, when behavioral control is immediately necessary, olanzapine in an injectable form (2.5–10 mg intramuscularly) or haloperidol, 5–10 mg orally or intramuscularly repeated as needed until symptoms subside, may be used. The dosage of the antipsychotic may be gradually reduced after lithium or another mood stabilizer is started. Olanzapine, quetiapine, and aripiprazole are approved as maintenance treatments for bipolar disorder to prevent subsequent cycles of both mania and depression.

B. Valproic Acid

Valproic acid (divalproex) is a first-line treatment for mania because it has a broader index of safety than lithium. This issue is particularly important in AIDS or other medically ill patients prone to dehydration or malabsorption with wide swings in serum lithium levels. Valproic acid has also been used effectively in panic disorder and migraine headache. Treatment is often started at a dose of 750 mg/day orally in divided doses, and dosage is then titrated to achieve therapeutic serum levels. Oral loading in acutely manic bipolar patients in an inpatient setting (initiated at a dosage of 20 mg/kg/day) can safely achieve serum therapeutic levels in 2–3 days. Concomitant use of aspirin may increase valproate levels, carbamazepine or phenytoin may decrease valproate levels, while warfarin levels may be elevated by valproate. Gastrointestinal symptoms and weight gain are the main side effects. Liver function tests, complete blood counts, glucose levels, and weight should be monitored at 2 weeks, 4 weeks, and at 3 months initially and annually or more frequently thereafter based on clinical judgment. Significant teratogenic effects are a concern so pregnancy should be ruled out prior to initiation. In utero exposure to valproate has been associated with adversely affecting intellectual development in the fetus and there is an FDA warning to that effect. Thus, alternatives to valproate should be considered in women of childbearing years who might become pregnant.

C. Lithium

As a prophylactic drug for bipolar affective disorder, lithium significantly decreases the frequency and severity of both manic and depressive attacks in about 50–70% of patients. Lithium appears to work best in patients with classic bipolar I disorder. Antipsychotics, valproate, lamotrigine, and carbamazepine may be more effective than lithium in the management of rapid cycling and mixed episodes. A positive response to lithium is more predictable if the patient has a low frequency of episodes (no more than two per year with intervals free of psychopathology). A positive response occurs more frequently in individuals who have blood relatives with a diagnosis of manic or hypomanic episodes.

In addition to its use in manic states, lithium is sometimes useful in the prophylaxis of recurrent unipolar depressions (perhaps undiagnosed bipolar disorder). Lithium may ameliorate nonspecific aggressive behaviors and dyscontrol syndromes. The dosages are the same as used in bipolar disorder. Most patients with bipolar disease can be managed long-term with lithium alone, although some will require continued or intermittent use of an antipsychotic, antidepressant, or carbamazepine. An excellent resource for information is the Lithium Information Center, http://www.miminc.org/aboutlithinfoctr.html.

Before treatment, the clinical workup should include a medical history and physical examination; complete blood count; T4, thyroid-stimulating hormone, blood urea nitrogen (BUN), serum creatinine, and serum electrolyte determinations; urinalysis; and electrocardiography (in patients over age 45 or with a history of cardiac disease). Compliance with lithium therapy is adversely affected by the loss of some hypomanic experiences valued by the patient. These include social extroversion and a sense of heightened enjoyment in many activities such as sex and business dealings, often with increased productivity in the latter.

1. Dosage—The common starting dosage of lithium carbonate is 300 mg orally two or three times daily, with trough blood levels measured after 5 days of treatment. In a small minority of patients, a slow release form or units of different dosage may be required. Lithium citrate is available as a syrup. The dosage is that required to maintain blood levels in the therapeutic range. For acute attacks, this ranges from 1 to 1.5 mEq/L. Although there is controversy about the optimal long-term maintenance dose, many clinicians reduce the acute level to 0.6–1 mEq/L in order to reduce side effects. The dose required to meet this need will vary in different individuals. For acute mania, doses of 1200–1800 mg/day are generally recommended. Augmentation of antidepressants is usually achieved with half of these doses. Once-a-day dosage is acceptable, but most patients have less nausea when they take the drug in divided doses with meals.

Lithium is readily absorbed, with peak serum levels occurring within 1–3 hours and complete absorption in 8 hours. Half of the total body lithium is excreted in 18–24 hours (95% in the urine). Blood for lithium levels should be drawn 12 hours after the last dose. Serum levels should be measured 5–7 days after initiation of treatment and changes in dose. For maintenance treatment, lithium levels should be monitored initially every 1–2 months but may be measured every 6–12 months in stable, long-term patients. Levels should be monitored more closely when there is any condition that causes volume depletion (eg, diarrhea, dehydration, use of diuretics).

2. Side effects—**Early side effects** include mild gastrointestinal symptoms (take lithium with food and in divided doses), fine tremors (treat with propranolol, 20–60 mg/day orally, only if persistent), slight muscle weakness, and some degree of somnolence can occur and are usually transient. Moderate polyuria (reduced renal responsiveness to ADH) and polydipsia (associated with increased plasma renin concentration) are often present. Potassium administration can blunt this effect, as may once-daily dosing of lithium. Weight gain (often a result of calories in fluids taken for polydipsia) and leukocytosis not due to infection are fairly common.

Thyroid side effects include goiter (3%; often euthyroid) and hypothyroidism (10%; concomitant administration of lithium and iodide or lithium and carbamazepine enhances the hypothyroid and goitrogenic effect of either drug). Most clinicians treat lithium-induced hypothyroidism (more common in women) with thyroid hormone while continuing lithium therapy. Changes in the glucose tolerance test toward a diabetes-like curve, nephrogenic diabetes insipidus (usually resolving about 8 weeks after cessation of lithium therapy), nephrotic syndrome, edema, folate deficiency, and pseudotumor cerebri (ophthalmoscopy is indicated if there are complaints of headache or blurred vision) can occur. Thyroid and kidney function should be checked at 4- to 6-month intervals. Hypercalcemia and elevated parathyroid hormone levels occur in some patients. Electrocardiographic abnormalities (principally T wave flattening or inversion) may occur during lithium administration but are not of major clinical significance. Sinoatrial block may occur, particularly in the elderly. Other medications that prolong intraventricular conduction, such as TCAs, must be used cautiously in conjunction with lithium. Lithium impairs ventilatory function in patients with airway obstruction. Lithium alone does not have a significant effect on sexual function, but when combined with benzodiazepines (clonazepam in most symptomatic patients) it causes sexual dysfunction in about 50% of men. Lithium may precipitate or exacerbate psoriasis in some patients. Most of these side effects subside when lithium is discontinued; when residual side effects exist, they are usually not serious.

Side effects from long-term lithium therapy include the development of cogwheel rigidity and, occasionally, other extrapyramidal signs. Lithium potentiates the parkinsonian effects of haloperidol. Long-term lithium therapy has also been associated with a relative lowering of the level of memory and perceptual processing (affecting compliance in some cases). Some impairment of attention and emotional reactivity has also been noted. Lithium-induced delirium with therapeutic lithium levels is an infrequent complication usually occurring in the elderly and may persist for several days after serum levels have become negligible. Encephalopathy has occurred in patients receiving combined lithium and antipsychotic therapy and in those who have cerebrovascular disease, thus requiring careful evaluation of patients who develop neurotoxic signs at subtoxic blood levels.

Some reports have suggested that the long-term use of lithium may have adverse effects on kidney function (with interstitial fibrosis, tubular atrophy, or nephrogenic diabetes insipidus). Persistent polyuria should require an investigation of the kidney's ability to concentrate urine. A rise in serum creatinine levels is an indication for in-depth evaluation of kidney function and consideration of alternative treatments if the individual can tolerate a change. Incontinence has been reported in women, apparently related to changes in bladder cholinergic-adrenergic balance.

Prospective studies suggest that the overall risk imposed by lithium in pregnancy may be overemphasized. However, lithium exposure in early pregnancy does increase the frequency of congenital anomalies, especially Ebstein and other major cardiovascular anomalies. For women who take psychotropic medications who become pregnant, the decision to make a change in medication is complex and requires informed consent regarding the relative risks to the patient and fetus. Indeed, the risk of untreated bipolar disorder carries its own risks for pregnancy. Formula feeding should be considered in mothers taking lithium, since concentration in breast milk is one-third to half that in serum.

Frank toxicity usually occurs at blood lithium levels greater than 2 mEq/L. Because sodium and lithium are reabsorbed at the same loci in the proximal renal tubules, any sodium loss (diarrhea, use of diuretics, or excessive perspiration) results in increased lithium levels. Symptoms and signs include vomiting and diarrhea, the latter exacerbating the problem since more sodium is lost and more lithium is absorbed. Other symptoms and signs, some of which may not be reversible, include tremors, marked muscle weakness, confusion, dysarthria, vertigo, choreoathetosis, ataxia, hyperreflexia, rigidity, lack of coordination, myoclonus, seizures, opisthotonos, and coma. Toxicity is more severe in the elderly, who should be maintained on slightly lower serum levels. Lithium overdosage may be accidental or intentional or may occur as a result of poor monitoring. Significant overdoses of lithium are typically managed with hemodialysis since the drug is excreted completely by the kidneys.

See Chapter 38 for the treatment of patients with massive ingestions of lithium or blood lithium levels greater than 2.5 mEq/L.

3. Drug interactions—Patients receiving lithium should use diuretics with caution and only under close medical supervision. The thiazide diuretics cause increased lithium reabsorption from the proximal renal tubules, resulting in increased serum lithium levels (Table 25–10), and adjustment of lithium intake must be made to compensate for this. Reduce lithium dosage by 25–40% when the patient is receiving 50 mg of hydrochlorothiazide daily. Potassium-sparing diuretics (spironolactone, amiloride, triamterene) may also increase serum lithium levels and require careful monitoring of lithium levels. Loop diuretics (furosemide, ethacrynic acid, bumetanide) do not appear to alter serum lithium levels. Concurrent use of lithium and

Table 25–10. Lithium interactions with other medications.

Drug	Effects
ACE inhibitors	↑ Lithium levels
Celecoxib	↑ Lithium levels
Fluoxetine	↑ Lithium levels
Ibuprofen	↑ Lithium levels
Indomethacin	↑ Lithium levels
Methyldopa	Rigidity, mutism, fascicular twitching
Osmotic diuretics (urea, mannitol)	↑ Lithium excretion
Phenylbutazone	↑ Lithium levels
Potassium-sparing diuretics (spironolactone, amiloride, triamterene)	↑ Lithium levels
Sodium bicarbonate	↑ Lithium excretion
Succinylcholine	↑ Duration of action of succinylcholine
Theophylline, aminophylline	↑ Lithium excretion
Thiazide diuretics	↑ Lithium levels
Valproic acid	↓ Lithium levels

ACE, angiotensin-converting enzyme.

angiotensin-converting enzyme inhibitors requires a 50–75% reduction in lithium intake.

D. Carbamazepine

Carbamazepine is used in the treatment of bipolar patients who cannot be satisfactorily treated with lithium (nonresponsive, excessive side effects, or rapid cycling). It is often effective at 800–1600 mg/day orally. It has also been used in the treatment of trigeminal neuralgias and alcohol withdrawal as well as in patients with behavioral dyscontrol. It suppresses some phases of kindling (see Stimulants) and has been used to treat residual symptoms in previous stimulant abusers (eg, PTSD with impulse control problems). Dose-related side effects include sedation and ataxia. Dosages start at 400–600 mg orally daily and are increased slowly to therapeutic levels. Skin rashes and a mild reduction in white count are common. SIADH occurs rarely. Nonsteroidal anti-inflammatory medications (except aspirin), the antibiotics erythromycin and isoniazid, the calcium channel blockers verapamil and diltiazem (but not nifedipine), fluoxetine, propoxyphene, and cimetidine all increase carbamazepine levels. Carbamazepine can be effective in conjunction with lithium, although there have been reports of reversible neurotoxicity with the combination. Carbamazepine stimulates hepatic microsomal enzymes and so tends to decrease levels of haloperidol and oral contraceptives. It also lowers T_4, free T_4, and T_3 levels. Cases of fetal malformation (particularly spina bifida) have been reported along with growth deficiency and

developmental delay. Liver tests and complete blood counts should be monitored in patients taking carbamazepine. Genetic studies suggest that screening for the HLA-B1502 allele in the Han Chinese population and the HLA-A3101 allele in northern Europeans may help target individuals more susceptible to a serious rash. **Oxcarbazepine,** a derivative of carbamazepine, does not appear to induce its own metabolism and is associated with fewer drug interactions, although it may impose a higher risk of hyponatremia. FDA-approved for partial seizures, oxcarbazepine may have efficacy in acute mania. It appears to be a safer alternative to carbamazepine due to its lower risk of hepatotoxicity.

E. Lamotrigine

Lamotrigine is thought to inhibit neuronal sodium channels and the release of the excitatory amino acids, glutamate and aspartate. It is FDA approved for the maintenance treatment of bipolar disorder. Two double-blind studies support its efficacy in the treatment of acute bipolar depression as adjunctive therapy or as monotherapy but several other controlled studies failed to demonstrate benefit. Likewise, lamotrigine has not proven effective in the management of acute mania. Its metabolism is inhibited by coadministration of valproic acid—doubling its half-life—and accelerated by hepatic enzyme-inducing agents such as carbamazepine. More frequent mild side effects include headache, dizziness, nausea, and diplopia. Rash occurring in 10% of patients is an indication for immediate cessation of dosing, since lamotrigine has been associated with Stevens-Johnson syndrome (1:1000) and, rarely, toxic epidermal necrolysis. Dosing starts at 25–50 mg/day orally and is titrated upward slowly to decrease the likelihood of rash. Slower titration and a lower total dose are indicated for patients taking valproic acid.

▶ **Prognosis**

Most depressive episodes are usually time-limited, and the prognosis with treatment is good if a pathologic pattern of adjustment does not intervene. Major affective disorders frequently respond well to a full trial of drug treatment. However, at least 20% of patients will have a more chronic illness lasting 2 or more years. Many patients do not sustain a complete remission of symptoms and most depressive episodes recur. At least 80% of patients who have a single major depressive episode will have one or more recurrences within 15 years of the index episode. Many patients, therefore, require long-term maintenance therapy with antidepressants.

Mania has a good prognosis with adequate treatment, although patient adherence to treatment is often quite challenging. Few effective treatments exist for bipolar depression, which include quetiapine, lurasidone, and the combination of fluoxetine and olanzapine. Most patients with bipolar disorder require treatment with two or more medications such as lithium, antipsychotics and sleeping agents. Breakthrough manic or depressive episodes are common, even with adherence to maintenance treatments, although maintenance therapy lessens the risk of recurrent episodes.

Geddes JR et al. Treatment of bipolar disorder. Lancet. 2013 May 11;381(9878):1672–82. [PMID: 23663953]

George MS et al. The expanding evidence base for rTMS treatment of depression. Curr Opin Psychiatry. 2013 Jan;26(1):13–8. [PMID: 23154644]

Gibbons RD et al. Suicidal thoughts and behavior with antidepressant treatment: reanalysis of the randomized placebo-controlled studies of fluoxetine and venlafaxine. Arch Gen Psychiatry. 2012 Jun;69(6):580–7. [PMID: 22309973]

Kéri S et al. Blood biomarkers of depression track clinical changes during cognitive-behavioral therapy. J Affect Disord. 2014 Aug;164:118–22. [PMID: 24856564]

Köhler S et al. The challenge of treatment in bipolar depression: evidence from clinical guidelines, treatment recommendations and complex treatment situations. Pharmacopsychiatry. 2014 Mar;47(2):53–9. [PMID: 24549861]

Malhi GS et al. Pharmacological management of unipolar depression. Acta Psychiatr Scand Suppl. 2013;(443):6–23. [PMID: 23586873]

Orsolini L et al. Serotonin reuptake inhibitors and breastfeeding: a systematic review. Hum Psychopharmacol. 2015 Jan;30(1):4–20. [PMID: 25572308]

Phillips ML et al. Bipolar disorder diagnosis: challenges and future directions. Lancet. 2013 May 11;381(9878):1663–71. [PMID: 23663952]

Robinson GE. Controversies about the use of antidepressants in pregnancy. J Nerv Ment Dis. 2015 Mar;203(3):159–63. [PMID: 25714252]

SLEEP-WAKE DISORDERS

Sleep consists of two distinct states as shown by electroencephalographic studies: (1) REM (rapid eye movement) sleep, also called dream sleep, D state sleep, paradoxic sleep, and (2) NREM (non-REM) sleep, also called S stage sleep, which is divided into stages 1, 2, 3, and 4 and is recognizable by different electroencephalographic patterns. Stages 3 and 4 are "delta" sleep. Dreaming occurs mostly in REM and to a lesser extent in NREM sleep.

Sleep is a cyclic phenomenon, with four or five REM periods during the night accounting for about one-fourth of the total night's sleep (1.5–2 hours). The first REM period occurs about 80–120 minutes after onset of sleep and lasts about 10 minutes. Later REM periods are longer (15–40 minutes) and occur mostly in the last several hours of sleep. Most stage 4 (deepest) sleep occurs in the first several hours.

Age-related changes in normal sleep include an unchanging percentage of REM sleep and a marked decrease in stage 3 and stage 4 sleep, with an increase in wakeful periods during the night. These normal changes, early bedtimes, and daytime naps play a role in the increased complaints of insomnia in older people. Variations in sleep patterns may be due to circumstances (eg, "jet lag") or to idiosyncratic patterns ("night owls") in persons who perhaps because of different "biologic rhythms" habitually go to bed late and sleep late in the morning. Creativity and rapidity of response to unfamiliar situations are impaired by loss of sleep. There are also rare individuals who have chronic difficulty in adapting to a 24-hour sleep-wake cycle (desynchronization sleep disorder), which can be resynchronized by altering exposure to light.

The three major sleep disorders are discussed below. Any persistent sleep disorder that is not attributable to another condition should be evaluated by a sleep specialist.

1. Dyssomnias (Insomnia)

► Classification & Clinical Findings

Patients may complain of difficulty getting to sleep or staying asleep, intermittent wakefulness during the night, early morning awakening, or combinations of any of these. Transient episodes are usually of little significance. Stress, caffeine, physical discomfort, daytime napping, and early bedtimes are common factors.

Psychiatric disorders are often associated with persistent insomnia. **Depression** is usually associated with fragmented sleep, decreased total sleep time, earlier onset of REM sleep, a shift of REM activity to the first half of the night, and a loss of slow wave sleep—all of which are nonspecific findings. In **manic disorders,** a reduced total sleep time and a decreased need for sleep are cardinal features and important early sign of impending mania. In addition to a decreased amount of sleep, manic episodes are characterized by a shortened REM latency and increased REM activity. Sleep-related panic attacks occur in the transition from stage 2 to stage 3 sleep in some patients with a longer REM latency in the sleep pattern preceding the attacks.

Abuse of alcohol may cause or be secondary to the sleep disturbance. There is a tendency to use alcohol as a means of getting to sleep without realizing that it disrupts the normal sleep cycle. Acute alcohol intake produces a decreased sleep latency with reduced REM sleep during the first half of the night. REM sleep is increased in the second half of the night, with an increase in total amount of slow wave sleep (stages 3 and 4). Vivid dreams and frequent awakenings are common. Chronic alcohol abuse increases stage 1 and decreases REM sleep (most medications delay or block REM sleep), with symptoms persisting for many months after the individual has stopped drinking. Acute alcohol or other sedative withdrawal causes delayed onset of sleep and REM rebound with intermittent awakening during the night.

Heavy smoking (more than a pack a day) causes difficulty falling asleep—apparently independently of the often associated increase in coffee drinking. Excess intake near bedtime of caffeine, cocaine, and other stimulants (eg, over-the-counter cold remedies) causes decreased total sleep time—mostly NREM sleep—with some increased sleep latency.

Sedative-hypnotics—specifically, the benzodiazepines, which are the most commonly prescribed medications to promote sleep—tend to increase total sleep time, decrease sleep latency, and decrease nocturnal awakening, with variable effects on NREM sleep. Nonbenzodiazepine hypnotics, such as zolpidem, have similar effects on sleep as do the benzodiazepines. Withdrawal causes just the opposite effects and results in continued use of the drug for the purpose of preventing withdrawal symptoms. Antidepressants decrease REM sleep (with marked rebound on withdrawal in the form of nightmares) and have varying effects on NREM sleep. The effect on REM sleep correlates with reports that REM sleep deprivation produces improvement in some depressions.

Persistent insomnias are also related to a wide variety of medical conditions, particularly delirium, pain, respiratory distress syndromes, uremia, asthma, thyroid disorders, and nocturia due to benign prostatic hyperplasia. Sleep apnea and restless leg movement are described below. Adequate analgesia and proper treatment of medical disorders will reduce symptoms and decrease the need for sedatives.

► Treatment

In general, there are two broad classes of treatment for insomnia, and the two may be combined: psychological (cognitive-behavioral) and pharmacologic. In situations of acute distress, such as a grief reaction, pharmacologic measures may be most appropriate. With primary insomnia, however, initial efforts should be psychologically based. This is particularly true in the elderly to avoid the potential adverse reactions of medications. The elderly population is at risk for complaints of insomnia because sleep becomes lighter and more easily disrupted with aging. Medical disorders that become more common with age may also predispose to insomnia.

A. Psychological

Psychological strategies should include educating the patient regarding good **sleep hygiene:** (1) Go to bed only when sleepy. (2) Use the bed and bedroom only for sleeping and sex. (3) If still awake after 20 minutes, leave the bedroom, pursue a restful activity (such as a bath or meditation), and only return when sleepy. (4) Get up at the same time every morning regardless of the amount of sleep during the night. (5) Discontinue caffeine and nicotine, at least in the evening if not completely. (6) Establish a daily exercise regimen. (7) Avoid alcohol as it may disrupt continuity of sleep. (8) Limit fluids in the evening. (9) Learn and practice relaxation techniques. (10) Establish a bedtime ritual and a routine time for going to sleep. Research suggests that cognitive behavioral therapy for insomnia is as effective as zolpidem with benefits sustained 1 year after treatment.

B. Medical

When the above measures are insufficient, medications may be useful. Lorazepam (0.5 mg orally nightly), temazepam (7.5–15 mg orally nightly) and the nonbenzodiazepine hypnotics, zolpidem (5–10 mg orally nightly), and zaleplon (5–10 mg orally nightly), are often effective for the elderly population and can be given in larger doses— twice what is prescribed for the elderly—in younger patients. Zolpidem is also available as a sublingual tablet to treat insomnia characterized by middle-of-the-night

awakening with difficulty falling back to sleep. The dose is 1.75 mg for women and 3.5 mg for men, taken once per night. A nonbenzodiazepine hypnotic, eszopiclone (2–3 mg orally), is similar in action to zolpidem and zaleplon and like oral zolpidem, is approved for long-term use. A lower dose of 1 mg is indicated in the elderly or those with hepatic impairment. It is important to note that short-acting agents like triazolam or zolpidem may lead to amnestic episodes if used on a daily ongoing basis. Longer-acting agents such as flurazepam (half-life of more than 48 hours) may accumulate in the elderly and lead to cognitive slowing, ataxia, falls, and somnolence. In general, it is appropriate to use medications for short courses of 1–2 weeks. The medications described above have largely replaced barbiturates as hypnotic agents because of their greater safety in overdose and their lesser hepatic enzyme induction effects. Antihistamines such as diphenhydramine (25 mg orally nightly) or hydroxyzine (25 mg orally nightly) may also be useful for sleep, as they produce no pharmacologic dependency; their anticholinergic effects may, however, produce confusion or urinary symptoms in the elderly. Trazodone, an atypical antidepressant, is a non–habit-forming, effective sleep medication in lower than antidepressant doses (25–150 mg orally at bedtime). Priapism is a rare side effect requiring emergent treatment. Ramelteon, 8 mg orally at bedtime, is a melatonin receptor agonist that helps with sleep onset and does not appear to have abuse potential. It appears to be safe for ongoing use without the development of tolerance.

The class of hypnotics dual orexin receptor antagonists (DORAs) are approved to help initiate and maintain sleep. DORAs such as suvorexant may be more effective than other hypnotics for some patients. However, the role of suvorexant has not been established relative to other hypnotics and is more expensive since it is not generically available. DORAs have shown a significant increase in depressive symptoms in a subset of patients, so other hypnotics may be a better choice in depressed patients. The dose of suvorexant is 10–20 mg orally given about 30 minutes before bedtime.

2. Hypersomnias (Disorders of Excessive Sleepiness)

► Classification & Clinical Findings

A. Breathing-Related Sleep Disorders

Obstructive sleep apnea hypopnea is by far the most common of the breathing-related sleep disorders that include central sleep apnea and sleep-related hypoventilation. Obstructive sleep apnea hypopnea is characterized by snoring, gasping, or breathing pauses during sleep and 5 or more apneas or hypopneas per hour or evidence by polysomnography or 15 or more apneas or hypopneas per hour. (See Chapter 9.)

B. Narcolepsy Hypocretin Deficiency Syndrome

Narcolepsy consists of a tetrad of symptoms: (1) sudden, brief (about 15 minutes) sleep attacks that may occur during any type of activity; (2) cataplexy—sudden loss of muscle tone involving specific small muscle groups or generalized muscle weakness that may cause the person to slump to the floor, unable to move, often associated with emotional reactions and sometimes confused with seizure disorder; (3) sleep paralysis—a generalized flaccidity of muscles with full consciousness in the transition zone between sleep and waking; and (4) hypnagogic hallucinations, visual or auditory, which may precede sleep or occur during the sleep attack. The attacks are characterized by an abrupt transition into REM sleep—a necessary criterion for diagnosis. The disorder begins in early adult life, affects both sexes equally, and usually levels off in severity at about 30 years of age.

REM sleep behavior disorder, characterized by motor dyscontrol and often violent dreams during REM sleep, may be related to narcolepsy.

C. Kleine-Levin Syndrome

This syndrome, which occurs mostly in young men, is characterized by hypersomnic attacks three or four times a year lasting up to 2 days, with hyperphagia, hypersexuality, irritability, and confusion on awakening. It has often been associated with antecedent neurologic insults. It usually remits after age 40.

D. Periodic Limb Movement Disorder

Periodic lower leg movements occur only during sleep with subsequent daytime sleepiness, anxiety, depression, and cognitive impairment. Restless leg syndrome includes movements while awake as well.

E. Shift Work Sleep Disorder

Shift work sleep disorder occurs when there is excessive fatigue as a consequence of work occurring during the normal sleep period.

▶ Treatment

Narcolepsy can be managed by daily administration of a stimulant such as dextroamphetamine sulfate, 10 mg orally in the morning, with increased dosage as necessary. Modafinil and its enantiomer armodafinil are schedule IV medications FDA-approved for treating the excessive daytime fatigue of narcolepsy, sleepiness associated with obstructive sleep apnea as well as for shift work sleep disorder. Usual dosing is 200–400 mg orally each morning for modafinil and 150–250 mg orally in the morning for armodafinil. The mechanism of action of modafinil and armodafil is unknown, yet they are thought to be less of an abuse risk than stimulants that are primarily dopaminergic. Common side effects include headache and anxiety; however, modafinil appears to be generally well tolerated. Modafinil may reduce the efficacy of cyclosporine, oral contraceptives, and other medications by inducing their hepatic metabolism. Imipramine, 75–100 mg orally daily, has been effective in treatment of cataplexy but not narcolepsy.

Periodic limb movement disorder and REM sleep behavior disorder can be treated with clonazepam with variable results. There is no treatment for Kleine-Levin syndrome.

Treatment of sleep apnea is discussed in Chapter 9.

3. Parasomnias (Abnormal Behaviors during Sleep)

These disorders (sleep terror, nightmares, sleepwalking, and enuresis) are fairly common in children and less so in adults.

Abbott SM et al. Circadian rhythm sleep-wake disorders. Psychiatr Clin North Am. 2015 Dec;38(4):805–23. [PMID: 26600110]

Khoury J et al. Primary sleep disorders. Psychiatr Clin North Am. 2015 Dec;38(4):683–704. [PMID: 26600103]

Mignot EJ. A practical guide to the therapy of narcolepsy and hypersomnia syndromes. Neurotherapeutics. 2012 Oct;9(4):739–52. [PMID: 23065655]

Reid KJ et al. Jet lag and shift work disorder. Sleep Med Clin. 2015 Dec;10(4):523–35. [PMID: 26568127]

Rhyne DN et al. Suvorexant in insomnia: efficacy, safety and place in therapy. Ther Adv Drug Saf. 2015 Oct;6(5):189–95. [PMID: 26478806]

Swanson LM et al. An open pilot of cognitive-behavioral therapy for insomnia in women with postpartum depression. Behav Sleep Med. 2013;11(4):297–307. [PMID: 23216373]

Trauer JM et al. Cognitive behavioral therapy for chronic insomnia: a systematic review and meta-analysis. Ann Intern Med. 2015 Aug 4;163(3):191–204. [PMID: 26054060]

Winkelman JW. Clinical practice. Insomnia disorder. N Engl J Med. 2015 Oct 8;373(15):1437–44. [PMID: 26444730]

DISORDERS OF AGGRESSION

Aggression and violence are symptoms rather than diseases, and most frequently they are not necessarily associated with an underlying medical condition. Clinicians are unable to predict dangerous behavior with greater than chance accuracy. Depression, schizophrenia, personality disorders, mania, paranoia, temporal lobe dysfunction, and organic mental states may be associated with acts of aggression. Impulse control disorders are characterized by physical abuse (usually of the aggressor's domestic partner or children), by pathologic intoxication, by impulsive sexual activities, and by reckless driving. Anabolic steroid usage by athletes has been associated with increased tendencies toward violent behavior.

In the United States, a significant proportion of all violent deaths are alcohol related. The ingestion of even small amounts of alcohol can result in pathologic intoxication that resembles an acute organic mental condition. Amphetamines, crack cocaine, and other stimulants are frequently associated with aggressive behavior. Phencyclidine is a drug commonly associated with violent behavior that is occasionally of a bizarre nature, partly due to lowering of the pain threshold. Domestic violence and rape are much more widespread than previously recognized. Awareness of the problem is to some degree due to increasing recognition of the rights of women and the understanding by women that they do not have to accept abuse. Acceptance of this kind of aggressive behavior inevitably leads to more, with the ultimate aggression being murder—20–50% of murders in the United States occur within the family. Police are called more for domestic disputes than all other criminal incidents combined. Children living in such family situations frequently become victims of abuse.

Features of individuals who have been subjected to long-term physical or sexual abuse are as follows: trouble expressing anger, staying angry longer, general passivity in relationships, feeling "marked for life" with an accompanying feeling of deserving to be victimized, lack of trust, and dissociation of affect from experiences. They are prone to express their psychological distress with somatization symptoms, often pain complaints. They may also have symptoms related to posttraumatic stress, as discussed above. The clinician should be suspicious about the origin of any injuries not fully explained, particularly if such incidents recur.

▶ Treatment

A. Psychological

Management of any violent individual includes appropriate psychological maneuvers. Move slowly, talk slowly with clarity and reassurance, and evaluate the situation. Strive to create a setting that is minimally disturbing, and eliminate people or things threatening to the violent individual. Do not threaten and do not touch or crowd the person. Allow no weapons in the area (an increasing problem in hospital emergency departments). Proximity to a door is comforting to both the patient and the examiner. Use a negotiator who the violent person can relate to comfortably. Food and drink are helpful in defusing the situation (as are cigarettes for those who smoke). Honesty is important. Make no false promises, bolster the patient's self-esteem, and continue to engage the subject verbally until the situation is under control. This type of individual does better with strong external controls to replace the lack of inner controls over the long term. Close probationary supervision and judicially mandated restrictions can be most helpful. There should be a major effort to help the individual avoid drug use (eg, Alcoholics Anonymous). Victims of abuse are essentially treated as any victim of trauma and, not infrequently, have evidence of PTSD.

B. Pharmacologic

Pharmacologic means are often necessary whether or not psychological approaches have been successful. This is particularly true in the agitated or psychotic patient. The drugs of choice in seriously violent or psychotic aggressive states are antipsychotics, given intramuscularly if necessary, every 1–2 hours until symptoms are alleviated. A number of second-generation intramuscular antipsychotics are FDA approved in the management of acute agitation, and include aripiprazole (9.75 mg/1.3 mL), ziprasidone (10-mg/0.5 mL), and olanzapine (10 mg/2 mL). The second-generation antipsychotics appear less likely than first-generation drugs like haloperidol (2.5–5 mg) to cause

acute extrapyramidal symptoms. However, the second-generation drugs appear no more effective than first-generation drugs and generally are more expensive. Benzodiazepine sedatives (eg, diazepam, 5 mg orally or intravenously every several hours) can be used for mild to moderate agitation but are sometimes associated with a disinhibition of aggressive impulses similar to alcohol. Chronic aggressive states, particularly in intellectual disabilities and brain damage (rule out causative organic conditions and medications such as anticholinergic medications in amounts sufficient to cause confusion), have been ameliorated with risperidone, 0.5–2 mg/day orally, propranolol, 40–240 mg/day orally, or pindolol, 5 mg twice daily orally (pindolol causes less bradycardia and hypotension than propranolol). Carbamazepine and valproic acid are effective in the treatment of aggression and explosive disorders, particularly when associated with known or suspected brain lesions. Lithium and SSRIs are also effective for some intermittent explosive outbursts. Buspirone (10–45 mg/day orally) is helpful for aggression, particularly in patients with intellectual disabilities.

C. Physical

Physical management is necessary if psychological and pharmacologic means are not sufficient. It requires the active and visible presence of an adequate number of personnel (five or six) to reinforce the idea that the situation is under control despite the patient's lack of inner controls. Such an approach often precludes the need for actual physical restraint. Seclusion rooms and restraints should be used only when necessary (ambulatory restraints are an alternative), and the patient must then be observed at frequent intervals. Narrow corridors, small spaces, and crowded areas exacerbate the potential for violence in an anxious patient.

D. Other Interventions

The treatment of victims (eg, battered women) is challenging and often complicated by their reluctance to leave the situation. Reasons for staying vary, but common themes include the fear of more violence because of leaving, the hope that the situation may ameliorate (in spite of steady worsening), and the financial aspects of the situation, which are seldom to the woman's advantage. Concerns for the children often finally compel the woman to seek help. An early step is to get the woman into a therapeutic situation that provides the support of others in similar straits. Al-Anon is frequently a valuable asset when alcohol is a factor. The group can support the victim while she gathers strength to consider alternatives without being paralyzed by fear. Many cities offer temporary emergency centers and counseling. Use the available resources, attend to any medical or psychiatric problems, and maintain a compassionate interest. Some states require physicians to report injuries caused by abuse or suspected abuse to police authorities.

Buckley P et al. Psychopharmacology of aggression in schizophrenia. Schizophr Bull. 2011 Sep;37(5):930–6. [PMID: 21860038]

Johnson DM et al. Cognitive behavioral treatment of PTSD in residents in battered women's shelters: results of a randomized clinical trial. J Consult Clin Psychol. 2011 Aug;79(4): 542–51. [PMID: 21787052]

Rees S et al. Lifetime prevalence of gender-based violence in women and the relationship with mental disorders and psychosocial function. JAMA. 2011 Aug 3;305(5):513–21. [PMID: 21813429]

SUBSTANCE USE DISORDERS

The term "dependency" was previously used to describe a severe form of substance abuse and drug addiction characterized by the triad of: (1) a **psychological dependence** or craving and the behavior involved in procurement of the drug; (2) **physiologic dependence,** with withdrawal symptoms on discontinuance of the drug; and (3) **tolerance,** ie, the need to increase the dose to obtain the desired effects. The terms "dependency" and "abuse" were dropped in *DSM-5* in favor of the single term "substance use disorder," ranging from mild to severe. Many patients could have a severe and life-threatening abuse problem without ever being dependent on a drug.

There is accumulating evidence that an impairment syndrome exists in many former (and current) drug users. It is believed that drug use produces damaged neurotransmitter receptor sites and that the consequent imbalance produces symptoms that may mimic other psychiatric illnesses. **"Kindling"**—repeated stimulation of the brain—renders the individual more susceptible to focal brain activity with minimal stimulation. Stimulants and depressants can produce kindling, leading to relatively spontaneous effects no longer dependent on the original stimulus. These effects may be manifested as mood swings, panic, psychosis, and occasionally overt seizure activity. The imbalance also results in frequent job changes, partner problems, and generally erratic behavior. Patients with PTSD frequently have treated themselves with a variety of drugs. Chronic abusers of a wide variety of drugs exhibit cerebral atrophy on CT scans, a finding that may relate to the above symptoms. Early recognition is important, mainly to establish realistic treatment programs that are chiefly symptom-directed.

The clinician faces three problems with substance use disorders: (1) the prescribing of substances such as sedatives, stimulants, or opioids that might produce dependency; (2) the treatment of individuals who have already abused drugs, most commonly alcohol; and (3) the detection of illicit drug use in patients presenting with psychiatric symptoms. The usefulness of urinalysis for detection of drugs varies markedly with different drugs and under different circumstances (pharmacokinetics is a major factor). Water-soluble drugs (eg, alcohol, stimulants, opioids) are eliminated in a day or so. Lipophilic substances (eg, barbiturates, tetrahydrocannabinol) appear in the urine over longer periods of time: several days in most cases, 1–2 months in chronic marijuana users. Sedative drug determinations are quite variable, amount of drug and duration of use being important determinants. False-positives can be a problem related to ingestion of some legitimate medications (eg, phenytoin for barbiturates, phenylpropanolamine for amphetamines, chlorpromazine for opioids) and some foods (eg, poppy seeds for opioids, coca leaf tea for cocaine). Manipulations can alter the legitimacy of the testing. Dilution, either in vivo or in vitro, can be detected by checking urine-specific gravity. Addition of ammonia, vinegar, or salt may invalidate the test, but odor and pH determinations are simple. Hair analysis can determine drug use over longer periods, particularly sequential drug-taking patterns. The sensitivity and reliability of such tests are considered good, and the method may be complementary to urinalysis.

Marlatt GA. Update on harm-reduction policy and intervention research. Annu Rev Clin Psychol. 2010 Apr 27;6:591–606. [PMID: 20192791]

ALCOHOL USE DISORDER (Alcoholism)

Meshell D. Johnson, MD

ESSENTIALS OF DIAGNOSIS

▶ Physiologic dependence as manifested by evidence of withdrawal when intake is interrupted.

▶ Tolerance to the effects of alcohol.

▶ Evidence of alcohol-associated illnesses, such as alcoholic liver disease, cerebellar degeneration.

▶ Continued drinking despite strong medical and social contraindications and life disruptions.

▶ Impairment in social and occupational functioning.

▶ Depression.

▶ Blackouts.

▶ General Considerations

Alcohol use disorder is a syndrome consisting of two phases: at-risk drinking and moderate to severe alcohol misuse. At-risk drinking is the repetitive use of alcohol, often to alleviate anxiety or solve other emotional problems. A moderate to severe alcohol use disorder is similar to that which occurs following the repeated use of other sedative-hypnotics and is characterized by recurrent use of alcohol despite disruption in social roles (family and work), alcohol-related legal problems, and taking safety risks by oneself and with others. The National Institute on Alcohol Abuse and Alcoholism formally defines at-risk drinking as **more than 4 drinks per day or 14 drinks per week for men or more than 3 drinks per day or 7 drinks per week for women.** A drink is defined by the CDC as 12 oz of beer, 8 oz of malt liquor, 5 oz of wine, or 1.3 oz or a "shot" of 80-proof distilled spirits of liquor. Individuals with at-risk drinking are at an increased risk for developing or are developing an alcohol use disorder. Alcohol and other drug abuse patients have a much higher prevalence of lifetime psychiatric disorders. While male-to-female ratios in alcoholic treatment agencies remain at 4:1, there is evidence that the rates are converging. Women delay seeking help, and when they do they tend to seek it in medical or mental health settings. Adoption and twin studies indicate some genetic influence. Ethnic distinctions are important—eg, 40% of Japanese have aldehyde dehydrogenase deficiency and are more susceptible to the effects of alcohol. Depression is often present and should be evaluated carefully. The majority of suicides and intrafamily homicides involve alcohol. Alcohol is a major factor in rapes and other assaults.

There are several screening instruments that may help identify an alcohol use disorder. One of the most useful is the Alcohol Use Disorder Identification Test (AUDIT) (see Table 1–7).

► Clinical Findings

A. Acute Intoxication

The signs of alcoholic intoxication are the same as those of overdosage with any other central nervous system depressant: drowsiness, errors of commission, psychomotor dysfunction, disinhibition, dysarthria, ataxia, and nystagmus. For a 70-kg person, an ounce of whiskey, a 4- to 6-oz glass of wine, or a 12-oz bottle of beer (roughly 15, 11, and 13 grams of alcohol, respectively) may raise the level of alcohol in the blood by 25 mg/dL. For a 50-kg person, the blood alcohol level would rise even higher (35 mg/dL) with the same consumption. Blood alcohol levels below 50 mg/dL rarely cause significant motor dysfunction (the legal limit for driving under the influence is commonly 80 mg/dL). Intoxication as manifested by ataxia, dysarthria, and nausea and vomiting indicates a blood level greater than 150 mg/dL, and lethal blood levels range from 350 to 900 mg/dL. In severe cases, overdosage is marked by respiratory depression, stupor, seizures, shock syndrome, coma, and death. Serious overdoses are frequently due to a combination of alcohol with other sedatives.

B. Withdrawal

There is a wide spectrum of manifestations of alcoholic withdrawal, ranging from anxiety, decreased cognition, and tremulousness, through increasing irritability and hyperreactivity to full-blown delirium tremens (DTs). **Alcohol withdrawal syndrome** can be categorized as mild, moderate, or severe withdrawal, withdrawal seizures, and DTs. Symptoms of mild withdrawal, including tremor, anxiety, tachycardia, nausea, vomiting, and insomnia begin within 6 hours after the last drink, often before the blood alcohol levels drop to zero, and usually have passed by day 2. Severe or major withdrawal occurs 48–96 hours after the last drink and is usually preceded by prolonged heavy alcohol use. Symptoms include disorientation, agitation, diaphoresis, whole body tremor, vomiting, hypertension, and visual and auditory hallucinations (visual>tactile>auditory). Moderate withdrawal signs and symptoms fall between those of minor and major withdrawal. **Withdrawal seizures** can occur as early as 8 hours after the last drink but usually do not manifest more than 48 hours after alcohol

cessation. Seizures are more prevalent in persons who have a history of withdrawal syndromes. These seizures are generalized tonic-clonic seizures, are brief in duration, and resolve spontaneously. If withdrawal is untreated, these seizures can recur in about 60% of patients. DTs will develop in approximately half of these patients. If seizures are focal, associated with trauma or fever, or have an onset more than 48 hours after the last drink, another etiology for seizures must be considered. DTs is the most severe form of alcohol withdrawal. It is an acute organic psychosis that usually manifests 48–72 hours after the last drink but may occur up to 7–10 days later. It is characterized by extreme mental confusion, agitation, tremor, diaphoresis, sensory hyperacuity, visual hallucinations (often of snakes, bugs, etc) and autonomic hyperactivity (tachycardia and hypertension). Complications of DTs include (1) dehydration, (2) electrolyte disturbances (hypokalemia, hypomagnesemia), (3) arrhythmias and seizures, and (4) cardiovascular collapse and death. The acute withdrawal syndrome is often completely unexpected and occurs when the patient has been hospitalized for some unrelated problem and presents as a diagnostic dilemma. Suspect alcohol withdrawal in every unexplained delirium. The mortality rate from DTs, which was upward of 35%, has steadily decreased with early diagnosis and improved treatment.

In addition to the immediate withdrawal symptoms, there is evidence of persistent longer-term ones, including sleep disturbances, anxiety, depression, excitability, fatigue, and emotional volatility. These symptoms may persist for 3–12 months, and in some cases they become chronic.

C. Alcoholic (Organic) Hallucinosis

This syndrome occurs either during heavy drinking or on withdrawal and is characterized by a paranoid psychosis without the tremulousness, confusion, and clouded sensorium seen in withdrawal syndromes. The patient appears normal except for the auditory hallucinations, which are frequently persecutory and may cause the patient to behave aggressively and in a paranoid fashion.

D. Chronic Alcoholic Brain Syndromes

These encephalopathies are characterized by increasing erratic behavior, memory and recall problems, and emotional instability—the usual signs of organic brain injury due to any cause. Wernicke-Korsakoff syndrome due to thiamine deficiency may develop with a series of episodes. Wernicke encephalopathy consists of the triad of confusion, ataxia, and ophthalmoplegia (typically sixth nerve). Early recognition and treatment with thiamine can minimize damage. One of the possible sequelae is Korsakoff psychosis, characterized by both anterograde and retrograde amnesia, with confabulation early in the course. Early recognition and treatment of the alcoholic with intravenous thiamine and B complex vitamins can minimize damage. Excessive alcohol consumption in men has been associated with faster cognitive decline compared with light to moderate alcohol consumption.

E. Laboratory Findings

Ethanol may contribute to the presence of an otherwise unexplained osmolar gap. There may also be elevated liver function tests, increased serum uric acid and triglycerides, and decreased serum potassium and magnesium. The most definitive biologic marker for chronic alcoholism is carbohydrate deficient transferrin, which can detect heavy use (60 mg/day over 7–10 days) with high specificity. Other useful tests for diagnosing alcohol use disorder are gamma-glutamyl transpeptidase measurement (levels greater than 30 units/L are suggestive of heavy drinking) and mean corpuscular volume (more than 95 fL in men and more than 100 fL in women). If both are elevated, a serious drinking problem is likely. Use of other recreational drugs with alcohol skews and negates the significance of these tests. Concomitant elevations of high-density lipoprotein cholesterol elevations and gamma-glutamyl transpeptidase concentrations also can help identify heavy drinkers.

▶ Differential Diagnosis

The differential diagnosis of **alcoholism** is essentially between primary alcohol use disorder (when no other major psychiatric diagnosis exists) and secondary alcohol use disorder (when alcohol is used as self-medication for major underlying psychiatric problems such as schizophrenia or affective disorder). The differentiation is important, since the latter group requires treatment for the specific psychiatric problem. In primary and secondary alcoholism, at-risk drinking can be distinguished from alcohol addiction by taking a careful psychiatric history and evaluating the degree to which recurrent drinking impacts the social role functioning and physical safety of the individual.

The differential diagnosis of **alcohol withdrawal** includes other sedative withdrawals and other causes of delirium. Acute alcoholic hallucinosis must be differentiated from other acute paranoid states such as amphetamine psychosis or paranoid schizophrenia. The form of the brain syndrome is of little help—eg, chronic brain syndromes from lupus erythematosus may be associated with confabulation similar to that resulting from long-standing alcoholism.

▶ Complications

The medical, economic, and psychosocial problems of alcoholism are staggering. The central and peripheral nervous system complications include chronic brain syndromes, cerebellar degeneration, cardiomyopathy, and peripheral neuropathies. Direct effects on the liver include cirrhosis, esophageal varices, and eventual hepatic failure. Indirect effects include protein abnormalities, coagulation defects, hormone deficiencies, and an increased incidence of liver neoplasms.

Fetal alcohol syndrome includes one or more of the following developmental defects in the offspring of alcoholic women: (1) low birth weight and small size with failure to catch up in size or weight, (2) mental retardation, with an average IQ in the 60s, and (3) a variety of birth defects, with a large percentage of facial and cardiac abnormalities. The risk is appreciably higher the more alcohol ingested by the mother each day. Cigarette and marijuana smoking as well as cocaine use can produce similar effects on the fetus.

▶ Treatment of At-Risk Drinking

A. Psychological

The most important consideration for the clinician is to suspect the problem early and take a nonjudgmental attitude, although this does not mean a passive one. The problem of denial must be faced, preferably with significant family members at the first meeting. This means dealing from the beginning with any enabling behavior of the spouse or other significant people. Enabling behavior allows the patient with an alcohol use disorder to avoid facing the consequences of his or her behavior.

There must be an emphasis on the things that can be done. This approach emphasizes the fact that the clinician cares and strikes a positive and hopeful note early in treatment. Valuable time should not be wasted trying to find out why the patient drinks; come to grips early with the immediate problem of how to stop the drinking. Although total abstinence should be the ultimate goal, a harm reduction model indicates that gradual progress toward abstinence can be a useful treatment stratagem.

Motivational interviewing, a model of counseling that addresses both the patient's ambivalence and motivation for change, may contribute to reduced consumption over time.

B. Social

Get the patient into Alcoholics Anonymous and the spouse into Al-Anon. Success is usually proportionate to the utilization of Alcoholics Anonymous, religious counseling, and other resources. The patient should be seen frequently for short periods and charged an appropriate fee.

Do not underestimate the importance of religion, particularly since the patient with alcohol use disorder is often a dependent person who needs a great deal of support. Early enlistment of the help of a concerned religious adviser can often provide the turning point for a personal conversion to sobriety.

One of the most important considerations is the patient's job—fear of losing a job is one of the most powerful motivations for giving up drink. The business community is aware of the problem; about 70% of the Fortune 500 companies offer programs to their employees to help with the problem of alcoholism. In the latter case, some specific recommendations to employers can be offered: (1) Avoid placement in jobs where the alcoholic patient must be alone, eg, as a traveling buyer or sales executive. (2) Use supervision but not surveillance. (3) Keep competition with others to a minimum. (4) Avoid positions that require quick decision-making on important matters (high-stress situations). In general, commitment to abstinence and avoidance of situations that might be conducive to drinking are most predictive of a good outcome.

C. Medical

Hospitalization is not usually necessary. It is sometimes used to dramatize a situation and force the patient to face the problem of alcoholism, but generally it should be used for medical indications. Alcohol is responsible for about 88,000 deaths in the United States each year.

Because of the many medical complications of alcoholism, a complete physical examination with appropriate laboratory tests is mandatory, with special attention to the liver and nervous system. Use of sedatives as a replacement for alcohol is not desirable. The usual result is concomitant use of sedatives and alcohol and worsening of the problem. Lithium is not helpful in the treatment of alcoholism.

Disulfiram (250–500 mg/day orally) has been used for many years as an aversive drug to discourage alcohol use. Disulfiram inhibits alcohol dehydrogenase, causing toxic reactions when alcohol is consumed. The results have generally been of limited effectiveness and depend on the motivation of the individual to be compliant.

Naltrexone, an opiate antagonist, in a dosage of 50 mg orally daily, lowers relapse rates over the 3–6 months after cessation of drinking, apparently by lessening the pleasurable effects of alcohol. One study suggests that naltrexone is most effective when given during periods of drinking in combination with therapy that supports abstinence but accepts the fact that relapses occur. Naltrexone is FDA-approved for maintenance therapy. Studies indicate that it reduces alcohol craving when used as part of a comprehensive treatment program. Acamprosate (333–666 mg orally three times daily) helps reduce craving and maintain abstinence and can be continued even during periods of relapse. Both acamprosate and oral naltrexone have been associated with reduction in return to drinking.

D. Behavioral

Conditioning approaches historically have been used in some settings in the treatment of alcoholism, most commonly as a type of aversion therapy. For example, the patient is given a drink of whiskey and then a shot of apomorphine, and proceeds to vomit. In this way a strong association is built up between the drinking and vomiting. Although this kind of treatment has been successful in some cases, after appropriate informed consent, many people do not sustain the learned aversive response.

▶ Treatment of Hallucinosis & Withdrawal

A. Hallucinosis

Alcoholic hallucinosis, which can occur either during or on cessation of a prolonged drinking period, is not a typical withdrawal syndrome and is handled differently. Since the symptoms are primarily those of a psychosis in the presence of a clear sensorium, they are handled like any other psychosis: hospitalization (when indicated) and adequate amounts of antipsychotic medications. Haloperidol, 5 mg orally twice a day for the first day or so, usually ameliorates symptoms quickly, and the drug can be decreased and discontinued over several days as the patient improves. It then becomes necessary to deal with the chronic alcohol abuse, which has been discussed.

B. Withdrawal

The onset of withdrawal symptoms is usually 6–36 hours and the peak intensity of symptoms is 48–72 hours after alcohol consumption is stopped. Providing adequate central nervous system depressants (eg, benzodiazepines) is important to counteract the excitability resulting from sudden cessation of alcohol intake. The choice of a specific sedative is less important than using adequate doses to bring the patient to a level of moderate sedation, and this will vary from person to person.

All patients should be evaluated for their risk of alcohol withdrawal. Mild dependency requires "drying out." For outpatients, in some instances, a short course of tapering long-acting benzodiazepines—eg, diazepam, 20 mg/day orally initially, decreasing by 5 mg daily—may be a useful adjunct. When the history or presentation suggests that patients are actively in withdrawal or at significant risk for withdrawal, they should be hospitalized. Risk factors include a recent drinking history; frequent alcohol consumption; a past history of withdrawal, seizures, hallucinosis, or DTs; a past history of needing medication for detoxification; or a history of benzodiazepine or barbiturate use, abuse, or dependency.

For all hospitalized patients, general management includes ensuring adequate hydration, correction of electrolyte imbalances (particularly magnesium, calcium, and potassium), and administering the vitamins thiamine (100 mg intravenously daily for 3 days then orally daily), folic acid (1 mg orally daily), and one multivitamin orally daily. **Thiamine should be given prior to any glucose-containing solutions to decrease the risk of precipitating Wernicke encephalopathy or Korsakoff syndrome.** Alcohol withdrawal is treated with benzodiazepines. Continual assessment is recommended to determine the severity of withdrawal and symptom-driven medication regimens, which have been shown to prevent undersedation and oversedation and reduce total benzodiazepine usage over fixed-dose schedules. The severity of withdrawal will determine a patient's level of care. For those at risk for withdrawal and with mild withdrawal symptoms, admission to a medical unit is adequate. For those with moderate withdrawal, a higher acuity hospital environment is recommended. Those with severe withdrawal should be admitted to the intensive care unit (ICU).

1. Assessing alcohol withdrawal symptom severity—The Clinical Institute Withdrawal Assessment for Alcohol, Revised (CIWA-Ar) is a validated tool that is widely used to determine severity of alcohol withdrawal. This survey assesses symptoms in 10 areas and can be administered relatively quickly (Figure 25–3). One caveat is that the patient must be able to communicate his or her symptoms to the provider. The maximum attainable score is 67. Clinical judgement should be used to determine final dosing of medications to patients who are in alcohol withdrawal because dosing can vary between patients and degrees of withdrawal.

Patient: _____ Date: _____ Time: _____ (24 hour clock, midnight = 00:00)

Pulse or heart rate, taken for 1 minute: _____ Blood pressure: _____

NAUSEA AND VOMITING — Ask "Do you feel sick to your stomach? Have you vomited?" Observation.

0 no nausea and no vomiting
1 mild nausea with no vomiting
2
3
4 intermittent nausea with dry heaves
5
6
7 constant nausea, frequent dry heaves and vomiting

TREMOR — Arms extended and fingers spread apart. Observation.

0 no tremor
1 not visible, but can be felt fingertip to fingertip
2
3
4 moderate, with patient's arms extended
5
6
7 severe, even with arms not extended

PAROXYSMAL SWEATS — Observation.

0 no sweat visible
1 barely perceptible sweating, palms moist
2
3
4 beads of sweat obvious on forehead
5
6
7 drenching sweats

ANXIETY — Ask "Do you feel nervous?" Observation.

0 no anxiety, at ease
1 mild anxious
2
3
4 moderately anxious, or guarded, so anxiety is inferred
5
6
7 equivalent to acute panic states as seen in severe delirium or acute schizophrenic reactions

TACTILE DISTURBANCES — Ask "Have you any itching, pins and needles sensations, any burning, any numbness, or do you feel bugs crawling on or under your skin?" Observation.

0 none
1 very mild itching, pins and needles, burning, or numbness
2 mild itching, pins and needles, burning, or numbness
3 moderate itching, pins and needles, burning, or numbness
4 moderately severe hallucinations
5 severe hallucinations
6 extremely severe hallucinations
7 continuous hallucinations

AUDITORY DISTURBANCES — Ask "Are you more aware of sounds around you? Are they harsh? Do they frighten you? Are you hearing anything that is disturbing to you? Are you hearing things you know are not there?" Observation.

0 not present
1 very mild harshness or ability to frighten
2 mild harshness or ability to frighten
3 moderate harshness or ability to frighten
4 moderately severe hallucinations
5 severe hallucinations
6 extremely severe hallucinations
7 continuous hallucinations

VISUAL DISTURBANCES — Ask "Does the light appear to be too bright? Is its color different? Does it hurt your eyes? Are you seeing anything that is disturbing to you? Are you seeing things you know are not there?" Observation.

0 not present
1 very mild sensitivity
2 mild sensitivity
3 moderate sensitivity
4 moderately severe hallucinations
5 severe hallucinations
6 extremely severe hallucinations
7 continuous hallucinations

HEADACHE, FULLNESS IN HEAD — Ask "Does your head feel different? Does it feel like there is a band around your head?" Do not rate for dizziness or lightheadedness. Otherwise, rate severity.

0 not present
1 very mild
2 mild
3 moderate
4 moderately severe
5 severe
6 very severe
7 extremely severe

▲ **Figure 25–3.** Alcohol withdrawal assessment. (Source: Clinical Institute Withdrawal Assessment of Alcohol Scale, Revised, *Br J Addict* 1989:84;1353.)

AGITATION — Observation.

0 normal activity
1 somewhat more than normal activity
2
3
4 moderately fidgety and restless
5
6
7 paces back and forth during most of the interview, or constantly thrashes about

ORIENTATION AND CLOUDING OF SENSORIUM — Ask "What day is this? Where are you? Who am I?"

0 oriented and can do serial additions
1 cannot do serial additions or is uncertain about date
2 disoriented for date by no more than 2 calendar days
3 disoriented for date by more than 2 calendar days
4 disoriented for place/or person

Total **CIWA-Ar** Score _____

Rater's Initials _____

Maximum Possible Score 67

This assessment for monitoring withdrawal symptoms requires approximately 5 minutes to administer. The maximum score is 67 (see instrument). Patients scoring less than 8 (or 10, according to some experts) do not usually need additional medication for withdrawal.

▲ **Figure 25–3.** (*Continued*).

2. Treating alcohol withdrawal symptoms based on CIWA-Ar score—

A. MINIMAL WITHDRAWAL SYMPTOMS (CIWA-AR SCORE LESS THAN 8)—Patients who have a history suggestive of alcohol withdrawal risk with minimal withdrawal symptoms are suitable for withdrawal prophylaxis. The recommended benzodiazepine options include chlordiazepoxide orally or lorazepam intravenously or orally, tapered over 3 days. The protocol calls for nursing assessment of sedation and withdrawal symptoms (CIWA-Ar) every 6 hours. If prophylactic medication is indicated, a sample tapering regimen may include lorazepam 1 mg orally every 6 hours for 1 day, then 1 mg orally every 8 hours for 1 day, then 1 mg orally every 12 hours for 1 day, then discontinue; or chlordiazepoxide 50 mg orally every 6 hours for 1 day, 25 mg orally every 6 hours for 2 days, then discontinue. Avoid chlordiazepoxide in elderly patients as well as patients with liver disease. Lorazepam is preferred in patients with liver disease. Sedation is assessed 30–60 minutes after each medication dose. The benzodiazepine dose is held for oversedation or if the respiratory rate is less than 10 breaths per minute. For CIWA-Ar score greater than 8, the provider must be notified, because this is suggestive of active withdrawal, and escalation of treatment must occur.

B. MILD WITHDRAWAL SYMPTOMS (CIWA-AR SCORE 8–15)—For patients in mild withdrawal, either chlordiazepoxide orally or lorazepam orally or intravenously can be used. Initially, chlordiazepoxide 50 mg orally or lorazepam 1 or 2 mg orally or intravenously is given hourly for 2 hours. Patients must be assessed for level of sedation and withdrawal symptoms (CIWA-Ar) every 4 hours. Dosing is adjusted as necessary to control symptoms without excessive sedation. After the first 2 hours, chlordiazepoxide or lorazepam is given every 4 hours and as needed. Typical dosing may include chlordiazepoxide 25–50 mg orally or lorazepam 0.5–1 mg orally or intravenously every 4 hours as needed. Additional doses of benzodiazepines should be given if the CIWA-Ar score remains between 8 and 15.

C. MODERATE WITHDRAWAL (CIWA-AR SCORE 16–20)—For patients in moderate withdrawal, chlordiazepoxide 100 mg orally or lorazepam 3 or 4 mg orally or intravenously is given every hour for the first 2 hours. CIWA-Ar monitoring should occur every 2 hours. Dosing is adjusted to control symptoms without excessive sedation. After initial dosing, continued treatment could include chlordiazepoxide 50 mg orally or lorazepam 1–2 mg orally or intravenously every 2 hours as needed for CIWA-Ar score between 16 and 20, and chlordiazepoxide 25 mg orally or lorazepam 0.5–1 mg orally or intravenously every 2 hours for CIWA-Ar score between 8 and 15. The maximum dose of chlordiazepoxide is 600 mg in 24 hours. Continuous pulse oximetry and cardiac monitoring should be considered. The degree of sedation should be monitored 30–60 minutes after each oral dose of medication and for 15 minutes after each parenteral dose.

D. SEVERE WITHDRAWAL (CIWA-AR SCORE GREATER THAN 21)—Patients with severe withdrawal are at risk for the development of DTs and should be transferred or admitted to the ICU. Intravenous lorazepam is the drug of choice for treating severe withdrawal. Lorazepam 1–2 mg intravenously every 15 minutes can be given until patient is calm and sedated but awake. Initial CIWA-Ar monitoring should occur every 30 minutes. The patient can then receive lorazepam 2 mg orally or intravenously every hour as needed when the CIWA-Ar score is between 16 and 20, and lorazepam 1–2 mg orally or intravenously every hour as needed when the CIWA-Ar score is between 8 and 15. If the patient requires more than 8 mg/h of lorazepam as an initial dose or continues to demonstrate observable agitation, tremors, tachycardia, or hypertension despite high doses of lorazepam, consider adding dexmedetomidine; it is not recommended as a sole agent for the treatment of alcohol withdrawal. Dexmedetomidine, an alpha-2-agonist, produces sedation with minimal effect on respiratory drive and lung function. The recommended dosing of dexmedetomidine is 0.2–0.7mcg/kg/h, with lorazepam 1–2 mg intravenously every 8 hours plus lorazepam 1–2 mg intravenously every hour as needed for agitation. In limited cases of severe withdrawal requiring frequent lorazepam boluses for at least 6 hours, continuous intravenous lorazepam infusion can be considered, but the patient must be monitored extremely carefully for signs of respiratory depression. Continuous pulse oximetry and close observance of the patient's respiratory status is required. Sedation is assessed 15 minutes after each intravenous dose. If withdrawal symptoms are refractory to escalating benzodiazepine usage, despite the addition of dexmedetomidine, patients often require intubation for airway protection, at which time initiation of propofol infusion for sedation is recommended.

In all cases, benzodiazepines should be held if the patient is too sedated or has a respiratory rate less than 10 breaths per minute. Do not bolus lorazepam in doses greater than 4 mg intravenously. Mixing benzodiazepines, eg, chlordiazepoxide orally every 8 hours with lorazepam, is not recommended. Instead, select a single agent and titrate as needed. Once a patient has been stable for 24 hours, the benzodiazepine dose can be reduced by 20% daily until withdrawal is complete.

3. Managing other withdrawal-associated conditions—
Meticulous examination for other medical problems is necessary. Alcoholic hypoglycemia can occur with low blood alcohol levels (see Chapter 27). Patients with severe alcohol use disorder commonly have liver disease with associated clotting disorders and are also prone to injury—and the combination all too frequently leads to undiagnosed subdural hematoma.

Phenytoin does not appear to be useful in managing alcohol withdrawal seizures per se. Sedating doses of benzodiazepines are effective in treating alcohol withdrawal seizures. Thus, other anticonvulsants are not usually needed unless there is a preexisting seizure disorder.

Chronic brain syndromes secondary to a long history of alcohol intake are not clearly responsive to thiamine and vitamin replenishment. Attention to the social and environmental care of this type of patient is paramount.

4. Initiating psychological and social measures—The
psychological and behavioral treatment methods outlined under Treatment of At-Risk Drinking become the primary considerations after successful treatment of alcoholic hallucinosis or withdrawal. Psychological and social measures should be initiated in the hospital prior to discharge. This increases the possibility of continued post-hospitalization treatment.

Bielka K et al. Addition of dexmedetomidine to benzodiazepines for patients with alcohol withdrawal syndrome in the intensive care unit: a randomized controlled study. Ann Intensive Care. 2015 Dec;5(1):33. [PMID: 26525052]

de Wit M et al. Alcohol-use disorders in the critically ill patient. Chest. 2010 Oct;138(4):994–1003. [PMID: 20923804]

Johnson BA. Medication treatment of different types of alcoholism. Am J Psychiatry. 2010 Jun;167(6):630–9. [PMID: 20516163]

Jonas DE et al. Pharmacotherapy for adults with alcohol use disorders in outpatient settings: a systematic review and meta-analysis. JAMA. 2014 May 14;311(18):1889–900. [PMID: 24825644]

Mayo-Smith MF et al; Practice Guidelines Committee, American Society of Addiction Medicine. Management of alcohol withdrawal delirium. An evidence-based practice guideline. Arch Intern Med. 2004 Jul 12;164(13):1405–12. Erratum in: Arch Intern Med. 2004 Oct 11;164(18):2068. Dosage error in article text. [PMID: 15249349]

Sabia S et al. Alcohol consumption and cognitive decline in early old age. Neurology. 2014 Jan 28;82(4):332–9. [PMID: 24431298]

Satre DD et al. Motivational interviewing to reduce hazardous drinking and drug use among depression patients. J Subst Abuse Treat. 2013 Apr;44(3):323–9. [PMID: 22999815]

OTHER DRUG & SUBSTANCE DEPENDENCIES

1. Opioids

While the terms "opioids" and "narcotics" both refer to a group of drugs with actions that mimic those of morphine, the term "opioids" is used when discussing medications prescribed in a controlled manner by a clinician, and the term "narcotics" is used to connote illicit drug use. All of the opioid analgesics can be reversed by the opioid antagonist naloxone.

The clinical symptoms and signs of mild narcotic intoxication include changes in mood, with feelings of euphoria; drowsiness; nausea with occasional emesis; needle tracks; and miosis. The incidence of snorting and inhaling heroin ("smoking") is increasing, particularly among cocaine users. This coincides with a decrease in the availability of methaqualone (no longer marketed) and other sedatives used to temper the cocaine "high" (see discussion of cocaine under Stimulants, below). Overdosage causes respiratory depression, peripheral vasodilation, pinpoint pupils, pulmonary edema, coma, and death.

Tolerance and withdrawal are major concerns when continued use of opioids occurs, although withdrawal causes only moderate morbidity (similar in severity to a bout of "flu"). Addicted patients sometimes consider themselves more addicted than they really are and may not require a withdrawal program. Grades of withdrawal are categorized from 0 to 4: grade 0 includes craving and anxiety; grade 1, yawning, lacrimation, rhinorrhea, and perspiration; grade 2, previous symptoms plus mydriasis, piloerection, anorexia, tremors, and hot and cold flashes with generalized aching; grades 3 and 4, increased intensity of previous symptoms and signs, with increased temperature, blood pressure, pulse, and respiratory rate and depth. In withdrawal from the most severe addiction, vomiting, diarrhea, weight loss, hemoconcentration, and spontaneous ejaculation or orgasm commonly occur.

Treatment for overdosage (or suspected overdosage) is discussed in Chapter 38.

Treatment for withdrawal begins if grade 2 signs develop. If a withdrawal program is necessary, use methadone, 10 mg orally (use parenteral administration if the patient is vomiting), and observe. If signs (piloerection, mydriasis, cardiovascular changes) persist for more than 4–6 hours, give another 10 mg; continue to administer methadone at 4- to 6-hour intervals until signs are not present (rarely greater than 40 mg of methadone in 24 hours). Divide the total amount of drug required over the first 24-hour period by 2 and give that amount every 12 hours. Each day, reduce the total 24-hour dose by 5–10 mg. Thus, a moderately addicted patient initially requiring 30–40 mg of methadone could be withdrawn over a 4- to 8-day period. Clonidine, 0.1 mg orally several times daily over a 10- to 14-day period, is both an alternative and an adjunct to methadone detoxification; it is not necessary to taper the dose. Clonidine is helpful in alleviating cardiovascular symptoms but does not significantly relieve anxiety, insomnia, or generalized aching. There is a protracted abstinence syndrome of metabolic, respiratory, and blood pressure changes over a period of 3–6 months.

Opioid antagonists (eg, naltrexone) can also be used successfully for treatment of the patient who has been free of opioids for 7–10 days. Naltrexone blocks the narcotic "high" of heroin when 50 mg is given orally every 24 hours initially for several days and then 100 mg is given every 48–72 hours. A monthly injectable form of naltrexone is available and may enhance compliance. Liver disorders are a major contraindication. Buprenorphine, a partial agonist, is a mainstay of office-based treatment of opiate dependency. Its use requires certified training.

Alternative strategies for the treatment of opioid withdrawal have included rapid and ultrarapid detoxification techniques. However, data do not support the use of either method. Methadone maintenance programs are of some value in chronic recidivism. Under carefully controlled supervision, the narcotic addict is maintained on fairly high doses of methadone (40–120 mg/day) that satisfy craving and block the effects of heroin to a great degree.

2. Sedatives (Anxiolytics)

See Anxiety Disorders, this chapter.

3. Psychedelics

All of the common psychedelics (LSD, mescaline, psilocybin, dimethyltryptamine, and other derivatives of phenylalanine and tryptophan) can produce similar behavioral and physiologic effects. An initial feeling of tension is followed by emotional release such as crying or laughing (1–2 hours). Later, perceptual distortions occur, with visual illusions and hallucinations, and occasionally there is fear of ego disintegration (2–3 hours). Major changes in time sense and mood lability then occur (3–4 hours). A feeling of detachment and a sense of destiny and control occur (4–6 hours). Of course, reactions vary among individuals, and some of the drugs produce markedly different time frames. Occasionally, the acute episode is terrifying (a "bad trip"), which may include panic, depression, confusion, or psychotic symptoms. Preexisting emotional problems, the attitude of the user, and the setting where the drug is used affect the experience.

Treatment of the acute episode primarily involves protection of the individual from erratic behavior that may lead to injury or death. A structured environment is usually sufficient until the drug is metabolized. In severe cases, antipsychotic medications with minimal side effects (eg, haloperidol, 5 mg intramuscularly) may be given every several hours until the individual has regained control. In cases where "flashbacks" occur (mental imagery from a "bad trip" that is later triggered by mild stimuli such as marijuana, alcohol, or psychic trauma), a short course of an antipsychotic drug—eg, olanzapine, 5–10 mg/day orally, or risperidone, 2 mg/day orally, initially, and up to 20 mg/day and 6 mg/day, respectively—is usually sufficient. Lorazepam or clonazepam, 1–2 mg orally every 2 hours as needed for acute agitation, may be a useful adjunct. An occasional patient may have "flashbacks" for much longer periods and may require small doses of antipsychotic medications over the longer term.

4. Phencyclidine

Phencyclidine (PCP, angel dust, peace pill, hog) is simple to produce and mimics to some degree the traditional psychedelic drugs. PCP is a common deceptive substitute for LSD, tetrahydrocannabinol, and mescaline. It is available in crystals, capsules, and tablets to be inhaled, injected, swallowed, or smoked (it is commonly sprinkled on marijuana).

Absorption after smoking is rapid, with onset of symptoms in several minutes and peak symptoms in 15–30 minutes. Mild intoxication produces euphoria accompanied by a feeling of numbness. Moderate intoxication (5–10 mg) results in disorientation, detachment from surroundings, distortion of body image, combativeness, unusual feats of strength (partly due to its anesthetic activity), and loss of ability to integrate sensory input, especially touch and proprioception. Physical symptoms include dizziness, ataxia, dysarthria, nystagmus, retracted upper eyelid with blank stare, hyperreflexia, and tachycardia. There are increases in blood pressure, respiration, muscle tone, and urine production. Usage in the first trimester of pregnancy is associated with an increase in spontaneous abortion and congenital defects. Severe intoxication (20 mg or more) produces an increase in degree of moderate symptoms, with the addition of seizures, deepening coma, hypertensive crisis, and severe psychotic ideation. The drug is particularly long-lasting (several days to several weeks) owing to high lipid solubility, gastroenteric recycling, and the production of active metabolites. Overdosage may be fatal, with the major causes of death being hypertensive crisis, respiratory arrest, and convulsions. Acute rhabdomyolysis has been reported and can result in myoglobinuric kidney failure.

Differential diagnosis involves the whole spectrum of street drugs, since in some ways phencyclidine mimics sedatives, psychedelics, and marijuana in its effects. Blood and urine testing can detect the acute problem.

Treatment is discussed in Chapter 38.

5. Marijuana

Cannabis sativa, a hemp plant, is the source of marijuana. Mercury may be a contaminant in marijuana grown in volcanic soil. The drug is usually inhaled by smoking. Effects occur in 10–20 minutes and last 2–3 hours. "Joints" of good quality contain about 500 mg of marijuana (which contains approximately 5–15 mg of tetrahydrocannabinol with a half-life of 7 days).

With moderate dosage, marijuana produces two phases: mild euphoria followed by sleepiness. In the acute state, the user has an altered time perception, less inhibited emotions, psychomotor problems, impaired immediate memory, and conjunctival injection. High doses produce transient psychotomimetic effects. No specific treatment is necessary except in the case of the occasional "bad trip," in which case the person is treated in the same way as for psychedelic usage. Marijuana frequently aggravates existing mental illness and adversely affects motor performance.

Studies of long-term effects have conclusively shown abnormalities in the pulmonary tree. Laryngitis and rhinitis are related to prolonged use, along with chronic obstructive pulmonary disease. Electrocardiographic abnormalities are common, but no chronic cardiac disease has been linked to marijuana use. Long-term usage has resulted in depression of plasma testosterone levels and reduced sperm counts. Abnormal menstruation and failure to ovulate have occurred in some women. Cognitive impairments are common. Health care utilization for a variety of health problems is increased in long-term marijuana smokers. Sudden withdrawal produces insomnia, nausea, myalgia, and irritability. Psychological effects of long-term marijuana usage are still unclear. Urine testing is reliable if samples are carefully collected and tested. Detection periods span 4–6 days in short-term users and 20–50 days in long-term users.

6. Stimulants: Amphetamines & Cocaine

Stimulant abuse is quite common, either alone or in combination with abuse of other drugs. The stimulants include illicit drugs such as methamphetamine ("speed")—one variant is a smokable form called "ice," which gives an intense and fairly long-lasting high—and methylphenidate and dextroamphetamine, which are under prescription control. Street availability of amphetamines remains high. Moderate usage of any of the stimulants produces hyperactivity, a sense of enhanced physical and mental capacity, and sympathomimetic effects. The clinical picture of acute stimulant intoxication includes sweating, tachycardia, elevated blood pressure, mydriasis, hyperactivity, and an acute brain syndrome with confusion and disorientation. Tolerance develops quickly, and, as the dosage is increased, hypervigilance, paranoid ideation (with delusions of parasitosis), stereotypy, bruxism, tactile hallucinations of insect infestation, and full-blown psychoses occur, often with persecutory ideation and aggressive responses. Stimulant withdrawal is characterized by depression with symptoms of hyperphagia and hypersomnia.

People who have used stimulants chronically (eg, anorexigenics) occasionally become sensitized (**"kindling"**) to future use of stimulants. In these individuals, even small amounts of mild stimulants such as caffeine can cause symptoms of paranoia and auditory hallucinations.

Cocaine is a stimulant. It is a product of the coca plant. The derivatives include seeds, leaves, coca paste, cocaine hydrochloride, and the free base of cocaine. Cocaine hydrochloride is the salt and the most commonly used form. Freebase, a purer (and stronger) derivative called "crack," is prepared by simple extraction from cocaine hydrochloride.

There are various modes of use. Coca leaf chewing involves toasting the leaves and chewing with alkaline material (eg, the ash of other burned leaves) to enhance buccal absorption. One achieves a mild high, with onset in 5–10 minutes and lasting for about an hour. Intranasal use is simply snorting cocaine through a straw. Absorption is slowed somewhat by vasoconstriction (which may eventually cause tissue necrosis and septal perforation); the onset of action is in 2–3 minutes, with a moderate high (euphoria, excitement, increased energy) lasting about 30 minutes. The purity of the cocaine is a major determinant of the high. Intravenous use of cocaine hydrochloride or "freebase" is effective in 30 seconds and produces a short-lasting, fairly intense high of about 15 minutes' duration. The combined use of cocaine and ethanol results in the metabolic production of cocaethylene by the liver. This substance produces more intense and long-lasting cocaine-like effects. Smoking freebase (volatilized cocaine because of the lower boiling point) acts in seconds and results in an intense high lasting several minutes. The intensity of the reaction is related to the marked lipid solubility of the freebase form and produces by far the most severe medical and psychiatric symptoms.

Cardiovascular collapse, arrhythmias, myocardial infarction, and transient ischemic attacks have been reported. Seizures, strokes, migraine symptoms, hyperthermia, and lung damage may occur, and there are several obstetric complications, including spontaneous abortion, abruptio placentae, teratogenic effects, delayed fetal growth, and prematurity. Cocaine can cause anxiety, mood swings, and delirium, and chronic use can cause the same problems as other stimulants (see above).

Clinicians should be alert to cocaine use in patients presenting with unexplained nasal bleeding or septal perforations, headaches, fatigue, insomnia, anxiety, depression, and chronic hoarseness. Sudden withdrawal of the drug is not life-threatening but usually produces craving, sleep disturbances, hyperphagia, lassitude, and severe depression (sometimes with suicidal ideation) lasting days to weeks.

Treatment is imprecise and difficult. Since the high is related to blockage of dopamine reuptake, the dopamine agonist bromocriptine, 1.5 mg orally three times a day, alleviates some of the symptoms of craving associated with acute cocaine withdrawal. Treatment of psychosis is the same as that of any psychosis: antipsychotic medications in dosages sufficient to alleviate the symptoms. Any medical symptoms (eg, hyperthermia, seizures, hypertension) are treated specifically. These approaches should be used in conjunction with a structured program, most often based on the Alcoholics Anonymous model. Hospitalization may be required if self-harm or violence toward others is a perceived threat (usually indicated by paranoid delusions).

7. Caffeine

Caffeine, along with nicotine and alcohol, is one of the most commonly used drugs worldwide. Tea, cocoa, and cola drinks also contribute to an intake of caffeine that is often astoundingly high in a large number of people. Low to moderate doses (30–200 mg/day) tend to improve some aspects of performance (eg, vigilance). The approximate content of caffeine in a (180-mL) cup of beverage is as follows: brewed coffee, 80–140 mg; instant coffee, 60–100 mg; decaffeinated coffee, 1–6 mg; black leaf tea, 30–80 mg; tea bags, 25–75 mg; instant tea, 30–60 mg; cocoa, 10–50 mg; and 12-oz cola drinks, 30–65 mg. A 2-oz chocolate candy bar has about 20 mg. Some herbal teas (eg, "morning thunder") contain caffeine. Caffeine-containing analgesics usually contain approximately 30 mg per unit. Symptoms of caffeinism (usually associated with ingestion of over 500 mg/day) include anxiety, agitation, restlessness, insomnia, a feeling of being "wired," and somatic symptoms referable to the heart and gastrointestinal tract. It is common for a case of caffeinism to present as an anxiety disorder. It is also common for caffeine and other stimulants to precipitate severe symptoms in compensated schizophrenic and manic-depressive patients. Chronically depressed patients often use caffeine drinks as self-medication. This diagnostic clue may help distinguish some major affective disorders. Discontinuation of caffeine (greater than 250 mg/day) can produce withdrawal symptoms, such as headaches, irritability, lethargy, and occasional nausea.

8. Miscellaneous Drugs & Solvents

The principal over-the-counter drugs of concern are an assortment of antihistaminic agents, frequently in combination with a mild analgesic promoted as cold remedies.

Antihistamines usually produce some central nervous system depression—thus their use as over-the-counter sedatives. Practically all of the so-called sleep aids are antihistamines. The mixture of antihistamines with alcohol usually exacerbates the central nervous system effects. Scopolamine and bromides have generally been removed from over-the-counter products.

The abuse of laxatives sometimes can lead to electrolyte disturbances that may contribute to the manifestations of a delirium. The greatest use of laxatives tends to be in the elderly and in those with eating disorders, both of whom are the most vulnerable to physiologic changes.

Anabolic steroids are abused by people who wish to increase muscle mass for cosmetic reasons or for greater strength. In addition to the medical problems, the practice is associated with significant mood swings, aggressiveness, and paranoid delusions. Alcohol and stimulant use is higher in these individuals. Withdrawal symptoms of steroid dependency include fatigue, depressed mood, restlessness, and insomnia.

Amyl nitrite is used as an "orgasm expander." The changes in time perception, "rush," and mild euphoria caused by the drug prompted its nonmedical use. Subjective effects last from 5 seconds to 15 minutes. Tolerance develops readily, but there are no known withdrawal symptoms. Abstinence for several days reestablishes the previous level of responsiveness. Long-term effects may include damage to the immune system and respiratory difficulties.

Sniffing of solvents and inhaling of gases (including aerosols) produce a form of inebriation similar to that of the volatile anesthetics. Agents include gasoline, toluene, petroleum ether, lighter fluids, cleaning fluids, paint thinners, and solvents that are present in many household products (eg, nail polish). Typical intoxication states include euphoria, slurred speech, hallucinations, and

confusion, and with high doses, acute manifestations are unconsciousness and cardiorespiratory depression or failure; chronic exposure produces a variety of symptoms related to the liver, kidney, bone marrow, or heart. Lead encephalopathy can be associated with sniffing leaded gasoline. In addition, studies of workers chronically exposed to jet fuel showed significant increases in neurasthenic symptoms, including fatigue, anxiety, mood changes, memory difficulties, and somatic complaints. These same problems have been noted in long-term solvent abuse.

The so-called designer drugs are synthetic substitutes for commonly used recreational drugs. Common designer drugs include methyl analogues of fentanyl used as heroin substitutes. MDMA (methylenedioxymethamphetamine), an amphetamine derivative sometimes called "ecstasy," is also a designer drug with high abuse potential and purported neurotoxicity. Often not detected by standard toxicology screens, these substances can present a vexing problem for clinicians faced with symptoms from a totally unknown cause.

Alford DP et al. Collaborative care of opioid-addicted patients in primary care using buprenorphine: five-year experience. Arch Intern Med. 2011 Mar 14;171(5):425–31. [PMID: 21403039]

Cicero TJ et al. The changing face of heroin use in the United States: a retrospective analysis of the past 50 years. JAMA Psychiatry. 2014 Jul 1;71(7):821–6. [PMID: 24871348]

Friedmann PD. Clinical practice. Alcohol use in adults. N Engl J Med. 2013 Jan 24;368(4):365–73. Erratum in: N Engl J Med. 2013 Apr 25;368(17):1661. N Engl J Med. 2013 Feb 21;368(8):781. [PMID: 23343065]

Hoch E et al. Efficacy of a targeted cognitive-behavioral treatment program for cannabis use disorders (CANDIS`). Eur Neuropsychopharmacol. 2012 Apr;22(4):267–80. [PMID: 21865014]

Merrill JO et al. Addiction disorders. Med Clin North Am. 2014 Sep;98(5):1097–122. [PMID: 25134875]

Mirijello A et al. Identification and management of alcohol withdrawal syndrome. Drugs. 2015 Mar;75(4):353–65. [PMID: 25666543]

Stehman CR et al. A rational approach to the treatment of alcohol withdrawal in the ED. Am J Emerg Med. 2013 Apr;31(4):734–42. [PMID: 23399338]

▼ DELIRIUM & OTHER COGNITIVE DISORDERS

ESSENTIALS OF DIAGNOSIS

► Transient or permanent brain dysfunction.

► Cognitive impairment to varying degrees.

► Impaired recall and recent memory, inability to focus attention and problems in perceptual processing, often with psychotic ideation.

► Random psychomotor activity such as stereotypy.

► Emotional disorders frequently present: depression, anxiety, irritability.

► Behavioral disturbances: impulse control, sexual acting-out, attention deficits, aggression, and exhibitionism.

General Considerations

The organic problem may be a primary brain disorder or a secondary manifestation of some general disorder. All of the cognitive disorders show some degree of impaired thinking depending on the site of involvement, the rate of onset and progression, and the duration of the underlying brain lesion. Emotional disturbances (eg, depression) are often present as significant comorbidities. The behavioral disturbances tend to be more common with chronicity, more directly related to the underlying personality or central nervous system vulnerability to drug side effects, and not necessarily correlated with cognitive dysfunction.

The causes of cognitive disorders are listed in Table 25–11.

Clinical Findings

The many manifestations include problems with orientation, short or fluctuating attention span, loss of recent memory and recall, impaired judgment, emotional lability, lack of initiative, impaired impulse control, inability to reason through problems, depression (worse in mild to moderate types), confabulation (not limited to alcohol organic brain syndrome), constriction of intellectual functions, visual and auditory hallucinations, and delusions.

Physical findings will vary according to the cause. The electroencephalogram usually shows generalized slowing in delirium.

A. Delirium

Delirium (acute confusional state) is a transient global disorder of attention, with clouding of consciousness, usually a result of systemic problems (eg, medications, hypoxemia). Onset is usually rapid. The mental status fluctuates (impairment is usually least in the morning), with varying inability to concentrate, maintain attention, and sustain purposeful behavior. There is a marked deficit of short-term memory and recall. Anxiety and irritability are common. Amnesia is retrograde (impaired recall of past memories) and anterograde (inability to recall events after the onset of the delirium). Orientation problems follow the inability to retain information. Perceptual disturbances (often visual hallucinations) and psychomotor restlessness with insomnia are common. Autonomic changes include tachycardia, dilated pupils, and sweating. The average duration is about 1 week, but delirium may be more persistent and can be associated with chronic deficits. Delirium can coexist with dementia. Delirium may be hypoactive, hyperactive, or mixed.

Table 25–11. Etiology of delirium and other cognitive disorders.

Disorder	Possible Causes
Intoxication	Alcohol, sedatives, bromides, analgesics (eg, pentazocine), psychedelic drugs, stimulants, and household solvents.
Drug withdrawal	Withdrawal from alcohol, sedative-hypnotics, corticosteroids.
Long-term effects of alcohol	Wernicke-Korsakoff syndrome.
Infections	Septicemia; meningitis and encephalitis due to bacterial, viral, fungal, parasitic, or tuberculous organisms or to central nervous system syphilis; acute and chronic infections due to the entire range of microbiologic pathogens.
Endocrine disorders	Thyrotoxicosis, hypothyroidism, adrenocortical dysfunction (including Addison disease and Cushing syndrome), pheochromocytoma, insulinoma, hypoglycemia, hyperparathyroidism, hypoparathyroidism, panhypopituitarism, diabetic ketoacidosis.
Respiratory disorders	Hypoxia, hypercapnia.
Metabolic disturbances	Fluid and electrolyte disturbances (especially hyponatremia, hypomagnesemia, and hypercalcemia), acid-base disorders, hepatic disease (hepatic encephalopathy), kidney failure, porphyria.
Nutritional deficiencies	Deficiency of vitamin B_1 (beriberi), vitamin B_{12} (pernicious anemia), folic acid, nicotinic acid (pellagra); protein-calorie malnutrition.
Trauma	Subdural hematoma, subarachnoid hemorrhage, intracerebral bleeding, concussion syndrome.
Cardiovascular disorders	Myocardial infarctions, cardiac arrhythmias, cerebrovascular spasms, hypertensive encephalopathy, hemorrhages, embolisms, and occlusions indirectly cause decreased cognitive function.
Neoplasms	Primary or metastatic lesions of the central nervous system, cancer-induced hypercalcemia.
Seizure disorders	Ictal, interictal, and postictal dysfunction.
Collagen-vascular and immunologic disorders	Autoimmune disorders, including systemic lupus erythematosus, Sjögren syndrome, and AIDS.
Degenerative diseases	Alzheimer disease, Pick disease, multiple sclerosis, parkinsonism, Huntington chorea, normal pressure hydrocephalus.
Medications	Anticholinergic medications, antidepressants, H_2-blocking agents, digoxin, salicylates (long-term use), and a wide variety of other over-the-counter and prescribed medications.

"Sundowning"—mild to moderate delirium at night- is more common in patients with preexisting dementia and may be precipitated by hospitalization, medications, and sensory deprivation.

Terminal delirium occurs commonly at the end of life. The delirium may be related to multiple medical causes, including organ failure, and may be unrecognized. Treatment must be based on a careful evaluation of the underlying etiology and the risks and benefits of available medical and nonmedical interventions.

B. Dementia

(See Chapters 4 and 24.) Dementia is characterized by chronicity and deterioration of selective mental functions. Specific cognitive assessment must be performed, since many patients are able to cover a deficit in routine conversation. The Mini-Mental State Examination produces a numerical score with up to 30 points given for correct answers to questions (likely organic less than 27 points).

In all types of dementia, loss of impulse control (sexual and language) is common. The tenuous level of functioning makes the individual most susceptible to minor physical and psychological stresses. **Pseudodementia** is a term previously applied to depressed patients who appear to be demented. These patients are often identifiable by their tendency to complain about memory problems vociferously rather than try to cover them up. They usually say they cannot complete cognitive tasks but with encouragement can often do so. They can be considered to have depression-induced reversible dementia that improves when the depression resolves. In many geriatrics patients, however, the depression appears to be an insult that often unmasks a progressive dementia. Thus, even though cognition tends to improve substantially in these patients, many go on to develop Alzheimer disease or other dementias.

C. Amnestic Syndrome

This is a memory disturbance without delirium or dementia. It is usually associated with thiamine deficiency and chronic alcohol use (eg, Korsakoff syndrome). There is an impairment in the ability to learn new information or recall previously learned information.

D. Substance-Induced Hallucinosis

This condition is characterized by persistent or recurrent hallucinations (usually auditory) without the other symptoms usually found in delirium or dementia. Alcohol or hallucinogens are often the cause. There does not have to be any other mental disorder, and there may be complete spontaneous resolution.

E. Personality Changes Due to a General Medical Condition (Formerly Organic Personality Syndrome)

This syndrome is characterized by emotional lability and loss of impulse control along with a general change in personality. Cognitive functions are preserved. Social inappropriateness is common. Loss of interest and lack of

concern with the consequences of one's actions are often present. The course depends on the underlying cause (eg, frontal lobe contusion may resolve completely).

▶ Differential Diagnosis

The differential diagnosis of dementia includes reversible causes of dementia such as hypothyroidism, vitamin B_{12} deficiency, and normal pressure hydrocephalus. Progressive dementias include Alzheimer disease, Lewy body, and frontotemporal dementias. Depression is sometimes confused with dementia.

Delirium can be confused with acute intoxication or withdrawal states, psychotic disorders, and depression in the hypoactive form.

▶ Complications

Chronicity may result from delayed correction of the defect, eg, subdural hematoma, low-pressure hydrocephalus. Accidents secondary to impulsive behavior and poor judgment are a major consideration. Secondary depression and impulsive behavior not infrequently lead to suicide attempts. Medications—particularly sedatives—may worsen thinking abilities and contribute to the overall problems.

▶ Treatment

A. Medical

Delirium should be considered a syndrome of acute brain dysfunction analogous to acute kidney failure. The first aim of treatment is to identify and correct the etiologic medical problem. Evaluation should consist of a comprehensive physical examination including a search for neurologic abnormalities, infection, or hypoxia. Laboratory tests may include serum electrolytes, serum glucose, BUN, serum creatinine, liver biochemical tests, thyroid function tests, arterial blood gases, complete blood count, serum calcium, phosphorus, magnesium, vitamin B_{12}, folate, blood cultures, urinalysis, and cerebrospinal fluid analysis. Discontinue medications that may be contributing to the problem (eg, analgesics, corticosteroids, cimetidine, lidocaine, anticholinergic medications, central nervous system depressants, mefloquine). Do not overlook any possibility of reversible organic disease. Electroencephalography, CT, and MRI evaluations of the brain may be helpful in diagnosis. Ideally, the patient should be monitored without further medications while the evaluation is carried out. There are, however, at least two indications for medication in delirious states: behavioral control (eg, pulling out lines) and subjective distress (eg, pronounced fear due to hallucinations). If these indications are present, medications may be used. If there is any hint of alcohol or substance withdrawal (the most common cause of delirium in the general hospital), a benzodiazepine such as lorazepam (1–2 mg every hour) can be given parenterally. If there is little likelihood of withdrawal syndrome, haloperidol is often used in doses of 1–10 mg every hour. Given intravenously under ECG monitoring, it appears to impose slight risk of extrapyramidal side effects. In addition to the medication, a pleasant, comfortable, nonthreatening, and physically safe environment with adequate nursing or attendant services should be provided. Once the underlying condition has been identified and treated, adjunctive medications can be tapered.

Treatment of the behavioral manifestations of the **dementia syndrome** usually involve trying to positively reinforce healthy behaviors and not reinforcing maladaptive behaviors (such as aggression). Arranging the physical environment to maximize autonomy as much as feasible and promote regularity of routine, helps the individual cope with their limited intellectual reserves. Simple, direct statements are more easily comprehended by these individuals. Understanding how their decreased cognitive function limits their abilities is important. For example, one elderly man in a residential apartment kept complaining that someone was stealing his ice cream at night. Realizing that he was unable to recall eating it himself, his "delusion" made a certain sense. Once his caregivers understood this, they were able to be more compassionate in listening to his complaints and less worried about an ice cream burglar.

Acetylcholinesterase inhibitors, such as donepezil, galantamine, and rivastigmine, and the glutamatergic agent memantine have modest effects on the cognitive symptoms of Alzheimer disease and may also help other dementias. The available agents may delay the progression of Alzheimer disease for 6–12 months and improve overall cognitive functioning in a subset of patients. Although the efficacy of these agents is not very robust, they are reasonably tolerated and many patients do find them helpful. The most common side effects of the acetylcholinesterase inhibitors are nausea, diminished appetite, and loose bowel movements; side effects of memantine include headache, constipation, and dizziness. The doses for these oral drugs are donepezil, 5–10 mg/day; rivastigmine, 1.5–6 mg twice daily; galantamine, 4–12 mg twice daily; and memantine, 5–10 mg daily to twice daily. Aggressiveness and rage states in dementia can be reduced with lipophilic beta-blockers (eg, propranolol, metoprolol) in moderate doses. Since the serotonergic system has been implicated in arousal conditions, medications that affect serotonin have been found to be of some benefit in aggression and agitation. Included in this group are lithium, trazodone, buspirone, and clonazepam. Dopamine blockers (eg, the antipsychotic medications such as haloperidol) have been used for many years to attenuate aggression. Likewise, second-generation antipsychotics may have a role in selected geriatric patients. However, no antipsychotic has been shown to be more beneficial than placebo in more rigorous controlled studies in the management of behavioral dyscontrol in dementia patients. In addition, both first- and second-generation agents have been associated with increased mortality in this population and carry FDA warnings to this effect. There are also reports of reduced agitation in Alzheimer disease from carbamazepine, 100–400 mg/day orally (with slow increase as needed). Emotional lability in some cases responds to fluoxetine (5–20 mg/day orally); depression, which often occurs early in the course of Alzheimer dementia, responds to the usual doses of antidepressant medications, preferably those with the least anticholinergic side effects (eg, SSRIs and SNRIs).

B. Social

Substitute home care, board and care, or convalescent home care may be most useful when the family is unable to care for the patient. The setting should include familiar people and objects, lights at night, and a simple schedule. Counseling may help the family to cope with problems and may help keep the patient at home as long as possible. Information about local groups can be obtained from the Alzheimer's Disease and Related Disorders Association, 70 East Lake Street, Suite 600, Chicago, IL 60601. Volunteer services, including homemakers, visiting nurses, and adult protective services, may be helpful in maintaining the patient at home.

C. Behavioral

Behavioral techniques include operant responses that can be used to induce positive behaviors, eg, paying attention to the patient who is trying to communicate appropriately, and extinction by ignoring inappropriate responses. Patients with Alzheimer disease can learn skills and retain them but do not recall the circumstances in which they were learned.

D. Psychological

Formal psychological therapies are not usually helpful and may make things worse by taxing the patient's limited cognitive resources.

► **Prognosis**

The prognosis is fair to good for recovery of mental functioning in delirium when the underlying condition is reversible. For most dementia syndromes, the prognosis is for gradual deterioration, although new drug treatments may prove helpful.

Barr J et al; American College of Critical Care Medicine. Clinical practice guidelines for the management of pain, agitation, and delirium in adult patients in the intensive care unit. Crit Care Med. 2013 Jan;41(1):263–306. [PMID: 23269131]

Deardorff WJ et al. The use of cholinesterase inhibitors across all stages of Alzheimer's Disease. Drugs Aging. 2015 Jul;32(7):537–47. [PMID: 26033268]

Gitlin LN et al. Nonpharmacologic management of behavioral symptoms in dementia. JAMA. 2012 Nov 21;308(19):2020–9. [PMID: 23168825]

Wong N et al. Managing delirium in the emergency department: tools for targeting underlying etiology. Emerg Med Pract. 2015 Oct;17(10):1–20. [PMID: 26367083]

▼ **PSYCHIATRIC PROBLEMS ASSOCIATED WITH HOSPITALIZATION & ILLNESS**

► **Diagnostic Categories**

A. Acute Problems

1. Delirium with psychotic features secondary to the medical or surgical problem, or compounded by effect of treatment.

2. Acute anxiety, often related to ignorance and fear of the immediate problem as well as uncertainty about the future.

3. Anxiety as an intrinsic aspect of the medical problem (eg, hyperthyroidism).

4. Denial of illness, which may present during acute or intermediate phases of illness.

B. Intermediate Problems

1. Depression as a function of the illness or acceptance of the illness, often associated with realistic or fantasied hopelessness about the future.

2. Behavioral problems, often related to denial of illness and, in extreme cases, causing the patient to leave the hospital against medical advice.

C. Recuperative Problems

1. Decreasing cooperation as the patient sees that improvement and compliance are not compelled.

2. Readjustment problems with family, job, and society.

▶ General Considerations

A. Acute Problems

1. "Intensive care unit psychosis"—The ICU environment may contribute to the etiology of delirium. Critical care unit factors include sleep deprivation, increased arousal, mechanical ventilation, and social isolation. Other causes include those common to delirium and require vigorous investigation (see Delirium).

2. Presurgical and postsurgical anxiety states—Anxiety before or after surgery is common and commonly ignored. Presurgical anxiety is very common and is principally a fear of death (many surgical patients make out their wills). Patients may be fearful of anesthesia (improved by the preoperative anesthesia interview), the mysterious operating room, and the disease processes that might be uncovered by the surgeon. Such fears frequently cause people to delay examinations that might result in earlier surgery and a greater chance of cure.

The opposite of this is **surgery proneness,** the quest for surgery to escape from overwhelming life stresses. Polysurgery patients may be classified as having factitious disorders. Dynamic motivations include the need to get medical care as a way of getting dependency needs met, the desire to outwit authority figures, unconscious guilt, or a masochistic need to suffer. Frequent surgery may also be related to a somatic symptom disorder, particularly body dysmorphic disorder (an obsession that a body part is disfigured). More apparent reasons may include an attempt to get relief from pain and a lifestyle that has become almost exclusively medically oriented, with all of the risks entailed in such an endeavor.

Postsurgical anxiety states are usually related to pain, procedures, and loss of body image. Acute pain problems are quite different from chronic pain disorders (see Chronic Pain Disorders, this chapter); the former are readily handled with adequate analgesic medication (see Chapter 5).

Alterations in body image, as with amputations, ostomies, and mastectomies, often raise concerns about relationships with others.

3. Iatrogenic problems—These usually pertain to medications, complications of diagnostic and treatment procedures, and impersonal and unsympathetic staff behavior. Polypharmacy is often a factor. Patients with unsolved diagnostic problems are at higher risk. They are desirous of relief, and the quest engenders more diagnostic procedures with a higher incidence of complications. The upset patient and family may be very demanding. Excessive demands usually result from anxiety. Such behavior is best handled with calm and measured responses.

B. Intermediate Problems

1. Prolonged hospitalization—Prolonged hospitalization presents unique problems in certain hospital services, eg, burn units or orthopedic services. The acute problems of the severely burned patient are discussed in Chapter 37. The problems often are behavioral difficulties related to length of hospitalization and necessary procedures. For example, in burn units, pain is a major problem in addition to anxiety about procedures. Disputes with staff are common and often concern pain medication or ward privileges. Some patients regress to infantile behavior and dependency. Staff members must agree about their approach to the patient in order to ensure the smooth functioning of the unit.

Denial of illness may present in some patients. Intervention by an authority figure (eg, immediate work supervisor) may help the patient accept treatment and eventually abandon the coping mechanism of denial.

2. Depression—Mood disorders ranging from mild adjustment disorder to major depressive disorder frequently occur during prolonged hospitalizations. A key to the diagnosis of depression in the medical setting is the individual's loss of self-esteem; they often think of themselves as worthless and are guilt ridden. Therapeutic medications (eg, corticosteroids) may be a factor. Depression can contribute to irritability and overt anger. Severe depression can lead to anorexia, which further complicates healing and metabolic balance. It is during this period that the issue of disfigurement arises—relief at survival gives way to concern about future function and appearance.

C. Recuperative Problems

1. Anxiety—Anxiety about return to the posthospital environment can cause regression to a dependent position. Complications increase, and staff forbearance again is tested. Anxiety occurring at this stage usually is handled more easily than previous behavior problems.

2. Posthospital adjustment—Adjustment difficulties after discharge are related to the severity of the deficits and the use of outpatient facilities (eg, physical therapy, rehabilitation programs, psychiatric outpatient treatment). Some patients may experience posttraumatic stress symptoms (eg, from traumatic injuries or even from necessary medical treatments). Lack of appropriate follow-up can contribute to depression in the patient, who may feel that he or she is making poor progress and may have thoughts of "giving up." Reintegration into work, educational, and social endeavors may be slow. Life is simply much more difficult when one is disfigured, disabled, or disenfranchised.

Clinical Findings

The symptoms that occur in these patients are similar to those discussed in previous sections of this chapter, eg, delirium, stress and adjustment disorders, anxiety, and depression. Behavior problems may include lack of cooperation, increased complaints, demands for medication, sexual approaches to nurses, threats to leave the hospital, and actual signing out against medical recommendations. The underlying personality structure of the individual is a major factor in coping styles (eg, the compulsive individual increases indecision, the hysterical individual increases dramatic behavior).

Differential Diagnosis

Delirium and dementia (including cases associated with HIV infection and drug abuse) must always be ruled out, since they often present with symptoms resembling anxiety, depression, or psychosis. Personality disorders existing prior to hospitalization often underlie the various behavior problems, but particularly the management problems.

Complications

Prolongation of hospitalization causes increased expense, deterioration of patient-staff relationships, and increased probabilities of iatrogenic and legal problems. The possibility of increasing posthospital treatment problems is enhanced.

Treatment

A. Medical

The most important consideration by far is to have one clinician in charge, a clinician whom the patient trusts and who is able to oversee multiple treatment approaches (see Somatic Symptom Disorders, above). In acute problems, attention must be paid to metabolic imbalance, alcohol withdrawal, and previous drug use—prescribed, recreational, or over-the-counter. Adequate sleep and analgesia are important in the prevention of delirium. When absolute behavioral control is urgently needed, agents such as propofol, dexmedetomidine, opioids, and midazolam have been used.

Many clinicians are attuned to the early detection of the surgery-prone patient. Plastic and orthopedic surgeons are at particular risk. Appropriate consultations may help detect some problems and mitigate future ones.

Postsurgical anxiety states can be alleviated by personal attention from the surgeon. Anxiety is not so effectively lessened by ancillary medical personnel, whom the patient perceives as lesser authorities, until after the clinician has reassured the patient. "Patient-controlled analgesia" can improve pain control, decrease anxiety, and minimize side effects.

Depression should be recognized early. If severe, it may be treated by antidepressant medications (see Antidepressant Medications, above). High levels of anxiety can be lowered with judicious use of anxiolytic agents. Unnecessary medications tend to reinforce the patient's impression that there must be a serious illness or medication would not be required.

B. Psychological

Prepare the patient and family for what is to come. This includes the types of units where the patient will be quartered, the procedures that will be performed, and any disfigurements that will result from surgery. Repetition improves understanding. The nursing staff can be helpful, since patients frequently confide a lack of understanding to a nurse but are reluctant to do so to the physician.

Denial of illness is frequently a block to acceptance of treatment. This too should be handled with family members present (to help the patient face the reality of the situation) in a series of short interviews (for reinforcement). Dependency problems resulting from long hospitalization are best handled by focusing on the changes to come as the patient makes the transition to the outside world. Key figures are teachers, vocational counselors, and physical therapists. Challenges should be realistic and practical and handled in small steps.

Depression is usually related to the loss of familiar hospital supports, and the outpatient therapists and counselors help to lessen the impact of the loss. Some of the impact can be alleviated by anticipating, with the patient and family, the signal features of the common depression to help prevent the patient from assuming a permanent sick role (invalidism).

Suicide is always a concern when a patient is faced with despair. An honest, compassionate, and supportive approach will help sustain the patient during this trying period.

C. Behavioral

Prior desensitization can significantly allay anxiety about medical procedures. A "dry run" can be done to reinforce the oral description. Cooperation during acute problem periods can be enhanced by the use of appropriate reinforcers such as a favorite nurse or helpful family member. People who are positive reinforcers are even more helpful during the intermediate phases when the patient becomes resistant to the seemingly endless procedures (eg, debridement of burned areas).

Specific situations (eg, psychological dependency on the respirator) can be corrected by weaning with appropriate reinforcers (eg, watching a favorite movie on a DVD player when disconnected from the ventilator). Behavioral approaches should be used in a positive and optimistic way for maximal reinforcement.

Relaxation techniques and attentional distraction can be used to block side effects of a necessary treatment (eg, nausea in cancer chemotherapy).

D. Social

A change in environment requires adaptation. Because of the illness, admission and hospitalization may be more easily handled than discharge. Reintegration into society can be difficult. In some cases, the family is a negative influence. A predischarge evaluation must be made to determine whether the family will be able to cope with the physical or mental changes in the patient. Working with the family while the patient is in the acute stage may presage a successful transition later on.

Development of a new social life can be facilitated by various self-help organizations (eg, the stoma club). Sharing problems with others in similar circumstances eases the return to a social life, which may be quite different from that prior to the illness.

▶ Prognosis

The prognosis is good in all patients who have reversible medical and surgical conditions. It is guarded when there is serious functional loss that impairs vocational, educational, or societal possibilities—especially in the case of progressive and ultimately life-threatening illness.

Katon WJ et al. Collaborative care for patients with depression and chronic illnesses. N Engl J Med. 2010 Dec 30; 363(27):2611–20. [PMID: 21190455]

Milani RV et al. Impact of exercise training and depression on survival in heart failure due to coronary heart disease. Am J Cardiol. 2011 Jan;107(1):64–8. [PMID: 21146688]

Endocrine Disorders

Paul A. Fitzgerald, MD

ANTERIOR HYPOPITUITARISM

 ESSENTIALS OF DIAGNOSIS

▸ Partial or complete deficiency of one or any combination of anterior pituitary hormones.

▸ **Adrenocorticotropic hormone deficiency:** reduced adrenal secretion of cortisol and epinephrine; aldosterone secretion remains intact.

▸ **Growth hormone (GH) deficiency:** short stature in children; asthenia, obesity, and increased cardiovascular risk in adults.

▸ **Prolactin deficiency:** postpartum lactation failure.

▸ **Thyroid-stimulating hormone (TSH) deficiency:** secondary hypothyroidism.

▸ **Luteinizing hormone (LH) and follicle-stimulating hormone (FSH) deficiency:** hypogonadism and infertility in men and women.

▶ General Considerations

Hypopituitarism can be caused by either hypothalamic or pituitary dysfunction. Patients with hypopituitarism may have single or multiple hormonal deficiencies (Table 26–1).

1. Hypopituitarism with mass lesions—Lesions in the hypothalamus, pituitary stalk, or pituitary can cause hypopituitarism. Pituitary adenomas can cause anterior hypopituitarism but rarely cause diabetes insipidus. Other mass lesions include granulomas, such as granulomatosis with polyangiitis (formerly Wegener granulomatosis), tuberculosis, cholesterol granuloma; cleft cysts; pituitary apoplexy; metastatic carcinomas or hematologic malignancies; aneurysms; and brain tumors (craniopharyngioma, meningioma, dysgerminoma, glioma, chondrosarcoma, chordoma of the clivus). Rare causes include postpartum pituitary necrosis (Sheehan syndrome), African trypanosomiasis, and Langerhans cell histiocytosis.

Lymphocytic hypophysitis is an autoimmune disorder that is more common in women (71%) and is associated with pregnancy in 11% of cases. Nearly 20% of cases are associated with other autoimmune conditions, such as systemic lupus erythematosus (SLE). Hypophysitis can also be caused by chemotherapy with ipilimumab. It typically presents with hypogonadotropic hypogonadism (62%), diabetes insipidus (54%), headache (50%), hypothyroidism (48%), adrenocorticotropic hormone (ACTH) deficiency (47%), growth hormone (GH) deficiency (37%), and hyperprolactinemia (36%), making clinicians often mistake it for a prolactinoma.

2. Hypopituitarism without mass lesions—Congenital hypopituitarism occurs in syndromes such as septo-optic dysplasia (de Morsier syndrome) and in patients with various gene mutations. Congenital isolated hypogonadotropic hypogonadism can be caused by mutations in any of the many genes that control the production or release of gonadotropin-releasing hormone (GnRH), LH, or FSH; it also occurs with the syndrome of congenital adrenal hypoplasia. Prader-Willi syndrome is a genetic disorder where genes on the paternal chromosome 15 are deleted or unexpressed. The incidence of this disorder is 1:15,000; both sexes are affected equally. Kallmann syndrome is caused by various gene mutations that impair the development or migration of GnRH-synthesizing neurons from the olfactory bulb to the hypothalamus. Congenital GH deficiency occurs as an isolated pituitary hormone deficiency in about one-third of cases.

Acquired hypopituitarism without mass lesions can result from cranial radiation therapy, pituitary surgery, encephalitis, cerebral malaria, hemochromatosis, autoimmunity, or coronary artery bypass grafting (CABG). Ipilimumab chemotherapy can induce hypophysitis with hypopituitarism that includes secondary adrenal insufficiency and an enlarged pituitary without a mass lesion on MRI. At least one pituitary hormone deficiency develops in about 25–30% of survivors of moderate to severe traumatic brain injury and in about 55% of survivors of aneurysmal subarachnoid hemorrhage. Some degree of hypopituitarism, most commonly GH deficiency and hypogonadotropic hypogonadism, occurs in one-third of ischemic stroke patients. Mitotane, given for adrenal

Table 26–1. Pituitary hormones.

Anterior pituitary
  Growth hormone (GH)[1]
  Prolactin (PRL)
  Adrenocorticotropic hormone (ACTH)
  Thyroid-stimulating hormone (TSH)
  Luteinizing hormone (LH)[2]
  Follicle-stimulating hormone (FSH)
Posterior pituitary
  Arginine vasopressin (AVP)[3]
  Oxytocin

[1]GH closely resembles human placental lactogen (hPL).
[2]LH closely resembles human chorionic gonadotropin (hCG).
[3]AVP is identical with antidiuretic hormone (ADH).

cortical carcinoma, can suppress TSH secretion and cause reversible secondary hypothyroidism.

Sheehan syndrome refers to hypopituitarism caused by postpartum pituitary necrosis, usually following severe postpartum uterine hemorrhage. It is characterized by postpartum amenorrhea and inability to lactate. Hypopituitarism can occur acutely, usually with severe secondary adrenal insufficiency that may be fatal unless recognized and treated. Acute hypopituitarism may also be associated with diabetes insipidus. However, hypopituitarism usually occurs gradually over 10–20 years and the diagnosis is typically delayed an average of 9 years. Panhypopituitarism or partial hypopituitarism, typically manifesting with hyponatremia, hypoglycemia, or anemia, may develop in affected women. In acute Sheehan syndrome, MRI shows an enlarged pituitary with only a thin rim of enhancement with gadolinium. After 1 year, MRI shows atrophy of the pituitary and a partially empty sella.

Functional hypopituitarism can occur with normal aging because of variable degrees of GH deficiency. Similarly, aging men develop variable degrees of hypogonadotropic hypogonadism, with serum free testosterone levels that are slightly low or near the lower end of normal reference ranges, while serum FSH and LH levels remain normal. Obesity also causes variable degrees of GH deficiency and male hypogonadotropic hypogonadism that are typically reversible with sufficient weight loss. Hypothalamic amenorrhea commonly occurs in women during severe emotional or physical stress, caloric restriction or eating disorders, or intense exercise. Hypogonadotropic hypogonadism also occurs with severe illness, alcoholism, opioid analgesics, anabolic steroids; hyperprolactinemia (drug-induced or spontaneous); anorexia nervosa; and malnutrition. Therapy with exogenous corticosteroids (parenteral, oral, inhaled, or topical) can suppress ACTH secretion and causes functional isolated secondary adrenal insufficiency.

▶ Clinical Findings

A. Symptoms and Signs

1. GH deficiency—**Congenital GH deficiency** typically presents with hypoglycemia in infancy and short stature in childhood.

Acquired GH deficiency is quite common. Also, when other more recognizable pituitary hormone deficits are present, there is a high likelihood of concurrent GH deficiency.

GH deficiency varies in severity from mild to severe, resulting in a variable spectrum of nonspecific symptoms that include mild to moderate central obesity, reduced physical and mental energy, impaired concentration and memory, and depression. Patients may also have variably reduced muscle and bone mass, increased low-density lipoprotein (LDL) cholesterol, and reduced cardiac output with exercise.

Laron syndrome is an autosomal recessive disorder that is mainly caused by mutations in the gene that encodes the GH receptor, resulting in GH-resistance. This causes a severe deficiency in serum insulin-like growth factor-1 (IGF-1), resulting in short stature (dwarfism). Affected individuals have a prominent forehead, depressed nasal bridge, small mandible, and central obesity. They may have recurrent hypoglycemic seizures. Partial resistance to GH may cause some cases of idiopathic short stature without features of Laron syndrome.

2. Gonadotropin deficiency (hypogonadotropic hypogonadism)—In gonadotropin deficiency, insufficiencies of LH and FSH cause hypogonadism and infertility.

Congenital gonadotropin deficiency is characterized by partial or complete lack of pubertal development. **Isolated hypogonadotropic hypogonadism** occurs with an estimated prevalence between 1 in 4000 and 1 in 10,000 males; it is less common in females. The sense of olfaction (smell) is entirely normal in 58% (normosmic isolated hypogonadotropic hypogonadism), or hyposmic or anosmic in 42% (Kallmann syndrome). Patients frequently have abnormal genitalia (25%), renal anomalies (28%), midline craniofacial defects (50%), neurologic deficits (42%), and musculoskeletal malformations, Some affected women have menarche followed by secondary amenorrhea. Some affected males also have **congenital adrenal hypoplasia** with X-linked inheritance. As adolescents, they fail to enter puberty; isolated hypogonadotropic hypogonadism and subtle signs of adrenal failure can present in adulthood.

Prader-Willi syndrome presents with cryptorchidism, mental retardation, short stature, hyperflexibility, autonomic dysregulation, cognitive impairment, hyperphagia with obesity, hypogonadotropic hypogonadism, or primary hypogonadism.

Acquired gonadotropin deficiency is characterized by the gradual loss of facial, axillary, pubic, and body hair. **Men** may note diminished libido, erectile dysfunction, muscle atrophy, infertility, and osteopenia. **Women** have amenorrhea, infertility, and osteoporosis.

3. TSH deficiency—TSH deficiency causes hypothyroidism with manifestations such as fatigue, weakness, weight change, and hyperlipidemia. Bexarotene and mitotane are drugs that suppress TSH.

4. ACTH deficiency—This results in diminished cortisol with symptoms of weakness, fatigue, weight loss, and hypotension. Patients with partial ACTH deficiency have some cortisol secretion and may not have symptoms until stressed by illness or surgery. Adrenal mineralocorticoid secretion continues, so manifestations of adrenal insufficiency in hypopituitarism are usually less striking than in bilateral adrenal gland destruction (Addison disease). Hyponatremia may occur, especially when ACTH and TSH deficiencies are both present.

5. Prolactin deficiency—This presents in women with failure to lactate in the puerperium.

6. Panhypopituitarism—This condition refers to a deficiency of several or all pituitary hormones. Congenital panhypopituitarism often develops gradually, usually presenting with short stature and growth failure due to GH and TSH deficiency; lack of pubertal development occurs due to deficiencies in FSH and LH. ACTH-cortisol deficiency tends to develop by age 18 years. Patients with long-standing hypopituitarism tend to have dry, pale, fine, wrinkled facial skin and an apathetic countenance.

7. Hypothalamic damage—This can cause obesity and cognitive impairment. Local tumor effects can cause headache or optic nerve compression with visual field impairment.

B. Laboratory Findings

Fasting hypoglycemia may be present with secondary hypoadrenalism, hypothyroidism, or GH deficiency. Hyponatremia is often present due to hypothyroidism or hypoadrenalism.

Men with hypogonadotropic hypogonadism have a low serum total or free testosterone and a normal or low serum LH. In such men, hyperprolactinemia may be seen with pituitary prolactinomas, acromegaly, or injury to the hypothalamus or pituitary infundibulum.

Women with hypogonadotropic hypogonadism have a low serum estradiol and a normal or low serum FSH. In nonpregnant women with amenorrhea or galactorrhea, hyperprolactinemia may be seen with a pituitary prolactinomas, acromegaly, or injury to the hypothalamus or pituitary infundibulum.

Patients with secondary hypothyroidism have a low serum free thyroxine (FT_4) and a normal or low serum TSH.

Patients with ACTH deficiency have secondary hypoadrenalism. There is functional atrophy of the adrenal cortex within 2 weeks of pituitary destruction. Therefore, the diagnosis of secondary hypoadrenalism can usually be confirmed with the cosyntropin test. For the cosyntropin test, patients should be either taking no corticosteroids or a short-acting corticosteroid (such as hydrocortisone), which is held after midnight on the morning of the test. At 8 AM, blood is drawn for serum cortisol, ACTH, and dehydroepiandrosterone (DHEA); then 0.25 mg of cosyntropin (synthetic $ACTH_{1-24}$) is administered intramuscularly or intravenously. Another serum cortisol is obtained 45 minutes after the cosyntropin injection; a stimulated serum cortisol of less than 20 mcg/dL (550 nmol/mL) indicates adrenal insufficiency. With gradual pituitary damage and early in the course of ACTH deficiency, patients can have a stimulated serum cortisol of 20 mcg/dL

or more but a baseline 8 AM serum cortisol less than 5 mcg/dL (137.5 nmol/L), which is suspicious for adrenal insufficiency. The baseline ACTH level is low or normal in secondary hypoadrenalism, distinguishing it from primary adrenal disease. The serum DHEA levels are usually low in patients with adrenal deficiency, helping confirm the diagnosis. For patients with signs of secondary adrenal insufficiency (hyponatremia, hypotension, pituitary tumor) but borderline cosyntropin test results, treatment can be instituted empirically and the test repeated at a later date.

The diagnosis of adult GH deficiency is difficult, since GH secretion is normally pulsatile and serum GH levels are nearly undetectable for most of the day. Also, adults (particularly men) physiologically tend to produce less GH when they are over age 50 or have abdominal obesity. Therefore, pathologic GH deficiency is often inferred by symptoms of GH deficiency in the presence of pituitary destruction or other pituitary hormone deficiencies. GH deficiency is present in 96% of patients with three or more other pituitary hormone deficiencies. While GH stimulates the production of IGF-1, the serum IGF-1 level is neither a sensitive (about 50%) nor specific test for GH deficiency in adults. While very low serum IGF-1 levels (less than 84 mcg/L) are usually indicative of GH deficiency, they also occur in malnutrition, prolonged fasting, oral estrogen, hypothyroidism, uncontrolled diabetes mellitus, and liver failure. In GH deficiency (but also in most adults over age 40), exercise-stimulated serum GH levels remain at less than 5 ng/mL and usually fail to rise.

Provocative GH stimulation testing to help diagnose adult GH deficiency has a sensitivity of only 66%. Therefore, a therapeutic trial of GH therapy should be considered for symptomatic patients who have either a serum IGF-1 less than 84 mcg/L or three other pituitary hormone deficiencies.

Provocative GH-stimulation tests are sometimes indicated or required for insurance coverage of GH therapy. In the absence of a serum IGF-1 level less than 84 mcg/L or multiple other pituitary hormone deficiencies, provocative GH-stimulation testing may be indicated for the following patients: (1) young adult patients who have completed GH therapy for childhood GH deficiency and have achieved maximal linear growth; (2) patients who have a hypothalamic or pituitary tumor or who have received surgery or radiation therapy to these areas; and (3) patients who have had prior head trauma, cerebrovascular accident, or encephalitis. When required, such testing usually entails measuring serum GH following provocative stimuli. The glucagon stimulation test is a practical alternative to traditional provocative GH stimulation testing to diagnose pathologic GH deficiency or functional GH deficiency due to aging or obesity. Glucagon 1.0 mg (or 1.5 mg if greater than 200 lbs [or 90 kg]) is administered intramuscularly to well-nourished patients who have not eaten for 8–9 hours. Serum GH is measured before the injection and every 30 minutes for 3 hours. In patients with GH deficiency, the maximum serum GH is usually less than 3 mcg/L. Late hypoglycemia can occur after glucagon, so patients are advised to eat following completion of the test.

Patients with lymphocytic hypophysitis frequently have elevated serum antinuclear or anticytoplasmic antibodies. Patients with hypopituitarism without an established etiology should be screened for hemochromatosis with a serum ferritin or iron and transferrin saturation.

C. Imaging

MRI of the hypothalamus and pituitary is indicated when a mass lesion suspected, such as men over age 16 with a serum testosterone less than 150 ng/dL and a low (or normal) serum LH, two or more pituitary hormone deficiencies, persistent hyperprolactinemia, or symptoms of a mass (headache, visual field defect). MRI is not indicated in cases of functional hypopituitarism associated with severe obesity, drugs, or nutritional disorders.

▶ Differential Diagnosis

The failure to enter puberty may simply reflect delayed puberty. Reversible hypogonadotropic hypogonadism may occur with serious illness, malnutrition, anorexia nervosa, or morbid obesity. Men typically develop partial secondary hypogonadism with aging. Profound hypogonadotropic hypogonadism develops in men who receive GnRH analog therapy (leuprolide) for prostate cancer; it usually persists following cessation of therapy. Hypogonadotropic hypogonadism can develop in patients receiving high-dose opioids, including long-term intrathecal opioid infusion; both GH deficiency and secondary adrenal insufficiency occur in 15% of such patients. Secondary adrenal insufficiency may persist for many months following high-dose corticosteroid therapy.

Suppression of TSH and T_4 can be caused by severe illness, hyperthyroxinemia, and administration of triiodothyronine (Cytomel) or bexarotene, resulting in temporary central hypothyroidism. Corticosteroids or megestrol reversibly suppress endogenous ACTH and cortisol secretion.

GH deficiency occurs normally with aging and physiologically with obesity (reversible with sufficient weight loss).

▶ Complications

Among patients with craniopharyngiomas, diabetes insipidus is found in 16% preoperatively and in 60% postoperatively. Hyponatremia often presents abruptly during the first 2 weeks following pituitary surgery. Visual field impairment may occur. Hypothalamic damage may result in morbid obesity as well as cognitive and emotional problems. Conventional radiation therapy results in an increased incidence of small vessel ischemic strokes and second tumors.

Patients with untreated hypoadrenalism and a stressful illness may become febrile and comatose and die of hyponatremia and shock.

Adults with GH deficiency have experienced an increased cardiovascular morbidity. Rarely, acute hemorrhage may occur in large pituitary tumors, manifested by rapid loss of vision, headache, and evidence of acute pituitary failure (pituitary apoplexy) requiring emergency decompression of the sella.

▶ Treatment

The therapy for hypopituitarism is lifetime hormone replacement.

A. Corticosteroid Replacement

Hydrocortisone tablets, 15–35 mg/day orally in divided doses, should be given. Most patients do well with 10–20 mg in the morning and 5–15 mg in the late afternoon. Patients with partial ACTH deficiency (basal morning serum cortisol above 8 mg/dL [220 mmol/L]) require hydrocortisone replacement in lower doses of about 5 mg orally twice daily. Some clinicians prefer prednisone (3–7.5 mg/day orally) or methylprednisolone (4–6 mg/day orally), given in divided doses. A mineralocorticoid is rarely needed. To determine the optimal corticosteroid replacement dosage, it is necessary to monitor patients carefully for over- or under-replacement. A white blood cell count (WBC) with a differential can be useful, since a relative neutrophilia and lymphopenia can indicate corticosteroid over-replacement, and vice versa. Additional corticosteroids must be given during stress, eg, infection, trauma, or surgical procedures. For mild illness, corticosteroid doses are doubled or tripled. For trauma or surgical stress, hydrocortisone 50 mg is given every 6 hours intravenously or intramuscularly and then reduced to usual doses as the stress subsides. Patients with adrenal insufficiency are advised to wear a medical alert bracelet describing their condition and treatment.

Patients with secondary adrenal insufficiency due to treatment with corticosteroids at supraphysiologic doses require their usual daily dose of corticosteroid during surgery and acute illness; supplemental hydrocortisone is not usually required.

B. Thyroid Hormone Replacement

Levothyroxine is given to correct hypothyroidism only after the patient is assessed for cortisol deficiency or is already receiving corticosteroids. The typical maintenance dose is about 1.6 mcg/kg body weight, averaging 125 mcg daily with a wide range of 25–300 mcg daily. The optimal replacement dose of thyroxine for each patient must be carefully assessed clinically. In patients receiving optimal thyroxine replacement, serum FT_4 levels are usually in the high-normal range while serum T_3 levels are in the low-normal range. Assessment of serum TSH is useless for monitoring patients with hypopituitarism, since TSH levels are always low or normal.

C. Gonadotropin Replacement

Hypogonadotropic hypogonadism often develops in patients with hyperprolactinemia and usually resolves with its treatment. See Male Hypogonadism and Female Hypogonadism.

Women with panhypopituitarism have profound androgen deficiency caused by the combination of both secondary hypogonadism and adrenal insufficiency. When serum DHEA levels are less than 400 ng/mL, women may also be treated with compounded USP-grade DHEA

50 mg/day orally. DHEA therapy tends to increase pubic and axillary hair and may modestly improve libido, alertness, stamina, and overall psychological well being.

For men with oligospermia, human chorionic gonadotropin (hCG) (equivalent to LH) may be given at a dosage of 2000–3000 units intramuscularly three times weekly and testosterone replacement discontinued. The dose of hCG is adjusted to normalize serum testosterone levels. After 6–12 months of hCG treatment, if the sperm count remains low, hCG injections are continued along with injections of follitropin beta (synthetic recombinant FSH) or urofollitropins (urine-derived FSH). An alternative for patients with an intact pituitary is the use of leuprolide (GnRH analog) by intermittent subcutaneous infusion. With treatment, testicular volumes increase within 5–12 months, and some spermatogenesis occurs in most cases. With persistent treatment and the use of intracytoplasmic sperm injection for some cases, the pregnancy success rate is about 70%. Men often feel better during hCG therapy than during testosterone replacement. Therefore, some men may elect to continue hCG therapy long-term.

Clomiphene, 25–50 mg/day orally, can sometimes stimulate a man's own pituitary gonadotropins (when his pituitary is intact), thereby increasing testosterone and sperm production. For fertility induction in females, ovulation may be induced with clomiphene, 50–100 mg/day orally for 5 days every 2 months. Ovulation induction with FSH and hCG can induce multiple births and should be used only by those experienced with their administration.

D. Human Growth Hormone (hGH) Replacement

Symptomatic adults with GH deficiency may be treated with a subcutaneous recombinant human growth hormone (rhGH, somatropin) injections starting at a dosage of about 0.2 mg/day (0.6 international units/day), administered three times weekly. The dosage of rhGH is increased every 2–4 weeks by increments of 0.1 mg (0.3 international units) until side effects occur or a sufficient salutary response and a normal serum IGF-1 level are achieved. In adults, if the desired effects (eg, improved energy and mentation, reduction in visceral adiposity) are not seen within 3–6 months at maximum tolerated dosage, rhGH therapy is discontinued.

During pregnancy, rhGH may be safely administered to women with hypopituitarism at their usual pregestational dose during the first trimester, tapering the dose during the second trimester, and discontinuing rhGH during the third trimester.

Oral estrogen replacement reduces hepatic IGF-1 production. Therefore, prior to commencing rhGH therapy, oral estrogen should be changed to transdermal or transvaginal estradiol.

Treatment of adult GH deficiency usually improves the patient's overall quality of life, with better emotional sense of well-being, increased muscle mass, and decreased visceral fat and waist circumference. Long-term treatment with rhGH does not appear to affect mortality.

Side effects of rhGH therapy may include peripheral edema, hand stiffness, arthralgias and myalgias, paresthesias, carpal tunnel syndrome, tarsal tunnel syndrome, headache, pseudotumor cerebri, gynecomastia,

hypertension, and proliferative retinopathy. Treatment with rhGH can also cause sleep apnea, insomnia, dyspnea, sweating, and fatigue. Side effects usually remit promptly after a sufficient reduction in dosage. Therapy with rhGH does not increase the risk of any malignancy or the regrowth of pituitary or brain neoplasms; serum IGF-1 levels should be kept in the normal range.

GH should not be administered during critical illness, since administration of very high doses of rhGH increased mortality in patients receiving intensive care. There is currently no proven role for GH replacement for the physiologic GH deficiency that is seen with abdominal obesity or normal aging.

E. Other Treatment

Selective transsphenoidal surgery is usually performed to resect non-prolactinoma pituitary masses and Rathke cleft cysts that cause local symptoms or hypopituitarism. Such surgery reverses hypopituitarism in a minority of cases. Patients with lymphocytic hypophysitis have been treated with glucocorticoid therapy and other immunosuppressants without much response and without reversing hypopituitarism.

▶ Prognosis

Hypopituitarism resulting from a pituitary tumor may be reversible with dopamine agonists or with careful selective resection of the tumor. Spontaneous recovery from hypopituitarism associated with pituitary stalk thickening has been reported. Patients can also recover from functional hypopituitarism. Spontaneous reversal of idiopathic isolated hypogonadotropic hypogonadism occurs in about 10% of patients after several years of hormone replacement therapy (HRT). However, hypopituitarism is usually permanent, and lifetime HRT is ordinarily required. There is an increased risk of death from infections with adrenal crisis in patients with untreated secondary insufficiency. Some pituitary tumors are locally invasive. In patients who have received pituitary radiation therapy, there is an increased risk of a second intracranial neoplasm and small-vessel stroke.

Asymptomatic Rathke cleft cysts may not require surgery, but do require endocrine, ophthalmic, and scan surveillance. Hypogonadism caused by a prolactinoma can be reversed with dopamine agonist therapy.

Functionally, most patients with hypopituitarism do very well with hormone replacement. Men with infertility who are treated with hCG/FSH or GnRH are likely to resume spermatogenesis if they have a history of sexual maturation, descended testicles, and a baseline serum inhibin B level over 60 pg/mL. Women under age 40 years, with infertility due to hypogonadotropic hypogonadism, can usually have successful ovulation induction.

Diri H et al. Sheehan's syndrome: new insights into an old disease. Endocrine. 2016 Jan;51(1):22–31. [PMID: 26323346]

Honegger J et al; Pituitary Working Group of the German Society of Endocrinology. Diagnosis of primary hypophysitis in Germany. J Clin Endocrinol Metab. 2015 Oct;100(10):3841–9. [PMID: 26262437]

Molitch ME et al. Evaluation and treatment of adult growth hormone deficiency: an Endocrine Society clinical practice guideline. J Clin Endocrinol Metab. 2011 Jun;96(6):1587–609. [PMID: 21602453]

Ntali G et al. Efficacy and complications of pituitary irradiation. Endocrinol Metab Clin North Am. 2015 Mar;44(1):117–26. [PMID: 25732648]

Pappachan JM et al. Excess mortality associated with hypopituitarism in adults: a meta-analysis of observational studies. J Clin Endocrinol Metab. 2015 Apr;100(4):1405–11. [PMID: 25658016]

Sundaram NK et al. The impact of traumatic brain injury on pituitary function. Endocrinol Metab Clin North Am. 2013 Sep; 42(3):565–86. [PMID: 24011887]

CENTRAL DIABETES INSIPIDUS

ESSENTIALS OF DIAGNOSIS

► Antidiuretic hormone (ADH) deficiency with polyuria (2–20 L/day) and polydipsia.

► Hypernatremia occurs if fluid intake is inadequate.

► General Considerations

Central diabetes insipidus is an uncommon disease caused by a deficiency in vasopressin (antidiuretic hormone [ADH]) from the posterior pituitary.

Primary central diabetes insipidus (without an identifiable lesion noted on MRI of the pituitary and hypothalamus) accounts for about one-third of all cases of diabetes insipidus. Familial diabetes insipidus occurs as a dominant genetic trait with symptoms developing at about 2 years of age. Diabetes insipidus also occurs in Wolfram syndrome, a rare autosomal recessive disorder that is also known by the acronym DIDMOAD (diabetes insipidus, type 1 diabetes mellitus, optic atrophy, and deafness). Although DIDMOAD manifestations usually present in childhood, they may not occur until adulthood, along with depression and cognitive problems. Central diabetes insipidus may also be due to autoimmunity against hypothalamic arginine vasopressin (AVP)-secreting cells. Reversible central diabetes insipidus can occur during chemotherapy with temozolomide and in the myelodysplastic preleukemic phase of acute myelogenous leukemia. **Secondary central diabetes insipidus** is due to damage to the hypothalamus or pituitary stalk by tumor, hypophysitis, infarction, hemorrhage, anoxic encephalopathy, surgical or accidental trauma, infection (eg, encephalitis, tuberculosis, syphilis), or granulomas (sarcoidosis or Langerhans cell granulomatosis). Metastases to the pituitary are more likely to cause diabetes insipidus (33%) than are pituitary adenomas (1%). Central diabetes insipidus can also be idiopathic.

► Clinical Findings

A. Symptoms and Signs

The symptoms of the disease are intense thirst, especially with a craving for ice water, the volume of ingested fluid varying from 2 L to 20 L daily, and polyuria, with large urine volumes and low urine specific gravity (usually less than 1.006 with ad libitum fluid intake). The urine is otherwise normal. Partial diabetes insipidus presents with less intense symptoms and should be suspected in patients with enuresis. Most patients with diabetes insipidus are able to maintain fluid balance by continuing to ingest large volumes of water. However, in patients without free access to water or with a damaged hypothalamic thirst center and altered thirst sensation, diabetes insipidus may present with hypernatremia and dehydration. Diabetes insipidus is aggravated by administration of high-dose corticosteroids, which increases renal free water clearance.

B. Laboratory Findings

Diagnosis of diabetes insipidus is a clinical one; there is no diagnostic laboratory test. Evaluation should include a 24-hour urine collection for volume and creatinine. A urine volume of less than 2 L/24 h (in the absence of hypernatremia) rules out diabetes insipidus. Hyperuricemia occurs in many patients with diabetes insipidus, since reduced vasopressin stimulation of the renal V1 receptor causes a reduction in the renal tubular clearance of urate.

A supervised "vasopressin challenge test" may be done: Desmopressin acetate 0.05–0.1 mL (5–10 mcg) intranasally (or 1 mcg subcutaneously or intravenously) is given, with measurement of urine volume for 12 hours before and 12 hours after administration. Patients with central diabetes insipidus notice a distinct reduction in thirst and polyuria; serum sodium usually remains normal. The dosage of desmopressin is doubled if the response is marginal. If symptoms of hyponatremia develop, serum sodium must be assayed immediately.

In **nonfamilial central diabetes insipidus**, MRI of the pituitary and hypothalamus is done to look for mass lesions. If the pituitary stalk is thickened, the cause may be Langerhans cell histiocytosis, sarcoidosis, or lymphocytic hypophysitis. With central diabetes insipidus, MRI T-1-weighted imaging shows an absence of the usual hyperintense signal (bright spot) in the posterior pituitary.

► Differential Diagnosis

Central diabetes insipidus must be distinguished from polyuria caused by psychogenic polydipsia, diabetes mellitus, Cushing syndrome, hypercalcemia, hypokalemia, and Parkinson disease. It must also be distinguished from vasopressinase-induced diabetes insipidus and from nephrogenic diabetes insipidus.

Vasopressinase-induced diabetes insipidus may be seen in the last trimester of pregnancy, associated with oligohydramnios, preeclampsia, or hepatic dysfunction, and in the puerperium. A circulating enzyme destroys native vasopressin; however, synthetic desmopressin is unaffected.

Nephrogenic diabetes insipidus is caused by unresponsiveness of the kidney tubules to the normal secretion of vasopressin, and the polyuria is due to unresponsiveness to it. A **congenital form** is familial and transmitted as an X-linked trait; it is caused by defective expression of renal vasopressin V2 receptors or vasopressin-sensitive water channels. Adults often also have hyperuricemia. **Acquired forms** are usually less severe and occur in pyelonephritis, renal amyloidosis, myeloma, potassium depletion, Sjögren syndrome, sickle cell anemia, chronic hypercalcemia, or recovery from acute tubular necrosis. Certain drugs (eg, corticosteroids, diuretics, demeclocycline, lithium, foscarnet, or methicillin) may induce nephrogenic diabetes insipidus. When nephrogenic diabetes insipidus is a diagnostic consideration, measurement of serum vasopressin is done during modest fluid restriction; typically, the vasopressin level is found to be high, distinguishing it from central diabetes insipidus.

▶ Complications

If water is not readily available, the excessive output of urine will lead to severe dehydration. Patients with an impaired thirst mechanism are very prone to hypernatremia, as are those with impaired mentation who forget to take their desmopressin. Excessive desmopressin acetate can induce water intoxication and hyponatremia.

▶ Treatment

Mild cases of diabetes insipidus require no treatment other than adequate fluid intake. Reduction of aggravating factors (eg, corticosteroids) will improve polyuria.

Desmopressin acetate is the treatment of choice for central diabetes insipidus. It is also useful in **vasopressinase-induced** diabetes insipidus associated with pregnancy or the puerperium, since desmopressin acetate is resistant to degradation by the circulating vasopressinase.

Desmopressin acetate (100 mcg/mL solution) is given intranasally every 12–24 hours as needed for thirst and polyuria. It may be administered via metered-dose nasal inhaler containing 0.1 mL (10 mcg/spray) or via a calibrated rhinal tube. The starting dose is one metered-dose spray or 0.05–0.1 mL every 12–24 hours, and the dose is then individualized according to response. Desmopressin nasal may cause rhinitis or conjunctivitis. If the generic preparation is ineffective, switching to the DDAVP brand may provide relief.

Oral desmopressin, 0.1 mg and 0.2 mg tablets, is given in a starting dose of 0.05 mg twice daily and increased to a maximum of 0.4 mg every 8 hours, if required. Sublingual desmopressin (DDAVP melt), 60, 120, or 250 mcg, is not available in the United States; hyponatremia has been reported with this formulation. Oral desmopressin is particularly useful for patients in whom rhinitis or conjunctivitis develops from the nasal preparation. Gastrointestinal symptoms, asthenia, and mild increases in hepatic enzymes can occur with the oral preparation.

Desmopressin can also be given intravenously, intramuscularly, or subcutaneously in doses of 1–4 mcg every 12–24 hours as needed.

Desmopressin may cause hyponatremia, but this is uncommon if minimum effective doses are used and the patient allows thirst to occur periodically. Desmopressin can sometimes cause agitation, emotional changes, and depression with an increased risk of suicide. Erythromelalgia occurs rarely.

▶ Prognosis

Central diabetes insipidus after pituitary surgery usually remits after days to weeks but may be permanent if the upper pituitary stalk is cut.

Chronic central diabetes insipidus is ordinarily more an inconvenience than a dire medical condition. Treatment with desmopressin allows normal sleep and activity. Hypernatremia can occur, especially when the hypothalamic thirst center is damaged, but diabetes insipidus does not otherwise reduce life expectancy, and the prognosis is that of the underlying disorder.

Bellastella A et al. Subclinical diabetes insipidus. Best Pract Res Clin Endocrinol Metab. 2012 Aug;26(4):471–83. [PMID: 22863389]

Oiso Y et al. Clinical review: treatment of neurohypophyseal diabetes insipidus. J Clin Endocrinol Metab. 2013 Oct; 98(10):3958–67. [PMID: 23884783]

ACROMEGALY & GIGANTISM

ESSENTIALS OF DIAGNOSIS

▶ Pituitary tumor.

▶ Gigantism before closure of epiphyses, excessive growth of hands, feet, jaw, and internal organs.

▶ Amenorrhea, headaches, visual field loss, weakness.

▶ Soft, doughy, sweaty handshake.

▶ Elevated serum IGF-1.

▶ Serum GH not suppressed following oral glucose.

▶ General Considerations

GH exerts much of its growth-promoting effects by stimulating the release of IGF-1 from the liver and other tissues.

Acromegaly is nearly always caused by a pituitary adenoma. Most are macroadenomas (over 1 cm in diameter). These tumors may be locally invasive, particularly into the cavernous sinus. Less than 1% are malignant. Acromegaly is usually sporadic but may rarely be familial, with less than 3% being due to multiple endocrine neoplasia (MEN) types 1 or 4. Acromegaly may also be seen rarely in McCune-Albright syndrome and Carney complex. Acromegaly is very rarely caused by ectopic secretion of GHRH or GH secreted by a lymphoma, hypothalamic tumor, bronchial carcinoid, or pancreatic tumor.

▶ Clinical Findings

A. Symptoms and Signs

Excessive GH causes tall stature and gigantism if it occurs in youth, before closure of epiphyses. Afterward, acromegaly develops. The term "acromegaly," meaning extremity enlargement, seriously understates the manifestations. The hands enlarge and a doughy, moist handshake is characteristic. The fingers widen, causing patients to enlarge their rings. Carpal tunnel syndrome is common. The feet also grow, particularly in shoe width. Facial features coarsen since the bones and sinuses of the skull enlarge; hat size increases. The mandible becomes more prominent, causing prognathism and malocclusion. Tooth spacing widens. Older photographs of the patient can be a useful comparison.

Macroglossia occurs, as does hypertrophy of pharyngeal and laryngeal tissue; this causes a deep, coarse voice and sometimes makes intubation difficult. Obstructive sleep apnea may occur. A goiter may be noted. Hypertension (50%) and cardiomegaly are common. At diagnosis, about 10% of acromegalic patients have overt heart failure, with a dilated left ventricle and a reduced ejection fraction. Weight gain is typical, particularly of muscle and bone. Insulin resistance is usually present and frequently causes diabetes mellitus (30%). Arthralgias and degenerative arthritis occur. Overgrowth of vertebral bone can cause spinal stenosis. Colon polyps are common, especially in patients with skin papillomas. The skin may also manifest hyperhidrosis, thickening, cystic acne, skin tags, and acanthosis nigricans.

GH-secreting pituitary tumors usually cause some degree of hypogonadism, either by cosecretion of prolactin (PRL) or by direct pressure upon normal pituitary tissue. Decreased libido and erectile dysfunction are common in men and irregular menses or amenorrhea in women. Women who become pregnant have an increased risk of gestational diabetes and hypertension. Secondary hypothyroidism sometimes occurs; hypoadrenalism is unusual. Headaches are frequent. Temporal hemianopia may occur as a result of the optic chiasm being impinged by a suprasellar growth of the tumor.

B. Laboratory Findings

For screening purposes, a random serum IGF-1 can be obtained. If it is normal for age, acromegaly is ruled out.

For further evaluation, the patient should be fasting for at least 8 hours (except for water), not be acutely ill, and not have exercised on the day of testing. Assay for the following: serum IGF-1 (increased and usually over five times normal in acromegalic patients), PRL (cosecreted by many GH-secreting tumors), glucose (diabetes mellitus is common in acromegaly), liver enzymes and serum creatinine or blood urea nitrogen (BUN) (liver failure or kidney disease can misleadingly elevate GH), serum calcium (to exclude hyperparathyroidism), serum inorganic phosphorus (frequently elevated), serum free T_4, and TSH (secondary hypothyroidism is common in acromegaly; primary hypothyroidism may increase PRL). Glucose syrup (100 g) is then administered orally, and serum GH is measured 60 minutes afterward; acromegaly is excluded if the serum GH is less than 1 ng/mL. For ultrasensitive GH assays, GH should be suppressed to less than 0.3 ng/mL. The serum IGF-1 and glucose-suppressed GH are usually complementary tests; however, disparities between the two occur in up to 30% of patients.

C. Imaging

MRI shows a pituitary tumor in 90% of acromegalic patients. MRI is generally superior to CT scanning,

especially in the postoperative setting. Radiographs of the skull may show an enlarged sella and thickened skull. Radiographs may also show tufting of the terminal phalanges of the fingers and toes. A lateral view of the foot shows increased thickness of the heel pad.

▶ Differential Diagnosis

Active acromegaly must be distinguished from familial coarse features, large hands and feet, and isolated prognathism and from inactive ("burned-out") acromegaly in which there has been a spontaneous remission due to infarction of the pituitary adenoma. GH-induced gigantism must be differentiated from familial tall stature and from aromatase deficiency.

Misleadingly high serum GH levels can be caused by exercise or eating just prior to the test; acute illness or agitation; liver failure or kidney disease; malnourishment; diabetes mellitus; or concurrent treatment with estrogens, beta-blockers, or clonidine. Acromegaly can be difficult to diagnose during pregnancy, since the placenta produces GH and commercial GH assays may not be able to distinguish between pituitary and placental GH. During normal adolescence, serum IGF-1 is usually elevated and GH may fail to be suppressed.

▶ Complications

Complications include hypopituitarism, hypertension, glucose intolerance or frank diabetes mellitus, cardiac enlargement, and heart failure. Carpal tunnel syndrome may cause thumb weakness and thenar atrophy. Arthritis of hips, knees, and spine can be troublesome. Cord compression may occur. Visual field defects may be severe and progressive. Acute loss of vision or cranial nerve palsy may occur if the tumor undergoes spontaneous hemorrhage and necrosis (pituitary apoplexy). Colon polyps are more likely to be found in patients with acromegaly.

▶ Treatment

A. Pituitary Microsurgery

Transsphenoidal pituitary microsurgery removes the adenoma while preserving anterior pituitary function in most patients. Postoperatively, GH levels fall immediately; diaphoresis and carpal tunnel syndrome often improve within a day after surgery. Transsphenoidal surgery is usually well tolerated, but complications occur in about 12% of patients, including infection, cerebrospinal fluid (CSF) leak, and hypopituitarism.

Fluid and electrolyte disturbances occur in most patients postoperatively. Diabetes insipidus can occur within 2 days postoperatively but is usually mild and self-correcting. Hyponatremia can occur abruptly 4–13 days postoperatively in 21% of patients; symptoms may include nausea, vomiting, headache, malaise, or seizure. It is treated with free water and hypotonic fluid restriction. It is prudent to monitor serum sodium levels postoperatively.

Corticosteroids are administered perioperatively and tapered to replacement doses over 1 week; hydrocortisone is discontinued and a cosyntropin stimulation test is performed about 6 weeks after surgery. At that time, the patient is screened for secondary hypothyroidism (by a serum FT_4) and secondary hypogonadism.

B. Medications

Acromegalic patients with an incomplete biochemical remission after pituitary surgery may benefit from medical therapy with dopamine agonists, somatostatin analogs, tamoxifen, or pegvisomant.

Cabergoline is the dopamine agonist of choice. It may be used first, since it is an oral medication. Cabergoline therapy is most successful for tumors that secrete both PRL and GH but can also be effective for patients with normal serum PRL levels. Therapy with cabergoline will shrink one-third of acromegaly-associated pituitary tumors by more than 50%. It appears to be safe during pregnancy. The initial dose is 0.25 mg orally twice weekly, which is gradually increased to a maximum dosage of 1 mg twice weekly (based on serum GH and IGF-1 levels). Side effects of cabergoline include nausea, fatigue, constipation, abdominal pain, and dizziness.

Octreotide and **lanreotide** are somatostatin analogs that are given by monthly subcutaneous injection. Such long-acting somatostatin analogs can achieve serum GH levels under 2 ng/mL in 79% of patients and normal serum IGF-1 levels in 53% of patients.

Tamoxifen is a selective estrogen receptor modulator (SERM) that may be particularly useful for persistent acromegaly in men and in women who are postmenopausal or who have had breast cancer. Tamoxifen in doses of 20–40 mg orally daily does not reduce serum GH levels but reduces serum IGF-1 levels in 82% of patients and normalizes serum IGF-1 levels in 47%. Serum testosterone levels increase in men.

Pegvisomant is a GH receptor antagonist that is given by daily subcutaneous injection. It blocks hepatic IGF-1 production, but does not shrink GH-secreting tumors. Patients need to be monitored carefully for growth of the pituitary tumor with visual field examinations, GH levels, and MRI scanning of the pituitary. Pegvisomant therapy produces symptomatic relief and normalizes serum IGF-1 levels in over 90% of patients.

C. Stereotactic Radiosurgery

Acromegalic patients who do not achieve a complete remission with transsphenoidal surgery or medical therapy may be treated with one or a combination of three types of stereotactic radiosurgery. **Linear accelerator** machines (eg, Cyberknife) administer x-rays to the tumor. **Gamma knife radiosurgery** administers gamma rays to the tumor. **Proton beam** therapy administers charged particles to the tumor. Stereotactic radiosurgery normalizes serum IGF-1 in up to 80% of treated patients. Following any pituitary radiation therapy, patients are advised to take lifelong daily low-dose aspirin because of the increased risk of small-vessel stroke. Stereotactic radiosurgery to pituitary tumors causes anterior hypopituitarism in 35–60% of patients within 5 years, so patients must have regular monitoring of their pituitary function.

Prognosis

Patients with acromegaly have increased morbidity and mortality from cardiovascular disorders and progressive acromegalic symptoms. Those who are treated and have a random serum GH under 1.0 ng/mL or a glucose-suppressed serum GH under 0.4 ng/mL with a normal age-adjusted serum IGF-1 level have reduced morbidity and mortality.

Transsphenoidal pituitary surgery achieves a remission in about 70% of patients followed over 3 years. In patients with tumors smaller than 2 cm in diameter and GH levels below 50 ng/mL, transsphenoidal pituitary surgery is successful in 80%. Extrasellar extension of the pituitary tumor, particularly cavernous sinus invasion, reduces the likelihood of surgical cure.

Adjuvant medical therapy has been quite successful in treating patients who are not cured by pituitary surgery. Postoperatively, normal pituitary function is usually preserved. Soft tissue swelling regresses but bone enlargement is permanent. Hypertension frequently persists despite successful surgery. Conventional radiation therapy (alone) produces a remission in about 40% of patients by 2 years and 75% of patients by 5 years after treatment. Gamma knife or cyberknife radiosurgery reduces GH levels an average of 77%, with 20% of patients having a full remission after 12 months. Heavy particle pituitary radiation produces a remission in about 70% of patients by 2 years and 80% of patients by 5 years. Radiation therapy eventually produces some degree of hypopituitarism in most patients. Conventional radiation therapy may cause some degree of organic brain syndrome and predisposes to small strokes. Patients must receive lifelong follow-up, with regular monitoring of serum GH and IGF-1 levels. Serum GH levels over 5 ng/mL and rising IGF-1 levels usually indicate a recurrent tumor. Most pregnant women with acromegaly do not have an increase in the size of the pituitary tumor and neonatal outcome is unaffected.

Anderson M. Management of endocrine disease: GH excess: diagnosis and medical therapy. Eur J Endocrinol. 2013 Nov; 170(1):R31–41. [PMID: 24144967]

Balili I et al. Tamoxifen as a therapeutic agent in acromegaly. Pituitary. 2014 Dec;17(6):500–4. [PMID: 24243064]

Katznelson L et al. Acromegaly: an Endocrine Society clinical practice guideline. J Clin Endocrinol Metab. 2014 Nov; 99(11):3933–51. [PMID: 25356808]

HYPERPROLACTINEMIA

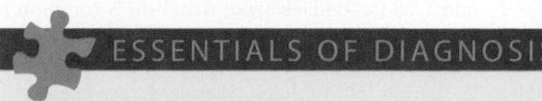

ESSENTIALS OF DIAGNOSIS

- ► **Women:** Oligomenorrhea, amenorrhea; galactorrhea; infertility.
- ► **Men:** Hypogonadism; decreased libido and erectile dysfunction; infertility.
- ► Elevated serum prolactin (PRL), though PRL is normally elevated during pregnancy.
- ► CT scan or MRI often demonstrates a pituitary adenoma.

▶ General Considerations

The causes of hyperprolactinemia are shown in Table 26–2. Augmentation or reduction mammoplasty, and mastectomy may stimulate PRL secretion. In acromegaly, there may be cosecretion of GH and PRL. Hyperprolactinemia (without a pituitary adenoma) may also be familial. PRL-secreting pituitary tumors are more common in women than in men and are usually sporadic but may rarely be familial as part of MEN type 1 or 4. Most are microadenomas (smaller than 1 cm in diameter) that do not grow even with pregnancy or oral contraceptives. However, some giant prolactinomas (over 3 cm in diameter) can spread into the cavernous sinuses and suprasellar areas; rarely, they may erode the floor of the sella to invade the paranasal sinuses.

▶ Clinical Findings

A. Symptoms and Signs

Hyperprolactinemia may cause hypogonadotropic hypogonadism and reduced fertility. Men usually have diminished libido and erectile dysfunction that may not respond to testosterone replacement; gynecomastia sometimes occurs but galactorrhea is rare. The diagnosis of a prolactinoma is often delayed in men, such that pituitary adenomas may grow and present with late manifestations of a pituitary macroprolactinoma (diameter 10 mm or larger).

About 90% of premenopausal women with prolactinomas experience amenorrhea, oligomenorrhea, or infertility. Estrogen deficiency can cause decreased vaginal lubrication, irritability, anxiety, and depression. Galactorrhea (lactation in the absence of nursing) is common. During pregnancy, clinically significant enlargement of a microprolactinoma (diameter smaller than 10 mm) occurs in less than 3%; clinically significant enlargement of a macroprolactinoma occurs in about 30%.

Pituitary prolactinomas may cosecrete GH and cause acromegaly. Large tumors may cause headaches, visual symptoms, and pituitary insufficiency.

Aside from pituitary tumors, some women secrete an abnormal form of prolactin that appears to cause peripartum cardiomyopathy. Suppression of prolactin secretion with dopamine agonists can reverse the cardiomyopathy.

B. Laboratory Findings

Evaluate for conditions known to cause hyperprolactinemia, particularly pregnancy (serum hCG), hypothyroidism (serum FT_4 and TSH), kidney disease (BUN and serum creatinine), cirrhosis (liver tests) and hyperparathyroidism (serum calcium). Men are evaluated for hypogonadism with determinations of serum total and free testosterone, LH, and FSH. Women who have amenorrhea are assessed for hypogonadism with determinations of serum estradiol, LH, and FSH. Patients with pituitary macroadenomas larger than 3 cm in diameter should have PRL measured on serial dilutions of serum, since immunoradiometric assay assays may otherwise report falsely low titers, the "high-dose hook effect." Patients with macroprolactinomas or manifestations of possible hypopituitarism should be evaluated for hypopituitarism. Patients with hyperprolactinemia who are relatively asymptomatic and have no apparent cause for hyperprolactinemia should have an assay for macroprolactinemia (discussed below).

C. Imaging

Patients with hyperprolactinemia not induced by drugs, hypothyroidism, or pregnancy should be examined by pituitary MRI. Small prolactinomas may thus be demonstrated, but clear differentiation from normal variants is not always possible. In the event that a woman with a macroprolactinoma becomes pregnant and elects not to take dopamine agonists during her pregnancy, MRI is usually not performed since the normal pituitary grows during pregnancy. However, if visual-field defects or other neurologic symptoms develop in a pregnant woman, a limited MRI study should be done, focusing on the pituitary without gadolinium contrast.

▶ Differential Diagnosis

The differential diagnosis for galactorrhea includes the small amount of breast milk that can be expressed from

Table 26–2. Causes of hyperprolactinemia.

Physiologic Causes	Pharmacologic Causes	Pathologic Causes
Exercise	Amoxapine	Acromegaly
Familial (mutant prolactin receptor)	Amphetamines	Chronic chest wall stimulation (post-thoracotomy, post-mastectomy, herpes zoster, breast problems, chest acupuncture, nipple rings, etc)
Idiopathic	Anesthetic agents	
Macroprolactin ("big prolactin")	Antipsychotics (conventional and atypical)	
Nipple stimulation	Butyrophenones	
Pregnancy	Cimetidine and ranitidine (not famotidine or nizatidine)	Cirrhosis
Puerperium	Cocaine	Hypothalamic disease
Sleep (REM phase)	Domperidone	Hypothyroidism
Stress (trauma, surgery)	Estrogens	Kidney disease (especially with zinc deficiency)
Suckling	Hydroxyzine	
	Locaserin	Multiple sclerosis
	Methyldopa	Optic neuromyelitis
	Metoclopramide	Pituitary stalk damage
	Opioids	Prolactin-secreting tumors
	Nicotine	
	Phenothiazines	Pseudocyesis (false pregnancy)
	Protease inhibitors	
	Progestins	Spinal cord lesions
	Reserpine	Systemic lupus erythematosus
	Risperidone	
	Selective serotonin reuptake inhibitors	
	Testosterone	
	Tricyclic antidepressants	
	Verapamil	

the nipple in many parous women that is not cause for concern. Nipple stimulation from nipple rings, chest surgery, or acupuncture can cause galactorrhea; serum PRL levels may be normal or minimally elevated. Some women can have galactorrhea with normal serum PRL levels and no discernible cause (idiopathic). Normal breast milk may be various colors besides white. However, bloody galactorrhea requires evaluation for breast cancer.

Other pituitary lesions besides prolactinomas can produce hyperprolactinemia, due to damage or pressure to the pituitary infundibulum reducing hypothalamic dopamine's inhibitory effect upon pituitary lactotrophes that produce PRL unless inhibited. About 40% of nonfunctional pituitary macroadenomas produce some degree of hyperprolactinemia. Similary, lesions that involve the infundibulum can also cause hyperprolactinemia. These and other lesions and malignancies can be misdiagnosed as prolactinomas. One distinguishing characteristic is that the serum PRL is usually only marginally elevated in the latter tumors, whereas with pituitary macroprolactinomas the serum PRL typically exceeds 100 mcg/L.

Pregnant women have high serum prolactin levels, with physiological hyperplastic enlargement of the pituitary on MRI. Increased pituitary size is a normal variant in young women. Macroprolactinemia is an increased circulating level of a high molecular weight PRL that is biologically inactive but is detected on assays. It occurs in 3.7% of the general population and accounts for 10–25% of all cases of hyperprolactinemia; pituitary MRI shows a nonpathological abnormality in 22% of such patients.

▶ **Treatment**

Medications known to increase PRL should be stopped if possible. Hyperprolactinemia due to hypothyroidism is corrected by thyroxine.

Women with microprolactinomas who have amenorrhea or are desirous of contraception may safely take oral contraceptives or estrogen replacement—there is minimal risk of stimulating enlargement of the microadenoma. Patients with infertility and hyperprolactinemia may be treated with a dopamine agonist in an effort to improve fertility. Women with amenorrhea who elect to receive no treatment have an increased risk of developing osteoporosis; such women require periodic bone densitometry.

Pituitary macroprolactinomas have a higher risk of progressive growth, particularly during estrogen or testosterone HRT or during pregnancy. Therefore, patients with macroprolactinomas should not be treated with HRT unless they are in remission with dopamine agonist medication or surgery.

Pregnant women with macroprolactinomas should continue to receive treatment with dopamine agonists throughout the pregnancy to prevent tumor growth. If dopamine agonists are not used during pregnancy in a woman with a macroprolactinoma, visual field testing is required in each trimester. Measurement of prolactin is not useful surveillance for tumor growth due to the fact that prolactin increases greatly during normal pregnancy.

A. Dopamine Agonists

Dopamine agonists (cabergoline, bromocriptine, or quinagolide) are the initial treatment of choice for patients with giant prolactinomas and those with hyperprolactinemia desiring restoration of normal sexual function and fertility. Cabergoline is the most effective and usually the best-tolerated ergot-derived dopamine agonist. The beginning dosage is 0.25 mg orally once weekly for 1 week, then 0.25 mg twice weekly for the next week, then 0.5 mg twice weekly. Further dosage increases may be required monthly, based on serum PRL levels, up to a maximum of 1.5 mg twice weekly. Bromocriptine (1.25–20 mg/day orally) is an alternative. Women who experience nausea with oral preparations may find relief with deep vaginal insertion of cabergoline or bromocriptine tablets; vaginal irritation sometimes occurs. Quinagolide (Norprolac; not available in the United States) is a non–ergot-derived dopamine agonist for patients intolerant or resistant to ergot-derived medications; the starting dosage is 0.075 mg/day orally, increasing as needed and tolerated to a maximum of 0.6 mg/day. Patients whose tumor is resistant to one dopamine agonist may be switched to another in an effort to induce a remission.

Dopamine agonists are given at bedtime to minimize side effects of fatigue, nausea, dizziness, and orthostatic hypotension. These symptoms usually improve with dosage reduction and continued use. Erythromelalgia is rare. Ergot-derived dopamine agonist treatment for prolactinomas has not been associated with cardiac valvulopathy. Dopamine agonists can cause a variety of psychiatric side effects that are not dose related and may take weeks to resolve once the drug is discontinued.

With dopamine agonist treatment, 90% of patients with prolactinomas experience a fall in serum PRL to 10% or less of pretreatment levels and about 80% of treated patients achieve a normal serum PRL level. Shrinkage of a pituitary adenoma occurs early, but the maximum effect may take up to a year. Nearly half of prolactinomas—even massive tumors—shrink more than 50%. Such shrinkage of invasive prolactinomas can result in CSF rhinorrhea.

Because dopamine agonists usually restore fertility promptly, many pregnancies have resulted; no increased risk of miscarriage or teratogenicity has been noted. However, women with microadenomas may have treatment withdrawn during pregnancy and may safely breastfeed postpartum without dopamine agonist therapy. Macroadenomas may enlarge significantly during pregnancy; if therapy is withdrawn, patients must be monitored with serum PRL determinations and computer-assisted visual fields. Women with macroprolactinomas who have responded to dopamine agonists may safely receive oral contraceptives as long as they continue receiving dopamine agonist therapy.

B. Surgical Treatment

Transsphenoidal pituitary surgery may be urgently required for large tumors undergoing apoplexy or those severely compromising visual fields. It is also used electively for patients who do not tolerate or respond to dopamine agonists. Surgery is generally well tolerated, with a mortality rate of less than 0.5%. For pituitary microprolactinomas, skilled neurosurgeons are successful in normalizing prolactin in 87% of patients. The 10-year recurrence rate is 13% and pituitary function can be preserved in over 95% of cases. However, the surgical success rate for macroprolactinomas is much lower, and the complication rates are higher. Craniotomy is rarely indicated.

Complications, such as CSF leakage, meningitis, stroke, or visual loss, occur in about 3% of cases; sinusitis, nasal septal perforation, or infection complicates about 6.5% of transsphenoidal surgeries. Diabetes insipidus can occur within 2 days postoperatively but is usually mild and self-correcting. Hyponatremia can occur abruptly 4–13 days postoperatively in 21% of patients; symptoms may include nausea, vomiting, headache, malaise, or seizure. It is treated with free water and hypotonic fluid restriction.

C. Stereotactic Radiosurgery

Stereotactic radiosurgery is seldom required for prolactinomas, since they usually respond to cabergoline or surgery. It is reserved for patients with macroadenomas that are growing despite treatment with dopamine agonists.

D. Chemotherapy

Some patients with aggressive pituitary macroadenomas or carcinomas are not surgical candidates and do not respond to dopamine agonists or radiation therapy. A small percentage of patients with aggressive tumors respond to temozolomide (150–200 mg/m^2 orally daily for 5 days of each 28-day cycle); after three cycles, treatment efficacy is determined by prolactin measurement and MRI scanning.

▶ Prognosis

Pituitary prolactinomas generally respond well to therapy with dopamine agonists. Women with microprolactinomas can take oral contraceptives with little risk of stimulating growth of the pituitary adenoma. During pregnancy, growth of a pituitary prolactinoma occurs in 2.7% of women with a microprolactinoma and in 22.9% of those with a macroprolactinoma. If cabergoline is stopped after 2 years of therapy, hyperprolactinemia recurs in 68% of patients with idiopathic hyperprolactinemia, 79% with microprolactinomas, and 84% with macroprolactinomas.

Losa M et al. Temozolomide therapy in patients with aggressive pituitary adenomas or carcinomas. J Neurooncol. 2016 Feb;126(3):519–25. [PMID: 26614517]
Melmed S et al. Diagnosis and treatment of hyperprolactinemia: an Endocrine Society clinical practice guideline. J Clin Endocrinol Metab. 2011 Feb;96(2):273–88. [PMID: 21296991]
Ntali G et al. Clinical review: functioning gonadotroph adenomas. J Clin Endocrinol Metab. 2014 Dec;99(12):4423–33. [PMID: 25166722]
Witek P et al. Management of prolactinomas during pregnancy. Minerva Endocrinol. 2013 Dec;38(4):351–63. [PMID: 24285103]

DISEASES OF THE THYROID GLAND

HYPOTHYROIDISM & MYXEDEMA

ESSENTIALS OF DIAGNOSIS

▶ Weakness, fatigue, cold intolerance, constipation, weight change, depression, menorrhagia, hoarseness.

▶ Dry skin, bradycardia, delayed return of deep tendon reflexes.

▶ Anemia, hyponatremia, hyperlipidemia.

▶ FT$_4$ level is usually low.

▶ TSH elevated in primary hypothyroidism.

▶ General Considerations

Hypothyroidism is common, affecting over 1% of the general population and about 5% of individuals over age 60 years. Thyroid hormone deficiency affects almost all body functions. The degree of severity ranges from mild and unrecognized hypothyroid states to striking myxedema.

Hypothyroidism may be due to failure or resection of the thyroid gland itself or deficiency of pituitary TSH. The condition must be distinguished from the functional hypothyroidism that occurs in severe nonthyroidal illness, which does not require treatment with thyroxine.

Maternal hypothyroidism during pregnancy results in offspring with IQ scores that are an average 7 points lower than those of euthyroid mothers.

Goiter may be present with thyroiditis, iodide deficiency, genetic thyroid enzyme defects, drug goitrogens (lithium, iodide, propylthiouracil or methimazole, sulfonamides, amiodarone, interferon-alpha, interferon-beta, interleukin-2), food goitrogens in iodide-deficient areas (eg, turnips, cassavas) or, rarely, peripheral resistance to thyroid hormone or infiltrating diseases (eg, cancer, sarcoidosis). A hypothyroid phase occurs in subacute (de Quervain) viral thyroiditis following initial hyperthyroidism. Hashimoto thyroiditis is the most common cause of hypothyroidism.

Goiter is usually absent when hypothyroidism is due to destruction of the gland by radiation therapy (to the head, neck, chest, and shoulder region) or ^{131}I therapy. Thyroidectomy causes hypothyroidism, and after hemithyroidectomy, hypothyroidism develops in 22% of patients. Goiter is often absent in patients with autoimmune thyroiditis.

Some malignancies that overexpress thyroid hormone inactivating enzyme D3 can cause "consumptive hypothyroidism." This has occurred with large hemangiomas or a heavy tumor burden of colon cancer, basal cell cancer, fibrous tumors, or gastrointestinal stromal tumors (GISTs).

Chemotherapeutic agents that can cause silent thyroiditis include the following: tyrosine kinase inhibitors (eg, sunitinib), denileukin diftitox, alemtuzumab, interferon-alpha, interleukin-2, ipilimumab, tremelimumab, thalidomide, and lenalidomide. This usually starts with hyperthyroidism (often unrecognized) and then progresses to hypothyroidism. Radioiodine-based chemotherapies can also cause hypothyroidism. Bexarotene causes a high rate of pituitary insufficiency with central hypothyroidism.

Amiodarone, because of its high iodine content, causes clinically significant hypothyroidism in about 15–20% of patients who receive it. Hypothyroidism occurs most often in patients with preexisting autoimmune thyroiditis and in patients who are not iodine-deficient. The T_4 level is low or low-normal, and the TSH is elevated, usually over 20 milli-international unit/L. Another 17% of patients are asymptomatic with normal serum T_4 levels despite elevations in serum TSH; they may be closely monitored without thyroxine therapy. Low-dose amiodarone is less likely to cause hypothyroidism. Cardiac patients with amiodarone-induced symptomatic hypothyroidism are treated with just enough thyroxine to relieve symptoms. Hypothyroidism usually resolves over several months if amiodarone is discontinued. Hypothyroidism may also develop in patients with a high iodine intake from other sources, especially if they have underlying lymphocytic thyroiditis.

Hepatitis C is associated with an increased risk of autoimmune thyroiditis, with 21% of affected patients having antithyroid antibodies and 13% having hypothyroidism.

▶ Clinical Findings

A. Symptoms and Signs

1. Common manifestations—Mild hypothyroidism often escapes detection without a screening serum TSH. Patients typically have nonspecific symptoms of hypothyroidism that include weight gain, fatigue, lethargy, depression, weakness, dyspnea on exertion, arthralgias or myalgias, muscle cramps, menorrhagia, constipation, dry skin, headache, paresthesias, cold intolerance, carpal tunnel syndrome, and Raynaud syndrome. Physical findings can include bradycardia; diastolic hypertension; thin, brittle nails; thinning of hair; peripheral edema; puffy face and eyelids; and skin pallor or yellowing (carotenemia). Delayed relaxation of deep tendon reflexes may be present. Patients often have a palpably enlarged thyroid (goiter) that arises due to elevated serum TSH levels or the underlying thyroid pathology, such as Hashimoto thyroiditis.

2. Less common manifestations—Less common symptoms of hypothyroidism include diminished appetite and weight loss, hoarseness, decreased sense of taste and smell, and diminished auditory acuity. Some patients may complain of dysphagia or neck discomfort. Although most menstruating women have menorrhagia, some women have scant menses or amenorrhea. Physical findings may include thinning of the outer halves of the eyebrows; thickening of the tongue; hard pitting edema; and effusions into the pleural and peritoneal cavities as well as into joints. Galactorrhea may also be present. Cardiac enlargement ("myxedema heart") and pericardial effusions may occur. Psychosis (myxedema madness) can occur from severe hypothyroidism or from toxicity of other drugs whose metabolism is slowed in hypothyroidism. Hypothermia

and stupor or myxedema coma, which is often associated with infection (especially pneumonia), may develop in patients with severe hypothyroidism. Pituitary enlargement due to hyperplasia of TSH-secreting cells, which is reversible following thyroid therapy, may be seen in long-standing hypothyroidism.

Some hypothyroid patients with Hashimoto thyroiditis have symptoms that are not due to hypothyroidism but rather to another associated disease. Some conditions that occur more commonly in patients with Hashimoto thyroiditis include Addison disease, hypoparathyroidism, diabetes mellitus, pernicious anemia, Sjögren syndrome, vitiligo, biliary cirrhosis, gluten sensitivity, and celiac disease.

B. Laboratory Findings

Hypothyroidism is a common disorder and thyroid function tests should be obtained for any patient with its nonspecific symptoms or signs. The single best screening test for hypothyroidism is the serum TSH (Table 26–3). In primary hypothyroidism, the serum TSH is increased, while the serum FT_4 is low or low-normal. Other laboratory abnormalities can include hyponatremia, hypoglycemia, or anemia (with normal or increased mean corpuscular volume). Additional frequent findings include increased serum levels of LDL cholesterol, triglycerides, lipoprotein (a), liver enzymes, creatine kinase, or prolactin. Semen analysis shows an increase in abnormal sperm morphology. In patients with autoimmune thyroiditis, titers of antibodies against thyroperoxidase and thyroglobulin are high; serum antinuclear antibodies may be present but are not usually indicative of lupus.

The normal reference range for ultrasensitive TSH levels is generally 0.4–4.0 milli-units/L. However, the normal range of TSH varies with age such that elderly patients have a mildly higher reference range. Over 95% of normal adults have serum TSH concentrations under 3.0 milli-units/L.

Subclinical hypothyroidism is defined as the state of having a normal serum FT_4 with a serum TSH that is above the reference range. It occurs most often in persons aged 65 years or older, in whom the prevalence is 13%. Subclinical hypothyroidism is often transient and the TSH normalizes spontaneously in about 35% of cases within 2 years. The likelihood of TSH normalization is higher in patients without antithyroid antibodies and those with a marginally elevated serum TSH. The term "subclinical" is somewhat misleading, since it does not refer to patients' symptoms but rather refers only to serum hormone levels; in fact, such patients can have subtle manifestations of hypothyroidism (eg, fatigue, depression, hyperlipidemia) that may improve with a trial of levothyroxine replacement. Patients without such symptoms do not require levothyroxine therapy but must be monitored regularly for the emergence of symptoms.

C. Imaging

Radiologic imaging is usually not necessary for patients with hypothyroidism. However, on CT or MRI, a goiter may be noted in the neck or in the mediastinum

Table 26–3. Appropriate use of thyroid tests.

	Test	Comment
Screening	Serum thyroid-stimulating hormone (TSH)	Most sensitive test for primary hypothyroidism and hyperthyroidism
	Free thyroxine (FT_4)	Excellent test
For hypothyroidism	Serum TSH	High in primary and low in secondary hypothyroidism
	Antithyroglobulin and antithyroperoxidase antibodies	Elevated in Hashimoto thyroiditis
For hyperthyroidism	Serum TSH	Suppressed except in TSH-secreting pituitary tumor or pituitary hyperplasia (rare)
	Triiodothyronine (T_3) or free triiodothyronine (FT_3)	Elevated
	^{123}I uptake and scan	Increased uptake; diffuse versus "hot" foci on scan
	Antithyroperoxidase and antithyroglobulin antibodies	Elevated in Graves disease
	Thyroid-stimulating immunoglobulin (TSI); TSH receptor antibody (TSH-R Ab [stim])	Usually (65%) positive in Graves disease
For thyroid nodules	Fine-needle aspiration (FNA) biopsy	Best diagnostic method for thyroid cancer
	^{123}I uptake and scan	Cancer is usually "cold"; less reliable than FNA biopsy
	^{99m}Tc scan	Vascular versus avascular
	Ultrasonography	Useful to assist FNA biopsy. Useful in assessing the risk of malignancy (multinodular goiter or pure cysts are less likely to be malignant). Useful to monitor nodules and patients after thyroid surgery for carcinoma.

(retrosternal goiter). An enlarged thymus is frequently seen in the mediastinum in cases of autoimmune thyroiditis. On MRI, the pituitary is often quite enlarged in primary hypothyroidism, due to reversible hyperplasia of TSH-secreting cells; concomitant hyperprolactinemia can lead to the mistaken diagnosis of a TSH-secreting or PRL-secreting pituitary adenoma.

▶ Differential Diagnosis

The differential diagnosis for subclinical hypothyroidism includes antibody interference with the serum TSH assay, macro-TSH, sleep deprivation, exercise, recovery from nonthyroidal illness, acute psychiatric emergencies, and other conditions and medications that can cause a low serum T_4 or high serum TSH in the absence of hypothyroidism (Table 26–4).

Euthyroid sick syndrome should be considered in patients without known thyroid disease who are found to have a low serum FT_4 with a serum TSH that is not elevated. This syndrome can be seen in patients with severe illness, caloric deprivation, or major surgery. Serum TSH tends to be suppressed in severe nonthyroidal illness, making the diagnosis of concurrent primary hypothyroidism quite difficult, although the presence of a goiter suggests the diagnosis.

The clinician must decide whether such severely ill patients (with a low serum T_4 but no elevated TSH) might have hypothyroidism due to hypopituitarism. Patients

without symptoms of prior brain lesion or hypopituitarism are very unlikely to suddenly develop hypopituitarism during an unrelated illness. Patients with diabetes insipidus, hypopituitarism, or other signs of a central nervous system (CNS) lesion may be given T_4 empirically.

Patients receiving prolonged dopamine infusions can develop true secondary hypothyroidism caused by dopamine's direct suppression of TSH-secreting cells.

▶ Complications

Patients with severe hypothyroidism have an increased susceptibility to bacterial pneumonia. Megacolon has been described in long-standing hypothyroidism. Organic psychoses with paranoid delusions may occur ("myxedema madness"). Rarely, adrenal crisis may be precipitated by thyroid therapy. Hypothyroidism is a rare cause of infertility, which may respond to thyroid replacement. Untreated hypothyroidism during pregnancy often results in miscarriage. Preexistent coronary artery disease and heart failure may be exacerbated by levothyroxine therapy.

Myxedema crisis refers to severe, life-threatening manifestations of hypothyroidism. Myxedema crisis particularly affects elderly women and can occur spontaneously in severely hypothyroid patients with prolonged exposure to the cold, with resultant hypothermia. It can also be induced by a stroke, heart failure, infection (particularly pneumonia), or trauma. Metabolism of drugs is slowed in hypothyroidism and myxedema crisis is often precipitated by the

Table 26–4. Factors that may cause aberrations in laboratory tests that may be mistaken for primary hypothyroidism.[1]

Low Serum T$_4$ or T$_3$	High Serum TSH
Laboratory error	Laboratory error
Acute psychiatric problems	Autoimmune disease (assay
Cirrhosis	interference)
Nephrotic syndrome	Heterophile antibodies
Familial thyroid-binding	Anti-mouse antibodies
globulin deficiency	Anti-thyrotropin antibodies
Severe illness	Macro-thyrotropin
Drugs	Strenuous exercise (acute)
Androgens	Sleep deprivation (acute)
Asparaginase	Recovery from nonthyroidal illness
Carbamazepine	(transient)
Chloral hydrate	Acute psychiatric admissions
Corticosteroids	(transient) (14%)
Diclofenac (T$_3$)	Elderly (especially women) (11%)
Didanosine	
Fenclofenac	
5-Fluorouracil	
Halofenate	
Mitotane	
Naproxen (T$_3$)	
Nicotinic acid	
Oxcarbazepine	
Phenobarbital	
Phenytoin (T$_4$ as low as	
2 mcg/dL)	
Salicylates in large doses	
(T$_3$ and T$_4$)	
Sertraline	
Stavudine	
T$_3$ therapy (T$_4$)	

[1]True primary hypothyroidism may coexist.
T$_4$, levothyroxine; T$_3$, triiodothyronine; TSH, thyroid-stimulating hormone.

administration of sedatives, antidepressants, hypnotics, anesthetics, or opioid analgesics. The drugs further impair cognition and respiratory drive and can precipitate respiratory arrest. Affected patients have impaired cognition, ranging from confusion to somnolence to coma (myxedema coma). Convulsions and abnormal CNS signs may occur. Patients have profound hypothermia, hypoventilation, hyponatremia, hypoglycemia, hypoxemia, hypercapnia, and hypotension. Rhabdomyolysis and acute kidney injury may occur. The mortality rate is high.

▶ **Treatment**

Before therapy with thyroid hormone is commenced, the hypothyroid patient requires at least a clinical assessment for adrenal insufficiency and angina, for which the patient would first require evaluation and treatment.

A. Treatment for Hypothyroidism

Synthetic levothyroxine has been the overwhelmingly preferred preparation for treating hypothyroid patients. However, some clinicians prescribe mixtures of levothyroxine and triiodothyronine for certain patients. Otherwise healthy young and middle-aged adults with hypothyroidism may be treated initially with levothyroxine in doses of 25–75 mcg orally daily. The lower doses are used for very mild hypothyroidism, while higher doses are given for more symptomatic hypothyroidism. Women who are pregnant with significant hypothyroidism may begin therapy with levothyroxine at higher doses of 100–150 mcg orally daily. The levothyroxine dosage may be increased according to clinical response and serum TSH, trying to keep the serum TSH level between 0.4 milli-units/L and 2.0 milli-units/L. Levothyroxine has traditionally been taken with water in the morning before breakfast. Taking levothyroxine at bedtime results in somewhat higher serum T$_4$ and lower TSH levels. Therefore, the administration timing for levothyroxine should be kept constant. After beginning daily administration, significant increases in serum T$_4$ levels are seen within 1–2 weeks, and near-peak levels are seen within 3–4 weeks.

Patients with coronary artery disease or those who are over age 60 years are treated with smaller initial doses of levothyroxine, 25–50 mcg orally daily; higher initial doses may be used if such patients are severely hypothyroid. The dose can be increased by 25 mcg every 1–3 weeks until the patient is euthyroid. Patients with hypothyroidism and known ischemic heart disease may begin thyroxine therapy following successful medical therapy or restoration of coronary perfusion by percutaneous coronary intervention (PCI) or CABG.

Myxedema crisis requires larger initial doses of levothyroxine intravenously, since myxedema itself can interfere with intestinal absorption of oral levothyroxine. Levothyroxine sodium 500 mcg is given intravenously as a loading dose, followed by 50–100 mcg intravenously daily; the lower dose is given to patients with suspected coronary artery disease. In patients with myxedema coma, liothyronine (T$_3$, Triostat) can be given intravenously with a loading dose of 10–20 mcg, followed by 10 mcg every 4–6 hours for the first 48 hours. The hypothermic patient is warmed only with blankets, since faster warming can precipitate cardiovascular collapse. Hypoglycemic patients are given 5% dextrose intravenously. Hyponatremic patients with a serum sodium 120–130 mEq/mL are administered 0.9% NaCl intravenously, while patients with a serum sodium below 120 mEq/mL are treated with boluses of 3% NaCl 100 mL intravenously with intravenous furosemide 20–40 mg to promote water diuresis; serum sodium levels must be followed closely and boluses of 3% NaCl can be repeated about every 6 hours until the serum sodium rises to 120 mmol/L or higher. When giving intravenous saline to myxedematous patients, care must be taken to avoid fluid overload.

Patients with hypercapnia require intubation and mechanical ventilation. Opioid medications must be stopped or used in very low doses. Infections must be detected and treated aggressively. Patients in whom concomitant adrenal insufficiency is suspected are treated with hydrocortisone, 100 mg intravenously, followed by 25–50 mg every 8 hours.

B. Monitoring and Optimizing Treatment of Hypothyroidism

Regular clinical and laboratory monitoring is critical to determine the optimal levothyroxine dose for each patient. An elevated serum TSH usually indicates the need for a higher dose of levothyroxine and the initial goal should be to normalize the serum TSH. The patient should be prescribed sufficient levothyroxine to restore a clinically euthyroid state, while maintaining the serum TSH, FT_4 and FT_3 within their reference ranges. For most patients with hypothyroidism, a stable maintenance dose of levothyroxine can usually be found.

Different levothyroxine preparations vary in their bioavailability by up to 14% and such differences may have a subtle but significant clinical impact. It is optimal for patients to consistently take the same manufacturer's brand of levothyroxine.

Increased levothyroxine dosage requirements can occur with drugs that increase the hepatic metabolism of levothyroxine (eg, carbamazepine, phenobarbital, primidone, phenytoin, rifabutin, rifampin, sunitinib, and other tyrosine kinase inhibitors). Sertraline can block the effect of thyroxine and increase the thyroxine dosage requirement. Imatinib chemotherapy can also increase dosage requirements. Amiodarone can cause an increase or decrease in thyroxine dose requirements. Malabsorption of thyroxine can be caused by coadministration of binding substances, such as iron (eg, in multivitamins); fiber; raloxifene; sucralfate; aluminum hydroxide antacids; sevelemer; orlistat; soy milk; bile acid-binding resins (cholestyramine and colesevelam); and calcium, magnesium, and soy protein supplements.

Proton pump inhibitors interfere slightly with the absorption of levothyroxine. Gastrointestinal disorders can interfere with thyroxine absorption, including celiac disease, inflammatory bowel disease, lactose intolerance, *Helicobacter pylori* gastritis, and atrophic gastritis. Nephrotic syndrome can increase the required dose of oral levothyroxine. Women with hypothyroidism may require increased doses of levothyroxine after commencing oral estrogen therapy.

Pregnancy usually increases the levothyroxine dosage requirement; an increase in levothyroxine requirement has been noted as early as the fifth week of pregnancy. Adequate levothyroxine is critical to the health of the fetus. Therefore, it is prudent to increase levothyroxine dosages by approximately 20–30% as soon as pregnancy is confirmed. The fetus is at least partially dependent on maternal T_4 for its CNS development—particularly in the second trimester. By mid pregnancy, women require an average of 47% increase in their levothyroxine dosage. Postpartum, levothyroxine replacement requirement ordinarily returns to prepregnancy level.

Decreased levothyroxine dose requirements occur in women after delivery, after bilateral oophorectomy or natural menopause, after cessation of oral estrogen replacement, or during therapy with GnRH agonists. Levothyroxine dosage may need to be titrated downward for patients who start taking teduglutide for short bowel syndrome.

1. Elevated serum TSH level—This usually indicates underreplacement with levothyroxine. However, before increasing the T_4 dosage, it is important to confirm that the patient is indeed taking the levothyroxine as directed and does not have angina. It is also important to exclude malabsorption of levothyroxine due to concurrent administration with binding substances (see above), with food (instead of fasting), or with gastrointestinal disorders (such as short bowel syndrome, celiac disease, regional enteritis, liver disease, or pancreatic exocrine insufficiency). Serum TSH may be elevated transiently in acute psychiatric illness, with antipsychotics and phenothiazines, and during recovery from nonthyroidal illness. Autoimmune disease can cause false elevations of TSH by interfering with the assay. Rarely, a high TSH can be caused by thyrotropin-secreting pituitary tumors.

2. Normal serum TSH level—Most patients may be given levothyroxine in doses sufficient to achieve a serum TSH in the low-normal range. However, for patients with coronary artery disease or recurrent atrial fibrillation, it may be prudent to administer lower doses of levothyroxine to keep their serum TSH in the high-normal range or even at a slightly elevated level.

Some otherwise healthy hypothyroid patients (taking levothyroxine with a normal serum TSH) continue to have hypothyroid-type symptoms, such as lethargy, weight gain, depression, or cognitive problems. Such patients must be carefully assessed for other concurrent conditions, such as an adverse drug reaction, Addison disease, depression, hypogonadism, anemia, celiac disease, or gluten sensitivity. If such conditions are not present or are treated and hypothyroid-type symptoms persist, a serum T_3 or free T_3 level is often helpful. Low serum T_3 levels may reflect inadequate peripheral deiodinase activity to convert inactive T_4 to active T_3. Such patients may be given a clinical trial of a higher dose of levothyroxine that results in a normal serum T_3 but a slightly low serum TSH. Alternatively, for such patients, some clinicians have found success with other strategies, such as supplementing levothyroxine with triiodothyronine (5–10 mcg/day) or using dessicated natural porcine thyroid preparations containing both T_4 and T_3 (eg, Armour Thyroid, Nature-Throid, NP Thyroid). For product conversion purposes, 100 mcg of levothyroxine is equivalent to about 65 mg (1 grain) of dessicated thyroid. The use of dessicated thyroid preparations has been discouraged by professional medical societies, but some patients prefer them.

3. Low or suppressed serum TSH level—A serum TSH level below the reference range (0.4–4.0 milli-units/L) is either "low" (0.04–0.4 milli-units/L) or "suppressed" (less than or equal to 0.03 milli-units/L). If a patient taking levothyroxine with a "suppressed" serum TSH has manifestations of hyperthyroidism, the dosage of levothyroxine must be reduced. However, if patients with "low" serum TSH levels exhibit no symptoms of hyperthyroidism, it is important to determine whether hypopituitarism or severe nonthyroidal illness is present. TSH can also be reduced by certain medications, such as nonsteroidal anti-inflammatory drugs;

opioids; nifedipine; verapamil; and high-dose (short-term) corticosteroids. Absent such conditions, a clinically euthyroid patient with a suppressed serum TSH should be given a lower dosage of levothyroxine. Patients who exhibit hypothyroid symptoms on the reduced dosage of levothyroxine may have the higher dose resumed.

As noted above, some hypothyroid patients continue to have hypothyroid-type symptoms despite receiving levothyroxine, even in doses that cause a low serum TSH. If the serum T_3 or FT_3 level is low, the patient may benefit from a slightly increased dose of levothyroxine. Patients who feel best with a levothyroxine dose that is associated with a "low" serum TSH (0.04–0.4 milli-units/L) may continue to take that dosage. Such patients who are clinically euthyroid but who have a mildly low serum TSH do not appear to suffer any long-term adverse consequences.

Patients with primary hypothyroidism who take levothyroxine and have a "suppressed" serum TSH (less than or equal to 0.03 milli-units/L) have an increased risk of atrial fibrillation and osteoporosis. Therefore, a lower dose of levothyroxine is prescribed for such patients. However, some patients feel unmistakably hypothyroid while taking the reduced dose of levothyroxine and have low serum T_3 or free T_3 levels. A higher levothyroxine dose may be resumed for such patients, but they require close long-term surveillance for atrial fibrillation, osteoporosis, and subtle hyperthyroidism.

▶ Prognosis

Patients with mild hypothyroidism caused by Hashimoto thyroiditis have a remission rate of 11%. Hypothyroidism caused by interferon-alpha resolves within 17 months of stopping the drug in 50% of patients. With levothyroxine treatment of hypothyroidism, striking transformations take place both in appearance and mental function. Return to a normal state is usually the rule, but relapses will occur if treatment is interrupted. However, untreated patients with myxedema crisis have a mortality rate approaching 100%; even with optimal treatment, the mortality rate is 20–50%.

▶ When to Refer

- Difficulty titrating levothyroxine replacement to normal TSH or clinically euthyroid state.
- Any patient with significant coronary artery disease needing levothyroxine therapy.

▶ When to Admit

- Suspected myxedema crisis.
- Hypercapnia.

De Groot L et al. Management of thyroid dysfunction during pregnancy and postpartum: an Endocrine Society clinical practice guideline. J Clin Endocrinol Metab. 2012 Aug; 97(8):2543–65. [PMID: 22869843]

Jonklaas J et al. Guidelines for the treatment of hypothyroidism: prepared by the American Thyroid Association Task Force on Thyroid Hormone Replacement. Thyroid. 2014 Dec; 24(12):1670–751. [PMID: 25266247]

Koulouri O et al. Pitfalls in the measurement and interpretation of thyroid function tests. Best Pract Res Clin Endocrinol Metab. 2013 Dec;27(6):745–62. [PMID: 24275187]

Rabin AS et al. Clinical problem-solving. Springing a leak. N Engl J Med. 2015 Oct;373(14):1362–7. [PMID: 26422727]

Salomo LH et al. Myxedema coma: an almost forgotten, yet still existing cause of multiorgan failure. BMJ Case Rep. 2014 Jan 30;2014:2013203223. [PMID: 24481020]

Wiersinga WM. Paradigm shifts in thyroid hormone replacement therapies for hypothyroidism. Nat Rev Endocrinol. 2014 Mar; 10(3):164–74. [PMID: 24419358]

HYPERTHYROIDISM (Thyrotoxicosis)

🧩 ESSENTIALS OF DIAGNOSIS

- ▶ Sweating, weight loss or gain, anxiety, palpitations, loose stools, heat intolerance, irritability, fatigue, weakness, menstrual irregularity.
- ▶ Tachycardia; warm, moist skin; stare; tremor.
- ▶ **Graves disease**: goiter (often with bruit); ophthalmopathy.
- ▶ Suppressed TSH in primary hyperthyroidism; increased T_4, FT_4, T_3, FT_3.

▶ General Considerations

The term "thyrotoxicosis" refers to the clinical manifestations associated with serum levels of T_4 or T_3 that are excessive for the individual (hyperthyroidism). Serum TSH levels are suppressed in primary hyperthyroidism. However, certain drugs and conditions can affect laboratory tests and lead to the erroneous diagnosis of hyperthyroidism in euthyroid individuals (Table 26–5). The causes of hyperthyroidism are many and diverse, as described below.

A. Graves Disease

Graves disease (known as Basedow disease in Europe) is the most common cause of thyrotoxicosis. It is an autoimmune disorder affecting the thyroid gland, characterized by an increase in synthesis and release of thyroid hormones. Graves disease is much more common in women than in men (8:1), and its onset is usually between the ages of 20 and 40 years. It may be accompanied by infiltrative ophthalmopathy (Graves exophthalmos) and, less commonly, by infiltrative dermopathy (pretibial myxedema). The thymus gland is typically enlarged and serum antinuclear antibody levels are usually elevated. Many patients with Graves disease have a family history of either Graves disease or Hashimoto thyroiditis. The pathogenesis of the hyperthyroidism of Graves disease involves the formation of autoantibodies that bind to the TSH receptor in thyroid cell membranes and stimulate the gland to hyperfunction. Such antibodies are called thyroid-stimulating immunoglobulins (TSI) or TSH receptor antibodies (TSHrAb).

Dietary iodine supplementation can trigger Graves disease. An increased incidence of Graves disease occurs in countries that have embarked on national programs to

Table 26–5. Factors that can cause aberrations in laboratory tests that may be mistaken for spontaneous clinical primary hyperthyroidism.[1]

High Serum T$_4$ or T$_3$	Low Serum TSH
Laboratory error	Laboratory error
Collection vial contains gel barrier for T$_3$	TSH variants not detected by commercial assays
Acute psychiatric problems (30%)	Autonomous thyroid or thyroid nodule
Acute medical illness (eg, acute intermittent porphyria)	Acute corticosteroid administration
	Biotin supplements
AIDS (increased thyroid-binding globulin)	Elderly euthyroid
	Nonthyroidal illness (severe)
Autoimmunity	Pregnancy (especially with morning sickness)
Biotin supplements	hCG-secreting trophoblastic tumors
Acute or chronic active hepatitis, primary biliary cirrhosis	Drugs
Pregnancy: morning sickness, hyperemesis gravidarum	Thyroid hormone
	Amphetamines
	Dopamine
Familial thyroid-binding abnormalities	Dopamine agonists
Familial resistance to thyroid (Refetoff syndrome)	Calcium channel blockers (nifedipine, verapamil)
Drugs	
Amiodarone	
Amphetamines	
Clofibrate	
Estrogens (oral)	
Heparin (dialysis method)	
Heroin	
Thyroid hormone therapy (excessive or factitious)	
Methadone	
Perphenazine	
Tamoxifen	

[1]True clinical hyperthyroidism may coexist.
hCG, human chorionic gonadotropin; NSAIDs, nonsteroidal anti-inflammatory drugs; T$_4$, levothyroxine; T$_3$, triiodothyronine; TSH, thyroid-stimulating hormone.

fortify commercial salt with potassium iodide; the increase in Graves disease lasts about 4 years. Similarly, patients being treated with potassium iodide or amiodarone (which contains iodine) have an increased risk of developing Graves disease.

Patients with Graves disease have an increased risk of other systemic autoimmune disorders, including Sjögren syndrome, celiac disease, pernicious anemia, Addison disease, alopecia areata, vitiligo, type 1 diabetes mellitus, hypoparathyroidism, myasthenia gravis, and cardiomyopathy.

B. Toxic Multinodular Goiter and Thyroid Nodules

Autonomous hyperfunctioning thyroid nodules that produce hyperthyroidism are known as toxic multinodular goiter (also called Plummer disease) and are more prevalent among the elderly and in iodine-deficient regions. A single hyperfunctioning nodule can also produce hyperthyroidism. Toxic multinodular goiter and Graves disease may sometimes coexist in the same gland (Marine-Lenhart syndrome). Thyroid cancer is found in about 4.7% of patients with toxic multinodular goiter.

C. Postpartum, Subacute, and Silent Thyroiditis

These conditions cause thyroid inflammation with release of stored hormone. They all produce a variable triphasic course: variable hyperthyroidism is followed by transient euthyroidism, and progresses to hypothyroidism.

Postpartum thyroiditis refers to Hashimoto thyroiditis that occurs in the first 12 months after delivery. Although this usually occurs after term pregnancies, it can also occur after miscarriages. It is common, occurring in 5% of postpartum women, with an increased incidence in women with preexistent type 1 diabetes mellitus and other autoimmune disorders. About 22% of affected women experience hyperthyroidism followed by hypothyroidism, whereas 30% of such women have isolated thyrotoxicosis and 48% have isolated hypothyroidism. The thyrotoxic phase typically occurs 2–6 weeks postpartum and lasts 2–3 months. Over 80% have antithyroid antibodies. Most women progress to a hypothyroid phase that usually lasts a few months but that can be permanent. The recurrence rate with subsequent pregnancies is about 70%.

Subacute thyroiditis is also known as "de Quervain" or "granulomatous" thyroiditis. It is typically caused by various viral infections. Women are affected four times more frequently than men. Patients typically experience a viral upper respiratory infection and develop an enlarged and extremely painful thyroid. About 50% of affected patients experience a symptomatic thyrotoxic phase that lasts 3–6 weeks. It is important to differentiate subacute thyroiditis from infectious (suppurative bacterial) thyroiditis. About 10% remain hypothyroid after 1 year. The recurrence rate is 1–4%.

Silent thyroiditis is also known as subacute lymphocytic thyroiditis or "Hashitoxicosis." It can occur spontaneously or be triggered by certain medications. Women are affected four times more frequently than men. About 50% have antithyroid antibodies and such patients have sometimes had chemotherapeutic agents (such as tyrosine kinase inhibitors, denileukin diftitox, alemtuzumab, interferon-alpha, interleukin-2, ipilimumab, tremelimumab, thalidomide, and lenalidomide). Other drugs can cause silent thyroiditis, including lithium and amiodarone. In those with spontaneous silent thyroiditis, about 10–20% remain hypothyroid after 1 year. There is a recurrence rate of 5–10%; this rate is higher in Japan.

D. Medication-Induced Hyperthyroidism

1. Amiodarone-induced thyrotoxicosis—Amiodarone is a widely used antiarrhythmic drug that is 37% iodine by weight. The half-life of amiodarone and its metabolites is about 100 days. In the short term, amiodarone increases the serum TSH, though usually not over 20 milli-units/L. Serum T$_4$ and FT$_4$ rise about 40% and may become frankly elevated in clinically euthyroid patients. Meanwhile, serum T_3 levels decline. Due to these short-term changes, it is best to not check thyroid function tests during the first 3 months of therapy with amiodarone, unless clinically indicated. After about 3 months, the serum TSH usually normalizes. Since serum T_4 levels can be misleadingly high, the serum TSH level must be suppressed to diagnose amiodarone-induced thyrotoxicosis. With amiodarone-induced thyrotoxicosis, the serum T_3 or FT_3 is usually high or high-normal. In the United States, amiodarone causes thyrotoxicosis in about 3% of patients taking the drug. In Europe and iodine-deficient geographic areas, amiodarone induces thyrotoxicosis in about 20%. Thyrotoxicosis can occur quite suddenly at any time during treatment with amiodarone and may even develop several months after it has been discontinued. The manifestations of amiodarone-induced thyrotoxicosis can be missed, particularly since amiodarone tends to cause bradycardia. Therefore, it is prudent to check thyroid function tests (TSH, FT_4, T_3) prior to commencing amiodarone, rechecking them in 3–6 months, and then every 6 months (or sooner if clinically indicated).

Amiodarone-induced thyrotoxicosis is categorized as type 1 or type 2; about 27% are mixed type 1–2. **Type 1** is caused by the active production of excessive thyroid hormone. Thyroid color-flow Doppler typically shows an enlarged gland with increased vascularity; scanning with ^{99m}Tc-sestamibi shows normal to increased thyroidal uptake. **Type 2** is caused by thyroiditis with the passive release of stored thyroid hormone. Thyroid color-flow Doppler shows a normal sized gland without increased vascularity; scanning with ^{99m}Tc-sestamibi scanning shows no thyroidal uptake.

2. Iodine-induced hyperthyroidism—This is also known as **Jod-Basedow disease**. The recommended iodine intake for nonpregnant adults is 150 mcg/day. Higher iodine intake can precipitate hyperthyroidism in patients with nodular goiters, autonomous thyroid nodules, or asymptomatic Graves disease, and less commonly in patients with no detectable underlying thyroid disorder. Common sources of excess iodine include intravenous iodinated radiocontrast dye, certain foods (eg, kelp, nori), topical iodinated antiseptics (eg, povidine iodine), and medications (eg, amiodarone or potassium iodide). Intravenous iodinated radiocontrast dye can rarely induce a painful, destructive subacute thyroiditis, similar to type 2 amiodarone-induced thyrotoxicosis.

3. Tyrosine kinase inhibitors—About 3.2% of patients receiving chemotherapy with tyrosine kinase inhibitors (eg, axitinib, sorafenib, sunitinib) develop silent thyroiditis that releases stored thyroid hormone, resulting in hyperthyroidism. While this hyperthyroidism may be subclinical, thyrotoxic crisis has been reported. Hypothyroidism usually follows hyperthyroidism and overall occurs in 19% of patients taking these drugs.

4. Alemtuzumab immunotherapy—Alemtuzumab is an anti-CD52 monoclonal antibody used to treat patients with multiple sclerosis. Graves disease with hyperthyroidism (usually mild) followed by hypothyroidism develops in about 22% of patients treated with alemtuzumab.

E. Pregnancy, hCG-Secreting Trophoblastic Tumors, and Testicular Choriocarcinoma

Human chorionic gonadotropin (hCG) can bind to the thyroid's TSH receptors, so very high levels of serum hCG, particularly during the first 4 months of pregnancy, may cause sufficient receptor activation to cause hyperthyroidism. About 18% of pregnant women have a low serum TSH during pregnancy, but only about 10% of such women have clinical hyperthyroidism that requires treatment. Pregnant women are more likely to have hCG-induced thyrotoxicosis if they have high levels of serum asialo-hCG, a subfraction of hCG that has a greater affinity for TSH receptors. Such women are also more likely to suffer from hyperemesis gravidarum. This condition must be distinguished from true Graves disease in pregnancy, which usually predates conception and may be associated with high serum levels of TSI and antithyroid antibodies or with exophthalmos.

High levels of hCG can also cause thyrotoxicosis in some cases of pregnancies with gestational trophoblastic disease (molar pregnancy, choriocarcinoma). Some such pregnancies have produced thyrotoxic crisis. Men have developed hyperthyroidism from high levels of serum hCG secreted by a testicular choriocarcinoma.

F. Rare Causes of Hyperthyroidism

Thyrotoxicosis factitia is due to intentional or accidental ingestion of excessive amounts of exogenous thyroid hormone. Isolated epidemics of thyrotoxicosis have been caused by consumption of ground beef contaminated with bovine thyroid gland. **Struma ovarii** refers to thyroid tissue contained in about 3% of ovarian dermoid tumors and teratomas. Such ectopic thyroid tissue can produce excess thyroid hormone from thyroid nodules or as a concomitant source of thyroid hormone excess with Graves disease. **Pituitary TSH hypersecretion** by a pituitary thyrotrophe tumor or hyperplasia can rarely cause hyperthyroidism. Serum TSH is elevated or inappropriately normal in the presence of true thyrotoxicosis. Pituitary hyperplasia may be detected on an MRI as a pituitary enlargement without a discrete adenoma being visible. **Metastatic functioning thyroid carcinoma** can cause hyperthyroidism in patients with a heavy tumor burden. Hyperthyroidism can be induced or aggravated by recombinant human thyroid-stimulating hormone (rhTSH) that is given prior to radio-iodine therapy or scanning.

▶ Clinical Findings

A. Symptoms and Signs

Thyrotoxicosis due to any cause produces nervousness, restlessness, heat intolerance, increased sweating, pruritus, fatigue, weakness, muscle cramps, frequent bowel movements, or weight change (usually loss). There may be palpitations or angina pectoris. Angina or atrial fibrillation may also be present, sometimes in the absence of other thyrotoxic symptoms (**apathetic hyperthyroidism**). Women frequently report menstrual irregularities. Women with postpartum thyroiditis are often asymptomatic or experience only minor symptoms, such as palpitations, heat intolerance, and irritability. Signs of thyrotoxicosis also include fine resting finger tremors, moist warm skin, fever, hyperreflexia, fine hair, and onycholysis. Chronic thyrotoxicosis may cause osteoporosis. Even subclinical hyperthyroidism (suppressed serum TSH with normal FT_4) may increase the risk of nonvertebral fractures. Clubbing and swelling of the fingers (acropachy) develop rarely.

Thyroid examination in patients with Graves disease usually reveals a diffusely enlarged thyroid, frequently asymmetric, often with a bruit. However, some patients have no palpable thyroid enlargement. The thyroid gland in subacute thyroiditis is usually moderately enlarged and tender. There is often dysphagia and pain that can radiate to the jaw or ear. In patients with toxic multinodular goiter, the thyroid usually has palpable nodules. Patients with silent thyroiditis or postpartum thyroiditis have either no palpable goiter or a small, nontender goiter. **Cardiopulmonary manifestations** of thyrotoxicosis commonly include a forceful heartbeat, premature atrial contractions, and sinus tachycardia. Patients often have exertional dyspnea. Atrial fibrillation or atrial tachycardia occurs in about 8% of patients with thyrotoxicosis, more commonly in men, the elderly, and those with ischemic or valvular heart disease. The ventricular response from the atrial fibrillation may be difficult to control. Thyrotoxicosis itself can cause a thyrotoxic cardiomyopathy, and the onset of atrial fibrillation can precipitate heart failure. Echocardiogram reveals pulmonary hypertension in 49% of patients with hyperthyroidism; of these, 71% have pulmonary artery hypertension while 29% have pulmonary venous hypertension. Even "subclinical hyperthyroidism" increases the risk for atrial fibrillation and overall mortality. Hemodynamic abnormalities and pulmonary hypertension are reversible with restoration of euthyroidism.

Graves eye manifestations, which can occur with hyperthyroidism of any etiology, include upper eyelid retraction, lid lag with downward gaze, and a staring appearance. Thyroid-associated orbitopathy (exophthalmos) is clinically apparent in 20–40% of patients with Graves disease and some cases of amiodarone-induced thyrotoxicosis. Aggravation of Graves eye disease has occurred after treatment with radioiodine or during therapy with thiazolidinediones (eg, pioglitazone). It usually consists of conjunctival edema (chemosis), conjunctivitis, and mild exophthalmos (proptosis). About 5–10% of patients experience more severe exophthalmos, with the eye being pushed forward by increased retro-orbital fat and eye muscles that have been thickened by lymphocytic infiltration. Such patients can experience diplopia from extraocular muscle entrapment. There may be weakness of upward gaze. The optic nerve may be compressed in severe cases, causing progressive loss of color vision, visual fields, and visual acuity. Corneal drying may occur with inadequate lid closure. Eye changes may sometimes be asymmetric or unilateral. The severity of eye disease is not closely correlated with the severity of thyrotoxicosis.

Exophthalmometry should be performed on all patients with Graves disease to document their degree of exophthalmos and detect progression of orbitopathy. The protrusion of the eye beyond the orbital rim is measured with a prism instrument (Hertel exophthalmometer). Maximum normal eye protrusion varies between kindreds and races, being about 22 mm for blacks, 20 mm for whites, and 18 mm for Asians.

Graves dermopathy (pretibial myxedema) occurs in about 3% of patients with Graves disease. It usually affects the pretibial region but can also affect the dorsal forearms and wrists and dorsum of the feet. It is more common in patients with high levels of serum TSI and severe Graves ophthalmopathy. Glycosaminoglycans accumulation and lymphoid infiltration occur in affected skin, which becomes erythematous with a thickened, rough texture. Elephantiasis of the legs is a rare complication.

Thyroid acropachy is an extreme and unusual manifestation of Graves disease. It presents with digital clubbing, swelling of fingers and toes, and a periosteal reaction of extremity bones. It is ordinarily associated with ophthalmopathy and thyroid dermopathy. Most affected patients are smokers.

Hyperthyroidism during pregnancy has a prevalence of about 0.2%. It may commence before conception or emerge during pregnancy, particularly the first trimester. Manifestations include many of the features of normal pregnancy: tachycardia, warm skin, heat intolerance, increased sweating, and a palpable thyroid. Pregnancy can have a beneficial effect on the thyrotoxicosis of Graves disease, with decreasing antibody titers and decreasing serum T_4 levels as the pregnancy advances; about 30% of affected women experience a remission by late in the second trimester. However, undiagnosed or undertreated hyperthyroidism in pregnancy carries an increased risk of miscarriage, preeclampsia-eclampsia, preterm delivery, abruptio placenta, maternal heart failure, and thyrotoxic crisis (thyroid storm). Such thyrotoxic crisis can be precipitated by trauma, infection, surgery, or delivery and confers a fetal/maternal mortality rate of about 25%.

TSI (TSHrAb) crosses the placenta and if maternal serum TSI levels reach greater than 500% in the third trimester, the risk of **transient neonatal Graves disease in the newborn** is increased. Such thyrotoxic newborns have an increased risk of intrauterine growth retardation and prematurity.

Hypokalemic periodic paralysis occurs in about 15% of Asian or Native American men with thyrotoxicosis. It usually presents abruptly with symmetric flaccid paralysis (and few thyrotoxic symptoms), often after intravenous dextrose, oral carbohydrate, or vigorous exercise. Attacks last 7–72 hours.

B. Laboratory Findings

Serum FT_4, T_3, FT_3, T_4, thyroid resin uptake, and FT_4 index are all usually increased. Sometimes the FT_4 level may be normal but with an elevated serum T_3 (T_3 toxicosis). Serum T_3 can be misleadingly elevated when blood is collected in tubes using a gel barrier, which causes certain immunoassays to report falsely elevated serum total T_3 levels in 24% of normal patients. Serum T_4 or T_3 can be elevated in other nonthyroidal conditions (Table 26–5).

Serum TSH is suppressed in hyperthyroidism (except in the very rare cases of pituitary inappropriate secretion of thyrotropin). Serum TSH may be misleadingly low in other nonthyroidal conditions (Table 26–5). The term "subclinical hyperthyroidism" is used to describe asymptomatic individuals with a low serum TSH but normal serum levels of FT_4 and T_3; progression to symptomatic thyrotoxicosis occurs at a rate of 1–2% per year in patients without a goiter and at a rate of 5% per year in patients with a multinodular goiter.

Hyperthyroidism can cause other laboratory abnormalities, including hypercalcemia, increased alkaline phosphatase, anemia, and decreased granulocytes. Hypokalemia and hypophosphatemia occur in thyrotoxic periodic paralysis.

Problems of diagnosis occur in patients with acute psychiatric disorders; about 30% of these patients have elevated serum T_4 levels without clinical thyrotoxicosis. The TSH is not usually suppressed, distinguishing psychiatric disorder from true hyperthyroidism. T_4 levels return to normal gradually.

In **Graves disease,** serum TSI is usually detectable (65%). Antithyroglobulin or antithyroperoxidase antibodies are usually elevated but are nonspecific. Serum antinuclear antibodies are also usually elevated without any evidence of SLE or other rheumatologic disease.

With **subacute thyroiditis,** patients often have an increased WBC, ESR, and C-reactive protein. About 25% have antithyroid antibodies (usually in low titer) and serum TSI (TSHrAb) levels are normal. Patients with iodine-induced hyperthyroidism also have undetectable serum TSI (or TSHrAb), an absence of serum antithyroperoxidase antibodies, and an elevated urinary iodine concentration. In thyrotoxicosis factitia, serum thyroglobulin levels are low, distinguishing it from other causes of hyperthyroidism.

With **hyperthyroidism during pregnancy,** women have an elevated serum total T_4 and FT_4 while the TSH is suppressed. However, about 18% of normal pregnant women have a low serum TSH. An apparent lack of full TSH suppression in hyperthyroidism can be seen due to misidentification of hCG as TSH in certain assays. The serum FT_4 assay is difficult in pregnancy. Although the serum T_4 is elevated in most pregnant women, values over 20 mcg/dL (257 nmol/L) are encountered only in hyperthyroidism. On treatment, serum total T_4 levels during pregnancy should be kept at about 1.5 × the pre-pregnancy level. The T_3 resin uptake, which is low in normal pregnancy because of high thyroxine-binding globulin (TBG) concentration, is normal or high in thyrotoxic persons.

Since high levels of T_4 and FT_4 are normally seen in patients taking **amiodarone, a** suppressed TSH must be present along with a greatly elevated T_4 (greater than 20 mcg/dL [257 nmol/L]) or T_3 (greater than 200 ng/dL [3.1 nmol/L]) in order to diagnose hyperthyroidism. In **type 1 amiodarone-induced thyrotoxicosis,** the presence of proptosis and serum TSI (TSHrAb) is diagnostic. In **type 2 amiodarone-induced thyrotoxicosis,** serum levels of interleukin-6 (IL-6) are usually quite elevated.

C. Imaging

Radioiodine (RAI) uptake and scanning can be helpful in determining the cause of hyperthyroidism. The isotope is administered orally and thyroidal radioiodone uptake is determined at about 4 hours and again at 24 hours, when a scan is also performed. RAI uptake and scanning is not necessary for patients with obvious Graves disease who have elevated serum TSI or associated Graves ophthalmopathy. Women with hyperthyroidism due to Graves disease should ideally have the RAI scan extended to include the pelvis in order to screen for concomitant struma ovarii (rare). A high RAI uptake is seen in Graves disease and toxic nodular goiter. Patients with **type 1 amiodarone-induced thyrotoxicosis** have RAI uptake that is usually detectable. A low RAI uptake is also characteristic of iodine-induced hyperthyroidism and thyroiditis (subacute, silent, or postpartum), distinguishing them from Graves disease. Low RAI uptake is also seen with interleukin-2 therapy and during hyperthyroidism that often follows neck surgery for hyperparathyroidism. In **type 2 amiodarone-induced thyrotoxicosis,** thyroid RAI uptake is usually below 3%.

Technetium (Tc- 99m) pertechnetate is given intravenously, and scanning is performed 20 minutes later. This scan is useful for distinguishing thyroiditis from Graves disease. Technetium (Tc- 99m) pertechnetate mimics radioiodine scanning but is more convenient, costs less, and confers less radiation exposure.

Thyroid ultrasound can be helpful in patients with hyperthyroidism, particularly in patients with palpable thyroid nodules. Thyroid ultrasound shows a variably heterogenous, hypoechoic gland in thyroiditis. **Color flow Doppler sonography** is helpful to distinguish type 1 amiodarone-induced thyrotoxicosis (normal to increased blood flow velocity and vascularity) from type 2 amiodarone-induced thyrotoxicosis (reduced vascularity).

99mTc-sestamibi scanning usually shows normal or increased uptake with type 1 amiodarone-induced thyrotoxicosis and decreased uptake in type 2.

MRI and CT scanning of the orbits are the imaging methods of choice to visualize Graves ophthalmopathy affecting the extraocular muscles. Imaging is required only in severe or unilateral cases or in euthyroid exophthalmos that must be distinguished from orbital pseudotumor, tumors, and other lesions.

▶ Differential Diagnosis

True thyrotoxicosis must be distinguished from those conditions that elevate serum T_4 and T_3 or suppress serum TSH without affecting clinical status. Biotin supplements can cause a false elevation in free T_4 and total T_3 and a false suppression of TSH in some assays that use a biotin-streptavidin fluorescent detection system (see Table 26–5). Biotin can also cause false-positives in some assays for thyrotropin receptor antibodies (TRAb), resulting in a misdiagnosis of Graves disease. Serum TSH is commonly suppressed in early pregnancy and only about 10% of pregnant women with a low TSH have clinical hyperthyroidism.

Some states of hypermetabolism without thyrotoxicosis—notably severe anemia, leukemia, polycythemia, cancer, and pheochromocytoma—rarely cause confusion. Acromegaly may also produce tachycardia, sweating, and thyroid enlargement. Appropriate laboratory tests will easily distinguish these entities.

The differential diagnosis for Graves ophthalmopathy includes an orbital tumor (eg, lymphoma) or pseudotumor. Ocular myasthenia gravis is another autoimmune condition that occurs more commonly in Graves disease but is usually mild, often with unilateral eye involvement. Acetylcholinesterase receptor antibody (AChR Ab) levels are elevated in only 36% of such patients, and a thymoma is present in 9%.

Diabetes mellitus and Addison disease may coexist with thyrotoxicosis.

Complications

Hypercalcemia, osteoporosis, and nephrocalcinosis may occur in hyperthyroidism. Decreased libido, erectile dysfunction, diminished sperm motility, and gynecomastia may be noted in men. Other complications include cardiac arrhythmias and heart failure, thyroid crisis, ophthalmopathy, dermopathy, and thyrotoxic hypokalemic periodic paralysis.

Treatment

A. Treatment of Graves Disease

1. Propranolol—Propranolol is generally used for symptomatic relief until the hyperthyroidism is resolved. It effectively relieves its accompanying tachycardia, tremor, diaphoresis, and anxiety. It is the initial treatment of choice for thyrotoxic crisis. Thyrotoxic hypokalemic periodic paralysis is also effectively treated with beta-blockade. It has no effect on thyroid hormone secretion. Treatment is usually begun with propranolol ER 60 mg orally once or twice daily, with dosage increases every 2–3 days to a maximum daily dose of 320 mg. Propranolol ER is initially given every 12 hours for patients with severe hyperthyroidism, due to accelerated metabolism of the propranolol; it may be given once daily as hyperthyroidism improves.

2. Thiourea drugs—Methimazole or propylthiouracil is generally used for young adults or patients with mild thyrotoxicosis, small goiters, or fear of isotopes. See Treatment of Hyperthyroidism during Pregnancy-Planning, Pregnancy, and Lactation. Elderly patients usually respond particularly well. These drugs are also useful for preparing hyperthyroid patients for surgery and elderly patients for RAI treatment. The drugs do not permanently damage the thyroid and are associated with a lower chance of posttreatment hypothyroidism (compared with RAI or surgery). When thiourea therapy is discontinued, there is a high recurrence rate for hyperthyroidism (about 50%). A better likelihood of long-term remission is seen in patients with small goiters or mild hyperthyroidism and those requiring small doses of thiourea. Patients whose thyroperoxidase and thyroglobulin antibodies remain high after 2 years of therapy have been reported to have only a 10% rate of relapse. Thiourea therapy may be continued long-term for patients who are tolerating it well.

All patients receiving thiourea therapy must be informed of the danger of agranulocytosis or pancytopenia and the need to stop the drug and seek medical attention immediately with the onset of any infection or unusual bleeding. Agranulocytosis (defined as an absolute neutrophil count below 500/mcL) or pancytopenia usually occurs abruptly in about 0.4% of patients taking either methimazole or propylthiouracil. Over 70% of agranulocytosis cases occur within the first 60 days and nearly 85% within 90 days of commencing therapy. But continued long-term vigilance for this side effect is required. About half the cases are discovered because of fever, pharyngitis, or bleeding, but the other cases are discovered with routine complete blood counts. There is a genetic tendency to develop agranulocytosis with thiourea therapy; if a close relative has had this adverse reaction, other therapies should be considered. Agranulocytosis generally remits spontaneously with discontinuation of the thiourea and during antibiotic treatment. Recovery has not been improved by filgrastim (granulocyte colony-stimulating factor [G-CSF]). Surveillance of the WBC can be done when blood is drawn to check thyroid levels during the first few months of treatment. Such surveillance may be helpful, since some cases of agranulocytosis occur gradually and many cases may be discovered while the patient is still asymptomatic.

Other side effects common to thiourea drugs include pruritus, allergic dermatitis, nausea, and dyspepsia. Antihistamines may control mild pruritus without discontinuation of the drug. Since the two thiourea drugs are similar, patients who have a major allergic reaction to one should not be given the other.

The patient may become clinically hypothyroid for 2 weeks or more before TSH levels rise, the pituitary gland having been suppressed by the preceding hyperthyroidism. Therefore, the patient's changing thyroid status is best monitored clinically and with serum FT_4 levels. Rapid growth of the goiter usually occurs if prolonged hypothyroidism is allowed to develop; the goiter may sometimes become massive but usually regresses rapidly with reduction or cessation of thiourea therapy or with thyroid hormone replacement.

A. Methimazole—Except during the first trimester of pregnancy, methimazole is generally preferred over propylthiouracil, since methimazole is more convenient to use and is less likely to cause fulminant hepatic necrosis. Methimazole therapy is also less likely to cause ^{131}I treatment failure. Methimazole is given orally in initial doses of 30–60 mg once daily. Some patients with very mild hyperthyroidism may respond well to smaller initial doses of methimazole (10–20 mg daily). Methimazole may also be administered twice daily to reduce the likelihood of gastrointestinal upset. Rare complications peculiar to methimazole include serum sickness, cholestatic jaundice, alopecia, nephrotic syndrome, hypoglycemia, and loss of taste. Methimazole use in pregnancy has been associated with an increased risk of major fetal anomalies (4.1% vs 2.1% in controls). If methimazole is used during pregnancy or breastfeeding, the dose should not exceed 20 mg daily. The dosage is reduced as manifestations of hyperthyroidism resolve and as the FT_4 level falls toward normal. For patients receiving ^{131}I therapy, methimazole is discontinued 4 days prior to receiving the ^{131}I and is resumed at a lower dose 3 days afterwards to avoid recurrence of hyperthyroidism. About 4 weeks after ^{131}I therapy, methimazole may be discontinued if the patient is euthyroid.

B. **Propylthiouracil**—Initially, propylthiouracil is given orally in doses of 300–600 mg daily in four divided doses. The dosage and frequency of administration are reduced as symptoms of hyperthyroidism resolve and the FT_4 level approaches normal. Rare complications peculiar to propylthiouracil include arthritis, lupus, aplastic anemia, thrombocytopenia, and hypoprothrombinemia. With propylthiouracil, acute hepatitis occurs rarely and is treated with prednisone. Acute liver failure occurs in about 1 in 10,000 patients, making this a second-line drug, usually reserved for pregnancy, since it is not known to cause fetal anomalies. During pregnancy, the dose of propylthiouracil is kept below 200 mg/day to avoid goitrous hypothyroidism in the infant; the patient may be switched to methimazole in the second trimester. Propylthiouracil has been the drug of choice during breastfeeding since it is not concentrated in the milk as much as methimazole. Propylthiouracil is also favored during pregnancy, possibly causing fewer problems in the newborn.

3. Iodinated contrast agents—These agents provide effective temporary treatment for thyrotoxicosis of any cause. Iopanoic acid (Telepaque) or ipodate sodium (Bilivist, Oragrafin) is given orally in a dosage of 500 mg twice daily for 3 days, then 500 mg once daily. These agents inhibit peripheral 5′-monodeiodination of T_4, thereby blocking its conversion to active T_3. Within 24 hours, serum T_3 levels fall an average of 62%. For patients with Graves disease, methimazole is begun first to block iodine organification; the next day, ipodate sodium or iopanoic acid may be added. The iodinated contrast agents are particularly useful for patients who are symptomatically very thyrotoxic. They offer a therapeutic option for patients with T_4 overdosage, subacute thyroiditis, and amiodarone-induced thyrotoxicosis; for those intolerant to thioureas; and for newborns with thyrotoxicosis (due to maternal Graves disease). Treatment periods of 8 months or more are possible, but efficacy tends to wane with time. In Graves disease, thyroid RAI uptake may be suppressed during treatment but typically returns to pretreatment uptake by 7 days after discontinuation of the drug, allowing ^{131}I treatment.

4. Radioactive iodine (^{131}I, RAI)—The administration of ^{131}I is an excellent method of destroying overactive thyroid tissue (either diffuse or toxic nodular goiter). Adolescent and adult patients who have been treated with RAI in adulthood do not have an increased risk of subsequent thyroid cancer, leukemia, or other malignancies. Children born to parents previously treated with ^{131}I show no increase in rates of congenital abnormalities.

Because radiation is harmful to the fetus and children, *RAI should not be given to pregnant or lactating women or to mothers who lack childcare.* A pregnancy test should be obtained within 48 hours before therapy for any woman with childbearing potential. RAI should not be given to women with Graves disease within 3 months prior to a planned conception.

Patients may receive ^{131}I while being symptomatically treated with propranolol ER, which is then reduced in dosage as hyperthyroidism resolves. A higher rate of ^{131}I treatment failure has been reported in patients with Graves disease who have been receiving methimazole or propylthiouracil. However, therapy with ^{131}I will usually be effective if the methimazole is discontinued at least 3–4 days before RAI therapy and if the therapeutic dosage of ^{131}I is adjusted (upward) according to RAI uptake on the pretherapy scan. Prior to ^{131}I therapy, patients are instructed against receiving intravenous iodinated contrast and should consume a low-iodine diet.

The presence of Graves ophthalmopathy is a relative contraindication to ^{131}I therapy. Following ^{131}I treatment for hyperthyroidism, Graves ophthalmopathy appears or worsens in 15% of patients (23% in smokers and 6% in nonsmokers) and improves in none, whereas during treatment with methimazole, ophthalmopathy worsens in 3% and improves in 2% of patients. Among patients receiving prednisone following ^{131}I treatment, preexistent ophthalmopathy worsens in none and improves in 67%. Therefore, patients with Graves ophthalmopathy who are to be treated with radioiodine should be considered for prophylactic prednisone (20–40 mg/day) for 2 months following administration of ^{131}I, particularly in patients who have severe orbital involvement.

Smoking increases the risk of having a flare in ophthalmopathy following ^{131}I treatment and also reduces the effectiveness of prednisone treatment. Patients who smoke are strongly encouraged to quit prior to RAI treatment. Smokers receiving RAI should be considered for prophylactic prednisone (see above).

FT_4 levels may sometimes drop within 2 months after ^{131}I treatment, but then rise again to thyrotoxic levels, at which time thyroid RAI uptake is low. This phenomenon is caused by a release of stored thyroid hormone from injured thyroid cells and does not indicate a treatment failure. In fact, serum FT_4 then falls abruptly to hypothyroid levels.

There is a high incidence of hypothyroidism in the months to years after ^{131}I, even when low activities are given. Patients with Graves disease treated with ^{131}I also have an increased lifetime risk of developing hyperparathyroidism, particularly when radioiodine therapy was administered in childhood or adolescence. Lifelong clinical follow-up is mandatory, with measurements of serum TSH, FT_4, and calcium when indicated.

5. Thyroid surgery—Thyroidectomy may be performed for pregnant women whose thyrotoxicosis is not controlled with low doses of thioureas, and for women who desire to become pregnant in the very near future. Surgery is also an option for nodular goiters, when there is a suspicion for malignancy.

The surgical procedure of choice for patients with Graves disease is a total resection of one lobe and a subtotal resection of the other lobe, leaving about 4 g of thyroid tissue (Hartley–Dunhill operation). Subtotal thyroidectomy of both lobes ultimately results in a 9% recurrence rate of hyperthyroidism. Total thyroidectomy of both lobes poses an increased risk of hypoparathyroidism and damage to the recurrent laryngeal nerves.

Patients are ordinarily rendered euthyroid preoperatively with a thiourea drug. Propranolol ER is given orally at initial doses of 60–80 mg twice daily and increased every 2–3 days until the heart rate is less than 90 beats per minute. Propranolol is continued until the serum T_3

(or free T_3) is normal preoperatively. If a patient undergoes surgery while thyrotoxic, larger doses of propranolol are given perioperatively to reduce the likelihood of thyroid crisis. Ipodate sodium or iopanoic acid (500 mg orally twice daily) may be used in addition to a thiourea to accelerate the decline in serum T_3. The patient should be euthyroid by the time of surgery.

To reduce thyroid vascularity preoperatively, the patient may be treated for 3 days prior to surgery with oral potassium iodide 25–50 mg (eg, ThyroShield 65 mg/mL, 0.5 mL, or SSKI [potassium iodide] 1 g/mL, 1 drop) three times daily or iodinated radiocontrast agents (eg, iopanoic acid 500 mg orally twice daily). However, preoperative potassium iodide often increases the volume of the thyroid, so the requirement for preoperative potassium iodide for Graves disease is debatable. Preoperative iodide supplementation is not recommended prior to surgery for multinodular goiter.

Surgical morbidity includes possible damage to a recurrent laryngeal nerve, with resultant vocal cord paralysis. If both recurrent laryngeal nerves are damaged, airway obstruction may develop, and the patient may require intubation and tracheostomy. Hypoparathyroidism also occurs; serum calcium levels must be checked postoperatively. Patients should be admitted for thyroidectomy surgery for at least an overnight observation period. When a competent, experienced neck surgeon performs a thyroidectomy, surgical complications are uncommon.

B. Treatment of Toxic Solitary Thyroid Nodules

Toxic solitary thyroid nodules are usually benign but may rarely be malignant. If a nonsurgical therapy is elected, the nodule should be evaluated with a fine-needle aspiration (FNA) biopsy. **Medical therapy** for hyperthyroidism caused by a single hyperfunctioning thyroid nodule may be treated symptomatically with propranolol ER and methimazole or propylthiouracil, as in Graves disease (see above). Patients who tolerate methimazole well may elect to continue it for long-term therapy. The dose of methimazole should be adjusted to keep the TSH slightly suppressed, so the risk of TSH-stimulated growth of the nodule is reduced. **Surgery** is usually recommended for patients under age 40 years and for healthy older patients; they are made euthyroid with a thiourea preoperatively and given several days of iodine, ipodate sodium, or iopanoic acid before surgery (see above). Postoperative hypothyroidism usually resolves spontaneously, but permanent hypothyroidism occurs in about 14% of patients by 6 years after surgery. **Radioiodine** (^{131}I) therapy may be offered to patients with a toxic solitary nodule who are over age 40 or in poor health. A pregnancy test should be obtained within 48 before therapy for any premenopausal woman. RAI should not be given to women with Graves disease within 3 months prior to a planned conception. If the patient has been receiving methimazole preparatory to ^{131}I, the TSH should be kept slightly suppressed in order to reduce the uptake of ^{131}I by the normal thyroid. Nevertheless, permanent hypothyroidism occurs in about one-third of patients by 8 years after ^{131}I therapy. The nodule remains palpable in 50% and may grow in 10% of patients after ^{131}I.

C. Treatment of Toxic Nodular Goiter

Medical therapy for patients with toxic nodular goiter consists of propranolol ER (while hyperthyroid) and a thiourea, as in Graves disease. Thioureas (methimazole or propylthiouracil) reverse hyperthyroidism but do not shrink the goiter. There is a 95% recurrence rate if the drug is stopped.

Surgery is the definitive treatment for patients with large toxic nodular goiter, following therapy with a thiourea to render them euthyroid. Surgery is particularly indicated to relieve pressure symptoms or for cosmetic indications. Patients with toxic nodular goiter are not treated preoperatively with potassium iodide. Total or near-total thyroidectomy is recommended, since surgical pathology reveals unsuspected differentiated thyroid cancer in 18.3% of cases.

Radioiodine (RAI, ^{131}I) therapy may be used to treat patients with toxic nodular goiter. RAI should not be given to women with a toxic multinodular goiter within 3 months prior to a planned conception. A pregnancy test should be obtained within 48 hours before therapy for any premenopausal woman. ^{131}I therapy is then administered within 2 days thereafter. Any suspicious nodules should be evaluated beforehand for malignancy with FNA cytology. Patients are rendered euthyroid with methimazole, which is stopped 3–4 days before a repeat RAI therapy.

Meanwhile, the patient follows a low-iodine diet in order to enhance the thyroid gland's uptake of RAI, which may be relatively low in this condition (compared to Graves disease). Relatively high doses of ^{131}I are usually required; hypothyroidism or recurrent thyrotoxicosis typically occurs, so patients must be monitored closely. Peculiarly, in about 5% of patients with diffusely nodular toxic goiter, the administration of ^{131}I therapy may induce Graves disease. Also, Graves eye disease has occurred rarely following ^{131}I therapy for multinodular goiter.

D. Treatment of Hyperthyroidism from Thyroiditis

Patients with thyroiditis (subacute, postpartum, or silent) are treated with propranolol during the hyperthyroid phase, which usually subsides spontaneously within weeks to months. For symptomatic relief, patients are treated with propranolol ER 60–80 mg twice daily and increased every 3 days until the heart rate is less than 90 beats per minute for symptomatic relief. Ipodate sodium or iopanoic acid, 500 mg orally daily, promptly corrects elevated T_3 levels and is continued for 15–60 days until the serum FT_4 level normalizes. Thioureas are ineffective, since thyroid hormone production is actually low in this condition. Patients are monitored carefully for the development of hypothyroidism and treated with levothyroxine as needed. With subacute thyroiditis, pain can usually be managed with nonsteroidal anti-inflammatory drugs and corticosteroids, but opioid analgesics are sometimes required.

E. Treatment of Hyperthyroidism during Pregnancy-Planning, Pregnancy, and Lactation

Both men and women with Graves disease who are planning pregnancy should not have RAI treatment within about 3 months of conception. Women with Graves disease who are planning to become pregnant are encouraged to consider definitive therapy with RAI or surgery well before conception. Dietary iodine must not be restricted for such women. There is an increased risk of fetal anomalies associated with methimazole in the first trimester. Therefore, women with Graves disease who are being treated with a thiourea should be treated with propylthiouracil through the first trimester and then switched to methimazole. Either thiourea should be given in the smallest dose possible, permitting mild subclinical hyperthyroidism to occur since it is usually well tolerated. About 30% of women with Graves disease experience a remission by the late second trimester.

Both propylthiouracil and methimazole cross the placenta and can induce hypothyroidism, with fetal TSH hypersecretion and goiter. Fetal ultrasound at 20–32 weeks gestation can visualize any fetal goiter, allowing fetal thyroid dysfunction to be diagnosed and treated. Thyroid hormone administration to the mother does not prevent hypothyroidism in the fetus, since T_4 and T_3 do not freely cross the placenta. Fetal hypothyroidism is rare if the mother's hyperthyroidism is controlled with small daily doses of propylthiouracil (50–150 mg/day orally) or methimazole (5–15 mg/day orally). Maternal serum TSI levels over 500% at term predict an increased risk of neonatal Graves disease in the infant.

Subtotal thyroidectomy is indicated for pregnant women with Graves disease under the following circumstances: (1) severe adverse reaction to thioureas; (2) high dosage requirement for thioureas (methimazole greater than or equal to 30 mg/day or propylthiouracil greater than or equal to 450 mg/day; (3) uncontrolled hyperthyroidism due to nonadherence to thiourea therapy. Surgery is best performed during the second trimester.

Both methimazole and propylthiouracil are secreted in breast milk, but not in amounts that affect the infant's thyroid hormone levels. No adverse reactions to these drugs (eg, rash, hepatic dysfunction, leukopenia) have been reported in breast-fed infants. Recommended doses are 20 mg orally daily or less for methimazole and 450 mg orally daily or less for propylthiouracil. It is recommended that the medication be taken just after breastfeeding.

F. Treatment of Amiodarone-Induced Thyrotoxicosis

Patients with any type of amiodarone-induced thyrotoxicosis require treatment with propranolol ER for symptomatic relief. Since it is difficult to accurately categorize patients as either type 1 or type 2 amiodarone-induced thyrotoxicosis, it is prudent to treat all patients with methimazole 30 mg orally daily. After two doses of methimazole, iopanoic acid or sodium ipodate may be added to the regimen to further block conversion of T_4 to T_3; the recommended dosage for each is 500 mg orally twice daily for 3 days, followed by 500 mg once daily until thyrotoxicosis is resolved. If iopanoic acid or sodium ipodate is not available, the alternative is potassium perchlorate; it is given in doses of less than or equal to 1000 mg daily (in divided doses) for a course not to exceed 30 days

in order to avoid the complication of aplastic anemia. Amiodarone may be withdrawn but this does not have a significant therapeutic impact for several months. For patients with type 1 amiodarone-induced thyrotoxicosis, therapy with ^{131}I may be successful, but only for those with sufficient RAI uptake. Patients with clear-cut type 2 amiodarone-induced thyrotoxicosis are usually also treated with prednisone at an initial dose of about 0.5–0.7 mg/kg orally daily; that dose of prednisone is continued for about 2 weeks and then slowly tapered and finally withdrawn after about 3 months. Subtotal thyroidectomy should be considered for patients with amiodarone-induced thyrotoxicosis that is resistant to treatment.

G. Treatment of Complications

1. Graves orbitopathy—The risk of having a "flare" of orbitopathy following ^{131}I treatment for hyperthyroidism is about 6% for nonsmokers and 23% for smokers. Graves orbitopathy can also be aggravated by thiazolidinediones (eg, pioglitazone, rosiglitazone); these oral diabetic agents should be avoided or withdrawn in patients with Graves disease. Patients with mild orbitopathy may be treated with selenium 100 mcg orally twice daily, which may slow its progression. For acute, progressive exophthalmos, intravenous methylprednisolone, begun promptly, is superior to oral prednisone, possibly due to improved compliance. Methylprednisolone is given in intravenous pulses, 500 mg weekly for 6 weeks, and then 250 mg weekly for 6 weeks. If oral prednisone is chosen for treatment, it must be given promptly in daily doses of 40–60 mg/day orally, with dosage reduction over several weeks. Higher initial prednisone doses of 80–120 mg/day are used when there is optic nerve compression. Prednisone alleviates acute eye symptoms in 64% of nonsmokers but in only 14% of smokers.

Patients with corticosteroid-resistant acute Graves orbitopathy may also be treated with rituximab. Rituximab may be given by retro-orbital injection, which limits systemic toxicity. The recommended dosing is rituximab 10 mg by retro-orbital injection into the affected eye weekly for 1 month, followed by a 1-month break, then another series of four weekly injections.

Progressive active exophthalmos may be treated with retrobulbar radiation therapy using a supervoltage linear accelerator (4–6 MeV) to deliver 20 Gy over 2 weeks to the extraocular muscles, avoiding the cornea and lens. Prednisone in high doses is given concurrently. Patients who respond well to orbital radiation include those with signs of acute inflammation, recent exophthalmos (less than 6 months), or optic nerve compression. Patients with chronic proptosis and orbital muscle restriction respond less well. Retrobulbar radiation does not cause cataracts or tumors; however, it can cause radiation-induced retinopathy (usually subclinical) in about 5% of patients overall, mostly in diabetics.

For severe cases, orbital decompression surgery may save vision, though diplopia often persists postoperatively. General eye protective measures include wearing glasses to protect the protruding eye and taping the lids shut during sleep if corneal drying is a problem. Methylcellulose drops and gels ("artificial tears") may also help. Tarsorrhaphy or canthoplasty can frequently help protect the cornea and provide improved appearance. Hypothyroidism and hyperthyroidism must be treated promptly.

2. Cardiac complications—

A. Sinus tachycardia—Treatment consists of treating the thyrotoxicosis. A beta-blocker such as propranolol is used in the interim unless there is an associated cardiomyopathy.

B. Atrial fibrillation—Hyperthyroidism must be treated immediately. Other drugs, including digoxin, beta-blockers, and anticoagulants, may be required. Electrical cardioversion is unlikely to convert atrial fibrillation to normal sinus rhythm while the patient is thyrotoxic. Spontaneous conversion to normal sinus rhythm occurs in 62% of patients with return of euthyroidism, but that likelihood decreases with age. Following conversion to euthyroidism, there is a 60% chance that atrial fibrillation will recur, despite normal thyroid function tests. Those with persistent atrial fibrillation may have elective cardioversion following anticoagulation 4 months after resolution of hyperthyroidism.

(1) Digoxin—Digoxin is used to slow a fast ventricular response to thyrotoxic atrial fibrillation; it must be used in larger than normal doses. Digoxin doses are reduced as hyperthyroidism is corrected.

(2) Beta-blockers—Beta-blockers may also reduce the ventricular rate, but they must be used with caution—particularly in patients with cardiomegaly or signs of heart failure—since their negative inotropic effect may precipitate overt heart failure. Therefore, an initial trial of a short-duration beta-blocker should be considered, such as esmolol intravenously. If a beta-blocker is used, doses of digoxin must be reduced.

(3) Anticoagulants—The doses of warfarin required in thyrotoxicosis are smaller than normal because of an accelerated plasma clearance of vitamin K–dependent clotting factors. Higher warfarin doses are usually required as hyperthyroidism subsides.

C. Heart failure—Thyrotoxicosis can cause heart failure due to extreme tachycardia, cardiomyopathy, or both. Very aggressive treatment of the hyperthyroidism is required in either case. The tachycardia from atrial fibrillation is treated with digoxin. If tachycardia appears to be the main cause of the patient's heart failure, beta-blockers are administered cautiously. Intravenous furosemide is typically required. Oral spironolactone or eplerenone may be helpful.

Heart failure may also occur as a result of low-output dilated cardiomyopathy. It is uncommon and may be caused by an idiosyncratic severe toxic effect of hyperthyroidism upon certain hearts. Cardiomyopathy may occur at any age and without preexisting cardiac disease. Emergency treatment may include afterload reduction, diuretics, digoxin, and other inotropic agents while the patient is being rendered euthyroid. However, the heart failure usually persists despite correction of the hyperthyroidism.

D. Apathetic hyperthyroidism—Apathetic hyperthyroidism may present with angina pectoris. Treatment is directed at reversing the hyperthyroidism as well as providing standard antianginal therapy. PCI or CABG can often be avoided by prompt diagnosis and treatment.

3. Thyroid crisis or "storm"—

This disorder, rarely seen today, is an extreme form of thyrotoxicosis that may be triggered by stressful illness, thyroid surgery, or RAI administration. Its manifestations often include marked delirium, severe tachycardia, vomiting, diarrhea, dehydration and very high fever. The mortality rate is high.

A thiourea drug is given (eg, methimazole, 15–25 mg orally every 6 hours or propylthiouracil, 150–250 mg orally every 6 hours). Ipodate sodium (500 mg/day orally) can be helpful if begun 1 hour after the first dose of thiourea. Iodide is given 1 hour later as potassium iodide (10 drops three times daily orally). Propranolol is given (cautiously in the presence of heart failure; see above) in a dosage of 0.5–2 mg intravenously every 4 hours or 20–120 mg orally every 6 hours. Hydrocortisone is usually given in doses of 50 mg orally every 6 hours, with rapid dosage reduction as the clinical situation improves. Aspirin is avoided since it displaces T_4 from thyroxine-binding globulin (TBG), raising FT_4 serum levels. Definitive treatment with ^{131}I or surgery is delayed until the patient is euthyroid.

4. Hyperthyroidism from postpartum thyroiditis—

Propranolol ER is given during the hyperthyroid phase followed by levothyroxine during the hypothyroidism phase.

5. Graves dermopathy—

Treatment involves application of a topical corticosteroid (eg, fluocinolone) with nocturnal plastic occlusive dressings. Compression stockings may improve any associated edema.

6. Thyrotoxic hypokalemic periodic paralysis—

Sudden symmetric flaccid paralysis, along with hypokalemia and hypophosphatemia can occur with hyperthyroidism despite few, if any, of the classic signs of thyrotoxicosis. It is most prevalent in Asian and Native Americans with hyperthyroidism and is 30 times more common in men than women. Therapy with oral propranolol, 3 mg/kg in divided doses, normalizes the serum potassium and phosphate levels and reverses the paralysis within 2–3 hours. No intravenous potassium or phosphate is ordinarily required. Intravenous dextrose and oral carbohydrate aggravate the condition and are to be avoided. Therapy is continued with propranolol, 60–80 mg orally every 8 hours (or sustained-action propranolol ER daily at equivalent daily dosage), along with a thiourea drug such as methimazole to treat the hyperthyroidism.

▶ Prognosis

Graves disease may rarely subside spontaneously, particularly when it is mild or subclinical. Graves disease that presents in early pregnancy has a 30% chance of spontaneous remission before the third trimester. The ocular, cardiac, and psychological complications can become serious and persistent even after treatment. Permanent hypoparathyroidism and vocal cord palsy are risks of surgical thyroidectomy. Recurrences are common following thiourea therapy but also occur after low-dose ^{131}I therapy or subtotal thyroidectomy. With adequate treatment and long-term follow-up, the results are usually good. However, despite treatment for their hyperthyroidism, women experience an increased long-term risk of death from thyroid disease, cardiovascular disease, stroke, and fracture of the femur. Posttreatment hypothyroidism is common. It may occur within a few months or up to several years after RAI therapy or subtotal thyroidectomy. Malignant exophthalmos has a poor prognosis unless treated aggressively.

Subclinical hyperthyroidism generally subsides spontaneously. Most patients do well without treatment. and the serum TSH usually reverts to normal within 2 years. Most such patients do not have accelerated bone loss. However, if a baseline bone density shows significant osteopenia, bone densitometry may be performed periodically. In persons over age 60 years, serum TSH is very low (less than 0.1 milli-units/L) in 3% and mildly low (0.1–0.4 milli-units/L) in 9%. The chance of developing atrial fibrillation is 2.8% yearly in elderly patients with very low TSH and 1.1% yearly in those with mildly low TSH. Asymptomatic persons with very low TSH are monitored closely but are not treated unless atrial fibrillation or other manifestations of hyperthyroidism develop.

▶ When to Admit

- Thyroid crisis.
- Hyperthyroidism-induced atrial fibrillation with severe tachycardia.
- Thyroidectomy.

Bahn RS et al. Hyperthyroidism and other causes of thyrotoxicosis: management guidelines of the American Thyroid Association and American Association of Clinical Endocrinologists. Thyroid. 2011 Jun;21(6):593–646. [PMID: 21510801]

Choong KC et al. Thyroid cancer in patients with toxic nodular goiter—is the incidence increasing? Am J Surg. 2015 Jun; 209(6):974–6. [PMID: 25896315]

De Groot L et al. Management of thyroid dysfunction during pregnancy and postpartum: an Endocrine Society clinical practice guideline. J Clin Endocrinol Metab. 2012 Aug; 97(8):2543–65. [PMID: 22869843]

Falhammar H et al. Thyrotoxic periodic paralysis: clinical and molecular aspects. Endocrine. 2013 Apr;43(2):274–84. [PMID: 22918841]

Pallais JC et al. Case records of the Massachusetts General Hospital. Case 38-2015. A 21-year-old man with fatigue and weight loss. N Engl J Med. 2015 Dec;373(24):2358–69. [PMID: 26650156]

Sundaresh V et al. Comparative effectiveness of therapies for Graves' hyperthyroidism: a systematic review and network meta-analysis. J Clin Endocrinol Metab. 2013 Sep;98(9):3671–7. [PMID: 23824415]

Zhu W et al. A prospective, randomized trial of intravenous glucocorticoids therapy with different protocols for patients with Graves' ophthalmopathy. J Clin Endocrinol Metab. 2014 Jun; 99(6):1999–2007. [PMID: 24606088]

THYROIDITIS

ESSENTIALS OF DIAGNOSIS

▶ **Acute and subacute forms:** thyroid gland swelling, sometimes causing pressure symptoms.

▶ **Chronic form:** thyroid gland may or may not be enlarged with rubbery firmness.

▶ Thyroid function tests variable.

▶ Serum antithyroperoxidase and antithyroglobulin antibody levels usually elevated in Hashimoto thyroiditis.

▶ General Considerations

Thyroiditis may be classified as follows: (1) Hashimoto thyroiditis (chronic lymphocytic thyroiditis due to autoimmunity), (2) subacute thyroiditis, (3) infectious (suppurative) thyroiditis, and (4) Riedel thyroiditis.

Hashimoto thyroiditis, an autoimmune condition, is the most common thyroid disorder in the United States. B-lymphocytes invade the thyroid gland, so the condition is also known as **chronic lymphocytic thyroiditis**. Elevated serum levels of antithyroid antibodies (antithyroperoxidase or antithyroglobulin antibodies, or both) are found in 3% of men and 13% of women. Women over the age of 60 years have a 25% incidence of elevated serum levels of antithyroid antibodies, yet only a small subset of such individuals ever develops thyroid dysfunction. However, 1% of the population has serum antithyroid antibody titers greater than 1:640 and they are at particular risk for thyroid dysfunction. The incidence of Hashimoto thyroiditis varies by kindred, race, and sex. It is commonly familial. In the United States, elevated levels of antithyroid antibodies are found in 14.3% of whites, 10.9% of Mexican-Americans, and 5.3% of blacks. Hashimoto thyroiditis is six times more common in women than in men.

Childhood or occupational exposure to head-neck external beam radiation increases the lifetime risk of Hashimoto thyroiditis. Women with gonadal dysgenesis (Turner syndrome) have a 15% incidence of thyroiditis by age 40 years. Thyroiditis is also commonly seen in patients with hepatitis C. Subclinical thyroiditis is extremely common; autopsy series have found focal thyroiditis in about 40% of women and 20% of men.

Dietary iodine supplementation (especially when excessive) increases the risk of Hashimoto thyroiditis. Certain drugs can trigger Hashimoto thyroiditis, including the following: tyrosine kinase inhibitors, denileukin diftitox, alemtuzumab, interferon-alpha, interleukin-2, ipilimumab, tremelimumab, thalidomide, lenalidomide, lithium, and amiodarone.

Hashimoto thyroiditis often progresses to hypothyroidism, which may be linked to thyrotropin receptor–blocking antibodies, detected in 10% of patients with Hashimoto thyroiditis. Hypothyroidism is more likely to develop in smokers than in nonsmokers, possibly due to the thiocyanates in cigarette smoke. High serum levels of thyroid peroxidase antibody also predict progression from subclinical to symptomatic hypothyroidism. Although the hypothyroidism is usually permanent, up to 11% of patients experience a remission after several years. Graves disease is often preceded by Hashimoto thyroiditis and most patients with Graves disease have concomitant antithyroid antibodies.

Hashimoto thyroiditis is sometimes associated with other endocrine deficiencies as part of polyglandular autoimmunity (PGA). Adults with type 2 PGA are prone to autoimmune thyroiditis, type 1 diabetes mellitus, autoimmune gonadal failure, hypoparathyroidism, and adrenal insufficiency. Thyroiditis is frequently associated with other autoimmune conditions: pernicious anemia, Sjögren syndrome, vitiligo, inflammatory bowel disease, celiac disease, and gluten sensitivity. It is less commonly associated with alopecia areata, hypophysitis, encephalitis, myocarditis, primary pulmonary hypertension, and membranous nephropathy.

Painless postpartum thyroiditis refers to autoimmune thyroiditis that occurs soon after delivery in 7.2% of women. Women in whom postpartum thyroiditis develops have a 70% chance of recurrence after subsequent pregnancies. It occurs most commonly in women who have high levels of thyroid peroxidase antibody in the first trimester of pregnancy or immediately after delivery. It is also more common in women with other autoimmunity or a family history of Hashimoto thyroiditis.

Painless sporadic thyroiditis is thought to be a subacute form of Hashimoto thyroiditis that is similar to painless postpartum thyroiditis, except that it is not related to pregnancy. It accounts for about 1% of cases of thyrotoxicosis.

Subacute thyroiditis—also called de Quervain thyroiditis, granulomatous thyroiditis, and giant cell thyroiditis—is relatively common. It is believed to be caused by a viral infection and often follows an upper respiratory tract infection. Its incidence peaks in the summer. It accounts for up to 5% of clinical thyroid disease and young and middle-aged women are most commonly affected.

Infectious (suppurative) thyroiditis refers to a nonviral infection of the thyroid gland. Infectious thyroiditis is quite rare among nonimmunosuppressed patients, since the thyroid is quite resistant to infection, due to its vasculature, encapsulation, and high iodine content. Congenital pyriform sinus fistulas are a cause for recurrent infectious thyroiditis. While infectious thyroiditis is usually bacterial, mycobacterial, fungal, and parasitic infections can occur, particularly in immunosuppressed individuals. In affected patients who are appropriately treated, when immunosuppression is reduced, the patient may experience an immune reconstitution inflammatory response (IRIS) from residual antigens triggering the normal immune response.

Riedel thyroiditis, also called invasive fibrous thyroiditis, Riedel struma, woody thyroiditis, ligneous thyroiditis, and invasive thyroiditis, is the rarest form of thyroiditis. It is found most frequently in middle-aged or elderly women and is usually part of a multifocal systemic fibrosis syndrome. It may occur as a thyroid manifestation of IgG$_4$-related systemic disease.

► Clinical Findings

A. Symptoms and Signs

In **Hashimoto thyroiditis,** the thyroid gland is usually diffusely enlarged, firm, and finely nodular. One thyroid lobe may be asymmetrically enlarged, raising concerns about neoplasm. Although patients may complain of neck tightness, pain and tenderness are not usually present. About 10% of cases are atrophic, the gland being fibrotic, particularly in elderly women.

Symptoms and signs are mostly related to ambient levels of thyroid hormone. However, depression and chronic fatigue are more common in such patients, even after correction of hypothyroidism. About one-third of patients have mild dry mouth (xerostomia) or dry eyes (keratoconjunctivitis sicca) related to Sjögren syndrome. Associated myasthenia gravis is usually of mild severity, mainly affecting the extraocular muscles and having a relatively low incidence of detectable AChR Ab or thymic disease. Associated celiac disease can produce fatigue or depression, often in the absence of gastrointestinal symptoms.

Postpartum thyroiditis is typically manifested by hyperthyroidism that begins 1–6 months after delivery and persists for only 1–2 months. Then, hypothyroidism tends to develop beginning 4–8 months after delivery.

Thyrotoxic symptoms in **painless sporadic thyroiditis** are usually mild; a small, nontender goiter may be palpated in about 50% of such patients. High serum thyroid peroxidase antibody concentrations are found in only 50%. The course is similar to painless postpartum thyroiditis.

Subacute thyroiditis presents with an acute, usually painful enlargement of the thyroid gland, often with dysphagia. The pain may radiate to the ears. Patients usually have a low-grade fever and fatigue. The manifestations may persist for weeks or months and may be associated with malaise. If there is no pain, it is called **silent thyroiditis.** Thyrotoxicosis develops in 50% of affected patients and tends to last for several weeks. Subsequently, hypothyroidism develops that lasts 4–6 months. Normal thyroid function typically returns within 12 months, but persistent hypothyroidism develops in 5% of patients.

Patients with **infectious thyroiditis** usually are febrile and have severe pain, tenderness, redness, and fluctuation in the region of the thyroid gland. In **Riedel thyroiditis,** thyroid enlargement is often asymmetric; the gland is stony hard and adherent to the neck structures, causing signs of compression and invasion, including dysphagia, dyspnea, pain, and hoarseness. Related conditions include retroperitoneal fibrosis, fibrosing mediastinitis, sclerosing cervicitis, subretinal fibrosis, and sclerosing cholangitis.

B. Laboratory Findings

In Hashimoto thyroiditis with clinically evident disease, there are usually increased circulating levels of antithyroid peroxidase (90%) or antithyroglobulin (40%) antibodies. However, some patients with autoimmune thyroiditis have no detectable antithyroid antibodies. Antithyroid antibodies decline during pregnancy and are often undetectable in the third trimester. Once

Hashimoto thyroiditis has been diagnosed, monitoring of these antibody levels is not helpful. The serum TSH level is elevated if thyroid hormone is not elaborated in adequate amounts by the thyroid gland.

Patients with Hashimoto thyroiditis have a 15% incidence of having serum antibodies (IgA tissue transglutaminase [tTG] antibody) associated with celiac disease and at least 5% have clinically significant celiac disease. Seronegative gluten sensitivity is even more common.

In subacute thyroiditis, the ESR is markedly elevated while antithyroid antibody titers are low, distinguishing it from autoimmune thyroiditis. In **infectious (suppurative) thyroiditis,** both the leukocyte count and ESR are usually elevated.

With hyperthyroidism due to Hashimoto thyroiditis or subacute thyroiditis, serum FT_4 levels tend to be proportionally higher than T_3 levels, since the hyperthyroidism is due to the passive release of stored thyroid hormone, which is predominantly T_4; this is in contrast to Graves disease and toxic nodular goiter, where T_3 is relatively more elevated. Because T_4 is less active than T_3, the hyperthyroidism seen in thyroiditis is usually less severe. Serum levels of TSH are suppressed in hyperthyroidism due to thyroiditis.

C. Imaging

Ultrasound in cases of Hashimoto thyroiditis typically shows a gland with characteristic diffuse heterogeneous density and hypoechogenicity. It helps distinguish thyroiditis from multinodular goiter or thyroid nodules that are suspicious for malignancy. It is also helpful in guiding FNA biopsy of small suspicious thyroid nodules. Color-flow Doppler ultrasonography can help distinguish thyroiditis from Graves disease, since patients with Graves disease have a hypervascular thyroid gland, whereas in thyroiditis there is normal or reduced vascularity.

RAI uptake and scan may be helpful in determining the cause of hyperthyroidism, distinguishing thyroiditis from Graves disease, since patients with subacute thyroiditis exhibit a very low RAI uptake. However, in patients with chronic Hashimoto thyroiditis (euthyroid or hypothyroid), RAI uptake may be normal or high with uneven uptake on the scan; scanning is not useful in diagnosis.

[18F] Fluorodeoxyglucose positron emission tomography (18FDG-PET) scanning frequently shows diffuse thyroid uptake of isotope in cases of thyroiditis. In fact, of all 18FDG-PET scans, about 3% show such uptake. However, discrete thyroid nodules can also be discovered on 18FDG-PET scanning; known as "thyroid PET incidentalomas," 50% are malignant.

D. Fine-Needle Aspiration Biopsy

Patients with **Hashimoto thyroiditis** who have a thyroid nodule should have an ultrasound-guided FNA biopsy, since the risk of papillary thyroid cancer is about 8% in such nodules. When **infectious (suppurative) thyroiditis** is suspected, an FNA biopsy with Gram stain and culture is required. FNA biopsy is usually not required for subacute thyroiditis but shows characteristic giant multinucleated cells.

► Complications

Hashimoto thyroiditis may lead to hypothyroidism or transient thyrotoxicosis. Hyperthyroidism may develop, either due to the emergence of Graves disease or due to the release of stored thyroid hormone, which is caused by inflammation. Variably termed "hashitoxicosis" or "painless sporadic thyroiditis," it is known as postpartum painless thyroiditis when it occurs in women after delivery. Pregnant women with Hashimoto thyroiditis have an increased risk of spontaneous miscarriage in the first trimester of pregnancy. Perimenopausal women with high serum levels of antithyroperoxidase antibodies have a higher relative risk of depression, independent of ambient thyroid hormone levels.

In the suppurative forms of thyroiditis, any of the complications of infection may occur. Subacute and chronic thyroiditis are complicated by the effects of pressure on the neck structures: dyspnea and, in Riedel struma, vocal cord palsy. Papillary thyroid carcinoma or thyroid lymphoma may rarely be associated with chronic thyroiditis and must be considered in the diagnosis of uneven painless enlargements that continue despite treatment; such patients require FNA biopsy.

► Differential Diagnosis

Thyroiditis must be considered in the differential diagnosis of all types of goiters, especially if enlargement is rapid. The very low RAI uptake in subacute thyroiditis with elevated T_4 and T_3 is helpful. Thyroid autoantibody tests have been of help in the diagnosis of Hashimoto thyroiditis, but the tests are not specific (positive in patients with multinodular goiters, malignancy [eg, thyroid carcinoma, lymphoma], and concurrent Graves disease). The subacute and suppurative forms of thyroiditis may resemble any infectious process in or near the neck structures. Chronic thyroiditis, especially if the enlargement is uneven and if there is pressure on surrounding structures, may resemble thyroid carcinoma, and both disorders may be present in the same gland.

► Treatment

A. Hashimoto Thyroiditis

If hypothyroidism is present, levothyroxine should be given in the usual replacement doses (0.05–0.2 mg orally daily). In patients with a large goiter and normal or elevated serum TSH, an attempt is made to shrink the goiter by administering levothyroxine in doses sufficient to drive the serum TSH below the reference range while maintaining clinical euthyroidism. Suppressive doses of T_4 tend to shrink the goiter an average of 30% over 6 months. If the goiter does not regress, lower replacement doses of levothyroxine may be given. If the thyroid gland is only minimally enlarged and the patient is euthyroid, regular observation is in order, since hypothyroidism may develop subsequently—often years later.

B. Subacute Thyroiditis

All treatment is empiric and must be continued for several weeks. Recurrence is common. The drug of choice is aspirin, which relieves pain and inflammation. Thyrotoxic symptoms are treated with propranolol, 10–40 mg every 6 hours. Iodinated contrast agents cause a prompt fall in serum T_3 levels and a dramatic improvement in thyrotoxic symptoms. Sodium ipodate (Oragrafin, Bilivist) or iopanoic acid (Telepaque) is given orally in doses of 500 mg orally daily until serum FT_4 levels return to normal. Transient hypothyroidism is treated with T_4 (0.05–0.1 mg orally daily) if symptomatic.

C. Suppurative Thyroiditis

Treatment is with antibiotics and with surgical drainage when fluctuation is marked. Immunocompromised individuals are particularly at risk and coccidioidomycosis thyroiditis has been reported. Surgical thyroidectomy may be required.

D. Riedel Struma

The treatment of choice is tamoxifen, 20 mg orally twice daily, which must be continued for years. Tamoxifen can induce partial to complete remissions in most patients within 3–6 months. Its mode of action appears to be unrelated to its antiestrogen activity. Short-term corticosteroid treatment may be added for partial alleviation of pain and compression symptoms. Surgical decompression usually fails to permanently alleviate compression symptoms; such surgery is difficult due to dense fibrous adhesions, making surgical complications more likely. Rituximab may be useful for Riedel thyroiditis that is refractory to tamoxifen and corticosteroids.

▶ Prognosis

Hashimoto thyroiditis is occasionally associated with other autoimmune disorders (celiac disease, diabetes mellitus, Addison disease, pernicious anemia, etc). In general, however, patients with Hashimoto thyroiditis have an excellent prognosis, since the condition either remains stable for years or progresses slowly to hypothyroidism, which is easily treated. Although 80% of women with postpartum thyroiditis subsequently recover normal thyroid function, permanent hypothyroidism eventually develops in about 50% within 7 years, more commonly in women who are multiparous or who have had a spontaneous abortion. In subacute thyroiditis, spontaneous remissions and exacerbations are common; the disease process may smolder for months. Papillary thyroid carcinoma carries a relatively good prognosis when it occurs in patients with Hashimoto thyroiditis.

Luo Y et al. Iodine excess as an environmental risk factor for autoimmune thyroid disease. Int J Mol Sci. 2014 Jul 21; 15(7):12895–912. [PMID: 25050783]

Samuels MH. Subacute, silent, and postpartum thyroiditis. Med Clin North Am. 2012 Mar;96(2):223–33. [PMID: 22443972]

Stagnaro-Green A. Approach to the patient with postpartum thyroiditis. J Clin Endocrinol Metab. 2012 Feb;97(2):334–42. [PMID: 22312089]

THYROID NODULES & MULTINODULAR GOITER

ESSENTIALS OF DIAGNOSIS

▶ Single or multiple thyroid nodules are commonly found with careful thyroid examinations.

▶ Thyroid function tests mandatory.

▶ Thyroid biopsy for single or dominant nodules or for a history of prior head–neck or chest–shoulder radiation.

▶ Ultrasound examination useful for biopsy and follow-up.

▶ Clinical follow-up required.

▶ General Considerations

Thyroid nodules are extremely common. Palpable nodules occur in 4–7% of all adults in the United States. They are much more common in women than men and become more prevalent with age. About 90% of palpable thyroid nodules are benign adenomas, colloid nodules, or cysts, but some are primary thyroid malignancies or (less frequently) metastatic malignancy. In recent years, an increased general use of scanning has led to an increased rate of incidentally detecting nonpalpable thyroid nodules. The detection rate for thyroid nodules on ultrasound is about 30%; of these, 20% are larger than 1 cm in diameter. Thyroid nodules are even more common in iodine-deficient regions. Thyroid nodules 1 cm or larger in diameter warrant follow-up and further testing for function and malignancy. An occasional nodule smaller than 1 cm in diameter requires follow-up if it has high-risk characteristics on ultrasound or if the patient is at high-risk for thyroid cancer due to prior head-neck radiation therapy during childhood. Thyroid nodules that are incidentally discovered with increased standard uptake value (SUV) on ^{18}FDG-PET scanning have a 33% risk for being malignant and definitely require FNA cytology.

Most patients with a thyroid nodule are euthyroid, but there is a high incidence of hypothyroidism or hyperthyroidism. Patients with multiple thyroid nodules have the same overall risk of thyroid cancer as patients with solitary nodules. The risk of a thyroid nodule being malignant is higher in males and among patients with a history of head-neck radiation, total body radiation for bone marrow transplantation, exposure to radioactive fallout as a child or teen, a family history of thyroid cancer or a thyroid cancer syndrome (eg, Cowden syndrome, multiple endocrine neoplasia type 2, familial polyposis, Carney syndrome), or a personal history of another malignancy. The risk of malignancy is also higher if there is hoarseness or vocal fold paralysis, adherence to the trachea or strap muscles, cervical lymphadenopathy. The malignancy risk is also higher for thyroid nodules that are solitary or 4.5 cm or larger in diameter. The presence of Hashimoto thyroiditis does not reduce the risk of malignancy; a nodule of 1 cm or larger in a gland with thyroiditis carries an 8% chance of malignancy.

Table 26–6. Clinical evaluation of thyroid nodules.[1]

Clinical Evidence	Low Index of Suspicion	High Index of Suspicion
History	Family history of goiter; residence in area of endemic goiter	Previous therapeutic radiation of head, neck, or chest; hoarseness
Physical characteristics	Older women; soft nodule; multinodular goiter	Young adults, men; solitary, firm nodule; vocal cord paralysis; enlarged lymph nodes; distant metastatic lesions
Serum factors	High titer of antithyroperoxidase antibody; hypothyroidism; hyperthyroidism	Elevated serum calcitonin
Fine-needle aspiration biopsy	Colloid nodule or adenoma	Papillary carcinoma, follicular lesion, medullary or anaplastic carcinoma
Scanning techniques		
Uptake of ^{123}I	Hot nodule	Cold nodule
Ultrasonogram	Cystic lesion	Solid lesion
Roentgenogram	Shell-like calcification	Punctate calcification
Response to thyroxine therapy	Regression after 0.05–0.1 mg/day for 6 months or more	Increase in size

[1]Clinically suspicious nodules should be evaluated with fine-needle aspiration biopsy.

▶ Clinical Findings

Table 26–6 illustrates the approach to the evaluation of thyroid nodules based on the index of suspicion for malignancy.

A. Symptoms and Signs

Most small thyroid nodules cause no symptoms. They may sometimes be detected only by having the patient swallow during careful inspection and palpation of the thyroid.

A thyroid nodule or multinodular goiter can grow to become visible and of concern to the patient. Particularly large nodular goiters can become a cosmetic embarrassment. Nodules can grow large enough to cause discomfort, hoarseness, or dysphagia. Nodules that cause ipsilateral recurrent laryngeal nerve palsy are more likely to be malignant. Retrosternal large multinodular goiters can cause dyspnea due to tracheal compression. Large substernal goiters may cause superior vena cava syndrome, manifested by facial erythema and jugular vein distention that progress to cyanosis and facial edema when both arms are kept raised over the head.

Depending on their cause, goiters and thyroid nodules may be associated with hypothyroidism (Hashimoto thyroiditis, endemic goiter) or hyperthyroidism (Graves disease, toxic nodular goiter, subacute thyroiditis, and thyroid cancer with metastases).

B. Laboratory Findings

A serum TSH level should be obtained for all patients with a thyroid nodule. Patients with a subnormal serum TSH must have a radionuclide (^{123}I or ^{99m}Tc pertechnetate) thyroid scan to determine whether the nodule is hyperfunctioning; hyperfunctioning nodules are rarely malignant. Very high levels of antithyroperoxidase antibodies and antithyroglobulin

antibodies are found in Hashimoto thyroiditis. However, thyroiditis frequently coexists with malignancy, so suspicious nodules should always be biopsied. Serum calcitonin is obtained if a medullary thyroid carcinoma is suspected in a patient with a family history of medullary thyroid carcinoma or MEN types 2 or 3.

C. Imaging

Neck ultrasonography should be performed to measure the size of a nodule and to determine its characteristics and whether a palpable nodule is part of a multinodular goiter. The following ultrasound characteristics of thyroid nodules increase the likelihood of malignancy: irregular or indistinct margins, heterogenous nodule echogenicity, intranodular vascular images, microcalcifications, complex cyst, being taller than wider, or diameter over 1 cm. Nodules that appear spongiform or cystic are more likely benign. Ultrasonography is generally preferred over CT and MRI. CT scanning is helpful for larger thyroid nodules and multinodular goiter; it can determine the degree of tracheal compression and the degree of extension into the mediastinum.

RAI (^{123}I or ^{131}I) scans are not helpful for assessing whether a thyroid nodule is benign or malignant. Hyperfunctioning (hot) nodules are ordinarily benign (but may sometimes be malignant). RAI uptake and scanning is helpful mainly for assessing patients who are hyperthyroid.

D. Incidentally Discovered Thyroid Nodules

Thyroid nodules are frequently discovered as an incidental finding, with an incidence that depends on the imaging modality: MRI, 50%; CT, 13%; and ^{18}FDG-PET, 2%. When such scanning detects a thyroid nodule, an ultrasound is performed to better determine the nodule's risk for malignancy and the need for FNA biopsy, and to establish a baseline for ultrasound follow-up. The malignancy risk is about 17% for nodules discovered incidentally on CT or MRI, and 25–50% for nodules discovered incidentally by ^{18}FDG-PET. For incidentally discovered thyroid nodules of borderline concern, follow-up thyroid ultrasound in 3–6 months may be helpful; growing lesions should be biopsied or resected.

E. Fine-Needle Aspiration of Thyroid Nodules

FNA is the best method to assess a thyroid nodule for malignancy. FNA can be done while patients continue taking anticoagulants or aspirin. For multinodular goiters, the four largest nodules (1 cm or larger in diameter) are usually biopsied to minimize the risk of missing a malignancy. For solitary thyroid nodules, FNA is indicated for: (1) nodules larger than 0.5 cm diameter with a suspicious appearance on ultrasound; (2) nodules associated with abnormal cervical lymph nodes; (3) nodules 1 cm diameter or larger that are solid or have microcalcifications; (4) mixed cystic-solid nodules 1.5 cm diameter or larger with any suspicious features on ultrasound or 2 cm diameter or larger with benign features on ultrasound; (5) spongiform nodules 2 cm diameter or larger. Pure cystic nodules are benign and do not require FNA biopsy. Using ultrasound guidance for FNA biopsy improves the diagnostic accuracy for both palpable and nonpalpable thyroid nodules. FNA cytology is typically reported using the Bethesda system, which divides results into six categories:

1. **Nondiagnostic or unsatisfactory:** The malignancy risk is 1–4%. The usual management is a repeat FNA under ultrasound guidance.
2. **Benign:** The malignancy risk is about 2.5%. The usual management is clinical follow-up with palpation or ultrasound at 6–18 month intervals.
3. **Atypia of undetermined significance (AUS):** The malignancy risk is about 14%%, higher with sonographic features of malignancy. The usual management is clinical correlation and a repeat FNA.
4. **Suspicious for follicular neoplasm (SFN) or follicular neoplasm (FN):** The malignancy risk is about 25%, higher when Hürthle cells are present and in patients over age 50. The usual management is either gene mutation analysis of the specimen *or* direct surgical lobectomy.
5. **Suspicious for malignancy (SFM):** The malignancy risk is about 70%. The usual management is either gene mutation analysis of the specimen *or* direct thyroid lobectomy or near-total thyroidectomy.
6. **Malignant:** The malignancy risk is about 99%. The usual management is a near-total thyroidectomy.

For FNA samples with Bethesda system cytopathology classified as FN or SFM the diagnostic accuracy can be improved with the use of molecular analysis. One molecular method is to analyze the residual FNA material using a gene-expression classifier, which examines messenger RNA. Another molecular approach is to assess for genetic abnormalities associated with thyroid cancer. *BRAF* or *RAS* mutations, *RET/PTC* translocations, PIK3A mutations,

and *PAX8-PPARγ* translocations are associated with follicular thyroid cancer and *TERT* promoter mutations are associated with papillary thyroid cancer. If a sample is positive for a *RAS* mutation, the chance of malignancy is about 85%. If the sample is positive for a *BRAF* mutation, the chance of malignancy is nearly 100%.

▶ Treatment

All thyroid nodules, including those that are benign, need to be monitored by regular periodic palpation and ultrasound about every 6 months initially. After several years of stability, yearly examinations are sufficient. Thyroid nodules should be rebiopsied if growth occurs. A toxic multinodular goiter and hyperthyroidism may develop in patients who have had exposure to large amounts of iodine, either orally (eg, amiodarone) or intravenously (eg, radiographic contrast). Therefore, excessive iodine intake should be minimized. Patients found to have hyperthyroidism may have a RAI uptake and scan, especially if ^{131}I is a therapeutic consideration. Patients with toxic multinodular goiters may also be treated with methimazole, propranolol, or surgery.

A. Levothyroxine Suppression Therapy

Patients with elevated levels of serum TSH are treated with levothyroxine replacement. Patients with nodules larger than 2 cm and elevated or normal TSH levels may be considered for TSH suppression with levothyroxine (starting doses of 50 mcg orally daily). Levothyroxine suppression therapy is not recommended for small benign thyroid nodules. Thyroxine suppression therapy is more successful in iodine-deficient areas of the world. Long-term levothyroxine suppression of TSH tends to keep nodules from enlarging but only 20% shrink more than 50%. Thyroid nodule size increased in 29% of patients treated with levothyroxine versus 56% of patients not receiving levothyroxine. Levothyroxine suppression also reduces the emergence of new nodules: 8% with levothyroxine and 29% without levothyroxine. Levothyroxine suppression therapy is not usually given to patients with coronary heart disease, since it increases the risk for angina and atrial fibrillation. Levothyroxine suppression causes a small loss of bone density, particularly in postmenopausal women if the serum TSH is suppressed to less than 0.05 milli-units/L. Such patients are advised to have bone density testing every 3–5 years. For patients with a low baseline TSH level, levothyroxine should not be administered, since that is an indication of autonomous thyroid secretion; levothyroxine will be ineffective and could cause thyrotoxicosis.

Levothyroxine suppression needs to be carefully monitored, since it carries a 17% risk of inducing hyperthyroidism. All patients receiving levothyroxine suppression therapy should have serum TSH levels monitored at least annually, with the levothyroxine dose adjusted to keep the serum TSH mildly suppressed (between 0.1 milli-units/L and 0.8 milli-units/L).

B. Surgery

Total thyroidectomy is required for thyroid nodules that are malignant on FNA biopsy. More limited thyroid surgery is indicated for benign nodules with indeterminate or suspicious cytologic test results, compression symptoms, discomfort, or cosmetic embarrassment. Surgery may also be used to remove hyperfunctioning "hot" thyroid adenomas or toxic multinodular goiter causing hyperthyroidism.

C. Percutaneous Ethanol Injection

Percutaneous ethanol injection can shrink pure cysts; the success rate is 80%, although it must often be repeated. Percutaneous ethanol injection can also be used to shrink biopsy-proven benign nodules. While complications occur in about 9%, serious or permanent complications are rare. Thyroid cysts can be aspirated, but cystic fluid recurs in 75% of patients.

D. Radioiodine (^{131}I) Therapy

Radioactive ^{131}I is a treatment option for hyperthyroid patients with toxic thyroid adenomas, multinodular goiter, or Graves disease. Therapy with ^{131}I shrinks benign nontoxic thyroid nodules by an average of 40% by 1 year and 59% by 2 years after ^{131}I therapy. Nodules that shrink after ^{131}I therapy generally remain palpable and become firmer; they may develop unusual cytologic characteristics on FNA biopsy. ^{131}I therapy may be used to shrink large multinodular goiter but may rarely induce Graves disease. Hypothyroidism is a risk and may occur years after ^{131}I therapy, so it is advisable to assess thyroid function every 3 months for the first year, every 6 months thereafter, and immediately for symptoms of hypothyroidism or hyperthyroidism.

▶ Prognosis

Benign thyroid nodules may involute but usually persist or grow slowly. About 90% of thyroid nodules will increase their volume by 15% or more over 5 years; about 11% of nodules increase their volume by more than 50% on follow-up. Growth is more common with multinodular goiter and larger nodules and in males; nodules are less likely to grow when they are solitary or cystic and when patients are over age 60. Multinodular goiters tend to persist or grow slowly. Cytologically benign nodules that grow are unlikely to be malignant; in one series, only 1 of 78 rebiopsied nodules was found to be malignant. The prognosis for patients with thyroid nodules that prove to be malignant is determined by the histologic type and other factors. Iodine supplementation in iodine-deficient areas does not usually shrink established goiters. Patients with very small (less than 1 cm diameter), incidentally discovered, nonpalpable thyroid nodules that have a benign ultrasound appearance require no FNA cytology and only yearly palpation and clinical follow-up, whereas such small nodules that have a slightly suspicious ultrasound appearance may require FNA cytology or thyroid ultrasound every 1–2 years. Such nodules, if malignant and excised, have a minimal effect upon morbidity and mortality.

Brito JP et al. The accuracy of thyroid nodule ultrasound to predict thyroid cancer: systematic review and meta-analysis. J Clin Endocrinol Metab. 2014 Apr;99(4):1253–63. [PMID: 24276450]

Burman KD et al. Clinical practice. Thyroid nodules. N Engl J Med. 2015 Dec 10;373(24):2347–56. [PMID: 26650154]
Durante C et al. The natural history of benign thyroid nodules. JAMA. 2015 Mar;313(9):926–35. [PMID: 25734734]
Renshaw AA et al. Reducing indeterminate thyroid FNAs. Cancer Cytopathol. 2015 Apr;123(4):237–43. [PMID: 25644425]
Straccia P et al. A meta-analytic review of the Bethesda System for Reporting Thyroid Cytopathology: has the rate of malignancy in indeterminate lesions been underestimated? Cancer Cytopathol. 2015 Dec;123(12):713–22. [PMID: 26355876]

THYROID CANCER

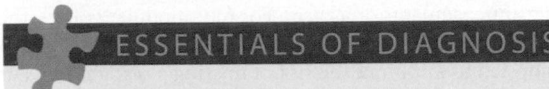

ESSENTIALS OF DIAGNOSIS

▶ Painless swelling in region of thyroid.

▶ Thyroid function tests usually normal.

▶ Past history of irradiation to head and neck region may be present.

▶ Positive thyroid FNA biopsy.

▶ General Considerations

The incidence of differentiated (papillary and follicular) thyroid carcinomas increases with age. The overall female:male ratio is 3:1. The yearly incidence of thyroid cancer has been increasing in the United States, with the number of cases diagnosed annually reaching 37,200, probably as a result of the wider use of ultrasound, CT, MRI, and PET that incidentally find small thyroid malignancies. Thyroid cancer mortality has been stable, accounting for about 1500 deaths in the United States annually. In routine autopsy series, thyroid microcarcinoma (10 mm diameter or smaller) is found with the surprising frequency of 35%. Clearly, most thyroid cancers remain microscopic and indolent. However, larger thyroid cancers (palpable or greater than or equal to 1 cm in diameter) are more malignant and require treatment.

Papillary thyroid carcinoma is the most common thyroid malignancy (Table 26–7). Pure papillary (and mixed papillary-follicular) carcinoma comprises about 80% of all thyroid cancers. It usually presents as a single thyroid nodule, but it can arise out of a multinodular goiter. Papillary thyroid carcinoma is commonly multifocal within the gland, with other foci usually arising de novo rather than representing intraglandular metastases. Papillary thyroid carcinoma is generally the least aggressive thyroid malignancy. It tends to grow slowly and often remains confined to the thyroid and regional lymph nodes for years. However, it may become more aggressive, especially in patients over age 45 years, and most particularly in the elderly. The cancer may invade the trachea and local muscles and may spread to the lungs.

Exposure to head and neck radiation therapy poses a particular threat to children who then have an increased lifetime risk of developing thyroid cancer, including papillary carcinoma. These cancers may emerge between 10 and 40 years after exposure, with a peak occurrence

Table 26–7. Some characteristics of thyroid cancer.

	Papillary	Follicular	Medullary	Anaplastic
Incidence	Most common	Common	Uncommon	Uncommon
Average age	42	50	50	57
Females	70%	72%	56%	56%
Invasion				
Juxtanodal	+++++	+	++++++	+++
Blood vessels	+	+++	+++	+++++
Distant sites	+	+++	++	++++
^{123}I uptake	+	++++	0	0
10-year disease-specific survival	97%	92%	78%	7.3%

20–25 years later. After an explosion at the Chernobyl Nuclear Power Plant in Ukraine in 1986, the risk of developing papillary thyroid carcinoma was highest among children who were under age 5 at the time of exposure to radiation; emergence of more aggressive papillary thyroid carcinoma occurred within 6–7 years after exposure.

Papillary thyroid carcinoma can occur in familial syndromes as an autosomal dominant trait, caused by loss of various tumor suppressor genes. Such syndromes (with associated features) include familial papillary carcinoma (with papillary renal carcinoma), familial nonmedullary thyroid carcinoma, familial polyposis (with large intestine polyps and gastrointestinal tumors), Gardner syndrome (with small and large intestine polyps, fibromas, lipomas, osteomas), Turcot syndrome (with large intestine polyps and brain tumors), and Cowden syndrome (with nodular goiter, benign or malignant breast lesions, macrocephaly, mental retardation, mucocutaneous lesions, benign or malignant uterine neoplasms, or gastrointestinal hamartomas or ganglioneuromas).

Papillary carcinoma is the least aggressive thyroid malignancy. However, the tumor involves both lobes in 30% of patients and in about 80% of patients there are microscopic metastases to cervical lymph nodes. Occult metastases to the lung occur in 10–15% of papillary thyroid cancer.

Microscopic "micropapillary" carcinoma (1 mm or smaller and invisible on thyroid ultrasound) is a variant of normal, being found in 24% of thyroidectomies performed for benign thyroid disease when 2-mm sections were carefully examined. Thus, the overwhelming majority of these microscopic foci never become clinically significant. The surgical pathology report of such a tiny papillary carcinoma does not justify aggressive measures. All that may be required is yearly follow-up with palpation of the neck and mild TSH suppression by thyroxine.

Follicular thyroid carcinoma and its variants (eg, Hürthle cell carcinoma) account for about 14% of thyroid malignancies; follicular carcinomas are generally more aggressive than papillary carcinomas. Rarely, some follicular carcinomas secrete enough T_4 to cause thyrotoxicosis.

Metastases commonly are found in neck nodes, bones, and lungs. Most follicular thyroid carcinomas avidly absorb iodine, making possible diagnostic scanning and treatment with ^{131}I after total thyroidectomy. The follicular histopathologic features that are associated with a high risk of metastasis and recurrence are poorly differentiated and Hürthle cell (oncocytic) variants. The latter variants do not take up RAI.

Medullary thyroid carcinoma represents 2–3% of thyroid cancers. About one-third of cases are sporadic, one-third are familial, and one-third are associated with MEN type 2A or 2B. Medullary thyroid carcinoma is often caused by an activating mutation of the *ret* protooncogene on chromosome 10. Mutation analysis of the *ret* protooncogene exons 10, 11, 13, and 14 detects 95% of the mutations causing MEN 2A and 90% of the mutations causing familial medullary thyroid carcinoma. Patients with MEN 2B have activating mutations in exon 16 of the *ret* protooncogene. These germline mutations can be detected by DNA analysis of peripheral WBCs. Therefore, discovery of a medullary thyroid carcinoma makes genetic analysis mandatory. If a gene defect is discovered, related family members must have genetic screening for that specific gene defect. When a family member with MEN 2 or 3 or familial medullary thyroid carcinoma does not have an identifiable *ret* protooncogene mutation, gene carriers may still be identified using family linkage analysis. Even when no gene defect is detectable, family members should have thyroid surveillance every 6 months. Medullary thyroid carcinoma arises from thyroid parafollicular cells that can secrete calcitonin, prostaglandins, serotonin, ACTH, corticotropin-releasing hormone (CRH), and other peptides. These peptides can cause symptoms and can be used as tumor markers.

Anaplastic thyroid carcinoma represents about 2% of thyroid cancers. It usually presents in an older patient as a rapidly enlarging mass in a multinodular goiter. It is the most aggressive thyroid carcinoma and metastasizes early to surrounding nodes and distant sites. Local pressure symptoms include dysphagia or vocal cord paralysis. This tumor does not concentrate iodine.

Other thyroid malignancies together represent about 3% of thyroid cancers. **Lymphoma** of the thyroid is more common in older women. Thyroid lymphomas are most commonly B cell lymphomas (50%) or mucosa-associated lymphoid tissue (MALT; 23%); other types include follicular, small lymphocytic, and Burkitt lymphoma and Hodgkin disease. Thyroidectomy is rarely required. **Other cancers** may sometimes metastasize to the thyroid, particularly bronchogenic, breast, and renal carcinomas and malignant melanoma.

▶ **Clinical Findings**

A. Symptoms and Signs

Thyroid carcinoma usually presents as a palpable, firm, nontender nodule in the thyroid. Most thyroid carcinomas are asymptomatic, but large thyroid cancers can cause neck discomfort, dysphagia, or hoarseness (due to pressure on the recurrent laryngeal nerve). **Papillary thyroid cancer** presents with palpable lymph node involvement in 10%; it may invade the trachea and local muscles. Occult metastases to the lung occur in 10–15%. **Follicular thyroid carcinoma** commonly metastasizes to neck nodes, bones, and lung, but nearly every organ can be involved. Metastatic functioning differentiated thyroid carcinoma can sometimes secrete enough thyroid hormone to produce thyrotoxicosis.

Medullary thyroid carcinoma typically metastases to local nodes and adjacent muscle and trachea as well as mediastinal lymph nodes. Eventually, metastases may appear in the bones, lungs, adrenals, or liver. Medullary thyroid carcinoma frequently causes flushing and persistent diarrhea (30%), which may be the initial clinical feature. Patients with metastases often experience fatigue as well as other symptoms. Cushing syndrome develops in about 5% of patients from secretion of ACTH or CRH.

Anaplastic thyroid carcinoma may sometimes be discovered while they are still relatively small and localized. However, they are more apt to be advanced at the time of diagnosis, presenting with signs of pressure or invasion of surrounding tissue, resulting in dysphagia, hoarseness, or recurrent laryngeal nerve palsy. Patients may also have dyspnea with metastases to the lungs. **Lymphoma** usually presents as a rapidly enlarging, painful mass arising out of a multinodular or diffuse goiter affected by autoimmune thyroiditis, with which it may be confused microscopically. About 20% of cases have concomitant hypothyroidism.

B. Laboratory Findings

Thyroid function tests are generally normal unless there is concomitant thyroiditis. Follicular carcinoma may secrete enough T_4 to suppress TSH and cause clinical hyperthyroidism. (FNA biopsy is discussed above in Thyroid Nodules.)

Serum thyroglobulin is high in most metastatic papillary and follicular tumors, making this a useful marker for recurrent or metastatic disease. Caution must be exercised for the following reasons: (1) Circulating antithyroglobulin antibodies can cause erroneous thyroglobulin determinations. However, declining levels of antithyroglobulin antibodies are a good prognostic sign after treatment for differentiated thyroid carcinoma. (2) Thyroglobulin levels may be misleadingly elevated in thyroiditis, which often coexists with carcinoma. (3) Certain thyroglobulin assays falsely report the continued presence of thyroglobulin after total thyroidectomy and tumor resection, causing undue concern about possible metastases. Therefore, unexpected thyroglobulin levels should prompt a repeat assay in another reference laboratory.

Serum calcitonin levels are usually elevated in **medullary thyroid carcinoma**, making this a marker for metastatic disease. However, serum calcitonin may be elevated in many other conditions, such as thyroiditis; pregnancy; azotemia; hypercalcemia; and other malignancies, including pheochromocytomas, carcinoid tumors, and carcinomas of the lung, pancreas, breast, and colon. Serum calcitonin and carcinoembryonic antigen (CEA) determinations should be obtained before surgery, then regularly in postoperative follow-up: every 4 months for 5 years, then every 6 months for life. In patients with extensive metastases, serum calcitonin should be measured in the laboratory with serial dilutions. Calcitonin levels remain elevated in patients with persistent tumor but also in some patients with apparent cure or indolent disease. Therefore, serum calcitonin levels greater than 250 ng/L (73 pmol/L) or rising levels of calcitonin are the best indication for recurrence or metastatic disease. Serum CEA levels are usually elevated with medullary carcinoma, making this a useful second marker; however, it is not specific for this carcinoma.

C. Imaging

1. Ultrasound of the neck—Ultrasound of the neck should be performed routinely on all patients with thyroid cancer for the initial diagnosis and for follow-up. Ultrasound is useful in determining the size and location of the malignancy as well as the location of any neck metastases.

2. Radioactive iodine scanning—RAI (^{131}I or ^{123}I) thyroid and whole-body scanning is used after thyroidectomy for differentiated thyroid cancer utilizing the protocol described later. (See Radioactive Iodine (^{131}I) Therapy for Differentiated Thyroid Cancer, later.)

3. CT and MRI scanning—CT scanning may demonstrate metastases and is particularly useful for localizing and monitoring lung metastases but is less sensitive than ultrasound for detecting metastases within the neck. Medullary carcinoma in the thyroid, nodes, and liver may calcify, but lung metastases rarely do so. MRI is particularly useful for imaging bone metastases.

4. PET scanning—PET scanning is particularly useful for detecting thyroid cancer metastases that do not have sufficient iodine uptake to be visible on RAI scans. Metastases are best detected using ^{18}FDG-PET whole-body scanning. The sensitivity of ^{18}FDG-PET scanning for differentiated thyroid cancer is enhanced if the patient is hypothyroid or receiving thyrotropin, which increases the metabolic activity of differentiated thyroid cancer. Disadvantages of PET scanning include its lack of specificity for thyroid cancer as well as its expense and lack of availability in some locations. [18]FDG-PET scanning has prognostic implications, since differentiated thyroid cancer metastases with low SUV scores are associated with a better prognosis.

Differential Diagnosis

RAI uptake occurs in many different tissues and can be mistaken for metastatic differentiated thyroid carcinoma. Head-neck RAI uptake is seen in normal thyroid, salivary glands, nasal mucosa, thyroglossal duct remnants, and sinusitis. Chest RAI uptake can occur in the breasts, infections, and pleural effusions. Gastrointestinal RAI uptake occurs with esophageal disease, normal gastric mucosa, gallbladder, diffuse liver disease, and poorly dissolved ^{131}I capsules. Skin RAI uptake occurs with external contamination, burns, and wound healing. Pelvic RAI uptake occurs with normal menses, fibroids, ovarian cysts, struma ovarii, inguinal hernia, and scrotal hydrocele. RAI uptake also occurs with certain nonthyroidal neoplasms, such as meningioma and salivary gland, lung, gastric, or ovarian carcinoma.

Negative RAI scans are common in early metastatic differentiated thyroid carcinoma. Unfortunately, negative RAI scans also occur frequently with more advanced metastatic thyroid carcinoma, making it more difficult to detect and to distinguish from nonthyroidal neoplasms. An elevated serum thyroglobulin in patients with a clear RAI scan should arouse suspicion for metastases that are not avid for radioiodine. Medullary thyroid carcinoma does not concentrate iodine.

Complications

The complications vary with the type of carcinoma. Differentiated thyroid carcinomas may have local or distant metastases, and hyperthyroidism can develop in patients with a heavy tumor burden. One-third of medullary thyroid carcinomas secrete serotonin and prostaglandins, producing flushing and diarrhea. The management of patients with medullary carcinomas may be complicated by the coexistence of pheochromocytomas or hyperparathyroidism.

Treatment of Differentiated Thyroid Carcinoma

A. Surgical Treatment

Surgical removal is the treatment of choice for thyroid carcinomas. Neck ultrasound is obtained preoperatively, since suspicious cervical lymphadenoapathy is detected in about 25%. For differentiated papillary and follicular carcinoma larger than 1 cm diameter, total thyroidectomy is performed with limited removal of cervical lymph nodes.

Surgery consists of a thyroid lobectomy for an indeterminate "follicular lesion" that is 4 cm diameter or smaller. If malignancy is diagnosed on pathology, a completion thyroidectomy is performed. For indeterminate follicular lesions larger than 4 cm diameter that are at higher risk for being malignant, a bilateral thyroidectomy is performed as the initial surgery. Higher risk lesions include those with a FNA biopsy that shows marked atypia or that are suspicious for papillary carcinoma and those that occur in

patients with a history of radiation exposure or a family history of thyroid carcinoma.

For biopsies that are diagnostic of malignancy, surgery involves lobectomy alone for papillary thyroid carcinomas smaller than 1 cm in diameter in patients under age 45 years who have no history of head and neck irradiation and no evidence of lymph node metastasis on ultrasonography. Other patients should have a total or near total thyroidectomy. The advantage of near-total thyroidectomy for differentiated thyroid carcinoma is that multicentric foci of carcinoma are more apt to be resected. Also, there is less normal thyroid tissue to compete with cancer for ^{131}I administered later for scans or treatment. A central neck lymph node dissection is performed at the time of thyroidectomy for patients with nodal metastases that are clinically evident. A lateral neck dissection is performed for patients with biopsy-proven lateral cervical lymphadenopathy. Neck muscle resections are usually avoided for differentiated thyroid carcinoma. However, patients with the Hürthle cell variant of follicular carcinoma may benefit from a modified radical neck dissection. Metastases to the brain are best treated surgically, since treatment with radiation or RAI is ineffective. Levothyroxine is prescribed in doses of 0.05–0.1 mg orally daily immediately postoperatively. About 2–4 months after surgery, patients require reevaluation and often ^{131}I therapy.

Permanent injury to one recurrent laryngeal nerve occurs in between 1–2% and 7% of patients, depending on the experience of the surgeon. Bilateral nerve palsies are rare. Temporary recurrent laryngeal nerve palsies occur in another 5% but often resolve within 6 months. After total thyroidectomy, temporary hypoparathyroidism occurs in 20% and becomes permanent in about 2%. The incidence of hypoparathyroidism may be reduced if accidentally resected parathyroids are immediately autotransplanted into the neck muscles. Thyroidectomy requires at least an overnight hospital admission, since late bleeding, airway problems, and tetany can occur. *Ambulatory thyroidectomy is potentially dangerous and should not be done.* Following surgery, staging (Table 26–8) should be done to help determine prognosis and to plan therapy and follow-up.

Table 26–8. Staging and prognosis for patients with papillary thyroid carcinoma using MACIS scoring.

Total Score[1] - Group	Percent of Patients with Papillary Thyroid Carcinoma	20-Year Survival
< 6.0 = Group I	74.2%	96–99%
6.0–6.99 = Group II	8.5%	68–89%
7.0–7.99 = Group III	9.2%	55–56%
≥ 8.0 = Group IV	8.1%	17–24%

[1]Total score = 3.1 × age (if aged ≤ 39 years) *or* 0.08 × age (if aged ≥ 40 yr) + 0.3 × tumor size (cm, if not completely resected), +1 (if locally invasive), +3 (if distant metastases).
MACIS, metastases, age, complete resection, invasion, size.

In pregnant women with thyroid cancer, surgery is usually delayed until after delivery, except for fast-growing tumors that may be resected after 24 weeks gestation; there has been no difference in survival or tumor recurrence rates in women who underwent surgery during or after their pregnancy. Differentiated thyroid carcinoma does not behave more aggressively during pregnancy. But there is a higher risk of complications in pregnant women undergoing thyroid surgery, compared to nonpregnant women.

B. Thyroxine Suppression for Differentiated Thyroid Cancer

Patients who have had a thyroidectomy for differentiated thyroid cancer must take thyroxine replacement for life. Oral thyroxine should be given in doses that suppress serum TSH without causing clinical thyrotoxicosis. Serum TSH should be suppressed below 0.1 milli-units/L for patients with stage II disease and below 0.05 milli-units/L for patients with stage III–IV disease. (See Table 26–8.) Although patients receiving thyroxine suppression therapy (TSH less than 0.05 milli-units/L) are at risk for a lower bone density than age-matched controls, the adverse effect upon bone density and fracture risk is relatively minor for patients who remain clinically euthyroid. Nevertheless, patients receiving thyroxine suppression therapy should have periodic bone densitometry.

C. Radioactive Iodine (^{131}I) Therapy for Differentiated Thyroid Cancer

Differentiated thyroid cancers variably retain the normal thyroid's ability to respond to TSH, secrete thyroglobulin, and concentrate iodine. There are two reasons to treat patients with ^{131}I after thyroidectomy: (1) thyroid remnant ablation and (2) treatment of known or suspected thyroid cancer. ^{131}I is usually administered 2–4 months after surgery. However, the indications and optimal activity (dose) for ^{131}I therapy for differentiated thyroid cancer remain controversial since there is an overwhelmingly good prognosis for most patients with differentiated thyroid cancer.

Before starting ^{131}I therapy, patients should follow a low iodine diet for at least 2 weeks. Patients must not be given amiodarone or intravenous radiologic contrast dyes containing iodine. Radioiodine administration is contraindicated in women who are pregnant or nursing.

1. RAI thyroid remnant ablation—A low activity[1] of 30 mCi (1.1 GBq) ^{131}I is given for "remnant ablation" of residual normal thyroid tissues after surgery for differentiated thyroid cancer. This small amount of ^{131}I is given to patients with no known lymph node involvement who are at low risk for metastases. There are several advantages to thyroid remnant ablation using ^{131}I: (1) There is usually remnant normal tissue that can produce thyroglobulin (a useful tumor marker); (2) It may destroy microscopic

deposits of cancer; (3) The post-therapy scan may visualize metastatic cancer that would otherwise have been invisible. However, ^{131}I remnant ablation is not required for patients with stage I papillary thyroid carcinomas smaller than 1 cm in diameter (whether unifocal or multifocal), except for patients with unfavorable histopathology (tall-cell, columnar cell, insular cell, Hürthle cell, or diffuse sclerosing subtypes).

2. RAI treatment of metastases—Therapy with ^{131}I improves survival and reduces recurrence rates for patients with stage III–IV cancer and those with stage II cancer having gross extrathyroidal extension. RAI therapy is also given to patients with stage II cancer who have distant metastases, a primary tumor larger than 4 cm in diameter, or primary tumors 1–4 cm diameter with lymph node metastases or other high-risk features. Brain metastases do not usually respond to ^{131}I and are best resected or treated with gamma knife radiosurgery (Table 26–8). A post-therapy whole-body scan is performed 2–10 days after ^{131}I therapy. About 70% of small lung metastases resolve following ^{131}I therapy; however, larger pulmonary metastases have only a 10% remission rate.

Staging with RAI scanning or ^{18}FDG-PET/CT scanning assists with determining the activity of ^{131}I to be administered. Treatment protocols vary among institutions. Generally, patients with higher-risk stage I cancer or stage II cancer are treated with ^{131}I activities of 50–100 mCi (1.8–3.7 GBq). Patients with stage III–IV cancers typically receive ^{131}I activities of 100–150 mCi (3.7–5.5 GBq). Repeated treatments may be required for persistent radioiodine-avid metastatic disease. Patients with differentiated thyroid carcinoma who have little or no uptake of RAI into metastases (about 35% of cases) should not be treated with ^{131}I. Patients with asymptomatic, stable, radioiodine-resistant metastases should receive levothyroxine to suppress serum TSH and should be carefully monitored for tumor progression.

Some patients have elevated serum thyroglobulin levels but a negative whole-body radioiodine scan and a negative neck ultrasound. In such patients, an ^{18}F-FDG PET/CT scan is obtained. If all scans are negative, the patient has a good prognosis and empiric therapy with ^{131}I is not useful.

Activities of ^{131}I over 100 mCi (3.7 GBq) can cause gastritis, temporary oligospermia, sialadenitis, and xerostomia. Therapy with ^{131}I can cause neurologic decompensation in patients with brain metastases; such patients are treated with prednisone 30–40 mg orally daily for several days before and after ^{131}I therapy. Cumulative doses of ^{131}I over 500 mCi (18.5 GBq) can cause infertility, pancytopenia (4%), and leukemia (0.3%). Pulmonary fibrosis can occur in patients with diffuse lung metastases after receiving cumulative ^{131}I activities over 600 mCi (22 GBq). The kidneys excrete RAI, so patients receiving dialysis require only 20% of the usual ^{131}I activity.

3. Recombinant human TSH (rhTSH)-stimulated ^{131}I therapy—Recombinant human thyroid stimulating hormone (rhTSH, Thyrogen) is given to increase the sensitivity of serum thyroglobulin for residual cancer and to increase the uptake of ^{131}I into residual thyroid tissue (thyroid remnant "ablation") or cancer. Thyrogen must be

---

[1] The amount of radioiodine radioactivity given in a procedure is referred to as radioactivity or "activity" and is expressed as Curies (Ci) or Becquerels (Bq), whereas the term "dose" is reserved to describe the amount of radiation absorbed by a given organ or tumor and is expressed as Gray (Gy) or radiation-absorbed dose (RAD).

kept refrigerated and is administered according to the following protocol: Thyroxine replacement is held for 2 days before rhTSH and for 3 days afterward. For 2 consecutive days, rhTSH (0.9 mg/day, reconstituted with 0.2 mL sterile saline) should be administered intragluteally (not intravenously). On the third day, blood is drawn: serum TSH is assayed to confirm that it is greater than 30 microunits/mL; serum hCG is measured in reproductive-age women to exclude pregnancy; and serum thyroglobulin is measured as a tumor marker. RAI is then administered at the prescribed activity (see above).

Thyrogen should not be administered to patients with an intact thyroid gland because it can cause severe thyroid swelling and hyperthyroidism. Hyperthyroidism can also occur in patients with significant metastases or residual normal thyroid. Other side effects include nausea (11%) and headache (7%). Thyrotropin has caused neurologic deterioration in 7% of patients with CNS metastases.

4. Thyroxine-withdrawal stimulated ^{131}I therapy—Thyroxine withdrawal is sometimes used because of its lower cost, despite the discomforts of becoming hypothyroid. Thyroxine is withdrawn for 14 days and the patient is allowed to become hypothyroid; high levels of endogenous TSH stimulate the uptake of RAI and production of thyroglobulin by thyroid cancer or residual thyroid. Just prior to ^{131}I therapy, the following blood tests are obtained: serum TSH to confirm it is greater than 30 microunits/mL, serum hCG in reproductive-age women to screen for pregnancy, serum thyroglobulin as a tumor marker. Three days after ^{131}I therapy, thyroxine therapy may be resumed at full replacement dose.

5. Side effects and contraindications to ^{131}I therapy—National Cancer Institute surveillance data for thousands of patients with thyroid cancer indicate that patients with differentiated thyroid cancer, treated with only surgery, have a 5% increased risk of developing a second non-thyroid malignancy (especially breast cancer). Patients with thyroid cancer who received ^{131}I therapy have a 20% increased risk of developing a second non-thyroid malignancy (especially leukemia and lymphoma). The risk of second cancers peaks about 5 years following ^{131}I therapy.

Women must not receive RAI therapy if they are pregnant, lactating, or lack childcare. Women are advised to avoid pregnancy for at least 4 months following ^{131}I therapy. Men have been found to have abnormal spermatozoa for up to 6 months following ^{131}I therapy and are advised to use contraceptive methods during that time.

D. Other Therapy for Differentiated Thyroid Cancer

Patients with asymptomatic osteolytic metastases to bone from differentiated thyroid cancer are treated with zoledronate, 4 mg intravenously every 6 months; those with symptomatic osteolytic metastases, are treated with zoledronate, 4 mg intravenously every 3 months for the first year and then every 6 months.

Patients with aggressive differentiated thyroid cancers may have metastases that are refractory to RAI therapy. Recurrence in the neck may be treated with surgical debulking and external beam radiation therapy. Patients with RAI-refractory differentiated thyroid cancer metastases that are advanced and rapidly progressive may be treated with certain tyrosine kinase inhibitors. Vandetanib and sunitinib induce partial responses in about 40%, while lenvatinib induced partial responses in about 65%; however, median progression-free survival has only been about 18 months and all tyrosine kinase inhibitors can cause serious adverse reactions, so the patient and clinician must decide whether this chemotherapy is worthwhile.

▶ Treatment of Other Thyroid Malignancies

Anaplastic thyroid carcinoma is treated with local resection and radiation. Lovastatin has been demonstrated to cause differentiation and apoptosis of anaplastic thyroid carcinoma cells in vitro, but clinical studies have not been performed. Anaplastic thyroid carcinoma does not respond to ^{131}I therapy and is resistant to most chemotherapy. Anaplastic thyroid cancers with mTOR mutations may be inhibited by everolimus.

Thyroid MALT lymphomas have a low risk of recurrence after simple thyroidectomy. Patients with other thyroid lymphomas are best treated with external radiation therapy; chemotherapy is added for extensive lymphoma.

Medullary thyroid carcinoma is best treated with surgery for the primary tumor and metastases. Patients with a *ret* protooncogene mutation should have a prophylactic total thyroidectomy, ideally by age 6 years (MEN 2A) or at age 6 months (MEN 2B). Medullary thyroid carcinoma does not respond to ^{131}I therapy and is relatively resistant to chemotherapy. Patients should be monitored closely, with serum calcitonin levels checked about every 3 months. Since medullary thyroid carcinoma can be indolent, patients should be considered for chemotherapy only if they have rapidly progressive metastases, as evidenced by a doubling time of serum calcitonin or CEA doubling time is within 3 years. Scanning with ^{18}FDG-PET is also useful for identifying rapidly progressive metastases. Vandetanib and cabozantinib are approved for use against rapidly progressive metastatic medullary thyroid carcinoma; both require close observation to avoid toxicity. Vandetanib should usually not be administered to patients with cardiac disease or a prolonged QT interval. Cabozantinib should usually not be administered to patients with gastrointestinal disease or prior radiation to the neck or mediastinum, since it increases the risk for gastrointestinal perforation and tracheoesophageal fistula. Patients with medullary thyroid carcinoma and diabetes should not receive diabetic therapy with glucagon-like peptide-1 (GLP-1) agonists because they may stimulate the growth of medullary thyroid carcinoma.

External beam radiation therapy may be delivered to bone metastases, especially those that are without radioiodine uptake or are RAI-refractory. Local neck radiation therapy may also be given to patients with anaplastic thyroid carcinoma. Brain metastases can be treated with gamma knife radiosurgery.

▶ Follow-Up

Most differentiated thyroid carcinoma recurs within the first 5–10 years after thyroidectomy. While lifetime monitoring is recommended, the follow-up protocol can be tailored to the staging and aggressiveness of the malignancy. All patients require at least a yearly thyroid ultrasound and serum thyroglobulin level (while taking levothyroxine). Patients at higher risk have traditionally required at least two annual consecutively negative stimulated serum thyroglobulin determinations less than 1 ng/mL and normal RAI scans (if done) and neck ultrasound scans before they are considered to be in remission. The first surveillance occurs with stimulated postoperative serum thyroglobulin, ^{131}I therapy, and post-therapy scanning about 2–4 months after surgery. At 9–12 months postoperatively, patients may receive another stimulated serum thyroglobulin and RAI scan. Patients need not have repeated ^{131}I therapies if persistent RAI uptake is confined to the thyroid bed and if neck ultrasounds appear normal and stimulated serum thyroglobulin levels remain less than 2 ng/mL. Patients with differentiated thyroid carcinoma must be monitored long-term for recurrent or metastatic disease. Further radioiodine or other scans may be required for patients with more aggressive differentiated thyroid cancer, prior metastases, rising serum thyroglobulin levels, or other evidence of metastases.

1. Serum TSH suppression—Patients with differentiated thyroid cancer are treated with thyroxine doses that are sufficient to suppress the serum TSH below the normal range. For intermediate- or high-risk patients, the serum TSH should be suppressed below 0.1 milli-units/L, while the target TSH for low-risk patients is 0.1–0.5 milli-units/mL. Patients who are considered cured should nevertheless be treated with sufficient thyroxine to keep the serum TSH less than 2 milli-units/L. Follow-up must include physical examinations and laboratory testing to ensure that patients remain clinically euthyroid with serum TSH levels in the target range. To achieve suppression of serum TSH, the required dose of thyroxine may be such that serum FT_4 levels may be slightly elevated; in that case, measurement of serum T_3 or free T_3 can be useful to ensure the patient is not frankly hyperthyroid. Thyrotoxicosis can be caused by over-replacement with thyroxine or by the growth of functioning metastases.

2. Serum thyroglobulin—Thyroglobulin is produced by normal thyroid tissue and by most differentiated thyroid carcinomas. It is only after a total or near-total thyroidectomy and ^{131}I remnant ablation that thyroglobulin becomes a useful tumor marker for patients with differentiated papillary or follicular thyroid cancer, particularly for patients who do not have serum antithyroglobulin antibodies.

Detectable thyroglobulin levels do not necessarily indicate the presence of residual or metastatic thyroid cancer. Conversely, baseline serum thyroglobulin levels are insensitive markers for disease recurrence. However, baseline or stimulated serum thyroglobulin levels 2 ng/mL or higher indicate the need for a repeat neck ultrasound and further scanning with RAI or ^{18}FDG-PET. If serum thyroglobulin levels remain 2 ng/mL or higher in the presence of normal scanning, it is prudent to repeat the serum thyroglobulin in a national reference laboratory. In one series of patients with differentiated thyroid cancer following thyroidectomy,

there was a 21% incidence of metastases in patients with serum thyroglobulin less than 1 ng/mL (while receiving thyroxine for TSH suppression). Therefore, *baseline* serum thyroglobulin levels are inadequately sensitive and *stimulated* serum thyroglobulin measurements should be used and *always* with neck ultrasound. The usefulness of routinely doing a radioiodine scan in low-risk patients is controversial but continues to be done in many centers during stimulation following either rhTSH or thyroid hormone withdrawal.

3. Neck ultrasound—Neck ultrasound should be used in all patients with thyroid carcinoma to supplement neck palpation; it should be performed preoperatively, 3 months postoperatively, and regularly thereafter. Ultrasound is more sensitive for lymph node metastases than either CT or MRI scanning. Small inflammatory nodes may be detected postoperatively and do not necessarily indicate metastatic disease, but follow-up is necessary. Ultrasound-guided FNA biopsy should be performed on suspicious lesions.

4. Radioactive iodine (RAI: ^{131}I or ^{123}I) neck and whole-body scanning—Despite its limitations, RAI scanning has traditionally been used to detect metastatic differentiated thyroid cancer and to determine whether the cancer is amenable to treatment with ^{131}I. RAI scanning is particularly useful for high-risk patients and those with persistent antithyroglobulin antibodies that make serum thyroglobulin determinations unreliable.

The ^{131}I radioisotope may be used in scanning activities provided it is given less than 2 weeks before scheduled ^{131}I treatment to avoid "stunning" metastases such that they take up less of the RAI therapy activity. Alternatively, the ^{123}I radioisotope may also be used and does not stun tumors; it allows single-photon emission computed tomography (SPECT) to better localize metastases. Initial RAI scanning is typically performed about 2–4 months following surgery for differentiated thyroid carcinoma. Whole-body scanning should be performed for at least 30 minutes for at least 140,000 counts and spot views of the neck should be obtained for at least 35,000 counts.

About 65% of metastases are detectable by RAI scanning, but only after optimal preparation: Patients should ideally have a total or near-total thyroidectomy, since any residual normal thyroid competes for RAI with metastases, which are less avid for iodine. It is reasonable to perform a rhTSH-stimulated scan and thyroglobulin level 2–3 months after the initial neck surgery; if the scan is negative and the serum thyroglobulin is less than 2 ng/mL, low-risk patients may not require further scanning but should continue to be monitored with neck ultrasound and serum thyroglobulin levels every 6–12 months. For higher-risk patients, the rhTSH-stimulated thyroglobulin and RAI scan may be repeated about 1 year after surgery and then again if warranted. Serum thyroglobulin and radioiodine scanning are stimulated by either rhTSH or thyroid hormone withdrawal according to the protocols described above for ^{131}I treatment.

The combination of rhTSH-stimulated scanning and thyroglobulin levels detects a thyroid remnant or cancer with a sensitivity of 84%. However, the presence of antithyroglobulin antibodies renders the serum thyroglobulin determination uninterpretable. In about 21% of low-risk patients, rhTSH stimulates serum thyroglobulin to above 2 ng/mL; such patients have a 23% risk of local neck metastases and a 13% risk of distant metastases. The rhTSH-stimulated radioiodine neck and whole-body scan detects only about half of these metastases because they are small or not avid for iodine. Some patients have persistent radioiodine uptake in the neck on diagnostic scanning but have no visible tumor on neck ultrasound; such patients do not require additional radioiodine therapy, especially if the serum thyroglobulin level is very low.

5. Positron emission tomography scanning—[18]FDG-PET scanning is particularly useful for detecting thyroid cancer metastases in patients with a detectable serum thyroglobulin (especially serum thyroglobulin levels greater than 10 ng/mL and rising) who have a normal whole-body RAI scan and an unrevealing neck ultrasound. It is also sensitive for detecting metastases from medullary thyroid carcinoma. Diabetic patients with serum glucose less than 200 mg/dL (11.2 mmol/L) may be scanned. [18]FDG-PET scanning can be combined with a CT scan; the resultant [18]FDG-PET/CT fusion scan is 60% sensitive for detecting metastases that are not visible by other methods. This scan is less sensitive for small brain metastases. [18]FDG-PET scanning detects the metabolic activity of tumor tissue; for differentiated thyroid carcinoma, this scan is more sensitive when the patient's thyroid cancer is stimulated with rhTSH (Thyrogen). One problem with [18]FDG-PET scanning is its lack of specificity. False-positives can occur with benign hepatic tumors, sarcoidosis, radiation therapy, suture granulomas, reactive lymph nodes, or inflammation at surgical sites that can persist for months.

6. Other scanning—Thallium-201 (^{201}Tl) scans may be useful for detecting metastatic differentiated thyroid carcinoma when the ^{131}I scan is normal but serum thyroglobulin is elevated. MRI scanning is particularly useful for imaging metastases in the brain, mediastinum, or bones. CT scanning is useful for imaging and monitoring pulmonary metastases.

▶ **Prognosis**

In the United States in 2014, there were an estimated 63,000 new diagnoses of thyroid cancer and about 1900 deaths, yielding an overall mortality rate of 3%. However, certain thyroid cancers behave aggressively.

Papillary thyroid cancer is best staged using the MACIS (metastasis, age, completeness of resection, invasion, size) scoring system. Scoring and survival data are shown in Table 26–8. [18]FDG-PET scanning independently predicts survival, with patients having few PET-avid metastases and low SUV_{max} (highest image-pixel standardized uptake value) having a better prognosis. There is generally a good prognosis, particularly for adults under age 45 years. Unlike other forms of cancer, patients with papillary thyroid carcinoma who have palpable lymph node metastases do not have a particularly increased mortality rate; however, their risk of local recurrence is increased. The

following characteristics imply a worse prognosis: age over 45 years, male sex, bone or brain metastases, macronodular (greater than 1 cm) pulmonary metastases, and lack of ^{131}I uptake into metastases. Younger patients with pulmonary metastases tend to respond better to ^{131}I therapy than do older adults. Certain papillary histologic types are associated with a higher risk of recurrence and reduced survival: tall cell, columnar cell, and diffuse sclerosing types. Brain metastases are detected in 1%; they reduce median survival to 12 months, but the patient's prognosis is improved by surgical resection. Patients with a **follicular variant of papillary carcinoma** have a prognosis somewhere between that of papillary and follicular thyroid carcinoma.

Patients with **follicular carcinoma** have a cancer mortality rate that is 3.4 times higher than patients with papillary carcinoma. The **Hürthle cell variant** of follicular carcinoma is even more aggressive. Both follicular carcinoma and its Hürthle cell variant tend to present at a more advanced stage than papillary carcinoma. However, at a given stage, the different types of differentiated thyroid carcinoma have a similar prognosis. Patients with primary tumors larger than 1 cm in diameter who undergo limited thyroid surgery (subtotal thyroidectomy or lobectomy) have a 2.2-fold increased mortality over those having total or near-total thyroidectomies. Patients who have not received ^{131}I ablation have mortality rates that are increased twofold by 10 years and threefold by 25 years (over those who have received ablation). The risk of cancer recurrence is twofold higher in men than in women and 1.7-fold higher in multifocal than in unifocal tumors.

Patients with a normal [18]FDG-PET scan have a 98% 5-year survival, while those having more than 10 metastases have a 20% 5-year survival. Those with a SUV_{max} of 0.1-4.6 have a 5-year survival of 85%, while those with a SUV_{max} greater than 13.3 have a 5-year survival of 20%. Patients with only local metastases have a 5-year survival of 95%, while those with regional (supraclavicular, mediastinal) metastases have a 5-year survival of 70%, and those with distant metastases have a 5-year survival of 35%.

Medullary thyroid carcinoma is more aggressive than differentiated thyroid cancer but is typically fairly indolent. The overall 10-year survival rate is 90% when the tumor is confined to the thyroid, 70% for those with metastases to cervical lymph nodes, and 20% for those with distant metastases. When postoperative serum calcitonin levels are below 150 pg/mL (44 pmol/L), residual disease is likely confined to the neck, whereas when postoperative serum calcitonin levels above 500 pg/mL (146 pmol/L) distant metastases are likely. Patients with sporadic disease usually have lymph node involvement noted at the time of diagnosis, whereas distal metastases may not be noted for years. For patients who have metastases to lymph nodes, modified radical neck dissection is recommended. Familial cases and those associated with MEN 2A tend to be less aggressive; the 10-year survival rate is higher, in part due to earlier detection. Patients with metastatic medullary thyroid carcinoma whose serum calcitonin doubling time is over 2 years also have a good prognosis.

Medullary thyroid carcinoma that is seen in MEN 2B (MEN 3) is more aggressive, arises earlier in life, and carries a worse overall prognosis, especially when associated with a germline *M918T* mutation. The elderly tend to have more aggressive medullary thyroid carcinomas. Women with medullary thyroid carcinoma who are under age 40 years have a better prognosis. A better prognosis is also obtained in patients undergoing total thyroidectomy and neck dissection; radiation therapy reduces recurrence in patients with metastases to neck nodes. The mortality rate is increased 4.5-fold when primary or metastatic tumor tissue stains heavily for myelomonocytic antigen M-1. Conversely, tumors with heavy immunoperoxidase staining for calcitonin are associated with prolonged survival even in the presence of significant metastases.

Anaplastic thyroid carcinoma carries a 1-year survival rate of about 10% and a 5-year survival rate of about 5%. Patients with fully localized tumors on MRI have a better prognosis.

Localized lymphoma carries a 5-year survival of nearly 100%. Those with disease outside the thyroid have a 63% 5-year survival. However, the prognosis is better for those with MALT lymphomas. Patients presenting with stridor, pain, laryngeal nerve palsy, or mediastinal extension tend to fare worse.

Choi H et al. Papillary thyroid carcinoma: prognostic significance of cancer presentation. Am J Surg. 2015 Aug;210(2): 298–301. [PMID: 25997714]

Klein Hesselink EN et al. Therapy of endocrine disease: response and toxicity of small-molecule tyrosine kinase inhibitors in patients with thyroid carcinoma: a systematic review and meta-analysis. Eur J Endocrinol. 2015 May;172(5):R215–25. [PMID: 25572389]

Links TP et al. Endocrine tumours: progressive metastatic medullary thyroid carcinoma: first- and second-line strategies. Eur J Endocrinol. 2015 Jun;172(6):R241–51. [PMID: 25627652]

Rowland KJ et al. Hereditary thyroid cancer syndromes and genetic testing. J Surg Oncol. 2015 Jan;111(1):51–60. [PMID: 25351655]

Ruel E et al. Adjuvant radioactive iodine therapy is associated with improved survival for patients with intermediate-risk papillary thyroid cancer. J Clin Endocrinol Metab. 2015 Apr; 100(4):1529–36. [PMID: 25642591]

Tuttle RM et al. Thyroid carcinoma, version 2.2014. J Natl Compr Canc Netw. 2014 Dec;12(12):1671–880. [PMID: 25505208]

Yoo DC et al. Controversy over radioiodine ablation in thyroid cancer: who benefits? Surg Clin North Am. 2014 Jun; 94(3):573–86. [PMID: 24857577]

IODINE DEFICIENCY DISORDER & ENDEMIC GOITER

ESSENTIALS OF DIAGNOSIS

▸ Common in regions with low-iodine diets.

▸ High rate of congenital hypothyroidism and cretinism.

▸ Goiters may become multinodular and enlarge.

▸ Most adults with endemic goiter are found to be euthyroid; however, some are hypothyroid or hyperthyroid.

► General Considerations

Considerable progress has been made to improve global iodine nutrition. However mild-to-moderate and sometimes severe iodine deficiency persists in 30 countries. Severe iodine deficiency increases the risk of miscarriage and stillbirth. Cretinism occurs in about 0.5% of live births in iodine-deficient areas. Moderate iodine deficiency during gestation and infancy causes other manifestations of congenital hypothyroidism, such as deafness and short stature and permanently lowers a child's IQ by 10–15 points. Even mild-to-moderate iodine deficiency appears to impair a child's perceptual reasoning and global cognitive index.

Although iodine deficiency is the most common cause of endemic goiter, there are other natural goitrogens, including certain foods (eg, sorghum, millet, maize, cassava), mineral deficiencies (selenium, iron, zinc), and water pollutants, which can themselves cause goiter or aggravate a goiter proclivity caused by iodine deficiency. In iodine-deficient patients, smoking can induce goiter growth. Pregnancy aggravates iodine deficiency and is associated with an increase in size of thyroid nodules and the emergence of new nodules. Some individuals are particularly susceptible to goiter owing to congenital partial defects in thyroid enzyme activity.

► Clinical Findings

A. Symptoms and Signs

Endemic goiters may become multinodular and very large. Growth often occurs during pregnancy and may cause compressive symptoms.

Substernal goiters are usually asymptomatic but can cause tracheal compression, respiratory distress and failure, dysphagia, superior vena cava syndrome, gastrointestinal bleeding from esophageal varices, palsies of the phrenic or recurrent laryngeal nerves, or Horner syndrome. Cerebral ischemia and stroke can result from arterial compression or thyrocervical steal syndrome. Substernal goiters can rarely cause pleural or pericardial effusions. The incidence of significant malignancy is less than 1%.

Some patients with endemic goiter may become hypothyroid. Others may become thyrotoxic as the goiter grows and becomes more autonomous, especially if iodine is added to the diet.

B. Laboratory Findings

The serum T_4 and TSH are generally normal. TSH falls in the presence of hyperthyroidism if a multinodular goiter has become autonomous in the presence of sufficient amounts of iodine for thyroid hormone synthesis. TSH rises with hypothyroidism. Thyroid RAI uptake is usually elevated, but it may be normal if iodine intake has improved. Serum levels of antithyroid antibodies are usually either undetectable or in low titers. Serum thyroglobulin is often elevated.

► Differential Diagnosis

Endemic goiter must be distinguished from all other forms of nodular goiter that may coexist in an endemic region.

Prevention

Adding iodine to commercial salt helps prevent iodine deficiency. Other sources of iodine include commercial bread, milk, and seafood. The minimum dietary requirement for iodine is about 50 mcg daily, with optimal iodine intake being 150–300 mcg daily. Iodine sufficiency is assessed by measurement of urinary iodide excretion, the target being more than 10 mcg/dL. Initiating iodine supplementation in an iodine-deficient area greatly reduces the emergence of new goiters but causes an increased frequency of hyperthyroidism during the first year.

Treatment

The addition of potassium iodide to table salt greatly reduces the prevalence of endemic goiter and cretinism but is less effective in shrinking established goiter. One iodine-depleted area was Pescopagano, Italy, where 46% of adults had goiters. Salt was iodized (30 mg of potassium iodate per kg salt) and made available in 1985. After 15 years, the incidence of goiter declined to 23%. However, the prevalence of Hashimoto thyroiditis rose from 3.5% to 14.5% after 15 years of iodine supplementation.

Iodine supplementation has not proven effective for treating adults with large multinodular goiter and actually increases their risk of developing thyrotoxicosis. Thyroidectomy may be required for cosmesis, compressive symptoms, or thyrotoxicosis. There is a high goiter recurrence rate in iodine-deficient geographic areas, so near-total thyroidectomy is preferred when surgery is indicated. Certain patients may be treated with ^{131}I for large compressive goiters.

Complications

Dietary iodine supplementation increases the risk of autoimmune thyroid dysfunction, which may cause hypothyroidism or hyperthyroidism. Excessive iodine supplementation increases the risk of goiter. Suppression of TSH by administering thyroxine carries the risk of inducing hyperthyroidism, particularly in patients with autonomous multinodular goiters; therefore, thyroxine suppression should not be started in patients with a low TSH level. Treating patients with ^{131}I for large multinodular goiter may shrink the gland; however, Graves disease develops in some patients 3–10 months following therapy.

Aghini Lombardi F et al. The effect of voluntary iodine prophylaxis in a small rural community: the Pescopagano survey 15 years later. J Clin Endocrinol Metab. 2013 Mar;98(3):1031–9. [PMID: 23436921]
Carlé A et al. Epidemiology of nodular goiter. Influence of iodine intake. Best Pract Res Clin Endocrinol Metab. 2014 Aug; 28(4):465–79. [PMID: 25047199]

DISEASES OF THE PARATHYROIDS

Parathyroid hormone (PTH) increases osteoclastic activity in bone, increases the renal tubular reabsorption of calcium, and stimulates the synthesis of 1,25-dihydroxycholecalciferol by the kidney. Meanwhile, PTH inhibits the absorption of phosphate and bicarbonate by the renal tubule. All of these actions cause a net increase in serum calcium.

HYPOPARATHYROIDISM & PSEUDOHYPOPARATHYROIDISM

ESSENTIALS OF DIAGNOSIS

► Tetany, carpopedal spasms, tingling of lips and hands, muscle and abdominal cramps, psychological changes.

► Positive Chvostek sign and Trousseau phenomenon.

► Serum calcium low; serum phosphate high; alkaline phosphatase normal; urine calcium excretion reduced.

► Low or low-normal serum PTH in presence of hypocalcemia.

► Serum magnesium may be low.

General Considerations

Acquired hypoparathyroidism occurs in about 18% of patients after thyroidectomy, with about 9.5% of such patients being symptomatic. The risk of hypoparathyroidism is much higher in patients undergoing total thyroidectomy and for patients over age 50. Postoperative hypoparathyroidism is usually transient and permanent hypoparathyroidism develops in less than half of such patients. Permanent hypoparathyroidism may occur after the resection of multiple parathyroid adenomas. It also occurs transiently after the surgical removal of a single parathyroid adenoma for primary hyperparathyroidism due to suppression of the remaining normal parathyroids and accelerated remineralization of the skeleton. This is known as "hungry bone syndrome." In such cases, hypocalcemia can be quite severe, particularly in patients with preoperative hyperparathyroid bone disease and vitamin D or magnesium deficiency. *All patients undergoing thyroidectomy or parathyroidectomy must be observed closely overnight.* Neck irradiation is a rare cause of hypoparathyroidism.

Autoimmune hypoparathyroidism may be isolated or combined with other endocrine deficiencies in polyglandular autoimmunity (PGA), which is also known as autoimmune polyendocrinopathy-candidiasis-ectodermal dystrophy (APECED). PGA type 1 presents in childhood with at least two of the following manifestations: candidiasis, hypoparathyroidism, or Addison disease. Cataracts, uveitis, alopecia, vitiligo, or autoimmune thyroid disease may also develop. Fat malabsorption occurs in 20% of patients with PGA-1 and may present as weight loss, diarrhea, or malabsorption of vitamin D. Hypoparathyroidism can also occur in SLE caused by antiparathyroid antibodies.

Parathyroid deficiency may also be the result of damage from heavy metals such as copper (Wilson disease) or iron (hemochromatosis, transfusion hemosiderosis), granulomas, Riedel thyroiditis, tumors, or infection.

Functional hypoparathyroidism may also occur as a result of magnesium deficiency (malabsorption, chronic alcoholism), which prevents the secretion of PTH. Correction of hypomagnesemia results in rapid disappearance of the condition. Hypermagnesemia can also suppress PTH secretion; it may occur in patients with kidney disease who take magnesium-containing antacids, laxatives, or dietary supplements.

Congenital hypoparathyroidism causes hypocalcemia beginning in infancy. However, it may not be diagnosed for many years. Since hypoparathyroidism can be familial, genetic testing and family screening is suggested for family members of any patient with idiopathic hypoparathyroidism.

▶ Clinical Findings

A. Symptoms and Signs

Acute hypoparathyroidism and hypocalcemia can occur spontaneously or may be precipitated when a patient with untreated hypoparathyroidism receives a proton pump inhibitor. Manifestations of hypocalcemia include tetany, muscle cramps, carpopedal spasm, irritability, altered mental status, convulsions, and stridor; tingling of the circumoral area, hands, and feet is almost always present. Symptoms of the chronic disease are lethargy, personality changes, anxiety, premature cataracts, Parkinsonism, and mental retardation. Some patients with chronic hypocalcemia are asymptomatic, even with very low levels of serum calcium.

Chvostek sign (facial muscle contraction on tapping the facial nerve in front of the ear) is positive, and Trousseau phenomenon (carpal spasm after application of a sphygmomanometer cuff) is present. Cataracts may occur; the nails may be thin and brittle; the skin is dry and scaly, at times with fungus infection (candidiasis), and there may be loss of eyebrows; and deep tendon reflexes may be hyperactive. Papilledema and elevated CSF pressure are occasionally seen. Teeth may be defective if the onset of the disease occurs in childhood.

B. Laboratory Findings

Serum calcium is low, serum phosphate high, urinary calcium low, and alkaline phosphatase normal. Serum calcium is largely bound to albumin. In patients with hypoalbuminemia, the serum ionized calcium may be determined; it should be 4.6–5.3 mg/dL (1.15–1.32 mmol/L). Alternatively, the serum calcium level can be corrected for serum albumin level as follows:

$$\text{“Corrected” serum } Ca^{2+} = \text{Serum } Ca^{2+} \text{ mg/dL} + (0.8 \times [4.0 - \text{Albumin g/dL}])$$

PTH levels are low. Hypomagnesemia may exacerbate symptoms and decrease parathyroid function.

C. Imaging

Radiographs or CT scans of the skull may show basal ganglia calcifications; the bones may be denser than normal. Cutaneous calcification may occur.

D. Other Examinations

Slit-lamp examination may show early posterior lenticular cataract formation. The electrocardiogram (ECG) may show prolonged QT intervals and T wave abnormalities. Patients with chronic hypoparathyroidism tend to have increased bone mineral density, particularly in the lumbar spine.

▶ Complications

Acute tetany with stridor, especially if associated with vocal cord palsy, may lead to respiratory obstruction requiring tracheostomy. Pseudotumor cerebri has been reported. Heart failure may rarely occur. The complications of chronic hypoparathyroidism largely depend on the duration of the disease. There may be associated autoimmunity causing celiac disease, pernicious anemia, or Addison disease. In long-standing cases, cataract formation and calcification of the basal ganglia are seen. Occasionally, parkinsonian symptoms or choreoathetosis develop. Ossification of the paravertebral ligaments may occur with nerve root compression; surgical decompression may be required. Seizures are common in untreated patients. Overtreatment with vitamin D and calcium may produce nephrocalcinosis and impairment of kidney function. Chronic hypocalcemia can cause heart failure.

▶ Differential Diagnosis

Paresthesias, muscle cramps, or tetany due to respiratory alkalosis, in which the serum calcium is normal, can be confused with hypocalcemia. In fact, hyperventilation tends to accentuate hypocalcemic symptoms.

At times hypoparathyroidism is misdiagnosed as idiopathic epilepsy, choreoathetosis, or brain tumor (on the basis of brain calcifications, convulsions, choked disks) or, more rarely, as "asthma" (on the basis of stridor and dyspnea). Hypocalcemia may also be due to malabsorption of calcium, magnesium, or vitamin D; patients do not always have diarrhea. Hypocalcemia may also be caused by certain drugs: loop diuretics, plicamycin, phenytoin, foscarnet, denosumab, and bisphosphonates (eg, alendronate, zoledronate). In addition, hypocalcemia may be seen in cases of rapid intravascular volume expansion or due to chelation from transfusions of large volumes of citrated blood. It is also observed in patients with acute pancreatitis. Hypocalcemia may develop in some patients with certain osteoblastic metastatic carcinomas (especially breast, prostate) instead of the expected hypercalcemia. Hypocalcemia with hyperphosphatemia (simulating hypoparathyroidism) is seen in azotemia but may also be caused by large doses of intravenous, oral, or rectal phosphate preparations and by chemotherapy of responsive lymphomas or leukemias.

Hypocalcemia with hypercalciuria may be due to a familial syndrome involving a mutation in the calcium-sensing receptor; such patients have levels of serum PTH that are in the normal range, distinguishing it from hypoparathyroidism. It is transmitted as an autosomal dominant disorder. Such patients are hypercalciuric; treatment with calcium and vitamin D may cause nephrocalcinosis.

Congenital **pseudohypoparathyroidism** is a group of disorders characterized by hypocalcemia due to resistance to PTH. There are several subtypes caused by different mutations involving the PTH receptor or its G protein or adenylyl cyclase.

▶ Treatment

A. Prophylaxis Against Severe Postoperative Hypocalcemia

Post-thyroidectomy hypocalcemia can be detected early by closely monitoring the serum calcium. The risk of severe hypocalcemia after thyroidectomy can be reduced by the postoperative administration of oral calcium (500 mg three times daily) and calcitriol (1 mcg twice daily) for 1 week. The same regimen is initiated for post-parathyroidectomy hypocalcemia and adjusted according to the patient's response.

B. Emergency Treatment for Acute Hypocalcemia (Hypoparathyroid Tetany)

1. Airway—Be sure an adequate airway is present.

2. Intravenous calcium gluconate—Calcium gluconate, 10–20 mL of 10% solution intravenously, may be given *slowly* until tetany ceases. Ten to 50 mL of 10% calcium gluconate may be added to 1 L of 5% glucose in water or saline and administered by slow intravenous drip. The rate should be adjusted so that the serum calcium is maintained in the range of 8–9 mg/dL (2–2.25 mmol/L).

3. Oral calcium—Calcium salts should be given orally as soon as possible to supply 1–2 g of calcium daily. Liquid calcium carbonate, 500 mg/5 mL, may be especially useful. The dosage is 1–3 g calcium orally daily. Calcium citrate contains 21% calcium, but a higher proportion is absorbed with less gastrointestinal intolerance.

4. Vitamin D preparations—(Table 26–9.) Therapy should be started as soon as oral calcium is begun. The active metabolite of vitamin D, 1,25-dihydroxycholecalciferol (calcitriol), has a very rapid onset of action and is not long-lasting if hypercalcemia occurs. It is of great use in the treatment of acute hypocalcemia. Therapy is commenced at a dosage of 0.25 mcg orally each morning with upward dosage titration to near normocalcemia. Ultimately, doses of 0.5–2 mcg/day are usually required.

5. Magnesium—If hypomagnesemia is present (chronic alcoholism, malnutrition, renal loss, drugs such as cisplatin, etc), it must be corrected to treat the resulting hypocalcemia. Acutely, magnesium sulfate is given intravenously, 1–2 g every 6 hours. Long-term magnesium replacement may be given as magnesium oxide tablets (600 mg), one or two per day, or as a combined magnesium and calcium preparation (CalMag, others).

C. Maintenance Treatment of Hypoparathyroidism

Patients with mild hypoparathyroidism may require no therapy but need close monitoring for manifestations of hypocalcemia. Therapy is ordinarily required for patients with symptomatic hypocalcemia or serum calcium levels below 8.0 mg/dL (2 mmol/L).

Vitamin D and calcium therapy: Patients with hypoparathyroidism have a reduced renal tubular reabsorption of calcium and are thus prone to hypercalciuria and kidney stones if the serum calcium is normalized with calcium and vitamin D therapy. Therefore, the goal is to maintain the serum calcium in a slightly low but asymptomatic range of 8–8.6 mg/dL (2–2.15 mmol/L). This minimizes the hypercalciuria that occurs with normocalcemia and provides a margin of safety against hypercalcemia that can permanently damage kidney function. It is prudent to monitor urine calcium with "spot" urine determinations and keep the level below 30 mg/dL (7.5 mmol/L), if possible. Hypercalciuria may respond to oral hydrochlorothiazide, usually given with a potassium supplement. Serum magnesium should be monitored and kept in the normal range with supplemental magnesium, if required. Serum phosphate should also be monitored and the serum calcium × phosphate product kept below 55 mg^2/dL^2 (4.4 mmol^2/L^2).

Calcium supplements can be given as elemental calcium in doses of 800–1000 mg orally daily. (Calcium carbonate 1 g contains 400 mg of elemental calcium; calcium citrate 1 g contains 211 mg of elemental calcium.) Patients with chronic hypoparathyroidism usually require some type of vitamin D (Table 26–9). Monitoring of serum calcium at regular intervals (at least every 3–4 months) is recommended. **Calcitriol,** a short-acting preparation, is given in doses that range from 0.25 mcg/day to 2.0 mcg orally daily. **Ergocalciferol** (vitamin D$_2$) is derived from plants and is commercially available. The usual dose ranges from 25,000 to 150,000 units/day. It is a slow-acting

Table 26–9. Vitamin D preparations used in the treatment of hypoparathyroidism.

	Available Preparations	Daily Dose	Duration of Action
Ergocalciferol, ergosterol (vitamin D$_2$, calciferol)	50,000 international units capsules; 8000 international units/mL oral solution	2000–200,000 units	1–2 weeks
Cholecalciferol (vitamin D$_3$)	50,000 international units capsules, not available commercially in United States; may be compounded	10,000–50,000 units	4–8 weeks
Calcitriol (Rocaltrol)	0.25 and 0.5 mcg capsules; 1 mcg/mL oral solution; 1 mcg/mL for injection	0.25–4 mcg	½–2 weeks

preparation that is stored in fat, giving it a long duration of action. If toxicity develops, hypercalcemia—treatable with hydration and prednisone—may persist for weeks after it is discontinued. Despite this risk, ergocalciferol usually produces a more stable serum calcium level than do the shorter-acting preparations.

PTH is effective for treating patients with hypoparathyroidism but is restricted to patients whose hypocalcemia cannot be adequately treated with calcium and vitamin D analogs (see above). **Recombinant human parathyroid hormone (rhPTH)** is an 84-amino acid polypeptide that is identical to native PTH. It is FDA-approved as an adjunct to calcium and vitamin D analogs to control symptomatic hypocalcemia in patients with hypoparathyroidism. Side effects of rhPTH include nausea, vomiting, diarrhea, arthralgias, and paresthesias. Also, osteosarcoma has occurred in rats receiving very high-dose PTH. The FDA requires that prescribers be certified before prescribing the drug and that patients and prescribers formally acknowledge the risk of osteosarcoma. rhPTH is extremely expensive, which limits its use.

Transplantation of cryopreserved parathyroid tissue, removed during prior surgery, restores normocalcemia in about 23% of cases.

Hypoparathyroidism in pregnancy presents special challenges. Maternal hypocalcemia can adversely affect the skeletal development of the fetus and cause compensatory hyperparathyroidism in the newborn. Maternal hypercalcemia can suppress fetal parathyroid development, resulting in neonatal hypocalcemia. This requires very close clinical and biochemical monitoring during pregnancy.

Caution: Phenothiazine drugs should be administered with caution, since they may precipitate extrapyramidal symptoms in hypocalcemic patients. Furosemide should be avoided, since it may worsen hypocalcemia.

Prognosis

The outlook is good if the diagnosis is made promptly and treatment instituted. Any dental changes, cataracts, and brain calcifications are permanent. Periodic serum calcium levels are required, since changes may call for modification of the treatment schedule. Hypercalcemia that develops in patients with seemingly stable, treated hypoparathyroidism may be a presenting sign of Addison disease.

Despite optimal therapy, patients with hypoparathyroidism have been reported to have an overall reduced quality of life. Affected patients have a high risk of mood and psychiatric disorders and a reduced overall sense of well being.

Bollerslev J et al. European Society of Endocrinology Clinical Guideline: treatment of chronic hypoparathyroidism in adults. Eur J Endocrinol. 2015 Aug;173(2):G1–20. [PMID: 26160136]

Cusano NE et al. Use of parathyroid hormone in hypoparathyroidism. J Endocrinol Invest. 2013 Dec;36(11):1121–7. [PMID: 24445125]

Fong J et al. Hypocalcemia: updates in diagnosis and management for primary care. Can Fam Physician. 2012 Feb;58(2):158–62. [PMID: 22439169]

HYPERPARATHYROIDISM

 ESSENTIALS OF DIAGNOSIS

▶ Frequently detected incidentally by routine blood testing.

▶ Renal calculi, polyuria, hypertension, constipation, fatigue, mental changes.

▶ Bone pain; rarely, cystic lesions and pathologic fractures.

▶ Elevated PTH, serum and urine calcium, and urine phosphate; serum phosphate low to normal; alkaline phosphatase normal to elevated.

▶ General Considerations

Primary hyperparathyroidism is the most common cause of hypercalcemia, with a prevalence of 1–4 cases per 1000 persons. It occurs at all ages but most commonly in the seventh decade and in women (74%). Before age 45, the prevalence is similar in men and women. It is more prevalent in blacks, followed by whites, then other races.

Parathyroid glands vary in number and location and ectopic parathyroid glands have been found within the thyroid gland, high in the neck or carotid sheath, in the retroesophageal space, and within the thymus or mediastinum. Hyperparathyroidism is caused by hypersecretion of PTH, usually by a single parathyroid adenoma (80%), and less commonly by hyperplasia by two or more parathyroid glands (20%), or carcinoma (1% or less). However, when hyperparathyroidism presents before age 30 years, there is a higher incidence of multiglandular disease (36%) and parathyroid carcinoma (5%). The size of the parathyroid adenoma correlates with the serum PTH level.

Hyperparathyroidism is familial in about 10% of cases. However, hyperparathyroidism presenting before age 45 has a higher chance of being familial. Parathyroid hyperplasia may arise in MEN types 1, 2 (2A), and 4. (See Table 26–14.) In MEN 1, multiglandular hyperparathyroidism is usually the initial manifestation and ultimately occurs in 90% of affected individuals. Hyperparathyroidism in MEN 2 (2A) is less frequent that in MEN 1 and is usually milder. Familial hyperparathyroidism can also occur in the hyperparathyroidism-jaw tumor syndrome, a rare autosomal dominant familial condition in which parathyroid cystic adenomas or carcinomas are associated with ossifying fibromas of the mandible and maxilla as well as renal lesions (cysts, hamartomas, Wilms tumors). Affected individuals usually present with severe hypercalcemia as teenagers or young adults; the pathology is usually a single parathyroid adenoma.

Hyperparathyroidism results in the excessive excretion of calcium and phosphate by the kidneys. PTH stimulates renal tubular reabsorption of calcium; however, hyperparathyroidism causes hypercalcemia and an increase in calcium in the glomerular filtrate that overwhelms tubular reabsorption capacity, resulting in hypercalciuria. At least

5% of renal calculi are associated with this disease. Diffuse parenchymal calcification (nephrocalcinosis) is seen less commonly. Excessive PTH can cause cortical demineralization that is particularly evident at the wrist and hip; trabecular bone is usually spared as evidenced by relatively higher spinal bone density compared to the wrist. Severe, chronic hyperparathyroidism can cause diffuse demineralization, pathologic fractures, and cystic bone lesions throughout the skeleton, a condition known as **osteitis fibrosa cystic**.

Parathyroid carcinoma is a rare cause of hyperparathyroidism, accounting for less than 1% of hyperparathyroidism. However, it occurs in about 15% of patients with hyperparathyroidism jaw-tumor syndrome and is also more common in patients with familial hyperparathyroidism or MEN. There is typically a palpable neck mass (75%). About 90% of parathyroid carcinomas are functional and present with serum calcium levels greater than or equal to 14.0 mcg/dL (3.5 mmol/L) or serum PTH levels greater than 5 times normal. However, some cases present with smaller tumors, less severe hypercalcemia, and benign-appearing histologic features. Local recurrence is the rule if surgical margins are positive. Distant metastases arise most commonly in the lungs but also in bones, liver, brain, and mediastinum. Although parathyroid carcinoma is typically indolent, an increasing tumor burden is associated with critically severe hypercalcemia and death.

Secondary and tertiary hyperparathyroidism usually occurs in patients with chronic kidney disease, in which hyperphosphatemia and decreased renal production of 1,25-dihydroxycholecalciferol ($1,25[OH]_2D_3$) initially produce a decrease in ionized calcium. The parathyroid glands are stimulated (secondary hyperparathyroidism) and may enlarge, becoming autonomous (tertiary hyperparathyroidism). The bone disease seen in this setting is known as **renal osteodystrophy.** See Disorders of Mineral Metabolism, Chapter 22. Hypercalcemia often occurs after kidney transplant. Secondary hyperparathyroidism predictably develops in patients with a deficiency in vitamin D. Serum calcium levels are typically in the normal range, but may rise to become borderline elevated with time, with tertiary hyperparathyroidism due to parathyroid glandular hyperplasia.

▶ **Clinical Findings**

A. Symptoms and Signs

In the developed world, hypercalcemia is typically discovered incidentally by routine chemistry panels. Many patients are asymptomatic or have mild symptoms that may be elicited only upon questioning. Parathyroid adenomas are usually so small and deeply located in the neck that they are almost never palpable; when a mass is palpated, it usually turns out to be an incidental thyroid nodule.

Symptomatic patients are said to have problems with "bones, stones, abdominal groans, psychic moans, with fatigue overtones."

1. Skeletal manifestations—Hyperparathyroidism causes a loss of cortical bone and a gain of trabecular bone. Low bone density is typically most prominent at the wrist. Postmenopausal women are prone to asymptomatic vertebral fractures. Although significant bone demineralization is uncommon in mild hyperparathyroidism, osteitis fibrosa cystica may present as pathologic fractures or as "brown tumors" or cysts of the jaw. More commonly, patients experience arthralgias and bone pain, particularly involving the legs.

2. Hypercalcemia manifestations—Mild hypercalcemia may be asymptomatic. However, hypercalcemia of hyperparathyroidism usually causes a variety of manifestations whose severity is not entirely predictable by the level of serum calcium or PTH. In fact, patients with only mild hypercalcemia can have significant symptoms, particularly depression, constipation, and bone and joint pain. **Neuromuscular** manifestations include paresthesias, muscle cramps and weakness, and diminished deep tendon reflexes. **Central nervous system** manifestations include malaise, headache, fatigue, intellectual weariness, insomnia, irritability, and depression. Patients may have cognitive impairment that can vary from intellectual weariness to more severe disorientation, psychosis, or stupor. **Cardiovascular** symptoms include hypertension, palpitations, prolonged P-R interval, shortened Q-T interval, bradyarrhythmias, heart block, asystole, and sensitivity to digitalis. **Renal** manifestations include polyuria and polydipsia, caused by hypercalcemia-induced nephrogenic diabetes insipidus. Among all patients with newly discovered hyperparathyroidism, calcium-containing renal calculi have occurred or are detectable in about 18%. Patients with asymptomatic hyperparathyroidism have a 7% incidence of asymptomatic calcium nephrolithiasis, compared to 1.6% incidence in age-matched controls. **Gastrointestinal** symptoms include anorexia, nausea, heartburn, vomiting, abdominal pain, weight loss, constipation, and obstipation. Pancreatitis occurs in 3%. **Pruritus** may be present. Calcium may precipitate in the corneas ("band keratopathy"), in extravascular tissues (calcinosis) and in small arteries, causing small vessel thrombosis and skin necrosis (calciphylaxis).

3. Normocalcemic primary hyperparathyroidism—Patients with normocalcemic primary hyperparathyroidism generally have few symptoms. However, on average, such patients have higher blood pressures (systolic blood pressure 10 mm Hg higher and diastolic blood pressure 7 mm Hg higher) than controls. Also, affected patients can have very subtle symptoms, such as mild fatigue, that may not be appreciated as abnormal.

4. Hyperparathyroidism during pregnancy—Pregnant women having mild hyperparathyroidism with a serum calcium below 11.0 mg/dL (less than 2.75 mmol/L) generally tolerate pregnancy well with normal outcomes. However, the majority of women with more severe hypercalcemia during pregnancy experience complications such as nephrolithiasis, hyperemesis, pancreatitis, muscle weakness, and cognitive changes. Hypercalcemic crisis may occur, especially postpartum. About 80% of fetuses experience complications of maternal hyperparathyroidism, including fetal demise, preterm delivery, and low birth weight. Newborns have hypoparathyroidism that can be permanent.

Hypocalcemia in the infant can present with tetany even 2–3 months after delivery.

5. Parathyroid carcinoma—Parathyroid carcinoma must always be suspected in patients with a serum calcium greater than or equal to 14.0 mcg/dL (3.5 mmol/L), a serum PTH greater than or equal to 5 times normal, or hyperparathyroidism with a large neck mass. FNA biopsy is not recommended because it may seed the biopsy tract with tumor and cytologic distinction between benign and malignant tumors is problematic.

B. Laboratory Findings

The hallmark of primary hyperparathyroidism is hypercalcemia, with the serum adjusted total calcium greater than 10.5 mg/dL (10.6 mmol/L) (Figure 26–1). The adjusted total calcium = measured serum calcium in mg/dL + [0.8 × (4.0 – patient's serum albumin in g/dL)]. Serum ionized calcium levels should be in the 4.6–5.3 mg/dL (1.15–1.32 mmol/L) range.

The urine calcium excretion may be high or normal (averaging 250 mg/g creatinine) but it is usually low for the degree of hypercalcemia. The serum phosphate is often less than 2.5 mg/dL (0.8 mmol/L). There is an excessive loss of phosphate in the urine in the presence of hypophosphatemia (25% of cases), whereas the serum phosphate may be high in kidney disease, which causes secondary hyperparathyroidism. The alkaline phosphatase is elevated only if

bone disease is present. The plasma chloride and uric acid levels may be elevated. Vitamin D deficiency is common in patients with hyperparathyroidism, and it is prudent to screen for vitamin D deficiency with a serum 25-OH vitamin D determination. Serum 25-OH vitamin D levels below 20 mcg/L (50 nmol/L) can aggravate hyperparathyroidism and its bone manifestations; vitamin D replacement may be helpful in treating such patients with hyperparathyroidism.

Elevated serum levels of intact PTH (immunoradiometric assay) confirm the diagnosis of hyperparathyroidism. Patients with apparent hyperparathyroidism should be screened for familial benign hypocalciuric hypercalcemia with a 24-hour urine for calcium and creatinine. Patients should discontinue thiazide diuretics prior to this test. Calcium excretion of less than 50 mg/24 hours (12.5 mmol/24 hours) or less than 5 mg/dL (1.25 mmol/L) on a random urine is not typical for primary hyperparathyroidism and indicates possible familial benign hypocalciuric hypercalcemia.

Patients with low bone density who have an elevated serum PTH but a normal serum calcium must be evaluated for causes of secondary hyperparathyroidism (eg, vitamin D or calcium deficiency, hyperphosphatemia, renal failure). In the absence of secondary hyperparathyroidism, patients with an elevated serum PTH but normal serum calcium are determined to have normocalcemic hyperparathyroidism. Such individuals require monitoring, since hypercalcemia develops in about 19% of patients over 3 years of follow-up.

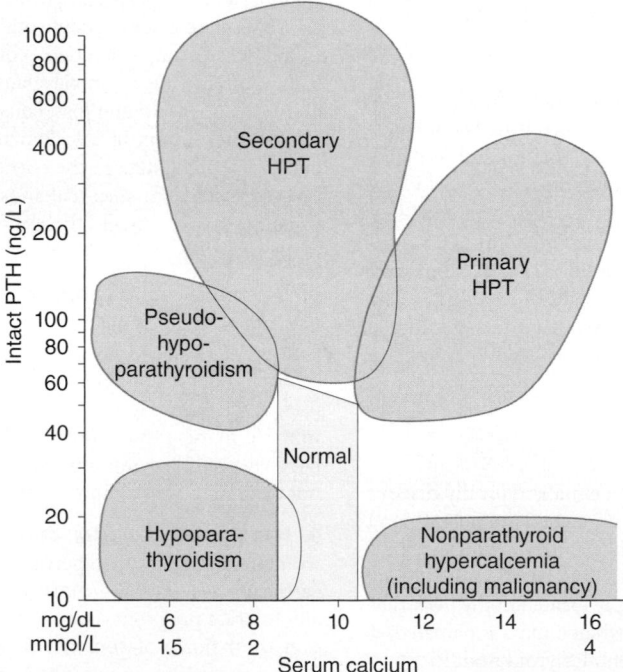

▲ **Figure 26–1.** Parathyroid hormone and calcium nomogram. Relationship between serum intact parathyroid hormone (PTH) and serum calcium levels in patients with hypoparathyroidism, pseudohypoparathyroidism, nonparathyroid hypercalcemia, primary hyperparathyroidism (HPT), and secondary hyperparathyroidism. (Used with permission from GJ Strewler, MD.) Note: A multivariate model that adds clinical and demographic information may perform better than the nomogram alone. (See O'Neill SS et al. Multivariate analysis of clinical, demographic, and laboratory data for classification of disorders of calcium homeostasis. Am J Clin Pathol. 2011 Jan;135(1):100–7. [PMID: 21173131])

C. Imaging

Parathyroid imaging is not necessary for the diagnosis of hyperparathyroidism, which depends on serum parathyroid and calcium levels. Imaging is performed for most patients prior to parathyroid surgery and is particularly important for patients who have had prior neck surgery. The visualization of an apparent parathyroid adenoma helps secure the diagnosis when there is occasional diagnostic difficulty and often allows for minimally invasive surgery.

Ultrasound of the neck should be performed with a high-resolution transducer (5–15 MHz) and should scan the neck from the mandible to the superior mediastinum in an effort to locate ectopic parathyroid adenomas. Ultrasound has a sensitivity of 79% for single adenomas but only 35% for multiglandular disease.

Sestamibi scintigraphy **with ^{99m}Tc-sestamibi and single-photon emission computed tomography (SPECT)** is most useful for localizing parathyroid adenomas. However, false-positive scans are common, caused by thyroid nodules, thyroiditis, or cervical lymphadenopathy. Sestamibi-SPECT imaging improves sensitivity for single parathyroid adenomas. Small benign thyroid nodules are discovered incidentally in nearly 50% of patients with hyperparathyroidism who have imaging with ultrasound or MRI.

Conventional CT and MRI imaging are not usually required prior to a first neck surgery for hyperparathyroidism, since they are generally inferior to ultrasound and sestamibi imaging. However, a four-dimensional CT (4D-CT), with the fourth dimension referring to time, captures the rapid uptake and washout of contrast from parathyroid adenomas; it is particularly useful for preoperative imaging when ultrasonography and sestamibi scans are negative. It can also be helpful for patients who have had prior neck surgery and for those with ectopic glands. In such patients, 4D-CT has a sensitivity of 88%, versus 54% for sestamibi SPECT and 21% for ultrasound. However, 4D-CT delivers more radiation to the thyroid and so is used mostly for older patients. MRI may also be useful for repeat neck operations and when ectopic parathyroid glands are suspected. MRI has the advantages of delivering no radiation and showing better soft tissue contrast than CT.

Patients with hyperparathyroidism have a high risk of calcium nephrolithiasis. Therefore, it has been suggested that all patients with hyperparathyroidism have noncontrast-enhanced CT scanning of the kidneys to determine whether calcium-containing stones are present. For patients with apparently asymptomatic hyperparathyroidism, the presence or absence of calcium nephrolithiasis can be a deciding factor about whether to have parathyroidectomy surgery.

Bone density measurements by dual energy x-ray absorptiometry (DXA) are helpful in determining the amount of bone loss in patients with hyperparathyroidism. Bone loss occurs mostly in long bones, and DXA should ideally include three areas: lumbar spine, hip, and distal radius.

Bone radiographs are usually normal and are not required to make the diagnosis of hyperparathyroidism. There may be demineralization, subperiosteal resorption of bone (especially in the radial aspects of the fingers), or loss of the lamina dura of the teeth. There may be cysts throughout the skeleton, mottling of the skull ("salt-and-pepper appearance"), or pathologic fractures. Articular cartilage calcification (chondrocalcinosis) is sometimes found.

Patients with renal osteodystrophy may have ectopic calcifications around joints or in soft tissue. Such patients may exhibit radiographic changes of osteopenia, osteitis fibrosa cystica, or osteosclerosis, alone or in combination. Osteosclerosis of the vertebral bodies is known as "rugger jersey spine."

▶ Complications

Pathologic long bone fractures are more common in patients with hyperparathyroidism than in the general population. Urinary tract infection due to stone and obstruction may lead to kidney disease and uremia. If the serum calcium level rises rapidly, clouding of sensorium, kidney disease, and rapid precipitation of calcium throughout the soft tissues may occur. Peptic ulcer and pancreatitis may be intractable before surgery. Insulinomas or gastrinomas may be associated, as well as pituitary tumors (MEN type 1). Pseudogout may complicate hyperparathyroidism both before and after surgical removal of tumors. Hypercalcemia during gestation produces neonatal hypocalcemia.

In tertiary hyperparathyroidism due to chronic kidney disease, high serum calcium and phosphate levels may cause disseminated calcification in the skin, soft tissues, and arteries (calciphylaxis); this can result in painful ischemic necrosis of skin and gangrene, cardiac arrhythmias, and respiratory failure. The actual serum levels of calcium and phosphate have not correlated well with calciphylaxis, but a calcium (mg/dL) × phosphate (mg/dL) product over 70 is usually present.

▶ Differential Diagnosis

Artifactual hypercalcemia is common, so a report of hypercalcemia should always prompt a confirmatory serum calcium level that is drawn after an overnight fast along with a serum protein, albumin, and triglyceride while ensuring that the patient is well-hydrated. Hypercalcemia may be due to high serum protein concentrations; in the presence of very high or low serum albumin concentrations, an adjusted serum calcium or a serum ionized calcium is more dependable than the total serum calcium concentration. Hypercalcemia may also be seen with dehydration. Spurious elevations in serum calcium have also been reported with severe hypertriglyceridemia, when the calcium assay uses spectrophotometry.

Hypercalcemia of malignancy occurs most frequently with breast, lung, pancreatic, uterine, and renal cell carcinoma, and paraganglioma. Most of these tumors secrete PTH-related protein (PTHrP), which has tertiary structural homologies to PTH and causes bone resorption and hypercalcemia similar to those caused by PTH. Serum phosphate is often low. Other tumors can secrete excessive 1,25 (OH)$_2$ vitamin D$_3$, particularly lymphoproliferative and ovarian malignancies. The clinical features of malignant hypercalcemia can closely simulate hyperparathyroidism. However, serum PTH levels are usually low. Serum PTHrP or 1,25 (OH)$_2$ vitamin D$_3$ may be elevated.

Multiple myeloma causes hypercalcemia in older individuals. Many other hematologic cancers, such as monocytic leukemia, T cell leukemia and lymphoma, and Burkitt lymphoma, have also been associated with hypercalcemia.

Sarcoidosis and other granulomatous disorders, such as tuberculosis, berylliosis, histoplasmosis, coccidioidomycosis, leprosy, and foreign-body granuloma, can cause hypercalcemia. Macrophages and perhaps other cells present in granulomatous tissue have the ability to synthesize 1,25(OH)$_2$D$_3$. Increased intestinal calcium absorption and hypercalciuria are more common than hypercalcemia. Serum levels of 1,25(OH)$_2$D$_3$ are elevated. Sarcoid granulomas can also secrete PTHrP.

Excessive calcium or vitamin D ingestion can cause hypercalcemia, especially in patients who concurrently take thiazide diuretics, which reduce urinary calcium loss. Hypercalcemia is reversible following withdrawal of calcium and vitamin D supplements. If hypercalcemia persists, the possibility of associated hyperparathyroidism should be considered. In vitamin D intoxication, hypercalcemia may persist for several weeks. Serum levels of 25-hydroxycholecalciferol (25[OH]D$_3$) are helpful to confirm the diagnosis. A brief course of corticosteroid therapy may be necessary if hypercalcemia is severe.

Familial benign hypocalciuric hypercalcemia can be easily mistaken for mild hyperparathyroidism. It is a common autosomal dominant inherited disorder (prevalence: 1 in 16,000) caused by a loss-of-function mutation in the gene encoding the calcium sensing receptor. Calcium sensing receptors are found on the surface of the parathyroid glands and allow the parathyroid glands to vary PTH secretion according to serum calcium levels. Reduced function of the calcium sensing receptor causes the parathyroid glands to falsely "sense" hypocalcemia and inappropriately release slightly excessive amounts of PTH. The renal tubule calcium sensing receptors are also affected, causing hypocalciuria. Familial benign hypocalciuric hypercalcemia is characterized by hypercalcemia, hypocalciuria (usually less than 50 mg/24 h), variable hypermagnesemia, and normal or minimally elevated serum levels of PTH. These patients do not normalize their hypercalcemia after subtotal parathyroid removal and should not be subjected to surgery. The condition has an excellent prognosis and is easily diagnosed with a family history and urinary calcium determination.

Prolonged immobilization at bed rest commonly causes hypercalcemia, particularly in adolescents, critically ill patients, and patients with extensive Paget disease of bone. Hypercalcemia develops in about one-third of acutely ill patients being treated in intensive care units, particularly patients with acute kidney injury. Serum calcium elevations are typically mild but may reach 15 mg/dL (3.75 mmol/L). Serum PTH levels are usually slightly elevated, consistent with mild hyperparathyroidism but may be suppressed or normal.

Rare causes of hypercalcemia include untreated adrenal insufficiency. Modest hypercalcemia is occasionally seen in patients taking thiazide diuretics or lithium; such patients may have an inappropriately nonsuppressed PTH level with hypercalcemia. Hyperthyroidism causes increased turnover of bone and occasional hypercalcemia. Bisphosphonates can increase serum calcium in 20% and serum PTH becomes high in 10%, mimicking hyperparathyroidism. Hypercalcemia may also occur following liver transplantation. Other causes of hypercalcemia are shown in Table 21–8.

▶ **Treatment**

A. "Asymptomatic" Primary Hyperparathyroidism

Patients with mild hyperparathyroidism should only be considered "asymptomatic" after very close questioning. Many patients may not realize they have manifestations, such as cognitive slowing, having become accustomed to such symptoms over years. It is important to assess blood pressure, kidney function with a serum BUN and creatinine, and to determine the presence of nephrolithiasis or nephrocalcinosis by radiography, ultrasonography, or CT scan of the kidneys. Truly asymptomatic patients may be closely monitored and advised to keep active, avoid immobilization, and drink adequate fluids. For postmenopausal women with hyperparathyroidism, estrogen replacement therapy reduces serum calcium by an average of 0.75 mg/dL (0.19 mmol/L) and slightly improves bone density.

Affected patients should avoid thiazide diuretics, large doses of vitamin A, and calcium-containing antacids or supplements. Serum calcium and albumin are checked at least twice yearly, kidney function and urine calcium once yearly, and three-site bone density (distal radius, hip, and spine) every 2 years. Rising serum calcium should prompt further evaluation and determination of serum PTH levels.

If it is not clear whether a patient with primary hyperparathyroid is symptomatic, it is reasonable to consider a trial of medical therapy with cinacalcet.

B. Medical Measures

1. Fluids—Hypercalcemia is treated with a large fluid intake unless contraindicated. Severe hypercalcemia requires hospitalization and intensive hydration with intravenous saline.

2. Cinacalcet—Cinacalcet hydrochloride is a calcimimetic agent that binds to sites of the parathyroid glands' extracellular calcium sensing receptors to increase the glands' affinity for extracellular calcium, thereby decreasing PTH secretion. Cinacalcet may be used as the initial therapy for patients with hyperparathyroidism or for failed surgical parathyroidectomy. For mild hypercalcemia, an initial dose of 15 mg (one-half of a 30 mg tablet) is advisable with weekly monitoring of serum calcium and an increased dose every 2 weeks if hypercalcemia persists until the patient becomes normocalcemic, which is successful in 73% of patients. Patients with parathyroid carcinoma and severe hypercalcemia are treated with cinacalcet in addition to zoledronate. For parathyroid cancer, cinacalcet is administered in doses of 30 mg orally twice daily, increased progressively to 60 mg twice daily, then 90 mg twice daily to a maximum of 90 mg every 6–8 hours. Cinacalcet is usually well tolerated but may cause nausea and vomiting, which are usually transient. Hypocalcemia has occurred, even at 30 mg/day.

About 50% of azotemic patients with secondary or tertiary hyperparathyroidism are resistant to vitamin D analogs. Cinacalcet is given orally in starting doses of 30 mg daily to a maximum of 250 mg daily, with dosage adjustments to keep the serum PTH in the range of 150–300 pg/mL (15–30 pmol/L).

3. Bisphosphonates—Intravenous bisphosphonates are potent inhibitors of bone resorption and can temporarily treat the hypercalcemia of hyperparathyroidism. Pamidronate in doses of 30–90 mg (in 0.9% saline) is administered intravenously over 2–4 hours. Zoledronate 5 mg is administered intravenously over 15–20 minutes. These drugs cause a gradual decline in serum calcium over several days that may last for weeks to months. Such intravenous bisphosphonates are used generally for patients with severe hyperparathyroidism in preparation for surgery. Oral bisphosphonates, such as alendronate, are not effective for treating the hypercalcemia or hypercalciuria of hyperparathyroidism. However, oral alendronate has been shown to improve bone mineral density in the lumbar spine and hip (not distal radius) and may be used for asymptomatic patients with hyperparathyroidism who have a low bone mineral density. It may also be combined with cinacalcet for the medical treatment of osteoporosis in patients with persistent hyperparathyroidism.

4. Denosumab—For patients with severe hypercalcemia due to parathyroid carcinoma, denosumab 120 mcg subcutaneously monthly may be effective.

5. Vitamin D and vitamin D analogs—

A. PRIMARY HYPERPARATHYROIDISM—For patients with vitamin D deficiency, vitamin D replacement may be beneficial to patients with hyperparathyroidism. Aggravation of hypercalcemia does not ordinarily occur. Serum PTH levels may fall with vitamin D replacement in doses of 800–2000 international units daily or more to achieve serum 25-OH vitamin D levels 30 ng/mL or more (50 nmol/L or more).

B. SECONDARY AND TERTIARY HYPERPARATHYROIDISM ASSOCIATED WITH AZOTEMIA—**Calcitriol,** given orally or intravenously after dialysis, suppresses parathyroid hyperplasia of kidney disease. For patients with normal serum calcium levels, it is given orally in starting doses of 0.25 mcg on alternate days or daily. Calcitriol often causes hypercalcemia, so that serum levels of calcium and phosphate must be monitored to ensure that the serum $Ca^{2+} \times PO_4^3$ product remains no greater than 70. If the product exceeds 70, the dose of calcitriol is decreased or the patient is switched to therapy with vitamin D analogs or cinacalcet.

The vitamin D analogs **paricalcitol** and **doxercalciferol** suppress PTH secretion and cause less hypercalcemia than calcitriol. The doses are adjusted to keep serum PTH levels in the range of 150–300 pg/mL (15–30 pmol/L). **Paricalcitol** is administered intravenously during dialysis three times weekly in starting doses of 0.04–0.1 mcg/kg to a maximum dose of 0.24 mcg/kg three times weekly. Alternatively, paricalcitol may be administered orally at doses of 1–2 mcg daily for serum PTH levels 100–500 pg/mL (10–50 pmol/L) or 2–4 mcg daily for serum PTH levels greater than 500 pg/mL (50 pmol/L). Dialysis patients receiving paricalcitol have improved survival compared with patients receiving calcitriol. **Doxercalciferol** is administered intravenously three times weekly during hemodialysis to patients with azotemic secondary hyperparathyroidism in starting doses of 4 mcg three times weekly to a maximum dose of 18 mcg three times weekly. Alternatively, doxercalciferol may be administered orally three times weekly at dialysis, starting with 10 mcg three times weekly at dialysis to a maximum of 60 mcg/wk.

6. Other measures—Estrogen replacement reduces hypercalcemia slightly in postmenopausal women with hyperparathyroidism. Similarly, oral raloxifene (60 mg/day) may be given to postmenopausal women with hyperparathyroidism; it reduces serum calcium an average of 0.4 mg/dL (0.1 mmol/L), while having an anti-estrogenic effect on breast tissue. Beta-blockers, such as propranolol, may also be useful for preventing the adverse cardiac effects of hypercalcemia. Parathyroid carcinoma metastases may be treated with radiofrequency ablation or arterial embolization.

C. Surgical Parathyroidectomy

Parathyroidectomy is recommended for patients with hyperparathyroidism who are symptomatic or who have nephrolithiasis or bone disease. During pregnancy, parathyroidectomy is performed in the second trimester for women who are symptomatic or have a serum calcium above 11 mg/dL (2.75 mmol/L).

Some patients with seemingly **asymptomatic hyperparathyroidism** may be surgical candidates for other reasons such as (1) serum calcium 1 mg/dL (0.25 mmol/L) above the upper limit of normal with urine calcium excretion greater than 50 mg/24 h (off thiazide diuretics), (2) urine calcium excretion greater than 400 mg/day (10 mmol/day), (3) creatinine clearance less than 60 mL/min, (4) nephrolithiasis or nephrocalcinosis, (5) cortical bone density (wrist, hip) indicating osteoporosis (T score below –2.5) or previous fragility bone fracture, (6) relative youth (under age 50 years), (7) difficulty ensuring medical follow-up, or (8) pregnancy.

Surgery for patients with "asymptomatic" hyperparathyroidism may improve bone mineral density and confer modest benefits in social and emotional well being and overall quality of life in comparison to similar patients being monitored without surgery. Cognitive function may benefit with improvements in nonverbal abstraction and memory.

Preoperative parathyroid imaging has been used in an attempt to allow unilateral minimally invasive neck surgery (see Imaging, above). The reported success rates vary considerably. Even in patients with concordant sestamibi and ultrasound scans, and an intraoperative PTH drop of more than 50%, hyperparathyroidism may persist postoperatively in up to 15% of patients.

Without preoperative localization studies, bilateral neck exploration is usually advisable for the following: (1) patients with a family history of hyperparathyroidism, (2) patients with a personal or family history of MEN, and (3) patients wanting an optimal chance of success with a single surgery. Patients undergoing unilateral neck exploration can have the incision widened for bilateral neck exploration if two abnormal glands are found or if the serum quick PTH falls by less than 63% within 10 minutes of the parathyroid resection. Parathyroid glands are not uncommonly supernumerary (five or more) or ectopic (eg, intrathyroidal, carotid sheath, mediastinum). The optimal surgical management for patients with MEN type 1 is subtotal parathyroidectomy that usually results in a cure, although recurrent hyperparathyroidism develops in 18% and the rate of postoperative hypoparathyroidism is high.

Intraoperative near-infrared autofluorescence spectroscopy imaging may improve intraoperative localization of parathyroid glands in primary hyperparathyroidism. The parathyroid glands have intrinsic near-infrared fluorescence that can be detected with a specialized camera. Near-infrared imaging may improve localization of parathyroid adenomas, particularly when preoperative localization studies have been negative or discrepant. However, operating lights must be turned off during image capture.

Parathyroid hyperplasia is commonly seen with secondary or tertiary hyperparathyroidism associated with uremia. Cinacalcet is an alternative to surgery. When surgery is performed, a subtotal parathyroidectomy is optimal; three and one-half glands are usually removed, and a metal clip is left to mark the location of residual parathyroid tissue.

Parathyroid carcinoma surgery consists of en bloc resection of the tumor and ipsilateral thyroid lobe with care to avoid rupturing the tumor capsule. If the surgical margins are not clear of tumor, postoperative neck radiation therapy may be given. Local and distant metastases may be debulked or irradiated. Preoperative MRI scanning is required to delineate the tumor. Zoledronate is given preoperatively. Severe hypercalcemia requires multiple medical measures, including hydration, furosemide, cinacalcet, and zoledronate.

Complications—Serum PTH levels fall below normal in 70% of patients within hours after successful surgery, commonly causing hypocalcemic paresthesias or even tetany. Hypocalcemia tends to occur the evening after surgery or on the next day. Therefore, frequent postoperative monitoring of serum calcium (or serum calcium plus albumin) is advisable beginning the evening after surgery. Once hypercalcemia has resolved, liquid or chewable calcium carbonate is given orally to reduce the likelihood of hypocalcemia. Symptomatic hypocalcemia is treated with larger doses of calcium; calcitriol (0.25–1 mcg daily orally) may be added, with the dosage depending on symptom severity. Magnesium salts are sometimes required postoperatively, since adequate magnesium is required for functional recovery of the remaining suppressed parathyroid glands.

In about 12% of patients having successful parathyroid surgery, PTH levels rise above normal (while serum calcium is normal or low) by 1 week postoperatively. This secondary hyperparathyroidism is probably due to "hungry bones" and is treated with calcium and vitamin D preparations. Such therapy is usually needed only for 3–6 months but is required long-term by some patients.

Hyperthyroidism commonly occurs immediately following parathyroid surgery. It is caused by release of stored thyroid hormone during surgical manipulation of the thyroid. In symptomatic patients, short-term treatment with propranolol may be required for several days.

▶ Prognosis

Patients with symptomatic hyperparathyroidism usually experience worsening disease (eg, nephrolithiasis) unless they have treatment. Conversely, the majority of completely asymptomatic patients with a serum calcium below 11.0 mg/dL (2.75 mmol/L) remain stable with follow-up. However, worsening hypercalcemia, hypercalciuria, and reductions in cortical bone mineral density develop in about one-third of asymptomatic patients. Therefore, asymptomatic patients must be monitored carefully and treated with oral hydration and mobilization.

Surgical removal of apparently single sporadic parathyroid adenomas is successful in 94%. Patients with MEN 1 undergoing subtotal parathyroidectomy may experience long remissions, but hyperparathyroidism frequently recurs. Despite treatment for hyperparathyroidism, patients remain at increased risk for all-cause mortality, cardiovascular disease, renal calculi, and renal failure. These increased risks are likely the residuals of pretreatment hypertension and nephrolithiasis.

Spontaneous cure due to necrosis of the tumor has been reported but is exceedingly rare. The bones, in spite of severe cyst formation, deformity, and fracture, will heal if hyperparathyroidism is successfully treated. The presence of pancreatitis increases the mortality rate. Acute pancreatitis usually resolves with correction of hypercalcemia, whereas subacute or chronic pancreatitis tends to persist. Significant renal damage may progress even after removal of a parathyroid adenoma.

Parathyroid carcinoma is associated with a 5-year survival of about 80% if surgical margins are clear and there are no detectable metastases postoperatively. Conversely, positive surgical margins or metastases predict a very poor 5-year survival. Repeat surgical debulking procedures may improve survival. Aggressive medical management can also prolong life. Metastases are relatively radiation-resistant, but additional therapies such as radiofrequency ablation or arterial embolization may be palliative.

▶ When to Refer

Refer to parathyroid surgeon for parathyroidectomy.

▶ When to Admit

Patients with severe hypercalcemia for intravenous hydration.

Bilezikian JP et al. Guidelines for the management of asymptomatic primary hyperparathyroidism: summary statement from the Fourth International Workshop. J Clin Endocrinol Metab. 2014 Oct;99(10):3561–9. [PMID: 25162665]

Chen G et al. Is normocalcemic primary hyperparathyroidism harmful or harmless? J Clin Endocrinol Metab. 2015 Jun; 100(6):2420–4. [PMID: 25668199]

Cheng SP et al. Quality of life after surgery or surveillance for asymptomatic primary hyperparathyroidism: a meta-analysis of randomized controlled trials. Medicine (Baltimore). 2015 Jun;95(23):e931. [PMID: 26061318]

Hirsch D et al. Pregnancy outcomes in women with primary hyperparathyroidism. J Clin Endocrinol Metab. 2015 May; 100(5):2115–22. [PMID: 25751112]

Khan A et al. Cinacalcet normalizes serum calcium in a double-blind randomized, placebo-controlled study in patients with primary hyperparathyroidism with contraindications to surgery. Eur J Endocrinol. 2015 May;172(5):527–35. [PMID: 25637076]

Lundstam K et al; SIPH Study Group. Effects of parathyroidectomy versus observation on the development of vertebral fractures in mild primary hyperparathyroidism. J Clin Endocrinol Metab. 2015 Apr;100(4):1359–67. [PMID: 25636048]

Marcocci C et al. Medical management of primary hyperparathyroidism: proceedings of the Fourth International Workshop on the management of asymptomatic primary hyperparathyroidism. J Clin Endocrinol Metab. 2014 Oct; 99(10):3607–18. [PMID: 25162668]

Table 26–10. Causes of osteoporosis.[1]

Aging	**Genetic disorders**
Hormone deficiency	Aromatase deficiency
Estradiol (women)	Collagen disorders
Testosterone (men)	Ehlers-Danlos syndrome
Hormone excess	Homocystinuria
Cushing syndrome or	Hypophosphatasia
corticosteroid	Idiopathic juvenile and adult
administration	osteoporosis
Thyrotoxicosis	Marfan syndrome
Hyperparathyroidism	Osteogenesis imperfecta
Alcoholism	**Miscellaneous conditions**
Immobilization and	Anorexia nervosa
microgravity	Celiac disease
Inflammatory bowel disease	Copper deficiency
Malignancy, especially	Diabetes mellitus
multiple myeloma	(uncontrolled)
Tobacco	Hyponatremia (chronic)
Medications (long-term)	Liver disease (chronic)
Aromatase inhibitors	Mastocytosis (systemic)
Heparin	Protein-calorie malnutrition
Pioglitazone	Rheumatoid arthritis
Selective serotonin	Vitamin C deficiency
reuptake inhibitors	
SGLT2 inhibitors	
Vitamin A excess	
Vitamin D excess	

[1]See Table 26–11 for causes of osteomalacia.

METABOLIC BONE DISEASE

The term "metabolic bone disease" denotes those conditions producing diffusely decreased bone density and diminished bone strength. It is categorized by histologic appearance: osteoporosis (bone matrix and mineral both decreased) and osteomalacia (bone matrix intact, mineral decreased). Osteoporosis and osteomalacia often coexist in the same patient.

OSTEOPOROSIS

ESSENTIALS OF DIAGNOSIS

► Fracture propensity of spine, hip, pelvis, and wrist from demineralization.

► Serum PTH, calcium, phosphorus, and alkaline phosphatase usually normal.

► Serum 25-hydroxyvitamin D levels often low as a comorbid condition.

► General Considerations

Osteoporosis is a skeletal disorder characterized by a loss of bone osteoid that reduces bone integrity and bone strength, predisposing to an increased risk of fracture. In the United States, osteoporosis causes over 1.5 million fractures annually, most commonly vertebral fractures, followed by hip fractures (300,000 annually) and pelvic fractures. Vertebral fractures are associated with increased mortality, pain, and spinal kyphosis. Hip fractures are also associated with increased mortality, pain, reduced independence, and diminished quality of life.

The frequency of fragility fractures varies with ethnicity, sex, and age. The lifetime risk of hip fracture in the United States is 15.8% in white women and 6.0% in white men, 2.4% in Chinese women and 1.9% in Chinese men, 8.5% in Hispanic women and 3.8% in Hispanic men. Blacks also have a much lower risk for fracture due to higher bone mineral density and hip morphology that is less fracture-prone. There is much less ethnic variability for vertebral fractures. The prevalence of vertebral fractures in women older than 65 years is 70% for white women, 68% for Japanese women, 55% for Mexican women, and 50% in African American women.

Osteoporosis can be caused by a variety of factors, which are listed in Table 26–10. The most common causes include aging, sex hormone deficiency, alcoholism, smoking, and high-dose glucocorticoid administration. Hypogonadal men frequently develop osteoporosis. Anti-androgen therapy for prostate cancer can cause osteoporosis and such men should be monitored with bone densitometry.

► Clinical Findings

A. Symptoms and Signs

Osteoporosis is usually asymptomatic until fractures occur. It may present as backache of varying degrees of severity or as a spontaneous fracture or collapse of a vertebra. Loss of height is common. Once osteoporosis is identified, a carefully directed history and physical examination must be performed to determine its cause (Table 26–10).

B. Laboratory Findings

Serum calcium, phosphate, and PTH are normal. The alkaline phosphatase is usually normal but may be slightly elevated, especially following a fracture. Vitamin D deficiency is very common and serum determination of 25-hydroxyvitamin D should be obtained for every individual with low bone density. Serum 25-hydroxyvitamin D levels below 20 ng/mL (50 nmol/L) are considered frank vitamin D deficiency. Lesser degrees of vitamin D deficiency (serum 25-hydroxyvitamin D levels in the range of 20–30 ng/mL (50–75 nmol/L) may also increase the risk for hip fracture. Testing for thyrotoxicosis and hypogonadism may be required. Celiac disease may be screened for with serum tissue transglutaminase antibody determinations.

C. Bone Densitometry

Dual-energy x-ray absorptiometry (DXA) is used to determine the bone density of the lumbar spine, hip, and distal radius. Bone densitometry should be performed on all patients who are at risk for osteoporosis or osteomalacia, including all postmenopausal women age 65 years and older and all men age 70 years and older. DXA screening should also be considered for younger postmenopausal women with elevated risk, especially women with early menopause and those with a family history of osteoporosis. It should also be performed in younger patients who have had pathologic fractures or radiographic evidence of diminished bone density. DXA delivers negligible radiation, and the measurements are quite accurate. However, DXA cannot distinguish osteoporosis from osteomalacia; in fact, both are often present. Also, the bone mineral density does not directly measure bone quality and is only fairly successful at predicting fractures. Vertebral bone mineral density may be misleadingly high in compressed vertebrae and in patients with extensive arthritis. DXA also overestimates the bone mineral density of taller persons and underestimates the bone mineral density of smaller persons.

Bone mineral density is typically expressed in g/cm^2, for which there are different normal ranges for each bone and for each type of DXA-measuring machine. The "T score" is a simplified way of reporting bone density in which the patient's bone mineral density is compared to the young normal mean and expressed as a standard deviation score. The World Health Organization has established criteria for defining osteoporosis based upon the T score:

T score ≥ –1.0: Normal.

T score –1.0 to –2.5: Osteopenia ("low bone density").

T score < –2.5: Osteoporosis.

T score < –2.5 with a fracture: Severe osteoporosis.

It is prudent to obtain DXA bone density measurements at two or three sites, including total lumbar spine and total hip. DXA bone density of the non-dominant distal radius is helpful for patients with hyperparathyroidism, for men receiving androgen deprivation therapy, and for patients with conditions causing other DXA measurement artifacts. Such artifacts can be caused by hip arthroplasties, spinal orthopedic hardware, severe spinal arthritis, or lumbar vertebral compression fractures; in such patients, only noncompressed vertebrae are relevant. Any bone density classification is somewhat arbitrary and there really is no bone mineral density fracture threshold; instead, the fracture risk increases about twofold for each standard deviation drop in bone mineral density. Surveillance DXA bone densitometry is recommended for postmenopausal women and elderly men with a frequency according to their T scores: obtain DXA every 5 years for T scores –1.0 to –1.5, every 3–5 years for scores –1.5 to –2.0, and every 1–2 years for scores under –2.0.

The "Z score" is used to express bone density in premenopausal women and young adult men. The Z score is a statistical term expressing an individual's bone density as standard deviation from age-matched, race-matched, and sex-matched means.

Fracture Risk Assessment Tool (FRAX) was developed by the World Health Organization to better predict an individual's 10-year risk of hip or other major osteoporotic fracture. It takes into consideration age, sex, ethnicity, bone mineral density, and other risk factors. It is available for use online at www.shef.ac.uk/frax/.

▶ Differential Diagnosis

Osteopenia and fractures can be caused by osteomalacia and bone marrow neoplasia such as myeloma or metastatic bone disease. These conditions coexist in many patients and cannot be distinguished with bone densitometry.

▶ Prevention & Treatment

A. Nonpharmacologic Measures

For prevention and treatment of osteoporosis, the diet should be adequate in protein, total calories, calcium, and vitamin D. Pharmacologic corticosteroid (oral, parenteral, or inhaled) should be reduced or discontinued if possible. Cigarette smoking cessation is strongly urged. Excessive alcohol intake must be avoided. Exercise is strongly recommended to increase both bone density and strength, thereby reducing the risk of fractures due to frailty falls. Walking increases the bone density at both the spine and hip. Resistance exercise increases spine density. The patient must choose an enjoyable exercise regimen to facilitate long-term compliance. Other fall prevention measures include adequate home lighting, handrails on stairs, handholds in bathrooms, and physical therapy training in fall prevention and balance exercises. Patients who have weakness or balance problems must use a cane or a walker; rolling walkers should have a brake mechanism. Medications that cause orthostasis, dizziness, or confusion should also be avoided.

B. Pharmacologic Measures

Many treatment options are available, so a regimen is tailored to each patient. Generally, treatment is indicated for all patients with osteoporosis (DXA T scores below –2.5), women with previous fragility fractures of the hip or vertebra, or a DXA T score between –2.5 and –1.5 with FRAX-determined (see above) 10-year hip fracture risk greater than 3% or major osteoporotic fracture risk greater than 20%.

1. Vitamin D and calcium—Deficiency of vitamin D or calcium causes osteomalacia, rather than osteoporosis, but they often coexist and cannot be distinguished by DXA bone densitometry; it is crucial to ensure sufficient vitamin D and calcium intake. Recommended daily vitamin D intake of 600–800 units/day is difficult to achieve by diet (unless high in fish) and sun exposure, particularly during winter months and for patients with intestinal malabsorption or during prolonged hospitalization or nursing home care. Oral vitamin D_3 (cholecalciferol) is given either as a universal supplement of 800–2000 units/day or in doses titrated to achieve 25-hydroxyvitamin D (25-OHD) serum levels greater than or equal to 20 ng/mL (50 nmol/L) for most of the population. However, the 25-OHD serum levels should be maintained at 30 ng/mL (75 nmol/L) or higher for those "at risk": pregnant women, older adults, and those with osteoporosis or fragility fractures. There is early observational data of adverse outcomes (increased heart disease and all-cause mortality) at 25-OHD serum levels greater than 50 ng/mL (125 nmol/L), so the optimal therapeutic range for 25-OHD serum levels appears to about 30–50 ng/mL (75–125 nmol/L).

A total elemental calcium intake at least 1000 mg/day is recommended for all adults and 1200 mg/day for postmenopausal women and men older than 70 years. Most healthy individuals do not require calcium supplementation, and 74% of cohort studies showed no association between dietary calcium intake and fracture risk. Other studies have reported that associated calcium supplementation (1 g/day or more) showed no reduced risk for hip or forearm fractures and a mere 14% reduction in vertebral fractures. Calcium supplements are generally reserved for patients with intestinal malabsorption or calcium-deficient diets that do not include dairy products, dark leafy greens, sardines, tofu, or fortified foods. Calcium citrate does not require acid for absorption and is preferred for patients receiving acid blockers. Calcium carbonate should be taken with food to enhance calcium absorption. Calcium supplements are usually taken along with vitamin D_3, and many commercial supplements contain the combination.

Some reports have indicated that calcium supplements increase the risk of myocardial infarction. However, the Women's Health Initiative found that 7 years of vitamin D and calcium supplementation did not increase cardiovascular disease but did increase the risk of nephrolithiasis by 13%. Taking calcium supplements with meals can reduce the risk of nephrolithiasis. Although calcium supplements are usually tolerated, some patients experience intestinal bloating and constipation.

2. Sex hormones—Sex hormone replacement can prevent osteoporosis in hypogonadal women and men but is not an effective therapy for established osteoporosis. Low-dose transdermal systemic estrogen prevents osteoporosis in women with hypogonadism; however, it is not covered by medical insurance for women over age 64 in the United States (see Estrogen Replacement Therapy). Testosterone replacement therapy prevents osteoporosis in hypogonadal men (see Male Hypogonadism).

3. Bisphosphonates—Bisphosphonate therapy is indicated for patients with a pathologic spine fracture or a low-impact hip fracture, and for patients with osteoporosis, defined as a DXA T score of –2.5 or less in the spine, total hip, or femoral neck. They are also indicated for patients with osteopenia (DXA T score between –2.5 and –1.5) and a FRAX-determined (see above) 10-year hip fracture risk greater than 3% or major osteoporotic fracture risk greater than 20%. Bisphosphonates all work similarly, inhibiting osteoclast-induced bone resorption. They increase bone density significantly and all reduce the incidence of vertebral fractures; all but ibandronate have been demonstrated to also reduce the risk of nonvertebral fractures. Bisphosphonates have also been effective in preventing corticosteroid-induced osteoporosis. To ensure intestinal absorption, oral bisphosphonates must be taken in the morning with at least 8 oz of plain water at least 40 minutes before consumption of anything else. The patient must remain upright after taking bisphosphonates to reduce the risk of esophagitis. These medications are excreted in the urine. However, no dosage adjustments are required for patients with creatinine clearances above 35 mL/min. There has been little experience giving bisphosphonates to patients with severe kidney disease; if given, the dose would need to be greatly reduced and serum phosphate levels monitored. Bone density falls in 18% of patients during their first year of treatment with bisphosphonates, but 80% of such patients gain bone density with continued bisphosphonate treatment. The half-life of bisphosphonates in bone is about 10 years. Therefore, after 3 years, a DXA bone densitometry may be obtained. If the patient's T score has risen above –2.5 and the patient has a relatively low fracture risk, the bisphosphonate may be discontinued. However, for patients with continued osteoporosis and a high fracture risk, the bisphosphonate may be continued another 2 years.

Alendronate is administered orally once weekly as either a 70-mg standard tablet (Fosamax) or a 70-mg effervescent tablet (Binosto). The effervescent tablet must be dissolved in 4 oz plain water over at least 5 minutes and stirred 10 seconds before drinking; it is easier to swallow for some patients and may reduce esophageal injury, but there have been no studies comparing it to standard alendronate tablets. **Risedronate** (Actonel) may be given once monthly as a 150 mg tablet. Both medications reduce the risk of vertebral and nonvertebral fractures, but alendronate appears to be superior to risedronate in preventing nonvertebral fractures. **Ibandronate sodium** (Boniva) is taken once monthly in a dose of 150 mg orally. It reduces the risk of vertebral fractures but not nonvertebral fractures; its effectiveness has not been directly compared with other bisphosphonates. Oral bisphosphonates can cause nausea, chest pain, and hoarseness. Erosive esophagus can occur, particularly in patients with hiatal hernia and gastroesophageal reflux. Although no increased risk of esophageal cancer has been conclusively demonstrated, the FDA recommends that bisphosphonates not be used by patients with Barrett esophagus.

For patients who cannot tolerate oral bisphosphonates or for whom oral bisphosphonates are contraindicated, intravenous bisphosphonates are available. Zoledronate (Zometa, Reclast) is a third-generation bisphosphonate and a potent osteoclast inhibitor. It can be given every 12 months in doses of 2–5 mg intravenously over at least

15–30 minutes. **Pamidronate** (Aredia) can be given in doses of 30–60 mg by slow intravenous infusion in normal saline solution every 3–6 months.

Bisphosphonate therapy can cause several side effects that are collectively known as the acute-phase response. Such a response occurs in 42% of patients following the first infusion of zoledronate and usually starts within the first few days following the infusion. Among patients receiving their first infusion of zoledronate, these adverse side effects have included fever, chills, or flushing (20%); musculoskeletal pain (20%); nausea, vomiting, or diarrhea (8%); nonspecific symptoms, such as fatigue, dyspnea, edema, headache, or dizziness (22%); and ocular inflammation (0.6%). Loratadine may reduce musculoskeletal pain. Intravenous zoledronate has caused seizures that may be idiosyncratic or due to hypocalcemia. The acute-phase response tends to diminish with time. Symptoms are transient, lasting several days and usually resolving spontaneously but typically recurring with subsequent doses. For patients experiencing a severe acute-phase response with zoledronate, intravenous pamidronate can be substituted for subsequent treatment. Symptoms may be treated with acetaminophen or NSAIDs. In addition, patients who experience an especially severe acute-phase response can be given prophylactic corticosteroids and ondansetron prior to subsequent bisphosphonate infusions.

Osteonecrosis of the jaw is a rare complication of bisphosphonate therapy for osteoporosis. A painful, necrotic, nonhealing lesion of the jaw occurs, particularly after tooth extraction. About 95% of jaw osteonecrosis cases have occurred with high-dose therapy with zoledronate or pamidronate for patients with myeloma or solid tumor osteolytic metastases. Only about 5% of cases have occurred in patients receiving oral (or, less frequently, intravenous) bisphosphonates for osteoporosis. The incidence of osteonecrosis is estimated to be about 1:100,000 patients treated for osteoporosis and 1:100 patients being treated for cancer. In a prospective 3-year trial of 7714 women who received intravenous zoledronate 5 mg/year, there were no cases of osteonecrosis. For patients with painful osteonecrotic exposed bone, treatment is 90% effective (without resolution of the exposed bone) using antibiotics along with 0.12% chlorhexidine antiseptic mouthwash. Patients receiving bisphosphonates must receive regular dental care and try to avoid dental extraction.

Atypical low-impact "chalkstick" fractures of the femoral shaft are a rare complication of bisphosphonate therapy. Atypical fractures are subtrochanteric or diaphyseal, occur with little trauma, and are usually transverse as opposed to the more typical comminuted or spiral femoral shaft fractures. In more than 52,000 postmenopausal women taking bisphosphonates for 5 years or longer, a subtrochanteric fracture occurred in 0.22% during the subsequent 2 years; 27% of such fractures were bilateral. About 70% of affected patients have had prodromal thigh pain prior to the fracture. The risk for atypical femoral fractures is particularly increased among Asian women and among patients taking high-dose corticosteroids and those receiving bisphosphonate treatment for more than 5 years. Teriparatide may be helpful to promote healing of such fractures. Despite this rare complication, the overall risk of hip fracture is reduced among patients taking bisphosphonates for up to 5 years.

In patients taking bisphosphonates, hypercalcemia is seen in 20% and serum PTH levels increase above normal in 10%, mimicking primary hyperparathyroidism. Hypocalcemia occurs frequently, resulting in secondary hyperparathyroidism; such patients may be treated with oral calcium supplements (500–1000 mg/day) and with oral vitamin D_3 (starting at 1000 units/day).

4. Denosumab—Denosumab (Prolia, Xgeva) is a monoclonal antibody that inhibits the proliferation and maturation of preosteoclasts into mature osteoclast bone-resorbing cells. It does this by binding to the osteoclast receptor activator of nuclear factor-kappa B ligand (RANKL). It is indicated for treatment of osteoporosis, major fragility fractures, or osteopenia with a high FRAX score in both men and women. It is also used for patients with high fracture risk who are receiving sex hormone suppression therapy for breast cancer or prostate cancer. Treatment reduces vertebral fractures by 68% and reduces hip fractures by 40%. Denosumab is administered in doses of 60 mg subcutaneously every 6 months. It increases bone mineral density more than oral alendronate. Unlike bisphosphonates, denosumab can be given to patients with severe kidney disease. It has been relatively well tolerated, with an 8% incidence of flu-like symptoms. It can decrease serum calcium and should not be administered to patients with hypocalcemia. Other side effects include hypercholesterolemia, eczema and dermatitis, serious infections, new malignancies, and pancreatitis. Its efficacy is comparable to bisphosphonates. With prolonged use, it predisposes to atypical femoral fractures and osteonecrosis of the jaw and is additive to bisphosphonates in that regard. As with bisphosphonates, denosumab is usually administered for a 3–5 year course.

5. Teriparatide—Teriparatide (Forteo, Parathar) is an analog of PTH. Teriparatide stimulates the production of new collagenous bone matrix that must be mineralized. Patients receiving teriparatide must have sufficient intake of vitamin D and calcium. When administered to patients with osteoporosis in doses of 20 mcg/day subcutaneously for 2 years, teriparatide dramatically improves bone density in most bones except the distal radius. Teriparatide may also be used to promote healing of atypical femoral chalkstick fractures associated with bisphosphonate therapy. The recommended dose should not be exceeded, since teriparatide has caused osteosarcoma in rats when administered in very high doses. Due to the potential risk for osteosarcoma, patients are excluded from receiving teriparatide if they have an increased risk of osteosarcoma due to the following: Paget disease of bone, unexplained elevations in serum alkaline phosphatase, prior radiation therapy to bones, open epiphyses, or a past history of osteosarcoma or chondrosarcoma. Side effects may include injection site reactions, orthostatic hypotension, arthralgia, muscle cramps, depression, or pneumonia. Hypercalcemia can occur and manifest as nausea, constipation, asthenia, or muscle weakness. Teriparatide is approved for only a 2-year course of treatment.

Teriparatide should not be used for patients with hypercalcemia. Similarly, teriparatide should be used with caution in patients if they are also taking corticosteroids and thiazide diuretics along with oral calcium supplementation because hypercalcemia may develop.

Following a course of teriparatide, bisphosphonates should be considered in order to retain the improved bone density. Alternatively, for severe osteoporosis, teriparatide may be administered along with denosumab; combined treatment for 2 years is more effective than any other single therapy.

6. Selective estrogen receptor modulators (SERMs)— SERMs can prevent osteoporosis but are not effective therapy for established osteoporosis. **Raloxifene** 60 mg/day orally may be taken by postmenopausal women in place of estrogen for prevention of osteoporosis. Bone density increases about 1% over 2 years in postmenopausal women versus 2% increases with estrogen replacement. It reduces the risk of vertebral fractures by about 40% but does not appear to reduce the risk of nonvertebral fractures. Raloxifene produces a reduction in LDL cholesterol but not the rise in high-density lipoprotein (HDL) cholesterol seen with estrogen. It has no direct effect on coronary plaque. Unlike estrogen, raloxifene does not reduce hot flushes; in fact, it often intensifies them. It does not relieve vaginal dryness. Unlike estrogen, however, raloxifene does not cause endometrial hyperplasia, uterine bleeding, or cancer, nor does it cause breast soreness. The risk of breast cancer is reduced 76% in women taking raloxifene for 3 years. Since it is a potential teratogen, it is relatively contraindicated in women capable of pregnancy. Raloxifene increases the risk for thromboembolism and should not be used by women with such a history. Leg cramps can also occur. **Tamoxifen** is another SERM that is commonly administered to women for up to 5 years after resection of breast cancer that is estrogen receptor positive.

Bazedoxifene is a SERM that is available as a fixed-dose combination medication with conjugated estrogens (Duavee). It is FDA-approved for the prevention of osteoporosis in postmenopausal women with an intact uterus. However, unlike raloxifene, it has not been shown to reduce the risk of breast cancer. It is expected that women taking this combination medication long-term will experience an increased risk of thromboembolic disease.

7. Calcitonin—Calcitonin therapy is much less effective than other treatments for osteoporosis. Long-term calcitonin therapy increases the risk of liver cancer but reduces the risk of breast cancer. Calcitonin is used primarily for its analgesic effect for the pain of acute osteoporotic vertebral compression fractures. It is ineffective for chronic pain. Its analgesic effect may be seen within 2–4 weeks. If it appears to be effective for analgesia, it is continued for up to 3 months. A nasal spray of calcitonin-salmon (Miacalcin) is available that contains 2200 units/mL in 2-mL metered-dose bottles. The usual dose is one puff (0.09 mL, 200 international units) once daily, alternating nostrils. Nasal symptoms such as rhinitis and epistaxis occur commonly; other less common adverse reactions include flu-like symptoms, allergy, arthralgias, back pain, and headache. Calcitonin reduces the incidence of vertebral fractures, but its effect upon nonvertebral fractures has not been established. If calcitonin is administered, other more effective treatments for osteoporosis should be given simultaneously.

8. Orthopedic surgery—Percutaneous vertebroplasty or kyphoplasty may be considered for patients with vertebral compression fractures who fail conservative pain management. However, no prospective randomized study has adequately compared the effectiveness of these orthopedic procedures compared to conservative therapy.

▶ Prognosis

Bone mineral density densitometries can detect whether progressive osteopenia or frank osteoporosis is developing. Osteoporosis should ideally be prevented, since it can be only partially reversed. Measures noted above are reasonably effective in preventing and treating osteoporosis and reducing fracture risk.

Black DM et al. Clinical practice. Postmenopausal osteoporosis. N Engl J Med. 2016 Jan 21;374(3):254–62. [PMID: 26789873]

Ensrud KE et al; Osteoporotic Fractures in Men Study Group. Implications of expanding indications for drug treatment to prevent fracture in older men in United States: cross sectional and longitudinal analysis of prospective cohort study. BMJ. 2014 Jul 3;349:g4120. [PMID: 24994809]

Golob AL et al. Osteoporosis: screening, prevention, and management. Med Clin North Am. 2015 May;99(3):587–606. [PMID: 25841602]

Langdahl BL et al. A 24-month study evaluating the efficacy and safety of denosumab for the treatment of men with low bone mineral density: results from the ADAMO trial. J Clin Endocrinol Metab. 2015 Apr;100(4):1335–42. [PMID: 25607608]

Moyer VA et al. Vitamin D and calcium supplementation to prevent fractures in adults: U.S. Preventive Services Task Force recommendation statement. Ann Intern Med. 2013 May 7;158(9):691–6. [PMID: 23440163]

Sugerman DT. JAMA patient page. Osteoporosis. JAMA. 2014 Jan 1;311(1):104. [PMID: 24381978]

Taylor CL et al. Questions about vitamin D for primary care practice: input from an NIH Conference. Am J Med. 2015 Nov; 128(11):1167–70. [PMID: 26071820]

Watts NB et al. Osteoporosis in men: an Endocrine Society clinical practice guideline. J Clin Endocrinol Metab. 2012 Jun; 97(6):1802–22. [PMID: 22675062]

OSTEOMALACIA

 ESSENTIALS OF DIAGNOSIS

▶ Painful proximal muscle weakness (especially pelvic girdle); bone pain and tenderness.

▶ Decreased bone density from defective mineralization.

▶ Increased alkaline phosphatase, decreased 25-hydroxy-vitamin D, hypocalcemia, hypocalciuria, hypophosphatemia, secondary hyperparathyroidism.

▶ Classic radiologic features may be present.

General Considerations

Defective mineralization of the growing skeleton in childhood causes permanent bone deformities (rickets). Defective skeletal mineralization in adults is known as osteomalacia. It is caused by any condition that results in inadequate calcium or phosphate mineralization of bone osteoid.

Etiology (Table 26–11)

A. Vitamin D Deficiency and Resistance

Vitamin D deficiency is the most common cause of osteomalacia and its incidence is increasing throughout the world as a result of diminished exposure to sunlight caused by urbanization, automobile and public transportation, modest clothing, and sunscreen use. Significant vitamin D deficiency, with serum 25OHD less than 20 ng/mL (50 nmol/L), was found in 24.3% of postmenopausal women from 25 countries. The incidence varied: less than 1% in Southeast Asia, 29% in the United States, and 36% in Italy. Patients in whom clinically severe osteomalacia develops typically have had chronic severe vitamin D deficiency (serum 25OHD under 25 nmol/L or under 10 ng/mL). The prevalence of severe vitamin D deficiency is 3.5% in the United States and 12.5% in Italy. Among US men over age 65 years, 25% have serum 25OHD levels below 20 ng/mL; men over age 75 with such low vitamin D levels have particularly accelerated bone loss. Vitamin D deficiency is particularly common in the institutionalized elderly, with the incidence exceeding 60% in some groups not receiving vitamin D supplementation. Deficiency of vitamin D may arise from insufficient sun exposure, malnutrition, or malabsorption (due to pancreatic insufficiency, cholestatic liver disease, celiac disease, inflammatory bowel disease, jejunoileal bypass, Billroth type II gastrectomy). Orlistat is a weight-loss medication that causes fat malabsorption and reduced serum 25OHD levels. Cholestyramine binds bile acids necessary for vitamin D absorption. Patients with severe nephrotic syndrome lose large amounts of vitamin D–binding protein in the urine.

Anticonvulsants (eg, phenytoin, carbamazepine, valproate, phenobarbital) inhibit the hepatic production of 25OHD and sometimes cause osteomalacia. Phenytoin can also directly inhibit bone mineralization.

Vitamin D–dependent rickets type I is caused by a rare autosomal recessive disorder with a defect in the renal enzyme 1-alpha-hydroxylase leading to defective synthesis of $1,25(OH)_2D$. It presents in childhood with rickets and alopecia; osteomalacia develops in adults with this condition unless treated with oral calcitriol in doses of 0.5–1 mcg daily.

Vitamin D–dependent rickets type II (better known as hereditary $1,25[OH]_2D$-resistant rickets) is caused by a genetic defect in the $1,25(OH)_2D$ receptor. Patients have hypocalcemia with childhood rickets and adult osteomalacia. Alopecia is common. These patients respond variably to oral calcitriol in very large doses (2–6 mcg daily).

B. Deficient Calcium Intake

The total daily consumption of calcium should be at least 1000 mg daily. Patients who have deficient calcium intake develop rickets (childhood) or osteomalacia (adulthood) despite sufficient vitamin D. A nutritional deficiency of calcium can occur in any severely malnourished patient. Some degree of calcium deficiency is common in the elderly, since intestinal calcium absorption declines with age. Ingestion of excessive wheat bran also causes calcium malabsorption.

C. Phosphate Deficiency

Hypophosphatemia can cause severe major muscle weakness, dysphagia, diplopia, cardiomyopathy, and respiratory muscle weakness. Patients may have impaired cognition. Chronic hypophosphatemia can cause bone pain and affect bone integrity. Phosphate deficiency in childhood causes classic rickets, whereas phosphate deficiency in adulthood causes osteomalacia.

1. Genetic disorders—Fibroblast growth factor-23 (FGF23) is a phosphaturic factor (phosphatonin) that is secreted by bone osteoblasts in response to elevated serum phosphate levels. Families with autosomal dominant hypophosphatemic rickets have a gain-of-function mutation in the gene encoding FGF23 that makes it resistant

Table 26–11. Causes of osteomalacia.[1]

Vitamin disorders
  Decreased availability of vitamin D
  Insufficient sunlight exposure
  Nutritional deficiency of vitamin D
  Malabsorption: aging, excess wheat bran, bariatric surgery, pancreatic enzyme deficiency
  Nephrotic syndrome
  Vitamin D–dependent rickets type I
  Liver disease
  Chronic kidney disease
  Kidney transplantation
  Phenytoin, carbamazepine, valproate, or barbiturate therapy (chronic)
Dietary calcium deficiency
Phosphate deficiency
  Intestinal malabsorption
  Nutritional deficiency of phosphorus
  Phosphate-binding antacid therapy
  Increased renal loss
  Adefovir therapy
  X-linked hypophosphatemic rickets
  Tumoral hypophosphatemic osteomalacia
  Association with other disorders, including paraproteinemias, glycogen storage diseases, neurofibromatosis, Wilson disease, Fanconi syndrome, renal tubular acidosis, and alcoholism
Inhibitors of mineralization
  Aluminum
  Bisphosphonates
Disorders of bone matrix
  Hypophosphatasia
  Fibrogenesis imperfecta
  Axial osteomalacia

[1]See Table 26–10 for causes of osteoporosis.

to proteolytic cleavage, thereby increasing serum FGF23 levels. In X-linked hypophosphatemic rickets, there is a mutation in the gene encoding PHEX endopeptidase, which fails to cleave FGF23, resulting in elevated serum FGF23 levels. An autosomal recessive form of hypophosphatemic rickets is caused by mutations in DMP1, a transcription factor that regulates FGF23 production in bone. All three conditions have high serum FGF23 levels causing hypophosphatemia and bone mineral depletion.

2. Tumor-induced osteomalacia—A variety of mesenchymal tumors (87% benign) secrete fibroblast growth factor-23 (FGF23) and cause marked hypophosphatemia due to renal phosphate wasting. Such tumors are usually small and are often difficult to locate. The condition is characterized by hypophosphatemia, excessive phosphaturia, reduced or normal serum $1,25(OH)_2D$ concentrations, and osteomalacia. Serum levels of FGF23 are elevated. Such tumors are often small and difficult to find, frequently lying in extremities. Imaging with ^{111}In-octreotide or ^{18}FDG-PET should include the entire body and may help localize the tumor.

3. Other causes of hypophosphatemia—Osteomalacia from hypophosphatemia can be caused by severe intestinal malabsorption or poor nutrition. Severe hypophosphatemia can occur with refeeding after starvation (eg, concentration camp victims, malnourished alcoholics). Other causes of hypophosphatemia include respiratory alkalosis, glucose infusions, salicylate intoxication, mannitol, and bisphosphonate therapy. Additional causes include chelation of phosphate in the gut by aluminum hydroxide antacids, calcium acetate (Phos-Lo), or sevelamer hydrochloride (Renagel). Excessive renal phosphate losses are also seen in proximal renal tubular acidosis and Fanconi syndrome.

D. Aluminum Toxicity

Bone mineralization is inhibited by aluminum. Osteomalacia may occur in patients receiving long-term renal hemodialysis with tap water dialysate or from aluminum-containing antacids used to reduce phosphate levels. Osteomalacia may develop in patients being maintained on long-term total parenteral nutrition if the casein hydrolysate used for amino acids contains high levels of aluminum.

E. Hypophosphatasia

Hypophosphatasia must not be confused with hypophosphatemia. Hypophosphatasia refers to a severe deficiency of bone alkaline phosphatase. It is a rare genetic cause of osteomalacia that is commonly misdiagnosed as osteoporosis. The incidence in the United States is about 1 in 100,000 live births; about 1 in 300 adults is a carrier. The phenotypic presentation of hypophosphatasia is extremely variable. At its mildest, hypophosphatasia can present in middle age with premature loss of teeth, foot pain (due to metatarsal stress fractures), thigh pain (due to femoral pseudofractures), or arthritis (due to chondrocalcinosis). Serum alkaline phosphatase is low. To confirm the diagnosis, a 24-hour urine should be assayed for phosphoethanolamine, a

substrate for tissue-nonspecific alkaline phosphatase, whose excretion is always elevated in patients with hypophosphatasia. Prenatal genetic testing is available for the infantile form of hypophosphatasia. There is no proven therapy for hypophosphatasia, except for supportive care. Teriparatide has been ineffective for treatment.

F. Fibrogenesis Imperfecta Ossium

This rare condition sporadically affects middle-aged patients, who present with progressive bone pain and pathologic fractures. Bones have a dense "fishnet" appearance on radiographs. Serum alkaline phosphatase levels are elevated. Some patients have a monoclonal gammopathy, indicating a possible plasma cell dyscrasia causing an impairment in osteoblast function and collagen disarray. Remission has been reported after repeated courses of melphalan, corticosteroids, and vitamin D analog over 3 years.

▶ **Clinical Findings**

The clinical manifestations of defective bone mineralization depend on the age at onset and the severity. In adults, osteomalacia is typically asymptomatic at first. Eventually, bone and joint pain occurs, along with reduced muscle strength and endurance. Pathologic fractures may occur with little or no trauma. These manifestations can occur with either hypocalcemia or hypophosphatemia.

▶ **Diagnostic Tests**

Serum is obtained for calcium, albumin, phosphate, alkaline phosphatase, PTH, and $25[OH]D_3$ determinations. Bone densitometry helps document the degree of osteopenia. Radiographs may show diagnostic features.

In one series of biopsy-proved osteomalacia, alkaline phosphatase was elevated in 94% of patients; the calcium or phosphorus was low in 47% of patients; $25(OH)D_3$ was low in 29% of patients; pseudofractures were seen in 18% of patients; and urinary calcium was low in 18% of patients. $1,25(OH)_2D_3$ may be low even when $25(OH)D_2$ levels are normal.

Genetic testing can confirm the diagnosis of autosomal dominant hypophosphatemic rickets (*FGF23*), X-linked hypophosphatemic rickets (*PHEX*), and autosomal recessive hypophosphatemic rickets (*DMP1*).

▶ **Differential Diagnosis**

Osteomalacia is often seen together with osteoporosis. The relative contribution of the two entities to diminished bone density may not be apparent until treatment, since a dramatic rise in bone density is often seen with therapy for osteomalacia. Phosphate deficiency must be distinguished from hypophosphatemia seen in hyperparathyroidism.

▶ **Prevention & Treatment**

To obtain adequate sunshine vitamin D, the face, arms, hands, or back must have sun exposure without sunscreen for 15 minutes at least twice weekly. The main natural food source of vitamin D is fish, particularly salmon, mackerel, cod liver oil, and sardines or tuna canned in oil. Most commercial cow's milk is fortified with vitamin D at about 400 international units per quart; however, skim milk and other dairy products contain much less vitamin D.

Many vitamin supplements contain plant-derived vitamin D_2, which has less biologic availability than once believed. Over-the-counter multivitamin/mineral supplements contain variable amounts of vitamin D, and vitamin D toxicity has occurred from two different multivitamins sold in the United States. Therefore, it is prudent to recommend that patients take a dedicated vitamin D supplement from a reliable manufacturer.

In sunlight-deprived individuals (eg, veiled women, confined patients, or residents of higher latitudes during winter), the recommended daily allowance should be vitamin D_3 1000 international units daily. In such individuals, vitamin D_3 supplements should be given prophylactically. Patients receiving long-term phenytoin therapy should also receive vitamin D_3 supplementation.

Frank vitamin D deficiency is treated with ergocalciferol (D_2), 50,000 international units orally once weekly for 8 weeks. Following that, vitamin D_3 (cholecalciferol) supplementation is used at a dose of 2000 international units daily. Vitamin D_3 is more effective than vitamin D_2 in raising serum levels of 25(OH)D. Some patients require long-term supplementation with ergocalciferol of up to 50,000 international units weekly. In patients with intestinal malabsorption, oral doses of 25,000–100,000 international units of vitamin D_3 daily may be required. Some patients with steatorrhea respond better to oral 25(OH)D_3 (calcifediol), 50–100 mcg/day. Serum levels of 25(OH)D should be monitored and the dosage of vitamin D adjusted to maintain serum 25(OH)D levels above 30 ng/mL. During treatment with high-dose vitamin D, serum calcium should also be monitored to avoid hypercalcemia.

Beyond increasing the intestinal absorption of calcium, vitamin D supplementation may have additional effects. Vitamin D supplementation has been associated with improved muscle strength and a reduced fall risk, factors that reduce the risk of bone fracture.

The addition of calcium supplements to vitamin D is probably not necessary for the prevention of osteomalacia in the majority of otherwise well-nourished patients. However, patients with malabsorption or poor nutrition should receive calcium supplementation. Recommended doses of calcium are as follows: calcium citrate (eg, Citracal), 0.4–0.6 g elemental calcium per day, or calcium carbonate (eg, OsCal, Tums), 1–1.5 g elemental calcium per day. Calcium supplements are best administered with meals.

In hypophosphatemic rickets or osteomalacia, nutritional deficiencies are corrected, aluminum-containing antacids are discontinued, and patients with renal tubular acidosis are given bicarbonate therapy. In patients with sporadic adult-onset hypophosphatemia, hyperphosphaturia, and low serum 1,25(OH)$_2$D levels, a search is conducted for occult tumors that may be resected; whole-body MRI scanning may be required.

For those with X-linked or idiopathic hypophosphatemia and hyperphosphaturia, oral phosphate supplements must be given long-term. Calcitriol, 0.25–0.5 mcg/day, is given also to improve the impaired calcium absorption caused by the oral phosphate. If necessary, rhGH may be added to the above regimen to reduce phosphaturia. The hypophosphatemia of autosomal dominant hypophosphatemic rickets has been reported to resolve with high-dose dietary iron supplementation.

Patients with hypophosphatasia have been treated with teriparatide with improvement in bone pain and fracture healing.

Hollick MF et al. Evaluation, treatment, and prevention of vitamin D deficiency: an Endocrine Society clinical practice guideline. J Clin Endocrinol Metab. 2011 Jul;96(7):1911–30. [PMID: 21646368]

Sahoo J et al. Tumor(s) induced osteomalacia—a curious case of double trouble. J Clin Endocrinol Metab. 2014 Feb;99(2):395–8. [PMID: 24297794]

PAGET DISEASE OF BONE (Osteitis Deformans)

ESSENTIALS OF DIAGNOSIS

► Often asymptomatic.

► Bone pain may be the first symptom.

► Kyphosis, bowed tibias, large head, deafness, and frequent fractures.

► Serum calcium and phosphate normal; alkaline phosphatase elevated; urinary hydroxyproline elevated.

► Dense, expanded bones on radiographs.

► General Considerations

Paget disease is manifested by one or more bony lesions having high bone turnover and disorganized osteoid formation. The involved bone first has increased osteoclast activity, causing lytic lesions in bone that may progress at about 1 cm/year. Increased osteoblastic activity follows, producing a high rate of disorganized bone formation. Involved bones become vascular, weak, and deformed. Eventually, there appears to be a final burned-out phase with markedly reduced bone cell activity and abnormal bones that may be enlarged with skeletal deformity.

The prevalence of Paget disease has declined by about 36% over the past 20 years. However, it remains a common disease in certain countries, with striking geographic variation in prevalence. It is most common in the United Kingdom and in areas of European migration, particularly New Zealand, Australia, the United States, South Africa, Quebec, and Brazil. Interestingly, the disease appears equally common among different races in these countries. In the United States, Paget disease occurs in 2–3% of all individuals over age 55 years, with its prevalence increasing with age. It is uncommon in Africa, Asia, and Scandinavia. Usually diagnosed in patients over age 40 years, its prevalence doubles with each decade thereafter, reaching an incidence of about 10% after age 80. It is most often discovered incidentally during radiology imaging or because of incidentally discovered elevations in serum alkaline phosphatase.

The cause of Paget disease is unknown. However, there is believed to be a genetic component with autosomal dominant transmission; about 20% of affected patients have a first-degree relative with the disease. Mutations in the *SQSTM1* gene have been discovered in 25–50% of cases with familial Paget disease and in 5–10% of patients with apparently sporadic Paget disease.

► Clinical Findings

A. Symptoms and Signs

Paget disease is often mild and asymptomatic. Only 27% of affected individuals are symptomatic at the time of diagnosis. Paget disease involves multiple bones (polyostotic) in 72% and only a single bone (monostotic) in 28%. It occurs most commonly in the pelvis, vertebrae, femur, humerus, and skull. The affected bones are typically involved right away and the disease tends not to involve additional bones during its course. Pain is the usual first symptom. It may occur in the involved bone or in an adjacent joint, which can be involved with degenerative arthritis. The pain is usually described as aching and deep and often worse at night. Paget disease typically first affects long bones proximally and then advances distally, with bone pain at the osteolytic front being aggravated by weight bearing. Joint surfaces (such as the knee) can be involved and cause arthritic pain. The bones can become soft, leading to bowed tibias, kyphosis, and frequent "chalkstick" fractures with slight trauma. If the skull is involved, the patient may report headaches and an increased hat size. Involvement of the petrous temporal bone frequently damages the cochlea and causes hearing loss (mixed sensorineural and conductive) and occasionally tinnitus or vertigo. Increased vascularity over the involved bones causes increased warmth and can cause vascular "steal" syndromes.

B. Laboratory Findings

Serum alkaline phosphatase is usually markedly elevated. However, some patients with limited monostotic involvement may have normal serum alkaline phosphatase levels. A serum bone-specific alkaline phosphatase is usually high and is useful for patients with a normal serum alkaline phosphatase and to distinguish the source of an elevated alkaline phosphatase as being from bone (rather than liver). Other useful measures for bone turnover are serum N-terminal propeptide of type 1 collagen (NTx) and serum betaC-terminal propeptide of type 1 collagen (betaCTx). However, such bone turnover markers may overestimate or underestimate the response to treatment. Serum calcium may be elevated, particularly if the patient is at bed rest. A serum 25-OH vitamin D determination should be obtained to screen for vitamin D deficiency, which can also present with an increased serum alkaline phosphatase and bone pain. Also, any vitamin D deficiency should be corrected before prescribing a bisphosphonate.

C. Imaging

On radiographs, the initial lesions are typically osteolytic, with focal radiolucencies ("osteoporosis circumscripta") in the skull or advancing flame-shaped lytic lesions in long bones. Bone lesions may subsequently become sclerotic and have a mixed lytic and sclerotic appearance. The affected bones eventually become thickened and deformed. Technetium pyrophosphate bone scans are helpful in delineating activity of bone lesions even before any radiologic changes are apparent.

► Differential Diagnosis

Certain rare familial types of sclerosing bone dysplasias share phenotypic homologies with Paget disease of bone. Familial expansile osteolysis, familial early-onset Paget disease, and familial skeletal hyperphosphatasia are autosomal dominant disorders caused by different tandem duplications of the gene encoding RANK, resulting in its constitutive activation. The differential diagnosis also includes myelofibrosis, intramedullary osteosclerosis, Erdheim-Chester disease, Langerhans cell histiocytosis, and sickle cell disease.

Paget disease must be differentiated from primary bone lesions such as osteogenic sarcoma, multiple myeloma, and fibrous dysplasia and from secondary bone lesions such as osteitis fibrosa cystica and metastatic carcinoma to bone. Fibrogenesis imperfecta ossium is a rare symmetric disorder that can mimic the features of Paget disease; serum alkaline phosphatase is likewise elevated. This condition may be associated with paraproteinemias.

► Complications

If immobilization occurs, hypercalcemia and renal calculi may develop. With severe polyostotic disease, the increased vascularity may give rise to high-output heart failure. Arthritis frequently develops in joints adjacent to involved bone.

Extensive skull involvement may cause cranial nerve palsies from impingement of the neural foramina. **Skull involvement** can also cause a vascular steal syndrome with somnolence or ischemic neurologic events; the optic nerve may be affected, resulting in loss of vision. Jaw involvement can cause the teeth to spread intraorally and become misaligned. Vertebral collapse can cause compression of spinal cord or spinal nerves, resulting in radiculopathy or paralysis. **Vertebral involvement** can also cause a vascular steal syndrome with paralysis. Surgery for fractured long bones is often complicated by excessive blood loss from these vascular lytic lesions.

A sarcoma or giant cell tumor may develop in longstanding lesions but is rare (less than 1%). Sarcomatous change is suggested by a marked increase in bone pain, sudden rise in alkaline phosphatase, and appearance of a new lytic lesion.

► Treatment

Asymptomatic patients may require only clinical surveillance and no treatment. However, treatment should be considered for asymptomatic patients who have significant involvement of the skull, long bones, or vertebrae. Patients must be monitored carefully before, during, and after treatment with clinical examinations and serial serum alkaline phosphatase determinations.

Bisphosphonates are used to treat patients with Paget disease. Intravenous zoledronate is the treatment of choice. Administered intravenously as a single 5 mg dose, it normalizes the serum alkaline phosphatase in 89% of patients by 6 months and in 98% by 2 years. Oral bisphosphonate regimens are frankly inferior to intravenous zolendronate.

In order to reduce the risk of intraoperative hemorrhaging and loosening of the prosthesis postoperatively, intravenous zoledronate should be administered prior to total arthroplasty for a Paget-involved joint. Similarly, intravenous zolendronate should be administered before osteotomy for severe bowing of a lower extremity caused by Paget disease. For patients with paraplegia due to vertebral involvement, intravenous zolendronate should be given while neurosurgical consultation is obtained.

Patients frequently experience a paradoxical increase in pain at sites of disease soon after commencing bisphosphonate therapy; this is the "first dose effect" and the pain usually subsides with further treatment. Flu-like symptoms occur fairly frequently. Following intravenous zoledronate, patients frequently experience fever, fatigue, myalgia, bone pain, and ocular problems. Serious side effects are rare but include seizures, uveitis, and acute kidney disease. Hypocalcemia is common and may be severe, especially if intravenous bisphosphonates are given along with loop diuretics. Therefore, it is advisable to administer calcium and vitamin D supplements, especially during the first 2 weeks following treatment. Asthma may occur in aspirin-sensitive patients. To prevent esophageal complications, oral bisphosphonates should be taken with 8 oz of plain water only; they are relatively contraindicated in patients with a history of esophagitis, esophageal stricture, dysphagia, hiatal hernia, or achalasia.

▶ Prognosis

The prognosis in general is good, but relapse can occur after an initial successful treatment with bisphosphonate. By 6.5 years after initial therapy, the recurrence rate is 12.5% after treatment with zoledronate and 62% after risedronate. Therefore, patients must be monitored long-term, measuring serum alkaline phosphatase at least yearly. In general, the prognosis is worse the earlier in life the disease starts. Fractures usually heal well. In the severe forms, marked deformity, intractable pain, and heart failure occur. These complications should become rare with prompt bisphosphonate treatment. Osteosarcoma that arises at sites of Paget disease results in a 2-year survival of only 25%.

Shah M et al. Paget's disease: a clinical review. Br J Hosp Med (Lond). 2015 Jan;76(1):25–30. [PMID: 25585180]
Singer FR et al. Paget's disease of bone: an Endocrine Society clinical practice guideline. J Clin Endocrinol Metab. 2014 Dec; 99(12):4408–22. [PMID: 25406796]

Tan A et al. Clinical presentation of Paget's disease: evaluation of a contemporary cohort and systematic review. Calcif Tissue Int. 2014 Nov;95(5):385–92. [PMID: 25160936]

▼ DISEASES OF THE ADRENAL CORTEX

PRIMARY ADRENAL INSUFFICIENCY (Addison Disease)

ESSENTIALS OF DIAGNOSIS

▶ Weakness, fatigue, anorexia, weight loss; nausea, vomiting, diarrhea; abdominal pain, muscle and joint pains; amenorrhea.

▶ Sparse axillary hair; increased skin pigmentation, especially of creases, pressure areas, and nipples.

▶ Hypotension, small heart.

▶ Serum sodium low; potassium, calcium, and BUN elevated; mild anemia and relative neutropenia, lymphocytosis, and eosinophilia.

▶ Plasma ACTH level elevated; cosyntropin ($ACTH_{1-24}$) unable to stimulate an increase in serum cortisol to 20 mcg/dL or more.

▶ Acute adrenal crisis: above manifestations become critical, along with fever, shock, confusion, coma, death.

▶ General Considerations

Primary adrenal insufficiency (Addison disease) is caused by dysfunction or absence of the adrenal cortices. It is distinct from secondary adrenal insufficiency caused by deficient secretion of ACTH.

Addison disease is an uncommon disorder with a prevalence of about 140 per million and an annual incidence of about 4 per million in the United States. Addison disease is characterized by a chronic deficiency of cortisol. Serum ACTH and alpha-MSH levels are consequently elevated, causing pigmentation that ranges from none to strikingly dark. Patients with destruction of the adrenal cortices or with classic 21-hydroxylase deficiency also have mineralocorticoid deficiency, typically with hyponatremia, volume depletion, and hyperkalemia. In contrast, mineralocorticoid deficiency is not present in patients with familial glucocorticoid deficiency and Allgrove syndrome.

Acute adrenal (addisonian) crisis is an emergency caused by insufficient cortisol. Crisis may occur in the course of treatment of chronic adrenal insufficiency, or it may be the presenting manifestation of adrenal insufficiency. Acute adrenal crisis is more commonly seen in primary adrenal insufficiency than in secondary adrenal insufficiency.

Adrenal crisis may occur in the following situations: (1) during stress, (eg, infection, trauma, surgery, hyperthyroidism, or prolonged fasting) in a patient with latent or treated adrenal insufficiency; (2) following sudden withdrawal of adrenocortical hormone in a patient with chronic insufficiency or in a patient with temporary insufficiency due to suppression by exogenous corticosteroids or megestrol; (3) following bilateral adrenalectomy or removal of a functioning adrenal tumor that had suppressed the other adrenal gland; (4) following sudden destruction of the pituitary gland (pituitary necrosis), or when thyroid hormone is given to a patient with adrenal insufficiency; (5) following injury to both adrenals (by trauma, hemorrhage, anticoagulant therapy, thrombosis, infection or, rarely, metastatic carcinoma); and (6) following administration of intravenous etomidate (used for rapid anesthesia induction or intubation).

▶ Etiology

Autoimmunity is the most common cause of Addison disease in the United States (accounting for about 80% of spontaneous cases). With such autoimmunity, adrenal function decreases over several years as it progresses to overt adrenal insufficiency. It may occur alone or as part of a **polyglandular autoimmune (PGA) syndrome. Type 1 PGA,** also known as autoimmune polyendocrinopathy-candidiasis-ectodermal dystrophy (APECED) syndrome, is caused by a defect in T cell–mediated immunity inherited as an autosomal recessive trait. Type 1 PGA usually presents in early childhood with mucocutaneous candidiasis, followed by hypoparathyroidism and dystrophy of the teeth and nails; Addison disease usually appears by age 15 years. Partial or late expression of the syndrome is common. A varied spectrum of associated diseases may be seen in adulthood, including hypogonadism, hypothyroidism, pernicious anemia, alopecia, vitiligo, hepatitis, malabsorption, and Sjögren syndrome.

Type 2 PGA usually presents in young adults aged 20–40 years, usually women (female:male ratio is 3:1). The following conditions occur in type 2 PGA: autoimmune adrenal insufficiency, type 1 diabetes mellitus, and autoimmune thyroid disease (usually hypothyroidism, sometimes hyperthyroidism). The combination of Addison disease and hypothyroidism is known as Schmidt syndrome. Patients may also have vitiligo, alopecia areata, Sjögren syndrome, or celiac disease. Type 2 PGA is also associated with autoimmune primary ovarian failure; testicular failure (5%); pernicious anemia (4%); and, rarely, autoimmune hypophysitis, encephalitis, or hypoparathyroidism (late-onset).

Infection is a relatively rare cause of Addison disease in the United States but is common in much of the world. Tuberculosis is the most common infection of the adrenals, and parallels its prevalence worldwide. Coccidioidomycosis and other infections are rare causes, particularly in immunocompetent patients.

Bilateral adrenal hemorrhage may occur with sepsis, heparin-associated thrombocytopenia, anticoagulation, or the antiphospholipid antibody syndrome. It may occur in association with major surgery or trauma, presenting about 1 week later with pain, fever, and shock. It may also occur spontaneously and present with flank pain; MRI may show adrenal enlargement with increased T2-weighted imaging. Meningococcemia may be associated with purpura and

adrenal insufficiency secondary to adrenal infarction (Waterhouse-Friderichsen syndrome).

Adrenoleukodystrophy is an X-linked peroxisomal disorder causing accumulation of very long-chain fatty acids in the adrenal cortex, testes, brain, and spinal cord. It may present at any age and accounts for one-third of cases of Addison disease in boys. Aldosterone deficiency occurs in 9%. Hypogonadism is common. Psychiatric symptoms often include mania, psychosis, or cognitive impairment. Neurologic deterioration may be severe or mild (particularly in heterozygote women), mimics symptoms of multiple sclerosis, and can occur years after the onset of adrenal insufficiency.

Rare causes of adrenal insufficiency include lymphoma, metastatic carcinoma, coccidioidomycosis, histoplasmosis, cytomegalovirus infection (more frequent in patients with AIDS), syphilitic gummas, scleroderma, amyloidosis, and hemochromatosis.

Congenital adrenal insufficiency occurs in several conditions. **Familial glucocorticoid deficiency** is an autosomal recessive disease that is caused by mutations in the adrenal ACTH receptor (melanocortin 2 receptor, MC2R). It is characterized by isolated cortisol deficiency and ACTH resistance and may present with neonatal hypoglycemia, frequent infections, and dark skin pigmentation. **Triple A (Allgrove) syndrome** is caused by a mutation in the *AAAS* gene that encodes a protein known as ALADIN (*al*achrima, *a*chalasia, *a*drenal *i*nsufficiency, *n*eurologic disorder). It is characterized by variable expression of the following: adrenal ACTH resistance with cortisol deficiency, achalasia, alacrima, nasal voice, autonomic dysfunction, and neuromuscular disease of varying severity (hyperreflexia to spastic paraplegia). Cortisol deficiency usually presents in infancy but may not occur until the third decade of life. **Congenital adrenal hypoplasia** causes adrenal insufficiency due to absence of the adrenal cortex; patients may also have hypogonadotropic hypogonadism, myopathy, and high-frequency hearing loss.

Congenital adrenal hyperplasia is caused by various genetic defects in the enzymes responsible for steroid synthesis. Due to defective cortisol synthesis, patients have variable degrees of adrenal insufficiency and increased levels of ACTH that causes hyperplasia of the adrenal cortex. The most common enzyme defect is *P450c21 (21-hydroxylase deficiency)*. Patients with severely defective P450c21 (classic congenital adrenal hyperplasia) manifest a deficiency of mineralocorticoids (salt wasting) in addition to deficient cortisol and excessive androgens. Hypertension commonly develops in older adult patients with classic congenital adrenal hyperplasia. Testicular adrenal rests can be found in 44% of men with the condition. Women with milder enzyme defects have adequate cortisol but develop hirsutism in adolescence or adulthood and are said to have "late-onset" congenital adrenal hyperplasia.

Patients with deficient *P450c17 (17-hydroxylase deficiency)* have varying degrees of cortisol deficiency with associated hypertension, hypokalemia, and primary hypogonadism. Severely affected genetic 46 XY males may present with female genitalia at birth (pseudohermaphroditism). The diagnosis is confirmed with high serum levels of

11-deoxycorticosterone and corticosterone. The absence of sex hormones results in primary amenorrhea.

Patients with deficient *P450c11 (11-hydroxylase deficiency)* present at birth with partial virilization and ambiguous genitalia in genetically female infants, childhood virilization in both sexes, and virilization and reduced fertility in adult women. Most patients have hypertension and variable degrees of cortisol deficiency. The diagnosis is established with elevated serum levels of 11-deoxycorticosterone and 11-deoxycortisol.

Drugs that cause primary adrenal insufficiency include mitotane (for adrenocortical carcinoma) and abiraterone acetate (a P450c17 inhibitor used for prostate cancer).

▶ Clinical Findings

A. Symptoms and Signs

The onset of symptoms can present suddenly but usually develops gradually over months or years. The diagnosis is often delayed, since many early symptoms are nonspecific. Nearly all patients complain of fatigue, reduced stamina, weakness, anorexia, and weight loss. Abdominal pain, nausea, and vomiting eventually develop in most patients; diarrhea can occur. Fevers and lymphoid tissue hyperplasia may also occur. Patients often have significant pain: arthralgias, myalgias, chest pain, abdominal pain, back pain, leg pain, or headache. Psychiatric symptoms include anxiety, irritability and depression. Cerebral edema can cause headache, vomiting, gait disturbance, and intellectual dysfunction that may progress to coma. Hypoglycemia can occur and worsen the patient's weakness and mental functioning. Patients often have salt craving and complain of orthostatic light-headedness. Blood pressure is usually low and orthostatic; about 90% have systolic blood pressures under 110 mm Hg; blood pressure over 130 mm Hg is rare. Hypotension is aggravated by dehydration caused by nausea or vomiting.

Skin hyperpigmentation eventually occurs in most patients due to increased pituitary secretion of alpha-MSH (melanocyte-stimulating hormone). Skin hyperpigmentation varies among affected patients (eg, from none to increased freckling to diffuse darkening that resembles a suntan or a bronze appearance). Sun-exposed areas darken the most, but nonexposed areas darken as well. Hyperpigmentation is often especially prominent over the knuckles, elbows, knees, posterior neck, palmar creases, gingival mucosa, and vermilion border of the lips. Nail beds may develop longitudinal pigmented bands. Nipples and areolas tend to darken. The skin also darkens in pressure areas, such as the belt or brassiere lines and the buttocks. Skin folds and new scars may also become pigmented. Conversely, patches of autoimmune vitiligo can be found in about 10% of patients. Scant axillary and pubic hair typically develops in women.

In pregnancy, undiagnosed adrenal insufficiency is rare, since the condition tends to cause anovulation and reduced fertility. In the first trimester, symptoms such as fatigue, nausea, vomiting, abdominal pain, and orthostasis are typically attributed to the pregnancy, thus delaying the diagnosis. Worse, the increased skin pigmentation of adrenal insufficiency may be mistaken for chloasma (melasma). Undiagnosed adrenal insufficiency can cause intrauterine growth retardation and fetal loss. Pregnant women with undiagnosed adrenal insufficiency can experience shock from adrenal crisis, particularly during the first trimester, concurrent illness, labor, or postpartum.

Patients with preexistent type 1 diabetes experience more frequent hypoglycemia with the onset of adrenal insufficiency, such that their insulin dosage must be reduced.

Acute adrenal crisis is an immediate threat to life. Nausea, vomiting, fever, dehydration, and profound hypotension progresses to life-threatening shock that does not fully respond to intravenous fluids and vasopressors.

B. Laboratory Findings

The WBC count typically shows moderate neutropenia, lymphocytosis, and eosinophilia (total eosinophil count over 300/mcL). Among patients with chronic adrenal insufficiency, the serum sodium is usually low (88%) and the potassium usually elevated (64%). (Patients with vomiting or diarrhea may not be hyperkalemic.) Fasting hypoglycemia is common. Hypercalcemia may be present.

A plasma cortisol less than 3 mcg/dL (83 nmol/L) at 8 AM is diagnostic, especially if accompanied by simultaneous elevation of the plasma ACTH level greater than 200 pg/mL (44 pmol/L). The diagnosis is confirmed by a simplified cosyntropin stimulation test: (1) Synthetic $ACTH_{1-24}$ (cosyntropin), 0.25 mg, is given intramuscularly. (2) Serum cortisol is obtained 45 minutes after cosyntropin is administered. Normally, serum cortisol rises to at least 20 mcg/dL (550 pmol/L), whereas patients with adrenal insufficiency have stimulated serum cortisol levels less than 20 mcg (550 pmol/L). For patients receiving corticosteroid treatment, hydrocortisone must not be given for at least 8 hours before the test. Other corticosteroids (eg, prednisone, dexamethasone) do not interfere with specific assays for cortisol. Cortrosyn is a pregnancy class C drug and may be used during pregnancy. However, the test may lack sensitivity, since adrenal ACTH-responsiveness increases during pregnancy.

Serum DHEA levels are less than 1000 ng/mL (350 nmol/L) in 100% of patients with adrenal insufficiency but also in about 15% of the population, so the test is very sensitive but not specific.

Anti-adrenal antibodies are found in the serum in about 50% of cases of autoimmune Addison disease. The presence of serum antibodies to 21-hydroxylase helps secure the diagnosis of autoimmune adrenal insufficiency. Antibodies to thyroid (45%) and other tissues may be present.

Salt-wasting congenital adrenal hyperplasia due to 21-hydroxylase deficiency is usually diagnosed at birth in females due to ambiguous genitalia. Males and patients with milder enzyme defects may present later. The diagnosis of adrenal insufficiency is made as above. The specific diagnosis requires elevated serum levels of 17-OH progesterone.

Elevated plasma renin activity (PRA) indicates the presence of depleted intravascular volume and the need for fludrocortisone administration. Serum epinephrine levels are low in patients with adrenal insufficiency, since these patients do not have the high local concentrations of cortisol that are required to induce the enzyme PNMT in adrenal medulla for the synthesis of epinephrine from norepinephrine.

Young men with idiopathic Addison disease are screened for X-linked adrenoleukodystrophy by determining plasma very long-chain fatty acid levels; affected patients have high levels.

In acute adrenal crisis, blood, sputum, or urine cultures may be positive if bacterial infection is the precipitating cause.

C. Imaging

When adrenal insufficiency is not clearly autoimmune, a CT scan of the adrenal glands should be obtained. Small, noncalcified adrenals are seen in autoimmune Addison disease. The adrenals are enlarged in about 85% of cases related to metastatic or granulomatous disease. Adrenal calcifications occur in about 50% of cases of tuberculous Addison disease but are also seen with hemorrhage, fungal infection, pheochromocytoma, and melanoma.

▶ Differential Diagnosis

Patients with secondary adrenal insufficiency (see Hypopituitarism) lack ACTH and have normal to decreased skin pigmentation that has been described as "alabaster skin". This contrasts with the increased skin pigmentation in patients with Addison disease. The hyperpigmentation may be confused with that due to ethnic or racial factors. Patients with ACTH deficiency have normal mineralocorticoid production and do not develop hyperkalemia. Addison disease should be considered in any patient with unexplained hypotension, but acute adrenal insufficiency must be distinguished from other causes of shock (eg, septic, hemorrhagic, cardiogenic).

Unexplained weight loss, weakness, and anorexia may be mistaken for occult cancer. Nausea, vomiting, diarrhea, and abdominal pain may be misdiagnosed as intrinsic gastrointestinal disease. Acute adrenal insufficiency must be distinguished from an acute abdomen in which neutrophilia is the rule, whereas in adrenal insufficiency there is lymphocytosis and eosinophilia. Weight loss may simulate anorexia nervosa or emotional stress. The neurologic manifestations of Allgrove syndrome and adrenoleukodystrophy (especially in women) may mimic multiple sclerosis. Hemochromatosis also causes bronze skin hyperpigmentation, but hemochromatosis may in fact be the cause of Addison disease. About 17% of patients with AIDS have symptoms of cortisol resistance. AIDS can also cause frank adrenal insufficiency.

Hyperkalemia can be caused by hyporeninemic hypoaldosteronism related to type IV renal tubular acidosis. Hyperkalemia is also seen with gastrointestinal bleeding, rhabdomyolysis, hyperkalemic paralysis, and certain drugs (eg, angiotensin-converting enzyme [ACE] inhibitors, spironolactone, and drospirenone).

Hyponatremia is seen in many other conditions (eg, hypothyroidism, diuretic use, heart failure, cirrhosis, vomiting, diarrhea, severe illness, or major surgery). Nearly 40% of critically ill patients have low serum cortisol levels due to low serum albumin levels, such that their total serum cortisol levels may be low but their serum free cortisol levels are normal.

▶ Complications

Any of the complications of the underlying disease (eg, tuberculosis) are more likely to occur in adrenal insufficiency, and intercurrent infections may precipitate an acute adrenal crisis. Associated autoimmune diseases are common (see above).

▶ Treatment

A. General Measures

Patients with Addison disease must be thoroughly informed about their condition. Patients are advised to wear a medical alert bracelet or medal reading, "Adrenal insufficiency—takes hydrocortisone." All infections should be treated immediately and vigorously, with hydrocortisone administered at appropriately increased doses.

B. Specific Therapy

Replacement therapy should include a combination of glucocorticoids and mineralocorticoids. In mild cases, glucocorticoids alone may be adequate.

1. Glucocorticoid replacement therapy—Maintenance therapy for most patients with Addison disease involves 15–30 mg of hydrocortisone orally daily in two divided doses, two-thirds in the morning and one-third in the late afternoon or early evening. Some patients respond better to prednisone (available in 1 mg tablets) or methylprednisolone (4 mg tablets) in doses of about 2–4 mg orally in the morning and 1–2 mg in the evening. Adjustments in dosage are made according to the clinical response. Plenadren (5 or 20 mg modified-release tablets) is a once-daily dual-release preparation of hydrocortisone that may be administered once daily in the morning (usual dose range is 20–30 mg); it is not available in the United States.

A proper glucocorticoid dose usually results in clinical improvement, a normal WBC count differential, and no manifestations of Cushing syndrome. Serum ACTH levels vary substantially and should not be used to determine dosing. The dose of glucocorticoid should be raised in case of infection, trauma, surgery, stressful diagnostic procedures, or other forms of stress. With infection, note that rifampin increases the clearance of hydrocortisone and necessitates increased dosing of hydrocortisone by up to 50%. During the third trimester of pregnancy, glucocorticoid requirements are higher, so usual glucocorticoid doses are increased by 50%. For severe stress of major illness, surgery, or delivery, a maximum stress dose of hydrocortisone is given as 50–100 mg intravenously or intramuscularly, followed by 50 mg every 6 hours. Lower doses, oral or parenteral, are used for less severe stress. The dose is reduced back to normal as the stress subsides.

2. Mineralocorticoid replacement therapy—**Fludrocortisone acetate** has a potent sodium-retaining effect. The dosage is 0.05–0.3 mg orally daily or every other day. In the presence of postural hypotension, hyponatremia, or hyperkalemia, the dosage is increased. Similarly, in patients with fatigue, an elevated PRA indicates the need for a higher replacement dose of fludrocortisone. If edema, hypokalemia, or hypertension ensues, the dose is decreased. During treatment with hydrocortisone with maximum doses appropriate for stress, fludrocortisone replacement is not required. Some patients cannot tolerate fludrocortisone and must substitute NaCl tablets to replace renal sodium loss.

DHEA is given to some women with adrenal insufficiency. In a double-blind clinical trial, women taking DHEA 50 mg orally each morning experienced an improved sense of well-being, increased muscle mass, and a reversal in bone loss at the femoral neck. DHEA replacement did not improve fatigue, cognitive problems, or sexual dysfunction; however, its placebo effect may be significant in that regard. Older women who receive DHEA should be monitored for androgenic effects. Because over-the-counter preparations of DHEA have variable potencies, it is best to have the pharmacy formulate this with pharmaceutical-grade micronized DHEA.

3. Acute adrenal crisis therapy—If acute adrenal crisis is suspected but the diagnosis of adrenal insufficiency is not yet established, blood is drawn for routine emergency laboratory tests and blood cultures, as well as serum cortisol and ACTH levels. Without waiting for the results, treatment is initiated *immediately* with hydrocortisone phosphate or hydrocortisone sodium succinate 100–300 mg intravenously along with saline solution. Thereafter, hydrocortisone is continued as intravenous infusions of 50–100 mg every 6 hours for the first day. The dosage may then be reduced according to the clinical picture and laboratory test results.

Since bacterial infection frequently precipitates acute adrenal crisis, broad-spectrum antibiotics should be administered empirically while waiting for the results of initial cultures. The patient must also be treated for electrolyte abnormalities, hypoglycemia, and dehydration, as indicated.

When the patient is able to take food by mouth, hydrocortisone is administered orally in doses of 10–20 mg every 6 hours, and the dosage is reduced to maintenance levels as needed. Most patients ultimately require hydrocortisone twice daily (10–20 mg in am; 5–10 mg in pm). Mineralocorticoid replacement is not needed when large amounts of hydrocortisone are being given, but as its dose is reduced it is usually necessary to add fludrocortisone acetate, 0.05–0.2 mg orally daily. Some patients never require fludrocortisone or become edematous at doses of more than 0.05 mg once or twice weekly. Once the crisis has passed, the patient must be evaluated to assess the degree of permanent adrenal insufficiency and to establish the cause, if possible.

▶ Prognosis

The life expectancy of patients with Addison disease is reasonably normal, as long as they are compliant with their medications and knowledgeable about their condition.

However, one retrospective Swedish study of 1675 patients with Addison disease found an unexpected increase in all-cause mortality, mostly from cardiovascular disease, malignancy, and infection. Associated conditions can pose additional health risks. For example, patients with adrenoleukodystrophy or Allgrove syndrome may suffer from neurologic disease. Patients with adrenal tuberculosis have a serious systemic infection that requires treatment. Adrenal crisis can occur in patients who stop their medication or who experience stress such as infection, trauma, or surgery without appropriately higher doses of corticosteroids. Patients who take excessive doses of corticosteroid replacement can develop Cushing syndrome, which imposes its own risks.

Most patients with Addison disease are able to live fully active lives. However, some patients feel residual fatigue, despite glucocorticoid and mineralocorticoid replacement. This may be due, in part, to the inadequacy of oral replacement to duplicate cortisol's normal circadian rhythm. Also, patients with Addison disease are deficient in epinephrine, but replacement epinephrine is not available. Fatigue may also be an indication of suboptimal dosing of medication, electrolyte imbalance, or concurrent hypothyroidism or diabetes mellitus.

For patients with acute adrenal crisis, rapid treatment is usually lifesaving. However, if adrenal crisis is unrecognized and untreated, shock that is unresponsive to fluid replacement and vasopressors can result in death.

Allolio B. Extensive expertise in endocrinology. Adrenal crisis. Eur J Endocrinol. 2015 Mar;172(3):R115–24. [PMID: 25288693]

Charmandari E et al. Adrenal insufficiency. Lancet. 2014 Jun 21; 383(9935):2152–67. [PMID: 24503135]

Husebye ES et al. Consensus statement on the diagnosis, treatment and follow-up of patients with primary adrenal insufficiency. J Intern Med. 2014 Feb;275(2):104–15. [PMID: 24330030]

Tiemensma J et al. Psychological morbidity and impaired quality of life in patients with stable treatment for primary adrenal insufficiency: cross-sectional study and review of the literature. Eur J Endocrinol. 2014 Aug;171(2):171–82. [PMID: 24801589]

Yuen KC et al. Adrenal insufficiency in pregnancy: challenging issues in diagnosis and management. Endocrine. 2013 Oct; 44(2):283–92. [PMID: 23377701]

CUSHING SYNDROME (Hypercortisolism)

ESSENTIALS OF DIAGNOSIS

▶ Central obesity, muscle wasting, thin skin, hirsutism, purple striae.

▶ Psychological changes.

▶ Osteoporosis, hypertension, poor wound healing.

▶ Hyperglycemia, glycosuria, leukocytosis, lymphocytopenia, hypokalemia.

▶ Elevated serum cortisol and urinary free cortisol. Lack of normal suppression by dexamethasone.

General Considerations

The term Cushing "syndrome" refers to the manifestations of excessive corticosteroids, commonly due to supraphysiologic doses of corticosteroid drugs and rarely due to spontaneous production of excessive corticosteroids by the adrenal cortex. Cases of spontaneous Cushing syndrome are rare (2.6 new cases yearly per million population in the United States) and have several possible causes.

About 40% of cases are due to Cushing "disease," by which is meant the manifestations of hypercortisolism due to ACTH hypersecretion by the pituitary. Cushing disease is caused by a benign pituitary adenoma that is typically smaller than 5 mm and usually located in the anterior pituitary (98%) or in the posterior pituitary (2%). It is at least three times more frequent in women than men. Excessive ingestion of gamma-hydroxybutyric acid (GHB, sodium oxybate) can also induce ACTH-dependent Cushing syndrome that resolves after the drug is stopped.

About 10% of cases are due to nonpituitary ACTH-secreting neuroendocrine neoplasms that produce excessive amounts of ectopic ACTH. Hypokalemia and hyperpigmentation are commonly found in this group. Ectopic locations include the lungs (55%), pancreas (9%), mediastinum-thymus (8%), adrenal (6%), gastrointestinal tract (5%), thyroid (4%), and other sites (13%). About 15% of cases are due to ACTH from a source that cannot be initially located.

About 30% of cases are due to excessive autonomous secretion of cortisol by the adrenals—independently of ACTH, serum levels of which are usually low. Most such cases are due to a unilateral adrenal tumor. Benign adrenal adenomas are generally small and produce mostly cortisol; adrenocortical carcinomas are usually large when discovered and can produce excessive cortisol as well as androgens but may be nonsecretory. ACTH-independent macronodular adrenal hyperplasia can also produce hypercortisolism due to the adrenal cortex cells' abnormal stimulation by hormones such as catecholamines, arginine vasopressin, serotonin, hCG/LH, or gastric inhibitory polypeptide; in the latter case, hypercortisolism may be intermittent and food dependent and serum ACTH may not be completely suppressed. Bilateral primary pigmented adrenal macronodular adrenocortical disease is a rare cause of Cushing syndrome in children and young adults. Bilateral primary pigmented adrenal macronodular adrenocortical disease may be an isolated condition or part of the **Carney complex,** an autosomal dominant condition with additional features consisting of myxomas of the heart and skin with spotty skin pigmentation and facial freckles.

Clinical Findings

A. Symptoms and Signs

The manifestations of Cushing syndrome vary considerably. Early in the course of the disease, patients frequently complain of fatigue or reduced endurance but may have few, if any, of the physical stigmata described below. Central obesity with a plethoric "moon face," "buffalo hump," supraclavicular fat pads, protuberant abdomen, and thin extremities eventually develop in most patients with Cushing syndrome. Muscle atrophy causes weakness, with difficulty standing up from a seated position or climbing stairs. Patients may also experience backache, headache, hypertension, osteoporosis, avascular necrosis of bone, acne, superficial skin infections, and oligomenorrhea or amenorrhea in women or erectile dysfunction in men. Patients may have thirst and polyuria (with or without glycosuria), renal calculi, glaucoma, purple striae (especially around the thighs, breasts, and abdomen), and easy bruisability. Unusual bacterial or fungal infections are common. Wound healing is impaired. Mental symptoms may range from diminished ability to concentrate to increased lability of mood to frank psychosis. Patients are susceptible to opportunistic infections.

Adrenocortical carcinomas can usually be distinguished from benign adrenal adenomas since they are usually larger (average 11 cm diameter) and many have metastases that are visible on preoperative scans. However, some adrenal carcinomas are smaller and the histopathologic diagnosis can be difficult. Some adrenal carcinomas have microscopic metastases that can only be inferred from the presence of detectable cortisol levels following removal of the primary adrenal tumor. The ENSAT staging system is used: stage 1 is a localized tumor 5 cm or smaller; stage 2 is a localized tumor larger than 5 cm; stage 3, tumor with local metastases; stage 4, tumor with distant metastases.

B. Laboratory Findings

Glucose tolerance is impaired as a result of insulin resistance. Polyuria is present as a result of increased free water clearance; diabetes mellitus with glycosuria may worsen it. Patients with Cushing syndrome often have leukocytosis with relative granulocytosis and lymphopenia. Hypokalemia may be present, particularly in cases of ectopic ACTH secretion.

Tests for Hypercortisolism

The biochemical evaluation for Cushing syndrome can be difficult, since test results are often misleading or conflicting. The **dexamethasone suppression test** is the easiest screening test for Cushing syndrome. Dexamethasone 1 mg is given orally at 11 PM and serum is collected for cortisol determination at 8 AM the next morning; a cortisol level less than 5 mcg/dL (135 nmol/L, fluorometric assay) or less than 1.8 mcg/dL (49 nmol/L, high-performance liquid chromatography [HPLC] assay) excludes Cushing syndrome with some certainty. However, 8% of established patients with pituitary Cushing disease have dexamethasone-suppressed cortisol levels less than 2 mcg/dL (55 nmol/L). Therefore, when other clinical criteria suggest hypercortisolism, further evaluation is warranted even in the face of normal dexamethasone-suppressed serum cortisol. Antiseizure drugs (eg, phenytoin, phenobarbital, primidone) and rifampin accelerate the metabolism of dexamethasone, causing a lack of cortisol suppression by dexamethasone. Estrogens—during pregnancy or as oral contraceptives or HRT—may also cause lack of dexamethasone suppressibility.

A 24-hour urinary free cortisol and creatinine is the usual confirmatory test for patients with an abnormal dexamethasone suppression test. An abnormally high 24-hour urine free cortisol (or free cortisol to creatinine ratio of greater than 95 mcg cortisol/g creatinine helps confirm hypercortisolism. A misleadingly high urine free cortisol excretion occurs with high fluid intake. In pregnancy, urine free cortisol is increased, while 17-hydroxycorticosteroids remain normal and diurnal variability of serum cortisol is normal. Carbamazepine and fenofibrate cause false elevations of urine free cortisol when determined by HPLC. **Late-night salivary cortisol** assays are useful due to the inconvenience of obtaining a midnight blood specimen for serum cortisol. Late-night salivary cortisol levels are normally less than 150 ng/dL (4.0 nmol/L). Late-night salivary cortisol levels that are consistently greater than 250 ng/dL (7.0 nmol/L) are considered very abnormal. The late-night salivary cortisol test has a relatively high sensitivity and specificity for Cushing syndrome, but false-positive and false-negative tests occur.

Midnight serum cortisol levels greater than 7.5 mcg/dL (200 nmol/L) are indicative of Cushing syndrome and distinguish it from other conditions associated with a high urine free cortisol (pseudo-Cushing states). Requirements for this test include being in the same time zone for at least 3 days, being without food for at least 3 hours, and having an indwelling intravenous line established in advance for the blood draw.

Finding the Cause of Hypercortisolism

Once hypercortisolism is confirmed, a plasma or serum ACTH is obtained. It must be collected properly in a plastic tube on ice and processed quickly by a laboratory with a reliable, sensitive assay. A level of ACTH below 20 pg/mL (4.4 pmol/L) indicates a probable adrenal tumor, whereas higher levels are produced by pituitary or ectopic ACTH-secreting tumors.

Localizing Techniques

In ACTH-independent Cushing syndrome, CT of the adrenals usually detects a mass lesion. Most such lesions are benign adrenal adenomas, but an adrenal carcinoma is suspected in the following circumstances: (1) diameter of 4 cm or more; (2) nodule growth; or (3) atypical imaging: density on noncontrast CT greater than 10 Hounsfield units (HU) or CT contrast washout 60% or more or relative contrast washout 40% or more at 15 minutes after intravenous administration.

In ACTH-dependent Cushing syndrome, MRI of the pituitary demonstrates a pituitary lesion in about 50% of cases. Premature cerebral atrophy is often noted. When the pituitary MRI is normal or shows a tiny (less than 5 mm diameter) irregularity that may be incidental, selective catheterization of the inferior petrosal sinus veins draining the pituitary is performed. ACTH levels in the inferior petrosal sinus that are more than twice the simultaneous peripheral venous ACTH levels are indicative of pituitary Cushing disease. Inferior petrosal sinus sampling is also done during ovine CRH (oCRH or Acthrel) administration, which

ordinarily causes the ACTH levels in the inferior petrosal sinus to be over three times the peripheral ACTH level when the pituitary is the source of ACTH.

When inferior petrosal sinus ACTH concentrations are not above the requisite levels, a search for an ectopic source of ACTH is undertaken. Location of ectopic sources of ACTH commences with CT scanning of the chest and abdomen, with special attention to the lungs (for carcinoid or small cell carcinomas), the thymus, the pancreas, and the adrenals. In patients with ACTH-dependent Cushing syndrome, chest masses should not be assumed to be the source of ACTH, since opportunistic infections are common, so it is prudent to biopsy a chest mass to confirm the pathologic diagnosis prior to resection.

For Cushing syndrome due to ectopic ACTH, CT scanning fails to detect the source of ACTH in about 34% of cases. In such cases, the most sensitive (82%) scanning technique is whole-body imaging with ^{68}Ga-somatostatin receptor-PET/CT (either ^{68}Ga-DOTATOTATE-PET/CT or ^{68}Ga-DOTATOC-PET/CT). The next most sensitive (58%) scanning technique is whole-body imaging with ^{18}F-DOPA-PET/CT.

In non-ACTH-dependent Cushing syndrome, a CT scan of the adrenals can localize the adrenal tumor in most cases.

Differential Diagnosis

Alcoholic patients can have hypercortisolism and many clinical manifestations of Cushing syndrome. Pregnant women have elevated serum ACTH levels, increased urine free cortisol, and high serum cortisol levels due to high serum levels of cortisol-binding globulin. Critically ill patients frequently have hypercortisolism, usually with suppression of serum ACTH. Regular use of gamma hydroxybutyrate (GHB, sodium oxybate) has been reported to cause reversible ACTH-dependent Cushing syndrome. Depressed patients also have hypercortisolism that can be nearly impossible to distinguish biochemically from Cushing syndrome but without clinical signs of Cushing syndrome. Cushing syndrome can be misdiagnosed as anorexia nervosa (and vice versa) owing to the muscle wasting and extraordinarily high urine free cortisol levels found in anorexia. Patients with severe obesity frequently have an abnormal dexamethasone suppression test, but the urine free cortisol is usually normal, as is diurnal variation of serum cortisol. Patients with familial cortisol resistance have hyperandrogenism, hypertension, and hypercortisolism without actual Cushing syndrome.

Some adolescents develop violaceous striae on the abdomen, back, and breasts; these are known as "striae distensae" and are not indicative of Cushing syndrome. Patients with familial partial lipodystrophy type I develop central obesity and moon facies, along with thin extremities due to atrophy of subcutaneous fat. However, these patients' muscles are strong and may be hypertrophic, distinguishing this condition from Cushing syndrome. Patients receiving antiretroviral therapy for HIV-1 infection frequently develop partial lipodystrophy with thin extremities and central obesity with a dorsocervical fat pad ("buffalo hump") causing pseudo-Cushing syndrome.

Adrenal nodules are discovered incidentally on up to 4% of abdominal CT or MRI scans obtained for other reasons; they have been dubbed **"adrenal incidentalomas."** It is always necessary to determine whether such masses are malignant or secretory. Although the overwhelming majority of adrenal incidentalomas are benign adrenal adenomas, the differential diagnosis includes adrenal carcinoma, pheochromocytoma, metastases, lymphoma, myelolipoma, infection, and cysts. When an adrenal incidentaloma larger than 4 cm in diameter is detected in a patient without a history of malignancy, it should be resected, unless it is an unmistakably benign myelolipoma, hemorrhage, or adrenal cyst. Masses 3–4 cm in diameter may be resected if they have suspicious features (heterogeneity or irregularity). Smaller adrenal incidentalomas are usually observed. A noncontrast CT scan can determine the density of the mass; adrenal incidentalomas with a density less than 10 HU on CT are unlikely to be a pheochromocytoma or metastasis. An adrenal intravenous contrast "washout" CT scan is obtained; the density of the adrenal incidentaloma in HU is calculated 60 seconds after contrast and again 15 minutes after contrast; a reduction (washout) of 40% or more is consistent with a benign adrenal adenoma. However, such testing is never absolutely accurate; so if the adrenal incidentaloma is not resected, a follow-up CT of the adrenals in 6–12 months is recommended to look for growth.

All patients with an adrenal nodule require a clinical assessment for Cushing syndrome and hyperaldosteronism. In particular, patients with hypertension or any possible manifestations of Cushing syndrome require an appropriate biochemical evaluation. All (even normotensive) patients with an adrenal incidentaloma require testing for pheochromocytoma with plasma fractionated free metanephrines.

▶ Treatment

Patients with Cushing syndrome of any etiology face a high complication rate after treatment and all patients require intensive clinical care and close follow-up. All patients and their families must receive thorough education about the effects of Cushing syndrome and its treatment. Patients must receive treatment for cortisol-dependent comorbidities, including osteoporosis, psychiatric disorders, diabetes mellitus, hypertension, hypokalemia, muscle weakness, and infections. Affected patients should also receive vaccinations against influenza, pneumococcus, and herpes zoster. All patients undergoing surgery should have prophylaxis against venous thromboembolism.

A. Surgical Therapy

Pituitary Cushing disease is best treated with transsphenoidal selective resection of the pituitary adenoma. With an experienced pituitary neurosurgeon, reported remission rates range from 65% to 90%. Postoperative hyponatremia occurs frequently, so serum sodium should be monitored frequently for the first 2 weeks postoperatively. The patient should be screened for secondary hypothyroidism with a serum free T_4 within 1–2 weeks after surgery. After successful pituitary surgery, the rest of the pituitary usually returns to normal function; however, the pituitary corticotrophs remain suppressed and require 6–36 months to recover normal function. Therefore, patients receive empiric replacement-dose hydrocortisone postoperatively. Postoperative secondary adrenal insufficiency is a mark of successful pituitary surgery; screening may include a morning serum cortisol 6–8 hours following the prior evening dose of hydrocortisone. The cosyntropin test becomes abnormal by 2 weeks following successful pituitary surgery. Patients with secondary adrenal insufficiency require patient education about the condition and must continue glucocorticoid replacement until a cosyntropin stimulation test is normal. A pituitary MRI should be obtained within 2–3 months postoperatively and repeated as indicated for clinical evidence of recurrent Cushing disease or Nelson syndrome.

Cushing disease may persist after pituitary surgery, particularly when there has been cavernous sinus involvement. After apparent successful pituitary surgery, Cushing disease recurs in 16% after a mean of 38 months. Patients must have repeated evaluations for recurrent Cushing disease for years postoperatively. For patients with persistent or recurrent Cushing disease, repeat transsphenoidal pituitary surgery may be warranted if the recurrent tumor is visible and deemed resectable. Otherwise, bilateral laparoscopic adrenalectomy is usually the best treatment option, particularly for patients with very severe disease, since it renders an immediate remission in a condition with significant morbidity and mortality. Residual or recurrent ACTH-secreting pituitary tumors may also be treated with stereotactic radiosurgery, which normalizes urine free cortisol in 70% of patients within a mean of 17 months, compared with a 23% remission rate with conventional radiation therapy. Pituitary radiosurgery can also be used to treat Nelson syndrome, the progressive enlargement of ACTH-secreting pituitary tumors following bilateral adrenalectomy.

Benign adrenal adenomas may be resected laparoscopically if they are smaller than 6 cm in diameter; cure is achieved in most patients. However, most patients experience prolonged secondary adrenal insufficiency. Patients with bilateral adrenal macronodular hyperplasia usually require bilateral adrenalectomies and an evaluation for Carney complex that can be confirmed with a genetic evaluation for activating mutations in the gene *PRKAR1A* or genetic changes at chromosome 2p16. Such patients require regular screening for testicular and thyroid tumors and frequent echocardiogram screening for atrial myxomas.

Adrenal carcinomas are resected surgically. Postoperative secondary adrenal insufficiency is a good prognostic sign, with an increased chance that the tumor was completely resected without metastases. However, the postoperative presence of detectable cortisol indicates metastases or residual tumor. Most patients are treated postoperatively with mitotane for 2–5 years, since it improves survival. Mitotane is given orally with meals, beginning with 0.5 g twice daily, increasing to 1 g twice daily within 2 weeks, with subsequent increased doses every 2–3 weeks to reach serum levels of 14–20 mcg/mL. Unfortunately, only half the patients are able to reach these levels due to side effects. Mitotane can cause hypogonadism and can suppress TSH and cause hypothyroidism. Mitotane often causes primary adrenal insufficiency. Replacement hydrocortisone or prednisone should be started when mitotane doses reach 2 g daily. The replacement dose of hydrocortisone starts at 15 mg in the morning and 10 mg in the afternoon, but must often be doubled or tripled because mitotane increases cortisol metabolism and cortisol binding globulin levels; the latter can artifactually raise serum cortisol levels. Other chemotherapy regimens have been used, usually adding etoposide to mitotane. When this regimen fails, chemotherapy with cisplatin (alone or with other agents) is usually used.

Ectopic ACTH-secreting tumors should be located, when possible, and surgically resected. If that cannot be done, laparoscopic bilateral adrenalectomy is usually recommended. Medical treatment with a combination of mitotane (3–5 g/24 h), ketoconazole (0.4–1.2 g/24 h), and metyrapone (3–4.5 g/24 h) often suppresses the hypercortisolism. Octreotide LAR, 20–40 mg injected intramuscularly every 28 days, suppresses ACTH secretion in about one-third of such cases. Pasireotide may prove more effective. Potassium-sparing diuretics are often helpful.

Patients who are successfully surgically treated for Cushing syndrome typically develop "cortisol withdrawal syndrome," even when given replacement corticosteroids for adrenal insufficiency. Manifestations can include hypotension, nausea, fatigue, arthralgias, myalgias, pruritus, and flaking skin. Increasing the hydrocortisone replacement to 30 mg orally twice daily can improve these symptoms; the dosage is then reduced slowly as tolerated. Patients with Cushing syndrome are prone to develop osteoporosis. Bone densitometry is recommended for all patients and treatment is commenced for patients with osteoporosis.

B. Medical Therapy

1. Cushing syndrome—For patients with Cushing syndrome who decline surgery or for whom surgery has been unsuccessful, medical therapy is available. Mineralocorticoid hypertension can be treated with spironolactone, eplerenone, and dihydroperidine calcium channel blockers. Women with hyperandrogenism may be treated with flutamide. Cabergoline, 0.5–3.5 mg orally twice weekly, was successful in 40% of patients with Cushing disease in one small study. Pasireotide, a multireceptor-targeting somatostatin analog, is another potential treatment for refractory ACTH-secreting pituitary tumors causing Cushing disease or Nelson syndrome. Ketoconazole inhibits adrenal steroidogenesis and is another treatment option when given in doses of about 200 mg orally every 6 hours; however, it is marginally effective and can cause liver toxicity.

2. Hypercortisolism—Metyrapone can also suppress hypercortisolism; required median daily doses were 1250-1500 mg/d in divided doses. It may be combined with ketoconazole. Metyrapone also may be used for patients with secretory adrenalcortical carcinoma whose hypercortisolism is not fully controlled with mitotane.

► Prognosis

The manifestations of Cushing syndrome regress with time, but patients are often left with residual cognitive or psychiatric impairment, muscle weakness, osteoporosis, and sequelae from vertebral fractures. Continued impaired quality of life is more common in women compared to men. Younger patients have a better chance for full recovery.

Patients with Cushing syndrome from a benign adrenal adenoma experience a 5-year survival of 95% and a 10-year survival of 90%, following a successful adrenalectomy. Patients with Cushing disease from a pituitary adenoma experience a similar survival if their pituitary surgery is successful, which can be predicted if the postoperative nonsuppressed serum cortisol is less than 2 mcg/dL (55 nmol/L). Following successful treatment, overall mortality remains particularly higher for patients with older age at diagnosis, higher preoperative ACTH concentrations, and longer duration of hypercortisolism.

Transsphenoidal surgery incurs a failure rate of about 10–20%, often due to the adenoma's ectopic position or invasion of the cavernous sinus. Those patients who have a complete remission after transsphenoidal surgery have about a 15–20% chance of recurrence over the next 10 years. Patients with failed pituitary surgery may require pituitary radiation therapy, which has its own morbidity. Laparoscopic bilateral adrenalectomy may be required. Recurrence of hypercortisolism may occur as a result of growth of an adrenal remnant stimulated by high levels of ACTH. The prognosis for patients with ectopic ACTH-producing tumors depends on the aggressiveness and stage of the particular tumor. Patients with ACTH of unknown source have a 5-year survival rate of 65% and a 10-year survival rate of 55%.

In patients with adrenocortical carcinoma, 5-year survival rates of treated patients have correlated with the ENSAT stage. For stage 1, the 5-year survival was 81%; for stage 2, 61%; for stage 3, 50%; and for stage 4, 13%. In patients with stage 1 or 2 disease, long-term survival does occur. However, despite apparent complete resection in stage 1, 2 or 3 tumors, visible metastases develop in about 40% of patients within 2 years. Adjuvant therapy with mitotane appears to improve the prognosis. Patients with stage 4 disease at the time of surgery have a poorer prognosis, but debulking surgery and therapy with mitotane may be beneficial.

► Complications

Cushing syndrome, if untreated, produces serious morbidity and even death. The patient may suffer from the complications of hypertension or diabetes mellitus. Susceptibility to infections is increased. Compression fractures of the osteoporotic spine and aseptic necrosis of the femoral head may cause marked disability. Nephrolithiasis and psychosis may occur. Following bilateral adrenalectomy for Cushing disease, a pituitary adenoma may enlarge progressively (Nelson syndrome), causing local destruction (eg, visual field impairment, cranial nerve palsy) and hyperpigmentation. Following successful therapy for Cushing syndrome, secondary adrenal insufficiency occurs and requires long-term glucocorticoid replacement. Five years after successful surgery, secondary hypoadrenalism resolves in about 58% of patients with pituitary Cushing disease, 82% of those with ectopic ACTH, and only 38% of those who had an adrenal tumor.

▶ When to Refer

Dexamethasone suppression test is abnormal.

▶ When to Admit

- Transsphenoidal hypophysectomy.
- Adrenalectomy.
- Resection of ectopic ACTH-secreting tumor.

Bansal V et al. Pitfalls in the diagnosis and management of Cushing's syndrome. Neurosurg Focus. 2015 Feb;38(2):E4. [PMID: 25639322]

Berr CM et al. Time to recovery of adrenal function after curative surgery for Cushing's syndrome depends on etiology. J Clin Endocrinol Metab. 2015 Apr;100(4):1300–8. [PMID: 25546155]

Bons J et al. Adrenal disorders in human immunodeficiency virus (HIV) infected patients. Ann Endocrinol (Paris). 2013 Dec; 74(5–6):508–14. [PMID: 24262982]

Bronstein MD et al. Management of endocrine disease: Management of pregnant patients with Cushing's syndrome. Eur J Endocrinol. 2015 Aug;173(2):R85–91. [PMID: 25872515]

Isidori AM et al; ABC Study Group. Conventional and nuclear medicine imaging in ectopic Cushing's syndrome: a systematic review. J Clin Endocrinol Metab. 2015 Sep;100(9):3231–44. [PMID: 26158607]

Nieman LK et al. Treatment of Cushing's syndrome: an Endocrine Society clinical practice guideline. J Clin Endocrinol Metab. 2015 Aug;100(8):2807–31. [PMID: 26222757]

Starkman MN. Neuropsychiatric findings in Cushing syndrome and exogenous glucocorticoid administration. Endocrinol Metab Clin North Am. 2013 Sep;42(3):477–88. [PMID: 24011881]

Tritos NA et al. Update on radiation therapy in patients with Cushing's disease. Pituitary. 2015 Apr;18(2):263–8. [PMID: 25359445]

PRIMARY ALDOSTERONISM

ESSENTIALS OF DIAGNOSIS

- ▶ Hypertension that may be severe or drug-resistant.
- ▶ Hypokalemia (in minority of patients) may cause polyuria, polydipsia, muscle weakness.
- ▶ Low plasma renin; elevated plasma and urine aldosterone levels.

▶ General Considerations

Primary aldosteronism (hyperaldosteronism) refers to an inappropriately high aldosterone secretion that does not suppress adequately with sodium loading. Most affected patients have hypertension, although some may be normotensive. Primary aldosteronism is believed to account for 8–10% of all cases of hypertension and 20% of cases of resistant hypertension. It should be suspected with early-onset hypertension or stroke before age 50 years (or both). It may be difficult to distinguish primary aldosteronism from cases of low renin essential hypertension, with which it may overlap. Patients of all ages may be affected, but the peak incidence is between 30 years and 60 years. Excessive aldosterone production increases sodium retention and suppresses plasma renin. It increases renal potassium excretion, which can lead to hypokalemia. Cardiovascular events are more prevalent in patients with aldosteronism (35%) than in those with essential hypertension (11%). Primary aldosteronism may be caused by a unilateral aldosterone-producing adrenal adenoma (Conn syndrome), 40% of which have been found to have somatic mutations in a gene involved with the potassium channel. Primary aldosteronism is most commonly caused by unilateral or bilateral adrenal hyperplasia. Bilateral aldosteronism may be corticosteroid suppressible, due to an autosomal-dominant genetic defect allowing ACTH stimulation of aldosterone production. Malignant ovarian tumors are a rare cause of hyperaldosteronism.

▶ Clinical Findings

A. Symptoms and Signs

Primary aldosteronism is the most common cause of refractory hypertension in youths and middle-aged adults. Patients have hypertension that is typically moderate but may be severe. Some patients have only diastolic hypertension, without other symptoms and signs. Edema is rarely seen in primary aldosteronism. About 37% of patients have hypokalemia that may be spontaneous or triggered by diuretic therapy. Hypokalemia can produce muscle weakness (at times with paralysis simulating periodic paralysis), paresthesias with frank tetany, headache, polyuria, and polydipsia.

B. Laboratory Findings

Plasma potassium should be determined in hypertensive individuals. However, hypokalemia, once thought to be the hallmark of hyperaldosteronism, is present in only 37% of affected patients: 50% of those with an adrenal adenoma and 17% of those with adrenal hyperplasia. Besides hypokalemia, many patients with primary aldosteronism have metabolic alkalosis with an elevated serum bicarbonate (HCO_3) concentration.

Testing for primary aldosteronism should be done for all hypertensive patients with (1) hypokalemia, whether spontaneous or diuretic induced; (2) treatment-resistant hypertension (despite three drugs); (3) severe hypertension: greater than 160 mm Hg systolic or greater than 100 mm Hg diastolic; (4) early-onset hypertension; (5) low-renin hypertension; (6) hypertension with an adrenal mass; (7) hypertension with a family history of early-onset hypertension or cerebrovascular accident before age 40 years; and (8) a first-degree relative who has aldosteronism.

For at least 2 weeks prior to testing, patients should consume a diet high in NaCl (more than 6 g/day) and ideally hold certain medications: all diuretics, ACE inhibitors, ARBs (stimulate PRA); beta-blockers, clonidine, NSAIDs (suppress PRA); oral estrogens and oral contraceptives should also ideally be held. Medications that are allowed include slow-release verapamil, hydralazine, terazosin, and doxazosin.

For blood testing, the patient should be out of bed for at least 2 hours and seated for 15–60 minutes before the blood draw, which should preferably be obtained between 8 AM and 10 AM. Proper phlebotomy technique is important to avoid spurious increases in potassium. The blood should be drawn slowly with a syringe and needle (rather than a vacutainer) at least 5 seconds after tourniquet release and without fist clenching. Plasma potassium, rather than the routine serum potassium, should be measured in cases of unexpected hyperkalemia, with the separation of plasma from cells within 30 minutes of collection. (Serum potassium levels must be normal, since hypokalemia suppresses aldosterone.) For practical purposes, the same blood draw can be used for simultaneous assays for plasma potassium, PRA, and direct renin assay (DRA). Patients with primary aldosteronism have a suppressed PRA less than 0.65 ng/mL/h or DRA less than 0.36 ng/mL. **PRA of 1 ng/mL/h (12.8 pmol/L/min) is equivalent to a DRA of 5.2 ng/mL (8.2 milli-units/L).** Blood specimens for PRA must be transported to the laboratory at room temperature for prompt separation and freezing of plasma. Serum aldosterone should ideally be measured with tandem mass spectrometry. Suppressed PRA or DRA with a serum aldosterone concentration greater than15 ng/dL (416 pmol/L) indicates hyperaldosteronism. Serum aldosterone (ng/dL): PRA (ng/mL/h) ratios less than 24 exclude primary aldosteronism, whereas ratios between 24 and 67 are suspicious and ratios greater than 67 are very suggestive of primary aldosteronism. Such elevated ratios are not diagnostic; rather, they indicate the need to document increased aldosterone secretion with a 24-hour urine collection. To confirm the diagnosis, a 24-hour urine is collected in an acidified container for aldosterone, cortisol, and creatinine; urine aldosterone greater than 20 mcg/24 h (55 nmol/24 h) confirms primary aldosteronism.

C. Imaging

Some patients with undiagnosed primary aldosteronism are incidentally found to have an adrenal nodule (incidentaloma) during abdominal or chest imaging. All patients with biochemically confirmed primary aldosteronism require a thin-section CT scan of the adrenals to screen for a rare adrenal carcinoma. In the absence of a large adrenal carcinoma, adrenal CT scanning cannot reliably distinguish unilateral from bilateral aldosterone excess, having a sensitivity of 78% and a specificity of 78% for unilateral aldosteronism. Therefore, the decision to perform a unilateral adrenalectomy should not be based solely on the adrenal CT scan. Adrenal vein sampling is often required.

E. Adrenal Vein Sampling

Unfortunately, bilateral selective adrenal vein sampling is invasive, expensive, not widely available, and often unsuccessful. The procedure (and surgery) may not be required for patients whose blood pressure is well controlled with spironolactone or eplerenone and for those with familial hyperaldosteronism. It is indicated only if surgery is contemplated in order to direct the surgeon to the correct adrenal gland. Adrenal vein sampling is probably not required in patients who have a classic adrenal adenoma (Conn syndrome), which is characterized by hypokalemia and a unilateral adrenal adenoma 10 mm or larger in diameter on CT.

Before this procedure, the patient must be properly prepared (see Laboratory Findings). However, patients with a persistently suppressed PRA may continue mineralocorticoid blockade. To ensure proper catheterization of both adrenal veins, the blood samples are assayed for both aldosterone and cortisol following cosyntropin administration. Aldosterone hypersecretion on one side usually indicates that adrenal has a unilateral aldosteronoma or hyperplasia, particularly when aldosterone secretion from the contralateral adrenal is suppressed, in which case unilateral surgery improves hypertension in 96%. The procedure has a sensitivity of 95% and a specificity of 100% but only when performed by an experienced radiologist. This procedure entails a 0.57% risk of major complications.

▶ Differential Diagnosis

The differential diagnosis of primary aldosteronism includes other causes of hypokalemia in patients with essential hypertension, especially diuretic therapy; chronic depletion of intravascular volume stimulates renin secretion and secondary hyperaldosteronism.

Real (black) licorice (derived from anise) or anise-flavored drinks (sambuca, pastis) contain glycyrrhizinic acid, which has a metabolite that inhibits the enzyme that normally inactivates cortisol in the renal tubule. Oral contraceptives may increase aldosterone secretion in some patients. Renal vascular disease can cause severe hypertension with hypokalemia but PRA is high. Excessive adrenal secretion of other corticosteroids (besides aldosterone), certain congenital adrenal enzyme disorders, and primary cortisol resistance may also cause hypertension with hypokalemia. The differential diagnosis also includes Liddle syndrome, an autosomal dominant cause of hypertension and hypokalemia resulting from excessive sodium absorption from the renal tubule; renin and aldosterone levels are low.

▶ Complications

Cardiovascular complications occur more frequently in primary aldosteronism than in idiopathic hypertension. Following unilateral adrenalectomy for Conn syndrome, suppression of the contralateral adrenal may result in temporary postoperative hypoaldosteronism, characterized by hyperkalemia and hypotension.

▶ Treatment

The unilateral adrenal adenoma of Conn syndrome is usually treated by laparoscopic adrenalectomy. During pregnancy, such surgery is best performed during the second trimester. However, long-term medical therapy is an option for unilateral hyperaldosteronism, if adequate blood pressure control can be maintained. Bilateral adrenal hyperplasia is best treated with medical therapy. Medical treatment must include a potassium-sparing diuretic, particularly spironolactone, eplerenone, or amiloride. Spironolactone is the most effective drug but also has antiandrogen activity and men frequently experience breast tenderness, gynecomastia, or reduced libido; it is given at initial doses of 12.5–25 mg orally once daily; the dose may be titrated upward to 200 mg daily. Spironolactone might lead to undervirilization of male infants and is contraindicated in pregnancy; reproductive-age women are cautioned to use contraception during therapy. Eplerenone is favored during pregnancy and for men, since it does not have antiandrogen effects; it must be taken orally twice daily in doses of 25–50 mg. Blood pressure must be monitored daily when beginning these anti-mineralocorticoid medications; significant drops in blood pressure have occurred when these drugs are added to other antihypertensives. Other antihypertensive drugs may be required, particularly amlodipine, and ACE inhibitors or ARBs. Glucocorticoid-remediable aldosteronism is very rare but may respond well to suppression with low-dose dexamethasone.

► Prognosis

The hypertension is reversible in about two-thirds of cases but persists or returns despite surgery in the remainder. The prognosis is much improved by early diagnosis and treatment. Only 2% of aldosterone-secreting adrenal tumors are malignant.

Chao CT et al. Diagnosis and management of primary aldosteronism: an updated review. Ann Med. 2013 Jun;45(4):375–83. [PMID: 23701121]

Piaditis G et al. Progress in aldosteronism: a review of the prevalence of primary aldosteronism in pre-hypertension and hypertension. Eur J Endocrinol. 2015 May;172(5):R191–203. [PMID: 25538205]

Riester A et al. Progress in primary aldosteronism: mineralocorticoid receptor antagonists and management of primary aldosteronism in pregnancy. Eur J Endocrinol. 2015 Jan; 172(1):R23–30. [PMID: 25163723]

Rossi GP et al. Clinical management of primary aldosteronism: 2013 Practical Recommendations of the Italian Society of Hypertension (SIIA). High Blood Press Cardiovasc Prev. 2014 Mar;21(1):71–5. [PMID: 24464387]

Zennaro MC et al. An update on novel mechanisms of primary aldosteronism. J Endocrinol. 2015 Feb;224(2):R63–77. [PMID: 25424518]

PHEOCHROMOCYTOMA & PARAGANGLIOMA

ESSENTIALS OF DIAGNOSIS

► "Attacks" of headache, perspiration, palpitations, anxiety. Multisystem crisis.

► Hypertension, frequently sustained but often paroxysmal, especially during surgery or delivery.

► Elevated urinary plasma free metanephrines. Normal serum T_4 and TSH.

► Frequent germline mutations.

► General Considerations

Both pheochromocytomas and non–head-neck paragangliomas are tumors of the sympathetic nervous system. Pheochromocytomas arise from the adrenal medulla and usually secrete both epinephrine and norepinephrine. Paragangliomas ("extra-adrenal pheochromocytomas") arise from sympathetic paraganglia, often metastasize, and secrete norepinephrine or are nonsecretory. Excessive levels of norepinephrine or neuropeptide Y cause hypertension, while epinephrine causes tachyarrhythmias. These tumors may be located in either or both adrenals or anywhere along the sympathetic nervous chain, and sometimes in the mediastinum, heart, or bladder.

These tumors are particularly dangerous and deceptive, although they account for less that 0.4% of hypertension cases. The incidence is higher in patients with moderate to severe hypertension, particularly in the presence of suspicious symptoms of headache, significant palpitations, or diaphoretic episodes. They account for about 4% of adrenal incidentalomas. The yearly incidence is 2 to 4 new cases per million population. However, many cases are undiagnosed during life, since the prevalence of pheochromocytomas and paragangliomas in autopsy series is 1 in 2000.

Nonsecretory paragangliomas arise in the head or neck, particularly in the carotid body, jugular-tympanic region, or vagal body; only about 4% secrete catecholamines. They often arise in patients who harbor *SDHD*, *SDHC*, or *SDHB* germline mutations.

Over 30% of patients with pheochromocytomas or paragangliomas harbor a germline mutation in 1 of at least 14 genes that makes them prone to develop the tumor, usually in an autosomal dominant manner with incomplete penetrance. For a patient with a pheochromocytoma or paraganglioma, the chance of harboring a germline mutation is nearly 100% with a family history of pheochromocytoma or paraganglioma or with multiple sites of primary tumor, compared to 17% in patients without such family history.

Pheochromocytomas develop in about 20% of patients with **von Hippel–Lindau (VHL) disease type 2** (hemangiomas of the retina, cerebellum, brainstem, and spinal cord; hyperparathyroidism; pancreatic cysts; endolymphatic sac tumors; cystadenomas of the adnexa or epididymis; pancreatic neuroendocrine tumors; renal cysts, adenomas, and carcinomas); inheritance is autosomal dominant. Patients with VHL develop pheochromocytomas that are less likely to be extra-adrenal, less likely to be malignant (3.5%), more likely to be bilateral, and more likely to present at an early age. Pheochromocytomas that arise in patients with VHL secrete exclusively norepinephrine and its metabolite normetanephrine. Therefore, individuals who carry type 2 VHL mutations should be screened for pheochromocytoma with plasma normetanephrine levels.

MEN 2 is associated with pheochromocytomas, hyperparathyroidism, cutaneous lichen amyloidosis, and medullary thyroid carcinoma. **MEN 3** may be familial but usually arises from a de novo *ret* mutation; MEN 3 is associated with pheochromocytoma (50%), aggressive medullary thyroid carcinoma, mucosal neuromas, and marfinoid habitus. **von Recklinghausen neurofibromatosis type 1***(NF-1)* is associated with an increased risk of pheochromocytomas/

paragangliomas as well as cutaneous neurofibromas, optic and brainstem gliomas, astrocytomas, vascular anomalies, hamartomas, malignant nerve sheath tumors, and smooth-bordered café au lait spots. **Familial paraganglioma** can be caused by mutations in the genes encoding succinate dehydrogenase (SDH) subunits B, C, or D. Patients with such germline mutations are more apt to have bilateral pheochromocytomas or multicentric paragangliomas. Patients with *SDHB* germline mutations are particularly prone to develop paragangliomas that metastasize aggressively; they are also prone to develop renal cell carcinomas and neuroblastomas.

Some kindreds are prone to develop pheochromocytomas and paragangliomas due to less common germline mutations in other tumor susceptibility genes: *SDHA, SDHAF2, TMEM127, MAX, KIF1B, HIF2A,* and *PHD2.* Pheochromocytomas are also more common in patients with Carney triad, Sturge-Weber syndrome, and tuberous sclerosis.

▶ Clinical Findings

A. Symptoms and Signs (Table 26–12)

Pheochromocytomas can be lethal unless they are diagnosed and treated appropriately. Catastrophic hypertensive crisis and fatal cardiac arrhythmias can occur spontaneously or may be triggered by needle biopsy or manipulation of the mass, intravenous contrast dye or glucagon injection, vaginal delivery, trauma, anesthesia, or surgery (both unrelated to the tumor or for its removal). Exercise, bending, lifting, or emotional stress can trigger paroxysms. Certain drugs can precipitate attacks: fluoxetine and other selective serotonin reuptake inhibitors (SSRIs), monoamine oxidase (MAO) inhibitors, caffeine, nicotine, decongestants, amphetamines, cocaine, ionic intravenous contrast, and epinephrine. Bladder paragangliomas may present with paroxysms during micturition.

Paroxysms typically produce hypertension (90%), severe headache (80%), perspiration (70%), and palpitations (60%); other symptoms may include anxiety (50%), a sense of impending doom, or tremor (40%). Vasomotor changes during an attack cause mottled cyanosis and facial pallor. As the attack subsides, facial flushing may occur as a result of reflex vasodilation. Epinephrine secretion by an adrenal pheochromocytoma may cause episodic tachyarrhythmias, hypotension, or even syncope. Acute coronary syndrome can be caused by coronary vasoconstriction. Confusion, psychosis, seizures, transient ischemic attacks, or stroke may occur with cerebrovascular vasoconstriction or hemorrhagic stroke. Aortic aneurysms may dissect and

Table 26–12. Clinical manifestations of pheochromocytoma and paraganglioma.

Blood pressure	Hypertension: severe or mild, paroxysmal or sustained; orthostasis; hypotension/shock; normotension
Vasospasm	Cyanosis, Raynaud syndrome, gangrene; severe radial artery vasospasm with thready pulse; falsely low blood pressure by radial artery transducer
Multisystem crisis	ARDS, severe hypertension/hypotension, acute heart failure, fever, renal failure, hepatic failure, encephalopathy, death
Cardiovascular	Palpitations, dysrhythmias, chest pain, acute coronary syndrome, cardiomyopathy, heart failure, cardiac paragangliomas
Gastrointestinal	Abdominal pain, nausea, vomiting, weight loss, intestinal ischemia; pancreatitis, cholecystitis, jaundice; rupture of abdominal aneurysm; constipation, toxic megacolon
Metabolic	Hyperglycemia/diabetes, lactic acidosis, fevers
Neurologic	Headache, paresthesias, numbness, dizziness, CVA, TIA, hemiplegia, hemianopsia, seizures, hemorrhagic stroke; skull metastases may impinge on brain structures, optic nerve, or other cranial nerves; spinal metastases may impinge on cord or nerve roots
Pulmonary	Dyspnea; hypoxia from ARDS
Psychiatric	Anxiety attacks or constant anxiety; depression; chronic fatigue; psychosis
Renal	Renal insufficiency, nephrotic syndrome, malignant nephrosclerosis; large tumors often involve the kidneys and renal vessels
Skin	Apocrine sweating during paroxysms, drenching sweats as attack subsides; eczema; mottled cyanosis during paroxysm
Thyroid	Paroxysmal thyroid swelling
Ectopic hormones	ACTH (Cushing syndrome); VIP (Verner-Morrison syndrome); PTHrP (hypercalcemia); erythropoietin (erythrocytosis)
Children	More commonly have sustained hypertension, diaphoresis, visual changes, polyuria/polydipsia, seizures, edematous or cyanotic hands; more commonly harbor germline mutations, multiple tumors, and paragangliomas
Women	More symptomatic than men: more frequent headache, weight loss, numbness, dizziness, tremor, anxiety, and fatigue
Pregnancy	Hypertension mimicking eclampsia; hypertensive multisystem crisis during vaginal delivery; postpartum shock or fever; high mortality
General laboratory	Leukocytosis, erythrocytosis, eosinophilia

ACTH, adrenocorticotropic hormone; ARDS, acute respiratory distress syndrome; CVA, cerebrovascular accident; PTHrP, parathyroid hormone–related protein; TIA, transient ischemic attack; VIP, vasoactive intestinal peptide.
Used, with permission, from Gardner D, Shoback D (editors). *Greenspan's Basic and Clinical Endocrinology.* 9th edition, McGraw-Hill, 2011.

rupture. Abdominal pain, nausea, vomiting, and even ischemic bowel can be due to splanchnic vasoconstriction. Large or hemorrhagic abdominal tumors can also cause abdominal pain. Peripheral vasoconstriction can cause Raynaud phenomenon or even gangrene. Patients may experience nervousness and irritability, increased appetite, and loss of weight. Other patients have pulmonary edema and heart failure due to cardiomyopathy. Although most patients are symptomatic, some patients are normotensive and asymptomatic, particularly when the tumor is nonsecretory or discovered at an early stage.

Cytokine release from pheochromocytomas or paragangliomas can cause proteinuria and nephrotic syndrome. Such patients have an increased risk of **multisystem crisis:** acute respiratory distress syndrome (ARDS), acute heart failure, severe hypotension, kidney failure, liver failure, and death. Multisystem crisis can occur spontaneously, or it may be provoked by surgery, vaginal delivery, or treatment of metastatic disease.

B. Laboratory Findings

Plasma fractionated free metanephrines is the single most sensitive test for secretory pheochromocytomas and paragangliomas. The blood specimen may be obtained after sitting quietly in the laboratory for at least 15 minutes. Normal levels rule out pheochromocytoma and paraganglioma with some certainty and the work-up can usually end there. However, misleading elevations in plasma metanephrines or normetanephrines occur at a rate of about 10–20% and can be caused by drawing blood in a sitting position. Therefore, patients with elevated levels drawn in the sitting position should have the test repeated while lying supine in a quiet room for 30 minutes before the blood is drawn. Other causes for misleading elevations with all assay methods include physical or emotional stress, sleep apnea, and certain drugs: sympathomimetics, cocaine, MAO inhibitors, tricyclic antidepressants, and phenoxybenzamine. Patients with confirmed elevations in plasma metanephrines or normetanephrines require further evaluation.

Assay of urinary fractionated metanephrines and creatinine effectively confirms most pheochromocytomas that were detected by elevated plasma fractionated metanephrines. A 24-hour urine specimen is usually obtained, although an overnight or shorter collection may be used; patients with pheochromocytomas generally have more than 2.2 mcg of total metanephrine per milligram of creatinine, and more than 135 mcg total catecholamines per gram creatinine. Urinary assay for total metanephrines is about 97% sensitive for detecting functioning pheochromocytomas.

Some drugs, foods, and stresses can cause misleading elevations in catecholamine excretion (Table 26–13). About 10% of hypertensive patients have a misleadingly elevated level of one or more tests.

Serum chromogranin A (CgA) is elevated in 90% of patients with pheochromocytoma and the levels correlate with tumor size, being higher in patients with metastatic disease. Serum CgA must be assayed in the fasting state, since levels rise after meals. Misleading CgA levels also

Table 26–13. Factors that can cause misleading catecholamine or metanephrine results.[1]

Drugs	Foods	Conditions
Acetaminophen[2]	Bananas[3]	Age (children and
Aldomet[2]	Caffeine[3]	elderly)[6]
Amphetamines[3]	Coffee[2]	Amyotrophic lateral
Anesthetics (local)[6]	Peppers[2]	sclerosis[3]
Bronchodilators[3]	Pineapples[3]	Brain lesions[3]
Buspirone[2]	Walnuts[3]	Anxiety[3,6]
Captopril[2]		Carcinoid[3]
Cimetidine[2]		Drug withdrawal
Cocaine[3]		(narcotic, alcohol,
Codeine[2]		clonidine)[3,6]
Contrast media (meglu-		Eclampsia[3]
mine acetrizoate,		Emotion (severe)[3,6]
meglumine		Essential hypertension[3]
diatrizoate)[5]		Exercise (vigorous)[3,6]
Decongestants[3]		Guillain-Barré
Ephedrine and		syndrome[3]
epinephrine[3]		Hypoglycemia[3]
Halothane anesthesia[6]		Lead poisoning[3]
Fenfluramine[4]		Myocardial infarction
Isoproterenol[3]		(acute)[3]
Labetalol[2,3]		Pain (severe)[3]
Levodopa[2]		Porphyria (acute)[3]
Mandelamine[2]		Psychosis (acute)[3]
Methenamine[4]		Quadriplegia
Mesalamine[2]		Renal failure[3,4,6]
Metoclopramide[2]		Sleep apnea[3,6]
Monoamine oxidase		Winter[6]
inhibitors[6]		
Nitroglycerin[3]		
Phenoxybenzamine[2,3]		
Serotonin-norepineph-		
rine reuptake inhibi-		
tors (SNRI):		
venlafaxine, desven-		
lafaxine, duloxetine,		
levomilnacipran[3]		
Smoking[6]		
Sulfasalazine[2]		
Tricyclic		
antidepressants[2,3]		

[1]Note that assays for metanephrine using tandem mass spectroscopy (MS/MS) are not prone to interference from drugs or foods, except those that increase catecholamine excretion.
[2]May cause confounding peaks for catecholamines or metanephrines with an HPLC-ECD chromatogram.
[3]Increases measured catecholamine excretion.
[4]Decreases measured catecholamine excretion.
[5]May decrease urine metanephrine excretion.
[6]Increases plasma and urinary normetanephrine and metanephrine.

occur in patients with azotemia or hypergastrinemia, and in those treated with corticosteroids or proton pump inhibitors.

Initial testing results are frequently inconclusive. When metanephrines are elevated but less than three times the upper limit of normal, there is a significant chance of the test result being falsely positive. False-positive test results should be particularly suspected when the ratio of normeta-nephrine to norepinephrine is less than 0.52 or the ratio of metanephrine to epinephrine is less than 4.2. In such cases, it is best to repeat biochemical testing under optimal conditions, eg, after eliminating potentially interfering drugs. Pharmacologic provocative and suppressive tests that evaluate the rise or fall in blood pressure are usually not required or recommended.

Hyperglycemia is present in about 35% of patients but is usually mild. Proteinuria is present in about 10–20% of patients. Leukocytosis is common. Eosinophilia occurs rarely. The ESR is sometimes elevated. PRA may be increased by catecholamines. Genetic testing should ideally be performed on all patients with pheochromocytoma or paraganglioma. Testing for VHL, *ret* protooncogene, and *SDHB/SDHC/SDHD* mutations is advisable. Family members may then be screened for the specific gene mutation.

C. Imaging

1. CT and MRI scanning—Imaging should only be performed in patients with suggestive laboratory findings, since adrenal pheochromocytomas can appear similar to benign adrenal adenomas that are very common (2–4% of all scans). When a pheochromocytoma is suspected because of biochemical testing or a genetic condition predisposing to pheochromocytoma, a noncontrast CT scan of the abdomen is performed, with thin sections through the adrenals. The CT usually shows an adrenal mass with a density greater than 10 HU. If an adrenal mass is present, another CT is immediately performed, infusing nonionic contrast (to reduce the risk of stimulating catecholamine release from a pheochromocytoma) with a "washout" protocol. Pheochromocytomas are usually avid for contrast and 84% of tumors retain greater than 40% of contrast after 15 minutes. Glucagon should not be used during scanning, since it can provoke hypertensive crisis.

MRI scanning has the advantage of not requiring intravenous contrast dye; its lack of radiation makes it the imaging of choice during pregnancy and childhood and for serial imaging. Both CT and MRI scanning have a sensitivity of about 90% for adrenal pheochromocytoma and a sensitivity of 95% for adrenal tumors over 0.5 cm in diameter. However, both CT and MRI are less sensitive for detecting recurrent tumors, metastases, and extra-adrenal paragangliomas. If no adrenal tumor is found, the scan is extended to include the entire abdomen, pelvis, and chest.

2. Nuclear imaging—A whole-body ^{123}I-meta-iodobenzyl-guanidine (^{123}I-MIBG) scan can localize tumors with a sensitivity of 94% and a specificity of 92%. However, it is less sensitive for MEN 2– or MEN 3–related pheochromocytomas and for metastases. Preoperative ^{123}I-MIBG scanning may help confirm that a mass is a pheochromocytoma or paraganglioma. Whole-body ^{123}I-MIBG scanning can also be useful to search for a nonadrenal paraganglioma when the adrenals and abdomen appear normal on CT scan in patients in whom a secretory paraganglioma is suspected. It is also prudent to perform a whole-body ^{123}I-MIBG scan about 3 months postoperatively to determine if metastatic or recurrent tumor is present. Drugs that reduce ^{123}I-MIBG uptake should be avoided, including tricyclic antidepressants and cyclobenzaprine (6 weeks). Other drugs, such as amphetamines, diet pills, decongestants, cocaine, phenothiazines, haloperidol, labetalol, and serotonin and norepinephrine reuptake inhibitors (venlafaxine, desvenlafaxine, duloxetine), can potentially reduce ^{123}I-MIBG uptake for up to 2 weeks. Drug interference is suspected in negative ^{123}I-MIBG scans that do not show normal uptake in salivary glands.

Somatostatin receptor imaging using ^{111}In-labeled octreotide is only 25% sensitive for detecting an adrenal pheochromocytoma. However, ^{111}In-labeled octreotide scanning is quite sensitive for detecting extra-adrenal pheochromocytomas (paragangliomas) and metastatic pheochromocytomas, sometimes locating tumors that were missed by ^{123}I-MIBG scanning.

PET/CT scanning usually detects tumors and metastases using ^{18}F-labeled deoxyglucose ([18]FDG-PET) or ^{18}F-labeled dopamine ([18]FDA-PET), and may demonstrate tumors that are not visible on ^{123}I-MIBG scanning.

▶ Differential Diagnosis

Certain conditions mimic pheochromocytoma: thyrotoxicosis, essential hypertension, myocarditis, glomerulonephritis or other renal lesions, eclampsia, acute intermittent porphyria, hypogonadal vascular instability (hot flushes), anxiety attacks, and cocaine or amphetamine use, and clonidine withdrawal.

Patients taking nonselective MAO inhibitor antidepressants can have hypertensive crisis after eating foods that contain tyramine. Patients with erythromelalgia can have hypertensive crises. Pheochromocytomas can cause chest pain and ECG changes that mimic acute cardiac ischemia. Renal artery stenosis can cause severe hypertension and may coexist with pheochromocytoma.

False-positive testing for catecholamines and metabolites occurs in about 10–20% of hypertensive patients, but levels are usually less than 50% above normal and typically normalize with repeat testing.

▶ Complications

All of the complications of severe hypertension may be encountered. In addition, a catecholamine-induced cardiomyopathy may develop. Severe heart failure and cardiovascular collapse may develop in patients during a paroxysm. Sudden death may occur due to cardiac arrhythmia. Multisystem crisis and ARDS can occur acutely and thus the initial manifestation of pheochromocytoma may be hypotension or even shock. Hypertensive crises with sudden blindness or cerebrovascular accidents are not uncommon.

After removal of the tumor, a state of severe hypotension and shock (resistant to epinephrine and norepinephrine) may ensue with precipitation of acute kidney injury or myocardial infarction. Hypotension and shock may occur from spontaneous infarction or hemorrhage of the tumor.

Malignant pheochromocytomas may metastasize. Cells can also be seeded within the peritoneum, either spontaneously or as a complication during surgical resection. Such seeding of the abdomen can result in multifocal recurrent intra-abdominal tumors, a condition known as pheochromocytomatosis.

▶ Medical Treatment

Patients must receive adequate treatment for hypertension and tachyarrhythmias prior to surgery for pheochromocytoma/paraganglioma. Patients are advised to measure their blood pressures daily and immediately during paroxysms. Some patients with pheochromocytoma or paraganglioma are not hypertensive and do not require preoperative antihypertensive management. Alpha-blockers or calcium channel blockers can be used, either alone or in combination. Blood pressure should be controlled before cardioselective beta-blockers are added for control of tachyarrhythmias. Normotensive patients with pheochromocytoma or sympathetic paraganglioma do not require preoperative alpha blockade, which increases their requirement for vasopressors and colloid after the tumor resection.

Alpha-blockers are typically administered preparatory to surgery. Phenoxybenzamine is a long-acting nonselective alpha-blocker with a half-life of 24 hours; it is given initially in a dosage of 10 mg orally every 12 hours, increasing gradually by about 10 mg/day about every 3 days until hypertension is controlled. Maintenance doses range from 10 mg/day to 120 mg/day. Doxazosin (half-life 22 hours), a selective alpha-1-blocker, may also be used in doses of 2–32 mg daily. Preoperative preparation with phenoxybenzamine reduces intraoperative hypertension but may increase the risk post-resection compared to patients given a preoperative selective alpha-1-blocker. Optimal alpha-blockade is achieved when supine arterial pressure is below 140/90 mm Hg or as low as possible for the patient to have a standing arterial pressure above 80/45 mm Hg.

Calcium channel blockers (nifedipine ER or nicardipine ER) are very effective and are usually added to alpha-blockers, but may be used alone. Nifedipine ER is initially given orally at a dose of 30 mg/day, increasing the dose gradually to a maximum of 60 mg twice daily. Calcium channel blockers are superior to phenoxybenzamine for long-term use, since they cause less fatigue, nasal congestion, and orthostatic hypotension. However, they should not be used for patients with severe heart failure. For acute hypertensive crisis (systolic blood pressure higher than 170 mm Hg) a nifedipine 10-mg capsule may be chewed and swallowed. Nifedipine is quite successful for treating acute hypertension in patients with pheochromocytoma/paraganglioma, even at home; it is reasonably safe as long as the blood pressure is carefully monitored.

Beta-blockers (eg, metoprolol XL) are often required after institution of alpha-blockade or calcium channel blockade. The use of a beta-blocker as initial antihypertensive therapy has resulted in an "unopposed alpha" status that causes paradoxical worsening of hypertension. Labetalol has combined alpha- and beta-blocking activity and is an effective agent but can cause paradoxical hypertension

if used as the initial antihypertensive agent. Labetalol can also interfere with catecholamine determinations in some laboratories and reduces the tumor's uptake of radioisotopes, such that it must be discontinued for at least 4–7 days before ^{123}I-MIBG or [18]FDG-PET scanning or therapy with high-dose ^{131}I-MIBG.

▶ Surgical Treatment

Surgical removal of pheochromocytomas or abdominal paragangliomas is the treatment of choice. For surgery, a team approach—endocrinologist, anesthesiologist, and surgeon—is critically important. Laparoscopic surgery is preferred, but large and invasive tumors require open laparotomy. Patients with small familial or bilateral pheochromocytomas may undergo selective resection of the tumors, sparing the adrenal cortex; however, there is a recurrence rate of 10% over 10 years.

Prior to surgery, blood pressure control should be maintained for a minimum of 4–7 days or until optimal cardiac status is established. The ECG should be monitored until it becomes stable. (It may take a week or even months to correct ECG changes in patients with catecholamine myocarditis, and it may be prudent to defer surgery until then in such cases.) Patients must be very closely monitored during surgery to promptly detect sudden changes in blood pressure or cardiac arrhythmias.

Intraoperative severe hypertension is managed with continuous intravenous nicardipine (a short-acting calcium channel blocker), 2–6 mcg/kg/min, or nitroprusside, 0.5–10 mcg/kg/min. Prolonged nitroprusside administration can cause cyanide toxicity. Tachyarrhythmia is treated with intravenous atenolol (1 mg boluses), esmolol, or lidocaine.

Autotransfusion of 1–2 units of blood at 12 hours preoperatively plus generous intraoperative volume replacement reduces the risk of postresection hypotension and shock caused by desensitization of the vascular alpha-1-receptors. Shock is treated with intravenous saline or colloid and high doses of intravenous norepinephrine. Intravenous 5% dextrose is infused postoperatively to prevent hypoglycemia.

▶ Detecting & Managing Metastatic Pheochromocytoma & Paraganglioma

Surgical histopathology for pheochromocytoma and paraganglioma cannot reliably determine whether a tumor is malignant. Therefore, all pheochromocytomas and paragangliomas must be approached as possibly malignant. Even if no metastases are visible at the time of surgery, they may become apparent years later. So all patients require lifetime follow-up. Therefore, it is essential to recheck blood pressure and plasma fractionated metanephrine levels about 4–6 weeks postoperatively, at least every 6 months for 5 years, then once yearly for life and immediately if hypertension, suspicious symptoms, or metastases become evident. With familial pheochromocytoma, carriers of germline mutations also require close lifetime surveillance Patients with nonsecretory tumors frequently have elevated serum levels of chromogranin A that can also be used as a tumor marker. It is also prudent to perform a whole-body ^{123}I-MIBG scan about 3 months postoperatively, since previously undetected metastases may become visible.

Since some metastases are indolent, it is important to tailor treatment to each individual according to their tumor's aggressiveness. Most surgeons resect the main tumor and larger metastases (debulking). Asymptomatic, indolent metastases may be kept under close surveillance without treatment.

A. Chemotherapy

Various chemotherapy regimens have been used, but there have been no controlled clinical trials to prove the effectiveness of one regimen over another or whether any regimen actually improves overall survival. The most common chemotherapy regimen combines intravenous cyclophosphamide, vincristine, and dacarbazine over 2 days in cycles that are repeated every 3 weeks (Table 39–11). About one-third of patients experience some degree of temporary remission. Sunitinib, a tyrosine kinase inhibitor, can also produce remissions, given orally in doses of 50 mg/day for 4 weeks on and then 2 weeks off; alternatively, a dose of 37.5 mg/day can be given continuously. Another chemotherapy regimen uses temozolomide, 250 mg/day orally for 5 days, repeating the cycle every 28 days; this is usually the best-tolerated chemotherapy and is particularly effective for metastatic pheochromocytoma or paraganglioma in patients with *SDHB* germline mutations. Each chemotherapy regimen has toxicities.

Metyrosine reduces catecholamine synthesis but does not impede the progressive growth of metastases; the initial metyrosine dosage is 250 mg four times daily, increased daily by increments of 250–500 mg to a maximum of 4 g/day. Metyrosine causes CNS side effects and crystalluria; hydration must be ensured.

B. ^{131}I-MIBG Therapy

About 60% of patients with metastatic pheochromocytoma or paraganglioma have tumors with sufficient uptake of ^{123}I-MIBG on diagnostic scanning to allow for therapy with high-activity ^{131}I-MIBG. Medications that reduce MIBG uptake must be avoided, particularly labetalol, phenothiazines, tricyclics, and sympathomimetics. Activities of 125–500 mCi are infused, with many centers administering repeated infusions of 2 mCi/kg to cumulative activities of at least 500–800 mCi. Radioisotope therapy can suppress the bone marrow temporarily. Myelodysplastic syndrome and leukemia can develop several years after ^{131}I-MIBG therapy, with the risk proportional to the cumulative amount of isotope. ARDS and multisystem failure occur rarely after ^{131}I-MIBG therapy, particularly in patients with pretreatment proteinuria.

C. Treatment for Bone Metastases

Patients with significant osteolytic bone metastases may be treated with external beam radiation therapy, which is often helpful in relieving pain and stabilizing local osseous disease. Patients with vertebral metastases and spinal cord compression require surgical decompression and kyphoplasty. Intravenous zoledronate or subcutaneous denosumab may also be administered to patients with osteolytic bone metastases.

► Prognosis

A pheochromocytoma or sympathetic paraganglioma is considered malignant if metastases are present, but metastases may take many years to become clinically evident. Therefore, lifetime surveillance is required (see above). Malignancy is more likely for larger tumors and for sympathetic paragangliomas. The prognosis is good for patients with pheochromocytomas that are resected before causing cardiovascular damage. Hypertension usually resolves after successful surgery but may persist or return in 25% of patients despite successful surgery. Although this may be essential hypertension, biochemical reevaluation is nonetheless required, looking for a second or metastatic pheochromocytoma.

The surgical mortality is under 3% with the use of laparoscopic surgical techniques, intraoperative monitoring, and preoperative blood pressure control with alpha-blockers or calcium channel blockers.

Patients with metastatic pheochromocytoma and paraganglioma have an extremely variable prognosis. Patients with a heavy and progressive tumor burden and distant metastases have a worse prognosis. Patients harboring *SDHB* germline mutations tend to have more aggressive tumors as do patients with pulmonary metastases. Patients with metastases limited to bones or the abdomen tend to have a better prognosis. Patients with intraperitoneal seeding (pheochromocytomatosis) rather than true metastases seem to have a better prognosis.

Patients who receive surgery and chemotherapy have a median 5-year survival of about 44%. Patients receiving surgery followed by high-activity ^{131}I-mIBG therapy have been reported to have a 5-year survival rate of 75%. Some patients have an indolent malignancy; prolonged survivals of up to 30 years have been reported with no treatment.

Deutschbein T et al. Treatment of malignant phaeochromocytoma with a combination of cyclophosphamide, vincristine and dacarbazine: own experience and overview of the contemporary literature. Clin Endocrinol (Oxf). 2015 Jan; 82(1):84–90. [PMID: 25143180]

Fishbein L et al. Pheochromocytoma/paraganglioma: review of perioperative management of blood pressure and update on genetic mutations associated with pheochromocytoma. J Clin Hypertens (Greenwich). 2013 Jun;15(6):428–34. [PMID: 23730992]

Lenders JW et al. Pheochromocytoma and paraganglioma: an Endocrine Society Clinical Practice Guideline. J Clin Endocrinol Metab. 2014 Jun;99(6):1915–42. [PMID: 24893135]

Van Berkel A et al. Biochemical diagnosis of phaeochromocytoma and paraganglioma. Eur J Endocrinol. 2014 Feb 4; 170(3):R109–19. [PMID: 24347425]

GASTROENTEROPANCREATIC NEUROENDOCRINE TUMORS (GEP-NETS) & CARCINOID TUMORS

ESSENTIALS OF DIAGNOSIS

▶ GEP-NETs are a subset of neuroendocrine tumors (NETs) that arise from the stomach, intestines, and endocrine pancreas. They may release monogenic amines or polypeptide hormones.

▶ Secretory GEP-NETs present with different manifestations depending on the hormones secreted.

▶ Half of GEP-NETs are nonsecretory or secretory without clinical manifestations; they may be detected incidentally on scans or may present with weight loss, abdominal pain, or jaundice.

▶ Carcinoid tumors arise from either the intestines or lung, secrete serotonin, and may metastasize.

▶ General Considerations

GEP-NETs are a subset of neuroendocrine tumors that arise from the stomach, intestines, or endocrine pancreas. Pancreatic neuroendocrine tumors (pNETs) arise from different islet cells, each with distinct chemical and microscopic features: the A cells (20%) secrete glucagon, the B cells (70%) secrete insulin,[1] the D cells (5%) secrete somatostatin or gastrin, and the F cells secrete pancreatic polypeptide. Gastrin-producing cells also found in the duodenum. Serotonin-producing cells are found throughout the gut, particularly near the terminal ileum.

The reported incidence of GEP-NETs has increased to about 37 per million yearly in the United States due to the incidental detection of small tumors on abdominal scans. About 40% are functional, producing hormones that also serve as tumor markers, important for diagnosis and follow-up. Up to 25% of GEP-NETs are associated with one of four different inherited disorders: MEN 1, von Hippel-Lindau disease (VHL), neurofibromatosis 1 (NF-1), and tuberous sclerosis complex (TSC). At presentation, 65% of GEP-NETs are unresectable or metastatic. In MEN 1, GEP-NETs are usually gastrinomas, carcinoids, or nonfunctioning tumors and are a common cause of death. In VHL, GEP-NETs are usually benign and multiple.

Insulinomas are the most common functional type of GEP-NET and are usually small, intrapancreatic, and benign (90%) and secrete excessive amounts of insulin. Insulinomas also produce proinsulin and C-peptide. Insulinomas are solitary in 95% of sporadic cases but are multiple in about 90% of cases arising in MEN 1. (See Chapter 27.)

Gastrinomas secrete excessive quantities of the hormone gastrin (as well as "big" gastrin). About 50% of gastrinomas are malignant and metastasize to the liver. Gastrinomas are typically found in the duodenum (49%),

pancreas (24%), or lymph nodes (11%). Sporadic gastrinoma is rarely suspected at the onset of symptoms; typically, there is a 5-year delay in diagnosis. About 22% of gastrinomas arise in patients with MEN 1, who usually present at a younger age, often with multiple tumors; hyperparathyroidism can occur many years before or after the discovery of a gastrinoma.

Glucagonomas are rare and usually malignant, despite their benign histologic appearance. They usually arise as a large intrapancreatic tumor with 60% having liver metastases apparent by the time of diagnosis. Besides glucagon, they usually secrete additional hormones, including gastrin.

Somatostatinomas are very rare and usually single. They arise in the pancreas (50%) or small intestine. They secrete somatostatin.

VIPomas are very rare and usually single intrapancreatic tumors with metastases usually evident (80%) at diagnosis. They produce vasoactive intestinal polypeptide (VIP).

CCKomas are rare tumors of the endocrine pancreas that secrete cholecystokinin.

Carcinoid tumors can arise from the small bowel (53%, particularly terminal ileum), colon (12%), esophagus through duodenum (6%), or lung (bronchial carcinoid [5%]). About 20% of cases present with metastases without a known primary location. Carcinoids are multiple in about 28% of cases. Although tumors are usually indolent, metastases are common, particularly to liver, lymph nodes, and peritoneum.

Nonfunctional pancreatic neuroendocrine tumors produce no significant hormones and usually grow to large size prior to detection. They may secrete chromogranin A (CgA) or pancreatic polypeptide, which can be used as tumor markers.

▶ Clinical Findings

A. Symptoms and Signs

Nonfunctioning tumors typically present with mass effect and metastases, such as pancreatitis, jaundice, abdominal pain, or weight loss.

Insulinomas secrete insulin and present with the symptoms of fasting hypoglycemia. (See Chapter 27.)

Gastrinomas usually present with peptic ulcer disease—abdominal pain (75%), heartburn (44%), bleeding (25%)—or weight loss (17%) (Zollinger-Ellison syndrome). Endoscopy usually shows hyperplastic gastric rugae (94%).

Glucagonomas usually present with weight loss caused by glucagon-stimulated protein hepatic gluconeogenesis and related protein catabolism. Other common manifestations include diarrhea, nausea, peptic ulcer, hypoaminoacidemia, or necrolytic migratory erythema, known as "glucagonoma syndrome". Diabetes mellitus develops in about 35% of patients. The median survival is 34 months after diagnosis.

Somatostatinomas can present with a classic triad of symptoms: diabetes mellitus due to its inhibition of insulin and glucagon secretion; cholelithiasis due to its inhibition of gallbladder motility; and steatorrhea due to its inhibition

---

[1] Insulinomas and hypoglycemia are discussed in Chapter 27.

of pancreatic exocrine function. Diarrhea, hypochlorhydria, and anemia can also occur.

VIPomas present with profuse *w*atery *d*iarrhea, (unremitting) *h*ypokalemia, and *achlorhydria* ("WDHA"), the so-called Verner-Morrison syndrome.

CCKomas may present with liver metastases and symptoms of diarrhea, peptic ulcer disease, and weight loss. Patients have elevated serum levels of cholecystokinin and chromogranin A.

Carcinoid tumors can produce "carcinoid syndrome": episodes of abdominal pain, diarrhea, bronchospasm, and weight loss. Skin flushing typically affects the upper body, neck, and face and lasts from 30 seconds to 30 minutes, although flushing with bronchial carcinoids can persist for days. Flushing can be unprovoked or precipitated by exercise, anesthesia, emotional stimuli, or foods (bananas, tomatoes, cheese, kiwi, eggplant, and alcohol). However, the full-blown carcinoid syndrome occurs with only about 10% of tumors. Other manifestations include carcinoid heart disease caused by endocardial fibrotic plaques. Tumor-induced fibrosis can also occur in the retroperitoneum causing ureteral obstruction or in the penis causing Peyronie disease. Pellagra (glossitis, confusion, dry skin), which results from the conversion of tryptophan (a precursor to niacin) to serotonin by tumor cells, may develop in affected patients with widespread metastases. Affected patients have high serum levels of chromogranin A and serotonin as well as elevated urinary excretion of 5-HIAAA, a renally-excreted product of serotonin metabolism.

Bronchial carcinoids secrete serotonin and can produce carcinoid syndrome even without hepatic metastases. Foregut carcinoids secrete serotonin that is metabolized by the liver and only produce carcinoid syndrome when they have metastasized to the liver. Hindgut carcinoids rarely produce serotonin and do not cause carcinoid syndrome.

Ectopic hormones can be secreted by GEP-NETs. Ectopic ACTH secretion from bronchial carcinoids or pNETs can produce Cushing syndrome.

B. Imaging

Localization of noninsulinoma GEP-NETs and their metastases is best done with somatostatin receptor scintigraphy (SRS) with ^{111}In-DTPA-octreotide (Octreoscan), which detects about 75% of noninsulinomas. PET scanning with 68Ga-DOTA-TATE, a radiolabeled somatostatin analog, is more sensitive. ^{18}F-DOPA PET/CT may be helpful in detecting occult carcinoid tumors. CT and MRI are also useful.

For insulinomas, preoperative localization studies are less successful and have the following sensitivities: ultrasonography 25%, CT 25%, endoscopic ultrasonography 27%, transhepatic portal vein sampling 40%, and arteriography 45%. Nearly all insulinomas can be successfully located at surgery by the combination of intraoperative palpation (sensitivity 55%) and ultrasound (sensitivity 75%). An abdominal CT scan is usually obtained, but extensive preoperative localization procedures, especially with invasive methods, are not required. Tumors may be located in the pancreatic head or neck (57%), body (15%), or tail (19%) or in the duodenum (9%). MRI is used to screen members

of kindreds with genetic syndromes that predispose them to GEP-NETs.

▶ Treatment

Surgery is the primary initial treatment for all types of GEP-NETs and is a reasonable option even for patients with stage IV disease. The aggressiveness of the surgery may vary from conservative debulking to radical resection and even liver transplantation.

With gastrinomas, the gastric hyperacidity of Zollinger-Ellison syndrome is treated with a proton pump inhibitor at quadruple the usual doses. Proton pump inhibitors increase serum gastrin, which would otherwise be useful as a tumor marker for gastrinoma recurrence after surgical resection.

Tumor visualization on octreotide scanning indicates that they may respond to long-acting preparations of somatostatin analogs, including lanreotide (Somatuline Depot) and octreotide (Sandostatin LAR Depot). Subcutaneous injections of Octreotide LAR 20–30 mg are required every 4 weeks. Treatment improves symptoms in patients with functioning tumors and also appears to improve progression-free survival in patients with either functioning or nonfunctioning GEP-NETs. Enlarging hepatic metastases may be embolized with ^{90}Y-labeled resin or glass microspheres. For patients with progressive metastatic disease, chemotherapy with everolimus or sunitinib improves progression-free survival when added to somatostatin analog therapy. Other chemotherapeutic agents such as dasatinib may also prove effective. Chemotherapy with combined streptozocin, 5-fluorouracil and doxorubicin or combined capecitabine with streptozocin can also produce remissions.

▶ Prognosis

The prognosis for patients with GEP-NETs is variable, depending on the tumor grade and stage. Patients with well or moderately-well differentiated GEP-NETs (Ki-67 less than 20%) have a much better survival than those with poorly differentiated tumors. Smaller tumors without detectable metastases have a much lower chance of recurrence after surgery. However, most patients with GEP-NETs are stage IV with hepatic metastases by the time of diagnosis. Nevertheless, low-grade metastases may be indolent or slow-growing and may respond to octreotide or lanreotide. The overall prognosis for patients with GEP-NETs is much better than that for adenocarcinomas that arise from the same organs.

The surgical complication rate for GEP-NETs is about 40%, with patients commonly developing fistulas and infections. Extensive pancreatic resection may cause diabetes mellitus. The overall 5-year survival is higher with functional tumors (77%) than with nonfunctional ones (55%) and higher with benign tumors (91%) than with malignant ones (55%). For patients with gastrinomas, the 5-, 10-, and 20-year survival rates with MEN 1 are 94%, 75%, and 58%, respectively, while the survival rates for patients with sporadic gastrinomas are 62%, 50%, and 31%, respectively.

Jung JG et al. Behavior of small, asymptomatic, nonfunctioning pancreatic neuroendocrine tumors (NF-PNETs). Medicine (Baltimore). 2015 Jul;94(26):e983. [PMID: 26131843]

Kunz PL et al; North American Neuroendocrine Tumor Society. Consensus guidelines for the management and treatment of neuroendocrine tumors. Pancreas. 2013 May;42(4):557–77. [PMID: 23591432]

Valle JW et al. A systematic review of non-surgical treatments for pancreatic neuroendocrine tumours. Cancer Treat Rev. 2014 Apr;40(3):376–89. [PMID: 24296109]

MULTIPLE ENDOCRINE NEOPLASIA (MEN)

MEN TYPES 1–4

ESSENTIALS OF DIAGNOSIS

► **MEN 1:** tumors of the parathyroid glands, endocrine pancreas and duodenum, anterior pituitary, adrenal, thyroid; carcinoid tumors; lipomas and facial angiofibromas.

► **MEN 2 (MEN 2A):** medullary thyroid cancers, pheochromocytomas, Hirschsprung disease.

► **MEN 3 (MEN 2B):** medullary thyroid cancers, pheochromocytomas, Marfan-like habitus, mucosal neuromas, intestinal ganglioneuroma, delayed puberty.

► **MEN 4:** tumors of the parathyroid glands, anterior pituitary gland, adrenal gland, ovary, testicle, kidney.

Syndromes of MEN are inherited as autosomal dominant traits that cause a predisposition to the development of tumors of two or more different endocrine glands (Table 26–14). MEN syndromes are caused by different germline mutations and tumors arising when certain additional somatic mutations occur in predisposed organs. Patients with MEN should have genetic testing so that their first-degree relatives may then be tested for the specific mutation.

1. MEN 1

Multiple endocrine neoplasia type 1 (MEN 1, Wermer syndrome) is a tumor syndrome with a prevalence of 2–10 per 100,000 persons in the United States. About 90% of affected patients harbor a detectable germline mutation in the *menin* gene. Genetic testing is able to detect the specific mutation in 60–95% of cases.

The presentation of MEN 1 is quite variable, even in the same kindred. Affected patients are prone to many different tumors, particularly involving the parathyroids, endocrine pancreas and duodenum, and anterior pituitary. With close endocrine surveillance of affected individuals, the initial biochemical manifestations (usually hypercalcemia) can often be detected as early as age 14–18 years in patients with a MEN 1 gene mutation, although clinical manifestations usually present in the third or fourth decade.

Hyperparathyroidism is the first clinical manifestation of MEN 1 in two-thirds of affected patients, but it may present at any time of life. The hyperparathyroidism of MEN 1 is notoriously difficult to treat surgically, due to multiple gland involvement and the frequency of supernumerary glands and ectopic parathyroid tissue. Typically, three and one-half glands are resected, leaving one-half of the most normal-appearing gland intact. Also, during neck surgery, a thymectomy is performed to resect any intrathymic parathyroid glands or occult thymic carcinoid tumors. Nevertheless, the surgical failure rate is about 38%, and there is a recurrence rate of about 16%, with hypercalcemia often recurring many years after neck surgery. Aggressive parathyroid resection can cause permanent hypoparathyroidism. Patients with persistent or recurrent hyperparathyroidism should avoid oral calcium supplements and thiazide diuretics; oral therapy with a calcimimetic drug, such as cinacalcet, may be effective.

Table 26–14. Multiple endocrine neoplasia (MEN) syndromes: Incidence of tumor types.

Tumor Type	MEN 1	MEN 2 (MEN 2A)	MEN 3 (MEN 2B)	MEN 4
Parathyroid	95%	20–50%	Rare	Common
Pancreatic	54%			Common
Pituitary	42%			Common
Medullary thyroid carcinoma		> 90%	80%	
Pheochromocytoma	Rare	20–35%	60%	
Mucosal and gastrointestinal ganglioneuromas		Rare	> 90%	
Subcutaneous lipoma	30%			
Adrenocortical adenoma	30%			Common
Thoracic carcinoid	15%			
Thyroid adenoma	55%			Common
Facial angiofibromas and collagenomas	85%			

GEP-NETs and carcinoids occur in up to 70% of patients with MEN 1. The GEP-NETs may secrete only pancreatic polypeptide or be nonsecretory altogether (20–55%). **Gastrinomas** occur in about 40% of patients with MEN 1. Concurrent hypercalcemia, due to hyperparathyroidism in MEN 1, stimulates gastrin and worsens gastric acid secretion; control of the hypercalcemia often reduces serum gastrin levels and gastric acid secretion. Gastrinomas of MEN 1 tend to be small, multiple, and ectopic; they are frequently found outside the pancreas, usually in the duodenum. They can metastasize to the liver; but in patients with MEN 1 (depending on the kindred), hepatic metastases tend to be less aggressive than those from sporadic gastrinomas. Treatment of gastrinomas of MEN 1 is usually conservative, using long-term high-dose proton pump inhibitor therapy and control of hypercalcemia; surgery is palliative and usually reserved for aggressive gastrinomas and those tumors arising in the duodenum. Carcinoid tumors can arise in the lung or abdomen and can metastasize, especially to liver.

Insulinomas occur in about 10% of patients with MEN 1. Surgery is usually attempted, but the tumors can be small, multiple, and difficult to detect. **Glucagonomas** occur in 1.6% of patients with MEN 1, **VIPomas** in 1%, and **somatostatinomas** in 0.7%. **Extrapancreatic NETs** are common in MEN 1, are frequently malignant, and include carcinoid tumors usually in foregut locations (69%), such as the lung, thymus, duodenum, or stomach.

Pituitary adenomas are the presenting tumor in 29% of patients with MEN 1 and eventually are found in about 42% of patients with MEN 1. About 78% of these pituitary adenomas occur in women. In MEN 1 patients with a pituitary adenoma, hyperparathyroidism is more common (92%). The majority of pituitary adenomas are found on routine screening of patients with known MEN 1. About 42% of the pituitary adenomas secrete prolactin, while others secrete GH (6%), ACTH (3%), gonadotrophins (2%), or multiple hormones (5%). The prolactinomas usually respond to medical therapy with cabergoline. In MEN 1, about 42% of pituitary adenomas are nonsecretory. While nonsecretory pituitary microadenomas (less than 1 cm diameter and detected on routine MRI screening) are usually indolent, about 25% of nonsecretory pituitary adenomas are macroadenomas (1 cm or more in diameter) and more aggressive.

Adrenal adenomas or **hyperplasia** occurs in about 40% of patients with MEN 1 and 50% are bilateral. They are generally benign and nonfunctional. These adrenal lesions are ACTH-independent.

Thymic NETs occur in 3.4% of affected patients, mostly in males, with a 10-year survival of 25%. **Lung NETs** occur in 13%, with a 10-year survival of 71%.

Benign thyroid adenomas or multinodular goiter occurs in about 55% of MEN 1 patients. Patients may undergo a thyroidectomy at the time of parathyroidectomy.

Nonendocrine tumors occur commonly in MEN 1, particularly small head-neck angiofibromas (85%) and lipomas (30%). Collagenomas are common (70%), presenting as firm dermal nodules. Affected patients may also be more prone to meningiomas, breast cancer, colorectal cancers, prostate cancer, and malignant melanomas.

Variants of MEN 1 also occur. Kindreds with MEN 1 Burin variant have a high prevalence of prolactinomas, late-onset hyperparathyroidism, and carcinoid tumors, but rarely enteropancreatic tumors. Overall, patients with MEN 1 have an increased mortality rate with a mean life expectancy of only 55 years.

2. MEN 2 (MEN 2A)

Multiple endocrine neoplasia type 2 (MEN 2A, Sipple syndrome) is a rare autosomal-dominant tumor syndrome that arises in patients with a germline *ret* protooncogene mutation. Genetic testing identifies about 95% of affected individuals. Each kindred has a certain *ret* codon mutation that correlates with a particular variation in the MEN 2 (2A) syndrome. However, there is incomplete penetrance, and about 30% of those with germline *ret* protooncogene mutations never manifest any of the following endocrine tumors.

Medullary thyroid carcinoma (greater than 90%); **hyperparathyroidism** (20–50%), with hyperplasia or adenomas of multiple parathyroid glands developing in over 70% of cases; **pheochromocytomas** (20–35%), which are often bilateral; or **Hirschsprung disease** may develop in patients with MEN 2 (2A). The medullary thyroid carcinoma is of mild to moderate aggressiveness. Children harboring an MEN 2A ret mutation are advised to have a prophylactic total thyroidectomy by age 6 years. No patients with MEN 2 should receive therapy for diabetes with glucagon-like peptide 1 (GLP 1) agonists that may increase the risk for medullary thyroid carcinoma. Before any surgical procedure, MEN 2 (2A) carriers should be screened for pheochromocytoma (see above) and for medullary thyroid carcinoma. The latter screening involves a thyroid ultrasound and a serum calcitonin drawn after 3 days of omeprazole, 20 mg orally twice daily; in medullary thyroid carcinoma, calcitonin levels usually rise to greater than 80 pg/mL (23 pmol/L) in women or greater than 190 pg/mL (56 pmol/L) in men.

3. MEN 3 (MEN 2B)

Multiple endocrine neoplasia type 3 (MEN 2B) is a familial, autosomal dominant multiglandular syndrome that is also caused by a mutation of the *ret* protooncogene. MEN 3 (2B) is characterized by mucosal neuromas (in more than 90% of affected patients) with bumpy and enlarged lips and tongue, Marfan-like habitus (75% of cases), adrenal pheochromocytomas (60%) that are rarely malignant and often bilateral, and medullary thyroid carcinoma (80%). Patients also have intestinal abnormalities (75%) such as intestinal ganglioneuromas, skeletal abnormalities (87%), and delayed puberty (43%). Medullary thyroid carcinoma is aggressive and presents early in life. Therefore, infants having a parent with MEN 3 (2B) must receive early genetic screening, with those carrying the *ret* protooncogene mutation undergoing a prophylactic total thyroidectomy by age 6 months.

4. MEN 4

Multiple endocrine neoplasia type 4 (MEN 4) is a rare autosomal-dominant familial tumor syndrome caused by germline mutations in the gene *CDKN1B*. Affected patients are particularly prone to adenomas of the pituitary, parathyroid glands, and NETs of the pancreas. Unlike patients with MEN 1, those with MEN 4 are also appear to be prone to adrenal tumors, renal tumors, testicular cancer, and neuroendocrine cervical carcinoma.

OTHER SYNDROMES OF MULTIPLE ENDOCRINE NEOPLASIA

Tumors in the adrenal cortex, pituitary, thyroid, and gonads as well as cardiac myxomas and hyperpigmentation are seen in patients with **Carney complex**. In patients with **Cowden disease** thyroid abnormalities (66%) such as benign adenomas and follicular adenocarcinomas, along with breast cancer (20–36% in women), and multiple hamartomas that affect the skin and multiple other organs develop. Precocious puberty (particularly girls) due to gonadal hypersecretion, Cushing syndrome caused by multiple adrenal nodules, hyperthyroidism from autonomously functioning thyroid nodules, and acromegaly caused by GH-secreting pituitary tumors are seen in patients with **McCune-Albright syndrome**. Patients have fibrous dysplasia of bones and hypophosphatemia, and bone fractures are common. Sudden death has been reported.

de Laat JM et al. Natural course and survival of neuroendocrine tumors of thymus and lung in MEN1 patients. J Clin Endocrinol Metab. 2014 Sep;99(9):3325–33. [PMID: 24915123]

Thakker RV et al; Endocrine Society. Clinical practice guidelines for multiple endocrine neoplasia type 1 (MEN 1). J Clin Endocrinol Metab. 2012 Sep;97(9):2990–3011. [PMID: 22723327]

Thakker RV. Multiple endocrine neoplasia type 1 (MEN 1) and type 4 (MEN 4). Mol Cell Endocrinol. 2014 Apr 5;386(1–2): 2–15. [PMID: 23933118]

DISEASES OF THE TESTES & MALE BREAST

MALE HYPOGONADISM

ESSENTIALS OF DIAGNOSIS

▶ Diminished libido and erections.

▶ Fatigue, depression, reduced exercise endurance.

▶ Decreased growth of body hair.

▶ Testes small or normal in size.

▶ Serum total testosterone or free testosterone level is decreased.

▶ Serum gonadotropin (LH and FSH) levels are decreased or normal in hypogonadotropic hypogonadism; they are increased in testicular failure (hypergonadotropic hypogonadism).

Table 26–15. Causes of male hypogonadism.

Hypogonadotropic (Low or Normal LH)	Hypergonadotropic (High LH)
Aging	Aging
Alcohol	Antitumor chemotherapy
Chronic illness	Bilateral anorchia
Congenital syndromes	Idiopathic
Constitutional delay	Klinefelter syndrome
Cushing syndrome	Leprosy
Drugs	Lymphoma
Estrogen	Male climacteric
GnRH agonist (leuprolide)	Mumps
Ketoconazole	Myotonic dystrophy
Marijuana	Noonan syndrome
Prior androgens	Orchitis
Spironolactone	Radiation therapy
Hemochromatosis	Sertoli cell-only syndrome
Hypopituitarism	Testicular trauma
Hypothyroidism	Tuberculosis
Idiopathic	Uremia
Kallmann syndrome	
17-Ketosteroid reductase deficiency	
Major medical or surgical illnesses	
Malnourishment	
Obesity (BMI > 30)	
Prader-Willi syndrome	

BMI, body mass index; GnRH, gonadotropin-releasing hormone; LH, luteinizing hormone.

▶ General Considerations

Male hypogonadism is caused by deficient testosterone secretion by the testes. It may be classified according to whether it is due to (1) insufficient gonadotropin secretion by the pituitary (hypogonadotropic); (2) pathology in the testes themselves (hypergonadotropic); or (3) both (Table 26–15). Partial male hypogonadism may be difficult to distinguish from the physiologic reduction in serum testosterone seen in normal aging, obesity, and illness.

▶ Etiology

A. Hypogonadotropic Hypogonadism (Low Testosterone with Normal or Low LH)

A deficiency in FSH and LH may be isolated or associated with other pituitary hormonal abnormalities. (See Hypopituitarism.) Hypogonadotropic hypogonadism can be **primary**, defined as failure to enter puberty by age 14, with causes including isolated hypogonadotropic hypogonadism, hypopituitarism, or simple constitutional delay of growth and puberty; or it can be **acquired**, with causes including pituitary or hypothalamic tumors, granulomatous diseases, lymphocytic hypophysitis, or hemochromatosis; Cushing syndrome; adrenal insufficiency; and thyroid hormone excess or deficiency. Genetic conditions (eg, Kallmann syndrome or *PROKR2* mutations) account for about 40% of cases of isolated, and apparently idiopathic, acquired hypogonadotropic hypogonadism with a serum testosterone level less than 150 ng/dL (5.2 nmol/L).

Partial male hypogonadotropic hypogonadism is defined as a serum testosterone in the range of 150–300 ng/dL (5.2–10.4 nmol/L). The main causes of acquired partial male hypogonadotropic hypogonadism include obesity, poor health, or normal aging, such that it is termed **age-related hypogonadism**. Spermatogenesis is usually preserved. After age 40, serum total testosterone declines variably by an average of 1–2% annually; serum free testosterone levels decline even faster, since sex hormone binding globulin increases with age. Serum levels of free testosterone are lower in men aged 40–70 compared with younger men, without any increase in serum LH. A problem with the diagnosis of age-related hypogonadism is that many laboratories provide reference ranges for testosterone that are derived from young men and may not provide age-adjusted reference ranges for serum testosterone and free testosterone. Consequently, among men ages 60–79 years, 20% have low serum total testosterone levels less than 317 ng/dL (11 nmol/L) and 25% have low serum free testosterone levels less than 65 pg/mL (225 pmol/L). Among men over age 80 years, 25% have low serum total testosterone levels and 45% have low serum free testosterone levels. Increasing obesity is the main reversible condition that contributes to the general decline in serum free testosterone with aging. After age 70, LH levels tend to rise, indicating a contribution of primary gonadal dysfunction with advancing age.

B. Hypergonadotropic Hypogonadism (Testicular Failure with High LH)

A failure of the testicular Leydig cells to secrete adequate testosterone causes a rise in LH. If testicular Sertoli cell function is deficient, FSH will also be elevated. Conditions that can cause testicular failure include viral infection (eg, mumps), irradiation, cancer chemotherapy or radioisotope therapy, autoimmunity, myotonic dystrophy, uremia, XY gonadal dysgenesis, partial 17-ketosteroid reductase deficiency, Klinefelter syndrome, and male climacteric. In men who have had a unilateral orchiectomy for cancer, the remaining testicle frequently fails, even in the absence of radiation or chemotherapy. Male hypergonadotropic hypogonadism can also be caused by a congenital partial deficiency in the steroidogenic enzyme CYP17 (17-hydroxylase). CYP17 may be deliberately inhibited by abiraterone acetate, a drug for prostate cancer.

Klinefelter syndrome (47,XXY and its variants) is the most common chromosomal abnormality among males, with an incidence of about 1:500. It is caused by the expression of an abnormal karyotype, classically 47,XXY. Other karyotypes occur, eg, 46,XY/47,XXY mosaicism, 48,XXYY, 48,XXXY, or 46,XX males. The manifestations of Klinefelter syndrome are variable and diagnosed in less than 25% of patients. Testes feel normal during childhood, but during adolescence they usually become firm, fibrotic, small, and nontender to palpation. Affected children have an increased risk of cryptorchidism, decreased penile size,

delayed speech, learning disabilities, psychiatric disturbances, and mediastinal malignancies. Up to 75% of affected boys experience some gynecomastia at puberty. Although puberty occurs at the normal time, the degree of virilization is variable. Serum testosterone is usually low and gonadotropins are elevated. Adult men usually have somewhat reduced facial and pubic hair. Over 95% have azoospermia or severe oligospermia, although some sperm production is often present in their early teens. Men with 46,XY/47,XXY mosaicism may have spontaneous fertility. Also, testicular biopsy reveals sperm in up to 50% of affected patients, allowing some men to be fertile with the use of in vitro fertilization using intracytoplasmic sperm injection (ICSI). Other common findings include tall stature and abnormal body proportions that are unusual for hypogonadal men (eg, height more than 3 cm greater than arm span). Patients with multiple X or Y chromosomes are more apt to have mental deficiency and other abnormalities such as clinodactyly or synostosis. They may also exhibit problems with coordination and social skills. Other problems include a higher incidence of breast cancer, chronic pulmonary disease, varicosities of the legs, osteoporosis, and diabetes mellitus (8% of patients) and impaired glucose tolerance (in another 19%).

The diagnosis of Klinefelter syndrome is confirmed by karyotyping or by determining the presence of RNA for X-inactive-specific transcriptase (XIST) in peripheral blood leukocytes by polymerase chain reaction. On semen analysis, most men (about 95%) with classic Klinefelter syndrome have azoospermia. **XY gonadal dysgenesis** describes several conditions that result in the failure of the testes to develop normally. *SRY* is a gene on the Y chromosome that initiates male sexual development. Mutations in *SRY* result in testicular dysgenesis. Affected individuals lack testosterone, which results in sex reversal: female external genitalia with a blind vaginal pouch, no uterus, and intra-abdominal dysgenetic gonads. Affected individuals are raised as girls and appear normal until their lack of pubertal development and amenorrhea leads to the diagnosis. Intra-abdominal rudimentary testes have an increased risk of developing a malignancy and are usually resected. Patients are considered women and receive estrogen replacement therapy.

C. Androgen Insensitivity

Partial resistance to testosterone is a rare condition in which phenotypic males have variable degrees of apparent hypogonadism, hypospadias, cryptorchism, and gynecomastia. Serum testosterone levels are normal.

▶ Clinical Findings

A. Symptoms and Signs

Hypogonadism that is congenital or acquired during childhood presents as delayed puberty. Men with acquired hypogonadism have variable manifestations, known as "testosterone deficiency syndrome." Most men experience decreased libido. Others complain of erectile dysfunction, poor morning erection, or hot sweats. Men often have depression, fatigue, or decreased ability to perform vigorous physical activity. The presenting complaint may also be infertility, gynecomastia, headache, fracture, or other symptoms related to the cause or result of the hypogonadism. The patient's history often gives a clue to the cause (Table 26–15).

Physical signs associated with hypogonadism may include decreased body, axillary, beard, or pubic hair, but only after years of severe hypogonadism. Men with hypogonadism lose muscle mass and gain weight due to an increase in subcutaneous fat. Examination should include measurements of arm span and height. Testicular size should be assessed with an orchidometer (normal volume is about 10–25 mL; normal length is usually over 6 cm). Testicular size may decrease but usually remains within the normal range in men with postpubertal hypogonadotropic hypogonadism, but it may be diminished with testicular injury or Klinefelter syndrome. The testes must also be carefully palpated for masses, since Leydig cell tumors may secrete estrogen and present with hypogonadism. The testicles must be carefully examined for evidence of trauma, infiltrative lesions (eg, lymphoma), or infection (eg, leprosy, tuberculosis).

B. Laboratory Findings

The evaluation for hypogonadism begins with a morning serum testosterone or free testosterone measurement (or both). Serum testosterone levels are considered low if they are confirmed to be less than 320 ng/dL (11 nmol/L). Serum free testosterone levels are considered low if they are confirmed to be less than 64 pg/mL (220 pmol/L).

Normal ranges for serum testosterone have been derived from nonfasting morning blood specimens, which tend to be the highest of the day. Later in the day, serum testosterone levels can be 25–50% lower. Therefore, a serum testosterone drawn fasting or late in the day may be misleadingly below the "normal range." Serum testosterone levels in men are highest at age 20–30 years and slightly lower at age 30–40 years; testosterone falls gradually but progressively after age 40 years. Testing for serum free testosterone is especially important for detecting hypogonadism in elderly men, who generally have high levels of sex hormone binding globulin. A low serum testosterone should be verified with a repeat assay and further evaluated with serum LH and FSH levels. LH and FSH are high in patients with hypergonadotropic hypogonadism but low or inappropriately normal in men with hypogonadotropic hypogonadism or normal aging. High serum estradiol levels are seen in men with obesity-related hypogonadotropic hypogonadism; sufficient weight loss causes a decrease in serum estradiol in such men.

Testosterone stimulates erythropoiesis in men, causing the normal red blood count range to be higher in men than in women; mild anemia is common in men with hypogonadism. For men with long-standing male hypogonadism, bone densitometry is recommended. Men with severe osteoporosis may require treatment with bisphosphonates and vitamin D, in addition to testosterone replacement therapy.

1. Hypogonadotropic hypogonadism—A serum PRL determination is obtained but may be elevated for many reasons (see Table 26–2). Men with gynecomastia may be screened for partial 17-ketosteroid reductase deficiency with serum determinations for androstenedione and estrone, which are elevated in this condition. Hypogonadotropic hypogonadism can also be seen with X-linked congenital adrenal hypoplasia, which causes hypogonadotropic hypogonadism and arrested puberty, azoospermia, and primary adrenal insufficiency; adrenal insufficiency usually presents in childhood but may remain undiagnosed into adulthood. The serum estradiol level may be elevated in patients with cirrhosis and in rare cases of estrogen-secreting tumors (testicular Leydig cell tumor or adrenal carcinoma). Men with no discernible definite cause for hypogonadotropic hypogonadism should be screened for hemochromatosis and have an MRI of the pituitary and hypothalamic region to look for a tumor or other lesion.

2. Hypergonadotropic hypogonadism—Men with hypergonadotropic hypogonadism have low serum testosterone levels with a compensatory increase in FSH and LH. Klinefelter syndrome can be confirmed by karyotyping or by measurement of leukocyte XIST. Testicular biopsy is usually reserved for younger patients in whom the reason for primary hypogonadism is unclear.

▶ Treatment

Testosterone replacement is reasonable for boys who have not entered puberty by age 14 years. It is also beneficial for most men with primary testicular failure (hypergonadotropic hypogonadism). Testosterone replacement is also warranted for men with severe hypogonadotropic hypogonadism of any etiology with serum testosterone levels less than 150 ng/mL (5.2 nmol/L). Many men have partial hypogonadotropic hypogonadism ("age-related hypogonadism") with serum testosterone levels low but greater than 150 ng/mL (5.2 nol/L) or serum free testosterone level low but greater than 40 pg/mL (140 pmol/L). Testosterone therapy should be considered for men with age-related hypogonadism if they have at least three of the following six symptoms: erectile dysfunction, poor morning erection, low libido, depression, fatigue, and inability to perform vigorous activity; testosterone replacement should be continued only if they clearly derive clinical benefit from therapy.

Testosterone therapy carries certain risks. The FDA has registered concern over the use of testosterone therapy for age-related hypogonadism, since there have been no controlled trials to determine the effects of testosterone therapy on cardiovascular outcomes. Due to such potential risks, testosterone therapy should not be given to men unless they have had a documented low serum total or free testosterone. Testosterone therapy should not be given to men with active breast cancer or prostate cancer. In men over age 50 years, a digital prostate examination and serum prostate-specific antigen (PSA) level should be done before beginning testosterone therapy. Men with symptoms of prostatic hypertrophy, a palpable prostate nodule, or a PSA greater than 4 ng/mL (greater than 3 ng/mL in men of

African ancestry) should have a urologic evaluation prior to treatment. Although serum PSA screening has not reduced prostate cancer-related mortality, many clinicians monitor serum PSA levels regularly in men receiving testosterone therapy. It is also prudent to monitor the hematocrit and lipid profile of men receiving testosterone, since therapy can cause erythrocytosis and hyperlipidemia. Testosterone therapy can also cause gynecomastia. Testosterone therapy is not given to men with untreated sleep apnea or heart failure. In men who have coronary risk factors or are over age 65, special attention should be given to improving cardiac risk factors (eg, controlling hypertension or hyperlipidemia) and administering low-dose aspirin while receiving testosterone replacement.

Drug interactions can occur. Testosterone should be administered cautiously to men receiving coumadin, since the combination can increase the INR and risk of bleeding. Similarly, testosterone therapy can increase serum levels of cyclosporine, tacrolimus, and tolvaptan. Testosterone can predispose to hypoglycemia in diabetic men receiving insulin or oral hypoglycemic agents, so close monitoring of blood sugars is advisable during initiation of testosterone therapy.

Oral androgen therapy with methyltestosterone is not advisable due to the potential for causing liver tumors, peliosis hepatis, and cholestatic jaundice.

A. Therapies for Male Hypogonadism

1. Testosterone topical gels—Topical testosterone is usually applied once daily in the morning after showering. Topical testosterone should not be applied to the breast or genitals. The gel should be allowed to air-dry (about 10 minutes) before donning a shirt. The patient should avoid swimming, showering, or washing the application area for at least 2 hours following application. **Testosterone topical generic 1%** gel is available in packets (12.5 mg/1.25 g, 25 mg/2.5 g, or 50 mg/5g) or tubes (50 mg/5 g). The recommended dose is 50–100 mg daily. **Testosterone topical generic 2%** gel is available in a gel pump (10 mg/0.5 g actuation). The recommended dose is 40–70 mg daily. **Androgel 1%** gel is available in 2.5-g packets (25 mg testosterone) and 5-g packets (50 mg testosterone) and in a pump that dispenses 12.5 mg testosterone per pump actuation: the recommended dose is 50–100 mg applied daily to the shoulders. **Androgel 1.6%** gel is available in a pump that dispenses 20.25 mg testosterone per pump actuation; the recommended dose is 40.5–81 mg daily. **Testim** 1% gel is available in 5-g tubes (50 mg testosterone); the recommended dose is 50–100 mg applied daily. **Fortesta** 2% gel is available in a pump that dispenses 10 mg testosterone per pump actuation; the recommended dose is 40–70 mg daily. **Testogel** is distributed in 5-g sachets (50 mg testosterone); this brand is not available in the United States. Testim, Fortesta, and Testogel may be applied to shoulders, upper arms, or abdomen. **Axiron** 2% solution is available in a pump that dispenses 30 mg per actuation; the recommended dose is 30–60 mg applied to each axilla daily. **Vogelxo** is a 1% testosterone gel that is available in packets or tubes (50 mg/5 g) or a gel pump (12.5 mg/1.25 g); it is applied to the shoulders in doses of 50–100 mg once daily.

The serum testosterone level should be determined about 14 days after starting therapy; if the level remains below normal or the clinical response is inadequate, the daily dose may be increased to 1.5 to 2 times the initial dose. Unfortunately, serum testosterone levels vary considerably during the day after topical testosterone gel application, such that a single serum testosterone level may not accurately reflect the average serum testosterone for that individual. After the application of topical testosterone, the hands should be washed. The application site should be allowed to dry for 10 minutes before dressing. Before close contact with women or children, a shirt must be worn or the areas of application washed with soap and water to prevent transfer of testosterone to them.

2. Transdermal testosterone patches—Testosterone transdermal systems (skin patches) are applied to nongenital skin. Androderm (2 or 4 mg/day) patches may be applied at bedtime in doses of 4–8 mg; it adheres tightly to the skin and may cause skin irritation.

3. Parenteral testosterone—The dose and injection intervals of injections are adjusted according to the patient's clinical response and serum testosterone levels drawn just before the next injection is due. A target serum testosterone level of 500 ng/dL (17.3 nmol/L) is suggested. **Testosterone cypionate** has been in use for decades; it is an intramuscular testosterone formulation that is available in solutions containing 200 mg/mL. Its main advantage is low cost. The usual dose is 200 mg every 2 weeks or 300 mg every 3 weeks. It is usually injected into the gluteus medius muscle in the upper lateral buttock, alternating sides.

Testosterone pellets (Testopel) is a very long-lasting depot testosterone formulation that is available as individual vials containing a single 75 mg implantable pellet in each vial. With sterile technique, the skin of the upper-outer buttock is anesthetized with lidocaine; using a trochar, the pellets are injected subcutaneously in doses of 150–450 mg every 3–6 months as an in-office procedure.

Testosterone undecanoate (Aveed, Nebido) is a long-lasting depot testosterone formulation. Its use is restricted to qualified healthcare facilities. It is usually injected into the gluteus medius muscle in the upper lateral buttock, alternating sides. Care must be taken to avoid intravascular injection by pulling back on the syringe plunger before injection; if any blood appears in the syringe, the needle is withdrawn and the syringe is discarded. Testosterone undecanoate (Aveed) is formulated as individual vials containing 750 mg/3 mL oily solution for intramuscular injection. The initial injection of 750 mg is followed by another 750 mg injection 4 weeks later and maintenance doses of 750 mg every 10 weeks. Testosterone undecanoate (Nebido) is formulated as individual vials containing 1000 mg/4 mL oily solution for intramuscular injection. The initial injection of 1000 mg is followed by another 1000 mg injection 6 weeks later and maintenance doses of 1000 mg every 12 weeks. A serum testosterone level is measured before the fourth dose; if the serum testosterone remains low, the dosing interval is shortened to every 10 weeks.

Caution: Testosterone undecanoate injections have caused serious pulmonary oil microembolism reactions that present with cough, dyspnea, tight throat, chest pain, and syncope. Anaphylaxis can also occur. *Patients must be observed in the healthcare setting for 30 minutes after the injection in order to provide appropriate medical care for the complication.*

4. Buccal testosterone—Testosterone buccal tablets (Striant) are placed between the upper lip and gingivae. One or two 30-mg tablets are thus retained and changed every 12 hours. They should not be chewed or swallowed.

5. Testosterone nasal gel—An intranasal gel formulation of testosterone (Natesto) is available. It is self-administered by a metered-dose nasal pump: one pump actuation (5.5 mg) into each nostril three times daily. The nasal pump needs to be primed by inverting it and pressing the pump 10 times before it is used the first time. It should not be used concurrently with intranasal sympathomimetic decongestants. Adverse effects include nasopharyngitis, sinusitis, bronchitis, epistaxis, nasal discomfort, and headache.

6. Oral methyltestosterone—Oral testosterone supplementation is available as methyltestosterone 10 mg tablets. The usual dose is 10–50 mg daily, given either once daily or given in divided doses. Oral methyltestosterone can produce acute hepatitis and chronic high-dose use can cause peliosis hepatis, cholestatic hepatitis, and hepatocellular carcinoma. Therefore, its use is not recommended, and it is no longer available in some countries.

7. Clomiphene citrate—Men with functional hypogonadotropic hypogonadism usually respond well to clomiphene citrate that is administered orally in doses that are titrated to achieve the desired clinical response with a serum testosterone level of about 500 ng/dL (17.3 nmol/L). Treatment with clomiphene is commenced with 25 mg on alternate days and increased to 50 mg on alternate days if necessary, with a maximum dose of 50 mg daily. Serum testosterone levels usually normalize while spermatogenesis usually improves.

8. Gonadotropins—Patients with hypogonadotropic hypogonadism may require therapy with gonadotropins, particularly to induce fertility. Men may receive hCG 1000 units subcutaneously three times weekly for 6 months; if the semen analysis shows inadequate sperm, FSH 75 units subcutaneously three times weekly is added. Many men prefer long-term therapy with hCG over testosterone therapy, but cost is an issue.

9. Weight loss—When hypogonadotropic hypogonadism is due to morbid obesity, significant weight loss will improve serum testosterone levels. The rise in serum testosterone is proportionate to the weight loss. Although diet-induced weight loss is beneficial, bariatric surgery has been much more effective and serum testosterone levels may normalize after dramatic weight loss.

B. Benefits of Testosterone Replacement Therapy

Testosterone therapy usually benefits men with low serum testosterone and at least three manifestations of hypogonadism. Testosterone therapy can improve overall mood, sense of well-being, sexual desire, and erectile function. It also increases physical vigor and muscle strength as manifested in measurements of leg-press and chest-press strength. Testosterone replacement also improves exercise endurance and stair climbing ability. Long-term testosterone replacement causes significant weight loss and a reduction in waist circumference. After 2 years of testosterone replacement, muscle mass increases about 4.5%, while fat mass decreases by about 9.1%. Testosterone replacement therapy also appears to improve overall survival.

C. Risks of Testosterone Replacement Therapy

Testosterone therapy can **aggravate benign prostatic hyperplasia** (BPH). However, aggravation of voiding problems is uncommon. In men with BPH, finasteride may be coadministered with testosterone to reduce prostate size. There have been no sufficient long-term trials studying the effect of testosterone supplementation on the incidence and mortality from prostate cancer. However, a meta-analysis of 19 smaller studies showed no statistically significant increased risk for prostate cancer among men receiving testosterone supplementation. Nevertheless, concern remains. Testosterone therapy is contraindicated in the presence of active prostate cancer, and it is prudent to screen for prostate cancer with a serum PSA before commencing therapy. Hypogonadal men who have had a prostatectomy for low-grade prostate cancer, and who have remained in complete remission for several years, may have testosterone therapy given cautiously while monitoring serum PSA levels.

Erythrocytosis develops in some men who are treated with testosterone. Erythrocytosis is more common with intramuscular injections of testosterone enanthate than with transcutaneous testosterone. However, no increase in the incidence of thromboembolic events has been reported.

Testosterone therapy tends to **aggravate sleep apnea** in older men, likely through CNS effects. Surveillance for sleep apnea is recommended during testosterone therapy and a formal evaluation with nocturnal pulse oximetry recording is recommended for all high-risk patients with snoring, obesity, partner's report of apneic episodes, nocturnal awakening, unrefreshing sleep with daytime fatigue, or hypertension.

Men who are treated with testosterone frequently experience some increase in **acne** that is usually mild and tolerated; topical antiacne therapy or a reduction in testosterone replacement dosage may be required. **Increases in intraocular pressure** have occurred during testosterone therapy. During the initiation of testosterone replacement therapy, **gynecomastia** develops in some men, which usually is mild and tends to resolve spontaneously; switching from testosterone injections to testosterone transdermal gel may help this condition.

D. Risks of Performance-enhancing Anabolic Steroids

Performance-enhancing agents, particularly androgenic anabolic steroids, are used by up to 2% of young athletes and by 20–65% of power sport athletes. They are often used as part of a "stacking" polypharmacy that may include nandrolone decanoate, dimethandrolone, testosterone propionate, or testosterone enanthate. These androgens are usually illegal and often contaminated by toxic substances and can produce toxic hepatitis, dependence, aggression, depression, dyslipidemias, gynecomastia, acne, male pattern baldness, hepatitis, thromboembolism, and cardiomyopathy. Shared needles may transmit hepatitis or HIV. Arsenic contamination has been reported to cause multiorgan failure and death.

▶ Prognosis of Male Hypogonadism

If hypogonadism is due to a pituitary lesion, the prognosis is that of the primary disease (eg, tumor, necrosis). The prognosis for restoration of virility is good if testosterone is given.

Basaria S. Male hypogonadism. Lancet. 2014 Apr 5; 383(9924):1250–63. [PMID: 24119423]

Dean J et al. Diagnosing secondary hypogonadism: important consequences for fertility and reversibility. BJU Int. 2016 Apr; 117(4):552–4. [PMID: 26360119]

Finkelstein JS et al. Gonadal steroids and body composition, strength, and sexual function in men. N Engl J Med. 2013 Sep 12;369(11):1011–22. [PMID: 24024838]

Groth KA et al. Clinical review. Klinefelter syndrome—a clinical update. J Clin Endocrinol Metab. 2013 Jan;98(1):20–30. [PMID: 23118429]

Klotz L. Testosterone therapy and prostate cancer—safety concerns are well founded. Nat Rev Urol. 2015 Jan;12(1):48–54. [PMID: 25563848]

Nguyen CP et al. Testosterone and "age-related hypogonadism"—FDA Concerns. N Engl J Med. 2015 Aug 20;373(8): 689–91. [PMID: 26287846]

Ramasamy R et al. Association between testosterone supplementation therapy and thrombotic events in elderly men. Urology. 2015 Aug;86(2):283–5. [PMID: 26299630]

Seftel AD et al. Critical update of the 2010 Endocrine Society clinical practice guidelines for male hypogonadism: a systematic analysis. Mayo Clin Proc. 2015 Aug;90(8):1104–15. [PMID: 26205546]

Sugerman DT. JAMA patient page. Low testosterone. JAMA. 2013 Nov 6;310(17):1872. [PMID: 24193092]

Swerdloff RS et al. Serum testosterone (T) level variability in T gel-treated older hypogonadal men: treatment monitoring implications. J Clin Endocrinol Metab. 2015 Sep;100(9):3280–7. [PMID: 26120790]

CRYPTORCHISM

One or both testes may be absent from the scrotum at birth in about 20% of premature or low-birth-weight male infants and in 3–6% of full term infants. Cryptorchism is found in 1–2% of males after 1 year of age but must be distinguished from retractile testes, which require no treatment. Infertility or subfertility occurs in up to 75% of men with bilateral cryptorchism and in 50% of men with unilateral cryptorchism. Some patients have underlying hypogonadism, including hypogonadotropic hypogonadism.

If the testes are not palpable, it is important to determine whether they are cryptorchid or intra-abdominal. MRI is more reliable than ultrasound for locating cryptorchid testes. Surgery for cryptorchid testes (orchiopexy)

should be performed by age 12–24 months and is generally successful. Alternatively, hCG, 1500 units intramuscularly daily for 3 days, causes a significant rise in testosterone if the testes are present. Therapy with hCG results in a testicular descent rate of about 25%.

The lifetime risk of testicular neoplasia is 0.002% in normal males. The risk of malignancy is higher for cryptorchid testes (0.06%) and for intra-abdominal testes (5%). Orchiopexy decreases the risk of neoplasia when performed before 10 years of age. Orchiectomy after puberty is an option for intra-abdominal testes.

GYNECOMASTIA

ESSENTIALS OF DIAGNOSIS

▶ Palpable enlargement of the male breast, often asymmetric or unilateral.

▶ Glandular gynecomastia characterized by tenderness.

▶ Fatty gynecomastia typically nontender.

▶ Must be distinguished from carcinoma or mastitis.

▶ General Considerations

Gynecomastia is defined as the presence of palpable glandular breast tissue in males. Pubertal gynecomastia develops in about 60% of boys; the swelling usually subsides spontaneously within a year. Gynecomastia is particularly common in teenagers who are very tall or overweight. Gynecomastia develops in about 50% of athletes who abuse androgens and anabolic steroids. About 20% of adult gynecomastia is caused by drug therapy. Gynecomastia can develop in HIV-infected patients treated with antiretroviral therapy, especially in men receiving efavirenz or didanosine; breast enlargement resolves spontaneously in 73% of patients within 9 months. Fatty pseudogynecomastia is common among elderly men, particularly when there is associated weight gain. However, true glandular gynecomastia can be the first sign of a serious disorder in older men.

The causes of gynecomastia are multiple and diverse (Table 26–16).

▶ Clinical Findings

A. Symptoms and Signs

The male breasts must be palpated carefully to distinguish true glandular gynecomastia from fatty pseudogynecomastia in which only adipose tissue is felt. The breasts are best examined both seated and supine. Using the thumb and forefinger as pincers, the subareolar tissue is compared to nearby adipose tissue. Fatty tissue is usually diffuse and nontender. True glandular enlargement beneath the areola may be tender. Pubertal gynecomastia is characterized by tender discoid enlargement of breast tissue 2–3 cm in diameter beneath the areola. The following characteristics

Table 26–16. Causes of gynecomastia.

Idiopathic	Clomiphene
Physiologic causes	Cyclophosphamide
Neonatal period	Diazepam
Puberty	Diethylstilbestrol
Aging	Digitalis preparations
Obesity	Dutasteride
Endocrine diseases	Estrogens (oral or topical)
Androgen resistance	Ethionamide
syndromes	Famotidine (rare)
Aromatase excess syndrome	Fenofibrate (rare)
(sporadic or familial)	Finasteride
Diabetic lymphocytic	Flutamide
mastitis	Goserelin
Hyperprolactinemia	Growth hormone
Hyperthyroidism	Haloperidol
Klinefelter syndrome	Hydroxyzine
Male hypogonadism	Isoniazid
Partial 17-ketosteroid	Ketoconazole
reductase deficiency	Lavender oil (topical)
Systemic diseases	Leuprolide and other GnRH
Androgen insensitivity	analogs
Chronic liver disease	Marijuana
Chronic kidney disease	Meprobamate
Hansen disease (leprosy)	Methadone
Neurologic disorders	Methotrexate (rare)
Refeeding after starvation	Methyldopa
Spinal cord injury	Metoclopramide
Neoplasms	Metronidazole
Adrenal tumors	Mirtazapine
Bronchogenic carcinoma	Nucleotide reverse
Carcinoma of the breast	transcriptase inhibitors
Ectopic hCG: lung,	Nilutamide
hepatocellular, gastric, renal	Omeprazole
carcinomas	Opioids
Pituitary prolactinoma	Penicillamine
Testicular hCG-secreting	Phenothiazines
tumors	Progestins
Drugs (partial list)	Protease inhibitors
Alcohol	Proton pump inhibitors
Alkylating agents	(uncommon)
Amiodarone	Ranitidine (rare)
Anabolic steroids	Reserpine
Androgens	Risperidone
Anti-androgens	Somatropin (growth hormone)
Antiretroviral agents	Soy ingestion
Bicalutamide	Statins (rare)
Busulfan	Spironolactone
Calcium channel blockers	Tea tree oil (topical)
(rare)	Testosterone
Chorionic gonadotropin	Thioridazine
Cimetidine	Tricyclic antidepressants
	Verapamil

are worrisome for malignancy: asymmetry; location not immediately below the areola; unusual firmness; or nipple retraction, bleeding, or discharge.

B. Laboratory Findings

In the presence of true glandular gynecomastia, serum determinations for PRL and beta-hCG are obtained. Detectable levels of beta-hCG implicate a testicular tumor

(germ cell or Sertoli cell) or other malignancy (usually lung or liver), though detectable low levels (less than 5 milli-units/mL) may be reported in primary hypogonadism and high serum LH levels if the assay for beta-hCG cross-reacts with LH. Measurements of serum free testosterone and LH are valuable in the diagnosis of primary or secondary hypogonadism. A low serum free testosterone and high LH are seen in primary hypogonadism. High testosterone levels plus high LH levels characterize partial androgen resistance. Serum estradiol is determined but is usually normal; increased levels may result from testicular tumors, increased beta-hCG, liver disease, obesity, adrenal tumors (rare), true hermaphroditism (rare), or aromatase gene gain-of-function mutations (rare). Serum TSH and FT$_4$ levels are also recommended. A karyotype (for Klinefelter syndrome) is obtained in men with persistent gynecomastia without obvious cause.

Investigation of unclear cases should include a chest radiograph to search for bronchogenic or metastatic carcinoma. Needle biopsy with cytologic examination may be performed on suspicious male breast enlargement (especially when unilateral or asymmetric) to distinguish gynecomastia from breast cancer or mastitis.

▶ Treatment

Pubertal gynecomastia often resolves spontaneously within 1–2 years. Drug-induced gynecomastia resolves after the offending drug is removed (eg, spironolactone stopped, with substitution of eplerenone). Patients with painful or persistent gynecomastia may be treated with medical therapy, usually for 9–12 months. Generally, it is prudent to treat patients for gynecomastia only when it becomes a troubling and continuing problem for them.

Selective estrogen receptor modulator (SERM) therapy is effective for true glandular gynecomastia. Raloxifene, 60 mg orally daily, may be somewhat more effective than tamoxifen, 10–20 mg orally daily.

Aromatase inhibitor (AI) therapy is also reasonably effective. For example, anastrozole reduces breast volume significantly over 6 months in adolescents given in a dose of 1 mg orally daily. Serum estradiol levels fall slightly while serum testosterone levels rise. Long-term AI therapy in adolescents is not recommended because of the possibility of inducing osteoporosis and of delaying epiphyseal fusion, which could cause an increase in adult height.

Testosterone therapy for men with hypogonadism may improve or worsen preexistent gynecomastia.

Radiation therapy has been used prophylactically to prevent gynecomastia in men with prostate cancer being treated with antiandrogen therapy. Low-dose prophylactic radiation therapy reduces its incidence from 71% to 28%. Existing gynecomastia improves in 33% with radiation therapy. However, the long-term breast and other cancer risks of such radiation are unknown.

Surgical correction is reserved for patients with persistent or severe gynecomastia.

Deepinder F et al. Drug-induced gynecomastia: an evidence-based review. Expert Opin Drug Saf. 2012 Sep;11(5):779–95. [PMID: 22862307]

Morcos RN et al. Gynecomastia: when is treatment indicated? J
Fam Pract. 2012 Dec;61(12):719–25. [PMID: 23313989]

Narula HS et al. Gynaecomastia—pathophysiology, diagnosis
and treatment. Nat Rev Endocrinol. 2014 Nov;10(11):684–98.
[PMID: 25112235]

Pallais JC et al. Case records of the Massachusetts General Hospital. Case 38-2015. A 21-year-old man with fatigue and
weight loss. N Engl J Med. 2015 Dec 10;373(24):2358–69.
[PMID: 26650156]

HIRSUTISM & VIRILIZATION

ESSENTIALS OF DIAGNOSIS

► Hirsutism, acne, menstrual disorders.

► Virilization: increased muscularity, androgenic alopecia, deepening of the voice, clitoromegaly.

► Rarely, a palpable pelvic tumor.

► Urinary 17-ketosteroids and serum DHEAS and
androstenedione elevated in adrenal disorders;
variable in others.

► Serum testosterone is often elevated.

► General Considerations

Hirsutism is defined as cosmetically unacceptable terminal
hair growth that appears in women in a male pattern. Significant hirsutism affects about 5–10% of non-Asian
women of reproductive age and over 40% of women at
some point during their life. The amount of hair growth
deemed unacceptable depends on a woman's ethnicity and
familial and cultural norms. Virilization is defined as the
development of male physical characteristics, such as pronounced muscle development, deep voice, male pattern
baldness, and more severe hirsutism.

► Etiology

Hirsutism may be idiopathic or familial or be caused by the
following disorders: polycystic ovary syndrome (PCOS),
ovarian hyperthecosis, steroidogenic enzyme defects, neoplastic disorders; or rarely by medications, acromegaly, or
ACTH-induced Cushing disease.

A. Idiopathic or Familial

Most women with hirsutism or androgenic alopecia have no
detectable hyperandrogenism. Patients often have a strong
familial predisposition to hirsutism that may be considered
normal in the context of their genetic background. Such
patients may have elevated serum levels of androstenediol
glucuronide, a metabolite of dihydrotestosterone that is
produced by skin in cosmetically unacceptable amounts.

B. Polycystic Ovary Syndrome (PCOS, Hyperthecosis, Stein-Leventhal Syndrome)

PCOS is a common functional disorder of the ovaries,
affecting about 4–6% of premenopausal women in the
United States and accounting for at least 50% of all cases of
hirsutism associated with elevated testosterone levels. It is
familial and transmitted as a modified autosomal dominant trait. Affected women have elevated serum testosterone or free testosterone level and have signs of androgen
excess, including hirsutism, acne, and male-pattern thinning of scalp hair. About 50% of affected women have oligomenorrhea or amenorrhea with anovulation.
Hyperandrogenism persists after natural menopause.
Despite the syndrome's name, the presence of ovarian cysts
is not helpful diagnostically and is actually a misnomer,
since about 30% of women with PCOS do *not* have cystic
ovaries and 25–30% of normal menstruating women *have*
cystic ovaries. Obesity and high serum insulin levels (due
to insulin resistance) contribute to the syndrome in 70% of
women. The serum LH:FSH ratio is often greater than 2.0.
Both adrenal and ovarian androgen hypersecretion are
commonly present. Women with PCOS have a 35% risk of
depression, compared with 11% in age-matched controls.
Diabetes mellitus is present in about 13% of cases. Obstructive sleep apnea is particularly common, even in slender
women with PCOS. Untreated women with amenorrhea
have a slightly increased risk of endometrial carcinoma.
Hypertension and hyperlipidemia are often present,
increasing the risk of cardiovascular disease. Women frequently regain normal menstrual cycles with aging.

C. Steroidogenic Enzyme Defects

Congenital adrenal steroidogenic enzyme defects result in
reduced cortisol secretion with a compensatory increase in
ACTH that causes adrenal hyperplasia. The most common
enzyme defect is 21-hydroxylase deficiency, with a prevalence of about 1:18,000.

Partial deficiency in adrenal 21-hydroxylase can present in women as hirsutism. About 2% of patients with
adult-onset hirsutism have been found to have a partial
defect in adrenal 21-hydroxylase. The condition is more
common in Ashkenazi Jews, Yupic Alaskans, and natives of
La Reunion Island. The phenotypic expression is delayed
until adolescence or adulthood; such patients do not have
salt wasting. Polycystic ovaries and adrenal adenomas are
more likely to develop in these women.

Some rare patients with hyperandrogenism and hypertension have 11-hydroxylase deficiency. This is distinguished from cortisol resistance by high cortisol serum
levels in the latter and by high serum 11-deoxycortisol
levels in the former.

Patients with an XY karyotype and a deficiency in
17-beta-hydroxysteroid dehydrogenase-3 or a deficiency in
5-alpha-reductase-2 may present as phenotypic girls in
whom virilization develops at puberty.

D. Neoplastic Disorders

Ovarian tumors are very uncommon causes of hirsutism
(0.8%) and include arrhenoblastomas, Sertoli-Leydig cell
tumors, dysgerminomas, and hilar cell tumors. Adrenal carcinoma is a rare cause of Cushing syndrome and hyperandrogenism that can be quite virilizing. Pure androgen-secreting
adrenal tumors occur very rarely; about 50% are malignant.

E. Rare Causes of Hirsutism & Virilization

Acromegaly and ACTH-induced Cushing syndrome are rare causes of hirsutism and virilization. Porphyria cutanea tarda can cause periorbital hair growth in addition to dermatitis in sun-exposed areas. Maternal virilization during pregnancy may occur as a result of a luteoma of pregnancy, hyperreactio luteinalis, or polycystic ovaries. In postmenopausal women, diffuse stromal Leydig cell hyperplasia is a rare cause of hyperandrogenism. Acquired hypertrichosis lanuginosa is manifested by the appearance of diffuse fine lanugo hair growth on the face and body along with stomatologic symptoms; the disorder is usually associated with an internal malignancy, especially colorectal cancer, and may regress after tumor removal. Pharmacologic causes include minoxidil, cyclosporine, phenytoin, anabolic steroids, interferon, cetuximab, diazoxide, and certain progestins.

▶ Clinical Findings

A. Symptoms and Signs

Modest androgen excess from any source increases sexual hair (chin, upper lip, abdomen, and chest) and increases sebaceous gland activity, producing acne. Menstrual irregularities, anovulation, and amenorrhea are common. If androgen excess is pronounced, defeminization (decrease in breast size, loss of feminine adipose tissue) and virilization (frontal balding, muscularity, clitoromegaly, and deepening of the voice) occur. Virilization points to the presence of an androgen-producing neoplasm. Hirsutism is quantitated using the Ferriman-Gallwey score in which hirsutism is graded from 0 (none) to 4 (severe) in nine areas of the body with a maximum possible score of 36; scores 8–15 indicate moderate hirsutism, while scores over 15 indicate severe hirsutism.

A pelvic examination may disclose clitoromegaly or ovarian enlargement that may be cystic or neoplastic. Hypertension may be present and should prompt consideration for the possible diagnosis of Cushing syndrome, adrenal 11-hydroxylase deficiency, or cortisol resistance syndrome.

B. Laboratory Testing and Imaging

Serum androgen testing is mainly useful to screen for rare occult adrenal or ovarian neoplasms. Some general guidelines are presented here, though exceptions are common.

Serum is assayed for total testosterone and free testosterone. A serum testosterone level greater than 200 ng/dL (6.9 nmol/L) or free testosterone greater than 40 ng/dL (140 pmol/L) indicates the need for pelvic examination and ultrasound. If that is negative, an adrenal CT scan is performed.

Most radioimmunoassays and enzyme-linked immunosorbent assays (ELISAs) for testosterone are inaccurate when serum testosterone levels are less than 300 ng/dL (10.4 nmol/L). The more accurate testosterone assays rely on extraction and chromatography, followed by mass spectrometry or immunoassay. Free testosterone is best measured by calculation, using accurate assays for testosterone and sex hormone–binding globulin. A serum androstenedione level greater than 1000 ng/dL (34.9 nmol/L) also points to an ovarian or adrenal neoplasm. Patients with milder elevations of serum testosterone or androstenedione usually are treated with an oral contraceptive.

Patients with a serum DHEAS greater than 700 mcg/dL (35 nmol/L) have an adrenal source of androgen. This usually is due to adrenal hyperplasia and rarely to adrenal carcinoma. An adrenal CT scan is performed.

No firm guidelines exist as to which patients (if any) with hyperandrogenism should be screened for "late-onset" 21-hydroxylase deficiency. The evaluation requires levels of serum 17-hydroxyprogesterone to be drawn at baseline and at 30–60 minutes after the intramuscular injection of 0.25 mg of cosyntropin (ACTH$_{1-24}$). Ideally, this test should be done during the follicular phase of a woman's menstrual cycle. Patients with congenital adrenal hyperplasia will usually have a baseline 17-hydroxyprogesterone level greater than 300 ng/dL (9.1 nmol/L) or a stimulated level greater than 1000 ng/dL (30.3 nmol/L). Patients with any clinical signs of Cushing syndrome should receive a screening test.

Serum levels of FSH and LH are elevated if amenorrhea is due to ovarian failure. An LH:FSH ratio greater than 2.0 is common in patients with PCOS. On abdominal ultrasound, about 25–30% of normal young women have polycystic ovaries, so the appearance of ovarian cysts on ultrasound is not helpful. Pelvic ultrasound or MRI can usually detect virilizing tumors of the ovary. However, small virilizing ovarian tumors may not be detectable on imaging studies; selective venous sampling for testosterone may be used for diagnosis in such patients.

▶ Treatment

Any drugs causing hirsutism (see above) should be stopped. Any underlying medical causes of hirsutism (eg, Cushing syndrome, acromegaly) should be treated.

A. Surgery

Androgenizing tumors of the adrenal or ovary are resected laparoscopically. Postmenopausal women with severe hyperandrogenism should undergo laparoscopic bilateral oophorectomy (if CT scan of the adrenals and ovaries is normal), since small hilar cell tumors of the ovary may not be visible on scans. Women with classic salt-wasting congenital adrenal hyperplasia and infertility or treatment-resistant hyperandrogenism may be treated with laparoscopic bilateral adrenalectomy.

B. Laser and Topical Treatments

Laser therapy (photoepilation) can be a very effective treatment for facial hirsutism, particularly for women with dark hair and light skin; longer-wavelength lasers are used for women with darker skin. In such women, laser removal of facial hair significantly improves their appearance and quality of life. However, laser does not remove nonpigmented hairs. Potential side effects include local pain, erythema, and hyperpigmentation (20%) that usually resolves; skin hypopigmentation occurs rarely. A paradoxical increase in hair growth occurs infrequently. Repeated laser treatments are usually required.

Local treatment of facial hirsutism by shaving or depilatories, waxing, electrolysis, or bleaching should be encouraged. **Eflornithine** (Vaniqa) 13.9% topical cream retards hair growth when applied twice daily to unwanted facial hair; improvement is noted within 4–8 weeks. However, local skin irritation may occur. Hirsutism returns with discontinuation. It may be used in conjunction with laser therapy.

Topical minoxidil may be used to treat androgenic alopecia and is mildly effective when applied to the scalp twice daily. Only the 2% formulation is FDA-approved for women.

C. Medications

Spironolactone is effective for reducing hirsutism, acne, and androgenic alopecia in women and is a first-line medical strategy for these women. It may be taken in doses of 100–200 mg orally daily (taken as a single dose or in two divided doses) on days 5–25 of the menstrual cycle or daily if used concomitantly with an oral contraceptive. Spironolactone is contraindicated in pregnancy, so reproductive-age women must use reliable contraception during this therapy. Hyperkalemia is an uncommon side effect, but serum potassium should be checked 1 month after beginning therapy or after dosage increases. Spironolactone should be avoided or used cautiously in women who are prone to hyperkalemia, including women with kidney disease or who are taking an ACE inhibitor or ARB for hypertension. Trimethoprim-sulfamethoxazole should not be taken along with high-dose spironolactone due to the risk of hyperkalemia and sudden death. Side effects of spironolactone include breast tenderness, menstrual irregularity, headaches, nausea, and fatigue, which may improve with continued treatment or dose reduction; paradoxical scalp hair loss has been reported at higher doses. If necessary, metformin can be added and may enhance the anti-hirsutism effect of low-dose spironolactone.

Flutamide inhibits testosterone binding to androgen receptors and also suppresses serum testosterone. It is given orally in a dosage of 250 mg once or twice daily for the first year and then 125–250 mg/day for maintenance. Used with an oral contraceptive, it appears to be more effective than spironolactone in improving hirsutism, acne, and male pattern baldness. Flutamide decreases cortisol renal clearance and corticosteroid replacement doses (eg, in congenital adrenal hyperplasia) should be reduced when flutamide is added. Hepatotoxicity has been reported but is rare. Flutamide must be given only to nonpregnant women. Women must be counseled to take strict contraceptive measures, since antiandrogen drug use during pregnancy causes malformations and disorders of sexual development (pseudohermaphroditism) in male infants.

Finasteride inhibits 5-alpha-reductase, the enzyme that converts testosterone to active dihydrotestosterone in the skin. Given as 5 mg doses orally daily, it provides modest reduction in hirsutism and androgenic alopecia over 6 months. Side effects are rare, but the drug is contraindicated in pregnancy and contraceptive measures are mandatory in reproductive age women.

Newer combined oral contraceptives that contain antiandrogenic progestins such as desogestrel (Azurette, Kariva), drospirenone (Yaz, Gianvi), norgestimate (Ortho Tri-Cyclen Lo), or cyproterone acetate (Diane 35, not available in United States) reduce hirsutism and acne. These newer antiandrogenic oral contraceptives confer a six-fold risk of deep venous thromboembolism, particularly when combined with higher doses of ethinyl estradiol, and therefore, oral contraceptives with the lowest possible dose of ethinyl estradiol (less than 50 mcg) should be selected. Older combined oral contraceptives that contain the progestins norethindrone, norgestrel, or levonorgestrel are relatively ineffective for hirsutism and acne. The risk for arterial thrombosis is increased by 50–100% for all combined oral contraceptives. For this reason, combined oral contraceptives are relatively contraindicated for women who are predisposed to thromboembolism: women who are smokers or who have migraines, hypertension or a personal history thromboembolism. However, progestin-only oral contraceptives do not confer any increased risk for venous or arterial thromboembolism. Metabolic syndrome and hypertriglyceridemia are seen, particularly with antiandrogenic progestins. The risks of metabolic syndrome may be offset by metformin.

Metformin may improve menstrual function in women with PCOS and amenorrhea or oligomenorrhea but is less effective than oral contraceptives. Metformin is not effective in promoting fertility in women with PCOS. Metformin alone is ineffective in improving hirsutism, but can enhance the anti-hirsutism effect of spironolactone. Metformin therapy is usually given orally with meals and is started at a dose of 500 mg/day with breakfast for 1 week, then increased to 500 mg with breakfast and dinner. If this dose is clinically insufficient but tolerated, the dose may be increased to 850–1000 mg twice daily. The most common side effects are dose-related gastrointestinal upset and diarrhea or constipation. Metformin appears to be nonteratogenic. Although metformin reduces insulin resistance, it does not cause hypoglycemia in nondiabetic patients. Metformin is contraindicated in kidney and liver disease.

Simvastatin can reduce hirsutism in women with PCOS. In one study, simvastatin 20 mg orally daily was given to women receiving an oral contraceptive for PCOS. Besides improving their serum lipid profiles, women receiving simvastatin had greater decreases in hirsutism and serum free testosterone levels than the women receiving an oral contraceptive alone. Atorvastatin also reduced serum testosterone by an average of 25% in women with PCOS.

Clomiphene is the treatment of choice for women with PCOS and infertility. Over 6 months, clomiphene therapy resulted in a 22.5% rate of conception with live births. The rate of pregnancy with multiple fetuses is 6%.

Women with classic congenital adrenal hyperplasia (21-hydroxylase deficiency) have hirsutism and adrenal insufficiency that requires glucocorticoid and mineralocorticoid replacement. However, women with partial "late onset" 21-hydroxylase deficiency do not require hormone replacement. Treating such women with dexamethasone risks iatrogenic Cushing syndrome and is not particularly more effective than other treatments for hirsutism.

GnRH agonist therapy has been successful in treating postmenopausal women with severe ovarian hyperandrogenism when laparoscopic oophorectomy is contraindicated or declined by the patient.

Buzney E et al. Polycystic ovary syndrome: a review for dermatologists: Part II. Treatment. J Am Acad Dermatol. 2014 Nov;71(5):859.e1–15. [PMID: 25437978]

Escobar-Morreale HF et al. Epidemiology, diagnosis and management of hirsutism: a consensus statement by the Androgen Excess and Polycystic Ovary Syndrome Society. Hum Reprod Update. 2012 Mar–Apr;18(2):146–70. [PMID: 22064667]

Loriaux DL. An approach to the patient with hirsutism. J Clin Endocrinol Metab. 2012 Sep;97(9):2957–68. [PMID: 22962669]

McMahon GT et al. Case records of the Massachusetts General Hospital. Case 33-2015. A 57-year-old woman with hair loss and deepening voice. N Engl J Med. 2015 Oct 22;373(17):1660–6. [PMID: 26488697]

Oliveira-Soares R et al. Finasteride 5 mg/day treatment of patterned hair loss in normo-androgenetic postmenopausal women. Int J Trichology. 2013 Jan;5(1):22–5. [PMID: 23960392]

van Zuuren EJ et al. Interventions for hirsutism (excluding laser and photoepilation therapy alone). Cochrane Database Syst Rev. 2015 Apr 28;4:CD010334. [PMID: 25918921]

AMENORRHEA & MENOPAUSE

PRIMARY AMENORRHEA

Menarche ordinarily occurs between ages 11 and 15 years (average in the United States: 12.7 years) (see also Chapter 18). The failure of any menses to appear is termed "primary amenorrhea," and evaluation is commenced (1) at age 14 years if neither menarche nor any breast development has occurred or if height is in the lowest 3%, or (2) at age 16 years if menarche has not occurred.

▶ Etiology of Primary Amenorrhea

The differential diagnoses for primary amenorrhea include hypothalamic-pituitary causes, hyperandrogenism, ovarian causes, disorders of sexual development (pseudohermaphroditism), uterine causes, and pregnancy.

A. Hypothalamic-Pituitary Causes (with Low or Normal FSH)

The most common cause of primary amenorrhea is a variant of normal known as constitutional delay of growth and puberty, which accounts for about 30% of delayed puberty cases. There is a strong genetic basis for this condition, such that over 50% of girls with it have a family history of delayed puberty. However, constitutional delay of growth and puberty is a diagnosis of exclusion and other etiologies must be considered.

A genetic deficiency of GnRH and gonadotropins may be isolated or associated with other pituitary deficiencies or diminished olfaction (Kallmann syndrome). Hypothalamic lesions, particularly craniopharyngioma, may be present. Pituitary tumors may be nonsecreting or may secrete PRL or GH. Cushing syndrome may be caused by

corticosteroid treatment, a cortisol-secreting adrenal tumor, or an ACTH-secreting pituitary tumor. Hypothyroidism can delay adolescence. Head trauma or encephalitis can cause gonadotropin deficiency. Primary amenorrhea may also be caused by severe illness, vigorous exercise (eg, ballet dancing, running), stressful life events, dieting, or anorexia nervosa; however, these conditions should not be assumed to account for amenorrhea without a full physical and endocrinologic evaluation.

B. Uterine Causes (with Normal FSH)

Müllerian agenesis results in a missing uterus and variable degrees of upper vaginal hypoplasia. It is the most common cause of permanent primary amenorrhea and is also known as Mayer-Rokitansky-Küster-Hauser syndrome. Affected women have intact ovaries and undergo an otherwise normal puberty. Such women ovulate and fertility is possible with in vitro fertilization and surrogacy.

An imperforate hymen is occasionally the reason for the absence of visible menses.

C. Hyperandrogenism (with Low or Normal FSH)

Polycystic ovaries and ovarian tumors can secrete excessive testosterone. Excess testosterone can also be secreted by adrenal tumors or by adrenal hyperplasia caused by steroidogenic enzyme defects such as P450c21 deficiency (salt-wasting) or P450c11 deficiency (hypertension). Androgenic steroid abuse may also cause this syndrome.

D. Ovarian Causes (with High FSH)

Gonadal dysgenesis (Turner syndrome and variants) is a frequent cause of primary amenorrhea. Autoimmune ovarian failure is another cause. Rare deficiencies in certain ovarian steroidogenic enzymes are causes of primary hypogonadism without virilization: 3-beta-hydroxysteroid dehydrogenase deficiency (adrenal insufficiency with low serum 17-hydroxyprogesterone) and P450c17 deficiency (hypertension and hypokalemia with high serum 17-hydroxyprogesterone). Deficiency in P450 aromatase (P450arom) activity produces female hypogonadism associated with polycystic ovaries, tall stature, osteoporosis, and virilization.

E. 46 XY Disorders of Sexual Development (Pseudohermaphroditism)

Complete androgen insensitivity syndrome is caused by homozygous inactivating mutations in the androgen receptor. 46 XY individuals with complete androgen insensitivity syndrome are born with completely normal external female genitalia, although some may have labial or inguinal swellings due to cryptorchid testes. Affected individuals are phenotypic girls and experience normal breast development at puberty, but fail to develop sexual hair and have primary amenorrhea. Investigation of the amenorrhea reveals an absent uterus, short vagina, and intra-abdominal gonads (testes). Serum testosterone levels are high and karyotype is 46 XY. Such individuals function as normal but infertile women but may require vaginal dilatation or surgery. Intra-abdominal testes have a low risk of developing germ cell tumors through adolescence, but the risk increases to about 5% during adulthood, when it is advisable that they be surgically removed. Following gonadectomy, such women require replacement estrogen.

Partial androgen insensitivity syndrome in 46 XY individuals results in variable degrees of ambiguous genitalia. Newborns have micropenis, hypospadias, and bifid scrotum.

F. Pregnancy (with High hCG)

Pregnancy may be the cause of primary amenorrhea even when the patient denies ever having had sexual intercourse.

▶ Clinical Findings

A. Symptoms and Signs

Patients with primary amenorrhea require a thorough history and physical examination to look for signs of the conditions noted above. Headaches or visual field abnormalities implicate a hypothalamic or pituitary tumor. Signs of pregnancy may be present. Blood pressure elevation, acne, and hirsutism should be noted. Short stature may be seen with an associated GH or thyroid hormone deficiency. Short stature with manifestations of gonadal dysgenesis indicates Turner syndrome. Olfactory deficits are seen in Kallmann syndrome. Obesity and short stature may be signs of Cushing syndrome. Tall stature may be due to eunuchoidism or acromegaly. Hirsutism or virilization suggests excessive testosterone.

An external pelvic examination plus a rectal examination should be performed to assess hymen patency and the presence of a uterus.

B. Laboratory and Radiologic Findings

The initial endocrine evaluation should include serum determinations of FSH, LH, PRL, testosterone, TSH, FT_4, and beta-hCG (pregnancy test). Patients who are virilized or hypertensive require serum electrolyte determinations and further hormonal evaluation. MRI of the hypothalamus and pituitary is used to evaluate teens with primary amenorrhea and low or normal FSH and LH—especially those with high PRL levels. Pelvic duplex/color sonography is very useful. Girls who have a normal uterus and high FSH without the classic features of Turner syndrome may require a karyotype to diagnose X chromosome mosaicism.

▶ Treatment

Treatment of primary amenorrhea is directed at the underlying cause. Girls with permanent hypogonadism are treated with HRT.

Klein DA et al. Amenorrhea: an approach to diagnosis and management. Am Fam Physician. 2013 Jun 1;87(11):781–8. [PMID: 23939500]

Marsh CA et al. Primary amenorrhea: diagnosis and management. Obstet Gynecol Surv. 2014 Oct;69(10):603–12. [PMID: 25336070]

SECONDARY AMENORRHEA & MENOPAUSE

Secondary amenorrhea is defined as the absence of menses for 3 consecutive months in women who have passed menarche. Menopause is defined as the terminal episode of naturally occurring menses; it is a retrospective diagnosis, usually made after 6 months of amenorrhea.

▶ Etiology

The causes of secondary amenorrhea include pregnancy, hypothalamic-pituitary causes, hyperandrogenism, uterine causes, premature ovarian failure, and menopause.

A. Pregnancy (High hCG)

Pregnancy is the most common cause for secondary amenorrhea in premenopausal women. The differential diagnosis includes rare ectopic secretion of hCG by a choriocarcinoma or bronchogenic carcinoma.

B. Hypothalamic-Pituitary Causes (with Low or Normal FSH)

The hypothalamus must release GnRH in a pulsatile manner for the pituitary to secrete gonadotropins. GnRH pulses occurring more than once per hour favor LH secretion, while less frequent pulses favor FSH secretion. In normal ovulatory cycles, GnRH pulses in the follicular phase are rapid and favor LH synthesis and ovulation; ovarian luteal progesterone is then secreted that slows GnRH pulses, causing FSH secretion during the luteal phase. Most women with hypothalamic amenorrhea have a persistently low frequency of GnRH pulses.

Secondary "hypothalamic" amenorrhea may be caused by stressful life events such as school examinations or leaving home. Such women usually have a history of normal sexual development and irregular menses since menarche. Amenorrhea may also be the result of strict dieting, vigorous exercise, organic illness, or anorexia nervosa. Intrathecal infusion of opioids causes amenorrhea in most women. These conditions should not be assumed to account for amenorrhea without a full physical and endocrinologic evaluation. Young women in whom the results of evaluation and progestin withdrawal test are normal have noncyclic secretion of gonadotropins resulting in anovulation. Such women typically recover spontaneously but should have regular evaluations and a progestin withdrawal test about every 3 months to detect loss of estrogen effect.

PRL elevation due to any cause may cause amenorrhea. Pituitary tumors or other lesions may cause hypopituitarism. Corticosteroid excess of any cause suppresses gonadotropins.

C. Hyperandrogenism (with Low-Normal FSH)

Elevated serum levels of testosterone can cause hirsutism, virilization, and amenorrhea. In PCOS, GnRH pulses are persistently rapid, favoring LH synthesis with excessive androgen secretion; reduced FSH secretion impairs follicular maturation. Progesterone administration can slow the GnRH pulses, thus favoring FSH secretion that induces follicular maturation. Rare causes of secondary amenorrhea include adrenal P450c21 deficiency, ovarian or adrenal malignancies, and Cushing syndrome. Anabolic steroids also cause amenorrhea.

D. Uterine Causes (with Normal FSH)

Infection of the uterus commonly occurs following delivery or D&C but may occur spontaneously. Endometritis due to tuberculosis or schistosomiasis should be suspected in endemic areas. Endometrial scarring may result, causing amenorrhea (Asherman syndrome). Such women typically continue to have monthly premenstrual symptoms. The vaginal estrogen effect is normal.

E. Early and Premature Menopause (with High FSH)

Early menopause refers to primary ovarian failure that occurs before age 45. It affects approximately 5% of women. About 1% of women experience **premature menopause** that is defined as ovarian failure before age 40; about 30% of such cases are due to autoimmunity against the ovary. X chromosome mosaicism accounts for 8% of cases of premature menopause. Other causes include surgical bilateral oophorectomy, radiation therapy for pelvic malignancy, and chemotherapy. Women who have undergone hysterectomy are prone to premature ovarian failure even though the ovaries were left intact. Myotonic dystrophy, galactosemia, and mumps oophoritis are additional causes. Early or premature menopause is frequently familial. Ovarian failure is usually irreversible.

F. Normal Menopause (with High FSH)

Normal menopause refers to primary ovarian failure that occurs after age 45. "Climacteric" is defined as the period of natural physiologic decline in ovarian function, generally occurring over about 10 years. By about age 40 years, the remaining ovarian follicles are those that are the least sensitive to gonadotropins. Increasing titers of FSH are required to stimulate estradiol secretion. Estradiol levels may actually rise during early climacteric.

The normal age for menopause in the United States ranges between 48 and 55 years, with an average of about 51.5 years. Serum estradiol levels fall and the remaining estrogen after menopause is estrone, derived mainly from peripheral aromatization of adrenal androstenedione. Such peripheral production of estrone is enhanced by obesity and liver disease. Individual differences in estrone levels partly explain why the symptoms noted above may be minimal in some women but severe in others.

► Clinical Findings

A. Symptoms and Signs

Vasomotor symptoms (hot flushes) are experienced by 60–80% of women at menopause. The duration of vasomotor symptoms can vary from seconds to many minutes. The severity can vary from mild to debilitating and many women experience drenching nocturnal sweats. Hot flushes peak in early menopause and then usually decline

gradually over a median of 10 years, but some women experience persistent severe vasomotor symptoms. African-American women tend to experience more severe vasomotor symptoms, whereas Asian women are less affected. Smokers tend to experience worse symptoms. Sleep disturbances are common and include problems initiating sleep, staying asleep, and early morning awakening. Other common symptoms of menopause include fatigue, headache, diminished libido, and rheumatologic symptoms. Psychological symptoms may include depression and irritability. Some women report mild cognitive impairment at menopause, which may be related to decreased cerebral blood flow noted in hypogonadal women, particularly during hot flushes. Estrogen deficiency causes vulvovaginal atrophy, with symptoms of vaginal dryness, dyspareunia, and irritation. Increased bone osteoclastic activity increases the risk for osteoporosis and fractures. The skin becomes more wrinkled. Increases in the LDL:HDL cholesterol ratio cause an increased risk for atherosclerosis.

A careful pelvic examination is useful to check for uterine or adnexal enlargement and to obtain a Papanicolaou smear and a vaginal smear for assessment of estrogen effect. Vulvovaginal complaints are not always due to estrogen deficiency and direct inspection of the vulva is necessary to detect other conditions, such as lichen sclerosis, contact dermatitis, squamous hyperplasia, or malignancy.

B. Laboratory Findings

1. Premature amenorrhea—An elevated hCG overwhelmingly indicates pregnancy; false-positive testing may occur very rarely with ectopic hCG secretion (eg, choriocarcinoma or bronchogenic carcinoma). Further laboratory evaluation for women who are not pregnant includes serum PRL, FSH, LH, and TSH. Hyperprolactinemia or hypopituitarism (without obvious cause) should prompt an MRI study of the pituitary region. Routine testing of kidney and liver function (BUN, serum creatinine, bilirubin, alkaline phosphatase, and alanine aminotransferase) is also performed. A serum testosterone level is obtained in hirsute or virilized women. Patients with manifestations of hypercortisolism receive a 1-mg overnight dexamethasone suppression test for initial screening. Nonpregnant women without any laboratory abnormality may receive a 10-day course of a progestin (eg, medroxyprogesterone acetate, 10 mg/day); absence of withdrawal menses typically indicates a lack of estrogen or a uterine abnormality.

2. Typical menopause—No laboratory testing is required to diagnose menopause, when amenorrhea occurs at the expected age. The expected age of menopause correlates with a woman's mother's age at menopause and varies among different kindreds and ethnic groups. An elevated serum FSH with a low or low-normal serum estradiol helps confirm the diagnosis.

► Treatment

A. Nonpharmacologic Approaches

Hot flushes may be reduced with low room temperatures, dressing coolly, and consuming cold beverages. Night sweats may be reduced by sleeping in a cool room and by avoiding the use of excessively warm blankets or down comforters. Slow, deep breathing can ameliorate hot flushes. Women may try avoiding known triggers for hot flushes, such as smoking, alcohol, caffeine, and hot spicy foods. Idiosyncratic triggers for hot flushes may be discerned and avoided. **Aerobic training** for 50 minutes four times weekly reduced all menopausal symptoms except vaginal dryness in a randomized controlled trial. **Clinical hypnosis** reduced hot flushes over 12 weeks in one study. Acupuncture may help alleviate symptoms in some women. **Replens** is a vaginal lubricant that can be used daily or 2 hours prior to intercourse. It improves vaginal moisture and elasticity and reduces vaginal irritation and dyspareunia.

B. Nonhormonal Medications

For women with severe hot flushes who cannot take estrogen, SSRIs may offer modest relief effective within a week; escitalopram (10–20 mg/day) can reduce hot flushes significantly, but must not be used by women taking tamoxifen for breast cancer, since it inhibits its metabolism to its active metabolite. Venlafaxine extended release (75 mg/day) may also be effective and does not have a drug interaction with tamoxifen. Sexual dysfunction has not been as significant with the latter drugs when used for vasomotor symptoms, compared to their use for depression. Gabapentin is also quite effective in oral doses titrated up to 200–800 mg every 8 hours. Side effects such as drowsiness, fatigue, dizziness, and headache, which are most pronounced during the first 2 weeks of therapy, often improve within 4 weeks. An herb, black cohosh, may possibly relieve hot flushes. Tamoxifen and raloxifene offer bone protection but aggravate hot flushes. Women with postmenopausal osteoporosis may be treated with bisphosphonates or denosumab. Women with low serum testosterone levels may experience hypoactive sexual desire disorder that may respond to low-dose testosterone replacement.

▶ Hormone Replacement Therapy (HRT)

Overall survival is improved among women who begin HRT before age 60 or within 10 years of menopause. However, no survival advantage was found in older women, according to a meta-analysis of 43 randomized controlled trials. Specifically, HRT does not increase the risk of cardiac death or stroke. **Breast cancer risk** is increased among women taking combined daily estrogen and progestin HRT, whereas breast cancer risk is reduced in women taking estrogen alone. **Venous thromboembolic disease** and **stroke** are increased by oral but not transdermal estrogen. **Osteoporosis risk** is reduced by even low-dose systemic estrogen replacement.

In light of these considerations, estrogen replacement is most commonly prescribed for women in early menopause, when symptoms are worst and the benefits are greatest. Transdermal estrogen is favored over oral therapy to reduce the risk of thromboembolism. In women with an intact uterus, estrogen replacement without a progestin risks endometrial hypertrophy and dysfunctional uterine bleeding. The addition of a progestin, however, increases the risk of breast cancer. Therefore, only the smallest effective dose of estrogen should be used to avoid the need for progestins or use them in lower doses or intermittently. Also, progestin may be delivered directly to uterus with progesterone-eluting intrauterine devices. The decision to prescribe menopausal hormonal therapy and its type and duration are dictated by individual symptoms, risk profile, and personal preferences, while considering potential benefits and risks.

A. Benefits of HRT

Estrogen replacement is the best treatment for hot flushes and sweats and eliminates these symptoms or improves them by more than 70%, usually within a month. Vaginal moisture is improved and libido is enhanced in some women. Estradiol vaginal rings can improve symptoms of an overactive bladder and vaginal dryness. Sleep disturbances are common in menopause and can be reversed with estrogen replacement. Some women notice a mild impairment in memory and cognitive function at menopause that may improve with HRT that is commenced soon after menopause. HRT does not reduce the risk of Alzheimer dementia. However, short-term transdermal estradiol has been demonstrated to slightly improve memory in women with existent mild to moderate Alzheimer disease. Estrogen replacement may also improve the body pain and reduced physical function experienced by some women at the time of menopause. Women with perimenopausal depression typically experience a significantly improved mood and overall sense of well being with estrogen replacement. Estrogen replacement does not prevent facial skin wrinkling; however, it may improve facial skin moisture and thickness, reducing seborrhea and atrophy.

Estrogen replacement prevents postmenopausal osteoporosis. The WHI study also found that women who received estrogen therapy experienced a reduced number of hip fractures (six fewer fractures/year per 10,000 women) compared with placebo. Even "microdose" transdermal estradiol (0.014 mg/day) preserves bone density.

Women aged 50–59 years in the WHI who received estrogen alone developed significantly lower CT coronary calcium scores (a marker for coronary atherosclerosis) than women receiving placebo. In the California Teachers Study, HRT in women under age 60 was associated with a dramatic 46% reduction in all-cause mortality, particularly cardiovascular disease. This association of HRT and lower mortality may suffer from self-selection bias. Nevertheless, there appears to be a survival advantage of HRT that requires longer-term administration (more than 5 years) to become apparent. The survival advantage is particularly strong for women under age 60 and diminishes with age; no reduction in mortality was noted in the group of women aged 85–94 years. The reduction in cardiovascular disease among younger postmenopausal women taking HRT may be explained by the reduction in serum levels of atherogenic lipoprotein(a) with HRT, with or without a progestin. Improvement in serum HDL cholesterol is greatest with unopposed estrogen but is also seen with the addition of a progestin.

1. Estrogen replacement without progestin (unopposed HRT)—Interestingly, the WHI study found that postmenopausal women taking unopposed estrogen had a 23% *reduction* in breast cancer risk. Unopposed estrogen replacement improves glycemic control in women with type 2 diabetes mellitus. Perimenopause-related depression is improved by unopposed estrogen replacement; the addition of a progestin may negate this effect. A 20-year study of 8801 women living in a retirement community found that estrogen use was associated with improved survival. Age-adjusted mortality rates were 56.4 (per 1000 person-years) among nonusers and 50.4 among women who had used estrogen for 15 years or longer.

2. Estrogen replacement therapy with progestins (combined HRT)—Women receiving conventional-dose daily conjugated estrogen and medroxyprogesterone acetate (0.625 mg and 2.5 mg, respectively) for an average of 5.6 years, experienced a lower risk of developing diabetes mellitus (3.5%) versus those taking a placebo (4.2%).

B. Risks of HRT

Oral estrogen increases the risk of arterial and venous thrombotic events in a dose-dependent manner, although the absolute risk is small. The WHI study found that women who received long-term conventional oral combined HRT had an increased risk of deep venous thrombosis (3.5 per 1000 person-years) compared with women receiving placebo (1.7 per 1000 person-years). Oral estrogen also increases the risk of ischemic stroke by about 30%. Oral estrogen causes a particularly increased risk for thromboembolic disease among older women and those with increased stroke proclivity (current smokers and those with hypertension, atrial fibrillation, prior thromboembolic event). Long-term use of oral conjugated estrogens in women over age 65 has been associated with poorer cognitive performance, perhaps due to small strokes. Transdermal or vaginal estrogen administration avoids this risk. Urinary stress incontinence appears to be increased by conventional-dose oral estrogen replacement, whereas topical vaginal estrogen may have a beneficial effect. Estrogen replacement may cause mastalgia that typically responds to dose reduction. Estrogen replacement also appears to increase the risk of seizures in women with epilepsy. Estrogen can stimulate the growth of untreated large pituitary prolactinomas. Oral estrogen and SERMs also increase the risk of gastroesophageal reflux disease. Oral HRT can increase the size of hepatic hemangiomas, but significant enlargement is uncommon. Conventional doses of estrogen carry higher risks than lower doses. The risks for HRT also depend on whether estrogen is administered alone (unopposed HRT) or with a progestin (combined HRT).

1. Estrogen replacement without progestin (unopposed HRT)—Surprisingly, the WHI study found that postmenopausal women who received conventional-dose estrogen-only therapy had a reduced risk of breast cancer (7 fewer cases/year per 10,000 women) compared with a placebo group. However, the California Teachers Study monitored women for a longer period; a group of 37,000 women who had been taking conventional-dose estrogen-only therapy for 20 years or longer did have a slightly increased risk of breast cancer. Women taking lower-dose unopposed estrogen therapy would be expected to have lower long-term risk of breast cancer.

Conventional-dose unopposed conjugated estrogen replacement (0.625–1.25 mg daily) increases the risk of endometrial hyperplasia and dysfunctional uterine bleeding, which often prompts patients to stop the estrogen. However, lower-dose unopposed estrogen confers a much lower risk of dysfunctional uterine bleeding. Recurrent dysfunctional bleeding necessitates a pelvic examination and possibly an endometrial biopsy. There has been considerable concern that unopposed estrogen replacement might increase the risk for endometrial carcinoma. However, a Cochrane Database Review found no increased risk of endometrial carcinoma in a review of 30 randomized controlled trials. Therefore, lower-dose unopposed estrogen replacement does not appear to confer any significant increased risk for endometrial cancer.

Long-term conventional-dose unopposed estrogen increases the mortality risk from ovarian cancer, although the absolute risk is small. The annual age-adjusted ovarian cancer death rates for women taking estrogen replacement for 10 years or longer are 64:100,000 for current users, 38:100,000 for former users, and 26:100,000 for women who had never taken estrogen. Lower-dose estrogen replacement is believed to confer a negligible increased risk for ovarian cancer.

The WHI trial was stopped in 2002 because of an increased risk of stroke among women taking conjugated oral estrogens in doses of 0.625 mg daily; the risk was about 44 strokes per 10,000 person-years versus about 32 per 10,000 person-years in women taking placebo. Transdermal or transvaginal estrogen is not thought to increase the risk of stroke.

Oral estrogens can cause hypertriglyceridemia, particularly in women with preexistent hyperlipidemia, rarely resulting in pancreatitis. Postmenopausal estrogen therapy also slightly increases the risk of gallstones and cholecystitis. These side effects may be reduced or avoided by using transdermal or vaginal estrogen replacement.

2. Estrogen replacement with a progestin (combined HRT)—Long-term conventional-dose oral combined HRT increases breast density and the risk for abnormal mammograms (9.4% versus 5.4% for placebo). There is also a higher risk of breast cancer (8 cases per 10,000 women/year versus 6.5 cases per 10,000 women/year for placebo); the increased risk of breast cancer is highest shortly after menopause (about 2 cases per 1000 women annually). This increased risk for breast cancer appears to mostly affect relatively thin women with a BMI less than 24.4. The Iowa Women's Health Study reported an increase in breast cancer with HRT only in women consuming more than 1 oz of alcohol weekly. No accelerated risk of breast cancer has been seen in users of HRT who have benign breast disease or a family history of breast cancer. Women in whom new-onset breast tenderness develops with combined HRT have an increased risk of breast cancer, compared with women without breast tenderness.

The Women's Health Initiative Mental Study (WHIMS) followed the effect of combined conventional-dose oral HRT on cognitive function in women 65–79 years old. HRT did not protect these older women from cognitive decline. In fact, they experienced an increased risk for severe dementia at a rate of 23 more cases/year for every 10,000 women over age 65 years. It is unknown whether this finding applies to younger postmenopausal women.

In the WHI study, women receiving conventional-dose combined oral HRT experienced an increased risk of stroke (31 strokes per 10,000 women/year versus 26 strokes per 10,000 women/year for placebo). Stroke risk was also increased by hypertension, diabetes, and smoking.

Women taking combined oral estrogen–progestin replacement do not experience an increased risk of ovarian cancer. They do experience a slightly increased risk of developing asthma.

Progestins may cause moodiness, particularly in women with a history of premenstrual dysphoric disorder. Cycled progestins may trigger migraines in certain women. Many other adverse reactions have been reported, including breast tenderness, alopecia, and fluid retention. Contraindications to the use of progestins include thromboembolic disorders, liver disease, breast cancer, and pregnancy.

C. HRT Agents

Hormone replacement needs to be individualized. Ideally, in women with an intact uterus, very low-dose transdermal estradiol may be used alone or with intermittent progestin or a progesterone-eluting intrauterine device, in order to reduce the risk of endometrial hyperplasia, while avoiding the need for daily oral progestin. Vaginal estrogen can be added if low-dose systemic estradiol replacement is insufficient to relieve symptoms of vulvovaginal atrophy. Women who have had a hysterectomy may receive transdermal estrogen at whatever is the lowest dose that adequately relieves symptoms. However, some women cannot find sufficient relief with transdermal estradiol and must use an oral preparation.

1. Transdermal estradiol—Estradiol can be delivered systemically with different systems of skin patches, mists, or gels. Transdermal estradiol works for most women, but some women have poor transdermal absorption. If a woman has a skin reaction to an estradiol patch, then a gel or mist may be tried at different doses until the ideal formulation is found.

A. ESTRADIOL PATCHES MIXED WITH ADHESIVE—These systems tend to cause minimal skin irritation. Generic estradiol transdermal (0.025, 0.0375, 0.05, 0.06, 0.075, 0.1 mg/day) is replaced weekly. Brand products include: Vivelle-Dot (0.025) or Minivivelle (0.0375, 0.05, 0.075, or 0.1 mg/day) or Alora (0.025, 0.05, 0.075, or 0.1 mg/day), replaced twice weekly; Climara (0.025, 0.0375, 0.05, 0.06, 0.075, or 0.1 mg/day), replaced weekly; and Menostar (0.014 mg/day), replaced weekly. This type of estradiol skin patch can be cut in half and applied to the skin without proportionately greater loss of potency. Minivivelle patches are the smallest.

B. ESTRADIOL MISTS AND GELS—Evamist is available as a topical mist dispenser that dispenses 1.53 mg estradiol/spray; 1–3 sprays are applied to the inner forearm daily; a single daily spray may provide sufficiently low-dose estradiol to possibly obviate the need for daily progestin in women with an intact uterus. EstroGel 0.06% is available in a metered-dose pump that dispenses 1.25 g gel per actuation (half–2 actuations/day). Elestrin 0.06% is available in a metered-dose pump that dispenses 0.87 g gel per activation (half–2 actuations/day). These gels are applied daily to one arm from the wrist to the shoulder after bathing. Divigel 0.1% gel (0.25, 0.5, 1 g/packet) is applied to the upper thigh daily. Estrasorb 2.5% is available in 1.74 g pouches (4.35 mg estradiol); 1–2 pouches of lotion are applied to the thigh/calf daily. To avoid spreading topical estradiol to others, the hands should be washed and precautions taken to avoid prolonged skin contact with children. Application of sunscreen prior to estradiol gel has been reported to *increase* the transdermal absorption of estradiol.

C. ESTRADIOL PATCHES WITH PROGESTIN MIXED WITH ADHESIVE—These preparations mix estradiol with either norethindrone acetate or levonorgestrel. Combipatch (0.05 mg E with 0.14 mg norethindrone acetate daily or 0.05 mg E with 0.25 mg norethindrone acetate daily) is replaced twice weekly. Climara Pro (0.045 mg E with 0.015 mg levonorgestrel daily) is replaced once weekly. The addition of a progestin reduces the risk of endometrial hyperplasia, but breakthrough bleeding occurs commonly. The combined patch increases the risk of breast cancer. Scalp hair loss, acne, weight gain, skin reactions, and poor skin adherence have been reported with these patches.

2. Oral estrogen—

A. ORAL ESTROGEN-ONLY PREPARATIONS—These preparations include conjugated equine estrogens that are available as Premarin (0.3, 0.45, 0.625, 0.9, and 1.25 mg), conjugated plant-derived estrogens (eg, Menest, 0.3, 0.625, and 2.5 mg), and conjugated synthetic estrogens that are available as Cenestin (0.3, 0.45, 0.625, 0.9, and 1.25 mg) and Enjuvia (0.3, 0.45, 0.625, 0.9, and 1.25 mg). Other preparations include estradiol (0.5, 1, and 2 mg), and estropipate (0.75, 1.5, and 3 mg).

B. ORAL ESTROGEN PLUS PROGESTIN PREPARATIONS—Conjugated equine estrogens with medroxyprogesterone acetate is available as Prempro (0.3/1.5, 0.45/1.5, 0.625/2.5, and 0.625 mg/5 mg); conjugated equine estrogens for 14 days cycled with conjugated equine estrogens plus medroxyprogesterone acetate for 14 days is available as Premphase (0.625/0, then 0.625 mg/5 mg); estradiol with norethindrone acetate (0.5/0.1 and 1 mg/0.5 mg); ethinyl estradiol with norethindrone acetate is available as Femhrt (2.5/0.5 and 5 mcg/1 mg) and Jinteli (5 mcg/1 mg); estradiol with drospirenone is available as Angeliq (0.5 mg/0.25 mg, and 1.0 mg/0.5 mg); estradiol with norgestimate is available as Prefest (estradiol 1 mg/day for 3 days, alternating with 1 mg estradiol/0.09 mg norgestimate daily for 3 days). Oral contraceptives can also be used for combined HRT.

3. Vaginal estrogen

Urogenital atrophy commonly develops in postmenopausal women and can cause dryness of the vagina, genital itching, burning, dyspareunia, and recurrent urinary tract infections. Urinary symptoms can include urgency and dysuria. Vaginal estrogen is intended to deliver estrogen directly to local tissues and is moderately effective in reducing these symptoms, while minimizing systemic estrogen exposure. Some estrogen is absorbed systemically and can relieve menopausal symptoms. Manufacturers recommend that these preparations be used for only 3–6 months in women with an intact uterus, since vaginal estrogen can cause endometrial proliferation. However, most clinicians use them for longer periods. Vaginal estrogen can be administered in three different ways: creams, tablets, and rings.

A. ESTROGEN VAGINAL CREAMS—These creams are administered intravaginally with a measured-dose applicator daily for 2 weeks for atrophic vaginitis, then administered one to three times weekly. Available preparations include conjugated equine estrogens, which is available as Premarin Vaginal (0.625 mg/g cream), dosed as 0.25–2 g cream administered vaginally one to three times weekly. Estradiol is available as Estrace Vaginal (0.1 mg/g cream), 1 g cream administered vaginally one to two times weekly.

B. ESTRADIOL VAGINAL TABLETS—These tablets are sold prepackaged in a disposable applicator and can be administered deep intravaginally daily for 2 weeks for atrophic vaginitis, then twice weekly. The tablets dissolve into a gel that gradually releases estradiol. This preparation is available as Vagifem (10 mcg/tablet), administered vaginally two times weekly.

C. ESTRADIOL VAGINAL RINGS—These rings are inserted manually into the upper third of the vagina, worn continuously, and replaced every 3 months. Only a small amount of the released estradiol enters the systemic circulation. Vaginal rings do not usually interfere with sexual intercourse. If a ring is removed or descends into the introitus, it may be washed in warm water and reinserted. Estring (2 mg estradiol/ring) releases estradiol 7.5 mcg/day; Femring releases estradiol acetate 0.05 mg/day or 0.1 mg/day. Both rings are replaced every 90 days. For women with postmenopausal urinary urgency and frequency, even the low-dose Estring can successfully reduce urinary symptoms.

D. ESTRADIOL WITH PROGESTIN VAGINAL RINGS—The available preparation is NuvaRing that releases a mixture of ethinyl estradiol 0.015 mg/day and etonogestrel 0.12 mg/day. It is a contraceptive vaginal ring that is placed in the vagina on or before day 5 of the menstrual cycle, left for 3 weeks, removed for 1 week, and then replaced.

4. Estradiol injections

Parenteral estradiol should be used only for particularly severe menopausal symptoms when other measures have failed or are contraindicated. Estradiol cypionate (Depo-Estradiol 5 mg/mL) may be administered intramuscularly in doses of 1–5 mg every 3–4 weeks. Estradiol valerate (20 or 40 mg/mL) may be administered intramuscularly in doses of 10–20 mg every 4 weeks. Women with an intact uterus should receive a progestin for the last 10 days of each cycle.

5. Oral progestins

For a woman with an intact uterus, long-term conventional-dose unopposed systemic estrogen therapy can cause endometrial hyperplasia, which typically results in dysfunctional uterine bleeding and might rarely lead to endometrial cancer. Progestin therapy transforms proliferative into secretory endometrium, causing a possible menses when given intermittently or no bleeding when given continuously.

The type of progestin preparation, its dosage, and the timing of administration may be tailored to the given situation. Progestins may be given daily, monthly, or at longer intervals. When given episodically, progestins are usually administered for 7–14 day periods. Bedtime administration may improve sleep. Some women find that progestins produce adverse effects, such as irritability, nausea, fatigue, or headache; long-term progestins given with estrogen replacement increase the risk for breast cancer.

Oral progestins are available in different formulations: Micronized progesterone (100 mg and 200 mg/capsule), medroxyprogesterone (2.5, 5.0, and 10 mg/tablet), norethindrone acetate (5 mg/tablet), and norethindrone (0.35 mg/tablet). Topical progesterone (20–50 mg/day) may reduce hot flushes in women who are intolerant to oral HRT. It may be applied to the upper arms, thighs, or inner wrists daily. It may be compounded as micronized progesterone 250 mg/mL in a transdermal gel. Its effects upon the breast and endometrium are unknown. Progesterone is also available as vaginal gels (eg, Prochieve, 4% = 45 mg/applicatorful, and 8% = 90 mg/applicatorful) that are typically given for secondary amenorrhea and administered vaginally every other day for six doses.

6. Progestin-releasing intrauterine devices

Intrauterine devices that release progestins can be useful for women receiving ERT, since they can reduce the incidence of dysfunctional uterine bleeding and endometrial carcinoma without exposing women to the significant risks of systemic progestins. The Mirena intrauterine device releases levonorgestrel and is inserted into the uterus by a clinician within 7 days of the onset of menses. It is equally effective at reducing endometrial hyperplasia as cycled medroxyprogesterone acetate and is associated with less hirsutism. It remains effective for up to 5 years. Parous women are generally better able to tolerate the Mirena intrauterine device than nulliparous women.

7. Selective estrogen receptor modulators

SERMs (eg, raloxifene, ospemifene, tamoxifen) are an alternative to estrogen replacement for hypogonadal women at risk for osteoporosis who prefer not to take estrogens because of their contraindications (eg, breast or uterine cancer) or side effects. Raloxifene (Evista) does not reduce hot flushes, vaginal dryness, skin wrinkling, or breast atrophy; it does not improve cognition. However, in doses of 60 mg/day orally, it inhibits bone loss without stimulating effects upon the breasts or endometrium. Raloxifene does not stimulate the endometrium and actually reduces the risk of endometrial carcinoma, so concomitant progesterone therapy is not required. Another advantage to raloxifene is that it reduces the risk of invasive breast cancer by about 50%. Raloxifene slightly increases the risk of venous thromboembolism (though less so than tamoxifen), so it should not be used by women at prolonged bed rest or otherwise prone to thrombosis. Ospemifene (Osphena) is a SERM that has unique estrogen-like effects on the vaginal epithelium and is indicated for the treatment of postmenopausal dyspareunia when other therapies are ineffective. Given orally in doses of 60 mg/day, it commonly aggravates hot flushes, increases the risks of thromboembolism, and increases endometrial hyperplasia. Ospemifene has unknown long-term effects upon bone and breast.

Tibolone (Livial) is an SERM whose metabolites have mixed estrogenic, progestogenic, and weak androgenic activity. It is comparable to HRT for the treatment of climacteric-related complaints. It does not appear to significantly stimulate proliferation of breast or endometrial tissue. It depresses both serum triglycerides and HDL cholesterol. Long-term studies are lacking. It is not available in the United States.

8. Testosterone replacement therapy in women—In premenopausal women, serum testosterone levels decline with age. Between 25 and 45 years of age, women's testosterone levels fall 50%. After natural menopause, the ovaries remain a significant source for testosterone and serum testosterone levels do not fall abruptly. In contrast, very low serum testosterone levels are found in women after bilateral oophorectomy, autoimmune ovarian failure, or adrenalectomy, and in hypopituitarism. Testosterone deficiency contributes to hot flushes, loss of sexual hair, muscle atrophy, osteoporosis, and diminished libido, also known as hypoactive sexual desire disorder. **Flibanserin** is a drug that is modestly effective for treating premenopausal women with acquired hypoactive sexual desire disorder. It is administered orally 100 mg at bedtime; side effects may include hypotension, appendicitis, nausea, xerostomia, sleep disorders, and fatigue.

In women, diminished libido is common and multifactorial. Although low serum testosterone levels may contribute to hypoactive sexual desire disorder, hysterectomy and sexual isolation are major causes. Low serum testosterone levels may also cause fatigue, a diminished sense of well being, and a dulled enthusiasm for life. Androgen replacement may improve these problems.

Selected women may be treated with low-dose testosterone. Methyltestosterone can be compounded into capsules and taken orally in doses of 1.25–2.5 mg daily. Testosterone can also be compounded as a cream containing 1 mg/mL, with 1 mL applied to the abdomen daily. Methyltestosterone also is available combined with esterified estrogens: 1.25 mg methyltestosterone/0.626 mg esterified estrogens or 2.5 mg methyltestosterone/1.25 mg esterified estrogens. The latter formulations are convenient but carry the same disadvantages as oral estrogen—particularly an increased risk of thromboembolism.

Women receiving testosterone therapy must be monitored for the appearance of any acne or hirsutism, and serum testosterone levels are determined periodically if women feel that they are benefitting and long-term testosterone therapy is instituted. Side effects of low-dose testosterone therapy are usually minimal but may include erythrocytosis, emotional changes, hirsutism, acne, an adverse effect on lipids, and potentiation of warfarin anticoagulation therapy. Testosterone therapy tends to reduce both triglyceride and HDL cholesterol levels. Hepatocellular neoplasms and peliosis hepatis, rare complications of oral androgens at higher doses, have not been reported with oral methyltestosterone doses of 2.5 mg or less daily.

Vaginal testosterone is an option for postmenopausal women who cannot use systemic or vaginal estrogen due to breast cancer. Testosterone 150–300 mcg/day vaginally appears to reduce vaginal dryness and dyspareunia without increasing systemic estrogen levels.

Caution: Androgens should not be given to women with liver disease or during pregnancy or breastfeeding. Testosterone replacement therapy for women should be used judiciously, since long-term prospective clinical trials are lacking. An analysis of the Nurses' Health Study found that women who had been taking conjugated equine estrogens plus methyltestosterone experienced an increased risk of breast cancer, so breast cancer screening is recommended.

Benkhadra K et al. Menopausal hormone therapy and mortality: a systematic review and meta-analysis. J Clin Endocrinol Metab. 2015 Nov;100(11):4021–8. [PMID: 26544652]

Cherry N et al. Long-term safety of unopposed estrogen used by women surviving myocardial infarction: 14-year follow-up of the ESPRIT randomised controlled trial. BJOG. 2014 May; 121(6):700–5. [PMID: 24533510]

Dhanuka I et al. Flibanserin for the treatment of hypoactive sexual desire disorder in premenopausal women. Expert Opin Pharmacother. 2015 Nov;16(16):2523–9. [PMID: 26395164]

Gurney EP et al. The Women's Health Initiative trial and related studies: 10 years later: a clinician's view. J Steroid Biochem Mol Biol. 2014 Jul;142:4–11. [PMID: 24172877]

Joffe H et al. Low-dose estradiol and the serotonin-norepinephrine reuptake inhibitor venlafaxine for vasomotor symptoms: a randomized clinical trial. JAMA Intern Med. 2014 Jul; 174(7):1058–66. [PMID: 24861828]

Klein DA et al. Amenorrhea: an approach to diagnosis and management. Am Fam Physician. 2013 Jun 1;87(11):781–8. [PMID: 23939500]

Mohammed K et al. Oral vs transdermal estrogen therapy and vascular events: a systematic review and meta-analysis. J Clin Endocrinol Metab. 2015 Nov;100(11):4012–20. [PMID: 26544651]

Nelson HD et al. Menopausal hormone therapy for the primary prevention of chronic conditions: a systematic review to update the U.S. Preventive Services Task Force recommendations. Ann Intern Med. 2012 Jul 17;157(2):104–13. [PMID: 22786830]

Palacios S et al. An update on drugs for the treatment of menopausal symptoms. Expert Opin Pharmacother. 2015 Nov; 16(16):2437–47. [PMID: 26395223]

Schmidt PJ et al. Effects of estradiol withdrawal on mood in women with past perimenopausal depression: a randomized clinical trial. JAMA Psychiatry. 2015 Jul;72(7):714–26. [PMID: 26018333]

Shapiro S et al. Risks and benefits of hormone therapy: has medical dogma now been overturned? Climacteric. 2014 Jun; 17(3):215–22. [PMID: 24654673]

Shifren JL. Testosterone for midlife women: the hormone of desire? Menopause. 2015 Oct;22(10):1147–9. [PMID: 26397145]

Stuenkel CA et al. Treatment of symptoms of the menopause: an Endocrine Society clinical practice guideline. J Clin Endocrinol Metab. 2015 Nov;100(11):3975–4011. [PMID: 26444994]

TURNER SYNDROME (Gonadal Dysgenesis)

ESSENTIALS OF DIAGNOSIS

► Short stature with normal GH levels.

► Primary amenorrhea or early ovarian failure.

► Epicanthal folds, webbed neck, short fourth metacarpals.

► Renal and cardiovascular anomalies.

Turner syndrome comprises a group of X chromosome disorders that are associated with spontaneous abortion, primary hypogonadism, short stature, and other phenotypic anomalies (Table 26–17). It affects 1–2% of fetuses, of which about 97% abort, accounting for about 10% of all spontaneous abortions. Nevertheless, it affects about 1 in every 2500 live female births. Patients with the classic syndrome (about 50% of cases) lack one of the two X chromosomes (45,XO karyotype). Other patients with Turner syndrome have X chromosome abnormalities, such as ring X or Xq (X/abnormal X) or X chromosome deletions affecting all or some somatic cells (mosaicism, XX/XO).

1. Classic Turner Syndrome (45,XO Gonadal Dysgenesis)

► Clinical Findings

A. Symptoms and Signs

Features of Turner syndrome are variable and may be subtle in girls with mosaicism. Turner syndrome may be diagnosed in infant girls at birth, since they tend to be small and may exhibit severe lymphedema. Evaluation for childhood short stature often leads to the diagnosis. Girls and women with Turner syndrome have an increased risk of aortic coarctation (11%) and bicuspid aortic valves (16%); these cardiac abnormalities are more common in patients with a webbed neck. If a woman with Turner syndrome becomes pregnant, there is a 2% risk of death from aortic dissection or rupture. Typical manifestations in adulthood include short stature, hypogonadism, webbed neck, high-arched palate, wide-spaced nipples, hypertension, and renal abnormalities (Table 26–17). Emotional disorders are common. Affected women are also more prone to autoimmune disease, particularly thyroiditis (37%), inflammatory bowel disease (4%), and celiac disease (3%).

Hypogonadism presents as "delayed adolescence" (primary amenorrhea, 80%) or early ovarian failure (20%); girls with 45,XO Turner (blood karyotyping) who enter puberty are typically found to have mosaicism if other tissues are karyotyped.

Table 26–17. Manifestations of Turner syndrome.

Short stature
Distinctive facial features
   Ptosis
   Micrognathia
   Low-set ears
   Epicanthal folds
Sexual infantilism due to gonadal dysgenesis with primary
   amenorrhea (80%)
Early ovarian failure with secondary amenorrhea (20%)
Webbed neck (40%)
Low hairline
High-arched palate
Cubitus valgus
Short fourth metacarpals (50%)
Lymphedema of hands and feet (30%)
Hypoplastic widely spaced nipples
Hyperconvex nails
Pigmented nevi
Keloid formation (eg, surgical scars or after ear piercing)
Recurrent otitis media
Renal abnormalities (60%)
   Horseshoe kidney
   Hydronephrosis
Hypertension (idiopathic or due to coarctation or kidney disease)
Cardiovascular anomalies
   Coarctation of the aorta (10–20%)
   Partial anomalous pulmonary venous connection
   Bicuspid aortic valve (with aortic stenosis or regurgitation)
   Aortic dissection due to coarctation and cystic medial necrosis
     of the aorta
Gastrointestinal disorders
   Telangiectasias with bleeding
   Celiac disease
   Inflammatory bowel disease
   Colon carcinoma
   Liver disease
Impaired space-form recognition, direction sense, and
   mathematical reasoning
Associated conditions
   Obesity
   Diabetes mellitus (types 1 and 2)
   Dyslipidemia
   Hyperuricemia
   Hashimoto thyroiditis
   Achlorhydria
   Cataracts, corneal opacities
   Neuroblastoma (1%)
   Rheumatoid arthritis

B. Laboratory Findings

Hypogonadism is confirmed in girls who have high serum levels of FSH and LH. A blood karyotype showing 45,XO (or X chromosome abnormalities or mosaicism) establishes the diagnosis. GH and IGF-1 levels are normal.

C. Imaging

An ultrasound and MRI scan of the chest and abdomen should be done in all patients with Turner syndrome to determine whether cardiac, aortic, and renal abnormalities are present.

Treatment

Treatment of short stature with daily injections of GH (0.1 unit/kg/day) plus an androgen (eg, oxandrolone) for at least 4 years before epiphyseal fusion increases final height by a mean of about 10.3 cm over the mean predicted height of 144.2 cm. Rarely, such GH treatment causes pseudotumor cerebri. After age 12 years, estrogen therapy is begun with low doses of conjugated estrogens (0.3 mg) or ethinyl estradiol (5 mcg) given on days 1–21 per month. When growth stops, HRT is begun with estrogen and progestin; transdermal estrogen may be used to initiate pubertal development.

Complications & Surveillance

Bicuspid aortic valves are associated with an increased risk of infective endocarditis, aortic valvular stenosis or regurgitation, and ascending aortic aneurysm and dissection. Partial anomalous pulmonary vein connections occur in 13% and can lead to left-to-right shunting of blood. Adults with Turner syndrome have a high incidence of ECG abnormalities.

Women with Turner syndrome have a reduced life expectancy due in part to their increased risk of diabetes mellitus (types 1 and 2), hypertension, dyslipidemia, and osteoporosis.

Diagnostic vigilance and aggressive treatment of these conditions reduce the risk of aortic aneurysm dissection, ischemic heart disease, stroke, and fracture. Patients are prone to keloid formation after surgery or ear piercing. Yearly ocular examinations and periodic thyroid evaluations are recommended.

Repeat cardiovascular evaluations should be done every 3–4 years. Patients with the classic 45,XO karyotype have a high risk of renal structural abnormalities, whereas those with 46 X/abnormal X are more prone to malformations of the urinary collecting system. The risk of aortic dissection is increased more than 100-fold in women with Turner syndrome, particularly those with pronounced neck webbing and shield chest. Patients with aortic root enlargement are usually treated with beta-blockade and serial imaging. About 5% of women with Turner syndrome experience natural pregnancy and even more can become pregnant with oocyte donation. Such pregnancies are very high-risk, with high rates of fetal morbidity, preeclampsia, and aortic dissection. Women are usually advised to deliver via cesarean section because of the risk of aortic aneurysm rupture during vaginal delivery.

2. Turner Syndrome Variants

A. 46,X (Abnormal X) Karyotype

Patients with small distal short arm deletions of the X chromosome (Xp-) that include the *SHOX* gene often have short stature and skeletal abnormalities but have a low risk of ovarian failure. Transmission of Turner syndrome from mother to daughter can occur. There may be an increased risk of trisomy 21 in the conceptuses of women with Turner syndrome. Patients with deletions of the long arm of the X chromosome (distal to Xq24) often have amenorrhea without short stature or other features of Turner syndrome.

Abnormalities or deletions of other genes located on both the long and short arms of the X chromosome can produce gonadal dysgenesis with few other somatic features.

B. 45,XO/46,XX and 45,XO/46, XY Mosaicism

45,XO/46,XX mosaicism results in a modified form of Turner syndrome. Such girls tend to be taller and may have more gonadal function and fewer other manifestations of Turner syndrome.

45,XO/46,XY mosaicism can produce some manifestations of Turner syndrome. Patients may have ambiguous genitalia or male infertility with an otherwise normal phenotype. Germ cell tumors, such as gonadoblastomas and seminomas, develop in about 10% of patients with 45,XO/46,XY mosaicism; most such tumors are benign.

Bondy C. Pregnancy and cardiovascular risk for women with Turner syndrome. Womens Health (Lond Engl). 2014 Jul; 10(4):469–76. [PMID: 25259906]

Levitsky LL et al. Turner syndrome: update on biology and management across the life span. Curr Opin Endocrinol Diabetes Obes. 2015 Feb;22(1):65–72. [PMID: 25517026]

Pinsker JE. Clinical review. Turner syndrome: updating the paradigm of clinical care. J Clin Endocrinol Metab. 2012 Jun; 97(6):E994–1003. [PMID: 22472565]

Practice Committee of American Society for Reproductive Medicine. Increased maternal cardiovascular mortality associated with pregnancy in women with Turner syndrome. Fertil Steril. 2012 Feb;97(2):282–4. [PMID: 22192347]

Trolle C et al. Sex hormone replacement in Turner syndrome. Endocrine. 2012 Apr;41(2):200–19. [PMID: 22147393]

Wasniewska M et al. Adult height in girls with Turner syndrome treated from before 6 years of age with a fixed per kilogram GH dose. Eur J Endocrinol. 2013 Sep 13;169(4):439–43. [PMID: 23904278]

CLINICAL USE OF CORTICOSTEROIDS

Prolonged treatment with systemic high-dose corticosteroids causes a variety of adverse effects that can be life threatening. Patients should be thoroughly informed of the major possible side effects of treatment such as insomnia, cognitive and personality changes, weight gain with central obesity, bruising, striae, muscle weakness, polyuria, renal calculi, diabetes mellitus, glaucoma, cataracts, sex hormone suppression, candidiasis and opportunistic infections. High-dose corticosteroids have adverse cardiovascular effects, increasing the risk of hypertension, dyslipidemia, myocardial infarction, stroke, atrial fibrillation or flutter, and heart failure. Prolonged corticosteroid therapy for systemic inflammatory disorders commonly suppresses pituitary ACTH secretion, causing secondary adrenal insufficiency.

In pregnancy, maternal corticosteroids are transmitted across the placenta to the fetus, causing adverse effects on fetal growth and development as well as childhood cognition and behavior. Therefore, women who are to receive high-dose corticosteroids should be screened for pregnancy and counseled to use contraception.

Bone fractures (especially spine and hip) ultimately occur in about 40% of patients receiving long-term corticosteroid therapy. Osteoporotic fractures can also occur in patients who receive extensive topical, inhaled, or intermittent oral

Table 26–18. Management of patients receiving systemic corticosteroids.

Recommendations for prescribing
- Do not administer corticosteroids unless absolutely indicated or more conservative measures have failed.
- Keep dosage and duration of administration to the minimum required for adequate treatment.

Monitoring recommendations
- Screen for tuberculosis with a purified protein derivative (PPD) test or chest radiograph before commencing long-term corticosteroid therapy.
- Screen for pregnancy in reproductive age women; recommend contraceptive measures.
- Screen for diabetes mellitus before treatment and at each clinician visit.
- Teach patient about the symptoms of hyperglycemia.
- Screen for hypertension before treatment and at each clinician visit.
- Screen for glaucoma and cataracts before treatment, 3 months after treatment inception, and then at least yearly.
- Monitor plasma potassium for hypokalemia and treat as indicated.
- Obtain bone densitometry before treatment and then periodically. Treat osteoporosis.
- Weigh daily. Use dietary measures to avoid obesity and optimize nutrition.
- Measure height frequently to document the degree of axial spine demineralization and compression.
- Watch for fungal or yeast infections of skin, nails, mouth, vagina, and rectum, and treat appropriately.
- With dosage reduction, watch for signs of adrenal insufficiency or corticosteroid withdrawal syndrome.

Patient information
- Prepare the patient and family for possible adverse effects on mood, memory, and cognitive function.
- Inform the patient about other possible side effects, particularly weight gain, osteoporosis, and aseptic necrosis of bone.
- Counsel to avoid smoking and excessive ethanol consumption.

Prophylactic measures
- Institute a vigorous physical exercise and isometric regimen tailored to each patient's abilities or disabilities.
- Administer calcium (1 g elemental calcium) and vitamin D_3, 400–800 units orally daily.
  - Check spot morning urines for calcium; alter dosage to keep urine calcium concentration < 30 mg/dL (< 7.5 mmol/L).
  - If the patient is receiving thiazide diuretics, check for hypercalcemia, and administer only 500 mg elemental calcium daily.
- If the patient has pre-existent osteoporosis or has been receiving glucocorticoids for ≥ 3 months, consider prophylaxis:
  - Bisphosphonate such as alendronate (70 mg every week orally), zoledronate (5 mg every year intravenously) for up to 3–5 years;

  Or

  - Denosumab (60 mg every 6 months subcutaneously) for up to 3–5 years.
- Avoid prolonged bed rest that will accelerate muscle weakness and bone mineral loss. Ambulate early after fractures.
- Avoid elective surgery, if possible. Vitamin A in a daily dose of 20,000 units orally for 1 week may improve wound healing, but it is not prescribed in pregnancy.
- Fall prevention strategies: walking assistance (cane, walker, wheelchair, handrails) when required due to weakness or balance problems; avoid activities that could cause falls or other trauma.
- For ulcer prophylaxis, if administering corticosteroids with nonsteroidals, prescribe a proton pump inhibitor (not required for corticosteroids alone). Avoid large doses of antacids containing aluminum hydroxide (many popular brands) because aluminum hydroxide binds phosphate and may cause a hypophosphatemic osteomalacia that can compound corticosteroid osteoporosis.
- Treat hypogonadism.
- Treat infections aggressively. Consider unusual pathogens.
- Treat edema as indicated.

corticosteroids (eg, prednisone 10 mg/day or more and cumulative dose greater than 1 g). Osteoporotic fractures can occur even in patients receiving long-term corticosteroid therapy at relatively low doses (eg, 5–7.5 mg prednisone daily). Vertebral fractures occur at higher bone densities compared to patients without corticosteroid exposure. Patients at increased risk for corticosteroid osteoporotic fractures include those who are over age 60 or who have a low body mass index, pretreatment osteoporosis, a family history of osteoporosis, or concurrent disease that limits mobility. Avascular necrosis of bone (especially hips) develops in about 15% of patients who receive corticosteroids at high doses (eg, prednisone 15 mg daily or more) for more than 1 month with cumulative prednisone doses of 10 g or more.

Bisphosphonates (eg, alendronate, 70 mg orally weekly) prevent the development of osteoporosis among patients receiving prolonged courses of corticosteroids. For patients who are unable to tolerate oral bisphosphonates

(due to esophagitis, hiatal hernia, or gastritis), periodic intravenous infusions of pamidronate, 60–90 mg, or zoledronate, 4 mg, should also be effective. Teriparatide, 20 mcg subcutaneously daily for up to 2 years, is also effective against corticosteroid-induced osteoporosis. It is wise to follow an organized treatment plan such as the one outlined in Table 26–18.

Buehring B et al. Glucocorticoid-induced osteoporosis: an update on effects and management. J Allergy Clin Immunol. 2013 Nov;132(5):1019–30. [PMID: 24176682]

Fardet L et al. Systemic glucocorticoid therapy: a review of its metabolic and cardiovascular adverse events. Drugs. 2014 Oct; 74(15):1731–45. [PMID: 25204470]

Sacre K et al. Pituitary-adrenal function after prolonged glucocorticoid therapy for systemic inflammatory disorders: an observational study. J Clin Endocrinol Metab. 2013 Aug; 98:3199–205. [PMID: 23760625]

Diabetes Mellitus & Hypoglycemia

Umesh Masharani, MB, BS, MRCP(UK)

DIABETES MELLITUS

ESSENTIALS OF DIAGNOSIS

Type 1 diabetes

▶ Polyuria, polydipsia, and weight loss associated with random plasma glucose of 200 mg/dL (11.1 mmol/L) or more.

▶ Plasma glucose of 126 mg/dL (7.0 mmol/L) or more after an overnight fast, documented on more than one occasion.

▶ Ketonemia, ketonuria, or both.

▶ Islet autoantibodies are frequently present.

Type 2 diabetes

▶ Many patients are over 40 years of age and obese.

▶ Polyuria and polydipsia. Ketonuria and weight loss generally are uncommon at time of diagnosis. Candidal vaginitis in women may be an initial manifestation. Many patients have few or no symptoms.

▶ Plasma glucose of 126 mg/dL or more after an overnight fast on more than one occasion. Two hours after 75 g oral glucose, diagnostic values are 200 mg/dL (11.1 mmol) or more.

▶ HbA$_{1c}$ 6.5% or more.

▶ Hypertension, dyslipidemia, and atherosclerosis are often associated.

▶ Epidemiologic Considerations

An estimated 29.1 million people (9.3%) in the United States have diabetes mellitus, of which approximately 1.25 million have type 1 diabetes and most of the rest have type 2 diabetes. A third group designated as "other specific types" by the American Diabetes Association (ADA) (Table 27–1) number only in the thousands.

▶ Classification & Pathogenesis

Diabetes mellitus is a syndrome with disordered metabolism and inappropriate hyperglycemia due to either a deficiency of insulin secretion or to a combination of insulin resistance and inadequate insulin secretion to compensate for the resistance.

A. Type 1 Diabetes Mellitus

This form of diabetes is due to pancreatic islet B cell destruction predominantly by an autoimmune process in over 95% of cases (type 1A) and idiopathic in less than 5% (type 1B). The rate of pancreatic B cell destruction is quite variable, being rapid in some individuals and slow in others. Type 1 diabetes is usually associated with ketosis in its untreated state. It occurs at any age but most commonly arises in children and young adults with a peak incidence before school age and again at around puberty. It is a catabolic disorder in which circulating insulin is virtually absent, plasma glucagon is elevated, and the pancreatic B cells fail to respond to all insulinogenic stimuli. Exogenous insulin is therefore required to reverse the catabolic state, prevent ketosis, reduce the hyperglucagonemia, and reduce blood glucose.

1. Immune-mediated type 1 diabetes mellitus (type 1A)—Approximately one-third of the disease susceptibility is due to genes and two-thirds to environmental factors. Genes that are related to the HLA locus contribute about 40% of the genetic risk. About 95% of patients with type 1 diabetes possess either HLA-DR3 or HLA-DR4, compared with 45–50% of white controls. *HLA-DQ* genes are even more specific markers of type 1 susceptibility, since a particular variety *(HLA-DQB1*0302)* is found in the DR4 patients with type 1, while a "protective" gene *(HLA-DQB1*0602)* is often present in the DR4 controls. The other important gene that contributes to about 10% of the genetic risk is found at the 5′ polymorphic region of the insulin gene. Mutations in genes associated with T cell tolerance can also cause autoimmune diabetes. The autoimmune regulatory gene *(AIRE)* product regulates the expression of several proteins in the thymus causing the

Table 27–1. Other specific types of diabetes mellitus.

Genetic defects of pancreatic B cell function
  MODY 1 (HNF-4alpha); rare
  MODY 2 (glucokinase); less rare
  MODY 3 (HNF-1alpha); accounts for two-thirds of all MODY
  MODY 4 (PDX1); very rare
  MODY 5 (HNF-1beta); very rare
  MODY 6 (neuroD1); very rare
  Mitochondrial DNA
Genetic defects in insulin action
  Type A insulin resistance
  Leprechaunism
  Rabson-Mendenhall syndrome
  Lipoatrophic diabetes
Diseases of the exocrine pancreas
Endocrinopathies
Drug- or chemical-induced diabetes
Other genetic syndromes (Down, Klinefelter, Turner, others)
  sometimes associated with diabetes

MODY, maturity-onset diabetes of the young; PDX1, pancreatic duodenal homeobox 1.

deletion of self-reactive T cells. Type 1 diabetes mellitus as well as other autoimmune disorders (autoimmune polyglandular syndrome 1) develop in 20% of individuals with homozygote mutations in *AIRE*. Most patients with type 1 diabetes mellitus have circulating antibodies to islet cells (ICA), glutamic acid decarboxylase 65 (GAD65), insulin (IAA), tyrosine phosphatase IA2 (ICA-512), and zinc transporter 8 (ZnT8) at the time the diagnosis is made (Table 27–2). These antibodies facilitate screening for an autoimmune cause of diabetes, particularly screening siblings of affected children, as well as adults with atypical features of type 2 diabetes mellitus. Also, low levels of anti-insulin antibodies develop in almost all patients once they are treated with insulin.

Family members of diabetic probands are at increased lifetime risk for developing type 1 diabetes mellitus. A child whose mother has type 1 diabetes has a 3% risk of developing the disease and a 6% risk if the child's father has it. The risk in siblings is related to the number of HLA haplotypes that the sibling shares with the diabetic proband. If one haplotype is shared, the risk is 6% and if two haplotypes are

shared, the risk increases to 12–25%. The highest risk is for identical twins, where the concordance rate is 25–50%.

Some patients with a milder expression of type 1 diabetes mellitus initially retain enough B cell function to avoid ketosis, but as their B cell mass diminishes later in life, dependence on insulin therapy develops. Islet cell antibody surveys among northern Europeans indicate that up to 15% of "type 2" diabetic patients may actually have this mild form of type 1 diabetes (latent autoimmune diabetes of adulthood; LADA). Evidence for environmental factors playing a role in the development of type 1 diabetes include the observation that the disease is more common in Scandinavian countries and becomes progressively less frequent in countries nearer and nearer to the equator. Also, the risk for type 1 diabetes increases when individuals who normally have a low risk emigrate to the Northern Hemisphere. For example, Pakistani children born and raised in Bradford, England have a higher risk for developing type 1 diabetes compared with children who lived in Pakistan all their lives.

Which environmental factor is responsible for the increased risk is not known. There have been a number of different hypotheses including infections with certain viruses (mumps, rubella, Coxsackie B4) and consumption of cow's milk. Also, in developed countries, childhood infections have become less frequent and so perhaps the immune system becomes dysregulated with development of autoimmunity and conditions such as asthma and diabetes. This theory is referred to as the **hygiene hypothesis**. Part of the difficulty in determining the causative environmental factor is that autoimmune injury is initiated many years before the clinical presentation of diabetes.

2. Idiopathic type 1 diabetes mellitus (type 1B)—Approximately 5% of subjects have no evidence of pancreatic B cell autoimmunity to explain their insulinopenia and ketoacidosis. This subgroup has been classified as "idiopathic type 1 diabetes" and designated as "type 1B." Although only a minority of patients with type 1 diabetes fall into this group, most of these individuals are of Asian or African origin. About 4% of the West Africans with ketosis-prone diabetes are homozygous for a mutation in *PAX-4* (*Arg133Trp*)—a transcription factor that is essential for the development of pancreatic islets.

B. Type 2 Diabetes Mellitus

This represents a heterogeneous group of conditions that used to occur predominantly in adults, but it is now more frequently encountered in children and adolescents. Circulating endogenous insulin is sufficient to prevent ketoacidosis but is inadequate to prevent hyperglycemia in the face of increased needs owing to tissue insensitivity (insulin resistance).

Genetic and environmental factors combine to cause both the insulin resistance and the beta cell loss. Most epidemiologic data indicate strong genetic influences, since in monozygotic twins over 40 years of age, concordance develops in over 70% of cases within a year whenever type 2 diabetes develops in one twin. So far, more than 30

Table 27–2. Diagnostic sensitivity and specificity of autoimmune markers in patients with newly diagnosed type 1 diabetes mellitus.

	Sensitivity	Specificity
ICA antibody	44–100%	96%
Glutamic acid decarboxylase (GAD65)	70–90%	99%
Insulin (IAA)	40–70%	99%
Tyrosine phosphatase (IA-2)	50–70%	99%
Zinc transporter 8 (ZnT8)	50–70%	99%

genetic loci have been associated with an increased risk of type 2 diabetes. A significant number of the identified loci appear to code for proteins that have a role in beta cell function or development. One of the genetic loci with the largest risk effect is *TCF7L2*. This gene codes for a transcription factor involved in the WNT signaling pathway that is required for normal pancreatic development.

Early in the disease process, hyperplasia of pancreatic B cells occurs and probably accounts for the fasting hyperinsulinism and exaggerated insulin and proinsulin responses to glucose and other stimuli. With time, chronic deposition of amyloid in the islets may combine with inherited genetic defects progressively to impair B cell function.

Obesity is the most important environmental factor causing insulin resistance. The degree and prevalence of obesity varies among different racial groups with type 2 diabetes. While obesity is apparent in no more than 30% of Chinese and Japanese patients with type 2, it is found in 60–70% of North Americans, Europeans, or Africans with type 2 and approaches 100% of patients with type 2 among Pima Indians or Pacific Islanders from Nauru or Samoa.

Visceral obesity, due to accumulation of fat in the omental and mesenteric regions, correlates with insulin resistance; subcutaneous abdominal fat seems to have less of an association with insulin insensitivity. There are many patients with type 2 diabetes who, while not overtly obese, have increased visceral fat; they are termed the "metabolically obese." Exercise may affect the deposition of visceral fat as suggested by CT scans of Japanese wrestlers, whose extreme obesity is predominantly subcutaneous. Their daily vigorous exercise program prevents accumulation of visceral fat, and they have normal serum lipids and euglycemia despite daily intakes of 5000–7000 kcal and development of massive subcutaneous obesity.

C. Other Specific Types of Diabetes Mellitus

1. Maturity-onset diabetes of the young (MODY)—This subgroup is a relatively rare monogenic disorder characterized by non–insulin-dependent diabetes with **autosomal dominant inheritance** and an age at onset of 25 years or younger. Patients are nonobese, and their hyperglycemia is due to impaired glucose-induced secretion of insulin. Six types of MODY have been described (Table 27–1). Except for MODY 2, in which a glucokinase gene is defective, all other types involve mutations of a nuclear transcription factor that regulates islet gene expression.

2. Diabetes due to mutant insulins or insulin receptors—Less than 10 families have been described with a subtype of nonobese type 2 diabetes from mutant insulins. Since affected individuals were heterozygous and possessed one normal insulin gene, diabetes was mild, did not appear until middle age, and showed autosomal dominant genetic transmission. Defects in one of their insulin receptor genes have been found in more than 40 people with diabetes, and most have extreme insulin resistance associated with acanthosis nigricans (Figure 27–1). In very rare instances when both insulin receptor genes are abnormal, newborns present with a leprechaun-like phenotype and seldom live through infancy.

▲ **Figure 27–1.** Acanthosis nigricans of the nape of the neck, with typical dark and velvety appearance. (Used, with permission, from Umesh Masharani, MB, BS, MRCP (UK).)

3. Diabetes mellitus associated with a mutation of mitochondrial DNA—Since sperm do not contain mitochondria, only the mother transmits mitochondrial genes to her offspring. Diabetes due to mutations of mitochondrial DNA occurs in less than 2% of patients with diabetes. The most common cause is the A3243G mutation in the gene coding for the tRNA (Leu, UUR). Diabetes usually develops in these patients in their late 30s, and characteristically, they also have hearing loss (maternally inherited diabetes and deafness [MIDD]).

4. Wolfram syndrome—Wolfram syndrome is an autosomal recessive neurodegenerative disorder first evident in childhood. It consists of diabetes insipidus, diabetes mellitus, optic atrophy, and deafness, hence the acronym DID-MOAD. It is due to mutations in a gene named *WFS1*, which encodes a 100.3 KDa transmembrane protein localized in the endoplasmic reticulum. Cranial diabetes insipidus and sensorineural deafness develop during the second decade in 60–75% of patients. Ureterohydronephrosis, neurogenic bladder, cerebellar ataxia, peripheral neuropathy, and psychiatric illness develop later in many patients.

5. Autosomal recessive syndromes—Homozygous mutations in a number of pancreatic transcription factors, *NEUROG3*, *PTF1A*, *RFX6*, and *GLI-similar 3 (GLIS3)*, cause neonatal or childhood diabetes. Homozygous *PTF1A* mutations result in absent pancreas and cerebellar atrophy; *NEUROG3* mutations cause severe malabsorption and diabetes before puberty. Homozygous mutations in *RFX6* cause the Mitchell-Riley syndrome characterized by absence of all islet cell types apart from pancreatic polypeptide cells, hypoplasia of the pancreas and gallbladder, and intestinal atresia. *GLIS3* gene plays a role in transcription of insulin gene, and homozygous mutations cause neonatal diabetes and congenital hypothyroidism. The gene *EIF2AK3* encodes PKR-like ER kinase (PERK), which controls one of the pathways of the unfolded protein response. Absence of PERK leads to inadequate response to

ER stress and accelerated beta cell apoptosis. Patients with mutation in this gene have neonatal diabetes, epiphyseal dysplasia, developmental delay, and hepatic and renal dysfunction (Wolcott-Rallison syndrome).

6. Diabetes mellitus secondary to other causes—Endocrine tumors secreting growth hormone, glucocorticoids, catecholamines, glucagon, or somatostatin can cause glucose intolerance (Table 27–3). In the first four of these situations, peripheral responsiveness to insulin is impaired. With excess of glucocorticoids, catecholamines, or glucagon, increased hepatic output of glucose is a contributory factor; in the case of catecholamines, decreased insulin release is an additional factor in producing carbohydrate intolerance, and with somatostatin, inhibition of insulin secretion is the major factor. Diabetes mainly occurs in individuals with underlying defects in insulin secretion, and hyperglycemia typically resolves when the hormone excess is resolved.

High-titer anti-insulin receptor antibodies that inhibit insulin binding cause a clinical syndrome characterized by severe insulin resistance, glucose intolerance or diabetes mellitus, and acanthosis nigricans. These patients usually have other autoimmune disorders. There are reports of spontaneous remission or remission with cytotoxic therapy.

Many medications are associated with carbohydrate intolerance or frank diabetes (Table 27–3). The medications act by decreasing insulin secretion or by increasing insulin resistance or both. Cyclosporine and tacrolimus impair insulin secretion; sirolimus principally increases insulin resistance. These agents contribute to the development of new-onset diabetes after transplantation. Corticosteroids increase insulin resistance but may also have an effect on beta cell function; in a case control study and a large population cohort study, oral corticosteroids doubled the risk for development of diabetes. Thiazide diuretics and beta-blockers modestly increase the risk for diabetes. Treating the hypokalemia due to thiazides may reverse the hyperglycemia. Atypical antipsychotics, particularly olanzapine and clozapine, have been associated with increased risk of glucose intolerance. These medications cause weight gain and insulin resistance but may also impair beta cell function; an increase in rates of diabetic ketoacidosis has been reported.

Chronic pancreatitis or subtotal pancreatectomy reduces the number of functioning B cells and can result in a metabolic derangement very similar to that of genetic type 1 diabetes except that a concomitant reduction in pancreatic A cells may reduce glucagon secretion so that relatively lower doses of insulin replacement are needed.

Insulin Resistance Syndrome (Syndrome X; Metabolic Syndrome)

Twenty-five percent of the general nonobese, nondiabetic population has insulin resistance of a magnitude similar to that seen in type 2 diabetes. These insulin-resistant nondiabetic individuals are at much higher risk for developing type 2 diabetes than insulin-sensitive persons. In addition to diabetes, these individuals have a cluster of abnormalities termed **syndrome X** or **metabolic syndrome** that significantly increases their risk of atherosclerotic disease: elevated plasma triglycerides and small, dense, low-density lipoproteins (LDL); lower high-density lipoproteins (HDLs); higher blood pressure; hyperuricemia; abdominal obesity; prothrombotic state with increased levels of plasminogen activator inhibitor type 1 (PAI-1); and proinflammatory state.

It has been postulated that hyperinsulinemia and insulin resistance play a direct role in these metabolic abnormalities, but supportive evidence is inconclusive. Although hyperinsulinism and hypertension often coexist in whites, that is not the case in blacks or Pima Indians. Moreover, patients with hyperinsulinism due to insulinoma are not hypertensive, and there is no fall in blood pressure after surgical removal of the insulinoma restores normal insulin levels. The main value of grouping these disorders as a syndrome, however, is to remind clinicians that the therapeutic goals are not only to correct hyperglycemia but also to manage the elevated blood pressure and dyslipidemia that result in increased cerebrovascular and cardiac morbidity and mortality in these patients.

American Diabetes Association. Standards of medical care in diabetes—2016. Diabetes Care. 2016 Jan;39(Suppl):S1–119. [PMID: 26696680]

Clinical Findings

A. Symptoms and Signs

1. Type 1 diabetes—A characteristic symptom complex of hyperosmolality and hyperketonemia from the accumulation of circulating glucose and fatty acids typically presents in patients with type 1 diabetes who have an absolute deficiency of insulin. Increased urination and thirst are consequences of osmotic diuresis secondary to sustained hyperglycemia. The diuresis results in a loss of glucose as well as free water and electrolytes in the urine. Blurred vision often develops as the lenses are exposed to hyperosmolar fluids.

Table 27–3. Secondary causes of hyperglycemia.

Hyperglycemia due to tissue insensitivity to insulin
  Hormonal tumors (acromegaly, Cushing syndrome, glucagonoma, pheochromocytoma)
  Pharmacologic agents (corticosteroids, sympathomimetic drugs, niacin)
  Liver disease (cirrhosis, hemochromatosis)
  Muscle disorders (myotonic dystrophy)
  Adipose tissue disorders (lipodystrophy, truncal obesity)
  Insulin receptor disorders (acanthosis nigricans syndromes, leprechaunism)
Hyperglycemia due to reduced insulin secretion
  Hormonal tumors (somatostatinoma, pheochromocytoma)
  Pancreatic disorders (pancreatitis, hemosiderosis, hemochromatosis)
  Pharmacologic agents (thiazide diuretics, phenytoin, pentamidine, calcineurin inhibitors)

Weight loss despite normal or increased appetite is a common feature of type 1 when it develops subacutely. The weight loss is initially due to depletion of water, glycogen, and triglycerides; thereafter, reduced muscle mass occurs as amino acids are diverted to form glucose and ketone bodies.

Lowered plasma volume produces symptoms of postural hypotension. Total body potassium loss and the general catabolism of muscle protein contribute to the weakness.

Paresthesias may be present at the time of diagnosis, particularly when the onset is subacute. They reflect a temporary dysfunction of peripheral sensory nerves, which clears as insulin replacement restores glycemic levels closer to normal, suggesting neurotoxicity from sustained hyperglycemia.

When absolute insulin deficiency is of acute onset, the above symptoms develop abruptly. Ketoacidosis exacerbates the dehydration and hyperosmolality by producing anorexia and nausea and vomiting, interfering with oral fluid replacement.

The patient's level of consciousness can vary depending on the degree of hyperosmolality. When insulin deficiency develops relatively slowly and sufficient water intake is maintained, patients remain relatively alert and physical findings may be minimal. When vomiting occurs in response to worsening ketoacidosis, dehydration progresses and compensatory mechanisms become inadequate to keep serum osmolality below 320–330 mOsm/L. Under these circumstances, stupor or even coma may occur. The fruity breath odor of acetone further suggests the diagnosis of diabetic ketoacidosis.

Hypotension in the recumbent position is a serious prognostic sign. Loss of subcutaneous fat and muscle wasting are features of more slowly developing insulin deficiency. In occasional patients with slow, insidious onset of insulin deficiency, subcutaneous fat may be considerably depleted.

2. Type 2 diabetes—While increased urination and thirst may be presenting symptoms in some patients with type 2 diabetes, many other patients have an insidious onset of hyperglycemia and are asymptomatic initially. This is particularly true in obese patients, whose diabetes may be detected only after glycosuria or hyperglycemia is noted during routine laboratory studies. Occasionally, when the disease has been occult for some time, patients with type 2 diabetes may have evidence of neuropathic or cardiovascular complications at the time of presentation. Chronic skin infections are common. Generalized pruritus and symptoms of vaginitis are frequently the initial complaints of women. Diabetes should be suspected in women with chronic candidal vulvovaginitis as well as in those who have delivered babies larger than 9 lb (4.1 kg) or have had polyhydramnios, preeclampsia, or unexplained fetal losses. Balanoposthitis (inflammation of the foreskin and glans in uncircumcised males) may occur.

Many patients with type 2 diabetes are overweight or obese. Even those who are not significantly obese often have characteristic localization of fat deposits on the upper segment of the body (particularly the abdomen, chest, neck, and face) and relatively less fat on the appendages, which may be quite muscular. This centripetal fat distribution is characterized by a high waist circumference; a waist circumference larger than 40 inches (102 cm) in men and 35 inches (88 cm) in women is associated with an increased risk of diabetes. Some patients may have acanthosis nigricans, which is associated with significant insulin resistance; the skin in the axilla, groin, and back of neck is hyperpigmented and hyperkeratotic (Figure 27–1). Mild hypertension is often present in obese patients with diabetes. Eruptive xanthomas on the flexor surface of the limbs and on the buttocks and lipemia retinalis due to hyperchylomicronemia can occur in patients with uncontrolled type 2 diabetes who also have a familial form of hypertriglyceridemia.

Hyperglycemic hyperosmolar coma can also be present; in these cases, patients are profoundly dehydrated, hypotensive, lethargic or comatose but without Kussmaul respirations.

B. Laboratory Findings

1. Urine glucose—A specific and convenient method to detect glucosuria is the paper strip impregnated with glucose oxidase and a chromogen system (Clinistix, Diastix), which is sensitive to as little as 100 mg/dL (5.5 mmol) glucose in urine. Diastix can be directly applied to the urinary stream, and differing color responses of the indicator strip reflect glucose concentration.

A normal renal threshold for glucose as well as reliable bladder emptying is essential for interpretation.

Nondiabetic glycosuria (renal glycosuria) is a benign asymptomatic condition wherein glucose appears in the urine despite a normal amount of glucose in the blood, either basally or during a glucose tolerance test. Its cause may vary from mutations in the *SGLT2* gene coding for sodium-glucose transporter 2 (familial renal glycosuria) to one associated with dysfunction of the proximal renal tubule (Fanconi syndrome, chronic kidney disease), or it may merely be a consequence of the increased load of glucose presented to the tubules by the elevated glomerular filtration rate (GFR) during pregnancy. As many as 50% of pregnant women normally have demonstrable sugar in the urine, especially during the third and fourth months. This sugar is practically always glucose except during the late weeks of pregnancy, when lactose may be present.

2. Urine and blood ketones—Qualitative detection of ketone bodies can be accomplished by nitroprusside tests (Acetest or Ketostix). Although these tests do not detect beta-hydroxybutyric acid, which lacks a ketone group, the semiquantitative estimation of ketonuria thus obtained is nonetheless usually adequate for clinical purposes. Many laboratories measure beta-hydroxybutyric acid, and there are meters available (Precision Xtra; Nova Max Plus) for patient use that measures beta-hydroxybutyric acid levels in capillary glucose samples. Beta-hydroxybutyrate levels greater than 0.6 mmol/L require evaluation. Patients with levels greater than 3.0 mmol/L, equivalent to very large urinary ketones, require hospitalization.

3. Plasma or serum glucose—The glucose concentration is 10–15% higher in plasma or serum than in whole blood

Table 27–4. Criteria for the diagnosis of diabetes.

	Normal Glucose Tolerance	Impaired Glucose Tolerance	Diabetes Mellitus[2]
Fasting plasma glucose mg/dL (mmol/L)	< 100 (5.6)	100–125 (5.6–6.9)	≥ 126 (7.0)
Two hours after glucose load[1] mg/dL (mmol/L)	< 140 (7.8)	≥ 140–199 (7.8–11.0)	≥ 200 (11.1)
HbA$_{1c}$ (%)	< 5.7	5.7–6.4	≥ 6.5

[1]Give 75 g of glucose dissolved in 300 mL of water after an overnight fast in persons who have been receiving at least 150–200 g of carbohydrate daily for 3 days before the test.
[2]A fasting plasma glucose ≥ 126 mg/dL (7.0 mmol) or HbA$_{1c}$ of ≥ 6.5% is diagnostic of diabetes if confirmed by repeat testing.

because structural components of blood cells are absent. A plasma glucose level of 126 mg/dL (7 mmol/L) or higher on more than one occasion after at least 8 hours of fasting is diagnostic of diabetes mellitus (Table 27–4). Fasting plasma glucose levels of 100–125 mg/dL (5.6–6.9 mmol/L) are associated with increased risk of diabetes (impaired fasting glucose tolerance).

4. Oral glucose tolerance test—If the fasting plasma glucose level is less than 126 mg/dL (7 mmol/L) when diabetes is nonetheless suspected, then a standardized oral glucose tolerance test may be done (Table 27–4). In order to optimize insulin secretion and effectiveness, especially when patients have been on a low-carbohydrate diet, a minimum of 150–200 g of carbohydrate per day should be included in the diet for 3 days preceding the test. The patient should eat nothing after midnight prior to the test day. On the morning of the test, adults are then given 75 g of glucose in 300 mL of water; children are given 1.75 g of glucose per kilogram of ideal body weight. The glucose load is consumed within 5 minutes. The test should be performed in the morning because there is some diurnal variation in oral glucose tolerance, and patients should not smoke or be active during the test.

Blood samples for plasma glucose are obtained at 0 and 120 minutes after ingestion of glucose. An oral glucose tolerance test is normal if the fasting venous plasma glucose value is less than 100 mg/dL (5.6 mmol/L) and the 2-hour value falls below 140 mg/dL (7.8 mmol/L). A fasting value of 126 mg/dL (7 mmol/L) or higher or a 2-hour value of greater than 200 mg/dL (11.1 mmol/L) is diagnostic of diabetes mellitus. Patients with 2-hour value of 140–199 mg/dL (7.8–11.1 mmol/L) have impaired glucose tolerance. False-positive results may occur in patients who are malnourished, bedridden, or afflicted with an infection or severe emotional stress.

5. Glycated hemoglobin (hemoglobin A1) measurements—Hemoglobin becomes glycated by ketoamine reactions between glucose and other sugars and the free

amino groups on the alpha and beta chains. Only glycation of the N-terminal valine of the beta chain imparts sufficient negative charge to the hemoglobin molecule to allow separation by charge dependent techniques. These charge separated hemoglobins are collectively referred to as hemoglobin A$_1$ (HbA$_1$). The major form of HbA$_1$ is hemoglobin A$_{1c}$ (HbA$_{1c}$) where glucose is the carbohydrate. HbA$_{1c}$ comprises 4–6% of total hemoglobin A$_1$. HbA$_{1c}$ is abnormally elevated in diabetic persons with chronic hyperglycemia. Office-based immunoassays using capillary blood give a result in about 9 minutes and this allows for nearly immediate feedback to the patients regarding their glycemic control.

Since glycohemoglobins circulate within red blood cells whose life span lasts up to 120 days, they generally reflect the state of glycemia over the preceding 8–12 weeks, thereby providing an improved method of assessing diabetic control. The HbA$_{1c}$ value, however, is weighted to more recent glucose levels (previous month) and this explains why significant changes in HbA$_{1c}$ are observed with short-term (1 month) changes in mean plasma glucose levels. Measurements should be made in patients with either type of diabetes mellitus at 3- to 4-month intervals. In patients monitoring their own blood glucose levels, HbA$_{1c}$ values provide a valuable check on the accuracy of monitoring. In patients who do not monitor their own blood glucose levels, HbA$_{1c}$ values are essential for adjusting therapy. There is a linear relationship between the HbA$_{1c}$ and the average glucose levels in the previous 3 months. In a study using a combination of intermittent seven-point capillary blood glucose profiles (preprandial, postprandial, and bedtime) and intermittent continuous glucose monitoring data, the change in glucose values was 28.7 mg/dL for every 1% change in HbA$_{1c}$. Substantial individual variability exists, however, between HbA$_{1c}$ and mean glucose concentration. For HbA$_{1c}$ values between 6.9% and 7.1%, the glucose levels ranged from 125 mg/dL to 205 mg/dL (6.9–11.4 mmol/L; 95% CIs). For HbA$_{1c}$ of 6%, the mean glucose levels ranged from 100 mg/dL to 152 mg/dL (5.5–8.5 mmol/L); and for 8% they ranged from 147 mg/dL to 217 mg/dL (8.1–12.1 mmol/L). For this reason, caution should be exercised in estimating average glucose levels from measured HbA$_{1c}$.

The accuracy of HbA$_{1c}$ values can be affected by hemoglobin variants or traits; the effect depends on the specific hemoglobin variant or derivative and the specific assay used. In patients with high levels of hemoglobin F, immunoassays give falsely low values of HbA$_{1c}$. The National Glycohemoglobin Standardization Program website (www. ngsp.org) has information on the impact of frequently encountered hemoglobin variants and traits on the results obtained with the commonly used HbA$_{1c}$ assays.

Any condition that shortens erythrocyte survival or decreases mean erythrocyte age (eg, recovery from acute blood loss, hemolytic anemia) will falsely lower HbA$_{1c}$ irrespective of the assay method used. Intravenous iron and erythropoietin therapy for treatment of anemia in chronic kidney disease also falsely lower HbA$_{1c}$ levels. Alternative methods such as fructosamine should be considered for these patients. Vitamins C and E are reported to falsely lower test results possibly by inhibiting glycation of hemoglobin. Conditions that increase erythrocyte survival such as splenectomy for hereditary spherocytosis will falsely raise HbA$_{1c}$ levels. Iron deficiency anemia is also associated with higher HbA$_{1c}$ levels.

HbA$_{1c}$ is endorsed by the ADA as a diagnostic test for type 1 and type 2 diabetes (Table 27–4). A cutoff value of 6.5% was chosen because the risk for retinopathy increases substantially above this value. The advantages of using the HbA$_{1c}$ to diagnose diabetes is that there is no need to fast; it has lower intraindividual variability than the fasting glucose test and the oral glucose tolerance test; and it provides an estimate of glucose control for the preceding 2–3 months. People with HbA$_{1c}$ levels of 5.7–6.4% should be considered at high risk for developing diabetes (prediabetes). The diagnosis should be confirmed with a repeat HbA$_{1c}$ test, unless the patient is symptomatic with plasma glucose levels greater than 200 mg/dL (11.1 mmol/L). This test is not appropriate to use in populations with high prevalence of hemoglobinopathies or in conditions with increased red cell turnover. Also, the testing is performed using a National Glycohemoglobin Standardization Program (NGSP) certified method and standardized to the Diabetes Control and Complication Trial assay. In the European Union, the tests are standardized to the International Federation of Clinical Chemistry (IFCC), which defines HbA$_{1c}$ as mmol glycated hexapeptide per mol (glycated and nonglycated hexapeptides) and reported as mmol HbA$_{1c}$/mol Hb. The conversion factor for NGSP and IFCC results is NGSP (USA) result = (0.09148*IFCC result) + 2.152. There is worldwide consensus that HbA$_{1c}$ should be reported in both NGSP (%) and IFCC (mmol/mol) units.

6. Serum fructosamine—Serum fructosamine is formed by nonenzymatic glycosylation of serum proteins (predominantly albumin). Since serum albumin has a much shorter half-life than hemoglobin, serum fructosamine generally reflects the state of glycemic control for only the preceding 1–2 weeks. Reductions in serum albumin (eg, nephrotic state, protein-losing enteropathy, or hepatic disease) will lower the serum fructosamine value. When abnormal hemoglobins or hemolytic states affect the interpretation of glycohemoglobin or when a narrower time frame is required, such as for ascertaining glycemic control at the time of conception in a diabetic woman who has recently become pregnant, serum fructosamine assays offer some advantage. Normal values vary in relation to the serum albumin concentration and are 200–285 mcmol/L when the serum albumin level is 5 g/dL. HbA$_{1c}$ values and serum fructosamine are highly correlated. Serum fructosamine levels of 300, 367, and 430 mcmol/L approximate to HbA$_{1c}$ values of 7%, 8%, and 9%, respectively. Substantial individual variability exists, though, when estimating the likely HbA$_{1c}$ value from the fructosamine measurement.

7. Self-monitoring of blood glucose—Capillary blood glucose measurements performed by patients themselves, as outpatients, are extremely useful. In type 1 patients in whom "tight" metabolic control is attempted, they are indispensable. There are several paper strip (glucose oxidase, glucose dehydrogenase, or hexokinase) methods for measuring glucose on capillary blood samples. A reflectance photometer or an amperometric system is then used to measure the reaction that takes place on the reagent strip. A large number of blood glucose meters are now available. All are accurate, but they vary with regard to speed, convenience, size of blood samples required, reporting capability, and cost. Popular models include those manufactured by LifeScan (One Touch), Bayer Corporation (Breeze, Contour), Roche Diagnostics (Accu-Chek), Sanofi Aventis (iBGStar), and Abbott Laboratories (Precision, FreeStyle). These blood glucose meters are relatively inexpensive, ranging from $50 to $100 each. Test strips remain a major expense, costing about $.25 to $1.50 apiece. Each glucose meter also comes with a lancet device and disposable 26- to 33-gauge lancets. Most meters can store from 100 to 1000 glucose values in their memories and have capabilities to download the values into a computer spreadsheet for review by the patients and their health care team. iBGStar is a glucose meter that connects directly to the iPhone. Some meters are designed to communicate with a specific insulin pump. Contour Next Link meter, for example, communicates with the MiniMed Medtronic pump). The accuracy of data obtained by home glucose monitoring does require education of the patient in sampling and measuring procedures as well as in properly calibrating the instruments.

The clinician should be aware of the limitations of the self-monitoring glucose systems. The strips have limited lifespans and improper storage (high temperature; open vial) can affect their function. Patients should also be advised not to use expired strips. Some of the older meters require input of a code for each batch of strips and failure to enter the code can result in misleading results. The newer meters no longer require this step. Increases or decreases in hematocrit can decrease or increase the measured glucose values. The mechanism underlying this effect is not known but presumably it is due to the impact of red cells on the diffusion of plasma into the reagent layer. Meters and the test strips are calibrated over the glucose concentrations ranging from 60 mg/dL (3.3 mmol/L) to 160 mg/dL (8.9 mmol/L) and the accuracy is not as good for higher and lower glucose levels. When the glucose is less than 60 mg/dL (3.3 mmol/L), the difference between the meter and the laboratory value may be as much as 20%. Glucose oxidase–based amperometric systems underestimate glucose levels in the presence of high oxygen tension. This may be important in the critically ill who are receiving supplemental oxygen; under these circumstances, a glucose dehydrogenase–based system may be preferable. Glucose-dehydrogenase pyrroloquinoline quinone (GDH-PQQ) systems may report falsely high glucose levels in patients who are receiving parenteral products containing nonglucose sugars such as maltose, galactose, or xylose or their metabolites. Some meters have been approved for measuring glucose in blood samples obtained at alternative sites such as the forearm and thigh. There is, however, a 5- to 20-minute lag in the glucose response on the arm with respect to the glucose response on the finger. Forearm blood glucose measurements could therefore result in a delay in detection of rapidly developing hypoglycemia. Impaired circulation to the fingers (for example, in patients with Raynaud disease) will artificially lower finger-stick glucose measurements (pseudohypoglycemia).

8. Continuous glucose monitoring systems—A number of continuous glucose monitoring systems are available for clinical use. The systems manufactured by Medtronic Minimed, DexCom systems, and Abbott Diagnostics (outside the United States), involve inserting a subcutaneous sensor (rather like an insulin pump cannula) that measures glucose concentrations in the interstitial fluid for 3–7 days. The MiniMed system can only be used in conjunction with the Minimed pump and the glucose data are displayed on the screen of the pump. The DexCom system transmits glucose data wirelessly to a separate pager-like device with a screen. The DexCom system also has the option of displaying data on smart phones or smart watches or on the screens of several insulin pumps. The systems allow the patient to set "alerts" for low and high glucose values and rate of change of glucose levels. Patients still have to calibrate the devices with periodic fingerstick glucose levels, and since there are concerns regarding reliability, it is still necessary to confirm the displayed glucose level with a fingerstick glucose before making interventions such as injecting extra insulin or eating extra carbohydrates. A 6-month randomized controlled study of type 1 patients showed that adults (25 years and older) using these systems had improved glycemic control without an increase in the incidence of hypoglycemia. A randomized controlled study of continuous glucose monitoring during pregnancy showed improved glycemic control in the third trimester, lower birth weight, and reduced risk of macrosomia. The individual glucose values are not that critical—what matters is the direction and the rate at which the glucose is changing, allowing the user to take corrective action. The wearer also gains insight into the way particular foods and activities affect their glucose levels. The other main benefit is the low glucose alert warning. The MiniMed insulin pump can be programmed to automatically suspend insulin delivery for up to 2 hours when the glucose levels on its continuous glucose monitoring device falls to a preset level and the patient does not respond to the alert. This insulin suspension feature has been shown to reduce the amount of time patients are in the hypoglycemic range at night. Many of these systems are covered by insurance. The initial cost is about $800 to $1000, and the sensor, which has to be changed every 3 to 7 days, costs $35 to $60; the out-of-pocket expense of about $4000 annually.

There is great interest in using the data obtained from these continuous glucose monitoring systems to automatically deliver insulin by continuous subcutaneous insulin infusion pump. Algorithms have been devised to link continuous glucose monitoring to insulin delivery. These closed loop systems (artificial pancreas) have been shown in short-term clinical studies to improve nighttime glucose control and reduce the risk of nocturnal hypoglycemia.

9. Lipoprotein abnormalities in diabetes—Circulating lipoproteins are just as dependent on insulin as is the plasma glucose. In type 1 diabetes, moderately deficient control of hyperglycemia is associated with only a slight elevation of LDL cholesterol and serum triglycerides and little if any change in HDL cholesterol. Once the hyperglycemia is corrected, lipoprotein levels are generally normal. However, in patients with type 2 diabetes, a distinct "diabetic dyslipidemia" is characteristic of the insulin resistance syndrome. Its features are a high serum triglyceride level (300–400 mg/dL [3.4–4.5 mmol/L]), a low HDL cholesterol (less than 30 mg/dL [0.8 mmol/L]), and a qualitative change in LDL particles, producing a smaller dense particle whose membrane carries supranormal amounts of free cholesterol. These smaller dense LDL particles are more susceptible to oxidation, which renders them more atherogenic. Since a low HDL cholesterol is a major feature predisposing to macrovascular disease, the term "dyslipidemia" has preempted the term "hyperlipidemia," which mainly denoted the elevated triglycerides. Measures designed to correct the obesity and hyperglycemia, such as exercise, diet, and hypoglycemic therapy, are the treatment of choice for diabetic dyslipidemia, and in occasional patients in whom normal weight was achieved, all features of the lipoprotein abnormalities cleared. Since primary disorders of lipid metabolism may coexist with diabetes, persistence of lipid abnormalities after restoration of normal weight and blood glucose should prompt a diagnostic workup and possible pharmacotherapy of the lipid disorder. Chapter 28 discusses these matters in detail.

Haidar A et al. Comparison of dual-hormone artificial pancreas, single-hormone artificial pancreas, and conventional insulin pump therapy for glycaemic control in patients with type 1 diabetes: an open-label randomised controlled crossover trial. Lancet Diabetes Endocrinol. 2015 Jan;3(1):17–26. [PMID: 25434967]

► Clinical Trials in Diabetes

Findings of the Diabetes Complications and Control Trial (DCCT) and of the United Kingdom Prospective Diabetes Study (UKPDS), have confirmed the beneficial effects of improved glycemic control in both type 1 and type 2 diabetes.

The Diabetes Control and Complications Trial, a long-term therapeutic study involving 1441 patients with type 1 diabetes mellitus, reported that "near" normalization of blood glucose resulted in a delay in the onset and a major slowing of the progression of established microvascular and neuropathic complications of diabetes during a follow-up period of up to 10 years. Multiple insulin injections (66%) or insulin pumps (34%) were used in the intensively treated group, who were trained to modify their therapy in response to frequent glucose monitoring. The conventionally treated groups used no more than two insulin injections, and clinical well-being was the goal with no attempt to modify management based on HbA_{1c} determinations or the glucose results.

In half of the patients, a mean hemoglobin A_{1c} of 7.2% (normal: less than 6%) and a mean blood glucose of 155 mg/dL (8.6 mmol/L) were achieved using intensive therapy, while in the conventionally treated group HbA_{1c} averaged 8.9% with an average blood glucose of 225 mg/dL

(12.5 mmol/L). Over the study period, which averaged 7 years, there was an approximately 60% reduction in risk between the two groups in regard to diabetic retinopathy, nephropathy, and neuropathy. The intensively treated group also had a nonsignificant reduction in the risk of macrovascular disease of 41% (95% CI, –10 to 68). Intensively treated patients had a threefold greater risk of serious hypoglycemia as well as a greater tendency toward weight gain. However, there were no deaths definitely attributable to hypoglycemia in any persons in the DCCT study, and no evidence of posthypoglycemic cognitive damage was detected.

Subjects participating in the DCCT study were subsequently enrolled in a follow-up observational study, the Epidemiology of Diabetes Interventions and Complications (EDIC) study. Even though the between-group differences in mean HbA$_{1c}$ narrowed over 4 years, the group assigned to intensive therapy had a lower risk of retinopathy at 4 years, microalbuminuria at 7 to 8 years, and impaired GFR (less than 60 mL/min/1.73 m^2) at 22 years of continued study follow-up. Moreover, by the end of the 11-year follow-up period, the intensive therapy group had significantly reduced their risk of any cardiovascular disease events by 42% (95% CI, 9% to 23%; $P = 0.02$). Thus, it seems that the benefits of good glucose control persist even if control deteriorates at a later date.

The general consensus of the ADA is that intensive insulin therapy associated with comprehensive self-management training should become standard therapy in patients with type 1 diabetes mellitus after the age of puberty. Exceptions include those with advanced chronic kidney disease and the elderly, since in these groups the detrimental risks of hypoglycemia outweigh the benefits of tight glycemic control.

The Diabetes Prevention Program was aimed at discovering whether treatment with either diet and exercise or metformin could prevent the onset of type 2 diabetes in people with impaired glucose tolerance; 3234 overweight men and women aged 25–85 years with impaired glucose tolerance participated in the study. Intervention with a low-fat diet and 150 minutes of moderate exercise (equivalent to a brisk walk) per week reduced the risk of progression to type 2 diabetes by 71% compared with a matched control group. Participants taking 850 mg of metformin twice a day reduced their risk of developing type 2 diabetes by 31%, but this intervention was relatively ineffective in those who were either less obese or in the older age group.

With the demonstration that intervention can be successful in preventing progression to diabetes in these subjects, a recommendation has been made to change the terminology from the less comprehensible "impaired glucose tolerance" to "prediabetes." The latter is a term that the public can better understand and thus respond to by implementing healthier diet and exercise habits.

The United Kingdom Prospective Diabetes Study, a multicenter study, was designed to establish, in type 2 diabetic patients, whether the risk of macrovascular or microvascular complications could be reduced by intensive blood glucose control with oral hypoglycemic agents or insulin and whether any particular therapy was of advantage.

Intensive treatment with either sulfonylureas, metformin, combinations of those two, or insulin achieved mean HbA$_{1c}$ levels of 7%. This level of glycemic control decreased the risk of microvascular complications (retinopathy and nephropathy) in comparison with conventional therapy (mostly diet alone), which achieved mean levels of HbA$_{1c}$ of 7.9%. Weight gain occurred in intensively treated patients except when metformin was used as monotherapy. No adverse cardiovascular outcomes were noted regardless of the therapeutic agent. In the overweight or obese subgroup, metformin therapy was more beneficial than diet alone in reducing the number of cases that progressed to diabetes as well as decreasing the number of patients who suffered myocardial infarctions and strokes. Hypoglycemic reactions occurred in the intensive treatment groups, but only one death from hypoglycemia was documented during 27,000 patient-years of intensive therapy.

Tight control of blood pressure (median value 144/82 mm Hg vs 154/87 mm Hg) substantially reduced the risk of microvascular disease and stroke but not myocardial infarction. In fact, reducing blood pressure by this amount had substantially greater impact on microvascular outcomes than that achieved by lowering HbA$_{1c}$ from 7.9% to 7%. An epidemiologic analysis of the UKPDS data did show that every 10 mm Hg decrease in updated mean systolic blood pressure was associated with 11% reduction in risk for myocardial infarction. More than half of the patients needed two or more medications for adequate therapy of their hypertension, and there was no demonstrable advantage of angiotensin-converting enzyme (ACE) inhibitor therapy over therapy with beta-blockers with regard to diabetes end points. Use of a calcium channel blocker added to both treatment groups appeared to be safe over the long term in this diabetic population despite some controversy in the literature about its safety in patients with diabetes.

Like the DCCT trialists, the UKPDS researchers performed post-trial monitoring to determine whether there were long-term benefits of having been in the intensively treated glucose and blood pressure arms of the study. The intensively treated group had significantly reduced risk of myocardial infarction (15%, $P = 0.01$) and death from any cause (13%, $P = 0.007$) during the follow-up period. The subgroup of overweight or obese subjects who were initially randomized to metformin therapy showed sustained reduction in risk of myocardial infarction and death from any cause in the follow-up period. Unlike the sustained benefits seen with glucose control, there were no sustained benefits from having been in the more tightly controlled blood pressure group. Both blood pressure groups were at similar risk for microvascular events and diabetes-related end points during the follow-up period.

Thus, the follow-up of the UKPDS type 2 diabetes cohort showed that, as in type 1 diabetes, the benefits of good glucose control persist even if control deteriorates at a later date. Blood pressure benefits, however, last only as long as the blood pressure is well controlled.

The Steno-2 study was designed in 1990 to validate the efficacy of targeting multiple concomitant risk factors (diet, smoking cessation, exercise, and pharmacologic interventions) for both microvascular and macrovascular disorders in type 2 diabetes. A prospective, randomized, open, blinded end point design was used where 160 patients with type 2 diabetes and microalbuminuria were assigned to conventional therapy with their general practitioner or to intensive care at the Steno Diabetes Center. The intensively treated group had stepwise introduction of lifestyle and pharmacologic interventions aimed at keeping glycated hemoglobin less than 6.5%, blood pressure lower than 130/80 mm Hg; total cholesterol under 175 mg/dL (4.5 mmol/L), and triglycerides less than 150 mg/dL (1.7 mmol/L). All the intensively treated group received ACE inhibitors and if intolerant, an angiotensin II-receptor blocker. The lifestyle component of intensive intervention included reduction in dietary fat intake to less than 30% of total calories; smoking cessation program; light to moderate exercise; daily vitamin-mineral supplement of vitamin C, E, and chromium picolinate. Initially, aspirin was only given as secondary prevention to patients with a history of ischemic cardiovascular disease; later, all patients received aspirin. After a mean follow-up of 7.8 years, cardiovascular events (eg, myocardial infarction, angioplasties, coronary bypass grafts, strokes, amputations, vascular surgical interventions) developed in 44% of patients in the conventional arm and only in 24% in the intensive multifactorial arm—about a 50% reduction. Rates of nephropathy, retinopathy, and autonomic neuropathy were also lower in the multifactorial intervention arm by 62% and 63%, respectively.

The data from the UKPDS and this study provide support for guidelines recommending vigorous treatment of concomitant microvascular and cardiovascular risk factors in patients with type 2 diabetes.

Results from three subsequent trials, the ACCORD, ADVANCE, and VADT, do not provide support for the hypothesis that near-normal glucose control in patients with type 2 diabetes will reduce cardiovascular events. It is, however, important not to over-interpret the results of these three studies. The results do not exclude the possibility that cardiovascular benefits might accrue with longer duration of near-normal glucose control. In the UKPDS, risk reductions for myocardial infarction and death from any cause were only observed during 10 years of post-trial follow-up. Specific subgroups of type 2 diabetic patients may also have different outcomes. The ACCORD, ADVANCE, and VADT studies recruited patients who had diabetes for 8–10 years and one-third of them already had established cardiovascular disease. Patients in the UKPDS, in contrast, had newly diagnosed diabetes and only 7.5% had a history of macrovascular disease. It is possible that the benefits of tight glycemic control on macrovascular events are attenuated in patients with longer duration of diabetes or with established vascular disease. Specific therapies used to lower glucose may also affect cardiovascular event rate or mortality. Severe hypoglycemia occurred more frequently in the intensively treated groups of the ACCORD, ADVANCE, and VADT studies; the ACCORD investigators were not able to exclude undiagnosed hypoglycemia as a potential cause for the increased death rate in the intensive treatment group.

A formal meta-analysis performed of the raw trial data from the ACCORD, ADVANCE, VADT, and UKPDS studies found that allocation to more intensive glucose control reduced the risk of myocardial infarction by 15% (hazard ratio 0.85, 95% CI 0.76–0.94). This benefit occurred in patients who did not have preexisting macrovascular disease.

The Diabetes Control and Complications Trial Research Group. The effect of intensive treatment of diabetes on the development and progression of long-term complications in insulin-dependent diabetes mellitus. N Engl J Med. 1993 Sep 30; 329(14):977–86. [PMID: 8366922]

UK Prospective Diabetes Study (UKPDS) Group. Intensive blood-glucose control with sulphonylureas or insulin compared with conventional treatment and risk of complications in patients with type 2 diabetes (UKPDS 33). Lancet. 1998 Sep 12;352(9131):837–53. [PMID: 9742976]

▶ **Treatment Regimens**

A. Diet

A well-balanced, nutritious diet remains a fundamental element of therapy. There is no specific recommendation on the percentage of calories that should come from carbohydrate, protein, and fat. The macronutrient proportions should be individualized based on the patient's eating patterns, preferences, and metabolic goals. In general, most patients with diabetes consume about 45% of their total daily calories in the form of carbohydrates, 25–35% in the form of fat, and 10–35% in the form of protein. In patients with type 2 diabetes, limiting the carbohydrate intake and substituting some of the calories with monounsaturated fats, such as olive oil, rapeseed (canola) oil, or the oils in nuts and avocados, can lower triglycerides and increase HDL cholesterol. A Mediterranean-style eating pattern (a diet supplemented with walnuts, almonds, hazelnuts, and olive oil) has been shown to improve glycemic control and lower combined endpoints for cardiovascular events and stroke. In those patients with obesity and type 2 diabetes, weight reduction by caloric restriction is an important goal of the diet (see Chapter 29). Patients with type 1 diabetes or type 2 diabetes who take insulin should be taught "carbohydrate counting," so they can administer their insulin bolus for each meal based on its carbohydrate content.

The current recommendations for saturated fats and dietary cholesterol intake for people with diabetes are the same as for the general population. Saturated fats should be limited to less than 10% of daily calories and dietary cholesterol intake should be less than 300 mg/day. For those patients with kidney disease, dietary protein should be maintained at the recommended daily allowance of 0.8g/kg/day. Exchange lists for meal planning can be obtained from the American Diabetes Association and its affiliate associations or from the American Dietetic Association (http://www.eatright.org), 216 W. Jackson Blvd., Chicago, IL 60606 (312-899-0040).

1. Dietary fiber—Plant components such as cellulose, gum, and pectin are indigestible by humans and are termed dietary "fiber." Insoluble fibers such as cellulose or hemicellulose, as found in bran, tend to increase intestinal transit and may have beneficial effects on colonic function. In contrast, soluble fibers such as gums and pectins, as found in beans, oatmeal, or apple skin, tend to retard nutrient absorption rates so that glucose absorption is slower and hyperglycemia may be slightly diminished. Although its recommendations do not include insoluble fiber supplements such as added bran, the ADA recommends food such as oatmeal, cereals, and beans with relatively high soluble fiber content as staple components of the diet in diabetics. High soluble fiber content in the diet may also have a favorable effect on blood cholesterol levels.

2. Glycemic index—The glycemic index of a carbohydrate containing food is determined by comparing the glucose excursions after consuming 50 g of test food with glucose excursions after consuming 50 g of reference food (white bread):

$$\text{Glycemic index} = \frac{\text{Blood glucose area under the curve (3h) for test food}}{\text{Blood glucose area under the curve (3h) for reference food}} \times 100$$

Eating low glycemic index foods results in lower glucose levels after meals. Low glycemic index foods have values of 55 or less and include many fruits, vegetables, grainy breads, pasta, and legumes. High glycemic index foods have values of 70 or greater and include baked potato, white bread, and white rice. Glycemic index is lowered by presence of fats and protein when food is consumed in a mixed meal. Even though it may not be possible to accurately predict the glycemic index of a particular food in the context of a meal, it is reasonable to choose foods with low glycemic index.

3. Artificial and other sweeteners—Saccharin (Sweet 'N Low), sucralose (Splenda), acesulfame potassium (Sweet One), and rebiana (Truvia) are "artificial" sweeteners that can be used in cooking and baking. Aspartame (NutraSweet) lacks heat stability, so it cannot be used in cooking. None of these sweeteners raise blood glucose levels.

Fructose represents a "natural" sugar substance that is a highly effective sweetener, induces only slight increases in plasma glucose levels, and does not require insulin for its metabolism. However, because of potential adverse effects of large amounts of fructose on raising serum cholesterol, triglycerides, and LDL cholesterol, it does not have any advantage as a sweetening agent in the diabetic diet. This does not preclude, however, ingestion of fructose-containing fruits and vegetables or fructose-sweetened foods in moderation.

Sugar alcohols, also known as polyols or polyalcohol, are commonly used as sweeteners and bulking agents. They occur naturally in a variety of fruits and vegetables but are also commercially made from sucrose, glucose, and starch. Examples are sorbitol, xylitol, mannitol, lactitol, isomalt, maltitol, and hydrogenated starch hydrolysates (HSH). They are not as easily absorbed as sugar, so they do not raise blood glucose levels as much. Therefore, sugar

alcohols are often used in food products that are labeled as "sugar free," such as chewing gum, lozenges, hard candy, and sugar-free ice cream. However, if consumed in large quantities, they will raise blood glucose and can cause bloating and diarrhea.

B. Medications for Treating Hyperglycemia

The medications for treating type 2 diabetes are listed in Table 27–5.

1. Medications that primarily stimulate insulin secretion by binding to the sulfonylurea receptor on the beta cell—

A. SULFONYLUREAS—The primary mechanism of action of the sulfonylureas is to stimulate insulin release from pancreatic B cells. Specific receptors on the surface of pancreatic B cells bind sulfonylureas in the rank order of their insulinotropic potency (glyburide with the greatest affinity and tolbutamide with the least affinity). It has been shown that activation of these receptors closes potassium channels, resulting in depolarization of the B cell. This depolarized state permits calcium to enter the cell and actively promote insulin release.

Sulfonylureas are used in patients with type 2 but not type 1 diabetes, since these medications require functioning pancreatic B cells to produce their effect on blood glucose. Sulfonylureas are metabolized by the liver and apart from acetohexamide, whose metabolite is more active than the parent compound, the metabolites of all the other sulfonylureas are weakly active or inactive. The metabolites are excreted by the kidney and, in the case of the second-generation sulfonylureas, partly excreted in the bile. Sulfonylureas are generally contraindicated in patients with severe liver or kidney impairment. Idiosyncratic reactions are rare, with skin rashes or hematologic toxicity (leukopenia, thrombocytopenia) occurring in less than 0.1% of users.

(1) First-generation sulfonylureas (tolbutamide, tolazamide, acetohexamide, chlorpropamide)—**Tolbutamide** is rapidly oxidized in the liver to inactive metabolites, and its approximate duration of effect is relatively short (6–10 hours). Tolbutamide is probably best administered in divided doses (eg, 500 mg before each meal and at bedtime); however, some patients require only one or two tablets daily with a maximum dose of 3000 mg/day. Because of its short duration of action, which is independent of kidney function, tolbutamide is relatively safe to use in kidney impairment. Prolonged hypoglycemia has been reported rarely with tolbutamide, mostly in patients receiving certain antibacterial sulfonamides (sulfisoxazole), phenylbutazone for arthralgias, or the oral azole antifungal medications to treat candidiasis. These medications apparently compete with tolbutamide for oxidative enzyme systems in the liver, resulting in maintenance of high levels of unmetabolized, active sulfonylurea in the circulation.

Tolazamide, acetohexamide, and chlorpropamide are rarely used. Chlorpropamide has a prolonged biologic effect, and severe hypoglycemia can occur especially in the elderly as their renal clearance declines with aging. Its other side effects include alcohol-induced flushing and hyponatremia due to its effect on vasopressin secretion and action.

Table 27–5. Drugs for treatment of type 2 diabetes mellitus.

Drug	Tablet Size	Daily Dose	Duration of Action
Sulfonylureas			
Acetohexamide (Dymelor)	250 and 500 mg	0.25–1.5 g as single dose or in two divided doses	8–24 hours
Chlorpropamide (Diabinese)	100 and 250 mg	0.1–0.5 g as single dose	24–72 hours
Gliclazide (not available in United States)	80 mg	40–80 mg as single dose; 160–320 mg as divided dose	12 hours
Glimepiride (Amaryl)	1, 2, and 4 mg	1–4 mg once a day is usual dose; 8 mg once a day is maximal dose	Up to 24 hours
Glipizide			
(Glucotrol)	5 and 10 mg	2.5–40 mg as a single dose or in two divided doses 30 minutes before meals	6–12 hours
(Glucotrol XL)	2.5, 5, and 10 mg	2.5 to 10 mg once a day is usual dose; 20 mg once a day is maximal dose	Up to 24 hours
Glyburide			
(Dia Beta, Micronase)	1.25, 2.5, and 5 mg	1.25–20 mg as single dose or in two divided doses	Up to 24 hours
(Glynase)	1.5, 3, and 6 mg	1.5–12 mg as single dose or in two divided doses	Up to 24 hours
Tolazamide (Tolinase)	100, 250, and 500 mg	0.1–1 g as single dose or in two divided doses	Up to 24 hours
Tolbutamide (Orinase)	250 and 500 mg	0.5–2 g in two or three divided doses	6–12 hours
Meglitinide analogs			
Mitiglinide (available in Japan)	5 and 10 mg	5 or 10 mg three times a day before meals	2 hours
Repaglinide (Prandin)	0.5, 1, and 2 mg	0.5 to 4 mg three times a day before meals	3 hours
D-Phenylalanine derivative			
Nateglinide (Starlix)	60 and 120 mg	60 or 120 mg three times a day before meals	1.5 hours
Biguanides			
Metformin (Glucophage)	500, 850, and 1000 mg	1–2.5 g; 1 tablet with meals two or three times daily	7–12 hours
Extended-release metformin (Glucophage XR)	500 and 750 mg	500–2000 mg once a day	Up to 24 hours
Thiazolidinediones			
Pioglitazone (Actos)	15, 30, and 45 mg	15–45 mg daily	Up to 24 hours
Rosiglitazone (Avandia)	2, 4, and 8 mg	4–8 mg daily (can be divided)	Up to 24 hours
Alpha-glucosidase inhibitors			
Acarbose (Precose)	50 and 100 mg	25–100 mg three times a day just before meals	4 hours
Miglitol (Glyset)	25, 50, and 100 mg	25–100 mg three times a day just before meals	4 hours
Voglibose (not available in United States)	0.2 and 0.3 mg	0.2–0.3 mg three times a day just before meals	4 hours
GLP-1 receptor agonists			
Exenatide (Byetta)	1.2 mL and 2.4 mL pre-filled pens containing 5 mcg and 10 mcg (subcutaneous injection)	5 mcg subcutaneously twice a day within 1 hour of breakfast and dinner. Increase to 10 mcg subcutaneously twice a day after about a month. Do not use if calculated creatinine clearance is < 30 mL/min.	6 hours
Exenatide, long-acting release (Byetta LAR, Bydureon)	2 mg (powder)	Suspend in provided diluent and inject subcutaneously.	1 week
Liraglutide (Victoza)	Pre-filled, multi-dose pen that delivers doses of 0.6 mg, 1.2 mg, or 1.8 mg	0.6 mg subcutaneously once a day (starting dose). Increase to 1.2 mg after a week if no adverse reactions. Dose can be further increased to 1.8 mg, if necessary.	24 hours
Albiglutide (Tanzeum)	30, 50 mg single dose pen (powder)	Mix with diluent and inject subcutaneously. 30 mg is usual dose. Dose can be increased to 50 mg if necessary.	1 week

(continued)

Table 27–5. Drugs for treatment of type 2 diabetes mellitus. (Continued)

Drug	Tablet Size	Daily Dose	Duration of Action
Dulaglutide (Trulicity)	0.75, 1.5 mg single dose pen or prefilled syringe	0.75 mg subcutaneously. Dose can be increased to 1.5 mg if necessary.	1 week
DPP-4 inhibitors			
Alogliptin (Nesina)	6.25, 12.5, and 25 mg	25 mg once daily; dose is 12.5 mg daily if calculated creatinine clearance is 30–59 mL/min and 6.25 mg daily if clearance < 30 mL/min.	24 hours
Saxagliptin (Onglyza)	2.5 and 5 mg	2.5 mg or 5 mg once daily. Use 2.5 mg dose if calculated creatinine clearance is ≤ 50 mL/min or if also taking drugs that are strong CYP3A4/5 inhibitors such as ketoconazole.	24 hours
Sitagliptin (Januvia)	25, 50, and 100 mg	100 mg once daily is usual dose; dose is 50 mg once daily if calculated creatinine clearance is 30 to 50 mL/min and 25 mg once daily if clearance is < 30 mL/min.	24 hours
Vildagliptin (Galvus) (not available in United States)	50 mg	50 mg once or twice daily. Contraindicated in patients with calculated creatinine clearance ≤ 60 mL/min or AST/ALT three times upper limit of normal.	24 hours
Linagliptin (Tradjenta)	5 mg	5 mg daily	24 hours
SGLT2 inhibitors			
Canagliflozin (Invokana)	100 and 300 mg	100 mg daily is usual dose. Do not use if eGFR < 45 mL/min/1.72 m². 300 mg dose can be used if normal eGFR, resulting in lowering the HbA$_{1c}$ an additional ~ 0.1–0.25%.	24 hours
Dapagliflozin (Farxiga)	5 and 10 mg	10 mg daily. Use 5 mg dose in hepatic failure.	24 hours
Empagliflozin (Jardiance)	10 and 25 mg	10 mg daily. 25 mg dose can be used if necessary.	24 hours
Others			
Bromocriptine (Cycloset)	0.8 mg	0.8 mg daily. Increase weekly by 1 tablet until maximal tolerated dose of 1.6–4.8 mg daily.	24 hours
Colesevelam (Welchol)	625 mg	3 tablets twice a day	24 hours
Pramlintide (Symlin)	5 mL vial containing 0.6 mg/mL; also available as prefilled pens. Symlin pen 60 or Symlin pen 120 (subcutaneous injection)	For insulin-treated type 2 patients, start at 60 mcg dose three times a day (10 units on U100 insulin syringe). Increase to 120 mcg three times a day (20 units on U100 insulin syringe) if no nausea for 3–7 days. Give immediately before meal.

For type 1 patients, start at 15 mcg three times a day (2.5 units on U100 insulin syringe) and increase by increments of 15 mcg to a maximum of 60 mcg three times a day, as tolerated. | 2 hours |
| | | To avoid hypoglycemia, lower insulin dose by 50% on initiation of therapy. | |

AST/ALT, aspartate aminotransferase/alanine aminotransferase; eGFR, estimated glomerular filtration rate.

(2) Second-generation sulfonylureas (glyburide, glipizide, gliclazide, glimepiride)—Glyburide, glipizide, gliclazide, and glimepiride are 100–200 times more potent than tolbutamide. These medications should be used with caution in patients with cardiovascular disease or in elderly patients, in whom prolonged hypoglycemia would be especially dangerous.

The usual starting dose of **glyburide** is 2.5 mg/day, and the average maintenance dose is 5–10 mg/day given as a single morning dose; maintenance doses higher than 20 mg/day are not recommended. Some reports suggest that 10 mg is a maximum daily therapeutic dose, with 15–20 mg having no additional benefit in poor responders and doses over 20 mg actually worsening hyperglycemia.

A "Press Tab" formulation of "micronized" glyburide—easy to divide in half with slight pressure if necessary—is available. Glyburide is metabolized in the liver into products with hypoglycemic activity, which probably explains why assays specific for the unmetabolized compound suggest a plasma half-life of only 1–2 hours, yet the biologic effects of glyburide are clearly persistent 24 hours after a single morning dose in diabetic patients. Glyburide is unique among sulfonylureas in that it not only binds to the pancreatic B cell membrane sulfonylurea receptor but also becomes sequestered within the B cell. This may also contribute to its prolonged biologic effect despite its relatively short circulating half-life.

Glyburide has few adverse effects other than its potential for causing hypoglycemia, which at times can be prolonged. Flushing has rarely been reported after ethanol ingestion. It does not cause water retention, as chlorpropamide does, but rather slightly enhances free water clearance. Glyburide should not be used in patients with liver failure and chronic kidney disease because of the risk of hypoglycemia. Elderly patients are at particular risk for hypoglycemia even with relatively small daily doses.

The recommended starting dose of **glipizide** is 5 mg/day, with up to 15 mg/day given as a single daily dose before breakfast. When higher daily doses are required, they should be divided and given before meals. The maximum dose recommended by the manufacturer is 40 mg/d, although doses above 10–15 mg probably provide little additional benefit in poor responders and may even be *less* effective than smaller doses. For maximum effect in reducing postprandial hyperglycemia, glipizide should be ingested 30 minutes before meals, since rapid absorption is delayed when the medication is taken with food.

At least 90% of glipizide is metabolized in the liver to inactive products, and 10% is excreted unchanged in the urine. Glipizide therapy should therefore not be used in patients with liver failure. Because of its lower potency and shorter duration of action, it is preferable to glyburide in elderly patients and for those patients with kidney disease. Glucotrol-XL provides extended release of glipizide during transit through the gastrointestinal tract with greater effectiveness in lowering prebreakfast hyperglycemia than the shorter-duration immediate-release standard glipizide tablets. However, this formulation appears to have sacrificed its lower propensity for severe hypoglycemia compared with longer-acting glyburide without showing any demonstrable therapeutic advantages over glyburide.

Gliclazide (not available in the United States) is another intermediate duration sulfonylurea with a duration of action of about 12 hours. The recommended starting dose is 40–80 mg/day with a maximum dose of 320 mg. Doses of 160 mg and above are given as divided doses before breakfast and dinner. The medication is metabolized by the liver; the metabolites and conjugates have no hypoglycemic effect. An extended release preparation is available.

Glimepiride has a long duration of effect with a half-life of 5 hours allowing once or twice daily dosing. Glimepiride achieves blood glucose lowering with the lowest dose of any sulfonylurea compound. A single daily dose of 1 mg/day has been shown to be effective, and the maximal recommended dose is 8 mg. It is completely metabolized by the liver to relatively inactive metabolic products.

B. Meglitinide analogs—**Repaglinide** is structurally similar to glyburide but lacks the sulfonic acid-urea moiety. It acts by binding to the sulfonylurea receptor and closing the adenosine triphosphate (ATP)-sensitive potassium channel. It is rapidly absorbed from the intestine and then undergoes complete metabolism in the liver to inactive biliary products, giving it a plasma half-life of less than 1 hour. The medication therefore causes a brief but rapid pulse of insulin. The starting dose is 0.5 mg three times a day 15 minutes before each meal. The dose can be titrated to a maximum daily dose of 16 mg. Like the sulfonylureas, repaglinide can be used in combination with metformin. Hypoglycemia is the main side effect. In clinical trials, when the medication was compared with a long-duration sulfonylurea (glyburide), there was a trend toward less hypoglycemia. Like the sulfonylureas, repaglinide causes weight gain. Metabolism is by cytochrome P450 3A4 isoenzyme, and other medications that induce or inhibit this isoenzyme may increase or inhibit (respectively) the metabolism of repaglinide. The medication may be useful in patients with kidney impairment or in the elderly.

Mitiglinide is a benzylsuccinic acid derivative that binds to the sulfonylurea receptor and is similar to repaglinide in its clinical effects. It is approved for use in Japan.

C. d-Phenylalanine derivative—**Nateglinide** stimulates insulin secretion by binding to the sulfonylurea receptor and closing the ATP-sensitive potassium channel. This compound is rapidly absorbed from the intestine, reaching peak plasma levels within 1 hour. It is metabolized in the liver and has a plasma half-life of about 1.5 hours. Like repaglinide, it causes a brief rapid pulse of insulin, and when given before a meal it reduces the postprandial rise in blood glucose. For most patients, the recommended starting and maintenance dose is 120 mg three times a day before meals. Use 60 mg in patients who have mild elevations in HbA_{1c}. Like the other insulin secretagogues, its main side effects are hypoglycemia and weight gain.

2. Medications that primarily lower glucose levels by their actions on the liver, muscle, and adipose tissue—

A. Metformin—Metformin (1,1-dimethylbiguanide hydrochloride) is used, either alone or in conjunction with other oral agents or insulin, in the treatment of patients with type 2 diabetes.

Metformin's therapeutic effects primarily derive from the increasing hepatic adenosine monophosphate-activated protein kinase activity, which reduces hepatic gluconeogenesis and lipogenesis.

Metformin has a half-life of 1.5–3 hours, is not bound to plasma proteins or metabolized, being excreted unchanged by the kidneys.

Metformin is the first-line therapy for patients with type 2 diabetes. The current recommendation is to start this medication at diagnosis. A side benefit of metformin therapy is its tendency to improve both fasting and postprandial hyperglycemia and hypertriglyceridemia in obese patients with diabetes without the weight gain associated with insulin or sulfonylurea therapy. Metformin is ineffective in patients with type 1 diabetes. Patients with chronic kidney disease should not be given this medication because failure to excrete it would produce high blood and tissue levels of metformin that could stimulate lactic acid overproduction. In the United States, metformin use is not recommended at or above a serum creatinine level of 1.4 mg/dL in women and 1.5 mg/dL in men. In the United Kingdom, the recommendations are to review metformin use when the serum creatinine exceeds 130 mcmol/L (1.5 mg/dL) or the estimated glomerular filtration rate (eGFR) falls below 45 mL/min per 1.73 m². The medication should be stopped if the serum creatinine exceeds 150 mcmol/L (1.7mg/dL) or the eGFR is below 30 mL/min per 1.73 m². Patients with liver failure or persons with excessive alcohol intake should not receive this medication—lactic acid production from the gut and other tissues, which rises during metformin therapy, could result in lactic acidosis when defective hepatocytes cannot remove the lactate or when alcohol-induced reduction of nucleotides interferes with lactate clearance.

The maximum dosage of metformin is 2550 mg, although little benefit is seen above a total dose of 2000 mg. It is important to begin with a low dose and increase the dosage very gradually in divided doses—taken with meals—to reduce minor gastrointestinal upsets. A common schedule would be one 500 mg tablet three times a day with meals or one 850 mg or 1000 mg tablet twice daily at breakfast and dinner. Up to 2000 mg of the extended-release preparation can be given once a day. Lower doses should be used in patients with eGFRs between 30 and 45 mL/min per 1.73 m².

The most frequent side effects of metformin are gastrointestinal symptoms (anorexia, nausea, vomiting, abdominal discomfort, diarrhea), which occur in up to 20% of patients. These effects are dose-related, tend to occur at onset of therapy, and often are transient. However, in 3–5% of patients, therapy may have to be discontinued because of persistent diarrheal discomfort. In a retrospective analysis, it has been reported that patients switched from immediate-release metformin to comparable dose of extended-release metformin experienced fewer gastrointestinal side effects.

Hypoglycemia does not occur with therapeutic doses of metformin, which permits its description as a "euglycemic" or "antihyperglycemic" medication rather than an oral hypoglycemic agent. Dermatologic or hematologic toxicity is rare. Metformin interferes with the calcium dependent absorption of vitamin B_{12}-intrinsic complex in the terminal ileum; vitamin B_{12} deficiency can occur after many years of metformin use. Periodic screening with vitamin B_{12} levels should be considered, especially in patients with peripheral neuropathy or if a macrocytic anemia develops. Increased intake of dietary calcium may prevent the metformin-induced B_{12} malaborption.

Lactic acidosis has been reported as a side effect but is uncommon with metformin in contrast to phenformin. Almost all reported cases have involved persons with associated risk factors that should have contraindicated its use (kidney, liver, or cardiorespiratory insufficiency; alcoholism; advanced age). Acute kidney injury can occur rarely in certain patients receiving radiocontrast agents. Metformin therapy should therefore be temporarily halted on the day of radiocontrast administration and restarted a day or two later after confirmation that renal function has not deteriorated.

B. Thiazolidinediones—Two medications of this class, rosiglitazone and pioglitazone, are available for clinical use. These medications sensitize peripheral tissues to insulin. They bind a nuclear receptor called peroxisome proliferator-activated receptor gamma (PPAR-gamma) and affect the expression of a number of genes. Like the biguanides, this class of medications does not cause hypoglycemia.

Both rosiglitazone and pioglitazone are effective as monotherapy and in combination with sulfonylureas or metformin or insulin, lowering HbA_{1c} by 1–2%. When used in combination with insulin, they can result in a 30–50% reduction in insulin dosage, and some patients can come off insulin completely. The dosage of rosiglitazone is 4–8 mg daily and of pioglitazone, 15–45 mg daily, and the medications do not have to be taken with food. Rosiglitazone is primarily metabolized by the CYP 2C8 isoenzyme and pioglitazone is metabolized by CYP 2C8 and CYP 3A4.

The combination of a thiazolidinedione and metformin has the advantage of not causing hypoglycemia. Patients inadequately managed on sulfonylureas can do well on a combination of sulfonylurea and rosiglitazone or pioglitazone.

These medications have some additional effects apart from glucose lowering. Rosiglitazone therapy is associated with increases in total cholesterol, LDL cholesterol (15%), and HDL cholesterol (10%). There is a reduction in free fatty acids of about 8–15%. The changes in triglycerides were generally not different from placebo. Pioglitazone in clinical trials lowered triglycerides (9%) and increased HDL cholesterol (15%) but did not cause a consistent change in total cholesterol and LDL cholesterol levels. A prospective randomized comparison of the metabolic effects of pioglitazone and rosiglitazone showed similar effects on HbA_{1c} and weight gain. Pioglitazone-treated persons, however, had lower total cholesterol, LDL cholesterol, and triglycerides when compared with rosiglitazone-treated persons. Small prospective studies have demonstrated that treatment with these medications leads to improvements in the biochemical and histologic features of nonalcoholic fatty liver disease. The thiazolidinediones also may limit vascular smooth muscle proliferation after injury, and there are reports that pioglitazone can reduce neointimal proliferation after coronary stent placement. In one double-blind, placebo-controlled study, rosiglitazone was shown to be associated with a decrease in the ratio of urinary albumin to creatinine excretion.

Safety concerns and some troublesome side effects have emerged about this class of medications that significantly limit their use. A meta-analysis of 42 randomized clinical trials with rosiglitazone suggested that this medication increases the risk of angina pectoris or myocardial infarction. A meta-analysis of clinical trials with pioglitazone did not show similar findings. Although conclusive data were lacking, the European Medicines Agency suspended the use of rosiglitazone in Europe. In the United States, the FDA established a restricted distribution program. A subsequent large prospective clinical trial (the RECORD study) failed to confirm the meta-analysis finding and the restrictions were lifted in the United States. It is unlikely, however, that there is going to be a resurgence in its use and pioglitazone is likely to remain the preferred agent.

Edema occurs in about 3–4% of patients receiving monotherapy with rosiglitazone or pioglitazone. The edema occurs more frequently (10–15%) in patients receiving concomitant insulin therapy and may result in heart failure. The medications are contraindicated in diabetic individuals with New York Heart Association class III and IV cardiac status. Thiazolidinediones have also been reported as being associated with new onset or worsening macular edema. Apparently, this is a rare side effect, and most of these patients also had peripheral edema. The macular edema resolved or improved once the medication was discontinued.

An increase in fracture risk in women (but not men) has been reported with both rosiglitazone and pioglitazone. The fracture risk is in the range of 1.9 per 100 patient-years with the thiazolidinedione compared to 1.1 per 100 patient years on comparison treatment. In at least one study of rosiglitazone, the fracture risk was increased in premenopausal as well as postmenopausal women.

Other side effects include anemia, which occurs in 4% of patients treated with these medications; it may be due to a dilutional effect of increased plasma volume rather than a reduction in red cell mass. Weight gain occurs, especially when the medication is combined with a sulfonylurea or insulin. Some of the weight gain is fluid retention, but there is also an increase in total fat mass. Initial reports in male rats and humans raised concern about bladder tumors. A 10-year observational cohort study of patients taking pioglitazone, however, failed to find an association with bladder cancer. Reassuringly, a large multipopulation pooled analysis (1.01 million persons over 5.9 million person years) also failed to find an association between cumulative exposure of pioglitazone or rosiglitazone and incidence of bladder cancer.

Troglitazone, the first medication in this class to go into widespread clinical use, was withdrawn from clinical use because of medication-associated fatal liver failure. Although rosiglitazone and pioglitazone have not been reported to cause liver injury, the FDA recommends that they should not be used in patients with clinical evidence of active liver disease or pretreatment elevation of the alanine aminotransferase (ALT) level that is 2.5 times greater than the upper limit of normal. Liver biochemical tests should be performed prior to initiation of treatment and periodically thereafter.

3. Medications that affect absorption of glucose—Alpha-glucosidase inhibitors competitively inhibit the alpha-glucosidase enzymes in the gut that digest dietary starch and sucrose. Two of these medications—acarbose and miglitol—are available for clinical use in the United States. Voglibose, another alpha-glucosidase inhibitor is available in Japan, Korea, and India. Acarbose and miglitol are potent inhibitors of glucoamylase, alpha-amylase, and

sucrase but have less effect on isomaltase and hardly any on trehalase and lactase. Acarbose binds 1000 times more avidly to the intestinal disaccharidases than do products of carbohydrate digestion or sucrose. A fundamental difference between acarbose and miglitol is in their absorption. Acarbose has the molecular mass and structural features of a tetrasaccharide, and very little (about 2%) crosses the microvillar membrane. Miglitol, however, has a structural similarity with glucose and is absorbable. Both medications delay the absorption of carbohydrate and lower postprandial glycemic excursion.

A. Acarbose—The recommended starting dose of acarbose is 50 mg twice daily, gradually increasing to 100 mg three times daily. For maximal benefit on postprandial hyperglycemia, acarbose should be given with the first mouthful of food ingested. In diabetic patients, it reduces postprandial hyperglycemia by 30–50%, and its overall effect is to lower the HbA_{1c} by 0.5–1%.

The principal adverse effect, seen in 20–30% of patients, is flatulence. This is caused by undigested carbohydrate reaching the lower bowel, where gases are produced by bacterial flora. In 3% of cases, troublesome diarrhea occurs. This gastrointestinal discomfort tends to discourage excessive carbohydrate consumption and promotes improved compliance of type 2 patients with their diet prescriptions. When acarbose is given alone, there is no risk of hypoglycemia. However, if combined with insulin or sulfonylureas, it might increase the risk of hypoglycemia from these agents. A slight rise in hepatic aminotransferases has been noted in clinical trials with acarbose (5% versus 2% in placebo controls, and particularly with doses greater than 300 mg/day). The levels generally return to normal on stopping the medication.

B. Miglitol—Miglitol is similar to acarbose in terms of its clinical effects. It is indicated for use in diet- or sulfonylurea-treated patients with type 2 diabetes. Therapy is initiated at the lowest effective dosage of 25 mg three times a day. The usual maintenance dose is 50 mg three times a day, although some patients may benefit from increasing the dose to 100 mg three times a day. Gastrointestinal side effects occur as with acarbose. The medication is not metabolized and is excreted unchanged by the kidney. Miglitol should not be used in end-stage chronic kidney disease, when its clearance would be impaired.

4. Incretins—Oral glucose provokes a threefold to fourfold higher insulin response than an equivalent dose of glucose given intravenously. This is because the oral glucose causes a release of gut hormones, principally glucagon-like peptide 1 (GLP-1) and glucose-dependent insulinotropic polypeptide (GIP1), that amplify the glucose-induced insulin release. This "incretin effect" of GLP-1 secretion (but not GIP1 secretion) is reduced in patients with type 2 diabetes and when GLP-1 is infused in patients with type 2 diabetes, it stimulates insulin secretion and lowers glucose levels. GLP-1, unlike the sulfonylureas, has only a modest insulin stimulatory effect at normoglycemic concentrations. This means that GLP-1 has a lower risk for hypoglycemia than the sulfonylureas.

In addition to its insulin stimulatory effect, GLP-1 also has a number of other pancreatic and extrapancreatic effects. It suppresses glucagon secretion and so may ameliorate the hyperglucagonemia that is present in people with diabetes and improve postprandial hyperglycemia. GLP-1 acts on the stomach delaying gastric emptying; the importance of this effect on glucose lowering is illustrated by the observation that antagonizing the deceleration of gastric emptying markedly reduces the glucose lowering effect of GLP-1. GLP-1 receptors are present in the central nervous system and may play a role in the anorectic effect of the drugs. Type 2 diabetic patients undergoing GLP-1 infusion are less hungry; it is unclear whether this is mainly due to a deceleration of gastric emptying or whether there is a central nervous system effect as well.

A. GLP-1 RECEPTOR AGONISTS—GLP-1 is rapidly proteolyzed by dipeptidyl peptidase 4 (DPP-4) and by other enzymes, such as endopeptidase 24.11, and is also cleared rapidly by the kidney. As a result, GLP-1's half-life is only 1–2 minutes. The native peptide, therefore, cannot be used therapeutically and the approach taken has been to develop metabolically stable analogs or derivatives of GLP-1 that are not subject to the same enzymatic degradation or renal clearance. Four GLP-1 receptor agonists, exenatide, liraglutide, albiglutide, and dulaglutide are available for clinical use.

Exenatide (Exendin 4) is a GLP-1 receptor agonist isolated from the saliva of the Gila monster (a venomous lizard) that is more resistant to DPP-4 action and cleared by the kidney. Its half-life is 2.4 hours, and its glucose lowering effect is about 6 hours. Exenatide is dispensed as two fixed-dose pens (5 mcg and 10 mcg). It is injected 60 minutes before breakfast and before dinner. Patients with type 2 diabetes should be prescribed the 5 mcg pen for the first month and, if tolerated, the dose can then be increased to 10 mcg twice a day. The medication is not recommended in patients with GFR less than 30 mL/min. In clinical trials, adding exenatide therapy to patients with type 2 diabetes already taking metformin or a sulfonylurea, or both, further lowered the HbA$_{1c}$ value by 0.4% to 0.6% over a 30-week period. These patients also experienced a weight loss of 3–6 pounds. Exenatide LAR is a once weekly preparation that is dispensed as a powder (2 mg). It is suspended in the provided diluent just prior to injection. In comparative clinical trials, the long-acting drug lowers the HbA$_{1c}$ level a little more than the twice daily drug. Low-titer antibodies against exenatide develop in over one-third (38%) of patients, but the clinical effects are not attenuated. High-titer antibodies develop in a subset of patients (~6%), and in about half of these cases, an attenuation of glycemic response has been seen.

Liraglutide is a soluble fatty acid acylated GLP-1 analog (with replacement of lysine with arginine at position 34 and the attachment of a C16 acyl chain to a lysine at position 26). The fatty-acyl GLP-1 retains affinity for GLP-1 receptors but the addition of the C16 acyl chain allows for noncovalent binding to albumin, both hindering DPP-4 access to the molecule and contributing to a prolonged half-life and duration of action. The half-life is approximately 12 hours, allowing the medication to be injected once a day. The dosing is initiated at 0.6 mg daily, increased

after 1 week to 1.2 mg daily. Some patients may benefit from increasing the dose to 1.8 mg. In clinical trials lasting 26 and 52 weeks, adding liraglutide to the therapeutic regimen (metformin, sulfonylurea, thiazolidinedione) of patients with type 2 diabetes further lowered the HbA$_{1c}$ value. Depending on the dose and design of the study, the HbA$_{1c}$ decline was in the range of 0.6% to 1.5%. The patients had sustained weight loss of 1–6 pounds. Liraglutide at a dose of 3 mg daily has been approved for weight loss.

Albiglutide is a human GLP-1 dimer fused to human albumin. It is rendered resistant to DPP-4 action by a glycine substitution for alanine at position 8. The half-life of albiglutide is about 5 days and a steady state is reached after 4–5 weeks of once weekly administration. The usual dose is 30 mg weekly by subcutaneous injection. The dose can be increased to 50 mg weekly if necessary. The pen contains a lyophilized powder that is reconstituted just prior to administration. Albiglutide monotherapy and combination therapy lowers HbA$_{1c}$ by about 0.8%. Weight loss is much less than with exenatide and liraglutide.

Dulaglutide consists of two GLP-1 analog molecules covalently linked to an Fc fragment of human IgG$_4$. The GLP-1 molecule has amino acid substitutions that resist DPP-4 action. The half-life of dulaglutide is about 5 days. The usual dose is 0.75 mg weekly by subcutaneous injection. The maximum recommended dose is 1.5 mg weekly. Dulaglutide monotherapy and combination therapy lowers HbA$_{1c}$ by about 0.7% to 1.6%. Weight loss ranged from 2 pounds to 7 pounds.

The most frequent adverse reactions of the GLP1 receptor agonists are nausea (11–40%), vomiting (4–13%), and diarrhea (9–17%). The reactions are more frequent at the higher doses. Albiglutide tends to have the lowest rates of these reactions. In clinical trials about 1–5% of participants withdrew from the studies because of the gastrointestinal symptoms.

All the GLP-1 receptor agonists are associated with increased risk of pancreatitis. The FDA reported 30 postmarketing reports of acute pancreatitis in patients taking exenatide. The pancreatitis was severe (hemorrhagic or necrotizing) in 6 instances, and 2 of these patients died. In the liraglutide, albiglutide, and dulaglutide clinical trials, there were 13, 6, and 5 cases of pancreatitis in the drug-treated groups versus 1, 2, and 1 case(s) in the comparator groups, respectively. This translates to about 1.4–2.2 vs 0.6–0.9 cases of pancreatitis per 1000 patient years. Patients taking GLP-1 receptor agonists should be advised to seek immediate medical care if they experience unexplained persistent severe abdominal pain.

There have been rare reports of acute kidney injury in patients taking exenatide. Some of these patients had pre-existing kidney disease, and others had one or more risk factors for kidney disease. A number of the patients reported nausea, vomiting, and diarrhea, and it is possible that these side effects caused volume depletion and contributed to the development of the kidney injury. For this reason, the GLP-1 receptors agonists should be prescribed cautiously in patients with kidney impairment.

GLP-1 receptor agonists stimulate C-cell neoplasia and cause medullary thyroid carcinoma in rats. Human C-cells express very few GLP1-receptors, and the relevance to human therapy is unclear. The medications, however, should not be used in patients with personal or family history of medullary thyroid carcinoma or multiple endocrine neoplasia (MEN) syndrome type 2.

B. DPP-4 INHIBITORS—An alternate approach to the use of GLP-1 receptor agonists is to inhibit the enzyme DPP-4 and prolong the action of endogenously released GLP-1 and GIP. Four oral DPP-4 inhibitors, sitagliptin, saxagliptin, linagliptin, and alogliptin, are available in the United States for the treatment of type 2 diabetes. An additional DPP-4 inhibitor, vildagliptin, is available in Europe.

Sitagliptin, when used in clinical trials alone and in combination with metformin and pioglitazone, improved HbA_{1c} from 0.5% to 1.4%. The usual dose of sitagliptin is 100 mg once daily, but the dose is reduced to 50 mg daily if the calculated creatinine clearance is 30–50 mL/min and to 25 mg for clearances less than 30 mL/min. Unlike exenatide, sitagliptin does not cause nausea or vomiting. It also does not result in weight loss. The main adverse effect appears to be a predisposition to nasopharyngitis or upper respiratory tract infection. A small increase in neutrophil count of ~200 cells/mcL has also occurred. Since its FDA approval and clinical use, there have been reports of serious allergic reactions to sitagliptin, including anaphylaxis, angioedema, and exfoliative skin conditions including Stevens-Johnson syndrome. There have also been reports of pancreatitis (88 cases including 2 cases of hemorrhagic or necrotizing pancreatitis). The frequency of these events is unclear.

Saxagliptin, when added to the therapeutic regimen (metformin, sulfonylurea, thiazolidinedione) of patients with type 2 diabetes, further lowered the HbA_{1c} value by about 0.7–0.9%. The dose is 2.5 mg or 5 mg orally once a day. The 2.5-mg dose should be used in patients with calculated creatinine clearance less than 50 mL/min. It lowers HbA_{1c} by about 0.6% when added to metformin or glyburide or thiazolidine in various 24-week clinical trials. The medication does not cause weight gain or loss. The main adverse reactions were upper respiratory tract infection, nasopharyngitis, headache, and urinary tract infection. There is also small reversible dose-dependent reduction in absolute lymphocyte count, which remains within normal limits. Hypersensitivity reactions, such as urticaria and facial edema, occurred in 1.5% of patients taking the medication compared with 0.4% receiving placebo. The metabolism of saxagliptin is by CYP3A4/5; thus, strong inhibitors or inducers of CYP3A4/5 will affect the pharmacokinetics of saxagliptin and its active metabolite. Saxagliptin may increase the risk of heart failure. In a post marketing study of 16,492 type 2 diabetes patients, there were 289 cases of heart failure in the saxagliptin group (3.5%) and 228 cases in the placebo group (2.8%)—a hazard ratio of 1.27. Patients at the highest risk for failure were those who had a history of heart failure or had elevated levels of N-terminal of the prohormone brain natriuretic peptide (NT-pBNP) or had kidney impairment.

Alogliptin lowers HbA_{1c} by about 0.5–0.6% when added to metformin, sulfonylurea, or pioglitazone. The usual dose is 25 mg orally daily. The 12.5-mg dose is used in patients with calculated creatinine clearance of 30 to 60 mLs/min; and 6.25 mg for clearance less than 30 mL/min. In clinical trials, pancreatitis occurred in 11 of 5902 patients on alogliptin (0.2%) and in 5 of 5183 patients receiving all comparators (<0.1%). There have been reports of hypersensitivity reactions (anaphylaxis, angioedema, Stevens-Johnson syndrome). Cases of hepatic failure have been reported but it is unclear if alogliptin was the cause. The medication, however, should be discontinued in the event of liver failure.

In a large post-marketing study, alogliptin, like saxagliptin, was associated with a slightly increased rate of heart failure.

Linagliptin lowers HbA_{1c} by about 0.4–0.6% when added to metformin, sulfonylurea, or pioglitazone. The dose is 5 mg orally daily, and, since it is primarily excreted unmetabolized via the bile, no dose adjustment is needed in patients with renal failure. The adverse reactions include nasopharyngitis and hypersensitivity reactions (urticaria, angioedema, localized skin exfoliation, bronchial hyperreactivity). In one study, there were eight cases of pancreatitis in 4687 patients exposed to drug (4311 patient years) with 0 cases in 1183 patients receiving placebo (433 patient years).

Vildagliptin lowers HbA_{1c} by about 0.5–1% when added to the therapeutic regimen of patients with type 2 diabetes. The dose is 50 mg once or twice daily. Adverse reactions include upper respiratory tract infections, nasopharyngitis, dizziness, and headache. Rare cases of hepatic dysfunction, including hepatitis, have been reported. Liver function testing is recommended quarterly during the first year of use and periodically thereafter.

5. Sodium-glucose co-transporter 2 inhibitors—Glucose is freely filtered by the renal glomeruli and is reabsorbed in the proximal tubules by the action of sodium-glucose co-transporters (SGLT). Sodium-glucose co-transporter 2 (SGLT2) accounts for about 90% of glucose reabsorption and its inhibition causes glycosuria in people with diabetes, lowering plasma glucose levels. The SGLT2 inhibitors canagliflozin, dapagliflozin, and empagliflozin are approved for clinical use in the United States.

Canagliflozin reduces the threshold for glycosuria from a plasma glucose threshold of ~180 mg/dL to 70–90 mg/dL. It has been shown to reduce HbA_{1c} by 0.6–1% when used alone or in combination with other oral agents or insulin. It also results in modest weight loss of 2–5 kg. The usual dose is 100 mg daily but up to 300 mg daily can be used in patients with normal kidney function.

Dapagliflozin is an SGLT2 inhibitor that has been shown to reduce HbA_{1c} levels by 0.5–0.8% when used alone or in combination with other oral agents or insulin. It also results in modest weight loss of about 2–4 kg. The usual dose is 10 mg daily but 5 mg daily is the recommended initial dose in patients with hepatic failure.

Empagliflozin reduces HbA_{1c} by 0.5–0.7% when used alone or in combination with other oral agents or insulin. It also results in modest weight loss of about 2–3 kg. The usual dosage is 10 mg daily but a higher dose of 25 mg daily can be used. In a postmarketing multinational study of

7020 patients with type 2 diabetes with known cardiovascular disease, the addition of empagliflozin was associated with a lower primary composite outcome of death from cardiovascular causes, nonfatal myocardial infarction, or nonfatal stroke (hazard ratio 0.86, $P = 0.04$). The mechanisms regarding the benefit remain unclear. Weight loss, lower blood pressure, and diuresis may have played a role since there were fewer deaths from heart failure in the treated group whereas the rates of myocardial infarction were unaltered. Additional studies with empagliflozin and other SGLT2 inhibitors are needed to confirm this result.

As might be expected, the efficacy of the SGLT2 inhibitors is reduced in chronic kidney disease. They can also increase creatinine and decrease eGFR, especially in patients with kidney impairment. Canagliflozin is contraindicated in patients with eGFR less than 45 mL/min/1.73 m². The main side effects are increased incidence of genital mycotic infections and urinary tract infections affecting ~8–9% of patients. There have also been reports of cases of pyelonephritis and septicemia requiring hospitalization. The glycosuria can cause intravascular volume contraction and hypotension.

Canagliflozin has been reported to cause a decrease in bone mineral density at the lumbar spine and the hip. In a pooled analysis of eight clinical trials (mean duration 68 weeks), a 30% increase in fractures was observed in patients taking canagliflozin. It is likely that the effect on the bones is a class effect and not restricted to canagliflozin. All the SGLT2 inhibitors cause a modest increase in LDL cholesterol levels (3–8%). Also, in clinical trials, patients taking dapagliflozin had higher rates of breast cancer (nine cases vs none in comparator arms) and bladder cancer (10 cases vs 1 in placebo arm). These cancer rates exceeded the expected rates in age-matched reference diabetes population.

Cases of diabetic ketoacidosis have been reported with off-label use of SGLT2 inhibitors in patients with type 1 diabetes. Type 1 patients are taught to give less insulin if their glucose levels are not elevated. SGLT2 inhibitors lower glucose levels by changing the renal threshold and not by insulin action. Type 1 patients taking an SGLT2 inhibitor, because the glucose levels are not elevated, may either withhold or reduce their insulin doses to such a degree as to induce ketoacidoisis. SGLT2 inhibitors should not be used in patients with type 1 diabetes and in those patients labelled as having type 2 diabetes but who are very insulin deficient and ketosis-prone.

6. Others—Pramlintide is a synthetic analog of islet amyloid polypeptide (IAPP or amylin). When given subcutaneously, it delays gastric emptying, suppresses glucagon secretion, and decreases appetite. It is approved for use both in type 1 diabetes and in insulin-treated type 2 diabetes. In 6-month clinical studies with type 1 and insulin-treated type 2 patients, those taking the medication had an approximately 0.4% reduction in HbA$_{1c}$ and about 1.7 kg weight loss compared with placebo. The HbA$_{1c}$ reduction was sustained for 2 years but some of the weight was regained. The medication is given by injection immediately before the meal. Hypoglycemia can occur, and it is recommended that the short-acting or premixed insulin doses be reduced by 50% when the medication is started. Since the medication slows gastric emptying, recovery from hypoglycemia can be a problem because of delay in absorption of fast-acting carbohydrates. Nausea was the other main side effect, affecting 30–50% of persons but tended to improve with time. In patients with type 1 diabetes, the initial dose of pramlintide is 15 mcg before each meal and titrated up by 15 mcg increments to a maintenance dose of 30 mcg or 60 mcg before each meal. In patients with type 2 diabetes, the starting dose is 60 mcg premeals increased to 120 mcg in 3 to 7 days if no significant nausea occurs.

Bromocriptine, a dopamine 2 receptor agonist, has been shown to modestly lower HbA$_{1c}$ by 0.1 0.5% when compared to baseline and 0.4–0.5% compared to placebo. The tablet dose is 0.8 mg and the daily dose is 2 (1.6 g) to 6 (4.8 mg) tablets as tolerated. Common side effects are nausea, vomiting, dizziness, and headache.

Colesevelam, the bile acid sequesterant, when added to metformin or sulfonylurea or insulin lowered HbA$_{1c}$ 0.3–0.4 % when compared to baseline and 0.5–0.6% compared to placebo. HbA$_{1c}$ lowering, however, was not observed in a single monotherapy clinical trial comparing colesevelam to placebo. Colesevelam use is associated with ~20% increase in triglyceride levels. Other adverse effects include constipation and dyspepsia.

With their modest glucose lowering and significant side effects, using bromocriptine or colesevelam to treat diabetes is not recommended.

7. Medication combinations—Several medication combinations are available in different dose sizes, including glyburide and metformin (Glucovance); glipizide and metformin (Metaglip); repaglinide and metformin (PrandiMet); rosiglitazone and metformin (Avandamet); pioglitazone and metformin (ACTOplusMet); rosiglitazone and glimepiride (Avandaryl); pioglitazone and glimepiride (Duetact); sitagliptin and metformin (Janumet); saxagliptin and metformin XR (Kombiglyze XR); linagliptin and metformin (Jentadueto); alogliptin and metformin (Kazano); alogliptin and pioglitazone (Oseni); dapagliflozin and metformin (Xigduo); canagliflozin and metformin (Invokamet); empagliflozin and metformin (Synjardy); and empagliflozin and linagliptin (Glyxambi). These medication combinations, however, limit the clinician's ability to optimally adjust dosage of the individual medications and for that reason are not recommended.

8. Safety of the antihyperglycemic agents—The UKPDS has put to rest previous concerns regarding the safety of sulfonylureas. It did not confirm any cardiovascular hazard among over 1500 patients treated intensively with sulfonylureas for over 10 years, compared with a comparable number who received either insulin or diet therapy. Analysis of a subgroup of obese patients receiving metformin also showed no hazard and even a slight reduction in cardiovascular deaths compared with conventional therapy.

C. Insulin

Insulin is indicated for type 1 diabetes as well as for type 2 diabetic patients with insulinopenia whose hyperglycemia does not respond to diet therapy either alone or combined with other hypoglycemic medications.

Table 27–6. Summary of bioavailability characteristics of the insulins.

Insulin Preparations	Onset of Action	Peak Action	Effective Duration
Insulins lispro, aspart, glulisine	5–15 minutes	1–1.5 hours	3–4 hours
Human regular	30–60 minutes	2 hours	6–8 hours
Human NPH	2–4 hours	6–7 hours	10–20 hours
Insulin glargine	0.5–1 hour	Flat	~24 hours
Insulin detemir	0.5–1 hour	Flat	17 hours
Insulin degludec	0.5–1.5 hours	Flat	More than 42 hours
Technosphere inhaled insulin	5–15 minutes	1 hour	3 hours

1. Characteristics of available insulin preparations— Commercial insulin preparations differ with respect to the time of onset and duration of their biologic action (Table 27–6).

Human insulin is dispensed as either regular (R) or NPH (N) formulations. Six analogs of human insulin— three rapidly acting (insulin lispro, insulin aspart, insulin glulisine) and three long-acting (insulin glargine, insulin detemir, and insulin degludec)—are approved by the FDA for clinical use (Table 27–7). Animal insulins are no longer available in the United States. All currently available insulins contain less than 10 ppm of proinsulin and are labeled as "purified." These purified insulins preserve their potency, so that refrigeration is recommended but not crucial.

Table 27–7. Insulin preparations available in the United States.[1]

Rapidly acting human insulin analogs
Insulin lispro (Humalog, Lilly)
Insulin aspart (Novolog, Novo Nordisk)
Insulin glulisine (Apidra, Sanofi Aventis)
Short-acting regular insulin
Regular insulin (Lilly, Novo Nordisk)
Technosphere inhaled regular insulin (Afrezza)
Intermediate-acting insulins
NPH insulin (Lilly, Novo Nordisk)
Premixed insulins
70% NPH/30% regular (70/30 insulin—Lilly, Novo Nordisk)
70% NPL/25% insulin lispro (Humalog Mix 75/25—Lilly)
50% NPL/50% insulin lispro (Humalog Mix 50/50—Lilly)
70% insulin aspart protamine/30% insulin aspart (Novolog Mix 70/30—Novo Nordisk)
70% insulin degludec/30 insulin aspart (Ryzodeg, Novo Nordisk)
Long-acting human insulin analogs
Insulin glargine (Lantus (U100), Toujeo (U300), Sanofi Aventis; Basaglar (U100), Lilly)
Insulin detemir (Levemir, Novo Nordisk)
Insulin degludec (Tresiba, Novo Nordisk)

[1]All insulins available in the United States are recombinant human or human insulin analog origin. All the above insulins are dispensed at U100 concentration. There is an additional U500 preparation of regular insulin; U300 preparation of insulin glargine; U200 preparation of insulin lispro; U200 preparation of insulin degludec. NPH, neutral protamine Hagedorn.

During travel, reserve supplies of insulin can be readily transported for weeks without losing potency if protected from extremes of heat or cold. All the insulins in the United States are available in a concentration of 100 units/ mL (U100) and dispensed in 10 mL vials or 0.3 mL cartridges or prefilled disposable pens. Several insulins are available at higher concentrations: insulin glargine, 300 units/mL (U300); insulin degludec, 200 units/mL (U200); insulin lispro, 200 units/mL (U200); and regular insulin, 500 units/mL (U500).

2. Insulin preparations—The short-acting preparations are regular insulin and the rapidly acting insulin analogs (Table 27–7). They are dispensed as clear solutions at neutral pH and contain small amounts of zinc to improve their stability and shelf life. The long-acting preparations are NPH insulin and the long-acting insulin analogs. NPH insulin is dispensed as a turbid suspension at neutral pH with protamine in phosphate buffer. The long-acting insulin analogs are also dispensed as clear solutions; insulin glargine is at acidic pH and insulin detemir is at neutral pH. The rapidly acting insulin analogs and the long-acting insulins are designed for subcutaneous administration, while regular insulin can also be given intravenously.

A. Short-Acting Insulin Preparations—

*(1) Regular insulin—*Regular insulin is a short-acting soluble crystalline zinc insulin whose effect appears within 30 minutes after subcutaneous injection and lasts 5–7 hours when usual quantities are administered. Intravenous infusions of regular insulin are particularly useful in the treatment of diabetic ketoacidosis and during the perioperative management of patients with diabetes who require insulin. Regular insulin is indicated when the subcutaneous insulin requirement is changing rapidly, such as after surgery or during acute infections—although the rapidly acting insulin analogs may be preferable in these situations.

For markedly insulin-resistant persons who would otherwise require large volumes of insulin solution, a U500 preparation of human regular insulin is available in a 10 mL vial. Since a U500 syringe is not available, when U500 insulin is required in cases of severe insulin resistance, a U100 insulin syringe or tuberculin syringe must be used to measure doses. The clinician should carefully note dosages in both units and volume to avoid overdosage. The U500 preparation is much more expensive and is rarely needed.

(2) Rapidly acting insulin analogs—Insulin lispro (Humalog), is an insulin analog where the proline at position B28 is reversed with the lysine at B29. Insulin aspart (Novolog), is a single substitution of proline by aspartic acid at position B28. In insulin glulisine (Apidra) the asparagine at position B3 is replaced by lysine and the lysine in position B29 by glutamic acid. These three analogs have less of a tendency to form hexamers, in contrast to human insulin. When injected subcutaneously, the analogs quickly dissociate into monomers and are absorbed very rapidly, reaching peak serum values in as soon as 1 hour—in contrast to regular human insulin, whose hexamers require considerably more time to dissociate and become absorbed. The amino acid changes in these analogs do not interfere with their binding to the insulin receptor, with the circulating half-life, or with their immunogenicity, which are all identical with those of human regular insulin.

Clinical trials have demonstrated that the optimal times of preprandial subcutaneous injection of comparable doses of the rapidly acting insulin analogs and of regular human insulin are 20 minutes and 60 minutes, respectively, before the meal. While this more rapid onset of action has been welcomed as a great convenience by diabetic patients who object to waiting as long as 60 minutes after injecting regular human insulin before they can begin their meal, patients must be taught to ingest adequate absorbable carbohydrate early in the meal to avoid hypoglycemia during the meal. Another desirable feature of rapidly acting insulin analogs is that their duration of action remains at about 4 hours irrespective of dosage. This contrasts with regular insulin, whose duration of action is prolonged when larger doses are used.

The rapidly acting analogs are also commonly used in pumps. In a double-blind crossover study comparing insulin lispro with regular insulin in insulin pumps, persons using insulin lispro had lower HbA_{1c} values and improved postprandial glucose control with the same frequency of hypoglycemia. In the event of pump failure, however, users of the rapidly acting insulin analogs will have more rapid onset of hyperglycemia and ketosis.

While insulin aspart has been approved for intravenous use (eg, in hyperglycemic emergencies), there is no advantage in using insulin aspart over regular insulin by this route. A U200 concentration of insulin lispro is available in a disposable prefilled pen. The only advantage of the U200 over the U100 insulin lispro preparation is that it delivers the same dose in half the volume.

B. Long-acting insulin preparations—

(1) NPH (neutral protamine Hagedorn or isophane) insulin—NPH is an intermediate-acting insulin whose onset of action is delayed by combining 2 parts soluble crystalline zinc insulin with 1 part protamine zinc insulin. This produces equivalent amounts of insulin and protamine, so that neither is present in an uncomplexed form ("isophane").

Its onset of action is delayed to 2–4 hours, and its peak response is generally reached in about 6–7 hours. Because its duration of action is often less than 24 hours (with a range of 10–20 hours), most patients require at least two injections daily to maintain a sustained insulin effect.

(2) Insulin glargine—In this insulin, the asparagine at position 21 of the insulin A chain is replaced by glycine and two arginines are added to the carboxyl terminal of the B chain. The arginines raise the isoelectric point of the molecule closer to neutral making it more soluble in an acidic environment. In contrast, human insulin has an isoelectric point of pH 5.4. Insulin glargine is a clear insulin, which, when injected into the neutral pH environment of the subcutaneous tissue, forms microprecipitates that slowly release the insulin into the circulation. It lasts for about 24 hours without any pronounced peaks and is given once a day to provide basal coverage. This insulin cannot be mixed with the other human insulins because of its acidic pH. When this insulin was given as a single injection at bedtime to type 1 patients in clinical trials, fasting hyperglycemia was better controlled with less nocturnal hypoglycemia when compared to NPH insulin.

A more concentrated form of insulin glargine (U300) is available as an insulin pen. In pharmacodynamic studies in type 1 patients, the U300 compared to the U100 preparation had approximately 5 hours longer duration of action. In clinical trials in type 1 patients, U300 use did not result in better control or reduce the rates of hypoglycemia. Although limited clinical data suggest that insulin glargine is safe in pregnancy, it is not approved for this use.

(3) Insulin detemir—In this insulin analog, the threonine at position B30 has been removed and a 14-C fatty acid chain (tetradecanoic acid) is attached to the lysine at position 29 by acylation. Its prolonged action is due to dihexamerization and binding of hexamers and dimers to albumin at the injection site as well as binding of the monomer via its fatty acid side chain to albumin in the circulation. The affinity of insulin detemir is fourfold to fivefold lower than that of human soluble insulin and therefore the U100 formulation of insulin detemir has an insulin concentration of 2400 nmol/mL compared with 600 nmol/mL for NPH. The duration of action for insulin detemir is about 17 hours at therapeutically relevant doses. It is recommended that the insulin be injected once or twice a day to achieve a stable basal coverage. It has been approved for use during pregnancy.

(4) Insulin degludec—In this insulin analog, the threonine at position B30 has been removed, and the lysine at position B29 is conjugated to hexdecanoic acid via a gamma-L-glutamyl spacer. In the vial, in the presence of phenol and zinc, the insulin is in the form of dihexamers but when injected subcutaneously, it self associates into large multihexameric chains consisting of thousands of dihexamers. The chains slowly dissolve in the subcutaneous tissue and insulin monomers are steadily released into the systemic circulation. The half-life of the insulin is 25 hours. Its onset of action is in 30–90 minutes and its duration of action is more than 42 hours. It is recommended that the insulin be injected once or twice a day to achieve a stable basal coverage. Insulin degludec is available in two concentrations, U100 and U200, and dispensed in prefilled disposable pens.

C. Mixed insulin preparations—Patients with type 2 diabetes can sometimes achieve reasonable glucose control with just pre-breakfast and pre-supper injections of mixtures of short acting and NPH insulins. The regular insulin or rapidly acting insulin analog is withdrawn first, then the NPH insulin and then injected immediately. Stable premixed insulins (70% NPH and 30% regular) are available as a convenience to patients who have difficulty mixing insulin because of visual problems or impairment of manual dexterity. Premixed preparations of insulin lispro and NPH insulins are unstable. In an attempt to remedy this, an intermediate insulin composed of isophane complexes of protamine with insulin lispro was developed called NPL (neutral protamine lispro). This insulin has the same duration of action as NPH insulin. Premixed combinations of NPL and insulin lispro (75% NPL/25% insulin lispro mixture [Humalog Mix 75/25] and 50% NPL/50% insulin lispro mixture [Humalog Mix 50/50]) are available for clinical use. Similarly, a 70% insulin aspart protamine/30% insulin aspart (NovoLog Mix 70/30) is available. The main advantages of these mixtures are that they can be given within 15 minutes of starting a meal and they are superior in controlling the postprandial glucose rise after a carbohydrate rich meal. These benefits have not translated into improvements in HbA_{1c} levels when compared with the usual 70% NPH/30% regular mixture. The longer-acting insulin analogs, insulin glargine and insulin detemir, cannot be mixed with either regular insulin or the rapidly acting insulin analogs. Insulin degludec, however, can be mixed and is available as 70% insulin degludec/30% insulin aspart and is injected once or twice a day.

3. Methods of insulin administration—

A. INSULIN SYRINGES AND NEEDLES—Plastic disposable syringes are available in 1 mL, 0.5 mL, and 0.3 mL sizes. The "low-dose" 0.3 mL syringes are popular, because many patients with diabetes do not take more than 30 units of insulin in a single injection except in rare instances of extreme insulin resistance. Three lengths of needles are available: 6 mm, 8 mm, and 12.7 mm. Long needles are preferable in obese patients to reduce variability of insulin absorption. The needles are of 28, 30, and 31 gauges. The 31 gauge needles are almost painless. "Disposable" syringes may be reused until blunting of the needle occurs (usually after three to five injections). Sterility adequate to avoid infection with reuse appears to be maintained by recapping syringes between uses. Cleansing the needle with alcohol may not be desirable since it can dissolve the silicone coating and can increase the pain of skin puncturing.

Any part of the body covered by loose skin can be used, such as the abdomen, thighs, upper arms, flanks, and upper buttocks. Preparation with alcohol is not required prior to injection as long as the skin is clean. Rotation of sites is recommended to avoid delayed absorption when fibrosis or lipohypertrophy occurs from repeated use of a single site. However, considerable variability of absorption rates from different sites, particularly with exercise, may contribute to the instability of glycemic control in certain type 1 patients if injection sites are rotated too frequently in different areas of the body. Consequently, it is best to limit injection sites to a single region of the body and rotate sites within that region. The abdomen is recommended for subcutaneous injections, since regular insulin has been shown to absorb more rapidly from there than from other subcutaneous sites. The effect of anatomic regions appears to be much less pronounced with the analog insulins.

B. INSULIN PEN INJECTOR DEVICES—Insulin pens eliminate the need for carrying insulin vials and syringes. Cartridges of insulin lispro and insulin aspart are available for reusable pens (Eli Lilly, Novo Nordisk, and Owen Mumford). Disposable prefilled pens are also available for insulin lispro, insulin aspart, insulin glulisine, insulin detemir, insulin glargine, insulin degludec, NPH, 70% NPH/30% regular, 75% NPL/25% insulin lispro, 50% NPL/50% insulin lispro, 70% insulin aspart protamine/30% insulin aspart, and 70% insulin degludec/30% insulin aspart. Pen needles are available in 29, 31, and 32 gauges and 4, 5, 6, 8, and 12.7 mm lengths (Novofine; BD).

C. INSULIN PUMPS—In the United States, Medtronic MiniMed, Animas, Insulet, Roche, and Tandem make battery operated continuous subcutaneous insulin infusion (CSII) pumps. These pumps are small (about the size of a pager) and very easy to program. They offer many features, including the ability to set a number of different basal rates throughout the 24 hours and to adjust the time over which bolus doses are given. They also are able to detect pressure build-up if the catheter is kinked. The catheter connecting the insulin reservoir to the subcutaneous cannula can be disconnected, allowing the patient to remove the pump temporarily (eg, for bathing). Ominpod (Insulet Corporation) is an insulin infusion system in which the insulin reservoir and infusion set are integrated into one unit (pod), so there is no catheter (electronic patch pump). The pod, placed on the skin, delivers subcutaneous basal and bolus insulin based on wirelessly transmitted instructions from a personal digital assistant. The great advantage of continuous subcutaneous insulin infusion (CSII) is that it allows for establishment of a basal profile tailored to the patient. The patient therefore is able to eat with less regard to timing because the basal insulin infusion should maintain constant blood glucose between meals. Also the ability to adjust the basal insulin infusion makes it easier for the patient to manage glycemic excursions that occur with exercise. The pumps also have software that can assist the patient to calculate boluses based on glucose reading and carbohydrates to be consumed. They keep track of the time elapsed since last insulin bolus and the patient is reminded of this when he or she attempts to give additional correction bolus before the effect of the previous bolus has worn off ("insulin on board" feature). This feature reduces the risk of overcorrecting and subsequent hypoglycemia.

CSII therapy is appropriate for patients with type 1 diabetes who are motivated, mechanically inclined, educated about diabetes (diet, insulin action, treatment of hypoglycemia and hyperglycemia), and willing to monitor their blood glucose four to six times a day. Known complications of CSII include ketoacidosis, which can occur when insulin delivery is interrupted, and skin infections. Another disadvantage is its cost and the time demanded of the clinician and staff in initiating therapy.

V-go (Valeritas) is a mechanical patch pump designed specifically for people with type 2 diabetes who employ a basal/bolus insulin regimen. The device is preset to deliver one of three fixed and flat basal rates (20, 30, or 40 units) for 24 hours (at which point it must be replaced) and there is a button that delivers two units per press to help cover meals.

D. INHALED INSULIN—The dry-powder formulation of recombinant human regular insulin that is delivered by inhalation (technosphere insulin, Afrezza) is approved for use in adults with diabetes. Pharmacokinetic studies show that technosphere insulin is rapidly absorbed with peak insulin levels reached in 12–15 minutes and declining to baseline in 3 hours. Pharmacodynamic studies show that median time to maximum effect with inhaled insulin is approximately 1 hour and declines to baseline by about 3 hours. In contrast, the median time to maximum effect with subcutaneous insulin lispro is about 2 hours and declines to baseline by 4 hours. In clinical trials, technosphere insulin combined with basal insulin was as effective in glucose lowering as rapid-acting insulin analogs combined with basal insulin. It is formulated as a single-use, color-coded cartridge delivering 4, 8, or 12 units immediately before the meal. The manufacturer provides a dose conversion table; patients injecting up to 4 units of rapid-acting insulin analog should use the 4-unit cartridge. Those injecting 5 to 8 units should use the 8-unit cartridge. If the dose is 9–12 units of rapid-acting insulin premeal then one 4-unit cartridge and one 8-unit cartridge or one 12-unit cartridge should be used. The inhaler is about the size of a referee's whistle.

The most common adverse reaction of the inhaled insulin was a cough affecting about 27% of patients. A small decrease in pulmonary function (forced expiratory volume in 1 second [FEV_1]) was seen in the first 3 months of use, which persisted over 2 years of follow-up. Inhaled insulin is contraindicated in smokers and patients with chronic lung disease, such as asthma and chronic obstructive pulmonary disease. Spirometry should be performed to identify potential lung disease prior to initiating therapy. During the clinical trials, there were two cases of lung cancer in patients who were taking inhaled insulin and none in the comparator-treated patients. All the patients in whom lung cancer developed had a history of prior cigarette smoking. There were also two cases of squamous cell carcinoma of the lung in nonsmokers exposed to inhaled insulin; these cases occurred after completion of the clinical trials. Cases of lung cancer were also reported in cigarette smokers using a previously available inhaled insulin preparation (Exubera). The incidence rate in the Exubera treated group was 0.13 per 1000 patient years and 0.03 per 1000 patient years in the comparator-treated group.

D. Transplantation

1. Pancreas transplantation—All uremic patients with type 1 diabetes who are candidates for a kidney transplant should be considered potential candidates for a pancreas transplant. Eligibility criteria include age younger than 55 and minimal cardiovascular risk. Contraindications include noncorrectable coronary artery disease, extensive peripheral vascular disease, and significant obesity (weight greater than 100 kg). The pancreas transplant may occur at the same time as kidney transplant or after kidney

transplant. Patients undergoing simultaneous pancreas and kidney transplantation have an 83% chance of pancreatic graft survival at 1 year and 69% at 5 years. Solitary pancreatic transplantation in the absence of a need for kidney transplantation is considered only in those rare patients who do not respond to all other insulin therapeutic approaches and who have frequent severe hypoglycemia or who have life-threatening complications related to their lack of metabolic control. Pancreas transplant alone graft survival is 78% at 1 year and 54% at 5 years.

2. Islet transplantation—Total pancreatectomy is curative for severe pain syndrome associated with chronic pancreatitis. The pancreatectomy, however, results in surgical diabetes. Harvesting islets from the removed pancreas and autotransplanting them into the liver (via portal vein) can prevent the development of diabetes or result in "mild" diabetes (partial islet function) that is easier to manage. Since the islets are autologous no immunosuppression is required. The number of islets transplanted is the main predictor of insulin independence.

People with type 1 diabetes can become insulin independent after receiving islets isolated from a donor pancreas (alloislet transplant). The islets are infused into the portal vein using a percutaneous transhepatic approach, and they lodge in the liver releasing insulin in response to physiologic stimuli. Long-term immunosuppression is necessary to prevent allograft rejection and to suppress the autoimmune process that led to the disease in the first place. Insulin independence for more than 5 years has been demonstrated in patients who got anti-CD3 antibody or anti-thymocyte globulin induction immunosuppression and calcineurin inhibitors, mTor inhibitors, and mycophenolate mofetil as maintenance immunosuppression. One major limitation is the need for more than one islet infusion to achieve insulin independence. This is because of significant loss of islets during isolation and the period prior to engraftment. Alloislet transplantation is currently an experimental procedure and widespread application will depend on improving insulin independence rates with one infusion and also demonstrating that the long-term outcomes are as good as those of pancreas transplant alone.

Bennett WL et al. Comparative effectiveness and safety of medications for type 2 diabetes: an update including new drugs and 2-drug combinations. Ann Intern Med. 2011 May 3; 154(9):602–13. Erratum in: Ann Intern Med. 2011 Jul 5; 155(1):67–8. [PMID: 21403054]

Bolli GB et al. New long-acting insulin analogs: from clamp studies to clinical practice. Diabetes Care. 2015 Apr;38(4):541–3. [PMID: 25805863]

Nauck MA. A critical analysis of the clinical use of incretin-based therapies: The benefits by far outweigh the potential risks. Diabetes Care. 2013 Jul;36(7):2126–32. [PMID: 23645884]

▶ Steps in the Management of the Diabetic Patient

A. Diagnostic Examination

An attempt should be made to characterize the diabetes as type 1 or type 2, based on the clinical features present and on whether or not ketonuria accompanies the glycosuria.

Features that suggest end-organ insulin insensitivity to insulin, such as visceral obesity, acanthosis nigricans, or both, must be identified. The family history should document not only the incidence of diabetes in other members of the family but also the age at onset, association with obesity, the need for insulin, and whether there were complications. For the occasional patient, measurement of GAD65, IAA, ICA 512, and zinc transporter 8 antibodies can help distinguish between type 1 and type 2 diabetes. Many patients with newly diagnosed type 1 diabetes still have significant endogenous insulin production, and C peptide levels do not reliably distinguish between type 1 and type 2 diabetes. Other factors that increase cardiac risk, such as smoking history, presence of hypertension or hyperlipidemia, or oral contraceptive pill use, should be recorded.

Laboratory diagnosis of diabetes should document fasting plasma glucose levels above 126 mg/dL (7 mmol/L) or postprandial values consistently above 200 mg/dL (11.1 mmol/L) or HbA$_{1c}$ of at least 6.5% and whether ketonuria accompanies the glycosuria. An HbA$_{1c}$ measurement is also useful for assessing the effectiveness of future therapy. Baseline values include fasting plasma triglycerides, total cholesterol and HDL-cholesterol, electrocardiography, kidney function studies, peripheral pulses, and neurologic, podiatric, and ophthalmologic examinations to help guide future assessments.

B. Patient Education (Self-Management Training)

Since diabetes is a lifelong disorder, education of the patient and the family is probably the most important obligation of the clinician who provides initial care. The best persons to manage a disease that is affected so markedly by daily fluctuations in environmental stress, exercise, diet, and infections are the patients themselves and their families. The "teaching curriculum" should include explanations by the clinician or nurse of the nature of diabetes and its potential acute and chronic hazards and how they can be recognized early and prevented or treated. Self-monitoring of blood glucose should be emphasized, especially in insulin-requiring diabetic patients, and instructions must be given on proper testing and recording of data.

Patients taking insulin should have an understanding of the actions of basal and bolus insulins. They should be taught to determine whether the basal dose is appropriate and how to adjust the rapidly acting insulin dose for the carbohydrate content of a meal. Patients and their families and friends should be taught to recognize signs and symptoms of hypoglycemia and how to treat low glucose reactions. Strenuous exercise can precipitate hypoglycemia, and patients must therefore be taught to reduce their insulin dosage in anticipation of strenuous activity or to take supplemental carbohydrate. Injection of insulin into a site farthest away from the muscles most involved in the exercise may help ameliorate exercise-induced hypoglycemia, since insulin injected in the proximity of exercising muscle may be more rapidly mobilized. Exercise training also increases the effectiveness of insulin and insulin doses should be adjusted accordingly. Infections can cause insulin resistance, and patients should be instructed on how to manage the hyperglycemia with supplemental rapidly acting insulin.

The targets for blood glucose control should be elevated appropriately in elderly patients since they have the greatest risk if subjected to hypoglycemia and the least long-term benefit from more rigid glycemic control. Advice on personal hygiene, including detailed instructions on foot and dental care, should be provided. All infections (especially pyogenic ones) provoke the release of high levels of insulin antagonists, such as catecholamines or glucagon, and thus bring about a marked increase in insulin requirements. Patients who are taking oral agents may decompensate and temporarily require insulin. Patients should be told about community agencies, such as Diabetes Association chapters, that can serve as a continuing source of instruction.

Finally, vigorous efforts should be made to persuade patients with newly diagnosed diabetes who smoke to give up the habit, since large vessel peripheral vascular disease and debilitating retinopathy are less common in nonsmoking diabetic patients.

C. Therapy

Treatment must be individualized on the basis of the type of diabetes and specific needs of each patient. However, certain general principles of management can be outlined for hyperglycemic states of different types.

1. Type 1 diabetes—Traditional once- or twice-daily insulin regimens are usually ineffective in type 1 patients without residual endogenous insulin. In these patients, information and counseling based on the findings of the DCCT (see above) should be provided about the advantages of taking multiple injections of insulin in conjunction with self-blood glucose monitoring. If near-normalization of blood glucose is attempted, at least four measurements of capillary blood glucose and three or four insulin injections are necessary.

A combination of rapidly acting insulin analogs and long-acting insulin analogs allows for more physiologic insulin replacement. The rapidly acting insulin analogs have been advocated as a safer and much more convenient alternative to regular human insulin for preprandial use. However, because of their relatively short duration (no more than 3–4 hours), the rapidly acting insulin analogs need to be combined with longer-acting insulins to provide basal coverage and avoid hyperglycemia prior to the next meal. In addition to carbohydrate content of the meal, the effect of simultaneous fat ingestion must also be considered a factor in determining the rapidly acting insulin analog dosage required to control the glycemic increment during and just after the meal. With low-carbohydrate content and high-fat intake, there is an increased risk of hypoglycemia from insulin lispro within 2 hours after the meal. Table 27–8 illustrates a regimen with a rapidly acting insulin analog and insulin detemir or insulin glargine that might be appropriate for a 70-kg person with type 1 diabetes eating meals providing standard carbohydrate intake and moderate to low fat content.

Table 27–8. Examples of intensive insulin regimens using rapidly acting insulin analogs (insulin lispro, aspart, or glulisine) and insulin detemir, or insulin glargine or degludec in a 70-kg man with type 1 diabetes.[1-3]

	Pre-Breakfast	Pre-Lunch	Pre-Dinner	At Bedtime
Rapidly acting insulin analog	5 units	4 units	6 units	
Insulin detemir	6–7 units			8–9 units
OR				
Rapidly acting insulin analog	5 units	4 units	6 units	—
Insulin glargine or degludec		—		15–16 units

[1]Assumes that patient is consuming approximately 75 g carbohydrate at breakfast, 60 g at lunch, and 90 g at dinner.
[2]The dose of rapidly acting insulin can be raised by 1 or 2 units if extra carbohydrate (15–30 g) is ingested or if premeal blood glucose is > 170 mg/dL (9.4 mmol/L).
[3]Insulin glargine or insulin detemir must be given as a separate injection.

Insulin glargine is usually given once in the evening to provide 24-hour coverage. This insulin *cannot be mixed* with any of the other insulins and must be given as a separate injection. There are occasional patients in whom insulin glargine does not seem to last for 24 hours, and in such cases it needs to be given twice a day. As shown, insulin detemir may also need to be given twice a day to get adequate 24-hour basal coverage. Alternatively, small doses of NPH (~3–4 units) can be given with each meal to provide daytime basal coverage with a larger dose at night. Unlike the long-acting insulin analogs, NPH can be mixed in the same syringe as the insulin lispro, insulin aspart, and insulin glulisine.

Continuous subcutaneous insulin infusion (CSII) by portable battery-operated "open loop" devices currently provides the most flexible approach, allowing the setting of different basal rates throughout the 24 hours and permitting patients to delay or skip meals and vary meal size and composition. The dosage is usually based on providing 50% of the estimated insulin dose as basal and the remainder as intermittent boluses prior to meals. For example, a 70-kg man requiring 35 units of insulin per day may require a basal rate of 0.7 units per hour throughout the 24 hours with the exception of 3 AM to 8 AM, when 0.8 units per hour might be appropriate (given the "dawn phenomenon"—reduced tissue sensitivity to insulin between 5 AM and 8 AM). The meal bolus would depend on the carbohydrate content of the meal and the premeal blood glucose value. **One unit per 15 g of carbohydrate plus 1 unit for 50 mg/dL (2.8 mmol/L) of blood glucose above a target value (eg, 120 mg/dL [6.7 mmol/L]) is a common starting point.** Further adjustments to basal and bolus dosages would depend on the results of blood glucose monitoring. The majority of patients use the rapidly acting insulin analogs in the pumps. One of the more difficult therapeutic problems in managing patients with type 1 diabetes is determining the proper adjustment of insulin dose when the prebreakfast blood glucose level is high. Occasionally, the prebreakfast hyperglycemia is due to the Somogyi effect, in which nocturnal hypoglycemia leads to a surge of counterregulatory hormones to produce high blood glucose levels by 7 AM. However, a more common cause for prebreakfast hyperglycemia is the waning of circulating insulin levels by the morning. Also, the dawn phenomenon is present in as many as 75% of type 1 patients and can aggravate the hyperglycemia.

The diagnosis of the cause of prebreakfast hyperglycemia can be facilitated by self-monitoring of blood glucose at 3 AM in addition to the usual bedtime and 7 AM measurements (Table 27–9). This is required for only a few nights, and when a particular pattern emerges from monitoring blood glucose levels overnight, appropriate therapeutic measures can be taken. The Somogyi effect can be treated by eliminating the dose of intermediate insulin at dinnertime and giving it at a lower dosage at bedtime or by supplying more food at bedtime. When a waning insulin level is the cause, then either increasing the evening dose or shifting it from dinnertime to bedtime (or both) can be effective. A bedtime dose either of insulin glargine or insulin detemir provides more sustained overnight insulin levels than human NPH and may be effective in managing refractory prebreakfast hyperglycemia. If this fails, insulin pump therapy may be required.

Table 27–9. Prebreakfast hyperglycemia: Classification by blood glucose and insulin levels.

	Blood Glucose (mg/dL) [mmol/L]			Free Immunoreactive Insulin (microunit/mL)		
	10:00 PM	3:00 AM	7:00 AM	10:00 PM	3:00 AM	7:00 AM
Somogyi effect	90 [5]	40 [2.2]	200 [11.1]	High	Slightly high	Normal
Dawn phenomenon	110 [6.1]	110 [6.1]	150 [8.3]	Normal	Normal	Normal
Waning of insulin dose plus dawn phenomenon	110 [6.1]	190 [10.6]	220 [12.2]	Normal	Low	Low
Waning of insulin dose plus dawn phenomenon plus Somogyi effect	110 [6.1]	40 [2.2]	380 [21.1]	High	Normal	Low

2. Type 2 diabetes—Therapeutic recommendations are based on the relative contributions of beta cell insufficiency and insulin insensitivity in individual patients. The possibility that the individual patient has a specific etiologic cause for their diabetes should always be considered, especially when the patient does not have a family history of type 2 diabetes or does not have any evidence of central obesity or insulin resistance. Such patients should be evaluated for other types of diabetes such as LADA or MODY. Patients with LADA should be prescribed insulin when the disease is diagnosed and treated like patients with type 1 diabetes. It is also important to note that many patients with type 2 diabetes mellitus have a progressive loss of beta cell function and will require additional therapeutic interventions with time.

A. WEIGHT REDUCTION—One of the primary modes of therapy in the obese patient with type 2 diabetes is weight reduction. Normalization of glycemia can be achieved by weight loss and improvement in tissue sensitivity to insulin. A combination of caloric restriction, increased exercise, and behavior modification is required if a weight reduction program is to be successful. Understanding the risks associated with the diagnosis of diabetes may motivate the patient to lose weight.

For selected patients, medical or surgical options for weight loss should be considered. Orlistat, phentermine/topiramate, lorcaserin, naltrexone/extended-release bupropion, and high-dose liraglutide (3 mg daily) are weight loss medications approved for use in combination with diet and exercise (see Chapter 29).

Bariatric surgery (Roux-en-Y, gastric banding, gastric sleeve, biliopancreatic diversion/duodenal switch) typically results in substantial weight loss and improvement in glucose levels. A meta-analysis examining the impact of bariatric surgery on patients with diabetes and BMI of 40 kg/m^2 or greater noted that 82% of patients had resolution of clinical and laboratory manifestations of diabetes in the first 2 years after surgery and 62% remained free of diabetes more than 2 years after surgery. The improvement was most marked in the procedure that caused the greatest weight loss (biliopancreatic diversion/duodenal switch). There was, however, a high attrition of patients available for follow-up, and there was little information about different ethnic types. Weight regain does occur after bariatric surgery, and it can be expected that 20–25% of the lost weight will be regained over 10 years. The impact of this weight gain on diabetes recurrence depends principally on the degree of beta cell dysfunction.

Nonobese patients with type 2 diabetes frequently have increased visceral adiposity—the so-called metabolically obese normal weight patient. There is less emphasis on weight loss, but exercise remains an important aspect of treatment.

B. GLUCOSE LOWERING AGENTS—Figure 27–2 outlines the treatment approach based on the consensus algorithm proposed by the American Diabetes Association and the European Association for the Study of Diabetes. The current recommendation is to start **metformin** therapy at diagnosis and not wait to see whether the patient can

Weight loss + exercise + metformin

↓ If HbA$_{1c}$ target not reached after ~ 3 months

Metforrmin + another agent

↓ If HbA$_{1c}$ target not reached after ~ 3 months

Metformin + two other agents

↓ If HbA$_{1c}$ target not reached after ~ 3 months

Metformin + more complex insulin regimen ± other noninsulin agent

↓

Seven main classes of agents
- Metformin
- Sulfonylureas (includes nateglinide, repaglinide)
- Pioglitazone
- GLP-1 receptor agonists
- DPP-4 inhibitors
- SGLT2 inhibitors
- Insulins

↓

Factors in Therapeutic Decision (single agent or combination)

↓

Efficacy
- DPP-4 inhibitors are of moderate efficacy
- All other agents are of high efficacy

Hypoglycemic risk
- Sulfonylureas and insulins have increased risk of hypoglycemia

Effect on weight
- Metformin and DPP-4 inhibitors are weight neutral
- GLP-1 receptor agonists and SGLT2 inhibitors promote weight loss
- Sulfonylureas, insulins, and pioglitazone are associated with weight gain

Major side effects
- Metformin can cause lactic acidosis
- Pioglitazone is associated with fluid retention, fracture risk, and possibly bladder cancer
- GLP-1 receptor agonists are associated with nausea and vomiting and pancreatitis
- DPP-4 inhibitors may be associated with pancreatitis risk
- SGLT2 inhibitors can cause urinary tract infections; genital mycotic infections; dehydration; cannot use in renal impairment

Cost
- All agents except metformin and sulfonylureas are expensive
- Insulins are expensive if the additional cost of monitoring is taken into consideration

▲ **Figure 27–2.** Algorithm for the treatment of type 2 diabetes based on the 2012 and 2015 recommendations of the consensus panel of the American Diabetes Association/European Association for the Study of Diabetes.

achieve target glycemic control with weight management and exercise. See discussion of the individual medications, above.

When diabetes is not well controlled with initial therapy (usually metformin), then a second agent should be added. **Sulfonylureas** have been available for many years and their use in combination with metformin is well established. They do, however, have the propensity of causing hypoglycemia and weight gain. In patients who experience hyperglycemia after a carbohydrate-rich meal (such as dinner), a short-acting secretagogue (repaglinide or nateglinide) before meals may suffice to get the glucose levels into the target range. Patients with severe insulin resistance may be candidates for pioglitazone. Patients who are very concerned about weight gain may benefit from a trial of GLP-1 receptor agonist or DPP-4 inhibitor or SGLT2 inhibitor. If two agents are inadequate, then a third agent is added, although data regarding efficacy of such combined therapy are limited.

When the combination of oral agents (and injectable GLP-1 receptor agonists) fail to achieve euglycemia in patients with type 2 diabetes, then insulin treatment should be instituted. Various insulin regimens may be effective. One proposed regimen is to continue the oral combination therapy and then simply add a bedtime dose of NPH or long-acting insulin analog (insulin glargine or insulin detemir) to reduce excessive nocturnal hepatic glucose output and improve fasting glucose levels. If the patient does not achieve target glucose levels during the day, then daytime insulin treatment can be initiated. A convenient insulin regimen under these circumstances is a split dose of 70/30 NPH/regular mixture (or Humalog Mix 75/25 or NovoLogMix 70/30) before breakfast and before dinner. If this regimen fails to achieve satisfactory glycemic goals or is associated with unacceptable frequency of hypoglycemic episodes, then a more intensive regimen of multiple insulin injections can be instituted as in patients with type 1 diabetes. Metformin principally reduces hepatic glucose output, and it is reasonable to continue with this medication when insulin therapy is instituted. Pioglitazone, which improves peripheral insulin sensitivity, can be used together with insulin but this combination is associated with more weight gain and peripheral edema. The sulfonylureas also continue to be of benefit. There is limited information on the benefits of continuing the GLP1-receptor agonists or the DPP-4 inhibitors or the SGLT2 inhibitors once insulin therapy is initiated. Weight-reducing interventions should continue even after initiation of insulin therapy and may allow for simplification of the therapeutic regimen in the future.

D. Acceptable Levels of Glycemic Control

A reasonable aim of therapy is to approach normal glycemic excursions without provoking severe or frequent hypoglycemia. **Criteria for "acceptable" control** includes the following: (1) blood glucose levels of 90–130 mg/dL (5–7.2 mmol/L) before meals and after an overnight fast, (2) levels no higher than 180 mg/dL (10 mmol/L) 1 hour after meals and 150 mg/dL (8.3 mmol/L) 2 hours after meals, and (3) HbA_{1c} levels less than 7% for nonpregnant adults. Less

stringent HbA_{1c} goals may be appropriate in children, those with a history of severe hypoglycemia, limited life expectancy, and advanced microvascular and macrovascular disease. In the elderly frail patient, an HbA_{1c} target of approximately 8% (preprandial blood glucose levels in the range of the 150–159 mg/dL) may be reasonable although formal evidence is lacking. **The UKPDS study demonstrated that blood pressure control was as significant or more significant than glycemic control in patients with type 2 diabetes regarding the prevention of microvascular as well as macrovascular complications.**

Inzucchi SE et al. Management of hyperglycemia in type 2 diabetes, 2015: a patient-centered approach: update to a position statement of the American Diabetes Association and the European Association for the Study of Diabetes. Diabetes Care. 2015 Jan;38(1):140–9. [PMID: 25538310]

Jin J. JAMA patient page. Starting insulin treatment for diabetes. JAMA. 2014 Jun 11;311(22):2347. [PMID: 24915279]

Switzer SM et al. Intensive insulin therapy in patients with type 1 diabetes mellitus. Endocrinol Metab Clin North Am. 2012 Mar;41(1):89–104. [PMID: 22575408]

E. Complications of Insulin Therapy

1. Hypoglycemia—Hypoglycemic reactions are the most common complications that occur in patients with diabetes who are treated with insulin. The signs and symptoms of hypoglycemia may be divided into those resulting from stimulation of the autonomic nervous system and those from neuroglycopenia (insufficient glucose for normal central nervous system function). When the blood glucose falls to around 54 mg/dL (3 mmol/L), the patient starts to experience both sympathetic (tachycardia, palpitations, sweating, tremulousness) and parasympathetic (nausea, hunger) nervous system symptoms. If these autonomic symptoms are ignored and the glucose levels fall further (to around 50 mg/dL [2.8 mmol/L]), then neuroglycopenic symptoms appear, including irritability, confusion, blurred vision, tiredness, headache, and difficulty speaking. A further decline in glucose can then lead to loss of consciousness or even a seizure. With repeated episodes of hypoglycemia, there is adaptation, and autonomic symptoms do not occur until the blood glucose levels are much lower and so the first symptoms are often due to neuroglycopenia. This condition is referred to as "hypoglycemic unawareness." It has been shown that hypoglycemic unawareness can be reversed by keeping glucose levels high for a period of several weeks. Except for sweating, most of the sympathetic symptoms of hypoglycemia are blunted in patients receiving beta-blocking agents. Though not absolutely contraindicated, these medications must be used with caution in patients with diabetes who require insulin, and beta-1-selective blocking agents are preferred.

Hypoglycemia can occur in patient taking sulfonylureas, repaglinide, and nateglinide, particularly if the patient is elderly, has kidney or liver disease, or is taking certain other medications that alter metabolism of the sulfonylureas (eg, phenylbutazone, sulfonamides, or warfarin). It occurs more frequently with the use of long-acting sulfonylureas than when shorter-acting agents are used. Otherwise, hypoglycemia in insulin-treated patients with diabetes occurs as a consequence of three factors: behavioral issues, impaired counterregulatory systems, and complications of diabetes.

Behavioral issues include injecting too much insulin for the amount of carbohydrates ingested. Drinking alcohol in excess, especially on an empty stomach, can also cause hypoglycemia. In patients with type 1 diabetes, hypoglycemia can occur during or even several hours after exercise, and so glucose levels need to be monitored and food and insulin adjusted. Some patients do not like their glucose levels to be high, and they treat every high glucose level aggressively. These individuals who "stack" their insulin—that is, give another dose of insulin before the first injection has had its full action—can develop hypoglycemia.

Counterregulatory issues resulting in hypoglycemia include impaired glucagon response, sympatho-adrenal responses, and cortisol deficiency. Patients with diabetes of greater than 5 years duration lose their glucagon response to hypoglycemia. As a result, they are at a significant disadvantage in protecting themselves against falling glucose levels. Once the glucagon response is lost, their sympatho-adrenal responses take on added importance. Unfortunately, aging, autonomic neuropathy, or hypoglycemic unawareness due to repeated low glucose levels further blunts the sympatho-adrenal responses. Occasionally, Addison disease develops in persons with type 1 diabetes mellitus; when this happens, insulin requirements fall significantly, and unless insulin dose is reduced, recurrent hypoglycemia will develop.

Complications of diabetes that increase the risk for hypoglycemia include autonomic neuropathy, gastroparesis, and end-stage chronic kidney disease. The sympathetic nervous system is an important system alerting the individual that the glucose level is falling by causing symptoms of tachycardia, palpitations, sweating, and tremulousness. Failure of the sympatho-adrenal responses increases the risk of hypoglycemia. In addition, in patients with gastroparesis, if insulin is given before a meal, the peak of insulin action may occur before the food is absorbed causing the glucose levels to fall. Finally, in end-stage chronic kidney disease, hypoglycemia can occur presumably because of decreased insulin clearance as well as loss of renal contribution to gluconeogenesis in the postabsorptive state.

To prevent and treat insulin-induced hypoglycemia, the diabetic patient should carry glucose tablets or juice at all times. For most episodes, ingestion of 15 grams of carbohydrate is sufficient to reverse the hypoglycemia. The patient should be instructed to check the blood glucose in 15 minutes and treat again if the glucose level is still low. A parenteral glucagon emergency kit (1 mg) should be provided to every patient with diabetes who is receiving insulin therapy. Family or friends should be instructed how to inject it subcutaneously or intramuscularly into the buttock, arm, or thigh in the event that the patient is unconscious or refuses food. The medication can occasionally cause vomiting, and the unconscious patient should be turned on his or her side to protect the airway. The glucagon mobilizes glycogen from the liver, raising the blood glucose by about 36 mg/dL (2 mmol/L) in about 15 minutes. After the patient recovers consciousness, additional oral carbohydrate should be given. People with diabetes receiving hypoglycemic medication therapy should also wear an identification MedicAlert bracelet or necklace or carry a card in his or her wallet (1-800-ID-ALERT, www.medicalert.org).

Medical personnel treating severe hypoglycemia can give 50 mL of 50% glucose solution by rapid intravenous infusion. If intravenous access is not available, 1 mg of glucagon can be injected intramuscularly.

2. Immunopathology of insulin therapy—At least five molecular classes of insulin antibodies are produced during the course of insulin therapy in diabetes, including IgA, IgD, IgE, IgG, and IgM. With the switch to human and purified pork insulin, the various immunopathologic syndromes such as insulin allergy, immune insulin resistance, and lipoatrophy have become quite rare since the titers and avidity of these induced antibodies are generally quite low.

A. Insulin allergy—Insulin allergy, or immediate-type hypersensitivity, is a rare condition in which local or systemic urticaria is due to histamine release from tissue mast cells sensitized by adherence of anti-insulin IgE antibodies. In severe cases, anaphylaxis results. When only human insulin has been used from the onset of insulin therapy, insulin allergy is exceedingly rare. Antihistamines, corticosteroids, and even desensitization may be required, especially for systemic hypersensitivity. There have been case reports of successful use of insulin lispro in those rare patients who have a generalized allergy to human insulin or insulin resistance due to a high titer of insulin antibodies.

B. Immune insulin resistance—A low titer of circulating IgG anti-insulin antibodies that neutralize the action of insulin to a small extent develops in most insulin-treated patients. With the old animal insulins, a high titer of circulating antibodies sometimes developed, resulting in extremely high insulin requirements—often more than 200 units daily. This is now rarely seen with the switch to human or highly purified pork insulins and has not been reported with the analogs.

C. Lipodystrophy—Atrophy of subcutaneous fatty tissue leading to disfiguring excavations and depressed areas may rarely occur at the site of injection. This complication results from an immune reaction, and it has become rarer with the development of human and highly purified insulin preparations. Lipohypertrophy, on the other hand, is a consequence of the pharmacologic effects of insulin being deposited in the same location repeatedly. It can occur with purified insulins as well. Rotation of injection sites will prevent lipohypertrophy.

Cryer PE. Mechanisms of hypoglycemia-associated autonomic failure in diabetes. N Engl J Med. 2013 Jul 25;369(4):362–72. [PMID: 23883381]

▶ Chronic Complications of Diabetes

Late clinical manifestations of diabetes mellitus include a number of pathologic changes that involve small and large blood vessels, cranial and peripheral nerves, the skin, and the lens of the eye. These lesions lead to hypertension, end-stage chronic kidney disease, blindness, autonomic and peripheral neuropathy, amputations of the lower extremities, myocardial infarction, and cerebrovascular accidents. These late manifestations correlate with the duration of the diabetic state subsequent to the onset of puberty. In type 1 diabetes, end-stage chronic kidney disease develops in up to 40% of patients, compared with less than 20% of patients with type 2 diabetes. Proliferative retinopathy ultimately develops in both types of diabetes but has a slightly higher prevalence in type 1 patients (25% after 15 years' duration). In patients with type 1 diabetes, complications from end-stage chronic kidney disease are a major cause of death, whereas patients with type 2 diabetes are more likely to have macrovascular diseases leading to myocardial infarction and stroke as the main causes of death. Cigarette use adds significantly to the risk of both microvascular and macrovascular complications in diabetic patients.

A. Ocular Complications

1. Diabetic cataracts—Premature cataracts occur in diabetic patients and seem to correlate with both the duration of diabetes and the severity of chronic hyperglycemia. Nonenzymatic glycosylation of lens protein is twice as high in diabetic patients as in age-matched nondiabetic persons and may contribute to the premature occurrence of cataracts.

2. Diabetic retinopathy—There are two main categories of diabetic retinopathy: nonproliferative and proliferative (see Chapter 7). Diabetic macular edema can occur at any stage. **Nonproliferative ("background") retinopathy** represents the earliest stage of retinal involvement by diabetes and is characterized by such changes as microaneurysms, dot hemorrhages, exudates, and retinal edema. The prevalence of nonproliferative retinopathy in patients with type 2 diabetes is 60% after 16 years.

Proliferative retinopathy involves the growth of new capillaries and fibrous tissue within the retina and into the vitreous chamber. It is a consequence of small vessel occlusion, which causes retinal hypoxia; this in turn stimulates new vessel growth. New vessel formation may occur at the optic disk or elsewhere on the retina. Prior to proliferation of new capillaries, a preproliferative phase often occurs in which arteriolar ischemia is manifested as cotton-wool spots (small infarcted areas of retina). Vision is usually normal until vitreous hemorrhage or retinal detachment occurs.

Proliferative retinopathy can occur in both types of diabetes but is more common in type 1, developing about 7–10 years after onset of symptoms, with a prevalence of 25% after 15 years' duration. Vision-threatening retinopathy virtually never appears in type 1 patients in the first 3–5 years of diabetes or before puberty. Up to 20% of patients with type 2 diabetes have retinopathy at the time of diagnosis, because many were probably diabetic for an extensive period of time before diagnosis. Annual consultation with an ophthalmologist should be arranged for patients who have had type 1 diabetes for more than 3–5 years and for all patients with type 2 diabetes. Chapter 7 describes the treatment of retinopathy and macular edema. There is no contraindication to using aspirin in patients with proliferative retinopathy.

3. Glaucoma—Glaucoma occurs in approximately 6% of persons with diabetes. It is responsive to the usual therapy for open-angle disease. Neovascularization of the iris in patients with diabetes can predispose to closed-angle glaucoma, but this is relatively uncommon except after cataract extraction, when growth of new vessels has been known to progress rapidly, involving the angle of the iris and obstructing outflow.

B. Diabetic Nephropathy

As many as 4000 cases of end-stage chronic kidney disease occur each year among diabetic people in the United States.

The cumulative incidence of nephropathy differs between the two major types of diabetes. Patients with type 1 diabetes have a 30–40% chance of having nephropathy after 20 years—in contrast to the much lower frequency in type 2 diabetes patients, in whom only about 15–20% develop clinical kidney disease. However, since there are many more individuals affected with type 2 diabetes, end-stage chronic kidney disease is much more prevalent in type 2 than in type 1 diabetes in the United States and especially throughout the rest of the world.

Diabetic nephropathy is initially manifested by proteinuria; subsequently, as kidney function declines, urea and creatinine accumulate in the blood. Sensitive radioimmunoassay methods detect small amounts of urinary albumin—in contrast to the less sensitive dipstick strips, whose minimal detection limit is 0.3–0.5%. Conventional 24-hour urine collections, in addition to being inconvenient for patients, also show wide variability of albumin excretion, since several factors such as sustained erect posture, dietary protein, and exercise tend to increase albumin excretion rates. For these reasons, an albumin-creatinine ratio in an early morning spot urine collected upon awakening is preferable. In the early morning spot urine, a ratio of albumin (mcg/L) to creatinine (mg/L) of less than 30 mcg/mg creatinine is normal, and a ratio of 30–300 mcg/mg creatinine suggests abnormal microalbuminuria. At least two early morning spot urine collections over a 3- to 6-month period should be abnormal before a diagnosis of microalbuminuria is justified. Short-term hyperglycemia, exercise, urinary tract infections, heart failure, and acute febrile illness can cause transient albuminuria and so testing for microalbuminuria should be postponed until resolution of these problems.

Subsequent end-stage chronic kidney disease can be predicted by persistent urinary albumin excretion rates exceeding 30 mcg/mg creatinine. Glycemic control as well as a protein diet of 0.8 g/kg/day may reduce both the hyperfiltration and the elevated microalbuminuria in patients in the early stages of diabetes and those with incipient diabetic nephropathy. Antihypertensive therapy also decreases microalbuminuria. Evidence from some studies—but not the UKPDS—supports a specific role for ACE inhibitors in reducing intraglomerular pressure in addition to their lowering of systemic hypertension. An ACE inhibitor (captopril, 50 mg twice daily) in normotensive diabetic patients impedes progression to proteinuria and prevents the increase in albumin excretion rate. Since microalbuminuria has been shown to correlate with elevated *nocturnal* systolic blood pressure, it is possible that "normotensive" diabetic patients with microalbuminuria have slightly elevated systolic blood pressure during sleep, which is lowered during antihypertensive therapy. This action may contribute to the reported efficacy of ACE inhibitors in reducing microalbuminuria in "normotensive" patients.

If treatment is inadequate, then the disease progresses with proteinuria of varying severity occasionally leading to nephrotic syndrome with hypoalbuminemia, edema, and an increase in circulating LDL cholesterol, as well as progressive azotemia. In contrast to all other kidney disorders, the proteinuria associated with diabetic nephropathy does not diminish with progressive end-stage chronic kidney disease (patients continue to excrete 10–11 g daily as creatinine clearance diminishes). As end-stage chronic kidney disease progresses, there is an elevation in the renal threshold at which glycosuria appears (see Chapter 22).

C. Diabetic Neuropathy

Diabetic neuropathies are the most common complications of diabetes affecting up to 50% of older patients with type 2 diabetes.

1. Peripheral neuropathy—

A. DISTAL SYMMETRIC POLYNEUROPATHY—This is the most common form of diabetic peripheral neuropathy where loss of function appears in a stocking-glove pattern and is due to an axonal neuropathic process. Longer nerves are especially vulnerable, hence the impact on the foot. Both motor and sensory nerve conduction is delayed in the peripheral nerves, and ankle jerks may be absent.

Sensory involvement usually occurs first and is generally bilateral, symmetric, and associated with dulled perception of vibration, pain, and temperature. The pain can range from mild discomfort to severe incapacitating symptoms. The sensory deficit may eventually be of sufficient degree to prevent patients from feeling pain. Patients who have a sensory neuropathy should therefore be examined with a 5.07 Semmes-Weinstein filament and those who cannot feel the filament must be considered at risk for unperceived neuropathic injury.

The denervation of the small muscles of the foot results in clawing of the toes and displacement of the submetatarsal fat pads anteriorly. These changes, together with the joint and connective tissue changes, alter the biomechanics of the foot and increase plantar pressures. This combination of decreased pain threshold, abnormally high foot pressures, and repetitive stress (such as from walking) can lead to calluses and ulcerations in the high-pressure areas such as over the metatarsal heads (Figure 27–3). Peripheral neuropathy, autonomic neuropathy, and trauma also predisposes to the development of Charcot arthropathy. An acute case of Charcot foot arthropathy presents with pain and swelling, and if left untreated, leads to a "rocker

▲ **Figure 27–3.** Diabetic foot ulcer over head of first metatarsal (arrow). (Used, with permission, from Dean SM, Satiani B, Abraham WT. *Color Atlas and Synopsis of Vascular Diseases.* McGraw-Hill, 2014.)

bottom" deformity and ulceration. The early radiologic changes show joint subluxation and periarticular fractures. As the process progresses, there is frank osteoclastic destruction leading to deranged and unstable joints particularly in the midfoot. Not surprisingly, the key issue for the healing of neuropathic ulcers in a foot with good vascular supply is mechanical unloading. In addition, any infection should be treated with debridement and appropriate antibiotics; healing duration of 8–10 weeks is typical. Occasionally, when healing appears refractory, **platelet-derived growth factor** (becaplermin [Regranex]) should be considered for local application. A post-marketing epidemiologic study showed increased cancer deaths in patients who had used three or more tubes of becaplermin on their leg or feet ulcers, resulting in a "black box" warning on the medication label. Once ulcers are healed, therapeutic footwear is key to preventing recurrences. Custom molded shoes are reserved for patients with significant foot deformities. Other patients with neuropathy may require accommodative insoles that distribute the load over as wide an area as possible. Patients with foot deformities and loss of their protective threshold should get regular care from a podiatrist. Patients should be educated on appropriate footwear and those with loss of their protective threshold should be instructed to inspect their feet daily for reddened areas, blisters, abrasions, or lacerations.

In some patients, hypersensitivity to light touch and occasionally severe "burning" pain, particularly at night, can become physically and emotionally disabling. Nortriptyline or desipramine in doses of 25–150 mg/day orally may provide dramatic relief for pain from diabetic neuropathy, often within 48–72 hours. This rapid response is in contrast to the 2 or 3 weeks required for an antidepressive effect. Patients often attribute the benefit to having a full night's sleep. Mild to moderate morning drowsiness is a side effect that generally improves with time or can be lessened by giving the medication several hours before bedtime. This medication should not be continued if improvement has not occurred after 5 days of therapy.

Amitriptyline, 25–75 mg orally at bedtime can also be used but has more anticholinergic effects. Tricyclic antidepressants, in combination with the phenothiazine, fluphenazine, have been shown in two studies to be efficacious in painful neuropathy, with benefits unrelated to relief of depression. Gabapentin (900–1800 mg orally daily in three divided doses) has also been shown to be effective in the treatment of painful neuropathy and should be tried if the tricyclic medications prove ineffective. Pregabalin, a congener of gabapentin, has been shown in an 8-week study to be more effective than placebo in treating painful diabetic peripheral neuropathy. However, this medication was not compared with an active control. Also, because of its abuse potential, it has been categorized as a schedule V controlled substance. Duloxetine (60–120 mg), a serotonin and norepinephrine reuptake inhibitor, has been approved for the treatment of painful diabetic neuropathy. In clinical trials, this medication reduced the pain sensitivity score by 40–50%. Capsaicin, a topical irritant, has been found to be effective in reducing local nerve pain; it is dispensed as a cream (Zostrix 0.025%, Zostrix-HP 0.075%) to be rubbed into the skin over the painful region two to four times daily. Gloves should be used for application since hand contamination could result in discomfort if the cream comes in contact with eyes or sensitive areas such as the genitalia. Application of a 5% lidocaine patch over an area of maximal pain has been reported to be of benefit. It is approved for treatment of postherpetic neuralgia and is in clinical trials for the treatment of painful diabetic neuropathy.

Diabetic neuropathic cachexia is a syndrome characterized by a symmetric peripheral neuropathy associated with profound weight loss (up to 60% of total body weight) and painful dysesthesias affecting the proximal lower limbs, the hands, or the lower trunk. Treatment is usually with insulin and analgesics. The prognosis is generally good, and patients typically recover their baseline weight with resolution of the painful sensory symptoms within 1 year.

B. Isolated peripheral neuropathy—Involvement of the distribution of only one nerve ("mononeuropathy") or of several nerves ("mononeuropathy multiplex") is characterized by sudden onset with subsequent recovery of all or most of the function. This neuropathology has been attributed to vascular ischemia or traumatic damage. Cranial and femoral nerves are commonly involved, and motor abnormalities predominate. The patient with cranial nerve involvement usually has diplopia and single third, fourth, or sixth nerve weakness on examination but the pupil is spared. A full recovery of function occurs in 6–12 weeks. Diabetic amyotrophy presents with onset of severe pain in the front of the thigh. Within a few days or weeks of the onset of pain, weakness and wasting of the quadriceps develops. As the weakness appears, the pain tends to improve. Management includes analgesia and improved diabetes control. The symptoms improve over 6–18 months.

2. Autonomic neuropathy—Neuropathy of the autonomic system occurs principally in patients with diabetes of long duration. It affects many diverse visceral functions including blood pressure and pulse, gastrointestinal activity,

bladder function, and erectile dysfunction. Treatment is directed specifically at each abnormality.

Involvement of the gastrointestinal system may be manifested by nausea, vomiting, postprandial fullness, reflux or dysphagia, constipation or diarrhea (or both), and fecal incontinence. Gastroparesis should be considered in type 1 diabetic patients in whom unexpected fluctuations and variability in their blood glucose levels develops after meals. Metoclopramide has been of some help in treating diabetic gastroparesis. It is given in a dose of 10 mg orally three or four times a day, 30 minutes before meals and at bedtime. Drowsiness, restlessness, fatigue, and lassitude are common adverse effects. Tardive dyskinesia and extrapyramidal effects can occur, especially when used for longer than 3 months, and the FDA has cautioned against the long-term use of metoclopramide.

Erythromycin appears to bind to motilin receptors in the stomach and has been found to improve gastric emptying over the short term in doses of 250 mg three times daily, but its effectiveness seems to diminish over time. In selected patients, injections of botulinum toxin into the pylorus can reduce pylorus sphincter resistance and enhance gastric emptying. Gastric electrical stimulation has been reported to improve symptoms and quality of life indices in patients with gastroparesis refractory to pharmacologic therapy.

Diarrhea associated with autonomic neuropathy has occasionally responded to broad-spectrum antibiotic therapy (such as rifaximin, metronidazole, amoxicillin/clavulanate, ciprofloxacin, or doxycycline), although it often undergoes spontaneous remission. Refractory diabetic diarrhea is often associated with impaired sphincter control and fecal incontinence. Therapy with loperamide, 4–8 mg daily, or diphenoxylate with atropine, two tablets up to four times a day, may provide relief. In more severe cases, tincture of paregoric or codeine (60 mg tablets) may be required to reduce the frequency of diarrhea and improve the consistency of the stools. Clonidine has been reported to lessen diabetic diarrhea; however, its usefulness is limited by its tendency to lower blood pressure in these patients who already have autonomic neuropathy, resulting in orthostatic hypotension. Constipation usually responds to stimulant laxatives such as senna.

Incomplete emptying of the bladder can sometimes occur. Bethanechol in doses of 10–50 mg orally three times a day has occasionally improved emptying of the atonic urinary bladder. Catheter decompression of the distended bladder has been reported to improve its function, and considerable benefit has been reported after surgical severing of the internal vesicle sphincter.

Use of Jobst fitted stockings, tilting the head of the bed, and arising slowly from the supine position can be helpful in treating symptoms of orthostatic hypotension. When such measures are inadequate, then treatment with fludrocortisone 0.1–0.2 mg orally daily can be considered. This medication, however, can result in supine hypertension and hypokalemia. Midodrine (10 mg orally three times a day), an alpha-agonist, can also be used.

Erectile dysfunction can result from neurologic, psychological or vascular causes, or a combination of these causes. Sildenafil (Viagra), vardenafil (Levitra), and tadalafil (Cialis) have been shown in placebo-controlled clinical trials to improve erections in response to sexual stimulation. The recommended dose of sildenafil for most patients is one 50-mg tablet taken approximately 1 hour before sexual activity. The peak effect is at 1.5–2 hours, with some effect persisting for 4 hours. Patients with diabetes mellitus using sildenafil reported 50–60% improvement in erectile function. The maximum recommended dose is 100 mg. The recommended dose of both vardenafil and tadalafil is 10 mg. The doses may be increased to 20 mg or decreased to 5 mg based on efficacy and side effects. Tadalafil has been shown to improve erectile function for up to 36 hours after dosing. Low doses are available for daily use. In clinical trials, only a few adverse effects have been reported—transient mild headache, flushing, dyspepsia, and some altered color vision. Priapism can occur with these medications, and patients should be advised to seek immediate medical attention if an erection persists for longer than 4 hours. These phosphodiesterase type 5 (PDE5) inhibitors potentiate the hypotensive effects of nitrates and their use is contraindicated in patients who are concurrently using organic nitrates in any form. Caution is advised for men who have suffered a heart attack, stroke, or life-threatening arrhythmia within the previous 6 months; men who have resting hypotension or hypertension; and men who have a history of heart failure or have unstable angina. Rarely, a decrease in vision or permanent visual loss has been reported after PDE5 inhibitor use.

Intracorporeal injection of vasoactive medications causes penile engorgement and erection. Medications most commonly used include papaverine alone, papaverine with phentolamine, and alprostadil (prostaglandin E_1). Alprostadil injections are relatively painless, but careful instruction is essential to prevent local trauma, priapism, and fibrosis. Intraurethral pellets of alprostadil avoid the problem of injection of the medication.

External vacuum therapy (Erec-Aid System) is a nonsurgical treatment consisting of a suction chamber operated by a hand pump that creates a vacuum around the penis. This draws blood into the penis to produce an erection that is maintained by a specially designed tension ring inserted around the base of the penis and which can be kept in place for up to 20–30 minutes. While this method is generally effective, its cumbersome nature limits its appeal.

Surgical implants of penile prostheses remain an option for those patients in whom the nonsurgical approaches are ineffective.

D. Cardiovascular Complications

1. Heart disease—Microangiopathy occurs in the heart and may explain the etiology of congestive cardiomyopathies in diabetic patients who do not have demonstrable coronary artery disease. More commonly, however, heart disease in patients with diabetes is due to coronary atherosclerosis. Myocardial infarction is three to five times more common in diabetic patients and is the leading cause of death in patients with type 2 diabetes. Cardiovascular disease risk is increased in patients with type 1 diabetes as

well, although the absolute risk is lower than in patients with type 2 diabetes. Premenopausal women who normally have lower rates of coronary artery disease lose this protection once diabetes develops. The increased risk in patients with type 2 diabetes reflects the combination of hyperglycemia, hyperlipidemia, abnormalities of platelet adhesiveness, coagulation factors, hypertension, oxidative stress, and inflammation. Large intervention studies of risk factor reduction in diabetes are lacking, but it is reasonable to assume that reducing these risk factors would have a beneficial effect. Lowering LDL cholesterol reduces first events in patients without known coronary disease and secondary events in patients with known coronary disease. These intervention studies included some patients with diabetes, and the benefits of LDL cholesterol lowering was apparent in this group. The National Cholesterol Education Program clinical practice guidelines have designated diabetes as a coronary risk equivalent and have recommended that patients with diabetes should have an LDL cholesterol goal of less than 100 mg/dL (2.6 mmol/L). Lowering LDL cholesterol to 70 mg/dL (1.8 mmol/L) may have additional benefit and is a reasonable target for most patients with type 2 diabetes who have multiple risk factors for cardiovascular disease.

The ADA also recommends lowering systolic blood pressure to less than 140 mm Hg and diastolic pressure to less than 90 mm Hg in patients with diabetes. The systolic target of 130 mm Hg or less and diastolic of 80 mm Hg or less is recommended for the younger patient if it can be achieved without undue treatment burden. The Systolic Blood Pressure Intervention Trial (SPRINT) reported that treating to a systolic blood pressure of less than 120 mm Hg reduced cardiovascular events by 25% and death from cardiovascular causes by 43% during 3.26 years of follow-up. People with diabetes, however, were excluded from this study, and it is unclear if the results are applicable to this population. Patients with type 2 diabetes who already have cardiovascular disease or microalbuminuria should be considered for treatment with an ACE inhibitor. More clinical studies are needed to address the question of whether patients with type 2 diabetes who do not have cardiovascular disease or microalbuminuria would specifically benefit from ACE inhibitor treatment.

Aspirin at a dose of 81–325 mg daily is effective in reducing cardiovascular morbidity and mortality in patients who have a history of myocardial infarction or stroke (secondary prevention). It is unclear if aspirin prevents primary cardiovascular events in people with diabetes. The current recommendation is to give aspirin to people with diabetes who have a greater than 10% 10-year risk of cardiovascular events. Typically, this includes most diabetic men aged 50 years or older and diabetic women aged 60 years or older with one or more additional risk factors (smoking, hypertension, dyslipidemia, family history of premature cardiovascular disease, or albuminuria). Contraindications for aspirin therapy are patients with aspirin allergy, bleeding tendency, recent gastrointestinal bleeding, or active hepatic disease. Based on the Early Treatment Diabetic Retinopathy Study (ETDRS), there does not appear to be a contraindication to aspirin use to achieve cardiovascular benefit in diabetic patients who have proliferative retinopathy. Aspirin also does not seem to affect the severity of vitreous/preretinal hemorrhages or their resolution.

2. Peripheral vascular disease—Atherosclerosis is markedly accelerated in the larger arteries. It is often diffuse, with localized enhancement in certain areas of turbulent blood flow, such as at the bifurcation of the aorta or other large vessels. Clinical manifestations of peripheral vascular disease include ischemia of the lower extremities, erectile dysfunction, and intestinal angina.

The incidence of **gangrene of the feet** in patients with diabetes is 30 times that in age-matched controls. The factors responsible for its development, in addition to peripheral vascular disease, are small vessel disease, peripheral neuropathy with loss of both pain sensation and neurogenic inflammatory responses, and secondary infection. In two-thirds of patients with ischemic gangrene, pedal pulses are not palpable. In the remaining one-third who have palpable pulses, reduced blood flow through these vessels can be demonstrated by plethysmographic or Doppler ultrasound examination. Prevention of foot injury is imperative. Agents that reduce peripheral blood flow such as tobacco should be avoided. Control of other risk factors such as hypertension is essential. Beta-blockers are relatively contraindicated because of presumed negative peripheral hemodynamic consequences but data that support this are lacking. Cholesterol-lowering agents are useful as adjunctive therapy when early ischemic signs are detected and when dyslipidemia is present. Patients should be advised to seek immediate medical care if a diabetic foot ulcer develops. Improvement in peripheral blood flow with endarterectomy and bypass operations is possible in certain patients.

E. Skin and Mucous Membrane Complications

Chronic pyogenic infections of the skin may occur, especially in poorly controlled diabetic patients. **Candidal infection** can produce erythema and edema of intertriginous areas below the breasts, in the axillas, and between the fingers. It causes vulvovaginitis in women with chronically uncontrolled diabetes who have persistent glucosuria and is a frequent cause of pruritus. While antifungal creams containing miconazole or clotrimazole offer immediate relief of vulvovaginitis, recurrence is frequent unless glucosuria is reduced.

In some patients with type 2 diabetes, poor glycemic control can cause a severe hypertriglyceridemia, which can present as **eruptive cutaneous xanthomas** and pancreatitis. The skin lesions appear as yellow morbilliform eruptions 2–5 mm in diameter with erythematous areolae. They occur on extensor surfaces (elbows, knees, buttocks) and disappear after triglyceride levels are reduced.

Necrobiosis lipoidica diabeticorum is usually located over the anterior surfaces of the legs or the dorsal surfaces of the ankles. They are oval or irregularly shaped plaques with demarcated borders and a glistening yellow surface and occur in women two to four times more frequently than in men. Pathologically, the lesions show degeneration

of collagen, granulomatous inflammation of subcutaneous tissues and blood vessels, capillary basement membrane thickening and obliteration of vessel lumina. The condition is associated with type 1 diabetes, although it can occur in patients with type 2 diabetes, and also in patients without diabetes. First-line therapy includes topical and subcutaneous corticosteroids. Improving glycemic control may help the condition.

"Shin spots" are not uncommon in adults with diabetes. They are brownish, rounded, painless atrophic lesions of the skin in the pretibial area.

F. Bone and Joint Complications

Long-standing diabetes can cause progressive stiffness of the hand secondary to contracture and tightening of skin over the joints (diabetic cheiroarthropathy), frozen shoulder (adhesive capsulitis), carpal tunnel syndrome, and Dupuytren contractures. These complications are believed to be due to glycosylation of collagen and perhaps other proteins in connective tissue. There may also be an inflammatory component.

Data on bone mineral density and fracture risk in people with diabetes are contradictory. Patients with type 2 diabetes do appear to be at increased risk for nonvertebral fractures. Women with type 1 diabetes have an increased risk of fracture when compared with women without diabetes. Other factors, such as duration of diabetes, and diabetes complications, such as neuropathy and kidney disease, likely affect both the bone mineral density and fracture risk.

Diffuse idiopathic skeletal hyperostosis (DISH) is characterized by ossification of the anterior longitudinal ligaments of the spine and various extraspinal ligaments. It causes stiffness and decreased range of spinal motion. The peripheral joints most commonly affected are the metacarpophalangeal joints, elbows, and shoulders. Diabetes, obesity, hypertension, and dyslipidemia are risk factors for this condition.

Hyperuricemia and acute and tophaceous gout are more common in type 2 diabetes.

Bursitis, particularly of the shoulders and hips, occurs more frequently than expected in patients with diabetes.

Chin JA et al. Diabetes mellitus and peripheral vascular disease: diagnosis and management. Clin Podiatr Med Surg. 2014 Jan; 31(1):11–26. [PMID: 24296015]

Razmaria AA. Diabetic neuropathy. JAMA Patient Page. JAMA. 2015 Nov 24;314(20):2202. [PMID: 26599195]

Singleton JR et al. The diabetic neuropathies: practical and rational therapy. Semin Neurol. 2012 Jul;32(3):196–203. [PMID: 23117944]

Stitt AW et al. The progress in understanding and treatment of diabetic retinopathy. Prog Retin Eye Res. 2016 Mar;51:156–86. [PMID: 26297071]

Waanders F et al. Current concepts in the management of diabetic nephropathy. Neth J Med. 2013 Nov;71(9):448–58. [PMID: 24218418]

Wright JT Jr et al; SPRINT research group. A randomized trial of intensive versus standard blood-pressure control. N Engl J Med. 2015 Nov 26;373(22):2103–16. [PMID: 26551272]

▶ Special Situations

A. Diabetes Management in the Hospital

Most patients with diabetes are hospitalized for reasons other than their diabetes. Indeed, up to 10–15% of all hospitalized patients have diabetes. Audits suggest that as many as a 30% of these hospitalized patients have inappropriate management of their diabetes, with such errors as being given metformin where contraindicated, failure to act on high blood glucose levels, omission of diabetes medication, no record of diabetes complications, and inappropriate insulin management or blood glucose monitoring. It is challenging using outpatient oral therapies or insulin regimens in the hospital because patients are not eating as usual; they are often fasting for procedures; clinical events increase adverse reactions associated with diabetes medicines, eg, thiazolidinediones can cause fluid retention and worsen heart failure; metformin should not be used in patients with significant chronic kidney or liver disease, or those getting contrast for radiographic studies. Subcutaneous or intravenous insulin therapy is frequently substituted for other diabetes medicines because the insulin dose can be adjusted to match changing inpatient needs and it is safe to use insulin in patients with heart, kidney, and liver disease.

Surgery represents a stress situation during which most of the insulin antagonists (eg, catecholamines, growth hormone, and corticosteroids) are mobilized. In the diabetic patient, this can lead to a worsening of hyperglycemia and perhaps even ketoacidosis. The aim of medical management of people with diabetes during the perioperative period is to minimize these stress-induced changes. Recommendations for management depend both on the patient's usual diabetic regimen and on the type of surgery (major or minor) to be done (see also Chapter 3).

For people with diabetes controlled with diet alone, no special precautions must be taken unless diabetic control is markedly disturbed by the procedure. If this occurs, small doses of short-acting insulin as needed will correct the hyperglycemia.

Patients taking oral agents should not take them on the day of surgery. If there is significant hyperglycemia, small doses of short-acting insulin are given as needed. If this approach does not provide adequate control, an insulin infusion should be started in the manner indicated below. The oral agents can be restarted once the patient is eating normally after the operation. It is important to order a postoperative serum creatinine level to ensure adequate kidney function prior to restarting metformin therapy.

Patients taking insulin represent the only serious challenge to management of diabetes when surgery is necessary. However, with careful attention to changes in the clinical or laboratory picture, glucose control can be managed successfully. The protocol used to control the glucose depends on the kind of diabetes (type 1 or type 2); whether it is minor surgery (lasting less than 2 hours and patient eating afterwards) or major surgery (lasting more than 2 hours, with invasion of a body cavity, and patient not eating afterwards); and the preoperative insulin regimen (basal bolus or premixed insulin twice a day or premeal bolus only or regular insulin before meals and NPH at bedtime). Patients with type 1 diabetes must be receiving some insulin to prevent the development of diabetic ketoacidosis. Many patients with type 2 diabetes who are taking insulin do well perioperatively without insulin for a few hours. Ideally, patients with diabetes should undergo surgery early in the morning. Table 27–10 summarizes the approach for these patients.

One insulin infusion method adds 10 units of regular insulin to 1 L of 5% dextrose in 0.45% saline, and this is infused intravenously at a rate of 100–180 mL/h. This gives the patient 1–1.8 units of insulin per hour which, except in the most severe cases, generally keeps the blood glucose within the range of 100–250 mg/dL (5.5–13.9 mmol/L). The infusion may be continued for several days, if necessary. Perioperatively, plasma glucose or blood glucose should be determined every 2–4 hours to be sure metabolic control is adequate. If it is not, adjustments in the ratio of insulin to dextrose in the intravenous solution can be made.

An alternative method consists of separate infusions of insulin and glucose delivered by pumps to permit independent adjustments of each infusion rate, depending on hourly variation of blood glucose values. There are a number of different algorithms available for insulin infusions (see http://www.hospitalmedicine.org).

Table 27–10. Recommendations for management of insulin-treated diabetes during surgery.

Type of Diabetes	Minor Surgical Procedures (< 2 hours; eating afterwards)	Major Surgical Procedures (> 2 hours; invasion of body cavity; not eating immediately after recovery)
Type 2: Patients taking basal bolus insulin regimen; twice daily premixed insulin	No insulin on the day of operation. Start 5% dextrose infusion; monitor fingerstick blood glucose and give subcutaneous short-acting insulin every 4 or 6 hours	Same regimen as minor procedure. If control is not satisfactory, then intravenous insulin infusion
Type 1: Patients taking basal bolus insulin regimen or using insulin pump	Patients using pump should discontinue the pump the evening before procedure and given 24-hour basal insulin. On day of procedure, start 5% dextrose; monitor blood glucose and give subcutaneous short-acting insulin every 4 or 6 hours	Initiate insulin infusion on morning of procedure and transition back to usual regimen when eating

After surgery, when the patient has resumed an adequate oral intake, subcutaneous administration of insulin can be resumed and intravenous administration of insulin and dextrose can be stopped 30 minutes after the first subcutaneous dose. Insulin needs may vary in the first several days after surgery because of continuing postoperative stresses and because of variable caloric intake. In this situation, multiple doses of short-acting insulin plus some long-acting basal insulin, guided by blood glucose determinations, can keep the patient in acceptable metabolic control.

In the **intensive care units (ICUs),** glucose levels are controlled most frequently using insulin infusions. Patients receiving total parenteral nutrition can have insulin added to the bag. Standard total parenteral nutrition contains 25% dextrose so an infusion rate of 50 mL/h delivers 12.5 g of dextrose per hour.

On the **general surgical and medical wards,** most patients are treated with subcutaneous insulin regimens. Limited cross-sectional and prospective studies suggest that the best glucose control is achieved on a combination of basal and bolus regimen with 50% of daily insulin needs provided by intermediate- or long-acting insulins. Standardized order sets can reduce errors, and they often include algorithms for recognition and treatment of hypoglycemia (see http://ucsfinpatientdiabetes.pbworks.com for examples).

The morbidity and mortality in diabetic patients is twice that of nondiabetic patients. Those with new-onset hyperglycemia (ie, those without a preadmission diagnosis of diabetes) have even higher mortality—almost eightfold that of nondiabetic patients in one study. These observations have led to the question of whether tight glycemic control in the hospital improves outcomes.

A large multicenter, multinational study (NICE-SUGAR) recruited 6104 surgical and medical ICU patients with hyperglycemia (20% had diabetes) and randomized them to tight control (blood glucose levels of 81–108 mg/dL [4.5–6 mmol/L]) or less tight control (glucose levels less than 180 mg/dL [10 mmol/L]). The tight group achieved blood glucose levels of 115 ± 18 mg/dL (6.4 ± 1.0 mmol/L) and the conventional group, 144 ± 23 mg/dL (8 ± 1.3 mmol/L). There were more deaths (829 versus 751 deaths) in the tight glucose control group compared with the less tight glucose control group ($P = 0.02$). The excess deaths in the intensive group were due to cardiovascular events. The intensively treated group also had more cases of severe hypoglycemia (206 versus 15 cases).

A study on tight intraoperative glycemic control during cardiac surgery also failed to show any benefit; if anything, the intensively treated group had more events. The United Kingdom Glucose Insulin in Stroke Trial (GIST-UK) failed to show beneficial effect of tight glycemic control in stroke patients; however, the investigators acknowledged that, because of slow recruitment, the study was underpowered.

Thus, based on the evidence available, ICU patients with diabetes and new-onset hyperglycemia with blood glucose levels above 180 mg/dL (10 mmol/L) should be treated with insulin, aiming for target glucose levels between 140 mg/dL (7.8 mmol/L) and 180 mg/dL

(10 mmol/L). In the ICU setting, aiming for blood glucose levels close to 100 mg/dL (5.6 mmol/L) is not beneficial and may even be harmful. When patients leave the ICU, target glucose values between 100 mg/dL (5.6 mmol/L) and 180 mg/dL (10 mmol/L) may be appropriate, although this view is based on clinical observations rather than conclusive evidence.

B. Pregnancy and the Diabetic Patient

Tight glycemic control with normal HbA$_{1c}$ levels is very important during pregnancy. Early in pregnancy, poor control increases the risk of spontaneous abortion and congenital malformations. Late in pregnancy, poor control can result in polyhydramnios, preterm labor, stillbirth, and fetal macrosomia with its associated problems. Diabetes complications can impact both maternal and fetal health. Diabetic retinopathy can first develop during pregnancy or retinopathy that is already present can worsen. Diabetic women with microalbuminuria can have worsening albuminuria during pregnancy and are at higher risk for preeclampsia. Patients who have preexisting kidney failure (prepregnancy creatinine clearance less than 80 mL/min) are at high risk for further decline in kidney function during the pregnancy, and this may not reverse after delivery. Diabetic gastroparesis can severely exacerbate the nausea and vomiting of pregnancy and some patients may require fluid and nutritional support.

Although there is evidence that glyburide is safe during pregnancy, the current practice is to control diabetes with insulin therapy. Every effort should be made, utilizing multiple injections of insulin or a continuous infusion of insulin by pump, to maintain near-normalization of fasting and preprandial blood glucose values while avoiding hypoglycemia.

Regular and NPH insulin and the insulin analogs lispro, aspart, and detemir are labeled pregnancy category B. Insulin glargine, glulisine, and degludec are labeled category C because of lack of clinical safety data. A small study using insulin glargine in 32 pregnancies did not reveal any problems.

Unless there are fetal or maternal complications, diabetic women should be able to carry the pregnancy to full-term, delivering at 38 to 41 weeks. Induction of labor before 39 weeks may be considered if there is concern about increasing fetal weight. See Chapter 19 for further details.

Blumer I et al. Diabetes and pregnancy: an endocrine society clinical practice guideline. J Clin Endocrinol Metab. 2013 Nov; 98(11):4227–49. [PMID: 24194617]

Kansagara D et al. Intensive insulin therapy in hospitalized patients: a systematic review. Ann Intern Med. 2011 Feb 15; 154(4):268–82. [PMID: 21320942]

▶ Prognosis

The DCCT showed that the previously poor prognosis for as many as 40% of patients with type 1 diabetes is markedly improved by optimal care. DCCT participants were generally young and highly motivated and were cared for in academic centers by skilled diabetes educators and endocrinologists who were able to provide more attention and services than are usually available. Improved training of primary care providers may be beneficial.

For type 2 diabetes, the UKPDS documented a reduction in microvascular disease with glycemic control, although this was not apparent in the obese subgroup. Cardiovascular outcomes were not improved by glycemic control, although antihypertensive therapy showed benefit in reducing the number of adverse cardiovascular complications as well as in reducing the occurrence of microvascular disease among hypertensive patients. In patients with visceral obesity, successful management of type 2 diabetes remains a major challenge in the attempt to achieve appropriate control of hyperglycemia, hypertension, and dyslipidemia. Once safe and effective methods are devised to prevent or manage obesity, the prognosis of type 2 diabetes with its high cardiovascular risks should improve considerably.

In addition to poorly understood genetic factors relating to differences in individual susceptibility to development of long-term complications of hyperglycemia, it is clear that in both types of diabetes, the diabetic patient's intelligence, motivation, and awareness of the potential complications of the disease contribute significantly to the ultimate outcome.

▶ When to Refer

- All patients should receive self-management education when diabetes is diagnosed and at intervals thereafter. The instructional team must include a registered dietitian and registered nurse; they must be Certified Diabetes Educators (CDEs).
- Patients with type 1 diabetes should be referred to an endocrinologist for comanagement with a primary care provider.
- Patients with type 2 diabetes should be referred to an endocrinologist if treatment goals are not met or if the patient requires an increasingly complex regimen to maintain glycemic control.
- Patients with type 2 diabetes should be referred to an ophthalmologist or optometrist for a dilated eye examination when the diabetes is diagnosed, and patients with type 1 diabetes should be referred 5 years after the diagnosis is made.
- Patients with peripheral neuropathy, especially those with loss of protective threshold (unable to detect 5.07 Semmes-Weinstein filament) or structural foot problems, should be referred to a podiatrist.
- Referrals to other specialists may be required for management of chronic complications of diabetes.

American Association of Diabetes Educators http://www.aad-enet.org/
American Diabetes Association http://www.diabetes.org/home
American Diabetes Association. Standards of Medical Care in Diabetes—2015. Diabetes Care. 2015 Jan;38(Suppl 1):S11–90. [PMID: 25537706]
American Dietetic Association http://www.eatright.org
Juvenile Diabetes Foundation http://www.jdf.org/index.html

DIABETIC COMA

Coma may be due to a variety of causes not directly related to diabetes. Certain causes directly related to diabetes require differentiation: (1) Hypoglycemic coma resulting from excessive doses of insulin or oral hypoglycemic agents. (2) Hyperglycemic coma associated with either severe insulin deficiency (diabetic ketoacidosis) or mild to moderate insulin deficiency (hyperglycemic hyperosmolar state). (3) Lactic acidosis associated with diabetes, particularly in patients with diabetes stricken with severe infections or with cardiovascular collapse.

DIABETIC KETOACIDOSIS

ESSENTIALS OF DIAGNOSIS

- ▶ Hyperglycemia greater than 250 mg/dL (13.9 mmol/L).
- ▶ Acidosis with blood pH < 7.3.
- ▶ Serum bicarbonate less than 15 mEq/L.
- ▶ Serum positive for ketones.

▶ General Considerations

Diabetic ketoacidosis may be the initial manifestation of type 1 diabetes or may result from increased insulin requirements in type 1 diabetes patients during the course of infection, trauma, myocardial infarction, or surgery. It is a life-threatening medical emergency with a mortality rate just under 5% in individuals under 40 years of age, but with a more serious prognosis in the elderly, who have mortality rates over 20%. The National Data Group reports an annual incidence of five to eight episodes of diabetic ketoacidosis per 1000 diabetic persons. Ketoacidosis may develop in patients with type 2 diabetes when severe stress such as sepsis or trauma is present. Diabetic ketoacidosis has been found to be one of the more common serious complications of insulin pump therapy, occurring in approximately 1 per 80 patient-months of treatment. Many patients who monitor capillary blood glucose regularly ignore urine ketone measurements, which would signal the possibility of insulin leakage or pump failure before serious illness develops. Poor compliance, either for psychological reasons or because of inadequate education, is one of the most common causes of recurrent diabetic ketoacidosis.

▶ Clinical Findings

A. Symptoms and Signs

The appearance of diabetic ketoacidosis is usually preceded by a day or more of polyuria and polydipsia associated with marked fatigue, nausea, and vomiting. If untreated, mental stupor ensues that can progress to coma. Drowsiness is fairly common, but frank coma only occurs in about 10% of patients. On physical examination, evidence of dehydration in a stuporous patient with rapid deep breathing and a "fruity" breath odor of acetone would strongly suggest the diagnosis. Hypotension with tachycardia indicates profound fluid and electrolyte depletion, and mild hypothermia is usually present. Abdominal pain and even tenderness may be present in the absence of abdominal disease. Conversely, cholecystitis or pancreatitis may occur with minimal symptoms and signs.

B. Laboratory Findings

Typically, the patient with moderately severe diabetic ketoacidosis has a plasma glucose of 350–900 mg/dL (19.4–50 mmol/L), serum ketones at a dilution of 1:8 or greater or beta-hydroxybutyrate more than 4 nmol/L, hyperkalemia (serum potassium level of 5–8 mEq/L), slight hyponatremia (serum sodium of approximately 130 mEq/L), hyperphosphatemia (serum phosphate level of 6–7 mg/dL [1.9–2.3 mmol/L]), and elevated blood urea nitrogen and serum creatinine levels (Table 27–11). Acidosis may be severe (pH ranging from 6.9 to 7.2 and serum bicarbonate ranging from 5 mEq/L to 15 mEq/L); PCO_2 is low (15–20 mm Hg) related to hyperventilation. Fluid depletion is marked, typically about 100 mL/kg.

The difference between venous and arterial pH is 0.02 to 0.15 pH units and venous and arterial bicarbonate is 1.88 mEq/L. These small differences will not affect either the diagnosis or the management of diabetic ketoacidosis, and there is no need to collect arterial blood for measuring the acid-base status.

The hyperkalemia occurs despite total body potassium depletion because of the shift of potassium from the intracellular to extracellular spaces that occurs in systemic acidosis. The average total body potassium deficit resulting from osmotic diuresis, acidosis, and gastrointestinal losses is about 3–5 mEq/kg. Similarly, despite the elevated serum phosphate, total body phosphate is generally depleted. Serum sodium is generally reduced due to loss of sodium ions (7–10 mEq/kg) by polyuria and vomiting and because

severe hyperglycemia shifts intracellular water into the interstitial compartment. There is some controversy about the correction factor for the serum sodium in the presence of hyperglycemia. Many guidelines recommend a correction factor, whereby the serum sodium concentration decreases by 1.6 mEq/L for every 100 mg/dL (5.56 mmol/L) rise in plasma glucose above normal, but there is evidence that the decrease may be greater when patients have more severe hyperglycemia (greater than 400 mg/dL or 22.2 mmol/L) and/or volume depletion. One group has suggested (based on short-term exposure of normal volunteers to markedly elevated glucose levels) that, when the serum glucose is greater than 200 mg/dL (11.1 mmol/L), the serum sodium concentration decreases by at least 2.4 mEq/L. Serum osmolality can be directly measured by standard tests of freezing point depression or can be estimated by calculating the molarity of sodium, chloride, and glucose in the serum. A convenient method of estimating effective serum osmolality is as follows (normal values in humans are 280–300 mOsm/kg):

$$mOsm/kg = 2\,[\text{measured Na}^+] + \frac{\text{Glucose (mg/dL)}}{18}$$

These calculated estimates are usually 10–20 mOsm/kg lower than values measured by standard cryoscopic techniques. Central nervous system depression or coma occurs when the effective serum osmolality exceeds 320–330 mOsm/L. Coma in a diabetic patient with a lower osmolality should prompt a search for cause of coma other than hyperosmolality (see Chapter 21).

Ketoacidemia represents the effect of insulin lack at multiple enzyme loci. Insulin lack associated with elevated levels of growth hormone, catecholamines, and glucagon contributes to increases in lipolysis from adipose tissue and in hepatic ketogenesis. In addition, reduced ketolysis by insulin-deficient peripheral tissues

Table 27–11. Laboratory diagnosis of coma in diabetic patients.

	Urine Glucose	Urine Ketones	Plasma Glucose	Plasma Bicarbonate	Plasma Ketones
Related to diabetes					
Hypoglycemia	0[1]	0 or +	Low	Normal	0
Diabetic ketoacidosis	++++	++++	High	Low	++++
Hyperglycemic hyperosmolar state coma	++++	0	High	Normal or slightly low	0
Lactic acidosis	0 or +	0 or +	Normal or low or high	Low	0 or +
Unrelated to diabetes					
Alcohol or other toxic drugs	0 or +	0 or +	May be low	Normal or low[2]	0 or +
Cerebrovascular accident or head trauma	+ or 0	0	Often high	Normal	0
Uremia	0 or +	0	High or normal	Low	0 or +

[1]Leftover urine in bladder might still contain glucose from earlier hyperglycemia.
[2]Alcohol can elevate plasma lactate as well as keto acids to reduce pH.

contributes to the ketoacidemia. The only true "keto" acid present is acetoacetic acid which, along with its by-product acetone, is measured by nitroprusside reagents (Acetest and Ketostix). The sensitivity for acetone, however, is poor, requiring over 10 mmol/L, which is seldom reached in the plasma of ketoacidotic patients—although this detectable concentration is readily achieved in urine. Thus, in the plasma of ketotic patients, only acetoacetate is measured by these reagents. The more prevalent beta-hydroxybutyric acid has no ketone group and is therefore not detected by conventional nitroprusside tests. This takes on special importance in the presence of circulatory collapse during diabetic ketoacidosis, wherein an increase in lactic acid can shift the redox state to increase beta-hydroxybutyric acid at the expense of the readily detectable acetoacetic acid. Bedside diagnostic reagents are then unreliable, suggesting no ketonemia in cases where beta-hydroxybutyric acid is a major factor in producing the acidosis. Combined glucose and ketone meter (Precision Xtra, Nova Max Plus) that measure blood beta-hydroxybutyrate concentration on capillary blood are now available. Many clinical laboratories also offer direct blood beta-hydroxybutyrate measurement.

Nonspecific elevations of serum amylase and lipase occurs in about 16–25% of cases of diabetic ketoacidosis, and an imaging study may be necessary if the diagnosis of acute pancreatitis is being seriously considered. Leukocytosis as high as 25,000/mcL with a left shift may occur with or without associated infection. The presence of an elevated or even a normal temperature would suggest the presence of an infection, since patients with diabetic ketoacidosis are generally hypothermic if uninfected.

▶ **Treatment**

Patients with mild diabetic ketoacidosis are alert and have pH levels between 7.25 and 7.30 and beta-hydroxybutyrate levels of 3–4 mmol/L; those with moderate ketoacidosis are either alert or little drowsy and have pH levels between 7.0 and 7.24 and beta-hydroxybutyrate levels of 4–8 mmol/L; and those with severe ketoacidosis are stuporose and have a pH < 7.0 and beta-hydroxybutyrate levels of greater than 8 mmol/L. Those with mild ketoacidosis can be treated in the emergency department, but those with moderate or severe ketoacidosis require admission to the ICU or step-down unit. Therapeutic goals are to restore plasma volume and tissue perfusion, reduce blood glucose and osmolality toward normal, correct acidosis, replenish electrolyte losses, and identify and treat precipitating factors. Gastric intubation is recommended in the comatose patient to prevent vomiting and aspiration that may occur as a result of gastric atony, a common complication of diabetic ketoacidosis. An indwelling catheter may also be necessary. In patients with preexisting heart or kidney failure or those in severe cardiovascular collapse, a central venous pressure catheter should be inserted to evaluate the degree of hypovolemia and to monitor subsequent fluid administration.

A comprehensive flow sheet that includes vital signs, serial laboratory data, and therapeutic interventions (eg, fluids, insulin) should be meticulously maintained by the clinician responsible for the patient's care. Plasma glucose should be recorded hourly and electrolytes and pH at least every 2–3 hours during the initial treatment period. Bedside glucose meters should be used to titrate the insulin therapy. The patient should not receive sedatives or opioids in order to avoid masking signs and symptoms of impeding cerebral edema.

A. Fluid Replacement

In most patients, the fluid deficit is 4–5 L. Initially, 0.9% saline solution is the solution of choice to help reexpand the contracted vascular volume and should be started in the emergency department as soon as the diagnosis is established. The saline should be infused rapidly to provide 1 L/h over the first 1–2 hours. After the first 2 L of fluid have been given, the intravenous infusion should be at the rate of 300–400 mL/h. Use 0.9% ("normal") saline unless the serum sodium is greater than 150 mEq/L, when 0.45% ("half normal") saline solution should be used. The volume status should be very carefully monitored. Failure to give enough volume replacement (at least 3–4 L in 8 hours) to restore normal perfusion is one of the most serious therapeutic shortcomings adversely influencing satisfactory recovery. Excessive fluid replacement (more than 5 L in 8 hours) may contribute to acute respiratory distress syndrome or cerebral edema. When blood glucose falls to approximately 250 mg/dL (13.9 mmol/L), the fluids should be changed to a 5% glucose-containing solution to maintain serum glucose in the range of 250–300 mg/dL (13.9–16.7 mmol/L). This will prevent the development of hypoglycemia and will also reduce the likelihood of cerebral edema, which could result from too rapid decline of blood glucose.

B. Insulin Replacement

Immediately after initiation of fluid replacement, regular insulin should be given intravenously in a loading dose of 0.1 unit/kg as a bolus to prime the tissue insulin receptors. Following the initial bolus, intravenous doses of insulin as low as 0.1 unit/kg/h are continuously infused or given hourly as an intramuscular injection; this is sufficient to replace the insulin deficit in most patients. A prospective randomized study showed that a bolus dose is not required if patients are given hourly insulin infusion at 0.14 unit/kg. Replacement of insulin deficiency helps correct the acidosis by reducing the flux of fatty acids to the liver, reducing ketone production by the liver, and also improving removal of ketones from the blood. Insulin treatment reduces the hyperosmolality by reducing the hyperglycemia. It accomplishes this by increasing removal of glucose through peripheral utilization as well as by decreasing production of glucose by the liver. This latter effect is accomplished by direct inhibition of gluconeogenesis and glycogenolysis as well as by lowered amino acid flux from muscle to liver and reduced hyperglucagonemia.

The insulin dose should be "piggy-backed" into the fluid line so the rate of fluid replacement can be changed without altering the insulin delivery rate. If the plasma glucose level fails to fall at least 10% in the first hour, a repeat loading dose (0.1 or 0.14 unit/kg) is recommended. Rarely, a patient with immune insulin resistance is encountered, and this requires doubling the insulin dose every 2–4 hours if hyperglycemia does not improve after the first two doses of insulin. The insulin dose should be adjusted to lower the glucose concentration by about 50–70 mg/dL (2.8–3.9 mmol/L). Patients who are normally take insulin glargine or insulin detemir can be given their usual maintenance doses during initial treatment of their diabetic ketoacidosis. The continuation of their subcutaneous basal insulins means that lower doses of intravenous insulin will be needed, and there will be a smoother transition from intravenous insulin infusion to the subcutaneous regimen.

C. Potassium

Total body potassium loss from polyuria and vomiting may be as high as 200 mEq. However, because of shifts of potassium from cells into the extracellular space as a consequence of acidosis, serum potassium is usually normal to slightly elevated prior to institution of treatment. As the acidosis is corrected, potassium flows back into the cells, and hypokalemia can develop if potassium replacement is not instituted. If the patient is not uremic and has an adequate urinary output, potassium chloride in doses of 10–30 mEq/h should be infused during the second and third hours after beginning therapy as soon as the acidosis starts to resolve. Replacement should be started sooner if the initial serum potassium is inappropriately normal or low and should be delayed if serum potassium fails to respond to initial therapy and remains above 5 mEq/L, as in cases of chronic kidney disease. Occasionally, a patient may present with a serum potassium level less than 3.5 mEq/L, in which case insulin therapy should be delayed until the potassium level is corrected to greater than 3.5 mEq/L. An ECG can be of help in monitoring the patient's potassium status: High peaked T waves are a sign of hyperkalemia, and flattened T waves with U waves are a sign of hypokalemia. Foods high in potassium content should be prescribed when the patient has recovered sufficiently to take food orally. Tomato juice has 14 mEq of potassium per 240 mL, and a medium-sized banana provides about 10 mEq.

D. Sodium Bicarbonate

The use of sodium bicarbonate in management of diabetic ketoacidosis has been questioned since clinical benefit was not demonstrated in one prospective randomized trial and because of the following potentially harmful consequences: (1) development of hypokalemia from rapid shift of potassium into cells if the acidosis is overcorrected; (2) tissue anoxia from reduced dissociation of oxygen from hemoglobin when acidosis is rapidly reversed (leftward shift of the oxygen dissociation curve); and (3) cerebral acidosis resulting from lowering of cerebrospinal fluid pH. It must be emphasized, however, that these considerations are less important when very severe acidosis exists. Therefore, it is recommended that bicarbonate be administered to diabetic patients in ketoacidosis if the arterial blood pH is 7.0 or less, with careful monitoring to prevent overcorrection.

One or two ampules of sodium bicarbonate (one ampule contains 44 mEq/50 mL) should be added to 1 L of 0.45% saline with 20 mEq KCl or to 400 mL of sterile water with 20 mEq KCl and infused over 1 to 2 hours. (**Note:** Addition of sodium bicarbonate to 0.9% saline would produce a markedly hypertonic solution that could aggravate the hyperosmolar state already present.) It can be repeated until the arterial pH reaches 7.1, but *it should not be given if the pH is 7.1 or greater* since additional bicarbonate would increase the risk of rebound metabolic alkalosis as ketones are metabolized. Alkalosis shifts potassium from serum into cells, which could precipitate a fatal cardiac arrhythmia.

E. Phosphate

Phosphate replacement is seldom required in treating diabetic ketoacidosis. However, if severe hypophosphatemia of less than 1 mg/dL (0.32 mmol/L) develops during insulin therapy, a small amount of phosphate can be replaced per hour as the potassium salt. However, three randomized studies in which phosphate was replaced in patients with diabetic ketoacidosis did not show any apparent clinical benefit from phosphate administration. Moreover, attempts to use potassium phosphate as the sole means of replacing potassium have led to a number of reported cases of severe hypocalcemia with tetany. To minimize the risk of inducing tetany from too-rapid replacement of phosphate, the average deficit of 40–50 mmol of phosphate should be replaced intravenously at a rate *no greater than 3–4 mmol/h* in a 60–70-kg person. A stock solution (Abbott) provides a mixture of 1.12 g KH_2PO_4 and 1.18 g K_2HPO_4 in a 5-mL single-dose vial (this equals 22 mmol of potassium and 15 mmol of phosphate). One-half of this vial (2.5 mL) should be added to 1 L of either 0.45% saline or 5% dextrose in water. Two liters of this solution, infused at a rate of 400 mL/h, will correct the phosphate deficit at the optimal rate of 3 mmol/h while providing 4.4 mEq of potassium per hour. (Additional potassium should be administered as potassium chloride to provide a total of 10–30 mEq of potassium per hour, as noted above.) If the serum phosphate remains below 2.5 mg/dL (0.8 mmol/L) after this infusion, a repeat 5-hour infusion can be given.

F. Hyperchloremic Acidosis During Therapy

Because of the considerable loss of keto acids in the urine during the initial phase of therapy, substrate for subsequent regeneration of bicarbonate is lost and correction of the total bicarbonate deficit is hampered. A portion of the bicarbonate deficit is replaced with chloride ions infused in large amounts as saline to correct the dehydration. In most patients, as the ketoacidosis clears during insulin replacement, a hyperchloremic, low-bicarbonate pattern emerges with a normal anion gap. This is a relatively benign condition that reverses itself over the subsequent 12–24 hours once intravenous saline is no longer being administered. Using a balanced electrolyte solution similar to serum in chloride concentration and pH during resuscitation instead of normal saline has been reported to prevent the hyperchloremic acidosis.

G. Treatment of Associated Infection

Antibiotics are prescribed as indicated. Cholecystitis and pyelonephritis may be particularly severe in these patients.

H. Transition to Subcutaneous Insulin Regimen

Once the diabetic ketoacidosis is controlled and the patient is awake and able to eat, subcutaneous insulin therapy can be initiated. The patient with type 1 diabetes may have persistent significant tissue insulin resistance and may require a total daily insulin dose of approximately 0.6 units/kg. The amount of insulin required in the previous 8 hours can also be helpful in estimating the initial insulin doses. Half the total daily dose can be given as a long-acting basal insulin and the other half as short-acting insulin premeals. The patient should receive subcutaneous basal insulin and rapid-acting insulin analog with the first meal and the insulin infusion discontinued an hour later. The overlap of the subcutaneous insulin action and insulin infusion is necessary to prevent relapse of the diabetic ketoacidosis. The increased insulin resistance is only present for a few days, and it is important to reduce both the basal and bolus insulins to avoid hypoglycemia. A patient with new-onset type 1 diabetes usually still has significant beta cell function and may not need any basal insulin and only very low doses of rapid-acting insulin before meals after recovery from the ketoacidosis. Patients with type 2 diabetes and diabetes ketoacidosis due to severe illness may initially require insulin therapy but can often transition back to oral agents during outpatient follow-up.

► Prognosis

Low-dose insulin infusion and fluid and electrolyte replacement combined with careful monitoring of patients' clinical and laboratory responses to therapy have dramatically reduced the mortality rates of diabetic ketoacidosis to less than 5%. However, this complication remains a significant risk in the aged who have mortality rates greater than 20% and in patients in profound coma in whom treatment has been delayed. Acute myocardial infarction and infarction of the bowel following prolonged hypotension worsen the outlook. A serious prognostic sign is end-stage chronic kidney disease, and prior kidney dysfunction worsens the prognosis considerably because the kidney plays a key role in compensating for massive pH and electrolyte abnormalities. Symptomatic cerebral edema occurs primarily in the pediatric population. Risk factors for its development include severe baseline acidosis, rapid correction of hyperglycemia, and excess volume administration in the first 4 hours. Onset of headache or deterioration in mental status during treatment should lead to consideration of this complication. Intravenous mannitol at a dosage of 1–2 g/kg given over 15 minutes is the mainstay of treatment. Excess crystalloid infusion can precipitate pulmonary edema. Acute respiratory distress syndrome is a rare complication of treatment of diabetic ketoacidosis.

After recovery and stabilization, patients should be instructed on how to recognize the early symptoms and signs of ketoacidosis. Urine ketones or capillary blood beta-hydroxybutyrate should be measured in patients with signs of infection or in insulin pump-treated patients when capillary blood glucose remains unexpectedly and persistently high. When heavy ketonuria and glycosuria persist on several successive examinations, supplemental rapid acting insulin should be administered and liquid foods such as lightly salted tomato juice and broth should be ingested to replenish fluids and electrolytes. The patient should be instructed to contact the clinician if ketonuria persists, and especially if there is vomiting and inability to keep down fluids. Recurrent episodes of severe ketoacidosis often indicate poor compliance with the insulin regimen, and these patients will require intensive counseling.

Savage MW et al. Joint British Diabetes Societies guideline for the management of diabetic ketoacidosis. Diabet Med. 2011 May;28(5):508–15. [PMID: 21255074]

HYPERGLYCEMIC HYPEROSMOLAR STATE

ESSENTIALS OF DIAGNOSIS

- ► Hyperglycemia greater than 600 mg/dL (33.3 mmol/L).
- ► Serum osmolality greater than 310 mOsm/kg.
- ► No acidosis; blood pH > 7.3.
- ► Serum bicarbonate greater than 15 mEq/L.
- ► Normal anion gap (less than 14 mEq/L).

► General Considerations

This second most common form of hyperglycemic coma is characterized by severe hyperglycemia in the absence of significant ketosis, with hyperosmolality and dehydration. It occurs in patients with mild or occult diabetes, and most patients are typically middle-aged to elderly. Accurate figures are not available as to its true incidence, but from data on hospital discharges it is rarer than diabetic ketoacidosis even in older age groups. Underlying chronic kidney disease or heart failure is common, and the presence of either worsens the prognosis. A precipitating event such as infection, myocardial infarction, stroke, or recent operation is often present. Certain medications such as phenytoin, diazoxide, corticosteroids, and diuretics have been implicated in its pathogenesis, as have procedures associated with glucose loading such as peritoneal dialysis.

► Pathogenesis

A partial or relative insulin deficiency may initiate the syndrome by reducing glucose utilization of muscle, fat, and liver while inducing hyperglucagonemia and increasing hepatic glucose output. With massive glycosuria, obligatory water loss ensues. If a patient is unable to maintain adequate fluid intake because of an associated acute or chronic illness or has suffered excessive fluid loss, marked dehydration results. As the plasma volume contracts, kidney function becomes impaired, limiting the urinary glucose losses and exacerbating the hyperglycemia. Severe hyperosmolality develops that causes mental confusion and finally coma. It is not clear why ketosis is virtually absent under these conditions of insulin insufficiency, although reduced levels of growth hormone may be a factor, along with portal vein insulin concentrations sufficient to restrain ketogenesis.

▶ Clinical Findings

A. Symptoms and Signs

Onset may be insidious over a period of days or weeks, with weakness, polyuria, and polydipsia. The lack of features of ketoacidosis may retard recognition of the syndrome and delay therapy until dehydration becomes more profound than in ketoacidosis. Reduced intake of fluid is not an uncommon historical feature, due to either inappropriate lack of thirst, nausea, or inaccessibility of fluids to elderly, bedridden patients. Lethargy and confusion develop as serum osmolality exceeds 310 mOsm/kg, and convulsions and coma can occur if osmolality exceeds 320–330 mOsm/kg. Physical examination confirms the presence of profound dehydration in a lethargic or comatose patient without Kussmaul respirations.

B. Laboratory Findings

Severe hyperglycemia is present, with blood glucose values ranging from 800 mg/dL to 2400 mg/dL (44.4 mmol/L to 133.2 mmol/L) (Table 27–11). In mild cases, where dehydration is less severe, dilutional hyponatremia as well as urinary sodium losses may reduce serum sodium to 120–125 mEq/L, which protects to some extent against extreme hyperosmolality. However, as dehydration progresses, serum sodium can exceed 140 mEq/L, producing serum osmolality readings of 330–440 mOsm/kg. Ketosis and acidosis are usually absent or mild. Prerenal azotemia is the rule, with serum urea nitrogen elevations over 100 mg/dL (35.7 mmol/L) being typical.

▶ Treatment

A. Fluid Replacement

Fluid replacement is of paramount importance in treating nonketotic hyperglycemic coma. The onset of hyperosmolarity is more insidious in elderly people without ketosis than in younger individuals with high serum ketone levels, which provide earlier indicators of severe illness (vomiting, rapid deep breathing, acetone odor, etc). Consequently, diagnosis and treatment are often delayed until fluid deficit has reached levels of 6–10 L.

If hypovolemia is present as evidenced by hypotension and oliguria, fluid therapy should be initiated with 0.9% saline. In all other cases, 0.45% saline appears to be preferable as the initial replacement solution because the body fluids of these patients are markedly hyperosmolar. As much as 4–6 L of fluid may be required in the first 8–10 hours. Careful monitoring of the patient is required for proper sodium and water replacement. Once blood glucose reaches 250 mg/dL (13.9 mmol/L), fluid replacement should include 5% dextrose in either water, 0.45% saline solution, or 0.9% saline solution. The rate of dextrose infusion should be adjusted to maintain glycemic levels of 250–300 mg/dL (13.9–16.7 mmol/L) in order to reduce the risk of cerebral edema. An important end point of fluid therapy is to restore urinary output to 50 mL/h or more.

B. Insulin

Less insulin may be required to reduce the hyperglycemia in nonketotic patients as compared to those with diabetic ketoacidotic coma. In fact, fluid replacement alone can reduce hyperglycemia considerably by correcting the hypovolemia, which then increases both glomerular filtration and renal excretion of glucose. Insulin treatment should therefore be delayed unless the patient has significant ketonemia (beta-hydroxybutyrate more than 1 mmol/L). Start the insulin infusion rate at 0.05 units/kg/h (bolus is not needed) and titrate to lower blood glucose levels by 50–70 mg/dL per hour (2.8–3.9 mmol/L/h). Once the patient has stabilized and the blood glucose falls to around 250 mg/dL (13.9 mmol/L), insulin can be given subcutaneously.

C. Potassium

With the absence of acidosis, there may be no initial hyperkalemia unless associated end-stage chronic kidney disease is present. This results in less severe total potassium depletion than in diabetic ketoacidosis, and less potassium replacement is therefore needed. However, because initial serum potassium is usually not elevated and because it declines rapidly as a result of insulin's effect on driving potassium intracellularly, it has been recommended that potassium replacement be initiated earlier than in ketotic patients, assuming that no chronic kidney disease or oliguria is present. Potassium chloride (10 mEq/L) can be added to the initial bottle of fluids administered if the patient's serum potassium is not elevated.

D. Phosphate

If severe hypophosphatemia (serum phosphate less than 1 mg/dL [0.32 mmol/L]) develops during insulin therapy, phosphate replacement can be given as described for ketoacidotic patients (at 3 mmol/h).

▶ Prognosis

The severe dehydration and low output state may predispose the patient to complications such as myocardial infarction, stroke, pulmonary embolism, mesenteric vein thrombosis, and disseminated intravascular coagulation. Fluid replacement remains the primary approach to the prevention of these complications. Low-dose heparin prophylaxis is reasonable but benefits of routine anticoagulation remain doubtful. Rhabdomyolysis is a recognized complication and should be looked for and treated.

The overall mortality rate of hyperglycemic hyperosmolar state coma is more than ten times that of diabetic ketoacidosis, chiefly because of its higher incidence in older patients, who may have compromised cardiovascular systems or associated major illnesses and whose dehydration is often excessive because of delays in recognition and treatment. (When patients are matched for age, the prognoses of these two hyperglycemic emergencies are reasonably comparable.) When prompt therapy is instituted, the mortality rate can be reduced from nearly 50% to that related to the severity of coexistent disorders.

After the patient is stabilized, the appropriate form of long-term management of the diabetes must be determined. Insulin treatment should be continued for a few weeks but patients usually recover sufficient endogenous insulin secretion to make a trial of diet or diet plus oral agents worthwhile. When the episode occurs in a patient who has known diabetes, then education of the patient and caregivers should be instituted. They should be taught how to recognize situations (nausea and vomiting, infection) that predispose to recurrence of the hyperglycemic, hyperosmolar state, as well as detailed information on how to prevent the escalating dehydration that culminates in hyperosmolar coma (small sips of sugar-free liquids, increase in usual hypoglycemic therapy, or early contact with the clinician).

Nyenwe EA et al. Evidence-based management of hyperglycemic emergencies in diabetes mellitus. Diabetes Res Clin Pract. 2011 Dec;94(3):340–51. [PMID: 21978840]

Scott AR; Joint British Diabetes Societies (JBDS) for Inpatient Care; JBDS hyperosmolar hyperglycaemic guidelines group. Management of hyperosmolar hyperglycaemic state in adults with diabetes. Diabet Med. 2015 Jun;32(6):714–24. [PMID: 25980647]

LACTIC ACIDOSIS

ESSENTIALS OF DIAGNOSIS

► Severe acidosis with hyperventilation.

► Blood pH below 7.30.

► Serum bicarbonate less than 15 mEq/L.

► Anion gap greater than 15 mEq/L.

► Absent serum ketones.

► Serum lactate greater than 5 mmol/L.

► General Considerations

Lactic acidosis is characterized by accumulation of excess lactic acid in the blood. Normally, the principal sources of this acid are the erythrocytes (which lack enzymes for aerobic oxidation), skeletal muscle, skin, and brain. Conversion of lactic acid to glucose and its oxidation principally by the liver but also by the kidneys represent the chief pathways for its removal. Overproduction of lactic acid (tissue hypoxia), deficient removal (hepatic failure), or both (circulatory collapse) can cause accumulation. Lactic acidosis is not uncommon in any severely ill patient suffering from cardiac decompensation, respiratory or hepatic failure, septicemia, or infarction of bowel or extremities. Lactic acidosis in patients with diabetes mellitus is uncommon but occasionally occurs in metformin-treated patients (see above) and it still must be considered in the acidotic diabetic patient, especially if the individual is seriously ill. Most cases of metformin-associated lactic acidosis occur in patients in whom there were contraindications to the use of metformin, in particular kidney failure.

► Clinical Findings

A. Symptoms and Signs

The main clinical feature of lactic acidosis is marked hyperventilation. When lactic acidosis is secondary to tissue hypoxia or vascular collapse, the clinical presentation is variable, being that of the prevailing catastrophic illness. However, in the idiopathic, or spontaneous, variety, the onset is rapid (usually over a few hours), blood pressure is normal, peripheral circulation is good, and there is no cyanosis.

B. Laboratory Findings

Plasma bicarbonate and blood pH are quite low, indicating the presence of severe metabolic acidosis. Ketones are usually absent from plasma and urine or at least not prominent. The first clue may be a high anion gap (serum sodium minus the sum of chloride and bicarbonate anions [in mEq/L] should be no greater than 15). A higher value indicates the existence of an abnormal compartment of anions. If this cannot be clinically explained by an excess of keto acids (diabetes), inorganic acids (uremia), or anions from medication overdosage (salicylates, methyl alcohol, ethylene glycol), then lactic acidosis is probably the correct diagnosis. (See also Chapter 21.) In the absence of azotemia, hyperphosphatemia may be a clue to the presence of lactic acidosis for reasons that are not clear. The diagnosis is confirmed by demonstrating, in a sample of blood that is promptly chilled and separated, a plasma lactic acid concentration of 5 mmol/L or higher (values as high as 30 mmol/L have been reported). Normal plasma values average 1 mmol/L, with a normal lactate/pyruvate ratio of 10:1. This ratio is greatly exceeded in lactic acidosis.[1]

► Treatment

Aggressive treatment of the precipitating cause of lactic acidosis is the main component of therapy, such as ensuring adequate oxygenation and vascular perfusion of tissues. Empiric antibiotic coverage for sepsis should be given after culture samples are obtained in any patient in whom the cause of the lactic acidosis is not apparent.

Alkalinization with intravenous sodium bicarbonate to keep the pH above 7.2 has been recommended by some in the emergency treatment of lactic acidosis; as much as 2000 mEq in 24 hours has been used. However, there is no evidence that the mortality rate is favorably affected by

---

[1] In collecting samples, it is essential to rapidly chill and separate the blood in order to remove red cells, whose continued glycolysis at room temperature is a common source of error in reports of high plasma lactate. Frozen plasma remains stable for subsequent assay.

administering bicarbonate, and its use remains controversial. Hemodialysis may be useful in cases where large sodium loads are poorly tolerated and in cases associated with metformin toxicity.

▶ Prognosis

The mortality rate of spontaneous lactic acidosis is high. The prognosis in most cases is that of the primary disorder that produced the lactic acidosis.

Lalau JD. Lactic acidosis induced by metformin: incidence, management and prevention. Drug Saf. 2010 Sep 1;33(9):727–40. [PMID: 20701406]

◢ THE HYPOGLYCEMIC STATES

Spontaneous hypoglycemia in adults is of two principal types: fasting and postprandial. Symptoms begin at plasma glucose levels in the range of 60 mg/dL (3.3 mmol/L) and impairment of brain function at approximately 50 mg/dL (2.8 mmol/L). Fasting hypoglycemia is often subacute or chronic and usually presents with neuroglycopenia as its principal manifestation; postprandial hypoglycemia is relatively acute and is often heralded by symptoms of neurogenic autonomic discharge (sweating, palpitations, anxiety, tremulousness).

▶ Differential Diagnosis (Table 27–12)

Fasting hypoglycemia may occur in certain endocrine disorders, such as hypopituitarism, Addison disease, or myxedema; in disorders related to liver malfunction, such as acute alcoholism or liver failure; and in instances of end-stage chronic kidney disease, particularly in patients requiring dialysis. These conditions are usually obvious, with hypoglycemia being only a secondary feature. When fasting hypoglycemia is a primary manifestation developing in adults without apparent endocrine disorders or

Table 27–12. Common causes of hypoglycemia in adults.[1]

Fasting hypoglycemia
Pancreatic B cell tumor
Surreptitious administration of insulin or sulfonylureas
Extrapancreatic tumors
Postprandial hypoglycemia
Alimentary
Noninsulinoma pancreatogenous hypoglycemia syndrome
Functional
Occult diabetes mellitus
Alcohol-related hypoglycemia
Immunopathologic hypoglycemia
Idiopathic anti-insulin antibodies (which release their bound insulin)
Antibodies to insulin receptors (which act as agonists)
Drug-induced hypoglycemia

[1]In the absence of clinically obvious endocrine, renal, or hepatic disorders and exclusive of diabetes mellitus treated with hypoglycemic agents.

inborn metabolic diseases from childhood, the principal diagnostic possibilities include: (1) hyperinsulinism, due to either pancreatic B cell tumors, iatrogenic or surreptitious administration of insulin or sulfonylurea and (2) hypoglycemia due to extrapancreatic tumors.

Postprandial (reactive) hypoglycemia may be seen after gastrointestinal surgery and is particularly associated with the dumping syndrome after gastrectomy and Roux-en-Y gastric bypass surgery. Occult diabetes very occasionally present with postprandial hypoglycemia. Rarely, it occurs with islet cell hyperplasia—the so-called noninsulinoma pancreatogenous hypoglycemia syndrome.

Alcohol-related hypoglycemia is due to hepatic glycogen depletion combined with alcohol-mediated inhibition of gluconeogenesis. It is most common in malnourished alcohol abusers but can occur in anyone who is unable to ingest food after an acute alcoholic episode followed by gastritis and vomiting.

Immunopathologic hypoglycemia is an extremely rare condition in which anti-insulin antibodies or antibodies to insulin receptors develop spontaneously. In the former case, the mechanism appears to relate to increasing dissociation of insulin from circulating pools of bound insulin. When antibodies to insulin receptors are found, most patients do not have hypoglycemia but rather severe insulin-resistant diabetes and acanthosis nigricans. However, during the course of the disease in these patients, certain anti-insulin receptor antibodies with agonist activity mimicking insulin action may develop, producing severe hypoglycemia.

HYPOGLYCEMIA DUE TO PANCREATIC B CELL TUMORS

ESSENTIALS OF DIAGNOSIS

▶ Hypoglycemic symptoms—frequently neuroglycopenic (confusion, blurred vision, diplopia, anxiety, convulsions).

▶ Immediate recovery upon administration of glucose.

▶ Blood glucose less than 45 mg/dL (2.5 mmol/L) with a serum insulin level of 6 microunit/mL or more.

▶ General Considerations

Fasting hypoglycemia in an otherwise healthy, well-nourished adult is rare and is most commonly due to an adenoma of the islets of Langerhans. Ninety percent of such tumors are single and benign, but multiple adenomas can occur as well as malignant tumors with functional metastases. Adenomas may be familial, and multiple adenomas have been found in conjunction with tumors of the parathyroids and pituitary (MEN type 1 [MEN 1]). It has been reported that about 30% of sporadic insulinoma tumors have a somatic mutation in the YY1 gene (T372R) that encodes the transcriptional repressor YY1. Over 99% of insulinomas are located within the pancreas and less than 1% in ectopic pancreatic tissue.

▶ Clinical Findings

A. Symptoms and Signs

The most important prerequisite to diagnosing an insulinoma is simply to consider it, particularly in relatively healthy-appearing persons who have fasting hypoglycemia associated with some degree of central nervous system dysfunction such as confusion or abnormal behavior. A delay in diagnosis can result in unnecessary treatment for psychomotor epilepsy or psychiatric disorders and may cause irreversible brain damage. In long-standing cases, obesity can result as a consequence of overeating to relieve symptoms.

The so-called Whipple triad is characteristic of hypoglycemia regardless of the cause. It consists of (1) a history of hypoglycemic symptoms, (2) an associated fasting blood glucose of 45 mg/dL (2.5 mmol/L) or less, and (3) immediate recovery upon administration of glucose. The hypoglycemic symptoms in insulinoma often develop in the early morning or after missing a meal. Occasionally, they occur after exercise. They typically begin with evidence of central nervous system glucose lack and can include blurred vision or diplopia, headache, feelings of detachment, slurred speech, and weakness. Personality and mental changes vary from anxiety to psychotic behavior, and neurologic deterioration can result in convulsions or coma. Sweating and palpitations may not occur.

Hypoglycemic unawareness is very common in patients with insulinoma. They adapt to chronic hypoglycemia by increasing their efficiency in transporting glucose across the blood-brain barrier, which masks awareness that their blood glucose is approaching critically low levels. Counterregulatory hormonal responses as well as neurogenic symptoms such as tremor, sweating, and palpitations are therefore blunted during hypoglycemia. If lack of these warning symptoms prevents recognition of the need to eat to correct the problem, patients can lapse into severe hypoglycemic coma. However, symptoms and normal hormone responses during experimental insulin-induced hypoglycemia have been shown to be restored after successful surgical removal of the insulinoma. Presumably with return of euglycemia, adaptive effects on glucose transport into the brain are corrected, and thresholds of counterregulatory responses and neurogenic autonomic symptoms are therefore restored to normal.

B. Laboratory Findings

B cell adenomas do not reduce secretion of insulin in the presence of hypoglycemia, and the critical diagnostic test is to demonstrate inappropriately elevated serum insulin, proinsulin, and C-peptide levels at a time when plasma glucose level is below 45 mg/dL.

The diagnostic criteria for insulinoma after a 72-hour fast are listed in Table 27–13. Other causes of hyperinsulinemic hypoglycemia must be considered, including factitious

Table 27–13. Diagnostic criteria for insulinoma after a 72-hour fast.

Laboratory Test	Result
Plasma glucose	< 45 mg/dL (2.5 mmol/L)
Plasma insulin (RIA)[1]	≥ 6 microunit/mL (36 pmol/L)
Plasma insulin (ICMA)[1]	≥ 3 microunit/mL (18 pmol/L)
Plasma C-peptide	≥ 200 pmol/L (0.2 nmol/L, 0.6 ng/mL)
Plasma proinsulin	≥ 5 pmol/L
Beta-hydroxybutyrate	≤ 2.7 mmol/L
Sulfonylurea screen (including repaglinide and nateglinide)	Negative

[1]Conversion factors: insulin microunit/mL × 6.0 = pmol/L; C-peptide ng/mL × 0.333 = nmol/L
RIA, radioimmunoassay; ICMA, immunochemiluminometric assays.

administration of insulin or sulfonylureas. Factitious use of insulin will result in suppression of endogenous insulin secretion and low C-peptide levels. In patients who have injected insulin, the insulin/C-peptide ratio (pmol/L) will be greater than 1. An elevated circulating proinsulin level in the presence of fasting hypoglycemia is characteristic of most B cell adenomas and does not occur in factitious hyperinsulinism. Thus, C-peptide levels (by immunochemiluminometric assays [ICMA]) of greater than 200 pmol/L and proinsulin levels (by radioimmunoassay [RIA]) of greater than 5 pmol/L are characteristic of insulinomas. In patients with insulinoma, plasma beta-hydroxybutyrate levels are suppressed to 2.7 mmol/L or less. No single hormone measurement (insulin, proinsulin, C-peptide) is 100% sensitive and specific for the diagnosis of insulinoma, and insulinoma cases have been reported with insulin levels below 3 microunit/mL (ICMA assay) or proinsulin level below 5 pmol/L. These hormonal assays are also not standardized between laboratories, and there can be significant variation in the results. Therefore, the diagnosis should be based on multiple biochemical parameters.

In patients with epigastric distress, a history of renal calculi, or menstrual or erectile dysfunction, a serum calcium, gastrin, or prolactin level may be useful in screening for MEN 1 associated with insulinoma.

C. Diagnostic Tests

If the history is consistent with episodic spontaneous hypoglycemia, patients should be given a home blood glucose monitor and advised to monitor blood glucose levels at the time of symptoms and before consumption of carbohydrates, if this can be done safely. Patients with insulinomas frequently report fingerstick blood glucose levels between 40 mg/dL (2.2 mmol/L) and 50 mg/dL (2.8 mmol/L) at the time of symptoms. The diagnosis, however, cannot be made based on a fingerstick blood glucose. It is necessary to have a low laboratory glucose concomitantly with elevated plasma insulin, proinsulin, and C-peptide levels and a negative sulfonylurea screen. When patients give a history of symptoms after only a short period of food withdrawal or with exercise, then an outpatient assessment can be attempted. The patient should be brought by a family member to the office after an overnight fast and observed in the office. Activity such as walking should be encouraged and fingerstick blood glucose measured repeatedly during observation. If symptoms occur or fingerstick blood glucose is below 50 mg/dL (2.8 mmol/L) then samples for plasma glucose, insulin, C-peptide, proinsulin, sulfonylurea screen, serum ketones, and antibodies to insulin should be sent. If outpatient observation does not result in symptoms or hypoglycemia and if the clinical suspicion remains high, then the patient should undergo an inpatient supervised 72-hour fast. A suggested protocol for the supervised fast is shown in Table 27–14.

In 30% of patients with insulinoma, the blood glucose levels often drop below 45 mg/dL (2.5 mmol/L) after an overnight fast, but some patients require up to 72 hours to develop symptomatic hypoglycemia. However, the term "72-hour fast" is actually a misnomer in most cases since the fast should be immediately terminated as soon as symptoms appear and laboratory confirmation of hypoglycemia is available. In normal male subjects, the blood glucose does not fall below 55–60 mg/dL (3.1–3.3 mmol/L) during a 3-day fast. In contrast, in normal premenopausal women who have fasted for only 24 hours, the plasma glucose may fall normally to such an extent that it can reach values as low as 35 mg/dL (1.9 mmol/L). In these cases,

however, the women are not symptomatic, presumably owing to the development of sufficient ketonemia to supply energy needs to the brain. Insulinoma patients, on the other hand, become symptomatic when plasma glucose drops to subnormal levels, since inappropriate insulin secretion restricts ketone formation. Moreover, the demonstration of a nonsuppressed insulin level of 6 microunit/mL or more using a RIA assay (greater than 3 microunit/mL using an ICMA assay) in the presence of hypoglycemia suggests the diagnosis of insulinoma. If hypoglycemia does not develop in a male patient after fasting for up to 72 hours—and particularly when this prolonged fast is terminated with a period of moderate exercise—insulinoma must be considered an unlikely diagnosis.

Stimulation with pancreatic B cell secretagogues such as tolbutamide, glucagon, or leucine has been devised to demonstrate exaggerated and prolonged insulin secretion in the presence of insulinomas. However, because insulin-secreting tumors have a wide range of granule content and degrees of differentiation, they are variably responsive to these secretagogues; and a negative response does not necessarily rule out an insulinoma. For these reasons, stimulation tests are not recommended in the diagnostic work-up of insulinoma.

An oral glucose tolerance test is of no value in the diagnosis of insulin secreting tumors. HbA$_{1c}$ levels may be low but there is considerable overlap with normal patients and no particular value is diagnostic.

D. Preoperative Localization of B Cell Tumors

After the diagnosis of insulinoma has been unequivocally made by clinical and laboratory findings, studies to localize the tumor should be initiated. The focus of attention should be directed to the pancreas since that is where virtually all insulinomas originate.

Because of the small size of these tumors (averaging 1.5 cm in diameter in one large series), imaging studies do not necessarily identify all of them. A pancreatic dual phase helical CT scan with thin section can identify 82–94% of the lesions. MRI scans with gadolinium can be helpful in detecting a tumor in 85% of cases. One case report suggests that diffusion-weighted MRI can be useful for detecting and localizing small insulinomas, especially for those with no hypervascular pattern. The imaging study used will depend on local availability and local radiologic skill. If the imaging study is normal, then an endoscopic ultrasound should be performed. In experienced hands, about 80–90% of tumors can be detected with this procedure. Fine-needle aspiration of the identified lesion can be attempted to confirm the presence of a neuroendocrine tumor. If the tumor is not identified or the imaging result is equivocal, then the patient should undergo selective calcium-stimulated angiography, which has been reported to localize the tumor to a particular region of the pancreas approximately 90% of the time. In this test, angiography is combined with injections of calcium gluconate into the gastroduodenal, splenic, and superior mesenteric arteries, and insulin levels are measured in the hepatic vein effluent. The procedure is performed after an overnight fast. Calcium gluconate 10% solution diluted to a volume

Table 27–14. Suggested hospital protocol for supervised fast in diagnosis of insulinoma.

(1) Obtain baseline plasma glucose, insulin, proinsulin, and C-peptide measurements at onset of fast and place intravenous cannula.

(2) Permit only calorie-free and caffeine-free fluids and encourage supervised activity (such as walking).

(3) Measure urine for ketones at the beginning and every 12 hours and at end of fast.

(4) Obtain capillary glucose measurements with a reflectance meter every 4 hours until values < 60 mg/dL are obtained. Then increase the frequency of fingersticks to each hour, and when capillary glucose value is < 45 mg/dL send a venous blood sample to the laboratory for plasma glucose,[1] insulin, proinsulin, and C-peptide measurements. Check frequently for manifestations of neuroglycopenia.

(5) If symptoms of hypoglycemia occur **or** if a laboratory value of serum glucose is < 45 mg/dL, or if 72 hours have elapsed then conclude the fast with a final blood sample for plasma glucose,[1] insulin, proinsulin, C-peptide, beta-hydroxybutyrate and sulfonylurea measurements. Then give oral fast-acting carbohydrate followed by a meal. If the patient is confused or unable to take oral agents, then administer 50 mL of 50% dextrose intravenously over 3 to 5 minutes. Do not conclude a fast based simply on a capillary blood glucose measurement—wait for the laboratory glucose value—unless the patient is very symptomatic and it would be dangerous to wait.

[1]Glucose sample should be collected in sodium fluoride containing tube on ice to prevent glycolysis and the plasma separated immediately upon receipt at the laboratory. Arrange for the laboratory to run the glucose samples "stat."

of 5 mL with 0.95% saline is bolused into the selected artery at a dose of 0.0125 mmol calcium/kg (0.005 mmol calcium/kg for obese patients). Small samples of blood (5 mL) are taken from the hepatic effluent at times 0, 30, 60, 90, 120, and 180 seconds after the calcium injection. Fingerstick blood glucose levels are measured at intervals and a dextrose infusion is maintained throughout the procedure to prevent hypoglycemia. Calcium stimulates insulin release from insulinomas but not normal islets, and so a step-up from baseline in insulin levels at 30 or 60 seconds (twofold or greater) regionalizes the source of the hyperinsulinism to the head of the pancreas for the gastroduodenal artery, the uncinate process for the superior mesenteric artery, and the body and tail of the pancreas for the splenic artery calcium infusions. A less than twofold elevation of insulin in the 120-second sample may represent effects of recirculating calcium and is not considered a positive localization. In a single insulinoma, the response is in one artery alone unless the tumor resides in an area fed by two arteries or if there are multiple insulinomas (eg, in MEN 1). Patients who have diffuse islet hyperplasia (the noninsulinoma pancreatogenous hypoglycemia syndrome) will have positive responses in multiple arteries. Because diazoxide may interfere with this test, it should be discontinued for at least 48–72 hours before sampling. Patients should be closely monitored during the procedure to avoid hypoglycemia (as well as hyperglycemia, which could affect insulin gradients). These studies combined with careful intraoperative ultrasonography and palpation by a surgeon experienced in insulinoma surgery identifies up to 98% of tumors.

▶ **Treatment**

The treatment of choice for insulin-secreting tumors is surgical resection. While waiting for surgery, patients should be given oral diazoxide. Divided doses of 300–400 mg/day usually suffice although an occasional patient may require up to 800 mg/day. Side effects include edema due to sodium retention, gastric irritation, and mild hirsutism. Hydrochlorothiazide, 25–50 mg daily, can be used to counteract the sodium retention and edema as well potentiate diazoxide's hyperglycemic effect.

In patients with a single benign pancreatic B cell adenoma, 90–95% have a successful cure at the first surgical attempt when intraoperative ultrasound is used by a skilled surgeon. Diazoxide should be administered on the day of the surgery because it reduces the risk of hypoglycemia during surgery. Typically, it does not mask the glycemic rise indicative of surgical cure. Blood glucose should be monitored throughout surgery, and 5% or 10% dextrose infusion should be used to maintain euglycemia. In cases where the diagnosis has been established but no adenoma is located after careful palpation and use of intraoperative ultrasound, it is no longer advisable to blindly resect the body and tail of the pancreas, since a nonpalpable tumor missed by ultrasound is most likely embedded within the fleshy head of the pancreas that is left behind with subtotal resections. Most surgeons prefer to close the incision and schedule a selective arterial calcium stimulation with hepatic venous sampling to locate the tumor site prior to a repeat operation. Laparoscopy using ultrasound and enucleation has been successful with a single tumor of the body or tail of the pancreas, but open surgery remains necessary for tumors in the head of the pancreas.

In patients with inoperable functioning islet cell carcinoma with and without hepatic metastasis and in approximately 5–10% of MEN 1 cases when subtotal removal of the pancreas has failed to produce cure, the treatment approach is the same as for other types of pancreatic neuroendocrine tumors (pNETs). Diazoxide is the treatment of choice in preventing hypoglycemia. Frequent carbohydrate feedings (every 2–3 hours) can also be helpful, although weight gain can become a problem. If patients are unable to tolerate diazoxide because of gastrointestinal upset, hirsutism, or edema, verapamil (which inhibits insulin release from insulinoma cells) can be tried. Somatostatin analogs, octreotide or lanreotide, should be considered if diazoxide is ineffective or if there is tumor progression. These drugs not only inhibit insulin secretion but also have antiproliferative activity. Surgery or embolization (bland, chemo- and radio-) or thermal ablation (radiofrequency, microwave, and cryoablation) can be used to reduce tumor burden and also provide symptomatic relief. There are also chemotherapy regimens that can be considered. Regimens include combination of streptozocin, 5–fluorouracil, and doxorubicin; capecitabine and oxaliplatin; and capecitabine and temozolomide. There is only limited data regarding efficacy of these regimens. Targeted therapies against multiple steps in PI3K/AKT/mTor pathway have been shown to be helpful; everoliumus, an inhibitor of mTor, has been approved for treatment of advanced pNETs. Sunitinib, a monoclonal antibody against VEGF receptors 2 and 3, PDGFR alpha and beta and c-kit, has been shown to slow growth of pNETs. Treatment with radioisotopes (indium -111 or yttrium-90 or lutetium-177) linked to a somatostatin analog have been reported to show benefit in a proportion of patients.

Cryer PE et al. Evaluation and management of adult hypoglycemic disorders: an Endocrine Society Clinical Practice Guideline. J Clin Endocrinol Metab. 2009 Mar;94(3):709–28. [PMID: 19088155]

Mathur A et al. Insulinoma. Surg Clin North Am. 2009 Oct; 89(5):1105–21. [PMID: 19836487]

NONISLET CELL TUMOR HYPOGLYCEMIA

These rare causes of hypoglycemia include mesenchymal tumors such as retroperitoneal sarcomas, hepatocellular carcinomas, adrenocortical carcinomas, and miscellaneous epithelial-type tumors. The tumors are frequently large and readily palpated or visualized on CT scans or MRI.

In many cases the hypoglycemia is due to the expression and release of an incompletely processed insulin-like growth factor 2 (IGF-2) by the tumor. This immature form of the IGF-II molecule (pro-IGF-2 or "big IGF-2") binds IGF-binding protein-3 (IGFBP-3) but not to the acid-labile subunit. As a consequence, this pro-IGF-II remains active and binds to insulin receptors in muscle to promote glucose transport and to insulin receptors in liver and kidney to reduce glucose output. It also binds to receptors for IGF-1 in the pancreatic B cell to inhibit insulin secretion and in the pituitary to suppress growth hormone release. With the reduction of growth hormone, there is a consequent lowering of IGF-1 levels as well as IGFBP-3 and acid-labile subunit.

The diagnosis is supported by laboratory documentation of serum insulin levels below 5 microunit/mL with plasma glucose levels of 45 mg/dL (2.5 mmol/L) or lower. Values for growth hormone and IGF-1 are also decreased. Levels of IGF-2 may be increased but often are "normal" in quantity, despite the presence of the immature, higher-molecular-weight form of IGF-2, which can only be detected by special laboratory techniques.

Not all the patients with nonislet cell tumor hypoglycemia have elevated pro-IGF-II. Ectopic insulin production has been described in bronchial carcinoma, ovarian carcinoma, and small cell carcinoma of the cervix. Hypoglycemia due to IgF-1 released from a metastatic large cell carcinoma of the lung has also been reported. GLP-1 secreting tumors (ovarian and pNETs) can also cause hypoglycemia by stimulating insulin release from normal pancreatic islets.

The prognosis for these tumors is generally poor, and surgical removal should be attempted when feasible. Dietary management of the hypoglycemia is the mainstay of medical treatment, since diazoxide is usually ineffective.

Bodnar TW et al. Management of non-islet-cell tumor hypoglycemia: a clinical review. J Clin Endocrinol Metab. 2014 Mar; 99(3):713–22. [PMID: 24423303]

POSTPRANDIAL HYPOGLYCEMIA

1. Hypoglycemia Following Gastric Surgery

Hypoglycemia sometimes develops in patients who have undergone gastric surgery (eg, gastrectomy, vagotomy, pyloroplasty, gastrojejunostomy, Nissan fundoplication, Bilroth II procedure and Roux-en-Y), especially when they consume foods containing high levels of carbohydrates. This late dumping syndrome occurs about 1–3 hours after a meal and is a result of rapid delivery of high concentration of carbohydrates in the proximal small bowel and rapid absorption of glucose. The hyperinsulinemic response to the high carbohydrate load causes hypoglycemia. The symptoms include lightheadedness, sweating, confusion and even loss of consciousness after eating a high carbohydrate meal. It is likely that excessive release of gastrointestinal hormones such as GLP-1 play a role in the hyperinsulinemic response. It has been reported that treatment with exendin 9-39, a GLP-1 receptor agonist can prevent post gastric bypass hypoglycemia. The incidence of secondary dumping syndrome declined with the advent of medical therapy for peptic ulcer disease. There has been resurgence of cases, however, with the popularity of Roux-en-Y gastric bypass surgery for the treatment of morbid obesity. Patients typically complain of symptoms that are more severe after consumption of large amounts of readily absorbable carbohydrates. In terms of documenting hypoglycemia, it is reasonable to request the patient to consume a meal that leads to symptoms during everyday life. An oral glucose tolerance test is not recommended because many normal persons have false-positive test results. There have been case reports of insulinoma and noninsulinoma pancreatogenous hypoglycemia syndrome in patients with hypoglycemia post Roux-en-Y surgery. It is unclear how often this occurs. A careful history may identify patients who have a history of hypoglycemia with exercise or missed meals, and these individuals may require a formal 72-hour fast to rule out an insulinoma.

Treatment for secondary dumping includes dietary modification, but this may be difficult to sustain. Patients can try more frequent meals with smaller portions of less rapidly digested carbohydrates. Alpha-glucosidase therapy may be a useful adjunct to a low carbohydrate diet. Octreotide 50 mcg administered subcutaneously two or three times a day 30 minutes prior to each meal has been reported to improve symptoms due to late dumping syndrome. Various surgical procedures to delay gastric emptying have been reported to improve symptoms but long-term efficacy studies are lacking.

2. Noninsulinoma Pancreatogenous Hypoglycemia Syndrome (Islet Cell Hyperplasia)

In a very small number of patients with organic hyperinsulinism, islet cell hyperplasia is present rather than an adenoma. This condition is referred to as noninsulinoma pancreatogenous hypoglycemia syndrome. These patients typically have documented hyperinsulinemic hypoglycemia after meals but not with fasting up to 72 hours. The patients have a positive response to calcium-stimulated angiography. A gradient-guided partial pancreatectomy leads to clinical remission, and the pathology of the pancreas shows evidence of islet cell hyperplasia and nesidioblastosis. These patients do not have mutations in the pancreatic islet beta-cell ATP-sensitive potassium channel inward rectifier (Kir 6.2) and the sulfonylurea receptor-1 (SUR1) genes, which have been reported in children with familial hyperinsulinemic hypoglycemia.

3. Functional Alimentary Hypoglycemia

Patients have symptoms suggestive of increased sympathetic activity, including anxiety, weakness, tremor, sweating or palpitations after meals. Physical examination and laboratory tests are normal. It is not recommended that patients with symptoms suggestive of increased sympathetic activity undergo either a prolonged oral glucose tolerance test or a mixed meal test. Instead, the patients should be given home blood glucose monitors (with memories) and instructed to monitor fingerstick glucose levels at the time of symptoms. Only patients who have symptoms when their fingerstick blood glucose is low (less than 50 mg/dL) and who have resolution of symptoms when the glucose is raised by eating rapidly released carbohydrate need additional evaluation. Patients who do not have evidence for low glucose levels at time of symptoms are generally reassured by their findings. Counseling and support should be the mainstays in therapy, with dietary manipulation only an adjunct.

4. Occult Diabetes

This condition is characterized by a delay in early insulin release from pancreatic B cells, resulting in initial exaggeration of hyperglycemia during a glucose tolerance test. In response to this hyperglycemia, an exaggerated insulin release produces a late hypoglycemia 4–5 hours after ingestion of glucose. These patients are often obese and frequently have a family history of diabetes mellitus.

Patients with this type of postprandial hypoglycemia often respond to reduced intake of refined sugars with multiple, spaced, small feedings high in dietary fiber. In the obese, treatment is directed at weight reduction to achieve ideal weight. These patients should be considered to have prediabetes or early diabetes (type 1 or 2) and advised to have periodic medical evaluations.

5. Autoimmune Hypoglycemia

Patients with autoimmune hypoglycemia have early postprandial hyperglycemia followed by hypoglycemia 3–4 hours later. The hypoglycemia is attributed to a dissociation of insulin-antibody immune complexes, releasing free insulin.

The disorder is associated with methimazole treatment for Graves disease, although it can also occur in patients treated with various other sulfhydryl-containing medications (captopril, penicillamine) as well as other drugs such as hydralazine, isoniazid, and procainamide. In addition, it has been reported in patients with autoimmune disorders such as rheumatoid arthritis, systemic lupus erythematosus, and polymyositis as well as in multiple myeloma and other plasma cell dyscrasias where paraproteins or antibodies cross-react with insulin. There is also an association with the HLA class II alleles (DRB1*0406, DQA1*0301, and DQB1*0302). These alleles are 10 to 20 times more common in Japanese and Korean populations, which explains why the disorder has been reported mostly in Japanese patients.

High titers of insulin autoantibodies, usually IgG class, can be detected. Insulin, proinsulin, and C-peptide levels may be elevated, but the results may be erroneous because of the interference of the insulin antibodies with the immunoassays for these peptides.

In most cases, the hypoglycemia is transient and usually resolves spontaneously within 3–6 months of diagnosis, particularly when the offending medications are stopped. The most consistent therapeutic benefit in management of this syndrome has been achieved by dietary treatment with small, frequent low-carbohydrate meals. Prednisone (30–60 mg orally daily) has been used to lower the titer of insulin antibodies.

Lupsa BC et al. Autoimmune forms of hypoglycemia. Medicine (Baltimore). 2009 May;88(3):141 53. [PMID: 19440117]

FACTITIOUS HYPOGLYCEMIA

Factitious hypoglycemia may be difficult to document. A suspicion of self-induced hypoglycemia is supported when the patient is associated with the health professions or has access to insulin or sulfonylurea medications taken by a diabetic member of the family. The triad of hypoglycemia, high immunoreactive insulin, and suppressed plasma C peptide immunoreactivity is pathognomonic of exogenous insulin administration. Insulin and C peptide is secreted in a 1:1 molar ratio. A large fraction of the endogenous insulin is cleared by the liver whereas C peptide, which is cleared by the kidney, has a lower metabolic clearance rate. For this reason, the molar ratio of insulin and C peptide in a hypoglycemic patient should be less than 1.0 in cases of insulinoma and is greater than 1.0 in cases of exogenous insulin administration. When sulfonylureas, repaglinide and nateglinide are suspected as a cause of factitious hypoglycemia, a plasma level of these medications to detect their presence may be required to distinguish laboratory findings from those of insulinoma.

HYPOGLYCEMIA DUE TO INSULIN RECEPTOR ANTIBODIES

Hypoglycemia due to insulin receptor autoantibodies is an extremely rare syndrome; most cases have occurred in women often with a history of autoimmune disease. Almost all of these patients have also had episodes of insulin-resistant diabetes and acanthosis nigricans. Their hypoglycemia may be either fasting or postprandial and is often severe and is attributed to an agonistic action of the antibody on the insulin receptor. Balance between the antagonistic and agonistic effects of the antibodies determines whether insulin-resistant diabetes or hypoglycemia occurs. Hypoglycemia was found to respond to corticosteroid therapy but not to plasmapheresis or immunosuppression.

Kim CH et al. Autoimmune hypoglycemia in a type 2 diabetic patient with anti-insulin and insulin receptor antibodies. Diabetes Care. 2004 Jan;27(1):288–9. [PMID: 14694017]

MEDICATION-INDUCED HYPOGLYCEMIA

A number of medications apart from the sulfonylureas can occasionally cause hypoglycemia. Common offenders include the fluoroquinolones such as gatifloxacin and levofloxacin, pentamidine, quinine, ACE inhibitors, salicylates and beta-adrenergic blocking agents. The fluoroquinolones, particularly gatifloxacin, have been associated with both hypoglycemia and hyperglycemia. It is thought that the drug acts on the ATP sensitive potassium channels in the beta cell. Hypoglycemia is an early event, and hyperglycemia occurs several days into therapy. Intravenous pentamidine is cytotoxic to beta cells and causes acute hyperinsulinemia and hypoglycemia followed by insulinopenia and hyperglycemia. Fasting patients taking noncardioselective beta-blockers can have an exaggerated hypoglycemic response to starvation. The beta-blockade inhibits fatty acids and gluconeogenesis substrate release and reduces plasma glucagon response. Therapy with ACE inhibitors increases the risk of hypoglycemia in patients who are taking insulin or sulfonylureas presumably because these drugs increase sensitivity to circulating insulin by increasing blood flow to the muscle.

Ethanol-associated hypoglycemia may be due to hepatic depletion of NADH and altered NADH:NAD ratio. This in turn limits conversion of lactate to pyruvate, the main substrate for hepatic gluconeogenesis. With prolonged starvation, glycogen reserves become depleted within 18–24 hours and hepatic glucose output becomes totally dependent on gluconeogenesis. Under these circumstances, a blood concentration of ethanol as low as 45 mg/dL (9.8 mmol/L) can induce profound hypoglycemia by blocking gluconeogenesis. Neuroglycopenia in a patient whose breath smells of alcohol may be mistaken for alcoholic stupor. Prevention consists of adequate food intake during ethanol ingestion. Therapy consists of glucose administration to replenish glycogen stores until gluconeogenesis resumes.

When sugar-containing soft drinks are used as mixers to dilute alcohol in beverages (gin and tonic, rum and cola), there seems to be a greater insulin release than when the soft drink alone is ingested and a tendency for more of a late hypoglycemic overswing to occur 3–4 hours later. Prevention would consist of avoiding sugar mixers while ingesting alcohol and ensuring supplementary food intake to provide sustained absorption.

Vue MH et al. Drug-induced glucose alterations part 1: drug-induced hypoglycemia. Diabetes Spectrum. 2011 Aug; 24(3):171–7.

Lipid Disorders

Robert B. Baron, MD, MS

For patients with known cardiovascular disease (secondary prevention), cholesterol lowering leads to a consistent reduction in total mortality and recurrent cardiovascular events in men and women and in middle-aged and older patients. Among patients without cardiovascular disease (primary prevention), the data are less conclusive, with rates of cardiovascular events, heart disease mortality, and all-cause mortality differing among studies. Nonetheless, treatment guidelines have been designed to assist clinicians in selecting patients for cholesterol-lowering therapy based on their overall risk of developing cardiovascular disease.

Hooper AJ et al. Update on primary hypobetalipoproteinemia. Curr Atheroscler Rep. 2014 Jul;16(7):423. [PMID: 24781598]

Rached FH et al. An overview of the new frontiers in the treatment of atherogenic dyslipidemias. Clin Pharmacol Ther. 2014 Jul;96(1):57–63. [PMID: 24727469]

Santos RD et al. What is new in familial hypercholesterolemia? Curr Opin Lipidol. 2014 Jun;25(3):183–8. [PMID: 24699416]

Sniderman AD et al. The severe hypercholesterolemia phenotype: clinical diagnosis, management, and emerging therapies. J Am Coll Cardiol. 2014 May 20;63(19):1935–47. [PMID: 24632267]

Sugerman DT. JAMA patient page. Blood lipids. JAMA. 2013 Oct 23;310(16):1751;. Erratum in: JAMA. 2013 Dec 11; 310(22):2460. [PMID: 24150481]

LIPID FRACTIONS & THE RISK OF CORONARY HEART DISEASE

In fasting serum, cholesterol is carried primarily on three different lipoproteins—the VLDL, LDL, and HDL molecules. Total cholesterol equals the sum of these three components:

$$\text{Total cholesterol} = \text{HDL cholesterol} + \text{VLDL cholesterol} + \text{LDL cholesterol}$$

Most clinical laboratories measure the total cholesterol, the total triglycerides, and the amount of cholesterol found in the HDL fraction, which is easily precipitated from serum. Most triglyceride is found in VLDL particles, which contain five times as much triglyceride by weight as

cholesterol. The amount of cholesterol found in the VLDL fraction can be estimated by dividing the triglyceride by 5:

$$\text{VLDL cholesterol} = \frac{\text{Triglycerides}}{5}$$

Because the triglyceride level is used as a proxy for the amount of VLDL, this formula works only in fasting samples and when the triglyceride level is less than 400 mg/dL (4.52 mmol/L). At higher triglyceride levels, LDL and VLDL cholesterol levels can be determined after ultracentrifugation or by direct chemical measurement.

The total cholesterol is reasonably stable over time; however, measurements of HDL and especially triglycerides may vary considerably because of analytic error in the laboratory and biologic variation in a patient's lipid level. Thus, the LDL should always be estimated as the mean of at least two determinations; if those two estimates differ by more than 10%, a third lipid profile is obtained. The LDL is estimated as follows:

$$\begin{array}{l} \text{LDL} \\ \text{choles-} \\ \text{terol} \end{array} = \begin{array}{l} \text{Total} \\ \text{cholesterol} \\ \text{(mg/dL)} \end{array} - \begin{array}{l} \text{HDL} \\ \text{cholesterol} \\ \text{(mg/dL)} \end{array} - \frac{\begin{array}{c}\text{Triglycerides}\\\text{(mg/dL)}\end{array}}{5}$$

When using SI units, the formula becomes

$$\begin{array}{l} \text{LDL} \\ \text{choles-} \\ \text{terol} \end{array} = \begin{array}{l} \text{Total} \\ \text{cholesterol} \\ \text{(mmol/L)} \end{array} - \begin{array}{l} \text{HDL} \\ \text{cholesterol} \\ \text{(mmol/L)} \end{array} - \frac{\begin{array}{c}\text{Triglycerides}\\\text{(mmol/L)}\end{array}}{2.2}$$

Some authorities use the ratio of the total to HDL cholesterol as an indicator of lipid-related coronary risk: the lower this ratio is, the better. Although ratios are useful predictors within populations of patients, they may obscure important information in individual patients. (A total cholesterol of 300 mg/dL [7.76 mmol/L] and an HDL of 60 mg/dL [1.56 mmol/L] result in the same ratio as a total cholesterol of 150 mg/dL [3.88 mmol/L] with an HDL of 30 mg/dL [0.78 mmol/L].) Moreover, the total cholesterol-to-HDL cholesterol ratio will magnify the importance of variations in HDL measurement.

There is no true "normal" range for serum lipids. In Western populations, cholesterol values are about 20% higher than in Asian populations and exceed 300 mg/dL (7.76 mmol/L) in nearly 5% of adults. About 10% of adults have LDL cholesterol levels above 200 mg/dL (5.17 mmol/L). Total and LDL cholesterol levels tend to rise with age in persons who are otherwise in good health.

Declines are seen in acute illness, and lipid studies in such patients are of little value with the exception of the serum triglyceride level in a patient with pancreatitis. Cholesterol levels (even when expressed as an age-matched percentile rank, such as the highest 20%) do not remain constant over time, especially from childhood through adolescence and young adulthood. Thus, children and young adults with relatively high cholesterol may have lower levels later in life, whereas those with low cholesterol may show increases.

THERAPEUTIC EFFECTS OF LOWERING CHOLESTEROL

Reducing cholesterol levels in healthy middle-aged men without CHD (primary prevention) reduces their risk in proportion to the reduction in LDL cholesterol. Treated adults have statistically significant and clinically important reductions in the rates of myocardial infarctions, strokes, new cases of angina, and need for coronary artery bypass procedures. The West of Scotland Study showed a 31% decrease in myocardial infarctions in middle-aged men treated with pravastatin compared with placebo. The Air Force/Texas Coronary Atherosclerosis Prevention Study (AFCAPS/TexCAPS) study showed similar results with lovastatin. As with any primary prevention interventions, large numbers of healthy patients need to be treated to prevent a single event. The numbers of patients needed to treat (NNT) to prevent a nonfatal myocardial infarction or a coronary artery disease death in these two studies were 46 and 50, respectively. The Anglo-Scandinavian Cardiac Outcomes Trial (ASCOT) study of atorvastatin in persons with hypertension and other risk factors but without CHD demonstrated a 36% reduction in CHD events. The Justification for the Use of Statins in Prevention: an Intervention Trial Evaluating Rosuvastatin (JUPITER) showed a 44% reduction in a combined end point of myocardial infarction, stroke, revascularization, hospitalization for unstable angina, or death from cardiovascular causes in both men and women. The NNT for 1 year to prevent one event was 169.

Primary prevention studies have found a less consistent effect on total mortality. The West of Scotland study found a 20% decrease in total mortality, tending toward statistical significance. The AFCAPS/TexCAPS study with lovastatin showed no difference in total mortality. The Antihypertensive and Lipid-Lowering Treatment to Prevent Heart Attack Trial (ALLHAT-LLT) also showed no reduction either in all-cause mortality or in CHD events when pravastatin was compared with usual care. Subjects treated with atorvastatin in the ASCOT study had a 13% reduction in mortality, but the result was not statistically

significant. This study, however, was stopped early due to the marked reduction in CHD events. The JUPITER trial demonstrated a statistically significant 20% reduction in death from any cause. The NNT for 1 year was 400.

In patients with CHD, the benefits of cholesterol lowering are clearer. Major studies with statins have shown significant reductions in cardiovascular events, cardiovascular deaths, and all-cause mortality in men and women with coronary artery disease. The NNT to prevent a nonfatal myocardial infarction or a coronary artery disease death in these studies was between 12 and 34. Aggressive cholesterol lowering with these agents causes regression of atherosclerotic plaques in some patients, reduces the progression of atherosclerosis in saphenous vein grafts, and can slow or reverse carotid artery atherosclerosis. Results with other classes of medications have been less consistent. For example, patients treated with gemfibrozil had fewer cardiovascular events, but there was no benefit in all-cause mortality when compared with placebo.

The disparities in results between primary and secondary prevention studies highlight several important points. The benefits and adverse effects of cholesterol lowering may be specific to each type of drug; the clinician cannot assume that the effects will generalize to other classes of medication. Second, the net benefits from cholesterol lowering depend on the underlying risk of CHD and of other disease. In patients with atherosclerosis, morbidity and mortality rates associated with CHD are high, and measures that reduce it are more likely to be beneficial even if they have no effect—or even slightly harmful effects—on other diseases.

Hirsh BJ et al. Utilization of and adherence to guideline-recommended lipid-lowering therapy after acute coronary syndrome: opportunities for improvement. J Am Coll Cardiol. 2015 Jul 14;66(2):184–92. [PMID: 26160634]

Jin J. JAMA patient page. PCSK9 inhibitors for treating high cholesterol. JAMA. 2015 Dec 1;314(21):2320. [PMID: 26624842]

Rader DJ et al. HDL and cardiovascular disease. Lancet. 2014 Aug 16;384(9943):618–25. [PMID: 25131981]

Ridker PM. LDL cholesterol: controversies and future therapeutic directions. Lancet. 2014 Aug 16;384(9943):607–17. [PMID: 25131980]

Savarese G et al. Benefits of statins in elderly subjects without established cardiovascular disease: a meta-analysis. J Am Coll Cardiol. 2013 Dec 3;62(22):2090–9. [PMID: 23954343]

Stone NJ et al. Treatment of blood cholesterol to reduce atherosclerotic cardiovascular disease risk in adults: synopsis of the 2013 American College of Cardiology/American Heart Association cholesterol guideline. Ann Intern Med. 2014 Mar 4; 160(5):339–43. [PMID: 24474185]

Stone NJ et al. 2013 ACC/AHA guideline on the treatment of blood cholesterol to reduce atherosclerotic cardiovascular risk in adults: a report of the American College of Cardiology/American Heart Association Task Force on Practice Guidelines. J Am Coll Cardiol. 2014 Jul 1;63(25 Pt B):2889–934. [PMID: 24239923]

Wang X et al. Cholesterol levels and risk of hemorrhagic stroke: a systematic review and meta-analysis. Stroke. 2013 Jul; 44(7):1833–9. [PMID: 23704101]

Wilkins JT et al. Coronary heart disease risks associated with high levels of HDL cholesterol. J Am Heart Assoc. 2014 Mar 13; 3(2):e000519. [PMID: 24627418]

SECONDARY CONDITIONS THAT AFFECT LIPID METABOLISM

Several factors, including drugs, can influence serum lipids. These are important for two reasons: abnormal lipid levels (or changes in lipid levels) may be the presenting sign of some of these conditions, and correction of the underlying condition may obviate the need to treat an apparent lipid disorder. Diabetes and alcohol use, in particular, are commonly associated with high triglyceride levels that decline with improvements in glycemic control or reduction in alcohol use, respectively. Thus, secondary causes of high blood lipids should be considered in each patient with a lipid disorder before lipid-lowering therapy is started. In most instances, special testing is not needed: a history and physical examination are sufficient.

CLINICAL PRESENTATIONS

Most patients with high cholesterol levels have no specific symptoms or signs. The vast majority of patients with lipid abnormalities are detected by the laboratory, either as part of the workup of a patient with cardiovascular disease or as part of a preventive screening strategy. Extremely high levels of chylomicrons or VLDL particles (triglyceride level above 1000 mg/dL or 10 mmol/L) result in the formation of **eruptive xanthomas** (Figure 28–1) (red-yellow papules, especially on the buttocks). High LDL concentrations result in **tendinous xanthomas** on certain tendons (Achilles, patella, back of the hand). Such xanthomas usually indicate one of the underlying genetic hyperlipidemias. **Lipemia retinalis** (cream-colored blood vessels in the fundus) is seen with extremely high triglyceride levels (above 2000 mg/dL or 20 mmol/L).

SCREENING & TREATMENT OF HIGH BLOOD CHOLESTEROL

All patients with cardiovascular disease and diabetes should have their lipids measured. The only exceptions are patients in whom lipid lowering is not indicated for other

▲ **Figure 28–1.** Eruptive xanthoma on the arm of a man with untreated hyperlipidemia and diabetes mellitus. (Reproduced, with permission, from Richard P. Usatine, MD.)

reasons. Patients who already have evidence of atherosclerosis are the group at highest risk for suffering additional manifestations in the near term and thus have the most to gain from lipid lowering. Additional risk reduction measures for atherosclerosis are discussed in Chapter 10; lipid lowering should be just one aspect of a program to reduce the progression and effects of the disease.

In patients with cardiovascular disease, a complete lipid profile (total cholesterol, HDL cholesterol, and triglyceride levels) after an overnight fast should be obtained. According to the 2013 American College of Cardiology/American Heart Association (ACC/AHA) guidelines, however, such patients are treated with statins independent of their lipid levels. Similarly, patients aged 40–75 with diabetes should also have a complete lipid profile. Those with diabetes and LDL greater than or equal to 70 mg/dL (1.81 mmol/L) should be treated with statins.

The best screening and treatment strategy for adults who do not have atherosclerotic cardiovascular disease is less clear. Several algorithms have been developed to guide the clinician in treatment decisions, but management decisions are individualized based on the patient's risk.

Although the 2013 ACC/AHA guidelines recommend screening of all adults aged 21 years or older for high blood cholesterol, the United States Preventive Services Task Force (USPSTF) suggests beginning at age 20 years only if there are other cardiovascular risk factors such as tobacco use, diabetes, hypertension, obesity, or a family history of premature cardiovascular disease. For men without other risk factors, screening is recommended beginning at age 35 years. For women and for men aged 20 to 35 without increased risk, the USPSTF makes no recommendation for or against routine screening for lipid disorders. Although there is no established interval for screening, screening can be repeated every 5 years for those with average or low risk and more often for those whose levels are close to therapeutic thresholds.

Individuals without cardiovascular disease should have their 10-year risk of CHD calculated. Although those with LDL cholesterol greater than 190 mg/dL (4.91 mmol/L) are recommended for treatment independent of their 10-year risk of cardiovascular disease, all other patients are recommended for treatment based on their overall cardiovascular risk. The best method for estimating 10-year risk is controversial. The 2013 ACC/AHA guidelines include a risk calculator that measures cardiovascular risk. It can be downloaded at myamericanheart.org under Statements & Guidelines and then Prevention Guidelines. It has been criticized by some authors as overestimating risk. The older Framingham 10-year calculator includes CHD but not stroke risk. One approach is to use both risk calculators until better data are available.

Numerous other risk factors have been studied in an attempt to better predict future CHD events. These include high-sensitivity C-reactive protein (hs-CRP), electron beam computed tomography (EBCT), homocysteine, fibrinogen, lipoprotein (a), LDL subfractions, ankle-brachial index, and others. Several of these, particularly hs-CRP and EBCT, may add additional prognostic ability after accounting for traditional risk factors, but no clinical trials have adequately examined the effect of these on health outcomes. Clinical guidelines suggest limiting the use of additional risk factors such as hs-CRP to selected patients if additional data are likely to change a therapeutic decision.

Several strategies for obtaining the initial cholesterol measurement have been proposed, including: (1) measuring total cholesterol alone, (2) measuring total cholesterol and HDL cholesterol, or (3) measuring LDL cholesterol. Initial measurement of the LDL cholesterol is least likely to lead to patient misinformation and misclassification and is the strategy recommended by the 2013 ACC/AHA guidelines.

Treatment decisions are based on the presence of clinical cardiovascular disease or diabetes, patient age, LDL cholesterol greater than 190 mg/dL (4.91 mmol/L), and the estimated 10-year risk of developing cardiovascular disease. The 2013 ACC/AHA guidelines define four groups of patients who benefit from statin medications: (1) individuals with clinical atherosclerotic cardiovascular disease; (2) individuals with primary elevation of LDL cholesterol greater than 190 mg/dL (4.91 mmol/L); (3) individuals aged 40–75 with diabetes and LDL greater than or equal to 70 mg/dL (1.81 mmol/L); and (4) individuals aged 40–75 without clinical atherosclerotic cardiovascular disease or diabetes, with LDL 70–189 mg/dL (1.81–4.91 mmol/L), and estimated 10-year CVD risk of 7.5% or higher.

► Screening & Treatment in Women

The foregoing screening and treatment guidelines are designed for both men and women. Yet several observational studies suggest that a low HDL cholesterol is a more important risk factor for CHD in women than a high LDL cholesterol. Meta-analysis of studies including women with known heart disease, however, has found that statins prevent recurrent myocardial infarctions in women. There is insufficient evidence to be certain of a similar effect from statins in women without evidence of CHD. Although most experts recommend application of the same primary prevention guidelines for women as for men, clinicians should be aware of the uncertainty in this area. Estimating the 10-year cardiovascular risk is particularly important in women since a larger percentage of women than men will have estimated 10-year cardiovascular risks below 7.5% per year and be advised not to take statins unless their LDL is very high (greater than 190 mg/dL [4.91 mmol/L]).

► Screening & Treatment in Older Patients

Meta-analysis of evidence relating cholesterol to CHD in the elderly suggests that cholesterol is not a risk factor for CHD for persons over age 75 years. Clinical trials have rarely included such individuals. One exception is the Prospective Study of Pravastatin in the Elderly at Risk (PROSPER). In this study, elderly patients with cardiovascular disease (secondary prevention) benefited from statin therapy, whereas those without cardiovascular disease (primary prevention) did not. The 2013 ACC/AHA guidelines suggest continuing statin treatment in patients over age 75 who have cardiovascular disease. The guidelines, however,

suggest not screening or treating patients over the age of 75 who do not have evidence of cardiovascular disease. Individual patient decisions to discontinue statin therapy should be based on overall functional status and life expectancy, comorbidities, and patient preference and should be made in context with overall therapeutic goals and end-of-life decisions.

Goff DC Jr et al. 2013 ACC/AHA Guideline on the Assessment of Cardiovascular Risk: a report of the American College of Cardiology/American Heart Association Task Force on Practice Guidelines. J Am Coll Cardiol. 2014 Jul 1;63(25 Pt B):2935–59. [PMID: 24239921]

Kavousi M et al. Comparison of application of the ACC/AHA guidelines, Adult Treatment Panel III guidelines, and European Society of Cardiology guidelines for cardiovascular disease prevention in a European cohort. JAMA. 2014 Apr 9; 311(14):1416–23. [PMID: 24681960]

Keaney JF Jr et al. A pragmatic view of the new cholesterol treatment guidelines. N Engl J Med. 2014 Jan 16;370(3):275–8. [PMID: 24283199]

Krumholz HM. Target cardiovascular risk rather than cholesterol concentration. BMJ. 2013 Nov 27;347:f7110. [PMID: 24284344]

Martin SS et al. 2013 ACC/AHA cholesterol treatment guideline: what was done well and what could be done better. J Am Coll Cardiol. 2014 Jun 24;63(24):2674–8. [PMID: 24681146]

Pencina MJ et al. Application of new cholesterol guidelines to a population-based sample. N Engl J Med. 2014 Apr 10; 370(15):1422–31. [PMID: 24645848]

Ridker PM et al. Statins: new American guidelines for prevention of cardiovascular disease. Lancet. 2013 Nov 30; 382(9907):1762–5. [PMID: 24268611]

Rubenfire M et al. HDL cholesterol and cardiovascular outcomes: what is the evidence? Curr Cardiol Rep. 2013 Apr; 15(4):349. [PMID: 23420445]

Singh S et al. Familial hypercholesterolemia–epidemiology, diagnosis, and screening. Curr Atheroscler Rep. 2015;17(2):482. [PMID: 25612857]

Stone NJ et al. 2013 ACC/AHA Guideline on the Treatment of Blood Cholesterol to Reduce Atherosclerotic Cardiovascular Risk in Adults: a report of the American College of Cardiology/American Heart Association Task Force on Practice Guidelines. J Am Coll Cardiol. 2014 Jul 1;63(25 Pt B):2889–934. [PMID: 24239923]

TREATMENT OF HIGH LDL CHOLESTEROL

Reduction of LDL cholesterol with statins is just one part of a program to reduce the risk of cardiovascular disease. Other measures—including smoking cessation, hypertension control, and aspirin—are also of central importance. Less well studied but of potential value is raising the HDL cholesterol level. Quitting smoking reduces the effect of other cardiovascular risk factors (such as a high cholesterol level); it may also increase the HDL cholesterol level. Exercise (and weight loss) may reduce the LDL cholesterol and increase the HDL. Modest alcohol use (1–2 ounces a day) also raises HDL levels and appears to have a salutary effect on CHD rates.

The use of medications to raise the HDL cholesterol has not been demonstrated to provide additional benefit. For example, cholesteryl ester transfer protein inhibitors are a class of medicines being investigated to raise HDL levels. Agents in this class, however, have not been shown to be effective. The use of niacin in addition to statins has also been carefully studied in the AIM-HIGH study and the HPS2-THRIVE study and shown not to be effective.

► Diet Therapy

Studies of nonhospitalized adults have reported only modest cholesterol-lowering benefits of dietary therapy, typically in the range of a 5–10% decrease in LDL cholesterol, with even less in the long term. The effect of diet therapy, however, varies considerably among individuals, as some patients will have striking reductions in LDL cholesterol—up to a 25–30% decrease—whereas others will have clinically important increases. Thus, the results of diet therapy should be assessed about 4 weeks after initiation.

Cholesterol-lowering diets may also have a variable effect on lipid fractions. Diets very low in total fat or in saturated fat may lower HDL cholesterol as much as LDL cholesterol. It is not known how these diet-induced changes affect coronary risk.

Several nutritional approaches to diet therapy are available. Most Americans currently eat over 35% of calories as fat, of which 15% is saturated fat. A traditional cholesterol-lowering diet recommends reducing total fat to 25–30% and saturated fat to less than 7% of calories. These diets replace fat, particularly saturated fat, with carbohydrate. In most instances, this approach will also result in fewer total calories consumed and will facilitate weight loss in overweight patients. Other diet plans, including the Dean Ornish Diet, the Pritikin Diet, and most vegetarian diets, restrict fat even further. Low-fat, high-carbohydrate diets may, however, result in reductions in HDL cholesterol.

An alternative strategy is the Mediterranean diet, which maintains total fat at approximately 35–40% of total calories but replaces saturated fat with monounsaturated fat such as that found in canola oil and in olives, peanuts, avocados, and their oils. This diet is equally effective at lowering LDL cholesterol but is less likely to lead to reductions in HDL cholesterol. Several studies have suggested that this approach may also be associated with reductions in endothelial dysfunction, insulin resistance, and markers of vascular inflammation and may result in better resolution of the metabolic syndrome than traditional cholesterol-lowering diets. A clinical trial demonstrated reduced cardiovascular events in persons on a Mediterranean diet supplemented with additional nuts or extra-virgin olive oil compared to persons on a less intensive Mediterranean diet.

Other dietary changes may also result in beneficial changes in blood lipids. Soluble fiber, such as that found in oat bran or psyllium, may reduce LDL cholesterol by 5–10%. Plant stanols and sterols can reduce LDL cholesterol by 10%. Intake of garlic, soy protein, vitamin C, and pecans, may also yield modest reductions of LDL cholesterol. Because oxidation of LDL cholesterol is a potential initiating event in atherogenesis, diets rich in antioxidants, found primarily in fruits and vegetables, may be helpful (see Chapter 29). Studies have suggested that when all of these elements are combined into a single dietary prescription, the impact of diet on LDL cholesterol may approach that of statin medications, lowering LDL cholesterol by close to 30%.

Eckel RH et al. 2013 AHA/ACC Guideline on Lifestyle Management to Reduce Cardiovascular Risk: a report of the American College of Cardiology/American Heart Association Task Force on Practice Guidelines. Circulation. 2014 Jun 24; 129(25 Suppl 2):S76–99. [PMID: 24222015]

Estruch R et al; PREDIMED Study Investigators. Primary prevention of cardiovascular disease with a Mediterranean Diet. N Engl J Med. 2013 Apr 4;368(14):1279–90. [PMID: 23432189]

Griffin BA. Nonpharmacological approaches for reducing serum low-density lipoprotein cholesterol. Curr Opin Cardiol. 2014 Jul; 29(4):360–5. [PMID: 24837072]

Kelley GA et al. Comparison of aerobic exercise, diet or both on lipids and lipoproteins in adults: a meta-analysis of randomized controlled trials. Clin Nutr. 2012 Apr;31(2):156–67. [PMID: 22154987]

Rees K et al. "Mediterranean" dietary pattern for the primary prevention of cardiovascular disease. Cochrane Database Syst Rev. 2013 Aug 12;8:CD009825. [PMID: 23939686]

Rubenfire M et al. HDL cholesterol and cardiovascular outcomes: what is the evidence? Curr Cardiol Rep. 2013 Apr; 15(4):349. [PMID: 23420445]

► Pharmacologic Therapy

Most patients whose risk from CHD is considered high enough to warrant pharmacologic therapy of an elevated LDL cholesterol should be given aspirin prophylaxis at a dose of 81 mg/day unless there are contraindications such as aspirin sensitivity, bleeding diatheses, or active peptic ulcer disease. Other CHD risk factors, such as hypertension and smoking, should also be controlled.

The 2013 ACC/AHA guidelines suggest treatment with statins for all patients who require drug treatment. As discussed above, the guidelines define four groups of patients who benefit from statin medications.

A. Statins (Hydroxymethylglutaryl-Coenzyme A [HMG-CoA] Reductase Inhibitors)

The statins (HMG-CoA reductase inhibitors) work by inhibiting the rate-limiting enzyme in the formation of cholesterol. They reduce myocardial infarctions and total mortality in secondary prevention, as well as in older middle-aged men free of CHD. A meta-analysis has demonstrated significant reduction in risk of stroke. Cholesterol synthesis in the liver is reduced, with a compensatory increase in hepatic LDL receptors (presumably so that the liver can take more of the cholesterol that it needs from the blood) and a reduction in the circulating LDL cholesterol level by up to 35%. There are also modest increases in HDL levels and decreases in triglyceride levels.

The 2013 ACC/AHA guidelines divide statins into high-intensity and moderate-intensity statin therapy (Table 28–1). High intensity statins lower LDL cholesterol by approximately 50%. Examples include atorvastatin 40–80 mg and rosuvastatin 20–40 mg/day (Table 28–2). Moderate intensity statins lower LDL cholesterol by approximately 30–50%. Examples include atorvastatin 10–20 mg, rosuvastatin 5–10 mg, simvastatin 20–40 mg, pravastatin 40–80 mg, and lovastatin 40 mg. All statins are given once daily in the morning or evening. The most common side effects are muscle aches, occurring in up to 10% of patients, and mild gastrointestinal effects. Statins are

Table 28–1. Indications for high intensity and moderate intensity statins: Recommendations of the 2013 ACC/AHA Guidelines.

Indications	Treatment Recommendation
Presence of clinical atherosclerotic cardiovascular disease	High intensity statin **or** moderate intensity statin if over age 75
Primary elevation of LDL cholesterol ≥ 190 mg/dL (4.91 mmol/L)	High intensity statin
Age 40–75 Presence of diabetes LDL ≥ 70 mg/dL (1.81 mmol/L)	Moderate intensity statin **or** high intensity statin if 10-year CVD risk 7.5% or higher
Aged 40–75 No clinical atherosclerotic cardiovascular disease or diabetes LDL 70–189 mg/dL (1.81–4.91 mmol/L) Estimated 10-year CVD risk 7.5% or higher	Treat with moderate-to-high intensity statin

ACC/AHA, American College of Cardiology/American Heart Association; CVD, cardiovascular disease; HDL, high-density lipoprotein; LDL, low-density lipoprotein.

associated with a 10% increase in the risk of diabetes. Other serious, but extremely uncommon, side effects include liver failure and muscle disease including myositis and rhabdomyolysis. Some patients experience muscle pain even when the serum creatine kinase levels are normal. Liver disease is more common in patients who are also taking fibrates or niacin. Manufacturers of statins recommend monitoring liver enzymes before initiating therapy and as clinically indicated thereafter. Muscle disease is more common with statins and fibrates and niacin as well as with erythromycin, antifungal medications, nefazadone, and cyclosporine. Simvastatin at the highest approved dose—80 mg—is associated with a higher risk of muscle injury or myopathy. This dose should only be used in those who have been taking the medication for longer than 1 year without muscle toxicity.

B. Niacin (Nicotinic Acid)

Niacin was the first lipid-lowering agent that was associated with a reduction in total mortality. Long-term follow-up of a secondary prevention trial of middle-aged men with previous myocardial infarction disclosed that about half of those who had been previously treated with niacin had died, compared with nearly 60% of the placebo group. This favorable effect on mortality was not seen during the trial itself, though there was a reduction in the incidence of recurrent coronary events. A meta-analysis of 10 randomized trials using niacin has also shown a 27% reduction in cardiovascular events.

Niacin reduces the production of VLDL particles, with secondary reduction in LDL and increases in HDL

cholesterol levels. The average effect of full-dose niacin therapy, 3–4.5 g/day, is a 15–25% reduction in LDL cholesterol and a 25–35% increase in HDL cholesterol. Full doses are required to obtain the LDL effect, but the HDL effect is observed at lower doses, eg, 1 g/day. Niacin will also reduce triglycerides by half and will lower lipoprotein(a) (Lp[a]) levels and will increase plasma homocysteine levels. Intolerance to niacin is common; only 50–60% of patients can take full doses. Niacin causes a prostaglandin-mediated flushing that patients may describe as "hot flashes" or pruritus and that can be decreased with aspirin (81–325 mg/day) or other nonsteroidal anti-inflammatory agents taken during the same day. Flushing may also be decreased by initiating niacin therapy with a very small dose, eg, 100 mg with the evening meal. The dose can be doubled each week until 1.5 g/day is tolerated. After rechecking blood lipids, the dose is increased and divided over three meals until the goal of 3–4.5 g/day is reached (eg, 1 g with each meal). Extended-release niacin is better tolerated by most patients. It is not known whether routine monitoring of liver enzymes results in early detection and thus reduced severity of hepatocellular hepatitis with jaundice. Niacin can also exacerbate gout and peptic ulcer disease. Although niacin may increase blood sugar in some patients, clinical trials have shown that niacin can be safely used in diabetic patients.

C. Bile Acid–Binding Resins

The bile acid–binding resins include cholestyramine, colesevelam, and colestipol. Treatment with these agents reduces the incidence of coronary events in middle-aged men by about 20%, with no significant effect on total mortality. The resins work by binding bile acids in the intestine. The resultant reduction in the enterohepatic circulation causes the liver to increase its production of bile acids, using hepatic cholesterol to do so. Thus, hepatic LDL receptor activity increases, with a decline in plasma LDL levels. The triglyceride level tends to increase slightly in some patients treated with bile acid–binding resins; they should be used with caution in those with elevated triglycerides and probably not at all in patients who have triglyceride levels above 500 mg/dL. The clinician can anticipate a reduction of 15–25% in the LDL cholesterol level, with insignificant effects on the HDL level.

The usual dose of cholestyramine is 12–36 g of resin per day in divided doses with meals, mixed in water or, more palatably, juice. Doses of colestipol are 20% higher (each packet contains 5 g of resin). The dose of colesevelam is 625 mg, 6–7 tablets per day.

These agents often cause gastrointestinal symptoms, such as constipation and gas. They may interfere with the absorption of fat-soluble vitamins (thereby complicating the management of patients receiving warfarin) and may bind other drugs in the intestine. Concurrent use of psyllium may ameliorate the gastrointestinal side effects.

D. Fibric Acid Derivatives

The fibrates are peroxisome proliferative-activated receptor-alpha (PPAR-alpha) agonists that result in potent reductions of plasma triglycerides and increases in HDL

Table 28–2. Effects of selected lipid-modifying drugs.

Drug	Lipid-Modifying Effects			Initial Daily Dose	Maximum Daily Dose	Cost for 30 Days Treatment with Dose Listed[1]
	LDL	HDL	Triglyceride			
Alirocumab (Praluent)	−45 to −60%	±	±	75 mg once every 2 weeks	150 mg once every 2 weeks	$1344.00 (75 mg every 2 weeks)
Atorvastatin (Lipitor)	−25 to −40%	+5 to 10%	↓↓	10 mg once	80 mg once	$164.70 (20 mg once)
Cholestyramine (Questran, others)	−15 to −25%	+5%	±	4 g twice a day	24 g divided	$201.06 (8 g divided)
Colesevelam (WelChol)	−10 to −20%	+10%	±	625 mg, 6–7 tablets once	625 mg, 6–7 tablets once	$622.08 (6 tablets once)
Colestipol (Colestid)	−15 to −60%	+5%	±	5 g twice a day	30 g divided	$236.00 (10 g divided)
Evolocumab (Repatha)	−50 to −60%	±	±	140 mg once every 2 weeks	420 mg once monthly	$1301.54 (140 mg every 2 weeks)
Ezetimibe (Zetia)	−20%	+5%	±	10 mg once	10 mg once	$311.95 (10 mg once)
Fenofibrate (Tricor, others)	−10 to −15%	+15 to 25%	↓↓	48 mg once	145 mg once	$171.60 (145 mg once)
Fenofibric Acid (Trilipix)	−10 to −15%	+15 to 25%	↓↓	45 mg once	135 mg once	$180.00 (135 mg once)
Fluvastatin (Lescol)	−20 to −30%	+5 to 10%	↓	20 mg once	40 mg once	$113.40 (20 mg once)
Gemfibrozil (Lopid, others)	−10 to −15%	+15 to 20%	↓↓	600 mg once	1200 mg divided	$71.40 (600 mg twice a day)
Lovastatin (Mevacor, others)	−25 to −40%	+5 to 10%	↓	10 mg once	80 mg divided	$71.10 (20 mg once)
Niacin (OTC, Niaspan)	−15 to −25%	+25 to 35%	↓↓	100 mg once	3–4.5 g divided	$22.20 (1.5 g twice a day, OTC) $449.40 (2 g Niaspan)
Pitavastatin (Livalo)	−30 to 40%	+10 to 25%	↓↓	2 mg once	4 mg once	$252.00 (2 mg once)
Pravastatin (Pravachol)	−25 to −40%	+5 to 10%	↓	20 mg once	80 mg once	$98.10 (20 mg once)
Rosuvastatin (Crestor)	−40 to −50%	+10 to 15%	↓↓	10 mg once	40 mg once	$298.20 (20 mg once)
Simvastatin (Zocor, others)	−25 to −40%	+5 to 10%	↓↓	5 mg once	80 mg once	$84.60 (10 mg once)

[1]Average wholesale price (AWP, for AB-rated generic when available) for quantity listed. Source: *Red Book (electronic version)*, Truven Health Analytics Information. http://www.micromedexsolutions.com/ accessed April 8, 2016. AWP may not accurately represent the actual pharmacy cost because wide contractual variations exist among institutions.
HDL, high-density lipoprotein; LDL, low-density lipoprotein; ± variable, if any; others, indicates availability of less expensive generic preparations; OTC, over the counter.

cholesterol. They reduce LDL levels by about 10–15%, although the result is quite variable, and triglyceride levels by about 40% and raise HDL levels by about 15–20%. The fibric acid derivatives or fibrates approved for use in the United States are gemfibrozil and fenofibrate. Ciprofibrate and bezafibrate are also available for use internationally.

Gemfibrozil reduced CHD rates in hypercholesterolemic middle-aged men free of coronary disease in the Helsinki Heart Study. The effect was observed only among those who also had lower HDL cholesterol levels and high triglyceride levels. In a VA study, gemfibrozil was also shown to reduce cardiovascular events in men with existing CHD whose primary lipid abnormality was a low HDL cholesterol. There was no effect on all-cause mortality.

The usual dose of gemfibrozil is 600 mg once or twice a day. Side effects include cholelithiasis, hepatitis, and myositis. The incidence of the latter two conditions may be higher among patients also taking other lipid-lowering agents. In the largest clinical trial that used clofibrate, there were significantly more deaths—especially due to cancer—in the treatment group; it should not be used.

E. Ezetimibe

Ezetimibe is a lipid-lowering drug that inhibits the intestinal absorption of dietary and biliary cholesterol by blocking passage across the intestinal wall by inhibiting a cholesterol transporter. The usual dose of ezetimibe is

10 mg/day orally. Ezetimibe reduces LDL cholesterol between 15% and 20% when used as monotherapy and can further reduce LDL in patients taking statins who are not yet at therapeutic goal. However, beneficial effects of ezetimibe monotherapy on cardiovascular outcomes has not been demonstrated.

One study has shown that adding ezetimibe to a statin resulted in a small incremental benefit on cardiovascular outcomes. At the end of 7 years of study, patients taking ezetimibe-simvastatin had a 2% absolute reduction in cardiovascular events compared to patients taking simvastatin alone.

F. Proprotein Convertase Subtilisin/Kexin Type 9 (PCSK9) Inhibitors

PCSK9 inhibitors are monoclonal antibodies that reduce liver LDL-receptor degradation and lower LDL cholesterol levels by 50–60%. Two agents, alirocumab and evolocumab, are approved for use in the United States for patients with familial hypercholesterolemia or cardiovascular disease who require additional lowering of LDL cholesterol. The medications are injected subcutaneously every 2–4 weeks. No significant increase in adverse events has been observed compared to placebo. Studies designed to demonstrate a reduction in cardiovascular events have not been published, but analysis of existing studies does suggest a substantial reduction in death from cardiovascular disease and myocardial infarction. However, cost effectiveness models suggest that these medications, at current prices, are not cost-effective.

▶ Initial Selection of Medication

For patients who require a lipid-modifying medication, an HMG-CoA reductase inhibitor is recommended. Although other medications will also have beneficial effects on lipids, there is little evidence demonstrating the desired effects on cardiovascular disease and all-cause mortality. Resins are the only lipid-modifying medication considered safe in pregnancy.

Combination therapy is rarely indicated. Despite improvements in the lipid profile, there are few data demonstrating improved clinical outcomes of combination therapy when compared with HMG-CoA reductase inhibitors alone. The AIM-High Study of niacin added to simvastatin, for example, was stopped early due to a lack of efficacy. The use of extended-release niacin with laropiprant (a prostaglandin antagonist) in high-risk patients taking a statin also did not reduce the risk of cardiovascular events. The addition of ezetimibe to simvastatin in the IMPROVE-IT study resulted in a statistically significant benefit on cardiovascular events but the absolute reduction was small.

Combinations may also increase the risk of complications of drug therapy. The combination of gemfibrozil and HMG-CoA reductase inhibitors increases the risk of muscle and liver disease more than either drug alone. An increase in adverse events was also seen when niacin plus laropiprant was added to statins.

AIM-HIGH Investigators; Boden WE et al. Niacin in patients with low HDL cholesterol levels receiving intensive statin therapy. N Engl J Med. 2011 Dec 15;365(24):2255–67. [PMID: 22085343]

Blom DJ et al; DESCARTES Investigators. A 52-week placebo-controlled trial of evolocumab in hyperlipidemia. N Engl J Med. 2014 May 8;370(19):1809–19. [PMID: 24678979]

Choi HD et al. Safety and efficacy of statin treatment alone and in combination with fibrates in patients with dyslipidemia: a meta-analysis. Curr Med Res Opin. 2014 Jan;30(1):1–10. [PMID: 24063624]

Cholesterol Treatment Trialists' (CTT) Collaboration. Efficacy and safety of LDL-lowering therapy among men and women: meta-analysis of individual data from 174,000 participants in 27 randomised trials. Lancet. 2015 Apr 11;385(9976): 1397–405. [PMID: 25579834]

Hayek S et al. Effect of ezetimibe on major atherosclerotic disease events and all-cause mortality. Am J Cardiol. 2013 Feb 15; 111(4):532–9. [PMID: 23219178]

HPS2-THRIVE Collaborative Group. Effects of extended-release niacin with laropiprant in high-risk patients. N Engl J Med. 2014 Jul 17;371(3):203–12. [PMID: 25014686]

Julius U et al. Nicotinic acid as a lipid-modifying drug—a review. Atheroscler Suppl. 2013 Jan;14(1):7–13. [PMID: 23357134]

Lavigne PM et al. The current state of niacin in cardiovascular disease prevention: a systematic review and meta-regression. J Am Coll Cardiol. 2013 Jan 29;61(4):440–6. [PMID: 23265337]

Naci H et al. Comparative tolerability and harms of individual statins: a study level network meta-analysis of 246,955 participants from 135 randomized, controlled trials. Circ Cardiovasc Qual Outcomes. 2013 Jul;6(4):390–9. [PMID: 23838105]

Raal FJ et al; RUTHERFORD-2 Investigators. PCSK9 inhibition with evolocumab (AMG 145) in heterozygous familial hypercholesterolaemia (RUTHERFORD-2): a randomised, double-blind, placebo-controlled trial. Lancet. 2015 Jan 24;385 (9965):331–40. [PMID: 25282519]

Robinson JG et al; LAPLACE-2 Investigators. Effect of evolocumab or ezetimibe added to moderate- or high-intensity statin therapy on LDL-C lowering in patients with hypercholesterolemia: the LAPLACE-2 randomized clinical trial. JAMA. 2014 May 14;311(18):1870–82. [PMID: 24825642]

Tice JA et al. Proprotein convertase subtilisin/kexin type 9 (PCSK9) inhibitors for treatment of high cholesterol levels: effectiveness and value. JAMA Intern Med. 2016 Jan 1; 176(1):107–8. [PMID: 26662572]

Wilkinson MJ et al. Overcoming toxicity and side-effects of lipid-lowering therapies. Best Pract Res Clin Endocrinol Metab. 2014 Jun;28(3):439–52. [PMID: 24840269]

HIGH BLOOD TRIGLYCERIDES

Patients with very high levels of serum triglycerides (greater than 1000 mg/dL) are at risk for pancreatitis. The pathophysiology is not certain, since pancreatitis never develops in some patients with very high triglyceride levels. Most patients with congenital abnormalities in triglyceride metabolism present in childhood; hypertriglyceridemia-induced pancreatitis first presenting in adults is more commonly due to an acquired problem in lipid metabolism.

Although there are no clear triglyceride levels that predict pancreatitis, most clinicians treat fasting levels above 500 mg/dL (5 mmol/L). The risk of pancreatitis may be more related to the triglyceride level following consumption of a fatty meal. Because postprandial increases in triglyceride are inevitable if fat-containing foods are eaten, fasting triglyceride levels in persons prone to pancreatitis should be kept well below that level.

The primary therapy for high triglyceride levels is dietary, avoiding alcohol, simple sugars, refined starches, saturated and trans fatty acids, and restricting total calories. Control of secondary causes of high triglyceride levels may also be helpful. In patients with fasting triglycerides greater than or equal to 500 mg/dL (5 mmol/L) despite adequate dietary compliance—and certainly in those with a previous episode of pancreatitis—therapy with a triglyceride-lowering drug (eg, niacin, a fibric acid derivative, omega-3-acid ethyl esters, or an HMG-CoA reductase inhibitor) is indicated. Combinations of these medications may also be used.

Whether patients with triglycerides greater than 150 mg/dL (1.5 mmol/L) should be treated to prevent CHD is not known. Meta-analysis of 17 observational studies suggests that after adjustment for other risk factors, elevated triglycerides increased CHD risk in men by 14% and in women by 37%. Elevated triglycerides are also an important feature of the metabolic syndrome. Other data, however, suggest that triglyceride measurements do not improve discrimination between those with and without CHD events, and clinical trial data are not available to support the routine treatment of high triglycerides in all patients.

Berglund L et al. Evaluation and treatment of hypertriglyceridemia: an Endocrine Society clinical practice guideline. J Clin Endocrinol Metab. 2012 Sep;97(9):2969–89. [PMID: 22962670]

Lewis GF et al. Hypertriglyceridemia in the genomic era: a new paradigm. Endocr Rev. 2015 Feb;36(1):131–47. [PMID: 25554923]

Nordestgaard BG et al. Triglycerides and cardiovascular disease. Lancet. 2014 Aug 16;384(9943):626–35. [PMID: 25131982]

Rana JS et al. The role of non-HDL cholesterol in risk stratification for coronary artery disease. Curr Atheroscler Rep. 2012 Apr; 14(2):130–4. [PMID: 22203405]

Schaefer EW et al. Management of severe hypertriglyceridemia in the hospital: a review. J Hosp Med. 2012 May–Jun; 7(5):431–8. [PMID: 22128096]

Singh A et al. What should we do about hypertriglyceridemia in coronary artery disease patients? Curr Treat Options Cardiovasc Med. 2013 Feb;15(1):104–17. [PMID: 23109123]

Tenenbaum A et al. Hypertriglyceridemia: a too long unfairly neglected major cardiovascular risk factor. Cardiovasc Diabetol. 2014 Dec 4;13:159. [PMID: 25471221]

Valdivielso P et al. Current knowledge of hypertriglyceridemic pancreatitis. Eur J Intern Med. 2014 Oct;25(8):689–94. [PMID: 25269432]

Weintraub HS. Overview of prescription omega-3 fatty acid products for hypertriglyceridemia. Postgrad Med. 2014 Nov;126(7):7–18. [PMID: 25387209]

Nutritional Disorders

Robert B. Baron, MD, MS

PROTEIN–ENERGY MALNUTRITION

ESSENTIALS OF DIAGNOSIS

▶ Decreased intake of energy or protein, increased nutrient losses, or increased nutrient requirements.

▶ **Kwashiorkor:** caused by protein deficiency.

▶ **Marasmus:** caused by combined protein and energy deficiency.

▶ Protein loss correlates with weight loss: 35–40% total body weight loss is usually fatal.

▶ General Considerations

Protein–energy malnutrition occurs as a result of a relative or absolute deficiency of energy and protein. It may be primary, due to inadequate food intake, or secondary, as a result of other illness. For most developing nations, primary protein–energy malnutrition remains among the most significant health problems. It occurs in two distinct syndromes. **Kwashiorkor,** caused by a deficiency of protein in the presence of adequate energy, is typically seen in weaning infants at the birth of a sibling in areas where foods containing protein are insufficient. **Marasmus,** caused by combined protein and energy deficiency, is seen where adequate quantities of food are simply not available.

In industrialized societies, protein–energy malnutrition is most often secondary to other diseases. **Kwashiorkor-like secondary protein–energy malnutrition** occurs primarily in association with hypermetabolic acute illnesses such as trauma, burns, and sepsis. **Marasmus-like secondary protein–energy malnutrition** typically results from chronic diseases such as chronic obstructive pulmonary disease (COPD), heart failure, cancer, or AIDS. These two syndromes are estimated to be present in at least 20% of hospitalized patients. A substantially greater number of patients have risk factors that could result in them. In both syndromes, protein–energy malnutrition is caused either by decreased intake of energy and protein or by increased nutrient losses or increased nutrient requirements from the underlying illness. For example, diminished energy intake may result from poor dentition or various gastrointestinal disorders. Increased nutrient losses result from malabsorption, diarrhea, and glycosuria. Increased nutrient requirements occur with fever, surgery, neoplasia, and burns.

▶ Clinical Findings

Clinical manifestations of protein–energy malnutrition range from mild growth retardation and weight loss to a number of distinct clinical syndromes. In the developing world, children manifest marasmus and kwashiorkor. In industrialized nations, clinical manifestations of secondary protein–energy malnutrition are affected by the patient's nutritional status prior to illness, illness resulting in the protein and energy deficiency, and degree of the deficiency.

Progressive wasting that begins with weight loss and proceeds to more severe cachexia typically develops in most patients with marasmus-like secondary protein–energy malnutrition. In the most severe form of this disorder, most body fat stores disappear and muscle mass decreases, most noticeably in the temporalis and interosseous muscles. Laboratory studies may be unremarkable—serum albumin, for example, may be normal or slightly decreased, rarely decreasing to less than 2.8 g/dL (28 g/L). In contrast, owing to its rapidity of onset, kwashiorkor-like secondary protein–energy malnutrition may develop in patients with normal subcutaneous fat and muscle mass or, if the patient is obese, even in patients with excess fat and muscle. The serum protein level, however, typically declines and the serum albumin is often less than 2.8 g/dL (28 g/L). Dependent edema, ascites, or anasarca may develop. As with primary protein–energy malnutrition, combinations of the marasmus-like and kwashiorkor-like syndromes can occur simultaneously, typically in patients with progressive chronic disease in whom a superimposed acute illness develops.

▶ Treatment

The treatment of severe protein–energy malnutrition is a slow process requiring great care. Initial efforts should be directed at correcting fluid and electrolyte abnormalities and infections. Of particular concern are depletion of potassium, magnesium, and calcium and acid–base abnormalities. The second phase of treatment is directed at repletion of protein, energy, and micronutrients. Treatment is started with modest quantities of protein and calories calculated based on the patient's actual body weight. Adult patients are given 1 g/kg of protein and 30 kcal/kg of calories. Concomitant administration of vitamins and minerals is obligatory. Either the enteral or parenteral route can be used, although the former is preferable. Enteral fat and lactose are withheld initially. Patients with less severe protein–calorie undernutrition can be given calories and protein simultaneously with the correction of fluid and electrolyte abnormalities. Similar quantities of protein and calories are recommended for initial treatment.

Patients treated for protein–energy malnutrition require close follow-up. In adults, both calories and protein are advanced as tolerated, adults to 1.5 g/kg/day of protein and 40 kcal/kg/day of calories.

Patients who are re-fed too rapidly may develop a number of untoward clinical sequelae. During refeeding, circulating potassium, magnesium, phosphorus, and glucose move intracellularly and can result in low serum levels of each. The administration of water and sodium with carbohydrate refeeding can result in heart failure in persons with depressed cardiac function. Enteral refeeding can lead to malabsorption and diarrhea due to abnormalities in the gastrointestinal tract.

Refeeding edema is a benign condition to be differentiated from heart failure. Changes in renal sodium reabsorption and poor skin and blood vessel integrity result in the development of dependent edema without other signs of heart disease. Treatment includes reassurance, elevation of the dependent area, and modest sodium restriction. Diuretics are usually ineffective, may aggravate electrolyte deficiencies, and should not be used.

The prevention and early detection of protein–energy malnutrition in hospitalized patients require awareness of its risk factors and early symptoms and signs. Patients at risk require formal assessment of nutritional status and close observation of dietary intake, body weight, and nutritional requirements during the hospital stay.

Bell CL et al. Malnutrition in the nursing home. Curr Opin Clin Nutr Metab Care. 2015 Jan;18(1):17–23. [PMID: 25394167]

Jeejeebhoy KN. Malnutrition, fatigue, frailty, vulnerability, sarcopenia and cachexia: overlap of clinical features. Curr Opin Clin Nutr Metab Care. 2012 May;15(3):213–9. [PMID: 22450775]

Jensen GL et al. A new approach to defining and diagnosing malnutrition in adult critical illness. Curr Opin Crit Care. 2012 Apr;18(2):206–11. [PMID: 22322266]

Morley JE. Undernutrition in older adults. Fam Pract. 2012 Apr; 29(Suppl 1):i89–93. [PMID: 22399563]

Mueller C et al. A.S.P.E.N. clinical guidelines: nutrition screening, assessment, and intervention in adults. JPEN J Parenter Enteral Nutr. 2011 Jan;35(1):16–24. [PMID: 21224430]

Pereira GF et al. Malnutrition among cognitively intact, noncritically ill older adults in the emergency department. Ann Emerg Med. 2015 Jan;65(1):85–91. [PMID: 25129819]

White JV et al. Consensus statement of the Academy of Nutrition and Dietetics/American Society for Parenteral and Enteral Nutrition: characteristics recommended for the identification and documentation of adult malnutrition (undernutrition). J Acad Nutr Diet. 2012 May;112(5):730–8. Erratum in: J Acad Nutr Diet. 2012 Nov;112(11):1899. [PMID: 22709779]

William JH et al. Secondary kwashiorkor: a rare complication of gastric bypass surgery. Am J Med. 2015 May;128(5):e1–2. [PMID: 25498166]

OBESITY

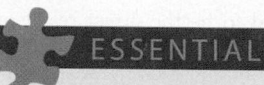

ESSENTIALS OF DIAGNOSIS

- ► Excess adipose tissue; body mass index (BMI) greater than 30.
- ► Upper body obesity (abdomen and flank) of greater health consequence than lower body obesity (buttocks and thighs).
- ► Associated with health consequences, including diabetes mellitus, hypertension, and hyperlipidemia.

► General Considerations

Obesity is one of the most common disorders in medical practice and among the most frustrating and difficult to manage. Little progress has been made in prevention or treatment, yet major changes have occurred in our understanding of its causes and its implications for health.

► Definition & Measurement

Obesity is defined as an excess of adipose tissue. Physical examination is usually sufficient to detect excess body fat. More quantitative evaluation is performed by calculating the BMI.

The **BMI** closely correlates with excess adipose tissue. It is calculated by dividing measured body weight in kilograms by the height in meters squared.

The National Institutes of Health (NIH) define a normal BMI as 18.5–24.9. Overweight is defined as BMI = 25–29.9. Class I obesity is 30–34.9, class II obesity is 35–39.9, and class III (extreme) obesity is BMI greater than 40. Factors other than total weight, however, are also important. Upper body obesity (excess fat around the waist and flank) is a greater health hazard than lower body obesity (fat in the thighs and buttocks). Obese patients with increased abdominal circumference (greater than 102 cm in men and 88 cm in women) or with high waist–hip ratios (greater than 1.0 in men and 0.85 in women) have a greater risk of diabetes mellitus, stroke, coronary artery disease, and early death than equally obese patients with lower ratios. Furthermore, visceral fat within the abdominal cavity is more hazardous to health than subcutaneous fat around the abdomen.

US survey data demonstrate that 68% of Americans are overweight and 33.8% are obese. Women in the

United States are more apt to be obese than men, and African-American and Mexican-American women are more obese than whites. The poor are more obese than the rich regardless of race. Approximately 60% of individuals with obesity in the United States have the metabolic syndrome (including three or more of the following factors: elevated abdominal circumference, blood pressure, blood triglycerides, and fasting blood sugar, and low high-density lipoprotein [HDL] cholesterol).

▶ Etiology

Obesity has been considered to be the direct result of a sedentary lifestyle plus chronic ingestion of excess calories. Yet, as much as 40–70% of obesity may be explained by genetic influences. Twin studies demonstrate substantial genetic influences on BMI with little influence from the childhood environment.

Five genes affecting control of appetite have been identified in mice. Mutations of each gene result in obesity, and each has a human homolog. One gene codes for a protein expressed by adipose tissue—leptin—and another for the leptin receptor in the brain. The other three genes affect brain pathways downstream from the leptin receptor. Numerous other candidate genes for human obesity have been identified. Only a small percentage of human obesity is thought to be due to single gene mutations. Most human obesity undoubtedly develops from the interactions of multiple genes, environmental factors, and behavior. The rapid increase in obesity in the last several decades clearly points to major roles for environmental and behavioral factors in its development.

▶ Medical Evaluation of the Obese Patient

Historical information should be obtained about age at onset, recent weight changes, family history of obesity, occupational history, eating and exercise behavior, cigarette and alcohol use, previous weight loss experience, and psychosocial factors including assessment for depression and eating disorders. Particular attention should be directed at use of laxatives, diuretics, hormones, nutritional supplements, and over-the-counter medications.

Physical examination should assess the BMI, degree and distribution of body fat, overall nutritional status, and signs of secondary causes of obesity.

Less than 1% of obese patients have an identifiable secondary, nonpsychiatric, cause of obesity. Hypothyroidism and Cushing syndrome are important examples that can usually be diagnosed by physical examination in patients with unexplained recent weight gain. Such patients require further endocrinologic evaluation, including serum thyroid-stimulating hormone (TSH) determination and dexamethasone suppression testing (see Chapter 26).

All obese patients should be assessed for medical consequences of their obesity by screening for the metabolic syndrome. Blood pressure, waist circumference, fasting glucose, low-density lipoprotein (LDL) and HDL cholesterol, and triglycerides should be measured.

▶ Treatment

Using conventional dietary techniques, only 20% of patients will lose 20 lb and maintain the loss for over 2 years; only 5% maintain a 40-lb loss. Average weight loss is approximately 7% of baseline weight. Continued close provider–patient contact appears to be more important for success of treatment than the specific features of any given treatment regimen. Careful patient selection improves success rates and decreases frustration of both patients and therapists. Only sufficiently motivated patients should enter active treatment programs. Specific attempts to identify motivated patients—eg, requesting a 3-day diet record—are often useful.

Most successful programs employ a multidisciplinary approach to weight loss, with hypocaloric diets, behavior modification to change eating behavior, aerobic exercise, and social support. Emphasis must be on *maintenance* of weight loss.

Dietary instructions for most patients incorporate the same principles that apply to healthy people who are not obese. These instructions emphasize intake of a wide variety of predominantly "unprocessed" foods, with special attention to limiting foods that provide large amounts of calories without other nutrients, ie, fat, sucrose, and alcohol. There is no physiologic advantage to diets that restrict carbohydrates, advocate relatively larger amounts of protein or fats, or recommend ingestion of foods one at a time. Diets that are restricted in carbohydrates (such as the Atkins and South Beach diets), however, can be effective in achieving a lower total calorie intake. Several studies have demonstrated that low-carbohydrate diets can be used safely and effectively for weight loss without adverse effects on lipids or other metabolic parameters. Meal replacement diets can also be used effectively and safely to achieve weight loss.

Long-term changes in eating behavior are required to maintain weight loss. Although formal **behavior modification** programs are available to which patients can be referred, the clinician caring for obese patients can teach a number of useful behavioral techniques. The most important technique is to emphasize planning and record keeping. Patients can be taught to plan menus and exercise sessions and to record their actual behavior. Record keeping not only aids in behavioral change, but also helps the provider to make specific suggestions for problem solving. Patients can be taught to recognize "eating cues" (emotional, situational, etc) and how to avoid or control them. Regular self-monitoring of weight is also associated with improved long-term weight maintenance.

Exercise offers a number of advantages to patients trying to lose weight and keep it off. Aerobic exercise directly increases the daily energy expenditure and is particularly useful for long-term weight maintenance. Exercise will also preserve lean body mass and partially prevent the decrease in basal energy expenditure (BEE) seen with semistarvation. Compared to no treatment, exercise alone results in small amounts of weight loss. Exercise plus diet results in slightly greater weight loss than diet alone. A greater intensity of exercise is associated with a greater amount of weight loss. Up to 1 hour of moderate exercise per day is associated with long-term weight maintenance in individuals who have successfully lost weight. **Social support** is essential for a successful weight loss program. Continued close contact with clinicians and involvement of the family and peer group are useful techniques for reinforcing behavioral change and preventing social isolation.

Patients with severe obesity may require more aggressive treatment regimens. **Very-low-calorie diets** (typically 800–1000 kcal/day) result in rapid weight loss and marked initial improvement in obesity-related metabolic complications. Patients are commonly maintained on such programs for 4–6 months. Patients who adhere to the program lose an average of 2 lb per week. Average maximum weight loss is approximately 15% of initial weight. Most programs use meal replacement diets to achieve the very-low-calorie intake. Long-term weight maintenance following meal replacement programs is less predictable and requires concurrent behavior modification, long-term use of low-calorie diets, careful self-monitoring, and regular exercise. Side effects such as fatigue, orthostatic hypotension, cold intolerance, and fluid and electrolyte disorders are observed in proportion to the degree of calorie reduction and require regular supervision by a clinician. Other less common complications include gout, gallbladder disease, and cardiac arrhythmias. Although weight loss is more rapidly achieved with very-low-calorie diets as compared with traditional diets, long-term outcomes are equivalent.

Medications for the treatment of obesity are available both over the counter and by prescription. Considerable controversy exists as to the appropriate use of medications for obesity. NIH clinical obesity guidelines state that obesity drugs may be used as part of a comprehensive weight loss program for patients with BMI greater than 30 or those with BMI greater than 27 with obesity-related risk factors. However, few data suggest that medications can improve long-term outcomes associated with obesity.

Several medications are approved by the US Food and Drug Administration (FDA) for treatment of obesity. Catecholaminergic medications (eg, phentermine, diethylpropion, benzphetamine, and phendimetrazine) are approved for short-term use only and have limited utility. **Orlistat** (120 mg orally up to three times daily with each fat-containing meal) is available by prescription for longer-term treatment of obesity. A nonprescription lower-dose formulation (60 mg) is available. Rather than in the central nervous system, orlistat works in the gastrointestinal tract to inhibit intestinal lipase, reducing fat absorption. Not unexpectedly, it may cause diarrhea, gas, and cramping and perhaps reduced absorption of fat-soluble vitamins. In randomized trials with up to 2 years of follow-up, orlistat resulted in 2–4 kg greater weight loss than placebo. A beneficial impact on long-term obesity-related clinical outcomes has not been established.

Four additional medications are approved for use in the United States. **Lorcaserin,** a selective serotonin receptor agonist given in a dose of 10 mg orally twice daily, is associated with modest weight loss, about 3% of initial weight more than placebo. Approximately twice as many patients (38% vs 16%) lose more than 5% of initial weight on lorcaserin compared to placebo. Post-marketing surveillance is focused on concerns about increased breast tumors in animal studies, valvular heart disease in patients receiving earlier drugs of this class, and psychiatric side effects.

The combination of **phentermine hydrochloride** and **topiramate** (3.75 mg/23 mg orally daily for 14 days, then 7.5 mg/46 mg orally daily, to a maximum dosage of 15 mg/92 mg orally daily) results in dose-dependent weight loss. In clinical trials, patients receiving the lowest dose lost 7.8% more weight than those receiving placebo; with the higher dose, 9.8% more weight was lost. Common side effects include mood changes, fatigue, and insomnia. Since the medications increase heart rate, a large clinical trial to assess cardiovascular risk is being conducted. The combination is also associated with increased birth defects and should not be used during pregnancy. Its distribution is restricted in the United States (telephone 1-888-998-4887 or visit www.QsymiaREMS.com).

The combination of **naltrexone** and **bupropion hydrochloride** (8 mg ER/90 mg ER, increasing from 1 tablet orally daily by 1 additional daily tablet each week to a maximum of 2 tablets twice daily) is also approved by the FDA for weight loss. Clinical trials demonstrated a 2–4% weight loss compared to placebo after 1 year. Concerns include an increased risk of suicidal thoughts and behaviors, other neuropsychiatric events, seizures, and elevation of blood pressure and heart rate. Other side effects include nausea and vomiting, diarrhea and constipation, headache, and dry mouth. A cardiovascular outcome trial to further assess safety is in progress.

Liraglutide (Saxenda), an injectable incretin (a glucagon-like peptide-1 receptor agonist), is FDA approved for obesity treatment in a dose of 0.6 mg subcutaneously daily, increasing by 0.6 mg daily each week to a maximum of 3 mg subcutaneously daily. Clinical trials demonstrated a 3.7–4.5% weight loss compared to placebo at 1 year. Concerns include thyroid tumors in animal studies, pancreatitis, gallbladder disease, renal impairment, increased heart rate, and suicidal thoughts. Common side effects include nausea and vomiting, diarrhea and constipation, and hypoglycemia. A cardiovascular outcomes trial is being conducted.

Bariatric surgery is an increasingly prevalent treatment option for patients with severe obesity. In the United States, gastric operations are considered the procedures of choice. Most popular is the Roux-en-Y gastric bypass (RYGB). In most centers, the operation can be done laparoscopically. RYGB typically results in substantial amounts of weight loss—over 30% of initial body weight in some studies. Complications occur in up to 40% of persons undergoing RYGB surgery and include peritonitis due to anastomotic leak; abdominal wall hernias; staple line disruption; gallstones; neuropathy; marginal ulcers; stomal stenosis; wound infections; thromboembolic disease; gastrointestinal symptoms; and nutritional deficiencies, including iron, vitamin B_{12}, folate, calcium, and vitamin D. Operative mortality rates within 30 days are nil to 1% in low-risk populations but have been reported to be substantially higher in Medicare beneficiaries. One-year mortality rates have been reported as high as 7.5% in men with Medicare. Surgical volume (number of cases performed by the surgeon or hospital) has been demonstrated to be an important predictor of outcome.

Another operation is gastric banding. Gastric banding results in less dramatic weight loss than RYGB and has fewer short-term complications. Frequent follow-up, however, is required to adjust the gastric band. Longer-term follow-up has shown a 39% rate of major complications and a 60% rate of re-operation.

A third operation, sleeve gastrectomy, is gaining in popularity. With this procedure, approximately three-quarters of the stomach is resected, but the gastrointestinal tract is otherwise left intact. Weight loss results are somewhat less than RYGB but greater than gastric banding.

NIH consensus panel recommendations are to limit obesity surgery to patients with BMIs over 40, or over 35 if obesity-related comorbidities are present. The procedure is cost-effective for patients with severe obesity and most third-party payers cover the procedure in selected patients. A large Swedish study suggested that bariatric surgery is associated with a significant reduction in deaths at 11-year follow-up. The number needed to treat to prevent one death in 11 years was 77 operations. A US Veterans Administration study, however, did not show a mortality benefit.

▶ When to Refer

Patients with BMI over 40 (or over 35 with obesity-related morbidities) who are interested in considering weight loss surgery.

Baron RB. Telling patients they are overweight or obese: an insult or an effective intervention? Arch Intern Med. 2011 Feb 28; 171(4):321–2. [PMID: 21357808]

Berra K et al. Making physical activity counseling a priority in clinical practice: the time for action is now. JAMA. 2015 Dec 22–29;314(24):2617–8. [PMID: 26662069]

Booth HP et al. Effectiveness of behavioural weight loss interventions delivered in a primary care setting: a systematic review and meta-analysis. Fam Pract. 2014 Dec;31(6):643–53. [PMID: 25298510]

Chang SH et al. The effectiveness and risks of bariatric surgery: an updated systematic review and meta-analysis, 2003–2012. JAMA Surg. 2014 Mar;149(3):275–87. [PMID: 24352617]

Colquitt JL et al. Surgery for weight loss in adults. Cochrane Database Syst Rev. 2014 Aug 8;8:CD003641. [PMID: 25105982]

Dietz WH et al. Management of obesity: improvement of healthcare training and systems for prevention and care. Lancet. 2015 Jun 20;385(9986):2521–33. [PMID: 25703112]

Gloy VL et al. Bariatric surgery versus non-surgical treatment for obesity: a systematic review and meta-analysis of randomised controlled trials. BMJ. 2013 Oct 22;347:f5934. [PMID: 24149519]

Gray LJ et al. A systematic review and mixed treatment comparison of pharmacological interventions for the treatment of obesity. Obes Rev. 2012 Jun;13(6):483–98. [PMID: 22288431]

Jensen MD et al. 2013 AHA/ACC/TOS guideline for the management of overweight and obesity in adults: a report of the American College of Cardiology/American Heart Association Task Force on Practice Guidelines and The Obesity Society. Circulation. 2014 Jun 24;129(25 Suppl 2):S102–38. [PMID: 24222017]

Jin J. JAMA patient page. Medications for weight loss: indications and usage. JAMA. 2015 Jun 2;313(21):2196. [PMID: 26034970]

Johansson K et al. Effects of anti-obesity drugs, diet, and exercise on weight-loss maintenance after a very-low-calorie diet or low-calorie diet: a systematic review and meta-analysis of randomized controlled trials. Am J Clin Nutr. 2014 Jan; 99(1):14–23. [PMID: 24172297]

Johnston BC et al. Comparison of weight loss among named diet programs in overweight and obese adults: a meta-analysis. JAMA. 2014 Sep 3;312(9):923–33. [PMID: 25182101]

Kumar RB et al. Efficacy comparison of medications approved for chronic weight management. Obesity (Silver Spring). 2015 Apr;23(Suppl 1):S4–7. [PMID: 25900871]

Kushner RF et al. Assessment and lifestyle management of patients with obesity: clinical recommendations from systematic reviews. JAMA. 2014 Sep 3;312(9):943–52. Erratum in: JAMA. 2014 Oct 15;312(15):1593. [PMID: 25182103]

Ogden CL et al. Prevalence of obesity in the United States. JAMA. 2014 Jul;312(2):189–90. [PMID: 25005661]

Pucci A et al. New medications for treatment of obesity: metabolic and cardiovascular effects. Can J Cardiol. 2015 Feb; 31(2): 142–52. [PMID: 25661549]

Tsai AG et al. In the clinic: obesity. Ann Intern Med. 2013 Sep 3; 159(5):ITC3-1–15. [PMID: 24026335]

Unick JL et al; Look AHEAD Research Group. The long-term effectiveness of a lifestyle intervention in severely obese individuals. Am J Med. 2013 Mar;126(3):236–42. [PMID: 23410564]

Yanovski SZ et al. Long-term drug treatment for obesity: a systematic and clinical review. JAMA. 2014 Jan 1;311(1):74–86. [PMID: 24231879]

▼ EATING DISORDERS

ANOREXIA NERVOSA

ESSENTIALS OF DIAGNOSIS

▶ Disturbance of body image and intense fear of becoming fat.

▶ Weight loss leading to body weight 15% below expected.

▶ In females, absence of three consecutive menstrual cycles.

▶ General Considerations

Anorexia nervosa typically begins in the years between adolescence and young adulthood. Ninety percent of patients are females, most from the middle and upper socioeconomic strata.

The prevalence of anorexia nervosa is greater than previously suggested. In Rochester, Minnesota, for example, the prevalence per 100,000 population is estimated to be 270 for females and 22 for males. Many other adolescent girls have features of the disorder without the severe weight loss.

The cause of anorexia nervosa is not known. Although multiple endocrinologic abnormalities exist in these patients, most authorities believe they are secondary to malnutrition and not primary disorders. Most experts favor a primary psychiatric origin, but no hypothesis explains all cases. The patient characteristically comes from a family whose members are highly goal and achievement oriented. Interpersonal relationships may be inadequate or destructive. The parents are usually overly directive and concerned with slimness and physical fitness, and much of the family conversation centers around dietary matters. One theory holds that the patient's refusal to eat is an attempt to regain control of her body in defiance of parental control. The patient's unwillingness to inhabit an "adult body" may also represent a rejection of adult responsibilities and the implications of adult interpersonal relationships. Patients are commonly perfectionistic in behavior and exhibit obsessional personality characteristics. Marked depression or anxiety may be present.

▶ Clinical Findings

A. Symptoms and Signs

Patients with anorexia nervosa may exhibit severe emaciation and may complain of cold intolerance or constipation. Amenorrhea is almost always present. Bradycardia, hypotension, and hypothermia may be present in severe cases. Examination demonstrates loss of body fat, dry and scaly skin, and increased lanugo body hair. Parotid enlargement and edema may also occur.

B. Laboratory Findings

Laboratory findings are variable but may include anemia, leukopenia, electrolyte abnormalities, and elevations of blood urea nitrogen (BUN) and serum creatinine. Serum cholesterol levels are often increased. Endocrine abnormalities include depressed levels of luteinizing and follicle-stimulating hormones and impaired response of luteinizing hormone to luteinizing hormone-releasing hormone.

▶ Diagnosis & Differential Diagnosis

The diagnosis is based on weight loss to a body weight 15% below expected, distorted body image, fear of weight gain or of loss of control over food intake and, in females, absence of at least three consecutive menstrual cycles. Other medical or psychiatric illnesses that can account for anorexia and weight loss must be excluded.

Behavioral features required for the diagnosis include intense fear of becoming obese, disturbance of body image, and refusal to exceed a minimal normal weight.

The differential diagnosis includes endocrine and metabolic disorders (eg, panhypopituitarism, Addison disease, hyperthyroidism, and diabetes mellitus); gastrointestinal disorders (eg, Crohn disease and gluten enteropathy); chronic infections (eg, tuberculosis); cancers, (eg, lymphoma); and rare central nervous system disorders (eg, hypothalamic tumor).

▶ Treatment

The goal of treatment is restoration of normal body weight and resolution of psychological difficulties. Hospitalization may be necessary. Treatment programs conducted by experienced teams are successful in about two-thirds of cases, restoring normal weight and menstruation. One-half continue to experience difficulties with eating behavior and psychiatric problems. Two to 6% of patients die of the complications of the disorder or commit suicide.

Various treatment methods have been used without clear evidence of superiority of one over another. Supportive care by clinicians and family is probably the most important feature of therapy. Cognitive behavioral therapy, intensive psychotherapy, and family therapy may be tried. A variety of medications including tricyclic antidepressants, selected serotonin reuptake inhibitors (SSRIs), and lithium carbonate are effective in some cases; overall, however, clinical trial results have been disappointing. Patients with severe malnutrition must be hemodynamically stabilized and may require enteral or parenteral feeding. Forced feedings should be reserved for life-threatening situations, since the goal of treatment is to reestablish normal eating behavior.

▶ When to Refer

- Adolescents and young adults with otherwise unexplained weight loss should be evaluated by a psychiatrist.
- All patients with diagnosed anorexia nervosa should be co-managed with a psychiatrist.

▶ When to Admit

- Signs of hypovolemia, major electrolyte disorders, and severe protein–energy malnutrition.
- Failure to improve with outpatient management.

Dalle Grave R et al. Cognitive behavioral therapy for anorexia nervosa: an update. Curr Psychiatry Rep. 2016 Jan;18(1):2. [PMID: 26689208]

Flament MF et al. Evidence-based pharmacotherapy of eating disorders. Int J Neuropsychopharmacol. 2012 Mar;15(2):189–207. [PMID: 21414249]

Franko DL et al. A longitudinal investigation of mortality in anorexia nervosa and bulimia nervosa. Am J Psychiatry. 2013 Aug 1;170(8):917–25. [PMID: 23771148]

Galsworthy-Francis L et al. Cognitive Behavioural Therapy for anorexia nervosa: a systematic review. Clin Psychol Rev. 2014 Feb;34(1):54–72. [PMID: 24394285]

Ozier AD et al. Position of the American Dietetic Association: nutrition intervention in the treatment of eating disorders. J Am Diet Assoc. 2011 Aug;111(8):1236–41. [PMID: 21802573]

Sachs KV et al. Cardiovascular complications of anorexia nervosa: a systematic review. Int J Eat Disord. 2016 Mar;49(3):238–48. [PMID: 26710932]

Smink FR et al. Epidemiology, course, and outcome of eating disorders. Curr Opin Psychiatry. 2013 Nov;26(6):543–8. [PMID: 24060914]

Sy R et al. Quality of life in anorexia nervosa: a review of the literature. Eat Disord. 2013;21(3):206–22. [PMID: 23600552]

BULIMIA NERVOSA

ESSENTIALS OF DIAGNOSIS

▶ Uncontrolled episodes of binge eating at least twice weekly for 3 months.

▶ Recurrent inappropriate compensation to prevent weight gain such as self-induced vomiting, laxatives, diuretics, fasting, or excessive exercise.

▶ Overconcern with weight and body shape.

General Considerations

Bulimia nervosa is the episodic uncontrolled ingestion of large quantities of food followed by recurrent inappropriate compensatory behavior to prevent weight gain such as self-induced vomiting, diuretic or cathartic use, or strict dieting or vigorous exercise.

Like anorexia nervosa, bulimia nervosa is predominantly a disorder of young, white, middle- and upper-class women. It is more difficult to detect than anorexia, and some studies have estimated that the prevalence may be as high as 19% in college-aged women.

Clinical Findings

Patients with bulimia nervosa typically consume large quantities of easily ingested high-calorie foods, usually in secrecy. Some patients may have several such episodes a day for a few days; others report regular and persistent patterns of binge eating. Binging is usually followed by vomiting, cathartics, or diuretics and accompanied by feelings of guilt or depression. Periods of binging may be followed by intervals of self-imposed starvation. Body weights may fluctuate but generally are within 20% of desirable weights.

Some patients with bulimia nervosa also have a cryptic form of anorexia nervosa with significant weight loss and amenorrhea. Family and psychological issues are generally similar to those of patients with anorexia nervosa. Bulimic patients, however, have a higher incidence of premorbid obesity, greater use of cathartics and diuretics, and more impulsive or antisocial behavior. Menstruation is usually preserved.

Medical complications are numerous. Gastric dilatation and pancreatitis have been reported after binges. Vomiting can result in poor dentition, pharyngitis, esophagitis, aspiration, and electrolyte abnormalities. Cathartic and diuretic abuse also cause electrolyte abnormalities or dehydration. Constipation and hemorrhoids are common.

Treatment

Treatment of bulimia nervosa requires supportive care and psychotherapy. Individual, group, family, and behavioral therapy have all been utilized. Antidepressant medications may be helpful. The best results have been with fluoxetine hydrochloride and other SSRIs. Although death from bulimia is rare, the long-term psychiatric prognosis in severe bulimia is worse than that in anorexia nervosa.

When to Refer

All patients with diagnosed bulimia should be co-managed with a psychiatrist.

Chacko SA et al. Recognizing disordered eating in primary care patients with obesity. Prev Med. 2015 Mar;72:89–94. [PMID: 25572624]

Jordan J et al. Bulimia nervosa-nonpurging subtype: closer to the bulimia nervosa-purging subtype or to binge eating disorder? Int J Eat Disord. 2014 Apr;47(3):231–8. [PMID: 24282157]

Poulsen S et al. A randomized controlled trial of psychoanalytic psychotherapy or cognitive-behavioral therapy for bulimia nervosa. Am J Psychiatry. 2014 Jan;171(1):109–16. [PMID: 24275909]

Waller G et al. Cognitive-behavioral therapy for bulimia nervosa and atypical bulimic nervosa: effectiveness in clinical settings. Int J Eat Disord. 2014 Jan;47(1):13–7. [PMID: 23996224]

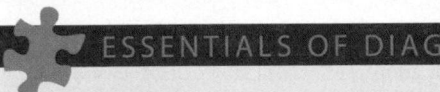

DISORDERS OF VITAMIN METABOLISM

THIAMINE (B₁) DEFICIENCY

$$\text{THIAMINE (B}_1\text{) DEFICIENCY}$$

ESSENTIALS OF DIAGNOSIS

▶ Most common in patients with chronic alcoholism.

▶ Early symptoms of anorexia, muscle cramps, paresthesias, irritability.

▶ Advanced syndromes of high output heart failure ("wet beriberi"), peripheral nerve disorders, and Wernicke-Korsakoff syndrome ("dry beriberi").

General Considerations

Most thiamine deficiency in the United States is due to chronic alcoholism, with poor dietary intake of thiamine and impaired thiamine absorption, metabolism, and storage. Thiamine deficiency is also associated with malabsorption, dialysis, and other causes of chronic protein–calorie undernutrition. Thiamine deficiency can be precipitated in patients with marginal thiamine status with intravenous dextrose solutions.

Clinical Findings

Early manifestations of thiamine deficiency include anorexia, muscle cramps, paresthesias, and irritability. Advanced deficiency primarily affects the cardiovascular system ("wet beriberi") or the nervous system ("dry beriberi"). Wet beriberi occurs in thiamine deficiency accompanied by severe physical exertion and high carbohydrate intake. Dry beriberi occurs in thiamine deficiency accompanied by inactivity and low calorie intake.

Wet beriberi is characterized by marked peripheral vasodilation resulting in high-output heart failure with dyspnea, tachycardia, cardiomegaly, and pulmonary and peripheral edema, with warm extremities mimicking cellulitis.

Dry beriberi involves both the peripheral and the central nervous systems. Peripheral nerve involvement is typically a symmetric motor and sensory neuropathy with pain, paresthesias, and loss of reflexes. The legs are affected more than the arms. Central nervous system involvement results in Wernicke-Korsakoff syndrome. Wernicke encephalopathy consists of nystagmus progressing to ophthalmoplegia, truncal ataxia, and confusion. Korsakoff syndrome includes amnesia, confabulation, and impaired learning.

▶ Diagnosis

In most instances, the clinical response to empiric thiamine therapy is used to support a diagnosis of thiamine deficiency. The most commonly used biochemical tests measure erythrocyte transketolase activity and urinary thiamine excretion. A transketolase activity coefficient greater than 15–20% suggests thiamine deficiency.

▶ Treatment

Thiamine deficiency is treated with large parenteral doses of thiamine. Fifty to 100 mg/day is administered intravenously for the first few days, followed by daily oral doses of 5–10 mg/day. All patients should simultaneously receive therapeutic doses of other water-soluble vitamins. Although treatment results in complete resolution in half of patients (one-fourth immediately and another one-fourth over days), the other half obtain only partial resolution or no benefit.

▶ When to Refer

Patients with signs of beriberi or Wernicke-Korsakoff syndrome should be referred to a neurologist.

THIAMINE TOXICITY

There is no known toxicity of thiamine.

Chisolm-Straker M et al. Altered and unstable: wet beriberi, a clinical review. J Emerg Med. 2013 Sep;45(3):341–4. [PMID: 23849362]

Lough ME. Wernicke's encephalopathy: expanding the diagnostic toolbox. Neuropsychol Rev. 2012 Jun;22(2):181–94. [PMID: 22577001]

Milone M et al. Wernicke encephalopathy in subjects undergoing restrictive weight loss surgery: a systematic review of literature data. Eur Eat Disord Rev. 2014 Jul;22(4):223–9. [PMID: 24764323]

Sriram K et al. Thiamine in nutrition therapy. Nutr Clin Pract. 2012 Feb;27(1):41–50. [PMID: 22223666]

ter Borg S et al. Micronutrient intakes and potential inadequacies of community-dwelling older adults: a systematic review. Br J Nutr. 2015 Apr 28;113(8):1195–206. [PMID: 25822905]

Yang JD et al. Beriberi disease: is it still present in the United States? Am J Med. 2012 Oct;125(10):e5. [PMID: 22800868]

RIBOFLAVIN (B₂) DEFICIENCY

▶ Clinical Findings

Riboflavin deficiency almost always occurs in combination with deficiencies of other vitamins. Dietary inadequacy, interactions with a variety of medications, alcoholism, and other causes of protein–calorie undernutrition are the most common causes of riboflavin deficiency.

Manifestations of riboflavin deficiency include cheilosis, angular stomatitis, glossitis, seborrheic dermatitis, weakness, corneal vascularization, and anemia.

▶ Diagnosis

Riboflavin deficiency can be confirmed by measuring the riboflavin-dependent enzyme erythrocyte glutathione reductase. Activity coefficients greater than 1.2–1.3 are suggestive of riboflavin deficiency. Urinary riboflavin excretion and serum levels of plasma and red cell flavins can also be measured.

▶ Treatment

Riboflavin deficiency is usually treated empirically when the diagnosis is suspected. It is easily treated with foods such as meat, fish, and dairy products or with oral preparations of the vitamin. Administration of 5–15 mg/day until clinical findings are resolved is usually adequate. Riboflavin can also be given parenterally, but it is poorly soluble in aqueous solutions.

RIBOFLAVIN TOXICITY

There is no known toxicity of riboflavin.

Aubuchon-Endsley NL et al. Relationships among socioeconomic status, dietary intake, and stress in breastfeeding women. J Acad Nutr Diet. 2015 Jun;115(6):939–46.e1. [PMID: 25687029]

Shi Z et al. Inadequate riboflavin intake and anemia risk in a Chinese population: five-year follow up of the Jiangsu Nutrition Study. PLoS One. 2014 Feb 12;9(2):e88862. [PMID: 24533156]

Whitfield KC et al. Poor thiamin and riboflavin status is common among women of childbearing age in rural and urban Cambodia. J Nutr. 2015 Mar;145(3):628–33. [PMID: 25733481]

NIACIN DEFICIENCY

▶ General Considerations

Niacin is a generic term for nicotinic acid and other derivatives with similar nutritional activity. Unlike most other vitamins, niacin can be synthesized from the amino acid tryptophan. Niacin is an essential component of the coenzymes nicotinamide adenine dinucleotide (NAD) and nicotinamide adenine dinucleotide phosphate (NADP), which are involved in many oxidation-reduction reactions. The major food sources of niacin are protein foods containing tryptophan and numerous cereals, vegetables, and dairy products.

Historically, niacin deficiency occurred when corn, which is relatively deficient in both tryptophan and niacin, was the major source of calories. Currently, niacin deficiency is more commonly due to alcoholism and nutrient–drug interactions. Niacin deficiency can also occur in inborn errors of metabolism. Niacin in the form of nicotinic acid is used therapeutically for the treatment of hypercholesterolemia and hypertriglyceridemia. Niacinamide (the form of niacin usually used to treat niacin deficiency) does not exhibit the lipid-lowering effects of nicotinic acid.

Clinical Findings

As with other B vitamins, early manifestations of niacin deficiency are nonspecific—anorexia, weakness, irritability, mouth soreness, glossitis, stomatitis, and weight loss. More advanced deficiency results in the classic triad of pellagra: dermatitis, diarrhea, and dementia. The dermatitis is symmetric, involving sun-exposed areas. Skin lesions are dark, dry, and scaling. The dementia begins with insomnia, irritability, and apathy and progresses to confusion, memory loss, hallucinations, and psychosis. The diarrhea can be severe and may result in malabsorption due to atrophy of the intestinal villi. Advanced pellagra can result in death.

Diagnosis

In early deficiency, diagnosis requires a high index of suspicion and attempts at confirmation of niacin deficiency. Niacin metabolites, particularly *N*-methylnicotinamide, can be measured in the urine. Low levels suggest niacin deficiency but may also be found in patients with generalized under-nutrition. Serum and red cell levels of NAD and NADP are also low but are similarly nonspecific. In advanced cases, the diagnosis of pellagra can be made on clinical grounds.

Treatment

Niacin deficiency can be effectively treated with oral niacin, usually given as nicotinamide (10–150 mg/day).

NIACIN TOXICITY

At the high doses of niacin used to treat hyperlipidemia, side effects are common. These include cutaneous flushing (partially prevented by pretreatment with aspirin, 81–325 mg/day, and use of extended-release preparations) and gastric irritation. Elevation of liver enzymes, hyperglycemia, and gout are less common untoward effects.

HPS2-THRIVE Collaborative Group; Landray MJ et al. Effects of extended-release niacin with laropiprant in high-risk patients. N Engl J Med. 2014 Jul 17;371(3):203–12. [PMID: 25014686]

Jackevicius CA et al. Use of niacin in the United States and Canada. JAMA Intern Med. 2013 Jul 22;173(14):1379–81. [PMID: 23753308]

Lavigne PM et al. The current state of niacin in cardiovascular disease prevention: a systematic review and meta-regression. J Am Coll Cardiol. 2013 Jan 29;61(4):440–6. [PMID: 23265337]

López M et al. Pellagra encephalopathy in the context of alcoholism: review and case report. Alcohol Alcohol. 2014 Jan–Feb; 49(1):38–41. [PMID: 23926211]

Sharma B et al. A rare case of alcoholic pellagra encephalopathy with startle myoclonus and marked response to niacin therapy: time for a new dictum? BMJ Case Rep. 2013 Apr 22; 2013:bcr2013008906. [PMID: 23608853]

Villaverde Doménech ME et al. Pellagra. A challenging differential diagnosis in burn injuries. J Tissue Viability. 2014 Feb; 23(1):37–41. [PMID: 24405724]

VITAMIN B$_6$ DEFICIENCY

Vitamin B$_6$ deficiency most commonly occurs as a result of interactions with medications—especially isoniazid, cycloserine, penicillamine, and oral contraceptives—or of alcoholism. A number of inborn errors of metabolism and other pyridoxine-responsive syndromes, particularly pyridoxine-responsive anemia, are not clearly due to vitamin deficiency but commonly respond to high doses of the vitamin. Patients with common variable immunodeficiency may have concomitant vitamin B$_6$ deficiency.

Clinical Findings

Vitamin B$_6$ deficiency results in clinical symptoms similar to those of other B vitamin deficiencies, including mouth soreness, glossitis, cheilosis, weakness, and irritability. Severe deficiency can result in peripheral neuropathy, anemia, and seizures. Studies have suggested a potential relationship of low vitamin B$_6$ levels and a variety of clinical conditions including cardiovascular diseases, inflammatory diseases, and certain cancers.

Diagnosis

The diagnosis of vitamin B$_6$ deficiency can be confirmed by measurement of pyridoxal phosphate in blood. Normal levels are greater than 50 ng/mL.

Treatment

Vitamin B$_6$ deficiency can be effectively treated with vitamin B$_6$ supplements (10–20 mg/day orally). Some patients taking medications that interfere with pyridoxine metabolism (such as isoniazid) may need doses as high as 50–100 mg/day orally to prevent vitamin B$_6$ deficiency. This is particularly true for patients who are more likely to have diets marginally adequate in vitamin B$_6$, such as the elderly, alcoholic patients, or the urban poor. Inborn errors of metabolism and pyridoxine-responsive syndromes often require doses up to 600 mg/day orally.

VITAMIN B$_6$ TOXICITY

A sensory neuropathy, at times irreversible, occurs in patients receiving large doses of vitamin B$_6$ (200–2000 mg/day).

Choi SW et al. Vitamins B$_6$ and cancer. Subcell Biochem. 2012;56:247–64. [PMID: 22116703]

Kjeldby IK et al. Vitamin B$_6$ deficiency and diseases in elderly people—a study in nursing homes. BMC Geriatr. 2013 Feb 8; 13:13. [PMID: 23394203]

Kulkantrakorn K. Pyridoxine-induced sensory ataxic neuronopathy and neuropathy: revisited. Neurol Sci. 2014 Nov;35(11):1827–30. [PMID: 25056196]

VITAMIN B$_{12}$ & FOLATE

Vitamin B$_{12}$ (cobalamin) and folate are discussed in Chapter 13.

VITAMIN C (Ascorbic Acid) DEFICIENCY

Most cases of vitamin C deficiency seen in the United States are due to dietary inadequacy in the urban poor, the elderly, and patients with chronic alcoholism. Patients with chronic illnesses such as cancer and chronic kidney disease and individuals who smoke cigarettes are also at risk.

▶ Clinical Findings

Early manifestations of vitamin C deficiency are nonspecific and include malaise and weakness. In more advanced stages, the typical features of scurvy develop. Manifestations include perifollicular hemorrhages, perifollicular hyperkeratotic papules, petechiae and purpura, splinter hemorrhages, bleeding gums, hemarthroses, and subperiosteal hemorrhages. Anemia is common, and wound healing is impaired. The late stages of scurvy are characterized by edema, oliguria, neuropathy, intracerebral hemorrhage, and death.

▶ Diagnosis

The diagnosis of advanced scurvy can be made clinically on the basis of the skin lesions in the proper clinical situation. Atraumatic hemarthrosis is also highly suggestive. The diagnosis can be confirmed with decreased plasma ascorbic acid levels, typically below 0.1 mg/dL.

▶ Treatment

Adult scurvy can be treated with ascorbic acid 300–1000 mg/day orally. Improvement typically occurs within days.

VITAMIN C TOXICITY

Very large doses of vitamin C can cause gastric irritation, flatulence, or diarrhea. Oxalate kidney stones are of theoretic concern because ascorbic acid is metabolized to oxalate, but stone formation has not been frequently reported. Vitamin C can also confound common diagnostic tests by causing false-negative results for some fecal occult blood tests and both false-negative and false-positive results for urine glucose.

Fossitt DD et al. Classic skin findings of scurvy. Mayo Clin Proc. 2014 Jul;89(7):e61. [PMID: 24996243]
Hoffer LJ. Ascorbic acid supplements and kidney stone risk. JAMA Intern Med. 2013 Jul 22;173(14):1384. [PMID: 23877084]
Kluesner NH et al. Scurvy: malnourishment in the land of plenty. J Emerg Med. 2014 Apr;46(4):530–2. [PMID: 24440620]

VITAMIN A DEFICIENCY

▶ Clinical Findings

Vitamin A deficiency is one of the most common vitamin deficiency syndromes, particularly in developing countries. In many such regions, it is the most common cause of blindness. In the United States, vitamin A deficiency is usually due to fat malabsorption syndromes or mineral oil laxative abuse and occurs most commonly in the elderly and urban poor.

Night blindness is the earliest symptom. Dryness of the conjunctiva (xerosis) and the development of small white patches on the conjunctiva (Bitot spots) are early signs. Ulceration and necrosis of the cornea (keratomalacia), perforation, endophthalmitis, and blindness are late manifestations. Xerosis and hyperkeratinization of the skin and loss of taste may also occur.

▶ Diagnosis

Abnormalities of dark adaptation are strongly suggestive of vitamin A deficiency. Serum levels below the normal range of 30–65 mg/dL are commonly seen in advanced deficiency.

▶ Treatment

Night blindness, poor wound healing, and other signs of early deficiency can be effectively treated with vitamin A 30,000 international units orally daily for 1 week. Advanced deficiency with corneal damage calls for administration of 20,000 international units/kg orally for at least 5 days. The potential antioxidant effects of beta-carotene can be achieved with supplements of 25,000–50,000 international units of beta-carotene.

VITAMIN A TOXICITY

Excess intake of beta-carotenes (hypercarotenosis) results in staining of the skin a yellow-orange color but is otherwise benign. Skin changes are most marked on the palms and soles, while the scleras remain white, clearly distinguishing hypercarotenosis from jaundice.

Excessive vitamin A (hypervitaminosis A), on the other hand, can be quite toxic. Chronic toxicity usually occurs after ingestion of daily doses of over 50,000 international units/day for more than 3 months. Early manifestations include dry, scaly skin, hair loss, mouth sores, painful hyperostoses, anorexia, and vomiting. More serious findings include hypercalcemia; increased intracranial pressure, with papilledema, headaches, and decreased cognition; and hepatomegaly, occasionally progressing to cirrhosis. Excessive vitamin A is also related to increased risk of hip fracture. Acute toxicity can result from ingestion of massive doses of vitamin A, such as in drug overdoses or consumption of polar bear liver. Manifestations include nausea, vomiting, abdominal pain, headache, papilledema, and lethargy.

The diagnosis can be confirmed by elevations of serum vitamin A levels. The only treatment is withdrawal of vitamin A from the diet. Most symptoms and signs improve rapidly.

Fok JS et al. Visual deterioration caused by vitamin A deficiency in patients after bariatric surgery. Eat Weight Disord. 2012 Jun;17(2):e144–6. [PMID: 23010786]
Haskell MJ. The challenge to reach nutritional adequacy for vitamin A: beta-carotene bioavailability and conversion—evidence in humans. Am J Clin Nutr. 2012 Nov;96(5):1193S–203S. [PMID: 23053560]

Sommer A et al. A global clinical view on vitamin A and carotenoids. Am J Clin Nutr. 2012 Nov;96(5):1204S–6S. [PMID: 23053551]

VITAMIN D

Vitamin D is discussed in Chapter 26.

VITAMIN E DEFICIENCY

▶ Clinical Findings

Clinical deficiency of vitamin E is most commonly due to severe malabsorption or abetalipoproteinemia in adults or chronic cholestatic liver disease, biliary atresia, or cystic fibrosis in children. Manifestations of deficiency include areflexia, disturbances of gait, decreased vibration and proprioception, and ophthalmoplegia.

▶ Diagnosis

Plasma vitamin E levels can be measured; normal levels are 0.5–0.7 mg/dL or higher. Since vitamin E is normally transported in lipoproteins, the serum level should be interpreted in relation to circulating lipid levels.

▶ Treatment

The optimum therapeutic dose of vitamin E has not been clearly defined. Large doses, often administered parenterally, can be used to improve the neurologic complications seen in abetalipoproteinemia and cholestatic liver disease. Several trials of supplemental vitamin E have shown slower cognitive decline in patients with Alzheimer disease.

VITAMIN E TOXICITY

Clinical trials have suggested an increase in all-cause mortality with high dose (400 international units/day or more) vitamin E supplements. Large doses of vitamin E can also increase the vitamin K requirement and can result in bleeding in patients taking oral anticoagulants.

Ashor AW et al. Effect of vitamin C and vitamin E supplementation on endothelial function: a systematic review and meta-analysis of randomised controlled trials. Br J Nutr. 2015 Apr 28; 113(8):1182–94. [PMID: 25919436]

Curtis AJ et al. Vitamin E supplementation and mortality in healthy people: a meta-analysis of randomised controlled trials. Cardiovasc Drugs Ther. 2014 Dec;28(6):563–73. [PMID: 25398301]

Dysken MW et al. Effect of vitamin E and memantine on functional decline in Alzheimer disease: the TEAM-AD VA cooperative randomized trial. JAMA. 2014 Jan 1;311(1):33–44. [PMID: 24381967]

Fortmann SP et al. Vitamin and mineral supplements in the primary prevention of cardiovascular disease and cancer: an updated systematic evidence review for the U.S. Preventive Services Task Force. Ann Intern Med. 2013 Dec 17; 159(12):824–34. [PMID: 24217421]

Wang L et al. Vitamin E and C supplementation and risk of cancer in men: posttrial follow-up in the Physicians' Health Study II randomized trial. Am J Clin Nutr. 2014 Sep; 100(3):915–23. [PMID: 25008853]

VITAMIN K

Vitamin K is discussed in Chapter 14.

▼ DIET THERAPY

In consultation with a registered dietician, specific therapeutic diets can be designed to facilitate the medical management of most common illnesses. Diet therapy is a difficult process, though, and not all patients are able to cooperate fully. Requesting the patient to record dietary intake for 3–5 days may provide useful insight into the patient's motivation as well as providing nutrient information about the current diet.

Therapeutic diets can be divided into three groups: (1) diets that alter the consistency of food, (2) diets that restrict or otherwise modify dietary components, and (3) diets that supplement dietary components.

DIETS THAT ALTER CONSISTENCY

▶ Clear Liquid Diet

This diet provides adequate water, 500–1000 kcal as simple sugar, and some electrolytes. It is fiber free and requires minimal digestion or intestinal motility.

A clear liquid diet is useful for patients with resolving postoperative ileus, acute gastroenteritis, partial intestinal obstruction, and as preparation for diagnostic gastrointestinal procedures. It is commonly used as the first diet for patients who have been taking nothing by mouth for long periods. Because of the low calorie and minimal protein content of the clear liquid diet, it is used only for short periods.

▶ Full Liquid Diet

The full liquid diet provides adequate water and can be designed to provide adequate calories and protein. Vitamins and minerals—especially folic acid, iron, and vitamin B_6—may be inadequate and should be provided in the form of supplements. Dairy products, soups, eggs, and soft cereals are used to supplement clear liquids. Commercial oral supplements can also be incorporated into the diet or used alone.

This diet is low in residue and can be used in many instances instead of the clear liquid diet described above—especially in patients with difficulty in chewing or swallowing, with partial obstructions, or in preparation for some diagnostic procedures. Full liquid diets are commonly used following clear liquid diets to advance diets in patients who have been taking nothing by mouth for long periods.

▶ Soft Diets

Soft diets are designed for patients unable to chew or swallow hard or coarse food. Tender foods are used, and most raw fruits and vegetables and coarse breads and cereals are eliminated. Soft diets are commonly used to assist in progression from full liquid diets to regular diets in postoperative patients, in patients who are too weak or those whose dentition is too poor to handle a general diet, in head and neck surgical patients, in patients with esophageal strictures, and in other patients who have difficulty with chewing or swallowing.

The soft diet can be designed to meet all nutritional requirements.

DIETS THAT RESTRICT NUTRIENTS

Diets can be designed to restrict (or eliminate) virtually any nutrient or food component. The most commonly used restricted diets are those that limit sodium, fat, and protein. Other restrictive diets include gluten restriction in gluten enteropathy, potassium and phosphate reduction in chronic kidney disease, and various elimination diets for food allergies.

▶ Sodium-Restricted Diets

Low-sodium diets are useful in the management of hypertension and in conditions in which sodium retention and edema are prominent features, particularly heart failure, chronic liver disease, and chronic kidney disease. Sodium restriction is beneficial with or without diuretic therapy. When used in conjunction with diuretics, sodium restriction allows lower dosage of the diuretic medication and may prevent side effects. Potassium excretion, in particular, is directly related to distal renal tubule sodium delivery, and sodium restriction will decrease diuretic-related potassium losses.

Typical American diets contain 4–6 g (175–260 mEq) of sodium per day. A no-added-salt diet contains approximately 3 g (132 mEq) of sodium per day. Further restriction can be achieved with diets of 2 or 1 g of sodium per day. Diets with more severe restriction are poorly accepted by patients and are rarely used. Current Institute of Medicine guidelines recommend 2.3 g of sodium per day, which is approximately 1 teaspoon of salt.

Dietary sodium includes sodium naturally occurring in foods, sodium added during food processing, and sodium added by the consumer during cooking and at the table. About 80% of the current US dietary intake is from processed and pre-prepared foods. Diets designed for 2.3 g of sodium per day require elimination of most processed foods, added salt, and foods with particularly high sodium content. Patients who follow such diets for 2–3 months lose their craving for salty foods and can often continue to restrict their sodium intake indefinitely. Many patients with mild hypertension will achieve significant reductions in blood pressure (approximately 5 mm Hg diastolic) with this degree of sodium restriction.

Diets allowing 1 g of sodium require further restriction of commonly eaten foods. Special "low-sodium" products are available to facilitate such diets. These diets are difficult for most people to follow and are generally reserved for hospitalized patients, most commonly those with severe liver disease and ascites.

▶ Fat-Restricted Diets

Traditional fat-restricted diets are useful in the treatment of fat malabsorption syndromes. Such diets will improve the symptoms of diarrhea with steatorrhea independently of the primary physiologic abnormality by limiting the quantity of fatty acids that reach the colon. The degree of fat restriction necessary to control symptoms must be individualized. Patients with severe malabsorption can be limited to 40–60 g of fat per day. Diets containing 60–80 g of fat per day can be designed for patients with less severe abnormalities.

In general, fat-restricted diets require broiling, baking, or boiling meat and fish; discarding the skin of poultry and fish and using those foods as the main protein source; using nonfat dairy products; and avoiding desserts, sauces, and gravies.

▶ Low-Cholesterol, Low-Saturated-Fat Diets

Fat-restricted diets that specifically restrict saturated fats and dietary cholesterol are the mainstay of dietary treatment of hyperlipidemia (see Chapter 28). Similar diets are often recommended for diabetes mellitus (see Chapter 27) and for the prevention of coronary artery disease (see Chapter 10). The large Women's Health Initiative Dietary Modification Trial, however, did not show any significant benefit of a low-fat diet on weight control or prevention of cardiovascular disease or cancer. In contrast, a study of Mediterranean diets, supplemented by nuts or extra-virgin olive oil, did demonstrate a reduction in cardiovascular events.

The aim of low-cholesterol, low-fat diets is to restrict total fat to less than 30% of calories and to achieve a normal body weight by caloric restriction and increased physical activity. Saturated fat is restricted to 7% of calories and dietary cholesterol to 200 mg/day. Saturated fat can be replaced either with complex carbohydrates or, if energy balance permits, with monounsaturated fats. Saturated fat, total fat, and dietary cholesterol can be restricted further, but studies suggest that more extreme restriction offers little further advantage in overall modification of serum lipids. Cholesterol-lowering diets can be further augmented with the addition of plant stanols and sterols and with soluble dietary fiber.

▶ Protein-Restricted Diets

Protein-restricted diets are most commonly used in patients with hepatic encephalopathy due to chronic liver disease and in patients with advanced chronic kidney disease to slow the progression of early disease and to decrease symptoms of uremia in more severe disease. Patients with selected inborn errors of amino acid metabolism and other abnormalities resulting in hyperammonemia also require restriction of protein or of specific amino acids.

Protein restriction is intended to limit the production of nitrogenous waste products. Energy intake must be adequate to facilitate the efficient use of dietary protein. Proteins must be of high biologic value and be provided in sufficient quantity to meet minimal requirements. For most patients, the diet should contain at least 0.6 g/kg/day of protein. Patients with encephalopathy who do not respond to this degree of restriction are unlikely to respond to more severe restriction.

DIETS THAT SUPPLEMENT NUTRIENTS

▶ High-Fiber Diet

Dietary fiber is a diverse group of plant constituents that is resistant to digestion by the human digestive tract. Guidelines suggest that men eat 30–38 g/day and women 21–25 g/day. Typical US diets, however, contain about half of that amount. Epidemiologic evidence has suggested that populations consuming greater quantities of fiber have a lower incidence of certain gastrointestinal disorders, including diverticulitis and, in some studies, colon cancer and a lower risk of cardiovascular disease. A meta-analysis of 22 studies suggested that each 7 g of dietary fiber was associated with a 9% decrease in first cardiovascular events.

Diets high in dietary fiber (21–38 g/day) are also commonly used in the management of a variety of gastrointestinal disorders, particularly irritable bowel syndrome and recurrent diverticulitis. Diets high in fiber, particularly soluble fiber, may also be useful to reduce blood sugar in patients with diabetes and to reduce cholesterol levels in patients with hypercholesterolemia. Good sources of soluble fiber are oats, nuts, seeds, legumes and most fruits. Foods with insoluble fiber include whole wheat, brown rice, other whole grains, and most vegetables. For some patients, the addition of psyllium seed (2 tsp per day) or natural bran (one-half cup per day) may be a useful adjunct to increase dietary fiber.

▶ High-Potassium Diets

Potassium-supplemented diets are used most commonly to compensate for potassium losses caused by diuretics. Although potassium losses can be partially prevented by using lower doses of diuretics, concurrent sodium restriction, and potassium-sparing diuretics, some patients require additional potassium to prevent hypokalemia. High-potassium diets may also have a direct antihypertensive effect. Typical American diets contain about 3 g (80 mEq) of potassium per day. High-potassium diets commonly contain 4.5–7 g (120–180 mEq) of potassium per day.

Most fruits, vegetables, and their juices contain high concentrations of potassium. Supplemental potassium can also be provided with potassium-containing salt substitutes (up to 20 mEq in one-quarter tsp) or as potassium chloride in solution or capsules, but this is rarely necessary if the above measures are followed to prevent potassium losses and supplement dietary potassium.

▶ High-Calcium Diets

Additional intakes of dietary calcium have been recommended for the prevention of postmenopausal osteoporosis, the prevention and treatment of hypertension, and the prevention of colon cancer. The Women's Health Initiative, however, suggested that calcium and vitamin D supplementation did not prevent fractures or colon cancer. Observational studies have also suggested that calcium supplements, especially when taken without vitamin D, may be associated with an increased risk of coronary heart disease. The recommended dietary allowance for the total calcium intake (from food and supplements) in adults ranges from 1000 mg/day to 1200 mg/day. Average American daily intakes are approximately 700 mg/day.

Dairy products are the primary dietary sources of calcium in the United States. An 8-ounce glass of milk, for example, contains approximately 300 mg of calcium. Patients with lactose intolerance who cannot tolerate liquid dairy products may be able to use lactose-free milk, take supplemental lactase enzyme supplements, or tolerate non-liquid products such as cheese and yogurt. Leafy green vegetables and canned fish with bones also contain high concentrations of calcium, although the latter is also high in sodium.

Albenberg LG et al. Diet and the intestinal microbiome: associations, functions, and implications for health and disease. Gastroenterology. 2014 May;146(6):1564–72. [PMID: 24503132]

Bao Y et al. Association of nut consumption with total and cause-specific mortality. N Engl J Med. 2013 Nov 21; 369(21):2001–11. [PMID: 24256379]

Baron RB. Eat more fibre. BMJ. 2013 Dec 19;347:f7401. [PMID: 24355540]

Baron RB. Should we all be vegetarians? JAMA Intern Med. 2013 Jul 8;173(13):1238–9. [PMID: 23836265]

Estruch R et al; PREDIMED Study Investigators. Primary prevention of cardiovascular disease with a Mediterranean diet. N Engl J Med. 2013 Apr 4;368(14):1279–90. Erratum in: N Engl J Med. 2014 Feb 27;370(9):886. [PMID: 23432189]

Imamura F et al. Consumption of sugar sweetened beverages, artificially sweetened beverages, and fruit juice and incidence of type 2 diabetes: systematic review, meta-analysis, and estimation of population attributable fraction. BMJ. 2015 Jul 21; 351:h3576. [PMID: 26199070]

Orlich MJ et al. Vegetarian dietary patterns and mortality in Adventist Health Study 2. JAMA Intern Med. 2013 Jul 8; 173(13):1230–8. [PMID: 23836264]

Sabaté J et al. A perspective on vegetarian dietary patterns and risk of metabolic syndrome. Br J Nutr. 2015 Apr;113(Suppl 2): S136–43. [PMID: 26148917]

Threapleton DE et al. Dietary fibre intake and risk of cardiovascular disease: systematic review and meta-analysis. BMJ. 2013 Dec 19;347:f6879. [PMID: 24355537]

Valls-Pedret C et al. Mediterranean diet and age-related cognitive decline: a randomized clinical trial. JAMA Intern Med. 2015 Jul;175(7):1094–103. [PMID: 25961184]

Vazquez-Roque MI et al. A controlled trial of gluten-free diet in patients with irritable bowel syndrome-diarrhea: effects on bowel frequency and intestinal function. Gastroenterology. 2013 May;144(5):903–11.e3. [PMID: 23357715]

▼ NUTRITIONAL SUPPORT

Nutritional support is the provision of nutrients to patients who cannot meet their nutritional requirements by eating standard diets. Nutrients may be delivered enterally, using oral nutritional supplements, nasogastric and nasoduodenal feeding tubes, and tube enterostomies, or parenterally, using lines or catheters placed in peripheral or central veins, respectively. Current nutritional support techniques permit adequate nutrient delivery to most patients. Nutrition support should be utilized, however, only if it is likely to improve the patient's clinical outcome. The financial costs and risks of side effects must be balanced against the potential advantages of improved nutritional status in each clinical situation.

INDICATIONS FOR NUTRITIONAL SUPPORT

The precise indications for nutritional support remain controversial. Most authorities agree that nutritional support is indicated for at least four groups of adult patients: (1) those with inadequate bowel syndromes, (2) those with severe prolonged hypercatabolic states (eg, due to extensive burns, multiple trauma, mechanical ventilation), (3) those requiring prolonged therapeutic bowel rest, and (4) those with severe protein–calorie undernutrition with a treatable disease who have sustained a loss of over 25% of body weight.

It has been difficult to prove the efficacy of nutritional support in the treatment of most other conditions. In most cases it has not been possible to show a clear advantage of treatment by means of nutritional support over treatment without such support.

The American Society for Parenteral and Enteral Nutrition (ASPEN) has published recommendations for the rational use of nutritional support. The recommendations emphasize the need to individualize the decision to begin nutritional support, weighing the risks and costs against the benefits to each patient. They also reinforce the need to identify high-risk malnourished patients by nutritional assessment.

▶ Nutritional Support Methods

Selection of the most appropriate nutritional support method involves consideration of gastrointestinal function, the anticipated duration of nutritional support, and the ability of each method to meet the patient's nutritional requirements. The method chosen should meet the patient's nutritional needs with the lowest risk and lowest cost possible. For most patients, enteral feeding is safer and cheaper and offers significant physiologic advantages. An algorithm for selection of the most appropriate nutritional support method is presented in Figure 29–1.

Prior to initiating specialized enteral nutritional support, efforts should be made to supplement food intake. Attention to patient preferences, timing of meals and diagnostic procedures and use of medications, and the use of foods brought to the hospital by family and friends can often increase oral intake. Patients unable to eat enough at regular mealtimes to meet nutritional requirements can be given **oral supplements** as snacks or to replace low-calorie beverages. Oral supplements of differing nutritional composition are available for the purpose of individualizing the diet in accordance with specific clinical requirements. Fiber and lactose content, caloric density, protein level, amino acid profiles, vitamin K, and calcium can all be modified as necessary.

Patients unable to take adequate oral nutrients who have functioning gastrointestinal tracts and who meet the criteria for nutritional support are candidates for **liquid artificial nutrition ("tube feedings")**. Small-bore feeding tubes are placed via the nose into the stomach or duodenum. Patients able to sit up in bed who can protect their airways can be fed into the stomach. Because of the increased risk of aspiration, patients who cannot adequately protect their airways should be fed nasoduodenally (though, as noted below, this may not prevent all aspirations, particularly if the pylorus is patulous). Feeding tubes can usually be passed into the duodenum by leaving an extra length of tubing in the stomach and placing the patient in the right decubitus position. Metoclopramide, 10 mg intravenously, can be given 20 minutes prior to insertion and continued every 6 hours thereafter to facilitate passage through the pylorus. Occasionally, patients will require fluoroscopic or endoscopic guidance to insert the tube distal to the pylorus. Placement of nasogastric and, particularly, nasoduodenal tubes should be confirmed radiographically before delivery of feeding solutions.

Feeding tubes can also be placed directly into the gastrointestinal tract using **tube enterostomies**. Most tube enterostomies are placed in patients who require long-term enteral nutritional support. Gastrostomies have the advantage of allowing bolus feedings, while jejunostomies require

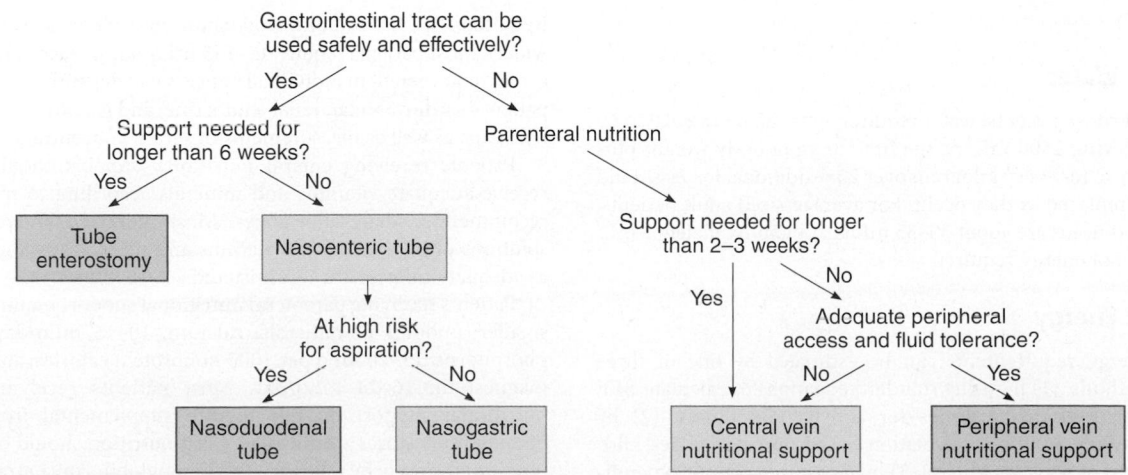

▲ **Figure 29–1.** Nutritional support method decision tree.

continuous infusions. Gastrostomies—like nasogastric feeding—should be used only in patients at low risk for aspiration. Gastrostomies can also be placed percutaneously with the aid of endoscopy. These tubes can then be advanced to jejunostomies. Tube enterostomies can also be placed surgically.

Patients who require nutritional support but whose gastrointestinal tracts are nonfunctional should receive **parenteral nutritional support**. Most patients receive parenteral feedings via a central vein—most commonly the subclavian vein. Peripheral veins can be used in some patients, but because of the high osmolality of parenteral solutions this is rarely tolerated for more than a few weeks.

Peripheral vein nutritional support is most commonly used in patients with nonfunctioning gastrointestinal tracts who require immediate support but whose clinical status is expected to improve within 1–2 weeks, allowing enteral feeding. Peripheral vein nutritional support is administered via standard intravenous lines. Solutions should always include lipid and dextrose in combination with amino acids to provide adequate nonprotein calories. Serious side effects are infrequent, but there is a high incidence of phlebitis and infiltration of intravenous lines.

Central vein nutritional support is delivered via intravenous catheters placed percutaneously using aseptic technique. Proper placement in the superior vena cava is documented radiographically before the solution is infused. Catheters must be carefully maintained by experienced nursing personnel and used solely for nutritional support to prevent infection and other catheter-related complications.

NUTRITIONAL REQUIREMENTS

Each patient's nutritional requirements should be determined independently of the method of nutritional support. In most situations, solutions of equal nutrient value can be designed for delivery via enteral and parenteral routes, but differences in absorption must be considered. A complete nutritional support solution must contain water, energy, amino acids, electrolytes, vitamins, minerals, and essential fatty acids.

▶ Water

For most patients, water requirements can be calculated by allowing 1500 mL for the first 20 kg of body weight plus 20 mL for every kilogram over 20. Additional losses should be replaced as they occur. For average-sized adult patients, fluid needs are about 30–35 mL/kg, or approximately 1 mL/kcal of energy required.

▶ Energy

Energy requirements can be estimated by one of three methods: (1) by using standard equations to calculate BEE plus additional calories for activity and illness, (2) by applying a simple calculation based on calories per kilogram of body weight, or (3) by measuring energy expenditure with indirect calorimetry.

BEE can be estimated by the **Harris–Benedict equation**: for men, BEE = 666 + (13.7 × weight in kg) + (5 × height in cm) – (6.8 × age in years). For women, BEE = 655 + (9.5 × weight in kg) + (1.8 × height in cm) – (4.7 × age in years). For undernourished patients, actual body weight should be used; for obese patients, ideal body weight should be used. For most patients, an additional 20–50% of BEE is administered as nonprotein calories to accommodate energy expenditures during activity or relating to the illness. Occasional patients are noted to have energy expenditures greater than 150% of BEE.

Energy requirements can be estimated also by multiplying actual body weight in kilograms (for obese patients, ideal body weight) by 30–35 kcal.

Both of these methods provide imprecise estimates of actual energy expenditures, especially for the markedly underweight, overweight, and critically ill patient. Studies using indirect calorimetry have demonstrated that as many as 30–40% of patients will have measured expenditures 10% above or below estimated values. For accurate determination of energy expenditure, indirect calorimetry should be used.

▶ Protein

Protein and energy requirements are closely related. If adequate calories are provided, most patients can be given 0.8–1.2 g of protein per kilogram per day. Patients undergoing moderate to severe stress should receive up to 1.5 g/kg/day. As in the case of energy requirements, actual weights should be used for normal and underweight patients and ideal weights for patients with significant obesity.

Patients who are receiving protein without adequate calories will catabolize protein for energy rather than utilizing it for protein synthesis. Thus, when energy intake is low, excess protein is needed for nitrogen balance. If both energy and protein intakes are low, extra energy will have a more significant positive effect on nitrogen balance than extra protein.

▶ Electrolytes & Minerals

Requirements for sodium, potassium, and chloride vary widely. Most patients require 45–145 mEq/day of each. The actual requirement in individual patients will depend on the patient's cardiovascular, renal, endocrine, and gastrointestinal status as well as measurements of serum concentration.

Patients receiving enteral nutritional support should receive adequate vitamins and minerals according to the recommended daily allowances. Most premixed enteral solutions provide adequate vitamins and minerals as long as adequate calories are administered.

Patients receiving parenteral nutritional support require smaller amounts of minerals: calcium, 10–15 mEq/day; phosphorus, 15–20 mEq per 1000 nonprotein calories; and magnesium, 16–24 mEq/day. Most patients receiving nutritional support do not require supplemental iron because body stores are adequate. Iron nutrition should be monitored closely by following the hemoglobin concentration, mean corpuscular volume, and iron studies.

Parenteral administration of iron is associated with a number of adverse effects and should be reserved for iron-deficient patients unable to take oral iron.

Patients receiving parenteral nutritional support should be given the trace elements zinc (about 5 mg/day) and copper (about 2 mg/day). Patients with diarrhea will require additional zinc to replace fecal losses. Additional trace elements—especially chromium, manganese, and selenium—are provided to patients receiving long-term parenteral nutrition.

Parenteral vitamins are provided daily. Standardized multivitamin solutions are currently available to provide adequate quantities of vitamins A, B_{12}, C, D, E, thiamine, riboflavin, niacin, pantothenic acid, pyridoxine, folic acid, and biotin. Vitamin K is not given routinely but administered when the prothrombin time becomes abnormal.

▶ Essential Fatty Acids

Patients receiving nutritional support should be given 2–4% of their total calories as linoleic acid to prevent essential fatty acid deficiency. Most prepared enteral solutions contain adequate linoleic acid. Patients receiving parenteral nutrition should be given at least 250 mL of a 20% intravenous fat (emulsified soybean or safflower oil) about two or three times a week. Intravenous fat can also be used as an energy source in place of dextrose.

ENTERAL NUTRITIONAL SUPPORT SOLUTIONS

Most patients who require enteral nutritional support can be given commercially prepared enteral solutions (Table 29–1). Nutritionally complete solutions have been designed to provide adequate proportions of water, energy, protein, and micronutrients. Nutritionally incomplete solutions are also available to provide specific macronutrients (eg, protein, carbohydrate, and fat) to supplement complete solutions for patients with unusual requirements or to design solutions that are not available commercially.

Nutritionally complete solutions are characterized as follows: (1) by osmolality (isotonic or hypertonic), (2) by lactose content (present or absent), (3) by the molecular form of the protein component (intact proteins; peptides or amino acids), (4) by the quantity of protein and calories provided, and (5) by fiber content (present or absent). For most patients, isotonic solutions containing no lactose or fiber are preferable. Such solutions generally contain moderate amounts of fat and intact protein. Most commercial isotonic solutions contain 1000 kcal and about 37–45 g of protein per liter.

Solutions containing hydrolyzed proteins or crystalline amino acids and with no significant fat content are called elemental solutions, since macronutrients are provided in their most "elemental" form. These solutions have been designed for patients with malabsorption, particularly pancreatic insufficiency and limited fat absorption. Elemental diets are extremely hypertonic and often result in more severe diarrhea. Their use should be limited to patients who cannot tolerate isotonic solutions.

Table 29–1. Enteral solutions.

Complete
  Blenderized (eg, Compleat Regular, Compleat Modified,[1] Vitaneed[1])
  Whole protein, lactose-containing (eg, Mentene, Carnation and Delmark Instant Breakfast, Forta Shake)
  Whole protein, lactose-free, low-residue:
    1 kcal/mL (eg, Ensure, Isocal, Osmolite, Nutren 1.0,[1] Nutrilan, Isolan,[1] Sustacal, Resource)
    1.5 kcal/mL (eg, Ensure Plus, Sustacal HC, Comply, Nutren 1.5, Resource Plus)
    2 kcal/mL (eg, Isocal HCN, Magnacal, TwoCal HN)
    High-nitrogen: > 15% total calories from protein (eg, Ensure HN, Attain,[1] Osmolite HN,[1] Replete, Entrition HN,[1] Isolan,[1] Isocal HN,[1] Sustacal HC, Isosource HN,[1] Ultralan)
  Whole protein, lactose-free, high-residue:
    1 kcal/mL (eg, Jevity,[1] Profiber,[1] Nutren 1.0 with fiber,[1] Fiberlan,[1] Sustacal with fiber, Ultracal,[1] Ensure with fiber, Fibersource)
  Chemically defined peptide- or amino acid-based (eg, Accupep HPF, CriticareHN, Peptamen,[1] Reabfin, Vital HN, AlitraQ, Tolerex, Vivonex TEN)
"Disease-specific" formulas
  Advanced chronic kidney disease: with essential amino acids (eg, Amin-Aid, Travasorb Renal, Aminess)
  Malabsorption: with medium-chain triglycerides (eg, Portagen,[1] Travasorb MCT)
  Respiratory failure: with > 50% calories from fat (eg, Pulmocare, NutriVent)
  Hepatic encephalopathy: with high amounts of branched-chain amino acids (eg, Hepatic-Acid II, Travasorb Hepatic)
Incomplete (modular)
  Protein (eg, Nutrisource Protein, Promed, Propac)
  Carbohydrate (eg, Nutrisource Carbohydrate, Polycose, Sumacal)
  Fat (eg, MCT Oil, Microlipid, Nutrisource Lipid)
  Vitamins (eg, Nutrisource Vitamins)
  Minerals (eg, Nutrisource Minerals)

[1]Isotonic.

Although formulas have been designed for specific clinical situations—solutions containing primarily essential amino acids (for advanced chronic kidney disease), medium-chain triglycerides (for fat malabsorption), more fat (for respiratory failure and CO_2 retention), and more branched-chain amino acids (for hepatic encephalopathy and severe trauma)—they have not been shown to be superior to standard formulas for most patients.

Enteral solutions should be administered via continuous infusion, preferably with an infusion pump. Isotonic feedings should be started at full strength at about 25–33% of the estimated final infusion rate. Feedings can be advanced by similar amounts every 12 hours as tolerated. Hypertonic feedings should be started at half strength. The strength and the rate can then be advanced every 6 hours as tolerated.

COMPLICATIONS OF ENTERAL NUTRITIONAL SUPPORT

Minor complications of tube feedings occur in 10–15% of patients. Gastrointestinal complications include diarrhea (most common), inadequate gastric emptying, emesis, esophagitis, and occasionally gastrointestinal bleeding.

Diarrhea associated with tube feeding may be due to intolerance to the osmotic load or to one of the macronutrients (eg, fat, lactose) in the solution. Patients being fed in this way may also have diarrhea from other causes (as side effects of antibiotics or other drugs, associated with infection, etc), and these possibilities should always be investigated in appropriate circumstances.

Mechanical complications of tube feedings are potentially the most serious. Of particular importance is aspiration. All patients receiving nasogastric tube feedings are at risk for this life-threatening complication. Limiting nasogastric feedings to those patients who can adequately protect their airway and careful monitoring of patients being fed by tube should limit these serious complications to 1–2% of cases. Minor mechanical complications are common and include tube obstruction and dislodgment.

Metabolic complications during enteral nutritional support are common but in most cases are easily managed. The most important problem is hypernatremic dehydration, most commonly seen in elderly patients given excessive protein intake who are unable to respond to thirst. Abnormalities of potassium, glucose, CO_2 production, and acid–base balance may also occur.

PARENTERAL NUTRITIONAL SUPPORT SOLUTIONS

Parenteral nutritional support solutions can be designed to deliver adequate nutrients to most patients. The basic parenteral solution is composed of dextrose, amino acids, and water. Electrolytes, minerals, trace elements, vitamins, and medications can also be added. Most commercial solutions contain the monohydrate form of dextrose that provides 3.4 kcal/g. Crystalline amino acids are available in a variety of concentrations, so that a broad range of solutions can be made up that will contain specific amounts of dextrose and amino acids as required.

Typical solutions for central vein nutritional support contain 25–35% dextrose and 2.75–6% amino acids depending upon the patient's estimated nutrient and water requirements. These solutions typically have osmolalities in excess of 1800 mOsm/L and require infusion into a central vein. A typical formula for patients without organ failure is shown in Table 29–2.

Solutions with lower osmolalities can also be designed for infusion into peripheral veins. Typical solutions for peripheral infusion contain 5–10% dextrose and 2.75–4.25% amino acids. These solutions have osmolalities between 800 and 1200 mOsm/L and result in a high incidence of thrombophlebitis and line infiltration. These solutions will provide adequate protein for most patients but inadequate energy. Additional energy must be provided in the form of emulsified soybean or safflower oil. Such intravenous fat solutions are currently available in 10% and 25% solutions providing 1.1 and 2.2 kcal/mL, respectively. Intravenous fat solutions are isosmotic and well tolerated by peripheral veins.

Typical patients are given 200–500 mL of a 20% solution each day. As much as 60% of total calories can be administered in this manner.

Table 29–2. Typical parenteral nutrition solution (for stable patients without organ failure).

Dextrose (3.4 kcal/g)	25%
Amino acids (4 kcal/g)	6%
Na^+	50 mEq/L
K^+	40 mEq/L
Ca^{2+}	5 mEq/L
Mg^{2+}	8 mEq/L
Cl^-	60 mEq/L
P	12 mEq/L
Acetate	Balance
MVI-12 (vitamins)	10 mL/day
MTE (trace elements)	5 mL/day
Fat emulsion 20%	250 mL five times a week
Typical rate	Day 1: 30 mL/h
	Day 2: 60 mL/h
By day 2, solution provides:	Calories: 1925 kcal total
	Protein: 86 g
	Fat: 19% of total kcal
	Fluid: 1690 mL

Intravenous fat can also be provided to patients receiving central vein nutritional support. In this instance, dextrose concentrations should be decreased to provide a fixed concentration of energy. Intravenous fat has been shown to be equivalent to intravenous dextrose in providing energy to spare protein. Intravenous fat is associated with less glucose intolerance, less production of carbon dioxide, and less fatty infiltration of the liver and has been increasingly utilized in patients with hyperglycemia, respiratory failure, and liver disease. Intravenous fat has also been increasingly used in patients with large estimated energy requirements. The maximum glucose utilization rate is approximately 5–7 mg/min/kg. Patients who require additional calories can be given them as fat to prevent excess administration of dextrose. Intravenous fat can also be used to prevent essential fatty acid deficiency. The optimal ratio of carbohydrate and fat in parenteral nutritional support has not been determined.

Infusion of parenteral solutions should be started slowly to prevent hyperglycemia and other metabolic complications. Typical solutions are given initially at a rate of 50 mL/h and advanced by about the same amount every 24 hours until the desired final rate is reached.

COMPLICATIONS OF PARENTERAL NUTRITIONAL SUPPORT

Complications of central vein nutritional support occur in up to 50% of patients. Although most are minor and easily managed, significant complications will develop in about 5% of patients. Complications of central vein nutritional support can be divided into catheter-related complications and metabolic complications.

Table 29–3. Metabolic complications of parenteral nutritional support.

Complication	Common Causes	Possible Solutions
Hyperglycemia	Too rapid infusion of dextrose, "stress," corticosteroids	Decrease glucose infusion; insulin; replacement of dextrose with fat
Hyperosmolar nonketotic dehydration	Severe, undetected hyperglycemia	Insulin, hydration, potassium
Hyperchloremic metabolic acidosis	High chloride administration	Decrease chloride
Azotemia	Excessive protein administration	Decrease amino acid concentration
Hyperphosphatemia, hypokalemia, hypomagnesemia	Extracellular to intracellular shifting with refeeding	Increase solution concentration
Liver enzyme abnormalities	Lipid trapping in hepatocytes, fatty liver	Decrease dextrose
Acalculous cholecystitis	Biliary stasis	Oral fat
Zinc deficiency	Diarrhea, small bowel fistulas	Increase concentration
Copper deficiency	Biliary fistulas	Increase concentration

Catheter-related complications can occur during insertion or while the catheter is in place. Pneumothorax, hemothorax, arterial laceration, air emboli, and brachial plexus injury can occur during catheter placement. The incidence of these complications is inversely related to the experience of the physician performing the procedure but will occur in at least 1–2% of cases even in major medical centers. Each catheter placement should be documented by chest radiograph prior to initiation of nutritional support.

Catheter thrombosis and catheter-related sepsis are the most important complications of indwelling catheters. Patients with indwelling central vein catheters in whom fever develops without an apparent source should have their lines changed over a wire or removed immediately, the tip quantitatively cultured, and antibiotics begun empirically. Quantitative tip cultures and blood cultures will help guide further antibiotic therapy. Catheter-related sepsis occurs in 2–3% of patients even if maximal efforts are made to prevent infection.

Metabolic complications of central vein nutritional support occur in over 50% of patients (Table 29–3). Most are minor and easily managed, and termination of support is seldom necessary.

PATIENT MONITORING DURING NUTRITIONAL SUPPORT

Every patient receiving enteral or parenteral nutritional support should be monitored closely. Formal nutritional support teams composed of a physician, a nurse, a dietitian, and a pharmacist have been shown to decrease the rate of complications.

Patients should be monitored both for the adequacy of treatment and to prevent complications or detect them early when they occur. Because estimates of nutritional requirements are imprecise, frequent reassessment is necessary. Daily intakes should be recorded and compared with estimated requirements. Body weight, hydration status, and overall clinical status should be followed. Patients who do not appear to be responding as anticipated can be evaluated for nitrogen balance by means of the following equation:

$$\text{Nitrogen balance} = \frac{\dfrac{24\text{-hour protein intake (g)}}{6.25}} - \left(\dfrac{24\text{-hour urinary nitrogen (g)}} + 4 \right)$$

Patients with positive nitrogen balances can be continued on their current regimens; patients with negative balances should receive moderate increases in calorie and protein intake and then be reassessed. Monitoring for metabolic complications includes daily measurements of electrolytes; serum glucose, phosphorus, magnesium, calcium, and creatinine; and BUN until the patient is stabilized. Once the patient is stabilized, electrolytes, phosphorus, calcium, magnesium, and glucose should be obtained at least twice weekly. Red blood cell folate, zinc, and copper should be checked at least once a month.

Alhazzani W et al. Small bowel feeding and risk of pneumonia in adult critically ill patients: a systematic review and meta-analysis of randomized trials. Crit Care. 2013 Jul 2;17(4):R127. [PMID: 23820047]

Arabi YM et al; PermiT Trial Group. Permissive underfeeding or standard enteral feeding in critically ill adults. N Engl J Med. 2015 Jun 18;372(25):2398–408. Erratum in: N Engl J Med. 2015 Sep 24;373(13):1281. [PMID: 25992505]

Bally MR et al. Nutritional support and outcomes in malnourished medical inpatients: a systematic review and meta-analysis. JAMA Intern Med. 2016 Jan 1;176(1):43–53. [PMID: 26720894]

Boelens PG et al. Reduction of postoperative ileus by early enteral nutrition in patients undergoing major rectal surgery: prospective, randomized, controlled trial. Ann Surg. 2014 Apr; 259(4):649–55. [PMID: 24169163]

Codner PA. Enteral nutrition in the critically ill patient. Surg Clin North Am. 2012 Dec;92(6):1485–501. [PMID: 23153881]

Davies AR et al. A multicenter, randomized controlled trial comparing early nasojejunal with nasogastric nutrition in critical illness. Crit Care Med. 2012 Aug;40(8):2342–8. [PMID: 22809907]

Desai SV et al. Nutrition in the ICU: an evidence-based approach. Chest. 2014 May;145(5):1148–57. [PMID: 24798840]

Marik PE. Enteral nutrition in the critically ill: myths and misconceptions. Crit Care Med. 2014 Apr;42(4):962–9. [PMID: 24296860]

Reignier J et al; Clinical Research in Intensive Care and Sepsis (CRICS) Group. Effect of not monitoring residual gastric volume on risk of ventilator-associated pneumonia in adults receiving mechanical ventilation and early enteral feeding: a randomized controlled trial. JAMA. 2013 Jan 16;309(3):249–56. [PMID: 23321763]

Ross VM et al. National clinical guidelines and home parenteral nutrition. Nutr Clin Pract. 2011 Dec;26(6):656–64. [PMID: 22205553]

Schulman RC et al. Metabolic and nutrition support in the chronic critical illness syndrome. Respir Care. 2012 Jun; 57(6):958–77. [PMID: 22663970]

van Zanten AR et al. High-protein enteral nutrition enriched with immune-modulating nutrients vs standard high-protein enteral nutrition and nosocomial infections in the ICU: a randomized clinical trial. JAMA. 2014 Aug 6;312(5):514–24. [PMID: 25096691]

Vincent JL et al. When should we add parenteral to enteral nutrition? Lancet. 2013 Feb 2;381(9864):354–5. [PMID: 23218814]

Wernerman J. Combined enteral and parenteral nutrition. Curr Opin Clin Nutr Metab Care. 2012 Mar;15(2):161–5. [PMID: 22261951]

Yi F et al. Meta-analysis: total parenteral nutrition versus total enteral nutrition in predicted severe acute pancreatitis. Intern Med. 2012;51(6):523–30. [PMID: 22449657]

Common Problems in Infectious Diseases & Antimicrobial Therapy

Peter V. Chin-Hong, MD

B. Joseph Guglielmo, PharmD

COMMON PROBLEMS IN INFECTIOUS DISEASES

FEVER OF UNKNOWN ORIGIN (FUO)

ESSENTIALS OF DIAGNOSIS

▸ Illness of at least 3 weeks duration.

▸ Fever over 38.3°C on several occasions.

▸ Diagnosis has not been made after 3 outpatient visits or 3 days of hospitalization.

▸ General Considerations

The intervals specified in the criteria for the diagnosis of FUO are arbitrary ones intended to exclude patients with protracted but self-limited viral illnesses and to allow time for the usual radiographic, serologic, and cultural studies to be performed. Because of costs of hospitalization and the availability of most screening tests on an outpatient basis, the original criterion requiring 1 week of hospitalization has been modified to accept patients in whom a diagnosis has not been made after 3 outpatient visits or 3 days of hospitalization.

Several additional categories of FUO have been added: (1) **Hospital-associated FUO** refers to the hospitalized patient with fever of 38.3°C or higher on several occasions, due to a process not present or incubating at the time of admission, in whom initial cultures are negative and the diagnosis remains unknown after 3 days of investigation (see Health care-associated Infections below). (2) **Neutropenic FUO** includes patients with fever of 38.3°C or higher on several occasions with less than 500 neutrophils per microliter in whom initial cultures are negative and the diagnosis remains uncertain after 3 days (see Chapter 2 and Infections in the Immunocompromised Patient, below). (3) **HIV-associated FUO** pertains to HIV-positive patients with fever of 38.3°C or higher who have been febrile for 4 weeks or more as an outpatient or 3 days as an inpatient, in whom the diagnosis remains uncertain after 3 days of investigation with at least 2 days for cultures to incubate (see Chapter 31). Although not usually

considered separately, FUO in solid organ transplant recipients and FUO in the returning traveler are common scenarios, each with a unique differential diagnosis, and are also discussed in this chapter.

For a general discussion of fever, see the section on fever and hyperthermia in Chapter 2.

A. Common Causes

Most cases represent unusual manifestations of common diseases and not rare or exotic diseases—eg, tuberculosis, endocarditis, gallbladder disease, and HIV (primary infection or opportunistic infection) are more common causes of FUO than Whipple disease or familial Mediterranean fever.

B. Age of Patient

In adults, infections (25–40% of cases) and cancer (25–40% of cases) account for the majority of FUOs. In children, infections are the most common cause of FUO (30–50% of cases) and cancer a rare cause (5–10% of cases). Autoimmune disorders occur with equal frequency in adults and children (10–20% of cases), but the diseases differ. Juvenile rheumatoid arthritis is particularly common in children, whereas systemic lupus erythematosus, granulomatosis with polyangiitis (formerly Wegener granulomatosis), and polyarteritis nodosa are more common in adults. Still disease, giant cell arteritis, and polymyalgia rheumatica occur exclusively in adults. In the elderly (over 65 years of age), multisystem immune-mediated diseases such as temporal arteritis, polymyalgia rheumatica, sarcoidosis, rheumatoid arthritis, and granulomatosis with polyangiitis account for 25–30% of all FUOs.

C. Duration of Fever

The cause of FUO changes dramatically in patients who have been febrile for 6 months or longer. Infection, cancer, and autoimmune disorders combined account for only 20% of FUOs in these patients. Instead, other entities such as granulomatous diseases (granulomatous hepatitis, Crohn disease, ulcerative colitis) and factitious fever become important causes. One-fourth of patients who say they have been febrile for 6 months or longer actually have no true fever or underlying disease. Instead, the usual normal circadian variation in temperature (temperature 0.5–1°C higher in the afternoon than in the morning) is interpreted as abnormal. Patients with episodic or recurrent fever (ie, those who meet the criteria for FUO but have fever-free periods of 2 weeks or longer) are similar to those with prolonged fever. Infection, malignancy, and autoimmune disorders account for only 20–25% of such fevers, whereas various miscellaneous diseases (Crohn disease, familial Mediterranean fever, allergic alveolitis) account for another 25%. Approximately 50% of cases remain undiagnosed but have a benign course with eventual resolution of symptoms.

D. Immunologic Status

In the neutropenic patient, fungal infections and occult bacterial infections are important causes of FUO. In the patient taking immunosuppressive medications (particularly organ transplant patients), cytomegalovirus (CMV) infections are a frequent cause of fever, as are fungal infections, nocardiosis, *Pneumocystis jirovecii* pneumonia, and mycobacterial infections.

E. Classification of Causes of FUO

Most patients with FUO will fit into one of five categories.

1. Infection—Both systemic and localized infections can cause FUO. Tuberculosis and endocarditis are the most common systemic infections, but mycoses, viral diseases (particularly infection with Epstein-Barr virus and CMV), toxoplasmosis, brucellosis, Q fever, cat-scratch disease, salmonellosis, malaria, and many other less common infections have been implicated. Primary infection with HIV or opportunistic infections associated with AIDS—particularly mycobacterial infections—can also present as FUO. The most common form of localized infection causing FUO is an occult abscess. Liver, spleen, kidney, brain, and bone abscesses may be difficult to detect. A collection of pus may form in the peritoneal cavity or in the subdiaphragmatic, subhepatic, paracolic, or other areas. Cholangitis, osteomyelitis, urinary tract infection, dental abscess, or paranasal sinusitis may cause prolonged fever.

2. Neoplasms—Many cancers can present as FUO. The most common are lymphoma (both Hodgkin and non-Hodgkin) and leukemia. Posttransplant lymphoproliferative disorders may also present with fever. Other diseases of lymph nodes, such as angioimmunoblastic lymphoma and Castleman disease, can also cause FUO. Primary and metastatic tumors of the liver are frequently associated with fever, as are renal cell carcinomas. Atrial myxoma is an often forgotten neoplasm that can result in fever. Chronic lymphocytic leukemia and multiple myeloma are rarely associated with fever, and the presence of fever in patients with these diseases should prompt a search for infection.

3. Autoimmune disorders—Still disease, systemic lupus erythematosus, cryoglobulinemia, and polyarteritis nodosa are the most common causes of autoimmune-associated FUO. Giant cell arteritis and polymyalgia rheumatica are

seen almost exclusively in patients over 50 years of age and are nearly always associated with an elevated erythrocyte sedimentation rate (greater than 40 mm/h).

4. Miscellaneous causes—Many other conditions have been associated with FUO but less commonly than the foregoing types of illness. Examples include thyroiditis, sarcoidosis, Whipple disease, familial Mediterranean fever, recurrent pulmonary emboli, alcoholic hepatitis, drug fever, and factitious fever.

5. Undiagnosed FUO—Despite extensive evaluation, the diagnosis remains elusive in 15% or more of patients. Of these patients, the fever abates spontaneously in about 75% with no diagnosis; in the remainder, more classic manifestations of the underlying disease appear over time.

► Clinical Findings

Because the evaluation of a patient with FUO is costly and time-consuming, it is imperative to first document the presence of fever. This is done by observing the patient while the temperature is being taken to ascertain that fever is not factitious (self-induced). Associated findings that accompany fever include tachycardia, chills, and piloerection. A thorough history—including family, occupational, social (sexual practices, use of injection drugs), dietary (unpasteurized products, raw meat), exposures (animals, chemicals), and travel—may give clues to the diagnosis. Repeated physical examination may reveal subtle, evanescent clinical findings essential to diagnosis.

A. Laboratory Tests

In addition to routine laboratory studies, blood cultures should always be obtained, preferably when the patient has not taken antibiotics for several days, and should be held by the laboratory for 2 weeks to detect slow-growing organisms. Cultures on special media are requested if *Legionella, Bartonella,* or nutritionally deficient streptococci are possible pathogens. "Screening tests" with immunologic or microbiologic serologies ("febrile agglutinins") are of low yield and should not be done. If the history or physical examination suggests a specific diagnosis, specific serologic tests with an associated fourfold rise or fall in titer may be useful. Because infection is the most common cause of FUO, other body fluids are usually cultured, ie, urine, sputum, stool, cerebrospinal fluid, and morning gastric aspirates (if one suspects tuberculosis). Direct examination of blood smears may establish a diagnosis of malaria or relapsing fever (*Borrelia*).

B. Imaging

All patients with FUO should have a chest radiograph. Studies such as sinus films, upper gastrointestinal series with small bowel follow-through, barium enema, proctosigmoidoscopy, and evaluation of gallbladder function are reserved for patients who have symptoms, signs, or a history that suggest disease in these body regions. CT scan of the abdomen and pelvis is also frequently performed and is particularly useful for looking at the liver, spleen, and retroperitoneum. When the CT scan is abnormal, the findings often lead to a specific diagnosis. A normal CT scan is not quite as useful; more invasive procedures such as biopsy or exploratory laparotomy may be needed. The role of MRI in the investigation of FUO has not been evaluated. In general, however, MRI is better than CT for detecting lesions of the nervous system and is useful in diagnosing various vasculitides. Ultrasound is sensitive for detecting lesions of the kidney, pancreas, and biliary tree. Echocardiography should be used if one is considering endocarditis or atrial myxoma. Transesophageal echocardiography is more sensitive than surface echocardiography for detecting valvular lesions, but even a negative transesophageal study does not exclude endocarditis (10% false-negative rate). The usefulness of radionuclide studies in diagnosing FUO is variable. Some experts use positron emission tomography (PET) in conjunction with CT scans early in the investigation of FUO. However, more studies are needed before this practice can be more fully integrated into clinical practice. Theoretically, a gallium or PET scan would be more helpful than an indium-labeled white blood cell scan because gallium and fluorodeoxyglucose may be useful for detecting infection, inflammation, and neoplasm whereas the indium scan is useful only for detecting infection. Indium-labeled immunoglobulin may prove to be useful in detecting infection and neoplasm and can be used in the neutropenic patient. It is not sensitive for lesions of the liver, kidney, and heart because of high background activity. In general, radionuclide scans are plagued by high rates of false-positive and false-negative results that are not useful when used as screening tests and, if done at all, are limited to those patients whose history or examination suggests local inflammation or infection.

C. Biopsy

Invasive procedures are often required for diagnosis. Any abnormal finding should be aggressively evaluated: Headache calls for lumbar puncture to rule out meningitis; skin rash should be biopsied for cutaneous manifestations of collagen vascular disease or infection; and enlarged lymph nodes should be aspirated or biopsied for neoplasm and sent for culture. Bone marrow aspiration with biopsy is a relatively low-yield procedure (15–25%; except in HIV-positive patients, in whom mycobacterial infection is a common cause of FUO), but the risk is low and the procedure should be done if other less invasive tests have not yielded a diagnosis, particularly in persons with hematologic abnormalities. Liver biopsy will yield a specific diagnosis in 10–15% of patients with FUO and should be considered in any patient with abnormal liver tests even if the liver is normal in size. CT scanning and MRI have decreased the need for exploratory laparotomy; however, surgical visualization and biopsies should be considered when there is continued deterioration or lack of diagnosis.

► Treatment

Although it is tempting to begin an empiric course of antimicrobials for FUO, it is rarely helpful and may delay diagnosis if the etiology is infectious (eg, by reducing the sensitivity of blood cultures).

Empiric administration of corticosteroids should be discouraged because they can suppress fever and exacerbate many infections.

► When to Refer

- Any patient with FUO and progressive weight loss and other constitutional signs.
- Any immunocompromised patient (eg, transplant recipients and HIV-infected patients).
- Infectious diseases specialists may also be able to coordinate and interpret specialized testing (eg, Q fever serologies) with outside agencies, such as the US Centers for Disease Control and Prevention.

► When to Admit

- Any patient who is rapidly declining with weight loss where hospital admission may expedite work-up.
- If FUO is present in immunocompromised patients, such as those who are neutropenic from recent chemotherapy or those who have undergone transplantation (particularly in the previous 6 months).

Ben-Baruch S et al. Predictive parameters for a diagnostic bone marrow biopsy specimen in the work-up of fever of unknown origin. Mayo Clin Proc. 2012 Feb;87(2):136–42. [PMID: 22226833]

Brown M. Pyrexia of unknown origin 90 years on: a paradigm of modern clinical medicine. Postgrad Med J. 2015 Dec; 91(1082):665–9. [PMID: 26489766]

Cunha BA et al. Fever of unknown origin: a clinical approach. Am J Med. 2015 Oct;128(10):1138.e1–15. [PMID: 26093175]

Hayakawa K et al. Fever of unknown origin: an evidence-based review. Am J Med Sci. 2012 Oct;344(4):307–16. [PMID: 22475734]

Horowitz HW. Fever of unknown origin or fever of too many origins? N Engl J Med. 2013 Jan 17;368(3):197–9. [PMID: 23323894]

Manohar K et al. F-18 FDG-PET/CT in evaluation of patients with fever of unknown origin. Jpn J Radiol. 2013 May; 31(5):320–7. [PMID: 23456545]

Naito T et al. Diagnostic workup for fever of unknown origin: a multicenter collaborative retrospective study. BMJ Open. 2013 Dec 20;3(12):e003971. [PMID: 24362014]

INFECTIONS IN THE IMMUNOCOMPROMISED PATIENT

ESSENTIALS OF DIAGNOSIS

- ► Fever and other symptoms may be blunted because of immunosuppression.

- ► A contaminating organism in an immunocompetent individual may be a pathogen in an immunocompromised one.

- ► The interval since transplantation and the degree of immunosuppression can narrow the differential diagnosis.

- ► Empiric broad-spectrum antibiotics may be appropriate in high-risk patients whether or not symptoms are localized.

General Considerations

Immunocompromised patients have defects in their natural defense mechanisms resulting in an increased risk for infection. In addition, infection is often severe, rapidly progressive, and life threatening. Organisms that are not usually problematic in the immunocompetent person may be important pathogens in the compromised patient (eg, *Staphylococcus epidermidis, Corynebacterium jeikeium, Propionibacterium acnes, Bacillus* species). Therefore, culture results must be interpreted with caution, and isolates should not be disregarded as merely contaminants. Although the type of immunodeficiency is associated with specific infectious disease syndromes, any pathogen can cause infection in any immunosuppressed patient at any time. Thus, a systematic evaluation is required to identify a specific organism.

A. Impaired Humoral Immunity

Defects in humoral immunity are often congenital, although hypogammaglobulinemia can occur in multiple myeloma, chronic lymphocytic leukemia, small lymphocyte lymphoma, and in patients who have undergone splenectomy. Patients with ineffective humoral immunity lack opsonizing antibodies and are at particular risk for infection with encapsulated organisms, such as *Haemophilus influenzae, Neisseria meningitides,* and *Streptococcus pneumoniae.* Although rituximab is normally thought of as being linked to impaired cellular immunity, it has been associated with the development of *Pneumocystis jirovecii* infection as well as with hepatitis B reactivation.

B. Granulocytopenia (Neutropenia)

Granulocytopenia is common following hematopoietic cell transplantation ("stem cell transplantation") and among patients with solid tumors—as a result of myelosuppressive chemotherapy—and in acute leukemias. The risk of infection begins to increase when the absolute granulocyte count falls below 1000/mcL, with a dramatic increase in frequency and severity when the granulocyte count falls below 100/mcL. The infection risk is also increased with a rapid rate of decline of neutrophils and with a prolonged period of neutropenia. The granulocytopenic patient is particularly susceptible to infections with gram-negative enteric organisms, *Pseudomonas,* gram-positive cocci (particularly *Staphylococcus aureus, S epidermidis,* and viridans streptococci), *Candida, Aspergillus,* and other fungi that have recently emerged as pathogens such as *Trichosporon, Scedosporium, Fusarium,* and the mucormycoses.

C. Impaired Cellular Immunity

Patients with cellular immune deficiency encompass a large and heterogeneous group, including patients with HIV infection (see Chapter 31); patients with lymphoreticular malignancies, such as Hodgkin disease; and patients receiving immunosuppressive medications, such as corticosteroids, cyclosporine, tacrolimus, and other cytotoxic drugs. This latter group—those who are immunosuppressed as a result of medications—includes patients who have undergone solid organ transplantation, many patients receiving therapy for solid tumors, and patients receiving prolonged high-dose corticosteroid treatment (eg, for asthma, temporal arteritis, systemic lupus erythematosus). Patients taking tumor necrosis factor (TNF) inhibitors, such as etanercept and infliximab, are also included in this category. Patients with cellular immune dysfunction are susceptible to infections by a large number of organisms, particularly ones that replicate intracellularly. Examples include bacteria, such as *Listeria, Legionella, Salmonella,* and *Mycobacterium;* viruses, such as herpes simplex, varicella, and CMV; fungi, such as *Cryptococcus, Coccidioides, Histoplasma,* and *Pneumocystis;* and protozoa, such as *Toxoplasma.* Patients taking TNF inhibitors have specific defects that increase risk of bacterial, mycobacterial (particularly tuberculosis), viral (HBV reactivation and HCV progression), and fungal infections (primary and reactivation).

D. Hematopoietic Cell Transplant Recipients

The length of time it takes for complications to occur in hematopoietic cell transplant recipients can be helpful in determining the etiologic agent. In the early (preengraftment) posttransplant period (day 1–21), patients will become severely neutropenic for 7–21 days. Patients are at risk for gram-positive (particularly catheter-related) and gram-negative bacterial infections, as well as herpes simplex virus, respiratory syncytial virus, and fungal infections. In contrast to solid organ transplant recipients, the source of fever is unknown in 60–70% of hematopoietic cell transplant patients. Between 3 weeks and 3 months posttransplant, infections with CMV, adenovirus, *Aspergillus,* and *Candida* are most common. *P jirovecii* pneumonia is possible, particularly in patients who receive additional immunosuppression for treatment of graft-versus-host disease. Patients continue to be at risk for infectious complications beyond 3 months following transplantation, particularly those who have received allogeneic transplantation and those who are taking immunosuppressive therapy for chronic graft-versus-host disease. Varicella-zoster is common, and *Aspergillus* and CMV infections are increasingly seen in this period as well.

E. Solid Organ Transplant Recipients

The length of time it takes for infection to occur following solid organ transplantation can also be helpful in determining the infectious origin. Immediate postoperative infections often involve the transplanted organ. Following lung transplantation, pneumonia and mediastinitis are particularly common; following liver transplantation, intra-abdominal abscess, cholangitis, and peritonitis may be seen; after kidney transplantation, urinary tract infections, perinephric abscesses, and infected lymphoceles can occur.

Most infections that occur in the first 2–4 weeks posttransplant are related to the operative procedure and to hospitalization itself (wound infection, intravenous catheter infection, urinary tract infection from a Foley catheter) or are related to the transplanted organ. In rare instances, donor-derived infections (eg, West Nile virus, tuberculosis) may present during this time period. Compensated organ transplants obtained abroad through "medical tourism" can introduce additional risk of infections, which vary by country and by transplant setting. Infections that occur between the first and sixth months are often related to immunosuppression. During this period, reactivation of viruses, such as herpes simplex, varicella-zoster, and CMV is quite common. Opportunistic infections with fungi (eg, *Candida, Aspergillus, Cryptococcus, Pneumocystis*), *Listeria monocytogenes, Nocardia,* and *Toxoplasma* are also common. After 6 months, if immunosuppression has been reduced to maintenance levels, infections that would be expected in any population occur. Patients with poorly functioning allografts receiving long-term immunosuppression therapy continue to be at risk for opportunistic infections.

F. Other Immunocompromised States

A large group of patients who are not specifically immunodeficient are at increased risk for infection due to debilitating injury (eg, burns or severe trauma), invasive procedures (eg, chronic central intravenous catheters, Foley catheters, dialysis catheters), central nervous system dysfunction (which predisposes patients to aspiration pneumonia and decubitus ulcers), obstructing lesions (eg, pneumonia due to an obstructed bronchus, pyelonephritis due to nephrolithiasis, cholangitis secondary to cholelithiasis), and use of broad-spectrum antibiotics. Patients with diabetes mellitus have alterations in cellular immunity, resulting in mucormycosis, emphysematous pyelonephritis, and foot infections.

▶ Clinical Findings

A. Laboratory Findings

Routine evaluation includes complete blood count with differential, chest radiograph, and blood cultures; urine and respiratory cultures should be obtained if indicated clinically or radiographically. Any focal complaints (localized pain, headache, rash) should prompt imaging and cultures appropriate to the site.

Patients who remain febrile without an obvious source should be evaluated for viral infection (serum CMV antigen test or polymerase chain reaction), abscesses (which usually occur near previous operative sites), candidiasis involving the liver or spleen, or aspergillosis. Serologic evaluation may be helpful if toxoplasmosis or an endemic fungal infection (coccidioidomycosis, histoplasmosis) is a possible cause. Antigen-based assays may be useful for the diagnosis of aspergillosis (detected by galactomannan level in serum or bronchoalveolar lavage fluid), or other invasive fungal disease, including *Pneumocystis* infection (serum $(1{\rightarrow}3)$-beta-D-glucan level).

B. Special Diagnostic Procedures

Special diagnostic procedures should also be considered. The cause of pulmonary infiltrates can be easily determined with simple techniques in some situations—eg, induced sputum yields a diagnosis of *Pneumocystis* pneumonia in 50–80% of AIDS patients with this infection. In other situations, more invasive procedures may be required (bronchoalveolar lavage, transbronchial biopsy, open lung biopsy). Skin, liver, or bone marrow biopsy may be helpful in establishing a diagnosis. Next generation DNA-sequencing analysis is being evaluated as an option for diagnosis of infectious diseases in immunocompromised persons.

▶ Differential Diagnosis

Transplant rejection, organ ischemia and necrosis, thrombophlebitis, and lymphoma (posttransplant lymphoproliferative disease) may all present as fever and must be considered in the differential diagnosis.

▶ Prevention

There is great interest in preventing infection with prophylactic antimicrobial regimens but no uniformity of opinion about optimal drugs or dosage regimens. Hand washing is the simplest and most effective means of decreasing hospital-associated infections, especially in the compromised patient. Invasive devices such as central and peripheral lines and Foley catheters are potential sources of infection. Some centers use laminar airflow isolation or high-efficiency particulate air (HEPA) filtering in hematopoietic cell transplant patients. Rates of infection and episodes of febrile neutropenia, but not mortality, are decreased if colony-stimulating factors are used (typically in situations where the risk of febrile neutropenia is 20% or higher) during chemotherapy or during stem-cell transplantation.

A. *Pneumocystis* & Herpes Simplex Infections

Trimethoprim-sulfamethoxazole (TMP-SMZ), one double-strength tablet orally three times a week, one double-strength tablet twice daily on weekends, or one single-strength tablet daily for 3–6 months, is frequently used to prevent *Pneumocystis* infections in transplant patients. In patients allergic to TMP-SMZ, dapsone, 50 mg orally daily or 100 mg three times weekly, is recommended. Glucose-6-phosphate dehydrogenase (G6PD) levels should be determined before therapy when the latter is instituted. Acyclovir prevents herpes simplex infections in bone marrow and solid organ transplant recipients and is given to seropositive patients who are not receiving ganciclovir or valganciclovir for CMV prophylaxis. The usual dose is 200 mg orally three times daily for 4 weeks (hematopoietic cell transplants) to 12 weeks (other solid organ transplants).

B. CMV

No uniformly accepted approach has been adopted for prevention of CMV. Prevention strategies often depend on the serologic status of the donor and recipient and the organ transplanted, which determines the level of immunosuppression after transplant. In solid organ transplants (liver, kidney, heart, lung), the greatest risk of developing CMV disease is in seronegative patients who receive organs from seropositive donors. These high-risk patients usually receive oral valganciclovir, 900 mg daily for 3–6 months (longer in lung transplant recipients). Other solid organ transplant recipients (seropositive recipients) are at lower risk for developing CMV disease but still usually receive oral valganciclovir for 3 months. The lowest risk group for the development of CMV disease is in seronegative patients who receive organs from seronegative donors. Typically, no CMV prophylaxis is used in this group. Ganciclovir and valganciclovir also prevent herpes virus reactivation. Because immunosuppression is increased during periods of rejection, patients treated for rejection usually receive CMV prophylaxis during rejection therapy. Alternatively, in a preemptive approach, patients can be monitored without specific prophylaxis by having blood sampled weekly to look for CMV by polymerase chain reaction techniques. If CMV is detected, then therapy is instituted with oral valganciclovir, 900 mg orally twice daily for a minimum of 2–3 weeks.

Recipients of hematopoietic cell transplants are more severely immunosuppressed than recipients of solid organ transplants, are at greater risk for developing serious CMV infection (usually CMV reactivation), and thus usually receive more aggressive prophylaxis. Like in solid organ transplant recipients, two approaches have been used: universal prophylaxis or preemptive therapy. In the former, all high-risk patients (seropositive patients who receive allogeneic transplants) may receive oral valganciclovir, 900 mg daily to day 100. This method is costly and associated with significant bone marrow toxicity. Because of this, many clinicians prefer the preemptive approach for recipients of hematopoietic stem cell transplants. However, while this preemptive approach is effective, it does miss a small number of patients in whom CMV disease would have been prevented had prophylaxis been used. Other preventive strategies include use of CMV-negative or leukocyte-depleted blood products for CMV-seronegative recipients.

C. Other Organisms

Routine decontamination of the gastrointestinal tract to prevent bacteremia in the neutropenic patient is not recommended. Prophylactic administration of antibiotics in the afebrile, asymptomatic neutropenic patient is controversial, although many centers have adopted this strategy. Rates of bacteremia are decreased, but overall mortality is not affected and emergence of resistant organisms is a risk. Use of intravenous immunoglobulin is reserved for the small number of patients with severe hypogammaglobulinemia following bone marrow transplantation and should not be routinely administered to all transplant patients.

Prophylaxis with antifungal agents to prevent invasive mold (primarily *Aspergillus*) and yeast (primarily *Candida*) infections is routinely used, but the optimal agent, dose, and duration have not been standardized. Lipid-based preparations of amphotericin B, aerosolized amphotericin B, intravenous and oral fluconazole or voriconazole, and oral posaconazole solution and tablets are all prophylactic options in the neutropenic patient. Because voriconazole is superior to amphotericin for documented *Aspergillus* infections and because posaconazole prophylaxis (compared with fluconazole) has been shown to result in fewer cases of invasive aspergillosis among allogeneic stem cell transplant recipients with graft-versus-host disease, one approach to prophylaxis is to use oral fluconazole (400 mg/day) for

patients at low risk for developing fungal infections (those who receive autologous bone marrow transplants) and oral voriconazole (200 mg twice daily) or oral posaconazole (200 mg solution three times daily) for those at high risk (allogeneic transplants, graft-versus-host disease) at least until engraftment (usually 30 days). In solid organ transplant recipients, the risk of invasive fungal infection varies considerably (1–2% in liver, pancreas, and kidney transplants and 6–8% in heart and lung transplants). Whether universal prophylaxis or observation with preemptive therapy is the best approach has not been determined. Although fluconazole is effective in preventing yeast infections, emergence of fluconazole-resistant *Candida* and molds (*Fusarium, Aspergillus, Mucor*) has raised concerns about its routine use as a prophylactic agent in the general solid organ transplant population. However, liver transplant recipients with additional risk factors, such as having undergone a choledochojejunostomy, having had a high transfusion requirement or having developed renal failure, may benefit from abbreviated *Candida* prophylaxis while in the ICU postoperatively.

Given the high risk of reactivation of tuberculosis in patients taking TNF inhibitors, all patients should be screened for latent tuberculosis infection (LTBI) with a tuberculin skin test or an interferon-gamma release assay prior to the start of therapy. If LTBI is diagnosed, treatment with the TNF inhibitors should be delayed until treatment for LTBI is completed. There is also a marked risk of reactivation of hepatitis B and hepatitis C in patients taking TNF inhibitors; patients should also be screened for these viruses when TNF inhibitor treatment is being considered.

▶ Treatment

A. General Measures

Because infections in the immunocompromised patient can be rapidly progressive and life-threatening, diagnostic procedures must be performed promptly, and empiric therapy is usually instituted.

While reduction or discontinuation of immunosuppressive medication may jeopardize the viability of the transplanted organ, this measure may be necessary if the infection is life-threatening. Hematopoietic growth factors (granulocyte and granulocyte-macrophage colony-stimulating factors) stimulate proliferation of bone marrow stem cells, resulting in an increase in peripheral leukocytes. These agents shorten the period of neutropenia and have been associated with reduction in infection.

B. Specific Measures

Antimicrobial drug therapy ultimately should be tailored to culture results. While combinations of antimicrobials may be used with the intent of providing synergy or preventing resistance, the primary reason for empiric combination therapy is broad-spectrum coverage of multiple pathogens (since infections in these patients are often polymicrobial).

Empiric therapy is often instituted at the earliest sign of infection in the immunosuppressed patient because prompt therapy favorably affects outcome. The antibiotic or combination of antibiotics used depends on the degree of immune compromise and the site of infection. For example, in the febrile neutropenic patient, an algorithmic approach to therapy is often used. Febrile neutropenic patients should be empirically treated with broad-spectrum agents active against selected gram-positive bacteria, *Pseudomonas aeruginosa*, and other aerobic gram-negative bacilli (such as cefepime 2 g every 8 hours intravenously). The addition of vancomycin, 10–15 mg/kg/dose intravenously every 12 hours, should be considered in those patients with suspected infection due to methicillin-resistant *Staphylococcus aureus* (MRSA), *S epidermidis*, enterococcus, and resistant viridans streptococci. Continued neutropenic fever necessitates broadening of antibacterial coverage from cefepime to agents such as imipenem 500 mg every 6 hours or meropenem 1 g every 8 hours intravenously with or without tobramycin 5–7 mg/kg intravenously every 24 hours. Antifungal agents (such as voriconazole, 200 mg intravenously or orally every 12 hours, or caspofungin, 50 mg daily intravenously) should be added if fevers continue after 5–7 days of broad-spectrum antibacterial therapy. Regardless of whether the patient becomes afebrile, therapy is continued until resolution of neutropenia. Failure to continue antibiotics through the period of neutropenia has been associated with increased morbidity and mortality.

Patients with fever and low-risk neutropenia (neutropenia expected to persist for less than 10 days, no comorbid complications requiring hospitalization, and cancer adequately treated) can be treated with oral antibiotic regimens, such as ciprofloxacin, 750 mg every 12 hours, plus amoxicillin-clavulanic acid, 500 mg every 8 hours. Antibiotics are continued as long as the patient is neutropenic even if a source is not identified. In the organ transplant patient with interstitial infiltrates, the main concern is infection with *Pneumocystis* or *Legionella* species, so that empiric treatment with a macrolide or fluoroquinolone (*Legionella*) and TMP-SMZ, 15 mg/kg/day orally or intravenously, based on trimethoprim component (*Pneumocystis*) would be reasonable in those patients not receiving TMP-SMZ prophylaxis. If the patient does not respond to empiric treatment, a decision must be made to add more antimicrobial agents or perform invasive procedures (see above) to make a specific diagnosis. By making a definite diagnosis, therapy can be specific, thereby reducing selection pressure for resistance and superinfection.

▶ When to Refer

- Any immunocompromised patient with an opportunistic infection.
- Patients with potential drug toxicities and drug interactions related to antimicrobials where alternative agents are sought.
- Patients with latent tuberculosis, HBV, and HCV infection in whom therapy with TNF inhibitors is planned.

▶ When to Admit

Immunocompromised patients who are febrile, or those without fevers in whom an infection is suspected, particularly in the following groups: solid-organ or hematopoietic stem cell transplant recipient (particularly in the first 6 months), neutropenic patients, patients receiving TNF inhibitors, transplant recipients who have had recent rejection episodes (including graft-versus-host disease).

Hocevar SN et al; Microsporidia Transplant Transmission Investigation Team. Microsporidiosis acquired through solid organ transplantation: a public health investigation. Ann Intern Med. 2014 Feb 18;160(4):213–20. [PMID: 24727839]

Marr KA et al. Combination antifungal therapy for invasive aspergillosis: a randomized trial. Ann Intern Med. 2015 Jan 20; 162(2):81–9. Erratum in: Ann Intern Med. 2015 Mar 17; 162(6):463. [PMID: 25599346]

Martin-Garrido I et al. *Pneumocystis* pneumonia in patients treated with rituximab. Chest. 2013 Jul;144(1):258–65. [PMID: 23258406]

Muller E et al. HIV-positive-to-HIV-positive kidney transplantation—results at 3 to 5 years. N Engl J Med. 2015 Feb 12; 372(7):613–20. [PMID: 25671253]

Shoham S et al. Invasive fungal infections in solid organ transplant recipients. Future Microbiol. 2012 May;7(5):639–55. [PMID: 22568718]

Smith TJ et al. Recommendations for the use of WBC growth factors: American Society of Clinical Oncology Clinical Practice Guideline Update. J Clin Oncol. 2015 Oct 1;33(28):3199–212. [PMID: 26169616]

Sun HY et al. Predictors of immune reconstitution syndrome in organ transplant recipients with cryptococcosis: implications for the management of immunosuppression. Clin Infect Dis. 2015 Jan 1;60(1):36–44. [PMID: 25210020]

Wilson MR et al. Actionable diagnosis of neuroleptospirosis by next-generation sequencing. N Engl J Med. 2014 Jun 19; 370(25):2408–17. [PMID: 24896819]

HEALTH CARE–ASSOCIATED INFECTIONS

 ESSENTIALS OF DIAGNOSIS

- ▶ Health care–associated infections are acquired during the course of receiving health care treatment for other conditions.
- ▶ Hospital-associated infections are a subset of health care–associated infections defined as those not present or incubating at the time of hospital admission and developing 48 hours or more after admission.
- ▶ Most health care–associated infections are preventable.
- ▶ Hand washing is the most effective means of preventing health care–associated infections and should be done routinely even when gloves are worn.

▶ General Considerations

In the United States, approximately 5% of patients acquire a health care–associated infection, resulting in prolongation of the hospital stay, increase in cost of care, significant morbidity, and a 5% mortality rate. The most common infections are urinary tract infections, usually associated with Foley catheters or urologic procedures; bloodstream infections, most commonly from indwelling catheters but also from secondary sites, such as surgical wounds, abscesses, pneumonia, the genitourinary tract, and the gastrointestinal tract; pneumonia in intubated patients or those with altered levels of consciousness; surgical wound infections; MRSA infections; and *Clostridium difficile* colitis.

Some general principles are helpful in preventing, diagnosing, and treating health care–associated infections:

1. Many infections are a direct result of the use of invasive devices for monitoring or therapy, such as intravenous catheters, Foley catheters, shunts, surgical drains, catheters placed by interventional radiology for drainage, nasogastric tubes, and orotracheal or nasotracheal tubes for ventilatory support. Early removal of such devices reduces the possibility of infection.

2. Patients in whom health care–associated infections develop are often critically ill, have been hospitalized for extended periods, and have received several courses of broad-spectrum antibiotic therapy. As a result, health care–associated infections are often due to multidrug resistant pathogens and are different from those encountered in community-acquired infections. For example, *S aureus* and *S epidermidis* (a frequent cause of prosthetic device infection) are often resistant to nafcillin and cephalosporins and require vancomycin for therapy; *Enterococcus faecium* resistant to ampicillin and vancomycin; gram-negative infections caused by *Pseudomonas, Citrobacter, Enterobacter, Acinetobacter,* and *Stenotrophomonas* may be resistant to most antibacterials. When choosing antibiotics to treat the seriously ill patient with a health care–associated infection, antimicrobial history and the "local ecology" must be considered. In the most seriously ill patients, broad-spectrum coverage with vancomycin and a carbapenem with or without an aminoglycoside is recommended. Once a pathogen is isolated and susceptibilities are known, the most narrow spectrum, least toxic, most cost-effective drug should be used.

Widespread use of antimicrobial drugs contributes to the selection of drug-resistant organisms, thus every effort should be made to limit the spectrum of coverage and unnecessary duration. All too often, unreliable or uninterpretable specimens are obtained for culture that result in unnecessary use of antibiotics. The best example of this principle is the diagnosis of line-related or bloodstream infection in the febrile patient. To avoid unnecessary use of antibiotics, thoughtful consideration of culture results is mandatory. A positive wound culture without signs of inflammation or infection, a positive sputum culture without pulmonary infiltrates on chest radiograph, or a positive urine culture in a catheterized patient without symptoms or signs of pyelonephritis are all likely to represent colonization, not infection.

▶ **Clinical Findings**

A. Symptoms and Signs

Catheter-associated infections have a variable presentation, depending on the type of catheter used (peripheral or central venous catheters, nontunneled or tunneled). Local signs of infection may be present at the insertion site, with pain, erythema, and purulence. Fever is often absent in uncomplicated infections and if present, may indicate more disseminated disease such as bacteremia, cellulitis and septic thrombophlebitis. Often signs of infection at the insertion site are absent.

1. Fever in an intensive care unit patient—Fever complicates up to 70% of patients in intensive care units, and the etiology of the fever may be infectious or noninfectious. Common infectious causes include catheter-associated infections, hospital-acquired and ventilator-associated pneumonia (see Chapter 9), surgical site infections, urinary tract infections, and sepsis. Clinically relevant sinusitis is relatively uncommon in the patient in the intensive care unit.

An important noninfectious cause is thromboembolic disease. Fever in conjunction with refractory hypotension and shock may suggest sepsis; however, adrenal insufficiency, thyroid storm, and transfusion reaction may have a similar clinical presentation. Drug fever is difficult to diagnose and is usually a diagnosis of exclusion unless there are other signs of hypersensitivity, such as a typical maculopapular rash.

2. Fever in the postoperative patient—Postoperative fever is very common and in many cases resolves spontaneously. Etiologies are both infectious and noninfectious. Timing of the fever in relation to the surgery and the nature of the surgical procedure may help diagnostically.

A. IMMEDIATE FEVER (IN THE FIRST FEW HOURS AFTER SURGERY)—Immediate fever can be due to medications that were given perioperatively, to the trauma of surgery itself, or to infections that were present before surgery. Necrotizing fasciitis due to group A streptococci or mixed organisms may present in this period. Malignant hyperthermia is rare and presents 30 minutes to several hours following inhalational anesthesia and is characterized by extreme hyperthermia, muscle rigidity, rhabdomyolysis, electrolyte abnormalities, and hypotension. Aggressive cooling and dantrolene are the mainstays of therapy. Aspiration of acidic gastric contents during surgery can cause a chemical pneumonitis (Mendelson syndrome) that rapidly develops but is transient and does not require antibiotics. Fever due to the trauma of surgery itself usually resolves in 2–3 days, longer in more complicated operative cases and in patients with head trauma.

B. ACUTE FEVER (WITHIN 1 WEEK OF SURGERY)—Acute fever is usually due to common causes of hospital-associated infections, such as ventilator-associated pneumonia (including aspiration pneumonia in patients with decreased gag reflex) and line infections. Noninfectious causes include alcohol withdrawal, gout, pulmonary embolism, and pancreatitis. Atelectasis following surgery is commonly invoked as a cause of postoperative fever but there is no good evidence to support a causal association between the presence or degree of atelectasis and fever.

C. SUBACUTE FEVER (AT LEAST 1 WEEK AFTER SURGERY)—Surgical site infections commonly present at least 1 week after surgery. The type of surgery that was performed predicts specific infectious etiologies. Patients undergoing cardiothoracic surgery may be at higher risk for pneumonia and deep and superficial sternal wound infections. Meningitis without typical signs of meningismus may complicate neurosurgical procedures. Abdominal surgery may result in deep abdominal abscesses that require drainage.

B. Laboratory Findings

Blood cultures are universally recommended, and chest radiographs are frequently obtained. A properly prepared sputum Gram stain and semi-quantitative sputum cultures may be useful in selected patients where there is a high pretest probability of pneumonia but multiple exclusion criteria probably limit generalizability in most patients, such as immunocompromised patients and those with drug resistance. Other diagnostic strategies will be dictated by the clinical context (eg, transesophageal echocardiogram in a patient with S aureus bacteremia).

Any fever in a patient with a central venous catheter should prompt the collection of blood. The best method to evaluate bacteremia is to gather at least two peripherally obtained blood cultures. Blood cultures from unidentified sites, a single blood culture from any site, or a blood culture through an existing line will often be positive for S epidermidis, resulting in the inappropriate use of vancomycin. Unless two separate venipuncture cultures are obtained—not through catheters—interpretation of results is impossible and unnecessary therapy may be given. Every such "pseudobacteremia" increases laboratory costs, antibiotic use, and length of stay. Microbiologic evaluation of the removed catheter can sometimes be helpful, but only in addition to (not instead of) blood cultures drawn from peripheral sites. The differential time to positivity measures the difference in time that cultures simultaneously drawn through a catheter and a peripheral site become positive. A positive test (about 120 minutes' difference in time) supports a catheter-related bloodstream infection, and a negative test may permit catheters to be retained.

▶ Complications

Patients who have persistent bacteremia and fever despite removal of the infected catheter may have complications such as septic thrombophlebitis, endocarditis, or metastatic foci of infection (particularly with S aureus). Additional studies such as venous Doppler studies, transesophageal echocardiogram, and chest radiographs may be indicated, and 4–6 weeks of antibiotics may be needed. In the case of septic thrombophlebitis, anticoagulation with heparin is also recommended if there are no contraindications.

▶ Differential Diagnosis

Although most fevers are due to infections, about 25% of patients will have fever of noninfectious origin, including drug fever, nonspecific postoperative fevers (tissue damage or necrosis), hematoma, pancreatitis, pulmonary embolism, myocardial infarction, and ischemic bowel disease.

▶ Prevention

The concept of universal precautions emphasizes that all patients are treated as though they have a potential blood-borne transmissible disease, and thus all body secretions are handled with care to prevent spread of disease. Body substance isolation requires use of gloves whenever a health care worker anticipates contact with blood or other body secretions. Even though gloves are worn, health care workers should routinely wash their hands, since it is the easiest and most effective means of preventing hospital-associated infections. Application of a rapid drying, alcohol-based antiseptic is simple, takes less time than traditional hand washing with soap and water, is more effective at reducing hand colonization, and promotes compliance with hand decontamination. For prevention of transmission of C difficile infection, hand-washing is more effective than alcohol-based antiseptics. Even after removing gloves, providers should always wash hands in cases of proven or suspected C difficile infection.

Peripheral intravenous lines should be replaced every 3 days. Arterial lines and lines in the central venous circulation (including those placed peripherally) can be left in place indefinitely and are changed or removed when they are clinically suspected of being infected, when they are nonfunctional, or when they are no longer needed. Using sterile barrier precautions (including cap, mask, gown, gloves, and drape) is recommended while inserting central venous catheters. Silver alloy–impregnated Foley catheters reduce the incidence of catheter-associated bacteriuria, and antibiotic-impregnated (minocycline plus rifampin or chlorhexidine plus silver sulfadiazine) venous catheters reduce line infections and bacteremia. Silver-coated endotracheal tubes may reduce the incidence of ventilator-associated pneumonia. Whether the increased cost of these devices justifies their routine use should be determined by individual institutions. Catheter-related urinary tract infections and intravenous catheter-associated infections are not Medicare-reimbursable conditions. Preoperative skin preparation with chlorhexidine and alcohol (versus povidone-iodine) has been shown to reduce the incidence of infection following surgery. Another strategy that can prevent surgical-site infections is the identification and treatment of S aureus nasal carriers with 2% mupirocin nasal ointment and chlorhexidine soap. Daily bathing of ICU patients with chlorhexidine-impregnated washcloths versus soap and water results in lower risk of MRSA-associated clinical cultures and catheter-associated bloodstream infections. Selective decontamination of the digestive tract with nonabsorbable or parenteral antibiotics, or both, may prevent hospital-acquired pneumonia and decrease mortality.

Attentive nursing care (positioning to prevent decubitus ulcers, wound care, elevating the head during tube feedings to prevent aspiration) is critical in preventing hospital-associated infections. In addition, monitoring of high-risk areas by hospital epidemiologists is critical in the prevention of infection. Some guidelines advocate rapid screening (active surveillance cultures) for MRSA on admission to acute care facilities among certain subpopulations of patients (eg, those recently hospitalized, admission to the intensive care unit, patients undergoing hemodialysis).

However, outside the setting of an MRSA outbreak, it is not clear whether this strategy decreases the incidence of hospital-associated MRSA infections.

Vaccines, including hepatitis A, hepatitis B, and the varicella, pneumococcal, and influenza vaccinations, are important adjuncts. (See section below on Immunization against Infectious Diseases.)

► Treatment

A. Fever in an Intensive Care Unit Patient

Unless the patient has a central neurologic injury with elevated intracranial pressure or has a temperature higher than 41°C, there is less physiologic need to maintain euthermia. Empiric broad-spectrum antibiotics (see Table 30–5) are recommended for neutropenic and other immunocompromised patients and in patients who are clinically unstable.

B. Catheter-Associated Infections

Factors that inform treatment decisions include the type of catheter, the causative pathogen, the availability of alternate catheter access sites, the need for ongoing intravascular access, and the severity of disease.

In general, catheters should be removed if there is purulence at the exit site; if the organism is *S aureus,* gram-negative rods, or *Candida* species; if there is persistent bacteremia (more than 48 hours while receiving antibiotics); or if complications, such as septic thrombophlebitis, endocarditis, or other metastatic disease exist. Central venous catheters may be exchanged over a guidewire provided there is no erythema or purulence at the exit site and the patient does not appear to be septic. Methicillin-resistant, coagulase-negative staphylococci are the most common pathogens; thus, empiric therapy with vancomycin, 15 mg/kg intravenously twice daily, should be given assuming normal kidney function. Empiric gram-negative coverage may be considered in patients who are immunocompromised or who are critically ill (see Table 30–5).

Antibiotic treatment duration depends on the pathogen and the extent of disease. For uncomplicated bacteremia, 5–7 days of therapy is usually sufficient for coagulase-negative staphylococci, even if the original catheter is retained. Fourteen days of therapy is generally recommended for uncomplicated bacteremia caused by gram-negative rods, *Candida* species, and *S aureus.* Antibiotic lock therapy involves the instillation of supratherapeutic concentrations of antibiotics with heparin in the lumen of catheters. The purpose is to achieve adequate concentrations of antibiotics to kill microbes in the biofilm. Antibiotic lock therapy can be used for catheter-related bloodstream infections caused by coagulase-negative staphylococci or enterococci and when the catheter is being retained in a salvage situation.

► When to Refer

- Any patient with multidrug-resistant infection.
- Any patient with fungemia or persistent bacteremia.
- Patients with multisite infections.

- Patients with impaired or fluctuating kidney function for assistance with dosing of antimicrobials.
- Patients with refractory or recurrent *C difficile* colitis.

Baron EJ et al. A guide to utilization of the microbiology laboratory for diagnosis of infectious diseases: 2013 recommendations by the Infectious Diseases Society of America (IDSA) and the American Society for Microbiology (ASM)(a). Clin Infect Dis. 2013 Aug;57(4):e22–e121. [PMID: 23845951]

Cannon CM et al. The GENESIS Project (GENeralized Early Sepsis Intervention Strategies): a multicenter quality improvement collaborative. J Intensive Care Med. 2013 Nov–Dec; 28(6):355–68. [PMID: 22902347]

Drekonja D et al. Fecal microbiota transplantation for *Clostridium difficile* infection: a systematic review. Ann Intern Med. 2015 May 5;162(9):630–8. [PMID: 25938992]

Ferrer R et al. Empiric antibiotic treatment reduces mortality in severe sepsis and septic shock from the first hour: results from a guideline-based performance improvement program. Crit Care Med. 2014 Aug;42(8):1749–55. [PMID: 24717459]

Harris AD et al. Universal glove and gown use and acquisition of antibiotic-resistant bacteria in the ICU: a randomized trial. JAMA. 2013 Oct 16;310(15):1571–80. [PMID: 24097234]

Huang SS et al; CDC Prevention Epicenters Program; AHRQ DECIDE Network and Healthcare-Associated Infections Program. Targeted versus universal decolonization to prevent ICU infection. N Engl J Med. 2013 Jun 13;368(24):2255–65. Erratum in: N Engl J Med. 2013 Aug 8;369(6):587. [PMID: 23718152]

Lessa FC et al. Burden of *Clostridium difficile* infection in the United States. N Engl J Med. 2015 Feb 26;372(9):825–34. [PMID: 25714160]

Lo E et al. Strategies to prevent catheter-associated urinary tract infections in acute care hospitals: 2014 update. Infect Control Hosp Epidemiol. 2014 Sep;35(Suppl 2):S32–47. [PMID: 25376068]

Mimoz O et al; CLEAN trial investigators. Skin antisepsis with chlorhexidine-alcohol versus povidone iodine-alcohol, with and without skin scrubbing, for prevention of intravascular-catheter-related infection (CLEAN): an open-label, multicentre, randomised, controlled, two-by-two factorial trial. Lancet. 2015 Nov 21;386(10008):2069–77. [PMID: 26388532]

Oostdijk EA et al. Effects of decontamination of the oropharynx and intestinal tract on antibiotic resistance in ICUs: a randomized clinical trial. JAMA. 2014 Oct 8;312(14):1429–37. [PMID: 25271544]

Sawyer RG et al. Trial of short-course antimicrobial therapy for intraabdominal infection. N Engl J Med. 2015 May 21; 372(21):1996–2005. [PMID: 25992746]

Sinuff T et al; Canadian Critical Care Trials Group. Implementation of clinical practice guidelines for ventilator-associated pneumonia: a multicenter prospective study. Crit Care Med. 2013 Jan;41(1):15–23. [PMID: 23222254]

INFECTIONS OF THE CENTRAL NERVOUS SYSTEM

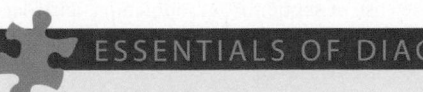

ESSENTIALS OF DIAGNOSIS

- ► Central nervous system infection is a medical emergency.
- ► Symptoms and signs common to all central nervous system infections include headache, fever, sensorial disturbances, neck and back stiffness, positive Kernig and Brudzinski signs, and cerebrospinal fluid abnormalities.

Table 30–1. Typical cerebrospinal fluid findings in various central nervous system diseases.

Diagnosis	Cells/mcL	Glucose (mg/dL)	Protein (mg/dL)	Opening Pressure
Normal	0–5 lymphocytes	45–85[1]	15–45	70–180 mm H$_2$O
Purulent meningitis (bacterial)[2] community-acquired	200–20,000 polymorphonuclear neutrophils	Low (< 45)	High (> 50)	Markedly elevated
Granulomatous meningitis (mycobacterial, fungal)[3]	100–1000, mostly lymphocytes[3]	Low (< 45)	High (> 50)	Moderately elevated
Spirochetal meningitis	100–1000, mostly lymphocytes[3]	Normal	High (> 50)	Normal to slightly elevated
Aseptic meningitis, viral or meningoencephalitis[4]	25–2000, mostly lymphocytes[3]	Normal or low	High (> 50)	Slightly elevated
"Neighborhood reaction"[5]	Variably increased	Normal	Normal or high	Variable

[1]Cerebrospinal fluid glucose must be considered in relation to blood glucose level. Normally, cerebrospinal fluid glucose is 20–30 mg/dL lower than blood glucose, or 50–70% of the normal value of blood glucose.
[2]Organisms in smear or culture of cerebrospinal fluid; counterimmunoelectrophoresis or latex agglutination may be diagnostic.
[3]Polymorphonuclear neutrophils may predominate early.
[4]Viral isolation from cerebrospinal fluid early; antibody titer rise in paired specimens of serum; polymerase chain reaction for herpesvirus.
[5]May occur in mastoiditis, brain abscess, epidural abscess, sinusitis, septic thrombus, brain tumor. Cerebrospinal fluid culture results usually negative.

General Considerations

Infections of the central nervous system can be caused by almost any infectious agent, including bacteria, mycobacteria, fungi, spirochetes, protozoa, helminths, and viruses.

Etiologic Classification

Central nervous system infections can be divided into several categories that usually can be readily distinguished from each other by cerebrospinal fluid examination as the first step toward etiologic diagnosis (Table 30–1).

A. Purulent Meningitis

Patients with bacterial meningitis usually seek medical attention within hours or 1–2 days after onset of symptoms. The organisms responsible depend primarily on the age of the patient as summarized in Table 30–2. The diagnosis is usually based on the Gram-stained smear (positive in 60–90%) or culture (positive in over 90%) of the cerebrospinal fluid.

Table 30–2. Initial antimicrobial therapy for purulent meningitis of unknown cause.

Population	Usual Microorganisms	Standard Therapy
18–50 years	*Streptococcus pneumoniae, Neisseria meningitidis*	Vancomycin[1] **plus** ceftriaxone[2]
Over 50 years	*S pneumoniae, N meningitidis, Listeria monocytogenes,* gram-negative bacilli, group B streptococcus	Vancomycin[1] **plus** ampicillin,[3] **plus** ceftriaxone[2]
Impaired cellular immunity	*L monocytogenes,* gram-negative bacilli, *S pneumoniae*	Vancomycin[1] **plus** ampicillin[3] **plus** cefepime[4]
Postsurgical or posttraumatic	*Staphylococcus aureus, S pneumoniae,* aerobic gram-negative bacilli, coagulase-negative staphylococci, diphtheroids (eg, *Propionibacterium acnes*) (uncommon)	Vancomycin[1] **plus** cefepime[4]

[1] Given to cover highly penicillin- or cephalosporin-resistant pneumococci. The dose of vancomycin is 15 mg/kg/dose intravenously every 8 hours. Vancomycin trough levels should be maintained at > 15 mcg/mL. Stopped if the causative organism is susceptible to ceftriaxone.
[2] Ceftriaxone can often be used safely in meningitis patients with a history of penicillin allergy (aztreonam can be considered for empiric coverage of gram-negative bacilli in patients with serious penicillin and cephalosporin allergy). The usual dose of ceftriaxone is 2 g intravenously every 12 hours. If the organism is sensitive to penicillin, 3–4 million units intravenously every 4 hours is given.
[3]In severely ill patients, ampicillin is used when *L monocytogenes* infection is a consideration. For confirmed infection due to *L monocytogenes,* gentamicin is sometimes added to ampicillin. (For patients allergic to penicillin, trimethoprim-sulfamethoxazole [TMP-SMZ] in a dosage of 15–20 mg/kg/day of TMP in 3 or 4 divided doses can be considered.) The dose of ampicillin is usually 2 g intravenously every 4 hours.
[4]Cefepime is given in a dose of 2–3 g intravenously every 8 hours.
Adapted from *Treat Guide Med Lett.* 2013 Jul; 11(131):65–73.

B. Chronic Meningitis

The presentation of chronic meningitis is less acute than purulent meningitis. Patients with chronic meningitis usually have a history of symptoms lasting weeks to months. The most common pathogens are *Mycobacterium tuberculosis*, atypical mycobacteria, fungi (*Cryptococcus, Coccidioides, Histoplasma*), and spirochetes (*Treponema pallidum* and *Borrelia burgdorferi*). The diagnosis is made by culture or in some cases by serologic tests (cryptococcosis, coccidioidomycosis, syphilis, Lyme disease).

C. Aseptic Meningitis

Aseptic meningitis—a much more benign and self-limited syndrome than purulent meningitis—is caused principally by viruses, especially herpes simplex virus and the enterovirus group (including coxsackieviruses and echoviruses). Infectious mononucleosis may be accompanied by aseptic meningitis. Leptospiral infection is also usually placed in the aseptic group because of the lymphocytic cellular response and its relatively benign course. This type of meningitis also occurs during secondary syphilis and disseminated Lyme disease. Prior to the routine administration of measles-mumps-rubella (MMR) vaccines, mumps was the most common cause of viral meningitis. Drug-induced aseptic meningitis has been reported with nonsteroidal anti-inflammatory drugs, sulfonamides, and certain monoclonal antibodies.

D. Encephalitis

Encephalitis (due to herpesviruses, arboviruses, rabies virus, flaviviruses [West Nile encephalitis, Japanese encephalitis]), and many others, produces disturbances of the sensorium, seizures, and many other manifestations. Patients are more ill than those with aseptic meningitis. Cerebrospinal fluid may be entirely normal or may show some lymphocytes and in some instances (eg, herpes simplex) red cells as well. Influenza has been associated with encephalitis, but the relationship is not clear. An autoimmune form of encephalitis associated with N-methyl-D-aspartate receptor antibodies should be suspected in younger patients with encephalitis and associated seizures, movement disorders, and psychosis.

E. Partially Treated Bacterial Meningitis

Previous effective antibiotic therapy given for 12–24 hours will decrease the rate of positive Gram stain results by 20% and culture by 30–40% of the cerebrospinal fluid but will have little effect on cell count, protein, or glucose. Occasionally, previous antibiotic therapy will change a predominantly polymorphonuclear response to a lymphocytic pleocytosis, and some of the cerebrospinal fluid findings may be similar to those seen in aseptic meningitis.

F. Neighborhood Reaction

As noted in Table 30–1, this term denotes a purulent infectious process in close proximity to the central nervous system that spills some of the products of the inflammatory process—white blood cells or protein—into the cerebrospinal fluid. Such an infection might be a brain abscess, osteomyelitis of the vertebrae, epidural abscess, subdural empyema, or bacterial sinusitis or mastoiditis.

G. Noninfectious Meningeal Irritation

Carcinomatous meningitis, sarcoidosis, systemic lupus erythematosus, chemical meningitis, and certain drugs—nonsteroidal anti-inflammatory drugs, OKT3, TMP-SMZ, and others—can also produce symptoms and signs of meningeal irritation with associated cerebrospinal fluid pleocytosis, increased protein, and low or normal glucose. Meningismus with normal cerebrospinal fluid findings occurs in the presence of other infections such as pneumonia and shigellosis.

H. Brain Abscess

Brain abscess presents as a space-occupying lesion; symptoms may include vomiting, fever, change of mental status, or focal neurologic manifestations. When brain abscess is suspected, a CT scan should be performed. If positive, lumbar puncture should *not* be performed since results rarely provide clinically useful information and herniation can occur. The bacteriology of brain abscess is usually polymicrobial and includes *S aureus*, gram-negative bacilli, streptococci, and mouth anaerobes (including anaerobic streptococci and *Prevotella* species).

I. Health Care–Associated Meningitis

This infection may arise as a result of invasive neurosurgical procedures (eg, craniotomy, internal or external ventricular catheters, external lumbar catheters), complicated head trauma, or from hospital-acquired bloodstream infections. Outbreaks have been associated with contaminated epidural or paraspinal corticosteroid injections. In general, the microbiology is distinct from community-acquired meningitis, with gram-negative organisms (eg, *Pseudomonas*), *S aureus,* and coagulase-negative staphylococci and, in the outbreaks associated with contaminated corticosteroids, mold and fungi (*Exserohilum rostratum* and *Aspergillus fumigatus*) playing a larger role.

▶ Clinical Findings

A. Symptoms and Signs

The classic triad of fever, stiff neck, and altered mental status has a low sensitivity (44%) for bacterial meningitis. However, nearly all patients with bacterial meningitis have at least two of the following symptoms—fever, headache, stiff neck, or altered mental status.

B. Laboratory Tests

Evaluation of a patient with suspected meningitis includes a blood count, blood culture, lumbar puncture followed by careful study and culture of the cerebrospinal fluid, and a chest film. The fluid must be examined for cell count, glucose, and protein, and a smear stained for bacteria (and acid-fast organisms when appropriate) and cultured for pyogenic organisms and for mycobacteria and fungi when indicated. Latex agglutination tests can detect antigens of encapsulated organisms (*S pneumoniae, H influenzae,*

N meningitidis, and *Cryptococcus neoformans*) but are rarely used except for detection of *Cryptococcus* or in partially treated patients. Polymerase chain reaction (PCR) testing of cerebrospinal fluid has been used to detect bacteria (*S pneumoniae*, *H influenzae*, *N meningitidis*, *M tuberculosis*, *B burgdorferi*, and *Tropheryma whipplei*) and viruses (herpes simplex, varicella-zoster, CMV, Epstein-Barr virus, and enteroviruses) in patients with meningitis. The greatest experience is with PCR for herpes simplex and varicella-zoster, and the tests are very sensitive (greater than 95%) and specific. Tests to detect the other organisms may not be any more sensitive than culture, but the real value is the rapidity with which results are available, ie, hours compared with days or weeks. In patients at risk for infection possibly following a contaminated corticosteroid injection, a negative fungal culture or negative PCR test from a diagnostic specimen obtained from the central nervous system or a parameningeal site does not rule out infection. Active fungal infection may be present even when these tests are negative. Consultation with an infectious disease expert is recommended.

C. Lumbar Puncture and Imaging

Since performing a lumbar puncture in the presence of a space-occupying lesion (brain abscess, subdural hematoma, subdural empyema, necrotic temporal lobe from herpes encephalitis) may result in brainstem herniation, a CT scan is performed prior to lumbar puncture if a space-occupying lesion is suspected on the basis of papilledema, seizures, or focal neurologic findings. Other indications for CT scan are an immunocompromised patient or moderate to severely impaired level of consciousness. If delays are encountered in obtaining a CT scan and bacterial meningitis is suspected, blood cultures should be drawn and antibiotics and corticosteroids administered even before cerebrospinal fluid is obtained for culture to avoid delay in treatment (Table 30–1). Antibiotics given within 4 hours before obtaining cerebrospinal fluid probably do not affect culture results. MRI with contrast of the epidural injection site and surrounding areas is recommended (sometimes repeatedly) for those with symptoms following a possibly contaminated corticosteroid injection to exclude epidural abscess, phlegmon, vertebral osteomyelitis, discitis, or arachnoiditis.

▶ Treatment

Although it is difficult to prove with existing clinical data that early antibiotic therapy improves outcome in bacterial meningitis, prompt therapy is still recommended. In purulent meningitis, the identity of the causative microorganism may remain unknown or doubtful for a few days and initial antibiotic treatment as set forth in Table 30–2 should be directed against the microorganisms most common for each age group.

The duration of therapy for bacterial meningitis varies depending on the etiologic agent: *H influenzae*, 7 days; *N meningitidis*, 3–7 days; *S pneumoniae*, 10–14 days; *L monocytogenes*, 14–21 days; and gram-negative bacilli, 21 days.

For adults with pneumococcal meningitis, dexamethasone 10 mg administered intravenously 15–20 minutes before or simultaneously with the first dose of antibiotics and continued every 6 hours for 4 days decreases morbidity and mortality. Patients most likely to benefit from corticosteroids are those infected with gram-positive organisms (*Streptococcus pneumoniae* or *S suis*), and those who are HIV negative. It is unknown whether patients with meningitis due to *N meningitidis* and other bacterial pathogens benefit from the use of adjunctive corticosteroids. Increased intracranial pressure due to brain edema often requires therapeutic attention. Hyperventilation, mannitol (25–50 g intravenously as a bolus), and even drainage of cerebrospinal fluid by repeated lumbar punctures or by placement of intraventricular catheters have been used to control cerebral edema and increased intracranial pressure. Dexamethasone (4 mg intravenously every 4–6 hours) may also decrease cerebral edema.

Therapy of brain abscess consists of drainage (excision or aspiration) in addition to 3–4 weeks of systemic antibiotics directed against organisms isolated. An empiric regimen often includes metronidazole, 500 mg intravenously or orally every 8 hours, plus ceftriaxone, 2 g intravenously every 12 hours, with or without vancomycin, 10–15 mg/kg/dose intravenously every 12 hours. Vancomycin trough serum levels should be greater than 15 mcg/mL in such patients. In cases where abscesses are smaller than 2 cm, where there are multiple abscesses that cannot be drained, or if an abscess is located in an area where significant neurologic sequelae would result from drainage, antibiotics for 6–8 weeks can be used without drainage.

In addition to antibiotics, in cases of health care–associated meningitis associated with an external intraventricular catheter, the probability of cure is increased if the catheter is removed. In infections associated with internal ventricular catheters, removal of the internal components and insertion of an external drain is recommended. After collecting cerebrospinal fluid, epidural aspirate, or other specimens for culture, empiric antifungal therapy with voriconazole as well as routine empiric treatment for other pathogens (as above) is recommended until the specific cause of the patient's central nervous system or parameningeal infection has been identified. In addition, early consultation with a neurosurgeon is recommended for those found to have an epidural abscess, phlegmon, vertebral osteomyelitis, discitis, or arachnoiditis to discuss possible surgical management (eg, debridement).

Therapy of other types of meningitis is discussed elsewhere in this book (fungal meningitis, Chapter 36; syphilis and Lyme borreliosis, Chapter 34; tuberculous meningitis, Chapter 33; herpes encephalitis, Chapter 32).

▶ When to Refer

- Patients with acute meningitis, particularly if culture negative or atypical (eg, fungi, syphilis, Lyme disease, *M tuberculosis*), or if the patient is immunosuppressed.
- Patients with chronic meningitis.
- All patients with brain abscesses and encephalitis.
- Patients with suspected hospital-acquired meningitis (eg, in patients who have undergone recent neurosurgery or epidural or paraspinal corticosteroid injection).
- Patients with recurrent meningitis.

When to Admit

- Patients with suspected acute meningitis, encephalitis, and brain or paraspinous abscess should be admitted for urgent evaluation and treatment.

- There is less urgency to admit patients with chronic meningitis; these patients may be admitted to expedite diagnostic procedures and coordinate care, particularly if no diagnosis has been made in the outpatient setting.

Centers for Disease Control and Prevention (CDC). West Nile virus and other arboviral diseases—United States, 2012. MMWR Morb Mortal Wkly Rep. 2013 Jun 28;62(25):513–7. [PMID: 23803959]

Day JN et al. Combination antifungal therapy for cryptococcal meningitis. N Engl J Med. 2013 Apr 4;368(14):1291–302. [PMID: 23550668]

Gelfand JM et al. Encephalitis of unclear origin diagnosed by brain biopsy: a diagnostic challenge. JAMA Neurol. 2015 Jan 1; 72(1):66–72. [PMID: 25365755]

John CC et al. Global research priorities for infections that affect the nervous system. Nature. 2015 Nov 19;527(7578):S178–86. [PMID: 26580325]

McCotter OZ et al. Update on multistate outbreak of fungal infections associated with contaminated methylprednisolone injections, 2012–2014. MMWR Morb Mortal Wkly Rep. 2015 Oct 30;64(42):1200–1. [PMID: 26513534]

Thakur KT et al. Predictors of outcome in acute encephalitis. Neurology. 2013 Aug 27;81(9):793–800. [PMID: 23892708]

ANIMAL & HUMAN BITE WOUNDS

ESSENTIALS OF DIAGNOSIS

- ► Cat and human bites have higher rates of infection than dog bites.

- ► Hand bites are particularly concerning for the possibility of closed-space infection.

- ► Antibiotic prophylaxis indicated for noninfected bites of the hand and hospitalization required for infected hand bites.

- ► All infected wounds need to be cultured to direct therapy.

General Considerations

About 1000 dog bite injuries require emergency department attention each day in the United States, most often in urban areas. Dog bites occur most commonly in the summer months. Biting animals are usually known by their victims, and most biting incidents are provoked (ie, bites occur while playing with the animal or after surprising the animal while eating or waking it abruptly from sleep). Failure to elicit a history of provocation is important, because an unprovoked attack raises the possibility of rabies. Human bites are usually inflicted by children while playing or fighting; in adults, bites are associated with alcohol use and closed-fist injuries that occur during fights.

The animal inflicting the bite, the location of the bite, and the type of injury inflicted are all important determinants of whether they become infected. Cat bites are more likely to become infected than human bites—between 30% and 50% of all cat bites become infected. Infections following human bites are variable. Bites inflicted by children rarely become infected because they are superficial, and bites by adults become infected in 15–30% of cases, with a particularly high rate of infection in closed-fist injuries. Dog bites, for unclear reasons, become infected only 5% of the time. Bites of the head, face, and neck are less likely to become infected than bites on the extremities. "Through and through" bites (eg, involving the mucosa and the skin) have an infection rate similar to closed-fist injuries. Puncture wounds become infected more frequently than lacerations, probably because the latter are easier to irrigate and debride.

The bacteriology of bite infections is polymicrobial. Following dog and cat bites, over 50% of infections are caused by aerobes and anaerobes and 36% are due to aerobes alone. Pure anaerobic infections are rare. *Pasteurella* species are the single most common isolate (75% of infections caused by cat bites and 50% of infections caused by dog bites). Other common aerobic isolates include streptococci, staphylococci, *Moraxella*, and *Neisseria;* the most common anaerobes are *Fusobacterium, Bacteroides, Porphyromonas,* and *Prevotella.* The median number of isolates following human bites is four (three aerobes and one anaerobe). Like dog and cat bites, infections caused by most human bites are a mixture of aerobes and anaerobes (54%) or are due to aerobes alone (44%). Streptococci and *S aureus* are the most common aerobes. *Eikenella corrodens* (found in up to 30% of patients), *Prevotella,* and *Fusobacterium* are the most common anaerobes. Although the organisms noted are the most common, innumerable others have been isolated—including *Capnocytophaga* (dog and cat), *Pseudomonas,* and *Haemophilus*—emphasizing the point that all infected bites should be cultured to define the microbiology.

HIV can be transmitted from bites (either from biting or receiving a bite from an HIV-infected patient) but has rarely been reported.

Treatment

A. Local Care

Vigorous cleansing and irrigation of the wound as well as debridement of necrotic material are the most important factors in decreasing the incidence of infections. Radiographs should be obtained to look for fractures and the presence of foreign bodies. Careful examination to assess the extent of the injury (tendon laceration, joint space penetration) is critical to appropriate care.

B. Suturing

If wounds require closure for cosmetic or mechanical reasons, suturing can be done. However, one should never suture an infected wound, and wounds of the hand should generally not be sutured since a closed-space infection of the hand can result in loss of function.

C. Prophylactic Antibiotics

Prophylaxis is indicated in high-risk bites and in high-risk patients. Cat bites in any location and hand bites by any animal, including humans, should receive prophylaxis. Individuals with certain comorbidities (diabetes, liver disease) are at increased risk for severe complications and should receive prophylaxis even for low-risk bites, as should patients without functional spleens who are at increased risk for overwhelming sepsis (primarily with *Capnocytophaga* species). Amoxicillin-clavulanate (Augmentin) 500 mg orally three times daily for 5–7 days is the regimen of choice. For patients with serious allergy to penicillin, a combination of clindamycin 300 mg orally three times daily together with one of the following is recommended for 5–7 days: doxycycline 100 mg orally twice daily, or double-strength TMP-SMZ orally twice daily, or a fluoroquinolone (ciprofloxacin 500 mg orally twice daily or levofloxacin 500–750 mg orally once daily). Moxifloxacin, a fluoroquinolone with good aerobic and anaerobic activity, may be suitable as monotherapy at 400 mg orally once daily for 5–7 days. Agents such as dicloxacillin, cephalexin, erythromycin, and clindamycin should not be used alone because they lack activity against *Pasteurella* species. Doxycycline and TMP-SMZ have poor activity against anaerobes and should only be used in combination with clindamycin.

Because the risk of HIV transmission is so low following a bite, routine postexposure prophylaxis is not recommended. Each case should be evaluated individually and consideration for prophylaxis should be given to those who present within 72 hours of the incident, the source is known to be HIV infected, and the exposure is high risk.

D. Antibiotics for Documented Infection

For wounds that are infected, antibiotics are clearly indicated. How they are given (orally or intravenously) and the need for hospitalization are individualized clinical decisions. The most commonly encountered pathogens require treatment with either a combination of a beta-lactam plus a beta-lactamase inhibitor (ampicillin-sulbactam [Unasyn], 1.5–3.0 g intravenously every 6–8 hours; or piperacillin-tazobactam [Zosyn], 3.375 g intravenously every 6–8 hours; or amoxicillin-clavulanate [Augmentin], 500 mg orally three times daily); or with a carbapenem (ertapenem, 1 g intravenously daily; imipenem, 500 mg intravenously every 6–8 hours; or meropenem, 1 g intravenously every 8 hours). For the patient with severe penicillin allergy, a combination of clindamycin 600–900 mg intravenously every 8 hours plus a fluoroquinolone (ciprofloxacin, 400 mg intravenously every 12 hours; levofloxacin, 500–750 mg intravenously once daily) or TMP-SMZ (10 mg/kg of trimethoprim daily in two or three divided doses) is indicated. Duration of therapy is usually 2–3 weeks unless complications such as septic arthritis or osteomyelitis are present; if these complications are present, therapy should be extended to 4 and 6 weeks, respectively.

E. Tetanus and Rabies

All patients must be evaluated for the need for tetanus (see Chapter 33) and rabies (see Chapter 32) prophylaxis.

When to Refer

- If septic arthritis or osteomyelitis is suspected.
- For exposure to bites by dogs, cats, reptiles, amphibians, and rodents.
- When rabies is a possibility.

When to Admit

- Patients with infected hand bites.
- Deep bites, particularly if over joints.

Giordano A et al. Clinical features and outcomes of *Pasteurella multocida* infection. Medicine (Baltimore). 2015 Sep; 94(36):e1285. [PMID: 26356688]

Wilde H et al. Worldwide rabies deaths prevention—a focus on the current inadequacies in postexposure prophylaxis of animal bite victims. Vaccine. 2016 Jan 4;34(2):187–9. [PMID: 26626211]

SEXUALLY TRANSMITTED DISEASES

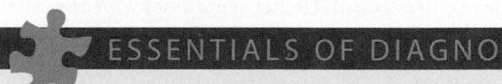

ESSENTIALS OF DIAGNOSIS

- ► All sexually transmitted diseases (STDs) have subclinical or latent periods, and patients may be asymptomatic.
- ► Simultaneous infection with several organisms is common.
- ► All patients who seek STD testing should be screened for syphilis and HIV.
- ► Partner notification and treatment are important to prevent further transmission and reinfection of the index case.

General Considerations

The most common STDs are gonorrhea,[*] syphilis,[*] human papillomavirus (HPV)–associated condyloma acuminatum, chlamydial genital infections,[*] herpesvirus genital infections, trichomonas vaginitis, chancroid,[*] granuloma inguinale, scabies, louse infestation, and bacterial vaginosis (among women who have sex with women). However, shigellosis[*]; hepatitis A, B, and C[*]; amebiasis; giardiasis[*]; cryptosporidiosis[*]; salmonellosis[*]; and campylobacteriosis may also be transmitted by sexual (oral-anal) contact, especially in men who have sex with men. Both homosexual and heterosexual contact are risk factors for the transmission of HIV (see Chapter 31). All STDs have subclinical or latent phases that play an important role in long-term persistence of the infection or in its transmission from infected (but largely asymptomatic) persons to other contacts. Simultaneous infection by several different agents is common.

---

[*] Reportable to public health authorities.

Infections typically present in one of several ways, each of which has a defined differential diagnosis, which should prompt appropriate diagnostic tests.

A. Genital Ulcers

Common etiologies include herpes simplex virus, primary syphilis, and chancroid. Other possibilities include lymphogranuloma venereum (see Chapter 33), granuloma inguinale caused by *Klebsiella granulomatis* (see Chapter 33), as well as lesions caused by infection with Epstein-Barr virus and HIV. Noninfectious causes are Behçet disease (see Chapter 20), neoplasm, trauma, drugs, and irritants.

B. Urethritis with or without Urethral Discharge

The most common infections causing urethral discharge are *Neisseria gonorrhoeae* and *Chlamydia trachomatis*. *N gonorrhoeae* and *C trachomatis* are also frequent causes of prostatitis among sexually active men. Other sexually transmitted infections that can cause urethritis include *Mycoplasma genitalium*, *Ureaplasma urealyticum*, and *Trichomonas vaginalis*. Noninfectious causes of urethritis include reactive arthritis (Reiter syndrome) with associated urethritis.

C. Vaginal Discharge

Common causes of vaginitis are bacterial vaginosis (caused by overgrowth of anaerobes such as *Gardnerella vaginalis*), candidiasis, and *T vaginalis* (see Chapter 18). Less common infectious causes of vaginitis include HPV-associated condylomata acuminata and group A streptococcus. Noninfectious causes are physiologic changes related to the menstrual cycle, irritants, and lichen planus. Even though *N gonorrhoeae* and *C trachomatis* are frequent causes of cervicitis, they rarely produce vaginal discharge.

▶ Screening & Prevention

All persons who seek STD testing should undergo routine screening for HIV infection, using rapid HIV-testing (if patients may not follow up for results obtained by standard methods) or nucleic acid amplification followed by confirmatory serology (if primary HIV infection may be a possibility) as indicated. Patients in whom certain STDs have been diagnosed and treated (chlamydia or gonorrhea, and trichomonas in women) are at a high risk for reinfection and should be encouraged to be rescreened for STDs at 3 months following the initial STD diagnosis.

Asymptomatic patients often request STD screening at the time of initiating a new sexual relationship. Routine HIV testing and hepatitis B serology testing should be offered to all such patients. In sexually active women who have not been recently screened, cervical Papanicolaou testing and nucleic acid amplification testing of a urine specimen for gonorrhea and chlamydia are recommended. Among men who have sex with men, additional screening is recommended for syphilis; hepatitis A; urethral, pharyngeal, and rectal gonorrhea; as well as urethral and rectal chlamydia. Nucleic acid amplification testing is recommended for gonorrhea or chlamydia. There are no recommendations to screen heterosexual men for urethral chlamydia but this could be considered in STD clinics, adolescent clinics, or correctional facilities. The periodicity of screening thereafter depends on sexual risk, but most screening should be offered at least annually to sexually active adults (particularly to those 25 years old and under). Clinicians should also evaluate transgender men and women for STD screening, based on current anatomy and behaviors practiced. If not immune, hepatitis B vaccination is recommended for all sexually active adults, and hepatitis A vaccination in men who have sex with men. Persons between the ages of 9 and 26 should be routinely offered vaccination against HPV (quadrivalent or 9-valent).

The risk of developing an STD following a **sexual assault** is difficult to accurately ascertain given high rates of baseline infections and poor follow-up. Victims of assault have a high baseline rate of infection (*N gonorrhoeae*, 6%; *C trachomatis*, 10%; *T vaginalis*, 15%; and bacterial vaginosis, 34%), and the risk of acquiring infection as a result of the assault is significant but is often lower than the preexisting rate (*N gonorrhoeae*, 6–12%; *C trachomatis*, 4–17%; *T vaginalis*, 12%; syphilis, 0.5–3%; and bacterial vaginosis, 19%). Victims should be evaluated within 24 hours after the assault, and nucleic acid amplification tests for *N gonorrhoeae* and *C trachomatis* should be performed. Vaginal secretions are obtained for *Trichomonas* wet mount and culture, or point-of-care testing. If a discharge is present, if there is itching, or if secretions are malodorous, a wet mount should be examined for *Candida* and bacterial vaginosis. In addition, a blood sample should be obtained for immediate serologic testing for syphilis, hepatitis B, and HIV. Follow-up examination for STDs should be repeated within 1–2 weeks, since concentrations of infecting organisms may not have been sufficient to produce a positive test at the time of initial examination. If prophylactic treatment was given (may include postexposure hepatitis B vaccination without hepatitis B immune globulin; treatment for chlamydial, gonorrheal, or trichomonal infection; and emergency contraception), tests should be repeated only if the victim has symptoms. If prophylaxis was not administered, the individual should be seen in 1 week so that any positive tests can be treated. Follow-up serologic testing for syphilis and HIV infection should be performed in 6, 12, and 24 weeks if the initial tests are negative. The usefulness of presumptive therapy is controversial, some feeling that all patients should receive it and others that it should be limited to those in whom follow-up cannot be ensured or to patients who request it.

Although seroconversion to HIV has been reported following sexual assault when this was the only known risk, this risk is believed to be low. The likelihood of HIV transmission from vaginal or anal receptive intercourse when the source is known to be HIV positive is 1 per 1000 and 5 per 1000, respectively. Although prophylactic antiretroviral therapy has not been studied in this setting, the Department of Health and Human Services recommends the prompt institution of postexposure prophylaxis with antiretroviral therapy if the person seeks care within 72 hours of the assault, the source is known to be HIV positive, and the exposure presents a substantial risk of transmission.

In addition to screening asymptomatic patients with STDs, other strategies for preventing further transmission include evaluating sex partners and administering preexposure vaccination of preventable STDs to individuals at risk; other strategies include the consistent use of male and female condoms and male circumcision. Adult male circumcision has been shown to decrease the transmission of HIV by 50%, and of herpes simplex virus and HPV by 30% in heterosexual couples in sub-Saharan Africa. For each patient, there are one or more sexual contacts who require diagnosis and treatment. Prompt treatment of contacts by giving antibiotics to the index case to distribute to all sexual contacts (patient-delivered therapy) is an important strategy for preventing further transmission and to prevent reinfection of the index case.

Note that vaginal spermicides and condoms containing nonoxynol-9 provide no additional protection against STDs. Early initiation of antiretroviral therapy in HIV-infected individuals can prevent HIV acquisition in an uninfected sex partner. Also, preexposure prophylaxis with a once-daily pill containing tenofovir plus emtricitabine has been shown to be effective in preventing HIV infection among high-risk men who have sex with men.

▶ **When to Refer**

- Patients with a new diagnosis of HIV.
- Patients with persistent, refractory or recurrent STDs, particularly when drug resistance is suspected.

Allen VG et al. *Neisseria gonorrhoeae* treatment failure and susceptibility to cefixime in Toronto, Canada. JAMA. 2013 Jan 9; 309(2):163–70. [PMID: 23299608]

Baeten JM et al; Partners PrEP Study Team. Antiretroviral prophylaxis for HIV prevention in heterosexual men and women. N Engl J Med. 2012 Aug 2;367(5):399–410. [PMID: 22784037]

Centers for Disease Control and Prevention, Center for HIV/AIDS, Viral Hepatitis, STD, and TB Prevention, Division of HIV/AIDS Prevention. Male Circumcision. http://www.cdc.gov/hiv/pdf/prevention_research_malecircumcision.pdf

Gottlieb SL et al. Screening and treating *Chlamydia trachomatis* genital infection to prevent pelvic inflammatory disease: interpretation of findings from randomized controlled trials. Sex Transm Dis. 2013 Feb;40(2):97–102. [PMID: 23324973]

Juusola JL et al. The cost-effectiveness of preexposure prophylaxis for HIV prevention in the United States in men who have sex with men. Ann Intern Med. 2012 Apr 17;156(8): 541–50. [PMID: 22508731]

LeFevre ML. Behavioral counseling interventions to prevent sexually transmitted infections: U.S. Preventive Services Task Force recommendation statement. Ann Intern Med. 2014 Dec 16; 161(12):894–901. [PMID: 25244227]

Liu A et al. Early experiences implementing pre-exposure prophylaxis (PrEP) for HIV prevention in San Francisco. PLoS Med. 2014 Mar 4;11(3):e1001613. [PMID: 24595035]

Markowitz LE et al. Reduction in human papillomavirus (HPV) prevalence among young women following HPV vaccine introduction in the United States, National Health and Nutrition Examination Surveys, 2003–2010. J Infect Dis. 2013 Aug 1; 208(3):385–93. [PMID: 23785124]

Mayer KH et al. Raltegravir, tenofovir DF, and emtricitabine for postexposure prophylaxis to prevent the sexual transmission of HIV: safety, tolerability, and adherence. J Acquir Immune Defic Syndr. 2012 Apr 1;59(4):354–9. [PMID: 22267017]

Moyer VA. Screening for HIV: U.S. Preventive Services Task Force Recommendation Statement. Ann Intern Med. 2013 Jul 2; 159(1):51–60. [PMID: 23698354]

Seña AC et al. Sexual assault and sexually transmitted infections in adults, adolescents, and children. Clin Infect Dis. 2015 Dec 15; 61(Suppl 8):S856–64. [PMID: 26602623]

Volk JE et al. No new HIV infections with increasing use of HIV preexposure prophylaxis in a clinical practice setting. Clin Infect Dis. 2015 Nov 15;61(10):1601–3. [PMID: 26334052]

Wandeler G et al. Hepatitis C virus infections in the Swiss HIV Cohort Study: a rapidly evolving epidemic. Clin Infect Dis. 2012 Nov 15;55(10):1408–16. [PMID: 22893583]

Workowski KA et al; Centers for Disease Control and Prevention (CDC). Sexually transmitted diseases treatment guidelines, 2015. MMWR Recomm Rep. 2015 Jun 5;64(RR–03):1–137. Erratum in: MMWR Recomm Rep. 2015 Aug 28;64(33):924. [PMID: 26042815]

INFECTIONS IN DRUG USERS

ESSENTIALS OF DIAGNOSIS

▶ Common infections that occur with greater frequency in drug users include:

 – Skin infections, aspiration pneumonia, tuberculosis.

 – Hepatitis A, B, C, D; STDs; HIV/AIDS.

 – Pulmonary septic emboli, infective endocarditis.

 – Osteomyelitis and septic arthritis.

▶ **General Considerations**

There is a high incidence of infection among drug users, particularly those who inject drugs. Increased risk of infection is likely associated with poor hygiene and colonization with potentially pathogenic organisms, contamination of drugs and equipment, increased sexual risk behaviors, and impaired immune defenses. The use of parenterally administered recreational drugs has increased enormously in recent years. There are now an estimated 300,000 or more injection drug users in the United States.

Skin infections are associated with poor hygiene and use of nonsterile technique when injecting drugs. *S aureus* (including community-acquired methicillin-resistant strains) and oral flora (streptococci, *Eikenella, Fusobacterium, Peptostreptococcus*) are the most common organisms, with enteric gram-negatives generally more likely seen in those who inject into the groin. Cellulitis and subcutaneous abscesses occur most commonly, particularly in association with subcutaneous ("skin-popping") or intramuscular injections and the use of cocaine and heroin mixtures (probably due to ischemia). Myositis, clostridial myonecrosis, and necrotizing fasciitis occur infrequently but are life-threatening. Wound botulism in association with black tar heroin occurs sporadically but often in clusters.

Aspiration pneumonia and its complications (lung abscess, empyema, brain abscess) result from altered consciousness associated with drug use. Mixed aerobic and anaerobic mouth flora are usually involved.

Tuberculosis also occurs in drug users, and infection with HIV has fostered the spread of tuberculosis in this population. Morbidity and mortality rates are increased in HIV-infected individuals with tuberculosis. Classic radiographic findings are often absent; tuberculosis is suspected in any patient with infiltrates who does not respond to antibiotics.

Hepatitis is very common among habitual drug users and is transmissible both by the parenteral (hepatitis B, C, and D) and by the fecal-oral route (hepatitis A). Multiple episodes of hepatitis with different agents can occur.

Pulmonary septic emboli may originate from venous thrombi or right-sided endocarditis.

STDs are not directly related to drug use, but the practice of exchanging sex for drugs has resulted in an increased frequency of STDs. Syphilis, gonorrhea, and chancroid are the most common.

HIV/AIDS has a high incidence among injection drug users and their sexual contacts and among the offspring of infected women (see Chapter 31).

Infective endocarditis in persons who use drugs intravenously is most commonly caused by *S aureus*, *Candida* (usually *C albicans* or *C parapsilosis*), *Enterococcus faecalis*, other streptococci, and gram-negative bacteria (especially *Pseudomonas* and *Serratia marcescens*). See Chapter 33.

Other vascular infections include septic thrombophlebitis and mycotic aneurysms. Mycotic aneurysms resulting from direct trauma to a vessel with secondary infection most commonly occur in femoral arteries and less commonly in arteries of the neck. Aneurysms resulting from hematogenous spread of organisms frequently involve intracerebral vessels and thus are seen in association with endocarditis.

Osteomyelitis and septic arthritis involving vertebral bodies, sternoclavicular joints, the pubic symphysis, the sacroiliac joints, and other sites usually results from hematogenous distribution of injected organisms or septic venous thrombi. Pain and fever precede radiographic changes, sometimes by several weeks. While staphylococci—often methicillin-resistant—are common organisms, *Serratia*, *Pseudomonas*, *Candida* (often not *C albicans*), and other pathogens rarely encountered in spontaneous bone or joint disease are found in injection drug users.

▶ Treatment

A common and difficult clinical problem is management of the parenteral drug user who presents with fever. In general, after obtaining appropriate cultures (blood, urine, and sputum if the chest radiograph is abnormal), empiric therapy is begun. If the chest radiograph is suggestive of a community-acquired pneumonia (consolidation), therapy for outpatient pneumonia is begun with a third-generation cephalosporin, such as ceftriaxone, 1 g intravenously every 24 hours, plus azithromycin, 500 mg orally or intravenously every 24 hours, or doxycycline, 100 mg orally or

intravenously twice daily. If the chest radiograph is suggestive of septic emboli (nodular infiltrates), therapy for presumed endocarditis is initiated, usually with vancomycin 15 mg/kg/dose every 12 hours intravenously (due to the high prevalence of MRSA and the possibility of enterococcus). If the chest radiograph is normal and no focal site of infection can be found, endocarditis is presumed. While awaiting the results of blood cultures, empiric treatment with vancomycin is started. If blood cultures are positive for organisms that frequently cause endocarditis in drug users (see above), endocarditis is presumed to be present and treated accordingly. If blood cultures are positive for an organism that is an unusual cause of endocarditis, evaluation for an occult source of infection should go forward. In this setting, a transesophageal echocardiogram may be quite helpful since it is 90% sensitive in detecting vegetations and a negative study is strong evidence against endocarditis. If blood cultures are negative and the patient responds to antibiotics, therapy should be continued for 7–14 days (oral therapy can be given once an initial response has occurred). In every patient, careful examination for an occult source of infection (eg, genitourinary, dental, sinus, gallbladder) should be done.

▶ When to Refer

- Any patient with suspected or proven infective endocarditis.
- Patients with persistent bacteremia.

▶ When to Admit

- Injection drug users with fever.
- Patients with abscesses or progressive skin and soft tissue infection that require debridement.

Bachhuber MA et al. Changes in testing for human immunodeficiency virus, sexually transmitted infections, and hepatitis C virus in opioid treatment programs. JAMA. 2013 Dec 25; 310(24):2671–2. [PMID: 24368468]

Choopanya K et al. Antiretroviral prophylaxis for HIV infection in injecting drug users in Bangkok, Thailand (the Bangkok Tenofovir Study): a randomised, double-blind, placebo-controlled phase 3 trial. Lancet. 2013 Jun 15;381(9883):2083–90. [PMID: 23769234]

Conrad C et al; Centers for Disease Control and Prevention (CDC). Community outbreak of HIV infection linked to injection drug use of oxymorphone—Indiana, 2015. MMWR Morb Mortal Wkly Rep. 2015 May 1;64(16):443–4. [PMID: 25928470]

Ip EJ et al. Infectious disease, injection practices, and risky sexual behavior among anabolic steroid users. AIDS Care. 2016 Mar; 28(3):294–9. [PMID: 26422090]

McCance-Katz EF et al. Hepatitis C virus treatment and injection drug users: it is time to separate fact from fiction. Ann Intern Med. 2015 Aug 4;163(3):224–5. [PMID: 26120801]

North CS et al. Hepatitis C and substance use: new treatments and novel approaches. Curr Opin Psychiatry. 2012 May; 25(3):206–12. [PMID: 22395769]

Rabkin DG et al. Long-term outcome for the surgical treatment of infective endocarditis with a focus on intravenous drug users. Ann Thorac Surg. 2012 Jan;93(1):51–7. [PMID: 22054655]

ACUTE INFECTIOUS DIARRHEA

ESSENTIALS OF DIAGNOSIS

▶ **Acute diarrhea:** lasts less than 2 weeks

▶ **Chronic diarrhea:** lasts longer than 2 weeks.

▶ **Mild diarrhea:** 3 or fewer stools per day.

▶ **Moderate diarrhea:** 4 or more stools per day with local symptoms (abdominal cramps, nausea, tenesmus).

▶ **Severe diarrhea:** 4 or more stools per day with systemic symptoms (fever, chills, dehydration).

▶ General Considerations

Acute diarrhea can be caused by a number of different factors, including emotional stress, food intolerance, inorganic agents (eg, sodium nitrite), organic substances (eg, mushrooms, shellfish), drugs, and infectious agents (including viruses, bacteria, and protozoa) (Table 30–3). From a diagnostic and therapeutic standpoint, it is helpful to classify infectious diarrhea into syndromes that produce inflammatory or bloody diarrhea and those that are noninflammatory, nonbloody, or watery. In general, the term "inflammatory diarrhea" suggests colonic involvement by invasive bacteria or parasites or by toxin production. Patients complain of frequent bloody, small-volume stools, often associated with fever, abdominal cramps, tenesmus, and fecal urgency. Common causes of this syndrome include *Shigella, Salmonella, Campylobacter, Yersinia,* invasive strains of *Escherichia coli,* and other Shiga-toxin–producing strains of *coli* (STEC), *Entamoeba histolytica,* and *C difficile.* Tests for fecal leukocytes or the neutrophil marker lactoferrin are frequently positive, and definitive etiologic diagnosis requires stool culture. Noninflammatory diarrhea is generally milder and is caused by viruses or toxins that affect the small intestine and interfere with salt and water balance, resulting in large-volume watery diarrhea, often with nausea, vomiting, and cramps. Common causes of this syndrome include viruses (eg, rotavirus, norovirus, astrovirus, enteric adenoviruses), vibriones *(Vibrio cholerae, Vibrio parahaemolyticus),* enterotoxin-producing *E coli, Giardia lamblia,* cryptosporidia, and agents that can cause foodborne gastroenteritis. In developed countries, viruses (particularly norovirus) are an important cause of hospitalizations due to acute gastroenteritis among adults.

The term "food poisoning" denotes diseases caused by toxins present in consumed foods. When the incubation period is short (1–6 hours after consumption), the toxin is usually preformed. Vomiting is usually a major complaint, and fever is usually absent. Examples include intoxication from *S aureus* or *Bacillus cereus,* and toxin can be detected in the food. When the incubation period is longer—between 8 hours and 16 hours—the organism is present in the food and produces toxin after being ingested. Vomiting is less prominent, abdominal cramping is frequent, and fever is often absent. The best example of this disease is that due to *Clostridium perfringens.* Toxin can be detected in food or stool specimens.

The inflammatory and noninflammatory diarrheas discussed above can also be transmitted by food and water and usually have incubation periods between 12 and 72 hours. *Cyclospora,* cryptosporidia, and *Isospora* are protozoans capable of causing disease in both immunocompetent and immunocompromised patients. Characteristics of disease include profuse watery diarrhea that is prolonged but usually self-limited (1–2 weeks) in the immunocompetent patient but can be chronic in the compromised host. Epidemiologic features may be helpful in determining etiology. Recent hospitalization or antibiotic use suggests *C difficile;* recent foreign travel suggests *Salmonella, Shigella, Campylobacter, E coli,* or *V cholerae;* undercooked hamburger suggests STEC; outbreak in long-term care facility, school, or cruise ship suggests norovirus (including newly identified strains, eg, GII.4 Sydney); and fried rice consumption is associated with *B cereus* toxin. Prominent features of some of these causes of diarrhea are listed in Table 30–3.

▶ Treatment

A. General Measures

In general, most cases of acute gastroenteritis are self-limited and do not require therapy other than supportive measures. Treatment usually consists of replacement of fluids and electrolytes and, very rarely, management of hypovolemic shock and respiratory compromise. In mild diarrhea, increasing ingestion of juices and clear soups is adequate. In more severe cases of dehydration (postural lightheadedness, decreased urination), oral glucose-based rehydration solutions can be used (Ceralyte, Pedialyte).

B. Specific Measures

When symptoms persist beyond 3–4 days, initial presentation is accompanied by fever or bloody diarrhea, or if the patient is immunocompromised, cultures of stool are usually obtained. Symptoms have often resolved by the time cultures are completed. In this case, even if a pathogen is isolated, therapy is not needed (except for *Shigella,* since the infecting dose is so small that therapy to eradicate organisms from the stool is indicated for epidemiologic reasons). If symptoms persist and a pathogen is isolated, it is reasonable to institute specific treatment even though therapy has not been conclusively shown to alter the natural history of disease for most pathogens. Exceptions include infection with *Shigella* where antibiotic therapy has been shown to shorten the duration of symptoms by 2–3 days, and *Campylobacter* infections (early therapy, within 4 days of onset of symptoms, shortens the course of disease). Conversely, antibiotic therapy for infections with STEC does not ameliorate symptoms and may increase the risk of developing hemolytic-uremic syndrome. Uncomplicated gastroenteritis due to *Salmonella* does not require therapy because the disease is usually self-limited and therapy may prolong carriage and perhaps increase

Table 30–3. Acute bacterial diarrheas and "food poisoning."

Organism	Incubation Period	Vomiting	Diarrhea	Fever	Associated Foods	Diagnosis	Clinical Features and Treatment
Staphylococcus (preformed toxin)	1–8 hours	+++	±	±	Staphylococci grow in meats, dairy, and bakery products and produce enterotoxin.	Clinical. Food and stool can be tested for toxin.	Abrupt onset, intense nausea and vomiting for up to 24 hours, recovery in 24–48 hours. Supportive care.
Bacillus cereus (preformed toxin)	1–8 hours	+++	±	–	Reheated fried rice causes vomiting or diarrhea.	Clinical. Food and stool can be tested for toxin.	Acute onset, severe nausea and vomiting lasting 24 hours. Supportive care.
B cereus (diarrheal toxin)	10–16 hours	±	+++	–	Toxin in meats, stews, and gravy.	Clinical. Food and stool can be tested for toxin.	Abdominal cramps, watery diarrhea, and nausea lasting 24–48 hours. Supportive care.
Clostridium perfringens	8–16 hours	±	+++	–	Clostridia grow in rewarmed meat and poultry dishes and produce an enterotoxin.	Stools can be tested for enterotoxin or cultured.	Abrupt onset of profuse diarrhea, abdominal cramps, nausea; vomiting occasionally. Recovery usual without treatment in 24–48 hours. Supportive care; antibiotics not needed.
C. botulinum	12–72 hours	±	–	–	Clostridia grow in anaerobic acidic environment eg, canned foods, fermented fish, foods held warm for extended periods.	Stool, serum, and food can be tested for toxin. Stool and food can be cultured.	Diplopia, dysphagia, dysphonia, respiratory embarrassment. Treatment requires clear airway, ventilation, and intravenous polyvalent antitoxin (see text). Symptoms can last for days to months.
C. difficile	Usually occurs after 7–10 days of antibiotics. Can occur after a single dose or several weeks after completion of antibiotics.	–	+++	++	Associated with antimicrobial drugs; clindamycin and beta-lactams most commonly implicated. Fluoroquinolones associated with hypervirulent strains.	Stool tested for toxin.	Abrupt onset of diarrhea that may be bloody; fever. Oral metronidazole for mild to moderate cases. Oral vancomycin for more severe disease.
Enterohemorrhagic Escherichia coli, including Shiga-toxin producing E coli strains (STEC)	1–8 days	+	+++	–	Undercooked beef, especially hamburger, unpasteurized milk and juice; raw fruits and vegetables.	Shiga-toxin–producing E coli can be cultured on special medium. Other toxins can be detected in stool.	Usually abrupt onset of diarrhea, often bloody; abdominal pain. In adults, it is usually self-limited to 5–10 days. In children, it is associated with hemolytic-uremic syndrome (HUS). Antibiotic therapy may increase risk of HUS. Plasma exchange may help patients with STEC-associated HUS.

Organism	Incubation Period	Vomiting	Diarrhea	Fever	Associated Foods	Diagnosis	Clinical Features, Diagnosis, and Treatment
Enterotoxigenic E coli (ETEC)	1–3 days	±	+++	±	Water, food contaminated with feces.	Stool culture. Special tests required to identify toxin-producing strains.	Watery diarrhea and abdominal cramps, usually lasting 3–7 days. In travelers, fluoroquinolones shorten disease.
Vibrio parahaemolyticus	2–48 hours	+	+	±	Undercooked or raw seafood.	Stool culture on special medium.	Abrupt onset of watery diarrhea, abdominal cramps, nausea and vomiting. Recovery is usually complete in 2–5 days.
V cholerae	24–72 hours	+	+++	–	Contaminated water, fish, shellfish, street vendor food.	Stool culture on special medium.	Abrupt onset of liquid diarrhea in endemic area. Needs prompt intravenous or oral replacement of fluids and electrolytes. Tetracyclines and azithromycin shorten excretion of vibrios.
Campylobacter jejuni	2–5 days	±	+++	+	Raw or undercooked poultry, unpasteurized milk, water.	Stool culture on special medium.	Fever, diarrhea that can be bloody, cramps. Usually self-limited in 2–10 days. Treat with azithromycin or fluoroquinolones for severe disease. May be associated with Guillain-Barré syndrome.
Shigella species (mild cases)	24–48 hours	±	+	+	Food or water contaminated with human feces. Person to person spread.	Routine stool culture.	Abrupt onset of diarrhea, often with blood and pus in stools, cramps, tenesmus, and lethargy. Stool cultures are positive. Therapy depends on sensitivity testing, but the fluoroquinolones are most effective. Do not give opioids. Often mild and self-limited.
Salmonella species	1–3 days	–	++	+	Eggs, poultry, unpasteurized milk, cheese, juices, raw fruits and vegetables.	Routine stool culture.	Gradual or abrupt onset of diarrhea and low-grade fever. No antimicrobials unless high risk (see text) or systemic dissemination is suspected, in which case give a fluoroquinolone. Prolonged carriage can occur.
Yersinia enterocolitica	24–48 hours	±	+	+	Undercooked pork, contaminated water, unpasteurized milk, tofu.	Stool culture on special medium.	Severe abdominal pain (appendicitis-like symptoms), diarrhea, fever. Polyarthritis, erythema nodosum in children. If severe, give tetracycline or fluoroquinolone. Without treatment, self-limited in 1–3 weeks.
Rotavirus	1–3 days	++	+++	+	Fecally contaminated foods touched by infected food handlers.	Immunoassay on stool.	Acute onset, vomiting, watery diarrhea that lasts 4–8 days. Supportive care.
Noroviruses and other caliciviruses	12–48 hours	++	+++	+	Shellfish and fecally contaminated foods touched by infected food handlers.	Clinical diagnosis with negative stool cultures. PCR available on stool.	Nausea, vomiting (more common in children), diarrhea (more common in adults), fever, myalgias, abdominal cramps. Lasts 12–60 hours. Supportive care.

PCR, polymerase chain reaction.

relapses. Because bacteremia with complications can occur in high-risk patients, some experts have recommended therapy for *Salmonella* in patients over the age of 50, in organ transplant recipients, in those with HIV, in patients taking corticosteroids, in those with lymphoproliferative diseases, and in those with vascular grafts. Ciprofloxacin, 500 mg orally every 12 hours for 5 days, is effective in shortening the course of illness compared with placebo in patients presenting with diarrhea, whether a pathogen is isolated or not. However, because of concerns about selecting for resistant organisms (especially *Campylobacter*, where increasing resistance to fluoroquinolones has been documented and erythromycin is the drug of choice) coupled with the fact that most infectious diarrhea is self-limited, routine use of antibiotics for all patients with diarrhea is not recommended. Antibiotics should be considered in patients with evidence of invasive disease (white cells in stool, dysentery), with symptoms 3–4 days or more in duration, with multiple stools (eight to ten or more per day), and in those with impaired immune responses. Antimotility drugs are useful in mild cases. Their use should be limited to patients without fever and without dysentery (bloody stools), and they should be used in low doses because of the risk of producing toxic megacolon. Postinfectious irritable bowel syndrome can follow infection and is approached in a similar fashion as in non-infectious irritable bowel syndrome.

Therapeutic recommendations for specific agents can be found elsewhere in this book.

Ahmed SM et al. Global prevalence of norovirus in cases of gastroenteritis: a systematic review and meta-analysis. Lancet Infect Dis. 2014 Aug;14(8):725–30. [PMID: 24981041]

Cardemil CV et al; Rotavirus Investigation Team. Two rotavirus outbreaks caused by genotype G2P[4] at large retirement communities: cohort studies. Ann Intern Med. 2012 Nov 6; 157(9):621–31. [PMID: 23128862]

Gaffga NH et al. Outbreak of salmonellosis linked to live poultry from a mail-order hatchery. N Engl J Med. 2012 May 31; 366(22):2065–73. [PMID: 22646629]

Hensgens MP et al. Diarrhoea in general practice: when should a *Clostridium difficile* infection be considered? Results of a nested case-control study. Clin Microbiol Infect. 2014 Dec; 20(12):O1067–74. [PMID: 25040463]

Kirk MD et al. World Health Organization estimates of the global and regional disease burden of 22 foodborne bacterial, protozoal, and viral diseases, 2010: a data synthesis. PLoS Med. 2015 Dec 3;12(12):e1001921. [PMID: 26633831]

Konijeti GG et al. Cost-effectiveness of competing strategies for management of recurrent *Clostridium difficile* infection: a decision analysis. Clin Infect Dis. 2014 Jun;58(11):1507–14. [PMID: 24692533]

Pfeiffer ML et al. The patient presenting with acute dysentery–a systematic review. J Infect. 2012 Apr;64(4):374–86. [PMID: 22266388]

Torpy JM et al. JAMA patient page. Viral gastroenteritis. JAMA. 2012 Aug 1;308(5):528. [PMID: 22851123]

Wikswo ME et al. Outbreaks of acute gastroenteritis transmitted by person-to-person contact, environmental contamination, and unknown modes of transmission—United States, 2009–2013. MMWR Surveill Summ. 2015 Dec 11;64(12):1–16. [PMID: 26656915]

INFECTIOUS DISEASES IN THE RETURNING TRAVELER

 ESSENTIALS OF DIAGNOSIS

- ▶ Most infections are common and self-limited.
- ▶ Identify patients with transmissible diseases that require isolation.
- ▶ The incubation period may be helpful in diagnosis.
- ▶ Less than 3 weeks following exposure may suggest dengue, leptospirosis, and yellow fever; more than 3 weeks suggest typhoid fever, malaria, and tuberculosis.

▶ **General Considerations**

The differential diagnosis of fever in the returning traveler is broad, ranging from self-limited viral infections to life-threatening illness. The evaluation is best done by identifying whether a particular syndrome is present, then refining the differential diagnosis based on an exposure history. The travel history should include directed questions regarding geography (rural versus urban, specific country visited), animal or arthropod contact, unprotected sexual intercourse, ingestion of untreated water or raw foods, historical or pretravel immunizations, and adherence to malaria prophylaxis.

▶ **Etiologies**

The most common infectious causes of fever—excluding simple causes such as upper respiratory infections, bacterial pneumonia and urinary tract infections—in returning travelers are malaria (see Chapter 35), diarrhea (see next section), and dengue (see Chapter 32). Others include respiratory infections, including seasonal influenza, influenza A/H1N1 "swine" influenza, and influenza A/H5N1 or A/H7N9 "avian" influenza (see Chapter 32); leptospirosis (see Chapter 34); typhoid fever (see Chapter 33); and rickettsial infections (see Chapter 32). Foreign travel is increasingly recognized as a risk factor for colonization and disease with resistant pathogens, such as extended-spectrum beta-lactamases (ESBL)–producing gram-negative organisms. Systemic febrile illnesses without a diagnosis also occur commonly, particularly in travelers returning from sub-Saharan Africa or Southeast Asia.

A. Fever and Rash

Potential etiologies include dengue, Ebola, Chikungunya, and Zika viruses, viral hemorrhagic fever, leptospirosis, meningococcemia, yellow fever, typhus, *Salmonella typhi*, and acute HIV infection.

B. Pulmonary Infiltrates

Tuberculosis, ascaris, *Paragonimus*, and *Strongyloides* can all cause pulmonary infiltrates.

C. Meningoencephalitis

Etiologies include *N meningitidis*, leptospirosis, arboviruses, rabies, and (cerebral) malaria.

D. Jaundice

Consider hepatitis A, yellow fever, hemorrhagic fever, leptospirosis, and malaria.

E. Fever without Localizing Symptoms or Signs

Malaria, typhoid fever, acute HIV infection, rickettsial illness, visceral leishmaniasis, trypanosomiasis, and dengue are possible etiologies.

F. Traveler's Diarrhea

See next section.

▶ Clinical Findings

Fever and rash in the returning traveler should prompt blood cultures and serologic tests based on the exposure history. The work-up of a **pulmonary infiltrate** should include the placement of a PPD or use of an interferon-gamma release assay, examination of sputum for acid-fast bacilli and possibly for ova and parasites. Patients with evidence of **meningoencephalitis** should receive lumbar puncture, blood cultures, thick/thin smears of peripheral blood, history-guided serologies, and a nape biopsy (if rabies is suspected). **Jaundice** in a returning traveler should be evaluated for hemolysis (for malaria), and the following tests should be performed: liver tests, thick/thin smears of peripheral blood, and directed serologic testing. The work-up of **traveler's diarrhea** is presented in the following section. Finally, patients with **fever** but no localizing signs or symptoms should have blood cultures performed. Routine laboratory studies usually include complete blood count with differential, electrolytes, liver tests, urinalysis, and blood cultures. Thick and thin peripheral blood smears should be done (and repeated in 12–24 hours if clinical suspicion remains high) for malaria if there has been travel to endemic areas. Other studies are directed by the results of history, physical examination, and initial laboratory tests. They may include stool for ova and parasites, chest radiograph, HIV test, and specific serologies (eg, dengue, leptospirosis, rickettsial disease, schistosomiasis, *Strongyloides*). Bone marrow biopsy to diagnose typhoid fever could be helpful in the appropriate patient.

▶ When to Refer

Travelers with fever, particularly if immunocompromised.

▶ When to Admit

Any evidence of hemorrhage, respiratory distress, hemodynamic instability, and neurologic deficits.

Dye C; WHO Ebola Response Team. Ebola virus disease in West Africa—the first 9 months. N Engl J Med. 2015 Jan 8; 372(2):189. [PMID: 25564903]

Farmakiotis D et al. Typhoid fever in an inner city hospital: a 5-year retrospective review. J Travel Med. 2013 Jan–Feb; 20(1):17–21. [PMID: 23279226]

Fischer M et al; Arboviral Diseases Branch, National Center for Emerging and Zoonotic Infectious Diseases, CDC. Notes from the field: chikungunya virus spreads in the Americas—Caribbean and South America, 2013-2014. MMWR Morb Mortal Wkly Rep. 2014 Jun 6;63(22):500–1. [PMID: 24898168]

Gautret P et al; GeoSentinel Surveillance Network. Travel-associated illness in older adults (>60 y). J Travel Med. 2012 May–Jun;19(3):169–77. [PMID: 22530824]

Jensenius M et al; GeoSentinel Surveillance Network. Acute and potentially life-threatening tropical diseases in western travelers—a GeoSentinel multicenter study, 1996–2011. Am J Trop Med Hyg. 2013 Feb;88(2):397–404. [PMID: 23324216]

Johnson BA et al. Prevention of malaria in travelers. Am Fam Physician. 2012 May 15;85(10):973–7. Erratum in: Am Fam Physician. 2012 Aug 1;86(3):222. [PMID: 22612048]

Kantele A et al. Antimicrobials increase travelers' risk of colonization by extended-spectrum betalactamase-producing Enterobacteriaceae. Clin Infect Dis. 2015 Mar 15;60(6):837–46. [PMID: 25613287]

Li Q et al. Epidemiology of human infections with avian influenza A(H7N9) virus in China. N Engl J Med. 2014 Feb 6; 370(6):520–32. [PMID: 23614499]

Matteelli A et al. Travel-associated sexually transmitted infections: an observational cross-sectional study of the GeoSentinel surveillance database. Lancet Infect Dis. 2013 Mar;13(3): 205–13. [PMID: 23182931]

Ruppé E et al. High rate of acquisition but short duration of carriage of multidrug-resistant Enterobacteriaceae after travel to the tropics. Clin Infect Dis. 2015 Aug 15;61(4):593–600. [PMID: 25904368]

TRAVELER'S DIARRHEA

ESSENTIALS OF DIAGNOSIS

▶ Usually a benign, self-limited disease occurring about 1 week into travel.

▶ Prophylaxis not recommended unless there is a comorbid disease (inflammatory bowel syndrome, HIV, immunosuppressive medication).

▶ Single-dose therapy of a fluoroquinolone usually effective if significant symptoms develop.

▶ General Considerations

Whenever a person travels from one country to another—particularly if the change involves a marked difference in climate, social conditions, or sanitation standards and facilities—diarrhea may develop within 2–10 days. Bacteria cause 80% of cases of traveler's diarrhea, with enterotoxigenic *E coli*, *Shigella* species, and *Campylobacter jejuni* being the most common pathogens. Less common are *Aeromonas*, *Salmonella*, noncholera vibriones, *E histolytica*, and *G lamblia*. Contributory causes include unusual food and drink, change in living habits, occasional viral infections (adenoviruses or rotaviruses), and change in bowel flora. Chronic watery diarrhea may be due to amebiasis or giardiasis or, rarely, tropical sprue.

Clinical Findings

A. Symptoms and Signs

There may be up to ten or even more loose stools per day, often accompanied by abdominal cramps and nausea, occasionally by vomiting, and rarely by fever. The stools are usually watery and not associated with fever when caused by enterotoxigenic *E coli*. With invasive bacterial pathogens (*Shigella, Campylobacter, Salmonella*) stools can be bloody and fever may be present. The illness usually subsides spontaneously within 1–5 days, although 10% remain symptomatic for 1 week or longer, and symptoms persist for longer than 1 month in 2%. Traveler's diarrhea is also a significant risk factor for developing irritable bowel syndrome.

B. Laboratory Findings

In patients with fever and bloody diarrhea, stool culture is indicated, but in most cases, cultures are reserved for those who do not respond to antibiotics.

Prevention

A. General Measures

Avoidance of fresh foods and water sources that are likely to be contaminated is recommended for travelers to developing countries, where infectious diarrheal illnesses are endemic.

B. Specific Measures

Because not all travelers will have diarrhea and because most episodes are brief and self-limited, the currently recommended approach is to provide the traveler with a supply of antimicrobials to be taken if significant diarrhea occurs during the trip. In areas where toxin-producing bacteria are the major cause of diarrhea (Latin America and Africa), loperamide (4 mg oral loading dose, then 2 mg after each loose stool to a maximum of 16 mg/day) with a single oral dose of ciprofloxacin (750 mg), levofloxacin (500 mg), or ofloxacin (200 mg), cures most cases of traveler's diarrhea. If diarrhea is associated with bloody stools or persists despite a single dose of a fluoroquinolone, 1000 mg of azithromycin should be taken. In pregnant women and in areas where invasive bacteria more commonly cause diarrhea (Indian subcontinent, Asia, especially Thailand where fluoroquinolone-resistant *Campylobacter* is prevalent), azithromycin is the drug of choice. Rifaximin, a nonabsorbable agent, is also approved for therapy of traveler's diarrhea at a dose of 200 mg orally three times per day or 400 mg twice a day for 3 days. Because luminal concentrations are high, but tissue levels are insufficient, it should not be used in situations where there is a high likelihood of invasive disease (eg, fever, systemic toxicity, or

bloody stools). Prophylaxis is recommended for those with significant underlying disease (inflammatory bowel disease, AIDS, diabetes mellitus, heart disease in the elderly, conditions requiring immunosuppressive medications) and for those whose full activity status during the trip is so essential that even short periods of diarrhea would be unacceptable.

Prophylaxis is started upon entry into the destination country and is continued for 1 or 2 days after leaving. For stays of more than 3 weeks, prophylaxis is not recommended because of the cost and increased toxicity. For prophylaxis, numerous oral antimicrobial once-daily regimens are effective, such as norfloxacin, 400 mg; ciprofloxacin, 500 mg; or rifaximin, 200 mg. Bismuth subsalicylate is effective but turns the tongue and the stools black and can interfere with doxycycline absorption, which may be needed for malaria prophylaxis; it is rarely used.

Treatment

For most individuals, the affliction is short-lived, and symptomatic therapy with loperamide is all that is required, provided the patient is not systemically ill (fever 39°C or higher) and does not have dysentery (bloody stools), in which case antimotility agents should be avoided. Packages of oral rehydration salts to treat dehydration are available over the counter in the United States (Infalyte, Pedialyte, others) and in many foreign countries.

When to Refer

- Cases refractory to treatment.
- Persistent infection.
- Immunocompromised patient.

When to Admit

Patients who are severely dehydrated or hemodynamically unstable should be admitted to the hospital.

Kollaritsch H et al. Traveler's diarrhea. Infect Dis Clin North Am. 2012 Sep;26(3):691–706. [PMID: 22963778]
Steffen R et al. Traveler's diarrhea: a clinical review. JAMA. 2015 Jan 6;313(1):71–80. [PMID: 25562268]

ANTIMICROBIAL THERAPY

SELECTED PRINCIPLES OF ANTIMICROBIAL THERAPY

Specific steps (outlined below) are required when considering antibiotic therapy for patients. Drugs within classes, drugs of first choice, and alternative drugs are presented in Table 30–4.

A. Etiologic Diagnosis

Based on the organ system involved, the organism causing infection can often be predicted. See Tables 30–5 and 30–6.

Table 30–4. Drugs of choice for suspected or proved microbial pathogens.

Suspected or Proved Etiologic Agent	Drug(s) of First Choice	Alternative Drug(s)
Gram-negative cocci		
Moraxella catarrhalis	Cefuroxime, a fluoroquinolone[1]	Ceftriaxone, cefuroxime axetil, an erythromycin,[2] a tetracycline,[3] azithromycin, amoxicillin-clavulanic acid, TMP-SMZ[4]
Neisseria gonorrhoeae (gonococcus)	Ceftriaxone plus azithromycin or doxycycline	Cefixime plus azithromycin or doxycycline[5]
Neisseria meningitidis (meningococcus)	Penicillin[6]	Ceftriaxone, ampicillin
Gram-positive cocci		
Streptococcus pneumoniae[7] (pneumococcus)	Penicillin[6]	An erythromycin,[2] a cephalosporin,[8] vancomycin, clindamycin, azithromycin, a tetracycline,[3] respiratory fluoroquinolones[1]
Streptococcus, hemolytic, groups A, B, C, G	Penicillin[6]	An erythromycin,[2] a cephalosporin,[8] vancomycin, clindamycin, azithromycin
Viridans streptococci	Penicillin[6] ± gentamicin	Cephalosporin,[8] vancomycin
Staphylococcus, methicillin-resistant	Vancomycin	TMP-SMZ,[4] doxycycline, minocycline, linezolid,[11] tedizolid,[11] daptomycin,[11] televancin,[11] dalbavancin,[11] oritavancin,[11] ceftaroline
Staphylococcus, non-penicillinase-producing	Penicillin[6]	A cephalosporin,[8] clindamycin
Staphylococcus, penicillinase-producing	Penicillinase-resistant penicillin[9]	Vancomycin, a cephalosporin,[8] clindamycin, amoxicillin-clavulanic acid, ampicillin-sulbactam, piperacillin-tazobactam, TMP-SMZ[4]
Enterococcus faecalis	Ampicillin ± gentamicin[10]	Vancomycin ± gentamicin
Enterococcus faecium	Vancomycin ± gentamicin[10]	Linezolid,[11] quinupristin-dalfopristin,[11] daptomycin,[11] tigecycline,[11] tedizolid,[11] oritavancin[11]
Gram-negative rods		
Acinetobacter	Imipenem, meropenem	Tigecycline, minocycline, doxycycline, aminoglycosides,[12] colistin
Prevotella, oropharyngeal strains	Clindamycin	Metronidazole
Bacteroides, gastrointestinal strains	Metronidazole	Ticarcillin-clavulanate, ampicillin-sulbactam, piperacillin-tazobactam, carbapenem
Brucella	Doxycycline + rifampin[3]	TMP-SMZ[4] ± gentamicin; ciprofloxacin + rifampin
Campylobacter jejuni	Erythromycin[2] or azithromycin	Tetracycline,[3] a fluoroquinolone[1]
Enterobacter	Ertapenem, imipenem, meropenem, cefepime	Aminoglycoside, a fluoroquinolone,[1] TMP-SMZ[4]
Escherichia coli (sepsis)[13]	Cefotaxime, ceftriaxone	Ertapenem,[13] imipenem[13] or meropenem,[13] aminoglycosides,[12] a fluoroquinolone,[1] aztreonam, ticarcillin-clavulanate, piperacillin-tazobactam, ceftazidime-avibactam,[13] ceftolozane-tazobactam[13]
Escherichia coli (uncomplicated outpatient urinary infection)	Nitrofurantoin, fosfomycin	Fluoroquinolones,[1] TMP-SMZ,[4] oral cephalosporin
Haemophilus (meningitis and other serious infections)	Ceftriaxone	Aztreonam
Haemophilus (respiratory infections, otitis)	Ampicillin-clavulanate	Doxycycline, azithromycin, ceftriaxone, cefuroxime, cefuroxime axetil, TMP-SMZ[4]
Helicobacter pylori	Amoxicillin, clarithromycin and PPI	Bismuth subsalicylate, tetracycline, metronidazole and PPI
Klebsiella[13]	A cephalosporin	TMP-SMZ,[4] aminoglycoside,[12] ertapenem,[13] imipenem[13] or meropenem,[13] a fluoroquinolone,[1] aztreonam, ticarcillin-clavulanate, piperacillin-tazobactam, ceftazidime-avibactam,[13] ceftolozane-tazobactam[13]
Legionella species (pneumonia)	Azithromycin, or fluoroquinolones[1] ± rifampin	Doxycycline ± rifampin

(continued)

Table 30–4. Drugs of choice for suspected or proved microbial pathogens. (continued)

Suspected or Proved Etiologic Agent	Drug(s) of First Choice	Alternative Drug(s)
Proteus mirabilis	Ampicillin	An aminoglycoside,[12] TMP-SMZ,[4] a fluoroquinolone,[1] a cephalosporin[8]
Proteus vulgaris and other species (Morganella, Providencia)	Ceftriaxone	Aminoglycoside,[12] ertapenem, imipenem or meropenem, TMP-SMZ,[4] a fluoroquinolone[1]
Pseudomonas aeruginosa	Piperacillin-tazobactam or ceftazidime or cefepime, or imipenem or meropenem or doripenem or aztreonam ± aminoglycoside[12]	Ciprofloxacin (or levofloxacin) ± piperacillin-tazobactam; ciprofloxacin (or levofloxacin) ± ceftazidime; ciprofloxacin (or levofloxacin) ± cefepime; ceftazidime-avibactam[13]; ceftolozane-tazobactam[13]
Burkholderia pseudomallei (melioidosis)	Ceftazidime	Tetracycline,[3] TMP-SMZ,[4] amoxicillin-clavulanic acid, imipenem or meropenem
Burkholderia mallei (glanders)	Streptomycin + tetracycline[3]	Chloramphenicol + streptomycin
Salmonella (bacteremia)	Ceftriaxone	A fluoroquinolone[1]
Serratia	Carbapenem	TMP-SMZ,[4] aminoglycosides,[12] a fluoroquinolone,[1] ceftriaxone
Shigella	A fluoroquinolone[1]	Azithromycin, ampicillin, TMP-SMZ,[4] ceftriaxone
Vibrio (cholera, sepsis)	A tetracycline[3]	TMP-SMZ,[4] a fluoroquinolone[1]
Yersinia pestis (plague)	Streptomycin ± a tetracycline[3]	Chloramphenicol, TMP-SMZ[5]
Gram-positive rods		
Actinomyces	Penicillin[6]	Tetracycline,[3] clindamycin
Bacillus (including anthrax)	Penicillin[6]	Erythromycin,[2] a fluoroquinolone[1]
Clostridium (eg, gas gangrene, tetanus)	Penicillin[6]	Metronidazole, clindamycin, imipenem or meropenem
Corynebacterium diphtheria	Erythromycin[2]	Penicillin[6]
Corynebacterium jeikeium	Vancomycin	Linezolid
Listeria	Ampicillin ± aminoglycoside[12]	TMP-SMZ[4]
Acid-fast rods		
Mycobacterium tuberculosis[15]	Isoniazid (INH) + rifampin + pyrazinamide ± ethambutol	Other antituberculous drugs (see Tables 9–15 and 9–16)
Mycobacterium leprae	Dapsone + rifampin ± clofazimine	Minocycline, ofloxacin, clarithromycin
Mycobacterium kansasii	INH + rifampin ± ethambutol	Clarithromycin, azithromycin, ethionamide, cycloserine
Mycobacterium avium complex	Clarithromycin or azithromycin + ethambutol, ± rifabutin	Amikacin, ciprofloxacin
Mycobacterium fortuitum-chelonei	Cefoxitin + clarithromycin	Amikacin, rifampin, sulfonamide, doxycycline, linezolid
Nocardia	TMP-SMZ[4]	Minocycline, imipenem or meropenem, linezolid
Spirochetes		
Borrelia burgdorferi (Lyme disease)	Doxycycline, amoxicillin, cefuroxime axetil	Ceftriaxone, penicillin, azithromycin
Borrelia recurrentis (relapsing fever)	Doxycycline[3]	Penicillin[6]
Leptospira	Penicillin[6]	Doxycycline,[3] ceftriaxone
Treponema pallidum (syphilis)	Penicillin[6]	Doxycycline, ceftriaxone
Treponema pertenue (yaws)	Penicillin[6]	Doxycycline

(continued)

Table 30–4. Drugs of choice for suspected or proved microbial pathogens. (continued)

Suspected or Proved Etiologic Agent	Drug(s) of First Choice	Alternative Drug(s)
Mycoplasmas	Clarithromycin or azithromycin or doxycycline	A fluoroquinolone,[1] erythromycin[2]
Chlamydiae		
C psittaci	Doxycycline	Chloramphenicol
C trachomatis (urethritis or pelvic inflammatory disease)	Doxycycline or azithromycin	Levofloxacin, ofloxacin
C pneumoniae	Doxycycline[3]	Erythromycin,[2] azithromycin, a fluoroquinolone[1,16]
Rickettsiae	Doxycycline[3]	Chloramphenicol, a fluoroquinolone[1]

[1]Fluoroquinolones include ciprofloxacin, ofloxacin, levofloxacin, moxifloxacin, and others (see text). Gemifloxacin, levofloxacin, and moxifloxacin, the so-called "respiratory fluoroquinolones," demonstrate the most reliable activity against gram-positive organisms, including penicillin-resistant S pneumoniae and methicillin-sensitive S aureus. Activity against enterococci and S epidermidis is variable.

[2]Erythromycin estolate is best absorbed orally but carries the highest risk of hepatitis; erythromycin stearate and erythromycin ethylsuccinate are also available.

[3]All tetracyclines have similar activity against most microorganisms. Minocycline (the most active tetracycline), doxycycline, have increased activity over tetracycline against S aureus.

[4]TMP-SMZ is a mixture of 1 part trimethoprim and 5 parts sulfamethoxazole.

[5]Test of cure required if ceftriaxone not used.

[6]Penicillin G is preferred for parenteral injection; penicillin V for oral administration—to be used only in treating infections due to highly sensitive organisms.

[7]Infections caused by isolates with intermediate resistance may respond to high doses of penicillin or ceftriaxone, as well as the respiratory fluoroquinolones (gemifloxacin, levofloxacin, and moxifloxacin). Infections caused by highly resistant strains should be treated with vancomycin. Many strains of penicillin-resistant pneumococci are resistant to macrolides, cephalosporins, tetracyclines, and TMP-SMZ.

[8]Most intravenous cephalosporins (with the exception of ceftazidime) have good activity against streptococci and staphylococci.

[9]Parenteral nafcillin or oxacillin; oral dicloxacillin, cloxacillin, or oxacillin.

[10]Addition of gentamicin indicated only for severe enterococcal infections (eg, endocarditis, meningitis).

[11]Linezolid, tedizolid, daptomycin, televancin, dalbavancin, oritavancin should be reserved for the treatment of vancomycin-resistant isolates or in patients intolerant of vancomycin. Daptomycin, tigecycline, tedizolid, and oritavancin are not approved by FDA for treatment of vancomycin-resistant strains of enterococci but are frequently active in vitro.

[12]Aminoglycosides—gentamicin, tobramycin, amikacin, netilmicin—should be chosen on the basis of local patterns of susceptibility.

[13]Extended beta-lactamase–producing isolates should be treated with a carbapenem. If a carbapenem cannot be used, either ceftazidime-avibactam or ceftolozane-tazobactam can be considered.

[14]Ceftazidime-avibactam and ceftolozane-tazobactam often active in multidrug-resistant P aeruginosa.

[15]Resistance is common and susceptibility testing should be done.

[16]Ciprofloxacin has inferior antichlamydial activity compared with levofloxacin or ofloxacin.

Adapted, with permission, and updated, from *Treat Guide Med Lett.* 2010 June;6(94):43–52; *Med Lett Drugs Therapeut.* 2012 Jul 23(1395); *Treat Guide Med Lett.* 2013 Jul;11(131):65; and *Med Lett Drugs Therapeut.* 2014 May 12 (1442). www.medicalletter.org

Key: ±, alone or combined with.

B. "Best Guess"

Select an empiric regimen that is likely to be effective against the suspected pathogens.

C. Laboratory Control

Specimens for laboratory examination should be obtained before institution of therapy to determine susceptibility.

D. Clinical Response

Based on clinical response and other data, the laboratory reports are evaluated and then the desirability of changing the regimen is considered. If the specimen was obtained from a normally sterile site (eg, blood, cerebrospinal fluid, pleural fluid, joint fluid), the recovery of a microorganism in significant amounts is meaningful even if the organism recovered is different from the clinically suspected agent,

and this may force a change in treatment. Isolation of unexpected microorganisms from the respiratory tract, gastrointestinal tract, or surface lesions (sites that have a complex flora) may represent colonization or contamination, and cultures must be critically evaluated before drugs are abandoned that were judiciously selected on a "best guess" basis.

E. Drug Susceptibility Tests

Some microorganisms are predictably inhibited by certain drugs; if such organisms are isolated, they need not be tested for drug susceptibility. For example, all group A hemolytic streptococci are inhibited by penicillin. Other organisms (eg, enteric gram-negative rods) are variably susceptible and generally require susceptibility testing whenever they are isolated. Organisms that once had predictable susceptibility patterns have now become resistant

Table 30–5. Examples of initial antimicrobial therapy for acutely ill, hospitalized adults pending identification of causative organism.

Suspected Clinical Diagnosis	Likely Etiologic Diagnosis	Drugs of Choice
Meningitis, bacterial, community-acquired	*Streptococcus pneumoniae* (pneumococcus),[1] *Neisseria meningitidis* (meningococcus)	Ceftriaxone, 2 g intravenously every 12 hours[2]; **plus** vancomycin, 15 mg/kg intravenously every 8 hours
Meningitis, bacterial, age > 50, community-acquired	Pneumococcus, meningococcus, *Listeria monocytogenes*,[2] gram-negative bacilli, group B streptococcus	Ampicillin, 2 g intravenously every 4 hours, **plus** ceftriaxone, 2 g intravenously every 12 hours, **plus** vancomycin, 15 mg/kg intravenously every 8 hours
Meningitis, postoperative (or posttraumatic)	*S aureus*, gram-negative bacilli, coagulase-negative staphylococci, diphtheroids (eg, *Propionibacterium acnes*) (uncommon) pneumococcus (in posttraumatic)	Vancomycin, 15 mg/kg intravenously every 8 hours, **plus** cefepime, 3 g intravenously every 8 hours
Brain abscess	Mixed anaerobes, pneumococci, streptococci	Ceftriaxone, 2 g intravenously every 12 hours **plus** metronidazole, 500 mg orally every 8 hours **plus** vancomycin, 15 mg/kg intravenously every 8 hours
Pneumonia, acute, community-acquired, non-ICU hospital admission	Pneumococci, *M pneumoniae*, *Legionella*, *C pneumoniae*	Ceftriaxone, 1 g intravenously every 24 hours or ampicillin 2 g intravenously every 6 hours) **plus** azithromycin 500 mg intravenously every 24 hours; **or** a respiratory fluoroquinolone[3] alone
Pneumonia, postoperative or nosocomial	*S aureus*, mixed anaerobes, gram-negative bacilli	Cefepime, 1 g intravenously every 8 hours; **or** ceftazidime, 2 g intravenously every 8 hours; **or** piperacillin-tazobactam, 4.5 g intravenously every 6 hours; **or** imipenem, 500 mg intravenously every 6 hours; **or** meropenem, 1 g intravenously every 8 hours **plus** tobramycin, 5–7 mg/kg intravenously every 24 hours; **or** ciprofloxacin, 400 mg intravenously every 12 hours; **or** levofloxacin, 500 mg intravenously every 24 hours **plus** vancomycin, 15 mg/kg intravenously every 12 hours
Endocarditis, acute (including injection drug user)	*S aureus*, *E faecalis*, gram-negative aerobic bacteria, viridans streptococci	Vancomycin, 15 mg/kg intravenously every 12 hours, **plus** gentamicin, 1 mg/kg every 8 hours
Septic thrombophlebitis (eg, IV tubing, IV shunts)	*S aureus*, gram-negative aerobic bacteria	Vancomycin, 15 mg/kg intravenously every 12 hours, **plus** ceftriaxone, 1 g intravenously every 24 hours
Osteomyelitis	*S aureus*	Nafcillin, 2 g intravenously every 4 hours; **or** cefazolin, 2 g intravenously every 8 hours
Septic arthritis	*S aureus*, *N gonorrhoeae*	Ceftriaxone, 1–2 g intravenously every 24 hours
Pyelonephritis with flank pain and fever (recurrent urinary tract infection)	*E coli*, *Klebsiella*, *Enterobacter*, *Pseudomonas*	Ceftriaxone, 1 g intravenously every 24 hours; **or** ciprofloxacin, 400 mg intravenously every 12 hours (500 mg orally); **or** levofloxacin, 500 mg once daily (intravenously/orally)
Fever in neutropenic patient receiving cancer chemotherapy	*S aureus*, *Pseudomonas*, *Klebsiella*, *E coli*	Ceftazidime, 2 g intravenously every 8 hours; **or** cefepime, 2 g intravenously every 8 hours
Intra-abdominal sepsis (eg, postoperative, peritonitis, cholecystitis)	Gram-negative bacteria, *Bacteroides*, anaerobic bacteria, streptococci, clostridia	Piperacillin-tazobactam, 4.5 g intravenously every 6 hours, **or** ertapenem, 1 g every 24 hours

[1]Some strains may be resistant to penicillin.
[2]TMP-SMZ can be used to treat *Listeria monocytogenes* in patients allergic to penicillin in a dosage of 15–20 mg/kg/day of TMP in three or four divided doses.
[3]Levofloxacin 750 mg/day, moxifloxacin 400 mg/day.

Table 30–6. Examples of empiric choices of antimicrobials for adult outpatient infections.

Suspected Clinical Diagnosis	Likely Etiologic Agents	Drugs of Choice	Alternative Drugs
Erysipelas, impetigo, cellulitis, ascending lymphangitis	Group A streptococcus	Phenoxymethyl penicillin, 0.5 g orally four times daily for 7–10 days	Cephalexin, 0.5 g orally four times daily for 7–10 days; **or** azithromycin, 500 mg on day 1 and 250 mg on days 2–5
Furuncle with surrounding cellulitis	*Staphylococcus aureus*	Dicloxacillin, 0.5 g orally four times daily for 7–10 days for MSSA. However, in many areas of the United States, CA-MRSA has become predominant: TMP-SMZ two double-strength tablets twice daily for 7–10 days; **or** clindamycin 0.3 g orally four times daily for 7–10 days	Cephalexin, 0.5 g orally four times daily for 7–10 days for MSSA. For CA-MRSA, tetracyclines, but not fluoroquinolones, are reasonable alternatives
Pharyngitis	Group A streptococcus	Phenoxymethyl penicillin, 0.5 g orally four times daily, **or** amoxicillin, 0.5–1 g orally three times daily, for 10 days	For patients with history of non-anaphylactic penicillin allergy, cephalexin, 0.5 g orally four times daily for 10 days; for patients with more severe penicillin allergy, clindamycin, 300 mg orally four times daily for 10 days; **or** azithromycin, 500 mg on day 1 and 250 mg on days 2–5; **or** azithromycin for susceptible isolates
Otitis media	*Streptococcus pneumoniae, Haemophilus influenzae, Moraxella catarrhalis*	Amoxicillin, 0.5–1 g orally three times daily for 10 days	Augmentin,[2] 0.875 g orally twice daily; **or** cefuroxime, 0.5 g orally twice daily; **or** cefpodoxime, 0.2–0.4 g daily; **or** doxycycline, 100 mg twice daily; **or** TMP-SMZ,[1] one double-strength tablet twice daily (all regimens for 10 days)
Acute sinusitis	*S pneumoniae, H influenzae, M catarrhalis*	Augmentin,[2] 0.875 g orally twice daily,	For patients allergic to penicillin, doxycycline, 100 mg twice daily for 10 days, or some fluoroquinolones[5] can be considered. Due to increasing resistance among pneumococci, monotherapy with a macrolide, a cephalosporin, or TMP-SMZ is not recommended
Aspiration pneumonia	Mixed oropharyngeal flora, including anaerobes	Clindamycin, 0.3 g orally four times daily for 10–14 days	Phenoxymethyl penicillin, 0.5 g orally four times daily for 10–14 days
Pneumonia	*S pneumoniae, Mycoplasma pneumoniae, Legionella pneumophila, Chlamydophila pneumoniae*	Doxycycline, 100 mg orally twice daily, **or** azithromycin (erythromycin, clarithromycin), 0.5 g orally on day 1 and 0.25 g on days 2–5	Amoxicillin, 0.5–1.0 g orally three times daily. A respiratory fluoroquinolone[5] for patients at high risk for infection due to resistant pneumococci
Cystitis	*Escherichia coli, Staphylococcus saprophyticus, Klebsiella pneumoniae, Proteus* species, other gram-negative rods or enterococci	Nitrofurantoin monohydrate macrocrystals 100 mg twice daily for 5–7 days (unless pregnant); fosfomycin 3 g orally as a single dose	Cephalexin, 0.5 g orally four times daily for 7 days, for uncomplicated cystitis. Due to increasing resistance, TMP-SMZ and fluoroquinolones should not be used as first-line therapy for empiric treatment
Pyelonephritis	*E coli, K pneumoniae, Proteus* species, *S saprophyticus*	Fluoroquinolones[4] for 7 days if prevalence of resistance among uropathogens is < 10%	TMP-SMZ,[1] one double-strength tablet twice daily for 7–14 days for susceptible pathogens. Oral beta-lactams are considered less effective
Gastroenteritis	*Salmonella, Shigella, Campylobacter, Entamoeba histolytica*	See footnote 3	

(continued)

Table 30–6. Examples of empiric choices of antimicrobials for adult outpatient infections. (continued)

Suspected Clinical Diagnosis	Likely Etiologic Agents	Drugs of Choice	Alternative Drugs
Urethritis, epididymitis	Neisseria gonorrhoeae, Chlamydia trachomatis	Ceftriaxone, 250 mg intramuscularly once **plus** azithromycin (or doxycycline) for N gonorrhoeae; azithromycin 1 g orally once, **or** doxycycline, 100 mg orally twice daily for 7 days, for C trachomatis	Cefixime 400 mg orally once for N gonorrhoeae[6]
Pelvic inflammatory disease	N gonorrhoeae, C trachomatis, anaerobes, gram-negative rods	Levofloxacin 500 mg orally daily, **or** ofloxacin, 400 mg orally twice daily, for 14 days, **plus** metronidazole, 500 mg orally twice daily, for 14 days	Cefoxitin, 2 g intramuscularly, with probenecid, 1 g orally, followed by doxycycline, 100 mg orally twice daily for 14 days; **or** ceftriaxone, 250 mg intramuscularly once, followed by doxycycline, 100 mg orally twice daily for 14 days
Syphilis			
Early syphilis (primary, secondary, or latent of < 1 year's duration)	Treponema pallidum	Benzathine penicillin G, 2.4 million units intramuscularly once	Doxycycline, 100 mg orally twice daily for 2 weeks
Latent syphilis of > 1 year's duration or cardiovascular syphilis	T pallidum	Benzathine penicillin G, 2.4 million units intramuscularly once a week for 3 weeks (total: 7.2 million units)	Doxycycline, 100 mg orally twice daily, for 4 weeks
Neurosyphilis	T pallidum	Aqueous penicillin G, 12–24 million units/day intravenously for 10–14 days	

[1]TMP-SMZ is a fixed combination of 1 part trimethoprim and 5 parts sulfamethoxazole. Single-strength tablets: 80 mg TMP, 400 mg SMZ; double-strength tablets: 160 mg TMP, 800 mg SMZ.

[2]Augmentin is a combination of amoxicillin, 250 mg, 500 mg, or 875 mg, plus 125 mg of clavulanic acid. Augmentin XR is a combination of amoxicillin 1 g and clavulanic acid 62.5 mg.

[3]The diagnosis should be confirmed by culture before therapy. Salmonella gastroenteritis does not require therapy. For susceptible Shigella isolates, give ciprofloxacin, 0.5 g orally twice daily for 5 days; or TMP-SMZ double-strength tablets twice daily for 5 days; or ampicillin, 0.5 g orally four times daily for 5 days. For Campylobacter infection, give azithromycin, 1 g orally times one dose, or ciprofloxacin, 0.5 g orally twice daily for 5 days. For E histolytica infection, give metronidazole, 750 mg orally three times daily for 5–10 days, followed by diiodohydroxyquinoline, 600 mg orally three times daily for 3 weeks.

[4]Fluoroquinolones and dosages include ciprofloxacin, 500 mg orally twice daily; ofloxacin, 400 mg orally twice daily; levofloxacin, 500 mg orally daily.

[5]Fluoroquinolones with activity against S pneumoniae, including penicillin-resistant isolates, include gemifloxacin (320 mg orally once daily), levofloxacin (500–750 mg orally once daily) and moxifloxacin (400 mg orally once daily). Use fluoroquinolones as drug of choice if recent antibiotic use within 3 months or comorbidities present.

[6]Test of cure recommended if ceftriaxone is not used.

Adapted from Treat Guide Med Lett. 2013 Jul; 11(131):65–73.

CA-MRSA, community-acquired methicillin-resistant Staphylococcus aureus; MRSA, methicillin-resistant S aureus; MSSA, methicillin-sensitive S aureus; TMP-SMZ, trimethoprim-sulfamethoxazole.

and require testing. Examples include the pneumococci, which may be resistant to multiple drugs (including penicillin, macrolides, and TMP-SMZ); the enterococci, which may be resistant to penicillin, aminoglycosides, and vancomycin; and extended-spectrum beta-lactamase producing–E coli resistant to third-generation cephalosporins and fluoroquinolones.

Over the past several years, the pharmaceutical industry has shifted away from developing and producing antibacterial medications, particularly those active against

gram-negative pathogens. However, in 2015, two beta-lactamase inhibitor combinations have been approved by the FDA which offer much-needed options in the treatment of resistant Pseudomonas aeruginosa and ESBL-producing Enterobacteriaceae. Nonetheless, the paucity of new drugs and increasing bacterial resistance reinforce the need to use all antimicrobials judiciously. When culture and susceptibility results have been finalized, it is important to utilize the most narrow spectrum agent possible to decrease the selection pressure for antibacterial resistance.

Antimicrobial drug susceptibility tests may be performed on solid media as disk diffusion tests, in broth, in tubes, in wells of microdilution plates, or as E-tests (strips with increasing concentration of antibiotic). The latter three methods yield results expressed as MIC (minimal inhibitory concentration). In most infections, the MIC is the appropriate in vitro test to guide selection of an antibacterial agent. When there appear to be marked discrepancies between susceptibility testing and clinical response, the following possibilities must be considered:

1. Selection of an inappropriate drug, drug dosage, or route of administration.

2. Failure to drain a collection of pus or to remove a foreign body.

3. Failure of a poorly diffusing drug to reach the site of infection (eg, central nervous system) or to reach intracellular phagocytosed bacteria.

4. Superinfection in the course of prolonged chemotherapy.

5. Emergence of drug resistance in the original pathogen or superinfection with a new more resistant organism.

6. Participation of two or more microorganisms in the infectious process, of which only one was originally detected and used for drug selection.

7. Inadequate host defenses, including immunodeficiencies and diabetes mellitus.

8. Noninfectious causes, including drug fever, malignancy, and autoimmune disease.

F. Promptness of Response

Response depends on a number of factors, including the patient (immunocompromised patients respond slower than immunocompetent patients), the site of infection (deep-seated infections such as osteomyelitis and endocarditis respond more slowly than superficial infections such as cystitis or cellulitis), the pathogen (virulent organisms such as S aureus respond more slowly than viridans streptococci; mycobacterial and fungal infections respond slower than bacterial infections), and the duration of illness (in general, the longer the symptoms are present, the longer it takes to respond). Thus, depending on the clinical situation, persistent fever and leukocytosis several days after initiation of therapy may not indicate improper choice of antibiotics but may be due to the natural history of the disease being treated. In most infections, either a bacteriostatic or a bactericidal agent can be used. In some infections (eg, infective endocarditis and meningitis), a bactericidal agent should be used. When potentially toxic drugs (eg, aminoglycosides, flucytosine) are used, serum levels of the drug are measured to minimize toxicity and ensure appropriate dosage. In patients with altered renal or hepatic clearance of drugs, the dosage or frequency of administration must be adjusted; it is best to measure levels in the elderly, morbidly obese patients, or those with altered kidney function when possible and adjust therapy accordingly.

G. Duration of Antimicrobial Therapy

Generally, effective antimicrobial treatment results in reversal of the clinical and laboratory parameters of active infection and marked clinical improvement. However, varying periods of treatment may be required for cure. Key factors include (1) the type of infecting organism (bacterial infections generally can be cured more rapidly than fungal or mycobacterial ones), (2) the location of the process (eg, endocarditis and osteomyelitis require prolonged therapy), and (3) the immunocompetence of the patient. Recommendations about duration of therapy are often given based on clinical experience, not prospective controlled studies of large numbers of patients.

H. Adverse Reactions and Toxicity

These include hypersensitivity reactions, direct toxicity, superinfection by drug-resistant microorganisms, and drug interactions. If the infection is life threatening and treatment cannot be stopped, the reactions are managed symptomatically or another drug is chosen that does not cross-react with the offending one (Table 30–4). If the infection is less serious, it may be possible to stop all antimicrobials and monitor the patient closely.

I. Route of Administration

Intravenous therapy is preferred for acutely ill patients with serious infections (eg, endocarditis, meningitis, sepsis, severe pneumonia) when dependable levels of antibiotics are required for successful therapy. Certain drugs (eg, fluconazole, voriconazole, rifampin, metronidazole, TMP-SMZ, and fluoroquinolones) are so well absorbed that they generally can be administered orally in seriously ill—but not hemodynamically unstable—patients.

Food does not significantly influence the bioavailability of most oral antimicrobial agents. However, the tetracyclines and the quinolones chelate multivalent cations resulting in decreased antibacterial absorption. Azithromycin capsules are associated with decreased bioavailability when taken with food and should be given 1 hour before or 2 hours after meals. Posaconazole solution should always be administered with food.

A major complication of intravenous antibiotic therapy is catheter infections. Peripheral catheters are changed every 48–72 hours to prevent phlebitis, and antimicrobial-coated central venous catheters (minocycline and rifampin, chlorhexidine and sulfadiazine) have been associated with a decreased incidence of catheter-related infections. Most of these infections present with local signs of infection (erythema, tenderness) at the insertion site. In a patient with fever who is receiving intravenous therapy, the catheter must always be considered a potential source. Small-gauge (20–23F) peripherally inserted silicone or polyurethane catheters (Per Q Cath, A-Cath, Ven-A-Cath, and others) are associated with a low infection rate and can be maintained for 3–6 months without replacement. Such catheters are ideal for long-term outpatient antibiotic therapy.

J. Cost of Antibiotics

The cost of these agents can be substantial. In addition to acquisition costs and monitoring costs (drug levels, liver tests, electrolytes, etc), the cost of treating adverse reactions, the cost of treatment failure, and the costs associated with drug administration must be considered.

Chambers HF et al. Antibacterial resistance leadership group: open for business. Clin Infect Dis. 2014 Jun;58(11):1571–6. [PMID: 24610430]

Jenkins SG et al. Current concepts in laboratory testing to guide antimicrobial therapy. Mayo Clin Proc. 2012 Mar;87(3):290–308. [PMID: 22386185]

Rivera AM et al. Current concepts in antimicrobial therapy against select gram-positive organisms: methicillin-resistant *Staphylococcus aureus*, penicillin-resistant pneumococci, and vancomycin-resistant enterococci. Mayo Clin Proc. 2011 Dec; 86(12):1230–43. [PMID: 22134942]

HYPERSENSITIVITY TESTS & DESENSITIZATION

► Penicillin Allergy

All penicillins are cross-sensitizing and cross-reacting. Skin tests with penicilloyl-polylysine, with minor antigenic determinants, and with undegraded penicillin can identify most individuals with IgE-mediated reactions (hives, bronchospasm). Among positive reactors to skin tests, the incidence of subsequent immediate severe penicillin reactions is high. A history of a penicillin reaction in the past is often not reliable. Only a small proportion (less than 20%) of patients with a history of penicillin allergy have an adverse reaction when challenged with the drug. The decision to administer penicillin or related drugs (other beta-lactams) to patients with an allergic history depends on the severity of the reported reaction, the severity of the infection being treated, and the availability of alternative drugs. For patients with a history of severe reaction (anaphylaxis), alternative drugs should be used. In the rare situations when there is a strong indication for using penicillin (eg, syphilis in pregnancy) in allergic patients, desensitization can be performed. If the reaction is mild (nonurticarial rash), the patient may be rechallenged with penicillin or may be given another beta-lactam antibiotic.

Allergic reactions include anaphylaxis, serum sickness (urticaria, fever, joint swelling, angioedema 7–12 days after exposure), skin rashes, fever, interstitial nephritis, eosinophilia, hemolytic anemia, other hematologic disturbances, and vasculitis. The incidence of hypersensitivity to penicillin is estimated to be 1–5% among adults in the United States. Life-threatening anaphylactic reactions are very rare (0.05%). Ampicillin produces maculopapular skin rashes more frequently than other penicillins, but many ampicillin (and other beta-lactam) rashes are not allergic in origin. The non-allergic ampicillin rash usually occurs after 3–4 days of therapy, is maculopapular, is more common in patients with coexisting viral illness (especially Epstein-Barr infection), and resolves with continued therapy. The maculopapular rash may or may not reappear with rechallenge. Rarely, penicillins can induce nephritis with primary tubular lesions associated with anti-basement membrane antibodies.

If the intradermal test described below is negative, desensitization is not necessary, and a full dose of the material may be given. If the test is positive, alternative drugs should be strongly considered. If that is not feasible, desensitization is necessary.

Patients with a history of allergy to penicillin are also at an increased risk for having a reaction to **cephalosporins** or **carbapenems**. A common approach to these patients is to assess the severity of the reaction. If an IgE-mediated reaction to penicillin can be excluded by history, a cephalosporin can be administered. When the history justifies concern about an immediate-type reaction, penicillin skin testing should be performed. If the test is negative, the cephalosporin or carbapenem can be given. If the test is positive, there is a 5–10% chance of cross reactivity with cephalosporins, and the decision whether to use cephalosporins depends on the availability of alternative agents and the severity of the infection. While carbapenems historically have been considered highly cross reactive with penicillins, the cross reactivity appears to be minimal (1%).

► Intradermal Test for Hypersensitivity

Penicillin is the drug that most frequently serves as an indication for sensitivity testing and desensitization. A clinical history of penicillin allergy has a positive predictive value of only 15%. IgG-mediated delayed reactions such as erythematous or maculopapular skin rash or serum sickness should be distinguished from immediate-type IgE-mediated reactions, such as urticaria, angioedema, and anaphylaxis.

► Desensitization

A. Precautions

1. The desensitization procedure is not innocuous— deaths from anaphylaxis have been reported. If extreme hypersensitivity is suspected, it is advisable to use an alternative structurally unrelated drug and to reserve desensitization for situations when treatment cannot be withheld and no alternative drug is available.

2. An antihistaminic drug (25–50 mg of hydroxyzine or diphenhydramine intramuscularly or orally) should be administered before desensitization is begun in order to lessen any reaction that occurs.

3. Desensitization should be conducted in an intensive care unit where cardiac monitoring and emergency endotracheal intubation can be performed.

4. Epinephrine, 1 mL of 1:1000 solution, must be ready for immediate administration.

B. Desensitization Method

Several methods of desensitization have been described for penicillin, including use of both oral and intravenous preparations. All methods start with very small doses of drug and gradually increase the dose until therapeutic doses are achieved. For penicillin, 1 unit of drug is given intravenously and the patient observed for 15–30 minutes. If there is no reaction, some recommend doubling the dose while others recommend increasing it tenfold every 15–30 minutes until a dosage of 2 million units is reached; then give the remainder of the desired dose.

For recommendations on skin testing and desensitization for other preparations (eg, botulism antitoxin and diphtheria antitoxin), the manufacturer's package inserts should be consulted.

Blumenthal KG et al. Peripheral blood eosinophilia and hypersensitivity reactions among patients receiving outpatient parenteral antibiotics. J Allergy Clin Immunol. 2015 Nov; 136(5):1288–94.e1. [PMID: 25981739]
Chang C et al. Overview of penicillin allergy. Clin Rev Allergy Immunol. 2012 Aug;43(1–2):84–97. [PMID: 21789743]
Romano A et al. Antibiotic allergies in children and adults: from clinical symptoms to skin testing diagnosis. J Allergy Clin Immunol Pract. 2014 Jan–Feb;2(1):3–12. [PMID: 24565763]

IMMUNIZATION AGAINST INFECTIOUS DISEASES

RECOMMENDED IMMUNIZATION OF INFANTS, CHILDREN, & ADOLESCENTS

The recommended schedules and dosages of vaccination change often, so the manufacturer's package inserts should always be consulted.

The schedule for active immunizations in children can be accessed at www.cdc.gov/travel/destinations/list. All adolescents should see a health care provider to ensure vaccination of those who have not received varicella or hepatitis B vaccine, to make certain that a second dose of MMR has been given, to receive a booster of tetanus toxoid, reduced diphtheria toxoid and acellular pertussis vaccine (Tdap adolescent preparation), to receive meningococcal vaccine conjugate vaccine, to obtain HPV vaccine if not given previously, and to receive immunizations (influenza and pneumococcal vaccines) that may be indicated for certain high-risk individuals.

RECOMMENDED IMMUNIZATION FOR ADULTS

Immunization is one of the most important tools (along with sanitation) used to prevent morbidity and mortality from infectious diseases. In general, the administration of most vaccinations induces a durable antibody response (active immunity). In contrast, passive immunization occurs when preformed antibodies are given (eg, immune globulin from pooled serum), resulting in temporary protection which is a less durable response. The two variants of active immunization are live attenuated vaccines (which are believed to result in an immunologic response more like natural infection), and inactivated or killed vaccines.

The schedule of vaccinations varies based on the risk of the disease being prevented by vaccination, whether a vaccine has been given previously, the immune status of the patient (probability of responding to vaccine) and safety of the vaccine (live versus killed product, as well as implications for the fetus in pregnant women). Recommendations for healthy adults as well as special populations based on medical conditions are summarized in Table 30–7, which can be accessed online at www.cdc.gov/vaccines/schedules.

1. Healthy Adults

Vaccination recommendations are made by the Advisory Committee on Immunization Practices (ACIP) of the US Centers for Disease Control and Prevention (Table 30–7).

2. Pregnant Women

Given the uncertainty of risks to the fetus, vaccination during pregnancy is generally avoided with the following exceptions: tetanus (transfer of maternal antibodies across the placenta important to prevent neonatal tetanus), diphtheria, and influenza. Live vaccines are avoided during pregnancy.

Influenza can be a serious infection if acquired in pregnancy, and all pregnant women should be offered influenza (inactivated) vaccination. The live attenuated (intranasal) influenza vaccine is not recommended during pregnancy.

3. HIV-Infected Adults

HIV-infected patients have impaired cellular and B cell responses. Inactivated or killed vaccinations can generally be given without any consequence, but the recipient may not be able to mount an adequate antibody response. Live or attenuated vaccines are generally avoided with some exceptions (ie, in patients with CD4+ T lymphocytes greater than 200 cells/mcL). Guidelines for vaccinating HIV-infected patients have been issued jointly by the Centers for Disease Control and Prevention, the US National Institutes of Health, and the HIV Medical Association of the Infectious Diseases Society of America. Timing of vaccination is important to optimize response. If possible, vaccination should be given early in the course of HIV disease or following immune reconstitution.

4. Hematopoietic Cell Transplant Recipients

Hematopoietic cell transplant (HCT) recipients have varying rates of immune reconstitution following transplantation, depending on (1) the type of chemotherapy or radiotherapy used pretransplant (in autologous HCT), (2) the preparative regimen used for the transplant, (3) whether graft-versus-host disease is present, and (4) the type of immunosuppression used posttransplantation (in allogeneic HCT). Vaccines may not work immediately in the posttransplant period. B cells may take 3–12 months to return to normal posttransplant, and naïve T cells that can respond to new antigens only appear 6–12 months posttransplant. B cells of posttransplant patients treated with rituximab may take up to 6 months to fully recover after the last dose of the drug. Vaccines are therefore administered 6–12 months following transplantation with a minimum of 1 month between doses to maximize the probability of response.

5. Solid Organ Transplant Recipients

Solid organ transplant recipients demonstrate a broad spectrum of immunosuppression, depending on the reason for and type of organ transplantation and the nature of the immunosuppression (including T-cell-depleting agents

Table 30–7. Recommended adult immunization schedule—United States, 2016.

Recommended Adult Immunization Schedule—United States - 2016

Note: These recommendations must be read with the footnotes that follow containing number of doses, intervals between doses, and other important information.

Figure 1. Recommended immunization schedule for adults aged 19 years or older, by vaccine and age group[1]

VACCINE ▼ AGE GROUP ▶	19-21 years	22-26 years	27-49 years	50-59 years	60-64 years	≥ 65 years
Influenza[*,2]	1 dose annually					
Tetanus, diphtheria, pertussis (Td/Tdap)[*,3]	Substitute Tdap for Td once, then Td booster every 10 yrs					
Varicella[*,4]	2 doses					
Human papillomavirus (HPV) Female[*,5]	3 doses	3 doses				
Human papillomavirus (HPV) Male[*,5]	3 doses	3 doses				
Zoster[6]					1 dose	
Measles, mumps, rubella (MMR)[*,7]	1 or 2 doses depending on indication					
Pneumococcal 13-valent conjugate (PCV13)[*,8]	1 or 2 doses depending on indication				1 dose	
Pneumococcal 23-valent polysaccharide (PPSV23)[8]	1 or 2 doses depending on indication					1 dose
Hepatitis A[*,9]	2 or 3 doses depending on vaccine					
Hepatitis B[*,10]	3 doses					
Meningococcal 4-valent conjugate (MenACWY) or polysaccharide (MPSV4)[*,11]	1 or more doses depending on indication					
Meningococcal B (MenB)[11]	2 or 3 doses depending on vaccine					
Haemophilus influenzae type b (Hib)[*,12]	1 or 3 doses depending on indication					

*Covered by the Vaccine Injury Compensation Program

Recommended for all persons who meet the age requirement, lack documentation of vaccination, or lack evidence of past infection; zoster vaccine is recommended regardless of past episode of zoster

Recommended for persons with a risk factor (medical, occupational, lifestyle, or other indication)

No recommendation

Report all clinically significant postvaccination reactions to the Vaccine Adverse Event Reporting System (VAERS). Reporting forms and instructions on filing a VAERS report are available at www.vaers.hhs.gov or by telephone, 800-822-7967.

Information on how to file a Vaccine Injury Compensation Program claim is available at www.hrsa.gov/vaccinecompensation or by telephone, 800-338-2382. To file a claim for vaccine injury, contact the U.S. Court of Federal Claims, 717 Madison Place, N.W., Washington, D.C. 20005; telephone, 202-357-6400.

Additional information about the vaccines in this schedule, extent of available data, and contraindications for vaccination is also available at www.cdc.gov/vaccines or from the CDC-INFO Contact Center at 800-CDC-INFO (800-232-4636) in English and Spanish, 8:00 a.m. - 8:00 p.m. Eastern Time, Monday - Friday, excluding holidays.

Use of trade names and commercial sources is for identification only and does not imply endorsement by the U.S. Department of Health and Human Services.

The recommendations in this schedule were approved by the Centers for Disease Control and Prevention's (CDC) Advisory Committee on Immunization Practices (ACIP), the American Academy of Family Physicians (AAFP), the American College of Physicians (ACP), the American College of Obstetricians and Gynecologists (ACOG), and the American College of Nurse-Midwives (ACNM).

Figure 2. Vaccines that might be indicated for adults aged 19 years or older based on medical and other indications[1]

VACCINE ▼ / INDICATION ▶	Pregnancy	Immuno-compromising conditions (excluding HIV infection)[4,6,7,8,13]	HIV infection CD4+ count (cells/μL)[4,6,7,8,13] <200	HIV infection CD4+ count (cells/μL)[4,6,7,8,13] ≥200	Men who have sex with men (MSM)	Kidney failure, end-stage renal disease, on hemodialysis	Heart disease, chronic lung disease, chronic alcoholism	Asplenia and persistent complement component deficiencies[8,11,12]	Chronic liver disease	Diabetes	Healthcare personnel
Influenza[*,2]	1 dose annually										
Tetanus, diphtheria, pertussis (Td/Tdap)[*,3]	1 dose Tdap each pregnancy	Substitute Tdap for Td once, then Td booster every 10 yrs									
Varicella[*,4]		Contraindicated	Contraindicated	2 doses							
Human papillomavirus (HPV) Female[*,5]		3 doses through age 26 yrs	3 doses through age 26 yrs		3 doses through age 26 yrs						
Human papillomavirus (HPV) Male[*,5]		3 doses through age 26 yrs	3 doses through age 26 yrs		3 doses through age 21 yrs						
Zoster[6]		Contraindicated	Contraindicated		1 dose						
Measles, mumps, rubella (MMR)[*,7]		Contraindicated	Contraindicated		1 or 2 doses depending on indication						
Pneumococcal 13-valent conjugate (PCV13)[*,8]						1 dose					
Pneumococcal polysaccharide (PPSV23)[8]						1, 2, or 3 doses depending on indication					
Hepatitis A[*,9]					2 or 3 doses depending on vaccine						
Hepatitis B[*,10]					3 doses						
Meningococcal 4-valent conjugate (MenACWY) or polysaccharide (MPSV4)[*,11]						1 or more doses depending on indication					
Meningococcal B (MenB)[11]						2 or 3 doses depending on vaccine					
Haemophilus influenzae type b (Hib)[*,12]		3 doses post-HSCT recipients only				1 dose					

*Covered by the Vaccine Injury Compensation Program

Legend:
- Recommended for all persons who meet the age requirement, lack documentation of vaccination, or lack evidence of past infection; zoster vaccine is recommended regardless of past episode of zoster
- Recommended for persons with a risk factor (medical, occupational, lifestyle, or other indication)
- No recommendation
- Contraindicated

U.S. Department of Health and Human Services
Centers for Disease Control and Prevention

These schedules indicate the recommended age groups and medical indications for which administration of currently licensed vaccines is commonly recommended for adults aged ≥19 years, as of February 2016. For all vaccines being recommended on the Adult Immunization Schedule: a vaccine series does not need to be restarted, regardless of the time that has elapsed between doses. Licensed combination vaccines may be used whenever any components of the combination are indicated and when the vaccine's other components are not contraindicated. For detailed recommendations on all vaccines, including those used primarily for travelers or that are issued during the year, consult the manufacturers' package inserts and the complete statements from the Advisory Committee on Immunization Practices (www.cdc.gov/vaccines/hcp/acip-recs/index.html). Use of trade names and commercial sources is for identification only and does not imply endorsement by the U.S. Department of Health and Human Services.

(continued)

Table 30–7. Recommended adult immunization schedule—United States, 2016. (continued)

Footnotes

Recommended Immunization Schedule for Adults Aged 19 Years or Older: United States, 2015

1. Additional information

- Additional guidance for the use of the vaccines described in this supplement is available at www.cdc.gov/vaccines/hcp/acip-recs/index.html.
- Information on vaccination recommendations when vaccination status is unknown and other general immunization information can be found in the General Recommendations on Immunization at www.cdc.gov/mmwr/preview/mmwrhtml/rr6002a1.htm.
- Information on travel vaccine requirements and recommendations (e.g., for hepatitis A and B, meningococcal, and other vaccines) is available at wwwnc.cdc.gov/travel/destinations/list.
- Additional information and resources regarding vaccination of pregnant women can be found at www.cdc.gov/vaccines/adults/rec-vac/pregnant.html.

2. Influenza vaccination

- Annual vaccination against influenza is recommended for all persons aged ≥6 months. A list of currently available influenza vaccines can be found at http://www.cdc.gov/flu/protect/vaccine/vaccines.htm.
- Persons aged ≥6 months, including pregnant women, can receive the inactivated influenza vaccine (IIV). An age-appropriate IIV formulation should be used.
- Intradermal IIV is an option for persons aged 18 through 64 years.
- High-dose IIV is an option for persons aged ≥65 years.
- Live attenuated influenza vaccine (LAIV [FluMist]) is an option for healthy, non-pregnant persons aged 2 through 49 years.
- Recombinant influenza vaccine (RIV [Flublok]) is approved for persons aged ≥18 years.
- RIV, which does not contain any egg protein, may be administered to persons aged ≥18 years with egg allergy of any severity; IIV may be used with additional safety measures for persons with hives-only allergy to eggs.
- Health care personnel who care for severely immunocompromised persons who require care in a protected environment should receive IIV or RIV; health care personnel who receive LAIV should avoid providing care for severely immunosuppressed persons for 7 days after vaccination.

3. Tetanus, diphtheria, and acellular pertussis (Td/Tdap) vaccination

- Administer 1 dose of Tdap vaccine to pregnant women during each pregnancy (preferably during 27–36 weeks' gestation) regardless of interval since prior Td or Tdap vaccination.
- Persons aged ≥11 years who have not received Tdap vaccine or for whom vaccine status is unknown should receive a dose of Tdap followed by tetanus and diphtheria toxoids (Td) booster doses every 10 years thereafter. Tdap can be administered regardless of interval since the most recent tetanus or diphtheria-toxoid-containing vaccine.
- Adults with an unknown or incomplete history of completing a 3-dose primary vaccination series with Td-containing vaccines should begin or complete a primary vaccination series including a Tdap dose.
- For unvaccinated adults, administer the first 2 doses at least 4 weeks apart and the third dose 6–12 months after the second.
- For incompletely vaccinated (i.e., less than 3 doses) adults, administer remaining doses.
- Refer to the ACIP statement for recommendations for administering Td/Tdap as prophylaxis in wound management (see footnote 1).

4. Varicella vaccination

- All adults without evidence of immunity to varicella (as defined below) should receive 2 doses of single-antigen varicella vaccine or a second dose if they have received only 1 dose.
- Vaccination should be emphasized for those who have close contact with persons at high risk for severe disease (e.g., health care personnel and family contacts of persons with immunocompromising conditions) or are at high risk for exposure or transmission (e.g., teachers; child care employees; residents and staff members of institutional settings, including correctional institutions; college students; military personnel; adolescents and adults living in households with children; nonpregnant women of childbearing age; and international travelers).
- Pregnant women should be assessed for evidence of varicella immunity. Women who do not have evidence of immunity should receive the first dose of varicella vaccine upon completion or termination of pregnancy and before discharge from the health care facility. The second dose should be administered 4–8 weeks after the first dose.
- Evidence of immunity to varicella in adults includes any of the following:
  — documentation of 2 doses of varicella vaccine at least 4 weeks apart;
  — U.S.-born before 1980, except health care personnel and pregnant women;
  — history of varicella based on diagnosis or verification of varicella disease by a health care provider;
  — history of herpes zoster based on diagnosis or verification of herpes zoster disease by a health care provider; or
  — laboratory evidence of immunity or laboratory confirmation of disease.

5. Human papillomavirus (HPV) vaccination

- Three HPV vaccines are licensed for use in females (bivalent HPV vaccine [2vHPV], quadrivalent HPV vaccine [4vHPV], and 9-valent HPV vaccine [9vHPV]) and two HPV vaccines are licensed for use in males (4vHPV and 9vHPV).
- For females, 2vHPV, 4vHPV, or 9vHPV is recommended in a 3-dose series for routine vaccination at age 11 or 12 years and for those aged 13 through 26 years, if not previously vaccinated.

- For males, 4vHPV or 9vHPV is recommended in a 3-dose series for routine vaccination at age 11 or 12 years and for those aged 13 through 21 years, if not previously vaccinated. Males aged 22 through 26 years may be vaccinated.
- HPV vaccination is recommended for men who have sex with men through age 26 years who did not get any or all doses when they were younger.
- Vaccination is recommended for immunocompromised persons (including those with HIV infection) through age 26 years who did not get any or all doses when they were younger.
- A complete HPV vaccination series consists of 3 doses. The second dose should be administered 4–8 weeks (minimum interval of 4 weeks) after the first dose; the third dose should be administered 24 weeks after the first dose and 16 weeks after the second dose (minimum interval of 12 weeks).
- HPV vaccines are not recommended for use in pregnant women. However, pregnancy testing is not needed before vaccination. If a woman is found to be pregnant after initiating the vaccination series, no intervention is needed; the remainder of the 3-dose series should be delayed until completion or termination of pregnancy.

6. Zoster vaccination
- A single dose of zoster vaccine is recommended for adults aged ≥60 years regardless of whether they report a prior episode of herpes zoster. Although the vaccine is licensed by the U.S. Food and Drug Administration for use among and can be administered to persons aged ≥50 years, ACIP recommends that vaccination begin at age 60 years.
- Persons aged ≥60 years with chronic medical conditions may be vaccinated unless their condition constitutes a contraindication, such as pregnancy or severe immunodeficiency.

7. Measles, mumps, rubella (MMR) vaccination
- Adults born before 1957 are generally considered immune to measles and mumps. All adults born in 1957 or later should have documentation of 1 or more doses of MMR vaccine unless they have a medical contraindication to the vaccine or laboratory evidence of immunity to each of the three diseases. Documentation of provider-diagnosed disease is not considered acceptable evidence of immunity for measles, mumps, or rubella.

Measles component:
- A routine second dose of MMR vaccine, administered a minimum of 28 days after the first dose, is recommended for adults who:
  — are students in postsecondary educational institutions,
  — work in a health care facility, or
  — plan to travel internationally.
- Persons who received inactivated (killed) measles vaccine or measles vaccine of unknown type during 1963–1967 should be revaccinated with 2 doses of MMR vaccine.

Mumps component:
- A routine second dose of MMR vaccine, administered a minimum of 28 days after the first dose, is recommended for adults who:
  — are students in a postsecondary educational institution,
  — work in a health care facility, or
  — plan to travel internationally.
- Persons vaccinated before 1979 with either killed mumps vaccine or mumps vaccine of unknown type who are at high risk for mumps infection (e.g., persons who are working in a health care facility) should be considered for revaccination with 2 doses of MMR vaccine.

Rubella component:
- For women of childbearing age, regardless of birth year, rubella immunity should be determined. If there is no evidence of immunity, women who are not pregnant should be vaccinated. Pregnant women who do not have evidence of immunity should receive MMR vaccine upon completion or termination of pregnancy and before discharge from the health care facility.

Health care personnel born before 1957:
- For unvaccinated health care personnel born before 1957 who lack laboratory evidence of measles, mumps, and/or rubella immunity or laboratory confirmation of disease, health care facilities should consider vaccinating personnel with 2 doses of MMR vaccine at the appropriate interval for measles and mumps or 1 dose of MMR vaccine for rubella.

8. Pneumococcal vaccination
- General information
  — Adults are recommended to receive 1 dose of 13-valent pneumococcal conjugate vaccine (PCV13) and 1, 2, or 3 doses (depending on indication) of 23-valent pneumococcal polysaccharide vaccine (PPSV23).
  — PCV13 should be administered at least 1 year after PPSV23.
  — PPSV23 should be administered at least 1 year after PCV13, except among adults with immunocompromising conditions, anatomical or functional asplenia, cerebrospinal fluid leak, or cochlear implant, for whom the interval should be at least 8 weeks; the interval between PPSV23 doses should be at least 5 years.
  — No additional dose of PPSV23 is indicated for adults vaccinated with PPSV23 at age ≥65 years.
  — When both PCV13 and PPSV23 are indicated, PCV13 should be administered first; PCV13 and PPSV23 should not be administered during the same visit.
  — When indicated, PCV13 and PPSV23 should be administered to adults whose pneumococcal vaccination history is incomplete or unknown.
- Adults aged ≥65 years (immunocompetent) who:
  — have not received PCV13 or PPSV23: administer PCV13 followed by PPSV23 at least 1 year after PCV13.
  — have not received PCV13 but have received a dose of PPSV23 at age ≥65 years: administer PCV13 at least 1 year after PPSV23.

(continued)

Table 30–7. Recommended adult immunization schedule—United States, 2016. (continued)

- —have not received PCV13 but have received 1 or more doses of PPSV23 at age <65 years: administer PCV13 at least 1 year after the most recent dose of PPSV23. Administer a dose of PPSV23 at least 1 year after PCV13 and at least 5 years after the most recent dose of PPSV23.
  - —have received PCV13 but not PPSV23 at age <65 years: administer PPSV23 at least 1 year after PCV13.
  - —have received PCV13 and 1 or more doses of PPSV23 at age <65 years: administer PPSV23 at least 1 year after PCV13 and at least 5 years after the most recent dose of PPSV23.

- Adults aged ≥19 years with immunocompromising conditions or anatomical or functional asplenia (defined below) who:
  - —have not received PCV13 or PPSV23: administer PCV13 followed by PPSV23 at least 8 weeks after PCV13. Administer a second dose of PPSV23 at least 5 years after the first dose of PPSV23.
  - —have not received PCV13 but have received 1 dose of PPSV23: administer PCV13 at least 1 year after the PPSV23. Administer a second dose of PPSV23 at least 8 weeks after PCV13 and at least 5 years after the first dose of PPSV23.
  - —have not received PCV13 but have received 2 doses of PPSV23: administer PCV13 at least 1 year after the most recent dose of PPSV23.
  - —have received PCV13 but not PPSV23: administer PPSV23 at least 8 weeks after PCV13. Administer a second dose of PPSV23 at least 5 years after the first dose of PPSV23.
  - —have received PCV13 and 1 dose of PPSV23: administer a second dose of PPSV23 at least 8 weeks after PCV13 and at least 5 years after the first dose of PPSV23.
  - —If the most recent dose of PPSV23 was administered at age <65 years, at age ≥65 years, administer a dose of PPSV23 at least 8 weeks after PCV13 and at least 5 years after the last dose of PPSV23.

  Immunocompromising conditions that are indications for pneumococcal vaccination are: congenital or acquired immunodeficiency (including B- or T-lymphocyte deficiency, complement deficiencies, and phagocytic disorders excluding chronic granulomatous disease), HIV infection, chronic renal failure, nephrotic syndrome, leukemia, lymphoma, Hodgkin disease, generalized malignancy, multiple myeloma, solid organ transplant, and iatrogenic immunosuppression (including long-term systemic corticosteroids and radiation therapy).

  Anatomical or functional asplenia that are indications for pneumococcal vaccination are: sickle cell disease and other hemoglobinopathies, congenital or acquired asplenia, splenic dysfunction, and splenectomy. Administer pneumococcal vaccines at least 2 weeks before immunosuppressive therapy or an elective splenectomy, and as soon as possible to adults who are newly diagnosed with asymptomatic or symptomatic HIV infection.

- Adults aged ≥19 years with cerebrospinal fluid leaks or cochlear implants: administer PCV13 followed by PPSV23 at least 8 weeks after PCV13; no additional dose of PPSV23 is indicated if aged <65 years. If PPSV23 was administered at age <65 years, at age ≥65 years, administer another dose of PPSV23 at least 5 years after the last dose of PPSV23.

- Adults aged 19 through 64 years with chronic heart disease (including congestive heart failure and cardiomyopathies, excluding hypertension), chronic lung disease (including chronic obstructive lung disease, emphysema, and asthma), chronic liver disease (including cirrhosis), alcoholism, or diabetes mellitus, or who smoke cigarettes: administer PPSV23. At age ≥65 years, administer PCV13 at least 1 year after PPSV23, followed by another dose of PPSV23 at least 1 year after PCV13 and at least 5 years after the last dose of PPSV23.

- Routine pneumococcal vaccination is not recommended for American Indian/Alaska Native or other adults unless they have an indication as above; however, public health authorities may consider recommending the use of pneumococcal vaccines for American Indians/Alaska Natives or other adults who live in areas with increased risk for invasive pneumococcal disease.

9. Hepatitis A vaccination

- Vaccinate any person seeking protection from hepatitis A virus (HAV) infection and persons with any of the following indications:
  - —men who have sex with men;
  - —persons who use injection or noninjection illicit drugs;
  - —persons working with HAV-infected primates or with HAV in a research laboratory setting;
  - —persons with chronic liver disease and persons who receive clotting factor concentrates;
  - —persons traveling to or working in countries that have high or intermediate endemicity of hepatitis A (see footnote 1); and
  - —unvaccinated persons who anticipate close personal contact (e.g., household or regular babysitting) with an international adoptee during the first 60 days after arrival in the United States from a country with high or intermediate endemicity of hepatitis A (see footnote 1). The first dose of the 2-dose hepatitis A vaccine series should be administered as soon as adoption is planned, ideally 2 or more weeks before the arrival of the adoptee.

- Single-antigen vaccine formulations should be administered in a 2-dose schedule at either 0 and 6–12 months (Havrix), or 0 and 6–18 months (Vaqta). If the combined hepatitis A and hepatitis B vaccine (Twinrix) is used, administer 3 doses at 0, 1, and 6 months; alternatively, a 4-dose schedule may be used, administered on days 0, 7, and 21–30 followed by a booster dose at 12 months.

10. Hepatitis B vaccination

- Vaccinate any person seeking protection from hepatitis B virus (HBV) infection and persons with any of the following indications:
  - —sexually active persons who are not in a long-term, mutually monogamous relationship (e.g., persons with more than 1 sex partner during the previous 6 months); persons seeking evaluation or treatment for a sexually transmitted disease (STD); current or recent injection drug users; and men who have sex with men;
  - —health care personnel and public safety workers who are potentially exposed to blood or other infectious body fluids;
  - —persons who are aged <60 years with diabetes as soon as feasible after diagnosis; persons with diabetes who are aged ≥60 years at the discretion of the treating clinician based on the likelihood of acquiring HBV infection, including the risk posed by an increased need for assisted blood glucose monitoring in long-term care facilities, the likelihood of experiencing chronic sequelae if infected with HBV, and the likelihood of immune response to vaccination;
  - —persons with end-stage renal disease (including patients receiving hemodialysis), persons with HIV infection, and persons with chronic liver disease;

— household contacts and sex partners of hepatitis B surface antigen–positive persons, clients and staff members of institutions for persons with developmental disabilities, and international travelers to regions with high or intermediate levels of endemic HBV infection (see footnote 1); and

— all adults in the following settings: STD treatment facilities, HIV testing and treatment facilities, facilities providing drug abuse treatment and prevention services, health care settings targeting services to injection drug users or men who have sex with men, correctional facilities, end-stage renal disease programs and facilities for chronic hemodialysis patients, and institutions and nonresidential day care facilities for persons with developmental disabilities.

- Administer missing doses to complete a 3-dose series of hepatitis B vaccine to those persons not vaccinated or not completely vaccinated. The second dose should be administered at least 1 month after the first dose; the third dose should be administered at least 2 months after the second dose (and at least 4 months after the first dose). If the combined hepatitis A and hepatitis B vaccine (Twinrix) is used, give 3 doses at 0, 1, and 6 months; alternatively, a 4-dose Twinrix schedule may be used, administered on days 0, 7, and 21–30, followed by a booster dose at 12 months.

- Adult patients receiving hemodialysis or with other immunocompromising conditions should receive 1 dose of 40 mcg/mL (Recombivax HB) administered on a 3-dose schedule at 0, 1, and 6 months or 2 doses of 20 mcg/mL (Engerix-B) administered simultaneously on a 4-dose schedule at 0, 1, 2, and 6 months.

11. Meningococcal vaccination

- General information

— Serogroup A, C, W, and Y meningococcal vaccine is available as a conjugate (MenACWY [Menactra, Menveo]) or a polysaccharide (MPSV4 [Menomune]) vaccine.

— Serogroup B meningococcal (MenB) vaccine is available as a 2-dose series of MenB-4C vaccine (Bexsero) administered at least 1 month apart or a 3-dose series of MenB-FHbp (Trumenba) vaccine administered at 0, 2, and 6 months; the two MenB vaccines are not interchangeable, i.e., the same MenB vaccine product must be used for all doses.

— MenACWY vaccine is preferred for adults with serogroup A, C, W, and Y meningococcal vaccine indications who are aged ≤55 years, and for adults aged ≥56 years: 1) who were vaccinated previously with MenACWY vaccine and are recommended for revaccination or 2) for whom multiple doses of vaccine are anticipated; MPSV4 vaccine is preferred for adults aged ≥56 years who have not received MenACWY vaccine previously and who require a single dose only (e.g., persons at risk because of an outbreak).

— Revaccination with MenACWY vaccine every 5 years is recommended for adults previously vaccinated with MenACWY or MPSV4 vaccine who remain at increased risk for infection (e.g., adults with anatomical or functional asplenia or persistent complement component deficiencies, or microbiologists who are routinely exposed to isolates of *Neisseria meningitidis*).

— MenB vaccine is approved for use in persons aged 10 through 25 years; however, because there is no theoretical difference in safety for persons aged >25 years compared to those aged 10 through 25 years, MenB vaccine is recommended for routine use in persons aged >10 years who are at increased risk for serogroup B meningococcal disease.

— There is no recommendation for MenB revaccination at this time.

— MenB vaccine may be administered concomitantly with MenACWY vaccine but at a different anatomic site, if feasible.

— HIV infection is not an indication for routine vaccination with MenACWY or MenB vaccine; if an HIV-infected person of any age is to be vaccinated, administer 2 doses of MenACWY vaccine at least 2 months apart.

- Adults with anatomical or functional asplenia or persistent complement component deficiencies: administer 2 doses of MenACWY vaccine at least 2 months apart and revaccinate every 5 years. Also administer a series of MenB vaccine.

- Microbiologists who are routinely exposed to isolates of *Neisseria meningitidis*: administer a single dose of MenACWY vaccine; revaccinate with MenACWY vaccine every 5 years if remain at increased risk for infection. Also administer a series of MenB vaccine.

- Persons at risk because of a meningococcal disease outbreak: if the outbreak is attributable to serogroup A, C, W, or Y, administer a single dose of MenACWY vaccine; if the outbreak is attributable to serogroup B, administer a series of MenB vaccine.

- Persons who travel to or live in countries in which meningococcal disease is hyperendemic or epidemic: administer a single dose of MenACWY vaccine and revaccinate with MenACWY vaccine every 5 years if the increased risk for infection remains (see footnote 1); MenB vaccine is not recommended because meningococcal disease in these countries is generally not caused by serogroup B.

- Military recruits: administer a single dose of MenACWY vaccine.

- First-year college students aged ≤21 years who live in residence halls: administer a single dose of MenACWY vaccine if they have not received a dose on or after their 16th birthday.

- Young adults aged 16 through 23 years (preferred age range is 16 through 18 years): may be vaccinated with a series of MenB vaccine to provide short-term protection against most strains of serogroup B meningococcal disease.

12. *Haemophilus influenzae* type b (Hib) vaccination

- One dose of Hib vaccine should be administered to persons who have anatomical or functional asplenia or sickle cell disease or are undergoing elective splenectomy if they have not previously received Hib vaccine. Hib vaccination 14 or more days before splenectomy is suggested.

- Recipients of a hematopoietic stem cell transplant (HSCT) should be vaccinated with a 3-dose regimen 6–12 months after a successful transplant, regardless of vaccination history; at least 4 weeks should separate doses.

- Hib vaccine is not recommended for adults with HIV infection since their risk for Hib infection is low.

13. Immunocompromising conditions

- Inactivated vaccines (e.g., pneumococcal, meningococcal, and inactivated influenza vaccines) generally are acceptable and live vaccines generally should be avoided in persons with immune deficiencies or immunocompromising conditions. Information on specific conditions is available at www.cdc.gov/vaccines/hcp/acip-recs/index.html.

during treatment of organ rejection). These factors affect the propensity for infection posttransplantation and the ability to develop antibody responses to vaccination. In many cases, the time between placing a patient on a transplant list and undergoing the transplantation takes months or years. Providers should take this opportunity to ensure that indicated vaccines are given during this pretransplant period to optimize antibody responses. If this is not possible, most experts give vaccines 3–6 months following transplantation. Live vaccines are contraindicated in the posttransplant period.

RECOMMENDED IMMUNIZATIONS FOR TRAVELERS

Individuals traveling to other countries frequently require immunizations in addition to those routinely recommended and may benefit from chemoprophylaxis against various diseases. Vaccinations against yellow fever and meningococcus are the only ones required by certain countries. These and other travel-specific vaccines are listed at http://wwwnc.cdc.gov/travel/destinations/list.

Various vaccines can be given simultaneously at different sites. Some, such as cholera, plague, and typhoid vaccine, cause significant discomfort and are best given at different times. In general, live attenuated vaccines (measles, mumps, rubella, yellow fever, and oral typhoid vaccine) should not be given to immunosuppressed individuals or household members of immunosuppressed people or to pregnant women. Immunoglobulin should not be given for 3 months before or at least 2 weeks after live virus vaccines, because it may attenuate the antibody response.

Chemoprophylaxis of malaria is discussed in Chapter 35.

Cholera

Because cholera among travelers is rare and the vaccine marginally effective, the World Health Organization (WHO) does not require immunization for persons traveling to endemic areas or to areas with recent outbreaks (eg, Haiti). No country requires vaccination for entry, but some local authorities may require documentation for entry. In such cases, a medical waiver will suffice or a single dose of the oral vaccine is usually sufficient.

Hepatitis B

The risk of hepatitis B infection for most international travelers is low. Hepatitis B vaccination should be considered for those traveling to areas with high (8% or higher) or intermediate (2–7%) rates of endemic hepatitis B infection if the individual will have contact with blood or secretions, will have unprotected sex, or will be using illicit drugs. Examples of high and intermediate risk areas include all of Africa and most of South Asia and the Middle East. Vaccination should begin at least 6 months before travel to allow for completion of the series.

Hepatitis A

Protection is recommended for susceptible persons traveling to areas where sanitation is poor and the risk of exposure to hepatitis A high because of contaminated food and water supplies and contact with infected persons (eg, anywhere except Canada, western Europe, Japan, Australia, and New Zealand). Either hepatitis A vaccine or immunoglobulin can be used, although vaccination is preferred. The first dose of vaccine should be given as soon as travel is considered. In healthy individuals, a single dose of vaccine administered any time prior to travel will provide adequate protection. In older patients, those who are immunocompromised, and those with chronic liver disease or other chronic medical problems who are planning to travel in 2 weeks or less should receive hepatitis A vaccine and immunoglobulin 0.02 mL/kg simultaneously at different anatomic sites. Those who choose not to receive vaccine should receive immunoglobulin.

Meningococcal Meningitis

If travel is contemplated to an area where meningococcal meningitis is epidemic (Nepal, sub-Saharan Africa, the "meningitis belt" from Senegal in the west to Ethiopia in the east, northern India) or highly endemic, vaccination with MCV4 is indicated for those 2–55 years of age, otherwise MPSV should be used. (Saudi Arabia requires immunization for pilgrims to Mecca.)

Plague

The risk of plague is so small to travelers that vaccine is no longer commercially available and vaccination is not required for entry into any country. Travelers at unavoidable high risk of exposure to rodents should consider chemoprophylaxis with doxycycline or TMP-SMZ.

Poliomyelitis

Polio remains endemic in three countries (Afghanistan, Pakistan, and Nigeria), and sporadic outbreaks or environmental evidence of infection continues to occur in Cameroon, Ethiopia, Equatorial Guinea, Iraq, Israel, Somalia, and Syria. Adults traveling to endemic or epidemic areas (now termed "polio infected" countries) who have not previously been immunized against poliomyelitis should receive a primary series of three doses of inactivated enhanced-potency poliovaccine (IPV). Travelers who have previously been fully immunized with oral polio vaccine (OPV) or inactivated polio vaccine (IPV) should receive a one-time booster dose with IPV. Travelers departing polio infected countries must now provide evidence of vaccination or booster within the past 1 year. Live attenuated poliovaccine is no longer recommended because of the risk of vaccine-associated disease and is no longer available in the United States, although it continues to be used in many other countries.

Rabies

For travelers to areas where rabies is common in domestic animals (eg, India, Asia, Mexico, Africa, areas of Central and South America), with extensive outdoor activities or certain professional activities (veterinarians, animal handlers, field biologists), preexposure prophylaxis with human diploid cell vaccine (HDCV), rabies vaccine adsorbed (RVA), or purified chick embryo cell culture (PCEC) vaccine should be considered. Chloroquine can blunt the immunologic response to rabies vaccine. If malaria prophylaxis with chloroquine (or mefloquine) is required, vaccination should be given intramuscularly (*not* intradermally) to ensure adequate antibody response.

Typhoid

Typhoid vaccination is recommended for travelers to developing countries (especially the Indian subcontinent, Asia, Africa, Central and South America, and the Caribbean) who will have prolonged exposure to contaminated food and water. Two preparations of approximately equal efficacy (50–75% effective) are available in the United States: (1) an oral live attenuated Ty21a vaccine supplied as enteric-coated capsules, and (2) a Vi capsular polysaccharide (Vi CPS) vaccine for parenteral use. The Ty21a vaccine is given as one capsule every other day for four doses. The capsules must be refrigerated and taken with cool liquids (37°C or less) at least 1 hour before meals. All four doses must be taken for maximum protection and should be completed 1 week before travel. It is not recommended for infants or children younger than 6 years. The Vi CPS vaccine is given as a single intramuscular injection at least 2 weeks prior to travel. It is not recommended for infants younger than 2 years. If continued or repeated exposures are anticipated, boosters are recommended every 2 years for the Vi CPS and every 5 years for the Ty21a. The live attenuated vaccine should not be used in immunosuppressed patients, including those with HIV infection.

Yellow Fever

The live attenuated yellow fever virus vaccine is administered once subcutaneously. Although the risk of yellow fever is low for most travelers, a number of countries require vaccination for all visitors and others require it for travelers to or from endemic areas (mainly equatorial Africa and parts of South and Central America). The WHO certificate requires registration of the manufacturer and the batch number of the vaccine. Vaccination is available in the United States only at approved centers; the local health department should be contacted for available resources. Reimmunization is no longer recommended for most travelers.

Because it is a live attenuated vaccine prepared in embryonated eggs, the yellow fever vaccine should not be given to immunosuppressed individuals or those with a history of anaphylaxis to eggs. Pregnancy is a relative contraindication to vaccination.

Two very severe adverse reactions have been associated with yellow fever vaccination. Viscerotropic disease presents with fever, jaundice, and multiple organ system failure within 30 days of yellow fever vaccination. Clinically and histopathologically, the illness is identical to yellow fever and is associated with a high mortality rate. The other adverse reaction is neurotropic disease and presents as encephalitis, encephalomyelitis, or Guillain-Barré syndrome.

Japanese B Encephalitis

Japanese B encephalitis is a mosquito-borne viral encephalitis that affects primarily children and older adults (65 years and older) and usually occurs from May to September. It is the leading cause of encephalitis in Asia. Because the risk of infection is low and because adverse effects of the vaccine can be serious, not all travelers to Asia should be vaccinated. Vaccine should be given to travelers to endemic areas who will be staying at least 30 days and who are traveling during the transmission season, particularly if they are visiting rural areas. Travelers who spend less than 30 days in the region should be considered for vaccination if they intend to visit areas of epidemic transmission or if extensive outdoor activities are planned in rural rice-growing areas. Of the two vaccines currently available in the United States, only one (inactivated Vero cell derived vaccine, IXIARO) is for adults aged 17 and older. The schedule is 0.5 mL intramuscularly at 0 and 28 days. Only children are eligible to receive the other vaccine (inactivated mouse brain derived vaccine, JE-VAX) given its limited supply in the United States.

VACCINE SAFETY

Most vaccines are safe to administer. In general, it is recommended that the use of live vaccines be avoided in immunocompromised patients, including pregnant women. Vaccines are generally not contraindicated in the following situations: mild, acute illness with low-grade fevers (less than 40.5°C); concurrent antibiotic therapy; soreness or redness at the site; family history of adverse reactions to vaccinations. Absolute contraindications to vaccines are rare (Table 30–8).

Bridges CB et al; Immunization Services Division, National Center for Immunization and Respiratory Diseases, CDC. Advisory Committee on Immunization Practices recommended immunization schedule for adults aged 19 years or older—United States, 2014. MMWR Morb Mortal Wkly Rep. 2014 Feb 7;63(5):110–2. [PMID: 24500291]

Centers for Disease Control and Prevention (CDC). Adult immunization schedules—United States, 2016. http://www.cdc.gov/vaccines/schedules/hcp/adult.html

Centers for Disease Control and Prevention (CDC). Health Information for International Travel 2014. http://wwwnc.cdc.gov/travel/page/yellowbook-home

Centers for Disease Control and Prevention (CDC). Vaccine safety. http://www.cdc.gov/vaccinesafety/index.html

Danziger-Isakov L et al; AST Infectious Diseases Community of Practice. Vaccination in solid organ transplantation. Am J Transplant. 2013 Mar;13 (Suppl 4):311–7. [PMID: 23465023]

Ferreira I et al. Vaccines and biologics. Ann Rheum Dis. 2014 Aug;73(8):1446–54. [PMID: 24845388]

Grijalva CG et al. Association between hospitalization with community-acquired laboratory-confirmed influenza pneumonia and prior receipt of influenza vaccination. JAMA. 2015 Oct 13;314(14):1488–97. [PMID: 26436611]

LaRocque RC et al; Global TravEpiNet Consortium. Pre-travel health care of immigrants returning home to visit friends and relatives. Am J Trop Med Hyg. 2013 Feb;88(2):376–80. Erratum in: Am J Trop Med Hyg. 2013 Mar;88(3):606. [PMID: 23149585]

Rubin LG et al. 2013 IDSA clinical practice guideline for vaccination of the immunocompromised host. Clin Infect Dis. 2014 Feb;58(3):309–18. [PMID: 24421306]

Shefer A et al. Updated recommendations of the Advisory Committee on Immunization Practices for healthcare personnel vaccination: a necessary foundation for the essential work that remains to build successful programs. Infect Control Hosp Epidemiol. 2012 Jan;33(1):71–4. [PMID: 22173525]

Table 30–8. Adverse effects and contraindications to commonly used vaccines in adults.

Vaccine	Adverse Effects	Contraindications[1]
Haemophilus influenzae Type b (Hib)	Minimal Consist mainly of pain at the injection site	Any severe allergic reaction (eg, anaphylaxis) after a previous dose or to a vaccine component.
Hepatitis A	Minimal Consist mainly of pain at the injection site	Any severe allergic reaction (eg, anaphylaxis) after a previous dose or to a vaccine component.
Hepatitis B	Minimal Consist mainly of pain at the injection site	Any severe allergic reaction (eg, anaphylaxis) after a previous dose or to a vaccine component.
Human papillomavirus	Minimal Consists mainly of mild to moderate localized pain, erythema, swelling Systemic reactions, mainly fever, seen in 4% of recipients	Any severe allergic reaction (eg, anaphylaxis) after a previous dose or to a vaccine component.

Influenza (intramuscular inactivated and intra-nasal live attenuated vaccines)	**Intramuscular, inactivated vaccine:** Local reactions (erythema and tenderness) at the site of injection are common, but fevers, chills, and malaise (which last in any case only 2–3 days) are rare.
	Either inactivated or live attenuated vaccine: A potential association between Guillain-Barré syndrome (3000–6000 cases per year in the United States, usually following respiratory infections) and vaccination with intramuscular, inactivated influenza vaccine has been reported (possibly, 1–2 persons per million persons vaccinated), but this rate is lower than the risk of the syndrome developing after influenza itself (given that approximately 750 persons per million adults are hospitalized annually with influenza, and many more cases remain as outpatients). Influenza vaccination may be associated with multiple false-positive serologic tests to HIV, HTLV-1, and hepatitis C, but it is self-limited, lasting 2–5 months.
		Contraindication to both inactivated and live attenuated vaccine:
		  History of Guillain-Barré syndrome, especially within 6 weeks of receiving a previous influenza vaccine.
		  Any severe allergic reaction (eg, anaphylaxis) after a previous dose or to a vaccine component, including egg protein.[2]
		Intranasal, live attenuated vaccine [FluMist] should not be used in:
		People 50 years of age and over
		Immunosuppressed individuals and those on immunosuppressive therapy
		Household members of immunosuppressed individuals
		Health care workers, or others with close contact with immunosuppressed persons
		Presence of reactive airway disease (eg, asthma) or chronic underlying metabolic (eg, kidney), pulmonary, or heart diseases (use intramuscular inactivated vaccine)
		Pregnancy[3]
		It is recommended that salicylates should be avoided for 6 weeks following vaccination (to prevent Reye syndrome).

Measles, mumps, and rubella (MMR)[4]	Fever will develop in about 5–15% of unimmunized individuals, and a mild rash will develop in about 5% 5–12 days after vaccination. Fever and rash are self-limited, lasting only 2–3 days. Local swelling and induration are particularly common in individuals previously vaccinated with inactivated vaccine.	Pregnancy[5] Known severe immunodeficiency (eg, from hematologic and solid cancers, receipt of chemotherapy, congenital immunodeficiency, long-term immunosuppressive therapy (eg, > 2 weeks of prednisone 20 mg daily or higher), other disease- or therapy-related immune suppression, or patients with HIV infection who are severely immunocompromised. May be used in asymptomatic HIV-infected individuals whose CD4 count is > 200/mcL. Severe allergic reaction (eg, anaphylaxis) to a previous dose or to a vaccine component, (eg, neomycin or to related agents such as streptomycin).
Meningococcal, oligosaccharide conjugate; (MCV4 or MenACWY [Menactra, Menveo]; meningococcal polysaccharide conjugate MPSV4 [Menomune]); meningococcal group B, recombinant (MenB [Bexsero, Trumenba])	Minor reactions (fever, redness, swelling, erythema, pain) occur slightly more commonly with MCV4. Major reactions are rare. A potential association between Guillain-Barré syndrome (3000–6000 cases per year in the United States, usually following respiratory infections) and vaccination with MCV4 has been reported, but current recommendations favor continued use of MCV4, since the benefits of preventing the serious consequences of meningococcal infection outweigh the theoretical risk of Guillain-Barré syndrome.	Any severe allergic reaction (eg, anaphylaxis) to a previous dose or to a vaccine component, (eg, persons with history of adverse reaction to diphtheria toxoid should not receive meningococcal oligosaccharide conjugate and polysaccharide conjugate vaccines since the protein conjugate used in them is diphtheria toxoid).

(continued)

Table 30–8. Adverse effects and contraindications to commonly used vaccines in adults. (continued)

Vaccine	Adverse Effects	Contraindications[1]
Pneumococcal conjugate (PCV13 [Prevnar]); Pneumococcal polysaccharide (PPSV23) [Pneumovax])	Mild local reactions (erythema and tenderness) occur in up to 50% of recipients, but systemic reactions are uncommon. Similarly, revaccination at least 5 years after initial vaccination is associated with mild self-limited local but not systemic reactions.	Any severe allergic reaction (eg, anaphylaxis) after a previous dose or to a vaccine component (eg, for PCV13 to any vaccine containing diphtheria toxoid).
Tetanus, diphtheria, and pertussis (DTP, Tdap); tetanus, diphtheria (Td)	Minimal Consist mainly of pain at the injection site	Any severe allergic reaction (eg, anaphylaxis) after a previous dose or to a vaccine component. For pertussis-containing vaccines: any history of unexplained encephalopathy (eg, coma, decreased level of consciousness, or prolonged seizures) within 7 days of administration of a previous dose of Tdap or diphtheria and tetanus toxoids and pertussis (DTP) or diphtheria and tetanus toxoids and acellular pertussis (Tdap) vaccine.
Varicella	Can occur as late as 4–6 weeks after vaccination. Tenderness and erythema at the injection site are seen in 25%, fever in 10–15%, and a localized maculopapular or vesicular rash in 5%; a diffuse rash, usually with five or fewer vesicular lesions, develops in a smaller percentage. Spread of virus from vaccinees to susceptible individuals is possible, but the risk of such transmission even to immunocompromised patients is small and disease, when it develops, is mild and treatable with acyclovir.	Known severe immunodeficiency (eg, from hematologic and solid cancers, receipt of chemotherapy, congenital immunodeficiency, long-term immunosuppressive therapy [eg, > 2 weeks of prednisone 20 mg daily or higher; other immunosuppressive medications], other disease- or therapy-related immune suppression, or patients with HIV infection who are severely immunocompromised). Pregnancy. Severe allergic reaction (eg, anaphylaxis) after a previous dose or to a vaccine component (eg, neomycin). For theoretic reasons, it is recommended that salicylates should be avoided for 6 weeks following vaccination (to prevent potential for Reye syndrome).
Zoster	Mild and limited to local reactions Although it is theoretically possible to transmit the virus to susceptible contacts, no such cases have been reported.	Known severe immunodeficiency (eg, from hematologic and solid cancers, receipt of chemotherapy, congenital immunodeficiency, long-term immunosuppressive therapy (eg, > 2 weeks of prednisone 20 mg daily or higher; other immunosuppressive medications), other disease- or therapy-related immune suppression, or patients with HIV infection who are severely immunocompromised. May be used in asymptomatic HIV-infected individuals whose CD4 count is > 200/mcL). Pregnancy. Any severe allergic reaction (eg, anaphylaxis) after a previous dose or to a vaccine component (eg, gelatin or neomycin).

[1]Adapted from CDC, Table 6. Contraindications and precautions to commonly used vaccines. General recommendations on immunization: recommendations of the Advisory Committee on Immunization Practices. MMWR. 2011;60(No. RR-2):40-1; and from Hamborsky J et al (editors). Appendix A. Epidemiology and prevention of vaccine preventable diseases. 13th edition. Washington, DC, Public Health Foundation, 2015. Available at www.cdc.gov/vaccines/pubs/pinkbook/index.html.

[2]The vaccine has typically been prepared using embryonated chicken eggs. However, a new vaccine using mammalian cell culture is now FDA-approved.

[3]The inactivated influenza vaccine can be given during any trimester.

[4]MMR vaccine can be safely given to patients with a history of egg allergy even when severe.

[5]Although vaccination of pregnant women is *not* recommended, with the currently available RA27/3 vaccine strain the congenital rubella syndrome does not occur in the offspring of those inadvertently vaccinated during pregnancy or within 3 months before conception.

31

HIV Infection & AIDS

Mitchell H. Katz, MD

General Considerations

The Centers for Disease Control and Prevention (CDC) AIDS case definition (Table 31–1) includes opportunistic infections and malignancies that rarely occur in the absence of severe immunodeficiency (eg, *Pneumocystis* pneumonia, central nervous system lymphoma). It also classifies persons as having AIDS if they have positive HIV serology and certain infections and malignancies that can occur in immunocompetent hosts but that are more common among persons infected with HIV (pulmonary tuberculosis, invasive cervical cancer). Several nonspecific conditions, including dementia and wasting (documented weight loss)—in the presence of a positive HIV serology—are considered AIDS. The definition includes criteria for both definitive and presumptive diagnoses of certain infections and malignancies. Finally, persons with positive HIV serology who have ever had a CD4 lymphocyte count below 200 cells/mcL or a CD4 lymphocyte percentage below 14% are considered to have AIDS. Inclusion of persons with low CD4 counts as AIDS cases reflects the recognition that **immunodeficiency is the defining characteristic of AIDS.** The choice of a cutoff point at 200 cells/mcL is supported by several cohort studies showing that AIDS will develop within 3 years in over 80% of persons with counts below this level in the absence of effective antiretroviral therapy (ART). The prognosis of persons with HIV/AIDS has dramatically improved due to the development of effective ART. One consequence is that fewer persons with HIV ever develop an infection or malignancy or have a low enough CD4 count to classify them as having AIDS, which means that the CDC definition has become a less useful measure of the impact of HIV/AIDS in the United States. Conversely, persons in whom AIDS had been diagnosed based on a serious opportunistic infection, malignancy, or immunodeficiency may now be markedly healthier, with high CD4 counts, due to the use of ART. Therefore, **the Social Security Administration as well as most social service agencies focus on functional assessment for determining eligibility for benefits rather than the simple presence or absence of an AIDS-defining illness.**

Epidemiology

The modes of transmission of HIV are similar to those of hepatitis B, in particular with respect to sexual, parenteral, and vertical transmission. Although certain sexual practices (eg, receptive anal intercourse) are significantly riskier than other sexual practices (eg, oral sex), it is difficult to quantify per-contact risks. The reason is that studies of sexual transmission of HIV show that most people at risk for HIV infection engage in a variety of sexual practices and have sex with multiple persons, only some of whom may actually be HIV infected. Thus, it is difficult to determine which practice with which person actually resulted in HIV transmission.

Nonetheless, the best available estimates indicate that the risk of HIV transmission with receptive anal intercourse is between 1:100 and 1:30, with insertive anal intercourse 1:1000, with receptive vaginal intercourse 1:1000, with insertive vaginal intercourse 1:10,000, and with receptive fellatio with ejaculation 1:1000. The per-contact risk of HIV transmission with other behaviors, including receptive fellatio without ejaculation, insertive fellatio, and cunnilingus, is not known.

A number of cofactors are known to increase the risk of HIV transmission during a given encounter, including the presence of ulcerative or inflammatory sexually transmitted diseases, trauma, menses, and lack of male circumcision.

Table 31–1. CDC AIDS case definition for surveillance of adults and adolescents.

Definitive AIDS diagnoses (with or without laboratory evidence of HIV infection)

1. Candidiasis of the esophagus, trachea, bronchi, or lungs.

2. Cryptococcosis, extrapulmonary.

3. Cryptosporidiosis with diarrhea persisting longer than 1 month.

4. Cytomegalovirus disease of an organ other than liver, spleen, or lymph nodes.

5. Herpes simplex virus infection causing a mucocutaneous ulcer that persists longer than 1 month; or bronchitis, pneumonitis, or esophagitis of any duration.

6. Kaposi sarcoma in a patient younger than 60 years of age.

7. Lymphoma of the brain (primary) in a patient younger than 60 years of age.

8. *Mycobacterium avium* complex or *Mycobacterium kansasii* disease, disseminated (at a site other than or in addition to lungs, skin, or cervical or hilar lymph nodes).

9. *Pneumocystis jirovecii* pneumonia

10. Progressive multifocal leukoencephalopathy.

11. Toxoplasmosis of the brain.

Definitive AIDS diagnoses (with laboratory evidence of HIV infection)

1. Coccidioidomycosis, disseminated (at a site other than or in addition to lungs or cervical or hilar lymph nodes).

2. HIV encephalopathy.

3. Histoplasmosis, disseminated (at a site other than or in addition to lungs or cervical or hilar lymph nodes).

4. Isosporiasis with diarrhea persisting longer than 1 month.

5. Kaposi sarcoma at any age.

6. Lymphoma of the brain (primary) at any age.

7. Other non-Hodgkin lymphoma of B cell or unknown immunologic phenotype.

8. Any mycobacterial disease caused by mycobacteria other than *Mycobacterium tuberculosis*, disseminated (at a site other than or in addition to lungs, skin, or cervical or hilar lymph nodes).

9. Disease caused by extrapulmonary *M tuberculosis*.

10. *Salmonella* (nontyphoid) septicemia, recurrent.

11. HIV wasting syndrome.

12. CD4 lymphocyte count below 200 cells/mcL or a CD4 lymphocyte percentage below 14%.

13. Pulmonary tuberculosis.

14. Recurrent pneumonia.

15. Invasive cervical cancer.

Presumptive AIDS diagnoses (with laboratory evidence of HIV infection)

1. Candidiasis of esophagus: (a) recent onset of retrosternal pain on swallowing; and (b) oral candidiasis.

2. Cytomegalovirus retinitis. A characteristic appearance on serial ophthalmoscopic examinations.

3. Mycobacteriosis. Specimen from stool or normally sterile body fluids or tissue from a site other than lungs, skin, or cervical or hilar lymph nodes, showing acid-fast bacilli of a species not identified by culture.

4. Kaposi sarcoma. Erythematous or violaceous plaque-like lesion on skin or mucous membrane.

5. *Pneumocystis jirovecii* pneumonia: (a) a history of dyspnea on exertion or nonproductive cough of recent onset (within the past 3 months); and (b) chest film evidence of diffuse bilateral interstitial infiltrates or gallium scan evidence of diffuse bilateral pulmonary disease; and (c) arterial blood gas analysis showing an arterial oxygen partial pressure of less than 70 mm Hg or a low respiratory diffusing capacity of less than 80% of predicted values or an increase in the alveolar-arterial oxygen tension gradient; and (d) no evidence of a bacterial pneumonia.

6. Toxoplasmosis of the brain: (a) recent onset of a focal neurologic abnormality consistent with intracranial disease or a reduced level of consciousness; and (b) brain imaging evidence of a lesion having a mass effect or the radiographic appearance of which is enhanced by injection of contrast medium; and (c) serum antibody to toxoplasmosis or successful response to therapy for toxoplasmosis.

7. Recurrent pneumonia: (a) more than one episode in a 1-year period; and (b) acute pneumonia (new symptoms, signs, or radiologic evidence not present earlier) diagnosed on clinical or radiologic grounds by the patient's clinician.

8. Pulmonary tuberculosis. (a) apical or miliary infiltrates and (b) radiographic and clinical response to antituberculous therapy.

The risk of acquiring HIV infection from a needlestick with infected blood is approximately 1:300. Factors known to increase the risk of transmission include depth of penetration, hollow bore needles, visible blood on the needle, and advanced stage of disease in the source. The risk of HIV transmission from a mucosal splash with infected blood is unknown but is assumed to be significantly lower.

The risk of acquiring HIV infection from illicit drug use with sharing of needles from an HIV-infected source is estimated to be 1:150. Use of clean needles markedly decreases the chance of HIV transmission but does not eliminate it if other drug paraphernalia are shared (eg, cookers).

When blood transfusion from an HIV-infected donor occurs, the risk of transmission is 95%. Fortunately, since 1985, blood donor screening using the HIV enzyme-linked immunosorbent assay (ELISA) has been universally practiced in the United States. Also, persons who have recently engaged in unsafe behaviors (eg, sex with a person at risk for HIV, injection drug use) are not allowed to donate. This essentially eliminates donations from persons who are HIV infected but have not yet developed antibodies (ie, persons in the "window" period). HIV antigen and viral load testing have been added to the screening of blood to further lower the chance of HIV transmission. With these precautions, the chance of HIV transmission with receipt of blood transfusion in the United States is about 1:1,000,000. Between 13% and 40% of children born to HIV-infected mothers contract HIV infection when the mother has not received treatment or when the child has not received perinatal HIV prophylaxis. The risk is higher with vaginal than with cesarean delivery, higher among mothers with high viral loads, and higher among those who breast-feed their children. The combination of prenatal HIV testing and counseling, antiretroviral treatment for infected mothers during pregnancy and for the infant immediately after birth, scheduled cesarean delivery when the mother has a viral load of greater than 1000 copies/mL, and avoidance of breastfeeding has reduced the rate of perinatal transmission of HIV to less than 2% in the United States and Europe.

HIV has not been shown to be transmitted by respiratory droplet spread, by vectors such as mosquitoes, or by casual nonsexual contact. Saliva, sweat, stool, and tears are not considered infectious fluids.

There are an estimated 1,218,400 Americans aged 13 years or older living with HIV infection, of whom 156,300 do not know that they are infected. About 50,000 new infections occur each year. There are an estimated 516,401 persons in the United States living with AIDS. Of those, 76% are men, of whom 65% were exposed through male-to-male sexual contact, 14% were exposed through injection drug use, 12% were exposed through heterosexual contact, and 8% were exposed through male-to-male sexual contact and injection drug use. Women account for 24% of living persons with AIDS, of whom 71% were infected through heterosexual contact and 26% were exposed through injection drug use. Children under the age of 13 account for less than 0.1% of living cases. African Americans have been disproportionately hard hit by the epidemic. The estimated rate of new HIV diagnoses in the United States per 100,000 is 49.4 among African Americans, 18.4 among Latinos, 15.4 among persons of multiple races, 10.6 among native Hawaiians and Pacific Islanders, 9.5 among American Indians/Alaskan natives, 6.2 among whites, and 6.1 among Asians.

In general, the progression of HIV-related illness is similar in men and women. However, there are some important differences. Women are at risk for gynecologic complications of HIV, including recurrent candidal vaginitis, pelvic inflammatory disease, and cervical dysplasia. Violence directed against women, pregnancy, and frequent occurrence of drug use and poverty all complicate the treatment of HIV-infected women.

Worldwide there are an estimated 37 million persons infected with HIV, with heterosexual spread being the most common mode of transmission for men and women. The reason for the greater risk for transmission with heterosexual intercourse in Africa and Asia than in the United States may relate to cofactors such as general health status, the presence of genital ulcers, relative lack of male circumcision, the number of sexual partners, and different HIV serotypes.

Centers for Disease Control and Prevention. HIV Surveillance Report. 2014;26. http://www.cdc.gov/hiv/library/reports/surveillance
Panel on treatment of HIV-infected pregnant women and prevention of perinatal transmission. Recommendations for use of antiretroviral drugs in pregnant HIV-1-infected women for maternal health and interventions to reduce perinatal HIV-1 transmission in the United States. July 31, 2012 Guideline. http://aidsinfo.nih.gov/contentfiles/lvguidelines/PerinatalGL.pdf
World Health Organization. HIV/AIDS. Fact sheet N°. 360. November 2015. http://www.who.int/mediacentre/factsheets/fs360/en/

▶ Pathophysiology

Clinically, the syndromes caused by HIV infection are usually explicable by one of three known mechanisms: immunodeficiency, autoimmunity, and allergic and hypersensitivity reactions.

A. Immunodeficiency

Immunodeficiency is a direct result of the effects of HIV upon immune cells as well as the indirect impact of a generalized state of inflammation and immune activation due to chronic viral infection. A spectrum of infections and neoplasms is seen, as in other congenital or acquired immunodeficiency states. Two remarkable features of HIV immunodeficiency are the low incidence of certain infections such as listeriosis and aspergillosis and the frequent occurrence of certain neoplasms such as lymphoma or Kaposi sarcoma. This latter complication has been seen primarily in MSM or in bisexual men, and its incidence steadily declined through the first 15 years of the epidemic. A herpesvirus (KSHV or HHV-8) is the cause of Kaposi sarcoma.

B. Autoimmunity/Allergic and Hypersensitivity Reactions

Autoimmunity can occur as a result of disordered cellular immune function or B lymphocyte dysfunction. Examples of both lymphocytic infiltration of organs (eg, lymphocytic interstitial pneumonitis) and autoantibody production (eg, immunologic thrombocytopenia) occur. These phenomena may be the only clinically apparent disease or may coexist with obvious immunodeficiency. Moreover, HIV-infected individuals appear to have higher rates of allergic reactions to unknown allergens as seen with eosinophilic pustular folliculitis ("itchy red bump syndrome") as well as increased rates of hypersensitivity reactions to medications (for example, the fever and sunburn-like rash seen with trimethoprim-sulfamethoxazole reactions).

► Clinical Findings

The complications of HIV-related infections and neoplasms affect virtually every organ. The general approach to the HIV-infected person with symptoms is to evaluate the organ systems involved, aiming to diagnose treatable conditions rapidly. As can be seen in Figure 31–1, the CD4 lymphocyte count result enables the clinician to focus on the diagnoses most likely to be seen at each stage of immunodeficiency. Certain infections may occur at any CD4 count, while others rarely occur unless the CD4 lymphocyte count has dropped below a certain level. For example, a patient with a CD4 count of 600 cells/mcL, cough, and fever may have a bacterial pneumonia but would be very unlikely to have *Pneumocystis* pneumonia.

A. Symptoms and Signs

Many individuals with HIV infection remain asymptomatic for years even without ART, with a mean time of approximately 10 years between infection and development of AIDS. When symptoms occur, they may be remarkably protean and nonspecific. Since virtually all the findings may be seen with other diseases, a combination of complaints is more suggestive of HIV infection than any one symptom.

Physical examination may be entirely normal. Abnormal findings range from completely nonspecific to highly specific for HIV infection. Those that are specific for HIV infection include hairy leukoplakia of the tongue, disseminated Kaposi sarcoma, and cutaneous bacillary angiomatosis. Generalized lymphadenopathy is common early in infection.

The specific presentations and management of the various complications of HIV infection are discussed under the Complications section below.

B. Laboratory Findings

Specific tests for HIV include antibody and antigen detection (Table 31–2). Conventional HIV antibody testing is done by ELISA. Positive specimens are then confirmed by a different method (eg, Western blot). The sensitivity of screening serologic tests is greater than 99.9%. The specificity of positive results by two different techniques approaches 100% even in low-risk populations. False-positive screening tests may occur as normal biologic variants or in association with recent influenza vaccination or other disease states, such as connective tissue disease. These are usually detected by negative confirmatory tests. Antibodies will be detectable with current screening serologic tests in 95% of persons within 6 weeks after infection.

▲ **Figure 31–1.** Relationship of CD4 count to development of opportunistic infections. MAC, *Mycobacterium avium* complex; CMV, cytomegalovirus; CNS, central nervous system.

Table 31–2. Laboratory findings with HIV infection.

Test	Significance
HIV enzyme-linked immunosorbent assay (ELISA)	Screening test for HIV infection. Of ELISA tests 50% are positive within 22 days after HIV transmission; 95% are positive within 6 weeks after transmission. Sensitivity greater than 99.9%; to avoid false-positive results, repeatedly reactive results must be confirmed with Western blot.
Western blot	Confirmatory test for HIV. Specificity when combined with ELISA greater than 99.99%. Indeterminate results with early HIV infection, HIV-2 infection, influenza vaccine, autoimmune disease, pregnancy, and recent tetanus toxoid administration.
HIV rapid antibody test	Screening test for HIV. Produces results in 10–20 minutes. Can be performed by personnel with limited training. Positive results must be confirmed with standard HIV tests (ELISA and Western blot).
Complete blood count	Anemia, neutropenia, and thrombocytopenia common with advanced HIV infection.
Absolute CD4 lymphocyte count	Most widely used predictor of HIV progression. Risk of progression to an AIDS opportunistic infection or malignancy is high with CD4 less than 200 cells/mcL in the absence of treatment.
CD4 lymphocyte percentage	Percentage may be more reliable than the CD4 count. Risk of progression to an AIDS opportunistic infection or malignancy is high with percentage less than 14% in the absence of treatment.
HIV viral load tests	These tests measure the amount of actively replicating HIV virus. Correlate with disease progression and response to antiretroviral medications. Best tests available for diagnosis of acute HIV infection (prior to seroconversion); however, caution is warranted when the test result shows low-level viremia (ie, less than 500 copies/mL) as this may represent a false-positive test.

Rapid HIV antibody tests of blood or oral fluid provide results within 10–20 minutes and can be performed in clinician offices, including by personnel without laboratory training and without a Clinical Laboratory Improvement Amendment (CLIA)-approved laboratory. Persons who test positive on a rapid test should be told that they may be HIV-infected or their test may be falsely reactive. Standard testing (ELISA with Western blot confirmation) should be performed to distinguish these two possibilities. Rapid testing is particularly helpful in settings where a result is needed immediately (eg, a woman in labor who has not recently been tested for HIV) or when the patient is unlikely to return for a result. Rapid HIV home tests that allow the testers to learn their status privately by simply swabbing along their gum lines are also available (www.oraquick.com).

Nonspecific laboratory findings with HIV infection may include anemia, leukopenia (particularly lymphopenia), and thrombocytopenia in any combination, elevation of the erythrocyte sedimentation rate, polyclonal hypergammaglobulinemia, and hypocholesterolemia. Cutaneous anergy is common.

The most widely used marker is the absolute CD4 lymphocyte count to provide prognostic information and guide therapy decisions (Table 31–2). As counts decrease, the risk of serious opportunistic infection over the subsequent 3–5 years increases (Figure 31–1). There are many limitations to using the CD4 count, including diurnal variation, depression with intercurrent illness, and intralaboratory and interlaboratory variability. Therefore, the trend is more important than a single determination. The frequency of performance of counts depends on the patient's health status and whether or not they are receiving antiretroviral treatment. **All patients regardless of CD4 count should be offered ART; CD4 counts should be monitored every 3–6 months in patients taking ART consistently.** Initiation of *Pneumocystis jirovecii* prophylactic therapy is recommended when the CD4 count drops below 200 cells/mcL, and initiation of *Mycobacterium avium* prophylaxis is recommended when the CD4 count drops below 75–100 cells/mcL. Some studies suggest that the percentage of CD4 lymphocytes is a more reliable indicator of prognosis than the absolute counts because the percentage does not depend on calculating a manual differential. While the CD4 count measures immune dysfunction, it does not provide a measure of how actively HIV is replicating in the body. **HIV viral load** tests assess the level of viral replication and provide useful prognostic information that is independent of the information provided by CD4 counts.

▶ Differential Diagnosis

HIV infection may mimic a variety of other medical illnesses. Specific differential diagnosis depends on the mode of presentation. In patients presenting with constitutional symptoms such as weight loss and fevers, differential considerations include cancer, chronic infections such as tuberculosis and endocarditis, and endocrinologic diseases such as hyperthyroidism. When pulmonary processes dominate the presentation, acute and chronic lung infections must be considered as well as other causes of diffuse interstitial pulmonary infiltrates. When neurologic disease is the mode of presentation, conditions that cause mental status changes or neuropathy—eg, alcoholism, liver disease, kidney dysfunction, thyroid disease, and vitamin deficiency—should be considered. If a patient presents with headache and a cerebrospinal fluid pleocytosis, other causes of chronic meningitis enter the differential. When diarrhea is a prominent complaint, infectious enterocolitis, antibiotic-associated colitis, inflammatory bowel disease, and malabsorptive symptoms must be considered.

Complications

A. Systemic Complaints

Fever, night sweats, and weight loss are common symptoms in HIV-infected patients and may occur without a complicating opportunistic infection. Patients with persistent fever and no localizing symptoms should nonetheless be carefully examined, and evaluated with a chest radiograph (*Pneumocystis* pneumonia can present without respiratory symptoms), bacterial blood cultures if the fever is greater than 38.5°C, serum cryptococcal antigen, and mycobacterial cultures of the blood. Sinus CT scans or sinus radiographs should be considered to evaluate occult sinusitis. If these studies are normal, patients should be observed closely. Antipyretics are useful to prevent dehydration.

1. Weight loss and wasting syndrome—Weight loss is a particularly distressing complication of long-standing HIV infection. Patients typically have disproportionate loss of muscle mass, with maintenance or less substantial loss of fat stores. The mechanism of HIV-related weight loss is not completely understood but appears to be multifactorial.

A. PRESENTATION—AIDS patients frequently suffer from anorexia, nausea, and vomiting, all of which contribute to weight loss by decreasing caloric intake. In some cases, these symptoms are secondary to a specific infection, such as viral hepatitis. In other cases, however, evaluation of the symptoms yields no specific pathogen, and it is assumed to be due to a primary effect of HIV. Malabsorption also plays a role in decreased caloric intake. Patients may suffer diarrhea from infections with bacterial, viral, or parasitic agents.

Exacerbating the decrease in caloric intake, many AIDS patients have an increased metabolic rate. This increased rate has been shown to exist even among asymptomatic HIV-infected persons, but it accelerates with disease progression and secondary infection. AIDS patients with secondary infections also have decreased protein synthesis, which makes maintaining muscle mass difficult.

B. MANAGEMENT—Several strategies have been developed to slow AIDS wasting. In the long term, nothing is as effective as ART, since it treats the underlying HIV infection. In the short term, effective fever control decreases the metabolic rate and may slow the pace of weight loss, as does treating the underlying opportunistic infection. Food supplementation with high-calorie drinks may enable patients with not much appetite to maintain their intake. Selected patients with otherwise good functional status and weight loss due to unrelenting nausea, vomiting, or diarrhea may benefit from total parenteral nutrition (TPN). It should be noted, however, that TPN is more likely to increase fat stores than to reverse the muscle wasting process.

Two pharmacologic approaches for increasing appetite and weight gain are the progestational agent **megestrol acetate** (80 mg orally four times a day) and the antiemetic agent **dronabinol** (2.5–5 mg orally three times a day), but neither of these agents increases lean body mass. Side effects from megestrol acetate are rare, but thromboembolic phenomena, edema, nausea, vomiting, and rash have been reported. Euphoria, dizziness, paranoia, and somnolence

and even nausea and vomiting have been reported in 3–10% of patients using dronabinol. Dronabinol contains only one of the active ingredients in marijuana, and many patients report better relief of nausea and improvement of appetite with **medical cannabis** (administered via smoking, vaporization, essential oils or cooked in food). In the United States, at least 23 states and the District of Columbia have legalized medical marijuana. However, the use and sale of marijuana is still illegal under federal law.

Two regimens that have resulted in increases in lean body mass are growth hormone and anabolic steroids. **Growth hormone** at a dose of 0.1 mg/kg/day (up to 6 mg) subcutaneously for 12 weeks has resulted in modest increases in lean body mass. Treatment with growth hormone can cost as much as $10,000 per month. **Anabolic steroids** also increase lean body mass among HIV-infected patients. They seem to work best for patients who are able to do weight training. The most commonly used regimens are testosterone enanthate or testosterone cypionate (100–200 mg intramuscularly every 2–4 weeks). Testosterone transdermal system (apply 5 mg system each evening) and testosterone gel (1%; apply a 5-g packet [50 mg testosterone] to clean, dry skin daily) are also available. The anabolic steroid oxandrolone (20 mg orally in two divided doses) has also been found to increase lean body mass.

2. Nausea—Nausea leading to weight loss is sometimes due to esophageal candidiasis. Patients with oral candidiasis and nausea should be empirically treated with an oral antifungal agent. Patients with weight loss due to nausea of unclear origin may benefit from use of antiemetics prior to meals (prochlorperazine, 10 mg three times daily; metoclopramide, 10 mg three times daily; or ondansetron, 8 mg three times daily). Dronabinol (5 mg three times daily) or medical cannabis can also be used to treat nausea. Depression and adrenal insufficiency are two potentially treatable causes of weight loss.

B. Pulmonary Disease

1. *Pneumocystis* pneumonia—(See also Chapter 36.) *P jirovecii* pneumonia is the most common opportunistic infection associated with AIDS. *Pneumocystis* pneumonia may be difficult to diagnose because the symptoms—fever, cough, and shortness of breath—are nonspecific. Furthermore, the severity of symptoms ranges from fever and no respiratory symptoms through mild cough or dyspnea to frank respiratory distress.

Hypoxemia may be severe, with a PO_2 less than 60 mm Hg. The cornerstone of diagnosis is the chest radiograph. Diffuse or perihilar infiltrates are most characteristic, but only two-thirds of patients with *Pneumocystis* pneumonia have this finding. Normal chest radiographs are seen in 5–10% of patients with *Pneumocystis* pneumonia, while the remainder have atypical infiltrates. Apical infiltrates are commonly seen among patients with *Pneumocystis* pneumonia who have been receiving aerosolized pentamidine prophylaxis. Large pleural effusions are uncommon with *Pneumocystis* pneumonia; their presence suggests bacterial pneumonia, other infections such as tuberculosis, or pleural Kaposi sarcoma.

Definitive diagnosis can be obtained in 50–80% of cases by Wright-Giemsa stain or direct fluorescence antibody (DFA) test of induced sputum. Sputum induction is performed by having patients inhale an aerosolized solution of 3% saline produced by an ultrasonic nebulizer. Patients should not eat for at least 8 hours and should not use toothpaste or mouthwash prior to the procedure since they can interfere with test interpretation. The next step for patients with negative sputum examinations in whom *Pneumocystis* pneumonia is still suspected should be bronchoalveolar lavage. This technique establishes the diagnosis in over 95% of cases.

In patients with symptoms suggestive of *Pneumocystis* pneumonia but with negative or atypical chest radiographs and negative sputum examinations, other diagnostic tests may provide additional information in deciding whether to proceed to bronchoalveolar lavage. Elevation of serum lactate dehydrogenase occurs in 95% of cases of *Pneumocystis* pneumonia, but the specificity of this finding is at best 75%. A serum beta-glucan test is more sensitive and specific test for *Pneumocystis* pneumonia compared with serum lactate dehydrogenase and may avoid more invasive tests when used in the appropriate clinical setting. Either a normal diffusing capacity of carbon monoxide (DL_{CO}) or a high-resolution CT scan of the chest that demonstrates no interstitial lung disease makes the diagnosis of *Pneumocystis* pneumonia very unlikely. In addition, a CD4 count greater than 250 cells/mcL within 2 months prior to evaluation of respiratory symptoms makes a diagnosis of *Pneumocystis* pneumonia unlikely; only 1–5% of cases occur above this CD4 count level (Figure 31–1). This is true even if the patient previously had a CD4 count lower than 200 cells/mcL but has had an increase with ART. Pneumothoraces can be seen in HIV-infected patients with a history of *Pneumocystis* pneumonia.

Trimethoprim-sulfamethoxazole is the preferred treatment of *Pneumocystis* pneumonia (Table 31–3). In addition to specific anti-*Pneumocystis* treatment, corticosteroid therapy has been shown to improve the course of patients with moderate to severe *P jirovecii* pneumonia (PaO_2 less than 70 mm Hg on room air or alveolar-arterial O_2 gradient greater or equal to 35 mm Hg) when administered within 72 hours of the start of anti-*Pneumocystis* treatment. It should be started as early as possible after initiation of treatment, using prednisone 40 mg orally twice daily for days 1–5, 40 mg daily for days 6–10, and 20 mg daily for days 11–21 (for patients who cannot take oral medication, intravenous methylprednisolone can be substituted at 75% of the dose). The mechanism of action is presumed to be a decrease in alveolar inflammation.

2. Other infectious pulmonary diseases—

A. PRESENTATION—Other infectious causes of pulmonary disease in AIDS patients include bacterial, mycobacterial, and viral pneumonias. **Community-acquired pneumonia is the most common cause of pulmonary disease in HIV-infected persons.** An increased incidence of pneumococcal pneumonia with septicemia and *Haemophilus influenzae* pneumonia has been reported. *Pseudomonas aeruginosa* is an important respiratory pathogen in advanced disease

and, more rarely, pneumonia from *Rhodococcus equi* infection can occur. The incidence of infection with *Mycobacterium tuberculosis* has markedly increased in metropolitan areas because of HIV infection as well as homelessness. Tuberculosis occurs in an estimated 4% of persons in the United States who have AIDS. Apical infiltrates and disseminated disease occur more commonly than among immunocompetent persons. Although a purified protein derivative (PPD) test should be performed on all HIV-infected persons in whom a diagnosis of tuberculosis is being considered, the lower the CD4 cell count, the greater the likelihood of anergy. Because "anergy" skin test panels do not accurately classify those patients who are infected with tuberculosis but unreactive to the PPD, they are not recommended. **Interferon gamma release assays** (including the QuantiFERON and T-SPOT tests) are likely to be more sensitive than skin testing in HIV-infected patients in whom tuberculosis infection is suspected.

B. MANAGEMENT—Treatment of HIV-infected persons with active tuberculosis is similar to treatment of HIV-uninfected tubercular individuals. However, rifampin should not be given to patients receiving a boosted protease inhibitor (PI)-regimen. In these cases, rifabutin may be substituted, but it may require dosing modifications depending on the antiretroviral regimen. Multidrug-resistant tuberculosis has been a major problem in several metropolitan areas of the developed world, and reports from South Africa of "extremely resistant" tuberculosis in AIDS patients is a growing global concern. Noncompliance with prescribed antituberculous medications is a major risk factor. Several of the reported outbreaks appear to implicate nosocomial spread. The emergence of medication resistance makes it essential that antibiotic sensitivities be performed on all positive cultures. Medication therapy should be individualized. Patients with multidrug-resistant *M tuberculosis* infection should receive at least three medications to which their organism is sensitive. Atypical mycobacteria can cause pulmonary disease in AIDS patients with or without preexisting lung disease and responds variably to treatment. Making a distinction between *M tuberculosis* and atypical mycobacteria requires culture of sputum specimens. If culture of the sputum produces acid-fast bacilli, definitive identification may take several weeks using traditional techniques. DNA probes allow for presumptive identification usually within days of a positive culture. **While awaiting definitive diagnosis, clinicians should err on the side of treating patients as if they have *M tuberculosis* infection.** In cases in which the risk of atypical mycobacteria is very high (eg, a person without risk for tuberculosis exposure with a CD4 count under 50 cells/mcL—see Figure 31–1), clinicians may wait for definitive diagnosis if the person is smear-negative for acid-fast bacilli, clinically stable, and not living in a communal setting. Isolation of cytomegalovirus (CMV) from bronchoalveolar lavage fluid occurs commonly in AIDS patients but does not establish a definitive diagnosis. Diagnosis of CMV pneumonia requires biopsy; response to treatment is poor. Histoplasmosis, coccidioidomycosis, and cryptococcal disease as well as more common respiratory viral infections should

Table 31–3. Treatment of AIDS-related opportunistic infections and malignancies.[1]

Infection or Malignancy	Treatment	Complications[2]
Pneumocystis jirovecii infection[3]	Preferred regimen: Trimethoprim-sulfamethoxazole, 15 mg/kg/day (based on trimethoprim component) intravenously or one double-strength tablet orally three times a day for 21 days. Add prednisone when PaO_2 < 70 mm Hg on room air or alveolar-arterial O_2 gradient > 35 mm Hg: 40 mg orally twice a day on days 1–5, 40 mg orally daily on days 6–10, 20 mg orally daily on days 11–21	Nausea, neutropenia, anemia, hepatitis, rash, Stevens-Johnson syndrome
	Pentamidine, 3–4 mg/kg/day intravenously for 21 days plus prednisone when indicated as above	Hypotension, hypoglycemia, anemia, neutropenia, pancreatitis, hepatitis
	Primaquine, 30 mg/day orally, and clindamycin, 600 mg every 8 hours orally, for 21 days plus prednisone when indicated as above	Primaquine: hemolytic anemia in G6PD-deficient patients,[3] methemoglobinemia, neutropenia, colitis Clindamycin: rash, nausea, abdominal pain, colitis
	Not recommended for severe disease: Trimethoprim, 15 mg/kg/day orally in three divided doses, with dapsone, 100 mg/day orally, for 21 days,[3] plus prednisone when indicated as above	Nausea, rash, hemolytic anemia in G6PD[3]-deficient patients; methemoglobinemia (weekly levels should be less than 10% of total hemoglobin)
	Not recommended for severe disease: Atovaquone, 750 mg orally three times daily with food for 21 days, plus prednisone when indicated as above	Rash, elevated aminotransferases, anemia, neutropenia
Mycobacterium avium complex infection	Clarithromycin, 500 mg orally twice daily with ethambutol, 15 mg/kg/day orally (maximum, 1 g). May also add:	Clarithromycin: hepatitis, nausea, diarrhea; ethambutol: hepatitis, optic neuritis
	Rifabutin, 300 mg orally daily.	Rash, hepatitis, uveitis
Toxoplasmosis	Preferred regimen: Pyrimethamine, 200 mg orally as loading dose, followed by 50 mg daily (weight ≤ 60 kg) or 75 mg daily (weight > 60 kg), combined with sulfadiazine, 1000 mg orally four times daily (weight ≤ 60 kg) or 500 mg orally four times daily (weight > 60 kg) and leucovorin 10–25 mg orally daily for at least 6 weeks. Longer courses are necessary for extensive disease or incomplete clinical or radiographic resolution. Maintenance therapy with pyrimethamine 25–50 mg orally plus sulfadiazine 2000–4000 mg in two to four divided doses plus leucovorin 10–25 mg orally daily. Long-term treatment should be maintained until immune reconstitution with ART occurs.	Pyrimethamine: leukopenia, anorexia, vomiting Sulfadiazine: nausea, vomiting, Stevens-Johnsons syndrome
	For patients who are intolerant of sulfa who cannot be desensitized: substitute clindamycin 600 mg intravenously or orally every 6 hours for the sulfadiazine in the above regimen	Pyrimethamine: leukopenia, anorexia, vomiting Clindamycin: rash, nausea, abdominal pain, colitis
	If pyrimethamine not available: trimethoprim-sulfamethoxazole, 10 mg/kg/day (based on trimethoprim component)	Nausea, neutropenia, anemia, hepatitis, rash, Stevens-Johnson syndrome
Non-Hodgkin lymphoma	Combination chemotherapy (eg, EPOCH with rituximab and G-CSF) Central nervous system disease: radiation treatment with dexamethasone for edema	Nausea, vomiting, anemia, neutropenia, thrombocytopenia cardiac toxicity (with doxorubicin)
Cryptococcal meningitis	Preferred regimen: Liposomal amphotericin B, 3–4 mg/kg/day intravenously, with flucytosine, 25 mg/kg/day orally in four divided doses for 2 weeks (adjust dose for renal function), then fluconazole, 400 mg orally daily for 8 weeks, then 200 mg orally daily to complete 1 year of therapy	Liposomal amphotericin: fever, chills, hypokalemia, renal failure Flucytosine: bone marrow suppression, renal failure, hepatitis Fluconazole: hepatitis
	Amphotericin B, 0.7 mg/kg/day intravenously, with flucytosine, 100 mg/kg/day orally in four divided doses for 2 weeks (adjust dose for renal function), then fluconazole, 400 mg orally daily for 8 weeks, then 200 mg orally daily to complete 1 year of therapy	Amphotericin: fever, chills, hypokalemia, renal failure Flucytosine: bone marrow suppression, renal failure, hepatitis Fluconazole: hepatitis
	Fluconazole, 400 mg orally daily for 8 weeks, then 200 mg orally daily to complete 1 year of therapy	Hepatitis

(continued)

Table 31–3. Treatment of AIDS-related opportunistic infections and malignancies.[1] (continued)

Infection or Malignancy	Treatment	Complications[2]
Cytomegalovirus retinitis (immediate sight-threatening)	Preferred regimen: Intravitreal ganciclovir (2 mg/injection) or foscarnet (2.4 mg/injection) for 1–4 doses for 7–10 days plus valganciclovir, 900 mg orally twice a day for 14–21 days with food followed by 900 mg daily (maintenance)	Neutropenia, anemia, thrombocytopenia
	Ganciclovir, 10 mg/kg/day intravenously in two divided doses for 14 days, followed by 5 mg/kg daily or valganciclovir 900 mg orally daily (maintenance)	Neutropenia (especially when used concurrently with zidovudine), anemia, thrombocytopenia Adjust ganciclovir dose for renal function
	Foscarnet, 60 mg/kg intravenously every 8 hours or 90 mg/kg intravenously every 12 hours for 14–21 days, followed by 90–120 mg/kg once daily. (Adjust dose for renal function.)	Nausea, hypokalemia, hypocalcemia, hyperphosphatemia, azotemia
	Cidofovir, 5 mg/kg/week intravenously for 2 weeks then 5 mg/kg every other week with probenecid 2 g orally 3 hours before dose, 1 g orally 2 hours after dose, and 1 g orally 8 hours after dose	Nephrotoxicity (to reduce likelihood, pre and post saline hydration, along with probenecid), neutropenia Avoid in patients with sulfa allergy because of cross hypersensitivity with probenecid
Esophageal candidiasis or recurrent vaginal candidiasis	Fluconazole, 100–200 mg orally daily for 14–21 days for esophageal disease and > 7 days for recurrent vaginal disease	Hepatitis, development of azole resistance
Herpes simplex infection	Acyclovir, 400 mg orally three times daily for 5–10 days; or acyclovir, 5 mg/kg intravenously every 8 hours for severe cases	Resistant herpes simplex with long-term therapy
	Famciclovir, 500 mg orally twice daily for 5–10 days	Nausea
	Valacyclovir, 1 g orally twice daily for 5–10 days	Nausea
	Foscarnet, 40 mg/kg intravenously every 8 hours, for acyclovir–resistant cases. (Adjust dose for renal function.)	Nausea, hypokalemia, hypocalcemia, hyperphosphatemia, azotemia
Herpes zoster	Preferred regimen: Valacyclovir, 500 mg orally three times daily for 7–10 days	Resistant herpes simplex with long-term therapy
	Preferred regimen: Famciclovir, 500 mg orally three times daily for 7–10 days	Nausea
	Acyclovir, 800 mg orally four or five times daily for 7–10 days. Intravenous therapy at 10 mg/kg every 8 hours for ocular involvement, visceral disease until clinical improvement then switch to oral therapy to complete a 10- to 14-day course	Nausea
Kaposi sarcoma		
Mild to moderate	Initiation or optimization of ART	Side effects of ART
Advanced disease	Combination chemotherapy (eg, daunorubicin, bleomycin, vinblastine)	Bone marrow suppression, cardiac toxicity, fever

[1] Recommendations drawn from Centers for Disease Control. Guidelines for the prevention and treatment of opportunistic infections in HIV-infected adults and adolescents. 2015. http://aidsinfo.nih.gov/contentfiles/lvguidelines/adult_oi.pdf

[2]List of complications is not exhaustive.

[3]Prior to use of primaquine or dapsone, check glucose-6-phosphate dehydrogenase (G6PD) level in black patients and those of Mediterranean origin.

EPOCH, etoposide, prednisolone, vincristine (Oncovin), cyclophosphamide, doxorubicin (hydroxydaunomycin); G-CSF, granulocyte-colony stimulating factor (filgrastim).

also be considered in the differential diagnosis of unexplained pulmonary infiltrates.

3. Noninfectious pulmonary diseases—

A. PRESENTATION—Noninfectious causes of lung disease include Kaposi sarcoma, non-Hodgkin lymphoma, interstitial pneumonitis, and increasingly, in the current ART era, lung cancer. In patients with known Kaposi sarcoma, pulmonary involvement complicates the course in approximately one-third of cases. However, pulmonary involvement is rarely the presenting manifestation of Kaposi sarcoma. Non-Hodgkin lymphoma may involve the lung as the sole site of disease but more commonly involves other organs as well, especially the brain, liver, and gastrointestinal tract. Both of these processes may show nodular or diffuse parenchymal involvement, pleural effusions, and mediastinal adenopathy on chest radiographs.

Nonspecific interstitial pneumonitis may mimic *Pneumocystis* pneumonia. Lymphocytic interstitial pneumonitis seen in lung biopsies has a variable clinical course. Typically, these patients present with several months of mild cough and dyspnea; chest radiographs show interstitial infiltrates. Many patients with this entity undergo transbronchial biopsies in an attempt to diagnose *Pneumocystis* pneumonia. Instead, the tissue shows interstitial inflammation ranging from an intense lymphocytic infiltration (consistent with lymphoid interstitial pneumonitis) to a mild mononuclear inflammation.

B. MANAGEMENT—Corticosteroids may be helpful in some cases refractory to ART.

4. Sinusitis—

A. PRESENTATION—Chronic sinusitis can be a frustrating problem for HIV-infected patients. Symptoms include sinus congestion and discharge, headache, and fever. Some patients may have radiographic evidence of sinus disease on sinus CT scan or sinus x-ray in the absence of significant symptoms.

B. MANAGEMENT—Nonsmoking patients with purulent drainage should be treated with amoxicillin (500 mg orally three times a day). Patients who smoke cigarettes should be treated with amoxicillin-potassium clavulanate (500 mg orally three times a day) to cover *H influenzae*. A 7-day course of pseudoephedrine 60 mg twice daily may be helpful in decreasing congestion. Prolonged treatment (3–6 weeks) with an antibiotic and guaifenesin (600 mg orally twice daily) is sometimes necessary. For patients not responding to amoxicillin-potassium clavulanate, levofloxacin may be tried (400 mg orally daily). In patients with advanced immunodeficiency, *Pseudomonas* infections should be suspected, especially if there is not a response to first-line antibiotics. Some patients may require referral to an otolaryngologist for sinus drainage.

C. Central Nervous System Disease

Central nervous system disease in HIV-infected patients can be divided into intracerebral space-occupying lesions, encephalopathy, meningitis, and spinal cord processes. Many of these complications have declined markedly in prevalence in the era of effective ART. Cognitive declines, however, may be more common in HIV patients especially as they age (older than 50 years), even those who are taking fully suppressive ART.

1. **Toxoplasmosis**—Toxoplasmosis is the most common space-occupying lesion in HIV-infected patients. Headache, focal neurologic deficits, seizures, or altered mental status may be presenting symptoms. The diagnosis is usually made presumptively based on the characteristic appearance of cerebral imaging studies in an individual known to be seropositive for *Toxoplasma*. Typically, toxoplasmosis appears as multiple contrast-enhancing lesions on CT scan. Lesions tend to be peripheral, with a predilection for the basal ganglia.

Single lesions are atypical of toxoplasmosis. When a single lesion has been detected by CT scanning, MRI scanning may reveal multiple lesions because of its greater sensitivity. If a patient has a single lesion on MRI and is neurologically stable, clinicians may pursue a 2-week empiric trial of toxoplasmosis therapy. A repeat scan should be performed at 2 weeks. If the lesion has not diminished in size, biopsy of the lesion should be performed. A positive *Toxoplasma* serologic test does not confirm the diagnosis because many HIV-infected patients have detectable titers without having active disease. Conversely, less than 3% of patients with toxoplasmosis have negative titers. Therefore, negative *Toxoplasma* titers in an HIV-infected patient with a space-occupying lesion should be a cause for aggressively pursuing an alternative diagnosis. The preferred treatment of toxoplasmosis is with pyrimethamine and sulfadiazine (Table 31–3). If pyrimethamine is not available, patients can be treated with trimethoprim-sulfamethoxazole.

2. **Central nervous system lymphoma**—Primary non-Hodgkin lymphoma is the second most common space-occupying lesion in HIV-infected patients. Symptoms are similar to those with toxoplasmosis. While imaging techniques cannot distinguish these two diseases with certainty, lymphoma more often is solitary. Other less common lesions should be suspected if there is preceding bacteremia, positive tuberculin test, fungemia, or injection drug use. These include bacterial abscesses, cryptococcomas, tuberculomas, and *Nocardia* lesions.

Stereotactic brain biopsy should be strongly considered if lesions are solitary or do not respond to toxoplasmosis treatment, especially if they are easily accessible. Diagnosis of lymphoma is important because many patients benefit from treatment (radiation therapy). Although a positive polymerase chain reaction (PCR) assay of cerebrospinal fluid for Epstein–Barr virus DNA is consistent with a diagnosis of lymphoma, the sensitivity and specificity of the test are not high enough to obviate the need for a brain biopsy.

3. **HIV-associated dementia**—Patients with HIV-associated dementia typically have difficulty with cognitive tasks (eg, memory, attention), exhibit diminished motor function, and have emotional or behavioral problems. Patients may first notice a deterioration in their handwriting. The manifestations of dementia may wax and wane, with persons exhibiting periods of lucidity and confusion over the course of a day. The diagnosis of HIV-associated dementia is one of exclusion based on a brain imaging study and on spinal fluid analysis that excludes other pathogens. Neuropsychiatric testing is helpful in distinguishing patients with dementia from those with depression. Many patients improve with effective ART. However, slowly progressive neurocognitive deficits may still develop in patients taking ART as they age.

Metabolic abnormalities may also cause changes in mental status: hypoglycemia, hyponatremia, hypoxia, and drug overdose are important considerations in this population. Other less common infectious causes of encephalopathy include progressive multifocal leukoencephalopathy (discussed below), CMV, syphilis, and herpes simplex encephalitis.

4. Cryptococcal meningitis—Cryptococcal meningitis typically presents with fever and headache. Less than 20% of patients have meningismus. Diagnosis is based on a positive latex agglutination test of serum that detects cryptococcal antigen (or "CRAG") or positive culture of spinal fluid for *Cryptococcus*. Seventy to 90% of patients with cryptococcal meningitis have a positive serum CRAG. Thus, a negative serum CRAG test makes a diagnosis of cryptococcal meningitis unlikely and can be useful in the initial evaluation of a patient with headache, fever, and normal mental status. HIV meningitis, characterized by lymphocytic pleocytosis of the spinal fluid with negative culture, is common early in HIV infection. The preferred treatment is liposomal amphotericin with flucytosine (Table 31–3).

5. HIV myelopathy—Spinal cord function may also be impaired in HIV-infected individuals. HIV myelopathy presents with leg weakness and incontinence. Spastic paraparesis and sensory ataxia are seen on neurologic examination. Myelopathy is usually a late manifestation of HIV disease, and most patients will have concomitant HIV encephalopathy. Pathologic evaluation of the spinal cord reveals vacuolation of white matter. Because HIV myelopathy is a diagnosis of exclusion, symptoms suggestive of myelopathy should be evaluated by lumbar puncture to rule out CMV polyradiculopathy (described below) and an MRI or CT scan to exclude epidural lymphoma.

6. Progressive multifocal leukoencephalopathy (PML)—PML is a viral infection of the white matter of the brain seen in patients with very advanced HIV infection. It typically results in focal neurologic deficits such as aphasia, hemiparesis, and cortical blindness. Imaging studies are strongly suggestive of the diagnosis if they show nonenhancing white matter lesions without mass effect. Extensive lesions may be difficult to differentiate from the changes caused by HIV. Several patients have stabilized or improved after the institution of effective ART, and due to wide use of ART, PML is now rarely seen.

D. Peripheral Nervous System

A. Presentation—Peripheral nervous system syndromes include inflammatory polyneuropathies, sensory neuropathies, and mononeuropathies.

An **inflammatory demyelinating polyneuropathy** similar to Guillain-Barré syndrome occurs in HIV-infected patients, usually prior to frank immunodeficiency. The syndrome in many cases improves with plasmapheresis, supporting an autoimmune basis of the disease. CMV can cause an ascending polyradiculopathy characterized by lower extremity weakness and a neutrophilic pleocytosis on spinal fluid analysis with a negative bacterial culture. Transverse myelitis can be seen with herpes zoster or CMV.

Peripheral neuropathy is common among HIV-infected persons. Patients typically complain of numbness, tingling, and pain in the lower extremities. Symptoms are disproportionate to findings on gross sensory and motor evaluation. Beyond HIV infection itself, the most common cause is prior ART with stavudine or didanosine. Although not used commonly in Western countries, stavudine is still

being used in resource-limited settings through national ART programs. Caution should be used when administering these agents to patients with a history of peripheral neuropathy. Unfortunately, medication-induced neuropathy is not always reversed when the offending agent is discontinued. Patients with advanced disease may also develop peripheral neuropathy even if they have never taken ART. Evaluation should rule out other causes of sensory neuropathy such as alcoholism, thyroid disease, vitamin B_{12} deficiency, and syphilis.

B. Management—Treatment of peripheral neuropathy is aimed at symptomatic relief. Patients should be initially treated with gabapentin (start at 300 mg at bedtime and increase to 300–900 mg orally three times a day) or other co-analgesics for neuropathic pain (see Chapter 5). Opioid analgesics should be avoided because the condition tends to be chronic and patients are likely to become dependent on these agents without significant improvement in their well-being.

E. Rheumatologic and Bone Manifestations

Arthritis, involving single or multiple joints, with or without effusion, has been commonly noted in HIV-infected patients. Involvement of large joints is most common. Although the cause of HIV-related arthritis is unknown, most patients will respond to nonsteroidal anti-inflammatory medications. Patients with a sizable effusion, especially if the joint is warm or erythematous, should have the joint aspirated, followed by culture of the fluid to rule out suppurative arthritis as well as fungal and mycobacterial disease.

Several rheumatologic syndromes, including reactive arthritis, psoriatic arthritis, sicca syndrome, and systemic lupus erythematosus, have been reported in HIV-infected patients (see Chapter 20). However, it is unclear if the prevalence is greater than in the general population. Cases of avascular necrosis of the femoral heads have been reported sporadically, generally in the setting of advanced disease with long-standing infection and in patients receiving long-term ART. The etiology is not clear but is probably multifactorial in nature.

Osteoporosis and osteopenia appear to be more common in HIV-infected patients with chronic infection and perhaps associated with long-term use of ART. Vitamin D deficiency appears to be quite common among HIV-infected populations and monitoring vitamin D levels and replacement therapy for detected deficiency are recommended. Bone mineral density scans for postmenopausal women and for men over the age of 50 is also recommended.

F. Myopathy

Myopathies are infrequent in the era of effective ART but can be related to either HIV-infection or ART, particularly with use of zidovudine (azidothymidine [AZT]). Proximal muscle weakness is typical, and patients may have varying degrees of muscle tenderness. Given its long-term toxicities, zidovudine is no longer recommended when alternative treatments are available.

G. Retinitis

Complaints of visual changes must be evaluated immediately in HIV-infected patients by an ophthalmologist familiar with the manifestations of HIV disease. CMV retinitis, characterized by perivascular hemorrhages and white fluffy exudates, is the most common retinal infection in AIDS patients and can be rapidly progressive. In contrast, cotton wool spots, which are also common in HIV-infected people, are benign, remit spontaneously, and appear as small indistinct white spots without exudation or hemorrhage. Other rare retinal processes include other herpesvirus infections or toxoplasmosis. Choice of treatment for CMV retinitis (Table 31–3) depends on severity of lesions, their location, as well as the patient's overall condition and circumstances.

H. Oral Lesions

A. PRESENTATION—The presence of oral candidiasis or hairy leukoplakia is significant for several reasons. First, these lesions are highly suggestive of HIV infection in patients who have no other obvious cause of immunodeficiency. Second, several studies have indicated that patients with candidiasis have a high rate of progression to AIDS even with statistical adjustment for CD4 count.

Hairy leukoplakia is caused by the Epstein-Barr virus. The lesion is not usually troubling to patients and sometimes regresses spontaneously. Hairy leukoplakia is commonly seen as a white lesion on the lateral aspect of the tongue. It may be flat or slightly raised, is usually corrugated, and has vertical parallel lines with fine or thick ("hairy") projections. **Oral candidiasis** can be bothersome to patients, many of whom report an unpleasant taste or mouth dryness. The two most common forms of oral candidiasis seen are pseudomembranous (removable white plaques) and erythematous (red friable plaques).

B. MANAGEMENT—Treatment of oral candidiasis is with topical agents such as clotrimazole 10-mg troches (one troche four or five times a day). Patients with candidiasis who do not respond to topical antifungals can be treated with fluconazole (50–100 mg orally once a day for 3–7 days). Angular cheilitis—fissures at the sides of the mouth—is usually due to *Candida* as well and can be treated topically with ketoconazole cream (2%) twice a day.

Gingival disease is common in HIV-infected patients and is thought to be due to an overgrowth of microorganisms. It usually responds to professional dental cleaning and chlorhexidine rinses. A particularly aggressive gingivitis or periodontitis will develop in some HIV-infected patients; these patients should be given antibiotics that cover anaerobic oral flora (eg, metronidazole, 250 mg four times a day for 4 or 5 days) and referred to oral surgeons with experience with these entities.

Aphthous ulcers are painful and may interfere with eating. They can be treated with fluocinonide (0.05% ointment mixed 1:1 with plain Orabase and applied six times a day to the ulcer). For lesions that are difficult to reach, patients should use dexamethasone swishes (0.5 mg in 5 mL elixir three times a day). The pain of the ulcers can be relieved with use of an anesthetic spray (10% lidocaine).

Other lesions seen in the mouths of HIV-infected patients include Kaposi sarcoma (usually on the hard palate) and warts.

I. Gastrointestinal Manifestations

1. Candidal esophagitis—(See also Chapter 15.) Esophageal candidiasis is a common AIDS complication. In a patient with characteristic symptoms, empiric antifungal treatment is begun with fluconazole (100–200 mg orally daily for 14–21 days). Improvement in symptoms should be apparent within 1–2 days of antifungal treatment. If there is no improvement, further evaluation to identify other causes of esophagitis (herpes simplex, CMV) is recommended.

2. Hepatic disease—

A. PRESENTATION—Autopsy studies have demonstrated that the liver is a frequent site of infections and neoplasms in HIV-infected patients. However, many of these infections are not clinically symptomatic. Mild elevations of alkaline phosphatase and aminotransferases are often noted on routine chemistry panels. Mycobacterial disease, CMV, hepatitis B virus, hepatitis C virus, and lymphoma cause liver disease and can present with varying degrees of nausea, vomiting, right upper quadrant abdominal pain, and jaundice. Sulfonamides, imidazole medications, antituberculous medications, pentamidine, clarithromycin, and didanosine have also been associated with hepatitis. All nucleoside reverse transcriptase inhibitors cause lactic acidosis, which can be fatal. Lactic acidosis, however, occurs most commonly when didanosine is used with stavudine; this combination is no longer recommended in ART regimens. HIV-infected patients with chronic hepatitis may have more rapid progression of liver disease because of the concomitant immunodeficiency or hepatotoxicity of ART. Percutaneous liver biopsy may be helpful in diagnosing liver disease, but some common causes of liver disease (eg, *M avium* complex, lymphoma) can be determined by less invasive measures (eg, blood culture, biopsy of a more accessible site).

B. MANAGEMENT—With patients living longer as a result of advances in ART, advanced liver disease and hepatic failure due to chronic active hepatitis B and/or C are increasing causes of morbidity and mortality. HIV-infected individuals who are coinfected with hepatitis B should be treated with antiretroviral regimens that include medications with activity against both viruses (eg, lamivudine [3TC], emtricitabine [FTC], tenofovir [TDF]). It is important to be extremely cautious about discontinuing these medications in coinfected patients as sudden discontinuation could lead to a fatal flare of hepatitis B infection.

Hepatitis C is more virulent in persons with HIV and should be treated using the new HCV direct-acting antivirals. For treatment-naïve coinfected patients with genotype 1a (the most common hepatitis C genotype in the United States) the recommended regimens are (1) fixed-dose ledipasvir (90 mg)/sofosbuvir (400 mg) daily for 12 weeks, (2) fixed-dose paritaprevir (150 mg)/ritonavir (100 mg)/ombitasvir (25 mg) plus dasabuvir (250 mg twice daily) and weight-based ribavirin (1000 mg for patients weighing less than 75 kg and 1200 mg for patients weighing more than 75 kg) for 12 weeks (24 weeks for patients with cirrhosis), (3) sofosbuvir (400 mg) plus simeprevir (150 mg) with or without weight-based ribavirin (see previous regimen) for 12 weeks (24 weeks in patients with cirrhosis). Because there are no data to support one regimen over another, the least expensive regimen may be preferred. At the moment, all are very expensive, but it is hoped that competition between the regimens will ultimately reduce the price. Acid-reducing medicines should be avoided with ledipasvir and paritaprevir/ritonavir/ombitasvir/dasabuvir.

Although the recommended regimens are the same for HIV-infected patients potential drug interactions with ART may complicate treatment. Ledipasvir increases tenofovir levels. These two medications should be avoided in patients with creatinine clearance below 60 mL/min or in those taking these two medications and a ritonavir-boosted PI. Paritaprevir/ritonavir/ombitasvir/dasabuvir can be used safely with raltegravir, enfuvirtide, tenofovir, emtricitabine, lamivudine, and atazanavir. Simeprevir can be used safely with raltegravir, rilpivirine, maraviroc, enfuvirtide, tenofovir, emtricitabine, lamivudine, and abacavir. For hepatitis C treatment recommendations in patients with other scenarios (other medication interactions, genotypes, prior treatment, renal impairment), clinicians should consult the guidelines listed in the references below (see also Table 16–6).

Liver transplants have been performed successfully in HIV-infected patients. This strategy is most likely to be successful in persons who have CD4 counts greater than 100 cells/mcL and nondetectable viral loads.

3. Biliary disease—Cholecystitis presents with manifestations similar to those seen in immunocompetent hosts but is more likely to be acalculous. Sclerosing cholangitis and papillary stenosis have also been reported in HIV-infected patients. Typically, the syndrome presents with severe nausea, vomiting, and right upper quadrant pain. Liver function tests generally show alkaline phosphatase elevations disproportionate to elevation of the aminotransferases. Although dilated ducts can be seen on ultrasound, the diagnosis is made by endoscopic retrograde cholangiopancreatography, which reveals intraluminal irregularities of the proximal intrahepatic ducts with "pruning" of the terminal ductal branches. Stenosis of the distal common bile duct at the papilla is commonly seen with this syndrome. CMV, *Cryptosporidium*, and microsporidia are thought to play inciting roles in this syndrome but these conditions are rarely seen unless the patient is suffering with very advanced HIV-related immunodeficiency.

4. Enterocolitis—

A. PRESENTATION—Enterocolitis is a common problem in HIV-infected individuals. Organisms known to cause enterocolitis include bacteria (*Campylobacter*, *Salmonella*, *Shigella*), viruses (CMV, adenovirus), and protozoans (*Cryptosporidium*, *Entamoeba histolytica*, *Giardia*, *Isospora*, microsporidia). HIV itself may cause enterocolitis. Several of the organisms causing enterocolitis in HIV-infected individuals also cause diarrhea in immunocompetent

persons. However, HIV-infected patients tend to have more severe and more chronic symptoms, including high fevers and severe abdominal pain that can mimic acute abdominal catastrophes. Bacteremia and concomitant biliary involvement are also more common with enterocolitis in HIV-infected patients. Relapses of enterocolitis following adequate therapy have been reported with both *Salmonella* and *Shigella* infections.

Because of the wide range of agents known to cause enterocolitis, a stool culture and multiple stool examinations for ova and parasites (including modified acid-fast staining for *Cryptosporidium*) should be performed. Those patients who have *Cryptosporidium* in one stool with improvement in symptoms in less than 1 month should not be considered to have AIDS, as *Cryptosporidium* is a cause of self-limited diarrhea in HIV-negative persons. More commonly, HIV-infected patients with *Cryptosporidium* infection have persistent enterocolitis with profuse watery diarrhea.

B. MANAGEMENT—To date, no consistently effective treatments have been developed for *Cryptosporidium* infection. The most effective treatment of cryptosporidiosis is to improve immune function through the use of effective ART. The diarrhea can be treated symptomatically with diphenoxylate with atropine (one or two tablets orally three or four times a day). Those who do not respond may be given paregoric with bismuth (5–10 mL orally three or four times a day). Octreotide in escalating doses (starting at 0.05 mg subcutaneously every 8 hours for 48 hours) has been found to ameliorate symptoms in approximately 40% of patients with cryptosporidia or idiopathic HIV-associated diarrhea although the benefit is often short-lived.

Patients with a negative stool examination and persistent symptoms should be evaluated with colonoscopy and biopsy. Patients whose symptoms last longer than 1 month with no identified cause of diarrhea are considered to have a presumptive diagnosis of AIDS enteropathy. Patients may respond to institution of effective ART. Upper endoscopy with small bowel biopsy is not recommended as a routine part of the evaluation.

5. Other disorders—Two other important gastrointestinal abnormalities in HIV-infected patients are **gastropathy** and malabsorption. It has been documented that some HIV-infected patients do not produce normal levels of stomach acid and therefore are unable to absorb medications that require an acid medium. This decreased acid production may explain, in part, the susceptibility of HIV-infected patients to *Campylobacter*, *Salmonella*, and *Shigella*, all of which are sensitive to acid concentration. There is no evidence that *Helicobacter pylori* is more common in HIV-infected persons.

A **malabsorption** syndrome occurs commonly in AIDS patients. It can be due to infection of the small bowel with *M avium* complex, *Cryptosporidium*, or microsporidia.

J. Endocrinologic Manifestations

Hypogonadism is probably the most common endocrinologic abnormality in HIV-infected men. The adrenal gland is also a commonly afflicted endocrine gland in patients with AIDS. Abnormalities demonstrated on autopsy include infection (especially with CMV and *M avium* complex), infiltration with Kaposi sarcoma, and injury from hemorrhage and presumed autoimmunity. The prevalence of clinically significant adrenal insufficiency is low. Patients with suggestive symptoms should undergo a cosyntropin stimulation test.

Although frank deficiency of cortisol is rare, an isolated defect in mineralocorticoid metabolism may lead to salt-wasting and hyperkalemia. Such patients should be treated with fludrocortisone (0.1–0.2 mg orally daily).

AIDS patients appear to have abnormalities of thyroid function tests different from those of patients with other chronic diseases. AIDS patients have been shown to have high levels of triiodothyronine (T_3), thyroxine (T_4), and thyroid-binding globulin and low levels of reverse triiodothyronine (rT_3). The causes and clinical significance of these abnormalities are unknown.

K. Skin Manifestations

The skin manifestations that commonly develop in HIV-infected patients can be grouped into viral, bacterial, fungal, neoplastic, and nonspecific dermatitides.

1. Viral dermatitides—

A. Herpes simplex infections—These infections occur more frequently, tend to be more severe, and are more likely to disseminate in AIDS patients than in immunocompetent persons. Because of the risk of progressive local disease, **all herpes simplex attacks should be treated** for 5–10 days with acyclovir (400 mg orally three times a day), famciclovir (500 mg orally twice daily), or valacyclovir (500 mg orally twice daily) (Table 31–3). To avoid the complications of attacks, many clinicians recommend suppressive therapy for HIV-infected patients with a history of recurrent herpes. Options for suppressive therapy include acyclovir (400 mg orally twice daily), famciclovir (250 mg orally twice daily), and valacyclovir (500 mg orally daily). Long-term suppressive herpes prophylaxis with acyclovir does not reduce HIV transmission between heterosexual men and women from developing countries.

B. Herpes zoster—This is a common manifestation of HIV infection. As with herpes simplex infections, patients with zoster should be treated for 7–10 days with famciclovir (500 mg orally three times a day) or valacyclovir (500 mg three times a day). Acyclovir can also be used, but it requires very frequent dosing (800 mg orally four or five times per day for 7 days). Vesicular lesions should be cultured if there is any question about their origin, since herpes simplex responds to much lower doses of acyclovir. Disseminated zoster and cases with ocular involvement should be treated with intravenous (10 mg/kg every 8 hours for 7–10 days) rather than oral acyclovir. The **zoster vaccine** appears to be safe and immunogenic in HIV-infected patients over the age of 50 years with CD4 greater than 200/mcL, although the long-term benefit in preventing recurrences has yet to be established.

C. Molluscum contagiosum—This infection is caused by a pox virus and is seen in HIV infected patients, as in other immunocompromised patients. The characteristic umbilicated fleshy papular lesions have a propensity for spreading widely over the patient's face and neck and should be treated with topical liquid nitrogen.

2. Bacterial dermatitides

A. Staphylococcal infection—*Staphylococcus* is the most common bacterial cause of skin disease in HIV-infected patients; it usually presents as **folliculitis, superficial abscesses (furuncles),** or **bullous impetigo**. These lesions should be treated aggressively since sepsis can occur. Folliculitis is initially treated with topical clindamycin or mupirocin, and patients may benefit from regular washing with an antibacterial soap such as chlorhexidine. Intranasal mupirocin has been used successfully for staphylococcal decolonization in other settings. In HIV-infected patients with recurrent staphylococcal infections, weekly intranasal mupirocin should be considered in addition to topical care and systemic antibiotics. Abscesses often require incision and drainage. Patients may need anti-staphylococcal antibiotics as well. Due to high frequency of methicillin-resistant *Staphylococcus aureus* (MRSA) skin infections in HIV-infected populations, lesions should be cultured prior to initiating empiric antistaphylococcal therapy. Recommendations for empiric treatment are either (1) trimethoprim-sulfamethoxazole (one double-strength tablet orally twice daily) with or without clindamycin (500 mg orally three times daily); or (2) doxycycline (100 mg orally twice daily) with close follow-up.

B. Bacillary angiomatosis—It is caused by two closely related organisms: *Bartonella henselae* and *Bartonella quintana*. The epidemiology of these infections suggests zoonotic transmission from fleas of infected domestic cats. The most common manifestation is raised, reddish, highly vascular skin lesions that can mimic the lesions of Kaposi sarcoma. Fever is a common manifestation of this infection; involvement of bone, lymph nodes, and liver has also been reported. The infection responds to doxycycline, 100 mg orally twice daily, or erythromycin, 250 mg orally four times daily. Therapy is continued for at least 14 days, and patients who are seriously ill with visceral involvement may require months of therapy.

3. Fungal rashes—

A. Rashes due to dermatophytes and candida—The majority of **fungal rashes** afflicting AIDS patients are due to dermatophytes and *Candida*. These are particularly common in the inguinal region but may occur anywhere on the body. Fungal rashes generally respond well to topical clotrimazole (1% cream twice a day) or ketoconazole (2% cream twice a day).

B. Seborrheic dermatitis—This is more common in HIV-infected patients. Scrapings of seborrhea have revealed *Malassezia furfur (Pityrosporum ovale)*, implying that the seborrhea is caused by this fungus. Consistent with the isolation of this fungus is the clinical finding that seborrhea responds well to topical clotrimazole (1% cream) as well as hydrocortisone (1% cream).

4. Neoplastic dermatitides—See Chapter 6 and the Kaposi sarcoma section below.

5. Nonspecific dermatitides—

A. Xerosis—This condition presents in HIV-infected patients with severe pruritus. The patient may have no rash, or nonspecific excoriations from scratching. Treatment is with emollients (eg, absorption base cream) and antipruritic lotions (eg, camphor 9.5% and menthol 0.5%).

B. Psoriasis—Psoriasis can be very severe in HIV-infected patients. Phototherapy and etretinate (0.25–9.75 mg/kg/day orally in divided doses) may be used for recalcitrant cases in consultation with a dermatologist.

L. HIV-Related Malignancies

Four cancers are currently included in the CDC classification of AIDS: Kaposi sarcoma, non-Hodgkin lymphoma, primary lymphoma of the brain, and invasive cervical carcinoma. Epidemiologic studies have shown that between 1973 and 1987 among single men in San Francisco, the risk of Kaposi sarcoma increased more than 5000-fold and the risk of non-Hodgkin lymphoma more than 10-fold. The increase in incidence of malignancies is probably a function of impaired cell-mediated immunity. **In the current treatment era, cancers not classified as AIDS-related, such as lung cancer, are being increasingly diagnosed in aging HIV-infected individuals despite optimal ART treatment.** Cohort studies suggest that HIV-infected adults are at increased risk for a variety of cancers compared to age-matched uninfected populations. Mortality secondary to malignancies represents an increasing cause of death in HIV-infected populations.

1. Kaposi sarcoma—

A. Presentation—Lesions may appear anywhere; careful examination of the eyelids, conjunctiva, pinnae, palate, and toe webs is mandatory to locate potentially occult lesions. In light-skinned individuals, Kaposi lesions usually appear as purplish, nonblanching lesions that can be papular or nodular. In dark-skinned individuals, the lesions may appear more brown. In the mouth, lesions are most often palatal papules, though exophytic lesions of the tongue and gingivae may also be seen. Kaposi lesions may be confused with other vascular lesions such as angiomas and pyogenic granulomas. Kaposi sarcoma lesions can occur shortly after initiating ART, especially in patients starting ART who have advanced immunodeficiency. In this situation, Kaposi sarcoma is likely to be an immune reconstitution reaction (see Inflammatory Reactions below). Kaposi sarcoma can also cause visceral disease (eg, gastrointestinal, pulmonary).

B. Management—Patients with mild to moderate forms of Kaposi sarcoma do not require specific treatment as the lesions usually resolve with effective ART. However, it should be noted that the lesions may flare when ART is first initiated—probably as a result of an immune reconstitution process. Advanced disease is treated with combination chemotherapy (Table 31–3).

2. Non-Hodgkin lymphoma—

A. Presentation—Non-Hodgkin lymphoma in HIV-infected persons tends to be very aggressive. The malignancies are usually of B cell origin and characterized as diffuse large-cell tumors. Over 70% of the malignancies are extranodal.

B. Management—The prognosis of patients with systemic non-Hodgkin lymphoma depends primarily on the degree of immunodeficiency at the time of diagnosis. Patients with high CD4 counts do markedly better than those diagnosed at a late stage of illness. Patients with primary central nervous system lymphoma are treated with radiation. Response to treatment is good, but prior to the availability of ART, most patients died within a few months after diagnosis due to their underlying disease. Systemic disease is treated with combination chemotherapy (eg, EPOCH [etoposide, prednisolone, vincristine, cyclophosphamide, doxorubicin]) with rituximab. Granulocyte colony-stimulating factor (G-CSF; filgrastim) is used to maintain white blood counts.

3. Hodgkin disease—
Although Hodgkin disease is not included as part of the CDC definition of AIDS, studies have found that HIV infection is associated with a fivefold increase in the incidence of Hodgkin disease. HIV-infected persons with Hodgkin disease are more likely to have mixed cellularity and lymphocyte depletion subtypes of Hodgkin disease and to seek medical attention at an advanced stage of disease.

4. Anal dysplasia and squamous cell carcinoma—
These lesions have been strongly correlated with previous infection by human papillomavirus (HPV) and have been noted in HIV-infected men and women. Although many of the infected MSM report a history of anal warts or have visible warts, a significant percentage have silent papillomavirus infection. Cytologic (using Papanicolaou smears) and papillomavirus DNA studies can easily be performed on specimens obtained by anal swab. Because of the risk of progression from dysplasia to cancer in immunocompromised patients, **some experts suggest that annual anal swabs for cytologic examination should be done in all HIV-infected persons.** An anal Papanicolaou smear is performed by rotating a moistened Dacron swab about 2 cm into the anal canal. The swab is immediately inserted into a cytology bottle. However, there is no evidence that screening for anal cancer with Papanicolaou smears decreases the incidence of invasive cancer.

HPV also appears to play a causative role in **cervical dysplasia** and **neoplasia**. The incidence and clinical course of cervical disease in HIV-infected women are discussed below.

M. Gynecologic Manifestations

Vaginal candidiasis, cervical dysplasia and neoplasia, and pelvic inflammatory disease are more common in HIV-infected women than in uninfected women. These manifestations also tend to be more severe when they occur in association with HIV infection. Therefore, HIV-infected women need frequent gynecologic care. Vaginal candidiasis may be treated with topical agents or a single dose of oral fluconazole (150 mg) (see Chapter 36). Recurrent vaginal candidiasis should be treated with fluconazole (100–200 mg) for at least 7 days.

The incidence of cervical dysplasia in HIV-infected women is 40%. Because of this finding, recommended screening for **HIV-infected women is more extensive than for uninfected women** (see Chapter 18). For women younger than 30 years, a Papanicolaou smear should be performed within a year of the onset of sexual activity but no later than 21 years of age. If normal, Papanicolaou smears should be performed yearly. After three negative examinations, screening should be done every 3 years. HPV DNA testing of the cervical specimen is not recommended for women younger than 30 years of age.

For women 30 and older, screening should continue beyond age 65 unlike the general population. There are two accepted screening protocols, one using cytology alone, the other using cytology with HPV DNA cotesting. A Papanicolaou smear is done when HIV is diagnosed and every 12 months thereafter and after three negative examinations, ongoing screening should be performed every 3 years. Alternatively, a Papanicolaou smear with cotesting for HPV DNA can be performed when HIV is diagnosed or starting when patients are 30 years old. If Papanicolaou is normal and HPV test is negative, then the next screening would be in 3 years.

The management of abnormal Papanicolaou tests and positive HPV tests is the same in infected women as in uninfected women. Treatment should follow the consensus guidelines in the references below.

While pelvic inflammatory disease appears to be more common in HIV-infected women, the bacteriology of this condition appears to be the same as among HIV-uninfected women. HIV-infected women with pelvic inflammatory disease should be treated with the same regimens as uninfected women (see Chapter 18).

N. Coronary Artery Disease

HIV-infected persons are at higher risk for coronary artery disease than age- and sex-matched controls. Part of this increase in coronary artery disease is due to changes in lipids caused by antiretroviral agents (see Treatment section on Antiretroviral Therapy below), especially stavudine and several of the PIs. However, some of the risk appears to be due to HIV infection, independent of its therapy. It is important that clinicians pay close attention to this issue because myocardial infarctions tend to present at a younger age in HIV-infected individuals than in HIV-uninfected individuals. HIV-infected patients with symptoms of coronary artery disease such as chest pain or dyspnea should be rapidly evaluated. Clinicians should aggressively treat conditions that result in increased risk of heart disease, especially smoking, hypertension, hyperlipidemia, obesity, diabetes mellitus, and sedentary lifestyle.

O. Inflammatory Reactions (Immune Reconstitution Inflammatory Syndromes)

With initiation of ART, some patients experience inflammatory reactions that appear to be associated with immune reconstitution as indicated by a rapid increase in CD4 count. These inflammatory reactions may present with generalized signs of fevers, sweats, and malaise with or without more localized manifestations that usually represent unusual presentations of opportunistic infections. For example, vitreitis has developed in patients with CMV retinitis after they have been treated with ART.

M avium can present as focal even suppurative lymphadenitis or granulomatous masses in patients receiving ART. Tuberculosis may paradoxically worsen with new or evolving pulmonary infiltrates and lymphadenopathy. PML and cryptococcal meningitis may also behave atypically. Clinicians should be alert to these syndromes, which are most often seen in patients who have initiated ART in the setting of advanced disease and who show rapid increases in CD4 counts with treatment. The diagnosis of immune reconstitution inflammatory syndrome (IRIS) is one of exclusion and can be made only after recurrence or new opportunistic infection has been ruled out as the cause of the clinical deterioration. Management of IRIS is conservative and supportive with use of corticosteroids only for severe reactions. Most authorities recommend that ART be continued unless the reaction is life-threatening.

American Association for the Study of Liver Diseases and Infectious Diseases Society of America. HCV Guidance: Recommendations for testing, managing, and treating hepatitis C 2015. http://www.hcvguidelines.org/full-report-view

Massad LS et al. 2012 updated consensus guidelines for the management of abnormal cervical cancer screening tests and cancer precursors. J Low Genit Tract Dis. 2013 Apr;17 (5 Suppl 1):S1–27. Erratum in: J Low Genit Tract Dis. 2013 Jul;17(3):367. [PMID: 23519301]

Silverberg MJ et al; North American AIDS Cohort Collaboration on Research and Design of the International Epidemiologic Databases to Evaluate AIDS. Cumulative incidence of cancer among persons with HIV in North America: a cohort study. Ann Intern Med. 2015 Oct 6;163(7):507–18. [PMID: 26436616]

► Prevention

A. Primary Prevention

Until vaccination is a reality, prevention of HIV infection will depend on HIV testing and counseling, including precautions regarding sexual practices and injection drug use, initiation of ART as a prevention tool for transmission to others, preexposure and postexposure use of ART, perinatal management including ART therapy for the mother, screening of blood products, and infection control practices in the health care setting.

1. HIV testing and counseling—Primary care clinicians should routinely obtain a sexual history and provide risk factor assessment of their patients. Because approximately one-fifth of the HIV-infected persons in the United States do not know they are infected, the **USPSTF recommends that clinicians screen for HIV infection in adolescents and adults ages 15 to 65 years. Younger adolescents and older adults who are at increased risk should also be screened**. Clinicians should review the risk factors for HIV infection with the patient and discuss safer sex and safer needle use as well as the meaning of a positive test. Although the CDC recommends "opt-out" testing in medical settings, some states require specific written consent.

For persons whose test results are positive, it is critically important that they be connected to ongoing medical care. Referrals for partner-notification services, social services, mental health services, and HIV-prevention services should also be provided. Prevention interventions focused on the importance of HIV-infected persons not putting others at risk have been successful.

For patients whose test results are negative, clinicians should review safer sex and needle use practices, including counseling not to exchange bodily fluids unless they are in a long-term mutually monogamous relationship with someone who has tested HIV antibody-negative and has not engaged in unsafe sex, injection drug use, or other HIV risk behaviors for at least 6 months prior to or at any time since the negative test.

To prevent sexual transmission of HIV, only latex condoms should be used, along with a water-soluble lubricant. Although nonoxynol-9, a spermicide, kills HIV, it is contraindicated because in some patients it may cause genital ulcers that could facilitate HIV transmission. Patients should be counseled that condoms are not 100% effective. They should be made familiar with the use of condoms, including, specifically, the advice that condoms must be used every time, that space should be left at the tip of the condom as a receptacle for semen, that intercourse with a condom should not be attempted if the penis is only partially erect, that men should hold on to the base of the condom when withdrawing the penis to prevent slippage, and that condoms should not be reused. Although anal intercourse remains the sexual practice at highest risk for transmitting HIV, seroconversions have been documented with vaginal and oral intercourse as well. Therefore, condoms should be used when engaging in these activities. Women as well as men having sex with men should understand how to use condoms to be sure that their partners are using them correctly. Partners of HIV-infected women should use latex barriers such as dental dams (available at dental supply stores) to prevent direct oral contact with vaginal secretions. Several randomized trials in Africa demonstrated that male circumcision significantly reduced HIV incidence in men, but there are a number of barriers to performing widespread circumcisions among men in Africa.

Persons using injection drugs should be cautioned never to share needles or other drug paraphernalia. When sterile needles are not available, bleach does appear to inactivate HIV and should be used to clean needles.

2. ART for decreasing transmission of HIV to others— Besides preventing progression of HIV disease, effective ART likely decreases the risk of HIV transmission between sexual partners. Among serodiscordant couples, **early ART almost completely eliminates the risk of HIV transmission to the uninfected partner.** Although HIV-negative persons in stable long-term partnerships with HIV-infected persons represent only one group of at risk persons, theoretically increasing the use of ART among the population of HIV-infected persons could decrease community wide transmission of HIV. However, even patients who have been treated with antiretrovirals and have undetectable viral loads must practice safer sex and not share needles so as to avoid the possibility of transmitting HIV.

3. Preexposure ART prophylaxis—Several large randomized double-blind placebo-controlled trials demonstrated that administering emtricitabine/tenofovir (Truvada) can reduce the risk of sexual transmission of HIV among uninfected individuals at high risk for infection; one study was of HIV-negative men and transgender women who have sex with men, two studies were of heterosexual HIV-discordant couples. Preexposure tenofovir has also been shown to reduce HIV infection among injection drug users from Thailand. The combination of emtricitabine/tenofovir is recommended for preexposure prophylaxis (PrEP) by the CDC for use in HIV-negative persons at risk for infection.

4. Postexposure prophylaxis for sexual and drug use exposures to HIV—The goal of postexposure prophylaxis is to reduce or prevent local viral replication prior to dissemination such that the infection can be aborted. Although there is no proof that administration of antiretroviral medications following a sexual or parenteral drug use exposure reduces the likelihood of infection, there is suggestive data from animal models, perinatal experience, and a case-control study of health care workers who experienced a needle stick.

The choice of antiretroviral agents and the duration of treatment are the same as those for exposures that occur through the occupational route; the preferred regimen is tenofovir 300 mg with emtricitabine 200 mg daily with raltegravir 400 mg twice a day. Some clinicians prescribe a two-drug regimen of tenofovir 300 mg and emtricitabine 200 mg (Truvada) because it is simpler for patients to take (single pill once a day), and more affordable for individuals and for public entities that provide this service to uninsured persons. In contrast to those with occupational exposures, some individuals may present very late after exposure. Because the likelihood of success declines with length of time from HIV exposure, **treatment should be provided as soon as possible, and it is not recommended that treatment be offered more than 72 hours after exposure.** In addition, because the psychosocial issues involved with postexposure prophylaxis for sexual and drug use exposures are complex, it should be offered with prevention counseling. Counseling should focus on how to prevent future exposures. Clinicians needing more information on postexposure prophylaxis for occupational or nonoccupational exposures should contact the National Clinicians' Postexposure Hotline (1-888-448-4911; http://nccc.ucsf.edu/clinician-consultation/pep-post-exposure-prophylaxis/).

5. Prevention of perinatal transmission of HIV—Prevention of perinatal transmission of HIV begins by offering HIV counseling and testing to all women who are pregnant or considering pregnancy. HIV-infected women who are pregnant should start ART with at least three medications. Recommended regimens are zidovudine and lamivudine with either ritonavir-boosted lopinavir or ritonavir-boosted atazanavir. Cesarean delivery should be planned if HIV viral load is greater than 1000 copies near the time of delivery. Zidovudine should be given to the infant after birth for 6 weeks. When possible, breastfeeding should be avoided.

6. Prevention of HIV transmission in health care settings— In health care settings, universal body fluid precautions should be used, including use of gloves when handling body fluids and the addition of gown, mask, and goggles for procedures that may result in splash or droplet spread, and use of specially designed needles with sheath devices to decrease the risk of needle sticks. Because transmission of tuberculosis may occur in health care settings, all patients with cough should be encouraged to wear masks. Hospitalized HIV-infected patients with cough should be placed in respiratory isolation until tuberculosis can be excluded by chest radiograph and sputum smear examination.

Epidemiologic studies show that needle sticks occur commonly among health care professionals, especially among surgeons performing invasive procedures, inexperienced hospital housestaff, and medical students. Efforts to reduce needle sticks should focus on avoiding recapping needles and use of safety needles whenever doing invasive procedures under controlled circumstances. **The risk of HIV transmission from a needle stick with blood from an HIV-infected patient is about 1:300.** The risk is higher with deep punctures, large inoculum, and source patients with high viral loads. The risk from mucous membrane contact is too low to quantitate.

Health care professionals who sustain needle sticks should be counseled and offered HIV testing as soon as possible. HIV testing is done to establish a negative baseline for worker's compensation claims in case there is a subsequent conversion. Follow-up testing is usually performed at 6 weeks, 3 months, and 6 months. With the patient's permission, their blood can be tested for HIV antibody and HIV viral load.

A case-control study by the CDC indicates that administration of zidovudine following a needle stick decreases the rate of HIV seroconversion by 79%. Therefore, **providers should be offered ART as soon as possible after exposure and continued for 4 weeks.** The preferred regimen is tenofovir 300 mg with emtricitabine 200 mg (Truvada) daily with raltegravir 400 mg twice a day. Providers who have exposures to persons who are likely to have antiretroviral medication resistance (eg, persons receiving therapy who have detectable viral loads) should have their therapy individualized, using at least two medications to which the source is unlikely to be resistant. Because reports have noted hepatotoxicity due to nevirapine in this setting, this agent should be avoided. Unfortunately, there have been documented cases of seroconversion following potential parenteral exposure to HIV despite prompt use of zidovudine prophylaxis. Counseling of the provider should include "safer sex" guidelines.

7. Prevention of transmission of HIV through blood or blood products—Current efforts in the United States to screen blood and blood products have lowered the risk of HIV transmission with transfusion of a unit of blood to 1:1,000,000. Use of blood and blood products should be judicious, with patients receiving the least amount necessary, and patients should be encouraged to donate their own blood prior to elective procedures.

8. HIV vaccine—Primate model data have suggested that development of a protective vaccine may be possible, but clinical trials in humans have been disappointing. Only one vaccine trial has shown any degree of efficacy. In this randomized, double-blind, placebo-controlled trial, a recombinant canarypox vector vaccine plus two booster injections of a recombinant gp120 vaccine was moderately efficacious (26–31%) in reducing the risk of HIV among a primarily heterosexual population in Thailand. Vaccine development efforts are aimed at identifying broadly neutralizing antibodies to the highly conserved regions of the HIV envelope.

Gallo RC. Developing a successful HIV vaccine. J Infect Dis. 2015 Jul 15;212(Suppl 1):S40–1. [PMID: 26116730]

Kuhar DT et al. Updated US Public Health Service guidelines for the management of occupational exposures to human immunodeficiency virus and recommendations for postexposure prophylaxis. Infect Control Hosp Epidemiol. 2013 Sep;34 (9):875–92. [PMID: 23917901]

Marrazzo JM et al. HIV prevention in clinical care settings: 2014 recommendations of the International Antiviral Society-USA Panel. JAMA. 2014 Jul 23–30;312(4):390–409. Erratum in: JAMA. 2014 Aug 13;312(6):652. [PMID: 25038358]

McCormack S et al. Pre-exposure prophylaxis to prevent the acquisition of HIV-1 infection (PROUD): effectiveness results from the pilot phase of a pragmatic open-label randomised trial. Lancet. 2016 Jan 2;387(10013):53–60. [PMID: 26364263]

New York State Department of Health AIDS Institute. HIV prophylaxis following non-occupational exposure. October 2014 update. http://www.hivguidelines.org/wp-content/uploads/ 2014/12/hiv-prophylaxis-following-non-occupational-exposure.pdf

U.S. Preventive Services Task Force. Screening for HIV: U.S. Preventive Services Task Force Recommendation Statement. April 2013. http://www.uspreventiveservicestaskforce.org/uspstf13/hiv/hivfinalrs.htm

U.S. Public Health Service. Preexposure prophylaxis for the prevention of HIV infection in the United States—2014: a clinical practice guideline. http://www.cdc.gov/hiv/pdf/PrEPguidelines2014.pdf

Volk JE et al. No new HIV infections with increasing use of HIV preexposure prophylaxis in a clinical practice setting. Clin Infect Dis. 2015 Nov 15;61(10):1601–3. [PMID: 26334052]

B. Secondary Prevention

In the era prior to the development of effective ART, cohort studies of individuals with documented dates of seroconversion demonstrate that AIDS developed within 10 years in approximately 50% of untreated seropositive persons. With currently available treatment, progression of disease has been markedly decreased. In addition to antiretroviral treatment, prophylactic regimens can prevent opportunistic infections and improve survival. Prophylaxis and early intervention prevent several infectious diseases, including tuberculosis and syphilis, which are transmissible to others. Recommendations for screening tests, vaccinations, and prophylaxis are listed in Table 31–4.

1. Tuberculosis—Because of the increased occurrence of tuberculosis among HIV-infected patients, all such individuals should undergo **annual PPD testing.** Although anergy is common among AIDS patients, the likelihood of a false-negative result is much lower when the test is done early in infection. Those with positive tests (defined for HIV-infected patients as greater than 5 mm of induration) need a chest radiograph. Patients with an infiltrate in any location, especially if accompanied by

Table 31–4. Health care maintenance and monitoring of HIV-infected individuals.

For all HIV-infected individuals:
CD4 counts every 3–6 months (Can decrease to every 12 months if viral load suppressed on ART for 2 years and CD4 count greater than 300 cells/mcL)
Viral load tests every 3–6 months and 1 month following a change in therapy
Genotypic resistance testing at baseline and if viral load not fully suppressed and patient taking ART
Complete blood count, chemistry profile, transaminases and total bilirubin, at baseline and every 3–6 months
Urinalysis at baseline and annually during ART (every 6 months if ART regimen includes TDF)
Fasting glucose or hemoglogin A$_{1c}$ at baseline and annually during ART
Fasting lipid panel at baseline, 4–8 weeks after starting or changing an ART regimen that affects lipids, and annually for everyone over 40 years of age
PPD annually
INH for those with positive PPD and normal chest radiograph
RPR or VDRL at entry and periodically based on sexual activity
Toxoplasma IgG serology at baseline
Hepatitis serologies: hepatitis A antibody, hepatitis B surface antigen, hepatitis B surface antibody, hepatitis B core antibody, hepatitis C antibody
Pneumococcal vaccine
Inactivated influenza vaccine annually in season
Hepatitis A vaccine for those without immunity to hepatitis A
Hepatitis B vaccine for those who are hepatitis B surface antigen and antibody negative. (Use 40 mcg formulation at 0, 1, and 6 months; repeat if no immunity 1 month after three-vaccine series.)
Combined tetanus, diphtheria, pertussis vaccine
Human papillomavirus vaccine for HIV-infected women age 26 years or less
Haemophilus influenzae type b vaccination
Bone mineral density monitoring for postmenopausal women and men 50 years of age or older
Papanicolaou smears annually; if three smears are negative, can switch to longer intervals (see Complications, Section M)
Consider anal swabs for cytologic evaluation
For HIV-infected individuals with CD4 less than 200 cells/mcL:
Pneumocystis jirovecii prophylaxis (see Prophylactic Treatment of Complications of HIV Infection section under Treatment and Table 31–5)
For HIV-infected individuals with CD4 less than 75 cells/mcL:
Mycobacterium avium complex prophylaxis (see Prophylaxis of Opportunistic Infections section under Treatment)
For HIV-infected individuals with CD4 less than 50 cells/mcL:
Consider CMV prophylaxis

ART, antiretroviral therapy; BUN, blood urea nitrogen; CMV, cytomegalovirus; IgG, immunoglobulin G; INH, isoniazid; PPD, purified protein derivative; RPR, rapid plasma reagin; VDRL, Venereal Disease Research Laboratories.

mediastinal adenopathy, should have sputum sent for acid-fast staining. Patients with a positive PPD but negative evaluations for active disease should receive isoniazid (300 mg orally daily) with pyridoxine (50 mg orally daily) for 9 months to a year. Blood tests can also be used to assess prior tuberculosis exposure. Blood samples are mixed with synthetic antigens representing *M tuberculosis*. Patients infected with *M tuberculosis* produce interferon-gamma in response to contact with the antigens. Unlike the PPD, the patient does not have to return for a second visit. The test is less likely to result in false-positive results than a PPD. HIV-infected persons with a CD4 count less than 100 cells may not respond to the Mitogen positive control; their results will be reported as indeterminate by QuantiFERON.

2. Syphilis—Because of the increased number of cases of syphilis among MSM, including those who are HIV infected, **all such men should be screened for syphilis by rapid plasma reagin (RPR) or Venereal Disease Research Laboratories (VDRL) test every 6 months.** Increases of syphilis cases among HIV-infected persons are of particular concern because these individuals are at increased risk for reactivation of syphilis and progression to tertiary syphilis despite standard treatment. Because the only widely available tests for syphilis are serologic and because HIV-infected individuals are known to have disordered antibody production, there is concern about the interpretation of these titers. This concern has been fueled by a report of an HIV-infected patient with secondary syphilis and negative syphilis serologic testing. Furthermore, HIV-infected individuals may lose fluorescent treponemal antibody absorption (FTA-ABS) reactivity after treatment for syphilis, particularly if they have low CD4 counts. Thus, in this population, a nonreactive treponemal test does not rule out a past history of syphilis. In addition, persistence of treponemes in the spinal fluid after one dose of benzathine penicillin has been demonstrated in HIV-infected patients with primary and secondary syphilis. Therefore, **the CDC has recommended an aggressive diagnostic approach to HIV-infected patients with reactive RPR or VDRL tests of longer than 1 year or unknown duration.** All such patients should have a lumbar puncture with cerebrospinal fluid cell count and cerebrospinal fluid VDRL. Those with a normal cerebrospinal fluid evaluation are treated as having late latent syphilis (benzathine penicillin G, 2.4 million units intramuscularly weekly for 3 weeks) with follow-up titers. Those with a pleocytosis or a positive cerebrospinal fluid-VDRL test are treated as having neurosyphilis (aqueous penicillin G, 2–4 million units intravenously every 4 hours, or procaine penicillin G, 2.4 million units intramuscularly daily, with probenecid, 500 mg four times daily, for 10 days) followed by weekly benzanthine penicillin G 2.4 million units intramuscularly for 3 weeks. Some clinicians take a less aggressive approach to patients who have low titers (less than 1:8), a history of having been treated for syphilis, and a normal neurologic examination. Close follow-up of titers is mandatory if such a course is taken. For a more detailed discussion of this topic, see Chapter 34.

3. Immunizations—HIV-infected individuals should receive immunizations as outlined in Table 31–4. Patients without evidence of hepatitis B surface antigen or surface antibody should receive hepatitis B vaccination, using the 40 mcg formulation; the higher dose is to increase the chance of developing protective immunity. If the patient does not have immunity 1 month after the three-shot series, then the series should be repeated. HIV-infected persons should also receive the standard inactivated vaccines such as tetanus and diphtheria boosters that would be given to uninfected persons. **Most live vaccines, such as yellow fever vaccine, should be avoided.** Measles vaccination, while a live virus vaccine, appears relatively safe when administered to HIV-infected individuals and should be given if the patient has never had measles or been adequately vaccinated. The herpes zoster vaccine, two doses 6 weeks apart, has been found to be reasonably safe for HIV-infected persons with CD4 counts greater than 200 cells/mL and undetectable viral loads even though it is a live vaccine. However, it is not known if it is efficacious in preventing herpes zoster in this population.

4. Other measures—A randomized study found that multivitamin supplementation decreased HIV disease progression and mortality in HIV-infected women in Africa. However, supplementation is unlikely to be as effective in well-nourished populations.

HIV-infected individuals should be counseled with regard to the importance of practicing safer sex even with other HIV-infected persons because of the possibility of contracting a sexually transmitted disease, such as gonorrhea or syphilis. There is also the possibility of transmission of a particularly virulent or a drug-resistant strain between HIV infected persons. Substance abuse treatment should be recommended for persons who are using recreational drugs. They should be warned to avoid consuming raw meat, eggs, or shellfish to avoid infections with *Toxoplasma*, *Campylobacter*, and *Salmonella*. HIV-infected patients should wash their hands thoroughly after cleaning cat litter or should forgo this household chore to avoid possible exposure to toxoplasmosis. To reduce the likelihood of infection with *Bartonella* species, patients should avoid activities that might result in cat scratches or bites. Although the data are not conclusive, many clinicians recommend that HIV-infected persons—especially those with low CD4 counts—drink bottled water instead of tap water to prevent cryptosporidia infection.

Because of the emotional impact of HIV infection and subsequent illness, many patients will benefit from supportive counseling.

▶ Treatment

Treatment for HIV infection can be broadly divided into the following categories: (1) prophylaxis for opportunistic infections, malignancies, and other complications of HIV infection; (2) treatment of opportunistic infections, malignancies, and other complications of HIV infection; and (3) treatment of the HIV infection itself with combination ART.

A. Prophylactic Treatment of Complications of HIV Infection

In general, decisions about prophylaxis of opportunistic infections are based on the CD4 count, recent HIV viral load, and a history of having had the infection in the past. In the era prior to ART, patients who started taking prophylactic regimens were maintained on them indefinitely. However, **studies have shown that in patients with robust improvements in immune function—as measured by increases in CD4 counts above the levels that are used to initiate treatment—prophylactic regimens can safely be discontinued.**

Because individuals with advanced HIV infection are susceptible to a number of opportunistic pathogens, the use of agents with activity against more than one pathogen is preferable.

1. Prophylaxis against *Pneumocystis* pneumonia—Patients with CD4 counts below 200 cells/mcL, a CD4 lymphocyte percentage below 14%, or weight loss or oral candidiasis should be offered primary prophylaxis for *Pneumocystis* pneumonia. Patients with a history of *Pneumocystis* pneumonia should receive secondary prophylaxis until their viral load is undetectable and they have maintained a CD4 count of 200 cells/mcL or more while receiving ART for longer than 3 months. Regimens for *Pneumocystis* prophylaxis are given in Table 31–5.

Table 31–5. *Pneumocystis jirovecii* prophylaxis, in order of preference.

Medication	Dose	Side Effects	Limitations
Trimethoprim–sulfamethoxazole	One double-strength tablet three times a week to one tablet daily	Rash, neutropenia, hepatitis, Stevens-Johnson syndrome	Hypersensitivity reaction is common but, if mild, it may be possible to treat through.
Dapsone	50–100 mg orally daily or 100 mg two or three times per week	Anemia, nausea, methemoglobinemia, hemolytic anemia	Less effective than above. Glucose-6-phosphate dehydrogenase (G6PD) level should be checked prior to therapy. Check methemoglobin level after 1 month of treatment.
Atovaquone	1500 mg orally daily with a meal	Rash, diarrhea, nausea	Less effective than suspension trimethoprim-sulfamethoxazole; equal efficacy to dapsone, but more expensive.
Aerosolized pentamidine	300 mg monthly	Bronchospasm (pretreat with bronchodilators); rare reports of pancreatitis	Apical *P jirovecii* pneumonia, extrapulmonary *P jirovecii* infections, pneumothorax.

2. Prophylaxis against *M avium* complex infection—
Patients whose CD4 counts fall to below 75–100 cells/mcL should be given prophylaxis against *M avium* complex infection. Clarithromycin (500 mg orally twice daily) and azithromycin (1200 mg orally weekly) have both been shown to decrease the incidence of disseminated *M avium* complex infection by approximately 75%, with a low rate of breakthrough of resistant disease. The azithromycin regimen is generally preferred based on high compliance and low cost. Prophylaxis against *M avium* complex infection may be discontinued in patients whose CD4 counts rise above 100 cells/mcL in response to ART for longer than 3 months.

3. Prophylaxis against *M tuberculosis* infection—Isoniazid, 300 mg orally daily, plus pyridoxine, 50 mg orally daily, for 9–12 months should be given to all HIV-infected patients with positive PPD reactions (defined as greater than 5 mm of induration for HIV-infected patients) without evidence of active disease.

4. Prophylaxis against toxoplasmosis—Toxoplasmosis prophylaxis is desirable in patients with a positive IgG toxoplasma serology and CD4 counts below 100 cells/mcL. Trimethoprim-sulfamethoxazole (one double-strength tablet daily) offers good protection against toxoplasmosis, as does a combination of pyrimethamine, 25 mg orally once a week, plus dapsone, 50 mg orally daily, plus leucovorin, 25 mg orally once a week. A glucose-6-phosphate dehydrogenase (G6PD) level should be checked prior to dapsone therapy, and a methemoglobin level should be checked at 1 month. Prophylaxis can be discontinued when the CD4 cells have increased to greater than 200 cells/mcL for more than 3 months.

B. Treatment of Complications of HIV Infection

Treatment of common AIDS-related complications is detailed above and in Table 31–3. In the era prior to the use of ART, patients required lifelong treatment for many infections, including CMV retinitis, toxoplasmosis, and cryptococcal meningitis. However, **among patients who have a good response to ART, maintenance therapy for some opportunistic infections can be terminated.** For example, in consultation with an ophthalmologist, maintenance treatment for CMV infection can be discontinued when persons receiving ART have had a sustained increase in CD4 count to greater than 100 cells/mcL for at least 3–6 months. Similar results have been observed in patients with *M avium* complex bacteremia, who have completed a year or more of therapy for *M avium* complex and have an increase in their CD4 count for greater than 6 months while receiving ART. Cessation of secondary prophylaxis for *Pneumocystis* pneumonia is described above.

Treating patients with repeated episodes of the same opportunistic infection can pose difficult therapeutic challenges. For example, patients with second or third episodes of *Pneumocystis* pneumonia may have developed allergic reactions to standard treatments with a prior episode. Fortunately, there are several alternatives available for the treatment of *Pneumocystis* infection. Trimethoprim with dapsone and primaquine with clindamycin are two

combinations that often are tolerated in patients with a prior allergic reaction to trimethoprim-sulfamethoxazole and intravenous pentamidine. Patients in whom second episodes of *Pneumocystis* pneumonia develop while taking prophylaxis tend to have milder courses.

Adjunctive Treatments—Epoetin alfa (erythropoietin) is approved for use in HIV-infected patients with anemia, including those with anemia secondary to zidovudine use. As zidovudine is rarely used now, especially at high doses, the use of epoetin alfa has also decreased. An erythropoietin level greater than 500 milli-units/mL should be demonstrated before starting therapy. The starting dose of epoetin alfa is 8000 units subcutaneously three times a week. Hypertension is the most common side effect.

Human G-CSF (filgrastim) and **granulocyte-macrophage colony-stimulating factor (GM-CSF [sargramostim])** have been shown to increase the neutrophil counts of HIV-infected patients. Because of the high cost of this therapy, the dosage should be closely monitored and minimized, aiming for a neutrophil count of 1000/mcL. When the medication is used for indications other than cytotoxic chemotherapy, one or two doses at 5 mcg/kg per week subcutaneously are usually sufficient.

C. Antiretroviral Therapy

The availability of agents that in combination suppress HIV replication (Table 31–6) has had a profound impact on the natural history of HIV infection. Indeed, **with the advent of effective ART, the life expectancy of HIV-infected persons approaches that of uninfected persons when treatment is initiated early in the course of the disease.**

The recognition that HIV damages the immune system from the beginning of infection, even when the damage is not easily measured by conventional tests, combined with the greater potency, the improved side effect profile, and the decreased pill burden of modern HIV regimens, have led to the recommendation to **start treatment for all HIV-infected persons regardless of CD4 count,** which is supported by the World Health Organization. The START trial demonstrated that immediate treatment is associated with a greater than 50% reduction in risk for serious illness or death, compared to delaying treatment until the CD4 count falls below 350 cells/mcL. Because 5–20% of patients in developed countries who are treatment-naïve have a virus that is resistant to some medications, **resistance testing is recommended for all patients prior to initiating ART.**

Once a decision to initiate therapy has been made, several important principles should guide therapy. First, because medication resistance to antiretroviral agents develops in HIV-infected patients, **a primary goal of therapy should be complete suppression of viral replication as measured by the serum viral load.** Therapy that achieves undetectable viral load has been shown to provide a durable response to the therapy. To achieve this and maintain virologic control over time, **combination therapy with at least three medications from at least two different classes is necessary,** and partially suppressive combinations such as dual nucleoside therapy should be

Table 31–6. Antiretroviral therapy.

Medication	Dose	Common Side Effects	Special Monitoring[1]	Cost[2]	Cost/Month
Nucleoside reverse transcriptase inhibitors					
Abacavir (Ziagen)	300 mg orally twice daily	Rash, fever—if occur, rechallenge may be fatal	No special monitoring	$10.04/300 mg	$602.40
Didanosine (ddI) (Videx)	400 mg orally daily (enteric-coated capsule) for persons greater or equal to 60 kg 250 mg orally daily (enteric-coated capsule) for persons 30–59 kg	Peripheral neuropathy, pancreatitis, dry mouth, hepatitis	Bimonthly neurologic questionnaire for neuropathy, potassium, amylase, bilirubin, triglycerides	$12.29/400 mg	$368.72
Emtricitabine (Emtriva)	200 mg orally once daily	Skin discoloration palms/soles (mild)	No special monitoring	$21.46/200 mg	$643.82
Lamivudine (3TC) (Epivir)	150 mg orally twice daily or 300 mg daily	Rash, peripheral neuropathy	No special monitoring	$7.16/150 mg	$429.60
Stavudine (d4T) (Zerit)	40 mg orally twice daily for persons ≥ 60 kg 30 mg orally twice daily for persons < 60 kg	Peripheral neuropathy, hepatitis, pancreatitis	Monthly neurologic questionnaire for neuropathy, amylase	$6.85/40 mg	$410.70
Zidovudine (AZT) (Retrovir)	600 mg orally daily in two divided doses	Anemia, neutropenia, nausea, malaise, headache, insomnia, myopathy	CBC with differential 4–8 weeks after starting AZT	$6.02/300 mg	$360.97
Nucleotide reverse transcriptase inhibitors					
Tenofovir TDF (Viread)	300 mg orally once daily	Renal failure, bone resorption, gastrointestinal distress	Creatinine every 3–4 months, urine analysis every 6 months	$39.91/300 mg	$1197.32
Nonnucleoside reverse transcriptase inhibitors (NNRTIs)					
Delavirdine (Rescriptor)	400 mg orally three times daily	Rash	No special monitoring	$2.75/200 mg	$494.62
Efavirenz (Sustiva)	600 mg orally daily	Neurologic disturbances, rash	No special monitoring	$37.00/600 mg	$1110.13
Etravirine (Intelence)	200 mg orally twice daily	Rash, peripheral neuropathy	No special monitoring	$10.90/100 mg	$1308.06
Nevirapine (Viramune)	200 mg orally daily for 2 weeks, then 200 mg orally twice daily	Rash	No special monitoring	$10.83/200 mg	$649.80
Rilpivirine (Edurant)	25 mg daily	Depression, rash	No special monitoring	$35.84/25 mg	$1075.15
Protease inhibitors (PIs)					
Fosamprenavir (Lexiva)	**For PI-experienced patients:** 700 mg orally twice daily and 100 mg of ritonavir orally twice daily **For PI-naïve patients:** 1400 mg orally twice daily or 1400 mg orally once daily and 200 mg of ritonavir orally once daily	Gastrointestinal, rash	No special monitoring	$21.47/700 mg	$1288.02–2576.04 (plus cost of ritonavir for lower dose)
Indinavir (Crixivan)	800 mg orally three times daily	Renal calculi	Bilirubin level every 3–4 months	$3.05/400 mg	$548.12

(continued)

Table 31–6. Antiretroviral therapy. (continued)

Medication	Dose	Common Side Effects	Special Monitoring[1]	Cost[2]	Cost/Month
Lopinavir/ritonavir (Kaletra)	400 mg/100 mg orally twice daily	Diarrhea	No special monitoring	$9.22/200 mg (lopinavir)	$1106.29
Nelfinavir (Viracept)	750 mg orally three times daily or 1250 mg twice daily	Diarrhea	No special monitoring	$4.16/250 mg $10.42/625 mg	$1250.36 $1250.36
Ritonavir (Norvir)	600 mg orally twice daily or in lower doses (eg, 100 mg orally once or twice daily) for boosting other PIs	Gastrointestinal distress, peripheral parestheslas	No special monitoring	$10.29/100 mg	$3703.20 ($617.20 in lower doses)
Saquinavir hard gel (Invirase)	1000 mg orally twice daily with 100 mg ritonavir orally twice daily	Gastrointestinal distress	No special monitoring	$11.45/500 mg	$1373.41 (plus cost of ritonavir)
Atazanavir (Reyataz)	400 mg orally once daily or 300 mg atazanavir with 100 mg ritonavir daily	Hyperbilirubinemia	Bilirubin level every 3–4 months	$27.61/200 mg	$1656.52 (plus cost of ritonavir)
Atazanavir/cobicistat (Evotaz)	300 mg of atazanavir with 150 mg cobicistat orally once daily	Hyperbilirubinemia	Bilirubin level every 3–4 months.	60.58/tablet	$1817.51
Darunavir/ritonavir (Prezista/Norvir)	**For PI-experienced patients:** 600 mg of darunavir and 100 mg of ritonavir orally twice daily **For PI-naïve patients:** 800 mg of darunavir and 100 mg of ritonavir orally daily	Rash	No special monitoring	$27.15/600 mg (darunavir) $10.29/100 mg (ritonavir) $25.16/400 mg (darunavir)	$2246.26 (for combination) $1818.40 (for combination)
Darunavir/cobicistat (Prezcobix)	800 mg of darunavir and 150 mg of cobicistat orally once daily	Rash	No special monitoring	$62.07/tablet	$1862.12
Tipranavir/ritonavir (Aptivus/Norvir)	500 mg of tipranavir and 200 mg of ritonavir orally twice daily	Gastrointestinal, rash	No special monitoring	$14.04/250 mg (tipranavir) $10.29/100 mg (ritonavir)	$2920.00 (for combination)
Entry inhibitors					
Enfuvirtide (Fuzeon)	90 mg subcutaneously twice daily	Injection site pain and allergic reaction	No special monitoring	$68.30/90 mg	$4097.78
Maraviroc (Selzentry)	150–300 mg orally daily	Cough, fever, rash	No special monitoring	$25.94/150 mg or 300 mg	$1556.12
Integrase inhibitors					
Raltegravir (Isentress)	400 mg orally twice daily	Diarrhea, nausea, headache	No special monitoring	$25.75/400 mg	$1545.07
Elvitegravir (Vitekta)	Elvitegravir 85 or 150 mg once daily depending on combination regimen used OR 85 mg once daily when administered with atazanavir and ritonavir, or lopinavir and ritonavir 150 mg once daily when administered with darunavir and ritonavir, or fosamprenavir and ritonavir or tipranavir and ritonavir	Diarrhea, rash		$48.18/Tablet	$1445.34

(continued)

Table 31–6. Antiretroviral therapy. (continued)

Medication	Dose	Common Side Effects	Special Monitoring[1]	Cost[2]	Cost/Month
Dolutegravir (Tivicay)	Treatment-naïve or integrase-naïve patients: 50 mg daily. When administered with efavirenz, fosamprenavir/ritonavir, tipranavir/ritonavir, or rifampin: 50 mg twice daily. When administered to integrase-experienced patients with suspected integrase resistance: 50 mg twice daily.	Hypersensitivity, rash	No special monitoring	$56.91/50 mg	$1707.26

[1]Standard monitoring is complete blood count (CBC) and differential, basic chemistries, serum aminotransferases and total bilirubin every 3–6 months, urinalysis at baseline and annually during ART, fasting glucose or hemoglogin A$_{1c}$ at baseline and annually during ART, fasting lipid profile at baseline, 4–8 weeks after starting an ART regimen that affects lipids, and annually for everyone over 40 years of age.
[2]Average wholesale price (AWP, for AB-rated generic when available) for quantity listed. Source: *Red Book* (electronic version), Truven Health Analytics Information, http://www.micromedexsolutions.com/ accessed April 8, 2016. AWP may not accurately represent the actual pharmacy cost because wide contractual variations exist among institutions.

avoided. Similarly, if toxicity develops, it is preferable to change the offending medication rather than reduce individual doses.

The presence of an acute opportunistic infection in most cases does not preclude the initiation of ART. Randomized trials compared early initiation of ART (within 2 weeks of starting treatment for an opportunistic infection or tuberculosis) with ART that was deferred until after treatment of the opportunistic infection was completed (6 weeks after its start); results demonstrated that early initiation reduced death or AIDS progression by 50%. The reduced progression rates were related to more rapid improvements in CD4 counts in patients with advanced immunodeficiency. Furthermore, IRIS and other adverse events were no more frequent in the early ART arm.

Several randomized studies have also demonstrated improved clinical outcomes in HIV/tuberculosis coinfected patients who initiate ART early in the setting of active treatment for tuberculosis and whose CD4 counts are less than 50 cells/mcL. The exception to early ART in the setting of active infections may be in patients with a CNS-associated infection, such as cryptococcal or tuberculosis meningitis. Several studies from low-income countries have shown high mortality rates with early ART initiation in this setting.

For hospitalized patients, initiating treatment in patients with opportunistic infections requires close coordination between inpatient and outpatient clinicians to ensure that treatment is continued once patients are discharged.

D. Choosing an ART Regimen

Although the ideal combination of medications has not yet been defined for all possible clinical situations, possible regimens can be better understood after a review of the available agents. These medications can be grouped into five major categories: nucleoside and nucleotide reverse transcriptase inhibitors (NRTI); nonnucleoside reverse transcriptase inhibitors (NNRTI); PIs; entry inhibitors, which include a fusion inhibitor and CCR5 antagonists; and integrase inhibitors.

1. Nucleoside and nucleotide reverse transcriptase inhibitors (NRTI)—There are currently seven NRTI agents available and approved for use. The choice of which agent to use depends primarily on the patient's prior treatment experience, results of resistance testing, medication side effects, other underlying conditions, and convenience of formulation. However, most clinicians use fixed-dose combinations (see Table 31–7) of either tenofovir/emtricitabine (TDF/FTC) or abacavir/lamivudine (ABC/3TC), both of which can be given once a day. Abacavir should only be given to HLA-B*5701-negative persons. In patients with viral loads greater than 100,000 copies/mL, ABC/3TC was less effective than tenofovir/emtricitabine when combined with efavirenz or ritonavir-boosted atazanavir. However, ABC/3TC appears to be equally efficacious as tenofovir/emtricitabine in patients with viral loads greater than 100,000 copies/mL when combined with dolutegravir or raltegravir. In some studies, abacavir increased risks of myocardial infarction, and therefore should be avoided in patients at high risk for cardiovascular disease. Zidovudine/lamivudine (AZT/3TC) is usually reserved for second- or third-line regimens because of toxicity and dosing schedule. Of the available agents, zidovudine is the most likely to cause anemia. Zidovudine and didanosine are the most likely to cause neutropenia. Stavudine is the most likely to cause lipoatrophy (loss of fat in the face, extremities, and buttocks) followed by zidovudine. Didanosine is the most likely to cause peripheral neuropathy. Lamivudine, emtricitabine, and tenofovir have activity against hepatitis B. Didanosine, lamivudine, emtricitabine, and tenofovir can be administered daily. Information specific to each medication is given below.

A. ZIDOVUDINE—Zidovudine was the first approved antiviral medication for HIV infection. It is administered at a dose of 300 mg orally twice daily. A combination of zidovudine 300 mg and lamivudine 150 mg (Combivir;

Table 31–7. Fixed dose antiretroviral combinations.

Name	Components	Dosing and Special Considerations	Cost per month
Truvada	TDF 300 mg Emtricitabine 200 mg	One pill daily with a NNRTI, protease inhibitor, integrase inhibitor, or maraviroc (entry inhibitor). Most commonly used nucleoside/nucleotide reverse transcriptase inhibitor backbone.	$1759.73
Epzicom	Abacavir 600 mg Lamivudine 300 mg	One pill daily with a NNRTI, protease inhibitor, integrase inhibitor, or maraviroc (entry inhibitor).	$1550.05
Trizivir	Abacavir 300 mg Lamivudine 150 mg Zidovudine 300 mg	One tablet twice daily with a NNRTI, protease inhibitor, integrase inhibitor, or maraviroc (entry inhibitor). Although it contains three medications it *does not* constitute a complete treatment.	$1931.64
Atripla	TDF 300 mg Emtricitabine 200 mg Efavirenz 600 mg	One pill daily constitutes a complete regimen.	$2869.86
Stribild	TDF 300 mg Emtricitabine 200 mg Elvitegravir 150 mg Cobicistat 150 mg	One pill daily constitutes a complete regimen. Although it contains four medications, one component (Cobicistat) is a medication booster only.	$3244.76
Genvoya	TAF 10 mg Emtricitabine 200 mg Elvitegravir 150 mg Cobicistat 150 mg	One pill daily constitutes a complete regimen. Although it contains four medications, one component (cobicistat) is a medication booster only. The only difference between Stribild and Genvoya is that Genvoya has a different form of tenofovir (TAF) that appears to be safer than tenofovir (TDF) with less effect on renal function and bone mineral density.	$3093.19
Triumeq	Abacavir 600 mg Lamivudine 300 mg Dolutegravir 50 mg	One pill constitutes a complete regimen.	$2889.22
Complera	TDF 300 mg Emtricitabine 200 mg Rilpivirine 25 mg	One pill daily constitutes complete regimen. Only for patients with HIV viral load less than 100,000/mL.	$2815.04

TAF, tenofovir alafenamide; TDF, tenofovir disoproxil fumarate. Average wholesale price (AWP, for AB-rated generic when available) for quantity listed. Source: Red Book (electronic version), Truven Health Analytics Information, http://www.micromedexsolutions.com/ accessed April 8, 2016. AWP may not accurately represent the actual pharmacy cost because wide contractual variations exist among institutions.

see Table 31–7) is available. Side effects seen with zidovudine are listed in Table 31–6. Approximately 40% of patients experience subjective side effects that usually remit within 6 weeks. The common dose-limiting side effects are anemia and neutropenia, which require ongoing laboratory monitoring. Long-term use has been associated with lipoatrophy.

B. Lamivudine—Lamivudine (3TC) is a safe and well-tolerated agent. The dosage is 150 mg orally twice daily or 300 mg orally once a day. The dose should be reduced with chronic kidney disease. There are no significant side effects with lamivudine, and it has activity also against hepatitis B.

C. Emtricitabine—Emtricitabine is a nucleoside analog that is dosed at 200 mg orally. It was developed primarily as a once a day alternative to lamivudine. However, lamivudine can be dosed daily, eliminating the special indication for emtricitabine. As is true of lamivudine, emtricitabine has activity against hepatitis B and its dosage should be reduced in patients with chronic kidney disease.

D. Abacavir—A daily dose of 300 mg orally twice daily results in potent antiretroviral activity. Prior to initiation of abacavir, patients should undergo testing for HLA typing. Those with the B*5701 allele should not be treated with abacavir because the likelihood of a hypersensitivity

reaction developing is high; the reaction is characterized by a flu-like syndrome with rash and fever that worsens with successive doses. Unfortunately, the absence of this allele does not guarantee that the patient will avoid the hypersensitivity reaction. Individuals in whom the hypersensitivity reaction develops *should not* be rechallenged with this agent because subsequent hypersensitivity reactions can be fatal. Abacavir has also been associated with an increased risk of myocardial infarction in some cohort studies. This increased risk is generally seen in patients who have underlying risks of cardiovascular disease. Consequently, abacavir should not be used in such patients if effective alternative nucleoside or nucleotide analog agents exist. Abacavir is usually prescribed as a fixed-dose combination pill with lamivudine for use as a once daily pill (Epzicom; Table 31–7).

Abacavir is also formulated with zidovudine and lamivudine in a single pill (Trizivir, one tablet orally twice daily; Table 31–7). Trizivir is not recommended as solo treatment for HIV because it is not as efficacious as combining two nucleoside/nucleotide analogs with a ritonavir-boosted PI, an NNRTI, or an integrase inhibitor.

E. Tenofovir—Tenofovir is the only licensed nucleotide analog. It comes in two forms: tenofovir disoproxil fumarate (TDF) and tenofovir alafenamide (TAF). TDF is the older form and is available both as a single medication with a daily oral dose of 300 mg and as a fixed-dose combination pill with emtricitabine (Truvada; Table 31–7) for daily dosing. Several single-tablet once-a-day complete regimens that include TDF (Atripla, Complera, Stribild) are available (Table 31–7). Tenofovir is active against hepatitis B, including isolates that have resistance to lamivudine. TDF is associated with a clinically modest loss of kidney function, a small increased risk of acute renal injury, and increased rate of bone resorption.

TAF is the newer form of the medication; it attains higher levels in cells with a much lower plasma level. For this reason, it appears to cause less harm to kidneys, less bone resorption, and appears to have stronger antiviral properties than TDF. It is available in a combination tablet with elvitegravir, covicistat, and emtricitabine (Genvoya, Table 31–7). It is likely that the FDA will approve combinations containing TAF with emtricitabine, and TAF with rilpivirine and emtricitabine.

F. Didanosine—The most convenient formulation of didanosine (ddI) is the enteric-coated capsule. For adults weighing at least 60 kg, the dose is one 400-mg enteric-coated capsule orally daily; for those 30–59 kg, the dose is one 250-mg enteric-coated capsule orally daily. Didanosine should be taken on an empty stomach.

Didanosine has been associated with pancreatitis. The incidence of pancreatitis with didanosine is 5–10%—of fatal pancreatitis, less than 0.4%. Patients with a history of pancreatitis, as well as those taking other medications associated with pancreatitis (including trimethoprim-sulfamethoxazole and intravenous pentamidine) are at higher risk for this complication. Other common side effects with didanosine include a dose-related, reversible, painful peripheral neuropathy, which occurs in about 15% of patients, and dry mouth. Fulminant hepatic failure and electrolyte abnormalities, including hypokalemia, hypocalcemia, and hypomagnesemia, have been reported in patients taking didanosine. Because of the side-effect profile, didanosine is rarely used today.

G. Stavudine—Because of its side effects including lipoatrophy, lipodystrophy, peripheral neuropathy and, rarely, lactic acidosis and hepatitis, stavudine (d4T) should no longer be used except when there is no alternative.

2. Nonnucleoside reverse transcriptase inhibitors—NNRTI inhibit reverse transcriptase at a site different from that of the nucleoside and nucleotide agents described above. All five NNRTI have shown antiviral activity as measured by HIV viral load and CD4 responses. The major advantage of the NNRTI is that three of them (efavirenz, rilpivirine, and nevirapine) have potencies comparable to that of PI (next section), at least for patients with viral loads under 100,000 copies/mL—with lower pill burden and fewer side effects. In particular, they do not appear to cause lipodystrophy; patients with cholesterol and triglyceride elevations who are switched from a PI to an NNRTI may have improvement in their lipids. The resistance patterns of the NNRTI are distinct from those of the PI, so their use still leaves open the option for future PI use.

The NNRTI can be used with PI in patients who are difficult to suppress on simpler regimens or when it is difficult to identify at least two NRTI agents to which the patient is not resistant. Because these agents may cause alterations in the clearance of PIs, dose modifications may be necessary when these two classes of medications are administered concomitantly. There is a high degree of cross-resistance among the "first-generation" NNRTIs, such that resistance to one medication in this class uniformly predicts resistance to other medications. However, the "second-generation" NNRTI etravirine appears to have consistent antiviral activity in patients with prior exposure and resistance to nevirapine, efavirenz, or delavirdine. In particular, the K103N mutation does not appear to have an impact on etravirine (or rilpivirine). There is no therapeutic reason for using more than one NNRTI at the same time.

A. Efavirenz—The major advantages of efavirenz is that it can be given once daily in a single dose (600 mg orally), and it is available in a once-daily fixed-dose combination with tenofovir and emtricitabine in a single pill (Atripla; Table 31–7). The major side effects are rash and psychiatric/neurologic complaints, with patients reporting symptoms ranging from lack of concentration and strange dreams to delusions and mania. These side effects tend to wane over time, usually within a month or so; however, there are some patients who cannot tolerate these effects, especially if they persist longer than a month. Participant level data from four randomized trials of efavirenz regimens versus non-efavirenz containing regimens found increased suicidality (hazard ratio of 2.6) among those taking efavirenz. Administration of efavirenz with food, especially fatty food, may increase its serum levels and consequent neurotoxicity. Therefore, it should be taken on an empty stomach; taking before bedtime may also reduce patients' experience of neuropsychiatric symptoms.

B. Rilpivirine—This medication, dosed at 25 mg once daily, is equal in efficacy to efavirenz in patients with HIV viral loads below 100,000 copies/mL. Rilpivirine should not be used in patients with baseline viral loads of 100,000 copies/mL or greater or those with CD4 counts below 200 cells/mcL because of greater risk of viral failure. As is true of efavirenz, rilpivirine is available in a once-daily fixed-dose combination with tenofovir and emtricitabine (Complera; Table 31–7) to be taken with a fatty meal (at least 290 calories). Proton pump inhibitors should not be given with rilpivirine. Rilpivirine has fewer neurologic side effects than efavirenz.

C. Nevirapine—The dose of nevirapine is 400 mg orally daily (extended release) but it is initiated at a dose of 200 mg once a day to decrease the incidence of rash, which is as high as 40% when full doses are begun immediately. If rash develops while the patient is taking 200 mg daily, liver enzymes should be checked and the dose should not be increased until the rash resolves. Patients with mild rash and no evidence of hepatotoxicity can continue to be treated with nevirapine. Nevirapine should not be used in treatment-naïve women with CD4 counts greater than 250 cells/mcL or in males with CD4 counts greater than 400 cells/mcL because they have greater risk of hepatotoxicity.

In general, because of the risk of fatal hepatotoxicity, nevirapine should be used only when there is not a better alternative.

D. DELAVIRDINE—Of the available NNRTIs, delavirdine is used the least largely because of its inconvenient dosing and pill burden compared with the other available NNRTIs. Unlike nevirapine and efavirenz, delavirdine inhibits P450 cytochromes rather than inducing these enzymes. This means that delavirdine can act like ritonavir and boost other antiretrovirals, although delavirdine is not as potent as ritonavir in this capacity. The dosage is 400 mg orally three times a day. The major side effect is rash.

E. ETRAVIRINE—Etravirine is an NNRTI approved for the treatment of patients with prior NNRTI intolerance or resistance. Etravirine has been shown to be effective even when some degree of NNRTI-resistance is present, making it a true "second generation" medication in this class. Etravirine dosage is one 200-mg tablet twice daily. It should be used with a PI and an NRTI and not just with two NRTI. The most common side effects are nausea and rash; rarely, the rash can be severe (toxic epidermal necrolysis). Patients with signs of severe rash or hypersensitivity reactions should immediately discontinue the medication. Prior rash due to treatment with one of the other NNRTIs does not make rash more likely with etravirine. Etravirine should not be taken by people with severe liver disease or administered with tipranavir/ritonavir, fosamprenavir/ritonavir, atazanavir/ritonavir, full-dose ritonavir, or PI without low-dose ritonavir.

3. Protease inhibitors—Ten PIs—indinavir, nelfinavir, ritonavir, saquinavir, amprenavir, fosamprenavir, lopinavir (in combination with ritonavir), atazanavir, darunavir, and tipranavir are available. PIs are potent suppressors of HIV replication and are administered as part of a combination regimen.

All the PIs—to differing degrees—are metabolized by the cytochrome P450 system, and each can inhibit and induce various P450 isoenzymes. Therefore, medication interactions are common and difficult to predict. Clinicians should consult the product inserts before prescribing PIs with other medications. Medications such as rifampin that are known to induce the P450 system should be avoided.

The fact that the PIs are dependent on metabolism through the cytochrome P450 system has led to the use of ritonavir to boost the medication levels of saquinavir, lopinavir, indinavir, atazanavir, tipranavir, darunavir and amprenavir, allowing use of lower doses and simpler dosing schedules of these PIs. A second boosting agent, cobicistat, is coformulated with the PI atazanavir (Evotaz) and darunavir (Prescobix). Similar to ritonavir, cobicistat also inhibits liver enzymes that metabolize other HIV medications.

In fact, **guidelines recommend that all PI-containing regimens except nelfinavir use boosting if possible.**

When choosing which PI to use, prior patient experience, resistance patterns, side effects, and ease of administration are the major considerations. The first three PIs to be developed—indinavir, saquinavir, and ritonavir (as single agents)—are now rarely used because of the superiority

of the second generation of PIs. Amprenavir has been almost entirely replaced by its prodrug, fosamprenavir. Unfortunately, all PIs, with the exception of unboosted atazanavir have been linked to a constellation of metabolic abnormalities, including elevated cholesterol levels, elevated triglyceride levels, insulin resistance, diabetes mellitus, and changes in body fat composition (eg, buffalo hump, abdominal obesity). The lipid abnormalities and body habitus changes are referred to as **lipodystrophy.** Although lipodystrophy is commonly associated with PIs, it has been seen also in HIV-infected persons who have never been treated with these agents. In particular, the lipoatrophy effects seen in patients receiving ART appears to be more related to the nucleoside toxicity and in particular to the thymidine analogs (stavudine and zidovudine).

Of the different manifestations of lipodystrophy, the dyslipidemias that occur are of particular concern because of the likelihood that increased levels of cholesterol and triglycerides will result in increased prevalence of heart disease. **All patients taking PIs or NRTIs should have fasting serum cholesterol, low-density lipoprotein (LDL) cholesterol, and triglyceride levels performed every 12 months.** Clinicians should assess for coronary heart disease risk (see Chapter 28) and consider initiating dietary changes or medication therapy (or both). PIs inhibit statin metabolism. Lovastatin and simvastatin should be avoided. In general, the least interaction is with pravastatin (20 mg daily orally). Atorvastatin (10 mg daily orally) or rosuvastatin (5 mg/day orally initially; maximum 10 mg/day) may also be used cautiously. Fish oil (3000 mg daily) combined with exercise and dietary counseling has been found to decrease triglyceride levels by 25%. Patients with persistently elevated fasting serum triglyceride levels of 500 mg/dL or more who do not respond to dietary intervention should be treated with gemfibrozil (600 mg twice daily prior to the morning and evening meals). PIs are associated with abnormalities in cardiac conduction, especially prolongation of the PR interval.

A. INDINAVIR—Indinavir is usually dosed at 800 mg twice daily in combination with 100 mg of ritonavir twice daily. Nausea and headache are common complaints with this medication. Indinavir crystals are present in the urine in approximately 40% of patients; this results in clinically apparent nephrolithiasis in about 15% of patients receiving indinavir. Lower urinary tract symptoms and acute kidney injury also have been reported. Patients taking this medication should be instructed to drink at least 48 ounces of fluid a day to ensure adequate hydration in an attempt to limit these complications. Mild indirect hyperbilirubinemia is also commonly observed in patients taking indinavir but is not an indication for discontinuation of the medication.

B. SAQUINAVIR—Saquinavir is formulated only as a hard-gel capsule (Invirase). It should only be used with ritonavir (1000 mg of hard-gel saquinavir with 100 mg of ritonavir orally twice daily). The most common side effects with saquinavir are diarrhea, nausea, dyspepsia, and abdominal pain.

C. RITONAVIR—Use of this potent PI at full dose (600 mg orally twice daily) has been limited by its inhibition of the cytochrome P450 pathway causing a large number of drug–drug interactions and by its frequent side effects of fatigue, nausea, and paresthesias. However, it is widely used in lower dose (eg, 100 mg daily to 100 mg twice daily) as a booster of other PIs.

D. NELFINAVIR—Nelfinavir is the only PI for which ritonavir boosting is not recommended. Unboosted nelfinavir is generally not as potent as a boosted PI regimen (eg, lopinavir plus ritonavir). The dose of nelfinavir is 1250 mg orally twice daily. Diarrhea is a side effect in 25% of patients taking nelfinavir, but this symptom may be controlled with over-the-counter antidiarrheal agents in most patients.

E. AMPRENAVIR—Amprenavir has efficacy and side effects similar to those of other PIs. Common side effects are nausea, vomiting, diarrhea, rash, and perioral paresthesia. The dose is 1200 mg orally twice daily. The concentration of amprenavir decreases when coadministered with ethinyl estradiol; therefore, amprenavir should be used with circumspection in the treatment of transgender persons requiring high-dose estrogen.

F. FOSAMPRENAVIR—Fosamprenavir is a prodrug of amprenavir. Its major advantage over using amprenavir is a much lower pill burden. For PI-naïve patients, it can be dosed at 1400 mg orally twice daily (four capsules a day) or at 1400 mg orally daily (two capsules) with ritonavir 200 mg orally daily (two capsules) or at 700 mg orally with ritonavir 100 mg orally twice daily. Patients previously treated with a PI should receive 700 mg orally with ritonavir 100 mg orally twice daily. Side effects are similar to those with amprenavir—most commonly gastrointestinal distress and hyperlipidemia. As with amprenavir, the concentration of fosamprenavir decreases when coadministered with ethinyl estradiol; therefore, fosamprenavir should be used with circumspection in the treatment of transgender persons requiring high-dose estrogen.

G. LOPINAVIR/R—Lopinavir/r is lopinavir (200 mg) coformulated with a low dose of ritonavir (50 mg) to maximize the bioavailability of lopinavir. It has been shown to be more effective than nelfinavir when used in combination with stavudine and lamivudine. The usual dose is 400 mg lopinavir with 100 mg of ritonavir (two tablets) orally twice daily with food. When given along with efavirenz or nevirapine, a higher dose (600 mg/150 mg—three tablets) is usually prescribed. The most common side effect is diarrhea, and lipid abnormalities are frequent. Because of these side effects, lopinavir/r has fallen off the list of medications recommended as part of first-line treatment regimens.

H. ATAZANAVIR—Atazanavir is available alone and coformulated with cobicistat (Evotaz). Atazanavir can be dosed as 400 mg (two 200-mg capsules) daily with food or it can be dosed as 300 mg in combination with 100 mg of ritonavir once daily with food. When coformulated with cobicistat, it is dosed at 300 mg atazanavir and 150 mg cobicistat. The most common side effect is mild hyperbilirubinemia that resolves with discontinuation of the medication. Nephrolithiasis and cholelithiasis have also been reported with this PI. Both tenofovir and efavirenz lower the serum concentration of atazanavir. Therefore, when either of

these two medications is used with atazanavir, it should be boosted by administering ritonavir or given coformulated with cobicistat. Proton pump inhibitors are contraindicated in patients taking atazanavir because atazanavir requires an acidic pH to remain in solution.

I. TIPRANAVIR—Tipranavir is the only nonpeptidic PI approved by the US Food and Drug Administration (FDA). Because of its unique structure, it is active against some strains of HIV that are resistant to other PIs. It is dosed with ritonavir (two 250 mg capsules of tipranavir with two 100 mg capsules of ritonavir orally twice daily with food). The most common side effects are nausea, vomiting, diarrhea, fatigue, and headache. Tipranavir/ritonavir has been also associated with liver damage and should be used very cautiously in patients with underlying liver disease. Reports of intracranial hemorrhage in patients taking tipranavir-containing regimens have raised additional safety concerns about this potent PI. Because it is a sulfa-containing medication, its use should be closely monitored in patients with sulfa allergy.

J. DARUNAVIR—Darunavir has impressive antiviral activity in the setting of significant PI resistance and in treatment-naïve patients. It is formulated by itself and coformulated with cobicistat (Prezcobix). When formulated without cobicistat it requires boosting with ritonavir. For initial treatment of HIV or for treatment-experienced patients without darunavir-related resistance mutations, daily dosing is 800 mg of darunavir with 100 mg of ritonavir or with 150 mg of cobicistat. For patients with prior PI treatment experience or PI resistance (with mutations known to impact darunavir), darunavir should be dosed at 600 mg orally twice daily, with ritonavir, 100 mg orally twice daily. Darunavir has a safety profile similar to other PIs, such as ritonavir-boosted lopinavir, but is generally better tolerated. Like tipranavir, darunavir is a sulfa-containing medication, and its use should be closely monitored in patients with sulfa allergy.

4. Entry inhibitors—

A. ENFUVIRTIDE—Enfuvirtide (Fuzeon) is known as a fusion inhibitor; it blocks the entry of HIV into cells by blocking the fusion of the HIV envelope to the cell membrane. The addition of enfuvirtide to an optimized antiretroviral regimen improved CD4 counts and lowered viral loads in heavily pretreated patients with multidrug-resistant HIV. Unfortunately, resistance develops rapidly in patients receiving nonsuppressive treatment. The dose is 90 mg by subcutaneous injection twice daily; unfortunately, painful injection site reactions develop in most patients, which makes long-term use problematic.

B. MARAVIROC—Maraviroc is a CCR5 co-receptor antagonist. Medications in this class prevent the virus from entering uninfected cells by blocking the CCR5 co-receptor. Before starting therapy, a viral tropism assay should be performed because this class of entry inhibitors is only active against "CCR5-tropic virus." This form of the HIV-1 virus tends to predominate early in infection, while so-called "dual/mixed tropic virus" (which utilizes either R5 or CXCR4 co-receptors) emerges later as infection progresses. Approximately 50–60% of previously treated HIV-infected patients have circulating CCR5-tropic HIV. The medication has been shown to be effective in HIV-infected persons with ongoing viral replication despite being heavily treated and who have CCR5-tropic virus. The dose of maraviroc is 150–300 mg orally twice daily, based on the other medications the patient is taking at the time—in combination with a ritonavir boosted PI, 150 mg daily of maraviroc has been used successfully. Common side effects are cough, fever, rash, musculoskeletal problems, abdominal pain, and dizziness; however, maraviroc is generally well tolerated with limited impact on serum lipids.

5. Integrase inhibitors—Integrase inhibitors slow HIV replication by blocking the HIV integrase enzyme needed for the virus to multiply. Three integrase inhibitors are available: raltegravir, elvitegravir, and dolutegravir. Clinical trials of all integrase inhibitors reveal a consistent pattern of more rapid decline in viral load compared with more standard PI/r or NNRTI-based regimens. The clinical significance of this observation is unclear. Integrase inhibitors are effective (when combined with other active medications) in the treatment of HIV-infected patients with documented resistance to each of the three main classes of antiretroviral medications (nucleoside analogs, PIs, NNRTIs). Avoid administering with antacids or other medications with divalent cations (Ca^{2+}, Mg^{2+}, Al^{2+}, Fe^{2+}) because chelation of the integrase inhibitor by the cation reduces absorption. When these medications must be taken with integrase inhibitors, consult a pharmacist to determine the best separation of times of administration.

A. Raltegravir—The dose of raltegravir is 400 mg orally twice daily. It has been found to be superior to efavirenz and ritonavir-boosted darunavir and ritonavir-boosted atazanavir. Common side effects are diarrhea, nausea, and headache, but overall it is well tolerated and has the additional advantage over PI-based regimens and efavirenz-based regimens in that it appears to have little impact on lipid profiles or glucose metabolism.

B. Elvitegravir—Elvitegravir has been studied only in treatment naïve patients. It has the advantage of being available in a combination pill (Stribild) (Table 31–7) that contains 125 mg of elvitegravir and 150 mg of cobicistat, a boosting agent, along with standard doses of TDF and emtricitabine. Stribild has been shown to be noninferior to two preferred first-line regimens: Atripla and boosted atazanavir with tenofovir/emtricitabine. The main side effects include increases in serum creatinine levels which has been shown to be related to the cobicistat inhibition of tubular secretion of creatinine by the kidney and is thought to be nonpathologic and reversible. However, because of this effect, Stribild is recommended in treatment-naïve patients with estimated creatinine clearance greater than 70 mL/min. A urine analysis should be done at baseline and at initial follow-up to look for proteinuria and glycosuria, which are signs of tubulopathy. Diarrhea and rash may also occur, although overall the medication is well tolerated. Elvitegravir is also coformulated with TAF along with emtricitabine and cobicistat boosting in a single once a day

pill (Genvoya). Since TAF appears to have greater activity and fewer side effects than TDF, this is likely to become the preferred elvitegravir regimen.

C. Dolutegravir—Dolutegravir shows excellent potency and tolerability and is dosed once-a-day in most circumstances. Unlike elvitegravir, dolutegravir does not require a boosting agent. Similar to cobicistat, it inhibits tubular secretion of creatinine by the kidney, resulting in small increases in serum creatinine levels. The standard dosage used in treatment-naïve, integrase-naïve patients is 50 mg/day. It is available combined with abacavir and lamivudine in a single once a day tablet (Triumeq, Table 31–7). In patients receiving efavirenz, fosamprenavir/ritonavir, tipranavir/ritonavir, or rifampin, the dose should be increased to 50 mg twice daily. It should also be dosed at 50 mg twice daily in integrase-experienced patients in whom integrase resistance is suspected. Indeed, when combined with other active medications, it has been shown to provide some activity in patients with integrase resistance who have not responded to prior raltegravir- or elvitegravir-containing regimens. Dolutegravir has demonstrated impressive results from clinical trials of treatment-naïve patients when compared with the more standard NNRTI, boosted PI, and raltegravir-containing regimens.

6. Constructing regimens—Only combinations of three or more medications from two or more classes have been able to decrease HIV viral load by 2–3 logs and provide durable suppression of HIV RNA to below the threshold of detection.

Six antiretroviral regimes are recommended for initiating treatment (Table 31–8). These regimens are recommended because of their combination of antiviral potency and tolerability as well as dosing convenience. Of note, five out of the six regimens use integrase inhibitors, indicating the greater efficacy and tolerability of this class compared to other classes that can be combined with NRTI backbones. Studies have shown dolutegravir/abacavir/lamivudine to be superior to efavirenz/TDF/emtricitabine and have shown dolutegravir to be superior to ritonavir-boosted darunavir (both combined with either abacavir/lamivudine or TDF/emtricitabine). A network meta-analysis adjusting for NRTI backbone found that dolutegravir had superior efficacy in suppressing viral load compared with regimens containing ritonavir-boosted atazanavir, ritonavir-boosted darunavir, efavirenz, or ritonavir-boosted lopinavir. Discontinuation due to adverse events was also statistically lower in the dolutegravir regimens.

The integrase inhibitor raltegravir has done well in comparative studies. Among treatment-naïve patients, raltegravir in combination with TDF/emtricitabine is as effective as efavirenz/TDF/emtricitabine for daily treatment and has fewer side effects. In a 5-year follow-up to the double-blind trial, the raltegravir arm out-performed the efavirenz combination regimen largely due to better long-term tolerability. Furthermore, the CD4 response appeared better in patients treated with the raltegravir combination.

Three of the recommended integrase inhibitor/NRTI regimens are available in a single pill that can be dosed just

Table 31–8. Recommended and alternative initial antiretroviral regimens.[1] (continued)

Regimen	Advantages	Disadvantages
Recommended		
Dolutegravir + abacavir + lamivudine[2] (Triumeq)	Single pill once-a-day regimen Has activity in some patients with integrase resistance Superior to Atripla Dolutegravir plus either abacavir/lamivudine or emtricitabine/TDF superior to darunavir/ritonavir plus either of the NRTI backbones	Abacavir should be used only in HLA-B*5701-negative persons When used in patients with integrase resistance or combined with certain other medications, requires twice a day dosing Avoid antacids and other medications with divalent cations (Ca^{2+}, Mg^{2+}, Al^{2+}+, Fe^{2+})
Dolutegravir (50 mg daily) + emtricitabine/TDF (Truvada)	Has activity in some patients with integrase resistance Once-a-day regimen	No single tablet available When used in patients with integrase resistance or combined with certain other medications, requires twice a day dosing Avoid antacids and other medications with divalent cations (Ca^{2+}, Mg^{2+}, Al^{2+}, Fe^{2+})
Emtricitabine/TAF/elvitegravir with cobicistat boosting (Genvoya)	Single tablet once-a-day regimen Excellent response across broad range of CD4 and viral loads Contains TAF instead of TDF and is therefore less nephrotoxic and less likely to lead to bone resorption when compared with Stribild	Cobicistat boosting causes similar drug-drug interactions as ritonavir; increases in serum creatinine (nonpathologic) No dosage adjustment with estimated creatinine clearance > 30 mL/min Avoid antacids and other medications with divalent cations (Ca^{2+}, Mg^{2+}, Al^{2+}, Fe^{2+})
Emtricitabine/TDF/elvitegravir with cobicistat boosting (Stribild)	Single tablet once-a-day regimen Excellent response across broad range of CD4 and viral loads	Cobicistat boosting causes similar drug-drug interactions as ritonavir; increases in serum creatinine (nonpathologic) Requires estimated creatinine clearance ≥ 70 mL/min Avoid antacids and other medications with divalent cations (Ca^{2+}, Mg^{2+}, Al^{2+}, Fe^{2+})
Raltegravir (400 mg twice daily) + emtricitabine/TDF (Truvada)	Superior to Atripla over 5 years of follow-up	Requires twice a day dosing No single tablet available Avoid antacids and other medications with divalent cations (Ca^{2+}, Mg^{2+}, Al^{2+}, Fe^{2+})
Darunavir (800 mg daily) with ritonavir (100 mg daily) boosting + emtricitabine/TDF (Truvada)	Potent boosted PI Can be given once daily Limited risk of resistance with poor adherence	Not available as a single tablet. May cause rash in patients with sulfa allergy. Ritonavir boosting required. Has metabolic side effects.
Alternative regimens		
TDF/emtricitabine/efavirenz (Atripla)	Single tablet once-a-day regimen Longest term clinical experience Highly effective across broad range of initial CD4 counts and viral loads	Avoid in patients with transmitted K103N Neuropsychiatric symptoms common and can be persistent
TDF/emtricitabine/rilpivirine (Complera)	Single tablet once-a-day regimen Noninferior to Atripla in patients with baseline viral load < 100,000/mcL Limited metabolic side-effects	Requires taking with a meal Cannot be used with proton pump inhibitors Use only in patients with viral loads < 100,000/mL and CD4 counts > 200 cells/mcL
Atazanavir (300 mg daily) coformulated with 150 mg cobicistat + emtricitabine/TDF (Truvada)	Once-a-day regimen. Limited risk of resistance with poor adherence Resistance to atazanavir generally does not confer resistance to other PI	Not available as a single tablet Increases in bilirubin (nonpathologic) Increased risk of cholelithiasis, nephrolithiasis, and chronic kidney injury Has metabolic side effects Should be taken with food and H_2-blockers and proton pump inhibitors should be avoided Requires estimated creatinine clearance > 70 mL/min
Atazanavir (300 mg daily) with ritonavir (100 mg daily) boosting + emtricitabine/TDF (Truvada)	Once-a-day regimen Limited risk of resistance with poor adherence Resistance to atazanavir generally does not confer resistance to other PI	Not available as a single tablet Increases in bilirubin (nonpathologic) Increased risk of cholelithiasis, nephrolithiasis, and chronic kidney injury Has metabolic side effects Should be taken with food and H_2-blockers and proton pump inhibitors should be avoided

(continued)

Table 31–8. Recommended and alternative initial antiretroviral regimens.[1] (continued)

Regimen	Advantages	Disadvantages
Darunavir (800 mg daily) coformulated with cobicistat (150 mg daily) + abacavir/lamivudine (Epzicom)	Potent boosted PI Can be given once daily Limited risk of resistance with poor adherence	Not available as a single tablet May cause rash in patients with sulfa allergy Has metabolic side effects
Darunavir (800 mg daily) with ritonavir (100 mg daily) boosting + abacavir/lamivudine (Epzicom)	Potent boosted PI Can be given once daily Limited risk of resistance with poor adherence	Not available as a single tablet May cause rash in patients with sulfa allergy Has metabolic side effects
Darunavir (800 mg daily) coformulated with cobicistat (150 mg daily + emtricitabine/TDF (Truvada)	Potent boosted PI Can be given once daily Limited risk of resistance with poor adherence	Not available as a single tablet Requires creatinine clearance >70 mL/min May cause rash in patients with sulfa allergy Has metabolic side effects

[1]Recommendations drawn from US Department of Health and Human Services. Guidelines for the use of antiretroviral agents in HIV-1-infected adults and adolescents.2015. http://aidsinfo.nih.gov/ContentFiles/lvguidelines/AdultandAdolescentGL.pdf
[2]Usual medication doses are supplied when not part of a fixed-dose preparation.
TAF, tenofovir alafenamide; TDF, tenofovir disoproxil fumarate.

once a day (Triumeq, Genvoya, and Stribild). Seven alternative regimens that are generally not as good but may be indicated in certain populations are also listed in Table 31–8. **Resistance testing should be performed prior to starting ART.** Of newly infected persons in some urban areas of the United States, 8–10% have NNRTI resistance (primarily K103N). Patients with NNRTI resistance would not be expected to respond fully to an efavirenz-based regimen. The boosted PI regimens require more pills, have many drug-drug interactions and may have additional undesirable metabolic impacts. In patients with increased risk of metabolic abnormalities or comorbidities, the dolutegravir or raltegravir integrase regimens should be considered preferred choices.

In constructing regimens, toxicities should be nonoverlapping and agents that are either virologically antagonistic or incompatible in terms of drug-drug interactions should be avoided. For example, the combination of stavudine plus didanosine should be avoided, since there is increased risk of toxicities, in particular in pregnant women because of the increased risk of lactic acidosis, which can be fatal. Moreover, the nucleoside pair of zidovudine and stavudine should be avoided because of increased toxicity and the potential for antagonism that results from intracellular competition for phosphorylation. The combination of didanosine with tenofovir should be avoided because of observed declines in CD4 counts. Etravirine should not be used with boosted tipranavir because of drug-drug interactions. Lamivudine and emtricitabine are essentially the same medication and so are not used together.

The most important determinant of treatment efficacy is adherence to the regimen. Therefore, it is vitally important that the regimen chosen be one to which the patient can easily adhere (Figure 31–2). In general, patients are more compliant with medication regimens (Table 31–8) that offer a complete regimen in one pill that needs to be taken only once or twice a day, do not require special timing with regard to meals, can be taken at the same time as other medications, do not require refrigeration or special preparation, and do not have bothersome side effects. Given the high level of effectiveness of recommended regimens, patients for whom the viral load does not fully suppress are likely noncompliant. Pharmacists and other specially trained clinicians can be very effective in helping patients improve their adherence by taking the time to understand why patients miss their medications and problem solve (eg, take medicine at same time every day, keep a supply in the car or at work in case you forget.) For certain populations (eg, unstably housed individuals), specially tailored programs that include medication dispensing are needed.

E. Monitoring ART

1. Goals of monitoring ART—Monitoring of ART has two goals: evaluate for toxicity and measure efficacy using objective markers. Laboratory evaluation for toxicity depends on the specific medications in the combination but generally should be done approximately every 3–4 months once a patient is on a stable regimen. Patients who are intolerant of their initial regimen (eg, patients who cannot tolerate the neurologic side effects of efavirenz) should be changed to an alternative medication or regimen. The second aspect of monitoring is to regularly measure objective markers of efficacy. The CD4 cell count and HIV viral load should be repeated 1–2 months after the initiation or change of antiretroviral regimen and every 3–6 months thereafter in clinically stable patients. (Patients receiving ART with undetectable viral load for 2 years and CD4 counts 300 cells/mcL or more may have CD4 testing only every 12 months.)

2. The challenge of compliance—In a patient who is adherent to an effective regimen, viral loads should be

▲ **Figure 31–2.** Approach to initial and subsequent antiretroviral therapy.

undetectable within 12–24 weeks. For patients in whom viral loads are not suppressed or who have viral rebound after suppression, the major question facing the clinician is **whether the patient is nonadherent or has resistance to the regimen, or both.** The issue is complicated because many patients report being more compliant than they really are. Patients who are having trouble adhering to their treatment should receive counseling on how to better comply with their treatment. In patients who are adherent or who have missed enough doses to make resistance possible, resistance testing should be performed. Based on the results of resistance testing, and assessment of the patient's ability to comply with complicated regimens or to tolerate predictable side effects, the clinician should prescribe a combination of three medications to which there is no or only minimal resistance.

Once ART has been initiated, it is not advisable to stop the therapy unless there is a compelling reason (eg, toxicity, poor adherence, etc). So-called "drug holidays" or "structured treatment interruptions" have been shown to increase risk of AIDS-related complications, increase CD4 declines, and increase morbidity from non–AIDS-related complications (eg, myocardial infarctions and liver failure) and are not recommended.

3. The challenge of medication resistance—HIV-1 medication resistance limits the ability to fully control HIV replication and remains an important cause for antiretroviral regimen failure. **Resistance has been documented for all currently available antiretrovirals including the newer classes of fusion inhibitor, CCR5 inhibitors, and integrase inhibitors.** The problem of medication resistance is widespread in HIV-infected patients undergoing treatment in countries where ART is widely available. However, reports suggest that the degree of high level resistance is declining in the past few years, which is likely related to better tolerated, easier to use, and more efficacious antiretroviral agents. Resistance also occurs in patients who are ART-naïve, but who have been infected with a medication resistant strain—primary resistance or transmitted medication resistance. Cohort studies of ART-naïve patients entering care in North America and Western Europe show that roughly 10–12% (and as high as 25%) of recently infected individuals have been infected with a medication-resistant strain of HIV-1.

In addition to being performed as part of a standard baseline, resistance testing is also recommended for patients who are receiving ART and have suboptimal viral suppression (ie, viral loads greater than 200 copies/mL). Both genotypic and phenotypic tests are commercially available and in randomized controlled studies their use has been shown to result in improved short-term virologic outcomes compared to making treatment choices without resistance testing. Furthermore, multiple retrospective studies have conclusively demonstrated that resistance tests provide prognostic information about virologic response to newly initiated therapy that cannot be gleaned from standard clinical information (ie, treatment history, examination, CD4 count, and viral load tests).

Because of the complexity of resistance tests, many clinicians require expert interpretation of results. In the case of genotypic assays, results may show that the mutations that are selected for during ART are medication-specific or contribute to broad cross-resistance to multiple medications within a therapeutic class. An example of a medication-specific mutation for the reverse transcriptase inhibitors would be the M184V mutation that is selected for by lamivudine or emtricitabine therapy—this mutation causes resistance only to those two medications. Conversely, the thymidine analog mutations ("TAMs") of M41L, D67N, K70R, L210W, T215Y/F, and T219Q/K/E are selected for by either zidovudine or stavudine therapy, but cause resistance to all the medications in the class and often extend to the nucleotide inhibitor tenofovir when three or more of these TAMs are present. Further complicating the interpretation of genotypic tests is the fact that some mutations that cause resistance to one medication can actually make the virus that contains this mutation more sensitive to another medication. The M184V mutation, for example, is associated with increased sensitivity to zidovudine, stavudine, and tenofovir. The most common mutations associated with medication resistance and cross-resistance patterns for NRTIs, NNRTIs, PIs, and integrase inhibitors can be found at http://hivdb.stanford.edu. Phenotypic tests also require interpretation in that the distinction between a resistant virus and sensitive one is not fully defined for all available medications.

Both methods of resistance testing are limited by the fact that they may measure resistance in only some of the viral strains present in an individual. Resistance results may also be misleading if a patient is not taking antiretroviral medications at the time of testing because the dominant virus is likely the wild-type, even if there are resistant viruses in the body that can become dominant with the selective pressure of antivirals. Thus, resistance results do not replace a careful history of what medications a patient has taken in the past and for how long. Also, the results of resistance testing should be viewed cumulatively—ie, if resistance is reported to an agent on one test, it should be presumed to be present thereafter even if subsequent tests do not give the same result.

In designing second-line regimens for patients with resistance to initial therapy, the goal is to identify three medications from at least two different classes to which the virus is not resistant. Even without resistance testing certain forms of cross-resistance between medications within a class can be assumed. For example, the resistance patterns of lopinavir/ritonavir and indinavir are overlapping, and patients with virus resistant to these agents are unlikely to respond to nelfinavir or saquinavir even though they have never received treatment with these agents. Similarly, the resistance patterns of nevirapine and efavirenz are overlapping–as are the resistance patterns between raltegravir and elvitegravir.

Given the availability of new class medications and new generation medications, **a combination of ART can successfully treat virtually all patients—no matter how much resistance is present.**

► Course & Prognosis

With improvements in therapy, patients who are compliant with treatment should have near normal life spans. A population-based study conducted in Denmark found that HIV-infected persons at age 25 years without hepatitis C had a life expectancy similar to that of an uninfected 25-year-old. Unfortunately, not all HIV-infected persons have access to treatment. Studies consistently show less access to treatment for blacks, the homeless, and injection drug users. For patients whose disease progresses even though they are receiving appropriate treatment, meticulous palliative care must be provided (see Chapter 5), with attention to pain control, spiritual needs, and family (biologic and chosen) dynamics.

► When to Refer

- HIV-infected patients should be referred to specialists, given the increasing number of treatment regimens available.

- Extra efforts should be made to obtain specialty consultation for those patients with detectable viral loads on ART; those intolerant of standard medications; those in need of systemic chemotherapy; and those with complicated opportunistic infections, particularly when invasive procedures or experimental therapies are needed.

► When to Admit

Patients with opportunistic infections who are acutely ill (eg, who are febrile, who have had rapid change of mental status, or who are in respiratory distress) or who require intravenous medications.

Eron JJ et al; BENCHMRK Study Teams. Efficacy and safety of raltegravir for treatment of HIV for 5 years in the BENCHMRK studies: final results of two randomised, placebo-controlled trials. Lancet Infect Dis. 2013 Jul;13(7):587–96. [PMID: 23664333]

Günthard HF et al. Antiretroviral treatment of adult HIV infection: 2014 recommendations of the International Antiviral Society-USA Panel. JAMA. 2014 Jul 23–30;312(4):410–25. [PMID: 25038359]

INSIGHT START Study Group; Lundgren JD et al. Initiation of antiretroviral therapy in early asymptomatic HIV infection. N Engl J Med. 2015 Aug 27;373(9):795–807. [PMID: 26192873]

Jin J. JAMA patient page. Medications to prevent HIV infection. JAMA. 2014 Jul 23–30;312(4):452. [PMID: 25038373]

Patel DA et al. 48-week efficacy and safety of dolutegravir relative to commonly used third agents in treatment-naive HIV-1-infected patients: a systematic review and network meta-analysis. PLoS One. 2014 Sep 4;9(9):e105653. [PMID: 25188312]

Raffi F et al; extended SPRING-2 Study Group. Once-daily dolutegravir versus twice-daily raltegravir in antiretroviral-naive adults with HIV-1 infection (SPRING-2 study): 96 week results from a randomised, double-blind, non-inferiority trial. Lancet Infect Dis. 2013 Nov;13(11):927–35. [PMID: 24074642]

Rockstroh JK et al. A randomized, double-blind comparison of coformulated elvitegravir/cobicistat/emtricitabine/tenofovir DF vs ritonavir-boosted atazanavir plus coformulated emtricitabine and tenofovir DF for initial treatment of HIV-1 infection: analysis of week 96 results. J Acquir Immune Defic Syndr. 2013 Apr 15;62(5):483–6. [PMID: 23337366]

U.S. Department of Health and Human Services. Guidelines for the prevention and treatment of opportunistic infections in HIV-infected adults and adolescents. 2015. http://aidsinfo.nih.gov/contentfiles/lvguidelines/adult_oi.pdf

U.S. Department of Health and Human Services. Guidelines for the use of antiretroviral agents in HIV-1-infected adults and adolescents. 2015. http://aidsinfo.nih.gov/ContentFiles/lvguidelines/AdultandAdolescentGL.pdf

U.S. Food and Drug Administration. FDA Drug Safety Communication: interactions between certain HIV or hepatitis C drugs and cholesterol-lowering statin drugs can increase the risk of muscle injury. http://www.fda.gov/Drugs/DrugSafety/ucm293877.htm

Walmsley SL et al; SINGLE Investigators. Dolutegravir plus abacavir-lamivudine for the treatment of HIV-1 infection. N Engl J Med. 2013 Nov 7;369(19):1807–18. [PMID: 24195548]

Zolopa A et al; GS-US-236-0102 Study Team. A randomized double-blind comparison of coformulated elvitegravir/cobicistat/emtricitabine/tenofovir disoproxil fumarate versus efavirenz/emtricitabine/tenofovir disoproxil fumarate for initial treatment of HIV-1 infection: analysis of week 96 results. J Acquir Immune Defic Syndr. 2013 May 1;63(1):96–100. [PMID: 23392460]

Viral & Rickettsial Infections

32

Wayne X. Shandera, MD

Natalie J. M. Dailey Garnes, MD, MPH

VIRAL DISEASES

HUMAN HERPESVIRUSES

1. Herpesviruses 1 & 2

ESSENTIALS OF DIAGNOSIS

► Spectrum of illness from stomatitis and urogenital lesions to facial nerve paralysis (Bell palsy) and encephalitis.

► Variable intervals between exposure and clinical disease, since HSV causes both primary (often subclinical) and reactivation disease.

► General Considerations

Herpes simplex viruses 1 and 2 affect primarily the oral and genital areas, respectively. Asymptomatic shedding of either virus is common and may be responsible for transmission. Asymptomatic HSV-2–infected individuals shed the virus less frequently than those with symptomatic infection. Disease typically indicates reactivation. Total and subclinical shedding of HSV-2 virus decreases after the first year of initial infection, although viral shedding continues for years thereafter.

Although HSV-2 is the most common cause of genital ulcers in the developed world, epidemiologic studies show that HSV-1 is a more common cause of both genital and oral lesions than HSV-2 in young women in the United States. Most HSV-2 infected persons in the United States are unaware that they are infected.

HSV-2 seropositivity increases the risk of HIV acquisition (it is threefold higher among persons who are HSV-2 seropositive than among those who are HSV-2 seronegative), and reactivates more often in advanced HIV infection. HIV replication is increased by interaction with HSV proteins. Suppression of HSV-2 decreases HIV-1 plasma levels and genital tract shedding of HIV, which can contribute to a reduction in the sexual transmission of HIV-1.

► Clinical Findings

A. Symptoms and Signs

1. Mucocutaneous disease—See Chapter 6 for **HSV-1 mucocutaneous disease** involving the mouth and oral cavity ("herpes labialis" or "gingivostomatitis;" the latter largely in children). Digital lesions **(whitlows)** (Figure 32–1) are an occupational hazard in medicine and dentistry. Contact sports (eg, wrestling) are associated with outbreaks of skin infections ("herpes gladiatorum"). Asymptomatic shedding of HSV-1 is frequent, with most infected individuals shedding virus at least once a month.

Vesicles form moist ulcers after several days and epithelialize over 1–2 weeks if untreated. Primary infection is usually more severe than recurrences but may be asymptomatic. Recurrences often involve fewer lesions, tend to be labial, heal faster, and are induced by stress, fever, infection, sunlight, chemotherapy (eg, fludarabine, azathioprine) or other undetermined factors.

HSV-2 lesions largely involve the genital tract, with the virus remaining latent in the presacral ganglia (see Chapter 6). Occasionally, lesions arise in the perianal region or on the buttocks and upper thighs. Dysuria, cervicitis, and urinary retention may occur in women. Proctitis and extensive, ulcerating, weeping sacral lesions may be presenting symptoms in HIV-infected persons with CD4 cytopenia. Large ulcerations and atypical lesions suggest drug-resistant isolates.

2. Ocular disease—HSV can cause keratitis, blepharitis, and keratoconjunctivitis. Keratitis is usually unilateral and is often associated with impaired visual acuity. Lesions limited to the epithelium usually heal without affecting vision, whereas stromal involvement can cause uveitis, scarring, and eventually blindness. Recurrences of ocular disease are frequent. HSV is the second most common cause, after VZV, of acute retinal necrosis.

3. Neonatal and congenital infection—Both herpesviruses rarely infect the fetus and induce congenital malformations (organomegaly, bleeding, and central nervous system [CNS] abnormalities). Maternal infection during the third trimester is associated with the highest risk of neonatal transmission, but about 70% of these infections are asymptomatic or

▲ **Figure 32–1.** Herpetic whitlow. (Reproduced, with permission, from Richard P. Usatine, MD.)

unrecognized. Neonatal transmission during delivery, however, is more common than intrauterine infection. Invasive fetal monitoring and vacuum or forceps delivery increase the risk of herpesvirus transmission.

4. CNS disease—Traditionally, herpes simplex encephalitis is associated with HSV-1 infection and aseptic meningitis with HSV-2. However, both viruses can cause encephalitis. Encephalitis presents with nonspecific symptoms: a flu-like prodrome, followed by headache, fever, behavioral and speech disturbances, and focal or generalized seizures. The temporal lobe is often involved. Untreated disease and presentation with coma carry a high mortality rate. Many survivors suffer neurologic sequelae, which are observed more frequently among patients with HSV-1. Both HSV-1 and HSV-2 are increasingly recognized as causes of mild, nonspecific neurologic symptoms and are also associated with benign recurrent lymphocytic (Mollaret) meningitis.

5. Disseminated infection—Disseminated HSV infection occurs in the setting of immunosuppression, either primary or iatrogenic, or rarely with pregnancy. In disseminated disease, skin lesions are not always present. Disseminated skin lesions are a particular complication in patients with atopic eczema (eczema herpeticum) and burns. Pneumonia can occur regardless of immune status.

6. Bell palsy—HSV-1 is a cause of Bell palsy.

7. Esophagitis and proctitis—HSV-1 can cause esophagitis in immunocompromised patients, particularly those with AIDS. The lesions are smaller and deeper than those observed in patients with cytomegalovirus (CMV) esophagitis or with other herpesviruses known to cause esophagitis in immunocompromised persons. Proctitis occurs mainly in men who have sex with men.

8. Erythema multiforme—Herpes simplex viruses remain, along with certain drugs, a leading cause of erythema multiforme minor ("herpes-associated erythema multiforme") and of the more severe condition Stevens-Johnson syndrome/toxic epidermal necrolysis (see also Chapter 6).

9. Other—HSV is the cause of approximately 1% of cases of acute liver failure, particularly in pregnant women and immunosuppressed patients. The mortality of such rare fulminant hepatitis is nearly 75%. An HSV lower respiratory tract infection of unknown clinical significance is common in mechanically ventilated patients. Evidence suggests that this finding is usually an indicator rather than the cause of a poor clinical condition. HSV-1 pneumonia is associated with high morbidity in patients with solid tumors. HSV-1 is reported to be a cause of perinephric abscess, febrile neutropenia, chronic urticaria, and esophagitis and enteritis in systemic lupus erythematosus. HSV is also associated with *Helicobacter pylori*–negative upper gastrointestinal tract ulcers.

B. Laboratory Findings

1. Mucocutaneous disease—See Chapter 6.

2. Ocular disease—Herpes keratitis is diagnosed by branching (dendritic) ulcers that stain with fluorescein. The extent of epithelial injury in herpes keratitis correlates well with polymerase chain reaction (PCR) positivity.

3. Encephalitis and recurrent meningitis—Cerebrospinal fluid pleocytosis is common, with a similar increase in the number of red cells although cerebrospinal fluid findings may be atypical in immunosuppressed patients. HSV DNA PCR of the cerebrospinal fluid is a rapid, sensitive, and specific tool for early diagnosis and can be included in a multiple rapid array panel. Viral detection by this method can be delayed and should be repeated if the clinical picture is consistent. Antibodies to HSV in cerebrospinal fluid can confirm the diagnosis but appear late in disease. Viral culture shows a sensitivity of only 10%. MRI scanning is often a useful adjunct showing increased signal in the temporal and frontal lobes. Temporal lobe seizure foci may be shown on electroencephalograms (EEGs).

4. Esophagitis and proctitis—Esophagitis is diagnosed by endoscopic biopsy with real-time PCR and cultures. Proctitis may be diagnosed by rectal swab for PCR, culture, or both. Complicated cases may require biopsy.

5. Pneumonia—Pneumonia is diagnosed by clinical, pathologic, and radiographic findings. The CT findings include diffuse or multifocal areas of ground-glass attenuation or consolidative changes or both and are best confirmed by using high-resolution CT techniques.

▶ **Treatment & Prophylaxis**

Medications that inhibit replication of HSV-1 and HSV-2 include trifluridine and vidarabine (both for keratitis), acyclovir and related compounds, foscarnet, and cidofovir (Table 32–1).

A. Mucocutaneous Disease

See Chapter 6.

B. Keratitis

For the treatment of acute epithelial keratitis, oral antiviral agents such as valacyclovir or famciclovir are first-line therapies. Alternatives include topical antiviral agents (ophthalmic

Table 32–1. Agents for viral infections.[1]

Drug	Dosing	Spectrum	Toxicities
Acyclovir	200–800 mg orally five times daily; 250–500 mg/m^2 intravenously every 8 hours for 7 days	HSV, VZV	Neurotoxic reactions, reversible renal dysfunction, local reactions
Amantadine	200 mg daily orally, once daily in the elderly	Influenza A (not H1N1)	Confusion
Cidofovir	5 mg/kg intravenously weekly for 2 weeks, then every other week	CMV	Neutropenia, renal failure, ocular hypotonia
Famciclovir	500 mg orally three times daily for 7 days for acute VZV; 250 mg three times daily for 7–10 days for genital or cutaneous HSV-1/HSV-2 infection; 125 mg twice daily for 5 days for recurrences (500 mg twice daily for 7 days if HIV-infected)	HSV, VZV	Early angioedema; later rarely, gastrointestinal symptoms, headaches, rashes
Fomivirsen	165 mcg by intravitreal injection once weekly for 3 weeks, then every other week	CMV	Ocular inflammation, retinal detachment
Foscarnet	20 mg/kg intravenous bolus, then 120 mg/kg intravenously every 8 hours for 2 weeks; maintain with 60 mg/kg/day intravenously for 5 days each week	CMV, HSV resistant to acyclovir, VZV, HIV-1	Nephrotoxicity, genital ulcerations, calcium disturbances
Ganciclovir	5 mg/kg intravenous bolus every 12 hours for 14–21 days; maintain with 3.75 mg/kg/day intravenously for 5 days each week	CMV	Neutropenia, thrombocytopenia, CNS side effects
Idoxuridine	Topical, 0.1% every 1–2 hours for 3–5 days	HSV keratitis	Local reactions
Interferon alpha-2b	3–5 million international units subcutaneously three times weekly to daily. Intralesionally: 1 million international units per 0.1 mL in up to five warts three times weekly for 3 weeks	HBV, HCV, HPV	Influenza-like syndrome, myelosuppression, neurotoxicity
Interferon alpha-n3	0.05 mL/wart biweekly up to 8 weeks 3 milli-units intravenously three times per week	HPV HCV	Local reactions Influenza-like syndrome, myelosuppression, neurotoxicity
Laninamivir (CS-8958)	40 mg single inhaled dose	Influenza A and B	Under study (medication is marketed in Japan)
Oseltamivir	75 mg orally twice daily for 5 days beginning 48 hours after onset of symptoms	Influenza A and B	Few
Palivizumab	15 mg/kg intramuscularly every month in RSV season	RSV	Upper respiratory infection symptoms
Penciclovir	Topical 1% cream every 2 hours for 4 days	HSV	Local reactions
Peramivir	Intravenous, 600 mg single dose	Influenza (H1N1)	Nausea, vomiting, diarrhea, neutropenia
Ribavirin	Aerosol: 1.1 g/day as 20 mg/mL dilution over 12–18 hours for 3–7 days (See text for Lassa fever doses.)	RSV, severe influenza A or B, Lassa fever	Wheezing
Rimantadine	100 mg twice daily orally, once daily in the elderly	Influenza A (not H1N1)	Confusion
Trifluridine	Topical, 1% drops every 2 hours to 9 drops/day	HSV keratitis	Local reactions
Valacyclovir	1 g orally three times daily for 7 days for acute VZV; 1 g twice daily for primary genital HSV-1/HSV-2 infection with 500 mg three times daily for recurrences	VZV, HSV	Thrombotic thrombocytopenic purpura or hemolytic-uremic syndrome in AIDS
Valganciclovir	900 mg orally twice daily for 3 weeks; 900 mg daily as maintenance	CMV	See ganciclovir
Vidarabine	15 mg/kg/day intravenously for 10 days	HSV, VZV	Teratogenic, megaloblastosis, neurotoxicity
Zanamivir	2–5 mg inhalations twice daily for 5 days	Influenza A and B	Few

[1]Agents used exclusively in the management of HIV infection and AIDS are found in Chapter 31. Agents used in the management of HBV and HCV infections are found in Chapter 16.

CMV, cytomegalovirus; CNS, central nervous system; CSF, cerebrospinal fluid; HBV, hepatitis B virus; HCV, hepatitis C virus; HPV, human papillomavirus; HSV, herpes simplex virus; RSV, respiratory syncytial virus; VZV, varicella-zoster virus.

trifluridine, vidarabine, acyclovir, and ganciclovir), which are all nearly equivalent in efficacy. Intravenous acyclovir is used for acute retinal necrosis. The usage of topical corticosteroids may exacerbate the infection, although systemic corticosteroids may help with selected cases of stromal infection. Long-term treatment (more than 1 year) with acyclovir at a dosage of 800 mg/day orally decreases recurrence rates of keratitis, conjunctivitis or blepharitis due to HSV.

C. Neonatal Disease

Intravenous acyclovir (20 mg/kg every 8 hours for 14–21 days) is effective for the treatment of disseminated lesions in neonatal disease. Counseling with serologic screening should be offered to pregnant mothers. The use of maternal antenatal suppressive therapy with acyclovir (typically, 400 mg three times daily) beginning at 36 weeks gestation decreases the presence of detectable HSV, the rates of recurrence at delivery, and the need for cesarean delivery. Cesarean delivery is recommended for pregnant women with active genital lesions or typical prodromal symptoms.

D. Encephalitis and CNS Meningitis

Because of the need for rapid treatment to decrease mortality and neurologic sequelae, intravenous acyclovir (10 mg/kg every 8 hours for 10 days or more, adjusting for kidney dysfunction) should be started in those patients with suspected HSV encephalitis, stopping only if another diagnosis is established. If the PCR of cerebrospinal fluid is negative but clinical suspicion remains high, treatment should be continued for 10 days because the false-negative rate for PCR can be as high as 25% (especially in children) and acyclovir is relatively nontoxic. HSV viral load does not appear to correlate with outcome of meningitis, and it is not recommended to follow viral load over time.

Long-term neurologic sequelae of HSV encephalitis are common and late pediatric relapse is recognized. Acyclovir resistance in a case of herpes simplex encephalitis is reported. Aseptic meningitis may also require a course of intravenous acyclovir or valacyclovir. Long-term oral prophylaxis with valacyclovir, however, does not appear to prevent recurrences of aseptic meningitis with HSV-2.

E. Disseminated Disease

Disseminated disease responds best to parenteral acyclovir when treatment is initiated early.

F. Bell Palsy

Prednisolone, 25 mg orally twice daily for 10 days started within 72 h of onset, significantly increases the rate of recovery. Data on antiherpes antiviral agents are equivocal; according to one study, valacyclovir (but not acyclovir), 1 g orally daily for 5 days, plus corticosteroid therapy may be beneficial if started within 7 days of symptom onset. In patients with severe or complete facial paralysis, such antiviral therapy is often administered but without proof of efficacy.

G. Esophagitis and Proctitis

Patients with esophagitis should receive either intravenous acyclovir (5–10 mg/kg every 8 hours) or oral acyclovir (400 mg five times daily) through resolution of symptoms, typically 3–5 days; however, longer treatment may be necessary for immunosuppressed patients. Maintenance therapy for AIDS patients is also with acyclovir (400 mg three to five times daily). Proctitis is treated with similar dosages and usually responds within 5 days.

H. Erythema Multiforme

Suppressive therapy with oral acyclovir (400 mg twice a day for 6 months) decreases the recurrence rate of HSV-associated erythema multiforme. Valacyclovir (500 mg twice a day) may be effective in cases unresponsive to acyclovir.

▶ Prevention

Besides antiviral suppressive therapy (see above and Chapter 6), prevention also requires counseling and the use of condom barrier precautions during sexual activity. Disclosure to sexual partners of HSV-seropositive status is associated with about a 50% reduction in HSV-2 acquisition. Male circumcision is associated with a lower incidence of acquiring HSV-2 infection.

Preventing spread to hospital staff and other patients from cases with mucocutaneous, disseminated, or genital disease requires isolation and the usage of handwashing and gloving–gowning precautions. Staff with active lesions (eg, whitlows) should not have contact with patients. There is no approved herpes vaccine.

Cao S et al. Herpes simplex virus type 2 and the risk of cervical cancer: a meta-analysis of observational studies. Arch Gynecol Obstet. 2014 Dec;290(6):1059–66. [PMID: 25030659]

Kleines M et al. Clinical application of viral cerebrospinal fluid PCR testing for diagnosis of central nervous system disorders: a retrospective 11-year experience. Diagn Microbiol Infect Dis. 2014 Nov;80(3):207–15. [PMID: 25178670]

Workowski KA et al; Centers for Disease Control and Prevention. Sexually transmitted diseases treatment guidelines, 2015. MMWR Recomm Rep. 2015 Jun 5;64(RR-03):1–137. Erratum in: MMWR Recomm Rep. 2015 Aug 28;64(33):924. [PMID: 26042815]

Yi TJ et al. A randomized controlled pilot trial of valacyclovir for attenuating inflammation and immune activation in HIV/herpes simplex virus 2-coinfected adults on suppressive antiretroviral therapy. Clin Infect Dis. 2013 Nov;57(9):1331–8. [PMID: 23946220]

2. Varicella (Chickenpox) & Herpes Zoster (Shingles)

ESSENTIALS OF DIAGNOSIS

▶ **Varicella rash:** pruritic, centrifugal, papular changing to vesicular ("dewdrops on a rose petal"), pustular, and finally crusting.

▶ **Zoster rash:** tingling, pain, eruption of vesicles in a dermatomal distribution, evolving to pustules and then crusting.

General Considerations

Varicella zoster virus (VZV), or HHV-3, disease manifestations include chickenpox (varicella) and shingles (herpes zoster). Chickenpox generally presents during childhood; has an incubation period of 10–20 days (average 2 weeks); and is highly contagious, spreading by inhalation of infective droplets or contact with lesions.

The incidence and severity of herpes zoster ("shingles"), which affects up to 25% of persons during their lifetime, increases with age due to an age-related decline in immunity against VZV. More than half of all patients in whom herpes zoster develops are older than 60 years, and the incidence of herpes zoster reaches 10 cases per 1000 patient-years by age 80 (by which time 50% are infected with VZV). The annual incidence in the United States of 1 million cases is increasing as the population ages. Populations at increased risk for varicella-zoster–related diseases include immunosuppressed persons and persons receiving biologic agents (eg, tumor necrosis factor [TNF] inhibitors).

Clinical Findings

A. Varicella

1. Symptoms and signs—Fever and malaise are mild in children and more marked in adults. The pruritic rash begins prominently on the face, scalp, and trunk, and later involves the extremities (Table 32–2). Maculopapules change in a few hours to vesicles that become pustular and eventually form crusts (Figures 32–2 and 32–3). New lesions may erupt for 1–5 days, so that different stages of

Table 32–2. Diagnostic features of some acute exanthems.

Disease	Prodromal Signs and Symptoms	Nature of Eruption	Other Diagnostic Features	Laboratory Tests
Atypical measles	Same as measles.	Maculopapular centripetal rash, becoming confluent.	History of measles vaccination.	Measles antibody present in past, with titer rise during illness.
Chikungunya fever	2–4 (sometimes 1–12) days, fever, headaches, abdominal complaints, myalgias, arthralgias.	Maculopapular, centrally distributed, pruritus, can be bullous with sloughing in children, occasional facial edema and petechiae.	History of mosquito bites, epidemiologic factors.	ELISA-based IgM or IgG (fourfold increase in titers); PCR and cultures are infrequently available.
Eczema herpeticum	None.	Vesiculopustular lesions in area of eczema.		Herpes simplex virus isolated in cell culture. Multinucleate giant cells in smear of lesion.
Ehrlichiosis	Headache, malaise.	Rash in one-third, similar to Rocky Mountain spotted fever.	Pancytopenia, elevated liver function tests.	Polymerase chain reaction, immunofluorescent antibody.
Enterovirus infections	1–2 days of fever, malaise.	Maculopapular rash resembling rubella, rarely papulovesicular or petechial.	Aseptic meningitis.	Virus isolation from stool or cerebrospinal fluid; complement fixation titer rise.
Erythema infectiosum (parvovirus B19)	None. Usually in epidemics.	Red, flushed cheeks; circumoral pallor; maculopapules on extremities.	"Slapped face" appearance.	White blood count normal.
Exanthema subitum (HHV-6, 7; roseola)	3–4 days of high fever.	As fever falls, pink maculopapules appear on chest and trunk; fade in 1–3 days.		White blood count low.
Infectious mononucleosis (EBV)	Fever, adenopathy, sore throat.	Maculopapular rash resembling rubella, rarely papulovesicular.	Splenomegaly, tonsillar exudate.	Atypical lymphocytes in blood smears; heterophile agglutination (Monospot test).
Kawasaki disease	Fever, adenopathy, conjunctivitis.	Cracked lips, strawberry tongue, maculopapular polymorphous rash, peeling skin on fingers and toes.	Edema of extremities. Angiitis of coronary arteries.	Thrombocytosis, electrocardiographic changes.
Measles (rubeola)	3–4 days of fever, coryza, conjunctivitis, and cough.	Maculopapular, brick red; begins on head and neck; spreads downward and outward, in 5–6 days rash brownish, desquamating. See Atypical Measles, above.	Koplik spots on buccal mucosa.	White blood count low. Virus isolation in cell culture. Antibody tests by hemagglutination inhibition or neutralization.

(continued)

Table 32–2. Diagnostic features of some acute exanthems. (continued)

Disease	Prodromal Signs and Symptoms	Nature of Eruption	Other Diagnostic Features	Laboratory Tests
Meningococcemia	Hours of fever, vomiting.	Maculopapules, petechiae, purpura.	Meningeal signs, toxicity, shock.	Cultures of blood, cerebrospinal fluid. White blood count high.
Rocky Mountain spotted fever	3–4 days of fever, vomiting.	Maculopapules, petechiae, initial distribution centripetal (extremities to trunk, including palms).	History of tick bite.	Indirect fluorescent antibody; complement fixation.
Rubella	Little or no prodrome.	Maculopapular, pink; begins on head and neck, spreads downward, fades in 3 days. No desquamation.	Lymphadenopathy, postauricular or occipital.	White blood count normal or low. Serologic tests for immunity and definitive diagnosis (hemagglutination inhibition).
Scarlet fever	One-half to 2 days of malaise, sore throat, fever, vomiting.	Generalized, punctate, red; prominent on neck, in axillae, groin, skin folds; circumoral pallor; fine desquamation involves hands and feet.	Strawberry tongue, exudative tonsillitis.	Group A beta-hemolytic streptococci in cultures from throat; antistreptolysin O titer rise.
Smallpox	Fever, malaise, prostration.	Maculopapules to vesicles to pustules to scars (lesions develop at the same pace).	Centrifugal rash; fulminant sepsis in small percentage of patients, gastrointestinal and skin hemorrhages.	Contact CDC[1] for suspicious rash; EM and gel diffusion assays.
Typhus	3–4 days of fever, chills, severe headaches.	Maculopapules, petechiae, initial distribution centrifugal (trunk to extremities).	Endemic area, lice.	Complement fixation.
Varicella (chickenpox)	0–1 day of fever, anorexia, headache.	Rapid evolution of macules to papules, vesicles, crusts; all stages simultaneously present; lesions superficial, distribution centripetal.	Lesions on scalp and mucous membranes.	Specialized complement fixation and virus neutralization in cell culture. Fluorescent antibody test of smear of lesions.

[1]http://www.bt.cdc.gov/agent/smallpox/response-plan/.
EBV, Epstein-Barr virus; ELISA, enzyme-linked immunosorbent assay; EM, electron microscopy; HHV, human herpesvirus; Ig, immunoglobulin; PCR, polymerase chain reaction.

the eruption are usually present simultaneously. The crusts slough in 7–14 days. The vesicles and pustules are superficial and elliptical, with slightly serrated borders. Pitted scars are frequent. Although the disease is often mild, complications (such as secondary bacterial infection, pneumonitis, and encephalitis) occur in about 1% of cases and often lead to hospitalization.

After the primary infection, the virus remains dormant in cranial nerve sensory ganglia and spinal dorsal root ganglia. Latent VZV will reactivate as herpes zoster in about 10–30% of persons (see below). Varicella is more severe in older patients and immunocompromised persons. In the latter, atypical presentations, including widespread dissemination in the absence of skin lesions, are often described.

There is a small increased risk of Guillain-Barré syndrome for at least 2 months after an acute herpes zoster attack.

2. Laboratory findings—Diagnosis is usually made clinically, with confirmation by direct immunofluorescent antibody staining or PCR of scrapings from lesions. Multinucleated giant cells are usually apparent on a Tzanck smear of material from the vesicle base. Leukopenia and subclinical transaminase elevation are often present and thrombocytopenia occasionally occurs. A varicella skin test and interferon-gamma enzyme-linked immunospot (ELISPOT) can screen for VZV susceptibility.

B. Herpes Zoster

Herpes zoster (**"shingles"**) usually occurs among adults, but cases are reported among infants and children. Skin lesions resemble those of chickenpox. Pain is often severe and commonly precedes the appearance of rash. Lesions follow a dermatomal distribution, with thoracic and lumbar roots being the most common. In most cases, a single

▲ **Figure 32–2.** Primary varicella (chickenpox) skin lesions. (Public Health Image Library, CDC.)

unilateral dermatome is involved, but occasionally, neighboring and distant areas are involved. Lesions on the tip of the nose, inner corner of the eye, and root and side of the nose (**Hutchinson sign**) indicate involvement of the

▲ **Figure 32–3.** Chickenpox (varicella) with classic "dew drop on rose petal" appearance. (Reproduced, with permission, from Richard P. Usatine, MD.)

trigeminal nerve (**herpes zoster ophthalmicus**). Facial palsy, lesions of the external ear with or without tympanic membrane involvement, vertigo and tinnitus, or deafness signify geniculate ganglion involvement (**Ramsay Hunt syndrome** or **herpes zoster oticus**). Shingles is a particularly common and serious complication among immunosuppressed patients. Other rare risk factors include statin therapy and possibly anti-TNF therapy. Contact with patients who have varicella does not appear to be a risk factor for zoster.

► **Complications**

A. Varicella

Secondary bacterial skin superinfections, particularly with group A streptococcus and *Staphylococcus aureus*, are the most common complications. Cellulitis, erysipelas, and scarlet fever are described. Bullous impetigo and necrotizing fasciitis are less often seen. Other associations with varicella include epiglottitis, necrotizing pneumonia, osteomyelitis, septic arthritis, epidural abscess, meningitis, endocarditis, pancreatitis, and purpura fulminans. Toxic shock syndrome can also develop.

Interstitial VZV pneumonia is more common in adults (especially smokers, HIV-infected patients, and pregnant women) and may result in acute respiratory distress syndrome (ARDS). After healing, numerous densely calcified lesions are seen throughout the lung fields on chest radiographs.

Historically, neurologic complications developed in about 1 in 2000 children. Cerebellar ataxia occurs at a frequency of 1:4000 in the young. A limited course and complete recovery are the rule. Encephalitis is similarly infrequent, occurs mostly in adults, and is characterized by delirium, seizures, and focal neurologic signs. The rates for both mortality and long-term neurologic sequelae are about 10%. Ischemic strokes in the wake of acute VZV infection present at a mean of 4 months after rashes and may be due to an associated vasculitis. Multifocal encephalitis, ventriculitis, myeloradiculitis, arterial aneurysm formation, and arteritis are also described in immunosuppressed, especially HIV-infected, patients.

Clinical hepatitis is uncommon and mostly presents in the immunosuppressed patient but can be fulminant and fatal. Reye syndrome (fatty liver with encephalopathy) also complicates varicella (and other viral infections, especially influenza B virus), usually in childhood, and is associated with aspirin therapy (see Influenza, below).

When contracted during the first or second trimesters of pregnancy, varicella carries a very small risk of congenital malformations, including cicatricial lesions of an extremity, growth retardation, microphthalmia, cataracts, chorioretinitis, deafness, and cerebrocortical atrophy. If varicella develops around the time of delivery, the newborn is at risk for disseminated disease.

B. Herpes Zoster

Postherpetic neuralgia occurs in 60–70% of patients who have herpes zoster and are older than 60 years. The pain can be prolonged and debilitating. Risk factors for postherpetic neuralgia include advanced age, female sex, the presence of a prodrome, and severity of rash or pain but not family history.

Other complications include the following: (1) bacterial skin superinfections; (2) herpes zoster ophthalmicus, which occurs with involvement of the trigeminal nerve and is a sight-threatening complication (especially when it involves the iris), and is a marker for stroke over the ensuing year (Hutchinson sign is a marker of ocular involvement in the HIV-positive population); (3) rarely, unilateral ophthalmoplegia; (4) involvement of the geniculate ganglion of cranial nerve VII as well as cranial nerves V, VIII, IX, and X; (5) aseptic meningitis; (6) peripheral motor neuropathy; (7) transverse myelitis; (8) encephalitis; (9) acute cerebellitis; (10) stroke; (11) vasculopathy; (12) acute retinal necrosis; (13) progressive outer retinal necrosis (largely among HIV infected persons); (14) temporal arteritis; and (15) sacral meningoradiculitis (Elsberg syndrome). VZV is a major cause of Bell palsy in patients who are HSV seronegative.

Diagnosis of neurologic complications requires the detection of VZV DNA in cerebrospinal fluid or the detection of VZV DNA in tissue. Diagnosis by examination of saliva may be possible. *Zoster sine herpete* (pain without rash) can also be associated with most of the above complications.

▶ **Treatment**

A. General Measures

In general, patients with varicella should be isolated until primary lesions have crusted. The skin is kept clean. Pruritus can be relieved with antihistamines, calamine lotion, and colloidal oatmeal baths. Fever can be treated with acetaminophen (not aspirin). Fingernails can be closely cropped to avoid skin excoriation and infection.

B. Antiviral Therapy

1. Varicella—Acyclovir, 20 mg/kg (up to 800 mg per dose) orally four times daily for 5 days, should be given within the first 24 hours after the onset of varicella rash and should be considered for patients older than 12 years, secondary household contacts (disease tends to be more severe in secondary cases), patients with chronic cutaneous and cardiopulmonary diseases, and children receiving long-term therapy with salicylates (to decrease the risk of Reye syndrome). Acyclovir hastens defervescence and healing of lesions but does not impact complication rates. Experience with valacyclovir and famciclovir in these settings is scant and while these agents are often used, their use is not FDA-approved in the United States.

In immunocompromised patients, in pregnant women during the third trimester, and in patients with extracutaneous disease (encephalitis, pneumonitis), antiviral therapy with high-dose acyclovir (30 mg/kg/day in three divided doses intravenously for at least 7 days) should be started once the diagnosis is suspected. Corticosteroids may be useful in the presence of pneumonia. Prolonged prophylactic acyclovir is important to prevent VZV reactivation in profoundly immunosuppressed patients.

2. Herpes zoster—For uncomplicated herpes zoster, valacyclovir or famciclovir is preferable to acyclovir due to dosing convenience and higher drug levels in the body. Therapy should start within the first 72 hours of the onset of the lesions and be continued for 7 days or until the lesions crust over. Antiviral therapy reduces the duration of herpetic lesions and associated episodes of acute pain but does not in all studies decrease the risk of postherpetic neuralgia. Corticosteroids (a tapering course starting at 60 mg/day, for 2–3 weeks) are safe in immunocompetent patients and may be useful in the acute management of disease to hasten the resolution of acute lesions. Corticosteroids do not prevent the development of postherpetic neuralgia.

Intravenous acyclovir is used for extradermatomal complications of zoster. Adjunctive therapy may be considered in retinal disease (foscarnet) and acute herpes zoster (sorivudine, a topical antiviral). In cases of prolonged or repeated acyclovir use, immunosuppressed patients may require a switch to foscarnet due to the development of acyclovir-resistant VZV infections. The Ramsay Hunt syndrome is more resistant to antiviral therapy.

C. Treatment of Postherpetic Neuralgia

Once established, postherpetic neuralgia may respond to neuropathic pain agents such as gabapentin or lidocaine patches. Tricyclic antidepressants, opioids, and capsaicin cream are also widely used and effective. The epidural injection of corticosteroids and local anesthetics appears to modestly reduce herpetic pain at 1 month but, as with oral corticosteroids, is not effective for prevention of long-term postherpetic neuralgia. There is reported success using transcutaneous electrical nerve stimulation.

▶ **Prognosis**

The total duration of varicella from onset of symptoms to disappearance of crusts rarely exceeds 2 weeks. Fatalities are rare except in immunosuppressed patients.

Herpes zoster resolves in 2–6 weeks. Antibodies persist longer and at higher levels than with primary varicella. Eye involvement with herpes zoster necessitates periodic future examinations.

▶ **Prevention**

Health care workers should be screened for varicella and vaccinated if seronegative. Patients with active varicella or herpes zoster are promptly separated from seronegative patients. For patients with varicella, airborne and contact isolation is recommended, whereas for those with zoster, contact precautions are sufficient. For immunosuppressed patients with zoster, precautions should be the same as if the patient had varicella. Exposed serosusceptible patients should be placed in isolation and exposed serosusceptible employees should stay away from work between days 10 and 21 after exposure. Health care workers with zoster should receive antiviral agents during the first 72 hours of disease and withdraw from work until lesions are crusted. Postexposure prophylaxis should be evaluated (see below).

A. Varicella

1. Vaccination—Universal childhood vaccination against varicella is effective. The varicella vaccine (Varilrix) is live and attenuated, safe, and over 98.1% effective when given after 13 months of age. A single antigen live attenuated vaccine (VARIVAX) or a quadrivalent measles, mumps, rubella, and varicella vaccine (ProQuad) are available. The first dose should be administered at 12–15 months of age and the second at 4–6 years. Aspirin should be avoided for at least 6 weeks because of the risk of Reye syndrome. This vaccine is safe, well tolerated, but the quadrivalent vaccine is associated with a small risk of febrile seizures 5–12 days after vaccination among infants aged 12–23 months. Rashes, when secondary to the varicella vaccine, appear 15–42 days after vaccination.

For serosusceptible individuals older than 13 years, two doses of varicella vaccine (single antigen) administered 4–8 weeks apart are recommended. For those who received a single dose in the past, a catch-up second dose is advised, especially in the epidemic setting (where it is effective when it can be given during the first 5 days postexposure). Household contacts of immunocompromised patients should adhere to these recommendations. Susceptible pregnant women (who should not be vaccinated with live varicella-zoster vaccines during pregnancy) need to receive the first dose of vaccine before discharge after delivery and the second dose 4–8 weeks later. The quadrivalent vaccine MMRV can be used for the second doses of MMR and varicella in patients aged 15 months to 12 years and for the first dose in patients aged 48 months or older. The vaccine, administered as two doses 3 months apart, should also be considered for HIV-infected adolescents and adults with CD4 T lymphocyte counts 200 cells/mcL or more. The vaccine may also be given to patients with impaired humoral immunity, to patients receiving corticosteroids, and to patients with juvenile rheumatoid arthritis who receive methotrexate. Patients receiving high doses of corticosteroids for over 2 weeks may be vaccinated a month after discontinuation of the therapy. Patients with leukemia, lymphoma, or other malignancies whose disease is in remission and who have not undergone chemotherapy for at least 3 months may be vaccinated. Kidney and liver transplant patients should be vaccinated if they are susceptible to varicella.

The incidence of varicella in the United States is significantly reduced with the varicella vaccine. Meanwhile, the varicella vaccine is associated with a small increase in the incidence of herpes zoster, with the latter occurring more often in warm months. It is thought that vaccination against varicella provides less protection against future zoster than does natural varicella.

The FDA no longer maintains a registry for exposed pregnant women because of the low rate of such incidents and the general safety of varicella vaccines. Incidents can be reported to Merck (877-888-4231) or through the Vaccine Adverse Events Registry System Vaccine (https://vaers.hhs.gov/index).

2. Postexposure—Postexposure vaccination is recommended for unvaccinated persons without other evidence of immunity. Varicella-zoster immune globulin available in the United States only as VariZIG should be considered for susceptible exposed patients (for up to 10 days after exposure but as soon as feasible) who cannot receive the vaccine, including immunosuppressed patients, neonates from mothers with varicella around the time of delivery, exposed premature infants born from serosusceptible mothers at greater than 28 weeks of gestation, neonates born at less than 28 weeks of gestation regardless of maternal serostatus, and pregnant women. No controlled studies have evaluated the use of acyclovir in this setting. VariZIG is given by intramuscular injection in a dosage of 125 international units/10 kg, to a maximum of 625 international units with a weight-based (2 kg cutoff) minimum dose of 62.5 or 125 international units), with a repeat identical dose in 3 weeks if a high-risk patient remains exposed. VariZIG has no place in therapy of established disease; however, it reduces severity of varicella in high-risk children or adults (ie, those with impaired immunity, pregnant women, and infants exposed peripartum) if given within 4 days of exposure. Varicella vaccination should be delayed at least 5 months after VariZIG administration.

Further information may be obtained by calling the Centers for Disease Control and Prevention's Immunization Information Hotline (800-232-2522).

B. Herpes Zoster

A live attenuated VZV vaccine (ZOSTAVAX, 19,400 plaque forming units [pfu] of Oka/Merck strain) contains at least 14 times the concentration of varicella virus found in VARIVAX. It is recommended for persons 60 years and older because it reduces the incidence of herpes zoster and postherpetic neuralgia by 51% and 67%, respectively. **Even if the person has had a prior episode of herpes zoster, the vaccine has efficacy and can be administered.** No specific recommendations exist regarding how long to wait between a zoster outbreak and administering the vaccine; the CDC recommends waiting at least until the outbreak has resolved. An adjuvanted recombinant subunit vaccine (HZ/su, GlaxoSmithKline Biologicals) is in trials. Two doses of this vaccine given 2 months apart had 97% efficacy with no significant decrease with age.

Concurrent administration of the live attenuated VZV vaccine with pneumococcal vaccine is safe. If a varicella vaccine is mistakenly administered to an adult instead of a live attenuated zoster vaccine, the dose should be considered invalid and the patient should be administered a dose of zoster vaccine at the same visit. On the other hand, the zoster vaccine cannot be used in children in place of varicella vaccine; if the vaccine is accidentally given to a child, the event should be reported to the CDC.

Centers for Disease Control and Prevention (CDC). Updated recommendations for use of VariZIG—United States, 2013. MMWR Morb Mortal Wkly Rep. 2013 Jul 19;62(28):574–6. [PMID: 23863705]

Chen N et al. Antiviral treatment for preventing postherpetic neuralgia. Cochrane Database Syst Rev. 2014 Feb 6;2: CD006866. [PMID: 24500927]

Cohen JI. Clinical practice: herpes zoster. N Engl J Med. 2013 Jul 18; 369(3):255–63. [PMID: 23863052]

Han Y et al. Corticosteroids for preventing postherpetic neuralgia. Cochrane Database Syst Rev. 2013 Mar 28;3:CD005582. [PMID: 23543541]

Lal H et al; ZOE-50 Study Group. Efficacy of an adjuvanted herpes zoster subunit vaccine in older adults. N Engl J Med. 2015 May 28;372(22):2087–96. [PMID: 25916341]

Wu PY et al. Varicella vaccination alters the chronological trends of herpes zoster and varicella. PLoS One. 2013 Oct 30;8(10): e77709. [PMID: 24204928]

Yawn BP et al. The global epidemiology of herpes zoster. Neurology. 2013 Sep 3;81(10):928–30. [PMID: 23999562]

3. Epstein-Barr Virus & Infectious Mononucleosis

▲ **Figure 32–4.** Conjunctival hemorrhage of the eye due to infectious mononucleosis. (From Dr. Thomas F. Sellers, Emory University, Public Health Image Library, CDC.)

ESSENTIALS OF DIAGNOSIS

► Malaise, fever, and sore throat, sometimes with exudates.

► Palatal petechiae, lymphadenopathy, splenomegaly, and, occasionally, a maculopapular rash.

► Positive heterophile agglutination test (Monospot).

► Atypical large lymphocytes in blood smear; lymphocytosis.

► Complications: hepatitis, myocarditis, neuropathy, encephalitis, airway obstruction secondary to lymph node enlargement, hemolytic anemia, thrombocytopenia.

General Considerations

Epstein-Barr virus (EBV, or human herpes virus-4 [HHV-4]) is one of the most ubiquitous human viruses, infecting more than 95% of the adult population worldwide and persisting for the lifetime of the host. Infectious mononucleosis is a common manifestation of EBV and may occur at any age. In the United States the incidence of EBV infection is declining although prevalence of EBV remains high for those aged 12–19 years. In the developing world, infectious mononucleosis occurs at younger ages and tends to be less symptomatic. Rare cases in the elderly occur usually without the full symptomatology. EBV is largely transmitted by saliva but can also be recovered from genital secretions. Saliva may remain infectious during convalescence, for 6 months or longer after symptom onset. The incubation period lasts several weeks (30–50 days).

Clinical Findings

A. Symptoms and Signs

The protean manifestations of infectious mononucleosis reflect the dissemination of the virus in the oral cavity and through peripheral blood lymphocytes and cell-free plasma. Fever, sore throat, fatigue, malaise, anorexia, and myalgia typically occur in the early phase of the illness.

Physical findings include lymphadenopathy (discrete, non-suppurative, slightly painful, especially along the posterior cervical chain), transient bilateral upper lid edema (Hoagland sign), and splenomegaly (in up to 50% of patients). A maculopapular or occasionally petechial rash occurs in less than 15% of patients unless ampicillin is given (in which case rash is seen in more than 90%). Conjunctival hemorrhage (Figure 32–4), exudative pharyngitis, uvular edema, tonsillitis, or gingivitis may occur and soft palatal petechiae may be noted.

Other manifestations include hepatitis, interstitial pneumonitis, cholestasis, gastritis, acute interstitial nephritis, nervous system involvement in 1–5% (mononeuropathies and occasionally aseptic meningitis, encephalitis, cerebellitis, peripheral and optic neuritis, transverse myelitis, or Guillain-Barré syndrome), kidney disease (mostly interstitial nephritis), pneumonia, pleural involvement, and myocarditis. Vaginal ulcers are rare but may be present. Airway obstruction from lymph node enlargement, pericarditis, life-threatening thrombocytopenia, severe CNS complications, and massive splenomegaly are all considered indications for hospitalization or close observation.

B. Laboratory Findings

An initial phase of granulocytopenia is followed within 1 week by lymphocytic leukocytosis (greater than 50% of all leukocytes) with atypical lymphocytes (larger than normal mature lymphocytes, staining more darkly, and showing vacuolated, foamy cytoplasm and dark nuclear chromatin) comprising more than 10% of the leukocyte count. Hemolytic anemia, with anti-i antibodies, occurs occasionally as does thrombocytopenia (at times marked).

Diagnosis is made on the basis of characteristic manifestations and serologic evidence of infection (the heterophile sheep cell agglutination [HA] antibody tests or the correlated mononucleosis spot test [Monospot]). These tests usually become positive within 4 weeks after onset of illness and are specific but often not sensitive in early illness. Heterophile antibodies may be absent in young children and in as many as 20% of adults. During acute illness, there is a rise and fall in immunoglobulin M (IgM) antibody to EB virus capsid antigen (VCA) and a rise in IgG antibody to VCA, which persists for life. Antibodies (IgG) to EBV nuclear antigen (EBNA) appear after 4 weeks of onset and also persist. Absence of IgG and IgM VCA or the presence of IgG EBNA should make one reconsider the diagnosis of acute EBV infection.

PCR for EBV DNA is useful in the evaluation of malignancies associated with EBV. For instance, detection of EBV DNA in cerebrospinal fluid shows a sensitivity of 90% and specificity of nearly 100% for the diagnosis of primary CNS lymphoma in patients with AIDS.

▶ Differential Diagnosis

CMV infection, toxoplasmosis, acute HIV infection, secondary syphilis, HHV-6, rubella, and drug hypersensitivity reactions may be indistinguishable from infectious mononucleosis due to EBV, but exudative pharyngitis is usually absent and the heterophile antibody tests are negative. With acute HIV infection, rash and mucocutaneous ulceration are common but atypical lymphocytosis is much less common. Heterophile-negative infectious mononucleosis with nonsignificant lymphocytosis (especially if rash or mucocutaneous ulcers are present) should prompt investigation for acute HIV infection. CMV, toxoplasmosis and, on occasion, EBV can cause heterophile-negative infectious mononucleosis with atypical lymphocytosis. Mycoplasma infection may also present as pharyngitis, though lower respiratory symptoms usually predominate. A hypersensitivity syndrome induced by carbamazepine or phenytoin may mimic infectious mononucleosis.

The differential diagnosis of acute exudative pharyngitis includes gonococcal and streptococcal infections, and infections with adenovirus and herpes simplex. Head and neck soft tissue infections (pharyngeal and tonsillar abscesses) may occasionally be mistaken as the lymphadenopathy of mononucleosis.

▶ Complications

Secondary bacterial pharyngitis can occur and is often streptococcal. Splenic rupture (0.5–1%) is a rare but dramatic complication, and a history of preceding trauma can be elicited in 50% of the cases. Acalculous cholecystitis, fulminant hepatitis with massive necrosis, pericarditis and myocarditis are also infrequent complications. Neurologic involvement—including transverse myelitis, encephalitis, and Guillain-Barré syndrome—is infrequent.

▶ Treatment

A. General Measures

Over 95% of patients with acute EBV-associated infectious mononucleosis recover without specific antiviral therapy. Treatment is symptomatic with acetaminophen or other nonsteroidal anti-inflammatory drugs and warm saline throat irrigations or gargles three or four times daily. Acyclovir decreases viral shedding but shows no clinical benefit. Corticosteroid therapy, although widespread, is not recommended in uncomplicated cases; its use is reserved

for impending airway obstruction from enlarged lymph nodes, hemolytic anemia, and severe thrombocytopenia. The value of corticosteroid therapy in impending splenic rupture, pericarditis, myocarditis, and nervous system involvement is less well established. If a throat culture grows beta-hemolytic streptococci, a 10-day course of penicillin or azithromycin is indicated. **Ampicillin and amoxicillin are avoided because of the frequent association with rash.**

B. Treatment of Complications

Hepatitis, myocarditis, and encephalitis are treated symptomatically. Rupture of the spleen requires splenectomy and is most often caused by deep palpation of the spleen or vigorous activity. Patients should avoid contact or collision sports for at least 4 weeks to decrease the risk of splenic rupture (even if splenomegaly is not detected by physical examination, which can be insensitive).

▶ Prognosis & Prevention

In uncomplicated cases, fever disappears in 10 days and lymphadenopathy and splenomegaly in 4 weeks. The debility sometimes lingers for 2–3 months.

Death is uncommon and is usually due to splenic rupture, hypersplenic phenomena (severe hemolytic anemia, thrombocytopenic purpura), or encephalitis.

A glycoprotein vaccine and a protein vaccine are under development with the former reducing the rate of infectious mononucleosis in EBV seronegative recipients. Neither vaccine is currently commercially available. Handwashing after contact and avoidance of close personal contact with active cases is prudent.

4. Other EBV-Associated Syndromes

EBV viral antigens are found in more than 90% of patients with endemic (African) Burkitt lymphoma and nasopharyngeal carcinoma (among whom quantified EBV DNA can be used to follow disease). Risk factors for Burkitt lymphoma include a history of malaria (which may decrease resistance to EBV infection) while risk factors for nasopharyngeal carcinoma include long-term heavy cigarette smoking and seropositive EBV serologies (VCA and deoxyribonuclease [DNase]). VCA-IgA in peripheral blood is a sensitive and specific predictor for nasopharyngeal carcinoma in endemic areas.

Chronic EBV infection is associated with aberrant cellular immunity (a low frequency of EBV-specific CD8+ T cells), an X-linked lymphoproliferative syndrome (Duncan disease), lymphomatoid granulomatosis, and a fatal T cell lymphoproliferative disorder in children.

EBV is an important trigger for hemophagocytic lymphohistiocytosis among immunodeficient patients and causes B-cell lymphomas (such as primary CNS lymphoma in HIV-infected individuals), natural killer/T cell lymphoma, and posttransplant lymphoproliferative disorders. Posttransplant lymphoproliferative states are commonly associated with EBV, especially in children. EBV-naïve patients who receive a donor organ from an EBV-infected donor are at the highest risk for the development of posttransplant lymphoproliferative disorder. Decreasing the iatrogenic immunosuppression given to prevent graft rejection is the initial step in managing such patients, while rituximab (CD20 monoclonal antibody) is effective in treating more than two-thirds of cases. The efficacy of rituximab or traditional chemotherapy often can be assessed by monitoring levels of EBV DNA load in the blood and, if indicated, CNS. Infusion of EBV-specific cytotoxic T cell lymphocytes (adoptive cell therapy) is also used but with a less established role.

Age is a major determinant of the type of tumor associated with EBV. T and NK cell lymphoma caused by chronic active EBV infections are more frequent in childhood while peripheral T cell lymphomas and diffuse large B cell lymphomas are more common in the elderly due to waning immunity. EBV is also associated with leiomyomas in children with AIDS and with nasal T cell lymphomas.

When to Admit

Severe complications of EBV disease, including the following conditions:

- Acute meningitis, encephalitis, or acute Guillain-Barré syndrome.
- Severe thrombocytopenia; significant hemolysis.
- Potential splenic rupture.
- Airway obstruction from severe adenitis.
- Pericarditis.
- Abdominal findings mimicking an acute abdomen.

Balfour HH Jr et al. Age-specific prevalence of Epstein-Barr virus infection among individuals aged 6–19 years in the United States and factors affecting its acquisition. J Infect Dis. 2013 Oct 15;208(8):1286–93. [PMID: 23868878]

Draborg AH et al. Epstein-Barr virus in systemic autoimmune diseases. Clin Dev Immunol. 2013;2013:535738. [PMID: 24062777]

Green M et al. Epstein-Barr virus infection and posttransplant lymphoproliferative disorder. Am J Transplant. 2013 Feb; 13(Suppl 3):41–54. [PMID: 23347213]

Mailankody S et al. HIV, EBV, and monoclonal gammopathy. Blood. 2013 Oct 24;122(17):2924–5. [PMID: 24159162]

Vouloumanou EK et al. Current diagnosis and management of infectious mononucleosis. Curr Opin Hematol. 2012 Jan; 19(1):14–20. [PMID: 22123662]

5. Cytomegalovirus Disease

ESSENTIALS OF DIAGNOSIS

- ► Mononucleosis-like syndrome.
- ► Frequent pathogen seen in transplant populations.
- ► Diverse clinical syndromes in HIV (retinitis, esophagitis, pneumonia, encephalitis).
- ► Major pathogen to consider in neonates in the differential of maternally transmitted agents.

General Considerations

Most cytomegalovirus (CMV) infections are asymptomatic. After primary infection, the virus remains latent in most body cells. Seroprevalence in adults of Western developed countries is about 60–80% but is higher in developing countries. CMV seroprevalence increases with age and lower socioeconomic status and is higher among persons employed in child-care centers. Seroprevalence further increases with the number of sexual partners and a history of prior sexually transmitted infections. The virus can be isolated from a variety of tissues under nonpathogenic conditions. Transmission occurs through sexual contact, breastfeeding, blood products, or transplantation; it may also occur person-to-person (eg, day care centers) or be congenital. Serious disease occurs primarily in immunocompromised persons.

There are three recognizable clinical syndromes: (1) perinatal disease and CMV inclusion disease; (2) diseases in immunocompetent persons; and (3) diseases in immunocompromised persons. **Congenital CMV infection** is the most common congenital infection in developed countries (about 0.6% of live births, with higher rates in underdeveloped areas and among lower socioeconomic groups). Transmission is much higher from mothers with primary disease than those with reactivation (40% vs 0.2–1.8%). About 10% of infected newborns will be symptomatic with CMV inclusion disease.

In **immunocompetent persons**, acute CMV infection is the most common cause of the mononucleosis-like syndrome with negative heterophile antibodies. In critically ill immunocompetent adults, CMV reactivation is associated with prolonged hospitalization and death.

In **immunocompromised persons**, solid organ and bone marrow transplant patients are at highest risk for a year after allograft transplantation (but especially during the first 100 days afterward) and in particular when graft-versus-host disease is present or when the donor is CMV seropositive and the recipient is seronegative. Depending on the serostatus of the donor and recipient, disease may present as primary infection or reactivation. The risk of CMV disease is proportionate to the degree of immunosuppression and manifestations may differ by the cause. CMV may contribute to transplanted organ dysfunction, which often mimics organ rejection. CMV retinitis may develop after solid organ or bone marrow transplantation. CMV disease in HIV-infected patients (retinitis, serious gastrointestinal disease) occurs most prominently when the CD4 count is less than 50 cells/mcL and can be a marker for increased mortality. Antiretroviral therapy (ART) reduces the frequency of retinitis and may reverse active disease. Patients with immune recovery with CD4 cell count greater than 100 cells/mcL show decreased mortality. CMV retinitis associated with intravitreal delivery of corticosteroids (injections or implants) or systemic anti-TNF antibodies is also described. Occasionally, CMV retinitis presents in immunocompetent persons. Serious gastrointestinal CMV disease also occurs after organ transplantation, cancer chemotherapy, or corticosteroid therapy. CMV may exist alongside other pathogens, such as *Cryptosporidium*, in up to 15% of patients with AIDS cholangiopathy. CMV pneumonitis occurs in transplant recipients (mainly bone marrow and lung) with a mortality rate up to 60–80%, and less often in AIDS patients. CMV pneumonitis in hematologic malignancies (eg, lymphoma) is increasingly reported. Neurologic CMV in patients with advanced AIDS is usually associated with disseminated CMV infection.

▶ Clinical Findings

A. Symptoms and Signs

1. Perinatal disease and CMV inclusion disease—CMV inclusion disease in infected newborns is characterized by jaundice, hepatosplenomegaly, thrombocytopenia, purpura, microcephaly, periventricular CNS calcifications, mental retardation, and motor disability. Hearing loss develops in more than 50% of infants who are symptomatic at birth. Most infected neonates are asymptomatic, but neurologic deficits may ensue later in life, including hearing loss in 15% and mental retardation in 10–20%. Perinatal infection acquired through breastfeeding or blood products typically shows a benign clinical course.

2. Disease in immunocompetent persons—Acute acquired CMV infection is characterized by fever, malaise, myalgias, arthralgias, and splenomegaly. Exudative pharyngitis or cervical lymphadenopathies are uncommon, but cutaneous rashes (including the typical maculopapular rash after exposure to ampicillin) are common. The mean duration of symptoms is 7–8 weeks. Complications include mucosal gastrointestinal damage, encephalitis, severe hepatitis, thrombocytopenia (on occasion, refractory), the Guillain-Barré syndrome, pericarditis, and myocarditis. A mononucleosis-like syndrome due to CMV can also occur postsplenectomy, often years later and associated with a protracted fever, marked lymphocytosis, and impaired anti-CMV IgM response.

3. Disease in immunocompromised persons—Distinguishing between CMV infection (with evidence of CMV replication) and CMV disease (evidence for systemic symptoms or organ invasion by pathologic diagnosis) is important. In addition to patients infected with HIV, those who have undergone transplantation (solid organ or hematopoietic stem cell) show a wide spectrum of disease including gastrointestinal (eg, acute cholecystitis), renal, and CNS disease, as outlined above. CMV viral loads serve as an important predictor of disease presence.

A. CMV RETINITIS—A funduscopic examination reveals neovascular, proliferative lesions ("pizza-pie" retinopathy). Immune restoration with ART is associated with CMV vitritis and cystoid macular edema. Infants with CMV retinitis tend to have more macular than peripheral disease.

B. GASTROINTESTINAL AND HEPATOBILIARY CMV—Esophagitis presents with odynophagia. Gastritis can occasionally cause bleeding, and small bowel disease may mimic inflammatory bowel disease or may present as ulceration or perforation. Colonic CMV disease causes diarrhea, hematochezia, abdominal pain, fever, and weight loss and may mimic inflammatory bowel disease. CMV

hepatitis commonly complicates liver transplantation and appears to be increased in those with hepatitis B or hepatitis C viral infection.

C. RESPIRATORY CMV—CMV pneumonitis is characterized by cough, dyspnea, and relatively little sputum production.

D. NEUROLOGIC CMV—Neurologic syndromes associated with CMV include polyradiculopathy, transverse myelitis, ventriculoencephalitis (suspected with ependymitis), and focal encephalitis. These manifestations are more prominent in patients with advanced AIDS in whom the encephalitis has a subacute onset.

B. Laboratory Findings

1. Mothers and newborns—Pregnant women should be tested for CMV viremia every 3 months if an assay during the first trimester is seropositive. Congenital CMV disease is confirmed by presence of the virus in amniotic fluid or an IgM assay from fetal blood. Amniocentesis is less reliable before 21 weeks of gestation (due to inadequate fetal urinary development and release into the amniotic fluid), but amniocentesis is attendant with greater risk when performed after 21 weeks of gestation. PCR assays of dried blood samples from newborns, micro-enzyme-linked immunosorbent assay (ELISA), shell-vial culture, or culture of urine, saliva, or blood specimens obtained during the first 3 weeks of life are used to diagnose congenital CMV infection.

2. Immunocompetent persons—The acute mononucleosis-like syndrome is characterized by initial leukopenia; within 1 week, it is followed by absolute lymphocytosis with atypical lymphocytes. Abnormal liver function tests are common in the first 2 weeks of the disease (often 2 weeks after the fever). Detection of CMV DNA, specific IgM, or a fourfold increase of specific IgG levels support the diagnosis of acute infection.

3. Immunocompromised persons—CMV retinitis is diagnosed on the basis of the characteristic ophthalmoscopic findings. In HIV-infected patients, negative CMV serologies lower the possibility of the diagnosis but do not eliminate it. Cultures alone are of little use in diagnosing AIDS-related CMV infections, since viral shedding of CMV is common. PCR analysis should be used to diagnose CNS infection since cultures are not specific for disease.

Detection of CMV by quantitative DNA PCR is used in posttransplant patients for guidance on both treatment and prevention and should be interpreted in the context of clinical and pathologic findings. CMV viral loads are internationally standardized and have replaced conventional CMV antigenemia tests in many settings. The PCR is sensitive in predicting clinical disease. Serial PCR should be performed and compared using the same specimen type (ie, whole blood or plasma).

Rapid shell-vial cultures detect early CMV antigens with fluorescent antibodies in 24–48 hours. Shell-vial cultures are more useful on bronchoalveolar lavage fluid than in routine blood monitoring. CMV colitis can occur in the absence of a detectable viremia.

C. Imaging

The chest radiographic findings of CMV pneumonitis are consistent with interstitial pneumonia.

D. Biopsy

Tissue confirmation is especially useful in diagnosing CMV pneumonitis and CMV gastrointestinal disease; the diagnosis of colonic CMV disease is made by mucosal biopsy showing characteristic CMV histopathologic findings of intranuclear ("owl's eye") and intracytoplasmic inclusions. In situations where histopathologic or immunohistochemical findings are not seen but CMV colitis is suspected, CMV DNA PCR can be used to identify additional cases.

► Treatment

In congenital CMV infection, treatment with ganciclovir or valganciclovir for 6 months (or as little as 6 weeks in one study) is associated with improved hearing and with some improvement in developmental outcomes up to 24 months of age.

Sight-threatening CMV retinitis (lesions close to the fovea or optic nerve head) is treated with ganciclovir induction therapy (5 mg/kg intravenously every 12 hours for 14–21 days) followed by maintenance therapy at lower doses (5 mg/kg intravenously daily) (Table 32–1). Intravitreal injections of ganciclovir or foscarnet may be used as adjunct therapy. Treatment is effective in improving survival and preventing dissemination. In less severe retinal disease, valganciclovir (900 mg orally twice daily for 14–21 days followed by 900 mg/day maintenance) is preferred. Due to potential toxicities, foscarnet and cidofovir are usually reserved for CMV infections resistant to ganciclovir. Combinations of ganciclovir and foscarnet are shown to be safe and effective in treating clinically resistant CMV retinitis. The role of ART in reducing the need for CMV antiviral agents is essential. Because recurrence occurs even at high CD4 cell counts, ongoing ophthalmologic surveillance is necessary. Other forms of CMV disease in AIDS are managed initially with intravenous ganciclovir and subsequently with oral valganciclovir; alternative agents (listed above) are used when resistance evolves.

The treatment of other systemic CMV infection (colitis, encephalitis, pneumonia) involves valganciclovir, ganciclovir with foscarnet, and cidofovir reserved for treatment of resistant infections; the efficacy of ganciclovir is established in childhood pneumonia. The length of therapy depends on the state of immunosuppression, and secondary prophylaxis is typically maintained until immune restoration with two CD4 T-cell counts greater than 100 cells/mcL is present for at least 6 months in the setting of HIV infection. Prolonged prophylaxis may be necessary in other immunosuppressed patients, such as those receiving TNF inhibitors.

For non-severe, posttransplant CMV disease, oral valganciclovir (900 mg twice daily) or intravenous ganciclovir (5 mg/kg every 12 hours) are the recommended first-line agents. Valganciclovir has been shown to be noninferior to intravenous ganciclovir-based therapy in solid organ transplant patients and is associated with less clinical resistance than ganciclovir. **For severe CMV disease**, intravenous ganciclovir remains the treatment of choice. Dosage adjustments of all medications are needed for kidney dysfunction. Reduction of immunosuppression should be attempted when possible (especially for muromonab, azathioprine, or mycophenolate mofetil). Treatment should be continued for at least 2 weeks until viral clearance is achieved. Two consecutive negative results from CMV DNA PCR or antigenemia-based assay ensure viral clearance. Other agents that may be useful in resistant CMV infections include leflunomide, sirolimus-based therapy, artesunate and adoptive immunotherapy.

► Prevention

A multitude of humoral and cellular immunity vaccines against CMV are under study and development. An experimental CMV glycoprotein B with MF59 adjuvant vaccine shows efficacy of 50% in preventing primary infection in pregnant women and in reducing viremia in kidney transplant recipients.

A major source of CMV for pregnant women is their own young children, particularly those in childcare. These women can decrease their risk of contracting primary CMV just before pregnancy or during pregnancy by practicing hand hygiene after changing diapers and after contact with respiratory secretions; avoiding kissing young children on the face; and avoiding sharing utensils, food, and cleansing objects that have been in contact with children's secretions.

ART is effective in preventing CMV infections in HIV-infected patients. Primary prevention is best accomplished by good hand hygiene and use of barrier methods during sexual contacts with persons who are members of high prevalence groups (ie, men who have sex with men, injection drug users, and those who have exposure to children in child care).

The use of leukocyte-depleted blood products effectively reduces the incidence of CMV disease in patients who have undergone transplantation. Prophylactic and preemptive strategies (eg, antiviral agents only when antigen detection or PCR assays show evidence of active CMV replication) appear equally effective in preventing invasive disease and mortality after hematopoietic stem cell transplant. The appropriate management of transplant patients is based on the serostatus of the donor and the recipient. All effective anti-CMV agents can serve as prophylactic agents for CMV-seropositive transplants or for CMV-seronegative recipients of CMV-positive organ transplants. Acyclovir may also be used. The dose for valganciclovir prophylaxis is 450 mg orally twice daily. Brincidofovir (CMX001, Chimerix of Durham NC), under study, appears to be effective when given 100 mg twice a week in preventing CMV infections among hematopoietic stem cell transplant recipients.

CMV immune globulin may also be useful in reducing the incidence of bronchiolitis obliterans in the bone marrow transplant population and is used in some centers as part of the prophylaxis in kidney, liver, and lung transplantation patients. CMV immune globulin as prophylaxis is not recommended in hematopoietic stem cell transplant recipients.

When to Refer

- Neonatal infections consistent with CMV inclusion disease.
- AIDS patients with retinitis, esophagitis, colitis, hepatobiliary disease, or encephalitis.
- Organ and hematopoietic stem cell transplants with suspected reactivation CMV.

When to Admit

- Escalating CMV viral load at the onset of illness.
- Risk of colonic perforation.
- Evaluation of unexplained, advancing encephalopathy.
- Initiation of treatment with intravenous anti-CMV agents.

Boekh M et al. Valganciclovir for the prevention of complications of late cytomegalovirus infection after allogeneic hematopoietic cell transplantation: a randomized trial. Ann Intern Med. 2015 Jan 6;162(1):1–10. [PMID: 25560711]

Hirsch HH et al. An international multicenter performance analysis of cytomegalovirus load tests. Clin Infect Dis. 2013 Feb;56(3):367–73. [PMID: 23097587]

Jabs DA et al; Studies of the Ocular Complications of AIDS Research Group. Long-term outcomes of cytomegalovirus retinitis in the era of modern antiretroviral therapy: results from a United States cohort. Ophthalmology. 2015 Jul; 122(7):1452–63. [PMID: 25892019]

Kimberlin DW et al; National Institute of Allergy and Infectious Diseases Collaborative Antiviral Study Group. Valganciclovir for symptomatic congenital cytomegalovirus disease. N Engl J Med. 2015 Mar 5;372(10):933–43. [PMID: 25738669]

Marty FM et al; CMX001-201 Clinical Study Group. CMX001 to prevent cytomegalovirus disease in hematopoietic-cell transplantation. N Engl J Med. 2013 Sep 26;369(13):1227–36. [PMID: 24066743]

Price SM et al. Educating women about congenital cytomegalovirus: assessment of health education materials through a web-based survey. BMC Womens Health. 2014 Nov 30;14:144. [PMID: 25433837]

U.S. Department of Health and Human Services (HHS). AIDSinfo. Guidelines for the prevention and treatment of opportunistic infections in HIV-infected adults and adolescents. Cytomegalovirus. 2015 Nov 4. https://aidsinfo.nih.gov/guidelines/html/4/adult-and-adolescent-oi-prevention-and-treatment-guidelines/337/cmv

6. Human Herpesviruses 6, 7, & 8

HHV-6 is a B cell lymphotropic virus that is the principal cause of exanthema subitum (roseola infantum, sixth disease). Primary HHV-6 infection occurs most commonly in children under 2 years of age and is a major cause of infantile febrile seizures. HHV-6 is also associated with encephalitis (symptoms may include insomnia, seizures, and hallucinations) and with acute liver failure. Primary infection in immunocompetent adults is rare and can produce a mononucleosis-like illness. Reactivation of HHV-6 in immunocompetent adults is rare and can present as encephalitis. Imaging studies in HHV-6 encephalitis typically show lesions in the hippocampus, amygdala, and limbic structures.

Infection during pregnancy and congenital transmission is recognized. Most cases of reactivation, however, occur in immunocompromised persons. Reactivation is associated with graft rejection, graft-versus-host disease, and bone marrow suppression in transplant patients and with encephalitis and pneumonitis in AIDS patients. In recipients of hematopoietic stem cell transplants, HHV-6–induced encephalitis is associated strongly with umbilical cord hematopoietic cell transplants (in the absence of an HHV-6 association with survival in such patients surveillance for the virus may not be needed).

HHV-6 is on occasion also associated with drug-induced hypersensitivity syndromes. HHV-6 may cause fulminant hepatic failure and acute decompensation of chronic liver disease in children. Purpura fulminans and corneal inflammation are reported with HHV-6 infection. Two variants (A and B) of HHV-6 have been identified. HHV-6B is the predominant strain found in both normal and immunocompromised persons. Ganciclovir, cidofovir, and foscarnet (but not acyclovir) appear to be clinically active against HHV-6.

HHV-7 is a T cell lymphotropic virus that is associated with roseola (serologically), seizures and, rarely, encephalitis. Pregnant women are often infected. Infection with HHV-7 is synergistic with CMV in kidney transplant recipients.

HHV-8 (see also Chapter 31) is associated with Kaposi sarcoma, multicentric Castleman disease, and primary effusion (body cavity) lymphoma. HHV-8 infection is endemic in Africa; transmission seems to be primarily horizontal in childhood from intrafamilial contacts and continues through adulthood possibly by nonsexual routes.

Husain Z et al. DRESS syndrome: part I. Clinical perspectives. J Am Acad Dermatol. 2013 May;68(5):693.e1–14. [PMID: 23602182]

Ogata M et al. Human herpesvirus 6 (HHV-6) reactivation and HHV-6 encephalitis after allogeneic hematopoietic cell transplantation: a multicenter, prospective study. Clin Infect Dis. 2013 Sep;57(5):671–81. [PMID: 23723198]

MAJOR VACCINE-PREVENTABLE VIRAL INFECTIONS[1]

1. Measles

ESSENTIALS OF DIAGNOSIS

- ▶ Exposure 10–14 days before onset in an unvaccinated patient.[1]
- ▶ Prodrome of fever, coryza, cough, conjunctivitis, malaise, irritability, photophobia, Koplik spots.
- ▶ Rash: brick red, irregular, maculopapular; onset 3–4 days after onset of prodrome; begins on the face and proceeds "downward and outward," affecting the palms and soles last.
- ▶ Leukopenia.

---

[1]A general guide for vaccine preventable diseases is available at http://www.who.int/influenza/vaccines/en/.

General Considerations

Measles is a reportable acute systemic paramyxoviral infection transmitted by inhalation of infective droplets. It is a major worldwide cause of pediatric morbidity and mortality, although vaccination programs successfully reduced this number. Despite encouraging vaccination reports in 2013 with 91.9% of children aged 19–35 months in the United States having received one or more doses of measles, mumps, and rubella vaccine (MMR) between January 1 and September 18, 2015, 189 cases of measles were reported to the CDC from 24 states and the District of Columbia in at least 5 outbreaks with 113 (60%) part of a multi-state outbreak associated with an amusement park in Southern California. Low vaccine uptake in children aged 10–19 years drives these outbreaks and is rooted in unfounded concerns over the potential link between MMR and autism.

The 668 confirmed measles cases reported to CDC in 2014 was the highest number reported since the United States declared elimination of measles in 2000. Many countries struggle with measles, including the United Kingdom, France, Bosnia, and the Philippines (the likely source of the Southern California outbreak) with all reporting recent outbreaks. Reassuringly, however, the caseloads appear to be decreasing in four of six World Health Organization (WHO) areas, and the WHO anticipates elimination of measles globally by 2020.

Illness confers permanent immunity. It is highly contagious and communicability is greatest during the preeruptive and catarrhal stages but continues as long as the rash remains. Despite high community vaccination coverage, rising rates of intentional undervaccination lead to sporadic outbreaks among clusters of intentionally undervaccinated children and can undermine measles elimination programs. Therefore, laboratory testing and confirmation of suspected measles infection is especially important in countries that report the elimination of measles. Sporadic outbreaks of the disease in adults, adolescents, and unvaccinated preschool children in dense urban areas, and sporting event participants emphasize the need for specific recommendations concerning prevention.

Clinical Findings

A. Symptoms and Signs

Fever is often as high as 40–40.6°C. It persists through the prodrome and early rash (about 5–7 days) (Table 32–2). Malaise may be marked. Coryza (nasal obstruction, sneezing, and sore throat) resembles that seen with upper respiratory infections. Cough is persistent and nonproductive. Conjunctivitis manifests as redness, swelling, photophobia, and discharge. These symptoms intensify over 2–4 days before onset of the rash and peak on the first day of the rash. **Koplik spots** (small, irregular, and red with whitish center on the mucous membranes) are pathognomonic of measles. They appear about 2 days before the rash and last 1–4 days as tiny "table salt crystals" on the buccal mucosa opposite the molars and vaginal membranes. The rash lasts for 3–7 days and fades in the same manner it appeared.

Hyperpigmentation remains in fair-skinned individuals and severe cases. Slight desquamation may follow.

Other findings in measles include pharyngeal erythema, tonsillar yellowish exudate, coating of the tongue in the center with a red tip and margins, moderate generalized lymphadenopathy and, at times, splenomegaly.

B. Laboratory Findings

Leukopenia is usually present unless secondary bacterial complications exist. A lymphocyte count under 2000/mcL is a poor prognostic sign. Thrombocytopenia is common. Proteinuria is often observed. Although technically difficult, virus can be cultured from nasopharyngeal washings and from blood. Detection of IgM measles antibodies with ELISA or a fourfold rise in serum hemagglutination inhibition antibody supports the diagnosis. Fluorescent antibody staining of respiratory or urinary epithelial cells can also confirm the diagnosis.

IgM assays can be falsely negative the first few days of infection and falsely positive in the presence of rheumatoid factor or with acute rubella, erythrovirus (parvovirus) B19, or HHV-6 infection. Reverse transcriptase-PCR (RT-PCR) techniques, typically available in research settings, can help establish a diagnosis. The virologic clearance of measles can take months, leading to false-positive results.

Differential Diagnosis

Measles is usually diagnosed clinically but may be mistaken for other exanthematous infections (Table 32–2). Frequent difficulty in establishing a diagnosis suggests that measles may be more prevalent than is recognized.

Complications

A. Central Nervous System

Postinfectious encephalomyelitis occurs in about 0.05–0.1% of cases. Higher rates of encephalitis occur in adolescents and adults than in school-aged children. Its onset is usually 3–7 days after the rash. Vomiting, convulsions, coma, and diverse, severe neurologic symptoms and signs may develop. Treatment is symptomatic and supportive. Virus is usually not found in the CNS, though demyelination is prominent. There is an appreciable mortality (10–20%) and morbidity (33% of survivors are left with neurologic deficit).

A similar form, "inclusion body encephalitis," occurs months after exposure. This complication is reported to occur after measles vaccination in patients with inadequate cellular immunity but is associated with isolation of the measles virus.

Subacute sclerosing panencephalitis (SSPE) is a very rare, late CNS complication (5–15 years after infection; the measles virus acts as a "slow virus" to produce degenerative CNS disease years after the initial infection.

Measles virus can opportunistically invade the CNS. An acute progressive encephalitis (subacute measles encephalitis), characterized by seizures, neurologic deficits, and stupor progressing to death, can occur among immunosuppressed patients. Treatment is supportive, withholding immunosuppressive chemotherapy when feasible. Interferon and ribavirin are variably successful.

B. Respiratory Tract Disease

Early in the course of the disease, bronchopneumonia or bronchiolitis due to the measles virus may occur in up to 5% of patients and result in serious respiratory difficulties. Bronchiectasis may occur in up to a quarter of nonvaccinated children.

C. Secondary Bacterial Infections

Immediately following measles, secondary bacterial infection, particularly cervical adenitis, otitis media (the most common complication), and pneumonia, occurs in about 15% of patients.

D. Immune Reactivity

Measles produces temporary anergy to cell-mediated skin tests.

E. Gastroenteritis

Diarrhea and protein-losing enteropathy (prodromal rectal Koplik spots may be seen) are significant complications among malnourished children.

F. Other Complications

Other complications include conjunctivitis, keratitis, and otosclerosis.

▶ Treatment

A. General Measures

The patient should be isolated for the week following onset of rash and kept at bed rest until afebrile. Treatment is symptomatic including antipyretics and fluids as needed. Vitamin A, 200,000 units/day orally for 2 days (the benefit being maintenance of gastrointestinal and respiratory epithelial mucosa) reduces pediatric morbidity (diarrhea, night blindness, xerophthalmia) and measles-associated mortality for infants between 6 months and 5 years of age, although high-dose vitamin A exposure increases the severity and risk of antibiotic failure in non-measles pneumonia. Measles virus is susceptible to ribavirin in vitro and has been used in selected severe cases of pneumonitis (35 mg/kg/day intravenously in three divided doses for 2 days, followed by 20 mg/kg/day intravenously in three divided doses for 5 days).

B. Treatment of Complications

Secondary bacterial infections, including pneumonia, are treated with appropriate antibacterial antibiotics. Post-measles encephalitis, including SSPE, can only be managed symptomatically.

Repeated studies fail to show an association between vaccination and autism. The prevalence of asthma-like diseases in childhood appears to be reduced among vaccinated children. Some data implicate the measles virus in the pathogenesis of rheumatoid arthritis.

▶ Prognosis

Between 2000 and 2008, the measles mortality rate declined by 78%. In the last decade, the case-fatality rate in the United States stayed around 3 per 1000 reported cases, with deaths principally due to encephalitis (15% mortality rate) and secondary bacterial pneumonia. Deaths in the developing world are mainly related to diarrhea and protein-losing enteropathy.

▶ Prevention

In the United States, children receive their first vaccine dose at 12–15 months and a second at age 4–6 years, prior to entry into school. Combination measles-mumps-rubella-varicella vaccines (MMRV) can be used in place of the traditional measles, mumps, and rubella (MMR) vaccine. The median coverage with at least one dose of MMR vaccine nationally in 2013 was 91.9% among children 19–35 months of age; however, there is considerable geographic disparity in this value (in the US Virgin Islands the coverage is only 59% and in Ohio and West Virginia it is 86%). The clustering of unvaccinated individuals also increases the likelihood of an outbreak. Susceptibility to measles is 2.4-fold higher if the vaccine is given prior to 15 months, suggesting that administration before that age may not be optimal for measles eradication. The evidence is not convincing that routine anthelmintic treatment affects the immune response to childhood vaccination.

American students beyond high school and medical staff starting employment require documentation of the above vaccination schedule or must show serologic evidence of immunity if they were born after 1956. For individuals born before 1957, herd immunity is assumed. Health care workers, immigrants, and refugees should be screened and vaccinated if necessary regardless of date of birth. International travelers (if immunocompetent and born after 1956) to the developing world and teachers should receive booster doses of vaccination.

At 6 months of age, more than 99% of infants of vaccinated women and 95% of infants of naturally immune women lose maternal antibodies. Therefore, in outbreaks that include infants less than 1 year of age, initial vaccination may be given at 6 months, with repeat at 15 months. When outbreaks take place in day care centers, K–12 institutions, or colleges and universities, revaccination is probably indicated for all, in particular for students and their siblings born after 1956 who do not have documentation of immunity as defined above. Susceptible personnel who were exposed should be isolated from patient contact between the fifth and the twenty-first day after exposure regardless of whether they were vaccinated or given immune globulin. If measles develops in these persons, they should be isolated from patient contact until 7 days after the rash develops.

When susceptible individuals are exposed to measles, live virus vaccine can prevent disease if given within 5 days of exposure. In addition, immune globulin (0.25 mL/kg [0.11 mL/lb] body weight) can be injected intramuscularly for prevention or modification of clinical illness if given within 6 days after exposure. This must be followed by active immunization with live measles vaccine 3 months later. In the developing world, the use of a second vaccine dose is an important aspect of achieving control of measles. Health care settings can be a source of continuing exposure in measles outbreaks, particularly in the developing world, and the mandatory two-dose immunization of health care workers is a means of control recommended in South Asia, with other means of control being postexposure prophylaxis of the immunocompromised, and strict triage of admissions.

Pregnant women and immunosuppressed persons should *not* receive this vaccine. Exception to this contraindication is asymptomatic HIV-infected patients (with normal CD4 counts), including children, who have not shown adverse effects from measles vaccination. In asymptomatic HIV-infected children, vaccination improves survival after measles, and ART is associated with an improved vaccine response. Repeat vaccination may be necessary in HIV-infected children after immune restoration. Immune globulin should be administered within 6 days of exposure for postexposure prophylaxis in any high-risk person exposed to measles. Such high-risk persons include children with malignancy and patients with AIDS who are at risk for developing severe or fatal disease.

Severe allergic reactions including anaphylaxis to the MMR vaccine are rare, though fever and rash appear to occur slightly more often among female recipients. Quadrivalent MMRV vaccine is associated with an increased risk of seizures that appears to be age-related; the risk is highest when MMRV is given to infants under 15 months of age.

When to Refer

- Any suspect cases should be reported to public health authorities.
- HIV infection.
- Pregnancy.

When to Admit

- Meningitis, encephalitis, or myelitis.
- Severe pneumonia.
- Diarrhea that significantly compromises fluid or electrolyte status.

Clemmons NS et al; Centers for Disease Control and Prevention (CDC). Measles—United States, January 4–April 2, 2015. MMWR Morb Mortal Wkly Rep. 2015 Apr 17;64(14):373–6. [PMID: 25879894]

Durrheim DN et al. Measles—the epidemiology of elimination. Vaccine. 2014 Dec 5;32(51):6880–3. [PMID: 25444814]

Feenstra B et al. Common variants associated with general and MMR vaccine-related febrile seizures. Nat Genet. 2014 Dec; 46(12):1274–82. [PMID: 25344690]

Jin J. JAMA patient page. Measles vaccination. JAMA. 2015 Apr 7; 313(13):1386. [PMID: 25686026]

Perry RT et al; Centers for Disease Control and Prevention (CDC). Progress toward regional measles elimination—worldwide, 2000–2013. MMWR Morb Mortal Wkly Rep. 2014 Nov 14;63(45):1034–8. [PMID: 25393223]

Strikas RA; Centers for Disease Control and Prevention (CDC); Advisory Committee on Immunization Practices (ACIP); ACIP Child/Adolescent Immunization Work Group. Advisory committee on immunization practices recommended immunization schedules for persons aged 0 through 18 years—United States, 2015. MMWR Morb Mortal Wkly Rep. 2015 Feb 6;64(4):93–4. [PMID: 25654610]

2. Mumps

ESSENTIALS OF DIAGNOSIS

- ▶ Exposure 14–21 days before onset.
- ▶ Painful, swollen salivary glands, usually parotid.
- ▶ Frequent involvement of testes, pancreas, and meninges in unvaccinated individuals.
- ▶ Mumps occurs in appropriately vaccinated persons in the majority of cases in highly vaccinated communities.

General Considerations

Mumps is a paramyxoviral disease spread by respiratory droplets. Children are the age group most affected, although in some outbreaks, patients are in the late second or early third decades of life. Mumps can spread rapidly in congregate settings, such as colleges and schools. The incidence is highest in spring. The incubation period is 14–21 days (average, 18 days). Infectivity occurs via saliva and urine and precedes the symptoms by about 1 day and is maximal for 3 days, although it may last a week. Up to one-third of affected individuals have subclinical infection. Despite high vaccination rates in America, Europe, and other regions, several mumps outbreaks were reported in these places over the past few years. More than half of these mumps cases reported appropriate MMR vaccination histories.

Clinical Findings

A. Symptoms and Signs

Mumps is more serious in adults than in children. Parotid tenderness and overlying facial edema (Figure 32–5) are the most common physical findings and typically develop within 48 hours of the prodromal symptoms. Usually, one parotid gland enlarges before the other, but unilateral parotitis alone occurs in 25% of patients. The orifice of Stensen duct may be red and swollen. Trismus may result from parotitis. The parotid glands return to normal within a week. Involvement of other salivary glands (submaxillary and sublingual) occurs in 10% of cases.

Fever and malaise are variable but often minimal in young children. High fever accompanies meningitis or orchitis. Neck stiffness, headache, and lethargy suggest meningitis. Testicular swelling and tenderness (unilateral in 75% of cases) denote orchitis; the testes are the most common extrasalivary disease site in adults. Orchitis develops 7–10 days after the onset of parotitis in about 25–40% of postpubertal men but occurred in only 7% of males

▲ **Figure 32–5.** Mumps. (Public Health Image Library, CDC.)

above age 12 in the Orthodox Jewish outbreaks in New York. Sterility is rare. Acute hormonal disturbances are prevalent, including decreased levels of testosterone and inhibin B with low or normal levels of gonadotropins in up to 35% cases with mumps orchitis. Upper abdominal pain, nausea, and vomiting suggest pancreatitis. Mumps is the leading cause of pancreatitis in children. Lower abdominal pain and ovarian enlargement suggest oophoritis (which occurs in 5% of postpubertal women, usually unilateral); it is a difficult diagnosis to establish.

B. Laboratory Findings

Mild leukopenia with relative lymphocytosis may be present. Serum amylasemia usually reflects salivary gland involvement rather than pancreatitis. Lymphocytic pleocytosis and hypoglycorrhachia of the cerebrospinal fluid in meningitis may be asymptomatic. Mild kidney function abnormalities are found in up to 60% of patients.

Characteristic clinical picture is usually sufficient for diagnosis. An elevated serum IgM is considered diagnostic and a repeat test 2–3 weeks after the onset of symptoms is recommended if the first assay is negative due to a delay in IgM rise, especially in vaccinated persons. A fourfold rise in complement-fixing antibodies to mumps virus in paired serum IgG also confirms infection. Confirmatory diagnosis of mumps is also made by isolating the virus preferably from a swab of the duct of the parotid or other affected salivary gland. The virus can also be isolated from cerebrospinal fluid early in the course of aseptic meningitis. Isolation from urine is no longer advised. Nucleic acid amplification techniques are more sensitive than viral cultures but their availability is limited.

▶ Differential Diagnosis

Swelling of the parotid gland may be due to calculi in the parotid ducts, tumors, or cysts, or to a reaction to iodides.

Other causes include starch ingestion, sarcoidosis, cirrhosis, diabetes, bulimia, pilocarpine usage, and Sjögren syndrome. Parotitis may be produced by pyogenic organisms (eg, *S aureus*, gram-negative organisms [particularly in debilitated individuals with poor oral intake]), drug reaction (phenothiazines, propylthiouracil), and other viruses (influenza A, parainfluenza, EBV infection, coxsackieviruses, adenoviruses, HHV-6). Swelling of the parotid gland must be differentiated from inflammation of the lymph nodes located more posteriorly and inferiorly than the parotid gland.

▶ Complications

Other manifestations of the disease are less common and usually follow parotitis but may precede it or occur without salivary gland involvement. Such manifestations include meningitis (30%), priapism or testicular infarction from orchitis, thyroiditis, neuritis, hepatitis, myocarditis, thrombocytopenia, migratory arthralgias (infrequently among adults and even rarer in children), and nephritis. Mumps has also been associated with cases of endocardial fibroelastosis and a hemophagocytosis syndrome. Rare neurologic complications include encephalitis, Guillain-Barré syndrome, cerebellar ataxia, facial palsy, and transverse myelitis. Encephalitis is associated with cerebral edema, serious neurologic manifestations, and sometimes death. Deafness from eighth nerve neuritis develops in about 0.1%; it is typically unilateral, severe, and permanent.

▶ Treatment

The patient should be isolated until swelling subsides (about 9 days from onset) and kept on bed rest while febrile. Treatment is symptomatic. Topical compresses may relieve parotid discomfort. Some clinicians advocate intravenous immunoglobulin (IVIG) for complicated disease (eg, thrombocytopenia) although its definitive role is unproven.

▶ Prognosis

The entire course of mumps rarely exceeds 2 weeks. Rare fatalities are usually due to encephalitis.

▶ Prevention

Mumps live virus vaccine is safe and effective (there is some variability among vaccines, the Jeryl Lynn strain being highly effective, the Urabe intermediate, the Rubini less so) with long lasting immunity. It is recommended for routine immunization for children older than 12 months, either alone or in combination with other virus vaccines (eg, in the MMR vaccine or as a quadrivalent vaccine with varicella). A second dose is recommended for children (ages 4–6 years) before starting school. Two doses of the vaccine should also be considered for high-risk adults (eg, health care workers) born before 1957 and without evidence of immunity. In a recent summer camp outbreak, a single, third dose of the mumps vaccine has shown efficacy.

There are no known cases of long-term sequelae associated with mumps vaccination and the currently used mumps strain (Jeryl Lynn) shows the lowest associated incidence of post vaccine aseptic meningitis (from 1 in 150,000 to 1 in 1.8 million). This vaccine is less effective in epidemic settings. Reactions are reviewed in the measles section. It should not be given to pregnant women or to immunocompromised individuals. The vaccine can be given to HIV-infected persons who show immune restoration with ART.

▶ When to Refer

Any suspect cases should be reported to public health authorities.

▶ When to Admit

- Trismus; meningitis, encephalitis; myocarditis; pancreatitis.
- Severe testicular pain; priapism.
- Severe thrombocytopenia.

Maillet M et al. Mumps outbreak and laboratory diagnosis. J Clin Virol. 2015 Jan;62:14–9. [PMID: 25542464]

McLean HQ et al; Centers for Disease Control and Prevention. Prevention of measles, rubella, congenital rubella syndrome, and mumps, 2013: summary recommendations of the Advisory Committee on Immunization Practices (ACIP). MMWR Recomm Rep. 2013 Jun 14;62(RR-04):1–34. [PMID: 23760231]

Sane J et al. Epidemic of mumps among vaccinated persons, The Netherlands, 2009–2012. Emerg Infect Dis. 2014 Apr; 20(4):643–8. [PMID: 24655811]

3. Poliomyelitis

ESSENTIALS OF DIAGNOSIS

- ▶ Incubation period 9–12 days from exposure.
- ▶ Muscle weakness, headache, stiff neck, fever, nausea and vomiting, sore throat.
- ▶ Lower motor neuron lesion (flaccid paralysis) with decreased deep tendon reflexes and muscle wasting.
- ▶ Cerebrospinal fluid shows lymphocytic pleocytosis but rarely greater than 500/mcL.

▶ General Considerations

Poliomyelitis virus, an enterovirus, is present in throat washings and stools (excretion may last for weeks after infection). It is highly contagious through fecal-oral route, especially during the first week of infection. By 2013, all but two countries (Afghanistan, Pakistan with Africa considered now poliomyelitis-free) had eliminated indigenous transmission of wild poliovirus (WPV) type 1. Only type 1 remains endemic currently and 359 cases were reported in 2014. As of October 20, 2015, there were 51 cases of poliomyelitis in the two endemic countries, and 14 circulating vaccine-derived type 1 cases, 9 of which were in Madagascar. The last type 2 case of poliomyelitis

occurred in 1999 in India and the last type 3 in 2012 in Nigeria. At least 80% of the world now lives in polio-free regions, which include the Americas (since 1994), the Western Pacific (since 2000), Europe (since 2002), Southeast Asia (since 2014), and possibly Africa (since 2015).

▶ Clinical Findings

A. Symptoms and Signs

At least 95% of infections are asymptomatic, but in those who become ill, manifestations include abortive poliomyelitis (minor illness), nonparalytic poliomyelitis, and paralytic poliomyelitis.

1. Abortive poliomyelitis (minor illness)—Such minor illness occurs in 4–8% of infections and the symptoms are fever, headache, vomiting, diarrhea, constipation, and sore throat lasting 2–3 days. This entity is suspected clinically only during an epidemic.

2. Nonparalytic poliomyelitis—In addition to the above symptoms, signs of meningeal irritation and muscle spasm occur in the absence of frank paralysis. This disease is indistinguishable from aseptic meningitis caused by other viruses.

3. Paralytic poliomyelitis—Paralytic poliomyelitis represents 0.1% of all poliomyelitis cases (the incidence is higher when infections are acquired later in life). Paralysis may occur at any time during the febrile period. Tremors, muscle weakness, constipation, and ileus may appear. Paralytic poliomyelitis is divided into two forms, which may coexist: (1) **spinal poliomyelitis**, with involvement of the muscles innervated by the spinal nerves, and (2) **bulbar poliomyelitis**, with weakness of the muscles supplied by the cranial nerves (especially nerves IX and X) and of the respiratory and vasomotor centers.

In spinal poliomyelitis, paralysis of the shoulder girdle often precedes intercostal and diaphragmatic paralysis, which leads to diminished chest expansion and decreased vital capacity. The paralysis occurs over 2–3 days, is flaccid, has an asymmetric distribution, and affects the proximal muscles of the lower extremities more frequently. Sensory loss is very rare.

In bulbar poliomyelitis, symptoms include diplopia (uncommonly), facial weakness, dysphagia, dysphonia, nasal voice, weakness of the sternocleidomastoid and trapezius muscles, difficulty in chewing, inability to swallow or expel saliva, and regurgitation of fluids through the nose. The most life-threatening aspect of bulbar poliomyelitis is respiratory paralysis. Lethargy or coma may be due to hypoxia, most often from hypoventilation. Vasomotor disturbances in blood pressure and heart rate may occur. Convulsions are rare. Bulbar poliomyelitis is more common in adults. Bulbar and spinal disease can coexist (bulbospinal poliomyelitis).

B. Laboratory Findings

The virus may be recovered from throat washings (early) and stools (early and late) and PCR of washings, stool, or cerebrospinal fluid can also facilitate diagnosis. Cerebrospinal fluid findings include the following: (1) normal or slightly increased pressure and protein, (2) glucose is not decreased, and (3) white blood cells usually number less than 500/mcL and are principally lymphocytes after the first 24 hours. Cerebrospinal fluid is normal in 5% of patients. Neutralizing and complement-fixing antibodies appear during the first or second week of illness. Serologic testing cannot distinguish between wild type and vaccine-related virus infections.

Differential Diagnosis

Nonparalytic poliomyelitis is similar to other forms of enteroviral meningitis; the distinction is made serologically. **Acute flaccid paralysis** is the term used in the developing world for the variety of neurologic illnesses that both include and mimic poliomyelitis. Acute flaccid paralysis due to poliomyelitis is distinguished by the greater frequency of fever and asymmetric neurologic signs. Acute inflammatory polyneuritis (Guillain-Barré syndrome), Japanese virus encephalitis, West Nile virus infection, and tick paralysis may resemble poliomyelitis. In Guillain-Barré syndrome (see Chapter 24), the weakness is more symmetric and ascending in most cases, but the Miller Fisher variant is quite similar to bulbar polio. Paresthesias are uncommon in poliomyelitis but common in Guillain-Barré syndrome. The cerebrospinal fluid usually has high protein content but normal cell count in Guillain-Barré syndrome.

Complications

Urinary tract infection, atelectasis, pneumonia, myocarditis, paralytic ileus, gastric dilation, and pulmonary edema may occur. Respiratory failure may be a result of paralysis of respiratory muscles, airway obstruction from involvement of cranial nerve nuclei, or lesions of the respiratory center.

Treatment

In the acute phase of paralytic poliomyelitis patients should be hospitalized. Strict bed rest in the first few days of illness reduces the rate of paralysis. Comfortable but rotating positions should be maintained. In cases of respiratory weakness or paralysis, intensive care is needed. Intensive physiotherapy may help recover some motor function with paralysis. Attention to psychological disorders in long-standing disease is also important. Physical therapy is essential.

Prognosis

During the febrile period, paralysis may develop or progress. Mild weakness of small muscles is more likely to regress than severe weakness of large muscles. Bulbar poliomyelitis carries a mortality rate of up to 50%. Long-term sequelae include pain, weakness, fatigue, and obesity, factors often worsened by age and comorbidities. When new muscle weakness and pain develop and progress slowly years after recovery from acute paralytic poliomyelitis, the entity is called **postpoliomyelitis syndrome**. Risk factors for the syndrome include female gender, respiratory symptoms during the acute polio syndrome, and the need for orthoses and aids during the rehabilitation phase. The syndrome presents with signs of chronic and new

denervation, is associated with increasing dysfunction of surviving motor neurons, and is not infectious in origin; patients do not shed the virus. Immune modulators, such as prednisone, interferon, and IVIG, do not show any clear benefit in the treatment of postpoliomyelitis syndrome.

Prevention

Given the epidemiologic distribution of poliomyelitis and the continued concern about vaccine-associated disease (estimated in 1:750,000 recipients) with the trivalent oral live poliovirus vaccine (OPV), the inactive (Salk) parenteral vaccination is currently used in the United States for all four recommended doses (at ages 2 months, 4 months, 6–18 months, and at 4–6 years). Inactivated vaccine is also routinely used elsewhere in the developed world where one dose is often administered although immunogenicity is improved with additional doses. Oral vaccines have been limited to usage for outbreak control, for travel to endemic areas within the ensuing month, and for protection of children whose parents do not comply with the recommended number of immunizations. The advantages of oral vaccination are the ease of administration, low cost, effective local gastrointestinal and circulating immunity, and herd immunity. They are known to attenuate the response to BCG vaccination. Because of the risks with oral vaccination of vaccine-derived poliomyelitis, there is currently a global movement toward the total elimination of oral vaccines by the end of this decade.

Routine immunization of adults in the United States is no longer recommended because of the low incidence of the disease. Exceptions include adults not vaccinated within the prior decade who are exposed to poliomyelitis or who plan to travel to endemic areas (currently only Afghanistan and Pakistan). Vaccination should also be considered for adults engaged in high-risk activities (eg, laboratory workers handling stools). Such adults should be given inactivated poliomyelitis vaccine (Salk) as should immunodeficient or immunosuppressed individuals and members of their households. Ancillary useful control measures ("supplementary immunization activities") in polio-endemic countries include national immunization days (mass campaigns in which all children are vaccinated twice, 4–6 weeks apart, regardless of vaccine history); cross-border vaccination activities; surveillance for acute flaccid paralysis, an indicator for poliomyelitis; and aggressive outbreak responses as well as intensified immunization activities in countries impacted by armed conflicts.

When to Refer

- Neurologic compromise.
- Any suspicious cases should be referred to public health authorities.

Centers for Disease Control and Prevention (CDC); Immunization Systems Management Group of the Global Polio Eradication Initiative. Introduction of inactivated poliovirus vaccine and switch from trivalent to bivalent oral poliovirus vaccine—worldwide, 2013–2016. MMWR Morb Mortal Wkly Rep. 2015 Jul 3;64(25):699–702. [PMID: 26135591]

Grassly NC. Immunogenicity and effectiveness of routine immunization with 1 or 2 doses of inactivated poliovirus vaccine: systematic review and meta-analysis. J Infect Dis. 2014 Nov 1;210(Suppl 1):S439–46. [PMID: 24634499]

Hagan JE et al; Centers for Disease Control and Prevention (CDC). Progress toward polio eradication—worldwide, 2014–2015. MMWR Morb Mortal Wkly Rep. 2015 May 22; 64(19):527–31. [PMID: 25996095]

World Health Organization; Global Polio Eradication Initiative. Data and monitoring: polio this week. http://www.polioeradication.org/Dataandmonitoring/Poliothisweek.aspx

4. Rubella

ESSENTIALS OF DIAGNOSIS

► Exposure 14–21 days before onset.

► Arthralgia, particularly in young women.

► No prodrome in children, mild prodrome in adults; mild symptoms (fever, malaise, coryza) coinciding with eruption.

► Posterior cervical and postauricular lymphadenopathy 5–10 days before rash.

► Fine maculopapular rash of 3 days duration; face to trunk to extremities.

► Leukopenia, thrombocytopenia.

General Considerations

Rubella is a systemic disease caused by a togavirus transmitted by inhalation of infective droplets. It is moderately communicable. One attack usually confers permanent immunity but reinfection is possible, albeit rarely. The incubation period is 14–21 days (average, 16 days). The disease is transmissible from 1 week before the rash appears until 15 days afterward.

The clinical picture of rubella is difficult to distinguish from other viral illnesses such as infectious mononucleosis, measles, echovirus infections, and coxsackievirus infections; however, arthritis is more prominent in rubella. The principal importance of rubella lies in its devastating effects on the fetus in utero, producing teratogenic effects and a continuing congenital infection (**congenital rubella syndrome**). The burden of congenital rubella continues to drop, with fewer than 100 cases reported in 2014 compared with 103,000 cases reported in 2010 and 121,344 cases in 2009. This precipitous drop is due to widespread implementation of rubella-containing vaccines, currently used in 68% of countries as of 2013, with 58% of countries showing over 90% of the population showing immunization coverage. The United States reported elimination of rubella in 2004, although a median of 11 cases of rubella occurred annually through 2011. As of April 25, 2015, PAHO declared that the Americas are free of congenital rubella syndrome. The six US cases of congenital rubella syndrome between 2004 and 2012 were associated with overseas maternal acquisition of rubella. Globally, the remaining cases of congenital rubella syndrome were reported from Bangladesh (66), Romania (26), Nepal (16), Zambia (10), Japan (9), Sri Lanka (4), Cambodia and Zimbabwe (2 each), with one each from Jordan, Mauritius, the Republic of South Africa, Sweden, Tunisia, and Vietnam. The large unknown is sub-Saharan Africa where rates of immunization coverage are known in only a few countries. The WHO currently anticipates global elimination of rubella along with measles by 2020.

Clinical Findings

A. Symptoms and Signs

While fetal rubella can be devastating, postnatally acquired rubella is usually innocuous and asymptomatic in up to 50% of cases. In the postnatally acquired infection, fever and malaise, usually mild, accompanied by tender suboccipital adenitis, may precede the eruption by 1 week. Mild coryza may be present. Polyarticular arthritis occurs in about 25% of adult cases and involves the fingers, wrists, and knees. Rarely does chronic arthritis develop. The polyarthritis usually subsides within 7 days but may persist for weeks. Early posterior cervical and postauricular lymphadenopathy is very common. Erythema of the palate and throat, sometimes patchy, may be noted.

A fine, pink maculopapular rash appears on the face, trunk, and extremities in rapid progression (2–3 days) and fades quickly, usually lasting 1 day in each area (Table 32–2). Rubella without rash may be at least as common as the exanthematous disease. When rubella is suspected because of disease in the community, the diagnosis requires serologic confirmation.

B. Laboratory Findings

Leukopenia may be present early and may be followed by an increase in plasma cells. The definitive diagnosis of acute rubella infection is based on elevated IgM antibody, fourfold or greater rise in IgG antibody titers, or isolation of the virus. False-positive IgM antibodies, however, are associated with EBV, CMV, erythrovirus (parvovirus), and rheumatoid factor. Detection of antibodies against rubella in other body fluids, such as urine and saliva, are promising diagnostic aids. An interferon-gamma-ELISPOT can provide valuable additional information in seronegative individuals. PCR techniques are also available.

Complications

A. Exposure During Pregnancy

When a pregnant woman is exposed to a possible case of rubella, an immediate hemagglutination-inhibiting rubella antibody level should be obtained to document immunity, since fetal infection during the first trimester leads to congenital rubella in at least 80% of fetuses.

Positive tests for IgG antibodies alone indicate past infection or vaccination. High-avidity anti-rubella IgG assays may distinguish past infection from vaccination. If no antibodies are found, clinical observation and serologic follow-up are essential. An isolated IgM-positive test needs to be interpreted with caution, because it does not necessarily imply acute infection. Confirmation of rubella in the expectant mother raises the question of therapeutic abortion, an alternative to be considered in light of personal, religious, legal, and other factors.

The immune status of the mother needs to be evaluated because titers fall to seronegativity in about 10% by 12 years after vaccination.

B. Congenital Rubella

An infant acquiring the infection in utero may be normal at birth but probably—50% in a series of nearly 70 pregnant women with rubella in Mexico—will have a wide variety of manifestations, including early-onset cataracts and glaucoma, microphthalmia, hearing deficits, psychomotor retardation, congenital heart defects (patent ductus arteriosus, branch pulmonary artery stenosis), organomegaly, and maculopapular rash. In general, the younger the fetus when infected, the more severe the illness. Deafness is the primary complication in the second trimester. Viral excretion in the throat and urine persists for many months despite high antibody levels. A specific test for IgM rubella antibody is useful for diagnosis in the newborn. A confirmatory diagnosis is made by isolation of the virus or PCR detection of viral RNA in tissues. Treatment is directed toward the many anomalies.

C. Postinfectious Encephalopathy

In 1:6000 cases, postinfectious encephalopathy develops 1–6 days after the rash; the virus cannot always be isolated. The mortality rate is 20%, but residual deficits are rare among the recovered. The mechanism is unknown.

Other unusual complications of rubella include hemorrhagic manifestations due to thrombocytopenia and vascular damage, duodenal stenosis, and mild hepatitis.

▶ Treatment

Rubella and its complications should be treated symptomatically.

▶ Prognosis

Rubella is a mild illness and rarely lasts more than 3–4 days. Congenital rubella, on the other hand, has a high mortality rate, and the associated congenital defects are largely permanent.

▶ Prevention

Live attenuated rubella virus vaccine should be given to all infants and a second dose should be given to children of school age. It is important that girls in particular are immune to rubella prior to the menarche. When women are immunized, they should not be pregnant, and the absence of antibodies should be established. (In the United States, about 80% of 20-year-old women are immune to rubella.) Postpartum administration to susceptible female hospital employees is recommended. It is recommended that women not become pregnant for at least 3 months

after vaccine administration. Nonetheless, there are no reports of congenital rubella syndrome after rubella immunization, and inadvertent immunization of a pregnant woman is not considered an indication for therapeutic abortion. Arthritis is more marked after rubella vaccination than in native disease and appears to be immunologically mediated. A flare of juvenile rheumatoid arthritis after rubella vaccination is reported. The association between chronic arthropathies and rubella vaccination is controversial. Anaphylactoid reactions following vaccination are rare, and a self-limited thrombotic thrombocytopenic purpura is a reported but very rare (2.6 per 100,000 doses) complication.

MMR may be given in conjunction with DPT or varicella boosters as adequate serologic responses are documented. The administration of two or more doses appears to overcome an immunogenetic risk for vaccine failure in some vaccinees. Immunogenicity is similar with intramuscular and intracutaneous infection, for MMR and varicella vaccinations. Children with biliary atresia in particular show impaired responses to MMR and varicella vaccinations, although children with juvenile rheumatoid arthritis show intact responses to MMR boosters. Preliminary data suggests that vaccination may be safe for patients receiving immunosuppressive therapy in the setting of solid organ, bone marrow, or stem cell transplantation. Immigrants, especially the HIV-positive, should be vaccinated if CD4 counts show immune restoration.

Geographic areas with high birth rates and transmission rates of rubella may require baseline societal coverage rates for rubella higher than the conventional 80% often used.

▶ When to Refer

- Pregnancy.
- Meningitis/encephalitis.
- Significant vaccination reactions.
- Any suspect cases should be reported to public health authorities.

Centers for Disease Control and Prevention (CDC). Three cases of congenital rubella syndrome in the postelimination era—Maryland, Alabama, and Illinois, 2012. MMWR Morb Mortal Wkly Rep. 2013 Mar 29;62(12):226–9. [PMID: 23535689]

McCarthy M. Imported measles and rubella pose threat to US elimination of the diseases, says CDC report. BMJ. 2013 Dec 9; 347:f7373. [PMID: 24324216]

Papania MJ et al. Elimination of endemic measles, rubella, and congenital rubella syndrome from the Western hemisphere: the US experience. JAMA Pediatr. 2014 Feb;168(2):148–55. [PMID: 24311021]

Strikas RA; Centers for Disease Control and Prevention (CDC); Advisory Committee on Immunization Practices (ACIP); ACIP Child/Adolescent Immunization Work Group. Advisory committee on immunization practices recommended immunization schedules for persons aged 0 through 18 years—United States, 2015. MMWR Morb Mortal Wkly Rep. 2015 Feb 6;64(4):93–4. [PMID: 25654610]

World Health Organization. Measles & Rubella Initiative. Annual Report 2012. WHO 2013. http://www.who.int/immunization/diseases/MRI_2012_Annual_Report.pdf

OTHER NEUROTROPIC VIRUSES

1. Rabies

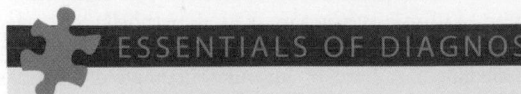

ESSENTIALS OF DIAGNOSIS

▶ History of animal bite.

▶ Paresthesias, hydrophobia, rage alternating with calm.

▶ Convulsions, paralysis, thick tenacious saliva.

▶ General Considerations

Rabies is a viral (rhabdovirus) encephalitis transmitted by infected saliva that gains entry into the body by an animal bite or an open wound. Worldwide, 17.4 million cases of animal bites are reported every year, and it is estimated that between 26,400 and 61,000 deaths annually are attributable to rabies. Most of these cases occur in rural areas of Africa and Asia. India has the highest incidence, accounting for 36% of global deaths. In developing countries, more than 90% of human cases and 99% of human deaths from rabies are secondary to bites from infected dogs. Many victims are children. Rabies among travelers to rabies-endemic areas is usually associated with animal injuries (including dogs in North Africa and India, cats in the Middle East, and non-human primates in sub-Saharan Africa and Asia), with most travel-associated cases occurring within 10 days of arrival. Rare but related viruses are the Australian lyssavirus, transmitted by bats including one referred to as the black flying fox, and which has caused 3 deaths over the last 20 years, and the European lyssavirus, with cases from Germany and the United Kingdom.

In the United States, domestically acquired rabies cases are rare (approximately 92% of cases are associated with wildlife) but probably underreported. Reports largely from the East Coast show an increase in rabies among cats, with about 1% of tested cats showing rabies seropositivity. In 2013, 3 cases of rabies were reported among United States citizens, one in Maryland transmitted by organ transplantation, a second in North Carolina identified retrospectively in the organ donor, and the third a Guatemalan refugee under detention in Texas. Surveillance for animal rabies showed 5865 cases occurring in 39 states and Puerto Rico. Wildlife reservoirs, with each species having its own rabies variant(s), follow a unique geographic distribution in the United States: raccoons on the East Coast; skunks in the Midwest, Southwest, and California; and foxes in the Southwest and in Alaska. Hawaii is the only rabies-free state to date. Most of Western Europe and much of Oceania is rabies-free.

Raccoons and bats were the most commonly reported rabid animals during 2013. Raccoons, bats, and skunks account for 84% of the rabid animals found in the United States; other rabid animals include foxes, cats, cattle, and dogs. Rodents and lagomorphs (eg, rabbits) are unlikely to spread rabies because they cannot survive the disease long enough to transmit it (woodchucks and groundhogs are exceptions). Wildlife epizootics present a constant public health threat in addition to the danger of reintroducing rabies to domestic animals. Vaccination is the key to controlling rabies in small animals and preventing rabies transmission to human beings.

The virus gains entry into the salivary glands of dogs 5–7 days before their death from rabies, thus limiting their period of infectivity. Less common routes of transmission include contamination of mucous membranes with saliva or brain tissue, aerosol transmission, and corneal transplantation. Transmission through solid organ and vascular segment transplantation from donors with unrecognized infection is also reported. A number of transplantation–associated cases are reported, including two clusters in the United States. Postexposure prophylaxis can be administered in these patients and may prevent development of disease.

The incubation period may range from 10 days to many years but is usually 3–7 weeks depending in part on the distance of the wound from the CNS. The virus travels in the nerves to the brain, multiplies there, and then migrates along the efferent nerves to the salivary glands. Rabies virus infection forms cytoplasmic inclusion bodies similar to Negri bodies. These Negri body-like structures are thought to be the sites of viral transcription and replication.

▶ Clinical Findings

A. Symptoms and Signs

While there is usually a history of animal bite, bat bites may not be recognized. The prodromal syndrome consists of pain at the site of the bite in association with fever, malaise, headache, nausea, and vomiting. The skin is sensitive to changes of temperature, especially air currents (aerophobia). Percussion myoedema can be present and persist throughout the disease. The CNS stage begins about 10 days after the prodrome and may be either encephalitic ("furious") or paralytic ("dumb"). The encephalitic form (about 80% of the cases) produces the classic rabies manifestations of delirium alternating with periods of calm, extremely painful laryngeal spasms on attempting drinking (hydrophobia), autonomic stimulation (hypersalivation), and seizures. In the less common paralytic form, an acute ascending paralysis resembling Guillain-Barré syndrome predominates with relative sparing of higher cortical functions initially. Both forms progress relentlessly to coma, autonomic nervous system dysfunction, and death.

B. Laboratory Findings

Biting animals that appear well should be quarantined and observed for 10 days. Sick or dead animals should be tested for rabies. A wild animal, if captured, should be sacrificed and the head shipped on ice to the nearest laboratory qualified to examine the brain for evidence of rabies virus. When the animal cannot be examined, raccoons, skunks, bats, and foxes should be presumed to be rabid.

Direct fluorescent antibody testing of skin biopsy material from the posterior neck (where hair follicles are highly innervated) has a sensitivity of 60–80%.

Quantitative RT-PCR, nucleic acid sequence-based amplification, direct rapid immunohistochemical test and viral isolation from the cerebrospinal fluid or saliva are advocated as definitive diagnostic assays. Antibodies can be detected in the serum and the cerebrospinal fluid. Pathologic specimens often demonstrate round or oval eosinophilic inclusion bodies (Negri bodies) in the cytoplasm of neuronal cells, but the finding is neither sensitive nor specific. MRI signs are diffuse and nonspecific.

Treatment & Prognosis

Management requires intensive care with attention to the airway, maintenance of oxygenation, and control of seizures. Universal precautions are essential. Corticosteroids are of no use.

If postexposure prophylaxis (discussed below) is given expediently, before clinical signs develop, it is nearly 100% successful in prevention of disease. Once the symptoms have appeared, death almost inevitably occurs after 7 days, usually from respiratory failure. Most deaths occur in persons with unrecognized disease who do not seek medical care or in individuals who do not receive postexposure prophylaxis. The very rare cases in which patients recover without intensive care are referred to as "abortive rabies."

Prevention

Immunization of household dogs and cats and active immunization of persons with significant animal exposure (eg, veterinarians) are important. The most important decisions, however, concern animal bites. Animals that are frequent sources of infection to travelers are dogs, cats, and non-human primates.

In the developing world, education, surveillance, and animal (particularly dog) vaccination programs (at recurrent intervals) are preferred over mass destruction of dogs, which is followed typically by invasion of susceptible feral animals into urban areas. In some Western European countries, campaigns of oral vaccination of wild animals led to the elimination of rabies in wildlife. Human contact with animal vaccine baits is a recent public health concern although no new cases of rabies from such contact have been reported.

A. Local Treatment of Animal Bites and Scratches

Thorough cleansing, debridement, and repeated flushing of wounds with soap and water are important. Rabies immune globulin or antiserum should be given as stated below. Wounds caused by animal bites should not be sutured.

B. Postexposure Immunization

The decision to treat should be based on the circumstances of the bite, including the extent and location of the wound, the biting animal, the history of prior vaccination, and the local epidemiology of rabies. **Any contact or suspect contact with a bat, skunk, or raccoon is usually deemed a sufficient indication to warrant prophylaxis.** Consultation with state and local health departments is recommended. Postexposure treatment including both immune globulin and vaccination should be administered as promptly as possible when indicated.

The optimal form of passive immunization is human rabies immune globulin (HRIG; 20 international units/kg),

administered once. As much as possible of the full dose should be infiltrated around the wound, with any remaining injected intramuscularly at a site distant from the wound. Finger spaces can be safely injected without development of a compartment syndrome. If HRIG is not available and appropriate tests for horse serum sensitivity are done, equine rabies antiserum (40 international units/kg) can be used. As much as possible of the rabies immune globulin should be injected at the wound site and the remainder injected intramuscularly at a site distant from vaccine administration.

Two vaccines are licensed and available for use in humans in the United States: a human diploid cell vaccine and a purified chick embryo cell vaccine. The current vaccines may be given as four injections of 1 mL intramuscularly in the deltoid or, in small children, into the anterolateral thigh muscles on days 0, 3, 7, and 14 after exposure. (The fifth dose at 28 days after exposure is no longer recommended except among immunosuppressed patients.) The vaccine should not be given in the gluteal area due to suboptimal response. An alternative vaccination strategy that only takes 1 week, with injections on days 0, 3, and 7 after exposure with a verocell vaccine is reportedly successful in achieving adequate neutralizing titers at days 14 and 28 in a study from Thailand.

Rabies vaccines and HRIG should never be given in the same syringe or at the same site. Allergic reactions to the vaccine are rare, although local reactions (pruritus, erythema, tenderness) occur in about 25% and mild systemic reactions (headaches, myalgias, nausea) in about 20% of recipients. Adverse reactions to HRIG seem to be more frequent in women and rare in young children. The vaccine is commercially available or can be obtained through health departments.

Globally, diverse anti-rabies vaccines are used. In some countries, the full spectrum of vaccines, from human diploid rabies to chromatographically purified rabies vaccine are available, whereas in others, the gamut is smaller and intradermal application of smaller vaccine doses at multiple sites and at different times is commonly practiced in an attempt to lower costs, and is deemed safe and effective by the WHO.

In patients with history of past vaccination, the need for HRIG is eliminated (RIG is in short supply worldwide), but postexposure vaccination is still required. The vaccine should be given 1 mL in the deltoid twice (on days 0 and 3). Neither the passive nor the active form of postexposure prophylaxis is associated with fetal abnormalities and thus pregnancy is not considered a contraindication to vaccination.

C. Preexposure Immunization

Preexposure prophylaxis with three injections of human diploid cell vaccine intramuscularly (1 mL on days 0, 7, and 21 or 28) is recommended for persons at high risk for exposure: veterinarians (who should have rabies antibody titers checked every 2 years and be boosted with 1 mL intramuscularly); animal handlers; laboratory workers; Peace Corps workers; and travelers with stays over 1 month to remote areas in endemic countries in Africa, Asia, and Latin America. An intradermal route is also available (0.1 mL on days 0, 7, and 21 over the deltoid) but not in the United States. Immunosuppressive illnesses and agents including corticosteroids as well as antimalarials—in particular chloroquine—may diminish the antibody response. A single dose booster at 10 years after initial immunization increases the level of antibody titers. Unfortunately, data from travel services indicate that only a small proportion of travelers with anticipated lengthy stays in rabies-impacted areas receive the vaccine as recommended.

▶ When to Refer

Suspicion of rabies requires contact with public health personnel to initiate appropriate passive and active prophylaxis and observation of suspect cases.

▶ When to Admit

- Respiratory, neuromuscular, or CNS dysfunction consistent with rabies.

- Patients with suspect rabies require initiation of therapy until the disease is ruled out in suspect animals, and this requires coordination of care based on likelihood of patient compliance, availability of inpatient and outpatient facilities, and response of local public health teams.

Centers for Disease Control and Prevention (CDC). Human contacts with oral rabies vaccine baits distributed for wildlife rabies management—Ohio, 2012. MMWR Morb Mortal Wkly Rep. 2013 Apr 12;62(14):267–9. [PMID: 23575240]

Dolan SB et al. Pre-exposure rabies vaccination among US international travelers: findings from the global TravEpiNet consortium. Vector Borne Zoonotic Dis. 2014 Feb;14(2):160–7. [PMID: 24359420]

Dyer JL et al. Rabies surveillance in the United States during 2013. J Am Vet Med Assoc. 2014 Nov 15;245(10):1111–23. Erratum in: J Am Vet Med Assoc. 2014 Dec 15;245(12):1358. [PMID: 25356711]

Lankau EW et al. Prevention and control of rabies in an age of global travel: a review of travel- and trade-associated rabies events—United States, 1986–2012. Zoonoses Public Health. 2014 Aug;61(5):305–16. [PMID: 23870674]

Vora NM et al. Clinical management and humoral immune responses to rabies post-exposure prophylaxis among three patients who received solid organs from a donor with rabies. Transpl Infect Dis. 2015 Jun;17(3):389–95. [PMID: 25851103]

World Health Organization. WHO Expert Consultation on rabies. Second report. World Health Organ Tech Rep Ser. 2013;(982):1–139, back cover. [PMID: 24069724]

2. Arbovirus Encephalitides

ESSENTIALS OF DIAGNOSIS

- ▶ Fever, malaise, stiff neck, sore throat, and vomiting, progressing to stupor, coma, and convulsions.

- ▶ Upper motor neuron lesion signs: exaggerated deep tendon reflexes, absent superficial reflexes, and spastic paralysis.

- ▶ Cerebrospinal fluid opening pressure and protein are often increased, with lymphocytic pleocytosis.

▶ General Considerations

The arboviruses are arthropod-borne pathogens that produce clinical manifestations in humans. The **mosquito-borne pathogens** that cause encephalitis include three togaviruses (causing Western, Eastern, and Venezuelan equine encephalitis), six flaviviruses (causing West Nile fever, St. Louis encephalitis, Japanese encephalitis, dengue (see below under Hemorrhagic Viruses), Murray Valley encephalitis, and Zika virus (see below under Other Systemic Viruses) and bunyaviruses (the California serogroup of viruses, including the La Crosse agent of California encephalitis). The **tick-borne** causes of encephalitis include the flavivirus of the Powassan encephalitis (northeastern United States and Canada), tick-borne encephalitis virus of Europe, and the Colorado tick fever reovirus. Tick-borne encephalitis virus, Colorado tick fever, and the arboviruses associated with viral hemorrhagic fever (including dengue) are discussed below, and only those viruses causing primarily encephalitis in the United States will be discussed here, although West Nile agent is being reported in many other areas, including Italy, Greece, Portugal, and Hungary as well as in Africa (Madagascar and South Africa), Canada, the Middle East, and West Asia.

West Nile virus is the leading cause of domestically acquired arboviral disease in the United States. Infection with West Nile virus was first identified in the United States in the New York City area in 1999. The virus spread rapidly, and current cases are reported throughout the continental United States. As of October 13, 2015 CDC surveillance data identified 1332 cases of West Nile virus infection in 48 states (all but Alaska and Hawaii) and the District of Columbia. The total caseload from 1999 through 2014 includes 41,762 cases; of these, neuroinvasive disease was present in 18,810. The mortality of the collected cases through the end of 2014 was 4.2% but 8.7% among neuroinvasive cases. In the United States, the highest incidence of neuroinvasive disease is among the Rocky Mountain states, the upper Midwest and the lower Mississippi River valley, while the largest numbers of cases occur in Texas, Colorado, and California. Outbreaks with West Nile infection tend to occur between mid-July and early September. Climatic factors, including elevated mean temperatures and rainfall, correlate with increased West Nile infection.

La Crosse virus was the second most commonly reported cause of arboviral disease in 2013 with 77 reported cases of neuroinvasive disease and the highest caseloads between 2004 and 2013 occurring in North Carolina, Ohio, and Tennessee. Other recognized and reported arbovirus infections in 2013 include Jamestown Canyon virus (22 cases, 7 in Wisconsin), Powassan virus (15 cases, 4 in New York), and eastern equine encephalitis virus (8 cases, 3 in Florida), and St. Louis encephalitis (1 case in Texas). These arboviruses can also cause sporadic cases, neuroinvasive disease, and seasonal outbreaks.

Pathogen-specific reservoirs (typically small mammals or birds) are responsible for maintaining the encephalitis-producing viruses in nature. For the eastern equine encephalitis virus, cotton rats and house sparrows serve as amplifying reservoirs. Birds are the main reservoir for West Nile virus and substantial avian mortality accompanies

West Nile fever outbreaks (monitoring chickens is recommended and a possible mode of disease surveillance). The mosquito species associated with transmission is different in the Western vs Eastern United States (*Culex tarsalis* vs *Culex pipiens*) and consequently the terrain associated with high prevalence areas differs (open grasslands vs urban areas).

Only dengue and Venezuelan equine encephalitis viruses produce viremias high enough to allow continued transmission to other mosquitoes and ticks between humans and vectors (mosquitoes of distinct species). Human to human transmission of the other arboviruses is usually related to blood (including granulocyte) transfusion or organ transplantation (although most infected donors give a history of clinically significant disease). Perinatal, transplacental, breastfeeding (rarely), laboratory, solid organ transplant, and possibly aerosol transmission of West Nile virus can also occur. St. Louis encephalitis and Powassan encephalitis occur among adults; western equine encephalitis, Venezuelan equine encephalitis, La Crosse and California encephalitis occur primarily among children. West Nile fever and eastern equine encephalitis are diseases of both children and adults.

▶ Clinical Findings

A. Symptoms and Signs

The human incubation period for arboviral encephalitides is 2–14 days. Symptoms include fever, malaise, sore throat, headache, gastrointestinal upset, lethargy, and stupor progressing to coma. Using blood donor surveys, it is estimated that only about 26% of infections are symptomatic (women and the highly viremic are more symptomatic). A nonpruritic maculopapular rash is variably present. Stiff neck and mental status changes are the most common neurologic signs. It is estimated that West Nile fever develops in 20–25% of those infected with West Nile virus, while neuroinvasive disease occurs in less than 1%, but has a mortality rate of at least 10%. About 50% of hospitalized patients with West Nile virus infection in the United States have significant muscle weakness that may be initially confused with the Guillain-Barré syndrome. Acute flaccid (poliomyelitis-like) paralysis is seen in 10% of West Nile virus neuroinvasive disease and less commonly with the other arboviruses. Other signs include tremors, seizures, cranial nerve palsies, and pathologic reflexes. Myocarditis, pancreatitis, and hearing loss are also reported. The disease manifestations associated with West Nile virus infection are strongly age-dependent: the acute febrile syndrome and mild neurologic symptoms (but on occasion meningitis) are more common in the young, aseptic meningitis and poliomyelitis-like syndromes are seen in the middle aged, and frank encephalopathy is seen more often in the elderly. All forms of disease tend to be severe in immunocompromised persons in whom neuroinvasive manifestations and associated high mortality are more apt to develop.

Host genetic variation in the interferon response pathway is associated with both risk for symptomatic West Nile virus infection and West Nile virus disease progression.

B. Laboratory Findings

The peripheral white blood cell count is variable. Cerebrospinal fluid protein is elevated; cerebrospinal fluid glucose is normal; there is usually a lymphocytic pleocytosis; and polymorphonuclear cells may predominate early. The diagnosis of arboviral encephalitides depends on serologic tests. Antibodies to arboviruses persist for life and the presence of IgG in the absence of a rising titer of IgM may indicate past exposure rather than acute infection. Individuals with chronic symptoms after West Nile virus infection may show persistent renal infection for up to 6 years with West Nile virus RNA present in urine. Documentation of a fourfold increase in acute/convalescence titers IgG or the presence of IgM antibodies is confirmatory. For West Nile virus, an IgM capture ELISA in serum or cerebrospinal fluid is almost always positive by the time the disease is clinically evident, and the presence of IgM in cerebrospinal fluid indicates neuroinvasive disease. These tests are available commercially but also through local or state health departments. Cross-reactivity exists among the different flaviviruses, so a plaque reduction assay may be needed to definitively distinguish between West Nile fever and St. Louis encephalitis (with possible seroreactivity now in the United States against dengue as well). PCR assays (also available through the CDC) are less sensitive than serologic tests for the diagnosis of acute infections but are the preferred method for screening blood products and may be particularly useful in immunocompromised patients with abnormal antibody responses. CT scans of the brain usually show no acute disease, but MRI may reveal leptomeningeal, basal ganglia, thalamic, or periventricular enhancement.

▶ Differential Diagnosis

Mild forms of encephalitis must be differentiated from aseptic meningitis, lymphocytic choriomeningitis, and nonparalytic poliomyelitis.

Severe forms of arbovirus encephalitides are to be differentiated from other causes of viral encephalitis (HSV, mumps virus, poliovirus or other enteroviruses, HIV), encephalitis accompanying exanthematous diseases of childhood (measles, varicella, infectious mononucleosis, rubella), encephalitis following vaccination (a demyelinating type following rabies, measles, pertussis), toxic encephalitis (from drugs, poisons, or bacterial toxins such as *Shigella dysenteriae* type 1), Reye syndrome, and severe forms of stroke, brain tumors, brain abscess, autoimmune processes such as lupus cerebritis, and intoxications. In the California Encephalitis Project, anti-*N*-methyl-D-aspartate receptor (anti-NMDAR) encephalitis is a more common cause of encephalitis than viral diseases especially in the young, with 65% of encephalitis due to anti-NMDAR occurring among patients 18 or younger.

▶ Complications

Bronchial pneumonia, urinary retention and infection, prolonged weakness, and decubitus ulcers may occur. A chronic syndrome consisting of myalgias, arthralgias, and difficulty with concentration and memory is reported in over half the symptomatic cases.

Treatment

Although specific antiviral therapy is not available for most causative entities, vigorous supportive measures can be helpful. Such measures include reduction of intracranial pressure (mannitol) and monitoring of intraventricular pressure. The efficacy of corticosteroids in these infections is not established. Ribavirin is commonly used to treat some tick-borne viral hemorrhagic diseases such as Crimean-Congo hemorrhagic fever, although the effectiveness of ribavirin is unclear. Other potentially beneficial therapeutic options include IVIG, interferon-alpha, and hyperimmune plasma and gamma globulin. Poor therapeutic options propel the search for an effective vaccine.

Prognosis

Although most infections are mild or asymptomatic, the prognosis is always guarded, especially at the extremes of age. Most fatalities occur with neuroinvasive disease. In 2014, one of the largest prospective clinical investigations of West Nile virus neuroinvasive disease in the United States revealed that 7 (12%) of 55 patients died. Most presented in a coma. Otherwise, age older than 50 years is an important risk factor for severe disease and death. Other risk factors for mortality include black race, chronic kidney disease, hepatitis C virus infection, and immunosuppression. Recovery of persons with severe neurologic compromise may take months; in a cohort of 157 persons infected with West Nile virus, 40% continued to experience symptoms related to their infection up to 8 years later. Sequelae of West Nile virus infection include a poliomyelitis-like syndrome, cognitive complaints, movement disorders, epilepsy, and depression; and they may become apparent late in the course of what appears to be a successful recovery.

The long-term prognosis is generally better for Western equine than for Eastern equine or St. Louis encephalitis.

Prevention

No human vaccine is currently available for the arboviruses prevalent in North America, although phase I studies of a peroxide inactivated vaccine for West Nile are currently under way. Mosquito control (repellents, protective clothing, and insecticide spraying) is effective in prevention. Since 2003, all blood donations in the United States are screened with nucleic acid amplification tests for West Nile virus. Laboratory precautions are indicated for handling all these pathogens, in particular the West Nile virus. Because of reports of poor pregnancy outcomes possibly associated with Zika virus infection, pregnant women are advised to postpone travel to areas where Zika virus is circulating if possible. If they must travel, pregnant women are advised to follow recommendations to avoid mosquito bites while traveling.

Dyer O. Zika virus spreads across Americas as concerns mount over birth defects. BMJ. 2015 Dec 23;351:h6983. [PMID: 26698165]

Enserink M. An obscure mosquito-borne disease goes global. Science. 2015 Nov 27;350(6264):1012–3. [PMID: 26612926]

Hart J Jr et al; NIAID Collaborative Antiviral Study Group West Nile Virus 210 Protocol Team. West Nile virus neuroinvasive disease: neurological manifestations and prospective longitudinal outcomes. BMC Infect Dis. 2014 May 9;14:248. [PMID: 24884681]

Lindsey NP et al; Division of Vector-Borne Diseases, National Center for Emerging and Zoonotic Infectious Diseases, CDC. West Nile virus and other arboviral diseases—United States, 2013. MMWR Morb Mortal Wkly Rep. 2014 Jun 20; 63(24):521–6. [PMID: 24941331]

Murray KO et al. Survival analysis, long-term outcomes, and percentage of recovery up to 8 years post-infection among the Houston West Nile virus cohort. PLoS One. 2014 Jul 23; 9(7):e102953. [PMID: 25054656]

3. Japanese Encephalitis

> **ESSENTIALS OF DIAGNOSIS**
>
> ▶ Major cause of summertime encephalitis in East Asia.
> ▶ Vector-borne, with Aedes mosquito the carrier.
> ▶ Wide spectrum of symptoms with many asymptomatic infections.
> ▶ Vaccine available but no effective antiviral therapy.

General Considerations

The Japanese encephalitis virus is a flavivirus akin to those causing West Nile infection and St. Louis encephalitis. It is the most common cause of encephalitis in East Asia with over 68,000 estimated annual cases. It is geographically contained to East Asia but the area of distribution includes 24 countries, extending from Pakistan to Japan and from Northern China to Indonesia, Malaysia, and Northern Australia. Most cases occur in the summer and late fall, although in tropical and subtropical areas transmission occurs throughout the year. Major outbreaks every 2–15 years often correlate with patterns of agricultural development. The vector is the *Culex* species of mosquito, especially *Culex tritaeniorhynchus*. Wading birds and pigs more commonly sustain the infection as reservoirs in nature, since the viremia in man is transient and not usually high enough to sustain transmission.

Clinical Findings

Most persons asymptomatically seroconvert. The 1% of patients in whom meningitis develops report the usual symptoms of headaches, nausea, mental status changes, movement disorders, and in a smaller percentage, seizures, typically in children. Infections that most clinically mimic Japanese encephalitis are St. Louis encephalitis and West Nile encephalitis, although epidemiologic data readily distinguishes these infections in most instances. Cases among travelers to the Orient are rare.

Suspicion of disease is based on epidemiologic data, with laboratory confirmation of cases based on serum of cerebrospinal fluid examination of antibodies at reference laboratories.

Complications

A variety of cognitive, neurologic, and psychiatric complications are recognized to occur in as many as 50% of survivors. The mortality is reportedly as high as 30%.

Treatment

Treatment is only supportive, including antipyretics, analgesics, bedrest, and fluids.

Prevention

Four effective types of vaccine against Japanese encephalitis are available. A live attenuated vaccine made in China (referred to as SA14-14-2) is the most common. Other vaccine types include inactivated mouse brain-derived vaccines, live recombinant vaccines, and inactivated Vero cell–derived vaccines. In the United States, a vaccine licensed as inactivated Vero-cell culture-derived Japanese encephalitis vaccine (IXIARO, also based on the SA14-14-2 vaccine) has been available for those age 17 years and older since 2009 and a pediatric vaccine for those age 7–16 years since 2013. Travelers who plan to spend time (typically at least 1 month) in rural East Asia during the summer or fall should receive the two-course vaccine, given at a 1-month interval. The risk of serious reactions, including potential encephalitis, with live vaccines is very low (1:1,000,000 or less), with the newer vaccines being safer. Booster doses can be given for anticipated near future exposures.

Use of mosquito repellents, wearing long sleeves, long pants, and socks, and use of air conditioned facilities and bed nets are essential means of protection.

Centers for Disease Control and Prevention (CDC). Japanese encephalitis. 2015 Aug 5. http://www.cdc.gov/japaneseencephalitis/index.html

Chen HL et al. Current recommendations for the Japanese encephalitis vaccine. J Chin Med Assoc. 2015 May;78(5):271–5. [PMID: 25841620]

Firbas C et al. Product review on the JE vaccine IXIARO. Hum Vaccin Immunother. 2015;11(2):411–20. [PMID: 25621812]

World Health Organization. Japanese encephalitis: fact sheet No. 386. December 2015. http://www.who.int/mediacentre/factsheets/fs386/en/

4. Tick-Borne Encephalitis

ESSENTIALS OF DIAGNOSIS

- ▶ Flaviviral encephalitis found in Eastern, Central, and occasionally Northern Europe and Asia.
- ▶ Transmitted via ticks or ingestion of unpasteurized milk.
- ▶ Long-term neurologic sequelae occur in 2–25% of cases.
- ▶ Therapy is largely supportive.
- ▶ Prevention is based on avoiding tick exposure, pasteurization of milk, and vaccination.

General Considerations

Tick-borne encephalitis (TBE), a flaviviral infection caused by TBE virus, is the most common arbovirus infection transmitted by ticks in Europe. An estimated 10,000 to 12,000 cases occur each year in parts of Eurasia (from eastern France to northern Japan, from northern Siberia to Albania), with annual increases thought to be a function of increased recognition, climatic changes, and personal or social habits. TBE is endemic in Japan and parts of China as well. TBE occurs predominantly in the late spring through fall. It is usually a consequence of exposure to infected ticks, although unpasteurized milk from viremic livestock is also a recognized form of transmission. Surges in cases over the last 20 years are thought to be a consequence of agricultural policies that alter land cover, host prevalence, climatic factors, and human behavior (including pesticide usage and travel to endemic areas). The maximum altitude for occurrence of cases has increased to 5000 feet (about 1500 meters). The incubation period is 7–14 days for tick-borne exposures but only 3–4 days for milk ingestion. The principal reservoirs for TBE virus are small rodents; humans are an accidental host. The vectors for most cases are *Ixodes ricinus* (most of Europe, including Turkey, Iran, and the Caucasus) and *Ixodes persulcatus* (in the belt from Eastern Europe to China and Japan).

Related viruses found in Eastern and mid-Western North America are the Powassan agent and the deer tick virus. In Germany during 2015, an unrelated bornavirus, variegated squirrel bornavirus-1, was thought to have caused fatal encephalitis in three breeders of variegated squirrels.

Clinical Findings

A. Symptoms and Signs

Most cases are subclinical and many resemble a flu-like syndrome. There are two variants of clinical presentation: the Western subtype occurs mainly in the fall (but as early as April) and is most severe among the elderly, and the Eastern subtype is more severe among children.

Western subtype disease is biphasic in which after 2–10 days of fever (usually with malaise, headache, and myalgias), a 1–21 day symptom-free interval leads to a second phase with resumed fevers followed by neurologic symptoms. **Eastern subtype disease** is progressive without an asymptomatic interval. The neurologic manifestations range from febrile headache (accounting for up to 50% of Eastern subtype cases) to aseptic meningitis and encephalitis with or without myelitis (preferentially of the cervical anterior horn) and spinal paralysis (usually flaccid). A myeloradiculitic form can also develop but is less common. Peripheral facial palsies, sometimes bilaterally, tend to occur infrequently, late in the course of infection, usually after encephalitis, and usually are associated with a favorable outcome within 30–90 days. Double infection with *Borrelia burgdorferi* (the agent of Lyme disease; transmitted by the same tick vector) may result in a more severe disease. Mortality in TBE is usually a consequence of brain edema or bulbar involvement.

B. Diagnosis

Leukocytosis and neutrophilia are common. Abnormal cerebrospinal fluid findings include an inconsistent pleocytosis that may persist for up to 4 months. Neuroimaging shows hyperintense lesions in the thalamus, brainstem, and basal ganglia. TBE virus IgM and IgG are detected by ELISA techniques when neurologic symptoms occur. Cross-reactivity with other flaviviruses or a vaccinated state may require confirmation by detection of TBE virus–specific antibodies in cerebrospinal fluid. RT-PCR of blood (at earlier stages of the disease) or cerebrospinal fluid can sometimes, if available, assist with the diagnosis. Viral detection in the urine has been reported in a small group of cases. TBE virus can be differentiated from serologically indistinguishable viruses (Powassan agent and deer tick virus) by plaque-reduction neutralization tests.

► Complications

The main sequela of disease is paresis, which occurs in up to 10% of Western and up to 25% of Eastern subtype disease. Other causes of long-term morbidity include protracted cognitive dysfunction and persistent spinal nerve paralysis. The **postencephalitic syndrome**, characterized by headache, difficulties concentrating, balance disorders, dysphasia, hearing defects, and chronic fatigue, occurs with both subtypes. A progressive motor neuron disease and partial continuous epilepsy are complications seen with the Eastern subtype. Cognitive impairments may develop in children after infection. Long-standing psychiatric complications are reported and these include attention deficits, slowness of thought and learning impairment, depression, lability, and mutism.

► Differential Diagnosis

The differential diagnosis includes other causes of aseptic meningitis such as enteroviral infections, herpes simplex encephalitis, and a variety of tick-borne pathogens including tularemia, the rickettsial diseases, babesiosis, Lyme disease, poliomyelitis (no longer reported from Eastern Europe), and other flaviviral infections. Coinfections are documented with *Anaplasma, Babesia,* and *Borrelia* infections.

► Treatment

Therapy is largely supportive. Some clinicians believe corticosteroids may be useful, although no controlled clinical trials exist.

► Prognosis

TBE usually has a good prognosis. In Switzerland, the mortality rate was of 0.7% between 2005 and 2011. A 1–2% mortality rate was reported from Croatia in 2015. Worse outcomes are associated with older age.

► Prevention

There are two inactivated TBE virus vaccines for adults and two vaccines for children licensed in Europe. Their effectiveness is about 99%. They were developed in Austria and Germany and in Russia, and there appears to be cross-reactivity against isolates from diverse geographic areas although concomitant administration of the two different vaccines may result in immune interference. The initial vaccination schedule requires three doses given over 1 year with boosters every 3–5 years. There are decreased antibody titers (quantity not quality) and booster response in recipients of TBE vaccines who are over 50 years of age, indicating the need for a modified immunization strategy in older patients.

Poor uptake of the vaccine in endemic countries is responsible for limited abilities to control the disease. Other prevention recommendations include avoidance of tick exposure and pasteurization of cow and goat milk.

Šmit R et al. Review of tick-borne encephalitis and vaccines: clinical and economical aspects. Expert Rev Vaccines. 2015 May;14(5):737–47. [PMID: 25427237]
Stupica D et al. Tick borne encephalitis without cerebrospinal fluid pleocytosis. BMC Infect Dis. 2014 Nov 18;14:614. [PMID: 25403498]
Więdłocha M et al. Psychiatric aspects of herpes simplex encephalitis, tick-borne encephalitis and herpes zoster encephalitis among immunocompetent patients. Adv Clin Exp Med. 2015 Mar–Apr;24(2):361–71. [PMID: 25931371]

5. Lymphocytic Choriomeningitis

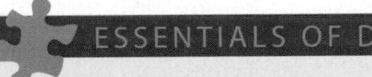

ESSENTIALS OF DIAGNOSIS

► "Influenza-like" prodrome of fever, chills, and cough, followed by a meningeal phase.

► Aseptic meningitis with stiff neck, headache, nausea, vomiting, and lethargy.

► Cerebrospinal fluid: slight increase of protein, lymphocytic pleocytosis (500–3000/mcL); low glucose in 25% of patients.

► Complement-fixing antibodies within 2 weeks.

► General Considerations

The lymphocytic choriomeningitis virus is an arenavirus (related to the pathogen causing Lassa fever, discussed below) that primarily infects the CNS. Its main reservoir is the house mouse (*Mus musculus*). Other rodents (such as rats, guinea pigs, and even pet hamsters), monkeys, dogs, and swine are also potential reservoirs. The infected animal sheds lymphocytic choriomeningitis virus in nasal secretions, urine, and feces; transmission to humans probably occurs through aerosolized particles and mucosal exposure, direct contact, or animal bites. The disease in humans is underdiagnosed and occurs most often in autumn. The lymphocytic choriomeningitis virus is typically not spread person to person, although vertical transmission is reported, and it is considered as an underrecognized teratogen. Rare cases related to solid organ transplantation and autopsies of infected individuals are also reported. All reported cases were donor derived. Outbreaks are uncommon, and usually occur in laboratory settings among those workers with significant rodent exposure.

The ubiquitous nature of its reservoir and the wide distribution of the reported cases suggest a widespread geographic risk for lymphocytic choriomeningitis virus infection. Serologic surveys in the southern and eastern United States suggest past infection in approximately 3–5% of those tested, although more recent data from upstate New York showed less than 1% seroprevalence. The risk of infection can be reduced by limiting contact with pet rodents and rodent trappings.

▶ Clinical Findings

A. Symptoms and Signs

The incubation period is 8–13 days to the appearance of systemic manifestations and 15–21 days to the appearance of meningeal symptoms. Symptoms are biphasic, with a prodromal illness characterized by fever, chills, headache, myalgia, cough, and vomiting, occasionally with lymphadenopathy and maculopapular rash. After 3–5 days the fever subsides only to return after 2–4 days alongside the meningeal phase, characterized by headache, nausea and vomiting, lethargy, and variably present meningeal signs. Arthralgias can develop late in the course. Transverse myelitis, deafness, Guillain-Barré syndrome, and transient and permanent hydrocephalus are reported. Lymphocytic choriomeningitis virus is a well-known, albeit underrecognized, cause of congenital infection frequently complicated with obstructive hydrocephalus and chorioretinitis. In fetuses and newborns with ventriculomegaly or other abnormal neuroimaging findings, screening for congenital lymphocytic choriomeningitis may be considered; mothers are asymptomatic half the time. In over one-third of cases, rodent exposure is reported retrospectively. Occasionally, a syndrome resembling the viral hemorrhagic fevers is described in transplant recipients of infected organs and in patients with lymphoma.

B. Laboratory Findings

Leukocytosis or leukopenia and thrombocytopenia may be initially present. During the meningeal phase, cerebrospinal fluid analysis frequently shows lymphocytic pleocytosis (total count is often 500–3000/mcL) alongside a slight increase in protein, while a low to normal glucose is seen in at least 25%. The virus may be recovered from the blood and cerebrospinal fluid by mouse inoculation. Complement-fixing antibodies appear during or after the second week. Detection of specific IgM by ELISA is widely used. Detection of lymphocytic choriomeningitis virus by PCR is available in research settings.

▶ Differential Diagnosis

The influenza-like prodrome and latent period may distinguish this from other aseptic meningitides, and bacterial and granulomatous meningitis. A history of exposure to mice or other potential vectors is an important diagnostic clue.

▶ Treatment

Treatment is supportive. In the survivor of a transplant-associated outbreak, ribavirin (which is effective against other arenaviruses) was used successfully along with decreasing immunosuppression.

▶ Prognosis

Complications and fatalities are rare in the general population. The illness usually lasts 1–2 weeks, though convalescence may be prolonged. Congenital infection is more severe with about 30% mortality rate among infected infants, and more than 90% of survivors suffering long-term neurologic abnormalities. Lymphocytic choriomeningitis in solid organ transplant recipients is associated with a poor prognosis; of reported cases, the mortality rate is more than 80%.

▶ Prevention

Pregnant women should be advised of the dangers to their unborn children inherent in exposure to rodents.

Anderson JL et al. Congenital lymphocytic choriomeningitis virus: when to consider the diagnosis. J Child Neurol. 2013 May 10;29(6):837–42. [PMID: 23666045]

Lapošová K et al. Lymphocytic choriomeningitis virus: invisible but not innocent. Acta Virol. 2013;57(2):160–70. [PMID: 23600874]

6. Prion Diseases

ESSENTIALS OF DIAGNOSIS

- ▶ Rare in humans.
- ▶ Cognitive decline.
- ▶ Myoclonic fasciculations, ataxia, visual disturbances, pyramidal and extrapyramidal symptoms.
- ▶ Variant form presents in younger persons with prominent psychiatric or sensory symptoms.
- ▶ Specific EEG patterns.

▶ General Considerations

The transmissible spongiform encephalopathies are a group of fatal neurodegenerative diseases affecting humans and animals. They are caused by **proteinaceous infectious particles** or **prions.** These agents show slow replicative capacity and long latent intervals in the host. They induce the conformational change of a normal brain protein (prion protein; PrP[C]) into an abnormal isoform (PrP[Sc]) that accumulates and causes neuronal vacuolation (spongiosis), reactive proliferation of astrocytes and microglia and, in some cases, the deposition of beta-amyloid oligomeric plaques.

Prion disease can be hereditary, sporadic, or transmissible in humans. Hereditary disorders are caused by germ line mutations in the PrP[C] gene causing **familial**

Creutzfeldt–Jakob disease (fCJD), Gerstmann-Sträussler-Scheinker syndrome (GSS), and **fatal familial insomnia.** Another uncommon hereditary disorder is PrP systemic amyloidosis.

Sporadic Creutzfeldt-Jakob disease (sCJD) is the most common of the human prion diseases, accounting for approximately 85% of cases; it has no known cause. Transmissible prion disease is only described for kuru and Creutzfeldt-Jakob disease in its **iatrogenic (iCJD)** and **variant (vCJD)** form. Iatrogenic transmission of CJD is associated with prion contaminated human corneas, dura mater grafts, growth hormone, gonadotropins, stereotactic electroencephalography, electrodes, and neurosurgical instruments.

Kuru, once prevalent in central New Guinea, is now rare, a decline in prevalence that started after the abandonment of cannibalism in the late 1950s (a protective allele of the PrP gene is now identified at codon 127).

More than 200 cases of vCJD (**bovine spongiform encephalopathy [BSE]** or **"mad cow disease"**) were reported in the United Kingdom since the first documented cases there in the mid-1990s. It is far less common in North America, with only four cases reported in the United States (the last one in 2014) and two deaths in Canada from definite or probably vCJD. Of the US-reported cases, none are confirmed to have acquired the disease locally (two of them acquired the infection in the United Kingdom, one in Saudi Arabia, one possibly in a Middle Eastern or Eastern European country). This disease is characterized by its bovine-to-human transmission through ingestion of meat from cattle infected with BSE. There is no animal-to-animal spread of BSE, and milk and its derived products are not considered infectious. Reports of secondary transmission of vCJD due to blood transfusions from asymptomatic donors are reported in the United Kingdom. Although iCJD and vCJD are not associated with a known PrP gene mutation, a polymorphism in codon 129 is prevalent and seems to determine susceptibility and expression of clinical disease.

The overall annual incidence of prion disease worldwide is approximately 1–2 in 1 million persons per year. In the United States, among the 3285 cases reported through August 25, 2015 to the US National Prion Disease Pathology Surveillance Center, 2929 (89.2%) were sporadic, 333 (10.1%) familial, 7 (0.2%) iatrogenic, and 4 (0.1%) vCJD.

▶ Clinical Findings

A. Symptoms and Signs

Both sCJD and fCJD usually present in the sixth or seventh decade of life, whereas the iCJD form tends to occur in a much younger population. Clinical features of these three forms of disease usually involve mental deterioration (dementia, behavioral changes, loss of cortical function) progressive over several months, as well as myoclonus, extrapyramidal (hypokinesia) and cerebellar manifestations (ataxia, dysarthria). Finally, coma ensues, usually associated with an akinetic state and less commonly decerebrate/decorticate posturing. Like iCJD, vCJD usually affects younger patients (averaging ~28 years), but the

duration of disease is longer (about 1 year). The degree of organ involvement is often extensive, and the clinical symptoms are unique, mainly characterized by prominent psychiatric and sensory symptoms.

B. Laboratory Findings

CJD should be considered as a diagnosis in the proper clinical scenario, in the absence of alternative diagnoses after routine investigations. Abnormalities in cerebrospinal fluid are subtle and rarely helpful. The detection of 14-3-3 protein in the cerebrospinal fluid is helpful for the diagnosis of sCJD but not in vCJD and fCJD. Its sensitivity and specificity are widely variable among different studies. Cerebrospinal fluid detection of total PrP can differentiate CJD from atypical Alzheimer disease with 82.1% sensitivity and 91.3% specificity.

A blood-based assay and PCR in cerebrospinal fluid show promising results in the diagnosis of vCJD with high specificity but 71% sensitivity. The assay is available through academic specialty prion clinics in the United Kingdom. It is also recognized that a variant with low titers ("very low peripheral prion colonization") in peripheral tissue, including frequently biopsied tonsillar tissue, may lead to underrecognition of vCJD.

In sCJD, EEG typically shows a pattern of paroxysms with high voltages and slow waves, while MRI is characteristic for bilateral areas of increased signal intensity, predominantly in the caudate and putamen. MRI has great potential for improving early diagnosis of sCJD because clinical findings are often missed. When an experienced neuroradiologist or a prion disease expert reviews the MRI, diagnostic sensitivity of MRI for sCJD increases to 91%. Cortical findings associated with sCJD often are not documented by referring centers. In contrast, vCJD shows a diffusely abnormal but nondiagnostic EEG. MRI characteristically reveals hyperintensity of the posterior thalamus ("pulvinar sign"). Positron emission tomography can help distinguish GSS disease. The differentiation and definitive diagnosis of these neurodegenerative diseases are established by neuropathologic confirmation.

▶ Differential Diagnosis

Autoimmune encephalitis can have a similar clinical picture. The presence of high titer autoantibodies (eg, to the NMDA receptor) in the cerebrospinal fluid is consistent with autoimmune encephalitis.

▶ Treatment & Prevention

There is no specific treatment for CJD. Once symptoms appear, the infection invariably leads to death. Flupirtine (an analgesic drug) is sometimes useful in slowing the associated cognitive decline but does not affect survival. Studies are in progress to identify vaccines, but no promising candidates exist to date.

Iatrogenic CJD can be prevented by limiting patient exposure to potentially infectious sources as mentioned above. Prevention of vCJD relies on monitoring livestock for possible infection. The American Red Cross does not accept blood donations from persons with a family history of CJD or with a history of dural grafts or pituitary-derived growth hormone injections.

An international referral and database for CJD is available at: http://www.cjdsurveillance.com.

Reference centers are available at Case Western Reserve University in the United States and the University College London Hospitals in the United Kingdom.

Dorey A et al. Association of cerebrospinal fluid prion protein levels and the distinction between Alzheimer disease and Creutzfeldt-Jacob disease. JAMA Neurol. 2015 Mar;72(3):267–75. [PMID: 25559883]

Mead S et al. A new prion disease: relationship with central and peripheral amyloidoses. Nat Rev Neurol. 2015 Feb;11(2):90–7. [PMID: 25623792]

Mead S et al. Variant Creutzfeldt-Jakob disease with extremely low lymphoreticular deposition of prion protein. JAMA Neurol. 2014 Mar;71(3):340–3. [PMID: 24445428]

Rossi M et al. Neuronal antibodies in patients with suspected or confirmed sporadic Creutzfeldt-Jakob disease. J Neurol Neurosurg Psychiatry. 2015 Jun;86(6):692–4. [PMID: 25246643]

7. Progressive Multifocal Leukoencephalopathy (PML)

PML is a rare demyelinating CNS disorder caused by the reactivation of the JC virus (John Cunningham virus or JCV). This polyomavirus usually causes its primary infection during childhood with about 80% of adults typically being seropositive. The virus remains latent in the kidneys, lymphoid tissues, epithelial cells, peripheral blood leukocytes, bone marrow, and possibly brain until reactivation occurs and symptoms become evident. This reactivation is usually seen in adults with impaired cell-mediated immunity, especially AIDS patients (5–10% of whom develop PML), as well as those with idiopathic CD4 lymphopenia syndrome. It is also reported among those with lymphoproliferative and myeloproliferative disorders; granulomatous, inflammatory, and rheumatic diseases (systemic lupus erythematosus and rheumatoid arthritis in particular); as well as in those who have undergone solid and hematopoietic cell transplantation; and occasionally in those who have other medical states, including cirrhosis and kidney disease.

Diagnostic criteria that use clinical, imaging, pathologic, and virologic manifestations of JCV are available from the American Academy of Neurology.

Medication-associated PML is described with the use of natalizumab, rituximab, infliximab (one case), azathioprine with corticosteroids (one case), and mycophenolate mofetil. Natalizumab, a monoclonal antibody used in the treatment of multiple sclerosis, is associated with the risk of PML developing in 1.35 cases per 1000 patients treated for more than a year and 1.78 per 1000 for patients treated for longer than 2 years. The risk of clinical PML appears to increase up to 36 months of therapy and levels off thereafter. The virus is detected in the cerebrospinal fluid of up to one-half all patients treated with natalizumab although the exact relationship between latent JCV and frank PML remains unclear, with higher JC viral loads detected among patients who are immunosuppressed and among those who have HIV with lower CD4 counts.

Although an immune reconstitution inflammatory state may follow cessation of monoclonal antibody therapy, the JCV presence and the residual neurologic deficits may not clear for years after therapy is stopped. The risk of developing PML associated with rituximab is at least 1 in 25,000 exposed patients with cases reported in various autoimmune conditions (systemic lupus erythematosus, rheumatoid arthritis, multiple sclerosis). The mean interval between use of the drug to the diagnosis of PML is 5.5 months. Smoking is reportedly associated with an increased risk of PML.

▶ Clinical Findings

A. Symptoms and Signs

JCV causes lytic infection of oligodendrocytes in the white matter and symptoms presenting subacutely reflect the diverse areas of CNS involvement. Symptoms include altered mental status, aphasia, ataxia, hemiparesis or hemiplegia and visual field disturbances. Seizures occur in about 18%. Involvement of cranial nerves and the cervical spine is rare.

B. Laboratory Findings

PCR for JCV in cerebrospinal fluid is used for diagnosis in patients with compatible clinical and radiologic findings. A quantitative PCR is more sensitive. Persistent JC viremia and increasing urinary JCV DNA may be predictive of PML. An anti-JCV immunoglobuin G (IgG) was higher 6 months before diagnosis but was not predictive of PML in a cohort of HIV-infected persons.

MRI of the brain shows multifocal areas of white matter demyelination without mass effect or, usually, contrast enhancement. These findings may not be distinguishable from immune reconstitution inflammatory syndrome. Increased uptake of methionine with concomitant decreased uptake of fluorodeoxyglucose in positron emission tomography may be helpful for diagnosis. In HIV-infected patients, a syndrome of cerebellar degeneration is described.

▶ Treatment & Prevention

Limiting the immunosuppressed state represents the mainstay of therapy for PML. Treatment of HIV with ART reduces the incidence of PML, improves the clinical symptoms, reverses some of the radiographic abnormalities, and improves the 1-year mortality rate, regardless of baseline CD4 count. Immune restoration can induce worsening of the clinical picture in a small number of cases. Immune reconstitution syndromes do not alter mortality but are associated with a form of PML called non-determined leukoencephalopathy associated with a distinct chemokine polymorphism. Significant neurologic sequelae to PML infections are the rule. Deficits associated with PML, including monoclonal associated forms, may persist for years.

Decreasing immunosuppression in non-AIDS patients with PML (eg, transplant patients) is also typically beneficial. Cidofovir may be beneficial in non-AIDS related cases while corticosteroids may be useful with immune reconstitution. Because the JCV infects cells through serotonin receptors, some clinicians recommend the use of risperidone and mirtazapine. Plasma exchange, which theoretically reduces the plasma level of agents associated with PML, may be useful in natalizumab-associated PML.

Berger JR et al. PML diagnostic criteria: consensus statement from the AAN Neuroinfectious Disease Section. Neurology. 2013 Apr 9;80(15):1430–8. [PMID: 23568998]

Major EO et al. JC viremia in natalizumab-treated patients with multiple sclerosis. N Engl J Med. 2013 Jun 6;368(23):2240–1. [PMID: 23738566]

Shirai S et al. Usefulness of 11C-methionine-positron emission tomography for the diagnosis of progressive multifocal leuko-encephalopathy. J Neurol. 2014 Dec;261(12):2314–8. [PMID: 25223960]

8. Human T Cell Lymphotropic Virus (HTLV)

HTLV-1 and -2 are retroviruses that infect CD4 and CD8 T cells respectively, where they persist as a lifelong latent infection. HTLV-1 currently infects approximately 20 million individuals worldwide. It is endemic to many regions in the world including southern Japan, the Caribbean, much of sub-Saharan Africa, South America, Eastern Europe, and Oceania. The Caribbean basin and southwestern Japan show the highest prevalence of infection (4–37%). Conversely, HTLV-2 is mainly found in native populations of South (1–58%), Central (8–10%), and North America (2–13%) as well as African pygmy tribes.

In the United States, studies done in blood donors show a seroprevalence of HTLV-1 of 0.005% and HTLV-2 of 0.014%, a decline since the early 1990s. Over 85% of cases found in the United States are located in the West or Southwest. The virus is transmitted horizontally (sex), vertically (intrauterine, peripartum, and breast feeding), and parenterally (injection drug use and blood transfusion). Hence, a higher prevalence is seen among injection drug users. Coinfection with HIV-1 occurs but is often underrecognized. Transmission via organ transplant has been reported.

▶ Clinical Findings

A. Symptoms and Signs

HTLV-1 infection is associated with **HTLV-1 adult T cell lymphoma/leukemia (ATL)** and **HTLV-1 associated myelopathy/tropical spastic paraparesis (HAM/TSP)**. In contrast, HTLV-2 is significantly less pathogenic, with few reported cases of HAM/TSP as well as other neurologic manifestations. The causative association of HTLV-1 with ATL, attributed to the virally encoded oncoprotein *tax*, is well established. The lifetime risk of developing ATL among seropositive persons is estimated to be 3% in women and 7% in men, with an incubation period of at least 15 years. The mean age of diagnosis of ATL is 40–50 years in Central and South America and 60 years in Japan.

ATL clinical syndromes may be classified as chronic, acute (leukemic), smoldering, or lymphomatous. A primary cutaneous tumor is also described and shows a worse prognosis compared with the smoldering type. Clinical features of ATL include diffuse lymphadenopathy, maculo-papular skin lesions that may evolve into erythroderma,

organomegaly, lytic bone lesions, and hypercalcemia. Opportunistic infections, such as *Pneumocystis jirovecii* pneumonia and cryptococcal meningitis, are common.

HAM/TSP, associated with both HTLV-1 and HTLV-2, develops in 0.3–4% of seropositive individuals and is more common in women. A chronic inflammation of the spinal cord leads to progressive motor weakness and symmetric spastic paraparesis, nociceptive low back pain, and paraplegia with hyperreflexia. Bladder and sexual disorders (eg, dyspareunia, erectile dysfunction), sensory disturbances, and constipation are also common. A progressive cognitive impairment is seen with HAM/TSP in children. Both viruses can also induce motor abnormalities, such as leg weakness, impaired tandem walk, and vibration sense, without overt HTLV-associated myelopathy.

An HTLV-1 provirus load in peripheral blood mononuclear cells and cerebrospinal fluid cells, and an HTLV-1 mRNA load are proposed as markers of HAM risk and progression. HTLV positivity is associated with erythrocytosis, lymphocytosis (HTLV-2) and with thrombocytosis (HTLV-1).

HTLV-1 seropositivity is associated with an increased risk of tuberculosis, *Strongyloides stercoralis* hyperinfection, crusted scabies, and infective dermatitis. Inflammatory states associated with HTLV-1 infection include arthropathy, polymyositis, uveitis, Sjögren syndrome, vasculitis, cryoglobulinemia, infiltrative pneumonitis, and ichthyosis. Bronchioloalveolar carcinoma is increased in frequency in the presence of HTLV-1.

HTLV-2 appears to cause a myelopathy that is milder and slower to progress than HAM. All-cause and cancer mortality is higher among HTLV-2 seropositive patients.

HTLV-1/HIV coinfection is associated both with higher CD4 counts and a higher risk of HAM.

B. Laboratory Findings

The peripheral smear can show atypical lymphoid cells with basophilic cytoplasm and convoluted nuclei (flower cells) but the diagnostic standard is evidence of clonal integration of the proviral DNA genome into tumor cell. The identification of HTLV-1 antibodies supports the diagnosis.

▶ Treatment, Prevention, & Prognosis

Management of ATL consists mainly of chemotherapy, with allogeneic stem cell transplantation and the use of monoclonal antibodies (anti-CCR4 and anti-CD25). A chemotherapy regimen in Japan using eight different agents shows a higher response rate than traditional biweekly CHOP (40% vs 25%). Combination therapy with interferon-alpha has been used with success. A therapeutic vaccine is in early clinical trials. Prophylaxis against infections is needed in ATL because patients show a profound immunodeficiency.

HAM is treated with a variety of immune-modulating agents (including corticosteroids) without consistent results. Combination therapy with antiretrovirals does not show benefit. Interferon-alpha may be of some efficacy. Small, uncontrolled studies suggest plasmapheresis results in improvement in gait and sensory disturbance among some patients. Screening of the blood supply for HTLV-1 is required in the United States. There is significant cross-reactivity between HTLV-1 and HTLV-2 by serologic studies, but PCR can distinguish the two. Improved assays to screen organ donors for HTLV-1 and -2 infections are needed although such screening is not currently required.

Patients who are coinfected with HIV-1 and HTLV require underlying management of each individually because HTLV does not respond to ART.

Nagamine Y et al. Human T lymphotropic virus type-1-associated myelopathy manifesting shortly after living-donor renal transplantation. Intern Med. 2015;54(1):75–8. [PMID: 25742898]

Okajima R et al. High prevalence of skin disorders among HTLV-1 infected individuals independent of clinical status. PLoS Negl Trop Dis. 2013 Nov 7;7(11):e2546. [PMID: 24244779]

Suehiro Y et al. Clinical outcomes of a novel therapeutic vaccine with Tax peptide-pulsed dendritic cells for adult T cell leukaemia/lymphoma in a pilot study. Br J Haematol. 2015 May; 169(3):356–67. [PMID: 25612920]

VIRAL HEMORRHAGIC FEVERS

1. Ebola Viral Disease (EVD)

ESSENTIALS OF DIAGNOSIS

▶ Early stage EVD presents as a nonspecific febrile illness.

▶ Later stage EVD typically includes severe gastrointestinal symptoms, followed by neurologic symptoms and hypovolemic shock.

▶ Hemorrhagic manifestations are rare.

▶ Travel and contact history from an Ebola-affected country raise suspicion.

▶ Diagnosis is confirmed by detection of virus with a real-time RT-PCR.

▶ General Considerations

Genus *Ebolavirus* is a single-stranded RNA virus in the Filoviridae family. Five species of *Ebolavirus* have been identified, and each species has an associated virus:

1. Species, *Tai Forest ebolavirus;* virus, Tai Forest (TAFV).
2. Species, *Reston ebolavirus;* virus, Reston virus (RESTV).
3. Species, *Sudan ebolavirus;* virus, Sudan virus (SUDV).
4. Species, *Zaire ebolavirus;* virus, Ebola virus (EBOV or ZEBOV).
5. Species, *Bundibugyo ebolavirus;* virus, Bundibugyo virus (BDBV).

Only three viruses are clinically relevant in humans (EBOV, SUDV, and TAFV). "Ebola" as discussed in this section refers to the clinically relevant viruses.

While the zoonotic reservoir is unknown, evidence from Marbug suggests fruit bats as a possible vector. After

a zoonotic transmission to a human occurs, Ebola can continue to be transmitted among humans who directly contact infected body fluids (droplet and contact precautions advised). There is no evidence supporting airborne transmission; however, the virus aerosolizes, meaning that certain settings such as health care facilities carry additional risk.

To acquire EVD, the virus must enter the body via mucous membranes, nonintact skin, sexual intercourse, breastfeeding, or needlestick. Ebola has a 2–21 day incubation period, and over 95% of cases present with symptoms during the first 14 days. **Prior to manifestation of symptoms, Ebola is not transmissible.** Even at symptom onset, the risk of transmission is extremely low but increases over time. Traditional burial practices (which entail considerable contact with the corpse) and unprotected direct care of persons with EVD are associated with highest transmission risk.

The first Ebola outbreak occurred in 1976 as a simultaneous epidemic in Congo and Sudan. The first cases were identified along the Ebola River, in Congo but near the Sudanese border, resulting in naming of the disease. This was the second largest Ebola outbreak in history. Subsequent outbreaks had been confined to Congo, Uganda, and Sudan until March 2014 when the first Ebola case in West Africa was identified in Gueckedou, Guinea, near the borders of Sierra Leone and Liberia. *Zaire ebolavirus* was the species identified, more specifically referred to as a novel variant of Ebola virus (EBOV) called "Makona." Subsequently, this Ebola outbreak grew to be larger than all prior Ebola outbreaks.

As of October 18, 2015, there were 28,476 reported EVD cases in eight affected countries, with 11,298 reported deaths. The number of EVD cases in the highly affected countries during this outbreak is as follows: 3803 persons in Guinea, 10,666 persons in Liberia, and 14,001 persons in Sierra Leone. There were 881 cases with 531 deaths in these three countries among health care workers. Other EVD cases were reported from Italy, Mali, Nigeria, Senegal, Spain, the United Kingdom, and the United States. Significant underreporting of cases, estimated at 2.5-fold, is noted across the highly affected countries.

Several factors led to the unprecedented magnitude of the 2014–2015 Ebola epidemic. Although Côte d'Ivoire did have one EVD case (TAFV) in 1994, the 2014–2015 epidemic was the first significant outbreak in West Africa. These countries with fragile health systems were recovering from civil wars and a coup d'etat and had no Ebola surveillance systems. Another compounding factor was the size of the epidemic at the time it was uncovered, with the epidemic already having reached Conakry, the capital of Guinea, and having progressed into Sierra Leone and Liberia. Aside from the earlier Kikwik outbreak in Congo, which occurred in an isolated, quarantine city, this epidemic has been recognized as the first truly urbanized outbreak, making traditional public health measure such as contact tracing more difficult. Liberia was declared free of EVD on September 15, 2015. As of October 18, 2015, Sierra Leone reported no new cases for 5 weeks. Cases continue at 1–3 per week in Guinea. Besides Liberia, the following countries as of October 20, 2015, with prior cases are free of EVD (42 days without evidence for an infection): Italy, Mali, Nigeria, Spain, the United Kingdom, and the United States.

► Clinical Findings

A. Symptoms and Signs

At symptom onset, early stage EVD most typically presents as a nonspecific febrile illness. Along with fevers, patients tend to experience malaise, fatigue, myalgia, and arthralgia. After 3–5 days, later stage EVD may develop with nausea, vomiting, abdominal pain, diarrhea, and other gastrointestinal symptoms accompanying the febrile illness. Nausea and vomiting continue to worsen until the patient can no longer tolerate oral intake, and diarrhea becomes large volume (5 or more liters per day). This stage of the illness may continue for a week during which time neurologic symptoms gain prominence. Encephalitis is commonly observed and includes the symptoms of confusion, slowed cognition, agitation, and occasional seizures. Shock develops in most patients, but hemorrhagic manifestations develop in only 1–5% of patients. Respiratory symptoms (ie, cough) are not typical for EVD.

B. Laboratory Findings

Although several novel point-of-care diagnostic technologies are available, EBOV continues to be diagnosed with RT-PCR. Blood samples obtained within the first 3 days of illness should be repeated if the results are negative and clinical symptoms and signs persist. After about 10 days, IgM antibodies begin to develop and, after approximately 2 weeks, an IgG antibody response develops.

Given that filoviruses infect dendritic cells and then hepatocytes and renal cortical cells, laboratory findings typically include a low platelet count, leukopenia, transaminitis (aspartate aminotransferase [AST] greater than alanine aminotransferase [ALT]), and increased serum creatinine level. The nature of this illness and its significant fluid loss tend to cause electrolyte abnormalities and accelerate acute kidney injury. For many patients in highly affected countries, non-Ebola diagnostic testing is inaccessible.

C. Imaging

Radiographic findings can be used to suggest alternative diagnoses.

► Differential Diagnosis

The differential diagnosis varies with the stage of illness. Early stage EVD is commonly mistaken for malaria, typhoid, and other viral illnesses. Myriad illnesses, though, could present as a nonspecific febrile illness. As gastrointestinal symptoms develop, health providers should also consider viral hepatitis, toxins, leptospirosis, and rickettsial diseases. In later stage EVD, health providers need to consider bacterial, viral, and parasitic illnesses, including cholera and, in children, rotavirus infection, which can present with severe gastroenteritis and shock. Encephalitis

must be differentiated from the confusion associated with acute kidney injury and other neurologic manifestations. Hemorrhagic manifestations raise suspicion for EVD but could be due to leukemia, thrombotic thrombocytopenic purpura, hemolytic-uremic syndrome, or disseminated intravascular coagulation. Travel and contact history are crucial when considering the differential diagnosis in areas where Ebola is not endemic. If such histories are present, patients need to be asked if they had unprotected exposures to persons with Ebola.

► Complications

Hypovolemic shock and multiorgan failure are the most common complications of EVD. Coinfections with malaria or bacteria (or both) are important considerations and can occur before presentation and during treatment of EVD.

► Treatment

Treatment is supportive. In the presence of oral rehydration salts, mortality rates are approximately 70%. Several studies have shown that intravenous fluids can reduce the mortality rates to less than 50%. In these studies, the amount of intravenous fluid replacement was relatively less than what would be used in countries with developed health systems. According to the CDC and other agencies, as of October 20, 2015, 10 persons have been treated for Ebola in the United States. Most were healthcare workers who were evacuated to biocontainment units in the United States and received intensive care and experimental therapies. All but two patients survived.

In addition to supportive care, two particular antivirals used in the EVD outbreak are the monoclonal antibody combination referred to as **ZMapp** (the supply of which is easily exhausted) and an RNA inference agent referred to as **TKM-Ebola**, which appears ineffective in phase II trials. Other antiviral agents under study include brincidofovir (whose trial was discontinued because of low caseload in Liberia) and favipiravir, an RNA-dependent RNA polymerase inhibitor, which showed preliminary encouraging antiviral activity among patients with low viremia in Guinea; it cannot be given during pregnancy.

Aside from Ebola treatment and experimental therapies, patients typically receive empiric antimalarial agents and broad-spectrum antibiotics. Empiric therapies are important at presentation because the risk associated with non-Ebola diagnostics prevents studies from being conducted until results are obtained.

► Prognosis

The prognosis depends greatly on patient, exposure, and clinical characteristics. Children under the age of 5 and adults older than 40 years have a high risk of death from EVD. In prior Ebola outbreaks, pregnant women all died. In the 2014–2015 epidemic, a small but significant percentage of pregnant women survived. Immunosuppressed patients show a poor prognosis. All persons who had a needlestick of a confirmed Ebola case died. Clinical characteristics indicating a poor prognosis include a short incubation time, rapid progression of symptoms, hepatic dysfunction, and hemorrhagic manifestations. In general, poor overall medical care confers a poor prognosis.

▶ Prevention

Disinfection, hygiene, and sanitation are the cornerstones to infection prevention and control measures.

At least nine vaccines are under clinical development. A summary of these vaccines is available at http://www.who.int/medicines/emp_ebola_q_as/en/.

▶ When to Admit

- Persons living in or returning from a country with high rates of Ebola transmission should be monitored for 21 days and admitted to a healthcare facility when symptoms meeting the WHO case definition of a suspected EVD case develop, in accordance with the screening protocol designated by the respective country's governmental health decision-making body. For example, the screening procotol from the Ministry of Health and Sanitation in Sierra Leone includes:

  - Any person suffering from a fever (or history of fever) and having had contact with suspected, probable, or confirmed Ebola case; **or**

  - Any person with a fever (or history of fever) and at least three of the following symptoms: headaches, vomiting, anorexia/loss of appetite, diarrhea, lethargy, stomach pain, aching muscles or joints, difficulty swallowing, breathing difficulties, or hiccups; **or**

  - Any person with inexplicable bleeding.

Bai EI et al. Clinical presentation of patients with Ebola viral disease in Conakry, Guinea. N Engl J Med. 2015 Jan 1; 372(1):40–7. [PMID: 25372658]

Bishop BM. Potential and emerging treatment options for Ebola virus disease. Ann Pharmacother. 2015 Feb;49(2):196–206. [PMID: 25414384]

Centers for Disease Control and Prevention (CDC). MMWR Ebola Reports. http://www.cdc.gov/mmwr/ebola_reports.html

Henao-Restrepo AM et al. Efficacy and effectiveness of an rVSV-vectored vaccine expressing Ebola surface glycoprotein: interim results from the Guinea ring vaccination cluster-randomised trial. Lancet. 2015 Aug 29;386(9996):857–66. [PMID: 26248676]

Kuhn JH et al. Nomenclature- and database-compatible names for the two Ebola virus variants that emerged in Guinea and the Democratic Republic of the Congo in 2014. Viruses. 2014 Nov 24;6(11):4760–99. [PMID: 25421896]

Schibler M et al. Clinical features and viral kinetics in a rapidly cured patient with Ebola virus disease: a case report. Lancet Infect Dis. 2015 Sep;15(9):1034–40. [PMID: 26201298]

Schieffelin JS et al; KGH Lassa Fever Program; Viral Hemorrhagic Fever Consortium; WHO Clinical Response Team. Clinical illness and outcomes in patients with Ebola in Sierra Leone. N Engl J Med. 2014 Nov 27;371(22):2092–100. [PMID: 25353969]

Van Herp M et al. Favipiravir—a prophylactic treatment for Ebola contacts? Lancet. 2015 Jun 13;385(9985):2350. [PMID: 26088635]

World Health Organization. Ebola situation report. Weekly reports available at: http://who.int/csr/disease/ebola/en/

2. Other Hemorrhagic Fevers

This diverse group of illnesses results from infection with one of several single-stranded RNA viruses (members of the families Arenaviridae, Bunyaviridae, Filoviridae, and Flaviviridae). Flaviviruses, such as the pathogens causing dengue and yellow fever (both with occasional hemorrhagic complications), and Filoviridae, causing Ebola and Marburg, are discussed in separate sections.

Lassa fever (an Old World arenavirus) is rodent associated and transmission usually occurs through aerosolized particles (from rodents or infected individuals). Transmission through direct contact with infected biologic fluids or tissues is also documented and food-borne transmission, while considered, is not definitively proven. Similar modes of transmission are assumed for **Junin virus** and other members of the New World Arenaviridae (Machupo virus, Sabia virus, Guanarito virus, Whitewater Arroyo virus).

The bunyaviruses include the **Crimean-Congo hemorrhagic fever** (transmitted by infected animal exposure or tick bite), the **Rift Valley fever** (transmitted by exposure to infected animal products or bite of an infected mosquito or flea), and the **hantaviruses** (associated with rodent exposure and discussed separately below). The geographic distribution of Crimean-Congo hemorrhagic fever, like that of its tick vector, is widespread with cases reported in Asia, the Middle East, and Eastern Europe. In 2002, Turkey experienced the largest reported outbreak with over 2500 cases. An outbreak occurred with 22 cases in the country of Georgia. Rift Valley fever causes outbreaks in sub-Saharan and Northern Africa. The last reported outbreak was in 2010 in Sudan. Rift Valley cases have also been confirmed outside the African continent, in Saudi Arabia and Yemen.

A new bunyavirus, a phlebovirus, associated with fever and thrombocytopenia, was identified in 2010 in Central and Northeastern China and is named for its symptoms: the **severe fever with thrombocytopenia syndrome (SFTS)** virus. Its differential diagnosis includes anaplasmosis, hemorrhagic fever with renal syndrome, or leptospirosis. The current candidate vector is a tick of the Ixodidae family. A mortality of 12% was noted among the first 171 patients. A new pathogenic virus **(Heartland virus)** similar to the SFTS virus was isolated in Missouri in 2009 from two farmers who had fever, diarrhea, and fatigue. The virus appears to be amplified in deer and raccoons. Transmission occurs via the Lone Star tick (*Amblyomma americanum*). There is no evidence for the transmission of viral hemorrhagic fever through air travel.

▶ Clinical Findings

A. Symptoms and Signs

The incubation period can be as short as 2 days for the Rift Valley fever or as long as 21 days for Lassa fever. The clinical symptoms in the early phase of a viral hemorrhagic fever are very similar, irrespective of the causative virus, and resemble a flu-like illness or gastroenteritis. Hepatitis is common.

The late phase is more specific and is characterized by organ failure, persistent leukopenia, altered mental status, and hemorrhage. Exanthemas and mucosal lesions can occur. The range of pathology described with Crimean-Congo hemorrhagic fever continues to grow and includes cardiac failure, bilateral alveolar hemorrhages, and retinal hemorrhages. Rift Valley fever is reportedly associated with encephalitis and also retinitis. Adrenal dysfunction is a common sequela of this class of infections and a cause for the development of the late-stage shock associated with these infections. The case-fatality rate ranges from 5% to 30%. The convalescence period can be long and complicated. There is no evidence of chronic infection among survivors. Risk factors for complications in patients with Crimean-Congo hemorrhagic fever include advanced age, thrombocytopenia, prolonged clotting factor parameters, and hepatitis while risk factors for mortality include altered sensorium and prolonged international normalized ratio. Risk factors for acquiring Rift Valley fever include male sex; working with abortive animal tissue; slaughtering, skinning, or sheltering animals; and drinking raw milk; complications of Rift Valley fever are more common among older men and among persons with a history of herding or slaughtering livestock and having poor visual acuity.

B. Laboratory Findings

Laboratory features usually include thrombocytopenia, leukopenia, (although with Lassa fever leukocytosis is noted), anemia, increased hematocrit, elevated liver function tests, and findings consistent with disseminated intravascular coagulation (although less prominently in Lassa fever). Urinalysis can reveal proteinuria and hematuria.

Special care should be taken for handling clinical specimens of suspected cases. Laboratory personnel should be warned about the diagnostic suspicion and the CDC must be contacted for guidance (Special Pathogens Branch, 404-639-1115). Diagnosis may be made by antigen detection (by ELISA), nucleic acid amplification (PCR techniques), or by demonstration of a significant specific fourfold or greater rise in antibody titer. Crimean-Congo hemorrhagic fever is best diagnosed with an IgM serology, although IgG ELISA or immunofluorescence and quantitative reverse transcription PCR are nearly as effective. These viruses can be isolated in culture, but this testing should be done at a biosafety level 4 laboratory facility.

Differential Diagnosis

The differential diagnosis for hemorrhagic fever includes meningococcemia or other septicemias, Rocky Mountain spotted fever, dengue, typhoid fever, and malaria. The likelihood of acquiring hemorrhagic fevers among travelers is low.

Treatment

Patients should be placed in private rooms with standard contact and droplet precautions. Barrier precautions to prevent contamination of skin or mucous membranes should also be adopted by the caring personnel. Airborne precautions should be considered in patients with significant pulmonary involvement or undergoing procedures that stimulate cough.

Certain arenaviruses (the Lassa pathogen, Junin virus in its viscerotropic phase, Machupo virus) and bunyaviruses (the Congo-Crimean hemorrhagic fever and Rift Valley fever pathogens) respond to oral ribavirin if it is started promptly. Patients rarely survive without ribavirin therapy. The efficacy for postexposure ribavirin in the management of Lassa fever, other arenaviruses, or hospital-associated Crimean-Congo hemorrhagic fever remains anecdotal; its successful use in a German hospital on a soldier infected in Afghanistan is encouraging. If ribavirin is used, expert experience suggests a high loading dose (35 mg/kg orally followed by 15 mg/kg three times daily for 10 days) and only for high-risk settings (eg, needlestick injury, mucous membrane contamination, emergency resuscitative contact, or prolonged intimate exposure during transport). The anti-trypanosomal agent suramin may be effective against the Rift Valley fever virus.

The flaviviruses do not respond to ribavirin. Live attenuated vaccines are available for Junin hemorrhagic fever and the Rift Valley fever, and they are under study for Crimean-Congo hemorrhagic fever. In addition, recombinant and virus-like particle vaccines are under development for most of these pathogens (including the Lassa fever virus but not the Junin hemorrhagic fever virus). Therapeutic interventions that target the hematologic system are at most only marginally effective.

When to Admit

- Persons with symptoms compatible with those of any hemorrhagic fever and who have travelled from a possible endemic area should be isolated for diagnosis and symptomatic treatment.
- Isolation is particularly important because diseases due to some of these agents, such as Lassa virus, are highly transmissible to healthcare workers.

Ajayi NA et al. Lassa fever—full recovery without ribavarin treatment: a case report. Afr Health Sci. 2014 Dec;14(4):1074–7. [PMID: 25834520]

Aradaib IE et al. Rift Valley fever, Sudan, 2007 and 2010. Emerg Infect Dis. 2013 Feb;19(2):246–53. [PMID: 23347790]

LaBeaud AD et al. Factors associated with severe human Rift Valley fever in Sangailu, Garissa County, Kenya. PLoS Negl Trop Dis. 2015 Mar 12;9(3):e0003548. [PMID: 25764399]

Mamuchishvili N et al; Centers for Disease Control and Prevention (CDC). Notes from the field: increase in reported Crimean-Congo hemorrhagic fever cases—country of Georgia, 2014. MMWR Morb Mortal Wkly Rep. 2015 Mar 6; 64(8):228–9. [PMID: 25742385]

Mertens M et al. The impact of Crimean-Congo hemorrhagic fever virus on public health. Antiviral Res. 2013 May; 98(2):248–60. [PMID: 23458713]

Nicholas DE et al. Risk factors associated with human Rift Valley fever infection: systematic review and meta-analysis. Trop Med Int Health. 2014 Dec;19(12):1420–9. [PMID: 25252137]

Russier M et al. Immune responses and Lassa virus infection. Viruses. 2012 Nov 5;4(11):2766–85. [PMID: 23202504]

3. Dengue

▶ General Considerations

Dengue is due to a flavivirus transmitted by the bite of the *Aedes* mosquito. It may be caused by one of four, possibly five, distinct serotypes widely distributed globally between the tropics of Capricorn and Cancer. An estimated 70–500 million cases of dengue fever and several hundred thousand cases of dengue hemorrhagic fever occur each year with numbers growing in both dengue fever and dengue hemorrhagic fever as a consequence of climatic factors, travel, and urbanization. **It is thus along with malaria one of the two most common and important vector-borne diseases of humans**, with 2.5 billion persons living in dengue-infected regions and regions of major intermittent outbreaks. In the Philippines, for example, there are over 117,000 cases annually. The incubation period is 3–15 days (usually 7–10 days). When the virus is introduced into susceptible populations, usually by viremic travelers, epidemic attack rates range from 50% to 70%.

Dengue is endemic in the lower Rio Grande Valley and adjacent border towns, with 40% of Brownsville, Texas residents showing serologic evidence of past infection and the virus being detected in mosquito larvae among 30% of households. In other areas of the world, the seroprevalence of southern Indians is 21%, of Haitians by age 3 is over 53%, and of residents of the French West Indies islands of Guadeloupe and Martinique, 93.5%. In some areas of endemicity there is cyclicity (in China, cases surge every 4–7 years). Surveillance systems for dengue are relatively undeveloped in much of sub-Saharan Africa.

Severe epidemics of dengue hemorrhagic fever (serotype 3) occurred over the past 20 years in East Africa, Sri Lanka, and Latin America. In 2014, an unexpected large outbreak of more than 40,000 dengue virus serotype 2 infections occurred in Guangdong province, China. Other significant regional outbreaks include the Portuguese archipelago of Madeira (Europe) in 2012 with over 2000 persons infected.

Dengue is the second overall cause of a febrile illness (after malaria) in travelers returning from developing countries. The high transmission rates of malaria compared to dengue and high numbers of travelers with a febrile illness returning from sub-Saharan Africa drive the global statistic. Yet on other continents (and regions), dengue is more common than malaria, except for Central America where slightly more malaria transmission is reported. In one US series based on CDC reports, the highest proportion of laboratory-confirmed and probable cases were among travelers returning from the Dominican Republic (121 cases, 20% of total), Mexico (55 cases, 9% of total) and India (43 cases, 7% of total). Since the 1980s, domestically acquired cases of dengue are reported from Guam, Puerto Rico, Samoa, the US Virgin Islands, and in the continental United States at the Texas-Mexico border, and Key West, Florida. Health care–associated transmission (needlestick, mucocutaneous exposure or transplant related) and vertical transmission occur rarely. Cases among returning missionaries from Jamaica emphasize that even short trips (in this case, 1 week) to endemic areas are sufficient intervals of exposure for acquiring dengue.

▶ Clinical Findings

A. Symptoms and Signs

A history of travel to a dengue-endemic area within 14 days of symptom onset is helpful in establishing a diagnosis of dengue. Dengue infection may range from asymptomatic to severe hemorrhagic fever to fatal shock (**dengue shock syndrome**). Dengue fever is usually a nonspecific, self-limited biphasic febrile illness. More than half of infected children are asymptomatic. The illness is more severe and begins more suddenly in adults. After an incubation period of 4–5 days, there is a sudden onset of high fever, chills, and "break bone" aching of the head, back, and extremities accompanied by sore throat, prostration, and malaise. The fever is usually cleared by day 8. There may be conjunctival redness, particularly with serotype 1. Initially, the skin appears flushed or blotched, but 3–4 days after the lysis of the fever, a maculopapular rash, which spares palms and soles, appears in over 50% of cases. As the rash fades, localized clusters of petechiae on the extensor surface of the limbs become apparent. Up to 25% may manifest signs of cardiac involvement. Arthralgias are commonly seen among serotype 2 cases. Hepatitis frequently complicates dengue fever with acute fulminant hepatitis in up to 5%.

Severe dengue, often with hemorrhage, usually affects children living in endemic areas and is most likely to occur in secondary infections and in infections with serotype 2. A few days into the illness, signs of hemorrhage such as ecchymoses, gastrointestinal bleeding, and epistaxis appear. Symptoms found more often among the dengue hemorrhagic fever subset of patients include restlessness, epistaxis, and abdominal pain. Gastroenterologic complications, including hemorrhage, tenderness, and ascites, are more common with dengue hemorrhagic fever and often require intensive care observation. Severe dengue occurs more commonly among HIV-infected persons, although initial presentations do not differ by HIV status.

A subset of patients (more often girls than boys) often with secondary infection, may progress to severe dengue, which is defined by the presence of serum leakage, hemorrhage, or organ involvement (typically liver, heart, CNS). Acute fever, hemorrhagic manifestations, and marked capillary leak may be prominent, with the latter manifesting as pleural effusions and ascites, and there is a tendency for shock to develop. In infants, even primary infection can lead to dengue shock syndrome. While the infection is difficult to distinguish from malaria, yellow fever, or influenza, the rash makes dengue far more likely. Continuous abdominal pain with vomiting, bleeding, a decrease in the level of consciousness, rash, conjunctival congestion, and hypothermia should raise concern about dengue shock syndrome. Acute kidney injury in dengue largely occurs with dengue shock syndrome and shows a high mortality. While acute severe hepatitis can occur with dengue, concomitant other hepatotropic agents are usually responsible.

B. Laboratory Findings

Leukopenia is characteristic, and elevated transaminases are found frequently in dengue fever. Thrombocytopenia (seen more often with serotype 2 and more severe among diabetic patients in whom dengue develops), increased fibrinolysis, and hemoconcentration occur more often in the hemorrhagic form of the disease. Liver biochemical test abnormalities are nearly universal. Thrombocytopenia, plasma leakage, and acute hepatitis are identified as predictors of severe manifestations of dengue and higher mortality. The nonspecific nature of the illness mandates laboratory verification for diagnosis, usually with IgM and IgG ELISAs after the febrile phase. Virus may be recovered from the blood during the acute phase. PCR or detection of the specific viral protein NS1 by ELISA may be diagnostic during the first few days of infection and may be appropriate for febrile travelers. Immunohistochemistry for antigen detection in tissue samples and dried blood spots can also be used. Because the erythrocyte sedimentation rate is normal in most cases, elevation may suggest an alternative diagnosis. Chest radiographs in dengue hemorrhagic fever show infiltrates and effusions, which follow the course of laboratory abnormalities.

Differential Diagnosis

Distinguishing between dengue and other causes of febrile illness in endemic areas is difficult. Fevers due to dengue are more often associated with neutropenia and thrombocytopenia and with myalgias, arthralgias/arthritis, and lethargy among adults. Chikungunya is more apt to develop a chronic arthritis and the arboviral forms of encephalitis require assistance with epidemiologic information and serologic data. Influenza and malaria are easily confused early in disease although the rhinitis and malaise should help distinguish influenza, and the cyclicity of fevers and presence of splenomegaly should suggest malaria.

Complications

Usual complications include pneumonia, bone marrow failure, hepatitis, iritis, retinal hemorrhages and maculopathy, orchitis, and oophoritis. Depression and chronic fatigue, occurring more often in older women, are also

reported. Neurologic complications (such as encephalitis, Guillain-Barré syndrome, phrenic neuropathy, subdural hematoma, and transverse myelitis) are less common, although encephalitic complications are increasingly recognized. Aplastic anemia and hemophagocytosis syndrome are very rare complications. Dengue is rarely associated with stroke in patients with focal neurologic deficit and encephalopathy. Maternal infection poses a risk for premature birth and hemorrhage in both the mother and the infant if infection occurs near term. While placental transmission is not usually considered detrimental, vertical transmission is documented.

Bacterial superinfection occurs more commonly with advanced age, higher fever, gastrointestinal bleeding, kidney disease, and altered consciousness.

Treatment

Treatment entails the appropriate use of volume support, blood products, and pressor agents, and acetaminophen rather than nonsteroidal anti-inflammatory drugs for analgesia. Activities are gradually restored during prolonged convalescences. Endoscopic therapy is useful in evaluating and managing gastrointestinal hemorrhage, although injection therapy with sclerosing agents is not beneficial in most dengue hemorrhagic states. Platelet counts do not usefully predict clinically significant bleeding. Platelet transfusions, however, should be considered for severe thrombocytopenia (less than 10,000/mcL) or when there is evidence of bleeding. Monitoring vital signs and blood volume may help in anticipating the complications of dengue hemorrhagic fever or shock syndrome.

There are no specific therapeutic options for the clinical management of dengue, besides supportive care. Statins show a strong therapeutic potential because lovastatin has in vitro evidence of antiviral effects in dengue and may provide protective anti-inflammatory benefits in the disease pathophysiology.

Prognosis

Fatalities are rare but do occur (and more often among girls and the very young), especially during epidemic outbreaks, with occasional patients dying of fulminant hepatitis. Acute kidney injury in dengue shock syndrome portends an especially poor prognosis. Convalescence for most patients is slow. Factors associated with development of severe disease in Sri Lanka included elevated AST, lymphopenia, and thrombocytopenia, while factors associated with mortality in Brazil included age 50 years or older, limited education, need for hospitalization, rural residency, male gender, and elevated hematocrit (but not moderate thrombocytopenia). In general, the more advanced forms of disease (hemorrhagic fever and shock) occur less often in the Americas than in Asia.

Prevention

A recombinant, live, attenuated, tetravalent dengue vaccine (CYD-TDV) showed 64.7% efficacy with a reduction in hospitalization in healthy children between the ages of 9 and 16 years which were conducted in five Latin American countries and later in Southeast Asia. A follow-up study showed an anomalous increase in hospitalization among recipients younger than age 9 when they were infected 2–5 years after vaccination. There was no difference in safety profiles of the vaccine and placebo. The dengue vaccine Dengvaxia, made by Sanofi Pasteur, was approved for use in Mexico in December 2015 for persons aged 9–45 years.

Preventive measures should be encouraged such as control of mosquitoes by screening and insect repellents including long-lasting insecticides, particularly during early morning and late afternoon exposures. Screening blood transfusions for dengue is of increasing importance, especially in endemic areas. Stochastic models using rainfall and temperature are useful in predicting geographic areas at increased risk for dengue.

Huang SY et al. Use of simple clinical and laboratory predictors to differentiate influenza from dengue and other febrile illnesses in the emergency room. BMC Infect Dis. 2014 Nov 25;14:623. [PMID: 25421019]

Pang J et al. Differential clinical outcome of dengue infection among patients with and without HIV infection: a matched case-control study. Am J Trop Med Hyg. 2015 Jun;92(6):1156–62. [PMID: 25825389]

Sinhabahu VP et al. Perinatal transmission of dengue: a case report. BMC Res Notes. 2014 Nov 14;7:795. [PMID: 25394748]

Taylor WR et al. Dengue in adults admitted to a referral hospital in Hanoi, Vietnam. Am J Trop Med Hyg. 2015 Jun;92(6):1141–9. [PMID: 25918201]

World Health Organization. Dengue and severe dengue: fact sheet No. 117. February 2014. http://www.who.int/mediacentre/factsheets/fs117/en/

Yung CF et al. Dengue serotype-specific differences in clinical manifestation, laboratory parameters and risk of severe disease in adults, Singapore. Am J Trop Med Hyg. 2015 May;92(5): 999–1005. [PMID: 25825386]

4. Hantaviruses

ESSENTIALS OF DIAGNOSIS

► Transmitted by rodents and cause two clinical syndromes.

► Hantavirus pulmonary syndrome (HPS): 40% mortality rate.

► Hemorrhagic fever with renal syndrome (HFRS): mild to severe illness.

► Ribavirin is used with some success in HFRS.

General Considerations

Hantaviruses are enveloped RNA bunyaviruses naturally hosted in rodents, moles, and shrews. Over 21 hantavirus strains are known to cause human disease. These differ in rodent hosts, geographic distribution, and degree of pathogenicity. Two major clinical syndromes are described: **hemorrhagic fever with renal syndrome (HFRS)** and **hantavirus pulmonary syndrome (HPS)**. Each year, over 150,000 cases of these two syndromes occur globally, with HPS being far less common. While they share many

clinical features, a specific strain is not associated with a specific syndrome and overlap is seen between the syndromes. Usually seen in the southwestern United States, **Sin Nombre virus** (Muerto Canyon, Four Corners) is the most common hantavirus infection in the United States and is the main North American virus responsible for HPS. The presence of antibodies in Mexican rodents suggests HPS is probably unrecognized in Mexico. While retrospective diagnostics show that the disease occurred decades earlier in the United States, it was not until 1993 when the first outbreak was recognized. Through December 31, 2013, 637 cases were reported in 34 states; 95% of the cases were reported from states west of the Mississippi River, including all continental states west of the Mississippi River except Missouri, with over one-half the cases from the Four Corners area and another focus recognized in Yosemite National Park, California. Other strains native to North America known to cause HPS include Bayou, Black Creek Canal, New York, and Monongahela viruses. Outbreaks of HPS associated with other hantavirus types are also reported in Central and South America, and nearly two-thirds of cases from a series in Panama experienced little or no pulmonary disease.

Hantaviruses are ubiquitous, with infections described in North and South America (New World hantaviruses) as well as Europe, Africa, and Asia (Old World hantaviruses). The Hantaan viruses cause severe hemorrhagic fever with renal syndrome and are found primarily in Korea, China, and eastern Russia. The Seoul viruses produce a less severe form of disease and are found primarily in Korea and China. Cases of autochthonous Seoul hantavirus infections are described in the United States. The Puumala and Dobrava-Belgrade viruses are found in Scandinavia and Europe and are associated with a mild form of the syndrome termed "nephropathia epidemica," which presents with fever, headache, gastrointestinal symptoms, and impaired kidney function. Between 16% and 48% of Dobrova-Belgrade virus cases, however, may require dialysis.

Aerosols of virus-contaminated rodent urine and feces are thought to be the main vehicle for transmission to humans. Person-to-person transmission is observed only with the Andes virus. Occupation is the main risk factor for transmission of all hantaviruses: animal trappers, forestry workers, laboratory personnel, farmers, and military personnel are considered to be at highest risk. Climate change appears to be impacting the incidence of hantavirus infection mainly through effects on reservoir ecology.

► Clinical Findings

A. Symptoms and Signs

Vascular leakage is the hallmark of the disease for both syndromes, with lungs being the main target of HPS and the kidneys on HFRS.

HPS is a more severe disease than HFRS, with a mortality rate of about 40%. The clinical course of HPS is divided into a febrile prodrome, a cardiopulmonary stage, oliguric and diuretic phase followed by convalescence. A 14- to 17-day incubation period is followed by a prodromal phase, typically lasting 3–6 days, that is associated with myalgia, malaise, gastrointestinal disturbance, headache, chills, and fever of abrupt onset. An ensuing cardiopulmonary phase is characterized by the acute onset of pulmonary edema. In this stage, cough is generally present, gastrointestinal manifestations may dominate the clinical presentation, and in severe cases, significant myocardial depression occurs. Acute kidney injury and myositis may occur. Sequelae include neuropsychological impairments in some HPS survivors.

HFRS manifests as mild, moderate, or severe illness depending on the causative strain, with a mortality rate of up to 12%. A 2- to 3-week incubation period is followed by a protracted clinical course, typically consisting of five distinct phases: febrile period, hypotension, oliguria, diuresis, and convalescence phase. Various degrees of renal involvement are usually seen, occasionally with frank hemorrhage. Pulmonary edema is not typically seen but when present usually occurs in the final stages of disease (oliguric and diuretic phase). Encephalitis and pituitary involvement are rare findings with hantavirus infection, although a few cases are reported with Puumala virus. Patients may have persistent hematuria, proteinuria, or hypertension up to 35 months after infection.

B. Laboratory Findings

Laboratory features include hemoconcentration and elevation in lactate dehydrogenase, serum lactate, and hepatocellular enzymes. Early thrombocytopenia and leukocytosis (as high as 90,000 cells/mcL in HPS) are seen in both HFRS and HPS. In HPS, immunoblasts (activated lymphocytes with plasmacytoid features) can be seen in blood, lungs, kidneys, bone marrow, liver, and spleen. The severity of "nephropathia epidemica" correlates with plasma interleukin-6 levels.

The viremia of human hantavirus infections is short-term, and therefore, viral RNA cannot be readily detected in the blood or urine of patients. An indirect fluorescent assay and enzyme immunoassay are available for detection of specific IgM or low-avidity IgG virus-specific antibodies. Seroconversion in the absence of pulmonary symptoms probably occurs often and is documented to be common in Panama.

A plaque reduction neutralization test is considered the gold standard serologic assay and distinguishes between the different hantavirus species, although cross reaction between Old and New World viruses exist. This test needs to be performed in a laboratory with appropriate biosafety (level 3).

▶ Differential Diagnosis

The differential diagnosis of the acute febrile syndrome seen with HFRS or early HPS includes scrub typhus, leptospirosis, and dengue. HPS requires differentiation from other respiratory infections caused by such pathogens as *Legionella*, *Chlamydia*, and *Mycoplasma*. Coxsackievirus infections should also be considered in the differential diagnosis.

▶ Treatment

Treatment is mainly supportive. Cardiorespiratory support with vasopressors is frequently needed; extracorporeal membrane oxygenation may be required in severe cases of

HPS. Intravenous ribavirin is used in HFRS (Hantaan virus) with some success in decreasing the severity of the kidney injury. Its effectiveness in HPS, however, is not established. The bradykinin receptor antagonist icatibant was used successfully in two cases of Puumala virus infection in Germany.

▶ Prognosis

The outcome is highly variable depending on severity of disease. In Sin Nombre virus infections, the persistence of elevated IgG titers correlates with a favorable outcome.

▶ Prevention

Because infection is thought to occur by inhalation of rodent waste, prevention is aimed at eradication of rodents in houses and avoidance of exposure to rodent excreta, including forest service facilities. Multiple vaccines, inactivated, virus-like particles, and recombinant remain under development.

Hartline J et al. Hantavirus infection in North America: a clinical review. Am J Emerg Med. 2013 Jun;31(6):978–82. [PMID: 23680331]

Knust B et al. Twenty-year summary of surveillance for human hantavirus infections, United States. Emerg Infect Dis. 2013 Dec;19(12):1934–7. [PMID: 24274585]

Laine O et al. Severe Puumala virus infection in a patient with a lymphoproliferative disease treated with icatibant. Infect Dis (Lond). 2015 Feb;47(2):107–11. [PMID: 25496418]

Latus J et al. Clinical course and long-term outcome of hantavirus-associated nephropathia epidemica, Germany. Emerg Infect Dis. 2015 Jan;21(1):76–83. [PMID: 25533268]

Manigold T et al. Human hantavirus infections: epidemiology, clinical features, pathogenesis and immunology. Swiss Med Wkly. 2014 Mar 20;144:w13937. [PMID: 24652684]

5. Yellow Fever

 ESSENTIALS OF DIAGNOSIS

- ▶ Endemic area exposure (tropical South and Central America, Africa, but not Asia).
- ▶ Sudden onset of severe headache, aching in legs, and tachycardia.
- ▶ Brief (1 day) remission, followed by bradycardia, hypotension, jaundice, hemorrhagic tendency.
- ▶ Proteinuria, leukopenia, bilirubinemia, bilirubinuria.
- ▶ Rare and potentially fatal reactions to vaccination.

▶ General Considerations

Yellow fever is a zoonotic flavivirus infection transmitted by *Aedes* mosquitoes. It occurs in urban, intermediate (involving small outbreaks in villages in humid savannahs), and sylvatic cycles in Africa, while in South America only the urban and sylvatic cycles are recognized. Genetic studies suggest it arose in South America through the slave trade 300–400 years ago. Epidemics have extended into unvaccinated populations. There are only seven countries in Latin America that struggle with endemic disease and a partially unvaccinated population. Yellow fever outbreaks continue to occur in Africa and South America, although the 21 recognized cases in 2014 among 3 outbreaks (Peru (1), the Democratic Republic of Congo [2]) suggest an encouraging decrease in total global caseload.

Infection is transmitted by an infected mosquito bite. The incubation period in humans is 3–6 days. Adults and children are equally susceptible, though attack rates are highest among adult males because of their work habits. Between 5% and 50% of infections are asymptomatic.

Clinical Findings

A. Symptoms and Signs

1. Mild form—Symptoms are malaise, headache, fever, retroorbital pain, nausea, vomiting, and photophobia. Relative bradycardia, conjunctival injection, and facial flushing may be present.

2. Severe form—Severe illness develops in about 15%. Initial symptoms are similar to the mild form, but a brief fever remission lasting hours to a few days is followed by a "period of intoxication" manifested by fever and relative bradycardia (Faget sign), hypotension, jaundice, hemorrhage (gastrointestinal, nasal, oral), and delirium that may progress to coma.

B. Laboratory Findings

Leukopenia occurs, although it may not be present at the onset. Kidney disease with proteinuria is present, sometimes as high as 5–6 g/L, and usually disappears completely with recovery. Levels of liver enzymes and bilirubin can be remarkably abnormal with the levels of AST usually doubling those of ALT. Prothrombin time may be elevated as well. Serologic diagnosis is made by using capture ELISA to measure IgM during the acute and convalescent phases. Viral culture is used in epidemic settings. Rapid test involving PCR and monoclonal antibody assays against circulating viral antigens are available through reference laboratories. The plaque reduction neutralization assay is the most frequently used. IgM antibodies are shown to persist in up to 73% of recipients 3–4 years after vaccination.

Differential Diagnosis

It may be difficult to distinguish yellow fever from hepatitis, malaria, leptospirosis, louse-borne relapsing fever, dengue, and other hemorrhagic fevers on clinical evidence alone. **Albuminuria is a constant feature in yellow fever patients** and its presence helps differentiate yellow fever from other viral hepatitides. Serologic confirmation is often needed.

Treatment

No specific antiviral therapy is available. Treatment is directed toward symptomatic relief and management of complications.

Prognosis

The mortality rate of the severe form is 20–50%, with death occurring most commonly between the sixth and the tenth days. In survivors, the temperature returns to normal by the seventh or eighth day. The prognosis in any individual case is guarded at the onset, since sudden changes for the worse are common. Intractable hiccups, copious black vomitus, melena, anuria, jaundice, and elevated AST are unfavorable signs. Convalescence is prolonged, including 1–2 weeks of asthenia. Infection confers lifelong immunity to those who recover.

Prevention

The yellow fever vaccine, which is derived from the live attenuated 17D strain, and currently given as a single dose for a lifetime, is the most effective way to prevent and control disease. A single dose of vaccine provides life-long immunity. WHO recommends that all endemic countries should include yellow fever vaccine in their national immunization programs. Yellow fever vaccines can be given to immunocompetent persons over 9 months of age living in or traveling to endemic areas. In one study of US travelers visiting a yellow fever endemic country to provide humanitarian service, over 90% were vaccinated at their pretravel health consultation or reported a yellow fever vaccination within the past 10 years.

The vaccine is contraindicated in severely immunocompromised populations and persons with severe egg allergies. HIV-infected persons with CD4 cell counts at least 200 cells/mL can safely receive the vaccine, while pregnant women should receive the vaccine only if they cannot defer travel to endemic areas (Chapter 30). Clinicians should be aware of rare but frequently fatal vaccine-induced reactions, including neurotropic (encephalitis-like syndrome) and viscerotropic (yellow fever–like) diseases; persons at risk include older men, women 19–34, patients who have undergone thymectomy, infants and children 11 years or younger (especially at risk for the neurologic complications), and immunocompromised patients (including those with autoimmune diseases).

The best personal protective measures are to avoid mosquito bites. Eradication of mosquitoes is difficult because of the sylvatic cycle (mainly maintained by nonhuman primates). If not in an endemic area, the patient should be isolated from mosquitoes to prevent transmission, since blood in the acute phase is potentially infectious.

Seligman SJ et al. Defining risk groups to yellow fever vaccine—associated viscerotropic disease in the absence of denominator data. Am J Trop Med Hyg. 2014 Feb;90(2):267–71. [PMID: 24394480]

Staples JE et al; Centers for Disease Control and Prevention (CDC). Yellow fever vaccine booster doses: recommendations of the Advisory Committee on Immunization Practices, 2015. MMWR Morb Mortal Wkly Rep. 2015 Jun 19;64(23):647–50. [PMID: 26086636]

Stoney RJ et al. Pre-travel preparation of US travelers going abroad to provide humanitarian service, Global TravEpiNet 2009–2011. Am J Trop Med Hyg. 2014 Mar;90(3):553–9. [PMID: 24445203]

World Health Organization. Vaccines and vaccination against yellow fever: WHO Position Paper, June 2013—recommendations. Vaccine. 2015 Jan 1;33(1):76–7. [PMID: 2485272]
Yellow fever in Africa and the Americas, 2014. Wkly Epidemiol Rec. 2015 Jun 26;90(26):323–34. [PMID: 26121768]

OTHER SYSTEMIC VIRAL DISEASES

1. Zika Virus

ESSENTIALS OF DIAGNOSIS

- ▶ Most infected persons asymptomatically seroconvert.
- ▶ Clinical symptoms are akin to those of chikungunya virus infection.
- ▶ Complications include Guillain-Barré and possibly microcephaly, the latter among infants born to mothers infected during pregnancy.
- ▶ There is no effective antiviral or vaccine.

▶ General Considerations

Zika virus is a flavivirus, akin to the viruses that cause dengue fever, Japanese encephalitis, and West Nile infection. It was originally isolated from macaques in 1947, in the Zika forest near the Entebbe airport of Uganda. The virus was named Zika in 1952, and the first human cases were noted in Nigeria in 1968 although earlier cases probably occurred in Uganda and Tanzania.

The virus was noted in Africa and Asia during the 1950s–1980s but first spread beyond those two continents during 2007 when an outbreak occurred in Yap State, Federated States of Micronesia. A large outbreak occurred in French Polynesia in 2013. A smaller outbreak occurred on Easter Island during 2014. The virus then spread to the Western hemisphere and was first noted in northeastern Brazil in 2015. Up to 1.3 million cases occurred in Brazil during that year. Zika virus then spread rapidly throughout South America, Central America, the Caribbean, and Mexico. An area of particular concern is northeastern Brazil where it is associated with microcephaly among infants born to women infected during the first trimester.

Aedes species mosquitoes, particularly *Aedes aegypti*, are responsible for transmission of Zika virus. The biodistribution of the species largely determines the area of prevalence for Zika virus. *Aedes* species mosquitoes are found primarily in the southeastern United States, but one species *Aedes albopictus* (the Asian tiger mosquito known to sequester in tires) may be seen as far north as Pennsylvania. As of May 4, 2016, there were reported in the fifty US states no locally-acquired vector borne Zika cases, but there were 472 imported, travel-associated Zika cases, among whom 44 were pregnant. Sexual transmission was deemed to have occurred among 10 cases and 1 had the Guillain Barré syndrome. In the US territories (largely Puerto Rico but also American Samoa and the US Virgin Islands) there were only 3 travel-associated cases reported, but there were 658 locally acquired cases, among whom 59 were pregnant and 5 had developed the Guillain-Barré syndrome.

▶ Clinical Findings

A. Symptoms and Signs

The incubation period is about 10 days. Symptoms include acute onset fever, maculopapular rash, nonpurulent conjunctivitis, and arthralgias, the latter mimicking the symptoms of the chikungunya virus. Rash may outlast the fever but is not always present. Symptoms last up to 7 days. Most infections are asymptomatic. Viral infections most often confused with Zika include dengue and chikungunya virus infections.

B. Laboratory Findings and Diagnostic Studies

The CDC recommends that everyone with symptoms of Zika infection be tested if they have traveled to an endemic area in the past two weeks, as well as all pregnant women who have lived or visited affected regions. Men should be tested if they have lived in, or visited, an affected region, in case of sexual transmission of the virus. Infants born to mothers who while pregnant lived or traveled to transmission areas should also be tested.

Diagnosis is made with RT-PCR or neutralizing antibody, IgM early in infection, IgG after 4 days of symptoms. A commercially available RT-PCR test of blood samples for the Zika virus provides results in one to two days. This molecular testing detects the virus when it is in blood. A negative test does not exclude the presence of the virus in other tissues. Other diagnostic modalities are available from the CDC and at some state health department laboratories. Zika virus RNA can be detected in urine for at least 2 weeks after onset of symptoms. A CDC Trioplex rRT-PCR assay is the only diagnostic tool authorized by the FDA for Zika virus testing of urine. The CDC recommends Zika virus rRT-PCR be performed on urine collected <14 days after onset of symptoms in patients with suspected Zika virus disease. Tests of amniotic fluid are of indeterminate accuracy but may be very suggestive of active infection. Amniocentesis is attendant with the small risk of fetal loss, especially early in pregnancy. Infants in whom infection is suspected should have umbilical cord blood or blood from the infant within 2 days of birth collected and serum tested by RT-PCR for the virus and by neutralizing antibody assay. Neutralizing antibodies can cross-react with dengue and other flaviviruses, so public health laboratories may perform specialized testing to definitively make the diagnosis. Cerebrospinal fluid and placental tissue may also be tested by RT-PCR. Ophthalmologic evaluation is recommended in infants in whom congenital Zika virus infection is diagnosed. Pregnant women with suspected Zika virus infection can be monitored by serial ultrasounds at 3–4 week intervals, assessing the fetus for intracranial calcifications and head size.

▶ Complications

Two neurologic complications are of particular concern: (1) Guillain-Barré syndrome, first noted during the outbreak in French Polynesia where 73 cases were reported; and (2) microcephaly, an association noted in Brazil but without firmly documented data regarding pathogenicity.

Macular atrophy, diffuse brain calcifications, and other abnormalities in brain development are reported to accompany microcephaly. A possible contributory role of pesticides or other teratogenic viruses is under investigation, in part because the selective geographic distribution of microcephalic cases in northeastern Brazil is not fully explained. Nonetheless, the isolation of the viral tissue from the brain of infected fetal material supports the role of Zika virus in the pathogenesis of microcephalic infants.

Treatment

There are no effective antivirals against Zika virus. Aspirin is not used for another flavivirus, dengue, because of its propensity toward hemorrhage on reinfection. Zika virus infections, however, do not appear to be associated with major hemorrhagic complications.

Prevention

The most effective means is environmental control of mosquitoes and removal of areas where water is stagnant or builds up. Such measures include screens on houses; removal of old tires and debris from endemic areas of infection; and movement toward better living conditions, including air conditioning in impoverished areas. Because of the association between microcephaly and Zika virus infection during pregnancy, pregnant women are advised to avoid travel to areas where Zika virus is circulating. Guidelines for testing of pregnant women potentially exposed are available through CDC. Infected individuals should refrain from blood donations for several months.

There is no current vaccine against Zika virus, although there is hope that one will become available because other flavivirus vaccines exist, including the effective Japanese encephalitis vaccine and dengue virus vaccines which are both commercially available (for those aged 9–45 years in Mexico) and under considerable study.

Fauci AS et al. Zika virus in the Americas—yet another arbovirus threat. N Engl J Med. 2016 Feb 18;374(7):601–4. [PMID: 26761185]

Hennessey M et al. Zika virus spreads to new areas—region of the Americas, May 2015–January 2016. MMWR Morb Mortal Wkly Rep. 2016 Jan 29;65(3):55–8. [PMID: 26820163]

Musso D. Zika virus transmission from French Polynesia to Brazil. Emerg Infect Dis. 2015 Oct;21(10):1887. [PMID: 26403318]

Oduyebo T et al. Update: interim guidelines for health care providers caring for pregnant women and women of reproductive age with possible Zika virus exposure—United States, 2016. MMWR Morb Mortal Wkly Rep. 2016 Feb 12;65(5):122–7. [PMID: 26866840]

Oehler E et al. Zika virus infection complicated by Guillain-Barre syndrome—case report, French Polynesia, December 2013. Euro Surveill. 2014 Mar 6;19(9):20720. [PMID: 24626205]

Petersen EE et al. Interim guidelines for pregnant women during a Zika virus outbreak—United States, 2016. MMWR Morb Mortal Wkly Rep. 2016 Jan 22;65(2):30–3. [PMID: 26796813]

Ventura CV et al. Zika virus in Brazil and macular atrophy in a child with microcephaly. Lancet. 2016 Jan 16;387(10015):228. [PMID: 26775125]

2. Chikungunya Fever

Chikungunya ("that which bends up" in the Bantu language Makonde) fever is an alphavirus infection transmitted to humans by *A aegypti* and *A albopictus* and is considered a classic "arthritogenic" virus. The virus is indigenous to tropical Africa and Asia. Outbreaks originated in Kenya in 2004 and subsequently were reported from areas that adjoin the Indian Ocean, Southeast Asia and its neighboring islands (2005–2007), South India (2005), the island of La Réunion (2005–2006), with subsequent spread with autochthonous cases in Italy and France (2007). In 2013, the first autochthonous case of chikungunya occurred on Saint Martin in the Caribbean. As of October 23, 2015, a total of 1,118,578 suspected and 25,627 laboratory-confirmed autochthonous cases have been reported in the Americas, including 12 confirmed cases in Florida during 2014. The incidence rate in the Caribbean decreased during 2015—the highest incidence rate was reported in Central America 400/100,000 population. Travel-associated cases are reported widely with 2799 cases from 46 states (all but Alaska, Nebraska, North Dakota, and Wyoming). The US Caribbean territories reported 4622 locally acquired cases. Among naïve populations, attack rates are often as high as 50%. Vertical transmission is documented if the mother is viremic during parturition. Endemicity of *A aegypti* in the Americas and the introduction of *A albopictus* into Europe and the New World raise concern for global extension of the epidemic. There are reports of cases of chikungunya coinfection with yellow fever, malaria, and dengue fever. Statistics on chikungunya virus infection in the Western hemisphere may be found at http://www.paho.org/hq/index.php?option=com_topics&view=readall&cid=5927&Itemid=40931&lang=en. Statistics for the United States may be found at: http://www.cdc.gov/chikungunya/geo/united-states-2014.html.

Clinical Findings

A. Symptoms and Signs

After an incubation period of 1–12 days (average 2–4), there is an abrupt onset of fever; headache; intestinal complaints; myalgias; and arthralgias/arthritis affecting small, large, and axial joints. The simultaneous involvement of more than 10 joints and the presence of tenosynovitis (especially in the wrist) are characteristic. The stooped posture of patients gives the disease its name. Joint symptoms persist for 4 months in 33% and linger for years in about 10%. A centrally distributed pigmented or pruritic maculopapular rash is reported in 10–40% of patients; it can be bullous with sloughing in children. Mucosal disease occurs in about 15%. Facial edema and localized petechiae are reported. Neurologic complications, including encephalitis, myelopathy, peripheral neuropathy, myeloneuropathy, and myopathy, are usually associated with a good outcome. In infants, primary manifestations of disease include fever, lethargy, acrocyanosis, and erythema evolving into vesiculobullous lesions. Hemorrhagic fever-like presentations are exceptional. Coinfection with other respiratory viruses and with dengue is common. Death is rare and usually related to underlying comorbidities.

B. Laboratory Findings

Diagnosis is made epidemiologically and clinically. Mild leukopenia occurs as does thrombocytopenia, which is seldom severe. Elevated inflammatory markers do not correlate well with the severity of arthritis. Radiographs of affected joints are normal during the acute phase. Bone lesions are visible in some patients with chronic symptoms.

Serologic confirmation requires elevated IgM titers or fourfold increase in convalescent IgG levels using an ELISA. RT-PCR and ELISA are commercially available; no ELISA kit is FDA-cleared. Culture techniques (viral isolation in insect or mammalian cell lines or by inoculation of mosquitoes or mice) require BSL-3 containment. Suspected cases in the United States should be promptly reported to public health authorities including the CDC Arboviral Diseases Branch, 970-221-6400. The differential includes other tropical febrile diseases, such as malaria, leishmaniasis, or dengue.

▶ Complications & Prognosis

A major complication of chikungunya fever is long-term weakness, asthenia, and arthritis, noted to occur in up to 66.5% of cases at 1-year in a series from Italy but in between 4% and 25% in series from India. Risk factors for long-term arthralgias include the presence of such symptoms at 4 months after onset of disease and age over 35 years. Persons with preexisting arthritis are also at increased risk for prolonged symptoms after chikungunya infection. Children with symptomatic congenital chikungunya infection may have adverse neurocognitive outcomes.

▶ Treatment & Prevention

Treatment is supportive with nonsteroidal anti-inflammatory drugs. Chloroquine may be useful for managing refractory arthritis. In a retrospective study on La Réunion, methotrexate was associated with a positive response. No licensed vaccine exists. However, a live recombinant measles virus–based vaccine and a virus-like particle vaccine are in early clinical trials. At this time, prevention relies on avoidance of the mosquito vectors.

Chang LJ et al; VRC 311 Study Team. Safety and tolerability of chikungunya virus-like particle vaccine in healthy adults: a phase 1 dose-escalation trial. Lancet. 2014 Dec 6;384(9959):2046–52. [PMID: 25132507]

Gérardin P et al. Neurocognitive outcome of children exposed to perinatal mother-to-child chikungunya virus infection: the CHIMERE cohort study on Reunion Island. PLoS Negl Trop Dis. 2014 Jul 17;8(7):e2996. [PMID: 25033077]

Javelle E et al. Specific management of post-chikungunya rheumatic disorders: a retrospective study of 159 cases in Reunion Island from 2006–2012. PLoS Negl Trop Dis. 2015 Mar 11; 9(3):e0003603. [PMID: 25760632]

Kendrick K et al. Notes from the field: transmission of chikungunya virus in the continental United States—Florida, 2014. MMWR Morb Mortal Wkly Rep. 2014 Dec 5;63(48):1137. [PMID: 25474035]

Lindsey NP et al. Chikungunya virus infection among travelers—United States, 2010–2013. Am J Trop Med Hyg. 2015 Jan; 92(1):82–7. [PMID: 25349374]

Ramsauer K et al. Immunogenicity, safety and tolerability of a recombinant measles-virus-based chikungunya vaccine: a randomized, double-blind, placebo-controlled, active-comparator, first-in-man trial. Lancet Infect Dis. 2015 May;15(5):519–27. [PMID: 25739878]

Schilte C et al. Chikungunya virus-associated long-term arthralgia: a 36-month prospective longitudinal study. PLoS Negl Trop Dis. 2013;7(3):e2137. [PMID: 23556021]

3. Colorado Tick Fever

ESSENTIALS OF DIAGNOSIS

▶ Onset 1–19 days (average, 4 days) following tick bite.

▶ Fever, chills, myalgia, headache, prostration.

▶ Leukopenia, thrombocytopenia.

▶ Second attack of fever after remission lasting 2–3 days.

▶ General Considerations

Colorado tick fever is a reportable biphasic, febrile illness caused by a reovirus infection transmitted by *Dermacentor andersoni* tick bite. About five cases occur annually, largely among men over age 40. The disease is limited to the western United States and Canada and is most prevalent during the tick season (March to November). There is a discrete history of tick bite or exposure in 90% of cases. The virus infects the marrow erythrocyte precursors. Despite frequent exposure among national park and forest employees to ticks and reported bites, Colorado tick fever rarely develops in these persons. Most cases occur in late spring and early summer.

▶ Clinical Findings

A. Symptoms and Signs

The incubation period is 3–6 days, rarely as long as 19 days. The onset is usually abrupt with a high fever. Severe myalgia, headache, photophobia, anorexia, nausea and vomiting, and generalized weakness are prominent. Physical findings are limited to an occasional faint rash. The acute symptoms resolve within a week. Remission is followed in 50% of cases by recurrent fever and a full recrudescence lasting 2–4 days. In an occasional case, there may be three bouts of fever.

The differential diagnosis includes influenza, Rocky Mountain spotted fever, numerous other viral infections and, in the right setting, relapsing fevers.

B. Laboratory Findings

Leukopenia (2000–3000/mcL) with a shift to the left and atypical lymphocytes occurs, reaching a nadir 5–6 days after the onset of illness. Thrombocytopenia may occur. Viremia may be demonstrated by inoculation of blood into mice or by fluorescent antibody staining of the patient's red cells (with adsorbed virus). An RT-PCR assay may be used to detect early viremia. Detection of IgM by capture ELISA or plaque reduction neutralization is possible after 2 weeks from symptom onset and is the most frequently used diagnostic tool.

▶ Complications

Aseptic meningitis (particularly in children), encephalitis, and hemorrhagic fever occur rarely. Malaise may last weeks to months. Fatalities are very uncommon. Rarely, spontaneous abortion or multiple congenital anomalies may complicate Colorado tick fever infection acquired during pregnancy.

Treatment

No specific treatment is available. Ribavirin has shown efficacy in an animal model. Antipyretics are used, although salicylates should be avoided due to potential bleeding with the thrombocytopenia seen in patients with Colorado tick fever.

Prognosis

The disease is usually self-limited and benign.

Prevention

Tick avoidance is the best prevention. The tick season is primarily from March to November, and the ticks mostly live at high altitudes (over 7000 feet) in sagebrush.

Geissler AL et al. Infection with Colorado tick fever virus among humans and ticks in a national park and forest, Wyoming, 2010. Vector Borne Zoonotic Dis. 2014 Sep;14(9):675–80. [PMID: 25229706]

Yendell SJ et al. Colorado tick fever in the United States, 2002–2012. Vector Borne Zoonotic Dis. 2015 May;15(5):311–6. [PMID: 25988440]

COMMON VIRAL RESPIRATORY INFECTIONS

1. Respiratory Syncytial Virus (RSV) & Other Paramyxoviruses

> ### ESSENTIALS OF DIAGNOSIS
>
> ▶ RSV is a major cause of morbidity and mortality at the extremes of age.
>
> ▶ Care for patients with RSV infections is largely supportive.
>
> ▶ A monoclonal antibody against RSV, palivizumab, is good but expensive prophylaxis among patients with certain at-risk cardiopulmonary conditions.
>
> ▶ No active vaccination for RSV is available.

General Considerations

Respiratory syncytial virus (RSV) is a paramyxovirus that causes annual outbreaks during the wintertime with usual onset of pulmonary symptoms between mid-October and early January in the continental United States (excluding Florida). Outside the United States, RSV usually peaks during wet months in areas with high annual precipitation and during cooler months in hot and dry areas. There are two major subtypes, A and B, and it appears that the A genotype is associated with disease severity. **RSV is the leading cause of hospitalization in US children**, with annual hospitalization rates of 6 per 1000 children under 5 years of age. Risk factors for infection in children include prematurity, low birth weight, younger age (especially younger than 6 months), bronchopulmonary dysplasia, congenital heart disease, later birth order, and day care exposure. HIV-infected children are at higher risk for hospitalization and

poorer outcomes than uninfected children. RSV infection in children is associated with persistence of airway reactivity later in life.

RSV also causes upper and lower respiratory tract infection in adults with increasingly recognized severity in those with comorbid conditions, the elderly (accounting for a rate of 4 per 1000 hospitalizations and 14,000 deaths annually), persons with severe combined immunodeficiency, and following lung or bone marrow transplantation (because CD8 T cells are not available for viral clearance). Recurrent infections occur throughout life. The virus enters through contact with mucosal surfaces. The average incubation period is 5 days. Up to 10% of disease classified as invasive pneumococcal disease is thought to be RSV or influenza (above).

In immunocompromised patients, such as bone marrow transplant recipients, serious pneumonia can occur, and outbreaks with a high mortality rate (greater than 70%) are reported.

Other paramyxoviruses important in human disease include human metapneumovirus, parainfluenza virus, and Nipah virus.

Human metapneumovirus is a seasonal virus circulating during late winter to early spring. It is divided into subgroups A and B. Clinical presentations range from mild upper respiratory tract infections to severe lower respiratory tract infections (eg, bronchiolitis, croup, and pneumonia). Lower respiratory tract (sometimes severe) infections have been observed among immunocompromised and elderly adults. In lung transplant recipients, human metapneumovirus is a common cause of respiratory illness and is thought to increase the risk of acute and chronic graft rejection.

Human parainfluenza viruses (HPIVs) are commonly seen in children and are the most common cause of laryngotracheitis (croup). Four different serotypes are described, and they differ in their clinical presentations as well as epidemiology. HPIV-1 and HPIV-2 are responsible for croup. HPIV-3 is associated with bronchiolitis and pneumonia. HPIV-4 is a less frequently reported pathogen. Reinfections are common throughout life. HPIVs can also cause severe disease in the elderly, immunocompromised persons, and those with chronic illnesses.

Nipah virus, is a highly virulent paramyxovirus first described in 1999. Cases are concentrated mainly in Southeast Asia (Malaysia, Singapore, Bangladesh and India). Fruit bats are identified as the natural host of the virus. Direct pig-human, cow-human, human-human, and nosocomial transmission are reported. Nipah virus causes acute encephalitis with a high fatality rate (67–92%), although respiratory symptoms are also described. Cranial nerve palsies, encephalopathy, and dystonia are among neurologic sequelae (15–32%) seen in infected individuals. Relapses occurring weeks and months after initial infection are described (3.4–7.5%).

Bocavirus infections are discussed under Erythrovirus (parvovirus) infections below.

Clinical Findings

A. Symptoms and Signs

In RSV bronchiolitis, proliferation and necrosis of bronchiolar epithelium develop, producing obstruction from sloughed epithelium and increased mucus secretion. An interleukin-1 receptor polymorphism is shown to be associated with more severe bronchiolitis. Signs of infection include low-grade fever, tachypnea, and wheezes. Apnea is a common presenting symptom. Hyperinflated lungs, decreased gas exchange, and increased work of breathing are present. In children, RSV is globally the most common cause of acute lower respiratory infection and also a common cause of acute and recurrent otitis media. In patients with Down syndrome, RSV develops at a later age and is associated with more protracted hospitalizations.

B. Laboratory Findings

A rapid diagnosis of RSV infection is made by viral antigen identification of nasal washings using an ELISA or immunofluorescent assay. PCR is increasingly used. RSV viral load assay values at day 3 of infection may correlate with requirement of intensive care and respiratory failure in children.

Human metapneumovirus is best diagnosed by PCR. Tests for rapid detection of viral antigens with immunofluorescence or ELISA, and PCR techniques are also widely available for detection of HPIV. Culture may also be used. ELISA (serum and cerebrospinal fluid) and PCR (urine, respiratory secretions but not blood) are both used for Nipah virus infection diagnosis.

▶ Treatment & Prevention

Treatment of RSV consists of supportive care, including hydration, humidification of inspired air, and ventilatory support as needed. Neither bronchodilating agents nor corticosteroids have demonstrated efficacy in bronchiolitis although individual patients with significant bronchospasm or history of asthma might respond to them. Oral antiviral agents are being studied through healthy adult challenge experiments.

The use of aerosolized ribavirin can be considered in high-risk patients, such as those with a history of bone marrow transplantation, and appears to lessen mortality. Pregnant women, including hospital staff, should avoid ribavirin exposure. Prophylactic administration of palivizumab, an anti-RSV monoclonal antibody, (15 mg/kg intramuscularly monthly during the season of high transmission) is recommended for infants at high-risk for complication, including those with chronic lung disease of prematurity and hemodynamically significant congenital heart disease. Data support the use of palivizumab in upper airway anomalies, other pulmonary diseases, and cystic fibrosis as well as in children with Down syndrome.

No RSV vaccine is available but a promising live attenuated intranasal vaccine candidate is under study. It was associated with decreased shedding of the vaccine virus, increasing titers of neutralizing antibodies, and antibody responses in previously seronegative individuals. Vaccines for use in pregnant women designed to protect infants during their period of highest vulnerability are in early clinical trials.

Prevention in hospitals entails rapid diagnosis, handwashing, contact isolation, and perhaps passive immunization. The use of conjugated pneumococcal vaccination appears to decrease the incidence of concomitant pneumonia associated with viral infections in children in some countries.

Therapeutic modalities for human metapneumovirus and parainfluenza virus infections under investigation include intravenous ribavirin administration.

DeVicenzo JP et al. Activity of oral ALS-008176 in a respiratory syncytial virus challenge study. N Engl J Med. 2015 Nov 19; 373(21):2048–58. [PMID: 26580997]

Jain S et al; CDC EPIC Study Team. Community-acquired pneumonia requiring hospitalization among U.S. children. N Engl J Med. 2015 Feb 26;372(9):835–45. [PMID: 25714161]

Karron RA et al. A gene deletion that up-regulates viral gene expression yields an attenuated RSV vaccine with improved antibody responses in children. Sci Transl Med. 2015 Nov 4; 7(312):312ra175. [PMID: 26537255]

Muñoz FM. Respiratory syncytial virus in infants: is maternal vaccination a realistic strategy? Curr Opin Infect Dis. 2015 Jun; 28(3):221–4. [PMID: 25918956]

Volling C et al. Respiratory syncytial virus infection-associated hospitalization in adults: a retrospective cohort study. BMC Infect Dis. 2014 Dec 13;14:665. [PMID: 25494918]

2. Seasonal Influenza

ESSENTIALS OF DIAGNOSIS

▶ Cases usually in epidemic pattern.

▶ Onset with fever, chills, malaise, cough, coryza, and myalgias.

▶ Aching, fever, and prostration out of proportion to catarrhal symptoms.

▶ Leukopenia.

▶ General Considerations

Influenza (an orthomyxovirus) is a highly contagious disease transmitted by the respiratory route in humans. Transmission occurs primarily by droplet nuclei rather than fomites or direct contact. There are three types of influenza viruses. While type A can infect a variety of mammals (humans, swine, horses, etc) and birds, types B and C almost exclusively infect humans. Type A viruses are further divided into subtypes based on the hemagglutinin (H) and the neuraminidase (N) expressed on their surface. There are 18 subtypes of hemagglutinin and 11 subtypes of neuraminidase.

Annual epidemics usually appear in the fall or winter in temperate climatic areas (although sporadic cases occur as summer outbreaks in northern areas such as Alaska or the southern hemisphere). Up to 5 million cases of severe influenza are estimated by the WHO to occur annually, with up to 0.5 million annual deaths. Influenza epidemics affect 10–20% of the global population on average each year and are typically the result of frequent minor antigenic variations of the virus, or antigenic drift, which are more common in influenza A virus. On the other hand, pandemics—associated with higher mortality—appear at longer and varying intervals (decades) as a consequence of a major genetic reassortment of the virus (antigenic shift) or the mutation of an avian virus that adapts to the human (as with the pandemic virus of 1918 with H1N1 properties).

The highly pathogenic avian (H5N1) and the H7N9 subtypes are discussed in the next section. The novel swine-origin influenza A (pandemic H1N1) virus emerged in Mexico in March 2009 and quickly spread throughout North America. This virus originated from triple-reassortment of North American swine, human and avian virus lineages and Eurasian swine virus lineages and has now replaced the previous H1N1 seasonal strain and is subsequently referred to here as seasonal H1N1. This virus, as with other pathogenic influenza viruses, is of particular concern for pregnant women and immunosuppressed persons.

▶ Clinical Findings

A. Symptoms and Signs

Seasonal influenza viruses of types A and B produce clinically indistinguishable infections, whereas type C usually causes a minor illness. The incubation period is 1–4 days. In unvaccinated persons, uncomplicated influenza often begins abruptly. Symptoms range widely from a nearly asymptomatic state to a constellation of symptoms including fever, chills, malaise, myalgias, substernal soreness, headache, nasal stuffiness, and occasionally nausea. Fever lasts 1–7 days (usually 3–5). Coryza, nonproductive cough, and sore throat are present. Elderly patients especially may present with only lassitude and confusion, often without fever or respiratory symptoms. Signs include mild pharyngeal injection, flushed face, and conjunctival redness. Moderate enlargement of the cervical lymph nodes may be observed. The presence of fever (higher than 38.2°C) and cough during influenza season is highly predictive of influenza infection in those older than 4 years of age.

Other symptoms particularly noted during the 2009 H1N1 pandemic included gastrointestinal (especially diarrhea) and respiratory (pneumonia) manifestations. Hospitalization or ICU admission for influenza is often a consequence of diffuse viral pneumonitis with severe hypoxemia and sometimes shock. Neurologic complications, including seizures and encephalopathy, and cardiac dysfunction, including myocarditis and pulmonary thromboemboli, may occur. Asthmatic patients with pneumonia are at higher risk for ICU admission and death. H1N1-associated hemophagocytic syndromes are reported. Most patients with mild disease recover fully, but 9–31% of hospitalized cases require ICU admission, where the mortality was as high as 46% during the 2009 pandemic.

Attack rates for influenza are highest in children and young adults of certain ethnic backgrounds, particularly Hispanics, blacks, and Native Americans, with relative sparing of adults older than 60 years of age presumably due to previous exposure with related strains (conferring some degree of cross-protection). High-risk groups include patients with severe obesity, asthma, immunosuppression, or neurologic disorders, and pregnant and postpartum women. Infection during pregnancy increases the risk for hospitalization and may be associated with severe illness, sepsis, pneumothorax and respiratory failure, spontaneous abortion, preterm labor, and fetal distress. Overall case fatality rate is < 0.5% with 90% of deaths in those under 65 years of age and higher mortality recognized among men and patients with liver disease or a cancer diagnosis within the last year.

B. Laboratory Findings

Leukopenia is common, but leukocytosis can occur. Proteinuria may be present. The virus may be isolated from throat swabs or nasal washings by inoculation of embryonated eggs or cell cultures. Rapid immunofluorescence assays and enzyme immunoassays for detection of influenza antigens from nasal or throat swabs are widely available. The sensitivity of such assays is suboptimal (at most 60–80%), especially among adults, and with very significant intertest variability, only a few can distinguish between influenza A and B. More sensitive nucleic acid amplification (PCR) techniques are increasingly accessible although their sensitivity is compromised early in the season during low prevalence periods. Complement-fixing and hemagglutination-inhibiting antibodies (for which fourfold or greater rises in levels are needed to establish diagnosis) appear during the second week. A nasopharyngeal swab, nasal aspirate, combined nasopharyngeal swab with oropharyngeal swab, or material from a bronchoalveolar lavage can be tested for any influenza strain.

Local laboratories can perform rapid influenza antigen enzyme or direct immunofluorescent assays to distinguish influenza viruses types A and B, but the results of these assays should be interpreted with caution due to a limited sensitivity (11–70%). Test material can be kept at 4°C up to 4 days (not frozen) and shipped with an ice pack. The CDC or many state public health laboratories can then perform a real-time PCR or viral culture, when needed, such as during a pandemic. Chest radiographic findings rarely show lobular infiltrates and pathologic findings show similar particular propensities toward diffuse alveolar damage.

▶ Differential Diagnosis

The differential diagnoses for influenza-like infections include a variety of viral infections (parainfluenza infections, RSV infections, dengue, adenovirus, echoviruses, CMV, EBV infection, acute HIV infection, as well as bacterial infections such as mycobacterial infection (atypical pneumonia), pertussis, and Legionnaire disease. Epidemiologic factors can suggest Legionnaire (elderly smokers), chronicity of cough may support adenovirus, mycobacterial and pertussis infections, leukocytosis initially supports CMV, and lymphadenopathy is more common with EBV or CMV infection. Distinguishing influenza from dengue requires attention to rhinitis (influenza) and thrombocytopenia (dengue).

▶ Complications

Influenza causes necrosis of the respiratory epithelium, which predisposes to secondary bacterial infections. In turn, bacterial enzymes (eg, proteases, trypsin-like compounds, and streptokinase) activate influenza viruses. Frequent complications are acute sinusitis, otitis media, purulent bronchitis, and pneumonia. Children under 5 years of age, pregnant women, residents of nursing homes and long-term–care facilities, the elderly (aged 65 years or older), children and teens under 19 years of age who are receiving long-term aspirin therapy, and persons with underlying medical conditions (pulmonary, renal, cardiovascular, hepatic, hematologic, neurologic and neurodevelopmental conditions and immune-deficient conditions such as HIV) are at high risk for complications. Persons who are morbidly obese (body mass index greater than 40), American Indians, and Alaskan natives are also at high risk for complications.

Cardiovascular diseases are a particular complication of influenza infection, in particular among the elderly, and influenza is postulated to be a significant trigger for myocardial infarction, cerebrovascular diseases, and sudden death.

Primary influenza pneumonia may occur, particularly in young children with cardiovascular disease and pregnant women, and is associated with high mortality. Secondary bacterial pneumonia due to pneumococci, staphylococci, or *Haemophilus* spp is not uncommon. Pericarditis and myocarditis occur rarely. There is an association of acute myocardial infarction with preceding respiratory infection, including influenza; a UK study showed that influenza vaccination is associated with a lower rate of acute myocardial infarction. Rhabdomyolysis and leukocytoclastic vasculitis are rare complications of influenza.

Reye syndrome (fatty liver with encephalopathy) is a rare and severe complication of influenza (usually B type) and other viral diseases (especially varicella), particularly in young children. It consists of rapidly progressive hepatic failure and encephalopathy, and there is a 30% mortality rate. The pathogenesis is unknown, but the syndrome is associated with aspirin use in the management of viral infections.

Encephalopathic complications of influenza are uncommon and include an acute necrotizing encephalopathy associated with disseminated intravascular coagulation and cytokine storm, with worsening when treated with certain nonsteroidal anti-inflammatory medications (diclofenac and mefenamic acid), and an acute encephalopathy associated with febrile seizures and the use of theophylline. An analysis of Medicare utilization data shows no increase in the Guillain-Barré syndrome following influenza vaccination.

► **Treatment**

Many patients with influenza prefer to rest in bed. Analgesics and a cough mixture may be used. Treatment should be considered for all persons with acute illness, in particular those with a suggestive clinical presentation or with laboratory confirmed influenza and at high risk for developing complications (nursing home residents; patients with chronic pulmonary, cardiovascular, kidney, or liver disease; those with diabetes mellitus, active malignancy, immunosuppression, or impairment for managing respiratory secretions), or living with persons at significant risk for them. Maximum benefit is expected with the earliest initiation of therapy. Although the benefit of antiviral therapy after 48 hours of illness is reduced, it should be considered if the patient is hospitalized. There is no benefit to double-dose oseltamivir in severe influenza infections although some influenza experts continue to recommend double-dose therapy among immunocompromised patients.

The neuraminidase inhibitors, inhaled **zanamivir**, 10 mg (2 inhalations) twice daily for 5 days, oral **oseltamivir**, 75 mg twice daily for 5 days, or intravenous **peramivir**, 600 mg single dose, are equally effective in the treatment of susceptible strains of influenza. Clinical trials show a reduction in the duration of symptoms as well as secondary complications, such as otitis, sinusitis, or pneumonia, but not in the rate of hospitalizations or mortality when using these agents. When administered early (within the first 2 days of illness), antiviral medications (neuraminidase inhibitors) are most effective. Patients with asthma who are hospitalized with pneumonia should be treated early with antivirals.

Since high levels of resistance to the adamantanes (amantadine and rimantadine) persist among seasonal H1N1 and H3N2 influenza A viruses and these agents are not effective against influenza B viruses, adamantanes are generally not recommended for treatment.

Resistance to neuraminidase inhibitors (oseltamivir, zanamivir, and peramivir) can occur with prolonged use in immunocompromised patients. With the previous seasonal H1N1 strain, oseltamivir resistance was reported at rates as high as 25% in Europe and Africa due to a genetic mutation (H275Y). With the current seasonal H1N1 strain, rates of oseltamivir resistance have been low (~1%) but are associated with the same H275Y mutation, and person-to-person transmission is documented. An outbreak with a resistant strain may have occurred in Austrialia in 2011. Increasing rates of oseltamivir resistance should be expected over time.

Zanamivir is relatively contraindicated among persons with asthma because of the risk of bronchospasm and is not formulated for use in mechanically ventilated patients. Transient neuropsychiatric events, occasionally resulting in self-injury and death, have been reported post marketing for both neuraminidase inhibitors. Patients receiving these medications should be closely monitored for any unusual behavior, and healthcare professionals should be notified immediately if such signs occur. Laninamivir is a long-acting inhaled neuraminidase inhibitor used for the treatment of seasonal influenza, including infection caused by oseltamivir-resistant virus. It is licensed in Japan (RAPIACTA) and South Korea (PERAMIFLU) and was used in the past for severe H1N1 influenza during the 2009 pandemic under an Emergency Authorization Use but remains under clinical study. The license for its clinical use in the United States expired in 2010. Antibacterial antibiotics should be reserved for treatment of bacterial complications. Acetaminophen or ibuprofen rather than aspirin should be used for fever in children to avoid Reye syndrome.

Oseltamivir-resistant virus usually remains sensitive to zanamivir. Intravenous zanamavir is available for patients unable to take medication by mouth through compassionate use programs available through GlaxoSmithKline at 877-626-8019 or 866-341-9160 or gskclinicalsupportHD@gsk.com (http://www.clinicalsupporthd.gsk.com/) (http://www.flu.nc.gov/providers/documents/IVzanamivirRequestInformation.pdf).

Peramivir is FDA approved for intravenous therapy of influenza infections. It does not have activity against oseltamivir-resistant virus.

For oseltamivir-resistant seasonal H1N1 viral infection, intravenous zanamivir is preferred. While a case of multidrug-resistant seasonal H1N1 virus with resistance to oseltamivir, zanamivir, and peramivir is reported, this particular isolate is less pathogenic in animal studies than susceptible H1N1 strains.

The use of high frequency oscillatory ventilation and extracorporeal membrane oxygenation can improve oxygenation but the impact on mortality is unknown. Corticosteroids for an associated ARDS are not useful and may increase the mortality except that the use of corticosteroids is associated with a lower rate of mechanical ventilation if used in high doses (1 mg/kg prednisone equivalence orally at the time of diagnosis) in patients with a history of hematopoietic stem cell transplantation.

Updated advice is available at http://www.cdc.gov/flu/index.htm.

▶ Prognosis

The duration of the uncomplicated illness is 1–7 days, and the prognosis is excellent in healthy, nonelderly adults. Hospitalization typically occurs in those with underlying medical disease, at the extremes of age and in pregnant woman. Young adults and obese individuals were also at increased risk for hospitalization during the 2009 pandemic. With the current H1N1 strain, elevated alkaline phosphatase, creatine kinase, creatinine, thrombocytopenia and metabolic acidosis suggest a poor prognosis. Purulent bronchitis and bronchiectasis may result in chronic pulmonary disease and fibrosis that persist throughout life. Most fatalities are due to bacterial pneumonia although exacerbations of other disease processes, in particular cardiac diseases, occur which contributed to the overall increase in fatalities. Pneumonia resulting from influenza has a high mortality rate among pregnant women and persons with a history of rheumatic heart disease. Mortality among adults hospitalized with influenza ranges from 4% to 8%, although higher mortality (greater than 10–15%) may be seen during pandemics and among immunocompromised individuals. An increase in mortality among the elderly in Europe from influenza was attributed to the return to pandemic status of H3N2 strains.

If the fever recurs or persists for more than 4 days with productive cough and white cell count over 10,000/mcL, secondary bacterial infection should be suspected. Pneumococcal pneumonia is the most common secondary infection, and staphylococcal pneumonia is the most serious.

▶ Prevention

Annual administration of influenza vaccine is the most effective measure for preventing influenza and its complications (Table 30–7). The main circulating seasonal influenza viruses that are the target of 2015–16 vaccines are an A/California/7/2009 (H1N1)pdm09-like virus, an A/Switzerland/9715293/2013 (H3N2)-like virus, and a B/Phuket/3073/2013-like virus (a B/Yamagata lineage virus),

with quadrivalent preparations also including a B/Brisbane/60/2008-like virus. For the Southern Hemisphere, recommendations include two differences: replacing the second A influenza strain and inverting the order of the B strains: an A/California/7/2009 (H1N1)pdm09-like virus, an A/Hong Kong/4801/2014 (H3N2)-like virus, and the B/Brisbane/60/2008-like virus (a B/Victoria-lineage virus), with use in the quadrivalent vaccines of a B/Phuket/3073/2013-like virus (a B/Yamagata-lineage virus).

Currently 12 vaccines are available for use in the United States. These include seven trivalent inactivated influenza vaccines (including one cell-culture based, one recombinant, one high-dose recommended for those 65 and older, and one adjuvanted vaccine also recommended for those 65 and older) and five quadrivalent influenza vaccines (four inactivated, one of which is given intradermally, and one live attenuated vaccine [LAIV] given intranasally) (Table 32–3). All vaccines contain antigens from one strain each of influenza A (H1N1), influenza A (H3N2), and influenza B. Persons with a history of egg allergy with hives only may receive inactivated influenza vaccine under close observation for adverse effects or trivalent recombinant influenza vaccine (RIV3 or FluBlok) for those 18 or older. For those with severe egg allergies, RIV3 can be administered in those age 18 or over. Administration in the deltoid is recommended for older children and adults, in the anterolateral thigh for children. Influenza vaccine recommendations can be found at http://www.cdc.gov/flu/professionals/vaccination/index.htm.

Chemotherapeutic regimens containing rituximab show persistent perturbations of B cell and Ig synthesis, and these modifications decrease humoral responses to the influenza vaccine.

The Advisory Committee on Immunization Practices (ACIP) and the American College of Obstetricians and Gynecologists' Committee recommend annual influenza vaccination for all persons over 6 months of age. In particular, vaccination is emphasized for women who will be pregnant through the influenza season (October through May with peak activity during December to March in the United States) with vaccination early in the season regardless of gestational age. No study to date has shown any major adverse consequence of inactivated influenza vaccine in pregnant women or their offspring.

Fluzone High-Dose is an FDA-approved trivalent influenza vaccine (TIV) containing four times more hemagglutinin than standard TIV and is recommended for persons age 65 or older. Fluzone intradermal trivalent vaccine (15 mcg hemagglutinin per strain given to those aged 18–64, with current data suggesting 60 mg is the appropriate dose) is an intradermal vaccine that is equally immunogenic and safe but more expensive than the traditional intramuscular vaccine (given to those over age 2 years). Fluad is the first seasonal influenza vaccine containing an adjuvant approved in the United States. It contains MF59®, an oil-in-water squalene oil emulsion, as an adjuvant and is recommended for persons 65 years and older.

The LAIV is available for use in healthy individuals between 2 and 49 years of age; it should not be given to asthmatic patients, pregnant women, or those who have

Table 32–3. Current influenza vaccination preparations available in the United States.

Trade name	Manufacturer	Presentation	Mercury (from thimerosal) mcg/0.5 mL	Ovalbumin mcg/0.5 mL	Age Indications	Latex	Route
Inactivated influenza vaccine, quadrivalent (IIV4), standard dose							
Contraindications*: Severe allergic reaction to any vaccine component, including egg protein, or after previous dose of any influenza vaccine.							
Precautions*: Moderate to severe acute illness with or without fever; history of Guillain-Barré syndrome within 6 weeks of receipt of influenza vaccine.							
Fluarix Quadrivalent	GlaxoSmithKline	0.5 mL single-dose prefilled syringe	—	≤ 0.05	≥ 3 yrs	No	IM†
FluLaval Quadrivalent	ID Biomedical Corp. of Quebec (distributed by GlaxoSmithKline)	5.0 mL multi-dose vial	< 25	≤ 0.3	≥ 3 yrs	No	IM†
Fluzone Quadrivalent	Sanofi Pasteur	0.25 mL single-dose prefilled syringe	—	§	6 through 35 mos	No	IM†
		0.5 mL single-dose prefilled syringe	—	§	≥ 36 mos	No	IM†
		0.5 mL single-dose vial	—	§	≥ 36 mos	No	IM†
		5.0 mL multi-dose vial	25	§	≥ 6 mos	No	IM†
Fluzone Intradermal¶ Quadrivalent	Sanofi Pasteur	0.1 mL single-dose prefilled microinjection system	—	§	18 through 64 yrs	No	ID**
Inactivated influenza vaccine, trivalent (IIV3), standard dose							
Contraindications*: Severe allergic reaction to any vaccine component, including egg protein, or after previous dose of any influenza vaccine.							
Precautions*: Moderate to severe acute illness with or without fever; history of Guillain-Barré syndrome within 6 weeks of receipt of influenza vaccine.							
Afluria	bioCSL	0.5 mL single-dose prefilled syringe	—	< 1	≥ 9 yrs††	No	IM†
		5.0 mL multi-dose vial	24.5	< 1	≥ 9 yrs†† via needle; 18 through 64 yrs via jet injector	No	IM†
Fluvirin	Novartis Vaccines and Diagnostics	0.5 mL single-dose prefilled syringe	≤ 1	≤ 1	≥ 4 yrs	Yes§§	IM†
		5.0 mL multi-dose vial	25	≤ 1	≥ 4 yrs	No	IM†
Fluzone	Sanofi Pasteur	5.0 mL multi-dose vial	25	§	≥ 6 mos	No	IM†
Inactivated influenza vaccine, cell-culture-based (ccIIV3), standard dose							
Contraindications*: Severe allergic reaction to any vaccine component, including egg protein, or after previous dose of any influenza vaccine.							
Precautions*: Moderate to severe acute illness with or without fever; history of Guillain-Barré syndrome within 6 weeks of receipt of influenza vaccine.							
Flucelvax	Novartis Vaccines and Diagnostics	0.5 mL single-dose prefilled syringe	—	¶¶	≥ 18 yrs	Yes§§	IM†
Inactivated influenza vaccine, trivalent (IIV3), high dose							
Contraindications*: Severe allergic reaction to any vaccine component, including egg protein, or after previous dose of any influenza vaccine.							
Precautions*: Moderate to severe acute illness with or without fever; history of Guillain-Barré syndrome within 6 weeks of receipt of influenza vaccine.							
Fluzone High-Dose***	Sanofi Pasteur	0.5 mL single-dose prefilled syringe	—	§	≥ 65 yrs	No	IM†

(continued)

Table 32–3. Current influenza vaccination preparations available in the United States.(continued)

Trade name	Manufacturer	Presentation	Mercury (from thi-merosal) mcg/0.5 mL	Ovalbumin mcg/0.5 mL	Age Indications	Latex	Route
Recombinant influenza vaccine, trivalent (RIV3), standard dose Contraindications*: Severe allergic reaction to any vaccine component. Precautions*: Moderate to severe acute illness with or without fever; history of Guillain-Barré syndrome within 6 weeks of receipt of influenza vaccine.							
Flublok	Protein Sciences	0.5 mL single-dose vial	—	0	≥ 18 yrs	No	IM†
Live attenuated influenza vaccine, quadrivalent (LAIV4) Contraindications*: Severe allergic reaction to any vaccine component, including egg protein, or after previous dose of any influenza vaccine. Concomitant use of aspirin or aspirin-containing medications in children and adolescents. In addition, ACIP recommends LAIV4 not be used for pregnant women, immunosuppressed persons, persons with egg allergy, and children aged 2 through 4 years who have asthma or who have had a wheezing episode noted in the medical record within the past 12 months, or for whom parents report that a health care provider stated that they had wheezing or asthma within the last 12 months. LAIV4 should not be administered to persons who have taken influenza antiviral medications within the previous 48 hours. Persons who care for severely immunosuppressed persons who require a protective environment should not receive LAIV4, or should avoid contact with such persons for 7 days after receipt. Precautions*: Moderate to severe acute illness with or without fever; history of Guillain-Barré syndrome within 6 weeks of receipt of influenza vaccine; asthma in persons aged 5 years and older; medical conditions that might predispose to higher risk for complications attributable to influenza.							
FluMist Quadrivalent†††	MedImmune	0.2 mL single-dose prefilled intranasal sprayer	—	< 0.24 (per 0.2 mL)	2 through 49 yrs	No	IN

ACIP, Advisory Committee on Immunization Practices; ID, intradermal; IM, intramuscular; IN, intranasal.

* Immunization providers should check Food and Drug Administration-approved prescribing information for 2015–16 influenza vaccines for the most complete and updated information, including (but not limited to) indications, contraindications, warnings, and precautions. Package inserts for U.S.-licensed vaccines are available at www.fda.gov/BiologicsBloodVaccines/Vaccines/ApprovedProducts/ucm093833.htm.

† For adults and older children, the recommended site for intramuscular influenza vaccination is the deltoid muscle. The preferred site for infants and young children is the anterolateral aspect of the thigh. Specific guidance regarding site and needle length for intramuscular administration may be found in the ACIP General Recommendations on Immunization, available at www.cdc.gov/mmwr/preview/mmwrhtml/rr6002a1.htm.

§ Available upon request from Sanofi Pasteur (1–800–822–2463 or MIS.Emails@sanofipasteur.com).

¶ Quadrivalent inactivated influenza vaccine, intradermal: a 0.1-mL dose contains 9 mcg of each vaccine antigen (36 mcg total).

** The preferred injection site is over the deltoid muscle. Fluzone Intradermal Quadrivalent is administered using the delivery system included with the vaccine.

†† Age indication per package insert is ≥5 years; however, ACIP recommends Afluria not be used in children aged 6 months through 8 years because of increased risk of febrile reactions noted in this age group with bioCSL's 2010 Southern Hemisphere IIV3. If no other age-appropriate, licensed inactivated seasonal influenza vaccine is available for a child aged 5 through 8 years who has a medical condition that increases the child's risk for influenza complications, Afluria can be used; however, providers should discuss with the parents or caregivers the benefits and risks of influenza vaccination with Afluria before administering this vaccine. Afluria may be used in persons aged ≥9 years.

§§ Syringe tip cap may contain natural rubber latex.

¶¶ Information not included in package insert. Estimated to contain <50 femtograms (5×10^{-8} mcg) of total egg protein (of which ovalbumin is a fraction) per 0.5 mL dose of Flucelvax.

*** Trivalent inactivated influenza vaccine, high-dose: a 0.5-mL dose contains 60 mcg of each vaccine antigen (180 mcg total).

††† FluMist is shipped refrigerated and stored in the refrigerator at 35°F–46°F (2°C–8°C) after arrival in the vaccination clinic. The dose is 0.2 mL divided equally between each nostril. Health care providers should consult the medical record, when available, to identify children aged 2 through 4 years with asthma or recurrent wheezing that might indicate asthma. In addition, to identify children who might be at greater risk for asthma and possibly at increased risk for wheezing after receiving LAIV, parents or caregivers of children aged 2 through 4 years should be asked: "In the past 12 months, has a health care provider ever told you that your child had wheezing or asthma?" Children whose parents or caregivers answer "yes" to this question and children who have asthma or who had a wheezing episode noted in the medical record within the past 12 months should not receive FluMist.

Reproduced with permission from Grohskopf LA et al. Prevention and control of influenza with vaccines: recommendations of the Advisory Committee on Immunization Practices, United States, 2015–16 Influenza Season. MMWR Morb Mortal Wkly Rep. 2015 Aug 7;64(30):818–25. [PMID: 26247435] taken neuraminidase inhibitors within the prior 48 hours. For children, the CDC no longer preferentially recommends the LAIV.

Among the HIV-infected and the elderly, preliminary data suggest that a quadruple-dose influenza vaccine is associated with higher seroconversion rates. Data are limited supporting particular protective efficacy in vaccinating those with end-stage renal disease, although annual vaccination continues to be recommended, with benefits present even with low rates of efficacy considering the high risks of influenza in this population.

The seasonal influenza vaccines can reduce influenza hospitalizations by an estimated 61%. Vaccine efficacy is greater by serologic indices of infection rather than clinical disease or days of work lost. New recombinant and cell culture vaccines are available for those with a hypersensitivity to chicken eggs or other components of the vaccine, although inactivated vaccines can safely be given to most patients with suspected egg allergies. Determination of the degree of egg allergy (only skin reactions or frank angioedema) as well as consultation with CDC sources and infectious disease physicians and allergists may be prudent in cases of severe egg allergy. Patients with significant egg allergies should be vaccinated only in physicians' (or for severe cases, allergists') offices.

Vaccination remains contraindicated for persons with a history of vaccine-associated Guillain-Barré syndrome, or in persons with an acute febrile illness until symptomatic improvement. Concomitant warfarin or corticosteroid therapy is not a contraindication to influenza vaccination. Statin therapy at the time of influenza vaccination may adversely affect vaccine effectiveness in the elderly. Side effects are infrequent and include tenderness, redness, or induration at the intramuscular site of the TIV and mild upper respiratory symptoms for the LAIV. There is great inequity globally in the distribution of influenza vaccine with only 3.7% of the vaccine available to the 47% of the population living in Africa, Eastern Europe, and Southeast Asia.

Chemoprophylaxis is considered for individuals who are unvaccinated, for those in whom vaccination is contraindicated, and in those exposed to an infected patient within 2 weeks after vaccination with TIV. Chemoprophylaxis is not necessary and is contraindicated for those vaccinated with the LAIV, since this vaccine confers more rapid protection. Other circumstances that warrant consideration of chemoprophylaxis include outbreaks in long-term–care facilities, persons living with or in close contact with high-risk individuals, persons with immune deficiencies who might not respond to vaccination, unvaccinated staff during response to an outbreak in a closed institutional setting with residents at high risk, and first responders to epidemic situations.

Winter school breaks during periods of high influenza transmission appear to decrease rates of visits to primary care practitioners for influenza illness among children and adults.

Chemoprophylaxis against influenza A and B is accomplished with a single daily dose of the neuraminidase inhibitors oseltamivir (75 mg/day, oral) or zanamivir (10 mg/day, inhaled). These agents reduce the attack rate among unvaccinated individuals if begun within 48 hours after exposure. The CDC recommends chemoprophylaxis for up to 10 days after exposure. For outbreak control in long-term–care facilities and hospitals, a minimum of 2 weeks is recommended, including in vaccinated persons, and until 1 week after identification of the last known case. Zanamivir should not be given as chemoprophylaxis to asthmatic persons, nursing home residents, or children under 5 years of age. A Cochrane review on the effects of usage and stockpiling of neuraminidase inhibitors showed that adverse effects of the agents might limit the cost-benefit balance of their usage. Attendant recommendations that question the use of these agents in both prophylaxis and treatment of influenza have been met with controversy.

Breakthrough infections with influenza occur with neuraminidase inhibitors (in a study with zanamivir) with vaccination. The efficacy of chemoprophylaxis is proven for individual and household but not community settings.

Hand hygiene and surgical facemasks appear to prevent household transmission of influenza virus isolates when implemented within 36 hours of recognition of symptoms in an index patient. Such nonpharmaceutical interventions assist in mitigating the spread of pandemic and interpandemic influenza to nonvaccinated persons. Patients with seasonal H1N1 influenza infection should be considered potentially infectious from 1 day before to about 7 days following illness onset. Children and immunosuppressed persons exhibit prolonged viral shedding and may be infectious longer.

Any hospital patient in whom the infection is suspected should be isolated in individual rooms with standard and droplet precautions. CDC guidelines recommend the equivalent of N95 masks for aerosol generating procedures (eg, bronchoscopy, elective intubation, suctioning, administering nebulized medications). For such procedures, an airborne infection isolation room can be used, with air exhausted directly outside or recirculated after filtration by a high efficiency particulate air (HEPA) filter. Strict adherence to hand hygiene with soap and water or an alcohol-based hand sanitizer and immediate removal of gloves and other equipment after contact with respiratory secretions is essential. Precautions should be maintained until 7 days from symptom onset or until symptom resolution, whichever is longer. Postexposure prophylaxis should be considered for close contacts of patients (confirmed, probable, or suspected) who are at high risk for complications of influenza as well as for healthcare personnel, public health workers, or first responders who experienced a recognized, unprotected close contact exposure to a person with influenza virus infection (confirmed, probable, or suspected) during that person's infectious period. The CDC continues to recommend considering postexposure prophylaxis with neuraminidase inhibitors to contacts of the infected person.

► **When to Admit**

- Limited availability of supporting services.
- Pneumonia or decreased oxygen saturation.
- Changes in mental status.
- Consider with pregnancy.

Black S et al. Influence of statins on influenza vaccine response in elderly individuals. J Infect Dis. 2016 Apr 15;213(8):1224–8. [PMID: 26516142]

Centers for Disease Control and Prevention (CDC). FluView: a weekly influenza surveillance report. http://www.cdc.gov/flu/weekly

Coleman BL et al. Zanamivir versus trivalent split virus influenza vaccine: a pilot randomized trial. Influenza Other Respir Viruses. 2015 Mar;9(2):78–84. [PMID: 25557838]

Grohskopf LA et al. Prevention and control of influenza with vaccines: recommendations of the Advisory Committee on Immunization Practices, United States, 2015–16 Influenza Season. MMWR Morb Mortal Wkly Rep. 2015 Aug 7;64(30):818–25. [PMID: 26247435]

Jefferson T et al. Neuraminidase inhibitors for preventing and treating influenza in healthy adults and children. Cochrane Database Syst Rev. 2014 Apr 10;4:CD008965. [PMID: 24718923]

Jin J. JAMA patient page. Influenza vaccine. JAMA. 2014 Oct 8; 312(14):1482. [PMID: 25291598]

Okoli GN et al. Use of neuraminidase inhibitors for rapid containment of influenza: a systematic review and meta-analysis of individual and household transmission studies. PLoS One. 2014 Dec 9;9(12):e113633. [PMID: 25490762]

Omer SB et al. Impact of statins on influenza vaccine effectiveness against medically attended acute respiratory illness. J Infect Dis. 2016 Apr 15;213(8):1216–23. [PMID: 26516141]

Remschmidt C et al. Influenza vaccination in patients with end-stage renal disease: systematic review and assessment of quality of evidence related to vaccine efficacy, effectiveness, and safety. BMC Med. 2014 Dec 19;12:244. [PMID: 25523432]

3. Avian Influenza (H5N1 & Analogs)

ESSENTIALS OF DIAGNOSIS

► Cases to date in humans, mostly from Southeast Asia and Egypt.

► Clinically indistinguishable from seasonal influenza.

► Epidemiologic factors assist in diagnosis.

► Rapid antigen assays confirm diagnosis but do not distinguish avian from seasonal influenza.

General Considerations

The normal hosts for avian influenza viruses are aquatic waterfowl. Although avian influenza was first recognized in Italy in 1878, the current outbreak of highly pathogenic influenza A subtype (H5N1) in poultry was recognized in 1997 in Hong Kong and was followed by the first documented human cases. A massive slaughter of poultry contained the disease. Outbreaks of H5N1 influenza in poultry reemerged in 2003 and now involve more than 65 countries of East and Southeast Asia, Eurasia, Western and Eastern Europe, Northern Africa, and Haiti. The 884 confirmed human cases as of October 15, 2015 include 449 deaths (51% of cases and 94% of deaths are reported from China, Cambodia, Egypt, Indonesia, Turkey, and Vietnam) (the details are maintained and updated by the Global Outbreak Alert and Response Network, WHO: http://www.who.int/influenza/human_animal_interface/EN_GIP_20151015cumulativeNumberH5N1cases.pdf?ua=1

Although highly contagious among birds, the transmission of this H5N1 strain from human-to-human is inefficient and not sustained although studies documented transmissibility of laboratory mutated virus via aerosols between ferrets. Evidence from cluster outbreaks suggests that host genetic susceptibility limits human-to-human transmission. The result is only rare cases of person-to-person infection. Occasional transmission to other mammals, including domestic cats and dogs, is also documented. Most human cases of H5N1 and analogous viruses occur after exposure to infected poultry or surfaces contaminated with poultry droppings. Because infection in humans is associated with a mortality rate greater than 50% and the avian H5N1 subtype continues to spread among birds (with many parts of Southeast Asia now considered endemic for the virus), there is worldwide concern that the virus may undergo genetic reassortment or mutation (as with the 1918 strain) and develop greater human-to-human transmissibility with the potential to produce a global pandemic.

Cases of H7 influenza viruses are sporadic and global and usually occur among poultry handlers. Infections with several of these H7 avian influenza viruses (H7N2, H7N3, and H7N7) have occurred in Australia, Canada, Italy, Mexico, the Netherlands, the United Kingdom, and the United States (New York). Cases of H7N9 are significantly reported from Canada, Taiwan, and Malaysia, with 571 to date, and associated with 212 deaths (a mortality of 37%). Unique characteristics were bilateral ground-glass opacities, lymphocytopenia, and thrombocytopenia. ARDS developed in patients who had underlying coexisting medical conditions. Person-to-person transmission was also documented. Rare cases of influenza H9N2, another poultry pathogen, are reported from Bangladesh, and human-to-human transmission of this pathogen is not documented. Poultry infected with H5N2 have been detected in 13 American states and with H5N8 in 2 states with most leading poultry-importing foreign countries having banned at least partially the importation of American poultry. Rates of bird-to-human transmission are low, although serologic data for H5 and H7 infection are high among poultry and slaughterhouse workers.

Clinical Findings

A. Symptoms and Signs

Distinguishing avian influenza from regular influenza is difficult. History of exposure to dead or ill poultry in the prior 10 days, recent travel to Southeast Asia or Egypt, or contact with known cases should be investigated. The symptoms and signs include fever and predominantly respiratory symptoms (cough and dyspnea), but a variety of other systems may be involved, producing headaches and gastrointestinal complaints in particular. Subclinical disease is relatively rare. With cytokines responsible for much of the pathology, prolonged febrile states and generalized malaise are common. Children are preferentially impacted. Respiratory failure is the usual cause of death.

B. Laboratory Findings

Current commercial rapid antigen tests are not optimally sensitive or specific for detection of H5N1 influenza but are still first-line diagnostic tests because of their widespread availability. Diagnostic yield can be improved by early collection of samples. More sensitive RT-PCR assays are available through many hospitals and state health departments. An initial negative result in the right clinical setting warrants retesting. Throat or lower respiratory swabs may provide higher yield of detection than nasal swabs. When highly pathogenic strains (eg, H5N1) are suspected, extreme care in the handling of these samples must be observed during preliminary testing. Positive samples must then be forwarded to the appropriate public health authorities for further investigations (eg, culture) in laboratories with the adequate level of biosafety (level 3).

► Treatment

Resistance of avian H5N1 influenza strains to amantadine and rimantadine is present in most geographic areas. Resistance to neuraminidase inhibitors (oseltamivir, zanamivir, and peramivir) can occur in avian (H5N1)-infected patients. The current first-line recommendation is to use the neuraminidase inhibitor oseltamivir, 75 mg orally twice daily for 5 days administered within 48 hours from onset of illness. Overall oseltamivir, by modeling, is associated with a 49% reduction in mortality from H5N1 infections. A higher dose (150 mg twice daily), longer duration (7–10 days), and possible combination therapy with amantadine or rimantadine (in countries where A [H5N1] viruses are likely to be susceptible to adamantanes) may be considered in patients with pneumonia or progressive disease, although in general the adamantanes are no longer recommended for influenza infections. Twice daily oseltamivir is also recommended for H7N9 influenza infections. Evidence of resistance to oseltamivir is reported. Although inhaled zanamivir is proven effective in treating seasonal influenza, no data of its efficacy against H5N1 strains are available. Zanamivir is recommended, intravenously, for patients not improving with oseltamivir after 2 days of treatment. Peramivir was used through an Emergency Use Act with the FDA during the 2009–2010 outbreak. It is now approved for treatment of seasonal influenza.

► Prevention

Postexposure prophylaxis with 75 mg of oseltamivir orally once daily for 7–10 days should be given to close contacts and considered for moderate contacts of documented cases of H5N1 and H7N9 influenza infections although human-to-human transmission appears to be limited. Personnel exposed to patients should be monitored for symptoms. Careful surveillance for human cases and prudent stockpiling of medications with establishment of an infrastructure for dissemination are essential modalities of control. Nonpharmacologic means of control include masks, social distancing, quarantine, travel limitations, and infrastructure development, particularly for emergency departments.

An adjuvanted human vaccine against H5N1 influenza is licensed by Sanofi Pasteur (but not marketed) in the United States with the government stockpiling supplies in the event of need. It appears to be only moderately immunogenic. Other vaccines are licensed by GlaxoSmithKline in Europe and CS Limited in Australia. Vaccine candidates include one made with an oil-in-water emulsion-based adjuvant that is highly immunogenic and well tolerated. A major concern with H5N1 vaccinology is the evolution of the virus in vaccinated poultry, especially in the endemic nations of Egypt and Indonesia, and the need to maintain current surveillance and update vaccine development should avian influenza become more pathogenic in humans. Seasonal and H5N1 vaccines in phase II studies can be given either combined or in sequence safely and without affecting immunogenicity. An intranasal H5N1 vaccine trial is under development. Prevention of exposure to avian influenza strains also includes hygienic practices during handling of poultry products, including hand washing and prevention of crosscontamination, as well as thorough cooking of poultry products (to 70°C). There is no risk of acquiring avian influenza through the consumption of cooked poultry products, although there is a risk associated with handling feathers or birds from endemic areas, and the US government bans the importation of poultry from infected areas. Culling of infected H7 poultry is difficult because most animals are asymptomatic.

Because the potential for pandemic influenza for many of the new reassortment viruses is not fully known, continued surveillance is essential, and stockpiling of vaccines, adjuvant, and medications (oseltamivir and zanamivir) is warranted at the public health level.

Gao HN et al. Clinical findings in 111 cases of influenza A (H7N9) virus infection. N Engl J Med. 2013 Jun 13;368(24):2277–894. [PMID: 23697469]

Herfst S et al. The future of research and publication on altered H5N1 viruses. J Infect Dis. 2012 Jun;205(11):1628–31. [PMID: 22454474]

Hsieh YH et al. Quantification of bird-to-bird and bird-to-human infections during 2013 novel H7N9 avian influenza outbreak in China. PLoS One. 2014 Dec 5;9(12):e111834. [PMID: 25479054]

Jhung MA et al; Centers for Disease Control and Prevention (CDC). Outbreaks of avian influenza A (H5N2), (H5N8), and (H5N1) among birds—United States, December 2014–January 2015. MMWR Morb Mortal Wkly Rep. 2015 Feb 6;64(4):111. [PMID: 25654614]

Qi X et al. Probable person to person transmission of novel avian influenza A (H7N9) virus in Eastern China, 2013: epidemiological investigation. BMJ. 2013 Aug 6;347:f4752. [PMID: 23920350]

Yang Y et al. Household transmissibility of avian influenza A (H7N9) virus, China, February to May 2013 and October 2013 to March 2014. Euro Surveill. 2015 Mar 12;20(10):21056. [PMID: 25788253]

4. Middle East Respiratory Syndrome–Coronavirus (MERS-CoV)

ESSENTIALS OF DIAGNOSIS

▶ Mild, moderate, or severe respiratory illness.

▶ Travel to endemic area, including Saudi Arabia, United Arab Emirates, Qatar, and Jordan, within 14 days before symptom onset.

▶ Contact with camels reported in many cases.

▶ Fever, cough, and dyspnea are most common symptoms.

▶ CDC can assist with real time-PCR using serum and lower and upper respiratory samples, or serology.

▶ No specific treatment available; mortality as high as 45%.

▶ General Considerations

Middle East respiratory syndrome (MERS) is a syndrome associated with a coronavirus similar to the cause of severe acute respiratory syndrome (SARS). Patients with MERS have had a history of residence or travel in the Middle East, in particular Saudi Arabia, or contact with such patients. The virus is probably transmitted through direct or indirect contact of mucous membranes with infectious respiratory droplets. The virus is shed in stool, but the role of fecal–oral transmission is unknown. The earliest cases were identified in 2012 in the Kingdom of Saudi Arabia, and 75% of all cases have occurred there. Additional cases from the Middle East have occurred in Iran, Jordan, Kuwait, Lebanon, Oman, Qatar, United Arab Emirates (UAE), and Yemen; in Africa, cases are reported from Algeria, Egypt, and Tunisia; from Europe, in Austria, France, Germany, Greece, Italy, the Netherlands, and the United Kingdom; from Asia in China, Malaysia, South Korea, Philippines, Thailand, and Turkey; and from North America in the United States. During 2015, a large outbreak began in South Korea from a single patient with travel history to multiple countries in the Middle East. As of October 25, 2015, this outbreak included 186 cases, including 36 deaths. As of October 25, 2015, 1599 laboratory-confirmed cases have been recognized worldwide with at least 574 deaths (36%). Among 163 laboratory-associated cases, as of May 2014, 138 (84%) were reported from the Kingdom of Saudi Arabia, although laboratory-associated cases also occurred in the UAE, Iran, Jordan, Lebanon, the Netherlands, and the United States.

Person-to-person transmission can occur within families; hospital-associated cases comprise 25% of cases. The median incubation period is 5.2 days (range, 2–13) with the mean age of 50 (range 9 months to 99 years) and 65% occurring among men. Over 90% of patients have an underlying medical condition, including diabetes mellitus (68%), hypertension (34%), or chronic heart or kidney disease. Those with diabetes, renal failure, chronic lung disease, or other immunocompromising conditions are considered to be at highest risk for severe disease.

Camels appear to be the principal reservoir, and several studies show that contact with dromedary herds of camels is greater among cases than controls. Raw camel milk is considered a potential source. Persons who work with camels are more likely to have antibody evidence of past infection.

▶ Clinical Findings

A. Symptoms and Signs

MERS is an acute respiratory syndrome, with the most common symptoms being fever (98%), cough (83%), and dyspnea (72%). Chills and rigors are common (87%). Gastrointestinal symptoms may occur with diarrhea being most common (26%), followed by nausea and abdominal pain, and may precede respiratory symptoms. Mild and asymptomatic cases have been reported.

B. Laboratory Findings and Imaging

Hematologic findings in the largest series to date include thrombocytopenia (36%), lymphopenia (34%), and lymphocytosis (11%). Moderate elevations in lactate dehydrogenase (49%), AST (15%), and ALT (11%) are recognized. Chest radiograph abnormalities are nearly universal and include increased bronchovascular markings, patchy infiltrates or consolidations, interstitial changes, opacities (reticular and nodular) as well as pleural effusions and total lung opacification. Ground-glass opacities and consolidation are most commonly seen. The findings mimic those of many other causes of pneumonia.

Serum serologies and RT-PCR are available through CDC (contact information below, on MMWR reference site). Highest viral loads are found in lower respiratory tract specimens, including bronchoalveolar lavage fluid, sputum, and tracheal aspirates. These samples are preferred for diagnosis. The CDC recommends sending lower respiratory tract specimens, nasopharyngeal and oropharyngeal swabs, and serum for testing. In confirmed cases, serial sample collection (perhaps every 2–4 days) from multiple sites is recommended to increase understanding of virus shedding kinetics. In cases in which symptom onset occurred more than 14 days prior and symptoms are ongoing, serum should be sent to the CDC for serologic testing and the above specimens should be sent for RT-PCR.

C. Case Definition

A patient with **severe illness** shows the following characteristics: fever (38°C, 100.4°F or higher) and pneumonia or ARDS (based on clinical or radiologic evidence); and **either** history of travel in or near the Arabian Peninsula (Bahrain, Iraq, Iran, Israel, Jordan, Kuwait, Lebanon, Oman, Palestinian territories, Qatar, Saudi Arabia, Syria, the United Arab Emirates (UAE), and Yemen) within 14 days before symptom onset; **or** close contact with a symptomatic traveler in whom fever and acute respiratory illness (not necessarily pneumonia) developed within 14 days after travelling in or near the Arabian Peninsula (above); **or** is a member of a cluster of patients with severe acute respiratory illness (eg, fever and pneumonia requiring hospitalization) of unknown etiology in which MERS-CoV is being evaluated, in consultation with state and local health departments.

In milder illness, patients have fever and symptoms of respiratory illness (not necessarily pneumonia; eg, cough, shortness of breath) and history of having close contact with a confirmed MERS case as well as a history of being in a healthcare facility (as a patient, worker, or visitor) within 14 days of symptom onset in a country or territory within the Arabian Peninsula in which recent healthcare-associated cases of MERS have been identified.

Of note, fever may not be present in certain patients, including the very young, elderly, immunosuppressed, or those taking certain medications.

▶ Complications

Respiratory failure is such a common complication that in a series from Saudi Arabia, 89% of patients required intensive care and mechanical ventilation. Patients with MERS-CoV appear to advance faster to respiratory failure than do those with SARS.

▶ Treatment

Respiratory support is essential. A small retrospective study found improved survival at 14 days with ribavirin and interferon-alpha but not at 28 days.

▶ Prognosis

The overall mortality rate of identified cases is about 45%. Advanced age is associated with a poor prognosis.

▶ Prevention

Isolation and quarantine of cases is authorized by CDC. Strict infection control measures are essential as well as care and management of household contacts and hospital workers engaged in the care of patients. Travelers to Saudi Arabia (including the many pilgrims to the holy sites) should practice frequent hand washing and avoid contact with those who have respiratory symptoms. Evaluation of patients with suspect symptoms within 14 days of return from Saudi Arabia is essential. Because health care workers engaged in procedures that involve contact with respiratory droplets are at risk, isolation of high-risk patients is essential, as are simple hygienic measures. Control measures, including quarantining in the home for high-risk exposed persons and the use of facemasks for preventing hospital-acquired infections, are important. Assisting public health authorities with case reporting and surveillance is essential.

Camel workers including slaughterhouse and market workers, veterinarians, and racing personnel should wear facial protection and protective clothing and practice good personal hygiene, including frequent hand washing after touching animals. Family members of such personnel

should not be exposed to work paraphernalia including clothing and shoes and workers should shower at the site of employment rather than the home. Avoid direct contact with camels (who may be asymptomatic but who can transmit the virus though nasal or ocular discharge, milk, urine, and feces). All infected animals should be kept off the market, including their meat products, and buried or destroyed.

MMWR and the WHO periodically update the infection control recommendations and the status of ongoing outbreaks.

Bialek SR et al; Centers for Disease Control and Prevention (CDC). First confirmed cases of Middle East respiratory syndrome coronavirus (MERS-CoV) infection in the United States, updated information on the epidemiology of MERS-CoV infection, and guidance for the public, clinicians, and public health authorities—May 2014. MMWR Morb Mortal Wkly Rep. 2014 May 16;63(19):431–6. Erratum in: MMWR Morb Mortal Wkly Rep. 2014 Jun 27;63(25):554. [PMID: 24827411]

Das KM et al. Acute Middle East respiratory syndrome coronavirus: temporal lung changes observed on the chest radiographs of 55 patients. AJR Am J Roentgenol. 2015 Sep; 205(3):W267–74. [PMID: 26102309]

Omrani AS et al. Ribavirin and interferon alfa-2a for severe Middle East respiratory syndrome coronavirus infection: a retrospective cohort study. Lancet Infect Dis. 2014 Nov; 14(11):1090–5. [PMID: 25278221]

World Health Organization. Middle East repiratory syndrome coronavirus (MERS-CoV): summary of current situation, literature update and risk assessment as of 7 July 2015. http://apps.who.int/iris/bitstream/10665/179184/2/WHO_MERS_RA_15.1_eng.pdf

ADENOVIRUS INFECTIONS

▶ General Considerations

At least 56 serotypes of adenovirus are described to date and divided into 7 subgroups A–G. About half of these subgroups produce a variety of clinical syndromes. Adenoviruses show a worldwide distribution and occur throughout the year. These infections are usually self-limited or clinically inapparent and occur most commonly among infants, young children, and military recruits. However, these infections may cause significant morbidity and mortality in immunocompromised persons, such as HIV-infected persons and COPD patients, as well as in patients who have undergone solid organ and hematopoietic stem cell transplantation or cardiac surgery or in those who have received cancer chemotherapy. A few cases of donor-transmitted adenoviral infection have been reported in past years. Adenoviruses, although a common cause of human disease, also receive particular recognition through their role as vectors in gene therapy.

▶ Clinical Findings

A. Symptoms and Signs

The incubation period is 4–9 days. Clinical syndromes of adenovirus infection, often overlapping, include the following. The **common cold** (Chapter 8) is characterized by rhinitis, pharyngitis, and mild malaise without fever. Conjunctivitis is often present. **Nonstreptococcal exudative pharyngitis** is characterized by fever lasting 2–12 days and accompanied by malaise and myalgia. **Lower respiratory tract infection** may occur, including bronchiolitis, suggested by cough and rales, or pneumonia. (Types 1, 2, 3, 4, and 7 commonly cause acute respiratory disease and atypical pneumonia; coinfections or serial infections are documented to occur.) Infections are especially severe in Native American children. Adenovirus type 14 is increasingly reported as a cause of severe and sometimes fatal pneumonia in those with chronic lung disease but is also seen in healthy young adults and military recruit outbreaks. Viral or bacterial coinfections occur with adenovirus in 15–20% of cases. **Pharyngoconjunctival fever** is manifested by fever and malaise, conjunctivitis (often unilateral), mild pharyngitis, and cervical adenitis. **Epidemic keratoconjunctivitis** (transmissible person-to-person, most often types 8 [and showing considerable variation by season], 19, and 37) occurs in adults and is manifested by bilateral conjunctival redness, pain, tearing, and an enlarged preauricular lymph node (multiple types may be involved in a single outbreak). Various outbreaks (types 3, 8, 19) were reported from four US states in 2008–2010. Keratitis may lead to subepithelial opacities (especially with the above types). **Acute hemorrhagic cystitis** is a disorder of children often associated with adenovirus type 11 and 21. **Sexually transmitted genitourinary ulcers and urethritis** may be caused by types 2, 8, and 37 in particular. Adenoviruses also cause **acute gastroenteritis** (types 40 and 41), **mesenteric adenitis, acute appendicitis,** and **intussusception**. Rarely, they are associated with encephalitis, meningitis, acute flaccid paralysis, and pericarditis. Adenovirus is commonly identified in endomyocardial tissue of patients with **myocarditis** and dilated cardiomyopathy. Risk factors associated with severity of infection include youth, chronic underlying infections, recent transplantation, and serotypes 5 or 21.

Hepatitis (type 5 adenovirus), **pneumonia,** and **hemorrhagic cystitis** (types 11 and 34) tend to develop in infected liver, lung, or kidney transplant recipients, respectively. Syndromes that may develop in hematopoietic stem cell transplant patients include hepatitis, pneumonia, hemorrhagic cystitis, tubulointerstitial nephritis, colitis, and encephalitis.

B. Laboratory Findings and Imaging

Antigen detection assays including direct fluorescence assay or enzyme immunoassay are rapid and show sensitivity of 40–60% compared with viral culture (considered the standard). Samples with negative rapid assays require PCR assays or viral cultures for diagnosis. Quantitative real-time rapid-cycle PCR is useful in distinguishing disease from colonization, especially in hematopoietic stem cell transplant patients. Multiplex nucleic acid amplification assays are increasingly used to test for multiple respiratory viruses simultaneously with increased sensitivity. Adenovirus differs from other viral and bacterial respiratory infections seen on chest CT imaging, appearing as a multifocal consolidation or ground-glass opacity without airway inflammatory findings.

▶ Treatment & Prognosis

Treatment is symptomatic. Ribavirin or cidofovir is used in immunocompromised individuals with occasional success, although cidofovir is attendant with significant renal toxicity. IVIG is also used in immunocompromised patients and can be used in combination with other therapies, but data are still limited. Reduced immunosuppression is often required. Adoptive immunotherapy with transfusion of adenovirus-specific T cells is being investigated and has been associated with improved mortality. Typing of isolates is useful epidemiologically and in distinguishing transmission from endogenous reactivation. Topical steroids or tacrolimus may be used to treat adenoviral keratoconjunctivitis. Complications of adenovirus pneumonia in children include bronchiolitis obliterans. Deaths are reported on occasion (eight in one season among the American military).

The control of epidemic adenoviral conjunctivitis is often difficult and requires meticulous attention to hand hygiene, use of disposable gloves, sterilization of equipment (isopropyl alcohol is insufficient, recommendations of manufacturers are preferred), cohorting of cases, and furloughing of employees.

Vaccines are not available for general use. Use of live oral vaccines containing attenuated type 4 and type 7 was reinstated in military personnel in 2013 and has been associated with significant decrease in adenoviral disease.

Centers for Disease Control and Prevention (CDC). Adenovirus-associated epidemic keratoconjunctivitis outbreaks—four states, 2008–2010. MMWR Morb Mortal Wkly Rep. 2013 Aug 16; 62(32):637–41. [PMID: 23945769]

Feucht J et al. Adoptive T-cell therapy with hexon-specific Th1 cells as a treatment of refractory adenovirus infection after HSCT. Blood. 2015 Mar 19;125(12):1986–94. [PMID: 25617426]

Huang YC et al. Adenovirus infection associated with central nervous system dysfunction in children. J Clin Virol. 2013 Aug; 57(4):300–4. [PMID: 23619053]

Lu MP et al. Clinical characteristics of adenovirus associated lower respiratory tract infection in children. World J Pediatr. 2013 Nov;9(4):346–9. [PMID: 24235068]

Radin JM et al. Dramatic decline of respiratory illness among US military recruits after the renewed use of adenovirus vaccines. Clin Infect Dis. 2014 Oct;59(7):962–8. [PMID: 24991024]

OTHER EXANTHEMATOUS VIRAL INFECTIONS

1. Erythrovirus (Parvovirus) Infections

Erythrovirus, formerly parvovirus B19, infects human erythroid precursor cells. It is quite widespread (by age 15 years about 50% of children have detectable IgG), and its transmission occurs through respiratory secretions and saliva, through the placenta (vertical transmission with 30–50% of pregnant women nonimmune), and through administration of blood products. The incubation period is 4–14 days. Chronic forms of the infection can occur. Bocavirus, another erythrovirus (parvovirus), is a cause of winter acute respiratory disease in children and adults.

► Clinical Findings

A. Symptoms and Signs

Erythrovirus (parvovirus B19) causes several syndromes and manifests differently in various populations.

1. Children—In children, an exanthematous illness ("fifth disease," erythema infectiosum) is characterized by a fiery red "slapped cheek" appearance, circumoral pallor, and a subsequent lacy, maculopapular, evanescent rash on the trunk and limbs. Malaise, headache, pruritus (especially on the palms and soles), and diarrhea (rarely) occur. Systemic symptoms and fever are mostly abated by the time of rash appearance. Eosinophilic cellulitis (Well syndrome) is also reported with parvovirus. Parvovirus is also one of the most common causes of myocarditis in childhood.

2. Immunocompromised patients—A transient aplastic crisis and pure red blood cell aplasia may occur. Bone marrow aspirates reveal absence of mature erythroid precursors and characteristic giant pronormoblasts. The parvovirus B19 gene is detected in 16–19% of acute leukemia and chronic myeloid leukemia patients.

3. Adults—A limited nonerosive symmetric polyarthritis that mimics lupus erythematosus and rheumatoid arthritis, which may in some cases be a type II mixed cryoglobulinemia, can develop in middle-aged persons (especially women) but can also occur in children. Rashes, especially facial, are less common in adults.

Chloroquine and its derivatives exacerbate erythrovirus (parvovirus)-associated anemia and are linked with significantly lower hematocrit in hospital admissions in malaria endemic areas. Rare reported presentations include myocarditis with infarction, constrictive pericarditis, chronic dilated cardiomyopathy, hepatitis, pneumonitis, neutropenia, thrombocytopenia, a lupus-like syndrome, glomerulopathy, CNS vasculitis, papular-purpuric "gloves and socks" syndrome, and a chronic fatigue syndrome. A subclinical infection is documented among patients with sickle cell disease. Other CNS manifestations of erythrovirus (parvovirus) include encephalitis, meningitis, stroke (usually in sickle cell anemia patients with aplastic crises), and peripheral neuropathy (brachial plexitis and carpal tunnel syndrome) with occasional chronic residua.

The symptoms of erythrovirus (parvovirus) infection can mimic those of autoimmune states such as lupus, systemic sclerosis, antiphospholipid syndrome, or vasculitis. The molecular mimicry of erythrovirus (parvovirus) to human cytokeratin and transcription factors engaged in hematopoiesis is the basis for theories that implicate erythrovirus (parvovirus) in the pathogenesis of these autoimmune states.

In pregnancy, premature labor, hydrops fetalis, and fetal loss are reported sequelae. Pregnant women with a recent exposure or with suggestive symptoms should be tested for the disease and carefully monitored if results are positive.

B. Laboratory Findings

The diagnosis is clinical (Table 32–2) but may be confirmed by either an elevated titer of IgM anti-erythrovirus (parvovirus) antibodies in serum or with PCR in serum or bone marrow. By the time common presenting symptoms manifest, in particular a rash or polyarthropathy in an immunocompetent patient, the viremia may have cleared but IgM antibodies are likely present. In immunocompromised patients, RT-PCR is the optimal test. Autoimmune antibodies (antiphospholipid and antineutrophil cytoplasmic antibodies) can be present and are thought to be a consequence of molecular mimicry. False-positive serologies also occur in the presence of recent IVIG and anti-B cell therapy. Assays on marrow tissue are indicated only if a marrow is deemed necessary for other hematologic reasons.

► Complications

Uncommon complications include the CNS diseases listed above, chronic hemolytic anemia, thrombotic thrombocytopenic purpuric syndrome, acute postinfectious glomerulonephritis, and hepatitis.

► Treatment

Treatment in healthy persons is symptomatic (nonsteroidal anti-inflammatory drugs are used to treat arthralgias, and transfusions are used to treat transient aplastic crises). In immunosuppressed patients including those infected with HIV, IVIG is very effective in the short-term reduction of anemia. Relapses tend to occur about 4 months after administration of IVIG. There is no reduction in encephalitic complications with IVIG. Intrauterine blood transfusion can be considered in severe fetal anemia, although such transfusions have been linked to impaired neurologic development.

► Prevention & Prognosis

Several nosocomial outbreaks are documented. In these cases, standard containment guidelines, including handwashing after patient exposure and avoiding contact with pregnant women are paramount.

The prognosis is generally excellent in immunocompetent individuals. In immunosuppressed patients, persistent anemia may require prolonged transfusion dependence. Remission of erythrovirus (parvovirus) infection in AIDS patients may occur with ART, though the immune restoration syndrome is also reported.

ARUP Consult. The physician's guide to laboratory test selection and interpretation: parvovirus B19. http://www.arupconsult.com/Topics/ParvovirusB19.html

Bihari C et al. Parvovirus B19 associated hepatitis. Hepat Res Treat. 2013;2013:472027. [PMID: 24232179]

Crabol Y et al; Groupe d'experts de l'Assistance Publique-Hôpitaux de Paris. Intravenous immunoglobulin therapy for pure red cell aplasia related to human parvovirus b19 infection: a retrospective study of 10 patients and review of the literature. Clin Infect Dis. 2013 Apr;56(7):968–77. [PMID: 23243178]

da Costa AC et al. Investigation of human parvovirus B19 occurrence and genetic variability in different leukaemia entities. Clin Microbiol Infect. 2013 Jan;19(1):E31–43. [PMID: 23167493]

Molina KM et al. Parvovirus B19 myocarditis causes significant morbidity and mortality in children. Pediatr Cardiol. 2013 Feb; 34(2):390–7. [PMID: 22872019]

Phan TG et al. New parvovirus in child with unexplained diarrhea, Tunisia. Emerg Infect Dis. 2014 Nov;20(11):1911–3. [PMID: 25340816]

Wolfromm A et al. Spectrum of adult Parvovirus B19 infection according to the underlying predisposing condition and proposals for clinical practice. Br J Haematol. 2015 Jul;170(2):192–9. [PMID: 25920561]

2. Poxvirus Infections

Among the nine poxviruses causing disease in humans, the following are the most clinically important: variola/vaccinia, molluscum contagiosum, orf and paravaccinia, and monkeypox.

1. Variola/vaccinia—Smallpox (variola) was a highly contagious disease associated with high mortality and disabling sequelae. Its manifestations include severe headache, acute onset of fever, prostration and a rash characterized by the uniform progression from macules to papules to firm, deep-seated vesicles or pustules. The synchronous progression in smallpox readily differentiates lesions from those of varicella (see also Chapter 6).

Complications of smallpox include bacterial superinfections (cellulitis and pneumonia), encephalitis, and keratitis with corneal ulcerations (risk factor for blindness). **Effective vaccination led to its global elimination by 1979 and routine vaccination stopped in 1985.** Despite the recommendation of destroying remaining samples of this virus, significant concern exists for the potential misuse of these repositories in military or terrorist activities.

Smallpox should be considered, in concordance with the CDC's Smallpox Response Plan (www.bt.cdc.gov/agent/smallpox/response-plan/index.asp), in any patient with fever and a characteristic rash (see above) for which other etiologies—such as herpes infections, erythema multiforme, drug reactions (eczema herpeticum may be differentiated from suspect smallpox by appropriate serologic stains), or other infections—are unlikely. One hundred and fifteen cases of vaccine-related disease from contact with a smallpox vaccinee in the United States between 2003 and 2011 (including sexual transmission) were reported. Two cases of vaccinia infection after contact with oral rabies animal baits (which uses the vaccinia vector) are reported. Patients with suspected infection should be placed in airborne and contact isolation and the official agency contacted (CDC Emergency Preparedness and Response Branch; 770-488-7100).

Cidofovir may be considered for treatment of poxviral conditions and intravenous human vaccinia immunoglobulin may be useful for vaccinia. In the event of accidental smallpox exposure, a guideline for the use of the three vaccinia-based smallpox vaccinations and their contraindications in immunosuppressive states, including HIV and atopic eczema, is available at http://www.cdc.gov/ncidod/monkeypox/treatmentguidelines.htm.

2. Molluscum contagiosum—Molluscum contagiosum may be transmitted sexually or by other close contact. It may occur also in an extensive form in children with genetic defects in dendritic and T cell migration (the DOCK8 [dedicator of cytokinesis] deficiency). The disease is manifested by pearly, raised, umbilicated skin nodules sparing the palms and soles. Keratoconjunctivitis can occur. There may be an association with atopic dermatitis or eczema. Marked and persistent lesions in AIDS patients respond readily to combination ART. Treatment options include destructive therapies (curettage, cryotherapy, cantharidin, and keratolytics, among others), immunomodulators (imiquimod, cimetidine, and *Candida* antigen), and antiviral agents (topical cidofovir is effective anecdotally in refractory cases and there is some efficacy suggested for a new lipid acyclic nucleoside phosphonate called CMX001, an agent used for other viral infections, including in particular CMV). No treatment is uniformly effective and multiple courses of therapy are often needed. There is anecdotal evidence that intralesional MMR vaccination may expedite resolution. Cryptococcal skin lesions can mimic molluscum contagiosum.

3. Orf and paravaccinia—Orf (contagious pustular dermatitis, or ecthyma contagiosa) and paravaccinia (milker's nodules) are occupational diseases acquired by contact with sheep and cattle, respectively. Household meat processing and animal slaughter have been implicated as nontraditional risk factors. A new poxvirus akin to parapoxviruses was reported in 2015 in two patients, from rural Tennessee and Missouri (the latter had also traveled to Tanzania). The use of nonporous gloves for persons with animal handling is recommended, especially if the persons are immunosuppressed.

4. Monkeypox—First identified in 1970, monkeypox is enzootic in the rain forests of equatorial Africa and presents in humans as a syndrome similar to smallpox. The incubation period is about 12 days, and limited person-to-person spread occurs. African mortality rates vary from 3% to 11% depending on the immune status of the patient. Secondary attack rates appear to be about 10%. The first community-acquired outbreak in the United States of monkeypox occurred in 2003 in Wisconsin and other states of the upper Midwest. African outbreaks have been reported from the Sudan and the Democratic Republic of Congo. The source appeared to be imported Gambian giant rats via consequent exposure of prairie dogs. Other susceptible animals include nonhuman primates, rabbits, and rodents. Confusion with smallpox and varicella occurs; however, both lymphadenopathy (seen in up to 90% of unvaccinated persons) and a febrile prodrome are prominent features in monkeypox infection. Distinguishing characteristics of the monkeypox rash are its deep seated and well-circumscribed nature, it appears at the same stage of development (unlike varicella but like smallpox), and is centrifugal (including the palms and soles). Suspected cases should be placed on standard, contact and droplet precautions; and local and state public health officials and the CDC should be notified for assistance with confirmation of the diagnosis (electron microscopy, viral culture, ELISA, PCR). Cidofovir is effective against monkeypox, and IVIG can be used in selected cases.

Other general precautions that should be taken are avoidance of contact with prairie dogs and Gambian giant rats (whose illness is manifested by alopecia, rash, and ocular or nasal discharge), appropriate care and isolation of those exposed within 3 prior weeks to such animals, and veterinary examination and investigation of suspect animals through health departments. Vaccinia immunization is effective against monkeypox and is recommended, if no contraindication exists (outlined above), for those involved in the investigation of the outbreak and for healthcare workers caring for those infected with monkeypox. Post exposure vaccination is also advised for documented contacts of infected persons or animals. US federal agencies currently prohibit the importation of African rodents.

5. A new orthopox virus—Two cases in the country of Georgia with a novel orthopox virus occurred in 2013 with a third diagnosed serologically from 2010. All cases had animal contact, cattle for two, and serologic data showed possible associations with rodents and shrews as well as cattle. None had been vaccinated for smallpox (routine smallpox vaccinations ceased before their births).

Centers for Disease Control and Prevention (CDC). Updated interim CDC guidance for use of smallpox vaccine, cidofovir, and vaccinia immune globulin (VIG) for prevention and treatment in the setting of an outbreak of monkeypox infections. http://www.cdc.gov/ncidod/monkeypox/treatmentguidelines.htm

Chen X et al. Molluscum contagiosum virus infection. Lancet Infect Dis. 2013 Oct;13(10):877–88. [PMID: 23972567]

Levy Y et al. Estimated size of the population at risk of severe adverse events after smallpox vaccination in Israel. Vaccine. 2012 Oct 19;30(47):6632–5. [PMID: 22963804]

Nougairede A et al. Sheep-to-human transmission of Orf virus during Eid al-Adha religious practices, France. Emerg Infect Dis. 2013 Jan;19(1):102–5. [PMID: 23260031]

Osadebe LU et al. Novel poxvirus infection in 2 patients from the United States. Clin Infect Dis. 2015 Jan 15;60(2):195–202. [PMID: 25301210]

Petersen BW et al. Clinical guidance for smallpox vaccine use in a postevent vaccination program. MMWR Recomm Rep. 2015 Feb 20;64(RR-02):1–26. [PMID: 25695372]

Vora NM et al. Human infection with a zoonotic orthopoxvirus in the country of Georgia. N Engl J Med. 2015 Mar 26;372(13):1223–30. [PMID: 25806914]

Wertheimer ER et al. Contact transmission of vaccinia virus from smallpox vaccinees in the United States, 2003–2011. Vaccine. 2012 Feb 1;30(6):985–8. [PMID: 22192851]

VIRUSES & GASTROENTERITIS

Viruses are responsible for at least 30–40% of cases of infectious diarrhea in the United States. These agents include rotaviruses; caliciviruses, including noroviruses such as Norwalk virus; astroviruses; enteric adenoviruses; and, less often, toroviruses, coronaviruses, picornaviruses (including the Aichi virus), and pestiviruses. Rotaviruses and noroviruses are responsible for most nonbacterial cases of gastroenteritis.

Rotaviruses are reoviruses with eight species and significant animal reservoirs. They are the leading worldwide cause of dehydrating gastroenteritis in young children and are associated with significant morbidity and mortality (an estimated 20,000 to 35,000 pediatric hospitalizations annually from rotavirus infection, a fall from 70,000 annually in 2006). Each year, about 400,000 children die of rotavirus infection worldwide. Children aged 6 months to 2 years are the most affected, although adults are affected occasionally as well. By age 5, virtually every child has been infected with this pathogen. The diverse set of rotaviruses (classified by glycoproteins and protease-sensitive proteins [G-type and P-type antigens] which segregate independently) results in a constellation of phenotypes although only about four of these are responsible for over 90% of disease. Rotavirus infections follow an endemic pattern, especially in the tropics and low-income countries, although they peak during the winter in temperate regions. The virus is transmitted by fecal-oral route and can be shed in feces for up to 3 weeks in severe infections. In outbreak settings (eg, daycare centers), the virus is ubiquitously found in the environment, and secondary attack rates are between 16% and 30% (including household contacts). Nosocomial outbreaks are reported.

The disease is usually mild and self-limiting. A 2- to 3-day prodrome of fever and vomiting is followed by non-bloody diarrhea (up to 10–20 bowel movements per day) lasting for 1–4 days. It is thought that rarely systemic disease occurs and rare reported presentations include cerebellitis and pancreatitis. Children with gastroenteritis are not routinely tested for rotavirus because the results do not alter treatment. If confirmatory testing is required, stool PCR is the most sensitive tool for diagnosing rotavirus. Antigen detection by enzyme immunoassay is another option. Oral and intravenous rehydration solutions are the primary treatment options, but effective adjunctive therapies include specific probiotics (eg, *Lactobacillus* GG or *Saccharomyces boulardii*), nitazoxanide, diosmectite, or racecadotril. Adjunctive therapies shorten the median duration of diarrhea and hospitalization. Local intestinal immunity gives protection against successive infection.

Two oral rotavirus vaccines are available in the United States: a live, oral, pentavalent human-bovine reassortment rotavirus vaccine (PRV, RotaTeq; to be given at 2, 4, and 6 months of age) and a live, oral attenuated monovalent human rotavirus vaccine (HRV, Rotarix; to be given at 2 and 4 months of age). The vaccines showed 85–98% efficacy against severe rotavirus gastroenteritis in trials based in the Americas and Europe. Reduced efficacy (50–64%) has been noted in studies conducted in Asia and Africa. One advantage of these vaccines is the evidence of heterotypic immunity (prevention against rotavirus strains not included in the vaccine). RotaTeq showed efficacy even with incomplete two-dose regimens. Contraindications include allergy to any of the vaccine ingredients, previous allergic reaction to the vaccine, and immunodeficiency. The risk of intussusception, which is far lower with this than earlier rotavirus preparations, is small (1:51,000 to 1:68,000 vaccinated infants) and is considered significantly lower than the risk associated with untreated rotavirus gastroenteritis. Vaccine coverage is inadequate in the United States for rotavirus (68% in the 2012 National Immunization Study), particularly among the poor. As of October 2015, national immunization programs of 79 countries include rotavirus vaccine.

Several other rotavirus vaccines are available throughout the world. Examples include live, oral vaccines such as Rotavin-M1 (approved in Vietnam in 2012) and RotaVac or the new Indian vaccine, 116E, which was approved in 2014.

Noroviruses, such as Norwalk virus (one of a variety of small round viruses divided into 5 genogroups and at least 34 genotypes), are major causes of severe diarrhea in adults and are recognized as the major cause of epidemic gastroenteritis (with food handlers largely responsible and associated foods most often leafy vegetables, fruits/nuts, and molluscs). They are responsible for a significant percentage of childhood hospitalizations for gastroenteritis in the developing world (15% in surveys from India, 31% from Peru) and about 13% of gastroenteritis-associated ambulatory visits in the United States. In the United States, noroviruses are responsible for over 90% of reported nonbacterial gastroenteritis outbreaks during cold weather intervals (hence the colloquial name "gastric flu").

Norovirus gastroenteritis is responsible for an estimated 800 deaths annually in the United States and 200,000 deaths globally. The efficacy of the rotavirus vaccination is increasing the percentage of gastroenteritis caused by norovirus. The noroviruses appear to evolve by antigenic drift (similar to influenza). While 90% of young adults show serologic evidence of past infection, no long-lasting protective immunity develops and reinfections are common.

Outbreak environments include long-term–care facilities (nursing homes in particular), restaurants, hospitals, schools, daycare centers, vacation destinations (including cruise ships), and military bases. Persons at particular risk are the young, the elderly, the institutionalized, and the immunosuppressed. A strain that began in Australia (GII.4 Sydney) is responsible for increasing proportions of US cases and is transmitted most often in long-term–care facilities. Although transmission is usually fecal-oral, airborne, person-to-person, and waterborne transmission are also documented. A short incubation period (24–48 hours), a short symptomatic illness (12–60 hours, but up to 5 days in hospital-associated cases and in children younger than 11 years), a high frequency (greater than 50%) of vomiting, and absence of bacterial pathogens in stool samples are highly predictive of norovirus gastroenteritis.

RT-PCR of stool samples is used for diagnostic and epidemiologic purposes. Several licensed multiple pathogen platform assays are available, but they are expensive and interpretation of the cause of illness in a given patient may be difficult. Treatment options are similar to rotavirus (see above) and rely mostly on oral and intravenous rehydration. Deaths are rare in the developed world, and the more common associated diseases are aspiration pneumonia, septicemia, and necrotizing enterocolitis.

A number of vaccines for norovirus are under development and all entail the use of Norwalk viral-like proteins (VLP).

Outbreak control for both **rotavirus and norovirus infections** include strict adherence to general hygienic measures. Despite the promise of alcohol-based sanitizers for the control of pathogen transmission, such cleansers may be relatively ineffective against the noroviruses compared with antibacterial soap and water, reinforcing the need for new hygienic agents against this prevalent group of viruses. Cohorting of sick patients, contact precautions for symptomatic hospitalized patients, exclusion from work of symptomatic staff until symptom resolution (or 48–72 h after this for norovirus disease), and proper decontamination procedures are crucial.

Aliabadi N et al; Centers for Disease Control and Prevention (CDC). Sustained decrease in laboratory detection of rotavirus after implementation of routine vaccination—United States, 2000–2014. MMWR Morb Mortal Wkly Rep. 2015 Apr 10; 64(13):337–42. [PMID: 25856253]

Anderson EJ. Time to begin a new chapter and expand rotavirus immunization. Clin Infect Dis. 2014 Oct;59(7):982–6. [PMID: 24944227]

Bhandari N et al; India Rotavirus Vaccine Group. Efficacy of a monovalent human-bovine (116E) rotavirus vaccine in Indian children in the second year of life. Vaccine. 2014 Aug 11; 32(Suppl 1):A110–6. [PMID: 25091663]

Gastañaduy PA et al. Burden of norovirus gastroenteritis in the ambulatory setting—United States, 2001–2009. J Infect Dis. 2013 Apr;207(7):1058–65. [PMID: 23300161]

Guarino A et al. European Society for Pediatric Gastroenterology, Hepatology, and Nutrition/European Society for Pediatric Infectious Diseases evidence-based guidelines for the management of acute gastroenteritis in children in Europe: update 2014. J Pediatr Gastroenterol Nutr. 2014 Jul;59(1): 132–52. [PMID: 24739189]

Lopman B et al; Centers for Disease Control and Prevention (CDC). Global burden of norovirus and prospects for vaccine development. 2015 Aug. http://www.cdc.gov/norovirus/downloads/global-burden-report.pdf

Payne DC et al. Norovirus and medically attended gastroenteritis in U.S. children. N Engl J Med. 2013 Mar 21;368(12):1121–30. [PMID: 23514289]

ENTEROVIRUSES THAT PRODUCE SEVERAL SYNDROMES

The most famous enterovirus, the poliomyelitis virus, is discussed above under Major Vaccine-Preventable Viral Infections. Other clinically relevant enteroviral infections are discussed in this section.

1. Coxsackievirus Infections

Coxsackievirus infections cause several clinical syndromes. As with other enteroviruses, infections are most common during the summer. Two groups, A and B, are defined either serologically or by mouse bioassay. There are more than 50 serotypes.

► Clinical Findings

A. Symptoms and Signs

The clinical syndromes associated with coxsackievirus infection are summer grippe; herpangina; epidemic pleurodynia; aseptic meningitis and other neurologic syndromes; acute nonspecific pericarditis; myocarditis; hand, foot, and mouth disease; epidemic conjunctivitis; and other syndromes.

1. Summer grippe (A and B)—A febrile illness, principally of children, summer grippe usually lasts 1–4 days. Minor symptoms of upper respiratory tract infection are often present.

2. Herpangina (A2–6, 10: B3)—There is sudden onset of fever, which may be as high as 40.6°C, sometimes with febrile convulsions. Other symptoms are headache, myalgia, and vomiting. The sore throat is characterized early by petechiae or papules on the soft palate that ulcerate in about 3 days and then heal. An outbreak in Taiwan with A2 was associated with herpangina and coincided with an enterovirus 71 (below) outbreak, characterized by hand, foot, and mouth disease. Dual A6/A10 outbreaks are reported from Europe. Treatment is symptomatic.

3. Epidemic pleurodynia (Bornholm disease) (B1–5)—Pleuritic pain is prominent. Tenderness, hyperesthesia, and muscle swelling are present over the area of diaphragmatic attachment. Other findings include headache, sore throat, malaise, nausea, and fever. Orchitis and aseptic meningitis occur in less than 10% of patients. Most patients are ill for 4–6 days.

4. Aseptic meningitis (A and B) and other neurologic syndromes—Fever, headache, nausea, vomiting, stiff neck, drowsiness, and cerebrospinal fluid lymphocytosis without chemical abnormalities may occur, and pediatric clusters of group B (especially B5) meningitis are reported. Focal encephalitis and transverse myelitis are reported with coxsackievirus group A. Disseminated encephalitis occurs after group B infection, and acute flaccid paralysis is reported with both coxsackievirus groups A and B. An outbreak of aseptic meningitis occurred in central China (Gansu Province) in 2008, with 85 cases reported of coxsackie A9 disease. Severe neonatal illnesses are reported with B1 infections, including encephalomyocarditis and neonatal deaths due to multiorgan failure.

5. Acute nonspecific pericarditis (B types)—Sudden onset of anterior chest pain, often worse with inspiration and in the supine position, is typical. Fever, myalgia, headache, and pericardial friction rub appear early and these symptoms are often transient. Evidence for pericardial effusion on imaging studies is often present, and the occasional patient has a paradoxical pulse. Electrocardiographic evidence of pericarditis is often present. Relapses may occur.

6. Myocarditis (B1–5)—Heart failure in the neonatal period secondary to in utero myocarditis and over 20% of adult cases of myocarditis and dilated cardiomyopathy are associated with group B (especially B3) infections.

7. Hand, foot, and mouth disease (A5, 6, 10, 12, and 16, B5)—This disease is sometimes epidemic and is characterized by stomatitis, a vesicular rash on hands and feet, nail dystrophies and onychomadesis (nail shedding). Enterovirus 71 is also a causative agent.

8. Epidemic conjunctivitis—As with enterovirus 70, the A24 variant of coxsackievirus is associated with acute epidemic hemorrhagic conjunctivitis in tropical areas with outbreaks reported in the last few years in southern China,

Pakistan, southern Sudan, the Comoros, Uganda, Cuba, and Thailand. It is also reported as a cause of corneal endothelitis after cataract surgery.

9. Other syndromes associated with coxsackievirus infections—These include rhabdomyolysis, fulminant neonatal hepatitis (occurs rarely), pancreatitis with concomitant hepatitis and myocarditis (A4), infant sepsis (A10), glomerulopathy (group B infections), onychomadesis (B1), neonatal hemophagocytic lymphohistiocytosis (B1), types 1 and 2 diabetes mellitus (mainly group B infections), and thyroid disease (group B4), although definitive causality is not established. A pathogenic role in primary Sjögren syndrome and acute myocardial infarction has also been proposed for group B coxsackievirus infections. A report of confirmed infective endocarditis due to coxsackievirus B2 in a patient with a prosthetic cardiac device suggests that viral etiologies of culture-negative infective endocarditis should be considered.

B. Laboratory Findings

Routine laboratory studies show no characteristic abnormalities. Neutralizing antibodies appear during convalescence. The virus may be isolated from throat washings or stools inoculated into suckling mice. Viral culture is expensive, labor intensive, and requires several days for results. A PCR test for enterovirus RNA is available and, although it cannot identify the serotype, appears to be useful, particularly in cases of meningitis.

▶ **Treatment & Prognosis**

Treatment is symptomatic. With the exception of meningitis, myocarditis, pericarditis, diabetes, and rare illnesses such as pancreatitis or poliomyelitis-like states, the syndromes caused by coxsackieviruses are benign and self-limited. Two controlled trials showed a potential clinical benefit with pleconaril for patients with enteroviral meningitis although the compassionate use of this medication has stopped. There are anecdotal reports of success with IVIG in severe disease. Coxsackie A16 and enterovirus 71 in outbreaks of hand, foot, and mouth disease can be controlled with 5 minutes of exposure to 3120 ppm sodium hypochlorite. Vaccine development for Coxsackie-associated hand, foot, and mouth disease is underway in China.

Abzug MJ. The enteroviruses: problems in need of treatments. J Infect. 2014 Jan;68(Suppl 1):S108–14. [PMID: 24119825]
Chansaenroj J et al. Epidemic outbreak of acute haemorrhagic conjunctivitis caused by coxsackievirus A24 in Thailand, 2014. Epidemiol Infect. 2015 Oct;143(14):3087–93. [PMID: 25824006]
Greninger AL et al. A novel outbreak enterovirus D68 strain associated with acute flaccid myelitis cases in the USA (2012–14): a retrospective cohort study. Lancet Infect Dis. 2015 Jun; 15(6):671–82. [PMID: 25837569]

2. Echovirus Infections

Echoviruses are enteroviruses that produce several clinical syndromes, particularly in children. Infection is most common during summer. Among reported specimens, death ensues in about 3%. Males younger than 20 years are more commonly infected than other persons.

Over 30 serotypes of echoviruses are recognized and the most common serotypes for disease are types 6, 9, 11, and 30. Most can cause aseptic meningitis, which may be associated with a rubelliform rash. Transmission is primarily fecal–oral. Handwashing is an effective control measure in outbreaks of aseptic meningitis. Outbreaks related to fecal contamination of water sources, including drinking water and swimming and bathing pools, were reported in the past.

Besides meningitis, other conditions associated with echoviruses range from common respiratory diseases (bronchiolitis occurs often in children) and epidemic diarrhea to myocarditis, a hemorrhagic obstetric syndrome, keratoconjunctivitis, severe hepatitis with coagulopathy, leukocytoclastic vasculitis, and neonatal as well as adult cases of encephalitis and sepsis, interstitial pneumonitis, pleurodynia, hemophagocytic syndromes (in children with cancer), sudden deafness, encephalitis, acute flaccid paralysis (a current leading cause in India), optic neuritis, uveitis, and septic shock. Echoviruses and enteroviruses are also a common cause of nonspecific exanthems.

As with other enterovirus infections, diagnosis is best established by correlation of clinical, epidemiologic, and laboratory evidence. Cytopathic effects are produced in tissue culture after recovery of virus from throat washings, blood, or cerebrospinal fluid. An enterovirus PCR of the cerebrospinal fluid can assist in the diagnosis and is associated with a shorter duration of hospitalization in febrile neonates. Fourfold or greater rises in antibody titer signify systemic infection.

Treatment is usually symptomatic, and the prognosis is excellent, though there are reports of mild paralysis after CNS infection. In vitro data suggest some role for amantadine or ribavirin but clinical studies supporting these findings are not available.

From a public health standpoint, clustered illnesses such as swimming in sewage-infested seawater in travelers suggest point-source exposure. Prevention of fecal–oral contamination and maintenance of pool hygiene through chlorination and pH control are important public health control measures.

Maan HS et al. Genetic variants of echovirus 13, northern India, 2010. Emerg Infect Dis. 2013 Feb;19(2):293–6. [PMID: 23343581]

Su T et al. Molecular characterization of a new human echovirus 11 isolate associated with severe hand, foot, and mouth disease in Yunnan, China, in 2010. Arch Virol. 2015 Sep;160(9):2343–7. [PMID: 26100404]

3. Enteroviruses 68, 70, 71, & Related Agents

Several distinct clinical syndromes are being described in association with enteroviruses.

Enterovirus 68 (EV-D68) is a unique enterovirus that shares epidemiologic characteristics with human rhinovirus and is typically associated with respiratory illness. Several clusters are reported from the Netherlands, Japan, the Philippines, the United States, and Thailand. An outbreak was reported during August 2014–January 2015, with 1153 cases reported from 49 states. Respiratory illness was caused by EV-D68. The outbreak was also associated with cases of acute flaccid myelitis but not definitively linked thus far. The agent is implicated also in aseptic meningitis, and encephalitis.

Enterovirus 70 (EV-70), a ubiquitous agent first identified in 1969 and responsible for abrupt bilateral eye discharge and subconjunctival hemorrhage with occasional systemic symptoms, is most commonly associated with acute hemorrhagic conjunctivitis. Enterovirus infection of the pancreas can trigger cell-mediated autoimmune destruction of beta cells resulting in diabetes. Enterovirus myocarditis can be a serious infection in neonates, complicated by cardiac dysfunction and arrhythmias.

Enterovirus 71 (EV-71) almost always occurs in the Asia-Pacific region and is associated with hand, foot, and mouth disease (HFMD), which can be severe or even fatal, herpangina as well as a form of epidemic encephalitis associated on occasion with pulmonary edema, and acute flaccid paralysis often mimicking poliomyelitis. A recombinant virus (between EV-71 and coxsackievirus A16) caused an outbreak of HFMD in Fuyang China in 2008. In Taiwan, 29% of EV-71 in children is asymptomatic. There is an association reported between gastrointestinal enterovirus infection and type 1 diabetes.

Human enteroviruses are neurotropic. They may have a role in amyotropic lateral sclerosis. EV-68 has been reported in a case of fatal meningitis/encephalitis.

Mortality is especially high in enterovirus 71-associated brainstem encephalitis, which is often complicated by pulmonary edema, particularly when it occurs in children younger than 5 years. A complication is autonomic nervous system dysregulation, which may develop prior to the pulmonary edema. Because of lower herd immunity, HFMD tends to infect the very young (under age 5) in nonendemic areas. Disease is usually more severe and sequelae more common than with other enteroviruses. Some children with enterovirus-associated cardiopulmonary failure require the usage of extracorporeal life support, which can improve the outcome. Recognized sequelae include central hypoventilation, dysphagia, and limb weakness.

Clinical and epidemiologic findings aided by isolation of the suspect agent from conjunctival scraping for enterovirus 70; vesicle swabs, body secretions, or cerebrospinal fluid for enterovirus 71; and respiratory secretions for D68 facilitate diagnosis of these enteroviral entities. Enzyme immunoassays and complement fixation tests show good specificity but poor sensitivity (less than 80%). RT-PCR may increase the detection rate in enterovirus infections and is useful in the analysis of cerebrospinal fluid samples among patients with meningitis and of blood samples among infants with a sepsis-like illness.

Treatment of these entities remains largely symptomatic. There is anecdotal success in managing myocarditis with immunoglobulins. The major complication associated with enterovirus 70 is the rare development of an acute neurologic illness with motor paralysis akin to poliomyelitis. Attention-deficit with hyperactivity occurs in about

20% with confirmed infection. Treatment of acute flaccid paralysis related to enterovirus 71 with IVIG does not appear to improve neurologic outcomes.

EV-D68 requires supportive care with particular attention to respiratory support. The CDC's National Enterovirus Surveillance System should receive reports of disease at wnix@cdc.gov.

Household contacts, especially children under 6 months of age, are at particular risk for enterovirus 71 acquisition. A commercial disinfectant, Virkon S, at 1–2% application, appears to reduce infectivity titers. A stage-based supportive treatment for enterovirus 71 infections, recognizing the potential for late onset CNS disease and cardiopulmonary failure is important. There is no commercial EV-71 vaccine in the United States although vaccines produced in China appear to be successful against EV-71–associated hand, foot, and mouth disease and herpangina. Decreases in antibody titers suggest booster doses of these vaccines may be needed.

Enterovirus 72 (EV-72) is another term for hepatitis A virus (see Chapter 16). Enterovirus EV-104A is related to rhinoviruses and associated with respiratory illness in reports from Italy and Switzerland.

Greninger AL et al. A novel outbreak enterovirus D68 strain associated with acute flaccid myelitis cases in the USA (2012–14): a retrospective cohort study. Lancet Infect Dis. 2015 Jun; 15(6):671–82. [PMID: 25837569]

Lee HF et al. Enterovirus 71 infection-associated acute flaccid paralysis: a case series of long-term neurologic follow-up. J Child Neurol. 2014 Oct;29(10):1283–90. [PMID: 24453152]

Messacar K et al. A cluster of acute flaccid paralysis and cranial nerve dysfunction temporally associated with an outbreak of enterovirus D68 in children in Colorado, USA. Lancet. 2015 Apr 25;385(9978):1662–71. [PMID: 25638662]

Midgley CM et al. Severe respiratory illness associated with enterovirus D68—Missouri and Illinois, 2014. MMWR Morb Mortal Wkly Rep. 2014 Sep 12;63(36):798–9. [PMID: 25211545]

Tan CW et al. Recent developments in antiviral agents against enterovirus 71 infection. J Biomed Sci. 2014 Feb 12;21:14. [PMID: 24521134]

Zhu F et al. Efficacy, safety, and immunogenicity of an enterovirus 71 vaccine in China. N Engl J Med. 2014 Feb 27;370(9):818–28. [PMID: 24571754]

4. Human Parechovirus Infection (HPeV)

HPeV is one of six members of the Picornaviridae family that cause disease in humans. The pathogen mainly affects small children during the summer and early fall, although disease can also occur in older adults. Cases are reported worldwide, and 16 genotypes are recognized. During 2009–2013, HPeV3 was most commonly reported among isolates in the United States. Clinical presentation is mainly driven by gastrointestinal and respiratory illness, although otitis, neonatal sepsis, flaccid paralysis, myalgias, diffuse maculopapular and palmar-plantar rashes, aseptic meningitis, and encephalitis are described in the literature.

Screening with a human parechovirus-specific PCR provides a significant increase in determining the viral cause of neonatal sepsis or CNS symptoms in children younger than 5 years but is not widely performed. Human parechoviruses are one of the leading causes of viral sepsis and meningitis in young children. HPeV1 is the most prevalent genotype found among stool and nasopharyngeal samples in children (under 2 years old) but may particularly cause severe disease among neonates. HPeV6 affects individuals older than 20 years. HPeV3 is responsible for meningitis/encephalitis, neonatal sepsis, and was reported in association with necrotizing enterocolitis and hepatitis. It is the most prevalent picornavirus type found in cerebrospinal fluid samples of CNS-related infections in very young children. Cerebrospinal fluid parameters may be normal. CNS infection may be seen with HPeV4 as well. Respiratory and gastrointestinal illnesses are seen with types HPeV4–HPeV6, HPeV10, HPeV13-HPeV15. Neonatal deaths are reported with HPeV3 and HPeV6.

Treatment is largely supportive and rapid identification of the viral antigen by PCR in stools, respiratory samples, and cerebrospinal fluid may decrease use of unnecessary antibiotics and shorten hospital stay, although current PCR assays are not always sufficiently sensitive to exclude parechoviruses. Intravenous immunoglobulin was anecdotally successful in one case of parechovirus dilated cardiomyopathy. Reported complications of neonatal cerebral infections include learning disabilities, epilepsy, and cerebral palsy.

Abedi GR et al. Enterovirus and human parechovirus surveillance—United States, 2009–2013. MMWR Morb Mortal Wkly Rep. 2015 Sep 4;64(34):940–3. [PMID: 26334674]

Kolehmainen P et al. Human parechovirus type 3 and 4 associated with severe infections in young children. Pediatr Infect Dis J. 2014 Nov;33(11):1109–13. [PMID: 25361406]

Wildenbeest JG et al. Clinical relevance of positive human parechovirus type 1 and 3 PCR in stool samples. Clin Microbiol Infect. 2014 Oct;20(10):O640–7. [PMID: 24438366]

▼ RICKETTSIAL DISEASES

TYPHUS GROUP

1. Epidemic Louse-Borne Typhus

 ESSENTIALS OF DIAGNOSIS

- ▸ Prodrome of headache, then chills and fever.
- ▸ Severe, intractable headaches, prostration, persisting high fever.
- ▸ Macular rash appearing on the fourth to seventh days on the trunk and in the axillae, spreading to the rest of the body but sparing the face, palms, and soles.
- ▸ Diagnosis confirmed by specific antibodies using complement fixation, microagglutination, or immunofluorescence.

▸ General Considerations

Epidemic louse-borne typhus is caused by *Rickettsia prowazekii*, an obligate parasite of the body louse *Pediculus humanus corporis* (Table 32–4). Transmission is favored by

Table 32–4. Rickettsial diseases.

Disease	Rickettsial Pathogen	Geographic Areas of Prevalence	Insect Vector	Mammalian Reservoir	Travel Association
Typhus group					
Epidemic (louse-borne) typhus	*Rickettsia prowazekii*	South America, Northeastern and Central Africa	Louse	Humans, flying squirrels	Rare
Endemic (murine) typhus	*Rickettsia typhi*	Worldwide; small foci (United States: southeastern Gulf coast)	Flea	Rodents, opossums	Often
Scrub typhus group					
Scrub typhus	*Orientia tsutsugamushi*	Southeast Asia, Japan, Australia, Western Siberia	Mite[1]	Rodents	Often
Spotted fever group					
Rocky Mountain spotted fever	*Rickettsia rickettsii*	Western Hemisphere; United States (especially mid-Atlantic coast region)	Tick[1]	Rodents, dogs, porcupines	Rare
California flea rickettsiosis	*Rickettsia felis*	Worldwide	Flea	Cats, opossums	
Mediterranean spotted fever, Boutonneuse fever, Kenya tick typhus, South African tick fever, Indian tick typhus	*Rickettsia conorii*	Africa, India, Mediterranean regions	Tick[1]	Rodents, dogs	Often
Queensland tick typhus	*Rickettsia australis*	Eastern Australia	Tick[1]	Rodents, marsupials	Rare
Siberian Asian tick typhus	*Rickettsia sibirica*	Siberia, Mongolia	Tick[1]	Rodents	Rare
African tick bite fever	*Rickettsia africae*	Rural sub-Saharan Africa, Eastern Caribbean	Tick[1]	Cattle	Often
Lymphangitis associated rickettsiosis	*R sibirica mongolitimonae*	Europe, Africa, Mongolia	Tick[1]	Unknown	Unknown
Tick-borne lymphadenopathy/Dermacentor-borne necrosis erythema lymphadenopathy/scalp eschar neck lymphadenopathy	*R slovaca, R raoultii, Candidatus R rioja*	Europe	Tick	Unknown	Occasional
Rickettsialpox	*Rickettsia akari*	United States, Korea, former USSR	Mite[1]	Mice	Occasional
Other					
Ehrlichiosis and anaplasmosis, human Monocytic	*Ehrlichia chaffeensis, Anaplasma equi, Ehrlichia canis*	Southeastern United States	Tick[1]	Dogs	Occasional
Granulocytic	*Anaplasma phagocytophilum, Ehrlichia ewingii*	Northeastern United States	Tick[1]	Rodents, deer, sheep	Occasional
Q fever	*Coxiella burnetii*	Worldwide	None[2]	Cattle, sheep, goats	Occasional

[1]Also serve as arthropod reservoirs by maintaining rickettsiae through transovarian transmission.
[2]Human infection results from inhalation of dust.

crowded, unsanitary living conditions, famine, war, or any circumstances that predispose to heavy infestation with lice. After biting a person infected with *R prowazekii*, the louse becomes infected by the organism, which persists in the louse gut and is excreted in its feces. When the same louse bites an uninfected individual, the feces gain entry into the bloodstream when the person scratches the itching wound. Dry, infectious louse feces may also enter via the respiratory tract. Cases can be acquired by travel to pockets of infection (eg, central and northeastern Africa, Central and South America). Outbreaks have been reported from Peru, Burundi, and Russia. Because of aerosol transmissibility,

R prowazekii is considered a possible bioterrorism agent. In the United States, cases occur among the homeless, refugees, and the unhygienic, most often in the winter.

R prowazekii can survive in lymphoid and adipose (in endothelial reservoirs) tissues after primary infection, and years later, produce recrudescence of disease (**Brill-Zinsser disease**) without exposure to infected lice. This phenomenon can serve as a point source for future outbreaks.

An extrahuman reservoir of *R prowazekii* in the United States is flying squirrels, *Glaucomys volans*. Transmission to humans can occur through their ectoparasites, usually causing atypical mild disease. A case of recrudescent (Brill-Zinsser) disease 11 years after disease acquired by contact with flying squirrels is reported. Foci of sylvatic typhus are found in the eastern United States and are reported to occur in Brazil, Ethiopia, and Mexico.

▶ Clinical Findings

A. Symptoms and Signs

(Table 32–2). Prodromal malaise, cough, headache, backache, arthralgia, and chest pain begin after an incubation period of 10–14 days, followed by an abrupt onset of chills, high fever, and prostration, with flu-like symptoms progressing to delirium and stupor. The headache is severe and the fever is prolonged.

Other findings consist of conjunctivitis, mild vitritis, retinal lesions, optic neuritis, and hearing loss from neuropathy of the eighth cranial nerve, flushed facies, rales at the lung bases, abdominal pain, myalgias, and often splenomegaly. A macular rash (that may become confluent) appears first in the axillae and then over the trunk, spreading to the extremities but rarely involving the face, palms, or soles. In severely ill patients, the rash becomes hemorrhagic, and hypotension becomes marked. There may be acute kidney injury, stupor, seizures, and delirium. Improvement begins 13–16 days after onset with a rapid drop of fever and typically a spontaneous recovery.

B. Laboratory Findings

The white blood cell count is variable. Thrombocytopenia, elevated liver enzymes, proteinuria and hematuria commonly occur. Serum obtained 5–12 days after onset of symptoms usually shows specific antibodies for *R prowazekii* antigens as demonstrated by complement fixation, microagglutination, or immunofluorescence. In primary rickettsial infection, early antibodies are IgM; in recrudescence (Brill-Zinsser disease), early antibodies are predominantly IgG. A PCR test exists, but its availability is limited. *R prowazekii* is differentiated into 7 genotypes.

C. Imaging

Radiographs of the chest may show patchy consolidation.

▶ Differential Diagnosis

The prodromal symptoms and the early febrile stage lack enough specificity to permit diagnosis in nonepidemic situations. The rash is sufficiently distinctive for diagnosis, but it may be absent in up to 50% of cases or may be difficult to observe in dark-skinned persons. A variety of other acute febrile diseases should be considered, including typhoid fever, meningococcemia, and measles.

▶ Complications

Pneumonia, thromboses, vasculitis with major vessel obstruction and gangrene, circulatory collapse, myocarditis, and uremia may occur.

▶ Treatment

Treatment consists of either doxycycline (100 mg orally twice daily) or chloramphenicol (50–100 mg/kg/day in four divided doses, orally or intravenously) for 4–10 days. Chloramphenicol is considered less effective than doxycycline, but it is still the drug of choice in pregnancy. In epidemic conditions, a single dose of doxycycline can be effective and is less costly.

▶ Prognosis

The prognosis depends greatly on the patient's age and immune status. In children under age 10 years, the disease is usually mild. The mortality rate is 10% in the second and third decades but in the past reached 60% in the sixth decade. Brill-Zinsser disease has a more gradual onset than primary *R prowazekii* infection, fever and rash are of shorter duration, and the disease is milder and rarely fatal.

▶ Prevention

Prevention consists of louse control with insecticides, particularly by applying chemicals to clothing or treating it with heat, and frequent bathing.

A deloused and bathed typhus patient is not infectious. The disease is not transmitted from person to person. Patients are infectious from the lice during the febrile period and perhaps 2–3 days after the fever returns to normal. Infected lice pass rickettsiae in their feces within 2–6 days after the blood meal and can be infectious earlier if crushed. Rickettsiae remain viable in a dead louse for weeks.

No vaccine is available for the prevention of *R prowazekii* infection.

Badiaga S et al. Human louse-transmitted infectious diseases. Clin Microbiol Infect. 2012 Apr;18(4):332–7. [PMID: 22360386]

Sahni SK et al. Recent molecular insights into rickettsial pathogenesis and immunity. Future Microbiol. 2013 Oct;8(10):1265–88. [PMID: 24059918]

2. Endemic Flea-Borne Typhus (Murine Typhus)

Rickettsia typhi, a ubiquitous pathogen recognized on all continents, is transmitted from rat to rat through the rat flea (Table 32–4). Serosurveys of animals show high prevalence of antibodies to *R typhi* in opossums, followed by dogs and cats. Humans usually acquire the infection in an urban or suburban setting when bitten by an infected flea, which releases infected feces while sucking blood. Rare human cases in the developed world follow travel, usually

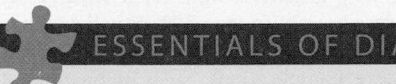

to Southeast Asia (in Bangladesh 67% of patients with febrile illness in one series showed IgM seropositivity), Africa (Burundi and Ethiopia have foci of infection), or the Mediterranean area although other pockets of infection are also known to occur in the Andes and the Yucatán. In the United States, cases are mainly reported from Texas and Southern California.

Endemic typhus resembles recrudescent epidemic typhus in that it has a gradual onset, less severe symptoms, and a shorter duration of illness than epidemic typhus (7–10 days versus 14–21 days). The presentation is nonspecific, including fever, headache, and chills. Maculopapular rash occurs in around 50% of cases; it is concentrated on the trunk and fades fairly rapidly. Liver dysfunction occurs in the majority of cases. Peripheral facial paralysis and splenic infarction are reported to occur. Severe disease with mental confusion and signs of hepatic, cardiac, renal, and pulmonary involvement may develop. Postinfectious optic neuritis is rare and may occur weeks after successful treatment. Rare complications include a respiratory distress syndrome and a hemophagocytosis syndrome. Jaundice, bradycardia, and the absence of a headache are correlated with a delayed defervescence (in both epidemic and endemic typhus).

The most common entity in the differential diagnosis is Rocky Mountain spotted fever, usually occurring after a rural exposure and with a different rash (centripetal versus centrifugal for epidemic or endemic typhus). Serologic confirmation may be necessary for differentiation, with complement-fixing or immunofluorescent antibodies detectable within 15 days after onset, with specific *R typhi* antigens. A fourfold rise in serum antibody titers between the acute and the convalescent phase is diagnostic.

Antibiotic treatment is the same as for epidemic typhus (see above). Ciprofloxacin (500–750 mg orally twice a day) and ampicillin (500 mg orally three times a day) are reportedly successful in pregnant women. Mortality is usually low with (1%) or without (4%) appropriate antibiotics. Preventive measures are directed at control of rats and ectoparasites (rat fleas) with insecticides, rat poisons, and rat-proofing of buildings.

Anyfantakis D et al. Liver function test abnormalities in murine typhus in Greece: a retrospective study of 165 cases. Infez Med. 2013 Sep;21(3):207–10. [PMID: 24008853]

Badiaga S et al. Murine typhus in the homeless. Comp Immunol Microbiol Infect Dis. 2012 Jan;35(1):39–43. [PMID: 22093517]

Blanton LS et al. Reemergence of murine typhus in Galveston, Texas, USA, 2013. Emerg Infect Dis. 2015 Mar;21(3):484–6. [PMID: 25695758]

Maude RR et al. Serosurveillance of *Orientia tsutsugamushi* and *Rickettsia typhi* in Bangladesh. Am J Trop Med Hyg. 2014 Sep;91(3):580–3. [PMID: 25092819]

Peniche-Lara G et al. *Rickettsia typhi* in rodents and *R. felis* in fleas in Yucatán as a possible causal agent of undefined febrile cases. Rev Inst Med Trop Sao Paulo. 2015 Mar–Apr;57(2):129–32. [PMID: 25923891]

Raby E et al. Endemic (murine) typhus in returned travelers from Asia, a case series: clues to early diagnosis and comparison with dengue. Am J Trop Med Hyg. 2013 Apr;88(4):701–3. [PMID: 23358638]

3. Scrub Typhus (Tsutsugamushi Fever)

► Exposure to mites in endemic area of Southeast Asia, the western Pacific (including Korea), and Australia.

► Black eschar at site of the bite, with regional and generalized lymphadenopathy.

► High fever, headache, myalgia, and a short-lived macular rash.

► Frequent pneumonitis, encephalitis, and cardiac failure.

► General Considerations

Scrub typhus is caused by *Orientia tsutsugamushi*, which is principally a parasite of rodents and is transmitted by larval trombiculid mites (chiggers). The disease is endemic in Korea, China, Taiwan, Japan, Pakistan, India, Thailand, Malaysia and Queensland, Australia (Table 32–4), which form an area known as the "tsutsugamushi triangle." Scrub typhus is an increasingly recognized cause of acute febrile illness in India, being responsible for about 24% of cases in one series and is a recognized cause of fever of unknown origin. Transmission is often more common at higher altitudes. The mites live on vegetation but complete their maturation cycle by biting humans who come in contact with infested vegetation. Therefore, the disease is more common in rural areas within these countries, although an outbreak was reported among users of an urban park in Guangzhou, China. Vertical transmission occurs, and blood transfusions may transmit the pathogen as well. Rare occupational transmission via inhalation is documented among laboratory workers. Increasingly cases with travel to endemic areas are recognized.

► Clinical Findings

A. Symptoms and Signs

After a 1- to 3-week incubation period, malaise, chills, severe headache and backache develop. At the site of the bite, a papule evolves into a flat black eschar (the groin and the abdomen being the most common sites followed by the chest and axilla), a finding that is usually helpful for diagnosis and reported in 55% of a large Indian series. The regional lymph nodes are commonly enlarged and tender, and sometimes a more generalized adenopathy occurs. Fever rises gradually during the first week of infection, and the rash is usually macular and primarily on the trunk area. The rash can be fleeting or more severe, peaking at 8 days but lasting up to 21 days after onset of infection. The patient may become obtunded. Gastrointestinal symptoms, including nausea, vomiting, and diarrhea, occur in nearly two-thirds of patients and correspond to the presence of superficial mucosal hemorrhage, multiple erosions, or ulcers in the gastrointestinal tract. Both acalculous cholecystitis and acute abdominal attacks are reported. An acute kidney injury is increasingly reported and renal abnormalities were present in over 80% of patients in one series. Transient parkinsonism, opsoclonus, or myoclonus may occur. Severe complications, such as pneumonitis, myocarditis and heart failure, encephalitis or aseptic meningitis, acute abdominal pain, peritonitis, granulomatous hepatitis, a hemophagocytic syndrome, disseminated intravascular coagulation, cerebrovascular hemorrhage or infarction, cranial nerve palsies, parkinsonian symptoms, ARDS, hemophagocytosis, or acute kidney disease may develop during the second or third week. An attack confers prolonged immunity against homologous strains and transient immunity against heterologous strains. Heterologous strains produce mild disease if infection occurs within a year after the first episode.

B. Laboratory Findings

Thrombocytopenia and elevation of liver enzymes, bilirubin, and creatinine are common. Serologic testing with immunofluorescence and immunoperoxidase assays or commercial dot-blot ELISA dipstick assays are convenient diagnostic aids, but a conclusive diagnosis requires documentation of a fourfold increase between acute and convalescence titers of antibodies. An indirect immunofluorescence assay is the mainstay of serologic diagnosis and titers quickly lose sensitivity so should be read as soon as possible after collection. A rapid immunochromatographic test for IgM and IgG detection is more sensitive and specific than the standard immunofluorescence assay. PCR (from the eschar or blood) may be the most sensitive diagnostic test but remains positive even after the initiation of treatment. Culture of the organism (by mouse inoculation) from blood obtained in the first few days of illness is another diagnostic modality but requires a specialized BioSafety Level 3 laboratory. Filter paper immunofluorescent assays are as sensitive and specific as paired sera and may be especially useful in field settings.

▶ Differential Diagnosis

Leptospirosis, typhoid, dengue, malaria, Q fever, hemorrhagic fevers, and other rickettsial infections should be considered. The headache may mimic trigeminal neuralgia. Scrub typhus is a recognized cause of obscure tropical fevers, especially in children.

▶ Treatment & Prognosis

Without treatment, fever subsides spontaneously after 2 weeks, but the mortality rate may be 10–30%. Empiric treatment for 3 days with doxycycline, 100 mg orally twice daily, or with minocyline, 100 mg intravenously twice daily, or for 7 days with chloramphenicol, 25 mg/kg/day orally or intravenously in four divided doses, eliminates most deaths and relapses. Chloramphenicol- and tetracycline-resistant strains have been reported from Southeast Asia, where azithromycin or roxithromycin may become the medication of choice for children, pregnant women, and patients with refractory disease. Azithromycin is reportedly successfully given as 500 mg intravenously daily for 5 days.

Rifampin reduces the duration of fever by 1 day when used with doxycycline.

Poor prognostic factors include hypotension requiring vasopressors, ICU care, high APACHE-II scores, age over 60 years, absence of an eschar (making the diagnosis difficult) and laboratory findings such as leukocytosis or hypoalbuminemia. HIV infection does not appear to influence the severity of scrub typhus.

▶ Prevention

Repeated application of long-acting miticides can make endemic areas safe. Insect repellents on clothing and skin as well as protective clothing are effective preventive measures. For short exposure, chemoprophylaxis with doxycycline (200 mg weekly) can prevent the disease but permits infection. No effective vaccines are available.

Aung AK et al. Rickettsial infections in Southeast Asia: implications for local populace and febrile returned travelers. Am J Trop Med Hyg. 2014 Sep;91(3):451–60. [PMID: 24957537]

Jang MO et al. Outcome of intravenous azithromycin therapy in patients with complicated scrub typhus compared with that of doxycycline therapy using propensity-matched analysis. Antimicrob Agents Chemother. 2014;58(3):1488–93. [PMID: 24366734]

Kumar V et al. Scrub typhus is an under-recognized cause of acute febrile illness with acute kidney injury in India. PLoS Negl Trop Dis. 2014 Jan 30;8(1):e2605. [PMID: 24498445]

McGready R et al. Pregnancy outcome in relation to treatment of murine typhus and scrub typhus infection: a fever cohort and a case series analysis. PLoS Negl Trop Dis. 2014 Nov 20; 8(11):e3327. [PMID: 25412503]

Wei Y et al. A city park as a potential epidemic site of scrub typhus: a case-control study of an outbreak in Guangzhou, China. Parasit Vectors. 2014 Nov 18;7:513. [PMID: 25403988]

SPOTTED FEVERS

1. Rocky Mountain Spotted Fever

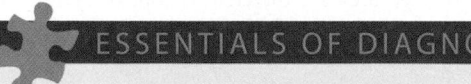

ESSENTIALS OF DIAGNOSIS

▶ Exposure to tick bite in an endemic area.

▶ An influenza-like prodrome followed by chills, fever, severe headache, and myalgias; occasionally, delirium and coma.

▶ Red macular rash appears between the second and sixth days of fever, first on the wrists and ankles and then spreading centrally; it may become petechial.

▶ Serial serologic examinations by indirect fluorescent antibody confirm the diagnosis retrospectively.

▶ General Considerations

Despite its name, most cases of Rocky Mountain spotted fever (RMSF) occur outside the Rocky Mountain area. Passive surveillance data from 2002 to 2007 reported cases from 46 states and the District of Columbia. More than half (64%) of these cases were from only five states: North Carolina, Tennessee, Oklahoma, Missouri, and Arkansas. RMSF is endemic in Central and South America with a small fatal familiar cluster reported from Panama (Table 32–4). Native Americans are at high risk for infection. The causative agent, *R rickettsii*, is transmitted to humans by the bite of ticks, including the Rocky Mountain wood tick, *Dermacentor andersoni*, in the western United States, and the American dog tick, *D variabilis*, in the eastern United States. Several hours of contact between the tick and the human host are required for transmission. The brown dog tick, *Rhipicephalus sanguineus*, is a vector in eastern Arizona and responsible for many Native American cases. Other hard-bodied ticks transmit the organism in the southern United States and in Central and South America and are responsible for transmitting it among rodents, dogs, porcupines, and other animals. There are 25 genotypes of *R rickettsii* in four different groups, and potential genomic-clinical correlations are underway. Several other rickettsial species cause mild, nonlethal infections in the United States, including *R parkeri*, *R phillipi*, and *R massiliae*. These are discussed in the "tick typhus" section.

In the United States, the estimated annual incidence of RMSF is increasing to as high as seven cases per million persons (primarily occurring from April through September), with a higher incidence among children and men. Better diagnostic capacity and improved surveillance are thought responsible for the changing epidemiology.

A Brazilian spotted fever with higher mortality than RMSF is now thought to be due to a virulent strain of *Rickettsia rickettsii*.

► Clinical Findings

A. Symptoms and Signs

RMSF can cause severe multiorgan dysfunction and fatality rates of up to 73% if left untreated, making it the most serious rickettsial disease. Two to 14 days (mean, 7 days) after the bite of an infectious tick, symptoms begin with the abrupt onset of high fever, chills, headache, nausea and vomiting, myalgias, restlessness, insomnia, and irritability. The characteristic rash (faint macules that progress to maculopapules and then petechiae) appears between days 2 and 6 of fever. It initially involves the wrists and ankles, spreading *centrally* to the arms, legs, and trunk over the next 2–3 days. Involvement of the palms and soles is characteristic. Facial flushing, conjunctival injection, and hard palatal lesions (Figure 32–6) may occur. In about 10% of cases, however, no rash or only a minimal rash is seen. Cough and pneumonitis may develop and delirium, lethargy, seizures, stupor, and coma may also appear in more severe cases. Splenomegaly, hepatomegaly, jaundice, myocarditis (which may mimic an acute coronary syndrome), adrenal hemorrhage, polyarticular arthritis, or uremia is occasionally present. ARDS and necrotizing vasculitis, when present, are of greatest concern.

B. Laboratory Findings

Thrombocytopenia, hyponatremia, elevated aminotransferases, and hyperbilirubinemia are common. Cerebrospinal

▲ **Figure 32–6.** Hard palate lesion caused by Rocky Mountain spotted fever. (Public Health Image Library, CDC.)

fluid may show hypoglycorrhachia and mild pleocytosis. Disseminated intravascular coagulation is observed in severe cases. Diagnosis during the acute phase of the illness can be made by immunohistologic or PCR demonstration of *R rickettsii* in skin biopsy specimens (or cutaneous swabs of eschars or skin lesions). Performing such studies as soon as skin lesions become apparent and before antibiotics commence maximizes sensitivity. Children with fatal disease frequently have platelet counts less than 50,000 cells/mcL.

Serologic studies confirm the diagnosis, but most patients do not mount an antibody response until the second week of illness. The indirect fluorescent antibody test is most commonly used. No commercial PCR technique is validated.

► Differential Diagnosis

The diagnosis is challenging because early symptoms resemble those of many other infections. The classic triad of fever, rash, and tick bite is rarely recognized, with up to 40% of patients not recalling a tick bite. Moreover, the rash may be confused with that of measles, typhoid, and ehrlichiosis, or—most importantly—meningococcemia. Coinfections may mask the diagnosis. Blood cultures and examination of cerebrospinal fluid establish the latter. Some spotted fever rickettsioses may also mimic RMSF but will not be detected by routine serologic testing for RMSF.

► Treatment & Prognosis

Treatment with doxycycline at similar doses and duration as for epidemic typhus (100 mg orally twice daily for 4–10 days) is recommended, including for children. Similarly, chloramphenicol (50–100 mg/kg/day in four divided doses, orally or intravenously for 4–10 days) is the preferred alternative during pregnancy. Patients usually defervesce within 48–72 hours and therapy should be maintained for at least 3 days after defervescence occurs. Mild cases in low-risk individuals may be observed without treatment.

The reported mortality rate in the United States is about 3–5%. The following features are associated with increased mortality: (1) infection in very young children, the elderly, or Native Americans; (2) the presence of atypical clinical features (absence of headache, no history of tick attachment, gastrointestinal symptoms) and underlying chronic diseases; and (3) a delay in initiation of appropriate antibiotic therapy. Hemorrhage and acute kidney injury are associated with mortality in children. The usual cause of death is pneumonitis with respiratory or cardiac failure. Sequelae may include seizures, encephalopathy, peripheral neuropathy, paraparesis, bowel and bladder incontinence, cerebellar and vestibular dysfunction, hearing loss, and motor deficits.

► **Prevention**

Protective clothing, tick-repellent chemicals, and the removal of ticks at frequent intervals are helpful measures. The effectiveness of aggressive campaigns to decrease ticks in the community is under investigation in Native American communities with high RMSF attack rates. Prophylactic therapy after a tick bite is not currently recommended.

Alvarez-Hernandez G et al. Clinical profile and predictors of fatal Rocky Mountain spotted fever in children from Sonora, Mexico. Pediatr Infect Dis J. 2015 Feb;34(2):125–30. [PMID: 25126856]

Chaudhry MA et al. Atypical Rocky Mountain spotted fever with polyarticular arthritis. Am J Med Sci. 2013 Nov;346(5):427–9. [PMID: 24157965]

Drexler N et al. Community-based control of the brown dog tick in a region with high rates of Rocky Mountain spotted fever, 2012–2013. PLoS One. 2014 Dec 5;9(12):e112368. [PMID: 25479289]

Vaughn MF et al. Seroepidemiologic study of human infections with spotted fever group Rickettsiae in North Carolina. J Clin Microbiol. 2014 Nov;52(11):3960–6. [PMID: 25187639]

2. Rickettsialpox

Rickettsialpox is an acute, self-limiting, febrile illness caused by *Rickettsia akari*, a parasite of mice, transmitted by the mite *Liponyssoides sanguineus* (Table 32–4). Infections are reported globally. Seroprevalence studies done on injection drug users in inner Baltimore showed antibody positivity as high as 16%. In New York, its association with poverty is very strong. The illness has also been found in farming communities. Crowded conditions and mouse-infested housing allow transmission of the pathogen to humans. The primary lesion is a painless red papule that vesiculates and forms a black eschar followed by an incubation period of 7–12 days. Onset of symptoms is sudden, with chills, fever, headache, photophobia, and disseminated aches and pains. Two to 4 days later, a widespread papular eruption appears. The rash becomes vesicular and forms crusts that are shed in about 10 days. Early lesions may resemble those of chickenpox (typically vesicular versus papulovesicular in rickettsialpox). Pathologic findings include dermal edema, subepidermal vesicles, and at times a lymphocytic vasculitis.

Transient leukopenia and thrombocytopenia and acute hepatitis can occur. A fourfold rise in serum antibody titers to rickettsial antigen, detected by complement fixation or indirect fluorescent assays, is diagnostic. Conjugated anti-rickettsial globulin can identify antigen in punch biopsies of skin lesions. PCR detection of rickettsial DNA in fresh tissue also appears of value. *R akari* can reportedly also be isolated from eschar biopsy specimens.

Treatment consists of oral doxycycline (200 mg/day) for 7 days. The disease is usually mild and self-limited without treatment, but occasionally severe symptoms may require hospitalization. Control requires the elimination of mice from human habitations and insecticide applications.

Eremeeva ME et al. Investigation of an outbreak of rickettsial febrile illness in Guatemala, 2007. Int J Infect Dis. 2013 May;17(5):e304–11. [PMID: 23266334]

Greene SK et al. Disparities in reportable communicable disease incidence by census tract-level poverty, New York City, 2006–2013. Am J Public Health. 2015 Sep;105(9):e27–34. [PMID: 26180961]

3. Tick Typhus (Rickettsial Fever)

The term "tick typhus" denotes a variety of spotted rickettsial fevers, often named by their geographic location (eg, Mediterranean spotted fever, Queensland tick typhus, Oriental spotted fever, African tick bite fever, Siberian tick typhus, North Asian tick typhus), or by morphology (eg, boutonneuse fever). These illnesses are caused by various rickettsial organisms (eg, *R africae*, *R australis*, *R conorii*, *R japonica*, *R massiliae*, *R parkeri*, and *R sibirica*, and *R 364D*—recognized in California in 2013) and are transmitted by various tick species. Lymphangitis-associated rickettsiosis (LAR), caused by *R sibirica mongolitimonae*, was first described in 1996 and has been reported in Europe only thus far, including a small outbreak in Spain) (Table 32–4). Dogs and wild animals, usually rodents and even reptiles, may serve as reservoirs for rickettsial fevers. Travel is a risk factor for disease, particularly among elderly ecotourists. In a series of 280 international travelers with rickettsial disease, the most common cause was spotted fever rickettsiosis (231 cases, 82.5% of the total) followed by scrub typhus (16, 5.7%).

Tick-borne rickettsioses are the main source of rickettsia infections in Europe and cause a syndrome similar to that seen in Mediterranean spotted fever. Newly recognized species include *R helvetica*, *R monacensis*, *R massiliae*, and *R aeschlimannii*. Another described syndrome is tick-borne lymphadenopathy/Dermacentor-borne-necrosis-erythema-lymphadenopathy/scalp eschar neck lymphadenopathy (TIBOLA/DEBONEL/SENLAT) associated with *R slovaca*, *Candidatus R rioja*, and *R raoultii* and characterized by tick bite, eschar on the scalp, and cervical lymphadenopathy.

The pathogens usually produce an eschar or black spot (tâche noire) at the site of the tick bite that may be useful in diagnosis, though spotless boutonneuse fever occurs. Symptoms include fever, headache, myalgias, and rash. Painful lymphadenopathy or lymphangitis may also occur. Rarely, papulovesicular lesions may resemble rickettsialpox. Endothelial injury produces perivascular edema and dermal necrosis. Regional adenopathy, disseminated lesions, kidney disease, splenic rupture, and focal hepatic necrosis are observed. Neurologic manifestations, including encephalitis, internuclear ophthalmoplegia, coronary involvement, and the hemophagocytic syndrome, are rare.

The diagnosis is clinical, with serologic or PCR (culture can be used but is less sensitive than either) of the buffy coat of blood, or an eschar if one is available, used for confirmation. Treatment should be started upon clinical suspicion since delayed therapy is the usual cause of increased morbidity. Oral treatment with doxycycline (200 mg/day) or chloramphenicol (50–75 mg/kg/day in four divided doses) for 7–10 days is indicated. Caution is advised with the use of ciprofloxacin because it is associated with a poor outcome and increases the severity of disease in Mediterranean spotted fever. The combination of azithromycin and rifampin is effective and safe in pregnancy. Prevention entails protective clothing, repellents, and inspection for and removal of ticks.

Formerly classified as an endemic or murine typhus, the cat-flea typhus, caused by *Rickettsia felis* is now more properly classified as a spotted fever. The causative agent has been linked to the cat flea and opossum exposure. Most cases in the United States (southern Texas and California, and possibly Hawaii) occur in the spring and summer. Treatment is the same as for other rickettsial fevers.

Drexler NA et al. National surveillance of spotted fever group rickettsioses in the United States, 2008–2012. Am J Trop Med Hyg. 2016 Jan 6;94(1):26–34. [PMID: 26324732]

Myers T et al. Detecting *Rickettsia parkeri* infection from eschar swab specimens. Emerg Infect Dis. 2013 May;19(5):778–80. [PMID: 23647926]

Portillo A et al. Rickettsioses in Europe. Microbes Infect. 2015 Nov–Dec;17(11-12):834–8. [PMID: 26384814]

OTHER RICKETTSIAL & RICKETTSIAL-LIKE DISEASES

1. Ehrlichiosis & Anaplasmosis

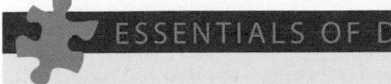

ESSENTIALS OF DIAGNOSIS

► Infection of monocyte or granulocyte by tick-borne gram-negative bacteria.

► Nine-day incubation period, with variable clinical illness, ranging from asymptomatic to persistent or life threatening.

► Common symptoms are malaise, nausea, fever, and headaches.

► US cases are largely in elderly white men in the summer.

► Excellent response to therapy with tetracyclines.

General Considerations

Ehrlichiae and anaplasmae are small tick-borne gram-negative obligate intracellular bacteria that infect monocytes or granulocytes. Human monocytic ehrlichiosis is caused by *Ehrlichia chaffeensis* (Table 32–4). Human granulocytic anaplasmosis is caused by *Anaplasma phagocytophilium*. *Ehrlichia ewingii* (infecting primarily dogs) can rarely cause human granulocytic ehrlichiosis (also referred to as *E ewingii* ehrlichiosis) similar to human granulocytic anaplasmosis. A third *Ehrlichia* species that infects humans appears to be related to *Ehrlichia muris*. An *Ehrlichia*-like organism, *Neorickettsia sennetsu*, is the etiologic agent of sennetsu fever, which is confined to western Japan.

Human monocytic ehrlichiosis is seen primarily in the south central states (especially Arkansas, Missouri, and Oklahoma) of the United States, although cases are also recognized in Israel, Japan, Mexico, South America, and Europe. Human granulocytic anaplasmosis is more frequent in the upper midwestern United States with most cases reported from Minnesota and Wisconsin although there is a secondary focus along the New England coast, especially in Rhode Island. Infections in Europe and China are also well documented with a newly diagnosed species from China being named *Anaplasma capra*. Human infection with *E ewingii* is limited to the Midwest and Southeast and occurs mainly among the immunocompromised with an infection identified from bone marrow in a resident of Arkansas with fever and pancytopenia. In North America, the major vectors for these pathogens are the Lone Star tick (*Amblyomma americanus* for *E chaffeensis* and *E ewingii*), the western blacklegged tick (*Ixodes pacificus* for *E chaffeensis*), and *Ixodes scapularis* (the same vector for Lyme disease and babesiosis for *A phagocytophilum*). Reported incidences of both human monocytic and granulocytic ehrlichiosis are increasing and both are now at about 3 per million, respectively, with higher rates in the summer among whites and among men. Up to 4.9% of *Amblyomma americanus* and *D variabilis* ticks are seropositive for *Ehrlichia*.

The principal reservoirs for human monocytic ehrlichiosis and human granulocytic anaplasmosis are the white tail deer and the white-footed mouse, respectively. Other mammals are implicated as well. A nosocomial outbreak was reported from China (where nine patients had exposure to body fluids and none reported tick bites). Perinatal and blood product transmission of human granulocytic anaplasmosis is also documented.

Clinical Findings

A. Symptoms and Signs

Clinical disease of human monocytic ehrlichiosis ranges from mild to life threatening. Typically, after about a 9-day incubation period and a prodrome consisting of malaise, rigors, and nausea, worsening fever and headache develop. A pleomorphic rash may occur. Presentation in immunosuppressed patients (including transplant patients) and the elderly tends to be more severe. Serious sequelae include acute respiratory failure and ARDS, encephalopathy, and acute kidney disease, which may mimic thrombotic thrombocytopenic purpura.

The symptoms of human granulocytic ehrlichiosis and *E ewingii* infection are similar to those seen with human monocytic ehrlichiosis. Rash, however, is infrequent in human granulocytic ehrlichiosis and should prompt the consideration of other infections (eg, Lyme disease). Persistent fever and malaise are reported to occur for 2 or more years.

The clinical manifestations of anaplasmosis are similar to those of ehrlichiosis. Coinfection with anaplasmosis and Lyme disease or babesiosis may occur, but the clinical manifestations (including fever and cytopenias) are greater with anaplasmosis than with Lyme disease. A spirochete, *Borrelia miyamotoi*, may mimic anaplasmosis in its clinical manifestations.

B. Laboratory Findings

Diagnosis can be made by the history of tick exposure followed by a characteristic clinical presentation. Leukopenia, absolute lymphopenia, thrombocytopenia, and transaminitis occur often. Thrombocytopenia occurs more often than leukopenia in human granulocytic ehrlichiosis. Examination of peripheral blood with Giemsa stain may reveal characteristic intraleukocytic vacuoles (morulae). An indirect fluorescent antibody assay is available through the CDC and requires acute and convalescent sera. A PCR assay, if available, is a rapid diagnostic tool, especially for early disease.

▶ Treatment & Prevention

Treatment for all forms of ehrlichiosis is with doxycycline, 100 mg twice daily (orally or intravenously) for at least 10 days or until 3 days of defervescence. Rifampin is an alternative in pregnant women and children. Treatment should not be withheld while awaiting confirmatory serology when suspicion is high. Lack of clinical improvement and defervescence 48 hours after doxycycline initiation suggests an alternate diagnosis. Tick control is the essence of prevention and, as foci of new infection are identified (eg, Northern China), the area for such heightened control broadens. Transmission of *Ehrlichia chaffeensis* by renal transplantation is documented.

Allen MB et al. First reported case of *Ehrlichia ewingii* involving human bone marrow. J Clin Microbiol. 2014 Nov;52(11):4102–4. [PMID: 25187638]

Dahlgren FS et al. Human granulocytic anaplasmosis in the United States from 2008 to 2012: a summary of national surveillance data. Am J Trop Med Hyg. 2015 Jul;93(1):66–72. [PMID: 25870428]

Sachdev SH et al. Severe life-threatening *Ehrlichia chaffeensis* infections transmitted through solid organ transplantation. Transpl Infect Dis. 2014 Feb;16(1):119–24. [PMID: 24330198]

2. Q Fever

 ESSENTIALS OF DIAGNOSIS

▶ Exposure to sheep, goats, cattle, or their products; some infections are laboratory acquired.

▶ An acute or chronic febrile illness with severe headache, cough, prostration, and abdominal pain.

▶ Extensive pneumonitis, hepatitis, or encephalopathy; less often, endocarditis, vascular infections, or chronic fatigue syndrome.

▶ A common cause of culture-negative endocarditis.

▶ General Considerations

Q fever (for "query" in view of its formerly unknown cause), a reportable and significantly underestimated disease in the United States, is caused by *Coxiella burnetii*, an organism previously classified as a rickettsia but now considered a proteobacterium. Unlike rickettsiae, *C burnetii* is usually transmitted to humans not by arthropods but by inhalation or ingestion. *Coxiella* infections occur globally, mostly in cattle, sheep, and goats, in which they cause mild or subclinical disease (Table 32–4). In these animals, reactivation of the infection occurs during pregnancy and causes abortions or low birth weight offspring. *Coxiella* is resistant to heat and drying and remains infective in the environment for months.

Humans become infected by inhalation of aerosolized bacteria (in dust or droplets) from feces, urine, milk (in particular raw milk), or products of conception of infected animals. Ingestion and skin penetration are other recognized routes of transmission. Outbreaks associated with other mammals such as cats and dogs are also described. A major outbreak in the Netherlands that began in 2007 was thought to be due to exposure to aborting ruminants and was associated with over 3000 cases. A common source outbreak occurred in Germany in 2014 among recipients of xenotransfusion entailing intramuscular injections of animal cells, given for diverse health reasons.

There is a known occupational risk for animal handlers, slaughterhouse workers, veterinarians, laboratory workers, and other workers exposed to animal products. Outbreaks in military personnel returning from Iraq and Afghanistan were described. Transmission through aerosols is possible in that *Coxiella* can be pathogens of other organisms (free living amoebae), which are transmitted through air ducts and intrahospital transmission to a pregnant woman presumably from aerosols is documented. In the United States, over 60% of cases do not report an exposure to potentially infectious animals, but cases are more than twice as likely as noncases to report drinking raw milk. An epidemiologic study suggests that in French Guiana three-toed sloths may be a reservoir for *Coxiella* organisms. Seroprevalence studies show ubiquity of infection, with rates of 24% in French Guiana, 10% in China, 10–32% in Egypt where contact with camels is deemed responsible and significant under recognition throughout sub-Saharan Africa.

Endocarditis, an uncommon but serious form of *Coxiella* infection, is linked to preexisting valvular conditions, immunocompromised states, urban residence, and raw milk ingestion. Delays in diagnosis often occur. Horizontal spread from one human to another does not seem to occur even in the presence of florid pneumonitis, but maternal–fetal infection can occur.

▶ Clinical Findings

A. Symptoms and Signs

Asymptomatic infection is common. For the remaining cases, a febrile illness develops after an incubation period of 2–3 weeks, usually accompanied by headache, relative bradycardia, prostration, and muscle pains. The clinical course may be acute, chronic (duration 6 months or longer), or relapsing. Pneumonia and granulomatous hepatitis are the predominant manifestations in the acute form (3.5% of community-acquired pneumonia in a German series was due to Q fever), whereas other less common manifestations include skin rashes (maculopapular or purpuric), fever of unknown origin, myocarditis, pericarditis, aortic aneurysms, aseptic meningitis, encephalitis, hemolytic anemia, orchitis, acute kidney disease, iliopsoas abscess, spondylodiscitis, tenosynovitis, and regional (mediastinal) or diffuse lymphadenopathies. Cases of Q fever mimicking autoimmune and systemic inflammatory disease are reported. The most common presentation of chronic Q fever is culture-negative endocarditis, which occurs in less than 1% of infected individuals. It is found mainly in the setting of preexisting valve disease. Vascular infections, particularly of the aorta (causing mycotic aneurysms), are the second most common form of Q fever and are associated with a high mortality (25%). A post-Q fever chronic fatigue syndrome (1 year after acute infection with chronic symptoms not explained by chronic Q fever) is controversial and of unknown pathophysiology although the basis may be immunogenetic.

Reactivation of Q fever in pregnant women may cause spontaneous abortions, intrauterine growth retardation, intrauterine fetal death, premature delivery, and oligohydramnios.

B. Laboratory Findings

Laboratory examination during the acute phase may show elevated liver function tests and occasional leukocytosis. Patients with acute Q fever usually produce antibodies to *C burnetii* phase II antigen. A fourfold rise between acute and convalescent sera by indirect immunofluorescence is diagnostic. Realtime PCR for *C burnetii* DNA is helpful only in early diagnosis of Q fever with *C burnetii* DNA becoming undetectable in serum as serologic responses develop. The positive predictive value of antibodies to phase II antigens in acute disease is at most 65%.

While chronic Q fever can be diagnosed on the basis of serologic tests done at 3- and 6-month intervals (with an IgG titer against phase I antigen of 1:1600 or greater), the sensitivity of such serologies is often low, and it is recommended that clinical criteria be used for diagnosis of chronic disease. Diagnosis is often made at the time of valve replacement with PCR of tissue samples. *C burnetti* may also be isolated from affected valves using the shell-vial technique. The organism is highly transmissible to laboratory workers and culture techniques require a biosafety level 3 setting. In one series, at 6 years after infection, reversion to seronegativity occurred in 7 of 38 patients, and none showed the organism in peripheral blood mononuclear cells. Antiphospholipid antibodies and anti-ADAMTS 13 antibodies may be present and account for thrombotic and other clinical symptoms.

C. Imaging

Radiographs of the chest show patchy pulmonary infiltrates, often more prominent than the physical signs suggest.

▶ Differential Diagnosis

Viral, mycoplasmal, and bacterial pneumonias, viral hepatitis, brucellosis, Legionnaire disease, Kawasaki disease, tuberculosis, psittacosis, and other animal-borne diseases must be considered. Q fever should be considered in cases of unexplained fevers with negative blood cultures in association with embolic or cardiac disease.

▶ Treatment & Prognosis

For acute infection, treatment with doxycycline (100 mg orally twice daily) for 14 days or at least 3 full days after defervescence is recommended. Even in untreated patients, the mortality rate is usually low, except when endocarditis develops. In a Dutch series, long-term fatigue is documented after acute infection.

For chronic infection, there is no agreement on the type and duration of antimicrobial therapy. Most experts recommend a combination oral therapy with doxycycline (100 mg twice a day) plus ciprofloxacin (typically 750 mg twice a day) or rifampin (300 mg twice a day) or hydroxychloroquine (200 mg three times a day) for approximately 2 years or more for the treatment of endocarditis. A study reported in 1999 of 35 patients with Q fever endocarditis showed favorable outcomes with oral doxycycline (100 mg twice a day) plus oral hydroxychloroquine (200 mg three times a day) for 18 months for native valves and 24 months for prosthetic valves. There are rare reports of doxycycline resistance.

Serologic responses can be monitored during and after completion of therapy and treatment extended in the absence of favorable serologic response (considered a titer of 1:1600 or greater to phase I antigen). The general variability of serologic data, however, limits their usefulness and providers usually rely on clinical criteria. Patients should be monitored for at least 5 years due to risk of relapse. Heart valve replacement may be necessary in refractory disease. **Given the difficulty in treating endocarditis, transthoracic echocardiography is recommended for all patients with acute Q fever, and the same aforementioned therapy for 1 year should be offered in**

the presence of valvulopathy. In addition, patients undergoing routine valve surgery should have routine Q fever serologies in endemic countries and appropriate treatment if tests are positive for Q fever.

Because of the obstetric complications (which appear to have strain specificity) that occur among pregnant women in whom Q fever develops, a regimen of long-term trimethoprim-sulfamethoxazole (320/1600 mg orally for the duration of pregnancy) should be given to all infected pregnant women. However, a randomized controlled study of pregnant women in Holland did not show that serologic surveillance and treatment of seropositive women were effective in preventing obstetric complications. Other data from Denmark among pregnant women exposed in the past to *Coxiella* also suggest the risk of obstetric complications may not be high. The official recommendations nonetheless remain as stated.

► **Prevention**

Prevention is based on detection of the infection in livestock, including camels in the Middle East; reduction of contact with infected and, in particular, parturient animals or contaminated dust; special care when working with animal tissues; and effective pasteurization of milk. No vaccine is approved for use in the United States, although a whole-cell Q fever vaccine, with a 5-year efficacy of greater than 95%, is available in Australia for persons with high-risk exposures where some seroprevalence studies show 7% seropositivity.

C burnetii is a category B bioterrorism agent. In the setting of a bioterrorist attack, postexposure prophylaxis with doxycycline (100 mg orally twice daily) for 5 days should be started 8–12 days after exposure.

Pregnant women should take trimethoprim-sulfamethoxazole (160 mg/800 mg orally twice daily) for the duration of the pregnancy.

Anderson A et al. Diagnosis and management of Q fever—United States, 2013: recommendations from CDC and the Q Fever Working Group. MMWR Recomm Rep. 2013 Mar 29; 62(RR-03):1–30. Erratum in: MMWR Recomm Rep. 2013 Sep 6;62(35):730. [PMID: 23535757]

Dahlgren FS et al. Q fever is underestimated in the United States: a comparison of fatal Q fever cases from two national reporting systems. Am J Trop Med Hyg. 2015 Feb;92(2):244–6. [PMID: 25404074]

Eldin C et al. Rainfall and sloth births in may, Q fever in July, Cayenne, French Guiana. Am J Trop Med Hyg. 2015 May; 92(5):979–81. [PMID: 25802429]

Grisoli D et al. Latent Q fever endocarditis in patients undergoing routine valve surgery. J Heart Valve Dis. 2014 Nov; 23(6):735–43. [PMID: 25790621]

Robyn MP et al. Q fever outbreak among travelers to Germany who received live cell therapy—United States and Canada, 2014. MMWR Morb Mortal Wkly Rep. 2015 Oct 2; 64(38):1071–3. [PMID: 26421460]

Tyler R et al. Delayed diagnosis of Q fever: finally diagnosed after elective cardiac surgery. Ann Thorac Surg. 2015 Jul; 100(1):325–6. [PMID: 26140783]

Vanderburg S et al. Epidemiology of *Coxiella burnetii* infection in Africa: a OneHealth systematic review. PLoS Negl Trop Dis. 2014 Apr 10;8(4):e2787. [PMID: 24722554]

van Loenhout JA et al. Serious long-term health consequences of Q-fever and Legionnaires' disease. J Infect. 2014 Jun; 68(6):527–33. [PMID: 24468188]

Wegdam-Blans MC et al. Serology in chronic Q fever is still surrounded by question marks. Eur J Clin Microbiol Infect Dis. 2014 Jul;33(7):1089–94. [PMID: 24430618]

KAWASAKI DISEASE

ESSENTIALS OF DIAGNOSIS

► Fever, conjunctivitis, oral mucosal changes, rash, cervical lymphadenopathy, peripheral extremity changes.

► Elevated erythrocyte sedimentation rate and C-reactive protein levels.

► **General Considerations**

Kawasaki disease is a worldwide multisystemic disease. It is also known as the "mucocutaneous lymph node syndrome." It occurs mainly in children between the ages of 3 months and 5 years but can occur occasionally in adults as well. Kawasaki disease occurs significantly more often in Asians or native Pacific Islanders than in whites. Its incidence appears to be increasing in Japan, where it was first described in 1967. Children with a history of allergic diseases are at increased risk for Kawasaki disease. It is an acute, self-limiting, mucocutaneous vasculitis characterized by the infiltration of vessel walls with mononuclear cells and later by IgA secreting plasma cells that can result in the destruction of the tunica media and aneurysm formation. Several infectious agents (New Haven coronavirus, parvovirus, bocavirus, CMV, *Yersinia pseudotuberculosis*, meningococcus), bacterial superantigens, and genetic polymorphisms (confirmed in whole genome analysis) in components of the immune system (interleukin 10 and 18) are implicated in its pathogenesis. A "new" RNA virus was considered a trigger of the disease, based on the finding of intracytoplasmic inclusion bodies in ciliated bronchial epithelium of Kawasaki patients. Epidemiologic studies from Seattle show an increased risk with advanced maternal age, mother of foreign birth, maternal group B streptococcus colonization, and early infancy hospitalization. Whole genomic analysis, mostly from China, is identifying target gene products.

► **Clinical Findings**

A clinical diagnosis of "complete" Kawasaki disease requires, in the absence of other processes, explaining the current illness of fever and four of the following criteria for at least 5 days: bilateral nonexudative conjunctivitis, mucous membrane changes of at least one type (injected pharynx, erythema, swelling and fissuring of the lips, strawberry tongue), peripheral extremity changes of at least one type (edema, desquamation, erythema of the palms and soles, induration of the hands and feet, Beau lines [transverse grooves of the nails]), a polymorphous rash, and cervical lymphadenopathy greater than 1.5 cm (most worrisome when retropharyngeal with edema is present). An "incomplete" form is diagnosed when only two criteria are met and accompanied by other laboratory or imaging findings. The classic syndrome is often preceded by nonspecific symptoms including irritability, vomiting, anorexia, cough, and diarrhea for up to 10 days. A Kawasaki shock syndrome is a presentation and a complication often misdiagnosed that occurs more often among children with neutrophilia, high C-reactive protein levels, and thrombocytopenia.

Major complications include arteritis and aneurysms of the coronary vessels, occurring in about 25% of untreated patients (and slightly over 10% of treated patients in a Danish review), on occasion causing myocardial infarction. The "incomplete" form appears more frequently to result in cardiac complications. The pathogenesis of infarction is often thrombus formation, vasospasm, stenosis, or aneurysm rupture. Coronary complications are more common among patients older than 6 years or younger than 1 year of age. Noninvasive diagnosis of coronary complications can be made with CT coronary angiography (the most sensitive test), magnetic resonance angiography or transthoracic echocardiography (advocated for early screening). Other factors associated with the development of coronary artery aneurysms are male sex, relentless fever (even after the administration of IVIG), high C-reactive protein, urticarial exanthems, anemia, hypoalbuminemia, hyponatremia, and thrombocytopenia or thrombocytosis. Pericardial effusions, myocarditis, and mitral regurgitation (usually mild) are also common. Coronary artery fistulas occur in up to 5% of patients and diastolic dysfunction is also reported. Systemic arteritis and aneurysms (often symmetric and in younger children), peripheral gangrene, syndrome of inappropriate secretion of antidiuretic hormone (SIADH), a parapharyngeal abscess, and the hemophagocytic syndrome are also reported. Cases of pancreatitis and bile duct stenosis due to underlying vasculitis are reported. Cerebrospinal fluid pleocytosis is found in one-third of cases, and encephalitis is rarely reported. Other CNS complications include seizures, oculomotor palsies, and sensorineural hearing loss which, when sought, can be found in as many as 55% of cases. Rare case reports of atypical presentations (eg, retropharyngeal abscess) are described.

Differentiation from disseminated adenovirus infection is important and can be performed with rapid adenovirus assays.

► Treatment & Prevention

Every patient with a clinical diagnosis of Kawasaki disease (complete or incomplete) should be treated. IVIG (2 g/kg over 10–12 hours) is given within the first 10 days of illness. Patients in whom persistent fever, ongoing systemic inflammation, or aneurysm formation presents later should be offered IVIG as well. Concomitant aspirin should be started at 80–100 mg/kg/day orally (divided into four doses and not exceeding 4 g/day) until the patient is afebrile for 48 hours and then reduced to 3–5 mg/kg/day

until markers of acute inflammation normalize. Aspirin therapy is continued if coronary aneurysm develops. If fevers persist beyond 36 hours after the initial IVIG infusion, a second dose of IVIG at 2 g/kg should be given if no other source of fever is found. Rare cases of aseptic meningitis are reported with IVIG, and this complication may be hard to distinguish from the occasional CNS disease associated with Kawasaki syndrome itself although the time course and the cerebrospinal fluid differential (more polymorphonuclear with IVIG, more lymphocytic with Kawasaki syndrome) may help differentiate the two. Hemolytic anemia is another rare complication of IVIG. Methylprednisolone (30 mg/kg/day intravenously if possible for a maximum of 3 days) followed by tapering dose of corticosteroids in addition to IVIG administration improve coronary artery outcomes in severe Kawasaki disease. Routine childhood vaccinations should be given and live vaccines (eg, MMR) should be delayed for at least 9 months only if IVIG was administered (IVIG can block the immune response to live vaccines). If vaccine-preventable disease endemicity requires urgent vaccination, it is prudent to revaccinate 11 months after the IVIG and first vaccination were given.

Further options for refractory cases include TNF blockers (infliximab or etanercept), cyclophosphamide or cyclosporine, methotrexate, and plasmapheresis, but not further pulse corticosteroid or IVIG. Abciximab therapy may be associated with coronary vessel remodeling in large coronary artery aneurysms. An echocardiogram is essential in the acute phase of illness and 6–8 weeks after onset. Anticoagulation with warfarin or low-molecular-weight heparin (the latter is preferable for children where dosage adjustments are difficult using warfarin) is indicated along with aspirin, 81 mg orally daily, in patients with aneurysms greater than 8 mm in diameter. If myocardial infarction occurs, therapy with thrombolytics, percutaneous coronary intervention, coronary artery bypass grafts, and even cardiac transplantation should be considered. Manifestations of coronary artery aneurysms can occur as late as in the third or fourth decade of life with a study showing a prevalence of 5% coronary sequelae from Kawasaki disease among young adults evaluated with angiography. Data are equivocal on the development of accelerated atherosclerosis among those with a history of Kawasaki disease.

While secondary prevention of complications entails the modalities described above, primary prevention is difficult in the absence of a clear explanation for the disease.

► Prognosis

Cases that develop recurrent disease tend to more often show cardiac complications. Patients with a parental history of Kawasaki disease show more recurrent disease and more cardiac complications. Pregnant women with a history of Kawasaki disease have an increased risk of complications during pregnancy and of Kawasaki disease in their children. The long-term prognosis for adults with a history of Kawasaki disease but without coronary artery aneurysms is excellent. A heart-healthy lifestyle, however, is essential. The prognosis of patients with a history of cardiac complications requires regular follow-up (using transthoracic echocardiography) with risk stratification based on published guidelines and under cardiologic supervision. The coronary artery severity in patients 1 month after the onset of disease is a correlate of late coronary outcomes. Children with Kawasaki disease show an increased prevalence of multiple other viral infections including adenoviruses, enteroviruses, rhinoviruses, and coronaviruses.

▶ **When to Refer**

All cases of Kawasaki disease merit referral to specialists.

Chen PS et al. Clinical manifestations of Kawasaki disease shock syndrome: a case-control study. J Microbiol Immunol Infect. 2015 Feb;48(1):43–50. [PMID: 23927822]

Gordon CT et al. Pregnancy in women with a history of Kawasaki disease: management and outcomes. BJOG. 2014 Oct; 121(11):1431–8. [PMID: 24597833]

Kuwabara M et al. Cardiac lesions and initial laboratory data in Kawasaki disease: a nationwide survey in Japan. J Epidemiol. 2015;25(3):189–93. [PMID: 25716055]

Sundel RP. Kawasaki disease. Rheum Dis Clin North Am. 2015;41(1):63–73. [PMID: 25399940]

Bacterial & Chlamydial Infections

33

Brian S. Schwartz, MD

INFECTIONS CAUSED BY GRAM-POSITIVE BACTERIA

STREPTOCOCCAL INFECTIONS

1. Pharyngitis

> ### ESSENTIALS OF DIAGNOSIS

> ▶ Abrupt onset of sore throat, fever, malaise, nausea, and headache.
> ▶ Throat red and edematous, with or without exudate; cervical nodes tender.
> ▶ Diagnosis confirmed by culture of throat.

▶ General Considerations

Group A beta-hemolytic streptococci *(Streptococcus pyogenes)* are the most common bacterial cause of pharyngitis. Transmission occurs by droplets of infected secretions. Group A streptococci producing erythrogenic toxin may cause scarlet fever in susceptible persons.

▶ Clinical Findings

A. Symptoms and Signs

"Strep throat" is characterized by a sudden onset of fever, sore throat, pain on swallowing, tender cervical adenopathy, malaise, and nausea. The pharynx, soft palate, and tonsils are red and edematous. There may be a purulent exudate. The Centor clinical criteria for the diagnosis of streptococcal pharyngitis are temperature greater than 38°C, tender anterior cervical adenopathy, lack of a cough, and pharyngotonsillar exudate.

The rash of scarlet fever is diffusely erythematous, resembling a sunburn, with superimposed fine red papules, and is most intense in the groin and axillas. It blanches on pressure, may become petechial, and fades in 2–5 days, leaving a fine desquamation. The face is flushed, with circumoral pallor, and the tongue is coated with enlarged red papillae (strawberry tongue).

B. Laboratory Findings

Leukocytosis with neutrophil predominance is common. Throat culture onto a single blood agar plate has a sensitivity of 80–90%. Rapid diagnostic tests based on detection of streptococcal antigen are slightly less sensitive than culture. Clinical criteria, such as the Centor criteria, are useful for identifying patients in whom a rapid antigen test or throat culture is indicated. Patients who meet two or more of these criteria merit further testing. When three of the four are present, laboratory sensitivity of rapid antigen testing exceeds 90%. When only one criterion is present, streptococcal pharyngitis is unlikely. In high-prevalence settings or if clinical suspicion for streptococcal pharyngitis is high, a negative antigen test or culture should be confirmed by a follow-up culture.

▶ Complications

Suppurative complications include sinusitis, otitis media, mastoiditis, peritonsillar abscess, and suppuration of cervical lymph nodes.

Nonsuppurative complications are rheumatic fever and glomerulonephritis. Rheumatic fever may follow recurrent episodes of pharyngitis beginning 1–4 weeks after the onset of symptoms. Glomerulonephritis follows a single infection with a nephritogenic strain of streptococcus group A (eg, types 4, 12, 2, 49, and 60), more commonly on the skin than in the throat, and begins 1–3 weeks after the onset of the infection.

▶ Differential Diagnosis

Streptococcal sore throat resembles (and cannot be reliably distinguished clinically from) pharyngitis caused by viruses such as adenoviruses, Epstein-Barr virus, primary HIV, or other bacteria such as *Fusobacterium necrophorum* and *Arcanobacterium haemolyticum* (which also may cause a rash). Pharyngitis and lymphadenopathy are common findings in primary HIV infection. Generalized lymphadenopathy, splenomegaly, atypical lymphocytosis, and a positive serologic test distinguish mononucleosis from streptococcal pharyngitis. Diphtheria is characterized by a pseudomembrane; oropharyngeal candidiasis shows white patches of exudate and less erythema; and necrotizing ulcerative gingivostomatitis (Vincent fusospirochetal gingivitis or stomatitis) presents with shallow ulcers in the mouth. Retropharyngeal abscess or bacterial epiglottitis should be considered when odynophagia and difficulty in handling secretions are present and when the severity of symptoms is disproportionate to findings on examination of the pharynx. *F necrophorum* causes pharyngitis at a similar rate as group A beta-hemolytic streptococci in adolescents and young adults. *F necrophorum* pharyngitis is associated with the Lemierre syndrome, suppurative thrombophlebitis of the internal jugular vein, bacteremia, and metastatic infections. Early recognition and treatment of this syndrome is important.

Treatment

Antimicrobial therapy has a modest effect on resolution of symptoms and primarily is administered for prevention of complications. Antibiotic therapy can be safely delayed until the diagnosis is established on the basis of a positive antigen test or culture. Empiric therapy usually is not a cost-effective approach to the management of most adults with pharyngitis because the prevalence of streptococcal pharyngitis is likely to be no more than 10–20% in typical clinical settings. The positive predictive value of clinical criteria is low. Since macrolides are not reliable against *F necrophorum* infection, adolescents or young adults with pharyngitis, which is not confirmed to be due to group A beta-hemolytic streptococci, should be given penicillin or amoxicillin preferentially at the doses listed below. If the pharyngitis does not resolve quickly, symptoms worsen, or unilateral neck swelling develops, clinicians should consider suppurative complications such as peritonsillar abscess and the Lemierre syndrome.

A. Benzathine Penicillin G

Benzathine penicillin G, 1.2 million units intramuscularly as a single dose, is optimal therapy.

B. Penicillin VK

Penicillin VK, 250 mg orally four times daily or 500 mg orally twice daily for 10 days, is effective.

C. Amoxicillin

Amoxicillin, 1000 mg orally once daily or 500 mg orally twice daily for 10 days is another option.

D. Cephalosporins

Cephalexin, 500 mg orally twice daily for 10 days, cefdinir, 300 mg orally twice daily for 5–10 days or 600 mg orally once daily for 10 days, and cefpodoxime, 100 mg orally twice daily for 5–10 days, should be reserved for penicillin-allergic patients who do not have immediate-type hypersensitivity to penicillin.

E. Macrolides

Erythromycin, 500 mg orally four times a day, or azithromycin, 500 mg orally once daily for 5 days, is an alternative for the penicillin-allergic patient. Macrolides are less effective than penicillins and are considered second-line agents. Macrolide-resistant strains almost always are susceptible to clindamycin, a suitable alternative to penicillins; a 10-day course of 300 mg orally twice daily is effective.

Prevention of Recurrent Rheumatic Fever

Effectively controlling rheumatic fever depends on identification and treatment of primary streptococcal infection and secondary prevention of recurrences. Patients who have had rheumatic fever should be treated with a continuous course of antimicrobial prophylaxis for at least 5 years. Effective regimens are erythromycin, 250 mg orally twice daily, or penicillin G, 500 mg orally daily.

When to Refer

Patients with peritonsillar or retropharyngeal abscess should be referred to an otolaryngologist.

When to Admit

- Odynophagia resulting in dehydration.
- Suspected or known epiglottitis.

Cirilli AR. Emergency evaluation and management of the sore throat. Emerg Med Clin North Am. 2013 May;31(2):501–15. [PMID: 23601485]

Shulman ST et al. Clinical practice guideline for the diagnosis and management of group A streptococcal pharyngitis: 2012 update by the Infectious Diseases Society of America. Clin Infect Dis. 2012 Nov 15;55(10):1279–82. [PMID: 23091044]

van Driel ML et al. Different antibiotic treatments for group A streptococcal pharyngitis. Cochrane Database Syst Rev. 2013 Apr 30;4:CD004406. [PMID: 23633318]

2. Streptococcal Skin Infections

Group A beta-hemolytic streptococci are not normal skin flora. Streptococcal skin infections result from colonization of normal skin by contact with other infected individuals or by preceding streptococcal respiratory infection.

Clinical Findings

A. Symptoms and Signs

Impetigo is a focal, vesicular, pustular lesion with a thick, amber-colored crust with a "stuck-on" appearance (see Chapter 6).

Erysipelas is a painful superficial cellulitis that frequently involves the face. It is well demarcated from the surrounding normal skin. It affects skin with impaired lymphatic drainage, such as edematous lower extremities or wounds.

B. Laboratory Findings

Cultures obtained from a wound or pustule are likely to grow group A streptococci. Blood cultures are occasionally positive.

▶ **Treatment**

Parenteral antibiotics are indicated for patients with facial erysipelas or evidence of systemic infection. Penicillin, 2 million units intravenously every 4 hours, is the drug of choice. However, staphylococcal infections may at times be difficult to differentiate from streptococcal infections. In practice, initial therapy for patients with risk factors for *Staphylococcus aureus* (eg, injection drug use, diabetes mellitus, wound infection) should cover this organism. Nafcillin, 1–2 g every 4–6 hours intravenously, and cefazolin, 1 g intravenously or intramuscularly every 8 hours, are reasonable choices. In the patient at risk for methicillin-resistant *S aureus* infection or with a serious penicillin allergy (ie, anaphylaxis), vancomycin, 1 g intravenously every 12 hours, or daptomycin 4 mg/kg intravenously daily, should be used (Table 33–1).

Patients who do not require parenteral therapy may be treated with amoxicillin, 875 mg twice daily for 7–10 days. A first-generation oral cephalosporin, eg, cephalexin, 500 mg four times daily, or clindamycin, 300 mg orally three times daily, is an alternative to amoxicillin. In patients with recurrent cellulitis of the leg, maintenance therapy (for at least 1 year) with penicillin, 250 mg orally twice daily, can reduce the likelihood of relapse.

Stevens DL et al. Practice guidelines for the diagnosis and management of skin and soft tissue infections: 2014 update by the Infectious Diseases Society of America. Clin Infect Dis. 2014 Jul 15;59(2):147–59. [PMID: 24947530]

Thomas KS et al; U.K. Dermatology Clinical Trials Network's PATCH I Trial Team. Penicillin to prevent recurrent leg cellulitis. N Engl J Med. 2013 May 2;368(18):1695–703. [PMID: 23635049]

3. Other Group A Streptococcal Infections

Arthritis, pneumonia, empyema, endocarditis, and necrotizing fasciitis are relatively uncommon infections that may be caused by group A streptococci. Toxic shock-like syndrome also occurs.

Arthritis generally occurs in association with cellulitis. In addition to intravenous therapy with penicillin G, 2 million units every 4 hours (or cefazolin or vancomycin in doses recommended above for penicillin-allergic patients), frequent percutaneous needle aspiration should be performed to remove joint effusions. Open surgical drainage may be necessary in many cases.

Pneumonia and **empyema** often are characterized by extensive tissue destruction and an aggressive, rapidly progressive clinical course associated with significant morbidity and mortality. High-dose penicillin and chest tube drainage are indicated for treatment of empyema. Vancomycin is an acceptable substitute in penicillin-allergic patients.

Group A streptococci can cause **endocarditis.** Endocarditis should be treated with 4 million units of penicillin G intravenously every 4 hours for 4–6 weeks. Vancomycin, 1 g intravenously every 12 hours, is recommended for persons allergic to penicillin.

Table 33–1. Empiric treatment of common skin and soft tissue infections (SSTI).

SSTI Type	Common Pathogens	Treatment
Purulent (abscess, furuncle, carbuncle, cellulitis with purulence)	*Staphylococcus aureus*	Incision and drainage is the primary treatment Consider the addition of antibiotics in select situations[1] **Oral antibiotic regimens** 　Cephalexin 500 mg four times daily *or* dicloxacillin 500 mg four times daily 　Clindamycin 300–450 mg three or four times daily[2] *or* one double-strength tablet of 　　trimethoprim-sulfamethoxazole twice daily[2] *or* doxycycline 100 mg twice daily[2] **Intravenous antibiotic regimens**[3] 　Cefazolin 1 g three times daily *or* nafcillin 1–2 g four to six times daily 　Vancomycin 1 g twice daily[2] *or* daptomycin 4 mg/kg once daily[2]
Nonpurulent (cellulitis, erysipelas)	Beta-hemolytic streptococci (*S aureus* less likely)	**Oral antibiotic regimens** 　Cephalexin 500 mg four times daily *or* dicloxacillin 500 mg four times daily 　Clindamycin 300–450 mg three or four times daily[2] *or* amoxicillin 875 mg twice daily 　　*plus* one double-strength tablet of trimethoprim-sulfamethoxazole twice daily[2] **Intravenous antibiotic regimens**[3] 　Cefazolin 1 g three times daily *or* nafcillin 1–2 g four to six times daily 　Vancomycin 1 g twice daily[2] *or* daptomycin 4 mg/kg once daily

[1]Antibiotic therapy should be given in addition to incision and drainage for purulent SSTI if the patient has any of the following: severe or extensive disease, symptoms and signs of systemic illness, purulent cellulitis/wound infection, comorbidities and extremes of age, abscess in area difficult to drain or on face/hand, associated septic phlebitis, or lack of response to incision and drainage alone.
[2]Regimens with activity against methicillin-resistant *S aureus*.
[3]Other regimens approved by the FDA for treatment of complicated skin and soft tissue infections include tigecycline at 100 mg intravenously once followed by 50 mg intravenously twice a day, ceftaroline at 600 mg twice a day for 7–14 days, dalbavancin at 1 g intravenously on day 1 and then 500 mg intravenously on day 8, oritavancin as a single intravenous dose of 1200 mg, and telavancin at 10 mg/kg intravenously once daily for 7–14 days.

Necrotizing fasciitis is a rapidly spreading infection involving the fascia of deep muscle. The clinical findings at presentation may be those of severe cellulitis, but the presence of systemic toxicity and severe pain, which may be followed by anesthesia of the involved area due to destruction of nerves as infection advances through the fascial planes, is a clue to the diagnosis. Surgical exploration is mandatory when the diagnosis is suspected. Early and extensive debridement is essential for survival.

Any streptococcal infection—and necrotizing fasciitis in particular—can be associated with **streptococcal toxic shock syndrome**, typified by invasion of skin or soft tissues, acute respiratory distress syndrome, and kidney failure. The very young, the elderly, and those with underlying medical conditions are at particularly high risk for invasive disease. Bacteremia occurs in most cases. Skin rash and desquamation may not be present. Mortality rates can be up to 80%. The syndrome is due to elaboration of pyrogenic erythrotoxin (which also causes **scarlet fever**), a superantigen that stimulates massive release of inflammatory cytokines believed to mediate the shock. A beta-lactam, such as penicillin, remains the drug of choice for treatment of serious streptococcal infections, but clindamycin, which is a potent inhibitor of toxin production, should also be administered at a dose of 600 mg every 8 hours intravenously for invasive disease, especially in the presence of shock. Intravenous immune globulin should be considered for streptococcal toxic shock syndrome for possible therapeutic benefit from specific antibody to streptococcal exotoxins in immune globulin preparations. Many dosing regimens have been used, including 0.5 g/kg once daily for 5–6 days or a single dose of 2 g/kg with a repeat dose at 48 hours if the patient remains unstable.

Outbreaks of invasive disease have been associated with colonization by invasive clones that can be transmitted to close contacts who, though asymptomatic, may be a reservoir for disease. Tracing contacts of patients with invasive disease is controversial.

Carapetis JR et al. Effectiveness of clindamycin and intravenous immunoglobulin, and risk of disease in contacts, in invasive group A streptococcal infections. Clin Infect Dis. 2014 Aug 1; 59(3):358–65. [PMID: 24785239]

Linnér A et al. Clinical efficacy of polyspecific intravenous immunoglobulin therapy in patients with streptococcal toxic shock syndrome: a comparative observational study. Clin Infect Dis. 2014 Sep 15;59(6):851–7. [PMID: 24928291]

Stevens DL et al. Practice guidelines for the diagnosis and management of skin and soft tissue infections: 2014 update by the Infectious Diseases Society of America. Clin Infect Dis. 2014 Jul 15;59(2):147–59. [PMID: 24947530]

Waddington CS et al. Management of invasive group A streptococcal infections. J Infect. 2014 Nov;69(Suppl 1):S63–9. [PMID: 25307276]

4. Non-Group A Streptococcal Infections

Non-group A hemolytic streptococci (eg, groups B, C, and G) produce a spectrum of disease similar to that of group A streptococci. The treatment of infections caused by these strains is the same as for group A streptococci.

Group B streptococci are an important cause of sepsis, bacteremia, and meningitis in the neonate. Antepartum screening to identify carriers and peripartum antimicrobial prophylaxis are recommended in pregnancy. This organism, part of the normal vaginal flora, may cause septic abortion, endometritis, or peripartum infections and, less commonly, cellulitis, bacteremia, and endocarditis in adults. Treatment of infections caused by group B streptococci is with either penicillin or vancomycin in doses recommended for group A streptococci. Because of in vitro synergism, some experts recommend the addition of low-dose gentamicin, 1 mg/kg every 8 hours.

Viridans streptococci, which are nonhemolytic or alpha-hemolytic (ie, producing a green zone of hemolysis on blood agar), are part of the normal oral flora. Although these strains may produce focal pyogenic infection, they are most notable as the leading cause of native valve endocarditis.

Group D streptococci include *Streptococcus gallolyticus (bovis)* and the enterococci. *S gallolyticus (bovis)* is a cause of endocarditis in association with bowel neoplasia or cirrhosis and is treated like viridans streptococci.

Baddour LM et al. Infective endocarditis in adults: diagnosis, antimicrobial therapy, and management of complications: a scientific statement for healthcare professionals from the American Heart Association. Circulation. 2015 Oct 13; 132(15):1435–86. Erratum in: Circulation. 2015 Oct 27; 132(17):e215. [PMID: 26373316]

Ohlsson A et al. Intrapartum antibiotics for known maternal Group B streptococcal colonization. Cochrane Database Syst Rev. 2013 Jan 31;1:CD007467. [PMID: 23440815]

ENTEROCOCCAL INFECTIONS

Two species, *Enterococcus faecalis* and *Enterococcus faecium*, are responsible for most human enterococcal infections. Enterococci cause wound infections, urinary tract infections, bacteremia, and endocarditis. Infections caused by penicillin-susceptible strains should be treated with ampicillin 2 g every 4 hours or penicillin 3–4 million units every 4 hours; if the patient is penicillin-allergic, vancomycin 15 mg/kg every 12 hours intravenously can be given. If the patient has endocarditis or meningitis, gentamicin 1 mg/kg every 8 hours intravenously should be added to the regimen in order to achieve the bactericidal activity that is required to cure these infections. In cases of endocarditis, ceftriaxone 2 g every 12 hours may be given instead of gentamicin in combination with the ampicillin.

Resistance to vancomycin, penicillin, and gentamicin is common among enterococcal isolates, especially *E faecium*; it is essential to determine antimicrobial susceptibility of isolates. Infection control measures that may be indicated to limit their spread include isolation, barrier precautions, and avoidance of overuse of vancomycin and gentamicin. Consultation with an infectious diseases specialist is strongly advised when treating infections caused by resistant strains of enterococci. Quinupristin/dalfopristin and linezolid are approved by the FDA for treatment of infections caused by vancomycin-resistant strains of enterococci. Daptomycin, tigecycline, tedizolid, and oritavancin are not approved by the FDA for the treatment for vancomycin-resistant strains of enterococci, although they are frequently active in vitro.

Quinupristin/dalfopristin is not active against strains of *E faecalis* and should be used only for infections caused by *E faecium*. The dose is 7.5 mg/kg intravenously every 8–12 hours. Phlebitis and irritation at the infusion site (often requiring a central line) and an arthralgia-myalgia syndrome are relatively common side effects. Linezolid, an oxazolidinone, is active against both *E faecalis* and *E faecium*. The dose is 600 mg twice daily, and both intravenous and oral preparations are available. Its two principal side effects are thrombocytopenia and bone marrow suppression; however, peripheral neuropathy, optic neuritis, and lactic acidosis have been observed with prolonged use due to mitochondrial toxicity. Emergence of resistance has occurred during therapy with both quinupristin/dalfopristin and linezolid.

Baddour LM et al. Infective endocarditis in adults: diagnosis, antimicrobial therapy, and management of complications: a scientific statement for healthcare professionals from the American Heart Association. Circulation. 2015 Oct 13; 132(15):1435–86. Erratum in: Circulation. 2015 Oct 27; 132(17):e215. [PMID: 26373316]

Barber KE et al. Therapeutic options for vancomycin-resistant enterococcal bacteremia. Expert Rev Anti Infect Ther. 2015 Mar;13(3):363–77. [PMID: 25661903]

Patel R et al. Vancomycin-resistant enterococcal bacteremia pharmacotherapy. Ann Pharmacother. 2015 Jan;49(1):69–85. [PMID: 25352037]

PNEUMOCOCCAL INFECTIONS

1. Pneumococcal Pneumonia

ESSENTIALS OF DIAGNOSIS

► Productive cough, fever, rigors, dyspnea, early pleuritic chest pain.

► Consolidating lobar pneumonia on chest radiograph.

► Gram-positive diplococci on Gram stain of sputum.

General Considerations

The pneumococcus is the most common cause of community-acquired pyogenic bacterial pneumonia. Alcoholism, asthma, HIV infection, sickle cell disease, splenectomy, and hematologic disorders are predisposing factors. The mortality rate remains high in the setting of advanced age, multilobar disease, severe hypoxemia, extrapulmonary complications, and bacteremia.

Clinical Findings

A. Symptoms and Signs

Presenting symptoms and signs include high fever, productive cough, occasionally hemoptysis, and pleuritic chest pain. Rigors occur within the first few hours of infection but are uncommon thereafter. Bronchial breath sounds are an early sign.

B. Laboratory Findings

Pneumococcal pneumonia classically is a lobar pneumonia with radiographic findings of consolidation and occasionally effusion. However, differentiating it from other pneumonias is not possible radiographically or clinically because of significant overlap in presentations. Diagnosis requires isolation of the organism in culture, although the Gram stain appearance of sputum can be suggestive. Sputum and blood cultures, positive in 60% and 25% of cases of pneumococcal pneumonia, respectively, should be obtained prior to initiation of antimicrobial therapy in patients who are admitted to the hospital. A good-quality sputum sample (less than 10 epithelial cells and greater than 25 polymorphonuclear leukocytes per high-power field) shows gram-positive diplococci in 80–90% of cases. A rapid urinary antigen test for *Streptococcus pneumoniae*, with sensitivity of 70–80% and specificity greater than 95%, can assist with early diagnosis.

Complications

Parapneumonic (sympathetic) effusion is common and may cause recurrence or persistence of fever. These sterile fluid accumulations need no specific therapy. Empyema occurs in 5% or less of cases and is differentiated from sympathetic effusion by the presence of organisms on Gram-stained fluid or positive pleural fluid cultures.

Pneumococcal pericarditis is a rare complication that can cause tamponade. Pneumococcal arthritis also is uncommon. Pneumococcal endocarditis usually involves the aortic valve and often occurs in association with meningitis and pneumonia (sometimes referred to as Austrian or Osler triad). Early heart failure and multiple embolic events are typical.

Treatment

A. Specific Measures

Initial antimicrobial therapy for pneumonia is empiric (see Chapter 9 for specific recommendations) pending isolation and identification of the causative agent. Once *S pneumoniae* is identified as the infecting pathogen, any of several antimicrobial agents may be used depending on the clinical setting, community patterns of penicillin resistance, and susceptibility of the particular isolate. Uncomplicated pneumococcal pneumonia (ie, arterial PO_2 greater than 60 mm Hg, no coexisting medical problems, and single-lobe disease without signs of extrapulmonary infection) caused by penicillin-susceptible strains of pneumococcus may be treated on an outpatient basis with amoxicillin, 750 mg orally twice daily for 7–10 days. For penicillin-allergic patients, alternatives are azithromycin, one 500-mg dose orally on the first day and 250 mg for the next 4 days; clarithromycin, 500 mg orally twice daily for 10 days; doxycycline, 100 mg orally twice daily for 10 days;

levofloxacin, 750 mg orally for 5 days; or moxifloxacin, 400 mg orally for 7–14 days. Patients should be monitored for clinical response (eg, less cough, defervescence within 2–3 days) because pneumococci have become increasingly resistant to penicillin and the second-line agents.

Parenteral therapy is generally recommended for the hospitalized patient at least until there has been clinical improvement. Aqueous penicillin G, 2 million units intravenously every 4 hours, or ceftriaxone, 1 g intravenously every 24 hours, is effective for strains that are not highly penicillin-resistant (ie, strains for which the minimum inhibitory concentration [MIC] of penicillin is 1 mcg/mL or less). For serious penicillin allergy or infection caused by a highly penicillin-resistant strain, vancomycin, 1 g intravenously every 12 hours, is effective. Alternatively, a respiratory fluoroquinolone (eg, levofloxacin, 750 mg) can be used. The total duration of therapy is not well defined but 5–7 days is appropriate for patients who have an uncomplicated infection and demonstrate a good clinical response.

B. Treatment of Complications

Pleural effusions developing after initiation of antimicrobial therapy usually are sterile, and thoracentesis need not be performed if the patient is otherwise improving. Thoracentesis is indicated for an effusion present prior to initiation of therapy and in the patient who has not responded to antibiotics after 3–4 days. Chest tube drainage may be required if pneumococci are identified by culture or Gram stain, especially if aspiration of the fluid is difficult.

Echocardiography should be done if pericardial effusion is suspected. Patients with pericardial effusion who are responding to therapy and have no signs of tamponade may be monitored and treated with indomethacin, 50 mg orally three times daily, for pain. In patients with increasing effusion, unsatisfactory clinical response, or evidence of tamponade, pericardiocentesis will determine whether the pericardial space is infected. Infected fluid must be drained either percutaneously (by tube placement or needle aspiration), by placement of a pericardial window, or by pericardiectomy. Pericardiectomy eventually may be required to prevent or treat constrictive pericarditis, a common sequela of bacterial pericarditis.

Endocarditis should be treated for 4 weeks with 3–4 million units of penicillin G every 4 hours intravenously; ceftriaxone, 2 g once daily intravenously; or vancomycin, 15 mg/kg every 12 hours intravenously. Mild heart failure from endocarditis may respond to medical therapy, but moderate to severe heart failure is an indication for prosthetic valve implantation, as are systemic emboli or large friable vegetations as determined by echocardiography.

C. Penicillin-Resistant Pneumococci

Resistance breakpoints for parenterally administered penicillin and high-dose oral amoxicillin (2 g twice daily) are as follows: susceptible, penicillin MIC 2 mcg/mL or less; intermediate, MIC = 4 mcg/mL; resistant, MIC 8 mcg/mL or more. This change reflected results from studies demonstrating equivalent cure rates when high doses of parenteral penicillin were used for treatment of pneumococcal

pneumonia due to isolates with penicillin MIC 2 mcg/mL or less. Note, however, that these new breakpoints do not apply to orally administered penicillin, which are the same as for use of penicillin in treatment of meningitis. In cases of pneumococcal pneumonia where the isolate has a penicillin MIC greater than 2 mcg/mL, cephalosporin cross-resistance is common, and a non–beta-lactam antimicrobial, such as vancomycin, 1 g intravenously every 12 hours or a fluoroquinolone with enhanced gram-positive activity (eg, levofloxacin, 750 mg intravenously or orally once daily or moxifloxacin, 400 mg intravenously or orally once daily), is recommended. Penicillin-resistant strains of pneumococci may be resistant to macrolides, trimethoprim-sulfamethoxazole, and chloramphenicol, and susceptibility must be documented prior to their use. All blood and cerebrospinal fluid isolates should still be tested for resistance to penicillin. There has been no change to the penicillin susceptibility breakpoint for pneumococcal isolates causing meningitis, nor any change in treatment recommendations.

▶ Prevention

See Chapter 30 for discussion of pneumococcal vaccines.

▶ When to Refer

- All patients with suspected pneumococcal endocarditis or meningitis to an infectious disease specialist.
- Extensive disease.
- Seriously ill patient with pneumonia, particularly in the setting of comorbid conditions (eg, liver disease).
- Progression of pneumonia or failure to improve on antibiotics.

▶ When to Admit

- All patients in whom pneumococcal endocarditis or meningitis is suspected or documented should be admitted for observation and empiric therapy.
- All patients with pneumococcal pneumonia that is multilobar or associated with significant hypoxemia.
- Failure of outpatient pneumonia therapy, including inability to maintain oral intake and medications.
- Exacerbations of underlying disease (eg, heart failure) by pneumonia that would benefit from hospitalization.

Jain S et al; CDC EPIC Study Team. Community-acquired pneumonia requiring hospitalization among U.S. adults. N Engl J Med. 2015 Jul 30;373(5):415–27. [PMID: 26172429]

Moran GJ et al. Emergency management of community-acquired bacterial pneumonia: what is new since the 2007 Infectious Diseases Society of America/American Thoracic Society guidelines. Am J Emerg Med. 2013 Mar;31(3):602–12. [PMID: 23380120]

Postma DF et al; CAP-START Study Group. Antibiotic treatment strategies for community-acquired pneumonia in adults. N Engl J Med. 2015 Apr 2;372(14):1312–23. [PMID: 25830421]

2. Pneumococcal Meningitis

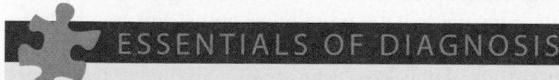

- ▶ Fever, headache, altered mental status.
- ▶ Meningismus.
- ▶ Gram-positive diplococci on Gram stain of cerebrospinal fluid.

▶ General Considerations

S pneumoniae is the most common cause of meningitis in adults. Head trauma with cerebrospinal fluid leaks, sinusitis, and pneumonia may precede it.

▶ Clinical Findings

A. Symptoms and Signs

The onset is rapid, with fever, headache, meningismus, and altered mentation. Pneumonia may be present. Compared with meningitis caused by the meningococcus, pneumococcal meningitis lacks a rash, and focal neurologic deficits, cranial nerve palsies, and obtundation are more prominent features.

B. Laboratory Findings

The cerebrospinal fluid typically has greater than 1000 white blood cells per microliter, over 60% of which are polymorphonuclear leukocytes; the glucose concentration is less than 40 mg/dL (2.22 mmol/L), or less than 50% of the simultaneous serum concentration; and the protein usually exceeds 150 mg/dL (1500 mg/L) (see Chapter 30). Not all cases of meningitis will have these typical findings, and alterations in cerebrospinal fluid cell counts and chemistries may be surprisingly minimal, overlapping with those of aseptic meningitis.

Gram stain of cerebrospinal fluid shows gram-positive cocci in 80–90% of cases, and in untreated cases, blood or cerebrospinal fluid cultures are almost always positive.

▶ Treatment

Antibiotics should be given as soon as the diagnosis is suspected. If lumbar puncture must be delayed (eg, while awaiting results of an imaging study to exclude a mass lesion), the patient should be treated empirically for presumed meningitis with intravenous ceftriaxone, 2 g, plus vancomycin, 15 mg/kg, plus dexamethasone, 0.15 mg/kg administered concomitantly after blood cultures (positive in 50% of cases) have been obtained. Once susceptibility to penicillin has been confirmed, penicillin, 24 million units intravenously daily in six divided doses, or ceftriaxone, 2 g every 12 hours intravenously, is continued for 10–14 days in documented cases.

The best therapy for penicillin-resistant strains is not known. Penicillin-resistant strains (MIC greater than 0.06 mcg/mL) are often cross-resistant to the third-generation

cephalosporins as well as other antibiotics. Susceptibility testing is essential to proper management of this infection. If the MIC of ceftriaxone or cefotaxime is 0.5 mcg/mL or less, single-drug therapy with either of these cephalosporins is likely to be effective; when the MIC is 1 mcg/mL or more, treatment with a combination of ceftriaxone, 2 g intravenously every 12 hours, plus vancomycin, 30 mg/kg/day intravenously in two or three divided doses, is recommended. If a patient with a penicillin-resistant organism is slow to respond clinically, repeat lumbar puncture may be indicated to assess bacteriologic response.

Dexamethasone administered with antibiotic to adults has been associated with a 60% reduction in mortality and a 50% reduction in unfavorable outcomes. It is recommended that dexamethasone, 10 mg intravenously, be given immediately prior to or concomitantly with the first dose of appropriate antibiotic and continued in those with pneumococcal disease every 6 hours thereafter for a total of 4 days. Patients with pneumococcal meningitis and AIDS who do not have access to resources may not benefit from dexamethasone. The effect of dexamethasone on outcome of meningitis caused by penicillin-resistant organisms is not known.

Erdem H et al. Mortality indicators in pneumococcal meningitis: therapeutic implications. Int J Infect Dis. 2014 Feb;19:13–9. [PMID: 24211227]

Glimåker M et al. Adult bacterial meningitis: earlier treatment and improved outcome following guideline revision promoting prompt lumbar puncture. Clin Infect Dis. 2015 Apr 15; 60(8):1162–9. [PMID: 25663160]

van de Beek D et al. Advances in treatment of bacterial meningitis. Lancet. 2012 Nov 10;380(9854):1693–702. [PMID: 23141618]

STAPHYLOCOCCUS AUREUS INFECTIONS

1. Skin & Soft Tissue Infections

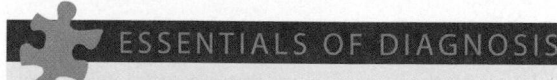

- ▶ Localized erythema with induration and purulent drainage.
- ▶ Abscess formation.
- ▶ Folliculitis commonly observed.
- ▶ Gram stain of pus with gram-positive cocci in clusters; cultures usually positive.

▶ General Considerations

Approximately one-quarter of people are asymptomatic nasal carriers of *S aureus*, which is spread by direct contact. Carriage often precedes infection, which occurs as a consequence of disruption of the cutaneous barrier or impairment of host defenses. *S aureus* tends to cause more localized skin infections than streptococci, and abscess formation is common. The prevalence of methicillin-resistant

▲ **Figure 33–1.** Methicillin-resistant *Staphylococcus aureus* (MRSA) abscess of the neck. (From Edward Wright, MD; Reproduced, with permission, from Usatine RP, Smith MA, Mayeaux EJ Jr, Chumley H, Tysinger J. *The Color Atlas of Family Medicine.* McGraw-Hill, 2009.)

strains in community settings is increasing, and these strains have been associated with recurrent and severe skin and soft tissue infections, including necrotizing fasciitis.

► Clinical Findings

A. Symptoms and Signs

S aureus skin infections may begin around one or more hair follicles, causing folliculitis; may become localized to form boils (or furuncles); or may spread to adjacent skin and deeper subcutaneous tissue (ie, a carbuncle) (Figure 33–1). Deep abscesses involving muscle or fascia may occur, often in association with a deep wound or other inoculation or injection. Necrotizing fasciitis, a rare form of *S aureus* skin and soft tissues infection, has been reported with community strains of methicillin-resistant *S aureus*.

B. Laboratory Findings

Cultures of the wound or abscess material will almost always yield the organism. In patients with systemic signs of infection, blood cultures should be obtained because of potential endocarditis, osteomyelitis, or metastatic seeding of other sites. Patients who are bacteremic should have blood cultures taken early during therapy to exclude persistent bacteremia, an indicator of severe or complicated infection.

► Treatment

Proper drainage of abscess fluid or other focal infections is the mainstay of therapy. Incision and drainage alone may be sufficient for cutaneous abscess. For uncomplicated skin infections, oral antimicrobial therapy is satisfactory. Before the emergence of community methicillin-resistant strains of *S aureus*, an oral penicillinase-resistant penicillin or cephalosporin, such as dicloxacillin or cephalexin, 500 mg four times a day for 7–10 days, was the drug of choice for

empiric therapy. However, increasing prevalence of methicillin-resistant strains of *S aureus* among community isolates may necessitate use of other oral agents to which the isolate is susceptible in vitro, such as clindamycin, 300 mg three times daily; doxycycline or minocycline, 100 mg twice daily; or trimethoprim-sulfamethoxazole, given in two divided doses based on 5–10 mg/kg/day of the trimethoprim component. Because of the high prevalence of macrolide resistance among *S aureus* strains, these agents should not be used unless susceptibility is documented (see Table 33–1).

For more complicated infections with extensive cutaneous or deep tissue involvement or fever, parenteral therapy is indicated initially. A penicillinase-resistant penicillin such as nafcillin or oxacillin in a dosage of 1.5 g every 6 hours intravenously or cefazolin 1 g intravenously or intramuscularly is preferred for infections caused by methicillin-susceptible isolates. In patients with a serious allergy to beta-lactam antibiotics or if the strain is methicillin-resistant, vancomycin, 1 g intravenously every 12 hours, is a drug of choice. If the local prevalence of methicillin resistance is high (eg, 10% or more), and particularly if the patient is seriously ill, vancomycin is indicated empirically pending strain isolation and determination of susceptibility.

Linezolid is FDA-approved for treatment of skin and skin-structure infections as well as hospital-acquired pneumonia caused by methicillin-resistant strains of *S aureus* and clinically is as effective as vancomycin. The dose is 600 mg orally (bioavailability of 100%) or intravenously twice a day for 10–14 days. Its considerable cost makes it an unattractive choice for most routine outpatient infections, and its safety in treatment courses lasting longer than 2–3 weeks is not well characterized. Tedizolid, (an oxazolidinone, like linezolid) is also approved for treating skin and soft tissue infection at a dose of 200 mg orally once daily for 6 days. Other drugs FDA approved for treating skin and soft tissue infections include daptomycin, 4 mg/kg intravenously once daily for 7–14 days; tigecycline (a glycylcycline class antimicrobial), 100 mg intravenously once followed by 50 mg intravenously twice a day for 5–14 days; ceftaroline (a novel cephalosporin with activity against methicillin-resistant *S aureus*), 600 mg twice a day for 7–14 days; dalbavancin (a lipoglycopeptide), 1 g intravenously on day 1 and then 500 mg intravenously on day 8; oritavancin (a lipoglycopeptide), a single intravenous dose of 1200 mg; and telavancin (a lipoglycopeptide), 10 mg/kg intravenously once daily for 7–14 days. Telavancin is also approved for the treatment of hospital-acquired *S aureus* pneumonia but has been associated with nephrotoxicity.

Boucher HW et al. Once-weekly dalbavancin versus daily conventional therapy for skin infection. N Engl J Med. 2014 Jun 5; 370(23):2169–79. [PMID: 24897082]

Corey GR et al; SOLO I Investigators. Single-dose oritavancin in the treatment of acute bacterial skin infections. N Engl J Med. 2014 Jun 5;370(23):2180–90. [PMID: 24897083]

Moran GJ et al. Tedizolid for 6 days versus linezolid for 10 days for acute bacterial skin and skin-structure infections (ESTABLISH-2): a randomised, double-blind, phase 3, non-inferiority trial. Lancet Infect Dis. 2014 Aug;14(8):696–705. [PMID: 24909499]

Stevens DL et al. Practice guidelines for the diagnosis and management of skin and soft tissue infections: 2014 update by the Infectious Diseases Society of America. Clin Infect Dis. 2014 Jul 15;59(2):147–59. [PMID: 24947530]

2. Osteomyelitis

S aureus causes approximately 60% of all cases of osteomyelitis. Osteomyelitis may be caused by direct inoculation, eg, from an open fracture or as a result of surgery; by extension from a contiguous focus of infection or open wound; or by hematogenous spread. Long bones and vertebrae are the usual sites. Epidural abscess is a common complication of vertebral osteomyelitis and should be suspected if fever and severe back or neck pain are accompanied by radicular pain or symptoms or signs indicative of spinal cord compression (eg, incontinence, extremity weakness, pathologic extremity reflexes).

▶ Clinical Findings

A. Symptoms and Signs

The infection may be acute, with abrupt development of local symptoms and systemic toxicity, or indolent, with insidious onset of vague pain over the site of infection, progressing to local tenderness and constitutional symptoms (fever, malaise, anorexia, night sweats). Fever is absent in one-third or more of cases. Back pain is often the only symptom in vertebral osteomyelitis and may be associated with an epidural abscess and spinal cord compression. Draining sinus tracts occur in chronic infections or infections of foreign body implants.

B. Laboratory Findings

The diagnosis is established by isolation of S aureus from the blood, bone, or a contiguous focus of a patient with symptoms and signs of focal bone infection. Blood culture will be positive in approximately 60% of untreated cases. Bone biopsy and culture are indicated if blood cultures are sterile.

C. Imaging

Bone scan and gallium scan, each with a sensitivity of approximately 95% and a specificity of 60–70%, are useful in identifying or confirming the site of bone infection. Plain bone films early in the course of infection are often normal but will become abnormal in most cases even with effective therapy. Spinal infection (unlike malignancy) traverses the disk space to involve the contiguous vertebral body. CT is more sensitive than plain films and helps localize associated abscesses. MRI is slightly less sensitive than bone scan but has a specificity of 90%. It is indicated when epidural abscess is suspected in association with vertebral osteomyelitis.

▶ Treatment

Prolonged therapy is required to cure staphylococcal osteomyelitis. Durations of 4–6 weeks or longer are recommended. Intravenous therapy is preferred, particularly during the acute phase of the infection for patients with systemic toxicity. Cefazolin, 2 g every 8 hours, or alternatively, nafcillin or oxacillin, 9–12 g/day in six divided doses, are the drugs of choice for infection with methicillin-sensitive isolates. Patients with infections due to methicillin-resistant strains of S aureus or who have severe penicillin allergies should be treated with vancomycin, 30 mg/kg/day intravenously divided in two or three doses. Doses should be adjusted to achieve a vancomycin trough level of 15–20 mcg/mL. In patients with S aureus isolates susceptible to a fluoroquinolone and rifampin, that combination has been shown to be effective if given for 4 weeks following 2 weeks of induction therapy with an intravenous agent as above. Consultation with an infectious diseases specialist is recommended. The role of newer agents, such as daptomycin or linezolid, remains to be defined.

Surgical treatment is often indicated under the following circumstances: (1) staphylococcal osteomyelitis with associated epidural abscess and spinal cord compression, (2) other abscesses (psoas, paraspinal), (3) extensive disease, or (4) recurrent infection following standard medical therapy. Follow-up imaging may not be needed in patients who demonstrate clinical response to disease with improvement in symptoms and normalization of inflammatory markers.

Berbari EF et al. 2015 Infectious Diseases Society of America (IDSA) clinical practice guidelines for the diagnosis and treatment of native vertebral osteomyelitis in adults. Clin Infect Dis. 2015 Sep 15;61(6):e26–46. [PMID: 26229122]

Bernard L et al; Duration of Treatment for Spondylodiscitis (DTS) study group. Antibiotic treatment for 6 weeks versus 12 weeks in patients with pyogenic vertebral osteomyelitis: an open-label, non-inferiority, randomised, controlled trial. Lancet. 2015 Mar 7;385(9971):875–82. [PMID: 25468170]

Vardakas KZ et al. Incidence, characteristics, and outcomes of patients with bone and joint infections due to community-associated methicillin-resistant Staphylococcus aureus: a systematic review. Eur J Clin Microbiol Infect Dis. 2013 Jun; 32(6):711–21. [PMID: 23334662]

3. Staphylococcal Bacteremia

S aureus readily invades the bloodstream and infects sites distant from the primary site of infection. Whenever S aureus is recovered from blood cultures, the possibility of endocarditis, osteomyelitis, or other metastatic deep infection must be considered. Bacteremia that persists for more than 48–96 hours after initiation of therapy is strongly predictive of worse outcome and complicated infection. Given the relatively high risk of infective endocarditis in patients with S aureus bacteremia, transesophageal echocardiography is recommended for most patients as a sensitive and cost-effective method for excluding underlying endocarditis. However, transthoracic echocardiography may be sufficient in select patients considered to be at low risk for endocarditis, namely those who meet all the following criteria: (1) no permanent intracardiac device, (2) sterile follow-up blood cultures within 4 days after the initial set, (3) no hemodialysis dependence, (4) nosocomial acquisition of S aureus bacteremia, and (5) no clinical signs of infective endocarditis or secondary foci of infection.

Empiric therapy of staphylococcal bacteremia should be with vancomycin, 15–20 mg/kg/dose intravenously every 8–12 hours, or daptomycin 6 mg/kg/day intravenously until results of susceptibility tests are known. If the *S aureus* isolate is methicillin-susceptible, treatment should be narrowed to cefazolin, 2 g every 8 hours or nafcillin or oxacillin, 2 g intravenously every 4 hours. Cefazolin is as effective as nafcillin or oxacillin and has been associated with fewer adverse events during treatment. In patients with methicillin-resistant *S aureus*, treatment should be with vancomycin, 15–20 mg/kg/dose intravenously every 8–12 hours. Maintaining a vancomycin trough concentration of 15–20 mcg/mL may improve outcomes and is recommended. Daptomycin 6 mg/k/day is also an FDA-approved option as long as the patient does not require treatment for concomitant *S aureus* pneumonia. Duration of therapy for *S aureus* bacteremia is 4–6 weeks of antibiotic therapy but a subset of patients with uncomplicated infection may be able to be treated for 14 days. A patient with uncomplicated bacteremia must meet all the following criteria: (1) infective endocarditis has been excluded, (2) no implanted prostheses are present, (3) follow-up blood cultures drawn 2–4 days after the initial set are sterile, (4) the patient defervesces within 72 hours of initiation of effective antibiotic therapy, and (5) no evidence of metastatic infection is present on examination. When present, infected central venous catheters should also be removed. Vancomycin treatment failures are relatively common, particularly for complicated bacteremia and among infections involving foreign bodies. Consultation with an infectious diseases specialist should be considered in all cases of *S aureus* bacteremia and particularly when vancomycin treatment fails.

▲ **Figure 33–2.** Morbilliform rash in toxic shock syndrome caused by *Staphylococcus aureus*. (Public Health Image Library, CDC.)

shock syndrome is characterized by abrupt onset of high fever, vomiting, and watery diarrhea. Sore throat, myalgias, and headache are common. Hypotension with kidney and heart failure is associated with a poor outcome. A diffuse macular erythematous rash (Figure 33–2) and nonpurulent conjunctivitis are common, and desquamation, especially of palms and soles, is typical during recovery. Fatality rates may be as high as 15%. Although originally associated with tampon use, any focus (eg, nasopharynx, bone, vagina, rectum, abscess, or wound) harboring a toxin-producing *S aureus* strain can cause toxic shock syndrome and nonmenstrual cases of toxic shock syndrome are common. Classically, blood cultures are negative because symptoms are due to the effects of the toxin and not systemic infection.

Important aspects of treatment include rapid rehydration, antistaphylococcal drugs, management of kidney or heart failure, and addressing sources of toxin, eg, removal of tampon or drainage of abscess.

Holland TL et al. Clinical management of *Staphylococcus aureus* bacteremia: a review. JAMA. 2014 Oct 1;312(13):1330–41. [PMID: 25268440]

Kalil AC et al. Association between vancomycin minimum inhibitory concentration and mortality among patients with *Staphylococcus aureus* bloodstream infections: a systematic review and meta-analysis. JAMA. 2014 Oct 15;312(15):1552–64. [PMID: 25321910]

Liu C et al. Clinical practice guidelines by the Infectious Diseases Society of America for the treatment of methicillin-resistant *Staphylococcus aureus* infections in adults and children. Clin Infect Dis. 2011 Feb 1;52(3):e18–55. [PMID: 21208910]

Rao SN et al. Treatment outcomes with cefazolin versus oxacillin for deep-seated methicillin-susceptible *Staphylococcus aureus* bloodstream infections. Antimicrob Agents Chemother. 2015 Sep;59(9):5232–8. Erratum in: Antimicrob Agents Chemother. 2015 Nov;59(11):7159. [PMID: 26077253]

Youngster I et al. Comparative evaluation of the tolerability of cefazolin and nafcillin for treatment of methicillin-susceptible *Staphylococcus aureus* infections in the outpatient setting. Clin Infect Dis. 2014 Aug 1;59(3):369–75. [PMID: 24785233]

4. Toxic Shock Syndrome

S aureus produces toxins that cause three important entities: "scalded skin syndrome" in children, toxic shock syndrome in adults, and enterotoxin food poisoning. Toxic

5. Infections Caused by Coagulase-Negative Staphylococci

Coagulase-negative staphylococci are an important cause of infections of intravascular and prosthetic devices and of wound infection following cardiothoracic surgery. These organisms infrequently cause infections such as osteomyelitis and endocarditis in the absence of a prosthesis, but rates may be increasing. Most human infections are caused by *Staphylococcus epidermidis*, *S haemolyticus*, *S hominis*, *S warnerii*, *S saprophyticus*, *S saccharolyticus*, and *S cohnii*. These common hospital-acquired pathogens are less virulent than *S aureus*, and infections caused by them tend to be more indolent.

Because coagulase-negative staphylococci are normal inhabitants of human skin, it is difficult to distinguish infection from contamination, the latter perhaps accounting for three-fourths of blood culture isolates. Infection is more likely if the patient has a foreign body (eg, sternal wires, prosthetic joint, prosthetic cardiac valve, pacemaker, intracranial pressure monitor, cerebrospinal fluid shunt, peritoneal dialysis catheter) or an intravascular device in place. Purulent or serosanguineous drainage, erythema, pain, or tenderness at the site of the foreign body or device suggests infection. Instability and pain are signs of prosthetic joint infection. Fever, a new murmur, instability of the prosthesis, or signs of systemic embolization are evidence of prosthetic valve endocarditis. Immunosuppression and recent antimicrobial therapy are risk factors.

Infection is also more likely if the same strain is consistently isolated from two or more blood cultures (particularly if samples were obtained at different times) and from the foreign body site. Contamination is more likely when a single blood culture is positive or if more than one strain is isolated from blood cultures. The antimicrobial susceptibility pattern and speciation are used to determine whether one or more strains have been isolated. More sophisticated typing methods, eg, pulse-field gel electrophoresis of restriction enzyme digested chromosomal DNA, may be required to identify distinct strains.

Whenever possible, the intravascular device or foreign body suspected of being infected by coagulase-negative staphylococci should be removed. However, removal and replacement of some devices (eg, prosthetic joint, prosthetic valve, cerebrospinal fluid shunt) can be a difficult or risky procedure, and it may sometimes be preferable to treat with antibiotics alone with the understanding that the probability of cure is reduced and that surgical management may eventually be necessary.

Coagulase-negative staphylococci are commonly resistant to beta-lactams and multiple other antibiotics. For patients with normal kidney function, vancomycin, 1 g intravenously every 12 hours, is the treatment of choice for suspected or confirmed infection caused by these organisms until susceptibility to penicillinase-resistant penicillins or other agents has been confirmed. Duration of therapy has not been established for relatively uncomplicated infections, such as those secondary to intravenous devices, which may be eliminated by simply removing the infected device. Infection involving bone or a prosthetic valve should be treated for 6 weeks. A combination regimen of vancomycin plus rifampin, 300 mg orally twice daily, plus gentamicin, 1 mg/kg intravenously every 8 hours, is recommended for treatment of prosthetic valve endocarditis caused by methicillin-resistant strains.

Baddour LM et al. Infective endocarditis in adults: diagnosis, antimicrobial therapy, and management of complications: a scientific statement for healthcare professionals from the American Heart Association. Circulation. 2015 Oct 13; 132(15):1435–86. Erratum in: Circulation. 2015 Oct 27; 132(17):e215. [PMID: 26373316]

May L et al. Trends in antibiotic resistance in coagulase-negative staphylococci in the United States, 1999 to 2012. Antimicrob Agents Chemother. 2014;58(3):1404–9. [PMID: 24342646]

CLOSTRIDIAL DISEASES

1. Clostridial Myonecrosis (Gas Gangrene)

> ### ESSENTIALS OF DIAGNOSIS
>
> ▶ Sudden onset of pain and edema in an area of wound contamination.
>
> ▶ Prostration and systemic toxicity.
>
> ▶ Brown to blood-tinged watery exudate, with skin discoloration of surrounding area.
>
> ▶ Gas in the tissue by palpation or radiograph.
>
> ▶ Gram-positive rods in culture or smear of exudate.

▶ General Considerations

Gas gangrene or clostridial myonecrosis is produced by any one of several clostridia (*Clostridium perfringens, C ramosum, C bifermentans, C histolyticum, C novyi*, etc). Trauma and injection drug use are common predisposing conditions. Toxins produced in devitalized tissues under anaerobic conditions result in shock, hemolysis, and myonecrosis.

▶ Clinical Findings

A. Symptoms and Signs

The onset is usually sudden, with rapidly increasing pain in the affected area, hypotension, and tachycardia. Fever is present but is not proportionate to the severity of the infection. In the last stages of the disease, severe prostration, stupor, delirium, and coma occur.

The wound becomes swollen, and the surrounding skin is pale. There is a foul-smelling brown, blood-tinged serous discharge. As the disease advances, the surrounding tissue changes from pale to dusky and finally becomes deeply discolored, with coalescent, red, fluid-filled vesicles. Gas may be palpable in the tissues.

B. Laboratory Findings

Gas gangrene is a clinical diagnosis, and empiric therapy is indicated if the diagnosis is suspected. Radiographic studies may show gas within the soft tissues, but this finding is not specific. The smear shows absence of neutrophils and the presence of gram-positive rods. Anaerobic culture confirms the diagnosis.

▶ Differential Diagnosis

Other bacteria can produce gas in infected tissue, eg, enteric gram-negative organisms, or anaerobes.

Treatment

Penicillin, 2 million units every 3 hours intravenously, is effective. Clindamycin may decrease the production of bacterial toxin, and some experts recommend the addition of clindamycin, 600–900 mg every 8 hours intravenously, to penicillin. Adequate surgical debridement and exposure of infected areas are essential, with radical surgical excision often necessary. Hyperbaric oxygen therapy has been used empirically but must be used in conjunction with administration of an appropriate antibiotic and surgical debridement.

Kaafarani HM et al. Necrotizing skin and soft tissue infections. Surg Clin North Am. 2014 Feb;94(1):155–63. [PMID: 24267503]
Stevens DL et al. Practice guidelines for the diagnosis and management of skin and soft tissue infections: 2014 update by the Infectious Diseases Society of America. Clin Infect Dis. 2014 Jul 15;59(2):147–59. [PMID: 24947530]
Yang Z et al. Interventions for treating gas gangrene. Cochrane Database Syst Rev. 2015 Dec 3;12:CD010577. [PMID: 26631369]

2. *Clostridium sordellii* Toxic Shock Syndrome

ESSENTIALS OF DIAGNOSIS

- ► Sudden onset after medical abortion.
- ► Abdominal pain.
- ► Absence of fever.
- ► Tachycardia, severe hypotension, capillary leak syndrome with edema.
- ► Profound leukocytosis, hemoconcentration.

General Considerations & Clinical Findings

C sordellii is a rare cause of endometritis and toxic shock syndrome following childbirth. Fatal cases of uterine infection following medically induced abortion with mifepristone have been reported. Onset of illness was within 4–5 days of ingestion of mifepristone and the clinical course fulminant. Infection appeared to be limited to the uterus, which showed necrosis, edema, hemorrhage, and acute inflammatory changes.

Treatment

Early recognition, aggressive resuscitation from shock, immediate surgical debridement with hysterectomy, and administration of an antimicrobial that is active against *C sordellii* are essential to survival. Based on in vitro susceptibility data, any of several agents should be active, including penicillin, ampicillin, a macrolide, clindamycin, a tetracycline, or metronidazole. Whether a protein synthesis inhibitor to block further toxin production offers any advantage over a beta-lactam is unknown.

3. Tetanus

ESSENTIALS OF DIAGNOSIS

- ► History of wound and possible contamination.
- ► Jaw stiffness followed by spasms of jaw muscles (trismus).
- ► Stiffness of the neck and other muscles, dysphagia, irritability, hyperreflexia.
- ► Finally, painful convulsions precipitated by minimal stimuli.

General Considerations

Tetanus is caused by the neurotoxin tetanospasmin, elaborated by *C tetani*. Spores of this organism are ubiquitous in soil and may germinate when introduced into a wound. The vegetative bacteria produce tetanospasmin, a zinc metalloprotease that cleaves synaptobrevin, a protein essential for neurotransmitter release. Tetanospasmin interferes with neurotransmission at spinal synapses of inhibitory neurons. As a result, minor stimuli result in uncontrolled spasms, and reflexes are exaggerated. The incubation period is 5 days to 15 weeks, with the average being 8–12 days.

Most cases occur in unvaccinated individuals. Persons at risk are the elderly, migrant workers, newborns, and injection drug users. While puncture wounds are particularly prone to causing tetanus, any wound, including bites or decubiti, may become colonized and infected by *C tetani*.

Clinical Findings

A. Symptoms and Signs

The first symptom may be pain and tingling at the site of inoculation, followed by spasticity of the muscles nearby. Stiffness of the jaw, neck stiffness, dysphagia, and irritability are other early signs. Hyperreflexia develops later, with spasms of the jaw muscles (trismus) or facial muscles and rigidity and spasm of the muscles of the abdomen, neck, and back. Painful tonic convulsions precipitated by minor stimuli are common. Spasms of the glottis and respiratory muscles may cause acute asphyxia. The patient is awake and alert throughout the illness. The sensory examination is normal. The temperature is normal or only slightly elevated.

B. Laboratory Findings

The diagnosis of tetanus is made clinically.

Differential Diagnosis

Tetanus must be differentiated from various acute central nervous system infections such as meningitis. Trismus may occasionally develop with the use of phenothiazines. Strychnine poisoning should also be considered.

Complications

Airway obstruction is common. Urinary retention and constipation may result from spasm of the sphincters. Respiratory arrest and cardiac failure are late, life-threatening events.

Prevention

Tetanus is preventable by active immunization (see Table 30–7). For primary immunization of adults, Td (tetanus and diphtheria toxoids vaccine) is administered as two doses 4–6 weeks apart, with a third dose 6–12 months later. For one of the doses, Tdap (tetanus toxoid, reduced-dose diphtheria toxoid, acellular pertussis vaccine) should be substituted for Td. Booster doses are given every 10 years or at the time of major injury if it occurs more than 5 years after a dose. A single dose of Tdap is preferred to Td for wound prophylaxis if the patient has not been previously vaccinated with Tdap.

Passive immunization should be used in nonimmunized individuals and those whose immunization status is uncertain whenever a wound is contaminated or likely to have devitalized tissue. Tetanus immune globulin, 250 units, is given intramuscularly. Active immunization with tetanus toxoid is started concurrently. Table 33–2 provides a guide to prophylactic management.

Treatment

A. Specific Measures

Human tetanus immune globulin, 500 units, should be administered intramuscularly within the first 24 hours of presentation. Whether intrathecal administration has any additional benefit is controversial. An unblinded, randomized trial comparing intramuscular tetanus immune globulin to intramuscular plus intrathecal tetanus immune globulin found more rapid resolution of spasms, fewer days of ventilatory support, and a shorter hospital stay in the intrathecal group. However, the exact immunoglobulin preparation that was used was not specified and the total dose was 4000 units.

Tetanus does not produce natural immunity, and a full course of immunization with tetanus toxoid should be administered once the patient has recovered.

B. General Measures

Minimal stimuli can provoke spasms, so the patient should be placed at bed rest and monitored under the quietest conditions possible. Sedation, paralysis with curare-like agents, and mechanical ventilation are often necessary to control tetanic spasms. Penicillin, 20 million units intravenously daily in divided doses, is given to all patients—even those with mild illness—to eradicate toxin-producing organisms.

Prognosis

High mortality rates are associated with a short incubation period, early onset of convulsions, and delay in treatment. Contaminated lesions about the head and face are more dangerous than wounds on other parts of the body.

Yen C et al; Centers for Disease Control and Prevention (CDC). Missed opportunities for tetanus postexposure prophylaxis—California, January 2008–March 2014. MMWR Morb Mortal Wkly Rep. 2015 Mar 13;64(9):243–6. [PMID: 25763876]

4. Botulism

ESSENTIALS OF DIAGNOSIS

► History of recent ingestion of home-canned or smoked foods or of injection drug use and demonstration of toxin in serum or food.

► Sudden onset of diplopia, dry mouth, dysphagia, dysphonia, and muscle weakness progressing to respiratory paralysis.

► Pupils are fixed and dilated in most cases.

Table 33–2. Guide to tetanus prophylaxis in wound management.

History of Absorbed Tetanus Toxoid	Clean, Minor Wounds		All Other Wounds[1]	
	Tdap or Td[2]	TIG[3]	Tdap or Td[2]	TIG[3]
Unknown or < 3 doses	Yes	No	Yes	Yes
3 or more doses	No[4]	No	No[5]	No

[1]Such as, but not limited to, wounds contaminated with dirt, feces, soil, saliva, etc; puncture wounds; avulsions; and wounds resulting from missiles, crushing, burns, and frostbite.
[2]Td indicates tetanus toxoid and diphtheria toxoid, adult form. Tdap indicates tetanus toxoid, reduced diphtheria toxoid, and acellular pertussis vaccine, which may be substituted as a single dose for Td. Unvaccinated individuals should receive a complete series of three doses, one of which is Tdap.
[3]Human tetanus immune globulin, 250 units intramuscularly.
[4]Yes if more than 10 years have elapsed since last dose.
[5]Yes if more than 5 years have elapsed since last dose. (More frequent boosters are not needed and can enhance side effects.) Tdap has been safely administered within 2 years of Td vaccination, although local reactions to the vaccine may be increased.

General Considerations

Botulism is a paralytic disease caused by botulinum toxin, which is produced by *C botulinum*, a ubiquitous, strictly anaerobic, spore-forming bacillus found in soil. Four toxin types—A, B, E, and F—cause human disease. Botulinum toxin is a zinc metalloprotease that cleaves a specific component of the synaptic vesicle membrane docking and fusion complex at the neuromuscular junction blocking release of the neurotransmitter acetylcholine. Botulinum toxin is extremely potent and is classified by the CDC as a high-priority agent because of its potential for use as an agent of bioterrorism. Naturally occurring botulism occurs in one of three forms: food-borne botulism, infant botulism, or wound botulism. Food-borne botulism is caused by ingestion of preformed toxin present in canned, smoked, or vacuum-packed foods such as home-canned vegetables, smoked meats, and vacuum-packed fish. Commercial foods have also been associated with outbreaks of botulism. Infant botulism (associated with ingestion of honey) and wound botulism (which typically occurs in association with injection drug use) result from organisms present in the gut or wound that elaborate toxin in vivo.

Clinical Findings

A. Symptoms and Signs

Twelve to 36 hours after ingestion of the toxin, visual disturbances appear, particularly diplopia and loss of accommodation. Ptosis, cranial nerve palsies with impairment of extraocular muscles, and fixed dilated pupils are characteristic signs. The sensory examination is normal. Other symptoms are dry mouth, dysphagia, and dysphonia. Nausea and vomiting may be present, particularly with type E toxin. The sensorium remains clear and the temperature normal. Paralysis progressing to respiratory failure and death may occur unless mechanical assistance is provided.

B. Laboratory Findings

Toxin in patients' serum and in suspected foods can be demonstrated by mouse inoculation and identified with specific antiserum.

Differential Diagnosis

Because the clinical presentation of botulism is so distinctive and the differential diagnosis limited, botulism once considered is not easily confused with other diseases. Cranial nerve involvement may be seen with vertebrobasilar insufficiency, the C. Miller Fisher variant of Guillain-Barré syndrome, myasthenia gravis, or any basilar meningitis (infectious or carcinomatous). Intestinal obstruction or other types of food poisoning are considered when nausea and vomiting are present.

Treatment

If botulism is suspected, the practitioner should contact the state health authorities or the CDC for advice and help with procurement of equine serum heptavalent botulism antitoxin and for assistance in obtaining assays for toxin in serum, stool, or food. Skin testing is recommended to exclude hypersensitivity to the antitoxin preparation. Antitoxin should be administered as early as possible, ideally within 24 hours of the onset of symptoms or signs, to arrest progression of disease; its administration should not be delayed for laboratory confirmation of the diagnosis. Respiratory failure is managed with intubation and mechanical ventilation. Parenteral fluids or alimentation should be given while swallowing difficulty persists. The removal of unabsorbed toxin from the gut may be attempted. Any remnants of suspected foods should be assayed for toxin. Persons who might have eaten the suspected food must be located and observed.

Adalja AA et al. Clinical management of potential bioterrorism-related conditions. N Engl J Med. 2015 Mar 5;372(10):954–62. [PMID: 25738671]

Chalk CH et al. Medical treatment for botulism. Cochrane Database Syst Rev. 2014 Feb 20;2:CD008123. [PMID: 24558013]

McCarty CL et al. Large outbreak of botulism associated with a church potluck meal—Ohio, 2015. MMWR Morb Mortal Wkly Rep. 2015 Jul 31;64(29):802–3. [PMID: 26225479]

ANTHRAX

ESSENTIALS OF DIAGNOSIS

► Appropriate epidemiologic setting, eg, exposure to animals or animal hides, or potential exposure from an act of bioterrorism.

► A painless cutaneous black eschar on exposed areas of the skin, with marked surrounding edema and vesicles.

► Nonspecific flu-like symptoms that rapidly progress to extreme dyspnea and shock; mediastinal widening and pleural effusions on chest radiograph.

General Considerations

The death of a Florida photo editor from inhalational anthrax acquired from a letter deliberately contaminated with spores of *Bacillus anthracis* thrust this extremely rare infection into the public awareness. Between September 18 and November 21 of 2001, there were 13 cases of cutaneous anthrax and 11 cases of inhalational anthrax associated with exposure to anthrax spores in contaminated mail.

Naturally occurring anthrax is a disease of sheep, cattle, horses, goats, and swine. *B anthracis* is a gram-positive spore-forming aerobic rod. Spores—not vegetative bacteria—are the infectious form of the organism. These are transmitted to humans from contact with contaminated animals, animal products, or animal hides, or from soil by inoculation of broken skin or mucous membranes; by inhalation of aerosolized spores; or, rarely, by ingestion resulting in cutaneous, inhalational, or gastrointestinal forms of anthrax, respectively. Spores germinate into vegetative bacteria that multiply locally in cutaneous and gastrointestinal anthrax but may also disseminate to cause systemic infection. Inhaled spores are ingested by pulmonary macrophages and carried via lymphatics to regional lymph nodes, where they germinate. The bacteria rapidly multiply within the lymphatics, causing a hemorrhagic lymphadenitis. Invasion of the bloodstream leads to overwhelming sepsis, killing the host.

▶ Clinical Findings

A. Symptoms and Signs

1. Cutaneous anthrax—This occurs within 2 weeks after exposure to spores; there is no latency period for cutaneous disease as there is with inhalational anthrax. The initial lesion is an erythematous papule, often on an exposed area of skin that vesiculates and then ulcerates and undergoes necrosis, ultimately progressing to a purple to black eschar. The eschar typically is painless; pain indicates secondary staphylococcal or streptococcal infection. The surrounding area is edematous and vesicular but not purulent. Regional adenopathy, fever, malaise, headache, and nausea and vomiting may be present. The infection is self-limited in most cases, but hematogenous spread with sepsis or meningitis may occur.

2. Inhalational anthrax—Illness occurs in two stages, beginning on average 10 days after exposure, but may have a latent onset 6 weeks after exposure. Nonspecific viral-like symptoms such as fever, malaise, headache, dyspnea, cough, and congestion of the nose, throat, and larynx are characteristic of the initial stage. Anterior chest pain is an early symptom of mediastinitis. Within hours to a few days, progression to the fulminant stage of infection occurs in which symptoms or signs of overwhelming sepsis predominate. Delirium, obtundation, or findings of meningeal irritation suggest an accompanying hemorrhagic meningitis.

3. Gastrointestinal anthrax—Fever, diffuse abdominal pain, rebound abdominal tenderness, vomiting, constipation, and diarrhea occur 2–5 days after ingestion of meat contaminated with anthrax spores. The primary lesion is ulcerative, producing emesis that may be blood-tinged or coffee-grounds and stool that may be blood-tinged or melenic. Bowel perforation can occur. The oropharyngeal form of the disease is characterized by local lymphadenopathy, cervical edema, dysphagia, and upper respiratory tract obstruction.

B. Laboratory Findings

Laboratory findings are nonspecific. The white blood cell count initially may be normal or modestly elevated, with polymorphonuclear predominance and an increase in early forms. Pleural fluid from patients with inhalational anthrax is typically hemorrhagic with few white cells. Cerebrospinal fluid from meningitis cases is also hemorrhagic. Gram stain of pleural fluid, cerebrospinal fluid, unspun blood, blood culture, or fluid from a cutaneous lesion may show the characteristic boxcar-shaped encapsulated rods in chains.

The diagnosis is established by isolation of the organism from culture of the skin lesion (or fluid expressed from it), blood, or pleural fluid—or cerebrospinal fluid in cases of meningitis. In the absence of prior antimicrobial therapy, cultures are invariably positive. Cultures obtained after initiation of antimicrobial therapy may be negative. If anthrax is suspected on clinical or epidemiologic grounds, immunohistochemical tests (eg, to detect capsular antigen), polymerase chain reaction assays, and serologic tests (useful for documenting past cutaneous infection) are available through the CDC and should be used to establish the diagnosis. Any suspected case of anthrax should be immediately reported to the CDC so that a complete investigation can be conducted.

C. Imaging

The chest radiograph is the most sensitive test for inhalational disease, being abnormal (though the findings can be subtle) initially in every case of bioterrorism-associated disease. Mediastinal widening due to hemorrhagic lymphadenitis, a hallmark feature of the disease, was present in 70% of the bioterrorism-related cases. Pleural effusions were present initially or occurred over the course of illness in all cases, and approximately three-fourths had pulmonary infiltrates or signs of consolidation.

▶ Differential Diagnosis

Cutaneous anthrax, despite its characteristic appearance, can be confused with a variety of other also uncommon or rare conditions such as ecthyma gangrenosum, rat-bite fever, ulceroglandular tularemia, plague, glanders, rickettsialpox, orf (parapoxvirus infection), or cutaneous mycobacterial infection. Inhalational anthrax must be differentiated from mediastinitis due to other bacterial causes, fibrous mediastinitis due to histoplasmosis, coccidioidomycosis, atypical or viral pneumonia, silicosis, sarcoidosis, and other causes of mediastinal widening (eg, superior vena cava syndrome or aortic aneurysm or dissection). Gastrointestinal anthrax shares clinical features with a variety of common intra-abdominal disorders, including bowel obstruction, perforated viscus, peritonitis, gastroenteritis, and peptic ulcer disease.

▶ Treatment

Strains of *B anthracis* (including the strain isolated in the bioterrorism cases) are susceptible in vitro to penicillin, amoxicillin, chloramphenicol, clindamycin, imipenem, doxycycline, ciprofloxacin (as well as other fluoroquinolones), macrolides, rifampin, and vancomycin. *B anthracis* may express beta-lactamases that confer resistance to cephalosporins and penicillins. For this reason, penicillin or amoxicillin is no longer recommended for use as a single agent in treatment of disseminated disease. Based on results of animal experiments and because of concern for engineered drug resistance in strains of *B anthracis* used in bioterrorism, ciprofloxacin is considered the drug of choice (Table 33–3) for treatment and for prophylaxis following exposure to anthrax spores. Other fluoroquinolones with activity against gram-positive bacteria (eg, levofloxacin, moxifloxacin) are likely to be just as effective as ciprofloxacin. Doxycycline is an alternative first-line

Table 33–3. Antimicrobial agents for treatment of anthrax or for prophylaxis against anthrax.

First-line agents and recommended doses
Ciprofloxacin, 500 mg twice daily orally or 400 mg every 12 hours intravenously
Doxycycline, 100 mg every 12 hours orally or intravenously

Second-line agents and recommended doses
Amoxicillin, 500 mg three times daily orally
Penicillin G, 2–4 million units every 4 hours intravenously

Alternative agents with in vitro activity and suggested doses
Rifampin, 10 mg/kg/day orally or intravenously
Clindamycin, 450–600 mg every 8 hours orally or intravenously
Clarithromycin, 500 mg orally twice daily
Erythromycin, 500 mg every 6 hours intravenously
Vancomycin, 1 g every 12 hours intravenously
Imipenem, 500 mg every 6 hours intravenously

agent. Combination therapy with at least one additional agent is recommended for inhalational or disseminated disease and in cutaneous infection involving the face, head, and neck or associated with extensive local edema or systemic signs of infection, eg, fever, tachycardia and elevated white blood cell count. Single-drug therapy is recommended for prophylaxis following exposure to spores.

The required duration of therapy is poorly defined. In naturally occurring disease, treatment for 7–10 days for cutaneous disease and for at least 2 weeks following clinical response for disseminated, inhalational, or gastrointestinal infection have been standard recommendations. Because of concern about relapse from latent spores acquired by inhalation of aerosol in bioterrorism-associated cases, the initial recommendation was treatment for 60 days. Raxibacumab, a human monoclonal antibody directed against the protective antigen component of lethal toxin, is FDA approved for the treatment of inhalation anthrax when used in combination with recommended antibacterial treatments.

Prevention

In 2001, the CDC offered one of two options for postal workers receiving prophylaxis for exposure to contaminated mail: (1) antibiotics for 100 days (fearing that even with 60 days of treatment late relapses might occur) or (2) vaccination with an investigative agent (three doses administered over a 1-month period) in conjunction with 40 days of antibiotic administration to cover the time required for a protective antibody response to develop. Insufficient information exists to favor one recommendation over the other.

The FDA has approved a vaccine for persons at high risk for exposure to anthrax spores. The vaccine is cell-free antigen prepared from an attenuated strain of *B anthracis*. Multiple injections over 18 months and an annual booster dose are required to achieve and maintain protection. Existing supplies have been reserved for vaccination of military personnel. Lastly, raxibacumab, a human

monoclonal antibody, is also approved for prevention of inhalation anthrax when other treatments are not available or appropriate.

Prognosis

The prognosis in cutaneous infection is excellent. Death is unlikely if the infection has remained localized, and lesions heal without complications in most cases. By contrast, the reported mortality rate for gastrointestinal and inhalational infections is up to 85%. Yet, the experience with bioterrorism-associated inhalational cases in which six of eleven victims survived suggests a somewhat better outcome with modern supportive care and antibiotics provided that treatment is initiated before the patient has progressed to the fulminant stage of disease. No cases of anthrax have occurred among the several thousand individuals receiving antimicrobial prophylaxis following exposure to spores.

Adalja AA et al. Clinical management of potential bioterrorism-related conditions. N Engl J Med. 2015 Mar 5;372(10):954–62. [PMID: 25738671]
Raxibacumab for anthrax. Med Lett Drugs Ther. 2013 Apr 1; 55(1413):27–8. [PMID: 23545582]

DIPHTHERIA

ESSENTIALS OF DIAGNOSIS

▶ Tenacious gray membrane at portal of entry in pharynx.

▶ Sore throat, nasal discharge, hoarseness, malaise, fever.

▶ Myocarditis, neuropathy.

▶ Culture confirms the diagnosis.

General Considerations

Diphtheria is an acute infection caused by *Corynebacterium diphtheriae* that usually attacks the respiratory tract but may involve any mucous membrane or skin wound. The organism is spread chiefly by respiratory secretions. Exotoxin produced by the organism is responsible for myocarditis and neuropathy.

Clinical Findings

A. Symptoms and Signs

Nasal, laryngeal, pharyngeal, and cutaneous forms of diphtheria occur. Nasal infection produces few symptoms other than a nasal discharge. Laryngeal infection may lead to upper airway and bronchial obstruction. In pharyngeal diphtheria, the most common form, a tenacious gray membrane covers the tonsils and pharynx. Mild sore throat, fever, and malaise are followed by toxemia and prostration.

Myocarditis and neuropathy are the most common and most serious complications. Myocarditis causes cardiac arrhythmias, heart block, and heart failure. The neuropathy usually involves the cranial nerves first, producing diplopia, slurred speech, and difficulty in swallowing.

B. Laboratory Findings

The diagnosis is made clinically but can be confirmed by culture of the organism.

▶ Differential Diagnosis

Diphtheria must be differentiated from streptococcal pharyngitis, infectious mononucleosis, adenovirus or herpes simplex infection, Vincent angina, pharyngitis due to *Arcanobacterium haemolyticum*, and candidiasis. A presumptive diagnosis of diphtheria should be made on clinical grounds without waiting for laboratory verification, since emergency treatment is needed.

▶ Prevention

Active immunization with diphtheria toxoid is part of routine childhood immunization with appropriate booster injections. The immunization schedule for adults is the same as for tetanus.

Susceptible persons exposed to diphtheria should receive a booster dose of diphtheria toxoid (or a complete series if previously unimmunized), as well as a course of penicillin or erythromycin.

▶ Treatment

Antitoxin, which is prepared from horse serum, must be given in all cases when diphtheria is suspected. For mild early pharyngeal or laryngeal disease, the dose is 20,000–40,000 units; for moderate nasopharyngeal disease, 40,000–60,000 units; for severe, extensive, or late (3 days or more) disease, 80,000–100,000 units. Diphtheria equine antitoxin can be obtained from the CDC.

Removal of membrane by direct laryngoscopy or bronchoscopy may be necessary to prevent or alleviate airway obstruction.

Either penicillin, 250 mg orally four times daily, or erythromycin, 500 mg orally four times daily, for 14 days is effective therapy, although erythromycin is slightly more effective in eliminating the carrier state. Azithromycin or clarithromycin is probably as effective as erythromycin. The patient should be isolated until three consecutive cultures at the completion of therapy have documented elimination of the organism from the oropharynx. Contacts to a case should receive erythromycin, 500 mg orally four times daily for 7 days, to eradicate carriage.

Centers for Disease Control and Prevention (CDC). Updated recommendations for use of tetanus toxoid, reduced diphtheria toxoid, and acellular pertussis vaccine (Tdap) in pregnant women—Advisory Committee on Immunization Practices (ACIP), 2012. MMWR Morb Mortal Wkly Rep. 2013 Feb 22; 62(7):131–5. [PMID: 23425962]

Koepke R et al. Estimating the effectiveness of tetanus-diphtheria-acellular pertussis vaccine (Tdap) for preventing pertussis: evidence of rapidly waning immunity and difference in effectiveness by Tdap brand. J Infect Dis. 2014 Sep 15;210(6):942–53. [PMID: 24903664]

LISTERIOSIS

ESSENTIALS OF DIAGNOSIS

- ▶ Ingestion of contaminated food product leads to primary infection.
- ▶ Undifferentiated fever in a pregnant woman in her third trimester.
- ▶ Altered mental status and fever in an elderly or immunocompromised patient.
- ▶ Obtain blood and cerebrospinal fluid cultures.
- ▶ Culture confirms the diagnosis.

▶ General Considerations

Listeria monocytogenes is a facultative, motile, gram-positive rod that is capable of invading several cell types and causes intracellular infection. Most cases of infection caused by *L monocytogenes* are sporadic, but outbreaks have been traced to eating contaminated food, including unpasteurized dairy products, hot dogs, and delicatessen meats. In 2011, a multistate outbreak of *Listeria* infection was traced to contaminated cantaloupes, and in 2012, a multistate outbreak was traced to ricotta cheese. Both outbreaks were associated with significant morbidity and mortality in infected persons.

▶ Clinical Findings

Five types of infection are recognized:

(1) **Infection during pregnancy**, usually in the last trimester, is a mild febrile illness without an apparent primary focus. This relatively benign disease for the mother may resolve without specific therapy. However, approximately one in five pregnancies complicated by listeriosis result in spontaneous abortion or stillbirth and surviving infants are at high risk for clinical neonatal listeriosis.

(2) **Granulomatosis infantisepticum** is a neonatal infection acquired in utero, characterized by disseminated abscesses, granulomas, and a high mortality rate.

(3) **Bacteremia** with or without sepsis syndrome is an infection of neonates or immunocompromised adults. The presentation is of a febrile illness without a recognized source.

(4) **Meningitis** caused by *L monocytogenes* affects infants under 2 months of age as well as older adults, ranking third after meningococcus and pneumococcus as common causes of bacterial meningitis. Cerebrospinal fluid shows a *neutrophilic* pleocytosis. Adults with meningitis are often immunocompromised, and cases have been associated with HIV infection and therapy with tumor necrosis factor (TNF) inhibitors such as infliximab.

(5) Finally, **focal infections**, including adenitis, brain abscess, endocarditis, osteomyelitis, and arthritis, occur rarely.

▶ Treatment

Ampicillin, 8–12 g/day intravenously in four to six divided doses (the higher dose for meningitis) is considered the treatment of choice. Gentamicin, 5 mg/kg/day intravenously once or in divided doses is synergistic with ampicillin against *Listeria* in vitro and in animal models, and the use of combination therapy may be considered during the first few days of treatment to enhance eradication of organisms. In patients with penicillin allergies, trimethoprim-sulfamethoxazole has excellent intracellular and cerebrospinal fluid penetration and is considered an appropriate alternative. The dose is 10–20 mg/kg/day intravenously of the trimethoprim component. Mortality and morbidity rates still are high. Therapy should be administered for at least 2–3 weeks. Longer durations—between 3 and 6 weeks—have been recommended for treatment of meningitis, especially in immunocompromised persons.

Allerberger F et al. Pregnancy related listeriosis: treatment and control. Expert Rev Anti Infect Ther. 2015 Mar;13(3):395–403. [PMID: 25604158]

Jackson BR et al; Centers for Disease Control and Prevention (CDC). Notes from the field: listeriosis associated with stone fruit—United States, 2014. MMWR Morb Mortal Wkly Rep. 2015 Mar 20;64(10):282–3. [PMID: 25789745]

Kourtis AP et al. Pregnancy and infection. N Engl J Med. 2014 Jun 5;370(23):2211–8. [PMID: 24897084]

INFECTIVE ENDOCARDITIS

ESSENTIALS OF DIAGNOSIS

- ▶ Fever.
- ▶ Preexisting organic heart lesion.
- ▶ Positive blood cultures.
- ▶ Evidence of vegetation on echocardiography.
- ▶ New or changing heart murmur.
- ▶ Evidence of systemic emboli.

▶ General Considerations

Endocarditis is a bacterial or fungal infection of the valvular or endocardial surface of the heart. The clinical presentation depends on the infecting organism and the valve or valves that are infected. More virulent organisms— *S aureus* in particular—tend to produce a more rapidly progressive and destructive infection. Endocarditis caused by more virulent organisms often presents as an acute febrile illnesses and is complicated by early embolization, acute valvular regurgitation, and myocardial abscess formation. Viridans strains of streptococci, enterococci, other bacteria, yeasts, and fungi tend to cause a more subacute picture.

Underlying valvular disease, less common than in the past, is present in about 50% of cases. Valvular disease alters blood flow and produces jet effects that disrupt the endothelial surface, providing a nidus for attachment and infection of microorganisms that enter the bloodstream. Predisposing valvular abnormalities include rheumatic involvement of any valve, bicuspid aortic valves, calcific or sclerotic aortic valves, hypertrophic subaortic stenosis, mitral valve prolapse, and a variety of congenital disorders such as ventricular septal defect, tetralogy of Fallot, coarctation of the aorta, or patent ductus arteriosus. Rheumatic disease is no longer the major predisposing factor in developed countries. Regurgitation lesions are more susceptible than stenotic ones.

The initiating event in native valve endocarditis is colonization of the valve by bacteria or yeast that gain access to the bloodstream. Transient bacteremia is common during dental, upper respiratory, urologic, and lower gastrointestinal diagnostic and surgical procedures. It is less common during upper gastrointestinal and gynecologic procedures. Intravascular devices are increasingly implicated as a portal of access of microorganisms into the bloodstream. A large proportion of cases of *S aureus* endocarditis are attributable to health care-associated bacteremia.

Native valve endocarditis is usually caused by *S aureus*, viridans streptococci, enterococci, or HACEK organisms (an acronym for *Haemophilus aphrophilus* [now *Aggregatibacter aphrophilus*], *Actinobacillus actinomycetemcomitans* [now *Aggregatibacter actinomycetemcomitans*], *Cardiobacterium hominis*, *Eikenella corrodens*, and *Kingella* species). Streptococcal species formerly accounted for the majority of native valve endocarditis cases, but the proportion of cases caused by *S aureus* has been increasing, and this organism is now the leading cause. Gram-negative organisms and fungi account for a small percentage.

In injection drug users, *S aureus* accounts for over 60% of all endocarditis cases and for 80–90% of cases in which the tricuspid valve is infected. Enterococci and streptococci comprise the balance in about equal proportions. Gram-negative aerobic bacilli, fungi, and unusual organisms may cause endocarditis in injection drug users.

The microbiology of prosthetic valve endocarditis also is distinctive. Early infections (ie, those occurring within 2 months after valve implantation) are commonly caused by staphylococci—both coagulase-positive and coagulase-negative—gram-negative organisms, and fungi. In late prosthetic valve endocarditis, streptococci are commonly identified, although coagulase-negative and coagulase-positive staphylococci still cause many cases.

▶ Clinical Findings

A. Symptoms and Signs

Virtually all patients have fever at some point in the illness, although it may be very low grade (less than 38°C) in elderly individuals and in patients with heart failure or kidney failure. Rarely, there may be no fever at all.

The duration of illness typically is a few days to a few weeks. Nonspecific symptoms are common. The initial symptoms and signs of endocarditis may be caused by

▲ **Figure 33–3.** Splinter hemorrhages appearing as red lineal streaks under the nail plate and within the nail bed, in endocarditis, psoriasis, and trauma. (Reproduced, with permission, from Richard P. Usatine, MD.)

▲ **Figure 33–4.** Osler node causing pain within the pulp of the big toe and multiple painless flat Janeway lesions over the sole of the foot. (From David A. Kasper, DO, MBA; Reproduced, with permission, from Usatine RP, Smith MA, Mayeaux EJ Jr, Chumley H, Tysinger J. *The Color Atlas of Family Medicine*. McGraw-Hill, 2009.)

direct arterial, valvular, or cardiac damage. Although a changing regurgitant murmur is significant diagnostically, it is the exception rather than the rule. Symptoms also may occur as a result of embolization, metastatic infection or immunologically mediated phenomena. These include cough; dyspnea; arthralgias or arthritis; diarrhea; and abdominal, back, or flank pain.

The characteristic peripheral lesions—petechiae (on the palate or conjunctiva or beneath the fingernails), subungual ("splinter") hemorrhages (Figure 33–3), Osler nodes (painful, violaceous raised lesions of the fingers, toes, or feet) (Figure 33–4), Janeway lesions (painless erythematous lesions of the palms or soles), and Roth spots (exudative lesions in the retina)—occur in about 25% of patients. Strokes and major systemic embolic events are present in about 25% of patients, and tend to occur before or within the first week of antimicrobial therapy. Hematuria and proteinuria may result from emboli or immunologically mediated glomerulonephritis, which can cause kidney dysfunction.

B. Imaging

Chest radiograph may show evidence for the underlying cardiac abnormality and, in right-sided endocarditis, pulmonary infiltrates. The electrocardiogram is nondiagnostic, but new conduction abnormalities suggest myocardial abscess formation. Echocardiography is useful in identifying vegetations and other characteristic features suspicious for endocarditis and may provide adjunctive information about the specific valve or valves that are infected. The sensitivity of transthoracic echocardiography is between 55% and 65%; it cannot reliably rule out endocarditis but may confirm a clinical suspicion. Transesophageal echocardiography is 90% sensitive in detecting vegetations and is particularly useful for identifying valve ring abscesses as well as prosthetic valve endocarditis.

C. Diagnostic Studies

1. Blood cultures—Blood cultures establish the diagnosis. Three sets of blood cultures at least 1 hour apart before starting antibiotics are recommended to maximize the opportunity for a microbiologic diagnosis. Approximately 5% of cases will be culture-negative, usually attributable to administration of antimicrobials prior to obtaining cultures. If antimicrobial therapy has been administered prior to obtaining cultures and the patient is clinically stable, it is reasonable to withhold further antimicrobial therapy for 2–3 days so that appropriate cultures can be obtained. Culture-negative endocarditis may also be due to organisms that require special media for growth (eg, *Legionella*,

Bartonella, Abiotrophia species, formerly referred to as nutritionally deficient streptococci), organisms that do not grow on artificial media (*Tropheryma whipplei*, or pathogens of Q fever or psittacosis), or those that are slow-growing and may require prolonged incubation (eg, *Brucella*, anaerobes, HACEK organisms). *Bartonella quintana* has emerged as an important cause of culture-negative endocarditis.

2. Modified Duke criteria—Clinical criteria, referred to as the Modified Duke criteria, have been proposed for the diagnosis of endocarditis. Major criteria include: (1) two positive blood cultures for a microorganism that typically causes infective endocarditis or persistent bacteremia; (2) evidence of endocardial involvement documented by echocardiography (eg, definite vegetation, myocardial abscess, or new partial dehiscence of a prosthetic valve); or (3) development of a new regurgitant murmur. Minor criteria include the presence of a predisposing condition; fever of 38°C or higher; vascular phenomena, such as cutaneous hemorrhages, aneurysm, systemic emboli, pulmonary infarction; immunologic phenomena, such as glomerulonephritis, Osler nodes, Roth spots, rheumatoid factor; and positive blood cultures not meeting the major criteria or serologic evidence of an active infection. A definite diagnosis can be made with 80% accuracy if two major criteria, one major criterion and three minor criteria, or five minor criteria are fulfilled. A possible diagnosis of endocarditis is made if one major and one minor criterion or three minor criteria are met. If fewer criteria are found, or a sound alternative explanation for illness is identified, or the patient's febrile illness has resolved within 4 days, endocarditis is unlikely.

► **Complications**

The course of infective endocarditis is determined by the degree of damage to the heart, by the site of infection (right-sided versus left-sided, aortic versus mitral valve), by the presence of metastatic foci of infection, by the occurrence of embolization, and by immunologically mediated processes. Destruction of infected heart valves is especially common and precipitous with *S aureus* but can occur with any organism and can progress even after bacteriologic cure. The infection can also extend into the myocardium, resulting in abscesses leading to conduction disturbances, and involving the wall of the aorta, creating sinus of Valsalva aneurysms.

Peripheral embolization to the brain and myocardium may result in infarctions. Embolization to the spleen and kidneys is also common. Peripheral emboli may initiate metastatic infections or may become established in vessel walls, leading to mycotic aneurysms. Right-sided endocarditis, which usually involves the tricuspid valve, causes septic pulmonary emboli, occasionally with infarction and lung abscesses.

► **Prevention**

In 2007, the American Heart Association made major revisions to their recommendation on antibiotic prophylaxis for infective endocarditis. The committee determined that

Table 33–4. Cardiac conditions with high risk of adverse outcomes from endocarditis for which prophylaxis with dental procedures is recommended.[1,2]

Prosthetic cardiac valve
Previous infective endocarditis
Congenital heart disease (CHD)[3]
Unrepaired cyanotic CHD, including palliative shunts and conduits
Completely repaired congenital heart defect with prosthetic material or device, whether placed by surgery or by catheter intervention, during the first 6 months after the procedure[4]
Repaired CHD with residual defects at the site or adjacent to the site of a prosthetic patch or prosthetic device
Cardiac transplantation recipients in whom cardiac valvulopathy develops

[1]Reproduced, with permission, from the American Heart Association. Circulation. 2007 Oct 9;116(15):1736–54.
[2]See Table 33–6 for prophylactic regimens.
[3]Except for the conditions listed above, antibiotic prophylaxis is no longer recommended for other forms of CHD.
[4]Prophylaxis is recommended because endothelialization of prosthetic material occurs within 6 months after procedure.

only a few cases of infective endocarditis would be prevented by antibiotic prophylaxis for dental procedures even if the prophylactic therapy were 100% effective. Therefore, they limited their recommendations for prophylaxis to a small group of patients with predisposing congenital or valvular anomalies (Table 33–4) undergoing select dental procedures, operations involving the respiratory tract, or operations of infected skin, skin structure, or musculoskeletal tissue (Table 33–5). Current antimicrobial recommendations are given in Table 33–6.

Table 33–5. Recommendations for administration of bacterial endocarditis prophylaxis for patients according to type of procedure.[1]

Prophylaxis Recommended	Prophylaxis Not Recommended
Dental procedures	**Dental procedures**
All dental procedures that involve manipulation of gingival tissue or the periapical region of the teeth or perforation of the oral mucosa	Routine anesthetic injections through noninfected tissue, taking dental radiographs, placement of removable prosthodontic or orthodontic appliances, adjustment of orthodontic appliances, placement of orthodontic brackets, shedding of deciduous teeth, and bleeding from trauma to the lips or oral mucosa
Respiratory tract procedures	
Only respiratory tract procedures that involve incision of the respiratory mucosa	
Procedures on infected skin, skin structure, or musculoskeletal tissue	**Gastrointestinal tract procedures**
	Genitourinary tract procedures

[1]Reproduced, with permission, from the American Heart Association. Circulation. 2007 Oct 9;116(15):1736–54.

Table 33–6. American Heart Association recommendations for endocarditis prophylaxis for dental procedures for patients with cardiac conditions.[1-3]

Oral	Amoxicillin	2 g 1 hour before procedure
Penicillin allergy	Clindamycin	600 mg 1 hour before procedure
	or	
	Cephalexin	2 g 1 hour before procedure (contraindicated if there is history of a beta-lactam immediate hypersensitivity reaction)
	or	
	Azithromycin or clarithromycin	500 mg 1 hour before procedure
Parenteral	Ampicillin	2 g intramuscularly or intravenously 30 minutes before procedure
Penicillin allergy	Clindamycin	600 mg intravenously 1 hour before procedure
	or	
	Cefazolin	1 g intramuscularly or intravenously 30 minutes before procedure (contraindicated if there is history of a beta-lactam immediate hypersensitivity reaction)

[1]Data from the American Heart Association. Circulation. 2007 Oct 9;116(15):1736–54.
[2]For patients undergoing respiratory tract procedures involving incision of respiratory tract mucosa to treat an established infection or a procedure on infected skin, skin structure, or musculoskeletal tissue known or suspected to be caused by *S aureus*, the regimen should contain an anti-staphylococcal penicillin or cephalosporin. Vancomycin can be used to treat patients unable to tolerate a beta-lactam or if the infection is known or suspected to be caused by a methicillin-resistant strain of *S aureus*.
[3]See Table 33–4 for list of cardiac conditions.

▶ Treatment

Empiric regimens for endocarditis while culture results are pending should include agents active against staphylococci, streptococci, and enterococci. Vancomycin 1 g every 12 hours intravenously plus ceftriaxone 2 g every 24 hours provides appropriate coverage pending definitive diagnosis. Consultation with an infectious disease expert is strongly recommended when initiating treatment for infective endocarditis.

A. Viridans Streptococci

For penicillin-susceptible viridans streptococcal endocarditis (ie, MIC 0.1 mcg/mL or less), penicillin G, 18 million units intravenously either continuously or in four to six equally divided doses or ceftriaxone 2 g intravenously once daily for 4 weeks, is recommended. The duration of therapy can be shortened to 2 weeks if gentamicin, 3 mg/kg intravenously every 24 hours, is used with penicillin or ceftriaxone. The 2-week regimen is reasonable and can be considered in patients with uncomplicated endocarditis, rapid response to therapy, and no underlying kidney disease. For the patient unable to tolerate penicillin or ceftriaxone, vancomycin, 15 mg/kg intravenously every 12 hours for 4 weeks, is given with a desired trough level of 10–15 mcg/mL. Prosthetic valve endocarditis is treated with a 6-week course of penicillin or ceftriaxone and the clinician can consider adding 2 weeks of gentamicin at the start of therapy.

Viridans streptococci relatively resistant to penicillin (ie, MIC greater than 0.12 mcg/mL but less than or equal to 0.5 mcg/mL) should be treated for 4 weeks. Penicillin G, 24 million units intravenously either continuously or in four to six equally divided doses, is combined with gentamicin, 3 mg/kg intravenously every 24 hours for the first 2 weeks. In the patient with IgE-mediated allergy to penicillin, vancomycin alone, 15 mg/kg intravenously every 12 hours for 4 weeks, should be administered. Prosthetic valve endocarditis is treated with a 6-week course of penicillin or ceftriaxone plus gentamicin as above.

Endocarditis caused by viridans streptococci with an MIC greater than 0.5 mcg/mL or by nutritionally deficient streptococci should be treated the same as enterococcal endocarditis.

B. Other Streptococci

Endocarditis caused by *S pneumoniae*, *S pyogenes* (group A streptococcus), or groups B, C, and G streptococci is unusual. *S pneumoniae* sensitive to penicillin (MIC less than 0.1 mcg/mL) can be treated with penicillin 18 million units intravenously either continuously or in four to six equally divided doses or cefazolin 6 g intravenously either continuously or in three equally divided doses, or ceftriaxone 2 g daily intravenously for 4 weeks. High-dose penicillin (24 million units) or a third-generation cephalosporin may be required for the treatment of endocarditis (without meningitis) caused by strains resistant to penicillin (MIC greater than 0.1 mcg/mL). The addition of vancomycin and rifampin to ceftriaxone may be considered in patients with *S pneumoniae* strains with cefotaxime MIC greater than 2 mcg/mL. Group A streptococcal infection can be treated with penicillin or ceftriaxone for 4–6 weeks. Groups B, C, and G streptococci tend to be more resistant to penicillin than group A streptococci, and some experts have recommended adding gentamicin, 3 mg/kg intravenously every

24 hours, to penicillin for the first 2 weeks of a 4- to 6-week course. Endocarditis caused by *S gallolyticus (bovis)* is associated with liver disease, especially cirrhosis, and gastrointestinal abnormalities, especially colon cancer. Colonoscopy should be performed to exclude the latter.

C. Enterococci

For enterococcal endocarditis, penicillin or ampicillin alone is inadequate. The combination of penicillin or ampicillin with gentamicin had been the treatment of choice but in vitro studies have identified synergy between ampicillin and ceftriaxone, presumably caused by saturation of different penicillin-binding proteins. Subsequently, several clinical studies of the combination of ampicillin plus ceftriaxone have demonstrated clinical outcomes equivalent to the combination of ampicillin plus gentamicin. Therefore, recommended regimens are now ampicillin, 2 g intravenously every 4 hours, or penicillin G, 18–30 million units intravenously continuously in six equally divided doses plus gentamicin, 1 mg/kg intravenously every 8 hours. Another acceptable option is ampicillin (2 g intravenously every 4 hours) plus ceftriaxone 2 g intravenously every 12 hours. The recommended duration of therapy is 4–6 weeks (the longer duration for patients with symptoms for more than 3 months, relapse, or prosthetic valve endocarditis). The combination of ampicillin plus ceftriaxone is recommended for patients with creatinine clearance less than 50 mL/min or whose enterococcal isolates are resistant to gentamicin. In patients intolerant of penicillin and ampicillin or who have enterococcal isolate resistant to these agents, vancomycin plus gentamicin can be used.

Endocarditis caused by strains resistant to penicillin and vancomycin are particularly difficult to treat. Such cases must always be managed in consultation with an infectious diseases specialist.

D. Staphylococci

For methicillin-susceptible *S aureus* isolates, nafcillin or oxacillin, 12 g intravenously daily given continuously or in four to six divided doses or cefazolin, 6 g intravenously daily given continuously or in three divided doses for 6 weeks, is the preferred therapy. For patients with history of immediate type hypersensitivity to beta-lactams, a desensitization protocol should be undertaken. For patients with a history of nonanaphylactoid reactions to penicillins, cefazolin should be used. Patients who are infected with methicillin-resistant *S aureus* or who are unable to tolerate beta-lactam therapy should receive vancomycin, 30 mg/kg/day intravenously divided in two or three doses to achieve a goal trough level of 15–20 mcg/kg, or daptomycin intravenously at greater than or equal to 8 mg/kg/day. Aminoglycoside combination regimens are not recommended. The effect of rifampin with antistaphylococcal drugs is variable, and its routine use is not recommended.

Because coagulase-negative staphylococci—a common cause of prosthetic valve endocarditis—are routinely resistant to methicillin, beta-lactam antibiotics should not be used for this infection unless the isolate is demonstrated to

be susceptible. A combination of vancomycin, 30 mg/kg/day intravenously divided in two or three doses for 6 weeks; rifampin, 300 mg every 8 hours for 6 weeks; and gentamicin, 3 mg/kg intravenously every 8 hours for the first 2 weeks is recommended for prosthetic valve infection. If the organism is sensitive to methicillin, either nafcillin or oxacillin or cefazolin can be used in combination with rifampin and gentamicin. Combination therapy with nafcillin or oxacillin (vancomycin or daptomycin for methicillin-resistant strains), rifampin, and gentamicin is also recommended for treatment of *S aureus* prosthetic valve infection.

E. HACEK Organisms

HACEK organisms are slow-growing, fastidious gram-negative coccobacilli or bacilli (*H aphrophilus* [now *A aphrophilus*], *A actinomycetemcomitans*, *C hominis*, *E corrodens*, and *Kingella* species) that are normal oral flora and cause less than 5% of all cases of endocarditis. They may produce beta-lactamase, and thus the treatment of choice is ceftriaxone (or some other third-generation cephalosporin), 2 g intravenously once daily for 4 weeks. Prosthetic valve endocarditis should be treated for 6 weeks. In the penicillin-allergic patient, experience is limited, but fluoroquinolones have in vitro activity and should be considered.

F. Culture-Negative Endocarditis

Failure to culture microorganisms from patients with suspected infective endocarditis may be due to infection from organisms not recovered in routine microbiology testing or previous administration of antimicrobial agents before blood cultures were obtained. These cases must be managed with the assistance of an infectious disease specialist. Pathogens that are not able to be cultured by commonly used techniques include *Bartonella* species, *Chlamydia* species, *Brucella* species, and *Tropheryma whipplei*. Serologic testing should be performed in patients who have epidemiologic risk factors for these infections. Treatment should be directed at likely pathogens while awaiting serologic results; treatment of patients given prior antimicrobials before cultures were obtained must also consider likely pathogens.

G. Role of Surgery

While many cases can be successfully treated medically, operative management is frequently required. Acute heart failure unresponsive to medical therapy is an indication for valve replacement even if active infection is present. Infections unresponsive to appropriate antimicrobial therapy after 7–10 days (ie, persistent fevers, positive blood cultures despite therapy) are more likely to be eradicated if the valve is replaced. Surgery is nearly always required for cure of fungal endocarditis and is more often necessary with highly-resistant bacteria. It is also indicated when the infection involves the sinus of Valsalva or produces septal abscesses. Recurrent infection with the same organism prompts an operative approach, especially with infected prosthetic valves. Continuing embolization presents a difficult problem when the infection is otherwise responding; surgery may be the proper approach. Particularly challenging is a large and fragile vegetation demonstrated by echocardiography in the absence of embolization. Most clinicians favor an operative approach, vegetectomy with valve repair if the patient is a good candidate. Embolization after bacteriologic cure does not necessarily imply recurrence of endocarditis.

H. Role of Anticoagulation

Anticoagulation is contraindicated in native valve endocarditis because of an increased risk of intracerebral hemorrhage. The role of anticoagulant therapy during active prosthetic valve endocarditis is more controversial. Reversal of anticoagulation may result in thrombosis of the mechanical prosthesis, particularly in the mitral position. On the other hand, anticoagulation during active prosthetic valve endocarditis caused by S aureus has been associated with fatal intracerebral hemorrhage. One approach is to discontinue anticoagulation during the septic phase of S aureus prosthetic valve endocarditis. In patients with S aureus prosthetic valve endocarditis complicated by a central nervous system embolic event, anticoagulation should be discontinued for the first 2 weeks of therapy. Indications for anticoagulation following prosthetic valve implantation for endocarditis are the same as for patients with prosthetic valves without endocarditis (eg, nonporcine mechanical valves and valves in the mitral position).

▶ Response to Therapy

If infection is caused by viridans streptococci, enterococci, or coagulase-negative staphylococci, defervescence occurs in 3–4 days on average; with S aureus or Pseudomonas aeruginosa, fever may persist for longer. Blood cultures should be obtained to document sterilization of the blood. Other causes of persistent fever are myocardial or metastatic abscess, sterile embolization, superimposed hospital-acquired infection, and drug reaction. Most relapses occur within 1–2 months after completion of therapy. Obtaining one or two blood cultures during this period is prudent.

▶ When to Refer

- Consider consulting an infectious diseases specialist in all cases of suspected infective endocarditis.
- Consult a cardiac surgeon in the situations mentioned in the Role of Surgery section above to prevent further embolic disease, heart failure, and other complications including death.

▶ When to Admit

Patients with infective endocarditis should be hospitalized for expedited evaluation and treatment.

Baddour LM et al. Infective endocarditis in adults: diagnosis, antimicrobial therapy, and management of complications: a scientific statement for healthcare professionals from the American Heart Association. Circulation. 2015 Oct 13; 132(15):1435–86. Erratum in: Circulation. 2015 Oct 27; 132(17):e215. [PMID: 26373316]

Wilson W et al. Prevention of infective endocarditis: guidelines from the American Heart Association: a guideline from the American Heart Association Rheumatic Fever, Endocarditis, and Kawasaki Disease Committee, Council on Cardiovascular Disease in the Young, and the Council on Clinical Cardiology, Council on Cardiovascular Surgery and Anesthesia, and the Quality of Care and Outcomes Research Interdisciplinary Working Group. Circulation. 2007 Oct 9;116(15):1736–54. [PMID: 17446442]

INFECTIONS CAUSED BY GRAM-NEGATIVE BACTERIA

BORDETELLA PERTUSSIS INFECTION (Whooping Cough)

ESSENTIALS OF DIAGNOSIS

- ▶ Predominantly in infants under age 2 years. Adolescents and adults are an important reservoir of infection.
- ▶ Two-week prodromal catarrhal stage of malaise, cough, coryza, and anorexia.
- ▶ Paroxysmal cough ending in a high-pitched inspiratory "whoop."
- ▶ Absolute lymphocytosis, often striking; culture confirms diagnosis.

▶ General Considerations

Pertussis is an acute infection of the respiratory tract caused by B pertussis that is transmitted by respiratory droplets. The incubation period is 7–17 days. Half of all cases occur before age 2 years. Neither immunization nor disease confers lasting immunity to pertussis. Consequently, adults are an important reservoir of the disease.

▶ Clinical Findings

The symptoms of classic pertussis last about 6 weeks and are divided into three consecutive stages. The catarrhal stage is characterized by its insidious onset, with lacrimation, sneezing, and coryza, anorexia and malaise, and a hacking night cough that becomes diurnal. The paroxysmal stage is characterized by bursts of rapid, consecutive coughs followed by a deep, high-pitched inspiration (whoop). The convalescent stage begins 4 weeks after onset of the illness with a decrease in the frequency and severity of paroxysms of cough. The diagnosis often is not considered in adults, who may not have a typical presentation. Cough persisting more than 2 weeks is suggestive. Infection may also be asymptomatic.

The white blood cell count is usually 15,000–20,000/mcL (rarely, as high as 50,000/mcL or more), 60–80% of which are lymphocytes. The diagnosis is established by isolating the organism from nasopharyngeal culture. A special medium (eg, Bordet-Gengou agar) must be requested. Polymerase chain reaction assays for diagnosis of pertussis may be available in some clinical or health department laboratories.

▶ Prevention

Acellular pertussis vaccine is recommended for all infants, combined with diphtheria and tetanus toxoids (DTaP). Infants and susceptible adults with significant exposure should receive prophylaxis with an oral macrolide. In recognition of their importance as a reservoir of disease, vaccination of adolescents and adults against pertussis is recommended (see Table 30–7 and www.cdc.gov/vaccines/schedules). The FDA licensed two tetanus toxoid, reduced diphtheria toxoid and acellular pertussis vaccine (Tdap) products (BOOSTRIX, GlaxoSmithKline and ADACEL, Sanofi Pasteur) in 2005. Adolescents aged 11–18 years (preferably between 11 and 12 years of age) who have completed the DTP or DTaP vaccination series should receive a single dose of either Tdap product instead of Td (tetanus and diphtheria toxoids vaccine) for booster immunization against tetanus, diphtheria, and pertussis. Adults of all ages (including those older than age 64 years) should receive a single dose of Tdap. In addition, pregnant women should receive a dose of Tdap during each pregnancy regardless of prior vaccination history. The optimal timing for such Tdap administration is between 27 and 36 weeks of gestation, in order to maximize the antibody response of the pregnant woman and the passive antibody transfer to the infant. For any woman who was not previously vaccinated with Tdap and for whom the vaccine was not given during her pregnancy, Tdap should be administered immediately postpartum. The CDC has eliminated the recommendation that a 2-year period window is needed between receiving the Td and Tdap vaccines based on data showing that there is not an increased risk of adverse events.

▶ Treatment

Antibiotic treatment should be initiated in all suspected cases. Treatment options include erythromycin, 500 mg four times a day orally for 7 days; azithromycin, 500 mg orally on day 1 and 250 mg for 4 more days; or clarithromycin, 500 mg orally twice daily for 7 days. Trimethoprim-sulfamethoxazole, 160 mg–800 mg orally twice a day for 7 days, also is effective. Treatment shortens the duration of carriage and may diminish the severity of coughing paroxysms. These same regimens are indicated for prophylaxis of contacts to an active case of pertussis that are exposed within 3 weeks of the onset of cough in the index case.

Centers for Disease Control and Prevention (CDC). Updated recommendations for use of tetanus toxoid, reduced diphtheria toxoid, and acellular pertussis (Tdap) vaccine in adults aged 65 years and older—Advisory Committee on Immunization Practices (ACIP), 2012. MMWR Morb Mortal Wkly Rep. 2012 Jun 29;61(25):468–70. Erratum in: MMWR Morb Mortal Wkly Rep. 2012 Jul 13;61(27):515. [PMID: 22739778]

Sukumaran L et al. Association of Tdap vaccination with acute events and adverse birth outcomes among pregnant women with prior tetanus-containing immunizations. JAMA. 2015 Oct 20;314(15):1581–7. [PMID: 26501534]

OTHER *BORDETELLA* INFECTIONS

Bordetella bronchiseptica is a pleomorphic gram-negative coccobacillus causing kennel cough in dogs. On occasion it causes upper and lower respiratory infection in humans, principally HIV-infected patients. Infection has been associated with contact with dogs and cats, suggesting animal-to-human transmission. Treatment of *B bronchiseptica* infection is guided by results of in vitro susceptibility tests.

MENINGOCOCCAL MENINGITIS

ESSENTIALS OF DIAGNOSIS

▶ Fever, headache, vomiting, confusion, delirium, convulsions.

▶ Petechial rash of skin and mucous membranes in many.

▶ Neck and back stiffness with positive Kernig and Brudzinski signs is characteristic.

▶ Purulent spinal fluid with gram-negative intracellular and extracellular diplococci.

▶ Culture of cerebrospinal fluid, blood, or petechial aspiration confirms the diagnosis.

▶ General Considerations

Meningococcal meningitis is caused by *Neisseria meningitidis* of groups A, B, C, Y, and W-135, among others. Meningitis due to serogroup A is uncommon in the United States. Serogroup B generally causes sporadic cases. The frequency of outbreaks of meningitis caused by group C meningococcus has increased, and this serotype is the most common cause of epidemic disease in the United States. Up to 40% of persons are nasopharyngeal carriers of meningococci, but disease develops in relatively few of these persons. Infection is transmitted by droplets. The clinical illness may take the form of meningococcemia (a fulminant form of septicemia without meningitis), meningococcemia with meningitis, or meningitis. Recurrent meningococcemia with fever, rash, and arthritis is seen rarely in patients with certain terminal complement deficiencies.

▶ Clinical Findings

A. Symptoms and Signs

High fever, chills, and headache; back, abdominal, and extremity pains; and nausea and vomiting are typical. Rapidly developing confusion, delirium, seizures, and coma occur in some. On examination, nuchal and back rigidity are typical. Positive Kernig and Brudzinski signs (Kernig sign is pain in the hamstrings upon extension of the knee with the hip at 90-degree flexion; Brudzinski sign is flexion of the knee in response to flexion of the neck) are specific but not sensitive findings. A petechial rash appearing in the lower extremities and at pressure points is found in most cases. Petechiae may vary in size from pinpoint lesions to large ecchymoses or even skin gangrene that may later slough if the patient survives.

B. Laboratory Findings

Lumbar puncture typically reveals a cloudy or purulent cerebrospinal fluid, with elevated pressure, increased protein, and decreased glucose content. The fluid usually contains greater than 1000 cells/mcL, with polymorphonuclear cells predominating and containing gram-negative intracellular diplococci. The absence of organisms in a Gram-stained smear of the cerebrospinal fluid sediment does not rule out the diagnosis. The capsular polysaccharide can be demonstrated in cerebrospinal fluid or urine by latex agglutination; this is useful in partially treated patients, though sensitivity is 60–80%. The organism is usually demonstrated by smear and culture of the cerebrospinal fluid, oropharynx, blood, or aspirated petechiae.

Disseminated intravascular coagulation is an important complication of meningococcal infection and is typically present in toxic patients with ecchymotic skin lesions.

▶ Differential Diagnosis

Meningococcal meningitis must be differentiated from other meningitides. In small infants and in the elderly, fever or stiff neck is often missing, and altered mental status may dominate the picture.

Rickettsial, echovirus and, rarely, other bacterial infections (eg, staphylococcal infections, scarlet fever) also cause petechial rash.

▶ Prevention

Four meningococcal vaccines are now available. There are two vaccines with coverage against meningococcal serogroups A, C, Y, and W-135 and two with coverage against meningococcal serogroup B. The two vaccines effective for meningococcal serogroups A, C, Y, and W-135 are the meningococcal polysaccharide vaccine (MPSV4) indicated for vaccination of persons over age 55 and the conjugate vaccine (MCV4) indicated for persons aged 2–55 years. The two vaccines against meningococcal serogroup B are MenB-FHbp and MenB-4C are approved for persons age 10–25 years and are not interchangeable.

The Advisory Committee on Immunization Practices recommends immunization with a dose of MCV4 for preadolescents ages 11–12 with a booster at age 16 (see www.cdc.gov/vaccines/schedules/hcp/child-adolescent.html). For ease of program implementation, persons aged 21 years or younger should have documentation of receipt of a dose of MCV4 not more than 5 years before enrollment to college. If the primary dose was administered before the sixteenth birthday, a booster dose should be administered before enrollment. Vaccine is also recommended as a two-dose primary series administered 2 months apart for persons aged 2 through 54 years with persistent complement deficiency, persons with functional or anatomic asplenia, and for adolescents with HIV infection. All other persons at increased risk for meningococcal disease (eg, military recruits, microbiologists, or travelers to an epidemic or highly endemic country) should receive a single dose. One of the meningococcal serogroup B vaccines may be administered to persons 10 years of age or older who are at increased risk for meningococcal disease. These persons include those with persistent complement component deficiencies; persons with anatomic or functional asplenia; microbiologists routinely exposed to isolates of *Neisseria meningitidis*; and persons identified to be at increased risk because of a serogroup B meningococcal disease outbreak. Vaccination of persons aged 16–23 years may provide short-term protection against most strains of serogroup B meningococcal disease; the MenB vaccine is preferred for persons aged 16–18 years.

Eliminating nasopharyngeal carriage of meningococci is an effective prevention strategy in closed populations and to prevent secondary cases in household or otherwise close contacts. Rifampin, 600 mg orally twice a day for 2 days, ciprofloxacin, 500 mg orally once, or one intramuscular 250-mg dose of ceftriaxone is effective. Cases of fluoroquinolone-resistant meningococcal infections have been identified in the United States. However, ciprofloxacin remains a recommended empiric agent for eradication of nasopharyngeal carriage. School and work contacts ordinarily need not be treated. Hospital contacts receive therapy only if intense exposure has occurred (eg, mouth-to-mouth resuscitation). Accidentally discovered carriers without known close contact with meningococcal disease do not require prophylactic antimicrobials.

▶ Treatment

Blood cultures must be obtained and intravenous antimicrobial therapy started immediately. This may be done prior to lumbar puncture in patients in whom the diagnosis is not straightforward and for those in whom MR or CT imaging is indicated to exclude mass lesions. Aqueous penicillin G is the antibiotic of choice (24 million units/24 h intravenously in divided doses every 4 hours). The prevalence of strains of *N meningitidis* with intermediate resistance to penicillin in vitro (MICs 0.1 to 1 mcg/mL) is increasing, particularly in Europe. At what level of resistance penicillin treatment failure can occur is not known. Penicillin-intermediate strains thus far remain fully susceptible to ceftriaxone and other third-generation cephalosporins used to treat meningitis, and these should be effective alternatives to penicillin. In penicillin-allergic patients or those in whom *Haemophilus influenzae* or gram-negative meningitis is a consideration, ceftriaxone, 2 g intravenously every 12 hours, should be used. Treatment should be continued in full doses by the intravenous route until the patient is afebrile for 5 days. Shorter courses—as few as 4 days if ceftriaxone is used—are also effective.

▶ When to Admit

All patients with suspected meningococcal infection including meningitis and meningococcemia should be admitted for evaluation and empiric intravenous antibiotic therapy.

Cohn AC et al; Centers for Disease Control and Prevention (CDC). Prevention and control of meningococcal disease: recommendations of the Advisory Committee on Immunization Practices (ACIP). MMWR Recomm Rep. 2013 Mar 22;62(RR-2): 1–28. [PMID: 23515099]

Folaranmi T et al; Centers for Disease Control (CDC). Use of serogroup B meningococcal vaccines in persons aged ≥10 years at increased risk for serogroup B meningococcal disease: recommendations of the Advisory Committee on Immunization Practices, 2015. MMWR Morb Mortal Wkly Rep. 2015 Jun 12;64(22):608–12. Erratum in: MMWR Morb Mortal Wkly Rep. 2015 Jul 31;64(29):806. [PMID: 26068564]

MacNeil JR et al. Use of serogroup B meningococcal vaccines in adolescents and young adults: recommendations of the Advisory Committee on Immunization Practices, 2015. MMWR Morb Mortal Wkly Rep. 2015 Oct 23;64(41):1171–6. [PMID: 26492381]

Simon MS et al. Invasive meningococcal disease in men who have sex with men. Ann Intern Med. 2013 Aug 20;159(4):300–1. [PMID: 23778867]

INFECTIONS CAUSED BY *HAEMOPHILUS* SPECIES

H influenzae and other *Haemophilus* species may cause sinusitis, otitis, bronchitis, epiglottitis, pneumonia, cellulitis, arthritis, meningitis, and endocarditis. Nontypeable strains are responsible for most disease in adults. Alcoholism, smoking, chronic lung disease, advanced age, and HIV infection are risk factors. *Haemophilus* species colonize the upper respiratory tract in patients with chronic obstructive pulmonary disease and frequently cause purulent bronchitis.

Beta-lactamase–producing strains are less common in adults than in children. For adults with sinusitis, otitis, or respiratory tract infection, oral amoxicillin, 750 mg twice daily for 10–14 days, is adequate. For beta-lactamase–producing strains, use of the oral fixed-drug combination of amoxicillin, 875 mg, with clavulanate, 125 mg, is indicated. For the penicillin-allergic patient, oral cefuroxime axetil, 250 mg twice daily; or a fluoroquinolone (ciprofloxacin, 500 mg orally twice daily; levofloxacin, 500–750 mg orally once daily; or moxifloxacin, 400 mg orally once daily) for 7 days is effective. Azithromycin, 500 mg orally once followed by 250 mg daily for 4 days, is preferred over clarithromycin when a macrolide is the preferred agent. Trimethoprim-sulfamethoxazole (160/800 mg orally twice daily) can be considered, but resistance rates have been reported to be up to 25%.

In the more seriously ill patient (eg, the toxic patient with multilobar pneumonia), ceftriaxone, 1 g/day intravenously is recommended pending determination of whether the infecting strain is a beta-lactamase producer. A fluoroquinolone (see above for dosages) can be used for the penicillin-allergic patients for a 10- to 14-day course of therapy.

Epiglottitis is characterized by an abrupt onset of high fever, drooling, and inability to handle secretions. An important clue to the diagnosis is complaint of a severe sore throat despite an unimpressive examination of the pharynx. Stridor and respiratory distress result from laryngeal obstruction. The diagnosis is best made by direct visualization of the cherry-red, swollen epiglottis at laryngoscopy. Because laryngoscopy may provoke laryngospasm and

obstruction, especially in children, it should be performed in an intensive care unit or similar setting, and only at a time when intubation can be performed promptly. Ceftriaxone, 1 g intravenously every 24 hours for 7–10 days, is the drug of choice. Trimethoprim-sulfamethoxazole or a fluoroquinolone (see above for dosage) may be used in the patient with serious penicillin allergy.

Meningitis, rare in adults, is a consideration in the patient who has meningitis associated with sinusitis or otitis. Initial therapy for suspected *H influenzae* meningitis should be with ceftriaxone, 4 g/day in two divided doses, until the strain is proved not to produce beta-lactamase. Meningitis is treated for 10–14 days. Dexamethasone, 0.15 mg/kg intravenously every 6 hours may reduce the incidence of long-term sequelae, principally hearing loss.

Collins S et al. Risk of invasive *Haemophilus influenzae* infection during pregnancy and association with adverse fetal outcomes. JAMA. 2014 Mar 19;311(11):1125–32. [PMID: 24643602]

INFECTIONS CAUSED BY *MORAXELLA CATARRHALIS*

M catarrhalis is a gram-negative aerobic coccus morphologically and biochemically similar to *Neisseria*. It causes sinusitis, bronchitis, and pneumonia. Bacteremia and meningitis have also been reported in immunocompromised patients. The organism frequently colonizes the respiratory tract, making differentiation of colonization from infection difficult. If *M catarrhalis* is the predominant isolate, therapy is directed against it. *M catarrhalis* typically produces beta-lactamase and therefore is usually resistant to ampicillin and amoxicillin. It is susceptible to amoxicillin-clavulanate, ampicillin-sulbactam, trimethoprim-sulfamethoxazole, ciprofloxacin, and second- and third-generation cephalosporins.

LEGIONNAIRES DISEASE

ESSENTIALS OF DIAGNOSIS

► Patients are often immunocompromised, smokers, or have chronic lung disease.
► Scant sputum production, pleuritic chest pain, toxic appearance.
► Chest radiograph: focal patchy infiltrates or consolidation.
► Gram stain of sputum: polymorphonuclear leukocytes and no organisms.

► General Considerations

Legionella infection ranks among the three or four most common causes of community-acquired pneumonia and is considered whenever the etiology of a pneumonia is in question. Legionnaires disease is more common in immunocompromised persons, in smokers, and in those with chronic lung disease. Outbreaks have been associated with contaminated water sources, such as showerheads and faucets in patient rooms and air conditioning cooling towers.

Clinical Findings

A. Symptoms and Signs

Legionnaires disease is one of the atypical pneumonias, so called because a Gram-stained smear of sputum does not show organisms. However, many features of Legionnaires disease are more like typical pneumonia, with high fevers, a toxic patient, pleurisy, and grossly purulent sputum. Classically, this pneumonia is caused by *Legionella pneumophila*, though other species can cause identical disease.

B. Laboratory Findings

Several laboratory abnormalities can be associated with Legionnaires disease, which include hyponatremia, elevated liver enzymes, and elevated creatine kinase. Culture of *Legionella* species onto charcoal-yeast extract agar or similar enriched medium is the most sensitive method (80–90% sensitivity) for diagnosis and permits identification of infections caused by species and serotypes other than *L pneumophila* serotype 1. Dieterle silver staining of tissue, pleural fluid, or other infected material is also a reliable method for detecting *Legionella* species. Direct fluorescent antibody stains and serologic testing are less sensitive because these will detect only *L pneumophila* serotype 1. In addition, making a serologic diagnosis requires that the host respond with sufficient specific antibody production. Urinary antigen tests, which are targeted for detection of *L pneumophila* serotype 1, are also less sensitive than culture.

Treatment

Azithromycin (500 mg orally once daily), clarithromycin (500 mg orally twice daily), or a fluoroquinolone (eg, levofloxacin, 750 mg orally once daily), and not erythromycin, are the drugs of choice for treatment of legionellosis because of their excellent intracellular penetration and in vitro activity, as well as desirable pharmacokinetic properties that permit oral administration and once or twice daily dosing. Duration of therapy is 10–14 days, although a 21-day course of therapy is recommended for immunocompromised patients.

Del Castillo M et al. Atypical presentation of *Legionella* pneumonia among patients with underlying cancer: a fifteen-year review. J Infect. 2016 Jan;72(1):45–51. [PMID: 26496794]

Haubitz S et al. Ruling out *Legionella* in community-acquired pneumonia. Am J Med. 2014 Oct;127(10):1010.e11–9. [PMID: 24813862]

GRAM-NEGATIVE BACTEREMIA & SEPSIS

Gram-negative bacteremia can originate in a number of sites, the most common being the genitourinary system, hepatobiliary tract, gastrointestinal tract, and lungs. Less common sources include intravenous lines, infusion fluids, surgical wounds, drains, and pressure ulcers.

Patients with potentially fatal underlying conditions in the short term such as neutropenia or immunoparesis have a mortality rate of 40–60%; those with serious underlying diseases likely to be fatal in 5 years, such as solid tumors, cirrhosis, and aplastic anemia, die in 15–20% of cases; and individuals with no underlying diseases have a mortality rate of 5% or less.

Clinical Findings

A. Symptoms and Signs

Most patients have fevers and chills, often with abrupt onset. However, 15% of patients are hypothermic (temperature 36.4°C or less) at presentation, and 5% never develop a temperature above 37.5°C. Hyperventilation with respiratory alkalosis and changes in mental status are important early manifestations. Hypotension and shock, which occur in 20–50% of patients, are unfavorable prognostic signs.

B. Laboratory Findings

Neutropenia or neutrophilia, often with increased numbers of immature forms of polymorphonuclear leukocytes, is the most common laboratory abnormality in septic patients. Thrombocytopenia occurs in 50% of patients, laboratory evidence of coagulation abnormalities in 10%, and overt disseminated intravascular coagulation in 2–3%. Both clinical manifestations and the laboratory abnormalities are nonspecific and insensitive, which accounts for the relatively low rate of blood culture positivity (approximately 20–40%). If possible, three blood cultures from separate sites should be obtained in rapid succession before starting antimicrobial therapy. The chance of recovering the organism in at least one of the three blood cultures is greater than 95%. The false-negative rate for a single culture of 5–10 mL of blood is 30%. This may be reduced to 5–10% (albeit with a slight false-positive rate due to isolation of contaminants) if a single volume of 30 mL is inoculated into several blood culture bottles. Because blood cultures may be falsely negative, when a patient with presumed septic shock, negative blood cultures, and inadequate explanation for the clinical course responds to antimicrobials, therapy should be continued for 10–14 days.

Treatment

Several factors are important in the management of patients with sepsis.

A. Removal of Predisposing Factors

This usually means decreasing or stopping immunosuppressive medications and, in certain circumstances, giving granulocyte colony-stimulating factor (filgrastim; G-CSF) to the neutropenic patient.

B. Identifying the Source of Bacteremia

By simply finding the source of bacteremia and removing it (central venous catheter) or draining it (abscess), a fatal disease becomes easily treatable.

C. Supportive Measures

The use of fluids, vasopressors, and corticosteroids in septic shock are discussed in Chapter 14; management of disseminated intravascular coagulation is discussed in Chapter 13.

D. Antibiotics

Antibiotics should be given as soon as the diagnosis is suspected, since delays in therapy have been associated with increased mortality rates, particularly once hypotension develops. In general, bactericidal antibiotics should be used and given intravenously to ensure therapeutic serum levels. Penetration of antibiotics into the site of primary infection is critical for successful therapy—ie, if the infection originates in the central nervous system, antibiotics that penetrate the blood-brain barrier should be used—eg, third- or fourth-generation cephalosporin—but not first-generation cephalosporins or aminoglycosides, which penetrate poorly. Sepsis caused by gram-positive organisms cannot be differentiated on clinical grounds from that due to gram-negative bacteria. Therefore, initial therapy should include antibiotics active against both types of organisms.

The number of antibiotics necessary remains controversial and depends on the cause. Table 30–4 provides a guide for empiric therapy. Although a combination of antibiotics is often recommended for "synergism," combination therapy has not been shown to be superior to a single-drug regimen with any of several broad-spectrum antibiotics (eg, a third-generation cephalosporin, piperacillin-tazobactam, carbapenem). If multiple drugs are used initially, the regimen should be modified and coverage narrowed based on the results of culture and sensitivity testing.

Ferrer R et al. Empiric antibiotic treatment reduces mortality in severe sepsis and septic shock from the first hour: results from a guideline-based performance improvement program. Crit Care Med. 2014 Aug;42(8):1749–55. [PMID: 24717459]

Zhang D et al. Time to appropriate antibiotic therapy is an independent determinant of postinfection ICU and hospital lengths of stay in patients with sepsis. Crit Care Med. 2015 Oct;43(10):2133–40. [PMID: 26121071]

SALMONELLOSIS

Salmonellosis includes infection by any of approximately 2000 serotypes of salmonellae. The taxonomy of *Salmonella* species has been confusing. All *Salmonella* serotypes are members of a single species, *Salmonella enterica*. Human infections are caused almost exclusively by *S enterica* subsp *enterica*, of which three serotypes—*typhi*, *typhimurium*, and *choleraesuis*—are predominantly isolated. Three clinical patterns of infection are recognized: (1) enteric fever, the best example of which is typhoid fever, due to serotype *typhi*; (2) acute enterocolitis, caused by serotype *typhimurium*, among others; and (3) the "septicemic" type, characterized by bacteremia and focal lesions, exemplified by infection with serotype *choleraesuis*. All types are transmitted by ingestion of the organism, usually from contaminated food or drink.

1. Enteric Fever (Typhoid Fever)

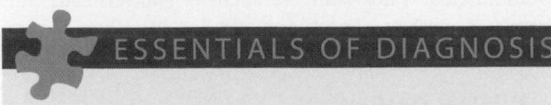

ESSENTIALS OF DIAGNOSIS

▶ Gradual onset of malaise, headache, nausea, vomiting, abdominal pain.

▶ Rose spots, relative bradycardia, splenomegaly, and abdominal distention and tenderness.

▶ Slow (stepladder) rise of fever to maximum and then slow return to normal.

▶ Leukopenia; blood, stool, and urine culture positive for salmonella.

▶ **General Considerations**

Enteric fever is a clinical syndrome characterized by constitutional and gastrointestinal symptoms and by headache. It can be caused by any *Salmonella* species. The term "typhoid fever" applies when serotype *typhi* is the cause. Infection is transmitted by consumption of contaminated food or drink. The incubation period is 5–14 days. *Salmonella* is an intracellular pathogen. Infection begins when organisms breach the mucosal epithelium of the intestines by transcytosis, an organism-mediated transport process through the cell via an endocytic vesicle. Having crossed the epithelial barrier, organisms invade and replicate in macrophages in Peyer patches, mesenteric lymph nodes, and the spleen. Serotypes other than *typhi* usually do not cause invasive disease, presumably because they lack the necessary human-specific virulence factors. Bacteremia occurs, and the infection then localizes principally in the lymphoid tissue of the small intestine (particularly within 60 cm of the ileocecal valve). Peyer patches become inflamed and may ulcerate, with involvement greatest during the third week of disease. The organism may disseminate to the lungs, gallbladder, kidneys, or central nervous system.

▶ **Clinical Findings**

A. Symptoms and Signs

During the prodromal stage, there is increasing malaise, headache, cough, and sore throat, often with abdominal pain and constipation, while the fever ascends in a stepwise fashion. After about 7–10 days, it reaches a plateau and the patient is much more ill, appearing exhausted and often prostrated. There may be marked constipation, especially early, or "pea soup" diarrhea; marked abdominal distention occurs as well. If there are no complications, the patient's condition will gradually improve over 7–10 days. However, relapse may occur for up to 2 weeks after defervescence.

During the early prodrome, physical findings are few. Later, splenomegaly, abdominal distention and tenderness, relative bradycardia, and occasionally meningismus appear. The rash (rose spots) commonly appears during the second week of disease. The individual spot, found principally on the trunk, is a pink papule 2–3 mm in diameter that fades on pressure. It disappears in 3–4 days.

B. Laboratory Findings

Typhoid fever is best diagnosed by blood culture, which is positive in the first week of illness in 80% of patients who have not taken antimicrobials. The rate of positivity declines thereafter, but one-fourth or more of patients still have positive blood cultures in the third week. Cultures of bone marrow occasionally are positive when blood cultures are not. Stool culture is unreliable because it may be positive in gastroenteritis without typhoid fever. Relative bradycardia and leukopenia are typical.

► Differential Diagnosis

Enteric fever must be distinguished from other gastrointestinal illnesses and from other infections that have few localizing findings. Examples include tuberculosis, infective endocarditis, brucellosis, lymphoma, and Q fever. Often there is a history of recent travel to endemic areas, and viral hepatitis, malaria, or amebiasis may be in the differential as well.

► Complications

Complications occur in about 30% of untreated cases and account for 75% of deaths. Intestinal hemorrhage, manifested by a sudden drop in temperature and signs of shock followed by dark or fresh blood in the stool, or intestinal perforation, accompanied by abdominal pain and tenderness, is most likely to occur during the third week. Appearance of leukocytosis and tachycardia should suggest these complications. Urinary retention, pneumonia, thrombophlebitis, myocarditis, psychosis, cholecystitis, nephritis, osteomyelitis, and meningitis are less often observed.

► Prevention

Immunization is not always effective but should be considered for household contacts of a typhoid carrier, for travelers to endemic areas, and during epidemic outbreaks. A multiple-dose oral vaccine and a single-dose parenteral vaccine are available. Their efficacies are similar, but oral vaccine causes fewer side effects. Boosters, when indicated, should be given every 5 years and 2 years for oral and parenteral preparations, respectively.

Adequate waste disposal and protection of food and water supplies from contamination are important public health measures to prevent salmonellosis. Carriers cannot work as food handlers.

► Treatment

A. Specific Measures

Because of increasing antimicrobial resistance, fluoroquinolones—such as ciprofloxacin 750 mg orally twice daily or levofloxacin 500 mg orally once daily, 5–7 days for uncomplicated enteric fever and 10–14 days for severe infection—have become the agents of choice for treatment of salmonella infections. Ceftriaxone, 2 g intravenously for 7 days, is also effective. Although resistance to fluoroquinolones or cephalosporins occurs uncommonly, the prevalence appears to be increasing. When an infection is caused by a multidrug-resistant strain, select an antibiotic to which the isolate is susceptible in vitro. Alternatively, increasing the dose of ceftriaxone to 4 g/day and treating for 10–14 days or using azithromycin 500 mg orally for 7 days in uncomplicated cases may be effective. In years past, ampicillin, chloramphenicol, and trimethoprim-sulfamethoxazole had been effective treatments but resistance has spread globally.

B. Treatment of Carriers

Chemotherapy often is unsuccessful in eradicating the carrier state. Ciprofloxacin, 750 mg orally twice a day for 4 weeks, has proved to be highly effective. Cholecystectomy may also achieve this goal. When the isolate is susceptible, treatment of carriage with ampicillin, trimethoprim-sulfamethoxazole, or chloramphenicol may be successful.

► Prognosis

The mortality rate of typhoid fever is about 2% in treated cases. Elderly or debilitated persons are likely to do poorly. With complications, the prognosis is poor. Relapses occur in up to 15% of cases. A residual carrier state frequently persists in spite of chemotherapy.

Anwar E et al. Vaccines for preventing typhoid fever. Cochrane Database Syst Rev. 2014 Jan 2;1:CD001261. [PMID: 24385413]
Wain J et al. Typhoid fever. Lancet. 2015 Mar 21;385(9973):1136–45. [PMID: 25458731]

2. *Salmonella* Gastroenteritis

By far the most common form of salmonellosis is acute enterocolitis caused by numerous *Salmonella* serotypes. The incubation period is 8–48 hours after ingestion of contaminated food or liquid.

Symptoms and signs consist of fever (often with chills), nausea and vomiting, cramping abdominal pain, and diarrhea, which may be grossly bloody, lasting 3–5 days. Differentiation must be made from viral gastroenteritis, food poisoning, shigellosis, amebic dysentery, and acute ulcerative colitis. The diagnosis is made by culturing the organism from the stool.

The disease is usually self-limited, but bacteremia with localization in joints or bones may occur, especially in patients with sickle cell disease.

In most cases, treatment of uncomplicated enterocolitis is symptomatic only. However, patients who are malnourished or severely ill, patients with sickle cell disease, and patients who are immunocompromised (including those who are HIV-positive) should be treated with ciprofloxacin, 500 mg orally twice a day; ceftriaxone, 1 g intravenously once daily; trimethoprim-sulfamethoxazole, 160 mg/80 mg orally twice a day; or azithromycin, 500 mg orally once daily for 7–14 days (14 days for immunocompromised patients).

Williams S et al. *Salmonella* in the tropical household environment—everyday, everywhere. J Infect. 2015 Dec;71(6):642–8. [PMID: 26416474]

3. *Salmonella* Bacteremia

Salmonella infection may be manifested by prolonged or recurrent fevers accompanied by bacteremia and local infection in bone, joints, pleura, pericardium, lungs, or other sites. Mycotic abdominal aortic aneurysms may also occur. Serotypes other than typhi usually are isolated. This complication tends to occur in immunocompromised persons and is seen in HIV-infected individuals, who typically have bacteremia without an obvious source. Treatment is the same as for typhoid fever, plus drainage of any abscesses. In HIV-infected patients, relapse is common, and lifelong suppressive therapy may be needed. Ciprofloxacin, 750 mg orally twice a day, is effective both for therapy of acute infection and for suppression of recurrence. Incidence of infections caused by drug-resistant strains may be on the rise.

Crump JA et al. Epidemiology, clinical presentation, laboratory diagnosis, antimicrobial resistance, and antimicrobial management of invasive salmonella infections. Clin Microbiol Rev. 2015 Oct;28(4):901–37. [PMID: 26180063]

Gibani MM et al. Control of invasive salmonella disease in Africa: is there a role for human challenge models? Clin Infect Dis. 2015 Nov 1;61(Suppl 4):S266–71. [PMID: 26449941]

SHIGELLOSIS

ESSENTIALS OF DIAGNOSIS

► Diarrhea, often with blood and mucus.

► Crampy abdominal pain and systemic toxicity.

► White blood cells in stools; organism isolated on stool culture.

▶ General Considerations

Shigella dysentery is a common disease, often self-limited and mild but occasionally serious. *S sonnei* is the leading cause in the United States, followed by *S flexneri*. *S dysenteriae* causes the most serious form of the illness. Shigellae are invasive organisms. The infective dose is 10^2–10^3 organisms. There has been a rise in strains resistant to multiple antibiotics.

▶ Clinical Findings

A. Symptoms and Signs

The illness usually starts abruptly, with diarrhea, lower abdominal cramps, and tenesmus. The diarrheal stool often is mixed with blood and mucus. Systemic symptoms are fever, chills, anorexia and malaise, and headache. The abdomen is tender. Sigmoidoscopic examination reveals an inflamed, engorged mucosa with punctate and sometimes large areas of ulceration.

B. Laboratory Findings

The stool shows many leukocytes and red cells. Stool culture is positive for shigellae in most cases, but blood cultures grow the organism in less than 5% of cases.

▶ Differential Diagnosis

Bacillary dysentery must be distinguished from salmonella enterocolitis and from disease due to enterotoxigenic *Escherichia coli, Campylobacter*, and *Yersinia enterocolitica*. Amebic dysentery may be similar clinically and is diagnosed by finding amoebas in the fresh stool specimen. Ulcerative colitis is also an important cause of bloody diarrhea.

▶ Complications

Temporary disaccharidase deficiency may follow the diarrhea. Reactive arthritis is an uncommon complication, usually occurring in HLA-B27 individuals infected by *Shigella*. Hemolytic-uremic syndrome occurs rarely.

▶ Treatment

Treatment of dehydration and hypotension is lifesaving in severe cases. Recommended empiric antimicrobial therapy is either a fluoroquinolone (ciprofloxacin, 750 mg orally twice daily for 7–10 days, or levofloxacin, 500 mg orally once daily for 3 days) or ceftriaxone, 1 g intravenously once daily for 5 days. If the isolate is susceptible, trimethoprim-sulfamethoxazole, 160/80 mg orally twice daily for 5 days or azithromycin, 500 mg orally once daily for 3 days, is also effective. High rates of resistance to amoxicillin make it a less effective treatment option.

Heiman KE et al; Centers for Disease Control and Prevention (CDC). Notes from the field: *Shigella* with decreased susceptibility to azithromycin among men who have sex with men—United States, 2002–2013. MMWR Morb Mortal Wkly Rep. 2014 Feb 14;63(6):132–3. [PMID: 24522098]

Serafino Wani RL et al. Invasive shigellosis in MSM. Int J STD AIDS. 2015 Oct 1. [Epub ahead of print] [PMID: 26429891]

GASTROENTERITIS CAUSED BY *ESCHERICHIA COLI*

E coli causes gastroenteritis by a variety of mechanisms. Enterotoxigenic *E coli* (ETEC) elaborates either a heat-stable or heat-labile toxin that mediates the disease. ETEC is an important cause of traveler's diarrhea. Enteroinvasive *E coli* (EIEC) differs from other *E coli* bowel pathogens in that these strains invade cells, causing bloody diarrhea and dysentery similar to infection with *Shigella* species. EIEC is uncommon in the United States. Neither ETEC nor EIEC strains are routinely isolated and identified from stool cultures because there is no selective medium. Antimicrobial therapy against *Salmonella* and *Shigella*, such as ciprofloxacin 500 mg orally twice daily, shortens the clinical course, but the disease is self-limited.

Shiga-toxin-producing *E coli* (STEC) infection can result in asymptomatic carrier stage, nonbloody diarrhea, hemorrhagic colitis, hemolytic-uremic syndrome, or thrombotic thrombocytopenic purpura. Although *E coli* O157:H7 is responsible for most cases of STEC infection in the United States, recently in Europe, other STEC strains (such as *E coli* O104:H4) have been reported to cause severe disease. *E coli* O157:H7 has caused several outbreaks of diarrhea and hemolytic-uremic syndrome related to consumption of undercooked hamburger, unpasteurized apple juice, and spinach, while *E coli* O145 was recently linked to the consumption of contaminated lettuce. Older individuals and young children are most affected, with hemolytic-uremic syndrome being more common in the latter group. STEC identification can be difficult and the CDC recommends that all stools submitted for routine testing from patients with acute community-acquired diarrhea be simultaneously cultured for *E coli* O157:H7 and tested with an assay that detects Shiga toxins to detect non-O157 STEC, such as *E coli* O145. Antimicrobial therapy does not alter the course of the disease and may increase the risk of hemolytic-uremic syndrome. Treatment is primarily supportive. Hemolytic-uremic syndrome or thrombotic thrombocytopenic purpura occurring in association with a diarrheal illness suggests the diagnosis and should prompt evaluation for STEC. Confirmed infections should be reported to public health officials.

Crim SM et al; Centers for Disease Control and Prevention (CDC). Preliminary incidence and trends of infection with pathogens transmitted commonly through food—Foodborne Diseases Active Surveillance Network, 10 U.S. sites, 2006–2014. MMWR Morb Mortal Wkly Rep. 2015 May 15; 64(18):495–9. [PMID: 25974634]

Lüth S et al. Prevention of hemolytic uremic syndrome with daily bowel lavage in patients with Shiga toxin-producing enterohemorrhagic *Escherichia coli* O104:H4 infection. JAMA Intern Med. 2014 Jun;174(6):1003–5. [PMID: 24781800]

Tobias J et al. Involvement of main diarrheagenic *Escherichia coli*, with emphasis on enteroaggregative *E. coli*, in severe non-epidemic pediatric diarrhea in a high-income country. BMC Infect Dis. 2015 Feb 21;15:79. [PMID: 25887696]

CHOLERA

ESSENTIALS OF DIAGNOSIS

▶ History of travel in endemic area or contact with infected person.

▶ Voluminous diarrhea.

▶ Stool is liquid, gray, turbid, and without fecal odor, blood, or pus ("rice water stool").

▶ Rapid development of marked dehydration.

▶ Positive stool cultures and agglutination of vibrios with specific sera.

▶ General Considerations

Cholera is an acute diarrheal illness caused by certain serotypes of *Vibrio cholerae*. The disease is toxin-mediated, and fever is unusual. The toxin activates adenylyl cyclase in intestinal epithelial cells of the small intestines, producing hypersecretion of water and chloride ion and a massive diarrhea of up to 15 L/day. Death results from profound hypovolemia. Cholera occurs in epidemics under conditions of crowding, war, and famine (eg, in refugee camps) and where sanitation is inadequate. Infection is acquired by ingestion of contaminated food or water. For over a century, cholera was rarely seen in the Western Hemisphere until an outbreak occurred in Peru, starting in the early 1990s and ending by 2001; the outbreak resulted in almost 400,000 cholera cases and more than 4000 deaths. Cholera again became a rare disease in the Western Hemisphere until late 2010. A massive earthquake in Haiti in January 2010 crumbled the country's already fragile infrastructure. Later that fall, a cholera outbreak erupted that has continued and resulted in thousands of deaths.

▶ Clinical Findings

Cholera is characterized by a sudden onset of severe, frequent watery diarrhea (up to 1 L/h). The liquid stool is gray; turbid; and without fecal odor, blood, or pus ("rice water stool"). Dehydration and hypotension develop rapidly. Stool cultures are positive, and agglutination of vibrios with specific sera can be demonstrated.

▶ Prevention

A vaccine is available that confers short-lived, limited protection and may be required for entry into or reentry after travel to some countries. It is administered in two doses 1–4 weeks apart. A booster dose every 6 months is recommended for persons remaining in areas where cholera is a hazard.

Vaccination programs are expensive and not particularly effective in managing outbreaks of cholera. When outbreaks occur, efforts should be directed toward establishing clean water and food sources and proper waste disposal.

▶ Treatment

Treatment is by replacement of fluids. In mild or moderate illness, oral rehydration usually is adequate. A simple oral replacement fluid can be made from 1 teaspoon of table salt and 4 heaping teaspoons of sugar added to 1 L of water. Intravenous fluids are indicated for persons with signs of severe hypovolemia and those who cannot take adequate fluids orally. Lactated Ringer infusion is satisfactory.

Antimicrobial therapy will shorten the course of illness. Several antimicrobials are active against *V cholerae*, including tetracycline, ampicillin, chloramphenicol, trimethoprim-sulfamethoxazole, fluoroquinolones, and azithromycin. Multiple drug-resistant strains are increasingly encountered, so susceptibility testing, if available, is advisable. A single 1 g oral dose of azithromycin is effective for severe cholera caused by strains with reduced susceptibility to fluoroquinolones, but resistance is emerging to this drug as well.

Luquero FJ et al. Use of *Vibrio cholerae* vaccine in an outbreak in Guinea. N Engl J Med. 2014 May 29;370(22):2111–20. [PMID: 24869721]

Schilling KA et al. Diarrheal illness among U.S. residents providing medical services in Haiti during the cholera epidemic, 2010 to 2011. J Travel Med. 2014 Jan;21(1):55–7. [PMID: 24383654]

INFECTIONS CAUSED BY OTHER *VIBRIO* SPECIES

Vibrios other than *V cholerae* that cause human disease are *Vibrio parahaemolyticus*, *V vulnificus*, and *V alginolyticus*. All are halophilic marine organisms. Infection is acquired by exposure to organisms in contaminated, undercooked, or raw crustaceans or shellfish and warm (greater than 20°C [82.4°F]) ocean waters and estuaries. Infections are more common during the summer months from regions along the Atlantic coast and the Gulf of Mexico in the United States and from tropical waters around the world. Oysters are implicated in up to 90% of food-related cases. *V parahaemolyticus* causes an acute watery diarrhea with crampy abdominal pain and fever, typically occurring within 24 hours after ingestion of contaminated shellfish. The disease is self-limited, and antimicrobial therapy is usually not necessary. *V parahaemolyticus* may also cause cellulitis and sepsis, though these findings are more characteristic of *V vulnificus* infection.

V vulnificus and *V alginolyticus*—neither of which is associated with diarrheal illness—are important causes of cellulitis and primary bacteremia following ingestion of contaminated shellfish or exposure to sea water. Cellulitis with or without sepsis may be accompanied by bulla formation and necrosis with extensive soft tissue destruction, at times requiring debridement and amputation. The infection can be rapidly progressive and is particularly severe in immunocompromised individuals—especially those with cirrhosis—with death rates as high as 50%. Patients with chronic liver disease and those who are immunocompromised should be cautioned to avoid eating raw oysters.

Tetracycline at a dose of 500 mg orally four times a day for 7–10 days is the drug of choice for treatment of suspected or documented primary bacteremia or cellulitis caused by *Vibrio* species. *V vulnificus* is susceptible in vitro to penicillin, ampicillin, cephalosporins, chloramphenicol, aminoglycosides, and fluoroquinolones, and these agents may also be effective. *V parahaemolyticus* and *V alginolyticus* produce beta-lactamase and therefore are resistant to penicillin and ampicillin, but susceptibilities otherwise are similar to those listed for *V vulnificus*.

Lee YC et al. Prognostic factor of mortality and its clinical implications in patients with necrotizing fasciitis caused by *Vibrio vulnificus*. Eur J Clin Microbiol Infect Dis. 2014 Jun; 33(6):1011–8. [PMID: 24419406]

Wong KC et al. Antibiotic use for *Vibrio* infections: important insights from surveillance data. BMC Infect Dis. 2015 Jun 11; 15:226. [PMID: 26062903]

INFECTIONS CAUSED BY *CAMPYLOBACTER* SPECIES

Campylobacter organisms are microaerophilic, motile, gram-negative rods. Two species infect humans: *Campylobacter jejuni*, an important cause of diarrheal disease, and *C fetus* subsp *fetus*, which typically causes systemic infection and not diarrhea. Dairy cattle and poultry are an important reservoir for campylobacters. Outbreaks of enteritis have been associated with consumption of raw milk. *Campylobacter* gastroenteritis is associated with fever, abdominal pain, and diarrhea characterized by loose, watery, or bloody stools. The differential diagnosis includes shigellosis, *Salmonella* gastroenteritis, and enteritis caused by *Y enterocolitica* or invasive *E coli*. The disease is self-limited, but its duration can be shortened with antimicrobial therapy. Either azithromycin, 1 g orally as a single dose, or ciprofloxacin, 500 mg orally twice daily for 3 days, is effective therapy. However, fluoroquinolone resistance among *C jejuni* isolates has been increasing, particularly in Southeast Asia, and susceptibility testing should be routinely performed.

C fetus causes systemic infections that can be fatal, including primary bacteremia, endocarditis, meningitis, and focal abscesses. It infrequently causes gastroenteritis. Patients infected with *C fetus* are often older, debilitated, or immunocompromised. Closely related species, collectively termed "campylobacter-like organisms," cause bacteremia in HIV-infected individuals. Systemic infections respond to therapy with gentamicin, chloramphenicol, ceftriaxone, or ciprofloxacin. Ceftriaxone or chloramphenicol should be used to treat infections of the central nervous system because of their ability to penetrate the blood-brain barrier.

Kaakoush NO et al. Global epidemiology of *Campylobacter* infection. Clin Microbiol Rev. 2015 Jul;28(3):687–720. [PMID: 26062576]

Ricotta EE et al. Epidemiology and antimicrobial resistance of international travel-associated *Campylobacter* infections in the United States, 2005–2011. Am J Public Health. 2014 Jul; 104(7):e108–14. [PMID: 24832415]

BRUCELLOSIS

ESSENTIALS OF DIAGNOSIS

► History of animal exposure, ingestion of unpasteurized milk or cheese.

► Insidious onset: easy fatigability, headache, arthralgia, anorexia, sweating, irritability.

► Intermittent and persistent fever.

► Cervical and axillary lymphadenopathy; hepatosplenomegaly.

► Lymphocytosis, positive blood culture, positive serologic test.

► General Considerations

The infection is transmitted from animals to humans. *Brucella abortus* (cattle), *B suis* (hogs), and *B melitensis* (goats) are the main agents. Transmission to humans occurs by contact with infected meat (slaughterhouse workers), placentae of infected animals (farmers, veterinarians), or ingestion of infected unpasteurized milk or cheese. The incubation period varies from a few days to several weeks. Brucellosis is a systemic infection that may become chronic. In the United States, brucellosis is very rare. Almost all US cases are imported from countries where brucellosis is endemic (eg, Mexico, Mediterranean Europe, Spain, South American countries).

Clinical Findings

A. Symptoms and Signs

The onset may be acute, with fever, chills, and sweats, but more often is insidious with symptoms of weakness, weight loss, low-grade fevers, sweats, and exhaustion upon minimal activity. Headache, abdominal or back pain with anorexia and constipation, and arthralgias are also common. The chronic form may assume an undulant nature, with periods of normal temperature between acute attacks; symptoms may persist for years, either continuously or intermittently.

Fever, hepatosplenomegaly, and lymphadenopathy are the most common physical findings. Infection may present with or be complicated by specific organ involvement with signs of endocarditis, meningitis, epididymitis, orchitis, arthritis (especially sacroiliitis), spondylitis, or osteomyelitis.

B. Laboratory Findings

The organism can be recovered from cultures of blood, cerebrospinal fluid, urine, bone marrow, or other sites. Modern automated systems have shortened the time to detection of the organism in blood culture. Cultures are more likely to be negative in chronic cases. The diagnosis often is made by serologic testing.

Differential Diagnosis

Brucellosis must be differentiated from any other acute febrile disease, especially influenza, tularemia, Q fever, mononucleosis, and enteric fever. In its chronic form it resembles Hodgkin disease, tuberculosis, HIV infection, malaria, and disseminated fungal infections such as histoplasmosis and coccidioidomycosis.

Complications

The most frequent complications are bone and joint lesions such as spondylitis and suppurative arthritis (usually of a single joint), endocarditis, and meningoencephalitis. Less common complications are pneumonitis with pleural effusion, hepatitis, and cholecystitis.

Treatment

Single-drug regimens are not recommended because the relapse rate may be as high as 50%. Combination regimens of two or three drugs are most effective. Regimens of doxycycline (200 mg/day orally for 6 weeks) plus rifampin (600 mg/day orally for 6 weeks) or streptomycin (1 g/day intramuscularly for 2 weeks) or gentamicin (240 mg intramuscularly once daily for 7 days) have the lowest recurrence

rates. Longer courses of therapy may be required to prevent relapse of meningitis, osteomyelitis, or endocarditis.

Herrick JA et al. *Brucella* arteritis: clinical manifestations, treatment, and prognosis. Lancet Infect Dis. 2014 Jun;14(6):520–6. [PMID: 24480149]

Rubach MP et al. Brucellosis in low-income and middle-income countries. Curr Opin Infect Dis. 2013 Oct;26(5):404–12. [PMID: 23963260]

TULAREMIA

ESSENTIALS OF DIAGNOSIS

▸ History of contact with rabbits, other rodents, and biting arthropods (eg, ticks in summer) in endemic area.

▸ Fever, headache, nausea, and prostration.

▸ Papule progressing to ulcer at site of inoculation.

▸ Enlarged regional lymph nodes.

▸ Serologic tests or culture of ulcer, lymph node aspirate, or blood confirm the diagnosis.

General Considerations

Tularemia is a zoonotic infection of wild rodents and rabbits caused by *Francisella tularensis*. Humans usually acquire the infection by contact with animal tissues (eg, trapping muskrats, skinning rabbits) or from a tick or insect bite. Hamsters and prairie dogs also may carry the organism. An investigation of an outbreak of pneumonic tularemia on Martha's Vineyard in Massachusetts implicated lawn-mowing and brush-cutting as risk factors for infection, underscoring the potential for probable aerosol transmission of the organism. *F tularensis* has been classified as a high-priority agent for potential bioterrorism use because of its virulence and relative ease of dissemination. Infection in humans often produces a local lesion and widespread organ involvement but may be entirely asymptomatic. The incubation period is 2–10 days.

Clinical Findings

A. Symptoms and Signs

Fever, headache, and nausea begin suddenly, and a local lesion—a papule at the site of inoculation—develops and soon ulcerates. Regional lymph nodes may become enlarged and tender and may suppurate. The local lesion may be on the skin of an extremity or in the eye. Pneumonia may develop from hematogenous spread of the organism or may be primary after inhalation of infected aerosols, which are responsible for human-to-human transmission. Following ingestion of infected meat or water, an enteric form may be manifested by gastrointestinal symptoms, stupor, and delirium. In any type of involvement, the spleen may be enlarged and tender and there may be nonspecific rashes, myalgias, and prostration.

B. Laboratory Findings

Culturing the organism from blood or infected tissue requires special media. For this reason and because cultures of *F tularensis* may be hazardous to laboratory personnel, the diagnosis is usually made serologically. A positive agglutination test (greater than 1:80) develops in the second week after infection and may persist for several years.

▶ Differential Diagnosis

Tularemia must be differentiated from rickettsial and meningococcal infections, cat-scratch disease, infectious mononucleosis, and various bacterial and fungal diseases.

▶ Complications

Hematogenous spread may produce meningitis, perisplenitis, pericarditis, pneumonia, and osteomyelitis.

▶ Treatment

Streptomycin is drug of choice for treatment of tularemia. The recommended dose is 7.5 mg/kg intramuscularly every 12 hours for 7–14 days. Gentamicin, which has good in vitro activity against *F tularensis*, is generally less toxic than streptomycin and probably just as effective. Doxycycline (200 mg/day orally) is also effective but has a higher relapse rate. A variety of other agents (eg, fluoroquinolones) are active in vitro but their clinical effectiveness is less well established.

Birdsell DN et al. *Francisella tularensis* subsp. *tularensis* group A.I, United States. Emerg Infect Dis. 2014 May;20(5):861–5. [PMID: 24755401]

Ulu-Kilic A et al. An overview: tularemia and travel medicine. Travel Med Infect Dis. 2014 Nov–Dec;12(6 Pt A):609–16. [PMID: 25457302]

PLAGUE

ESSENTIALS OF DIAGNOSIS

- ▶ History of exposure to rodents in endemic area.
- ▶ Sudden onset of high fever, malaise, muscular pains, and prostration.
- ▶ Axillary or inguinal lymphadenitis (bubo).
- ▶ Bacteremia, pneumonitis, and meningitis may occur.
- ▶ Positive smear and culture from bubo and positive blood culture.

▶ General Considerations

Plague is an infection of wild rodents with *Yersinia pestis*, a small bipolar-staining gram-negative rod. It is endemic in California, Arizona, Nevada, and New Mexico. It is transmitted among rodents and to humans by the bites of fleas or from contact with infected animals. Following a fleabite, the organisms spread through the lymphatics to the lymph nodes, which become greatly enlarged (buboes). They may then reach the bloodstream to involve all organs. When pneumonia or meningitis develops, the outcome is often fatal. The patient with pneumonia can transmit the infection to other individuals by droplets. The incubation period is 2–10 days. Because of its extreme virulence, its potential for dissemination and person-to-person transmission, and efforts to develop the organism as an agent of biowarfare, plague bacillus is considered a high-priority agent for bioterrorism.

▶ Clinical Findings

A. Symptoms and Signs

The onset is sudden, with high fever, malaise, tachycardia, intense headache, delirium, and severe myalgias. The patient appears profoundly ill. If pneumonia develops, tachypnea, productive cough, blood-tinged sputum, and cyanosis also occur. There may be signs of meningitis. A pustule or ulcer at the site of inoculation and lymphangitis may be observed. Axillary, inguinal, or cervical lymph nodes become enlarged and tender and may suppurate and drain. With hematogenous spread, the patient may rapidly become toxic and comatose, with purpuric spots (black plague) appearing on the skin.

Primary plague pneumonia is a fulminant pneumonitis with bloody, frothy sputum and sepsis. It is usually fatal unless treatment is started within a few hours after onset.

B. Laboratory Findings

The plague bacillus may be found in smears from aspirates of buboes examined with Gram stain. Cultures from bubo aspirate or pus and blood are positive but may grow slowly. In convalescing patients, an antibody titer rise may be demonstrated by agglutination tests.

▶ Differential Diagnosis

The lymphadenitis of plague is most commonly mistaken for the lymphadenitis accompanying staphylococcal or streptococcal infections of an extremity, sexually transmitted diseases such as lymphogranuloma venereum or syphilis, and tularemia. The systemic manifestations resemble those of enteric or rickettsial fevers, malaria, or influenza. The pneumonia resembles other bacterial pneumonias, and the meningitis is similar to those caused by other bacteria.

▶ Prevention

Avoiding exposure to rodents and fleas in endemic areas is the best prevention strategy. Drug prophylaxis may provide temporary protection for persons exposed to the risk of plague infection, particularly by the respiratory route. Doxycycline, 100 mg twice daily for 7 days, is effective. No vaccine is available at this time.

Treatment

Therapy should be started immediately once plague is suspected. Either streptomycin (the agent with which there is greatest experience), 1 g every 12 hours intravenously, or gentamicin, administered as a 2-mg/kg loading dose, then 1.7 mg/kg every 8 hours intravenously, is effective. Alternatively, doxycycline, 100 mg orally or intravenously, may be used. The duration of therapy is 10 days. Patients with plague pneumonia are placed in strict respiratory isolation, and prophylactic therapy is given to any person who came in contact with the patient.

Raoult D et al. Plague: history and contemporary analysis. J Infect. 2013 Jan;66(1):18–26. [PMID: 23041039]

Runfola JK et al; Centers for Disease Control and Prevention (CDC). Outbreak of human pneumonic plague with dog-to-human and possible human-to-human transmission—Colorado, June–July 2014. MMWR Morb Mortal Wkly Rep. 2015 May 1;64(16):429–34. [PMID: 25928467]

GONOCOCCAL INFECTIONS

ESSENTIALS OF DIAGNOSIS

- ▶ Purulent and profuse urethral discharge, especially in men, with dysuria, yielding positive smear.
- ▶ Men: epididymitis, prostatitis, periurethral inflammation, proctitis.
- ▶ Women: cervicitis with purulent discharge, or asymptomatic, yielding positive culture; vaginitis, salpingitis, proctitis also occur.
- ▶ Fever, rash, tenosynovitis, and arthritis with disseminated disease.
- ▶ Gram-negative intracellular diplococci seen in a smear or cultured from any site, particularly the urethra, cervix, pharynx, and rectum.

General Considerations

Gonorrhea is caused by *Neisseria gonorrhoeae*, a gram-negative diplococcus typically found inside polymorphonuclear cells. It is transmitted during sexual activity and has its greatest incidence in the 15- to 29-year-old age group. The incubation period is usually 2–8 days.

Classification

A. Urethritis and Cervicitis

In men, there is initially burning on urination and a serous or milky discharge. One to 3 days later, the urethral pain is more pronounced and the discharge becomes yellow, creamy, and profuse, sometimes blood-tinged. The disorder may regress and become chronic or progress to involve the prostate, epididymis, and periurethral glands with painful inflammation. Chronic infection leads to prostatitis and urethral strictures. Rectal infection is common in men who have sex with men. Atypical sites of primary infection (eg, the pharynx) must always be considered. Asymptomatic infection is common and occurs in both sexes.

Gonococcal infection in women often becomes symptomatic during menses. Women may have dysuria, urinary frequency, and urgency, with a purulent urethral discharge. Vaginitis and cervicitis with inflammation of Bartholin glands are common. Infection may be asymptomatic, with only slightly increased vaginal discharge and moderate cervicitis on examination. Infection may remain as a chronic cervicitis—an important reservoir of gonococci. It can progress to involve the uterus and tubes with acute and chronic salpingitis, with scarring of tubes and sterility. In pelvic inflammatory disease, anaerobes and chlamydiae often accompany gonococci. Rectal infection may result from spread of the organism from the genital tract or from anal coitus.

Gram stain of urethral discharge in men, especially during the first week after onset, shows gram-negative diplococci in polymorphonuclear leukocytes. Gram stain is less often positive in women. Nucleic acid amplification tests are the preferred method for diagnosing all types of gonorrhea given their excellent sensitivity and specificity. In women with suspected cervical infection, endocervical or vaginal swabs (clinician- or self-collected) as well as first catch AM urine specimen (later specimens have 10% reduced sensitivity) are options. In men with urethral infection, first catch AM urine is recommended. Nucleic acid amplification tests are also recommended by the CDC for oropharyngeal and rectal sites testing although they are not FDA approved for these specimen types. Cultures should still be obtained when evaluating a treatment failure to assess for antimicrobial resistance.

B. Disseminated Disease

Systemic complications follow the dissemination of gonococci from the primary site via the bloodstream. Two distinct clinical syndromes—either purulent arthritis or the triad of rash, tenosynovitis, and arthralgias—are commonly observed in patients with disseminated gonococcal infection, although overlap can be seen. The skin lesions can range from maculopapular to pustular or hemorrhagic, which tend to be few in number and peripherally located. The tenosynovitis is often found in the hands and wrists and feet and ankles. These unique findings can help distinguish among other infectious syndromes. The arthritis can occur in one or more joints. Gonococci are isolated by culture from less than half of patients with gonococcal arthritis. Rarely, gonococcal endocarditis or meningitis develops.

C. Conjunctivitis

The most common form of eye involvement is direct inoculation of gonococci into the conjunctival sac. In adults, this occurs by autoinoculation of a person with genital infection. The purulent conjunctivitis may rapidly progress to panophthalmitis and loss of the eye unless treated promptly. A single 1-g dose of ceftriaxone is effective.

▶ Differential Diagnosis

Gonococcal urethritis or cervicitis must be differentiated from nongonococcal urethritis; cervicitis or vaginitis due to *Chlamydia trachomatis, Gardnerella vaginalis, Trichomonas, Candida,* and many other pathogens associated with sexually transmitted diseases; and pelvic inflammatory disease, arthritis, proctitis, and skin lesions. Often, several such pathogens coexist in a patient. Reactive arthritis (urethritis, conjunctivitis, arthritis) may mimic gonorrhea or coexist with it.

▶ Prevention

Prevention is based on education and mechanical or chemical prophylaxis. The condom, if properly used, can reduce the risk of infection. Effective drugs taken in therapeutic doses within 24 hours of exposure can abort an infection. Partner notification and referral of contacts for treatment has been the standard method used to control sexually transmitted diseases. Expedited treatment of sex partners by patient-delivered partner therapy is more effective than partner notification in reducing persistence and recurrence rates of gonorrhea and chlamydia. This strategy is being increasingly adopted as a means of disease control.

▶ Treatment

Therapy typically is administered before antimicrobial susceptibilities are known. The choice of which regimen to use should be based on the national prevalences of antibiotic-resistant organisms. Nationwide, strains of gonococci that are resistant to penicillin, tetracycline, or ciprofloxacin have been increasingly observed. Consequently, these drugs can no longer be considered first-line therapy. All sexual partners should be treated and tested for HIV infection and syphilis, as should the patient.

A. Uncomplicated Gonorrhea

Due to increasing resistance of *N gonorrhoeae* to cephalosporins, the CDC has updated its treatment recommendation for gonorrhea. Treatment for gonorrhea should include a higher dose of intramuscular ceftriaxone in combination with a second drug (azithromycin or doxycycline) regardless of concern for possible secondary infection with chlamydia. For uncomplicated gonococcal infections of the cervix, urethra, and rectum, the recommended treatment is ceftriaxone (250 mg intramuscularly) plus azithromycin (1000 mg orally as a single dose). In cases where an oral cephalosporin is the only option, cefixime, 400 mg orally as a single dose, can be combined with azithromycin as above. When azithromycin is not an option, doxycycline at 100 mg orally twice daily for 7 days can be substituted. Fluoroquinolones are no longer recommended for treatment due to high rates of microbial resistance. Spectinomycin, 1 g intramuscularly once, may be used for the penicillin-allergic patient but is not currently available in the United States. Pharyngeal gonorrhea is also treated with ceftriaxone (250 mg intramuscularly) plus azithromycin (1000 mg orally as a single dose) but for conjunctival gonorrhea the recommendation is for ceftriaxone (1 g intramuscularly) plus azithromycin (1000 mg orally as a single dose).

B. Treatment of Other Infections

Disseminated gonococcal infection (including arthritis and arthritis-dermatitis syndromes) should be treated with ceftriaxone (1 g intravenously daily) plus azithromycin (1000 mg orally as a single dose), until 48 hours after improvement begins, at which time therapy may be switched to cefixime (400 mg orally daily) to complete at least 1 week of antimicrobial therapy. Endocarditis should be treated with ceftriaxone (2 g every 24 hours intravenously) for at least 4 weeks.

Pelvic inflammatory disease requires cefoxitin (2 g parenterally every 6 hours) or cefotetan (2 g intravenously every 12 hours) plus doxycycline (100 mg every 12 hours). Clindamycin (900 mg intravenously every 8 hours) plus gentamicin (administered intravenously as a 2-mg/kg loading dose followed by 1.5 mg/kg every 8 hours) is also effective. Ceftriaxone (250 mg intramuscularly as a single dose) or cefoxitin (2 g intramuscularly) plus probenecid (1 g orally as a single dose) plus doxycycline (100 mg twice a day for 14 days), with or without metronidazole (500 mg twice daily for 14 days) is an effective outpatient regimen.

Workowski KA et al; Centers for Disease Control and Prevention. Sexually transmitted diseases treatment guidelines, 2015. MMWR Recomm Rep. 2015 Jun 5;64(RR-03):1–137. Erratum in: MMWR Recomm Rep. 2015 Aug 28;64(33):924. [PMID: 26042815]
Zakher B et al. Screening for gonorrhea and *Chlamydia:* a systematic review for the U.S. Preventive Services Task Force. Ann Intern Med. 2014 Dec 16;161(12):884–93. [PMID: 25244000]

CHANCROID

Chancroid is a sexually transmitted disease caused by the short gram-negative bacillus *Haemophilus ducreyi.* The incubation period is 3–5 days. At the site of inoculation, a vesicopustule develops that breaks down to form a painful, soft ulcer with a necrotic base, surrounding erythema, and undermined edges. There may be multiple lesions due to autoinoculation. The adenitis is usually unilateral and consists of tender, matted nodes of moderate size with overlying erythema. These may become fluctuant and rupture spontaneously. With lymph node involvement, fever, chills, and malaise may develop. Balanitis and phimosis are frequent complications in men. Women may have no external signs of infection. The diagnosis is established by culturing a swab of the lesion onto a special medium.

Chancroid must be differentiated from other genital ulcers. The chancre of syphilis is clean and painless, with a hard base. Mixed sexually transmitted disease is very common (including syphilis, herpes simplex, and HIV infection), as is infection of the ulcer with fusiforms, spirochetes, and other organisms.

A single dose of either azithromycin, 1 g orally, or ceftriaxone, 250 mg intramuscularly, is effective treatment. Effective multiple-dose regimens are erythromycin,

500 mg orally four times a day for 7 days, or ciprofloxacin, 500 mg orally twice a day for 3 days.

Workowski KA et al; Centers for Disease Control and Prevention. Sexually transmitted diseases treatment guidelines, 2015. MMWR Recomm Rep. 2015 Jun 5;64(RR-03):1–137. Erratum in: MMWR Recomm Rep. 2015 Aug 28;64(33):924. [PMID: 26042815]

GRANULOMA INGUINALE

Granuloma inguinale is a chronic, relapsing granulomatous anogenital infection due to *Calymmatobacterium (Donovania) granulomatis*. The pathognomonic cell, found in tissue scrapings or secretions, is large (25–90 mcm) and contains intracytoplasmic cysts filled with bodies (Donovan bodies) that stain deeply with Wright stain.

The incubation period is 8 days to 12 weeks. The onset is insidious. The lesions occur on the skin or mucous membranes of the genitalia or perineal area. They are relatively painless infiltrated nodules that soon slough. A shallow, sharply demarcated ulcer forms, with a beefy-red friable base of granulation tissue. The lesion spreads by contiguity. The advancing border has a characteristic rolled edge of granulation tissue. Large ulcerations may advance onto the lower abdomen and thighs. Scar formation and healing occur along one border while the opposite border advances.

Superinfection with spirochete-fusiform organisms is common. The ulcer then becomes purulent, painful, foul-smelling, and extremely difficult to treat.

Several therapies are available. Because of the indolent nature of the disease, duration of therapy is relatively long. The following recommended regimens should be given for 3 weeks or until all lesions have healed: doxycycline, 100 mg orally twice daily; or azithromycin, 1 g orally once weekly; or ciprofloxacin, 750 mg orally twice daily; or erythromycin, 500 mg orally four times a day.

Workowski KA et al; Centers for Disease Control and Prevention. Sexually transmitted diseases treatment guidelines, 2015. MMWR Recomm Rep. 2015 Jun 5;64(RR-03):1–137. Erratum in: MMWR Recomm Rep. 2015 Aug 28;64(33):924. [PMID: 26042815]

BARTONELLA SPECIES

Bartonella species are responsible for a wide variety of clinical syndromes. **Bacillary angiomatosis**, an important manifestation of bartonellosis, is discussed in Chapter 31. A variety of atypical infections, including retinitis, encephalitis, osteomyelitis, and persistent bacteremia and endocarditis have been described.

Trench fever is a self-limited, louse-borne relapsing febrile disease caused by *B quintana*. The disease has occurred epidemically in louse-infested troops and civilians during wars and endemically in residents of scattered geographic areas (eg, Central America). An urban equivalent of trench fever has been described among the homeless. Humans acquire infection when infected lice feces enter sites of skin breakdown. Onset of symptoms is abrupt and fever lasts 3–5 days, with relapses. The patient complains of weakness and severe pain behind the eyes and typically in the back and legs. Lymphadenopathy, splenomegaly, and a transient maculopapular rash may appear. Subclinical infection is frequent, and a carrier state is recognized. The differential diagnosis includes other febrile, self-limited states such as dengue, leptospirosis, malaria, relapsing fever, and typhus. Recovery occurs regularly even in the absence of treatment.

Cat-scratch disease is an acute infection of children and young adults caused by *Bartonella henselae*. It is transmitted from cats to humans as the result of a scratch or bite. Within a few days, a papule or ulcer will develop at the inoculation site in one-third of patients. One to 3 weeks later, fever, headache, and malaise occur. Regional lymph nodes become enlarged, often tender, and may suppurate. Lymphadenopathy from cat scratches resembles that due to neoplasm, tuberculosis, lymphogranuloma venereum, and bacterial lymphadenitis. The diagnosis is usually made clinically. Special cultures for bartonellae, serology, or excisional biopsy, though rarely necessary, confirm the diagnosis. The biopsy reveals necrotizing lymphadenitis and is itself not specific for cat-scratch disease. Cat-scratch disease is usually self-limited, requiring no specific therapy. Encephalitis occurs rarely.

Disseminated forms of the disease—bacillary angiomatosis, peliosis hepatis, and retinitis—occur most commonly in immunocompromised patients such as persons with late stages of HIV or solid organ transplant recipients. The lesions are vasculoproliferative and histopathologically distinct from those of cat-scratch disease. Unexplained fever in patients with late stages of HIV infection is not uncommonly due to bartonellosis. *B quintana*, the agent of trench fever, can also cause bacillary angiomatosis and persistent bacteremia or endocarditis (which will be "culture-negative" unless specifically sought), the latter two entities being associated with homelessness. Due to the fastidious nature of the organism and its special growth requirements, serologic testing (eg, demonstration of a high antibody titer in an indirect immunofluorescence assay) or nucleic acid amplification tests are often required to establish a diagnosis.

The disseminated forms of the disease (bacillary angiomatosis, peliosis hepatis, and retinitis) require a prolonged course of antibiotic therapy often in combination with a second agent. Bacteremia and endocarditis can be effectively treated with a 6-week course of doxycycline (200 mg orally or intravenously in two divided doses per day) plus either gentamicin 3 mg/kg/day intravenously or rifampin 600 mg/day orally in two divided doses. Relapse may occur.

Edouard S et al. *Bartonella*, a common cause of endocarditis: a report on 106 cases and review. J Clin Microbiol. 2015 Mar; 53(3):824–9. [PMID: 25540398]
Zangwill KM. Cat scratch disease and other *Bartonella* infections. Adv Exp Med Biol. 2013;764:159–66. [PMID: 23654065]

ELIZABETHKINGIA SPECIES

Elizabethkingia species (previously known as *Flavobacterium* and *Chryseobacterium* species) are gram-negative rods that cause infection primarily in patients with compromised immune systems or multiple other comorbidities. Outbreaks due to the subspecies *E meningoseptica* and *E anopheles* have been associated with contaminated water sources and have often occurred in health-care facilities. Meningitis and bacteremia as well as skin and bone infections have developed in patients infected with *Elizabethkingia*. Empiric treatment is piperacillin/tazobactam 4.5 g intravenously four times daily. However, *Elizabethkingia* species can be resistant to multiple antimicrobials. When an outbreak of *Elizabethkingia* species infections occurs in a health-care setting, the facility's infection control specialists must search for and eliminate the contaminated water source.

Moore LS et al. Waterborne *Elizabethkingia meningoseptica* in adult critical care. Emerg Infect Dis. 2016 Jan;22(1):9–17. [PMID: 26690562]

ANAEROBIC INFECTIONS

Anaerobic bacteria comprise the majority of normal human flora. Normal microbial flora of the mouth (anaerobic spirochetes, *Prevotella*, fusobacteria), the skin (anaerobic diphtheroids), the large bowel (bacteroides, anaerobic streptococci, clostridia), and the female genitourinary tract (bacteroides, anaerobic streptococci, fusobacteria) produce disease when displaced from their normal sites into tissues or closed body spaces.

Anaerobic infections tend to be polymicrobial and abscesses are common. Pus and infected tissue often are malodorous. Septic thrombophlebitis and metastatic infection are frequent and may require incision and drainage. Diminished blood supply that favors proliferation of anaerobes because of reduced tissue oxygenation may interfere with the delivery of antimicrobials to the site of anaerobic infection. Cultures, unless carefully collected under anaerobic conditions, may yield negative results.

Important types of infections that are most commonly caused by anaerobic organisms are listed below. Treatment of all these infections consists of surgical exploration and judicious excision in conjunction with administration of antimicrobial drugs.

1. Head & Neck Infections

Prevotella melaninogenica (formerly *Bacteroides melaninogenicus*) and anaerobic spirochetes are commonly involved in periodontal infections. These organisms, fusobacteria, and peptostreptococci may cause chronic sinusitis, peritonsillar abscess, chronic otitis media, and mastoiditis. *F necrophorum* has been recognized as a common cause of pharyngitis in adolescents and young adults. *F necrophorum* infection has been associated with septic internal jugular thrombophlebitis (Lemierre syndrome) and causes septic pulmonary embolization. Hygiene, drainage, and surgical debridement are as important in treatment as antimicrobials. Oral anaerobic organisms have been uniformly susceptible to penicillin, but there has been a recent trend of increasing penicillin resistance, usually due to beta-lactamase production. Therefore, ampicillin/sulbactam 1.5-3 g intravenously

every 6 hours (if parenteral therapy is required) or amoxicillin/clavulanic acid 875 mg/125 mg orally twice daily, or clindamycin can be used (600 mg intravenously every 8 hours or 300 mg orally every 6 hours). Antimicrobial treatment is continued for a few days after symptoms and signs of infection have resolved. Indolent, established infections (eg, mastoiditis or osteomyelitis) may require prolonged courses of therapy, eg, 4–6 weeks or longer.

Brook I. Anaerobic bacteria in upper respiratory tract and head and neck infections: microbiology and treatment. Anaerobe. 2012 Apr;18(2):214–20. [PMID: 22197951]
Brook I. Spectrum and treatment of anaerobic infections. J Infect Chemother. 2016 Jan;22(1):1–13. [PMID: 26620376]

2. Chest Infections

Usually in the setting of poor oral hygiene and periodontal disease, aspiration of saliva (which contains 10^8 anaerobic organisms per milliliter in addition to aerobes) may lead to necrotizing pneumonia, lung abscess, and empyema. Polymicrobial infection is the rule and anaerobes—particularly *P melaninogenica*, fusobacteria, and peptostreptococci—are common etiologic agents. Most pulmonary infections respond to antimicrobial therapy alone. Percutaneous chest tube or surgical drainage is indicated for empyema.

Penicillin-resistant *Bacteroides fragilis* and *P melaninogenica* are commonly isolated and have been associated with clinical failures. Clindamycin, 600 mg intravenously once, followed by 300 mg orally every 6–8 hours, is the treatment of choice for these infections. Metronidazole does not cover facultative streptococci, which often are present, and if used, a second agent that is active against streptococci, such as ceftriaxone 1 g intravenously or intramuscularly daily, should be added. Penicillin, 2 million units intravenously every 4 hours, followed by amoxicillin, 500 mg every 8 hours orally, is an alternative; however, increasing prevalence of beta-lactamase producing organisms is a concern. Moxifloxacin, 400 mg orally or intravenously once daily, may be used. Because these infections respond slowly, a prolonged course of therapy (eg, 4–6 weeks) is generally recommended.

Bartlett JG. Anaerobic bacterial infection of the lung. Anaerobe. 2012 Apr;18(2):235–9. [PMID: 22209937]
Brook I. Spectrum and treatment of anaerobic infections. J Infect Chemother. 2016 Jan;22(1):1–13. [PMID: 26620376]

3. Central Nervous System

Anaerobes are a common cause of brain abscess, subdural empyema, or septic central nervous system thrombophlebitis. The organisms reach the central nervous system by direct extension from sinusitis, otitis, or mastoiditis or by hematogenous spread from chronic lung infections. Antimicrobial therapy—eg, ceftriaxone, 2 g intravenously every 12 hours, plus metronidazole, 500 mg intravenously every 8 hours—is an important adjunct to surgical drainage. Duration of therapy is 6–8 weeks but should be based on follow-up imaging. Some small multiple brain abscesses can be treated with antibiotics alone without surgical drainage.

Brook I. Spectrum and treatment of anaerobic infections. J Infect Chemother. 2016 Jan;22(1):1–13. [PMID: 26620376]

4. Intra-abdominal Infections

In the colon there are up to 10^{11} anaerobes per gram of content—predominantly B fragilis, clostridia, and peptostreptococci. These organisms play a central role in most intra-abdominal abscesses following trauma to the colon, diverticulitis, appendicitis, or perirectal abscess and may also participate in hepatic abscess and cholecystitis, often in association with aerobic coliform bacteria. The bacteriology includes anaerobes as well as enteric gram-negative rods and on occasion enterococci. Therapy should be directed both against anaerobes and gram-negative aerobes. Agents that are active against B fragilis include metronidazole, chloramphenicol, moxifloxacin, tigecycline, ertapenem, imipenem, doripenem, ampicillin-sulbactam, ticarcillin-clavulanic acid, piperacillin-tazobactam, and ceftolozane/tazobactam. Resistance to cefoxitin, cefotetan, and clindamycin is increasingly encountered. Most third-generation cephalosporins have poor efficacy.

Table 33–7 summarizes the antibiotic regimens for management of moderate to moderately severe infections (eg, patient hemodynamically stable, good surgical drainage possible or established, low APACHE score, no multiple organ failure) and severe infections (eg, major peritoneal soilage, large or multiple abscesses, patient hemodynamically unstable), particularly if drug-resistant organisms are suspected. An effective oral regimen for patients able to take it is presented also.

Table 33–7. Treatment of anaerobic intra-abdominal infections.

Community-onset
Oral therapy
Moxifloxacin 400 mg every 24 hours
Intravenous therapy
Moderate to moderately severe infections:
Ertapenem 1 g every 24 hours
or—
Ceftriaxone 1 g every 24 hours (or ciprofloxacin 400 mg every 12 hours, if penicillin allergic) plus metronidazole 500 mg every 8 hours
Severe infections:
Imipenem, 0.5 g every 6–8 hours or meropenem 1 g every 8 hours or doripenem 0.5 g every 8 hours or piperacillin/tazobactam 3.75 g every 6 hours
Health-care–associated
Intravenous therapy
Imipenem, 0.5 g every 6–8 hours or meropenem 1 g every 8 hours or doripenem 0.5 g every 8 hours or piperacillin/tazobactam 4.5 g every 6 hours
or—
Ceftazidime or cefepime 2 g every 8 hours plus metronidazole 0.5 g every 8 hours

Brand M et al. Prophylactic antibiotics for penetrating abdominal trauma. Cochrane Database Syst Rev. 2013 Nov 18;11: CD007370. [PMID: 24249389]

Brook I. Spectrum and treatment of anaerobic infections. J Infect Chemother. 2016 Jan;22(1):1–13. [PMID: 26620376]

Sawyer RG et al. Trial of short-course antimicrobial therapy for intraabdominal infection. N Engl J Med. 2015 May 21; 372(21):1996–2005. [PMID: 25992746]

5. Female Genital Tract & Pelvic Infections

The normal flora of the vagina and cervix includes several species of bacteroides, peptostreptococci, group B streptococci, lactobacilli, coliform bacteria, and, occasionally, spirochetes and clostridia. These organisms commonly cause genital tract infections and may disseminate from there.

While salpingitis is often caused by gonococci and chlamydiae, tubo-ovarian and pelvic abscesses are associated with anaerobes in most cases. Postpartum infections may be caused by aerobic streptococci or staphylococci, but anaerobes are often found, and the worst cases of postpartum or postabortion sepsis are associated with clostridia and bacteroides. These have a high mortality rate, and treatment requires both antimicrobials directed against anaerobes and coliforms and abscess drainage or early hysterectomy.

Brook I. Spectrum and treatment of anaerobic infections. J Infect Chemother. 2016 Jan;22(1):1–13. [PMID: 26620376]

Lapinsky SE. Obstetric infections. Crit Care Clin. 2013 Jul; 29(3):509–20. [PMID: 23830651]

Mackeen AD et al. Antibiotic regimens for postpartum endometritis. Cochrane Database Syst Rev. 2015 Feb 2;2:CD001067. [PMID: 25922861]

6. Bacteremia & Endocarditis

Anaerobic bacteremia usually originates from the gastrointestinal tract, the oropharynx, decubitus ulcers, or the female genital tract. Endocarditis due to anaerobic and microaerophilic streptococci and bacteroides originates from the same sites. Most cases of anaerobic or microaerophilic streptococcal endocarditis can be effectively treated with 12–20 million units of penicillin G daily for 4–6 weeks, but optimal therapy of other types of anaerobic bacterial endocarditis must rely on laboratory guidance. Propionibacteria, clostridia, and bacteroides occasionally cause endocarditis.

Brook I. Spectrum and treatment of anaerobic infections. J Infect Chemother. 2016 Jan;22(1):1–13. [PMID: 26620376]

7. Skin & Soft Tissue Infections

Anaerobic infections of the skin and soft tissue usually follow trauma, inadequate blood supply, or surgery and are most common in areas that are contaminated by oral or fecal flora. These infections also occur in injection drug users and persons sustaining animal bites. There may be progressive tissue necrosis (Figure 33–5) and a putrid odor.

▲ **Figure 33–5.** Left foot gangrene, with plantar extension. (Used, with permission, from Dean SM, Satiani B, Abraham WT. *Color Atlas and Synopsis of Vascular Diseases.* McGraw-Hill, 2014.)

Several terms, such as bacterial synergistic gangrene, synergistic necrotizing cellulitis, necrotizing fasciitis, and non-clostridial crepitant cellulitis, have been used to classify these infections. Although there are some differences in microbiology among them, their differentiation on clinical grounds alone is difficult. All are mixed infections caused by aerobic and anaerobic organisms and require aggressive surgical debridement of necrotic tissue for cure. Surgical consultation is obligatory to assist in diagnosis and treatment.

Broad-spectrum antibiotics active against both anaerobes and gram-positive and gram-negative aerobes (eg, vancomycin plus piperacillin-tazobactam) should be instituted empirically and modified by culture results (see Table 30–5). They are given for about a week after progressive tissue destruction has been controlled and the margins of the wound remain free of inflammation.

Brook I. Spectrum and treatment of anaerobic infections. J Infect Chemother. 2016 Jan;22(1):1–13. [PMID: 26620376]

Kaafarani HM et al. Necrotizing skin and soft tissue infections. Surg Clin North Am. 2014 Feb;94(1):155–63. [PMID: 24267503]

ACTINOMYCOSIS

 ESSENTIALS OF DIAGNOSIS

► History of recent dental infection or abdominal trauma.

► Chronic pneumonia or indolent intra-abdominal or cervicofacial abscess.

► Sinus tract formation.

► General Considerations

Actinomyces israelii and other species of *Actinomyces* occur in the normal flora of the mouth and tonsillar crypts. They are anaerobic, gram-positive, branching filamentous bacteria (1 mcm in diameter) that may fragment into bacillary forms. When introduced into traumatized tissue and associated with other anaerobic bacteria, these actinomycetes become pathogens.

The most common site of infection is the cervicofacial area (about 60% of cases). Infection typically follows extraction of a tooth or other trauma. Lesions may develop in the gastrointestinal tract or lungs following ingestion or aspiration of the organism from its endogenous source in the mouth. Interestingly, *T whipplei*, the causative agent of Whipple disease, is an actinomycete and therefore is related to the species that cause actinomycosis.

► Clinical Findings

A. Symptoms and Signs

1. Cervicofacial actinomycosis—Cervicofacial actinomycosis develops slowly. The area becomes markedly indurated, and the overlying skin becomes reddish or cyanotic. Abscesses eventually draining to the surface persist for long periods. "Sulfur granules"—masses of filamentous organisms—may be found in the pus. There is usually little pain unless there is secondary infection. Trismus indicates that the muscles of mastication are involved. Radiography may reveal bony involvement. Cervicofacial or thoracic disease may occasionally involve the central nervous system, most commonly brain abscess or meningitis.

2. Thoracic actinomycosis—Thoracic involvement begins with fever, cough, and sputum production with night sweats and weight loss. Pleuritic pain may be present. Multiple sinuses may extend through the chest wall, to the heart, or into the abdominal cavity. Ribs may be involved. Radiography shows areas of consolidation and in many cases pleural effusion.

3. Abdominal actinomycosis—Abdominal actinomycosis usually causes pain in the ileocecal region, spiking fever and chills, vomiting, and weight loss; it may be confused with Crohn disease. Irregular abdominal masses may be palpated. Pelvic inflammatory disease caused by actinomycetes has been associated with prolonged use of an intrauterine contraceptive device. Sinuses draining to the exterior may develop. CT scanning reveals an inflammatory mass extended to involve bone.

B. Laboratory Findings

The anaerobic, gram-positive organism may be demonstrated as a granule or as scattered branching gram-positive filaments in the pus. Anaerobic culture is necessary to distinguish actinomycetes from nocardiae because specific therapy differs for the two infections.

▶ Treatment

Penicillin G is the drug of choice. Ten to 20 million units are given via a parenteral route for 4–6 weeks, followed by oral penicillin V, 500 mg four times daily. Alternatives include ampicillin, 12 g/day intravenously for 4–6 weeks followed by oral amoxicillin 500 mg three times daily or doxycycline 100 mg twice daily intravenously or orally. Response to therapy is slow. Therapy should be continued for weeks to months after clinical manifestations have disappeared in order to ensure cure. Surgical procedures such as drainage and resection may be beneficial.

With penicillin and surgery, the prognosis is good. The difficulties of diagnosis, however, may permit extensive destruction of tissue before the diagnosis is identified and therapy is started.

Könönen E et al. *Actinomyces* and related organisms in human infections. Clin Microbiol Rev. 2015 Apr;28(2):419–42. [PMID: 25788515]

Sasaki Y et al. Actinomycosis in the mandible: CT and MR findings. AJNR Am J Neuroradiol. 2014 Feb;35(2):390–4. [PMID: 23928143]

◤ NOCARDIOSIS

Nocardia species are aerobic filamentous soil bacteria that can cause pulmonary and systemic nocardiosis. Common *Nocardia* species include members of the *Nocardia asteroides* complex and *Nocardia brasiliensis*. Bronchopulmonary abnormalities (eg, alveolar proteinosis) predispose to colonization, but infection is unusual unless the patient is also receiving systemic corticosteroids or is otherwise immunosuppressed.

▶ Clinical Findings

Pulmonary involvement usually begins with malaise, loss of weight, fever, and night sweats. Cough and production of purulent sputum are the chief complaints. Radiography may show infiltrates accompanied by pleural effusion. The lesions may penetrate to the exterior through the chest wall, invading the ribs.

Dissemination involves any organ. Brain abscesses and subcutaneous nodules are most frequent. Even in the absence of clinical symptoms and signs of central nervous system infection, clinicians should consider brain imaging in patients with nocardiosis to rule out an occult abscess.

Nocardia species are usually found as delicate, branching, gram-positive filaments. They may be weakly acid-fast, occasionally causing diagnostic confusion with tuberculosis. Identification is made by culture.

▶ Treatment

For isolated cutaneous infections, therapy is initiated with trimethoprim-sulfamethoxazole administered at a dosage of 5–10 mg/kg/day (based on trimethoprim) as an oral or intravenous formulation. Surgical procedures such as drainage and resection may be needed as adjunctive therapy. A higher dose of 15 mg/kg/day (based on trimethoprim) should be used for disseminated or pulmonary infections. Resistance to trimethoprim-sulfamethoxazole may be increasing and initiating treatment with two drugs while awaiting antibiotic susceptibilities in cases of disseminated or severe localized disease should be considered. Alternative agents or drugs that can be given in combination with trimethoprim-sulfamethoxazole include imipenem, 500 mg intravenously every 6 hours; amikacin, 7.5 mg/kg intravenously every 12 hours; or minocycline, 100–200 mg orally or intravenously twice daily. Consultation with an infectious diseases expert should be considered.

Response may be slow, and therapy should be continued for at least 6 months. The prognosis in systemic nocardiosis is poor when diagnosis and therapy are delayed.

Anagnostou T et al. Nocardiosis of the central nervous system: experience from a general hospital and review of 84 cases from the literature. Medicine (Baltimore). 2014 Jan;93(1):19–32. [PMID: 24378740]

Chen J et al. Clinical and radiographic characteristics of pulmonary nocardiosis: clues to earlier diagnosis. PLoS One. 2014 Mar 3; 9(3):e90724. [PMID: 24594890]

Wang HL et al. Nocardiosis in 132 patients with cancer: microbiological and clinical analyses. Am J Clin Pathol. 2014 Oct; 142(4):513–23. [PMID: 25239419]

◤ INFECTIONS CAUSED BY MYCOBACTERIA

NONTUBERCULOUS MYCOBACTERIAL DISEASES

About 10% of mycobacterial infections are caused by nontuberculous mycobacteria. Nontuberculous mycobacterial infections are among the most common opportunistic infections in advanced HIV disease. These organisms have distinctive laboratory characteristics, occur ubiquitously in the environment, are not communicable from person to person, and are often resistant to standard antituberculous drugs.

Egelund EF et al. Medications and monitoring in nontuberculous mycobacteria infections. Clin Chest Med. 2015 Mar; 36(1):55–66. [PMID: 25676519]

Henkle E et al. Nontuberculous mycobacteria infections in immunosuppressed hosts. Clin Chest Med. 2015 Mar; 36(1):91–9. [PMID: 25676522]

1. Pulmonary Infections

Mycobacterium avium complex (MAC) causes a chronic, slowly progressive pulmonary infection resembling tuberculosis in immunocompetent patients, who typically have underlying pulmonary disease. Susceptibility testing for macrolide-resistance should be performed on clinical isolates. Treatment of nodular or bronchiectatic pulmonary disease is clarithromycin (1000 mg orally three times per week) or azithromycin (500 mg orally three times per week) plus rifampin (600 mg orally three times per week) or rifabutin (300 mg orally three times per week) plus ethambutol (25 mg/kg orally three times per week). Patients with fibrocavitary lung disease or severe nodular or bronchiectatic disease should receive three-drug therapy with clarithromycin (500–1000 mg orally daily) or azithromycin (250 orally mg daily) plus rifampin (600 mg orally daily) or rifabutin (300 mg orally daily) plus ethambutol (15 mg/kg orally daily). Therapy is continued for at least 12 months after sterilization of cultures.

M kansasii can produce clinical disease resembling tuberculosis, but the illness progresses more slowly. Most such infections occur in patients with preexisting lung disease, though 40% of patients have no known pulmonary disease. Microbiologically, *M kansasii* is similar to *M tuberculosis* and is sensitive to the same drugs except pyrazinamide, to which it is resistant. Therapy with isoniazid, ethambutol, and rifampin for 2 years (or 1 year after sputum conversion) has been successful.

Less common causes of pulmonary disease include *M xenopi*, *M szulgai*, and *M gordonae*. These organisms have variable sensitivities, and treatment is based on results of sensitivity tests. The rapid growing mycobacteria, *M abscessus*, *M chelonae*, and *M fortuitum* also can cause pneumonia in the occasional patient.

Benwill JL et al. *Mycobacterium abscessus*: challenges in diagnosis and treatment. Curr Opin Infect Dis. 2014 Dec;27(6):506–10. [PMID: 25268925]

Martiniano SL et al. Nontuberculous mycobacterial infections in cystic fibrosis. Clin Chest Med. 2015 Mar;36(1):101–15. [PMID: 25676523]

Mitchell JD. Surgical approach to pulmonary nontuberculous mycobacterial infections. Clin Chest Med. 2015 Mar; 36(1):117–22. [PMID: 25676524]

Park IK et al. Nontuberculous mycobacteria in cystic fibrosis and non-cystic fibrosis bronchiectasis. Semin Respir Crit Care Med. 2015 Apr;36(2):217–24. [PMID: 25826589]

Philley JV et al. Treatment of slowly growing mycobacteria. Clin Chest Med. 2015 Mar;36(1):79–90. [PMID: 25676521]

van Ingen J. Microbiological diagnosis of nontuberculous mycobacterial pulmonary disease. Clin Chest Med. 2015 Mar; 36(1):43–54. [PMID: 25676518]

2. Lymphadenitis

Most cases of lymphadenitis (scrofula) in adults are caused by *M tuberculosis* and can be a manifestation of disseminated disease. In children, the majority of cases are due to nontuberculous mycobacterial species, with MAC being the most common followed by *M scrofulaceum* in the United States and *M malmoense* and *M haemophilum* in Northern Europe. *M kansasii*, *M bovis*, *M chelonae*, and *M fortuitum* are less commonly observed. Unlike disease caused by *M tuberculosis*, which requires systemic therapy for 6 months, infection with nontuberculous mycobacteria can be successfully treated by surgical excision without antituberculous therapy.

3. Skin & Soft Tissue Infections

Skin and soft tissue infections such as abscesses, septic arthritis, and osteomyelitis can result from direct inoculation or hematogenous dissemination or may occur as a complication of surgery.

M abscessus, *M chelonae*, and *M fortuitum* are frequent causes of these types of infections. Most cases occur in the extremities and initially present as nodules. Ulceration with abscess formation often follows. The organisms are resistant to the usual antituberculosis drugs and may have susceptibility to clarithromycin, azithromycin, doxycycline, amikacin, cefoxitin, sulfonamides, imipenem, and ciprofloxacin. Given the multidrug-resistant nature of these organisms, obtaining antibiotic susceptibility testing is recommended. Therapy often includes surgical debridement along with at least two active antibiotics. Antibiotic therapy is usually continued for 3 months, although this must be determined based on clinical response.

M marinum infection ("swimming pool granuloma") presents as a nodular skin lesion following exposure to nonchlorinated water. The lesions respond to therapy with clarithromycin, doxycycline, minocycline, or trimethoprim-sulfamethoxazole.

M ulcerans infection (Buruli ulcer) is seen mainly in Africa and Australia and produces a large ulcerative lesion. Therapy consists of surgical excision and skin grafting.

4. Disseminated *Mycobacterium avium* Infection

MAC causes disseminated disease in immunocompromised patients, most commonly in patients in the late stages of HIV infection, when the CD4 cell count is less than 50/mcL. Persistent fever and weight loss are the most common symptoms. The organism can usually be cultured from multiple sites, including blood, liver, lymph node, or bone marrow. Blood culture is the preferred means of establishing the diagnosis and has a sensitivity of 98%.

Agents with proved activity against MAC are rifabutin, azithromycin, clarithromycin, and ethambutol. Amikacin and ciprofloxacin work in vitro, but clinical results are inconsistent. A combination of two or more active agents should be used to prevent rapid emergence of secondary resistance. Clarithromycin, 500 mg orally twice daily, plus ethambutol, 15 mg/kg/day orally as a single dose, with or without rifabutin, 300 mg/day orally, is the treatment of choice. Azithromycin, 500 mg orally once daily, may be used instead of clarithromycin. Insufficient data are available to permit specific recommendations about second-line regimens for patients intolerant of macrolides or those with macrolide-resistant organisms. MAC therapy may be discontinued in patients wh o have been treated with 12 months of therapy for disseminated MAC, who have no evidence of active disease, and whose CD4 counts exceed 100 cells/mcL for 6 months while receiving antiretroviral therapy (ART).

Antimicrobial prophylaxis of MAC prevents disseminated disease and prolongs survival. It is the standard of care to offer it to all HIV-infected patients with CD4 counts of 50/mcL or less. In contrast to active infection, single-drug oral regimens of clarithromycin, 500 mg twice daily, azithromycin, 1200 mg once weekly, or rifabutin, 300 mg once daily, are appropriate. Clarithromycin or azithromycin is more effective and better tolerated than rifabutin, and therefore preferred. Primary prophylaxis for MAC infection can be stopped in patients who have responded to antiretroviral combination therapy with elevation of CD4 counts of greater than 100 cells/mcL for 3 months.

Aksamit TR et al. Nontuberculous mycobacterial (NTM) lung disease: the top ten essentials. Respir Med. 2014 Mar; 108(3):417–25. [PMID: 24484653]

Griffith DE et al; ATS Mycobacterial Diseases Subcommittee; American Thoracic Society; Infectious Disease Society of America. An official ATS/IDSA statement: diagnosis, treatment, and prevention of nontuberculous mycobacterial diseases. Am J Respir Crit Care Med. 2007 Feb 15;175(4):367–416. [PMID: 17277290]

Masur H et al. Prevention and treatment of opportunistic infections in HIV-infected adults and adolescents: updated guidelines from the Centers for Disease Control and Prevention, National Institutes of Health, and HIV Medicine Association of the Infectious Diseases Society of America. Clin Infect Dis. 2014 May;58(9):1308–11. [PMID: 24585567]

MYCOBACTERIUM TUBERCULOSIS INFECTIONS

Tuberculosis is discussed in Chapter 9. Further information and expert consultation can be obtained from the Francis J. Curry International Tuberculosis Center at the Web site www.currytbcenter.ucsf.edu or by telephone, 415-502-4600, or fax, 415-502-4620.

TUBERCULOUS MENINGITIS

ESSENTIALS OF DIAGNOSIS

► Gradual onset of listlessness, irritability, and anorexia.

► Headache, vomiting, and seizures common.

► Cranial nerve abnormalities typical.

► Tuberculosis focus may be evident elsewhere.

► Cerebrospinal fluid shows several hundred lymphocytes, low glucose, and high protein.

General Considerations

Tuberculous meningitis is caused by rupture of a meningeal tuberculoma resulting from earlier hematogenous seeding of tubercle bacilli from a pulmonary focus, or it may be a consequence of miliary spread.

Clinical Findings

A. Symptoms and Signs

The onset is usually gradual, with listlessness, irritability, anorexia, and fever, followed by headache, vomiting, convulsions, and coma. In older patients, headache and behavioral changes are prominent early symptoms. Nuchal rigidity and cranial nerve palsies occur as the meningitis progresses. Evidence of active tuberculosis elsewhere or a history of prior tuberculosis is present in up to 75% of patients.

B. Laboratory Findings

The spinal fluid is frequently yellowish, with increased pressure, 100–500 cells/mcL (predominantly lymphocytes, though neutrophils may be present early during infection), increased protein, and decreased glucose. Acid-fast stains of cerebrospinal fluid usually are negative, and cultures also may be negative in 15–25% of cases. Nucleic acid amplification tests for rapid diagnosis of tuberculosis have variable sensitivity and specificity and none are FDA-approved for use in meningitis. Chest radiographs often reveal abnormalities compatible with tuberculosis but may be normal.

Differential Diagnosis

Tuberculous meningitis may be confused with any other type of meningitis, but the gradual onset, the predominantly lymphocytic pleocytosis of the spinal fluid, and evidence of tuberculosis elsewhere often point to the diagnosis. The tuberculin skin test is usually (not always) positive. Fungal and other granulomatous meningitides, syphilis, and carcinomatous meningitis are in the differential diagnosis.

Complications

Complications of tuberculous meningitis include seizure disorders, cranial nerve palsies, stroke, and obstructive hydrocephalus with impaired cognitive function. These result from inflammatory exudate primarily involving the basilar meninges and arteries.

Treatment

Presumptive diagnosis followed by early, empiric antituberculous therapy is essential for survival and to minimize sequelae. Even if cultures are not positive, a full course of therapy is warranted if the clinical setting is suggestive of tuberculous meningitis.

Regimens that are effective for pulmonary tuberculosis are effective also for tuberculous meningitis (see Table 9–16). Rifampin, isoniazid, and pyrazinamide all penetrate into cerebrospinal fluid well. The penetration of ethambutol is more variable, but therapeutic concentrations can be achieved, and the drug has been successfully used for meningitis. Aminoglycosides penetrate less well. Regimens that do not include both isoniazid and rifampin may be effective but are less reliable and generally must be given for longer periods.

Many authorities recommend the addition of corticosteroids for patients with focal deficits or altered mental status. Dexamethasone, 0.15 mg/kg intravenously or orally four times daily for 1–2 weeks, then discontinued in a tapering regimen over 4 weeks, may be used.

Thwaites GE et al. Tuberculous meningitis: more questions, still too few answers. Lancet Neurol. 2013 Oct;12(10):999–1010. [PMID: 23972913]
Török ME. Tuberculous meningitis: advances in diagnosis and treatment. Br Med Bull. 2015 Mar;113(1):117–31. [PMID: 25693576]

LEPROSY (Hansen Disease)

ESSENTIALS OF DIAGNOSIS

▶ Pale, anesthetic macular—or nodular and erythematous—skin lesions.

▶ Superficial nerve thickening with associated anesthesia.

▶ History of residence in endemic area in childhood.

▶ Acid-fast bacilli in skin lesions or nasal scrapings, or characteristic histologic nerve changes.

General Considerations

Leprosy (Hansen disease) is a chronic infectious disease caused by the acid-fast rod *M leprae*. The mode of transmission probably is respiratory and involves prolonged exposure in childhood. The disease is endemic in tropical and subtropical Asia, Africa, Central and South America, and the Pacific regions, and rarely seen sporadically in the southern United States.

Clinical Findings

A. Symptoms and Signs

The onset is insidious. The lesions involve the cooler body tissues: skin, superficial nerves, nose, pharynx, larynx, eyes, and testicles. Skin lesions may occur as pale, anesthetic macular lesions 1–10 cm in diameter; discrete erythematous, infiltrated nodules 1–5 cm in diameter; or diffuse skin infiltration. Neurologic disturbances are caused by nerve infiltration and thickening, with resultant anesthesia, and motor abnormalities. Bilateral ulnar neuropathy is highly suggestive. In untreated cases, disfigurement due to the skin infiltration and nerve involvement may be extreme, leading to trophic ulcers, bone resorption, and loss of digits.

The disease is divided clinically and by laboratory tests into two distinct types: lepromatous and tuberculoid. The **lepromatous** type (also referred to as multibacillary leprosy) occurs in persons with defective cellular immunity. The course is progressive and malignant, with nodular skin lesions; slow, symmetric nerve involvement; abundant acid-fast bacilli in the skin lesions; and a negative lepromin skin test. In the **tuberculoid** type (paucibacillary leprosy), cellular immunity is intact and the course is more benign and less progressive, with macular skin lesions, severe asymmetric nerve involvement of sudden onset with few bacilli present in the lesions, and a positive lepromin skin test. Intermediate ("borderline") cases are frequent. Eye involvement (keratitis and iridocyclitis), nasal ulcers, epistaxis, anemia, and lymphadenopathy may occur.

B. Laboratory Findings

Laboratory confirmation of leprosy requires the demonstration of acid-fast bacilli in a skin biopsy. Biopsy of skin or of a thickened involved nerve also gives a typical histologic picture. *M leprae* does not grow in artificial media but does grow in the foot pads of armadillos.

Differential Diagnosis

The skin lesions of leprosy often resemble those of lupus erythematosus, sarcoidosis, syphilis, erythema nodosum, erythema multiforme, cutaneous tuberculosis, and vitiligo.

Complications

Kidney failure and hepatomegaly from secondary amyloidosis may occur with long-standing disease.

Treatment

Combination therapy is recommended for treatment of all types of leprosy. Single-drug treatment is accompanied by emergence of resistance, and primary resistance to dapsone also occurs. For borderline and lepromatous cases (ie, multibacillary disease), the World Health Organization recommends a triple oral drug-regimen of rifampin, 600 mg once a month; dapsone, 100 mg daily; and clofazimine, 300 mg once a month and 50 mg daily for 12 months although longer courses may be needed for patients with high burden of disease. For indeterminate and tuberculoid leprosy (paucibacillary disease), the recommendation is rifampin, 600 mg once a month, plus dapsone, 100 mg daily for 6 months.

Two reactional states—erythema nodosum leprosum and reversal reactions—may occur as a consequence of therapy. The reversal reaction, typical of borderline lepromatous leprosy, probably results from enhanced host immunity. Skin lesions and nerves become swollen and tender, but systemic manifestations are not seen. Erythema nodosum leprosum, typical of lepromatous leprosy, is a consequence of immune injury from antigen-antibody complex deposition in skin and other tissues; in addition to skin and nerve manifestations, fever and systemic involvement may be seen. Prednisone, 60 mg/day orally, or thalidomide, 300 mg/day orally (in the nonpregnant patient only), is effective for erythema nodosum leprosum. Improvement is expected within a few days after initiating prednisone, and thereafter the dose may be tapered over several weeks to avoid recurrence. Thalidomide is also tapered over several weeks to a 100-mg bedtime dose. Erythema nodosum leprosum is usually confined to the first year of therapy, and prednisone or thalidomide can be discontinued. Thalidomide is ineffective for reversal reactions, and prednisone, 60 mg/d, is indicated. Reversal reactions tend to recur, and the dose of prednisone should be slowly tapered over weeks to months. Therapy for leprosy should not be discontinued during treatment of reactional states.

Kamath S et al. Recognizing and managing the immunologic reactions in leprosy. J Am Acad Dermatol. 2014 Oct;71(4): 795–803. [PMID: 24767732]

Nolen L et al; Centers for Disease Control and Prevention (CDC). Incidence of Hansen's disease—United States, 1994–2011. MMWR Morb Mortal Wkly Rep. 2014 Oct 31; 63(43):969–72. [PMID: 25356604]

INFECTIONS CAUSED BY CHLAMYDIAE

Chlamydiaceae is a family of obligate intracellular parasites closely related to gram-negative bacteria. They include two important genera of human pathogens—*Chlamydia*, which includes the species of *Chlamydia trachomatis*, and *Chlamydophila*, which includes the species *Chlamydophila psittaci* (formerly known as *Chlamydia psittaci*) and *Chlamydophila pneumoniae* (formerly known as *Chlamydia pneumoniae*). The differentiation of genera is based on differences in intracellular inclusions, sulfonamide susceptibility, antigenic composition, and disease production. *C trachomatis* causes many different human infections involving the eye (trachoma, inclusion conjunctivitis), the genital tract (lymphogranuloma venereum, nongonococcal urethritis, cervicitis, salpingitis), or the respiratory tract in infants (pneumonitis). *C psittaci* causes psittacosis and *C pneumoniae* is a cause of respiratory tract infections.

CHLAMYDIA TRACHOMATIS INFECTIONS

1. Lymphogranuloma Venereum

ESSENTIALS OF DIAGNOSIS

▸ Evanescent primary genital lesion.

▸ Lymph node enlargement, softening, and suppuration, with draining sinuses.

▸ Proctitis and rectal stricture in women or in men who have sex with men.

▸ Positive complement fixation test.

General Considerations

Lymphogranuloma venereum (LGV) is an acute and chronic sexually transmitted disease caused by *C trachomatis* types L1–L3. The disease is acquired during intercourse or through contact with contaminated exudate from active lesions. The incubation period is 5–21 days. After the genital lesion disappears, the infection spreads to lymph channels and lymph nodes of the genital and rectal areas. Inapparent infections and latent disease are not uncommon.

Clinical Findings

A. Symptoms and Signs

In men, the initial vesicular or ulcerative lesion (on the external genitalia) is evanescent and often goes unnoticed. Inguinal buboes appear 1–4 weeks after exposure, are often bilateral, and have a tendency to fuse, soften, and break down to form multiple draining sinuses, with extensive scarring. In women, the genital lymph drainage is to the perirectal glands. Early anorectal manifestations are proctitis with tenesmus and bloody purulent discharge; late manifestations are chronic cicatrizing inflammation of the rectal and perirectal tissue. These changes lead to obstipation and rectal stricture and, occasionally, rectovaginal and perianal fistulas. They are also seen in homosexual men.

B. Laboratory Findings

The complement fixation test may be positive (titers greater than 1:64), but cross-reaction with other chlamydiae occurs. Although a positive reaction may reflect remote infection, high titers usually indicate active disease. Nucleic acid detection tests are sensitive, but not FDA-approved for rectal specimens and cannot differentiate LGV from non-LGV strains.

Differential Diagnosis

The early lesion of LGV must be differentiated from the lesions of syphilis, genital herpes, and chancroid; lymph node involvement must be distinguished from that due to tularemia, tuberculosis, plague, neoplasm, or pyogenic infection; and rectal stricture must be distinguished from that due to neoplasm and ulcerative colitis.

Treatment

If diagnostic testing for LGV is not available, patients with a clinical presentation suggestive of LGV should be treated empirically. The antibiotic of choice is doxycycline (contraindicated in pregnancy), 100 mg orally twice daily for 21 days. Erythromycin, 500 mg orally four times a day for 21 days, is also effective. Azithromycin, 1 g orally once weekly for 3 weeks, may also be effective.

de Vries HJ et al. 2013 European guideline on the management of lymphogranuloma venereum. J Eur Acad Dermatol Venereol. 2015 Jan;29(1):1–6. [PMID: 24661352]

Workowski KA et al; Centers for Disease Control and Prevention. Sexually transmitted diseases treatment guidelines, 2015. MMWR Recomm Rep. 2015 Jun 5;64(RR-03):1–137. Erratum in: MMWR Recomm Rep. 2015 Aug 28;64(33):924. [PMID: 26042815]

2. Chlamydial Urethritis & Cervicitis

ESSENTIALS OF DIAGNOSIS

▶ *C. trachomatis* is a common cause of urethritis, cervicitis, and post-gonococcal urethritis.

▶ Diagnosis made by nucleic acid amplification of urine or swab specimen.

General Considerations

C trachomatis immunotypes D–K are isolated in about 50% of cases of nongonococcal urethritis and cervicitis. In other cases, *Ureaplasma urealyticum* or *Mycoplasma genitalium* can be grown as a possible etiologic agent. *C trachomatis* is an important cause of postgonococcal urethritis. Coinfection with gonococci and chlamydiae is common, and postgonococcal (ie, chlamydial) urethritis may persist after successful treatment of the gonococcal component. Occasionally, epididymitis, prostatitis, or proctitis is caused by chlamydial infection. Chlamydiae are a leading cause of infertility in females in the United States.

Clinical Findings

A. Symptoms and Signs

Females infected with chlamydiae may be asymptomatic or may have symptoms and signs of cervicitis, salpingitis, or pelvic inflammatory disease. The urethral or cervical discharge due to *C trachomatis* tends to be less painful, less purulent, and watery compared with gonococcal infection.

B. Laboratory Findings

A patient with urethritis or cervicitis and absence of gram-negative diplococci on Gram stain and of *N gonorrhoeae* on culture is assumed to have chlamydial infection until proven otherwise. The diagnosis should be confirmed, whenever possible, by the FDA-approved, highly sensitive nucleic acid amplification tests for use with urine or vaginal swabs. A negative nucleic acid amplification test for chlamydia reliably excludes the diagnosis of chlamydial urethritis or cervicitis and therapy need not be administered.

C. Screening

Active screening for chlamydial infection is recommended in certain settings: pregnant women; all sexually active women 25 years of age and under; older women with risk factors for sexually transmitted diseases; and men with risk factors for sexually transmitted diseases, such as HIV-positive men or men who have sex with men.

Treatment

Recommended regimens are a single oral 1-g dose of azithromycin (preferred and safe in pregnancy), 100 mg of doxycycline orally for 7 days (contraindicated in pregnancy), or 500 mg of levofloxacin once daily for 7 days

(also contraindicated in pregnancy). Presumptively administered therapy still may be indicated for some patients (such as for an individual with gonococcal infection in whom no chlamydial testing was performed or a test other than a nucleic acid amplification test was used to exclude the diagnosis, or an individual for whom a test result is pending but is considered unlikely to follow up, and for sexual contacts of documented cases). As for all patients in whom sexually transmitted diseases are diagnosed, studies for HIV and syphilis should also be performed.

Geisler WM et al. Azithromycin versus doxycycline for urogenital *Chlamydia trachomatis* infection. N Engl J Med. 2015 Dec 24; 373(26):2512–21. [PMID: 26699167]

Workowski KA et al; Centers for Disease Control and Prevention. Sexually transmitted diseases treatment guidelines, 2015. MMWR Recomm Rep. 2015 Jun 5;64(RR-03):1–137. Erratum in: MMWR Recomm Rep. 2015 Aug 28;64(33):924. [PMID: 26042815]

CHLAMYDOPHILA PSITTACI & PSITTACOSIS (Ornithosis)

ESSENTIALS OF DIAGNOSIS

▶ Fever, chills, and cough; headache common.

▶ Atypical pneumonia with slightly delayed appearance of signs of pneumonitis.

▶ Contact with infected bird (psittacine, pigeons, many others) 7–15 days previously.

▶ Isolation of chlamydiae or rising titer of complement-fixing antibodies.

General Considerations

Psittacosis is acquired from contact with birds (parrots, parakeets, pigeons, chickens, ducks, and many others), which may or may not be ill. The history may be difficult to obtain if the patient acquired infection from an illegally imported bird.

Clinical Findings

The onset is usually rapid, with fever, chills, myalgia, dry cough, and headache. Signs include temperature-pulse dissociation, dullness to percussion, and rales. Pulmonary findings may be absent early. Dyspnea and cyanosis may occur later. Endocarditis, which is culture-negative, may occur. The radiographic findings in typical psittacosis are those of atypical pneumonia, which tends to be interstitial and diffuse in appearance, though consolidation can occur. Psittacosis is indistinguishable from other bacterial or viral pneumonias by radiography.

The organism is rarely isolated from cultures. The diagnosis is usually made serologically; antibodies appear during the second week and can be demonstrated by complement fixation or immunofluorescence. Antibody response may be suppressed by early chemotherapy.

Differential Diagnosis

The illness is indistinguishable from viral, mycoplasmal, or other atypical pneumonias except for the history of contact with birds. Psittacosis is in the differential diagnosis of culture-negative endocarditis.

Treatment

Treatment consists of giving tetracycline, 0.5 g orally every 6 hours or 0.5 g intravenously every 12 hours, for 14–21 days. Erythromycin, 500 mg orally every 6 hours, may be effective as well.

Lagae S et al. Emerging *Chlamydia psittaci* infections in chickens and examination of transmission to humans. J Med Microbiol. 2014 Mar;63(Pt 3):399–407. [PMID: 24324029]

CHLAMYDOPHILA PNEUMONIAE INFECTION

C pneumoniae causes pneumonia and bronchitis. The clinical presentation of pneumonia is that of an atypical pneumonia. The organism accounts for approximately 10% of community-acquired pneumonias, ranking second to mycoplasma as an agent of atypical pneumonia. A putative role in coronary artery disease has not held up to close scientific scrutiny.

Like *C psittaci*, strains of *C pneumoniae* are resistant to sulfonamides. Erythromycin or tetracycline, 500 mg orally four times a day for 10–14 days, appears to be effective therapy. Fluoroquinolones, such as levofloxacin (500 mg once daily for 7–14 days) or moxifloxacin (400 mg once daily for 7–14 days), are active in vitro against *C pneumoniae* and probably are effective. It is unclear if empiric coverage for atypical pathogens in hospitalized patients with community-acquired pneumonia provides a survival benefit or improves clinical outcome.

Choroszy-Król I et al. Infections caused by *Chlamydophila pneumoniae*. Adv Clin Exp Med. 2014 Jan–Feb;23(1):123–6. [PMID: 24596014]

Fajardo KA et al. Pneumonia outbreak caused by *Chlamydophila pneumoniae* among US Air Force Academy cadets, Colorado, USA. Emerg Infect Dis. 2015 Jun;21(6):1049–51. [PMID: 25988545]

Spirochetal Infections

Susan S. Philip, MD, MPH

SYPHILIS

NATURAL HISTORY & PRINCIPLES OF DIAGNOSIS & TREATMENT

Syphilis is a complex infectious disease caused by *Treponema pallidum*, a spirochete capable of infecting almost any organ or tissue in the body and causing protean clinical manifestations (Table 34–1). Transmission occurs most frequently during sexual contact (including oral sex); sites of inoculation are usually genital but may be extragenital. The risk of acquiring syphilis after unprotected sex with an individual with infectious syphilis is approximately 30–50%. Rarely, it can also be transmitted through nonsexual contact, blood transfusion, or via the placenta from mother to fetus (congenital syphilis).

The natural history of acquired syphilis is generally divided into two major stages: **early (infectious) syphilis** and **late syphilis**. Between these stages is a symptom-free latent phase. In **early latent syphilis**, which is defined as the symptom-free interval lasting up to 1 year after initial infection, infectious lesions can recur. Infectious syphilis includes primary lesions (chancre and regional lymphadenopathy) appearing during **primary syphilis,** secondary lesions (commonly involving skin and mucous membranes, occasionally bone, central nervous system [CNS], or liver) appearing during **secondary syphilis,** relapsing lesions during early latency, and congenital lesions. The hallmark of these lesions is an abundance of spirochetes; tissue reaction is usually minimal. Late syphilis consists of so-called benign (gummatous) lesions involving skin, bones, and viscera; cardiovascular disease (principally aortitis); and a variety of CNS and ocular syndromes. These forms of syphilis are not contagious. The lesions contain few demonstrable spirochetes, but tissue reactivity (vasculitis, necrosis) is severe and suggestive of hypersensitivity phenomena.

Public health efforts to control syphilis focus on the diagnosis and treatment of early (infectious) cases and their partners.

Most cases of syphilis in the United States continue to occur in men who have sex with men (MSM). Globally, the World Health Organization (WHO) estimates 6 million total incident syphilis infections in 2012, equally in both men and women, and a prevalence of 1% among pregnant women attending antenatal clinics. Preventing congenital syphilis is a major public health goal for the Centers for Disease Control (CDC) and WHO.

COURSE & PROGNOSIS

The lesions associated with primary and secondary syphilis are self-limiting, even without treatment, and resolve with few or no residua. Late syphilis may be highly destructive and permanently disabling and may lead to death. Many experts now believe that while infection is almost never completely eradicated in the absence of treatment, most infections remain latent without sequelae, and only a small number of latent infections progress to further disease.

CLINICAL STAGES OF SYPHILIS

1. Primary Syphilis

 ESSENTIALS OF DIAGNOSIS

▶ History of sexual contact (may be unreliable).

▶ Painless ulcer on genitalia, perianal area, rectum, pharynx, tongue, lip, or elsewhere.

▶ Nontender enlargement of regional lymph nodes.

▶ Fluid expressed from lesion contains *T pallidum* by immunofluorescence or darkfield microscopy.

▶ Serologic nontreponemal and treponemal tests.

▶ Clinical Findings

A. Symptoms and Signs

This is the stage of invasion and may pass unrecognized. The typical lesion is the **chancre** at the site or sites of inoculation, most frequently located on the penis (Figure 34–1), labia, cervix, or anorectal region. Anorectal lesions are especially common among MSM. Chancres also occur occasionally in the oropharynx (lip, tongue, or tonsil) and

Table 34–1. Stages of syphilis and common clinical manifestations.

Primary syphilis
Chancre: painless ulcer with clean base and firm indurated borders
Regional lymphadenopathy

Secondary syphilis
Skin and mucous membranes
Rash: diffuse (may include palms and soles), macular, papular, pustular, and combinations
Condylomata lata
Mucous patches: painless, silvery ulcerations of mucous membrane with surrounding erythema
Generalized lymphadenopathy
Constitutional symptoms
Fever, usually low-grade
Malaise
Anorexia
Arthralgias and myalgias
Central nervous system
Asymptomatic
Symptomatic
Headache
Meningitis
Cranial neuropathies (II–VIII)
Ocular
Iritis
Iridocyclitis
Other
Renal: glomerulonephritis, nephrotic syndrome
Liver: hepatitis
Bone and joint: arthritis, periostitis

Late syphilis
Late benign (gummatous): granulomatous lesion usually involving skin, mucous membranes, and bones but any organ can be involved
Cardiovascular
Aortic regurgitation
Coronary ostial stenosis
Aortic aneurysm
Neurosyphilis
Asymptomatic
Meningovascular
Seizures
Hemiparesis or hemiplegia
Tabes dorsalis
Impaired proprioception and vibratory sensation
Argyll Robertson pupil
Shooting pains
Ataxia
Romberg sign
Urinary and fecal incontinence
Charcot joint
Cranial neuropathies (II–VIII)
General paresis
Personality changes Hyperactive reflexes
Argyll Robertson pupil
Decreased memory
Slurred speech
Optic atrophy

Note: Central nervous system involvement may occur at any stage.

▲ **Figure 34–1.** Primary syphilis with a large chancre on the glans of the penis. (Used with permission from Joseph Engelman, MD; San Francisco City Clinic.)

rarely on the breast or finger or elsewhere. An initial small erosion appears 10–90 days (average, 3–4 weeks) after inoculation then rapidly develops into a painless superficial ulcer with a clean base and firm, indurated margins. This is associated with enlargement of regional lymph nodes, which are rubbery, discrete, and nontender. Bacterial infection of the chancre may occur and may lead to pain. Healing occurs without treatment, but a scar may form, especially with secondary bacterial infection. Multiple chancres may be present, particularly in HIV-positive patients. Although the "classic" ulcer of syphilis has been described as nontender, nonpurulent, and indurated, only 31% of patients have this triad.

B. Laboratory Findings

1. Microscopic examination—In early (infectious) syphilis, darkfield microscopic examination by a skilled observer of fresh exudate from moist lesions or material aspirated from regional lymph nodes is up to 90% sensitive for diagnosis but is usually only available in select clinics that specialize in sexually transmitted disease.

An immunofluorescent staining technique for demonstrating *T pallidum* in dried smears of fluid taken from early syphilitic lesions is available through some laboratories but is not widely available.

Polymerase chain reaction (PCR) testing is not yet commercially available in the United States but has many advantages as a tool for direct detection, including high sensitivity and ability to use a wide range of clinical specimen types.

2. Serologic tests for syphilis—(Table 34–2.) Serologic tests (the mainstay of syphilis diagnosis) fall into two general categories: (1) Nontreponemal tests detect antibodies to lipoidal antigens present in the host after modification by *T pallidum*. (2) Treponemal tests use live or killed *T pallidum* as antigen to detect antibodies specific for pathogenic treponemes.

A. NONTREPONEMAL ANTIGEN TESTS—The most commonly used nontreponemal antigen tests are the Venereal Disease Research Laboratory (VDRL) and rapid plasma

Table 34–2. Percentage of patients with positive serologic tests for syphilis.[1]

Test	Stage		
	Primary	Secondary	Tertiary
VDRL or RPR	75–85%	99–100%	40–95%
FTA-ABS, TPPA, or MHA-TP	69–100%	100%	94–98%
IgG EIA	100%	100%	NA
CIA	98%	100%	100%

[1]Based on untreated cases.
CIA, chemiluminescence assay; EIA, enzyme immunoassay; FTA-ABS, fluorescent treponemal antibody absorption assay; MHA-TP, microhemagglutination assay for *T pallidum*; RPR, rapid plasma reagin test; TPPA, *T pallidum* particle agglutination; VDRL, Venereal Disease Research Laboratory test.

reagin (RPR) tests, which measure the ability of heated serum to flocculate a suspension of cardiolipin–cholesterol–lecithin. The flocculation tests are inexpensive, rapid, and easy to perform and have therefore been commonly used for routine screening. Quantitative expression of the reactivity of the serum, based on titration of dilutions of serum, is valuable in establishing the diagnosis and in evaluating the efficacy of treatment, since **titers usually correlate with disease activity**. A different, enzyme immunoassay (EIA)-based screening algorithm is discussed below.

Nontreponemal tests generally become positive 4–6 weeks after infection or 1–3 weeks after the appearance of a primary lesion; they are almost invariably positive in the secondary stage, with titers 1:16 or higher. These serologic tests are not specific and must be confirmed with treponemal-specific tests and closely correlated with other clinical and laboratory findings. The tests are positive in patients with non–sexually transmitted treponematoses (see below). More important, false-positive serologic reactions are frequently encountered in a wide variety of other conditions, including connective tissue diseases, infectious mononucleosis, malaria, febrile diseases, leprosy, injection drug use, infective endocarditis, old age, hepatitis C viral infection, and pregnancy. False-positive reactions are usually of low titer and transient and may be distinguished from true positives by performing a treponemal specific-antibody test. False-negative results can be seen when very high antibody titers are present (**the prozone phenomenon**). If syphilis is strongly suspected and the nontreponemal test is negative, the laboratory should be instructed to dilute the specimen to detect a positive reaction. The RPR and VDRL tests are equally reliable, but RPR titers tend to be higher than the VDRL. Thus, when these tests are used to follow disease activity, the same testing method should be used and preferably performed at the same laboratory.

Nontreponemal antibody titers are used to assess adequacy of therapy. The rate of the VDRL or RPR decline depends on various factors. In general, persons with repeat infections, higher initial titers, more advanced stages of

disease, or those who are HIV-infected at the time of treatment have a slower seroconversion rate and are more likely to remain serofast (ie, titers decline but do not become nonreactive). Data based on recommended treatment regimens suggest that in primary and secondary syphilis it may take 6–12 months to see a fourfold decrease in titer.

B. TREPONEMAL ANTIBODY TESTS—These tests measure antibodies capable of reacting with *T pallidum* antigens. The *T pallidum* hemagglutination (TPHA) test and the *T pallidum* particle agglutination (TPPA) test are comparable in specificity and sensitivity to the fluorescent treponemal antibody absorption test (FTA-ABS). The TPPA test, because of ease of performance, has supplanted the FTA-ABS test as the means of confirming the diagnosis of syphilis following a positive nontreponemal test. Newer treponemal tests used in reverse screening algorithms include EIA and chemiluminescence assay (CIA).

In traditional screening, the treponemal tests are used to determine whether a positive nontreponemal antigen test is a false-positive result (see above) or is indicative of syphilis. Because of their great sensitivity, particularly in the late stages of the disease, these tests are also of value when there is clinical evidence of syphilis but the nontreponemal serologic test for syphilis is negative. Treponemal tests are reactive in many patients with primary syphilis and in almost all patients with secondary syphilis (Table 34–2). Although a reactive treponemal-specific serologic test remains reactive throughout a patient's life in most cases, it may (like nontreponemal antibody tests) revert to negative with adequate therapy. Final decisions about the significance of the results of serologic tests for syphilis must be based on a total clinical appraisal and may require expert consultation.

C. ENZYME IMMUNOASSAY (EIA)-OR CHEMILUMINESCENCE IMMUNOASSAY (CIA)-BASED SCREENING ALGORITHMS—Newer screening algorithms reverse the traditional test order and begin with an automated treponemal antibody test, (eg, EIA or CIA) and then follow up with a nontreponemal test (RPR or VDRL) if the treponemal test is positive. This algorithm is faster and decreases labor costs to laboratories when compared with traditional screening. Compared with traditional treponemal-specific tests, the EIAs have sensitivities of 95–100% and specificities of 99–100%.

The reverse algorithms can cause challenges in clinical management. A positive treponemal test with a negative RPR or VDRL may represent prior, treated syphilis; untreated latent syphilis; or a false-positive treponemal test. Such results should be evaluated with a second treponemal test as a "tie-breaker," but interpretation of discordant results is not yet fully standardized and a clinician may benefit from an expert opinion. Reverse algorithms are recommended by several international organizations including the International Union against Sexually Transmitted Infections (IUSTI), but the CDC still recommend the traditional algorithm.

D. RAPID TREPONEMAL TESTS—A single rapid point of care treponemal test is approved for use in the United States, including in outreach and other nonlaboratory settings. Other tests are available internationally and are commonly used in limited-resource settings. Sensitivity ranges from 62% to 100% and specificity from 83% to 95%.

3. Polymerase chain reaction—PCR has been increasingly evaluated and utilized worldwide for the diagnosis of genital ulcer disease, including syphilis, but these tests are not yet commercially available in the United States.

4. Cerebrospinal fluid examination—See Neurosyphilis section.

▶ Differential Diagnosis

The syphilitic chancre may be confused with genital herpes, chancroid (usually painful and uncommon in the United States), lymphogranuloma venereum, or neoplasm. **Any genital ulcer should be considered a possible primary syphilitic lesion.** Simultaneous evaluation for herpes simplex virus types 1 and 2 using PCR or culture should also be done in these cases.

▶ Prevention & Screening

Avoidance of sexual contact is the only completely reliable method of prevention but is an impractical public health measure. Latex or polyurethane condoms are effective but protect covered areas only. Men who have sex with men should be screened every 6–12 months, and as often as every 3 months in high-risk individuals (those who have multiple encounters with anonymous partners or who have sex in conjunction with the use of drugs). Pregnant women should be screened at the first prenatal visit and again in the third trimester; a third screen at delivery should be performed if there are risk indicators, including poverty, sex work, illicit drug use, history of other sexually transmitted diseases, and residing in a community with high syphilis morbidity. Patients treated for other sexually transmitted diseases should also be tested for syphilis, and persons who have known or suspected sexual contact with patients who have syphilis should be evaluated and presumptively treated to abort development of infectious syphilis (see Treating Syphilis Contacts below).

▶ Treatment

A. Antibiotic Therapy

Penicillin remains the preferred treatment for syphilis, since there have been no documented cases of penicillin-resistant *T pallidum* (Table 34–3). In pregnant women,

Table 34–3. Recommended treatment for syphilis.[1]

Stage of Syphilis	Treatment	Alternative[2]	Comment
Early			
Primary, secondary, or early latent	Benzathine penicillin G 2.4 million units intramuscularly once	Doxycycline 100 mg orally twice daily for 14 days or Tetracycline 500 mg orally four times daily for 14 days or Ceftriaxone 1 g intramuscularly or intravenously daily for 8–10 days[3]	
Late			
Late latent or uncertain duration	Benzathine penicillin G 2.4 million units intramuscularly weekly for 3 weeks	Doxycycline 100 mg orally twice daily for 28 days or Tetracycline 500 mg orally four times a day for 28 days	No routine cerebrospinal fluid evaluation unless neurologic, otologic or ocular abnormalities
Tertiary without neurosyphilis	Benzathine penicillin G 2.4 million units intramuscularly weekly for 3 weeks	Doxycycline 100 mg orally twice daily for 28 days or Tetracycline 500 mg orally four times a day for 28 days	Cerebrospinal fluid evaluation recommended in all patients
Neurosyphilis	Aqueous penicillin G 18–24 million units intravenously daily, given every 3–4 hours or as continuous infusion for 10–14 days	Procaine penicillin, 2.4 million units intramuscularly daily with probenecid 500 mg orally four times a day for 10–14 days or Ceftriaxone 2 g intramuscularly or intravenously daily for 10–14 days	Follow treatment with benzathine penicillin G 2.4 million units intramuscularly weekly for up to 3 weeks

[1]Penicillin is the only documented effective treatment in pregnancy, so pregnant patients with true allergy should be desensitized and treated with penicillin according to stage of disease as above.
[2]Patients treated with alternative therapies require close clinical and serologic monitoring.
[3]Fewer data for ceftriaxone treatment, optimal dose or duration not known.

penicillin is the only option because it reliably treats the fetus (see below).

There are some alternatives to penicillin for nonpregnant patients, including doxycycline. There are also limited data for ceftriaxone, although optimum dose and duration are not well defined. Azithromycin has been shown to be effective but should be used with caution; it should not be used at all in MSM due to demonstrated resistance. All patients treated with a non-penicillin regimen must have particularly close clinical and serologic follow up.

B. Managing Jarisch–Herxheimer Reaction

The Jarisch–Herxheimer reaction, manifested by fever and aggravation of the existing clinical picture in the hours following treatment, is ascribed to the sudden massive destruction of spirochetes and is not an IgE-mediated allergic reaction. It is most common in early syphilis, particularly secondary syphilis where it can occur in 66% of cases.

The reaction may be blunted by simultaneous administration of antipyretics, although no proven method of prevention exists. In cases with increased risk of morbidity due to the Jarisch–Herxheimer reaction (including CNS or cardiac involvement and pregnancy), consultation with an infectious disease expert is recommended. Patients should be reminded that the reaction does not signify an allergy to penicillin.

C. Local Measures (Mucocutaneous Lesions)

Local treatment is usually not necessary. No local antiseptics or other chemicals should be applied to a suspected syphilitic lesion until specimens for microscopy have been obtained.

D. Public Health Measures

Patients with infectious syphilis must abstain from sexual activity for 7–10 days after treatment. **All cases of syphilis must be reported to the appropriate local public health agency in order to identify and treat sexual contacts.** In addition, **all patients with syphilis should have an HIV test at the time of diagnosis.** In areas of high HIV prevalence, a repeat HIV test should be performed in 3 months if the initial test result was negative.

E. Treating Syphilis Contacts

Patients who have been sexually exposed to infectious syphilis within the preceding 3 months may be infected but seronegative and thus should be treated as for early syphilis even if serologic tests are negative. Persons exposed more than 3 months previously should be treated based on serologic results; however, if the patient is unreliable for follow-up, empiric therapy is indicated.

▶ Follow-Up Care

Because treatment failures and reinfection may occur, patients treated for syphilis should be monitored clinically and serologically every 6 months. **In primary and secondary syphilis, failure of nontreponemal antibody titers to**

decrease fourfold by 6–12 months may identify a group at high risk for treatment failure. Optimal management of these patients is unclear, but at a minimum, close clinical and serologic follow-up is indicated. In HIV-uninfected patients, an HIV test should be repeated (all patients with syphilis should have an HIV test at the time of diagnosis); a thorough neurologic history and examination should be performed and lumbar puncture considered since unrecognized neurosyphilis can be a cause of treatment failure; and, if careful follow-up cannot be ensured (3-month intervals for HIV-positive individuals and 6-month intervals for HIV-negative patients), treatment should be repeated with 2.4 million units of benzathine penicillin G intramuscularly weekly for 3 weeks. If symptoms or signs persist or recur after initial therapy or there is a fourfold or greater increase in nontreponemal titers, the patient has been reinfected (more likely) or the therapy failed (if a non-penicillin regimen was used). In those individuals, an HIV test should be performed, a lumbar puncture done (unless reinfection is a certainty), and re-treatment given as indicated above.

2. Secondary Syphilis

🧩 ESSENTIALS OF DIAGNOSIS

▶ Generalized maculopapular skin rash.

▶ Mucous membrane lesions, including patches and ulcers.

▶ Weeping papules (condyloma lata) in moist skin areas.

▶ Generalized nontender lymphadenopathy.

▶ Fever may be present.

▶ Meningitis, hepatitis, osteitis, arthritis, iritis may be present.

▶ Many treponemes in moist lesions by immunofluorescence or darkfield microscopy.

▶ Positive serologic tests for syphilis.

▶ Clinical Findings

The secondary stage of syphilis usually appears a few weeks (or up to 6 months) after development of the chancre, when **dissemination of *T pallidum* produces systemic signs (fever, lymphadenopathy) or infectious lesions at sites distant from the site of inoculation.** The most common manifestations are skin and mucosal lesions. The skin lesions are nonpruritic, macular, papular, pustular, or follicular (or combinations of any of these types, but generally *not* vesicular) and generalized; involvement of the palms and soles (Figure 34–2) occurs in 80% of cases. Annular lesions simulating ringworm may be observed in dark-skinned individuals. Mucous membrane lesions may include mucous patches (Figure 34–3), which can be found on the lips, mouth, throat, genitalia, and anus. Specific lesions—**condylomata lata**

▲ **Figure 34–2.** Secondary syphilis lesions on the soles of the feet. (From Dr. Gavin Hart, Public Health Image Library, CDC.)

▲ **Figure 34–4.** Secondary syphilis perianal condylomata lata. (Used with permission from Joseph Engelman, MD; San Francisco City Clinic.)

(Figure 34–4)—are fused, weeping papules on the moist areas of the skin and mucous membranes and are sometimes mistaken for genital warts. The mucous membrane lesions are highly infectious.

Meningeal (aseptic meningitis or acute basilar meningitis), hepatic, renal, bone, and joint invasion may occur, with resulting cranial nerve palsies, jaundice, nephrotic syndrome, and periostitis. Alopecia (moth-eaten appearance) and uveitis may also occur.

The serologic tests for syphilis are positive in almost all cases (see Primary Syphilis). The moist cutaneous and mucous membrane lesions often show *T pallidum* on dark-field microscopic examination. A transient cerebrospinal fluid (CSF) pleocytosis is seen in 40% of patients with secondary syphilis. There may be evidence of hepatitis or nephritis (immune complex type) as circulating immune complexes are deposited in blood vessel walls.

Skin lesions may be confused with the infectious exanthems, pityriasis rosea, and drug eruptions (Figure 34–5). Visceral lesions may suggest nephritis or hepatitis due to other causes.

► **Treatment**

Treatment is as for primary syphilis unless CNS or ocular disease is present, in which case a lumbar puncture should be performed and, if positive, treatment for neurosyphilis

▲ **Figure 34–5.** Secondary syphilis rash of the buttocks and legs. (From J. Pledger, BSS/VD, Public Health Image Library, CDC.)

▲ **Figure 34–3.** Secondary syphilis mucous patch of the tongue. (Used with permission from Kenneth Katz, MD, MSc, MSCE.)

given (Table 34–3). See Primary Syphilis for follow-up care and treatment of contacts.

3. Latent Syphilis

ESSENTIALS OF DIAGNOSIS

▶ Early latent syphilis: infection less than 1 year in duration.

▶ Late latent syphilis: infection more than 1 year in duration.

▶ No physical signs.

▶ History of syphilis with inadequate treatment.

▶ Positive serologic tests for syphilis.

▶ General Considerations

Latent syphilis is the clinically quiescent phase in the absence of primary or secondary lesions. **Early latent syphilis** is defined as the first year after primary infection and may relapse to secondary syphilis if undiagnosed or inadequately treated (see above). Relapse is almost always accompanied by a rising titer in quantitative serologic tests; indeed, a rising titer may be the first or only evidence of relapse. About 90% of relapses occur during the first year after infection.

Early latent infection can be diagnosed if there was documented seroconversion or a fourfold increase in non-treponemal titers in the past 12 months; the patient can recall symptoms of primary or secondary syphilis; or the patient had a sex partner with documented primary, secondary, or early latent syphilis.

After the first year of latent syphilis, the patient is said to be in the **late latent stage** and noninfectious to sex partners. Transmission to the fetus, however, can probably occur in any phase. There are (by definition) no clinical manifestations during the latent stage, and the only significant laboratory findings are positive serologic tests. A diagnosis of late latent syphilis is justified only when the history and physical examination show no evidence of tertiary disease or neurosyphilis. The latent stage may last from months to a lifetime.

▶ Treatment

Treatment of **early latent syphilis** and follow-up is as for primary syphilis unless CNS disease is present (Table 34–3). Treatment of **late latent syphilis** is shown in Table 34–3. The treatment of this stage of the disease is intended to prevent late sequelae. If there is evidence of CNS involvement, a lumbar puncture should be performed and, if positive, the patient should receive treatment for neurosyphilis. Titers may not decline as rapidly following treatment compared to early syphilis. Nontreponemal serologic tests should be repeated at 6, 12, and 24 months. If titers increase fourfold or if initially high titers (1:32 or higher) fail to decrease fourfold by 12–24 months or if symptoms or signs consistent with syphilis develop, an HIV test

should be repeated in HIV-uninfected patients, lumbar puncture should be performed, and re-treatment given according to the stage of the disease.

4. Late (Tertiary) Syphilis

ESSENTIALS OF DIAGNOSIS

▶ Infiltrative tumors of skin, bones, liver (gummas).

▶ Aortitis, aneurysms, aortic regurgitation.

▶ CNS disorders, including meningovascular and degenerative changes, paresthesias, shooting pains, abnormal reflexes, dementia, or psychosis.

▶ General Considerations

This stage may occur at any time after secondary syphilis, even after years of latency, and is rarely seen in developed countries in the modern antibiotic era. Late lesions are thought to represent a delayed hypersensitivity reaction of the tissue to the organism and are usually divided into two types: (1) a localized gummatous reaction, with a relatively rapid onset and generally prompt response to therapy and (2) diffuse inflammation of a more insidious onset that characteristically involves the CNS and large arteries, is often fatal if untreated, and is at best arrested by treatment. **Gummas** may involve any area or organ of the body but most often affect the skin or long bones. Cardiovascular disease is usually manifested by aortic aneurysm, aortic regurgitation, or aortitis. Various forms of diffuse or localized CNS involvement may occur.

Late syphilis must be differentiated from neoplasms of the skin, liver, lung, stomach, or brain; other forms of meningitis; and primary neurologic lesions.

Although almost any tissue and organ may be involved in late syphilis, the following are the most common types of involvement: skin, mucous membranes, skeletal system, eyes, respiratory system, gastrointestinal system, cardiovascular system, and nervous system.

▶ Clinical Findings

A. Symptoms and Signs

1. Skin—Cutaneous lesions of late syphilis are of two varieties: (1) multiple nodular lesions that eventually ulcerate (lues maligna) or resolve by forming atrophic, pigmented scars and (2) solitary gummas that start as painless subcutaneous nodules, then enlarge, attach to the overlying skin, and eventually ulcerate (Figure 34–6).

2. Mucous membranes—Late lesions of the mucous membranes are nodular gummas or leukoplakia, highly destructive to the involved tissue.

3. Skeletal system—Bone lesions are destructive, causing periostitis, osteitis, and arthritis with little or no associated redness or swelling but often marked myalgia and myositis of the neighboring muscles. The pain is especially severe at night.

▲ **Figure 34–6.** Gumma of the nose due to long-standing tertiary syphilis. (From J. Pledger, Public Health Image Library, CDC.)

▲ **Figure 34–7.** Ascending saccular aneurysm of the thoracic aorta in tertiary syphilis. (Public Health Image Library, CDC.)

4. Eyes—Late ocular lesions are gummatous iritis, chorioretinitis, optic atrophy, and cranial nerve palsies, in addition to the lesions of CNS syphilis.

5. Respiratory system—Respiratory involvement by late syphilis is caused by gummatous infiltrates into the larynx, trachea, and pulmonary parenchyma, producing discrete pulmonary densities. There may be hoarseness, respiratory distress, and wheezing secondary to the gummatous lesion itself or to subsequent stenosis occurring with healing.

6. Gastrointestinal system—Gummas involving the liver produce the usually benign, asymptomatic hepar lobatum. A picture resembling Laennec cirrhosis is occasionally produced by liver involvement. Gastric involvement can consist of diffuse infiltration into the stomach wall or focal lesions that endoscopically and microscopically can be confused with lymphoma or carcinoma. Epigastric pain, early satiety, regurgitation, belching, and weight loss are common symptoms.

7. Cardiovascular system—Cardiovascular lesions (10–15% of late syphilitic lesions) are often progressive, disabling, and life-threatening. CNS lesions are often present concomitantly. Involvement usually starts as an arteritis in the supracardiac portion of the aorta and progresses to one or more of the following: (1) narrowing of the coronary ostia, with resulting decreased coronary circulation, angina, and acute myocardial infarction; (2) scarring of the aortic valves, producing aortic regurgitation, and eventually heart failure; and (3) weakness of the wall of the aorta, with saccular aneurysm formation (Figure 34–7) and associated pressure symptoms of dysphagia, hoarseness, brassy cough, back pain (vertebral erosion), and occasionally rupture of the aneurysm. Recurrent respiratory infections are common as a result of pressure on the trachea and bronchi.

8. Nervous system (neurosyphilis)—See next section.

▶ **Treatment**

Treatment of tertiary syphilis (excluding neurosyphilis) is the same as late latent syphilis (Table 34–3); symptoms may not resolve after treatment. Positive serologic tests do not

usually become negative. Viable spirochetes are occasionally found in the eyes, in CSF, and elsewhere in patients with "adequately" treated syphilis, but claims for their capacity to cause progressive disease are speculative.

The pretreatment clinical and laboratory evaluation should include neurologic, ocular, cardiovascular, psychiatric, and CSF examinations. In the presence of definite CSF or neurologic abnormalities, one should treat for neurosyphilis.

5. Neurosyphilis

> ESSENTIALS OF DIAGNOSIS

▶ Can occur at any stage of disease.

▶ Consider both clinical presentation and laboratory data.

▶ Carefully evaluate the neurologic examination in all patients and consider CSF evaluation for atypical symptoms or lack of decrease in nontreponemal serology titers.

▶ **General Considerations**

Neurosyphilis can occur at any stage of disease and can be a progressive, disabling, and life-threatening complication. Asymptomatic CSF abnormalities and meningovascular syphilis occur earlier (months to years after infection, sometimes coexisting with primary and secondary syphilis) than tabes dorsalis and general paresis (2–50 years after infection).

▶ **Clinical Findings**

A. Classification

1. Asymptomatic neuroinvasion—This form has been reported in up to 40% of patients with early syphilis and is characterized by spinal fluid abnormalities (positive spinal fluid serology, increased cell count, occasionally increased protein) without symptoms or signs of neurologic involvement. There are no clear data to support that these asymptomatic CSF abnormalities have clinical significance.

2. Meningovascular syphilis—This form is characterized by meningeal involvement or changes in the vascular structures of the brain (or both), producing symptoms of acute or chronic meningitis (headache, irritability); cranial nerve palsies (basilar meningitis); unequal reflexes; irregular pupils with poor light and accommodation reflexes; and when large vessels are involved, cerebrovascular accidents. The CSF shows increased cells (100–1000/mcL), elevated protein, and may have a positive serologic test (CSF VDRL) for syphilis. The symptoms of acute meningitis are rare in late syphilis.

3. Tabes dorsalis—This form is a chronic progressive degeneration of the parenchyma of the posterior columns of the spinal cord and of the posterior sensory ganglia and nerve roots. The symptoms and signs are impairment of proprioception and vibration sense, **Argyll Robertson pupils** (which react poorly to light but accommodate for near focus), and muscular hypotonia and hyporeflexia. Impaired proprioception results in a wide-based gait and inability to walk in the dark. Paresthesias, analgesia, or sharp recurrent pains in the muscles of the leg ("shooting" or "lightning" pains) may occur. Crises are also common in tabes: gastric crises, consisting of sharp abdominal pains with nausea and vomiting (simulating an acute abdomen); laryngeal crises, with paroxysmal cough and dyspnea; urethral crises, with painful bladder spasms; and rectal and anal crises. Crises may begin suddenly, last for hours to days, and cease abruptly. Neurogenic bladder with overflow incontinence is also seen. Painless trophic ulcers may develop over pressure points on the feet. Joint damage may occur as a result of lack of sensory innervation (Charcot joint, Figure 34–8). The CSF may have a normal or increased cell count, elevated protein, and variable results of serologic tests.

▲ **Figure 34–8.** Neuropathic arthropathy (Charcot joint) from tertiary syphilis. (From Susan Lindsley, Public Health Image Library, CDC.)

4. General paresis—This is generalized involvement of the cerebral cortex with insidious onset of symptoms. There is usually a decrease in concentrating power, memory loss, dysarthria, tremor of the fingers and lips, irritability, and mild headaches. Most striking is the change of personality; the patient may become slovenly, irresponsible, confused, and psychotic. The CSF findings resemble those of tabes dorsalis. Combinations of the various forms of neurosyphilis (especially tabes and paresis) are not uncommon.

B. Laboratory Findings

See Serologic Tests for Syphilis, above; these tests should also be performed in cases of suspected neurosyphilis.

1. Indications for a lumbar puncture—In early syphilis (primary and secondary syphilis and early latent syphilis of less than 1 year's duration), invasion of the CNS by *T pallidum* with CSF abnormalities occurs commonly, but clinical neurosyphilis rarely develops in patients who have received standard therapy. Thus, unless clinical symptoms or signs of neurosyphilis or ophthalmologic involvement (uveitis, neuroretinitis, optic neuritis, iritis) are present, a lumbar puncture in *early syphilis* is not routinely recommended. In *latent syphilis*, routine lumbar puncture is not indicated since the yield is low and findings rarely influence therapeutic decisions. **CSF evaluation is recommended, however, if neurologic or ophthalmologic symptoms or signs are present, if there is evidence of treatment failure (see earlier discussion), or if there is evidence of active tertiary syphilis (eg, aortitis, iritis, optic atrophy, the presence of a gumma).**

2. Spinal fluid examination—CSF findings in neurosyphilis are variable. In "classic" cases, there is an elevation of total protein, lymphocytic pleocytosis, and a positive CSF reagin test (VDRL). The serum nontreponemal titers will be reactive in most cases. In later stages of syphilis, normal CSF analysis in the presence of infection can occur, but it is unusual. False-positive reagin tests rarely occur in the CSF; a positive test confirms the presence of neurosyphilis. Because the CSF VDRL may be negative in 30–70% of cases of neurosyphilis, *a negative test does not exclude neurosyphilis.* The CSF FTA-ABS is sometimes used; it is a highly sensitive test but lacks specificity, and a high serum titer of FTA-ABS may result in a positive CSF titer in the absence of neurosyphilis.

▶ Treatment

Neurosyphilis is treated with high doses of aqueous penicillin to achieve better penetration and higher levels of medication in the CSF than is possible with benzathine penicillin G (Table 34–3). There are limited data for using ceftriaxone to treat neurosyphilis as well, but because other regimens have not been adequately studied, patients with a history of an IgE-mediated reaction to penicillin may require skin testing for allergy to penicillin and, if positive, should be desensitized. Because of concerns about slowly dividing organisms that may persist after completing 10–14 days of therapy with short-acting aqueous penicillin G, many experts recommend subsequent administration of

2.4 million units of the longer-acting benzathine penicillin G intramuscularly once weekly for up to 3 weeks as additional therapy.

All patients treated for neurosyphilis should have nontreponemal serologic tests done every 3–6 months. Guidelines established by the CDC recommend spinal fluid examinations at 6-month intervals until the CSF cell count is normal; however, there are data to suggest that in certain patients normalization of serum titers are an acceptable surrogate for CSF response. In general, CSF white blood cell count and CSF VDRL normalize more quickly (usually in 12 months) than CSF protein concentration, which can remain abnormal for extended periods. If the serum nontreponemal titers do not normalize, the CSF analysis should be repeated. A second course of penicillin therapy may be given if the CSF cell count has not decreased at 6 months or is not normal at 2 years.

6. Syphilis in HIV-Infected Patients

Syphilis is common among HIV-infected individuals. Some data suggest that syphilis coinfection is associated with an increase in HIV viral load and a decrease in CD4 count that normalizes with therapy. Researchers from a prospective cohort study of HIV-infected individuals reported that they found no association with HIV disease progression in persons with syphilis coinfection. However, for optimal patient care as well as prevention of transmission to partners, **guidelines for the primary care of HIV-infected patients recommend routine syphilis screening.**

Interpretation of serologic tests should be the same for HIV-positive and HIV-negative persons. All HIV-positive patients in care should be screened at least annually to identify latent disease because by establishing a serologic history, unnecessary lumbar punctures and prolonged treatment for latent syphilis of uncertain duration can be avoided. If the diagnosis of syphilis is suggested on clinical grounds but reagin tests are negative, alternative tests should be performed. These tests include darkfield examination of lesions and direct fluorescent antibody staining for *T pallidum* of lesion exudate or biopsy specimens.

HIV-positive patients with primary and secondary syphilis should have careful clinical and serologic follow-up at 3, 6, 9, 12, and 24 months. HIV-infected patients with late latent syphilis, syphilis of uncertain duration, and neurosyphilis should be treated like HIV-negative individuals, with follow-up at 6, 12, 18, and 24 months. The use of antiretroviral therapy has been associated with reduced serologic failure rates after syphilis treatment.

The diagnosis of neurosyphilis in HIV-infected patients is complicated by the fact that CSF abnormalities are frequently seen if lumbar puncture is performed. The significance of these abnormalities is unknown, and similar abnormalities are frequently seen in non–HIV-infected patients with primary or secondary syphilis. Thus, **CSF testing is not recommended in those with uncomplicated disease and a normal neurologic examination.** In contrast, a lumbar puncture should be performed in all patients, regardless of HIV-infection status, if neurologic signs are present or if therapy has failed. Following treatment, CSF white blood cell counts normalize within 12 months

regardless of HIV status, while the CSF VDRL is slower to normalize in HIV-infected individuals, especially those with CD4 counts less than 200 cells/mcL. As discussed above, the same criteria for failure apply to HIV-positive and HIV-negative patients, and re-treatment regimens are the same.

Because clinical experience in treating HIV-infected patients with syphilis is based on penicillin regimens, few options exist for treating the penicillin-allergic patient. Doxycycline or tetracycline regimens can be used for primary, secondary, and early latent syphilis as well as for late latent syphilis and latent syphilis of unknown duration though with caution and close follow-up (Table 34–3). For neurosyphilis, limited efficacy data exist for ceftriaxone; therefore, penicillin regimens are optimal even if this requires skin testing and desensitization.

7. Syphilis in Pregnancy

All pregnant women should have a nontreponemal serologic test for syphilis at the time of the first prenatal visit (see Chapter 19). In women who may be at increased risk for syphilis or for populations in which there is a high prevalence of syphilis, additional nontreponemal tests should be performed during the third trimester at 28 weeks and again at delivery. The serologic status of all women who have delivered should be known before discharge from the hospital. Seropositive women should be considered infected and should be treated unless prior treatment with fall in antibody titer is medically documented.

The only acceptable treatment for syphilis in pregnancy is penicillin in dosage schedules appropriate for the stage of disease (see above). Penicillin prevents congenital syphilis in 90% of cases, even when treatment is given late in pregnancy. Tetracycline and doxycycline are contraindicated in pregnancy. Erythromycin should not be used because of failure to eradicate infection in the fetus, and insufficient data are available to justify a recommendation for ceftriaxone or azithromycin. Thus, women with a history of penicillin allergy should be skin tested and desensitized if necessary.

The infant should be evaluated immediately, as noted below, and at 6–8 weeks of age.

8. Congenital Syphilis

Congenital syphilis is a transplacentally transmitted infection that occurs in infants of untreated or inadequately treated mothers. The physical findings at birth are quite variable: The infant may have many or minimal signs or even no signs until 6–8 weeks of life (delayed form). The most common findings are on the mucous membranes and skin—maculopapular rash, condylomas, mucous membrane patches, and serous nasal discharge (snuffles). These lesions are infectious; *T pallidum* can easily be found microscopically, and the infant must be isolated. Other common findings are hepatosplenomegaly, anemia, or osteochondritis. These early active lesions subsequently heal, but if the disease is left untreated it produces the characteristic stigmas of congenital syphilis—interstitial keratitis, Hutchinson teeth, saddle nose, saber shins, deafness, and CNS involvement.

The presence of negative serologic tests at birth in both the mother and the infant usually means that the newborn is free of infection. However, recent infection near the time of delivery may result in negative tests because there has been insufficient time to develop a serologic response. Thus, it is necessary to maintain a high index of suspicion in infants born to high-risk mothers. All infants born to mothers with positive nontreponemal and treponemal antibody titers should have blood drawn for an RPR or VDRL test and, if positive, be referred to a pediatrician for further evaluation and therapy.

▶ When to Refer

- Consultation with the local public health department may help obtain all prior positive syphilis serologic results and may be helpful in complicated or atypical cases.
- Early (infectious) syphilis cases may be contacted for partner notification and treatment by local public health authorities.

▶ When to Admit

- Pregnant women with syphilis and true penicillin allergy should be admitted for desensitization and treatment.
- Women in late pregnancy treated for early syphilis should have close outpatient monitoring or be admitted because the Jarisch-Herxheimer reaction can induce premature labor.
- Patients with neurosyphilis usually require admission for treatment with aqueous penicillin.

Clement ME et al. Treatment of syphilis: a systematic review. JAMA. 2014 Nov 12;312(18):1905–17. [PMID: 25387188]

Tipple C et al. Syphilis testing, typing, and treatment follow-up: a new era for an old disease. Curr Opin Infect Dis. 2015 Feb; 28(1):53–60. [PMID: 25485649]

Workowski KA et al; Centers for Disease Control and Prevention. Sexually transmitted diseases treatment guidelines, 2015. MMWR Recomm Rep. 2015 Jun 5;64(RR-03):1–137. Erratum in: MMWR Recomm Rep. 2015 Aug 28;64(33):924. [PMID: 26042815]

NON–SEXUALLY TRANSMITTED TREPONEMATOSES

A variety of treponemal diseases other than syphilis occur endemically in many tropical areas of the world. They are distinguished from disease caused by *T pallidum* by their nonsexual transmission via direct skin contact, their relatively high incidence in certain geographic areas and among children, and their tendency to produce less severe visceral manifestations. As in syphilis, skin, soft tissue, and bone lesions may develop, organisms can be demonstrated in infectious lesions with darkfield microscopy or immunofluorescence but cannot be cultured in artificial media; the serologic tests for syphilis are positive; molecular methods such as PCR and genome sequencing are available but not widely used in endemic areas; the diseases have primary, secondary, and sometimes tertiary stages; and penicillin is the drug of choice. Treatment with penicillin in doses appropriate to primary syphilis (eg, 2.4 million units of benzathine penicillin G intramuscularly) is generally curative in any stage of the non–sexually transmitted treponematoses. In cases of penicillin hypersensitivity, tetracycline, 500 mg orally four times a day for 10–14 days, is usually the recommended alternative. In a randomized controlled trial, oral azithromycin (30 mg/kg once) was noninferior to benzathine penicillin G for the treatment of yaws in children.

YAWS (Frambesia)

Yaws is a contagious disease largely limited to tropical regions that is caused by *T pallidum* subspecies *pertenue*. It is characterized by granulomatous lesions of the skin, mucous membranes, and bone. Yaws is rarely fatal, though if untreated it may lead to chronic disability and disfigurement. Yaws is acquired by direct nonsexual contact, usually in childhood, although it may occur at any age. The "mother yaw," a painless papule that later ulcerates, appears 3–4 weeks after exposure. There is usually associated regional lymphadenopathy. Six to 12 weeks later, secondary lesions that are raised papillomas and papules that weep highly infectious material appear and last for several months or years. Painful ulcerated lesions on the soles are called "crab yaws" because of the resulting gait. Late gummatous lesions may occur, with associated tissue destruction involving large areas of skin and subcutaneous tissues. The late effects of yaws, with bone change, shortening of digits, and contractions, may be confused with similar changes occurring in leprosy. CNS, cardiac, or other visceral involvement is rare. See above for therapy. The World Health Organization has set a goal of eliminating yaws by the year 2020 using mass treatment with azithromycin.

PINTA

Pinta is a non–sexually transmitted spirochetal infection caused by *T pallidum* subspecies *carateum*. It occurs endemically in rural areas of Latin America, especially in Mexico, Colombia, and Cuba, and in some areas of the Pacific. A nonulcerative, erythematous primary papule spreads slowly into a papulosquamous plaque showing a variety of color changes (slate, lilac, black). Secondary lesions resemble the primary one and appear within a year after it. These appear successively, new lesions together with older ones; are most common on the extremities; and later show atrophy and depigmentation. Some cases show pigmentary changes and atrophic patches on the soles and palms, with or without hyperkeratosis, that are indistinguishable from "crab yaws." See above for therapy.

ENDEMIC SYPHILIS (Bejel)

Endemic syphilis is an acute or chronic infection caused by *T pallidum* subspecies *endemicum*. It has been reported in a number of countries, particularly in the eastern Mediterranean area, often with local names: bejel in Syria, Saudi

Arabia, and Iraq, and dichuchwa, njovera, and siti in Africa. It also occurs in Southeast Asia. The local forms have distinctive features. Moist ulcerated lesions of the skin or oral or nasopharyngeal mucosa are the most common manifestations. Generalized lymphadenopathy and secondary and tertiary bone and skin lesions are also common. Deep leg pain points to periostitis or osteomyelitis. In the late stages of disease, destructive gummatous lesions similar to those seen in yaws can develop, resulting in loss of cartilage and saber shin deformity. Cardiovascular and CNS involvement are rare. See above for therapy.

Marks M et al. Endemic treponemal diseases. Trans R Soc Trop Med Hyg. 2015 Sep;109(9):604. [PMID: 26286945]
Mitjà O et al. Advances in the diagnosis of endemic treponematoses: yaws, bejel, and pinta. PLoS Negl Trop Dis. 2013 Oct 24; 7(10):e2283. [PMID: 24205410]

▼ SELECTED SPIROCHETAL DISEASES

RELAPSING FEVER

The infectious organisms in relapsing fever are spirochetes of the genus *Borrelia*. The infection has two forms: tick-borne and louse-borne. The main reservoir for tick-borne relapsing fever is rodents, which serve as the source of infection for ticks. **Tick-borne** relapsing fever may be transmitted transovarially from one generation of ticks to the next. Humans can be infected by tick bites or by rubbing crushed tick tissues or feces into the bite wound. Tick-borne relapsing fever is endemic but is not transmitted from person to person. In the United States, infected ticks are found throughout the West, especially in mountainous areas, but clinical cases are uncommon in humans.

The **louse-borne** form is primarily seen in the developing world, and humans are the only reservoir. Large epidemics may occur in louse-infested populations, and transmission is favored by crowding, malnutrition, and cold climate.

▶ Clinical Findings

A. Symptoms and Signs

There is an abrupt onset of fever, chills, tachycardia, nausea and vomiting, arthralgia, and severe headache. Hepatomegaly and splenomegaly may develop, as well as various types of rashes (macular, papular, petechial) that usually occur at the end of a febrile episode. Delirium occurs with high fever, and there may be various neurologic and psychic abnormalities. The attack terminates, usually abruptly, after 3–10 days. After an interval of 1–2 weeks, relapse occurs, but often it is somewhat milder. Three to ten relapses may occur before recovery in tick-borne disease, whereas louse-borne disease is associated with only one or two relapses.

B. Laboratory Findings

During episodes of fever, large spirochetes are seen in blood smears stained with Wright or Giemsa stain. The organisms can be cultured in special media but rapidly lose pathogenicity. The spirochetes can multiply in injected rats or mice and can be seen in their blood.

A variety of anti-borrelia antibodies develop during the illness; sometimes the Weil–Felix test for rickettsioses and nontreponemal serologic tests for syphilis may also be falsely positive. Infection can cause false-positive indirect fluorescent antibody and Western blot tests for *Borrelia burgdorferi*, causing some cases to be misdiagnosed as Lyme disease. PCR assays have been developed but are not widely available. CSF abnormalities occur in patients with meningeal involvement. Mild anemia and thrombocytopenia are common, but the white blood cell count tends to be normal.

▶ Differential Diagnosis

The manifestations of relapsing fever may be confused with malaria, leptospirosis, meningococcemia, yellow fever, typhus, or rat-bite fever.

▶ Prevention

Prevention of tick bites (as described for rickettsial diseases) and delousing procedures applicable to large groups can prevent illness. Arthropod vectors should be controlled if possible.

Postexposure prophylaxis with doxycycline 200 mg orally on day 1 and 100 mg daily for 4 days has been shown to prevent recurrent fever following tick bites in highly endemic areas.

▶ Treatment

A single dose of tetracycline or erythromycin, 0.5 g orally, or a single dose of procaine penicillin G, 600,000–800,000 units intramuscularly (adults) or 400,000 units intramuscularly (children), probably constitutes adequate treatment for louse-borne relapsing fevers; however, some experts advocate for longer courses of treatment to prevent persistent infection. Because of higher relapse rates, tick-borne disease is routinely treated with 0.5 g of tetracycline or erythromycin given orally four times daily for 10 days. If CNS invasion is suspected, penicillin G, 3 million units intravenously every 4 hours, or ceftriaxone, 1 g intravenously daily, should be given for 10–14 days. Jarisch–Herxheimer reactions occur commonly following treatment and may be life-threatening, so patients should be closely monitored (see Syphilis, above). One study in patients with louse-borne relapsing fever showed that administration of anti-TNF antibodies prior to antibiotic therapy can be effective in preventing the reaction.

▶ Prognosis

The overall mortality rate is usually about 5%. Fatalities are most common in old, debilitated, or very young patients. With treatment, the initial attack is shortened and relapses are largely prevented.

Cutler SJ. Relapsing fever *Borreliae*: a global review. Clin Lab Med. 2015 Dec;35(4):847–65. [PMID: 26593261]

RAT-BITE FEVER

Rat-bite fever is an uncommon acute infectious disease caused by the treponeme *Spirillum minus* (Asia), or the bacteria *Streptobacillus moniliformis* (North America). It is transmitted to humans by the bite of a rat. Inhabitants of rat-infested dwellings, owners of pet rats, and laboratory workers are at greatest risk.

▶ Clinical Findings

A. Symptoms and Signs

In *Spirillum* infections, the original rat bite, unless secondarily infected, heals promptly, but 1 to several weeks later the site becomes swollen, indurated, and painful; assumes a dusky purplish hue; and may ulcerate. Regional lymphangitis and lymphadenitis, fever, chills, malaise, myalgia, arthralgia, and headache are present. Splenomegaly may occur. A sparse, dusky-red maculopapular rash appears on the trunk and extremities in many cases, and there may be frank arthritis.

After a few days, both the local and systemic symptoms subside, only to reappear several days later. This relapsing pattern of fever for 3–4 days alternating with afebrile periods lasting 3–9 days may persist for weeks. The other features, however, usually recur only during the first few relapses. Endocarditis is a rare complication of infection.

B. Laboratory Findings

Leukocytosis is often present, and the nontreponemal test for syphilis is often falsely positive. The organism may be identified in darkfield examination of the ulcer exudate or aspirated lymph node material; more commonly, it is observed after inoculation of a laboratory animal with the patient's exudate or blood. It has not been cultured in artificial media.

▶ Differential Diagnosis

Rat-bite fever must be distinguished from the rat-bite–induced lymphadenitis and rash of streptobacillary fever. Clinically, the severe arthritis and myalgias seen in streptobacillary disease are rarely seen in disease caused by *S minus*. Reliable differentiation requires an increasing titer of agglutinins against *S moniliformis* or isolation of the causative organism. Other diseases in the differential include tularemia, rickettsial disease, *Pasteurella multocida* infections, and relapsing fever.

▶ Treatment

Penicillin is given for 10–14 days. During the acute phase of illness, the intravenous route is used (1–2 million units every 4–6 hours) and once improvement has occurred, therapy is completed with oral medication, penicillin V 500 mg four times daily to complete 10–14 days of therapy. For the penicillin-allergic patient, tetracycline 500 mg orally four times daily or doxycycline 100 mg twice a day can be used.

▶ Prognosis

The reported mortality rate of about 10% should be markedly reduced by prompt diagnosis and antimicrobial treatment.

Budair B et al. Septic arthritis secondary to rat bite fever: a challenging diagnostic course. BMJ Case Rep. 2014 Apr 2; 2014:204086. [PMID: 24695665]

LEPTOSPIROSIS

ESSENTIALS OF DIAGNOSIS

▶ Clinical illness can vary from asymptomatic to fatal liver and kidney disease.

▶ Anicteric leptospirosis is the more common and milder form of the disease.

▶ Icteric leptospirosis (Weil syndrome) is characterized by impaired kidney and liver function, abnormal mental status, and hemorrhagic pneumonia and has a 5–40% mortality rate.

▶ General Considerations

Leptospirosis is an acute and sometimes severe treponemal infection that is caused by multiple serotypes of the spirochete, *Leptospira interrogans*. The disease is distributed worldwide, and it is among the most common zoonotic infections. The leptospires are often transmitted to humans by the ingestion of food and drink contaminated by the urine of an infected animal. The organism may also enter through minor skin lesions and probably via the conjunctiva. Reports of recreational cases in international travelers have been increasing, following swimming or rafting in contaminated water, and occupational cases occur among sewer workers, rice planters, abattoir workers, and farmers. Sporadic urban cases have been seen in the homeless exposed to rat urine.

▶ Clinical Findings

A. Symptoms and Signs

Anicteric leptospirosis, the more common and milder form of the disease, is often biphasic. After an incubation period of 2–20 days, the initial or "septicemic" phase begins with abrupt fever to 39–40°C, chills, abdominal pain, severe headache, and myalgias, especially of the calf muscles. There may be marked conjunctival suffusion. Leptospires can be isolated from blood, CSF, and tissues. Following a 1- to 3-day period of improvement in symptoms and absence of fever, the second or "immune" phase begins; however, in severe disease the phases may appear indistinct. Leptospires are absent from blood and CSF but are still present in the kidney, and specific antibodies appear. A recurrence of symptoms is seen as in the first phase of disease with the onset of meningitis. Uveitis (which can be unilateral or bilateral and usually involves the entire uveal tract), rash, and adenopathy may occur.

A rare but severe manifestation is hemorrhagic pneumonia. The illness is usually self-limited, lasting 4–30 days, and complete recovery is the rule.

Icteric leptospirosis (Weil syndrome) is the most severe form of the disease, characterized by impaired kidney and liver function, abnormal mental status, hemorrhagic pneumonia, hypotension, and a 5–40% mortality rate. Symptoms and signs often are continuous and not biphasic.

Leptospirosis with jaundice must be distinguished from hepatitis, yellow fever, rickettsial disease, and relapsing fever.

B. Laboratory Findings

The leukocyte count may be normal or as high as 50,000/mcL (0.05/L), with neutrophils predominating. The urine may contain bile, protein, casts, and red cells. Oliguria is common, and in severe cases uremia may occur. Elevated bilirubin and aminotransferases are seen in 75%, and elevated creatinine (greater than 1.5 mg/dL) (132.6 mcmol/L) is seen in 50% of cases. Serum creatine kinase is usually elevated in persons with leptospirosis and normal in persons with hepatitis. In cases with meningeal involvement, organisms may be found in the CSF during the first 10 days of illness. Early in the disease, the organism may be identified by darkfield examination of the patient's blood (a test requiring expertise since false-positives are frequent in inexperienced hands) or by culture on a semisolid medium (eg, Fletcher EMJH). Cultures take 1–6 weeks to become positive but may remain negative if antibiotics were started before culture was obtained. The organism may also be grown from the urine from the tenth day to the sixth week. Diagnosis is usually made by means of serologic tests, including the microscopic agglutination test (considered the gold standard but not widely available), and enzyme-linked immunosorbent assay (ELISA). PCR molecular diagnostics are not widely available but appear to be sensitive, specific, positive early in disease, and able to detect leptospiral DNA in blood, urine, CSF, and aqueous humor.

▶ Complications

Myocarditis, aseptic meningitis, acute kidney injury, and pulmonary infiltrates with hemorrhage are not common but are the usual causes of death. Iridocyclitis may occur.

▶ Prevention

The mainstay of prevention is avoidance of potentially contaminated food and water.

Prophylaxis with doxycycline has been effective in trials but is not routinely recommended. Human vaccine is used in some limited settings but is not available in the United States.

▶ Treatment

Many cases are self-limited without specific treatment. Various antimicrobial medications, including penicillin, ceftriaxone, and tetracyclines, show antileptospiral activity; however, meta-analysis has not demonstrated a clear survival benefit for any antibiotic. Doxycycline (100 mg every 12 hours orally or intravenously), penicillin (eg, 1.5 million units every 6 hours intravenously), and ceftriaxone (1 g daily intravenously) are used in severe leptospirosis. Jarisch–Herxheimer reactions may occur (see Syphilis, above). Although therapy for mild disease is controversial, most clinicians treat with doxycycline, 100 mg orally twice daily, for 7 days, or amoxicillin 50 mg/kg, divided into three doses daily. Azithromycin is also active, but clinical experience is limited.

▶ Prognosis

Without jaundice, the disease is almost never fatal. With jaundice, the mortality rate is 5% for those under age 30 years and 40% for those over age 60 years.

▶ When to Admit

Patients with jaundice or other evidence of severe disease should be admitted for close monitoring and may require admission to an intensive care unit.

Haake DA et al. Leptospirosis in humans. Curr Top Microbiol Immunol. 2015;387:65–97. [PMID: 25388133]

Musso D et al. Laboratory diagnosis of leptospirosis: a challenge. J Microbiol Immunol Infect. 2013 Aug;46(4):245–52. [PMID: 23639380]

LYME DISEASE (Lyme Borreliosis)

ESSENTIALS OF DIAGNOSIS

- ▶ Erythema migrans, a flat or slightly raised red lesion that expands with central clearing.
- ▶ Headache or stiff neck.
- ▶ Arthralgias, arthritis, and myalgias; arthritis is often chronic and recurrent.
- ▶ Wide geographic distribution, with most US cases in the Northeast, mid-Atlantic, upper Midwest, and Pacific coastal regions.

▶ General Considerations

This illness, named after the town of Old Lyme, Connecticut, is the most common tick-borne disease in the United States and Europe and is caused by genospecies of the spirochete *B burgdorferi*. In the United States, the causative genospecies is *B burgdorferi senu strictu*, whereas in Europe and Asia *B garinii* and *B afzelii* predominate. Most US cases are reported from the mid-Atlantic, northeastern, and north central regions of the country. The true incidence of Lyme disease is not known for a number of reasons: (1) serologic tests are not standardized (see below); (2) clinical manifestations are nonspecific; and (3) even with reliable testing, serology is insensitive in early disease.

The tick vector of Lyme disease varies geographically and is *Ixodes scapularis* in the northeastern, north central, and mid-Atlantic regions of the United States; *Ixodes pacificus* on the West Coast; *Ixodes ricinus* in Europe; and *Ixodes persulcatus* in Asia. The disease also occurs in Australia. Mice and deer make up the major animal reservoir of *B burgdorferi*, but other rodents and birds may also be infected. Domestic animals such as dogs, cattle, and horses can also develop clinical illness, usually manifested as arthritis.

Under experimental conditions, **ticks must feed for 24–36 hours or longer to transmit infections**. Most cases are reported in the spring and summer months. Human epidemiologic studies have indicated that the incidence of disease is significantly higher when tick attachment is for longer than 72 hours than if it is less than 72 hours, though rare cases have been documented with attachment of less than 24 hours. In addition, the percentage of ticks infected varies on a regional basis. In the northeastern and midwestern regions, 15–65% of *I scapularis* ticks are infected with the spirochete; in the western United States, only 2% of *I pacificus* are infected. These are important epidemiologic features in assessing the likelihood that tick exposure will result in disease. Eliciting a history of brushing a tick off the skin (ie, the tick was not feeding) or removing a tick on the same day as exposure (ie, the tick did not feed long enough) decreases the likelihood that infection will develop.

Because the *Ixodes* tick is so small, the bite is usually painless and goes unnoticed. After feeding, the tick drops off in 2–4 days. If a tick is found, it should be removed immediately. The best way to accomplish this is to use fine-tipped tweezers to pull firmly and repeatedly on the tick's mouth part—not the tick's body—until the tick releases its hold. Saving the tick in a bottle of alcohol for future identification may be useful, especially if symptoms develop.

► **Clinical Findings**

Prior clinical description of Lyme disease divided the illness into three stages: stage 1, flu-like symptoms and a typical skin rash (**erythema migrans,** see Figure 6–27); stage 2, weeks to months later, facial (cranial nerve VII) palsy or meningitis; and stage 3, months to years later, arthritis. The problem with this simplified scheme is that there is a great deal of overlap, and the skin, CNS, and musculoskeletal system can be involved early or late. A more accurate classification divides disease into early and late manifestations and specifies whether disease is localized or disseminated.

A. Symptoms and Signs

1. Stage 1, early localized infection—Stage 1 infection is characterized by erythema migrans. About 1 week after the tick bite (range, 3–30 days; median 7–10 days), a flat or slightly raised red lesion appears at the site, which is commonly seen in areas of tight clothing such as the groin, thigh, or axilla. This lesion expands over several days. Although originally described as a lesion that progresses with central clearing ("bulls-eye" lesion), often there is a

more homogeneous appearance or even central intensification. About 10–20% of patients either do not have typical skin lesions or the lesions go unnoticed. Most patients with erythema migrans will have a concomitant viral-like illness (the "summer flu") characterized by myalgias, arthralgias, headache, and fatigue. Fever may or may not be present. Even without treatment, the symptoms and signs of erythema migrans resolve in 3–4 weeks. Although the classic lesion of erythema migrans is not difficult to recognize, atypical forms can occur that may lead to misdiagnosis. Chemical reactions to tick and spider bites (these usually recede in 24–48 hours, whereas erythema migrans increases in size in this time period), drug eruptions, urticaria, and staphylococcal and streptococcal cellulitis have been mistaken for erythema migrans. Southern tick–associated rash illness (STARI) has a similar appearance, but it occurs in geographically distinct areas of the United States.

Completely asymptomatic disease, without erythema migrans or flu-like symptoms, can occur but is very uncommon in the United States.

2. Stage 2, early disseminated infection—Up to 50–60% of patients with erythema migrans are bacteremic and within days to weeks of the original infection, secondary skin lesions develop in about 50% of patients. These lesions are similar in appearance to the primary lesion but are usually smaller. Malaise, fatigue, fever, headache (sometimes severe), neck pain, and generalized achiness are common with the skin lesions. Most symptoms are transient, although fatigue may persist for months. After hematogenous spread, the organism may sequester itself in certain areas and produce focal symptoms. Some patients experience cardiac (4–10% of patients) or neurologic (10–15% of patients) manifestations. Cardiac involvement includes myopericarditis, with atrial or ventricular arrhythmias and heart block. Neurologic manifestations include both the central and peripheral nervous systems. The most common CNS manifestation is aseptic meningitis with mild headache and neck stiffness. The most common peripheral manifestation is a cranial nerve VII neuropathy, ie, facial palsy (usually unilateral but can be bilateral, see Figure 24–2). A sensory or motor radiculopathy and mononeuritis multiplex occur less frequently. Conjunctivitis, keratitis and, rarely, panophthalmitis can also occur. Rarely, skin involvement can be manifested as a cutaneous hypopigmented lesion called a **borrelial lymphocytoma**.

3. Stage 3, late persistent infection—Stage 3 infection occurs months to years after the initial infection and again primarily manifests itself as musculoskeletal, neurologic, and skin disease. In early reports, musculoskeletal complaints developed in up to 60% of patients, but with early recognition and treatment of disease, this has decreased to less than 10%. The classic manifestation of late disease is a monarticular or oligoarticular arthritis most commonly affecting the knee or other large weight bearing joints. While these joints may be quite swollen, these patients generally report less pain compared to patients with bacterial septic arthritis. Even if untreated, the arthritis is self-limited, resolving in a few weeks to months. Multiple recurrences are common but are usually less severe than the original disease. Joint fluid reflects an inflammatory arthritis with a mean white blood cell count of 25,000/mcL (0.025/L) with a predominance of neutrophils. Chronic arthritis develops in about 10% of patients. The pathogenesis of chronic Lyme arthritis may be an immunologic phenomenon rather than persistence of infection.

Rarely, the nervous system (both central and peripheral) can be involved in late Lyme disease. In the United States, a subacute encephalopathy, characterized by memory loss, mood changes, and sleep disturbance, is seen. In Europe, a more severe encephalomyelitis caused by *B garinii* is seen and presents with cognitive dysfunction, spastic paraparesis, ataxia, and bladder dysfunction. Peripheral nervous system involvement includes intermittent paresthesias, often in a stocking glove distribution, or radicular pain.

The cutaneous manifestation of late infection, which can occur up to 10 years after infection, is **acrodermatitis chronicum atrophicans**. It has been described mainly in Europe after infection with *B afzelii*, a genospecies that commonly causes disease in Europe but not the United States. There is usually bluish-red discoloration of a distal extremity with associated swelling. These lesions become atrophic and sclerotic with time and eventually resemble localized scleroderma. Cases of diffuse fasciitis with eosinophilia, an entity that resembles scleroderma, have been rarely associated with infection with *B burgdorferi*.

B. Laboratory Findings

The diagnosis of Lyme disease is based on both clinical manifestations and laboratory findings. The US Surveillance Case Definition specifies a person with **exposure to a potential tick habitat (within the 30 days just prior to developing erythema migrans) with (1) erythema migrans diagnosed by a physician or (2) at least one late manifestation of the disease and (3) laboratory confirmation as fulfilling the criteria for Lyme disease.**

Nonspecific laboratory abnormalities can be seen, particularly in early disease. The most common are an elevated sedimentation rate of more than 20 mm/h seen in 50% of cases, and mildly abnormal liver function tests are present in 30%. The abnormal liver function tests are transient and return to normal within a few weeks of treatment. A mild anemia, leukocytosis (11,000–18,000/mcL) (0.011–0.018/L), and microscopic hematuria have been reported in 10% or less of patients.

Laboratory confirmation requires **serologic tests** to detect specific antibodies to *B burgdorferi* in serum, preferably by ELISA and not by indirect immunofluorescence assay (IFA), which is less sensitive and specific and can cause misdiagnosis. A two-test approach is recommended for the diagnosis of active Lyme disease, with all specimens positive or equivocal by ELISA then confirmed with a Western immunoblot assay that can detect both IgM and IgG antibodies. A positive immunoblot requires that antibodies are detected against two (for IgM) or five (for IgG) specific protein antigens from *B burgdorferi*.

If a patient with suspected early Lyme disease has negative serologic studies, acute and convalescent titers should be obtained since up to 50% of patients with early disease can be antibody negative in the first several weeks of illness. **A fourfold rise in antibody titer would be diagnostic of recent infection.** In patients with later stages of disease, almost all are antibody positive. False-positive reactions in the ELISA and IFA have been reported in juvenile rheumatoid arthritis, rheumatoid arthritis, systemic lupus erythematosus, infectious mononucleosis, subacute infective endocarditis, syphilis, relapsing fever, leptospirosis, enteroviral and other viral illnesses, and patients with gingival disease (presumably because of cross-reactivity with oral treponemes). False-negative serologic reactions occur early in illness, and antibiotic therapy early in disease can abort subsequent seroconversion.

The diagnosis of late **nervous system Lyme disease** is often difficult since clinical manifestations, such as subtle memory impairment, may be difficult to document. Most patients have a history of previous erythema migrans or monarticular or polyarticular arthritis, and the vast majority have antibody present in serum. Patients with late disease and peripheral neuropathy almost always have positive serum antibody tests, usually have abnormal electrophysiology tests, and may have abnormal nerve biopsies showing perivascular collections of lymphocytes; however, the CSF is usually normal and does not demonstrate local antibody production.

Caution should be exercised in interpreting serologic tests because they are not subject to national standards, and inter-laboratory variation is a major problem. In addition, some laboratories perform tests that are entirely unreliable and should never be used to support the diagnosis of Lyme disease (eg, the Lyme urinary antigen test, immunofluorescent staining for cell wall–deficient forms of *B burgdorferi*, lymphocyte transformation tests, using PCR on inappropriate specimens such as blood or urine). Finally, testing is often done in patients with nonspecific symptoms such as headache, arthralgia, myalgia, fatigue, and palpitations. Even in endemic areas, the pretest probability of having Lyme disease is low in these patients, and the probability of a false-positive test result is greater than that of a true-positive result. For these reasons, the CDC has established guidelines for laboratory evaluation of patients with suspected Lyme disease:

1. The diagnosis of early Lyme disease is clinical (ie, exposure in an endemic area, with physician-documented erythema migrans), and does *not* require laboratory confirmation. (Tests are often negative at this stage.)

2. Late disease requires objective evidence of clinical manifestations (recurrent brief attacks of monarticular or oligoarticular arthritis of the large joints; lymphocytic meningitis, cranial neuritis [facial palsy], peripheral neuropathy or, rarely, encephalomyelitis—but *not* headache, fatigue, paresthesias, or stiff neck alone; atrioventricular conduction defects with or without myocarditis) and laboratory evidence of disease (two-stage testing with ELISA or IFA followed by Western blot, as described above).

3. Patients with nonspecific symptoms without objective signs of Lyme disease should *not* have serologic testing done. It is in this setting that false-positive tests occur more commonly than true-positive tests.

4. The role of serologic testing in nervous system Lyme disease is unclear, as sensitivity and specificity of CSF serologic tests have not been determined. However, it is rare for a patient to have positive serologic tests on CSF without positive tests on serum (see below).

5. Other tests such as the T cell proliferative assay and urinary antigen detection have not yet been studied well enough to be routinely used.

Cultures for *B burgdorferi* can be performed but are not routine and are usually reserved for clinical studies.

PCR is very specific for detecting the presence of *Borrelia* DNA, but sensitivity is variable and depends on which body fluid is tested, the stage of the disease, and collection and testing technique. In general, PCR is more sensitive than culture, especially in chronic disease but is not available in many clinical laboratories. Testing should not be done on blood or urine but has been successfully performed on synovial fluid and CSF. A negative PCR result does not rule out disease.

▶ Complications

Based on several observational studies, *B burgdorferi* infection in pregnant women has not been associated with congenital syndromes, unlike other spirochetal illnesses such as syphilis.

Some patients and advocacy groups have claimed either a post-Lyme syndrome (in the presence of positive laboratory tests and after appropriate treatment) or "chronic Lyme disease" in which tests may all be negative. Both entities include nonspecific symptoms such as fatigue, myalgias, and cognitive difficulties (see Prognosis below). Expert groups are in agreement that there are no data to support that ongoing infection is the cause of either syndrome.

▶ Prevention

There is no human vaccine currently available. Simple preventive measures such as avoiding tick-infested areas, covering exposed skin with long-sleeved shirts and wearing long trousers tucked into socks, wearing light-colored clothing, using repellents, and inspecting for ticks after exposure will greatly reduce the number of tick bites. Environmental controls directed at limiting ticks on residential property would be helpful, but trying to limit the deer, tick, or white-footed mouse populations over large areas is not feasible.

Prophylactic antibiotics following tick bites is recommended in certain high-risk situations if all of the following criteria are met: (1) a tick identified as an adult or nymphal *I scapularis* has been attached for at least 36 hours; (2) prophylaxis can be started within 72 hours of the time the tick was removed; (3) more than 20% of ticks in the area are known to be infected with *B burgdorferi;* and

(4) there is no contraindication to the use of doxycycline (not pregnant, age greater than 8 years, not allergic). The medication of choice for prophylaxis is a single 200-mg dose of doxycycline. If doxycycline is contraindicated, no prophylaxis should be given and the patient should be closely monitored for early disease, since short course prophylactic therapy with other agents has not been studied, and if early disease does develop, appropriate therapy is very effective in preventing long-term sequelae. Individuals who have removed ticks (including those who have had prophylaxis) should be monitored carefully for 30 days for possible coinfections.

▶ Coinfections

Lyme disease, **babesiosis** (see Chapter 35), and **human granulocytic anaplasmosis** (formerly human granulocytic ehrlichiosis) (see Chapter 32) are endemic in similar areas of the country and are transmitted by the same tick, *I scapularis*. Coinfection with two or even all three of these organisms can occur, causing a clinical picture that is not "classic" for any of these diseases. The presence of erythema migrans is highly suggestive of Lyme disease, whereas flu-like symptoms without rash are more suggestive of babesiosis or anaplasmosis. The complete blood count is usually normal in Lyme disease, but in patients with Lyme disease and babesiosis, anemia and thrombocytopenia are more common. Patients with Lyme disease and anaplasmosis are more likely to have leukopenia. Coinfection should be considered and excluded in patients who have persistent high fevers 48 hours after starting appropriate therapy for Lyme disease; in patients with persistent symptoms despite resolution of rash; and in those with anemia, leukopenia, or thrombocytopenia.

Even in patients with documented Lyme disease, immunity is not complete. Reinfection, although uncommon, is predominantly seen in patients successfully treated for early disease (erythema migrans) who do not develop antibody titers. Clinical manifestations and serologic response is similar to an initial infection.

▶ Treatment

Present recommendations for therapy are outlined in Table 34–4. For erythema migrans, antibiotic therapy shortens the duration of rash and prevents late sequelae. Doxycycline is most commonly used and has the advantage of being active against *Anaplasma phagocytophilum* (formerly *Ehrlichia*). Amoxicillin is also effective and is recommended for pregnant or lactating women and for those who cannot tolerate doxycycline. Cefuroxime axetil, is as effective as doxycycline, but because of its cost it should be considered an alternative choice for those who cannot tolerate doxycycline or amoxicillin or for those in whom the medications are contraindicated. Erythromycin and azithromycin are less effective, associated with higher rates of relapse, and are not recommended as first-line therapy.

Isolated facial palsy (without meningitis or peripheral neuropathy) can be treated with doxycycline, amoxicillin, or cefuroxime axetil for 2–3 weeks. Although therapy does

Table 34–4. Treatment of Lyme disease.

Manifestations	Drug and Dosage
Tick bite	No treatment in most circumstances (see text); observe
Erythema migrans	Doxycycline, 100 mg orally twice daily, or amoxicillin, 500 mg orally three times daily, or cefuroxime axetil, 500 mg orally twice daily—all for 2–3 weeks
Neurologic disease	
Facial palsy (without meningitis)	Doxycycline, amoxicillin, or cefuroxime axetil as above for 2–3 weeks
Other central nervous system disease	Ceftriaxone, 2 g intravenously once daily, or penicillin G, 18–24 million units daily intravenously in six divided doses, or cefotaxime, 2 g intravenously every 8 hours—all for 2–4 weeks
Cardiac disease	
Atrioventricular block and myopericarditis[1]	An oral or parenteral (if more severe disease) regimen as described above can be used
Arthritis	
Oral dosage	Doxycycline, amoxicillin, or cefuroxime axetil as above for 28 days (see text)
Parenteral dosage	Ceftriaxone, cefotaxime, or penicillin G as above for 2–4 weeks
Acrodermatitis chronicum atrophicans	Doxycycline, amoxicillin, or cefuroxime axetil as above for 3 weeks
"Chronic Lyme disease" or "post-Lyme disease syndrome"	Symptomatic therapy; prolonged antibiotics are *not* recommended

[1]Symptomatic patients, those with second- or third-degree block and those with first-degree block with a PR interval ≥ 300 milliseconds should be hospitalized for observation.

not affect the rate of resolution of the cranial neuropathy, it does prevent development of late manifestations of disease.

The need for a lumbar puncture in patients with seventh nerve palsy is controversial. Some clinicians perform lumbar puncture on all patients with facial palsy and others only if there are symptoms or signs of meningitis. If meningitis is present, therapy with a parenteral antibiotic is indicated. Ceftriaxone is most commonly used, but penicillin is equally efficacious. In European countries, doxycycline 400 mg/d orally for 14 days is frequently used and is comparable in efficacy to ceftriaxone.

Patients with atrioventricular block or myopericarditis (or both) can be treated with either oral or parenteral agents for 2–3 weeks. Hospitalization and observation is indicated for symptomatic patients, those with second- or third-degree block, and those with first-degree block with a PR interval of 300 milliseconds or more. Once stabilized,

hospitalized patients can be transitioned to one of the oral regimens to complete therapy.

Therapy of arthritis is difficult because some patients do not respond to any therapy, and those who do respond may do so slowly. Oral agents (doxycycline, amoxicillin, or cefuroxime axetil) are as effective as intravenous regimens (ceftriaxone, cefotaxime, or penicillin). A reasonable approach to the patient with Lyme arthritis is to start with oral therapy for 28 days, and if this fails (persistent or recurrent joint swelling), to re-treat with an oral regimen for 28 days or switch to an intravenous regimen for 2–4 weeks. If arthritis persists after re-treatment, symptomatic therapy with nonsteroidal anti-inflammatory drugs is recommended. For severe refractory pain, synovectomy may be required.

Based on the limited published data, therapy of Lyme disease in pregnancy should be the same as therapy in other patients with the exception that doxycycline should not be used.

Clinicians may encounter patients with nonspecific symptoms (such as fatigue and myalgias) and positive serologic tests for Lyme disease who request (or demand) therapy for their illness. It is important in managing these patients to remember (1) that nonspecific symptoms alone are not diagnostic; (2) that serologic tests are fraught with difficulty (as noted above), and in areas where disease prevalence is low, false-positive serologic tests are much more common than true-positive tests; and (3) that parenteral therapy with ceftriaxone for 2–4 weeks is costly and has been associated with significant adverse effects, including cholelithiasis and *Clostridium difficile* colitis. Parenteral therapy should be reserved for those most likely to benefit, ie, those with cutaneous, neurologic, cardiac, or rheumatic manifestations that are characteristic of Lyme disease.

► **Prognosis**

Most patients respond to appropriate therapy with prompt resolution of symptoms within 4 weeks. True treatment failures are thus uncommon, and in most cases re-treatment or prolonged treatment of Lyme disease is instituted because of misdiagnosis or misinterpretation of serologic results (both IgG and IgM antibodies can persist for prolonged periods despite adequate therapy) rather than inadequate therapy or response. Prolonged courses of antibiotic therapy for nonspecific symptoms that persist after completion of appropriate assessment (and treatment, if necessary) for Lyme disease is not recommended.

The long-term outcome of adult patients with Lyme disease is generally favorable, but some patients have chronic complaints. Joint pain, memory impairment, and poor functional status secondary to pain are common subjective complaints in patients with Lyme disease, but physical examination and neurocognitive testing fail to document the presence of these symptoms as objective sequelae. Similarly, in highly endemic areas, patients with a diagnosis of Lyme disease commonly complain of pain, fatigue, and an inability to perform certain physical activities when followed for several years. However, these complaints occur just as commonly in age-matched controls without a history of Lyme disease.

When to Refer

Consultation with an infectious diseases specialist with experience in diagnosing and treating Lyme disease can be helpful in atypical or prolonged cases.

When to Admit

Admission for parenteral antibiotics is indicated for any patient with symptomatic CNS or cardiac disease as well as those with second- or third-degree atrioventricular block, or first-degree block with a PR interval of 300 milliseconds or more.

Halperin JJ. Nervous system Lyme disease. Curr Infect Dis Rep. 2015 Jan;17(1):445. [PMID: 25421861]

Shapiro ED. Lyme disease. N Engl J Med. 2014 Aug 14;371(7):684. [PMID: 25119621]

Protozoal & Helminthic Infections

35

Philip J. Rosenthal, MD

PROTOZOAL INFECTIONS

AFRICAN TRYPANOSOMIASIS
(Sleeping Sickness)

ESSENTIALS OF DIAGNOSIS

- ▶ Exposure to tsetse flies; chancre at bite site uncommon.
- ▶ **Hemolymphatic disease:** Irregular fever, headache, joint pain, rash, edema, lymphadenopathy.
- ▶ **Meningoencephalitic disease:** Somnolence, severe headache, progressing to coma.
- ▶ Trypanosomes in blood or lymph node aspirates; positive serologic tests.
- ▶ Trypanosomes and increased white cells and protein in cerebrospinal fluid.

▶ General Considerations

African trypanosomiasis is caused by the hemoflagellates *Trypanosoma brucei rhodesiense* and *Trypanosoma brucei gambiense*. The organisms are transmitted by bites of tsetse flies (genus *Glossina*), which inhabit shaded areas along streams and rivers. Trypanosomes ingested in a blood meal develop over 18–35 days in the fly; when the fly feeds again on a mammalian host, the infective stage is injected. Human disease occurs in rural areas of sub-Saharan Africa from south of the Sahara to about 30 degrees south latitude. *T b gambiense* causes West African trypanosomiasis, and is transmitted in the moist sub-Saharan savannas and forests of west and central Africa. *T b rhodesiense* causes East African trypanosomiasis, and is transmitted in the savannas of east and southeast Africa.

T b rhodesiense infection is primarily a zoonosis of game animals and cattle; humans are infected sporadically. Humans are the principal mammalian host for *T b gambiense*, but domestic animals can be infected. The number of reported cases increased from the 1960s to the 1990s and

has since decreased by about 80%. Total incidence has been estimated at about 20,000 cases per year, most of which are due to *T b gambiense*, and the largest number in the Democratic Republic of the Congo. Infections are rare among travelers, including visitors to game parks.

▶ Clinical Findings

A. Symptoms and Signs

1. West African trypanosomiasis—Chancres at the site of the bite are uncommon. After an asymptomatic period that may last for months, **hemolymphatic disease** presents with fever, headache, myalgias, arthralgias, weight loss, and lymphadenopathy, with discrete, nontender, rubbery nodes, referred to as Winterbottom sign when in a posterior cervical distribution. Other common signs are mild splenomegaly, transient edema, and a pruritic erythematous rash. Febrile episodes may be broken by afebrile periods of up to several weeks. The hemolymphatic stage progresses over months to **meningoencephalitic disease**, with somnolence, irritability, personality changes, severe headache, and parkinsonian symptoms progressing to coma and death.

2. East African trypanosomiasis—Chancres at the bite site are more commonly recognized with *T b rhodesiense* infection, with a painful lesion of 3–10 cm and regional lymphadenopathy that appears about 48 hours after the tsetse fly bite and lasts 2–4 weeks. East African disease follows a much more acute course, with the onset of symptoms usually within a few days of the insect bite. The hemolymphatic stage includes intermittent fever and rash, but lymphadenopathy is less common than with West African disease. Myocarditis can cause tachycardia and death due to arrhythmias or heart failure. If untreated, East African trypanosomiasis progresses over weeks to months to meningoencephalitic disease, somnolence, coma, and death.

B. Laboratory Findings

Diagnosis can be difficult, and definitive diagnosis requires identification of trypanosomes. Microscopic examination of fluid expressed from a chancre or lymph node may show motile trypanosomes or, in fixed specimens, parasites stained with Giemsa. During the **hemolymphatic stage**, detection of parasites in Giemsa-stained blood smears is common in East African disease but difficult in West African disease. Serial specimens should be examined, since parasitemias vary greatly over time. **Meningoencephalitic (or second stage) disease** is defined by the World Health Organization (WHO) as cerebrospinal fluid (CSF) showing at least five mononuclear cells per microliter, elevated protein, or presence of trypanosomes. Concentration techniques can aid identification of parasites in blood or CSF. Serologic tests are also available. The card agglutination test for trypanosomes (CATT) has excellent sensitivity and specificity for West African disease and can be performed in the field, but the diagnosis should be confirmed by identification of the parasites. Field-applicable immunochromatographic lateral flow rapid diagnostic tests that cost less than CATT and are simpler to perform are available; combining tests improves sensitivity and specificity. Molecular diagnostic tests, including PCR and field-friendly loop-mediated isothermal amplification (LAMP) appear to have excellent sensitivity and specificity, but these are not yet standardized or routinely available.

▶ Treatment

Detection of trypanosomes is a prerequisite for treatment of African trypanosomiasis because of the significant toxicity of most available therapies. Treatment recommendations depend on the type of trypanosomiasis (Table 35–1), which is determined by geography, and stage of disease, which requires examination of CSF. Eflornithine, nifurtimox, suramin, and melarsoprol are available in the United States from the CDC Drug Service (www.cdc.gov/laboratory/drugservice).

A. West African Trypanosomiasis

1. Early stage infection—Pentamidine (4 mg/kg intramuscularly or intravenously every day or every other day for 7 days) is used to treat infection that does not involve the central nervous system (CNS). The side effects of pentamidine include immediate hypotension; tachycardia; gastrointestinal symptoms during administration; sterile abscesses; and pancreatic (hypoglycemia), liver, and kidney abnormalities. An alternate drug is eflornithine (100 mg/kg/day intravenously every 6 hours for 14 days).

2. Late stage infection—The treatment of choice for CNS infection is a combination of intravenous eflornithine (400 mg/kg/day in two doses for 7 days) and oral nifurtimox (15 mg/kg/day in three doses for 10 days), which has improved efficacy and less toxicity than older regimens. Eflornithine, though less toxic than older trypanocidal drugs, can cause gastrointestinal symptoms, bone marrow suppression, seizures, and alopecia. The alternative agent is melarsoprol.

B. East African Trypanosomiasis

Pentamidine and eflornithine are not reliably effective, and early disease is treated with suramin. The dosing regimens of suramin vary (eg, 100–200 mg test dose, then 20 mg/kg [maximum 1 g] intravenously on days 1, 3, 7, 14, and 21 or weekly for five doses). Suramin toxicities include vomiting and, rarely, seizures and shock during infusions as well as subsequent fever, rash, headache, neuropathy, and kidney and bone marrow dysfunction.

Suramin does not enter the CNS, so East African trypanosomiasis involving the CNS is treated with melarsoprol (three series of 3.6 mg/kg/day intravenously for 3 days, with 7-day breaks between the series or a 10-day intravenous course with 0.6 mg/kg on day 1, 1.2 mg/kg on day 2, and 1.8 mg/kg on days 3–10). Melarsoprol also acts against West African disease, but eflornithine plus nifurtimox is preferred due to its lower toxicity. Immediate side effects of melarsoprol include fever and gastrointestinal symptoms. The most important side effect is a reactive encephalopathy that can progress to seizures, coma, and death. To help avoid this side effect, corticosteroids are coadministered (dexamethasone 1 mg/kg/day intravenously for 2–3 days or oral prednisolone 1 mg/kg/day for 5 days, and then 0.5 mg/kg/day until treatment completion). In addition, increasing resistance to melarsoprol is a serious concern.

▶ Prevention & Control

Individual prevention in endemic areas should include long sleeves and pants, insect repellents, and mosquito nets. Control programs focusing on vector elimination and treatment of infected persons and animals have shown good success in many areas but suffer from limited resources.

Table 35–1. Treatment of African trypanosomiasis.

Disease	Stage	First Line	Alternative
West African	Early	Pentamidine	Suramin Eflornithine
	CNS involvement	Eflornithine + nifurtimox	Melarsoprol
East African	Early CNS involvement	Suramin Melarsoprol	Pentamidine

CNS, central nervous system.

Barrett MP et al. Management of trypanosomiasis and leishmaniasis. Br Med Bull. 2012;104:175–96. [PMID: 23137768]
Brun R et al. Human African trypanosomiasis. Infect Dis Clin North Am. 2012 Jun;26(2):261–73. [PMID: 22632638]
Eperon G et al. Treatment options for second-stage gambiense human African trypanosomiasis. Expert Rev Anti Infect Ther. 2014 Nov;12(11):1407–17. [PMID: 25204360]
Franco JR et al. Epidemiology of human African trypanosomiasis. Clin Epidemiol. 2014 Aug 6;6:257–75. [PMID: 25125985]
Jamonneau V et al. Accuracy of individual rapid tests for serodiagnosis of gambiense sleeping sickness in West Africa. PLoS Negl Trop Dis. 2015 Feb 2;9(2):e0003480. [PMID: 25642701]
Kennedy PG. Clinical features, diagnosis, and treatment of human African trypanosomiasis (sleeping sickness). Lancet Neurol. 2013 Feb;12(2):186–94. [PMID: 23260189]

AMERICAN TRYPANOSOMIASIS
(Chagas Disease)

> ### ESSENTIALS OF DIAGNOSIS
>
> **Acute stage**
> ► Inflammatory lesion at inoculation site.
> ► Fever.
> ► Hepatosplenomegaly; lymphadenopathy.
> ► Myocarditis.
> ► Parasites in blood is diagnostic.
>
> **Chronic stage**
> ► Heart failure, cardiac arrhythmias.
> ► Thromboembolism.
> ► Megaesophagus; megacolon.
> ► Serologic tests are usually diagnostic.

General Considerations

Chagas disease is caused by *Trypanosoma cruzi*, a protozoan parasite found only in the Americas; it infects wild animals and to a lesser extent humans from southern South America to the southern United States. An estimated 8–10 million people are infected, mostly in rural areas. Control efforts in endemic countries have decreased disease incidence to about 40,000 new infections and 12,500 deaths per year. The disease is often acquired in childhood. In many countries in South America, Chagas disease is the most important cause of heart disease. In the United States, the vector is found, some animals are infected, and a few instances of local transmission have been reported.

T cruzi is transmitted by reduviid (triatomine) bugs infected by ingesting blood from animals or humans who have circulating trypanosomes. Multiplication occurs in the digestive tract of the bug and infective forms are eliminated in feces. Infection in humans occurs when the parasite penetrates the skin through the bite wound, mucous membranes, or the conjunctiva. Transmission can also occur by blood transfusion, organ or bone marrow transplantation, congenital transfer, or ingestion of food contaminated with vector feces. From the bloodstream, *T cruzi* invades many cell types but has a predilection for myocardium, smooth muscle, and CNS glial cells. Multiplication causes cellular destruction, inflammation, and fibrosis, with progressive disease over decades.

Clinical Findings

A. Symptoms and Signs

As many as 70% of infected persons remain asymptomatic. The **acute stage** is seen principally in children and lasts 1–2 months. The earliest findings are at the site of inoculation either in the eye—Romaña sign (unilateral edema, conjunctivitis, and lymphadenopathy)—or in the skin—a chagoma (swelling with local lymphadenopathy).

Subsequent findings include fever, malaise, headache, mild hepatosplenomegaly, and generalized lymphadenopathy. Acute myocarditis and meningoencephalitis are rare but can be fatal.

An asymptomatic **latent period (indeterminate phase)** may last for life, but symptomatic disease develops in 10–30% of infected individuals, commonly many years after infection.

Chronic Chagas disease generally manifests as abnormalities in cardiac and smooth muscle. Cardiac disease includes arrhythmias, heart failure, and embolic disease. Smooth muscle abnormalities lead to mega esophagus and megacolon, with dysphagia, regurgitation, aspiration, constipation, and abdominal pain. These findings can be complicated by superinfections. In immunosuppressed persons, including AIDS patients and transplant recipients, latent Chagas disease may reactivate; findings have included brain abscesses and meningoencephalitis.

B. Diagnostic Testing

The diagnosis is made by detecting parasites in persons with suggestive findings who have resided in an endemic area. With **acute infection**, evaluation of fresh blood or buffy coats may show motile trypanosomes, and fixed preparations may show Giemsa-stained parasites. Trypanosomes may be identified in lymph nodes, bone marrow, or pericardial or spinal fluid. PCR is highly sensitive, and can be used to detect parasites in organ transplant recipients or after accidental exposure. When initial tests are unrevealing, xenodiagnosis using laboratory vectors, laboratory culture, or animal inoculation may provide a diagnosis, but these methods are expensive and slow.

Chronic Chagas disease is usually diagnosed serologically. Many different serologic assays are available, but sensitivity and specificity are not ideal; confirmatory assays are advised after an initial positive test, as is standard for blood bank testing in South America. The diagnosis of chronic disease with PCR remains suboptimal.

Treatment

Treatment is inadequate because the two drugs used, benznidazole and nifurtimox, often cause severe side effects, must be used for long periods, and are ineffective against chronic infection. In acute and congenital infections, the drugs can reduce the duration and severity of infection, but cure is achieved in only about 70% of patients. During the chronic phase of infection, although parasitemia may disappear in up to 70% of patients, treatment does not clearly alter the progression of the disease. In a recent trial for Chagas cardiomyopathy, benznidazole significantly reduced parasite detection but not progression of cardiac disease. Nevertheless, there is general consensus that treatment should be considered in all *T cruzi*-infected persons regardless of clinical status or time since infection. In particular, treatment is recommended for acute, congenital, and reactivated infections and for children and young adults with chronic disease. Both benznidazole and nifurtimox are available in the United States from the CDC Drug Service (www.cdc.gov/laboratory/drugservice).

Benznidazole is generally preferred due to better efficacy and safety profiles. It is given orally at a dosage of 5 mg/kg/day in two divided doses for 60 days. Its side effects include granulocytopenia, rash, and peripheral neuropathy. Nifurtimox is given orally in daily doses of 8–10 mg/kg in four divided doses after meals for 90–120 days. Side effects include gastrointestinal (anorexia, vomiting) and neurologic (headaches, ataxia, insomnia, seizures) symptoms, which appear to be reversible and to lessen with dosage reduction. Patients with chronic Chagas disease may also benefit from antiarrhythmic therapy, standard therapy for heart failure, and conservative and surgical management of megaesophagus and megacolon.

▶ Prevention & Control

In South America, a major eradication program based on improved housing, use of residual pyrethroid insecticides and pyrethroid-impregnated bed curtains, and screening of blood donors has achieved striking reductions in new infections. In endemic areas and ideally in donors from endemic areas, blood should not be used for transfusion unless at least two serologic tests are negative.

Bern C. Chagas' disease. N Engl J Med. 2015 Jul 30;373(5):456–66. [PMID: 26222561]

Montgomery SP et al. Neglected parasitic infections in the United States: Chagas disease. Am J Trop Med Hyg. 2014 May; 90(5):814–8. [PMID: 24808250]

Morillo CA et al; BENEFIT Investigators. Randomized trial of benznidazole for chronic Chagas' cardiomyopathy. N Engl J Med. 2015 Oct;373(14):1295–306. [PMID: 26323937]

Pérez-Molina JA et al. Old and new challenges in Chagas disease. Lancet Infect Dis. 2015 Nov;15(11):1347–56. [PMID: 26231478]

LEISHMANIASIS

ESSENTIALS OF DIAGNOSIS

- ▶ Sand fly bite in an endemic area.
- ▶ **Visceral leishmaniasis:** irregular fever, progressive hepatosplenomegaly, pancytopenia, wasting.
- ▶ **Cutaneous leishmaniasis:** chronic, painless, moist ulcers or dry nodules.
- ▶ **Mucocutaneous leishmaniasis:** destructive nasopharyngeal lesions.
- ▶ Amastigotes in macrophages in aspirates, touch preparations, or biopsies.
- ▶ Positive culture, serologic tests, PCR, or skin test.

▶ General Considerations

Leishmaniasis is a zoonosis transmitted by bites of sand flies of the genus *Lutzomyia* in the Americas and *Phlebotomus* elsewhere. When sand flies feed on an infected host, the parasitized cells are ingested with the blood meal. Leishmaniasis is caused by about 20 species of *Leishmania*;

taxonomy is complex. Clinical syndromes are generally dictated by the infecting species, but some species can cause more than one syndrome.

An estimated 350 million persons are at risk for leishmaniasis. The estimated annual incidence of disease is 1–1.5 million new cases of cutaneous and 400,000 cases of visceral disease, leading to an estimated 40,000 deaths.

Visceral leishmaniasis (kala azar) is caused mainly by *Leishmania donovani* in the Indian subcontinent and East Africa; *Leishmania infantum* in the Mediterranean, Middle East, China, parts of Asia, and Horn of Africa; and *Leishmania chagasi* in South and Central America. Other species may occasionally cause visceral disease. Over 90% of cases occur in five countries: India, Bangladesh, Nepal, Sudan, and Brazil. In each locale, the disease has particular clinical and epidemiologic features. The incubation period is usually 4–6 months (range: 10 days to 24 months). Without treatment, the fatality rate reaches 90%. Early diagnosis and treatment reduces mortality to 2–5%.

Old World cutaneous leishmaniasis is caused mainly by *Leishmania tropica*, *Leishmania major*, and *Leishmania aethiopica* in the Mediterranean, Middle East, Africa, Central Asia, and Indian subcontinent. **New World cutaneous leishmaniasis** is caused by *Leishmania mexicana*, *Leishmania amazonensis*, and the species listed below for mucocutaneous disease in Central and South America. **Mucocutaneous leishmaniasis** (espundia) occurs in lowland forest areas of the Americas and is caused by *Leishmania braziliensis*, *Leishmania panamensis*, and *Leishmania peruviana*.

▶ Clinical Findings

A. Symptoms and Signs

1. Visceral leishmaniasis (kala azar)—Most infections are subclinical, but a small number progress to full-blown disease. A local nonulcerating nodule at the site of the sand fly bite may precede systemic manifestations but usually is inapparent. The onset of illness may be acute, within 2 weeks of infection, or insidious. Symptoms and signs include fever, chills, sweats, weakness, anorexia, weight loss, cough, and diarrhea. The spleen progressively becomes greatly enlarged, firm, and nontender. The liver is somewhat enlarged, and generalized lymphadenopathy may occur. Hyperpigmentation of skin can be seen, leading to the name kala azar ("black fever"). Other signs include skin lesions, petechiae, gingival bleeding, jaundice, edema, and ascites. As the disease progresses, severe wasting and malnutrition are seen; death eventually occurs, often due to secondary infections, within months to a few years. **Post-kala azar dermal leishmaniasis** may appear after apparent cure in the Indian subcontinent and Sudan. It may simulate leprosy, with hypopigmented macules or nodules developing on preexisting lesions. **Viscerotropic leishmaniasis** has been reported in small numbers of American military personnel in the Middle East, with mild systemic febrile illnesses after *L tropica* infections.

2. Old World and New World cutaneous leishmaniasis—Cutaneous swellings appear 2 weeks to several months after sand fly bites and can be single or multiple. Characteristics

▲ **Figure 35–1.** Skin ulcer due to cutaneous leishmaniasis. (From D. S. Martin, Public Health Image Library, CDC.)

of lesions and courses of disease vary depending on the leishmanial species and host immune response. Lesions begin as small papules and develop into nonulcerated dry plaques or large encrusted ulcers with well-demarcated raised and indurated margins (Figure 35–1). Satellite lesions may be present. The lesions are painless unless secondarily infected. Local lymph nodes may be enlarged. Systemic symptoms are uncommon, but fever, constitutional symptoms, and regional lymphadenopathy may be seen. For most species, healing occurs spontaneously in months to a few years, but scarring is common.

Leishmaniasis recidivans is a relapsing form of *L tropica* infection associated with hypersensitivity, in which the primary lesion heals centrally, but spreads laterally, with extensive scarring. **Diffuse cutaneous leishmaniasis** involves spread from a central lesion to local dissemination of nodules and a protracted course. **Disseminated cutaneous leishmaniasis** involves multiple nodular or ulcerated lesions, often with mucosal involvement.

3. Mucocutaneous leishmaniasis (espundia)—In Latin America, mucosal lesions develop in a small percentage of persons infected with *L braziliensis* and some other species, usually months to years after resolution of a cutaneous lesion. Nasal congestion is followed by ulceration of the nasal mucosa and septum, progressing to involvement of the mouth, lips, palate, pharynx, and larynx. Extensive destruction can occur, and secondary bacterial infection is common.

4. Infections in patients with AIDS—Leishmaniasis is an opportunistic infection in persons with AIDS. Visceral leishmaniasis can present late in the course of HIV infection, with fever, hepatosplenomegaly, and pancytopenia. The gastrointestinal tract, respiratory tract, and skin may also be involved.

B. Laboratory Findings

Identifying amastigotes within macrophages in tissue samples provides a definitive diagnosis. In **visceral leishmaniasis**, fine-needle aspiration of the spleen for culture and tissue evaluation is generally safe, and yields a diagnosis in over 95% of cases. Bone marrow aspiration is less sensitive but safer and diagnostic in most cases, and Giemsa-stained buffy coat of peripheral blood may occasionally show organisms. Cultures with media available from the CDC will grow promastigotes within a few days to weeks. PCR can also identify the infection. Serologic tests may facilitate diagnosis, but none are sufficiently sensitive or specific to be used alone. Numerous antibody-based rapid diagnostic tests are available; these have shown good specificity but limitations in sensitivity outside of India. For **cutaneous lesions**, biopsies should be taken from the raised border of a skin lesion, with samples for histopathology, touch preparation, and culture. The histopathology shows inflammation with mononuclear cells. Macrophages filled with amastigotes may be present, especially early in infection. An intradermal leishmanin (Montenegro) skin test is positive in most individuals with cutaneous disease but negative in those with progressive visceral or diffuse cutaneous disease; this test is not approved in the United States. In **mucocutaneous leishmaniasis**, diagnosis is established by detecting amastigotes in scrapings, biopsy preparations, or aspirated tissue fluid, but organisms may be rare. Cultures from these samples may grow organisms. Serologic studies are often negative, but the leishmanin skin test is usually positive.

▶ Treatment

A. Visceral Leishmaniasis

The treatment of choice for visceral leishmaniasis is liposomal amphotericin B (approved by the FDA), which is generally effective and well tolerated but expensive. Standard dosing is 3 mg/kg/day intravenously on days 1–5, 14, and 21. Simpler regimens that have shown good efficacy in India include four doses of 5 mg/kg over 4–10 days and a single dose of 15 mg/kg, but efficacy appears to be lower in Africa. Conventional amphotericin B deoxycholate, which is much less expensive, is also highly effective but with more toxicity. It is administered as a slow intravenous infusion of 1 mg/kg/day for 15–20 days or 0.5–1 mg/kg every second day for up to 8 weeks. A single infusion of an amphotericin B lipid emulsion, which is more affordable than liposomal preparations, showed excellent efficacy, albeit lower than that of the liposomal formulation. Infusion-related side effects with conventional or liposomal amphotericin B include gastrointestinal symptoms, fever, chills, dyspnea, hypotension, and hepatic and renal toxicity.

Pentavalent antimonials remain the most commonly used drugs to treat leishmaniasis in most areas. Response rates are good outside India, but in India, resistance is a major problem. Two preparations are available, sodium stibogluconate in the United States and many other areas and meglumine antimonate in Latin America and francophone countries; the compounds appear to have comparable activities. In the United States, sodium stibogluconate can be obtained from the CDC Drug Service (www.cdc.gov/laboratory/drugservice).

Treatment with either antimonial is given once daily at a dose of 20 mg/kg/day intravenously (preferred) or intramuscularly for 20 days for cutaneous leishmaniasis and

28 days for visceral or mucocutaneous disease. Toxicity increases over time, with development of gastrointestinal symptoms, fever, headache, myalgias, arthralgias, pancreatitis, and rash. Intramuscular injections can cause sterile abscesses. Monitoring should include serial ECGs, and changes are indications for discontinuation to avoid progression to serious arrhythmias.

Miltefosine is the first oral drug for the treatment of leishmaniasis, and it is registered in India for this indication. It has demonstrated excellent results in India, but after over a decade of use, efficacy may be decreasing. It can be administered at a daily oral dose of 2.5 mg/kg in two divided doses for 28 days. A 28-day course of miltefosine (2.5 mg/kg/day) is also effective for the treatment of New World cutaneous leishmaniasis. Vomiting, diarrhea, and elevations in transaminases and kidney function studies are common, but generally short-lived, side effects.

The aminoglycoside paromomycin (11 mg/kg/day intramuscularly for 21 days) was shown to be similarly efficacious to amphotericin B for the treatment of visceral disease in India, where it is approved for this indication. It is much less expensive than liposomal amphotericin B or miltefosine. Paromomycin has shown relatively poor efficacy in Africa. The drug is well tolerated; side effects include ototoxicity and reversible elevations in liver enzymes.

The use of drug combinations to improve treatment efficacy, shorten treatment courses, and reduce the selection of resistant parasites has been actively studied. In India, compared to a standard 30-day (treatment on alternate days) course of amphotericin, noninferior efficacy and decreased adverse events were seen with a single dose of liposomal amphotericin plus a 7-day course of miltefosine, a single dose of liposomal amphotericin plus a 10-day course of paromomycin, or a 10-day course of miltefosine plus paromomycin. In East Africa, compared to a standard 30-day course of sodium stibogluconate, similar efficacy was seen with a 17-day course of sodium stibogluconate plus paromomycin.

B. Cutaneous Leishmaniasis

In the Old World, cutaneous leishmaniasis is generally self-healing over some months and does not metastasize to the mucosa, so it may be justified to withhold treatment in regions without mucocutaneous disease if lesions are small and cosmetically unimportant. Lesions on the face or hands are generally treated. New World leishmaniasis has a greater risk of progression to mucocutaneous disease, so treatment is more often warranted. Standard therapy is with pentavalent antimonials for 20 days, as described above. Other treatments include those discussed above for visceral disease, azole antifungals, and allopurinol. In studies in South America, a 28-day course of miltefosine was superior to a 20-day course of meglumine antimoniate, and oral fluconazole also showed good efficacy. Topical therapy has included intralesional antimony, intralesional pentamidine, paromomycin ointment, cryotherapy, local heat, and surgical removal. Diffuse cutaneous leishmaniasis and related chronic skin processes generally respond poorly to therapy.

C. Mucocutaneous Leishmaniasis

Cutaneous infections from regions where parasites include those that cause mucocutaneous disease (eg, *L braziliensis* in parts of Latin America) should all be treated to help prevent disease progression. Treatment of mucocutaneous disease with antimonials is disappointing, with responses in only about 60% in Brazil. Other therapies listed above for visceral leishmaniasis may also be used, although they have not been well studied for this indication.

▶ Prevention & Control

Personal protection measures for avoidance of sand fly bites include use of insect repellants, fine-mesh insect netting, long sleeves and pants, and avoidance of warm shaded areas where flies are common. Disease control measures include destruction of animal reservoir hosts, mass treatment of humans in disease-prevalent areas, residual insecticide spraying in dwellings, limiting contact with dogs and other domesticated animals, and use of permethrin-impregnated collars for dogs.

Burza S et al. Five-year field results and long-term effectiveness of 20 mg/kg liposomal amphotericin B (Ambisome) for visceral leishmaniasis in Bihar, India. PLoS Negl Trop Dis. 2014 Jan 2;8(1):e2603. [PMID: 24392168]

Goto H et al. Cutaneous and mucocutaneous leishmaniasis. Infect Dis Clin North Am. 2012 Jun;26(2):293–307. [PMID: 22632640]

Sundar S et al. An update on pharmacotherapy for leishmaniasis. Expert Opin Pharmacother. 2015 Feb;16(2):237–52. [PMID: 25346016]

Sundar S et al. Efficacy and safety of amphotericin B emulsion versus liposomal formulation in Indian patients with visceral leishmaniasis: a randomized, open-label study. PLoS Negl Trop Dis. 2014 Sep 18;8(9):e3169. [PMID: 25233346]

Sundar S et al. Single-dose indigenous liposomal amphotericin B in the treatment of Indian visceral leishmaniasis: a phase 2 study. Am J Trop Med Hyg. 2015 Mar 4;92(3):513–7. [PMID: 25510715]

van Griensven J et al. Visceral leishmaniasis. Infect Dis Clin North Am. 2012 Jun;26(2):309–22. [PMID: 22632641]

MALARIA

ESSENTIALS OF DIAGNOSIS

▶ Exposure to anopheline mosquitoes in a malaria-endemic area.

▶ Intermittent attacks of chills, fever, and sweating.

▶ Headache, myalgia, vomiting, splenomegaly; anemia, thrombocytopenia.

▶ Intraerythrocytic parasites identified in thick or thin blood smears.

▶ **Complications of falciparum malaria:** cerebral malaria, severe anemia, hypotension, pulmonary edema, acute kidney injury, hypoglycemia, acidosis, and hemolysis.

General Considerations

Malaria is the most important parasitic disease of humans, causing hundreds of millions of illnesses and hundreds of thousands of deaths each year. The disease is endemic in most of the tropics, including much of South and Central America, Africa, the Middle East, the Indian subcontinent, Southeast Asia, and Oceania. Transmission, morbidity, and mortality are greatest in Africa, where most deaths from malaria are in young children. Malaria is also common in travelers from nonendemic areas to the tropics.

Four species of the genus *Plasmodium* classically cause human malaria. *Plasmodium falciparum* is responsible for nearly all severe disease. It is endemic in most malarious areas and is by far the predominant species in Africa. *Plasmodium vivax* is about as common as *P falciparum*, except in Africa. *P vivax* uncommonly causes severe disease, although this outcome may be more common than previously appreciated. *Plasmodium ovale* and *Plasmodium malariae* are much less common causes of disease, and generally do not cause severe illness. *Plasmodium knowlesi*, a parasite of macaque monkeys, is now recognized to cause occasional illnesses, including some severe disease, in humans in Southeast Asia.

Malaria is transmitted by the bite of infected female anopheline mosquitoes. During feeding, mosquitoes inject sporozoites, which circulate to the liver, and rapidly infect hepatocytes, causing asymptomatic liver infection. Merozoites are subsequently released from the liver, and they rapidly infect erythrocytes to begin the asexual erythrocytic stage of infection that is responsible for human disease. Multiple rounds of erythrocytic development, with production of merozoites that invade additional erythrocytes, lead to large numbers of circulating parasites and clinical illness. Some erythrocytic parasites also develop into sexual gametocytes, which are infectious to mosquitoes, allowing completion of the life cycle and infection of others.

Malaria may uncommonly be transmitted from mother to infant (congenital malaria), by blood transfusion, and in nonendemic areas by mosquitoes infected after biting infected immigrants or travelers. In *P vivax* and *P ovale*, parasites also form dormant liver hypnozoites, which are not killed by most drugs, allowing subsequent relapses of illness after initial elimination of erythrocytic infections. For all plasmodial species, parasites may recrudesce following initial clinical improvement after suboptimal therapy.

In highly endemic regions, where people are infected repeatedly, antimalarial immunity prevents severe disease in most older children and adults. However, young children, who are relatively nonimmune, are at high risk for severe disease from *P falciparum* infection, and this population is responsible for most deaths from malaria. Pregnant women are also at increased risk for severe falciparum malaria. In areas with lower endemicity, individuals of all ages commonly present with uncomplicated or severe malaria. Travelers, who are generally nonimmune, are at high risk for severe disease from falciparum malaria at any age.

Clinical Findings

A. Symptoms and Signs

An acute attack of malaria typically begins with a prodrome of headache and fatigue, followed by fever. A classic malarial paroxysm includes chills, high fever, and then sweats. Patients may appear to be remarkably well between febrile episodes. Fevers are usually irregular, especially early in the illness, but without therapy may become regular, with 48-hour (*P vivax* and *P ovale*) or 72-hour (*P malariae*) cycles, especially with non-falciparum disease. Headache, malaise, myalgias, arthralgias, cough, chest pain, abdominal pain, anorexia, nausea, vomiting, and diarrhea are common. Seizures may represent simple febrile convulsions or evidence of severe neurologic disease. Physical findings may be absent or include signs of anemia, jaundice, splenomegaly, and mild hepatomegaly. Rash and lymphadenopathy are not typical in malaria, and thus suggestive of another cause of fever.

In the developed world, it is imperative that all persons with suggestive symptoms, in particular fever, who have traveled in an endemic area be evaluated for malaria. The risk for falciparum malaria is greatest within 2 months of return from travel; other species may cause disease many months—and occasionally more than a year—after return from an endemic area.

Severe malaria is characterized by signs of severe illness, organ dysfunction, or a high parasite load (peripheral parasitemia greater than 5% or greater than 200,000 parasites/mcL). It is principally a result of *P falciparum* infection because this species uniquely infects erythrocytes of all ages and mediates the sequestration of infected erythrocytes in small blood vessels, thereby evading clearance of infected erythrocytes by the spleen.

Severe falciparum malaria can include dysfunction of any organ system, including neurologic abnormalities progressing to alterations in consciousness, repeated seizures, and coma (cerebral malaria); severe anemia; hypotension and shock; noncardiogenic pulmonary edema and the acute respiratory distress syndrome; acute kidney injury due to acute tubular necrosis or, less commonly, severe hemolysis; hypoglycemia; acidosis; hemolysis with jaundice; hepatic dysfunction; retinal hemorrhages and other fundoscopic abnormalities; bleeding abnormalities, including disseminated intravascular coagulation; and secondary bacterial infections, including pneumonia and *Salmonella* bacteremia. In the developing world, severe malaria and deaths from the disease are mostly in young children, in particular from cerebral malaria and severe anemia. Cerebral malaria is a consequence of a single severe infection while severe anemia follows multiple malarial infections, intestinal helminths, and nutritional deficiencies. In a large trial of African children, acidosis, impaired consciousness, convulsions, renal impairment, and underlying chronic illness were associated with poor outcome.

Uncommon disorders resulting from immunologic responses to chronic infection are massive splenomegaly and, with *P malariae* infection, immune complex glomerulopathy with nephrotic syndrome. HIV-infected individuals are at increased risk for malaria and for severe disease, in particular with advanced immunodeficiency.

▲ **Figure 35–2.** Thin film Giemsa-stained micrograph with *Plasmodium falciparum* ring forms. (From Steven Glenn, Laboratory & Consultation Division, Public Health Image Library, CDC.)

▲ **Figure 35–4.** Thin film Giemsa-stained micrograph with *Plasmodium vivax* schizont. (From Steven Glenn, Laboratory & Consultation Division, Public Health Image Library, CDC.)

B. Laboratory Findings

Giemsa-stained blood smears remain the mainstay of diagnosis (Figures 35–2 through 35–5), although other routine stains (eg, Wright stain) will also demonstrate parasites. Thick smears provide efficient evaluation of large volumes of blood, but thin smears are simpler for inexperienced personnel and better for discrimination of parasite species. Single smears are usually positive in infected individuals, although parasitemias may be very low in nonimmune individuals. If illness is suspected, repeating smears at 8- to 24-hour intervals is appropriate. The severity of malaria correlates only loosely with the quantity of infecting parasites, but high parasitemias (especially greater than 10–20% of erythrocytes infected or greater than 200,000–500,000 parasites/mcL) or the presence of malarial pigment (a breakdown product of hemoglobin) in more than 5% of neutrophils is associated with a particularly poor prognosis.

A second means of diagnosis is rapid diagnostic tests to identify circulating plasmodial antigens with a simple "dipstick" format. These tests are not well standardized but are widely available. At best, they offer sensitivity and specificity near that of high-quality blood smear analysis and are simpler to perform.

Serologic tests indicate history of disease but are not useful for diagnosis of acute infection. PCR and related molecular tests (eg, LAMP) are highly sensitive but not available for routine diagnosis. In immune populations, highly sensitive tests, such as PCR, have limited value because subclinical infections, which are of uncertain significance and not routinely treated, are common.

Other diagnostic findings with uncomplicated malaria include thrombocytopenia, anemia, leukocytosis or leukopenia, liver function abnormalities, and hepatosplenomegaly. Severe malaria can present with the laboratory abnormalities expected for the advanced organ dysfunction discussed above.

▶ Treatment

Malaria is the most common cause of fever in much of the tropics and in travelers seeking medical attention after

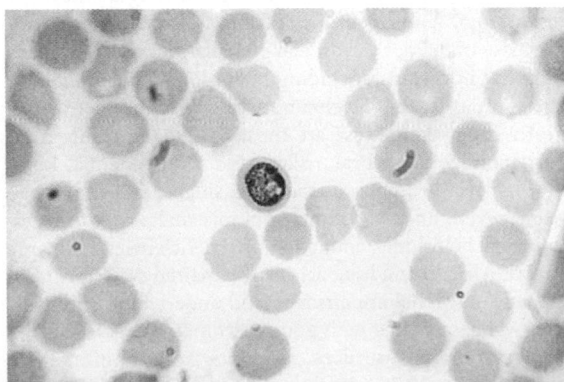

▲ **Figure 35–3.** Thin film Giemsa-stained micrograph with *Plasmodium malariae* trophozoite. (From Steven Glenn, Laboratory & Consultation Division, Public Health Image Library, CDC.)

▲ **Figure 35–5.** Thin film Giemsa-stained micrograph with *Plasmodium ovale* trophozoite. (From Steven Glenn, Laboratory & Consultation Division, Public Health Image Library, CDC.)

Table 35–2. Major antimalarial drugs.

Drug	Class	Use
Chloroquine	4-Aminoquinoline	Treatment and chemoprophylaxis of infection with sensitive parasites
Amodiaquine[1]	4-Aminoquinoline	Treatment of *Plasmodium falciparum*, optimally in fixed combination with artesunate
Piperaquine[1]	4-Aminoquinoline	Treatment of *P falciparum* in fixed combination with dihydroartemisinin
Quinine	Quinoline methanol	Oral and intravenous[1] (for severe infections) treatment of *P falciparum*
Quinidine	Quinoline methanol	Intravenous therapy of severe infections with *P falciparum*
Mefloquine	Quinoline methanol	Chemoprophylaxis and treatment of infections with *P falciparum*
Primaquine	8-Aminoquinoline	Radical cure and terminal prophylaxis of infections with *Plasmodium vivax* and *Plasmodium ovale*; alternative for malaria chemoprophylaxis
Sulfadoxine-pyrimethamine (Fansidar)	Folate antagonist combination	Treatment of *P falciparum*, optimally in combination with artesunate; intermittent preventive therapy
Atovaquone-proguanil (Malarone)	Quinone-folate antagonist combination	Treatment and chemoprophylaxis of *P falciparum* infection
Doxycycline	Tetracycline	Treatment (with quinine) of infections with *P falciparum*; chemoprophylaxis
Halofantrine[1]	Phenanthrene methanol	Treatment of infections with some chloroquine-resistant *P falciparum*
Lumefantrine	Amyl alcohol	Treatment of *P falciparum* malaria in fixed combination with artemether (Coartem)
Pyronaridine	Benzonaphthyridine	Treatment of *P falciparum* malaria in fixed combination artesunate
Artemisinins (Artesunate, artemether, dihydroartemisinin)	Sesquiterpene lactone endoperoxides	Treatment of *P falciparum* in oral combination regimens for uncomplicated disease and parenterally for severe malaria

[1]Not available in the United States.

Modified, with permission, from Katzung BG. *Basic & Clinical Pharmacology*. 11th edition. McGraw-Hill, 2009.

return from endemic areas. Fevers are often treated presumptively in endemic areas, but ideally, treatment should follow definitive diagnosis, especially in non-immune individuals.

Symptomatic malaria is caused only by the erythrocytic stage of infection. Available antimalarial drugs (Table 35–2) act against this stage, except for primaquine, which acts principally against hepatic parasites.

A. Non-Falciparum Malaria

The first-line drug for non-falciparum malaria from most areas remains chloroquine. Due to increasing resistance of *P vivax* to chloroquine, alternative therapies are recommended when resistance is suspected, particularly for infections acquired in Indonesia, Oceania, and South America. These infections can be treated with artemisinin-based combination therapies (ACTs) or other first-line regimens for *P falciparum* infections as discussed below. For *P vivax* or *P ovale*, eradication of erythrocytic parasites with chloroquine should be accompanied by treatment with primaquine (after evaluating for glucose-6-phosphate dehydrogenase [G6PD] deficiency; see below) to eradicate dormant liver stages (hypnozoites), which may lead to relapses with recurrent erythrocytic infection and malaria symptoms after weeks to months if left untreated. Tafenoquine, which is related to primaquine, appears to offer similar efficacy with simpler dosing, but it also engenders

potential toxicity in those with G6PD deficiency, and it remains under study. *P malariae* infections need only be treated with chloroquine.

B. Uncomplicated Falciparum Malaria

P falciparum is resistant to chloroquine and sulfadoxine-pyrimethamine in most areas, with the exceptions of Central America west of the Panama Canal and Hispaniola. Falciparum malaria from other areas should not be treated with these older drugs, and decisions regarding chemoprophylaxis should follow the same geographic considerations.

ACTs, all including a short-acting artemisinin and longer-acting partner drug, are first-line therapies in nearly all endemic countries. The WHO recommends six ACTs to treat falciparum malaria (Table 35–3), but the efficacy of these regimens varies. Other combination therapies are under development. Quinine generally remains effective for falciparum malaria, but it must be taken for an extended period to cure disease and is poorly tolerated, and should best be reserved for the treatment of severe malaria and for treatment after another regimen has failed (Table 35–4).

In developed countries, malaria is an uncommon but potentially life-threatening infection of travelers and immigrants, many of whom are nonimmune, so they are at risk for rapid progression to severe disease. Nonimmune individuals with falciparum malaria should generally be

Table 35–3. WHO recommendations for the treatment of uncomplicated falciparum malaria.

Regimen	Notes
Artemether-lumefantrine (Coartem, Riamet)	Coformulated, first-line therapy in many countries. Approved in the United States.
Artesunate-amodiaquine (ASAQ)	Coformulated, first-line therapy in multiple African countries.
Artesunate-mefloquine	First-line therapy in parts of Southeast Asia and South America but efficacy decreasing in parts of Thailand.
Artesunate- pyronaridine	Coformulated. Most recently approved regimen; used in some Southeast Asian countries.
Artesunate-sulfadoxine-pyrimethamine	First-line in some countries, but efficacy lower than other regimens in most areas.
Dihydroartemisinin–piperaquine	Coformulated. First-line in some Southeast Asian countries but efficacy decreasing in parts of Cambodia.

World Health Organization: Guidelines for the Treatment of Malaria. World Health Organization. Geneva 2010. *ISBN* 978 92 4 154792 5.

admitted to the hospital due to risks of rapid progression of disease. A number of options are available for the treatment of uncomplicated falciparum malaria in the United States (Table 35–4).

C. Severe Malaria

Severe malaria is a medical emergency. Parenteral treatment is indicated for severe malaria, as defined above, and with inability to take oral drugs. With appropriate prompt therapy and supportive care, rapid recoveries may be seen even in very ill individuals.

The standard of care for severe malaria is intravenous artesunate, which has demonstrated superior efficacy and better tolerability than quinine. In the United States, intravenous artesunate is available on an investigational basis through the CDC (for enrollment call 770-488-7788); if approved, the drug is provided emergently from CDC Quarantine Stations. The drug is administered in four doses of 2.4 mg/kg over 3 days, every 12 hours on day 1, and then daily. If artesunate cannot be obtained promptly, severe malaria should be treated with intravenous quinine (available in most countries but not the United States) or quinidine (available in the United States). In endemic regions, if parenteral therapy is not available, intrarectal administration of artemether or artesunate is also effective. Patients receiving intravenous quinine or quinidine should receive continuous cardiac monitoring; if QTc prolongation exceeds 25% of baseline, the infusion rate should be reduced. Blood glucose should be monitored every 4–6 hours, and 5–10% dextrose may be coadministered to decrease the likelihood of hypoglycemia.

Appropriate care of severe malaria includes maintenance of fluids and electrolytes; respiratory and hemodynamic support; and consideration of blood transfusions, anticonvulsants, antibiotics for bacterial infections, and hemofiltration or hemodialysis. With high parasitemia (greater than 5–10%), exchange transfusion has been used, but beneficial effects have not clearly been demonstrated, and it is generally no longer recommended.

D. Antimalarial Drugs

1. Chloroquine—Chloroquine remains the drug of choice for the treatment of sensitive *P falciparum* and other species of malaria parasites (Table 35–4). Chloroquine is active against erythrocytic parasites of all human malaria species. It does not eradicate hepatic stages, so must be used with primaquine to eradicate *P vivax* and *P ovale* infections. Chloroquine-resistant *P falciparum* is widespread in nearly all areas of the world with falciparum malaria, with the exceptions of Central America west of the Panama Canal, Mexico, and Hispaniola. Chloroquine-resistant *P vivax* has been reported from a number of areas, most notably Southeast Asia and Oceania.

Chloroquine is the drug of choice for the treatment of non-falciparum and sensitive falciparum malaria. It rapidly terminates fever (in 24–48 hours) and clears parasitemia (in 48–72 hours) caused by sensitive parasites. Chloroquine is also the preferred chemoprophylactic agent in malarious regions without resistant falciparum malaria.

Chloroquine is usually well tolerated, even with prolonged use. Pruritus is common, primarily in Africans. Nausea, vomiting, abdominal pain, headache, anorexia, malaise, blurring of vision, and urticaria are uncommon. Dosing after meals may reduce some adverse events.

2. Amodiaquine, piperaquine, and pyronaridine—Amodiaquine is a 4-aminoquinoline that is closely related to chloroquine. Amodiaquine has been widely used to treat malaria because of its low cost, limited toxicity and, in some areas, effectiveness against chloroquine-resistant strains of *P falciparum*. Use of amodiaquine decreased after recognition of rare but serious side effects, notably agranulocytosis, aplastic anemia, and hepatotoxicity. However, serious side effects are rare with short-term use, and artesunate-amodiaquine is one of the standard ACTs recommended to treat falciparum malaria (Table 35–3). Chemoprophylaxis with amodiaquine is best avoided because of increased toxicity with long-term use.

Piperaquine is another 4-aminoquinoline that was previously heavily used in China and has been coformulated with dihydroartemisinin in an ACT. Piperaquine appears to be well tolerated and in combination with dihydroartemisinin to offer a highly efficacious therapy for falciparum and vivax malaria. Due to the long half-life of piperaquine (~3 weeks), dihydroartemisinin-piperaquine offers the longest period of posttreatment prophylaxis of available ACTs. However, resistance to piperaquine appears to be emerging in southeast Asia, threatening the efficacy of dihydroartemisinin-piperaquine against *P falciparum*.

Pyronaridine is a benzonaphthyridine that was also previously used as a monotherapy to treat malaria in China.

Table 35–4. Treatment of malaria.

Clinical Setting	Drug Therapy[1]	Alternative Drugs
Chloroquine-sensitive *Plasmodium falciparum* and *Plasmodium malariae* infections	Chloroquine phosphate, 1 g at 0, followed by 500 mg at 6, 24, and 48 hours —or— Chloroquine phosphate, 1 g at 0 and 24 hours, then 0.5 g at 48 hours	
Plasmodium vivax and *Plasmodium ovale* infections	Chloroquine (as above), then (if G6PD normal) primaquine, 30 mg base daily for 14 days	For infections from Indonesia, Papua New Guinea, and other areas with suspected resistance: therapies listed for uncomplicated chloroquine-resistant *P falciparum* plus primaquine
Uncomplicated infections with chloroquine-resistant *P falciparum*	Coartem (artemether 20 mg, lumefantrine 120 mg), four tablets twice daily for 3 days —or— Malarone, four tablets (total of 1 g atovaquone, 400 mg proguanil) daily for 3 days —or— Quinine sulfate, 650 mg three times daily for 3–7 days Plus one of the following (when quinine given for < 7 days) Doxycycline, 100 mg twice daily for 7 days —or— Clindamycin, 600 mg twice daily for 7 days	Mefloquine, 15 mg/kg once or 750 mg, then 500 mg in 6–8 hours —or— Dihydroartemisinin-piperaquine[2] (dihydroartemisinin 40 mg, piperaquine 320 mg), 4 tablets daily for 3 days —or— ASAQ[2] (artesunate 100 mg, amodiaquine 270 mg), two tablets daily for 3 days
Severe or complicated infections with *P falciparum*	Artesunate 2.4 mg/kg intravenously every 12 hours for 1 day, then daily[3,6]	Quinidine gluconate,[4–6] 10 mg/kg intravenously over 1–2 hours, then 0.02 mg/kg intravenously/min —or— Quinidine gluconate,[4–6] 15 mg/kg intravenously over 4 hours, then 7.5 mg/kg intravenously over 4 hours every 8 hours —or— Quinine dihydrochloride,[2,4–6] 20 mg/kg intravenously over 4 hours, then 10 mg/kg intravenously every 8 hours —or— Artemether,[2,6] 3.2 mg/kg intramuscularly, then 1.6 mg/kg/day intramuscularly

[1]All dosages are oral and refer to salts unless otherwise indicated. See text for additional information on all agents, including toxicities and cautions. See Centers for Disease Control and Prevention's guidelines (phone: 877-FYI-TRIP; http://www.cdc.gov/malaria/) for additional information and pediatric dosing.
[2]Not available in the United States.
[3]Available in the United States only on an investigational basis through the CDC (phone: 770-488-7788).
[4]Cardiac monitoring should be in place during intravenous administration of quinidine or quinine.
[5]Avoid loading doses in persons who have received quinine, quinidine, or mefloquine in the prior 24 hours.
[6]With all parenteral regimens, change to an oral regimen as soon as the patient can tolerate it.
G6PD, glucose-6-phosphate dehydrogenase.

The medication acts against many drug-resistant strains of *P falciparum*, although resistance has been reported. The combination of artesunate plus pyronaridine has been well-tolerated and has shown excellent efficacy against falciparum and vivax malaria.

3. Mefloquine—Mefloquine is effective against many chloroquine-resistant strains of *P falciparum* and against other malarial species. Although toxicity is a concern, mefloquine is also a recommended chemoprophylactic drug. Resistance to mefloquine has been reported sporadically

from many areas, but it appears to be uncommon except in regions of Southeast Asia with high rates of multidrug resistance (especially border areas of Thailand).

For treatment of uncomplicated malaria, mefloquine can be administered as a single dose or in two doses over 1 day. It is used in combination with artesunate in Southeast Asia, where resistance to mefloquine has been seen but the combination remains effective in most areas. It should be taken with meals and swallowed with a large amount of water. Mefloquine is recommended by the CDC for chemoprophylaxis in all malarious areas except those with no chloroquine resistance (where chloroquine is preferred) and some rural areas of Southeast Asia with a high prevalence of mefloquine resistance.

Adverse effects with weekly dosing of mefloquine for chemoprophylaxis include nausea, vomiting, dizziness, sleep and behavioral disturbances, epigastric pain, diarrhea, abdominal pain, headache, rash and, uncommonly, seizures and psychosis. There is an FDA black box warning about neuropsychiatric toxicity, including possibly rare, irreversible effects. Mefloquine should be avoided in persons with histories of psychiatric disease or seizures.

Adverse effects are more common (up to 50% of treatments) with the higher dosages of mefloquine required for treatment. These effects may be lessened by splitting administration into two doses separated by 6–8 hours. Serious neuropsychiatric toxicities (depression, confusion, acute psychosis, or seizures) have been reported in less than 1 in 1000 treatments, but some authorities believe that these are more common. Mefloquine can also alter cardiac conduction, and so it should not be coadministered with quinine, quinidine, or halofantrine, and caution is required if these drugs are used to treat malaria after mefloquine chemoprophylaxis. Mefloquine is generally considered safe in young children and pregnant women.

4. Quinine and quinidine—Quinine dihydrochloride and quinidine gluconate remain first-line therapies for falciparum malaria, especially severe disease, although toxicity concerns complicate therapy (Table 35–4). Quinine acts rapidly against the four species of human malaria parasites. Quinidine, the dextrorotatory stereoisomer of quinine, is at least as effective as quinine in the treatment of severe falciparum malaria.

Resistance of *P falciparum* to quinine is common in some areas of Southeast Asia, where the drug may fail if used alone to treat falciparum malaria. However, quinine still provides at least a partial therapeutic effect in most patients.

Quinine and quinidine are effective treatments for severe falciparum malaria, although intravenous artesunate is the standard of care. The drugs can be administered in divided doses or by continuous intravenous infusion; treatment should begin with a loading dose to rapidly achieve effective plasma concentrations. Intravenous quinine and quinidine should be administered with cardiac monitoring because of their cardiac toxicity and the relative unpredictability of their pharmacokinetics. Therapy should be changed to an oral agent as soon as the patient has improved and can tolerate oral medications.

In areas without newer combination regimens, oral quinine sulfate is an alternative first-line therapy for uncomplicated falciparum malaria, although poor tolerance may limit compliance. Quinine is commonly used with a second drug (most often doxycycline) to shorten the duration of use (usually to 3 days) and to limit toxicity. Therapeutic dosages of quinine and quinidine commonly cause tinnitus, headache, nausea, dizziness, flushing, and visual disturbances. Hematologic abnormalities include hemolysis (especially with G6PD deficiency), leukopenia, agranulocytosis, and thrombocytopenia. Therapeutic doses may cause hypoglycemia through stimulation of insulin release; this is a particular problem in severe

infections and in pregnant patients, who have increased sensitivity to insulin. Overly rapid infusions can cause severe hypotension. ECG abnormalities (QT prolongation) are fairly common, but dangerous arrhythmias are uncommon when the drugs are administered appropriately. Quinine should not be given concurrently with mefloquine and should be used with caution in a patient who has previously received mefloquine.

5. Primaquine—Primaquine phosphate, a synthetic 8-aminoquinoline, is the drug of choice for the eradication of dormant liver forms of *P vivax* and *P ovale* (Table 35–4). Primaquine is active against hepatic stages of all human malaria parasites. This action is optimal soon after therapy with chloroquine or quinine. Primaquine also acts against erythrocytic stage parasites, although this activity is too weak for the treatment of active disease, and against gametocytes.

For *P vivax* and *P ovale* infections, chloroquine or other drugs are used to eradicate erythrocytic forms, and if the G6PD level is normal, a 14-day course of primaquine (52.6 mg primaquine phosphate [30 mg base] daily) is initiated to eradicate liver hypnozoites and prevent a subsequent relapse. Some strains of *P vivax*, particularly in New Guinea and Southeast Asia, are relatively resistant to primaquine, and the drug may fail to eradicate liver forms.

Standard chemoprophylaxis does not prevent a relapse of *P vivax* or *P ovale* infections, since liver hypnozoites are not eradicated by chloroquine or other standard treatments. To diminish the likelihood of relapse, some authorities advocate the use of a treatment course of primaquine after the completion of travel to an endemic area. Primaquine can also be used for chemoprophylaxis to prevent *P falciparum* and *P vivax* infection in persons with normal levels of G6PD.

Primaquine in recommended doses is generally well tolerated. It infrequently causes nausea, epigastric pain, abdominal cramps, and headache, especially when taken on an empty stomach. Rare adverse effects include leukopenia, agranulocytosis, leukocytosis, and cardiac arrhythmias. Standard doses of primaquine may cause hemolysis or methemoglobinemia (manifested by cyanosis), especially in persons with G6PD deficiency or other hereditary metabolic defects. Patients should be tested for G6PD deficiency before primaquine is prescribed. When a patient is deficient in G6PD, treatment strategies may consist of (1) withholding therapy and treating subsequent relapses, if they occur, with chloroquine; (2) treating patients with standard dosing, paying close attention to their hematologic status; or (3) treating with weekly primaquine (45 mg base) for 8 weeks. G6PD-deficient individuals of Mediterranean and Asian ancestry are most likely to have severe deficiency, while those of African ancestry usually have a milder biochemical defect. This difference can be taken into consideration in choosing a treatment strategy. Primaquine should be discontinued if there is evidence of hemolysis or anemia and should be avoided in pregnancy.

6. Inhibitors of folate synthesis—Inhibitors of two parasite enzymes involved in folate metabolism, dihydrofolate reductase (DHFR) and dihydropteroate synthase (DHPS), are used, generally in combination regimens, for the treatment and prevention of malaria, although the drugs are rather slow acting and now limited by resistance.

Fansidar is a fixed combination of sulfadoxine (500 mg) and pyrimethamine (25 mg). The long half-lives of its components allow weekly dosing for chemoprophylaxis, but due to rare serious side effects with long-term dosing, this drug is no longer recommended for this purpose. For treatment, advantages of sulfadoxine-pyrimethamine include ease of administration (a single oral dose) and low cost. However, resistance is now a major problem.

Sulfadoxine-pyrimethamine is a component of two combination regimens for uncomplicated malaria recommended by the WHO (Table 35–3). Sulfadoxine-pyrimethamine plus artesunate has shown efficacy in some areas but is best replaced by more effective combination regimens in most areas. Amodiaquine plus sulfadoxine-pyrimethamine has shown quite good efficacy in Africa, despite increasing resistance to both components. It is recommended monthly during the rainy season for chemoprophylaxis in regions with seasonal malaria transmission and limited drug resistance. Another antifolate combination, trimethoprim-sulfamethoxazole (TMP-SMZ), is widely used to prevent coinfections in patients infected with HIV, and it offers partial protection against malaria.

7. Artemisinins—Artemisinin (qinghaosu) is a sesquiterpene lactone endoperoxide, the active component of an herbal medicine that has been used for various indications in China for over 2000 years. Analogs have been synthesized to increase solubility and improve antimalarial efficacy. The most important of these analogs are artesunate, artemether, and dihydroartemisinin. The WHO encourages availability of oral artemisinins only in coformulated combination regimens.

Artemisinins act very rapidly against all erythrocytic-stage human malaria parasites. Of concern, delayed clearance of parasites and some clinical failures have been seen after treatment with artesunate in parts of Southeast Asia, heralding the emergence of artemisinin resistance in this region.

Artemisinins are playing an increasing role in the treatment of malaria, including multidrug-resistant *P falciparum* malaria. However, due to their short plasma half-lives, recrudescence rates are unacceptably high after short-course therapy, leading to use in conjunction with another agent. Also because of their short-half lives, they are not useful in chemoprophylaxis.

The ACTs that are currently most advocated in Africa are artesunate plus amodiaquine (ASAQ) and artemether plus lumefantrine (Coartem), each of which is available as a coformulated product. Another ACT, artesunate plus mefloquine is used mostly outside of Africa; its efficacy may be declining in parts of Asia. Dihydroartemisinin-piperaquine is a newer ACT that has shown excellent efficacy and is the first-line regimen in some countries in Southeast Asia, but recent studies have shown declining efficacy in Cambodia. The newest ACT, artesunate-pyronaridine, is approved in Cambodia.

In studies of severe malaria, intramuscular artemether was at least as effective as intramuscular quinine, and intravenous artesunate was superior to intravenous quinine in terms of efficacy and tolerability. Thus, the standard of care for severe malaria is intravenous artesunate, when it is available, although parenteral quinine and quinidine remain acceptable alternatives. Artesunate and artemether have also been effective in the treatment of severe malaria when administered rectally, offering a valuable treatment modality when parenteral therapy is not available.

Artemisinins are very well tolerated. The most commonly reported adverse effects have been nausea, vomiting, and diarrhea, which may often be due to acute malaria, rather than drug toxicity. Neutropenia, anemia, hemolysis, and elevated levels of liver enzymes have been noted rarely. Hemolysis may occur weeks after therapy with intravenous artesunate. Artemisinins are teratogenic in animals, and they should be avoided in the first trimester of pregnancy for uncomplicated malaria. However, for severe malaria, for which all available treatments entail some risk, the WHO endorses the use of intravenous artesunate or quinine while additional data are gathered on artesunate safety.

8. Atovaquone plus proguanil (Malarone)—Atovaquone, a hydroxynaphthoquinone, is not effective when used alone, due to rapid development of drug resistance. However, Malarone, a fixed combination of atovaquone (250 mg) and the antifolate proguanil (100 mg), is highly effective for both the treatment and chemoprophylaxis of falciparum malaria, and it is approved for both indications in the United States (Table 35–4). It also appears to be active against other species of malaria parasites. Unlike most other antimalarials, Malarone provides activity against both erythrocytic and hepatic stage parasites.

For treatment, Malarone is given at an adult dose of four tablets daily for 3 days. For chemoprophylaxis, Malarone must be taken daily. It has an advantage over mefloquine and doxycycline in requiring shorter durations of treatment before and after the period at risk for malaria transmission, due to activity against liver-stage parasites. It should be taken with food.

Malarone is generally well tolerated. Adverse effects include abdominal pain, nausea, vomiting, diarrhea, headache, and rash, and these are more common with the higher dose required for treatment. Reversible elevations in liver enzymes have been reported. The safety of atovaquone in pregnancy is unknown.

9. Antibiotics—A number of antibacterials in addition to the folate antagonists and sulfonamides are slow-acting antimalarials. None of the antibiotics should be used as single agents for the treatment of malaria due to their slow rate of action.

Doxycycline is commonly used in the treatment of falciparum malaria in conjunction with quinidine or quinine, allowing a shorter and better-tolerated course of those drugs (Table 35–4). Doxycycline is also a standard chemoprophylactic drug, especially for use in areas of Southeast Asia with high rates of resistance to other antimalarials, including mefloquine. Doxycycline side effects include gastrointestinal symptoms, candidal vaginitis, and photosensitivity. The drug should be taken while upright with a large amount of water to avoid esophageal irritation.

Clindamycin can be used in conjunction with quinine or quinidine in those for whom doxycycline is not recommended, such as children and pregnant women (Table 35–4). The most common toxicities with clindamycin are gastrointestinal.

10. Halofantrine and lumefantrine—Halofantrine, a phenanthrene-methanol related to quinine, is effective against erythrocytic stages of all four human malaria species, but it is rarely used due to toxicity concerns.

Lumefantrine, an aryl alcohol related to halofantrine, is available only as a fixed-dose combination with artemether (Coartem or Riamet). Oral absorption is highly variable and improved when the drug is taken with food. Use of Coartem with a fatty meal is recommended. Coartem is highly effective for the treatment of falciparum malaria, but it requires twice-daily dosing. Despite this limitation, due to its reliable efficacy against falciparum malaria, Coartem is the first-line therapy for malaria in many malarious countries. Coartem is well tolerated; side effects include headache, dizziness, loss of appetite, gastrointestinal symptoms, and palpitations. Importantly, Coartem does not generally cause QT prolongation or the serious cardiac toxicity seen with halofantrine.

▶ **Prevention**

Malaria is transmitted by night-biting anopheline mosquitoes. Bed nets, in particular nets treated with permethrin insecticides, are heavily promoted as inexpensive means of antimalarial protection, and improvement in mortality rates has been demonstrated. Extensive efforts are also underway to develop a malaria vaccine, and partial protection of African children has been demonstrated with the RTS,S vaccine, which is under development, but a vaccine offering a high level of protection is not anticipated in the near future. The availability of improved modalities to control mosquito

vectors and treat and prevent malaria has heightened enthusiasm for malaria elimination, and there have been important gains in some areas; however, control remains very challenging in highly endemic regions, and elimination is not expected in these areas in the foreseeable future.

When travelers from nonendemic to endemic countries are counseled on the prevention of malaria, it is imperative to emphasize measures to prevent mosquito bites (insect repellents, insecticides, and bed nets), since parasites are increasingly resistant to multiple drugs and no chemoprophylactic regimen is fully protective. Chemoprophylaxis is recommended for all travelers from nonendemic regions to endemic areas, although risks vary greatly for different locations, and some tropical areas entail no risk; specific recommendations for travel to different locales are available from the CDC (www.cdc.gov; 877-FYI-TRIP). Recommendations from the CDC include the use of chloroquine for chemoprophylaxis in the few areas with only chloroquine-sensitive malaria parasites (principally the Caribbean and Central America west of the Panama Canal), mefloquine or Malarone for most other malarious areas, and doxycycline for areas with a high prevalence of multidrug-resistant falciparum malaria (principally parts of Southeast Asia) (Table 35–5). Recommendations should be checked regularly because they may change in response to changing resistance patterns and increasing experience with new drugs. In some circumstances, it may be appropriate for travelers to not use chemoprophylaxis but to carry supplies of drugs with them in case a febrile illness develops and medical attention is unavailable. Regimens for self-treatment include ACTs, Malarone, and quinine. Most authorities do not recommend routine terminal chemoprophylaxis with primaquine to eradicate dormant hepatic stages of *P vivax* and *P ovale* after travel, but this may be appropriate in some circumstances, especially for travelers with major exposure to these parasites.

Table 35–5. Drugs for the prevention of malaria in travelers.[1]

Drug	Use[2]	Adult Dosage (all oral)[3]
Chloroquine	Areas without resistant *Plasmodium falciparum*	500 mg weekly
Malarone	Areas with multidrug-resistant *P falciparum*	1 tablet (250 mg atovaquone/100 mg proguanil) daily
Mefloquine	Areas with chloroquine-resistant *P falciparum*	250 mg weekly
Doxycycline	Areas with multidrug-resistant *P falciparum*	100 mg daily
Primaquine[4]	Terminal prophylaxis of *Plasmodium vivax* and *Plasmodium ovale* infections; alternative for *P falciparum* prophylaxis	30 mg base daily for 14 days after travel

[1]Recommendations may change, as resistance to all available drugs is increasing. See text for additional information on toxicities and cautions. For additional details and pediatric dosing, see Centers for Disease Control and Prevention's guidelines (phone: 800-CDC-INFO; http://wwwnc.cdc.gov/travel/). Travelers to remote areas should consider carrying effective therapy (see text) for use if a febrile illness develops, and they cannot reach medical attention quickly.
[2]Areas without known chloroquine-resistant *P falciparum* are Central America west of the Panama Canal, Haiti, Dominican Republic, Egypt, and most malarious countries of the Middle East. Malarone or mefloquine is currently recommended for other malarious areas except for border areas of Thailand, where doxycycline is recommended.
[3]For drugs other than primaquine, begin 1–2 weeks before departure (except 2 days before for doxycycline and Malarone) and continue for 4 weeks after leaving the endemic area (except 1 week for Malarone). All dosages refer to salts unless otherwise indicated.
[4]Screen for glucose-6-phosphate dehydrogenase deficiency before using primaquine.
Reproduced, with permission, from Katzung BG. *Basic & Clinical Pharmacology.* 11th edition. McGraw-Hill, 2009.

Regular chemoprophylaxis is not a standard management practice in developing world populations due to the expense and potential toxicities of long-term therapy. However, intermittent preventive therapy, whereby at-risk populations (in particular pregnant women and children) receive antimalarial therapy at set intervals, is of increasing interest. This strategy may decrease the incidence of malaria while allowing antimalarial immunity to develop. During pregnancy, intermittent preventive therapy with sulfadoxine-pyrimethamine, provided once during both the second and third trimesters, has improved pregnancy outcomes. In infants, therapy with sulfadoxine-pyrimethamine following standard immunization schedules has offered benefits. With increasing resistance the preventive efficacy of sulfadoxine-pyrimethamine is likely falling, and the long-acting ACT dihydroartemisinin-piperaquine is a promising replacement. In areas with seasonal malaria transmission and limited drug resistance, principally the Sahel sub-region of West Africa, the policy is to administer amodiaquine and sulfadoxine-pyrimethamine to children monthly during the transmission season.

Prognosis

When treated appropriately, uncomplicated malaria generally responds well, with resolution of fevers within 1–2 days and a mortality of about 0.1%. Severe malaria can commonly progress to death, but many children respond well to therapy. In the developed world, mortality from malaria is mostly in adults, and often follows extended illnesses and secondary complications long after eradication of the malarial infection. Pregnant women are at particular risk during their first pregnancy. Malaria in pregnancy also increases the likelihood of poor pregnancy outcomes, with increased prematurity, low birth weight, and mortality.

When to Refer

Referral to an expert on infectious diseases or travel medicine is important with all cases of malaria in the United States, and in particular for falciparum malaria; referral should not delay initial diagnosis and therapy, since delays in therapy can lead to severe illness or death.

When to Admit

- Admission for non-falciparum malaria is only warranted if specific problems that require hospital management are present.
- Patients with falciparum malaria are generally admitted because the disease can progress rapidly to severe illness; exceptions may be made with individuals who are from malaria-endemic areas, and thus expected to have a degree of immunity, who are without evidence of severe disease, and who are judged able to return promptly for medical attention if their disease progresses.

Ashley EA et al; Tracking Resistance to Artemisinin Collaboration (TRAC). Spread of artemisinin resistance in *Plasmodium falciparum* malaria. N Engl J Med. 2014 Jul 31;371(5):411–23. [PMID: 25075834]

Baird KJ et al. Diagnosis and treatment of *Plasmodium vivax* malaria. Adv Parasitol. 2012;80:203–70. [PMID: 23199489]
Dondorp AM et al; AQUAMAT Group. Artesunate versus quinine in the treatment of severe falciparum malaria in African children (AQUAMAT): an open-label, randomised trial. Lancet. 2010 Nov 13;376(9753):1647–57. [PMID: 21062666]
Nadjm B et al. Malaria: an update for physicians. Infect Dis Clin North Am. 2012 Jun;26(2):243–59. [PMID: 22632637]
Rolling T et al. Delayed hemolysis after treatment with parenteral artesunate in African children with severe malaria—a double-center prospective study. J Infect Dis. 2014 Jun 15; 209(12):1921–8. [PMID: 24376273]
RTS,S Clinical Trials Partnership. Efficacy and safety of RTS,S/AS01 malaria vaccine with or without a booster dose in infants and children in Africa: final results of a phase 3, individually randomised, controlled trial. Lancet. 2015 Jul 4; 386(9988):31–45. Erratum in: Lancet. 2015 Jul 4;386(9988):30. [PMID: 25913272]
Spring MD et al. Dihydroartemisinin-piperaquine failure associated with a triple mutant including *kelch13 C580Y* in Cambodia: an observational cohort study. Lancet Infect Dis. 2015 Jun;15(6):683–91. [PMID: 25877962]
White NJ et al. Malaria. Lancet. 2014 Feb 22;383(9918):723–35. [PMID: 23953767]
Whitty CJ et al. Investigation and treatment of imported malaria in non-endemic countries. BMJ. 2013 May 21;346:f2900. [PMID: 23693055]
World Health Organization. *Guidelines for the treatment of malaria*, 3rd edition. Geneva, Switzerland, 2015. http://www.who.int/malaria/publications/atoz/9789241549127/en/

BABESIOSIS

ESSENTIALS OF DIAGNOSIS

- History of tick bite or exposure to ticks.
- Fever, flu-like symptoms, anemia.
- Intraerythrocytic parasites on Giemsa-stained blood smears.
- Positive serologic tests.

General Considerations

Babesiosis is an uncommon intraerythrocytic infection caused mainly by two *Babesia* species and transmitted by *Ixodes* ticks. In the United States, hundreds of cases of babesiosis have been reported, and infection is caused by *Babesia microti*, which also infects wild mammals. Most babesiosis in the United States occurs in the coastal northeast, with some cases also in the upper midwest, following the geographic range of the vector *Ixodes scapularis*, and Lyme disease and anaplasmosis, which are spread by the same vector. The incidence of the disease appears to be increasing in some areas. Babesiosis is caused by *Babesia divergens* in Europe and by *Babesia venatorum* in China. Rare episodes of illnesses caused by other Babesia-like organisms have been reported from other areas. Babesiosis can also be transmitted by blood transfusion.

Clinical Findings

A. Symptoms and Signs

Serosurveys suggest that asymptomatic infections are common in endemic areas. With *B microti* infections, symptoms appear 1 to several weeks after a tick bite; parasitemia is evident after 2–4 weeks. Patients usually do not recall the tick bite. The typical flu-like illness develops gradually and is characterized by fever, fatigue, headache, arthralgia, and myalgia. Other findings may include nausea, vomiting, abdominal pain, sore throat, depression, emotional lability, anemia, thrombocytopenia, and splenomegaly. Parasitemia may continue for months to years, with or without symptoms, and the disease is usually self-limited. Severe complications are most likely to occur in older persons or in those who have had splenectomy. Serious complications include respiratory failure, hemolytic anemia, disseminated intravascular coagulation, heart failure, and acute kidney injury. In a study of hospitalized patients, the mortality rate was 6.5%. Most recognized *B divergens* infections in Europe have been in patients who have had splenectomy. These infections progress rapidly with high fever, severe hemolytic anemia, jaundice, hemoglobinuria, and acute kidney injury, with death rates over 40%.

B. Laboratory Findings

Identification of the intraerythrocytic parasite on Giemsa-stained blood smears establishes the diagnosis (Figure 35–6). These can be confused with malaria parasites, but the morphology is distinctive. Repeated smears are often necessary because well under 1% of erythrocytes may be infected, especially early in infection, although parasitemias can exceed 10%. An indirect immunofluorescent antibody test for *B microti* is available from the CDC; antibody is detectable within 2–4 weeks after the onset of symptoms and persists for months. Diagnosis can also be made by PCR or by inoculation of hamsters or gerbils.

▲ **Figure 35–6.** Blood smear showing *Babesia* spp. rings with basophilic stippling. (From Dr. Mae Melvin, Public Health Image Library, CDC.)

Treatment

Most patients have a mild illness and recover without therapy. Standard therapy for mild to moderate disease is a 7-day course of atovaquone (750 mg orally every 12 hours) plus azithromycin (600 mg orally once daily), which is equally effective and better tolerated than the alternative regimen, a 7-day course of quinine (650 mg orally three times daily) plus clindamycin (600 mg orally three times daily). However, there is more experience using quinine plus clindamycin, and this regimen is recommended for severe disease. Exchange transfusion has been used successfully in severely ill asplenic patients and those with parasitemia greater than 10%.

Vannier E et al. Human babesiosis. N Engl J Med. 2012 Jun 21; 366(25):2397–407. [PMID: 22716978]
Vannier EG et al. Babesiosis. Infect Dis Clin North Am. 2015 Jun; 29(2):357–70. [PMID: 25999229]

TOXOPLASMOSIS

> ### ESSENTIALS OF DIAGNOSIS
>
> ▶ Infection confirmed by isolation of *Toxoplasma gondii* or identification of tachyzoites in tissue or body fluids.
>
> **Primary infection**
> ▶ Fever, malaise, headache, sore throat.
> ▶ Lymphadenopathy.
> ▶ Positive IgG and IgM serologic tests.
>
> **Congenital infection**
> ▶ Follows acute infection of seronegative mothers and leads to CNS abnormalities and retinochoroiditis.
>
> **Infection in immunocompromised persons**
> ▶ Reactivation leads to encephalitis, retinochoroiditis, pneumonitis, myocarditis.
> ▶ Positive IgG but negative IgM serologic tests.

General Considerations

T gondii, an obligate intracellular protozoan, is found worldwide in humans and in many species of mammals and birds. The definitive hosts are cats. Humans are infected after ingestion of cysts in raw or undercooked meat, ingestion of oocysts in food or water contaminated by cats, transplacental transmission of trophozoites or, rarely, direct inoculation of trophozoites via blood transfusion or organ transplantation. *Toxoplasma* seroprevalence varies widely. It has decreased in the United States to 20–30% or less, but it is much higher in other countries in both the developed and developing worlds, where it may exceed 80%. In the United States, *T gondii* is estimated to infect 1.1 million persons each year, with resultant chorioretinitis developing in 21,000 and vision loss in 4800.

► Clinical Findings

A. Symptoms and Signs

The clinical manifestations of toxoplasmosis may be grouped into four syndromes.

1. Primary infection in the immunocompetent person— After ingestion, *T gondii* infection progresses from the gastrointestinal tract to lymphatics, and then dissemination. Most acute infections are asymptomatic. About 10–20% are symptomatic after an incubation period of 1–2 weeks. Acute infections in immunocompetent persons typically present as mild, febrile illnesses that resemble infectious mononucleosis. Nontender cervical or diffuse lymphadenopathy may persist for weeks to months. Systemic findings may include fever, malaise, headache, sore throat, rash, myalgias, hepatosplenomegaly, and atypical lymphocytosis. Rare severe manifestations are pneumonitis, meningoencephalitis, hepatitis, myocarditis, polymyositis, and retinochoroiditis. Symptoms may fluctuate, but most patients recover spontaneously within at most a few months.

2. Congenital infection— Congenital transmission occurs as a result of infection, which may be symptomatic or asymptomatic, in a nonimmune woman during pregnancy. Fetal infection follows maternal infection in 30–50% of cases, but this risk varies by trimester: 10–25% during the first, 30–50% during the second, and 60% or higher during the third trimester. In the United States, an estimated 400 to 4000 congenital infections occur yearly. While the risk of fetal infection increases, the risk of severe fetal disease decreases over the course of pregnancy. Early fetal infections commonly lead to spontaneous abortion, stillbirths, or severe neonatal disease, including neurologic manifestations. Neurologic findings can include seizures, psychomotor retardation, deafness, and hydrocephalus. Retinochoroiditis and other sight-threatening eye lesions may develop. Systemic findings include fever or hypothermia, jaundice, vomiting, diarrhea, hepatosplenomegaly, pneumonitis, myocarditis, and rash. Infections later in pregnancy less commonly lead to major fetal problems. Most infants appear normal at birth, but they may have subtle abnormalities and progress to symptoms and signs of congenital toxoplasmosis later in life. Hepatosplenomegaly and lymphadenopathy may develop in the first few months of life; CNS and eye disease often present later. The most common late presentation of congenital toxoplasmosis is retinochoroiditis.

3. Retinochoroiditis— This manifestation of congenital toxoplasmosis presents weeks to years after congenital infection, commonly in teenagers or young adults. Retinochoroiditis also is seen in persons who acquire infection early in life, and these patients more often present with unilateral disease. Uveitis is also seen. Disease presents with pain, photophobia, and visual changes, usually without systemic symptoms. Signs and symptoms eventually improve, but visual defects may persist. Rarely, progression may result in glaucoma and blindness.

4. Disease in the immunocompromised person— Reactivated toxoplasmosis occurs in patients with AIDS, cancer, or those given immunosuppressive drugs. In patients with advanced AIDS, the most common manifestation is encephalitis, with multiple necrotizing brain lesions. The encephalitis usually presents subacutely, with fever, headache, altered mental status, focal neurologic findings, and other evidence of brain lesions. Less common manifestations of toxoplasmosis in patients with AIDS are chorioretinitis and pneumonitis. Chorioretinitis presents with ocular pain and alterations in vision. Pneumonitis presents with fever, cough, and dyspnea. Toxoplasmosis can develop in seronegative recipients of solid organ or bone marrow transplants due to reactivation or, more rarely, transmission of infection. Reactivation also can occur in those with hematologic malignancies or treated with immunosuppressive drugs. With primary or reactivated disease in those with immunodeficiency due to malignancy or immunosuppressive drugs, toxoplasmosis is similar to that in individuals with AIDS, but pneumonitis and myocarditis are more common.

B. Diagnostic Testing

1. Identification of parasites— Organisms can be seen in tissue or body fluids, although they may be difficult to identify; special staining techniques can facilitate identification. The demonstration of tachyzoites indicates acute infection; cysts may represent either acute or chronic infection. With lymphadenopathy due to toxoplasmosis, examination of lymph nodes usually does not show organisms. Parasite identification can also be made by inoculation of tissue culture or mice. PCR can be used for sensitive identification of organisms in amniotic fluid, blood, CSF, aqueous humor, and bronchoalveolar lavage fluid.

2. Serologic diagnosis— Multiple serologic methods are used, including the Sabin-Feldman dye test, enzyme-linked immunosorbent assay (ELISA), indirect fluorescent antibody test, and agglutination tests. IgG antibodies are seen within 1–2 weeks of infection, and usually persist for life. IgM antibodies peak earlier than IgG and decline more rapidly, although they may persist for years. In immunocompromised individuals in whom reactivation is suspected, a positive IgG assay indicates distant infection, and thus the potential for reactivated disease; a negative IgG argues strongly against reactivation toxoplasmosis. With reactivation in immunocompromised persons, IgM tests are generally negative.

3. During pregnancy and in newborns— Conversion from a negative to positive serologic test or rising titers are suggestive of acute infection, but tests are not routinely performed during pregnancy. When pregnant women are screened, negative IgG and IgM assays exclude active infection, but indicate the risk of infection during the pregnancy. The pattern of positive IgG with negative IgM is highly suggestive of chronic infection, with no risk of congenital disease unless the mother is severely immunocompromised. A positive IgM test is concerning for new infection because of the risk of congenital disease. Confirmatory testing should be performed before consideration of treatment or possible termination of pregnancy due to the limitations of available tests. Tests of the avidity of anti-IgG antibodies can be helpful, but a battery of tests is needed for confirmation of acute infection during pregnancy. When acute infection during pregnancy is suspected, PCR of amniotic fluid offers a sensitive assessment for congenital disease; this test should optimally be performed at 18 weeks of gestation. In newborns, positive IgM or IgA antibody tests are indicative of congenital infection, although the diagnosis is not ruled out by a negative test. Positive IgG assays may represent transfer of maternal antibodies without infection of the infant. Organisms may be identified by PCR; smears; or culture of blood, CSF, or tissue.

4. In immunocompetent individuals—Individuals with a suggestive clinical syndrome should be tested for IgG and IgM antibodies. Seroconversion, a 16-fold rise in antibody titer, or an IgM titer greater than 1:64 are suggestive of acute infection, although false-positive results may occur. Acute infection can also be diagnosed by detection of tachyzoites in tissue, culture of organisms, or PCR of blood or body fluids. Histologic evaluation of lymph nodes can show characteristic morphology, with or without organisms.

5. In immunodeficient individuals—A presentation consistent with toxoplasmic encephalitis warrants imaging of the brain. CT and MRI scans typically show multiple ring-enhancing cerebral lesions, most commonly involving the corticomedullary junction and basal ganglia. MRI is the more sensitive imaging modality. In AIDS patients with a positive IgG serologic test and no recent antitoxoplasma or antiviral therapy, the predictive value of a typical imaging study is about 80%. The other common diagnosis in this setting is CNS lymphoma, which more typically causes a single brain lesion. The differential diagnosis also includes tuberculoma, bacterial brain abscess, fungal abscess, and carcinoma. Diagnosis of CNS toxoplasmosis is most typically made after a therapeutic trial, with clinical and radiologic improvement expected within 2–3 weeks. Definitive diagnosis requires brain biopsy and search for organisms and typical histology. In retinochoroiditis, funduscopic examination shows vitreous inflammatory reaction, white retinal lesions, and pigmented scars. Diagnosis of other clinical entities in immunocompromised individuals is generally based on histology.

▶ Treatment

A. Approach to Treatment

Therapy is generally not necessary in immunocompetent persons, since primary illness is self-limited. However, for severe, persistent, or visceral disease, treatment for 2–4 weeks may be considered. Treatment is appropriate for primary infection during pregnancy because the risk of fetal transmission or the severity of congenital disease may be reduced. For retinochoroiditis, most episodes are self-limited, and opinions vary on indications for treatment. Treatment is often advocated for episodes with decreases in visual acuity, multiple or large lesions, macular lesions, significant inflammation, or persistence for over a month. Immunocompromised patients with active infection must be treated. For those with transient immunodeficiency, therapy can be continued for 4–6 weeks after cessation of symptoms. For those with persistent immunodeficiency, such as AIDS patients, full therapy for 4–6 weeks is followed by maintenance therapy with lower doses of drugs. Immunodeficient patients who are asymptomatic but have a positive IgG serologic test should receive long-term chemoprophylaxis.

B. Medications

Drugs for toxoplasmosis are active only against tachyzoites, so they do not eradicate infection. Standard therapy is the combination of pyrimethamine (200 mg loading dose, then 50–75 mg [1 mg/kg] orally once daily) plus sulfadiazine (1–1.5 g orally four times daily), with folinic acid (10–20 mg orally once daily) to prevent bone marrow suppression. Patients should be screened for a history of sulfonamide sensitivity (skin rashes, gastrointestinal symptoms, hepatotoxicity). To prevent crystal-induced nephrotoxicity, good urinary output should be maintained. Pyrimethamine side effects include headache and gastrointestinal symptoms. Even with folinic acid therapy, bone marrow suppression may occur; platelet and white blood cell counts should be monitored at least weekly. A first-line alternative is clindamycin (600 mg orally four times daily) replacing sulfadiazine as the standard therapy regimen. Another alternative is replacement of sulfadiazine with TMP-SMZ. Pyrimethamine is not used during the first trimester of pregnancy due to its teratogenicity. Standard therapy for acute toxoplasmosis during pregnancy is spiramycin (1 g orally three times daily until delivery) to decrease the risk of fetal infection; it reduces the frequency of transmission to the fetus by about 60%. Spiramycin does not cross the placenta, so when fetal infection is documented or for acute infections late in pregnancy (which commonly lead to fetal transmission) treatment with combination regimens as described above is indicated.

▶ Prevention

Prevention of primary infection centers on avoidance of undercooked meat or contact with material contaminated by cat feces, particularly for seronegative pregnant women and immunocompromised persons. Irradiation, cooking to 66°C, or freezing to –20°C kills tissue cysts. Thorough cleaning of hands and surfaces is needed after contact with raw meat or areas contaminated by cats. Oocysts passed in cat feces can remain infective for a year or more, but fresh oocysts are not infective for 48 hours. For best protection, litter boxes should be changed daily and soaked in boiling water for 5 minutes, gloves should be worn when gardening, fruits and vegetables should be thoroughly washed, and ingestion of dried meat should be avoided.

Universal screening of pregnant women for *T gondii* antibodies is conducted in some countries but not the United States. Pregnant women should ideally have their serum examined for IgG and IgM antibody, and those with negative titers should adhere to the prevention measures described above. Seronegative women who continue to have environmental exposure should undergo repeat serologic screening several times during pregnancy.

For immunocompromised individuals, chemoprophylaxis to prevent primary or reactivated infection is warranted. For hematopoietic cell transplant recipients and advanced AIDS patients, chemoprophylaxis with TMP-SMZ (one double-strength tablet daily or two tablets three times weekly), used for protection against *Pneumocystis*, is effective against *T gondii*. Alternatives are pyrimethamine plus either sulfadoxine or dapsone (various regimens). In AIDS patients, chemoprophylaxis can be discontinued if antiretroviral therapy leads to immune reconstitution.

Gajurel K et al. *Toxoplasma* prophylaxis in haematopoietic cell transplant recipients: a review of the literature and recommendations. Curr Opin Infect Dis. 2015 Aug;28(4):283–92. [PMID: 26098500]

Jones JL et al. Neglected parasitic infections in the United States: toxoplasmosis. Am J Trop Med Hyg. 2014 May;90(5):794–9. [PMID: 24808246]

Robert-Gangneux F et al. Epidemiology of and diagnostic strategies for toxoplasmosis. Clin Microbiol Rev. 2012 Apr;25(2):264–96. [PMID: 22491772]

AMEBIASIS

ESSENTIALS OF DIAGNOSIS

► Organisms or antigen present in stools or abscess aspirate.

► Positive serologic tests with colitis or hepatic abscess, but these may represent prior infections.

► Mild to moderate colitis with recurrent diarrhea.

► Severe colitis including bloody diarrhea, fever, and abdominal pain, with potential progression to hemorrhage or perforation.

► Hepatic abscess with fever, hepatomegaly, and abdominal pain.

General Considerations

The *Entamoeba* complex contains three morphologically identical species: *Entamoeba dispar* and *Entamoeba moshkovskii*, which are avirulent, and *Entamoeba histolytica*, which may be an avirulent intestinal commensal or lead to serious disease. Disease follows penetration of the intestinal wall, resulting in diarrhea, and with severe involvement, dysentery or extraintestinal disease, most commonly liver abscess.

E histolytica infections are present worldwide but are most prevalent in subtropical and tropical areas under conditions of crowding, poor sanitation, and poor nutrition. Of the estimated 500 million persons worldwide infected with *Entamoeba*, most are infected with *E dispar* and an estimated 10% with *E histolytica*. The prevalence of *E moshkovskii* is unknown. Mortality from invasive *E histolytica* infections is estimated at 100,000 per year.

Humans are the only established *E histolytica* host. Transmission occurs through ingestion of cysts from fecally contaminated food or water, facilitated by person-to-person spread, flies and other arthropods as mechanical vectors, and use of human excrement as fertilizer. Urban outbreaks have occurred because of common-source water contamination.

Clinical Findings

A. Symptoms and Signs

1. Intestinal amebiasis—In most infected persons, the organism lives as a commensal, and the carrier is without symptoms. With symptomatic disease, diarrhea may begin within a week of infection, although an incubation period of 2–4 weeks is more common, with gradual onset of abdominal pain and diarrhea. Fever is uncommon. Periods of remission and recurrence may last days to weeks or longer. Abdominal examination may show distention, tenderness, hyperperistalsis, and hepatomegaly. Microscopic hematochezia is common. More severe presentations include colitis and dysentery, with more extensive diarrhea (10–20 stools per day) and bloody stools. With dysentery, physical findings include high fevers, prostration, vomiting, abdominal pain and tenderness, hepatic enlargement, and hypotension. Severe presentations are more common in young children, pregnant women, those who are malnourished, and those receiving corticosteroids. Thus, in endemic regions, corticosteroids should not be started for presumed inflammatory bowel disease without first ruling out amebiasis. Fulminant amebic colitis can progress to necrotizing colitis, intestinal perforation, mucosal sloughing, and severe hemorrhage, with mortality rates over 40%. More chronic complications of intestinal amebiasis include chronic diarrhea with weight loss, which may last for months to years; bowel ulcerations; and amebic appendicitis. Localized granulomatous lesions (amebomas) can present after either dysentery or chronic intestinal infection. Clinical findings include pain, obstructive symptoms, and hemorrhage and may suggest intestinal carcinoma.

2. Extraintestinal amebiasis—The most common extraintestinal manifestation is amebic liver abscess. This can occur with colitis, but more frequently presents without history of prior intestinal symptoms. Patients present with the acute or gradual onset of abdominal pain, fever, an enlarged and tender liver, anorexia, and weight loss. Diarrhea is present in a small number of patients. Physical examination may show intercostal tenderness. Abscesses are most commonly single and in the right lobe of the liver, and they are much more common in men. Without prompt treatment, amebic abscesses may rupture into the pleural, peritoneal, or pericardial space, which is often fatal. Amebic infections may rarely occur throughout the body, including the lungs, brain, and genitourinary system.

B. Laboratory Findings

Laboratory studies with intestinal amebiasis show leukocytosis and hematochezia, with fecal leukocytes not present in all cases. With extraintestinal amebiasis, leukocytosis and elevated liver function studies are seen.

C. Diagnostic Testing

Diagnosis is by finding *E histolytica* or its antigen or by serologic tests. However, each method has limitations.

1. Intestinal amebiasis—Diagnosis is most commonly made by identifying organisms in the stool. *E histolytica* and *E dispar* cannot be distinguished, but the identification of amebic trophozoites or cysts in a symptomatic patient is highly suggestive of amebiasis. Stool evaluation for organisms is not highly sensitive (~30–50% for amebic colitis), and at least three stool specimens should be evaluated after concentration and staining. Multiple serologic assays are available; these tests are fairly sensitive, although sensitivity is lower (~70% in colitis) early in illness, and they cannot distinguish recent and old disease, as they remain positive for years after infection. A commercially available stool antigen test (TechLab II) offers improved sensitivity (more than 90% for colitis); it requires fresh or frozen (not preserved) stool specimens. PCR-based tests are available but not used routinely. Colonoscopy of uncleansed bowel typically shows no specific findings in mild intestinal disease; in severe disease, ulcers may be found with intact intervening friable mucosa, resembling inflammatory bowel disease (Figure 35–7). Examination of fresh ulcer exudate for motile trophozoites and for *E histolytica* antigen may yield a diagnosis.

2. Hepatic abscess—Serologic tests for anti-amebic antibodies are almost always positive, except very early in the infection. Thus, a negative test in a suspicious case should be repeated in about a week. The TechLab II antigen test can be used to test serum, with good sensitivity if used before the initiation of therapy. Examination of stools for organisms or antigen is frequently negative; the antigen test is positive in ~40% of cases. As imaging studies cannot distinguish amebic and pyogenic abscesses, when a diagnosis is not available from serologic studies, percutaneous aspiration may be indicated, ideally with an image-guided needle. Aspiration typically yields brown or yellow fluid. Detection of organisms in the aspirate is uncommon, but detection of *E histolytica* antigen is very sensitive and diagnostic. The key risk of aspiration is peritoneal spillage leading to peritonitis from amebas or other (pyogenic or echinococcal) organisms.

D. Imaging

Liver abscesses can be identified by ultrasonography, CT, or MRI, typically with round or oval low-density nonhomogeneous lesions, with abrupt transition from normal liver to the lesion, and hypoechoic centers. Abscesses are most commonly single, but more than one may be present. The right lobe is usually involved.

▶ Treatment

Treatment of amebiasis generally entails the use of metronidazole or tinidazole to eradicate tissue trophozoites and a luminal amebicide to eradicate intestinal cysts (Table 35–6). Asymptomatic infection with *E dispar* does not require therapy. This organism cannot be differentiated morphologically from *E histolytica*, but with negative serology *E dispar* colonization is likely, and treatment is not indicated. Colonization with *E histolytica* is generally treated with a luminal agent. Effective luminal agents are diloxanide furoate (500 mg orally three times daily with meals for 10 days), iodoquinol (diiodohydroxyquin; 650 mg orally three times daily for 21 days), and paromomycin (30 mg/kg base orally, maximum 3 g, in three divided doses after meals daily for 7 days). Side effects associated with luminal agents are flatulence with diloxanide furoate, mild diarrhea with iodoquinol, and gastrointestinal symptoms with paromomycin. Relative contraindications are thyroid disease for iodoquinol and kidney disease for iodoquinol or paromomycin.

Treatment of intestinal amebiasis requires metronidazole (750 mg orally three times daily for 10 days) or tinidazole (2 g orally once daily for 3 days for mild disease and 5 days for serious disease) plus a luminal agent (Table 35–6). Metronidazole has most commonly been used in the United States, but tinidazole offers simpler dosing and less side effects. Metronidazole often induces transient nausea, vomiting, epigastric discomfort, headache, or a metallic taste. A disulfiram-like reaction may occur if alcohol is coingested. Metronidazole should be avoided in pregnant or nursing mothers if possible. The same toxicities and concerns probably apply for tinidazole, although it appears to be better tolerated. Fluid and electrolyte replacement is also important for patients with significant diarrhea. Surgical management of acute complications of intestinal amebiasis is best avoided whenever possible. Successful therapy of severe amebic colitis may be followed by postdysenteric colitis, with continued diarrhea without persistent infection; this syndrome generally resolves in weeks to months.

Alternatives for the treatment of intestinal amebiasis are tetracycline (250–500 mg orally four times daily for 10 days) plus chloroquine (500 mg orally daily for 7 days). Emetine or dehydroemetine, which are not available in the United States, can be given subcutaneously or intramuscularly in a dose of 1–1.5 mg/kg/day; the maximum daily dose is 90 mg for dehydroemetine and 65 mg for emetine). These agents are effective but cardiotoxic with a narrow therapeutic range and should be used only until severe disease is controlled. They cause nausea, vomiting, and pain at the injection site.

▲ **Figure 35–7.** Gross pathology showing intestinal ulcers due to amebiasis. (From Dr. Mae Melvin, Public Health Image Library, CDC.)

Table 35–6. Treatment of amebiasis.[1]

Clinical Setting	Drugs of Choice and Adult Dosage	Alternative Drugs and Adult Dosage
Asymptomatic intestinal infection	**Luminal agent:** Diloxanide furoate,[2] 500 mg orally three times daily for 10 days –or– Iodoquinol, 650 mg orally three times daily for 21 days –or– Paromomycin, 10 mg/kg orally three times daily for 7 days	
Mild to moderate intestinal infection	Metronidazole, 750 mg orally three times daily (or 500 mg intravenously every 6 hours) for 10 days –or– Tinidazole, 2 g orally daily for 3 days plus– Luminal agent (see above)	Luminal agent (see above) plus either– Tetracycline, 250 mg orally three times daily for 10 days –or– Erythromycin, 500 mg orally four times daily for 10 days
Severe intestinal infection	Metronidazole, 750 mg orally three times daily (or 500 mg intravenously every 6 hours) for 10 days –or– Tinidazole, 2 g orally daily for 3 days plus– Luminal agent (see above)	Luminal agent (see above) plus either– Tetracycline, 250 mg orally three times daily for 10 days –or– Dehydroemetine[2] or emetine,[2] 1 mg/kg subcutaneously or intramuscularly for 3–5 days
Hepatic abscess, ameboma, and other extraintestinal disease	Metronidazole, 750 mg orally three times daily (or 500 mg intravenously every 6 hours) for 10 days –or– Tinidazole, 2 g orally daily for 3 days plus– Luminal agent (see above)	Dehydroemetine[2] or emetine,[2] 1 mg/kg subcutaneously or intramuscularly for 8–10 days, followed by (liver abscess only) chloroquine, 500 mg orally twice daily for 2 days, then 500 mg daily for 21 days plus– Luminal agent (see above)

[1]See text for additional details and cautions.
[2]Not available in the United States.

Amebic liver abscess is also treated with metronidazole or tinidazole plus a luminal agent (even if intestinal infection is not documented; Table 35–6). Metronidazole can be used intravenously when necessary. With failure of initial response to metronidazole or tinidazole, chloroquine, emetine or dehydroemetine may be added. Needle aspiration may be helpful for large abscesses (over 5–10 cm), in particular if the diagnosis remains uncertain, if there is an initial lack of response, or if a patient is very ill, suggesting imminent abscess rupture. With successful therapy, abscesses disappear slowly (over months).

Prevention & Control

Prevention requires safe water supplies; sanitary disposal of human feces; adequate cooking of food; protection of food from fly contamination; handwashing; and, in endemic areas, avoidance of fruits and vegetables that cannot be cooked or peeled. Water supplies can be boiled, treated with iodine (0.5 mL tincture of iodine per liter for 20 minutes; cysts are resistant to standard concentrations of chlorine), or filtered.

Gonzales ML et al. Antiamoebic drugs for treating amoebic colitis. Cochrane Database Syst Rev. 2009 Apr 15;(2): CD006085. [PMID: 19370624]

Wright SG. Protozoan infections of the gastrointestinal tract. Infect Dis Clin North Am. 2012 Jun;26(2):323–39. [PMID: 22632642]

COCCIDIOSIS (Cryptosporidiosis, Isosporiasis, Cyclosporiasis, Sarcocystosis) & MICROSPORIDIOSIS

ESSENTIALS OF DIAGNOSIS

► Acute diarrhea, especially in children in developing countries.

► Outbreaks of diarrhea secondary to contaminated water or food.

► Prolonged diarrhea in immunocompromised persons.

► Diagnosis mostly by identifying organisms in specially stained stool specimens.

General Considerations

The causes of coccidiosis are *Cryptosporidium* species (*C parvum, C hominis,* and others); *Isospora belli; Cyclospora* cayetanensis; and *Sarcocystis* species. Microsporidiosis is caused by at least 14 species, most commonly *Enterocytozoon bieneusi* and *Encephalitozoon intestinalis*. These infections occur worldwide, particularly in the tropics and in regions where hygiene is poor. They are causes of endemic childhood gastroenteritis (particularly in malnourished children in developing countries); institutional and community outbreaks of diarrhea; traveler's diarrhea; and acute and chronic diarrhea in immunosuppressed patients, in particular those with AIDS. They are all notable for the potential to cause prolonged diarrhea, often lasting for a number of weeks. Clustering occurs in households, day care centers, and among sexual partners.

The infectious agents are oocysts (coccidiosis) or spores (microsporidiosis) transmitted from person to person or by contaminated drinking or swimming water or food. Ingested oocysts release sporozoites that invade and multiply in enterocytes, primarily in the small bowel. Coccidian oocysts and microsporidian cysts can remain viable in the environment for years.

I belli and *C cayetanensis* appear to infect only humans. *C cayetanensis* has caused a number of food-borne outbreaks in the United States in recent years, most commonly associated with imported fresh produce. *Sarcocystis* infects many species; humans are intermediate hosts (infected by ingestion of fecal sporocysts) for some species but definitive hosts for *Sarcocystis bovihominis* and *Sarcocystis suihominis* (infected by ingestion of tissue cysts in undercooked beef and pork, respectively).

Cryptosporidiosis is a zoonosis (*C parvum* principally infects cattle), but most human infections are acquired from humans, in particular with *C hominis*. Cryptosporidia are highly infectious and readily transmitted in day care settings and households. They have caused large community outbreaks due to contaminated water supplies (causing ~400,000 illnesses in Milwaukee in 1993) and are the leading cause of recreational water–associated outbreaks of gastroenteritis. In the developing world cryptosporidiosis is a leading cause of childhood diarrhea. In a study of causes of moderate-to-severe diarrhea in Asia and Africa, *Cryptosporidium* was the second most commonly identified pathogen in children under 2 years of age.

► Clinical Findings

A. Symptoms and Signs

1. Cryptosporidiosis—The incubation period appears to be 1–14 days. In developing countries, disease is primarily in children under 5 years of age, causing 5–10% of childhood diarrhea. Presenting symptoms in children include acute watery diarrhea, abdominal pain, and cramps, with rapid resolution in most patients; however, symptoms quite commonly persist for 2 weeks or more. In developed countries, most patients are adults. Diarrhea in immunocompetent individuals typically lasts from 5 to 10 days. It is usually watery, with accompanying abdominal pain and cramps, nausea, vomiting, and fever. Relapses may follow initial resolution of symptoms. Mild illness and asymptomatic infection are also common.

Cryptosporidiosis is a well-characterized cause of diarrhea in those with AIDS. It was common before the advent of highly active antiretroviral therapy, particularly with advanced immunosuppression. Clinical manifestations are variable, but patients commonly have chronic diarrhea with frequent foul smelling stools, malabsorption, and weight loss. Severe, life-threatening watery diarrhea may be seen. Cryptosporidiosis also causes extraintestinal disease with AIDS, including pulmonary infiltrates with dyspnea and biliary tract infection with sclerosing cholangitis and AIDS cholangiopathy.

2. Isosporiasis—The incubation period for *I belli* is about 1 week. In immunocompetent persons, it usually causes a self-limited watery diarrhea lasting 2–3 weeks, with abdominal cramps, anorexia, malaise, and weight loss. Fever is unusual. Chronic symptoms may persist for months. In immunocompromised patients, isosporiasis more commonly causes severe and chronic diarrhea, with complications including marked dehydration, malnutrition, and hemorrhagic colitis. Extraintestinal disease has been reported rarely.

3. Cyclosporiasis—*C cayetanensis* oocysts must undergo a period of sporulation of 7 days or more after shedding before they become infectious. Therefore, person-to-person spread is unlikely, and spread has typically been due to contaminated food (especially fresh produce) and water. The incubation period is 1–11 days. Infections can be asymptomatic. Cyclosporiasis causes an illness similar to that described for the other pathogens described in this section, with watery diarrhea, abdominal cramps, nausea, fatigue, and anorexia. Fever is seen in 25% of cases. Symptoms typically continue for 2 weeks or longer and may persist for months. Relapses of diarrhea are common. Diarrhea may be preceded by a flu-like prodrome and followed by persistent fatigue. In immunocompromised patients, cyclosporiasis is typically more severe and prolonged, with chronic fulminant watery diarrhea and weight loss.

4. Sarcocystosis—*Sarcocystis* infection may be common in some developing countries, but it is usually asymptomatic. Infection appears to most commonly follow the ingestion of undercooked beef or pork, leading to the development of cysts in muscle, with myalgias, fever, bronchospasm, pruritic rash, lymphadenopathy, and subcutaneous nodules. Ingestion of fecal sporocysts may lead to gastrointestinal symptoms.

5. Microsporidiosis—Microsporidia are obligate intracellular protozoans that cause a wide spectrum of diseases. Many infections are of zoonotic origin, but human-to-human transmission has been documented. Infection is mainly by ingestion of spores, but also by direct inoculation of the eyes. In immunocompetent hosts, microsporidian infections most commonly present as self-limited diarrhea. Ocular infections have also been described. Disease from microsporidia is seen mainly in immunocompromised persons, particularly those with AIDS. Infections in AIDS patients are most commonly with *E bieneusi* and *E intestinalis*. They cause chronic diarrhea, with anorexia, bloating, weight loss, and wasting, especially in those with advanced immunodeficiency. Fever is usually not seen. Other illnesses in immunocompromised persons associated with microsporidians (including the genera *Enterocytozoon*, *Encephalitozoon*, *Brachiola*, *Vittaforma*, *Pleistophora*, *Trachipleistophora*, and *Microsporidium*) include biliary tract disease (AIDS cholangiopathy), genitourinary infection with cystitis, kidney disease, hepatitis, peritonitis, myositis, respiratory infections including sinusitis, central nervous system infections including granulomatous encephalitis, and disseminated infections. Ocular infections with *Encephalitozoon* species cause conjunctivitis and keratitis, presenting as redness, photophobia, and loss of visual acuity.

B. Laboratory Findings

1. Cryptosporidiosis—Typically, stool is without blood or leukocytes. Diagnosis is traditionally made by detecting the organism in stool using a modified acid-fast stain; this technique is relatively insensitive, and multiple specimens should be evaluated before ruling out the diagnosis. Of note, routine evaluation for ova and parasites typically does not include a modified acid-fast stain, so this must be specifically requested in many laboratories. Various antigen detection methods, including immunofluorescence microscopy, ELISA, and immunochromatography, offer improved sensitivity and specificity, both over 90% with available assays, and these methods may be considered the optimal means of diagnosis.

2. Isosporiasis—Diagnosis of isosporiasis is by examination of stool wet mounts or after modified acid-fast staining, in which the organism is clearly distinguishable from other parasites. Other stains also show the organism. Shedding of oocysts may be intermittent, so the sensitivity of stool evaluation is not high, and multiple samples should be examined. The organism may also be identified in duodenal aspirates or small bowel biopsies.

3. Cyclosporiasis—Diagnosis is made by examination of stool wet mounts or after modified acid-fast staining. Multiple specimens may need to be examined to make a diagnosis. The organism can also be identified in small bowel aspirates or biopsy specimens.

4. Sarcocystosis—Eosinophilia and elevated creatine kinase may be seen. Diagnosis is by identification of the acid-fast organisms in stool or by identification of trophozoites or bradyzoites in tissue biopsies.

5. Microsporidiosis—Diagnosis can be made by identification of organisms in specially stained stool, fluid, or tissue specimens, for example with Weber chromotrope-based stain. Electron microscopy is helpful for confirmation of the diagnosis and speciation. PCR and culture techniques are available but not used routinely.

▶ Treatment

Most acute infections with these pathogens in immunocompetent persons are self-limited and do not require treatment. Supportive treatment for severe or chronic diarrhea includes fluid and electrolyte replacement and, in some cases, parenteral nutrition.

1. Cryptosporidiosis—Treatment of cryptosporidiosis is challenging. No agent is clearly effective. Modest benefits have been seen in some (but not other) studies with paromomycin, a nonabsorbed aminoglycoside (25–35 mg/kg orally for 14 days has been used), and nitazoxanide (500 mg–1 g orally twice daily for 3 days in nonimmunocompromised and 2–8 weeks in advanced AIDS patients), which is approved in the United States for this indication. Other agents that have been used with mixed success in AIDS patients with cryptosporidiosis include azithromycin, spiramycin, bovine hyperimmune colostrum, and octreotide. Reversing immunodeficiency with effective antiretroviral therapy is of greatest importance.

2. Isosporiasis—Isosporiasis is effectively treated in immunocompetent and immunosuppressed persons with TMP-SMZ (160 mg/800 mg orally two to four times daily for 10 days, with the higher dosage for patients with AIDS). An alternative therapy is pyrimethamine (75 mg orally in four divided doses) with folinic acid (10–25 mg/day orally). Maintenance therapy with low-dose TMP-SMZ (160 mg/800 mg daily or three times per week) or Fansidar (1 tablet weekly) prevents relapse in those with persistent immunosuppression.

3. Cyclosporiasis—Cyclosporiasis is also treated with TMP-SMZ (dosing as for isosporiasis). With AIDS, long-term maintenance therapy (160 mg/ 800 mg three times weekly) helps prevent relapse. For patients intolerant of TMP-SMZ, ciprofloxacin (500 mg orally twice daily for 7 days) showed efficacy, albeit with less ability to clear the organism than TMP-SMZ.

4. Sarcocystosis—For sarcocystosis, no specific treatment is established, but patients may respond to therapy with albendazole or TMP-SMZ.

5. Microsporidiosis—Treatment of microsporidiosis is complex. Infections with most species, including those causing gastrointestinal and other manifestations, should be treated with albendazole (400 mg orally twice daily for 2–4 weeks), which has activity against a number of species, but relatively poor efficacy (about 50%) against *E bieneusi*, the most common microsporidial cause of diarrhea in AIDS patients. Fumagillin, which is used to treat honeybees and fish with microsporidian infections, has shown benefit in clinical trials at a dose of 20 mg three times per day for 14 days; treatment was accompanied by reversible thrombocytopenia. As with cryptosporidiosis, the best means of controlling microsporidiosis in AIDS patients is to restore immune function with effective antiretroviral therapy. Ocular microsporidiosis can be treated with fumagillin solution (3 mg/mL); this probably should be given with concurrent systemic therapy with albendazole. Adjunctive management may include corticosteroids to decrease inflammation and keratoplasty.

▶ Prevention

Water purification is important for control of these infections. Chlorine disinfection is not effective against cryptosporidial oocysts, so other purification measures are needed. Immunocompromised patients should boil or filter drinking water and should consider avoidance of lakes and swimming pools. Routine precautions (handwashing, gloves, disinfection) should prevent institutional patient-to-patient spread. Optimal means of preventing microsporidial infections are not well understood, but water purification and body substance precautions for immunocompromised and hospitalized individuals are likely effective.

Checkley W et al. A review of the global burden, novel diagnostics, therapeutics, and vaccine targets for cryptosporidium. Lancet Infect Dis. 2015 Jan;15(1):85–94. [PMID: 25278220]
Didier ES et al. Microsporidiosis: not just in AIDS patients. Curr Opin Infect Dis. 2011 Oct;24(5):490–5. [PMID: 21844802]
Fayer R et al. Human infections with *Sarcocystis* species. Clin Microbiol Rev. 2015 Apr;28(2):295–311. [PMID: 25715644]
Marcos LA et al. Intestinal protozoan infections in the immunocompromised host. Curr Opin Infect Dis. 2013 Aug;26(4): 295–301. [PMID: 23806893]

GIARDIASIS

ESSENTIALS OF DIAGNOSIS

▶ Acute diarrhea; may be profuse and watery.

▶ Chronic diarrhea with greasy, malodorous stools.

▶ Abdominal cramps, distention, flatulence, and malaise.

▶ Cysts or trophozoites in stools.

▶ General Considerations

Giardiasis is a protozoal infection of the upper small intestine caused by the flagellate *Giardia lamblia* (also called *Giardia intestinalis* and *Giardia duodenalis*). The parasite occurs worldwide, most abundantly in areas with poor sanitation. In developing countries, young children are very commonly infected. In the United States and Europe, the infection is the most common intestinal protozoal pathogen; the US estimate is 100,000 to 2.5 million new infections leading to 5000 hospital admissions yearly. Groups at special risk include travelers to *Giardia*-endemic areas, those who swallow contaminated water during recreation or wilderness travel, men who have sex with men, and persons with impaired immunity. Outbreaks are common in households, children's day care centers, and residential facilities, and may occur as a result of contamination of water supplies.

The organism occurs in feces as a flagellated trophozoite and as a cyst. Only the cyst form is infectious by the oral route; trophozoites are destroyed by gastric acidity. Humans are a reservoir for the pathogen; dogs, cats, beavers, and other mammals have been implicated but not confirmed as reservoirs. Under suitable moist, cool conditions, cysts can survive in the environment for weeks to months. Cysts are transmitted as a result of fecal contamination of water or food, by person-to-person contact, or by anal-oral sexual contact. The infectious dose is low, requiring as few as ten cysts. After the cysts are ingested, trophozoites emerge in the duodenum and jejunum. Epithelial damage and mucosal invasion are uncommon. Hypogammaglobulinemia, low secretory IgA levels in the gut, achlorhydria, and malnutrition favor the development of infection.

▶ Clinical Findings

A. Symptoms and Signs

It is estimated that about 50% of infected persons have no discernable infection, about 10% become asymptomatic cyst passers, and 25–50% develop an acute diarrheal syndrome. Acute diarrhea may clear spontaneously but is commonly followed by chronic diarrhea. The incubation period is usually 1–3 weeks but may be longer. The illness may begin gradually or suddenly. Cysts may not be detected in the stool at the onset of the illness. The acute phase may last days or weeks, and is usually self-limited, although cyst excretion may be prolonged. The initial illness may include profuse watery diarrhea, and hospitalization may be required due to dehydration, particularly in young children. Typical symptoms of chronic disease are abdominal cramps, bloating, flatulence, nausea, malaise, and anorexia. Fever and vomiting are uncommon. Diarrhea is usually not severe in the chronic stage of infection; stools are greasy or frothy and foul smelling, without blood, pus, or mucus. The diarrhea may be daily or recurrent; intervening periods may include constipation. Symptoms can persist for weeks to months. Weight loss is frequent. Chronic disease can include malabsorption, including fat and protein-losing enteropathy and vitamin deficiencies.

B. Laboratory Findings

Most patients seek medical attention after having been ill for over a week, commonly with weight loss of 5 kg or more. Stool is generally without blood or leukocytes. Diagnosis is traditionally made by the identification of trophozoites or cysts in stool. A wet mount of liquid stool may identify motile trophozoites. Stained fixed specimens may show cysts or trophozoites. Sensitivity of stool analysis is not ideal, estimated at 50–80% for a single specimen and over 90% for three specimens. Sampling of duodenal contents with a string test or biopsy is no longer generally recommended, but biopsies may be helpful in very ill or immunocompromised patients. When giardiasis is suspected, antigen assays may be simpler and cheaper than repeated stool examinations, but these tests will not identify other stool pathogens. Multiple tests, which identify antigens of trophozoites or cysts, are available. They are generally quite sensitive (85–98%) and specific (90–100%).

▶ Treatment

The treatments of choice for giardiasis are metronidazole (250 mg orally three times daily for 5–7 days) or tinidazole (2 g orally once). The drugs are not universally effective; cure rates for single courses are typically about 80–95%. Toxicities are as described for treatment of amebiasis, but the lower dosages used for giardiasis limit side effects. Albendazole (400 mg orally once daily for 5 days) and nitazoxanide (500 mg orally twice daily for 3 days) both appear to have similar efficacy and fewer side effects compared with metronidazole, although data are limited, and a recent meta-analysis suggested superiority in efficacy of tinidazole over albendazole. Nitazoxanide is generally well tolerated but may cause mild gastrointestinal side effects. Other drugs with activity against *Giardia* include furazolidone (100 mg orally four times a day for 7 days), which is about as effective as the other named drugs but causes gastrointestinal side effects, and paromomycin (500 mg orally three times a day for 7 days), which appears to have somewhat lower efficacy but unlike metronidazole, tinidazole, and furazolidone is safe in pregnancy. Symptomatic giardiasis should always be treated. Treatment of asymptomatic patients should be considered, since they can transmit the infection. With a suggestive presentation but negative diagnostic studies, an empiric course of treatment may be appropriate. Household or day care contacts with an index case should be tested and treated if infected.

▶ Prevention

Community chlorination (0.4 mg/L) of water is relatively ineffective for inactivating cysts, so filtration is required. For wilderness or international travelers, bringing water to a boil for 1 minute or filtration with a pore size less than 1 mcm are adequate. In day care centers, appropriate disposal of diapers and frequent handwashing are essential.

Escobedo AA et al. A meta-analysis of the efficacy of albendazole compared with tinidazole as treatments for *Giardia* infections in children. Acta Trop. 2016 Jan;153:120–7. [PMID: 26476393]
Watkins RR et al. Treatment of giardiasis: current status and future directions. Curr Infect Dis Rep. 2014 Feb;16(2):396. [PMID: 24493628]

TRICHOMONIASIS

▶ ESSENTIALS OF DIAGNOSIS

- ▶ Copious vaginal discharge in women.
- ▶ Nongonococcal urethritis in men.
- ▶ Motile trichomonads on wet mounts.

▶ General Considerations

Trichomoniasis is caused by the protozoan *Trichomonas vaginalis* and is among the most common sexually transmitted diseases, causing vaginitis in women and nongonococcal urethritis in men. It can also occasionally be acquired by other means, since it can survive in moist environments for several hours.

▶ Clinical Findings

A. Symptoms and Signs

T vaginalis is often harbored asymptomatically. For women with symptomatic disease, after an incubation period of 5 days to 4 weeks, a vaginal discharge develops, often with vulvovaginal discomfort, pruritus, dysuria, dyspareunia, or abdominal pain. Examination shows a copious discharge, which is usually not foul smelling but is often frothy and yellow or green in color. Inflammation of the vaginal walls and cervix with punctate hemorrhages are common. Most men infected with *T vaginalis* are asymptomatic, but it can be isolated from about 10% of men with nongonococcal urethritis. In men with trichomonal urethritis, the urethral discharge is generally more scanty than with other causes of urethritis.

B. Diagnostic Testing

Diagnosis is typically made by identifying the organism in vaginal or urethral secretions. Examination of wet mounts will show motile organisms. Tests for bacterial vaginosis (pH > 4.5, fishy odor after addition of potassium hydroxide) are often positive with trichomoniasis. Newer diagnostic tests include point-of-care antigen tests and nucleic acid amplification assays, both of which offer improved sensitivity compared to wet mount microscopy and excellent specificity.

▶ Treatment

The treatment of choice is tinidazole or metronidazole, each as a 2 g single oral dose. Tinidazole may be better tolerated and active against some resistant parasites. Toxicities of these drugs are discussed in the section on amebiasis. If the large single dose cannot be tolerated, an alternative metronidazole dosage is 500 mg orally twice daily for 1 week. All infected persons should be treated, even if asymptomatic, to prevent subsequent symptomatic disease and limit spread. Treatment failure suggests reinfection, but metronidazole-resistant organisms have been reported. These may be treated with tinidazole, longer courses of metronidazole, furazolidone, or other experimental therapies (see Chapter 18).

Hobbs MM et al. Modern diagnosis of *Trichomonas vaginalis* infection. Sex Transm Infect. 2013 Sep;89(6):434–8. [PMID: 23633669]
Secor WE et al. Neglected parasitic infections in the United States: trichomoniasis. Am J Trop Med Hyg. 2014 May; 90(5):800–4. [PMID: 24808247]
Sobel R et al. Metronidazole for the treatment of vaginal infections. Expert Opin Pharmacother. 2015 May;16(7):1109–15. [PMID: 25887246]

TREMATODE (FLUKE) INFECTIONS

SCHISTOSOMIASIS (Bilharziasis)

ESSENTIALS OF DIAGNOSIS

▸ History of fresh water exposure in an endemic area.

▸ **Acute schistosomiasis:** fever, headache, myalgias, cough, urticaria, diarrhea, and eosinophilia.

▸ **Intestinal schistosomiasis:** abdominal pain, diarrhea, and hepatomegaly, progressing to anorexia, weight loss, and features of portal hypertension.

▸ **Urinary schistosomiasis:** hematuria and dysuria, progressing to hydroureter, hydronephrosis and urinary infections.

▸ Diagnosis based on characteristic eggs in feces or urine; biopsy of rectal or bladder mucosa; positive serology.

General Considerations

Schistosomiasis, which affects more than 200 million persons worldwide, leads to severe consequences in 20 million persons and about 100,000 deaths annually. The disease is caused by six species of trematode blood flukes. Five species cause intestinal schistosomiasis, with infection of mesenteric venules: *Schistosoma mansoni*, which is present in Africa, the Arabian peninsula, South America, and the Caribbean; *Schistosoma japonicum*, which is endemic in China and Southeast Asia; *Schistosoma mekongi*, which is endemic near the Mekong River in Southeast Asia; and *Schistosoma intercalatum* and *Schistosoma guineensis*, which occur in parts of Africa. *Schistosoma haematobium* causes urinary schistosomiasis, with infection of venules of the urinary tract, and is endemic in Africa and the Middle East. Transmission of schistosomiasis is focal, with greatest prevalence in poor rural areas. Control efforts have diminished transmission significantly in many areas, but high level transmission remains common in sub-Saharan Africa and some other areas. Prevalence of infection and illness typically peaks at about 15–20 years of age.

Humans are infected with schistosomes after contact with fresh water containing cercariae released by infected snails. Infection is initiated by penetration of skin or mucous membranes. After penetration, schistosomulae migrate to the portal circulation, where they rapidly mature. After about 6 weeks, adult worms mate, and migrate to terminal mesenteric or bladder venules, where females deposit their eggs. Some eggs reach the lumen of the bowel or bladder and are passed with feces or urine, while others are retained in the bowel or bladder wall or transported in the circulation to other tissues, in particular the liver. Disease in endemic areas is primarily due to a host response to eggs, with granuloma formation and

inflammation, eventually leading to fibrosis. Chronic infection can result in scarring of mesenteric or vesicular blood vessels, leading to portal hypertension and alterations in the urinary tract. In previously uninfected individuals, such as travelers with fresh water contact in endemic regions, acute schistosomiasis may occur, with a febrile illness 2–8 weeks after infection.

Clinical Findings

A. Symptoms and Signs

1. Cercarial dermatitis—Following cercarial penetration, localized erythema develops in some individuals, which can progress to a pruritic maculopapular rash that persists for some days. Dermatitis can be caused by human schistosomes and, in non-tropical areas, by bird schistosomes that cannot complete their life cycle in humans (swimmer's itch).

2. Acute schistosomiasis (Katayama syndrome)—A febrile illness may develop 2–8 weeks after exposure in persons without prior infection, most commonly after heavy infection with *S mansoni* or *S japonicum*. Presenting symptoms and signs include acute onset of fever; headache; myalgias; cough; malaise; urticaria; diarrhea, which may be bloody; hepatosplenomegaly; lymphadenopathy; and pulmonary infiltrates. Localized lesions may occasionally cause severe manifestations, including CNS abnormalities and death. Acute schistosomiasis usually resolves in 2–8 weeks.

3. Chronic schistosomiasis—Many infected persons have light infections and are asymptomatic, but an estimated 50–60% have symptoms and 5–10% have advanced organ damage. Asymptomatic infected children may suffer from anemia and growth retardation. Symptomatic patients with intestinal schistosomiasis typically experience abdominal pain, fatigue, diarrhea, and hepatomegaly. Over years, anorexia, weight loss, weakness, colonic polyps, and features of portal hypertension develop. Late manifestations include hematemesis from esophageal varices, hepatic failure, and pulmonary hypertension. Urinary schistosomiasis may present within months of infection with hematuria and dysuria, most commonly in children and young adults. Fibrotic changes in the urinary tract can lead to hydroureter, hydronephrosis, bacterial urinary infections and, ultimately, kidney disease or bladder cancer.

B. Laboratory Findings

Microscopic examination of stool or urine for eggs, evaluation of tissue, or serologic tests establish the diagnosis. Characteristic eggs can be identified on smears of stool or urine. The most widely used stool test is the Kato-Katz technique. Quantitative tests that yield more than 400 eggs per gram of feces or 10 mL of urine are indicative of heavy infections with increased risk of complications. Diagnosis can also be made by biopsy of the rectum, colon, liver, or bladder. Serologic tests include an ELISA available from the CDC that is 99% specific for all species, but cannot distinguish acute and past infection. Sensitivity of the test is 99% for *S mansoni*, 95% for *S haematobium*, but less than 50% for *S japonicum*. Serology is of limited use in endemic settings, but can be helpful in travelers from nonendemic regions. Point-of-care assays to detect circulating schistosome antigens in serum and urine are also available; the most widely used tests target circulating anodic and cathodic antigens. Antigen tests have better sensitivity than stool smears, especially for *S mansoni*; sensitivity is lower for *S haematobium*. Molecular tests for schistosomiasis have been developed but are not routinely used for diagnosis. In acute schistosomiasis, leukocytosis and marked eosinophilia may occur; serologic tests may become positive before eggs are seen in stool or urine. After therapy, eggs may be shed in stool or urine for months, and so the identification of eggs in fluids or tissue cannot distinguish past or active disease. With a diagnosis of schistosomiasis, evaluation for the extent of disease is warranted, including liver function studies and imaging of the liver with intestinal disease and ultrasound or other imaging studies of the urinary system in urinary disease.

▶ Treatment

Treatment is indicated for all schistosome infections. In areas where recurrent infection is common, treatment is valuable in reducing worm burdens and limiting clinical complications. The drug of choice for schistosomiasis is praziquantel. The drug is administered for 1 day at an oral dose of 40 mg/kg (in one or two doses) for *S mansoni*, *S haematobium, S intercalatum*, and *S guineensis* infections and a dose of 60 mg/kg (in two or three doses) for *S japonicum* and *S mekongi*. Cure rates are generally greater than 80% after a single treatment, and those not cured have marked reduction in the intensity of infection. Praziquantel is active against invading cercariae but not developing schistosomulae. Therefore, the drug may not prevent illness when given after exposure and, for recent infections, a repeat course after a few weeks may be appropriate. Praziquantel may be used during pregnancy. Resistance to praziquantel has been reported. Toxicities include abdominal pain, diarrhea, urticaria, headache, nausea, vomiting, and fever, and may be due both to direct effects of the drug and responses to dying worms. Alternative therapies are oxamniquine for *S mansoni* infection and metrifonate for *S haemotobium* infection. Both of these drugs currently have limited availability (they are not available in the United States), and resistance may be a problem. No second-line drug is available for *S japonicum* infections. The antimalarial drug artemether has activity against schistosomulae and adult worms and may be effective in chemoprophylaxis; however, it is expensive, and long-term use in malarious areas might select for resistant malaria parasites. With severe disease, use of corticosteroids in conjunction with praziquantel may decrease complications. Treatment should be followed by repeat examinations for eggs about every 3 months for 1 year after therapy, with re-treatment if eggs are seen.

▶ Prevention

Travelers to endemic areas should avoid fresh water exposure. Vigorous toweling after exposure may limit cercarial penetration. Chemoprophylaxis with artemether has

shown efficacy but is not standard practice. Community control of schistosomiasis includes improved sanitation and water supplies, elimination of snail habitats, and intermittent treatment to limit worm burdens.

Colley DG et al. Human schistosomiasis. Lancet. 2014 Jun 28;383(9936):2253–64. [PMID: 24698483]
Gryseels B. Schistosomiasis. Infect Dis Clin North Am. 2012 Jun;26(2):383–97. [PMID: 22632645]
Utzinger J et al. New diagnostic tools in schistosomiasis. Clin Microbiol Infect. 2015 Jun;21(6):529–42. [PMID: 25843503]
Weerakoon KG et al. Advances in the diagnosis of human schistosomiasis. Clin Microbiol Rev. 2015 Oct;28(4):939–67. [PMID: 26224883]

LIVER, LUNG, & INTESTINAL FLUKES

FASCIOLIASIS

Infection by *Fasciola hepatica*, the sheep liver fluke, results from ingestion of encysted metacercariae on watercress or other aquatic vegetables. Infection is prevalent in sheep-raising areas in many countries, especially parts of South America, the Middle East, and southern Europe, and it has increasingly been recognized in travelers to these areas. *Fasciola gigantica* has a more restricted distribution in Asia and Africa and causes similar findings. Eggs are passed from host feces into fresh water, leading to infection of snails, and then deposition of metacercariae on vegetation. In humans, metacercariae excyst, penetrate into the peritoneum, migrate through the liver, and mature in the bile ducts, where they cause local necrosis and abscess formation.

Two clinical syndromes are seen, related to acute migration of worms and chronic infection of the biliary tract. Symptoms related to migration of larvae present 6–12 weeks after ingestion. Typical findings are abdominal pain, fever, malaise, weight loss, urticaria, eosinophilia, and leukocytosis. Tender hepatomegaly and elevated liver function tests may be seen. Rarely, migration to other organs may lead to localized disease. The symptoms of worm migration subside after 2–4 months, followed by asymptomatic infection by adult worms or intermittent symptoms of biliary obstruction, with biliary colic and, at times, findings of cholangitis. Early diagnosis is difficult, as eggs are not found in the feces during the acute migratory phase of infection. Clinical suspicion should be based on clinical findings and marked eosinophilia in at risk individuals. CT and other imaging studies show hypodense migratory lesions of the liver. Definitive diagnosis is made by the identification of characteristic eggs in stool. Repeated examinations may be necessary. In chronic infection, imaging studies show masses obstructing the extrahepatic biliary tract. Serologic assays have sensitivity and specificity greater than 90%, but cannot distinguish between past and current infection. Antigen tests with excellent sensitivity and specificity are available in veterinary medicine and show promise for humans.

Fascioliasis is unusual among fluke infections, in that it does not respond well to treatment with praziquantel. The treatment of choice is triclabendazole, which is also used in veterinary medicine, but is not available in the United States. Standard dosing of 10 mg/kg orally in a single dose or two doses over 12 hours achieves a cure rate of about 80%, but repeat dosing is indicated if abnormal radiologic findings or eosinophilia do not resolve. Of concern, resistance to triclabendazole has been widely reported in animal infections. The second-line drug for fascioliasis is bithionol (30–50 mg/kg/day orally in three divided doses on alternate days for 10–15 days); this drug is no longer available in the United States. Treatment with either drug can be accompanied by abdominal pain and other gastrointestinal symptoms. Other potential therapies are emetine and dehydroemetine, both widely used in the past but quite toxic, and nitazoxanide. Prevention of fascioliasis involves avoidance of ingestion of raw aquatic plants.

CLONORCHIASIS & OPISTHORCHIASIS

Infection by *Clonorchis sinensis*, the Chinese liver fluke, is endemic in areas of Japan, Korea, China, Taiwan, Southeast Asia, and the far eastern part of Russia. An estimated 15 million people are infected (13 million in China); in some communities, prevalence can reach 80%. Opisthorchiasis is principally caused by *Opisthorchis felineus* (regions of the former Soviet Union) or *Opisthorchis viverrini* (Thailand, Laos, Vietnam). Clonorchiasis and opisthorchiasis are clinically indistinguishable. Parasite eggs are shed into water in human or animal feces, where they infect snails, which release cercariae, which infect fish. Human infection follows ingestion of raw, undercooked, or pickled freshwater fish containing metacercariae. These parasites excyst in the duodenum and ascend into the biliary tract, where they mature and remain for many years, shedding eggs in the bile.

Most patients harbor few parasites and are asymptomatic. An acute illness can occur 2–3 weeks after initial infection, with fever, abdominal pain, tender hepatomegaly, urticaria, and eosinophilia. The acute syndrome is difficult to diagnose, since ova may not appear in the feces until 3–4 weeks after onset of symptoms. In chronic heavy infections, findings include abdominal pain, anorexia, weight loss, and tender hepatomegaly. More serious findings can include recurrent bacterial cholangitis and sepsis, cholecystitis, liver abscess, and pancreatitis. An increased risk of cholangiocarcinoma has been documented.

Early diagnosis is presumptive, based on clinical findings and epidemiology. Subsequent diagnosis is made by finding characteristic eggs in stool or duodenal or biliary contents. The stool Kato-Katz test is widely used; performing repeated tests improves sensitivity. Imaging studies show characteristic biliary tract dilatations with filling defects due to flukes. Serologic assays for clonorchiasis with excellent sensitivity are available but cannot distinguish between past and current infection. Molecular tests have been developed but are not widely used.

The drug of choice is praziquantel, 25 mg/kg orally three times daily for 2 days, which provides cure rates over 95%. One day of treatment may be sufficient. Re-treatment may be required, especially in some areas with known decreased praziquantel efficacy. The second-line drug is albendazole (400 mg orally twice daily for 7 days), which

appears to be somewhat less effective. Tribendimidine, which is approved in China, has shown efficacy for clonorchiasis similar to that of praziquantel.

PARAGONIMIASIS

Eight species of *Paragonimus* lung flukes cause human disease. The most important is *Paragonimus westermani*. *Paragonimus* species are endemic in East Asia, Oceania, West Africa, and South America, where millions of persons are infected; rare infections caused by *Paragonimus kellicotti* have occurred in North America. Eggs are released into fresh water, where parasites infect snails, and then cercariae infect crabs and crayfish. Human infection follows consumption of raw, undercooked, or pickled freshwater shellfish. Metacercariae then excyst, penetrate into the peritoneum, and pass into the lungs, where they mature into adult worms over about 2 months.

Most persons have moderate worm burdens and are asymptomatic. In symptomatic cases, abdominal pain and diarrhea develop 2 days to 2 weeks after infection, followed by fever, cough, chest pain, urticaria, and eosinophilia. Acute symptoms may last for several weeks. Chronic infection can cause cough productive of brown sputum, hemoptysis, dyspnea, and chest pain, with progression to chronic bronchitis, bronchiectasis, bronchopneumonia, lung abscess, and pleural disease. Ectopic infections can cause disease in other organs, most commonly the CNS, where disease can present with seizures, headaches, and focal neurologic findings due to parasite meningitis and to intracerebral lesions.

The diagnosis of paragonimiasis is made by identifying characteristic eggs in sputum or stool or identifying worms in biopsied tissue. Multiple examinations and concentration techniques may be needed. Serologic tests may be helpful; an ELISA available from the CDC has sensitivity and specificity more than 95%. Chest radiographs may show varied abnormalities of the lungs or pleura, including infiltrates, nodules, cavities, and fibrosis, and the findings can be confused with those of tuberculosis. With CNS disease, skull radiographs can show clusters of calcified cysts, and CT or MRI can show clusters of ring-enhancing lesions.

Treatment is with praziquantel (25 mg/kg orally three times daily for 2 days), which provides efficacy of at least 90%. Alternative therapies are bithionol and triclabendazole. As with cysticercosis, for cerebral paragonimiasis, praziquantel should generally be used with corticosteroids. Chronic infection may lead to permanent lung dysfunction and pleural disease requiring drainage procedures.

INTESTINAL FLUKES

The large intestinal fluke, *Fasciolopsis buski*, is a common parasite of pigs and humans in eastern and southern Asia. Eggs shed in stools hatch in fresh water, followed by infection of snails, and release of cercariae that encyst on aquatic plants. Humans are infected by eating uncooked plants, including water chestnuts, bamboo shoots, and watercress. Adult flukes mature in about 3 months and live in the small intestine attached to the mucosa, leading to local inflammation and ulceration. Other intestinal flukes that cause similar syndromes include *Heterophyes* (North Africa and Turkey) and *Metagonimus* (East Asia) species; these species are transmitted by undercooked freshwater fish.

Infections with intestinal flukes are often asymptomatic, although eosinophilia may be marked. In symptomatic cases, after an incubation period of 1–2 months, manifestations include epigastric pain and diarrhea. Other gastrointestinal symptoms, ileus, edema, and ascites may be seen uncommonly. Diagnosis is based on identification of characteristic eggs or adult flukes in the stool. In contrast to other fluke infections, illness more than 6 months after travel in an endemic area is unlikely. The drug of choice is praziquantel, 25 mg/kg orally as a single dose. Alternative therapies are triclabendazole and niclosamide (for most species).

Ashrafi K et al. Fascioliasis: a worldwide parasitic disease of importance in travel medicine. Travel Med Infect Dis. 2014 Nov–Dec;12(6 Pt A):636–49. [PMID: 25287722]

Blair D. Paragonimiasis. Adv Exp Med Biol. 2014;766:115–52. [PMID: 24903365]

Fischer PU et al. North American paragonimiasis: epidemiology and diagnostic strategies. Expert Rev Anti Infect Ther. 2015 Jun; 13(6):779–86. [PMID: 25835312]

Fürst T et al. Manifestation, diagnosis, and management of food-borne trematodiasis. BMJ. 2012 Jun 26;344:e4093. [PMID: 22736467]

Qian MB et al. Clonorchiasis. Lancet. 2016 Feb 20; 387(10020):800–10. [PMID: 26299184]

Xu LL et al. Efficacy and safety of praziquantel, tribendimidine and mebendazole in patients with co-infection of *Clonorchis sinensis* and other helminths. PLoS Negl Trop Dis. 2014 Aug 14; 8(8):e3046. [PMID: 25122121]

CESTODE INFECTIONS

NONINVASIVE CESTODE INFECTIONS

The four major tapeworms that cause noninvasive infections in humans are the beef tapeworm *Taenia saginata*, the pork tapeworm *Taenia solium*, the fish tapeworm *Diphyllobothrium latum*, each of which can reach many meters in length, and the dwarf tapeworm *Hymenolepis nana*. *Taenia* and *Hymenolepis* species are broadly distributed, especially in the tropics; *D latum* is most prevalent in temperate regions. Other tapeworms that can cause noninvasive human disease include the rodent tapeworm *Hymenolepis diminuta*, the dog tapeworm *Dipylidium caninum*, and other *Taenia* and *Diphyllobothrium* species. Invasive tapeworm infections, including *T solium* (when infective eggs, rather than cysticerci are ingested) and *Echinococcus* species, will be discussed separately.

1. Beef Tapeworm

Infection is most common in cattle breeding areas. Humans are the definitive host. Gravid segments of *T saginata* are passed in human feces to soil, where they are ingested by grazing animals, especially cattle. The eggs then hatch to release embryos that encyst in muscle as cysticerci. Humans

are infected by eating raw or undercooked infected beef. Most individuals infected with *T saginata* are asymptomatic, but abdominal pain and other gastrointestinal symptoms may be present. Eosinophilia is common. The most common presenting finding is the passage of proglottids in the stool.

2. Pork Tapeworm

T solium is transmitted to pigs that ingest human feces. Humans can be either the definitive host (after consuming undercooked pork, leading to tapeworm infection) or the intermediate host (after consuming food contaminated with human feces containing *T solium* eggs, leading to cysticercosis, which is discussed under Invasive Cestode Infections). As with the beef tapeworm, infection with *T solium* adult worms is generally asymptomatic, but gastrointestinal symptoms may occur. Infection is generally recognized after passage of proglottids. Autoinfection with eggs can progress to cysticercosis.

3. Fish Tapeworm

Infection with *D latum* follows ingestion of undercooked freshwater fish, most commonly in temperate regions. Eggs from human feces are taken up by crustaceans, these are eaten by fish, which are then infectious to humans. Infection with multiple worms over many years can occur. Infections are most commonly asymptomatic, but nonspecific gastrointestinal symptoms, including diarrhea, may occur. Diagnosis usually follows passage of proglottids. Prolonged heavy infection can lead to megaloblastic anemia and neuropathy from vitamin B_{12} deficiency, which is due to infection-induced dissociation of the vitamin from intrinsic factor and to utilization of the vitamin by worms.

4. Dwarf Tapeworm

H nana is the only tapeworm that can be transmitted between humans. Infections are common in warm areas, especially with poor hygiene and institutionalized populations. Infection follows ingestion of food contaminated with human feces. Eggs hatch in the intestines, where oncospheres penetrate the mucosa, encyst as cysticercoid larvae, and then rupture after about 4 days to release adult worms. Autoinfection can lead to amplification of infection. Infection with *H nana*, the related rodent tapeworm *H diminuta*, or the dog tapeworm *D caninum* can also follow accidental ingestion of infected insects. *H nana* are dwarf in size relative to other tapeworms but can reach 5 cm in length. Heavy infection is common, especially in children, and can be accompanied by abdominal discomfort, anorexia, and diarrhea.

▶ Laboratory Findings

Diagnosis is usually made based on the identification of characteristic eggs or proglottids in stool. Egg release may be irregular, so examination of multiple specimens or concentration techniques may be needed.

► Treatment

The treatment of choice for noninvasive tapeworm infections is praziquantel. A single dose of praziquantel (5–10 mg/kg orally) is highly effective, except for *H nana*, for which the dosage is 25 mg/kg. Treatment of *H nana* is more difficult, as the drug is not effective against maturing cysts. Therefore, a repeat treatment after 1 week and screening after therapy to document cure are appropriate with heavy infections. Therapy can be accompanied by headache, malaise, dizziness, abdominal pain, and nausea.

The alternative therapy for these infections is niclosamide. A single dose of niclosamide (2 g chewed) is effective against *D latum, Taenia,* and *D caninum* infections. For *H nana*, therapy is continued daily for 1 week. Niclosamide may cause nausea, malaise, and abdominal pain.

Craig P et al. Intestinal cestodes. Curr Opin Infect Dis. 2007 Oct; 20(5):524–32. [PMID: 17762788]

INVASIVE CESTODE INFECTIONS

1. Cysticercosis

ESSENTIALS OF DIAGNOSIS

► Exposure to *T solium* through fecal contamination of food.

► Seizures, headache, and other findings of a focal CNS lesion.

► Brain imaging shows cysts; positive serologic tests.

► General Considerations

Cysticercosis is due to tissue infection with cysts of *T solium* that develop after humans ingest food contaminated with eggs from human feces, thus acting as an intermediate host for the parasite. Prevalence is high where the parasite is endemic, in particular Mexico, Central and South America, the Philippines, and Southeast Asia. An estimated 20 million persons are infected with cysticerci yearly, leading to about 400,000 persons with neurologic symptoms and 50,000 deaths. Antibody prevalence rates up to 10% are recognized in some endemic areas, and the infection is one of the most important causes of seizures in the developing world and in immigrants to the United States from endemic countries. In Latin America, it is estimated that 0.5–1.5 million people suffer from epilepsy secondary to cysticercosis.

► Clinical Findings

A. Symptoms and Signs

Neurocysticercosis can cause intracerebral, subarachnoid, and spinal cord lesions and intraventricular cysts. Single or multiple lesions may be present. Lesions may persist for years before symptoms develop, generally due to local inflammation or ventricular obstruction. Presenting symptoms include seizures, focal neurologic deficits, altered cognition, and psychiatric disease. Symptoms develop more quickly with intraventricular cysts, with findings of hydrocephalus and meningeal irritation, including severe headache, vomiting, papilledema, and visual loss. A particularly aggressive form of the disease, racemose cysticercosis, involves proliferation of cysts at the base of the brain, leading to alterations of consciousness and death. Spinal cord lesions can present with progressive focal findings.

Cysticercosis of other organ systems is usually clinically benign. Involvement of muscles can uncommonly cause discomfort and is identified by radiographs of muscle showing multiple calcified lesions. Subcutaneous involvement presents with multiple painless palpable skin lesions. Involvement of the eyes can present with ptosis due to extraocular muscle involvement or intraocular abnormalities.

B. Laboratory Findings

CSF examination may show lymphocytic or eosinophilic pleocytosis, decreased glucose, and elevated protein. Serology plays an important role in diagnosis. ELISAs and related immunoblot assays have excellent sensitivity and specificity, but sensitivity is lower with only single or calcified lesions.

C. Imaging

With neuroimaging by CT or MRI, multiple parenchymal cysts are most typically seen. Parenchymal calcification is also common. Ventricular cysts may be difficult to visualize, with MRI offering better sensitivity than CT.

► Treatment

The medical management of neurocysticercosis is controversial, as the benefits of cyst clearance must be weighed against potential harm of an inflammatory response to dying worms. Antihelminthic therapy hastens radiologic improvement in parenchymal cysticercosis, but some randomized trials have shown that corticosteroids alone are as effective as specific therapy plus corticosteroids for controlling seizures. Overall, most authorities recommend treatment of active lesions, in particular lesions with a high likelihood of progression, such as intraventricular cysts. At the other end of the spectrum, inactive calcified lesions probably do not benefit from therapy. When treatment is deemed appropriate, standard therapy consists of albendazole (10–15 mg/kg/day orally for 8 days) or praziquantel (50 mg/kg/day orally for 15–30 days). Albendazole is probably preferred, since it has shown better efficacy in some comparisons and since corticosteroids appear to lower circulating praziquantel levels but increase albendazole levels. Increasing the dosage of albendazole to 30 mg/kg/day orally may improve outcomes. Combining albendazole plus praziquantel improved outcomes compared to albendazole alone in patients with multiple viable intraparenchymal cysts. Corticosteroids are usually administered concurrently, but dosing is not standardized. Patients should be observed for evidence of localized inflammatory responses. Anticonvulsant therapy is provided if needed, and shunting is performed if required for elevated intracranial pressure. Surgical removal of cysts may be helpful for some difficult cases of neurocysticercosis and for symptomatic non-neurologic disease.

Brunetti E et al. Cestode infestations: hydatid disease and cysticercosis. Infect Dis Clin North Am. 2012 Jun;26(2):421–35. [PMID: 22632647]

Cantey PT et al. Neglected parasitic infections in the United States: cysticercosis. Am J Trop Med Hyg. 2014 May;90(5):805–9. [PMID: 24808248]

Garcia HH et al. Clinical symptoms, diagnosis, and treatment of neurocysticercosis. Lancet Neurol. 2014 Dec;13(12):1202–15. [PMID: 25453460]

Garcia HH et al; Cysticercosis Working Group in Peru. Efficacy of combined antiparasitic therapy with praziquantel and albendazole for neurocysticercosis: a double-blind, randomised controlled trial. Lancet Infect Dis. 2014 Aug; 14(8):687–95. [PMID: 24999157]

2. Echinococcosis

ESSENTIALS OF DIAGNOSIS

▶ History of exposure to dogs or wild canines in an endemic area.

▶ Large cystic lesions, most commonly of the liver or lung.

▶ Positive serologic tests.

General Considerations

Echinococcosis occurs when humans are intermediate hosts for canine tapeworms. Infection is acquired by ingesting food contaminated with canine feces containing parasite eggs. The principal species that infect humans are *Echinococcus granulosus*, which causes cystic hydatid disease, and *Echinococcus multilocularis*, which causes alveolar hydatid disease. *E granulosus* is transmitted by domestic dogs in areas with livestock (sheep, goats, camels, and horses) as intermediate hosts, including Africa, the Middle East, southern Europe, South America, Central Asia, Australia, New Zealand, and the southwestern United States. *E multilocularis*, which much less commonly causes human disease, is transmitted by wild canines, and endemic in northern forest areas of the northern hemisphere, including central Europe, Siberia, northern Japan, northwestern Canada, and western Alaska. An increase in the fox population in Europe has been associated with an increase in human cases. The disease range has also extended southward in Central Asia and China. Other species that cause limited disease in humans are endemic in South America and China.

After humans ingest parasite eggs, the eggs hatch in the intestines to form oncospheres, which penetrate the mucosa, enter the circulation, and encyst in specific organs as hydatid cysts. *E granulosus* forms cysts most commonly in the liver (65%) and lungs (25%), but the cysts may develop in any organ, including the brain, bones, skeletal muscles, kidneys, and spleen. Cysts are most commonly single. The cysts can persist and slowly grow for many years.

Clinical Findings

A. Symptoms and Signs

Infections are commonly asymptomatic and may be noted incidentally on imaging studies or present with symptoms caused by an enlarging or superinfected mass. Findings may include abdominal or chest pain, biliary obstruction, cholangitis, portal hypertension, cirrhosis, bronchial obstruction leading to segmental lung collapse, and abscesses. Cyst leakage or rupture may be accompanied by a severe allergic reaction, including fever and hypotension. Seeding of cysts after rupture may extend the infection to new areas.

E multilocularis generally causes a more aggressive disease than *E granulosus*, with initial infection of the liver, but then local and distant spread commonly suggesting a malignancy. Symptoms based on the areas of involvement gradually worsen over years, with the development of obstructive findings in the liver and elsewhere.

B. Laboratory Findings

Serologic tests, including ELISA and immunoblot, offer sensitivity and specificity over 80% for *E granulosus* liver infections, but lower sensitivity for involvement of other organs. Serologic tests may also distinguish the two major echinococcal infections.

C. Imaging

Diagnosis is usually based on imaging studies, including ultrasonography, CT, and MRI. In *E granulosus* infection, a large cyst containing daughter cysts is highly suggestive of the diagnosis. In *E multilocularis* infection, imaging shows an irregular mass, often with areas of calcification.

Treatment

Treatment of cystic hydatid disease has traditionally involved cautious surgical resection of cysts, with care not to rupture cysts during removal. Injection of a cysticidal agent was used to limit spread in the case of rupture. Newer management algorithms include treatment with albendazole, often in conjunction with surgery. When used alone, as in cases where surgery is not possible, albendazole (10–15 mg/kg/day orally) has demonstrated efficacy, with courses of 3 months or longer duration, in some cases with alternating cycles of treatment and rest. Mebendazole (40–50 mg/kg/day orally) is an alternative drug, and praziquantel may also be effective. In some cases, medical therapy is begun, with surgery performed if disease persists after some months of therapy. Another approach, in particular with inoperable cysts, is percutaneous aspiration, injection, and reaspiration (PAIR). In this approach (which should not be used if cysts communicate with the biliary tract), patients receive antihelminthic therapy, and the cyst is partially aspirated. After diagnostic confirmation by examination for parasite protoscolices, a scolicidal agent (95% ethanol, hypertonic saline, or 0.5% cetrimide) is injected, and the cyst is reaspirated after about 15 minutes. PAIR includes a small risk of anaphylaxis, which has been reported in about 2% of procedures, but death due to anaphylaxis has been rare. Treatment of alveolar cyst disease is challenging, generally relying on wide surgical resection of lesions. Therapy with albendazole before or during surgery may be beneficial and may also provide improvement or even cure in inoperable cases.

Gomez I Gavara C et al. Review of the treatment of liver hydatid cysts. World J Gastroenterol. 2015 Jan 7;21(1):124–31. [PMID: 25574085]
McManus DP et al. Diagnosis, treatment, and management of echinococcosis. BMJ. 2012 Jun 11;344:e3866. [PMID: 22689886]
Nasseri-Moghaddam S et al. Percutaneous needle aspiration, injection, and re-aspiration with or without benzimidazole coverage for uncomplicated hepatic hydatid cysts. Cochrane Database Syst Rev. 2011 Jan 19;(1):CD003623. [PMID: 21249654]

INTESTINAL NEMATODE (ROUNDWORM) INFECTIONS

ASCARIASIS

ESSENTIALS OF DIAGNOSIS

▶ Transient cough, urticaria, pulmonary infiltrates, eosinophilia.

▶ Nonspecific abdominal symptoms.

▶ Eggs in stool; adult worms occasionally passed.

General Considerations

Ascaris lumbricoides is the most common of the intestinal helminths, infecting about a quarter of the world's population, with estimates of about a billion infections, 12 million acute cases, and 10,000 or more deaths annually. Prevalence is high wherever there is poor hygiene and sanitation or where human feces are used as fertilizer. Heavy infections are most common in children.

Infection follows ingestion of eggs in contaminated food. Larvae hatch in the small intestine, penetrate into the bloodstream, migrate to the lungs, and then travel via airways back to the gastrointestinal tract, where they develop to adult worms, which can be up to 40 cm in length, and live for 1–2 years.

Clinical Findings

Most persons with *Ascaris* infection are asymptomatic. In a small proportion of patients, symptoms develop during migration of worms through the lungs, with fever, nonproductive cough, chest pain, dyspnea, and eosinophilia, occasionally with eosinophilic pneumonia. Rarely, larvae lodge

ectopically in the brain, kidney, eye, spinal cord, and other sites and may cause local symptoms.

Light intestinal infections usually produce no symptoms. With heavy infection, abdominal discomfort may be seen. Adult worms may also migrate and be coughed up, be vomited, or may emerge through the nose or anus. They may also migrate into the common bile duct, pancreatic duct, appendix, and other sites, which may lead to cholangitis, cholecystitis, pyogenic liver abscess, pancreatitis, obstructive jaundice, or appendicitis. With very heavy infestations, masses of worms may cause intestinal obstruction, volvulus, intussusception, or death. Although severe manifestations of infection are uncommon, the very high prevalence of ascariasis leads to large numbers of individuals, especially children, with important sequelae. Moderate to high worm loads in children are also associated with nutritional abnormalities due to decreased appetite and food intake, and also decreased absorption of nutrients.

The diagnosis of ascariasis is made after adult worms emerge from the mouth, nose, or anus, or by identifying characteristic eggs in the feces, usually with the Kato-Katz technique. Imaging studies demonstrate worms, with filling defects in contrast studies and at times evidence of intestinal or biliary obstruction. Eosinophilia is marked during worm migration but may be absent during intestinal infection.

▶ Treatment

All infections should ideally be treated. Treatments of choice are albendazole (single 400 mg oral dose), mebendazole (single 500 mg oral dose or 100 mg twice daily for 3 days), or pyrantel pamoate (single 11 mg/kg oral dose, maximum 1 g). These drugs are all well tolerated but may cause mild gastrointestinal toxicity. They are considered safe for children above 1 year of age and in pregnancy, although use in the first trimester is best avoided. In endemic areas, reinfection after treatment is common. Intestinal obstruction usually responds to conservative management and antihelminthic therapy. Surgery may be required for appendicitis and other gastrointestinal complications.

TRICHURIASIS

Trichuris trichiura, the whipworm, infects about a billion persons throughout the world, particularly in humid tropical and subtropical environments. Infection is heaviest and most frequent in children. Infections are acquired by ingestion of eggs. The larvae hatch in the small intestine and mature in the large bowel to adult worms of about 4 cm in length. The worms do not migrate through tissues.

Most infected persons are asymptomatic. Heavy infections may be accompanied by abdominal cramps, tenesmus, diarrhea, distention, nausea, and vomiting. The *Trichuris* dysentery syndrome may develop, particularly in malnourished young children, with findings resembling inflammatory bowel disease including bloody diarrhea and rectal prolapse. Chronic infections in children can lead to iron deficiency anemia, growth retardation, and clubbing of the fingers.

Trichuriasis is diagnosed by identification of characteristic eggs and sometimes adult worms in stools. Eosinophilia is common. Treatment is typically with albendazole (400 mg/day orally) or mebendazole (200 mg/day orally), for 1–3 days for light infections or 3–7 days for heavy infections, but cure rates are lower than for ascariasis or hookworm infection. Recent randomized trials showed albendazole plus oxantel pamoate (31% cure; 96% egg reduction) to be superior to mebendazole, and albendazole plus oxantel pamoate (69% cure; 99% egg reduction) and albendazole plus ivermectin (28% cure; 95% egg reduction) to be superior to albendazole plus mebendazole. Oxantel pamoate has low efficacy against *Ascaris* and hookworm infection.

HOOKWORM DISEASE

ESSENTIALS OF DIAGNOSIS

▸ Transient pruritic skin rash and pulmonary symptoms.

▸ Anorexia, diarrhea, abdominal discomfort.

▸ Iron deficiency anemia.

▸ Characteristic eggs and occult blood in the stool.

▸ General Considerations

Infection with the hookworms *Ancylostoma duodenale* and *Necator americanus* is very common, especially in most tropical and subtropical regions. Both worms are broadly distributed. Prevalence is estimated at about 1 billion, causing approximately 65,000 deaths each year. When eggs are deposited on warm moist soil they hatch, releasing larvae that remain infective for up to a week. With contact, the larvae penetrate skin and migrate in the bloodstream to the pulmonary capillaries. In the lungs, the larvae penetrate into alveoli and then are carried by ciliary action upward to the bronchi, trachea, and mouth. After being swallowed, they reach and attach to the mucosa of the upper small bowel, where they mature to adult worms. *Ancylostoma* infection can also be acquired by ingestion of the larvae in food or water. Hookworms attach to the intestinal mucosa and suck blood. Blood loss is proportionate to the worm burden.

▸ Clinical Findings

A. Symptoms and Signs

Most infected persons are asymptomatic. A pruritic maculopapular rash (ground itch) may occur at the site of larval penetration, usually in previously sensitized persons. Pulmonary symptoms may be seen during larval migration through the lungs, with dry cough, wheezing, and low-grade fever, but these symptoms are less common than with ascariasis. About 1 month after infection, as maturing worms attach to the small intestinal mucosa, gastrointestinal symptoms may develop, with epigastric pain, anorexia, and diarrhea, especially in previously unexposed individuals.

Persons chronically infected with large worm burdens may have abdominal pain, anorexia, diarrhea, and findings of marked iron-deficiency anemia and protein malnutrition. Anemia can lead to pallor, weakness, dyspnea, and heart failure, and protein loss can lead to hypoalbuminemia, edema, and ascites. These findings may be accompanied by impairment in growth and cognitive development in children. Infection with the dog hookworm *Ancylostoma caninum* can uncommonly lead to abdominal pain, diarrhea, and eosinophilia, with intestinal ulcerations and regional lymphadenitis.

B. Laboratory Findings

Diagnosis is based on the demonstration of characteristic eggs in feces; concentration techniques are usually not needed. Microcytic anemia, occult blood in the stool, and hypoalbuminemia are common. Eosinophilia is common, especially during worm migration.

▸ Treatment

Treatment is with albendazole (single 400 mg oral dose) or mebendazole (100 mg orally twice daily for 3 days). These drugs are teratogenic, but experience suggests that they are safe in children over 1 year of age and during the second and third trimesters of pregnancy. Occasional adverse effects are diarrhea and abdominal pain. Pyrantel pamoate and levamisole are also effective. Anemia should be managed with iron replacement and, for severe symptomatic anemia, blood transfusion. Mass treatment of children with single doses of albendazole or mebendazole at regular intervals limits worm burdens and the extent of disease and is advocated by the WHO.

STRONGYLOIDIASIS

ESSENTIALS OF DIAGNOSIS

▸ Transient pruritic skin rash and pulmonary symptoms.

▸ Anorexia, diarrhea, abdominal discomfort.

▸ Hyperinfection syndrome in the immunocompromised.

▸ Larvae detected in stool.

▸ With hyperinfection, larvae detected in sputum or other fluids.

▸ Eosinophilia.

▸ General Considerations

Strongyloidiasis is caused by infection with *Strongyloides stercoralis*. Although much less prevalent than ascariasis, trichuriasis, or hookworm infections, strongyloidiasis is nonetheless a significant problem, infecting tens of millions of individuals in tropical and subtropical regions. Infection is also endemic in some temperate regions of North America, Europe, Japan, and Australia. Of particular importance is the predilection of the parasite to cause severe infections in immunocompromised individuals due to its ability to replicate in humans. A related parasite, *Strongyloides fuelleborni*, infects humans in parts of Africa and New Guinea.

Among nematodes, *S stercoralis* is uniquely capable of maintaining its full life cycle both within the human host and in soil. Infection occurs when filariform larvae in soil penetrate the skin, enter the bloodstream, and are carried to the lungs, where they escape from capillaries into alveoli, ascend the bronchial tree, and are then swallowed and carried to the duodenum and upper jejunum, where maturation to the adult stage takes place. Females live embedded in the mucosa for up to 5 years, releasing eggs that hatch in the intestines as free rhabditiform larvae that pass to the ground via the feces. In moist soil, these larvae metamorphose into infective filariform larvae. Autoinfection can occur in humans, when some rhabditiform larvae develop into filariform larvae that penetrate the intestinal mucosa or perianal skin, and enter the circulation. The most dangerous manifestation of *S stercoralis* infection is the **hyperinfection syndrome**, with dissemination of large numbers of filariform larvae to the lungs and other tissues in immunocompromised individuals. Mortality with this syndrome approaches 100% without treatment and has been about 25% with treatment. The hyperinfection syndrome is seen in patients receiving corticosteroids and other immunosuppressive medications; patients with hematologic malignancies, malnutrition, or alcoholism; or persons with AIDS. The risk seems greatest for those receiving corticosteroids.

► Clinical Findings

A. Symptoms and Signs

As with other intestinal nematodes, most infected persons are asymptomatic. An acute syndrome can be seen at the time of infection, with a pruritic, erythematous, maculopapular rash, usually of the feet. These symptoms may be followed by pulmonary symptoms (including dry cough, dyspnea, and wheezing) and eosinophilia after a number of days, followed by gastrointestinal symptoms after some weeks, as with hookworm infections. Chronic infection may be accompanied by epigastric pain, nausea, diarrhea, and anemia. Maculopapular or urticarial rashes of the buttocks, perineum, and thighs, due to migrating larvae, may be seen. Large worm burdens can lead to malabsorption or intestinal obstruction. Eosinophilia is common but may fluctuate.

With **hyperinfection** large numbers of larvae can migrate to many tissues, including the lungs, CNS, kidneys, and liver. Gastrointestinal symptoms can include abdominal pain, nausea, vomiting, diarrhea, and more severe findings related to intestinal obstruction, perforation, or hemorrhage. Bacterial sepsis, probably secondary to intestinal ulcerations, is a common presenting finding. Pulmonary findings include pneumonitis, cough, hemoptysis, and respiratory failure. Sputum may contain adult worms, larvae, and eggs. CNS disease includes meningitis and brain abscesses; the CSF may contain larvae. Various presentations can progress to shock and death.

B. Laboratory Findings

The diagnosis of strongyloidiasis can be difficult, as eggs are seldom found in feces. Diagnosis is usually based on the identification of rhabditiform larvae in the stool or duodenal contents. These larvae must be distinguished from hookworm larvae, which may hatch after stool collection. Repeated examinations of stool or examination of duodenal fluid may be required for diagnosis because the sensitivity of individual tests is only about 30%. Hyperinfection is diagnosed by the identification of large numbers of larvae in stool, sputum, or other body fluids. An ELISA from the CDC offers about 90% sensitivity and specificity, but cross-reactions with other helminths may occur. Eosinophilia and mild anemia are common, but eosinophilia may be absent with hyperinfection. Hyperinfection may include extensive pulmonary infiltrates, hypoproteinemia, and abnormal liver function studies.

C. Screening

It is important to be aware of the possibility of strongyloidiasis in persons with even a distant history of residence in an endemic area, since the infection can be latent for decades. Screening of at-risk individuals for infection is appropriate before institution of immunosuppressive therapy. Screening can consist of serologic tests, with stool examinations in those with positive serologic tests, but consideration of presumptive treatment even if the stool evaluations are negative (see below).

► Treatment

Full eradication of *S stercoralis* is more important than with other intestinal helminths due to the ability of the parasite to replicate in humans. The treatment of choice for routine infection is ivermectin (200 mcg orally daily for 1–2 days). This treatment has replaced thiabendazole (25 mg/kg orally twice daily for 3 days), which is relatively poorly tolerated, and albendazole (400 mg orally twice daily for 3 days), which is less effective. For hyperinfection, ivermectin should be administered daily until the clinical syndrome has resolved and larvae have not been identified for at least 2 weeks. Follow-up examinations for larvae in stool or sputum are necessary, with repeat dosing if the infection persists. With continued immunosuppression, eradication may be difficult, and regular repeated doses of antihelminthic therapy (eg, monthly ivermectin) may be required.

ENTEROBIASIS

ESSENTIALS OF DIAGNOSIS

► Nocturnal perianal pruritus.
► Identification of eggs or adult worms on perianal skin or in stool.

General Considerations

Enterobius vermicularis, the pinworm, is a common cause of intestinal infections worldwide, with maximal prevalence in school-age children. Enterobiasis is transmitted person-to-person via ingestion of eggs after contact with the hands or perianal region of an infected individual, food or fomites that have been contaminated by an infected individual, or infected bedding or clothing. Autoinfection also occurs. Eggs hatch in the duodenum and larvae migrate to the cecum. Females mature in about a month, and remain viable for about another month. During this time, they migrate through the anus to deposit large numbers of eggs on the perianal skin. Due to the relatively short lifespan of these helminths, continuous reinfection, as in institutional settings, is required, for long-standing infection.

Clinical Findings

A. Symptoms and Signs

Most individuals with pinworm infection are asymptomatic. The most common symptom is perianal pruritus, particularly at night, due to the presence of the female worms or deposited eggs. Insomnia, restlessness, and enuresis are common in children. Perianal scratching may result in excoriation and impetigo. Many mild gastrointestinal symptoms have also been attributed to enterobiasis, but associations are not proven. Serious sequelae are uncommon. Rarely, worm migration results in inflammation or granulomatous reactions of the gastrointestinal or genitourinary tracts. Colonic ulceration and eosinophilic colitis have been reported.

B. Laboratory Findings

Pinworm eggs are usually not found in stool. Diagnosis is made by finding adult worms or eggs on the perianal skin. A common test is to apply clear cellophane tape to the perianal skin, ideally in the early morning, followed by microscopic examination for eggs. The sensitivity of the tape test is reported to be about 50% for a single test and 90% for three tests. Nocturnal examination of the perianal area or gross examination of stools may reveal adult worms, which are about 1 cm in length. Eosinophilia is rare.

Treatment

Treatment is with single oral doses of albendazole (400 mg), mebendazole (100 mg) or pyrantel pamoate (11 mg/kg, to a maximum of 1 g). The dose is repeated in 2 weeks due to frequent reinfection. Other infected family members should be treated concurrently, and treatment of all close contacts may be appropriate when rates of reinfection are high in family, school, or institutional settings. Standard handwashing and hygiene practices are helpful in limiting spread. Perianal scratching should be discouraged. Washing of clothes and bedding should kill pinworm eggs.

Greaves D et al. Strongyloides stercoralis infection. BMJ. 2013 Jul 30;347:f4610. [PMID: 23900531]
Knopp S et al. Nematode infections: soil-transmitted helminths and trichinella. Infect Dis Clin North Am. 2012 Jun;26(2):341–58. [PMID: 22632643]

Lamberton PH et al. Human ascariasis: diagnostics update. Curr Trop Med Rep. 2015;2(4):189–200. [PMID: 26550552]
Mejia R et al. Screening, prevention, and treatment for hyperinfection syndrome and disseminated infections caused by *Strongyloides stercoralis*. Curr Opin Infect Dis. 2012 Aug; 25(4):458–63. [PMID: 22691685]
Speich B et al. Efficacy and safety of albendazole plus ivermectin, albendazole plus mebendazole, albendazole plus oxantel pamoate, and mebendazole alone against *Trichuris trichiura* and concomitant soil-transmitted helminth infections: a four-arm, randomised controlled trial. Lancet Infect Dis. 2015 Mar; 15(3):277–84. [PMID: 25589326]
Speich B et al. Oxantel pamoate-albendazole for *Trichuris trichiura* infection. N Engl J Med. 2014 Feb 13;370(7):610–20. [PMID: 24521107]

INVASIVE NEMATODE (ROUNDWORM) INFECTIONS

TRICHINOSIS

ESSENTIALS OF DIAGNOSIS

▶ Ingestion of inadequately cooked pork or game.

▶ Transient intestinal symptoms followed by fever, myalgias, and periorbital edema.

▶ Eosinophilia and elevated serum muscle enzymes.

General Considerations

Trichinosis (or trichinellosis) is caused worldwide by *Trichinella spiralis* and related *Trichinella* species. The disease is spread by ingestion of undercooked meat, most commonly pork in areas where pigs feed on garbage. When infected raw meat is ingested, *Trichinella* larvae are freed from cyst walls by gastric acid and pass into the small intestine. The larvae then invade intestinal epithelial cells, develop into adults, and the adults release infective larvae. These parasites travel to skeletal muscle via the bloodstream. They invade muscle cells, enlarge, and form cysts. These larvae may be viable for years. Pigs and other animals become infected by eating infected uncooked food scraps or other animals, such as rats.

The worldwide incidence of trichinosis has decreased, but human infections continue to occur sporadically or in outbreaks, with estimates of ~10,000 cases annually. In addition to undercooked pork, infections have been transmitted by ingestion of game and other animals, including bear and walrus in North America and wild boar and horse in Europe. In the United States, about 20 infections are reported annually, mostly from ingesting wild game.

Clinical Findings

A. Symptoms and Signs

Most infections are asymptomatic. In symptomatic cases, gastrointestinal symptoms, including diarrhea, vomiting, and abdominal pain, develop within the week after ingestion of contaminated meat. These symptoms usually last for less than a week but can occasionally persist for much longer. During the following week, symptoms and signs related to migrating larvae are seen. These findings include, most notably, fever, myalgias, periorbital edema, and eosinophilia. Additional findings may include headache, cough, dyspnea, hoarseness, dysphagia, macular or petechial rash, and subconjunctival and retinal hemorrhages. Systemic symptoms usually peak within 2–3 weeks, and commonly persist for about 2 months. In severe cases, generally with large parasite burdens, muscle involvement can be pronounced, with severe muscle pain, edema, and weakness, especially in the head and neck. Muscle pain may persist for months. Uncommon severe findings include myocarditis, pneumonitis, and meningoencephalitis, sometimes leading to death.

B. Laboratory Findings

The clinical diagnosis is supported by findings of elevated serum muscle enzymes (creatine kinase, lactate dehydrogenase, aspartate aminotransferase). A commercial ELISA assay is available in the United States. Serologic tests become positive 2 or more weeks after infection, but cross-reactivity can be seen with other parasites. Rising antibody titers are highly suggestive of the diagnosis. Muscle biopsy can usually be avoided, but if the diagnosis is uncertain, biopsy of a tender, swollen muscle may identify *Trichinella* larvae. For maximal yield, biopsy material should be examined histologically, and a portion enzymatically digested to release larvae, but evaluation before 3 weeks after infection may not show muscle larvae. Serum and muscle biopsy analysis are available from the CDC.

▶ Treatment

No effective specific therapy for full-blown trichinosis has been identified. However, if infection is suspected early in the course of illness, treatment with mebendazole (2.5 mg/kg orally twice daily) or albendazole (5–7.5 mg/kg orally twice daily) will kill intestinal worms and may limit progression to tissue invasion. Supportive therapy for systemic disease consists of analgesics, antipyretics, bed rest and, in severe illness, corticosteroids. Infection is prevented by cooking to a temperature of at least 71°C for at least 1 minute. Irradiation of meat is also effective in eliminating *Trichinella* larvae, but freezing is not reliable.

Gottstein B et al. Epidemiology, diagnosis, treatment, and control of trichinellosis. Clin Microbiol Rev. 2009 Jan;22(1):127–45. [PMID: 19136437]

TOXOCARIASIS

▶ General Considerations

The dog roundworm *Toxocara canis*, the cat roundworm *Toxocara cati*, and less commonly other helminths may cause visceral larva migrans. *T canis* is highly prevalent in dogs. Humans are infected after ingestion of eggs in material contaminated by dog or other feces. Infection is spread principally by puppies and lactating females, and the eggs must be on the ground for several weeks before they are infectious. After ingestion by humans, larvae migrate to various tissues but cannot complete their life cycle.

▶ Clinical Findings

Visceral larva migrans is seen principally in young children. Most infections are asymptomatic. The most commonly involved organs are the liver and lungs. Presentations include cough, fever, wheezing, hepatomegaly, splenomegaly, lymphadenopathy, pulmonary infiltrates, and eosinophilia. Involvement of the CNS can occur rarely, leading to eosinophilic meningitis and other abnormalities. Ocular larva migrans is a distinct syndrome, usually in children older than is typical for visceral larva migrans. Children present with visual deficits, pain, and a retinal mass, which can be confused with retinoblastoma. *Baylisascaris procyonis*, a roundworm of raccoons, can rarely cause visceral larva migrans in humans, typically with similar, but more severe manifestations than *T canis*.

The diagnosis of visceral larva migrans is suggested by the finding of eosinophilia in a child with hepatomegaly or other signs of the disease, especially with a history of exposure to puppies. The diagnosis is confirmed by the identification of larvae in a biopsy of infected tissue, usually performed when other diseases are suspected. Serologic tests may be helpful; an ELISA against a group of excreted antigens has shown good sensitivity and specificity. Most patients recover without specific therapy, although symptoms may persist for months.

▶ Treatment

Treatment with antihelminthics or corticosteroids may be considered in severe cases. No drugs have been proven to be effective, but albendazole (400 mg orally twice daily for 5 days), mebendazole, thiabendazole, diethylcarbamazine, and ivermectin have been used, and albendazole has been recommended as the treatment of choice.

Moreira GM et al. Human toxocariasis: current advances in diagnostics, treatment, and interventions. Trends Parasitol. 2014 Sep;30(9):456–64. [PMID: 25089038]

CUTANEOUS LARVA MIGRANS (Creeping Eruption)

Cutaneous larva migrans is caused principally by larvae of the dog and cat hookworms, *Ancylostoma braziliense* and *A caninum*. Other animal hookworms, gnathostomiasis, and strongyloidiasis may also cause this syndrome. Infections are common in warm areas, including the southeastern United States. They are most common in children. The disease is caused by the migration of worms through skin; the non-human parasites cannot complete their life cycles, so only cause cutaneous disease.

▶ Clinical Findings

Intensely pruritic erythematous papules develop, usually on the feet or hands, followed within a few days by

▲ **Figure 35–8.** Cutaneous larva migrans on the foot. (Reproduced, with permission, from Richard P. Usatine, MD.)

serpiginous tracks marking the course of the parasite, which may travel several millimeters per day (Figure 35–8). Several tracks may be present. The process may continue for weeks, with lesions becoming vesiculated, encrusted, or secondarily infected. Systemic symptoms or eosinophilia are uncommon.

The diagnosis is based on the characteristic appearance of the lesions. Biopsy is usually not indicated.

 Treatment

Without treatment, the larvae eventually die and are absorbed. Mild cases do not require treatment. Thiabendazole (10% aqueous suspension) can be applied topically three times daily for 5 or more days. Systemic therapy with albendazole (400 mg orally once or twice daily for 3–5 days) or ivermectin (200 mcg/kg orally single dose) is highly effective.

Kincaid L et al. Management of imported cutaneous larva migrans: a case series and mini-review. Travel Med Infect Dis. 2015 Sep–Oct;13(5):382–7. [PMID: 26243366]

FILARIASIS

LYMPHATIC FILARIASIS

ESSENTIALS OF DIAGNOSIS

► Episodic attacks of lymphangitis, lymphadenitis, and fever.
► Chronic progressive swelling of extremities and genitals; hydrocele; chyluria; lymphedema.
► Microfilariae in blood, chyluria, or hydrocele fluid; positive serologic tests.

► **General Considerations**

Lymphatic filariasis is caused by three filarial nematodes: *Wuchereria bancrofti*, *Brugia malayi*, and *Brugia timori*,

and is among the most important parasitic diseases of man. Approximately 120 million people are infected with these organisms in tropical and subtropical countries, about a third of these suffer clinical consequences of the infections, and many are seriously disfigured. *W bancrofti* causes about 90% of episodes of lymphatic filariasis. It is transmitted by *Culex, Aedes,* and *Anopheles* mosquitoes and is widely distributed in the tropics and subtropics, including sub-Saharan Africa, Southeast Asia, the western Pacific, India, South America, and the Caribbean. *B malayi* is transmitted by *Mansonia* and *Anopheles* mosquitoes and is endemic in parts of China, India, Southeast Asia, and the Pacific. *B timori* is found only in islands of southeastern Indonesia. *Mansonella* are filarial worms transmitted by midges and other insects in Africa and South America.

Humans are infected by the bites of infected mosquitoes. Larvae then move to the lymphatics and lymph nodes, where they mature over months to thread-like adult worms, and then can persist for many years. The adult worms produce large numbers of microfilariae, which are released into the circulation, and infective to mosquitoes, particularly at night (except for the South Pacific, where microfilaremia peaks during daylight hours).

► **Clinical Findings**

A. Symptoms and Signs

Many infections remain asymptomatic despite circulating microfilariae. Clinical consequences of filarial infection are principally due to inflammatory responses to developing, mature, and dying worms. The initial manifestation of infection is often acute lymphangitis, with fever, painful lymph nodes, edema, and inflammation spreading peripherally from involved lymph nodes (in contrast to bacterial lymphangitis, which spreads centrally). Lymphangitis and lymphadenitis of the upper and lower extremities is common (Figure 35–9); genital involvement, including

▲ **Figure 35–9.** Elephantiasis of legs due to filariasis. (Public Health Image Library, CDC.)

epididymitis and orchitis, with scrotal pain and tenderness, occurs principally only with *W bancrofti* infection. Acute attacks of lymphangitis last for a few days to a week and may recur a few times per year. Filarial fevers may also occur without lymphatic inflammation.

The most common chronic manifestation of lymphatic filariasis is swelling of the extremities or genitals due to chronic lymphatic inflammation and obstruction. Extremities become increasingly swollen, with a progression over time from pitting edema, to nonpitting edema, to sclerotic changes of the skin that are referred to as elephantiasis. Genital involvement, particularly with *W bancrofti*, occurs more commonly in men, progressing from painful epididymitis to hydroceles that are usually painless but can become very large, with inguinal lymphadenopathy, thickening of the spermatic cord, scrotal lymphedema, thickening and fissuring of the scrotal skin, and occasionally chyluria. Lymphedema of the female genitalia and breasts may also occur.

Tropical pulmonary eosinophilia is a distinct syndrome principally affecting young adult males with either *W bancrofti* or *B malayi* infection but typically without microfilaremia. This syndrome is characterized by asthma-like symptoms, with cough, wheezing, dyspnea, and low-grade fevers, usually at night. Without treatment, tropical pulmonary eosinophilia can progress to interstitial fibrosis and chronic restrictive lung disease. *Mansonella* can inhabit serous cavities, the retroperitoneum, the eye, or the skin, and cause abnormalities related to inflammation at these sites.

B. Laboratory Findings

The diagnosis of lymphatic filariasis is strongly suggested by characteristic findings of lymphangitis or lymphatic obstruction in persons with risk factors for the disease. The diagnosis is confirmed by finding microfilariae, usually in blood, but microfilariae may be absent, especially early in the disease progression (first 2–3 years) or with chronic obstructive disease. To increase yields, blood samples are obtained at about midnight in most areas, but during daylight hours in the South Pacific. Smears are evaluated by wet mount to identify motile parasites and by Giemsa staining; these examinations can be delayed until the following morning, with storage of samples at room temperature. Of note, the periodicity of microfilaremia is variable, and daytime samples may yield positive results. Microfilariae may also be identified in hydrocele fluid or chylous urine. Eosinophilia is usually absent, except during acute inflammatory syndromes. Serologic tests may be helpful but cannot distinguish past and active infections. Rapid antigen tests with sensitivity and specificity over 90% are available for detection of *W bancrofti*. These can be considered the diagnostic tests of choice and are increasingly used to guide control programs. However, cross-reactivity with *Loa loa* infections has been described. Due to potential severe toxicity, caution is appropriate before treatment with ivermectin for positive *W bancrofti* antigen tests in areas also endemic for *L loa* infection. Multiple molecular tests, including field-friendly LAMP assays, have been developed. Adult worms may also be found in lymph node biopsy specimens (although biopsy is not usually clinically

indicated) or by ultrasound of a scrotal hydrocele or lymphedematous breast. When microfilaremia is lacking, especially if sophisticated techniques are not available, diagnoses may need to be made on clinical grounds.

▶ Treatment & Control

A. Drug Treatment

Diethylcarbamazine is the drug of choice, but it cannot cure infections due to its limited action against adult worms. Asymptomatic infection and acute lymphangitis are treated with this drug (2 mg/kg orally three times daily) for 10–14 days, leading to a marked decrease in microfilaremia. Therapy may be accompanied by allergic symptoms, including fever, headache, malaise, hypotension, and bronchospasm, probably due to release of antigens from dying worms. For this reason, treatment courses may begin with a lower dosage, with escalation over the first 4 days of treatment. Single annual doses of diethylcarbamazine (6 mg/kg orally), alone or with ivermectin (400 mcg/kg orally) or albendazole (400 mg orally) may be as effective as longer courses of diethylcarbamazine. When onchocerciasis or loiasis is suspected, it may be appropriate to withhold diethylcarbamazine to avoid severe reactions to dying microfilariae; rather, ivermectin plus albendazole may be given, although these drugs are less active than diethylcarbamazine against adult worms. Appropriate management of advanced obstructive disease is uncertain. Drainage of hydroceles provides symptomatic relief, although they will recur. Therapy with diethylcarbamazine cannot reverse chronic lymphatic changes but is typically provided to lower worm burdens. An interesting approach under study is to treat with doxycycline (100–200 mg/day orally for 4–6 weeks), which kills obligate intracellular *Wolbachia* bacteria, leading to death of adult filarial worms. Doxycycline was also effective at controlling *Mansonella perstans* infection, which does not respond well to standard antifilarial drugs. Secondary bacterial infections must be treated. Surgical correction may be helpful in some cases.

B. Disease Control

Avoidance of mosquitoes is a key measure; preventive measures include the use of screens, bed nets (ideally treated with insecticide), and insect repellents. Community-based treatment with single annual doses of effective drugs offers a highly effective means of control. The current WHO strategy for control includes mass treatment of at risk communities with single annual doses of diethylcarbamazine plus albendazole or, for areas with onchocerciasis, albendazole plus ivermectin; in some circumstances, more frequent dosing offers improved control.

Alhassan A et al. Expanding the MDx toolbox for filarial diagnosis and surveillance. Trends Parasitol. 2015 Aug;31(8):391–400. [PMID: 25978936]

Tisch DJ et al. Reduction in acute filariasis morbidity during a mass drug administration trial to eliminate lymphatic filariasis in Papua New Guinea. PLoS Negl Trop Dis. 2011 Jul; 5(7):e1241. [PMID: 21765964]

ONCHOCERCIASIS

- ▶ Severe pruritus; skin excoriations, thickening, and depigmentation; and subcutaneous nodules.
- ▶ Conjunctivitis progressing to blindness.
- ▶ Microfilariae in skin snips and on slit-lamp examination; adult worms in subcutaneous nodules.

▶ General Considerations

Onchocerciasis, or river blindness, is caused by *Onchocerca volvulus*. An estimated 37 million persons are infected, of whom 3–4 million have skin disease, 500,000 have severe visual impairment, and 300,000 are blinded. Over 99% of infections are in sub-Saharan Africa, especially the West African savanna, with about half of cases in Nigeria and Congo. In some hyperendemic African villages, close to 100% of individuals are infected, and 10% or more of the population is blind. The disease is also prevalent in the southwestern Arabian peninsula and Latin America, including southern Mexico, Guatemala, Venezuela, Colombia, Ecuador, and northwestern Brazil. Onchocerciasis is transmitted by simulium flies (blackflies). These insects breed in fast-flowing streams and bite during the day.

After the bite of an infected blackfly, larvae are deposited in the skin, where adults develop over 6–12 months. Adult worms live in subcutaneous connective tissue or muscle nodules for a decade or more. Microfilariae are released from the nodules and migrate through subcutaneous and ocular tissues. Disease is due to responses to worms and to intracellular *Wolbachia* bacteria.

▶ Clinical Findings

A. Symptoms and Signs

After an incubation period of up to 1–3 years, the disease typically produces an erythematous, papular, pruritic rash, which may progress to chronic skin thickening and depigmentation. Itching may be severe and unresponsive to medications, such that more disability-adjusted life years are lost to onchocercal skin problems than to blindness. Numerous firm, nontender, movable subcutaneous nodules of about 0.5–3 cm, which contain adult worms, may be present. Due to differences in vector habits, these nodules are more commonly on the lower body in Africa but on the head and upper body in Latin America. Inguinal and femoral lymphadenopathy is common, at times resulting in a "hanging groin," with lymph nodes hanging within a sling of atrophic skin. Patients may also have systemic symptoms, with weight loss and musculoskeletal pain.

The most serious manifestations of onchocerciasis involve the eyes. Microfilariae migrating through the eyes elicit host responses that lead to pathology. Findings include punctate keratitis and corneal opacities, progressing to sclerosing keratitis and blindness. Iridocyclitis, glaucoma, choroiditis, and optic atrophy may also lead to vision loss. The likelihood of blindness after infection varies greatly based on geography, with the risk greatest in savanna regions of West Africa.

B. Diagnostic Testing

The diagnosis is made by identifying microfilariae in skin snips, by visualizing microfilariae in the cornea or anterior chamber by slit-lamp examination, by identification of adult worms in a biopsy or aspirate of a nodule or, uncommonly, by identification of microfilariae in urine. Skin snips from the iliac crest (Africa) or scapula (Americas) are allowed to stand in saline for 2–4 hours or longer, and then examined microscopically for microfilariae. Deep punch biopsies are not needed, and if suspicion persists after a skin snip is negative, the procedure should be repeated. Ultrasound may identify characteristic findings suggestive of adult worms in skin nodules. When the diagnosis remains difficult, the Mazzotti test can be used; exacerbation of skin rash and pruritus after a 50-mg dose of diethylcarbamazine is highly suggestive of the diagnosis. This test should only be used after other tests are negative, since treatment can elicit severe skin and eye reactions in heavily infected individuals. A related and safer test using topical diethylcarbamazine is also available. Eosinophilia is a common, but inconsistent finding. Antigen and antibody detection tests are under study.

▶ Treatment & Control

The treatment of choice is ivermectin, which has replaced diethylcarbamazine due to a much lower risk of severe reactions to therapy. Ivermectin kills microfilariae, but not adult worms, so disease control requires repeat administrations. Treatment is with a single oral dose of 150 mcg/mL, but schedules for re-treatment have not been standardized. One regimen is to treat every 3 months for 1 year, followed by treatment every 6–12 months for the suspected lifespan of adult worms (about 15 years). Treatment results in marked reduction in numbers of microfilariae in the skin and eyes, although its impact on the progression of visual loss remains uncertain. Toxicities of ivermectin are generally mild; fever, pruritus, urticaria, myalgias, edema, hypotension, and tender lymphadenopathy may be seen, presumably due to reactions to dying worms. Ivermectin should be used with caution in patients also at risk for loiasis, since it can elicit severe reactions including encephalopathy. As with other filarial infections, doxycycline acts against *O volvulus* by killing intracellular *Wolbachia* bacteria. A course of 100 mg/day for 6 weeks kills the bacteria and prevents parasite embryogenesis for at least 18 months. Doxycycline shows promise as a first-line agent to treat onchocerciasis because of its improved activity against adult worms compared to other agents and limited toxicity due to the slow action of the drug.

Protection against onchocerciasis includes avoidance of biting flies. Major efforts are underway to control insect vectors in Africa. In addition, mass distribution of ivermectin for intermittent administration at the community level is ongoing, and the prevalence of severe skin and eye disease is decreasing.

Knopp S et al. Nematode infections: filariases. Infect Dis Clin North Am. 2012 Jun;26(2):359–81. [PMID: 22632644]

LOIASIS

ESSENTIALS OF DIAGNOSIS

► Subcutaneous swellings; adult worms migrating across the eye.

► Encephalitis, which may be brought on by treatment.

► Microfilariae in the blood.

► General Considerations

Loiasis is a chronic filarial disease caused by infection with *Loa loa*. The infection occurs in humans and monkeys in rainforest areas of West and central Africa. An estimated 3–13 million persons are infected. The disease is transmitted by chrysops flies, which bite during the day. Over 6–12 months after infection, larvae develop into adult worms, which migrate through subcutaneous tissues, including the subconjunctiva (leading to the term "eye worm"). Adults can live for up to 17 years.

► Clinical Findings

A. Symptoms and Signs

Many infected persons are asymptomatic, although they may have high levels of microfilaremia and eosinophilia. Transient subcutaneous swellings (Calabar swellings) develop in symptomatic persons. The swellings are nonerythematous, up to 20 cm in diameter, and may be preceded by local pain or pruritus. They usually resolve after 2–4 days but occasionally persist for several weeks. Calabar swellings are commonly seen around joints and may recur at the same or different sites. Visitors from nonendemic areas are more likely to have allergic-type reactions, including pruritus, urticaria, and angioedema. Adult worms may be seen to migrate across the eye, with either no symptoms or conjunctivitis, with pain and edema. The most serious complication of loiasis is encephalitis, which is most common in those with high level microfilaremia and microfilariae in the CSF. Symptoms may range from headache and insomnia to coma and death. Encephalitis may be brought on by treatment with diethylcarbamazine or ivermectin. Other complications of loiasis include kidney disease, with hematuria and proteinuria; endomyocardial fibrosis; and peripheral neuropathy.

B. Laboratory Findings

The diagnosis is established by identifying microfilariae in blood. Blood is evaluated as for lymphatic filariasis, but for loiasis blood should be obtained during the day. The failure to find microfilariae does not rule out the diagnosis. Identification of a migrating eye worm is also diagnostic. Serologic tests may be helpful in persons from nonendemic areas who may be acutely ill without detectable microfilaremia, but such tests have limited utility for residents of endemic areas because most of them will have positive test results. Molecular methods, including field-friendly LAMP assays, are available to rule out loiasis before administration of ivermectin for the control of other filarial infections.

► Treatment

The treatment of choice is diethylcarbamazine, which eliminates microfilariae and has some activity against adult worms. Treatment is with 8–10 mg/kg/day orally for 21 days; repeat courses may be needed. Mild side effects are common, including fever, pruritus, arthralgias, nausea, diarrhea, and Calabar swellings. These symptoms may be lessened by antihistamines or corticosteroids. Patients with large worm burdens are at greater risk for serious complications of therapy, including kidney injury, shock, encephalitis, coma, and death. Treatment with ivermectin, which is highly active against microfilariae, but not adult worms, entails a higher risk of severe reactions. To attempt to avoid these sequelae, pretreatment with corticosteroids and antihistamines, and escalating dosage of diethylcarbamazine have been used, but this strategy does not prevent encephalitis. The circulating parasite load that indicates particular risk for severe complications with therapy has been estimated at 2500/mL. Strategies to treat patients with high parasite loads include (1) no treatment; (2) apheresis, if available, to remove microfilariae prior to therapy with diethylcarbamazine; or (3) therapy with albendazole, which appears to be well tolerated due to its slow antiparasitic effects, prior to therapy with diethylcarbamazine or ivermectin. Doxycycline is not effective for loiasis.

Drame PM et al. Loop-mediated isothermal amplification for rapid and semiquantitative detection of *Loa loa* infection. J Clin Microbiol. 2014 Jun;52(6):2071–7. [PMID: 24696020]

Padgett JJ et al. Loiasis: African eye worm. Trans R Soc Trop Med Hyg. 2008 Oct;102(10):983–9. [PMID: 18466939]

Mycotic Infections

Samuel A. Shelburne, III, MD, PhD

Richard J. Hamill, MD

36

CANDIDIASIS

ESSENTIALS OF DIAGNOSIS

- ▶ Common normal flora but opportunistic pathogen.
- ▶ Gastrointestinal mucosal disease, particularly esophagitis, most common.
- ▶ Fungemia, arising from an intravenous catheter or the gastrointestinal tract occurs in patients who have sustained cutaneous or mucosal injury, undergone instrumentation, are receiving total parenteral nutrition, have kidney disease, or have received broad-spectrum antibiotics.

▶ General Considerations

Candida albicans can be cultured from the mouth, vagina, and feces of most people. Cutaneous and oral lesions are discussed in Chapters 6 and 8, respectively. The risk factors for invasive candidiasis include prolonged neutropenia, recent abdominal surgery, broad-spectrum antibiotic therapy, kidney disease, and the presence of intravascular catheters (especially when providing total parenteral nutrition). Cellular immunodeficiency predisposes to mucocutaneous disease. When no other underlying cause is found, persistent oral or vaginal candidiasis should arouse a suspicion of HIV infection.

▶ Clinical Findings

A. Mucosal Candidiasis

Esophageal involvement is the most frequent type of significant mucosal disease. Presenting symptoms include substernal odynophagia, gastroesophageal reflux, or nausea without substernal pain. Oral candidiasis, though often associated, is not invariably present. Diagnosis is best confirmed by endoscopy with biopsy and culture.

Vulvovaginal candidiasis occurs in an estimated 75% of women during their lifetime. Risk factors include pregnancy, uncontrolled diabetes mellitus, broad-spectrum antimicrobial treatment, corticosteroid use, and HIV infection. Symptoms include acute vulvar pruritus, burning vaginal discharge, and dyspareunia.

B. Candidal Funguria

Most cases of candidal funguria are asymptomatic and represent specimen contamination or bladder colonization. However, signs and symptoms of true *Candida* urinary tract infections are indistinguishable from bacterial urinary tract infections and can include urgency, hesitancy, fever, chills, or flank pain.

C. Invasive Candidiasis

Invasive candidiasis can be (1) candidemia without deep-seated infection; (2) candidemia with deep-seated infection (typically eyes, kidney, or abdomen); and (3) deep-seated candidiasis in the absence of bloodstream infection. Varying ratios of these clinical entities depends on the predominating risk factors for affecting patients (ie, neutropenia, dialysis, postsurgical). The clinical presentation of candidemia varies from minimal fever to septic shock that can resemble a severe bacterial infection. The diagnosis of invasive *Candida* infection is problematic because *Candida* species are often isolated from mucosal sites in the absence of invasive disease while blood cultures are positive only 50% of the time in invasive infection.

Hepatosplenic candidiasis can occur following prolonged neutropenia in patients with underlying hematologic cancers, but this entity is less common in the era of widespread antifungal prophylaxis. Typically, fever and variable abdominal pain present weeks after chemotherapy, when neutrophil counts have recovered. Blood cultures are generally negative.

D. Candidal Endocarditis

Candidal endocarditis is a rare infection that is most frequently associated with exposure to a healthcare setting. Candidal endocarditis occurs with increased frequency on prosthetic valves in the first few months following surgery.

The diagnosis is established definitively by culturing *Candida* from emboli or from vegetations at the time of valve replacement.

▶ Treatment

A. Mucosal Candidiasis

Therapy of **esophageal candidiasis** depends on the severity of disease. If patients are able to swallow and take adequate amounts of fluid orally, fluconazole, 100 mg/day (or itraconazole solution, 10 mg/mL, 200 mg/day), for 10–14 days usually suffices. In the individual who is more ill or in whom esophagitis has developed while taking fluconazole, options include oral or intravenous voriconazole, 200 mg twice daily; intravenous amphotericin B, 0.3 mg/kg/day; intravenous caspofungin, 50 mg/day; intravenous anidulafungin, 100 mg on day 1, then 50 mg/day; or intravenous micafungin, 150 mg/day. Relapse is common with all agents when there is underlying HIV infection without adequate immune reconstitution.

Various topical azole preparations (eg, clotrimazole, 100 mg vaginal tablet for 7 days, or miconazole, 200 mg vaginal suppository for 3 days) are effective against **vulvovaginal candidiasis**. One 150 mg oral dose of fluconazole has been shown to have equivalent efficacy with better patient acceptance. Disease recurrence is common but can be decreased with weekly fluconazole therapy (150 mg weekly).

B. Candidal Funguria

Candidal funguria frequently resolves with discontinuance of antibiotics or removal of bladder catheters. Clinical benefit from treatment of asymptomatic candiduria has not been demonstrated, but persistent funguria should raise the suspicion of invasive infection. When symptomatic funguria persists, oral fluconazole, 200 mg/day for 7–14 days, can be used.

C. Invasive Candidiasis

The 2016 guidelines for management of candidiasis recommend an echinocandin such as caspofungin (loading dose of 70 mg intravenously once, then 50 mg intravenously daily), micafungin (100 mg intravenously daily), or anidulafungin (loading dose of 200 mg intravenously once, then 100 mg intravenously daily). Fluconazole (loading dose of 800 mg [12 mg/kg] intravenously, then 400 mg [6 mg/kg] intravenously daily) is an acceptable alternative for less critically ill patients without recent azole exposure. Therapy for candidemia should be continued for 2 weeks after the last positive blood culture and resolution of symptoms and signs of infection. A dilated fundoscopic examination is recommended for all patients with candidemia to exclude endophthalmitis and repeat blood cultures should be drawn to demonstrate organism clearance. Once patients have become clinically stable, parenteral therapy can be discontinued and oral fluconazole, 200–800 mg orally given as one or two doses daily, is used to complete treatment for isolates known to be or likely to be susceptible to fluconazole.

Removal or exchange of intravascular catheters is generally recommended for patients with candidemia in whom the catheter is the suspected source of infection.

Non-*albicans* species of *Candida* account for over 50% of clinical bloodstream isolates and often have resistance patterns that are different from *C albicans*. An echinocandin is recommended for treatment of *Candida glabrata* infection with a transition to oral fluconazole or voriconazole reserved for patients whose isolates are known to be susceptible to these agents. *C glabrata* that is resistant to azoles and echinocandins is being increasingly reported. Similarly, *Candida krusei* is generally fluconazole-resistant and so should be treated with an alternative agent, such as echinocandin or voriconazole. Fluconazole may be optimal for *Candida parapsilosis* due to possible echinocandin resistance in such isolates.

Although the isolation of *Candida* species from mucosal sites raises the possibility of invasive candidiasis, randomized trials of empiric antifungal agents in such situations have not shown clear clinical benefit. Hepatosplenic candidiasis generally requires treatment for several months until lesion resolution.

D. Candidal Endocarditis

Best results are achieved with a combination of medical and surgical therapy. Lipid formulation amphotericin B (3–5 mg/kg/day) or high-dose echinocandin (caspofungin 150 mg/day, micafungin 150 mg/day, or anidulafungin 200 mg/day) is recommended as initial therapy. Step-down or long-term suppressive therapy for nonsurgical candidates may be done with fluconazole at 6–12 mg/kg/day for susceptible organisms.

In high-risk patients undergoing induction chemotherapy, bone marrow transplantation, or liver transplantation, prophylaxis with antifungal agents has been shown to prevent invasive fungal infections although the effect on mortality and the preferred agent remain debated.

Knitsch W et al. A randomized, placebo-controlled trial of preemptive antifungal therapy for the prevention of invasive candidiasis following gastrointestinal surgery for intraabdominal infections. Clin Infect Dis. 2015 Dec 1; 61(11):1671–8. [PMID: 26270686]

Pappas PG et al. Clinical practice guideline for the management of candidiasis: 2016 update by the Infectious Diseases Society of America. Clin Infect Dis. 2016 Feb 15;62(4):e1–50. [PMID: 26679628]

HISTOPLASMOSIS

ESSENTIALS OF DIAGNOSIS

▶ Epidemiologically linked with exposure to bird and bat droppings; common along river valleys (especially the Ohio River and the Mississippi River valleys).

▶ Most patients asymptomatic; respiratory illness most common clinical problem.

▶ Disseminated disease especially common in AIDS or other immunosuppressed states, with poor prognosis.

▶ Biopsy of affected organs with culture or urinary polysaccharide antigen most useful in disseminated disease.

General Considerations

Histoplasmosis is caused by *Histoplasma capsulatum,* a dimorphic fungus that has been isolated from soil contaminated with bird or bat droppings in endemic areas (central and eastern United States, eastern Canada, Mexico, Central America, South America, Africa, and Southeast Asia). Infection presumably takes place by inhalation of conidia. These convert into small budding cells that are engulfed by phagocytes in the lungs. The organism proliferates and undergoes lymphohematogenous spread to other organs.

Clinical Findings

A. Symptoms and Signs

Most cases of histoplasmosis are asymptomatic or mild and thus go unrecognized. Past infection is recognized by pulmonary and splenic calcification noted on incidental radiographs. Symptomatic infection may present with mild influenza-like illness, often lasting 1–4 days. Moderately severe infections are frequently diagnosed as atypical pneumonia. These patients have fever, cough, and mild central chest pain lasting 5–15 days.

Clinically evident infections occur in several forms: (1) **Acute pulmonary histoplasmosis** frequently occurs in epidemics, often when soil containing infected bird or bat droppings is disturbed. Clinical manifestations can vary from a mild influenza-like illness to severe pneumonia. The illness may last from 1 week to 6 months but is almost never fatal. (2) **Progressive disseminated histoplasmosis** is commonly seen in patients with underlying HIV infection (with CD4 cell counts usually less than 100 cells/mcL) or other conditions of impaired cellular immunity. Disseminated histoplasmosis has also been reported in patients from endemic areas taking tumor necrosis factor (TNF)-blocking agents. It is characterized by fever and multiple organ system involvement. Chest radiographs may show a miliary pattern. Presentation may be fulminant, simulating septic shock, with death ensuing rapidly unless treatment is provided. Symptoms usually consist of fever, dyspnea, cough, loss of weight, and prostration. Ulcers of the mucous membranes of the oropharynx may be present. The liver and spleen are nearly always enlarged, and all the organs of the body are involved, particularly the adrenal glands; this results in adrenal insufficiency in about 50% of patients. Gastrointestinal involvement may mimic inflammatory bowel disease. (3) **Chronic pulmonary histoplasmosis** is usually seen in older patients who have underlying chronic lung disease. Chest radiographs show various lesions including apical cavities, infiltrates, and nodules. (4) **Complications of pulmonary**

histoplasmosis include granulomatous mediastinitis characterized by persistently enlarged mediastinal lymph nodes and fibrosing mediastinitis in which an excessive fibrotic response to *Histoplasma* infection results in compromise of pulmonary vascular structures.

B. Laboratory Findings

Most patients with chronic pulmonary disease show anemia of chronic disease. Bone marrow involvement may be prominent in disseminated forms with pancytopenia. Marked lactate dehydrogenase (LD) and ferritin elevations are also common as mild elevations of serum aspartate aminotransferase.

With pulmonary involvement, sputum culture is rarely positive except in chronic disease; antigen testing of bronchoalveolar lavage fluid may be helpful in acute disease. The combination of a first morning urine and serum polysaccharide antigen assays has an 83% sensitivity for the diagnosis of acute pulmonary histoplasmosis. Blood or bone marrow cultures from immunocompromised patients with acute disseminated disease are positive more than 80% of the time but may take several weeks for growth. The urine antigen assay has a sensitivity of greater than 90% for disseminated disease in immunocompromised patients and a declining titer can be used to follow response to therapy.

Treatment

For progressive localized disease and for mild to moderately severe nonmeningeal disseminated disease in immunocompetent or immunocompromised patients, itraconazole, 200–400 mg/day orally divided into two doses, is the treatment of choice with an overall response rate of approximately 80%. The oral solution is better absorbed than the capsule formulation, which requires gastric acid for absorption. Duration of therapy ranges from weeks to several months depending on the severity of illness. Intravenous amphotericin B formulations are used in patients with more severe illness such as meningitis, with guidelines favoring the use of liposomal or lipid complex amphotericin formulations at a dose of 3 mg/kg/day over amphotericin B deoxycholate. Patients with AIDS-related histoplasmosis require lifelong suppressive therapy with itraconazole, 200 mg/day orally, although secondary prophylaxis may be discontinued if immune reconstitution occurs in response to antiretroviral therapy. There is no clear evidence that antifungal or anti-inflammatory agents are of benefit for patients with granulomatous mediastinitis or fibrosing mediastinitis although oral itraconazole is often used. Reported outcomes in patients with fibrosing mediastinitis treated with either surgical procedures or nonsurgical intravascular interventions appear to be relatively good.

Hage CA et al. Histoplasmosis: up-to-date evidence-based approach to diagnosis and management. Semin Respir Crit Care Med. 2015 Oct;36(5):729–45. [PMID: 26398539]

Vergidis P et al. Histoplasmosis complicating tumor necrosis factor-α blocker therapy: a retrospective analysis of 98 cases. Clin Infect Dis. 2015 Aug 1;61(3):409–17. [PMID: 25870331]

COCCIDIOIDOMYCOSIS

ESSENTIALS OF DIAGNOSIS

▶ Influenza-like illness with malaise, fever, backache, headache, and cough.

▶ Erythema nodosum common with acute infection.

▶ Dissemination may result in meningitis, bony lesions, or skin and soft tissue abscesses.

▶ Chest radiograph findings vary from pneumonitis to cavitation.

▶ Serologic tests useful; large spherules containing endospores demonstrable in sputum or tissues.

▶ General Considerations

Coccidioidomycosis should be considered in the diagnosis of any obscure illness in a patient who has lived in or visited an endemic area. Infection results from the inhalation of arthroconidia of *Coccidioides immitis* or *C posadasii*; both organisms are molds that grow in soil in certain arid regions of the southwestern United States, in Mexico, and in Central and South America. Less than 1% of immunocompetent persons show dissemination, but among these patients, the mortality rate is high.

In HIV-infected people in endemic areas, coccidioidomycosis is a common opportunistic infection. In these patients, disease manifestations range from focal pulmonary infiltrates to widespread miliary disease with multiple organ involvement and meningitis; severity is inversely related to the extent of control of the HIV infection.

▶ Clinical Findings

A. Symptoms and Signs

Symptoms of **primary coccidioidomycosis** occur in about 40% of infections. Symptom onset (after an incubation period of 10–30 days) is usually that of a respiratory tract illness with fever and occasionally chills. Coccidioidomycosis is a common, frequently unrecognized, etiology of community-acquired pneumonia in endemic areas.

Erythema nodosum may appear 2–20 days after onset of symptoms. Persistent pulmonary lesions, varying from cavities and abscesses to parenchymal nodular densities or bronchiectasis, occur in about 5% of diagnosed cases.

Disseminated disease occurs in about 0.1% of white and 1% of nonwhite patients. Filipinos and blacks are especially susceptible, as are pregnant women of all races. Any organ may be involved. Pulmonary findings usually become more pronounced, with mediastinal lymph node enlargement, cough, and increased sputum production. Lung abscesses may rupture into the pleural space, producing an empyema. These may also extend to bones and skin, and pericardial and myocardial involvement has been occasionally observed. Fungemia may occur and is characterized clinically by a diffuse miliary pattern on chest radiograph and by early death. The course may be

particularly rapid in immunosuppressed patients. Clinicians caring for immunosuppressed patients in endemic areas need to consider that patients may be latently infected.

Meningitis occurs in 30–50% of cases of dissemination. Subcutaneous abscesses and verrucous skin lesions are especially common in fulminating cases. HIV-infected persons with disseminated disease have a higher incidence of miliary infiltrates, lymphadenopathy, and meningitis, but skin lesions are uncommon.

B. Laboratory Findings

In **primary coccidioidomycosis,** there may be moderate leukocytosis and eosinophilia. Serologic testing is useful for both diagnosis and prognosis. The immunodiffusion tube precipitin test and enzyme-linked immunosorbent assay (ELISA) detect IgM antibodies and are both useful for diagnosis early in the disease process. Historically, a persistent rising IgG complement fixation titer (1:16 or more) has been considered suggestive of disseminated disease; in addition, immunodiffusion complement fixation titers can be used to assess the adequacy of therapy. Serum complement fixation titer may be low when there is meningitis but no other disseminated disease. In patients with HIV-related coccidioidomycosis, the false-negative rate may be as high as 30%.

Demonstrable complement-fixing antibodies in spinal fluid are diagnostic of coccidioidal meningitis. These are found in over 90% of cases; *Coccidioides* antigen testing may augment (not replace) CSF antibody testing. Spinal fluid findings include increased cell count with lymphocytosis and reduced glucose. Spinal fluid culture is positive in approximately 30% of meningitis cases. Spherules filled with endospores may be found in biopsy specimens of soft tissues and bone; though they are not infectious, they convert to the highly contagious arthroconidia when grown in culture media. Blood cultures are rarely positive.

C. Imaging

Radiographic findings vary, but patchy, nodular and lobar upper lobe pulmonary infiltrates are most common. Hilar lymphadenopathy may be visible and is seen in localized disease; mediastinal lymphadenopathy suggests dissemination. There may be pleural effusions and lytic lesions in bone with accompanying complicated soft-tissue collections.

▶ Treatment

General symptomatic therapy is given as needed for disease limited to the chest with no evidence of progression. For progressive pulmonary or extrapulmonary disease, amphotericin B intravenously is used although oral azoles may be used for mild cases (see Chapter 30). Duration of therapy is determined by a declining complement fixation titer and a favorable clinical response. For meningitis, treatment usually is with high-dose oral fluconazole (400–800 mg/day, or higher) although lumbar or cisternal intrathecal administration of amphotericin B daily in increasing doses up to 1–1.5 mg/day is used initially by some clinicians or in cases refractory to fluconazole. Systemic therapy with amphotericin B, 0.6 mg/kg/day intravenously, is generally given concurrently with intrathecal therapy but is not sufficient alone for the treatment of meningeal disease. Once the patient is clinically stable, oral therapy with an azole, usually with fluconazole (400 mg daily) and given lifelong, is the recommended alternative to intrathecal amphotericin B therapy.

Itraconazole, 400 mg orally daily divided into two doses, or fluconazole, 200–400 mg, or higher, orally once or twice daily should be given for disease in the chest, bones, and soft tissues; however, therapy must be continued for 6 months or longer after the disease is inactive to prevent relapse. Response to therapy should be monitored by following the clinical response and progressive decrease in serum complement fixation titers.

Surgical drainage is necessary for management of soft tissue abscesses, necrotic bone and complicated pulmonary disease (eg, rupture of coccidioidal cavity).

▶ Prognosis

The prognosis for patients with limited disease is good, but persistent pulmonary cavities may cause complications such as hemoptysis or rupture producing pyopneumothorax. Serial complement fixation titers should be performed after therapy for patients with coccidioidomycosis; rising titers warrant reinstitution of therapy because relapse is likely. Late central nervous system complications of adequately treated meningitis include cerebral vasculitis with stroke and hydrocephalus that may require shunting. Disseminated and meningeal forms still have mortality rates exceeding 50% in the absence of therapy.

Ampel NM. The treatment of coccidioidomycosis. Rev Inst Med Trop Sao Paulo. 2015 Sep;57(Suppl 19):51–6. [PMID: 26465370]
Bamberger DM et al. Cerebrospinal fluid *Coccidioides* antigen testing in the diagnosis and management of central nervous system coccidioidomycosis. Mycoses. 2015 Oct;58(10):598–602. [PMID: 26393436]
Twarog M et al. Coccidioidomycosis: recent updates. Semin Respir Crit Care Med. 2015 Oct;36(5):746–55. [PMID: 26398540]

PNEUMOCYSTOSIS
(*Pneumocystis jirovecii* Pneumonia)

ESSENTIALS OF DIAGNOSIS

▶ Fever, dyspnea, nonproductive cough.

▶ Bilateral diffuse interstitial disease without hilar adenopathy by chest radiograph.

▶ Bibasilar crackles on auscultation in many cases; others have no findings.

▶ Reduced partial pressure of oxygen.

▶ *P jirovecii* in sputum, bronchoalveolar lavage fluid, or lung tissue.

▶ General Considerations

Pneumocystis jirovecii, the *Pneumocystis* species that affects humans, is distributed worldwide. Although symptomatic *P jirovecii* disease is rare in the general population, serologic evidence indicates that asymptomatic infections have occurred in most persons by a young age. The mode of transmission in primary infection is unknown, but the evidence suggests airborne transmission. Following asymptomatic primary infection, latent and presumably inactive organisms are sparsely distributed in the alveoli. De novo infection and reactivation of latent disease likely contribute to the mechanism of acute disease in older children and adults.

The overt infection is an acute interstitial plasma cell pneumonia that occurs with high frequency among two groups: (1) as epidemics of primary infections among premature or debilitated or marasmic infants on hospital wards in underdeveloped parts of the world, and (2) as sporadic cases among older children and adults who have an abnormal or altered cellular immunity. Cases occur commonly in patients with cancer or severe malnutrition and debility, in patients treated with immunosuppressive or cytotoxic drugs or irradiation for the management of organ transplants and cancer and, most frequently, in patients with AIDS (Chapter 31).

Pneumocystis pneumonia occurs in up to 80% of AIDS patients not receiving prophylaxis and is a major cause of death. Its incidence increases in direct proportion to the fall in CD4 cells, with most cases occurring at CD4 cell counts less than 200/mcL. In non-AIDS patients receiving immunosuppressive therapy, symptoms frequently begin after corticosteroids have been tapered or discontinued.

▶ Clinical Findings

A. Symptoms and Signs

Findings are usually limited to the pulmonary parenchyma. In the sporadic form of the disease associated with deficient cell-mediated immunity, the onset is typically abrupt, with fever, tachypnea, shortness of breath, and usually nonproductive cough. Pulmonary physical findings may be slight and disproportionate to the degree of illness and the radiologic findings; many patients have bibasilar crackles, but others do not. Without treatment, the course is usually one of rapid deterioration and death. Adult patients may present with spontaneous pneumothorax, usually in patients with previous episodes or those receiving aerosolized pentamidine prophylaxis. Patients with AIDS will usually have other evidence of HIV-associated disease, including fever, fatigue, and weight loss, for weeks or months preceding the illness.

B. Laboratory Findings

Chest radiographs most often show diffuse "interstitial" infiltration, which may be heterogeneous, miliary, or patchy early in infection. There may also be diffuse or focal consolidation, cystic changes, nodules, or cavitation within nodules. Pleural effusions are not seen. About 5–10% of patients with *Pneumocystis* pneumonia have normal chest films. High-resolution chest CT scans may be quite suggestive of *P jirovecii* pneumonia, helping distinguish it from other causes of pneumonia.

Arterial blood gas determinations usually show hypoxemia with hypocapnia but may be normal; however, rapid desaturation occurs if patients exercise before samples are drawn. Serologic tests are not helpful in diagnosis. The organism cannot be cultured, and definitive diagnosis depends on morphologic demonstration of the organisms in respiratory specimens using specific stains. The use of monoclonal antibody with immunofluorescence increases the sensitivity of diagnosis beyond Giemsa or methenamine silver stains. Polymerase chain reaction (PCR) of bronchoalveolar lavage is overly sensitive in that the test is often positive in colonized, noninfected persons but quantitative values may help with identifying infected patients, although precise cutoffs have not been established and may vary between different patient populations. Open lung biopsy and needle lung biopsy are infrequently done but may need to be performed to diagnose a granulomatous form of *Pneumocystis* pneumonia.

► Treatment

(Table 31–5.) It is appropriate to start empiric therapy for *P jirovecii* pneumonia if the disease is suspected clinically; however, in both AIDS patients and non-AIDS patients with mild to moderately severe disease, continued treatment should be based on a proved diagnosis because of clinical overlap with other infections, the toxicity of therapy, and the possible coexistence of other infectious organisms. Oral trimethoprim-sulfamethoxazole (TMP-SMZ) is the preferred agent because of its low cost and excellent bioavailability in both AIDS patients and non-AIDS patients with mild to moderately severe disease. Patients suffering from nausea and vomiting or intractable diarrhea should be given intravenous TMP-SMZ until they can tolerate the oral formulation. The impact of resistance of *Pneumocystis* to TMP-SMZ is unclear, although increasing rates of mutations in the *DHPS* and *DHFR* genes that mediate TMP-SMZ resistance have been reported. The best-studied second-line option is a combination of primaquine and clindamycin, although dapsone/trimethoprim, pentamidine, and atovaquone have also been used. Therapy should be continued with the selected medication for at least 5–10 days before considering changing agents, as fever, tachypnea, and pulmonary infiltrates persist for 4–6 days after starting treatment. Some patients have a transient worsening of their disease during the first 3–5 days, which may be related to an inflammatory response secondary to the presence of dead or dying organisms. Early addition of corticosteroids may attenuate this response (see below). Some clinicians prefer to treat episodes of AIDS-associated *Pneumocystis* pneumonia for 21 days rather than the usual 14 days recommended for non-AIDS cases.

A. Trimethoprim-Sulfamethoxazole

The dosage of TMP/SMZ is 15–20 mg/kg/day (based on trimethoprim component) given orally or intravenously daily in three or four divided doses for 14–21 days. Patients with AIDS have a high frequency of hypersensitivity reactions (approaching 50%), which may include fever, rashes (sometimes severe), malaise, neutropenia, hepatitis, nephritis, thrombocytopenia, hyperkalemia, and hyperbilirubinemia.

B. Primaquine/Clindamycin

A meta-analysis suggested that primaquine, 15–30 mg/day, plus clindamycin, 600 mg three times daily, is the best second-line therapy with superior results when compared with pentamidine. Primaquine may cause hemolytic anemia in patients with glucose-6-phosphate dehydrogenase (G6PD)-deficiency.

C. Pentamidine Isethionate

The use of pentamidine has decreased as alternative agents have been studied. This medication is administered intravenously (preferred) or intramuscularly as a single dose of 3–4 mg (salt)/kg/day for 14–21 days. Pentamidine causes side effects in nearly 50% of patients. Hypoglycemia (often clinically inapparent), hyperglycemia, hyponatremia, and delayed nephrotoxicity with azotemia may occur.

D. Atovaquone

Atovaquone is approved by the US Food and Drug Administration (FDA) for patients with mild to moderate disease who cannot tolerate TMP-SMZ or pentamidine, but failure is reported in 15–30% of cases. Mild side effects are common, but no serious reactions have been reported. The dosage is 750 mg three times daily for 21 days. Atovaquone should be administered with a fatty meal.

E. Other Medications

Trimethoprim, 15 mg/kg/day in three divided doses daily, plus dapsone, 100 mg/day, is an alternative oral regimen for mild to moderate disease or for continuation of therapy after intravenous therapy is no longer needed.

F. Prednisone

Based on studies done in patients with AIDS, prednisone is given for moderate to severe pneumonia (when Pao$_2$ on admission is less than 70 mm Hg or oxygen saturation is less than 90%) in conjunction with antimicrobials. The dosage of prednisone is 40 mg twice daily orally for 5 days, then 40 mg daily for 5 days, and then 20 mg daily until therapy is completed. The role of prednisone in non-AIDS patients is unclear, especially in patients in whom symptoms developed following tapering doses of corticosteroids.

► Prevention

Primary prophylaxis for *Pneumocystis* pneumonia in HIV-infected patients should be given to persons with CD4 counts less than 200 cells/mcL, a CD4 percentage below 14%, or weight loss or oral candidiasis (see Table 31–4). Primary prophylaxis is often used in patients with hematologic malignancy and transplant recipients, although the clinical characteristics of persons with these conditions who would benefit from *Pneumocystis* prophylaxis have not been clearly defined. Patients with a history of *Pneumocystis* pneumonia should receive secondary prophylaxis until they have had a durable virologic response to antiretroviral therapy for at least 3–6 months and maintained a CD4 count of greater than 200 cells/mcL.

► Prognosis

In the absence of early and adequate treatment, the fatality rate for the endemic infantile form of *Pneumocystis* pneumonia is 20–50%; for the sporadic form in immunodeficient persons, the fatality rate is nearly 100%. Early treatment reduces the mortality rate to about 3% in the former and 10–20% in AIDS patients. The mortality rate in other immunodeficient patients is still 30–50%, probably because of failure to make a timely diagnosis. In immunodeficient patients who do not receive prophylaxis, recurrences are common (30% in AIDS).

Karageorgopoulos DE et al. Accuracy of β-D-glucan for the diagnosis of *Pneumocystis jirovecii* pneumonia: a meta-analysis. Clin Microbiol Infect. 2013 Jan;19(1):39–49. [PMID: 22329494]

Stern A et al. Prophylaxis for *Pneumocystis* pneumonia (PCP) in non-HIV immunocompromised patients. Cochrane Database Syst Rev. 2014 Oct 1;10:CD005590. [PMID: 25269391]

CRYPTOCOCCOSIS

ESSENTIALS OF DIAGNOSIS

► Most common cause of fungal meningitis.

► Predisposing factors: Chemotherapy for hematologic malignancies, Hodgkin lymphoma, corticosteroid therapy, transplant recipients, TNF inhibitor therapy, HIV infection.

► Symptoms of headache, abnormal mental status; meningismus seen occasionally, though rarely in HIV-infected patients.

► Demonstration of capsular polysaccharide antigen in cerebrospinal fluid is diagnostic.

► General Considerations

Cryptococcosis is mainly caused by *Cryptococcus neoformans*, an encapsulated budding yeast that has been found worldwide in soil and on dried pigeon dung. *C gattii* is a closely related species that also causes disease in humans although *C gattii* may affect more ostensibly immunocompetent persons. It is a major cause of cryptococcosis in the Pacific Northwestern region of the United States and may result in more severe disease than *C neoformans*.

Infections are acquired by inhalation. In the lung, the infection may remain localized, heal, or disseminate. Clinically apparent cryptococcal pneumonia rarely develops in immunocompetent persons. Progressive lung disease and dissemination most often occur in the setting of cellular immunodeficiency, including underlying hematologic malignancies under treatment, Hodgkin lymphoma, long-term corticosteroid therapy, solid-organ transplant, TNF-inhibitor therapy, or HIV infection.

► Clinical Findings

A. Symptoms and Signs

Pulmonary disease ranges from simple nodules to widespread infiltrates leading to respiratory failure. Disseminated disease may involve any organ, but central nervous system disease predominates. Headache is usually the first symptom of meningitis. Confusion and other mental status changes as well as cranial nerve abnormalities, nausea, and vomiting may be seen as the disease progresses. Nuchal rigidity and meningeal signs occur about 50% of the time but are uncommon in HIV-infected patients. Communicating hydrocephalus may complicate the course. *C gattii* infection frequently presents with respiratory symptoms along with neurologic signs caused by space-occupying lesions in the central nervous system. Primary *C neoformans* infection of the skin may mimic bacterial cellulitis, especially in persons receiving immunosuppressive therapy such as corticosteroids. Clinical worsening associated with improved immunologic status has been reported in HIV-positive and transplant patients with cryptococcosis; this entity has been labeled the immune reconstitution inflammatory syndrome (IRIS).

B. Laboratory Findings

Respiratory tract disease is diagnosed by culture of respiratory secretions or pleural fluid. For suspected meningeal disease, lumbar puncture is the preferred diagnostic procedure. Spinal fluid findings include increased opening pressure, variable pleocytosis, increased protein, and decreased glucose, though as many as 50% of AIDS patients have no pleocytosis. Gram stain of the cerebrospinal fluid usually reveals budding, encapsulated fungi. Cryptococcal capsular antigen in cerebrospinal fluid and culture together establish the diagnosis over 90% of the time. Patients with AIDS often have the antigen in both cerebrospinal fluid and serum, and extrameningeal disease (lungs, blood, urinary tract) is common. In patients with AIDS, the serum cryptococcal antigen is also a sensitive screening test for meningitis, being positive in over 95% of cases. MRI is more sensitive than CT in finding central nervous system abnormalities such as cryptococcomas. Antigen testing by lateral flow assay appears to have improved sensitivity and specificity over the conventional latex agglutination test and can provide more rapid diagnostic results.

► Treatment

Because of decreased efficacy, initial therapy with an azole alone is not recommended for treatment of acute cryptococcal meningitis. Liposomal amphotericin B, 3–4 mg/kg/day intravenously for 14 days is the preferred agent for induction therapy, followed by an additional 8 weeks of fluconazole, 400 mg/day orally. This regimen has been quite effective, achieving clinical responses and cerebrospinal fluid sterilization in about 70% of patients. The addition of flucytosine has been associated with improved survival, but toxicity is common. Flucytosine is administered orally at a dose of 100 mg/kg/day divided into four equal doses and given every 6 hours.

Hematologic parameters should be closely monitored during flucytosine therapy, and it is important to adjust the dose for any decreases in kidney function. Fluconazole (800–1200 mg orally daily) may be given with amphotericin B when flucytosine is not available or patients cannot tolerate it. Frequent, repeated lumbar punctures or ventricular shunting should be performed to relieve high cerebrospinal fluid pressures or if hydrocephalus is a complication. **Failure to adequately relieve raised intracranial pressure is a major cause of morbidity and mortality.** The end points for amphotericin B therapy and for switching to oral fluconazole are a favorable clinical response (decrease in temperature; improvement in headache, nausea, vomiting, and mini-mental status scores), improvement in cerebrospinal fluid biochemical parameters and, most importantly, conversion of cerebrospinal fluid culture to negative.

A similar approach is reasonable for patients with cryptococcal meningitis in the absence of AIDS, though the mortality rate is considerably higher. Therapy is generally continued until cerebrospinal fluid cultures become negative. Maintenance antifungal therapy is important after treatment of an acute episode in HIV-related cases, since otherwise the rate of relapse is greater than 50%. Fluconazole, 200 mg/day orally, is the maintenance therapy of choice, decreasing the relapse rate approximately tenfold compared with placebo and threefold compared with weekly amphotericin B in patients whose cerebrospinal fluid has been sterilized by the induction therapy. After successful therapy of cryptococcal meningitis, it is possible to discontinue secondary prophylaxis with fluconazole in individuals with AIDS who have had a satisfactory response to antiretroviral therapy (eg, CD4 cell count greater than 100–200 cells/mcL for at least 6 months). Among practitioners treating patients without AIDS, there has been a trend in recent years to prescribe a course (eg, 6–12 months) of fluconazole as maintenance therapy following successful treatment of the acute illness; published guidelines suggest this as an option.

► Prognosis

Factors that indicate a poor prognosis include the activity of the predisposing conditions, older age, organ failure, lack of spinal fluid pleocytosis, high initial antigen titer in either serum or cerebrospinal fluid, decreased mental status, increased intracranial pressure, and the presence of disease outside the nervous system.

Abassi M et al. Cryptococcal meningitis: diagnosis and management update. Curr Trop Med Rep. 2015 Jun 1;2(2):90–99. [PMID: 26279970]

Chang CC et al. Pulmonary cryptococcosis. Semin Respir Crit Care Med. 2015 Oct;36(5):681–91. [PMID: 26398535]

Chen SC et al. *Cryptococcus gattii* infections. Clin Microbiol Rev. 2014 Oct;27(4):980–1024. [PMID: 25278580]

Meya DB et al. The immunopathogenesis of cryptococcal immune reconstitution inflammatory syndrome: understanding a conundrum. Curr Opin Infect Dis. 2016 Feb;29(1):10–22. [PMID: 26658650]

ASPERGILLOSIS

ESSENTIALS OF DIAGNOSIS

▶ Most common cause of non-candidal invasive fungal infection in stem cell or organ transplant recipients and in patients with hematologic malignancies.

▶ Predisposing factors: leukemia, bone marrow or organ transplant, late HIV infection.

▶ Pulmonary, sinus, and central nervous system are most common disease sites.

▶ Detection of galactomannan by ELISA or PCR in serum or other body fluid samples is useful for early diagnosis and treatment.

► General Considerations

Aspergillus fumigatus is the usual cause of aspergillosis, though many species of *Aspergillus* may cause a wide spectrum of disease. The lungs, sinuses, and brain are the organs most often involved. Clinical illness results either from an aberrant immunologic response or tissue invasion.

► Clinical Findings

A. Allergic Forms of Aspergillosis

Allergic bronchopulmonary aspergillosis (ABPA) occurs in patients with preexisting asthma or cystic fibrosis who develop worsening bronchospasm and fleeting pulmonary infiltrates accompanied by eosinophilia, high levels of IgE, and IgG *Aspergillus* precipitins in the blood. It also may complicate cystic fibrosis. Allergic aspergillus sinusitis produces a chronic sinus inflammation characterized by eosinophilic mucus and noninvasive hyphal elements.

B. Chronic Aspergillosis

Chronic pulmonary aspergillosis produces a spectrum of disease that usually occurs when there is preexisting lung damage but not significant immunocompromise. Disease manifestations range from aspergillomas that develop in a lung cavity to chronic fibrosing pulmonary aspergillosis in which the majority of lung tissue is replaced with fibrosis. Longstanding (longer than 3 months) pulmonary and systemic symptoms such as cough, shortness of breath, weight loss, and malaise are common.

C. Invasive Aspergillosis

Invasive aspergillosis most commonly occurs in profoundly immunodeficient patients, particularly in patients who have undergone hematopoietic stem cell transplants; in those with prolonged, severe neutropenia; and in patients with chronic granulomatous disease. Specific risk factors in patients who have undergone a hematopoietic stem cell transplant include cytopenias, corticosteroid use, iron overload, cytomegalovirus disease, and graft-versus-host disease. Pulmonary disease is most common, with patchy infiltration leading to a severe necrotizing pneumonia. Invasive sinus disease also occurs. At any time, there may be hematogenous dissemination to the central nervous system, skin, and other organs. Early diagnosis and reversal of any correctable immunosuppression are essential. Blood cultures have very low yield. Detection of galactomannan by ELISA or *Aspergillus* DNA by PCR, or both, has been used for the early diagnosis of invasive disease, though multiple determinations should be done and usefulness is decreased in patients receiving anti-mold prophylaxis (ie, voriconazole or posaconazole). Galactomannan levels and *Aspergillus* DNA PCR can be tested in serum or in bronchoalveolar lavage fluid, which may be more sensitive than serum. Higher galactomannan levels are correlated with increased mortality, and failure of galactomannan levels to fall in response to therapy portends a worse outcome. Isolation of *Aspergillus* from pulmonary secretions does not necessarily imply invasive disease, although its positive predictive value increases with more advanced immunosuppression. Therefore, a definitive diagnosis requires demonstration of *Aspergillus* in tissue or culture from a sterile site. CT scan of the chest may show characteristics quite suggestive of invasive aspergillosis (eg, "halo sign").

▶ Prevention

The high mortality rate and difficulty in diagnosis of invasive aspergillosis often leads clinicians to institute prophylactic therapy for patients with profound immunosuppression. The best-studied agents include voriconazole and posaconazole, although patient and agent selection criteria remain undefined. Widespread use of broad-spectrum azoles raises concern for development of invasive disease by highly resistant fungi.

▶ Treatment

A. Allergic Forms of Aspergillosis

For acute exacerbations of ABPA, oral prednisone is begun at a dose of 1 mg/kg/day and then tapered slowly over several months. Itraconazole at a dose of 200 mg daily for 16 weeks appears to improve pulmonary function and decrease corticosteroid requirements in these patients, although voriconazole is increasingly being used. Itraconazole is the best studied agent for the treatment of allergic aspergillus sinusitis with topical corticosteroids being the cornerstone of therapy.

B. Chronic Aspergillosis

The most effective therapy for symptomatic aspergilloma remains surgical resection. Other forms of chronic aspergillosis are generally treated with at least 4–6 months of oral triazole therapy (itraconazole 200 mg twice daily, voriconazole 200 mg twice daily, or posaconazole 300 mg daily).

C. Invasive Aspergillosis

When invasive aspergillosis is considered clinically likely or is demonstrable by laboratory testing, rapid institution of voriconazole (6 mg/kg intravenously twice on day 1 and then 4 mg/kg every 12 hours thereafter) is considered optimal therapy. A randomized controlled trial did not find an overall benefit with the addition of anidulafungin (200 mg on day 1 and then 100 mg daily) to voriconazole, but patients in whom galactomannan was detected who received combination therapy had better outcomes. Isavuconazole (372 mg of prodrug on days 1 and 2 and then 372 mg once daily) was equivalent to voriconazole. Alternatives include a lipid formulation of amphotericin B (3–5 mg/kg/day), caspofungin (70 mg intravenously on day 1 and then 50 mg/day thereafter), and posaconazole oral tablets (300 mg twice daily on day 1 and then 300 mg daily thereafter). Oral dosing of voriconazole at 4 mg/kg twice daily can be used for less serious infections or as a step-down strategy after intravenous therapy. Therapeutic drug monitoring should be considered for both voriconazole and posaconazole given variations in metabolism and absorption.

Surgical debridement is generally done for sinusitis, and there is increasing data regarding resection of focal pulmonary lesions, especially for treatment of life-threatening hemoptysis. The mortality rate of pulmonary or disseminated disease in the immunocompromised patient remains high, particularly in patients with refractory neutropenia.

Denning DW et al; European Society for Clinical Microbiology and Infectious Diseases and European Respiratory Society. Chronic pulmonary aspergillosis: rationale and clinical guidelines for diagnosis and management. Eur Respir J. 2016 Jan;47(1):45–68. [PMID: 26699723]

Maertens JA et al. Isavuconazole versus voriconazole for primary treatment of invasive mould disease caused by *Aspergillus* and other filamentous fungi (SECURE): a phase 3, randomised-controlled, non-inferiority trial. Lancet. 2016 Feb 20; 387(10020):760–9. [PMID: 26684607]

Marr KA et al. Combination antifungal therapy for invasive aspergillosis: a randomized trial. Ann Intern Med. 2015 Jan 20; 162(2):81–9. Erratum in: Ann Intern Med. 2015 Mar 17; 162(6):463. [PMID: 25599346]

MUCORMYCOSIS

ESSENTIALS OF DIAGNOSIS

▶ Most common cause of non-*Aspergillus* invasive mold infection.

▶ Predisposing factors: poorly controlled diabetes, leukemia, bone marrow or organ transplant, trauma with wound contamination by soil.

▶ Pulmonary, rhinocerebral, and skin are most common disease sites.

▶ Rapidly fatal without multidisciplinary interventions.

▶ General Considerations

The term "mucormycosis" is applied to opportunistic infections caused by members of the genera *Rhizopus*,

Mucor, Lichtheimia (formerly *Absidia*), and *Cunningha-mella*. Predisposing conditions include hematologic malignancy, stem cell transplantation, solid organ transplantation, diabetic ketoacidosis, chronic kidney disease, desferoxamine therapy, and treatment with corticosteroids or cytotoxic drugs.

▶ Clinical Findings

Invasive disease of the sinuses, orbits, and the lungs may occur. Necrosis is common due to hyphal tissue invasion that may manifest as ulceration of the hard palate or nasal palate or hemoptysis. Widely disseminated disease can occur. No serologic or laboratory findings assist with diagnosis, and blood cultures are unhelpful. A reverse halo sign may be seen on chest CT. Biopsy of involved tissue remains the cornerstone of diagnosis, although cultures are frequently negative. The organisms appear in tissues as broad, branching nonseptate hyphae.

▶ Treatment

Optimal therapy of mucormycosis involves reversal of predisposing conditions (if possible), surgical debridement, and prompt antifungal therapy. A prolonged course of a lipid preparation of intravenous amphotericin B (5 mg/kg with higher doses possibly given for CNS disease) should be started early. Based on in vitro susceptibility, posaconazole tablets 300 mg/day orally is generally used after disease has been stabilized. Combination therapy with amphotericin and posaconazole is not proven but is commonly used because of the poor response to monotherapy. Isavuconazole has in vitro activity against some agents of mucormycosis. Other azoles are not effective. There are limited data suggesting beneficial synergistic activity when amphotericin and caspofungin are used in combination for mucormycosis. Despite favorable animal studies, a pilot study in humans incorporating adjunctive iron chelation therapy with deferasirox demonstrated a higher mortality rate than antifungal therapy alone. Control of diabetes and other underlying conditions, along with extensive repeated surgical removal of necrotic, nonperfused tissue, is essential. Even when these measures are introduced in a timely fashion, the prognosis remains guarded.

Danion F et al. Mucormycosis: new developments into a persistently devastating infection. Semin Respir Crit Care Med. 2015 Oct;36(5):692–705. [PMID: 26398536]

Dioverti MV et al. Gastrointestinal mucormycosis in immunocompromised hosts. Mycoses. 2015 Dec;58(12):714–8. [PMID: 26456920]

Jung J et al. Comparison of computed tomographic findings in pulmonary mucormycosis and invasive pulmonary aspergillosis. Clin Microbiol Infect. 2015 Jul;21(7):684.e11–8. [PMID: 25882362]

BLASTOMYCOSIS

Blastomycosis occurs most often in men infected during occupational or recreational activities out of doors and in a geographically limited area of the south central and midwestern United States and Canada. Disease usually occurs in immunocompetent individuals.

Chronic pulmonary infection is most common and may be asymptomatic. When dissemination takes place, lesions are most frequently seen in the skin, bones, and urogenital system.

Cough, moderate fever, dyspnea, and chest pain are common. These may resolve or progress, with purulent sputum production, pleurisy, fever, chills, loss of weight, and prostration. Radiologic studies, either chest radiographs or CT scans, usually reveal airspace consolidation or masses.

Raised, verrucous cutaneous lesions are commonly present in disseminated blastomycosis. Bones—often the ribs and vertebrae—are frequently involved. Epididymitis, prostatitis, and other involvement of the male urogenital system may occur. Although they do not appear to be at greater risk for acquisition of disease, infection in HIV-infected persons may progress rapidly, with dissemination common.

Laboratory findings usually include leukocytosis and anemia, though these are not specific. The organism is found in clinical specimens, such as expectorated sputum or tissue biopsies, as a thick-walled cell 5–20 mcm in diameter that may have a single broad-based bud. It grows readily on culture. A urinary antigen test is available, but it has considerable cross reactivity with *Histoplasma*; it may be useful in monitoring disease resolution or progression. A serum enzyme immunoassay based on the surface protein BAD-1 has much better sensitivity and specificity than the urinary antigen test, but it is not yet commercially available.

Itraconazole, 200–400 mg/day orally for at least 2–3 months, is the therapy of choice for nonmeningeal disease, with a response rate of over 80%. Amphotericin B, 0.7–1.0 mg/kg/day intravenously (or lipid formulation amphotericin B), is given for severe disease, treatment failures, or central nervous system involvement.

Clinical follow-up for relapse should be made regularly for several years so that therapy may be resumed or another drug instituted.

Smith JA et al. New developments in blastomycosis. Semin Respir Crit Care Med. 2015 Oct;36(5):715–28. [PMID: 26398538]

PARACOCCIDIOIDOMYCOSIS (South American Blastomycosis)

Paracoccidioides brasiliensis infections have been found only in patients who have resided in South or Central America or Mexico. Long asymptomatic periods enable patients to travel far from the endemic areas before developing clinical problems. Weight loss, pulmonary complaints, or mucosal ulcerations are the most common symptoms. Cutaneous papules may ulcerate and enlarge both peripherally and deeper into the subcutaneous tissue. Differential diagnosis includes mucocutaneous leishmaniasis and syphilis. Extensive coalescent ulcerations may eventually result in destruction of the epiglottis, vocal cords, and uvula. Extension to the lips and face may occur. Lymph node enlargement may follow mucocutaneous lesions, eventually ulcerating and forming draining sinuses; in some patients, it is the presenting symptom. Hepatosplenomegaly may be present as well. HIV-infected patients with paracoccidioidomycosis are more likely to have extrapulmonary dissemination and a more rapid clinical disease course.

Laboratory findings are nonspecific. Serology by immunodiffusion is positive in more than 80% of cases. Complement fixation titers correlate with progressive disease and fall with effective therapy. The fungus is found in clinical specimens as a spherical cell that may have many buds arising from it. If direct examination of secretions does not reveal the organism, biopsy with Gomori staining may be helpful.

Itraconazole, 100 mg twice daily orally, is the treatment of choice and generally results in a clinical response within 1 month and effective control after 2–6 months. TMP-SMZ (480 mg/1200 mg) twice daily orally is equally effective and less costly but associated with more adverse effects and longer time to clinical cure. Amphotericin B intravenously is the medication of choice for severe and life-threatening infection.

Shikanai-Yasuda MA. Paracoccidioidomycosis treatment. Rev Inst Med Trop Sao Paulo. 2015 Sep;57(Suppl 19):31–7. [PMID: 26465367]

SPOROTRICHOSIS

Sporotrichosis is a chronic fungal infection caused by organisms of the *Sporothrix schenckii* complex. It is worldwide in distribution; most patients have had contact with soil, sphagnum moss, or decaying wood. Infection takes place when the organism is inoculated into the skin—usually on the hand, arm, or foot, especially during gardening.

The most common form of sporotrichosis begins with a hard, nontender subcutaneous nodule. This later becomes adherent to the overlying skin and ulcerates. Within a few days to weeks, lymphocutaneous spread along the lymphatics draining this area occurs, which may result in ulceration. Cavitary pulmonary disease occurs in individuals with underlying chronic lung disease.

Disseminated sporotrichosis is rare in immunocompetent persons but may present with widespread cutaneous, lung, bone, joint, and central nervous system involvement in immunocompromised patients, especially those with cellular immunodeficiencies, including AIDS and alcohol abuse.

Cultures are needed to establish diagnosis. The usefulness of serologic tests is limited, but may be helpful in diagnosing disseminated disease, especially meningitis.

Itraconazole, 200–400 mg orally daily for several months, is the treatment of choice for localized disease and some milder cases of disseminated disease. Terbinafine, 500 mg orally twice daily, also appears to have good efficacy in lymphocutaneous disease. Amphotericin B intravenously, 0.7–1.0 mg/kg/day, or a lipid amphotericin B preparation, 3–5 mg/kg/day are used for severe systemic infection. Surgery may be indicated for complicated pulmonary cavitary disease, and joint involvement may require arthrodesis.

The prognosis is good for lymphocutaneous sporotrichosis; pulmonary, joint, and disseminated disease respond less favorably.

Mahajan VK. Sporotrichosis: an overview and therapeutic options. Dermatol Res Pract. 2014;2014:272376. [PMID: 25614735]

MYCETOMA (Eumycetoma & Actinomycetoma)

Mycetoma is a chronic local, slowly progressive destructive infection that usually involves the foot; it begins in subcutaneous tissues, frequently after localized trauma, and then spreads to contiguous structures with sinus tracts and extruding grains. Eumycetoma (also known as maduromycosis) is the term used to describe mycetoma caused by true fungi. The disease begins as a papule, nodule, or abscess that over months to years progresses slowly to form multiple abscesses and sinus tracts ramifying deep into the tissue. Secondary bacterial infection may result in large open ulcers. Radiographs may show destructive changes in the underlying bone. Causative species can often be suggested by the color of the characteristic grains and hyphal size within the infected tissues but definitive diagnosis requires culture.

The prognosis for eumycetoma is poor, though surgical debridement along with prolonged oral itraconazole therapy, 200 mg twice daily, or combination therapy including itraconazole and terbinafine may result in a response rate of 70%. The various etiologic agents may respond differently to antifungal agents, so culture results are invaluable. Amputation is necessary in far advanced cases.

Nenoff P et al. Eumycetoma and actinomycetoma—an update on causative agents, epidemiology, pathogenesis, diagnostics and therapy. J Eur Acad Dermatol Venereol. 2015 Oct;29(10): 1873–83. [PMID: 25726758]

OTHER OPPORTUNISTIC MOLD INFECTIONS

Fungi previously considered to be harmless colonizers, including *Pseudallescheria boydii (Scedosporium apiospermum), Scedosporium prolificans, Fusarium, Paecilomyces, Trichoderma longibrachiatium*, and *Trichosporon*, are now significant pathogens in immunocompromised patients. This occurs most often in patients being treated for hematopoietic malignancies and in those receiving broad-spectrum antifungal prophylaxis. Infection may be localized in the skin, lungs, or sinuses, or widespread disease may appear with lesions in multiple organs. Fusariosis should be suspected in severely immunosuppressed persons in whom multiple, painful skin lesions develop; blood cultures are often positive. Sinus infection may cause bony erosion. Infection in subcutaneous tissues following traumatic implantation may develop as a well-circumscribed cyst or as an ulcer.

Nonpigmented septate hyphae are seen in tissue and are indistinguishable from those of *Aspergillus* when infections are due to *S apiospermum* or species of *Fusarium, Paecilomyces, Penicillium*, or other hyaline molds. Spores or mycetoma-like granules are rarely present in tissue. The differentiation of *S apiospermum* and *Aspergillus* is particularly important, since the former is uniformly resistant to amphotericin B but may be sensitive to azole antifungals (eg, voriconazole). Infection by any of a number of black molds is designated as phaeohyphomycosis. These black molds (eg, *Exophiala, Bipolaris, Cladophialophora, Curvularia, Alternaria*) are common in the environment, especially on decaying vegetation. In tissues of patients with phaeohyphomycosis, the mold is seen as black or faintly brown hyphae, yeast cells, or both. Culture on appropriate medium is needed to identify the agent. Histologic demonstration of these organisms is definitive evidence of invasive infection; positive cultures must be interpreted cautiously and not assumed to be contaminants in immunocompromised hosts.

Köhler JR et al. The spectrum of fungi that infects humans. Cold Spring Harb Perspect Med. 2014 Nov 3;5(1):a019273. [PMID: 25367975]

HOUSEHOLD MOLDS

ESSENTIALS OF DIAGNOSIS

▶ Molds are very common indoors where moisture exists in enclosed spaces.

▶ Most common indoor molds are *Cladosporium, Penicillium, Aspergillus*, and *Alternaria*.

▶ People most at risk for health problems include those with allergies, asthma, and underlying immunocompromising conditions.

Molds are commonly present in homes, particularly in the presence of moisture, and patients will commonly seek assessment for whether their illness is due to molds. Invasive disease due to environmental fungi can occur in the immunocompromised patient (eg, see section on Invasive Aspergillosis), but there are no data that mold exposure can induce immune dysfunction. Similarly, the concept of toxic-mold syndrome or cognitive impairment due to inhalation of mycotoxins has not been validated despite scrutiny by expert panels. Allergic symptoms (eg, asthma, hypersensitivity pneumonitis) can be worsened by environmental mold exposure, and reduction of household mold in such patients may lead to clinical improvement. The presence of mold in the household is typically easily discernable with visual inspection or detection by odor; if present, predisposing conditions should be corrected by individuals experienced in mold remediation.

ANTIFUNGAL THERAPY

Table 36–1 summarizes the major properties of currently available antifungal agents. Two different lipid-based amphotericin B formulations are used to treat systemic invasive fungal infections. Their principal advantage appears to be substantially reduced nephrotoxicity, allowing administration of much higher doses. Three agents of the echinocandin class, caspofungin acetate, anidulafungin, and micafungin sodium, are approved for use. The echinocandins have relatively few adverse effects and are useful for the treatment of invasive *Candida* infections, although resistance is beginning to emerge clinically; *C glabrata* in particular has shown resistance to this class of antifungals. Caspofungin acetate is also approved for use in refractory

Table 36–1. Agents for systemic mycoses.

Drug	Dosing	Renal Clearance?	CSF Penetration?	Toxicities	Spectrum of Activity
Amphotericin B	0.3–1.5 mg/kg/day intravenously	No	Poor	Rigors, fever, azotemia, hypokalemia, hypomagnesemia, renal tubular acidosis, anemia	All major pathogens except *Scedosporium*
Amphotericin B lipid complex	5 mg/kg/day intravenously	No	Poor	Fever, rigors, nausea, hypotension, anemia, azotemia, tachypnea	Same as amphotericin B, above
Amphotericin B, liposomal	3–6 mg/kg/day intravenously	No	Poor	Fever, rigors, nausea, hypotension, azotemia, anemia, tachypnea, chest tightness	Same as amphotericin B, above
Anidulafungin	100 mg intravenous loading dose, followed by 50 mg/day intravenously in one dose	< 1%	Poor	Diarrhea, hepatic enzyme elevations, histamine-mediated reactions	Mucosal and invasive candidiasis
Caspofungin acetate	70 mg intravenous loading dose, followed by 50 mg/day intravenously in one dose	< 50%[1]	Poor	Transient neutropenia; hepatic enzyme elevations when used with cyclosporine	Aspergillosis, mucosal and invasive candidiasis, empiric antifungal therapy in febrile neutropenia

(continued)

Table 36–1. Agents for systemic mycoses. (continued)

Drug	Dosing	Renal Clearance?	CSF Penetration?	Toxicities	Spectrum of Activity
Fluconazole	100–800 mg/day in one or two doses intravenously or orally	Yes	Yes	Nausea, rash, alopecia, headache, hepatic enzyme elevations	Mucosal candidiasis (including urinary tract), cryptococcosis, histoplasmosis, coccidioidomycosis
Flucytosine (5-FC)	100–150 mg/kg/day orally in four divided doses	Yes	Yes	Leukopenia,[2] rash, diarrhea, hepatitis, nausea, vomiting	Cryptococcosis,[3] candidiasis,[3] chromomycosis
Isavuconazole	200 mg/day orally or intravenously once daily	No	Low in CSF, high in brain	Nausea, diarrhea, upper abdominal pain, dizziness	Broad range of activity including the *Mucorales*
Itraconazole	100–400 mg/day orally in one or two doses with a meal or carbonated beverage	No	Variable	Nausea, hypokalemia, edema, hypertension, peripheral neuropathy	Histoplasmosis, coccidioidomycosis, blastomycosis, paracoccidioidomycosis, mucosal candidiasis (except urinary), sporotrichosis, aspergillosis, chromomycosis
Ketoconazole	200–800 mg/day orally in one or two doses with a meal or carbonated beverage	No	Poor	Anorexia, nausea, suppression of testosterone and cortisol, rash, headache, hepatic enzyme elevations, hepatic failure	Nonmeningeal histoplasmosis and coccidioidomycosis, blastomycosis, paracoccidioidomycosis, mucosal candidiasis (except urinary)
Micafungin sodium	150 mg intravenously in one dose (treatment) 50 mg (prophylaxis)	No	Poor	Rash, rigors, headache, phlebitis	Mucosal and invasive candidiasis, prophylaxis in hematopoietic stem cell transplantation
Posaconazole	400–800 mg/day orally in one or two doses (oral suspension) or 300 mg orally once daily (tablets) or 300 mg intravenously twice daily for 2 days loading dose followed by 300 mg once daily	No	Yes	Nausea, vomiting, abdominal pain, diarrhea, and headache	Broad range of activity including the *Mucorales*
Terbinafine	250 mg/day orally in one dose	Yes	Poor	Nausea, abdominal pain, taste disturbance, rash, diarrhea, and hepatic enzyme elevations	Dermatophytes, sporotrichosis
Voriconazole	200–400 mg/day orally in two doses or 12 mg/kg intravenously as loading dose for 2 days followed by 6 mg/kg/day intravenously in two doses[5]	Yes	Yes	Transient visual disturbances, rash, photosensitivity, fluoride excess with periostitis, peripheral neuropathy, squamous cell skin cancers, hepatic enzyme elevations[4]	All major pathogens except the *Mucorales* and sporotrichosis

[1]No dosage adjustment required for chronic kidney disease; dosage adjustment necessary with moderate to severe hepatic dysfunction.
[2]Use should be monitored with blood levels to prevent this or the dose adjusted according to creatinine clearance.
[3]In combination with amphotericin B.
[4]Administration with drugs that are metabolized by the cytochrome P450 system is contraindicated or requires careful monitoring.
[5]Some authorities advocate therapeutic drug monitoring in patients who are not responding to therapy.

cases of invasive aspergillosis. Voriconazole has excellent activity against a broad range of fungal pathogens and has been FDA approved for use in invasive *Aspergillus* cases, *Fusarium* and *Scedosporium* infections, *Candida* esophagitis, deep *Candida* infections, and candidemia. Posaconazole has good activity against a broad range of filamentous fungi, including the *Mucorales*. Some experts now recommend therapeutic drug monitoring in individuals with severe invasive fungal infections receiving these newer azoles because of unreliable serum levels due to either metabolic alterations as a result of genetic polymorphisms (voriconazole) or erratic absorption (posaconazole). A delayed-release tablet preparation of posaconazole provides more reliable pharmacokinetics. Isavuconazole has been approved for the treatment of aspergillosis and mucormycosis; it is available in an intravenous form that does not utilize the cyclodextrin carrier like previous azoles as well as an oral form with relatively reliable pharmacokinetic properties.

Nett JE et al. Antifungal agents: Spectrum of activity, pharmacology, and clinical indications. Infect Dis Clin North Am. 2016 Mar;30(1):51–83. [PMID: 26739608]

Rybak JM et al. Isavuconazole: pharmacology, pharmacodynamics, and current clinical experience with a new triazole antifungal agent. Pharmacotherapy. 2015 Nov;35(11):1037–51. [PMID: 26598096]

Wiederhold NP et al. What's new in antifungals: an update on the in-vitro activity and in-vivo efficacy of new and investigational antifungal agents. Curr Opin Infect Dis. 2015 Dec;28(6): 539–45. [PMID: 26374950]

Disorders Related to Environmental Emergencies

37

Jacqueline A. Nemer, MD, FACEP

Melissa C. Clark, MD

COLD & HEAT

The human body maintains a steady temperature through the balance of internal heat production and environmental heat loss. Heat exchange between the body and environment occurs via four common processes: radiation, evaporation, conduction, and convection. In extreme temperatures, the body's thermoregulation may fail. This results in the core body temperature (CBT) moving toward the temperature of the external environment. Cold and heat exposure may cause a wide spectrum of conditions; the severity varies considerably among individuals. Many of these conditions are preventable with appropriate education and planning. Preventive measures should be implemented on an individual and population level.

The likelihood and severity of extreme temperature–related conditions depend on physiologic and environmental factors. Physiologic risk factors include extremes of age; cognitive impairment; poor physical conditioning/ sedentary lifestyle or immobility; poor acclimatization; concurrent injury; prior temperature-related injury, and underlying medical conditions. Underlying medical conditions include cardiopulmonary, vascular, neurologic, psychiatric, musculoskeletal, immunologic, hematologic, endocrine [hypothyroidism, adrenal insufficiency, hypopituitarism], renal, hepatic, skin, and infectious diseases. Pharmacologic risk factors include medications, holistic or alternative treatments, illicit drugs, tobacco, and alcohol. There is a subset of medications associated with a particularly high likelihood of worsening temperature-related conditions, such as those that impact sweating and the central nervous system (ie, anticholingerics, stimulants, and sedatives) and those that affect cutaneous blood flow (peripheral vasoconstrictors or vasodilators). Environmental risk factors include weather conditions (humidity, wind, rain, snow, etc), inadequate clothing, inadequate housing, (homelessness, or housing with inadequate temperature control), occupational or recreational exposure.

DISORDERS DUE TO HEAT

ESSENTIALS OF DIAGNOSIS

▶ Spectrum of preventable heat-related illnesses: heat cramps, heat exhaustion, heat syncope, and heat stroke.

▶ **Heat stroke:** hyperthermia with cerebral dysfunction in a patient with heat exposure.

▶ **Best outcome:** early recognition, initiation of rapid cooling, and avoidance of shivering during cooling.

▶ **Best choice of cooling method:** whichever can be instituted the fastest with the least compromise to the patient. Delays in cooling result in higher morbidity and mortality in heat stroke victims.

▶ General Considerations

Heat-related illnesses are the most commonly seen environmental emergencies in US emergency departments. An estimated 326,497 cases presented to US emergency departments between 2006 and 2010, translating to a rate of 21.5 visits per 100,000 population/year. The amount of heat retained in the body is determined by internal metabolic function and environmental conditions (temperature, humidity). Hyperthermia results from the body's inability to maintain normal internal temperature through heat loss. Hyperthermia results from either compromised heat dissipation mechanisms or abnormally high heat production. Heat loss occurs primarily through sweating and peripheral vasodilation. Conduction (convection)—the direct transfer of heat from the skin to the surrounding air—occurs with diminishing efficiency as ambient temperature rises, especially above 37.2°C, the point at which heat transfer reverses direction. At normal temperatures, evaporation accounts for approximately 20% of the body's heat loss, but at high temperatures it becomes the major mechanism for dissipation of heat; with vigorous exertion, sweat loss can be as much as 2.5 L/h. This mechanism diminishes as humidity rises.

There is a spectrum of preventable heat-related illnesses related to environmental exposure, ranging from mild forms, such as heat cramps, to severe forms, such as heat stroke. Risk factors related to exertion include longer duration of exertion, hot environment, insufficient acclimatization, and dehydration. Additional risk factors include skin disorders or other medical conditions that inhibit sweat production or evaporation, obesity, prolonged seizures, hypotension, reduced cutaneous blood flow (ie, vasoconstrictors, beta-adrenergic blocking agents, dehydration), reduced cardiac output, the use of drugs that increase metabolism or muscle activity or impair sweating, and withdrawal syndromes. Medications that impair sweating include anticholinergics, antihistamines, phenothiazines, tricyclic antidepressants, monoamine oxidase inhibitors, and diuretics. Reduced cutaneous blood flow results from use of vasoconstrictors and beta-adrenergic blocking agents and dehydration results from use of alcohol. Illicit drugs, including stimulants, some hallucinogens and antipsychotic agents, can cause increased muscle activity and thus generate increased body heat.

Classic (nonexertional) heat-related illness may occur in any individual in a hot relaxing environment (ie, hot bath, steam room, sunbathing, or sauna). It may also occur when a high-risk individual is in extreme heat environmental conditions (heat, humidity) even if that individual is not physically active.

Heat cramping results from dilutional hyponatremia as sweat losses are replaced with water alone. **Heat exhaustion** results from prolonged strenuous activity in a hot environment without adequate water or salt intake. It is characterized by dehydration, sodium depletion, or isotonic fluid loss with accompanying cardiovascular changes.

Heat syncope or sudden collapse may result in unconsciousness from volume depletion and cutaneous vasodilation with consequent systemic and cerebral hypotension. Exercise-associated postural hypotension is usually the cause of heat syncope: it may occur during or immediately following exercise. **Heat stroke,** the hallmark of which is cerebral dysfunction with CBT over 40°C, presents in one of two forms: classic and exertional. **Classic (nonexertional) heat stroke** occurs in patients with impaired thermoregulatory mechanisms or in extreme environmental conditions. **Exertional heat stroke** occurs in healthy persons undergoing strenuous exertion in a hot or humid environment. Persons at greatest risk are those who are at the extremes of age, chronically debilitated, and taking medications that interfere with heat-dissipating mechanisms (ie, anticholinergics, antihistamines, phenothiazines).

► Clinical Findings

For all types of heat related illnesses, skin temperature may not reflect core temperature; thus, it is important to use an internal rectal, foley, or esophageal thermometer when diagnosing and treating disorders due to heat. **Heat cramps**

are painful skeletal muscle contractions and severe muscle spasms with onset during or shortly after exercise. Examination findings typically include stable vital signs; normal or slightly increased CBT; moist and cool skin; and tender, hard, lumpy, painful muscles that may be twitching. The diagnosis is made clinically.

Heat exhaustion is diagnosed based on symptoms and clinical findings of a CBT slightly elevated but less than 40°C, increased pulse, and moist skin. Symptoms are similar to those of heat syncope and heat cramps. Additional symptoms include nausea, vomiting, malaise, myalgias, hyperventilation, thirst, and weakness. Central nervous system symptoms include headache, dizziness, fatigue, anxiety, paresthesias, impaired judgment, and occasionally psychosis. Heat exhaustion may progress to heat stroke if sweating ceases and mental status declines.

With **heat syncope**, there is usually a history of prolonged vigorous physical activity or prolonged standing in a hot humid environment followed by a sudden collapse. The skin is cool and moist, the pulse is weak, and the systolic blood pressure is low.

Heat stroke is a life-threatening emergency; **the hallmark of heat stroke is cerebral dysfunction when the CBT is over 40°C.** Presenting symptoms include all findings seen in heat exhaustion with additional neurologic symptoms such as dizziness, weakness, emotional lability, confusion, delirium, blurred vision, convulsions, collapse, and unconsciousness. Physical examination findings may be variable and therefore unreliable. Exertional heat stroke may present with sudden collapse and loss of consciousness followed by irrational behavior. Sweating may not be present. Providers should be vigilant in monitoring for kidney injury, liver failure, metabolic derangements, respiratory compromise, coagulopathy, and ischemia. Initial laboratory findings are nonspecific to this condition.

► Treatment

A. Heat Cramps

The patient must be moved to a shaded, cool environment and given oral rehydration solution to replace both electrolytes and water. *Oral salt tablets are not recommended.* The patient may have to rest for at least 2 days with continued dietary supplementation before returning to work or resuming strenuous activity in the heat.

B. Heat Exhaustion

Treatment consists of moving patient to a shaded, cool environment, providing adequate fluid and electrolyte replacement, and active cooling (ie, fans, cool packs) if necessary. Physiologic saline or isotonic glucose solution should be administered intravenously when oral administration is not appropriate. At least 48 hours of rest and rehydration are recommended.

C. Heat Syncope

Treatment consists of rest and recumbency in a shaded, cool place, and fluid and electrolyte replacement by mouth (or intravenously if necessary).

D. Heat Stroke

Initially, the patient's ABCs (airway, breathing, circulation) must be addressed and stabilized, then treatment is aimed at rapidly reducing the CBT (within 1 hour) while supporting circulation and perfusion. Monitoring includes vital signs, temperature, pulse oximetry, and cardiac rhythm. The patient should also be observed for complications such as hypovolemic or cardiogenic shock, metabolic abnormalities, cardiac arrhythmias, coagulopathy, acute respiratory distress syndrome (ARDS), hypoglycemia, rhabdomyolysis, seizures, organ dysfunction, infection, and severe edema that can progress to compartment syndrome. Circulatory failure in heat-related illness is mostly due to shock from relative or absolute hypovolemia. Oral or intravenous fluid administration must be provided to ensure adequate urinary output. Fluid input and output should be monitored closely. Clinicians must also assess for and treat concurrent conditions (infection; trauma; and drug effects).

Choice of cooling method depends on which can be instituted the fastest with the least compromise to the overall care of the patient. Evaporative cooling is preferred for nonexertional heat stroke and conductive-based cooling for exertional heat stroke. **Evaporative cooling** is a noninvasive, effective, quick and easy way to reduce temperature. This method is done by placing the undressed patient in lateral recumbent position or supported in a hands-and-knees position to expose maximum skin surface to the air. Large fans circulate the room air while the entire undressed body is sprayed with lukewarm water (20°C). Inhalation of cool air or oxygen is also effective. **Conductive-based cooling** involves cool fluid infusion, gastric or bladder lavage, ice packs, and immersion into ice water or cool water. When immersion in ice water or cold water is available in the field, it is the preferred method of cooling for exertional heat stroke. Ice packs are most effective when covering the whole body, as opposed to the traditional method of just the axilla and groin. Intravascular heat exchange catheter systems as well as hemodialysis using cold dialysate (30–35°C) have been successful in reducing CBT. Research suggests that brain cooling may lessen cerebrovascular injury from heat stroke.

Shivering must be avoided because it inhibits the effectiveness of cooling by increasing internal heat production. Medications can be used to suppress shivering including magnesium, quick-acting opioid analgesics, benzodiazepines, and quick-acting anesthetic agents. Skin massage is recommended to prevent cutaneous vasoconstriction. *Antipyretics (aspirin, acetaminophen) have no effect on environmentally induced hyperthermia and are contraindicated.* Treatment should be continued until the CBT drops to 39°C.

Prevention

Public education is necessary to improve prevention and early recognition of heat-related disorders. Individuals should take steps to reduce personal risk factors and to gradually acclimatize to the hot environment.

Coaches, athletic trainers, athletes, and parents of young athletes must be educated about heat-related illness, specifically about prevention, risks, signs and symptoms, and treatment. Medical evaluation and monitoring should be used to identify the individuals and the weather conditions that increase risk of heat-related disorders.

Those who are physically active in a hot environment should increase fluid consumption before, during, and after physical activities. Fluid consumption should include balanced electrolyte fluids and water. Water consumption alone may lead to electrolyte imbalance, particularly hyponatremia. *It is not recommended to have salt tablets available for use because of the risk of hypertonic hypernatremia.* Close monitoring of fluid and electrolyte intake and early intervention are recommended in situations necessitating exertion or activity in hot environments.

▶ Prognosis

Mortality is high from heat stroke; multiorgan dysfunction is the usual cause of heat stroke–related death. The patient is also at risk for rhabdomyolysis, ARDS, and inflammation even after temperature has normalized. Following heat stroke, immediate reexposure to ambient heat should be avoided.

▶ When to Refer

Potential consultants include surgeons for suspicion of compartment syndrome, nephrologist for kidney injury, and transplant surgeon for fulminant liver failure.

▶ When to Admit

All patients with suspected heat stroke must be admitted to the hospital with intensive care capability for close monitoring.

Horseman MA et al. A case of severe heatstroke and review of pathophysiology, clinical presentation, and treatment. J Intensive Care Med. 2013 Nov–Dec;28(6):334–40. [PMID: 22232203]

Lipman GS et al. Wilderness Medical Society practice guidelines for the prevention and treatment of heat-related illness: 2014 update. Wilderness Environ Med. 2014 Dec;25 (4 Suppl):S55–65. [PMID: 25498263]

Pryor RR et al. Exertional heat illness: emerging concepts and advances in prehospital care. Prehosp Disaster Med. 2015 Jun; 30(3):297–305. [PMID: 25860637]

ACCIDENTAL SYSTEMIC HYPOTHERMIA

ESSENTIALS OF DIAGNOSIS

▶ Systemic hypothermia is a CBT below 35°C.

▶ Accurate CBT measurement must be obtained using a low-reading core temperature probe that measures as low as 25°C.

▶ The CBT must be over 32°C before terminating resuscitation efforts.

▶ Extracorporeal membrane oxygenation (ECMO) or cardiopulmonary bypass should be considered in hypothermic patients with hemodynamic instability or cardiac arrest.

General Considerations

Systemic hypothermia is defined as CBT below 35°C. This may be primary (from exposure to prolonged ambient extremely low temperature) or secondary (due to thermoregulatory dysfunction). Both may be present at the same time.

Hypothermia should be considered in any patient with prolonged exposure to an ambient cold environment, especially in any patients with prior cold weather injury as well as risk factors listed in Cold & Heat section. In prolonged or repetitive cold exposure, hypothermia ensues if the body's thermoregulatory responses become impaired.

Clinical Findings

Symptoms and signs of hypothermia are typically nonspecific and markedly variable based on the patient's underlying health and circumstances of hypothermia. Laboratory studies should assess acid-base status, electrolyte derangements (particularly potassium and glucose), coagulopathy, kidney failure, rhabdomyolysis and liver or pancreas dysfunction. Inaccurate laboratory values will occur if the blood sample is warmed to 37°C for the testing. All patients should be evaluated for associated conditions (ie, hypoglycemia, trauma, infection, overdose, and peripheral cold injury).

Accurate CBT measurement must be obtained using a low-reading core temperature probe that measures as low as 25°C. **Hypothermia stage I** is typically seen when the CBT is between 32°C and 35°C and is defined by shivering and possibly poor judgement or coordination but hemodynamic stability and a normal level of consciousness. **Stage II** correlates with CBT 28–32°C. Shivering stops; bradycardia, dilated pupils, slowed reflexes, cold diuresis, and confusion and lethargy ensue. The electrocardiogram (ECG) may reveal a J wave or Osborn wave (positive deflection in the terminal portion of the QRS complex, most notable in leads II, V_5, and V_6) (Figure 37–1). When the CBT is below

28°C, the likelihood of hemodynamic instability and cardiac arrest increase dramatically.

Stage III (CBT 24–28°C) is characterized by loss of consciousness but present vital signs. **Stage IV** (CBT less than 24°C) is the loss of vital signs. Coma, loss of reflexes, rigor mortis, asystole, or ventricular fibrillation may falsely lead the clinician to assume that patient is dead despite reversible hypothermia.

Treatment

Rewarming is the initial, imperative treatment for all hypothermic patients. Resuscitation begins with rapid assessment and support of airway, breathing and circulation, simultaneously with the initiation of rewarming, and prevention of further heat loss. All cold, wet clothing must be removed and replaced with warm, dry clothing and blankets.

Mild or stage I hypothermia can be treated by passive external rewarming (ie, removing wet clothing and providing dry clothes) and active external rewarming (ie, a warm environment, warm blankets, and warm beverages). In contrast to those with more severe hypothermia, it is safe and recommended for the uninjured patient with mild hypothermia to become physically active to generate heat. **Active external rewarming** is highly effective and safe for mild hypothermia. This is a noninvasive method of applying external heat to the patient's skin. Examples include warm bedding, heated blankets, heat packs, and immersion into a 40°C bath. Warm bath immersion limits the ability to monitor the patient or treat other coexisting conditions. Patients with mild hypothermia and previous good health usually respond well to passive and active external warming.

Stage II and III hypothermia are treated with more aggressive rewarming in addition to external rewarming strategies. This requires close monitoring of vital signs, pulse oximetry and cardiac rhythm during rewarming. Warm intravenous fluids (38–42°C) are considered minimally invasive and effective.

As hypothermia becomes more severe there are increased complications of both hypothermia itself and rewarming. Complications of rewarming occur as colder peripheral blood returns to central circulation. This may result in core temperature afterdrop, rewarming lactic acidosis from shunting lactate into the circulation, rewarming shock from peripheral vasodilation and hypovolemia, ventricular fibrillation, and other cardiac arrhythmias. Afterdrop can be lessened by active external rewarming of the trunk but not the extremities and by avoiding any muscle movement by the patient. Extreme caution must be taken when handling the hypothermic patient to avoid triggering potentially fatal arrhythmias in a phenomenon known as rescue collapse.

Patients with hemodynamic instability or cardiac arrest should be transferred to a facility with extracorporeal membrane oxygenation (ECMO) or cardiopulmonary bypass capability.

In patients who go into cardiac arrest (stage IV), the presence of hypothermia calls for modification of typical resuscitation algorithms. *High quality CPR should be continued until the patient's CBT is at least 32°C.* There is a discrepancy between the recommendations on use and

▲ **Figure 37–1.** Electrocardiogram shows leads II and V5 in a patient whose body temperature is 24°C. Note the bradycardia and Osborn waves. These findings become more prominent as the body temperature lowers, and gradually resolve with rewarming. Osborn waves have an extra positive deflection in the terminal portion of the QRS complex and are best seen in the inferior and lateral precordial leads (most notably in leads II, V_5, and V_6).

dosing of epinephrine in cardiac arrest of the severely hypothermic patient. The European Resuscitation Council recommends withholding epinephrine until warmed to 30°C, and decreasing the frequency from 30°C to 35°C. The American Heart Association permits dosage as usual in conjunction with rewarming. ECMO or cardiopulmonary bypass should be done in patients with hypothermia who are in cardiac arrest except when patients have fatal hyperkalemia (10–12 mmol/L) or evidence of death from a traumatic cause such as decapitation or asphyxiation in an avalanche. Studies show great success with ECMO and bypass in such cases, documenting 47–63% of patients returning to full neurologic function.

Any hypothermic patient with return of spontaneous circulation must be monitored very closely because of the high likelihood of subsequent multiorgan system failure.

▶ When to Admit

Hypothermia patients must undergo close monitoring for potential complications. This is typically done during an inpatient admission or prolonged observation.

Brown DJ et al. Accidental hypothermia. N Engl J Med. 2012 Nov 15;367(20):1930–8. Erratum in: N Engl J Med. 2013 Jan 24; 368(4):394. [PMID: 23150960]

Gordon L et al. Severe accidental hypothermia. BMJ. 2014 Feb 21; 348:g1675. [PMID: 24563453]

Petrone P et al. Management of accidental hypothermia and cold injury. Curr Probl Surg. 2014 Oct;51(10):417–31. [PMID: 25242454]

Zafren K et al. Wilderness Medical Society practice guidelines for the out-of-hospital evaluation and treatment of accidental hypothermia: 2014 update. Wilderness Environ Med. 2014 Dec; 25(4 Suppl):S66–85. [PMID: 25498264]

HYPOTHERMIA OF THE EXTREMITIES

ESSENTIALS OF DIAGNOSIS

▶ Extremities suffering cold-induced injuries should not be exercised, rubbed, or massaged during rewarming.

▶ Rewarming of extremities affected by cold-induced injuries must be performed as soon as possible after there is no risk of refreezing.

▶ Clinical Findings

Cold-induced injuries to the extremities range from mild to severe. Cold exposure of the extremities produces immediate localized vasoconstriction followed by generalized vasoconstriction. Tissue damage may result from ischemia and intravascular thromboses, endothelial damage, or by actual freezing. Freezing (frostbite) may occur when the temperature drops or in the presence of wind, water, immobility, malnutrition, or vascular disease.

▶ Prevention

"Keep warm, keep dry, and keep moving." Individuals should wear warm, dry clothing. Arms, legs, fingers, and toes should be exercised to maintain circulation. Wet clothing, socks, and shoes should be replaced with dry ones. Those most at risk are people with underlying diseases or medications that decrease tissue perfusion and those with environmental exposure to a prolonged cold environment. Caution must be taken to avoid cramped positions; constrictive clothing; prolonged dependency of the feet; use of tobacco, alcohol, and sedative medications; and exposure to wet muddy ground and windy conditions.

FROSTNIP & CHILBLAIN (Erythema Pernio)

Frostnip is a mild temporary form of cold-induced injury causing local paresthesias of the involved area that completely resolve with passive external rewarming.

Chilblains or **erythema pernio** are inflammatory skin changes caused by exposure to cold without actual freezing of the tissues. These skin lesions may be red or purple papular lesions, which are painful or pruritic, with burning or paresthesias. They may be associated with edema or blistering and aggravated by warmth. With continued exposure, ulcerative or hemorrhagic lesions may appear and progress to scarring, fibrosis, and atrophy.

Treatment consists of elevating and passively externally rewarming the affected part. Caution must be taken to avoid rubbing or massaging injured tissues and to avoid applying ice or heat. The area must be protected from trauma, secondary infection, and further cold exposure.

IMMERSION FOOT OR TRENCH FOOT

Immersion foot (or hand) is caused by prolonged immersion in cold water or mud, usually below 10°C. **Prehyperemic stage** is marked by early symptoms of cold and anesthesia of the affected area. **Hyperemic stage** follows with hot sensation, intense burning, and shooting pains. **Posthyperemic stage** occurs with ongoing cold exposure; the affected part becomes pale or cyanotic with diminished pulsations due to vasospasm. This may result in blistering, swelling, redness, ecchymoses, hemorrhage, necrosis, peripheral nerve injury, or gangrene.

Treatment consists of air drying, protecting the extremities from trauma and secondary infection, and gradual rewarming by exposure to air at room temperature (not ice or heat). Caution must be taken to avoid massaging or moistening the skin and to avoid further cold injury and water immersion. Affected parts are elevated to aid in removal of edema fluid. Pressure sites (ie, heels) are protected with cushions. Bed rest is required until all ulcers have healed.

FROSTBITE

Frostbite is injury from tissue freezing and formation of ice crystals in the tissue. Most tissue destruction follows the reperfusion of the frozen tissues, with damaged endothelial cells and progressive microvascular thrombosis resulting in further tissue damage. In mild cases, only the skin and subcutaneous tissues are involved; the symptoms are numbness, prickling, itching, and pallor. With increasing severity, deep frostbite involves deeper structures. The skin appears white or yellow, loses its elasticity, and becomes immobile. Edema, hemorrhagic blisters, necrosis, gangrene, paresthesias and stiffness may occur.

► Treatment

A. Immediate Treatment

Evaluate and treat the patient for associated systemic hypothermia, concurrent conditions, and injury. Avoid secondary exposure to cold. Early use of systemic analgesics is recommended for nonfrozen injuries. The patient should be hydrated orally or parenterally to avoid hypovolemia and to improve perfusion.

1. Rewarming—Rapid rewarming at temperatures slightly above normal body temperature may significantly decrease tissue necrosis and reverse the tissue crystallization. **If there is any possibility of refreezing, the frostbitten part should not be thawed.** Ideally the frozen extremity should not be used. Rewarming is best accomplished by warm bath immersion. The frozen extremity is immersed for several minutes in a moving water bath heated to 40–42°C until the distal tip of the part being thawed flushes. In the absence of a thermometer, the temperature should be checked by an unaffected extremity, ideally of a caregiver rather than the patient. Water in this temperature range feels warm but not hot to the normal hand or wrist. If warm water is not available then passive thawing in a warm environment should be allowed. Dry heat (ie, stove or open fire) is not recommended because it is more difficult to regulate, and increases likelihood of accidental burns. Thawing may cause tenderness and burning pain. Once the frozen part has thawed and returned to normal temperature (usually in about 30 minutes), discontinue external heat. **In the early stage, rewarming by exercise, rubbing, or friction is contraindicated.** The patient must be kept at bed rest with the affected parts elevated and uncovered at room temperature. Casts, occlusive dressings, or bandages are not applied. Blisters should be left intact unless signs of infection supervene.

2. Anti-infective measures and wound care—Frostbite increases susceptibility to tetanus and infection. Tetanus prophylaxis must be considered. Infection risk may be reduced by aseptic wound care. Nonadherent sterile gauze and fluffy dressing should be loosely applied to wounds and cushions used for all areas of pressure. Antibiotics should not be administered empirically.

B. Medical and Surgical Treatment Options

With the availability of telemedicine, specialists are able to provide advice on early field treatment of cold-injured patients in remote areas, thereby improving outcome. Clinicians must watch for evidence of compartment syndrome and need for fasciotomy. Eschar formation without evidence of infection may be conservatively treated. The underlying skin may heal spontaneously with the eschar acting as a biologic dressing. Reduction of amputation rates have been shown from use of intravenous infusions of synthetic prostaglandins and from tissue plasminogen activators. Intra-arterial thrombolytic administration within 24 hours of exposure has resulted in improved tissue perfusion and has reduced amputation. There is insufficient evidence to recommend hyperbaric oxygen, heparin, or sympathectomy.

C. Follow-Up Care

Patient education must include ongoing care of the cold injury and prevention of future hypothermia and cold injury. Gentle, progressive physical therapy to promote circulation should be instituted as tolerated. Debridement and amputation should be considered only after it is established that the tissues are necrotic.

► Prognosis

Recovery from frostbite depends on the underlying comorbidities, the extent of initial tissue damage, the rewarming reperfusion injury, and the late sequelae. The involved extremity may be at increased susceptibility for discomfort and injury upon re-exposure to cold. Neuropathic sequelae include pain, numbness, tingling, hyperhidrosis, and cold sensitivity of the extremities, and nerve conduction abnormalities may persist for many years after the cold injury.

► When to Admit

- Management of tissue damage, comorbidities, associated injuries.
- Need for hospital-based interventions.
- Psychosocial factors (cognitive impairment, inadequate living situation) that could compromise patient safety or recovery.

Hutchison RL. Frostbite of the hand. J Hand Surg Am. 2014 Sep; 39(9):1863–8. [PMID: 25154574]

Ibrahim AE et al. The emerging role of tissue plasminogen activator in the management of severe frostbite. J Burn Care Res. 2015 Mar–Apr;36(2):e62–6. [PMID: 25687362]

Lantry J et al. Pathophysiology, management and complications of hypothermia. Br J Hosp Med (Lond). 2012 Jan;73(1):31–7. [PMID: 22241407]

McIntosh SE et al. Wilderness Medical Society practice guidelines for the prevention and treatment of frostbite: 2014 update. Wilderness Environ Med. 2014 Dec;25(4 Suppl):S43–54. [PMID: 25498262]

DROWNING

ESSENTIALS OF DIAGNOSIS

- ► The first requirement of rescue is immediate rescue breathing *and* CPR.
- ► Patient must also be assessed for hypothermia, hypoglycemia, concurrent injuries, and medical conditions.
- ► Clinical manifestations are hypoxemia, pulmonary edema, and hypoventilation.

▶ General Considerations

Drowning, as defined by the World Health Organization is the "process resulting in primary respiratory impairment from submersion in a liquid medium." Drowning may result in aspiration, laryngospasm, hypoxemia, and acidemia. Outcomes from drowning range from life without morbidity to death. Morbidity may be immediate or delayed. The asphyxia of drowning is usually due to aspiration of fluid but it may result from airway obstruction caused by laryngeal spasm while the victim is gasping under water. A patient may be deceptively asymptomatic during the initial recovery period only to deteriorate or die as a result of acute respiratory failure within the following 12–24 hours. Disseminated intravascular coagulation may also lead to bleeding after asphyxiation from drowning.

▶ Clinical Findings

A. Symptoms and Signs

The patient's appearance may vary from asymptomatic to marked distress with abnormal vital signs. Signs and symptoms include dyspnea, cough, wheezing, chest pain, dysrhythmia, hypotension, cyanosis, and apnea. The patient may experience headache, neurologic deficits, and altered level of consciousness. Hypothermia is highly likely with cold water or prolonged submersion.

B. Laboratory Findings

Arterial blood gas results are helpful in determining the degree of injury since initial clinical findings may appear benign. PaO_2 is usually decreased; $PaCO_2$ may be increased or decreased; pH is decreased. Bedside blood sugar must be checked rapidly. Other testing is based on clinical scenario. Metabolic acidosis is common.

▶ Prevention

Education and prevention are critical given the high burden of disease from drowning.

Preventive measures should be taken to reduce morbidity and mortality from drowning. Conditions that increase risk of submersion injury include the following: (1) use of alcohol or other drugs, (2) inadequate water safety skills, (3) poor physical health, (4) hyperventilation, (5) sudden acute illness (eg, hypoglycemia, seizure, dysrhythmia, myocardial infarction, asthma flare), (6) acute trauma (particularly brain or spinal cord injury, or both), (7) venomous stings or bites, (8) decompression sickness, (9) dangerous water conditions (temperature and turbulence), and (10) carbon monoxide exposure from boat motors.

▶ Treatment

A. First Aid

1. *The first requirement of rescue is immediate basic life support treatment and CPR.* At the scene, immediate measures to combat hypoxemia are critical to improve outcome.
2. Patient must be assessed for hypothermia, hypoglycemia, concurrent medical conditions and associated trauma, especially brain and cervical spine injury.

3. Rescuer should not attempt to drain water from the victim's lungs.
4. Resuscitation and basic life support efforts must be continued until CBT reaches 32°C.

B. Subsequent Management

1. Ensure optimal ventilation and oxygenation—The onset of hypoxemia exists even in the alert, conscious patient who appears to be breathing normally. Oxygen should be administered immediately at the highest available concentration. Oxygen saturation should be maintained at 90% or higher via supplemental oxygen, continuous positive airway pressure (CPAP), positive end-expiratory pressure (PEEP) or intubation and mechanical ventilation.

Serial physical examinations and chest radiographs should be performed to detect possible pneumonitis, atelectasis, and pulmonary edema. Bronchodilators may be used to treat wheezing. Nasogastric suctioning can decompress the stomach.

2. Cardiovascular support—Intravascular volume status must be monitored and supported by vascular fluid replacement, vasopressors, or diuretics as needed.

3. Correction of blood pH and electrolyte abnormalities—

Metabolic acidosis is present in 70% of drowning victims, but this typically corrects through adequate ventilation and oxygenation. Glycemic control improves outcome.

4. Cerebral and spinal cord injury—Central nervous system damage may progress despite apparently adequate treatment of hypoxia and shock.

5. Hypothermia—CBT should be measured and managed as appropriate (see Accidental Systemic Hypothermia, above).

▶ Course & Prognosis

Respiratory damage is often severe in the minutes to hours following a drowning. With respiratory supportive treatment, improvements typically occur quickly over the first few days following the drowning. Long-term complications of drowning may include neurologic impairment, seizure disorder, and pulmonary or cardiac damage. Prognosis is directly correlated with the patient's age, submersion time, rapid prehospital resuscitation and rapid transport to a medical facility, clinical status at time of arrival to hospital, Glasgow Coma Scale score, pupillary reactivity, and overall health assessment (APACHE II score).

▶ When to Admit

Most patients with significant drowning or concurrent medical or traumatic conditions require inpatient monitoring following the event. This includes continuous monitoring of cardiorespiratory, neurologic, renal and metabolic function. Pulmonary edema may not appear for 24 hours.

Dyson K et al. Drowning related out-of-hospital cardiac arrests: characteristics and outcomes. Resuscitation. 2013 Aug; 84(8):1114–8. [PMID: 23370162]

Engel SC. Drowning episodes: prevention and resuscitation tips. J Fam Pract. 2015 Feb;64(2):E1–6. [PMID: 25671539]

THERMAL BURNS

ESSENTIALS OF DIAGNOSIS

▶ Estimates of the burn location, size and depth greatly determine treatment plan.

▶ The first 48 hours of burn care offer the greatest impact on morbidity and mortality of a burn victim.

The first 48 hours after thermal burn injury offer the greatest opportunity to impact the survival of the patient. Early surgical intervention, wound care, enteral feeding, glucose control and metabolic management, infection control, and prevention of hypothermia and compartment syndrome have contributed to significantly lower mortality rates and shorter hospitalizations.

▶ General Considerations

A. Classification

Burns are classified by extent, depth, patient age, and associated illness or injury. Accurate estimation of burn size and depth is important since this figure will quantify the parameters of resuscitation.

1. Extent—In adults, the "rule of nines" (Figure 37–2) is useful for rapidly assessing the extent of a burn. It is important to view the entire patient to make an accurate assessment of skin findings on initial and subsequent examinations. One rule of thumb is that the palm of an open hand constitutes 1% total body surface area in adults. Only second- and third-degree burns are included in calculating the total burn surface area. First- or second-degree burns may convert to deeper burns, especially if treatment is delayed or bacterial colonization or superinfection occurs.

2. Depth—Judgment of depth of injury is difficult. The **first-degree burn** may be red or gray but will demonstrate excellent capillary refill. First-degree burns are not blistered initially. If the wound is blistered, this represents a partial-thickness injury to the dermis, which is referred to as a **second-degree burn**. As the degree of burn is progressively deeper, there is a progressive loss of adnexal structures, referred to as a **third-degree burn**. Hairs can be easily extracted or are absent, sweat glands become less visible, and the skin appears smoother.

Deep second- and third-degree burns are treated in a similar fashion. Neither will heal appropriately without early debridement and grafting; the resultant skin is thin and scarred.

B. Survival after Burn Injury

Transfer to a burn unit is indicated for large burn size, circumferential burn, or burn involving a joint or high-risk body part, and patients with comorbidities. Mortality rates have been significantly reduced due to treatment advances including improvements in wound care, treatment of infection, early burn excision, skin substitute usage, and early nutritional support through parenteral or enteral feeding.

C. Associated Injuries or Illnesses

Smoke inhalation, associated trauma, and electrical injuries are commonly associated with burns. Smoke inhalation (see Chapter 9) must be suspected when a burn victim is found in an enclosed space, or in close proximity to the fire. Clinical findings include singed nasal or facial hairs, carbonaceous sputum, or an elevated carboxyhemoglobin level. Severe burns from any source may result in similar complications (ie, infections, respiratory compromise, multiorgan dysfunction, venous thromboembolism, and gastrointestinal complications).

D. Systemic Reactions to Burn Injury

When burns greater than approximately 20% of total body surface area are present, systemic metabolic derangements may occur and require intensive support. The inflammatory cascade can result in shock. In addition, coagulopathy may develop.

▶ Treatment

A. Initial Resuscitation

The clinician must proceed with a full trauma assessment, starting with "ABCDE" (airway, breathing, circulation, disability, exposure). Serial assessments of airway and breathing are necessary since endotracheal intubation or cricothyotomy may be needed for major burn victims,

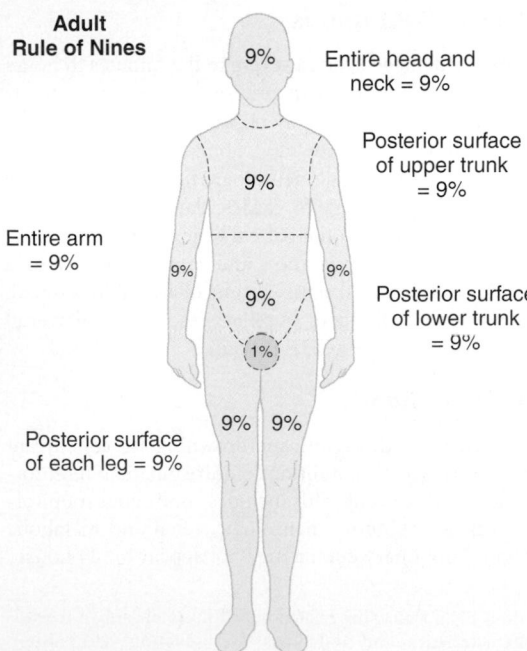

Adult Rule of Nines

Entire head and neck = 9%

Posterior surface of upper trunk = 9%

9%

Entire arm = 9%

9%   9%

9%

Posterior surface of lower trunk = 9%

1%

9%   9%

Posterior surface of each leg = 9%

▲ **Figure 37–2.** Estimation of body surface area in burns.

particularly those with possible inhalation injury. Generalized edema may develop during fluid resuscitation, including edema of the soft tissues of the upper airway and perhaps the lungs as well. Chest radiographs are typically normal initially but may develop an ARDS picture in 24–48 hours, especially with severe inhalation injury.

Generalized capillary leak results from burn injury over more than 20% of total body surface area. This often necessitates intravascular volume replacement with large volumes of crystalloid. There are many guidelines for fluid resuscitation. The most widely recognized is the **Parkland formula** (http://www.mdcalc.com/parkland-formula-for-burns/) in which the fluid requirement in the first 24 hours is estimated as 4 mL/kg × body weight per percent of body surface area burned. Half the calculated fluid is given in the first 8-hour period, based on the time of injury rather than time of arrival to medical care. The remaining fluid is delivered over the next 16 hours. An extremely large volume of fluid may be required. Deep electrical burns and inhalation injury may increase the fluid requirement.

B. Management

1. Pain control—Pain control is critical in these patients. Treatment is with opioids and nonsteroidal anti-inflammatory drugs.

2. Chemoprophylaxis—

A. Tetanus immunization—Tetanus status should be verified and updated in all burn patients. (See Chapter 33.)

B. Antibiotics—All nonsuperficial depth wounds should be covered with topical antibiotics. Prophylaxis with systemic antibiotics is not indicated.

3. Surgical management—

A. Escharotomy—As edema fluid accumulates, ischemia may develop under any constricting eschar if the full-thickness burn is circumferential. Escharotomy incisions through the anesthetic eschar can save life and limb.

B. Fasciotomy—Fasciotomy is indicated for any compartment syndrome. Clinicians must vigilantly monitor patients for early signs of compartment syndrome, particularly in those with circumferential burns.

C. Debridement, dressings, and topical and systemic antibiotic therapy—Minor burn wounds should be debrided at the bedside to determine the depth of the burn and then thoroughly cleansed. Thereafter, daily wound care should consist of debridements as needed, topical antibiotics, and wound dressing. Patient compliance and adequate pain control is essential for successful outpatient treatment. The wound should be reevaluated by the treating clinician within 24–72 hours to evaluate for signs of infection.

The goal of burn wound management is to protect the wound from desiccation and avoid further injury or infection. Regular and thorough cleansing of burned areas is a critically important intervention. Topical antibiotics should be applied. Silver nylon dressings have been shown to be beneficial in decreasing length of stay, controlling pain, and preventing infection.

Systemic infection remains a leading cause of morbidity among patients with major burn injuries. Healthcare-associated infections are increasingly common.

D. Wound management—The goal of therapy after fluid resuscitation is rapid and stable closure of the wound.

E. Abdominal compartment syndrome—Abdominal compartment syndrome is emerging as a potentially lethal condition in severely burned patients. Bladder pressures over 30 mm Hg establish the diagnosis in at-risk patients. Surgical abdominal decompression may be indicated to improve ventilation and oxygen delivery, but even after this surgery, survival remains low.

C. Patient Support

Burn patients require extensive supportive care, both physiologically and psychologically. It is important to maintain normal CBT and avoid hypothermia (by maintaining environmental temperature at or above 30°C) in patients with burns over more than 20% of total body surface area. Burn patients are at risk for many complications such as respiratory injury, ARDS or respiratory failure unresponsive to maximal ventilatory support, sepsis, multiorgan failure, and venous thromboembolism.

Burn patients require careful assessment and provision of optimal nutritional needs since their metabolism is higher and they require more energy, nutrients, and antioxidants for wound healing. Early aggressive nutrition (by parenteral or enteral routes) reduces infections, recovery time, noninfectious complications, length of hospital stay, long-term sequelae, and mortality.

► Prognosis

Prognosis depends on the extent and location of the burn tissue damage, associated injuries, comorbidities, and complications. Hyperglycemia from poor glucose control is a predictor of worse outcomes. Complications most commonly include sepsis; gangrene requiring limb amputation; or neurologic, cardiac, cognitive, or psychiatric dysfunction. Psychiatric support may be necessary following burn injury.

► When to Refer

- Transfer to a burn unit is indicated for large burn size, circumferential burn, or burn involving a joint or high-risk body part, and patients with comorbidities.

► When to Admit

- Significant burns (based on location and extent).
- Patients with significant comorbidities and suboptimal home situations.

Cancio LC et al. Evolving changes in the management of burns and environmental injuries. Surg Clin North Am. 2012 Aug; 92(4):959–86. [PMID: 22850157]

Wasiak J et al. Dressings for superficial and partial thickness burns. Cochrane Database Syst Rev. 2013 Mar 28;3:CD002106. [PMID: 23543513]

Wolf SE et al. The year in burns 2013. Burns. 2014 Dec; 40(8):1421–32. [PMID: 25454722]

ELECTRICAL INJURY

ESSENTIALS OF DIAGNOSIS

▶ Extent of injury is determined by the type, amount, duration, and pathway of electrical current.

▶ Resuscitation must be attempted before assuming the electrical injury victim is dead; clinical findings are unreliable.

▶ Skin findings may be misleading and are not indicative of the degree of deeper tissue injury.

General Considerations

Electricity-induced injuries are common and most are preventable. These inquiries occur by exposure to electrical current of low voltage, high voltage, or lightning. Electrical current type is either alternating current (AC) or direct current (DC). Electricity causes acute damage by direct tissue damage, muscle tetany, direct thermal injury and coagulation necrosis, and associated trauma.

Alternating current (AC) is bidirectional electrical flow that may cause muscle tetany, which prolongs the duration and amount of current exposure. AC current can be low voltage or high voltage. **Low voltage** (less than 1000 V) is typically household AC current that ranges in severity from minor injury to significant damage and death. **High voltage** (greater than 1000 V) is most often related to occupational exposure and is associated with deep tissue damage and higher morbidity and mortality. **Direct current (DC)** is unidirectional electrical flow (ie lightning, batteries, and automotive electrical systems). It is more likely to cause a single intense muscle contraction and asystole. **Lightning** differs from other high-voltage electrical shock in that lightning is massive DC current of millions of volts lasting a very brief duration (a small fraction of a second).

The extent of damage depends on the following factors: voltage (high or low, whether greater or less than 1000 volts), current type, tissue resistance, moisture, pathway; duration of exposure; associated trauma and comorbidities. Current is the most important determinant of tissue damage. Current passes through the tissues of least resistance, and this energy produces heat causing direct thermal injury. Tissue resistance varies throughout the body. Nerve cells are the most vulnerable, and bone is the most resistant to electrical current.

Clinical Findings

Electrical burns are of three distinct types: flash (arcing) burns, flame (clothing) burns, and the direct heating effect of tissues by the electrical current.

Skin damage does not correlate with the degree of injury. Not all electrical injuries cause skin damage; only very minor skin damage may be present with massive internal injuries. Symptoms and signs may range from tingling, superficial skin burns, and myalgias to coma, paralysis, massive tissue damage, or death. The presence of entrance and exit burns signifies an increased risk of deep tissue damage. The entrance and exit points on the skin are the most damaged. Current passing through skeletal muscle can cause muscle necrosis and contractions severe enough to result in bone fracture. If the current passes through the heart or brainstem, death may be immediate due to ventricular fibrillation, asystole, or apnea.

Resuscitation must be initiated on all victims of electrical injury since clinical findings are deceptive and unreliable and a viable victim of electrical current injury may appear dead on examination.

Complications

Complications include respiratory arrest; autonomic dysfunction (resulting in pupils that are fixed, dilated, or asymmetric); dysrhythmias; altered mental status; seizures; paralysis; headache; pneumothorax; vascular injury; tissue edema and necrosis; compartment syndrome; associated traumatic injuries (ruptured ear drums, fractures from falls or muscle contractions); rhabdomyolysis; acute kidney injury; hypovolemia from third spacing; infections; ocular complications (ie, acute or delayed cataract formation); sepsis; gangrene requiring limb amputation; neurologic, cognitive, or psychiatric dysfunction. Psychiatric support may be necessary following electrical injury.

Treatment

A. Emergency Measures

The patient must be assessed and treated as a trauma victim. The victim must be safely separated from the electrical current prior to initiation of CPR or other treatment. Resuscitation must then be initiated since clinical findings of death are unreliable.

B. Hospital Measures

The initial assessment involves airway, breathing, and circulation followed by a full trauma protocol. Fluid resuscitation is important to maintain adequate urinary output. Initial evaluation includes cardiac monitoring and ECG, complete blood count, electrolytes, renal function tests, liver biochemical tests, urinalysis, urine myoglobin, serum creatine kinase, and cardiac enzymes. ECG does not show typical patterns of ischemia since the electrical damage is epicardial. Victims must be evaluated for hidden injury (eg, ophthalmic, otologic, muscular, compartment syndromes), organ injury (myocardium, liver, kidney, pancreas), blunt trauma, dehydration, skin burns, hypertension, posttraumatic stress, acid-base disturbances, and neurologic damage.

Electrical burn injury remains the most underrecognized and devastating burn injury, sometimes leading to amputations (often because of unrecognized compartment syndromes) and acute kidney injury, resulting in part from rhabdomyolysis (see Chapter 22).

Superficial skin may appear deceivingly benign, leading to a delayed or completely overlooked diagnosis of deep tissue injury. When electrical injury occurs, extensive deep tissue necrosis should be suspected. Deep tissue necrosis leads to profound tissue swelling, which results in a high risk of a compartment syndrome. Early debridement of devitalized tissues and tetanus prophylaxis may reduce the risks of infection.

Pain management is important before, during, and after initial treatment and rehabilitation. Multimodal approach to pain is the most effective. Interventions include medications (opioids, acetaminophen, nonsteroidal anti-inflammatory drugs), heat therapy, massage, and cognitive-behavioral therapy.

Prognosis

Prognosis depends on the degree and location of electrical injury, initial tissue damage, associated injuries, comorbidities, and complications.

When to Refer

- Surgical specialists may be needed to perform fasciotomy for compartment syndrome or devitalized tissue debridement or microvascular reconstruction.
- Ophthalmologists should evaluate patients for possible ocular complications, and patients should be referred to ENT for tympanic membrane rupture or hearing loss.

When to Admit

Indications for hospitalization include high voltage exposure; dysrhythmia or ECG changes; large burn; neurologic, pulmonary, or cardiac symptoms; suspicion of significant deep tissue or organ damage; transthoracic current pathway; history of cardiac disease or other significant comorbidities or injuries; and need for surgery.

Davis C et al. Wilderness Medical Society practice guidelines for the prevention and treatment of lightning injuries: 2014 update. Wilderness Environ Med. 2014 Dec;25(4 Suppl):S86–95. [PMID: 25498265]
Forster SA et al. Lightning burn—review and case report. Burns. 2013 Mar;39(2):e8–12. [PMID: 22995421]

RADIATION EXPOSURE

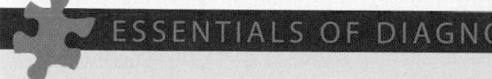

ESSENTIALS OF DIAGNOSIS

- Damage from radiation is determined by the source, type, quantity, duration, bodily location, and susceptibility and accumulation of exposures of the person.
- Clinicians and patients should be educated regarding the risks of medical diagnostic radiation. These radiation risks must be weighed against the benefits of the medical imaging needed.

Exposure to radiation may occur from environmental, occupational, medical care, accidental, or intentional (ie,

terrorism) exposure. With advancements in nuclear technology in the fields of medicine, energy, and industry, there is a growing risk of radiation exposure to patients, occupational workers, and the public. The extent of damage due to radiation exposure depends on the type, quantity, and duration of radiation exposure; the organs exposed; the degree of disruption to DNA; metabolic and cellular function; and the age, underlying condition, susceptibility, and accumulative exposures of the victim.

Radiation occurs from both nonionizing and ionizing radiation sources. **Nonionizing radiation** is low energy, resulting in injuries related to local thermal damage (ie, microwave, ultraviolet, visible light, and radiowave). **Ionizing radiation** is high energy, causing bodily damage in several ways (ie, cellular disruption, DNA damage, and mutations). Ionizing radiation is either electromagnetic (ie, x-rays and gamma rays) or particulate (ie, alpha or beta particles, neutrons, and protons). Exposure may be external, internal, or both.

International Commission on Radiological Protection (ICRP) website provides the most up-to-date recommendations for protection against ionizing radiation (http://www.icrp.org/index.asp).

Clinical Findings

Radiation exposure results in acute and delayed effects. Acute effects involve damage of the rapidly dividing cells (ie, the mucosa, skin, and bone marrow). This may be manifested as mucositis, nausea, vomiting, gastrointestinal edema and ulcers, skin burns, and bone marrow suppression over hours to days after exposure. Delayed effects include malignancy, reproduction abnormalities, liver, kidney, and central nervous system and immune system dysfunction.

Clinicians must be educated to recognize and treat acute radiation sickness also referred to as **acute radiation syndrome**. Acute radiation syndrome is due to an exposure to high doses of ionizing radiation over a brief time course. The symptom onset is within hours to days depending on the dose. Symptoms include anorexia, nausea, vomiting, weakness, exhaustion, lassitude and, in some cases, prostration; these symptoms may occur singly or in combination. Dehydration, anemia, and infection may follow. The Centers for Disease Control and Prevention offers web-based information for clinicians regarding acute radiation syndrome (http://emergency.cdc.gov/radiation/arsphysicianfactsheet.asp).

In **acute radiation exposure**, medical care includes close monitoring of the gastrointestinal, cutaneous, hematologic, cardiopulmonary, and cerebrovascular symptoms and signs from initial exposure and over time.

Therapeutic Radiation Exposure

Radiation therapy has been a successful component in the treatment of many malignancies. These radiation-treated cancer survivors have a higher risk of development of a second malignancy; obesity; and pulmonary, cardiac and thyroid dysfunction as well as an increased overall risk for chronic health conditions and mortality.

Medical Imaging Radiation Exposure

Medical imaging with ionizing radiation exposure (ie, computed tomography [CT] and nuclear medicine studies) has dramatically increased over the past few decades. Medical imaging radiation exposure has become a growing concern for the healthcare professionals and the public. Research has found significantly large variability in the radiation dose for the same study among different machines and different clinicians, within and across institutions, with radiation doses varying by as much as a factor of 10. These findings highlight the urgent safety need for standardization and regulation of radiation dosing for medical diagnostics and for clinician and public education.

American College of Radiology (ACR) offers "ACR Appropriateness Criteria" which are evidence-based guidelines created by expert panels to serve as a reference for best practices for imaging decisions by healthcare providers (http://www.acr.org/Quaity-Safety/Appropriateness-Criteria). Clinicians and patients must carefully weigh the risks and benefits of radiation exposure when deciding on an imaging test.

Occupational & Environmental Radiation Exposure

The National Nuclear Security Administration's Radiation Emergency Assistance Center provides 24-hour access to expert consultation services over the telephone or via email (telephone: 1-865-576-1005 or email: https://orise.orau.gov/reacts/). The National Nuclear Security Administration is part of the International Emergency Management and Cooperation, an international collaborative of foreign governments to establish an infrastructure worldwide for emergency preparedness and support, including radiation exposure. The Centers for Disease Control and Prevention "Radiation Emergency" website (http://emergency.cdc.gov/radiation/) is a useful resource for professionals.

Treatment

Treatment is focused on decontamination, symptomatic relief, supportive care, and psychosocial support. Specific treatments focus on the dose, route, and effects of exposure.

Prognosis

Prognosis is determined by the radiation dose, duration, and frequency as well as by the underlying condition of the victim. Death is usually due to hematopoietic failure gastrointestinal mucosal damage, central nervous system damage, widespread vascular injury, or secondary infection.

Carcinogenesis is related to the radiation type, total dose, duration, accumulation of exposure, and to the susceptibility of the victim. The younger the victim's age at the time of exposure, the greater the risk of acute and long-term damage from radiation. Radiation-related cancer risks persist throughout the exposed person's lifespan.

With the increased use of ionizing radiation for medical diagnostics and treatments, there is a growing concern for the iatrogenic increase in radiation-induced cancer risks.

There are age-related sensitivities to radiation; prenatal and younger age victims are more susceptible to carcinogenesis.

When to Admit

Most patients with significant ionizing radiation exposure require admission for close monitoring and supportive treatment.

Bui E et al. Contemporary management of radiation exposure and injury. J Trauma Acute Care Surg. 2014 Sep;77(3): 495–500. [PMID: 25159256]

Goodman DM. Initiatives focus on limiting radiation exposure to patients during CT scans. JAMA. 2013 Feb 20;309(7): 647–8. [PMID: 23423394]

Hasegawa A et al. Health effects of radiation and other health problems in the aftermath of nuclear accidents, with an emphasis on Fukushima. Lancet. 2015 Aug 1;386(9992): 479–88. [PMID: 26251393]

Kamiya K et al. Long-term effects of radiation exposure on health. Lancet. 2015 Aug 1;386(9992):469–78. [PMID: 26251392]

ENVIRONMENTAL DISORDERS RELATED TO ALTITUDE

DYSBARISM & DECOMPRESSION SICKNESS

ESSENTIALS OF DIAGNOSIS

▶ Symptoms temporally related to recent altitude or pressure changes (ie, scuba diving).

▶ Early recognition and prompt treatment of decompression sickness are extremely important.

▶ Patient must also be assessed for hypothermia, hypoglycemia, concurrent injuries, and medical conditions.

▶ Consultation with diving medicine or hyperbaric oxygen specialist is indicated.

General Considerations

Dysbarism and decompression sickness are physiologic problems that result from altitude changes and the effects of environmental pressure on gases in the body during underwater descent and ascent. These are most likely to occur when scuba diving is followed closely by travel to high altitudes, or when the scuba diver is not adherent to the conservative dive guidelines for dive duration, course, depth, and surface times.

As a diver descends, the gases in the body compress; gases dissolve in blood and tissues. During the ascent, gases in the body expand.

Dysbarism results from barotrauma when gas compression or expansion occurs in parts of the body that are noncompressible or have limited compliance. Pulmonary overinflation syndrome is one of the most serious and potentially fatal results of barotrauma. Pulmonary overinflation syndrome is due to an inappropriately rapid ascent causing alveoli rupture and air bubble extravasation into tissue planes or even the cerebral circulation.

Decompression sickness occurs when the ascent is too rapid and gas bubbles form and cause damage depending on their location (ie, coronary, pulmonary, spinal or cerebral blood vessels, joints, soft tissue). These gas bubbles cause damage due to mechanical disruption of tissue, local inflammatory response, occlusion of blood flow, platelet activation, endothelial dysfunction, and capillary leakage. Decompression sickness symptoms depends on the size and number and location of gas bubbles released (notably nitrogen). Risk of decompression sickness depends on the dive details (depth, duration, number of dives, and interval surface time between dives, water conditions) as well as the diver's age, weight, physical condition, physical exertion, the rate of ascent, and the length of time between the low altitude (scuba dive) and high altitude (air travel or ground ascent). Predisposing factors for decompression sickness include obesity, injury, hypoxia, lung or cardiac disease, right to left cardiac shunt (ie, patent foramen ovale), diver's overall health, dehydration, alcohol and medication effects, and panic attacks. Decompression sickness may also occur in those who take hot showers after cold dives.

Preventive measures include diver education; pre-dive medical screening and dive planning; strict adherence to dive course, timing, and depths; and a slow and controlled ascent plus proper control of buoyancy. Conservative recommendation is to avoid high altitudes (air travel or ground ascent) for at least 24 hours after surfacing from the dive, especially following multiple dives.

Clinical Findings

The range of clinical manifestations varies depending on the location of the gas bubble formation or the compressibility of gases in the body. Symptom onset may be immediate, within minutes or hours (in the majority), or present up to 36 hours later. Decompression sickness symptoms include pain in the joints ("the bends"); skin pruritus or burning (skin bends); cardiac symptoms (acute coronary syndrome, conduction abnormalities); spinal cord or cerebral symptoms (focal neurologic dysfunction or "dissociation" symptoms that do not follow typical distribution neuroanatomy patterns); labyrinthine decompression sickness ("the staggers," central vertigo); pulmonary decompression sickness ("the chokes," inspiratory pain, cough, and respiratory distress); arterial gas embolism (cerebral, pulmonary); barotrauma of the lungs, ear and sinus; coma and death.

Decompression sickness involving the brain and spinal cord may occur by different mechanisms due to air bubbles causing arterial occlusion, venous obstruction, or in situ toxicity.

The clinician must assess for associated conditions of hypothermia, hypoglycemia, hypovolemia, drowning, trauma, envenomations, or concurrent medical conditions.

Treatment

Early recognition and prompt treatment are extremely important. Decompression sickness must be considered if symptoms are temporally related to recent diving or altitude or pressure changes within the past 48 hours. Continuous administration of 100% oxygen is indicated and beneficial for all patients. Hyperbaric oxygen treatment is commonly recommended for decompression sickness symptoms. Immediate consultation with a diving medicine or hyperbaric oxygen specialist is indicated even if mild decompression sickness symptoms resolve. Nonsteroidal anti-inflammatory drugs, acetaminophen or aspirin may be given for pain control if there are no contraindications. Opioids should be used very cautiously, since these may obscure the response to recompression.

When to Admit

Rapid transportation to a hyperbaric treatment facility for recompression is imperative for decompression sickness. The Divers Alert Network is an excellent worldwide resource for emergency advice 24 hours daily for the management of diving-related conditions (www.diversalertnetwork.org).

Bove AA. Diving medicine. Am J Respir Crit Care Med. 2014 Jun 15;189(12):1479–86. [PMID: 24869752]

Hall J. The risks of scuba diving: a focus on decompression illness. Hawaii J Med Public Health. 2014 Nov;73(11 Suppl 2):13–6. [PMID: 25478296]

Moon RE. Hyperbaric oxygen treatment for decompression sickness. Undersea Hyperb Med. 2014 Mar–Apr;41(2):151–7. [PMID: 24851553]

Smart D et al. Joint position statement on persistent foramen ovale (PFO) and diving. South Pacific Underwater Medicine Society (SPUMS) and the United Kingdom Sports Diving Medical Committee (UKSDMC). Diving Hyperb Med. 2015 Jun;45(2):129–31. [PMID: 26165538]

HIGH-ALTITUDE ILLNESS

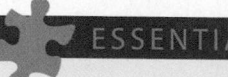

ESSENTIALS OF DIAGNOSIS

► The severity of the high-altitude illness is affected by the rate and height of ascent, and the individual's susceptibility.

► Prompt recognition and medical treatment of early symptoms of high-altitude illness may prevent progression.

► Clinicians should assess other conditions which may coexist or mimic symptoms of high altitude illness (severe dehydration, hyponatremia, or hypoglycemia, trauma, or infection).

► Immediate descent is the definitive treatment for high-altitude cerebral edema and high-altitude pulmonary edema.

General Considerations

As altitude increases, hypobaric hypoxia results due to a decrease in both barometric pressure and oxygen partial pressure. High-altitude medical problems are due to hypobaric hypoxia at high altitudes (usually greater than 2000 meters or 6560 feet). High-altitude illness includes a spectrum of disorders categorized by end-organ effects (mostly cerebral and pulmonary), and exposure duration (acute and long-term). Acute high-altitude conditions are **acute mountain sickness (AMS), high-altitude cerebral edema (HACE),** and **high-altitude pulmonary edema (HAPE).** Long-term exposure to high altitude over months or years with inadequate acclimatization can result in sub-acute mountain sickness and chronic mountain sickness (Monge disease).

Acclimatization occurs as a physiologic response to the rise in altitude and increasing hypobaric hypoxia. Physiologic changes include increases in alveolar ventilation and oxygen extraction by the tissues and increased hemoglobin level and oxygen binding. High-altitude illness results when the hypoxic stress is greater than the individual's ability to acclimatize. Risk factors for high-altitude illness include increased physical activity with insufficient acclimatization, inadequate education and preparation, and individual susceptibility, and previous high-altitude illness. The key determinants of high-altitude illness risk and severity include both individual susceptibility factors and altitudinal factors (rapid rate and height of ascent and total change in altitude).

Individual susceptibility factors include underlying conditions such as cardiac and pulmonary dysfunction, patent foramen ovale, blood disorders (ie, sickle cell disease), pregnancy, neurologic condition, recent surgery, and many other chronic medical conditions. Those with symptomatic cardiac or pulmonary disease should avoid high altitudes.

Patient assessment for high-altitude illness should also include evaluation for other conditions, which may coexist or may present in a similar manner.

1. High-Altitude–Associated Neurologic Conditions: AMS & HACE

There is a spectrum of neurologic conditions caused by high altitude, ranging from AMS to the more serious form HACE. Clinicians must rely on patient's report of symptoms to determine the severity of AMS. In addition to the patient's report of symptoms, HACE includes neurologic examination findings.

AMS includes symptoms such as headache (most severe and persistent symptom), lassitude, drowsiness, dizziness, chilliness, nausea and vomiting, difficulty sleeping. Later symptoms include irritability, difficulty concentrating, anorexia, insomnia, and increased headaches.

HACE includes the severe symptoms of AMS and results from cerebral vasogenic edema and cerebral cellular hypoxia. It usually occurs at elevations above 2500 meters (8250 feet) but may occur at lower elevations. Hallmarks are altered mental status, ataxia, severe lassitude, and encephalopathy. Examination findings may include confusion, ataxia, urinary retention or incontinence, focal neurologic deficits, papilledema, and seizures. Symptoms may progress to obtundation, coma, and death.

► Treatment

Definitive treatment is immediate descent. Descent should be at least 610 meters (2000 feet), and it should continue until symptoms improve. Descent is essential if the symptoms are persistent, severe, worsening or if HACE or HAPE are present. If immediate descent is not possible, portable hyperbaric chambers can provide symptomatic relief but they should not delay descent.

Initial treatment involves oxygen administration to keep the pulse oximetry S_pO_2 to greater than 90%.

Acetazolamide (250 mg twice daily) is an effective medication for treatment of mild symptoms of AMS.

Dexamethasone is most effective for moderate to severe AMS (4 mg orally every 6 hours). Dexamethasone is the primary treatment for HACE (8 mg once then 4 mg every 6 hours). Acetazolamide can be added as an adjunct in severe HACE cases. In most individuals, symptoms clear within 24–48 hours.

It is imperative that the clinician also assess for other conditions that may mimic or coexist with AMS and HACE (ie, dehydration, exhaustion, hypoglycemia, hypothermia, hyponatremia, trauma, infection).

If HAPE symptoms and signs are present along with HACE, nifedipine or a selective phosphodiesterase inhibitor may be added for pulmonary vasodilation. The clinician must be cautious when using combinations of vasodilators.

2. Acute HAPE

HAPE is the leading cause of death from high altitude illness. The hallmark is markedly elevated pulmonary artery pressure followed by pulmonary edema. It usually occurs at altitudes above 3000 meters (9840 feet), although it may occur at lower levels. Early symptoms may appear within 6–36 hours after arrival at a high-altitude area. These include incessant dry cough, shortness of breath disproportionate to exertion, headache, decreased exercise performance, fatigue, dyspnea at rest, and chest tightness. Recognition of the early symptoms may enable the patient to descend before incapacitating pulmonary edema develops. Strenuous exertion should be avoided. Later, wheezing, orthopnea, and hemoptysis may occur as pulmonary edema worsens.

Physical findings may include tachycardia, mild fever, tachypnea, cyanosis, prolonged respiration, rales, and rhonchi. The clinician must assess for other potential medical conditions because the clinical picture may resemble other etiologies (pneumonia, viral upper respiratory tract infection, mucous plugging, bronchospasm, or acute coronary syndrome). Diagnosis is usually clinical; ancillary tests are nonspecific or unavailable on site. Prompt recognition and medical attention of early symptoms of HAPE may prevent progression.

► Treatment

Immediate descent (at least 610 meters [2000 feet]) is essential although this may not be immediately possible, and may not alone improve symptoms.

The patient must rest, reclined with head elevated. Supplemental oxygen must be administered to maintain pulse oximetry reading S_pO_2 greater than 90%. Recompression in a portable hyperbaric bag will temporarily reduce symptoms if rapid or immediate descent is not possible, but should not delay descent.

Nifedipine (30 mg slow extended-release tablets every 12 hours) can be used as an adjunct if the other therapies (descent, oxygen, or portable hyperbarics) are not successful or available. Selective phosphodiesterase inhibitors (tadalafil, 10 mg orally every 12 hours; sildenafil, 50 mg orally every 8 hours) are used for HAPE prevention but may also provide effective symptom relief as an alternative or if nifedipine is not available. Administering nifedipine plus a phosphodiesterase inhibitor as pulmonary vasodilators is not recommended because this combination may also lower the mean arterial pressure and decrease cerebral perfusion. Treatment for ARDS (see Chapter 9) is required for some patients. If neurologic symptoms are present concurrently with HAPE and do not resolve with improved oxygenation, dexamethasone should be added according to HACE treatment guidelines.

3. Subacute Mountain Sickness

This occurs most frequently in unacclimatized individuals and at high altitudes (above 4500 meters) for a prolonged period of time. Symptoms of dyspnea and cough are probably due to hypoxic pulmonary hypertension and secondary heart failure. Treatment consists of rest, oxygen administration, diuretics, and return to lower altitudes.

4. Chronic Mountain Sickness (Monge Disease)

This uncommon condition is seen in residents of high-altitude communities who have lost their acclimatization to such a hypobaric hypoxic environment. It is difficult to differentiate from chronic pulmonary disease.

▶ Prevention of High-Altitude Disorders

Pre-trip preventive measures include participant education, medical prescreening, pre-trip planning, optimal physical conditioning before travel, and adequate rest and sleep the day before travel and during the trip. Preventive efforts during ascent include reduced food intake; avoidance of alcohol, tobacco, and unnecessary physical activity during travel.

Gradual ascent is the most effective way to allow acclimatization. Low-risk ascension rate is 2 or more days to arrive at 2500–3000 meters. The altitude reached during waking hours is not as important as the altitude at which this hiker sleeps. If the terrain does not allow a sleeping elevation increase below 500 meters, an extra rest day should be added before or after the increased sleep elevation more than 500 meters.

Drug prophylaxis may be prescribed for AMS and HACE if no contraindications exist. Prophylactic low-dose acetazolamide (125 mg twice daily orally) has been shown to reduce the incidence and severity of AMS and HACE when started 3 days prior to ascent and continued for 48–72 hours at high altitude. Dexamethasone is an alternative prophylactic medication for AMS and HACE (2 mg every 6 hours or 4 mg every 12 hours orally beginning on the day of ascent, continuing for 3 days at the higher altitude, and then tapering over 5 days).

Individuals with a past history of HAPE should use drug prophylaxis to reduce the risk of recurrence. Nifedipine, 30 mg extended-release every 12 hours started the day before ascent and continued through the fourth day at target elevation, or through the seventh day if the ascent rate was faster, is recommended. Salmeterol can be added at doses of 125 mcg by inhaler every 12 hours beginning 24 hours prior to ascent. This can be used as an adjunct to nifedipine but not as monotherapy.

Phosphodiesterase inhibitors (eg, tadalafil 10 mg orally twice a day or sildenafil 50 mg orally every 8 hours) may be beneficial in the treatment of HAPE based on their physiologic effects of decreased pulmonary arterial pressures and pulmonary vasodilation. This drug class may be used if nifedipine is not available but should not be administered along with nifedipine since the additive vasodilation effects may increase the patient's risk of hypotension and cerebral hypoperfusion.

▶ When to Admit

- All patients with HACE or HAPE must be hospitalized for further observation.

- Hospitalization must also be considered for any patient who remains symptomatic after treatment and descent.

- Pulmonary symptoms and hypoxia may be worsened by complications such as pulmonary embolism, secondary respiratory infection, bronchospasms, mucous plugging, or acute coronary syndrome.

Bärtsch P et al. Clinical practice: acute high-altitude illnesses. N Engl J Med. 2013 Jun 13;368(24):2294–302. [PMID: 23758234]

Luks AM et al. Wilderness Medical Society practice guidelines for the prevention and treatment of acute altitude illness: 2014 update. Wilderness Environ Med. 2014 Dec;25(4 Suppl):S4–14. [PMID: 25498261]

Yanamandra U et al. High-altitude cerebral oedema mimicking stroke. BMJ Case Rep. 2014 Mar 26;2014:201897. [PMID: 24671373]

Zafren K. Prevention of high altitude illness. Travel Med Infect Dis. 2014 Jan–Feb;12(1):29–39. [PMID: 24393671]

SAFETY OF AIR TRAVEL & SELECTION OF PATIENTS FOR AIR TRAVEL

The medical safety of air travel depends on the nature and severity of the traveler's preflight condition and factors such as travel duration, frequency and use of inflight exercise, cabin altitude pressure, availability of medical supplies, and presence of health care professionals on board. Air travel passengers are susceptible to a wide range of flight-related problems: pulmonary (hypoxemia, gas expansion), venous thromboembolism (VTE), infectious, cardiac, gastrointestinal, ocular, immunologic, syncope, neuropsychiatric, metabolic, trauma, and substance-related.

These air-travel risks are higher for those air travelers with preexisting medical conditions.

Hypobaric hypoxia is the underlying etiology of most serious medical emergencies in flight due to cabin altitude. Despite commercial aircraft pressurization requirements, there is significant hypoxemia, dyspnea, gas expansion, and stress in travelers.

Any form of prolonged travel involving immobilization has been associated with increased risk of VTE (referred to as "traveler's thrombosis"), although air travel has been the main focus of medical review. Conditions that place long-distance travelers at high risk for VTE include the following: (1) travel involving immobilization for 4 or more hours, (2) hypercoagulable disorders (ie, Factor V Leiden, deficiencies in proteins C and S or antithrombin, elevated factor VIII, hyperprothrombinemia, antiphospholipid syndrome), and (3) acquired risks (previous VTE, recent surgery, stroke or trauma, active malignancy, obesity, pregnancy or postpartum, oral contraceptives or hormone therapy, advanced age, immobilization or limited mobility,, inflammatory bowel disease, and nephrotic syndrome)

Air travel is not advised for anyone who is "incapacitated" or has any "unstable conditions." The Air Transport Association of America defines an **incapacitated passenger** as "one who is suffering from a physical or mental disability and who, because of such disability or the effect of the flight on the disability, is incapable of self-care; would endanger the health or safety of such person or other passengers or airline employees; or would cause discomfort or annoyance of other passengers." **Unstable conditions** include active pneumothorax, advanced pulmonary hypertension, acute worsening of an underlying lung disease, poorly controlled hypertension, dysrhythmias, angina, valvular disease, heart failure, or acute psychiatric condition; severe anemia or symptomatic sickle cell disease; recent myocardial infarction; cerebrovascular accident; poorly controlled seizure disorder; deep venous thrombosis; postsurgery, especially heart surgery (unless approved by surgeon); and any active communicable disease (influenza, tuberculosis, measles, chickenpox, zoster, or other communicable virulent infections).

► Pregnancy

Long travel increases risk of VTE for the pregnant traveler. Pregnant women may be permitted to fly during the first 8 months of pregnancy unless there is a history of pregnancy complications or premature birth. The clinician's authorization is required if travel is essential during the ninth month of pregnancy or earlier in a complicated pregnancy. Pregnant travelers are at higher risk for infection transmission and air travel radiation exposure.

► Prevention

Air travel complications may be reduced by the following preventive measures: passenger prescreening, passenger education, and in-flight positioning and activity. Prescreening evaluation is recommended for all high-risk patients including preexisting requirement of oxygen, continuous positive pressure or ventilator support, underlying restrictive or obstructive lung disease, comorbidities worsened by hypoxemia (pulmonary hypertension, cardiac or cerebrovascular disease), previous respiratory distress during air travel, recent pneumothorax, and being within 6 weeks of an acute respiratory illness.

Air travel education should include risk reduction of VTE, infectious diseases, and exacerbations of underlying medical conditions. Patients and clinicians can check the World Health Organization website for the most updated information on travel health risks and infectious diseases (http://www.who.int/ith/en/). Patients requiring oxygen therapy or CPAP must be reminded to make prior arrangements for oxygen provision prior to departure and upon arrival at their destinations.

All long-distance travelers can reduce VTE risk by avoiding constrictive clothing, staying well-hydrated, changing position frequently, avoiding cramped position, avoiding leg crossing, engaging in frequent in-flight leg stretching exercises at least every hour, and walking for 5 minutes every hour. Clinicians should assess those with high risk of VTE prior to air travel to determine whether anticoagulation is indicated (see Table 14–14).

Hu X et al. Air travel and pneumothorax. Chest. 2014 Apr;145(4):688–94. [PMID: 24687705]

Johnston RV et al; Aerospace Medical Association Air Transport Medicine Committee. Travelers' thrombosis. Aviat Space Environ Med. 2014 Feb;85(2):191–4. [PMID: 24597166]

Josephs LK et al; British Thoracic Society Air Travel Working Group. Managing patients with stable respiratory disease planning air travel: a primary care summary of the British Thoracic Society recommendations. Prim Care Respir J. 2013 Jun;22(2):234–8. [PMID: 23732637]

Nicholson TT et al. Fitness to fly in patients with lung disease. Ann Am Thorac Soc. 2014 Dec;11(10):1614–22. [PMID: 25393882]

Tucker R. Advising pregnant women on minimising travel risks. Nurs Times. 2014 Apr 2–8;110(14):19–21. [PMID: 24772798]

Poisoning

Kent R. Olson, MD

38

Patients with drug overdoses or poisoning may initially have no symptoms or they may have varying degrees of overt intoxication. The asymptomatic patient may have been exposed to or may have ingested a lethal dose but not yet exhibit any manifestations of toxicity. It is important to: (1) quickly assess the potential danger, (2) consider gut decontamination to prevent absorption, (3) treat complications if they occur, and (4) observe the asymptomatic patient for an appropriate interval.

▶ Assess the Danger

If the drug or poison is known, its danger can be assessed by consulting a text or computerized information resource or by calling a regional poison control center. (In the United States, dialing 1-800-222-1222 will direct the call to the regional poison control center.) Assessment will usually take into account the dose ingested; the time since ingestion; the presence of any symptoms or clinical signs; preexisting cardiac, respiratory, kidney, or liver disease; and, occasionally, specific serum drug or toxin levels. Be aware that the history given by the patient or family may be incomplete or unreliable.

IMMEDIATE 24-HOUR TOXICOLOGY CONSULTATION

Call your regional poison control center
U.S. toll-free 1-800-222-1222

▶ Observation of the Patient

Asymptomatic or mildly symptomatic patients should be observed for at least 4–6 hours. Longer observation is indicated if the ingested substance is a sustained-release preparation or is known to slow gastrointestinal motility (opioids, anticholinergics, salicylate) or may cause a delayed onset of symptoms (such as acetaminophen, colchicine, or hepatotoxic mushrooms). After that time, the patient may be discharged if no symptoms have developed. Before discharge,

psychiatric evaluation should be performed to assess suicide risk. Intentional ingestions in adolescents should raise the possibility of unwanted pregnancy or sexual abuse.

In symptomatic patients, treatment of life-threatening complications takes precedence over in-depth diagnostic evaluation. Patients with mild symptoms may deteriorate rapidly, which is why all potentially significant exposures should be observed in an acute care facility. The following complications may occur, depending on the type of poisoning.

COMA

▶ Assessment & Complications

Coma is commonly associated with ingestion of large doses of antihistamines (eg, diphenhydramine), benzodiazepines and other sedative-hypnotic drugs, ethanol, opioids, antipsychotic drugs, or antidepressants. The most common cause of death in comatose patients is respiratory failure, which may occur abruptly. Pulmonary aspiration of gastric contents may also occur, especially in victims who are deeply obtunded or convulsing. Hypoxia and hypoventilation may cause or aggravate hypotension, arrhythmias, and seizures. Thus, protection of the airway and assisted ventilation are the most important treatment measures for any poisoned patient.

▶ Treatment

A. Emergency Management

The initial emergency management of coma can be remembered by the mnemonic *ABCD*, for *A*irway, *B*reathing, *C*irculation, and *D*rugs (dextrose, thiamine, and naloxone or flumazenil), respectively.

1. Airway—Establish a patent airway by positioning, suction, or insertion of an artificial nasal or oropharyngeal airway. If the patient is deeply comatose or if airway reflexes are depressed, perform endotracheal intubation. These airway interventions may not be necessary if the patient is intoxicated by an opioid or a benzodiazepine and responds to intravenous naloxone or flumazenil.

2. Breathing—Clinically assess the quality and depth of respiration, and provide assistance if necessary with a bag-valve-mask device or mechanical ventilator. Administer supplemental oxygen, if needed. The arterial or venous blood CO_2 tension is useful in determining the adequacy of ventilation. The arterial blood PO_2 determination may reveal hypoxemia, which may be caused by respiratory depression, bronchospasm, pulmonary aspiration, or non-cardiogenic pulmonary edema. Pulse oximetry provides an assessment of oxygenation but is not reliable in patients with methemoglobinemia or carbon monoxide poisoning, unless a pulse oximetry device capable of detecting these forms of hemoglobin is used.

3. Circulation—Measure the pulse and blood pressure and estimate tissue perfusion (eg, by measurement of urinary output, skin signs, arterial blood pH). Place the patient on continuous ECG monitoring. Insert an intravenous line, and draw blood for glucose, electrolytes, serum creatinine and liver tests, and possible quantitative toxicologic testing.

4. Drugs—

A. DEXTROSE AND THIAMINE—Unless promptly treated, severe hypoglycemia can cause irreversible brain damage. Therefore, in all obtunded, comatose or convulsing patients, give 50% dextrose, 50–100 mL by intravenous bolus, unless a rapid point of care blood sugar test rules out hypoglycemia. In alcoholic or very malnourished patients who may have marginal thiamine stores, give thiamine, 100 mg intramuscularly or in the intravenous fluids.

B. OPIOID ANTAGONISTS—Naloxone, 0.4–2 mg intravenously, may reverse opioid-induced respiratory depression and coma. It is often given empirically to any comatose patient with depressed respirations. If opioid overdose is strongly suspected, give additional doses of naloxone (up to 5–10 mg may be required to reverse the effects of potent opioids). **Note:** Naloxone has a shorter duration of action (2–3 hours) than most common opioids; repeated doses may be required, and continuous observation for at least 3–4 hours after the last dose is mandatory.

C. FLUMAZENIL—Flumazenil, 0.2–0.5 mg intravenously, repeated as needed up to a maximum of 3 mg, may reverse benzodiazepine-induced coma. **Caution:** Flumazenil should **not** be given if the patient has coingested a potential convulsant drug, is a user of high-dose benzodiazepines, or has a seizure disorder because its use in these circumstances may precipitate seizures. *In most circumstances, use of flumazenil is not advised as the potential risks outweigh its benefits.* **Note:** Flumazenil has a short duration of effect (2–3 hours), and resedation requiring additional doses may occur.

HYPOTHERMIA

▶ Assessment & Complications

Hypothermia commonly accompanies coma due to opioids, ethanol, hypoglycemic agents, phenothiazines, barbiturates, benzodiazepines, and other sedative-hypnotics and central nervous system depressants. Hypothermic patients may have a barely perceptible pulse and blood pressure. Hypothermia may cause or aggravate hypotension, which will not reverse until the temperature is normalized.

▶ Treatment

Treatment of hypothermia is discussed in Chapter 37. Gradual rewarming is preferred unless the patient is in cardiac arrest.

HYPOTENSION

▶ Assessment & Complications

Hypotension may be due to poisoning by many different drugs and poisons, including antihypertensive drugs, beta-blockers, calcium channel blockers, disulfiram (ethanol interaction), iron, trazodone, quetiapine, and other antipsychotic agents and antidepressants. Poisons causing hypotension include cyanide, carbon monoxide, hydrogen sulfide, aluminum or zinc phosphide, arsenic, and certain mushrooms.

Hypotension in the poisoned or drug-overdosed patient may be caused by venous or arteriolar vasodilation, hypovolemia, depressed cardiac contractility, or a combination of these effects.

▶ Treatment

Most hypotensive patients respond to empiric treatment with repeated 200 mL intravenous boluses of 0.9% saline or other isotonic crystalloid up to a total of 1–2 L; much larger amounts may be needed if the victim is profoundly volume depleted (eg, as with *Amanita phalloides* mushroom poisoning). Monitoring the central venous pressure (CVP) can help determine whether further fluid therapy is needed. If fluid therapy is not successful after adequate volume replacement, give dopamine or norepinephrine by intravenous infusion. Consider bedside cardiac ultrasound or pulmonary artery catheterization (or both) if hypotension persists.

Hypotension caused by certain toxins may respond to specific treatment. For hypotension caused by overdoses of tricyclic antidepressants or other sodium channel blockers, administer sodium bicarbonate, 50–100 mEq by intravenous bolus injection. Norepinephrine 4–8 mcg/min by intravenous infusion is more effective than dopamine in some patients with overdoses of tricyclic antidepressants or of drugs with predominantly vasodilating effects. For beta-blocker overdose, glucagon (5–10 mg intravenously) may be of value. For calcium channel blocker overdose, administer calcium chloride, 1–2 g intravenously (repeated doses may be necessary; doses of 5–10 g and more have been given in some cases). High-dose insulin (0.5–1 units/kg/h intravenously) euglycemic therapy may also be used (see the sections on Beta-Adrenergic Blockers and Calcium Channel Blockers, below). Intralipid 20% lipid emulsion has been reported to improve hemodynamics in some cases of intoxication by highly lipid-soluble drugs such as bupivacaine, bupropion, clomipramine, and verapamil.

Kryshtal DO et al. In vitro studies indicate intravenous lipid emulsion acts as lipid sink in verapamil poisoning. J Med Toxicol. 2015 Nov 9. [Epub ahead of print] [PMID: 26553277]

Woodward C et al. High dose insulin therapy, an evidence-based approach to beta blocker/calcium channel blocker toxicity. Daru. 2014 Apr 8;22(1):36. [PMID: 24713415]

HYPERTENSION

Assessment & Complications

Hypertension may be due to poisoning with amphetamines, anticholinergics, cocaine, performance-enhancing products (containing caffeine, phenylephrine, ephedrine, or yohimbine), monoamine oxidase (MAO) inhibitors, and other drugs.

Severe hypertension (eg, diastolic blood pressure greater than 105–110 mm Hg in a person who does not have chronic hypertension) can result in acute intracranial hemorrhage, myocardial infarction, or aortic dissection.

Treatment

Treat hypertension if the patient is symptomatic or if the diastolic pressure is higher than 105–110 mm Hg—especially if there is no prior history of hypertension.

Hypertensive patients who are agitated or anxious may benefit from a sedative such as lorazepam, 2–3 mg intravenously. For persistent hypertension, administer phentolamine, 2–5 mg intravenously, or nitroprusside sodium, 0.25–8 mcg/kg/min intravenously. If excessive tachycardia is present, *add* propranolol, 1–5 mg intravenously, or esmolol, 25–100 mcg/kg/min intravenously, or labetalol 0.2–0.3 mg/kg intravenously. **Caution:** Do not give beta-blockers alone, since doing so may paradoxically worsen hypertension as a result of unopposed alpha-adrenergic stimulation.

Le Roux G et al. Recreational phenethylamine poisonings reported to a French poison control center. Drug Alcohol Depend. 2015 Sep 1;154:46–53. [PMID: 26205314]

ARRHYTHMIAS

Assessment & Complications

Arrhythmias may occur with a variety of drugs or toxins (Table 38–1). They may also occur as a result of hypoxia, metabolic acidosis, or electrolyte imbalance (eg, hyperkalemia, hypokalemia, hypomagnesemia or hypocalcemia), or following exposure to chlorinated solvents or chloral hydrate overdose. Atypical ventricular tachycardia (torsades de pointes) is often associated with drugs that prolong the QT interval.

Treatment

Hypoxia or electrolyte imbalance should be sought and treated. If ventricular arrhythmias persist, administer lidocaine or amiodarone at usual antiarrhythmic doses. **Note:**

Table 38–1. Common toxins or drugs causing arrhythmias.[1]

Arrhythmia	Common Causes
Sinus bradycardia	Beta-blockers, calcium channel blockers, clonidine, digitalis glycosides, organophosphates
Atrioventricular block	Beta-blockers, calcium channel blockers, class Ia antiarrhythmics (including quinidine), carbamazepine, clonidine, digitalis glycosides, lithium
Sinus tachycardia	Beta-agonists (eg, albuterol), amphetamines, anticholinergics, antihistamines, caffeine, cocaine, pseudoephedrine, tricyclic and other antidepressants
Wide QRS complex	Class Ia and class Ic antiarrhythmics, phenothiazines (eg, thioridazine), potassium (hyperkalemia), propranolol, tricyclic antidepressants, bupropion, lamotrigine, diphenhydramine (severe overdose)
QT interval prolongation and torsades de pointes	Arsenic, class Ia and class III antiarrhythmics, citalopram, droperidol, lithium, methadone, pentamidine, sertraline, sotalol, and many other drugs[2]
Ventricular premature beats and ventricular tachycardia	Amphetamines, cocaine, ephedrine, caffeine, chlorinated or fluorinated hydrocarbons, digoxin, aconite (found in some Chinese herbal preparations), fluoride, theophylline. QT prolongation can lead to atypical ventricular tachycardia (torsades de pointes).

[1]Arrhythmias may also occur as a result of hypoxia, metabolic acidosis, or electrolyte imbalance (eg, hyperkalemia or hypokalemia, hypocalcemia, hypomagnesemia).
[2]https://crediblemeds.org/

Wide QRS complex tachycardia in the setting of tricyclic antidepressant overdose (or diphenhydramine or class Ia antiarrhythmic drugs) should be treated with sodium bicarbonate, 50–100 mEq intravenously by bolus infusion. (See discussion of tricyclic antidepressant poisoning.) **Caution:** Avoid class Ia antiarrhythmic agents (eg, procainamide, disopyramide) and amiodarone, which may aggravate arrhythmias caused by tricyclic antidepressants. Torsades de pointes associated with prolonged QT interval may respond to intravenous magnesium (2 g intravenously over 2 minutes) or overdrive pacing. Treat digitalis-induced arrhythmias with digoxin-specific antibodies (see discussion of cardiac glycoside poisoning).

For tachyarrhythmias induced by chlorinated solvents, chloral hydrate, Freons, or sympathomimetic agents, use propranolol or esmolol (see doses given above in Hypertension section).

Laskowski LK et al. Start me up! Recurrent ventricular tachydys-rhythmias following intentional concentrated caffeine ingestion. Clin Toxicol (Phila). 2015;53(8):830–3. [PMID: 26279469]

Tormoehlen LM et al. Hydrocarbon toxicity: a review. Clin Toxicol (Phila). 2014 Jun;52(5):479–89. [PMID: 24911841]

SEIZURES

▶ Assessment & Complications

Seizures may be due to poisoning with many poisons and drugs, including amphetamines, antidepressants (especially tricyclic antidepressants, bupropion, and venlafaxine), antihistamines (especially diphenhydramine), antipsychotics, camphor, cocaine, isoniazid (INH), chlorinated insecticides, tramadol, and theophylline. The onset of seizures may be delayed for up to 18–24 hours after extended-released bupropion overdose.

Seizures may also be caused by hypoxia, hypoglycemia, hypocalcemia, hyponatremia, withdrawal from alcohol or sedative-hypnotics, head trauma, central nervous system infection, or idiopathic epilepsy.

Prolonged or repeated seizures may lead to hypoxia, metabolic acidosis, hyperthermia, and rhabdomyolysis.

▶ Treatment

Administer lorazepam, 2–3 mg, or diazepam, 5–10 mg, intravenously over 1–2 minutes, or—if intravenous access is not immediately available—midazolam, 5–10 mg intramuscularly. If convulsions continue, administer phenobarbital, 15–20 mg/kg slowly intravenously over no less than 30 minutes. (For drug-induced seizures, phenobarbital is preferred over phenytoin or levetiracetam.) Propofol infusion has also been reported effective for some resistant drug-induced seizures.

Seizures due to a few drugs and toxins may require antidotes or other specific therapies (as listed in Table 38–2).

Chen HY, Albertson TE, Olson KR. Treatment of drug-induced seizures. Br J Clin Pharmacol. 2016 Mar;81(3):412–9. [PMID: 26174744]

Reichert C et al. Seizures after single-agent overdose with pharmaceutical drugs: analysis of cases reported to a poison center. Clin Toxicol (Phila). 2014 Jul;52(6):629–34. [PMID: 24844578]

HYPERTHERMIA

▶ Assessment & Complications

Hyperthermia may be associated with poisoning by amphetamines (especially methylenedioxymethamphetamine [MDMA; "Ecstasy"]), atropine and other anticholinergic drugs, cocaine, salicylates, strychnine, tricyclic antidepressants, and various other medications. Overdoses of serotonin reuptake inhibitors (eg, fluoxetine, paroxetine, sertraline) or their use in a patient taking an MAO inhibitor may cause agitation, hyperactivity, myoclonus, and hyperthermia ("serotonin syndrome"). Antipsychotic agents can cause rigidity and hyperthermia (neuroleptic

Table 38–2. Seizures related to toxins or drugs requiring special consideration.[1]

Toxin or Drug	Comments
Methylenedioxymethamphetamine (MDMA; "Ecstasy")	Seizures may also be due to hyponatremia or hyperthermia.
Isoniazid	Administer pyridoxine.
Lithium	May indicate need for hemodialysis.
Organophosphates	Administer pralidoxime (2-PAM) and atropine in addition to usual anticonvulsants.
Strychnine	"Seizures" are actually spinally mediated muscle spasms and usually require neuromuscular paralysis and mechanical ventilation.
Theophylline	Seizures indicate need for hemodialysis.
Tricyclic antidepressants	Hyperthermia and cardiotoxicity are common complications of repeated seizures; paralyze early with neuromuscular blockers to reduce muscular hyperactivity.

[1]See text for dosages.

malignant syndrome [NMS]). (See section on schizophrenia and other psychotic disorders in Chapter 25.) Malignant hyperthermia is a rare disorder associated with general anesthetic agents.

Hyperthermia is a rapidly life-threatening complication. Severe hyperthermia (temperature higher than 40–41°C) can rapidly cause brain damage and multiorgan failure, including rhabdomyolysis, acute kidney injury, and coagulopathy (see Chapter 37).

▶ Treatment

Treat hyperthermia aggressively by removing the patient's clothing, spraying the skin with tepid water, and fanning. If this is not rapidly effective, as shown by a normal rectal temperature within 30–60 minutes, or if there is significant muscle rigidity or hyperactivity, induce neuromuscular paralysis with a nondepolarizing neuromuscular blocker (eg, rocuronium, vecuronium). Once paralyzed, the patient must be intubated and mechanically ventilated and sedated. While the patient is paralyzed, the absence of visible muscular convulsive movements may give the false impression that brain seizure activity has ceased; bedside electroencephalography may be useful in recognizing continued nonconvulsive seizures.

Dantrolene (2–5 mg/kg intravenously) may be effective for hyperthermia associated with muscle rigidity that does not respond to neuromuscular blockade (ie, malignant hyperthermia). Bromocriptine, 2.5–7.5 mg orally daily, has been recommended for neuroleptic malignant syndrome. Cyproheptadine, 4 mg orally every hour for three or four doses, or chlorpromazine, 25 mg intravenously or 50 mg intramuscularly, has been used to treat serotonin syndrome.

Hayes BD et al. Drug-induced hyperthermic syndromes: part I. Hyperthermia in overdose. Emerg Med Clin North Am. 2013 Nov;31(4):1019–33. [PMID: 24176476]

Paden MS et al. Hyperthermia caused by drug interactions and adverse reactions. Emerg Med Clin North Am. 2013 Nov;31(4):1035–44. [PMID: 24176477]

ANTIDOTES & OTHER TREATMENT

ANTIDOTES

Give an antidote (if available) when there is reasonable certainty of a specific diagnosis (Table 38–3). Be aware that some antidotes themselves may have serious side effects. The indications and dosages for specific antidotes are discussed in the respective sections for specific toxins.

Gasco L et al. Insufficient stocking of cyanide antidotes in US hospitals that provide emergency care. J Pharmacol Pharmacother. 2013 Apr;4(2):95–102. [PMID: 23761707]

Marraffa JM et al. Antidotes for toxicological emergencies: a practical review. Am J Health Syst Pharm. 2012 Feb 1; 69(3):199–212. [PMID: 22261941]

Table 38–3. Some toxic agents for which there are specific antidotes.[1]

Toxic Agent	Specific Antidote
Acetaminophen	N-Acetylcysteine
Anticholinergics (eg, atropine)	Physostigmine
Anticholinesterases (eg, organophosphate pesticides)	Atropine and pralidoxime (2-PAM)
Benzodiazepines	Flumazenil (rarely used)[2]
Carbon monoxide	Oxygen (hyperbaric oxygen of uncertain benefit)
Cyanide	Sodium nitrite, sodium thiosulfate; hydroxocobalamin
Digitalis glycosides	Digoxin-specific Fab antibodies
Heavy metals (eg, lead, mercury, iron) and arsenic	Specific chelating agents
Isoniazid	Pyridoxine (vitamin B_6)
Methanol, ethylene glycol	Ethanol (ethyl alcohol) or fomepizole (4-methylpyrazole)
Opioids	Naloxone, nalmefene
Snake venom	Specific antivenin
Sulfonylurea oral hypoglycemic drugs	Glucose, octreotide

[1]See text for indications and dosages.
[2]May induce seizures in patients with preexisting seizure disorder, benzodiazepine addiction, or concomitant tricyclic antidepressant or other convulsant overdose. If seizures occur, diazepam and other benzodiazepine anticonvulsants will not be effective. As with naloxone, the duration of action of flumazenil is short (2–3 hours) and resedation may occur, requiring repeated doses.

DECONTAMINATION OF THE SKIN

Corrosive agents rapidly injure the skin and eyes and must be removed immediately. In addition, many toxins are readily absorbed through the skin, and systemic absorption can be prevented only by rapid action.

Wash the affected areas with copious quantities of lukewarm water or saline. Wash carefully behind the ears, under the nails, and in skin folds. For oily substances (eg, pesticides), wash the skin at least twice with plain soap and shampoo the hair. Specific decontaminating solutions or solvents (eg, alcohol) are rarely indicated and in some cases may paradoxically enhance absorption. For exposure to chemical warfare poisons such as nerve agents or vesicants, some authorities recommend use of a dilute hypochlorite solution (household bleach diluted 1:10 with water), but not in the eyes.

DECONTAMINATION OF THE EYES

Act quickly to prevent serious damage. Flush the eyes with copious amounts of saline or water. (If available, instill local anesthetic drops in the eye before beginning irrigation.) Remove contact lenses if present. Direct the irrigating stream so that it will flow across the eyes after running off the nasal bridge. Lift the tarsal conjunctiva to look for undissolved particles and to facilitate irrigation. Continue irrigation for 15 minutes or until each eye has been irrigated with at least 1 L of solution. If the toxin is an acid or a base, check the pH of the tears after irrigation, and continue irrigation until the pH is between 6 and 8. An amphoteric decontamination solution (Diphoterine, Prevor) is used in some countries for treatment of alkali injuries to the eye.

After irrigation is complete, perform a careful examination of the eye, using fluorescein and a slit lamp or Wood lamp to identify areas of corneal injury. Patients with serious conjunctival or corneal injury should be immediately referred to an ophthalmologist.

GASTROINTESTINAL DECONTAMINATION

Removal of ingested poisons was a routine part of emergency treatment for decades. However, prospective randomized studies have failed to demonstrate improved clinical outcome after gastric emptying. For small or moderate ingestions of most substances, toxicologists generally recommend oral activated charcoal alone without prior gastric emptying; in some cases, when the interval after ingestion has been more than 1–2 hours and the ingestant is non–life-threatening, even charcoal is withheld (eg, if the estimated benefit is outweighed by the potential risk of pulmonary aspiration of charcoal). Exceptions are large ingestions of anticholinergic compounds and salicylates, which often delay gastric emptying, and ingestion of sustained-release or enteric-coated tablets, which may remain intact for several hours. In these cases, aggressive gut decontamination may be indicated.

Gastric emptying is not generally used for ingestion of corrosive agents or petroleum distillates, because further esophageal injury or pulmonary aspiration may result. However, in certain cases, removal of the toxin may be more important than concern over possible complications. Consult a medical toxicologist or regional poison control center (1-800-222-1222) for advice.

A. Emesis

Emesis using syrup of ipecac can partially evacuate gastric contents if given very soon after ingestion. However, it is no longer used in the routine management of ingestions because it increases the risk of pulmonary aspiration and may delay or prevent the use of oral activated charcoal.

B. Gastric Lavage

Gastric lavage is more effective for liquid poisons or small pill fragments than for intact tablets or pieces of mushroom. It is most useful when started within 60 minutes after ingestion. However, the lavage procedure may delay administration of activated charcoal and may stimulate vomiting and pulmonary aspiration in an obtunded patient.

1. Indications—Gastric lavage is sometimes used after very large ingestions (eg, massive aspirin overdose), for collection and examination of gastric contents for identification of the poison, and make it easier to administer charcoal and oral antidotes.

2. Contraindications—Do *not* use lavage for stuporous or comatose patients with depressed airway protective reflexes unless they are endotracheally intubated beforehand. Some authorities advise against lavage when caustic material has been ingested; others regard it as essential to remove liquid corrosives from the stomach.

3. Technique—In obtunded or comatose patients, the danger of aspiration pneumonia is reduced by performing endotracheal intubation with a cuffed tube before the procedure. Gently insert a lubricated, soft but noncollapsible stomach tube (at least 37–40 F) through the mouth or nose into the stomach. Aspirate and save the contents, and then lavage repeatedly with 50- to 100-mL aliquots of fluid until the return fluid is clear. Use lukewarm tap water or saline.

C. Activated Charcoal

Activated charcoal effectively adsorbs almost all drugs and poisons. Poorly adsorbed substances include iron, lithium, potassium, sodium, mineral acids, and alcohols.

1. Indications—Activated charcoal can be used for prompt adsorption of drugs or toxins in the stomach and intestine. However, evidence of benefit in clinical studies is lacking. Administration of charcoal, especially if mixed with sorbitol, can provoke vomiting, which could lead to pulmonary aspiration in an obtunded patient.

2. Contraindications—Activated charcoal should not be used for comatose or convulsing patients unless it can be given by gastric tube and the airway is first protected by a cuffed endotracheal tube. It is also contraindicated for patients with ileus or intestinal obstruction or those who have ingested corrosives for whom endoscopy is planned.

3. Technique—Administer activated charcoal, 60–100 g orally or via gastric tube, mixed in aqueous slurry. Repeated

doses may be given to ensure gastrointestinal adsorption or to enhance elimination of some drugs.

D. Catharsis

1. Indications—Cathartics are used by some toxicologists for stimulation of peristalsis to hasten the elimination of unabsorbed drugs and poisons and the activated charcoal slurry. There is no clinical evidence to support their use, and some agents (eg, sorbitol) can provoke vomiting, increasing the risk of pulmonary aspiration.

2. Contraindications and cautions—Do not give a cathartic to patients with suspected intestinal obstruction. Avoid sodium-based cathartics in patients with hypertension, advanced kidney disease, and heart failure and avoid magnesium-based cathartics in patients with advanced kidney disease. Sorbitol (an osmotic cathartic found in some prepackaged activated charcoal slurry products) can cause hypotension and dehydration due to third-spacing and also causes intestinal cramping and vomiting.

E. Whole Bowel Irrigation

Whole bowel irrigation uses large volumes of a balanced polyethylene glycol-electrolyte solution to mechanically cleanse the entire intestinal tract. Because of the composition of the irrigating solution, there is no significant gain or loss of systemic fluids or electrolytes.

1. Indications—Whole bowel irrigation is particularly effective for massive iron ingestion in which intact tablets are visible on abdominal radiographs. It has also been used for ingestions of lithium, sustained-release and enteric-coated tablets, and swallowed drug-filled packets.

2. Contraindications—Do not use in patients with suspected intestinal obstruction. Use with caution in patients who are obtunded or have depressed airway protective reflexes.

3. Technique—Administer a balanced polyethylene glycol-electrolyte solution (CoLyte, GoLYTELY) into the stomach via gastric tube at a rate of 1–2 L/h until the rectal effluent is clear. This may take several hours. It is most effective when patients are able to sit on a commode to pass the intestinal contents.

F. Increased Drug Removal

1. Urinary manipulation—Forced diuresis is hazardous; the risk of complications (pulmonary edema, electrolyte imbalance) usually outweighs its benefits. Some drugs (eg, salicylates, phenobarbital) are more rapidly excreted with an alkaline urine. To alkalinize the urine, add 100 mEq (two ampules) of sodium bicarbonate to 1 L of 5% dextrose in 0.2% saline, and infuse this solution intravenously at a rate of about 150–200 mL/h. Acidification (sometimes promoted for amphetamines, phencyclidine) is *not* very effective and is contraindicated in the presence of rhabdomyolysis or myoglobinuria.

2. Hemodialysis—The indications for dialysis are as follows: (1) Known or suspected potentially lethal amounts of a dialyzable drug (Table 38–4); (2) Poisoning with deep

Table 38–4. Recommended use of hemodialysis in poisoning.

Poison	Common Indications[1]
Carbamazepine	Seizures, severe cardiotoxicity; serum level > 60 mg/L
Ethylene glycol	Acidosis, serum level > 50 mg/dL
Lithium	Severe symptoms; level > 4–5 mEq/L, especially if renal impairment Note: dialysis of uncertain value; consult with medical toxicologist
Methanol	Acidosis, serum level > 50 mg/dL
Phenobarbital	Intractable hypotension, acidosis despite maximal supportive care
Salicylate	Severe acidosis, CNS symptoms, serum level > 100 mg/dL (acute overdose) or > 60 mg/dL (chronic intoxication)
Theophylline	Serum level > 90–100 mg/L (acute) or seizures and serum level > 40–60 mg/L (chronic)
Valproic acid	Serum level > 900–1000 mg/L or deep coma, severe acidosis

[1]See text for further discussion of indications.
CNS, central nervous system; CVVHD, continuous venovenous hemodialysis.

coma, apnea, severe hypotension, fluid and electrolyte or acid-base disturbance, or extreme body temperature changes that cannot be corrected by conventional measures; or (3) Poisoning in patients with severe kidney, cardiac, pulmonary, or hepatic disease who will not be able to eliminate toxin by the usual mechanisms.

Continuous renal replacement therapy (including continuous venovenous hemodiafiltration and similar techniques) is of uncertain benefit for elimination of most poisons but has the advantage of gradual removal of the toxin and correction of any accompanying acidosis, and its use has been reported in the management of lithium intoxication.

3. Repeat-dose charcoal—Repeated doses of activated charcoal, 20–30 g orally or via gastric tube every 3–4 hours, may hasten elimination of some drugs (eg, phenytoin, carbamazepine, dapsone) by absorbing drugs excreted into the gut lumen ("gut dialysis"). However, clinical studies have failed to prove better outcome using repeat dose charcoal. Sorbitol or other cathartics should *not* be used with each dose, or resulting large stool volumes may lead to dehydration or hypernatremia.

Benson BE et al; American Academy of Clinical Toxicology; European Association of Poisons Centres and Clinical Toxicologists. Position paper update: gastric lavage for gastrointestinal decontamination. Clin Toxicol (Phila). 2013 Mar; 51(3):140–6. [PMID: 23418938]

Ghannoum M et al. Enhanced poison elimination in critical care. Adv Chronic Kidney Dis. 2013 Jan;20(1):94–101. [PMID: 23265601]
Ouellet G et al. Available extracorporeal treatments for poisoning: overview and limitations. Semin Dial. 2014 Jul–Aug; 27(4):342–9. [PMID: 24697909]
Villarreal J et al. A retrospective review of the prehospital use of activated charcoal. Am J Emerg Med. 2015 Jan;33(1):56–9. [PMID: 25455049]

DIAGNOSIS OF POISONING

The identity of the ingested substance or substances is usually known, but occasionally a comatose patient is found with an unlabeled container or the patient is unable or unwilling to give a coherent history. By performing a directed physical examination and ordering common clinical laboratory tests, the clinician can often make a tentative diagnosis that may allow empiric interventions or may suggest specific toxicologic tests.

► Physical Examination

Important diagnostic variables in the physical examination include blood pressure, pulse rate, temperature, pupil size, sweating, and the presence or absence of peristaltic activity. Poisonings may present with one or more of the following common syndromes.

A. Sympathomimetic Syndrome

The blood pressure and pulse rate are elevated, though with severe hypertension reflex bradycardia may occur. The temperature is often elevated, pupils are dilated, and the skin is sweaty, though mucous membranes are dry. Patients are usually agitated, anxious, or frankly psychotic.

Examples: Amphetamines, cocaine, ephedrine, and pseudoephedrine.

B. Sympatholytic Syndrome

The blood pressure and pulse rate are decreased and body temperature is low. The pupils are small or even pinpoint. Patients are usually obtunded or comatose.

Examples: Barbiturates, benzodiazepines and other sedative hypnotics, gamma-hydroxybutyrate (GHB), clonidine and related antihypertensives, ethanol, opioids.

C. Cholinergic Syndrome

Stimulation of muscarinic receptors causes bradycardia, miosis, sweating, and hyperperistalsis as well as bronchorrhea, wheezing, excessive salivation, and urinary incontinence. Nicotinic receptor stimulation may produce initial hypertension and tachycardia as well as fasciculations and muscle weakness. Patients are usually agitated and anxious.

Examples: Carbamates, nicotine, organophosphates (including nerve agents), physostigmine.

D. Anticholinergic Syndrome

Tachycardia with mild hypertension is common, and the body temperature is often elevated. Pupils are widely dilated. The skin is flushed, hot, and dry. Peristalsis is decreased, and urinary retention is common. Patients may have myoclonic jerking or choreoathetoid movements. Agitated delirium is frequently seen, and severe hyperthermia may occur.

Examples: Atropine, scopolamine, other naturally occurring and pharmaceutical anticholinergics, antihistamines, tricyclic antidepressants.

▶ **Laboratory Tests**

The following clinical laboratory tests are recommended for screening of the overdosed patient: measured serum osmolality and osmol gap, electrolytes and anion gap, glucose, creatinine, blood urea nitrogen (BUN), creatine kinase, urinalysis (eg, oxalate crystals with ethylene glycol poisoning, myoglobinuria with rhabdomyolysis), and electrocardiography. Serum acetaminophen and ethanol quantitative levels should be determined in all patients with drug overdoses.

A. Osmol Gap

The osmol gap (Table 38–5) is increased in the presence of large quantities of low-molecular-weight substances, most commonly ethanol. Other common poisons associated with increased osmol gap are acetone, ethanol, ethylene glycol, isopropyl alcohol, methanol, and propylene glycol. **Note:** Severe alcoholic ketoacidosis and diabetic ketoacidosis can also cause an elevated osmol gap resulting from the production of ketones and other low-molecular-weight substances.

B. Anion Gap

Metabolic acidosis associated with an elevated anion gap is usually due to an accumulation of lactic acid or other acids (see Chapter 21). Common causes of elevated anion gap in poisoning include carbon monoxide, cyanide, ethylene glycol, medicinal iron, INH, methanol, metformin, ibuprofen and salicylates. Massive acetaminophen overdose can cause early-onset anion gap metabolic acidosis.

Table 38–5. Use of the osmol gap in toxicology.

The osmol gap (Delta osm) is determined by subtracting the calculated serum osmolality from the measured serum osmolality.

$$\text{Calculated osmolality (osm)} = 2[Na^+ (mEq/L)] + \frac{\text{Glucose (mg/dL)}}{18} + \frac{\text{BUN (mg/dL)}}{2.8}$$

Delta osm = Measured osmolality – Calculated osmolality = 0 ± 10

Serum osmolality may be increased by contributions of exogenous substances such as alcohols and other low-molecular-weight substances. Since these substances are not included in the calculated osmolality, there will be a gap proportionate to their serum concentration. Contact a medical toxicologist or poison control center for assistance in calculating and interpreting the osmol gap.

The osmol gap should also be checked; combined elevated anion and osmol gaps suggests poisoning by methanol or ethylene glycol, though this may also occur in patients with diabetic ketoacidosis and alcoholic ketoacidosis.

C. Toxicology Laboratory Testing

A comprehensive toxicology screen is of little value in the initial care of the poisoned patient because results usually do not return in time to influence clinical management. Specific quantitative levels of certain drugs may be extremely helpful (Table 38–6), however, especially if specific antidotes or interventions (eg, dialysis) would be indicated based on the results.

Table 38–6. Specific quantitative levels and potential therapeutic interventions.[1]

Drug or Toxin	Treatment
Acetaminophen	Specific antidote (*N*-acetylcysteine) based on serum level
Carbon monoxide	High carboxyhemoglobin level indicates need for 100% oxygen, consideration of hyperbaric oxygen
Carbamazepine	High level may indicate need for hemodialysis
Digoxin	On basis of serum digoxin level and severity of clinical presentation, treatment with Fab antibody fragments (eg, DigiFab) may be indicated
Ethanol	Low serum level may suggest nonalcoholic cause of coma (eg, trauma, other drugs, other alcohols); serum ethanol may also be useful in monitoring ethanol therapy for methanol or ethylene glycol poisoning
Iron	Level may indicate need for chelation with deferoxamine
Lithium	Serum levels can guide decision to institute hemodialysis
Methanol, ethylene glycol	Acidosis, high levels indicate need for hemodialysis, therapy with ethanol or fomepizole
Methemoglobin	Methemoglobinemia can be treated with methylene blue intravenously
Salicylates	High level may indicate need for hemodialysis, alkaline dieresis
Theophylline	Immediate hemodialysis or hemoperfusion may be indicated based on serum level
Valproic acid	Elevated levels may indicate need to consider hemodialysis or L-carnitine therapy, or both

[1]Some drugs or toxins may have profound and irreversible toxicity unless rapid and specific management is provided outside of routine supportive care. For these agents, laboratory testing may provide the serum level or other evidence required for administering a specific antidote or arranging for hemodialysis.

Many hospitals can perform a quick but limited urine screen for "drugs of abuse" (typically these screens include only opiates, amphetamines, and cocaine, and some add benzodiazepines, barbiturates, methadone, and tetrahydrocannabinol [marijuana]). There are numerous false-positive and false-negative results. For example, synthetic opioids, such as fentanyl, oxycodone, and methadone are often not detected by routine opioid immunoassays.

Abdominal Radiographs

A plain film of the abdomen may reveal radiopaque iron tablets, drug-filled condoms, or other toxic material. Studies suggest that few tablets are predictably visible (eg, ferrous sulfate, sodium chloride, calcium carbonate, and potassium chloride). Thus, the radiograph is useful only if abnormal.

When to Refer

Consultation with a regional poison control center (1-800-222-1222) or a medical toxicologist is recommended when the diagnosis is uncertain; there are questions about what laboratory tests to order; when dialysis is being considered to remove the drug or poison; or when advice is needed regarding the indications, dose, and side effects of antidotes.

When to Admit

- The patient has symptoms and signs of intoxication that are not expected to clear within a 6- to 8-hour observation period.
- Delayed absorption of the drug might be predicted to cause a later onset of serious symptoms (eg, after ingestion of a sustained-release product).
- Continued administration of an antidote is required (eg, N-acetylcysteine for acetaminophen overdose).
- Psychiatric or social services evaluation is needed for suicide attempt or suspected drug abuse.

Goldfrank LR (editor). Goldfrank's Toxicologic Emergencies, 10th ed. McGraw-Hill, 2014.
Holstege CP et al. Toxidromes. Crit Care Clin. 2012 Oct; 28(4):479–98. [PMID: 22998986]
Olson KR (editor). Poisoning & Drug Overdose, 6th ed. McGraw-Hill, 2011.

SELECTED POISONINGS

ACETAMINOPHEN

Acetaminophen (paracetamol in the United Kingdom, Europe) is a common analgesic found in many nonprescription and prescription products. After absorption, it is metabolized mainly by glucuronidation and sulfation, with a small fraction metabolized via the P450 mixed-function oxidase system (2E1) to a highly toxic reactive intermediate. This toxic intermediate is normally detoxified by cellular glutathione. With acute acetaminophen overdose (greater than 150–200 mg/kg, or 8–10 g in an average adult), hepatocellular glutathione is depleted and the reactive intermediate attacks other cell proteins, causing necrosis. Patients with enhanced P450 2E1 activity, such as those who chronically abuse alcohol and patients taking INH, are at increased risk for developing hepatotoxicity. Hepatic toxicity may also occur after overuse of acetaminophen—eg, as a result of taking two or three acetaminophen-containing products concurrently or exceeding the recommended maximum dose of 4 g/day for several days. The amount of acetaminophen in US oral prescription combination products (eg, hydrocodone/acetaminophen) is limited by the FDA to no more than 325 mg per tablet.

Clinical Findings

Shortly after ingestion, patients may have nausea or vomiting, but there are usually no other signs of toxicity until 24–48 hours after ingestion, when hepatic aminotransferase levels begin to increase. With severe poisoning, fulminant hepatic necrosis may occur, resulting in jaundice, hepatic encephalopathy, acute kidney injury, and death. Rarely, massive ingestion (eg, serum levels greater than 500–1000 mg/L [33–66 mmol/L]) can cause early onset of acute coma, seizures, hypotension, and metabolic acidosis unrelated to hepatic injury.

The diagnosis after acute overdose is based on measurement of the serum acetaminophen level. Plot the serum level versus the time since ingestion on the acetaminophen nomogram shown in Figure 38–1. Ingestion of sustained-release products or coingestion of an anticholinergic agent, salicylate, or opioid drug may cause delayed elevation of serum levels which can make it difficult to interpret the nomogram. The nomogram is also not useful after repeated overdose.

Treatment

A. Emergency and Supportive Measures

Administer activated charcoal (see p. 1582) if it can be given within 1–2 hours of the ingestion. Although charcoal may interfere with absorption of the oral antidote acetylcysteine, this is not considered clinically significant.

B. Specific Treatment

If the serum or plasma acetaminophen level falls above the line on the nomogram (Figure 38–1), treatment with N-acetylcysteine is indicated; it can be given orally or intravenously. Oral treatment begins with a loading dose of N-acetylcysteine, 140 mg/kg, followed by 70 mg/kg every 4 hours. Dilute the solution to about 5% with water, juice, or soda. If vomiting interferes with oral N-acetylcysteine administration, consider giving the antidote intravenously. The conventional oral N-acetylcysteine protocol in the United States calls for 72 hours of treatment. However, other regimens have demonstrated equivalent success with 20–48 hours of treatment.

The FDA-approved 21-hour intravenous regimen of acetylcysteine (Acetadote) calls for a loading dose of 150 mg/kg

▲ **Figure 38–1.** Nomogram for prediction of acetaminophen hepatotoxicity following acute overdosage. Patients with serum levels above the line after acute overdose should receive antidotal treatment. (Adapted, with permission, from Daly FF et al. Guidelines for the management of paracetamol poisoning in Australia and New Zealand–explanation and elaboration. A consensus statement from clinical toxicologists consulting to the Australasian poisons information centres. Med J Austr. 2008;188:296. © Copyright The Medical Journal of Australia. The Medical Journal of Australia does not accept responsibility for any errors in translation.)

given intravenously over 60 minutes, followed by a 4-hour infusion of 50 mg/kg, and a 16-hour infusion of 100 mg/kg. (If Acetadote is not available, the conventional oral formulation may also be given intravenously using a micropore filter and a slow rate of infusion. Call a regional poison control center or medical toxicologist for assistance.)

Treatment with *N*-acetylcysteine is most effective if it is started within 8–10 hours after ingestion.

Gosselin S et al. Extracorporeal treatment for acetaminophen poisoning: recommendations from the EXTRIP workgroup. Clin Toxicol (Phila). 2014 Sep–Oct;52(8):856–67. [PMID: 25133498]

Park BK et al. Paracetamol (acetaminophen) poisoning. BMJ Clin Evid. 2015 Oct 19;2015:2101. [PMID: 26479248]

ACIDS, CORROSIVE

The strong mineral acids exert primarily a local corrosive effect on the skin and mucous membranes. Symptoms include severe pain in the throat and upper gastrointestinal tract; bloody vomitus; difficulty in swallowing, breathing, and speaking; discoloration and destruction of skin and mucous membranes in and around the mouth; and shock. Severe systemic metabolic acidosis may occur both as a result of cellular injury and from systemic absorption of the acid.

Severe deep destructive tissue damage may occur after exposure to hydrofluoric acid because of the penetrating and highly toxic fluoride ion. Systemic hypocalcemia and hyperkalemia may also occur after fluoride absorption, even following skin exposure.

Inhalation of volatile acids, fumes, or gases such as chlorine, fluorine, bromine, or iodine causes severe irritation of the throat and larynx and may cause upper airway obstruction and noncardiogenic pulmonary edema.

► Treatment

A. Ingestion

Dilute immediately by giving a glass (4–8 oz) of water to drink. Do *not* give bicarbonate or other neutralizing agents, and do *not* induce vomiting. Some experts recommend immediate cautious placement of a small flexible gastric tube and removal of stomach contents followed by lavage, particularly if the corrosive is a liquid or has important systemic toxicity.

In symptomatic patients, perform flexible endoscopic esophagoscopy to determine the presence and extent of injury. CT scan or plain radiographs of the chest and abdomen may also reveal the extent of injury. Perforation, peritonitis, and major bleeding are indications for surgery.

B. Skin Contact

Flood with water for 15 minutes. Use no chemical antidotes; the heat of the reaction may cause additional injury.

For hydrofluoric acid burns, soak the affected area in benzalkonium chloride solution or apply 2.5% calcium gluconate gel (prepared by adding 3.5 g calcium gluconate to 5 oz of water-soluble surgical lubricant, eg, K-Y Jelly); then arrange immediate consultation with a plastic surgeon or other specialist. Binding of the fluoride ion may be achieved by injecting 0.5 mL of 5% calcium gluconate per square centimeter under the burned area. (**Caution:** *Do not use calcium chloride.*) Use of a Bier-block technique or intra-arterial infusion of calcium is sometimes required for extensive burns or those involving the nail bed; consult with a hand surgeon or poison control center (1-800-222-1222).

C. Eye Contact

Anesthetize the conjunctiva and corneal surfaces with topical local anesthetic drops (eg, proparacaine). Flood with water for 15 minutes, holding the eyelids open. Check pH with pH 6.0–8.0 test paper, and repeat irrigation, using 0.9% saline, until pH is near 7.0. Check for corneal damage with fluorescein and slit-lamp examination; consult an ophthalmologist about further treatment.

D. Inhalation

Remove from further exposure to fumes or gas. Check skin and clothing. Treat pulmonary edema.

Singh P et al. Ocular chemical injuries and their management. Oman J Ophthalmol. 2013 May;6(2):83–86. [PMID: 24082664]
Wu ML et al. Acute hydrofluoric acid exposure reported to Taiwan Poison Control Center, 1991–2010. Hum Exp Toxicol. 2014 May;33(5):449–54. [PMID: 23892993]
Zhang Y et al. Injuries following a serious hydrofluoric acid leak: First aid and lessons. Burns. 2015 Nov;41(7):1593–8. [PMID: 26188892]

ALKALIES

The strong alkalies are common ingredients of some household cleaning compounds and may be suspected by their "soapy" texture. Those with alkalinity above pH 12.0 are particularly corrosive. Disk (or "button") batteries are also a source. Alkalies cause liquefactive necrosis, which is deeply penetrating. Symptoms include burning pain in the upper gastrointestinal tract, nausea, vomiting, and difficulty in swallowing and breathing. Examination reveals destruction and edema of the affected skin and mucous membranes and bloody vomitus and stools. Radiographs may reveal evidence of perforation or the presence of radiopaque disk batteries in the esophagus or lower gastrointestinal tract.

▶ Treatment

A. Ingestion

Dilute immediately with a glass of water. Do *not* induce emesis. Some gastroenterologists recommend immediate cautious placement of a small flexible gastric tube and removal of stomach contents followed by gastric lavage after ingestion of liquid caustic substances, in order to remove residual material.

Prompt endoscopy is recommended in symptomatic patients to evaluate the extent of damage; CT scanning may also aid in assessment. If a radiograph reveals the location of ingested disk batteries in the esophagus, immediate endoscopic removal is mandatory.

The use of corticosteroids to prevent stricture formation is of no proved benefit and is definitely contraindicated if there is evidence of esophageal perforation.

B. Skin Contact

Wash with running water until the skin no longer feels soapy. Relieve pain and treat shock.

C. Eye Contact

Anesthetize the conjunctival and corneal surfaces with topical anesthetic (eg, proparacaine). Irrigate with water or saline continuously for 20–30 minutes, holding the lids open. Amphoteric solutions may be more effective than water or saline and some are available in Europe (Diphoterine, Prevor). Check pH with pH test paper, and repeat irrigation for additional 30-minute periods until the pH is near 7.0. Check for corneal damage with fluorescein and slit-lamp examination; consult an ophthalmologist for further treatment.

Brent J. Water-based solutions are the best decontaminating fluids for dermal corrosive exposures: a mini review. Clin Toxicol (Phila). 2013 Sep–Oct;51(8):731–6. [PMID: 24003912]
Demirören K et al. Gastrointestinal system lesions in children due to the ingestion of alkali and acid corrosive substances. Turk J Med Sci. 2015;45(1):184–90. [PMID: 25790550]

AMPHETAMINES & COCAINE

Amphetamines and cocaine are widely abused for their euphorigenic and stimulant properties. Both drugs may be smoked, snorted, ingested, or injected. Amphetamines and cocaine produce central nervous system stimulation and a generalized increase in central and peripheral sympathetic activity. The toxic dose of each drug is highly variable and depends on the route of administration and individual tolerance. The onset of effects is most rapid after intravenous injection or smoking. Amphetamine derivatives and related drugs include methamphetamine ("crystal meth," "crank"), MDMA ("Ecstasy"), ephedrine ("herbal ecstasy"), and methcathinone ("cat" or "khat"). Methcathinone derivatives and related synthetic chemicals such as methylenedioxypyrovalerone (MDPV) have become popular drugs of abuse and are often sold as purported "bath salts." Amphetamine-like reactions have also been reported after use of synthetic cannabinoids (eg, "Spice" and "K2"). Nonprescription medications and nutritional supplements may contain stimulant or sympathomimetic drugs such as ephedrine, yohimbine, or caffeine (see also Theophylline & Caffeine section).

▶ Clinical Findings

Presenting symptoms may include anxiety, tremulousness, tachycardia, hypertension, diaphoresis, dilated pupils, agitation, muscular hyperactivity, and psychosis. Muscle hyperactivity may lead to metabolic acidosis and rhabdomyolysis. In severe intoxication, seizures and hyperthermia may occur. Sustained or severe hypertension may result in intracranial hemorrhage, aortic dissection, or myocardial infarction. Ischemic colitis has been reported. Hyponatremia has been reported after MDMA use; the mechanism is not known but may involve excessive water intake, syndrome of inappropriate antidiuretic hormone (SIADH), or both.

The diagnosis is supported by finding amphetamines or the cocaine metabolite benzoylecgonine in the urine. Note that many drugs can give a false-positive result on the immunoassay for amphetamines.

▶ Treatment

A. Emergency and Supportive Measures

Maintain a patent airway and assist ventilation, if necessary. Treat seizures as described at the beginning of this chapter (see p. 1580). Rapidly lower the body temperature (see hyperthermia, p. 1580) in patients who are hyperthermic (temperature higher than 39–40°C). Give intravenous fluids to prevent myoglobinuric kidney injury in patients who have rhabdomyolysis.

B. Specific Treatment

Treat agitation, psychosis, or seizures with a benzodiazepine such as diazepam, 5–10 mg, or lorazepam, 2–3 mg intravenously. Add phenobarbital 15 mg/kg intravenously for persistent seizures. Treat hypertension with a vasodilator drug such as phentolamine (1–5 mg intravenously) or nitroprusside, or a combined alpha- and beta-adrenergic blocker such as labetalol (10–20 mg intravenously). Do *not* administer a pure beta-blocker such as propranolol alone, as this may result in paradoxic worsening of the hypertension as a result of unopposed alpha-adrenergic effects.

Treat tachycardia or tachyarrhythmias with a short-acting beta-blocker such as esmolol (25–100 mcg/kg/min by intravenous infusion). Treat hyperthermia as described above (see p. 1580). Treat hyponatremia as outlined in Chapter 21.

Jones P et al. Accidental death via intravaginal absorption of methamphetamine. Forensic Sci Med Pathol. 2014 Jun; 10(2):234–8. [PMID: 24515580]

Tait RJ et al. A systematic review of adverse events arising from the use of synthetic cannabinoids and their associated treatment. Clin Toxicol (Phila). 2016 Jan;54(1):1–13. [PMID: 26567470]

Tyndall JA et al. An outbreak of acute delirium from exposure to the synthetic cannabinoid AB-CHMINACA. Clin Toxicol (Phila). 2015 Dec;53(10):950–6. [PMID: 26555732]

ANTICOAGULANTS

Warfarin and related compounds (including ingredients of many commercial rodenticides, the so-called "superwarfarins" such as brodifacoum, difenacoum, and related compounds) inhibit the clotting mechanism by blocking hepatic synthesis of vitamin K–dependent clotting factors. After ingestion of "superwarfarins," inhibition of clotting factor synthesis may persist for several weeks or even months after a single dose. Newer oral anticoagulants include the direct thrombin inhibitor dabigatran and the factor Xa inhibitors rivaroxaban, apixiban, and edoxaban. Some of these, especially dabigatran, are largely eliminated by the kidney and may accumulate in patients with renal insufficiency.

Excessive anticoagulation may cause hemoptysis, gross hematuria, bloody stools, hemorrhages into organs, widespread bruising, and bleeding into joint spaces.

▶ Treatment

A. Emergency and Supportive Measures

Discontinue the drug at the first sign of gross bleeding, and determine the prothrombin time (international normalized ratio, INR). The prothrombin time is increased within 12–24 hours (peak 36–48 hours) after overdose of warfarin or "superwarfarins." **Note:** The newer oral anticoagulants (dabigatran, rivaroxaban, apixiban, and edoxaban) do not predictably alter the prothrombin time; however, a normal INR suggests no significant toxicity.

If the patient has ingested an acute overdose, administer activated charcoal (see p. 1582).

B. Specific Treatment

In cases of warfarin and "superwarfarin" overdose, do *not* treat prophylactically with vitamin K—wait for evidence of anticoagulation (elevated prothrombin time). If the INR is elevated, give phytonadione (vitamin K_1), 10–25 mg orally, and increase the dose as needed to restore the prothrombin time to normal. Doses as high as 200 mg/day have been required after ingestion of "superwarfarins." Give fresh-frozen plasma, prothrombin complex concentrate, or activated Factor VII as needed to rapidly correct the coagulation factor deficit if there is serious bleeding. If the patient is chronically anticoagulated and has strong medical indications for being maintained in that status (eg, prosthetic heart valve), give much smaller doses of vitamin K (1 mg orally) and fresh-frozen plasma (or both) to titrate to the desired prothrombin time. If the patient has ingested brodifacoum or a related superwarfarin, prolonged observation (over weeks) and repeated administration of large doses of vitamin K may be required.

Vitamin K does not reverse the anticoagulant effects of the direct-acting oral anticoagulants (dabigatran, rivaroxaban, apixiban, and edoxaban), but specific reversal agents have been developed and are now approved by the FDA: idarucizumab for dabigatran reversal and andexanet for reversal of the factor Xa inhibitors. The efficacy of fresh frozen plasma and clotting factor concentrates is uncertain.

Pollack CV Jr et al. Idarucizumab for dabigatran reversal. N Engl J Med. 2015 Aug 6;373(6):511–20. [PMID: 26095746]

Siegal DM et al. Andexanet alfa for the reversal of factor Xa inhibitor activity. N Engl J Med. 2015 Dec 17;373(25):2413–24. [PMID: 26559317]

Stevenson JW et al. An observational case series of dabigatran and rivaroxaban exposures reported to a poison control system. Am J Emerg Med. 2014 Sep;32(9):1077–84. [PMID: 24908445]

ANTICONVULSANTS

Anticonvulsants (carbamazepine, phenytoin, valproic acid, and many newer agents) are widely used in the management of seizure disorders and some are also used for treatment of mood disorders or pain.

Phenytoin can be given orally or intravenously. Rapid intravenous injection of phenytoin can cause acute myocardial depression and cardiac arrest owing to the solvent propylene glycol (fosphenytoin does not contain this diluent). Chronic phenytoin intoxication can occur following only slightly increased doses because of zero-order kinetics and a small toxic-therapeutic window. Phenytoin intoxication can also occur following acute intentional or accidental overdose. The overdose syndrome is usually mild even with high serum levels. The most common manifestations are ataxia, nystagmus, and drowsiness. Choreoathetoid movements have been described.

Carbamazepine intoxication causes drowsiness, stupor and, with high levels, atrioventricular block, coma, and seizures. Dilated pupils and tachycardia are common. Toxicity may be seen with serum levels over 20 mg/L (85 mcmol/L), although severe poisoning is usually associated with concentrations greater than 30–40 mg/L (127–169 mcmol/L). Because of erratic and slow absorption, intoxication may progress over several hours to days.

Valproic acid intoxication produces a unique syndrome consisting of hypernatremia (from the sodium component of the salt), metabolic acidosis, hypocalcemia, elevated serum ammonia, and mild liver aminotransferase elevation. Hypoglycemia may occur as a result of hepatic metabolic dysfunction. Coma with small pupils may be seen and can mimic opioid poisoning. Encephalopathy and cerebral edema can occur.

The newer anticonvulsants **gabapentin, levetiracetam, vigabatrin,** and **zonisamide** generally cause somnolence, confusion and dizziness; **felbamate** can cause crystalluria and kidney injury after overdose, and may cause idiosyncratic aplastic anemia with therapeutic use; **lamotrigine, topiramate,** and **tiagabine** have been reported to cause seizures after overdose.

▶ Treatment

A. Emergency and Supportive Measures

For recent ingestions, give activated charcoal orally or by gastric tube (see p. 1582). For large ingestions of carbamazepine or valproic acid—especially of sustained-release formulations—consider whole bowel irrigation (see p. 1582). Combined multiple-dose activated charcoal and whole-bowel irrigation may be beneficial in ensuring gut decontamination for selected large ingestions.

B. Specific Treatment

There are no specific antidotes. Naloxone was reported to have reversed valproic acid overdose in one anecdotal case. Carnitine may be useful in patients with valproic acid–induced hyperammonemia. Consider hemodialysis for massive intoxication with valproic acid or carbamazepine (eg, carbamazepine levels greater than 60 mg/L [254 mcmol/L] or valproic acid levels greater than 800 mg/L [5544 mcmol/L]).

Larkin TM et al. Overdose with levetiracetam: a case report and review of the literature. J Clin Pharm Ther. 2013 Feb;38(1): 68–70. [PMID: 22725831]

Ozhasenekler A et al. Benefit of hemodialysis in carbamazepine intoxications with neurological complications. Eur Rev Med Pharmacol Sci. 2012 Mar;16(Suppl 1):43–7. [PMID: 22582484]

Pons S et al. Acute overdose of enteric-coated valproic acid and olanzapine: unusual presentation and delayed toxicity. Clin Toxicol (Phila). 2012 Apr;50(4):268. [PMID: 22385067]

Spiller HA et al. Thirteen years of oxcarbazepine exposures reported to US poison centers: 2000 to 2012. Hum Exp Toxicol. 2015 Nov 26. [Epub ahead of print] [PMID: 26612556]

ANTIPSYCHOTIC DRUGS

Promethazine, prochlorperazine, chlorpromazine, haloperidol, droperidol, risperidone, olanzapine, ziprasidone, quetiapine, and aripiprazole are used as antipsychotic agents, and sometimes as antiemetics and potentiators of analgesic and hypnotic drugs.

Therapeutic doses of phenothiazines (particularly chlorpromazine) induce drowsiness and mild orthostatic hypotension in as many as 50% of patients. Larger doses can cause obtundation, miosis, severe hypotension, tachycardia, convulsions, and coma. Abnormal cardiac conduction may occur, resulting in prolongation of QRS or QT intervals (or both) and ventricular arrhythmias. Among the newer agents, quetiapine is more likely to cause coma and hypotension.

With therapeutic or toxic doses, an acute extrapyramidal dystonic reaction may develop in some patients, with spasmodic contractions of the face and neck muscles, extensor rigidity of the back muscles, carpopedal spasm, and motor restlessness. This reaction is more common with haloperidol and other butyrophenones and less common with newer atypical antipsychotics such as ziprasidone, lurasidone, olanzapine, aripiprazole, and quetiapine. Severe rigidity accompanied by hyperthermia and metabolic acidosis ("neuroleptic malignant syndrome") may occasionally occur and is life-threatening (see Chapter 25).

▶ Treatment

A. Emergency and Supportive Measures

Administer activated charcoal (see p. 1582) for large or recent ingestions. For severe hypotension, treatment with intravenous fluids and vasopressor agents may be necessary. Treat hyperthermia as outlined on p. 1580. Maintain cardiac monitoring.

B. Specific Treatment

Hypotension and cardiac arrhythmias associated with widened QRS intervals on the ECG in a patient with thioridazine poisoning may respond to intravenous sodium bicarbonate as used for tricyclic antidepressants.

Prolongation of the QT interval and torsades de pointes is usually treated with intravenous magnesium or overdrive pacing.

For extrapyramidal signs, give diphenhydramine, 0.5–1 mg/kg intravenously, or benztropine mesylate, 0.01–0.02 mg/kg intramuscularly. Treatment with oral doses of these agents should be continued for 24–48 hours.

Bromocriptine (2.5–7.5 mg orally daily) may be effective for mild or moderate neuroleptic malignant syndrome. Dantrolene (2–5 mg/kg intravenously) has also been used for muscle rigidity but is not a true antidote. For severe hyperthermia, rapid neuromuscular paralysis (see p. 1580) is preferred.

Berling I et al. Prolonged QT risk assessment in antipsychotic overdose using the QT nomogram. Ann Emerg Med. 2015 Aug;66(2):154–64. [PMID: 25639523]

George M et al. Acute dyskinesia, myoclonus, and akathisia in an adolescent male abusing quetiapine via nasal insufflation: a case study. BMC Pediatr. 2013 Nov 16;13:187. [PMID: 24238149]

ARSENIC

Arsenic is found in some pesticides and industrial chemicals and is used as a chemotherapeutic agent. Symptoms of acute poisoning usually appear within 1 hour after ingestion but may be delayed as long as 12 hours. They include abdominal pain, vomiting, watery diarrhea, and skeletal muscle cramps. Profound dehydration and shock may occur. In chronic poisoning, symptoms can be vague but often include pancytopenia, painful peripheral sensory neuropathy, and skin changes including melanosis, keratosis, and desquamating rash. Urinary arsenic levels may be falsely elevated after certain meals (eg, seafood) that contain large quantities of a nontoxic form of organic arsenic.

▶ Treatment

A. Emergency Measures

After recent ingestion (within 1–2 hours), perform gastric lavage (see p. 1582). Activated charcoal is of uncertain benefit because it binds arsenic poorly. Administer intravenous fluids to replace losses due to vomiting and diarrhea.

B. Antidote

For patients with severe acute intoxication, administer a chelating agent. The preferred drug is 2,3-dimercaptopropanesulfonic acid (DMPS, Unithiol) (3–5 mg/kg intravenously every 4 hours); although there is no FDA-approved commercial formulation of DMPS in the United States, it can be obtained from some compounding pharmacies. An alternative parenteral chelator is dimercaprol (British anti-Lewisite, BAL), which comes as a 10% solution in peanut oil, and is given 3–5 mg/kg intramuscularly every 4–6 hours for 2 days. The side effects include nausea, vomiting, headache, and hypertension. When gastrointestinal symptoms allow, switch to the oral chelator succimer (dimercaptosuccinic acid, DMSA), 10 mg/kg every 8 hours, for 1 week. Consult a medical toxicologist or regional poison control center (1-800-222-1222) for advice regarding chelation.

Hughes MF et al. Arsenic exposure and toxicology: a historical perspective. Toxicol Sci. 2011 Oct;123(2):305–32. [PMID: 21750349]

Pinto B et al. Chronic arsenic poisoning following ayurvedic medication. J Med Toxicol. 2014 Dec;10(4):395–8. [PMID: 24696169]

Shumy F et al. Acute arsenic poisoning diagnosed late. Trop Doct. 2015 Oct 27. [PMID: 26508422]

ATROPINE & ANTICHOLINERGICS

Atropine, scopolamine, belladonna, diphenoxylate with atropine, *Datura stramonium*, *Hyoscyamus niger*, some mushrooms, tricyclic antidepressants, and antihistamines are antimuscarinic agents with variable central nervous system effects. Symptoms of toxicity include dryness of the mouth, thirst, difficulty in swallowing, and blurring of vision. Physical signs include dilated pupils, flushed skin, tachycardia, fever, delirium, myoclonus, ileus, and flushed appearance. Antidepressants and antihistamines may induce convulsions.

Antihistamines are commonly available with or without prescription. Diphenhydramine commonly causes delirium, tachycardia, and seizures. Massive diphenhydramine overdose may mimic tricyclic antidepressant cardiotoxic poisoning.

▶ Treatment

A. Emergency and Supportive Measures

Administer activated charcoal (see p. 1582). External cooling and sedation, or neuromuscular paralysis in rare cases, are indicated to control high temperatures (see p. 1580).

B. Specific Treatment

For severe anticholinergic syndrome (eg, agitated delirium), give physostigmine salicylate, 0.5–1 mg slowly intravenously over 5 minutes, with ECG monitoring; repeat as needed to a total dose of no more than 2 mg. **Caution:** Bradyarrhythmias and convulsions are a hazard with physostigmine administration, and the drug should be avoided in patients with cardiotoxic effects from tricyclic antidepressants or other sodium channel blockers.

Dawson AH et al. Pharmacological management of anticholinergic delirium—theory, evidence and practice. Br J Clin Pharmacol. 2016 Mar;81(3):516–524. [PMID: 26589572]

Phillips MA et al. Use of a physostigmine continuous infusion for the treatment of severe and recurrent antimuscarinic toxicity in a mixed drug overdose. J Med Toxicol. 2014 Jun;10(2):205–9. [PMID: 24798647]

BETA-ADRENERGIC BLOCKERS

There are a wide variety of beta-adrenergic blocking drugs, with varying pharmacologic and pharmacokinetic properties (see Table 11–6). The most toxic beta-blocker is propranolol, which not only blocks beta-1 and beta-2 adrenoceptors but also has direct membrane-depressant and central nervous system effects.

Clinical Findings

The most common findings with mild or moderate intoxication are hypotension and bradycardia. Cardiac depression from more severe poisoning is often unresponsive to conventional therapy with beta-adrenergic stimulants such as dopamine and norepinephrine. In addition, with propranolol and other lipid-soluble drugs, seizures and coma may occur. Propranolol, oxprenolol, acebutolol, and alprenolol also have membrane-depressant effects and can cause conduction disturbance (wide QRS interval) similar to tricyclic antidepressant overdose.

The diagnosis is based on typical clinical findings. Routine toxicology screening does not usually include beta-blockers.

Treatment

A. Emergency and Supportive Measures

Attempts to treat bradycardia or heart block with atropine (0.5–2 mg intravenously), isoproterenol (2–20 mcg/min by intravenous infusion, titrated to the desired heart rate), or an external transcutaneous cardiac pacemaker are often ineffective, and specific antidotal treatment may be necessary.

For drugs ingested within an hour of presentation (or longer after ingestion of an extended-release formulation), administer activated charcoal (see p. 1582).

B. Specific Treatment

For persistent bradycardia and hypotension, give glucagon, 5–10 mg intravenously, followed by an infusion of 1–5 mg/h. Glucagon is an inotropic agent that acts at a different receptor site and is therefore not affected by beta-blockade. High-dose insulin (0.5–1 units/kg/h intravenously) along with glucose supplementation has been used to reverse severe cardiotoxicity. Membrane-depressant effects (wide QRS interval) may respond to boluses of sodium bicarbonate (50–100 mEq intravenously) as for tricyclic antidepressant poisoning. Intravenous lipid emulsion (Intralipid 20%, 1.5 mL/kg) has been used successfully in severe propranolol overdose.

Cole JB et al. A blinded, randomized, controlled trial of three doses of high-dose insulin in poison-induced cardiogenic shock. Clin Toxicol (Phila). 2013 May;51(4):201–7. [PMID: 23530460]
Graudins A et al. Calcium channel antagonist and beta-blocker overdose: antidotes and adjunct therapies. Br J Clin Pharmacol. 2016 Mar;81(3):453–461. [PMID: 26344579]

CALCIUM CHANNEL BLOCKERS

In therapeutic doses, nifedipine, nicardipine, amlodipine, felodipine, isradipine, nisoldipine, and nimodipine act mainly on blood vessels, while verapamil and diltiazem act mainly on cardiac contractility and conduction. However, these selective effects can be lost after acute overdose. Patients may present with bradycardia, atrioventricular (AV) nodal block, hypotension, or a combination of these effects. Hyperglycemia is common due to blockade of insulin release. With severe poisoning, cardiac arrest may occur.

Treatment

A. Emergency and Supportive Measures

For ingested drugs, administer activated charcoal (see p. 1582). In addition, whole bowel irrigation (see p. 1582) should be initiated as soon as possible if the patient has ingested a sustained-release product.

B. Specific Treatment

Treat symptomatic bradycardia with atropine (0.5–2 mg intravenously), isoproterenol (2–20 mcg/min by intravenous infusion), or a transcutaneous cardiac pacemaker. For hypotension, give calcium chloride 10%, 10 mL, or calcium gluconate 10%, 20 mL. Repeat the dose every 3–5 minutes. The optimum (or maximum) dose has not been established, but many toxicologists recommend raising the ionized serum calcium level to as much as twice the normal level. Calcium is most useful in reversing negative inotropic effects and is less effective for AV nodal blockade and bradycardia. High doses of insulin (0.5–1 units/kg intravenous bolus followed by 0.5–1 units/kg/h infusion) along with sufficient dextrose to maintain euglycemia have been reported to be beneficial but there are no controlled studies. Infusion of Intralipid 20% lipid emulsion has been reported to improve hemodynamics in animal models and case reports of calcium channel blocker poisoning. Methylene blue (1–2 mg/kg) was reported to reverse refractory shock due to profound vasodilation in a patient with amlodipine poisoning.

Graudins A et al. Calcium channel antagonist and beta-blocker overdose: antidotes and adjunct therapies. Br J Clin Pharmacol. 2016 Mar;81(3):453–61. [PMID: 26344579]
Laes JR et al. Improvement in hemodynamics after methylene blue administration in drug-induced vasodilatory shock: a case report. J Med Toxicol. 2015 Dec;11(4):460–3. [PMID: 26310944]
Olson KR. What is the best treatment for acute calcium channel blocker overdose? Ann Emerg Med. 2013 Sep;62(3):259–61. [PMID: 23567061]

CARBON MONOXIDE

Carbon monoxide is a colorless, odorless gas produced by the combustion of carbon-containing materials. Poisoning may occur as a result of suicidal or accidental exposure to automobile exhaust, smoke inhalation in a fire, or accidental exposure to an improperly vented gas heater, generator, or other appliance. Carbon monoxide avidly binds to hemoglobin, with an affinity approximately 250 times that of oxygen. This results in reduced oxygen-carrying capacity and altered delivery of oxygen to cells (see also Smoke Inhalation in Chapter 9).

Clinical Findings

At low carbon monoxide levels (carboxyhemoglobin saturation 10–20%), victims may have headache, dizziness, abdominal pain, and nausea. With higher levels, confusion, dyspnea, and syncope may occur. Hypotension, coma, and seizures are common with levels greater than 50–60%. Survivors of acute severe poisoning may develop permanent obvious or subtle neurologic and neuropsychiatric deficits. The fetus and newborn may be more susceptible because of high carbon monoxide affinity for fetal hemoglobin.

Carbon monoxide poisoning should be suspected in any person with severe headache or acutely altered mental status, especially during cold weather, when improperly vented heating systems may have been used. Diagnosis depends on specific measurement of the arterial or venous carboxyhemoglobin saturation, although the level may have declined if high-flow oxygen therapy has already been administered, and levels do not always correlate with clinical symptoms. Routine arterial blood gas testing and pulse oximetry are not useful because they give falsely normal PaO_2 and oxyhemoglobin saturation determinations, respectively. (A specialized pulse oximetry device, the Masimo pulse CO-oximeter, is capable of distinguishing oxyhemoglobin from carboxyhemoglobin.)

▶ **Treatment**

A. Emergency and Supportive Measures

Maintain a patent airway and assist ventilation, if necessary. Remove the victim from exposure. Treat patients with coma, hypotension, or seizures as described at the beginning of this chapter.

B. Specific Treatment

The half-life of the carboxyhemoglobin (CoHb) complex is about 4–5 hours in room air but is reduced dramatically by high concentrations of oxygen. Administer 100% oxygen by tight-fitting high-flow reservoir face mask or endotracheal tube. Hyperbaric oxygen (HBO) can provide 100% oxygen under higher than atmospheric pressures, further shortening the half-life; it may also reduce the incidence of subtle neuropsychiatric sequelae. Randomized controlled studies disagree about the benefit of HBO, but commonly recommended indications for HBO in patients with carbon monoxide poisoning include a history of loss of consciousness, CoHb greater than 25%, metabolic acidosis, age over 50 years, and cerebellar findings on neurologic examination.

Bleecker ML. Carbon monoxide intoxication. Handb Clin Neurol. 2015;131:191–203. [PMID: 26563790]
Weaver LK. Hyperbaric oxygen therapy for carbon monoxide poisoning. Undersea Hyperb Med. 2014 Jul–Aug;41(4):339–4. [PMID: 25109087]

CLONIDINE & OTHER SYMPATHOLYTIC ANTIHYPERTENSIVES

Overdosage with these agents (clonidine, guanabenz, guanfacine, methyldopa) causes bradycardia, hypotension, miosis, respiratory depression, and coma. (Transient hypertension occasionally occurs after acute overdosage, a result of peripheral alpha-adrenergic effects in high doses.) Symptoms are usually resolved in less than 24 hours, and deaths are rare. Similar symptoms may occur after ingestion of topical nasal decongestants chemically similar to clonidine (oxymetazoline, tetrahydrozoline, naphazoline). Brimonidine and apraclonidine are used as ophthalmic preparations for glaucoma. Tizanidine is a centrally acting muscle relaxant structurally related to clonidine; it produces similar toxicity in overdose.

▶ **Treatment**

A. Emergency and Supportive Measures

Give activated charcoal (see p. 1582). Maintain the airway and support respiration if necessary. Symptomatic treatment is usually sufficient even in massive overdose. Maintain blood pressure with intravenous fluids. Dopamine can also be used. Atropine is usually effective for bradycardia.

B. Specific Treatment

There is no specific antidote. Although tolazoline has been recommended for clonidine overdose, its effects are unpredictable and it should not be used. Naloxone has been reported to be successful in a few anecdotal and poorly substantiated cases.

Lowry JA et al. Significance of the imidazoline receptors in toxicology. Clin Toxicol (Phila). 2014 Jun;52(5):454–69. [PMID: 24666288]
Pomerleau AC et al. Dermal exposure to a compounded pain cream resulting in severely elevated clonidine concentration. J Med Toxicol. 2014 Mar;10(1):61–4. [PMID: 24129834]

COCAINE

See Amphetamines & Cocaine.

CYANIDE

Cyanide is a highly toxic chemical used widely in research and commercial laboratories and many industries. Its gaseous form, hydrogen cyanide, is an important component of smoke in fires. Cyanide-generating glycosides are also found in the pits of apricots and other related plants. Cyanide is generated by the breakdown of nitroprusside, and poisoning can result from rapid high-dose infusions. Cyanide is also formed by metabolism of acetonitrile, a solvent found in some over-the-counter fingernail glue removers. Cyanide is rapidly absorbed by inhalation, skin absorption, or ingestion. It disrupts cellular function by inhibiting cytochrome oxidase and preventing cellular oxygen utilization.

▶ **Clinical Findings**

The onset of toxicity is nearly instantaneous after inhalation of hydrogen cyanide gas but may be delayed for minutes to hours after ingestion of cyanide salts or cyanogenic plants or chemicals. Effects include headache, dizziness, nausea, abdominal pain, and anxiety, followed by confusion, syncope, shock, seizures, coma, and death. The odor of "bitter almonds" may be detected on the victim's breath or in vomitus, though this is not a reliable finding. The venous oxygen saturation may be elevated (greater than 90%) in severe poisonings because tissues have failed to take up arterial oxygen.

▶ **Treatment**

A. Emergency and Supportive Measures

Remove the victim from exposure, taking care to avoid exposure to rescuers. For suspected cyanide poisoning due to nitroprusside infusion, stop or slow the rate of infusion. (Metabolic acidosis and other signs of cyanide poisoning usually clear rapidly.)

For cyanide ingestion, administer activated charcoal (see p. 1582). Although charcoal has a low affinity for cyanide, the usual doses of 60–100 g are adequate to bind typically ingested lethal doses (100–200 mg).

B. Specific Treatment

In the United States, there are two available cyanide antidote regimens. The conventional cyanide antidote package (Nithiodote) contains sodium nitrite (to induce methemoglobinemia, which binds free cyanide) and sodium thiosulfate (to promote conversion of cyanide to the less toxic thiocyanate). Administer 3% sodium nitrite solution, 10 mL intravenously followed by 25% sodium thiosulfate solution, 50 mL intravenously (12.5 g). **Caution:** Nitrites may induce hypotension and dangerous levels of methemoglobin.

The other approved cyanide treatment in the United States is hydroxocobalamin (Cyanokit, EMD Pharmaceuticals), a newer and potentially safer antidote. The adult dose of hydroxocobalamin is 5 g intravenously (children's dose is 70 mg/kg). **Note:** Hydroxocobalamin causes red discoloration of skin and bodily fluids that may last several days and can interfere with some laboratory tests.

Anseeuw K et al. Cyanide poisoning by fire smoke inhalation: a European expert consensus. Eur J Emerg Med. 2013 Feb; 20(1):2–9. [PMID: 22828651]
Zakharov S et al. Successful use of hydroxocobalamin and sodium thiosulfate in acute cyanide poisoning: a case report with follow-up. Basic Clin Pharmacol Toxicol. 2015 Sep; 117(3):209–12. [PMID: 25645744]

DIETARY SUPPLEMENTS & HERBAL PRODUCTS

Unlike prescription and over-the-counter pharmaceuticals, dietary supplements do not require FDA approval, do not undergo the same premarketing evaluation of safety and efficacy as drugs, and purveyors may or may not adhere to good manufacturing practices and quality control standards. Supplements may cause illness as a result of intrinsic toxicity, misidentification or mislabeling, drug-herb reactions, or adulteration with pharmaceuticals. If you suspect a dietary supplement or herbal product may be the cause of an otherwise unexplained illness, contact the FDA (1-888-463-6332) or the regional poison control center (1-800-222-1222), or consult one of the following online databases: http://www.naturaldatabase.com and http://www.fda.gov/food/dietarysupplements/default.htm.

Table 38–7 lists selected examples of clinical toxicity from some of these products.

Table 38–7. Examples of potential toxicity associated with some dietary supplements and herbal medicines.

Product	Common Use	Possible Toxicity
Azarcon (Greta)	Mexican folk remedy for abdominal pain, colic	Contains lead (see pp. 1596–1597)
Comfrey	Gastric upset, diarrhea	Contains pyrrolizidine alkaloids, can cause hepatic veno-occlusive disease
Creatine	Athletic performance enhancement	Nausea, diarrhea, abdominal cramps; elevated serum creatinine
Ginkgo	Memory improvement, tinnitus	Antiplatelet effects, hemorrhage; abdominal pain, diarrhea
Ginseng	Immune system; stress	Decreased glucose; increased cortisol
Guarana	Athletic performance enhancement, appetite suppression	Contains caffeine: can cause tremor, tachycardia, vomiting
Kava	Anxiety, insomnia	Drowsiness, hepatitis, skin rash
Ma huang	Stimulant; athletic performance enhancement	Contains ephedrine: anxiety, insomnia, hypertension, tachycardia, seizures
Spirulina	Body building	Niacin-like flushing reaction
Yohimbine	Sexual enhancement	Hallucinations, hypertension, tachycardia
Zinc	Cold/flu symptoms	Nausea, oral irritation, anosmia

Adapted, with permission, from Table II-30 by Haller C in Herbal and Alternative Products In: Olson KR (ed.) *Poisoning & Drug Overdose*, 5th edition, McGraw Hill, 2007.

Cohen PA et al. Presence of banned drugs in dietary supplements following FDA recalls. JAMA. 2014 Oct 22–29; 312(16):1691–3. [PMID: 25335153]

Posadzki P et al. Contamination and adulteration of herbal medicinal products (HMPs): an overview of systematic reviews. Eur J Clin Pharmacol. 2013 Mar;69(3):295–307. [PMID: 22843016]

Teschke R et al. Herbal hepatotoxicity: a critical review. Br J Clin Pharmacol. 2013 Mar;75(3):630–6. [PMID: 22831551]

DIGITALIS & OTHER CARDIAC GLYCOSIDES

Cardiac glycosides paralyze the Na^+-K^+-ATPase pump and have potent vagotonic effects. Intracellular effects include enhancement of calcium-dependent contractility and shortening of the action potential duration. A number of plants (eg, oleander, foxglove, lily-of-the-valley) contain cardiac glycosides. Bufotenin, a cardiotoxic steroid found in certain toad secretions and used as an herbal medicine and a purported aphrodisiac, has pharmacologic properties similar to cardiac glycosides.

► Clinical Findings

Intoxication may result from acute single exposure or chronic accidental overmedication. After acute overdosage, nausea and vomiting, bradycardia, hyperkalemia, and AV block frequently occur. Patients in whom toxicity develops gradually during long-term therapy may be hypokalemic and hypomagnesemic owing to concurrent diuretic treatment and more commonly present with ventricular arrhythmias (eg, ectopy, bidirectional ventricular tachycardia, or ventricular fibrillation). Digoxin levels may be only slightly elevated in patients with intoxication from cardiac glycosides other than digoxin because of limited cross-reactivity of immunologic tests.

► Treatment

A. Emergency and Supportive Measures

After acute ingestion, administer activated charcoal (see p. 1582). Monitor potassium levels and cardiac rhythm closely. Treat bradycardia initially with atropine (0.5–2 mg intravenously) or a transcutaneous external cardiac pacemaker.

B. Specific Treatment

For patients with significant intoxication, administer digoxin-specific antibodies (digoxin immune Fab [ovine]; DigiFab). Estimation of the Digibind dose is based on the body burden of digoxin calculated from the ingested dose or the steady-state serum digoxin concentration, as described below. More effective binding of digoxin may be achieved if the dose is given partly as a bolus and the remainder as an infusion over a few hours.

1. From the ingested dose—Number of vials = approximately 1.5–2 × ingested dose (mg).

2. From the serum concentration—Number of vials = serum digoxin (ng/mL) × body weight (kg) × 10^{-2}. **Note:** This is based on the equilibrium digoxin level; after acute overdose, serum levels may be falsely high for several hours before tissue distribution is complete, and overestimation of the Digibind or DigiFab dose is likely.

3. Empiric dosing—Empiric titration of Digibind or DigiFab may be used if the patient's condition is relatively stable and an underlying condition (eg, atrial fibrillation) favors retaining a residual level of digitalis activity. Start with one or two vials and reassess the patient's clinical condition after 20–30 minutes. For cardiac glycosides other than digoxin or digitoxin, there is no formula for estimation of vials needed and treatment is entirely based on response to empiric dosing.

Note: After administration of digoxin-specific Fab antibody fragments, serum digoxin levels may be falsely elevated depending on the assay technique.

Chan BS et al. Digoxin-specific antibody fragments in the treatment of digoxin toxicity. Clin Toxicol (Phila). 2014 Sep–Oct; 52(8):824–36. [PMID: 25089630]

Roberts DM et al. Pharmacological treatment of cardiac glycoside poisoning. Br J Clin Pharmacol. 2016 Mar;81(3):488–95. [PMID: 26505271]

ETHANOL, BENZODIAZEPINES, & OTHER SEDATIVE-HYPNOTIC AGENTS

The group of agents known as sedative-hypnotic drugs includes a variety of products used for the treatment of anxiety, depression, insomnia, and epilepsy. Besides common benzodiazepines, such as lorazepam, alprazolam, clonazepam, diazepam, oxazepam, chlordiazepoxide, and triazolam, this group includes the newer benzodiazepine-like hypnotics zolpidem and zaleplon, and the muscle relaxant carisoprodol. Ethanol and other selected agents are also popular recreational drugs. All of these drugs depress the central nervous system reticular activating system, cerebral cortex, and cerebellum.

► Clinical Findings

Mild intoxication produces euphoria, slurred speech, and ataxia. Ethanol intoxication may produce hypoglycemia, even at relatively low concentrations, in children and in fasting adults. With more severe intoxication, stupor, coma, and respiratory arrest may occur. Carisoprodol (Soma) commonly causes muscle jerking or myoclonus. Death or serious morbidity is usually the result of pulmonary aspiration of gastric contents. Bradycardia, hypotension, and hypothermia are common. Patients with massive intoxication may appear to be dead, with no reflex responses and even absent electroencephalographic activity. Diagnosis and assessment of severity of intoxication are usually based on clinical findings. Ethanol serum levels over 300 mg/dL (0.3 g/dL; 65 mmol/L) can produce coma in persons who are not chronically abusing the drug, but regular users may remain awake at much higher levels.

▶ Treatment

A. Emergency and Supportive Measures

Administer activated charcoal if the patient has ingested a massive dose and the airway is protected (see p. 1582). Repeat-dose charcoal may enhance elimination of phenobarbital, but it has not been proved to improve clinical outcome. Hemodialysis may be necessary for patients with severe phenobarbital intoxication.

B. Specific Treatment

Flumazenil is a benzodiazepine receptor-specific antagonist; it has no effect on ethanol, barbiturates, or other sedative-hypnotic agents. If used, flumazenil is given slowly intravenously, 0.2 mg over 30–60 seconds, and repeated in 0.2–0.5 mg increments as needed up to a total dose of 3–5 mg. **Caution:** Flumazenil should rarely be used because it may induce seizures in patients with preexisting seizure disorder, benzodiazepine addiction, or concomitant tricyclic antidepressant or other convulsant overdose. If seizures occur, diazepam and other benzodiazepine anticonvulsants will not be effective. As with naloxone, the duration of action of flumazenil is short (2–3 hours) and resedation may occur, requiring repeated doses.

Penninga EI et al. Adverse events associated with flumazenil treatment for the management of suspected benzodiazepine intoxication—a systematic review with meta-analyses of randomised trials. Basic Clin Pharmacol Toxicol. 2016 Jan; 118(1):37–44. [PMID: 26096314]
Vallersnes OM et al. Patients presenting with acute poisoning to an outpatient emergency clinic: a one-year observational study in Oslo, Norway. BMC Emerg Med. 2015 Aug 13;15:18. [PMID: 26268351]
Zanoni S et al. Altered mental status due to pruno intoxication. J Emerg Med. 2014 Jun;46(6):767–8. [PMID: 24680101]

GAMMA-HYDROXYBUTYRATE (GHB)

GHB is a popular drug of abuse. It originated as a short-acting general anesthetic and is occasionally used in the treatment of narcolepsy. It gained popularity among bodybuilders for its alleged growth hormone stimulation and found its way into social settings, where it is consumed as a liquid. It has been used to facilitate sexual assault ("date-rape" drug). Symptoms after ingestion include drowsiness and lethargy followed by coma with respiratory depression. Muscle twitching and seizures are sometimes observed. Recovery is usually rapid, with patients awakening within a few hours. Other related chemicals with similar effects include butanediol and gamma-butyrolactone (GBL). A prolonged withdrawal syndrome has been described in some heavy users.

▶ Treatment

Monitor the airway and assist breathing if needed. There is no specific treatment. Most patients recover rapidly with supportive care. GHB withdrawal syndrome may require very large doses of benzodiazepines.

Schep LJ et al. The clinical toxicology of gamma-hydroxybutyrate, gamma-butyrolactone and 1,4-butanediol. Clin Toxicol (Phila). 2012 Jul;50(6):458–70. [PMID: 22746383]
Morse BL et al. Toxicokinetics/toxicodynamics of γ-hydroxybutyrate-ethanol intoxication: evaluation of potential treatment strategies. J Pharmacol Exp Ther. 2013 Sep; 346(3):504–13. [PMID: 23814094]

HYPOGLYCEMIC DRUGS

Medications used for diabetes mellitus include insulin, sulfonylureas and other insulin secretagogues, alpha-glucosidase inhibitors (acarbose, miglitol), biguanides (metformin), thiazolidinediones (pioglitazone, rosiglitazone), and newer peptide analogs (pramlintide, exenatide) or enhancers (sitagliptin) (see Chapter 27). Of these, insulin and the insulin secretagogues are the most likely to cause hypoglycemia. Metformin can cause lactic acidosis, especially in patients with impaired kidney function or after intentional drug overdose. Table 27–7 lists the duration of hypoglycemic effect of oral hypoglycemic agents and Figure 27–2 the extent and duration of various types of insulins.

▶ Clinical Findings

Hypoglycemia may occur quickly after injection of short-acting insulins or may be delayed and prolonged, especially if a large amount has been injected into a single area, creating a "depot" effect (see Figure 27–2). Hypoglycemia after sulfonylurea ingestion is usually apparent within a few hours but may be delayed several hours, especially if food or glucose-containing fluids have been given (see Table 27–8).

▶ Treatment

Give sugar and carbohydrate-containing food or liquids by mouth, or intravenous dextrose if the patient is unable to swallow safely. For severe hypoglycemia, start with D50W, 50 mL intravenously (25 g dextrose); repeat, if needed. Follow up with dextrose-containing intravenous fluids (D5W or D10W) to maintain a blood glucose greater than 70–80 mg/dL.

For hypoglycemia caused by sulfonylureas and related insulin secretagogues, consider use of octreotide, a synthetic somatostatin analog that blocks pancreatic insulin release. A dose of 50–100 mcg octreotide subcutaneously every 6–12 hours can reduce the need for exogenous dextrose and prevent rebound hypoglycemia from excessive dextrose dosing.

Admit all patients with symptomatic hypoglycemia after sulfonylurea overdose. Observe asymptomatic overdose patients for at least 12 hours.

Consider hemodialysis for patients with metformin overdose accompanied by severe lactic acidosis (lactate greater than 20 mmol/L or pH < 7.0).

Calello DP et al. Extracorporeal treatment for metformin poisoning: systematic review and recommendations from the extracorporeal treatments in poisoning workgroup. Crit Care Med. 2015 Aug;43(8):1716–30. [PMID: 25860205]

Glatstein M et al. Octreotide for the treatment of sulfonylurea poisoning. Clin Toxicol (Phila). 2012 Nov;50(9):795–804. [PMID: 23046209]

IRON

Iron is widely used therapeutically for the treatment of anemia and as a daily supplement in multiple vitamin preparations. Most children's preparations contain about 12–15 mg of iron (as sulfate, gluconate, or fumarate salt) per dose, compared with 60–90 mg in most adult-strength preparations. Iron is corrosive to the gastrointestinal tract and, once absorbed, has depressant effects on the myocardium and on peripheral vascular resistance. Intracellular toxic effects of iron include disruption of Krebs cycle enzymes. Carbonyl iron is a powdered form of elemental iron. It is not as irritating to the gastrointestinal tract as the iron salts and appears to be safer.

▶ Clinical Findings

Ingestion of less than 30 mg/kg of iron usually produces only mild gastrointestinal upset. Ingestion of more than 40–60 mg/kg may cause vomiting (sometimes with hematemesis), diarrhea, hypotension, and acidosis. Death may occur as a result of profound hypotension due to massive fluid losses and bleeding, metabolic acidosis, peritonitis from intestinal perforation, or sepsis. Fulminant hepatic failure may occur. Survivors of the acute ingestion may suffer permanent gastrointestinal scarring.

Serum iron levels greater than 350–500 mcg/dL are considered potentially toxic, and levels greater than 1000 mcg/dL are usually associated with severe poisoning. A plain abdominal radiograph may reveal radiopaque tablets.

▶ Treatment

A. Emergency and Supportive Measures

Treat hypotension aggressively with intravenous crystalloid solutions (0.9% saline or lactated Ringer solution). Fluid losses may be massive owing to vomiting and diarrhea as well as third-spacing into injured intestine.

Perform whole bowel irrigation to remove unabsorbed pills from the intestinal tract (see p. 1582). Activated charcoal is not effective but may be appropriate if other ingestants are suspected.

B. Specific Treatment

Deferoxamine is a selective iron chelator. It is not useful as an oral binding agent. For patients with established manifestations of toxicity—and particularly those with markedly elevated serum iron levels (eg, greater than 800–1000 mcg/dL)—administer 10–15 mg/kg/h by constant intravenous infusion; higher doses (up to 40–50 mg/kg/h) have been used in massive poisonings. Hypotension may occur. The presence of an iron-deferoxamine complex in the urine may give it a "vin rosé" appearance. Deferoxamine is safe for use in pregnant women with acute iron overdose. **Caution:** Prolonged infusion of deferoxamine (more than 36–48 hours) has been associated with development of

acute respiratory distress syndrome (ARDS)—the mechanism is not known.

Wolters JM et al. Fatal unsuspected iron ingestion. Emerg Med Australas. 2014 Apr;26(2):204–5. [PMID: 24708016]

ISONIAZID

INH is an antibacterial drug used mainly in the treatment and prevention of tuberculosis. It may cause hepatitis with long-term use, especially in alcoholic patients and elderly persons. It produces acute toxic effects by competing with pyridoxal 5-phosphate, resulting in lowered brain gamma-aminobutyric acid (GABA) levels. Acute ingestion of as little as 1.5–2 g of INH can cause toxicity, and severe poisoning is likely to occur after ingestion of more than 80–100 mg/kg.

▶ Clinical Findings

Confusion, slurred speech, and seizures may occur abruptly after acute overdose. Severe lactic acidosis—out of proportion to the severity of seizures—is probably due to inhibited metabolism of lactate. Peripheral neuropathy and acute hepatitis may occur with long-term use.

Diagnosis is based on a history of ingestion and the presence of severe acidosis associated with seizures. INH is not usually included in routine toxicologic screening, and serum levels are not readily available.

▶ Treatment

A. Emergency and Supportive Measures

Seizures may require higher than usual doses of benzodiazepines (eg, lorazepam, 3–5 mg intravenously) or administration of pyridoxine as an antidote.

Administer activated charcoal (see p. 1582) after large recent ingestion, but with caution because of the risk of abrupt onset of seizures.

B. Specific Treatment

Pyridoxine (vitamin B_6) is a specific antagonist of the acute toxic effects of INH and is usually successful in controlling convulsions that do not respond to benzodiazepines. Give 5 g intravenously over 1–2 minutes or, if the amount ingested is known, give a gram-for-gram equivalent amount of pyridoxine. Patients taking INH are usually given 25–50 mg of pyridoxine orally daily to help prevent neuropathy.

Skinner K et al. Isoniazid poisoning: pharmacokinetics and effect of hemodialysis in a massive ingestion. Hemodial Int. 2015 Oct;19(4):E37–40. [PMID: 25779481]

LEAD

Lead is used in a variety of industrial and commercial products, such as storage batteries, solders, paints, pottery, plumbing, and gasoline and is found in some traditional Hispanic and Ayurvedic ethnic medicines. Lead toxicity usually results from chronic repeated exposure and is rare after a single ingestion. Lead produces a variety of adverse effects on cellular function and primarily affects the nervous system, gastrointestinal tract, and hematopoietic system.

► Clinical Findings

Lead poisoning often goes undiagnosed initially because presenting symptoms and signs are nonspecific and exposure is not suspected. Common symptoms include colicky abdominal pain, constipation, headache, and irritability. Severe poisoning may cause coma and convulsions. Chronic intoxication can cause learning disorders (in children) and motor neuropathy (eg, wrist drop). Lead-containing bullet fragments in or near joint spaces can result in chronic lead toxicity.

Diagnosis is based on measurement of the blood lead level. Whole blood lead levels below 10 mcg/dL are usually considered nontoxic, although that limit has been lowered to 5 mcg/dL in children. Levels between 10 and 25 mcg/dL have been associated with impaired neurobehavioral development in children. Levels of 25–50 mcg/dL may be associated with headache, irritability, and subclinical neuropathy. Levels of 50–70 mcg/dL are associated with moderate toxicity, and levels greater than 70–100 mcg/dL are often associated with severe poisoning. Other laboratory findings of lead poisoning include microcytic anemia with basophilic stippling and elevated free erythrocyte protoporphyrin.

► Treatment

A. Emergency and Supportive Measures

For patients with encephalopathy, maintain a patent airway and treat coma and convulsions as described at the beginning of this chapter.

For recent acute ingestion, if a large lead-containing object (eg, fishing weight) is still visible in the stomach on abdominal radiograph, whole bowel irrigation (see p. 1582), endoscopy, or even surgical removal may be necessary to prevent subacute lead poisoning. (The acidic gastric contents may corrode the metal surface, enhancing lead absorption. Once the object passes into the small intestine, the risk of toxicity declines.)

Conduct an investigation into the source of the lead exposure.

Workers with a single lead level over 60 mcg/dL (or three successive monthly levels greater than 50 mcg/dL) or construction workers with any single blood lead level above 50 mcg/dL must by federal law be removed from the site of exposure. Contact the regional office of the United States Occupational Safety and Health Administration (OSHA) for more information. Several states mandate reporting of cases of confirmed lead poisoning.

B. Specific Treatment

The indications for chelation depend on the blood lead level and the patient's clinical state. A medical toxicologist or regional poison control center (1-800-222-1222) should be consulted for advice about selection and use of these antidotes.

Note: It is impermissible under the law to treat asymptomatic workers with elevated blood lead levels in order to keep their levels under 50 mcg/dL rather than remove them from the exposure.

1. Severe toxicity—Patients with severe intoxication (encephalopathy or levels greater than 70–100 mcg/dL) should receive edetate calcium disodium (ethylenediaminetetraacetic acid, EDTA), 1500 mg/m^2/kg/day (approximately 50 mg/kg/day) in four to six divided doses or as a continuous intravenous infusion. Most clinicians also add dimercaprol (BAL), 4–5 mg/kg intramuscularly every 4 hours for 5 days, for patients with encephalopathy.

2. Less severe toxicity—Patients with less severe symptoms and asymptomatic patients with blood lead levels between 55 and 69 mcg/dL may be treated with edetate calcium disodium alone in dosages as above. An oral chelator, succimer (DMSA), is available for use in patients with mild to moderate intoxication. The usual dose is 10 mg/kg orally every 8 hours for 5 days, then every 12 hours for 2 weeks.

Orchard GR et al. Lead poisoning in Australia associated with privately imported Ayurvedic complementary medicine. Anaesth Intensive Care. 2015 Sep;43(5):669–70. [PMID: 26310426]
Thihalolipavan S et al. Examining pica in NYC pregnant women with elevated blood lead levels. Matern Child Health J. 2013 Jan;17(1):49–55. [PMID: 22302239]

LITHIUM

Lithium is widely used for the treatment of bipolar depression and other psychiatric disorders. The only normal route of lithium elimination is via the kidney, so patients with chronic kidney disease are at risk for accumulation of lithium resulting in gradual onset (chronic) toxicity. Intoxication resulting from chronic accidental overmedication or renal impairment is more common and usually more severe than that seen after acute oral overdose.

► Clinical Findings

Mild to moderate toxicity causes lethargy, confusion, tremor, ataxia, and slurred speech. This may progress to myoclonic jerking, delirium, coma, and convulsions. Recovery may be slow and incomplete following severe intoxication. Laboratory studies in patients with chronic intoxication often reveal an elevated serum creatinine and an elevated BUN/creatinine ratio due to underlying volume contraction. The white blood cell count is often elevated. ECG findings include T-wave flattening or inversion, and sometimes bradycardia or sinus node arrest. Nephrogenic diabetes insipidus can occur with overdose or with therapeutic doses. Lithium levels may be difficult to interpret. Lithium has a low toxic: therapeutic ratio and chronic intoxication can be seen with levels only slightly above the therapeutic range (0.8–1.2 mEq/L). In contrast, patients with acute ingestion may have transiently very high levels (up to 10 mEq/L reported) without any symptoms before the lithium fully distributes into tissues. **Note:** Falsely high lithium levels (as high as 6–8 mEq/L) can be measured if a green-top blood specimen tube (containing lithium heparin) is used instead of a red- or marbled-top tube.

▶ Treatment

After acute oral overdose, consider gastric lavage (see p. 1582) or whole bowel irrigation (see p. 1582) to prevent systemic absorption (lithium is not adsorbed by activated charcoal). In all patients, evaluate renal function and volume status, and give intravenous saline-containing fluids as needed. Monitor serum lithium levels, and seek assistance with their interpretation and the need for dialysis from a medical toxicologist or regional poison control center (1-800-222-1222). Consider hemodialysis if the patient is markedly symptomatic or if the serum level exceeds 4–5 mEq/L, especially if renal function is impaired. Continuous renal replacement therapy may be an effective alternative to hemodialysis.

Chen WY et al. Reversible oro-lingual dyskinesia related to lithium intoxication. Acta Neurol Taiwan. 2013 Mar;22(1):32–5. [PMID: 23479244]
Decker BS et al. Extracorporeal treatment for lithium poisoning: systematic review and recommendations from the EXTRIP Workgroup. Clin J Am Soc Nephrol. 2015 May 7;10(5):875–87. [PMID: 25583292]
Lavonas EJ et al. Hemodialysis for lithium poisoning. Cochrane Database Syst Rev. 2015 Sep 16;9:CD007951. [PMID: 26374731]

LSD & OTHER HALLUCINOGENS

A variety of substances—ranging from naturally occurring plants and mushrooms to synthetic substances such as phencyclidine (PCP), toluene and other solvents, dextromethorphan, and lysergic acid diethylamide (LSD)—are abused for their hallucinogenic properties. The mechanism of toxicity and the clinical effects vary for each substance.

Many hallucinogenic plants and mushrooms produce anticholinergic delirium, characterized by flushed skin, dry mucous membranes, dilated pupils, tachycardia, and urinary retention. Other plants and mushrooms may contain hallucinogenic indoles such as mescaline and LSD, which typically cause marked visual hallucinations and perceptual distortion, widely dilated pupils, and mild tachycardia. PCP, a dissociative anesthetic agent similar to ketamine, can produce fluctuating delirium and coma, often associated with vertical and horizontal nystagmus. Toluene and other hydrocarbon solvents (butane, trichloroethylene, "chemo," etc) cause euphoria and delirium and may sensitize the myocardium to the effects of catecholamines, leading to fatal dysrhythmias. Newer drugs used for their psychostimulant effects include synthetic cannabinoid receptor agonists (street names include "spice" and "K2"), *Salvia divinorum*, and mephedrone and related cathinone derivatives. See www.erowid.org for very thorough descriptions of a variety of hallucinogenic substances.

▶ Treatment

A. Emergency and Supportive Measures

Maintain a patent airway and assist respirations if necessary. Treat coma, hyperthermia, hypertension, and seizures

as outlined at the beginning of this chapter. For recent large ingestions, consider giving activated charcoal orally or by gastric tube (see p. 1582).

B. Specific Treatment

Patients with anticholinergic delirium may benefit from a dose of physostigmine, 0.5–1 mg intravenously, not to exceed 1 mg/min. Dysphoria, agitation, and psychosis associated with LSD or mescaline intoxication may respond to benzodiazepines (eg, lorazepam, 1–2 mg orally or intravenously) or haloperidol (2–5 mg intramuscularly or intravenously) or another antipsychotic drug (eg, olanzapine or ziprasidone). Monitor patients who have sniffed solvents for cardiac dysrhythmias (most commonly premature ventricular contractions, ventricular tachycardia, ventricular fibrillation); treatment with beta-blockers such as propranolol (1–5 mg intravenously) or esmolol (250–500 mcg/kg intravenously, then 50 mcg/kg/min by infusion) may be more effective than lidocaine or amiodarone.

Bäckberg M et al. Phencyclidine analog use in Sweden—intoxication cases involving 3-MeO-PCP and 4-MeO-PCP from the STRIDA project. Clin Toxicol (Phila). 2015 Nov;53(9):856–64. [PMID: 26295489]
Harris CR et al. Synthetic cannabinoid intoxication: a case series and review. J Emerg Med. 2013 Feb;44(2):360–6. [PMID: 22989695]

MERCURY

Mercury poisoning may occur by ingestion of inorganic mercuric salts, organic mercury compounds, or inhalation of metallic mercury vapor. Ingestion of the mercuric salts causes a burning sensation in the throat, discoloration and edema of oral mucous membranes, abdominal pain, vomiting, bloody diarrhea, and shock. Direct nephrotoxicity causes acute kidney injury. Inhalation of high concentrations of metallic mercury vapor may cause acute fulminant chemical pneumonia. Chronic mercury poisoning causes weakness, ataxia, intention tremors, irritability, and depression. Exposure to alkyl (organic) mercury derivatives from highly contaminated fish or fungicides used on seeds has caused ataxia, tremors, convulsions, and catastrophic birth defects. Nearly all fish have some traces of mercury contamination; the US Environmental Protection Agency (EPA) advises consumers to avoid swordfish, shark, king mackerel, and tilefish because they contain higher levels. Fish and shellfish that are generally low in mercury content include shrimp, canned light tuna (not albacore "white" tuna), salmon, pollock, and catfish. Dental fillings composed of mercury amalgam pose a very small risk of chronic mercury poisoning and their removal is rarely justified. Some imported skin lightening creams contain toxic quantities of mercury.

▶ Treatment

A. Acute Poisoning

There is no effective specific treatment for mercury vapor pneumonitis. Remove ingested mercuric salts by lavage, and administer activated charcoal (see p. 1582). For acute ingestion of mercuric salts, give dimercaprol (BAL) at once, as for arsenic poisoning. Unless the patient has severe gastroenteritis, consider succimer (DMSA), 10 mg/kg orally every 8 hours for 5 days and then every 12 hours for 2 weeks. Unithiol (DMPS) is a chelator that can be given orally or parenterally, but is not commonly available in the United States; it can be obtained from some compounding pharmacies. Maintain urinary output. Treat oliguria and anuria if they occur.

B. Chronic Poisoning

Remove from exposure. Neurologic toxicity is not considered reversible with chelation, although some authors recommend a trial of succimer or unithiol (contact a regional poison center or medical toxicologist for advice).

Koirala S et al. Notes from the field: acute mercury poisoning after home gold and silver smelting—Iowa, 2014. MMWR Morb Mortal Wkly Rep. 2015 Dec 18;64(49):1365–6. [PMID: 26678598]
Mercer JJ et al. Acrodynia and hypertension in a young girl secondary to elemental mercury toxicity acquired in the home. Pediatr Dermatol. 2012 Mar–Apr;29(2):199–201. [PMID: 22409470]

METHANOL & ETHYLENE GLYCOL

Methanol (wood alcohol) is commonly found in a variety of products, including solvents, duplicating fluids, record cleaning solutions, and paint removers. It is sometimes ingested intentionally by alcoholic patients as a substitute for ethanol and may also be found as a contaminant in bootleg whiskey. Ethylene glycol is the major constituent in most antifreeze compounds. The toxicity of both agents is caused by metabolism to highly toxic organic acids—methanol to formic acid; ethylene glycol to glycolic and oxalic acids. Diethylene glycol is a nephrotoxic solvent that has been improperly substituted for glycerine in various liquid medications (cough syrup, teething medicine, acetaminophen) causing numerous deaths in Haiti, Panama, and Nigeria.

▶ Clinical Findings

Shortly after ingestion of methanol or ethylene glycol, patients usually appear "drunk." The serum osmolality (measured with the freezing point device) is usually increased, but acidosis is often absent early. After several hours, metabolism to toxic organic acids leads to a severe anion gap metabolic acidosis, tachypnea, confusion, convulsions, and coma. Methanol intoxication frequently causes visual disturbances, while ethylene glycol often produces oxalate crystalluria and acute kidney injury. **Note:** Point-of-care analytical devices common used in the emergency department may falsely measure glycolic acid (a toxic metabolite of ethylene glycol) as lactic acid.

▶ Treatment

A. Emergency and Supportive Measures

For patients presenting within 30–60 minutes after ingestion, empty the stomach by aspiration through a nasogastric tube (see p. 1582). Charcoal is not very effective but should be administered if other poisons or drugs have also been ingested.

B. Specific Treatment

Patients with significant toxicity (manifested by severe metabolic acidosis, altered mental status, and markedly elevated osmol gap) should undergo hemodialysis as soon as possible to remove the parent compound and the toxic metabolites. Treatment with folic acid, thiamine, and pyridoxine may enhance the breakdown of toxic metabolites.

Ethanol blocks metabolism of the parent compounds by competing for the enzyme alcohol dehydrogenase. Fomepizole (4-methylpyrazole; Antizol) blocks alcohol dehydrogenase and is much easier to use than ethanol. If started before onset of acidosis, fomepizole may be used as the sole treatment for ethylene glycol ingestion in some cases. A regional poison control center (1-800-222-1222) should be contacted for indications and dosing.

Imam YZ et al. Neurological manifestation of recreational fatal and near-fatal diethylene glycol poisonings: case series and review of literature. Medicine (Baltimore). 2014 Aug; 93(10):e62. [PMID: 25170933]
Riquier T et al. False hyperlactatemia in life-threatening ethylene glycol poisoning. Ann Fr Anesth Reanim. 2014 Apr; 33(4):e79–81. [PMID: 24630168]

METHEMOGLOBINEMIA-INDUCING AGENTS

A large number of chemical agents are capable of oxidizing ferrous hemoglobin to its ferric state (methemoglobin), a form that cannot carry oxygen. Drugs and chemicals known to cause methemoglobinemia include benzocaine (a local anesthetic found in some topical anesthetic sprays and a variety of nonprescription products), aniline, propanil (an herbicide), nitrites, nitrogen oxide gases, nitrobenzene, dapsone, phenazopyridine (Pyridium), and many others. Dapsone has a long elimination half-life and may produce prolonged or recurrent methemoglobinemia.

▶ Clinical Findings

Methemoglobinemia reduces oxygen-carrying capacity and may cause dizziness, nausea, headache, dyspnea, confusion, seizures, and coma. The severity of symptoms depends on the percentage of hemoglobin oxidized to methemoglobin; severe poisoning is usually present when methemoglobin fractions are greater than 40–50%. Even at low levels (15–20%), victims appear cyanotic because of the "chocolate brown" color of methemoglobin, but they have normal PO_2 results on arterial blood gas determinations. Conventional pulse oximetry gives inaccurate oxygen saturation measurements; the reading is often between 85% and 90%. (A newer pulse oximetry device [Masimo Pulse CO-oximeter] is capable of estimating the methemoglobin level.) Severe metabolic acidosis may be present. Hemolysis may occur, especially in patients susceptible to oxidant stress (ie, those with glucose-6-phosphate dehydrogenase deficiency).

▶ Treatment

A. Emergency and Supportive Measures

Administer high-flow oxygen. If the causative agent was recently ingested, administer activated charcoal (see p. 1582). Repeat-dose activated charcoal may enhance dapsone elimination.

B. Specific Treatment

Methylene blue enhances the conversion of methemoglobin to hemoglobin by increasing the activity of the enzyme methemoglobin reductase. For symptomatic patients, administer 1–2 mg/kg (0.1–0.2 mL/kg of 1% solution) intravenously. The dose may be repeated once in 15–20 minutes if necessary. Patients with hereditary methemoglobin reductase deficiency or glucose-6-phosphate dehydrogenase deficiency may not respond to methylene blue treatment. In severe cases where methylene blue is not available or is not effective, exchange blood transfusion may be necessary.

Messmer AS et al. P-chloroaniline poisoning causing methemoglobinemia: a case report and review of the literature. Case Rep Emerg Med. 2015;2015:208732. [PMID: 25861488]
Shahani L et al. Acquired methaemoglobinaemia related to phenazopyridine ingestion. BMJ Case Rep. 2012 Sep 17;2012. [PMID: 22987905]

MUSHROOMS

There are thousands of mushroom species that cause a variety of toxic effects. The most dangerous species of mushrooms are *Amanita phalloides* and related species, which contain potent cytotoxins (amatoxins). Ingestion of even a portion of one amatoxin-containing mushroom may be sufficient to cause death.

The characteristic pathologic finding in fatalities from amatoxin-containing mushroom poisoning is acute massive necrosis of the liver.

▶ Clinical Findings

A. Symptoms and Signs

Amatoxin-containing mushrooms typically cause a delayed onset (8–12 hours after ingestion) of severe abdominal cramps, vomiting and profuse diarrhea, followed by hepatic necrosis, hepatic encephalopathy, and frequently acute kidney injury in 1–2 days. Cooking the mushrooms does not prevent poisoning.

Monomethylhydrazine poisoning (*Gyromitra* and *Helvella* species) is more common following ingestion of uncooked mushrooms, as the toxin is water-soluble. Vomiting, diarrhea, hepatic necrosis, convulsions, coma, and hemolysis may occur after a latent period of 8–12 hours.

The clinical effects of these and other mushrooms are described in Table 38–8.

▶ Treatment

A. Emergency Measures

After the onset of symptoms, efforts to remove the toxic agent are probably useless, especially in cases of amatoxin or gyromitrin poisoning, where there is usually a delay of 12 hours or more before symptoms occur and patients seek medical attention. However, induction of vomiting or

Table 38–8. Poisonous mushrooms.

Toxin	Genus	Symptoms and Signs	Onset	Treatment
Amanitin	*Amanita (A ocreata, A phalloides, A verna, A virosa)*	Severe gastroenteritis followed by delayed hepatic failure and acute kidney injury after 48–72 hours	6–24 hours	Supportive. Correct dehydration. Give repeated doses of activated charcoal orally. Consider intravenous silibinin (Legalon-SIL).
Muscarine	*Inocybe, Clitocybe*	Muscarinic (salivation, miosis, bradycardia, diarrhea)	30–60 minutes	Supportive. Give atropine, 0.5–2 mg intravenously, for severe cholinergic symptoms and signs.
Ibotenic acid, muscimol	*Amanita muscaria* ("fly agaric")	Anticholinergic (mydriasis, tachycardia, hyperpyrexia, delirium)	30–60 minutes	Supportive. Give physostigmine, 0.5–2 mg intravenously, for severe anticholinergic symptoms and signs.
Coprine	*Coprinus*	Disulfiram-like effect occurs with ingestion of ethanol	30–60 minutes	Supportive. Abstain from ethanol for 3–4 days.
Monomethyl-hydrazine	*Gyromitra*	Gastroenteritis; occasionally seizures, hemolysis, hepatic failure, and acute kidney injury	6–12 hours	Supportive. Correct dehydration. Pyridoxine, 2.5 mg/kg intravenously, may be helpful for seizures.
Orellanine	*Cortinarius*	Nausea, vomiting; acute kidney injury after 1–3 weeks	2–14 days	Supportive.
Psilocybin	*Psilocybe*	Hallucinations	15–30 minutes	Supportive.
Gastrointestinal irritants	Many species	Nausea and vomiting, diarrhea	1/2–2 hours	Supportive. Correct dehydration.

administration of activated charcoal is recommended for any recent ingestion of an unidentified or potentially toxic mushroom (see p. 1582). Administer intravenous fluids to replace massive losses from vomiting and diarrhea.

B. Specific Treatment

A variety of purported antidotes (eg, thioctic acid, penicillin, corticosteroids) have been suggested for amatoxin-type mushroom poisoning, but controlled studies are lacking and experimental data in animals are equivocal. Aggressive fluid replacement for diarrhea and intensive supportive care for hepatic failure are the mainstays of treatment. Silymarin (silibinin), a derivative of milk thistle, is commonly used in Europe but is currently only commercially available in the United States as a nutritional supplement given orally. The European intravenous product (Legalon-SIL) can be obtained in the United States under an emergency IND provided by the FDA. Contact the regional poison control center (1-800-222-1222) for more information.

Liver transplant may be the only hope for survival in gravely ill patients—contact a liver transplant center early.

Garcia J et al. Amanita phalloides poisoning: mechanisms of toxicity and treatment. Food Chem Toxicol. 2015 Dec;86:41–55. [PMID: 26375431]
Ward J et al. Amatoxin poisoning: case reports and review of current therapies. J Emerg Med. 2013 Jan;44(1):116–21. [PMID: 22555054]

OPIATES & OPIOIDS

Prescription and illicit opiates and opioids (morphine, heroin, codeine, oxycodone, fentanyl, hydromorphone, etc) are popular drugs of misuse and abuse and the cause of frequent hospitalizations for overdose. These drugs have widely varying potencies and durations of action; for example, some of the illicit fentanyl derivatives are up to 2000 times more potent than morphine. All of these agents decrease central nervous system activity and sympathetic outflow by acting on opiate receptors in the brain. Tramadol is an analgesic that is unrelated chemically to the opioids but acts on opioid receptors. Buprenorphine is a partial agonist-antagonist opioid used for the outpatient treatment of opioid addiction.

▶ Clinical Findings

Mild intoxication is characterized by euphoria, drowsiness, and constricted pupils. More severe intoxication may cause hypotension, bradycardia, hypothermia, coma, and respiratory arrest. Pulmonary edema may occur. Death is usually due to apnea or pulmonary aspiration of gastric contents. Methadone is associated with QT interval prolongation and torsades de pointes. While the duration of effect for heroin is usually 3–5 hours, methadone intoxication may last for 48–72 hours or longer. Tramadol, dextromethorphan, and meperidine also occasionally cause seizures. With meperidine, the metabolite normeperidine is probably the cause of seizures and is most likely to accumulate with repeated

dosing in patients with chronic kidney disease. Propoxyphene prolongs the QRS interval and may cause seizures; it is no longer available in the United States. Wound botulism has been associated with skin-popping, especially involving "black tar" heroin. Buprenorphine added to an opioid regimen may produce acute narcotic withdrawal symptoms. Many opioids, including fentanyl, tramadol, oxycodone, and methadone, are not detected on routine urine toxicology "opiate" screening.

▶ Treatment

A. Emergency and Supportive Measures

Protect the airway and assist ventilation. Administer activated charcoal (see p. 1582) for recent large ingestions.

B. Specific Treatment

Naloxone is a specific opioid antagonist that can rapidly reverse signs of narcotic intoxication. Although it is structurally related to the opioids, it has no agonist effects of its own. Administer 0.2–2 mg intravenously, and repeat as needed to awaken the patient and maintain airway protective reflexes and spontaneous breathing. Very large doses (10–20 mg) may be required for patients intoxicated by some opioids (eg, codeine, fentanyl derivatives). **Caution:** The duration of effect of naloxone is only about 2–3 hours; repeated doses may be necessary for patients intoxicated by long-acting drugs such as methadone. Continuous observation for at least 3 hours after the last naloxone dose is mandatory.

Alford DP et al. JAMA patient page. Misuse of opioid medication. JAMA. 2013 May 15;309(19):2055. [PMID: 23677318]
Bowman S et al. Reducing the health consequences of opioid addiction in primary care. Am J Med. 2013 Jul;126(7):565–71. [PMID: 23664112]
Rudd RA et al. Increases in drug and opioid overdose deaths—United States, 2000–2014. MMWR Morb Mortal Wkly Rep. 2016 Jan 1;64(50–51):1378–82. [PMID: 26720857]
Vignali C et al. Methadone-related deaths. A ten year overview. Forensic Sci Int. 2015 Dec;257:172–6. [PMID: 26360592]

PESTICIDES: CHOLINESTERASE INHIBITORS

Organophosphorus and carbamate insecticides (organophosphates: parathion, malathion, etc; carbamates: carbaryl, aldicarb, etc) are widely used in commercial agriculture and home gardening and have largely replaced older, more environmentally persistent organochlorine compounds such as DDT and chlordane. The organophosphates and carbamates—also called anticholinesterases because they inhibit the enzyme acetylcholinesterase—cause an increase in acetylcholine activity at nicotinic and muscarinic receptors and in the central nervous system. There are a variety of chemical agents in this group, with widely varying potencies. Most of them are poorly water-soluble, are often formulated with an aromatic hydrocarbon solvent such as xylene, and are well absorbed through intact skin. Most chemical warfare "nerve agents" (such as GA [tabun], GB [sarin], GD [soman] and VX) are organophosphates.

► Clinical Findings

Inhibition of cholinesterase results in abdominal cramps, diarrhea, vomiting, excessive salivation, sweating, lacrimation, miosis (constricted pupils), wheezing and bronchorrhea, seizures, and skeletal muscle weakness. Initial tachycardia is usually followed by bradycardia. Profound skeletal muscle weakness, aggravated by excessive bronchial secretions and wheezing, may result in respiratory arrest and death. Symptoms and signs of poisoning may persist or recur over several days, especially with highly lipid-soluble agents such as fenthion or dimethoate.

The diagnosis should be suspected in patients who present with miosis, sweating, and hyperperistalsis. Serum and red blood cell cholinesterase activity is usually depressed at least 50% below baseline in those victims who have severe intoxication.

► Treatment

A. Emergency and Supportive Measures

If the agent was recently ingested, consider gut decontamination by aspiration of the liquid using a nasogastric tube followed by administration of activated charcoal (see p. 1582). If the agent is on the victim's skin or hair, wash repeatedly with soap or shampoo and water. Providers should take care to avoid skin exposure by wearing gloves and waterproof aprons. Dilute hypochlorite solution (eg, household bleach diluted 1:10) is reported to help break down organophosphate pesticides and nerve agents on equipment or clothing.

B. Specific Treatment

Atropine reverses excessive muscarinic stimulation and is effective for treatment of salivation, bronchial hypersecretion, wheezing, abdominal cramping, and sweating. However, it does not interact with nicotinic receptors at autonomic ganglia and at the neuromuscular junction and has no direct effect on muscle weakness. Administer 2 mg intravenously, and if there is no response after 5 minutes, give repeated boluses in rapidly escalating doses (eg, doubling the dose each time) as needed to dry bronchial secretions and decrease wheezing; as much as several hundred milligrams of atropine has been given to treat severe poisoning.

Pralidoxime (2-PAM, Protopam) is a more specific antidote that reverses organophosphate binding to the cholinesterase enzyme; therefore, it should be effective at the neuromuscular junction as well as other nicotinic and muscarinic sites. It is most likely to be clinically effective if started very soon after poisoning, to prevent permanent binding of the organophosphate to cholinesterase. However, clinical studies have yielded conflicting results regarding the effectiveness of pralidoxime in reducing mortality. Administer 1–2 g intravenously as a loading dose, and begin a continuous infusion (200–500 mg/h, titrated to clinical response). Continue to give pralidoxime as long as there is any evidence of acetylcholine excess. Pralidoxime is of questionable benefit for carbamate poisoning, because carbamates have only a transitory effect on

the cholinesterase enzyme. Other, unproven therapies for organophosphate poisoning include magnesium, sodium bicarbonate, clonidine, and extracorporeal removal.

King AM et al. Organophosphate and carbamate poisoning. Emerg Med Clin North Am. 2015 Feb;33(1):133–51. [PMID: 25455666]
Peter JV et al. Clinical features of organophosphate poisoning: a review of different classification systems and approaches. Indian J Crit Care Med. 2014 Nov;18(11):735–45. [PMID: 25425841]

PETROLEUM DISTILLATES & SOLVENTS

Petroleum distillate toxicity may occur from inhalation of the vapor or as a result of pulmonary aspiration of the liquid during or after ingestion. Acute manifestations of aspiration pneumonitis are vomiting, coughing, and bronchopneumonia. Some hydrocarbons—ie, those with aromatic or halogenated subunits—can also cause severe systemic poisoning after oral ingestion. Hydrocarbons can also cause systemic intoxication by inhalation. Vertigo, muscular incoordination, irregular pulse, myoclonus, and seizures occur with serious poisoning and may be due to hypoxemia or the systemic effects of the agents. Chlorinated and fluorinated hydrocarbons (trichloroethylene, Freons, etc) and many other hydrocarbons can cause ventricular arrhythmias due to increased sensitivity of the myocardium to the effects of endogenous catecholamines.

► Treatment

Remove the patient to fresh air. For simple aliphatic hydrocarbon ingestion, gastric emptying and activated charcoal are not recommended, but these procedures may be indicated if the preparation contains toxic solutes (eg, an insecticide) or is an aromatic or halogenated product. Observe the victim for 6–8 hours for signs of aspiration pneumonitis (cough, localized crackles or rhonchi, tachypnea, and infiltrates on chest radiograph). Corticosteroids are not recommended. If fever occurs, give a specific antibiotic only after identification of bacterial pathogens by laboratory studies. Because of the risk of arrhythmias, use bronchodilators with caution in patients with chlorinated or fluorinated solvent intoxication. If tachyarrhythmias occur, use esmolol intravenously 25–100 mcg/kg/min.

Phatak DR et al. Huffing air conditioner fluid: a cool way to die? Am J Forensic Med Pathol. 2012 Mar;33(1):64–7. [PMID: 22442834]
Tormoehlen LM et al. Hydrocarbon toxicity: a review. Clin Toxicol (Phila). 2014 Jun;52(5):479–89. [PMID: 24911841]

SALICYLATES

Salicylates (aspirin, methyl salicylate, bismuth subsalicylate, etc) are found in a variety of over-the-counter and prescription medications. Salicylates uncouple cellular oxidative phosphorylation, resulting in anaerobic metabolism and excessive production of lactic acid and heat, and they also interfere with several Krebs cycle enzymes. A single ingestion of more than 200 mg/kg of salicylate is likely to produce significant acute intoxication. Poisoning may also occur as a result of chronic excessive dosing over several days. Although the half-life of salicylate is 2–3 hours after small doses, it may increase to 20 hours or more in patients with intoxication.

▶ Clinical Findings

Acute ingestion often causes nausea and vomiting, occasionally with gastritis. Moderate intoxication is characterized by hyperpnea (deep and rapid breathing), tachycardia, tinnitus, and elevated anion gap metabolic acidosis. (A normal anion gap sometimes occurs due to salicylate interference with the chemistry analyzer, falsely raising the measured chloride.) Serious intoxication may result in agitation, confusion, coma, seizures, cardiovascular collapse, pulmonary edema, hyperthermia, and death. The prothrombin time is often elevated owing to salicylate-induced hypoprothrombinemia. Central nervous system intracellular glucose depletion can occur despite normal measured serum glucose levels.

Diagnosis of salicylate poisoning is suspected in any patient with metabolic acidosis and is confirmed by measuring the serum salicylate level. Patients with levels greater than 100 mg/dL (1000 mg/L or 7.2 mcmol/L) after an acute overdose are more likely to have severe poisoning. On the other hand, patients with subacute or chronic intoxication may suffer severe symptoms with levels of only 60–70 mg/dL (4.3–5 mcmol/L). The arterial blood gas typically reveals a respiratory alkalosis with an underlying metabolic acidosis.

▶ Treatment

A. Emergency and Supportive Measures

Administer activated charcoal orally (see p. 1582). Gastric lavage followed by administration of extra doses of activated charcoal may be needed in patients who ingest more than 10 g of aspirin (see p. 1582). The desired ratio of charcoal to aspirin is about 10:1 by weight; while this cannot always be given as a single dose, it may be administered over the first 24 hours in divided doses every 2–4 hours along with whole bowel irrigation (see p. 1583). Give glucose-containing fluids to reduce the risk of cerebral hypoglycemia. Treat metabolic acidosis with intravenous sodium bicarbonate. This is critical because acidosis (especially acidemia, pH < 7.40) promotes greater entry of salicylate into cells, worsening toxicity. **Warning:** Sudden and severe deterioration can occur after rapid sequence intubation and controlled ventilation if the pH is allowed to fall during the apneic period.

B. Specific Treatment

Alkalinization of the urine enhances renal salicylate excretion by trapping the salicylate anion in the urine. Add 100 mEq (two ampules) of sodium bicarbonate to 1 L of 5% dextrose in 0.2% saline, and infuse this solution intravenously at a rate of about 150–200 mL/h. Unless the patient is oliguric or hyperkalemic, add 20–30 mEq of potassium chloride to each liter of intravenous fluid. Patients who are volume-depleted often fail to produce an alkaline urine (paradoxical aciduria) unless potassium is given.

Hemodialysis may be lifesaving and is indicated for patients with severe metabolic acidosis, markedly altered mental status, or significantly elevated salicylate levels (eg, greater than 100–120 mg/dL [1000–1200 mg/L or 7.2–8.6 mcmol/L] after acute overdose or greater than 60–70 mg/dL [600–700 mg/L or 4.3–5 mcmol/L] with subacute or chronic intoxication).

Juurlink DN et al. Extracorporeal treatment for salicylate poisoning: systematic review and recommendations from the EXTRIP Workgroup. Ann Emerg Med. 2015 Aug;66(2):165–81. [PMID: 25986310]

Lim CS et al. Those Salicylate Cases—How Sweet Are They? Am J Ther. 2014 Sep 17. [Epub ahead of print] [PMID: 25233267]

SEAFOOD POISONINGS

A variety of intoxications may occur after eating certain types of fish or other seafood. These include scombroid, ciguatera, paralytic shellfish, and puffer fish poisoning. The mechanisms of toxicity and clinical presentations are described in Table 38–9. In the majority of cases, the seafood has a normal appearance and taste (scombroid may have a peppery taste).

▶ Treatment

A. Emergency and Supportive Measures

Caution: Abrupt respiratory arrest may occur in patients with acute paralytic shellfish and puffer fish poisoning. Observe patients for at least 4–6 hours. Replace fluid and electrolyte losses from gastroenteritis with intravenous saline or other crystalloid solution.

For recent ingestions, it may be possible to adsorb residual toxin in the gut with activated charcoal, 50–60 g orally (see p. 1582).

B. Specific Treatment

There is no specific antidote for paralytic shellfish or puffer fish poisoning.

1. Ciguatera—There are anecdotal reports of successful treatment of acute neurologic symptoms with mannitol, 1 g/kg intravenously, but this approach is not widely accepted.

2. Scombroid—Antihistamines such as diphenhydramine, 25–50 mg intravenously, and the H_2-blocker cimetidine, 300 mg intravenously, are usually effective.

Chan TY. Epidemiology and clinical features of ciguatera fish poisoning in Hong Kong. Toxins (Basel). 2014 Oct 20; 6(10):2989–97. [PMID: 25333356]

Table 38–9. Common seafood poisonings.

Type of Poisoning	Mechanism	Clinical Presentation
Ciguatera	Reef fish ingest toxic dinoflagellates, whose toxins accumulate in fish meat. Commonly implicated fish in the United States are barracuda, jack, snapper, and grouper.	1–6 hours after ingestion, victims develop abdominal pain, vomiting, and diarrhea accompanied by a variety of neurologic symptoms, including paresthesias, reversal of hot and cold sensation, vertigo, headache, and intense itching. Autonomic disturbances, including hypotension and bradycardia, may occur.
Scombroid	Improper preservation of large fish results in bacterial degradation of histidine to histamine. Commonly implicated fish include tuna, mahimahi, bonita, mackerel, and kingfish.	Allergic-like (anaphylactoid) symptoms are due to histamine, usually begin within 15–90 minutes, and include skin flushing, itching, urticaria, angioedema, bronchospasm, and hypotension as well as abdominal pain, vomiting, and diarrhea.
Paralytic shellfish poisoning	Dinoflagellates produce saxitoxin, which is concentrated by filter-feeding mussels and clams. Saxitoxin blocks sodium conductance and neuronal transmission in skeletal muscles.	Onset is usually within 30–60 minutes. Initial symptoms include perioral and intraoral paresthesias. Other symptoms include nausea and vomiting, headache, dizziness, dysphagia, dysarthria, ataxia, and rapidly progressive muscle weakness that may result in respiratory arrest.
Puffer fish poisoning	Tetrodotoxin is concentrated in liver, gonads, intestine, and skin. Toxic effects are similar to those of saxitoxin. Tetrodotoxin is also found in some North American newts and Central American frogs.	Onset is usually within 30–40 minutes but may be as short as 10 minutes. Initial perioral paresthesias are followed by headache, diaphoresis, nausea, vomiting, ataxia, and rapidly progressive muscle weakness that may result in respiratory arrest.

Feng C et al. Histamine (scombroid) fish poisoning: a comprehensive review. Clin Rev Allergy Immunol. 2016 Feb;50(1):64–9. [PMID: 25876709]

Goodman DM et al. JAMA patient page. Ciguatera fish poisoning. JAMA. 2013 Jun 26;309(24):2608. [PMID: 23800938]

SNAKE BITES

The venom of poisonous snakes and lizards may be predominantly neurotoxic (coral snake) or predominantly cytolytic (rattlesnakes, other pit vipers). Neurotoxins cause respiratory paralysis; cytolytic venoms cause tissue destruction by digestion and hemorrhage due to hemolysis and destruction of the endothelial lining of the blood vessels. The manifestations of rattlesnake envenomation are mostly local pain, redness, swelling, and extravasation of blood. Perioral tingling, metallic taste, nausea and vomiting, hypotension, and coagulopathy may also occur. Thrombocytopenia can persist for several days after a rattlesnake bite. Neurotoxic envenomation may cause ptosis, dysphagia, diplopia, and respiratory arrest.

▶ Treatment

A. Emergency Measures

Immobilize the patient and the bitten part in a neutral position. Avoid manipulation of the bitten area. Transport the patient to a medical facility for definitive treatment. Do *not* give alcoholic beverages or stimulants; do *not* apply ice; do *not* apply a tourniquet. The potential trauma to underlying tissues resulting from incision and suction performed by unskilled people is probably not justified in view of the small amount of venom that can be recovered.

B. Specific Antidote and General Measures

1. Pit viper (eg, rattlesnake) envenomation—For local signs such as swelling, pain, and ecchymosis but no systemic symptoms, give 4–6 vials of crotalid antivenin (CroFab) by slow intravenous drip in 250–500 mL saline. Repeated doses of 2 vials every 6 hours for up to 18 hours have been recommended, but many clinicians give additional doses only if needed. For more serious envenomation with marked local effects and systemic toxicity (eg, hypotension, coagulopathy), higher doses and additional vials may be required. Monitor vital signs and the blood coagulation profile. Type and cross-match blood. The adequacy of venom neutralization is indicated by improvement in symptoms and signs, and the rate that swelling slows. Prophylactic antibiotics are not indicated after a rattlesnake bite.

2. Elapid (coral snake) envenomation—Give 1–2 vials of specific antivenom as soon as possible. **Note:** Pfizer/Wyeth no longer makes coral snake antivenom in the United States and remaining supplies are dwindling. To locate antisera for this or exotic snakes, call a regional poison control center (1-800-222-1222).

Kanaan NC et al. Wilderness Medical Society practice guidelines for the treatment of pitviper envenomations in the United States and Canada. Wilderness Environ Med. 2015 Dec; 26(4):472–87. [PMID: 26433731]

Punguyire D et al. Bedside whole-blood clotting times: validity after snakebites. J Emerg Med. 2013 Mar;44(3):663–7. [PMID: 23047197]

Spano S et al. Snakebite Survivors Club: retrospective review of rattlesnake bites in Central California. Toxicon. 2013 Jul; 69:38–41. [PMID: 23200707]

Wood A et al. Review of Eastern coral snake (*Micrurus fulvius fulvius*) exposures managed by the Florida Poison Information Center Network: 1998-2010. Clin Toxicol (Phila). 2013 Sep–Oct;51(8):783–8. [PMID: 23962099]

SPIDER BITES & SCORPION STINGS

The toxin of most species of spiders in the United States causes only local pain, redness, and swelling. That of the more venomous black widow spiders (*Latrodectus mactans*) causes generalized muscular pains, muscle spasms, and rigidity. The brown recluse spider (*Loxosceles reclusa*) causes progressive local necrosis as well as hemolytic reactions (rare).

Stings by most scorpions in the United States cause only local pain. Stings by the more toxic *Centruroides* species (found in the southwestern United States) may cause muscle cramps, twitching and jerking, and occasionally hypertension, convulsions, and pulmonary edema. Stings by scorpions from other parts of the world are not discussed here.

► Treatment

A. Black Widow Spider Bites

Pain may be relieved with parenteral opioids or muscle relaxants (eg, methocarbamol, 15 mg/kg). Calcium gluconate 10%, 0.1–0.2 mL/kg intravenously, may transiently relieve muscle rigidity, though its effectiveness is unproven. *Latrodectus* antivenom is possibly more effective, but because of concerns about acute hypersensitivity reactions (horse serum-derived), it is often reserved for very young or elderly patients or those who do not respond promptly to the above measures. Horse serum sensitivity testing is required. (Instruction and testing materials are included in the antivenin kit.)

B. Brown Recluse Spider Bites

Because bites occasionally progress to extensive local necrosis, some authorities recommend early excision of the bite site, whereas others use oral corticosteroids. Anecdotal reports have claimed success with dapsone and colchicine. All of these treatments remain of unproved value.

C. Scorpion Stings

No specific treatment other than analgesics is required for envenomations by most scorpions found in the United States. An FDA-approved specific antivenom is available for *Centruroides* stings.

Boyer LV et al. Effectiveness of *Centruroides* scorpion antivenom compared to historical controls. Toxicon. 2013 Dec 15;76:377–85. [PMID: 23911733]

Dart RC et al. A randomized, double-blind, placebo-controlled trial of a highly purified equine F(ab)2 antibody black widow spider antivenom. Ann Emerg Med. 2013 Apr;61(4):458–67. [PMID: 23380292]

Isbister GK et al. Randomized controlled trial of intravenous antivenom versus placebo for latrodectism: the second Redback Antivenom Evaluation (RAVE-II) study. Ann Emerg Med. 2014 Dec;64(6):620–8.e2. [PMID: 24999282]

THEOPHYLLINE & CAFFEINE

Theophylline may cause intoxication after an acute single overdose, or intoxication may occur as a result of chronic accidental repeated overmedication or reduced elimination resulting from hepatic dysfunction or interacting drug (eg, cimetidine, erythromycin). The usual serum half-life of theophylline is 4–6 hours, but this may increase to more than 20 hours after overdose. Caffeine in energy drinks, herbal or dietary supplement products can produce similar toxicity.

► Clinical Findings

Mild intoxication causes nausea, vomiting, tachycardia, and tremulousness. Severe intoxication is characterized by ventricular and supraventricular tachyarrhythmias, hypotension, and seizures. Status epilepticus is common and often intractable to the usual anticonvulsants. After acute overdose (but not chronic intoxication), hypokalemia, hyperglycemia, and metabolic acidosis are common. Seizures and other manifestations of toxicity may be delayed for several hours after acute ingestion, especially if a sustained-release preparation such as Theo-Dur was taken.

Diagnosis is based on measurement of the serum theophylline concentration. Seizures and hypotension are likely to develop in acute overdose patients with serum levels greater than 100 mg/L (555 mcmol/L). Serious toxicity may develop at lower levels (ie, 40–60 mg/L [222–333 mcmol/L]) in patients with chronic intoxication.

► Treatment

A. Emergency and Supportive Measures

After acute ingestion, administer activated charcoal (see p. 1582). Repeated doses of activated charcoal may enhance theophylline elimination by "gut dialysis." Addition of whole bowel irrigation should be considered for large ingestions involving sustained-release preparations (see p. 1582).

Hemodialysis is effective in removing theophylline and is indicated for patients with status epilepticus or markedly elevated serum theophylline levels (eg, greater than 100 mg/L [555 mcmol/L] after acute overdose or greater than 60 mg/L [333 mcmol/L] with chronic intoxication).

B. Specific Treatment

Treat seizures with benzodiazepines (lorazepam, 2–3 mg intravenously, or diazepam, 5–10 mg intravenously) or phenobarbital (10–15 mg/kg intravenously). Phenytoin is not effective. Hypotension and tachycardia—which are mediated through excessive beta-adrenergic stimulation—may respond to beta-blocker therapy even in low doses. Administer esmolol, 25–50 mcg/kg/min by intravenous infusion, or propranolol, 0.5–1 mg intravenously.

Jabbar SB et al. Fatal caffeine overdose: a case report and review of literature. Am J Forensic Med Pathol. 2013 Dec;34(4):321–4. [PMID: 24196726]

Kneser J et al. Successful treatment of life threatening theophylline intoxication in a pregnant patient by hemodialysis. Clin Nephrol. 2013 Jul;80(1):72–4. [PMID: 22541679]

Laskowski LK et al. Start me up! Recurrent ventricular tachydys-rhythmias following intentional concentrated caffeine ingestion. Clin Toxicol (Phila). 2015;53(8):830–3. [PMID: 26279469]

TRICYCLIC & OTHER ANTIDEPRESSANTS

Tricyclic and related cyclic antidepressants are among the most dangerous drugs involved in suicidal overdose. These drugs have anticholinergic and cardiac depressant properties ("quinidine-like" sodium channel blockade). Tricyclic antidepressants produce more marked membrane-depressant cardiotoxic effects than the phenothiazines.

Newer generation antidepressants such as trazodone, fluoxetine, citalopram, paroxetine, sertraline, bupropion, venlafaxine, and fluvoxamine are not chemically related to the tricyclic antidepressant agents and do not generally produce quinidine-like cardiotoxic effects. However, they may cause seizures in overdoses and they may cause serotonin syndrome.

► Clinical Findings

Signs of severe intoxication may occur abruptly and without warning within 30–60 minutes after acute tricyclic overdose. Anticholinergic effects include dilated pupils, tachycardia, dry mouth, flushed skin, muscle twitching, and decreased peristalsis. Quinidine-like cardiotoxic effects include QRS interval widening (greater than 0.12 s; Figure 38–2), ventricular arrhythmias, AV block, and hypotension. Rightward-axis deviation of the terminal 40 ms of the QRS has also been described. Prolongation of the QT interval and torsades de pointes have been reported with several of the newer antidepressants. Seizures and coma are common with severe intoxication. Life-threatening hyperthermia

▲ **Figure 38–2.** Cardiac arrhythmias resulting from tricyclic antidepressant overdose. *A*: Delayed intraventricular conduction results in prolonged QRS interval (0.18 s). *B* and *C*: Supraventricular tachycardia with progressive widening of QRS complexes mimics ventricular tachycardia. (Reproduced, with permission, from Benowitz NL, Goldschlager N. Cardiac disturbances in the toxicologic patient. In: Haddad LM, Winchester JF [editors], *Clinical Management of Poisoning and Drug Overdose*, 3rd edition. Saunders/Elsevier, 1998.)

may result from status epilepticus and anticholinergic-induced impairment of sweating. Among newer agents, bupropion and venlafaxine have been associated with a greater risk of seizures.

The diagnosis should be suspected in any overdose patient with anticholinergic side effects, especially if there is widening of the QRS interval or seizures. For intoxication by most tricyclic antidepressants, the QRS interval correlates with the severity of intoxication more reliably than the serum drug level.

Serotonin syndrome should be suspected if agitation, delirium, diaphoresis, tremor, hyperreflexia, clonus (spontaneous, inducible, or ocular), and fever develop in a patient taking serotonin reuptake inhibitors.

► Treatment

A. Emergency and Supportive Measures

Observe patients for at least 6 hours, and admit all patients with evidence of anticholinergic effects (eg, delirium, dilated pupils, tachycardia) or signs of cardiotoxicity.

Administer activated charcoal (see p. 1582) and consider gastric lavage (see p. 1582) after recent large ingestions. All of these drugs are highly tissue-bound and are not effectively removed by hemodialysis procedures.

B. Specific Treatment

Cardiotoxic sodium channel-depressant effects of tricyclic antidepressants may respond to boluses of sodium bicarbonate (50–100 mEq intravenously). Sodium bicarbonate provides a large sodium load that alleviates depression of the sodium-dependent channel. Reversal of acidosis may also have beneficial effects at this site. Maintain the pH between 7.45 and 7.50. Alkalinization does not promote excretion of tricyclic antidepressants. Prolongation of the QT interval or torsades de pointes is usually treated with intravenous magnesium or overdrive pacing. Severe cardiotoxicity in patients with overdoses of lipid-soluble drugs (eg, amitriptyline, bupropion) has responded to intravenous lipid emulsion (Intralipid), 1.5 mL/kg repeated one or two times if needed. Plasma exchange using albumin has been reported successful in a few cases.

Mild serotonin syndrome may be treated with benzodiazepines and withdrawal of the antidepressant. Moderate cases may respond to cyproheptadine (4 mg orally or via gastric tube hourly for three or four doses) or chlorpromazine (25 mg intravenously). Severe hyperthermia should be treated with neuromuscular paralysis and endotracheal intubation in addition to external cooling measures.

Bruccoleri RE et al. A literature review of the use of sodium bicarbonate for the treatment of QRS widening. J Med Toxicol. 2016 Mar;12(1):121–9. [PMID: 26159649]
Kiberd MB et al. Lipid therapy for the treatment of a refractory amitriptyline overdose. CJEM. 2012 May;14(3):193–7. [PMID: 22575302]
Paksu S et al. Amitriptyline overdose in emergency department of university hospital: Evaluation of 250 patients. Hum Exp Toxicol. 2014 Feb 6;33(9):980–90. [PMID: 24505046]

Cancer

39

Patricia A. Cornett, MD
Tiffany O. Dea, PharmD

► Etiology

Cancer is the second most common cause of death in the United States. In 2015, an estimated 1,658,370 cases of cancer were diagnosed, and 589,430 persons died as a result of cancer. Based on current statistics, one in three Americans will be diagnosed with cancer in their lifetime. Table 39–1 lists the 10 leading cancer types in men and women by site.

However, the death rates from cancer are decreasing. Compared to the 1991 cancer death rate of 215.1 per 100,000 population, the 2009 rate of 173.1 per 100,000 represents a 20% reduction in its death rate. Importantly, death rates have declined in the four most common cancer types (lung, colon-rectum, breast, and prostate). The largest declines in death rates have been seen in chronic myeloid leukemia, stomach and colorectal cancer, and non-Hodgkin lymphoma.

Reductions in cancer mortality reflect a successful implementation of a broad strategy of prevention, detection, and treatment. Due to these improvements, the number of cancer survivors is increasing. In 2015, an estimated 14.5 million people were alive in whom cancer had been diagnosed at some point previously; that number is projected to grow to 18.9 million in 2024.

► Modifiable Risk Factors

Tobacco is the most common preventable cause of cancer death; it is estimated that at least 30% of all cancer deaths in the United States are directly linked to tobacco. In 2013, a total of 174,100 cancer deaths in the United States could be directly attributed to tobacco abuse. Clear evidence links at least 15 cancers to tobacco use. The most dramatic link is with lung cancer; 80% of lung cancer cases occur in smokers. Remarkably, among individuals who are long-term survivors of a tobacco-related cancer, almost 10% continue to use tobacco products, increasing their risk of yet another cancer.

Tobacco cessation directed toward the individual should start with the clinician providing counseling. Simple, concise advice from a clinician can yield cessation rates of 10–20%. Additive strategies include more intensive counseling; nicotine replacement therapy with patches, gum, or lozenges; and prescription medication with bupropion or varenicline (see Chapter 1).

On a societal level, state or local laws regulating tobacco use in restaurants, the workplace, and other public places have resulted in declines in tobacco use. Countermarketing with aggressive anti-tobacco advertisements has also contributed to tobacco cessation and abstinence. The key recipients of these messages are children; 80% of smokers will start by age 18.

There are encouraging signs of success with tobacco control. The prevalence of smoking for US adults based on the 2015 National Health Interview Survey is 17.0%, which is a remarkable reduction from the 1955 peak of 57% for males and the 1965 peak of 34% for females.

For those Americans who do not use tobacco, the most modifiable risk factors would be nutrition and physical activity. Prudent recommendations to reduce cancer risk are to (1) avoid tobacco, (2) be physically active, (3) maintain a healthy weight, (4) consume a diet rich in fruits, vegetables, and whole grains, (5) lower consumption of saturated and trans dietary fats, (6) limit alcohol use, and (7) avoid excess sun exposure.

Another modifiable risk factor is radiation from radiographic studies. A 2009 study reported that the use of computed tomography (CT) in diagnostic algorithms exposes individuals to significant radiation doses that may increase the lifetime risk of developing cancer. Both standardization of CT radiation doses and limiting testing have been important steps in minimizing this risk. Both the American Society of Hematology and the American Society of Clinical Oncology have guidelines, inspired by the American Board of Internal Medicine Foundation's "Choosing Wisely" campaign, for limiting radiographic testing, particularly when used in surveillance for treated cancer patients.

American Society of Clinical Oncology. http://www.asco.org

Department of Health and Human Services. Healthy People 2020. Tobacco use objectives: reduce tobacco use by adults. http://www.healthypeople.gov/2020/topicsobjectives2020/objectiveslist.aspx?topicId=41

National Cancer Institute. Cancer types. http://www.cancer.gov/types

Table 39–1. Estimated 10 most common cancer cases in the United States in males and females (all races).

Rank	Males — Total Cases = 848,200 (percent)	Females — Total Cases = 810,170 (percent)
1	Prostate (26)	Breast (29)
2	Lung and bronchus (14)	Lung and bronchus (13)
3	Colon and rectum (8)	Colon and rectum (8)
4	Urinary bladder (7)	Uterine corpus (7)
5	Lymphoma (5)	Thyroid (6)
6	Melanoma (5)	Lymphoma (4)
7	Kidney and renal pelvis (5)	Melanoma (4)
8	Oral cavity and pharynx (4)	Kidney and renal pelvis (3)
9	Leukemia (4)	Pancreas (3)
10	Liver and intrahepatic bile duct (3)	Leukemia (3)
	Other sites (19)	Other sites (20)

Data from the American Cancer Society, 2015.

National Comprehensive Cancer Network. http://www.nccn.org
Siegel RL et al. Cancer statistics, 2015. CA Cancer J Clin. 2015 Jan–Feb;65(1):5–29. [PMID: 25559415]
Weber WA et al. Surveillance of cancer patients with imaging: self-evident or evidence-based? J Nucl Med. 2013 Sep; 54(9):1513–5. [PMID: 23929825]

Staging

The most commonly used staging system at the time of diagnosis is the TNM (Tumor, Nodes, Metastasis) system (see www.cancerstaging.org). Rules for staging for individual cancers are established and published by the American Joint Committee on Cancer (AJCC). The elements used for staging are tumor location, size and level of tumor invasion (T), absence or presence and extent of nodal metastases (N), and presence or absence of systemic metastases (M). Once the TNM designations have been determined, an overall stage is assigned, stage I, II, III, or IV. Clinical staging utilizes physical examination, laboratory and imaging tests as well as results from biopsies; pathologic staging relies on the results from surgery. In some instances, other classifications may be used for certain cancers such as the Ann Arbor staging system for lymphomas.

Other characteristics of cancers, not reflected in the TNM stage, may be used as another indicator of prognosis and guidelines for treatment. Pathologic features seen on routine histologic examination for some cancers are very important; examples include the Gleason score for prostate cancer and the grade of sarcomas. Cancer specimens should also be sent for targeted molecular diagnostic testing, when appropriate. Examples include testing for *HER2* in breast and gastric cancers, *K-ras* and *BRAF* mutations in colorectal cancers, *BRAF* mutations in melanoma, and epidermal growth factor receptor (EGFR), *K-ras* mutations and the *ALK* fusion gene in lung cancer.

▼ **TYPES OF CANCER**

LUNG CANCER

Sunny Wang, MD

BRONCHOGENIC CARCINOMA

ESSENTIALS OF DIAGNOSIS

▶ New cough, or change in chronic cough.

▶ Dyspnea, hemoptysis, anorexia, weight loss.

▶ Enlarging nodule or mass; persistent opacity, atelectasis, or pleural effusion on chest radiograph or CT scan.

▶ Cytologic or histologic findings of lung cancer in sputum, pleural fluid, or biopsy specimen.

▶ **General Considerations**

Lung cancer is the leading cause of cancer deaths in both men and women. The American Cancer Society estimates 221,220 new diagnoses and 158,040 deaths from lung cancer in the United States in 2015, accounting for approximately 13% of new cancer diagnoses and 27% of all cancer deaths. More Americans die of lung cancer than of colorectal, breast, and prostate cancers combined.

Cigarette smoking causes 85–90% of cases of lung cancer. The causal connection between cigarettes and lung cancer is established not only epidemiologically but also through identification of carcinogens in tobacco smoke and analysis of the effect of these carcinogens on specific oncogenes expressed in lung cancer.

Other environmental risk factors for the development of lung cancer include exposure to environmental tobacco smoke, radon gas, asbestos, metals (arsenic, chromium, nickel, iron oxide), and industrial carcinogens (bis-chloromethyl ether). A familial predisposition to lung cancer is recognized. Certain diseases are associated with an increased risk of lung cancer, including pulmonary fibrosis, chronic obstructive pulmonary disease, and sarcoidosis.

The median age at diagnosis of lung cancer in the United States is 70; it is unusual under the age of 40. The combined relative 5-year survival rate for all stages of lung cancer is currently 17%.

Five histologic categories of bronchogenic carcinoma account for more than 90% of cases of primary lung cancer. **Squamous cell carcinomas** (22% of cases, based on US SEER data 2007–2011) arise from the bronchial epithelium and often present as an intraluminal mass. They are usually centrally located and more likely than other types of bronchogenic carcinoma to present with hemoptysis. Squamous cell carcinomas stain for P63 and P40 on immunohistochemistry. **Adenocarcinomas** (42% of cases) arise from mucous glands or from any epithelial cell within or distal to the terminal bronchioles. They usually present as peripheral nodules or masses and stain for TTF-1 and Napsin-A on immunohistochemistry. **Adenocarcinomas in situ** (formerly **bronchioloalveolar cell carcinomas**) spread along preexisting alveolar structures (lepidic growth) without evidence of invasion. **Large cell carcinomas** (2% of cases) are a heterogeneous group of undifferentiated cancers that share large cells and do not fit into other categories. Large cell carcinomas are typically aggressive and have rapid doubling times. They present as central or peripheral masses. Cancers that are not better differentiated on pathologic review other than non–small cell carcinomas (NSCLC) or carcinomas not otherwise specified make up about 16% of cases. **Small cell carcinomas** (13% of cases) are tumors of bronchial origin that typically begin centrally, infiltrating submucosally to cause narrowing of the bronchus without a discrete luminal mass. They are aggressive cancers that often involve regional or distant metastasis on presentation.

For purposes of staging and treatment, bronchogenic carcinomas are divided into small cell lung cancer (SCLC) and the other four types, labeled NSCLC. SCLC is prone to early hematogenous spread. It is rarely amenable to surgical resection and has a very aggressive course with a median survival (untreated) of 6–18 weeks. The four histologic categories comprising NSCLC spread more slowly. They may be cured in the early stages following resection, and for advanced disease, chemotherapy is tailored to specific histologies and molecular mutations.

▶ Clinical Findings

Lung cancer is symptomatic at diagnosis in over 75% of patients. The clinical presentation depends on the type and location of the primary tumor, the extent of local spread, and the presence of distant metastases and any paraneoplastic syndromes.

A. Symptoms and Signs

Anorexia, weight loss, or asthenia occurs in 55–90% of patients presenting with a new diagnosis of lung cancer. Up to 60% of patients have a new cough or a change in a chronic cough; 6–31% have hemoptysis; and 25–40% complain of pain, either nonspecific chest pain or pain from bony metastases to the vertebrae, ribs, or pelvis. Local spread may cause endobronchial obstruction with atelectasis and postobstructive pneumonia, pleural effusion (12–33%), change in voice (compromise of the recurrent laryngeal nerve), superior vena cava syndrome (obstruction of the superior vena cava with supraclavicular venous engorgement), and Horner syndrome (ipsilateral ptosis, miosis, and anhidrosis from involvement of the inferior cervical ganglion and the paravertebral sympathetic chain). Distant metastases to the liver are associated with asthenia and weight loss. Brain metastases (10% in NSCLC, more common in adenocarcinoma, and 20–30% in SCLC) may present with headache, nausea, vomiting, seizures, dizziness, or altered mental status.

Paraneoplastic syndromes are patterns of organ dysfunction related to immune-mediated or secretory effects of neoplasms. These syndromes occur in 10–20% of lung cancer patients. They may precede, accompany, or follow the diagnosis of lung cancer. In patients with small cell carcinoma, the syndrome of inappropriate antidiuretic hormone (SIADH) can develop in 10–15%; in those with squamous cell carcinoma, hypercalcemia can develop in 10%. Digital clubbing is seen in up to 20% of patients at diagnosis (see Figure 6–40). Other common paraneoplastic syndromes include increased ACTH production, anemia, hypercoagulability, peripheral neuropathy, and the Lambert-Eaton myasthenic syndrome. Their recognition is important because treatment of the primary tumor may improve or resolve symptoms even when the cancer is not curable.

B. Laboratory Findings

The diagnosis of lung cancer rests on examination of a tissue or cytology specimen. **Sputum cytology** is highly specific but insensitive; the yield is highest when there are lesions in the central airways. **Thoracentesis** (sensitivity 50–65%) can be used to establish a diagnosis of lung cancer in patients with malignant pleural effusions. Fine-needle aspiration (FNA) of palpable supraclavicular or cervical lymph nodes is frequently diagnostic. Serum tumor markers are neither sensitive nor specific enough to aid in diagnosis.

Fiberoptic bronchoscopy allows visualization of the major airways, cytology brushing of visible lesions or lavage of lung segments with cytologic evaluation of specimens, direct biopsy of endobronchial abnormalities, blind transbronchial biopsy of the pulmonary parenchyma or peripheral nodules, and FNA biopsy of mediastinal lymph nodes. Diagnostic yield varies widely (10–90%) depending on the size of the lesion and its location. The use of fluorescence bronchoscopy improves the ability to identify early endobronchial lesions, and endobronchial and transesophageal endoscopic ultrasound enhance the direction and yield of FNA of mediastinal nodes. Electromagnetic navigational bronchoscopy has emerged, allowing bronchoscopic approaches to small peripheral nodules. While the diagnostic yield of CT-guided FNA of peripheral nodules approaches 80–90%, the rates of pneumothorax are significant (15–30%), especially in those with emphysema. Mediastinoscopy, video-assisted thoracoscopic surgery (VATS), and thoracotomy are necessary in cases where less invasive techniques fail to yield a diagnosis.

C. Imaging

Nearly all patients with lung cancer have abnormal findings on chest radiography or CT scan. These findings are rarely specific for a particular diagnosis. Interpretation of characteristic findings in isolated nodules is described in Chapter 9.

D. Special Examinations

1. Staging—Accurate staging is crucial (1) to provide the clinician with information to guide treatment, (2) to provide the patient with accurate information regarding prognosis, and (3) to standardize entry criteria for clinical trials to allow interpretation of results.

There are two essential principles of staging **NSCLC**. First, the more extensive the disease, the worse the prognosis; second, surgical resection offers the best chance for cure. Staging of NSCLC uses two integrated systems. The **TNM international staging system** attempts a physical description of the neoplasm: T describes the size and location of the primary tumor; N describes the presence and location of nodal metastases; and M refers to the presence or absence of distant metastases. These TNM stages are grouped into summary stages I–IV, and these are used to guide therapy. Many patients with stage I and stage II disease are cured through surgery. Patients with stage IIIB and stage IV disease do not benefit from surgery (Table 39–2). Patients with stage IIIA disease have locally invasive disease that may benefit from surgery in selected cases as part of multimodality therapy.

SCLC is traditionally divided into two categories: **limited disease** (30%), when the tumor is limited to the unilateral hemithorax (including contralateral mediastinal nodes); or **extensive disease** (70%), when the tumor extends beyond the hemithorax (including pleural effusion). It is also recommended to stage SCLC according to the TNM staging system.

For both SCLC and NSCLC, staging begins with a thorough history and physical examination. A complete examination is essential to exclude obvious metastatic disease to lymph nodes, skin, and bone. A detailed history is essential because the patient's performance status is a powerful predictor of disease course. All patients should have measurement of a complete blood count (CBC), serum electrolytes, calcium, creatinine, liver tests, lactate dehydrogenase, and albumin.

NSCLC patients being considered for surgery require meticulous evaluation to identify those with resectable disease. CT imaging is key for staging candidates for resection. A chest CT scan precisely defines the size of parenchymal lesions and identifies atelectatic lung or pleural effusions. However, CT imaging is less accurate at determining invasion of the chest wall (sensitivity 62%) or mediastinum (sensitivity 60–75%). The sensitivity and specificity of CT imaging for identifying lung cancer metastatic to the mediastinal lymph nodes are 57% (49–66%) and 82% (77–86%), respectively. Therefore, chest CT imaging alone does not provide definitive staging information. CT imaging helps determine where to biopsy, and how the mediastinum should be sampled.

Positron emission tomography (PET) using 2-[^{18}F] fluoro-2-deoxyglucose (FDG) is an important modality for identifying metastatic foci in the mediastinum or distant sites. The sensitivity and specificity of PET for detecting mediastinal spread of primary lung cancer depend on the size of mediastinal nodes or masses. When mediastinal lymph nodes smaller than 1 cm are present, the sensitivity and specificity of PET for tumor involvement of nodes are 74% and 96%, respectively. When CT shows lymph nodes larger than 1 cm, the sensitivity and specificity are 95% and 76%, respectively.

The combination of PET and CT imaging has improved preoperative staging compared with CT or PET alone. Whole body fusion PET-CT imaging is most useful to confirm lack of regional or metastatic disease in NSCLC patients who are candidates for surgical resection. If regional lymph nodes are less than 1 cm and without FDG uptake with no distant metastases seen on PET-CT, the mediastinum is often sampled at surgical resection if the patient is a surgical candidate. If there are lymph nodes larger than 1–2 cm with or without FDG uptake, or if there are sites of potential metastatic disease, attempts to determine malignant involvement include endobronchial ultrasound, endoscopic ultrasound with transesophageal needle aspiration, mediastinoscopy, CT-guided FNA, or limited thoracotomy to biopsy suspected regional or metastatic disease.

Disadvantages of PET imaging include limited resolution below 1 cm and false-positive scans due to sarcoidosis, tuberculosis, or fungal infections. PET-CT scans are also inadequate for evaluating brain metastases due to the high FDG uptake there. Obtaining an MRI of the brain is important to rule out brain metastases in patients with SCLC and in patients with NSCLC with at least stage II disease or poorly differentiated histologies.

2. Preoperative assessment—See Chapter 3.

3. Pulmonary function testing—Many patients with NSCLC have moderate to severe chronic lung disease that increases the risk of perioperative complications as well as long-term pulmonary insufficiency following lung resection. All patients considered for surgery require spirometry. In the absence of other comorbidities, patients with

Table 39–2. Five-year survival rates for non–small cell lung cancer, based on TNM staging.

Stage	TNM subset	5-Year Survival for Clinical TNM	5-Year Survival for Pathologic TNM
0	Carcinoma in situ		
IA	T1a/T1b, N0M0	50–80%	73%
IB	T2aN0M0	47%	58%
IIA	T1a/T1b, N1M0 T2aN1M0 T2bN0M0	36%	46%
IIB	T2bN1M0 T3N0M0	26%	36%
IIIA	T1/T2, N2M0 T3, N1/N2, M0 T4, N0/N1, M0	19%	24%
IIIB	T4N2M0 Any T, N3, M0	7%	9%
IV	Any T, Any N, M1a/M1b	2%	13%

Data from multiple sources. Modified and reproduced, with permission, from Tsim S et al. Staging of non-small-cell lung cancer (NSCLC): a review. Respir Med. 2010 Dec;104(12):1767–74. and Goldstraw P et al. The IASLC Lung Cancer Staging Project: proposals for the revision of the TNM stage groupings in the forthcoming (seventh) edition of the TNM Classification of malignant tumours. J Thorac Oncol. 2007 Aug;2(8):706–14.

good lung function (preoperative $FEV_1$2 L or more) are at low risk for complications from lobectomy or pneumonectomy. If the FEV_1 is less than 2 L, then an estimated postoperative FEV_1 should be made. A predicted post-lung resection FEV_1 greater than 800 mL (or greater than 40% of predicted FEV_1) is associated with a low incidence of perioperative complications. High-risk patients include those with a predicted postoperative FEV_1 less than 700 mL (or less than 40% of predicted FEV_1). In these patients and in those with borderline spirometry, cardiopulmonary exercise testing may be helpful. A maximal oxygen uptake ($\dot{V}O_2$) of greater than 15 mL/kg/min identifies patients with an acceptable incidence of complications and mortality. Patients with a $\dot{V}O_2$ of less than 10 mL/kg/min have a very high mortality rate at thoracotomy.

4. Screening—Screening with low-dose helical CT scans has been shown to improve mortality rates for lung cancer. The National Lung Screening Trial, a multicenter randomized US trial involving over 53,000 current and former heavy smokers, showed that screening annually with low-dose helical CT for 3 years yielded a 20% relative reduction in lung cancer mortality and 6.7% reduction in all-cause mortality compared to chest radiography. Given these findings, US professional organizations, including the US Preventive Services Task Force, have recommended screening with low-dose helical CT for lung cancer. Recent analysis of the National Lung Screening Trial data showed cost-effective estimates of $81,000 per quality-adjusted life years (QALY) gained and $52,000 per life year gained, but with wide variation in estimates according to specific subsets. The results of ongoing European trials on lung cancer screening, in particular the NELSON trial in the Netherlands, are awaited. The implications of widespread screening of smokers raise issues of high rates of false positives, surgical and medical complications from additional testing, risks of cumulative exposure to radiation, and risks of increasing patient anxiety and stress on an already limited pool of resources. Improved risk stratification to target a higher risk population for low-dose CT screening may help alleviate these costs and concerns. Smoking cessation policies and efforts should be integrated with any screening program.

▶ **Treatment**

A. Non–Small Cell Lung Carcinoma

Cure of NSCLC is unlikely without resection. Therefore, the initial approach to the patient is determined by answering two questions: (1) Is complete surgical resection technically feasible? (2) If yes, is the patient able to tolerate the surgery with acceptable morbidity and mortality? Clinical features that preclude complete resection include extrathoracic metastases or a malignant pleural effusion; or tumor involving the heart, pericardium, great vessels, esophagus, recurrent laryngeal or phrenic nerves, trachea, main carina, or contralateral mediastinal lymph nodes. Accordingly, stage I and stage II patients are treated with surgical resection where possible. Stage II and select cases of stage IB are additionally recommended to receive adjuvant chemotherapy. Stage IIIA patients have poor outcomes when treated with resection alone. They should undergo multimodality treatment that includes chemotherapy or radiotherapy, or both. Stage IIIB patients treated with concurrent chemotherapy and radiation therapy have improved survival. Stage IV patients are treated with chemotherapy or symptom-based palliative therapy, or both.

Surgical approach affects outcome. In 1994, the North American Lung Cancer Study Group conducted a prospective trial of stage IA patients randomized to lobectomy versus limited resection. They reported a threefold increased rate of local recurrence in the limited resection group ($P = 0.008$) and a trend toward an increase in overall death rate (increase of 30%, $P = 0.08$) and increase in cancer-related death rate (increase of 50%, $P = 0.09$), compared with patients receiving lobectomy. However, for patients who cannot tolerate lobectomy, a sublobar resection (wedge resection or segmentectomy) may be considered. Given improved technology in detecting smaller tumors, a large randomized study is evaluating sublobar resection versus lobectomy for patients with peripheral tumors smaller than 2 cm. VATS has become an acceptable and reasonable alternative to standard thoracotomy, if there are no anatomic or surgical contraindications, based on large case series showing equivalent long-term outcomes and less short-term morbidity. Radiation therapy following surgery is considered for margin-positive disease or pathologic mediastinal lymph node involvement.

Patients with clinical stage I primary NSCLC, who are not candidates for surgery because of significant comorbidity or other surgical contraindication, may be candidates for stereotactic body radiotherapy. Stereotactic body radiotherapy, which is composed of multiple non-parallel radiation beams that converge, allows the delivery of a relatively large dose of radiation to a small, well-defined target. For clinical stage I NSCLC, 3-year local control rates with stereotactic body radiotherapy exceed 90%, and 3-year survival is estimated at over 55%. Patients with locally advanced disease (stages IIIA and IIIB) who are not surgical candidates have improved survival when treated with concurrent chemotherapy and radiation therapy compared with no therapy, radiation alone, or even sequential chemotherapy and radiation.

Neoadjuvant chemotherapy consists of giving antineoplastic drugs in advance of surgery or radiation therapy. There is no consensus on the impact of neoadjuvant therapy on survival in stage I/II NSCLC. Such therapy is not recommended outside of ongoing clinical trials. Neoadjuvant therapy is more widely used in selected patients with stage IIIA or select stage IIIB disease. Some studies suggest a survival advantage. This remains an area of active research.

Adjuvant chemotherapy consists of administering antineoplastic drugs following surgery or radiation therapy. Cisplatin-containing regimens have been shown to confer an overall survival benefit in at least stage II disease and a subset of stage IB disease where primary tumor size exceeds 4 cm. The Lung Adjuvant Cisplatin Evaluation Collaborative Group, a meta-analysis of the five largest cisplatin-based adjuvant trials, reported a 5% absolute benefit in 5-year overall survival with a cisplatin-containing doublet regimen following surgery ($P = 0.005$) in patients with at least stage II disease. For patients with poor performance status (Eastern Cooperative Oncology Group Score of 2 or more), there is no evidence of survival benefit for adjuvant chemotherapy; rather, it may be detrimental.

Although not curative, chemotherapy has been shown in multiple clinical trials to provide a modest increase in overall survival in patients with stage IIIB and stage IV NSCLC compared with supportive care alone, with median survival increased from 5 months to a range of 7–11 months. Palliative chemotherapy also leads to improved quality of life and symptom control, with first-line therapy involving a platinum-based regimen. Platinum-based doublet regimens consist of cisplatin or carboplatin (agents that bind DNA to form adducts that inhibit their synthesis and function) combined with another agent, such as pemetrexed, gemcitabine, taxane, or vinorelbine. The choice of chemotherapeutic agent should be tailored to histologic subtype in NSCLC. For nonsquamous histologies, patients have modestly improved overall survival when treated with a platinum agent plus pemetrexed (an inhibitor of folate-dependent enzymes important in purine and pyrimidine synthesis). Patients with squamous cell lung carcinomas have modestly improved overall survival when a platinum agent is combined with gemcitabine (a deoxycytidine analog that inhibits DNA synthesis). For good performance status patients with nonsquamous histologies, bevacizumab (a monoclonal antibody to vascular endothelial growth factor [VEGF]) can be added to a traditional platinum doublet regimen with further modest increase in survival benefit. Maintenance chemotherapy, that is, ongoing chemotherapy after an induction period of 4–6 cycles, has also been shown to improve overall survival. Finally, immune checkpoint inhibition with programmed cell-death-1 (PD-1) inhibitors (nivolumab and pembrolizumab) are playing important roles in the treatment of NSCLC. PD-1 inhibitors release T cells from the inhibitory signals they receive from tumor cells via the PD-1 pathway, restoring antitumor immunity. They are recommended as second-line treatment for both nonsquamous and squamous cell lung cancers.

With the advent of molecular profiling, targeted therapy has played a pivotal role in NSCLC. For patients with *EGFR* mutations, an EGFR tyrosine kinase inhibitor (erlotinib, gefitinib, or afatinib) rather than platinum-based chemotherapy is the first-line treatment. Response rates with EGFR inhibitors in patients with *EGFR* mutation are at least 70%, and median overall survival is estimated at 21–33 months. *EGFR* mutations are found in approximately 10–15% of the white population and 30–40% in the Asian population and are usually found among nonsmokers to light-smokers, females, and persons with nonsquamous histologies (particularly adenocarcinomas). Resistance to erlotinib or gefitinib generally occurs in 1 year, and a common mechanism of resistance is the development of a T790M mutation. Osimertinib, another EGFR tyrosine kinase inhibitor, has been FDA-approved for the treatment of patients with the T790M mutation, with response rates up to 60%. Approximately 5% of all patients with NSCLC carry another mutation, the *EML4-ALK* fusion gene product. This is usually found in a comparatively younger population, with adenocarcinoma histology, and nonsmoking to light-smoking history. In a phase III trial of *ALK*-rearranged lung cancer patients, treatment with crizotinib (an *ALK*, *cMET* and *ROS-1* tyrosine kinase inhibitor) showed a response rate over 70% compared with a rate of 45% among those treated with standard first-line chemotherapy, and an improvement in median progression-free survival of 10.9 vs 7 months, respectively. At 1 year, however, resistance develops in most patients taking crizotinib. Ceritinib and alectinib, second-generation *ALK* inhibitors, have been shown to induce response rates of 50% in those patients with *ALK*-rearranged lung cancers resistant to crizotinib. Approximately 1% of NSCLC harbor *ROS1* rearrangements, and are usually found among nonsmokers or light smokers and lung adenocarcinomas. *ROS1* rearranged lung cancers also respond to crizotinib with response rates over 70%. Finally, *K-ras* mutations are found among 25% of patients with adenocarcinomas, are associated with smoking, and indicate a poor prognosis. Unfortunately, there is still no effective targeted approach to therapy for *K-ras* mutated lung cancers. These mutations (*EGFR*, *EML4-ALK*, *ROS1*, and *K-ras*) are mutually exclusive. Difficulties may arise when only small fine-needle aspirate biopsies are obtained; clinicians are recommended to get at least core biopsies for sufficient tissue for molecular analysis.

B. Small Cell Lung Carcinoma

Response rates of SCLC to cisplatin and etoposide are excellent with 80–90% response in limited-stage disease (50–60% complete response), and 60–80% response in extensive stage disease (15–20% complete response). However, remissions tend to be short-lived with a median duration of 6–8 months. Once the disease has recurred, median survival is 3–4 months. Overall 2-year survival is 20–40% in limited-stage disease and 5% in extensive-stage disease (Table 39–3). Thoracic radiation therapy improves survival in patients with limited SCLC and is given concurrently with chemotherapy. Consolidative thoracic radiation therapy may be indicated for patients with extensive disease who have a significant response to chemotherapy and remain free of brain metastases. There is a high rate of brain metastasis in patients with SCLC, even following a good response to chemotherapy. Prophylactic cranial irradiation has been shown to decrease the incidence of central nervous system disease and improve survival in patients with limited stage disease who respond to chemotherapy

Table 39–3. Median survival for small cell lung carcinoma following treatment.

Stage	Mean 2-Year Survival	Median Survival
Limited	20–40%	15–20 months
Extensive	5%	8–13 months

Data from multiple sources, including Van Meerbeeck JP et al. Small-cell lung cancer. Lancet. 2011 Nov 12;378(9804):1741–55.

and a subset of patients with extensive stage disease who have had an excellent response to chemotherapy.

Occasionally, very early limited-stage disease (T1N0M0) may be detected on initial imaging. It may also be identified after a peripheral nodule proves to be SCLC on resection. These patients are recommended to receive adjuvant chemotherapy following surgery given the high risk of micrometastases in SCLC. Five-year survival following resection of and adjuvant chemotherapy for stage I SCLC can reach up to 50%.

C. Palliative Therapy

Photoresection with the Nd:YAG laser is sometimes performed on central tumors to relieve endobronchial obstruction, improve dyspnea, and control hemoptysis. External beam radiation therapy is also used to control dyspnea, hemoptysis, endobronchial obstruction, pain from bony metastases, obstruction from superior vena cava syndrome, and symptomatic brain metastases. Resection of a *solitary* brain metastasis improves quality of life and survival when combined with radiation therapy if there is no evidence of other metastatic disease. Intraluminal radiation (brachytherapy) is an alternative approach to endobronchial disease. Pain syndromes are very common in advanced disease. As patients approach the end of life, meticulous efforts at pain control are essential (see Chapter 5). In addition to standard oncologic care, early consultation with—or referral to—a palliative care specialist is recommended in advanced disease to aid in symptom management and can modestly improve survival.

► Prognosis

The 5-year survival rate for lung cancer is approximately 17%. Predictors of survival include the type of tumor (SCLC versus NSCLC), molecular typing, the stage of the tumor, the patient's performance status, and weight loss in the past 6 months. Patients with targetable mutations (*EGFR* and *ALK*) have better overall survival when compared with those without mutations due to superior efficacy of targeted drug therapy.

Borghaei H et al. Nivolumab versus docetaxel in advanced non-squamous non-small-cell lung cancer. N Engl J Med. 2015 Oct 22;373(17):1627–39. [PMID: 26412456]

Brahmer J et al. Nivolumab vs. docetaxel in advanced squamous cell non-small cell lung cancer. N Engl J Med. 2015 Jul 9; 373(2):123–35. [PMID: 26028407]

Gould MK. Clinical practice. Lung-cancer screening with low-dose computed tomography. N Engl J Med. 2014 Nov 6; 371(19):1813–20. [PMID: 25372089]

Howington JA et al. Treatment of stage I and II non-small cell lung cancer: diagnosis and management of lung cancer, 3rd ed: American College of Chest Physicians evidence-based clinical practice guidelines. Chest. 2013 May;143(5 Suppl): e278S–313S. [PMID: 23649443]

Jänne PA et al. AZD9291 in EGFR inhibitor-resistant non-small-cell lung cancer. N Engl J Med. 2015 Apr 30;372(18):1689–99. [PMID: 25923549]

Jett JR et al. Treatment of small cell lung cancer: diagnosis and management of lung cancer, 3rd ed: American College of Chest Physicians evidence-based clinical practice guidelines. Chest. 2013 May;143(5 Suppl):e400S–19S. [PMID: 23649448]

Masters GA et al. Systemic therapy for stage IV non-small cell lung cancer: American Society of Clinical Oncology Clinical Practice Guideline update. J Clin Oncol. 2015 Oct 20; 33(30):3488–515. [PMID: 26324367]

Ramnath N et al. Treatment of stage III non-small cell lung cancer: diagnosis and management of lung cancer, 3rd ed: American College of Chest Physicians evidence-based clinical practice guidelines. Chest. 2013 May;143(5 Suppl):e314S–40S. [PMID: 23649445]

Schmidt-Hansen M et al. FDG-PET/CT imaging for mediastinal staging in patients with potentially resectable non-small cell lung cancer. JAMA. 2015 Apr 14;313(14):1465–6. [PMID: 25871673]

Silvestri GA et al. The stage classification of lung cancer: diagnosis and management of lung cancer, 3rd edition: American College of Chest Physicians evidence-based clinical practice guidelines. Chest. 2013 May;143(5 Suppl):e191S–210S. [PMID: 23649438]

Slotman BJ et al. Use of thoracic radiotherapy for extensive stage small-cell lung cancer: a phase 3 randomised controlled trial. Lancet. 2015 Jan 3;385(9962):36–42. Erratum in: Lancet. 2015 Jan 3;385(9962):28. [PMID: 25230595]

Solomon BJ et al. First-line crizotinib versus chemotherapy in *ALK*-positive lung cancer. N Engl J Med. 2014 Dec 4; 371(23):2167–77. [PMID: 25470694]

PULMONARY METASTASIS

Pulmonary metastasis results from the spread of an extrapulmonary malignant tumor through vascular or lymphatic channels or by direct extension. Metastases usually occur via the pulmonary artery and typically present as multiple nodules or masses on chest radiography. The radiographic differential diagnosis of multiple pulmonary nodules also includes pulmonary arteriovenous malformation, infections (including abscesses, septic emboli, and atypical infections), sarcoidosis, rheumatoid nodules, and granulomatosis with polyangiitis. Metastases to the lungs are found in 20–55% of patients with various metastatic malignancies. Most are intraparenchymal. Carcinoma of the kidney, breast, rectum, colon, and cervix and malignant melanoma are the most likely primary tumors. Head and neck cancers with extensive or lower cervical nodal involvement have a 30% risk for distant metastasis; half of these metastases present in the lungs. Pulmonary metastases are common in patients with osteosarcomas and develop in approximately 20% of patients with soft tissue sarcomas.

Lymphangitic carcinomatosis denotes diffuse involvement of the pulmonary lymphatic network by primary or metastatic lung cancer, probably a result of extension of tumor from lung capillaries to the lymphatics. **Tumor embolization** from extrapulmonary cancer (renal cell carcinoma, hepatocellular carcinoma, choriocarcinoma) is an uncommon route for tumor spread to the lungs. Metastatic cancer may also present as a malignant pleural effusion.

► Clinical Findings

A. Symptoms and Signs

Symptoms are uncommon but include cough, hemoptysis and, in advanced cases, dyspnea and hypoxemia. Symptoms are more often referable to the site of the primary tumor.

B. Laboratory Findings

The diagnosis of metastatic cancer involving the lungs is usually established by identifying a primary tumor. Appropriate studies should be ordered if there is a suspicion of any primary cancer, such as breast, thyroid, testis, colorectal, or prostate, for which specific treatment is available. For example, an elevated prostate-specific antigen (PSA) may indicate prostate cancer, and beta-human chorionic gonadotropin (beta-hCG) and alpha-fetoprotein point to germ cell tumors. Based on the clinical setting, imaging studies should be ordered. If the history, physical examination, and initial studies fail to reveal the site of the primary tumor, attention is better focused on the lung, where tissue samples obtained by bronchoscopy, percutaneous needle biopsy, VATS, or thoracotomy may establish the histologic diagnosis and suggest the most likely primary cancer. Occasionally, cytologic studies of pleural fluid or pleural biopsy reveals the diagnosis.

To determine a primary diagnosis, immunohistochemical staining should be done on the biopsy specimen. For example, PSA and thyroglobulin staining are highly specific for prostate and thyroid cancer, respectively. Thyroid transcription factor-1 (TTF-1) and napsin-A are relatively specific for primary lung adenocarcinoma, while the former can be positive in cases of SCLC and thyroid carcinoma and the latter can be positive in papillary and clear cell renal cell carcinomas. An adenocarcinoma that demonstrates negative TTF-1 and napsin-A staining strongly suggests a nonpulmonary primary cancer. Positive estrogen receptor (ER) and progesterone receptor (PR) stains suggest primary breast cancer.

C. Imaging

Chest radiographs usually show multiple spherical densities with sharp margins. The size of metastatic lesions varies from a few millimeters (miliary densities) to large masses. The lesions are usually bilateral, pleural or subpleural in location, and more common in lower lung zones. Cavitation suggests squamous cell tumor; calcification suggests osteosarcoma. Lymphangitic spread and solitary pulmonary nodule are less common radiographic presentations of pulmonary metastasis. Mammography should be considered in women to search for possible primary breast cancer. CT imaging of the chest, abdomen, and pelvis may reveal the site of a primary tumor and will help determine feasibility of surgical resection of the metastatic lung tumors. PET-CT scan is helpful in identifying the site of a primary cancer and identifying other areas of extrathoracic metastasis.

▶ Treatment

Once the diagnosis has been established, management consists of treatment of the primary neoplasm and any pulmonary complications. Surgical resection of a *solitary* pulmonary nodule is often prudent in the patient with known current or previous extrapulmonary cancer. Local resection of one or more pulmonary metastases is feasible in a few carefully selected patients with various sarcomas and carcinomas (such as testis, colorectal, and kidney).

Surgical resection should be considered only if the primary tumor is under control, if the patient has adequate cardiopulmonary reserve to tolerate resection, if all of the metastatic tumor can be resected, if effective nonsurgical approaches are not available, and if any extrathoracic metastasis has been excluded. Relative contraindications to resection of pulmonary metastases include (1) malignant melanoma primary, (2) requirement for pneumonectomy, and (3) pleural involvement. Unfavorable prognostic factors also include shorter disease-free interval from primary tumor treatment to presentation of metastases and a larger number of metastases. To date, there have been no randomized data confirming the benefit of metastatectomy for pulmonary metastasis, with one randomized clinical trial in the UK currently enrolling patients (the Pulmonary Metastatectomy in Colorectal Cancer [PulMiCC] trial). Retrospective data from the International Registry of Lung Metastases report an overall 5-year survival rate of 36% and 10-year survival rate of 26% after complete resection of pulmonary metastases. Patients who are not surgical candidates but have solitary or limited metastatic disease to the lungs may be candidates for stereotactic radiotherapy, radioablation, or cryotherapy. For patients with unresectable progressive disease, chemotherapy tailored to the primary tumor can be offered, and diligent attention to palliative care is essential (see Chapter 5).

Gillams A et al. Survival after radiofrequency ablation in 122 patients with inoperable colorectal lung metastases. Cardiovasc Intervent Radiol. 2013 Jun;36(3):724–30. [PMID: 23070108]

Gonzalez M et al. Risk factors for survival after lung metastasectomy in colorectal cancer patients: a systematic review and meta-analysis. Ann Surg Oncol. 2013 Feb;20(2):572–9. [PMID: 23104709]

Moorcraft SY et al. Management of resectable colorectal lung metastases. Clin Exp Metastasis. 2016 Mar;33(3):285–96. [PMID: 26659389]

Ordóñez NG. Napsin A expression in lung and kidney neoplasia: a review and update. Adv Anat Pathol. 2012 Jan;19(1):66–73. [PMID: 22156835]

Treasure T et al. Pulmonary metastasectomy: what is the practice and where is the evidence for effectiveness? Thorax. 2014 Oct;69(10):946–9. [PMID: 24415715]

MESOTHELIOMA

ESSENTIALS OF DIAGNOSIS

▶ Unilateral, nonpleuritic chest pain and dyspnea.

▶ Distant (more than 20 years earlier) history of exposure to asbestos.

▶ Pleural effusion or pleural thickening or both on chest radiographs.

▶ Malignant cells in pleural fluid or tissue biopsy.

▶ General Considerations

Mesotheliomas are primary tumors arising from the surface lining of the pleura (80% of cases) or peritoneum

(20% of cases). About three-fourths of pleural mesotheliomas are diffuse (usually malignant) tumors, and the remaining one-fourth are localized (usually benign). Men outnumber women by a 3:1 ratio. Numerous studies have confirmed the association of **malignant pleural mesothelioma** with exposure to asbestos (particularly the amphibole form). The lifetime risk to asbestos workers of developing malignant pleural mesothelioma is as high as 10%. The latent period between exposure and onset of symptoms ranges from 20 to 40 years. The clinician should inquire about asbestos exposure through mining, milling, manufacturing, shipyard work, insulation, brake linings, building construction and demolition, roofing materials, and other asbestos products (pipes, textiles, paints, tiles, gaskets, panels). Although cigarette smoking significantly increases the risk of bronchogenic carcinoma in asbestos workers and aggravates asbestosis, there is no association between smoking and mesothelioma.

▶ Clinical Findings

A. Symptoms and Signs

The average interval between onset of symptoms and diagnosis is 2–3 months; the median age at diagnosis is 72–74 years in Western countries. Symptoms include the insidious onset of shortness of breath, nonpleuritic chest pain, and weight loss. Physical findings include dullness to percussion, diminished breath sounds and, in some cases, digital clubbing.

B. Laboratory Findings

Pleural fluid is exudative and often hemorrhagic. Cytologic tests of pleural fluid are often negative. VATS biopsy is usually necessary to obtain an adequate specimen for histologic diagnosis. The histologic variants of malignant pleural mesothelioma are epithelial (50–60%), sarcomatoid (10%), and biphasic (30–40%). Since distinction from benign inflammatory conditions and metastatic adenocarcinoma may be difficult, immunohistochemical stains are important to confirm the diagnosis.

C. Imaging

Radiographic abnormalities consist of nodular, irregular, unilateral pleural thickening and varying degrees of unilateral pleural effusion. Sixty percent of patients have right-sided disease, while only 5% have bilateral involvement. CT scans demonstrate the extent of pleural involvement. PET-CT is used to help differentiate benign from malignant pleural disease, improve staging accuracy, and identify candidates for aggressive surgical approaches.

▶ Complications

Malignant pleural mesothelioma progresses rapidly as the tumor spreads along the pleural surface to involve the pericardium, mediastinum, and contralateral pleura. The tumor may eventually extend beyond the thorax to involve abdominal lymph nodes and organs. Progressive pain and dyspnea are characteristic. Local invasion of thoracic structures may cause superior vena cava syndrome, hoarseness, Horner syndrome, arrhythmias, and dysphagia.

▶ Treatment

Chemotherapy is the mainstay of treatment, with surgery only included in multimodality treatment if there is localized disease that can be surgically resected and no evidence of mediastinal nodal involvement. The optimal surgical approach is still under debate. For localized disease, surgical options include pleurectomy and decortication (surgical stripping of the pleura and pericardium from apex of the lung to diaphragm) or extrapleural pneumonectomy (a radical surgical procedure involving removal of the ipsilateral lung, parietal and visceral pleura, pericardium, and most of the hemidiaphragm). Limited nonrandomized data have shown that a trimodality approach for localized disease with extrapleural pneumonectomy, adjuvant radiation, and (neoadjuvant or adjuvant) chemotherapy can prolong survival in highly selected patients. However, the benefit of extrapleural pneumonectomy has been brought into question with the results of the Mesothelioma and Radical Surgery (MARS) trial. This small randomized study, comparing extrapleural pneumonectomy with no extrapleural pneumonectomy after induction chemotherapy in 50 patients, showed that extrapleural pneumonectomy offers no survival benefit and may cause more harm. In advanced disease, palliative chemotherapy with cisplatin and pemetrexed can achieve response rates of 30–40%, extend median overall survival to 12 months, and improve quality of life. Other alternative chemotherapy regimens include gemcitabine, anthracyclines, or vinorelbine. Drainage of pleural effusions, pleurodesis, radiation therapy, and even surgical resection may offer palliative benefit in some patients.

▶ Prognosis

Most patients die of respiratory failure and complications of local extension. Median survival time from diagnosis ranges from 7 months to 17 months. Five-year survival is 5–10%. Tumors that are predominantly sarcomatoid are more resistant to therapy and have a worse prognosis, with median survivals less than 1 year. Poor prognostic features include poor performance status, non-epithelioid histology, male gender, nodal involvement, elevated lactate dehydrogenase, high white blood cell count, low hemoglobin, and high platelet count.

Ai J et al. Current issues in malignant pleural mesothelioma evaluation and management. Oncologist. 2014 Sep;19(9): 975–84. [PMID: 25061089]

Bovolato P et al. Does surgery improve survival of patients with malignant pleural mesothelioma?: a multicenter retrospective analysis of 1365 consecutive patients. J Thorac Oncol. 2014 Mar;9(3):390–6. [PMID: 24518090]

Husain AN et al. Guidelines for pathologic diagnosis of malignant mesothelioma: 2012 update of the consensus statement from the International Mesothelioma Interest Group. Arch Pathol Lab Med. 2013 May;137(5):647–67. [PMID: 22929121]

Meyerhoff RR et al. Impact of mesothelioma histologic subtype on outcomes in the Surveillance, Epidemiology, and End Results database. J Surg Res. 2015 Jun 1;196(1):23–32. [PMID: 25791825]

Pinto C et al. Second Italian Consensus Conference on Malignant Pleural Mesothelioma: state of the art and recommendations. Cancer Treat Rev. 2013 Jun;39(4):328–39. [PMID: 23244777]

van Zandwijk N et al. Guidelines for the diagnosis and treatment of malignant pleural mesothelioma. J Thorac Dis. 2013 Dec; 5(6):E254–307. [PMID: 24416529]

HEPATOBILIARY CANCERS

Lawrence S. Friedman, MD

HEPATOCELLULAR CARCINOMA

ESSENTIALS OF DIAGNOSIS

▶ In Western countries, usually a complication of cirrhosis.

▶ Characteristic CT and MRI features and elevated serum alpha-fetoprotein may obviate the need for a confirmatory biopsy.

▶ **General Considerations**

Malignant neoplasms of the liver that arise from parenchymal cells are called hepatocellular carcinomas; those that originate in the ductular cells are called cholangiocarcinomas.

Hepatocellular carcinomas are associated with cirrhosis in 80% of cases. In Africa and most of Asia, hepatitis B virus (HBV) infection is a major etiologic factor, and a family history of hepatocellular carcinoma increases the risk synergistically. In the United States and other Western countries, incidence rates have risen rapidly (over twofold since 1978, with slowing of the rate increase since 2006), presumably because of the increasing prevalence of cirrhosis caused by chronic hepatitis C virus (HCV) infection and nonalcoholic fatty liver disease. In Western countries, risk factors for hepatocellular carcinoma in patients known to have cirrhosis are male gender, age older than 55 years (although there has been an increase in the number of younger cases), Asian or Hispanic ethnicity, family history in a first-degree relative, overweight, obesity (especially in early adulthood), alcohol use (especially in combination with obesity), tobacco use, diabetes mellitus, hypothyroidism (in women), a prolonged prothrombin time, a low platelet count, and an elevated serum transferrin saturation. The risk of hepatocellular carcinoma is higher in persons with a viral rather than nonviral cause of cirrhosis and may be increased in persons with autoimmune diseases. Other associations include high levels of HBV replication; HBV genotype C; hepatitis D coinfection; elevated serum ALT levels in persons with chronic hepatitis B (in whom antiviral therapy to suppress HBV replication appears to reduce the risk); HCV genotypes 1b and 3; hemochromatosis (and possibly the C282Y carrier state); aflatoxin exposure (associated with mutation of the *TP53* gene); alpha-1-antiprotease (alpha-1-antitrypsin) deficiency; tyrosinemia; and radiation exposure. In patients with the metabolic syndrome, hepatocellular carcinoma may arise from a hepatocellular adenoma in the absence of cirrhosis. Evidence for an association with long-term use of oral contraceptives is inconclusive. While sulfonylurea and insulin use may increase the risk of hepatocellular carcinoma, consumption of coffee, vegetables, white meat, fish, and n-3 polyunsaturated fatty acids; aspirin use; and statin and metformin use in diabetic patients appear to be protective. The fibrolamellar variant of hepatocellular carcinoma generally occurs in young women and is characterized by a distinctive histologic picture, absence of risk factors, unique genomic profiles, and indolent course. Vinyl chloride exposure is associated with angiosarcoma of the liver. Hepatoblastoma, the most common malignant liver tumor in infants and young children, occurs rarely in adults.

▶ **Clinical Findings**

A. Symptoms and Signs

The presence of a hepatocellular carcinoma may be unsuspected until there is deterioration in the condition of a cirrhotic patient who was formerly stable. Cachexia, weakness, and weight loss are associated symptoms. The sudden appearance of ascites, which may be bloody, suggests portal or hepatic vein thrombosis by tumor or bleeding from a necrotic tumor.

Physical examination may show tender enlargement of the liver, occasionally with a palpable mass. In Africa, the typical presentation in young patients is a rapidly expanding abdominal mass. Auscultation may reveal a bruit over the tumor or a friction rub when the tumor has extended to the surface of the liver.

B. Laboratory Findings

Laboratory tests may reveal leukocytosis, as opposed to the leukopenia that is frequently encountered in cirrhotic patients. Anemia is common, but a normal or elevated hematocrit value may be found in up to one-third of patients owing to elaboration of erythropoietin by the tumor. Sudden and sustained elevation of the serum alkaline phosphatase in a patient who was formerly stable is a common finding. HBsAg is present in a majority of cases in endemic areas, whereas in the United States anti-HCV is found in up to 40% of cases. Alpha-fetoprotein levels are elevated in up to 70% of patients with hepatocellular carcinoma in Western countries (although the sensitivity is lower in blacks and levels are not elevated in patients with fibrolamellar hepatocellular carcinoma); however, mild elevations (10–200 ng/mL [10–200 mcg/L]) are also often seen in patients with chronic hepatitis. Serum levels of des-gamma-carboxy prothrombin are elevated in up to 90% of patients with hepatocellular carcinoma, but they may also be elevated in patients with vitamin K deficiency, chronic hepatitis, and metastatic cancer. Cytologic study of ascitic fluid rarely reveals malignant cells.

C. Imaging

Multiphasic helical CT and MRI with contrast enhancement are the preferred imaging studies for determining the location and vascularity of the tumor; MRI may be more sensitive than CT, and imaging with gadoxetic acid increases sensitivity. Lesions smaller than 1 cm may be difficult to characterize. Arterial phase enhancement of the lesion followed by delayed hypointensity ("washout") is most specific for hepatocellular carcinoma. Ultrasonography is less sensitive and more operator dependent but is used to screen for hepatic nodules in high-risk patients. Contrast-enhanced ultrasonography has sensitivity and specificity approaching those of arterial phase helical CT but, unlike CT and MRI, cannot image the entire liver during the short duration of the arterial phase and is thus associated with false-positive results. In selected cases, endoscopic ultrasonography (EUS) may be useful. PET is under study.

D. Liver Biopsy and Staging

Liver biopsy is diagnostic, although seeding of the needle tract by tumor is a potential risk (1–3%). For lesions smaller than 1 cm, ultrasonography may be repeated every 3 months followed by further investigation of enlarging lesions. For lesions 1 cm or larger, biopsy can be deferred when characteristic arterial hypervascularity and delayed washout are demonstrated on either multiphasic helical CT or MRI with contrast enhancement (or both) or if surgical resection is planned. Staging in the TNM classification includes the following definitions: T0: no evidence of primary tumor; T1: solitary tumor without vascular invasion; T2: solitary tumor with vascular invasion or multiple tumors none more than 5 cm; T3: multiple tumors more than 5 cm (3a) or tumor involving a major branch of the portal or hepatic vein (3b); and T4: tumor(s) with direct invasion of adjacent organs other than the gallbladder or with perforation of the visceral peritoneum; N1, regional lymph node metastasis; M1, distant metastasis; F0, no to moderate hepatic fibrosis; F1, severe hepatic fibrosis to cirrhosis. The Barcelona Clinic Liver Cancer (BCLC) staging system is preferred and includes the Child-Pugh stage, tumor stage, and liver tests and has the advantage of linking overall stage with preferred treatment modalities and with an estimation of life expectancy.

▶ Screening & Prevention

Surveillance for the development of hepatocellular carcinoma is recommended in patients with chronic hepatitis B (beginning as early as age 20 in Africans, age 40 in Asians or those with a family history of hepatocellular carcinoma, and age 50 in others) or cirrhosis caused by HCV, HBV, or alcohol. Whether surveillance for hepatocellular carcinoma leads to a survival advantage over clinical diagnosis is uncertain. The standard approach is ultrasonography and alpha-fetoprotein testing every 6 months, although the value of alpha-fetoprotein screening has been questioned because of its low sensitivity. CT and MRI are considered too expensive for screening, but the sensitivity of ultrasonography for detecting early hepatocellular carcinoma is only 63%. The risk of hepatocellular carcinoma in a patient with cirrhosis is 3–5% a year, and patients with tumors detected by surveillance have a less advanced stage on average and greater likelihood that treatment will prolong survival than those not undergoing surveillance. In a population of patients with cirrhosis, over 60% of nodules smaller than 2 cm in diameter detected on a screening ultrasonography prove to be hepatocellular carcinoma. Mass vaccination programs against HBV in developing countries are leading to reduced rates of hepatocellular carcinoma. Successful treatment of hepatitis B and of hepatitis C in patients with cirrhosis also reduces the subsequent risk of hepatocellular carcinoma.

▶ Treatment

Surgical resection of a solitary hepatocellular carcinoma may result in cure if liver function is preserved (Child-Pugh class A or possibly B) and portal vein thrombosis is not present. Laparoscopic liver resection has been performed in selected cases. Treatment of underlying chronic viral hepatitis, adjuvant chemotherapy, and adaptive immunotherapy may lower postsurgical recurrence rates. Liver transplantation may be appropriate for small unresectable tumors in a patient with advanced cirrhosis, with reported 5-year survival rates of up to 75%. The recurrence-free survival may be better for liver transplantation than for resection in patients with well-compensated cirrhosis and small tumors (one tumor less than 5 cm or three or fewer tumors each less than 3 cm in diameter [Milan criteria]) and in those with expanded (University of California, San Francisco) criteria of one tumor less than or equal to 6.5 cm or three or fewer tumors less than or equal to 4.5 cm. Patients with stage 2 hepatocellular carcinoma meeting the Milan criteria receive an additional 28 points on their Model for End-Stage Liver Disease (MELD) score after 6 months on the waiting list (see Chapter 16), markedly increasing their chances of undergoing transplantation. However, liver transplantation is often impractical because of the donor organ shortage, and living donor liver transplantation may be considered in these cases. Patients with larger tumors (3–5 cm), a serum alpha-fetoprotein level 455 ng/mL (455 mcg/L) or higher, or a MELD score 20 or more have poor posttransplantation survival. Chemotherapy, hormonal therapy with tamoxifen, and long-acting octreotide have not been shown to prolong life, but transarterial chemoembolization (TACE), TACE with drug-eluting beads, transarterial chemoinfusion (TACI), and transarterial radioembolization (TARE) via the hepatic artery are palliative and may prolong survival in patients with a large or multifocal tumor in the absence of extrahepatic spread. TACI and TARE are suitable for patients with portal vein thrombosis. Radiofrequency ablation of, cryotherapy of, microwave ablation of, or injection of absolute ethanol into tumors smaller than 2 cm may prolong survival in patients who are not candidates for resection and have tumors that are accessible; these interventions may also provide a "bridge" to liver transplantation. Radiofrequency ablation is superior to ethanol injection for tumors larger than 2 cm in diameter (but is not effective for those larger than 5 cm) and can be performed after TACE in select cases. Cryoablation may result in slower tumor progression than radiofrequency ablation for tumors that are 3.1–4 cm in diameter. Sorafenib (an oral multikinase inhibitor of Raf kinase, the VEGF receptor, and the platelet-derived growth factor receptor [and others]), prolongs median survival as well as the time to radiologic progression by 3 months in patients with advanced hepatocellular carcinoma; sorafenib is standard care in these patients. The modified Response Evaluation Criteria in Solid Tumors (mRECIST) are used to assess treatment response based on tumor shrinkage and viability after locoregional and antiangiogenic treatment. Meticulous efforts at palliative care are essential for patients in whom disease progresses despite treatment or in whom advanced tumors, vascular invasion, or extrahepatic spread are present. Severe pain may develop in such patients due to expansion of the liver capsule by the tumor and requires concerted efforts at pain management, including the use of opioids (see Chapter 5).

► **Prognosis**

In the United States, overall 1- and 5-year survival rates for patients with hepatocellular carcinoma are 23% and 5%, respectively. Five-year survival rates rise to 56% for patients with localized resectable disease (T1, T2, selected T3 and T4; N0; M0) but are virtually nil for those with locally unresectable or advanced disease. In patients with HCV-related hepatocellular carcinoma, the serum alpha-fetoprotein level at the time of diagnosis of cancer has been reported to be an independent predictor of mortality. A serum alpha-fetoprotein level greater than or equal to 200 ng/mL (200 milli-international units/mL) or increases of greater than 15 ng/mL/month predict worse outcomes in patients awaiting liver transplantation. In patients who are not eligible for surgery, an elevated serum C-reactive protein level is associated with poor survival. Contrary to traditional opinion, the fibrolamellar variant does not have a better prognosis than conventional hepatocellular carcinoma without cirrhosis.

► **When to Refer**

All patients with hepatocellular carcinoma should be referred to a specialist.

► **When to Admit**

- Complications of cirrhosis.
- Severe pain.
- For surgery and other interventions.

Bruix J et al. Hepatocellular carcinoma: clinical frontiers and perspectives. Gut. 2014 May;63(5):844–55. [PMID: 24531850]
Chou R et al. Imaging techniques for the diagnosis of hepatocellular carcinoma: a systematic review and meta-analysis. Ann Intern Med. 2015 May 19;162(10):697–711. [PMID: 25984845]
Cornella H et al. Unique genomic profile of fibrolamellar hepatocellular carcinoma. Gastroenterology. 2015 Apr;148(4):806–18. [PMID: 25557953]
Kim HD et al. Evaluation of early-stage hepatocellular carcinoma by magnetic resonance imaging with gadoxetic acid detects additional lesions and increases overall survival. Gastroenterology. 2015 Jun;148(7):1371–82. [PMID: 25733098]

Mokdad AA et al. JAMA Patient Page. Liver cancer. JAMA. 2015 Dec 22–29;314(24):2701. [PMID: 26720038]
Sieghart W et al. Transarterial chemoembolization: modalities, indication, and patient selection. J Hepatol. 2015 May;62(5):1187–95. [PMID: 25681552]
Wang C et al. Multicenter randomized controlled trial of percutaneous cryoablation versus radiofrequency ablation in hepatocellular carcinoma. Hepatology. 2015 May;61(5):1579–90. [PMID: 25284802]

CARCINOMA OF THE BILIARY TRACT

ESSENTIALS OF DIAGNOSIS

► Presents with obstructive jaundice, usually painless, often with dilated biliary tract.
► Pain is more common in gallbladder carcinoma than cholangiocarcinoma.
► A dilated gallbladder may be palpable (Courvoisier sign).
► Diagnosis by cholangiography with biopsy and brushings for cytology.

► **General Considerations**

Carcinoma of the gallbladder occurs in approximately 2% of all people operated on for biliary tract disease; the incidence may be decreasing in the United States. It is notoriously insidious, and the diagnosis is often made unexpectedly at surgery. Cholelithiasis (often large, symptomatic stones) is usually present. Other risk factors are chronic infection of the gallbladder with *Salmonella typhi*, gallbladder polyps over 1 cm in diameter (particularly with hypoecholic foci on EUS), mucosal calcification of the gallbladder (porcelain gallbladder), and anomalous pancreaticobiliary ductal junction. Genetic factors include *K-ras* and *TP53* mutations. Spread of the cancer—by direct extension into the liver or to the peritoneal surface—may be seen on initial presentation. The TNM classification includes the following stages: Tis, carcinoma in situ; T1a, tumor invades lamina propria, and T1b, tumor invades muscle layer; T2, tumor invades perimuscular connective tissue, no extension beyond serosa (visceral peritoneum) or into liver; T3, tumor perforates the serosa or directly invades the liver or adjacent organ or structure; T4, tumor invades the main portal vein or hepatic artery or invades multiple extrahepatic organs or structures; N1, regional lymph node metastasis; and M1, distant metastasis.

Carcinoma of the bile ducts (cholangiocarcinoma) accounts for 10–25% of all hepatobiliary malignancies and 3% of all cancer deaths in the United States. It is more prevalent in persons aged 50–70, with a slight male predominance, and more common in Asia. About 50% arise at the confluence of the hepatic ducts (perihilar, or so-called Klatskin, tumors), and 40% arise in the distal extrahepatic bile duct (the incidence of which has risen since 1990); the remainder are intrahepatic or peripheral (the incidence of which rose dramatically from the 1970s to the early 2000s).

Staging for extrahepatic cholangiocarcinoma is as follows: T1, tumor is confined to bile duct; T2, tumor spreads beyond the wall of the bile duct (2a) or to the adjacent liver (2b); T3, tumor spreads to unilateral branches of the portal vein or hepatic artery; T4, tumor spreads to main portal vein or its branches bilaterally, common hepatic artery, second-order biliary radicals bilaterally, or various combinations; N1, regional lymph node metastasis; M1, distant metastasis. Staging for intrahepatic cholangiocarcinoma is as follows: T1, solitary tumor without vascular invasion; T2, solitary tumor with vascular invasion or multiple tumors 5 cm or smaller; T3, multiple tumors larger than 5 cm or involving major branch of portal or hepatic veins; T4, tumor invades adjacent organ (except gallbladder) or perforation of visceral peritoneum; N1, regional lymph node metastasis; and M1, distant metastasis. Other staging systems consider the patient's performance status, tumor extent and form, vascular encasement, hepatic lobe atrophy, underlying liver disease, and peritoneal metastasis. The frequency of carcinoma in persons with a choledochal cyst has been reported to be over 14% at 20 years, and surgical excision is recommended. Most cases of cholangiocarcinoma are sporadic. There is an increased incidence of cholangiocarcinoma in patients with bile duct adenoma; biliary papillomatosis; Caroli disease; a biliary-enteric anastomosis; ulcerative colitis, especially those with primary sclerosing cholangitis; biliary cirrhosis; diabetes mellitus; hyperthyroidism; chronic pancreatitis; heavy alcohol consumption; smoking; and past exposure to Thorotrast, a contrast agent. In diabetic patients, metformin use is associated with a reduced risk of intrahepatic cholangiocarcinoma. In Southeast Asia, hepatolithiasis, chronic typhoid carriage, and infection of the bile ducts with helminths (Clonorchis sinensis, Opisthorchis viverrini) are associated with an increased risk of cholangiocarcinoma. Hepatitis C virus (and possibly hepatitis B virus) infection, cirrhosis, HIV infection, nonalcoholic fatty liver disease, diabetes mellitus, obesity, and tobacco smoking are risk factors for intrahepatic cholangiocarcinoma. Mixed hepatocellular carcinoma-cholangiocarcinoma is a tumor that is being recognized increasingly.

▶ Clinical Findings

A. Symptoms and Signs

Progressive jaundice is the most common and usually the first sign of obstruction of the extrahepatic biliary system. Pain in the right upper abdomen with radiation into the back is usually present early in the course of gallbladder carcinoma but occurs later in the course of bile duct carcinoma. Anorexia and weight loss are common and may be associated with fever and chills due to cholangitis. Rarely, hematemesis or melena results from erosion of tumor into a blood vessel (hemobilia). Fistula formation between the biliary system and adjacent organs may also occur. The course is usually one of rapid deterioration, with death occurring within a few months.

Physical examination reveals profound jaundice. Pruritus and skin excoriations are common. A palpable gallbladder with obstructive jaundice usually is said to signify malignant disease (Courvoisier sign); however, this clinical generalization has been proven to be accurate only about 50% of the time. Hepatomegaly due to hypertrophy of the unobstructed liver lobe is usually present and is associated with liver tenderness. Ascites may occur with peritoneal implants.

B. Laboratory Findings

With biliary obstruction, laboratory examination reveals predominantly conjugated hyperbilirubinemia, with total serum bilirubin values ranging from 5 to 30 mg/dL. There is usually concomitant elevation of the alkaline phosphatase and serum cholesterol. AST is normal or minimally elevated. The serum CA 19-9 level is elevated in up to 85% of patients and may help distinguish cholangiocarcinoma from a benign biliary stricture (in the absence of cholangitis) but is neither sensitive nor specific.

C. Imaging

Ultrasonography and contrast-enhanced, triple-phase, helical CT may show a gallbladder mass in gallbladder carcinoma and intrahepatic mass or biliary dilatation in carcinoma of the bile ducts. CT may also show involved regional lymph nodes and atrophy of a hepatic lobe because of vascular encasement with compensatory hypertrophy of the unaffected lobe. MRI with magnetic resonance cholangiopancreatography (MRCP) and gadolinium enhancement permits visualization of the entire biliary tract and detection of vascular invasion and obviates the need for angiography and, in some cases, direct cholangiography; it is the imaging procedure of choice but may understage malignant hilar strictures. The sensitivity and image quality can be increased with use of ferumoxide enhancement. The features of intrahepatic cholangiocarcinoma on MRI appear to differ from those of hepatocellular carcinoma, with contrast washout in the latter but not the former. In indeterminate cases, PET can detect cholangiocarcinomas as small as 1 cm and lymph node and distant metastases, but false-positive results occur. The most helpful diagnostic studies before surgery are either endoscopic retrograde or percutaneous transhepatic cholangiography with biopsy and cytologic specimens, although false-negative biopsy and cytology results are common. Digital image analysis and fluorescent in situ hybridization of cytologic specimens for polysomy improve sensitivity. EUS with FNA of tumors, peroral cholangioscopy, confocal laser endomicroscopy, and intraductal ultrasonography may confirm a diagnosis of cholangiocarcinoma in a patient with bile duct stricture and an otherwise indeterminate evaluation, but FNA can result in tumor seeding and is often avoided if the tumor is potentially resectable.

▶ Treatment

In young and fit patients, curative surgery for gallbladder carcinoma may be attempted if the tumor is well localized. The 5-year survival rate for carcinoma of the gallbladder invading the lamina propria or muscularis (stage 1, T1a or 1b, N0, M0) is as high as 85% with laparoscopic cholecystectomy but drops to 60%, even with a more extended open resection, if there is perimuscular invasion (T2). The role of radical surgery for T3 and T4 tumors is debatable. If the tumor is unresectable at laparotomy, biliary-enteric bypass (eg, Roux-en-Y hepaticojejunostomy) can be performed. Carcinoma of the bile ducts is curable by surgery in less than 10% of cases. If resection margins are negative, the 5-year survival rate may be as high as 47% for intrahepatic cholangiocarcinomas, 41% for hilar cholangiocarcinoma, and 37% for distal cholangiocarcinomas, but the perioperative mortality rate may be as high as 10%. Factors predicting shorter survival for intrahepatic cholangiocarcinoma include large tumor size, multiple tumors, lymph node metastasis, and vascular invasion. Palliation can be achieved by placement of a self-expandable metal stent via an endoscopic or percutaneous transhepatic route. Covered metal stents may be more cost-effective than uncovered metal stents because of a longer duration of patency, but they are associated with a higher rate of stent migration and cholecystitis due to occlusion of the cystic duct and are not associated with longer survival. For perihilar tumors, insertion of a unilateral stent rather than bilateral stents may suffice. Plastic stents are less expensive initially, but not in the long term, because they are more prone to occlude than metal ones; they may be considered in patients expected to survive only a few months. Photodynamic therapy in combination with stent placement prolongs survival when compared with stent placement alone in patients with nonresectable cholangiocarcinoma. Endoscopic retrograde cholangiopancreatography (ERCP)–directed radiofrequency ablation is another emerging option. Radiotherapy may relieve pain and contribute to biliary decompression. There is limited response to chemotherapy with gemcitabine alone, but the combination of cisplatin and gemcitabine prolongs survival by about 3 months in patients with locally advanced or metastatic cholangiocarcinoma. Few patients survive for more than 24 months. Although cholangiocarcinoma is generally considered to be a contraindication to liver transplantation because of rapid tumor recurrence, a 75% 5-year survival rate has been reported in patients with stage I and II perihilar cholangiocarcinoma undergoing chemoradiation and exploratory laparotomy followed by liver transplantation.

For those patients whose disease progresses despite treatment, meticulous efforts at palliative care are essential (see Chapter 5).

▶ When to Refer

All patients with carcinoma of the biliary tract should be referred to a specialist.

▶ When to Admit

- Biliary obstruction.
- Cholangitis.

Razumilava N et al. Cholangiocarcinoma. Lancet. 2014 Jun 21; 383(9935):2168–79. [PMID: 24581682]
Sawas T et al. Self-expandable metal stents versus plastic stents for malignant biliary obstruction: a meta-analysis. Gastrointest Endosc. 2015 Aug;82(2):256–67. [PMID: 25982849]

Singh A et al. The role of endoscopy in the diagnosis and management of cholangiocarcinoma. J Clin Gastroenterol. 2015 Oct; 49(9):725–37. [PMID: 26340677]
Walter D et al. Cost efficacy of metal stents for palliation of extrahepatic bile duct obstruction in a randomized controlled trial. Gastroenterology. 2015 Jul;149(1):130–8. [PMID: 25790742]

CARCINOMA OF THE PANCREAS & AMPULLA OF VATER

 ESSENTIALS OF DIAGNOSIS

- ▶ Obstructive jaundice (may be painless).
- ▶ Enlarged gallbladder (may be painful).
- ▶ Upper abdominal pain with radiation to back, weight loss, and thrombophlebitis are usually late manifestations.

▶ General Considerations

Carcinoma is the most common neoplasm of the pancreas. About 75% are in the head and 25% in the body and tail of the organ. Pancreatic carcinomas account for 2% of all cancers and 5% of cancer deaths. Risk factors include age, tobacco use (which is thought to cause 20–25% of cases), heavy alcohol use, obesity, chronic pancreatitis, diabetes mellitus, prior abdominal radiation, family history, and possibly gastric ulcer and exposure to arsenic and cadmium. New-onset diabetes mellitus after age 45 years occasionally heralds the onset of pancreatic cancer. In diabetic patients, metformin use may reduce the risk of pancreatic cancer slightly, but insulin use and glucagon-like peptide-1-based therapy (eg, sitagliptin) may increase the risk. About 7% of patients with pancreatic cancer have a family history of pancreatic cancer in a first-degree relative, compared with 0.6% of control subjects. In 5–10% of cases, pancreatic cancer occurs as part of a hereditary syndrome, including familial breast cancer (carriers of *BRCA-2* have a 7% lifetime risk of pancreatic cancer), hereditary pancreatitis (*PSS1* mutation), familial atypical multiple mole melanoma (*p16/CDKN2A* mutation), Peutz-Jeghers syndrome (*STK11/LKB1* mutation), ataxia-telangiectasia (*ATM* mutation), and Lynch syndrome (hereditary nonpolyposis colorectal cancer [*MLH1, MSH2, MSH6* mutations]). Neuroendocrine tumors account for 1–2% of pancreatic neoplasms and may be functional (producing gastrin, insulin, glucagon, vasoactive intestinal peptide, somatostatin, growth hormone–releasing hormone, adrenocorticotropic hormone, and others) or nonfunctional. Cystic neoplasms account for only 1% of pancreatic cancers, but they are important because they are often mistaken for pseudocysts. A cystic neoplasm should be suspected when a cystic lesion in the pancreas is found in the absence of a history of pancreatitis. At least 15% of all pancreatic cysts are neoplasms. Serous cystadenomas (which account for 32–39% of cystic pancreatic neoplasms and also occur in patients with von Hippel-Lindau disease) are benign. However, mucinous cystic neoplasms (defined by the presence of ovarian stroma) (10–45% of cystic pancreatic neoplasms), intraductal papillary mucinous neoplasms (21–33%), solid pseudopapillary tumors (less than 5%, primarily in young women), and cystic islet cell tumors (3–5%) may be malignant, although their prognoses are better than the prognosis of pancreatic adenocarcinoma, unless the cystic neoplasm is at least locally advanced.

▶ Clinical Findings

A. Symptoms and Signs

Pain is present in over 70% of cases and is often vague, diffuse, and located in the epigastrium or left upper quadrant when the lesion is in the tail. Radiation of pain into the back is common and sometimes predominates. Sitting up and leaning forward may afford some relief, and this usually indicates that the lesion has spread beyond the pancreas and is inoperable. Diarrhea, perhaps due to maldigestion, is an occasional early symptom. Migratory thrombophlebitis is a rare sign. Weight loss is a common but late finding and may be associated with depression. Occasional patients (often aged 40 years or older) present with acute pancreatitis in the absence of an alternative cause. Jaundice is usually due to biliary obstruction by a cancer in the pancreatic head. A palpable gallbladder is also indicative of obstruction by a neoplasm (Courvoisier sign), but there are frequent exceptions. A hard, fixed, occasionally tender mass may be present. In advanced cases, a hard periumbilical (Sister Joseph's) nodule may be palpable.

B. Laboratory Findings

There may be mild anemia. Glycosuria, hyperglycemia, and impaired glucose tolerance or true diabetes mellitus are found in 10–20% of cases. The serum amylase or lipase level is occasionally elevated. Liver biochemical tests may suggest obstructive jaundice. Steatorrhea in the absence of jaundice is uncommon. Occult blood in the stool is suggestive of carcinoma of the ampulla of Vater (the combination of biliary obstruction and bleeding may give the stools a distinctive silver appearance). CA 19-9, with a sensitivity of 70% and a specificity of 87%, has not proven useful for early detection of pancreatic cancer; increased values are also found in acute and chronic pancreatitis and cholangitis. Plasma chromogranin A levels are elevated in 88–100% of patients with pancreatic neuroendocrine tumors.

C. Imaging

Multiphase thin-cut helical CT is generally the initial diagnostic procedure and detects a mass in over 80% of cases. CT identifies metastases, delineates the extent of the tumor, and allows for percutaneous FNA for cytologic studies and tumor markers. MRI is an alternative to CT. Ultrasonography is not reliable because of interference by intestinal gas. PET is a sensitive technique for detecting pancreatic cancer and metastases, but PET-CT is not a routine staging procedure. Selective celiac and superior mesenteric arteriography may demonstrate vessel invasion by tumor, a finding that would preclude attempts at surgical resection, but it is used less commonly since the advent of multiphase helical CT.

EUS is more sensitive than CT for detecting pancreatic cancer and equivalent to CT for determining nodal involvement and resectability. A normal EUS excludes pancreatic cancer. EUS may also be used to guide FNA for tissue diagnosis, tumor markers, and DNA analysis. ERCP may clarify an ambiguous CT or MRI study by delineating the pancreatic duct system or confirming an ampullary or biliary neoplasm. MRCP appears to be at least as sensitive as ERCP in diagnosing pancreatic cancer. In some centers, pancreatoscopy or intraductal ultrasonography is used to evaluate filling defects in the pancreatic duct and assess resectability of intraductal papillary mucinous tumors. With obstruction of the splenic vein, splenomegaly or gastric varices are present, the latter detected by endoscopy, EUS, or angiography.

Cystic neoplasms can be distinguished by their appearance on CT, EUS, and ERCP and features of the cyst fluid on gross, cytologic, and genetic analysis. For example, serous cystadenomas may have a central scar or honeycomb appearance; mucinous cystadenomas are unilocular or multilocular and contain mucin-rich fluid with high carcinoembryonic antigen levels (greater than 200 ng/mL [200 mcg/L]) and K-ras mutations; and intraductal papillary mucinous neoplasms are associated with a dilated pancreatic duct and extrusion of gelatinous material from the ampulla.

▶ Staging

Staging of pancreatic cancer by the TNM classification includes the following definitions: Tis: carcinoma in situ; T1: tumor limited to the pancreas, 2 cm or less in greatest dimension; T2: tumor limited to the pancreas, more than 2 cm in greatest dimension; T3: tumor extends beyond the pancreas but without involvement of the celiac axis or the superior mesenteric artery; T4; tumor involves the celiac axis or the superior mesenteric artery (unresectable primary tumor); N1; regional lymph node metastasis; M1; distant metastasis.

▶ Treatment

Abdominal exploration is usually necessary when cytologic diagnosis cannot be made or if resection is to be attempted, which includes up to 30% of patients with pancreatic carcinoma. In a patient with a localized mass in the head of the pancreas and without jaundice, laparoscopy may detect tiny peritoneal or liver metastases and thereby avoid resection in 4–13% of patients. Radical pancreaticoduodenal (Whipple) resection is indicated for cancers strictly limited to the head of the pancreas, periampullary area, and duodenum (T1, N0, M0). Five-year survival rates are 20–25% in this group and as high as 40% in those with negative resection margins and without lymph node involvement. Preoperative endoscopic decompression of an obstructed bile duct is often achieved with a plastic stent or short metal stent but does not reduce operative mortality and is associated with complications. The best surgical results are achieved at centers that specialize in the multidisciplinary treatment of pancreatic cancer. Adjuvant or neoadjuvant chemotherapy with gemcitabine or fluorouracil (or both), possibly combined with irradiation, is of benefit (Table 39–4). Chemoradiotherapy downstages about 30% of patients with locally

Table 39–4. Treatment choices for cancers responsive to systemic agents.

Diagnosis	Current Treatment of Choice	Other Treatments
Acute lymphoblastic leukemia (ALL)	**Induction combination chemotherapy:** Vincristine, prednisone, daunorubicin, asparaginase, intrathecal methotrexate **Consolidation combination chemotherapy:** Cyclophosphamide, vincristine, doxorubicin, dexamethasone (hyper-CVAD) alternated with cytarabine, methotrexate **Maintenance chemotherapy:** Methotrexate, 6-mercaptopurine **Philadelphia chromosome–positive ALL:** Add imatinib or dasatinib to above regimen	Liposomal vincristine, blinatumomab, clofarabine, nelarabine (T cell ALL), nilotinib, bosutinib, ponatinib (Philadelphia chromosome-positive ALL), autologous or allogeneic transplantation for high risk or at relapse
Acute myeloid leukemia (AML)	**Combination chemotherapy:** Cytarabine, daunorubicin or Cytarabine, idarubicin or Cytarabine, daunomycin, cladrabine	Mitoxantrone, doxorubicin, cladribine, fludarabine, 5-azacytidine, decitabine, clofarabine
Chronic myeloid leukemia (CML)	Imatinib mesylate or nilotinib or dasatinib	Ponatinib, bosutinib, omacetaxine, allogeneic bone marrow transplantation
Chronic lymphocytic leukemia (CLL)	**Combination chemotherapy:** Fludarabine, cyclophosphamide, rituximab (FCR) or Bendamustine, rituximab **Single-agent chemotherapy:** Fludarabine, or Bendamustine or Chlorambucil	Alemtuzumab, ofatumumab, obinutuzumab, ibrutinib, idelalisib, lenalidomide, pentostatin, cladribine, cyclophosphamide, vincristine, doxorubicin, prednisone
Hairy cell leukemia	Cladribine (2-chlorodeoxyadenosine)	Pentostatin, rituximab, interferon-alpha, vemurafenib
Hodgkin lymphoma (stages III and IV)	**Combination chemotherapy:** Doxorubicin, bleomycin, vinblastine, dacarbazine (ABVD) or Doxorubicin, vinblastine, mechlorethamine, etoposide, vincristine, bleomycin, prednisone (Stanford V) or Bleomycin, etoposide, doxorubicin, cyclophosphamide, vincristine, procarbazine, prednisone (BEACOPP)	Combination chemotherapy second line: Dexamethasone, cisplatin, cytarabine (DHAP) or Etoposide, methylprednisolone, cytarabine, cisplatin (ESHAP) or Ifosfamide, carboplatin, etoposide (ICE) or Mesna, ifosfamide, mitoxantrone, etoposide (MIME); stem cell transplantation for high risk or first relapse Brentuximab vedotin
Non-Hodgkin lymphoma (intermediate and high grade)	**Combination chemotherapy:** Cyclophosphamide, doxorubicin, vincristine, prednisone, rituximab (CHOP-R) or Etoposide, prednisone, vincristine, cyclophosphamide, doxorubicin, rituximab (R-EPOCH) (for double rearrangements)	Combination chemotherapy second line: Dexamethasone, cisplatin, cytarabine (DHAP) or Etoposide, methylprednisolone, cytarabine, cisplatin (ESHAP) or Ifosfamide, carboplatin, etoposide (ICE) or Mesna, ifosfamide, mitoxantrone, etoposide (MIME); transplantation for high risk or first relapse
Non-Hodgkin lymphoma (low grade)	**Combination chemotherapy:** Fludarabine, cyclophosphamide, rituximab (FCR) or Fludarabine, rituximab (FR) or Bendamustine, rituximab or Cyclophosphamide, vincristine, doxorubicin, prednisone, rituximab (CHOP-R), or Cyclophosphamide, vincristine, prednisone, rituximab (CVP-R) or Lenalidomide, rituximab	Chlorambucil, rituximab, ^{131}I tositumomab, ^{90}Y ibritumomab tiuxetan, bendamustine, lenalidomide, idelalisib, ibrutinib, belinostat (T cell lymphoma), autologous or allogeneic transplantation
Multiple myeloma	**Combination chemotherapy (transplant candidates):** Bortezomib, dexamethasone, thalidomide or Bortezomib, dexamethasone, lenalidomide or Dexamethasone, lenalidomide Followed by autologous or miniallogeneic stem cell transplantation **Combination chemotherapy (non-transplant candidates):** Lenalidomide, dexamethasone, or Melphalan, prednisone, bortezomib, or Melphalan, prednisone, lenalidomide, or Melphalan, prednisone, thalidomide	Cyclophosphamide, liposomal doxorubicin, carfilzomib, pomalidomide, panobinostat, ixazomib, elotuzumab, daratumumab

(continued)

Table 39–4. Treatment choices for cancers responsive to systemic agents. (continued)

Diagnosis	Current Treatment of Choice	Other Treatments
Waldenström macroglobulin-emia	**Plasmapheresis alone or followed by combination chemotherapy:** Bortezomib with or without rituximab, or Thalidomide with or without rituximab, or Rituximab, cyclophosphamide, prednisone, or Carfilzomib, rituximab, dexamethasone	Cladribine, ibrutinib, ofatumumab, chlorambucil, bendamustine, alemtuzumab, everolimus, autologous bone marrow transplantation
Polycythemia vera	Phlebotomy, hydroxyurea, aspirin	Anagrelide, radiophosphorus ^{32}P, interferon-alpha
Non–small cell lung cancer	**Combination chemotherapy:** Cisplatin, vinorelbine, or Cisplatin, etoposide, or Paclitaxel, carboplatin, or Cisplatin, gemcitabine (squamous histology) Cisplatin, pemetrexed (nonsquamous histology) All regimens with or without bevacizumab Erlotinib, gefitinib or afatinib (*EGFR* mutation positive), or Crizotinib (*ALK* mutation positive)	Docetaxel, cetuximab, pembrolizumab, nivolumab, osimertinib, necitumumab, ramucirumab, cabozantinib (*RET* rearrangement), trastuzumab, afatinib (*HER2* mutation positive), crizotinib (*ROS1* rearrangement or *ALK* mutation positive), vemurafenib or dabrafenib or dabrafenib plus trametinib (*BRAF* V600E mutation positive)
Small cell lung cancer	**Combination chemotherapy:** Cisplatin, etoposide, or Carboplatin, etoposide, or Cisplatin, irinotecan	Irinotecan, cyclophosphamide, doxorubicin, vincristine, topotecan, gemcitabine, paclitaxel, bendamustine, temozolomide
Mesothelioma	**Combination chemotherapy:** Cisplatin, pemetrexed, or Carboplatin, pemetrexed, or Gemcitabine, cisplatin	Vinorelbine
Head and neck cancer	**Combination chemotherapy:** Cisplatin, fluorouracil, or Paclitaxel, carboplatin, or Docetaxel, cisplatin, fluorouracil, or Cisplatin or cetuximab with radiation therapy	Methotrexate
Esophageal and esophagogastric junction cancer	**Combination chemotherapy:** Cisplatin, fluorouracil, or Paclitaxel, carboplatin, or Oxaliplatin, fluorouracil	Irinotecan, oxaliplatin, capecitabine, epirubicin, docetaxel, ramucirumab (esophagogastric junction cancer)
Uterine cancer	**Hormone therapy:** Progestins, tamoxifen, aromatase inhibitors or **Combination chemotherapy:** Cisplatin, doxorubicin, or Docetaxel, carboplatin, or Carboplatin, paclitaxel	Liposomal doxorubicin, bevacizumab, topotecan, temsirolimus, docetaxel
Ovarian cancer	**Combination chemotherapy:** Paclitaxel, carboplatin with or without bevacizumab, or Docetaxel, carboplatin, or Paclitaxel, cisplatin	Gemcitabine, liposomal doxorubicin, topotecan, cyclophosphamide, etoposide, bevacizumab, pemetrexed, olaparib
Cervical cancer	**With radiation:** Cisplatin **Combination chemotherapy:** Cisplatin, paclitaxel with or without bevacizumab, or Cisplatin, topotecan, or Carboplatin, paclitaxel, or Cisplatin, gemcitabine, or Topotecan, paclitaxel with or without bevacizumab	Docetaxel, ifosfamide, vinorelbine, irinotecan, mitomycin, fluorouracil, docetaxel, pemetrexed, topotecan, altretamine
Breast cancer	**Adjuvant hormone therapy:** *Premenopausal:* Tamoxifen *Postmenopausal:* Aromatase inhibitors (anastrozole, letrozol, exemestane) **Adjuvant chemotherapy (without trastuzumab):** Doxorubicin, cyclophosphamide, paclitaxel, or Docetaxel, cyclophosphamide, or Doxorubicin, cyclophosphamide, or Doxorubicin, cyclophosphamide, docetaxel **Adjuvant chemotherapy (with trastuzumab):** Doxorubicin, cyclophosphamide, paclitaxel, trastuzumab with or without pertuzumab, or Docetaxel, carboplatin, trastuzumab with or without pertuzumab	Eribulin, capecitabine, mitoxantrone, cisplatin, etoposide, vinblastine, fluorouracil, ixabepilone, pertuzumab, gemcitabine, lapatinib, toremifene, fulvestrant, palbociclib raloxifene

(continued)

Table 39–4. Treatment choices for cancers responsive to systemic agents. (continued)

Diagnosis	Current Treatment of Choice	Other Treatments
Choriocarcinoma (trophoblastic neoplasms)	**Single-agent chemotherapy:** Methotrexate or dactinomycin for low-risk disease **Combination chemotherapy:** Etoposide, methotrexate, dactinomycin, cyclophosphamide, vincristine (EMA-CO) for high-risk disease	Vinblastine, cisplatin, mercaptopurine, chlorambucil, doxorubicin
Testicular cancer	**Combination chemotherapy:** Cisplatin, etoposide (EP), or Bleomycin, etoposide, cisplatin (BEP), or Etoposide, mesna, ifosfamide, cisplatin (VIP)	Vinblastine, paclitaxel, gemcitabine, oxaliplatin
Kidney (renal cell) cancer	**Single-agent chemotherapy:** Sunitinib or temsirolimus or bevacizumab or sorafenib or pazopanib or axitinib, or interleukin-2	Interferon-alpha, cabozantinib, nivolumab
Bladder cancer	**Combination chemotherapy:** Gemcitabine, cisplatin, or Methotrexate, vinblastine, doxorubicin, cisplatin (MVAC), or Cisplatin, methotrexate, vinblastine (CMV)	Carboplatin, paclitaxel, docetaxel, fluorouracil, pemetrexed
Prostate cancer	**Hormone therapy:** Luteinizing hormone-releasing agonist (leuprolide, goserelin, triptorelin, degarelix) with or without an antiandrogen (flutamide, bicalutamide, nilutamide)	Ketoconazole, docetaxel, abiraterone, enzalutamide, mitoxantrone, cabazitaxel, sipuleucel-T, prednisone, Radium (Ra)-223
Brain cancer (anaplastic astrocytoma and glioblastoma multiforme)	**Single-agent chemotherapy with radiation therapy:** Temozolomide	Bevacizumab, irinotecan, procarbazine, carmustine, lomustine, cyclophosphamide
Neuroblastoma	**Combination chemotherapy:** Cyclophosphamide, doxorubicin, cisplatin, etoposide	Vincristine, topetecan, irinotecan, ifosfamide, carboplatin, 13-cis-retinoic acid, ^{131}I-MIBG, dinutuximab, autologous or allogeneic transplantation
Thyroid cancer	**Single-agent chemotherapy:** Radioiodine (^{131}I) or sorafenib, or sunitinib or pazopanib or lenvatinib, vandetanib (medullary thyroid cancer)	Doxorubicin, dacarbazine, cabozantinib
Adrenal cancer	**Single-agent chemotherapy:** Mitotane	Doxorubicin, etoposide, cisplatin
Stomach (gastric) cancer	**Combination chemotherapy:** Epirubicin, cisplatin, fluorouracil, or Docetaxel, cisplatin, fluorouracil, or Fluorouracil, leucovorin, oxaliplatin Trastuzumab added for *HER2*-overexpressing adenocarcinomas	Capecitabine, irinotecan, paclitaxel, ramucirumab
Pancreatic cancer	**Combination chemotherapy:** Gemcitabine, cisplatin, or Gemcitabine, paclitaxel, or Gemcitabine, erlotinib, or Fluorouracil, leucovorin, irinotecan, oxaliplatin (FOLFIRINOX) **Single-agent chemotherapy:** Gemcitabine	Capecitabine
Colon cancer	**Combination chemotherapy:** Fluorouracil, leucovorin, oxaliplatin (FOLFOX6), or Capecitabine, oxaliplatin (CapeOx), or Fluorouracil, leucovorin, irinotecan (FOLFIRI) each regimen with or without bevacizumab	Cetuximab, panitumumab, regorafenib, ziv-aflibercept, trifluridine/tipiracil
Rectal cancer	**Chemotherapy with radiation:** Fluorouracil or capecitabine; For adjuvant or advanced disease treatment, same regimens used with colon cancer	Cetuximab, irinotecan, panitumumab, regorafenib, ziv-aflibercept, trifluridine/tipiracil
Anal cancer	**Combination chemotherapy with radiation:** Fluorouracil, mitomycin or capecitabine, mitomycin	Cisplatin
Carcinoid	Octreotide LAR or lanreotide	Doxorubicin, dacarbazine, temozolomide, streptozocin, oxaliplatin, fluorouracil, everolimus
Osteogenic sarcoma	**Combination chemotherapy:** Cisplatin, doxorubicin, or Methotrexate, cisplatin, doxorubicin or Doxorubicin, cisplatin, doxorubicin, or Ifosfamide, cisplatin, epirubicin	Cyclophosphamide, gemcitabine, docetaxel, etoposide, sorafinib, Radium (Ra)-233, Samarium (Sm)-153 (lexidronam)-ethylene diamine tetramethylene phosphate (EDTMP)

(continued)

Table 39–4. Treatment choices for cancers responsive to systemic agents. (continued)

Diagnosis	Current Treatment of Choice	Other Treatments
Soft tissue sarcomas	**Combination chemotherapy:** Doxorubicin, dacarbazine (AD), or Doxorubicin, ifosfamide, mesna (AIM), or Mesna, doxorubicin, ifosfamide, dacarbazine (MAID) **Single-agent chemotherapy:** Eribulin, pazopanib; imatinib or sunitinib or regorafenib (gastrointestinal stromal tumors)	Liposomal doxorubicin, methotrexate, gemcitabine, docetaxel, temozolomide, epirubicin, pazopanib; sorafenib, nilotinib, dasatinib, pazopanib (gastrointestinal stromal tumors)
Melanoma	**Combination chemotherapy** (non-*BRAF* mutation): nivolumab/ipilimumab **Combination chemotherapy** (*BRAF* mutation): dabrafenib/trametinib or vemurafenib/cobimetinib **Single-agent chemotherapy** (non-*BRAF* mutation): pembrolizumab or nivolumab **Single-agent chemotherapy** (*BRAF* mutation): vemurafenib or dabrafenib or cobimetinib	Dacarbazine, temozolomide, imatinib, paclitaxel, carboplatin
Hepatocellular cancer	**Single-agent chemotherapy:** Sorafenib	Doxorubicin
Kaposi sarcoma	**Single-agent chemotherapy:** Liposomal doxorubicin or liposomal daunorubicin	Paclitaxel, vinblastine, vincristine, etoposide, thalidomide

advanced disease to allow resection. When resection is not feasible, endoscopic stenting of the bile duct is performed to relieve jaundice. A plastic stent is generally placed if the patient's anticipated survival is less than 6 months (or surgery is planned). A metal stent is preferred when anticipated survival is 6 months or greater. Whether covered metal stents designed to prevent tumor ingrowth offer an advantage over uncovered stents is uncertain because covered stents are associated with higher rates of migration and acute cholecystitis due to occlusion of the cystic duct. Surgical biliary bypass may be considered in patients expected to survive at least 6 months. Surgical duodenal bypass may be considered in patients in whom duodenal obstruction is expected to develop; alternatively, endoscopic placement of a self-expandable duodenal stent may be feasible. Chemoradiation may be used for palliation of unresectable cancer confined to the pancreas. Chemotherapy has been disappointing in metastatic pancreatic cancer, although improved response rates have been reported with the combination of oxaliplatin, irinotecan, fluorouracil, and leucovorin (FOLFIRINOX) and with the combination of gemcitabine and albumin-bound paclitaxel. The addition of erlotinib (an inhibitor of the EGFR receptor), capecitabine (an oral fluoropyrimidine), or a platinum agent may improve survival but also increases toxicity. The high rate of *K-ras* mutations in pancreatic cancer limits the benefit of erlotinib. Celiac plexus nerve block (under CT or endoscopic ultrasound guidance) or thoracoscopic splanchnicectomy may improve pain control.

Surgical resection is the treatment of choice for neuroendocrine tumors, when feasible. Metastatic disease may be controlled with long-acting somatostatin analogs, interferon, peptide-receptor radionuclide therapy, and chemoembolization. There is a growing consensus that asymptomatic incidental pancreatic cysts 2 cm or smaller are at low risk for harboring invasive carcinoma; the cysts

may be monitored by imaging tests (MRI) in 1 year and then every 2 years for 5 years if no changes are observed, with EUS and FNA if a cyst enlarges to at least 3 cm and another high-risk feature (dilated main pancreatic duct, presence of a solid component) develops. Other guidelines have been proposed.

Surgical resection is indicated for mucinous cystic neoplasms, symptomatic serous cystadenomas, solid pseudopapillary tumors (which have a 15% risk of malignant transformation), and cystic tumors larger than 2 cm in diameter that remain undefined after helical CT, EUS, and diagnostic aspiration. All intraductal papillary mucinous neoplasms of the main pancreatic duct should be resected, but those of branch ducts may be monitored with serial imaging if they (1) are asymptomatic and exhibit benign features; (2) have a diameter less than 3 cm (some authorities recommend a diameter 1.5 cm or smaller, but even lesions 3 cm or larger may be monitored in elderly persons with no other worrisome cyst features); and (3) lack nonenhancing mural nodules, a thick wall, an abrupt change in the caliber of the pancreatic duct with distal pancreatic atrophy, or possibly bile duct dilatation and gallbladder adenomyomatosis. Most such lesions with benign features remain stable on follow-up, but the risk of pancreatic ductal carcinoma and of nonpancreatic cancers may also be increased in this group of patients. In the absence of locally advanced disease, survival is higher for malignant cystic neoplasms than for adenocarcinoma. Endoscopic resection or ablation, with temporary placement of a pancreatic duct stent, may be feasible for ampullary adenomas, but patients must be followed for recurrence.

▶ **Prognosis**

Carcinoma of the pancreas, especially in the body or tail, has a poor prognosis; 80–85% of patients present with advanced unresectable disease, and reported 5-year survival rates range from 2% to 5%. Tumors of the ampulla have a better prognosis, with reported 5-year survival rates of 20–40% after resection; jaundice and lymph node involvement are adverse prognostic factors. In carefully selected patients, resection of cancer of the pancreatic head is feasible and results in reasonable survival. In persons with a family history of pancreatic cancer in at least two first-degree relatives, or with a genetic syndrome associated with an increased risk of pancreatic cancer, screening with EUS and helical CT or MRI/MRCP should be considered beginning at age 40–45 or 10 years before the age at which pancreatic cancer was diagnosed in a family member.

For those patients whose disease progresses despite treatment, meticulous efforts at palliative care are essential (see Chapter 5).

▶ When to Refer

All patients with carcinoma involving the pancreas and the ampulla of Vater should be referred to a specialist.

▶ When to Admit

Patients who require surgery and other interventions should be hospitalized.

Bockhorn M et al. Borderline resectable pancreatic cancer: a consensus statement by the International Study Group of Pancreatic Surgery (ISGPS). Surgery. 2014 Jun;155(6):977–88. [PMID: 24856119]

Grant RC et al. Prevalence of germline mutations in cancer predisposition genes in patients with pancreatic cancer. Gastroenterology. 2015 Mar;148(3):556–64. [PMID: 25479140]

Kaimakliotis P et al. Sendai and Fukuoka Consensus Guidelines identify advanced neoplasia in patients with suspected mucinous cystic neoplasms of the pancreas. Clin Gastroenterol Hepatol. 2015 Oct;13(10):1808–15. [PMID: 25818077]

Ryan DP et al. Pancreatic adenocarcinoma. N Engl J Med. 2014 Sep 11;371(11):1039–49. [PMID: 25207767]

Vege SS et al. American Gastroenterological Association Institute guideline on the diagnosis and management of asymptomatic neoplastic pancreatic cysts. Gastroenterology. 2015 Apr;148(4):819–22. [PMID: 25805375]

ALIMENTARY TRACT CANCERS

Pelin Cinar, MD, MS
Kenneth R. McQuaid, MD

ESOPHAGEAL CANCER

ESSENTIALS OF DIAGNOSIS

- ▶ Progressive solid food dysphagia.
- ▶ Weight loss common.
- ▶ Endoscopy with biopsy establishes diagnosis.

▶ General Considerations

Esophageal cancer usually develops in persons between 50 and 70 years of age. The overall ratio of men to women is 3:1. There are two histologic types: squamous cell carcinoma and adenocarcinoma. In the United States, **squamous cell cancer** is much more common in blacks than in whites. Squamous cell cancer has a high incidence in certain regions of China and Southeast Asia. Half of all cases occur in the distal third of the esophagus. Chronic alcohol and tobacco use are strongly associated with an increased risk of squamous cell carcinoma. **Adenocarcinoma** is more common in whites. It is increasing dramatically in incidence and now is more common than squamous carcinoma in the United States. The majority of adenocarcinomas develop as a complication of Barrett metaplasia due to chronic gastroesophageal reflux. Thus, most adenocarcinomas arise in the distal third of the esophagus. Obesity also is strongly associated with adenocarcinoma, even after controlling for gastroesophageal reflux.

▶ Clinical Findings

A. Symptoms and Signs

Most patients with esophageal cancer present with advanced, incurable disease. Over 90% have solid food dysphagia, which progresses over weeks to months. Odynophagia is sometimes present. Significant weight loss is common. Local tumor extension into the tracheobronchial tree may result in a tracheo-esophageal fistula, characterized by coughing on swallowing or pneumonia. Chest or back pain suggests mediastinal extension. Recurrent laryngeal involvement may produce hoarseness. Physical examination is often unrevealing. The presence of supraclavicular or cervical lymphadenopathy or of hepatomegaly implies metastatic disease.

B. Laboratory Findings

Laboratory findings are nonspecific. Anemia related to chronic disease or occult blood loss is common. Elevated aminotransferase or alkaline phosphatase concentrations suggest hepatic or bony metastases. Hypoalbuminemia may result from malnutrition.

C. Imaging

A barium esophagogram may be the first study obtained to evaluate dysphagia. The appearance of a polypoid, obstructive, or ulcerative lesion is suggestive of carcinoma and requires endoscopic evaluation. However, even lesions believed to be benign by radiography warrant endoscopic evaluation. Chest radiographs may show adenopathy, a widened mediastinum, pulmonary or bony metastases, or signs of tracheo-esophageal fistula such as pneumonia.

D. Upper Endoscopy

Endoscopy with biopsy establishes the diagnosis of esophageal carcinoma with a high degree of reliability. In some cases, significant submucosal spread of the tumor may yield nondiagnostic mucosal biopsies. Repeated biopsy may be necessary.

Staging

After confirmation of the diagnosis of esophageal carcinoma, the stage of the disease should be determined since doing so influences the choice of therapy. Patients should undergo evaluation with CT of the chest and abdomen to look for evidence of pulmonary or hepatic metastases, lymphadenopathy, and local tumor extension. If there is no evidence of distant metastases or extensive local spread on CT, EUS with guided FNA biopsy of lymph nodes should be performed, which is superior to CT in demonstrating the level of local mediastinal extension and local lymph node involvement. PET with fluorodeoxyglucose or integrated PET-CT imaging is indicated to look for regional or distant spread in patients thought to have localized disease after other diagnostic studies, prior to invasive surgery. Bronchoscopy is sometimes required in esophageal cancers above the carina to exclude tracheobronchial extension. Laparoscopy to exclude occult peritoneal carcinomatosis should be considered in patients with tumors at or near the gastroesophageal junction (see Gastric Adenocarcinoma).

Differential Diagnosis

Esophageal carcinoma must be distinguished from other causes of progressive dysphagia, including peptic stricture, achalasia, and adenocarcinoma of the gastric cardia with esophageal involvement. Benign-appearing peptic strictures should be biopsied at presentation to exclude occult malignancy.

Treatment

The approach to esophageal cancer depends on the tumor stage, patient preference and functional status, and the expertise of the surgeons, oncologists, gastroenterologists, and radiotherapists. It is helpful to classify patients into two general categories.

A. Therapy for "Curable" Disease

Superficial esophageal cancers confined to the epithelium (high-grade dysplasia or carcinoma in situ [Tis]), lamina propria (T1a), or submucosal (T1b) are increasingly recognized in endoscopic screening and surveillance programs. Esophagectomy achieves high cure rates for superficial tumors but is associated with mortality (2%) and morbidity. If performed by experienced clinicians, endoscopic mucosal resection of Tis and T1a cancers achieves equivalent long-term survival with less morbidity (see Barrett Esophagus, Chapter 15). Patients with larger tumors or deeper tumors invasive to the submucosa (T1b) have higher rates of lymph node metastasis. Frequent posttreatment endoscopic surveillance is required to ensure no residual or recurrent tumor.

1. Surgery with or without neoadjuvant chemoradiation therapy—There are multiple surgical approaches to the resection of invasive (non-superficial) but potentially "curable" esophageal cancers (stage Ib, II, or IIIA). Accepted techniques include en bloc transthoracic excision of the esophagus with extended lymph node dissection, transhiatal esophagogastrectomy (entailing laparotomy with cervical anastamosis), and minimally invasive esophagectomy techniques. Meta-analysis data suggest equivalent oncologic outcomes from minimally invasive esophagectomy and conventional open techniques. Removal of at least 15 lymph nodes is recommended for optimal surgical staging in patients who have not received neoadjuvant therapy; the optimal number of lymph nodes after neoadjuvant therapy is not known though similar lymphadenectomy is recommended by expert guidelines.

Patients with stage I tumors have high cure rates with surgery alone and do not require radiation or chemotherapy. If regional lymph node metastases have occurred (stages IIB and III), the rate of cure with surgery alone is reduced to less than 20%. Meta-analysis of trials comparing neoadjuvant (preoperative) therapy followed by surgery with surgery alone suggests a 13% absolute improvement in 2-year survival with combined therapy. Preoperative (neoadjuvant) chemoradiation therapy is recommended for stage IIA, IIB, and III tumors in fit patients. The preferred neoadjuvant chemotherapy regimen used with radiation is weekly carboplatin plus paclitaxel, based on the 2012 randomized phase III CROSS trial that demonstrated improvement in median survival from 24 months with surgery alone to 49.4 months with neoadjuvant chemoradiation ($P = 0.003$). As an alternative, a combination of cisplatin plus 5-fluorouracil may be used along with radiation. Perioperative chemotherapy without radiation is also appropriate for tumors of the gastroesophageal junction based on the randomized, multicenter, phase III MAGIC trial.

2. Chemotherapy plus radiation therapy without surgery—Combined treatment with chemotherapy and radiation is superior to radiation alone and has achieved long-term survival rates in up to 25% of patients. Chemoradiation alone should be considered in patients with localized disease (stage II or IIIA) who are poor surgical candidates due to serious medical illness or poor functional status (Eastern Cooperative Oncology Group score greater than 2). Chemoradiation alone as definitive, nonsurgical therapy is more likely to achieve long-term disease-free survival in patients with squamous cell carcinoma than in patients with adenocarcinoma.

3. Supportive care during definitive therapy—Patients with significant tumor obstruction may require local measures such as esophageal stent placement or percutaneous feeding tube insertion to maintain adequate hydration and nutrition during neoadjuvant chemoradiation or chemotherapy. Multidisciplinary consultation is required to determine the optimal procedure. Consultation with a nutritionist also is appropriate to optimize nutrition perioperatively.

B. Therapy for Incurable Disease

More than half of patients have either locally extensive tumor spread (T4) that is unresectable or distant metastases (M1) (stage IIIB and stage IV). Surgery is not warranted in these patients. Since prolonged survival can be achieved in few patients, the primary goal is to provide relief from dysphagia and pain, optimize quality of life, and minimize treatment side effects. The optimal palliative approach depends on the presence or absence of metastatic disease, expected survival, patient preference, and institutional experience. Many patients with advanced disease may prefer concerted efforts at pain relief and care directed at symptom management (see Chapter 5).

1. Chemotherapy or chemoradiation—Combined radiation therapy and chemotherapy may achieve palliation in two-thirds of patients but is associated with significant side effects. It should be considered for patients with locally advanced tumors without distant metastases (stage IIIB) who have good functional status and no significant medical problems, in whom prolonged survival may be achieved. Improvement in dysphagia occurs within 2–4 weeks in almost 90% of patients.

Combination chemotherapy may be considered in those patients with metastatic disease who still have good functional status and expected survival of at least several months. Three-drug combinations commonly include a fluoropyrimidine (5-fluorouracil or capecitabine), a platinum drug (cisplatin or oxaliplatin), and either epirubicin or a taxane (docetaxel or paclitaxel). For patients with poor functional status, single-agent therapy with a fluoropyrimidine, a taxane, or irinotecan may be used. In patients with metastatic distal esophageal and gastroesophageal junction adenocarcinomas positive for amplification of the *HER2* gene (approximately 15% of cases), addition of the monoclonal antibody trastuzumab (see Chapter 17) to chemotherapy is associated with prolonged survival based on the randomized, phase III ToGA trial. In addition, ramucirumab, a monoclonal antibody targeting the VEGF receptor-2, demonstrated a survival advantage in patients with adenocarcinoma of the gastroesophageal junction after progression on first-line therapy when used both as monotherapy and in combination with paclitaxel.

2. Local therapy for esophageal obstruction—Patients with advanced esophageal cancer often have a poor functional and nutritional status. Radiation therapy alone to the area of esophageal obstruction may afford short-term relief of pain and dysphagia and may be suitable for patients with poor functional status or underlying medical problems. This can generally be performed in a short course over a few weeks or less but may be complicated by temporary worsening of dysphagia and odynophagia. For patients with frank obstruction or near obstruction, local antitumor therapies may be preferred. Rapid palliation of dysphagia may be achieved by peroral placement of permanent expandable wire stents (alone or followed by radiation). Palliative feeding tube placement may be considered for hydration and nutrition in selected cases if the obstruction is not amenable or if it is refractory to stenting, radiation, or other local therapies. Stents are most commonly used because of their relative ease of placement. Although dysphagia and quality of life are improved, patients seldom can eat normally after stent placement. Complications occur in 20–40% and include perforation, migration, and tumor ingrowth.

Prognosis

The overall 5-year survival rate of esophageal carcinoma is less than 20%. Apart from distant metastasis (M1b), the two most important predictors of poor survival are adjacent mediastinal spread (T4) and lymph node involvement. Whereas cure may be achieved in patients with regional lymph node involvement (stages IIB and III), involvement of nodes outside the chest (M1a) is indicative of metastatic disease (stage IV) that is incurable. For those patients whose disease progresses despite chemotherapy, meticulous efforts at palliative care are essential (see Chapter 5).

When to Refer

- Patients should be referred to a gastroenterologist for evaluation and staging (endoscopy with biopsy, EUS) and palliative endoscopic antitumor therapy (stent).

- Patients with metastatic disease and obstructive tumors not amenable or refractory to palliative radiation or stenting may require referral to an interventional radiologist, gastroenterologist, or surgeon for gastric or jejunal tube placement for liquid artificial nutrition.

- Patients with curable and resectable disease for whom neoadjuvant therapy may be appropriate (stage IIB or IIIA) and those with locally advanced or metastatic disease should be referred to an oncologist for consideration of neoadjuvant chemotherapy or chemoradiotherapy, or for palliative chemotherapy, respectively.

When to Admit

Patients with high-grade esophageal obstruction with inability to manage oral secretions or maintain hydration should be admitted. Acute complications such as perforation, bleeding, aspiration, or fistula also may require admission.

ASGE Standards of Practice Committee. The role of endoscopy in the assessment and treatment of esophageal cancer. Gastrointest Endosc 2013 Mar;77(3):328–34. [PMID: 23410694]

Blum Murphy MA et al. Current concepts and future potential in neoadjuvant chemotherapy for esophageal cancer. Expert Rev Gastroenterol Hepatol. 2016 Mar;10(3):383–92. [PMID: 26560689]

Dai Y et al. Interventions for dysphagia in oesophageal cancer. Cochrane Database Syst Rev. 2014 Oct 30;10:CD005048. [PMID: 25354795]

Fuchs CS et al. Ramucirumab monotherapy for previously treated advanced gastric or gastro-oesophageal junction adenocarcinoma (REGARD): an international, randomised, multicentre, placebo-controlled phase 3 trial. Lancet. 2014 Jan 4; 383(9911):31–9. [PMID: 24094768]

Glen P. The role of stents in the palliation of oesophageal cancer. BMJ Support Palliat Care. 2016 Mar;6(1):135–9. [PMID: 25573667]

Hofheinz RD et al. Ramucirumab as second-line treatment for patients with metastatic esophagogastric adenocarcinoma. Expert Rev Anticancer Ther. 2015 Jun;15(6):607–14. [PMID: 26035718]

Klevebro F et al. A randomised clinical trial of neoadjuvant chemotherapy vs. neoadjuvant chemoradiotherapy for cancer of the oesophagus or gastro-oesophageal junction. Ann Oncol. 2016 Apr;27(4):660–7. [PMID: 26782957]

Markar SR et al; FREGAT working group - FRENCH - AFC. Role of neoadjuvant treatment in clinical T2N0M0 oesophageal cancer: results from a retrospective multi-center European study. Eur J Cancer. 2016 Mar;56:59–68. [PMID: 26808298]

National Cancer Institute. Esophageal cancer treatment for health professionals. http://www.cancer.gov/types/esophageal/hp/esophageal-treatment-pdq

Rustgi AK et al. Esophageal carcinoma. N Engl J Med. 2014 Dec 25;371(26):2499–509. [PMID: 25539106]

Sihag S et al. Minimally invasive versus open esophagectomy for esophageal cancer: a comparison of early surgical outcomes from the Society of Thoracic Surgeons National Database. Ann Thorac Surg. 2016 Apr;101(4):1281–9. [PMID: 26704412]

Tani Y et al. 18F-Fluorodeoxyglucose positron emission tomography for evaluating the response to neoadjuvant chemotherapy in advanced esophageal cancer. Anticancer Res. 2016 Jan;36(1):367–73. [PMID: 26722067]

Umezawa R et al. Long-term results of chemoradiotherapy for stage II-III thoracic esophageal cancer in a single institution after 2000—with a focus on comparison of three protocols. BMC Cancer. 2015 Oct 27;15:813. [PMID: 26506988]

Wilke H et al; RAINBOW Study Group. Ramucirumab plus paclitaxel versus placebo plus paclitaxel in patients with previously treated advanced gastric or gastro-oesophageal junction adenocarcinoma (RAINBOW): a double-blind, randomised phase 3 trial. Lancet Oncol. 2014 Oct;15(11): 1224–35. [PMID: 25240821]

GASTRIC ADENOCARCINOMA

 ESSENTIALS OF DIAGNOSIS

▸ Dyspeptic symptoms with weight loss in patients over age 40 years.

▸ Iron deficiency anemia: occult blood in stools.

▸ Abnormality detected on upper gastrointestinal series or endoscopy.

▸ General Considerations

Gastric adenocarcinoma remains the second most common cause of cancer death worldwide. However, its incidence has declined rapidly over the last 70 years, especially in western countries, which may be attributable to changes in diet (more fruits and vegetables), food refrigeration (allowing more fresh foods and reduced salted, smoked, and preserved foods), reduced toxic environmental exposures, and a decline in *Helicobacter pylori*. The incidence of gastric cancer remains high (70/100,000) in Japan and many developing regions, including eastern Asia, Eastern Europe, Chile, Colombia, and Central America. In the United States, there are an estimated 22,220 new cases and 10,990 deaths/year. The incidence is higher in Latinos, African Americans, and Asian Americans.

There are two main histologic variants of gastric cancer: "intestinal-type" (which resembles intestinal cancers in forming glandular structures) and "diffuse" (which is poorly differentiated, has signet-ring cells, and lacks glandular formation). The incidence of **intestinal-type gastric cancer** has declined significantly but it is still the more common type (70–80%); it occurs twice as often in men as women, primarily affects older people (mean age 63 years), and is more strongly associated with environmental factors. It is believed to arise through a gradual, multi-step progression from inflammation (most commonly due to *H pylori*), to atrophic gastritis, to intestinal metaplasia, and finally dysplasia or cancer. Chronic *H pylori* gastritis is the strong risk factor for gastric carcinoma, increasing the relative risk 3.5- to 20-fold. It is estimated that 60–90% of cases of gastric carcinomas may be attributable to *H pylori*. Other risk factors for intestinal-type gastric cancer include pernicious anemia, a history of partial gastric resection more than 15 years previously, smoking, and diets that are high in nitrates or salt and low in vitamin C.

Diffuse gastric cancer accounts for 20–30% of gastric cancer. In contrast to intestinal-type cancer, it affects men and women equally, occurs more commonly in young people, is not as strongly related to *H pylori* infection, and has a worse prognosis than intestinal-type cancer. Most diffuse gastric cancers are attributable to acquired or hereditary mutations in the genes regulating the E-cadherin cell adhesion protein. Familial diffuse gastric cancer accounts for 1–3% of gastric cancers. The cancer may arise at a young age, is often multifocal and infiltrating with signet ring cell histology, and confers poor prognosis. Many of these families have a germline mutation of E-cadherin *CDH1*, which is inherited in an autosomal dominant pattern and carries a greater than 60% lifetime risk of gastric cancer. Prophylactic gastrectomy should be considered in patients known to carry this mutation.

Most gastric cancers arise in the body and antrum. These may occur in a variety of morphologic types: (1) polypoid or fungating intraluminal masses; (2) ulcerating masses; (3) diffusely spreading (linitis plastica), in which the tumor spreads through the submucosa, resulting in a rigid, atonic stomach with thickened folds (prognosis dismal); and (4) superficially spreading or "early" gastric cancer—confined to the mucosa or submucosa (with or without lymph node metastases) and associated with a favorable prognosis.

In contrast to the dramatic decline in cancers of the distal stomach, a rise in incidence of tumors of the gastric cardia has been noted. These tumors have demographic and pathologic features that resemble Barrett-associated esophageal adenocarcinomas (see Esophageal Cancer).

▸ Clinical Findings

A. Symptoms and Signs

Gastric carcinoma is generally asymptomatic until the disease is quite advanced. Symptoms are nonspecific and are determined in part by the location of the tumor. Dyspepsia, vague epigastric pain, anorexia, early satiety, and weight loss are the presenting symptoms in most patients. Patients may derive initial symptomatic relief from over-the-counter remedies, further delaying diagnosis. Ulcerating lesions can lead to acute gastrointestinal bleeding with hematemesis or melena. Pyloric obstruction results in postprandial vomiting. Lower esophageal obstruction causes progressive dysphagia. Physical examination is rarely helpful. A gastric mass is palpated in less than 20% of patients. Signs of metastatic spread include a left supraclavicular lymph node (Virchow node), an umbilical nodule (Sister Mary Joseph nodule), a rigid rectal shelf (Blumer shelf), and ovarian metastases (Krukenberg tumor). Guaiac-positive stools may be detectable.

B. Laboratory Findings

Iron deficiency anemia due to chronic blood loss or anemia of chronic disease is common. Liver test abnormalities, particularly elevation of alkaline phosphatase, may be present if there is metastatic liver spread. Circulating tumor markers do not have established clinical validity in screening, diagnosis, or management of gastric cancer.

C. Endoscopy

Upper endoscopy should be obtained in all patients over age 55 years with new onset of epigastric symptoms (dyspepsia) and in anyone with dyspepsia that is persistent or fails to respond to a short trial of antisecretory therapy. Endoscopy with biopsies of suspicious lesions is highly sensitive for detecting gastric carcinoma. It can be difficult to obtain adequate biopsy specimens in linitis plastica lesions.

D. Imaging

Once a gastric cancer is diagnosed, preoperative evaluation with CT of chest and abdomen (including pelvis in females) and EUS is indicated to delineate the local extent of the primary tumor as well as to evaluate for nodal or distant metastases. EUS is superior to CT in determining the depth of tumor penetration and is useful for evaluation of early gastric cancers that may be removed by endoscopic mucosal resection. PET or combined PET-CT imaging is recommended for detection of distant metastasis.

▶ Screening

Because of its unproven efficacy and cost-effectiveness, screening for *H pylori* infection and treating it to prevent gastric cancer is not recommended for asymptomatic adults in the general population but may be considered in patients who have immigrated from regions with a high incidence of gastric cancer or who have a family history of gastric cancer. Because of the high incidence of gastric carcinoma in Japan, screening upper endoscopy is performed there to detect early gastric carcinoma. Approximately 40% of tumors detected by screening are early, with a 5-year survival rate of almost 90%. Screening is not recommended in the United States.

▶ Staging

Staging is defined according to the TNM system, in which T1 tumors invade the lamina propria (T1a) or submucosa (T1b), T2 invade the muscularis propria, T3 penetrate the serosa, and T4 invade adjacent structures. Lymph nodes are graded as N0 if there is no involvement, and N1, N2, or N3 if there is involvement of 1–6, 7–15, or more than

15 regional nodes. M1 signifies the presence of metastatic disease. Sampling of at least 15 lymph nodes is recommended during surgical staging (see Curative Surgical Resection below). A staging laparoscopy prior to definitive surgery to exclude peritoneal carcinomatosis should be considered in patients with stage T1b or greater disease without radiographic evidence of distant metastases. Pathologic review should include (1) grade of tumor; (2) histologic subtype; (3) depth of invasion; (4) whether lymphatic or vascular invasion is present; and (5) if there is known metastatic disease, the status of HER2 protein expression by immunohistochemistry or fluorescent in situ hybridization or both.

▶ Differential Diagnosis

Ulcerating gastric adenocarcinomas are distinguished from benign gastric ulcers by biopsies. Approximately 3% of gastric ulcers initially believed to be benign later prove to be malignant. To exclude malignancy, all gastric ulcers identified at endoscopy should be biopsied. Ulcers that are suspicious for malignancy to the endoscopist or that have atypia or dysplasia on histologic examination warrant repeat endoscopy in 2–3 months to verify healing and exclude malignancy. Nonhealing ulcers should be considered for resection. Infiltrative carcinoma with thickened gastric folds must be distinguished from lymphoma and other hypertrophic gastropathies.

▶ Treatment

A. Curative Surgical Resection

Surgical resection is the only therapy with curative potential. Laparoscopic techniques achieve similar outcomes and lower overall complication rates as open gastrectomy. After preoperative staging, about two-thirds of patients will be found to have localized disease (ie, stages I–III). In Japan and in specialized centers in the United States, endoscopic mucosal resection is performed in selected patients with small (less than 1–2 cm), early (intramucosal or T1aN0) gastric cancers after careful staging with EUS. Approximately 25% of patients undergoing surgery will be found to have locally unresectable tumors or peritoneal, hepatic, or distant lymph node metastases that are incurable. The remaining patients with confirmed localized disease should undergo radical surgical resection with curative intent. For adenocarcinoma localized to the distal two-thirds of the stomach, a subtotal distal gastrectomy should be performed. For proximal gastric cancer or diffusely infiltrating disease, total gastrectomy is necessary. Vitamin B_{12} supplementation is required after gastrectomy. For patients with localized gastric cancer that is resectable, current National Comprehensive Cancer Network (NCCN) treatment guidelines recommend gastrectomy with extended (D1), or modified regional (D2), lymph node dissection and sampling of 15 or more lymph nodes.

B. Perioperative Chemotherapy or Chemoradiation

The use of perioperative chemotherapy or adjuvant chemoradiation is associated with improved survival in patients with localized or locoregional gastric adenocarcinoma who undergo surgical resection. The choice of treatment depends on the location and extent of tumor, type of surgery, patient comorbidities and performance status, and institutional experience. Treatment of tumors arising in the gastroesophageal junction may be treated following algorithms for esophageal primary tumors; multidisciplinary treatment decision-making involving the surgeon, radiation oncologist, and medical oncologist is imperative.

C. Palliative Modalities

Many patients will be found either preoperatively or at the time of surgical exploration to have advanced disease that is not amenable to "curative" surgery due to peritoneal or distant metastases or local invasion of other organs. In some of these cases, palliative resection of the tumor nonetheless may be indicated to alleviate pain, bleeding, or obstruction. For patients with unresectable disease, a surgical diversion with gastrojejunostomy may be indicated to prevent obstruction. Alternatively, unresected tumors may be treated with endoscopic laser or stent therapy, radiation therapy, or angiographic embolization to relieve bleeding or obstruction. Chemotherapy may be considered in patients with metastatic disease who still have good functional status and expected survival of at least several months. Multiple chemotherapy regimens have demonstrated activity in metastatic gastric adenocarcinoma. Two-drug combination regimens are preferred for first-line therapy, with most common regimens including a fluoropyrimidine or a taxane agent plus a platinum agent. A three-drug combination of epirubicin or docetaxel plus cisplatin and 5-fluorouracil, or a modification thereof, may be appropriate for first-line treatment in medically fit patients. A 2009 randomized, phase III study showed that addition of the biologic agent trastuzumab to standard chemotherapy prolonged survival in the subset (approximately 15%) of patients with advanced gastric adenocarcinomas harboring amplification of the EGFR-2 (HER2). Trastuzumab is not recommended for combination with anthracyclines such as epirubicin, however, due to risk for cardiotoxicity. After progression on first-line chemotherapy, treatment with irinotecan prolonged survival compared to best supportive care in a randomized, phase III trial. Ramucirumab, a monoclonal antibody targeting the VEGF receptor-2, demonstrated a survival advantage in patients with gastric or gastroesophageal junction adenocarcinoma after progression on first-line therapy when used both as monotherapy and in combination with paclitaxel.

▶ Prognosis

The long-term survival of gastric carcinoma is approximately 28%. However, 5-year survival in patients who undergo successful curative resection exceeds 45%. Survival is related to tumor stage, location, and histologic features. Stage I and stage II tumors resected for cure have a greater than 60% long-term survival. Patients with stage III tumors have a poor prognosis (less than 30% long-term survival) and should be considered for enrollment in clinical trials. Tumors of the diffuse type have a worse prognosis than the intestinal type. Tumors of the proximal stomach (fundus and cardia) carry a far worse prognosis than distal lesions. Even with apparently localized disease, proximal tumors have a 5-year survival of less than 15%. For those whose disease progresses despite therapy, meticulous efforts at palliative care are essential (see Chapter 5).

▶ When to Refer

- Patients with dysphagia, weight loss, protracted vomiting, iron deficiency anemia, melena, or new-onset of dyspepsia (especially if age 55 years or older or associated with other alarm symptoms) in whom gastric cancer is suspected should be referred for endoscopy.

- Patients should be referred to a surgeon for attempt at curative resection in stage I, II, or III cancer, including staging laparoscopy if indicated.

- Prior to surgery, patients should be referred to an oncologist to determine the role for neoadjuvant chemotherapy or adjuvant chemoradiation or chemotherapy.

- Patients who have undergone gastrectomy require consultation with a nutritionist due to propensity for malnutrition and complications, such as dumping syndrome and vitamin B_{12} deficiency, postoperatively.

- Patients with unresectable or metastatic disease should be referred to an oncologist for consideration of palliative chemotherapy or chemoradiation.

▶ When to Admit

Patients with protracted vomiting, inability to maintain hydration or nutrition, or acute bleeding.

Al-Batran SE et al. Quality-of-life and performance status results from the phase 3 RAINBOW study of ramucirumab plus paclitaxel versus placebo plus paclitaxel in patients with previously treated gastric or gastroesophageal junction adenocarcinoma. Ann Oncol. 2016 Apr;27(4):673–9. [PMID: 26747859]

Fuchs CS et al. Ramucirumab monotherapy for previously treated advanced gastric or gastro-oesophageal junction adenocarcinoma (REGARD): an international, randomised, multicentre, placebo-controlled phase 3 trial. Lancet. 2014 Jan 4; 383(9911):31–9. [PMID: 24094768]

Hecht JR et al. Lapatinib in combination with capecitabine plus oxaliplatin in human epidermal growth factor receptor 2-positive advanced or metastatic gastric, esophageal, or gastroesophageal adenocarcinoma: TRIO-013/LOGiC- a randomized phase III trial. J Clin Oncol. 2016 Feb 10;34(5):443–51. [PMID: 26628478]

Kamran SC et al. Advances in the management of gastric and gastroesophageal cancers. Curr Oncol Rep. 2016 Feb;18(2):13. [PMID: 26769118]

Lin JT. Screening of gastric cancer: who, when, and how. Clin Gastroenterol Hepatol. 2014 Jan;12(1):135–8. [PMID: 24107396]

National Cancer Institute. Stomach (Gastric) Cancer—Health Professional Version. http://www.cancer.gov/types/stomach/hp

Noh SH et al; CLASSIC trial investigators. Adjuvant capecitabine plus oxaliplatin for gastric cancer after D2 gastrectomy (CLASSIC): 5-year follow-up of an open-label, randomised phase 3 trial. Lancet Oncol. 2014 Nov;15(12):1389–96. [PMID: 25439693]

Park CH et al. Impact of carcinomatosis and ascites status on long-term outcomes of palliative treatment for patients with gastric outlet obstruction caused by unresectable gastric cancer: stent placement versus palliative gastrojejunostomy. Gastrointest Endosc. 2015 Feb;81(2):321–32. [PMID: 25085332]

Waddell T et al; European Society for Medical Oncology (ESMO); European Society of Surgical Oncology (ESSO); European Society of Radiotherapy and Oncology (ESTRO). Gastric cancer: ESMO-ESSO-ESTRO clinical practice guidelines for diagnosis, treatment and follow-up. Eur J Surg Oncol. 2014 May;40(5):584–91. [PMID: 24685156]

Wilke H et al; RAINBOW Study Group. Ramucirumab plus paclitaxel versus placebo plus paclitaxel in patients with previously treated advanced gastric or gastro-oesophageal junction adenocarcinoma (RAINBOW): a double-blind, randomised phase 3 trial. Lancet Oncol. 2014 Oct;15(11):1224–35. [PMID: 25240821]

Yazici O et al. Targeted therapies in gastric cancer and future perspectives. World J Gastroenterol. 2016 Jan 14;22(2):471–89. [PMID: 26811601]

GASTRIC LYMPHOMA

ESSENTIALS OF DIAGNOSIS

▶ Symptoms of dyspepsia, weight loss, or anemia.

▶ Variable abnormalities on upper gastrointestinal series or endoscopy including thickened folds, ulcer, mass or infiltrating lesions; diagnosis established by endoscopic biopsy.

▶ Abdominal CT and EUS required for staging.

▶ General Considerations

Gastric lymphomas may be primary (arising from the gastric mucosa) or may represent a site of secondary involvement in patients with nodal lymphomas. Distinguishing advanced primary gastric lymphoma with adjacent nodal spread from advanced nodal lymphoma with secondary gastric spread is essential because the prognosis and treatment of primary and secondary gastric lymphomas are different. Primary lymphoma is the second most common gastric malignancy, accounting for 3% of gastric cancers. More than 95% of these are non-Hodgkin B cell lymphomas. Most primary gastric lymphomas are believed to arise from mucosa-associated lymphoid tissue (MALT).

Infection with *H pylori* is an important risk factor for the development of primary gastric lymphoma. Chronic infection with *H pylori* causes an intense lymphocytic inflammatory response that may lead to the development of lymphoid follicles. Over 90% of low-grade primary gastric MALT-type lymphomas are associated with *H pylori* infection. It is hypothesized that chronic antigenic stimulation may result in a monoclonal lymphoproliferation that may culminate in low-grade or high-grade lymphoma.

▶ Clinical Findings & Staging

The clinical presentation and endoscopic appearance of gastric lymphoma are similar to those of adenocarcinoma.

Most patients have abdominal pain, weight loss, or bleeding. Patients with diffuse large B-cell lymphoma are more likely to have systemic symptoms and advanced tumor stage. At endoscopy, lymphoma may appear as an ulcer, mass, or diffusely infiltrating lesion. The diagnosis is established with endoscopic biopsy; FNA is not adequate. EUS is the most sensitive test for determining the level of invasion and presence of perigastric lymphadenopathy and should be performed, if available. All patients should undergo staging with CT scanning of chest, abdomen, and pelvis. For patients with diffuse large B-cell lymphomas involving the stomach, combination PET-CT imaging, bone marrow biopsy with aspirate, tumor lysis laboratory tests, and viral hepatitis and HIV serologies also may be required for staging and management (see Chapter 13).

▶ Treatment

Treatment of primary gastric lymphomas depends on the tumor histology, grade, and stage. Marginal B-cell lymphomas of the MALT type that are low-grade and localized to the stomach wall (stage IE) or perigastric lymph nodes (stage IIE_1) have an excellent prognosis. EUS should be performed to accurately determine tumor stage. Patients with primary gastric MALT-lymphoma should be tested for *H pylori* infection and treated if positive. Complete lymphoma regression after successful *H pylori* eradication occurs in approximately 75% of cases of stage IE and approximately 55% with stage II_1 low-grade lymphoma. Remission may take as long as a year, and relapse occurs in about 2% of cases per year. Endoscopic surveillance after *H pylori* eradication is recommended every 6 months for 2 years to look for recurrence. In patients whose tumors harbor specific gene translocations, including t(11;18) (API2-MALT1), t(1;14), or t(14;18), rates of remission after *H pylori* eradication are lower, and treatment with radiation may be required. Patients with localized marginal zone MALT-type lymphomas who either are not infected with *H pylori* or do not respond to eradication therapy may be treated with radiation therapy or rituximab, if not a candidate for radiation. Data from a 2010 study, however, suggest that many patients with minimal disease after successful *H pylori* eradication may be observed closely without further therapy. The long-term survival of low-grade MALT lymphoma for stage I is over 90% and for stage II is 35–65%. Because of a low risk of perforation with either radiation therapy or chemotherapy, surgical resection is no longer recommended. Diffuse large B-cell or other higher grade lymphomas with secondary gastrointestinal involvement usually present at an advanced stage with widely disseminated disease and are treated according to stage and subtype of lymphoma (see Chapter 13).

Ding W et al. Gastrointestinal lymphoma in Southwest China: subtype distribution of 1,010 cases using the WHO (2008) classification in a single institution. Acta Haematol. 2016;135(1):21–8. [PMID: 26303279]

Iwamuro M et al. Diagnosis of follicular lymphoma of the gastrointestinal tract: a better initial diagnostic workup. World J Gastroenterol. 2016 Jan 28;22(4):1674–83. [PMID: 26819532]

Nakamura S et al. Treatment strategy for gastric mucosa-associated lymphoid tissue lymphoma. Gastroenterol Clin North Am. 2015 Sep;44(3):649–60. [PMID: 26314674]

Pereira MI et al. Role of *Helicobacter pylori* in gastric mucosa-associated lymphoid tissue lymphomas. World J Gastroenterol. 2014 Jan 21;20(3):684–98. [PMID: 24574742]

Zullo A et al. Gastric MALT lymphoma: old and new insights. Ann Gastroenterol. 2014;27(1):27–33. [PMID: 24714739]

GASTRIC CARCINOID TUMORS

Gastric carcinoids are rare neuroendocrine tumors that make up less than 1% of gastric neoplasms. They may occur sporadically or secondary to chronic hypergastrinemia that results in hyperplasia and transformation of enterochromaffin cells in the gastric fundus. The majority of carcinoids are caused by hypergastrinemia and occur in association with either pernicious anemia (75%) (type 1) or Zollinger-Ellison syndrome (5%) (type 2). Initial diagnostic work-up includes serum gastrin level, upper endoscopy, and EUS. Gastrin level should be obtained 1 week after the patient has stopped taking protein pump inhibitors.

For patients with hypergastrinemia (suspected of type I or type II carcinoid), serum vitamin B_{12} and intrinsic factor antibody levels should be obtained to exclude pernicious anemia. Carcinoids associated with Zollinger-Ellison syndrome occur almost exclusively in patients with multiple endocrine neoplasia type 1 (MEN 1), in which chromosomal loss of 11q13 has been reported. Carcinoids caused by hypergastrinemia tend to be multicentric, smaller than 1 cm, have a low potential for metastatic spread, and thus are unlikely to cause development of the carcinoid syndrome. Small lesions may be successfully treated with endoscopic resection followed by periodic endoscopic surveillance, or with observation. Antrectomy reduces serum gastrin levels and may lead to regression of small tumors. Octreotide therapy may be appropriate for patients with underlying gastrinoma and Zollinger-Ellison syndrome. Patients with tumors larger than 2 cm should undergo endoscopic or surgical resection (see Small Intestinal Adenocarcinomas below).

Type 3 gastric carcinoid tumors arise sporadically, independent of gastrin production, and account for up to 20% of gastric carcinoids. Most sporadic gastric carcinoids are solitary, larger than 2 cm, and have a strong propensity for hepatic or pulmonary metastases and thus the carcinoid syndrome at initial presentation. CT or MRI should be obtained to evaluate for metastatic disease. Localized sporadic carcinoids should be treated with radical gastrectomy and regional lymphadenectomy.

Basuroy R et al. Review article: the investigation and management of gastric neuroendocrine tumours. Aliment Pharmacol Ther. 2014 May;39(10):1071–84. [PMID: 24628514]

Kidd M et al. Gastric carcinoids (neuroendocrine neoplasms). Gastroenterol Clin North Am. 2013 Jun;42(2):381–97. [PMID: 23639647]

Lahner E et al. Updated features associated with type 1 gastric carcinoids patients: a single-center study. Scand J Gastroenterol. 2014 Dec;49(12):1447–55. [PMID: 25309981]

Massironi S et al. Somatostatin analogs for gastric carcinoids: for many, but not all. World J Gastroenterol. 2015 Jun 14; 21(22):6785–93. [PMID: 26078554]

GASTROINTESTINAL MESENCHYMAL TUMORS

Gastrointestinal mesenchymal tumors (which include stromal tumors, leiomyomas, and schwannomas) derive from mesenchymal stem cells and have an epithelioid or spindle cell histologic pattern, resembling smooth muscle. The most common stromal tumors are gastrointestinal stromal tumors ("GISTs"), which originate from interstitial cells of Cajal. GISTs occur throughout the gastrointestinal tract but most commonly in the stomach (60%) and small intestine (30%). Approximately 85–90% of GISTs have mutations in *KIT*. Other mesenchymal tumors, such as leiomyomas, which derive from smooth muscle cells, generally stain negative for CD117. Mesenchymal tumors may be discovered incidentally on imaging studies or endoscopy or may cause symptoms (most commonly bleeding, pain, or obstruction). At endoscopy, they appear as a submucosal mass that may have central umbilication or ulceration. EUS with guided FNA biopsy is the optimal study for diagnosing gastric mesenchymal tumors and distinguishing them from other submucosal lesions. Percutaneous biopsy may confer risk of bleeding or intra-abdominal seeding. CT abdomen and pelvis, MRI and PET imaging are useful in the diagnosis and staging. PET imaging also may be useful to monitor response to treatment.

While almost all GISTs have malignant potential, the risk of developing metastasis is increased with tumor size greater than 2 cm, nongastric location, and mitotic index greater than 5 mitoses per 50 high-powered field. It is difficult to distinguish benign from malignant tumors before resection by endoscopic ultrasonographic appearance or FNA. In general, lesions are more likely benign if they are smaller than 2 cm, have a smooth border, and have a homogeneous echo pattern on endoscopic ultrasonogram.

Surgery is recommended for all patients with tumors that are 2 cm or larger, increasing in size, have an endoscopic ultrasonographic appearance suspicious for malignancy, or are symptomatic. The management of asymptomatic benign-appearing gastric lesions 2 cm or smaller in size is problematic. Because of the low but real long-term risk of malignancy, surgical resection should be considered in younger, otherwise healthy patients; however, other patients may be followed up with serial endoscopic ultrasonographic examinations or, in selected cases, endoscopic resections. After complete surgical resection, GISTs recur within 5 years in over half of patients. The majority of recurrences are within the first 3 years. Adjuvant therapy with the tyrosine kinase inhibitor imatinib delays recurrence and prolongs survival. Adjuvant imatinib is recommended for all high-risk patients for at least 1 year, though the 5-year recurrence-free survival rate is significantly better following 3 years than 1 year of such therapy (65.6% vs 47.9%). After surgical resection, patients should have surveillance with history and physical examination and CT of the abdomen and pelvis every 3–6 months. Neoadjuvant therapy with imatinib may be considered for patients with localized GIST tumors who are deemed to be at high risk for resection because of comorbidities, tumor size, or tumor location. A biopsy is required to confirm the diagnosis of GIST prior to initiation of neoadjuvant imatinib.

Untreated metastatic GIST tumors are aggressive and carry a poor prognosis. Imatinib induces disease control in up to 85% of patients with metastatic disease with a progression-free survival of 20–24 months and median overall survival of almost 5 years. Imatinib-resistant tumors may respond to high-dose imatinib or to sunitinib, another multi-targeted kinase inhibitor that is approved as second-line therapy for metastatic GIST. Patients in whom metastatic GIST develops after imatinib and sunitinib therapy may respond to the multi-targeted kinase inhibitor regorafenib. In the randomized, phase III GRID trial, patients treated with regorafenib had a significant improvement in progression-free survival compared to those receiving placebo (4.8 months vs 0.9 months). Regorafenib is now FDA approved to treat advanced GIST and is included in the NCCN guidelines for patients with treatment-refractory metastatic GIST.

Bae S et al. Personalized management: inoperable gastrointestinal stromal tumors. Clin Gastroenterol Hepatol. 2014 Jan; 12(1):130–4. [PMID: 23981520]

Balachandran VP et al. Gastrointestinal stromal tumors: who should get imatinib and for how long? Adv Surg. 2014;48: 165–83. [PMID: 25293614]

Bauer S et al. Emerging agents for the treatment of advanced, imatinib-resistant gastrointestinal stromal tumors: current status and future directions. Drugs. 2015 Aug;75(12):1323–34. [PMID: 26187774]

Demetri GD et al. Complete longitudinal analyses of the randomized, placebo-controlled phase III trial of sunitinib in patients with gastrointestinal stromal tumor following imatinib failure. Clin Cancer Res. 2012 Jun 1;18(11):3170–9. [PMID: 22661587]

Demetri GD et al; GRID study investigators. Efficacy and safety of regorafenib for advanced gastrointestinal stromal tumours after failure of imatinib and sunitinib (GRID): an international, multicentre, randomised, placebo-controlled, phase 3 trial. Lancet. 2013 Jan 26;381(9863):295–302. [PMID: 23177515]

Ferraro D et al. Regorafenib in gastrointestinal stromal tumors: clinical evidence and place in therapy. Ther Adv Med Oncol. 2014 Sep;6(5):222–8. [PMID: 25342989]

Joensuu H et al. Risk factors for gastrointestinal stromal tumor recurrence in patients treated with adjuvant imatinib. Cancer. 2014 Aug 1;120(15):2325–33. [PMID: 24737415]

Mullady DK et al. A multidisciplinary approach to the diagnosis and treatment of gastrointestinal stromal tumor. J Clin Gastroenterol. 2013 Aug;47(7):578–85. [PMID: 23751846]

Nishida T et al. The standard diagnosis, treatment, and follow-up of gastrointestinal stromal tumors based on guidelines. Gastric Cancer. 2016 Jan;19(1):3–14. [PMID: 26276366]

Rutkowski P et al. The safety of regorafenib for the treatment of gastrointestinal stromal tumors. Expert Opin Drug Saf. 2016 Jan; 15(1):105–16. [PMID: 26651387]

Serrano C et al. Recent advances in the treatment of gastrointestinal stromal tumors. Ther Adv Med Oncol. 2014 May; 6(3):115–27. [PMID: 24790651]

Vadakara J et al. Gastrointestinal stromal tumors: management of metastatic disease and emerging therapies. Hematol Oncol Clin North Am. 2013 Oct;27(5):905–20. [PMID: 24093167]

MALIGNANCIES OF THE SMALL INTESTINE

1. Small Intestinal Adenocarcinomas

These are aggressive tumors that occur most commonly in the duodenum or proximal jejunum. The incidence is rare, with approximately 6000 new diagnoses per year in the United States. Overall, prognosis is poor, with 5-year disease-specific survival of 65% for stage I, 48% for stage II, 35% for stage III, and 4% for stage IV disease (overall, 32% of patients are stage IV at diagnosis). The ampulla of Vater is the most common site of small bowel carcinoma. The incidence of ampullary carcinoma is increased more than 200-fold in patients with familial adenomatous polyposis. Periodic endoscopic surveillance to detect early ampullary neoplasms is therefore recommended. Ampullary carcinoma may present with jaundice due to bile duct obstruction or bleeding. Surgical resection of early lesions is curative in up to 40% of patients.

2. Small Intestinal Lymphomas

Lymphomas may arise primarily in the gastrointestinal tract or involve it secondarily in patients with disseminated disease. In Western countries, primary gastrointestinal lymphomas account for 5% of lymphomas and 20% of small bowel malignancies. They occur most commonly in the small intestine. There is an increased incidence of small intestinal lymphomas in patients with AIDS, immunosuppressive therapy, and Crohn disease. The most common histologic subtype is non-Hodgkin extranodal marginal zone (MALT) B cell lymphoma. Enteropathy-associated T cell lymphomas appear to be increasing in incidence in the United States. They are associated with the diagnosis of celiac disease. In the Middle East, lymphomas may arise in the setting of immunoproliferative small intestinal disease. Other types of intestinal lymphomas include primary intestinal follicular cell lymphoma, mantle cell lymphoma, and Burkitt lymphoma (see Chapter 13).

Presenting symptoms or signs of primary small bowel lymphoma include abdominal pain, weight loss, nausea and vomiting, distention, anemia, and occult blood in the stool. Fevers are unusual. Protein-losing enteropathy may result in hypoalbuminemia, but other signs of malabsorption are unusual. Barium radiography or CT enterography helps localize the site of the lesion. The diagnosis requires endoscopic, percutaneous, or laparoscopic biopsy. Imaging and bone marrow biopsy are required to determine stage.

Treatment depends on the tumor histologic subtype and stage of disease (see Chapter 13). Surgical resection of primary intestinal lymphoma, if feasible, may be appropriate for localized tumors. In patients with limited disease (stage IE) in whom resection is performed with negative margins, the role of adjuvant chemotherapy is unclear. Locoregional radiation should be considered if surgical margins are positive. Patients with more extensive disease generally are treated according to the tumor histology.

3. Intestinal Carcinoid Tumors

ESSENTIALS OF DIAGNOSIS

▶ Majority are asymptomatic and discovered incidentally at endoscopy or surgery.

▶ Carcinoid syndrome occurs in less than 10%; hepatic metastases are generally present.

▶ Risk of metastasis related to tumor size and location.

General Considerations

Gastrointestinal carcinoid tumors are generally slow growing neuroendocrine tumors that account for approximately one-third of tumors arising in the small bowel. Gastrointestinal carcinoid tumors most commonly occur in the small intestine (45%) but are also found in the rectum (20%), appendix (17%), and colon (11%), with the remainder occurring in the stomach (less than 10%; see Gastric Carcinoid Tumors above). Carcinoid tumors may contain a variety of hormones, including serotonin, somatostatin, gastrin, and substance P, each of which may or may not be secreted.

Small intestinal carcinoids most commonly arise in the distal ileum within 60 cm of the ileocecal valve. Up to 30% are multicentric. Although many carcinoids behave in an indolent fashion, the overall 5-year survival rates for patients with locoregional and metastatic small bowel carcinoids are approximately 65% and 35%, respectively. The risk of metastatic spread increases when the tumor is 1 cm or larger and when it is larger than 2 cm with invasion beyond muscularis propria. Appendiceal carcinoids are identified in 0.3% of appendectomies, usually as an incidental finding. Almost 80% of these tumors are smaller than 1 cm, and 90% are smaller than 2 cm. However, in patients with appendiceal carcinoid tumors larger than 2 cm, approximately 90% develop nodal and distant metastases; right hemicolectomy is recommended in these cases.

Rectal carcinoids are usually detected incidentally as submucosal nodules during proctoscopic examination and often locally excised by biopsy or snare polypectomy before the histologic diagnosis is known. Endorectal ultrasound is usually recommended to assess the size, presence and depth of invasion, and presence of lymph node metastases. Rectal carcinoids smaller than 1 cm virtually never metastasize and are treated effectively with local endoscopic or transanal excision. Larger tumors are associated with the development of metastasis in 10%. Hence, a more extensive cancer resection operation is warranted in fit patients with rectal carcinoid tumors larger than 1–2 cm or with high risk features (such as invasion of muscularis propria or evidence of nodal involvement), or both.

Clinical Findings

A. Symptoms and Signs

Most lesions smaller than 1–2 cm are asymptomatic and difficult to detect by endoscopy or imaging studies. Through local extension or metastasis to mesenteric lymph nodes, carcinoids engender a fibroblastic reaction with contraction and kinking of the bowel or encasement of mesenteric vessels. Small intestinal carcinoids may present with abdominal pain, bowel obstruction, bleeding, or bowel infarction. Appendiceal and rectal carcinoids usually are small and asymptomatic but large lesions can cause bleeding, obstruction, or altered bowel habits. **Carcinoid syndrome** occurs in less than 10% of patients. More than 90% of patients with carcinoid syndrome have hepatic metastases, usually from carcinoids of small bowel origin. About 10% of patients with carcinoid syndrome have primary bronchial or ovarian tumors without hepatic metastases.

Carcinoid syndrome is caused by tumor secretion of hormonal mediators. The manifestations include facial flushing, edema of the head and neck (especially with bronchial carcinoid), abdominal cramps and diarrhea, bronchospasm, cardiac lesions (pulmonary or tricuspid stenosis or regurgitation in 10–30%), and telangiectases.

B. Laboratory Findings

Serum chromogranin A (CgA) is elevated in the majority of neuroendocrine tumors, although its sensitivity for small, localized carcinoid tumors is unknown. CgA is elevated in almost 90% of patients with advanced small bowel carcinoid. Urinary 5-hydroxyindoleacetic acid (5-HIAA) and platelet serotonin levels are also elevated in patients with metastatic carcinoid; however, these tests are less sensitive than CgA. There is increased urinary 5-HIAA in carcinoid syndrome; symptomatic patients usually excrete more than 25 mg of 5-HIAA per day in the urine. Because certain foods and medications can interfere with 5-HIAA levels, these should be withheld for 48 hours prior to a 24-hour urine collection.

C. Imaging

Abdominal CT may demonstrate a mesenteric mass with tethering of the bowel, lymphadenopathy, and hepatic metastasis. Abdominal CT or enterography may reveal kinking of the bowel, but because the lesion is extraluminal, the diagnosis may be overlooked for several years. Somatostatin receptor scintigraphy, which is positive in up to 90% of patients with metastatic carcinoid, is routinely used in staging. Most patients with carcinoid syndrome have liver metastasis on abdominal imaging.

Treatment & Outcomes

Small intestinal carcinoids generally are indolent tumors with slow spread. Patients with disease confined to the small intestine should be treated with surgical excision. There is no proven role for adjuvant therapy after complete resection. Five-year survival rates for patients with stage I and II disease are 96% and 87%, respectively. In patients with resectable disease who have lymph node involvement (stage III), the 5-year survival is 74%; however, by 25 years, less than 25% remain disease free. Even patients with metastatic disease may have an indolent course with a 5-year survival of 43%.

In patients with advanced disease, therapy historically has been deferred until the patient is symptomatic, although one phase III, randomized, placebo-controlled trial demonstrated that early initiation of somatostatin analog therapy significantly delayed time to progression of hepatic metastases compared to placebo (14.3 vs 6 months, respectively). Conventional cytotoxic chemotherapy agents do not achieve significant responses in carcinoid tumors and have not been associated with improved outcomes. Radiolabeled somatostatin analogs are used in Europe but are currently under investigation in the United States as another treatment modality for patients with somatostatin-receptor positive advanced carcinoid tumors. In patients with metastatic disease, surgery should be directed toward palliation of obstructive symptoms or bleeding.

In patients with carcinoid syndrome, the somatostatin analog octreotide, 150–250 mcg subcutaneously three times daily or administered as a long-acting intramuscular depot formulation administered monthly, inhibits hormone secretion from the carcinoid tumor. This results in dramatic relief of symptoms of carcinoid syndrome, including diarrhea or flushing, in 90% of patients for a median period of 1 year. Thereafter, many patients stop responding to octreotide. In selected patients with refractory carcinoid syndrome, resection of hepatic metastases may provide dramatic improvement. Hepatic artery occlusion, liver-directed debulking procedures, and chemotherapy also may provide symptomatic improvement in some patients with hepatic metastases.

4. Small Intestine Sarcoma

Most small intestine sarcomas arise from stromal tumors (GISTs) that stain positive for CD117; a minority arise from smooth muscle tumors (leiomyosarcomas) (see Gastrointestinal Mesenchymal Tumors above).

Kaposi sarcoma was at one time a common complication in AIDS, but the incidence is declining with antiretroviral therapy. It can also occur in the setting of immunosuppression after organ transplant. It is caused by infection with human herpesvirus 8 (HHV8). Lesions may be present anywhere in the intestinal tract. Visceral involvement usually is associated with cutaneous disease. Most lesions are clinically silent; however, large lesions may be symptomatic. Widespread involvement may be best treated by systemic chemotherapy using single-agent therapy or combinations of pegylated-doxorubicin (Doxil), paclitaxel, vincristine, bleomycin, or etoposide. Surgery or radiation may be indicated for isolated high-risk lesions.

Ecker BL et al. Efficacy of adjuvant chemotherapy for small bowel adenocarcinoma: a propensity score-matched analysis. Cancer. 2016 Mar 1;122(5):693–701. [PMID: 26717303]

Faggian A et al. Small-bowel neoplasms: role of MRI enteroclysis. Gastroenterol Res Pract. 2016;2016:9686815. [PMID: 26819616]

Gleeson FC et al. Endoscopically identified well-differentiated rectal carcinoid tumors: impact of tumor size on the natural history and outcomes. Gastrointest Endosc. 2014 Jul; 80(1):144–51. [PMID: 24462168]

Hughes MS et al. Prospective evaluation and treatment of familial carcinoid small intestine neuroendocrine tumors (SI-NETs). Surgery. 2016 Jan;159(1):350–7. [PMID: 26454678]

Malamut G et al. Complications of coeliac disease. Best Pract Res Clin Gastroenterol. 2015 Jun;29(3):451–8. [PMID: 26060109]

Nakamura S et al. Gastrointestinal lymphoma: recent advances in diagnosis and treatment. Digestion. 2013;87(3):182–8. [PMID: 23635497]

Nijeboer P et al. Enteropathy-associated T-cell lymphoma: improving treatment strategies. Dig Dis. 2015;33(2):231–5. [PMID: 25925928]

Reynolds I et al. Malignant tumours of the small intestine. Surgeon. 2014 Oct;12(5):263–70. [PMID: 24637026]

Sandvik OM et al. Epidemiology and classification of gastroenteropancreatic neuroendocrine neoplasms using current coding criteria. Br J Surg. 2016 Feb;103(3):226–32. [PMID: 26511392]

Shah OJ et al. A selective approach to the surgical management of periampullary cancer patients and its outcome. Hepatobiliary Pancreat Dis Int. 2014 Dec;13(6):628–33. [PMID: 25475866]

Silverberg MJ et al; North American AIDS Cohort Collaboration on Research and Design of the International Epidemiologic Databases to Evaluate AIDS. Cumulative incidence of cancer among persons with HIV in North America: a cohort study. Ann Intern Med. 2015 Oct 6;163(7):507–18. [PMID: 26436616]

Toumpanakis C et al. Update on the role of somatostatin analogs for the treatment of patients with gastroenteropancreatic neuroendocrine tumors. Semin Oncol. 2013 Feb;40(1):56–68. [PMID: 23391113]

van Rijssen LB et al. National compliance to an evidence-based multidisciplinary guideline on pancreatic and periampullary carcinoma. Pancreatology. 2016 Jan–Feb;16(1):133–7. [PMID: 26560441]

Xing GS et al. Small bowel stromal tumors: different clinico-pathologic and computed tomography features in various anatomic sites. PLoS One. 2015 Dec 8;10(12):e0144277. [PMID: 26646242]

Yao JC et al; RAD001 in Advanced Neuroendocrine Tumours, Fourth Trial (RADIANT-4) Study Group. Everolimus for the treatment of advanced, non-functional neuroendocrine tumours of the lung or gastrointestinal tract (RADIANT-4): a randomised, placebo-controlled, phase 3 study. Lancet. 2016 Mar 5;387(10022):968–77. [PMID: 26703889]

Zaaimi Y et al. Advanced small bowel adenocarcinoma: molecular characteristics and therapeutic perspectives. Clin Res Hepatol Gastroenterol. 2016 Apr;40(2):154–60. [PMID: 26547136]

COLORECTAL CANCER

 ESSENTIALS OF DIAGNOSIS

► Personal or family history of adenomatous or serrated polyps or colorectal cancer are important risk factors.

► Symptoms or signs depend on tumor location.

► Proximal colon: fecal occult blood, anemia.

► Distal colon: change in bowel habits, hematochezia.

► Diagnosis established with colonoscopy.

► General Considerations

Colorectal cancer is the second leading cause of death due to malignancy in the United States. Colorectal cancer will develop in approximately 6% of Americans and 40% of those will die of the disease. In 2014, there were an estimated 96,830 new cases of colon cancer and 40,000 new cases of rectal cancer in the United States, with combined estimated 50,310 deaths. Between 1996 and 2010, the mortality has decreased by 46%. During this same period, the percent of patients 50 years or older who were screened for colorectal cancer has increased to 66.1%.

Colorectal cancers are almost all adenocarcinomas, which tend to form bulky exophytic masses or annular constricting lesions. The majority of colorectal cancers are thought to arise from malignant transformation of an adenomatous polyp (tubular, tubulovillous, or villous adenoma) or serrated polyp (hyperplastic polyp, traditional serrated adenoma, or sessile serrated adenoma). Polyps that are "advanced" (ie, polyps at least 1 cm in size, adenomas with villous features or high-grade dysplasia, or serrated polyps with dysplasia) are associated with a greater risk of cancer. Approximately 85% of sporadic colorectal cancers arise from adenomatous polyps and have loss of function of one or more tumor suppressor genes (eg, *p53*, *APC*, or *DCC*) due to a combination of spontaneous mutation of one allele combined with chromosomal instability and aneuploidy (abnormal DNA content) that leads to deletion and loss of heterozygosity of the other allele (eg, 5q, 17q, or 18p deletion). Activation of oncogenes such as *K-ras* and *B-raf* is present in a subset of colorectal cancers with prognostic and therapeutic implications discussed further below.

Approximately 10–20% of colorectal cancers arise from serrated polyps, most of which have hypermethylation of CpG-rich promoter regions that leads to inactivation of the DNA mismatch repair gene *MLH1*, resulting in microsatellite instability, and activation of mutations of the *BRAF* gene. Serrated colon cancers have distinct clinical and pathologic characteristics, including diploid DNA content, predominance in the proximal colon, poor differentiation, and more favorable prognosis.

Up to 5% of colorectal cancers are caused by inherited germline mutations resulting in polyposis syndromes (eg, familial adenomatous polyposis) or hereditary nonpolyposis colorectal cancer (HNPCC or Lynch syndrome). These conditions are discussed further in Chapter 15.

► Risk Factors

A number of factors increase the risk of developing colorectal cancer. Recognition of these has impact on screening strategies. However, 75% of all cases occur in people with no known predisposing factors.

A. Age

The incidence of colorectal cancer rises sharply after age 45 years, and 90% of cases occur in persons over the age of 50 years.

B. Family History of Neoplasia

A family history of colorectal cancer is present in approximately 20% of patients with colon cancer. Hereditary factors are believed to contribute to 20–30% of colorectal cancers; however, the genes responsible for most of these cases have not yet been identified. (See Chapter 15 for discussion of inherited polyposis syndromes.) Approximately 6% of the Ashkenazi Jewish population has a missense mutation in the *APC* gene (*APC I1307K*) that confers a modestly increased lifetime risk of developing colorectal cancer (OR 1.4–1.9) but phenotypically resembles sporadic colorectal cancer rather than familial adenomatous polyposis. Genetic screening is available, and patients harboring the mutation merit intensive screening.

A family history of colorectal cancer or adenomatous polyps is one of the most important risk factors for colorectal cancer. The risk of colon cancer is proportionate to the number and age of affected first-degree family members with colon neoplasia. People with one first-degree family member with colorectal cancer have an increased risk approximately two times that of the general population; however, the risk is almost four times if the family member was younger than 45 years when the cancer was diagnosed. Patients with two first-degree relatives have a fourfold increase, or 25–30% lifetime, risk of developing colon cancer. First-degree relatives of patients with adenomatous polyps also have a twofold increased risk for colorectal neoplasia, especially if they were younger than 60 years when the polyp was detected or if the polyp was 10 mm or larger.

C. Inflammatory Bowel Disease

The risk of adenocarcinoma of the colon begins to rise 8 years after disease onset in patients with ulcerative colitis and Crohn colitis (see Chapter 15).

D. Dietary and Lifestyle Factors and Chemoprevention in Colorectal Cancer Risk

In epidemiologic studies, diets rich in fats and red meat are associated with an increased risk of colorectal adenomas and cancer, whereas diets high in fruits, vegetables, and fiber are associated with a decreased risk. However, prospective studies have not shown a reduction in colon cancer or recurrence of adenomatous polyps with diets that are low in fat; are high in fiber, fruits or vegetables; or that include calcium, folate, beta-carotene, or vitamin A, C, D, or E supplements.

A US Preventive Services Task Force meta-analysis of cohort and case-control studies suggest that prolonged (more than 6 years) regular use of aspirin (at least 325 mg twice weekly) or NSAIDs is associated with a 22–33% relative risk reduction in the incidence of colorectal cancer. Two prospective, blinded clinical trials have shown that daily low-dose aspirin (80–325 mg) reduces the number of recurrent adenomas at 1–3 years in patients with a history of colorectal adenomas or cancer; however, two large randomized controlled trials in the United States did not demonstrate a reduction in colorectal cancer incidence in patients taking low-dose aspirin over 5–10 years. Because long-term aspirin use is associated with a low incidence of serious complications (gastrointestinal hemorrhage, stroke), the US Preventive Services Task Force concluded that it should not be prescribed as a chemopreventive agent in people without polyps or with small adenomas unless there are other medical indications. Long-term administration of low-dose aspirin may be considered in patients with a personal or family history of colorectal cancer or advanced adenomas; however, it does not obviate the need for colonoscopy screening and surveillance.

Retrospective analysis of randomized phase III trial data and a meta-analysis have shown that patients with higher levels of pre- and post-diagnosis physical activity experience reduced colorectal cancer–specific mortality and all-cause mortality. Maintaining a healthy body weight, a healthy diet, and a physically active lifestyle are recommended in colorectal cancer survivors.

E. Other Factors

The incidence of colon adenocarcinoma is higher in blacks than in whites. It is unclear whether this is due to genetic or socioeconomic factors (eg, diet or reduced access to screening).

▶ Clinical Findings

A. Symptoms and Signs

Adenocarcinomas grow slowly and may be present for several years before symptoms appear. However, some asymptomatic tumors may be detected by the presence of fecal occult blood (see Screening for Colorectal Neoplasms, below). Symptoms depend on the location of the carcinoma. Chronic blood loss from right-sided colonic cancers may cause iron deficiency anemia, manifested by fatigue and weakness. Obstruction, however, is uncommon because of the large diameter of the right colon and the liquid consistency of the fecal material. Lesions of the left colon often involve the bowel circumferentially. Because the left colon has a smaller diameter and the fecal matter is solid, obstructive symptoms may develop with colicky abdominal pain and a change in bowel habits. Constipation may alternate with periods of increased frequency and loose stools. The stool may be streaked with blood, though marked bleeding is unusual. With rectal cancers, patients note tenesmus, urgency, and recurrent hematochezia. Weight loss is uncommon. Physical examination is usually normal except in advanced disease. A mass may be palpable in the abdomen. The liver should be examined for hepatomegaly, suggesting metastatic spread. For cancers of the distal rectum, digital examination is necessary to determine whether there is extension into the anal sphincter or fixation, suggesting extension to the pelvic floor.

B. Laboratory Findings

A CBC is obtained to look for evidence of anemia. Elevated liver function tests, particularly the alkaline phosphatase, are suspicious for metastatic disease. Carcinoembryonic antigen (CEA) should be measured in all patients with proved colorectal cancer but is not appropriate for screening. A preoperative CEA level greater than 5 ng/mL is a poor prognostic indicator. After complete surgical resection, CEA levels should normalize; persistently elevated levels suggest the presence of persistent disease and warrant further evaluation.

C. Colonoscopy

Colonoscopy is the diagnostic procedure of choice in patients with a clinical history suggestive of colon cancer or in patients with an abnormality suspicious for cancer detected on radiographic imaging (Figure 39–1). Colonoscopy permits biopsy for pathologic confirmation of malignancy. In patients in whom the colonoscope is unable to reach the cecum (less than 5% of cases) or when a nearly

▲ **Figure 39–1.** Colon cancer. There is a large fungating mass within the right colon. This mass is hemicircumferential and nearly obstructing and occluding the lumen of the colon. (Used, with permission, from Michelle Nazareth, MD.)

obstructing tumor precludes passage of the colonoscope, barium enema or CT colonography examination should be performed.

D. Imaging

Chest, abdominal, and pelvic CT scans are required for preoperative staging. CT scans may demonstrate distal metastases but are less accurate in the determination of the level of local tumor extension (T stage) or lymphatic spread (N stage). Intraoperative assessment of the liver by direct palpation and ultrasonography is more accurate than CT scanning for the detection of hepatic metastases. For rectal cancers (generally defined as tumors arising 12 cm or less proximal to the anal verge), pelvic MRI or endorectal ultrasonography is required to determine the depth of penetration of the cancer through the rectal wall (T stage) and perirectal lymph nodes, informing decisions about preoperative (neoadjuvant) chemoradiotherapy and operative management. PET is not routinely used for staging or surveillance in colorectal cancers.

▶ Staging

The TNM system is the commonly used classification to stage colorectal cancer. Staging is important not only because it correlates with the patient's long-term survival but also because it is used to determine which patients should receive adjuvant therapy.

▶ Differential Diagnosis

The nonspecific symptoms of colon cancer may be confused with those of irritable bowel syndrome, diverticular disease, ischemic colitis, inflammatory bowel disease, infectious colitis, and hemorrhoids. Neoplasm must be excluded in any patient over age 40 years who reports a change in bowel habits or hematochezia or who has an unexplained iron deficiency anemia or occult blood in stool samples.

▶ Treatment

A. Surgery

Resection of the primary colonic or rectal cancer is the treatment of choice for almost all patients who have resectable lesions and can tolerate general anesthesia. For colon cancer, multiple studies demonstrate that minimally invasive, laparoscopically assisted colectomy results in similar outcomes and rates of recurrence to open colectomy. Regional dissection of at least 12 lymph nodes should be performed to determine staging, which guides decisions about adjuvant therapy.

For rectal carcinoma, preoperative (neoadjuvant) chemoradiation with 5-fluorouracil is recommended in all node-positive tumors, and in T3 and greater tumors, due to increased risk of local recurrence (see below). After neoadjuvant therapy, the operative approach depends on the level of the tumor above the anal verge, the size and depth of penetration, and the patient's overall condition. Clinical staging by endorectal ultrasound or MRI with endorectal coil is important in guiding the clinical approach. In carefully selected patients with small, mobile (less than 4 cm), well-differentiated T1 or T2 rectal tumors that are less than 8 cm from the anal verge, transanal excision may be considered. This approach avoids laparotomy and spares the rectum and anal sphincter, preserving normal bowel continence. All other patients will require either a low anterior resection with a colorectal anastomosis or an abdominoperineal resection with a colostomy, depending on how far above the anal verge the tumor is located and the extent of local tumor spread. Careful dissection of the entire mesorectum by either open or laparoscopic surgery reduces local recurrence to 5%. Although low anterior resections obviate a colostomy, they are associated with increased immediate postsurgical complications (eg, leak, dehiscence, stricture) and defecatory complaints (eg, increased stool frequency, and incontinence). With unresectable rectal cancer, the patient may be palliated with a diverting colostomy or placement of an expandable wire stent.

B. Systemic Chemotherapy for Colon Cancer

Chemotherapy and radiotherapy have been demonstrated to improve overall and tumor-free survival in selected patients with colorectal cancers depending on stage.

1. Stage I—Because of the excellent 5-year survival rate (90–100%), no adjuvant therapy is recommended.

2. Stage II (node-negative disease)—The 5-year survival rate is approximately 80%. A significant survival benefit from adjuvant chemotherapy has not been demonstrated in most randomized clinical trials for stage II colon cancer (see discussion for stage III disease). However, otherwise healthy patients with stage II disease who are at higher risk for recurrence (perforation, obstruction, T4 tumors, or fewer than 12 lymph nodes sampled) may benefit from adjuvant chemotherapy.

3. Stage III (node-positive disease)—With surgical resection alone, the expected 5-year survival rate is 30–50%. Postoperative adjuvant chemotherapy significantly increases disease-free survival as well as overall survival up to 30% and is recommended for all fit patients. Large, well-designed studies of adjuvant therapy for stage III colon cancer reported a higher rate of disease-free survival at 5 years for patients treated for 6 months postoperatively with a combination of oxaliplatin, 5-fluorouracil, and leucovorin (FOLFOX) (73.3%) than with 5-fluorouracil and leucovorin (FL) alone (67.4%). The addition of oxaliplatin is associated with an increased incidence of diarrhea, myelosuppression, and peripheral sensory neuropathy, all of which generally are reversible. Based on these studies, FOLFOX currently is the preferred adjuvant therapy for most patients with stage III colon cancer (see Table 39–11). The addition of a biologic agent (bevacizumab or cetuximab) to FOLFOX does not improve outcomes in the adjuvant setting.

4. Stage IV (metastatic disease)—Approximately 20% of patients have metastatic disease at the time of initial diagnosis, and an additional 30% eventually develop metastasis. A subset of these patients has limited disease that is potentially curable with surgical resection. Resection of isolated liver or lung metastases may result in long-term (over 5 years) survival in 35–55% of cases. For those with unresectable hepatic metastases, local ablative techniques (cryosurgery, radiofrequency or microwave coagulation, embolization, hepatic intra-arterial chemotherapy) may provide long-term tumor control. The majority of patients with metastatic disease do not have resectable (curable) disease. In the absence of other treatment, the median survival is less than 12 months; however, with current therapies, median survival approaches 24 months. The goals of therapy for patients with metastatic colorectal cancer are to slow tumor progression while maintaining a reasonable quality of life for as long as possible. Currently, either FOLFOX (the addition of oxaliplatin to 5-fluorouracil and folinic acid) or FOLFIRI (the addition of irinotecan to 5-fluorouracil and folinic acid) is the preferred first-line treatment regimens for fit patients. For convenience, oral capecitabine (instead of intravenous 5-fluorouracil and leucovorin) can be used in combination with oxaliplatin; however, combination with irinotecan is not recommended due to increased toxicity (diarrhea). Addition of a biologic agent to combination chemotherapy improves response rates and overall survival and is recommended in the first-line of treatment in suitable patients. Bevacizumab is a monoclonal antibody targeting VEGF. Combination therapy with bevacizumab and FOLFOX or FOLFIRI prolongs mean survival 2–5 months compared with either regimen alone (see Table 39–11). Cetuximab and panitumumab are monoclonal antibodies targeting EGFR. Activating codon 12 and 13 K-ras gene mutations downstream of EGFR are present in approximately 35% of patients with metastatic colorectal cancer and are a biomarker for nonresponse to cetuximab and panitumumab, for which reason the use of these agents is restricted to patients with tumors wild-type for K-ras. In stage IV patients with K-ras wild-type tumors, the addition of panitumumab or cetuximab to FOLFOX or FOLFIRI prolongs survival by approximately 4 months. Bevacizumab may cause serious side effects, including arterial thromboembolic events, bowel perforation, or serious bleeding, in up to 5% of patients. EGFR-targeted agents cause an acneiform rash in the majority of patients. Cetuximab is associated with severe infusion reactions in approximately 2–5%.

When disease progresses despite treatment either with FOLFOX or with FOLFIRI (often in conjunction with bevacizumab or an EGFR-targeted antibody), therapy is switched to the alternate regimen; patients may respond to the alternate regimen, prolonging mean survival to more than 20 months. The novel anti-angiogenic agent, aflibercept, is FDA-approved for use in second-line colorectal cancer in combination with FOLFIRI. Palliative therapy with cetuximab or panitumumab can benefit patients with *K-ras* wild-type tumors whose disease has progressed after first-line and second-line chemotherapies. The multi-targeted kinase inhibitor, regorafenib, was approved by the FDA in 2012 for patients with metastatic, refractory colorectal cancer after progression on standard regimens based on results of the randomized, phase III CORRECT trial showing improved overall survival compared to placebo. In 2015, trifluridine/tipiracil (TAS-102) was FDA approved for the treatment of patients with metastatic colorectal cancer who have been previously treated with fluoropyrimidine-, oxaliplatin-, and irinotecan-based chemotherapy, an anti-VEGF biologic product and, if KRAS wild-type cancer, an anti-EGFR monoclonal antibody. It was noted to result in improved overall survival (7.1 vs 5.3 months compared to placebo).

C. Neoadjuvant and Adjuvant Therapy for Rectal Cancer

Compared with colon cancer, rectal cancer has lower long-term survival rates and significantly higher rates of local tumor recurrence with surgery alone (approximately 25%) attributed in part to the difficulty of achieving adequate surgical resection margins and to lack of serosal encasement of the rectum. When initial imaging studies suggest stage I disease, surgery may be performed first (see Surgery above). For stage II and III tumors by clinical staging (including endorectal ultrasound or pelvic MRI), preoperative chemoradiation with 5-fluorouracil or capecitabine as a radiation-sensitizing agent improves disease-free survival and decreases pelvic recurrence rate (see Table 39–11). Preoperative chemoradiation has been shown to be superior to postoperative chemoradiation with lower local recurrence and toxicity rates in the randomized, phase III CAO/ARO/AIO-94 trial. Following surgical resection with total mesorectal excision (see Surgery above), adjuvant 5-fluorouracil–based therapy (generally with the FOLFOX regimen extrapolating from its benefit in patients with similarly-staged colon cancers) is recommended for a total of approximately 6 months of perioperative therapy inclusive of neoadjuvant chemoradiation.

▶ Follow-Up after Surgery

Patients who have undergone resections for cure are monitored closely to look for evidence of symptomatic or asymptomatic tumor recurrence that may be amenable to curative resection in a small number of patients. Patients should be evaluated every 3–6 months for 2 years and then every 6 months for a total of 5 years with history, physical examination, and laboratory surveillance, including serum CEA levels. The NCCN and ASCO guidelines recommend surveillance CT scans of chest, abdomen, and pelvis annually for up to 5 years post-resection in high-risk stage II and all stage III patients. Patients who had a complete preoperative colonoscopy should undergo another colonoscopy 1 year after surgical resection. Patients who did not undergo full colonoscopy preoperatively also should undergo colonoscopy within 3–6 months postoperatively to exclude other synchronous colorectal neoplasms. If a colonoscopy does not detect new adenomatous polyps 1 year postoperatively, surveillance colonoscopy should be performed every 3–5 years thereafter to look for metachronous polyps or cancer. Because of the high incidence of local tumor recurrence in patients with rectal cancer, proctoscopy surveillance of the low anterior resection anastomotic site may also be performed periodically. New onset of symptoms or a rising CEA warrants investigation with chest, abdominal, and pelvic CT and colonoscopy to look for a new primary tumor or recurrence, or metachronous metastatic disease that may be amenable to curative or palliative therapy. For patients with a rising CEA level with unrevealing CT imaging, a PET scan may be more sensitive for the detection of occult metastatic disease.

▶ Prognosis

The stage of disease at presentation is the most important determinant of long-term survival in colon cancer: stage I, greater than 90%; stage II, 70–85%; stage III with fewer than 4 positive lymph nodes, 67%; stage III with more than 4 positive lymph nodes, 33%; and stage IV, 5–7%. For each stage, rectal cancers have a worse prognosis. For those patients whose disease progresses despite therapy, meticulous efforts at palliative care are essential (see Chapter 5).

▶ Screening for Colorectal Neoplasms

Colorectal cancer is ideal for screening because it is a common disease that is fatal in almost 50% of cases yet is curable if detected at an earlier stage. Furthermore, most cases arise from benign adenomatous or serrated polyps that progress over many years to cancer, and removal of these polyps has been shown to prevent the majority of cancers. Colorectal cancer screening is endorsed by the US Preventive Services Task Force, the Agency for Health Care Policy and Research, the American Cancer Society, and every professional gastroenterology and colorectal surgery society. Although there is continued debate about the optimal cost-effective means of providing population screening, there is unanimous consent that screening of some kind should be offered to every patient over the age of 50 years. Several analyses suggest that screening is cost-effective.

It is important for primary care providers to understand the relative merits of various options and to discuss them with their patients. Discussion and encouragement by the primary care provider are the most important factors in achieving patient compliance with screening programs.

Table 39–5. Recommendations for colorectal cancer screening.[1]

Average-risk individuals ≥ 50 years old[2]
Annual fecal occult blood testing using higher sensitivity tests (Hemoccult SENSA)
Annual fecal immunochemical test (FIT)
Fecal DNA test (interval uncertain)
Flexible sigmoidoscopy every 5 years
Colonoscopy every 10 years
CT colonography every 5 years
Individuals with a family history of a first-degree member with colorectal neoplasia[3]
Single first-degree relative with colorectal cancer diagnosed at age ≥ 60 years: Begin screening at age 40. Screening guidelines same as average-risk individual; however, preferred method is colonoscopy every 10 years.
Single first-degree relative with colorectal cancer or advanced adenoma diagnosed at age<60 years, or two first-degree relatives: Begin screening at age 40 or at age 10 years younger than age at diagnosis of the youngest affected relative, whichever is first in time. Recommended screening: colonoscopy every 5 years.

[1]For recommendations for families with inherited polyposis syndromes or hereditary nonpolyposis colon cancer, see Chapter 15.
[2]Joint Guideline from the American Cancer Society, the US Multi-Society Task Force on Colorectal Cancer, and the American College of Radiology. Gastroenterology 2008 May;134(5):1570.
[3]American College of Gastroenterology. Guidelines for Colorectal Cancer Screening. Am J Gastroenterol. 2009 Mar;104(3):739.

Recommendations for screening from the US Multi-Society Task Force are listed in Table 39–5. Screening is recommended for all men and women ages 50 through 75 years of age who are at average risk for cancer. Some guidelines recommend screening for African Americans beginning at age 45. The potential for harm from screening must be weighed against the likelihood of benefit, especially in elderly patients with comorbid illnesses and shorter life expectancy. Although routine screening is not recommended in adults above age 75, it may be considered on a case-by-case basis in adults age 76 through 85 years who have excellent health and functional status. Patients with first-degree relatives with colorectal neoplasms (cancer or adenomatous polyps) are at increased risk; earlier and more frequent screening may be recommended (preferably with colonoscopy) for these individuals. Recommendations for screening in families with inherited cancer syndromes or inflammatory bowel disease are provided in Chapter 15. For patients at average risk for colorectal cancer, the recommendations of the Task Force are discussed below. Screening tests may be classified into two broad categories: stool-based tests and examinations that visualize the structure of the colon by direct endoscopic inspection or radiographic imaging.

A. Stool-Based Tests

1. Fecal occult blood test—Most colorectal cancers and some large adenomas result in increased chronic blood loss. A variety of tests for fecal occult blood are commercially available that have varying sensitivities and specificities for colorectal neoplasia. These include guaiac-based tests (Hemoccult I and II and Hemoccult SENSA) that detect the pseudoperoxidase activity of heme or hemoglobin and fecal immunochemical tests (FITs) that detect human globin.

When fecal occult blood test is administered to the general population as part of a screening program, 2–6% of tests are positive. Of those with positive tests, 5–18% have colorectal cancer that is more likely to be at an earlier stage (stage I or II).

For optimal detection, annual testing is required. In a meta-analysis of four large, prospective, longitudinal studies, annual or biennial screening with Hemoccult I or Hemoccult II reduced mortality from colorectal cancer by 25% among those who were compliant with regular testing.

Several FITs are commercially available. These tests are highly specific for detecting human globin and therefore eliminate the need for pretest dietary restrictions. In 19 clinical studies, the pooled sensitivity and specificity of FIT for colorectal cancer in average-risk patients were 79% and 94%, respectively. The optimal interval (yearly or every 2 years) and number of stool samples (one or two) required for optimal FIT testing is as yet undetermined. In clinical trials that compare FIT with guaiac-based tests, FIT had at least comparable sensitivity to Hemoccult SENSA for detection of cancers (60–85%) with higher specificity. Because FITs are not affected by diet or medications and have superior accuracy, they are increasingly preferred over guaiac-based tests despite a higher cost per test ($10–20). Randomized controlled trials comparing one-time colonoscopy with FIT testing for colorectal cancer screening are ongoing.

The US Multi-Society Task Force emphasizes that colon cancer prevention should be the primary goal of screening. For that reason, the lower sensitivity of fecal occult blood tests for advanced neoplasia (cancer and advanced adenomatous polyps) makes them a less attractive choice for population-based screening than endoscopic or radiographic tests. Currently, fecal occult blood tests are most suitable in settings where health care resources are limited or in patients who desire a noninvasive method of screening. Regardless of which stool-based test is used, patients should understand that annual testing is required to achieve the maximum screening benefit and that a positive test will require evaluation by colonoscopy accompanied by removal of any polyps identified. If colonoscopy reveals no colorectal neoplasm, further screening for colorectal cancer can be deferred for 10 years. In a meta-analysis of four large, prospective, longitudinal studies, annual or biennial screening with Hemoccult I or Hemoccult II reduced mortality from colorectal cancer by 25% among those who were compliant with regular testing. Long-term studies with more sensitive stool tests (Hemoccult SENSA or FIT) have not been performed.

2. Multitarget DNA assay—Stool DNA tests measure a variety of mutated genes and methylated gene markers from exfoliated tumor cells. The first-generation commercially available fecal DNA panel detected only one-half of cancers. In 2014, a newer generation assay (under the proprietary name "Cologuard") was approved by the FDA, which combines a fecal DNA panel with an immunochemical test for stool hemoglobin. In a prospective comparative trial conducted in persons at average risk for colorectal cancer undergoing colonoscopy, the sensitivity for colorectal cancer for "Cologuard" was 92.3% vs. 73.8% for FIT and the sensitivity for adenomas larger than 1 cm or serrated polyps for "Cologuard" was 42.4% vs. 23.8% for FIT. Although the Multi-Society Task Force concluded that fecal DNA is an acceptable option for colorectal cancer screening, population-based screening may be hampered by its high cost, cumbersome requirements for stool collection and mailing, and high false-positive rate (10.2%).

B. Endoscopic Examinations of the Colon

1. Flexible sigmoidoscopy—Use of a 60-cm flexible sigmoidoscope permits visualization of the rectosigmoid and descending colon. Adenomatous polyps are identified in 10–20% and colorectal cancers in 1% of patients. A 2012 US study of almost 155,000 participants randomized to sigmoidoscopy screening or usual care between 1993 and 2001 reported a 50% reduction in distal colorectal cancer mortality in the sigmoidoscopy group after 11 years median follow up.

The chief disadvantage of screening with flexible sigmoidoscopy is that is does not examine the proximal colon. The prevalence of proximal versus distal neoplasia is higher in people over age 65 years of age, African Americans, and women. In men, approximately 50% of advanced neoplasms (cancer, adenomas 1 cm or larger, polyps with villous histology, or high-grade dysplasia) are located in the proximal colon, compared with 60–70% in women. The finding at sigmoidoscopy of an adenomatous polyp in the distal colon increases the likelihood at least twofold that an advanced neoplasm is present in the proximal colon. Therefore, patients found on screening sigmoidoscopy to have an adenomatous polyp of any size should subsequently undergo colonoscopy to evaluate the proximal colon.

2. Colonoscopy—Colonoscopy permits examination of the entire colon. In addition to detecting early cancers, colonoscopy allows removal of adenomatous polyps by biopsy or polypectomy, which is believed to reduce the risk of subsequent cancer. Over the past decade, there has been a dramatic increase in screening colonoscopy and a similar decrease in screening sigmoidoscopy due to poor reimbursement and the perceived inferiority of sigmoidoscopy compared with colonoscopy. Almost 62% of US adults have undergone colonoscopy in the past 10 years. Colonoscopy requires aggressive bowel cleansing prior to the examination. To alleviate discomfort, intravenous sedation is used for most patients. The incidence of serious complications after colonoscopy (perforation, bleeding, cardiopulmonary events) is 0.1%. In asymptomatic individuals between 50 and 75 years of age undergoing screening colonoscopy, the prevalence of advanced neoplasia is 4–11% and of cancer is 0.1–1%.

Although colonoscopy is believed to be the most sensitive test for detecting adenomas and cancer, it is not infallible. In several studies, the rate of colorectal cancer within 3 years of a screening colonoscopy was 0.7–0.9%, ie, approximately 1 in 110 patients. This may be attributable to adenomatous and serrated polyps and early cancers that were overlooked during colonoscopy. Studies of back-to-back colonoscopies confirm that endoscopists overlook 6–12% of polyps greater than 1 cm in size and up to 25% of smaller adenomas. Polyps that are small, flat, or located behind folds are easily missed, especially if the bowel preparation is poor. Population-based case-control and cohort studies suggest that colonoscopy is associated with greater reduction in colorectal cancer incidence and mortality in the distal colon than the proximal colon. This may be attributable to incomplete examination of the proximal colon, and differences between the proximal and distal colon that include worse bowel preparation, suboptimal colonoscopic technique, and a higher prevalence of serrated polyps and flat adenomas. The latter are more common than previously recognized, are more likely to contain advanced pathology, and are more difficult to identify than raised (sessile or pedunculated) polyps. To optimize diagnostic accuracy as well as patient safety and comfort, colonoscopy should be performed after optimal bowel preparation by a well-trained endoscopist who spends sufficient time (at least 7 minutes) carefully examining the colon (especially the proximal colon) while withdrawing the endoscope.

C. Radiographic Examinations of the Colon

1. CT colonography—Using helical CT with computer-assisted image reconstruction, two- and three-dimensional views can be generated of the colon lumen that simulate the view of colonoscopy (virtual colonoscopy). CT colonography requires a similar bowel cleansing regimen as colonoscopy as well as insufflation of air into the colon through a rectal tube, which may be associated with discomfort. Nonetheless, this examination is performed rapidly and requires no sedation or intravenous contrast. It has minimal acute risk although there is controversy about potential long-term risks related to radiation exposure from CT examinations. Several large studies have compared the accuracy of virtual colonoscopy with colonoscopy for colorectal screening. Using current imaging software with multidetector helical scanners, the sensitivity is greater than 95% for the detection of cancer and greater than 84–92% for the detection of polyps 10 mm or larger. The sensitivity for polyps 6–9 mm in size ranges from 57% to 84%; for polyps 5 mm or less, the sensitivity is extremely poor.

Patients undergoing screening with CT colonography should be managed appropriately. If no polyps are found, the interval for repeat screening examination is uncertain; however, 5 years may be reasonable. All patients with polyps 10 mm or larger should be referred for colonoscopy with polypectomy because of the high prevalence (30%) of advanced pathology (cancer, high-grade dysplasia, or villous features) within these polyps. The optimal management of patients with polyps less than 10 mm in size is controversial. The US Multi-Society Task Force currently recommends that colonoscopy with polypectomy be offered to patients with one or more 6–9 mm polyps. Patients who refuse or who have increased risk of carcinoma should undergo surveillance CT colonography in 3–5 years. At the present time, there is no consensus on the management of patients with polyps smaller than 6 mm; however, some radiologists choose not even to report these findings.

2. Barium enema—Double-contrast barium enema was previously used as a screening technique because it was widely available, relatively inexpensive, and safe. However, compared to CT colonography, it is more time-consuming and difficult to perform, less comfortable, and less accurate. Although it continues to be included among recommended screening options, it has been supplanted by CT colonography, where available.

▶ When to Refer

- Patients with symptoms (change in bowel habits, hematochezia), signs (mass on abdominal examination or digital rectal examination [DRE]), or laboratory tests (iron deficiency anemia) suggestive of colorectal neoplasia should be referred for colonoscopy.
- Patients with suspected colorectal cancer or adenomatous polyps of any size should be referred for colonoscopy.
- Virtually all patients with proven colorectal cancer should be referred to a surgeon for resection. Patients with clinical stage T3 or node-positive rectal tumors (or both) also should be referred to medical and radiation oncologists preoperatively for neoadjuvant therapy. Patients with stage III or IV colorectal tumors should be referred to an oncologist.

▶ When to Admit

- Patients with complications of colorectal cancer (obstruction, acute bleeding) requiring urgent evaluation and intervention.
- Patients with severe complications of chemotherapy.
- Patients with advanced metastatic disease requiring palliative care.

Al-Hajeili M et al. Neoadjuvant treatment for surgically resectable metastatic colorectal cancer. Oncology (Williston Park). 2016 Jan 15;30(1):10–6. [PMID: 26791840]

André T et al. Adjuvant fluorouracil, leucovorin, and oxaliplatin in stage II to III colon cancer: updated 10-year survival and outcomes according to *BRAF* mutation and mismatch repair status of the MOSAIC Study. J Clin Oncol. 2015 Dec 10; 33(35):4176–87. [PMID: 26527776]

Bonjer HJ et al; COLOR II Study Group. A randomized trial of laparoscopic versus open surgery for rectal cancer. N Engl J Med. 2015 Apr 2;372(14):1324–33. [PMID: 25830422]

Bordaçahar B et al. Sessile serrated adenoma: from identification to resection. Dig Liver Dis. 2015 Feb;47(2):95–102. [PMID: 25445408]

Grothey A et al; CORRECT Study Group. Regorafenib monotherapy for previously treated metastatic colorectal cancer (CORRECT): an international, multicentre, randomised, placebo-controlled, phase 3 trial. Lancet. 2013 Jan 26; 381(9863):303–12. [PMID: 23177514]

Imperiale TF et al. Multitarget stool DNA testing for colorectal-cancer screening. N Engl J Med. 2014 Jul 10;371(2):187–8. [PMID: 25006736]

Jensen CD et al. Fecal immunochemical test program performance over 4 rounds of annual screening: a retrospective cohort study. Ann Intern Med. 2016 Apr 5;164(7):456–63. [PMID: 26811150]

Knight K et al; Lanarkshire Colorectal Study Group. Colorectal cancer in the elderly and the influence of lead time bias: better survival does not equate with improved life expectancy. Int J Colorectal Dis. 2016 Mar;31(3):553–9. [PMID: 26783116]

Lee JK et al. Accuracy of fecal immunochemical tests for colorectal cancer: systematic review and meta-analysis. Ann Intern Med. 2014 Feb 4;160(3):171. [PMID: 24658694]

Mayer RJ et al; RECOURSE Study Group. Randomized trial of TAS-102 for refractory metastatic colorectal cancer. N Engl J Med. 2015 May 14;372(20):1909–19. [PMID: 25970050]

Nishihara R et al. Long-term colorectal-cancer incidence and mortality after lower endoscopy. N Engl J Med. 2013 Sep 19; 369(12):1095–105. [PMID: 24047059]

Phipps AI et al. Association between molecular subtypes of colorectal cancer and patient survival. Gastroenterology. 2015 Jan;148(1):77–87. [PMID: 25280443]

Redwood DG et al. Stool DNA testing for screening detection of colorectal neoplasia in Alaska Native people. Mayo Clin Proc. 2016 Jan;91(1):61–70. [PMID: 26520415]

Shah MA et al. Impact of patient factors on recurrence risk and time dependency of oxaliplatin benefit in patients with colon cancer: analysis from modern-era adjuvant studies in the Adjuvant Colon Cancer End Points (ACCENT) database. J Clin Oncol. 2016 Mar 10;34(8):843–53. [PMID: 26811529]

Shaukat A et al. Long-term mortality after screening for colorectal cancer. N Engl J Med. 2013 Sept 19;369(12):1106–14. [PMID: 24047060]

Siegel RL et al. Cancer statistics, 2015. CA Cancer J Clin. 2015 Jan–Feb;65(1):5–29. [PMID: 25559415]

Singh S et al. Prevalence, risk factors, and outcomes of interval colorectal cancers: a systematic review and meta-analysis. Am J Gastroenterol. 2014 Sep;109(9):1375–89. [PMID: 24957158]

Sinicrope FA et al. Molecular markers identify subtypes of stage III colon cancer associated with patient outcomes. Gastroenterology. 2015 Jan;148(1):88–99. [PMID: 25305506]

Smith RA et al. Cancer screening in the United States, 2016: a review of current American Cancer Society guidelines and current issues in cancer screening. CA Cancer J Clin. 2016 Mar;66(2):95–114. [PMID: 26797525]

Van Cutsem E et al. Aflibercept plus FOLFIRI vs. placebo plus FOLFIRI in second-line metastatic colorectal cancer. Target Oncol. 2015 Dec 26. [Epub ahead of print] [PMID: 26706237]

Yang DX et al. Estimating the magnitude of colorectal cancers prevented during the era of screening: 1976 to 2009. Cancer. 2014 Sep 15;120(18):2893–901. [PMID: 24894740]

Zaniboni A. New active drugs for the treatment of advanced colorectal cancer. World J Gastrointest Surg. 2015 Dec 27; 7(12):356–9. [PMID: 26730280]

CARCINOMA OF THE ANUS

The anal canal is lined from its proximal to distal extent by columnar, transitional and non-keratinized squamous epithelium, which merges at the anal verge with the keratinized perianal skin. Tumors arising from the mucosa of the anal canal are relatively rare, comprising only 1–2% of all cancers of the anus and large intestine. Squamous cancers make up the majority of anal cancers. Anal cancer is increased among people practicing receptive anal intercourse and those with a history of anorectal warts. In over 80% of cases, HPV may be detected, suggesting that this virus is a major causal factor. In a large controlled trial, HPV vaccination of healthy men (16- to 26-years-old) who have sex with men decreased the incidence of anal intraepithelial neoplasia by 50%. Women with anal cancer are at increased risk for cervical cancer, which may be due to a field effect of oncogenic HPV infection, and require gynecologic screening and surveillance. Anal cancer is increased in HIV-infected individuals, possibly due to interaction with HPV. Bleeding, pain, and local tumor are the most common symptoms. The lesion is often confused with hemorrhoids or other common anal disorders. These tumors tend to become annular, invade the sphincter, and spread upward via the lymphatics into the perirectal mesenteric lymphatic nodes. CT or MRI scans of the abdomen and pelvis are required to identify regional lymphadenopathy or metastatic disease at diagnosis. PET imaging may be used in conjunction.

Treatment depends on the tumor location and histologic stage. Small (less than 3 cm) superficial lesions of the perianal skin may be treated with wide local excision. Adenocarcinoma of the anal canal is treated in similar fashion to rectal cancer (see above), commonly by abdominoperineal resection with neoadjuvant chemoradiotherapy and adjuvant chemotherapy. Squamous cancer of the anal canal and large perianal tumors invading the sphincter or rectum are treated with combined-modality therapy that includes external radiation with simultaneous chemotherapy (5-fluorouracil plus mitomycin). Local control is achieved in approximately 80% of patients. Radical surgery (abdominoperineal resection) is reserved for patients who fail chemotherapy and radiation therapy. Metastatic disease is generally treated with 5-fluorouracil in combination with cisplatin. The 5-year survival rate is 60–70% for localized tumors and over 25% for metastatic (stage IV) disease.

Alam NN et al. Systematic review of guidelines for the assessment and management of high-grade anal intraepithelial neoplasia (AIN II/III). Colorectal Dis. 2016 Feb;18(2):135–46. [PMID: 26559167]

Brickman C et al. Human papillomavirus in the HIV-infected host: epidemiology and pathogenesis in the antiretroviral era. Curr HIV/AIDS Rep. 2015 Mar;12(1):6–15. [PMID: 25644977]

Burgos J et al. Risk of progression to high-grade anal intraepithelial neoplasia in HIV-infected MSM. AIDS. 2015 Mar 27; 29(6):695–702. [PMID: 25849833]

Eng C et al. Optimal management of squamous cell carcinoma of the anal canal: where are we now? Expert Rev Anticancer Ther. 2014 Aug;14(8):877–86. [PMID: 24981728]

Gami B et al. Human papilloma virus and squamous cell carcinoma of the anus. Clin Med Insights Oncol. 2014 Sep 17; 8:113–9. [PMID: 25288893]

Ghosn M et al. Anal cancer treatment: current status and future perspectives. World J Gastroenterol. 2015 Feb 28;21(8): 2294–302. [PMID: 25741135]

Glynne-Jones R et al; European Society for Medical Oncology (ESMO); European Society of Surgical Oncology (ESSO); European Society of Radiotherapy and Oncology (ESTRO). Anal cancer: ESMO-ESSO-ESTRO clinical practice guidelines for diagnosis, treatment and follow-up. Eur J Surg Oncol. 2014 Oct;40(10):1165–76. [PMID: 25239441]

Musio D et al. Management of persistent anal canal carcinoma after combined-modality therapy: a clinical review. Radiat Oncol. 2014 Jan 28;9:39. [PMID: 24472223]

National Cancer Institute. Anal Cancer Treatment—Health Professional Version. www.cancer.gov/types/anal/hp/anal-treatment-pdq

Park IU et al. Human papillomavirus and genital warts: a review of the evidence for the 2015 Centers for Disease Control and Prevention Sexually Transmitted Diseases Treatment Guidelines. Clin Infect Dis. 2015 Dec 15;61(Suppl 8):S849–55. [PMID: 26602622]

Shiels MS et al. Anal cancer incidence in the United States, 1977–2011: distinct patterns by histology and behavior. Cancer Epidemiol Biomarkers Prev. 2015 Oct;24(10):1548–56. [PMID: 26224796]

Shridhar R et al. Anal cancer: current standards in care and recent changes in practice. CA Cancer J Clin. 2015 Mar; 65(2):139–62. [PMID: 25582527]

Stier EA et al. Prevalence of anal human papillomavirus infection and anal HPV-related disorders in women: a systematic review. Am J Obstet Gynecol. 2015 Sep;213(3):278–309. [PMID: 25797230]

CANCERS OF THE GENITOURINARY TRACT

Maxwell V. Meng, MD, FACS

PROSTATE CANCER

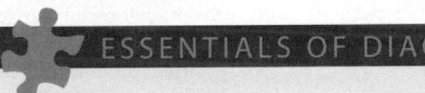
ESSENTIALS OF DIAGNOSIS

► Prostatic induration on DRE or elevation of PSA.

► Most often asymptomatic.

► Rarely: systemic symptoms (weight loss, bone pain).

▶ General Considerations

Prostatic cancer is the most common noncutaneous cancer detected in American men and the second leading cause of cancer-related death in men. In the United States, in 2015 an estimated 220,800 new cases of prostate cancer were diagnosed, and 27,540 deaths resulted. However, the clinical incidence of the disease does not match the prevalence noted at autopsy, where more than 40% of men over 50 years of age are found to have prostatic carcinoma. Most such occult cancers are small and contained within the prostate gland; few are associated with regional or distant disease. The incidence of prostatic cancer increases with age. Whereas 30% of men aged 60–69 years will have the disease at autopsy, its incidence increases to 67% in men aged 80–89 years. Although the global prevalence of prostatic cancer at autopsy is relatively consistent, the clinical incidence varies considerably (high in North America and European countries, intermediate in South America, and low in the Far East). A 50-year-old American man has a lifetime risk of 40% for latent cancer, 16% for developing clinically apparent cancer, and a 2.9% risk of death due to prostatic cancer. African American race, family history of prostatic cancer, and history of high dietary fat intake are risk factors for prostate cancer.

▶ Clinical Findings

A. Symptoms and Signs

Prostate cancer may manifest as focal nodules or areas of induration within the prostate at the time of DRE. However, currently most prostate cancers are detected because of elevations in serum PSA (not DRE findings).

Patients rarely present with signs of urinary retention or neurologic symptoms from epidural metastases and cord compression. Obstructive voiding symptoms are most often due to benign prostatic hyperplasia, which occurs in the same age group. Nevertheless, large or locally extensive prostatic cancers can cause obstructive voiding symptoms. Lymph node metastases can lead to lower extremity lymphedema. Because the axial skeleton is the most common site of metastases, patients may present with back pain or pathologic fractures.

B. Laboratory Findings

1. Serum tumor markers—PSA is a glycoprotein produced only by cells, either benign or malignant, of the prostate gland. The serum level is typically low and correlates with the volume of (benign and malignant) prostate tissue. Measurement of serum PSA is useful in detecting and staging prostate cancer, monitoring response to treatment, and detecting recurrence before it becomes clinically evident. As a screening test, PSA will be elevated (greater than 4.0 ng/mL [4.0 mcg/L]) in 10–15% of men. Approximately 18–30% of men with intermediate degrees of elevation (4.1–10 ng/mL [4.1–10 mcg/L]) and between 50% and 70% of men with elevations greater than 10 ng/mL (10 mcg/L) will be found to have prostate cancer. Patients with intermediate levels of PSA usually have localized and therefore potentially curable cancers. Interestingly, approximately 20% of patients who undergo radical prostatectomy for localized prostate cancers have normal levels of PSA.

In untreated patients with prostate cancer, the level of PSA correlates with the volume and stage of the disease. Whereas most organ-confined cancers are associated with PSA levels below 10 ng/mL (10 mcg/L), advanced disease (seminal vesicle invasion, lymph node involvement, or occult distant metastases) is more common in patients with PSA levels in excess of 40 ng/mL (40 mcg/L). Approximately 98% of patients with metastatic prostate cancer will have elevated PSA. However, there are rare cancers that are localized despite substantial elevations in PSA. Therefore, initial treatment decisions cannot be made on the basis of PSA testing alone. A rising PSA after therapy is usually consistent with progressive disease, either locally recurrent or metastatic.

2. Miscellaneous laboratory testing—Patients with urinary retention or with ureteral obstruction due to locoregionally advanced prostate cancers may present with elevations in blood urea nitrogen or serum creatinine. Patients with bony metastases may have elevations in serum alkaline phosphatase or calcium. Laboratory and clinical evidence of disseminated intravascular coagulation can occur in patients with advanced prostate cancers.

3. Prostate biopsy—Transrectal ultrasound-guided biopsy is the standard method for detection of prostate cancer. The use of a spring-loaded, 18-gauge biopsy needle has allowed transrectal biopsy to be performed with minimal patient discomfort and morbidity. Local anesthesia is routinely used and increases the tolerability of the procedure. The specimen preserves glandular architecture and permits accurate grading. Prostate biopsy specimens are taken from the apex, mid-portion, and base in men who have an abnormal DRE or an elevated serum PSA, or both. Extended-pattern biopsies, including a total of at least ten biopsies, are associated with improved cancer detection and risk stratification of patients with newly diagnosed disease. Patients with abnormalities of the seminal vesicles can have these structures specifically biopsied to identify local tumor invasion.

C. Imaging

Transrectal ultrasonography has primarily been used for the staging of prostate carcinomas, where tumors typically appear as hypoechoic areas. In addition, transrectal ultrasound-guided, rather than digitally-guided, biopsy of the prostate is a more accurate way to evaluate suspicious lesions. Use of imaging should be tailored to the likelihood of advanced disease in newly diagnosed cases. Asymptomatic patients with well-differentiated to moderately differentiated cancers, thought to be localized to the prostate on DRE and transrectal ultrasound and associated with modest elevations of PSA (ie, less than 10 ng/mL [10 mcg/L]), need no further imaging.

MRI allows for evaluation of the prostate as well as regional lymph nodes. The positive predictive value for detection of both capsular penetration and seminal vesicle invasion is similar for transrectal ultrasound and MRI, although newer multi-parametric MRI techniques may better stage patients considering treatment or, alternatively, active surveillance. MRI-guided biopsy may improve not only overall cancer detection but discovery of clinically relevant disease, and its use in routine clinical practice has increased. CT plays little role because of its inability to accurately identify or stage prostate cancers, but it can be used to detect regional lymphatic metastases and intraabdominal metastases.

Conventional radionuclide (99-technetium) bone scans are superior to conventional plain skeletal radiographs in detecting bony metastases. Most prostate cancer metastases are multiple and most commonly localized to the axial skeleton. Men with more advanced local lesions, symptoms of metastases (eg, bone pain), high-grade disease, or elevations in PSA greater than 20 ng/mL (20 mcg/L) should undergo radionuclide bone scan. PET (eg, ^{18}F-sodium fluoride [^{18}F-NaF] PET) and ^{18}F-NaF PET/CT hybrid imaging appear to be more sensitive than conventional bone scans. Because of the high frequency of abnormal scans in patients in this age group resulting from degenerative joint disease, plain films are often necessary in evaluating patients with indeterminate findings on bone scan. Cross-sectional imaging either by CT or MRI is usually indicated only in those patients in the latter group who have negative bone scans in an attempt to detect lymph node metastases. Patients found to have enlarged pelvic lymph nodes are candidates for FNA.

Intravenous urography and cystoscopy are not routinely needed to evaluate patients with prostate cancer.

Despite application of modern, sophisticated techniques, understaging of prostate cancer occurs in at least 20% of patients.

▶ Screening for Prostate Cancer

Whether screening for prostate cancer results in a decrease in its mortality rates is controversial. The screening tests currently available include DRE, PSA testing, and transrectal ultrasound. Prostate cancer detection rates using DRE alone vary from 1.5% to 7%, but unfortunately, most of these cancers are advanced (stage T3 or greater). Transrectal ultrasound should not be used as a first-line screening tool because of its expense, low specificity (and therefore high biopsy rate), and minimal improvement in detection rate when compared with the combined use of DRE and PSA testing.

PSA testing increases the detection rate of prostate cancers compared with DRE. Approximately 2–2.5% of men older than 50 years of age will be found to have prostate cancer using PSA testing compared with a rate of approximately 1.5% using DRE alone. The sensitivity, specificity, and positive predictive value of PSA and DRE are listed in Table 39–6. PSA-detected cancers are more likely to be localized compared with those detected by DRE alone. The Prostate Cancer Prevention Trial provided data demonstrating a significant risk of prostate cancer even in men with PSA less than 4.0 ng/mL (4.0 mcg/L) (Table 39–7) and a web-based calculator has been developed to estimate the risk of harboring both prostate cancer and high-grade cancer (http://deb.uthscsa.edu).

To improve the performance of PSA as a screening test, several investigators have developed alternative methods for its use. These include establishment of age- and race-specific reference ranges, measurement of free serum and protein-bound levels of PSA (percent free PSA), and

Table 39–7. Risk of prostate cancer in men with PSA ≤ 4.0 ng/mL (or mcg/L).

PSA level (ng/mL [or mcg/L])	Percentage with prostate cancer	Percentage with high-grade[1] prostate cancer
≤ 0.5	6.6	12.5
0.6–1.0	10.1	10.0
1.1–2.0	17.0	11.8
2.1–3.0	23.9	19.1
3.1–4.0	26.9	25.0

[1]High-grade cancer was defined as Gleason score ≥ 7.
Data from Thompson IM et al. Prevalence of prostate cancer among men with a prostate-specific antigen level ≤ 4.0 ng per milliliter. N Engl J Med. 2004 May 27;350(22):2239–46.

calculation of changes in PSA over time (PSA velocity). Generally, men with PSA free fractions exceeding 25% are unlikely to have prostate cancer, whereas those with free fractions less than 10% have an approximately 50% chance of having prostate cancer. The frequency of PSA testing also remains a matter of debate. The traditional yearly screening approach may not be the most efficient; rather, earlier PSA testing at younger age may allow less frequent testing later as well as provide information regarding PSA velocity. Studies from the Baltimore Longitudinal Study of Aging suggest that men with PSA above the age-based median when tested between 40 and 60 years are at significantly increased risk for subsequent cancer detection over 25 years. Men with lower PSA (0.6 ng/mL [0.6 mcg/L] ages 40–50 and 0.71 ng/mL [0.71 mcg/L] ages 50–60) may require less frequent PSA tests. In addition, men with PSA velocity greater than 0.35 ng/mL (0.35 mcg/L) per year measured 10–15 years before diagnosis had significantly worse cancer-specific survival compared with those with lower PSA velocity. The current NCCN guidelines (http://www.nccn.org/professionals/physician_gls/f_guidelines.asp) for prostate cancer early detection incorporate many of these factors (Figure 39–2). The current European Association of Urology (EAU) recommends offering a baseline serum PSA to all men aged 40–45 years and subsequently initiating a risk-adapted strategy.

Two large, randomized trials question the benefit of screening men for prostate cancer. In the US Prostate, Lung, Colorectal, and Ovarian (PLCO) Cancer Screening Trial, no mortality benefit was observed after combined screening with PSA testing and DRE during 13-year follow-up. Although screening resulted in a 12% increase in prostate cancer detection, the cancer-specific mortality rate was similar in the screening and control arms (3.7 and 3.4 deaths per 10,000 person-years, respectively). Similarly, in the European Randomized Study of Screening for Prostate Cancer (ERSPC) trial, the benefit of PSA screening was minimal with an absolute reduction of 1.28 prostate cancer deaths per 1000 men screened at 13-year follow-up. Based on these data, the US Preventive Services Task Force has recommended against PSA-based screening for prostate cancer in asymptomatic men (grade D recommendation)

Table 39–6. Screening for prostatic cancer: Test performance.

Test	Sensitivity	Specificity	Positive Predictive Value
Abnormal PSA (> 4 ng/ mL [mcg/L])	0.67	0.97	0.43
Abnormal DRE	0.50	0.94	0.24
Abnormal PSA or DRE	0.84	0.92	0.28
Abnormal PSA and DRE	0.34	0.995	0.49

DRE, digital rectal examination; PSA, prostate-specific antigen.
Modified, with permission, from Kramer BS et al. Prostate cancer screening: what we know and what we need to know. Ann Intern Med. 1993 Nov 1;119(9):914–23.

Figure 39–2. An algorithm for prostate cancer early detection. DRE, digital rectal examination; 5-ARI, 5-alpha-reductase inhibitor; PSAV, PSA velocity (ng/mL/year) calculated on at least three consecutive values over at least an 18–24 month period. (Based on NCCN guidelines, data from the Baltimore Longitudinal Study on Aging, and Prostate Cancer Prevention Trial.)

and early data already suggest a reduction in screening practice; further studies will reveal whether decreased or delayed detection of higher-grade tumors will impact cancer-specific mortality in the future.

▶ **Staging**

The majority of prostate cancers are adenocarcinomas. Most arise in the peripheral zone of the prostate, though a small percentage arise in the central (5–10%) and transition zones (20%) of the gland. Pathologists utilize the Gleason grading system whereby a "primary" grade is applied to the architectural pattern of malignant glands occupying the largest area of the specimen and a "secondary" grade is assigned to the next largest area of cancer. Grading is based on architectural rather than histologic criteria, and five "grades" are possible. Adding the score of the primary and secondary grades gives a Gleason score from 2 to 10. Gleason score correlates with tumor volume, pathologic stage, and prognosis.

► Treatment

A. Active Surveillance

The optimal treatment for patients with clinically localized prostate cancers remains controversial. A beneficial impact of treating localized prostate cancer has not been conclusively demonstrated with respect to survival. Patients need to be advised of all treatment options, including active surveillance, with the specific benefits, risks, and limitations. The goal of active surveillance is to avoid treatment in men who never experience disease progression while recognizing and effectively treating men with evidence of progression. Currently, treatment decisions are made based on stage and cancer grade (Gleason score) as well as the age and health of the patient. Given the observed significant migration to lower stage and grade resulting from screening using PSA testing, active surveillance alone may be appropriate management for selected patients. Such patients included are typically older with small volume, well-differentiated cancers. Depending on the age and health of the patient, some of these very low-volume, low-grade cancers may never become clinically relevant and can be monitored with active surveillance, that is, serial PSA levels, DREs, and periodic prostate biopsies to reassess grade and extent of cancer. Endpoints for intervention in patients on active surveillance, particularly PSA changes, have not been clearly defined and surveillance regimens remain an active area of research; nonetheless, they are increasingly accepted by patients and clinicians. Active surveillance, which is distinguished from mere observation, is featured prominently in the 2015 NCCN guidelines and may be the preferred management in most men with very low risk prostate cancer. This approach is increasingly accepted and incorporated in routine clinical practice.

B. Radical Prostatectomy

During radical prostatectomy, the seminal vesicles, prostate, and ampullae of the vas deferens are removed. Refinements in technique have allowed preservation of urinary continence in most patients and erectile function in selected patients. Radical prostatectomy can be performed via open retropubic, transperineal, or laparoscopic (with or without robotic assistance) surgery. Local recurrence is uncommon after radical prostatectomy and related to pathologic stage. Organ-confined cancers rarely recur; however, cancers with adverse pathologic features (capsular penetration, seminal vesicle invasion) are associated with higher local (10–25%) and distant (20–50%) relapse rates.

Ideal candidates for radical prostatectomy include healthy patients with stages T1 and T2 prostate cancers. Patients with advanced local tumors (T4) or lymph node metastases are rarely candidates for prostatectomy alone, although the surgery is sometimes used in combination with hormonal therapy and postoperative radiation therapy for select high-risk patients.

C. Radiation Therapy

Radiation can be delivered by a variety of techniques including use of external beam radiotherapy and transperineal implantation of radioisotopes. Morbidity is limited, and the survival of patients with localized cancers (T1, T2, and selected T3) approaches 65% at 10 years. As with surgery, the likelihood of local failure correlates with technique and cancer characteristics. The likelihood of a positive prostate biopsy more than 18 months after radiation varies between 20% and 60%. Patients with local recurrence are at an increased risk of cancer progression and cancer death compared with those who have negative biopsies. Ambiguous target definitions, inadequate radiation doses, and understaging of the cancer may be responsible for the failure noted in some series. Newer techniques of radiation (implantation, conformal therapy using three-dimensional reconstruction of CT-based tumor volumes, heavy particle, charged particle, and heavy charged particle) may improve local control rates. Three-dimensional conformal radiation delivers a higher dose because of improved targeting and appears to be associated with greater efficacy as well as lower likelihood of adverse side effects compared with previous techniques. Brachytherapy—the implantation of permanent or temporary radioactive sources (palladium, iodine, or iridium) into the prostate can be used as monotherapy in those with low-grade or low-volume malignancies or combined with external beam radiation in patients with higher-grade or higher-volume disease. The PSA may rise after brachytherapy because of prostate inflammation and necrosis. This transient elevation (PSA bounce) should not be mistaken for recurrence and may occur up to 20 months after treatment.

D. Cryosurgery

In cryosurgery, liquid nitrogen is circulated through small hollow-core needles inserted into the prostate under ultrasound guidance. The freezing process results in tissue destruction. The positive biopsy rate after cryoablation ranges between 7% and 23%.

E. Localized Disease

Although selected patients may be candidates for active surveillance based on age or health and evidence of small-volume or well-differentiated cancers, most men with an anticipated life expectancy in excess of 10 years should be considered for treatment. Newly introduced genomic tests may provide novel information to help guide treatment decisions. Both radiation therapy and radical prostatectomy result in acceptable levels of local control. A large, prospective, randomized trial compared active surveillance with radical prostatectomy in 695 men with clinically localized and well-differentiated to moderately differentiated cancers. Radical prostatectomy significantly reduced disease-specific mortality, overall mortality, and risks of metastasis and local progression. The relative reduction in the risk of death at 23 years was 0.56 in the prostatectomy group, with the number needed to treat to avert one death (NNT) = 8 patients; the benefit was largest in men younger than age 65 years (relative risk [RR] = 0.45) and with intermediate-risk prostate cancer (RR = 0.38). Surgery also reduced the risk of metastases in older men (RR = 0.68).

F. Locally and Regionally Advanced Disease

Patients with advanced pathologic stage or positive surgical margins are at an increased risk for local and distant tumor relapse. Such patients are candidates for adjuvant therapy (radiation for positive margins or androgen deprivation for lymph node metastases). Two randomized clinical trials (EORTC 22911 and SWOG 8794) have demonstrated improved progression-free and metastasis-free survival with early radiotherapy in these men, and subsequent analysis of SWOG 8794 showed improved overall survival in men receiving adjuvant radiation therapy. Evidence suggests that salvage radiotherapy after radical prostatectomy, within 2 years of PSA relapse, increases prostate cancer-specific survival in men with shorter PSA doubling time (less than 6 months).

Those with locally extensive cancers, including those with seminal vesicle and bladder neck invasion, are at increased risk for both local and distant relapse despite conventional therapy. Currently, a variety of investigational regimens are being tested in an effort to improve cancer outcomes in such patients. Combination therapy (androgen deprivation combined with surgery or irradiation), newer forms of irradiation, and hormonal therapy alone are being tested, as is neoadjuvant and adjuvant chemotherapy. Neoadjuvant and adjuvant androgen deprivation therapy combined with external beam radiation therapy have demonstrated improved survival compared with external beam radiation therapy alone.

G. Metastatic Disease

Since death due to prostate carcinoma is almost invariably the result of failure to control metastatic disease, research has emphasized efforts to improve control of distant disease. Most prostate carcinomas are hormone dependent and approximately 70–80% of men with metastatic prostate carcinoma will respond to various forms of androgen deprivation. Androgen deprivation may be affected at several levels along the pituitary–gonadal axis using a variety of methods or agents (Table 39–8). Use of luteinizing hormone-releasing hormone (LHRH) agonists (leuprolide, goserelin) achieves androgen deprivation without orchiectomy or administration of diethylstilbestrol and is currently the most common method of reducing testosterone levels. A single LHRH antagonist (degarelix) is FDA approved and has no short-term testosterone "flare" associated with LHRH agonists. Because of its rapid onset of action, ketoconazole should be considered in patients with advanced prostate cancer who present with spinal cord compression, bilateral ureteral obstruction, or disseminated intravascular coagulation. Although testosterone is the major circulating androgen, the adrenal gland secretes the androgens dehydroepiandrosterone, dehydroepiandrosterone sulfate, and androstenedione. Some investigators believe that suppressing both testicular and adrenal androgens allows for a better initial and longer response than methods that only inhibit production of testicular androgens. Complete androgen blockade can be achieved by combining an antiandrogen with use of an

Table 39–8. Androgen deprivation for prostatic cancer.

Level	Agent	Dose	Sequelae
Pituitary, hypothalamus	Diethylstilbestrol	1–3 mg orally daily	Gynecomastia, hot flushes, thromboembolic disease, erectile dysfunction
	LHRH agonists Leuprolide Goserelin Triptorelin Histrelin	Monthly to annual depot injection Subcutaneous implant	Erectile dysfunction, hot flushes, gynecomastia, rarely anemia
	LHRH antagonist Degarelix	240 mg subcutaneously initial dose, then 80 mg subcutaneously monthly	Hot flushes, weight gain, erectile dysfunction, increased liver tests
Adrenal	Ketoconazole	400 mg three times orally daily	Adrenal insufficiency, nausea, rash, ataxia
	Aminoglutethimide	250 mg four times orally daily	Adrenal insufficiency, nausea, rash, ataxia
	Corticosteroids Prednisone	20–40 mg orally daily 500 mg orally daily	Gastrointestinal bleeding, fluid retention
	CYP17a1 inhibitor Abiraterone		Weight gain, fluid retention, hypokalemia, hypertension
Testis	Orchiectomy		Gynecomastia, hot flushes, erectile dysfunction
Prostate cell	**Antiandrogens** Flutamide Bicalutamide Enzalutamide	250 mg three times orally daily 50 mg orally daily 160 mg orally daily	No erectile dysfunction when used alone; nausea, diarrhea Seizures, dizziness, asthenia

LHRH, luteinizing hormone-releasing hormone.

LHRH agonist/antagonist or orchiectomy. Nonsteroidal antiandrogen agents appear to act by competitively binding the receptor for dihydrotestosterone, the intracellular androgen responsible for prostate cell growth and development. A meta-analysis of trials comparing the use of either an LHRH agonist or orchiectomy alone or of either in combination with an antiandrogen agent showed little benefit of combination therapy. However, patients at risk for disease-related symptoms (bone pain, obstructive voiding symptoms) due to the initial elevation of serum testosterone that accompanies the use of an LHRH agonist should receive antiandrogens initially. Bisphosphonates can prevent osteoporosis associated with androgen deprivation, decrease bone pain from metastases, and reduce skeletal-related events. Denosumab, a RANK ligand inhibitor, is approved for the prevention of skeletal-related events in patients with bone metastases from prostate cancer and also appears to delay the development of these metastases.

Docetaxel is the first cytotoxic chemotherapy agent to improve survival in patients with hormone-refractory prostate cancer. Current research is underway combining docetaxel with androgen deprivation therapy, radiation therapy, and surgery to determine whether combinations are effective in patients with high-risk prostate cancer. Immune therapies are also under investigation and have shown promise for patients with advanced prostate cancer. Sipuleucel-T, an autologous cellular immunotherapy, is FDA approved in asymptomatic or minimally symptomatic men with metastatic hormone-refractory prostate cancer. Other agents—cabazitaxel, abiraterone, and enzalutamide—are also approved for advanced prostate cancer after clinical trials have demonstrated improvements in survival in men having received prior docetaxel. Both abiraterone and enzalutamide have been FDA approved for use in the pre-chemotherapy, metastatic setting. Radium-223 dichloride is approved for the treatment of men with castration-resistant, symptomatic bone metastases, with significant improvements in both overall survival and time to skeletal-related events (eg, fractures). A recent trial demonstrated the benefit of early combination treatment with chemotherapy and androgen deprivation therapy in men with newly diagnosed metastatic prostate cancer, with an overall survival advantage superior to chemotherapy given at the time of development of castration-resistant disease.

▶ Prognosis

The likelihood of success of active surveillance or treatment can be predicted using risk assessment tools that usually combine stage, grade, PSA level, and number and extent of positive prostate biopsies. Several tools are available on the Internet (eg, http://www.mskcc.org/nomograms/prostate). One of the most widely used is the Kattan nomogram; it incorporates cancer stage, grade, and PSA level to predict the likelihood that a patient will be disease-free after radical prostatectomy or radiation therapy.

The University of California San Francisco CAPRA nomogram uses serum PSA, Gleason score, clinical stage, percent positive biopsies, and patient age in a point system to risk stratify and predict the likelihood of PSA recurrence

Table 39–9. The UCSF Cancer of the Prostate Risk Assessment (CAPRA).

Variable	Level	Points
PSA (ng/mL [or mcg/L])	0–6	0
	6.1–10	1
	10.1–20	2
	20.1–30	3
	> 30	4
Gleason grade, primary/secondary	1–3/1–3	0
	1–3/4–5	1
	4–5/1–5	3
T-stage	T1 or T2	0
	T3a	1
% positive biopsies (biopsy cores positive divided by the number of biopsies obtained)	< 34%	0
	> 34%	1
Age	< 50 years	0
	> 50 years	1

3 and 5 years after radical prostatectomy (Tables 39–9 and 39–10) as well as metastasis, prostate cancer-specific, and overall survival. The CAPRA nomogram has been validated on large multicenter and international radical prostatectomy and radiation-treated cohorts.

The patterns of prostate cancer progression have been well defined. Small and well-differentiated cancers (Gleason grades 1 and 2) are usually confined within the prostate, whereas large-volume (greater than 4 mL) or poorly differentiated (Gleason grades 4 and 5) cancers are more often locally extensive or metastatic to regional lymph nodes or bone. Penetration of the prostate capsule by cancer is common and occurs along perineural spaces. Seminal vesicle invasion is associated with a high likelihood of

Table 39–10. CAPRA: Probability of freedom from PSA recurrence after radical prostatectomy by CAPRA point total.

CAPRA Score	3-Year Recurrence Free Survival (%) (95% CI)	5-Year Recurrence Free Survival (%) (95% CI)
0–1	91 (85–95)	85 (73–92)
2	89 (83–94)	81 (69–89)
3	81 (73–87)	66 (54–76)
4	81 (69–89)	59 (40–74)
5	69 (51–82)	60 (37–77)
6	54 (27–75)	34 (12–57)
7+	24 (9–43)	8 (0–28)

PSA, prostate-specific antigen.

regional or distant disease, and disease recurrence. The most common sites of lymph node metastases are the obturator and internal iliac lymph node chains and of distant metastases, the axial skeleton.

► When to Refer

- Refer all patients to a urologist.
- Active surveillance may be appropriate in selected patients with very low volume, low-grade prostate cancer.
- Localized disease may be managed by active surveillance, surgery, or radiation therapy.
- Locally extensive, regionally advanced, and metastatic disease often require multimodal treatment strategies.

Barry MJ et al. Evaluating an elevated screening PSA test. JAMA. 2015 Nov 17;314(19):2073–4. [PMID: 26575065]

Beer TM et al; PREVAIL Investigators. Enzalutamide in metastatic prostate cancer before chemotherapy. N Engl J Med. 2014 Jul 31;371(5):424–33. [PMID: 24881730]

Bill-Axelson A et al. Radical prostatectomy or watchful waiting in early prostate cancer. N Engl J Med. 2014 Mar 6;370(10):932–42. [PMID: 24597866]

Cooperberg MR et al. Trends in management for patients with localized prostate cancer, 1990–2013. JAMA. 2015 Jul 7; 314(1):80–2. [PMID: 26151271]

Eggener SE et al. Prostate cancer screening. JAMA. 2015 Aug 25; 314(8):825–6. [PMID: 26305653]

Filson CP et al. Expectant management for men with early stage prostate cancer. CA Cancer J Clin. 2015 Jul–Aug;65(4): 265–82. [PMID: 25958817]

Hoffman KE et al. Physician variation in management of low-risk prostate cancer: a population-based cohort study. JAMA Intern Med. 2014 Sep;174(9):1450–9. [PMID: 25023650]

Ilic D et al. Screening for prostate cancer. Cochrane Database Syst Rev. 2013 Jan 31;1:CD004720. [PMID: 23440794]

Jemal A et al. Prostate cancer incidence and PSA testing patterns in relation to USPSTF screening recommendations. JAMA. 2015 Nov 17;314(19):2054–61. [PMID: 26575061]

Meng MV et al. Treatment of patients with high risk localized prostate cancer: results from Cancer of the Prostate Strategic Urological Research Endeavor (CaPSURE). J Urol. 2005 May; 173(5):1557–61. [PMID: 15821485]

Moyer VA. Screening for prostate cancer: U.S. Preventive Services Task Force recommendation statement. Ann Intern Med. 2012 Jul 17;157(2):120–34. [PMID: 22801674]

Niraula S et al. Treatment of prostate cancer with intermittent versus continuous androgen deprivation: a systematic review of randomized trials. J Clin Oncol. 2013 Jun 1;31(16): 2029–36. [PMID: 23630216]

Razmaria AA. JAMA Patient Page. Prostate cancer screening. JAMA. 2015 Nov 17;314(19):2096. [PMID: 26575077]

Schröder FH et al; ERSPC Investigators. Screening and prostate cancer mortality: results of the European Randomised Study of Screening for Prostate Cancer (ERSPC) at 13 years of follow-up. Lancet. 2014 Dec 6;384(9959):2027–35. [PMID: 25108889]

Skolarus TA et al. American Cancer Society prostate cancer survivorship care guidelines. CA Cancer J Clin. 2014 Jul–Aug; 64(4):225–49. [PMID: 24916760]

Sweeney CJ et al. Chemohormonal therapy in metastatic hormone-sensitive prostate cancer. N Engl J Med. 2015 Aug 20; 373(8):737–46. [PMID: 26244877]

Thompson IM Jr et al. Long-term survival of participants in the prostate cancer prevention trial. N Engl J Med. 2013 Aug 15; 369(7):603–10. [PMID: 23944298]

Qaseem A et al. Screening for prostate cancer: a guidance statement from the Clinical Guidelines Committee of the American College of Physicians. Ann Intern Med. 2013 May 21; 158(10):761–9. [PMID: 23567643]

Violette PD et al. Decision aids for localized prostate cancer treatment choice: systematic review and meta-analysis. CA Cancer J Clin. 2015 May–Jun;65(3):239–51. [PMID: 25772796]

Wilt TJ et al; Prostate Cancer Intervention versus Observation Trial (PIVOT) Study Group. Radical prostatectomy versus observation for localized prostate cancer. N Engl J Med. 2012 Jul 19;367(3):203–13. Erratum in: N Engl J Med. 2012 Aug 9; 367(6):582. [PMID: 22808955]

BLADDER CANCER

ESSENTIALS OF DIAGNOSIS

- ► Gross or microscopic hematuria.
- ► Irritative voiding symptoms.
- ► Positive urinary cytology in most patients.
- ► Filling defect within bladder noted on imaging.

► General Considerations

Bladder cancer is the second most common urologic cancer; it occurs more commonly in men than women (3.1:1), and the mean age at diagnosis is 73 years. Cigarette smoking and exposure to industrial dyes or solvents are risk factors for the disease and account for approximately 60% and 15% of new cases, respectively. In the United States, almost all primary bladder cancers (98%) are epithelial malignancies, usually urothelial cell carcinomas (90%). Adenocarcinomas and squamous cell cancers account for approximately 2% and 7%, respectively. The latter is often associated with schistosomiasis, vesical calculi, or prolonged catheter use.

► Clinical Findings

A. Symptoms and Signs

Hematuria—gross or microscopic, chronic or intermittent—is the presenting symptom in 85–90% of patients with bladder cancer. Irritative voiding symptoms (urinary frequency and urgency) occur in a small percentage of patients as a result of the location or size of the cancer. Most patients with bladder cancer do not have signs of the disease because of its superficial nature. Abdominal masses detected on bimanual examination may be present in patients with large-volume or deeply infiltrating cancers. Hepatomegaly or palpable lymphadenopathy may be present in patients with metastatic disease, and lymphedema of the lower extremities results from locally advanced cancers or metastases to pelvic lymph nodes.

B. Laboratory Findings

Urinalysis reveals microscopic or gross hematuria in the majority of cases. On occasion, hematuria is accompanied by pyuria. Azotemia may be present in a small number of cases associated with ureteral obstruction. Anemia may occasionally be due to chronic blood loss or to bone marrow metastases. Exfoliated cells from normal and abnormal urothelium can be readily detected in voided urine specimens. Cytology can be useful to detect the disease initially or to detect its recurrence. Cytology is sensitive in detecting cancers of higher grade and stage (80–90%) but less so in detecting superficial or well-differentiated lesions (50%). There are numerous urinary tumor markers under investigation for screening, assessing recurrence, progression, prognosis or response to therapy.

C. Imaging

Bladder cancers may be identified using ultrasound, CT, or MRI as masses within the bladder. However, the presence of cancer is confirmed by cystoscopy and biopsy, with imaging primarily used to evaluate the upper urinary tract and to stage more advanced lesions.

D. Cystourethroscopy and Biopsy

The diagnosis and staging of bladder cancers are made by cystoscopy and transurethral resection. If cystoscopy—performed usually under local anesthesia—confirms the presence of bladder cancer, the patient is scheduled for transurethral resection under general or regional anesthesia. Random bladder and, on occasion, transurethral prostate biopsies are performed to detect occult disease in the bladder or elsewhere and potentially identify patients at greater risk for cancer recurrence and progression.

▶ Pathology & Staging

Grading is based on cellular features: size, pleomorphism, mitotic rate, and hyperchromatism. Bladder cancer staging is based on the extent (depth) of bladder wall penetration and the presence of regional or distant metastases.

The natural history of bladder cancer is based on two separate but related processes: cancer recurrence within the bladder and progression to higher-stage disease. Both are correlated with cancer grade and stage.

▶ Treatment

Patients with superficial cancers (Ta, T1) are treated with complete transurethral resection and selective use of intravesical chemotherapy. The subset of patients with carcinoma in situ and those undergoing resection of large, high-grade, recurrent Ta lesions or T1 cancers are good candidates for adjuvant intravesical therapy.

Patients with invasive (T2, T3) but still localized cancers are at risk for both nodal metastases and progression and require radical cystectomy, irradiation, or the combination of chemotherapy and selective surgery or irradiation due to the much higher risk of progression compared with patients with lower-stage lesions.

For patients with muscle invasive (T2 or greater) urothelial cell carcinoma, neoadjuvant systemic chemotherapy prior to radical cystectomy is superior to radical cystectomy alone. This is particularly important for higher stage or bulky tumors in order to improve their surgical resectability.

A. Intravesical Chemotherapy

Immunotherapeutic or chemotherapeutic agents delivered directly into the bladder via a urethral catheter can reduce the likelihood of recurrence in those who have undergone complete transurethral resection. Most agents are administered weekly for 6–12 weeks. Efficacy may be increased by prolonging contact time to 2 hours. The use of maintenance therapy after the initial induction regimen is beneficial. Common agents include thiotepa, mitomycin, doxorubicin, valrubicin, and BCG, the last being the most effective agent in reducing disease progression. Side effects of intravesical chemotherapy include irritative voiding symptoms and hemorrhagic cystitis. Patients in whom symptoms or infection develop from BCG may require antituberculous therapy.

B. Surgical Treatment

Although transurethral resection is the initial form of treatment for all bladder tumors since it is diagnostic, allows for proper staging, and controls superficial cancers, muscle-infiltrating cancers require more aggressive treatment. Partial cystectomy is indicated in selected patients with solitary lesions or those with cancers in a bladder diverticulum. Radical cystectomy entails removal of the bladder, prostate, seminal vesicles, and surrounding fat and peritoneal attachments in men and the uterus, cervix, urethra, anterior vaginal vault, and usually the ovaries in women. Bilateral pelvic lymph node dissection is performed in all patients.

Urinary diversion can be performed using a conduit of small or large bowel. However, continent forms of diversion have been developed that avoid the necessity of an external appliance and can be considered in a significant number of patients.

C. Radiotherapy

External beam radiotherapy delivered in fractions over a 6- to 8-week period is generally well tolerated, but approximately 10–15% of patients will develop bladder, bowel, or rectal complications. Local recurrence is common after radiotherapy alone (30–70%) and it is therefore combined with systemic chemotherapy in an effort to reduce the need for radical cystectomy or to treat patients who are poor candidates for radical cystectomy.

D. Chemotherapy

Metastatic disease is present in 15% of patients with newly diagnosed bladder cancer, and metastases develop within 2 years in up to 40% of patients who were believed to have localized disease at the time of cystectomy or definitive radiotherapy. Cisplatin-based combination chemotherapy results in partial or complete responses in 15–45% of patients (see Table 39–4).

Combination chemotherapy has been used to decrease recurrence rates with both surgery and radiotherapy and to attempt bladder preservation in those treated with radiation. Neoadjuvant chemotherapy appears to benefit all patients with muscle-invasive disease prior to planned cystectomy. Chemotherapy should also be considered before surgery in those with bulky lesions or those suspected of having regional disease. Chemoradiation is best suited for those with T2 or limited T3 disease without ureteral obstruction. Alternatively, chemotherapy has been used after cystectomy in patients at high risk for recurrence, such as those who have lymph node involvement or local invasion.

▶ Prognosis

The frequency of recurrence and progression are correlated with grade. Whereas progression may be noted in few low-grade cancers (19–37%), it is common with poorly differentiated lesions (33–67%). Carcinoma in situ is most often found in association with papillary bladder cancers. Its presence identifies patients at increased risk for recurrence and progression.

At initial presentation, approximately 50–80% of bladder cancers are superficial: stage Ta, Tis, or T1. When properly treated, lymph node metastases and progression are uncommon in such patients and survival is excellent (81%). Five-year survival of patients with T2 and T3 disease ranges from 50% to 75% after radical cystectomy. Long-term survival for patients with metastatic disease at presentation is rare.

▶ When to Refer

- Refer all patients to a urologist. Hematuria often deserves evaluation with both upper urinary tract imaging and cystoscopy, particularly in a high-risk group (eg, older men).
- Refer when histologic diagnosis and staging require endoscopic resection of cancer.

Bachir BG et al. Contemporary cost-effectiveness analysis comparing sequential bacillus Calmette-Guerin and electromotive mitomycin versus bacillus Calmette-Guerin alone for patients with high-risk non-muscle-invasive bladder cancer. Cancer. 2014 Aug 15;120(16):2424–31. [PMID: 24752448]

Burger M et al. ICUD-EAU International Consultation on Bladder Cancer 2012: non-muscle-invasive urothelial carcinoma of the bladder. Eur Urol. 2013 Jan;63(1):36–44. [PMID: 22981672]

Hautmann RE et al. ICUD-EAU International Consultation on Bladder Cancer 2012: urinary diversion. Eur Urol. 2013 Jan; 63(1):67–80. [PMID: 22995974]

Johnson DC et al. Surgical advances in bladder cancer: at what cost? Urol Clin North Am. 2015 May;42(2):235–52. [PMID: 25882565]

Jordan EJ et al. Targeted therapy in advanced bladder cancer: what have we learned? Urol Clin North Am. 2015 May; 42(2):253–62. [PMID: 25882566]

Kamat AM et al. ICUD-EAU International Consultation on Bladder Cancer 2012: screening, diagnosis, and molecular markers. Eur Urol. 2013 Jan;63(1):4–15. [PMID: 23083902]

Khurana KK et al. Multidisciplinary management of patients with localized bladder cancer. Surg Oncol Clin N Am. 2013 Apr; 22(2):357–73. [PMID: 23453340]

Lerner SP et al. Novel endoscopic diagnosis for bladder cancer. Cancer. 2015 Jan 15;121(2):169–78. [PMID: 25132313]

Lucca I et al. Novel biomarkers to predict response and prognosis in localized bladder cancer. Urol Clin North Am. 2015 May; 42(2):225–33. [PMID: 25882564]

Meeks JJ et al. Office-based management of nonmuscle invasive bladder cancer. Urol Clin North Am. 2013 Nov;40(4):473–9. [PMID: 24182970]

Razmaria AA. JAMA Patient Page. Bladder cancer. JAMA. 2015 Nov 3;314(17):1886. [PMID: 26529173]

Sandler HM et al. Current role of radiation therapy for bladder cancer. Semin Oncol. 2012 Oct;39(5):583–7. [PMID: 23040254]

Sternberg CN et al. ICUD-EAU International Consultation on Bladder Cancer 2012: chemotherapy for urothelial carcinoma-neoadjuvant and adjuvant settings. Eur Urol. 2013 Jan; 63(1):58–66. [PMID: 22917984]

CANCERS OF THE URETER & RENAL PELVIS

Cancers of the ureter and renal pelvis are rare and occur more commonly in patients with bladder cancer, with Balkan nephropathy, with Lynch syndrome, who smoke, who were exposed to Thorotrast (a contrast agent with radioactive thorium in use until the 1960s), and who have a long history of analgesic abuse. The majority are urothelial cell carcinomas. Gross or microscopic hematuria is present in most patients, and flank pain secondary to bleeding and obstruction occurs less commonly. Like bladder cancers, urinary cytology is often positive. The most common signs identified at the time of CT or intravenous urography include an intraluminal filling defect, unilateral nonvisualization of the collecting system, and hydronephrosis. Ureteral and renal pelvic tumors must be differentiated from calculi, blood clots, papillary necrosis, or inflammatory and infectious lesions. On occasion, upper urinary tract lesions are accessible for biopsy, fulguration, or resection using a ureteroscope. Treatment is based on the site, size, grade, depth of penetration, and number of cancers present. Most are excised with laparoscopic or open nephroureterectomy (renal pelvic and upper ureteral lesions) or segmental excision of the ureter (distal ureteral lesions). Endoscopic resection may be indicated in patients with limited renal function or focal, low-grade, cancers. Similar to urothelial bladder cancers, use of chemotherapy prior to surgery may improve outcomes.

Balar AV et al. Cytotoxic and DNA-targeted therapy in urothelial cancer: have we squeezed the lemon enough? Cancer. 2015 Jan 15;121(2):179–87. [PMID: 25091501]

Cordier J et al. Oncologic outcomes obtained after neoadjuvant and adjuvant chemotherapy for the treatment of urothelial carcinomas of the upper urinary tract: a review. World J Urol. 2013 Feb;31(1):77–82. [PMID: 23053212]

Grivas PD et al. Double-blind, randomized, phase 2 trial of maintenance sunitinib versus placebo after response to chemotherapy in patients with advanced urothelial carcinoma. Cancer. 2014 Mar 1;120(5):692–701. [PMID: 24249435]

Mooney D et al. Update in systemic therapy of urologic malignancies. Postgrad Med. 2014 Jan;126(1):44–54. [PMID: 24393751]

Porten S et al. Neoadjuvant chemotherapy improves survival of patients with upper tract urothelial carcinoma. Cancer. 2014 Jun 15;120(12):1794–9. [PMID: 24633966]

Rai BP et al. Surgical management for upper urinary tract transitional cell carcinoma (UUT-TCC): a systematic review. BJU Int. 2012 Nov;110(10):1426–35. [PMID: 22759317]

RENAL CELL CARCINOMA

ESSENTIALS OF DIAGNOSIS

▶ Gross or microscopic hematuria.

▶ Flank pain or mass in some patients.

▶ Systemic symptoms such as fever, weight loss may be prominent.

▶ Solid renal mass on imaging.

▶ General Considerations

Renal cell carcinoma accounts for 2.6% of all adult cancers. In the United States, approximately 63,920 cases of renal cell carcinoma are diagnosed and 13,860 deaths result annually. Renal cell carcinoma has a peak incidence in the sixth decade of life and a male-to-female ratio of 2:1. It may be associated with a number of paraneoplastic syndromes.

The cause is unknown. Cigarette smoking is the only significant environmental risk factor that has been identified. Familial causes of renal cell carcinoma have been identified (von Hippel–Lindau syndrome, hereditary papillary renal cell carcinoma, hereditary leiomyoma-renal cell carcinoma, Birt-Hogg-Dubé syndrome) and there is an association with dialysis-related acquired cystic disease and specific genetic aberrations (eg, Xp11.2 translocation), but sporadic carcinomas are far more common.

Renal cell carcinoma originates from the proximal tubule cells. Various histologic cell types are recognized (clear cell, papillary, chromophobe, collecting duct and sarcomatoid).

▶ Clinical Findings

A. Symptoms and Signs

Historically, 60% of patients presented with gross or microscopic hematuria. Flank pain or an abdominal mass was detected in approximately 30% of cases. The triad of flank pain, hematuria, and mass was found in only 10–15% of patients, and often a sign of advanced disease. Fever occurs as a paraneoplastic symptom. Symptoms of metastatic disease (cough, bone pain) occur in 20–30% of patients at presentation. Because of the widespread use of ultrasound and CT scanning, renal tumors are frequently detected incidentally in individuals with no urologic symptoms. There has been profound stage migration toward lower stages of disease over the past 10 years, likely due to the increased use of abdominal imaging. However, population mortality rates remain stable.

B. Laboratory Findings

Hematuria is present in 60% of patients. Erythrocytosis from increased erythropoietin production occurs in 5%, though anemia is more common; hypercalcemia may be present in up to 10% of patients. **Stauffer syndrome** is a reversible syndrome of hepatic dysfunction (with elevated liver tests) in the absence of metastatic disease.

C. Imaging

Solid renal masses are often first identified by abdominal ultrasonography or CT. CT and MRI scanning are the most valuable imaging tests for renal cell carcinoma. These scans confirm the character of the mass and further stage the lesion with respect to regional lymph nodes, renal vein, or liver. CT and MRI also provide valuable information regarding the contralateral kidney (function, bilaterality of neoplasm). Chest radiographs exclude pulmonary metastases, and bone scans should be performed for large tumors and in patients with bone pain or elevated serum alkaline phosphatase levels. MRI and duplex Doppler ultrasonography are excellent methods of assessing the presence and extent of tumor thrombus within the renal vein or vena cava.

▶ Differential Diagnosis

Solid lesions of the kidney are renal cell carcinoma until proved otherwise. Other solid masses include renal angiomyolipomas (fat density usually visible by CT), renal pelvis urothelial cancers (more central location, involvement of the collecting system, positive urinary cytology), renal oncocytomas (indistinguishable from renal cell carcinoma preoperatively), renal abscesses, and adrenal tumors (superoanterior to the kidney).

▶ Treatment

Surgical extirpation is the primary treatment for localized renal cell carcinoma. Patients with a single kidney, bilateral lesions, or significant medical renal disease should be considered for partial nephrectomy. Patients with a normal contralateral kidney and good renal function but a small cancer are also candidates for partial nephrectomy, while radical nephrectomy is indicated in patients with cancers larger than 7 cm and those in whom partial nephrectomy is not technically feasible. Radiofrequency and cryosurgical ablation are being studied; they likely yield equivalent short-term oncologic outcomes with reduced morbidity.

No effective chemotherapy is available for metastatic renal cell carcinoma. Vinblastine yields short-term partial response rates of 15%. Bevacizumab can prolong time to progression in patients with metastatic disease (see Table 39–4). With biologic response modifiers, such as interferon-alpha and interleukin-2, partial response rates of 15–20% and 15–35%, respectively, have been reported. Responders tend to have lower tumor burdens, metastatic disease confined to the lung, and a high performance status. Patients with metastatic renal cell carcinoma and good performance status who have resectable primary tumors should undergo cytoreductive nephrectomy. Two randomized trials have shown a survival benefit of surgery followed by the use of systemic therapy—specifically, biologic response modifiers—compared with the use of systemic therapy alone.

Several targeted drugs, specifically VEGF, Raf-kinase, and mTOR inhibitors, are effective (40% response rates) in patients with advanced kidney cancer. These drugs are oral agents, well tolerated, and particularly active for clear cell carcinoma. The appropriate timing and combination of these agents, with and without surgery and cytokine therapy, remains to be determined. To date, no benefit has been observed in the adjuvant use of these agents after complete surgical resection, even in those with adverse pathologic features. Nivolumab is a recently approved immunotherapy for treating metastatic disease that has progressed despite antiangiogenic therapy.

▶ Prognosis

After radical or partial nephrectomy, tumors confined to the renal capsule (T1–T2) demonstrate 5-year disease-free survivals of 90–100%. Tumors extending beyond the renal capsule (T3 or T4) and node-positive tumors have 50–60% and 0–15% 5-year disease-free survival, respectively. One subgroup of patients with nonlocalized disease has reasonable long-term survival, namely, those with solitary resectable metastases. In this setting, radical nephrectomy with resection of the solitary metastasis results in 5-year disease-free survival rates of 15–30%.

▶ When to Refer

- Refer patients with solid renal masses or complex cysts to a urologist for further evaluation.
- Refer patients with renal cell carcinoma to a urologic surgeon for surgical excision.
- Refer patients with metastatic disease to an oncologist and urologist.

Bowlin PR et al. Laparoscopic nephrectomy and partial nephrectomy: intraperitoneal, retroperitoneal, single site. Urol Clin North Am. 2015 Feb;42(1):31–42. [PMID: 25455170]
Cella D et al. Characterizing fatigue associated with sunitinib and its impact on health-related quality of life in patients with metastatic renal cell carcinoma. Cancer. 2014 Jun 15; 120(12):1871–80. [PMID: 24634003]
Escudier B et al. Randomized, controlled, double-blind, crossover trial assessing treatment preference for pazopanib versus sunitinib in patients with metastatic renal cell carcinoma: PISCES Study. J Clin Oncol. 2014 May 10;32(14):1412–8. [PMID: 24687826]
Halabi S et al. Progression-free survival as a surrogate endpoint of overall survival in patients with metastatic renal cell carcinoma. Cancer. 2014 Jan 1;120(1):52–60. [PMID: 24347384]
Jonasch E et al. Renal cell carcinoma. BMJ. 2014 Nov 10; 349:g4797. [PMID: 25385470]
Motzer RJ et al. Axitinib versus sorafenib as second-line treatment for advanced renal cell carcinoma: overall survival analysis and updated results from a randomised phase 3 trial. Lancet Oncol. 2013 May;14(6):552–62. Erratum in: Lancet Oncol. 2013 Jun;14(7):e254. [PMID: 23598172]
Motzer RJ et al; CheckMate 025 Investigators. Nivolumab versus everolimus in advanced renal-cell carcinoma. N Engl J Med. 2015 Nov 5;373(19):1803–13. [PMID: 26406148]
Motzer RJ et al. Pazopanib versus sunitinib in metastatic renal-cell carcinoma. N Engl J Med. 2013 Aug 22;369(8):722–31. [PMID: 23964934]

OTHER PRIMARY TUMORS OF THE KIDNEY

Oncocytomas account for 3–5% of renal tumors, are usually benign, and are indistinguishable from renal cell carcinoma on preoperative imaging. These tumors are seen in other organs, including the adrenals, salivary glands, and thyroid and parathyroid glands.

Angiomyolipomas are rare benign tumors composed of fat, smooth muscle, and blood vessels. They are most commonly seen in patients with tuberous sclerosis (often multiple and bilateral) or in young to middle-aged women. CT scanning may identify the fat component, which is diagnostic for angiomyolipoma. Asymptomatic lesions less than 5 cm in diameter usually do not require intervention; large lesions can spontaneously bleed. Acute bleeding can be treated by angiographic embolization or, in rare cases, nephrectomy. Lesions over 5 cm are often prophylactically treated with angioembolization to reduce the risk of bleeding.

SECONDARY CANCERS OF THE KIDNEY

The kidney is not an infrequent site for metastatic disease. Of the solid tumors, lung cancer is the most common (20%), followed by breast (10%), stomach (10%), and the contralateral kidney (10%). Lymphoma, both Hodgkin and non-Hodgkin, may also involve the kidney, although it tends to appear as a diffusely infiltrative process resulting in renal enlargement rather than a discrete mass.

TESTICULAR CANCERS (Germ Cell Tumors)

ESSENTIALS OF DIAGNOSIS

- ▶ Most common neoplasm in men aged 20–35 years.
- ▶ Patient typically discovers a painless nodule.
- ▶ Orchiectomy necessary for diagnosis.

▶ General Considerations

Malignant tumors of the testis are rare, with approximately five to six cases per 100,000 males reported in the United States each year. Ninety to 95 percent of all primary testicular tumors are germ cell tumors and can be divided into two major categories: **nonseminomas,** including embryonal cell carcinoma (20%), teratoma (5%), choriocarcinoma (less than 1%), and mixed cell types (40%); and **seminomas** (35%). The lifetime probability of developing testicular cancer is 0.3% for an American male.

Approximately 5% of testicular cancers develop in a patient with a history of cryptorchism, with seminoma being the most common. However, 5–10% of these tumors occur in the contralateral, normally descended testis. The relative risk of development of malignancy is higher for the intra-abdominal testis (1:20) and lower for the inguinal testis (1:80). Placement of the cryptorchid testis into the scrotum (orchidopexy) does not alter its malignant potential but does facilitate routine examination and cancer detection.

Testicular cancer is slightly more common on the right than the left, paralleling the increased incidence of cryptorchidism on the right side. One to 2 percent of primary testicular cancers are bilateral and up to 50% of these men have a history of unilateral or bilateral cryptorchidism. Primary bilateral testicular cancers may occur synchronously or asynchronously but tend to be of the same histology. Seminoma is the most common histologic finding in bilateral *primary* testicular cancers, while malignant lymphoma is the most common bilateral testicular tumor overall.

Clinical Findings

A. Symptoms and Signs

The most common symptom of testicular cancer is painless enlargement of the testis. Sensations of heaviness are not unusual. Patients are usually the first to recognize an abnormality, yet typical delay in seeking medical attention ranges from 3 to 6 months. Acute testicular pain resulting from intratesticular hemorrhage occurs in approximately 10% of cases. Ten percent of patients are asymptomatic at presentation, and 10% manifest symptoms relating to metastatic disease such as back pain (retroperitoneal metastases), cough (pulmonary metastases), or lower extremity edema (vena cava obstruction).

A discrete mass or diffuse testicular enlargement is noted in most cases. Secondary hydroceles may be present in 5-10% of cases. In advanced disease, supraclavicular adenopathy may be present, and abdominal examination may reveal a mass. Gynecomastia is seen in 5% of germ cell tumors.

B. Laboratory Findings

Several serum markers are important in the diagnosis and monitoring of testicular carcinoma, including human chorionic gonadotropin (hCG), alpha-fetoprotein, and lactate dehydrogenase. Alpha-fetoprotein is never elevated with pure seminomas, and while hCG is occasionally elevated in seminomas, levels tend to be lower than those seen with nonseminomas. Lactate dehydrogenase may be elevated with either type of tumor. Liver tests may be elevated in the presence of hepatic metastases, and anemia may be present in advanced disease.

C. Imaging

Scrotal ultrasound can readily determine whether a mass is intratesticular or extratesticular. Once the diagnosis of testicular cancer has been established by inguinal orchiectomy, clinical staging of the disease is accomplished by chest, abdominal, and pelvic CT scanning.

Staging

Testicular cancer is staged using the TNM system created based on extent of cancer in the testis, status of regional lymph nodes, the presence of metastases in distant lymph nodes or other viscera, and serum levels of tumor markers. Based on these features, germ cell tumors can be grouped to assign an overall stage: stage I lesion is confined to the testis; stage II demonstrates regional lymph node involvement in the retroperitoneum; and stage III indicates distant metastasis.

Differential Diagnosis

An incorrect diagnosis is made at the initial examination in up to 25% of patients with testicular tumors. Scrotal ultrasonography should be performed if any uncertainty exists with respect to the diagnosis. Although most intratesticular masses are malignant, a benign lesion—epidermoid cyst—may rarely be seen. Epidermoid cysts are usually very small benign nodules located just underneath the tunica albuginea; occasionally, however, they can be large. Testicular lymphoma is discussed below.

Treatment

Inguinal exploration with early vascular control of the spermatic cord structures is the initial intervention. If cancer cannot be excluded by examination of the testis, radical orchiectomy is warranted. Scrotal approaches and open testicular biopsies should be avoided. Further therapy depends on the histology of the tumor as well as the clinical stage.

Up to 75% of clinical stage I **nonseminomas** are cured by orchiectomy alone. Selected patients who meet specific criteria may be offered surveillance after orchiectomy. These criteria are as follows: (1) cancer is confined within the tunica albuginea; (2) cancer does not demonstrate vascular invasion; (3) tumor markers normalize after orchiectomy; (4) radiographic imaging of the chest and abdomen shows no evidence of disease; and (5) the patient is reliable. Patients most likely to experience relapse on a surveillance regimen include those with predominantly embryonal cancer and those with vascular or lymphatic invasion identified in the orchiectomy specimen.

Stage I, IIa, and IIb **seminomas** (retroperitoneal disease less than 2 cm diameter in IIa and 2-5 cm in IIb) are treated by radical orchiectomy and retroperitoneal irradiation. Patients with clinical stage I disease may be candidates for surveillance or single-agent carboplatin. Seminomas of stage IIc (greater than 5 cm diameter retroperitoneal nodes) and stage III receive primary chemotherapy (etoposide and cisplatin or cisplatin, etoposide, and bleomycin) (Table 39-4). Surgical resection of one or more residual retroperitoneal nodes is warranted if the node is greater than 3 cm in diameter and positive on PET scan, since 40% will harbor residual carcinoma.

Postoperative active surveillance by the clinician and patient means patients are followed up every 1-2 months for the first 2 years and quarterly in the third year. Tumor markers are obtained at each visit, and chest radiographs and CT scans are obtained every 3-4 months. Follow-up continues beyond the initial 3 years; however, 80% of relapses will occur within the first 2 years. With rare exceptions, patients who relapse can be cured by chemotherapy or surgery. Alternatives to surveillance for clinical stage I nonseminoma include adjuvant chemotherapy (bleomycin, etoposide, cisplatin) (see Table 39–4) or retroperitoneal lymph node dissection.

Patients with bulky retroperitoneal disease (greater than 5 cm nodes) or metastatic nonseminomas are treated with combination chemotherapy following orchiectomy (cisplatin and etoposide or cisplatin, etoposide, and bleomycin). If tumor markers normalize and a residual mass greater than 1 cm persists on imaging studies, it is resected because 15–20% will harbor residual cancer and 40% will harbor teratomas. Even if patients have a complete response to chemotherapy, some clinicians advocate retroperitoneal lymphadenectomy since 10% of patients may harbor residual carcinoma and 10%, retroperitoneal teratoma. If tumor markers fail to normalize following primary chemotherapy, salvage chemotherapy is required (cisplatin, etoposide, and ifosfamide).

▶ Prognosis

The 5-year disease-free survival rate for patients with stage A **nonseminomas** (includes all treatments) ranges from 96% to 100%. For low-volume stage B disease, 90% 5-year disease-free survival is expected. The 5-year disease-free survival rates for stage I and IIa **seminomas** (retroperitoneal disease less than 2 cm in diameter) treated by radical orchiectomy and retroperitoneal irradiation are 98% and 92–94%, respectively. Ninety-five percent of patients with stage III disease attain a complete response following orchiectomy and chemotherapy. Patients with bulky retroperitoneal or disseminated disease treated with primary chemotherapy followed by surgery have a 5-year disease-free survival rate of 55–80%.

▶ When to Refer

Refer all patients with solid masses of the testis to a urologist.

Ehrlich Y et al. Serum tumor markers in testicular cancer. Urol Oncol. 2013 Jan;31(1):17–23. [PMID: 20822927]

Hanna NH et al. Testicular cancer—discoveries and updates. N Engl J Med. 2014 Nov 20;371(21):2005–16. Erratum in: N Engl J Med. 2014 Dec 11;371(24):2342. [PMID: 25409373]

Nallu A et al. Testicular germ cell tumors: biology and clinical update. Curr Opin Oncol. 2013 May;25(3):266–72. [PMID: 23549473]

Tournaye H et al. Fertility preservation in men with cancer. Lancet. 2014 Oct 4;384(9950):1295–301. [PMID: 25283570]

SECONDARY CANCERS OF THE TESTIS

Secondary cancers of the testis are rare. In men over the age of 50 years, lymphoma is the most common. Overall, it is the most common secondary neoplasm of the testis, accounting for 5% of all testicular cancers. It may be seen in three clinical settings: (1) late manifestation of widespread lymphoma, (2) the initial presentation of clinically occult disease, and (3) primary extranodal disease. Radical orchiectomy is indicated to make the diagnosis. Prognosis is related to the stage of disease.

Metastasis to the testis is rare. The most common primary site of origin is the prostate, followed by the lung, gastrointestinal tract, melanoma, and kidney.

CANCER COMPLICATIONS & EMERGENCIES

SPINAL CORD COMPRESSION

ESSENTIALS OF DIAGNOSIS

▶ Complication of metastatic solid tumor, lymphoma, or multiple myeloma.

▶ Back pain is most common presenting symptom.

▶ Prompt diagnosis is essential because once a severe neurologic deficit develops, it is often irreversible.

▶ Emergent treatment may prevent or potentially reverse paresis and urinary and bowel incontinence.

▶ General Considerations

Cancers that cause spinal cord compression most commonly metastasize to the vertebral bodies, resulting in physical damage to the spinal cord from edema, hemorrhage, and pressure-induced ischemia to the vasculature of the spinal cord. Persistent compression can result in irreversible changes to the myelin sheaths resulting in permanent neurologic impairment.

Prompt diagnosis and therapeutic intervention are essential, since the probability of reversing neurologic symptoms largely depends on the duration of symptoms. Patients who are treated promptly after symptoms appear may have partial or complete return of function and, depending on tumor sensitivity to specific treatment, may respond favorably to subsequent anticancer therapy.

▶ Clinical Findings

A. Symptoms and Signs

Back pain at the level of the tumor mass occurs in over 80% of cases and may be aggravated by lying down, weight bearing, sneezing, or coughing; it usually precedes the development of neurologic symptoms or signs. Since involvement is usually epidural, a mixture of nerve root and spinal cord symptoms often develops. Progressive weakness and sensory changes commonly occur. Bowel and bladder symptoms progressing to incontinence are late findings.

The initial findings of impending cord compression may be quite subtle, and there should be a high index of suspicion when back pain or weakness of the lower extremities develops in cancer patients.

B. Imaging

MRI is usually the initial imaging procedure of choice in a cancer patient with new-onset back pain. If the back pain symptoms are nonspecific, a whole-body PET scan with ^{18}F-2-deoxyglucose may be useful as a screening procedure. Bone radiographs are neither sensitive nor specific for the evaluation of a cancer patient with back pain. When there are neurologic findings suggesting spinal cord compression, an emergent MRI should be obtained; the MRI should include a survey of the entire spine in order to define all areas of tumor involvement for treatment planning purposes.

▶ Treatment

Patients found to have epidural impingement of the spinal cord should be given corticosteroids immediately. The initial dexamethasone dose is 10–100 mg intravenously followed by 4–6 mg every 6 hours intravenously or orally. Patients without a known diagnosis of cancer should have emergent surgery to relieve the impingement and obtain a pathologic specimen. Patients with a single area of compression due to solid tumors are best treated with surgical decompression followed by radiation therapy. Better outcomes (ie, improved ability to ambulate and improved bladder and bowel function) are seen in patients who undergo surgery followed by radiation therapy than in those who receive radiation therapy alone. If multiple vertebral body levels are involved with cancer, fractionated radiation therapy is the preferred treatment option. Corticosteroids are generally tapered toward the end of radiation therapy. A scoring system exists for patients presenting with spinal cord metastases to identify those with poor survival times who would be best managed with supportive care or single fraction palliative radiation.

Kim JM et al. Clinical outcome of metastatic spinal cord compression treated with surgical excision +/– radiation versus radiation therapy alone: a systematic review of literature. Spine. 2012 Jan 1;37(1):78–84. [PMID: 21629164]

Loblaw DA et al. A 2011 updated systematic review and clinical practice guideline for the management of malignant extradural spinal cord compression. Int J Radiat Oncol Biol Phys. 2012 Oct 1;84(2):312–7. [PMID: 22420969]

Rades D et al. A score to identify patients with metastatic spinal cord compression who may be candidates for best supportive care. Cancer. 2013 Feb 15;119(4):897–903. [PMID: 23065671]

MALIGNANT EFFUSIONS

ESSENTIALS OF DIAGNOSIS

▶ Occur in pleural, pericardial, and peritoneal spaces.

▶ Caused by direct neoplastic involvement of serous surface or obstruction of lymphatic drainage.

▶ Half of undiagnosed effusions in patients not known to have cancer are malignant.

▶ General Considerations

The development of an effusion in the pleural, pericardial, or peritoneal space may be the initial finding in a patient with cancer, or an effusion may appear during the course of disease progression. Direct involvement of the serous surface with tumor is the most frequent initiating cause of the accumulation of fluid. The most common malignancies causing pleural and pericardial effusions are lung and breast cancers; the most common malignancies associated with malignant ascites are ovarian, colorectal, stomach, and pancreatic cancers.

▶ Clinical Findings

A. Symptoms and Signs

Patients with pleural and pericardial effusions complain of shortness of breath and orthopnea. Patients with ascites complain of abdominal distention and discomfort. Cardiac tamponade causing pressure equalization in the chambers impairing both filling and cardiac output can be a life-threatening event. Signs of tamponade include tachycardia, muffled heart sounds, pulsus paradoxus, and hypotension. Signs of pleural effusions include decreased breath sounds, egophony, and percussion dullness.

B. Laboratory Findings

Malignancy is confirmed as the cause of an effusion when analysis of the fluid specimen shows malignant cells in either the cytology or cell block specimen.

C. Imaging

The presence of effusions can be confirmed with radiographic studies or ultrasonography.

▶ Differential Diagnosis

The differential diagnosis of a malignant exudative pleural or pericardial effusion includes nonmalignant processes, such as infection, pulmonary embolism, heart failure, and trauma.

The differential diagnosis of malignant ascites includes similar benign processes, such as heart failure, cirrhosis, peritonitis, and pancreatic ascites.

Bloody effusions are usually due to cancer, but a bloody pleural effusion can also be due to pulmonary embolism, trauma and, occasionally, infection. Chylous pleural or ascitic fluid is generally associated with obstruction of lymphatic drainage as might occur in lymphomas.

▶ Treatment

In some cases, treatment of the underlying cancer with chemotherapy can cause regression of the effusions; however, not uncommonly, the presence of an effusion is an end-stage manifestation of the disease. In this situation, decisions regarding management are in large part dictated by the patient's symptoms and goals of care.

A. Pleural Effusion

A pleural effusion that is symptomatic may be managed initially with a **large volume thoracentesis.** With some patients, the effusion slowly reaccumulates, which allows for periodic thoracentesis when the patient becomes symptomatic. However, in many patients, the effusion reaccumulates quickly, causing rapid return of symptoms of shortness of breath. For those patients, two other options exist for management. **Chest tube drainage followed by pleurodesis** involves placement of a chest tube that is connected to closed water seal drainage. After lung expansion is confirmed on a chest radiograph, a sclerosing agent (such as talc slurry or doxycycline) is injected into the catheter. Patients should be premedicated with analgesics and placed in a variety of positions in order to distribute the drug through the pleural spaces. Pleurodesis will not be successful if the lung cannot be reexpanded. These patients are better managed with the second option of **placement of an indwelling catheter** that can be drained by a family member or a visiting nurse. This procedure may also be preferable for patients with short life expectancies or for those who do not respond to pleurodesis. Chest tube drainage followed by pleurodesis or placement of an indwelling catheter have essentially equivalent outcomes in terms of cost, relief of symptoms, and other measures of quality of life.

B. Pericardial Effusion

Fluid may be removed by a needle aspiration or by placement of a catheter for more thorough drainage. As with pleural effusions, most pericardial effusions will reaccumulate. Management options for recurrent, symptomatic effusions include prolonged catheter drainage for several days until drainage has decreased to 20–30 mL/day or pericardiectomy.

C. Malignant Ascites

Patients with malignant ascites not responsive to chemotherapy are generally treated with repeated large volume paracenteses. As the frequency of drainage to maintain comfort can compromise the patient's quality of life, other alternatives include placement of a catheter or port so that the patient, family member, or visiting nurse can drain fluid as needed at home.

Fysh ET et al. Predictors of clinical use of pleurodesis and/or indwelling pleural catheter therapy for malignant pleural effusion. Chest. 2015 Jun;147(6):1629–34. [PMID: 25474713]

Kastelik JA. Management of malignant pleural effusion. Lung. 2013 Apr;191(2):165–75. [PMID: 23315213]

Myers R et al. Tunneled pleural catheters: an update for 2013. Clin Chest Med. 2013 Mar;34(1):73–80. [PMID: 23411058]

Rahman NM et al. Effect of opioids vs NSAIDs and larger vs smaller chest tube size on pain control and pleurodesis efficacy among patients with malignant pleural effusion: the TIME1 randomized clinical trial. JAMA. 2015 Dec 22–29; 314(24):2641–53. [PMID: 26720026]

Saguil A et al. Diagnostic approach to pleural effusion. Am Fam Physician. 2014 Jul 15;90(2):99–104. [PMID: 25077579]

West HJ. JAMA Oncology Patient Page. Malignant pleural effusions. JAMA Oncol. 2015 May;1(2):260. [PMID: 26181036]

HYPERCALCEMIA

ESSENTIALS OF DIAGNOSIS

▸ Usually symptomatic and severe (15 mg/dL [3.75 mmol/L] or more).

▸ Most common paraneoplastic endocrine syndrome; accounts for most inpatients with hypercalcemia.

▸ The neoplasm is clinically apparent in nearly all cases when hypercalcemia is detected.

▸ General Considerations

Hypercalcemia affects 20–30% of cancer patients at some point during their illness. The most common cancers causing hypercalcemia are myeloma, breast carcinoma, and NSCLC. Hypercalcemia is caused by one of three mechanisms: systemic effects of tumor-released proteins, direct osteolysis of bone by tumor, or vitamin D–mediated osteoabsorption.

▸ Clinical Findings

A. Symptoms and Signs

Symptoms and signs of hypercalcemia can be subtle; more severe symptoms occur with higher levels of hypercalcemia and with a rapid rate at which the calcium level rises. Early symptoms typically include anorexia, nausea, fatigue, constipation, and polyuria; later findings may include muscular weakness and hyporeflexia, confusion, psychosis, tremor, and lethargy.

B. Laboratory Findings

Symptoms and signs are caused by free calcium; as calcium is bound by protein in the serum, the measured serum calcium will underestimate the free or ionized calcium in patients with low albumin levels. In the setting of hypoalbuminemia, the corrected serum calcium should be calculated by one of several available formulas (eg, corrected calcium = measured calcium – measured albumin + 4). Alternatively, the free ionized calcium can be measured. When the corrected serum calcium rises above 12 mg/dL (3 mmol/L), sudden death due to cardiac arrhythmia or asystole may occur. The presence of hypercalcemia does not invariably indicate a dismal prognosis, especially in patients with breast cancer, myeloma, or lymphoma.

In the absence of symptoms or signs of hypercalcemia, a laboratory finding of elevated serum calcium should be retested immediately to exclude the possibility of error.

C. ECG

Electrocardiography in hypercalcemia often shows a shortening of the QT interval.

Treatment

Emergency management should begin with the initiation of intravenous fluids with 0.9% saline at 100–300 mL/h to ensure rehydration with brisk urinary output of the often volume-depleted patient. If kidney function is normal or only marginally impaired, a bisphosphonate should be given. Choices include pamidronate, 60–90 mg intravenously over 2–4 hours, or zoledronic acid, 4 mg intravenously over 15 minutes. Zoledronic acid is more potent than pamidronate and has the advantage of a shorter administration time as well as a longer duration of effect, but with repeated dosing, it is more often associated with the very uncommon but serious side effect of osteonecrosis of the jaw. Once hypercalcemia is controlled, treatment directed at the cancer should be initiated if possible. Commonly, though, hypercalcemia occurs in patients with cancers that are unresponsive to treatment. In the event that the hypercalcemia becomes refractory to repeated doses of bisphosphonates, other agents that can help control hypercalcemia (at least temporarily) include calcitonin, denosumab, and gallium nitrate; corticosteroids can be useful in patients with myeloma and lymphoma. Salmon calcitonin, 4–8 international units/kg given subcutaneously or intramuscularly every 12 hours, can be used in patients with severe, symptomatic hypercalcemia; its onset of action is within hours but its hypocalcemic effect wanes in 2–3 days. Denosumab, 120 mg given subcutaneously weekly for 4 weeks followed by monthly administration, is a choice for long-term management of bisphosphonate-refractory hypercalcemia.

Ahmad S et al. Hypercalcemic crisis: a clinical review. Am J Med. 2015 Mar;128(3):239–45. [PMID: 25447624]

HYPERURICEMIA & TUMOR LYSIS SYNDROME

ESSENTIALS OF DIAGNOSIS

- ▶ Complication of treatment-associated tumor lysis of hematologic and rapidly proliferating malignancies.
- ▶ May be worsened by thiazide diuretics.
- ▶ Rapid increase in serum uric acid can cause acute urate nephropathy from uric acid crystallization.
- ▶ Reducing pre-chemotherapy serum uric acid is fundamental to preventing urate nephropathy.

General Considerations

Tumor lysis syndrome (TLS) is seen most commonly following treatment of hematologic malignancies, such as acute lymphoblastic leukemia and Burkitt lymphoma. However, TLS can develop from any tumor highly sensitive to chemotherapy. TLS is caused by the massive release of cellular material including nucleic acids, proteins, phosphorus, and potassium. If both the metabolism and excretion of these breakdown products are impaired, hyperuricemia, hyperphosphatemia, and hyperkalemia will develop abruptly. Acute kidney injury may then develop from the crystallization and deposition of uric acid and calcium phosphate within the renal tubules further exacerbating the hyperphosphatemia and hyperkalemia.

Clinical Findings

Symptoms of hyperphosphatemia include nausea and vomiting as well as seizures. Also, with high levels of phosphorus, co-precipitation with calcium can cause renal tubule blockage, further exacerbating the kidney injury. Hyperkalemia, due to release of intracellular potassium and impaired kidney excretion, can cause arrhythmias and sudden death.

Treatment

Prevention is the most important factor in the management of TLS. Published guidelines for TLS management include aggressive hydration prior to initiation of chemotherapy as well as during and after completion of the chemotherapy. Administration of fluid helps keep urine flowing and facilitates excretion of uric acid and phosphorus. For the patients with moderate risk of developing TLS, for instance, those with intermediate grade lymphomas and acute leukemias, allopurinol should be given before starting chemotherapy at an oral dose of 100 mg/m² every 8 hours (maximum 800 mg/day) with dose reductions for impaired kidney function. For patients at high risk for developing TLS, for instance, patients with high-grade lymphomas or patients with acute leukemias and markedly elevated white blood cell counts (with acute myeloid leukemia, white blood cell count greater than 50,000/mcL [50,000/10⁹/L]; with acute lymphoblastic leukemia, white blood cell count greater than 100,000/mcL [100,000/10⁹/L]) or in whom hyperuricemia develops despite treatment with allopurinol, rasburicase 0.1–0.2 mg/kg/day is given intravenously for 1–7 days. Rasburicase cannot be given to patients with known glucose 6-phosphate dehydrogenase (G6PD) deficiency nor can it be given to pregnant or lactating women. One of the historic mainstays of TLS management, systemic bicarbonate infusions to alkalinize the urine, is no longer routinely recommended. Laboratory values should be monitored following initiation of chemotherapy in addition to the hyperuricemia; elevated potassium or phosphorus levels need to be promptly managed.

When to Refer

Should urinary output drop, creatinine or potassium levels rise, or hyperphosphatemia persist, a nephrologist should be immediately consulted to evaluate the need for dialysis.

Firwana BM et al. Tumor lysis syndrome: a systematic review of case series and case reports. Postgrad Med. 2012 Mar; 124(2):92–101. [PMID: 22437219]

Wilson FP et al. Onco-nephrology: tumor lysis syndrome. Clin J Am Soc Nephrol. 2012 Oct;7(10):1730–9. [PMID: 22879434]

Wilson FP et al. Tumor lysis syndrome: new challenges and recent advances. Adv Chronic Kidney Dis. 2014 Jan;21(1): 18–26. [PMID: 24359983]

INFECTIONS

Chapters 30 and 31 provide more detailed discussions of infections in the immunocompromised patient.

ESSENTIALS OF DIAGNOSIS

▶ In patients with neutropenia, infection is a medical emergency.

▶ Although sometimes attributable to other causes, the presence of fever, defined as a single temperature greater than 38.3°C (101°F) or a temperature of greater than 38°C (100.4°F) for longer than 1 hour, must be assumed to be due to an infection.

▶ General Considerations

Many patients with disseminated neoplasms have increased susceptibility to infection. In some patients, this results from impaired defense mechanisms (eg, acute leukemia, Hodgkin lymphoma, multiple myeloma, chronic lymphocytic leukemia); in others, it results from the myelosuppressive and immunosuppressive effects of cancer chemotherapy or a combination of these factors. Complicating impaired defense mechanisms are the frequent presence of indwelling catheters, impaired mucosal surfaces, and colonization with more virulent hospital-acquired pathogens.

The source of a neutropenic febrile episode is determined in about 30% of cases through blood, urine, or sputum cultures. The bacterial organisms accounting for the majority of infections in cancer patients include gram-negative bacteria (*Escherichia coli*, *Klebsiella*, *Pseudomonas*, *Enterobacter*) and gram-positive bacteria (coagulase-negative *Staphylococcus*, *Staphylococcus aureus*, *Streptococcus pneumoniae*, *Corynebacterium*, and streptococci). There has been a trend over the last few decades of an increasing percentage of gram-positive organisms. The risk of bacterial infections rises when the neutrophil count is below 1000/mcL (1.0×10^9/L); the risk dramatically increases when the count falls below 100/mcL (0.1×10^9/L).

▶ Clinical Findings

A thorough physical examination should be performed. Routine DREs are generally avoided unless symptoms suggest a rectal abscess or prostatitis. If a DRE is necessary, antibiotics should be administered first. Appropriate cultures (eg, blood, sputum, urine and, if indicated, cerebrospinal fluid) should always be obtained. Two sets of blood cultures should be drawn before starting antibiotics; if the patient has an indwelling catheter, one of the cultures should be drawn from the line. A chest radiograph should also be obtained.

▶ Treatment

Empiric antibiotic therapy needs to be initiated immediately following the collection of blood cultures in the febrile, neutropenic patient. The choice of antibiotics depends on a number of different factors including the patient's clinical status and any localizing source of infection. If the patient is clinically well, monotherapy with an intravenous beta-lactam with anti-*Pseudomonas* activity (cefepime, ceftazidime, imipenem/cilastatin, piperacillin/tazobactam) should be started (see Infections in the Immunocompromised Patient, Chapter 30). If the patient is clinically ill with hypotension or hypoxia, an aminoglycoside or fluoroquinolone should be added for "double" gram-negative bacteria coverage. If there is a strong suspicion of a gram-positive organism, such as from *S aureus* catheter infection, vancomycin can be given empirically. In some instances, patients may be treated with oral antibiotics and potentially in the outpatient setting. The Infectious Diseases Society of America (IDSA) has published recommendations for antibiotic use in these low-risk patients. These patients must have an expected neutropenic timeframe of 7 days or less and not have comorbidities or signs of hemodynamic instability, gastrointestinal symptoms, altered mental status, pulmonary problems (infiltrate, hypoxia, or underlying chronic obstructive pulmonary disease), or liver or kidney disease or impairment. A validated risk index, such as the Multinational Association for Supportive Care in Cancer (MASCC) score, may be used to assess a patient for appropriateness of outpatient management. If a patient is to be treated as an outpatient, he or she must also have good support at home and easy access to returning to the hospital if the clinical status worsens.

Antibiotics should be continued until the neutrophil count is rising and greater than 500/mcL (0.5×10^9/L) for at least 1 day and the patient has been afebrile for 2 days. If an organism is identified through the cultures, the antibiotics should be adjusted to the antibiotic sensitivities of the isolate; treatment should be continued for the appropriate period of time and at least until the neutrophil count recovers.

For the neutropenic patient who is persistently febrile despite broad-spectrum antibiotics, an empiric antifungal drug should be added (amphotericin B, caspofungin, itraconazole, voriconazole, or liposomal amphotericin B).

Bow EJ. Infection in neutropenic patients with cancer. Crit Care Clin. 2013 Jul;29(3):411–41. [PMID: 23830647]

Flowers CR et al. Antimicrobial prophylaxis and outpatient management of fever and neutropenia in adults treated for malignancy: American Society of Clinical Oncology clinical practice guideline. J Clin Oncol. 2013 Feb 20;31(6):794–810. [PMID: 23319691]

Rolston KV. Neutropenic fever and sepsis: evaluation and management. Cancer Treat Res. 2014;161:181–202. [PMID: 24706225]

White L et al. Neutropenic fever. Emerg Med Clin North Am. 2014 Aug;32(3):549–61. [PMID: 25060249]

▼ PRIMARY CANCER TREATMENT

SYSTEMIC CANCER THERAPY

Detailed guidelines from the NCCN for cancer treatment can be found at www.nccn.org.

Use of cytotoxic drugs, hormones, antihormones, and biologic agents has become a highly specialized and increasingly effective means of treating cancer, with therapy administered and monitored by a medical oncologist or hematologist. Selection of specific drugs or protocols for various types of cancer is usually based on results of clinical trials. Increasingly, newer agents are being identified that target specific molecular pathways. Yet both initial and acquired drug resistance remains a challenge. Described mechanisms of drug resistance include impaired membrane transport of drugs, enhanced drug metabolism, mutated target proteins, and blockage of apoptosis due to mutations in cellular proteins.

TOXICITY & DOSE MODIFICATION OF CHEMOTHERAPEUTIC AGENTS

Use of chemotherapy to treat cancer is generally guided by results from clinical trials in individual tumor types. The complexity of treating cancer has increased over the last decade as more drugs, including those with novel mechanisms of action, have been approved by the Food and Drug Administration and introduced into general practice. Drug side effects and toxicities must be anticipated and carefully monitored. The short- and long-term toxicities of individual drugs are listed in Tables 39–11 and 39–12. Decisions on dose modifications for toxicities should be guided by the intent of therapy. In the palliative setting where the aim of therapy is to improve symptoms and quality of life, lowering doses to minimize toxicity is commonly done. However, when the goal of treatment is cure, dosing frequency and intensity should be maintained whenever possible.

A CBC including a differential count, with absolute neutrophil count and platelet count, and liver and kidney tests should be obtained before the initiation of chemotherapy. In patients with normal CBCs as well as normal liver and kidney function, drugs are started at their full dose. When the intent of chemotherapy is cure, including treatment in the adjuvant setting, every attempt should be made to schedule chemotherapy on time and at full dose. A CBC with differential may be checked at mid cycle (to determine the nadir of the absolute neutrophil and platelet counts), and liver and kidney function tests should be obtained immediately before the next cycle of chemotherapy.

Dose reductions may be necessary for patients with impaired kidney or liver function depending on the clearance mechanism of the drug. For patients receiving chemotherapy for palliation, bone marrow toxicity can be managed with dose reductions or delaying the next treatment cycle. A schema for dose modification is shown in Table 39–13.

1. Bone Marrow Toxicity

A. Neutropenia

Granulocyte colony-stimulating factor (G-CSF), given as either daily subcutaneous injections (filgrastim, 300 mcg or 480 mcg) or as a one-time dose (pegfilgrastim, 6 mg) beginning 24 hours after cytotoxic chemotherapy is completed, has been shown to reduce the duration and severity of granulocytopenia following cytotoxic chemotherapy (Table 39–12). The American Society of Clinical Oncology and NCCN guidelines recommend primary prophylaxis with a G-CSF when there is at least a 20% risk of febrile neutropenia or when the patient's age, medical history, and disease characteristics put the patient at high risk for complications related to myelosuppression.

B. Anemia

Erythropoiesis-stimulating agents (ESAs) ameliorate the anemia and its associated symptoms that are caused by cancer chemotherapy but these drugs have untoward effects, including an increased risk of thromboembolism, and even more concerning, potentially decreased survival due to cancer-related deaths as well as a shortened time to tumor progression. These findings have prompted the US Food and Drug Administration and other organizations (American Society of Hematology, American Society of Clinical Oncology, and NCCN) to issue advisories and guidelines limiting their use. The NCCN recommends that these drugs should not be used when the intent of chemotherapy is curative. Studies done in patients with potentially curable head and neck, breast, and cervical cancers have shown inferior outcomes when ESAs were used. However, the target hemoglobin used in these studies was higher than is currently recommended. Nonetheless, ESAs cannot be currently recommended when the intent of therapy is cure. The alternative to managing symptomatic anemia in these patients receiving curative chemotherapy is administration of red blood cell transfusions.

ESAs can be an option in cancer patients with symptomatic anemia undergoing palliative treatment; patient preference is important in determining when to use ESAs or transfusions. When using ESAs, treatment should not be initiated until the hemoglobin is less than 10 g/dL (100 g/L) with the medication held when the hemoglobin is greater than 12 g/dL (120 g/L). Epoetin alfa can be given subcutaneously at a dose of 40,000 units weekly or 150 units/kg three times weekly with a target hemoglobin of 11–12 g/dL (110–120 g/L). Darbepoetin alfa is given subcutaneously at a dose of 500 mcg every 3 weeks or 2.25 mcg weekly with the same target hemoglobin (see Table 39–12). Patients need to be iron replete to have maximum therapeutic effect. Uncontrolled hypertension is a contraindication to the use of ESAs; blood pressure must be controlled prior to initiation of this therapy. The FDA mandates that prescribing clinicians receive specific education on use of ESAs, and patients receiving ESAs must be provided written material describing the risks and benefits of the drug and sign an acknowledgment form that they talked with their provider about the risks of ESAs.

C. Thrombocytopenia

Drug management of chemotherapy-induced thrombocytopenia is more limited. The only available drug, oprelvekin or recombinant interleukin-11, has modest activity in improving thrombocytopenia associated with chemotherapy; however, it is rarely used due to the side effects of fluid

Table 39–11. Common chemotherapeutic agents.[1]

Chemotherapeutic Agent	Usual Adult Dosage	Adverse Effects
Alkylating Agents—Nitrogen Mustards		
Bendamustine (Treanda)	100–120 mg/m² intravenously every 3–4 weeks	Acute: hypersensitivity, nausea, vomiting Delayed: myelosuppression, rash, pyrexia, fatigue
Cyclophosphamide (Cytoxan)	500–1000 mg/m² intravenously every 3 weeks; 100 mg/m²/day orally for 14 days every 4 weeks; various doses	Acute: nausea and vomiting Delayed: myelosuppression, alopecia, hemorrhagic cystitis, cardiotoxicity (high dose)
Ifosfamide (Ifex)	1200 mg/m² intravenously daily for 5 days every 3 weeks; various doses	Acute: nausea and vomiting Delayed: alopecia, myelosuppression, hemorrhagic cystitis, neurotoxicity
Mechlorethamine (Mustargen)	0.4 mg/kg intravenously every 3–6 weeks	Acute: nausea and vomiting Delayed: myelosuppression
Melphalan (Alkeran)	0.25 mg/kg/day or 8–10 mg/m²/day orally for 4 days every 4–6 weeks; 16 mg/m² intravenously every 2–4 weeks; various doses	Acute: nausea, vomiting, diarrhea, hypersensitivity (intravenously) Delayed: mucositis (intravenously), myelosuppression, increased risk of secondary malignancies
Alkylating Agents—Platinum Analogs		
Carboplatin (Paraplatin)	Area under the curve (AUC)-based dosing use Calvert equation [Dose (mg) = AUC × (GFR + 25)] AUC = 2–7 mg/mL/min every 2–4 weeks	Acute: nausea and vomiting Delayed: myelosuppression, electrolyte disturbances, peripheral neuropathy, nephrotoxicity, hypersensitivity
Cisplatin (Platinol)	50–100 mg/m² intravenously every 3–4 weeks; 20 mg/m²/day intravenously for 5 days every 3 weeks; various doses	Acute: nausea and vomiting Delayed: nephrotoxicity, ototoxicity, neurotoxicity, myelosuppression, electrolyte disturbances
Oxaliplatin (Eloxatin)	85–130 mg/m² intravenously every 2–3 weeks	Acute: peripheral neuropathy exacerbated by cold, nausea, vomiting, diarrhea Delayed: myelosuppression, elevated transaminases
Alkylating Agents—Triazenes		
Dacarbazine (DTIC-Dome)	375 mg/m² intravenously on day 1 and 15 every 4 weeks; 900–1000 mg/m² intravenously over 3 to 4 days; various doses	Acute: nausea, vomiting, photosensitivity Delayed: myelosuppression, anorexia, hypotension, flu-like syndrome
Procarbazine (Matulane)	60–100 mg/m² orally for 14 days every 4 weeks; various doses	Acute: nausea and vomiting Delayed: myelosuppression, disulfiram-like reaction, MAO inhibition, rash
Temozolomide (Temodar)	75 mg/m² orally daily during radiation for 42 days; 150–200 mg/m² orally for 5 days every 4 weeks	Acute: nausea, vomiting, constipation Delayed: myelosuppression, fatigue
Alkylating Agents—Miscellaneous		
Busulfan (Myleran)	1–8 mg orally daily; 0.8 mg/kg intravenously every 6 hours for 4 days	Acute: nausea and vomiting Delayed: myelosuppression, mucositis, rash, edema, electrolyte disturbances, hepatic veno-occlusive disease (high dose)
Chlorambucil (Leukeran)	0.1–0.2 mg/kg/day orally for 3–6 weeks; 0.4 mg/kg pulse every 4 weeks	Acute: nausea Delayed: myelosuppression, rash
Antimetabolites—Folate Antagonists		
Methotrexate (MTX; Trexall)	**Intrathecal:** 12 mg **High dose:** 1000–12,000 mg/m² intravenously every 2–3 weeks	Acute: nausea, vomiting, mucositis Delayed: myelosuppression, nephrotoxicity, hepatotoxicity, neurotoxicity, photosensitivity, pulmonary toxicity
Pemetrexed (Alimta)	500 mg/m² intravenously every 3 weeks	Acute: nausea, vomiting, diarrhea, rash Delayed: myelosuppression, fatigue, mucositis
Antimetabolites—Purine Analogs		
Cladribine (Leustatin)	0.1 mg/kg/day subcutaneously daily for 5 days or 0.09 mg/kg/day intravenously via continuous infusion for 7 days	Acute: nausea, injection site reaction Delayed: myelosuppression, immunosuppression, fever, fatigue, rash

Table 39–11. Common chemotherapeutic agents.[1] (continued)

Chemotherapeutic Agent	Usual Adult Dosage	Adverse Effects
Clofarabine (Clolar)	52 mg/m^2 intravenously daily for 5 days every 2–6 weeks (for patients < 21 years of age)	Acute: nausea, vomiting, diarrhea Delayed: myelosuppression, hepatotoxicity, nephrotoxicity, rash, capillary leak syndrome
Fludarabine (Fludara)	25 mg/m^2 intravenously for 5 days every 4 weeks	Acute: fever, nausea, vomiting Delayed: asthenia, myelosuppression, immunosuppression, neurotoxicity, anorexia
Mercaptopurine (6-MP; Purinethol)	**Induction:** 2.5–5 mg/kg/day orally **Maintenance:** 1.5–2.5 mg/kg/day orally	Acute: nausea, vomiting, diarrhea, rash Delayed: myelosuppression, immunosuppression, hepatotoxicity, mucositis
Pentostatin (Nipent)	2–4 mg/m^2 intravenously every 2–3 weeks	Acute: nausea, vomiting, rash Delayed: myelosuppression, fever, myalgia, immunosuppression, hepatotoxicity, cough
Antimetabolites—Pyrimidine Analogs		
Azacitidine (Vidaza)	75–100 mg/m^2 subcutaneously or intravenously for 7 days every 4 weeks	Acute: injection site reaction (subcutaneously), nausea, diarrhea, fever Delayed: myelosuppression, dyspnea, arthralgia
Capecitabine (Xeloda)	1000–1250 mg/m^2 orally twice a day for 14 days every 3 weeks	Acute: nausea, vomiting, diarrhea Delayed: hand-foot syndrome, mucositis, hyperbilirubinemia, myelosuppression
Cytarabine (Ara-C, Cytosar U)	**Standard dose:** 100 mg/m^2/day intravenously via continuous infusion for 7 days **High dose:** 1000–3000 mg/m^2 intravenously every 12 hours for 2–6 days	Acute: nausea, vomiting, rash, flu-like syndrome Delayed: myelosuppression **High-dose:** neurotoxicity, ocular toxicities
Decitabine (Dacogen)	15 mg/m^2 intravenously every 8 hours for 3 days every 8 weeks; 20 mg m^2 intravenously daily for 5 days	Acute: nausea, vomiting, hyperglycemia Delayed: myelosuppression, fever, fatigue, cough
Fluorouracil (Adrucil)	400 mg/m^2 intravenous bolus followed by 2400 mg/m^2 intravenously over 46 hours every 2 weeks; 1000 mg/m^2 intravenously via continuous infusion for 4–5 days every 3–4 weeks; various doses	Acute: nausea, vomiting, diarrhea Delayed: myelosuppression, hand-foot syndrome, mucositis, photosensitivity, cardiotoxicity (rare)
Gemcitabine (Gemzar)	1000–1250 mg/m^2 intravenously on days 1 and 8 every 3 weeks or days 1, 8, 15 every 4 weeks	Acute: nausea, vomiting, rash, flu-like symptoms, fever, diarrhea Delayed: myelosuppression, edema, elevated transaminases
Antimicrotubules—Vinca Alkaloids		
Vinblastine (Velban)	6 mg/m^2 intravenously on days 1 and 15 every 4 weeks; various doses	Acute: constipation Delayed: myelosuppression, alopecia, bone pain, malaise
Vincristine (Oncovin)	0.5–1.4 mg/m^2 intravenously every 3 weeks; various doses; maximum single dose usually limited to 2 mg	Acute: constipation, nausea Delayed: peripheral neuropathy, alopecia
Liposomal Vincristine (Marqibo)	2.25 mg/m^2 intravenously every 7 days	Acute: constipation, nausea Delayed: fatigue, neurotoxicity, myelosuppression
Vinorelbine (Navelbine)	25–30 mg/m^2 intravenously weekly	Acute: nausea, vomiting Delayed: myelosuppression, peripheral neuropathy, constipation, alopecia, asthenia
Antimicrotubules—Taxanes		
Cabazitaxel (Jevtana)	25 mg/m^2 intravenously every 3 weeks	Acute: diarrhea, nausea, vomiting, hypersensitivity Delayed: myelosuppression, peripheral neuropathy, fatigue
Docetaxel (Taxotere)	60–100 mg/m^2 intravenously every 3 weeks	Acute: nausea, vomiting, diarrhea, hypersensitivity, rash Delayed: myelosuppression, asthenia, peripheral neuropathy, alopecia, edema, mucositis
Paclitaxel (Taxol)	135–175 mg/m^2 intravenously every 3 weeks; 50–80 mg/m^2 intravenously weekly; various doses	Acute: diarrhea, nausea, vomiting, hypersensitivity Delayed: myelosuppression, peripheral neuropathy, alopecia, mucositis, arthralgia

(continued)

Table 39–11. Common chemotherapeutic agents.[1] (continued)

Chemotherapeutic Agent	Usual Adult Dosage	Adverse Effects
Paclitaxel protein-bound (Abraxane)	100–125 mg/m^2 on days 1, 8, 15 every 3–4 weeks; 260 mg/m^2 intravenously every 3 weeks	Acute: nausea, vomiting, diarrhea Delayed: myelosuppression, peripheral neuropathy, alopecia, asthenia
Antimicrotubules—Epothilone		
Ixabepilone (Ixempra)	40 mg/m^2 intravenously every 3 weeks	Acute: nausea, vomiting, diarrhea, hypersensitivity Delayed: peripheral neuropathy, fatigue, alopecia, myelosuppression, mucositis, arthralgia
Enzyme Inhibitors—Anthracyclines		
Daunorubicin (Cerubidine)	30–60 mg/m^2 intravenously for 3 days	Acute: nausea, vomiting, diarrhea, red/orange discoloration of urine, infusion-related reactions (liposomal products) Delayed: myelosuppression, mucositis, alopecia, hand-foot syndrome (liposomal doxorubicin), cardiotoxicity (dose related)
Liposomal Daunorubicin (Daunoxome)	40 mg/m^2 intravenously every 2 weeks	
Doxorubicin (Adriamycin)	45–75 mg/m^2 intravenously every 3 weeks; various doses	
Liposomal Doxorubicin (Lipodox)	20–50 mg/m^2 intravenously every 3–4 weeks	
Epirubicin (Ellence)	60–120 mg/m^2 intravenously every 3–4 weeks	
Idarubicin (Idamycin)	10–12 mg/m^2 intravenously for 3 days	
Enzyme Inhibitors—Topoisomerase Inhibitors		
Etoposide (Vepesid)	50–100 mg/m^2 intravenously for 3–5 days every 3 weeks	Acute: nausea, vomiting, diarrhea, hypersensitivity, fever, hypotension Delayed: myelosuppression, alopecia, fatigue
Etoposide phosphate (Etopophos)	35–100 mg/m^2 intravenously for 3–5 days every 3–4 weeks	
Irinotecan (Camptosar)	180 mg/m^2 intravenously every other week; various doses	Acute: diarrhea, cholinergic syndrome, nausea, vomiting Delayed: myelosuppression, alopecia, asthenia
Irinotecan liposome (Onivyde)	70 mg/m^2 intravenously over 90 minutes every 2 weeks; prior to leucovorin and fluorouracil	Acute: diarrhea, nausea, vomiting Delayed: myelosuppression, fatigue, decrease in appetite
Topotecan (Hycamtin)	1.5 mg/m^2 intravenously for 5 days every 3 weeks; 2.3 mg/m^2 orally for 5 days every 3 weeks	Acute: nausea, vomiting, diarrhea Delayed: myelosuppression, alopecia, asthenia
Immunomodulatory Therapy		
Lenalidomide (Revlimid)	5–25 mg orally once daily on days 1–21 of 28-day cycle; or continuously	Acute: diarrhea, rash Delayed: myelosuppression, fatigue, venous thromboembolism, potential for birth defects
Pomalidomide (Pomalyst)	4 mg orally once daily on days 1–21 of 28-day cycle	Acute: nausea, diarrhea, dizziness Delayed: myelosuppression, fatigue, neuropathy, upper respiratory tract infections, venous thromboembolism, potential for birth defects
Thalidomide (Thalomid)	50–800 mg orally once daily	Acute: sedation, constipation, rash Delayed: edema, peripheral neuropathy, venous thromboembolism, potential for birth defects
Proteasome Inhibitor		
Bortezomib (Velcade)	1.3 mg/m^2 intravenous bolus or subcutaneously on days 1, 4, 8, 11 followed by a 10-day rest, or weekly for 4 weeks followed by 13-day rest	Acute: nausea, vomiting, diarrhea Delayed: peripheral neuropathy, fatigue, myelosuppression
Carfilzomib (Kyprolis)	20 mg/m^2 or 27 mg/m^2 intravenously on days 1, 2, 8, 9, 15, 16 followed by a 12-day rest (28-day cycle)	Acute: nausea, dyspnea, diarrhea, infusion-related reaction Delayed: fatigue, myelosuppression, elevated serum creatinine

(continued)

Table 39–11. Common chemotherapeutic agents.[1] (continued)

Chemotherapeutic Agent	Usual Adult Dosage	Adverse Effects
Ixazomib (Ninlaro)	4 mg orally on days 1, 8, 15 of a 28-day treatment cycle	Acute: diarrhea, constipation, nausea, vomiting Delayed: myelosuppression, peripheral neuropathy, peripheral edema, rash, hepatotoxicity (rare)
Targeted Therapy—Monoclonal Antibodies		
Ado-trastuzumab emtansine (Kadcyla)	3.6 mg/kg intravenously every 3 weeks	Acute: infusion-related reaction, nausea Delayed: fatigue, musculoskeletal pain, thrombocytopenia, cardiotoxicity, heptatotoxicity
Alemtuzumab (Campath)	3–10 mg intravenously or subcutaneously three times weekly	Acute: infusion-related reaction, nausea, vomiting, hypotension, rash Delayed: myelosuppression, immunosuppression
Bevacizumab (Avastin)	5–15 mg/kg intravenously every 2–3 weeks	Acute: infusion-related reaction Delayed: hypertension, proteinuria, wound healing complications, gastrointestinal perforation, hemorrhage
Blinatumomab (Blincyto)	9 mcg/day intravenously via continuous infusion on days 1 through 7; 28 mcg/day on days 8 through 28 of the first 42-day cycle; subsequent cycles: 28 mcg/day for 4 weeks followed by at least 2 weeks of no treatment	Acute: infusion-related reaction, nausea, headache, cytokine release syndrome, tumor lysis syndrome Delayed: pyrexia, peripheral edema, myelosuppression, hypokalemia, rash, neurologic toxicity, constipation
Brentuximab vedotin (Adcetris)	1.8 mg/kg intravenously every 3 weeks	Acute: infusion-related reaction, nausea, vomiting, diarrhea Delayed: myelosuppression, peripheral neuropathy, fatigue, rash, cough
Cetuximab (Erbitux)	Loading dose 400 mg/m² intravenously, maintenance dose 250 mg/m² intravenously weekly	Acute: infusion-related reaction, nausea, diarrhea Delayed: acneiform skin rash, hypomagnesemia, asthenia, paronychial inflammation, dyspnea
Elotuzumab (Empliciti)	10 mg/kg intravenously every week for the first 2 cycles and every 2 weeks thereafter	Acute: infusion-related reaction, diarrhea Delayed: fatigue, peripheral neuropathy, risk for opportunistic infections
Daratumumab (Darzalex)	16 mg/kg intravenously weekly for weeks 1–8, every 2 weeks for weeks 9–24, and every 4 weeks from week 25 until disease progression	Acute: infusion-related reaction, nausea Delayed: myelosuppression, fatigue, upper respiratory tract infection
Ipilimumab (Yervoy)	3 mg/kg intravenously every 3 weeks for a total of four doses	Acute: infusion-related reaction Delayed: immune-related reactions, fatigue
Necitumumab (Portrazza)	800 mg intravenously over 60 mins prior to gemcitabine and cisplatin on days 1 and 8 of 21-day cycle	Acute: infusion-related reaction, vomiting, diarrhea Delayed: electrolyte abnormalities (especially hypomagnesemia), rash, cardiopulmonary arrest (rare)
Nivolumab (Opdivo)	3 mg/kg intravenously over 1 hour every 2 weeks	Acute: vomiting Delayed: fatigue, musculoskeletal pain, rash, pruritus, cough, elevated transaminases
Obinutuzumab (Gazyva)	Cycle 1: 100 mg intravenously on day 1, 900 mg on day 2, 1000 mg on day 8 and 15 of a 28-day cycle; Cycles 2–6: 1000 mg intravenously on day 1	Acute: infusion-related reaction, tumor lysis syndrome Delayed: myelosuppression, pyrexia, cough, musculoskeletal disorder, potential hepatitis B reactivation
Ofatumumab (Arzerra)	300 mg initial dose intravenously, followed 1 week later by 2000 mg intravenously weekly for 7 doses, followed 4 weeks later by 2000 mg intravenously every 4 weeks for four doses; or 300 mg initial dose intravenously, followed 1 week later by 1000 mg intravenously, then 1000 mg intravenously every 4 weeks	Acute: infusion-related reaction, diarrhea, nausea Delayed: neutropenia, infections, pyrexia, rash, fatigue, potential hepatitis B reactivation
Panitumumab (Vectibix)	6 mg/kg intravenously every 2 weeks	Acute: infusion-related reaction, nausea Delayed: acneiform skin rash, hypomagnesemia, asthenia, paronychia, fatigue, dyspnea
Pembrolizumab (Keytruda)	2 mg/kg intravenously every 3 weeks	Acute: infusion-related reaction, nausea Delayed: immune-mediated reactions, fatigue, cough

(continued)

Table 39–11. Common chemotherapeutic agents.[1] (continued)

Chemotherapeutic Agent	Usual Adult Dosage	Adverse Effects
Pertuzumab (Perjeta)	840 mg intravenously once followed by 420 mg intravenously every 3 weeks	Acute: infusion-related reaction, diarrhea, nausea Delayed: fatigue, alopecia, neutropenia, rash, peripheral neuropathy, cardiomyopathy
Ramucirumab (Cyramza)	8 mg/kg intravenously every 2 weeks or 10 mg/kg intravenously every 3 weeks	Acute: infusion-related reaction, hypertension, diarrhea Delayed: fatigue, neutropenia, epistaxis
Rituximab (Rituxan)	375 mg/m^2 intravenously weekly for 4 weeks, or every 3–4 weeks	Acute: infusion-related reaction, tumor lysis syndrome Delayed: lymphopenia, asthenia, rash, potential hepatitis B reactivation
Siltuximab (Sylvant)	11 mg/kg intravenously every 3 weeks	Acute: infusion-related reaction, hyperuricemia Delayed: pruritus, edema, weight gain, rash, upper respiratory tract infection, diarrhea
Trastuzumab (Herceptin)	Initial dose 4 mg/kg intravenously, then 2 mg/kg intravenously weekly; or initial dose 8 mg/kg then 6 mg/kg, intravenously every 3 weeks	Acute: headache, nausea, diarrhea, infusion-related reaction Delayed: myelosuppression, pyrexia, cardiomyopathy, pulmonary toxicity (rare)
Targeted Therapy—Kinase Inhibitors		
Afatinib (Gilotrif)	40 mg orally once daily without food	Acute: diarrhea Delayed: acneiform rash, stomatitis, paronychia
Alectinib (Alecensa)	600 mg orally twice daily with food	Acute: none Delayed: myelosuppression, fatigue, edema, myalgia, dyspnea, elevated transaminases
Axitinib (Inlyta)	5–10 mg orally twice daily	Acute: diarrhea, nausea, vomiting Delayed: hypertension, fatigue, dysphonia, hand-foot syndrome, elevated transaminases
Bosutinib (Bosulif)	500–600 mg orally once daily with food	Acute: diarrhea, nausea, vomiting Delayed: myelosuppression, rash, abdominal pain, hepatotoxicity, fluid retention
Ceritinib (Zykadia)	740 mg orally once daily	Acute: diarrhea, nausea, vomiting Delayed: elevated transaminases, abdominal pain, fatigue, decreased appetite
Cobimetinib (Cotellic)	60 mg orally once daily on days 1 to 21 of a 28-day cycle	Acute: diarrhea, photosensitivity reaction, nausea, vomiting Delayed: myelosuppression, hepatotoxicity, rash, cardiomyopathy (with vemurafenib)
Crizotinib (Xalkori)	250 mg orally twice daily	Acute: nausea, vomiting, diarrhea, constipation Delayed: vision disorder, edema, elevated transaminases, fatigue
Dabrafenib (Tafinlar)	150 mg orally twice daily without food	Acute: headache Delayed: hyperkeratosis, fever, hand-foot syndrome, hyperglycemia, hypophosphatemia
Dasatinib (Sprycel)	100–180 mg orally once daily	Acute: diarrhea, nausea, vomiting Delayed: myelosuppression, fluid retention, fatigue, dyspnea, musculoskeletal pain, rash
Erlotinib (Tarceva)	100 or 150 mg orally once daily without food	Acute: diarrhea, nausea, vomiting Delayed: acneiform skin rash, fatigue, anorexia, dyspnea
Everolimus (Afinitor)	10 mg orally once daily	Acute: mucositis, diarrhea, nausea Delayed: myelosuppression, fatigue, edema, hypercholesterolemia, hypertriglyceridemia, hyperglycemia
Gefitinib (Iressa)	250 mg orally once daily	Acute: diarrhea Delayed: acneiform skin rash
Ibrutinib (Imbruvica)	420 mg or 560 mg orally once daily	Acute: diarrhea, nausea Delayed: myelosuppression, fatigue, edema, rash, elevated serum creatinine, hemorrhage

(continued)

Table 39–11. Common chemotherapeutic agents.[1] (continued)

Chemotherapeutic Agent	Usual Adult Dosage	Adverse Effects
Idelalisib (Zydelig)	150 mg orally twice daily	Acute: diarrhea, nausea Delayed: hepatotoxicity, pneumonitis, intestinal perforation, pyrexia, fatigue, neutropenia, hypertriglyceridemia, hyperglycemia
Imatinib (Gleevec)	100–800 mg orally once daily with food	Acute: nausea, vomiting, diarrhea Delayed: edema, muscle cramps, rash, myelosuppression, hepatotoxicity
Lapatinib (Tykerb)	1250 mg or 1500 mg orally once daily	Acute: diarrhea, nausea, vomiting Delayed: hand-foot syndrome, fatigue, hepatotoxicity (rare)
Lenvatinib (Lenvima)	24 mg orally daily	Acute: hypertension, nausea, vomiting, diarrhea Delayed: fatigue, arthralgia/myalgia, stomatitis, hand-foot syndrome
Nilotinib (Tasigna)	300 or 400 mg orally twice daily without food	Acute: nausea, vomiting, diarrhea Delayed: rash, fatigue, myelosuppression, prolonged QT interval (rare)
Osimertinib (Tagrisso)	80 mg orally once daily	Acute: diarrhea Delayed: myelosuppression, rash, dry skin, nail toxicity, cardiomyopathy (rare), QTc interval prolongation (rare)
Palbociclib (Ibrance)	125 mg orally daily with food for 21 days followed by 7 days off	Acute: nausea, diarrhea, vomiting Delayed: myelosuppression, fatigue, upper respiratory infection, stomatitis, alopecia
Pazopanib (Votrient)	800 mg orally once daily without food	Acute: diarrhea, nausea, vomiting Delayed: hypertension, hair color changes, hepatotoxicity, hemorrhage
Regorafenib (Stivarga)	160 mg orally once daily with food (low-fat breakfast)	Acute: diarrhea Delayed: asthenia, hand-foot syndrome, anorexia, hypertension, mucositis, myelosuppression, hepatotoxicity
Sorafenib (Nexavar)	400 mg orally twice daily without food	Acute: diarrhea and nausea Delayed: fatigue, hand-foot syndrome, rash, hypertension, hemorrhage
Sunitinib (Sutent)	50 mg orally once daily for 4 weeks followed by 2 weeks rest; 37.5 mg orally daily	Acute: diarrhea and nausea Delayed: hypertension, hand-foot syndrome, rash, yellow discoloration of skin, fatigue, hypothyroidism, mucositis, left ventricular dysfunction, bleeding, hepatotoxicity
Temsirolimus (Torisel)	25 mg intravenously weekly	Acute: hypersensitivity, rash Delayed: myelosuppression, asthenia, hyperglycemia, hyperlipidemia, elevated serum creatinine
Trametinib (Mekinist)	2 mg orally once daily without food	Acute: rash, diarrhea Delayed: elevated transaminases, lymphedema, cardiomyopathy
Vandetanib (Caprelsa)	300 mg orally once daily	Acute: diarrhea, nausea Delayed: acneiform skin rash, hypertension, prolonged QT interval
Vemurafenib (Zelboraf)	960 mg orally twice daily	Acute: nausea, hypersensitivity (rare) Delayed: photosensitivity, rash, arthralgia, alopecia, fatigue, prolonged QT interval, cutaneous squamous cell carcinoma
Miscellaneous Agents		
Arsenic trioxide (Trisenox)	0.15 mg/kg intravenously daily	Acute: nausea, dizziness Delayed: acute promyelocytic leukemia differentiation syndrome, prolonged QT interval

(continued)

Table 39–11. Common chemotherapeutic agents.[1] (Continued)

Chemotherapeutic Agent	Usual Adult Dosage	Adverse Effects
Asparaginase Erwinia chrysanthemi (Erwinaze)	25,000 international units/m² intramuscularly three times weekly	Acute: hypersensitivity, nausea, vomiting Delayed: coagulation abnormalities, hepatotoxicity, pancreatitis, neurotoxicity
Belinostat (Beleodaq)	1000 mg/m² intravenously on days 1 through 5, repeat every 21 days	Acute: nausea, vomiting Delayed: fatigue, pyrexia, anemia
Bleomycin (Blenoxane)	10 units/m² intravenously on days 1 and 15 every 28 days; 30 units intravenously on day 2, 9, and 16 every 21 days	Acute: hypersensitivity, fever Delayed: skin reaction (rash, hyperpigmentation of skin, striae), mucositis, pneumonitis
Dactinomycin (Cosmegen)	15 mcg/kg or 400–600 mcg/m² intravenously daily for 5 days	Acute: nausea, vomiting Delayed: myelosuppression, mucositis, rash, diarrhea, hepatoveno-occlusive disease (rare)
Hydroxyurea (Hydrea)	20–30 mg/kg orally daily	Acute: none Delayed: myelosuppression
Mitomycin (Mutamycin)	10–20 mg/m² intravenously every 4–8 weeks; 20–40 mg intravesically	Acute: cystitis (intravesically), nausea, vomiting Delayed: myelosuppression, mucositis, anorexia
Mitoxantrone (Novantrone)	12–14 mg/m² intravenously every 3 weeks; 12 mg/m² intravenously for 2–3 days	Acute: nausea, vomiting, diarrhea, mucositis, blue-green discoloration of urine Delayed: myelosuppression, alopecia, cardiotoxicity
Olaparib (Lynparza)	400 mg orally twice daily	Acute: nausea, vomiting, diarrhea Delayed: myelosuppression, elevated serum creatinine, MCV elevation, fatigue, abdominal pain
Omacetaxine mepesuccinate (Synribo)	Induction: 1.25 mg/m² subcutaneously twice daily for 14 days every 28 days Maintenance: 1.25 mg/m² subcutaneously twice daily for 7 days every 28 days	Acute: diarrhea, nausea, fatigue, injection site reaction Delayed: myelosuppression, infection
Panobinostat (Farydak)	20 mg orally per day on days 1, 3, 5, 8, 10, 12 of each 21-day cycle	Acute: diarrhea, nausea Delayed: myelosuppression, electrolyte abnormalities, infections
Tretinoin (All-Trans-Retinoic Acid, ATRA, Vesanoid)	45 mg/m² orally divided twice daily for 45–90 days or 30 days past complete remission	Acute: headache, nausea Delayed: vitamin A toxicity, retinoic acid-acute promyelocytic leukemia syndrome
Trifluridine/tipiracil (Lonsurf)	35 mg/m² based on trifluridine component orally twice daily within 1 hour of meal on days 1–5 and 8–12 (28-day cycle)	Acute: nausea, diarrhea, vomiting Delayed: myelosuppression, fatigue, anorexia
Ziv-aflibercept (Zaltrap)	4 mg/kg intravenously every 2 weeks	Acute: diarrhea Delayed: myelosuppression, proteinuria, elevated transaminases, stomatitis, fatigue, hypertension
Antiandrogens		
Bicalutamide (Casodex)	50 mg orally once daily	Acute: none Delayed: hot flashes, back pain, asthenia
Enzalutamide (Xtandi)	160 mg orally once daily	Acute: asthenia, diarrhea Delayed: hot flashes, arthralgia, peripheral edema
Flutamide (Eulexin)	250 mg orally every 8 hours	Acute: diarrhea Delayed: hot flashes, hepatotoxicity
Nilutamide (Nilandron)	300 mg orally for 30 days, then 150 mg orally once daily	Acute: none Delayed: visual disturbances (impaired adaptation to dark), hot flashes, disulfiram-like reaction
Selective Estrogen Receptor Modulators		
Tamoxifen (Nolvadex)	20–40 mg orally once daily	Acute: none Delayed: hot flashes, vaginal discharge, menstrual irregularities, arthralgia

(continued)

Table 39–11. Common chemotherapeutic agents.[1] (continued)

Chemotherapeutic Agent	Usual Adult Dosage	Adverse Effects
Toremifene (Fareston)	60 mg orally once daily	Acute: nausea Delayed: hot flashes, vaginal discharge
Aromatase Inhibitors		
Anastrozole (Arimidex)	1 mg orally once daily	Acute: nausea Delayed: hot flashes, peripheral edema, asthenia, hypercholesterolemia, arthralgia/myalgia, osteoporosis
Exemestane (Aromasin)	25 mg orally once daily	
Letrozole (Femara)	2.5 mg orally once daily	
Pure Estrogen Receptor Antagonist		
Fulvestrant (Faslodex)	500 mg intramuscularly on days 1, 15, 29, then monthly	Acute: injection site reaction, nausea Delayed: hot flashes, bone pain, elevated transaminases
LHRH Analogs		
Goserelin acetate (Zoladex)	3.6 mg subcutaneously every month; 10.8 mg subcutaneously every 3 months	Acute: injection site discomfort Delayed: hot flashes, tumor flare, edema, decreased libido, erectile dysfunction, osteoporosis
Leuprolide (Lupron)	7.5 mg intramuscularly or subcutaneously every month; 22.5 mg intramuscularly or subcutaneously every 3 months; 30 mg intramuscularly or subcutaneously every 4 months; 45 mg intramuscularly or subcutaneously every 6 months	
Triptorelin pamoate (Trelstar)	3.75 mg intramuscularly every 4 weeks; 11.25 mg intramuscularly every 12 weeks; 22.5 mg every 24 weeks	
LHRH Antagonist		
Degarelix (Firmagon)	240 mg subcutaneously once, then 80 mg subcutaneously every 28 days	Acute: injection site reaction Delayed: hot flashes, weight gain, elevated transaminases, QT prolongation
Adrenocorticosteroids		
Abiraterone (Zytiga)	1000 mg orally once daily	Acute: diarrhea, edema Delayed: adrenal insufficiency, hepatotoxicity, joint pain, hypokalemia
Ketoconazole	400 mg orally three times daily	Acute: nausea and vomiting Delayed: hepatotoxicity, adrenal insufficiency
Biologic Response Modifiers		
Aldesleukin (IL-2, Proleukin)	600,000 international units/kg intravenously every 8 hours for 14 doses, repeat after 9 days rest	Acute: hypotension, nausea, vomiting, diarrhea, flu-like syndrome, capillary leak syndrome Delayed: myelosuppression, confusion, somnolence, oliguria
Interferon-alpha-2b (Intron A)	20 million international units/m² intravenously 5 days a week for 4 weeks, then 10 million international units/m² subcutaneously three times a week for 48 weeks	Acute: flu-like syndrome, nausea, vomiting, diarrhea Delayed: myelosuppression, anorexia, alopecia, depression, elevated transaminases
Sipuleucel-T (Provenge)	One dose (minimum of 50 million autologous CD54 cells) intravenously every 2 weeks for three doses	Acute: infusion-related reaction, nausea, vomiting Delayed: fatigue, back pain, arthralgia

[1]For altretamine, denileukin diftitox, ibritumomab, lomustine, megestrol, pralatrexate, romidepsin, and vismodegib see Table 39–11 in *CMDT Online* at www.accessmedicine.com.
GFR, glomerular filtration rate; LHRH, luteinizing hormone–releasing hormone; MAO, monoamine oxidase; MCV, mean corpuscular volume.

Table 39–12. Commonly used supportive care agents.[1]

Agent	Indication	Usual Dose	Adverse Effects
Allopurinol (Xyloprim)	Prevent hyperuricemia from tumor lysis syndrome	600–800 mg/day orally	Acute: none Delayed: rash
Rasburicase (Elitek)	Prevent hyperuricemia from tumor lysis syndrome	3–6 mg intravenously once	Acute: hypersensitivity, nausea, vomiting, diarrhea, fever, headache Delayed: rash, peripheral edema
Mesna (Mesnex)	Prevent ifosfamide-induced hemorrhagic cystitis	20% of ifosfamide dose intravenously at 0, 4, and 8 hours; various doses	Acute: nausea, vomiting Delayed: fatigue
Leucovorin	Rescue after high-dose methotrexate; in combination with fluorouracil for colon cancer	10 mg/m^2 intravenously or orally every 6 hours; 20 mg/m^2 or 200–500 mg/m^2 intravenously before fluorouracil; various doses	Acute: nausea, vomiting, diarrhea Delayed: stomatitis, fatigue
Levoleucovorin (Fusilev)	Rescue after high-dose methotrexate; in combination with fluorouracil for colon cancer	7.5 mg intravenously every 6 hours for 10 doses; 100 mg/m^2 intravenously before fluorouracil	Acute: nausea, vomiting Delayed: stomatitis, diarrhea
Dexrazoxane (Zinecard)	Prevent cardiomyopathy secondary to doxorubicin; anthracycline-induced injection site extravasation	10 times the doxorubicin dose intravenously before doxorubicin; 1000 mg/m^2 intravenously on days 1 and 2, then 500 mg/m^2 intravenously on day 3	Acute: nausea Delayed: myelosuppression, elevated transaminases
Palifermin (Kepivance)	Prevent mucositis following chemotherapy	60 mcg/kg/day intravenously for 3 days before and 3 days after chemotherapy	Acute: none Delayed: rash, fever, elevated serum amylase, erythema, edema
Pilocarpine (Salagen)	Radiation-induced xerostomia	5–10 mg orally three times a day	Acute: flushing, sweating, nausea, dizziness Delayed: increased urinary frequency, rhinitis
Radium (Ra)-223 dichloride (Xofigo)	Symptomatic bone metastases	50 kilobecquerel/kg (1.35 microCurie/kg) intravenously every 4 weeks for 6 cycles	Acute: nausea, vomiting, diarrhea, peripheral edema Delayed: myelosuppression
Bone-Modifying Agents			
Denosumab (Xgeva)	Osteolytic bone metastasis	120 mg subcutaneously every 4 weeks	Acute: nausea Delayed: hypocalcemia, hypophosphatemia, fatigue, osteonecrosis of the jaw
Pamidronate (Aredia)	Osteolytic bone metastasis, hypercalcemia of malignancy	90 mg intravenously every 3–4 weeks; 60–90 mg intravenously, may repeat after 7 days	Acute: nausea Delayed: dyspnea, arthralgia, bone pain, osteonecrosis of the jaw, nephrotoxicity, hypocalcemia
Zoledronic acid (Zometa)	Osteolytic bone metastasis, hypercalcemia of malignancy	4 mg intravenously every 3–4 weeks; 4 mg intravenously once, may repeat after 7 days	
Growth Factors			
Epoetin alfa (Epogen, Procrit)	Chemotherapy-induced anemia	40,000 units subcutaneously once weekly; 150 units/kg subcutaneously three times a week	Acute: injection site reaction Delayed: hypertension, thromboembolic events, increased risk of tumor progression or recurrence
Darbepoetin alfa (Aranesp)	Chemotherapy-induced anemia	2.25 mcg/kg subcutaneously weekly; 500 mcg subcutaneously every 3 weeks	

(continued)

Table 39–12. Commonly used supportive care agents.[1] (continued)

Agent	Indication	Usual Dose	Adverse Effects
Filgrastim (Neupogen) Filgrastim-sndz (Zarxio)	Febrile neutropenia prophylaxis, mobilization of peripheral stem cells	5–10 mcg/kg/day subcutaneously or intravenously once daily, treat past nadir	Acute: injection site reaction Delayed: bone pain
Pegfilgrastim (Neulasta)	Febrile neutropenia prophylaxis	6 mg subcutaneously once per chemotherapy cycle	
Sargramostim (Leukine)	Myeloid reconstitution following bone marrow transplant, mobilization of peripheral blood stem cells	250 mcg/m^2 intravenously daily until the absolute neutrophil count is > 1500 cells/mcL for 3 consecutive days	Acute: fever, rash, pruritus, nausea, vomiting, diarrhea, injection site reaction, dyspnea Delayed: asthenia, bone pain, mucositis, edema, arrhythmia
Tbo-filgrastim (Neutroval)	Severe chemotherapy-induced neutropenia	5 mcg/kg subcutaneously once daily until neutrophil recovery	Acute: none Delayed: bone pain, leukocytosis

[1]For amifostine, samarium, and strontium, see Table 39–12 in CMDT Online at www.accessmedicine.com.

retention, heart failure, and arrhythmias (see Table 39–12). Thrombopoietin, the protein that stimulates megakaryopoiesis in vivo, was isolated in 1994. Despite much work attempting to produce a clinically effective thrombopoietin agent for therapeutic use, no such drug is commercially available for this indication. Two drugs that activate the thrombopoietin receptor and are approved for use in idiopathic thrombocytopenia, romiplostim and eltrombopag, have not been shown to be beneficial in patients receiving chemotherapy.

2. Chemotherapy-Induced Nausea & Vomiting

A number of cytotoxic anticancer drugs can induce nausea and vomiting, which can be the most anticipated and stressful side effects for patients. Chemotherapy-induced nausea and vomiting is mediated in part by the stimulation of at least two central nervous system receptors, 5-hydroxytryptamine subtype 3 (5HT$_3$) and neurokinin subtype 1 (NK$_1$). Anticipatory nausea and vomiting may even occur before the administration of chemotherapy. Chemotherapy-induced nausea and vomiting can be acute, occurring within minutes to hours of chemotherapy administration, or delayed until the second day and lasting up to 7 days. Chemotherapy drugs or drug regimens are classified into high, moderate, low, and minimal likelihoods of causing

Table 39–13. A common scheme for dose modification of cancer chemotherapeutic agents.

Granulocyte Count (cells/mcL)	Platelet Count (/mcL)	Suggested Drug Dosage (% of Full Dose)
> 2000	> 100,000	100%
1000–2000	75,000–100,000	50%
< 2000	< 50,000	0%

emesis (90%, 30–90%, 10–30%, less than 10%, respectively). Highly emetogenic chemotherapy drugs include cisplatin, carmustine, cyclophosphamide (at doses over 1.5 g/m^2), dacarbazine, mechlorethamine, and streptozocin, or a combination of regularly dosed cyclophosphamide and anthracyclines. Chemotherapy drugs that are moderately emetogenic include azacitidine, bendamustine, carboplatin, crizotinib, cyclophosphamide, cytarabine, daunomycin, doxorubicin, epirubicin, idarubicin, ifosfamide, irinotecan, mitotane, oxaliplatin, temozolomide, and vismodegib. Drugs with low emetic potential include bortezomib, brentuximab, capecitabine, cabozantinib, dabrafenib, dasatinib, docetaxel, erlotinib, etoposide, fludarabine, fluorouracil, gemcitabine, hydroxyurea, lenalidomide, methotrexate, mitomycin, mitoxantrone, omacetaxine, paclitaxel, pemetrexed, pomalidomide, ponatinib, temsirolimus, trametinib, and topotecan. Drugs with minimal risk of emesis include bevacizumab, bleomycin, cetuximab, cladribine, decitabine, fludarabine, panitumumab, rituximab, temsirolimus, trastuzumab, vinblastine, vincristine, and vinorelbine.

By understanding the physiology of chemotherapy-induced nausea and vomiting, major advances have occurred with the development of highly effective antiemetic drugs. Antagonists to the 5HT$_3$-receptor include ondansetron, granisetron, dolasetron, and palonosetron, as well as tropisetron and ramosetron (neither yet available in the United States). Ondansetron can be given either intravenously (8 mg or 0.15 mg/kg) or orally (24 mg for highly emetogenic chemotherapy, 8 mg twice daily for moderately emetogenic chemotherapy). Doses of 8 mg can be repeated parenterally or orally every 8 hours. Dosing of granisetron is 1 mg or 0.01 mg/kg intravenously or 1–2 mg orally. Dolasetron is given 1.8 mg/kg or a fixed dose of 100 mg intravenously or 100 mg can be given orally. Palonosetron, a long-acting 5HT$_3$ with high affinity for the 5HT$_3$-receptor given at a dose of 0.25 mg intravenously, is effective for not only acute but also delayed emesis. Where available, tropisetron is given at a dose of 5 mg either orally or intravenously. Ramosetron is given as a one time 300 mcg dose intravenously. The efficacy of the $5HT_3$-blockers is improved by adding 6–10 mg of either oral or intravenous dexamethasone. As a class of drugs, the $5HT_3$-receptor antagonists have the potential to cause electrocardiogram changes including QT prolongation. Before using these agents, any preexisting hypokalemia or hypomagnesemia should be corrected. In addition, clinicians should be cautious when using these agents in elderly patients, patients with preexisting bradyarrhymias or heart failure, and patients taking medications known to prolong the QT interval.

Aprepitant, fosaprepitant, and rolapitant are antagonists to the NK_1 receptor. Aprepitant is given as a 125-mg oral dose followed by 80 mg on the second and third day with a $5HT_3$-receptor antagonist (such as ondansetron or granisetron), the immediate and delayed protective effect for highly emetogenic chemotherapy is increased. Fosaprepitant, the intravenous formulation of aprepitant, can be given at a dose of 115 mg if followed by 2 days of aprepitant or at a dose of 150 mg if given alone. Rolapitant, a potent selective NK_1 receptor antagonist, has a 7-day half-life; it is given as a one-time oral dose of 180 mg 1–2 hours before the start of chemotherapy.

Standard therapy for highly emetogenic chemotherapy includes a $5HT_3$-antagonist given on the first day, and both dexamethasone and a neurokinin-1 receptor antagonist (aprepitant, fosaprepitant, or rolapitant) given on the first day as well as (if aprepitant) on the second and third days. Moderately emetogenic chemotherapy regimens are best managed with a two-drug regimen of a $5HT_3$-antagonist and dexamethasone. Palonosetron is now a preferred $5HT_3$-blocker due to its greater affinity for the $5HT_3$-receptor and its longer half-life. For low emetogenic chemotherapy drugs, a single agent such as a $5HT_3$-antagonist or prochlorperazine or dexamethasone should be given. A 25-mg suppository form of prochlorperazine may be used for patients unable to swallow oral medications. Another medication that may be helpful is lorazepam, 0.5–1.0 mg given orally every 6–8 hours.

The importance of treating chemotherapy-induced nausea and vomiting expectantly and aggressively beginning with the first course of chemotherapy cannot be overemphasized. Patients being treated in the clinic setting should always be given antiemetics for home use with written instructions as well as contact numbers to call for advice.

3. Gastrointestinal Toxicity

Untoward effects of cancer chemotherapy include damage to the more rapidly growing cells of the body such as the mucosal lining from the mouth through the gastrointestinal tract. Oral symptoms range from mild mouth soreness to frank ulcerations. Not uncommonly, mouth ulcerations will have superimposed candida or herpes simplex infections. In addition to receiving cytotoxic chemotherapy, a significant risk factor for development of oral mucositis is poor oral hygiene and existing caries or periodontal disease. Toxicity in the gastrointestinal tract usually manifests as diarrhea. Gastrointestinal symptoms can range from

mild symptoms of loose stools to life-threatening diarrhea leading to dehydration and electrolyte imbalances. Drugs most commonly associated with causing mucositis in the mouth and the gastrointestinal tract are cytarabine, 5-fluorouracil, and methotrexate.

Patients undergoing treatment for head and neck cancer with concurrent chemotherapy and radiation therapy have a very high risk of developing severe mucositis.

Preventive strategies for oral mucositis include a pretreatment dental examination, particularly for all head and neck cancer patients and any cancer patient with poor dental hygiene who will be receiving chemotherapy. For patients receiving fluorouracil, simple measures such as ice chips in the mouth for 30 minutes during infusion can reduce the incidence and severity of mucositis. Once mucositis is encountered, superimposed fungal infections should be treated with topical antifungal medications (oral nystatin mouth suspensions, or clotrimazole troches) or systemic therapy (fluconazole 100–400 mg orally daily). Suspected herpetic infections can be treated with acyclovir (up to 800 mg orally five times daily) or valacyclovir (1 g orally twice daily). Mucositis may also be managed with mouthwashes; it is also important to provide adequate pain medication.

Other strategies for prevention of oral mucositis include the use of the recombinant keratinocyte growth factor inhibitor, palifermin. Practice guidelines recommend prophylaxis with intravenous palifermin (60 mcg/kg/day) for patients receiving high-dose chemotherapy in order to reduce the incidence and duration of mucositis (Table 39–12).

Diarrhea is most associated with fluorouracil, capecitabine, and irinotecan as well as the tyrosine kinase inhibitors (sorafenib, sunitinib, regorafenib, imatinib, dasatinib, nilotinib) and epithelial growth factor inhibitors (cetuximab, panitumumab, and erlotinib). Mild to moderate diarrhea can be managed with oral antidiarrheal medication (loperamide, 4 mg initially followed by 2 mg every 2–4 hours until bowel movements are formed). Occasionally, the diarrhea will be overwhelming causing dehydration, electrolyte imbalances, and acute kidney injury. These patients require inpatient management with aggressive intravenous hydration and replacement of electrolytes. Octreotide, 100–150 mcg subcutaneously three times daily, can be used for severe diarrhea.

4. Skin Toxicity

Dermatologic complications from cancer chemotherapy can include hyperpigmentation (liposomal doxorubicin, busulfan, hydroxyurea), alopecia, photosensitivity, nail changes, acral erythema, and generalized rashes. Acral erythema (hand-foot syndrome), most commonly associated with administration of fluorouracil, capecitabine, and liposomal doxorubicin, manifests as painful palms or soles accompanied by erythema, progressing to blistering, desquamation, and ulceration in its worst forms. Strategies for prevention of acral erythema include oral pyridoxine, 200 mg daily, and applying cold packs to the extremities during chemotherapy administration. Agents targeting the epidermal growth factor pathway can cause an acne-like rash; the development of the rash may identify those who will respond to the drug. Inhibitors of the tyrosine kinase pathway are also associated with a high incidence of dermatologic complications, such as rash and acral erythema.

5. Miscellaneous Drug-Specific Toxicities

The toxicities of individual drugs are summarized in Tables 39–11 and 39–12; however, several of these warrant additional mention, since they occur with frequently administered agents, and special measures are often indicated.

A. Hemorrhagic Cystitis Induced by Cyclophosphamide or Ifosfamide

Metabolic products of cyclophosphamide that retain cytotoxic activity are excreted into the urine. Some patients appear to metabolize more of the drug to these active excretory products; if their urine is concentrated, severe bladder damage may result. Patients receiving cyclophosphamide must maintain a high fluid intake prior to and following the administration of the drug and be counseled to empty their bladders frequently. Early symptoms suggesting bladder toxicity include dysuria and increased frequency of urination. Should microscopic hematuria develop, it is advisable to stop the drug temporarily or switch to a different alkylating agent, to increase fluid intake, and to administer a urinary analgesic such as phenazopyridine. With severe cystitis, large segments of bladder mucosa may be shed, resulting in prolonged gross hematuria. Such patients should be observed for signs of urinary obstruction and may require cystoscopy for removal of obstructing blood clots. The cyclophosphamide analog ifosfamide can cause severe hemorrhagic cystitis when used alone. However, when its use is followed by a series of doses of the neutralizing agent mesna, bladder toxicity can be prevented (Table 39–12). Mesna can also be used for patients taking cyclophosphamide in whom cystitis develops.

B. Neuropathy Due to Vinca Alkaloids and Other Chemotherapy Drugs

Neuropathy is caused by a number of different chemotherapy drugs, the most common being vincristine. The peripheral neuropathy can be sensory, motor, autonomic, or a combination of these types. In its mildest form, it consists of paresthesias of the fingers and toes. Occasionally, acute jaw or throat pain can develop after vincristine therapy. This may be a form of trigeminal or glossopharyngeal neuralgia. With continued vincristine therapy, the paresthesias extend to the proximal interphalangeal joints, hyporeflexia appears in the lower extremities, and significant weakness can develop. Other drugs in the vinca alkaloid class as well as the taxane drugs (paclitaxel and docetaxel) and agents to treat myeloma (thalidomide and bortezomib) cause similar toxicity. The presence of neurologic symptoms is not in itself a reason to stop therapy; the severity of the symptoms must be balanced against the goals of therapy. Usually, though, the development of moderate to severe paresthesias or motor impairment results in the decision to discontinue the drug.

Constipation is the most common symptom of autonomic neuropathy associated with the vinca alkaloids. Patients receiving these drugs should be started on stool softeners and mild cathartics when therapy is begun; otherwise, severe impaction may result from an atonic bowel.

More serious autonomic involvement can lead to acute intestinal obstruction with signs indistinguishable from those of an acute abdomen. Bladder neuropathies are uncommon but may be severe. These two complications are absolute contraindications to continued vincristine therapy.

C. Methotrexate Toxicity

Methotrexate, a folate antagonist, is a commonly used component of regimens to treat patients with leptomeningeal disease, acute lymphoblastic leukemia, and sarcomas. Methotrexate is almost entirely eliminated by the kidney. Methotrexate toxicity affects cells with rapid turnover, including the bone marrow and mucosa resulting in myelosuppression and mucositis. Methotrexate can also damage the liver and kidney manifesting as elevated liver enzymes and creatinine. High-dose methotrexate, usually defined as a dose of 500 mg/m^2 or more given over 4–36 hours, would be lethal without "rescue" of the normal tissues. Leucovorin, a form of folate, will reverse the toxic effects of methotrexate and is given until serum methotrexate levels are in the safe range (less than 0.05 mmol/L). It is crucial that high-dose methotrexate and leucovorin are given precisely according to protocol as deviations of the timing of methotrexate delivery or delay in rescue can result in patient death. The dose used in intrathecal therapy is 12 mg. Lower doses of methotrexate can be problematic in patients with kidney disease who cannot clear the drug normally or with patients who have effusions in whom the drug distributes itself in effusions and leaks out continuously, exposing normal tissue to the drug. In patients with kidney disease or an effusion, prolonged rescue with leucovorin is necessary.

Vigorous hydration and bicarbonate loading can help prevent crystallization of high-dose methotrexate in the renal tubular epithelium and consequent nephrotoxicity. Daily monitoring of the serum creatinine is mandatory. Drugs impairing methotrexate excretion, such as aspirin, nonsteroidal anti-inflammatory drugs, amiodarone, omeprazole, penicillin, phenytoin, and sulfa, should be stopped if possible before methotrexate administration.

D. Anthracycline Cardiotoxicity

The anthracycline drugs, including doxorubicin, daunomycin, idarubicin, and epirubicin, are associated with cardiotoxicity. They can produce acute (during administration), subacute (days to months following administration), and delayed (years following administration) cardiac toxicity. The most feared complication is the delayed development of heart failure. Risk factors for this debilitating toxicity include the anthracycline cumulative dose, age over 70, previous or concurrent irradiation of the chest, preexisting cardiac disease, and concurrent administration of chemotherapy drugs such as trastuzumab. The problem is greatest with doxorubicin because it is the most commonly administered anthracycline due to its major role in the treatment of lymphomas, sarcomas, breast cancer, and certain other solid tumors. Patients receiving anthracyclines should have a baseline multiple-gated radionuclide cardiac scan (MUGA) to calculate the left ventricular-ejection fraction (LVEF). If the LVEF is greater than 50%, anthracyclines can be administered; if the LVEF is less than 30%, these drugs should not be given. For patients with intermediate cardiac function, anthracyclines should be cautiously given, if necessary, at lower doses with LVEF monitoring between doses. Changes in cardiac dynamics occur in most patients by the time they have received 300 mg/m^2 of doxorubicin. In general, patients should not receive a total dose of doxorubicin in excess of 450 mg/m^2; the dose should be lower if prior chest radiotherapy has been given. The appearance of a high resting pulse may herald the appearance of overt cardiac toxicity. Unfortunately, toxicity may be irreversible and frequently fatal at dosage levels above 550 mg/m^2. At lower doses (eg, 350 mg/m^2), the symptoms and signs of cardiac failure generally respond well to medical therapy and discontinuation of the anthracycline. Doxorubicin and daunomycin have been formulated as liposomal products; these drugs, approved for use in patients with Kaposi sarcoma and sometimes in other cancers as a substitute for the conventional anthracyclines, appear to have minimal potential for cardiac toxicity.

E. Cisplatin Nephrotoxicity and Neurotoxicity

Cisplatin is effective in treating testicular, bladder, head and neck, lung, and ovarian cancers. With cisplatin, the serious side effects of nephrotoxicity and neurotoxicity must be anticipated and aggressively managed. Patients must be vigorously hydrated prior to, during, and after cisplatin administration. Both kidney function and electrolytes must be monitored. Low serum magnesium, potassium, and sodium levels can develop. The neurotoxicity is usually manifested as a peripheral neuropathy of mixed sensorimotor type and may be associated with painful paresthesias. Development of neuropathy typically occurs after cumulative doses of 300 mg/m^2. Ototoxicity is a potentially serious manifestation of neurotoxicity and can progress to deafness. Amifostine, given intravenously at a dose of 910 mg/m^2 over 15 minutes prior to cisplatin, is used to protect against nephrotoxicity and neuropathy. Use of amifostine does not appear to compromise the antineoplastic effect of cisplatin. The second-generation platinum analog, carboplatin, is non-nephrotoxic, although it is myelosuppressive. In the setting of preexisting kidney disease or neuropathy, carboplatin is occasionally substituted for cisplatin.

PROGNOSIS

Patients receiving chemotherapy for curative intent will often tolerate side effects with the knowledge that the treatment may result in eradication of their cancer. Patients receiving therapy for palliative intent often have their therapy tailored to improve quality of life while minimizing major side effects. A valuable sign of clinical improvement is the general well-being of the patient. Although general well-being is a combination of subjective (possibly partly a placebo effect) and objective factors, it nonetheless serves as a sign of clinical improvement along with improved appetite and weight gain and increased "performance status" (eg, ambulatory versus bedridden). Evaluation of factors such as activity status enables the clinician to judge whether the net effect of chemotherapy is worthwhile palliation (see Chapter 5).

Basch E et al. Antiemetics use in oncology: updated guideline recommendations from ASCO. Am Soc Clin Oncol Educ Book. 2012:532–40. [PMID: 24451791]

Hershman DL et al; American Society of Clinical Oncology. Prevention and management of chemotherapy-induced peripheral neuropathy in survivors of adult cancers: American Society of Clinical Oncology clinical practice guideline. J Clin Oncol. 2014 Jun 20;32(18):1941–67. [PMID: 24733808]

Sugerman DT. JAMA Patient Page. Chemotherapy. JAMA. 2013 Jul 10;310(2):218. [PMID: 23839767]

West HJ et al. JAMA Oncology Patient Page. Neoadjuvant Therapy. JAMA Oncol. 2015 Jul;1(4):550. [PMID: 26181277]

Inherited Disorders

Reed E. Pyeritz, MD, PhD

ACUTE INTERMITTENT PORPHYRIA

ESSENTIALS OF DIAGNOSIS

▶ Unexplained abdominal crisis, generally in young women.

▶ Acute peripheral or central nervous system dysfunction; recurrent psychiatric illnesses.

▶ Hyponatremia.

▶ Porphobilinogen in the urine during an attack.

General Considerations

Though there are several different types of porphyrias, the one with the most serious consequences and the one that usually presents in adulthood is acute intermittent porphyria (AIP), which is inherited as an autosomal dominant, though it remains clinically silent in most patients who carry a mutation in *HMBS*. Clinical illness usually develops in women. Symptoms begin in the teens or 20s, but onset can begin after menopause in rare cases. The disorder is caused by partial deficiency of hydroxymethylbilane synthase activity, leading to increased excretion of aminolevulinic acid and porphobilinogen in the urine. The diagnosis may be elusive if not specifically considered. The characteristic abdominal pain may be due to abnormalities in autonomic innervation in the gut. In contrast to other forms of porphyria, cutaneous photosensitivity is absent in AIP. Attacks are precipitated by numerous factors, including drugs and intercurrent infections. Harmful and relatively safe drugs for use in treatment are listed in Table 40–1. Hyponatremia may be seen, due in part to inappropriate release of antidiuretic hormone, although gastrointestinal loss of sodium in some patients may be a contributing factor.

Clinical Findings

A. Symptoms and Signs

Patients show intermittent abdominal pain of varying severity, and in some instances it may so simulate acute

abdomen as to lead to exploratory laparotomy. Because the origin of the abdominal pain is neurologic, there is an absence of fever and leukocytosis. Complete recovery between attacks is usual. Any part of the nervous system may be involved, with evidence for autonomic and peripheral neuropathy. Peripheral neuropathy may be symmetric or asymmetric and mild or profound; in the latter instance, it can even lead to quadriplegia with respiratory paralysis. Other central nervous system manifestations include seizures, altered consciousness, psychosis, and abnormalities of the basal ganglia. Hyponatremia may further cause or exacerbate central nervous system manifestations.

B. Laboratory Findings

Often there is profound hyponatremia. The diagnosis can be confirmed by demonstrating an increased amount of porphobilinogen in the urine during an acute attack. Freshly voided urine is of normal color but may turn dark upon standing in light and air.

Most families have different mutations in *HMBS* causing AIP. Mutations can be detected in 90% of patients and used for presymptomatic and prenatal diagnosis.

Prevention

Avoidance of factors known to precipitate attacks of AIP—especially drugs—can reduce morbidity. Sulfonamides and barbiturates are the most common culprits; others are listed in Table 40–1 and on the Internet (www.drugs-porphyria.org). Starvation diets or prolonged fasting also cause attacks and so must be avoided. Hormonal changes during pregnancy can precipitate crises.

Treatment

Treatment with a high-carbohydrate diet diminishes the number of attacks in some patients and is a reasonable empiric gesture considering its benignity. Acute attacks may be life-threatening and require prompt diagnosis, withdrawal of the inciting agent (if possible), and treatment with analgesics and intravenous glucose in saline

Table 40–1. Some of the "unsafe" and "probably safe" drugs used in the treatment of acute porphyrias.

Unsafe	Probably Safe
Alcohol	Acetaminophen
Alkylating agents	Beta-adrenergic blockers
Barbiturates	Amitriptyline
Carbamazepine	Aspirin
Chloroquine	Atropine
Chlorpropamide	Chloral hydrate
Clonidine	Chlordiazepoxide
Dapsone	Corticosteroids
Ergots	Diazepam
Erythromycin	Digoxin
Estrogens, synthetic	Diphenhydramine
Food additives	Guanethidine
Glutethimide	Hyoscine
Griseofulvin	Ibuprofen
Hydralazine	Imipramine
Ketamine	Insulin
Meprobamate	Lithium
Methyldopa	Naproxen
Metoclopramide	Nitrofurantoin
Nortriptyline	Opioid analgesics
Pentazocine	Penicillamine
Phenytoin	Penicillin and derivatives
Progestins	Phenothiazines
Pyrazinamide	Procaine
Rifampin	Streptomycin
Spironolactone	Succinylcholine
Succinimides	Tetracycline
Sulfonamides	Thiouracil
Theophylline	
Tolazamide	
Tolbutamide	
Valproic acid	

Kuo HC et al. Neurological complications of acute intermittent porphyria. Eur Neurol. 2011;66(5):247–52. [PMID: 21986212]

Pischik E et al. An update of clinical management of acute intermittent porphyria. Appl Clin Genet. 2015 Sep 1;8:201–14. [PMID: 26366103]

Singal AK et al. Liver transplantation in the management of porphyria. Hepatology. 2014 Sep;60(3):1082–9. [PMID: 24700519]

Stein PE et al. Acute intermittent porphyria: fatal complications of treatment. Clin Med. 2012 Jun;12(3):293–4. [PMID: 22783787]

ALKAPTONURIA

 ESSENTIALS OF DIAGNOSIS

▶ Ochronosis (gray-black discoloration of connective tissue, including the sclerae, ears, and cartilage).

▶ Characteristic radiologic dense intervertebral disks in the spine.

▶ Arthropathy.

▶ Urine darkens on standing.

▶ Clinical Findings

A. Symptoms and Signs

Alkaptonuria is caused by a recessively inherited deficiency of the enzyme homogentisic acid oxidase. This acid derives from metabolism of both phenylalanine and tyrosine and is present in large amounts in the urine throughout the patient's life. A dark oxidation product accumulates slowly in cartilage and other connective tissues throughout the body, leading to degenerative joint disease of the spine and peripheral joints. Examination of patients in the third and fourth decades shows a slight darkish blue color below the skin in areas overlying cartilage, such as in the ears, a phenomenon called **ochronosis**. In some patients, a more severe hyperpigmentation can be seen in the sclera, conjunctiva, and cornea. Kidney, biliary, and salivary stones can occur. Accumulation of metabolites in heart valves can lead to aortic or mitral stenosis. A predisposition to coronary artery disease may also be present. Although the syndrome causes considerable morbidity, life expectancy is reduced only modestly. Symptoms are more often attributable to spondylitis with back pain, leading to a clinical picture difficult to distinguish from that of ankylosing spondylitis, though on radiographic assessment the sacroiliac joints are not fused in alkaptonuria. The disorder is uncommon in most populations (less than 1 per 100,000) but much more common in Slovakia and the Dominican Republic.

B. Laboratory Findings

The diagnosis is established by demonstrating homogentisic acid in the urine, which turns black spontaneously on exposure to the air; this reaction is particularly noteworthy

and hematin. A minimum of 300 g of carbohydrate per day should be provided orally or intravenously. Electrolyte balance requires close attention. Hematin therapy should be undertaken with full recognition of adverse consequences, especially phlebitis and coagulopathy. The intravenous dosage is up to 4 mg/kg once or twice daily. Liver transplantation may provide an option for patients with disease poorly controlled by medical therapy.

▶ When to Refer

• For management of severe abdominal pain, seizures, or psychosis.

• For preventive management when a patient with porphyria contemplates pregnancy.

• For genetic counseling and molecular diagnosis.

▶ When to Admit

The patient should be hospitalized when he or she has an acute attack accompanied by mental status changes, seizure, or hyponatremia.

if the urine is alkaline or when alkali is added to a specimen. Molecular analysis of the homogentisic acid oxidase gene (*HGD*) is available but not necessary for diagnosis.

▶ Prevention

Carrier screening and prenatal diagnosis are possible by testing for genetic mutations.

▶ Treatment

Treatment of the arthritis is similar to that for other arthropathies and joint replacement can be effective. Although, in theory, rigid dietary restriction or medications might reduce accumulation of the pigment, this has not proved to be of practical benefit. Since the aortic valve becomes involved by the fifth decade, screening echocardiography of affected adults is indicated. Nitisinone, a drug that inhibits the formation of homogentisic acid, reduces urinary homogentisic acid and shows clinical promise.

Ranganath LR et al. Suitability of nitisinone in alkaptonuria 1 (SONIA 1): an international, multicenter, randomized, open-label, no-treatment controlled, parallel-group, dose-response study to investigate the effect of once daily nitisinone on 24-h urinary homogentisic acid excretion in patients with alkaptonuria after 4 weeks of treatment. Ann Rheum Dis. 2016 Feb;75(2):362–7. [PMID: 25475116]

DOWN SYNDROME

ESSENTIALS OF DIAGNOSIS

- ▶ Typical craniofacial features (flat occiput, epicanthal folds, large tongue).
- ▶ Intellectual disability.
- ▶ Congenital heart disease (eg, atrioventricular canal defects) in 50% of patients.
- ▶ Dementia of the Alzheimer type in early-to-mid adulthood.
- ▶ Three copies of chromosome 21 (trisomy 21) or a chromosome rearrangement that results in three copies of a region of the long arm of chromosome 21.

▶ General Considerations

Nearly 0.5% of all human conceptions are trisomic for chromosome 21. Because of increased fetal mortality, birth incidence of Down syndrome is 1 per 700 but varies from 1 per 1000 in young mothers to more than three times as frequent in women of advanced maternal age. The presence of a fetus with Down syndrome can be detected in many pregnancies in the first or early second trimester through screening maternal serum for alpha-fetoprotein and other biomarkers ("multiple marker screening") and by detecting increased nuchal thickness and underdevelopment of the nasal bone on ultrasonography. Prenatal diagnosis with high sensitivity and specificity can be achieved by assaying fetal DNA that is circulating in maternal blood. The chance of bearing a child with Down syndrome increases exponentially with the age of the mother at conception and begins a marked rise after age 35. By age 45 years, the odds of having an affected child are as high as 1 in 40. The risk of other conditions associated with trisomy also increases, because of the predisposition of older oocytes to nondisjunction during meiosis. There is little risk of trisomy associated with increased paternal age. However, older men do have an increased risk of fathering a child with a new autosomal dominant condition. Because there are so many distinct conditions, though, the chance of fathering an offspring with any given one is extremely small.

▶ Clinical Findings

A. Symptoms and Signs

Down syndrome is usually diagnosed at birth on the basis of the typical craniofacial features, hypotonia, and single palmar crease. Several serious problems that may be evident at birth or may develop early in childhood include duodenal atresia, congenital heart disease (especially atrioventricular canal defects), and hematologic malignancy. The intestinal and cardiac anomalies usually respond to surgery. A transient neonatal leukemia generally responds to conservative management. The incidences of both acute lymphoblastic and myeloid leukemias are increased in childhood. Intelligence varies across a wide spectrum. Many people with Down syndrome do well in sheltered workshops and group homes, but few achieve full independence in adulthood. Other frequent complications include atlanto-axial instability, celiac disease, frequent infections due to immune deficiency, and hypothyroidism. An Alzheimer-like dementia usually becomes evident in the fourth or fifth decade. Patients with Down syndrome who survive childhood and who develop dementia have a reduced life expectancy; on average, they live to about age 55 years.

B. Laboratory Findings

Cytogenomic analysis should always be performed—even though most patients will have simple trisomy for chromosome 21—to detect unbalanced translocations; such patients may have a parent with a balanced translocation, and there will be a substantial recurrence risk of Down syndrome in future offspring of that parent and potentially that parent's relatives.

▶ Treatment

Duodenal atresia should be treated surgically. Congenital heart disease should be treated as in any other patient. As yet, no medical treatment has been proven to affect the neurodevelopmental or the neurodegenerative aspects. Based on the glutamatergic hypothesis for Alzheimer disease, studies have been initiated examining the potential benefit of the *N*-methyl-D-aspartate receptor antagonist memantine.

When to Refer

- For comprehensive evaluation of infants to investigate congenital heart disease, hematologic malignancy, and duodenal atresia.
- For genetic counseling of the parents.
- For signs of dementia in an adult patient.

When to Admit

An affected young patient should be hospitalized when he or she has failure to thrive, regurgitation, breathlessness, or easy bruising.

Costa AC. The glutamatergic hypothesis for Down syndrome: the potential use of *N*-methyl-D-aspartate receptor antagonists to enhance cognition and decelerate neurodegeneration. CNS Neurol Disord Drug Targets. 2014 Feb;13(1):16–25. [PMID: 24152324]

Ram G et al. Infections and immunodeficiency in Down syndrome. Clin Exp Immunol. 2011 Apr;164(1):9–16. [PMID: 21352207]

Ross WT et al. Care of the adult patient with Down syndrome. South Med J. 2014 Nov;107(11):715–21. [PMID: 25365441]

Taylor-Phillips S et al. Accuracy of non-invasive prenatal testing using cell-free DNA for detection of Down, Edwards and Patau syndromes: a systematic review and meta-analysis. BMJ Open. 2016 Jan 18;6(1):e010002. [PMID: 26781507]

Zemel BS et al. Growth charts for children with Down syndrome in the United States. Pediatrics. 2015 Nov;136(5):e1204–11. [PMID: 26504127]

FRAGILE X MENTAL RETARDATION

ESSENTIALS OF DIAGNOSIS

- ▶ Expanded trinucleotide repeat (more than 200) in the *FMR1* gene.
- ▶ Mental retardation and autism in males; large testes after puberty.
- ▶ Learning disabilities or mental retardation in females; premature ovarian failure.
- ▶ Late-onset tremor and ataxia in males and females with moderate trinucleotide repeat (55–200) expansion (premutation carriers).

Clinical Findings

A. Symptoms and Signs

This X-linked condition accounts for more cases of mental retardation in males than any condition except Down syndrome; about 1 in 4000 males is affected. The central nervous system phenotype includes autism spectrum, impulsivity and aggressiveness, and repetitive behaviors. The condition also affects intellectual function in females, although less severely and about 50% less frequently than in males. Affected (heterozygous) young women show no physical signs other than early menopause, but they may have learning difficulties, anxiety, sensory issues, or frank

retardation. Affected males show macro-orchidism (enlarged testes) after puberty, large ears and a prominent jaw, a high-pitched voice, autistic characteristics, and mental retardation. Some males show evidence of a mild connective tissue defect, with joint hypermobility and mitral valve prolapse.

Women who are premutation carriers (55–200 CGG repeats) are at increased risk for premature ovarian failure and mild cognitive abnormalities. Male and female premutation carriers are at risk for mood and anxiety disorders and the development of tremor and ataxia beyond middle age (fragile-X tremor-ataxia syndrome, FXTAS). Changes in the cerebellar white matter may be evident on MRI before symptoms appear. Because of the relatively high prevalence of premutation carriers in the general population (1/130–1/600), older people in whom any of these behavioral or neurologic problems develop should undergo testing of the *FMR1* locus.

B. Laboratory Findings

The first marker for this condition was a small gap, or fragile site, evident near the tip of the long arm of the X chromosome. Subsequently, the condition was found to be due to expansion of a trinucleotide repeat (CGG) near a gene called *FMR1*. All individuals have some CGG repeats in this location, but as the number increases beyond 52, the chances of further expansion during spermatogenesis or oogenesis increase.

Being born with one *FMR1* allele with 200 or more repeats results in mental retardation in most men, and in about 60% of women. The more repeats, the greater the likelihood that further expansion will occur during gametogenesis; this results in anticipation, in which the disorder can worsen from one generation to the next.

Prevention

DNA diagnosis for the number of repeats has supplanted cytogenetic analysis for both clinical and prenatal diagnosis. This should be done on any male or female who has unexplained mental retardation. Newborn screening based on hypermethylation of the *FMR1* gene is being considered as a means of early detection and intervention.

Treatment

Several treatments that address the imbalances in neurotransmission have been developed based on the mouse model and are in clinical trials. Valproic acid may reduce symptoms of hyperactivity and attention deficit, but standard therapies should be tried first.

When to Refer

- For otherwise unexplained mental retardation or learning difficulties in boys and girls.
- For otherwise unexplained tremor or ataxia in middle-aged individuals.
- For premature ovarian failure.
- For genetic counseling.

Gallagher A et al. Fragile X-associated disorders: a clinical overview. J Neurol. 2012 Mar;259(3):401–13. [PMID: 21748281]

Hagerman R et al. Advances in clinical and molecular understanding of the *FMR1* premutation and fragile X-associated tremor/ataxia syndrome. Lancet Neurol. 2013 Aug;12(8): 786–98. [PMID: 23867198]

Kidd SA et al. Fragile X syndrome: a review of associated medical problems. Pediatrics. 2014 Nov;134(5):995–1005. [PMID: 25287458]

Lozano R et al. Modulation of the GABAergic pathway for the treatment of fragile X syndrome. Neuropsychiatr Dis Treat. 2014 Sep 16;10:1769–79. [PMID: 25258535]

Nazareth T et al. Burden of illness among patients with fragile X syndrome (FXS): a Medicaid perspective. Curr Med Res Opin. 2016 Mar;32(3):405–16. [PMID: 26565934]

Tassone F et al. Fragile X premutation. J Neurodev Disord. 2014;6(1):22. [PMID: 25170346]

GAUCHER DISEASE

ESSENTIALS OF DIAGNOSIS

► Deficiency of beta-glucocerebrosidase.

► Anemia and thrombocytopenia; hypersplenism.

► Pathologic fractures.

► Clinical Findings

A. Symptoms and Signs

Gaucher disease has an autosomal recessive pattern of inheritance. A deficiency of beta-glucocerebrosidase causes an accumulation of sphingolipid within phagocytic cells throughout the body. Anemia and thrombocytopenia are common and may be symptomatic; both are due primarily to hypersplenism, but marrow infiltration with Gaucher cells may be a contributing factor. Cortical erosions of bones, especially the vertebrae and femur, are due to local infarctions, but the mechanism is unclear. Episodes of bone pain (termed "crises") are reminiscent of those in sickle cell disease. A hip fracture in a patient of any age with a palpable spleen—especially in a Jewish person of Eastern European origin—suggests the possibility of Gaucher disease. Peripheral neuropathy may develop in patients.

Two uncommon forms of Gaucher disease, called type II and type III, involve neurologic accumulation of sphingolipid and a variety of neurologic problems. Type II is of infantile onset and has a poor prognosis. Heterozygotes for Gaucher disease are at increased risk for developing Parkinson disease.

B. Laboratory Findings

Bone marrow aspirates reveal typical Gaucher cells, which have an eccentric nucleus and periodic acid–Schiff (PAS)-positive inclusions, along with wrinkled cytoplasm and inclusion bodies of a fibrillar type. In addition, the serum acid phosphatase is elevated. Definitive diagnosis requires the demonstration of deficient glucocerebrosidase activity in leukocytes. Hundreds of mutations have been found to cause Gaucher disease and some are highly predictive of the neuronopathic forms. Thus, mutation detection, especially in a young person, is of potential value. Only four mutations in glucocerebrosidase account for more than 90% of the disease among Ashkenazi Jews, in whom the carrier frequency is 1:15.

► Prevention

Most clinical complications can be prevented by early institution of enzyme replacement therapy. Carrier screening, especially among Ashkenazi Jews, detects those couples at 25% risk of having an affected child. Prenatal diagnosis through mutation analysis is feasible. Because of an increased risk of malignancy, especially multiple myeloma and other hematologic cancers, regular screening of adults with Gaucher disease is warranted.

► Treatment

A recombinant form of the enzyme glucocerebrosidase (imiglucerase) for intravenous administration on a regular basis reduces total body stores of glycolipid and improves orthopedic and hematologic manifestations. Unfortunately, the neurologic manifestations of types II and III have not improved with enzyme replacement therapy. The major drawback is the exceptional cost of imiglucerase, which can exceed $300,000 per year for a severely affected adult patient. More recently, an oral therapy that reduces substrate has been approved, but the annual cost is about the same. Early treatment of affected children normalizes growth and bone mineral density and improves liver and spleen size, anemia, and thrombocytopenia. In adults with thrombocytopenia due to splenic sequestration, enzyme replacement often obviates the need for splenectomy. Alternative or complementary therapies, including methods to reduce substrate and to provide a chaperone for a defective enzyme, are being developed. One approved medication, miglustat, does reduce the production of glucocerebroside in some patients, but can be poorly tolerated because of adverse effects.

Barkhuizen M et al. Advances in GBA-associated Parkinson's disease—pathology, presentation and therapies. Neurochem Int. 2016 Feb;93:6–25. [PMID: 26743617]

Baris HN et al. Gaucher disease: the metabolic defect, pathophysiology, phenotypes and natural history. Pediatr Endocrinol Rev 2014 Sep; 12 Suppl 1:72–81. [PMID: 25345088]

Linari S et al. Clinical manifestations and management of Gaucher disease. Clin Cases Miner Bone Metab. 2015 May–Aug; 12(2):157–64. [PMID: 26604942]

Suzuki Y. Chaperone therapy update: Fabry disease, GM1-gangliosidosis and Gaucher disease. Brain Dev. 2013 Jun; 35(6):515–23. [PMID: 23290321]

Utz J et al. Comorbidities and pharmacotherapies in patients with Gaucher disease type 1: The potential for drug-drug interactions. Mol Genet Metab. 2016 Feb;117(2):172–8. [PMID: 26674302]

Zimran A et al. Management of Gaucher disease: enzyme replacement therapy. Pediatr Endocrinol Rev. 2014 Sep; 12(Suppl 1):82–7. [PMID: 25345089]

DISORDERS OF HOMOCYSTEINE METABOLISM

ESSENTIALS OF DIAGNOSIS

► For homocystinuria, dislocated ocular lenses.
► Elevated homocysteine in the urine or plasma.

General Considerations

Considerable evidence has accumulated to support the observation that patients with clinical and angiographic evidence of coronary artery disease tend to have higher levels of plasma homocysteine than persons without coronary artery disease. The relationship has been extended to cerebrovascular and peripheral vascular diseases. Although this effect was initially thought to be due at least in part to heterozygotes for cystathionine beta-synthase deficiency (see below), there is little supporting evidence. Rather, an important factor leading to hyperhomocysteinemia is folate deficiency. Pyridoxine (vitamin B_6) and vitamin B_{12} are also important in the metabolism of methionine, and deficiency of any of these vitamins can lead to accumulation of homocysteine. A number of genes influence utilization of these vitamins and can predispose to deficiency. For example, having one—and especially two—copies of an allele that causes thermolability of methylene tetrahydrofolate reductase predisposes people to elevated fasting homocysteine levels. Both nutritional and most genetic deficiencies of these vitamins can be corrected by dietary supplementation of folic acid and, if serum levels are low, vitamins B_6 and B_{12}. In the United States, cereal grains are fortified with folic acid. However, therapy with B vitamins and folate lowers homocysteine levels significantly but does not reduce the risk of either venous thromboembolism or complications of coronary artery disease. The role of lowering homocysteine as primary prevention for cardiovascular disease has received modest direct support in clinical trials. Hyperhomocysteinemia occurs with end-stage chronic kidney disease.

Clinical Findings

A. Symptoms and Signs

Homocystinuria in its classic form is caused by cystathionine beta-synthase deficiency and exhibits an autosomal recessive pattern of inheritance. This results in extreme elevations of plasma and urinary homocystine levels, a basis for diagnosis of this disorder. Homocystinuria is similar in certain superficial aspects to Marfan syndrome, since patients may have a similar body habitus and ectopia lentis is almost always present. However, mental retardation is often present in homocystinuria, and the cardiovascular events are those of repeated venous and arterial thromboses whose precise cause remains obscure. Thus, the diagnosis should be suspected in patients in the second and third decades of life who have arterial or venous thromboses without other risk factors. Bone mineral density is reduced in untreated patients. Life expectancy is reduced, especially in untreated and pyridoxine-unresponsive patients; myocardial infarction, stroke, and pulmonary embolism are the most common causes of death. This condition is diagnosed by newborn screening for hypermethioninemia; however, pyridoxine-responsive infants may not be detected. In addition, homozygotes for a common mutant allele, p.I278T, show marked clinical variability, with some affected as adults.

B. Laboratory Findings

Although many mutations have been identified in the cystathionine beta-synthase gene (*CBS*), amino acid analysis of plasma remains the most appropriate diagnostic test. Patients should be studied after they have been off folate or pyridoxine supplementation for at least 1 week. Relatively few laboratories currently provide highly reliable assays for homocysteine. Processing of the specimen is crucial to obtain accurate results. The plasma must be separated within 30 minutes; otherwise, blood cells release the amino acid and the measurement will then be artificially elevated.

Prevention

About 50% of patients have a form of cystathionine beta-synthase deficiency that improves biochemically and clinically through pharmacologic doses of pyridoxine (50–500 mg/d) and folate (5–10 mg/d). For these patients, treatment from infancy can prevent retardation and the other clinical problems. Patients who are pyridoxine nonresponders must be treated with a dietary reduction in methionine and supplementation of cysteine, also from infancy. The vitamin betaine is also useful in reducing plasma methionine levels by facilitating a metabolic pathway that bypasses the defective enzyme.

Treatment

Patients with classic homocystinuria who have suffered venous thrombosis receive anticoagulation therapy, but there are no studies to support prophylactic use of warfarin or antiplatelet agents.

Debreceni B et al. The role of homocysteine-lowering B-vitamins in the primary prevention of cardiovascular disease. Cardiovasc Ther. 2014 Jun;32(3):130–8. [PMID: 24571382]

e Silva Ade S et al. Effects of physical activity and training programs on plasma homocysteine levels: a systematic review. Amino Acids. 2014 Aug;46(8):1795–804. [PMID: 24770903]

Sørensen JT et al. Molecular and biochemical investigations of patients with intermediate or severe hyperhomocysteinemia. Mol Genet Metab. 2016 Mar;117(3):344–50. [PMID: 26750749]

Weber DR et al. Low bone mineral density is a common finding in patients with homocystinuria. Mol Genet Metab. 2016 Mar;117(3):351–4. [PMID: 26689745]

Zeng R et al. The effect of folate fortification on folic acid-based homocysteine-lowering intervention and stroke risk: a meta-analysis. Public Health Nutr. 2015 Jun;18(8):1514–21. [PMID: 25323814]

KLINEFELTER SYNDROME

ESSENTIALS OF DIAGNOSIS

▶ Males with hypergonadotropic hypogonadism and small testes.

▶ 47,XXY karyotype.

▶ Clinical Findings

A. Symptoms and Signs

Boys with an extra X chromosome are normal in appearance before puberty; thereafter, they have disproportionately long legs and arms, sparse body hair, a female escutcheon, gynecomastia, and small testes. Infertility is due to azoospermia; the seminiferous tubules are hyalinized. The incidence is 1 in 660 newborn males, but the diagnosis is often not made until a man is evaluated for inability to conceive. Intellectual disability is somewhat more common than in the general population. Many men with Klinefelter syndrome have language-based learning problems. However, their intelligence usually tests within the broad range of normal. As adults, detailed psychometric testing may reveal a deficiency in executive skills. The risk of osteoporosis, breast cancer and diabetes mellitus is much higher in men with Klinefelter syndrome than in 46,XY men.

B. Laboratory Findings

Low serum testosterone is common. The karyotype is typically 47,XXY, but other sex chromosome anomalies cause variations of Klinefelter syndrome.

▶ Prevention

Screening for cancer (especially of the breast), deep venous thrombosis, and glucose intolerance are indicated.

▶ Treatment

Treatment with testosterone after puberty is advisable but will not restore fertility. However, men with Klinefelter syndrome have had mature sperm aspirated from their testes and injected into oocytes, resulting in fertilization. After the blastocysts have been implanted into the uterus of a partner, conception has resulted. However, men with Klinefelter syndrome do have an increased risk for aneuploidy in sperm, and therefore genomic analysis of a blastocyst should be considered before implantation.

Aksglaede L et al. Testicular function and fertility in men with Klinefelter syndrome: a review. Eur J Endocrinol. 2013 Mar 15; 168(4):R76–76. [PMID: 23504510]

Gies I et al. Management of Klinefelter syndrome during transition. Eur J Endocrinol. 2014 Aug;171(2):R67–77. [PMID: 24801585]

Gravholt CH. Sex chromosome abnormalities. In: Rimoin DL et al (editors). Emery and Rimoin's Principles and Practice of Medical Genetics, 6th ed. Philadelphia: Churchill Livingstone, 2013.

Nahata L et al. Sperm retrieval in adolescents and young adults with Klinefelter syndrome: a prospective, pilot study. J Pediatr. 2016 Mar;170:260–5.e2. [PMID: 26746120]

Sokol RZ. It's not all about the testes: medical issues in Klinefelter patients. Fertil Steril. 2012 Aug;98(2):261–5. [PMID: 22704628]

MARFAN SYNDROME

ESSENTIALS OF DIAGNOSIS

▶ Disproportionately tall stature, thoracic deformity, and joint laxity or contractures.

▶ Ectopia lentis and myopia.

▶ Aortic root dilation and dissection; mitral valve prolapse.

▶ Mutation in *FBN1*, the gene encoding fibrillin-1.

▶ General Considerations

Marfan syndrome, a systemic connective tissue disease, has an autosomal dominant pattern of inheritance. It is characterized by abnormalities of the skeletal, ocular, and cardiovascular systems; spontaneous pneumothorax; dural ectasia; and striae atrophicae. Of most concern is disease of the ascending aorta, which begins as a dilated aortic root. Histology of the aorta shows diffuse medial degeneration. Mitral valve leaflets are also abnormal and mitral prolapse and regurgitation may be present, often with elongated chordae tendineae, which on occasion may rupture.

▶ Clinical Findings

A. Symptoms and Signs

Affected patients are typically tall, with particularly long arms, legs, and digits (arachnodactyly). However, there can be wide variability in the clinical presentation. Commonly, scoliosis and anterior chest deformity, such as pectus excavatum, are found. Ectopia lentis is present in about half of patients; severe myopia is common and retinal detachment can occur. Mitral valve prolapse is seen in about 85% of patients. Aortic root dilation is common and leads to aortic regurgitation or dissection with rupture. To diagnose Marfan syndrome, people with an affected relative need features in at least two systems. People with no family history need features in the skeletal system, two other systems, and one of the major criteria of ectopia lentis, dilation of the aortic root, or aortic dissection. Patients with homocystinuria due to cystathionine beta-synthase deficiency also have dislocated lenses, tall, disproportionate stature, and thoracic deformity. They tend to have below normal intelligence, stiff joints, and a predisposition to arterial and venous occlusive disease. Males with Klinefelter syndrome do not show the typical ocular or cardiovascular features of Marfan syndrome and are generally sporadic occurrences in the family.

B. Laboratory Findings

Mutations in the fibrillin gene (*FBN1*) on chromosome 15 cause Marfan syndrome. Nonetheless, no simple laboratory test is available to support the diagnosis in questionable cases because related conditions may also be due to defects in fibrillin. The nature of the *FBN1* mutation has little predictive value in terms of prognosis. The pathogenesis of Marfan syndrome involves aberrant regulation of transforming growth factor (TGF)-beta activity. Mutations in either of two receptors for TGF-beta (TGFBR1 and TGFBR2) can cause conditions that resemble Marfan syndrome in terms of aortic aneurysm and dissection and autosomal dominant inheritance. Mutations in more than one dozen other genes can predispose adults to thoracic aortic aneurysm and dissection.

Prevention

There is prenatal and presymptomatic diagnosis for patients in whom the molecular defect in *FBN1* has been found.

Treatment

Children with Marfan syndrome require regular ophthalmologic surveillance to correct visual acuity and thus prevent amblyopia, and annual orthopedic consultation for diagnosis of scoliosis at an early enough stage so that bracing might delay progression. Patients of all ages require echocardiography at least annually to monitor aortic root diameter and mitral valve function. Long-term beta-adrenergic blockade, titrated to individual tolerance but enough to produce a negative inotropic effect (atenolol, 1–2 mg/kg orally daily) retards the rate of aortic dilation. A dozen clinical trials comparing the effectiveness of atenolol and losartan or other angiotensin receptor blockers (ARBs), drugs that reduces activity of TGF-beta, are underway or recently completed. Several trials suggested a benefit of an ARB over beta-blockade, but the largest found no difference in benefit when young subjects were treated with optimally titrated doses of atenolol or losartan. Restriction from vigorous physical exertion protects from aortic dissection. Prophylactic replacement of the aortic root with a composite graft when the diameter reaches 45–50 mm in an adult (normal: less than 40 mm) prolongs life. A procedure to resuspend the patient's native aortic valve and replace just the aneurysmal sinuses of Valsalva and ascending aorta avoids the need for lifelong anticoagulation. Women with Marfan syndrome are at heightened risk for aortic dissection in the peripartum and postpartum periods. Having an aortic root dimension greater than 40 mm should prompt consideration for prophylactic, valve-sparing aortic repair before undertaking a pregnancy.

Prognosis

People with Marfan syndrome who are untreated commonly die in the fourth or fifth decade from aortic dissection or heart failure secondary to aortic or mitral regurgitation. However, because of earlier diagnosis, lifestyle modifications, beta-adrenergic blockade, and prophylactic aortic and mitral valve surgery, life expectancy has increased by several decades.

When to Refer

- For detailed ophthalmologic examination.
- For at least annual cardiologic evaluation.
- For moderate scoliosis.
- For pregnancy in a woman with Marfan syndrome.
- For genetic counseling.

When to Admit

Any patient with Marfan syndrome in whom severe or unusual chest pain develops should be hospitalized to exclude pneumothorax and aortic dissection.

Bradley TJ et al. The expanding clinical spectrum of extracardiovascular and cardiovascular manifestations of heritable thoracic aortic aneurysm and dissection. Can J Cardiol. 2016 Jan; 32(1):86–99. [PMID: 26724513]

David TE et al. Long-term results of aortic root repair using the reimplantation technique. J Thorac Cardiovasc Surg. 2013 Mar; 145(3 Suppl):S22–5. [PMID: 23260437]

Lacro RV et al; Pediatric Heart Network Investigators. Atenolol versus losartan in children and young adults with Marfan's syndrome. N Engl J Med. 2014 Nov 27;371(22):2061–71. [PMID: 25405392]

Price J et al. Long-term outcomes of aortic root operations for Marfan syndrome: a comparison of Bentall versus aortic valve-sparing procedures. J Thorac Cardiovasc Surg. 2016 Feb; 151(2):330–8. [PMID: 26704057]

Pyeritz RE. Evaluation of the adolescent or adult with some features of Marfan syndrome. Genet Med. 2012 Jan;14(1):171–7. [PMID: 22237449]

Pyeritz RE. Marfan syndrome and related disorders. In: Rimoin DL et al (editors). *Emery and Rimoin's Principles and Practice of Medical Genetics*, 6th ed. Philadelphia: Churchill-Livingstone, 2013.

HEREDITARY HEMORRHAGIC TELANGIECTASIA

ESSENTIALS OF DIAGNOSIS

- ▸ Recurrent epistaxis.
- ▸ Mucocutaneous telangiectases.
- ▸ Visceral arteriovenous malformations (especially lung, liver, brain, bowel).

Clinical Findings

A. Symptoms and Signs

Hereditary hemorrhagic telangiectasia (HHT), formerly termed "Osler-Weber-Rendu syndrome," is an autosomal dominant disorder of development of the vasculature.

Epistaxis may begin in childhood or later in adolescence. Punctate telangiectases of the lips, tongue, fingers, and skin generally appear in later childhood and adolescence. Arteriovenous malformations (AVMs) can occur at any age in the brain, lungs, and liver. Bleeding from the gastrointestinal tract is due to mucosal vascular malformations and usually is not a problem until mid-adult years or later. Pulmonary AVMs can cause hypoxemia (with peripheral cyanosis, dyspnea, and clubbing) and right-to-left shunting (with embolic stroke or brain abscess). The criteria for diagnosis require presence of three of the following four features: (1) recurrent epistaxis, (2) visceral AVMs, (3) mucocutaneous telangiectases, and (4) being the near relative of a clearly affected individual. Mutation analysis can be used for presymptomatic diagnosis or exclusion of the worry of HHT.

B. Laboratory Findings

MR or CT arteriography detects AVMs. Mutations in at least five genes can cause HHT. Three have been identified, and molecular analysis to identify them is available; these mutations in *ENG, ALK1*, and *SMAD4* account for about 87% of families with HHT. When the familial mutation is known, molecular testing is far more cost effective than repeated clinical screening of relatives who are at risk.

▶ Prevention

Embolization of pulmonary AVMs with wire coils or other occlusive devices reduces the risk of stroke and brain abscess. Treatment of brain AVMs reduces the risk of hemorrhagic stroke. All patients with HHT with evidence of a pulmonary shunt should practice routine endocarditis prophylaxis (see Table 33–6). All intravenous lines (except those for transfusion of red blood cells and radiographic contrast) should have an air-filter to prevent embolization of an air bubble. Prenatal diagnosis through mutation detection is possible.

▶ Treatment

All patients in whom the diagnosis of HHT is considered should have an MRI of the brain with contrast. A contrast echocardiogram will detect most pulmonary AVMs when "bubbles" appear on the left side of the heart after 3–6 cardiac cycles. A positive contrast echocardiogram should be followed by a high-resolution CT angiogram for localization of pulmonary AVMs. Patients who have AVMs with a feeding artery of 1–2 mm diameter or greater should undergo embolization. After successful embolization of all treatable pulmonary AVMs, the CT angiogram should be repeated in 6 months and 3 years. A person with a negative contrast echocardiogram should have the test repeated every 5 years. Several recent studies suggest that treatment with anti-estrogenic agents (eg, tamoxifen), thalidomide or its relatives, or anti-vascular endothelial growth factor agents (eg, bevacizumab) can reduce epistaxis and gastrointestinal bleeding and improve hepatic shunting. Randomized, controlled clinical trials of these various therapies are ongoing.

Arizmendez NP et al. Intravenous bevacizumab for complications of hereditary hemorrhagic telangiectasia: a review of the literature. Int Forum Allergy Rhinol. 2015 Nov;5(11):1042–7. [PMID: 26202958]

Donaldson JW et al. Complications and mortality in hereditary hemorrhagic telangiectasia: A population-based study. Neurology. 2015 May 5;84(18):1886–93. [PMID: 25862798]

Faughnan ME et al; HHT Guidelines Working Group. International guidelines for the diagnosis and management of hereditary haemorrhagic telangiectasia. J Med Genet. 2011 Feb;48(2):73–87. [PMID: 19553198]

McDonald J et al. Hereditary hemorrhagic telangiectasia: genetics and molecular diagnostics in a new era. Front Genet. 2015 Jan 26;6:1. [PMID: 25674101]

McDonald J, Pyeritz RE. Hereditary hemorrhagic telangiectasia. GeneReviews 2014 Jul 14. http://www.ncbi.nlm.nih.gov/books/NBK1351/ [PMID: 20301525]

Sports Medicine & Outpatient Orthopedics

Anthony Luke, MD, MPH

C. Benjamin Ma, MD

Musculoskeletal problems account for about 10–20% of outpatient primary care clinical visits. Orthopedic problems can be classified as traumatic (ie, injury-related) or atraumatic (ie, degenerative or overuse syndromes) as well as acute or chronic. The mechanism of injury is usually the most helpful part of the history in determining the diagnosis.

SHOULDER

1. Subacromial Impingement Syndrome

ESSENTIALS OF DIAGNOSIS

- ▶ Shoulder pain with overhead motion.
- ▶ Night pain with sleeping on shoulder.
- ▶ Pain with internal rotation.
- ▶ Numbness and pain radiation below the elbow are usually due to cervical spine disease.

▶ General Considerations

The subacromial impingement syndrome describes a collection of diagnoses that cause mechanical inflammation in the subacromial space. Causes of impingement syndrome can be related to muscle strength imbalances, poor scapula control, rotator cuff tears, and subacromial bone spurs.

The chief complaints for shoulder problems are usually pain, instability, weakness, or loss of range of motion. With any shoulder problem, it is important to establish the patient's hand dominance, occupation, and recreational activities because shoulder injuries may present differently depending on the demands placed on the shoulder joint. For example, baseball pitchers with impingement syndrome may complain of pain while throwing. Alternatively, elders with even full thickness rotator cuff tears may not complain of any pain because the demands on the joint are low.

▶ Clinical Findings

A. Symptoms and Signs

Shoulder problems classically present with one or more of the following: pain with overhead activities, nocturnal pain with sleeping on the shoulder, or pain on internal rotation (eg, putting on a jacket or bra). On inspection, there may be appreciable atrophy in the supraspinatus or infraspinatus fossa. The patient with impingement syndrome can have mild scapula winging or "dyskinesis." The patient often has a rolled-forward shoulder posture or head-forward posture. On palpation, the patient can have tenderness over the anterolateral shoulder at the edge of the greater tuberosity. The patient may lack full active range of motion (Table 41–1) but should have preserved passive range of motion. Impingement symptoms can be elicited with the Neer and Hawkins impingement signs (Table 41–1).

B. Imaging

The following four radiographic views should be ordered to evaluate subacromial impingement syndrome: the anteroposterior (AP) scapula, the AP acromioclavicular joint, the lateral scapula (scapular Y), and the axillary lateral. The AP scapula view can rule out glenohumeral joint arthritis. The AP acromioclavicular view evaluates the acromioclavicular joint for inferior spurs. The scapula Y view evaluates the acromial shape, and the axillary lateral view visualizes the glenohumeral joint as well and for the presence of os acromiale.

MRI of the shoulder may demonstrate full or partial thickness tears or tendinosis. Ultrasound evaluation may demonstrate thickening of the rotator cuff tendons and tendinosis. Tears may also be visualized on ultrasound, although it is more difficult to identify partial tears from small full thickness than on MRI.

▶ Treatment

A. Conservative

The first-line treatment for impingement syndrome is usually a conservative approach with education, activity

Table 41–1. Shoulder examination.

Maneuver	Description
Rotator cuff strength testing	
Supraspinatus (open can) test 	Perform resisted shoulder abduction at 90 degrees with slight forward flexion to around 45 degrees to test for supraspinatus tendon strength ("open can" test), or with shoulder abduction at 30 degrees and flexion to 30 degrees ("empty can" test).
External rotation	The patient resists by externally rotating the arms with elbows at his or her side.
Internal rotation (lift off test)	A positive "lift-off" test is the inability of the patient to hold his or her hand away from the body when reaching toward the small of the back. The clinician pushes the patient's hand toward the back while the patient resists. A positive lift-off indicates subscapularis tendon insufficiency.

(continued)

Table 41–1. Shoulder examination. (continued)

Maneuver	Description
Internal rotation (belly press test)	A positive "belly-press" test is the inability to hold the elbow in front of the trunk while pressing down with the hand on the belly. A positive belly press test indicates subscapularis tendon insufficiency.
Impingement tests	
Neer impingement sign	Perform by having the clinician flex the shoulder maximally in an overhead position. The test is positive when pain is reproduced with full passive shoulder flexion. Sensitivity is 79%; specificity is 53%.
Hawkins impingement sign	Perform with the shoulder forward flexed 90 degrees and the elbow flexed at 90 degrees. The shoulder is then maximally internally rotated to impinge the greater tuberosity on the undersurface of the acromion. The test is considered positive when the patient's pain is reproduced by this maneuver. Sensitivity is 79%; specificity is 59%.

(continued)

Table 41–1. Shoulder examination. (continued)

Maneuver	Description
Stability tests	
Apprehension test 	With persistent anterior instability or a recent dislocation, the patient feels pain or guards when the shoulder is abducted and externally rotated at 90 degrees. With posterior instability, the patient is apprehensive with the shoulder forward flexed and internally rotated to 90 degrees with a posteriorly directed force.
Load and shift test 	Perform to determine shoulder instability by manually translating the humeral head anteriorly and posteriorly in relation to the glenoid. However, this test can be difficult to perform when the patient is not relaxed.
O'Brien test Palm down Palm up	Performed to rule out labral cartilage tears that often occur following a shoulder subluxation or dislocation. The test involves flexing the patient's arm to 90 degrees, fully internally rotating the arm so the thumb is facing down (palm down) and adducting the arm to 10 degrees. Once positioned properly, the clinician applies downward force and asks the patient to resist. The test is then repeated in the same position except that the patient has his arm fully supinated (palm up). A positive O'Brien test for labral tear is pain deep in the shoulder with palm down more than the palm up. The O'Brien test can also be used to identify AC joint pathology. The patient would typically complain equally of pain directly over the AC joint with the palm down or up.

modification, and physical therapy exercises. Impingement syndrome can be caused by muscle weakness or tear. Rotator cuff muscle strengthening can alleviate weakness or pain, unless the tendons are seriously compromised, which may cause more symptoms. Physical therapy is directed at rotator cuff muscle strengthening, scapula stabilization, and postural exercises. There is no strong evidence supporting the effectiveness of ice and NSAIDs as a prolonged therapy. In a Cochrane review, corticosteroid injections produced slightly better relief of symptoms in the short-term when compared with placebo. Most patients respond well to conservative treatment.

B. Surgical

Procedures include arthroscopic acromioplasty with coracoacromial ligament release, bursectomy, or debridement or repair of rotator cuff tears.

▶ When to Refer

- Failure of conservative treatment over 3 months.
- Young and active patients with impingement due to full thickness rotator cuff tears.

Hermans J et al. Does this patient with shoulder pain have rotator cuff disease? The Rational Clinical Examination systematic review. JAMA. 2013 Aug 28;310(8):837–47. [PMID: 23982370]

2. Rotator Cuff Tears

ESSENTIALS OF DIAGNOSIS

- ▶ A common cause of shoulder impingement syndrome after age 40.
- ▶ Difficulty lifting the arm with limited active range of motion.
- ▶ Weakness with resisted strength testing suggests full thickness tears.

▶ General Considerations

Rotator cuff tears can be caused by acute injuries related to falls on an outstretched arm or to pulling on the shoulder. It can also be related to chronic repetitive injuries with overhead movement and lifting. **Partial rotator cuff tears are one of the most common reasons for impingement syndrome.** Full thickness rotator cuff tears are usually more symptomatic and may require surgical treatment. The most commonly torn tendon is the supraspinatus.

▶ Clinical Findings

A. Symptoms and Signs

Most patients complain of weakness or pain with overhead movement. Night pain is also a common complaint. The clinical findings with rotator cuff tears include those of the impingement syndrome except that with full-thickness rotator cuff tears there may be more obvious weakness noted with light resistance testing of specific rotator cuff muscles. Supraspinatus tendon strength is tested with resisted shoulder abduction at 90 degrees with slight forward flexion to around 45 degrees ("open can" test) (Table 41–1). Infraspinatus/teres minor strength is tested with resisted shoulder external rotation with shoulder at 0 degrees abduction, elbow by side (Table 41–1). Subscapularis strength is tested with the "lift-off" or "belly-press" tests (Table 41–1). The affected patient usually also has positive Neer and Hawkins impingement tests.

B. Imaging

Recommended radiographs are very similar to impingement syndrome: AP scapula (glenohumeral), axillary lateral, supraspinatus outlet, and AP acromioclavicular joint views. The AP scapula view is useful in visualizing rotator cuff tears because degenerative changes can appear between the acromion and greater tuberosity of the shoulder. Axillary lateral views show superior elevation of the humeral head in relation to the center of the glenoid. Supraspinatus outlet views allow evaluation of the shape of the acromion. High-grade acromial spurs are associated with a higher incidence of rotator cuff tears. The AP acromioclavicular joint view evaluates for the presence of acromioclavicular joint arthritis, which can mimic rotator cuff tears, and for spurs that can cause rotator cuff injuries.

MRI is the best method for visualizing rotator cuff tears. The MR arthrogram can show partial or small (less than 1 cm) rotator cuff tears. For patients who cannot undergo MRI testing or when postoperative artifacts limit MRI evaluations, ultrasonography can be helpful.

▶ Treatment

Partial rotator cuff tears may heal with scarring. Most partial rotator cuff tears can be treated with physical therapy and scapular and rotator cuff muscle strengthening. However, research suggests that 40% of the partial thickness tears progress to full thickness tears in 2 years. Physical therapy can strengthen the remaining muscles to compensate for loss of strength and can have high rate of success for chronic tears. Physical therapy is also an option for older sedentary patients. On the contrary, full-thickness rotator cuff tears do not heal well and also have a tendency to increase in size with time. Forty-nine percent of the full thickness tears get bigger on an average of 2.8 years. When tears get larger, they are also associated with worsening pain. Fatty infiltration progresses in full thickness rotator cuff tears and it is a negative prognostic factor for successful surgical treatment. Fatty infiltration is an irreversible process so operative interventions are usually performed when the degree of infiltration is low. **Most young active patients with acute, full-thickness tears should be treated with operative fixation.** Full-thickness subscapularis tendon tears should undergo surgical repair as untreated tears usually lead to premature osteoarthritis (OA) of the shoulder.

When to Refer

- Young and active patients with full thickness rotator cuff tears.
- Partial tears with greater than 50% involvement and with significant pain.
- Older and sedentary patients with full-thickness rotator cuff tears who have not responded to nonoperative treatment.
- Full thickness subscapularis tears.

Gombera MM et al. Rotator cuff tear and glenohumeral instability: a systematic review. Clin Orthop Relat Res. 2014 Aug; 472(8):2448–56. [PMID: 24043432]

Keener JD et al. A prospective evaluation of survivorship of asymptomatic degenerative rotator cuff tears. J Bone Joint Surg Am. 2015 Jan 21;97(2):89–98. [PMID: 25609434]

Kuhn JE et al; MOON Shoulder Group. Effectiveness of physical therapy in treating atraumatic full-thickness rotator cuff tears: a multicenter prospective cohort study. J Shoulder Elbow Surg. 2013 Oct;22(10):1371–9. [PMID: 23540577]

3. Shoulder Dislocation & Instability

ESSENTIALS OF DIAGNOSIS

- ► Most dislocations (95%) are in the anterior direction.
- ► Pain and apprehension with an unstable shoulder that is abducted and externally rotated.
- ► Acute shoulder dislocations should be reduced as quickly as possible, using manual relocation techniques if necessary.

General Considerations

The shoulder is a ball and socket joint, similar to the hip. However, the bony contours of the shoulder bones are much different than the hip. Overall, the joint has much less stability than the hip, allowing greater movement and action. Stabilizing the shoulder joint relies heavily on rotator cuff muscle strength and also scapular control. If patients have poor scapular control or weak rotator cuff tendons or tears, their shoulders are more likely to have instability. Ninety-five percent of the shoulder dislocations/instability occur in the anterior direction. Dislocations usually are caused by a fall on an outstretched and abducted arm. Patients complain of pain and feeling of instability when the arm is in the abducted and externally rotated position. Posterior dislocations are usually caused by falls from a height, epileptic seizures, or electric shocks. Traumatic shoulder dislocation can lead to instability. The rate of repeated dislocation is directly related to the patient's age: patients age 21 years or younger have a 70–90% risk of redislocation, whereas patients age 40 years or older have a much lower rate (20–30%). Ninety percent of young active individuals who had traumatic shoulder dislocation have labral injuries often described as Bankart lesions when the anterior inferior labrum is torn, which can lead to continued instability. Older patients (over age 55 years) are more likely to have rotator cuff tears or fractures following dislocation. Atraumatic shoulder dislocations are usually caused by intrinsic ligament laxity or repetitive microtrauma leading to joint instability. This is often seen in swimmers, gymnasts, and pitchers as well as other athletes involved in overhead and throwing sports.

Clinical Findings

A. Symptoms and Signs

For acute traumatic dislocations, patients usually have an obvious deformity with the humeral head dislocated anteriorly. The patient holds the shoulder and arm in an externally rotated position. The patient complains of acute pain and deformity that are improved with manual relocation of the shoulder. Reductions are usually performed in the emergency department. Even after reduction, the patient will continue to have limited range of motion and pain for 4–6 weeks, especially following a first-time shoulder dislocation.

Patients with recurrent dislocations can have less pain with subsequent dislocations. Posterior dislocations can be easily missed because the patient usually holds the shoulder and arm in an internally rotated position, which makes the shoulder deformity less obvious. Patients complain of difficulty pushing open a door.

Atraumatic shoulder instability is usually well tolerated with activities of daily living. Patients usually complain of a "sliding" sensation during exercises or strenuous activities such as throwing. Such dislocations may be less symptomatic and can often undergo spontaneous reduction of the shoulder with pain resolving within days after onset. The clinical examination for shoulder instability includes the apprehension test (Table 41–1), the load and shift test (Table 41–1) and the O'Brien test (Table 41–1). Most patients with persistent shoulder instability have preserved range of motion.

B. Imaging

Radiographs for acute dislocations should include a standard trauma series of AP and axillary lateral scapula (glenohumeral) views to determine the relationship of the humerus and the glenoid and to rule out fractures. Orthogonal views are used to identify a posterior shoulder dislocation, which can be missed easily with one AP view of the shoulder. An axillary lateral view of the shoulder can be safely performed even in the acute setting of a patient with a painful shoulder dislocation. For chronic injuries or symptomatic instability, these recommended radiographic views are helpful to identify bony injuries and Hill-Sachs lesions (indented compression fractures at the posterior-superior part of the humeral head associated with anterior shoulder dislocation). MRI is commonly used to show soft tissue injuries to the labrum and to visualize associated rotator cuff tears. MRI arthrograms better identify labral tears and ligamentous structures. Three-dimensional CT scans are being used to determine the significance of bone loss.

Treatment

For **acute dislocations**, the shoulder should be reduced as soon as possible. The Stimson procedure is the least traumatic method and is quite effective. The patient lies prone with the dislocated arm hanging off the examination table with a weight applied to the wrist to provide traction for 20–30 minutes. Afterward, gentle medial mobilization can be applied manually to assist the reduction. The shoulder can also be reduced with axial "traction" on the arm with "counter-traction" along the trunk. The patient should be sedated and relaxed. The shoulder can then be gently internally and externally rotated to guide it back into the socket.

Initial treatment of acute shoulder dislocations should include sling immobilization for 2–4 weeks along with pendulum exercises. Early physical therapy can be used to maintain range of motion and strengthening of rotator cuff muscles. Patients can also modify their activities to avoid active and risky sports. For patients with a traumatic incident and unilateral shoulder dislocation, a Bankart lesion is commonly present. The risk of recurrence is dependent on the age of first shoulder dislocation. Young patients (less than 27 years of age) can have recurrence up to 70% whereas patients older than 40 years old have recurrences as low as 10%. However, once the patient has a second dislocation, the recurrence rate is extremely high, up to 95%. Operative intervention is the only treatment that has been shown to decrease recurrence. Open and arthroscopic stabilization can have very similar outcomes.

The treatment of **atraumatic shoulder instability** is different than traumatic shoulder instability. Patients with chronic, recurrent shoulder dislocations should be managed with physical therapy and a regular maintenance program, consisting of scapular stabilization and postural and rotator cuff strengthening exercises. Activities may need to be modified. Surgical reconstructions are less successful for atraumatic shoulder instability than for traumatic shoulder instability.

When to Refer

- Patients who are at risk for second dislocation, such as young patients, certain job holders (eg, police officers, fire fighters, and rock climbers) to avoid recurrent dislocation or dislocation while at work.
- Patients who have not responded to conservative approach or who have chronic instability.

Chahal J et al. Anatomic Bankart repair compared with nonoperative treatment and/or arthroscopic lavage for first-time traumatic shoulder dislocation. Arthroscopy. 2012 Apr; 28(4):565–75. [PMID: 22336435]

4. Adhesive Capsulitis ("Frozen Shoulder")

ESSENTIALS OF DIAGNOSIS

- ▶ Very painful shoulder triggered by minimal or no trauma.
- ▶ Pain out of proportion to clinical findings during the inflammatory phase.
- ▶ Stiffness during the "freezing" phase and resolution during the "thawing" phase.

General Considerations

Adhesive capsulitis ("frozen shoulder") is seen commonly in patients 40 to 65 years old. It is more commonly seen in women than men, especially in perimenopausal women or in patients with endocrine disorders, such as diabetes mellitus or thyroid disease. Adhesive capsulitis is a self-limiting but very debilitating disease.

Clinical Findings

A. Symptoms and Signs

Patients usually present with a painful shoulder that has a limited range of motion with both passive and active movements. A useful clinical sign is limitation of movement of external rotation with the elbow by the side of the trunk (Table 41–1). Strength is usually normal but it can appear diminished when the patient is in pain.

There are three phases: the inflammatory phase, the "freezing" phase, and the "thawing" phase. During the **inflammatory phase**, which usually lasts 4–6 months, patients complain of a very painful shoulder without obvious clinical findings to suggest trauma, fracture, or rotator cuff tear. During the **"freezing" phase**, which also usually lasts 4–6 months, the shoulder becomes stiffer and stiffer even though the pain is improving. The **"thawing" phase** can take up to a year as the shoulder slowly regains its motion. The total duration of an idiopathic frozen shoulder is usually about 24 months; it can be much longer for patients who have trauma or an endocrinopathy.

B. Imaging

Standard AP, axillary, and lateral glenohumeral radiographs are useful to rule out glenohumeral arthritis, which can also present with limited active and passive range of motion. However, adhesive capsulitis is usually a clinical diagnosis, and it does not need an extensive diagnostic work-up.

Treatment

Adhesive capsulitis is caused by acute inflammation of the capsule followed by scarring and remodeling. During the acute "freezing" phase, NSAIDs and physical therapy are recommended to maintain motion. There is also evidence of short-term benefit from intra-articular corticosteroid injection or oral prednisone. One study demonstrated improvement at 6 weeks but not 12 weeks following 30 mg of daily prednisone for 3 weeks. During the "freezing" phase, the shoulder is less painful but remains stiff. Anti-inflammatory medication is not as helpful during the "thawing" phase as it is during the "freezing" phase, and the shoulder symptoms usually resolve with time. Surgical treatments include manipulation under anesthesia and arthroscopic release.

► When to Refer

• When the patient does not respond after more than 6 months of conservative treatment.

• When there is no progress or worsening range of motion over 3 months.

Robinson CM et al. Frozen shoulder. J Bone Joint Surg Br. 2012 Jan;94(1):1–9. [PMID: 22219239]

SPINE PROBLEMS

1. Low Back Pain

ESSENTIALS OF DIAGNOSIS

► Nerve root impingement is suspected when pain is leg-dominant rather than back-dominant.

► Alarming signs for serious spinal disease include unexplained weight loss, failure to improve with treatment, severe pain for more than 6 weeks, and night or rest pain.

► The cauda equina syndrome often presents with bowel or bladder symptoms (or both) and is an emergency.

► General Considerations

Low back pain remains the most common cause of disability for patients under the age of 45 and is the second most common cause for primary care visits. The annual prevalence of low back pain is 15–45%, and the annual cost in the United States is over $50 billion. Low back pain is the condition associated with the highest years lived with disability. Approximately 80% of episodes of low back pain resolve within 2 weeks and 90% resolve within 6 weeks. The exact cause of the low back pain is often difficult to diagnose; its cause is often multifactorial, although there are usually degenerative changes in the lumbar spine.

Alarming symptoms for back pain caused by cancer include unexplained weight loss, failure to improve with treatment, pain for more than 6 weeks, and pain at night or rest. History of cancer and age older than 50 years are other risk factors for malignancy. Alarming symptoms for infection include fever, rest pain, recent infection (urinary tract infection, cellulitis, pneumonia), or history of immuno-compromise or injection drug use. The **cauda equina**

syndrome is suggested by urinary retention or incontinence, saddle anesthesia, decreased anal sphincter tone or fecal incontinence, bilateral lower extremity weakness, and progressive neurologic deficits. Risk factors for back pain due to vertebral fracture include use of corticosteroids, age over 70 years, history of osteoporosis, severe trauma, and presence of a contusion or abrasion. Back pain may also be the presenting symptom in other serious medical problems, including abdominal aortic aneurysm, peptic ulcer disease, kidney stones, or pancreatitis.

► Clinical Findings

A. Symptoms and Signs

The physical examination can be conducted with the patient in the standing, sitting, supine, and finally prone positions to avoid frequent repositioning of the patient. In the standing position, the patient's posture can be observed. Commonly encountered spinal asymmetries include scoliosis, thoracic kyphosis, and lumbar hyperlordosis. The active range of motion of the lumbar spine can be assessed while standing. The common directions include flexion, extension, rotation and lateral bending. The one-leg standing extension test assesses for pain as the patient stands on one leg while extending the spine. A positive test can be caused by pars interarticularis fractures (spondylolysis or spondylolisthesis) or facet joint arthritis.

With the patient sitting, motor strength, reflexes, and sensation can be tested (Table 41–2). The major muscles in the lower extremities are assessed for weakness by eliciting a resisted isometric contraction for approximately 5 seconds.

Table 41–2. Neurologic testing of lumbosacral nerve disorders.

Nerve Root	Motor	Reflex	Sensory Area
L1	Hip flexion	None	Groin
L2	Hip flexion	None	Thigh
L3	Extension of knee	Knee jerk	Knee
L4	Dorsiflexion of ankle	Knee jerk	Medial calf
L5	Dorsiflexion of first toe	Babinski reflex	First dorsal web space between first and second toes
S1	Plantar flexion of foot, knee flexors or hamstrings	Ankle jerk	Lateral foot
S2	Knee flexors or hamstrings	Knee flexor	Back of the thigh
S2–S4	External anal sphincter	Anal reflex, rectal tone	Perianal area

It is important to compare the strength bilaterally to detect subtle muscle weakness. Similarly, sensory testing to light touch can be checked in specific dermatomes for corresponding nerve root function. Knee (femoral nerve L2–4), ankle (deep peroneal nerve L4–L5), and Babinski (sciatic nerve L5–S1) reflexes can be checked with the patient sitting.

In the supine position, the hip should be evaluated for range of motion, particularly internal rotation. The straight leg raise test puts traction and compression forces on the lower lumbar nerve roots.

Finally, in the prone position, the clinician can carefully palpate each vertebral level of the spine and sacroiliac joints for tenderness. A rectal examination is required if the cauda equina syndrome is suspected. Superficial skin tenderness to a light touch over the lumbar spine, overreaction to maneuvers in the regular back examination, low back pain on axial loading of spine in standing, inconsistency in the straight leg raise test or on the neurologic examination suggest nonorthopedic causes for the pain or malingering.

B. Imaging

In the absence of alarming "red flag" symptoms suggesting infection, malignancy, or cauda equina syndrome, most patients do not need diagnostic imaging, including radiographs, in the first 6 weeks. The Agency for Healthcare Research and Quality guidelines for obtaining lumbar radiographs are summarized in Table 41–3. Most clinicians obtain radiographs for new back pain in patients older than 50 years. If done, radiographs of the lumbar spine should include AP and lateral views. Oblique views can be useful if the neuroforamina or bone lesions need to be visualized. MRI is the method of choice in the evaluation of symptoms

Table 41–3. AHRQ criteria for lumbar radiographs in patients with acute low back pain.

Possible fracture
 Major trauma
 Minor trauma in patients > 50 years
 Long-term corticosteroid use
 Osteoporosis
 > 70 years

Possible tumor or infection
 > 50 years
 < 20 years
 History of cancer
 Constitutional symptoms
 Recent bacterial infection
 Injection drug use
 Immunosuppression
 Supine pain
 Nocturnal pain

AHRQ, Agency for Healthcare Research and Quality.
Reproduced, with permission, from Suarez-Almazor et al. Use of lumbar radiographs for the early diagnosis of low back pain. Proposed guidelines would increase utilization. JAMA. 1997 Jun; 277:1782–6.

not responding to conservative treatment or in the presence of red flags of serious conditions.

C. Special Tests

Electromyography or nerve conduction studies may be useful in assessing patients with possible nerve root symptoms lasting longer than 6 weeks; back pain may or may not also be present. These tests are usually not necessary if the diagnosis of radiculopathy is clear.

▶ Treatment

A. Conservative

Nonpharmacologic treatments are key in the management of low back pain. Education alone improves patient satisfaction with recovery and recurrence. Patients require information and reassurance, especially when diagnostic procedures are not necessary. Discussion must include reviewing safe and effective methods of symptom control as well as how to decrease the risk of recurrence with proper lifting techniques, abdominal wall/core strengthening, weight loss, and smoking cessation.

Physical therapy exercise programs can be tailored to the patient's symptoms and pathology. Strengthening and stabilization exercises effectively reduce pain and functional limitation compared with usual care. Neither spinal manipulation nor traction have shown benefits for low back pain; however, the studies so far are low quality and limited by small sample sizes. Heat and cold treatments have not shown any long-term benefits but may be used for symptomatic treatment. The efficacy of transcutaneous electrical nerve stimulation (TENS), back braces, physical agents, and acupuncture is unproven. Improvements in posture, core stability strengthening, physical conditioning, and modifications of activities to decrease physical strain are keys for ongoing management.

NSAIDs are effective in the early treatment of low back pain (see Chapter 20). There is limited evidence that muscle relaxants provide short-term relief; since these medications have addictive potential, they should be used with care. Muscle relaxants are best used if there is true muscle spasm that is painful rather than simply a protective response. Opioids alleviate pain in the short term but have the usual side effects and concerns of long-term opioid use. Treatment of more chronic neuropathic pain with alpha-2-delta ligands (eg, gabapentin), serotonin-norepinephrine reuptake inhibitors (eg, duloxetine) or tricyclic antidepressants (eg, nortriptyline) may be helpful. Epidural injections may reduce pain in the short term, and appear to reduce the need for surgery in some patients within a 1-year period but not longer.

B. Surgical

Surgical indications for back surgery include cauda equina syndrome, ongoing morbidity with no response to more than 6 months of conservative treatment, cancer, infection, or severe spinal deformity. Prognosis is improved when there is an anatomic lesion that can be corrected and symptoms are neurologic. Spinal surgery has limitations. Patient selection is very important and the specific surgery recommended should have very clear indications. Patients should understand that surgery can improve their pain but is unlikely to cure it. Surgery is not generally indicated for radiographic abnormalities alone when the patient is relatively asymptomatic. Depending on the surgery performed, possible complications include persistent pain; surgical site pain, especially if bone grafting is needed; infection; neurologic damage; non-union; cutaneous nerve damage; implant failure; deep venous thrombosis; and death.

▶ When to Refer

- Patients with the cauda equina syndrome.
- Patients with cancer, infection, fracture, or severe spinal deformity.
- Patients who have not responded to conservative treatment.

Bicket MC et al. Epidural injections in prevention of surgery for spinal pain: systematic review and meta-analysis of randomized controlled trials. Spine J. 2015 Feb 1;15(2):348–62. [PMID: 25463400]

Deyo RA et al. Opioids for low back pain. BMJ. 2015 Jan 5; 350:g6380. [PMID: 25561513]

Downie A et al. Red flags to screen for malignancy and fracture in patients with low back pain: systematic review. BMJ. 2013 Dec 11;347:f7095. [PMID: 24335669]

2. Spinal Stenosis

ESSENTIALS OF DIAGNOSIS

- ▶ Pain is usually worse with back extension and relieved by sitting.
- ▶ Occurs in older patients.
- ▶ May present with neurogenic claudication symptoms with walking.

▶ General Considerations

OA in the lumbar spine can cause narrowing of the spinal canal. A large disk herniation can also cause stenosis and compression of neural structures or the spinal artery resulting in "claudication" symptoms with ambulation. The condition usually affects patients aged 50 years or older.

▶ Clinical Findings

Patients report pain that worsens with extension. They describe reproducible single or bilateral leg symptoms that are worse after walking several minutes and that are relieved by sitting ("neurogenic claudication"). On examination, patients often exhibit limited extension of the lumbar spine, which may reproduce the symptoms radiating

down the legs. A thorough neurovascular examination is recommended (Table 41–2).

▶ Treatment

Exercises, usually flexion-based as demonstrated by a physical therapist, can help relieve symptoms. Physical therapy showed similar results as surgical decompression in a randomized trial, though there was a 57% crossover rate from physical therapy to surgery. Facet joint corticosteroid injections can also reduce pain symptoms. A 2014 randomized trial found a benefit overall from epidural injection at 6 weeks but did not find a difference when patients received injections of corticosteroids plus lidocaine compared to lidocaine alone. The extended benefit of epidural lidocaine injection alone is not well studied, so present practice most likely will continue to include corticosteroids. Epidural corticosteroid injections similarly showed only modest but significant improvement compared to gabapentin in patients with worse leg symptoms.

Surgical treatments for spinal stenosis include spinal decompression (widening the spinal canal or laminectomy), nerve root decompression (freeing a single nerve), and spinal fusion (joining the vertebra to eliminate motion and diminish pain from the arthritic joints). In an ongoing multicenter randomized trial, subgroups initially improved significantly more with surgery than with nonoperative treatment. Variables associated with greater treatment effects included lower baseline disability scores, not smoking, neuroforaminal stenosis, predominant leg pain rather than back pain, not lifting at work, and the presence of a neurologic deficit. However, long-term follow-up of the patients with symptomatic spinal stenosis who received surgery in the multicenter randomized trial showed less benefit of surgery between 4 and 8 years, suggesting that the advantage of surgery for spinal stenosis likely does diminish over time.

▶ When to Refer

- If a patient exhibits radicular or claudication symptoms for longer than 12 weeks.
- MRI or CT confirmation of significant, symptomatic spinal stenosis.

Cohen SP et al. Epidural steroid injections compared with gabapentin for lumbosacral radicular pain: multicenter randomized double blind comparative efficacy study. BMJ. 2015 Apr 16;350:h1748. [PMID: 25883095]

Delitto A et al. Surgery versus nonsurgical treatment of lumbar spinal stenosis: a randomized trial. Ann Intern Med. 2015 Apr 7;162(7):465–73. [PMID: 25844995]

Friedly JL et al. A randomized trial of epidural glucocorticoid injections for spinal stenosis. N Engl J Med. 2014 Jul 3; 371(1):11–21. Erratum in: N Engl J Med. 2014 Jul 24; 371(4):390. [PMID: 24988555]

Lurie JD et al. Long-term outcomes of lumbar spinal stenosis: eight-year results of the Spine Patient Outcomes Research Trial (SPORT). Spine (Phila Pa 1976). 2015 Jan 15;40(2):63–76. [PMID: 25569524]

3. Lumbar Disk Herniation

ESSENTIALS OF DIAGNOSIS

▶ Pain with back flexion or prolonged sitting.

▶ Radicular pain into the leg due to compression of neural structures.

▶ Lower extremity numbness.

▶ Lower extremity weakness.

▶ General Considerations

Lumbar disk herniation is usually due to bending or heavy loading (eg, lifting) with the back in flexion, causing herniation or extrusion of disk contents (nucleus pulposus) into the spinal cord area. However, there may not be an inciting incident. Disk herniations usually occur from degenerative disk disease (dessication of the annulus fibrosis) in patients between 30 and 50 -years -old. The L5–S1 disk is affected in 90% of cases. Compression of neural structures, such as the sciatic nerve, causes radicular pain. Severe compression of the spinal cord can cause the cauda equina syndrome, a surgical emergency.

▶ Clinical Findings

A. Symptoms and Signs

Discogenic pain typically is localized in the low back at the level of the affected disk and is worse with activity. "Sciatica" causes electric shock-like pain radiating down the posterior aspect of the leg often to below the knee. Symptoms usually worsen with back flexion such as bending or sitting for long periods (eg, driving). A significant disk herniation can cause numbness and weakness, including weakness with plantar flexion of the foot (L5/S1) or dorsiflexion of the toes (L4/L5). The cauda equina syndrome should be ruled out if the patient complains of perianal numbness or bowel or bladder incontinence.

B. Imaging

Plain radiographs are helpful to assess spinal alignment (scoliosis, lordosis), disk space narrowing, and OA changes. MRI is the best method to assess the level and morphology of the herniation and is recommended if surgery is planned.

▶ Treatment

For an acute exacerbation of pain symptoms, bed rest is appropriate for up to 48 hours. Otherwise, first-line treatments include modified activities; NSAIDs and other analgesics; and physical therapy, including core stabilization and McKenzie exercises. Following nonsurgical treatment for a lumbar disk for over 1 year, the incidence of low back pain recurrence is at least 40% and is predicted by longer time to initial resolution of pain. In a randomized trial, oral prednisone caused a modest improvement in function at 3 weeks but there was no significant improvement in pain in patients with acute radiculopathy who were monitored for 1 year. The initial dose for oral prednisone is approximately 1 mg/kg once daily with tapering doses over 10–15 days. Analgesics for neuropathic pain, such as the calcium channel alpha-2-delta ligands (ie, gabapentin, pregabalin) or tricyclic antidepressants, may be helpful (see Chapter 5). Epidural and transforaminal corticosteroid injections can be beneficial. A systemic review demonstrated strong evidence that fluoroscopic-guided epidural injections gave short-term benefit (less than 6 months) in acute radicular pain for individuals. However, epidural injections have not shown any change in long-term surgery rates for disk herniations.

A large, ongoing trial has shown that patients who underwent surgery for a lumbar disk herniation achieved greater improvement than conservatively treated patients in all primary and secondary outcomes except return to work status after 4-year follow-up. Patients with sequestered fragments, symptom duration greater than 6 months, higher levels of low back pain, or who were neither working nor disabled at baseline showed greater surgical treatment effects. Microdiscectomy is the standard method of treatment with a low rate of complications and satisfactory results over 90% in the largest series. Minimally invasive techniques include percutaneous endoscopic discectomy, which involves using an endoscope to remove fragments of disk herniation fragments (interlaminar or transforaminal approaches) under local anesthesia, although results are less successful than microdiscectomy. So far, disk replacement surgery has not shown benefits beyond generally accepted clinically important differences in short-term pain relief, disability, and quality of life compared with spine fusion surgery.

▶ When to Refer

• Cauda equina syndrome.

• Progressive worsening of neurologic symptoms.

• Loss of motor function (sensory losses can be followed in the outpatient clinic).

Goldberg H et al. Oral steroids for acute radiculopathy due to a herniated lumbar disk: a randomized clinical trial. JAMA. 2015 May 19;313(19):1915–23. [PMID: 25988461]

Kerr D et al. What are long-term predictors of outcomes for lumbar disc herniation? A randomized and observational study. Clin Orthop Relat Res. 2015 Jun;473(6):1920–30. [PMID: 25057116]

Kreiner DS et al; North American Spine Society. An evidence-based clinical guideline for the diagnosis and treatment of lumbar disc herniation with radiculopathy. Spine J. 2014 Jan; 14(1):180–91. [PMID: 24239490]

Manchikanti L et al. Do epidural injections provide short- and long-term relief for lumbar disc herniation? A systematic review. Clin Orthop Relat Res. 2015 Jun;473(6):1940–56. [PMID: 24515404]

4. Neck Pain

▸ Most chronic neck pain is caused by degenerative joint disease and responds to conservative treatment.

▸ Cervical radiculopathy symptoms can be referred to the shoulder, arm, or upper back.

▸ Whiplash is the most common type of traumatic injury to the neck.

▸ Poor posture is often a factor for persistent neck pain.

▸ General Considerations

Most neck pain, especially in older patients, is due to mechanical degeneration involving the cervical disks, facet joints, and ligamentous structures and may occur in the setting of degenerative changes at other sites. Pain can also come from the supporting neck musculature, which often acts to protect the underlying neck structures. **Posture is a very important factor, especially in younger patients.** Many work-related neck symptoms are due to poor posture and repetitive motions over time. Acute injuries can also occur secondary to trauma. Whiplash occurs from rapid flexion and extension of the neck and affects 15–40% of people in motor vehicle accidents; chronic pain develops in 5–7%. Neck fractures are serious traumatic injuries acutely and can lead to OA in the long term. Ultimately, many degenerative conditions of the neck result in cervical canal stenosis or neural foraminal stenosis, sometimes affecting underlying neural structures.

Cervical radiculopathy can cause neurologic symptoms in the upper extremities usually involving the C5–C7 disks. Patients with neck pain may report associated headaches and shoulder pain. Thoracic outlet syndrome, in which there is mechanical compression of the brachial plexus and neurovascular structures with overhead positioning of the arm, should be considered in the differential diagnosis of neck pain. Other causes of neck pain include rheumatoid arthritis, fibromyalgia, osteomyelitis, neoplasms, polymyalgia rheumatica, compression fractures, pain referred from visceral structures (eg, angina), and functional disorders. Amyotrophic lateral sclerosis, multiple sclerosis, syringomyelia, spinal cord tumors, and tropical spastic paresis from HTLV-1 infection can mimic myelopathy from cervical arthritis.

▸ Clinical Findings

A. Symptoms and Signs

Neck pain may be limited to the posterior region or, depending on the level of the symptomatic joint, may radiate segmentally to the occiput, anterior chest, shoulder girdle, arm, forearm, and hand. It may be intensified by active or passive neck motions. The general distribution of pain and paresthesias corresponds roughly to the involved dermatome in the upper extremity.

The patient's posture should be assessed, checking for shoulder rolled forward or head forward posture as well as scoliosis in the thoracolumbar spine. Patients with discogenic neck pain often complain of pain with flexion, which causes cervical disks to herniate posteriorly. Extension of the neck usually affects the neural foraminal and facet joints of the neck. Rotation and lateral flexion of the cervical spine should be measured both to the left and the right. Limitation of cervical movements is the most common objective finding.

A detailed neurovascular examination of the upper extremities should be performed, including sensory input to light touch and temperature; motor strength testing, especially the hand intrinsic muscles (thumb extension strength [C6], opponens strength (thumb to pinky) [C7], and finger abductors and adductors strength [C8–T1]); and upper extremity reflexes (biceps, triceps, brachioradialis). True cervical radiculopathy symptoms should match an expected dermatomal or myotomal distribution. The **Spurling test** involves asking the patient to rotate and extend the neck to one side (Table 41–4). The clinician can apply a gentle axial load to the neck. Reproduction of the cervical radiculopathy symptoms is a positive sign of nerve root compression. Palpation of the neck is best performed with the patient in the supine position where the clinician can palpate each level of the cervical spine with the muscles of the neck relaxed.

Table 41–4. Spine: neck examination.

Maneuver	Description
Inspection	Check the patient's posture in the standing position. Assess for cervical hyperlordosis, head forward posture, kyphosis, scoliosis, torticollis.
Palpation	Include important landmarks: spinous process, facet joints, paracervical muscles (sternocleidomastoid, scalene muscles).
Range of motion testing	Check range of motion in the cervical spine, especially with flexion and extension. Rotation and lateral bending are also helpful to assess symmetric motion or any restrictions. Pain and radicular symptoms can be exacerbated by range of motion testing.
Neurologic examination	Check motor strength, reflexes and dermatomal sensation in the upper (and lower if necessary) extremities.
Spurling test	Involves asking the patient to rotate and extend the neck to one side. The clinician can apply a gentle axial load to the neck. Reproduction of the cervical radiculopathy symptoms is a positive sign of nerve root compression.

B. Imaging

Radiographs of the cervical spine include the AP and lateral view of the cervical spine. The odontoid view is usually added to rule out traumatic fractures and congenital abnormalities. Oblique views of the cervical spine can provide further information about arthritis changes and assess the neural foramina for narrowing. Plain radiographs can be completely normal in patients who have suffered an acute cervical strain. Comparative reduction in height of the involved disk space and osteophytes are frequent findings when there are degenerative changes in the cervical spine. Loss of cervical lordosis is commonly seen but is nonspecific.

MRI is the best method to assess the cervical spine since the soft tissue structures (such as the disks, spinal cord, and nerve roots) can be evaluated. If the patient has signs of cervical radiculopathy with motor weakness, these more sensitive imaging modalities should be obtained urgently. CT scanning is the most useful method if bony abnormalities, such as fractures, are suspected.

▶ Treatment

In the absence of trauma or evidence of infection, malignancy, neurologic findings, or systemic inflammation, the patient can be treated conservatively. More frequent observation of individuals in whom very severe symptoms are present early on after an injury is recommended because high pain-related disability is a predictor of poor outcome at 1 year even if individuals decline care. Ergonomics should be assessed at work and home. A course of neck stretching, strengthening and postural exercises in physical therapy have demonstrated benefit in relieving symptoms. A soft cervical collar can be useful for short-term use (up to 1–2 weeks) in acute neck injuries. Chiropractic manual manipulation and mobilization can provide short-term benefit for mechanical neck pain. Although the rate of complications is low (5–10/million manipulations), care should be taken whenever there are neurologic symptoms present. Specific patients may respond to use of home cervical traction. NSAIDs are commonly used and opioids may be needed in cases of severe neck pain. Muscle relaxants (eg, cyclobenzaprine 5–10 mg orally three times daily) can be used short-term if there is muscle spasm or as a sedative to aid in sleeping. Acute radicular symptoms can be treated with neuropathic medications (eg, gabapentin 300–1200 mg orally three times daily), and a short course of oral prednisone (5–10 days) can be considered (starting at 1 mg/kg). Cervical foraminal or facet joint injections can also reduce symptoms. Cervical spine surgery does not have clear evidence of benefit over conservative treatment. Surgeries are successful in reducing neurologic symptoms in 80–90% of cases but are still considered as treatments of last resort.

▶ When to Refer

- Patients with severe symptoms with motor weakness.
- Surgical decompression surgery if the symptoms are severe and there is identifiable, correctable pathology.

Åsenlöf P et al. The clinical course over the first year of whiplash associated disorders (WAD): pain-related disability predicts outcome in a mildly affected sample. BMC Musculoskelet Disord. 2013 Dec 21;14:361. [PMID: 24359208]

van Middelkoop M et al. Surgery versus conservative care for neck pain: a systematic review. Eur Spine J. 2013 Jan;22(1):87–95. [PMID: 23104514]

Verhagen AP et al. Conservative interventions for treating work-related complaints of the arm, neck or shoulder in adults. Cochrane Database Syst Rev. 2013 Dec 12;12:CD008742. [PMID: 24338903]

UPPER EXTREMITY

1. Lateral & Medial Epicondylosis

ESSENTIALS OF DIAGNOSIS

▶ Tenderness over the lateral or medial epicondyle.

▶ Diagnosis of tendinopathy is confirmed by pain with resisted strength testing and passive stretching of the affected tendon and muscle unit.

▶ Physical therapy and activity modification are more successful than anti-inflammatory treatments.

▶ General Considerations

Tendinopathy involving the wrist extensors, flexors, and pronators are very common complaints. The underlying mechanism is chronic repetitive overuse causing microtrauma at the tendon insertion, although acute injuries can occur as well if the tendon is strained due to excessive loading. The traditional term "epicondylitis" is a misnomer because histologically tendinosis or degeneration in the tendon is seen rather than acute inflammation. Therefore, these entities should be referred to as "tendinopathy" or "tendinosis." Lateral epicondylosis involves the wrist extensors, especially the extensor carpi radialis brevis. This is usually caused be lifting with the wrist and the elbow extended. Medial epicondylosis involves the wrist flexors and most commonly the pronator teres tendon. Ulnar neuropathy and cervical radiculopathy should be considered in the differential diagnosis.

▶ Clinical Findings

A. Symptoms and Signs

For lateral epicondylosis, the patient describes pain with the arm and wrist extended. For example, common complaints include pain while shaking hands, lifting objects, using a computer mouse, or hitting a backhand in tennis ("tennis elbow"). Medial epicondylosis presents with pain during motions in which the arm is repetitively pronated or the wrist is flexed. This is also known as "golfer's elbow" due to the motion of turning the hands over during the golf swing. On examination, tenderness directly over the epicondyle is present, especially over the posterior aspect where the tendon insertion occurs. The proximal tendon and musculotendinous junction can also be sore. To confirm that the pain is due to tendinopathy, pain can be reproduced over the epicondyle with resisted wrist extension and third digit extension for lateral epicondylosis and resisted wrist pronation and wrist flexion for medial epicondylosis. The pain is also often reproduced with passive stretching of the affected muscle groups, which can be performed with the arm in extension. It is useful to check the ulnar nerve (located in a groove at the posteromedial elbow) for tenderness as well as to perform a Spurling test for cervical radiculopathy.

B. Imaging

Radiographs are often normal, although a small traction spur may be present in chronic cases (enthesopathy). Diagnostic investigations are usually unnecessary, unless the patient does not improve after up to 3 months of conservative treatment. At that point, a patient who demonstrates significant disability due to the pain should be assessed with an MRI or ultrasound. Ultrasound and MRI can visualize the tendon and confirm tendinosis or tears.

▶ Treatment

Treatment is usually conservative, including patient education regarding activity modification and management of symptoms. Ice and NSAIDs can help with pain. The most important steps are to begin a good stretching program followed by strengthening exercises, particularly eccentric ones. Counterforce elbow braces might provide some symptomatic relief, although there is no published evidence to support their use. If the patient has severe or longstanding symptoms, the mainstay of treatment is a course of physical therapy. A randomized trial showed no differences with platelet-rich plasma, corticosteroid, or saline (placebo) injections at 3 months. Corticosteroid injection had improvement at 1 month as well as evidence of decreased tendon thickness and Doppler changes. Treatments such as extracorporeal shock wave therapy and other injections have not shown clear long-term benefit. A systematic review found strong evidence that platelet-rich plasma injections showed no effects for lateral epicondylitis. Unfortunately, pooled data from randomized controlled trials assessing the nonsurgical treatments of lateral epicondylitis lack evidence of intermediate- to long-term clinical benefit compared with observation only or placebo.

▶ When to Refer

Patients not responding to 6 months of conservative treatment should be referred for surgical debridement or repair of the tendon.

Ahmad Z et al. Lateral epicondylitis: a review of pathology and management. Bone Joint J. 2013 Sep;95-B(9):1158–64. [PMID: 23997125]
Amin NH et al. Medial epicondylitis: evaluation and management. J Am Acad Orthop Surg. 2015 Jun;23(6):348–55. [PMID: 26001427]

Moraes VY et al. Platelet-rich therapies for musculoskeletal soft tissue injuries. Cochrane Database Syst Rev. 2014 Apr 29; 4:CD010071. [PMID: 24782334]
Sayegh ET et al. Does nonsurgical treatment improve longitudinal outcomes of lateral epicondylitis over no treatment? A meta-analysis. Clin Orthop Relat Res. 2015 Mar;473(3):1093–107. [PMID: 25352261]

2. Carpal Tunnel Syndrome

 ESSENTIALS OF DIAGNOSIS

- ▶ Pain, burning, and tingling in the distribution of the median nerve.
- ▶ Initially, most bothersome during sleep.
- ▶ Late weakness or atrophy, especially of the thenar eminence.
- ▶ Can be caused by repetitive activities using the wrist.
- ▶ Commonly seen during pregnancy and in patients with diabetes mellitus or rheumatoid arthritis.

▶ General Considerations

An entrapment neuropathy, carpal tunnel syndrome is a painful disorder caused by compression of the median nerve between the carpal ligament and other structures within the carpal tunnel. The contents of the tunnel can be compressed by synovitis of the tendon sheaths or carpal joints, recent or malhealed fractures, tumors, tissue infiltration, and occasionally congenital syndromes (eg, mucopolysaccharidoses). Even though no anatomic lesion is apparent, flattening or even circumferential constriction of the median nerve may be observed during operative section of the overlying carpal ligament. The disorder may occur in fluid retention of pregnancy, in individuals with a history of repetitive use of the hands, or following injuries of the wrists. There is a familial type of carpal tunnel syndrome in which no etiologic factor can be identified. Carpal tunnel syndrome can also be a feature of many systemic diseases, such as rheumatoid arthritis and other rheumatic disorders (inflammatory tenosynovitis), myxedema, amyloidosis, sarcoidosis, leukemia, acromegaly, and hyperparathyroidism.

▶ Clinical Findings

A. Symptoms and Signs

The initial symptoms are pain, burning, and tingling in the distribution of the median nerve (the palmar surfaces of the thumb, the index and long fingers, and the radial half of the ring finger). Aching pain may radiate proximally into the forearm and occasionally proximally to the shoulder and over the neck and chest. Pain is exacerbated by manual activity, particularly by extremes of volar flexion or dorsiflexion of the wrist. It is most bothersome at night. Impairment of sensation in the median nerve distribution may or may not be demonstrable. Subtle disparity between

Table 41–5. Wrist examination.

Maneuver	Description
Inspection	Examine for the alignment of the wrist and fingers SEADS.
Palpation	Include important landmarks: scaphoid "snuff box," distal radius, scapholunate ligament, hook of hamate, ulnar joint line, distal radioulnar joint.
Range of motion testing	Check range of motion actively (patient performs) and passively (clinician performs) especially with flexion and extension of the wrist. Ulnar and radial deviation and circumduction of the wrist can be screened.
Neurovascular examination	Check motor strength and dermatomal sensation in the fingers in the radial (thumb), median (3rd finger) and ulnar distribution (5th finger). Check capillary refill to digits as well as radial pulse.
Tinel sign	Tingling or shock-like pain on volar wrist percussion. The carpal compression test, in which numbness and tingling are induced by the direct application of pressure over the carpal tunnel, may be more sensitive and specific than the Tinel and Phalen tests.
Phalen sign	Pain or paresthesia in the distribution of the median nerve when the patient flexes both wrists to 90 degrees for 60 seconds.
Carpel compression test	Performed by applying direct application of pressure over the carpal tunnel.

SEADS, swelling, erythema, atrophy, deformity, and (surgical) scars.

the affected and opposite sides can be shown by testing for two-point discrimination or by requiring the patient to identify different textures of cloth by rubbing them between the tips of the thumb and the index finger. A Tinel or Phalen sign may be positive. A **Tinel sign** is tingling or shock-like pain on volar wrist percussion (Table 41–5). The **Phalen sign** is pain or paresthesia in the distribution of the median nerve when the patient flexes both wrists to 90 degrees for 60 seconds (Table 41–5). The **carpal compression test**, in which numbness and tingling are induced by the direct application of pressure over the carpal tunnel, may be more sensitive and specific than the Tinel and Phalen tests (Table 41–5). Muscle weakness or atrophy, especially of the thenar eminence, can appear later than sensory disturbances as compression of the nerve worsens.

B. Imaging

Ultrasound can demonstrate flattening of the median nerve beneath the flexor retinaculum. Sensitivity of ultrasound for carpal tunnel syndrome is variable but estimated between 54% and 98%.

C. Special Tests

Electromyography and nerve conduction studies show evidence of sensory conduction delay before motor delay, which can occur in severe cases.

▶ Treatment

Treatment is directed toward relief of pressure on the median nerve. When a causative lesion is discovered, it should be treated appropriately. Otherwise, patients in whom carpal tunnel syndrome is suspected should modify their hand activities. The affected wrist can be splinted in the neutral position for up to 3 months, but a series of Cochrane reviews show limited evidence for splinting, therapeutic ultrasound, exercises, and ergonomic positioning. Oral corticosteroids or NSAIDs can also be tried. Methylprednisolone injections were found to have more effect at 10 weeks than placebo but the benefits diminished by 1 year. A randomized, controlled trial showed both corticosteroid injection and surgery resolved symptoms but only decompressive surgery led to resolution of neurophysiologic changes.

Compared to trigger finger management, which usually includes injections, as many as 71% of patients with carpal tunnel directly undergo surgery without first getting injections. Carpal tunnel release surgery can be beneficial if the patient has a positive electrodiagnostic test, at least moderate symptoms, high clinical probability, unsuccessful nonoperative treatment, and symptoms lasting longer than 12 months. Surgery can be done with an open approach or endoscopically, both yielding similar good improvements.

▶ When to Refer

- If symptoms persist more than 3 months despite conservative treatment, including the use of a wrist splint.
- If thenar muscle (eg, abductor pollicis brevis) weakness or atrophy develops.

Andreu JL et al. Local injection versus surgery in carpal tunnel syndrome: neurophysiologic outcomes of a randomized clinical trial. Clin Neurophysiol. 2014 Jul;125(7):1479–84. [PMID: 24321619]

Sears ED et al. National utilization patterns of steroid injection and operative intervention for treatment of common hand conditions. J Hand Surg Am. 2016 Mar;41(3):367–73.e2. [PMID: 26774548]

Vasiliadis HS et al. Endoscopic release for carpal tunnel syndrome. Cochrane Database Syst Rev. 2014 Jan 31;1:CD008265. [PMID: 24482073]

3. Dupuytren Contracture

ESSENTIALS OF DIAGNOSIS

- ▶ Benign fibrosing disorder of the palmar fascia.
- ▶ Contracture of one or more fingers can lead to limited hand function.

▶ General Considerations

This relatively common disorder is characterized by hyperplasia of the palmar fascia and related structures, with nodule formation and contracture of the palmar fascia. The cause is unknown, but the condition has a genetic predisposition and occurs primarily in white men over 50 years of age, particularly in those of Celtic descent. The incidence is higher among alcoholic patients and those with chronic systemic disorders (especially cirrhosis). It is also associated with systemic fibrosing syndrome, which includes plantar fibromatosis (10% of patients), Peyronie disease (1–2%), mediastinal and retroperitoneal fibrosis, and Riedel struma. The onset may be acute, but slowly progressive chronic disease is more common.

► Clinical Findings

Dupuytren contracture manifests itself by nodular or cord-like thickening of one or both hands, with the fourth and fifth fingers most commonly affected. The patient may complain of tightness of the involved digits, with inability to satisfactorily extend the fingers, and on occasion there is tenderness. The resulting cosmetic problems may be unappealing, but in general the contracture is well tolerated since it exaggerates the normal position of function of the hand.

► Treatment

If the palmar nodule is growing rapidly, injections of triamcinolone or collagenase into the nodule may be of benefit. The injection of collagenase *Clostridium histolyticum* is a nonoperative treatment option that lyses collagen disrupting the contracted cords. Surgical options include open fasciectomy, partial fasciectomy, or percutaneous needle aponeurotomy and are indicated in patients with significant flexion contractures. Recurrence is possible and there are more adverse events compared to nonoperative treatments. A multicenter study showed that collagenase injection and limited fasciectomy had similar improvements with contractures at the metacarpophalangeal joints, while surgery had better results for contractures involving the proximal interphalangeal joints.

► When to Refer

Referral can be considered when one or more digits are affected by severe contractures, which interfere with everyday activities and result in functional limitations.

Coleman S et al. Efficacy and safety of concurrent collagenase *Clostridium histolyticum* injections for multiple Dupuytren contractures. J Hand Surg Am. 2014 Jan;39(1):57–64. [PMID: 24315486]

Povlsen B et al. What is the better treatment for single digit Dupuytren's contracture: surgical release or collagenase *Clostridium histolyticum* (Xiapex) injection? Hand Surg. 2014;19(3):389–92. [PMID: 25155703]

Zhou C et al. Collagenase *Clostridium histolyticum* versus limited fasciectomy for Dupuytren's contracture: outcomes from a multicenter propensity score matched study. Plast Reconstr Surg. 2015 Jul;136(1):87–97. [PMID: 25829153]

4. Bursitis

ESSENTIALS OF DIAGNOSIS

► Often occurs around bony prominences where it is important to reduce friction.

► Typically presents with local swelling that is painful acutely.

► Septic bursitis can present without fever or systemic signs.

► General Considerations

Inflammation of bursae—the synovium-like cellular membranes overlying bony prominences—may be secondary to trauma, infection, or arthritic conditions such as gout, rheumatoid arthritis, or OA. Bursitis can result from infection. The two common sites are the olecranon (Figure 41–1) and prepatellar bursae; however, others include subdeltoid, ischial, trochanteric, and semimembranous-gastrocnemius (Baker cyst) bursae. The bursitis can be septic. Aseptic bursitis is usually afebrile.

► Clinical Findings

A. Symptoms and Signs

Bursitis presents with focal tenderness and swelling and is less likely to affect range of motion of the adjacent joint. Olecranon or prepatellar bursitis, for example, causes an oval (or, if chronic, bulbous) swelling at the tip of the elbow

▲ **Figure 41–1.** Aseptic olecranon bursitis secondary to repetitive trauma. (Reproduced, with permission, from Richard P. Usatine, MD.)

or knee and does not affect joint motion. Tenderness, erythema and warmth, cellulitis, a report of trauma, or evidence of a skin lesion are more common in septic bursitis but can be present in aseptic bursitis as well. Patients with septic bursitis can be febrile but the absence of fever does not exclude infection; **one-third of those with septic olecranon bursitis are afebrile**. A bursa can also become symptomatic when it ruptures. This is particularly true for Baker cyst, whose rupture can cause calf pain and swelling that mimic thrombophlebitis.

B. Imaging

Imaging is unnecessary unless there is concern for osteomyelitis, trauma or other underlying pathology. Ruptured Baker cysts are imaged easily by sonography or MRI. It may be important to exclude a deep venous thrombosis, which can be mimicked by a ruptured Baker cyst.

C. Special Tests

Acute swelling and redness at a bursal site calls for aspiration to rule out infection especially if the patient is either febrile (temperature more than 37.8°C) or has prebursal warmth (temperature difference greater than 2.2°C) or both. A bursal fluid white blood cell count of greater than 1000/mcL indicates inflammation from infection, rheumatoid arthritis, or gout. The bursal fluid of septic bursitis characteristically contains a purulent aspirate, fluid-to-serum glucose ratio less than 50%, white cell count more than 3000 cells/mcL, polymorphonuclear cells more than 50%, and a positive Gram stain for bacteria. Most cases are caused by *Staphylococcus aureus;* the Gram stain is positive in two-thirds.

▶ Treatment

Bursitis caused by trauma responds to local heat, rest, NSAIDs, and local corticosteroid injections. Chronic, stable olecranon bursa swelling usually does not require aspiration. Repetitive minor trauma to the olecranon bursa should be eliminated by avoiding resting the elbow on a hard surface or by wearing an elbow pad. For chronic aseptic bursitis or when there are athletic or occupational demands, aspiration with intrabursal steroid injection can be performed. Aspiration of the olecranon bursa runs the risk of creating a chronic drainage site, which can be reduced by using a "zig-zag" approach with a small needle (25-gauge if possible) and pulling the skin over the bursa before introducing it. Applying a pressure bandage may also help prevent chronic drainage. Ultrasound-guided aspiration and injection can improve the accuracy of the procedures. Treatment of a ruptured Baker cyst includes rest, leg elevation, and possibly injection of triamcinolone, 20–40 mg into the knee anteriorly (the knee compartment communicates with the cyst). However, corticosteroid injections in nonseptic bursitis have more complications and skin atrophy than simple symptomatic treatment.

Treatment for septic bursitis involves incision and drainage and antibiotics usually delivered intravenously.

▶ When to Refer

- Surgical removal of the bursa is indicated only for cases in which repeated infections occur.
- Elective removal for persistent symptoms affecting activities of daily living can be considered.

Baumbach SF et al. Prepatellar and olecranon bursitis: literature review and development of a treatment algorithm. Arch Orthop Trauma Surg. 2014 Mar;134(3):359–70. [PMID: 24305696]
Reilly D et al. Olecranon bursitis. J Shoulder Elbow Surg. 2016 Jan;25(1):158–67. [PMID: 26577126]

HIP

1. Hip Fractures

ESSENTIALS OF DIAGNOSIS

- ▶ Internal rotation of the hip is the best provocative diagnostic maneuver.
- ▶ Hip fractures should be surgically repaired as soon as possible (within 24 hours).
- ▶ Delayed treatment of hip fractures in the elderly leads to increased complications and mortality.

▶ General Considerations

Approximately 4% of the 7.9 million fractures that occur each year in the United States are hip fractures. There is a high mortality rate among elderly patients following hip fracture, with death occurring in 8–9% within 30 days and in approximately 25–30% within 1 year. Osteoporosis, female sex, height greater than 5-foot 8-inches, and age over 50 years are risk factors for hip fracture. Hip fractures usually occur after a fall. High velocity trauma is needed in younger patients. Stress fractures can occur in athletes or individuals with poor bone mineral density following repetitive loading activities.

▶ Clinical Findings

A. Symptoms and Signs

Patients typically report pain in the groin, though pain radiating to the lateral hip, buttock, or knee can also commonly occur. If a displaced fracture is present, the patient will not be able to bear weight and the leg may be externally rotated. Gentle logrolling of the leg with the patient supine helps rule out a fracture. Examination of the hip demonstrates pain with deep palpation in the area of the femoral triangle (similar to palpating the femoral artery). Provided the patient can tolerate it, the clinician can, with the patient supine, flex the hip to 90 degrees with the knee flexed to 90 degrees. The leg can then be internally and externally rotated to assess the range of motion on both sides. **Pain with internal rotation of the hip is the most sensitive test**

Table 41–6. Hip examination.

Maneuver	Description
Inspection	Examine for the alignment of the lower extremity, consider lumbar spine exam.
Palpation	Include important landmarks: ASIS and AIIS (proximal quadriceps muscle insertions), greater trochanter (gluteal tendon insertions and bursa), anterior femoral triangle (hip joint and hip flexion insertion), ischial tuberosity (hamstring tendon insertion), sacroiliac joints.
Range of motion testing	Check range of motion passively (clinician performs) especially internal and external rotation of the hip.
Hip strength testing	Test resisted hip flexion, extension, abduction and adduction strength manually.
Trendelenburg test	The patient balances first on one leg, raising the non-standing knee toward the chest. The clinician can stand behind the patient and observe for dropping of the pelvis and buttock on the non-stance side.

AIIS, anterior inferior iliac spine; ASIS, anterior superior iliac spine.

to identify intra-articular hip pathology. Hip flexion, extension, abduction, and adduction strength can be tested.

Patients with hip stress fractures have less pain on physical examination than described previously but typically have pain with weight bearing. The Trendelenburg test can be performed to examine for weakness or instability of the hip abductors, primarily the gluteus medius muscle (Table 41–6). Another functional test is asking the patient to hop or jump during the examination. If the patient has a compatible clinical history of pain and is unable or unwilling to hop, then a stress fracture should be ruled out. The back should be carefully examined in patients with hip complaints, including examining for signs for sciatica.

Following displaced hip fractures, a thorough medical evaluation and treatment should be pursued to maximize the patients' ability to undergo operative intervention. Patients who are unable to get up by themselves may have been immobile for hours or even days following their falls. Thus, clinicians must exclude rhabdomyolysis, hypothermia, deep venous thrombosis, pulmonary embolism, and other conditions that can occur with prolonged immobilization. Delay of operative intervention leads to an increased risk of perioperative morbidity and mortality.

B. Imaging

Useful radiographic views of the hip include AP views of the pelvis and bilateral hips and frog-leg-lateral views of the painful hip. A CT scan or MRI may be necessary to identify the hip fracture pattern or to evaluate nondisplaced fractures. Hip fractures are generally described by location, including femoral neck, intertrochanteric, or subtrochanteric.

▶ **Treatment**

Almost all patients with a hip fracture will require surgery and may need to be admitted to hospital for pain control while they await surgery. **Surgery is recommended within the first 24 hours** because studies have shown that delaying surgery 48 hours results in at least twice the rate of major and minor medical complications, including pneumonia, pressure ulcers, and deep venous thrombosis. High-volume centers have developed multidisciplinary teams (including orthopedic surgeons, internists, social workers, and specialized physical therapists) to comanage these patients, which improves perioperative medical care and expedites preoperative evaluation leading to reduced costs.

Stress fractures in active patients require a period of protected weight-bearing and a gradual return to activities, although it may take 4–6 months before a return to normal activities. Femoral neck fractures are commonly treated with hemiarthroplasty or total hip replacement. This allows the patient to begin weight-bearing immediately postoperatively. Peritrochanteric hip fractures are treated with open reduction internal fixation, where plate and screw construct or intramedullary devices are used. The choice of implant will depend on the fracture pattern. Since fracture fixation requires the fracture to proceed to union, the patient may need to have protected weight-bearing during the early postoperative period. Dislocation, periprosthetic fracture, and avascular necrosis of the hip are common complications after surgery. The surgical trends for treating femoral neck fractures show a rise in use of arthroplasty, which was possibly reflecting a rising trend toward specialty care (more arthroplasty surgeon care).

Patients should be mobilized as soon as possible postoperatively to avoid pulmonary complications and decubitus ulcers. Supervised physical therapy and rehabilitation are important for the patient to regain as much function as possible. Unfortunately, most patients following hip fractures will lose some degree of independence.

▶ **Prevention**

Bone density screening can identify patients at risk for osteopenia or osteoporosis, and treatment can be planned accordingly. There is strong evidence that bisphosphonates, denosumab, and teriparatide reduce fractures compared with placebo, with relative risk reductions of 0.60–0.80 for nonvertebral fractures. Nutrition (calcium and vitamin D intake) and bone health (bone densitometry, serum calcium and 25-OH vitamin D levels) should be reviewed with the patient (see Chapter 26). For patients with decreased mobility, systemic anticoagulation should be considered to avoid deep venous thrombosis (see Table 14–14). Fall prevention exercise programs are available for elderly patients at risk for falls and hip fractures. Hip protectors are uncomfortable and have less use in preventing fractures.

▶ **When to Refer**

- All patients in whom hip fracture is suspected.
- All patients with hip fracture or in whom the diagnosis is uncertain after radiographs.

Crandall CJ et al. Comparative effectiveness of pharmacologic treatments to prevent fractures: an updated systematic review. Ann Intern Med. 2014 Nov 18;161(10):711–23. [PMID: 25199883]

Miller BJ et al. Changing trends in the treatment of femoral neck fractures: a review of the American Board of Orthopaedic Surgery database. J Bone Joint Surg Am. 2014 Sep 3; 96(17):e149. [PMID: 25187593]

Swart E et al. Dedicated perioperative hip fracture comanagement programs are cost-effective in high-volume centers: an economic analysis. Clin Orthop Relat Res. 2016 Jan; 474(1):222–33. [PMID: 26260393]

2. Hip Osteoarthritis

ESSENTIALS OF DIAGNOSIS

▸ Pain deep in the groin on the affected side.

▸ Swelling.

▸ Degeneration of joint cartilage.

▸ Loss of active and passive range of motion in severe OA.

General Considerations

In the United States, the prevalence of OA will grow as the number of persons over age 65 years doubles to more than 70 million by 2030. Cartilage loss and OA symptoms are preceded by damage to the collagen-proteoglycan matrix. The etiology of OA is often multifactorial, including previous trauma, prior high-impact activities, genetic factors, obesity, and rheumatologic or metabolic conditions. Femoroacetabular impingement, which affects younger active patients, is considered an early development of hip OA.

Clinical Findings

A. Symptoms and Signs

OA usually causes pain in the affected joint with loading of the joint or at the extremes of motion. Mechanical symptoms—such as swelling, grinding, catching, and locking—suggest internal derangement, which is indicated by damaged cartilage or bone fragments that affect the smooth range of motion expected at an articular joint. Pain can also produce the sensation of "buckling" or "giving way" due to muscle inhibition. As the joint degeneration becomes more advanced, the patient loses active range of motion and may lose passive range of motion as well.

Patients complain of pain deep in the groin on the affected side and have problems with weight-bearing activities such as walking, climbing stairs, and getting up from a chair. They may limp and develop a lurch during their gait, leaning toward the unaffected side as they walk to reduce pressure on the hip.

B. Imaging

An anterior-posterior weight-bearing radiograph of the pelvis with a lateral view of the symptomatic hip are preferred views for evaluation of hip OA. Joint space narrowing and sclerosis suggest early OA, while osteophytes near the femoral head or acetabulum and subchondral bone cysts are more advanced changes. The sensitivity of radiographic hip OA for hip pain localized to the groin was 36.7%, specificity 90.5%, positive predictive value 6.0%, and negative predictive value 98.9%. However, not all patient with radiographic hip OA had hip or groin pain; the converse is also true because of the low sensitivity of the radiographs. After age 35, MRI of the hips already show labral changes in almost 70% of asymptomatic patients.

Treatment

A. Conservative

Changes in the articular cartilage are irreversible. Therefore, a cure for the diseased joint is not possible, although symptoms or structural issues can be addressed to try to maintain activity level. Conservative treatment for patients with OA includes activity modification, proper footwear, therapeutic exercises, weight loss, and use of assistive devices (such as a cane). A 2014 randomized study found that physical therapy did not lead to greater improvement in pain or function compared with sham treatment in patients with hip OA. Analgesics may be effective in some cases. Corticosteroid injections can be considered for short-term relief of pain; however, hip injections are best performed under fluoroscopic, ultrasound, or CT guidance to ensure accurate injection in the joint.

B. Surgical

Joint replacement surgeries are effective and cost-effective for patients with significant symptoms and functional limitations, providing improvements in pain, function, and quality of life. Minimally invasive surgeries and computer-assisted navigation during operation are being investigated as methods to improve techniques (eg, accurate placement of the hardware implant) and to reduce complication rates.

Hip resurfacing surgery is a newer joint replacement technique. Rather than use a traditional artificial joint implant of the whole neck and femur, only the femoral head is removed and replaced. Evidence to date suggests that hip resurfacing is comparable to total hip replacement and is a viable alternative for younger patients. The cumulative survival rate of this implant at 10 years is estimated to be 94%. Concerns following resurfacing surgery include the risk of femoral neck fracture and collapse of the head. In a systematic review of national databases, the average time to revision was 3.0 years for metal-on-metal hip resurfacing versus 7.8 years for total hip arthroplasty. Dislocations were more frequent with total hip arthroplasty than metal-on-metal hip resurfacing: 4.4 versus 0.9 per 1000 person-years, respectively.

Guidelines recommend prophylaxis for venous thromboembolic disease for a minimum of 14 days after arthroplasty of the hip or knee using warfarin, low-molecular-weight heparin, fondaparinux, aspirin, rivaroxaban, dabigatran, apixaban, or portable mechanical compression (see Table 14–14).

▶ When to Refer

Patients with sufficient disability, limited benefit from conservative therapy, and evidence of severe OA can be referred for joint replacement surgery.

Bennell KL et al. Effect of physical therapy on pain and function in patients with hip osteoarthritis: a randomized clinical trial. JAMA. 2014 May 21;311(19):1987–97. [PMID: 24846036]

Kim C et al. Association of hip pain with radiographic evidence of hip osteoarthritis: diagnostic test study. BMJ. 2015 Dec 2; 351:h5983. [PMID: 26631296]

Lieberman JR et al. Prevention of venous thromboembolic disease after total hip and knee arthroplasty. J Bone Joint Surg Am. 2013 Oct 2;95(19):1801–11. [PMID: 24088973]

Marshall DA et al. Hip resurfacing versus total hip arthroplasty: a systematic review comparing standardized outcomes. Clin Orthop Relat Res. 2014 Jul;472(7):2217–30. [PMID: 24700446]

Nwachukwu BU et al. Arthroscopic versus open treatment of femoroacetabular impingement: a systematic review of medium- to long-term outcomes. Am J Sports Med. 2016 Apr; 44(4):1062–8. [PMID: 26059179]

KNEE

1. Knee Pain

ESSENTIALS OF DIAGNOSIS

▶ Effusion can occur with intra-articular pathology, such as OA, and meniscus and cruciate ligament tears.

▶ Acute knee swelling (due to hemarthrosis) within 2 hours may indicate ligament injuries or patellar dislocation or fracture.

▶ General Considerations

The knee is the largest joint in the body and is susceptible to injury from trauma, inflammation, infection, and degenerative changes. The knee is a hinge joint. The joint line exists between the femoral condyles and tibial plateaus. Separating and cushioning these bony surfaces is the lateral and medial meniscal cartilage, which functions as a shock absorber during weight bearing, protecting the articular cartilage. The patella is a large sesamoid bone anterior to the joint. It is embedded in the quadriceps tendon, and it articulates with the trochlear groove of the femur. Poor patellar tracking in the trochlear groove is a common source of knee pain especially when the cause is atraumatic in nature. The knee is stabilized by the collateral ligaments against varus (lateral collateral ligament) and valgus (medial collateral ligament) stresses. The tibia is limited in its anterior movement by the anterior cruciate ligament (ACL) and in its posterior movement by the posterior cruciate ligament (PCL). The bursae of the knee are located between the skin and bony prominences. They are sac-like structures with a synovial lining. They act to decrease friction of tendons and muscles as they move over adjacent bony structures. Excessive external pressure or friction can lead to swelling and pain of the bursae. The **prepatellar bursae** (located between the skin and patella), and the **pes anserine bursa** (which is medial and inferior to the patella, just below the tibial plateau) are most commonly affected. Joint fluid, when excessive due to synovitis or trauma, can track posteriorly through a potential space, resulting in a popliteal cyst (also called a **Baker cyst**). Other structures that are susceptible to overuse injury and may cause knee pain following repetitive activity include the patellofemoral joint and the iliotibial band. OA of the knees is common after 50 years of age and can develop due to previous trauma, aging, activities, alignment issues, and genetic predisposition.

▶ Clinical Findings

A. Symptoms and Signs

Evaluation of knee pain should begin with general questions regarding duration and rapidity of symptom onset and the mechanism of injury or aggravating symptoms. Overuse or degenerative problems can occur with stress or compression from sports, hobbies, or occupation. A history of trauma, previous orthopedic problems with, or surgery to, the affected knee should also be specifically queried. Symptoms of infection (fever, recent bacterial infections, risk factors for sexually transmitted infections [such as gonorrhea] or other bacterial infections [such as staphylococcal infection]) should always be elicited.

Common symptom complaints include the following:

1. Presence of grinding, clicking, or popping with bending, may be indicative of OA or the patellofemoral syndrome.

2. "Locking" or "catching" when walking suggests an internal derangement, such as meniscal injury or a loose body in the knee.

3. Intra-articular swelling of the knee or an effusion indicates an internal derangement or a synovial pathology. Large swelling may cause a popliteal (Baker) cyst. Acute swelling within minutes to hours suggests a hemarthrosis, most likely due to an ACL injury, fracture or patellar dislocation, especially if trauma is involved.

4. Lateral "snapping" with flexion and extension of the knee may indicate inflammation of the iliotibial band.

5. Pain that is worsened with bending and walking downstairs suggests issues with the patellofemoral joint, usually degenerative such as chondromalacia of the patella or OA.

6. Pain that occurs when rising after prolonged sitting suggests a problem with tracking of the patella.

A careful history coupled with a physical examination that includes observation, palpation, and range of motion testing, as well as specific tests for particular anatomic structures is frequently sufficient to establish a diagnosis. When there is a knee joint effusion caused by increased fluid in the intra-articular space, physical examination will demonstrate swelling in the hollow or dimple around the patella and distention of the suprapatellar space.

Table 41–7. Differential diagnosis of knee pain.

Mechanical dysfunction or disruption
Internal derangement of the knee: injury to the menisci or ligaments
Degenerative changes caused by osteoarthritis
Dynamic dysfunction or misalignment of the patella
Fracture as a result of trauma

Intra-articular inflammation or increased pressure
Internal derangement of the knee: injury to the menisci or ligaments
Inflammation or infection of the knee joint
Ruptured popliteal (Baker) cyst

Peri-articular inflammation
Internal derangement of the knee: injury to the menisci or ligaments
Prepatellar or anserine bursitis
Ligamentous sprain

Table 41–7 shows the differential diagnosis of knee pain, and Table 41–8 outlines possible diagnoses based on the location of pain.

B. Laboratory Findings

Laboratory testing of aspirated joint fluid, when indicated, can lead to a definitive diagnosis in most patients (see Tables 20–2 and 20–3).

C. Imaging

Knee pain is evaluated with plain (weight-bearing) radiographs and MRI most commonly, but CT and ultrasound are sometimes useful.

Table 41–8. Location of common causes of knee pain.

Medial knee pain
Medial compartment osteoarthritis
Medial collateral ligament strain
Medial meniscal injury
Anserine bursitis (pain over the proximal medial tibial plateau)

Anterior knee pain
Patellofemoral syndrome (often bilateral)
Osteoarthritis
Prepatellar bursitis (associated with swelling anterior to the patella)
"Jumper's knee" (pain at the inferior pole of the patella)
Septic arthritis
Gout or other inflammatory disorder

Lateral knee pain
Lateral meniscal injury
Iliotibial band syndrome (pain superficially along the distal iliotibial band near lateral femoral condyle or lateral tibial insertion)
Lateral collateral ligament sprain (rare)

Posterior knee pain
Popliteal (Baker) cyst
Osteoarthritis
Meniscal tears
Hamstring or calf tendinopathy

An acute hemarthrosis represents bloody swelling that usually occurs within the first 1–2 hours following trauma. In situations where the trauma may be activity-related and not a result of a fall or collision, the differential diagnosis most commonly includes ACL tear (responsible for almost 50% of hemarthrosis in children and more than 70% in adults), fracture (patella, tibial plateau, femoral supracondylar, growth plate [physeal]), and patellar dislocation. Meniscal tears are unlikely to cause large hemarthrosis.

2. Anterior Cruciate Ligament Injury

 ESSENTIALS OF DIAGNOSIS

► An injury involving an audible pop when the knee buckles.

► Acute swelling immediately (or within 2 hours).

► Instability occurs with lateral movement activities and going down stairs.

► General Considerations

The anterior cruciate ligament (ACL) connects the posterior aspect of the lateral femoral condyle to the anterior aspect of the tibia. Its main function is to control anterior translation of the tibia on the femur. It also provides rotationally stability of the tibia on the femur. ACL tears are common with sporting injuries. They can result from both contact (valgus blow to the knee) and non-contact (jumping, pivoting, and deceleration) activities. The patient usually falls down following the injury, has acute swelling and difficulty with weight-bearing, and complains of instability. ACL injuries are common in skiing, soccer, football, and basketball among young adolescents and middle-age patients. Prepubertal and older patients usually sustain fractures instead of ligamentous injuries.

► Clinical Findings

A. Symptoms and Signs

Acute ACL injuries usually lead to acute swelling of the knee, causing difficulty with motion. After the swelling has resolved, the patient can walk with a "stiff-knee" gait or quadriceps avoidance gait because of the instability. More importantly, patients describe symptoms of instability while performing side-to-side maneuvers or descending stairs. Stability tests assess the amount of laxity of the knee while performing side-to-side maneuvers or descending stairs. The **Lachman test** (84–87% sensitivity and 93% specificity) is performed with the patient lying supine and the knee flexed to 20–30 degrees (Table 41–9). The clinician grasps the distal femur from the lateral side and the proximal tibia with the other hand on the medial side. With the knee in neutral position, stabilize the femur, and pull the tibia anteriorly using a similar force to lifting a

Table 41–9. Knee examination.

Maneuver	Description
Ligament stress tests	
Lachman test Fix femur	Performed with the patient lying supine, and the knee flexed to 20–30 degrees. The examiner grasps the distal femur from the lateral side, and the proximal tibia with the other hand on the medial side. With the knee in neutral position, stabilize the femur, and pull the tibia anteriorly using a similar force to lifting a 10–15 pound weight. Excessive anterior translation of the tibia compared with the other side indicates injury to the anterior cruciate ligament.
Anterior drawer	Performed with the patient lying supine and the knee flexed to 90 degrees. The clinician stabilizes the patient's foot by sitting on it and grasps the proximal tibia with both hands around the calf and pulls anteriorly. A positive test finds anterior cruciate ligament laxity compared with the unaffected side.
Pivot shift	Used to determine the amount of rotational laxity of the knee. The patient is examined while lying supine with the knee in full extension. It is then slowly flexed while applying internal rotation and a valgus stress. The clinician feels for a subluxation at 20–40 degrees of knee flexion. The patient must remain very relaxed to have a positive test.

(continued)

Table 41–9. Knee examination. (continued)

Maneuver	Description
Valgus stress 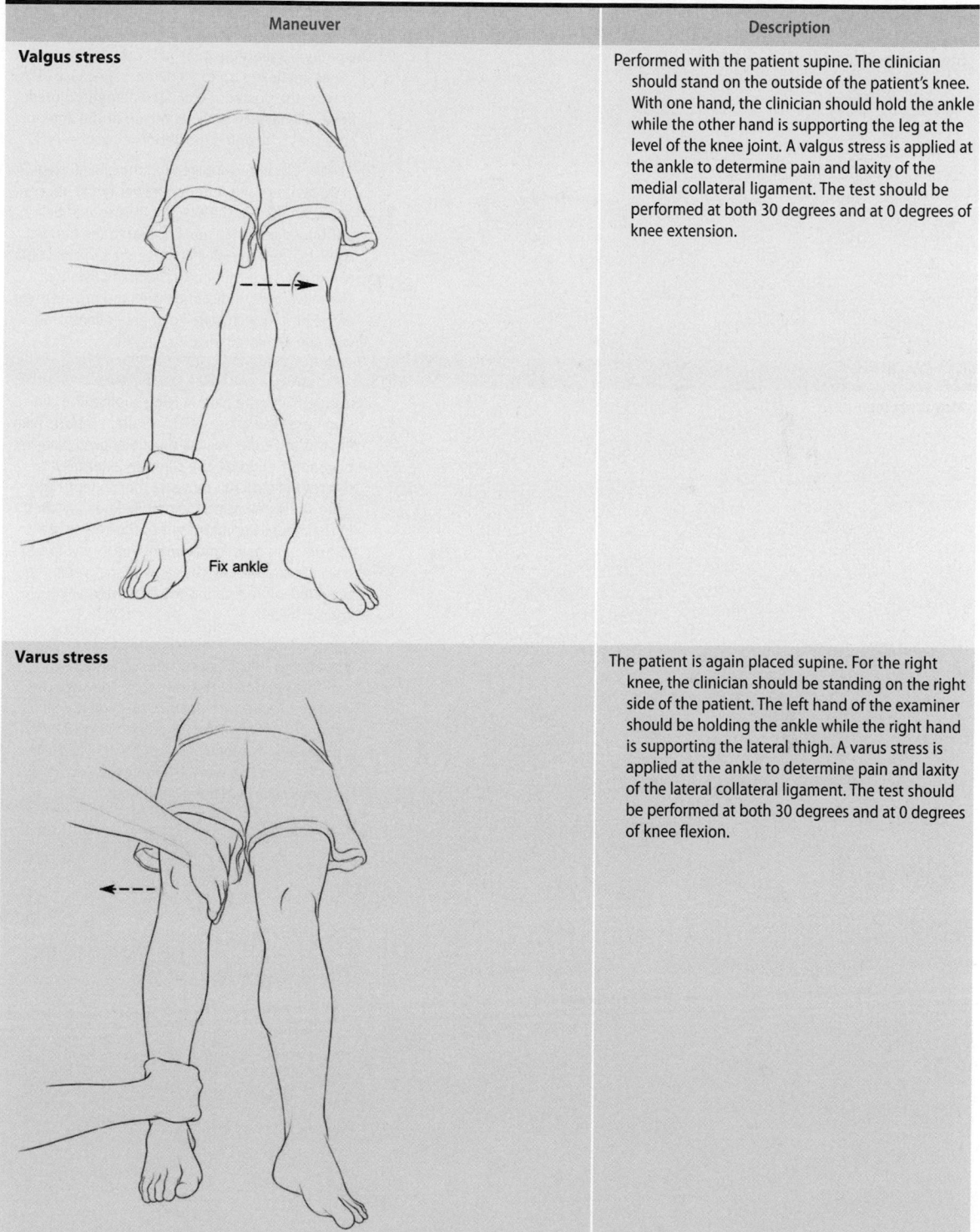 Fix ankle	Performed with the patient supine. The clinician should stand on the outside of the patient's knee. With one hand, the clinician should hold the ankle while the other hand is supporting the leg at the level of the knee joint. A valgus stress is applied at the ankle to determine pain and laxity of the medial collateral ligament. The test should be performed at both 30 degrees and at 0 degrees of knee extension.
Varus stress	The patient is again placed supine. For the right knee, the clinician should be standing on the right side of the patient. The left hand of the examiner should be holding the ankle while the right hand is supporting the lateral thigh. A varus stress is applied at the ankle to determine pain and laxity of the lateral collateral ligament. The test should be performed at both 30 degrees and at 0 degrees of knee flexion.

(continued)

Table 41–9. Knee examination. (continued)

Maneuver	Description
The sag sign	The patient is placed supine and both hips and knees are flexed up to 90 degrees. Because of gravity, the posterior cruciate ligament-injured knee will have an obvious set-off at the anterior tibia that is "sagging" posteriorly.
Posterior drawer	The patient is placed supine with the knee flexed at 90 degrees (see Anterior drawer figure above). In a normal knee, the anterior tibia should be positioned about 10 mm anterior to the femoral condyle. The clinician can grasp the proximal tibia with both hands and push the tibia posteriorly. The movement, indicating laxity and possible tear of the posterior cruciate ligament, is compared with the uninjured knee.
Meniscal signs	
McMurray test	Performed with the patient lying supine. The clinician flexes the knee until the patient reports pain. For this test to be valid, it must be flexed pain-free beyond 90 degrees. The clinician externally rotates the patient's foot and then extends the knee while palpating the medial knee for "click" in the medial compartment of the knee or pain reproducing pain from a meniscus injury. To test the lateral meniscus, the same maneuver is repeated while rotating the foot internally (53% sensitivity and 59–97% specificity).
Modified McMurray 	Performed with the hip flexed to 90 degrees. The knee is then flexed maximally with internal or external rotation of the lower leg. The knee can then be rotated with the lower leg in internal or external rotation to capture the torn meniscus underneath the condyles. A positive test is pain over the joint line while the knee is being flexed and internally or externally rotated.

(continued)

Table 41–9. Knee examination. (continued)

Maneuver	Description
Thessaly test 	Performed with the patient standing on one leg with knee slightly flexed. The patient is asked to twist the knee while standing on one leg. Pain can be elicited during twisting motion.
Patellofemoral joint test	
Apprehension sign	Suggests instability of the patellofemoral joint and is positive when the patient becomes apprehensive when the patella is deviated laterally.

10- to 15-pound weight. Excessive anterior translation of the tibia compared with the other side indicates injury to the ACL. The **anterior drawer test** (48% sensitivity and 87% specificity) is performed with the patient lying supine and the knee flexed to 90 degrees (Table 41–9). The clinician stabilizes the patient's foot by sitting on it and grasps the proximal tibia with both hands around the calf and pulls anteriorly. A positive test finds ACL laxity compared with the unaffected side. **The pivot shift** test is used to determine the amount of rotational laxity of the knee (Table 41–9). The patient is examined while lying supine with the knee in full extension. It is then slowly flexed while applying internal rotation and a valgus stress. The clinician feels for a subluxation at 20–40 degrees of knee flexion. The patient must remain very relaxed to have a positive test.

B. Imaging

Plain radiographs are usually negative in ACL tears but are useful to rule out fractures. A small avulsion injury can sometimes be seen over the lateral compartment of the knee. This is called a "Segond" fracture and is pathognomonic of an ACL injury. MRI is the best method to diagnose ACL tears and associated articular and meniscal cartilage issues. It has greater than 95% sensitivity and specificity for ACL tears.

▶ Treatment

Most young and active patients will require surgical reconstruction of the ACL. Some data suggest reconstruction within 5 months has better outcomes. However, a small randomized trial suggested that acute ACL injuries can be treated nonoperatively and delayed ACL reconstruction had similar outcomes to acute ACL reconstructions. Common surgical techniques use the patient's own tissues, usually the patellar or hamstring tendons (autograft) or a cadaver graft (allograft) to arthroscopically reconstruct the torn ACL. Different patients groups experienced improved results with specific surgical graft choices. However, allografts do have a higher failure rate when compared with autografts. Recovery from surgery usually requires 6 months.

Nonoperative treatments are usually reserved for older patients or those with a very sedentary lifestyle. Physical therapy can focus on hamstring strengthening and core stability. An ACL brace can help stability. Longitudinal studies have demonstrated that nonoperative management of an ACL tear can lead to a higher incidence of meniscus tears.

▶ When to Refer

- Almost all ACL tears should be referred to an orthopedic surgeon for evaluation.
- Individuals with instability in the setting of a chronic ACL tear (greater than 6 months) should be considered for surgical reconstruction.
- Patients with an ACL tear and associated meniscus or articular injuries may benefit from surgery to address the other injuries.

Frobell RB et al. Treatment for acute anterior cruciate ligament tear: five year outcome of randomised trial. BMJ. 2013 Jan 24; 346:f232. [PMID: 23349407]

Kaeding CC et al. Risk factors and predictors of subsequent ACL injury in either knee after ACL reconstruction: prospective analysis of 2488 primary ACL reconstructions from the Moon Cohort. Am J Sports Med. 2015 Jul;43(7):1583–90. [PMID: 25899429]

Shea KG et al. The American Academy of Orthopaedic Surgeons evidence-based guideline on management of anterior cruciate ligament injuries. J Bone Joint Surg Am. 2015 Apr 15; 97(8):672–4. [PMID: 25878313]

3. Collateral Ligament Injury

ESSENTIALS OF DIAGNOSIS

▶ Caused by a valgus or varus blow or stress to the knee.

▶ Pain and instability in the affected area.

▶ Limited range of motion.

▶ General Considerations

The medial collateral ligament (MCL) is the most commonly injured ligament in the knee. It is usually injured with a valgus stress to the partially flexed knee. It can also occur with a blow to the lateral leg. The MCL is commonly injured with acute ACL injuries. The lateral collateral ligament (LCL) is less commonly injured, but this can occur with a medial blow to the knee. Since both collateral ligaments are extra-articular, injuries to these ligaments may not lead to any intra-articular effusion. Affected patients may have difficulty walking initially, but this can improve when the swelling decreases.

▶ Clinical Findings

A. Symptoms and Signs

The main clinical findings for patients with collateral ligament injuries are pain along the course of the ligaments. The

patient may have limited range of motion due to pain, especially during the first 2 weeks following the injury. The best tests to assess the collateral ligaments are the varus and valgus stress tests. The sensitivity of the tests is as high as 86–96%.

The **valgus stress test** is performed with the patient supine (Table 41–9). The clinician should stand on the outside of the patient's knee. With one hand, the clinician should hold the ankle while the other hand is supporting the leg at the level of the knee joint. A valgus stress is applied at the ankle to determine pain and laxity of the MCL. The test should be performed at both 30 degrees and at 0 degrees of knee extension.

For the **varus stress test**, the patient is again placed supine (Table 41–9). For the right knee, the clinician should be standing on the right side of the patient. The clinician's left hand should be holding the ankle while the right hand is supporting the lateral thigh. A varus stress is applied at the ankle to determine pain and laxity of the LCL. The test should be performed at both 30 degrees and at 0 degrees of knee flexion.

The test results can be graded from 1–3. Grade 1 is when the patient has pain with varus/valgus stress test but no instability. With grade 2 injuries, the patient has pain, and the knee shows instability at 30 degrees of knee flexion. In grade 3 injuries, the patient has marked instability but not much pain. The knee is often unstable at both 30 degrees and 0 degrees of knee flexion.

B. Imaging

Radiographs are usually nondiagnostic except for avulsion injuries. However, radiographs should be used to rule out fractures that can occur with collateral ligament injuries. Isolated MCL injuries usually do not require evaluation by MRI, but MRI should be used to evaluate possible associated cruciate ligament injuries. LCL or posterolateral corner injuries should have MRI evaluation to exclude associated injuries and to determine their significance.

▶ Treatment

The majority of MCL injuries can be treated with protected weight-bearing and physical therapy. For grade 1 and 2 injuries, the patient can usually bear weight as tolerated with full range of motion. A hinged knee brace can be given to patients with grade 2 MCL tears to provide stability. Early physical therapy is recommended to protect range of motion and muscle strength. Grade 3 MCL injuries require long leg braces to provide stability. Patients can weight-bear but only with the knee locked in extension with a brace. The motion can then be increased with the brace unlocked. Grade 3 injuries can take up to 6–8 weeks to heal. MCL injuries rarely need surgery. LCL injuries usually require surgical repair or reconstruction.

▶ When to Refer

- Symptomatic instability with chronic MCL tears or acute MCL tears with other ligamentous injuries.

- LCL or posterolateral corner injuries require urgent surgical repair or reconstruction (within 1 week).

Pacheco RJ et al. Posterolateral corner injuries of the knee: a serious injury commonly missed. J Bone Joint Surg Br. 2011 Feb;93(2):194–7. [PMID: 21282758]

4. Posterior Cruciate Ligament Injury

ESSENTIALS OF DIAGNOSIS

- ▸ Usually follows an anterior trauma to the tibia, such as a dashboard injury during a motor vehicle accident.
- ▸ The knee may freely dislocate and reduce.
- ▸ One-third of multi-ligament injuries involving the PCL have neurovascular injuries.

▶ General Considerations

The posterior cruciate ligament (PCL) is the strongest ligament in the knee. PCL injuries usually represent significant trauma and are highly associated with multi-ligament injuries and knee dislocations. More than 70–90% of PCL injuries have associated injuries to the posterolateral corner, MCL, and ACL. Neurovascular injuries occur in up to one-third of all knee dislocations or PCL injuries. **There should be high suspicion for neurovascular injuries and a thorough neurovascular examination of the limb should be performed.**

▶ Clinical Findings

A. Symptoms and Signs

Most patients with acute injuries have difficulty with ambulation. Patients with chronic PCL injuries can ambulate without gross instability but may complain of subjective "looseness" and often report pain and dysfunction, especially with bending. Clinical examinations of PCL injuries include the **"sag sign"** (Table 41–9). The patient is placed supine and both hips and knees are flexed up to 90 degrees. Because of gravity, the PCL-injured knee will have an obvious set-off at the anterior tibia that is "sagging" posteriorly. The PCL ligament can also be examined using the **posterior drawer test** (90% sensitivity and 99% specificity) (Table 41–9). The patient is placed supine with the knee flexed at 90 degrees. In a normal knee, the anterior tibia should be positioned about 10 mm anterior to the femoral condyle. The clinician can grasp the proximal tibia with both hands and push the tibia posteriorly. The movement, indicating laxity and possible tear of the PCL, is compared with the uninjured knee. A PCL injury is sometimes mistaken for an ACL injury during the anterior drawer test since the tibia is subluxed posteriorly in a sagged position and can be abnormally translated forward, yielding a false-positive test for an ACL injury. Pain, swelling, pallor, and numbness in the affected extremity may suggest a knee dislocation with possible injury to the popliteal artery.

B. Imaging

Radiographs are often nondiagnostic but are required to diagnose any fractures. MRI is used to diagnose PCL and other associated injuries.

▶ Treatment

Isolated PCL injuries can be treated nonoperatively. Acute injuries are usually immobilized using a knee brace with the knee extension; the patient uses crutches for ambulation. Physical therapy can help achieve increased range of motion and improved ambulation. Many PCL injuries are associated with other injuries and may require operative reconstruction.

▶ When to Refer

- The patient should be seen urgently within 1–2 weeks.
- If the lateral knee is also unstable with varus stress testing, the patient should be assessed for a posterolateral corner injury, which may require an urgent surgical reconstruction.
- Isolated PCL tears may require surgery if the tear is complete (grade 3) and the patient is symptomatic.

5. Meniscus Injuries

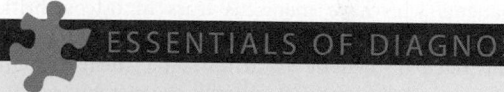

ESSENTIALS OF DIAGNOSIS

- ▸ Patient may or may not report an injury.
- ▸ Joint line pain and pain with deep squatting are the most sensitive signs.
- ▸ Difficulty with knee extension suggests an internal derangement that should be evaluated urgently with MRI.

▶ General Considerations

The menisci act as shock absorbers within the knee. Injuries to a meniscus can lead to pain, clicking, and locking sensation. Most meniscus injuries occur with acute injuries (usually in younger patients) or repeated microtrauma, such as squatting or twisting (usually in older patients).

▶ Clinical Findings

A. Symptoms and Signs

The patient may have an antalgic (painful) gait and difficulty with squatting. He or she may complain of catching or locking of the meniscal fragment. Physical findings can include effusion or joint line tenderness. Patients can usually point out the area of maximal tenderness along the joint line. Swelling usually occurs during the first 24 hours after the injury or later. Meniscus tears rarely lead to the immediate swelling that is commonly seen with fractures and ligament tears. Meniscus tears are commonly seen in arthritic knees. However, it is often unclear whether the pain is coming from the meniscus tear or the arthritis.

Provocative tests, including the **McMurray** test, the **modified McMurray test**, and the **Thessaly test**, can be performed to confirm the diagnosis (Table 41–9). Most symptomatic meniscus tears cause pain with deep squatting and when waddling (performing a "duck walk").

B. Imaging

Radiographs are usually normal but may show joint space narrowing, early OA changes, or loose bodies. MRI of the knee is the best diagnostic tool for meniscal injuries (93% sensitivity and 95% specificity). High signal through the meniscus (bright on T2 images) represents a meniscal tear.

▶ Treatment

Conservative treatment can be used for degenerative tears in older patients. The treatment is similar for patients with mild knee OA, including analgesics and physical therapy for strengthening and core stability. A randomized controlled trial showed that physical therapy compared to arthroscopic partial meniscectomy had similar outcomes at 6 months. However, 30% of the patients who were assigned to physical therapy alone underwent surgery within 6 months. Another randomized study has shown that arthroscopic surgery has no benefit over sham operation for patients who have meniscus tears in osteoarthritic knees. A 2013 randomized controlled study has further demonstrated no benefit for arthroscopic meniscectomy with sham operation for patients with degenerative meniscal tears.

Acute tears in young and active patients with signs of internal derangement and without signs of arthritis on imaging can be best treated arthroscopically with meniscus repair or debridement.

▶ When to Refer

- If the patient has symptoms of internal derangement suspected as meniscus injury. The patient should receive an MRI to confirm the injury.
- If the patient cannot extend the knee due to a mechanical block, the patient should be evaluated as soon as possible. Certain shaped tears on MRI, such as bucket handle tears, are amenable to meniscal repair surgery.

Katz JN et al. Surgery versus physical therapy for a meniscal tear and osteoarthritis. N Engl J Med. 2013 May 2;368(18):1675-84. Erratum in: N Engl J Med. 2013 Aug 15;369(7):683. [PMID: 23506518]

Khan M et al. Arthroscopic surgery for degenerative tears of the meniscus: a systematic review and meta-analysis. CMAJ. 2014 Oct 7;186(14):1057–64. [PMID: 25157057]

Sihvonen R et al; Finnish Degenerative Meniscal Lesion Study (FIDELITY) Group. Arthroscopic partial meniscectomy versus sham surgery for a degenerative meniscal tear. N Engl J Med. 2013 Dec 26;369(26):2515–24. [PMID: 24369076]

6. Patellofemoral Pain

 ESSENTIALS OF DIAGNOSIS

- ▶ Pain experienced with bending activities (kneeling, squatting, climbing stairs).
- ▶ Lateral deviation or tilting of the patella in relation to the femoral groove.

▶ General Considerations

Patellofemoral pain, also known as anterior knee pain, chondromalacia, or "runner's knee," describes any pain involving the patellofemoral joint. The pain affects any or all of the anterior knee structures, including the medial and lateral aspects of the patella as well as the quadriceps and patellar tendon insertions. The patella engages the femoral trochlear groove with approximately 30 degrees of knee flexion. Forces on the patellofemoral joint increase up to three times body weight as the knee flexes to 90 degrees (eg, climbing stairs), and five times body weight when going into full knee flexion (eg, squatting). Abnormal patellar tracking during flexion can lead to abnormal articular cartilage wear and pain. When the patient has ligamentous hyperlaxity, the patella can sublux out of the groove, usually laterally. Patellofemoral pain is also associated with muscle strength and flexibility imbalances as well as altered hip and ankle biomechanics.

▶ Clinical Findings

A. Symptoms and Signs

Patients usually complain of pain in the anterior knee with bending movements and less commonly in full extension. Pain from this condition is localized under the kneecap but can sometimes be referred to the posterior knee or over the medial or lateral inferior patella. Symptoms may begin after a trauma or after repetitive physical activity, such as running and jumping. When maltracking, palpable and sometimes audible crepitus can occur.

Intra-articular swelling usually does not occur unless there are articular cartilage defects or if OA changes develop. On physical examination, it is important to palpate the articular surfaces of the patella. For example, the clinician can use one hand to move the patella laterally, and use the fingertips of the other hand to palpate the lateral undersurface of patella. Patellar mobility can be assessed by medially and laterally deviating the patella (deviation by one-quarter of the diameter of the kneecap is consider normal; greater than one-half the diameter suggests excessive mobility). The **apprehension sign** suggests instability of the patellofemoral joint and is positive when the patient becomes apprehensive when the patella is deviated laterally

(Table 41–9). The **patellar grind test** is performed by grasping the knee superior to the patella and pushing it downward with the patient supine and the knee extended, pushing the patella inferiorly. The patient is asked to contract the quadriceps muscle to oppose this downward translation, with reproduction of pain or grinding being the positive sign for chondromalacia of the patella. There are two common presentations: (1) Patients whose ligaments and patella are too loose (hypermobility); (2) and patients who have soft tissues that are too tight leading to excessive pressure on the joint.

Evaluation of the quadriceps strength and hip stabilizers can be accomplished by having the patient perform a one-leg squat without support. Patients who are weak may display poor balance, with dropping of the pelvis (similar to a positive hip Trendelenburg sign) or excessive internal rotation of the knee medially. Normally, with a one-leg squat, the knee should align over the second metatarsal ray of the foot.

B. Imaging

Diagnostic imaging has limited use in younger patients and is more helpful in older patients to assess for OA or to evaluate patients who do not respond to conservative treatment. Radiographs may show lateral deviation or tilting of the patella in relation to the femoral groove. MRI may show thinning of the articular cartilage but is not clinically necessary, except prior to surgery or to exclude other pathology.

▶ Treatment

A. Conservative

For symptomatic relief, use of local modalities such as ice and anti-inflammatory medications can be beneficial. If the patient has signs of patellar hypermobility, physical therapy exercises are useful to strengthen the quadriceps (especially the vastus medialis obliquus muscle) to help stabilize the patella and improve tracking. There is consistent evidence that exercise therapy for **patellofemoral pain syndrome** may result in clinically important reduction in pain and improvement in functional ability. Lower quality research supports that hip and knee exercises are better than knee exercises alone. Strengthening the quadriceps and the posterolateral hip muscles such as the hip abductors that control rotation at the knee should be recommended. Support for the patellofemoral joint can be provided by use of a patellar stabilizer brace or special taping techniques (McConnell taping). Correcting lower extremity alignment (with appropriate footwear or over-the-counter orthotics) can help improve symptoms, especially if the patient has pronation or high arched feet. If the patient demonstrates tight peripatellar soft tissues, special focus should be put on stretching the hamstrings, iliotibial band, quadriceps, calves and hip flexors.

B. Surgical

Surgery is rarely needed and is considered a last resort for patellofemoral pain. Procedures performed include lateral release or patellar realignment surgery.

▶ When to Refer

Patients with persistent symptoms despite a course of conservative therapy.

Jin J. JAMA patient page. Running injuries. JAMA. 2014 Jul; 312(2):202. [PMID: 25005669]

Khayambashi K et al. Posterolateral hip muscle strengthening versus quadriceps strengthening for patellofemoral pain: a comparative control trial. Arch Phys Med Rehabil. 2014 May; 95(5):900–7. [PMID: 24440362]

van der Heijden RA et al. Exercise for treating patellofemoral pain syndrome. Cochrane Database Syst Rev. 2015 Jan 20; 1:CD010387. [PMID: 25603546]

7. Knee Osteoarthritis

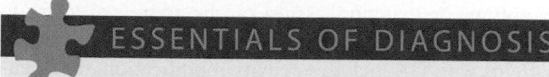
ESSENTIALS OF DIAGNOSIS

- ▶ Degeneration of joint cartilage.
- ▶ Pain with bending or twisting activities.
- ▶ Swelling.
- ▶ Loss of active and passive range of motion in severe OA.

▶ General Considerations

In the United States, the prevalence of OA will grow as the number of persons over age 65 years doubles to more than 70 million by 2030. The incidence of knee OA in the United States is 240 per 100,000 person-years.

Cartilage loss and OA symptoms are preceded by damage to the collagen-proteoglycan matrix. The etiology of OA is often multifactorial including previous trauma, prior high-impact activities, genetic factors, obesity, and rheumatologic or metabolic conditions.

▶ Clinical Findings

A. Symptoms and Signs

OA usually causes pain in the affected joint with loading of the joint or at the extremes of motion. Mechanical symptoms—such as swelling, grinding, catching, and locking—suggest internal derangement, which is indicated by damaged cartilage or bone fragments that affect the smooth range of motion expected at an articular joint. Pain can also produce the sensation of "buckling" or "giving way" due to muscle inhibition. As the joint degeneration becomes more advanced, the patient loses active range of motion and may lose passive range of motion as well.

As the condition worsens, patients with knee OA have an increasingly limited ability to walk. Symptoms include pain with bending or twisting activities, and going up and down stairs. Swelling, limping, and pain while sleeping are common complaints with OA, especially as it progresses.

B. Imaging

The most commonly recommended radiographs include bilateral weight-bearing 45-degree bent knee posteroanterior, lateral, and patellofemoral joint views (Merchant view). Radiographic findings include diminished width of the articular cartilage causing joint space narrowing, subchondral sclerosis, presence of osteophytes, and cystic changes in the subchondral bone. MRI of the knee is most likely unnecessary unless other pathology is suspected, including ischemic osteonecrosis of the knee.

▶ Treatment

A. Conservative

Changes in the articular cartilage are irreversible. Therefore, a cure for the diseased joint is not possible, although symptoms or structural issues can be addressed to try to maintain activity level. Conservative treatment for all patients with OA includes activity modification, therapeutic exercises, and weight loss. Lifestyle modifications also include proper footwear and avoidance of high impact activities. Optimal exercise programs for knee OA should focus on improving aerobic capacity, quadriceps muscle strength, or lower extremity performance. Ideally, the program should be supervised and carried out three times a week.

Use of a cane in the hand opposite to the affected side is mechanically advantageous. Knee sleeves or braces provide some improvement in subjective pain symptoms most likely due to improvements in neuromuscular function. If patients have unicompartmental OA in the medial or lateral compartment, joint unloader braces are available to offload the degenerative compartment. Cushioning footwear and appropriate orthotics or shoe adjustments are useful for reducing impact to the lower extremities.

There are several oral and intra-articular pharmacologic options. Treatments that have been shown to have small but robust differences include oral acetaminophen, diclofenac, ibuprofen, naproxen, celecoxib, and intra-articular corticosteroids and hyaluronic acid. All treatments except acetaminophen showed clinically significant improvement in pain. If a traditional NSAID is indicated, the choice should be based on cost, side-effect profile, and adherence. The cyclooxygenase (COX)-2 inhibitor celecoxib is no more effective than traditional NSAIDs; it may offer short-term, but probably not long-term, advantage in preventing gastrointestinal complications. Due to its cost and potential cardiovascular risk, celecoxib should be reserved for carefully selected patients. Topical NSAIDs or capsaicin can be effective in the treatment of OA, since they avoid many of the traditional NSAID complications. Opioids can be used appropriately in patients with severe OA (see Chapter 5). Glucosamine and chondroitin sulfate are supplements that have been widely used and marketed for OA. Evidence for their effectiveness in slowing or reversing cartilage loss is limited and any effect present appears to be small. Despite some initial promise, the best-controlled studies indicate these supplements are ineffective as analgesics in OA. However, they have minimal side effects and may be appropriate if the patient experiences subjective benefit.

Knee joint corticosteroid injections are options to help reduce pain and inflammation and can provide short-term pain relief, usually lasting about 6–12 weeks. Viscosupplementation by injections of hyaluronic acid–based products is controversial. Because reviews suggest that viscosupplementation has a questionably clinically relevant effect size, and has an increased risk of adverse events, the American Academy of Orthopedic Surgeons has recommended that viscosupplementation should not be used in the treatment of knee OA. However, the American College of Rheumatology's 2012 OA guidelines recommend the use of intra-articular hyaluronic acid injection for the treatment of OA of the knee in adults. Platelet-rich plasma injections contain high concentration of platelet-derived growth factors, which regulate some biologic processes in tissue repair. A meta-analysis of 10 studies demonstrated that platelet-rich plasma injections reduced pain in patients with knee OA more efficiently than placebo and hyaluronic acid injections. However, 9 of the 10 studies had a high risk of bias, and the underlying mechanism of biologic healing is unknown. The authors recommend further studies before recommending platelet-rich plasma for routine management of knee OA.

B. Surgical

Two randomized trials demonstrated that arthroscopy does not improve outcomes at 1 year over placebo or routine conservative treatment of OA. **Joint replacement surgeries are effective and cost-effective for patients with significant symptoms or functional limitations, providing improvements in pain, function, and quality of life.** The number of total knee arthroplasty procedures jumped 162% from 1991 to 2010, along with an increase in complications and hospital readmissions. Minimally invasive surgeries and computer-assisted navigation during operation are being investigated as methods to improve techniques (eg, accurate placement of the hardware implant) and to reduce complication rates; however, major improvements have yet to be demonstrated.

Knee realignment surgery, such as high tibial osteotomy or partial knee replacement surgery, is indicated in patients younger than age 60 with unicompartmental OA, who would benefit from delaying total knee replacement. Knee joint replacement surgery has been very successful in improving outcomes for patient with end-stage OA. Long-term series describe more than 95% survival rate of the implant at 15 years.

▶ When to Refer

Patients with sufficient disability, limited benefit from conservative therapy, and evidence of severe OA can be referred for joint replacement surgery.

Bannuru RR et al. Comparative effectiveness of pharmacologic interventions for knee osteoarthritis: a systematic review and network meta-analysis. Ann Intern Med. 2015 Jan 6; 162(1):46–54. [PMID: 25560713]

Jevsevar DS. Treatment of osteoarthritis of the knee: evidence-based guideline, 2nd edition. J Am Acad Orthop Surg. 2013 Sep;21(9):571–6. [PMID: 23996988]

Juhl C et al. Impact of exercise type and dose on pain and disability in knee osteoarthritis: a systematic review and meta-regression analysis of randomized controlled trials. Arthritis Rheumatol. 2014 Mar;66(3):622–36. [PMID: 24574223]

Laudy AB et al. Efficacy of platelet-rich plasma injections in osteoarthritis of the knee: a systematic review and meta-analysis. Br J Sports Med. 2015 May;49(10):657–72. [PMID: 25416198]

ANKLE INJURIES

1. Inversion Ankle Sprains

ESSENTIALS OF DIAGNOSIS

▸ Localized pain and swelling.

▸ The majority of ankle injuries involve inversion injuries affecting the lateral ligaments.

▸ Consider chronic ankle instability or associated injuries if pain persists for longer than 3 months following an ankle sprain.

▸ General Considerations

Ankle sprains are the most common sports injuries seen in outpatient clinics. Patients usually report "turning the ankle" during a fall or after landing on an irregular surface such as a hole or an opponent's foot. The most common mechanism of injury is an inversion and plantar flexion sprain, which injures the anterior talofibular ligament (ATF) ligament rather than the calcaneofibular ligament (CF) ligament. Other injuries that can occur with inversion ankle injuries are listed in Table 41–10. Women appear to sustain an inversion injury more frequently than men.

Table 41–10. Injuries associated with ankle sprains.

Ligaments
Subtalar joint sprain
Sinus tarsi syndrome
Syndesmotic sprain
Deltoid sprain
Lisfranc injury
Tendons
Posterior tibial tendon strain
Peroneal tendon subluxation
Bones
Osteochondral talus injury
Lateral talar process fracture
Posterior impingement (os trigonum)
Fracture at the base of the fifth metatarsal
Jones fracture
Salter fracture (fibula)
Ankle fractures

▸ Clinical Findings

A. Symptoms and Signs

The usual symptoms following a sprain include localized pain and swelling over the lateral aspect of the ankle, difficulty weight bearing, and limping. The patient's ankle may feel unstable. On examination, there may be swelling or bruising over the lateral aspect of the ankle. The anterior, inferior aspect below the lateral malleolus is most often the point of maximal tenderness consistent with ATF and CF ligament injuries. The swelling may limit motion of the ankle. Special stress tests for the ankle include the **anterior drawer test** (Table 41–11) and **subtalar tilt test**

Table 41–11. Ankle examination.

Maneuver	Description
Inspection	Examine for the alignment of the ankle (SEADS).
Palpation	Include important landmarks: Ottawa Ankle Rules (medial and lateral malleolus, base of fifth metatarsal and navicular area), anterior tibiofibular ligament, posterior talus; tendons (Achilles, peroneals, posterior tibialis, flexor hallucis longus).
Range of motion testing	Check range of motion actively (patient performs) and passively (clinician performs), especially with flexion and extension of the spine. Rotation and lateral bending are also helpful to assess symmetric motion or any restrictions.
Ankle strength testing	Test resisted ankle dorsiflexion, plantarflexion, inversion and eversion strength manually.
Ankle anterior drawer	The clinician keeps the foot and ankle in the neutral position with the patient sitting, then uses one hand to fix the tibia and the other to hold the patient's heel and draw the ankle forward. Normally, there may be approximately 3 mm of translation until an endpoint is felt. A positive test includes increased translation of one foot compared to the other with loss of the endpoint of the anterior talofibular ligament.
Subtalar tilt test	Performed with the foot in the neutral position with the patient sitting. The clinician uses one hand to fix the tibia and the other to hold and invert the calcaneus. Normal inversion at the subtalar joint is approximately 30 degrees. A positive test consists of increased subtalar joint inversion greater than 10 degrees on the affected side with loss of endpoint for the calcaneofibular ligament.
External rotation stress test	Performed when the clinician fixes the tibia with one hand and grasps the foot in the other with the ankle in the neutral position and then dorsiflexes and externally rotates the ankle, reproducing the patient's pain.

SEADS, swelling, erythema, atrophy, deformity, and (surgical) scars.

(Table 41–11). In order to grade the severity of ankle sprains, no laxity on stress tests is considered a grade 1 injury, laxity of the ATF ligament on anterior drawer testing but a negative tilt test is a grade 2 injury, and both positive drawer and tilt tests signify a grade 3 injury.

B. Imaging

Routine ankle radiographic views include the AP, lateral, and oblique (mortise) views. Less common views requested include the calcaneal view and subtalar view. **Ottawa Ankle Rules** are clinical prediction rules to guide the need for radiographs and have a 97% sensitivity and 99% negative predictive value. If the patient is unable to bear weight immediately in the office setting or emergency department for four steps, then the clinician should check for (1) bony tenderness at the posterior edge of the medial or lateral malleolus and (2) bony tenderness over the navicular (medial midfoot) or at the base of the fifth metatarsal. If either malleoli demonstrates pain or deformity, then ankle radiographs should be obtained. If the foot has bony tenderness, obtain foot radiographs. An MRI is helpful when considering the associated injuries.

▶ Treatment

Immediate treatment of an ankle sprain follows the MICE mnemonic: *m*odified activities, *i*ce, *c*ompression, and *e*levation. Subsequent treatment involves protected weight bearing with crutches and use of an ankle stabilizer brace, especially for grade 2 and 3 injuries. **Early motion is essential, and patients should be encouraged to do home exercises or physical therapy.** Proprioception and balance exercises (eg, "wobble board") are useful to restore function to the ankle and prevent future ankle sprains. Regular use of an ankle support with activities can reduce the risk of lateral ankle sprains. Chronic instability can develop after acute ankle sprain in 10–20% of people and may require surgical stabilization with ligament reconstruction surgery.

▶ When to Refer

- Ankle fractures.
- Recurrent ankle sprains or signs of chronic ligamentous ankle instability.
- No response after more than 3 months of conservative treatment.
- Suspicion of associated injuries.

Czajka CM. Ankle sprains and instability. Med Clin North Am. 2014 Mar;98(2):313–29. [PMID: 24559877]

Doherty C et al. The incidence and prevalence of ankle sprain injury: a systematic review and meta-analysis of prospective epidemiological studies. Sports Med. 2014 Jan;44(1):123–40. [PMID: 24105612]

Kemler E et al. A systematic review on the treatment of acute ankle sprain: brace versus other functional treatment types. Sports Med. 2011 Mar 1;41(3):185–97. [PMID: 21395362]

2. Eversion ("High") Ankle Sprains

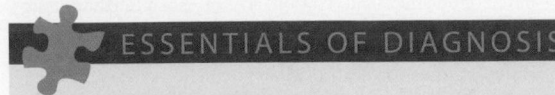

ESSENTIALS OF DIAGNOSIS

- ▶ Severe and prolonged pain.
- ▶ Limited range of motion.
- ▶ Mild swelling.
- ▶ Difficulty with weight bearing.

▶ General Considerations

A syndesmotic injury or "high ankle" sprain involves the anterior *tibio*fibular ligament in the anterolateral aspect of the ankle, superior to the anterior *talo*fibular (ATF) ligament. The injury mechanism often involves the foot being turned out or externally rotated and everted (eg, when being tackled). This injury is commonly missed or misdiagnosed as an ATF ligament sprain on initial visit.

▶ Clinical Findings

A. Symptoms and Signs

Symptoms of a high ankle sprain include severe and prolonged pain over the anterior ankle at the anterior tibiofibular ligament, worse with weight bearing. This is often more painful than the typical ankle sprain. The point of maximal tenderness involves the anterior tibiofibular ligament, which is higher than the ATF ligament. It is also important to palpate the proximal fibula to rule out any proximal syndesmotic ligament injury and associated fracture known as a "maisonneuve fracture." There is often some mild swelling in this area, and the patient may or may not have an ankle effusion. The patient usually has limited range of motion in all directions. The **external rotation stress test** reproduces the mechanism of injury (Table 41–11). (**Note:** The patient's foot should have an intact neurovascular examination before undertaking this test.)

B. Imaging

Radiographs of the ankle should include the AP, mortise, and lateral views. The mortise view may demonstrate loss of the normal overlap between the tibia and fibula, which should be at least 1–2 mm. Asymmetry in the joint space around the tibiotalar joint suggests disruption of the syndesmotic ligaments. If there is proximal tenderness in the lower leg especially around the fibula, an AP and lateral view of the tibia and fibula should be obtained to rule out a proximal fibula fracture. Radiographs during an external rotation stress test may visualize instability at the distal tibiofibular joint. MRI is the best method to visualize injury to the tibiofibular ligament and to assess status of the other ligaments and the articular cartilage.

Treatment

Whereas most ankle sprains are treated with early motion and weight bearing, treatment for a high ankle sprain should be conservative with a cast or walking boot for 4–6 weeks. Thereafter, protected weight bearing with crutches is recommended until the patient can walk pain-free. Physical therapy can start early to regain range of motion and maintain strength with limited weight-bearing initially.

When to Refer

If there is widening of the joint space and asymmetry at the tibiotalar joint, the patient should be referred urgently to a foot and ankle surgeon. Severe or prolonged persistent cases that do not heal may require internal fixation to avoid chronic instability at the tibiofibular joint. Screw fixation remains the gold standard, although newer techniques with bioabsorbable constructs are emerging.

Magan A et al. Evaluation and management of injuries of the tibiofibular syndesmosis. Br Med Bull. 2014 Sep;111(1):101–15. [PMID: 25190761]

Van Heest TJ et al. Injuries to the ankle syndesmosis. J Bone Joint Surg Am. 2014 Apr 2;96(7):603–13. [PMID: 24695928]

Index

NOTE: Page numbers in **boldface** type indicate a major discussion. A *t* following a page number indicates tabular material, and *f* following a page number indicates a figure. Drugs are listed under their generic names. When a drug trade name is listed, the reader is referred to the generic name.

A3243G mutation, in diabetes mellitus, 1212
A antigen, in compatibility testing, 542
A/California/7/2009 (H1N1) pdm09-like virus, 1413. *See also* Influenza
A cells, pancreatic, 1185
A/Hong Kong/4801/2014 (H3N2)-like virus, 1413. *See also* Influenza
A/Switzerland/9715293/2013 (H3N2)-like virus, 1413. *See also* Influenza
AA (Alcoholics Anonymous), 1084, 1094
AA (secondary) amyloidosis, 421, 538. *See also* Amyloidosis
  cardiac, 421
  renal, 946
AAA. *See* Abdominal aortic aneurysm
AAAS gene, in triple A (Allgrove) syndrome, 1169
Abacavir, 1351*t*, 1353, 1354. *See also* Antiretroviral therapy
  HLA-B-associated drug hypersensitivity and, 880, 1354
  with lamivudine (Epzicom), 1353, 1354, 1354*t*
    plus darunavir and cobicistat, 1360*t*
    plus darunavir and ritonavir, 1360*t*
  with lamivudine and dolutegravir (Triumeq), 1354*t*, 1358, 1359*t*, 1360
  with zidovudine and lamivudine (Trizivir), 1354, 1354*t*
Abatacept, for rheumatoid arthritis, 838
ABC/3TC. *See* Abacavir, with lamivudine
ABCB4 gene, in idiopathic adulthood ductopenia, 724
ABCD/ABCDE rule/features, in melanoma, 104
ABCD2 score, in transient ischemic attacks, 992
Abciximab. *See also* Glycoprotein IIb/IIIa receptors, drugs blocking
  for acute coronary syndromes, 368
  PCI and, 362
  platelet function affected by, 558*t*
Abdominal abscess/infection, 1314*t*
  actinomycosis, 1480–1481
  anaerobic, 1314*t*, **1479**, 1479*t*
  in Crohn disease, 653, 654
  in diverticulitis, 663, 664
  secondary peritonitis and, 603
Abdominal aortic aneurysm, **480–482**
  screening for, 6*t*, 7, 481
Abdominal compartment syndrome, in burn patient, 1569

Abdominal fistulas, in Crohn disease, 653, 654
Abdominal pain/tenderness, **578–580**. *See also specific cause*
  differential diagnosis of, 642
Abdominal paracentesis. *See* Paracentesis
Abdominal radiographs, in poisoning/drug overdose, 1585
Abdominal testes. *See* Cryptorchism
Abemaciclib, for breast cancer, 756
Abeta-2M (renal failure type) amyloidosis, 538
Abetalipoproteinemia, vitamin E deficiency and, 1025, 1278
ABI/ABPI. *See* Ankle-brachial index
ABIC score, in alcoholic liver disease, 695
Abilify. *See* Aripiprazole
Abiraterone, 1670*t*
  for prostate cancer, 1649*t*, 1650
abl gene, in chronic myeloid leukemia, 523
Abnormal illness behaviors, **1058–1060**
Abnormal movements. *See* Movement disorders
Abnormal sleep behaviors, **1090**
Abnormal uterine bleeding
  endometrial carcinoma and, 763, 764, 774
  ovulatory, 762, 763
  postmenopausal, **764**
    estrogen replacement therapy and, 764, 1203
  premenopausal, **762–764**
    in polycystic ovary syndrome, 780, 1196
ABO system
  compatibility testing for transfusion and, 542
  hemolytic transfusion reactions and, 542–543
Abortion
  anaerobic infection after, 1479
  clostridial infection after, 1452
  elective/induced, **791–792**
    breast cancer during pregnancy and, 745–747, 760
    heart disease during pregnancy and, 819
    hypertension during pregnancy and, 818
    rubella/rubella vaccination and, 1384, 1385
  IUD insertion after, 789
  recurrent (habitual), **805**
  spontaneous. *See* Spontaneous abortion
Abortive poliomyelitis, 1382
Abortive rabies, 1387

ABPA. *See* Allergic bronchopulmonary mycosis/aspergillosis
ABPI. *See* Ankle-brachial index
Abraxane. *See* Paclitaxel, protein-bound
Abscesses, 152–154, 1443*t*. *See also specific type and structure affected*
  anaerobic, 1314*t*, 1478–1479
    abdominal, 1314*t*, 1479, 1479*t*
    brain, 1314*t*, 1478–1479
    of lung, 268*t*, **274–276**, 1478
  in bacterial rhinosinusitis, 217
  brain, **1007–1008**, 1298, 1299, 1314*t*, 1478–1479. *See also* Brain abscess
  in Crohn disease, 652, 653, 654
  deep neck, 230
  in drug users, 1303
  epidural
    bacterial rhinosinusitis and, 217
    osteomyelitis and, 870, 871, 1449
    otitis media and, 206
  in HIV infection/AIDS, 1343
  intravascular (septic superficial thrombophlebitis), 488, 1314*t*. *See also* Septic thrombophlebitis
  liver
    amebic, 1525, 1526, 1527, 1527*t*
    pyogenic, **714–715**
  lung, **274–276**, 1478
    in coccidioidomycosis, 1550, 1551
  in mycetoma, 1557
  mycobacteria causing, 1482
  myocardial, endocarditis and, 1458
  perforated appendicitis and, 642
  perianal, 673
  peritonsillar, **229**
  soft tissue/subcutaneous, in coccidioidomycosis, 1550, 1551
  staphylococcal, 153, 1343, 1443*t*, 1447, 1448, 1448*f*
Absence (petit mal) seizures, 984–985, 984*t*. *See also* Seizures
  drug therapy for, 988*t*
Absidia (Lichtheimia) infection, 218, 1555–1556
Absorption (digestion), disorders of. *See* Malabsorption
Absorptive hypercalciuria, 962*t*, 963
Abstinence syndrome, in opioid withdrawal, 1099
Abuse
  aggression/violence/impulse control disorders and, 1090–1091
  child. *See* Child abuse
  drug/alcohol. *See* Alcohol use disorder; Substance use disorders

Abuse (*Cont.*):
  elder, 16, **70–71**, 71*t*
  partner/spousal (domestic violence), 16, 1090–1091, 1091
  prevention of, 16
ABVD regimen, 534
AC regimen, 751
AC-T regimen, 751, 752
AC-TH regimen, 752
Acamprosate, for alcohol use disorder, 17, 694, 1095
Acanthamoeba keratitis, **175–176**
Acanthosis nigricans, insulin resistance/diabetes and, 1212, 1212*f*, 1214
Acarbose, 1221*t*, 1225
  overdose/toxicity of, 1225, 1595
Accelerated idioventricular rhythm, **398**
  in myocardial infarction, 377, 398
Accessory atrioventricular pathways, supraventricular tachycardia and, 385, **387–388**
Accidental injury. *See* Trauma
Acclimatization, high-altitude illness and, 1574, 1575
ACCORD study, 1219
Accupril/Accuretic. *See* Quinapril
Accutane. *See* Isotretinoin
ACE. *See* Angiotensin-converting enzyme
ACE inhibitors. *See* Angiotensin-converting enzyme (ACE) inhibitors
Acebutolol, 452*t*
  overdose/toxicity of, 1591
Acellular pertussis vaccine, with tetanus-diphtheria toxoid (DTaP/Tdap vaccines), 4, 1320*t*, 1321*t*, 1322*t*, 1329*t*, 1453, 1453*t*, 1457, 1464. *See also* Tetanus and diphtheria toxoids and pertussis vaccines
Aceon. *See* Perindopril
Acetadote. *See* Acetylcysteine
Acetaminophen, **74**, 75*t*
  in analgesic nephropathy, 947
  contraindications to in heat stroke, 1563
  with opioid analgesics, 74, 80*t*
  for osteoarthritis, 828
  overdose/toxicity of, 74, 685, 686, 1581*t*, 1584*t*, **1585–1586**, 1586*f*
    anion gap acidosis and, 1584
    hepatotoxicity/liver failure and, 74, 685, 686, 1585, 1586*f*
Acetazolamide
  adverse ophthalmic effects of, 177*t*
  for glaucoma/ocular hypertension, 176, 180
  for high-altitude illness treatment/prevention, 1574, 1575
  for pseudotumor cerebri, 1009
Acetoacetate
  in alcoholic ketoacidosis, 905
  in diabetic ketoacidosis, 1247
Acetohexamide, 1220, 1221*t*
Acetonitrile, cyanide formed by metabolism of, 1592

Acetylcholine
  aminoglycosides affecting, 1047
  botulinum toxin affecting, 1046, 1454
  in myasthenic (Lambert-Eaton) syndrome, 1046
Acetylcholine receptor antibodies
  in cancer-related neuropathy, 1037
  in myasthenia gravis, 1045
Acetylcholinesterase inhibitors. *See* Anticholinesterases
Acetylcysteine
  for acetaminophen overdose/toxicity, 685, 1581*t*, 1584*t*, **1585–1586**
  contrast media nephrotoxicity mediated by, 919
Achalasia, 605*t*, **617–618**
Achlorhydria
  in bacterial overgrowth, 636
  in pernicious anemia gastritis, 622
  VIPomas causing, 1186
Achromycin. *See* Tetracycline
Acid, corrosive, **1586–1587**
  esophageal injury/ingestion and, 1586
  eye injury and, 198, 1581, 1587
  skin injury and, 1581, 1586–1587
Acid-antisecretory agents. *See also* Antacids; H_2 receptor blocking drugs; Proton pump inhibitors
  for dyspepsia, 580
  for GERD, 609
  for GI bleeding, 596–597
  for peptic ulcer disease, 625, 627
    bleeding control and, 629–630
Acid-base disorders, **903–911**, 904*t*. *See also* Acidosis; Alkalosis
  genetic, 892*t*
  in kidney disease/renal failure, 892*t*, 906–907, 906*t*, 908, 926*f*, 928
  mixed, **903–904**
  step-by-step analysis and, 903
Acid-fast rods, treatment of infections caused by, 1312*t*
Acidosis, 903. *See also specific type and* Ketoacidosis
  anion gap. *See* Anion gap/anion gap acidosis
  dilutional, 907
  drowning and, 1567
  hyperkalemia and, 893
  hypokalemia and, 891, 908
  hyporeninemic hypoaldosteronemic, 906*t*, 907
  in kidney disease/renal failure, 892*t*, 906–907, 906*t*, 908, 916, 926*f*, 928. *See also* Renal tubular acidosis
  lactic, 905, **1251–1252**. *See also* Lactic acidosis
  metabolic, 903, **904–905**, 904*t*. *See also* Metabolic acidosis
  nephrolithiasis/nephrocalcinosis/urolithiasis and, 906–907, 962
  normal anion gap. *See* Normal anion gap acidosis
  parenteral nutritional support and, 907, 1285*t*
  in poisoning/drug overdose, 1584
    corrosive acids and, 1586

  with methanol or ethylene glycol, 906, 908, 1584, 1599
  with salicylates, 906, 1603
  posthypocapnia, 907
  renal tubular, 892*t*, 906–907, 906*t*, 908. *See also* Renal tubular acidosis
  in tubulointerstitial disease, 948
  respiratory, 903, 904*t*, **910**. *See also* Respiratory acidosis
  in respiratory failure, 317–318, 910
  uremic, 906
Aciduria, paradoxic, in metabolic alkalosis, 909
Acinetobacter infections, 1311*t*
Acitretin
  adverse ophthalmic effects of, 179*t*
  for psoriasis, 108
ACL. *See* Anterior cruciate ligament
Aclidinum, for COPD, 260
Aclovate. *See* Alclometasone
Acne, **126–128**, 126*f*
  antibiotics for, 98*t*, 127–128
  folliculitis and, 127, 131
  inversa (hidradenitis suppurativa), 153
  rosacea differentiated from, 127, 129
  steroid (steroid folliculitis), 127, 130
  testosterone replacement therapy and, 1193, 1206
  vulgaris, **126–128**, 126*f*
Aconex. *See* Interferon-beta
Acoustic neuroma/neurinoma (vestibular schwannoma/eighth nerve tumors), 211*t*, **213–214**, 1004*t*, 1005
  in neurofibromatosis, 213, 1010
Acoustic trauma. *See* Noise trauma
Acquired immunodeficiency syndrome (AIDS). *See* HIV infection/AIDS
Acral erythema (hand-foot syndrome), chemotherapy-induced, 1673
Acral-lentiginous melanoma, 103, 104
Acrocyanosis, 844
Acrodermatitis chronicum atrophicans, 1503, 1505*t*
Acromegaly, **1114–1116**
  hirsutism/virilization and, 1197
  hyperprolactinemia and, 1117
Acromioclavicular joint, O'Brien test in evaluation of, 1688*t*
Acropachy, thyroid, 1127
ACS. *See* Acute coronary syndromes
ACT (artemisinin-based combination therapy), 1515, 1516*t*, 1519, 1521
  self-treatment and, 1520
ACTH. *See* Adrenocorticotropic hormone
Actinic dermatitis, chronic, 154
Actinic (ultraviolet) keratitis, **198**
Actinic keratoses, **117–118**
  squamous cell carcinoma arising from, 118, 144
Actinic prurigo, 154
Actinobacillus/Aggregatibacter actinomycetemcomitans. See HACEK organisms

Actinomyces/Actinomyces israelii
(actinomycosis), 1312*t*,
1480–1481
Actinomycetoma, **1557**
Actiq. *See* Fentanyl
Activated charcoal, for poisoning/drug
overdose, 1581, 1582
repeat-dose, 1583
Activated protein C, resistance to, DVT/
PE (venous thromboembolic
disease) and, 295
Activities of daily living–instrumental
activities of daily living
(ADLs–IADLs), assessment
of ability to perform, 55–56
Activity. *See* Exercise/activity
Actonel. *See* Risedronate
ACTOplus Met. *See* Pioglitazone, with
metformin
Actos. *See* Pioglitazone
Acular. *See* Ketorolac
Acupuncture, for migraine prophylaxis,
979
Acute adrenal crisis, 1168–1169, 1170,
1172
Acute angle-closure glaucoma/crisis.
See Angle-closure glaucoma
Acute arterial limb occlusion, **476–477**
Acute cardiogenic liver injury, 712–713
Acute colonic pseudo-obstruction
(Ogilvie syndrome), **639–640**
Acute coronary syndromes, 365
chest pain/discomfort in, 26–27, 27,
27*t*, 28
perioperative risk assessment/
management and, 46–47, 47*f*,
47*t*
without ST-segment elevation
(NSTEMI), 365, **365–370**,
367*f*, 369*t*. *See also* Non–
ST-segment elevation
syndromes
ST-segment elevation (STEMI), 26–27,
27, 27*t*, 28, 365, 369*t*,
370–381, 372*f*, 373*t*. *See also*
Myocardial infarction
Acute fatty liver of pregnancy, 697, **824**
liver failure and, 685, 824
Acute flaccid paralysis (AFP), 1383
coxsackievirus infection and, 1426
enterovirus 71 causing, 1427
Acute idiopathic polyneuropathy. *See*
Guillain-Barré syndrome
Acute intermittent porphyria, 1036,
1676–1677, 1677*t*
Acute interstitial pneumonia (AIP), 290,
291*t*
Acute kidney injury (acute renal failure),
913, **916–923**, 917*t*. *See also*
Kidney disease
acute tubular necrosis causing, 917*t*,
918–921
cardiorenal syndrome and, 923
cirrhosis and (hepatorenal syndrome),
702–703, 917
glomerulonephritis causing, 917*t*,
922–923
interstitial nephritis causing, 917*t*, **921**
intrinsic, 917*t*, 918, 921
postoperative, 54, 54*t*

postrenal, 916, 917*t*, 918
prerenal, 916, 917–918, 917*t*
in tumor lysis syndrome, 920, 1660
Acute leukemia, **527–529**. *See also specific*
type and Leukemias
bone marrow/stem cell transplantation
for, 528–529, 540, 541
chemotherapy choices for, 1622*t*
erythrovirus (parvovirus) infection in,
1422
Acute Liver Failure Early Dynamic
(ALFED) model, 686
Acute Liver Failure Study Group
(ALFSG) index, in liver
failure, 686
Acute lung injury
ARDS as, **319–321**, 320*t*
transfusion-related, 544
Acute lymphoblastic/lymphocytic
leukemia (ALL), 527, 528,
529, 1622*t*
bone marrow/stem cell transplantation
for, 529
Acute motor axonal neuropathy
(AMAN), 1038
Acute motor and sensory axonal
neuropathy (AMSAN),
1038
Acute mountain sickness (AMS), **1574**
Acute myeloid leukemia (AML), 519*t*,
527, 528, 528–529, 1622*t*
bone marrow/stem cell transplantation
for, 528–529, 540, 541
Acute-on-chronic liver failure, 686
Acute paralytic (adynamic) ileus,
638–639
Acute-phase response, bisphosphonates
causing, 1162
Acute Physiology and Chronic Health
Evaluation (APACHE II), in
pancreatitis, 726
Acute promyelocytic leukemia (APL),
527, 528
DIC associated with, 528, 554
Acute pulmonary histoplasmosis, 1549
Acute radiation syndrome (radiation
sickness), 1571
Acute renal failure, 913, **916–923**, 917*t*.
See also Acute kidney
injury
Acute respiratory distress syndrome
(ARDS), **319–321**, 320*t*. *See*
also Respiratory failure
acute gastric aspiration and, 305–306
in burn injury, 1569
in pancreatitis, 728, 729
smoke inhalation and, 305
Acute respiratory failure, **317–319**, 318*t*.
See also Acute respiratory
distress syndrome;
Respiratory failure
Acute retinal necrosis, 192
Acute tubular necrosis, 852, 917*t*,
918–921
in pancreatitis, 728
rhabdomyolysis and, 852, 920
Acyclovir, 119, 1365*t*, 1366
for herpes simplex infections, 119,
170*t*, 175, 1291, 1338*t*, 1343,
1365*t*, 1366

for herpes zoster/varicella infection,
121, 175, 982, 1338*t*, 1343,
1365*t*, 1370
nephrotoxicity of, 919
during pregnancy, 821, 823, 1366
AD. *See* Alzheimer disease
ADACEL. *See* Tdap vaccine
Adalat. *See* Nifedipine
Adalimumab. *See also* Anti-TNF agents
for inflammatory bowel disease,
651–652
Crohn disease, 656–657
ulcerative colitis, 660
for psoriasis, 108
for rheumatoid arthritis, 837–838
Adamantanes (amantadine and
rimantadine), influenza/
influenza resistance and,
1365*t*, 1412, 1418
ADAMTS-13 (von Willebrand factor
cleaving protease), in
thrombotic
thrombocytopenic purpura,
550, 551, 551*t*
Adapalene, for acne, 127
Adcetris. *See* Brentuximab vedotin
Addiction (drug), 1092. *See also*
Poisoning/drug overdose;
Substance use disorders
pain management and, 17, 73–74, 85
Addison disease (primary adrenal
insufficiency), 1110,
1168–1172. *See also* Adrenal
insufficiency
acute adrenal crisis and, 1168–1169,
1170, 1172
congenital, 1169
in diabetes, 1237
hyperkalemia and, 893, 1170, 1171
hyponatremia and, 886, 1111, 1170,
1171
perioperative corticosteroid
replacement and, 53
Addisonian (acute adrenal) crisis,
1168–1169, 1170, 1172
Adductor canal, femoral artery disease
and, 474
Adefovir, for hepatitis B, 687–688
Adenitis. *See also* Lymphadenitis
mesenteric, adenoviruses causing, 1421
Adenoid cystic carcinoma, salivary, 232
Adenoma sebaceum, 1010
Adenomas. *See specific type or structure*
affected
Adenomatous polyposis coli gene. *See*
APC gene
Adenomatous polyps, 665
colonoscopy/sigmoidoscopy/screening
tests in identification/
treatment of, 665–666, 666,
1642, 1642–1643
colorectal cancer and, 665, 666, 1637,
1640
familial, **666–667**, 1637. *See also*
Familial adenomatous
polyposis
gastric, 667
nonfamilial, **665–666**
Adenomyomatosis, biliary tract/
gallbladder, 717*t*, 719

Adenomyosis, uterine, 765, 766
Adenopathy. *See* Lymphadenopathy
Adenosine, 383*t*, 386
  for arrhythmias, 381, 383*t*
  for paroxysmal supraventricular
     tachycardia, 386
Adenosine deaminase, pleural fluid, in
     tuberculosis, 312
Adenosine deaminase 2, mutation in gene
     for, in polyarteritis nodosa,
     856
Adenosine triphosphatase, copper-
     transporting *(ATP7B)*, in
     Wilson disease, 710
Adenosylcobalamin, 506. *See also*
     Vitamin B$_{12}$
Adenovirus infections, **1420–1421**
  bronchiolitis, 266, 1421
  conjunctivitis/keratoconjunctivitis,
     166–167, 1421
  diarrhea/gastroenteritis, 1305, 1342,
     1421
ADH. *See* Antidiuretic hormone
Adherence/nonadherence, 1–2. *See also*
     specific disorder
  elderly patients and, 69
Adhesion molecule autoantibodies, in
     pemphigus, 139
Adhesive capsulitis (frozen shoulder),
     1691–1692
Adiana, for tubal interruption, 792
Adipose tissue. *See* Body fat
Adjustment (situational) disorders,
     1050–1051
  with depressed mood, 1075
  illness/hospitalization and, 1105
  posthospital, 1105, 1105–1106
  suicide risk and, 1076
Adjuvant chemotherapy. *See also*
     Chemotherapy
  for bladder cancer, 1652
  for breast cancer, 749, 750–751,
     751–752, 1623*t*
    in older women, 753
  for colorectal cancer, 1639–1640,
     1640
  for gastric adenocarcinoma, 1630–1631
  for lung cancer, 1611–1612, 1613
Adjuvant pain medications/treatments,
     84
ADLs–IADLs. *See* Activities of daily
     living–instrumental activities
     of daily living
Adnexal masses. *See* Ovarian cancer/
     tumors
Ado-trastuzumab emtansine, 1666*t*. *See
     also* Trastuzumab
  for breast cancer, 756
Adolescents
  antidepressant use/suicide risk and,
     1079
  immunization recommendations for,
     1319
    pertussis reimmunization and, 802,
      1464
ADPKD1/ADPKD2 genes, 949, 950
Adrenal adenoma, 1173, 1174, 1175, 1176
  hyperaldosteronism caused by,
     442–443, 1177, 1178
  in MEN, 1187*t*, 1188
Adrenal cortex

diseases of, **1168–1179**. *See also specific
     disorder*
  in hypopituitarism, 1109
  in HIV infection/AIDS, 1342–1343
  hyperplasia of
    aldosteronism caused by, 443,
      1178–1179
    amenorrhea and, 1170
    congenital, 1169–1170
    Cushing syndrome caused by, 1173,
      1175
    hirsutism/virilization and, 1169,
      1170, 1196, 1197
    in MEN, 1188
  hypoplasia of, congenital, 1108, 1109,
     1169
  tumors of. *See* Adrenal tumors
Adrenal crisis, 1168–1169, 1170, 1172
Adrenal hemorrhage, 1169
Adrenal incidentalomas, 1175, 1178, 1179
Adrenal insufficiency, 1108, 1109–1110,
     1110, 1111, **1168–1172**. *See
     also* Addison disease
  acute adrenal crisis and, 1168–1169,
     1170, 1172
  after adrenal carcinoma surgery, 1175,
     1176
  amenorrhea and, 1170
  congenital, 1169
  in diabetes mellitus, 1169, 1170
  in HIV infection/AIDS, 1171, 1343
  hyperkalemia and, 893, 1170, 1171
  hyponatremia and, 886, 1111, 1170,
     1171
  meningococcemia and
     (Waterhouse-Friderichsen
     syndrome), 1169
  perioperative corticosteroid
     replacement and, 53
  after pituitary surgery, 1175, 1176
Adrenal nodules, incidentally discovered,
     1175, 1178, 1179
Adrenal tumors
  amenorrhea caused by, 1199, 1201
  cancer, 1173, 1174, 1175–1176, 1176,
     1196, 1624*t*
  cortical
    ACTH-secreting, 1173, 1174
    aldosterone-secreting, 442–443,
      1177, 1178
    androgen-secreting, 1196, 1197
    cortisol-secreting, 1173
    estrogen-secreting, 1191
  medullary. *See* Pheochromocytoma
  in MEN, 1187*t*, 1188
Adrenal vein sampling, in aldosteronism,
     1178
Adrenalectomy
  adrenal crisis after, 1169
  for Conn syndrome, 1178
  for Cushing disease/syndrome, 1175,
     1176
Adrenergic drugs. *See* Alpha-adrenergic
     agonists; Alpha-adrenergic
     blocking drugs; Beta-
     adrenergic agonists; Beta-
     adrenergic blocking drugs
Adrenocortical carcinoma, 1173, 1174,
     1175–1176, 1176, 1624*t*
Adrenocortical deficiency/insufficiency.
     See Adrenal insufficiency

Adrenocorticosteroids. *See*
     Corticosteroids
Adrenocorticotropic hormone (ACTH),
     1109*t*
  adrenal adenoma secreting, 1173, 1174,
     1175, 1176
  in adrenal insufficiency/Addison
     disease, 1168, 1169, 1170,
     1171
  bronchial carcinoid secreting, 1186
  deficiency of, 1108, 1109–1110, 1110,
     1111, 1168, 1169. *See also*
     Adrenal insufficiency
  ectopic/hypersecretion of, 1169, 1173,
     1174, 1176
  in hypercortisolism/Cushing
     syndrome, 1173, 1174
  pituitary adenoma secreting, 1173,
     1174, 1175, 1176
Adrenoleukodystrophy, 1169, 1171, 1172
Adriamycin. *See* Doxorubicin
Adrucil. *See* Fluorouracil
Adson test, 1044
Adult Still disease, **838–839**
Adult T-cell deficiencies, 881*t*
Adult T cell lymphoma/leukemia (ATL),
     1396. *See also* Human T cell
     lymphotropic/leukemia virus
Adulthood ductopenia, idiopathic, 724
Advance care planning/advance
     directives, 90
ADVANCE study, 1219
Advil. *See* Ibuprofen
Adynamic bone disease, 927
Adynamic (paralytic) ileus, **638–639**
Aeroallergens. *See* Allergens
Aerobic training. *See also* Exercise/
     activity
  for menopausal symptoms, 1202
AeroBid. *See* Flunisolide
Aerodigestive tract. *See also specific
     structure*
  foreign bodies in, **238**
Aeromonas, diarrhea caused by, 588*t*, 592
Aerophagia, 587
Aerosols, sniffing, 1181
Afatinib, 1667*t*
  for lung cancer, 1612
Afeditab. *See* Nifedipine
Affect, in schizophrenia/psychotic
     disorders, 1066, 1067
Afinitor. *See* Everolimus
Aflatoxin exposure, hepatocellular
     carcinoma and, 1616
Aflibercept
  for age-related macular degeneration,
     185
  in cancer chemotherapy, 1669*t*
  for chronic macular edema in retinal
     vein occlusion, 186
  for colorectal cancer, 1640
  for diabetic macular edema, 190
Afluria, 1414*t*. *See also* Influenza virus
     vaccine
AFP. *See* Acute flaccid paralysis;
     Alpha-fetoprotein
Afrezza. *See* Technosphere inhaled
     insulin
African American patients. *See* Black
     patients
African tick bite fever, 1429*t*, 1434

African trypanosomiasis, **1507–1508**, 1508t
Afterdrop, in rewarming, 1564
Age/aging. *See also* Older adults
    anemia associated with, 502, 503
    breast cancer risk and, 738, 738t
    colorectal cancer risk and, 1637
    dementia and, 57–60, 1018–1019. *See also* Dementia
    entropion/ectropion and, 165, 165f
    hearing loss and (presbyacusis), **70**, 200, 208
    heart failure and, 402
    postoperative pulmonary complications and, 49
    preoperative screening tests and, 45
    testosterone levels and
        in men, 1190
        in women, 1206
    weight loss and, 35, **67**
Age-related hypogonadism, 1190, 1191
Age-related macular degeneration/ maculopathy, **185–186**
Agenerase. *See* Amprenavir
Agglutinins
    cold, 515
    febrile, 1288
Aggregatibacter actinomycetemcomitans. See HACEK organisms
Aggregatibacter aphrophilus. See HACEK organisms
Aggression, **1090–1092**. *See also* Violence
    alcohol use disorder and, 1090, 1093
    anabolic steroid use and, 1090, 1101
    in dementia, 1104
    phencyclidine use/abuse and, 1090, 1099
Aging. *See* Age/aging
Agitation. *See also* Delirium
    palliation of, **87**
Agnogenic myeloid metaplasia (primary myelofibrosis), 519t, 520t, **522–523**
Agnosia, intracranial tumors causing, 1005
Agoraphobia, 1053, 1056
Agranulocytosis. *See also* Neutropenia
    drug-induced, 518
        clozapine causing, 1014, 1072
        mirtazapine causing, 1081
        thiourea therapy causing, 1129
Agrin antibodies, in myasthenia gravis, 1045
AI. *See* Aromatase inhibitors
Aid to Capacity Evaluation, evaluation of decision-making ability and, 71
AIDS. *See* HIV infection/AIDS
AIDS cholangiopathy, 1529
AIDS enteropathy, 1342
AIDS wasting syndrome. *See* HIV wasting syndrome
AIP. *See* Acute intermittent porphyria; Acute interstitial pneumonia
Air pollution
    asthma and, 242
    COPD and, 257
Air travel
    dysbarism/decompression sickness and, 204, 1573

eustachian tube dysfunction/ barotrauma and, 203, 204
lower extremity edema/venous thromboembolism and, 33, 1576
medical safety/patient selection and, **1575–1576**
during pregnancy, 802, 1576
AIRE gene, in type 1 diabetes, 1210–1211
Airway disorders, **241–267**. *See also specific type*
    allergic bronchopulmonary mycosis, **264**, 879t
    asthma, **242–257**
    bronchiectasis, **263–264**
    bronchiolitis, **266–267**
    chronic obstructive pulmonary disease (COPD), **257–263**, 258t, 260t
    cystic fibrosis, **264–266**
    lower airway, **241–242**
    obstruction
        by food/"café coronary," 238, **306**
        foreign body causing, 238
        of lower airways, 241–242
        occupational disorders and, **308–309**
        during sleep (obstructive sleep apnea hypopnea), 230, 231, 316, 316–317, 1089
        tracheostomy and cricothyrotomy for, 237–238
        of upper airways, 238, 241
    respiratory failure caused by, 318t
    stridor and, 232
    thermal injury/smoke inhalation and, 305
    upper airways, **241**
Airway management. *See also* Intubation
    burn injury/smoke inhalation and, 305, 1568–1569
    for coma, 1577–1578
    in status epilepticus, 989
    tracheostomy and cricothyrotomy in, 237–238
AK-Poly. *See* Bacitracin/polymyxin
Akathisia
    antipsychotics causing, 1017, 1070, 1072
    SSRIs causing, 1079
Akinetic mutism (persistent vegetative state), **1028**
AL (primary) amyloidosis, 421, **538–539**. *See also* Amyloidosis
    cardiac, 421, 539
    renal, 946
Al-Anon, 1094
ALADIN protein, in triple A (Allgrove) syndrome, 1169
Alamast. *See* Pemirolast
Alanine aminotransferase (ALT). *See also specific disorder affecting*
    in liver disease/jaundice, 676, 676t, 694
    monitoring, during latent tuberculosis treatment, 4
    normal values for, 676t
Albendazole
    for ascariasis, 1538
    for clonorchiasis/opisthorchiasis, 1534
    for cutaneous larva migrans, 1543
    for cysticercosis, 1536

for enterobiasis/pinworms, 1541
for filariasis, 1544
for giardiasis, 1531
for hookworm disease, 1539
for hydatid disease, 1537, 1538
for microsporidiosis, 1529
for strongyloidiasis, 1540
for trichinosis, 1542
for trichuriasis/whipworm, 1539
for visceral larva migrans, 1542
Albiglutide, 1221t, 1226
Albinism, 157
Albinism-associated storage pool disease, 556
Albumin. *See also* Hypoalbuminemia
    ascitic fluid, 602, 701. *See also* Serum-ascites albumin gradient
    calcium levels and, 896
    in liver disease/jaundice, 676t
    normal values for, 676t
    in protein-losing enteropathy, 643
    in urine. *See* Albuminuria
Albuminuria, 914. *See also specific cause and* Proteinuria
    in yellow fever, 1405
Albuterol
    for asthma, 252, 253t
        with ipratropium, 253t
    for COPD, 260, 262
    for cystic fibrosis, 266
    for hyperkalemia, 895t
Alcaftadine, for allergic eye disease, 168, 170t
Alclometasone, 96t
Alcohol abuse, 17. *See also* Alcohol use disorder
Alcohol-based antiseptics/hand sanitizers, in infection control, 1295
Alcohol dependence, 17. *See also* Alcohol use disorder
Alcohol misuse, 17. *See also* Alcohol use disorder
Alcohol use disorder (alcoholism), **16–18, 1092–1098**, 1096–1097t
    acute intoxication/poisoning, 1093, 1584, 1584t
    aggressive/violent behavior and, 1090, 1093
    amnestic syndrome and, 1103
    anxiety self-treatment and, 1055
    at-risk drinking and, 1092, 1094–1095
    atrial fibrillation and, 388
    breast cancer risk and, 738
    cardiomyopathy and, 417
    cirrhosis and, 693, 694, 699, 700, 701, 705
        hepatocellular carcinoma and, 701, 705, 1616
    coma and, 1246t
    complications associated with, 1094
    Cushing syndrome/hypercortisolism and, 1174
    delirium caused by, 1093, 1102t
    depression and, 1076, 1084
    differential diagnosis of, 1094
    drug therapy for, 1095, 1097–1098
    fatty liver and, 694, 695
    folic acid deficiency and, 508
    gastritis/dyspepsia and, 580, 620, 621

Alcohol use disorder (alcoholism)
(*Cont.*):
hepatitis and, 693, 694
hyperosmolality caused by, 891
hypertension and, 441, 445, 446*t*
hypoglycemia associated with, 1098,
1236, 1252, 1252*t*, 1258,
1594–1595
hypophosphatemia and, 900
immunization recommendations in,
1321*t*
ketoacidosis and, 905–906, 908
lipid abnormalities and, 1261
liver disease associated with, **693–695**
Mallory-Weiss syndrome/tears and,
612
management of, 1094–1098,
1096–1097*f*
metabolic acidosis/osmolar gap and,
891, 1094, 1584
methotrexate use and, 837
neuropathy associated with, 1036, 1039
in pancreatitis, 725, 726, 730, 731, 732,
733
in panic disorder, 1053
platelet function affected by, 558*t*
pregnancy and, 799, 1094
preventable disease/deaths and, 3*t*
prevention of/screening tests for,
16–18, 18*t*, 1093
psychiatric/psychotic disorders
associated with, 1092, 1094
in PTSD, 1052
rhabdomyolysis and, 852
sleep-wake disorders and, 1088
suicide and, 1076, 1093
thiamine deficiency/supplement and,
694, 908, 1026, 1093, 1095,
1274, 1578
trauma outcome/incidence affected by,
16
Wernicke encephalopathy/
Wernicke-Korsakoff
syndrome and, 694, 908,
1026, 1093, 1095
withdrawal and, 1093, 1095–1098,
1096–1097*f*
delirium caused by, 1093, 1102*t*
differential diagnosis of, 1094
drug therapy for, 1095, 1097–1098
seizures caused by, 989, 1093, 1098
Alcohol Use Disorder Identification Test
(AUDIT), 17, 18*t*, 1093
Alcohol withdrawal syndrome, 1093
Alcoholic brain syndromes, chronic,
1093, 1098
Alcoholic cardiomyopathy, 417
Alcoholic (organic) hallucinosis, 1093,
1095
Alcoholic hepatitis, 693, 694
postoperative complications associated
with, 50
Alcoholic ketoacidosis, 905–906, 908
Alcoholics Anonymous, 1084, 1094
Aldactazide. *See* Spironolactone, for
hypertension, with
hydrochlorothiazide
Aldactone. *See* Spironolactone
Aldehyde dehydrogenase deficiency,
alcohol use disorder and,
1093

Aldesleukin, 1670*t*. *See also* Interleukin-2
Aldicarb poisoning, 1601–1602
Aldochlor. *See* Methyldopa
Aldosterone. *See also* Aldosteronism;
Hypoaldosteronism
adrenal adenoma/hyperplasia
secreting, 442–443, 1177,
1178, 1178–1179
drugs blocking receptors for. *See also*
Spironolactone
in cardiomyopathy, 416
for heart failure, 405*f*, 406
hypertension and, 449*t*
infarct-related, 376
for hypertension, 449*t*, 450*t*, 459
in hypertension, 441–442, 442–443,
444, 459, 1177
resistant disease and, 443, 467, 1177
potassium balance and, 891, 892, 1177
in primary aldosteronism, 442,
1177–1178
Aldosterone:plasma renin activity ratio,
442, 1178
Aldosteronism (hyperaldosteronism),
442–443, **1177–1179**
glucocorticoid-remediable, 441–442,
892*t*
hypertension and, 441–442, 442–443,
444, 1177
saline-unresponsive metabolic alkalosis
and, 909, 910, 1177
Alecensa. *See* Alectinib
Alectinib, 1667*t*
for lung cancer, 1612
Alemtuzumab, 1666*t*
hyperthyroidism/Graves disease caused
by, 1126
for multiple sclerosis, 1024*t*, 1025
Alendronate, 1161. *See also*
Bisphosphonates
adverse ophthalmic effects of, 179*t*
for hypercalcemia/
hyperparathyroidism, 1157
for osteoporosis prevention/
management, 1161
corticosteroid use and, 1209
Aleukemic leukemia, 528
Aleve. *See* Naproxen
ALFED (Acute Liver Failure Early
Dynamic) model, 686
Alfieri procedure, 340
ALFSG (Acute Liver Failure Study
Group) index, in liver failure,
686
Alfuzosin, 974, 974*t*
adverse ophthalmic effects of, 177*t*,
183, 974
Alginate, for unresponsive GERD, 610
Alimentary hypoglycemia, functional,
1256
Alimentary tract cancers, **1626–1644**.
*See also specific type or
structure affected*
Alimta. *See* Pemetrexed
Alirocumab, for lipid modification/
cardiovascular/heart disease
prevention, 353, 1265*t*, 1266
Aliskiren, 454, 455*t*, 465
with amlodipine, 455*t*
with amlodipine and
hydrochlorothiazide, 458*t*

with hydrochlorothiazide, 455*t*
with valsartan, 458*t*
Alisporivir, for hepatitis C, 691
ALK1 gene, in hereditary hemorrhagic
telangiectasia, 1684
ALK inhibitors, for lung cancer, 1612
ALK-rearranged lung cancer, 1612
Alkali administration. *See* Bicarbonate
Alkalies, caustic/corrosive, **1587**
esophageal injury/ingestion and, 1587
eye injury and, 198, 1581, 1587
skin injury and, 1587
Alkaline phosphatase
in hypophosphatasia, 1165
in liver disease/jaundice, 676, 676*t*, 694
normal values for, 676*t*
Alkalinization, urine. *See* Urine,
alkalinization of
Alkalosis, 903
contraction, 909
metabolic, 903, 904*t*, **908–910**, 910*t*.
See also Metabolic alkalosis
posthypercapnia, 909
respiratory, 903, 904*t*, **910–911**, 911*t*.
See also Respiratory alkalosis
salicylate overdose/toxicity causing,
1603
saline-responsive, 908–909, 909*t*, 910
saline-unresponsive, 909, 909*t*, 910
Alkaptonuria, **1677–1678**
Alkeran. *See* Melphalan
Alkylating agents, 1663*t*
breastfeeding and, 798*t*
ALL. *See* Acute lymphoblastic/
lymphocytic leukemia
All-trans-retinoic acid, 1669*t*. *See also*
Retinoic acid; Tretinoin
for acute promyelocytic leukemia, 527
Allergens. *See also* Allergies/allergic
disorders/reactions
asthma caused by, 242
desensitization therapy/
immunotherapy for, 250*t*,
251
avoidance of
for allergic contact dermatitis, 125
for allergic rhinitis, 219–220
Allergic alveolitis, extrinsic
(hypersensitivity
pneumonitis), **307–308**, 308*t*
Allergic bronchopulmonary mycosis/
aspergillosis, **264**, 879*t*, 1554,
1555
Allergic conjunctivitis, 168
Allergic contact dermatitis. *See* Contact
dermatitis
Allergic eye disease, **168–174**
Allergic rhinitis (hay fever), **218–220**
conjunctivitis and, 168
nasal polyps and, 219, 222
Allergic vasculitis, drugs causing, 162*t*
Allergies/allergic disorders/reactions,
876–881, 879*t*
anaphylactic, **876–877**
asthma and, 242
desensitization therapy/
immunotherapy for, 250*t*,
251
to drugs. *See* Drug allergy
eosinophilic esophagitis and, 613
in HIV infection/AIDS, 1332–1333

to insulin, 1237
in topical dermatologic therapy, 101
in topical ophthalmic therapy, 199
Allgrove (triple A) syndrome, 1169, 1171, 1172
Allodynia, opioid use and, 82
Allogeneic stem cell transplantation, **540–541**. *See also* Bone marrow/stem cell transplantation
Alloimmunization
platelet transfusion and, 544
Rhesus, 799, 800, **801**
stem cell transplantation and, 540, 541
Alloislet transplant, for diabetes, 1232
Allopurinol
adverse ophthalmic effects of, 179*t*
drug interactions of, 833
hypersensitivity reaction to, 833
HLA-B-associated, 880
for hyperuricemia/gout, 832, 833, 920
in cancer patients, 1660, 1671*t*
in polycythemia, 521
in transplant patients, 833
urinary stones and, 964
for tumor lysis syndrome, 1660, 1671*t*
Almotriptan, for migraine headache, 978
Alocril. *See* Nedocromil
Alogliptin, 1222*t*, 1227
with metformin, 1227, 1228
with pioglitazone, 1227, 1228
Alomide. *See* Lodoxamide
Alopecia, **158–159**
androgenetic (male pattern), 158–159
in women, 159
areata, 159
chemotherapy-induced, 1673
nonscarring, 158, 158–159
scarring (cicatricial), 158, 159
in syphilis, 1493
totalis, 159
universalis, 159
Alora, 1204
Alosetron, for irritable bowel syndrome, 646–647
Alpha-1a receptors, benign prostatic hyperplasia and, 974, 974*t*
Alpha-adrenergic agonists
for glaucoma/ocular hypertension, 180
for retrograde ejaculation, 970
for Tourette syndrome, 1018
Alpha-adrenergic blocking drugs, 462*t*
adverse ophthalmic effects/cataract surgery and, 177*t*, 183, 464, 974
for benign prostatic hyperplasia, 973*t*, 974, 974*t*
for hypertension, 459–464, 462*t*
pheochromocytoma/ pheochromocytoma surgery and, 1183
phosphodiesterase inhibitor interaction and, 967
ureteral stone expulsion and, 965
Alpha-1-antiprotease/antitrypsin
in COPD/emphysema, 259
replacement therapy and, 261–262
in hepatocellular carcinoma, 1616
in protein-losing enteropathy, 643
Alpha-delta storage pool disease, 556

Alpha-fetoprotein
in Down syndrome, 1678
in hepatocellular carcinoma, 1616, 1617
testicular tumors producing, 1656
Alpha-gal (galactose-alpha-1,3-galactose) hypersensitivity, 877
Alpha-globin gene/chain, 504
in thalassemia, 503, 504, 504*t*
Alpha-glucosidase inhibitors, 1221*t*, 1225
overdose/toxicity of, 1225, 1595
Alpha interferon. *See* Interferon-alpha
Alpha-melanocyte-stimulating hormone (alpha-MSH), in adrenal insufficiency/Addison disease, 1168, 1170
5-Alpha-reductase, deficiency of, 1196
5-Alpha-reductase inhibitors. *See also* Finasteride
for benign prostatic hyperplasia, 973*t*, 974
Alpha-synuclein gene, in parkinsonism/ Lewy body dementia, 1011
Alpha-thalassemia syndromes, 504, 504*t*, 505
sickle cell disease and, 512, 512*t*, 513
Alpha-thalassemia trait, 504, 504*t*, 505
sickle, 512, 512*t*
Alphagan/Alphagan P. *See* Brimonidine
Alprazolam, 1054*t*
overdose/toxicity of, 1594–1595
for panic disorders/attacks, 1055, 1056
Alprenolol, overdose/toxicity of, 1591
Alprostadil, for erectile dysfunction, 967
in diabetes, 1241
ALT. *See* Alanine aminotransferase
Altace. *See* Ramipril
Alteplase (tissue plasminogen activator/ tPA), 373*t*, 374, 996. *See also* Fibrinolytic therapy; Thrombolytic therapy
for acute arterial occlusion of limb, 477
for myocardial infarction, 373*t*, 374
for pulmonary embolism, 300–301, 576, 576*t*
for stroke, 996
Altered mental status. *See* Mental status, altered
Alternaria, phaeohyphomycosis caused by, 1558
Alternating current (AC) electrical injury, 1570
Altitude-related illness, **1572–1576**. *See also* Decompression sickness; High-altitude illness
Aluminum preparations
for hyperphosphatemia, 901, 927
osteomalacia caused by, 927, 1165
Alveolar hemorrhage syndromes, **304–305**
Alveolar hydatid disease, 1537, 1538
Alveolar hyperventilation, **316**
Alveolar hypoventilation, obesity and (Pickwickian syndrome), **315–316**
Alveolar proteinosis, **294**
Alveolitis, 289
extrinsic allergic (hypersensitivity pneumonitis), **307–308**, 308*t*
Alvimopan, for acute paralytic ileus, 639

Alzheimer disease, 57–60, 1019*t*, 1021. *See also* Dementia
deaths attributable to, 2*t*
neuroimaging in, 1020
seizures in, 983
treatment of, 59–60, 1104
Alzheimer's Association/Alzheimer's Disease and Related Disorders Association, 59, 1104
AMAN. *See* Acute motor axonal neuropathy
Amanita mushroom poisoning, 1600, 1600*t*, 1601
Amanitin toxin (amatoxin), poisoning with mushrooms containing, 1600, 1600*t*, 1601
Amantadine, 1365*t*, 1412. *See also* Antiparkinsonism drugs
for Huntington disease, 1015
influenza/influenza resistance and, 1365*t*, 1412, 1418
for neuroleptic malignant syndrome, 36, 1072
for parkinsonism/drug-induced parkinsonism, 1012, 1073
Amaryl. *See* Glimepiride
Amatoxin (amanitin toxin), poisoning with mushrooms containing, 1600, 1600*t*, 1601
Amaurosis fugax ("fleeting blindness"), 188–189, 477
Ambien. *See* Zolpidem
Ambiguous genitalia, 1170
AmBisome. *See* Liposomal amphotericin B
Ambulatory blood pressure monitoring, 439, 439–440, 440*f*
Ambulatory electrocardiographic monitoring
in angina, 358
in palpitation evaluation, 31
in syncope evaluation, 401
Ambulatory esophageal pH monitoring. *See* Esophageal pH monitoring
Amebiasis (entamoeba infection), **1525–1527**, 1526*f*, 1527*t*
extraintestinal/hepatic, 1525, 1526, 1527, 1527*t*
intestinal, 588*t*, 589, 592, 1305, 1315*t*, 1342, 1525, 1526, 1526*f*, 1527*t*
postdysenteric colitis and, 1526
Amebic liver abscess (hepatic amebiasis), 1525, 1526, 1527, 1527*t*
Amebic ulcers, 1525, 1526, 1526*f*
Amebicides, 1526–1527, 1527*t*
adverse ophthalmic effects of, 178*t*
Ameboma, 1525, 1527*t*
Amegakaryocytic thrombocytopenia, 546
Amen. *See* Progesterone
Amenorrhea, **1199–1207**
in anorexia nervosa, 1200, 1273
in hyperprolactinemia, 1110, 1118, 1200, 1201
hypothalamic, 1109, 1199, 1200
in polycystic ovary syndrome, 780, 1196, 1199, 1200–1201
primary, **1199–1200**

Amenorrhea (*Cont.*):
  secondary, **1200–1207**. *See also*
          Menopause; Pregnancy
  in Turner syndrome, 1199, 1200, 1208
American trypanosomiasis (Chagas
          disease), 30, **1509–1510**
  achalasia and, 617
American Urological Association (AUA)
          symptom index, 971–972,
          971*t*
Amifostine, cisplatin therapy toxicity and,
          1675
Amikacin
  for MAC infection, 286, 1482
  for pneumonia, 269*t*, 271, 275*t*
Amikin. *See* Amikacin
Amiloride
  for heart failure, 406
  hyperkalemia caused by, 894
  for hypertension, 450*t*
    with hydrochlorothiazide, 451*t*
  lithium interactions and, 1086, 1087*t*
Aminocaproic acid, for bleeding
          disorders, 559*t*, 560
Aminoglutethimide, for prostate cancer,
          1649*t*
Aminoglycosides
  contraindications to in myasthenia
          gravis, 1046, 1047
  nephrotoxicity/acute kidney injury
          and, 919
  neuromuscular transmission affected
          by, **1047**
  ototoxicity of, 208
  for pneumonia, 269*t*, 271, 275*t*
Aminophylline, lithium interactions and,
          1087*t*
5-Aminosalicylic acid, for inflammatory
          bowel disease, 650
  Crohn disease, 655
  ulcerative colitis, 659
Aminotransferase levels. *See also specific
          disorder affecting*
  in liver disease/jaundice, 676, 676*t*, 694
  normal values for, 676*t*
  in shock liver/cardiogenic liver injury,
          713
Amiodarone
  adverse ophthalmic effects of, 177*t*
  for arrhythmias, 381, 382*t*
    atrial fibrillation, 382*t*, 389–390, 393
    atrial flutter, 395
    in heart failure, 409
    infarct-related, 377, 380
    supraventricular tachycardia, 382*t*,
          386
    ventricular tachycardia, 382*t*, 397
  epididymitis and, 960
  hyperthyroidism/Graves disease caused
          by, 1124, 1125–1126, 1128,
          1132
  hyponatremia caused by, 886
  hypothyroidism caused by, 1120
  levothyroxine therapy affected by, 1123
Amitriptyline, 1078*t*, 1082. *See also*
          Antidepressants
  for dyspepsia, 580
  for interstitial cystitis, 961
  for migraine prophylaxis, 979*t*
  overdose/toxicity of, 979*t*, 1078*t*, 1082
  for painful diabetic neuropathy, 1240

AML. *See* Acute myeloid leukemia
Amlodipine, 461*t*. *See also* Calcium
          channel blocking drugs
  for angina, 361
  for hypertension, 459, 461*t*
    with aliskiren, 455*t*
    with atorvastatin, 461*t*
    with benazepril, 455*t*
    with hydrochlorothiazide and
          aliskiren, 458*t*
    with hydrochlorothiazide and
          olmesartan, 457*t*
    with hydrochlorothiazide and
          valsartan, 458*t*
    with olmesartan, 457*t*
    with perindopril, 456*t*
    with telmisartan, 458*t*
    with valsartan, 458*t*
  overdose/toxicity of, 459, 461*t*, 1591
  ophthalmic, 177*t*
Ammonia
  in liver failure/hepatic encephalopathy,
          685, 686, 703
  urinary, in acidosis, 906, 906*t*, 907
Ammonium tetrathiomolybdate, for
          Wilson disease, 711
Amnestic syndrome, 1103. *See also*
          Memory impairment
Amniocentesis, 800
  in Zika virus infection, 1406
Amodiaquine, 1515*t*, 1516–1517
  with artesunate (ASAQ), 1516, 1516*t*,
          1517*t*, 1519
  with sulfadoxine-pyrimethamine
          (Fansidar), 1519, 1521
Amoxapine, 1078*t*, 1081
Amoxicillin/amoxicillin-clavulanate
  for anaerobic infections, 276, 1478
  for anthrax, 1456*t*
  for bacterial rhinosinusitis, 216, 217*t*
  for endocarditis prophylaxis, 1461*t*
  in *H pylori* eradication therapy, 626,
          626*t*, 627
  for Lyme disease, 1504, 1505, 1505*t*
  for pharyngitis, 229, 1442
  pneumococcal resistance and, 1446
  for pneumonia, 269*t*, 270, 271, 1445
  rash caused by, in mononucleosis, 1373
  for rosacea, 129
  for sinusitis in HIV infection/AIDS,
          1339
  for skin and soft tissue infections,
          1443, 1443*t*
Amphetamines
  abuse/overdose of, **1100**, **1587–1588**
    during pregnancy, 799
    psychotic/violent behavior caused
          by, 1068
  adverse ophthalmic effects of, 177*t*
Amphoteric decontamination solution,
          for alkali eye injury, 1581,
          1587
Amphotericin B, 1558*t*
  for aspergillosis, 1555
  for blastomycosis, 1556
  for candidiasis, 1548
  for coccidioidomycosis, 1550,
          1550–1551
  for cryptococcal meningitis, 1337*t*,
          1340, 1553, 1554
  for histoplasmosis, 1549

  for leishmaniasis, 1511, 1512
  lipid-based preparations of. *See* Lipid-
          based amphotericin B
  for mucormycosis, 218, 1556
  nephrotoxicity/acute kidney injury
          and, 919
  for ophthalmic disorders, 170*t*, 175
  for paracoccidioidomycosis, 1557
  prophylactic, 1292
  for sporotrichosis, 1557
Amphotericin B lipid complex. *See*
          Lipid-based amphotericin B
Ampicillin
  allopurinol interactions and, 833
  for endocarditis/endocarditis
          prophylaxis, 1461*t*, 1462
  for meningitis, 1297*t*
  for pneumonia, 269*t*, 271
  rash caused by, 1318
    in mononucleosis, 228, 1372, 1373
  for urinary tract infection, 955*t*
Ampicillin-sulbactam
  for anaerobic infections, 1478, 1479
  for pneumonia, 269*t*, 271, 275*t*
  for spontaneous bacterial peritonitis,
          603
Amprenavir, 1356, 1357. *See also*
          Antiretroviral therapy
Ampulla of Vater, carcinoma of
          (ampullary/periampullary
          carcinoma), **1620–1626**,
          1634
Amputation
  in acute arterial limb occlusion, 477
  in electrical burns, 1570
  in tibial/pedal occlusive disease, 475
AMS. *See* Acute mountain sickness
AMSAN. *See* Acute motor and sensory
          axonal neuropathy
Amturnide. *See* Aliskiren, with
          amlodipine and
          hydrochlorothiazide
Amyl nitrite, abuse of, 1101
Amylase
  ascitic fluid, 602
  in pancreatic enzyme supplements,
          732*t*
  in pancreatitis, 312, 726, 731
  pleural fluid, 312
Amyloid angiopathy, cerebral, 997, 998
Amyloid protein, 538, 539. *See also*
          Amyloidosis
  in Alzheimer disease, 1020
Amyloidosis, **538–539**
  cardiac/cardiomyopathy and, 421–422,
          539
  hereditary (transthyretin/TTR), 421,
          422, 538
  localized, 538
  myeloma and, 535, 951
  nephrotic spectrum disorders and,
          934*t*, **946**
  neuropathy and, 1037
  primary (AL), 421, **538–539**, 946
  renal, 934*t*, **946**
  renal failure type (beta-2-
          microglobulin), 538
  secondary (AA), 421, 538, 946
  senile, 538
  systemic, 538, 538–539, 539
Amyotrophic lateral sclerosis, 1033, 1034

Amyotrophy
 diabetic, 1036
 neuralgic (idiopathic brachial plexus
  neuropathy), 1043
ANA. See Antinuclear antibody
Anabolic steroids
 abuse of, 1101, 1193–1194
  aggression/violence and, 1090, 1101
 for HIV wasting, 1335
Anaerobic infections, **1478–1480**, 1479t,
  1480f
 abdominal, 1314t, **1479**, 1479t
 pelvic/PID, 778, 1316t, **1479**
 pleuropulmonary (pneumonia/lung
  abscess), 268t, **274–276**,
  1314t, 1315t, 1478
 skin and soft tissue, **1479–1480**, 1480f
Anafranil. See Clomipramine
Anagrelide, for essential thrombocytosis,
  522
Anakinra
 for gout, 832
 for Still disease, 839
Anal candidiasis, 133
Anal dysplasia/cancer, 1624t, **1643–1644**
 in HIV infection/AIDS, 1344, 1644
Anal fissures, 672–673
 in Crohn disease, 652, 653, 654
 GI bleeding and, 598
Anal fistulas, 673
Anal sphincter, disorders of, fecal
  incontinence and, 671
Anal syphilis, 670
Anal warts. See Venereal (genital) warts
Analgesia/analgesics. See also specific type
  or disorder and Pain
  management
 breastfeeding and, 798t
 caffeine-containing, 1101
 in end-of-life care, 73–74
 for myocardial infarction, 375
 thrombocytopenia caused by, 555t
 tubulointerstitial disease caused by,
  947, 948
Analgesic nephropathy, 947, 948
 ureteral/renal pelvis cancer and, 1653
Analgesic rebound headache, **980**
Anaphylactoid reactions, 876, 879t
 to radiocontrast media, 878
Anaphylaxis/anaphylactic shock,
  876–877
 food, 877
 idiopathic (anaphylactoid reaction),
  876, 878, 879t
 insulin allergy causing, 1237
 penicillin allergy causing, 1318
 transfusion causing, 543
 venom allergy causing, 878
Anaplasma (anaplasmosis), 1429t,
  1435–1436
 babesiosis coinfection and, 1436, 1504
 capra, 1435
 equi, 1429t
 Lyme disease coinfection and, 1436,
  1504
 phagocytophilum, 1429t, 1435
Anaprox. See Naproxen
Anastrozole, 1670t
 adverse ophthalmic effects of, 178t
 for breast cancer prevention/treatment,
  739, 752, 755, 755t

for endometriosis, 776
 for gynecomastia, 1195
ANCA. See Antineutrophil cytoplasmic
  antibody
Ancef. See Cefazolin
Ancylostoma
 braziliense, 1542
 caninum, 1539, 1542
 cutaneous larva migrans caused by,
  1542
 duodenale, 1539
Andes virus, 1403
Andexanet, for DOAC overdose/toxicity,
  1588
Androderm, 1192
Androgel, 1192
Androgen deprivation, for prostate
  cancer, 1649, 1649–1650,
  1649t
Androgen insensitivity/resistance
 male hypogonadism caused by, 1190
 pseudohermaphroditism/amenorrhea
  in, 1199–1200
Androgenetic (male pattern) alopecia,
  158–159
 in women, 159
Androgenic steroids. See Anabolic
  steroids
Androgens. See also Antiandrogens;
  Testosterone
 for aplastic anemia, 517
 deficiency of. See also Hypogonadism
  pseudohermaphroditism/
  amenorrhea and, 1199–1200
 in women, 1206
 excess of. See Hyperandrogenism
 receptors for in cancer of male breast,
  760
 replacement therapy with. See
  Testosterone replacement
  therapy
Androstenedione, in hirsutism/
  virilization, 1197
Anejaculation, 966, 970, 1063. See also
  Erectile dysfunction/
  impotence
Anemias, **499–517**, 500t. See also specific
  cause or type
 aplastic, **516–517**, 516t
 in cancer chemotherapy, 1662
 of chronic disease, 501, **502–503**
 classification of, 499, 500t
 Cooley, 505
 of elderly, 502, 503
 in erythrovirus (parvovirus) infection,
  1422
 fish tapeworm infection and, 506–507,
  1535
 in folic acid deficiency, **508–509**, 508t,
  815
 hemolytic. See Hemolytic anemias/
  hemolysis
 of inflammation, 502, 503
 iron deficiency. See Iron, deficiency of/
  iron deficiency anemia
 in kidney disease, 503, 913, 916, 926f,
  928
 in malabsorption, 633t
 in myelodysplastic syndromes, 525,
  527
 in myeloma, 535

of organ failure, 502, 503
 perioperative evaluation/management
  and, 51
 pernicious, 506
 during pregnancy, **814–815**
 refractory, 525
 retinal/choroidal disease and, 191
 sickle cell. See Sickle cell anemia/
  syndromes
 thalassemias causing, **503–506**, 504t
 thiazolidinediones causing, 1225
 in vitamin B$_{12}$ deficiency, **506–508**,
  507t
 in Waldenström macroglobulinemia,
  537
Anergy testing. See Skin test anergy
Anesthesia/anesthetics
 liver function affected by, 50
 local, for eye disorders, precautions for
  use of, **198**
 malignant hyperthermia caused by, 35,
  1294, 1580
 for status epilepticus, 989–990
Aneuploidy screening, in prenatal testing,
  800
Aneurysms, **480–486**. See also specific
  type and artery involved
 aortic
  abdominal, **480–482**
   screening for, 6t, 7, 481
  dissection and, **484–486**
  in syphilis, 1495, 1495f
  thoracic, **482–483**
 intracranial, **1000**. See also Intracranial
  aneurysm
 mycotic
  drug use and, 1304
  intracranial, 1000
 peripheral arterial, **483–484**
Angeliq, 1204
Angiitis
 with granulomatosis (Wegener
  granulomatosis). See
  Granulomatosis, with
  polyangiitis
 primary, of central nervous system,
  862–863
Angina
 intestinal (visceral artery
  insufficiency), **479–480**
 Ludwig, 230
 pectoris, **355–364**, 360f, 363t. See also
  Coronary heart disease
  alteration in before myocardial
   infarction, 370
  aortic valve disease and, 341, 342,
   346
  in apathetic hyperthyroidism, 1126,
   1133
  chest pain/discomfort in, 26–27, 27,
   27t, 28, 356, 357
   change in before myocardial
    infarction, 370
  chronic stable, **355–364**, 360f, 363t
  coronary vasospasm and, 356,
   364–365
  drugs in management of, 359–362,
   360f
  jaw pain and, 983
  with normal arteriogram, **364–365**
  postinfarction, 376–377

Angina, pectoris (*Cont.*):
  Prinzmetal (variant), 365
  risk reduction and, 361–362
  thiazolidinedione use and, 1224
  unstable. See Acute coronary
    syndromes
  Vincent (necrotizing ulcerative
    gingivitis), **226**
Angiodysplasias, GI bleeding and, 595,
  597
Angioectasias, GI bleeding and,
  595, 597
Angioedema, **133–135**
  hereditary, 879*t*
Angiofibroma, in MEN, 1187*t*, 1188
Angiography/arteriography. *See also*
    specific disorder
  cardiac/coronary. *See also* Cardiac
      catheterization
    in angina/acute coronary
      syndromes/STEMI/chest
      pain evaluation, 28, 358–359,
      369, 369*t*, 376
      normal findings and, **364–365**
    in heart failure, 358, 404
  cerebral. *See* Cerebral angiography/
      arteriography; Neuroimaging
  CT. *See* Computed tomography;
      Helical (spiral) CT
  in GI bleeding
    diagnostic, 598–599, 600
    therapeutic, 597
  left ventricular, in angina, 359
  magnetic resonance. *See* Magnetic
      resonance angiography
  pulmonary, in pulmonary embolism,
    298
    helical CT, 23, 28, 296–297, 297*f*
  radionuclide
    in angina, 357
    in heart failure, 404
  in renal artery stenosis/renal vascular
    hypertension, 442, 931
Angiomas/angiomatosis
  bacillary, 1343, 1477
  in Sturge-Weber syndrome, 1010
Angiomyolipomas, of kidney, 1655
Angioplasty. *See also* Endovascular
    surgery/prostheses
  carotid, 478
  coronary
    for angina, 362–363
    rescue, 376
  for renal artery stenosis/renal vascular
    hypertension, 442, 932
Angiosarcoma, of liver, vinyl chloride
    causing, 697, 1616
Angiotensin II receptor blocking agents,
    457–458*t*, 459
  for cardiomyopathy, 416, 420*f*
  for diabetic nephropathy, 945
  for heart failure, 405*f*, 407, 410–411
    chronic kidney disease and, 926
    hypertension and, 449*t*, 459
    infarct-related, 376, 380
  hyperkalemia caused by, 459, 893–894,
    926
  for hypertension, 449*t*, 457–458*t*, 459,
    464
    in chronic kidney disease/renal
      failure, 449*t*, 466, 926

in combination regimen, 464–465,
    465*f*
  contraindications to during
    pregnancy, 818
  in diabetes, 449*t*, 459, 466
  for Marfan syndrome, 1683
  for nephrotic syndrome/nephrotic
    spectrum disorders, 942
Angiotensin-converting enzyme (ACE)
    inhibitors, 455–456*t*
  acute kidney injury/renal failure and,
    407, 917
  breastfeeding and, 798*t*
  for cardiomyopathy, 416, 420*f*
  in cardiovascular/heart disease
    prevention, 355, 464
  for diabetic nephropathy, 945,
    1238–1239
  for heart failure, 405*f*, 406, 406–407,
    410–411
    chronic kidney disease and, 926
    hypertension and, 449*t*, 454
    infarct-associated, 375–376, 380
  hyperkalemia caused by, 454, 893–894,
    926
  for hypertension, 449*t*, 454–459,
    455–456*t*, 464
    in chronic kidney disease, 449*t*, 454,
      466, 926
    in combination regimen, 464–465,
      465*f*
    contraindications to in pregnancy,
      459, 818
    in diabetes, 449*t*, 459, 465, 466,
      1218, 1241
    in urgencies/emergencies, 470*t*
  hypoglycemia caused by, 1257
  hyponatremia caused by, 886
  lithium interactions and, 1087, 1087*t*
  for myocardial infarction/STEMI,
    375–376, 380
    hypertension and, 449*t*
  for nephrotic syndrome/nephrotic
    spectrum disorders, 942
  pregnancy and, 434, 459, 818
Angle closure, pupillary dilation and, 176,
    198
Angle-closure glaucoma
  acute, 166*t*, **176–179**
    antipsychotics precipitating, 1071
    pupillary dilation and, 166*t*, 176, 198
  chronic, 179, 180, 180–181
Angular cheilitis, 225, 225*f*, 1341
Anhedonia, 1075. *See also* Depression
Anhidrosis and asthenia (tropical), 131
Anicteric leptospirosis, 1500–1501
Anidulafungin, 1558*t*
  for aspergillosis, 1555
  for candidiasis, 1548
Aniline, methemoglobinemia caused by,
    1599
Animal bites, **1300–1301**. *See also* Insect
      bites/stings
  anaerobic skin infections and, 1300,
    1301
  poisonous snake, 1581*t*, **1604–1605**
  rabies and, 1300, 1301, 1386, 1387
Anion gap/anion gap acidosis, 903,
    904–905, 904*t*. *See also*
      Urinary anion gap
  alcoholic ketoacidosis and, 905–906

decreased, 904*t*, 905
diabetic ketoacidosis and, 905, 1248
increased, 904*t*, **905–906**, 907–908,
    1584
  lactic acidosis and, 905, 1251, 1584
  normal, 904, 904*t*, **906–907**, 906*t*, 908.
      See also Normal anion gap
      acidosis
  with osmolar gap, 891, 1584
  in poisoning/drug overdose, 1584
    with methanol or ethylene glycol,
      906, 908, 1584, 1599
    with salicylates, 906, 1603
  in renal failure (uremic), 906
  in renal tubular acidosis, 892*t*,
    906–907, 906*t*, 908
  toxins causing, 906
Anisakiasis (*Anisakis marina*), 623
Anismus (pelvic floor dyssynergia), 584,
    584*t*, 585
Ankle injuries/sprains, **1715–1717**, 1715*t*
  eversion (high), 1715*t*, **1716–1717**
  inversion, **1715–1716**, 1715*t*
Ankle-brachial index (ABI/ABPI)
  in aortoiliac occlusive disease, 472
  in femoral/popliteal occlusive disease,
    474
  in tibial/pedal occlusive disease, 475
  in venous insufficiency, 33, 156,
    157
Ankylosing spondylitis, **863–864**
Annuloplasty, for tricuspid regurgitation,
    349
Anogenital/perianal pruritus, **147–148**,
    147*f*, 673
  in enterobiasis/pinworms, 147, 148,
    1541
Anogenital warts. *See* Venereal (genital)
      warts
Anorectal abscess, in Crohn disease, 652,
    653, 654
Anorectal disorders, **669–673**. *See also*
      specific cause and Genital
      ulcers
  anal cancer, 1344, 1624*t*, **1643–1644**
  bleeding in, 598. *See also* Rectal
      bleeding
  fecal incontinence and, **671–672**
  fissures/abscesses/fistula, 672–673
    in inflammatory bowel disease, 652,
      653, 654
  hemorrhoids, **669–670**
  infections, **670–671**
    lymphogranuloma venereum, 671,
      1485
  pruritus, **147–148**, 147*f*, 673
Anorectal manometry, in constipation,
    585
Anorexia
  in HIV infection/AIDS, 1335
  nervosa, **1272–1273**
    bulimia and, 1274
Anorexia-cachexia syndrome, 91
Anorgasmia. *See* Orgasm, loss of
Anoscopy
  in fecal incontinence, 672
  in GI bleeding, 598
Anosmia, 220–221
  intracranial tumors causing, 220
  in Kallmann syndrome, 1109, 1199,
    1200

Anosognosia, intracranial tumors causing, 1005
Anovulation
  abnormal uterine bleeding and, 762
  differential diagnosis of, 781
  infertility and, 783, 784, 784–785
  in polycystic ovary syndrome, 780, 781, 1196
Ansaid. See Flurbiprofen
Anserine (pes anserine) bursa/bursitis, 1704
Antacids. See also Acid-antisecretory agents
  antidepressant drug interactions and, 1083t
  benzodiazepine interactions and, 1056t
  for GERD, 609
Anterior blepharitis, 165
Anterior cerebral artery occlusion, in stroke, 995
Anterior chest wall syndrome, 359
Anterior cruciate ligament (ACL), 1704, 1705
  injury of, 1705–1710, 1706t
Anterior drawer sign/test
  ankle sprain and, 1715, 1715t
  knee stability/ACL injury and, 1706t, 1709
Anterior hypopituitarism, 1108–1113, 1109t. See also Hypopituitarism
Anterior interosseous syndrome, 1039–1040
Anterior ischemic optic neuropathy, 192
  in giant cell arteritis, 192, 854
Anterior (patellofemoral) knee pain, 1705t, 1712–1713
Anterior talofibular ligament, in ankle sprains, 1715
Anterior tibiofibular ligament, in ankle sprains, 1716
Anterior uveitis, 166t, 181, 181–182, 182. See also Uveitis
Anthracyclines, 1665t
  for breast cancer, 751
    during pregnancy, 747
  heart failure and, 414, 415, 1674–1675
  toxicity of, 414–415, 1674–1675
    dexrazoxane for, 415, 1671t
Anthrax, 1312t, 1454–1456, 1456t
Anthrax vaccine, 1456
Anti-140, in polymyositis/dermatomyositis, 848t
Anti-155/140, in polymyositis/dermatomyositis, 848, 848t
Anti-A antibodies, transfusion reactions and, 542
Anti-adrenal antibodies, in adrenal insufficiency/Addison disease, 1170
Anti-AMPA receptor antibody, in autoimmune paraneoplastic disorders, 1008
Anti-amphiphysin antibody, in autoimmune paraneoplastic disorders, 1008
Antiandrogenic progestins, for hirsutism/virilization, 1198
Antiandrogens
  for cancer chemotherapy, 1669t
  for hirsutism/virilization, 1198

for prostate cancer, 1649, 1649–1650, 1649t
  gynecomastia and, 1195
Antianginal drugs, 359–362, 360f
  perioperative management for patient taking, 46
Antianxiety drugs, 1054–1056, 1054t, 1056t. See also specific type
Antiarrhythmic drugs, 381–384, 382–383t. See also specific agent and specific arrhythmia
  for arrhythmias in poisoning/drug overdose, 1579
  in heart failure, 409
  for infarct-associated arrhythmias, 377, 380
  overdose/toxicity of, 381, 382–383t, 384
Anti-B antibodies, transfusion reactions and, 542
Antibacterial agents. See also Antibiotics; Antimicrobial therapy
  adverse ophthalmic effects of, 178t
  for ophthalmic disorders, 169–170t
Anti-beta-2-glycoprotein I antibodies
  in antiphospholipid syndrome, 815–816, 841, 843
  in SLE, 841
Antibiotic-associated/C difficile colitis/diarrhea, 589, 647–649, 1305, 1306t
Antibiotics, 1310–1319, 1311–1313t, 1314t, 1315–1316t. See also under Antimicrobial
  for acne, 98t, 127–128
  adverse reactions/toxicity and, 1317
    ophthalmic, 178t
  for asthma, 252
  for bite wounds, 1301
  breastfeeding and, 798t
  for bronchiectasis, 264
  for burn injury, 1569
  clinical response to, 1313
    promptness of, 1317
  colitis/diarrhea (C difficile) associated with use of, 589, 647–649, 1305, 1306t
  for COPD, 261, 262
  cost of, 1317–1318
  for Crohn disease, 655
  for cystic fibrosis, 265–266
  for diarrhea, 591, 1308
  duration of treatment and, 1296, 1317
  in fever management, 35, 1296, 1314t
  for frostbite, 1566
  for gram-negative infections, 1311t, 1311–1312t, 1468
  for gram-positive infections, 1311t, 1312t
  H pylori test results affected by, 622
  hypersensitivity tests/desensitization and, 1318–1319
  for impetigo, 98t, 124, 1315t
  infection in cancer patient and, 1661
  for malaria, 1519–1520
  for meningitis, 1297t, 1299
  in neutropenic patient, 35, 518, 1292, 1293, 1661
  for ophthalmic disorders, 169–170t
  perioperative, surgical site infections and, 54

for pharyngitis, 227, 229, 1315t, 1442
for pneumonia
  anaerobic, 276
  community-acquired pneumonia, 267–268, 269–270, 269t, 270–271, 1314t
  nosocomial pneumonia, 274, 275t, 1314t
  principles of use of, 1310–1318, 1311–1313t, 1314t, 1315–1316t
  prophylactic. See Antimicrobial chemoprophylaxis
  resistance to. See Drug resistance
  routes of administration for, 1317
  for septic shock, 497
  thrombocytopenia/platelet function and, 555t, 558t
  topical, 98t
  tubulointerstitial nephritis caused by, 947t
Antibodies. See Immunoglobulins
Anti-CADM 140 antibody, in polymyositis/dermatomyositis, 848t
Anticancer drugs. See Chemotherapy
Anticardiolipin antibodies
  in antiphospholipid antibody syndrome, 815, 840t, 841, 841t, 843
  in SLE, 841, 841t
Anti-Caspr2 antibody, in autoimmune paraneoplastic disorders, 1008
Anti-CCP antibodies, in rheumatoid arthritis, 835
Anticentromere antibody, 840t
  in CREST syndrome/scleroderma, 840t, 846
Anticholinergic agents
  for allergic disorders/rhinitis, 219
  antidepressant drug interactions and, 1083t
  for asthma
    long-acting, 249t, 251
    short-acting, 252, 253t
  for COPD, 260
  for irritable bowel syndrome, 646
  for nausea and vomiting, 87, 583
  overdose/toxicity of, 1581t, 1590
  ophthalmic, 177t
  for parkinsonism, 1014
Anticholinergic syndrome/effects, 1583–1584, 1590
  antidepressants causing, 1078t, 1082, 1606
  antipsychotics causing, 1068, 1069t, 1071
  hallucinogens causing, 1598
Anticholinergic-type mushroom poisoning, 1590
Anticholinesterases/acetylcholinesterase inhibitors
  for Alzheimer disease/dementia, 59, 1021, 1104
  for myasthenia gravis, 1045–1046
  overdose/toxicity/poisoning with, 1580t, 1581t, 1601–1602
Anticoagulants, lupus. See Lupus anticoagulant

Anticoagulation therapy, 563–575. *See also specific agent and* Direct-acting oral anticoagulants
for acute arterial limb occlusion, 476
for acute coronary syndromes/STEMI, 367f, 368
after fibrinolytic therapy, 372f, 375
antidepressant drug interactions and, 1083t
for antiphospholipid antibody syndrome, 842, 843
in pregnancy, 805, 816, 842, 843
for atrial fibrillation/stroke prevention, 388, 389, 389f, 390, 390–393, 390t, 391t, 392f, 997
in hyperthyroidism, 1133
in mitral stenosis, 336
for atrial flutter, 395
bleeding caused by, 300, 391, 391t, 393, 562, 628
bridging, 51, 51t, 351, 352t
after cardiac valve replacement, 337, 343, 350–351, 352t
endocarditis and, 352t, 1463
pregnancy and, 351, 352t
classes of drugs in, 563–567, 565–566t
for DVT/PE (venous thromboembolic disease), 300, 567–576, 570t, 571t, 572t, 573t, 574t, 575t
contraindications to, 569, 569t
drug selection and, 569, 570t, 571–575, 573t, 574t
duration of, 300, 573–574, 574t, 575t
patient selection and, 569–571, 571t
prevention and, 300, 567–569, 568t, 569t
treatment and, 300, 569–576, 570t, 571t, 572t, 573t, 574t, 575t
in endocarditis, 352t, 1463
GI bleeding/peptic ulcer disease and, 624, 628
for heart failure, 409
hematuria in patient taking, 953
heparin-induced thrombocytopenia and, 552–553, 553f, 555t
for hepatic vein obstruction (Budd-Chiari syndrome), 712
for intracranial venous thrombosis, 1002
in nephrotic syndrome/nephrotic spectrum disorders, 943
for noncirrhotic portal hypertension, 714
overdose/toxicity and, 300, **1588**
perioperative management of, 51–52, 51t, 52t, 392–393
prosthetic heart valves and, **350–351**, 352t
for portal vein thrombosis, 714
in pregnancy, **351**, 352t, 816, 842
for pulmonary hypertension, 303, 431, 432f
for stroke, 997
for superficial thrombophlebitis, 488
thrombocytopenia caused by, 552–553, 553f, 555t
for transient ischemic attacks, 993
Anticochlear antibodies, in autoimmune hearing loss, 209

Anticonstipation agents. *See* Fiber, dietary; Fiber laxatives; Laxatives
Anti-contactin associated protein-like 2 antibody, in autoimmune paraneoplastic disorders, 1008
Anticonvulsant therapy, 986–989, 987–988t
breastfeeding and, 798t
discontinuing, 988–989
drug selection and, 986, 987–988t
for glossopharyngeal neuralgia, 982
for migraine prophylaxis, 979t
monitoring serum levels during, 986–988, 987–988t
for myoclonus, 1017
nonadherence and, 988
status epilepticus and, 989
overdose/toxicity and, 987–988t, **1589**
for personality disorders, 1066
for postherpetic neuralgia, 982
during pregnancy, 820
for PTSD, 1052
for status epilepticus, 989–990
teratogenic effects of, 986
for trigeminal neuralgia, 981–982
Anti-CV2/CRMP5 antibody, in autoimmune paraneoplastic disorders, 1008
Anti-D, for immune thrombocytopenia, 549, 549f, 550
Anti-D antibodies, transfusion producing, 542
Antidepressants, 1077–1083, 1078t, 1080f, 1082t, 1083t. *See also specific type and agent*
with antipsychotic agents, 1070, 1079, 1083
for anxiety, 1054, 1055, 1055–1056, 1056
aripiprazole with, 1070, 1079, 1083
atypical, 1078t, 1079–1081
breastfeeding and, 798t
bupropion as augmenting agent for, 1079
buspirone as augmenting agent for, 1055, 1082
combination therapy and, 1079, 1082–1083
for dementia, 1021
dispensing, 1077, 1079
dose tapering and, 1083
drug interactions of, 1081, 1083t
for dyspepsia, 580
in elderly, 61
for irritable bowel syndrome, 646
lithium augmentation/interaction and, 1079
maintenance therapy with, 1083
for migraine prophylaxis, 979t
monoamine oxidase inhibitors (MAOIs), 1077, 1078t, 1082, 1082t, 1083t. *See also* Monoamine oxidase inhibitors
for neuropathic pain/painful diabetic neuropathy, 83, 83t, 1035, 1240
for OCD, 1057
overdose/toxicity of, 1590, **1606**

arrhythmias and, 1082, 1579, 1606, 1606f
hypotension caused by, 1082, 1578, 1606
ophthalmic, 178t
seizures and, 1082, 1580t, 1590, 1606
suicide and, 1077, 1079
for panic disorders/attacks, 1055, 1055–1056
for personality disorders, 1065
for phobic disorders, 1056
during pregnancy, 1081
for premenstrual syndrome, 765
for psychotic depression, 1070, 1079
for PTSD, 1052
selecting agent and, 1077–1079, 1080f
sexual dysfunction caused by, 1064, 1079, 1082
sleep cycle affected by, 1089
SNRIs, 1077, 1078t, 1079–1081. *See also* Serotonin (serotonin-selective) norepinephrine reuptake inhibitors
SSRIs, 1077, 1078t, 1079–1081. *See also* Serotonin-selective reuptake inhibitors
switching agents and, 1077–1079, 1082–1083
for terminally ill/dying patient, 92
thyroid medication/liothyronine as augmenting agent for, 1079
tricyclic, 1077, 1078t, 1081–1082, 1606. *See also* Tricyclic antidepressants
Antidiabetic agents, 1220–1228, 1221–1222t, 1235–1236, 1235f. *See also specific type and* Insulin therapy
adverse ophthalmic effects of, 179t
in chronic kidney disease, 929
combination regimens and, 1228
in HIV infection/AIDS, 1342
hospitalization/surgery and, 53, 1243
hypoglycemia and, 1236–1237, 1595
with insulin therapy, 1236
intensive therapy with, 1218
overdose/toxicity of, 1581t, **1595–1596**
during pregnancy, 817, 818, 1244
in prevention/delay of diabetes, 1218
safety of, 1228
Antidiarrheal agents, 590, 594, 1308
for Crohn disease, 655
for fecal incontinence, 672
for irritable bowel syndrome, 646
for microscopic colitis, 662
for short bowel syndrome, 637
for traveler's diarrhea, 590, 1310
for ulcerative colitis, 659
Antidiuretic hormone (ADH). *See also* Vasopressin
in diabetes insipidus/hypernatremia, 890, 1113
hyponatremia and, 885, 886, 887, 889
inappropriate secretion of (SIADH). *See* Syndrome of inappropriate ADH secretion
Antidotes, **1581**, 1581t. *See also specific agent*
Anti-double-stranded (anti-ds)-DNA, in lupus/SLE, 115, 841
Anti-DPPX encephalitis, 1008

Antidromic reentrant tachycardia, 387
Anti-EGFR therapy. *See* EGFR (epidermal growth factor) mutations/inhibitors
Antiemetics, 582–583, 582*t*
  for chemotherapy-induced nausea and vomiting, 582, 582*t*, 1672–1673
  for hyperemesis gravidarum, 803
  for opioid-induced nausea and vomiting, 83
Antiendomysial antibodies, in celiac disease, 634
Antiepilepsy drugs. *See* Anticonvulsant therapy
Antifibrinolytics. *See* Fibrinolytic therapy; Thrombolytic therapy
Antifolates. *See also* Methotrexate
  in cancer chemotherapy, 1663*t*
  for malaria, 1518–1519
Antifreeze. *See* Ethylene glycol poisoning
Antifungal agents, 98–99*t*, **1558–1560**, 1558–1559*t*. *See also specific agent or disorder*
  for candidiasis, 1548, 1560
    esophageal, 611, 1338*t*, 1548
    oral disease, 226, 1341
    vulvovaginal, 133, 767, 1338*t*, 1548
  for invasive sinusitis, 218
  monitoring blood levels of, 1560
  in neutropenia, 35, 518, 1292
  for ophthalmic disorders, 170*t*
  prophylactic, 1292
    in fever management, 35
  for skin disorders/topical, 98–99*t*
Anti-GABA$_B$ receptor antibody, in autoimmune paraneoplastic disorders, 1008
Anti-GalNAC-CD1a antibodies, in Guillain-Barré syndrome, 1038
Anti-GBM antibodies. *See* Anti-glomerular basement membrane antibodies
Anti-GD1a/GD1b antibodies, in Guillain-Barré syndrome, 1038
Antigen-antibody complexes
  in glomerulonephritis, 922, 935*f*, 940
  membranous nephropathy and, 944
Antigenic drift/shift
  influenza epidemics/pandemics and, 1410
  norovirus and, 1425
Antiglaucoma agents, 172–173*t*, 180
Antigliadin antibodies, in celiac disease, 634
Antiglobulin test. *See* Coombs test
Anti-glomerular basement membrane antibodies, in glomerulonephritis/Goodpasture syndrome, 304, 922, 933*t*, 935*f*, 940
Anti-GM1/GM1b antibodies, in Guillain-Barré syndrome, 1038
Anti-GQ1b antibodies, in Guillain-Barré syndrome, 1038
Anti-HAV, 678, 678*f*
Anti-HBc, 680–681, 680*f*, 681*t*, 687
  screening blood for, 543, 681
Anti-HBe, 680*f*, 681, 681*t*

Anti-HBs, 680, 680*f*, 681*t*
Anti-HCV, 683, 683*f*, 689
  screening blood for, 543
Anti-HDV, 684, 687
Anti-HEV, 684
Antihistamines, 95–100
  abuse/overdose/toxicity of, 1101, 1590
  for allergic eye disease, 168, 168–174, 170*t*, 170–171*t*
  for allergic rhinitis, 219
  breastfeeding and, 798*t*
  for desensitization reactions, 1318
  for insomnia, 1089
  MAOI interactions and, 1083*t*
  for nausea and vomiting, 87, 583
  nefazodone interactions and, 1081
  for pruritus, 95–100, 146, 147
  for scombroid poisoning, 1603
  for urticaria, 134
Anti-HMG-CoA reductase, in polymyositis/dermatomyositis, 848*t*, 849
Anti-Hu antibody
  in autoimmune paraneoplastic disorders, 1008
  in cancer-related neuropathy, 1008, 1037
  dysautonomia and, 990
Antihyperglycemic agents. *See* Antidiabetic agents
Antihypertensive drug therapy, 446–448, 447*f*, **448–467**, 448*t*, 449*t*, 450–451*t*, 452–453*t*, 455–458*t*, 460–461*t*, 462–463*t*, 465*f*, 466*t*. *See also specific class or agent*
  aldosterone receptor antagonists in, 449*t*, 450*t*, 459
  alpha-adrenoceptor antagonists in, 459–464, 462*t*
  angiotensin II receptor blocking agents in, 449*t*, 457–458*t*, 459, 464
  angiotensin-converting enzyme (ACE) inhibitors in, 449*t*, 454–459, 455–456*t*, 464
  in aortic dissection, 469*t*, 485
  arteriolar dilators in, 463*t*, 464
  beta-adrenergic blocking agents in, 449–454, 449*t*, 452–453*t*, 464
  in black patients, 466–467, 466*t*
  calcium channel blocking drugs in, 449*t*, 459, 460–461*t*, 464, 465
  cardiovascular/cardiac disease and, 10, 360*f*, 362, 446, 447*f*, 448*t*, 464
  cocaine use and, 469, 469*t*
  demography affecting choice of agent and, 465, 466*t*
  depression caused by, 1076
  developing regimen for, 464–465, 465*f*
  in diabetes mellitus, 446, 447*f*, 449*t*, 464, 465, 466, 1236
    complication rate/diabetic nephropathy and, 446, 945–946, 1218, 1236, 1238–1239
  diuretics in, 448, 449*t*, 450–451*t*, 464
  in elderly, 446, 467
  follow-up and, 467
  goals of, 446–448
    in aortic dissection, 485

  in chronic kidney disease/diabetic nephropathy, 466, 926, 945
  in diabetes, 446, 466, 1236, 1241
  in elderly, 446, 467
  in urgencies/emergencies, 468
  heart disease and, 10, 360*f*, 362, 446, 447*f*, 448*t*, 464
  initial treatment choices and, 448, 449*t*, 464–465, 465*f*
  nocturnal dosing and, 464
  nonadherence and, 465–466
    resistant hypertension and, 467
  patient selection for, 446, 447*f*, 448*t*
  peripheral sympathetic inhibitors in, 363*t*, 464
  pheochromocytoma/pheochromocytoma surgery and, 469, 469*t*, 1183
  in poisoning/drug overdose, 1579
  for preeclampsia/eclampsia, 810
  during pregnancy, 818
  for prehypertension, 447*f*
  preoperative/perioperative, 48
  in renal disease/failure, 449*t*, 466, 469*t*
  renin inhibitors in, 454, 455*t*
  stroke/stroke prevention and, 10, 446–447, 464, 996–997, 998
    in urgencies/emergencies, 468, 469*t*
  sympatholytics in, 462*t*, 464
  thresholds for, 446, 447*f*, 448*t*
  for urgencies/emergencies, 468–471, 469*t*, 470*t*
  vasodilators in, 463*t*, 464
Anti-IgA antibodies, IgA deficiency and, 882
Anti-inflammatory drugs. *See also* Corticosteroids; Nonsteroidal anti-inflammatory drugs
  for asthma, 248
  for ophthalmic disorders, 170–172*t*
Anti-insulin antibodies
  in autoimmune/immunopathologic hypoglycemia, 1252, 1257
  in diabetes mellitus, 1211, 1211*t*, 1233
  in immune insulin resistance, 1237
  insulin therapy causing, 1211, 1237
Anti-insulin receptor antibodies
  in diabetes mellitus, 1212
  in hypoglycemia, 1252, 1257
Anti-integrins, for inflammatory bowel disease, 652
  Crohn disease, 657
  ulcerative colitis, 660
Anti-intrinsic factor antibodies, in pernicious anemia gastritis, 622
Anti-Itch lotion. *See* Pramoxine
Anti-Jo-1 antibody, in polymyositis/dermatomyositis, 840*t*, 848, 848*t*
Anti-leucine rich glioma inactivated 1 antibody, in autoimmune paraneoplastic disorders, 1008
Antileukocyte antibodies, transfusion-related acute lung injury caused by, 544
Antileukotriene agents
  for allergic rhinitis, 219
  for asthma, 247*f*, 249–250*t*, 251

Anti-LKM1 (liver-kidney microsome type 1 antibodies), in autoimmune hepatitis, 692
Anti-Ma2 antibody, in autoimmune paraneoplastic disorders, 1008
Anti-MAG antibodies, in cancer-related neuropathy, 1037
Antimalarial agents, 1515t, 1516–1520, 1516t, 1517t
  adverse ophthalmic effects of, 178t
  for lupus/SLE, 115–116, 841
  for malaria, 1514–1516, 1515t, 1516–1520, 1516t, 1517t
    chemoprophylaxis, 1520–1521, 1520t
    non-falciparum, 1515
    in nonimmune individuals, 1515–1516
    self-treatment, 1520
    severe disease, 1516, 1517t, 1519
    treatment, 1514–1520, 1515t, 1516t, 1517t
    uncomplicated falciparum, 1515–1516, 1516, 1516t, 1517t, 1521
  rabies vaccination and, 1326–1327, 1388
  resistance to, 1515, 1516, 1517
  for rheumatoid arthritis, 837
Anti-MDA5 antibody, in polymyositis/dermatomyositis, 848t
Antimetabolites, in cancer chemotherapy, 1663–1664t
Anti-Mi-2 antibody, in polymyositis/dermatomyositis, 848, 848t
Antimicrobial chemoprophylaxis. *See also* Antimicrobial therapy
  for anthrax, 1455, 1456, 1456t
  for aspergillosis, 1292, 1555
  for bite wounds, 1301
  in bronchiectasis, 264
  in burn injury, 1569
  for candidiasis, 1548
  for CMV infection, 191, 1291–1292, 1376
  in COPD, 261
  for cystitis, 954
  for endocarditis, 1460, 1460t, 1461t
    in hereditary hemorrhagic telangiectasia, 1684
    during pregnancy, **436**, 819
  for esophageal varices, 615
  in fever management, 35
  for gonococcal infections, 1476
  for group B streptococcal infection, in pregnancy, 800–801, 1444
  for herpes simplex infection, 119
    in pregnancy, 823, 1366
  for histoplasmosis, 1549
  in HIV infection/AIDS, 1346–1347, 1347–1349, 1348t, 1349–1350, 1349t
  for influenza, 1416, 1418
  for Lyme disease, 1504
  for MAC infection, 1334, 1350, 1483
  for malaria, 1520–1521, 1520t. *See also* Antimalarial agents
    pregnancy and, 802, 1521
    rabies vaccination and, 1326–1327, 1388

in neutropenia, 518, 1292
for opportunistic infections, 1291–1292
for pertussis, 1464
for plague, 1326, 1474
for *Pneumocystis* infection/pneumonia, 1291, 1334, 1349, 1349t, 1552
for Q fever, 1438
for relapsing fever, 1499
for rheumatic fever, 424
sexual violence (rape/sexual assault) and, 793, 794, 1302
for spontaneous bacterial peritonitis, 702
for surgical site infections, 54
for syphilis contacts, 1492
for toxoplasmosis, 1350, 1525
for traveler's diarrhea, 1310
  pregnancy and, 802, 1310
for tuberculosis, in HIV infection/AIDS, 1348, 1350
Antimicrobial therapy, **1310–1319**, 1311–1313t, 1314t, 1315–1316t. *See also* Antibiotics; Antimicrobial chemoprophylaxis
  adverse reactions/toxicity and, 1317
  clinical response to, 1313
    promptness of, 1317
  cost of agents and, 1317–1318
  duration of, 1296, 1317
  empiric, 1313, 1314t, 1315–1316t
    in asthma, 252
    in bronchiectasis, 264
    for diarrhea, 591
    in febrile cancer patient, 1661
    in fever management, 35, 1296, 1314t
      in drug user, 1304
    in immunocompromised host, 1292–1293
    for pneumonia
      community-acquired pneumonia, 267–268, 269–270, 269t, 270–271, 1314t, 1445
      nosocomial pneumonia, 274, 275t
    for skin and soft tissue infections, 1315t
  in fever management, 35, 518, 1293, 1296, 1314t
  for frostbite, 1566
  hypersensitivity tests/desensitization and, **1318–1319**
  for meningitis, 1297t, 1299
  in neutropenic patient, 35, 518, 1292, 1293, 1661
  for opportunistic infection, 1292–1293
  principles of, **1310–1318**, 1311–1313t, 1314t, 1315–1316t
  resistance to. *See* Drug resistance
  routes of administration for, 1317
  susceptibility testing and, 1313–1317
  thrombocytopenia caused by, 555t
Antimicrotubule agents, in cancer chemotherapy, 1664–1665t
Antimitochondrial antibodies, in primary biliary cholangitis/cirrhosis, 706, 707

Antimitochondrial antibody-negative primary biliary cholangitis (autoimmune cholangitis), 707
Antimonials, pentavalent, for leishmaniasis, 1511–1512, 1512
Antimony. *See* Stibogluconate
Antimotility drugs. *See* Antidiarrheal agents
Antimullerian hormone, in infertility workup, 784
Antimuscarinic agents
  overdose/toxicity of, 1590
  for urinary incontinence, 66
Anti-nAChR, in cancer-related neuropathy, 1037
Anti-native DNA antibody, 840t, 841t
Antineoplastic agents. *See* Chemotherapy
Antineutrophil cytoplasmic antibody (ANCA), 840t
  in eosinophilic granulomatosis with polyangiitis (Churg-Strauss syndrome), 933t, 935f, 938
  in glomerulonephritis (pauci-immune), 858, 922, 933t, 935f, **938–939**
  in granulomatosis with polyangiitis (Wegener granulomatosis), 840t, 857, 858, 922, 933t, 935f, 938
  in microscopic polyangiitis, 859, 860, 935f, 938
  in primary sclerosing cholangitis, 724
Anti-NMDA receptor-associated encephalitis, 1008
Antinuclear antibody (ANA), 840t
  in biliary cholangitis, 707
  in granulomatosis with polyangiitis, 840t
  in hyperthyroidism/Graves disease, 1124, 1128
  in lupus/SLE, 115, 839, 839t, 840–841, 840t, 841t, 842, 935f
  in polymyositis/dermatomyositis, 840t, 848
  in rheumatoid arthritis, 840t
  in scleroderma/CREST syndrome, 840t, 846
  in Sjögren syndrome, 840t, 850
Antioxidants. *See also* Vitamin C; Vitamin E
  for age-related macular degeneration, 185
  in chemoprevention, 11
  lipid-lowering and, 1263
Antiparkinsonism drugs, 1012–1014
  for antipsychotic-induced side effects/parkinsonism, 1072–1073, 1073
Antiphlebitic stockings. *See* Compression stockings
Antiphospholipid antibody syndrome/antiphospholipid antibodies, 574, 575t, **815–816**, 841, 841t, 842, **842–843**
  factor II antibodies and, 561
  false-positive syphilis tests and, 841, 841t, 843
  livedo reticularis/racemosa and, 843, 863

pregnancy loss and, 805, 815, 816, 841, 842, 843
SLE and, 562–563, 841, 841*t*, 842
stroke and, 843, 996
Antiplatelet antibody
heparin-associated, 552
in immune thrombocytopenia, 548, 549
in posttransfusion purpura, 555
Antiplatelet therapy. *See also* Anticoagulation therapy; Aspirin
for acute coronary syndromes/STEMI, 366–368, 367*f*, 373, 374
postinfarction, 380
for angina, 360*f*, 361–362
for atrial fibrillation/stroke prevention, 390*t*, 392*f*, 393, 997
in cardiovascular/heart disease prevention, 355
after coronary artery bypass grafting, 363
coronary stent placement and, 362, 373, 374
GI bleeding/peptic ulcer disease and, 624, 628
perioperative discontinuation of, 51–52, 51*t*, 52*t*, 368
for stroke, 997
thrombocytopenia caused by, 555*t*
for transient ischemic attacks, 993
Antiprotease/antitrypsin, alpha-1. *See* Alpha-1-antiprotease/antitrypsin
Antiproteinase-3 ANCA. *See* Proteinase-3 ANCA
Antipruritic agents
systemic, 95–100
topical, 95, 99*t*
Antipsychotic drugs, 1068–1073, 1069*t*, 1071*t*. *See also specific type and agent*
abnormal movements caused by, 1017, 1072, 1073
adherence/nonadherence issues and, 1071
for aggressive/violent behavior, 1091
for alcoholic hallucinosis, 1095
with antidepressants, 1070, 1079, 1083
atypical. *See* Atypical antipsychotics
for bipolar disease/mania, 1084–1085, 1085
breast cancer and, 1072
catatonia caused by, 1073
clinical indications for, 1070
for delirium, 62, 87, 1071, 1103
delirium caused by, 58, 62, 1071
for dementia-associated behavior problems, 59, 1022, 1070, 1104
for depression, 1070, 1079, 1083
dosage forms and patterns for, 1069*t*, 1070–1071
for Huntington disease, 1015
intranasal administration of, 1071
long-acting forms of, 1071
neuroleptic malignant syndrome caused by, 35, 36, 1072, 1589, 1590
for OCD, 1057

overdose/toxicity/side effects of, 1068, 1069*t*, 1071–1073, 1071*t*, **1589–1590**
for parkinsonism, 1014
parkinsonism (reversible) caused by, 1011, 1017, 1073
for personality disorders, 1065–1066
in pregnancy, 1072
for psychedelic/hallucinogen abuse/toxicity, 1099, 1598
relative potencies of, 1069*t*
for Tourette syndrome, 1018, 1070
Antipyretic drugs, 35
contraindications to in heat stroke, 1563
Antireflux surgery. *See* Fundoplication
Antiretroviral therapy/HAART, 1350–1362, 1351–1353*t*, 1354*t*, 1359–1360*t*, 1361*f*. *See also specific agent*
adherence and, 1, 1360, 1360–1361, 1361*f*
antituberculous drug interactions and, 282, 1336, 1356
CD4 counts and, 1334, 1350
CMV disease control and, 191–192, 1374, 1376
combinations/regimens for, 1350–1353
alternative/second-line regimens and, 1359–1360*t*, 1360, 1362
choosing, 1353–1360, 1354*t*, 1359–1360*t*
constructing, 1358–1360, 1359–1360*t*
fixed dose preparations and, 1353, 1354*t*
recommended/first-line, 1358–1360, 1359*t*
drug-drug interactions and, 1360
drug holidays/structured treatment interruptions and, 1361
drug resistance and, 1350, 1360, 1361–1362
efficacy and, 1360–1362
gynecomastia and, 1195
hepatitis B and, 687–688
hepatitis C and, 683, 1342
HIV prognosis and, 1330, 1350, 1362
HIV transmission affected by, 1332, 1346
immune reconstitution disease and, 191–192, 1345
lactic acidosis caused by, 1341
lipid abnormalities/lipodystrophy/lipoatrophy and, 1174, 1345, 1353, 1355, 1356
monitoring, 1360–1362
myopathy caused by, 869, 1049, 1340
after needle stick, 1347
neuropathy caused by, 1340
opportunistic infection/malignancies and, 1353
oral contraceptive drug interaction and, 786
postexposure, 4, 1303, 1346
after needle stick, 1347
after sexual/drug use exposure, 1303, 1346
sexual violence (rape/sexual assault) and, 793, 1302

preexposure/prophylactic, 4, 1303, 1346
pregnancy/newborn and, 822, 1332, 1346
progressive multifocal leukoencephalopathy incidence and, 1340
sexual violence (rape/sexual assault) and, 793, 1302
syphilis and, 1497
toxicity and, 1360
tuberculosis outcomes and, 1353
Anti-Rh$_o$ (D) antibody
in hemolytic disease of newborn, 801
prenatal screening for, 799, 800
Anti-RNA polymerase III antibody, in scleroderma, 846
Anti-SAE, in polymyositis/dermatomyositis, 848*t*
Anti-SCL-70 antibody, 840*t*, 846
Antisecretory agents. *See* Acid-antisecretory agents
Antiseizure therapy. *See* Anticonvulsant therapy
Anti-signal recognition particle (anti-SRP) antibody, in polymyositis/dermatomyositis, 848, 848*t*
Anti-SLA, in autoimmune hepatitis, 692, 693
Anti-Smith (anti-Sm) antibody, in lupus/SLE, 115, 840*t*, 841, 841*t*
Antisocial personality disorder, 1064, 1065*t*, 1066
Antispasmodic agents, for irritable bowel syndrome, 646
Anti-SRP antibody, in polymyositis/dermatomyositis, 848, 848*t*
Anti-SS-A/Ro antibody, 840*t*
in lupus/SLE, 115, 840*t*
in Sjögren syndrome, 840*t*, 850
Anti-SS-B/La antibody, 840*t*
in lupus/SLE, 115, 840*t*
in Sjögren syndrome, 840*t*, 850
Antistreptolysin O (ASO) titers, in postinfectious glomerulonephritis, 936
Antisynthetase antibodies, in polymyositis/dermatomyositis, 848, 848*t*
Antisynthetase syndrome, 848
Antithrombin, deficiency of, DVT/PE (venous thromboembolic disease) and, 575*t*
Antithrombotic therapy, **563–577**. *See also* Anticoagulation therapy; Antiplatelet therapy; Fibrinolytic therapy; Thrombolytic therapy
for myocardial infarction, 376
after fibrinolytic therapy, 375
PCI and, 362, 373, 374
Antithymocyte globulin
for aplastic anemia, 517
for myelodysplastic syndromes, 526
Antithyroid (antithyroglobulin/antithyroperoxidase) antibodies, 1121*t*
in hyperthyroidism/Graves disease, 1121*t*, 1128
in hypothyroidism, 1120, 1121*t*

Antithyroid (antithyroglobulin/
antithyroperoxidase)
antibodies(*Cont.*):
in thyroid cancer, 1142
follow-up and, 1146
in thyroid nodules, 1138
in thyroiditis
Hashimoto, 1134, 1135, 1135–1136
postpartum, 1125
subacute, 1128
Anti-TNF agents. *See also specific agent*
for ankylosing spondylitis, 864
histoplasmosis in patient taking, 1549
for inflammatory bowel disease,
651–652
Crohn disease, 656–657, 657
with immunomodulating therapy,
650–651, 651, 656
ulcerative colitis, 660, 661
for psoriasis/psoriatic arthritis, 108,
865
for rheumatoid arthritis, 837–838
tuberculosis reactivation and, 652, 1292
Antitoxin
botulism, 1047, 1454
diphtheria, 1457
Anti-Tr antibody, in autoimmune
paraneoplastic disorders,
1008
Antitrypsin/antiprotease, alpha-1. *See*
Alpha-1-antiprotease/
antitrypsin
Anti-tTG (transglutaminase/tissue
transglutaminase) antibody
in celiac disease/dermatitis
herpetiformis, 123, 634
in Hashimoto thyroiditis, 1136
Antituberculous drugs, 280–284, 281t,
282t
adherence/nonadherence and,
280–281, 283, 1336
antiretroviral drug interactions and,
282, 1336, 1356
directly observed therapy (DOT) and,
280–281, 283
in drug-resistant tuberculosis, 281,
283
in HIV infection/AIDS, 282
drug-resistant disease and, 277, 278,
278t, 282–283, 284, 1336
treatment of contacts and, 284
for extrapulmonary disease, 283
in fixed dose combinations, 282
hepatotoxicity of, 4
in HIV-negative persons, 281–282
in HIV-positive persons, 282, 1336
drug-resistant disease and, 277,
282–283, 1336
prophylactic, 1348, 1350
in latent disease/chemoprophylactic,
283–284
monitoring therapy with, 283
during pregnancy/lactation, 282, 283,
821–822
in spinal tuberculosis, 872
treatment of contacts and, 284
for tuberculous pericarditis, 426
Anti-VEGF therapy. *See also specific agent*
for age-related macular degeneration,
185
for diabetic macular edema, 190

for iris neovascularization/macular
edema in retinal vein
occlusion, 186
for renal cell carcinoma, 1654–1655
Antivenin
for black widow spider bites, 1605
for scorpion stings, 1605
for snake bites, 1581t, 1604
Antiviral agents, 1365t. *See also specific*
agent or infection
adverse ophthalmic effects of, 178t
for ophthalmic disorders, 170t, 175
Anti-voltage-gated calcium channel
antibody, in autoimmune
paraneoplastic disorders,
1008
Anti-voltage-gated potassium channel
antibody, in autoimmune
paraneoplastic disorders,
1008
Anti-Yo antibody, in autoimmune
paraneoplastic disorders,
1008
Anti-Zic antibody, in autoimmune
paraneoplastic disorders,
1008
Antizol. *See* Fomepizole
Anton syndrome, 1005
Anus. *See also under Anal*
carcinoma of, 1624t, **1643–1644**
in HIV infection/AIDS, 1344, 1644
rectum protruding through (rectal
prolapse), 669
Anxiety/anxiety disorders, **1052–1057**
drugs for management of, 1054–1056,
1054t, 1056t
generalized, 1053, 1054–1055
hospitalization/illness and, 1105,
1105–1106, 1106
hyperventilation/respiratory alkalosis
and, 316, 910, 911
palpitations in, 30, 31
panic disorders and, 1053, 1055–1056
pre- and postsurgical, 1105,
1105–1106, 1106
Anxiolytic drugs, 1054–1056, 1054t,
1056t. *See also specific type*
Aorta. *See also under Aortic*
atherosclerotic/occlusive disease of,
472–473
coarctation of. *See* Coarctation of aorta
in Marfan syndrome, 1682, 1683
traumatic injury of, 434
Aortic aneurysms
abdominal, **480–482**
screening for, 6t, 7, 481
dissection and, **484–486**
in syphilis, 1495, 1495f
thoracic, **482–483**
Aortic arch
aneurysm of, 483
coarctation of, 323–324
Aortic dissection, **484–486**
chest pain/discomfort in, 27, 359, 485
hypertension/hypertension
management and, 27, 444,
469t, 484, 485
in pregnancy, 435
Aortic regurgitation, 332–334t, **345–347**,
347t. *See also* Valvular heart
disease

hypertension and, 445
in Marfan syndrome, 346, 1682, 1683
Aortic root disease/dilation
in aortic regurgitation, 345
in aortic stenosis, 341
in Marfan syndrome, 1682, 1683
in mitral valve prolapse, 340
Aortic sclerosis, 341
Aortic stenosis, 332–334t, **340–345**, 342t,
343t, 344f, 345t. *See also*
Valvular heart disease
interventions affecting murmur in,
335t
Aortic valve
repair/replacement of, 342–344, 343t,
344f, 345t, 346–347, 347t. *See*
also Valve replacement
in rheumatic fever/heart disease, 345,
422
traumatic rupture of, 434
Aortitis, in rheumatoid arthritis, 835
Aortoenteric fistula, GI bleeding and, 595
Aortoiliac occlusive disease, **472–473**
APACHE II, in pancreatitis, 726
Apallic state (persistent vegetative state),
1028
Apathetic hyperthyroidism, 1126, 1133
Apathy, in dementia, 1020, 1022
APC gene, 665, 667, 1637
APECED. *See* Autoimmune
polyendocrinopathy-
candidiasis-ectodermal
dystrophy
Aphasia. *See also specific cause*
dementia and, 1019t
intracranial tumors causing, 1003
nonfluent/agrammatic variant, 1019t
semantic variant, 1019t
stroke and, 995
Aphthous ulcer, **226–227**, 227f
in Behçet syndrome, 861, 862
in HIV infection/AIDS, 1341
API2-MALT1 gene translocation, in
gastric lymphoma, 1632
Apical ballooning syndrome. *See*
Tako-Tsubo (stress/
catecholamine-induced)
cardiomyopathy
Apicitis, petrous, 206
Apidra. *See* Insulin glulisine
Apixaban, 564, 565–566t, 567, 573
for atrial fibrillation/stroke prevention,
391–393, 391t, 564, 565t
for DVT/PE (venous thromboembolic
disease), 564, 565t, 568t,
570t, 573
overdose/toxicity of, 564, 1588
perioperative management of, 52t, 566t
for transient ischemic attacks, 993
APL. *See* Acute promyelocytic leukemia
Aplastic anemia, **516–517**, 516t
stem cell transplantation for, 517, 541,
547–548
thrombocytopenia and, 516, 517, 546,
547–548
Aplastic crises
erythrovirus (parvovirus) infection
and, 1422
in sickle cell disease, 512
in thalassemia, 505
Apnea, sleep. *See* Sleep apnea hypopnea

Apnea test, 1028
Apneustic breathing, in coma or stupor, 1027–1028
ApoE genotyping, in Alzheimer disease, 1021
APOL1 gene
    in chronic kidney disease, 440, 924
    in focal segmental glomerulosclerosis, 944
    in HIV-associated nephropathy, 946
Apparent mineralocorticoid excess, 442, 892*t*
Appearance, in schizophrenia/psychotic disorders, 1067
Appendectomy, 642
    in pregnant patient, 825
    ulcerative colitis risk and, 658
Appendiceal carcinoids, 1635
Appendicitis, **641–643**
    adenoviruses causing, 1421
    amebic, 1525
    PID differentiated from, 778
    in pregnancy, 642, **825**
Appetite, genes affecting control of, 1270
Apprehension sign/test
    for knee, 1709*t*, 1712–1713
    for shoulder, 1688*t*, 1690
Apraclonidine, 172*t*, 180
    overdose/toxicity of, 1592
Apraxia
    in dementia, 1020
    intracranial tumors causing, 1005
Apremilast, for psoriasis/psoriatic arthritis, 108, 865
Aprepitant, 582*t*, 583, 1673
Apresoline. *See* Hydralazine
Apriso. *See* Mesalamine
APS. *See* Antiphospholipid antibody syndrome
Aptivus/Norvir. *See* Tipranavir, with ritonavir
Aqua glycolic, 99*t*
Aquaphor, 95, 100*t*
Aquaporin-4, in neuromyelitis optica, 193, 1025
Aquinil. *See* Hydrocortisone
Ara-C. *See* Cytarabine
Aranesp. *See* Darbepoetin alfa
Arbovirus encephalitides, **1388–1390**
ARBs. *See* Angiotensin II receptor blocking agents
Arch aneurysms, 483
Arcing (flash) burns, 1570
ARDS. *See* Acute respiratory distress syndrome
Aredia. *See* Pamidronate
Arformoterol, for COPD, 260
Arg133Trp (PAX-4) mutation, in idiopathic type 1 diabetes mellitus, 1211
Argatroban, for heparin-induced thrombocytopenia, 552–553, 553*t*
Arginine vasopressin, 1109*t*
    in diabetes insipidus, 1113
Argyll Robertson pupils, in tabes dorsalis, 1496
Arimidex. *See* Anastrozole
Aripiprazole, 1068, 1069*t*, 1070, 1071, 1071*t*
    for aggressive/violent patient, 1091

for bipolar disease/mania, 1070, 1085
    for depression, 1070, 1079, 1083
    overdose/toxicity/side effects of, 1069*t*, 1071*t*, 1589–1590
Arm edema, in breast cancer/ postmastectomy, 742, 759
Armodafinil, for sleep-wake disorders, 1090
Arnold-Chiari malformation, 1023, 1032
    cough headache and, 980
    syringomyelia and, 1032
Aromasin. *See* Exemestane
Aromatase inhibitors/inactivators
    adverse effects of, 752, 755
        ophthalmic, 178*t*
    in cancer chemotherapy, 1670*t*
        for breast cancer treatment/ prevention, 738, 739, 752, 754, 755, 755*t*, 756
            in male, 760
    for endometriosis, 776
    for gynecomastia, 1195
Arousal (excitement) stage of sexual activity, 1062
    disorders related to, 1062, 1063–1064. *See also* Sexual dysfunction
    in female, 782
Arrhythmias, **381–398**, 382–383*t*. *See also specific type and* Electrocardiogram
    antidepressants causing, 1082
    in COPD, 262
    in heart failure, 403, 404, 409
    in hypercalcemia, 898
    in hypocalcemia, 897
    in hypothermia/rewarming, 1564, 1564*f*
    myocardial infarction and, 370, 377
    palpitations and, 30, 31
    perioperative evaluation/management of, 48
    in pheochromocytoma, 1179, 1180, 1182, 1183
    in poisoning/drug overdose, **1579–1580**, 1579*t*. *See also specific agent*
        with antidepressants, 1082, 1606, 1606*f*
        with antipsychotics, 1589, 1590
    seizures differentiated from cerebral hypoperfusion caused by, 986
    treatment of
        catheter ablation for, 384
        pharmacologic, 381–384, 382–383*t*. *See also* Antiarrhythmic drugs
Arsenic poisoning, 1581*t*, **1590**
Arsenic trioxide, 527, 1668*t*
Arsenical melanosis, 157
ART. *See* Antiretroviral therapy; Assisted reproductive technologies
Artemether
    for malaria, 1515*t*, 1517*t*
        with lumefantrine (Coartem/ Riamet), 1515*t*, 1516*t*, 1517*t*, 1519, 1520
        for severe disease, 1519
    for schistosomiasis chemoprophylaxis, 1533

Artemisinin-based combination therapy (ACT), 1515, 1516*t*, 1519, 1521
    self-treatment and, 1520
Artemisinins (qinghaosu)/artemisinin derivatives/combinations, 1515, 1515*t*, 1519
    self-treatment and, 1520
Arterial aneurysms, **480–486**. *See also specific type and* Aneurysms
Arterial blood gases
    in acid-base disorders, 903, 904*t*
    in ARDS, 320
    in asthma/asthma exacerbation, 245, 245*t*, 254, 256*f*
    in carbon monoxide poisoning, 23, 305, 1592
    COPD/home oxygen therapy and, 258, 258*t*, 259, 260*t*
    in cyanide poisoning, 23, 24
    in cystic fibrosis, 265
    in drowning, 1567
    in dyspnea evaluation, 23–24
    in metabolic acidosis, 904*t*, 907
    in metabolic alkalosis, 904*t*, 908, 910
    in *Pneumocystis* pneumonia, 1335, 1551–1552
    in pulmonary embolism, 295
    in pulmonary hypertension, 302, 303
    in respiratory acidosis, 904*t*, 910
    in respiratory alkalosis, 904*t*, 911
    in respiratory failure, 317
    ventilatory control and, 315
Arterial embolism. *See* Embolism; Thromboembolism
Arterial gas embolism, in decompression sickness, 1573
Arterial graft/prosthesis. *See* Bypass grafting
Arterial lines
    infection/infection prevention and, 1295
    in shock management, 495
Arterial occlusion
    acute limb, **476–477**
    atherosclerotic, **472–480**. *See also* Atherosclerosis
    peripheral artery aneurysms and, 484
Arterial puncture, femoral artery pseudoaneurysm caused by, 484
Arterial thrombosis. *See also* Thrombosis
    in antiphospholipid antibody syndrome, 815, 816, 841, 843
Arteriography. *See specific type and* Angiography
Arteriolar dilators. *See also* Vasodilator therapy
    for hypertension, 463*t*, 464
Arteriovenous fistulae, spinal dural, 1002–1003
Arteriovenous malformations
    gastrointestinal (angioectasias), bleeding from, 595, 597
    in hereditary hemorrhagic telangiectasia, 1684
    intracranial, 998, **1000–1002**. *See also* Stroke
Arteritic anterior ischemic optic neuropathy, 192

Arteritis. *See also* Polyarteritis
  coronary artery, in Kawasaki disease, 1439
  giant cell. *See* Giant cell (temporal/cranial) arteritis
  Takayasu, **855**
Artesunate, 1515*t*, 1517*t*
  with amodiaquine (ASAQ), 1516, 1516*t*, 1517*t*, 1519
  with mefloquine, 1516*t*, 1517, 1519
  with pyronaridine, 1515*t*, 1516*t*, 1517, 1519
  for severe malaria, 1516, 1517*t*, 1519
  with sulfadoxine-pyrimethamine (Fansidar), 1516*t*, 1519
Arthritis/arthralgia. *See also specific disorder causing*
  in alkaptonuria, 1677, 1678
  in ankylosing spondylitis, 863
  arthroplasty/joint replacement for, 829. *See also specific joint*
  in Behçet syndrome, 862
  cancer-associated, 875
  in chikungunya fever, 870, 1407, 1408
  chondroitin/glucosamine for, 829, 1714
  in Crohn disease, 653, 867
  crystal deposition, **829–834**, 830*t*, 831*f*, 832*t*
  degenerative, **826–829**, 828*f*. *See also* Osteoarthritis
  in erythrovirus (parvovirus) infection, 870, 1422
  extra-articular manifestations and, 826
  glucosamine/chondroitin for, 829, 1714
  gonococcal, **868–869**, 1314*t*, 1475, 1476
    reactive arthritis differentiated from, 866, 869, 1476
  gouty. *See* Gout/gouty arthritis
  in granulomatosis with polyangiitis, 836, 857, 858
  in hemophilia, 557, 558
  in hepatitis, 870
  of hip, **1703–1704**
  in HIV infection/AIDS, 869, 1340
  infectious, **867–870**
    in drug users, 867, 1304
  inflammatory intestinal diseases and, 653
  joint involvement pattern and, 826, 827*t*
  leukemic, 875
  Lyme. *See* Lyme disease (Lyme borreliosis), arthritis in
  mutilans, 865
  neck pain caused by, 1696
  nongonococcal bacterial (septic), **867–868**, 1314*t*
    in drug users, 867, 1304
  pneumococcal, 1445
  pseudoseptic, 867
  psoriatic, 107, **864–865**
  reactive. *See* Reactive arthritis
  in rheumatic fever, 422, 423, 423*t*
  rheumatoid. *See* Rheumatoid arthritis
  rubella/rubella vaccination and, 870, 1384, 1385
  in sarcoidosis, **872–873**
  septic. *See* Arthritis/arthralgia, nongonococcal bacterial
  in SLE, 839*t*, 840

staphylococcal, 867, 1314*t*
  in Still disease, 838–839
  streptococcal, 867, 1443
  tophaceous, 830, 831*f*, 833
  tuberculous, **872**
  in ulcerative colitis, 867
  viral, **870**
  in Whipple disease, 635
Arthritis-dermatitis syndromes, gonococcal infection and, 1475, 1476
Arthrocentesis, 826, 827*t*, 828*t*. *See also specific disorder*
Arthropathy, neurogenic. *See* Neurogenic arthropathy
Arthroplasty. *See* Joints, replacement of
Arthropods, skin lesions caused by, **150–151**
Arthroscopy, 829
Artificial insemination, 785, 970
Artificial nutrition. *See also* Nutritional support
  liquid (tube feedings), 1281–1282, 1281*f*. *See also* Enteral nutritional support
Artificial sweeteners, for diabetics, 1219
Artificial tears, for dry eye, 168
Aryepiglottic folds, cancer of, 235, 236
Arytenoid cartilage, contact ulcers/granulomas of, 234–235
Arzerra. *See* Ofatumumab
5-ASA. *See* 5-Aminosalicylic acid
Asacol. *See* Mesalamine
ASAQ (artesunate-amodiaquine), 1516, 1516*t*, 1517*t*, 1519
Asbestosis (asbestos exposure), 307, 307*t*
  lung cancer and, 307, 309, 1608
  mesothelioma and, 309, 1615
ASC-US. *See* Atypical squamous cells of unknown significance
Ascaris lumbricoides (ascariasis), **1538**
Ascites, **601–602**, 601*t*. *See also specific cause*
  bacterial peritonitis and, 601, 602, 602–604, 702
  chylous, 601, 701
  in cirrhosis, 701–702
  malignant, 601, 601*t*, **604**, 1658, 1659
  neutrocytic, 601–602, 603
  pancreatic, 602, 728
  portal hypertension and, 600, 601, 601*t*, 604
  in shock liver/cardiogenic liver injury, 713
  surgical risk in patients with, 50
Ascites albumin gradient, serum (SAAG), 601*t*, 602, 604, 701
Ascitic fluid analysis/examination, 601–602, 603, 604. *See also specific disorder and* Paracentesis
Ascorbic acid. *See* Vitamin C
ASCVD. *See* Atherosclerotic cardiovascular disease
ASD. *See* Atrial septal defect
Asenapine, 1068, 1069*t*, 1070, 1071*t*
Asendin. *See* Amoxapine
Aseptic meningitis, 1297*t*, 1298. *See also* Meningitis
  in Colorado tick fever, 1408
  coxsackieviruses causing, 1426

echoviruses causing, 1427
  herpes simplex causing, 1364, 1366
  leptospiral, 1500, 1501
  in Lyme disease, 1502, 1505
  mumps/mumps vaccine and, 1380, 1381
  in syphilis, 1493, 1496
Asherman syndrome, 1201
ASO titers. *See* Antistreptolysin O (ASO) titers
Asparaginase *Erwinia chrysanthemi*, 1669*t*
Aspartate aminotransferase (AST). *See also specific disorder affecting*
  in liver disease/jaundice, 676, 676*t*, 694
  normal values for, 676*t*
Aspergilloma, 1554, 1555
Aspergillus/Aspergillus fumigatus (aspergillosis), **1554–1555**
  allergic bronchopulmonary, **264**, 879*t*, 1554, 1555
  chemoprophylaxis for, 1292, 1555
  chronic pulmonary, 1554, 1555
  in immunocompromised host/HIV infection/AIDS, 1292, 1554–1555
  invasive, 1554–1555, 1555
  S apiospermum infection differentiated from, 1557
  sinusitis and, 218, 1555
Aspiration, **305–306**. *See also* Pneumonia, aspiration
  in drug users, 1304
  enteral nutritional support and, 1284
  of food/"café coronary," 238, **306**
  foreign body, **238**
    retention of, **306**
  of gastric contents
    acute (Mendelson syndrome), **305–306**, 1294
    chronic, **306**
    in pneumonia, 273, 1294
  gastrointestinal decontamination for poisoning/drug overdose and, 1581, 1582
  of inert material, **306**
  of toxic material, **306**
    petroleum distillates, 306, 1602
Aspirin, 74, 75*t*. *See also* Antiplatelet therapy; Salicylates
  for acute coronary syndromes/STEMI, 366, 367*f*, 371–372, 376
  after fibrinolytic therapy, 375
  postinfarction, 376, 380
  prevention and, 6*t*, 10–11
  in analgesic nephropathy, 947
  for angina, 360*f*, 361
  cardiac valve replacement and, 351, 352*t*
  in cardiovascular/heart disease prevention, 6*t*, 10–11, 355
    in diabetes, 1241–1242
  for chemoprevention, 6*t*, 10–11, 355. *See also specific disorder*
  in colorectal cancer prevention, 1637
  contraindications to in heat stroke, 1563
  after coronary artery bypass grafting, 363
  coronary stent thrombosis prevention and, 362, 374, 376

for DVT/PE (venous thromboembolic disease), 574
for essential thrombocytosis, 521, 522
GI/diverticular bleeding associated with, 74, 624
nasal polyps and asthma as contraindication to, 222
with opioid analgesics, 80t
overdose/toxicity of, 74, 1602–1603
for pain management, 74, 75t, 80t
in peptic ulcer disease, 624, 628. See also Peptic ulcer disease, NSAID-induced
for pericarditis, 426
perioperative use of, 46
platelet function affected by, 558t, 829
for polycythemia, 521
respiratory disease associated with sensitivity to, **878**
Reye syndrome and, 74, 1369, 1371, 1412
for rheumatic fever, 424
for stroke, 997
for thyroiditis, 1137
for transient ischemic attacks, 993
for transient monocular visual loss, 189
Aspirin (NSAID) exacerbated respiratory disease, **878**
Asplenia, immunization recommendations in, 1321t
meningococcal vaccine, 1325t, 1465
pneumococcal vaccine, 1324t
Assisted reproductive technologies, 785
Assistive devices, fall prevention and, 64
AST. See Aspartate aminotransferase
Astemizole, antidepressant drug interactions and, 1081, 1083t
Astereognosis, intracranial tumors causing, 1003
Asthenozoospermia, 969f
Asthma, **242–257**
allergic, 242
desensitization therapy/immunotherapy for, 250t, 251
allergic bronchopulmonary mycosis/aspergillosis and, 264, 1554
aspirin triggering (triad asthma), 222, 878
beta-adrenergic agents for
long-acting, 247f, 249t
oral sustained-release, 252
in pregnant patient, 819
short-acting, 244t, 247f, 248, 252, 253t, 254, 255f, 256f
"cardiac," 242
catamenial, 242
classification/diagnosis of, 242–246, 243f, 244t, 245t, 246–248, 247f
comorbid condition control and, 248
complications of, 246
controller medications for, 247f, 248, 248–252, 249–250t, 250t
COPD differentiated from, 246, 259
cough and, 19, 20, 20–21, 20t, 242
differential diagnosis of, 246
drugs causing, 242, 310t
exacerbations of

classification/assessment of severity of, 242–246, 243f, 244t, 245, 245t, 246–248, 247f, 252–257, 255f, 256f
treatment of, 243f, 244t, 245t, 248–257, 250t, 252, 253–254t, 255f, 256f
exercise-induced, 242, 243f, 244t, 247f
"functional," 246
mediator inhibitors/mast cell stabilizers for, 248–251, 249t
NAEPP 3 diagnosis/management guidelines for, 243f, 244t, 246–248, 247f, 248–257, 250t, 253–254t, 255f, 256f
occupational, 242, 308
perioperative pulmonary complications and, 49, 50
during pregnancy, **819–820**
pulmonary function testing in, 243f, 244t, 245–246, 245t, 251, 252, 254, 255f, 256f
reliever medications for, 244t, 247f, 248, 252, 253–254t
severity/control of, assessing/monitoring, 242–246, 243f, 244t, 245, 245t, 252–257, 255f, 256f
treatment of, 243f, 244t, 246–248, 247f, 248–257, 249–250t, 250t, 253–254t, 255f, 256f
desensitization/immunotherapy in, 250t, 251
in emergency department setting, 254–255, 255f
for exacerbations, 243f, 244t, 245t, 248–257, 250t, 252, 253–254t, 255f, 256f
inhalation therapy, 248, 249t, 250t, 252, 253t, 256f
in intensive care setting, 255–257, 256f
long-term control medications for, 247f, 248, 248–252, 249–250t, 250t
contraindications to for monotherapy, 251
NAEPP 3 guidelines for, 243f, 244t, 246–248, 247f, 248–257, 250t, 253–254t, 255f, 256f
pharmacologic, 243f, 244t, 246–248, 247f, 248, 248–257, 250t, 253–254t, 255f, 256f
in pregnant patient, 819
quick relief medications for, 244t, 247f, 248, 252, 253–254t
stepwise approach to, 243f, 244t, 247f
triad, 222
vaccinations for patients with, 251
zanamivir contraindicated in, 1412
Asthma action plan, 248
Astrocytoma, 1004t, 1624t
Astroviruses, diarrhea/gastroenteritis caused by, 1305
Asunaprevir, for hepatitis C, 690t, 691
ASXL1 mutation, in acute myeloid leukemia, 527
Asymmetric septal hypertrophy, 418
At-risk (problem) drinking, 17, 1092. See also Alcohol use disorder

differential diagnosis of, 1094
treatment of, 1094–1095
Atabrine. See Quinacrine
Atacand/Atacand HCT. See Candesartan
Atactic breathing, in coma or stupor, 1028
Ataxia
cerebellar tumors causing, 1005
fragile-X tremor-ataxia syndrome and, 1679
Friedreich, 1035–1036
Ataxia-telangiectasia mutation
breast cancer and, 738
pancreatic/periampullary carcinoma and, 1620
Atazanavir, 1352t, 1356, 1357. See also Antiretroviral therapy
with cobicistat, 1352t, 1356, 1357
plus Truvada (emtricitabine/tenofovir [TDF]), 1359t
with ritonavir, 1357
plus Truvada (emtricitabine and tenofovir [TDF]), 1359t
prophylactic, transmission to fetus/newborn and, 1346
Atelectasis
in bronchial obstruction, 242
mechanical ventilation and, 319
postoperative, 1294
in right middle lobe syndrome, 288
Atenolol, 452t
breastfeeding and, 798t
for hypertension, 452t
with chlorthalidone, 452t
for Marfan syndrome, 1683
ATF ligament. See Anterior talofibular ligament
ATG. See Antithymocyte globulin
Atherosclerosis, **472–480**. See also specific artery affected and Cardiovascular disorders; Vascular disorders
acute limb occlusion and, **476–477**
aortoiliac disease and, **472–473**
cerebrovascular occlusive disease and, **477–479**, 478f. See also Stroke
cholesterol/lipoproteins in, 10, 353, 1260
screening tests and, 6t, 10, 1261–1262
in women/older adults, 1261, 1262
coronary artery/heart disease and, **352–381**. See also Coronary heart disease
in diabetes mellitus, 475, 476, 1241–1242, 1242
estrogen replacement therapy and, 1202
femoral/popliteal artery disease and, **473–475**
homocysteine/hyperhomocysteinemia and, 1681
hypertension and, 442, 444
lipid-lowering therapy and, 353, 1260, **1262–1266**, 1264t, 1265t. See also Lipid-lowering therapy
mesenteric artery insufficiency and, 479
mesenteric vein occlusion and, **480**

Atherosclerosis (*Cont.*):
  renal artery stenosis/renal vascular
      hypertension and, 442, 931,
      932
  tibial/pedal artery disease and,
      475–476
  visceral artery insufficiency and,
      479–480
Atherosclerotic cardiovascular disease
      (ASCVD). *See also*
      Atherosclerosis; Coronary
      heart disease
  risks/statin benefits and, 353, 354*f*,
      355*t*, 361
Atherosclerotic cardiovascular disease
      risk calculator, 353
Athletes
  cardiovascular screening of, **436–437**,
      437*t*, 438*t*
  head injury/concussion in, 1030, 1031
  sports medicine injuries and,
      1685–1717
  sudden death of, 436–437, 437*t*, 438*t*
      cardiomyopathy causing, 421, 436,
          437, 438*t*
Athlete's foot, **113–114**, 113*f*
  cellulitis and, 113, 137
Ativan. *See* Lorazepam
ATL. *See* Adult T cell lymphoma/
      leukemia
Atlanta classification, revised, in
      pancreatitis, 727, 728
ATM mutation
  in chronic lymphocytic leukemia, 530
  in pancreatic/periampullary
      carcinoma, 1620
ATN1 gene, in dentatorubral-
      pallidoluysian atrophy, 1015
ATO. *See* Arsenic trioxide
Atonic seizures (epileptic drop attacks),
      984*t*, 985. *See also* Seizures
Atopic dermatitis, **104–106**
  herpes simplex infection (eczema
      herpeticum) and, 105, 106,
      1364, 1367*t*
  vesiculobullous of palms and soles
      (pompholyx), **121–122**, 122*f*
  tinea differentiated from, 114, 122
Atopic disease (atopy), 876. *See also*
      specific disorder and
      Allergies/allergic disorders/
      reactions
  allergic bronchopulmonary mycosis
      and, 264
  allergic rhinitis and, 220
  asthma and, 242
  eosinophilic esophagitis and, 613
Atopic keratoconjunctivitis, 168
Atorvastatin, 355*t*, 1260, 1263–1264,
      1265*t*. *See also* Statins
  with amlodipine, 461*t*
  in HIV infection/AIDS, 1356
  for polycystic ovary syndrome, 1198
Atovaquone
  for malaria, with proguanil (Malarone),
      1515*t*, 1517*t*, 1519
      for chemoprophylaxis, 1519, 1520,
          1520*t*
  self-treatment and, 1520
  for *P jirovecii* infection, 1337*t*, 1349*t*,
      1552

ATP1A2 gene, in familial hemiplegic
      migraine, 977
ATP7B, in Wilson disease, 710
ATRA. *See* All-trans-retinoic acid;
      Tretinoin
Atrial fibrillation, **388–394**, 389*t*, 390*t*,
      391*t*, 392*f*. *See also*
      Arrhythmias
  arterial emboli and, 388
  anticoagulation in prevention/
      management of, 351, 352*t*,
      388, 389, 389*t*, 390, 390–393,
      390*t*, 391*t*, 392*f*
  limb occlusion and, 476
  retinal artery occlusion and, 187,
      188
  stroke and, 388, 389*t*, 390, 390–391,
      390*t*, 996
  transient ischemic attacks and, 389*t*,
      390, 390*t*, 477, 991, 993
  with bradyarrhythmia ("tachy-brady
      syndrome"), 399
  cardiomyopathy and, 417, 419
  catheter ablation of, 384, 394
  in hyperthyroidism/thyrotoxicosis,
      388, 389, 1127, 1133
  in mitral regurgitation, 337, 338*f*
  in mitral stenosis, 335, 335–336, 336*f*
  in myocardial infarction, 377
  palpitations in, 30, 31
  prosthetic heart valves and, 351, 352*t*,
      392
  recurrent paroxysmal, 388, 394
  reentry/preexcitation and, 387
  refractory, 394
  treatment of, 382–383*t*, 389–394
Atrial flutter, **394–395**
  with bradyarrhythmia ("tachy-brady
      syndrome"), 399
  palpitations in, 30
  reentry/preexcitation and, 387, 394
  treatment of, 382–383*t*, 395
Atrial gallop. *See* Heart sounds
Atrial myxoma, 433
  fever/FUO and, 1288
Atrial natriuretic peptide, in senile
      amyloidosis, 538
Atrial (supraventricular) premature beats
      (atrial extrasystoles), **385**
  in myocardial infarction, 377
Atrial septal aneurysm, 325, 326
Atrial septal defect, **324–327**
Atrial septal lipoma, 433
Atrial tachycardia
  in hyperthyroidism, 1127
  multifocal, **395**
Atrioventricular (heart) block, **399–400**
  in atrial septal defect/patent foramen
      ovale, 325
  in Lyme disease, 1502, 1505, 1505*t*
  in myocardial infarction, 377
  palpitations in, 31
  in poisoning/drug overdose, 1579*t*
      antidepressants and, 1606, 1606*f*
Atrioventricular (AV) dissociation, **400**
Atrioventricular junctional rhythm, **395**
Atrioventricular nodal reentry
      tachycardia (AVNRT), 385
Atrioventricular pathways, accessory,
      supraventricular tachycardia
      caused by, 385, **387–388**

Atrioventricular reciprocating tachycardia
      (AVRT), 385, 387
Atripla (tenofovir [TDF]/emtricitabine/
      efavirenz), 1354*t*, 1355, 1359*t*
Atrophic age-related macular
      degeneration, 185
Atrophic gastritis
  gastric adenocarcinoma and, 622–623,
      1629
  H pylori infection and, 622
  in pernicious anemia, 622–623
Atrophic urethritis, urinary incontinence
      and, 43, 65
Atrophic vaginitis
  estrogen replacement therapy for, 795,
      1202, 1205
  in menopause, 794–795, 795
  urinary incontinence and, 43, 65
Atrophie blanche, 33
Atropine
  for cholinesterase inhibitor
      (anticholinesterase)
      poisoning, 1581*t*, 1602
  with diphenoxylate. *See* Diphenoxylate
      with atropine
  for infarction-related conduction
      disturbances, 377
  overdose/toxicity of, 1581*t*, **1590**
Atypical absence seizures, 984*t*, 985
Atypical antidepressants, 1078*t*,
      1079–1081. *See also*
      Antidepressants
Atypical antipsychotics, 1068–1070,
      1069*t*, 1070, 1071*t*. *See also*
      Antipsychotic drugs
  for bipolar disease/mania, 1084–1085,
      1085
  for dementia/dementia-associated
      behavior problems, 59, 1021,
      1070, 1104
  for depression, 1079, 1083
  diabetes and, 1071–1072, 1071*t*
  for Huntington disease, 1015
  overdose/toxicity/side effects of, 1069*t*,
      1071–1072, 1071*t*
  for parkinsonism, 1014
  for Tourette syndrome, 1018
Atypical facial pain, **982**
Atypical hemolytic-uremic syndrome,
      551, 551*t*
Atypical major depression, 1075, 1079
Atypical measles, 1367*t*
Atypical mycobacteria. *See*
      Nontuberculous (atypical)
      mycobacteria
Atypical nevi/mole, **102**, 102*f*
Atypical squamous cells of unknown
      significance (ASC-US), 769*t*,
      770
  screening guidelines and, 15
AUA symptom index, 971–972, 971*t*
AUB/AUB-O. *See* Abnormal uterine
      bleeding
Aubagio. *See* Teriflunomide
Audiology, 200–201
Audiovestibular disorders, 211*t*, **213–214**.
      See also Vestibular disorders
AUDIT (Alcohol Use Disorder
      Identification Test), 17, 18*t*,
      1093
Auditory canal. *See* Ear canal

Auditory system, central, diseases of, **213–214**, 213*t*
Auer rods, in acute leukemia, 528
Augmentation mammoplasty. *See* Breast implants
Augmentin. *See* Amoxicillin/amoxicillin-clavulanate
Aura
  in migraine headache, 977
  pre-seizure, 985
Auricle, **201**
Austin Flint murmur, 346
Austrian triad, 1445
Autism, vaccines and, 1379
Autofluorescence spectroscopy, near-infrared, during parathyroidectomy, 1158
Autoimmune adenopathy, 239
Autoimmune cholangitis, 707
Autoimmune cytopenia, common variable immunodeficiency and, 882
Autoimmune disorders, **834–853**. *See also specific disease*
  adrenal insufficiency/Addison disease and, 1169
  breast implants and, 737
  cognitive disorders/delirium caused by, 1102*t*
  common variable immunodeficiency and, 882
  diabetes and, 1210–1211, 1211*t*
  fever/FUO and, 1287, 1288
  hearing loss in, 209
  in HIV infection/AIDS, 1332–1333
Autoimmune hemolytic anemia, **513–515**
  with thrombocytopenia (Evans syndrome), 514
Autoimmune hepatitis, **692–693**
Autoimmune hypoglycemia, **1257**
Autoimmune hypoparathyroidism, 1149, 1150
Autoimmune myocarditis, 413, 413*t*
Autoimmune neutropenia, 518
Autoimmune pancreatitis, 731
Autoimmune paraneoplastic disorders, 1008
Autoimmune polyendocrinopathy-candidiasis-ectodermal dystrophy, 1149, 1169. *See also* Polyglandular autoimmune syndrome
Autoimmune regulatory gene, in type 1 diabetes, 1210–1211
Autoimmune thyroiditis. *See* Hashimoto (chronic lymphocytic/autoimmune) thyroiditis; Transient autoimmune thyroiditis
Autologous packed red blood cells, transfusion of, 542. *See also* Transfusion
Autologous serum eye drops, 168
Autologous stem cell transplantation, **540**. *See also* Bone marrow/stem cell transplantation
Automatism, postepileptic, 985
Automobile accidents
  cardiac injury and, 434
  prevention of injury caused by, 16

Automobile driving
  by patients with dementia, 59–60, 1022
  by patients with syncope/ventricular tachycardia/aborted sudden death, **402**
  by suicidal patients, 1077
Autonomic dysfunction (dysautonomia), **990–991**
  in enterovirus 71 infection, 1427
  in Guillain-Barré syndrome, 990, 1038
  neuropathy causing, 1035
  prenatal screening for, 800
Autonomic failure, pure, 990
Autonomic neuropathy
  cancer-related/chemotherapy-induced, 1038, 1674
  in diabetes, 1240–1241. *See also* Diabetic neuropathy
  dysautonomia and, 990
  in porphyria, 1036, 1676
Autonomic testing
  in dysautonomia, 991
  in syncope, 401
Autophony, patulous eustachian tube and, 203
Autopsy, 93–94
Autosomal dominant polycystic kidney disease, **949–950**, 949*t*
Autosomal recessive syndromes, diabetes mellitus in, 1212–1213
AV block. *See* Atrioventricular (heart) block
AV dissociation, **400**
AV junctional rhythm, **395**
AV nodal reentry tachycardia (AVNRT), 385
AV reciprocating tachycardia (AVRT), 385, 387
Avalide. *See* Irbesartan/irbesartan with hydrochlorothiazide
Avanafil, for erectile dysfunction diagnosis/treatment, 967
Avandamet. *See* Rosiglitazone, with metformin
Avandaryl. *See* Rosiglitazone, with glimepiride
Avandia. *See* Rosiglitazone
Avapro. *See* Irbesartan
Avascular necrosis of bone (osteonecrosis), **875–876**
  corticosteroid use and, 875, 1209
  in HIV infection/AIDS, 1340
  of jaw, bisphosphonate use and, 11, 875, 1162
Avastin. *See* Bevacizumab
Aveed. *See* Testosterone undecanoate
Aveeno, 99*t*
Aveeno Anti-Itch lotion. *See* Pramoxine
Avelox. *See* Moxifloxacin
Aventis. *See* Insulin glargine
Aventyl. *See* Nortriptyline
Avian influenza (H5N1 and analogs), **1417–1418**. *See also* Influenza
Avinza. *See* Morphine
Avita. *See* Tretinoin
AVM. *See* Arteriovenous malformations
AVNRT (AV nodal reentry tachycardia), 385
Avoidance therapy
  for allergic contact dermatitis, 125

  for allergic rhinitis, 219–220
  for rosacea, 129
Avoidant personality disorder, 1065*t*, 1066
AVP. *See* Arginine vasopressin
AVRT (AV reciprocating tachycardia), 385, 387
Axillary lymph nodes, in breast cancer, 741, 741*f*, 742
  adjuvant/neoadjuvant therapy and, 750, 751*t*
  dissection of, 749, 750, 750*f*
    arm edema and, 759
  irradiation of, 750, 754
  palpation for evaluation of, 741, 741*f*, 742
  prognosis/recurrence and, 750, 751*t*, 758
Axiron, 1192
Axitinib, 1667*t*
  thyroiditis caused by, 1126
Axonal injury, diffuse, 1030*t*
Axonal neuropathies, 1034, 1038. *See also specific type and* Guillain-Barré syndrome; Neuropathies
  in critically ill patient, 1037
  myeloma/paraproteinemias and, 1036
  toxic, 1037
Aygestin. *See* Norethindrone
Azacitidine, 1664*t*
  for myelodysplastic syndromes, 526
Azactam. *See* Aztreonam
Azarcon, toxicity of, 1593
Azarga. *See* Brinzolamide/timolol
AzaSite. *See* Azithromycin
Azathioprine
  for autoimmune hepatitis, 692–693
  for granulomatosis with polyangiitis, 859
  for inflammatory bowel disease, 650–651
    with anti-TNF agents, 650–651, 651, 656, 656–657
    Crohn disease, 656, 657
    ulcerative colitis, 659
  for myasthenia gravis, 1046
  for myasthenic (Lambert-Eaton) syndrome, 1046
  for neuromyelitis optica, 1025
  for pemphigus, 140
  thiopurine methyltransferase variants and, 651
Azelastine. *See also* Antihistamines
  for allergic eye disease, 168, 170*t*
  for allergic rhinitis, 219
Azidothymidine. *See* Zidovudine
Azilsartan/azilsartan with chlorthalidone, 457*t*
Azithromycin. *See also* Macrolides
  for endocarditis prophylaxis, 1461*t*
  for Lyme disease, 1504
  for MAC infection, 286, 1350, 1482, 1483
  for ophthalmic disorders, 169*t*
  for pharyngitis, 229
  for pneumonia, 269*t*, 271, 1445
  for syphilis, 1492
  for traveler's diarrhea, 1310
Azo compounds, for inflammatory bowel disease, 650

Azoospermia, 969, 969f
artificial insemination for infertility
caused by, 785
in cystic fibrosis, 265, 969, 970
in Klinefelter syndrome, 970, 1190,
1682
Y chromosome microdeletions
causing, 970
Azopt. See Brinzolamide
Azor (olmesartan and amlodipine). See
Olmesartan
Azotemia, 913. See also specific cause and
Kidney disease/injury
in hepatorenal syndrome, 702
in hyperglycemic hyperosmolar state,
1250
hyperparathyroidism and, 1157
hypocalcemia/hyperphosphatemia/
hypoparathyroidism and,
1150
pancreatitis and, 728
parenteral nutritional support and,
1285t
postrenal, 916, 917t, 918
prerenal, 916, 917–918, 917t
AZT. See Zidovudine
AZT/3TC. See Zidovudine (AZT), with
lamivudine
Aztreonam, for pneumonia, 269t, 275t

B19 parvovirus infection. See
Erythrovirus (parvovirus
B19) infection
B antigen, in compatibility testing, 542
B/Brisbane/60/2008-like virus, 1413. See
also Influenza
B-cell lymphoma, 531, 533. See also
Lymphoma; Non-Hodgkin
lymphoma
common variable immunodeficiency
and, 882
Epstein-Barr virus and, 1373
intestinal, 1634
stem cell transplantation for, 533, 540
B cells
defects in, common variable
immunodeficiency and, 882
pancreatic, 1185
in diabetes mellitus, 1210, 1211t
hypoglycemia caused by tumors of,
1185, **1252–1255**, 1253t,
1254t. See also Insulinomas;
Islet cell tumors
B/Phuket/3073/2013-like virus, 1413. See
also Influenza
B-raf/BRAF gene/mutations
colorectal cancer/HNPCC/Lynch
syndrome and, 665, 668,
1637
in thyroid cancer, 1139
B-type natriuretic peptide (BNP/beta)
in aortic regurgitation, 346
in aortic stenosis, 342
in cardiomyopathy, 415, 435
in dyspnea, 23
in heart failure, 23, 404
ascites and, 713
recombinant. See Nesiritide
Babesia divergens/microti/venatorum
(babesiosis), **1521–1522**,
1522f

ehrlichiosis/anaplasmosis coinfection
and, 1436, 1504
Lyme disease coinfection and, 1504
Bacillary angiomatosis, 1343, 1477
Bacillary dysentery (Shigella dysentery/
gastroenteritis), 588t, 589,
1305, 1307t, 1312t, 1315t,
1342, **1470**
Bacillus, 1312t
anthracis, 1312t, 1454, 1456. See also
Anthrax
cereus, diarrhea/food poisoning/
gastroenteritis caused by,
588t, 589, 1305, 1306t
Bacillus Calmette-Guérin (BCG), for
bladder cancer, 1652
Bacillus Calmette-Guérin (BCG) vaccine,
284
tuberculin skin test affected by, 4, 279,
284
tuberculosis blood tests/interferon
gamma release assays and, 4,
279–280
Bacitracin
for ophthalmic disorders, 169t
for staphylococcal carriage, 218
Bacitracin/polymyxin, for ophthalmic
disorders, 169t
Back pain, **1692–1694**, 1692t, 1693t. See
also specific cause
disk-related, 1695
spinal cord compression causing, 1657
spinal stenosis causing, 1694
Background (nonproliferative)
retinopathy, 189, 189–190,
189f, 1238
Baclofen
for alcohol use disorder, 694
for spasticity, 1026, 1034
Bacteremia. See also Sepsis/septic shock
anaerobic, **1479**
campylobacter causing, 1472
Elizabethkingia causing, 1478
gram-negative, **1467–1468**
health care-associated, 1293–1294,
1295
in listeriosis, 1457
neutropenia and, 1292
osteomyelitis from, 870
salmonella, 1308, 1312t, 1468, **1470**
staphylococcal, **1449–1450**
transfusion of contaminated blood
causing, 543
vibrios causing, 1312t, 1472
Bacterial infections, **1441–1485**. See also
specific type
actinomycosis, **1480–1481**
anaerobic, **1478–1480**, 1479t, 1480f
conjunctivitis, **167**
diarrhea in, 588t, 589, 592, 1305–1308,
1306–1307t, 1342. See also
Diarrhea, infectious
drugs for. See Antibiotics;
Antimicrobial therapy
endocarditis, 1314t, **1458–1463**, 1459f,
1460t, 1461t
folliculitis, 130–131, 130f
gram-negative, 1311t, 1311–1312t,
1463–1480
gram-positive, 1311t, 1312t,
1441–1458

keratitis, **174–175**
in measles, 1379
meningitis, 1297, 1297t, 1299, 1314t
mycobacterial, 1312t, **1481–1485**
myocarditis in, 413t
nocardiosis, 1312t, **1481**
pericarditis, 425, 426
peritonitis, 601, 602, **602–604**, 702
prostatitis, 955t, **957**, 957t, **958**
rhinosinusitis (sinusitis), **215–218**,
217t. See also Rhinosinusitis,
acute bacterial
shock and. See Sepsis/septic shock
tubulointerstitial nephritis, 947t
vaginosis, 767, 768, 1302
sexual violence (rape/sexual assault)
and, 1302
Bacterial overgrowth, **636–637**
diarrhea and, 588t, 592, 594, 636
irritable bowel syndrome and, 636, 644
vitamin B_{12} deficiency and, 506, 636
Bacterial synergistic gangrene, 1480
Bacteriuria, during pregnancy, 820
Bacteroides, 1311t, 1479
abdominal sepsis caused by, 1314t,
1479
fragilis, 1479
melaninogenicus. See Prevotella,
melaninogenica
Bactrim. See Trimethoprim-
sulfamethoxazole
Bactroban. See Mupirocin
BAD-1 protein, in blastomycosis
diagnosis, 1556
Bagassosis, 308t
Baker (popliteal) cyst, 1700, 1701, 1704
ruptured, lower extremity edema and,
32, 1701
BAL. See Dimercaprol
Balance. See Falls; Vestibular disorders
Balanitis
candidal, 133
in chancroid, 1476
in reactive arthritis, 866, 866f
Balanoposthitis, in diabetes, 1214
Baldness. See Alopecia
Balint syndrome, 1005
Balkan nephropathy, ureteral/renal pelvis
cancer and, 1653
Balloon angioplasty, coronary. See
Angioplasty, coronary;
Percutaneous coronary
intervention
Balloon expulsion test, 585
Balloon tube tamponade, for esophageal
varices, 615
Balloon valvuloplasty. See Valvuloplasty
Balsalazide, for inflammatory bowel
disease/ulcerative colitis, 650,
659
Bamboo spine, 864
Band keratopathy, in hypercalcemia/
hyperparathyroidism, 1153
Banding, gastric. See Bariatric surgery
Banding (band/variceal ligation)
for esophageal varices, 596, 599, 615
in noncirrhotic portal hypertension,
714
prevention of first bleeding episode
and, 616–617
prevention of rebleeding and, 616

for hemorrhoids, 670
for Mallory-Weiss syndrome, 612
Bankart lesion, 1690
Barbiturates. *See* Opioids/opioid
analgesics; Sedative-
hypnotics
Barcelona Clinic Liver Cancer (BCLC)
staging system, 1617
BARD score, in nonalcoholic fatty liver
disease, 698
Bariatric surgery, 1271–1272
hypoglycemia after, 1252, 1256
in type 2 diabetes, 1235
Baritosis, 307*t*
Barium enema, for cancer screening,
1643
Barium esophagography, 606
in esophageal cancer, 1626
in GERD, 607
in motility disorders, 617, 618
Barotrauma, **204**
dysbarism/decompression sickness
and, 204, 1572, 1573
mechanical ventilation and, 319
Barrett esophagus, 608, 609
esophageal carcinoma and, 608, 1626
Bartholin duct cyst/abscess, **768–769**,
768*f*
Bartonella henselae/quintana
(bartonellosis), **1477**
bacillary angiomatosis caused by, 1343,
1477
endocarditis caused by, 1460, 1462,
1477
in HIV infection/AIDS, 1343, 1477
lymphadenitis/lymphadenopathy in,
492, 1477
pediculosis and, 150, 1477
Bart's hemoglobin, 505
Bartter syndrome, 892*t*
Basal cell carcinoma
of skin, **143**, 143*f*
eyelid involvement and, 165–166
of vulva, 775
Basal cell nevus syndrome, 143
Basal energy expenditure (BEE), 1270,
1282
Basedow disease, 1124–1125. *See also*
Graves disease;
Hyperthyroidism
Basic activities of daily living (ADLs),
assessment of ability to
perform, 55–56
Basic life support, drowning and, 1567
Basilar artery migraine, 978
Basilar artery occlusion, stroke caused by,
995
Basilar meningitis, in syphilis, 1493, 1496
Basilar skull fracture, 1029
vertigo caused by, 212
"Bath salts," 1587
Bathing, in dermatologic therapy, 95
Battered child. *See* Child abuse
Battered elderly. *See* Elder abuse/
mistreatment
Battered woman. *See* Domestic violence
Batteries (disk/button), ingested, alkali
injuries caused by, 1587
Battle sign, 1029
Baylisascaris procyonis, visceral larva
migrans caused by, 1542

Bazedoxifene, for osteoporosis, 1163
BCG, for bladder cancer, 1652
BCG vaccine, 284
tuberculin skin test affected by, 4, 279,
284
tuberculosis blood tests/interferon
gamma release assays and, 4,
279–280
bcl-2 expression, in non-Hodgkin
lymphoma, 531, 533
BCLC (Barcelona Clinic Liver Cancer)
staging system, 1617
bcr/abl fusion gene
in acute lymphoblastic leukemia, 529
in chronic myeloid leukemia, 523–524,
524, 525
BDVV. *See* Bundibugyo virus
BEACOPP regimen, 534
Beau lines, 160
Becaplermin, for diabetic foot ulcers, 156,
1239
Becker muscular dystrophy, 1047, 1048*t*
Beclabuvir, for hepatitis C, 690*t*, 691
Beclomethasone
for allergic rhinitis, 219
for asthma, 250*t*
Bed rest. *See also* Immobility
for frostbite, 1566
hazards of, 62
hypercalcemia and, 1156
for threatened abortion, 804
Bedbugs, skin lesions caused by,
150, 151
Bedside Index for Severity in Acute
Pancreatitis (BISAP), 726
Bedside tracheotomy, 237
Bedsores. *See* Pressure ulcers
BEE. *See* Basal energy expenditure
Beef tapeworm (*T saginata*), **1535**, 1536
Beer potomania, hyponatremia caused by,
887
Behavioral problems, in dementia,
management of, 59,
1021–1022, 1104
Behavioral-variant frontotemporal
dementia, 1019*t*
Behçet syndrome, **861–862**
uveitis in, 181, 862
Bejel (endemic syphilis), **1498–1499**
Belching (eructation), 587
Beleodaq. *See* Belinostat
Belimumab, for SLE, 841
Belinostat, 1669*t*
Bell palsy, **1041**, 1041*f*. *See also* Facial
neuropathy/paralysis/palsy
herpes simplex/varicella zoster
infection and, 1041, 1364,
1366, 1369
Belladonna
MAOI interactions and, 1083*t*
overdose/toxicity of, 1590
Belly press test, 1687*t*, 1689
Belsomra. *See* Suvorexant
Benazepril/benazepril with
hydrochlorothiazide/
benazepril with amlodipine,
455*t*
Bence Jones proteinuria (light chain in
urine), in myeloma, 535,
535–536, 914, 951
renal toxicity and, 920, 951

Bendamustine, 1663*t*
for chronic lymphocytic leukemia, 530
Bendroflumethazide, with nadolol, 453*t*
Bends, 1573
Benicar/Benicar HCT. *See* Olmesartan
Benign essential (familial) tremor,
1010–1011
Benign mole, 101, 101*f*
Benign paroxysmal positioning vertigo
(BPPV), 211*t*, 212
Benign prostatic hyperplasia, **971–976**,
971*t*, 973*f*, 973*t*, 974*t*
kidney disease and, 918
testosterone replacement therapy and,
1191–1192, 1193
urinary incontinence and, 66, 67
Benign recurrent lymphocytic (Mollaret)
meningitis, 1364
Bentall procedure, 343
BenzaClin. *See* Clindamycin, with
benzoyl peroxide
Benzalkonium, for hydrofluoric acid
burns, 1586
Benzalkonium-free eye drops, for
glaucoma, 172*t*, 173*t*, 180
Benzamycin. *See* Erythromycin, with
benzoyl peroxide
Benzisoxazoles, 1068. *See also*
Antipsychotic drugs
Benznidazole, for Chagas disease, 1509,
1510
Benzocaine, methemoglobinemia caused
by, 1599
Benzodiazepines, 1054–1055, 1054*t*,
1055, 1056, 1056*t*. *See also*
specific agent
for aggressive/violent patient, 1091
for alcohol detoxification/withdrawal,
17, 989, 1095, 1097–1098,
1098
with antipsychotic agents, 1070
for anxiety, 1054–1055, 1054*t*, 1055,
1056, 1056*t*
for bipolar disease/mania, 1085
for delirium, 62, 1103
drug interactions of, 1056*t*
for hallucinogen overdose/toxicity,
1598
in older adult, 1055
overdose/toxicity of, 1055, 1578, 1581*t*,
1594
for panic disorders/attacks, 1055, 1056
for PTSD, 1052
sleep cycle affected by, 1088–1089
for sleep-wake disorders/insomnia,
1054*t*, 1055, 1089
withdrawal from, 1055
Benzoyl peroxide, for acne, 98*t*, 127
Benzoylecgonine, in cocaine abuse, 1588
Bepotastine. *See also* Antihistamines
for allergic eye disease, 168, 170*t*
Bepreve. *See* Bepotastine
Berger disease (IgA nephropathy), 933*t*,
935*f*, **937**
Beriberi, 1274–1275. *See also* Thiamine
(vitamin B$_1$), deficiency of
neuropathy associated with, 1036
Bernard-Soulier syndrome, 556
Berry aneurysms, 998, 1000. *See also*
Intracranial aneurysm
Berylliosis, 309

Besifloxacin, for ophthalmic disorders, 169t
Besivance. See Besifloxacin
Beta-adrenergic agonists
　for asthma
　　exacerbation management and, 252, 253t
　　long-acting, 247f, 249t, 251
　　　contraindications to for monotherapy, 251
　　oral sustained-release, 252
　　in pregnant patient, 819
　　short-acting, 244t, 247f, 248, 252, 253t, 254, 255f, 256f
　for COPD, 260, 262
Beta-adrenergic blocking drugs
　for acute coronary syndromes/STEMI, 368
　　postinfarction, 359, 375, 380
　　　hypertension and, 449t
　for angina, 359–361, 360f
　for anxiety/GAD, 1055, 1056
　for aortic dissection, 485
　for arrhythmias, 381, 382t
　　atrial fibrillation, 389, 390
　　in hyperthyroidism, 1133
　　infarct-related, 377
　　supraventricular tachycardia, 386
　　ventricular tachycardia, 397
　breastfeeding and, 798t
　for cardiomyopathy, 416, 418, 419, 420f, 422
　depression caused by, 1076
　for esophageal varices
　　prevention of first bleeding episode and, 616
　　prevention of rebleeding and, 616
　for glaucoma/ocular hypertension, 172t, 180
　in heart failure, 375, 405f, 407–408, 409, 454
　　hypertension and, 449t, 454
　　infarct-related, 375
　for hypertension, 449–454, 449t, 452–453t, 464
　　in aortic dissection, 485
　　in diabetes, 449t, 454, 466, 1218
　　in urgencies/emergencies, 470t
　hypoglycemia caused by, 1257
　hypoglycemia symptoms affected by, 1236
　for Marfan syndrome, 1683
　for mitral valve prolapse, 340
　overdose/toxicity of, 449–454, 1578, 1590–1591
　for panic attacks, 1056
　perioperative, 46
　pheochromocytoma/pheochromocytoma surgery and, 454, 469, 1183
　for phobic disorders, 1056
　during pregnancy, 434–435, 816
　for PTSD, 1052
Beta-carotene
　in chemoprevention, 11
　excess intake of, 1277
Beta-catenin, hepatocellular adenoma and, 716
Beta-globin gene/chain, 504
　in sickle cell syndromes, 511, 512
　in thalassemia, 503, 504, 504t

Beta-glucan levels, in Pneumocystis pneumonia, 1336
Beta-glucocerebrosidase, in Gaucher disease, 1680
Beta-2-glycoprotein antibodies
　in antiphospholipid syndrome, 815–816, 841, 843
　in SLE, 841
Beta-hCG. See Human chorionic gonadotropin
Beta-hemolytic streptococci. See specific type under Group
Beta-hydroxybutyrate/hydroxybutyric acid
　in alcoholic ketoacidosis, 905
　in diabetes mellitus/diabetic ketoacidosis, 905, 1214, 1246, 1247
　in insulinoma, 1253, 1253t
3-Beta-hydroxysteroid dehydrogenase deficiency, amenorrhea in, 1199
11-Beta-hydroxysteroid dehydrogenase deficiency, hypertension and, 442
17-Beta-hydroxysteroid dehydrogenase-3 deficiency, 1196
Beta interferon. See Interferon-beta
Beta-lactam antibiotics
　for pneumonia, 269t, 271, 1316
　for spontaneous bacterial peritonitis, 603
Beta-2-microglobulin, in amyloidosis, 538
Beta-natriuretic peptide. See B-type natriuretic peptide
Beta-thalassemia syndromes, 504, 504t, 505
　sickle cell disease and, 512, 512t, 513
Betagan. See Levobunolol
Betaine, for homocystinuria, 1681
Betamethasone/betamethasone valerate, 97t
　for fetal lung maturity, 810, 811
　topical, 97t
Betaseron. See Interferon-beta
Betaxolol
　for glaucoma/ocular hypertension, 172t, 180
　for systemic hypertension, 452t
Bethesda assay, 558, 561
Bethesda criteria, for HNPCC/Lynch syndrome, 668
Bethesda System
　for Pap smear classification, 769t, 770
　for thyroid nodules, 1139
Betimol. See Timolol
Betoptic/Betoptic S. See Betaxolol
Bevacizumab, 1666t
　for age-related macular degeneration, 185
　for breast cancer, 751, 753
　for colorectal cancer, 1639, 1640
　for diabetic macular edema, 190
　for intracranial tumors, 1005
　for iris neovascularization/macular edema in retinal vein occlusion, 186
　for lung cancer, 1612
　for renal cell carcinoma, 1654

Bexarotene, TSH/thyroid disorders and, 1109, 1111, 1120
Bezafibrate, 1265
Bezold-Jarisch reflex, 356
Biaxin. See Clarithromycin
Bicalutamide, 1669t
　for prostate cancer, 1649t
Bicarbonate
　in acid-base disorders, 903, 904, 904t
　for acidosis
　　diabetic ketoacidosis, 1248
　　increased anion gap acidosis, 908
　　lactic acidosis, 1251–1252
　　normal anion gap/renal tubular acidosis, 906t, 908
　in alcoholic ketoacidosis, 905
　in chronic kidney disease, 929
　　alkalosis and, 909
　contrast media nephrotoxicity mediated by, 919
　in diabetic ketoacidosis, 1246, 1246t
　in fluid management, 911t
　gastrointestinal loss of, acidosis caused by, 906, 906t, 907
　　urinary anion gap and, 906t, 907
　for hyperkalemia, 894, 895t, 908
　lithium interactions and, 1087t
　in metabolic acidosis, 904, 904t, 907
　in metabolic alkalosis, 904t, 908, 910
　in normal anion gap/renal tubular acidosis, 906, 907
　in respiratory acidosis, 904t, 910
　in respiratory alkalosis, 904t, 911
　for salicylate poisoning, 908, 1603
　for shock, 497
　for tricyclic antidepressant overdose, 1578, 1579, 1606
　for urinary alkalinization, 1582
Bicarbonaturia
　in alcoholic ketoacidosis, 906
　in metabolic alkalosis, 909
　in normal anion gap/renal tubular acidosis, 907
Bicuspid aortic valve, 341
Bier block, for hydrofluoric acid burns, 1587
Bifascicular block, 400
Bifidobacterium infantis probiotic, for irritable bowel syndrome, 647
"Big gastrin," gastrinoma secreting, 1185
"Big IGF-2," nonislet cell tumor hypoglycemia and, 1255
Bigeminy, 396
Biguanides, 1221t
　overdose/toxicity of, 1595
Bile acid-binding resins, for lipid modification, 1264
Bile ducts. See also under Biliary
　carcinoma of. See Cholangiocarcinoma; Periampullary/ampullary carcinoma
　stenosis of, in HIV infection/AIDS, 1342
　stones in (choledocholithiasis), 717t, 720–722
　　pancreatitis and, 729
　　in pregnancy, 824
Bile salt binders, for diarrhea, 594

Bile salts, malabsorption of
  in Crohn disease, 655
  in short bowel syndrome, 637
BiLE score, in liver failure, 686
Bilharziasis, **1532–1533**. *See also*
      Schistosoma
Biliary cholangitis
  primary (primary biliary cirrhosis),
      700, **706–707**
  secondary, autoimmune hepatitis and,
      692
Biliary obstruction
  in choledocholithiasis/cholangitis,
      721
  jaundice caused by, 674, 674–676, 675t,
      676t, 677, 721
Biliary pancreatitis, 723, 725–726, 726,
      728, 729, 732
Biliary sludge (microlithiasis), 717
  pancreatitis and, 726, 728, 729
Biliary stricture, **723**
  pancreatitis and, 731, 732
Biliary tract disease, **716–725**, 717t. *See*
      also specific disease
  carcinoma, **1618–1620**
  cholecystitis, 717t, **718–720**
    in pregnancy, **823–824**
  choledocholithiasis/cholangitis, 717t,
      720–722
  cholelithiasis (gallstones), **716–718**,
      717t
    during pregnancy, **823–824**
  CMV infection and, 1375
  dyspepsia and, 579
  in fascioliasis, 1533
  in HIV infection/AIDS, 1342
  inflammation. *See* Cholangitis
  nausea and vomiting in, 581t, 582
  pancreatitis and, 723, 725–726, 726,
      728, 729, 732
  pre- and postcholecystectomy
      syndromes, **720**
  pregnancy and, **823**
  primary sclerosing cholangitis,
      723–725
  strictures, **723**
Bilirubin levels, 674, 676t. *See also*
      Hyperbilirubinemia
  ascitic fluid, 602
  in liver disease/jaundice, 674, 676t,
      694
  normal values for, 674, 676t
  urine, 676t
Bilirubinate, calcium, in gallstones, 717
Bilivist. *See* Ipodate sodium
Billowing mitral valve. *See* Mitral valve
      prolapse
Biloma, 723
Bimatoprost, 173t
Bimatoprost/timolol, 173t
Binge eating. *See* Bulimia nervosa
Binosto. *See* Alendronate
Biologic response modifiers, 1670–1671t.
      See also specific agent
  for renal cell carcinoma, 1654
Biologic therapies, for inflammatory
      bowel disease, 651–652
Biomarkers
  in breast cancer, 748–749. *See also*
      Hormone receptor sites
    prognosis and, 750–751, 751t, 758

treatment and, 748–749, 752, 753,
      754–756, 755t
  cardiac. *See* Cardiac biomarkers/
      enzymes
Bioprostheses, for cardiac valve
      replacement, 337, 350–351,
      352t. *See also* Valve
      replacement
Bioterrorism
  anthrax and, 1454, 1455
  botulinum toxin and, 1454
  chemical warfare agents and
      nerve agents, 1601–1602
    skin decontamination and, 1581
  Coxiella burnetii and, 1438
  plague and, 1474
  Q fever and, 1438
  Rickettsia prowazekii and, 1430
  smallpox/smallpox vaccination and,
      1423
  tularemia (*Francisella tularensis*) and,
      1473
Biotin, thyroid tests affected by, 1128
Bipolar disorder, 1075–1076. *See also*
      Depression; Mania
  drug therapy for, 1084–1087, 1087t
  lithium for, 1084, 1085–1087, 1087t
  pregnancy risks and, 1086
  prognosis for, 1087–1088
  schizophrenia and, 1067
  sleep-wake disorders and, 1088
  suicide risk and, 1076
Bipolaris, phaeohyphomycosis caused by,
      1558
Bird-fancier's lung ("pigeon-breeder's
      disease"), 308t
Bird mites. *See* Mites
Birds
  avian influenza and, 1417
  bird-fancier's lung/"pigeon-breeder's
      disease" and, 308t
  histoplasmosis and, 1549
  psittacosis (ornithosis) and, 1486
  West Nile encephalitis and, 1388–1389
Birt-Hogg-Dube syndrome, renal cell
      carcinoma and, 1654
Birth classes, 799
Birth control pills. *See* Oral
      contraceptives
Bisacodyl/bisacodyl suppository, 585t,
      586
BISAP score, in pancreatitis, 726
Bismuth compounds
  for diarrhea, 590, 1342
    traveler's diarrhea and, 590, 1310
    pregnancy and, 802
  in *H pylori* eradication therapy, 626,
      626–627, 626t
  for peptic ulcer disease, 625, 626t
  salicylate overdose/toxicity and,
      1602–1603
Bismuth poisoning, tubulointerstitial
      disease and, 947
Bisoprolol
  for heart failure, 407–408
  for hypertension, 452t
  with hydrochlorothiazide, 452t
Bisphosphonates. *See also specific agent*
  adverse ophthalmic effects of, 179t
  in breast cancer management,
      752–753, 754

hypercalcemia associated with use of,
      1156, 1162
  for hypercalcemia/
      hyperparathyroidism, 898,
      1157, 1660
  hypocalcemia associated with use of,
      1150, 1162
  metabolic bone disorders/renal
      osteodystrophy and, 927
  osteonecrosis of jaw and, 11, 875, 1162
  for osteoporosis, 11, 1161–1162, 1702
    in androgen deprivation, 1650
    chronic corticosteroid treatment
      and, 1161, 1209
  for Paget disease of bone, 1168
"Bite" cells, in G6PD deficiency, 511
Bites. *See* Animal bites; Human bite
      wounds; Insect bites
Bithionol, for fascioliasis, 1534
Bitolterol, for asthma, 252
Bitot spots, in vitamin A deficiency, 1277
Bitter almonds, odor of in cyanide
      poisoning, 1593
Bivalirudin
  for acute coronary syndromes/STEMI,
      367f, 368, 373
  for heparin-induced
      thrombocytopenia, 552–553,
      553t
Biventricular pacing (resynchronization).
      See also Pacemaker
  for cardiomyopathy, 417, 419
  for heart failure, 405f, 409–410
Black eye, 197
  in nasal trauma, 222
Black fever. *See* Visceral leishmaniasis
Black molds, 1558
Black patients
  hypertension management and,
      466–467, 466t
  Kaposi sarcoma in, 146, 1344
  sickle cell anemia/syndromes in, 511
Black plague, 1474
Black widow spider bite, 150, 1605
  myocarditis caused by, 413t
Bladder
  biopsy of, in bladder cancer, 1652
  cancer of, 1608t, 1624t, **1651–1653**
    thiazolidinedione use and, 1225
  disorders/dysfunction of. *See specific*
      type and Urinary
      incontinence
  infection of. *See* Cystitis
  neuropathic, 1035
    chemotherapy-induced, 1674
  painful (interstitial cystitis), 43,
      960–961
  paraganglioma of, 1180
Bladder catheterization
  intermittent, for urinary incontinence,
      67
  urinary tract infection and, 1293, 1294,
      1295
Bladder toxicity
  cyclophosphamide/ifosfamide causing,
      1674
    mesna for, 1671t, 1674
  neuropathies, chemotherapy-induced,
      1674
Bladder training, for urinary
      incontinence, 66

Blalock shunt (classic/modified), for
tetralogy of Fallot, 329
Blast cells, refractory anemia with
(RAEB), 525
Blastomycosis, **1556**
South American
(paracoccidioidomycosis),
1556–1557
Bleeding/blood loss. *See also specific
cause and* Coagulopathy;
Thrombocytopenia
anticoagulation therapy and, 300, 391,
391*t*, 393, 628
in chronic kidney disease, 928
in cirrhosis/liver disease, 562, 700, 704
coagulation disorders causing,
557–577, 559*t*, 561*t*
acquired, 561–563
congenital, 557–561, 559*t*, 561*t*
in DIC, 553, 554
in essential thrombocytosis, 521
evaluation of, 547*t*
fibrinolytic therapy for myocardial
infarction and, 374, 375
gastrointestinal. *See* Gastrointestinal
bleeding
iron deficiency and, 499, 500, 599, 600
in malabsorption, 633*t*
perioperative risk evaluation/
management and, 45, 46*t*, 51
platelet count ranges and, 544, 547*t*,
549
platelet disorders causing, **546–557**,
547*t*, 549*f*, 551*t*, 553*t*, 554*t*,
555*t*, 558*t*. *See also* Platelet
disorders
in polycythemia vera, 519
during pregnancy, 547*t*, **812–813**
third-trimester, **812–813**
premenopausal/postmenopausal. *See*
Uterine bleeding
rectal. *See* Rectal bleeding
retinal disorders and, **191**
shock caused by, 493, 494*t*, 495
vaginal. *See* Menstruation; Vaginal
bleeding
Bleeding history, directed, preoperative,
45, 46*t*, 51
Bleeding scans, in GI bleeding, 598–599
Blenoxane. *See* Bleomycin
Bleomycin, 1669*t*
for Kaposi sarcoma, 1338*t*
for testicular cancer, 1656–1657, 1657
toxicity of, 1669*t*
for wart removal, 142
Blepharitis, 110, **165**
Blepharospasm, 1016
Blinatumomab, 1666*t*
Blincyto. *See* Blinatumomab
Blind loop syndrome, vitamin B$_{12}$
deficiency in, 506
Blindness. *See also disorders causing and*
Visual impairment/loss
age-related macular degeneration
causing, 185
cataract causing, 182
cortical, 1005
diabetic eye disease and, 189, 190
"fleeting" (amaurosis fugax), 188–189,
477
in giant cell arteritis, 854, 855

glaucoma causing, 179, 180, 181
ocular trauma causing, 196
river (onchocerciasis), **1545–1546**
snow, 198
trachoma causing, 167
vitamin A deficiency and, 1277
Blister, burn, 1568
"Blister" cells, in G6PD deficiency, 511
Blistering (bullous) skin disorders, 96*t*,
139–140. *See also specific
type*
Blocadren. *See* Timolol
Blood. *See also* Bleeding/blood loss
contaminated, transfusion of, 543
disorders of, **499–545**. *See also*
Hematologic disorders
screening, 543–544
for hepatitis, 543, 681, 683–684
for HIV, 543, 1332, 1347
for HTLV, 543, 1396, 1397
for West Nile virus, 543
in stool. *See* Diarrhea, bloody;
Dysentery; Fecal occult
blood testing
transfusion of. *See* Transfusion
in urine. *See* Hematuria;
Hemoglobinuria
Blood alcohol level, in acute intoxication,
1093, 1584*t*, 1594
Blood dyscrasias. *See also* Bleeding
retinal disorders associated with, **191**
Blood flukes, schistosomiasis caused by,
1532–1533
Blood gases. *See* Arterial blood gases;
Venous blood gases
Blood glucose levels. *See* Glucose, blood
levels of
Blood glucose meters, 1216
Blood loss. *See* Bleeding
Blood pressure. *See also* Hypertension;
Hypotension
cardiovascular/heart disease and, 356,
360*f*, 362, 439, 440, 446, 447*f*,
448*t*
in hypertension, 439, 440*f*, 444
treatment goals and, 446–448
urgencies/emergencies, 439, 440*f*,
468
measurement of, **439–440**, 440*f*
orthostatic changes in. *See* Orthostatic
(postural) hypotension
in prehypertension, 440
in shock, 494
Blood pressure screening/hypertension
assessment/diagnosis, 6*t*, 10,
439–440, 440*f*, 444
Blood transfusion. *See* Transfusion
Blood (compatibility) typing, for
transfusions, 542
Blood urea nitrogen (BUN), 915, 915*t*
in diabetic ketoacidosis, 1246
Blood urea nitrogen:creatinine ratio, 915,
917*t*
Blood vessels. *See specific type and under*
Vascular
Blowout fracture, of orbital floor, 197
"Blue bloaters," 257, 258*t*
Blue nevi, **102–103**, 102*f*
Blumer shelf, 1630
Blurred vision. *See* Visual impairment/
loss

BMI (body mass index), 12–13, 1269. *See
also* Obesity/overweight
preventable disease/deaths and, 3*t*,
12–13
BMPR1A gene, in familial juvenile
polyposis, 667
BNP. *See* B-type natriuretic peptide
Bocavirus, 1421
Boceprevir, for hepatitis C, 689, 690*t*
BODE index, 262
Body cavity (primary effusion)
lymphoma, 1377
Body fat. *See also* Obesity/overweight
distribution of in obesity, 1269
diabetes and, 1212, 1214, 1235
Body fluid precautions (universal). *See*
Body substance isolation
Body lice, 149–150. *See also* Lice
Body mass index (BMI), 12–13, 1269.
See also Obesity/overweight
preventable disease/deaths and, 3*t*,
12–13
Body substance isolation/universal
precautions, 1295
HIV infection/AIDS prevention and,
1346–1347
Body temperature
in burn injury, maintaining, 1569
in drowning, 1567
elevated, **34–36**. *See also* Fever;
Hyperthermia
cholinergic urticaria caused by, 134
in hyperthermia/heat exposure
syndrome, 1562, 1563
in hypothermia, 1564
maintenance of, 1561
normal, 34
Body water, 884, 885*t*. *See also* Fluid
management/hydration
water deficit calculation and, 890
Body weight. *See* Weight
Boerhaave syndrome, 582
Boils (furunculosis), **152–154**, 1315*t*,
1443*t*, 1448
in HIV infection/AIDS, 1343
Bone
adynamic disease of, 927
avascular necrosis of (osteonecrosis),
875–876
corticosteroid use and, 875, 1209
in HIV infection/AIDS, 1340
of jaw, bisphosphonate use and, 11,
875, 1162
defective mineralization of, in
osteomalacia, 1164, 1164*t*
in diabetes, 1242
in HIV infection/AIDS, 1340
in hypercalcemia/hyperparathyroidism,
898, 1153, 1155
infections of, **870–871**. *See also*
Osteomyelitis
in malabsorption, 633*t*
metabolic disease of, **1159–1168**. *See
also specific disorder*
in chronic kidney disease (renal
osteodystrophy), 927–928,
927*f*, 1153, 1155
myeloma involving, 535, 536
Paget disease of, **1166–1168**
pheochromocytoma/paraganglioma
involving, 1184

in syphilis, 1494
tuberculosis of, 283, **871–872**
Bone alkaline phosphatase, in
    hypophosphatasia, 1165
Bone density/bone density
    measurements/bone
    densitometry, 1160
in diabetes, 1242
in hyperparathyroidism, 1153, 1154,
    1155
in osteoporosis/osteoporosis
    prevention, 11, 795, 1160,
    1702
Bone marrow
depression/failure of
    antipsychotic drug use and, 1072
    in aplastic anemia, 516
    in cancer chemotherapy, **1662–1672**
        infections and, 1661
    methotrexate causing, 837, 1674
    in myelodysplastic syndromes, 525,
        526
    in neutropenia, 518, 518t, 1662
    in primary myelofibrosis, 519t, 522,
        522–523, 523
    thrombocytopenia caused by,
        546–548
infiltration of, thrombocytopenia
    caused by, **548**
Bone marrow/stem cell transplantation,
    540–541. *See also specific
    disorder*
adenovirus infection and, 1420
allogeneic, **540–541**
aspergillosis after, 1554–1555
autologous, **540**
for cancer, 540–541
chemotherapy and, 540, 541
CMV infection and, 1292, 1374, 1376
immunizations and, 1319
infection and, 1290
Bone-modifying agents, for
    chemotherapy-induced
    toxicity, 1671t
Bone morphogenic receptor protein 1A
    (BMPR1A) gene, in familial
    juvenile polyposis, 667
Bone scanning
for breast cancer metastases, 742
for prostate cancer metastases,
    1645–1646
Boniva. *See* Ibandronate
BOOP (bronchiolitis obliterans with
    organizing pneumonia). *See*
    Cryptogenic organizing
    pneumonia/pneumonitis
BOOSTRIX. *See* Tdap vaccine
Borderline personality disorder, 1064,
    1065, 1065t, 1066
Bordetella infection
bronchiseptica, 1464
pertussis (whooping cough), 19, 21,
    1463–1464
    prevention/immunization and, 4,
        1464. *See also* Pertussis
        vaccine
Boredom, in schizophrenia/psychotic
    disorders, 1067
Bornavirus-1, 1391
Bornholm disease (epidemic
    pleurodynia), 1426

Borrelia (borreliosis)
afzelii, 1501, 1503
burgdorferi, 1312t, 1501. *See also* Lyme
    disease
    senu strictu, 1501
garinii, 1501, 1503
miyamotoi, 1436
recurrentis, 1312t
relapsing fever caused by, 1312t, 1499
Borrelial lymphocytoma, 1502
Bortezomib, 1665t
for myeloma, 536
neuropathy caused by, 1674
Bosentan, for scleroderma, 847
Bosulif. *See* Bosutinib
Bosutinib, 1667t
for chronic myeloid leukemia, 525
Botox. *See* Botulinum toxin therapy
Botulinum toxin, 1046–1047, 1454
Botulinum toxin therapy
for achalasia, 617–618
for focal torsion dystonias, 1016
for migraine prophylaxis, 979, 979t
for Tourette syndrome, 1018
for urinary incontinence, 66
Botulism, **1046–1047,** 1306t,
    1453–1454
Botulism antitoxin, 1047, 1454
Bouchard nodes, 827, 828f
Bougie dilators. *See* Esophageal dilation
Boutonneuse fever, 1429t, 1434
Boutonnière deformity, 838
Bouveret syndrome, 717
Bovine spongiform encephalopathy
    (vCJD/mad cow disease),
    1394
Bowen disease, **118**
periungual/subungual, 160
BPH. *See* Benign prostatic hyperplasia
BPPV. *See* Benign paroxysmal positioning
    vertigo
Brachial plexus
lesions/neuropathy of, **1042–1043**
in thoracic outlet syndrome, 873, 1696
Brachytherapy. *See* Radiation therapy
Braden Scale, for pressure ulcers, 68
Bradycardia/bradyarrhythmias, **384,**
    399–402
in myocardial infarction, 370, 377
palpitations and, 31
persistent (sick sinus syndrome), **399**
in poisoning/drug overdose
    beta-adrenergic blockers and, 1591
    calcium channel blockers and, 1591
sinus. *See* Sinus bradycardia
BRAF/B-raf gene/mutations
colorectal cancer/HNPCC/Lynch
    syndrome and, 665, 668,
    1637
in thyroid cancer, 1139
Brain
vasculitis of (primary angiitis of central
    nervous system), **862–863**
Zika virus affecting development of,
    1406, 1407
Brain abscess, **1007–1008,** 1298, 1299,
    1314t
anaerobes causing, 1314t, 1478–1479
bacterial rhinosinusitis and, 217
in nocardiosis, 1481
otitis media and, 206

Brain cancer, 1624t. *See also* Intracranial
    masses/tumors
Brain death, **1028**
organ donation and, 93–94
Brain edema. *See* Cerebral edema
Brain imaging. *See* Neuroimaging
Brain natriuretic peptide. *See* B-type
    natriuretic peptide
Brain stimulation
for depression, 1084
for OCD, 1057
for parkinsonism, 1014
for seizures, 989
Brain tumors, **1003–1006,** 1004t, 1624t.
    See also Intracranial masses/
    tumors
Brainstem
arteriovenous malformations in, 1001
herniation of, lumbar puncture and,
    1299
ischemia of, seizures differentiated
    from, 986
lesions/tumors/infarction of, 1004t,
    1005
    coma or stupor caused by, 1027,
        1028
    gliomas, 1004t, 1005
    vertigo caused by, 213
Bran, dietary (bran powder), 585t, 1280.
    See also Fiber, dietary
Branch retinal artery occlusion,
    187–188
Branch retinal vein occlusion,
    186–187
Branchial cleft cysts, **238**
Brazilian spotted fever, 1433
BRCA1/BRCA2 genes
breast cancer and, 738, 738t, 739
    in male, 760
ovarian cancer and, 779
pancreatic/periampullary carcinoma
    and, 1620
Breast, **734–761**
abscess of, **736–737,** 737f
    nipple discharge caused by, 736
    puerperal mastitis and, 736, 814
augmented, 737. *See also* Breast
    implants
benign disorders of, **734–737**
biopsy of
    in breast mass evaluation, 740,
        742–744, 743f, 744f
    in fat necrosis, 736
    in fibroadenoma, 735
    in fibrocystic condition, 734
    mammographic localization, 744
    stereotactic, 744
    ultrasound-guided, 744
cancer of. *See* Breast cancer
density of, cancer risk and, 738
examination of
    in cancer follow-up, 758
    in cancer screening/early detection/
        mass evaluation, 14t, 739,
        740
fat necrosis of, **736**
fibroadenoma of, **735**
fibrocystic condition and, **734–735**
    breast cancer risk and, 734,
        735, 738
    nipple discharge in, 734, 736, 736t

Breast (*Cont.*):
male
carcinoma of, **760–761**
disorders/enlargement of, **1194–1196**, 1195t. *See also* Gynecomastia
mass/lump in. *See* Breast cancer; Lump (breast)
nipple discharge and, **735–736**, 736t
phyllodes tumor of, 735
reconstruction of after mastectomy, 737, 750, 759
local recurrence and, 737, 759
self-examination of, breast lump identification/cancer screening and, 14t, 740
Breast cancer, **737–761**, 1608t, 1623t
anatomic locations of, 741, 741f
antipsychotic drug use and, 1072
arm edema and, 742, 759
bilateral, 748
biomarkers/gene expression profiling and, 748–749
prognosis and, 750–751, 751t, 758
treatment and, 748–749, 752, 753, 754–756, 755t
biopsy in diagnosis of, 740, 742–744, 743f, 744f
breast reconstruction/implants and, 737, 759
clinical examination in detection/evaluation and, 739, 740, 741–742, 741f, 742f
follow-up care and, 758
cytologic evaluation of, 743–744, 744, 745
differential diagnosis of, 745
ductal
in situ, 748, 748t
invasive/infiltrating, 748t
early detection/screening for, 14–15, 14t, 739–745
clinical findings and, 741–745, 741f, 742f, 743f, 744f
genetic testing and, 738
pregnancy and, 745
estrogen replacement therapy and, 738, 758, 796, 1202, 1203
fibrocystic condition and, 734, 735, 738
genetic mutations associated with, 738, 738t, 739. *See also* BRCA1/ BRCA2 genes
gestational, 745–747
HER2 overexpression/*HER2* gene in, 748–749, 752, 753
in male, 760
prognosis and, 750, 751, 751t, 758
therapy and, 748–749, 751, 752, 753, 756
hypercalcemia and, 742, 1659
incidence/risk/mortality of, 737–739, 738t, 1608t
in male, 760
inflammatory, 745
in situ, 748, 748t
lactation and, 745–747
lobular
in situ, 748, 748t
invasive, 748t
in male, **760–761**, 1194–1195

mammography in detection/evaluation of, 14–15, 14t, 739–740, 740–741, 742, 743f, 744f
biopsy and, 744
breast implants and, 737
pregnancy and, 745
metastatic
evaluation of, 742
pregnancy and, 760
prognosis and, 751, 751t
treatment of, 749, 754–757, 755t
MRI in detection/evaluation of, 15, 740, 742, 745
nipple discharge in, 736, 736t
noninvasive, 748, 748t
oral contraceptive use and, 738, 786
Paget, 118, 118f, 745
pain/mastalgia and, 741, 745
pancreatic/periampullary carcinoma and, 1620
pathologic types of, 745, 748t
pregnancy affecting risk of, 758, 759–760
pregnancy and, 745–747, 758, 759–760
prevention of, 739
chemoprevention and, 11
genetic/family risk factors and, 738
prognosis for, 751t, 758, 758t
adjuvant systemic therapy and, 750–751, 751t
biomarkers and, 750–751, 751t
in male, 760–761
recurrence of, 750–751, 751t, 758–759. *See also* Breast cancer, prognosis for
breast reconstruction/implants and, 737, 759
self-examination in detection/ evaluation of, 14t, 740
staging of, 745, 746–747t
prognosis and, 750, 751t, 758, 758t
treatment choice and, 749
survivorship issues and, 759–760
treatment of, 1623t
adjuvant systemic, 749, 750–753, 751t, 1623t
in older women, 753
biomarkers/hormone receptor status and, 748–749, 752, 753, 754–756, 755t
bisphosphonates in, 752–753, 754
breast-conserving, 749–750, 750f
chemotherapy in, 749, 751–752, 756–757, 1623t
adjuvant/neoadjuvant, 749, 750–751, 751–752, 753, 1623t
palliative, 756–757
pregnancy and, 747
prognosis and, 751
choice/timing of primary therapy and, 749
curative, 749–754, 750f, 751t
endocrine therapy in, 752, 754–756, 755t. *See also* Hormone therapy, for breast cancer
follow-up, 758–760
in male, 760
mastectomy in, 749, 750
neoadjuvant, 749, 752, 753–754

palliative, 749, 754–757, 755t
during pregnancy/lactation, 747, 760
radiation therapy in, 750, 754
surgical resection, 749, 749–750, 750f. *See also* Lumpectomy; Mastectomy
targeted therapy in, 752, 754–756, 755t
"triple-negative," 749, 753, 756
ultrasonography in detection/ evaluation of, 740, 742, 744
Breast-conserving therapy, 749–750, 750f
local recurrence and, 737, 759
during pregnancy, 747
with radiation, 750
Breast implants, **737**
breast cancer in patient with, 737
for breast reconstruction, 737, 759
disorders associated with, **737**
Breast milk. *See* Lactation
Breast pain (mastalgia), 734, 735, 741, 745
Breast surgery, 749, 749–750, 750f. *See also* Lumpectomy; Mastectomy
for gynecomastia, 1195
reconstruction/implants after, 737, 750, 759
Breastfeeding. *See* Lactation
Breath tests
in bacterial overgrowth, 594, 636
for carbohydrate/lactose intolerance, 591, 638
in *H pylori* infection, 579, 622, 625
Breathing. *See also under* Respiratory
abnormalities of in coma or stupor, 1027–1028, 1028
assessment/support of
in burn injury, 1568–1569
in coma, 1027–1028, 1578
sleep-related disorders of, 230–231, **316**, 1089. *See also* Sleep apnea hypopnea
Breathing exercises, for COPD, 261
Brentuximab vedotin, 1666t
for Hodgkin lymphoma, 534
for non-Hodgkin lymphoma, 533
Brevibloc. *See* Esmolol
Bridging anticoagulation, 51, 51t, 351, 352t
Brief psychotic disorders, 1067
Brill-Zinsser disease, 1430
Brimonidine
for glaucoma/ocular hypertension, 172t, 180
overdose/toxicity of, 1592
for rosacea, 129
Brimonidine/brinzolamide, 173t
Brimonidine/timolol, 173t
Brincidofovir
for CMV prophylaxis, 1376
for Ebola viral disease, 1398
Brintellix. *See* Vortioxetine
Brinzolamide, 173t
Brinzolamide/brimonidine, 173t
Brinzolamide/timolol, 173t
British anti-Lewisite (BAL). *See* Dimercaprol
Brodalumab, for psoriasis, 108
Brodifacoum poisoning, 1588

"Broken heart syndrome," 418. *See also* Tako-Tsubo (stress/catecholamine-induced) cardiomyopathy
Bromfenac, for ophthalmic disorders, 168, 171*t*
Bromocriptine. *See also* Dopamine agonists
for cocaine withdrawal, 1100
for diabetes, 1222*t*, 1228
for hyperprolactinemia, 1118
for neuroleptic malignant syndrome, 36, 1072, 1580, 1590
for ovulation induction, 784
Brompheniramine, for allergic rhinitis, 219
Bronchi, foreign body in, **238**
Bronchial carcinoid tumors (bronchial adenomas), **288**, 1185, 1186
Bronchial gland carcinoma, 288
Bronchial obstruction, 241–242
Bronchial provocation testing, in asthma, 246
Bronchiectasis, **263–264**
COPD differentiated from, 259
cystic fibrosis and, 263, 265
in measles, 1379
Bronchiolitis, **266–267**
acute, 266
adenovirus causing, 266, 1421
constrictive (obliterative/bronchiolitis obliterans), 266, 267
with organizing pneumonia (BOOP/cryptogenic organizing pneumonia/pneumonitis/COP), 267, 291*t*, 292
diffuse panbronchiolitis, 267
follicular, 267
in measles, 1379
proliferative, 266, 267
respiratory, 267
interstitial lung disease associated with (RB-ILD), 291*t*, 292
RSV, 266, 1409–1410, 1410
Bronchioloalveolar cell carcinoma (adenocarcinoma in situ), 1609. *See also* Lung cancer
Bronchitis
chlamydial, 1487
chronic, 257, 258, 258–259, 258*t*, 261. *See also* Chronic obstructive pulmonary disease
industrial, 308
Bronchoconstriction. *See also* Asthma; Bronchospasm
exercise-induced, 242, 243*f*, 244*t*, 247*f*
Bronchodilators
adverse ophthalmic effects of, 177*t*
for asthma
assessment and, 245, 254–255, 255*f*
exacerbation management and, 252, 253*t*, 254–255, 255*f*
long-acting, 247*f*, 248–251
short-acting, 244*t*, 247*f*, 248, 252, 254, 255*f*, 256*f*
for COPD, 260
for cystic fibrosis, 266
Bronchogenic carcinoma, **1608–1613**, 1608*t*, 1610*t*, 1612*t*. *See also* Lung cancer

Bronchoprovocation testing. *See* Bronchial provocation testing
Bronchopulmonary mycosis/aspergillosis, allergic, **264**, 879*t*, 1554, 1555
Bronchoscopy
in interstitial (diffuse parenchymal) lung disease, 290
in lung cancer, 1609
Bronchospasm/bronchoconstriction. *See also* Asthma
exercise-induced, 242, 243*f*, 244*t*, 247*f*
in pulmonary edema, 412
transfusion causing, 543
Brown recluse spider bites, 150, 1605
Brown-Séquard syndrome, 1032
Brown tumors of bone, in hyperparathyroidism, 1153
Bruce protocol, for exercise testing, 363
Brucella abortus/melitensis/suis (brucellosis), 1311*t*, **1472–1473**
endocarditis caused by, 1462
Brudzinski sign, 1464
Brugada syndrome, 30, 31
sudden death of athlete and, 437, 438*t*
Brugia malayi/timori, 1543
Bruxism, earache and, 207
BSE. *See* Bovine spongiform encephalopathy; Breast, self-examination of
BSS. *See* Bernard-Soulier syndrome
Buboes
in lymphogranuloma venereum, 671, 1485
in plague, 1474
Budd-Chiari syndrome (hepatic vein obstruction), **711–712**
Budesonide
for allergic rhinitis, 219
for asthma, 250*t*
with formoterol, 249*t*
for autoimmune hepatitis, 692
for inflammatory bowel disease, 650
Crohn disease, 655
microscopic colitis, 662
ulcerative colitis, 659
Buerger disease (thromboangiitis obliterans), **480**
Raynaud disease/phenomenon and, 844
Bufotenin, toxicity of, 1594
Bulbar palsy, progressive, 1033
Bulbar poliomyelitis, 1382, 1383
Bulbospinal poliomyelitis, 1382
Bulimia nervosa, 581, **1274**
with anorexia nervosa, 1274
Bullectomy, for emphysema, 262
Bullous impetigo, 123–124, 124*f*, 1343
Bullous pemphigoid, **140**
Bullous (blistering) skin disorders, 96*t*, **139–140**. *See also specific type*
Bumetanide
for heart failure, 406, 412
infarct-related, 378
for hypertension, 450*t*
in urgencies/emergencies, 471
for pulmonary edema, 412
BUN. *See* Blood urea nitrogen

Bundibugyo virus, 1397
Bundle branch block, 399, 400
in myocardial infarction, 371, 377
ventricular tachycardia and, 397
Bunyaviruses, encephalitis caused by, 1388
Buprenorphine, 77*t*, 82
for heroin/opioid addiction/withdrawal, 17, 1099
overdose/toxicity of, 1601
Bupropion, 1077, 1078*t*, 1079–1081
for antidepressant drug augmentation, 1079
for anxiety, 1055
for drug-induced erectile dysfunction, 1079
with naltrexone, for obesity, 1271
in type 2 diabetes, 1235
overdose/toxicity of, 1078*t*, 1606
for smoking cessation, 7
during pregnancy, 799
Burin variant MEN 1, 1188
Burkholderia
mallei (glanders), 1312*t*
pseudomallei (melioidosis), 1312*t*
Burkitt lymphoma, 531, 532, 533
Epstein-Barr virus in, 1373
Burkitt-type ALL, 528
Burn dressings, 1569
Burn unit, 1568
Stevens Johnson syndrome/toxic epidermal necrolysis treatment and, 136
Burning mouth syndrome, **226**
Burns, **1568–1569**, 1568*f*
abdominal compartment syndrome and, 1569
chemical. *See* Chemical injury
depth of, 1568
electric, 1569
extent of, 1568, 1568*f*
flame (clothing), 1570
flash (arcing), 1570
infection and, 1569
injuries/illnesses associated with, 1568
patient assessment and, 1568
smoke inhalation and, 305, 1568
survival after, 1568
systemic reactions to, 1568
treatment of, 1568–1569
chemoprophylaxis in, 1569
patient support and, 1569
surgical management in, 1569
Bursa/bursitis, **1700–1701**, 1700*f*. *See also specific type or joint affected*
in diabetes, 1242
of knee, 1700–1701, 1704
Buruli ulcer, 1482
"Bush teas," sinusoidal obstruction syndrome caused by, 711
Buspar. *See* Buspirone
Buspirone, 1054*t*
antidepressant drug augmentation and, 1055, 1082
for anxiety, 1054*t*, 1055
for OCD, 1057
Busulfan, 1663*t*
Butane, toxicity of, 1598
Butanediol, overdose/toxicity of, 1595
Butenafine, 99*t*
for tinea corporis, 112

Butoconazole, for vulvovaginal candidiasis, 767
Butterbur, for migraine prophylaxis, 979t
Butterfly rash, in SLE, 839t, 840
Button batteries, ingested, alkali injuries caused by, 1587
Butyrolactone, gamma, overdose/toxicity of, 1595
Butyrophenones, 1068. See also Antipsychotic drugs; Haloperidol
overdose/toxicity of, 1589
Bydureon. See Exenatide
Byetta/Byetta LAR. See Exenatide
Bypass grafting
    for abdominal aortic aneurysm, 482
    for aortic dissection, 485–486
    for aortoiliac occlusive disease, 473
    coronary artery. See Coronary artery bypass grafting
    for erectile dysfunction, 968
    for femoral/popliteal occlusive disease, 474
    for intestinal ischemia, 479
    for tibial/pedal occlusive disease, 475
Bypass surgery, for obesity. See Bariatric surgery
Bypass tracts (accessory AV pathways), supraventricular tachycardia and, 385, 387–388
Byssinosis, 308–309
Bystolic. See Nebivolol

C3 glomerulonephropathies, 939–940
C5A, in familial Mediterranean fever, 604
C282Y mutation, in hemochromatosis, 708, 709
    cancer and, 708, 1616
C$_{cr}$. See Creatinine clearance
c-myc gene, in Burkitt lymphoma, 531
C-peptide
    in factitious hypoglycemia, 1257
    insulinoma secreting, 1253, 1253t
C-reactive protein, coronary heart disease risk and, 1261–1262
C-urea breath testing. See Urea breath testing
Ca. See Calcium
CA 15-3, in breast cancer, 742
CA 19-9
    in cholangiocarcinoma, 724, 1619
    in pancreatic/periampullary carcinoma, 1620
CA 27-29, in breast cancer, 742
CA 125, in ovarian tumors, 779, 779–780
CA-MRSA. See Community-associated methicillin-resistant S aureus
Cabazitaxel, 1664t
    for prostate cancer, 1650
Cabergoline
    adverse ophthalmic effects of, 178t
    for Cushing disease, 1176
    for GH-secreting tumors (acromegaly/ gigantism), 1116
    for hyperprolactinemia/prolactinoma, 1118, 1188
    for ovulation induction, 784
CABG. See Coronary artery bypass grafting
Cabozantinib, for thyroid cancer, 1145
Cachectin. See Tumor necrosis factor

Cachexia
    diabetic neuropathic, 1240
    in protein-energy malnutrition, 1268
    in terminally ill/dying patient, 91
CACNA1A gene, in familial hemiplegic migraine, 977
CACNA1S gene, in periodic paralysis, 1049
CACNL1A3 gene, in periodic paralysis, 1049
CAD (coronary artery disease). See Coronary heart disease
Cadherin cell adhesion protein, gastric cancer and, 1629
CADM 140 antibody, in polymyositis/ dermatomyositis, 848t
Cadmium, tubulointerstitial disease caused by, 947
Caduet. See Atorvastatin, with amlodipine
Café au lait spots, 1010
"Café coronary," 306
Cafergot, for migraine headache, 978
Caffeine, 1100–1101
    for migraine headache, 978
    overdose/toxicity of, 1100–1101, 1605–1606
    during pregnancy, 799
Caffeinism, 1101
cagA gene, in H pylori gastritis, 621
Cajal, interstitial cells of, gastrointestinal stromal tumors and, 1633
Calabar swellings, 1546
Calan. See Verapamil
Calcaneofibular ligament, ankle sprains and, 1715
Calcifediol, for vitamin D deficiency/ osteomalacia, 1166
Calciferol. See Ergocalciferol
Calcific (degenerative) aortic stenosis, 341
Calcimar. See Calcitonin
Calcimimetic agents. See Cinacalcet
Calcinosis, in hypercalcemia/ hyperparathyroidism, 1153
Calciphylaxis, in hypercalcemia/ hyperparathyroidism, 1153
Calcipotriene, for psoriasis, 108
Calcitonin (serum), in thyroid cancer, 1142, 1145
Calcitonin/nasal calcitonin-salmon
    for hypercalcemia, 898, 1660
    for osteoporosis, 1163
Calcitriol (1,25-dihydroxycholecalciferol)
    for hyperparathyroidism, 927, 1157
    for hypocalcemia/hypoparathyroidism/ tetany, 1151, 1151t
    for hypophosphatemic osteomalacia, 1166
    for metabolic bone disorders/renal osteodystrophy, 927
    after parathyroidectomy, 1158
Calcitriol ointment, for psoriasis, 108
Calcium
    albumin levels and, 896
    dietary/supplementary, 1280
        for calcium channel blocker overdose, 1578, 1591
        deficiency of in osteomalacia/rickets, 1164, 1164t

for hydrofluoric acid burns, 1586, 1587
        hypercalcemia caused by, 897, 1156
        hypercalciuria and, 963
        for hyperkalemia, 894, 895t
        for hypermagnesemia, 902, 903
        for hyperoxaluric calcium nephrolithiasis, 964
        for hyperphosphatemia, 901, 927
        for hypocalcemia/ hypoparathyroidism/tetany, 897, 1151
        for metabolic bone disorders/renal osteodystrophy, 927
        milk-alkali syndrome and, 897, 898
        for osteomalacia, 1166
        for osteoporosis prevention/ management, 11, 795, 1161, 1280, 1702
        after parathyroidectomy, 1158
        during pregnancy/lactation, 801
        requirements for in nutritional support, 1282
        urinary stone formation and, 963, 964, 1161
    disorders of concentration/metabolism of, 892t, 896–899, 896t, 898t. See also Hypercalcemia; Hypocalcemia
    in chronic kidney disease/renal osteodystrophy, 896, 927, 927f, 1153
    genetic disorders associated with, 892t
    magnesium balance and, 896, 897, 901
    normal values for, 896
    parathyroid hormone affecting, 896, 1149, 1152–1153, 1154, 1154f
    phosphorus/phosphate metabolism and, 896, 897, 899
    urinary excretion of. See Hypercalciuria
    in urinary stones, 961, 962, 963–964. See also Calcium nephrolithiasis; Hypercalciuria
Calcium acetate. See Calcium, dietary/ supplementary
Calcium bilirubinate, in gallstones, 717
Calcium carbonate. See Calcium, dietary/ supplementary
Calcium channel alpha2-delta ligands, for neuropathic pain, 83t, 84
Calcium channel blocking drugs, 383t, 460–461t
    for acute coronary syndromes/STEMI, 368, 376
        hypertension and, 449t
        postinfarction, 361, 380
    for angina, 360f, 361
    for arrhythmias, 381, 383t
        atrial fibrillation, 389, 390
        supraventricular tachycardia, 383t, 386
    for cardiomyopathy, 416, 419
    for hypertension, 449t, 459, 460–461t, 464, 465
        in combination regimen, 464–465, 465f
        in diabetes, 449t, 465, 466, 946, 1218
        in urgencies/emergencies, 470t

lower extremity edema caused by, 32–33
overdose/toxicity of, 459, 460–461t, 1578, **1591**
pheochromocytoma/ pheochromocytoma surgery and, 1183
pruritus caused by, 147
for pulmonary hypertension, 303, 431, 432f
for Raynaud phenomenon, 845
Calcium chloride. See Calcium, dietary/ supplementary
Calcium citrate. See Calcium, dietary/ supplementary
Calcium disodium edetate (EDTA), for lead poisoning, 1597
Calcium gluconate. See also Calcium, dietary/supplementary
for black widow spider bites, 1605
for calcium channel blocker overdose, 1591
for hydrofluoric acid burns, 1586, 1587
for hypocalcemia/hypoparathyroidism/ tetany, 897
Calcium nephrolithiasis, 962t, 963–964
calcium supplementation and, 963, 964, 1161
hypercalcemia/hypercalciuria/ hyperparathyroidism and, 897, 962t, 963–964, 1153, 1155, 1157
hyperoxaluria and, 963, 964
hyperuricosuria and, 964
hypocitraturia and, 963, 964
in polycystic kidney disease, 949, 950
Calcium polycarbophil, 585t. See also Fiber, dietary
Calcium pyrophosphate crystals, 826. See also Calcium pyrophosphate deposition disease
in pseudogout, 826, 831, 834
Calcium pyrophosphate deposition disease (CPPD), **834**
pseudogout, 826, 831, 834
pseudorheumatoid arthritis, 834, 836
Calcium-sensing receptor, 896
mutations in gene for, 892t, 896
in hypercalcemia, 892t, 896, 1156
in hypocalcemia/ hypoparathyroidism, 892t, 896, 1150
Calculus formation. See specific type or structure affected
Caliciviruses, gastroenteritis caused by, 1307t
California encephalitis, 1388, 1389
California flea rickettsiosis, 1429t
Calorie requirements, in nutritional support, 1282
Calorie restriction, in obesity management, 1270, 1271
CALR mutation. See Calreticulin gene (CALR) mutation
Calreticulin gene (CALR) mutation
in essential thrombocytosis, 521
in hepatic vein obstruction (Budd-Chiari syndrome), 711

in noncirrhotic portal hypertension, 714
in primary myelofibrosis, 523
Calymmatobacterium (Donovania) granulomatis, 1477
CAM. See Confusion assessment method
Camels, MERS-CoV transmission and, 1419, 1420
Cameron lesions, 628
Campath. See Alemtuzumab
Camphor/menthol preparations, 95, 99t
Camptosar. See Irinotecan/irinotecan liposome
Campylobacter, 1311t, **1472**
diarrhea/gastroenteritis caused by, 588t, 589, 1305, 1307t, 1315t, 1342, 1472
Guillain-Barré syndrome and, 1038
fetus subsp fetus, 1472
jejuni, 588t, 1307t, 1311t, 1472
Campylobacter-like organisms, 1472
Canagliflozin, 1222t, 1227, 1228
with metformin, 1228
Canakinumab
for gout, 832
for Still disease, 839
Canasa. See Mesalamine
Canavan disease, prenatal testing for, 800
Cancer, **1607–1675**. See also specific type and under Malignant
cognitive disorders/delirium and, 1102t
complications of, **1657–1661**
neurologic, **1008–1009**
DIC in, 553, 1008
early detection/screening tests for, 13–15, 14t. See also Cancer, prevention of
effusions associated with, 312, 312–313, 313t, 425, 426, 426–427, 428, **1658–1659**
emergencies associated with, **1657–1661**
Epstein-Barr virus infection and, 223, 1373
etiology of, 1607
exfoliative dermatitis/erythroderma and, 117
fever/FUO and, 1287, 1288, 1661
HIV infection/AIDS and, 1330, 1331t, 1332, 1337–1338t, 1344
hypercalcemia associated with, 897, 898, 1155–1156, **1659–1660**. See also Hypercalcemia
hyperuricemia associated with, 920, **1660**
incidence/risk/mortality of, 2t, 1607, 1607–1608, 1608t
obesity and, 12, 13, 1607
infectious complications of, **1661**
neuropathies associated with, **1037–1038**
nonmetastatic neurologic complications of, **1008–1009**
pericarditis/effusion associated with, 425, 426, 426–427, 428, 1658, 1659
periungual/subungual lesions, 160
pleural effusions in (malignant pleural effusions), 312, 312–313, 313t, 1658, 1659

polymyositis/dermatomyositis and, 847, 848, 848–849, 875
prevention of, **13–16**, 14t
chemoprevention and, 11
prognosis for, **1675**
radiation exposure and, 1571, 1572, 1607
rheumatologic manifestations of, **875**
SIADH and, 887, 887t
smoking/smoking cessation and, 7, 13, 1607
spinal cord compression and, 1007, **1657–1658**
staging of, 1608
stem cell transplants for, 540–541
treatment of, 1622–1625t, **1661–1675**, 1663–1670t, 1671–1672t, 1672t. See also Chemotherapy; Radiation therapy
tumor lysis syndrome and, 920, **1660**
Candesartan
for heart failure, 407
for hypertension, 457t
with hydrochlorothiazide, 457t
for migraine prophylaxis, 979t
Candida (candidiasis), **1547–1548**
albicans, 1547, 1548
chemoprophylaxis of, 1548
chorioretinitis caused by, 192
in diabetes, 1242
endocarditis in, 1547–1548, 1548
esophageal, 611, 1547, 1548
in HIV infection/AIDS, 611, 1335, 1338t, 1341
glabrata, 1548, 1558
hepatosplenic, 1547
in immunocompromised host/HIV infection/AIDS, 132, 192, 611, 1292, 1335, 1343
invasive, 1547, 1548
krusei, 1548
mucocutaneous/mucosal, **132–133**, 132f, 1547, 1548
nail infection and, 132f, 133, 159
non-albicans, 1548
oral (thrush), **225–226**, 225f
esophagitis and, 611, 1547
in HIV infection/AIDS, 226, 1335, 1341
parapsilosis, 1548
resistant strains of, 1548, 1558
tinea cruris differentiated from, 113
in urine, 1547, 1548
vulvovaginal, 133, 766, 766f, 767, 1302, 1547, 1548
in diabetes, 1214, 1242
in HIV infection/AIDS, 1338t, 1344
sexual violence (rape/sexual assault) and, 1302
Candida antigen, for wart removal, 142
Candidal funguria (candiduria), 1547, 1548
Candidatus R rioja, 1429t, 1434
Candidemia, 132, 1547, 1548
Candiduria, 1547, 1548
Canker sore (aphthous ulcer), **226–227**, 227f
in Behçet syndrome, 861, 862
in HIV infection/AIDS, 1341

Cannabidiol
  for nausea and vomiting, 583
  for neuropathic pain, 84
Cannabinoids
  for nausea and vomiting, 583. See also
        Dronabinol
  synthetic, toxicity/amphetamine-like
        reactions and, 1587, 1598
Cannabis sativa, 1099–1100. See also
        Marijuana
Cannon A waves, palpitations and, 30
CAP. See Community-acquired
        pneumonia
Capecitabine, 1664t
  for breast cancer, 753, 756, 757
  for colorectal cancer, 1639, 1640
  diarrhea caused by, 1673
  for pancreatic/periampullary
        carcinoma, 1625
Capillaria philippinensis (capillariasis),
        588t, 592
Capillary angiomas, in Sturge-Weber
        syndrome, 1010
Caplan syndrome, 307
Capoten. See Captopril
Capozide. See Captopril, for
        hypertension, with
        hydrochlorothiazide
CAPRA nomogram, for prostate cancer
        assessment, 1650, 1650t
Caprelsa. See Vandetanib
Capsaicin, 95, 99t
  for osteoarthritis, 829, 1714
  for painful diabetic neuropathy, 1240
  for postherpetic neuralgia, 982
  for pruritus, 95, 99t, 148, 673
Capsule imaging/endoscopy
  in colon polyp identification, 666
  in GI/small bowel bleeding, 599
Captopril
  for heart failure, 407
    infarct-related, 376
  for hypertension, 455t
    with hydrochlorothiazide, 455t
    in urgencies/emergencies, 470t, 471
Car accidents. See Automobile accidents
Car driving
  by patients with dementia, 59–60, 1022
  by patients with syncope/ventricular
        tachycardia/aborted sudden
        death, **402**
  by suicidal patients, 1077
Carac. See Fluorouracil
Carbamate poisoning, 1601–1602
Carbamazepine, 987t, 1087. See also
        Anticonvulsant therapy
  for bipolar disease/mania, 1087
  for dementia-associated behavior
        problems, 1104
  HLA-associated drug hypersensitivity
        and, 880, 1087
  for neuropathic pain, 1035
  overdose/toxicity of, 987t, 1087, 1584t,
        1589
    hemodialysis for, 1583t, 1584t, 1589
  pregnancy and, 820, 1087
  for seizures, 987t
Carbapenems, allergy to, penicillin
        allergy cross-reactivity and,
        1318
Carbaryl poisoning, 1601–1602

Carbidopa, 1012
Carbidopa/levodopa, 1012–1013
  with entacapone, 1013, 1014
Carbohydrate deficient transferrin,
        alcohol use disorder and,
        1094
Carbohydrates, dietary. See also
        High-carbohydrate diet
  in diabetes, 1219
    glycemic index and, 1219
  for hypoglycemia, 1237, 1595
  malabsorption of, diarrhea caused by,
        591
  in porphyria, 1036, 1676, 1677
Carbon dioxide. See also Arterial blood
        gases
  increased production of, respiratory
        failure and, 318t
Carbon dioxide laser therapy
  for CIN, 771
  for wart removal/condylomata
        acuminata, 142, 768
Carbon monoxide, diffusing capacity for
        (DL$_{CO}$), in *Pneumocystis*
        pneumonia, 1336
Carbon monoxide poisoning, 23, 1581t,
        1584t, **1591–1592**
  headache in, 40, 1591, 1592
  smoke inhalation and, 305
Carbonic anhydrase inhibitors, 173t, 180
  adverse ophthalmic effects of, 177t
Carboplatin, 1663t
  for breast cancer, 752, 753
  for lung cancer, 1612
  for testicular cancer, 1656
  toxicity of, 1675
Carboxyhemoglobin levels
  in carbon monoxide poisoning, 23, 24,
        305, 1591, 1592
  in smoke inhalation, 305
Carbuncles, **152–153**, 1443t, 1448, 1448f
Carcinoembryonic antigen (CEA)
  in breast cancer, 742
  in colorectal cancer, 1638, 1640
  in thyroid cancer, 1142, 1145
Carcinoid heart disease, 1186
  pulmonary valve regurgitation and,
        350
Carcinoid syndrome, 288, 1186, 1633,
        1635, 1636
Carcinoid tumors, **1185–1187**, 1624t
  bronchial, **288**, 1185, 1186
  gastric, **1633**
  intestinal, 1185, 1186, **1634–1636**
  in MEN, 1187t
  pernicious anemia gastritis and, 622,
        1633
Carcinoma in situ
  of bladder, 1652, 1653
  of breast, 748, 748t
  of cervix, 769–771, 769f, 769t, 771, 772
  of lung, 1609
  of vulva, 775
Carcinomatosis
  lymphangitic, 1613, 1614
  peritoneal, 604
Carcinomatous meningitis
        (leptomeningeal metastases),
        1006
Card agglutination test for trypanosomes
        (CATT), 1508

Cardene/Cardene SR. See Nicardipine
Cardiac amyloidosis, 421–422, 539
Cardiac angiography. See Angiography/
        arteriography, cardiac/
        coronary
Cardiac arrhythmias. See Arrhythmias
"Cardiac asthma," 242
Cardiac biomarkers/enzymes
  in acute coronary syndromes/STEMI/
        chest pain evaluation, 28,
        366, 371
  in cardiomyopathy, 415, 418
  in infectious myocarditis, 414
  in non-ST elevation acute coronary
        syndromes, 366
  in trauma, 434
Cardiac catheterization
  in acute coronary syndromes/STEMI,
        369, 369t
  in cardiomyopathy, 416t
  in heart failure, 404
  in pericarditis, 429
Cardiac cirrhosis, 700
Cardiac Disease in Pregnancy
        Investigation (CARPREG)
        scoring system, 434
Cardiac dysrhythmias. See Arrhythmias
Cardiac friction rub
  in chest pain evaluation, 28
  in pericarditis/effusion, 425, 427
Cardiac glycosides. See Digitalis/digitalis
        glycosides/digoxin
Cardiac index, in shock, 494, 496
Cardiac magnetic resonance imaging. See
        Magnetic resonance imaging
        (MRI), cardiac
Cardiac murmurs. See Heart murmurs
Cardiac output
  acute kidney injury and, 917
  in pregnancy, 819
  in shock liver/cardiogenic liver injury,
        712
Cardiac rehabilitation, 380
Cardiac resynchronization therapy
        (defibrillator/pacemaker).
        See also Pacemaker
  for cardiomyopathy, 417, 419
  for heart failure, 405f, 409–410
Cardiac risk assessment/reduction
  in angina management, 361–362
  in postinfarction management, 380
  preoperative, **45–48**, 46t, 47f, 47t
Cardiac Risk Index, Revised (RCRI), 45,
        46t
Cardiac rupture
  infarction and, 379
  traumatic, 434
Cardiac-specific markers (cardiac
        enzymes). See Cardiac
        biomarkers
Cardiac tamponade. See Tamponade
Cardiac transplantation, for heart failure,
        410
Cardiac trauma, **434**
  sudden death of athlete and, 437
Cardiac tumors, **433–434**
Cardiac valves. See Prosthetic heart
        valves; Valve replacement;
        Valvular heart disease
Cardiobacterium hominis. See HACEK
        organisms

Cardioembolism
  stroke and, 388, 389t, 390, 390t, 996
  transient ischemic attacks and, 477,
      991, 993
Cardiogenic liver injury, acute, 712–713
Cardiogenic pulmonary edema, **411–412**
Cardiogenic shock, 371, 372f, 378,
      493–494, 494t, 495, 497
  in infectious myocarditis, 414
Cardiogenic syncope, 401
Cardiomyopathy, 402–403, **415–422**,
      416t, 420f
  adenovirus infection and, 1421
  amyloidosis and, 421–422
  catecholamine-induced. *See*
      Cardiomyopathy,
      Tako-Tsubo
  cirrhotic, 700
  coxsackievirus infection and, 1426
  in diabetes, 1241
  dilated, 402–403, **415–417**, 416t
  heart failure and, 402–403, 415, 416,
      417, 420f, 422
  heart murmurs in, 335t, 415, 419
  in hyperthyroidism, 417, 1133
  hypertrophic, 416t, **419–421**, 420f
  infectious myocarditis and, 414
  ischemic, 416, 417
  mitral regurgitation and, 339
  of pregnancy (peripartum
      cardiomyopathy), 420, **435**
    prolactin causing, 435, 1117
  restrictive, 416t, **421–422**
    constrictive pericarditis
      differentiated from, 421, 429
    in sarcoidosis, 292, 293, 422
  sudden death of athlete and, 421, 436,
      437, 438t
  Tako-Tsubo (stress/
      catecholamine-induced),
      417–418
    myocardial infarction mimicked by,
      370, 418
    pheochromocytoma and, 1181, 1182
  trastuzumab causing, 752
Cardiomyotomy, Heller, for achalasia, 618
Cardiopulmonary resuscitation
  in drowning, 1567
  in hypothermia, 1564–1565
  orders regarding in end-of-life care, 90
Cardiorenal syndrome, **923**
Cardiotoxicity. *See also* Heart disease
  anthracycline, 414–415, 1674–1675
    dexrazoxane for, 415, 1671t
  antidepressants causing, 1606, 1606f
Cardiovascular disorders. *See also under*
      Cardiac; Coronary;
      Myocardial and Heart
      disease; Stroke
  adverse ophthalmic effects of drugs
      used in, 177t
  atherosclerotic (ASCVD). *See also*
      Atherosclerosis; Coronary
      heart disease
    risks/statin benefits and, 353, 354f,
      355t, 361
  in athletes, screening for, **436–437**,
      437t, 438t
  in Chagas disease, 1509, 1510
  chemoprevention in, 6t, **10–11**. *See
      also* Lipid-lowering therapy

chronic kidney disease/uremia and,
      404, 924t, 925–927
cocaine abuse and, 365, 370, 414, 1100
cognitive disorders/delirium caused by,
      1102t
coxibs (COX-2 inhibitors) and, 621,
      624, 829
in diabetes mellitus, 1241–1242
  glycemic control and, 361–362,
      1217, 1218, 1219
  hypertension control and, 446, 447f,
      464, 465, 466, 1218, 1236
  tibial and pedal artery disease and,
      475, 476
  in women, 1241
estrogen replacement therapy and,
      1202
homocysteine/hyperhomocysteinemia/
      homocystinuria and, 1681
in hypercalcemia/hyperparathyroidism,
      1153
hypertension/hypertension prevention/
      management and, 6t, **10**, 356,
      360f, 362, 439, 440, 443–444,
      446, 447f, 448t, 464
in hyperthyroidism, 1127
influenza and, 1412
lipid fractions/lipoproteins and, 6t, **10**,
      1259–1260
in Lyme disease, 425, 1502, 1505, 1505t
NSAID use and, 621, 624, 829
perioperative evaluation/management
      and, **45–48**, 46t, 47f, 47t
in pheochromocytoma/paraganglioma,
      1180, 1180t, 1181, 1182
pregnancy and, **434–436**, 819
prevention of, **5–11**, 6t, 8–9t, 9t,
      353–355, 354f, 355t, 1259,
      1260. *See also* Lipid-lowering
      therapy
  cholesterol screening and,
      1261–1262
  lipid-lowering therapy and,
      1262–1266, 1264t, 1265t. *See
      also* Lipid-lowering therapy
risk factors for, 5–6
smoking/smoking cessation and, 6t,
      7–9, 8–9t, 9t
syphilis and, 1316t, 1489t, 1494, 1495
thiamine deficiency and, 1274
Cardioversion
  for atrial fibrillation, 389, 391, 393
    infarct-related, 377
    rate control compared with, 393–394
  for atrial flutter, 394
  for supraventricular tachycardia, 386
  for ventricular tachycardia, 397
    infarct-related, 377
Cardioverter defibrillator, implantable.
      See Implantable cardioverter
      defibrillator
Carditis, rheumatic, 422, 422–423, 423t
Cardizem. *See* Diltiazem
Cardura/Cardura XL. *See* Doxazosin
Carey-Coombs murmur, in rheumatic
      carditis, 423
Carfilzomib, 1665t
  for myeloma, 536
Cariprazine, 1068, 1069t, 1070
Carisoprodol, overdose/toxicity of,
      1594–1595

Carney complex/syndrome, 433, 1175,
      1189
  acromegaly and, 1114
  Cushing syndrome and, 1173, 1175
  thyroid cancer and, 1137
L-Carnitine, for valproic acid overdose/
      toxicity, 1584t, 1589
Carotene/carotenoids
  for age-related macular degeneration,
      185
  in chemoprevention, 11
  excess intake of, 1277
Carotid angioplasty, 478
Carotid artery occlusive disease (carotid
      stenosis/insufficiency),
      477–479, 478f
  headache in, 981
  retinal artery occlusion and, 187, 188,
      477
  stroke/transient ischemic attacks
      caused by, 477, 477–478, 991,
      993, 994t, 995
    postoperative stroke and, 52–53
  transient monocular visual loss and,
      188, 189, 477
Carotid endarterectomy/
      thromboendarterectomy,
      478
  prophylactic/preoperative, 52–53,
      477–478
  retinal artery occlusion and, 188
  stroke as complication of, 478
  for transient ischemic attacks and
      stroke, 478, 993
Carotid insufficiency. *See* Carotid artery
      occlusive disease
Carotid sinus hypersensitivity, syncope
      in, 401
Carotid sinus massage/pressure
  for paroxysmal supraventricular
      tachycardia, 386
  in syncope evaluation, 401
Carotid stenosis. *See* Carotid artery
      occlusive disease
Carotid stenting, 478
Carpal compression test, 1699, 1699t
Carpal spasm. *See* Trousseau sign
Carpal tunnel syndrome, **1698–1699**,
      1699t
  in acromegaly, 1115
CARPREG (Cardiac Disease in
      Pregnancy Investigation)
      scoring system, 434
Carteolol, 172t
Cartia. *See* Diltiazem
Carvallo sign, 349
Carvedilol, 452t
  for heart failure, 407–408
    infarct-related, 375, 380
  for hypertension, 449, 452t, 454,
      464
Cascara, 585t, 586
Case management, in heart failure, 410
Casodex. *See* Bicalutamide
Caspofungin, 1558–1559, 1558t
  for aspergillosis, 1555, 1560
  for candidiasis, 1548
  for mucormycosis, 1556
Castleman disease, 1288, 1377
Casts, urinary, 913, 914t. *See also specific
      type and specific disorder*

Cat bites, 1300, 1301
  cat-scratch disease and, 1477
  rabies and, 1386, 1387
Cat exposure/feces
  bacillary angiomatosis and, 1343
  toxoplasmosis and, 1522, 1524
    pregnancy and, 799
Cat-flea typhus, 1435
Cat hookworm, cutaneous larva migrans
    caused by, 1542
Cat roundworm (T cati), toxocariasis/
    visceral larva migrans caused
    by, 1542
Cat-scratch disease, 1477. See also
    Bartonella henselae/quintana
  lymphadenitis/lymphadenopathy in,
    492, 1477
Cataflam. See Diclofenac
Catamenial asthma, 242
Catamenial pneumothorax, 314
Cataplexy, 1090
Catapres/Catapres TTS. See Clonidine
Cataract, 182–183
  diabetic, 1238
  hypoparathyroidism and, 897, 1150
Cataract surgery, 183
  alpha-blocker use and, 183, 464, 974
Catastrophic antiphospholipid syndrome,
    843
Catatonia, 1068, 1070
  antipsychotic-induced, 1073
Catcher's mitt hand, 874
Catecholamine-O-methyltransferase
    (COMT) inhibitors, for
    parkinsonism, 1013–1014
Catecholamine myocarditis, 1183
Catecholamines
  factors affecting levels of, 1181, 1181t
  in pheochromocytoma/paraganglioma,
    1179, 1181, 1181t, 1182
  in Tako-Tsubo cardiomyopathy, 418,
    1182
  tumors secreting, 1213
Catenin, beta, hepatocellular adenoma
    and, 716
Caterpillars, skin lesions caused by, 151
Cathartics, for poisoning/drug overdose,
    1582
Catheter ablation techniques, for
    arrhythmias, 384. See also
    specific arrhythmia
Catheterization
  bladder/urinary. See Bladder
    catheterization
  cardiac. See Cardiac catheterization
Catheters/intravenous lines
  health care–associated infection and,
    1285, 1290, 1291, 1294, 1295,
    1296, 1317
  for parenteral nutritional support,
    1282, 1285
  thrombophlebitis/septic phlebitis and,
    487–488, 488, 1295, 1314t
Cathinone derivatives, toxicity of, 1598
CATT (card agglutination test for
    trypanosomes), 1508
Cauda equina syndrome, 1692, 1695
Cauliflower ear (auricular hematoma),
    201
Caustic/corrosive agents
  acids, 1586–1587

alkalies, 1587
  esophageal injury and, 1586, 1587
  eye injury and, 1587
  skin injury and, 1581, 1586–1587,
    1587
Cavernoma, portal, 713
Cavernous hemangioma, of liver, 715
Cavernous sinus thrombosis, bacterial
    rhinosinusitis and, 217
CBS (cystathionine beta-synthase) gene,
    1681
CBT. See Core body temperature
CCFA (Crohn's and Colitis Foundation of
    America), 652
CCKomas, 1185, 1186
CCLE. See Chronic cutaneous lupus
    erythematosus
CCP antibodies, in rheumatoid arthritis,
    835
C_{cr}. See Creatinine clearance
CCR5 inhibitors, for HIV infection/
    AIDS, 1357–1358
  resistance to, 1361
CD markers. See also specific marker
  in acute leukemia, 528
  in chronic lymphocytic leukemia, 530
CD3-positive T-cell large granular
    lymphoproliferative disorder,
    518
CD4 lymphopenia syndrome, idiopathic,
    progressive multifocal
    leukoencephalopathy in,
    1395
CD4 T cells, in HIV infection/AIDS,
    1330, 1333f, 1334, 1334t
  absolute count, 1334, 1334t
  antiretroviral therapy initiation/
    monitoring and, 1334, 1350,
    1360
  CMV infection and, 191, 192, 1350,
    1374, 1376
  immune reconstitution and, 1345
  MAC infections and, 1334, 1350, 1482,
    1483
  opportunistic infection/course of
    disease and, 1333, 1333f,
    1334, 1348t, 1349, 1350
  percentage of, 1334, 1334t
  Pneumocystis pneumonia and, 1333,
    1334, 1336, 1349, 1552
  syphilis and, 1348, 1497
CD8 T cells, in drug-induced
    hypersensitivity, 880
CD10 (common ALL antigen), 528
CD34, in nephrogenic systemic fibrosis,
    952
CD55 deficiency, in paroxysmal
    nocturnal hemoglobinuria,
    510
CD59 deficiency, in paroxysmal
    nocturnal hemoglobinuria,
    510
CD117, in gastrointestinal stromal
    tumors, 1633
CDH-1 mutation, gastric cancer and,
    1629
CDK inhibition, for breast cancer, 756
CDKN1B gene, in MEN 4, 1189
CDKN2A gene, pancreatic/periampullary
    carcinoma and, 1620
CEA. See Carcinoembryonic antigen

Cecum, dilation of, in colonic
    pseudo-obstruction (Ogilvie
    syndrome), 639, 640
Cefazolin
  for endocarditis/endocarditis
    prophylaxis, 1461, 1461t,
    1462
  for group B streptococcal infection
    prophylaxis in pregnancy,
    800
  for ophthalmic disorders, 169t
  for skin and soft tissue infections,
    1443t, 1448
Cefdinir, for pharyngitis, 1442
Cefepime
  for anaerobic infections, 1479t
  for meningitis, 1297t
  for pneumonia, 269t, 271, 275t
Cefotaxime
  for Lyme disease, 1505, 1505t
  for pneumonia, 269t, 271
  for spontaneous bacterial peritonitis,
    603
Cefpodoxime
  for pharyngitis, 1442
  for pneumonia, 269t
Ceftaroline, for staphylococcal skin
    infections, 1448
Ceftazidime
  for anaerobic infections, 1479t
  for pneumonia, 275t
Ceftin. See Cefuroxime
Ceftolozane/tazobactam, for anaerobic
    infections, 1479
Ceftriaxone
  for anaerobic infections, 1478, 1479t
  for endocarditis, 1461, 1462
  for Lyme disease, 1505, 1505t
  for meningitis, 1297t, 1465
  for pneumonia, 269t, 271, 275t, 1446
  for spontaneous bacterial peritonitis,
    603
  for syphilis, 1491t, 1492, 1496
  for urinary tract infection, 955t
Cefuroxime/cefuroxime axetil
  for Lyme disease, 1504, 1505, 1505t
  for pharyngitis, 229
  for pneumonia, 269t
Celebrex. See Celecoxib
Celecoxib, 74, 75t, 621. See also Coxibs
  cardiovascular complications and, 621,
    624, 829
  for familial adenomatous polyposis,
    667
  gastritis and, 621
  lithium interactions and, 1087t
  for osteoarthritis, 828, 829, 1714
  for pain management, 74, 75t
  peptic ulcers/peptic ulcer prevention
    and, 74, 621, 626t, 829
Celexa. See Citalopram
Celiac disease/sprue (gluten enteropathy),
    632–635. See also
    Malabsorption
  dermatitis herpetiformis and, 123, 633
  Hashimoto's thyroiditis and, 1135,
    1136
  intestinal lymphoma and, 1634
  iron deficiency anemia and, 500, 634
  microscopic colitis and, 662
  pancreatitis and, 726

Cell-culture based influenza vaccine, 1413, 1414*t*

Cell-mediated (delayed/type IV) hypersensitivity, 876, **878–881**

Cell-mediated (cellular) immunity, infections associated with defects in, 1290

Cell surface antigens, immune cell. *See under CD*

Cellophane tape test, in enterobiasis/ pinworms, 1541

Cellular immunity, infections associated with defects in, 1290

Cellulitis, **137–139**, 138*f*, 1315*t*, 1443*t*
of auricle, 201
of breast, 737, 737*f*
puerperal mastitis and, 814
deep vein thrombosis differentiated from, 138
in drug users, 1303
erythrovirus (parvovirus) infection and, 1422
leg ulcers and, 137, 156, 489
lymphangitis/lymphadenitis and, 492, 1315*t*
lymphedema and, 493
necrotizing fasciitis/streptococcal gangrene differentiated from, 138, 492, 1444
non-clostridial crepitant, 1480
orbital, **195**
in bacterial rhinosinusitis, 195, 217
peritonsillar, **229**
sublingual/submaxillary space (Ludwig angina), 230
superficial (erysipelas), **136–137**, 1315*t*, 1442–1443, 1443*t*
synergistic necrotizing, 1480
tinea pedis and, 113, 137
vibrios causing, 1472

Cellulose phosphate, for absorptive hypercalciuria, 963

Cenesthetic hallucinations, 1067. *See also* Hallucinations

Cenestin, 1204

Centor criteria, for streptococcal pharyngitis, 228, 228–229, 1441

Central cord syndrome, 1032

"Central fever," 34

Central nervous system disorders. *See also* Neurologic disorders
adverse ophthalmic effects of drugs used in, 177–178*t*
in HIV infection/AIDS, 1339–1340
infections, **1296–1300**, 1297*t*. *See also* Encephalitis; Meningitis
anaerobic, **1478–1479**
otitis media and, 206
primary angiitis, **862–863**
vertigo and, 210*t*, 211, 211*t*, 213, 213–214

Central nervous system lymphoma, primary (primary cerebral lymphoma), 533, 1004*t*, 1006, 1337*t*, 1339, 1344

Central neurogenic hyperventilation, in coma or stupor, 316, 1027

Central pontine myelinolysis (cerebral osmotic demyelination), hyponatremia treatment and, 885, 888

Central retinal artery occlusion, **187–188**, 187*f*
in stroke, 995

Central retinal vein occlusion, **186–187**

Central sleep apnea, 316

Central vein nutritional support (total parenteral nutrition/ hyperalimentation), 1281*f*, 1282
acidosis caused by, 907, 1285*t*
in burn injury, 1569
complications of, 1284–1285, 1285*t*
in Crohn disease, 655
diabetes management/insulin therapy and, 1244
in HIV infection/AIDS, 1335
patient monitoring during, 1285–1286
solutions for, 1284, 1284*t*
for ulcerative colitis, 660

Central venous catheters
infection/infection prevention and, 1285, 1291, 1294, 1295, 1296
in shock management, 495–496

Central venous pressure, in shock, 495–496

Centruroides (scorpion) stings, 1605

Cephalexin
for endocarditis prophylaxis, 1461*t*
for pharyngitis, 1442
for skin and soft tissue infections, 1443, 1443*t*, 1448
for urinary tract infection, 954, 955*t*

Cephalosporins
allergy to, penicillin allergy cross-reactivity and, 1318
nephrotoxicity of, 919
for pharyngitis, 229, 1442
for spontaneous bacterial peritonitis, 603

Cephalothin, platelet function affected by, 558*t*

Ceratopic, 100*t*

Cercarial dermatitis, in schistosomiasis, 1532

Cerclage
for incompetent cervix, 805
for preterm birth prevention, 812

Cerebellar arteriovenous malformations, 1001

Cerebellar artery occlusion, in stroke, 995

Cerebellar degeneration
paraneoplastic, 1008
vertigo in, 211*t*

Cerebellar hemangioblastoma, 1003, 1004*t*, 1005

Cerebellar hemorrhage, 998

Cerebellar tonsils, herniation of, intracranial tumors causing, 1003

Cerebellar tumors, 1005

Cerebral amyloid angiopathy, 997, 998

Cerebral aneurysm. *See* Intracranial aneurysm

Cerebral angiography/arteriography. *See also* Neuroimaging
in brain death determination, 1028

Cerebral arteriovenous malformations, **1000–1001**

Cerebral artery occlusion, in stroke, 995

Cerebral circulation, absence of, brain death determination and, 1028

Cerebral contusions/lacerations, 1030*t*

Cerebral edema
head injury and, 1030
high-altitude (HACE), **1574**
hypernatremia treatment and, 890
in stroke, 996, 999

Cerebral hemorrhage. *See* Intracerebral hemorrhage

Cerebral hypoperfusion, arrhythmias causing, seizures differentiated from, 986

Cerebral infarction/ischemia, 994*t*, **995–997**. *See also* Stroke; Transient ischemic attacks

Cerebral injury, 1029, 1030*t*, 1031. *See also* Head injury
drowning and, 1567

Cerebral ischemia. *See* Cerebral infarction/ischemia; Stroke; Transient ischemic attacks

Cerebral lymphoma, primary (primary central nervous system lymphoma), 533, 1004*t*, 1006, 1337*t*, 1339, 1344

Cerebral malaria, 1513

Cerebral metastases, 1006

Cerebral osmotic demyelination, hyponatremia treatment and, 885, 888

Cerebral salt wasting, 886, 888

Cerebral toxoplasmosis, in HIV infection/AIDS, 1006, 1339. *See also Toxoplasma*

Cerebral vasoconstriction syndrome, headache caused by, 40

Cerebritis, lupus, 841

Cerebrospinal fluid analysis. *See also specific disorder*
in CNS infections, 1297*t*, 1298–1299
in headache evaluation, 41
in herpetic encephalitis/meningitis, 1364, 1366
in Lyme disease, 1505
in meningococcal meningitis, 1465
normal, 1297*t*
in pneumococcal meningitis, 1447
in syphilis, 1496
in HIV infection/AIDS, 1348, 1497
in tuberculous meningitis, 1483
in Zika virus infection, 1406

Cerebrospinal fluid leakage, in head injury, 1029, 1031

Cerebrovascular accident. *See* Stroke

Cerebrovascular disorders
cancer-related, 1008
deaths attributable to, 2*t*
headache in, 40, 981
homocysteine/hyperhomocysteinemia and, 1681
hypertensive, 444
occlusive, **477–479**, 478*f*. *See also* Stroke; Transient ischemic attacks
oral contraceptive use and, 786

Ceritinib, 1667t
for lung cancer, 1612
Certolizumab
for inflammatory bowel/Crohn disease, 652, 656–657
for rheumatoid arthritis, 837–838
Cerubidine. *See* Daunorubicin
Cerumen impaction, 200, **201**
Ceruminous gland adenoma, 203
Cervarix. *See* Human papillomavirus (HPV) vaccine
Cervical cap, **790**
Cervical carcinoma. *See* Cervix (uterine), cancer of
Cervical discharge, in chlamydial infection, 1486
Cervical intraepithelial neoplasia (CIN/ dysplasia of cervix), **769–771**, 769f, 769t, 771, 772
carcinoma of cervix and, 769, 769t, 770, 771, 772
HIV infection/AIDS and, 1344, 1345
HPV infection and, 769, 770, 1344, 1345
screening tests and, 769–770, 769t, 1345
vaccination in prevention and, 4, 13, 770, 772
Cervical lymphadenopathy, reactive, **239**
Cervical proprioceptive dysfunction, 213
Cervical radiculopathy, 1696
Cervical rib syndrome, 873, **1044–1045**
Cervical spine/disk disease, **1042**, 1043–1044f. *See also* Spine
chest pain and, 359
degenerative/cervical spondylosis, **1042**
herniation/protrusion, **1042**, 1043–1044f
neck pain and, **1696–1697**, 1696t
vertigo and, 213
Cervical spondylosis, **1042**
Cervical/cervical canal stenosis, 765
Cervical vertigo, 213
Cervical warts, 768. *See also* Venereal (genital) warts
Cervicitis
chlamydial, **1486**
gonococcal, 1475, 1476
postgonococcal, 1486
Cervicofacial actinomycosis, 1480
Cervix (uterine)
anaerobic flora/infection of, 1478, 1479
biopsy of
in abnormal uterine bleeding, 762–763
in CIN/cervical cancer, 769, 770, 772
cancer of, 769t, **771–772**, 1623t
HIV infection/AIDS and, 771, 1344
HPV infection and, 770, 771, 1344
screening tests for, 14t, 15, 769–770, 769t
vaccine in prevention of, 4, 13, 770, 772
invasive, 769t, 772
preinvasive (carcinoma in situ/CIN), **769–771**, 769f, 769t, 771, 772
prevention of/screening for, 14t, 15, 769–770, 769t, 772
conization of, for CIN/cervical cancer, 771, 772

dysplasia (CIN) of, **769–771**, 769f, 769t, 1344. *See also* Cervical intraepithelial neoplasia
incompetent, 804
cerclage/activity restriction for, 805
polyps of, **768**
stenosis of, 765
Cesarean delivery
in cardiac patient, 436, 819
morbidly adherent placenta and, 813
placenta previa and, 813
for prevention of disease transmission to fetus/newborn
hepatitis B, 681
herpes genitalis, 823, 1366
HIV, 822, 1332, 1346
puerperal infection and, 814, 820
Cestode infections, **1535–1538**. *See also specific type*
invasive, **1536–1538**
noninvasive, **1535–1536**
Cetirizine, 219. *See also* Antihistamines
Cetuximab, 1666t
for colorectal cancer, 1639, 1640
K-ras mutations and, 1639
CFTR. *See* Cystic fibrosis transmembrane conductance regulator (CFTR) protein
CgA. *See* Chromogranin A
CH50 (complement), in gonococcal arthritis, 869
CHA$_2$DS$_2$-VASc Risk Score, 390–391, 390t, 392f
CHADS$_2$ Risk Score, 389t, 390
Chagas disease (American trypanosomiasis), 30, **1509–1510**
achalasia and, 617
Chagoma, 1509
Chalazion, **165**
Chalkstick fractures
bisphosphonates causing, 1162
in Paget disease of bone, 1167
Chancre
syphilitic, 1488–1489, 1489f, 1489t
anal/anorectal, 670, 1488
differential diagnosis of, 1491
trypanosomal, 1507
Chancroid, **1476–1477**
Channelopathies, periodic paralysis, 1049
Charcoal, activated, for poisoning/drug overdose, 1581, 1582
repeat-dose, 1583
Charcot joint (neurogenic arthropathy), **875**
in diabetes mellitus, 875, 1239
in tabes dorsalis, 875, 1496, 1496f
Charcot-Marie-Tooth disease, 1035
Charcot triad, 721
CHD. *See* Coronary heart disease
Cheilitis, angular, 225, 225f, 1341
Cheiroarthropathy/cheiropathy, diabetic, 846, 1242
Chelation therapy. *See also specific type*
for absorptive hypercalciuria, 963
adverse ophthalmic effects of, 179t
for arsenic poisoning, 1581t, 1590
for heavy metal poisoning, 1581t
for hemochromatosis/iron poisoning/ overload, 709, 1581t, 1584, 1596

for lead poisoning, 1581t, 1597
for mercury poisoning, 1581t, 1599
for Wilson disease, 711
Chemical injury
acids causing, 198, 1581
alkalies causing, 198, 1581
of esophagus, 1586, 1587
of eye (conjunctivitis/keratitis), **198**, 1581, 1587
of lung
aspiration and, 305, 306
occupational, 290t
smoke inhalation and, 305
skin decontamination after, 1581
Chemical warfare agents. *See also* Bioterrorism
nerve agents, 1601–1602
skin decontamination after exposure to, 1581
Chemiluminescence (CIA) assay, in syphilis, 1490, 1490t
"Chemo brain," 759
Chemoprevention/chemoprophylaxis, 10–11
antibiotic/antimicrobial. *See* Antimicrobial chemoprophylaxis
for cancer, 11, 13
breast cancer and, 11
colorectal cancer and, 11, 1637
for cardiovascular disease, 6t, **10–11**. *See also* Lipid-lowering therapy
for cluster headache, 980
for DVT/PE (venous thromboembolic disease), 300, 567–569, 568t, 569t
contraindications to, 569, 569t
for migraine headache, 978–979, 979t
for stress gastritis, 319, 620–621
Chemoradiation therapy
for bladder cancer, 1652
for breast cancer, 754
for colorectal cancer, 1639, 1640
for esophageal cancer, 1627, 1628
for gastric adenocarcinoma, 1630–1631
for gliomas, 1005
for laryngeal cancer, 236
Chemoreceptor trigger zone, 580, 581t
Chemotherapy (cancer), 1622–1625t, **1661–1675**, 1663–1670t, 1671–1672t, 1672t. *See also specific agent and cancer type*
adverse ophthalmic effects of, 178t
anemia caused by, 1662
bone marrow/stem cell transplantation after, 540, 541
bone marrow toxicity of, **1662–1672**
fever and, 1314t
hyperuricemia/tumor lysis syndrome and, 920, 1660
leukemia caused by, 527
myocarditis and, 414–415
nausea and vomiting caused by, 87, 580, 581t, 582, 582t, **1672–1673**
neuropathies caused by, 1674
neutropenia caused by, 35, 518, 1290, 1662
infections and, 35, 1661
supportive agents for, 518, 1671t

ototoxicity and, 208
with radiation therapy. *See*
Chemoradiation therapy
supportive agents/care and, 518, 1671*t*
thrombocytopenia and, **548**, 555*t*,
1662–1672
toxicity/dose modification of agents
used in, **1662–1675**,
1663–1670*t*, 1671–1672*t*,
1672*t*
cardiac, 414–415
ophthalmic, 178*t*
Chest pain/discomfort, **26–29**, 27*t*,
365–366. *See also specific
cause*
in angina, 26–27, 27, 27*t*, 28, 356, 357
alteration in before myocardial
infarction, 370
coronary vasospasm causing, 356,
364–365
Prinzmetal (variant), 365
diagnosis/differential diagnosis of,
26–29, 27*t*, 365–366
in esophageal disorders, 27, 359, 611,
617, 618, 619
ischemic, 26–27, 27, 27*t*, 28, 356, 357,
365–366. *See also* Acute
coronary syndromes;
Angina
recurrent, 375, 376
in myocardial infarction, 26–27, 27,
27*t*, 28, 370
noncardiac, 27, 28, 29, 359, 611, 617,
618, **619**
palpitations and, 30
pleuritic, 22, 27, 27*t*
psychologic causes of, 29, 619
in pulmonary embolism, 26, 27, 28,
295, 296*t*
visceral sensitivity causing, 619
Chest pain observation units, 365–366
Chest tube drainage (tube thoracostomy)
for anaerobic pleuropulmonary
disease, 276, 1478
for malignant pleural effusion, 313,
1659
for parapneumonic pleural effusion,
313–314, 1446
for pneumothorax, 315
Chest wall
breast cancer recurrence in, 758–759
disorders of
chest pain/discomfort in, 27, 359,
619
anterior chest wall/Tietze
syndrome, 359
respiratory failure caused
by, 318*t*
Cheyne-Stokes respiration, in coma or
stupor, 1027, 1028
CHF (congestive heart failure). *See* Heart
(cardiac) failure
Chibroxin. *See* Norfloxacin
Chickenpox. *See* Varicella
Chiggers
in rickettsial disease transmission,
1431
skin lesions caused by, 151
Chikungunya fever, 1367*t*, **1407–1408**
arthritis in, 870, 1407, 1408
Chilblain (erythema pernio), **1565**

Child abuse
aggression/violence/impulse control
disorders and, 1090–1091
Munchausen by proxy and, 1059
PTSD and, 1052
Child-Turcotte-Pugh classification for
cirrhosis, 705, 705*t*
hepatocellular carcinoma and, 1617
postoperative complications and, 50
variceal hemorrhage and, 615, 616, 617
Childbirth. *See* Labor and delivery
Childbirth preparation classes, 799
Children
epilepsy/seizures in, 983
immunization recommendations for,
1319
parechovirus infection in, 1428
Chimera, allogeneic stem cell
transplantation producing,
541
Chinese liver fluke infection, 1534
Chlamydia (chlamydial infections), 1313*t*,
1485–1487. *See also
Chlamydophila*
diarrhea caused by, 588*t*
endocarditis, 1462
gonococcal coinfection and, 1486
inclusion conjunctivitis, **167**
keratoconjunctivitis, **167**
screening for, 1302, 1486
prenatal, 799, 800, 1486
in STD patients, 1302, 1486
trachoma, **167**
trachomatis, 1313*t*, 1485, **1485–1486**
anorectal involvement and, 671
epididymitis, 960, 1316*t*
lymphogranuloma venereum, 671,
1485
pelvic infection/PID, 778, 1313*t*,
1316*t*, 1486
pregnancy and, 799, 800, **823**, 1486
sexual violence (rape/sexual assault)
and, 793, 1302
urethritis/cervicitis/urinary tract
infection, 42, 1313*t*, 1316*t*,
1486
Chlamydophila, 1485. *See also Chlamydia
pneumoniae*, 268*t*, 1313*t*, 1314*t*, 1315*t*,
1485, **1487**
psittaci, 1313*t*, 1485, **1486–1487**
Chloasma (melasma), 157, 158
Chlorambucil, 1663*t*
adverse ophthalmic effects of, 178*t*
for chronic lymphocytic leukemia, 530
Chloramphenicol
adverse ophthalmic effects of, 178*t*
for anaerobic infections, 1479
for ophthalmic disorders, 169*t*
Chlordiazepoxide, 1054*t*
for alcohol withdrawal, 1097
overdose/toxicity of, 1594–1595
Chlorguanide. *See* Proguanil
Chloride
in fluid management, 911*t*
requirements for in nutritional
support, 1282
Chloride secretory agents, for
constipation, 586
Chloroquine, 1515*t*, 1516, 1517*t*
adverse ophthalmic effects of, 178*t*,
179*t*

for amebiasis, 1526, 1527*t*
erythrovirus (parvovirus)-associated
anemia and, 1422
for lupus, 116
for malaria, 1515*t*, 1516, 1517*t*
for chemoprophylaxis, 1516, 1520,
1520*t*
for non-falciparum malaria, 1515,
1515*t*, 1517*t*
in pregnancy, 802
resistance to, 1515, 1516
for uncomplicated falciparum
malaria, 1515
rabies vaccination affected by,
1326–1327, 1388
Chlorpheniramine, for allergic rhinitis,
219
Chlorpromazine, 1069*t*, 1072. *See also*
Antipsychotic drugs
for migraine headache, 978
overdose/toxicity of/side effects of,
1069*t*, 1072, 1589–1590
for serotonin syndrome, 36, 1580, 1606
Chlorpropamide, 1220, 1221*t*
adverse ophthalmic effects of, 179*t*
Chlorthalidone
for heart failure, 406
for hypertension, 448, 450*t*
with atenolol, 452*t*
with azilsartan, 457*t*
with clonidine, 462*t*
Chokes, 1573
Cholangiocarcinoma, 1608*t*, 1616,
1618–1619
clonorchiasis/opisthorchiasis and,
1534, 1619
with hepatocellular carcinoma, 1619
in primary sclerosing cholangitis, 724,
725, 1619
Cholangiography/
cholangiopancreatography,
677. *See also specific type*
pancreatitis after, 677
Cholangiopathy, AIDS, 1529
Cholangitis, **720–722**
autoimmune, 707
biliary stricture and, 723
choledocholithiasis and, **720–722**
IgG$_4$-associated, 724
liver abscess and, 714
pancreatitis and, 732
primary biliary (primary biliary
cirrhosis), 700, **706–707**
primary sclerosing, **723–725**
autoimmune hepatitis and, 692
cholangiocarcinoma and, 724, 725,
1619
in HIV infection/AIDS, 1342
pyogenic, 721
Cholecalciferol (vitamin D$_3$), 1151*t*. *See
also* Vitamin D
for hypoparathyroidism/tetany, 1151*t*
for vitamin D deficiency/osteoporosis/
osteomalacia, 1161, 1166
Cholecystectomy
for cholecystitis, 719, 824
for choledocholithiasis/cholangitis,
721–722
for cholelithiasis/gallstones, 717, 718
pancreatitis and, 729
for precholecystectomy syndrome, 720

Cholecystectomy (*Cont.*):
  pregnancy and, 824
  for primary sclerosing cholangitis, 725
  symptom persistence after
    (postcholecystectomy
    syndrome), 720
Cholecystitis, 717*t*, **718–720**, 1314*t*
  acalculous, 718, 719
    in HIV infection/AIDS, 1342
    parenteral nutritional support and,
      1285*t*
  acute, 717*t*, **718–720**
  choledocholithiasis (bile duct stones)
    and, 721
  cholelithiasis/gallstones and, 717, 718,
    719
  chronic, 717*t*, 719
  gallbladder cancer and, 719
  in HIV infection/AIDS, 1342
  during pregnancy, **823–824**
  xanthogranulomatous, 719
Cholecystokinin, tumors producing
  (CCKomas), 1185, 1186
Choledocholithiasis, 717*t*, **720–722**
  pancreatitis and, 729
  in pregnancy, 824
Cholelithiasis (gallstones), **716–718**, 717*t*
  cholecystitis and, 717, 718, 719
  choledocholithiasis (bile duct stones)
    and, 720, 721
  in Crohn disease, 653
  pancreatitis and, 725–726, 727, 729
  during pregnancy, 717, **823–824**
  in short bowel syndrome, 637
  somatostatinomas and, 1185
Cholera, 1312*t*, **1471**
  prevention/immunization and, 1326,
    1471
Cholera vaccine, 1326, 1471
Cholestasis, 674, 675*t*
  drugs/toxins causing, 696
  hereditary/intrahepatic, 674, 675*t*
  of pregnancy, 674, 675*t*, **824–825**
  in primary biliary cholangitis/cirrhosis,
    706
Cholestatic jaundice, 674, 675*t*
  antipsychotics causing, 1072
Cholesteatoma, 205–206, 205*f*
Cholesterol, 1259–1260. *See also specific*
  type and Lipoproteins
  antiretroviral therapy/protease
    inhibitors affecting, 1356
  in cardiovascular/coronary heart
    disease, 10, 353, **1259–1260**
  in diabetes mellitus, 1217, 1241, 1261
  dietary, 1263
  elevated levels of. *See also*
    Hypercholesterolemia; Lipid
    disorders
  screening tests for, 6*t*, **10**,
    1261–1262
    in women/older adults, 1261,
      1262
  estrogen replacement affecting, 1202
  in gallstones, 716, 717, 718
  lowering levels of. *See* Lipid-lowering
    therapy
  "normal"/reference values for, 1260
  thiazolidinediones affecting, 1224
  total, 1259, 1259–1260, 1261, 1262
Cholesterol-lowering diet, 1263, 1279

Cholesterolosis of gallbladder, 717*t*, 719
Cholesteryl ester transfer protein
    inhibitors, raising HDL levels
    and, 1262
Cholestyramine
  for diarrhea, 594
    in Crohn disease, 655
    in short bowel syndrome, 637
  for lipid modification, 1264, 1265*t*
Choline magnesium salicylate, 75*t*
Cholinergic rebound, 1082
Cholinergic syndrome, 1583
Cholinergic urticaria, 134
Cholinesterase inhibitors. *See*
    Anticholinesterases
Chondritis, 201. *See also* Polychondritis
Chondrocalcinosis, 834
  in hyperparathyroidism, 1155
Chondroitin/chondroitin plus
    glucosamine sulfate, in
    osteoarthritis, 829, 1714
Chondromalacia (patellofemoral knee
    pain), 1705*t*, **1712–1713**
Chorea
  drug-induced, 1017
  in Huntington disease, 1014, 1015
  in rheumatic fever (Sydenham), 422,
    423, 423*t*
Chorioamnionitis, **814**
Choriocarcinoma, **807–808**, 1624*t*
  hyperthyroidism and, 807, 1126
  testicular, 1655
Choriomeningitis, lymphocytic,
    1392–1393
Chorionic gonadotropin. *See* Human
    chorionic gonadotropin
Chorionic villus sampling, 800
Chorioretinitis, toxoplasmic, 1522, 1523
  in HIV infection/AIDS, 192, 1523
Chromoendoscopy, in ulcerative colitis,
    661
Chromogranin A (CgA)
  in carcinoid tumors, 1635
  pancreatic neuroendocrine tumors
    secreting, 1185, 1186
  in pheochromocytomas, 1181, 1184
Chronic actinic dermatitis, 154
Chronic bronchitis. *See* Bronchitis
Chronic cutaneous lupus erythematosus,
    115–116, 839*t*, 840
Chronic disease, anemia of, 501, **502–503**
Chronic fatigue syndrome, **37–39**, 38*f*
  fibromyalgia and, 873
  post-Q fever, 1437
Chronic inflammatory polyneuropathy,
    1039
Chronic intestinal pseudo-obstruction,
    640–641
Chronic kidney disease (CKD), 913,
    923–932, 923*t*, 924*t*, 925*f*,
    925*t*, 926*f*, 927*f*. *See also*
    Renal failure
  acid-base disorders and, 892*t*, 906–907,
    906*t*, 908, 926*f*, 928
  alkalosis in alkali administration and,
    909
  amyloidosis and, 538, 934*t*, **946**
  anemia in, 503, 913, 916, 926*f*, 928
  cardiorenal syndrome and, 923
  cardiovascular disorders and, 404,
    924*t*, 925–927

  coagulopathy of, 928
  complications of, 925–929, 926*f*, 927*f*
  diabetes and, 923, 929, 934*t*, 942,
    945–946, 1238, 1238–1239.
    See also Diabetic
    nephropathy
  dietary management in, 929
  drug/medication use and, 924, 929
  endocrine disorders and, 929
  gout and, 830, **952**
  heart failure and, 404, 923, 926
  hematologic complications and, 928
  hypercalcemia/hyperparathyroidism
    and, 898, 926*f*, 927, 927*f*,
    1153, 1155, 1157
  hyperkalemia and, 893, 894, 916, 920,
    926, 926*f*, 928
  hypermagnesemia and, 902, 903
  hyperphosphatemia in, 901, 916, 920,
    926*f*, 927, 927*f*
  hypertension/hypertension
    management and, 444, 449*t*,
    466, 923, 925, 926, 926*f*
  hypocalcemia and, 896, 927, 927*f*
  hypoglycemia and, 924, 929, 1237
  hypomagnesemia treatment and, 902
  hyponatremia in, 888
  immunization recommendations in,
    1321*t*
  metabolic bone disorders of (renal
    osteodystrophy), 927–928,
    927*f*, 1153, 1155
  nephrogenic systemic fibrosis and, 358,
    952
  neurologic complications of, 924*t*,
    928–929
  neuropathy associated with, 929, 1036
  pericarditis and (uremic pericarditis),
    425, 426, 924, 926–927
  reversible causes of, 925, 925*t*
  stages of, 923–924, 923*t*
  surgery in patient with, 54
Chronic kidney disease
    (CKD)-Epidemiology (EPI)
    Collaboration creatinine
    equation, 915
Chronic lymphocytic leukemia (CLL),
    529–531, 1622*t*
  stem cell transplantation for, 531, 541
Chronic lymphocytic thyroiditis. *See*
    Hashimoto (chronic
    lymphocytic/autoimmune)
    thyroiditis
Chronic mountain sickness (Monge
    disease), 1574, **1575**
Chronic myeloid leukemia (CML), 519,
    519*t*, 520*t*, **523–525**, 1622*t*
  bone marrow/stem cell transplantation
    for, 525, 541
  erythrovirus (parvovirus) infection in,
    1422
Chronic myelomonocytic leukemia
    (CMML), 525
Chronic noncancer pain (CNCP),
    1060–1062, 1061*f*
  management of, 72–73, 82, **84–86**,
    1061–1062
Chronic obstructive pulmonary disease
    (COPD), **257–263**, 258*t*,
    260*t*
  cor pulmonale and, 258, 262

cough in, 19, 21
immunization recommendations in, 259, 1321t
postoperative pulmonary complications and, 49, 50
smoking/smoking cessation and, 7, 257, 259
steroid-responsive, 261
Chronic pain disorders, **1060–1062**, 1061f. *See also* Pain
management of, 72–73, 82, **84–86**, 1061–1062
Chronic pelvic pain
in female, **765–766**
in male (nonbacterial prostatitis), 957t, **958–959**
Chronic prolymphocytic leukemia, 530
Chronic pulmonary histoplasmosis, 1549
Chronic renal failure, 913, **923–932**, 923t, 924t, 925f, 925t, 926f, 927f. *See also* Chronic kidney disease
Chronic thromboembolic pulmonary hypertension, 302, 303, 430, 430t, 433
Chronic traumatic encephalopathy, 1031
Chronic venous insufficiency. *See* Venous insufficiency/stasis
Chryseobacterium species. *See* Elizabethkingia (*Chryseobacterium*/ *Flavobacterium*) species
Churg-Strauss syndrome (eosinophilic granulomatosis with polyangiitis), 304
leukotriene modifiers for asthma and, 251
pulmonary involvement in, 304
renal involvement in, 933t, 935f, 938
Chvostek sign
in hypocalcemia/hypoparathyroidism, 897, 1150
in malabsorption, 633t
Chylous ascites, 601, 701
Chylous effusion, 312, 1658
CIA assay, in syphilis, 1490, 1490t
Cialis. *See* Tadalafil
Cicatricial (scarring) alopecia, 158, 159
Ciclopirox, 99t
Cidofovir, 1365t
adverse ophthalmic effects of, 178t
for CMV infection, 191, 1338t, 1365t, 1376
for poxviral infection, 1423
for recurrent respiratory papillomatosis, 234
Cigarette/cigar smoking. *See* Smoking
Cigarettes, electronic, as tobacco cessation aid, 259
Ciguatera poisoning, 1603, 1604t
Cilostazol, for transient ischemic attacks, 993
Ciloxan. *See* Ciprofloxacin
Cimetidine, 609. *See also* H_2 receptor blocking drugs
antidepressant drug interactions and, 1083t
antiplatelet therapy interactions and, 628
benzodiazepine interactions and, 1056t

CYP 2C19/ulcer complications and, 628
for scombroid poisoning, 1603
Cimex lectularius bites, 151
CIN. *See* Cervical intraepithelial neoplasia
Cinacalcet
for hypercalcemia/ hyperparathyroidism, 898, 927–928, 1156–1157, 1187
for metabolic bone disorders/renal osteodystrophy, 927–928
for parathyroid carcinoma, 1156–1157
for parathyroid hyperplasia, 1158
Cipro. *See* Ciprofloxacin
Ciprofibrate, 1265
Ciprofloxacin. *See also* Fluoroquinolones
for anaerobic infections, 1479t
for anthrax, 1455, 1456t
breastfeeding and, 798t
for Crohn disease, 655
for cyclosporiasis, 1529
for MAC infection, 1482
for ophthalmic disorders, 169t
for pneumonia, 269t, 271, 275t
for traveler's diarrhea, 1310
for typhoid fever/carriers, 1469
for urinary tract infection, 955t
Circulation assessment/support, in comatose patient, 1578
Circumcision, STD transmission risk and, 1303
HIV, 1303, 1346
HSV, 1303, 1366
Cirrhosis, **699–706**. *See also* Liver, disorders of
alcoholic liver disease/hepatitis and, 693, 694, 699, 700, 701, 705
biliary
primary (primary biliary cholangitis), 700, **706–707**
autoimmune hepatitis and, 692
secondary, 700
cardiac, 700
coagulopathy and, 562, 704
drugs/toxins causing, 697
esophageal varices and, 595, 596, 614, 615, 616, 617, 700. *See also* Esophageal varices
prevention of first bleeding episode and, 616–617
GI bleeding in, 595, 596, 614, 700
hemochromatosis and, 700, 708
hepatopulmonary syndrome/ portopulmonary hypertension and, 704
hepatorenal syndrome and, 702–703
hyponatremia in, 887
liver cancer and, 701, 705, 1616, 1617
methotrexate toxicity and, 837
nonalcoholic fatty liver disease and, 697, 698
hepatocellular carcinoma and, 699, 1616
portal hypertension and, 614, 699, 700, 701, 705
postoperative complications and, 50
spontaneous bacterial peritonitis and, 602–604, 702
viral hepatitis and, 682, 683, 684, 687, 688, 689

Cirrhotic cardiomyopathy, 700
CIS. *See* Clinically isolated syndrome
Cisapride, antidepressant drug interactions and, 1081, 1083t
Cisplatin, 1663t
for bladder cancer, 1652
for gastric adenocarcinoma, 1631
for lung cancer, 1611–1612, 1612
for testicular cancer, 1657
toxicity of, 1663t, 1675
amifostine for, 1675
ophthalmic toxicity, 178t
ototoxicity, 208, 1675
Citalopram, 1078t, 1079–1081
for Alzheimer disease/dementia, 59, 1021
overdose toxicity of, 1078t, 1079, 1606
during pregnancy, 1081
Citracal (calcium citrate). *See* Calcium, dietary/supplementary
Citrate, in hypocitraturic calcium nephrolithiasis, 963, 964
Civamide, for cluster headache prophylaxis, 980
CIWA-Ar (Clinical Institute Withdrawal Assessment for Alcohol Revised), 1095, 1096–1097f
treating alcohol withdrawal based on, 1097–1098
CJD. *See* Creutzfeldt-Jakob disease
CK. *See* Creatine kinase
CK-MB. *See* Creatine kinase-MB
CKD. *See* Chronic kidney disease
CKD-Epidemiology (EPI) Collaboration creatinine equation, 915
Cl⁻. *See* Chloride
Cladophialophora/Cladophialophora carrionii, phaeohyphomycosis caused by, 1558
Cladribine, 1663t
Clarithromycin. *See also* Macrolides
for anthrax, 1456t
for endocarditis prophylaxis, 1461t
in *H pylori* eradication therapy, 626, 626t, 627
for MAC infection, 286, 1337t, 1350, 1482, 1483
for pneumonia, 269t, 271, 1445
Classic (nonexertional) heat stroke, 1562
Claudication, 472. *See also specific cause*
spinal stenosis/disk herniation and, 1694
Cl_cr. *See* Creatinine clearance
Cleaning agents. *See* Caustic/corrosive agents
Clear liquid diet, 1278
Clemastine, for allergic rhinitis, 219
Clevidipine, for hypertensive urgencies/ emergencies, 469, 469t, 470t
Cleviprex. *See* Clevidipine
Clicks. *See* Heart murmurs; Heart sounds
Climacteric, 1201. *See also* Menopause
Climara/Climara Pro, 1204
Clindamycin
for acne, 98t, 127
for anaerobic infections, 276, 1478
for anthrax, 1456t
for bacterial vaginosis, 768
with benzoyl peroxide, 98t, 127
for endocarditis prophylaxis, 1461t

Clindamycin (*Cont.*):
for malaria, 1517t, 1520
for *P jirovecii* infection, 1337t, 1350, 1552
for rosacea, 129
for skin and soft tissue infections, 1343, 1443t, 1448
for toxoplasmosis, 1337t, 1524
Clinical Institute Withdrawal Assessment for Alcohol Revised (CIWA-Ar), 1095, 1096–1097f
treating alcohol withdrawal based on, 1097–1098
Clinically isolated syndrome (CIS), multiple sclerosis and, 1024
Clinoril. *See* Sulindac
Clitocybe (muscarine) mushroom poisoning, 1600t
CLL. *See* Chronic lymphocytic leukemia
Clobazam, 988t
Clobetasol, 97t
Clock drawing task, in dementia screening, 57–58
Clocortolone, 97t
Cloderm. *See* Clocortolone
Clofarabine, 1664t
Clofazimine, for leprosy, 1484
Clofibrate, 1265
Clolar. *See* Clofarabine
Clomiphene
in infertility workup, 784
for male hypogonadism/infertility, 1112, 1193
for ovulation induction, 784, 1112, 1198
Clomipramine, 1078t, 1081, 1082. *See also* Antidepressants
for OCD, 1057, 1081
Clonazepam, 988t. *See also* Benzodiazepines
for burning mouth syndrome, 226
overdose/toxicity of, 988t, 1594–1595
for panic disorders/attacks, 1055, 1056
for psychedelic/hallucinogen abuse/toxicity, 1099
for seizures, 988t
for sleep-wake disorders, 1090
Clonic seizures, 984t, 985. *See also* Seizures
Clonidine, 462t
antidepressant drug interactions and, 1083t
for diarrhea, 594
in diabetic autonomic neuropathy, 1240
for heroin/opioid withdrawal, 1099
for hypertension, 462t, 464
with chlorthalidone, 462t
in urgencies/emergencies, 470t, 471
for menopausal symptoms, 795
overdose/toxicity of, 462t, 464, 1592
perioperative use of, 46
for Tourette syndrome, 1018
Clonorchis sinensis (clonorchiasis), 1534
cholangiocarcinoma and, 1534, 1619
Clopidogrel
for acute coronary syndromes/STEMI, 366, 367f, 371
postinfarction, 380
for angina, 360f, 361

cardiac valve replacement and, 351, 352t
in cardiovascular/heart disease prevention, 355
coronary stent thrombosis prevention and, 362, 374, 376
CYP 2C19 and, 628
GI bleeding/peptic ulcer disease and, 624, 628
platelet function affected by, 558t
for transient ischemic attacks, 993
Clorazepate, 988t, 1054, 1054t
Clorpres. *See* Clonidine, for hypertension, with chlorthalidone
Clostridium (clostridial infections), 1312t, **1451–1454**
abdominal, 1314t, 1479
bifermentans, 1451
botulinum (botulism), **1046–1047,** 1306t, **1453–1454**
difficile
colitis/diarrhea caused by, 588t, 589, 592, **647–649,** 1305, 1306t
prevention of transmission of, 1295
histolyticum, 1451
myonecrosis/gas gangrene, 1312t, **1451–1452**
novyi, 1451
perfringens, 1451
diarrhea/food poisoning/gastroenteritis caused by, 588t, 589, 1305, 1306t
ramosum, 1451
sordellii/endometritis/toxic shock, **1452**
tetani, 1312t, 1453. *See also* Tetanus
Clothing (flame) burns, electrical, 1570
Clotrimazole, 98t
for candidiasis
cutaneous, 133
nail infection/paronychia, 133
oral, 226, 1341
vulvovaginal, 133, 767, 1548
topical, 98t
Clotting factors. *See* Coagulation factors
Clozapine, 1068, 1069t, 1071t, 1072, 1073. *See also* Antipsychotic drugs
agranulocytosis caused by, 1014, 1072
diabetes and, 1072, 1213
neuroleptic malignant syndrome and, 1072
overdose/toxicity/side effects of, 1014, 1069t, 1071t, 1072
in parkinsonism, 1014
Clozaril. *See* Clozapine
Clubbed fingers (digital clubbing), 160, 160f, 1609. *See also specific cause*
Clue cells, in bacterial vaginosis, 767
Cluster headache, **979–980**
Clusters of differentiation. *See* CD markers
CMF regimen, 751
CML. *See* Chronic myeloid leukemia
CMML. *See* Chronic myelomonocytic leukemia
CMV disease. *See* Cytomegalovirus (CMV) disease
CMV immune globulin, 1376
CMV inclusion disease, 1374, 1375

CNCP. *See* Chronic noncancer pain
CO_2 laser therapy. *See* Carbon dioxide laser therapy
Coagulase-negative staphylococci, **1450–1451**
endocarditis caused by, 1450, 1458, 1462
Coagulation disorders. *See* Bleeding; Coagulopathy
Coagulation factors. *See also specific type under Factor*
for anticoagulant overdose, 1588
deficiencies/defects of. *See* Bleeding; Coagulopathy
transfusion and, 544. *See also* Plasma/plasma fractions/components, transfusion of; Transfusion
Coagulopathy, **557–577,** 559t, 561t. *See also specific type and* Bleeding
acquired disorders causing, 561–563
of chronic kidney disease, 928
congenital disorders causing, 557–561, 559t, 561t
consumptive (DIC), **553–555,** 554t, **562.** *See also* Disseminated intravascular coagulation
of liver disease, **562,** 704
surgical complications associated with, 50
variceal hemorrhage and. *See* Esophageal varices
perioperative evaluation/management and, 45, 46t, 51
Coal worker's pneumoconiosis, 306–307, 307t
Coarctation of aorta, **323–324**
hypertension and, 324, 443
Coartem (artemether-lumefantrine/Riamet), 1515t, 1516t, 1517t, 1519, 1520
Cobalamin. *See* Vitamin B_{12}
Cobicistat, 1356. *See also* Antiretroviral therapy
with atazanavir, 1352t, 1356, 1357
plus Truvada (emtricitabine/tenofovir [TDF]), 1359t
with darunavir, 1352t, 1356, 1357
plus Epzicom (abacavir/lamivudine), 1360t
plus Truvada (emtricitabine/tenofovir [TDF]), 1360t
with tenofovir [TAF]/elvitegravir/emtricitabine (Genvoya), 1354t, 1355, 1358, 1359t, 1360
with tenofovir (TDF)/elvitegravir/emtricitabine (Stribild), 1354t, 1355, 1358, 1359t, 1360
Cobimetinib, 1667t
Cocaine/cocaine abuse, 17, **1100,** **1587–1588**
cardiac toxicity and, 365, 370, 414, 1100
epistaxis and, 221, 1100
granulomatosis with polyangiitis differentiated from, 858
heroin use and, 1098
hypertension caused by, 469, 469t
beta-blocker use and, 454, 469

levamisole-associated purpura and, 860
during pregnancy, 799, 1100
psychotic/violent behavior caused by, 1068, 1100
pulmonary disorders caused by, 309, 1100
rhabdomyolysis and, 852
Coccidioides immitis/posadasii (coccidioidomycosis), **1550–1551**
Coccidiosis, **1527–1530**
Cochlear disorders
hearing loss and, 200, 207–209. *See also* Sensory hearing loss
recruitment/hyperacusis and, 210
tinnitus and, 209
Cochlear implants, 201
"Cochlear otosclerosis," 207
Cockcroft-Gault formula, 915
Codeine, 74
with aspirin or acetaminophen, 74, 80t
breastfeeding and, 798t
for diarrhea, 594
overdose/toxicity of, 1601
in pain management, 74, 80t
Coffee grounds emesis/aspirate
in erosive/hemorrhagic gastritis (gastropathy), 620
in GI bleeding, 594, 595, 598
ulcer-related, 629
Cogan syndrome, 209
Cognitive ability
assessment of, 57–58
estrogen replacement therapy and, 796, 1202, 1203, 1204
impairment in. *See* Cognitive disorders
Cognitive disorders, 57–58, 59, 1018–1022, 1019t, **1101–1104**, 1102t. *See also specific type and* Delirium; Dementia
chemotherapy causing ("chemo brain"), 759
in elderly, 57–58, 59, 1018–1019
after head injury, 1029, 1031, 1102t
in HIV infection/AIDS, 1339
mild impairment, 58, 1018
postoperative, 52–53, 52t
Coin lesion. *See* Solitary pulmonary nodule
Coitus. *See* Sexual intercourse
Colchicine
for calcium pyrophosphate deposition/pseudogout, 834
for familial Mediterranean fever, 604
for gout, 831, 832
for pericarditis, 426
Cold (common cold/viral rhinosinusitis), **214–215**, 1420–1421
Cold, disorders caused by exposure to, **1561, 1563–1566**, 1564f. *See also* Hypothermia
livedo reticularis and, 863
Raynaud phenomenon and, 844, 845
Cold agglutinin disease, **515–516**
Cold/fever sore (herpes simplex), **118–120**, 119f, 1363. *See also* Herpes simplex infection
Cold urticaria, 134

Cold water, facial contact with, for paroxysmal supraventricular tachycardia, 386
Colesevelam
for diabetes, 1222t, 1228
for diarrhea, 594
in Crohn disease, 655
in short bowel syndrome, 637
for lipid modification, 1264, 1265t
Colestid. *See* Colestipol
Colestipol
for diarrhea, 594
in Crohn disease, 655
in short bowel syndrome, 637
for lipid modification, 1264, 1265t
Colitis. *See also* Diarrhea
amebic (intestinal amebiasis), 588t, 589, 592, 1305, 1315t, 1342, 1525, 1526, 1526f, 1527t
postdysenteric, 1526
antibiotic-associated/*C difficile*, 589, **647–649**, 1305, 1306t
CMV, 1342, 1375, 1376
collagenous, 662
Crohn, 652, 654, 655. *See also* Crohn disease
ischemic, 479, 598
lymphocytic, 662
microscopic, 588t, 592, **662**
postdysenteric, 1526
pseudomembranous, 648. *See also* Colitis, antibiotic-associated
ulcerative. *See* Ulcerative colitis
Collagenomas, in MEN, 1187t, 1188
Collagenous colitis, 662
Collateral ligaments of knee, 1704
injury of, 1707t, **1710–1711**
Colloids, for fluid management/volume replacement, 912
in shock, 496
Colography, CT (virtual colonoscopy), 15, 665, 1638, 1642–1643
Cologuard, in cancer screening, 1642
Colon
anaerobic flora of, 1478, 1479
biopsy of, in diarrhea, 593
cancer of, 1608t, 1624t, 1638, 1639. *See also* Colorectal cancer
chemotherapy for, 1624t, 1639–1640
GI bleeding and, 598
surgical excision and, 1639
dilation of. *See also* Megacolon
in acute colonic pseudo-obstruction (Ogilvie syndrome), 639, 640
disorders of, **643–669**. *See also specific disorder*
polyps of, **665–666**. *See also* Polyps/polyposis
colorectal cancer and, 665, 666, **666–669**, 1637, 1640
Colon cutoff sign, in pancreatitis, 727
Colonic CMV disease, 1375, 1376. *See also* Gastrointestinal system, disorders of, in CMV infection
Colonic inertia (slow colonic transit), constipation and, 584, 584t
Colonic pseudo-obstruction
acute (Ogilvie syndrome), **639–640**
chronic, **640–641**

Colonic transit time
constipation and, 584, 584t
normal, 584
Colonography, CT (virtual colonoscopy), 15, 665, 1638, 1642–1643
Colonoscopy
in cancer screening/evaluation, 14t, 15, 665–666, 666, 669, 1638, 1641t, 1642
after surgery, 1640
for colon decompression, 640
in diarrhea, 593
in GI bleeding
diagnostic, 598, 599, 600
therapeutic, 599
in HNPCC/Lynch syndrome, 669
in ischemic colitis, 479
in polyp identification/removal, 665–666, 666, 1642
bleeding after, 598, 666
surveillance, 666, 1640
in ulcerative colitis, 658
virtual, 15, 665, 1638, 1642–1643
Colorado tick fever, **1408–1409**
Colorectal cancer, 1624t, **1636–1643**, 1638f, 1641t
adjuvant/neoadjuvant therapy for, 1639–1640, 1640
aspirin/NSAIDs in prevention of, 1637
chemotherapy for, 1624t, 1639–1640
Crohn disease and, 654, 1637
diet and, 1637
familial adenomatous polyposis/family history and, 666, 667, 1637
genetic mutations associated with, 665, 667
fecal DNA assay in identification of, 665, 1641–1642
GI bleeding and, 598
hamartomatous polyposis syndromes and, **667–668**
hereditary, **666–669**, 1637
hereditary nonpolyposis (HNPCC/Lynch syndrome), **668–669**, 1637. *See also* Hereditary nonpolyposis colon cancer
incidence/risk/mortality of, 1608t, 1636, 1637–1638
inflammatory bowel disease and, 654, 661, 1637
metastatic, 1639–1640
nonfamilial adenomatous polyps and, 665, 666
pancreatic/periampullary carcinoma and, 1620
polyps/polyposis and, 665, 666, 1637, 1640
prevention of/screening for, 14t, 15, 665–666, 666, 669, 1638, 1640–1643, 1641t
chemoprevention and, 11, 1637
prophylactic surgery and, 667
primary sclerosing cholangitis and, 724, 725
prognosis for, 1640
staging of, 1638
surgery for, 1639
follow-up after, 1640
ulcerative colitis and, 661, 1637
Colostomy, 1639
Colostrum, 802

Colposcopy, 763t
in CIN, 770, 771
positive HPV tests and, 15
Columbia-Suicide Severity Risk Scale, 1077
CoLYTE. *See* Polyethylene glycol
Coma, **1026–1029**
assessment/emergency management of, 1027–1028, 1577, 1577–1578
diabetic/hyperglycemic, 1214, **1245**. *See also specific cause*
diabetic ketoacidosis and, 1214, 1245, 1246, 1246t, 1247
hyperglycemic hyperosmolar state and, 1214, 1245, 1246t, **1249–1251**
lactic acidosis and, 1245, 1246t, 1251
hypoglycemic, 1028, 1245, 1246t
in poisoning/drug overdose, 1578
hypothermia and, 1027, 1028, 1564, 1578
metabolic disturbances causing, 1027, **1028**. *See also* Metabolic encephalopathy
myxedema, 1120, 1122
in poisoning/drug overdose, 1246t, **1577–1578**
reversible, brain death differentiated from, 1028
in stroke, 995, 999, 1027, 1246t
structural lesions causing, 1027, **1028**
in subarachnoid hemorrhage, 999, 1027
Coma vigil (persistent vegetative state), **1028**
Combigan. *See* Brimonidine/timolol
Combination antiretroviral therapy. *See* Antiretroviral therapy
Combipatch, 1204
Combivir (zidovudine with lamivudine), 1353, 1353–1354
Comedones, in acne, 126, 127
Comfrey
sinusoidal obstruction syndrome caused by, 697, 711
toxicity of, 1593
Commissurotomy
mitral, 336, 336f
pulmonary valve, 323
Common ALL antigen, 528
Common cold (viral rhinosinusitis), **214–215**, 1420–1421
Common femoral artery, atherosclerotic/ occlusive disease of, 473–475
Common peroneal (fibular) nerve palsy, **1040**
Common variable immunodeficiency, 881t, **882–883**
Commotio cordis, 436–437, 438t
Community-acquired pneumonia, **267–272**, 269t, 1314t, 1445–1446. *See also* Pneumonia
chlamydial, 1487
in coccidioidomycosis, 1550
in HIV infection/AIDS, 1336
Legionnaires, 269, 1466–1467
Community-associated methicillin-resistant *S aureus* (CA-MRSA), 1447–1448, 1448f. *See also* Methicillin-resistant *S aureus* (MRSA) infections

impetigo caused by, 124
pneumonia caused by, 269, 269t, 271
Compartment syndrome
in burn patient
abdominal, 1569
fasciotomy for, 1569
in electrical burns, 1570, 1571
in frostbite, 1566
Compatibility testing, for transfusion, 542
Complement. *See also specific component*
disorders of, immunodeficiency and, 881t
in glomerulonephritis/ glomerulonephropathies, 922, 935f, **939–940**
in gonococcal arthritis, 869
immunization recommendations in deficiencies and, 1321t
in paroxysmal nocturnal hemoglobinuria, 509, 510
Complera (tenofovir [TDF]/ emtricitabine/rilpivirine), 1354t, 1355, 1359t
Complete abortion, 804
Complete (third-degree) heart block, 377, 399, 399–400. *See also* Atrioventricular (heart) block
Complete mole, 807
Complex 15, 100t
Complex drug eruptions, 161
Complex partial seizures (focal seizures with impairment of consciousness), 984, 984t. *See also* Seizures
schizophrenia differentiated from, 1068
Complex regional pain syndrome (reflex sympathetic dystrophy), **874–875**
Compliance/noncompliance (adherence/ nonadherence), 1–2. *See also specific disorder*
elderly patients and, 69
Compound nevi, 101, 101f
Compression chambers/centers. *See* Hyperbaric oxygen therapy; Recompression
Compression/entrapment neuropathy, 1039. *See also specific type or nerve affected and* Neuropathies
amyloidosis and, 1037
rheumatoid arthritis and, 835, 1037
Compression stockings
for leg ulcers, 156, 157, 490
for lower extremity edema/PE/DVT (venous thromboembolic disease), 33–34, 489, 490, 576
for lymphedema, 493
for varicose veins, 487
Compromised host. *See* Immunocompromised host
Compulsions, 1057. *See also* Obsessive-compulsive disorder
Compulsive water drinking. *See* Psychogenic polydipsia

Computed tomography (CT scans). *See also specific disorder and* Neuroimaging
in angina, 358
electron beam. *See* Electron beam CT
in hyperparathyroidism, 1155
in hyperthyroidism, 1128
in lung cancer screening, 14t, 15, 286, 1611
in pericarditis/effusion, 426, 428, 429
in pheochromocytoma/paraganglioma, 1182
in pulmonary embolism, 23, 28, 296–297, 297f
radiation exposure/cancer risk and, 1572, 1607
in thyroid cancer, 1142
Computed tomography angiography (CTA)
in angina/acute coronary syndromes/ STEMI/chest pain evaluation, 28, 358
in pulmonary embolism, 23, 28, 296–297, 297f
in renal artery stenosis/renal vascular hypertension, 442, 931
Computed tomography colography/ colonography (virtual colonoscopy), 15, 665, 1638, 1642–1643
Computerized stereotactic guided core needle breast biopsy, 744
COMT (catecholamine-*O*-methyltransferase) inhibitors, for parkinsonism, 1013–1014
Concussion, 1029, 1030, 1030t, 1031
labyrinthine, 211t, 212
Condoms, **790–791**
for contraception, **790–791**
for genital herpes prevention, 119, 1366
for gonorrhea prevention, 1476
for HIV infection/AIDS prevention, 4, 791, 1346
for STD prevention, 4, 791, 1303
for syphilis prevention, 1491
Conduction disturbances, **399–402**. *See also specific type and* Arrhythmias
in beta-blockers overdose/toxicity, 1591
intraventricular, **400**
in myocardial infarction, 27t, 377
Conduction velocity studies
in back pain evaluation, 1693
in motor neuron diseases, 1033
in neuropathies, 1034
Conductive-based cooling, for heat stroke, 1563
Conductive hearing loss, 200, 201. *See also* Hearing loss
Condylar groove, ulnar nerve lesions and, 1040
Condylomas (condylomata)
acuminata (venereal/genital warts), 140, 141–142, 141f, **768**
anal cancer and, 671, 1344, 1643–1644
anorectal involvement and, 141, 141f, 671, 768

cervical/vaginal/vulvar, **768**
HPV vaccination in prevention of, 141, 671, 768
lata, 141, 1489*t*, 1492–1493, 1493*f*
anorectal involvement and, 670, 1493*f*
Confusion, 1019, 1102. *See also* Cognitive disorders; Delirium
Confusion assessment method (CAM), 62
Congenital adrenal hyperplasia, 1169–1170
Congenital adrenal hypoplasia, 1108, 1109, 1169, 1191
Congenital adrenal insufficiency, 1169
Congenital heart disease, **322–331**. *See also specific disorder*
pregnancy and, 819
Congenital hypopituitarism, 1108
Congenital isolated hypogonadotropic hypogonadism, 1108, 1109
Congenital rubella syndrome, 1384, 1385
Congenital VZV syndrome, 821
Congestive heart failure. *See* Heart (cardiac) failure
Congo-Crimean hemorrhagic fever, 1390, 1399, 1400
Conivaptan, for hyponatremia/SIADH, 889
Conization of cervix, for CIN/cervical cancer, 771, 772
Conjugated equine estrogens. *See* Estrogen (hormone) replacement therapy
Conjunctiva
foreign body of, **196**
Kaposi sarcoma involving, 192
lacerations of, 197
Conjunctivitis, **166–174**, 166*t*. *See also specific type and* Keratoconjunctivitis
adenovirus causing, 166–167, 1421
allergic, 168
bacterial, **167**
chemical, **198**
coxsackievirus infection and, 167, 1426
enterovirus 70 causing, 167, 1427
gonococcal, **167**, 1475
inclusion, **167**
in loiasis, 1546
viral, **166–167**
Conn syndrome, 1177, 1178
Connective tissue disorders. *See also specific disorder*
cognitive disorders/delirium caused by, 1102*t*
Connexin-26 mutation, hearing loss and, 208
Consciousness
in absence seizures, 984
focal seizures with impairment of (complex partial seizures), 984, 984*t*
schizophrenia differentiated from, 1068
focal seizures without impairment of (simple partial seizures), 984, 984*t*
inconsistent evidence of, in minimally conscious state, 1029

in psychogenic nonepileptic/ pseudoepileptic seizures, 986, 1058
in tonic-clonic ("grand mal") seizures, 985
Constipation, **86**, **583–587**, 584*t*, 585*t*
anogenital pruritus and, 148
fecal impaction and, 586
opioid-induced, 82, 86, 586
palliation of, **86**
Constitutional delay in growth and puberty, 1189, 1199
Constrictive bronchiolitis, 266, 267. *See also* Bronchiolitis
Constrictive pericarditis, **428–429**
cardiac cirrhosis and, 700
restrictive cardiomyopathy differentiated from, 421, 429
Consumptive coagulopathy (DIC), **553–555**, 554*t*, **562**. *See also* Disseminated intravascular coagulation
"Consumptive hypothyroidism," 1119
Contact dermatitis, **124–126**, 125*f*
allergic, 124–126, 125*f*, 878–880
impetigo differentiated from, 124, 125
topical medications causing, 101, 124
urticaria in, 134
cellulitis differentiated from, 138
irritant, 124, 125
Contact lenses, 164
corneal infections/ulcers/ acanthamoeba keratitis and, 164, 174, 175
toxic/hypersensitivity reactions to cleaning solutions for, 199
Contact photosensitivity, 154. *See also* Photodermatitis
Contact ulcers, of arytenoid cartilage, 234–235
Contagious pustular dermatitis (orf), 1423
Continuous positive airway pressure (CPAP)
nasal, for sleep apnea, 317
postoperative pulmonary complication risk reduction and, 50
Continuous renal replacement therapy (continuous venovenous hemodiafiltration), for poisoning/drug overdose, 1583
Continuous subcutaneous insulin infusion (CSII) pumps, 1231–1232, 1234. *See also* Insulin infusion pumps
Contraception, **785–792**. *See also specific method*
emergency/postcoital, 785, **791**
IUD for, 789
for sexual violence (rape/sexual assault) victim, 791, 793, 794, 1302
fertility awareness and, **791**
sterilization for, **792**
Contraceptive foam/cream/film/sponge/ jelly/suppository, **790**
Contraceptive injections/implants, **788–789**

Contraceptive-related hypertension, 443, 786
Contraceptive transdermal patch, 789
Contraceptive vaginal ring, 789, 1205
Contraction alkalosis, 909
Contrast media
iodinated, for hyperthyroidism/Graves disease, 1130
thyroiditis and, 1124, 1137
nephrotoxicity/acute kidney injury and, 919
reactions to, 878
Contrast nephropathy, 919
Contrast venography, in DVT/PE (venous thromboembolic disease), 298
Contusions
cerebral, 1030*t*
of eye, **197**
myocardial, 434
Conversion disorder, 1058
psychogenic nonepileptic/ pseudoepileptic seizure and, 986, 1058
Convulsions. *See* Seizures
Cooley anemia, 505
Cooling
in heat exposure syndromes, 1562, 1563
for hyperthermia in poisoning/drug overdose, 1580
Coombs test/micro-Coombs test
in autoimmune hemolytic anemia, 514
in cold agglutinin disease, 515
in Waldenström macroglobulinemia, 538
CO-oximetry. *See* Pulse oximetry/ CO-oximetry
COP. *See* Cryptogenic organizing pneumonia/pneumonitis
Copaxone. *See* Glatiramer
COPD. *See* Chronic obstructive pulmonary disease
Copeptin, in acute coronary syndromes/ STEMI/chest pain evaluation, 28
Copper
accumulation of in Wilson disease, 710
parenteral nutritional support and, 1283, 1285*t*
Copper-containing IUD, 789
for emergency/postcoital contraception, 789, 791
Copper-transporting adenosine triphosphatase, in Wilson disease, 710
Coprine (*Coprinus*) mushroom poisoning, 1600*t*
Cor pulmonale, in COPD, 258, 262
Coral snake antivenom, 1604
Coral snake envenomation, 1604
Cord blood, stem cells in, for transplantation, 540–541
Cord cavitation (syringomyelia), **1032**
Corditis, polypoid, 234
Cordran. *See* Flurandrenolide
"Core-binding factor" leukemias, 527
Core body temperature (CBT), 1561. *See also* Body temperature
in burn injury, maintaining, 1569
in drowning, 1567

Core body temperature (CBT) (*Cont.*):
in hyperthermia/heat exposure
syndromes, 1562, 1563
in hypothermia, 1564
normal, 34
Core needle (large-needle) biopsy, for
breast lump evaluation, 743,
744. *See also* Breast, biopsy
of
Coreg/Coreg CR. *See* Carvedilol
Corgard. *See* Nadolol
Corlopam. *See* Fenoldopam
Cornea
foreign body of, **196**
infection of, 166*t*. *See also* Keratitis;
Keratoconjunctivitis
trauma to, 166*t*
abrasions, **197**
chemical burns (conjunctivitis and
keratitis), **198**
lacerations, 197–198, 197*f*
ulcers of, **174**. *See also* Keratitis
contact lens wear and, 164, 174
in herpes simplex keratitis, 175,
1363, 1364, 1364–1366
ultraviolet burns of (ultraviolet/actinic
keratitis), **198**
Corneoscleral lacerations, 197–198,
197*f*
Coronary angiography. *See* Angiography/
arteriography, cardiac/
coronary
Coronary angioplasty
for angina, 362–363
rescue, 376
Coronary arteries
disorders of
atherosclerotic, **352–381**. *See also*
Coronary heart disease
in Kawasaki syndrome, 1439
in pregnancy, **435–436**
sudden death and, 397
of athlete, 436, 437, 438*t*
traumatic injury to, 434
vasospasm of, 356, **364–365**
Coronary artery bypass grafting (CABG),
363
for acute coronary syndromes/STEMI,
367*f*, 380–381
for angina, 363
antiplatelet therapy/platelet function
and, 558*t*
for heart failure, 410
PCI compared with, 362–363
PCI for stenoses and, 362
prophylactic/preoperative,
46–47
Coronary artery disease (CAD). *See*
Coronary heart disease
Coronary artery revascularization
procedures. *See specific type*
and Revascularization
procedures
Coronary heart disease, **352–381**. *See also*
Acute coronary syndromes;
Angina; Myocardial
infarction
acute coronary syndromes without
ST-segment elevation
(NSTEMI) and, **365–370**,
367*f*, 369*t*

acute myocardial infarction with
ST-segment elevation
(STEMI) and, 26–27, 27, 27*t*,
28, 365, 369*t*, **370–381**, 372*f*,
373*t*. *See also* Myocardial
infarction
in alkaptonuria, 1677
angina pectoris (chronic stable) and,
355–364, 360*f*, 363*t*
antihypertensive drug therapy and, 10,
360*f*, 362, 446, 447*f*, 448*t*,
464
aortic stenosis and, 342
aspirin/chemoprevention for, 6*t*,
10–11, 355. *See also*
Lipid-lowering therapy
in diabetes, 1241–1242
cholesterol/lipoproteins in, 10, 353,
1259–1260
screening tests for levels of, 6*t*, 10,
1261–1262
in women/older adults, 1261,
1262
chronic kidney disease and, 926
in diabetes mellitus, 1241–1242
glycemic control and, 361–362
estrogen replacement therapy and,
1202
heart failure and, 358, 370, 377–378,
410
in HIV infection/AIDS, 1345, 1356
homocysteine/hyperhomocysteinemia
in, 1681
hypertension/hypertension prevention/
management and, 6*t*, 10, 356,
360*f*, 362, 439, 440, 443–444,
446, 447*f*, 448*t*, 464
lipid disorders and, 10, 353,
1259–1260
metabolic syndrome and, 353
myocardial hibernation/stunning and,
353
perioperative evaluation/management
and, 46–47, 47*f*, 47*t*
in pregnancy, **435–436**, 819
prevention of, **5–11**, 6*t*, 8–9*t*, 9*t*,
353–355, 354*f*, 355*t*, 1259,
1260. *See also* Lipid-lowering
therapy
cholesterol screening and,
1261–1262
lipid-lowering therapy and,
1262–1266, 1264*t*, 1265*t*. *See*
also Lipid-lowering therapy
revascularization procedures for,
358–359, 360*f*, 362–363,
380–381. *See also*
Revascularization procedures
risk/risk stratification for, 5–6,
352–353, 354*f*, 361–362
lipoproteins/lipid fractions and, 353,
1259–1260
sudden death and, 397
in athletes, 436, 437
vasospasm and, 356, **364–365**
Coronary reperfusion. *See* Reperfusion
therapy
Coronary sinus atrial septal defect, 325
Coronary stents, 362–363, 373. *See also*
Percutaneous coronary
intervention

antiplatelet therapy for patient with,
362, 373, 374
preoperative/perioperative risks and,
46–47
thrombotic events and, 362, 368, 373,
374, 376
Coronary vasospasm, 356, **364–365**
Coronavirus, Middle East respiratory
syndrome caused by,
1419–1420
Corrigan pulse, 346
Corrosive agents. *See* Caustic/corrosive
agents
Corti, organ of, hearing loss caused by
disorders of, 200
Cortical blindness, 1005
Corticobasal degeneration, parkinsonism
and, 1012
Corticosteroids, 95, 96–98*t*. *See also*
specific agent and disease
acne/folliculitis caused by, 127, 130
for adhesive capsulitis (frozen
shoulder), 1691–1692
for adrenal insufficiency/Addison
disease, 1111
adverse effects of, 650, 1208–1209
ophthalmic, 95, 178*t*
for allergic eye disease, 171–172*t*, 174
for allergic rhinitis, 219
for ARDS, 321
for aspergillosis, 1555
for asthma, 244*t*, 247*f*, 248, 249*t*, 250*t*,
252, 253–254*t*, 254, 255*f*
exacerbation management and, 244*t*,
247*f*, 248, 252, 253–254*t*, 254
inhaled, 247*f*, 248, 250*t*, 256*f*
in pregnant patient, 819
systemic, 244*t*, 247*f*, 248, 249*t*, 252,
253–254*t*, 254, 255*f*, 256*f*
for atopic dermatitis, 105, 106
for autoimmune hemolytic anemia,
514
for Bell palsy, 1041, 1366
in cancer chemotherapy, 1670*t*
for cancer-related hypercalcemia, 1660
for chronic inflammatory
polyneuropathy, 1039
clinical use of, **1208–1209**, 1209*t*
for contact dermatitis, 125–126
for COPD, 260–261, 262
Cushing syndrome caused by, 1172,
1173
for cysticercosis, 266, 1536
depression caused by, 1076
diabetes/insulin resistance and, 1213
for eosinophilic esophagitis, 613
for exfoliative dermatitis/
erythroderma, 117
for fetal lung maturity, 810, 811
for giant cell arteritis, 188, 854, 855
for gout, 831–832
for granulomatosis with polyangiitis,
859
for Graves ophthalmopathy, 195
for herpes zoster/varicella zoster
infection, 121
for immune thrombocytopenia,
549–550, 549*f*
for inflammatory bowel disease, 650
Crohn disease, 655–656
ulcerative colitis, 659, 660

intra-articular
  for gout, 832
  for osteoarthritis, 829, 1714
  for rheumatoid arthritis, 837
for lichen planus, 145
for lumbar disk herniation, 1695
for lupus/SLE, 115, 841, 842
management of patient receiving,
     1208–1209, 1209*t*
for meningitis, 1299, 1447, 1484
for minimal change disease, 943
for multiple sclerosis, 1024, 1024*t*
for myasthenia gravis, 1046
for nasal polyps, 222
for nausea and vomiting, 87, 582–583,
     582*t*
for ophthalmic disorders, 168,
     171–172*t*, 174
  precautions for use of, **198–199**
osteoporosis/osteoporosis prevention
     and, 650, 1160, 1208–1209
in pain management, 84
for pemphigus, 140
perioperative, 53
for *Pneumocystis* infection, 1336,
     1337*t*, 1552
for polyarteritis nodosa, 856
for polymyositis/dermatomyositis, 849
in pregnant patient, 819, 1208
for prostate cancer, 1649*t*
for psoriasis/psoriatic arthritis, 107,
     108, 865
for rheumatic fever/heart disease, 424
for rheumatoid arthritis, 836–837
rosacea caused by, 128
for shock, 497
for skin disorders, 95, 96–98*t*
for spinal stenosis, 1694
for spinal trauma/compression, 1032,
     1658
strongyloidiasis in patients taking,
     1540
for sudden sensory hearing loss, 200,
     201, 208
surgery in patients taking,
     perioperative replacement
     and, 53, 1111
for Takayasu arteritis, 855
for thyroid eye disease, 195
topical, 95, 96–98*t*
  for ophthalmic disorders, 168,
     171–172*t*, 174
  side effects of, 101
for urticaria, 134
Cortinarius mushroom poisoning, 1600*t*
Cortisol. *See also* Corticosteroids
  ACTH deficiency and, 1109–1110,
     1110
  in adrenal insufficiency/Addison
     disease, 1110, 1168, 1170,
     1171
  excess of, **1172–1177.** *See also* Cushing
     syndrome
  familial resistance to, 1174
  insufficiency of, 1109–1110, 1110. *See
     also* Adrenal insufficiency
    in acute adrenal (addisonian) crisis,
     1168–1169
    in adrenal insufficiency/Addison
     disease, 1109–1110, 1110,
     1168, 1171

  in HIV infection/AIDS, 1171, 1343
  hypoglycemia and, 1237
  levels of in Cushing syndrome
     diagnosis, 1174
Cortisol withdrawal syndrome, 1176
Corynebacterium
     diphtheriae, 1312*t*, 1456. *See also*
     Diphtheria
     jeikeium, 1312*t*
Corzide. *See* Nadolol, with
     bendroflumethazide
Cosmegen. *See* Dactinomycin
Cosopt/Cosopt PF. *See* Dorzolamide/
     dorzolamide and timolol
Cosyntropin test
  in adrenal insufficiency/Addison
     disease, 1110
  after pituitary surgery, 1175
  in hirsutism/virilization, 1197
Cotellic. *See* Cobimetinib
Cough, **19–22,** 20*t*. *See also specific cause*
  blood production and (hemoptysis),
     25–26
  drugs causing, 310*t*
  headache associated with, **980**
  in heart failure, 19, 20
Coumadin. *See* Warfarin
Counterpulsation, extracorporeal, for
     angina, 363
Courvoisier law/sign, 676
Coveram. *See* Perindopril, for
     hypertension, with
     amlodipine
Cowden syndrome/disease, 668, 1189
  thyroid cancer and, 1137, 1141
COX-1/COX-2, aspirin/NSAIDs
     affecting, 624, 828
  peptic ulcer disease and, 624, 829
COX-2 inhibitors. *See* Coxibs
Coxibs (COX-2 inhibitors), 74, 621
  cardiovascular complications
     associated with, 621, 624,
     829
  for familial adenomatous polyposis,
     667
  gastritis and, 74, 621
  lithium interactions and, 1087*t*
  for osteoarthritis, 828, 829, 1714
  in pain management, 74
  peptic ulcers/peptic ulcer prevention
     and, 74, 621, 624, 626*t*, 627,
     628, 829
Coxiella burnetii, 1429*t*, 1436–1437, 1437,
     1438
Coxsackievirus infections, **1425–1426**
  herpes stomatitis differentiated from,
     227
Cozaar. *See* Losartan
CPAP. *See* Continuous positive airway
     pressure
CPP. *See* Chronic pelvic pain
CPPD. *See* Calcium pyrophosphate
     deposition disease
CPR. *See* Cardiopulmonary resuscitation
Cr. *See* Creatinine
"Crab yaws," 1498
Crabs (pubic lice), 149–150. *See also*
     Lice
Crack cocaine. *See* Cocaine/cocaine abuse
Crackles (rales), in pulmonary embolism,
     296*t*

CRAG (cryptococcal antigen) test, 1340,
     1553
Cramps (menstrual). *See*
     Dysmenorrhea
Cranial arteritis. *See* Giant cell (temporal/
     cranial) arteritis
Cranial nerve VIII (acoustic nerve)
     lesions. *See* Schwannoma,
     vestibular
Cranial nerve palsies. *See also specific
     type*
  brainstem lesions causing, 1005
  in diabetes, 1240
  in head injury, 1029–1030
  in malignant external otitis, 202
  ocular motor palsies and, 194
  in sarcoidosis, 1037
  vertebrobasilar occlusion causing,
     995
Cranial neuropathies, glomus tumor
     causing, 207
Craniopharyngioma, 1003, 1004*t*, 1111,
     1199
CRB-65, 272
Creatine (supplement), toxicity of, 1593
Creatine kinase-MB (CK-MB), in acute
     coronary syndromes/STEMI,
     366, 371
Creatinine, 915
  ascitic fluid, 602
  in diabetic ketoacidosis, 1246
  urinary
    in Cushing syndrome diagnosis,
     1174
    ratio of to urinary protein, 914. *See
     also* Proteinuria
Creatinine:blood urea nitrogen ratio, 915,
     917*t*
Creatinine clearance, 915
  perioperative management of
     anticoagulation therapy and,
     52*t*
Creeping eruption, **1542–1543,**
     1543*f*
Crescentic glomerulonephritis, 933*t*, 935*f*,
     938
CREST syndrome, 840*t*, 845, 846. *See also*
     Scleroderma
  Raynaud phenomenon and, 844
Crestor. *See* Rosuvastatin
Cretinism, 1148, 1149. *See also*
     Hypothyroidism
Creutzfeldt-Jakob disease, 1022,
     1393–1394
  myoclonus in, 1017
  parkinsonism and, 1012
Cricothyrotomy, **237–238**
  for foreign body removal, 238
Crigler-Najjar syndrome, 674
Crimean-Congo hemorrhagic fever, 1390,
     1399, 1400
Critical illness
  community-acquired pneumonia and,
     269*t*, 271, 272
  diabetes management and, 1244
  fever/health care-associated infection
     and, 34, 1294, 1295, 1296
  hypercalcemia and, 1156
  hypercortisolism and, 1174
  neuropathy associated with, **1037**
  psychosis associated with, 1105

Critical illness (*Cont.*):
  shock liver/cardiogenic liver injury and, 712–713
  stress gastritis associated with, 319, 620, 620–621
Critical limb ischemia, 475
Crixivan. *See* Indinavir
Crizotinib, 1667*t*
  for lung cancer, 1612
CroFab, for snake bites, 1604
Crohn disease, 650, **652–657**. *See also* Inflammatory bowel disease
  arthritis in, 653, 867
  colorectal cancer and, 654, 1637
  diarrhea in, 592, 653, 655
  small intestine adenocarcinoma and, 654
  social support and, 652
  vitamin B$_{12}$ deficiency and, 507
Crohn's and Colitis Foundation of America (CCFA), 652
Crolom. *See* Cromolyn
Cromolyn
  for allergic eye disease, 168, 170*t*
  for allergic rhinitis, 219
  for asthma, 247*f*, 248–251, 249*t*
Crossmatching, in blood compatibility testing, 542
Cross-reactivity/sensitivity, in drug allergies, 1318
Cross-resistance, in antiretroviral therapy, 1355, 1361, 1362
Crotalid antivenin (CroFab), 1604
Croup, human parainfluenza virus causing, 1409
Crowned dens syndrome, 834
CRP. *See* C-reactive protein
Cruciate ligaments of knee, 1704
  injury of
    anterior cruciate (ACL), **1705–1710**, 1706*t*
    posterior cruciate (PCL), 1708*t*, **1711**
Crusted/weeping skin lesions, 96*t*, **123–126**. *See also specific type*
  drying agents for, 95
Cryoglobulins/cryoglobulinemia, **860–861**
  glomerulonephritis and, 860, 933*t*, 935*f*, **939**
  hepatitis C and, 683, 691, 860, 860–861, 939, 940
  neuropathies and, 860, 1037
  Raynaud phenomenon and, 845
Cryoprecipitate, 544
  for DIC, 554
Cryotherapy/cryosurgery. *See also* Liquid nitrogen
  for CIN/cervical cancer, 771, 772
  for prostate cancer, 1648
  for wart removal/condylomata acuminata, 141, 768
Cryptococcal antigen (CRAG) test, 1340, 1553
Cryptococcomas, 1553
Cryptococcus gattii/neoformans (cryptococcosis), **1553–1554**
  in HIV infection/AIDS, 1006, 1337*t*, 1340, 1553, 1554
  meningitis caused by, 1006, 1337*t*, 1553, 1553–1554

Cryptogenic organizing pneumonia/ pneumonitis (COP/ bronchiolitis obliterans with organizing pneumonia/ BOOP), 267, 291*t*, 292
Cryptogenic stroke. *See also* Stroke
  patent foramen ovale and, 326
Cryptorchism, **1194**
  pseudohermaphroditism and, 1200–1201
  testicular cancer and, 1190, 1194, 1655
Cryptosporidium hominis/parvum (cryptosporidiosis), 588*t*, 592, 1305, 1342, **1527–1530**
Crystal deposition arthritis, **829–834**, 830*t*, 831*f*, 832*t*
Crystalloids, for fluid management/ volume replacement, 912
  in burn injuries, 1569
  in shock, 496
CS-8958 (laninamivir), 1365*t*, 1412
CSF analysis. *See* Cerebrospinal fluid analysis
CSF FTA-ABS test, 1496
CSF-VDRL test, 1496
CSII. *See* Continuous subcutaneous insulin infusion (CSII) pumps
CT angiography. *See* Computed tomography; Helical (spiral) CT
CT colonography (virtual colonoscopy), 15, 665, 1638, 1642–1643
CT-FFR (fractional flow reserve), in angina, 358
  coronary revascularization and, 358–359
CT scans. *See* Computed tomography
CTA. *See* Computed tomography angiography
CTCL. *See* Cutaneous T-cell lymphoma
CTEPH. *See* Chronic thromboembolic pulmonary hypertension
Cubicin. *See* Daptomycin
Cubital tunnel, ulnar nerve lesions and, 1040
Cultural issues, in end-of-life care, 91
Culture-negative endocarditis, 1459–1460, 1462
Culture-negative neutrocytic ascites, 603
Cunninghamella infection, 1555–1556
Cup-disk ratio, in chronic glaucoma, 180
Cupping, optic disk, in chronic glaucoma, 179, 180
Cupulolithiasis, vertigo associated with, 211*t*, 212
Curative efforts, withdrawal of in terminally ill/dying patient, 91–92, 92*t*
  advance directives and, 90
CURB-65, 272
Curettage. *See* D&C; Endocervical curettage; Endometrial biopsy
Curvularia, phaeohyphomycosis caused by, 1558
Cushing disease, 1173, 1174, 1175, 1176. *See also* Cushing syndrome
  persistence/recurrence of after pituitary surgery, 1175, 1176

Cushing syndrome (hypercortisolism), **1172–1177**
  amenorrhea in, 1199
  hirsutism/virilization in, 1196, 1197
  hypertension and, 443, 1176
  medical therapy for, 1176
  pancreatic neuroendocrine tumors causing, 1173
Cutaneous anthrax, 1454, 1455, 1456
Cutaneous (mucocutaneous) candidiasis, **132–133**, 132*f*
Cutaneous drug reactions, **161–163**, 162–163*t*, **880**
  drug-induced hypersensitivity syndrome and, 161, 163, 880
Cutaneous larva migrans, **1542–1543**, 1543*f*
Cutaneous leishmaniasis, 1510, 1510–1511, 1511, 1511*f*, 1512
  post-kala azar, 1510
Cutaneous lupus erythematosus, discoid/ subacute/chronic, **115–116**, 839*t*, 840
Cutaneous T-cell lymphoma (mycosis fungoides), **116–117**
  exfoliative dermatitis/erythroderma and, 117
Cutaneous tests. *See specific type and* Skin tests
Cutting (self-mutilation), 1059
CVP. *See* Central venous pressure
Cyanide antidotes, 1581*t*, 1593
Cyanide poisoning, 23, 24, 305, 1581*t*, **1592–1593**
Cyanocobalamin. *See* Vitamin B$_{12}$
Cyanogenic plants, 1592
Cyanokit, 1593
Cyberknife surgery, for pituitary tumor, 1116
Cyclic citrullinated peptide (CCP) antibody, in rheumatoid arthritis, 835
Cyclic neutropenia, 518
Cyclic thrombocytopenia, **548**
Cyclin D1, in chronic lymphocytic leukemia, 530
Cyclin dependent kinase inhibition, for breast cancer, 756
Cycling, in bipolar disorder, 1076
  lithium use and, 1085
Cyclooxygenase-1 and 2 (COX-1/ COX-2), aspirin/NSAIDs affecting, 624, 828
  peptic ulcer disease and, 624, 829
Cyclooxygenase-2 (COX-2) inhibitors. *See* Coxibs
Cyclophosphamide, 1663*t*. *See also* Immunosuppressive therapy
  for breast cancer, 751, 753
  breastfeeding and, 798*t*
  for chronic lymphocytic leukemia, 530
  for granulomatosis with polyangiitis, 859
  hemorrhagic cystitis caused by, 1674
  interstitial cystitis caused by, 960, 961
  for lupus nephritis, 841, 941
  for microscopic polyangiitis, 860
  for scleroderma, 847
  toxicity of, 859, 1663*t*, 1674
Cycloserine (DCS), for phobic disorders, 1056

Cycloset. *See* Bromocriptine
Cyclospora cayetanensis (cyclosporiasis), 588*t*, 592, 1305, **1527–1530**
Cyclosporine
  adverse ophthalmic effects of, 178*t*
  for aplastic anemia, 517
  hyperkalemia caused by, 894
  insulin secretion affected by, 1213
  nefazodone interaction and, 1081
  nephrotoxicity/acute kidney injury/ graft rejection caused by, 919
  for ophthalmic disorders/dry eye, 168, 172*t*
  for psoriasis, 108
  for ulcerative colitis, 661
Cyclothymic disorders, 1076, 1085
Cycrin. *See* Progesterone
CYD-TDV vaccine, for dengue, 1403–1404
Cymbalta. *See* Duloxetine
CYP 2C9 variants, warfarin and, 572
CYP 2C19
  cimetidine and, 628
  clopidogrel and, 628
CYP17 (17-hydroxylase/P450c17) deficiency, 1169, 1190, 1199
CYP17a1 inhibition, for prostate cancer, 1190, 1649*t*
Cyproheptadine. *See also* Antihistamines
  for drug-induced anorgasmia, 1079
  for serotonin syndrome, 36, 1580, 1606
Cyproterone, for hirsutism/virilization, 1198
Cyramza. *See* Ramucirumab
Cystadenocarcinoma, of liver, 716
Cystadenoma
  of liver, 716
  pancreatic, 1620–1621, 1621, 1625
Cystathionine beta-synthase *(CBS)* gene, 1681
Cystathionine beta-synthase deficiency, in hypercysteinemia/ homocystinuria, 1681
Cysteine, supplementary, for homocystinuria, 1681
Cystic fibrosis, **264–266**
  bronchiectasis and, 263, 265
  COPD differentiated from, 259
  genetic/prenatal testing for, 265, 266, 800
  infertility and, 265, 969, 970
  pancreatitis and, 265, 731, 732
Cystic fibrosis transmembrane conductance regulator (CFTR) corrector therapy, 266
Cystic fibrosis transmembrane conductance regulator (CFTR) protein, 265
  mutations in gene for
    genetic/prenatal testing for, 265, 266
    in pancreatitis, 726, 731
Cystic hydatid disease, 1537, 1537–1538
Cystic inflammatory acne, 126–127, 126*f*, 127–128
Cystic medial necrosis, sudden death in athlete and, 436
Cysticercosis, 1535, **1536–1537**
Cystine urinary stones, 961, 962, 964
Cystinuria, 962
Cystitis, 42–44, 44*f*, **954–955**, 955*t*, 1315*t*

in female, 42–44, 44*f*, 954–955
  hemorrhagic. *See* Hemorrhagic cystitis
  interstitial, 43, **960–961**
  in male, 954, 955
Cystocele, 777
Cystoscopy, 953
  in benign prostatic hyperplasia, 972
  in hematuria, 953
  in interstitial cystitis, 961
Cystourethroscopy, in bladder cancer, 1652
Cytadren. *See* Aminoglutethimide
Cytarabine, 1664*t*
  mucositis caused by, 1673
Cytochrome P450 (CYP) 2C9 variants, warfarin and, 572
Cytochrome P450 (CYP) 2C19 variants
  cimetidine and, 628
  clopidogrel and, 628
Cytokine neutralization, immunodeficiency disorders caused by, 881
Cytolytic snake venom, 1604
Cytomegalovirus (CMV) disease, **1374–1377**
  esophageal, 611, 611–612, 1375
  gastritis/diarrhea, 588*t*, 589, 592, 623, 1342, 1375
  in immunocompetent host, 1374, 1375
  in immunocompromised host/HIV infection/AIDS, 611–612, 1291–1292, 1336–1338, 1338*t*, 1341, 1374–1375, 1375, 1376
    prophylaxis of, 191, 1291–1292, 1376
  mononucleosis, 1373, 1374, 1375
  perinatal/congenital, 1374, 1375, 1376
  posttransplant, 1291–1292, 1374, 1376
  prevention of, 1291–1292, 1376
  retinitis, 191–192, 1338*t*, 1341, 1374, 1375, 1376
  transfusion in transmission of, 543–544
Cytomegalovirus (CMV) immune globulin, 1376
Cytomegalovirus (CMV) inclusion disease, 1374, 1375
Cytomel. *See* Triiodothyronine
Cytopenia
  autoimmune, common variable immunodeficiency and, 882
  methotrexate causing, 837
  in myelodysplastic syndromes, 525, 526
Cytosar U. *See* Cytarabine
Cytotoxic drugs. *See specific agent and* Chemotherapy
Cytoxan. *See* Cyclophosphamide

d4T. *See* Stavudine
D antigen, in compatibility testing, 542
D&C, 763*t*
D cells, pancreatic, 1185
D-cycloserine (DCS), for phobic disorders, 1056
D-dimer fibrin
  in DIC, 554
  in DVT/PE (venous thromboembolic disease), 33, 295, 573
D state sleep, 1088

Dabigatran, 564, 565–566*t*, 567, 573
  for atrial fibrillation/stroke prevention, 391–393, 391*t*, 564, 565*t*
  cardiac valve replacement and, 351, 391
  for DVT/PE (venous thromboembolic disease), 564, 565*t*, 570*t*, 573
  overdose/toxicity of, 564, 566*t*, 1588
  perioperative management of, 52*t*, 566*t*
  for transient ischemic attacks, 993
Dabrafenib, 1667*t*
Dacarbazine, 1663*t*
Daclatasvir, for hepatitis C, 690*t*, 691
Dacogen. *See* Decitabine
Dacryocystitis, **166**
Dactinomycin, 1669*t*
Dalbavancin, for staphylococcal skin infections, 1448
Dalfampridine, for multiple sclerosis, 1025
Dalfopristin/quinupristin, for *E faecium* infection, 1444, 1445
Dalmane. *See* Flurazepam
Dalteparin, for DVT/PE (venous thromboembolic disease), 568*t*, 570*t*
Danazol
  for autoimmune hemolytic anemia, 514
  for endometriosis, 776
  for fibrocystic condition, 735
Dandruff, 110
Danoprevir, for hepatitis C, 691
Dantrolene
  for neuroleptic malignant syndrome/ malignant hyperthermia, 36, 1072, 1294, 1580, 1590
  for spasticity, 1025–1026
Dapagliflozin, 1222*t*, 1227
  with metformin, 1228
Dapsone
  for acne, 98*t*
  G6PD deficiency and, 511, 1291
  HLA-B-associated drug hypersensitivity and, 880
  for leprosy, 1484
  methemoglobinemia caused by, 1599
  for *P jirovecii* infection, 1291, 1337*t*, 1349*t*, 1350, 1552
    prophylactic, 1349*t*
  in toxoplasmosis, 1350, 1525
Daptomycin, for skin and soft tissue infections, 1443, 1443*t*
Daranide. *See* Dichlorphenamide
Daratumumab, 1666*t*
Darbepoetin alfa
  for anemia of chronic disease/chronic kidney disease, 503, 928
  for aplastic anemia, 517
  for chemotherapy-induced anemia, 1662, 1671*t*
Darkfield microscopic examination
  in non-sexually transmitted treponematoses, 1498
  in syphilis, 1489, 1493
Darunavir, 1357
  with cobicistat, 1352*t*, 1356, 1357
    and Epzicom (abacavir/lamivudine), 1360*t*
    and Truvada (emtricitabine/ tenofovir [TDF]), 1360*t*

Darunavir (*Cont.*):
  with ritonavir, 1352t, 1357
    plus Epzicom (abacavir/lamivudine), 1360t
    plus Truvada (emtricitabine/tenofovir [TDF]), 1359t
Darzalex. *See* Daratumumab
Dasabuvir, for hepatitis C, 690t, 691, 1341, 1342
Dasatinib, 1667t
  for chronic myeloid leukemia, 524–525
DASH diet, in hypertension/hypertension prevention, 445, 446t
"Date-rape" drug (gamma-hydroxybutyrate/GHB), **1595**
  Cushing syndrome and, 1173, 1174
Datril. *See* Acetaminophen
Datura stramonium, toxicity of, 1590
Daunorubicin/daunomycin, 1665t
  for Kaposi sarcoma, 1338t
  liposomal, 1665t
  toxicity of, 1665t, 1674–1675
Daunoxome. *See* Liposomal daunorubicin
Dawn phenomenon, 1234, 1234t
Daypro. *See* Oxaprozin
DC cardioversion. *See* Cardioversion
DCC gene, in colorectal cancer, 1637
DCCT (Diabetes Control and Complications Trial), 1217–1218, 1244–1245
DCIS. *See* Ductal carcinoma in situ
DCS. *See* D-cycloserine
DDAVP. *See* Desmopressin
ddI. *See* Didanosine
de Morsier syndrome (septo-optic dysplasia), 1108
De Quervain (subacute) thyroiditis, 1125, 1128, 1131, 1135, 1136–1137
  hypothyroid phase in, 1119, 1125, 1135
Deafness. *See* Hearing loss
Death. *See also* End of life; Sudden death
  Kübler-Ross' patterns of emotions and, 92
  leading/preventable causes of, 2, 2t, 3t. *See also* Preventive care
  patient expectations about, 88
  tasks after, **93–94**
Death certificate, 93
Debridement, in burn care, 1569
Decerebrate (extensor) posturing, 1027
Decision making, medical
  advance directives and, 90
  determination of older patient's capacity for, 58
  self neglect and, 70
  at end of life, 90
Decitabine, 1664t
  for myelodysplastic syndromes, 526
Decompression sickness, **1572–1573**
  barotrauma and, 204, 1572, 1573
Decongestants
  for bacterial rhinosinusitis, 216
  overdose/toxicity of, 1592
  ophthalmic, 177t
  for viral rhinosinusitis (common cold), 214–215
Decontamination
  eye, **1581**
    for caustic/corrosive burns, 1581, 1587

gastrointestinal, **1581–1583**
    caustic/corrosive agent ingestion and, 1586, 1587
  skin, **1581**
    for caustic/corrosive burns, 1581, 1586–1587, 1587
Decorticate (flexor) posturing, 1027
Decubitus ulcers. *See* Pressure ulcers
Dedicator of cytokinesis (DOCK8) deficiency, molluscum contagiosum in, 1423
De-efferented state (locked-in syndrome), **1029**
Deep brain stimulation
  for depression, 1084
  for OCD, 1057
  for parkinsonism, 1014
  for seizures, 989
Deep breathing exercises, postoperative pulmonary complications and, 50
Deep neck infections, **230**
"Deep sulcus" sign, in pneumothorax, 315
Deep venous thrombosis, 32, 33, 33t. *See also* Venous thromboembolic disease
  air travel and, 33, 1576
  in antiphospholipid antibody syndrome, 815, 816, 841, 843
  in Behçet syndrome, 862
  cellulitis differentiated from, 138
  estrogen replacement therapy and, 1202, 1203
  in granulomatosis with polyangiitis, 857
  hypercoagulability and, 295, 574, 575t
  joint replacement and, 298–300, 1703
  lower extremity edema and, 32, 33, 33t
  prevention of, 298–300, 567–569, 567t, 568t, 569t
    contraindications to, 569, 569t
  pulmonary embolism and, 294, 295, 297. *See also* Pulmonary venous thromboembolism
  risk/risk stratification for, 32, 33t, 295, 296t, 298, 298t, 299f, 299t, 567–568, 567t, 569–571, 571t, 573–574, 574t, 575t
  treatment of, 569–577, 570t, 571t, 572t, 573t, 574t, 575t, 576t
    anticoagulation, 300, 569–576, 570t, 571t, 572t, 573t, 574t, 575t
    nonpharmacologic, 301, 576–577
    thrombolytic therapy, 300–301, 576, 576t
  venous insufficiency/stasis and, 32, 33, 33t, 488
Deer tick virus, 1391
Defecation, dyssynergic (pelvic floor dyssynergia), 584, 584t, 585
Defecography, 585
Deferasirox
  adverse ophthalmic effects of, 179t
  for hemochromatosis/iron toxicity, 526, 709
  in mucormycosis, 1556
Deferiprone, for hemochromatosis/iron toxicity, 709

Deferoxamine
  adverse ophthalmic effects of, 179t
  for hemochromatosis/iron toxicity, 709, 1584t, 1596
Defibrillation. *See* Cardioversion
Defibrillator cardioverter, implantable. *See* Implantable cardioverter defibrillator
Defibrotide, for sinusoidal obstruction syndrome, 712
Degarelix, 1670t
  for prostate cancer, 1649, 1649t
Degenerative (calcific) aortic stenosis, 341
Degenerative joint disease, **826–829**, 828f. *See also* Arthritis; Osteoarthritis
  in alkaptonuria, 1677, 1678
Dehydration. *See* Volume status
Dehydroemetine, for amebiasis, 1526, 1527t
Dehydroepiandrosterone/dehydroepiandrosterone sulfate (DHEA/DHEAS)
  adrenal insufficiency/Addison disease and, 1110, 1170, 1172
  hirsutism/virilization and, 1197
  for hypopituitarism and hypogonadism, 1111–1112
Dejerine-Sottas disease, 1035
Delavirdine, 1351t, 1356. *See also* Antiretroviral therapy
Delayed adolescence/puberty. *See* Puberty
Delayed hypersensitivity, 876, **878–881**
Delirium, **61–62**, 87, 1019, 1102–1103, 1102t, 1103, 1103–1104
  alcohol use disorder/withdrawal and, 1093, 1102t
  anticholinergic, hallucinogens causing, 1598
  antipsychotics causing, 58, 62, 1071
  dementia and, 57, 58, 1019, 1102–1103, 1102t
  in elderly, **61–62**
    dementia and, 57, 58
    at end of life, **87**
    urinary incontinence and, 65
  hospitalization/illness and, 61, 62, 1104
  lithium causing, 1086
  palliation of, **87**
  postoperative, 52–53, 52t
  terminal (terminal restlessness), 87, 1103
Delirium tremens, 1093
Delivery (childbirth). *See* Labor and delivery
Delta agent (hepatitis D virus/HDV), D, 682, 684, 687. *See also* Hepatitis
"Delta" sleep, 1088
Delta⁹-tetrahydrocannabinol
  for HIV wasting, 1335
  for nausea and vomiting, 87, 583
    in HIV infection/AIDS, 1335
Delusional disorders, 1066
Delusions
  in psychotic major depression, 1075
  in schizophrenia/psychotic disorders, 1066, 1067
Demadex. *See* Torsemide
Demeclocycline, for hyponatremia, 889

Dementia, **57–60**, **1018–1022**, 1019*t*, 1103, 1103–1104. *See also* Alzheimer disease
　behavioral problems and, 59, 1021–1022, 1104
　behavioral variant frontotemporal, 1019*t*
　cognitive impairment assessment/ treatment and, 57–58, 59, 1020, 1021, 1102*t*
　delirium and, 57, 58, 1019, 1102–1103, 1102*t*
　depression and (pseudodementia), 57, 61, 1103
　in elderly, **57–60**
　estrogen replacement therapy and, 796, 1202, 1204
　frontotemporal, 1019*t*, 1020, 1021
　head injury and, 1031
　in HIV infection/AIDS, 1339
　in Huntington disease, 1014, 1015
　hypertension and, 444
　in Jakob-Creutzfeldt disease, 1022, 1394
　with Lewy bodies, 59, 1019*t*, 1021
　mood disorders and, 1021–1022
　in niacin deficiency, 1276
　rapidly progressive, 1022
　screening for, 57–58, 1020
　seizures in, 983
　treatment of, 59–60, 1021–1022, 1103–1104
　vascular, 57, 1019*t*
Demerol. *See* Meperidine
Demyelinating neuropathies/ polyneuropathies, 1034. *See also specific type and* Neuropathies
　chronic inflammatory, **1039**
　in HIV infection/AIDS, 1340
　myeloma/paraproteinemias and, 1036
　optic neuritis and, 193
Demyelination. *See also* Demyelinating neuropathies/ polyneuropathies
　hyponatremia complications/treatment and, 885, 888
　in multiple sclerosis, 1023
Dengue/dengue hemorrhagic fever, 1388, 1389, **1401–1403**
Dengue shock syndrome, 1401, 1402
Dengue vaccine, 1402–1403
Denial, at-risk drinking and, 1094
Denial of illness, 1105, 1106
Denosumab
　for breast cancer, 753
　for cancer-related hypercalcemia, 1157, 1660
　for chemotherapy-induced toxicity/ bone metastases, 1671*t*
　for osteoporosis, 1162
　for prostate cancer, 1650
"Dense deposit disease," 940
Dental disorders
　anaerobic pleuropulmonary infections and, 275, 1478
　bacterial rhinosinusitis and, 215
　bisphosphonate use and, 11, 875, 1162
　deep neck infections and, 230
　earache and, 207
　facial pain caused by, 982–983

Dental procedures, endocarditis prophylaxis and, 1460, 1460*t*
Dentatorubral-pallidoluysian atrophy, 1015
Dentition, poor. *See* Dental disorders
Deoxyribonuclease, human (rhDNase), for cystic fibrosis, 265
Dependency (drug), 1092. *See also specific drug and* Substance use disorders
　in opioid therapy, 73, 85
Dependent personality disorder, 1065*t*
Depigmentation disorders, 157. *See also* Hypopigmentation
DepoEstradiol, 1205
Depression, **60–61**, **1074–1088**
　adjustment disorder with, 1075
　alcohol dependency and, 1076, 1084
　with atypical features, 1075, 1079
　bipolar disorder and, 1075
　complications of, 1076–1077
　in cyclothymic disorders, 1076
　dementia and (pseudodementia), 57, 61, 1103
　differential diagnosis of, 1076
　dispensing medications and, 1077, 1079
　drug-induced, 1076
　drug therapy for, 1077–1083, 1078*t*, 1080*f*, 1082*t*, 1083*t*. *See also* Antidepressants
　dysthymia, 1075
　ECT for, 1077, 1079, 1083–1084
　in elderly, **60–61**
　at end of life, 92
　hospitalization/illness and, 1076, 1105, 1106
　hypercortisolism and, 1174
　lithium for, 1085
　major depressive disorder, 1075, 1079
　　in elderly, 60–61
　OCD and, 1057
　oral contraceptive use and, 786, 1076
　panic disorder and, 1053
　parkinsonism differentiated from, 1012
　perimenopausal, estrogen replacement therapy and, 1202, 1203
　phototherapy for, 1084
　with postpartum onset, 1075
　during pregnancy/prenatal, 1081
　in premenstrual dysphoric disorder, 764, 765, 1075
　prognosis for, 1087
　PTSD and, 1052
　reserpine causing, 463*t*, 464, 1076
　schizophrenic/psychotic disorders/ ideation and, 1066, 1067, 1070, 1075, 1079
　screening for, in elderly, 61
　with seasonal onset, 1075, 1079, 1084
　sleep-wake disorders and, 1088
　somatic symptom disorder and, 1058
　suicide and, 1076–1077, 1079
　treatment of, 1077–1084, 1080*f*. *See also* Antidepressants
　　in elderly, 61
Dermabrasion, for acne scars, 128
Dermacentor-borne-necrosis-erythema- lymphadenopathy/scalp eschar neck lymphadenopathy/ tick-borne lymphadenopathy, 1429*t*, 1434

Dermatitis. *See also* Skin disorders
　actinic, chronic, 154
　atopic. *See* Atopic dermatitis
　cercarial, in schistosomiasis, 1532
　contact. *See* Contact dermatitis
　contagious pustular (orf), 1423
　drugs causing, **161–163**, 162–163*t*, **880**
　　drug-induced hypersensitivity syndrome and, 161, 163, 880
　exfoliative (exfoliative erythroderma), **117**
　　drugs causing, 117, 162*t*
　　psoriatic, 107, 117. *See also* Psoriasis
　fungal, in HIV infection/AIDS, 1343
　herpetiformis, **123**, 633
　in HIV infection/AIDS, 1343–1344
　medicamentosa (drug eruption), **161–163**, 162–163*t*, **880**
　　drug-induced hypersensitivity syndrome and, 161, 163, 880
　in niacin deficiency, 1276
　seborrheic. *See* Seborrheic dermatitis
　stasis, 33. *See also* Venous insufficiency/stasis
　　cellulitis differentiated from, 138
　　leg ulcers and, 156, 156*f*
　vesiculobullous of palms and soles (pompholyx), **121–122**, 122*f*
　　tinea differentiated from, 114, 122
Dermatographism, 134
Dermatologic disorders. *See* Dermatitis; Skin disorders
Dermatologic therapy, **95–101**, 96–100*t*
　adverse ophthalmic effects of, 179*t*
　complications of, 101
Dermatomyositis, **847–850**, 848*f*, 848*t*
　autoantibodies in, 840*t*, 848, 848*t*
　cancer-related, 847, 848, 848–849, 875, 1008
　sine myositis, 847
Dermatop. *See* Prednicarbate
Dermatopathic lymphadenopathy, 116
Dermatophytosis, **113–114**. *See also* Tinea
　furunculosis/carbuncles differentiated from, 153
　in HIV infection/AIDS, 1343
Dermatoses. *See* Skin disorders
Dermopathy
　in Graves disease (pretibial myxedema), 1124, 1127, 1133
　nephrogenic fibrosing, 846
DES. *See* Diethylstilbestrol
Des-gamma-carboxy prothrombin, in hepatocellular carcinoma, 1616
Desensitization reprocessing
　for OCD, 1057
　for phobic disorders, 1056
　for psychiatric problems associated with hospitalization, 1106
　for PTSD, 1052
Desensitization therapy. *See also* Immunotherapy
　for asthma, 250*t*, 251
　for drug/penicillin allergies, 1318
Designer drugs, 17, 1101

Desipramine, 1078t, 1081. *See also*
  Antidepressants
  for neuropathic pain/painful diabetic
    neuropathy, 83t, 1239–1240
Desloratadine, for allergic rhinitis, 219
Desmoid tumors, in familial
    adenomatous polyposis, 667
Desmopressin (DDAVP)
  in diabetes insipidus diagnosis,
    1113
  in diabetes insipidus treatment, 1114
  for hemophilia, 558, 559t
  for von Willebrand disease, 559t, 560
Desogestrel, in oral contraceptives,
    787t
  for hirsutism/virilization, 1198
  thromboembolism and, 786, 1198
Desonide, 96t
Desoximetasone, 98t
Desvenlafaxine, 1078t, 1079–1081
  overdose/toxicity of, 1078t, 1081
Desynchronization sleep disorder, 1088
Desyrel. *See* Trazodone
Detergent worker's lung, 308t
Detrusor muscle disorders, urinary
    incontinence and, 65–66, 66,
    67
DeVega annuloplasty, 349
Devic disease/syndrome (neuromyelitis
    optica), **1025**
  optic neuritis in, 193, 1025
Dexamethasone. *See also*
    Corticosteroids
  for chronic macular edema in retinal
    vein occlusion, 186
  for fetal lung maturity, 810, 811
  for high-altitude illness treatment/
    prevention, 1574, 1575
  for immune thrombocytopenia, 549f
  for meningitis, 1299, 1447, 1484
  for multiple sclerosis, 1024t
  for nausea and vomiting, 87, 582–583,
    582t, 1673
  for ophthalmic disorders, 171t
  for spinal tumors/cord compression,
    1007, 1658
Dexamethasone implant, for diabetic
    macular edema, 190
Dexamethasone suppression test, in
    Cushing syndrome diagnosis,
    1173
Dexlansoprazole, 609, 625. *See also*
    Proton pump inhibitors
Dexmedetomidine, for alcohol
    withdrawal, 1097–1099
Dexrazoxane, for chemotherapy-induced
    cardiac toxicity, 415, 1671t
Dextroamphetamine
  abuse/overdose of, 1100
  for depression, 1082
  for narcolepsy, 1090
Dextromethorphan
  MAOI interactions and, 1083t
  overdose/toxicity of, 1598, 1601
Dextrose
  for coma, 1027, 1578
  in fluid management, 911, 911t
  for hypernatremia, 890
  for hypoglycemia, 1595
  for shock, 495
  for status epilepticus, 989

DHEA/DHEAS. *See*
    Dehydroepiandrosterone/
    dehydroepiandrosterone
    sulfate
DHFR gene, TMP-SMZ resistance and,
    1552
DHPS gene, TMP-SMZ resistance and,
    1552
DiaBeta. *See* Glyburide
Diabetes Control and Complications Trial
    (DCCT), 1217–1218,
    1244–1245
Diabetes insipidus, 1109, **1113–1114**
  craniopharyngioma and, 1111
  hypernatremia and, 890, 1114
  nephrogenic, 892t, 1113–1114
    hypercalcemia/hyperparathyroidism
      and, 897, 898, 1153
    lithium causing, 1086
  after pituitary microsurgery, 1115,
    1119
  in Wolfram syndrome, 1113, 1212
Diabetes mellitus, **1210–1252**. *See also*
    under Diabetic
  adrenal insufficiency/Addison disease
    and, 1237
  angina in patients with, 361–362
  antipsychotic drug use and,
    1071–1072, 1071t
  blood glucose levels in diagnosis of,
    1214–1215, 1215t, 1233
  blood glucose self/continuous-
    monitoring in, 1216–1217,
    1217
    in pregnant patient, 818, 1217
  bone/joint complications in, 1242
  cardiovascular/vascular complications
    of, 1241–1242
    cholesterol screening and,
      1261–1262
    glycemic control and, 361–362,
      1217, 1218, 1219
    hypertension control and, 446, 447f,
      464, 465, 466, 1218, 1236
    tibial and pedal artery disease and,
      475, 476
    in women, 1241
  chronic kidney disease and, 923, 929,
    934t, 942, 945–946, 1238,
    1238–1239. *See also* Diabetic
    nephropathy
  classification and pathogenesis of,
    1210–1213, 1211t, 1212f,
    1213t
  clinical trials in, 1217–1219
  coma in patient with, 1214, **1245**,
    1246t
  complications of, 1237–1242. *See also*
    *specific type or organ/system
    affected*
    clinical studies of glycemic control
      and, 1217–1219
    hypoglycemia and, 1237
    insulin therapy and, 1236–1237
  continuous glucose monitoring
    systems in, 1217
  deaths attributable to, 2t
  diagnosis of/diagnostic examination in,
    1214–1217, 1215t,
    1232–1233
  diuretic use and, 448, 449t

  drugs/medications associated with,
    1213, 1213t
  emphysematous pyelonephritis
    in, 956
  environmental factors in, 1211, 1212
  epidemiologic considerations in, 1210,
    1211t
  erectile dysfunction in, 1240–1241
  estrogen replacement affecting, 1203
  exercise and, 1218, 1219
    insulin requirements and, 1233
  foot disorders/foot care in, 475, 476,
    1239, 1239f, 1242
  gastroparesis in, 640, 641, 1240
  genetic factors in, 1210–1211, 1211t,
    1212
  gestational, 800, 817–818, 817t
  glucagonoma and, 1185
  glucose tolerance test in, 1215, 1215t
    in pregnant patient, 800, 817, 817t
  glucosuria/glycosuria in, 1214
  glycated hemoglobin (HbA$_{1c}$)
    measurements in,
      1215–1216, 1215t. *See also*
      Hemoglobin A$_1$/A$_{1c}$
  glycemic control in. *See also* Glycemic
    control in diabetes
    acceptable levels of, 1236
    blood glucose self/
      continuous-monitoring in,
      1216–1217, 1217
    in pregnant patient, 818, 1217
    cardiovascular disease and, 361–362,
      1217, 1218, 1219
    clinical studies in evaluation of,
      1217–1219
    hospitalization/surgery and, 53,
      1243–1244, 1243t
    intensive insulin therapy for. *See*
      Insulin therapy, intensive
    pregnancy and, 817, 818
  heart disease in, 1241–1242
  hepatitis B vaccination in, 4, 681,
    1321t, 1324t
  HLA in, 1210
  hospitalization/surgery and, 53,
    1243–1244, 1243t
  hypertension/hypertension
    management in, 446, 447f,
    449t, 464, 465, 466, 1236
    ACE inhibitors for, 449t, 454, 465,
      466, 1218, 1241
    benefits of control and, 945, 1218,
      1236
    beta-adrenergic blocking agents for,
      449t, 454, 466, 1218
    calcium channel blocking agents for,
      449t, 465, 466, 1218
  immunization recommendations in,
    1321t
  insulin resistance and, 1211t, 1212,
    1213. *See also* Insulin
    resistance/insensitivity
  ketones (urine/blood) in, 1214
  latent autoimmune of adulthood
    (LADA), 1211, 1235
  lipid/lipoprotein abnormalities in,
    1217, 1261
  lipoatrophic, 1211t
  maturity-onset of young (MODY),
    1211t, 1212, 1235

mitochondrial DNA mutations and, 1211*t*, 1212
mutant insulins/insulin receptors causing, 1212
nephrotic syndrome and. *See* Diabetic nephropathy
neurogenic arthropathy (Charcot joint) in, 875, 1239
neuropathy and, 1036, 1239–1241, 1239*f. See also* Diabetic neuropathy
nonalcoholic fatty liver disease and, 697, 698
occult, 1252, **1257**
ocular complications of, 189–190, 189*f*, 1238. *See also* Diabetic retinopathy
osteomyelitis in, 871
pancreatic disorders/cancer/ pancreatitis and, 728, 730, 731, 1211*t*, 1213, 1620
patient education (self-management training) in, 1233
perioperative evaluation/management and, 53
polycystic ovary syndrome and, 780, 1196
prebreakfast hyperglycemia in, 1234, 1234*t*
during pregnancy, 800, **817–818**, 817*t*, 1244
prevention/delay of, 1218
prognosis for, 1244–1245
screening for
   cardiovascular disease prevention and, 6*t*
   pregnancy and, 800
secondary, 1213, 1213*t*
self/continuous-monitoring of blood glucose and, 1216–1217, 1217, 1233, 1234
   in pregnant patient, 818, 1217
skin/mucous membrane disorders and, 1214, 1242
somatostatinomas and, 1185
surgery in patients with, 53, 1243–1244, 1243*t*
treatment of, 1219–1232, 1232–1237
   in chronic kidney disease, 929
   clinical studies in evaluation of, 1217–1219
   diet in, 1219–1220. *See also* Diet
   drugs in, 1220–1228, 1221–1222*t*, 1235–1236, 1235*f. See also* Antidiabetic agents
   hospitalization/surgery and, 1243–1244, 1243*t*
   insulin in, 1228–1232, 1229*t*, 1233–1234, 1234*t*, 1236–1237. *See also* Insulin therapy
   postoperative management and, 1244
   in pregnant patient, 818
   steps in, 1232–1237, 1234*t*, 1235*t*
   transplantation in, 1232
type 1, 1210–1211, 1213–1214, 1233–1234, 1234*t*
   HLA in, 1210
   idiopathic (type 1B), 1211
   immune-mediated (type 1A), 1210–1211

insulin therapy for, 1217–1218
prognosis for, 1244–1245
surgery in patient with, 53, 1243, 1243*t*
type 2, 1211–1212, 1214, 1235–1236, 1235*f*
   drugs for management of, 1220–1228, 1221–1222*t*, 1235–1236, 1235*f. See also* Antidiabetic agents
   insulin therapy for, 1218, 1230–1231, 1231–1232, 1235, 1235*f*, 1236
   in nonobese patients, 1235
   in obese patients, 1212, 1214, 1218, 1219, 1235
   prevention of, 1218
   prognosis for, 1245
   surgery in patient with, 53, 1243, 1243*t*
vascular disorders in. *See* Diabetes mellitus, cardiovascular/ vascular complications of
weight loss (unintended) in, 1214
   diabetic neuropathic cachexia and, 1240
in Wolfram syndrome, 1212
Diabetes Prevention Program (DPP), 1218
Diabetic amyotrophy, 1036
Diabetic cataracts, 1238
Diabetic cheiroarthropathy/cheiropathy, 846, 1242
Diabetic coma, 1214, **1245**, 1246*t. See also specific cause*
   diabetic ketoacidosis and, 1214, 1245, 1246, 1246*t*, 1247
   hyperglycemic hyperosmolar state and, 1214, 1245, 1246*t*, **1249–1251**
   lactic acidosis and, 1245, 1246*t*, 1251
Diabetic diarrhea, 1240
Diabetic dyslipidemia, 1217, 1261
Diabetic ketoacidosis, 905, 1214, **1245–1249**, 1246*t*
   coma caused by, 1214, 1245, 1246, 1246*t*, 1247
   hypophosphatemia in, 900, 1248
   increased anion gap acidosis and, 905
   insulin infusion pumps and, 1231, 1245, 1249
   insulin needs during surgery and, 1243
   insulin therapy for, 1229, 1247–1248, 1249
   normal anion gap acidosis and, 905, 1248
   SGLT2 inhibitor use and, 1228
Diabetic maculopathy/macular edema, 190, 1238
Diabetic nephropathy, 934*t*, 942, **945–946**, 1238–1239
   glycemic control affecting development/progression of, 945, 1218, 1219, 1238
   pregnancy and, 1244
Diabetic neuropathic cachexia, 1240
Diabetic neuropathy, 1036, 1239–1241, 1239*f*
   glycemic control affecting development/progression of, 1217, 1218, 1219

neurogenic arthropathy (Charcot joint) and, 875, 1239
Diabetic papillopathy, 192
Diabetic retinopathy, **189–190**, 189*f*, 1238
   glycemic control affecting development/progression of, 189, 1218, 1219
   during pregnancy, 1244
Diabetic shin spots, 1242
Diabinese. *See* Chlorpropamide
Diagnostic/laboratory tests. *See also specific disorder*
   in cancer screening, 13–15, 14*t*
   in poisoning/drug overdose, 1584–1585, 1584*t*
   in prenatal care, 799–801. *See also* Prenatal testing
   preoperative evaluation and, 45
Diagnostic and Statistical Manual (DSM-5), 1050
Dialysis, 930
   "gut" (repeat-dose charcoal), 1583
   for hypercalcemia, 898
   hypercalcemia/hyperphosphatemia associated with, 898
   for hyperkalemia, 894, 895*t*
   iron deficiency and, 502
   for kidney disease/injury
      acute injury/acute tubular necrosis, 921
      chronic/end-stage, 930
   nephrogenic systemic fibrosis and, 952
   for poisoning/drug overdose, 1582–1583, 1583*t. See also specific drug/toxin*
   pruritus associated with, 147
   renal cysts and, 949
      renal cell carcinoma and, 1654
   skin lesions and (porphyria cutanea tarda-like), 123
   surgery in patient receiving, 54
3,4-Diaminopyridine, for myasthenic (Lambert-Eaton) syndrome, 1046
Diamox. *See* Acetazolamide
Diaphragm, respiratory failure caused by disorders of, 318*t*
Diaphragm (contraceptive), **790**
DIAPPERS mnemonic, 65
Diarrhea, **587–594**, 588*t*, 590*f*, 593*f. See also specific cause and* Colitis; Gastroenteritis
   acute, **588–591**, 588*t*, 590*f*, 1305–1308, 1306–1307*t*
   in amebiasis. *See* Intestinal amebiasis
   antibiotic-associated, 589, 647–649, 1305, 1306*t*
   antibiotics for, 591, 1308
   in bacterial overgrowth, 588*t*, 592, 594, 636
   bloody, 589, 598. *See also* Dysentery
   chemotherapy-induced, 1673
   in cholera, 1471
   chronic, 588*t*, **591–594**, 593*f*
   diabetic, 1240
   drugs in management of, 590, 594. *See also* Antidiarrheal agents
   enteral nutritional support and, 1283, 1284
   fecal impaction and, 586
   fluid management in, 590, 911*t*

Diarrhea (*Cont.*):
Guillain-Barré syndrome and, 1038
hypokalemia caused by, 891
in immunocompromised host/HIV infection/AIDS, 588t, 589, 592, 1305, 1335, 1342
infectious
acute, 588t, 589, 598, **1305–1308**, 1306–1307t
chronic, 588t, 592
inflammatory, 588t, 589, 592, 1305. *See also* Dysentery
acute, 588t, 589, 1305
chronic, 588t, 592
in malabsorption, 588t, 591, 592, 633t
in measles, 1379
in niacin deficiency, 1276
noninflammatory, 589, 1305
osmotic, 588t, 591
secretory, 588t, 592, 594
toxins causing, 588t, 589, 1305, 1306t
traveler's, 589, 590, 1305, **1309–1310**
in typhoid fever, 1468
viral, 588t, 589, 1305, 1342, **1424–1425**. *See also specific virus*
Diastolic blood pressure. *See also* Blood pressure
in hypertension, 439, 440f
treatment goals and, 446. *See also* Antihypertensive drug therapy, goals of
in hypertensive urgencies/emergencies, 439, 440f, 468
in prehypertension, 440
Diastolic dysfunction/heart failure, 402, 403. *See also* Heart (cardiac) failure
Diastolic murmurs. *See* Heart murmurs
Diazepam, 1054, 1054t, 1055. *See also* Benzodiazepines
adverse ophthalmic effects of, 177t
for aggressive/violent behavior, 1091
for alcohol withdrawal, 1095
for anxiety, 1054, 1054t, 1055
overdose/toxicity of, 1594–1595
for seizures
in poisoning/drug overdose, 1580
status epilepticus and, 989
for spasticity, 1026
Diazoxide, for insulin-secreting tumors, 1255
Dibenzoxazepines, 1068. *See also* Antipsychotic drugs
DIC. *See* Disseminated intravascular coagulation
Dichlorphenamide, 180
Dichuchwa (endemic syphilis), **1498–1499**
Diclofenac, 75t, 829
for ophthalmic disorders, 168, 171t
Dicloxacillin
for pharyngitis, 229
for skin and soft tissue infections, 1443t, 1448
nasal vestibulitis, 218
Didanosine (ddI), 1351t, 1353, 1355, 1360. *See also* Antiretroviral therapy

lactic acidosis caused by, 1341, 1360
neuropathy caused by, 1340, 1353, 1355
DIDMOAD, 1113, 1212
Diet. *See also* Nutrition
acne and, 127
in acute tubular necrosis, 920
breast cancer risk and, 738
cancer/cancer prevention and, 1607
cardiovascular disease prevention and, 6t
cholelithiasis/gallstones and, 717
cholesterol/lipid-lowering, 1263, 1279
in cirrhosis, 701
colorectal cancer and, 1637
consistency alterations and, **1278–1279**
constipation and, 585–586, 585t
in Crohn disease, 655
in diabetes mellitus, 1219–1220
pregnant patient and, 817, 818
prevention/complications and, 1218
in diarrhea control, 590
diverticular disease and, 662–663, 663
in GERD management, 609
gluten-free, for celiac disease/dermatitis herpetiformis, 123, 634
in gout, 832, 832t
in heart failure management, 410
in hemochromatosis, 709
in hypertension/hypertension prevention, 445, 446t
in hypertriglyceridemia, 1267
in irritable bowel syndrome, 645–646
in kidney disease, 929, 942
lactation and, 802
lactose-free, 638
MAOI interactions and, 1082, 1082t
Mediterranean, 1263
nutrient-restricting, **1279**
nutrient-supplementing, **1280**
obesity management/prevention and, 12, 13, 1270
in osteoporosis, 1160
in pancreatitis, 729, 732
in porphyria, 1036, 1676, 1677
during pregnancy, 799, **801**
preventable disease/deaths and, 3t, 6t
therapeutic, **1278–1280**
in ulcerative colitis, 659
urinary stone formation and, 961, 962, 963, 964
in Wilson disease, 710
Diet therapy, **1278–1280**. *See also* Diet; Nutrition
Dietary supplements
oral nutritional supplements, 1281
for elderly, 67
toxicity of, **1593–1594**, 1593t
Diethylcarbamazine
for filariasis, 1544
for loiasis, 1546
Diethylene glycol, toxicity of, 1599
Diethylstilbestrol (DES)
for breast cancer, 755t
for prostate cancer, 1649t
Dieulafoy lesion, 595
Difenacoum poisoning, 1588
Diffuse axonal injury, 1030t
Diffuse cutaneous leishmaniasis, 1511
Diffuse esophageal spasm, 605t

Diffuse gastric cancer, 1629
Diffuse idiopathic skeletal hyperostosis (DISH), 864, 1242
Diffuse infiltrative lymphocytosis syndrome, 869
Diffuse interstitial pneumonias, **289–292**, 290t, 291t, 292f
Diffuse panbronchiolitis, 267
Diffuse parenchymal lung disease, **289–294**, 290t, 291t, 292f. *See also specific disorder and* Interstitial lung disease
Diffusing capacity for carbon monoxide (DL$_{CO}$), in *Pneumocystis* pneumonia, 1336
Diflorasone, 97t
Diflunisal, 75t
Digestion, disorders of. *See* Malabsorption
Digibind. *See* Digoxin-specific Fab antibody
DigiFab. *See* Digoxin-specific Fab antibody
Digital clubbing, 160, 160f, 1609. *See also specific cause*
Digital mammography, 15, 740
Digital rectal examination. *See* Rectal examination
Digitalis/digitalis glycosides/digoxin, 383t, 408
antidepressant drug interactions and, 1083t
for arrhythmias, 381, 383t
atrial fibrillation, 389, 390
in hyperthyroidism, 1133
benzodiazepine interactions and, 1056t
for cardiomyopathy, 417
for heart failure, 405f, 408
in myocardial infarction, 378
overdose/toxicity of, 383t, 1579, 1581t, 1584t, **1594**
chronic kidney disease and, 926
hypokalemia and, 891
ophthalmic, 177t
for pulmonary hypertension, 432f
thrombocytopenia caused by, 555t
Digoxin-specific Fab antibody (digoxin immune Fab), 1579, 1581t, 1584t, 1594
DIHS. *See* Drug-induced hypersensitivity syndrome
Dihydroartemisinin, 1515t
with piperaquine, 1516, 1516t, 1517t, 1519, 1521
Dihydroergotamine
for cluster headache, 980
for migraine headache, 978
Dihydroindolones, 1068. *See also* Antipsychotic drugs
1,25-Dihydroxycholecalciferol. *See* Calcitriol
Diiodohydroxyquin. *See* Iodoquinol
Dilacor. *See* Diltiazem
Dilated cardiomyopathy. *See* Cardiomyopathy
Dilation and curettage. *See* D&C
Dilaudid. *See* Hydromorphone
Diloxanide, for amebiasis, 1526, 1527t
Dilt-CD. *See* Diltiazem
Diltia. *See* Diltiazem

Diltiazem, 383t, 460t. *See also* Calcium channel blocking drugs
  for acute coronary syndromes, 368
  for angina, 361
  for arrhythmias, 383t
    atrial fibrillation, 389
    infarct-related, 377
    supraventricular tachycardia, 383t, 386
  for hypertension, 459, 460t
  overdose/toxicity of, 383t, 459, 460t, 1591
Dilutional acidosis, 907
Dimenhydrinate, 583
Dimercaprol (BAL)
  for arsenic poisoning, 1590
  for lead poisoning, 1597
  for mercury poisoning, 1599
Dimercaptosuccinic acid (DMSA). *See* Succimer
Dimethoate poisoning, 1602
Dimethyl fumarate, for multiple sclerosis, 1024t, 1025
1,1-Dimethylbiguanide hydrochloride. *See* Metformin
Dimethyltryptamine, 1099
Diovan/Diovan HCT. *See* Valsartan
Dipeptidyl peptidase 4 (DPP-4), 1227
Dipeptidyl peptidase 4 (DPP-4) inhibitors, 1222t, 1227, 1235f, 1236
Dipeptidyl-peptidase-like protein-6, in autoimmune paraneoplastic disorders, 1008
Diphenhydramine. *See also* Antihistamines
  breastfeeding and, 798t
  for insomnia, 1089
  for nausea and vomiting, 87
  overdose/toxicity of, 1590
  for scombroid poisoning, 1603
Diphenoxylate with atropine, 590, 594, 1342. *See also* Antidiarrheal agents
  for Crohn disease, 655
  overdose/toxicity of, 1590
  for ulcerative colitis, 659
Diphoterine, for alkali eye injury, 1587
Diphtheria, 1312t, **1456–1457**
  neuropathy in, 1037, 1457
  pharyngitis in, 228, 1441, 1456, 1457
  prevention/immunization and, 1457. *See also* Diphtheria and tetanus toxoids and pertussis vaccines
Diphtheria antitoxin, 1457
Diphtheria and tetanus toxoids and pertussis vaccines (DTaP/Tdap/Td vaccines), 4, 1320t, 1321t, 1322t, 1329t, 1453, 1453t, 1457, 1464
  adverse effects/contraindications and, 1329t
  bite wounds and, 1301
  booster and, 4, 1320t, 1322t, 1453, 1457, 1464
  burn injury and, 1569
  frostbite and, 1566
  in immunocompromised host/HIV infection/AIDS, 5, 1321t, 1349

pregnancy and, 802, 1319, 1321t, 1322t, 1464
  Tdap replacing Td and, 4, 1320t, 1453, 1464
Diphtheria toxoid, 1457. *See also* Diphtheria and tetanus toxoids and pertussis vaccines
Diphyllobothrium latum (fish tapeworm), **1535**, 1536
  vitamin B$_{12}$ deficiency and, 506–507, 1535
Dipivefrin, 180
Diprolene. *See* Betamethasone
Dipstick urinalysis, 913, 914. *See also* Urinalysis
Dipylidium caninum (dog tapeworm), 1535, 1536
  echinococcosis and, 1537
Dipyridamole
  platelet function affected by, 558t
  for transient ischemic attacks, 993
Dipyridamole-thallium scintigraphy. *See* Myocardial perfusion scintigraphy
Diquafasol, for dry eye, 168
Direct-acting oral anticoagulants (DOACs/new/novel oral anticoagulants [NOACs]), 564–567, 565–566t, 573. *See also specific drug*
  for atrial fibrillation/stroke prevention, 391–393, 391t, 392f, 564, 565t
  mitral stenosis and, 336
  cardiac valve replacement and, 351
  coagulopathy caused by, 391, 391t, 393, 562
  for DVT/PE (venous thromboembolic disease), 300, 564, 565t, 570t, 573
  overdose/toxicity and, 564, 566t, 1588
  perioperative management and, 51–52, 52t, 392–393, 566t
  reversal of, 393, 564
  switching to from warfarin, 392, 566t
  switching to warfarin from, 566t
Direct current (DC) electrical injury, 1570
Direct renin assay, in aldosteronism, 1178
Direct thrombin inhibitors
  for acute coronary syndromes, 368
  for heparin-induced thrombocytopenia, 552–553, 553t
  overdose/toxicity of, 1588
Directed bleeding history, preoperative, 45, 46t, 51
Directly observed therapy (DOT), for tuberculosis, 280–281, 283
  in drug-resistant tuberculosis, 281, 283
  in HIV infection/AIDS, 282
Disability assessment, in burn injury, 1568
Discogenic disease. *See* Cervical spine/disk disease; Lumbar spine/disk disease; Sacral spine/disk disease
Discoid lupus erythematosus, **115–116**, 839t, 840

Disease-modifying antirheumatic drugs (DMARDs), 836, 837, 837–838
Disease prevention. *See* Preventive care
DISH. *See* Diffuse idiopathic skeletal hyperostosis
Disk batteries, ingested, alkali injuries caused by, 1587
Disk disease. *See* Cervical spine/disk disease; Lumbar spine/disk disease; Sacral spine/disk disease
Dislocated shoulder, 1688t, **1690–1691**
  atraumatic, 1690, 1691
Disopyramide, 381, 382t
  for cardiomyopathy, 419, 420f
  overdose/toxicity of, 382t
Dissection. *See* Aortic dissection
Disseminated cutaneous leishmaniasis, 1511
Disseminated intravascular coagulation (DIC), **553–555**, 554t, **562**
  in acute leukemia, 528, 554
  in cancer, 553, 1008
  in meningococcal meningitis, 1465
Distal muscular dystrophy, 1048t
Distal renal tubular acidosis, 892t, 906–907, 906t. *See also* Renal tubular acidosis
  genetic defects associated with, 892t
  nephrolithiasis/nephrocalcinosis/urolithiasis and, 906–907, 962
  in tubulointerstitial disease, 948
Distal symmetric polyneuropathy, in diabetes, 1239–1240, 1239f
Distributive shock, 494, 494t, 495, 496–497, 497
Disulfiram
  for alcohol use disorder, 17, 1095
  antidepressant drug interactions and, 1083t
  benzodiazepine interactions and, 1056t
Diulo. *See* Metolazone
Diuretics. *See also specific agent*
  for acute tubular necrosis, 920
  adverse effects of, 448, 450t
    ophthalmic, 177t
  for cardiomyopathy, 416, 420f, 422
  for cirrhotic ascites, 701
  contraction alkalosis and, 909
  gout/hyperuricemia and, 448, 831, 832
  for heart failure, 405f, 406, 410, 412
    in chronic kidney disease, 926
    hypertension and, 449t
    left ventricular (infarct-related), 378
  for hyperkalemia, 894, 895t
  for hypernatremia, 890
  for hypertension, 448, 449t, 450–451t, 464
    in chronic kidney disease, 448, 449t, 466, 926
    in combination products, 451t, 452t, 453t, 455t, 456t, 457t, 458t
    in combination regimen, 464–465, 465f
    in urgencies/emergencies, 469t, 470t, 471
  hypokalemia caused by, 448, 892, 893
  hyponatremia caused by, 886
  lithium interactions and, 1086, 1087t

Diuretics (*Cont.*):
ototoxicity of, 208
for pericarditis, 429
during pregnancy, 435
for pulmonary edema, 412
for pulmonary hypertension, 431, 432*f*
for tricuspid regurgitation, 349
for tricuspid stenosis, 348
tubulointerstitial nephritis caused by,
947*t*
Divalproex. *See* Valproic acid/valproate
Diversion (medication), long-term opioid
therapy and, 74, 85
Diverticula
colonic, **662–664**
Zenker, **614**
Diverticular bleeding, 597, 598, 599, 662,
664
Diverticulitis, 662, **663–664**
Diverticulosis, 662, **663**
GI bleeding in, 597, 598, 599, 662, 664
infection and (diverticulitis), 662,
663–664
Divigel, 1204
Diving (underwater). *See* Scuba/deep sea
diving
Dix-Hallpike testing, 211
Dizziness. *See* Vertigo; Vestibular
disorders
DJ1 gene, in parkinsonism, 1011
DKA. *See* Diabetic ketoacidosis
DL_{CO} (diffusing capacity for carbon
monoxide), in *Pneumocystis*
pneumonia, 1336
DLE. *See* Discoid lupus erythematosus
DMARDs. *See* Disease-modifying
antirheumatic drugs
DML, 100*t*
DMP1 mutations, in osteomalacia/rickets,
1165
DMPA. *See* Medroxyprogesterone
DMPS. *See* Unithiol
DMSA. *See* Succimer
DNA
double-stranded, antibodies to, in
lupus/SLE, 115, 841
hepatitis B virus, 680*f*, 681, 687,
688
HPV, 770
mitochondrial, mutations in
in diabetes mellitus, 1211*t*, 1212
myopathies associated with, **1049**
native, antibodies to, 840*t*, 841*t*
DNA analysis/diagnosis/probes
in cancer screening/polyp
identification, 665,
1641–1642
in nontuberculous mycobacterial
infection, 285
in tuberculosis, 278, 278*t*
DNMT3A mutation, in acute myeloid
leukemia, 527
Do not attempt resuscitation (DNAR)
orders, 90
Dobrova-Belgrade virus, 1403
Dobutamine
for cardiogenic shock, 378, 497
for left ventricular (infarct-related)
heart failure, 378
Dobutamine stress echocardiography. *See*
Echocardiography/Doppler

Docetaxel, 1664*t*
adverse ophthalmic effects of, 178*t*
for breast cancer, 751, 752, 753, 756,
757
for gastric adenocarcinoma, 1631
neuropathy caused by, 1674
for prostate cancer, 1650
DOCK8 (dedicator of cytokinesis)
deficiency, molluscum
contagiosum in, 1423
Doctor-patient communication, in
end-of-life care, 88–89, 89*t*
Docusate sodium, 585*t*
Dofetilide, 381, 382*t*, 383*t*
for atrial fibrillation, 382*t*, 383*t*, 393
for atrial flutter, 382*t*, 383*t*, 395
Dog bites, 1300
rabies and, 1300, 1386, 1387
Dog hookworm, 1539
cutaneous larva migrans caused by,
1542
Dog roundworm (*T canis*), toxocariasis/
visceral larva migrans caused
by, 1542
Dog tapeworm (*D caninum*), 1535, 1536
echinococcosis and, 1537
Dolasetron, 582, 582*t*, 1672. *See also*
Antiemetics
Dolobid. *See* Diflunisal
Dolophine. *See* Methadone
Dolutegravir, 1353*t*, 1358
with lamivudine and abacavir
(Triumeq), 1354*t*, 1358,
1359*t*, 1360
with Truvada (emtricitabine and
tenofovir [TDF]), 1359*t*
Domestic violence, 16, 1090–1091, 1091
elder abuse and, 16, **70–71**, 71*t*
intimate partner, 16, 1090–1091, 1091
Donepezil, for dementia, 59, 1021, 1104
Donovan bodies, 1477
Dopamine
depletion of in parkinsonism, 1011
for hypotension/shock, 496–497
cardiogenic, 378, 497
for left ventricular (infarct-related)
failure, 378
receptors for, in nausea and vomiting,
580
in schizophrenia, 1066
Dopamine agonists
for acromegaly/gigantism, 1116
for hyperprolactinemia, 1117, 1118
for neuroleptic malignant syndrome,
1072
for parkinsonism, 1013
Dopamine antagonists, 1068. *See also*
Antipsychotic drugs
for nausea and vomiting, 582*t*, 583
Doppler. *See* Echocardiography/Doppler
Doral. *See* Quazepam
DORAs. *See* Dual orexin receptor
antagonists
Doripenem, for anaerobic infections,
1479, 1479*t*
Dornase alpha (rhDNase), for cystic
fibrosis, 265
Dorzolamide/dorzolamide and timolol,
173*t*
DOT. *See* Directly observed therapy
Double-chambered right ventricle, 322

Double outlet right ventricle, 328
Double-stranded DNA antibodies, in
lupus/SLE, 115, 841
Down syndrome (trisomy 21),
1678–1679
prenatal screening for, 800, 1678
Doxazosin, 462*t*
adverse ophthalmic effects of, 177*t*, 183
for benign prostatic hyperplasia, 974,
974–975, 974*t*
for hypertension, 459–464, 462*t*
pheochromocytoma/
pheochromocytoma surgery
and, 1183
Doxepin, 95, 99*t*, 1078*t*. *See also*
Antidepressants
for anogenital pruritus, 148
topical, 95, 99*t*
for urticaria, 134
Doxercalciferol, for hyperparathyroidism,
1157
Doxorubicin, 1665*t*
for breast cancer, 751, 753
liposomal, 1665*t*
for Kaposi sarcoma, 146
toxicity of, 1665*t*, 1674–1675
Doxycycline
for acne, 127–128
adverse ophthalmic effects of, 178*t*
for anthrax, 1455–1456, 1456*t*
for bacterial rhinosinusitis, 217*t*
breastfeeding and, 798*t*
for Lyme disease prophylaxis/
treatment, 1504, 1505, 1505*t*
for malaria, 1515*t*, 1517*t*, 1518, 1519
for chemoprophylaxis, 1519, 1520,
1520*t*
for pneumonia, 269*t*, 1445
for rosacea, 129
for skin and soft tissue infections,
1343, 1443*t*, 1448
for syphilis, 1491*t*, 1492
for urinary tract infection, 955*t*
for *Wolbachia* eradication
in filariasis, 1544
in onchocerciasis, 1545
Doxylamine, for vomiting during
pregnancy, 583, 803
DPI. *See* Dry powder inhalers
DPOA-HC. *See* Durable Power of
Attorney for Health Care
DPOAF. *See* Durable power of attorney
for finance matters
DPP-4, 1227
DPP-4 inhibitors, 1222*t*, 1227, 1235*f*,
1236
DPP (Diabetes Prevention Program),
1218
DRA. *See* Direct renin assay
Drawer sign/test
anterior
ankle sprain and, 1715, 1715*t*
knee stability/ACL injury and,
1706*t*, 1709
posterior, 1708*t*, 1711
DRE (digital rectal examination). *See*
Rectal examination
Dream sleep, 1088
DRESS. *See* Drug reaction with
eosinophilia and systemic
symptoms

Dressler syndrome (postmyocardial infarction/postcardiotomy pericarditis), 379, 425, 426
Drinking, at-risk/problem/risky, 17, 1094. *See also* Alcohol use disorder
    differential diagnosis of, 1094
    treatment of, 1094–1095
Driver rehabilitation specialist, 60
Driving (automobile)
    by patients with dementia, 59–60, 1022
    by patients with syncope/ventricular tachycardia/aborted sudden death, **402**
    by suicidal patients, 1077
Dronabinol (delta⁹-tetrahydrocannabinol)
    for HIV wasting, 1335
    for nausea and vomiting, 87, 583
    in HIV infection/AIDS, 1335
Dronedarone, 381, 383*t*
Drop attacks, epileptic (atonic seizures), 984*t*, 985. *See also* Seizures
Droperidol, overdose/toxicity of, 1589–1590
Drospirenone
    in estrogen replacement therapy, 1204
    in oral contraceptives, 787*t*
        for hirsutism/virilization, 1198
        thromboembolism and, 786, 1198
Drowning, **1566–1567**
Drug abuse, **16–18**. *See also* Poisoning/drug overdose; Substance use disorders
Drug addiction, 1092. *See also* Poisoning/drug overdose; Substance use disorders
    pain management and, 17, 73–74, 85
Drug allergy, **877**, 1318–1319. *See also specific agent*
    to antimicrobial agents, **1318–1319**
    delayed hypersensitivity and, **880**, **880–881**
    desensitization therapy for, 1318
    in HIV infection/AIDS, 1333
    HLA haplotypes and, 880
    in ophthalmic therapy, 199
Drug dependency, 1092. *See also specific drug and* Substance use disorders
    in opioid therapy, 73, 85
Drug eruptions, **161–163**, 162–163*t*, **880**
    drug-induced hypersensitivity syndrome and, 161, 163, 880
Drug fever, 1294
Drug-induced disorders/side effects
    abnormal movements, **1017**
    agranulocytosis, 518
    allergic reactions. *See* Drug allergy
    asthma, 242, 310*t*
    cognitive disorders/delirium, 58, 62, 1102*t*
    constipation, 82, 86, 584*t*, 586
    depression, 1076
    dermatitis (dermatitis medicamentosa), **161–163**, 162–163*t*, **880**
    diarrhea, 588*t*, 591
    in elderly, **69**
        falls and, 64, 64*t*
        incontinence and, 65
    with eosinophilia and systemic symptoms, 161, 163, **880–881**

erythema multiforme/Stevens-Johnson syndrome/toxic epidermal necrolysis, 135, 136, 161, 162*t*, 163
esophagitis, 612
exfoliative dermatitis/erythroderma, 117, 162*t*
fetotoxicity, 798*t*
G6PD deficiency, 511
headache (analgesic rebound/medication overuse headache), **980**
HLA haplotypes and, 880
hyperthyroidism, 1125–1126
hypoglycemia, 1252*t*, **1257–1258**
hyponatremia, 886
lichenoid/lichen planus-like, 145, 162*t*
liver disease/failure, 685, 686
lung disease, 290*t*, **309**, 310*t*
lupus/SLE, 115, 116, 162*t*, 310*t*, **842**
mood disorders, 1076
myocarditis, 413*t*, **414–415**
nausea and vomiting, 581*t*
neutropenia, 518, 1662
ocular, 177–179*t*, **199**
ototoxicity, 208
overdoses. *See* Poisoning/drug overdose
photodermatitis, 154, 155, 162*t*
pigmentary changes, 158, 163*t*
pityriasis rosea-like eruption, 109, 163*t*
porphyria, 122–123, 123, 1676, 1677*t*
progressive multifocal leukoencephalopathy, 652, 1024, 1395
pulmonary disorders, 290*t*, **309**, 310*t*
renal clearance and, 924, 929
rhinitis (rhinitis medicamentosa), 215
seizures, 1580, 1580*t*
SIADH, 887, 887*t*
teratogenicity, 798*t*
thrombocytopenia/platelet function, 552–553, 553*t*, **555**, 555*t*, 558*t*
tubulointerstitial nephritis, 946, 947*t*
urticaria, 134, 162*t*
Drug-induced hypersensitivity syndrome (drug reaction with eosinophilia and systemic symptoms), 161, 163, **880–881**
Drug overdose. *See* Poisoning/drug overdose
Drug reaction with eosinophilia and systemic symptoms (DRESS), 161, 163, **880–881**
Drug resistance, 1294, 1313–1317. *See also specific agent*
    in anthrax, 1455
    in antiretroviral therapy, 1350, 1360, 1361–1362
        for hepatitis B, 688
        for hepatitis C, 689, 690, 691
    in bacterial rhinosinusitis, 215, 216, 217*t*
    in coagulase-negative staphylococcal infection, 1451
    in enterococcal infections, 1316, 1444, 1445

in gonococcal infection, 1476
health care-associated infections and, 1294
    in HIV infection/AIDS, 1347, 1350, 1360, 1361–1362, 1361*f*
    in influenza, 1412
    in leishmaniasis, 1511, 1512
    in leprosy, 1484
    in malaria, 1515, 1516, 1517
    in nontuberculous mycobacterial infection, 285, 1482
    pharyngitis treatment and, 227, 229
    in pneumococcal infections, 1446
    in pneumonia
        community-acquired pneumonia, 269, 270–271, 271
        nosocomial pneumonia, 273
        pneumococcal pneumonia, 1446
        Pneumocystis jirovecii pneumonia, 1552
    Salmonella infection and, 1469, 1470
    in staphylococcal infections. *See* Methicillin-resistant *S aureus* (MRSA) infections
    susceptibility testing and, 1313–1317
        in HIV infection/AIDS, 1350, 1360, 1361–1362, 1361*f*
        in tuberculosis, 278, 278*t*, 1336
    in tuberculosis, 277, 278, 278*t*, 282–283, 284, 1336
        directly observed therapy (DOT) and, 281, 283
        treatment of contacts and, 284
Drug susceptibility testing, 1313–1317. *See also* Drug resistance
    in HIV infection/AIDS, 1350
    in nontuberculous mycobacterial infection, 285
    in tuberculosis, 278, 278*t*
Drug tolerance, 1092. *See also* Substance use disorders
    opioid, 73, 82, 1098
"Drugs of abuse" toxicology screen, 1585
Drusen
    optic disk, 194
    retinal, in age-related macular degeneration, 185
"Dry" age-related macular degeneration, 185
Dry beriberi, 1274, 1275
Dry eye (keratoconjunctivitis sicca), **167–168**
    in Sjögren syndrome, 167, 850, 851
Dry mouth
    antipsychotics causing, 1071
    in Sjögren syndrome, 850, 851
Dry powder inhalers, for asthma therapy, 248, 250*t*, 251
Dry skin, emollients for, 95, 99–100*t*
Drying agents, for weepy dermatoses, 95
DSM-5 (Diagnostic and Statistical Manual), 1050
DTaP vaccines. *See* Diphtheria and tetanus toxoids and pertussis vaccines
DTI. *See* Direct thrombin inhibitors
DTIC-Dome. *See* Dacarbazine
DTs. *See* Delirium tremens

Dual antiplatelet therapy. *See also* Aspirin; Clopidogrel
  for angina, 361
  after coronary stent placement, 374
  GI bleeding/peptic ulcer disease and, 624, 628
Dual-chamber pacing, 400. *See also* Pacemaker
  for atrioventricular block, 400
  for cardiomyopathy, 419
Dual energy x-ray absorptiometry (DXA)
  in hyperparathyroidism, 1155
  in osteoporosis, 1160
Dual orexin receptor antagonists (DORAs), for sleep-wake disorders, 1089
Duavee. *See* Bazedoxifene
Dubin-Johnson syndrome, 674, 675t
Duchenne muscular dystrophy, 1047, 1048t
Duct-centric chronic pancreatitis, idiopathic, 731
Ductal carcinoma in situ, 748, 748t
  Paget carcinoma and, 118, 118f, 745
Ductography, in nipple discharge/breast cancer, 736, 744–745
Ductopenia, idiopathic adulthood, 724
Ductoscopy, in nipple discharge/breast cancer, 736, 745
Ductus arteriosus, patent, **330–331**, 331t
Duetact. *See* Pioglitazone, with glimepiride
Duke criteria (modified), for endocarditis, 1460
Duke Treadmill Score, 363, 363t
Dulaglutide, for diabetes, 1222t, 1226
Duloxetine, 61, 1078t, 1079–1081
  for anxiety, 1055
  for neuropathic pain/diabetic neuropathy, 61, 83t, 84, 1035, 1240
  overdose/toxicity of, 1078t, 1081
Dumping syndrome, 1252, 1256
Duncan disease, 1373
Duodenal ulcers, 622, 623, 624, 626t, 627. *See also* Peptic ulcer disease
Duodenum. *See also* Small intestine disorders of, **619–632**
DuoTrav. *See* Travoprost
Dupuytren contracture, **1699–1700**
Durable power of attorney for finance matters (DPOAF), 60
Durable Power of Attorney for Health Care (DPOA-HC), 90
Duroziez sign, 346
Dutasteride, 974
DVT. *See* Deep venous thrombosis
Dwarf tapeworm (*H nana*), **1535**, 1536
Dwarfism, 1109
DXA. *See* Dual energy x-ray absorptiometry
Dyazide. *See* Triamterene, with hydrochlorothiazide
Dying patient, care of. *See* End of life, provision of care at
Dymelor. *See* Acetohexamide
DynaCirc. *See* Isradipine
Dysautonomia (autonomic dysfunction), **990–991**
  in enterovirus 71 infection, 1427
  in Guillain-Barré syndrome, 990, 1038

neuropathy causing, 1035
  prenatal screening for, 800
Dysbarism, **1572–1573**
  barotrauma and, 204
Dysentery, 589, 1305. *See also specific cause*
  amebic (intestinal amebiasis), 588t, 589, 592, 1305, 1315t, 1342, 1525, 1526, 1526f, 1527t
    colitis after (postdysenteric colitis), 1526
  bacillary (*Shigella*). *See* Bacillary dysentery
  reactive arthritis and, 866
  Trichuris, 1538
Dysequilibrium (imbalance). *See* Vertigo; Vestibular disorders
Dysfunctional uterine bleeding. *See* Abnormal uterine bleeding
Dysgeusia, **226**
Dyshidrosis/dyshidrotic eczema. *See* Pompholyx
Dyskeratosis congenita, 546
Dyskinesia
  in Huntington disease, 1015
  levodopa-induced, 1012, 1013
  tardive, 1073
Dyslipidemia. *See also* Hyperlipidemia; Lipid disorders/lipids
  antiretroviral therapy and, 1174, 1345, 1356
  in diabetes mellitus, 1217, 1261
  drug therapy for, 1263–1266, 1264t, 1265t
  polycystic ovary syndrome and, 781, 1196
Dysmenorrhea, **765**
  IUD use and, 790
Dysmetabolic iron overload syndrome, 698
Dysmotility. *See* Motility disorders
Dysnomia, intracranial tumors causing, 1003
Dysorgasmia. *See* Orgasm, loss of
Dyspareunia (painful intercourse), 782, 782–783
Dyspepsia, **578–580**, 625. *See also specific cause*
Dysphagia, 605, 605t. *See also specific cause*
  in esophageal cancer, 605t, 1626
  in esophageal motility disorders, 605, 605t, 617, 618, 618–619
  in GERD, 607, 619
Dysphonia, **232–233**
  in laryngeal cancer, 235
  laryngopharyngeal reflux causing, 233
  in vocal fold paralysis, 237
Dysphoric disorder, premenstrual, 764–765, 1075
Dysplastic nevi. *See* Atypical nevi/mole
Dyspnea, **22–24**, 23t, **86–87**. *See also specific cause*
  cough and, 19
  in heart failure, 23, 402, 403, 404, 408
  palliation of, **86–87**
Dysrhythmias. *See* Arrhythmias
Dyssomnias, **1088–1089**. *See also* Insomnia
Dyssynergia, pelvic floor (dyssynergic defecation), 584, 584t, 585

Dysthymia, 1075. *See also* Depression
Dystocia, maternal diabetes and, 817
Dystonia
  drug-induced, 1017
    antipsychotics causing, 1072–1073, 1589
  oromandibular, 1016
  torsion
    focal, **1016–1017**
    idiopathic, **1015–1016**
Dystrophin, in muscular dystrophy, 1047, 1048t
Dysuria (painful voiding), **42–44**, 44f
DYT6/DYT7 genes, in focal torsion dystonia, 1016

E-cadherin cell adhesion protein, gastric cancer and, 1629
E-cigarettes, as tobacco cessation aid, 259
E coli. *See Escherichia coli*
EACA. *See* Aminocaproic acid
Ear, **200–214**. *See also under* Hearing
  barotrauma affecting, **204**
  cauliflower, 201
  in HIV infection/AIDS, **214**
  inner, **207–213**, 210t, 211t
  middle, **204–207**, 205f, 207f
  painful. *See* Earache
Ear canal, **201–203**
  bony overgrowths (exostoses/ osteomas) of, **202–203**
  foreign body in, **202**
  neoplasia of, **203**
  pruritus of, **202**
Ear drops
  for cerumen removal, 201
  for external otitis, 202
  ototoxic, perforated tympanic membrane and, 208
Earache (otalgia), **207**
  in external otitis/malignant external otitis, 202
Early goal-directed therapy, for shock, 496
Early menopause, 1201
East African trypanosomiasis, 1507, 1508, 1508t
Eastern (equine) encephalitis, 1388, 1389
Eastern subtype tick-borne encephalitis, 1391
Eating disorders, **1272–1274**. *See also specific type*
Eaton-Lambert syndrome. *See* Lambert-Eaton (myasthenic) syndrome
EBCT. *See* Electron beam CT
Ebola viral disease (EVD), **1397–1399**
Ebola virus vaccine, 1399
Ebola virus (Zaire), 1397
Ebolavirus species, 1397
EBOV. *See* Ebola virus
Ebstein anomaly, 348, 349
  lithium use during pregnancy and, 1086
EBV. *See* Epstein-Barr virus
EC regimen, 751
Ecchymosis
  of eye (black eye), 197
    in nasal trauma, 222
  in malabsorption, 633t
ECG. *See* Electrocardiogram

Echinacea purpurea, for benign prostatic hyperplasia, 975
Echinocandins, 1548, 1558. *See also specific agent*
Echinococcus granulosus/multilocularis (echinococcosis), **1537–1538**
Echocardiography/Doppler. *See also* Ultrasonography
  in angina, 357–358
  in aortic regurgitation, 334*t*, 346
  in aortic stenosis, 334*t*, 342
  for athlete screening, 436
  in atrial septal defect/patent foramen ovale, 325–326
  in cardiomyopathy, 416, 416*t*, 418, 419, 421
  in coarctation of aorta, 324
  in heart failure, 404
  in hypertension, 442, 445
  in mitral regurgitation, 334*t*, 337
  in mitral stenosis, 334*t*, 335
  in mitral valve prolapse, 340
  in myocardial infarction, 371
  in patent ductus arteriosus, 330
  in pericarditis/effusion, 425–426, 426, 427–428, 428, 429
  in pulmonary valve regurgitation, 350
  in pulmonary valve stenosis, 323
  in tetralogy of Fallot, 329
  in tricuspid regurgitation, 334*t*, 349
  in tricuspid stenosis, 334*t*, 348
  in valvular heart disease, 334*t*
  in ventricular septal defect, 327
Echolalia, in schizophrenia/psychotic disorders, 1067
Echovirus infections, **1426–1427**
Eclampsia, 443. *See also* Preeclampsia-eclampsia
  hypermagnesemia associated with treatment of, 810, 901, 902–903
Econazole, 98*t*
ECP. *See* Extracorporeal counterpulsation
"Ecstasy," 1101, 1587
  "herbal" (ephedrine), 1587
  hyponatremia caused by, 886
  seizures caused by, 1580*t*
ECT. *See* Electroconvulsive therapy
Ectasias, GI bleeding in, 595, 597
Ecthyma, 124
  contagiosa (orf), 1423
Ectopia lentis, in Marfan syndrome, 1682
Ectopic pregnancy, **805–807**
  appendicitis differentiated from, 642
  hCG levels in, 797, 806
  IUDs and, 790
  minipill use and, 788
  PID and, 778
Ectropion, **165**, 165*f*
Eculizumab
  for atypical hemolytic-uremic syndrome, 552
  for paroxysmal nocturnal hemoglobinuria, 510
Eczema. *See also* Atopic dermatitis
  dyshidrotic. *See* Eczema, vesiculobullous hand
  herpeticum, 105, 106, 1364, 1367*t*
  vesiculobullous hand (pompholyx), **121–122**, 122*f*
  tinea differentiated from, 114, 122

Edarbi. *See* Azilsartan
Edarbychlor. *See* Azilsartan
Edecrin. *See* Ethacrynic acid
Edema. *See also specific cause*
  arm, in breast cancer/postmastectomy, 742, 759
  in cirrhosis, 701–702
  in filariasis, 1543, 1543*f*, 1544
  in heart failure, 403
  lower extremity, **32–34**, 33*t*
  in malabsorption, 633*t*
  in nephritic syndrome, 936
  in nephrotic syndrome, 942
  optic disk, 193–194
  refeeding, 1269
  Reinke, 234
  thiazolidinediones causing, 1225
  in venous insufficiency, 32–34, 33*t*, 489
    leg ulcers and, 32, 33, 156, 489, 490
Edetate calcium disodium (EDTA), for lead poisoning, 1597
EDIC (Epidemiology of Diabetes Interventions and Complications) study, 1218
Edoxaban, 564, 565–566*t*, 567, 573
  for atrial fibrillation/stroke prevention, 391–393, 391*t*, 564, 565*t*
  for DVT/PE (venous thromboembolic disease), 564, 565*t*, 568*t*, 570*t*, 573
  overdose/toxicity of, 564, 1588
  perioperative management of, 52*t*, 566*t*
EDTA. *See* Edetate calcium disodium
Efavirenz, 1351*t*, 1355. *See also* Antiretroviral therapy
  pregnancy and, 822
  with tenofovir (TDF) and emtricitabine (Atripla), 1354*t*, 1355, 1359*t*
Effexor. *See* Venlafaxine
Effusions. *See* Malignant effusions; Pericardial effusions; Pleural effusions
Effusive-constrictive pericarditis, 428
Efinaconazole, 99*t*
  for onychomycosis, 160
Eflornithine
  for African trypanosomiasis, 1508, 1508*t*
  for hirsutism/virilization, 781, 1198
EGDT. *See* Early goal-directed therapy
eGFR. *See* Estimated glomerular filtration rate
EGFR (epidermal growth factor) mutations/inhibitors
  in colorectal cancer, 1639, 1640
  in gastric adenocarcinoma, 1631
  in lung cancer, 1612
  in pancreatic/periampullary carcinoma, 1625
EHEC. *See Escherichia coli,* enterohemorrhagic
Ehlers–Danlos syndrome
  aortic disorders/aneurysm in, pregnancy and, 435
  mitral valve prolapse in, 340
Ehrlichia canis/chaffeensis/ewingii/muris (ehrlichiosis), 1367*t*, 1429*t*, **1435–1436**
EIA, in syphilis, 1490
EIB. *See* Exercise-induced bronchoconstriction/asthma

EICs. *See* Epidermal inclusion cysts
EIEC. *See Escherichia coli,* enteroinvasive
EIF2AK3 gene, in diabetes, 1212
Eighth nerve lesions. *See* Schwannoma, vestibular
Eikenella corrodens. See HACEK organisms
Eisenmenger physiology, 430
  in atrial septal defect, 325
  in patent ductus arteriosus, 330
  in ventricular septal defect, 327
Ejaculate, for semen analysis. *See* Semen analysis
Ejaculation disturbances, 966, 1063. *See also* Erectile dysfunction/impotence
  antidepressants causing, 1079, 1082
  antipsychotics causing, 1071
  in infertility, 970
Ejaculatory ducts, obstruction of, in infertility, 970
Ejection clicks. *See* Heart murmurs; Heart sounds
Ejection fraction. *See* Left ventricular ejection fraction
ELANE/ELA-2 gene defect, in neutropenia, 518
Elapid (coral snake) envenomation, 1604
Elastic compression stockings. *See* Compression stockings
Elavil. *See* Amitriptyline
Elbasvir, for hepatitis C, 690, 690*t*
Elbow
  bursitis of (olecranon bursitis), 1700–1701, 1700*f*
  tennis or golf, 1697
Elder abuse/mistreatment, 16, **70–71**, 71*t*
Elderly patients. *See* Geriatric medicine; Older adults
Electrical alternans, in pericardial effusion, 427
Electrical burns, 1569, **1570–1571**
Electrical cardioversion. *See* Cardioversion
Electrical injury, **1570–1571**
Electrocardiogram (ECG). *See also specific disorder*
  in acute coronary syndromes/STEMI, 27, 27*t*, 28, 366, 371
  ambulatory monitoring of. *See* Ambulatory electrocardiographic monitoring
  in angina, 356, 357
  antidepressants affecting, 1082
  antipsychotics affecting, 1071
  in aortic dissection, 485
  in aortic regurgitation, 333*t*, 346
  in aortic stenosis, 333*t*, 342
  for athlete screening, 436, 437
  in atrial fibrillation, 389
  in atrial septal defect/patent foramen ovale, 325
  in cancer-related hypercalcemia, 1659
  in cardiomyopathy, 415, 416*t*, 418, 419, 421
  in chest pain evaluation, 27, 27*t*, 28, 356, 357, 366
  in coarctation of aorta, 324
  in electrical injury, 1570
  in heart failure, 404

Electrocardiogram (ECG) (*Cont.*):
in hyperkalemia, 894
in hypertension, 445
in hypokalemia, 893
in hypothermia, 1564, 1564*f*
in infectious myocarditis, 413
in mitral regurgitation, 333*t*
in mitral stenosis, 333*t*
in myocardial infarction, 27, 27*t*, 28, 366, 371
in palpitations, 30*t*, 31
in paroxysmal supraventricular tachycardia, 385
in patent ductus arteriosus, 330
in pericarditis/effusion, 426, 427
preoperative, 46
in pulmonary embolism, 295
in pulmonary valve regurgitation, 350
in pulmonary valve stenosis, 323
in syncope, 401
in tetralogy of Fallot, 329
in tricuspid regurgitation, 333*t*, 349
in tricuspid stenosis, 333*t*, 348
in valvular heart disease, 333*t*
in ventricular septal defect, 327
Electroconvulsive therapy (ECT), 1083–1084
for catatonia, 1070
for depression, 1077, 1079, 1083–1084
for neuroleptic malignant syndrome, 1072
for schizophrenia/psychotic disorders, 1070, 1072, 1083
Electroencephalogram (EEG)
in epilepsy, 985, 989
isoelectric, in brain death determination, 1028
in psychogenic nonepileptic/ pseudoepileptic seizure identification, 986, 1058
Electrolytes, 884. *See also specific type*
disorders of concentration of, **884–903**, 892*t*
assessment of, **884–885**, 885*t*
drowning and, 1567
genetic disorders and, 892*t*
replacement guidelines for, 911–912, 911*t*
requirements for in nutritional support, 911–912, 1282–1283
Electromyography
in back pain evaluation, 1693
in motor neuron disease, 1033
Electron beam CT (EBCT)
in angina, 358
coronary heart disease risk and, 1261–1262
Electronic cigarettes, as tobacco cessation aid, 259
Electrophoresis. *See* Hemoglobin electrophoresis
Electrophysiologic testing, in syncope evaluation, 401
Electrovaporization of prostate, transurethral, 976
Elephantiasis, 1544
Elestat. *See* Epinastine
Elestrin, 1204
Eletriptan, for migraine headache, 978
Elevated intraocular pressure, 179, 180
agents for reduction of, 172–173*t*

in chronic glaucoma, 179, 180
testosterone replacement therapy and, 1193
Elidel. *See* Pimecrolimus
ELISA. *See* Enzyme-linked immunosorbent assay
Elizabethkingia (*Chryseobacterium/ Flavobacterium*) species, **1477–1478**
Ellence. *See* Epirubicin
Elmiron. *See* Pentosan
Elocon. *See* Mometasone
Elotuzumab, 1666*t*
Eloxatin. *See* Oxaliplatin
Elsberg syndrome, 1370
Eltrombopag
for aplastic anemia, 517, 548
for hepatic coagulopathy, 704
for myelodysplastic syndromes, 526, 548
for thrombocytopenia
chemotherapy-induced, 548, 1672
immune, 549*f*, 550
Elvitegravir, 1352*t*, 1358. *See also* Antiretroviral therapy
with tenofovir (TAF)/cobicistat/ emtricitabine (Genvoya), 1354*t*, 1355, 1358, 1359*t*, 1360
with tenofovir (TDF)/cobicistat/ emtricitabine (Stribild), 1354*t*, 1355, 1358, 1359*t*, 1360
Emadine. *See* Emedastine
Embolectomy
for acute arterial limb occlusion, 477
for stroke, 996
Embolism. *See also* Thromboembolism; Venous thromboembolic disease
acute arterial limb occlusion caused by, 476
in atrial fibrillation, 388
anticoagulation in prevention/ treatment of, 351, 352*t*, 388, 389, 389*t*, 390, 390–393, 390*t*, 391*t*, 392*f*
in atrial flutter, 395
carotid sources of, 477, 478
cerebrovascular occlusion and, 477, 478. *See also* Stroke
in endocarditis, 1459, 1460, 1462
gas, in decompression sickness, 1573
paradoxic, 991
peripheral arterial aneurysms and, 484
during pregnancy, 435
air travel and, 1576
pulmonary. *See* Pulmonary venous thromboembolism
in retinal artery occlusion, 187, 188
in transient ischemic attacks, 477, 991, 993
in transient monocular visual loss, 188, 189
Embolization
for GI bleeding, 597, 599
tumor, in lung cancer, 1613
Embryo. *See* Fetus
Embryonal cell carcinoma, of testis, 1556, 1655

Emedastine, for allergic eye disease, 168, 170*t*
Emergencies
cancer-related, **1657–1661**
hypertensive. *See* Hypertensive emergencies
in-flight (air travel), **1574–1576**
Emergency/postcoital contraception, 785, **791**
IUD for, 789, 791
for sexual violence (rape/sexual assault) victim, 791, 793, 794, 1302
Emery-Dreifuss muscular dystrophy, 1048*t*
Emesis, **87**, **580–583**, 581*t*, 582*t*. *See also* Nausea and vomiting
for poisoning/drug overdose, 1582
Emetine, for amebiasis, 1526, 1527*t*
Emission, loss of (anejaculation), 966, 1063. *See also* Erectile dysfunction/impotence
EML4-ALK mutation, in lung cancer, 1612
Emollients, 95, 99–100*t*
Emotional challenges, for terminally ill/ dying patient, 92
Empagliflozin, 1222*t*, 1227–1228
with linagliptin, 1228
with metformin, 1228
Emphysema, 257, 258, 258*t*, 259. *See also* Chronic obstructive pulmonary disease
alpha-1-antiprotease/antitrypsin deficiency in, 259
replacement therapy and, 261–262
bullectomy for, 262
lung volume reduction surgery for, 262
panacinar bibasilar, 259
Emphysematous pyelonephritis, 956
Empliciti. *See* Elotuzumab
Empty can test, 1686*t*
Empyema
anaerobes causing, 275, 276, 1478
in hepatic hydrothorax, 702
middle ear, 204. *See also* Otitis, media
pleural, 311, 312, 313, 313*t*
in pneumonia, 275, 276, 1445
streptococcal, 1443
subdural, 1478
Emsam. *See* Selegiline, transdermal
Emtricitabine, 1351*t*, 1354, 1360. *See also* Antiretroviral therapy
for hepatitis B, 1341, 1354
resistance to, 1361
with tenofovir (TDF) (Truvada), 1353, 1354*t*, 1355
after needle stick, 1347
plus atazanavir and cobicistat, 1359*t*
plus atazanavir and ritonavir, 1359*t*
plus darunavir and cobicistat, 1360*t*
plus darunavir and ritonavir, 1359*t*
plus dolutegravir, 1359*t*
plus raltegravir, 1358, 1359*t*
prophylactic, 4, 1346
with tenofovir (TAF)/elvitegravir/ cobicistat (Genvoya), 1354*t*, 1355, 1358, 1359*t*, 1360
with tenofovir (TDF) and efavirenz (Atripla), 1354*t*, 1355, 1359*t*

with tenofovir (TDF)/elvitegravir/ cobicistat (Stribild), 1354*t*, 1355, 1358, 1359*t*, 1360

with tenofovir (TDF) and rilpivirine (Complera), 1354*t*, 1355, 1359*t*

Emtriva. *See* Emtricitabine

Enalapril
  for heart failure, 407
  for hypertension, 455*t*
    with hydrochlorothiazide, 455*t*

Enalaprilat, for hypertensive urgencies/ emergencies, 470*t*, 471

Enbrel. *See* Etanercept

Encainide, toxicity of, 384

Encephalitis, 1298. *See also specific cause and* Meningoencephalitis
  anti-DPPX, 1008
  anti-NMDA receptor-associated, 1008
  arbovirus, **1388–1390**
  CMV, 1375, 1376
  in coxsackievirus infection, 1426
  enterovirus 71 causing, 1427
  herpes simplex, 1364, 1366
  HHV-6 causing, 1377
  inclusion body, measles and, 1378
  limbic, 1008
  in loiasis, 1546
  measles/measles vaccination and, 1378–1379
  Nipah virus causing, 1409
  parkinsonism after, 1011
  rabies, 1386
  tick-borne, 1388, **1391–1392**
  toxoplasmic, 1524
  varicella zoster virus, 1369
  yellow fever vaccine-associated, 1327, 1405

Encephalitozoon/Encephalitozoon intestinalis, 1528, 1529

Encephalomyelitis
  cancer-related, 1008
  in Lyme disease, 1503
  measles/measles vaccine and, 1378–1379
  optic neuritis and, 193
  yellow fever vaccine-associated, 1327, 1405

Encephalopathy
  alcohol use disorder and (chronic alcoholic brain syndromes), 1093, 1098
  bovine spongiform (vCJD/mad cow disease), 1394
  in cancer, 1008
  with fatty liver. *See* Reye syndrome
  hepatic. *See* Hepatic encephalopathy
  in HIV infection/AIDS, 1339
  hypertensive, 444, 468
  hyponatremic, 888
  in influenza, 1412
  lead, 1597
    gasoline sniffing and, 1101
  lithium causing, 1086
  in Lyme disease, 1503
  melarsoprol causing, 1508
  metabolic. *See* Metabolic encephalopathy
  in Reye syndrome. *See* Reye syndrome
  after rubella infection, 1385

spongiform (spongiosis/prion diseases), **1393–1395**
uremic, 925, 928
Wernicke, 908, **1026**, 1093, 1095, 1275

End of life
  Kübler-Ross' patterns of emotions and, 92
  patient expectations about, 88
  prognosis at, 88
  provision of care at, **88–94**. *See also* Palliative care
    advance care planning/advance directives and, 90
    care of family and, 89, 89*t*
    clinician self-care and, 89
    communicating with patient and, 88–89, 89*t*
    cultural issues in, 91
    decision-making and, 90
    DNAR orders and, 90
    follow-up/grieving and, 94
    in hospice/palliative care institution, 90–91
    nutrition/hydration needs and, 91
    pain management and, **73–74**
    patient's wishes regarding, 90
    psychologic/social/spiritual issues and, 92–93, 92*t*, 93*t*
    tasks after death and, **93–94**
    withdrawal/withholding curative efforts and, 91–92, 92*t*
    advance directives and, 90

End-stage renal disease (ESRD), 923, 923*t*, 929–930. *See also* Chronic kidney disease; Renal failure
  amyloidosis and, 946
  diabetic nephropathy and, 945, 1239
  immunization recommendations in, 1321*t*
  juvenile-nephronophthisis-medullary cystic disease and, 951
  kidney transplantation for. *See* Kidney transplantation
  polycystic kidney disease and, 949, 950

Endarterectomy, carotid. *See* Carotid endarterectomy/ thromboendarterectomy

Endemic flea-borne (murine) typhus, 1429*t*, **1430–1431**

Endemic goiter, **1148–1149**

Endemic hemolytic-uremic syndrome, 550, 551, 551*t*

Endemic syphilis, **1498–1499**

Endocarditis
  infective, 1314*t*, 1458–1463, 1459*f*, 1460*t*, 1461*t*
    anaerobic, **1479**
    anticoagulation and, 352*t*, 1463
    antimicrobial chemoprophylaxis and, 1460, 1460*t*, 1461*t*
    in hereditary hemorrhagic telangiectasia, 1684
    in patent ductus arteriosus, 330
    during pregnancy, **436**, 819
    prosthetic heart valves and, 337
    in tetralogy of Fallot, 329–330
    in ventricular septal defect, 327–328
    in bartonellosis, 1460, 1462, 1477
    candidal, 1547–1548, 1548

Coxiella/Q fever, 1429*t*, 1437, 1437–1438
  in drug user, 1304, 1314*t*, 1458
  enterococcal, 1314*t*, 1444, 1458, 1462
  gonococcal, 1475, 1476
  HACEK organisms causing, 1458, 1462
  native valve, 1458
    anticoagulation and, 1463
  pneumococcal, 1445, 1446, 1461
  prosthetic valve, 337, 1458, 1461
    anticoagulation and, 352*t*, 1463
  staphylococcal, 1314*t*, 1449, 1450, 1458, 1462, 1463
  streptococcal, 1443, 1458, 1461–1462
  surgical management of, 1462–1463
Libman-Sacks, in SLE, 840, 843

Endocervical curettage, 763*t*
  in CIN/cervical cancer, 772
  in endometrial carcinoma, 774

Endoclips, for GI bleeding, 596, 599
  in Mallory-Weiss syndrome/tears, 612
  in peptic ulcer disease, 630

Endocrine disorders, **1108–1209**. *See also specific gland and disorder and* Multiple endocrine neoplasia
  antipsychotic drug use and, 1072
  in chronic kidney disease, 929
  cognitive disorders/delirium caused by, 1102*t*
  in HIV infection/AIDS, 1342–1343
  in hyponatremia, 886
  in infertility. *See* Hypogonadism
  perioperative evaluation/management and, **53**

Endocrine therapy. *See* Hormone therapy

Endoleaks, after abdominal aneurysm repair, 482

Endolymphatic hydrops (Ménière disease), 211–212, 211*t*

Endometrial biopsy, 763*t*
  in abnormal uterine bleeding, 762–763
  in endometrial carcinoma, 774

Endometrial carcinoma/cancer of uterus, **774**, 1608*t*, 1623*t*
  abnormal premenopausal uterine bleeding and, 763
  breast cancer risk and, 738
  estrogen replacement therapy and, 774, 795, 1203
  HNPCC/Lynch syndrome and, 668, 669, 774
  incidence/mortality/risk of, 774, 1608*t*
  oral contraceptive use and, 774, 786
  polycystic ovary syndrome and, 774, 780, 1196
  postmenopausal bleeding and, 764, 774

Endometrial curettage. *See* Endometrial biopsy

Endometrial hyperplasia
  estrogen replacement therapy and, 795, 1203
  postmenopausal vaginal bleeding and, 764

Endometriosis, **776–777**
  infertility and, 776, 784
  pelvic pain and, 765, 776

Endometritis, **778–779**, 814. *See also*
  Pelvic inflammatory disease
amenorrhea and, 1201
clostridial, 1452
postpartum, 814, 820
Endomyocardial biopsy, in infectious
  myocarditis, 414
Endomyocardial fibrosis, 421
Endomyometritis, 814. *See also*
  Endometritis
Endomysial antibodies, in celiac disease,
  634
Endoscopic retrograde
  cholangiopancreatography
  (ERCP), 677
  cholangitis after, 677
  in choledocholithiasis, 721, 722
  in chronic pancreatitis evaluation, 731
  pancreatitis after, 677, 729
  in pregnant patient, 824
Endoscopic ultrasonography, 677
Endoscopy
  in achalasia, 617
  in cancer screening/polyp
    identification/removal,
    665–666, 1642. *See also*
    Colonoscopy; Sigmoidoscopy
  in diarrhea, 593
  in dyspepsia, 579
  in erosive/hemorrhagic gastritis
    (gastropathy), 620
  in esophageal disorders, 605
    Barrett esophagus, 608
    bleeding varices, 615
      prevention of first bleeding
        episode and, 616
    cancer, 608, 1626
    caustic/corrosive injury, 1586, 1587
    GERD, 607
    infectious esophagitis, 611
    Mallory-Weiss syndrome, 612
    motility disorders, 617, 618
    stricture, 608
  in gastric adenocarcinoma, 1630
  in GI bleeding, 596, 598, 599, 600
    peptic ulcer disease and, 630
  in *H pylori* detection/assessment,
    622
  in pancreatitis, 732
  in peptic ulcer disease, 624–625
    bleeding management and, 630
  in ulcerative colitis, 658
Endothelial erectile dysfunction, 966
Endothelin receptor blockers (ERBs), for
  pulmonary hypertension,
  303, 431, 432f
Endotracheal intubation. *See* Intubation
Endovascular surgery/prostheses. *See also*
  Angioplasty; Stents/stent
  grafts
  for abdominal aortic aneurysm, 482
  for acute arterial limb occlusion, 477
  for aortoiliac occlusive disease, 473
  for carotid occlusive disease, 478
  for femoral/popliteal occlusive disease,
    474
  for intestinal ischemia, 479
  for renal artery stenosis/renal vascular
    hypertension, 442, 932
  for subarachnoid hemorrhage, 999
  for thoracic aortic aneurysm, 483

for tibial/pedal occlusive disease, 475
for transient ischemic attacks, 993
Endurance exercise. *See also* Exercise/
  activity
  hyponatremia after, 887
Endurant. *See* Rilpivirine
Enemas
  barium, for cancer screening, 1643
  for constipation, 585t
Energy deficiency (protein–energy
  malnutrition), **1268–1269**
Energy requirements, in nutritional
  support, 1282
Enfuvirtide, 1352t, 1357. *See also*
  Antiretroviral therapy
ENG gene, in hereditary hemorrhagic
  telangiectasia, 1684
Engerix B. *See* Hepatitis B vaccine
Enjuvia, 1204
Enolase, neuron-specific, in
  Jakob-Creutzfeldt disease,
  1022
Enoxaparin
  for acute coronary syndromes, 367f
  for DVT/PE (venous thromboembolic
    disease), 568t, 570t
  after fibrinolytic therapy for
    myocardial infarction, 375
Entacapone, 1013–1014
  with levodopa and carbidopa, 1013,
    1014
Entamoeba, 1525. *See also* Amebiasis
  dispar, 1525, 1526
  histolytica, 588t, 589, 590, 592, 1305,
    1315t, 1342, 1525, 1526
  moshkovskii, 1525
Entecavir, for hepatitis B, 687–688
Enteral nutritional support (tube
    feedings), 1281–1282, 1281f.
    See also Nutritional support
  in burn injury, 1569
  complications of, **1283–1284**
  for Crohn disease, 655
  for elderly/dementia, 67, 91
  in end-of-life care, 91
  in pancreatitis, 729
  patient monitoring during, 1284
  for protein–energy malnutrition,
    1269
  solutions for, **1283**, 1283t
Enteric (typhoid) fever, **1468–1469**
  carrier state and, 1469
  prevention/immunization and, 1327,
    1469
Enteric infection/enteritis. *See also*
  Gastroenteritis
  irritable bowel syndrome after, 644,
    1308
Enterobacter infections, 1311t
  urinary, 1314t
Enterobius vermicularis (enterobiasis/
    pinworms), **1540–1541**
  anogenital pruritus and, 147, 148, 1541
Enterocele, 777
Enterococcus faecalis/faecium
    (enterococcal infection),
    1311t, 1315t, **1444–1445**
  drug resistance and, 1316, 1444, 1445
  endocarditis, 1314t, 1444, 1458, 1462
Enterocolitis. *See also* Diarrhea;
  Gastroenteritis

in HIV infection/AIDS, 588t, 589,
    1335, 1342
  salmonella, 588t, 589, 1305, 1307t,
    1308, 1315t, 1342, **1469**
Enterocytozoon/Enterocytozoon bieneusi,
    588t, 1528, 1529
Enteropancreatic tumors, **1185–1187**. *See*
    also specific type and
    Neuroendocrine
    tumors
  in MEN, 1185, 1187t, 1188, 1252
Enteropathy
  AIDS, 1342
  gluten-sensitive. *See* Celiac disease
  protein-losing, **643**. *See also* Protein-
    losing enteropathy
Enteropathy-associated T cell lymphoma,
    1634
Enterostomies, tube, 1281–1282, 1281f.
    See also Enteral nutritional
    support
Enterovirus infections, 1367t, **1425–1428**.
    See also specific virus
Enterovirus 68, **1427**, 1428
Enterovirus 70, **1427**
Enterovirus 71, **1427**, 1428
Enterovirus 72, 1428. *See also* Hepatitis A
    virus
Enterovirus EV-104A, 1428
Enthesopathy/enthesitis
  in ankylosing spondylitis, 863
  in lateral/medial epicondylosis, 1698
  in psoriatic arthritis, 864
Enthesophytes, in diffuse idiopathic
    skeletal hyperostosis, 864
Entocort. *See* Budesonide
Entrapment/compression neuropathy,
    1039. *See also specific type or*
    nerve affected and
    Neuropathies
  amyloidosis and, 1037
  rheumatoid arthritis and, 835, 1037
Entropion, **165**
Entry inhibitors, for HIV infection/AIDS,
    1352t, 1357–1358. *See also*
    Antiretroviral therapy
  resistance to, 1361
Environmental emergencies, disorders
    caused by, **1561–1576**. *See*
    also specific disorder
Environmental factors
  in asthma, 246
    control of, 248
  in diabetes, 1211, 1212
  in lung disease, 290t, **305–310**. *See also*
    specific disorder
Environmental radiation exposure,
    1572
Environmental tobacco smoke. *See*
    Passive smoking
Enzalutamide, 1669t
  for prostate cancer, 1649t, 1650
Enzyme immunoassay (EIA), in syphilis,
    1490
Enzyme inhibitors, in cancer
    chemotherapy, 1665t
Enzyme-linked immunosorbent assay
    (ELISA). *See also specific*
    disorder
  in HIV infection/AIDS, 1333, 1334,
    1334t

Eosinophilia
    drug-induced hypersensitivity/drug
        reaction and, 161, 163,
        880–881
    in pulmonary disorders. *See*
        Eosinophilic pulmonary
        syndromes
Eosinophilic esophagitis, 605t, **613**
Eosinophilic fasciitis, 846
Eosinophilic folliculitis, 130, 131, 1333
Eosinophilic granulomatosis with
        polyangiitis (Churg-Strauss
        syndrome), 304
    leukotriene modifiers for asthma and,
        251
    pulmonary involvement in, 304
    renal involvement in, 933t, 935f, 938
Eosinophilic meningitis/
        meningoencephalitis, in
        toxocariasis, 1542
Eosinophilic pneumonia, 294
Eosinophilic pulmonary syndromes,
        294
    tropical pulmonary eosinophilia, 1544
Ependymoma, 1004t
Ephedrine (decongestant), adverse
        ophthalmic effects of, 177t
Ephedrine ("herbal ecstasy"), 1587
Ephelides (freckles), **103**
Epicondylosis (epicondylitis), lateral and
        medial, **1697–1698**
Epidemic encephalitis, enterovirus 71
        causing, 1427
Epidemic keratoconjunctivitis
    adenovirus, 167, 1421
    coxsackievirus, 1426
Epidemic louse-borne typhus, 150,
        1428–1430, 1429t
Epidemic pleurodynia, 1426
Epidemiology of Diabetes Interventions
        and Complications (EDIC)
        study, 1218
Epidermal growth factor (EGFR)
        mutations/inhibitors
    in colorectal cancer, 1639, 1640
    in gastric adenocarcinoma, 1631
    in lung cancer, 1612
    in pancreatic/periampullary
        carcinoma, 1625
Epidermal inclusion cysts (EICs), **154**
    furuncles/carbuncles differentiated
        from, 153, 154
Epidermoid cyst, testicular, 1656
Epididymis, obstruction of, in infertility,
        970
Epididymitis, 955t, **959–960**, 1316t
    chlamydial, 960, 1316t
    in filariasis, 1544
    gonococcal, 960, 1316t
Epidural abscess
    bacterial rhinosinusitis and, 217
    osteomyelitis and, 870, 871, 1449
    otitis media and, 206
Epidural hemorrhage
    cerebral, 1030t
    spinal, 1002
Epifrin. *See* Epinephrine
Epigastric pain. *See* Abdominal pain/
        tenderness; Dyspepsia
Epiglottis, cancer of, 235, 236
Epiglottis "thumb sign," 234

Epiglottitis (supraglottitis), **234**
    Haemophilus causing, 234, 1466
Epilepsia partialis continua, 1017
Epilepsy, **983–990**, 984t, 987–988t. *See
        also* Seizures
    drug therapy for, 986–989, 987–988t.
        See also Anticonvulsant
        therapy
    genetic, 983
    myoclonic ragged red fiber (MERRF),
        1049
    myoclonus/myoclonic jerks and, 1017
    photosensitive, 985
    posttraumatic, 983, 1031
    pregnancy and, 820
    seizure classification in, 983–985, 984t
    solitary seizure and, 989
    structural/metabolic, 983
    surgical management of, 989
    vagal nerve stimulation in
        management of, 989
Epileptic drop attacks (atonic seizures),
        984t, 985. *See also* Seizures
Epinastine, for allergic eye disease, 168,
        171t
Epinephrine
    for anaphylaxis, 877
    for cardiac arrest in hypothermia,
        1565
    for desensitization reactions, 1318
    endoscopic injection of
        for GI bleeding/peptic ulcer, 599,
            630
        for Mallory-Weiss syndrome/tears,
            612
    for glaucoma/ocular hypertension, 180
    in pheochromocytoma, 1179, 1180
    for shock, 496
Epi-pen. *See* Epinephrine
Epirubicin, 1665t
    for breast cancer, 751, 753
    for gastric adenocarcinoma, 1631
    toxicity of, 1665t, 1674–1675
Episodic dyspnea, 24
Episodic vertigo, 211, 213
Epistaxis, **221–222**
    cocaine abuse and, 221, 1100
    in hereditary hemorrhagic
        telangiectasia, 221, 1684
    in malabsorption, 633t
Epithelial cells/renal tubular casts, 913,
        914t
Epivir. *See* Lamivudine
Eplerenone
    for adrenal hyperplasia, 1179
    for heart failure, 406, 407
        infarct-related, 376
    for hypertension, 450t, 459
EPO. *See* Erythropoietin
EPOCH regimen, 533, 1337t, 1344
Epoetin alfa. *See* Erythropoietin
Epogen. *See* Erythropoietin
Epoprostenol, for pulmonary
        hypertension, 303, 431–433
Epothilones, in cancer chemotherapy,
        1665t
Eprosartan/eprosartan with
        hydrochlorothiazide, 457t
Epsom salts. *See* Magnesium sulfate
Epstein-Barr virus, **1372–1374**
    Burkitt lymphoma and, 1373

mononucleosis caused by, 228, 1367t,
        1372–1373, 1372f
    nasopharyngeal carcinoma and, 223,
        1373
Eptifibatide
    for acute coronary syndromes, 367f,
        368
    PCI and, 362
    platelet function affected by, 558t
Epzicom (abacavir with lamivudine),
        1353, 1354, 1354t
    with darunavir and cobicistat,
        1360t
    with darunavir and ritonavir, 1360t
Equianalgesic dosing, 77–81t, 82
Equine encephalitis, 1388
Equine rabies antiserum, 1387
ERB. *See* Endothelin receptor blockers
Erb (limb-girdle) muscular dystrophy,
        849, 1047, 1048t
Erbitux. *See* Cetuximab
ERCP. *See* Endoscopic retrograde
        cholangiopancreatography
Erec-Aid System. *See* Vacuum erection
        device
Erectile dysfunction/impotence, **965–968**,
        1063, 1064. *See also* Sexual
        dysfunction
    in chronic kidney disease, 929
    in diabetes mellitus, 1240–1241
    drugs causing, 966
        antidepressants, 1064, 1079, 1082
        antipsychotics, 1071
    endocrine causes/hypogonadism and,
        967
    phosphodiesterase inhibitors/sildenafil
        for diagnosis/treatment of,
        967, 1064, 1079
    psychologic/psychogenic, 966,
        966–967, 967, 1063
    vascular disease and, 966, 967, 968
Erections, 966
    loss of, 966. *See also* Erectile
        dysfunction/impotence
    prolonged painful. *See* Priapism
Ergocalciferol (vitamin D₂), 1151–1152,
        1151t. *See also* Vitamin D
    for hypoparathyroidism/tetany,
        1151–1152, 1151t
    for vitamin D deficiency/osteomalacia,
        1166
Ergosterol. *See* Ergocalciferol
Ergotamine
    for cluster headache, 980
    for migraine headache, 978
Erlotinib, 1667t
    K-ras mutations and, 1625
    for lung cancer, 1612
    for pancreatic/periampullary
        carcinoma, 1625
Erosive esophagitis. *See* Esophagitis
Erosive gastritis. *See* Gastritis
Erosive skin disorders, 96t
Ertaczo. *See* Sertaconazole
Ertapenem
    for anaerobic infections, 1479, 1479t
    for pneumonia, 275t
Eructation (belching), 587
Eruptive psoriasis, 107. *See also* Psoriasis
Eruptive xanthoma, 1261, 1261f
    in diabetes, 1214, 1242, 1261, 1261f

Erwinaze. *See* Asparaginase *Erwinia chrysanthemi*
Erysipelas, **136–137**, 1315*t*, 1442–1443, 1443*t*
Erysipeloid, 137
Erythemas, 96*t*, **133–139**. *See also specific type*
  acral (hand-foot syndrome), chemotherapy-induced, 1673
  induratum, 152
  infectiosum, 1367*t*, 1422
  infectious, **136–139**
  marginatum, in rheumatic fever, 422, 423, 423*t*
  migrans, **136**, 137*f*, 1502, 1503, 1504, 1505*t*. *See also* Lyme disease
  multiforme, **135–136**, 135*f*
    drugs causing, 135, 136
    herpes-associated, 135, 136, 1364, 1366
    major. *See* Stevens-Johnson syndrome; Toxic epidermal necrolysis
  nodosum, **151–152**, 152*f*
    in coccidioidomycosis, 1550
    drugs causing, 152, 162*t*
    leprosum, 1484, 1484–1485
    in sarcoidosis, 292, 293
  pernio (chilblain), **1565**
  reactive, **133–136**, 134*f*, 135*f*
Erythrasma, 113, 147, 147*f*
Erythrocyte count, in pleural fluid, 313*t*
Erythrocytes. *See also under Red cell*
  in myeloproliferative neoplasms, 520*t*
  in pleural fluid, 313*t*
  in urine. *See* Hematuria; Red cell casts
Erythrocytosis, testosterone replacement therapy and, 1193
Erythroderma
  exfoliative, **117**
    drugs causing, 117, 162*t*
    psoriatic, 107, 117. *See also* Psoriasis
Erythrogenic toxin (pyrogenic erythrotoxin), 1444
Erythromelalgia, 845, 875
  in essential thrombocytosis, 521, 522, 875
Erythromycin. *See also* Macrolides
  for acne, 98*t*, 127
  for amebiasis, 1527*t*
  for anthrax, 1456*t*
  with benzoyl peroxide, 98*t*, 127
  for Lyme disease, 1504
  for ophthalmic disorders, 169*t*
  for pharyngitis, 229, 1442
Erythroplakia, 224
Erythropoiesis
  iron deficiency anemia and, 500
  iron-restricted, 502
Erythropoiesis-stimulating agents. *See also specific type*
  for anemia of chronic kidney disease, 928
  for chemotherapy-associated anemia, 1662, 1671–1672*t*
  toxicity of, 1662, 1671–1672*t*
Erythropoietin (epoetin alfa)
  for anemia of chronic disease/chronic kidney disease, 503, 928
  for aplastic anemia, 517

  for chemotherapy-induced anemia, 1662, 1671*t*
  for HIV infection/AIDS, 1350
  for myelodysplastic syndromes, 526
Erythrotoxin, pyrogenic (erythrogenic toxin), 1444
Erythrovirus (parvovirus B19) infection, **1421–1423**
  arthritis in, 870, 1422
    rheumatoid arthritis differentiated from, 836
  erythema infectiosum, 1367*t*, 1422
ESAs. *See* Erythropoiesis-stimulating agents
Eschar formation
  in burn injury, 1569
  in frostbite, 1566
  in rickettsialpox, 1434
  in scrub typhus, 1431
  in tick typhus, 1434
Escharotomy, in burn care, 1569
Escherichia coli, 1311*t*, 1315*t*
  cystitis/urinary tract infection caused by, 954, 1311*t*, 1314*t*, 1315*t*
  diarrhea/gastroenteritis/food poisoning caused by, 588*t*, 589, 1305, **1470–1471**
  enterohemorrhagic (EHEC), 588*t*, 589, 1306*t*. *See also* Shiga-toxin producing *E coli*
  enteroinvasive (EIEC), 588*t*, 1470
  enterotoxigenic (ETEC), 588*t*, 589, 1305, 1307*t*, 1470
  fever/neutropenia/chemotherapy and, 1314*t*
  hemolytic-uremic syndrome caused by, 550, 551, 551*t*, 1471
  pneumonia caused by, 268*t*
  shiga-toxin–producing (STEC), 589, 1305, 1306*t*, 1470–1471
Escherichia coli O104:H4, 589, 1470
Escherichia coli O145, 550, 551, 1471
Escherichia coli O157:H5, 588*t*
Escherichia coli O157:H7, 589, 1470–1471
  antibiotics contraindicated in diarrhea caused by, 1471
  hemolytic-uremic syndrome caused by, 550, 551, 551*t*, 1471
Escitalopram, 1078*t*, 1079–1081
  for dyspepsia, 580
  for menopausal symptoms, 1202
Esidrix. *See* Hydrochlorothiazide
Eslicarbazepine, 988*t*
Esmolol
  for arrhythmias, 382*t*
    atrial fibrillation, 389
    infarct-related, 377
    supraventricular tachycardia, 382*t*, 386
  for hypertension
    in aortic dissection, 469*t*, 485
    in urgencies/emergencies, 469, 469*t*, 470*t*
Esomeprazole, 609, 625. *See also* Proton pump inhibitors
Esophageal clearance, abnormal, in GERD, 607
Esophageal dilation
  for achalasia, 618
  for esophageal webs and rings, 613
  for stricture, 608–609

Esophageal dysphagia, 605, 605*t*. *See also* Dysphagia
Esophageal manometry, 606
  in motility disorders, 606, 618
Esophageal motility disorders, **617–619**
  chest pain in, 27, 359, 617, 618, 619
  dysphagia in, 605, 605*t*, 617, 618, 618–619
  in scleroderma, 846
Esophageal pH monitoring, 606, 607, 609–610
Esophageal (Schatzki) rings, 605*t*, **613–614**
Esophageal spasm, diffuse, 605*t*
Esophageal sphincter
  artificial, for GERD, 610
  lower, in GERD, 606
  upper, in Zenker diverticulum, 614
Esophageal varices, **614–617**
  cirrhosis and, 595, 596, 614, 615, 617, 700
  GI bleeding from, 594–595, 614–617
  noncirrhotic portal hypertension and, 714
  portal hypertension and, 594–595, 614
  prevention of first bleeding episode and, 616–617
  prevention of rebleeding from, 616
Esophageal webs, **613–614**
  iron deficiency anemia and (Plummer-Vinson syndrome), 501, 613
Esophagectomy, for esophageal cancer, 608, 1627
Esophagitis
  bisphosphonates and, 1161
  candidal, 611, 1547, 1548
    in HIV infection/AIDS, 611, 1335, 1338*t*, 1341
  CMV, 611, 611–612, 1375
  dysphagia in, 605*t*, 611
  eosinophilic, 605*t*, **613**
  erosive/reflux. *See also* Gastroesophageal reflux disease
    GERD and, 606, 607, 610
    GI bleeding and, 595
  herpetic, 611, 612, 1364, 1366
  in HIV infection/AIDS, 611, 1341
  infectious, **611–612**
  pill-induced, **612**
  stricture formation and, 608
Esophagography, barium. *See* Barium esophagography
Esophagus
  Barrett, 608, 609
    esophageal carcinoma and, 608, 1626
  cancer of, 1623*t*, **1626–1629**
    adenocarcinoma, 1626
    Barrett esophagus and, 608, 1626
    bisphosphonate use and, 1161
    dyspepsia and, 578
    dysphagia in, 605*t*, 1626
    squamous cell, 1626
  disorders of, **604–619**, 605*t*. *See also under Esophageal and* Esophagitis
    benign, **612–617**
    chest pain and, 27, 359, 611, 617, 618, 619

corrosive/caustic injury, 1586, 1587
dysphagia in, 605, 605t, 617, 618, 618–619
GERD, **606–611**
motility and, **617–619**. *See also* Esophageal motility disorders
in scleroderma, 846
foreign body in, **238**
nutcracker, 619
rupture of
pleural effusion in, 313t
vomiting and (Boerhaave syndrome), 582
"sigmoid," 617
strictures of
dysphagia in, 605t, 608–609
peptic, 605t, 608–609
Espundia (mucocutaneous leishmaniasis), 1510, 1511, 1512
ESRD. *See* End-stage renal disease
Essential fatty acids, in nutritional support, 1283
Essential hypertension, 441, 444. *See also* Hypertension
Essential thrombocytosis, 519t, 520t, **521–522**
Essure, for tubal interruption, 792
Estazolam, 1054t
Estimated glomerular filtration rate, 914–915. *See also* Glomerular filtration rate
Estrace, 1205
Estradiol/ethinyl estradiol
for abnormal uterine bleeding, 763
in estrogen replacement therapy, 795, 796, 1202, 1204, 1205
in male infertility, 970
in oral contraceptives, 785–786, 787t
parenteral, 1205
in vaginal rings
contraceptive, 789, 1205
for hormone replacement, 795, 1202, 1205
Estradiol gels/mists, 1204
Estradiol injections, 1205
Estradiol transdermal systems (skin patches)
for contraception, 789
in hormone replacement therapy, 795, 1204
Estradiol vaginal ring
contraceptive, 789, 1205
with progestin, 789, 1205
in estrogen replacement therapy, 795, 1202, 1205
Estradiol vaginal tablets, 1205
Estrasorb, 1204
Estring, 1205
EstroGel, 1204
Estrogen-progesterone therapy. *See* Estrogen (hormone) replacement therapy
Estrogen receptor modulators, selective (SERMs). *See* Selective estrogen receptor modulators
Estrogen (hormone) replacement therapy, 1202–1207. *See also* Estrogens; Selective estrogen receptor modulators
adverse ophthalmic effects of, 178t

agents used in, 1204–1206
for atrophic urethritis/vaginitis, 795, 1202, 1205
benefits of, 1202–1203
breast cancer/breast cancer risk and, 738, 758, 796, 1202, 1203
endometrial hyperplasia/carcinoma and, 774, 795, 1203
in hypercalcemia/hyperparathyroidism, 1157
hypertension and, 443
injections, 1205
lipid modification/heart disease and, 795, 796, 1202, 1203
nipple discharge caused by, 736
oral, 795, 1204
for osteoporosis prevention/management, 795, 796, 1161, 1202
ovarian cancer risk and, 1203, 1204
postmenopausal bleeding and, 764, 1203
with progestins (combined HRT), 795, 1203, 1203–1204
benefits of, 1203
risks of, 795–796, 1203–1204
without progestins (unopposed HRT), 795, 1203
benefits of, 1203
risks of, 796, 1203
risks of, 795–796, 1203–1204
after surgical menopause, 796
transdermal, 795, 1202, 1204
HRT risks and, 1202, 1203
in Turner syndrome, 1208
vaginal, 795, 1205
for vasomotor symptoms of menopause, 795
Estrogen vaginal creams/tablets, 795, 1205
Estrogens. *See also* Estrogen (hormone) replacement therapy
for abnormal uterine bleeding, 763
breast cancer/breast cancer risk and, 738, 758, 796, 1202, 1203
in male, 760
in fibrocystic breast condition, 734, 735
hypertension and, 443
in hypogonadotropic hypogonadism, 1110
in menopause, 794
oral, 795, 1204
in oral contraceptives, 785–786, 787t
plant-derived, 1204
with progestins (combined HRT), 795, 1203, 1203–1204
benefits of, 1203
risks of, 795–796, 1203–1204
without progestins (unopposed HRT), 795, 1203
benefits of, 1203
risks of, 796, 1203
receptors for
antagonists of, in cancer chemotherapy, 1670t
in breast cancer, 748
in male, 760
prognosis and, 750, 751t, 758
therapy and, 748, 754

transdermal, 795, 1202, 1204
HRT risks and, 1202, 1203
vaginal, 795, 1205
HRT risks and, 1203
Estrone, in estrogen replacement therapy, 795, 796
Estropipate, 1204
Eszopiclone, 1054t, 1089
Etanercept. *See also* Anti-TNF agents
for psoriasis, 108
for rheumatoid arthritis, 837–838
ETEC. *See* Escherichia coli, enterotoxigenic
Ethacrynic acid, 450t
Ethambutol, 281t, 282t
adverse ophthalmic effects of, 178t
for MAC infection, 286, 1337t, 1482
for tuberculosis, 281–282, 281t, 282t, 283
in pregnancy, 282, 283, 821
Ethanol (ethyl alcohol). *See also* Alcohol use disorder
blood levels of, in acute intoxication, 1093, 1584t, 1594
for methanol or ethylene glycol poisoning, 908, 1581t, 1584t, 1599
for thyroid nodules, 1140
Ethanol-associated hypoglycemia, 1098, 1236, 1252, 1252t, 1258, 1594–1595
Ethanol intoxication/poisoning, 1093, 1584t, **1594–1595**. *See also* Alcohol use disorder
metabolic acidosis/osmolar gap and, 891, 1094, 1584
Ethics, principles of care and, 2
Ethinyl estradiol. *See* Estradiol/ethinyl estradiol; Estrogens
Ethmoiditis/ethmoid sinusitis, 215
Ethosuximide, 988t
Ethyl alcohol. *See* Alcohol use disorder; Ethanol
Ethylene glycol poisoning, 1581t, 1584t, **1599**
anion gap/osmolar gap in, 891, 906, 1584, 1599
hemodialysis for, 1583t, 1584t, 1599
Ethylenediaminetetraacetic acid (EDTA), for lead poisoning, 1597
Ethynodiol diacetate, in oral contraceptives, 787t
Ethyol. *See* Amifostine
Etodolac, 75t, 621
Etonogestrel
in contraceptive implant, 789
in contraceptive vaginal ring, 789, 1205
in hormone replacement therapy, 1205
Etopophos. *See* Etoposide/etoposide phosphate
Etoposide/etoposide phosphate, 1665t
leukemia associated with, 527
for lung cancer, 1612
for testicular cancer, 1657
Etravirine, 1351t, 1356, 1360. *See also* Antiretroviral therapy
Etretinate
adverse ophthalmic effects of, 179t
for psoriasis in HIV infection/AIDS, 1344
Eucerin, 95, 100t

Euglycemic insulin therapy. *See*
    High-dose insulin
    euglycemic therapy
Eulexin. *See* Flutamide
Eumycetoma (maduromycosis), **1557**
EUS. *See* Endoscopic ultrasonography
Eustachian tube, **203–204**
    dysfunction of, 200, **203**
        barotrauma and, 204
        cholesteatoma and, 205–206
        hearing loss and, 200, 203
        in HIV infection/AIDS, 214
        serous otitis media development
            and, 203–204
    patulous, 203
Euthyroid sick syndrome, 1121
Euvolemic hypernatremia, 890
Euvolemic hypotonic hyponatremia, 885*f*,
    886–887, 888
EV-70. *See* Enterovirus 70
EV-71. *See* Enterovirus 71
EV-D68. *See* Enterovirus 68
Evamist, 1204
Evans syndrome, 514
Evaporative cooling, for heat stroke,
    1563
EVD. *See* Ebola viral disease
Event recording, 381
    in palpitation evaluation, 31
    in syncope evaluation, 401
Everolimus, 362, 1667*t*
    for breast cancer, 756
    for gastroenteropancreatic
        neuroendocrine tumors/
        insulinoma, 1186, 1255
Eversion (high) ankle sprain, 1715*t*,
    1716–1717
Evista. *See* Raloxifene
Evolocumab, for lipid modification/
    cardiovascular/heart disease
    prevention, 353, 1265*t*,
    1266
Evotaz. *See* Atazanavir, with cobicistat
Exalgo. *See* Hydromorphone
Exanthema subitum (roseola infantum),
    1367*t*, 1377
Exanthems, 1367–1368*t*, **1421–1424**. *See
    also* Rashes
    drugs causing (dermatitis
        medicamentosa), **161–163**,
        162–163*t*, 880
    drug-induced hypersensitivity
        syndrome and, 161, 163, 880
Exchange transfusion. *See* Transfusion
Excitement (arousal) stage of sexual
    activity, 1062
    disorders related to, 1062, 1063–1064.
        See also Sexual dysfunction
    in female, 782
Executive function, impaired, dementia
    causing, 1020
Exelderm. *See* Sulconazole
Exemestane, 1670*t*
    for breast cancer prevention/treatment,
        739, 752, 755*t*
Exenatide, 1221*t*, 1226
    overdose/toxicity of, 1595
Exendin 4. *See* Exenatide
Exercise/activity
    angina precipitated by, 356
    ankle sprain and, 1716

bronchoconstriction/asthma
    precipitated by, 242, 243*f*,
    244*t*, 247*f*. *See also* Asthma
cancer/cancer prevention and, 13,
    1607, 1637–1638
cardiovascular/heart disease
    prevention and, 6*t*, **11–12**
    postinfarction, 380
cholesterol reduction and, 1262
for COPD, 261
in dementia management, 1021
in diabetes
    insulin requirements and, 1233
    prevention/management and, 1218,
    1219
for fatigue/chronic fatigue syndrome,
    38, 39
in health maintenance, 3*t*, 6*t*, **11–12**
for heart failure, 410
heart murmurs affected by, 335*t*
heat exposure syndromes and, 1562
hypertension/hypertension
    management and, 441, 445,
    446*t*
hyponatremia and, 887
for knee osteoarthritis, 1714
for menopausal symptoms, 1202
migraine exacerbated by, 40, 40*t*
in obesity/overweight management/
    prevention, 11, 12, 13, 1270–
    1271
for osteoporosis prevention/
    management, 11, 795, 1160
patellofemoral pain syndrome and,
    1713
periodic paralysis precipitated by, 1049
during pregnancy, 799
for pulmonary hypertension, 431, 432*f*
reduced. *See* Bed rest; Immobility
Exercise challenge (bronchial
    provocation) testing, in
    asthma, 246
Exercise-induced bronchoconstriction/
    asthma, 242, 243*f*, 244*t*, 247*f*.
    See also Asthma
Exercise-induced hypoglycemia, 1233,
    1237
Exercise testing. *See also* Stress testing
    in asthma, 246
    in chest pain/angina, 28, 357
    electrocardiography, 357
    postinfarction, 380
Exertional heat stroke, 1562
Exfoliative dermatitis/erythroderma, **117**
    drugs causing, 117, 162*t*
    psoriatic, 107, 117. *See also* Psoriasis
Exforge/Exforge HCT. *See* Valsartan, for
    hypertension, with
    amlodipine
Existential challenges, for terminally ill/
    dying patient, 92–93, 93*t*
Exophiala, phaeohyphomycosis caused
    by, 1558
Exophthalmos, Graves, **194–195**, 1124,
    1127, 1129, 1130, 1132–1133
    RAI treatment for hyperthyroidism
        and, 195, 1127, 1130, 1132
Exostoses, ear canal, **202–203**
Exposure (cold). *See* Cold, disorders
    caused by exposure to
Exposure keratitis, 174

Extavia. *See* Interferon-beta
Extensively drug-resistant tuberculosis,
    277, 1336
Extensor (decerebrate) posturing,
    1027
External auditory canal. *See* Ear canal
External hordeolum (sty), 164–165
External otitis/malignant external otitis,
    202
External rewarming, active and passive,
    for hypothermia, 1564
External rotation, assessment of
    in ankle, 1715*t*, 1716
    in shoulder
        adhesive capsulitis (frozen shoulder)
            and, 1691
        rotator cuff strength and, 1686*t*,
        1689
External rotation stress test, in ankle
    sprain, 1716
Extracorporeal counterpulsation, for
    angina, 363
Extracorporeal shock wave lithotripsy
    for renal stones, 965
    for ureteral stones, 965
Extramammary Paget disease, 118
Extraocular movements. *See* Eye
    (extraocular) movements
Extrapancreatic neuroendocrine tumors,
    1188
Extrapyramidal disorders/effects,
    antipsychotics and, 1068,
    1069*t*, 1072–1073, 1589,
    1590
Extrasystoles. *See* Atrial
    (supraventricular) premature
    beats; Ventricular premature
    beats
Extrauterine pregnancy. *See* Ectopic
    pregnancy
Extremities. *See also* Lower extremity;
    Upper extremity
    acute arterial occlusion of, **476–477**
    hypothermia of, **1565–1566**
Extrinsic allergic alveolitis
    (hypersensitivity
    pneumonitis), **307–308**, 308*t*
Exubera, 1232
Exudates, pleural, 311, 311*t*, 312
Exudative age-related macular
    degeneration, 185
Eye, **164–199**. *See also under Ocular;
    Optic; Visual*
    chemical burns involving, 198, 1581,
    1587
    decontamination of, **1581**, 1587
    disorders of, **164–199**. *See also specific
        type or cause and Visual
        impairment/loss*
    age-related macular degeneration,
        185–186
    allergic, **168–174**
    in American trypanosomiasis
        (Chagas disease), 1509
    in Behçet syndrome, 181, 862
    in blood dyscrasias, **191**
    cataract, **182–183**
    chemical burns, 198, 1581, 1587
    chlamydial, 167
        in newborn, 823
    corneal ulcers, **174**

diabetes and, 189–190, 189f, 1238. *See also* Diabetic retinopathy
drugs (systemic) causing, 177–179t, **199**
glaucoma
    acute angle-closure, 166t, **176–179**
    chronic, **179–181**
gonococcal, 167, 1475
in granulomatosis with polyangiitis, 857, 857f
herpes simplex infection, 1363, 1364
herpes zoster infection, **175**, 192, 1369, 1370
in HIV infection/AIDS, **191–192**, 1341. *See also* HIV infection/AIDS, retinal disorders associated with
in hyperthyroidism/Graves disease, **194–195**, 1124, 1127, 1129, 1130, 1132–1133
inflammation. *See also* Conjunctivitis; Uveitis
    conjunctivitis, **166–174**, 166t
    uveitis, 166t, **181–182**, 182f
keratitis. *See also* Keratitis
    infectious, **174–176**
    ultraviolet/actinic, **198**
lids/lacrimal apparatus involvement and, **164–166**
management of
    drugs in, 169–173t, **198**. *See also* Ophthalmic medications
    precautions in, **198–199**
ocular motor palsies, **194**
optic disk swelling, **193–194**
optic neuritis, **193**
optic neuropathy (ischemic), **192**
orbital cellulitis, **195**
pinguecula/pterygium, **174**
refractive errors, **164**
retinal
    arterial occlusions, **187–188**, 187f
    detachment, **183–184**
    systemic disease associations and, **189–192**, 189f, 191f
    venous occlusions, **186–187**
in rheumatoid arthritis, 835
in syphilis, 1489t, 1495
thyroid (Graves ophthalmopathy), **194–195**, 1124, 1127, 1129, 1130, 1132–1133
transient monocular visual loss, **188–189**
traumatic, **196–198**, 196f, 197f
in uremia, 924t
in vitamin A deficiency, 1277
vitreous hemorrhage, **184–185**, 184f
dry (keratoconjunctivitis sicca), **167–168**
in Sjögren syndrome, 167, 850, 851
examination of
    in coma or stupor, 1027
    in diabetes patients, 190, 1238
    in elderly, 69
foreign body in
    conjunctival/corneal, **196**, 196f
    intraocular, **196**
melanoma of, 103
in SLE, 840

systemic drugs affecting, 177–179t, **199**
in toxoplasmosis, 192, 1522, 1523
traumatic injury of, **196–198**, 196f, 197f
Eye drops. *See also* Ophthalmic medications
    autologous serum, 168
    contaminated, **199**
    preservative-free, 172t, 173t, 180, 199
    systemic absorption/effects of, **199**
    toxic and hypersensitivity reactions to, 168, **199**
Eye (extraocular) movements
    in coma or stupor, 1027
    in ocular motor palsies, 194
"Eye worm" *(Loa loa)*, 1546
Eyelids
    blepharitis affecting margins of, 110, 165
    disorders of, **164–166**, 165f
    lacerations of, 197
    seborrheic dermatitis affecting margins of, 110, 165
    tumors of, **165–166**
Eylea. *See* Aflibercept
Ezetimibe, 353, 1265–1266, 1265t
    in combination therapy, 1266
Ezogabine, 987t

F cells, pancreatic, 1185
Face. *See also under* Facial
    fracture of in head injury, 1029
    herpes zoster affecting, 120, 214, 1041, 1369. *See also* Ramsay Hunt syndrome
    seborrheic dermatitis affecting, 110
Facial neuropathy/paralysis/palsy, 1041, **1041**, 1041f
    in herpes infection/Ramsay Hunt syndrome, 120, 214, 1041
    herpes zoster and, 1369, 1369–1370, 1370
    Lyme disease and, 1041, 1041f, 1502, 1504–1505, 1505t
    otitis media and, 206
Facial pain, **981–983**
Facioscapulohumeral muscular dystrophy, 1048t
Factitious disorders, 1059. *See also specific disorder*
Factor II antibodies, **561**
Factor II deficiency, 560–561
Factor V antibodies, **561–562**
Factor V deficiency, 560–561
Factor V Leiden, DVT/PE (venous thromboembolic disease) and, 295, 575t
Factor VII deficiency, 560–561
Factor VIII
    acquired antibodies to, **561**
    in cryoprecipitate, 544
    deficiency of
        in hemophilia, 557, 559t
        in von Willebrand disease, 560, 561t
    inhibitors of in hemophilia, 557, 558, 558–559
Factor VIII concentrate, for hemophilia, 558, 559t
Factor IX
    deficiency of in hemophilia, 557, 559t

inhibitors of in hemophilia, 557, 558, 558–559
Factor IX concentrate, for hemophilia, 558, 559t
Factor X deficiency, 560–561
Factor XI deficiency, 559t, **560**
Factor XIII deficiency, 561
Factor concentrates, for hemophilia, 558, 559t
Factor inhibitors, in hemophilia, 557, 558, 558–559
Faget sign, 1405
Fainting, 401. *See also* Syncope
Faldaprevir, for hepatitis C, 691
Fallot
    pentalogy of, 328
    tetralogy of, **328–330**
Falls, in elderly, **63–65**, 63t, 64t
False vocal folds, cancer of, 235, 236
Famciclovir, 1365t
    for herpes simplex infections, 119, 1338t, 1343, 1365t
    for herpes zoster/varicella infection, 121, 175, 1338t, 1343, 1365t, 1370
    prophylactic/suppressive, 1343
Familial adenomatous polyposis, **666–667**, 1637, 1640
    colorectal cancer and, 667, 1637, 1640
    genetic mutations associated with, 667
    thyroid cancer and, 1141
Familial cortisol resistance, 1174
Familial Creutzfeldt-Jakob disease, 1022, 1393–1394. *See also* Creutzfeldt-Jakob disease
Familial dysautonomia, prenatal testing for, 800
Familial glucocorticoid deficiency, 1169
Familial hemiplegic migraine, 977
Familial hirsutism, 1196
Familial hyperparathyroidism, 1152
Familial hypocalcemia, 892t
Familial hypocalciuric hypercalcemia, 892t, 898, 1156
Familial juvenile polyposis, 667
Familial Mediterranean fever, **604**
Familial medullary thyroid carcinoma, 1141
Familial melanoma, 102
Familial nonmedullary thyroid carcinoma, 1141
Familial papillary thyroid carcinoma, 1141
Familial paraganglioma, 1180
Familial partial lipodystrophy type, I, 1174
Familial renal glycosuria, 1214
Familial (benign essential) tremor, **1010–1011**
Family/significant others, of patient at end of life
    caring for, 89, 89t
    follow-up/grieving and, 94
Famotidine, 609. *See also* H_2 receptor blocking drugs
Fanapt. *See* Iloperidone
Fanconi anemia/syndrome, 546, 900, 951
Fanconi-like syndrome, tenofovir causing, 688

Fansidar (pyrimethamine-sulfadoxine), 1515*t*, 1519
   with amodiaquine, 1519, 1521
   with artesunate, 1516*t*, 1519
   for chemoprophylaxis, 1519
     in pregnancy/infants, 1521
   resistance to, 1515
   for uncomplicated falciparum disease, 1515
FAP. *See* Familial adenomatous polyposis
Fareston. *See* Toremifene
Farmer's lung, 308*t*
Farydak. *See* Panobinostat
Fasciitis
   eosinophilic, 846
   necrotizing. *See* Necrotizing fasciitis
   palmar, cancer and, 875
Fasciola hepatica/gigantica (fascioliasis), **1533–1534**
Fasciolopsis buski, 1534–1535
Fasciotomy, in burn care, 1569
Faslodex. *See* Fulvestrant
Fasting
   cholelithiasis/gallstones and, 717
   insulinoma diagnosis and, 1253, 1253*t*, 1254, 1254*t*
   porphyria and, 1676
Fasting hypoglycemia, 1252, 1252*t. See also* Hypoglycemia
Fat. *See also* Lipid disorders/lipids
   body. *See* Body fat; Obesity/overweight
   dietary, 1263. *See also* Lipid disorders/lipids
     lowering. *See* Lipid-lowering therapy
   intravenous. *See* Intravenous fat
Fat necrosis of breast, **736**
Fat-restricted diet, 1263, 1279. *See also* Low-fat diet
   for pancreatitis, 729, 732
Fatal familial insomnia, 1394
Fatigue, **37–39**, 38*f*, **87**
   post-Q fever, 1437
Fatty acid binding protein, heart, in acute coronary syndromes/STEMI/chest pain evaluation, 28
Fatty acids
   in nutritional support, 1283
   omega-3. *See* Omega-3 fatty acids
   trans, preventable disease/deaths associated with high intake of, 3*t*
Fatty liver (hepatic steatosis)
   alcoholic, 694, 695
   drugs/toxins causing, 697
   with encephalopathy. *See* Reye syndrome
   in hepatitis C, 683
   nonalcoholic, **697–699**
   of pregnancy, 697, **824**
     liver failure and, 685, 824
Favipiravir, for Ebola viral disease, 1398
FBN1 mutation, in Marfan syndrome, 1683
5-FC. *See* Flucytosine
fCJD. *See* Familial Creutzfeldt-Jakob disease
Fᴇ. *See* Fractional excretion
Febrile agglutinins, 1288
Febuxostat, for hyperuricemia/gout, 832, 833
   in transplant patients, 833

FEC regimen, 751, 753
Fecal antigen assay, in *H pylori* infection, 579, 622
Fecal DNA tests, in cancer screening/polyp identification, 665, 1641–1642
Fecal immunochemical test (FIT). *See also* Fecal occult blood testing
   in cancer screening/polyp identification, 15, 665, 1641
   constipation and, 584
   in GI bleeding, 599, 600
Fecal impaction, 586
   "overflow" fecal incontinence/diarrhea and, 586, 671
   urinary incontinence and, 65
Fecal incontinence, **671–672**
   fecal impaction and, 586, 671
Fecal microbiota transplant, for antibiotic-associated colitis relapse, 649
Fecal occult blood testing
   in cancer screening/polyp identification, 14*t*, 15, 665, 1638, 1641
   in constipation, 584
   in GI bleeding, 599, 600
Fecal osmolality, 591
Feeding tubes, 1281–1282, 1281*f. See also* Enteral nutritional support
   in elderly/dementia, 67, 91
Feet
   atherosclerotic/occlusive disease and, 475–476
   in diabetes mellitus, 475, 476, 1239, 1239*f*, 1242
   immersion/trench, **1565**
   tinea of, **113–114**, 113*f*
     cellulitis and, 113, 137
   vesiculobullous dermatitis of (pompholyx), **121–122**
     tinea differentiated from, 114, 122
Felbamate, 987*t*
   overdose/toxicity of, 987*t*, 1589
Feldene. *See* Piroxicam
Felodipine, 461*t*
   for angina, 361
   for hypertension, 459, 461*t*
   overdose/toxicity of, 459, 461*t*, 1591
Felty syndrome, 518
Female condom, 791
Female infertility. *See* Infertility
Female sex hormones. *See* Estrogens
Female sexual dysfunction, **781–783**
Femara. *See* Letrozole
Femhrt, 1204
Femoral arteries
   aneurysms of, 484
   atherosclerotic/occlusive disease of, **473–475**
Femoral cutaneous nerve, lateral, lesions of (meralgia paresthetica), 1040
Femoral neck fracture, 1702. *See also* Hip fracture
   atypical, bisphosphonate use causing, 1162
Femoral neuropathy/femoral nerve palsy, **1040**
Femring, 1205

Fenofibrate/fenofibric acid, for lipid modification, 1265, 1265*t*
Fenoldopam, for hypertensive urgencies/emergencies, 469*t*, 470*t*, 471
Fenoprofen, 75*t*
Fentanyl/fentanyl oral transmucosal and buccal/fentanyl transdermal, 74, 77–78*t*, 82
   overdose/toxicity of, 1601
Fenthion poisoning, 1602
Fentora. *See* Fentanyl
Ferric gluconate. *See* Iron, supplementary
Ferric pyrophosphate citrate, iron deficiency in dialysis patients and, 502
Ferriman-Gallwey scale, 1197
Ferritin, 499, 501
   in anemia of chronic disease/chronic kidney disease, 503, 928
   in hemochromatosis, 708, 709
   in iron deficiency anemia, 499, 500, 501, 503
Ferroportin, 499, 500
   gene encoding (*FPN1* gene), in hemochromatosis, 708
Ferrous sulfate. *See* Iron, supplementary
Fertility awareness, contraception based on, **791**
Fertility disorders. *See* Infertility
Fertilization, in vitro, 785, 970
Fetal alcohol syndrome, 799, 1094
Fetal fibronectin, preterm labor and, 811
Fetal goiter, 1132
Fetal hemoglobin. *See* Hemoglobin F
Fetal lung maturity
   delivery in preeclampsia/eclampsia and, 810
   preterm labor and, 811
Fetal-placental unit, in preeclampsia-eclampsia, 809*t*
Fetal testing, 799–801. *See also specific disorder and* Genetic testing
Fetal varicella infection, 821
Fetoprotein. *See* Alpha-fetoprotein
Fetotoxic drugs, 798*t*
Fetus. *See also* Pregnancy
   age of viability of, 811
   chikungunya fever transmission to, 1407
   CMV transmission to, 1374, 1375
   dengue transmission to, 1402
   hepatitis transmission to, 681, 822, 822–823
   herpes simplex transmission to, 823, 1363–1364, 1366
   HIV transmission to, 822, 1332, 1346
   hypercalcemia/hyperparathyroidism affecting, 1153
   malaria transmission to, 1513, 1521
   rubella affecting, 1384, 1385
   syphilis transmission to, 1488, 1497–1498
   thyroid disease affecting, 816, 1119, 1132. *See also* Pregnancy, thyroid disease and
   toxoplasmosis transmission to, 799, 1523, 1523–1524
   Zika virus infection affecting, 1406, 1407
Fetzima. *See* Levomilnacipran
FEV_1. *See* Pulmonary function tests

FEV$_1$/FVC ratio. *See* Pulmonary function tests
Fever, **34–36**. *See also specific disorder or cause*
  cancer-related, 1287, 1288, 1661
  "central," 34
  in critically ill patient, 34, 1294, 1295, 1296
  drug, 1294
  drug user presenting with, 1304
  factitious (self-induced), 1288
  in HIV infection/AIDS, 1287, 1288, 1335
  in neutropenic patient, 518, 1287, 1288
    antimicrobial therapy and, 35, 518, 1293, 1296, 1314t, 1661
  postoperative, 1294–1295
  severe, with thrombocytopenia, 1399
  travel and, 1308, 1309
    dengue causing, 1401, 1402
    without localizing signs/symptoms, 1309
  of unknown/undetermined origin (FUO), **1287–1289**
  in giant cell arteritis, 854, 1288
Fever/cold sore (herpes simplex), **118–120**, 119f, 1363. *See also* Herpes simplex infection
Fexofenadine, 219. *See also* Antihistamines
FFI. *See* Fatal familial insomnia
FFP. *See* Fresh-frozen plasma
FGF23. *See* Fibroblast growth factor-23
FHM. *See* Familial hemiplegic migraine
Fiber, dietary, 1219–1220, 1280
  constipation and, 585–586, 585t
  in diabetes mellitus, 1219–1220, 1280
  diverticular disease and, 662–663, 663, 1280
  for hemorrhoids, 670
  for irritable bowel syndrome, 646, 1280
  lipid-modifying effects of, 1263, 1280
Fiber laxatives, 585–586, 585t
Fiberoptic bronchoscopy. *See* Bronchoscopy
Fibric acid derivatives (fibrates), for lipid modification, 1264–1265
Fibrillation. *See* Atrial fibrillation; Ventricular fibrillation
Fibrillin, mutation in gene for, in Marfan syndrome, 1683
Fibrin D-dimer. *See* D-dimer fibrin
Fibrinogen
  in DIC, 553, 554
  replacement. *See* Cryoprecipitate
Fibrinolytic therapy, 373t, 374–375. *See also* Thrombolytic therapy
  after cardiac valve replacement, 351, 352t
  for myocardial infarction/STEMI, 372f, 373, 373t, 374–375
    contraindications to without ST-segment elevation, 366, 372
  PCI and, 362, 373, 374
  for stroke, 996
Fibroadenoma of breast, **735**
Fibroblast growth factor-23 (phosphatonin), 899, 927, 1164–1165, 1165
Fibrocystic breast condition, **734–735**

breast cancer risk and, 734, 735, 738
  nipple discharge in, 734, 736, 736t
Fibroelastoma, valvular papillary, 433
Fibrogenesis imperfecta ossium, 1165
Fibroid tumor of uterus, **772–774**
Fibromuscular dysplasia/hyperplasia
  renal artery stenosis/renal vascular hypertension and, 442, 931, 932
  transient ischemic attacks and, 991
Fibromyalgia, **873–874**
Fibronectin, fetal, preterm labor and, 811
Fibrosing cholestatic hepatitis, 688
Fibular (peroneal) nerve, common, injury to, **1040**
Fidaxomicin, for antibiotic-associated colitis, 649
Field defects/loss. *See* Visual field defects/loss; Visual impairment/loss
"Field treatment," for actinic keratoses, 118
Fifth disease (erythema infectiosum), 1367t, 1422
Figurate ("shaped") erythema, 96t. *See also specific type and* Erythemas
Filariasis, **1543–1546**, 1543f
  loiasis, **1546**
  lymphatic, **1543–1544**, 1543f
  onchocerciasis, **1545–1546**
Filgrastim (G-CSF)/filgrastim-sndz
  for aplastic anemia, 517
  for chemotherapy-induced toxicity, 1662, 1672t
  for HIV infection/AIDS, 1350
  for myelodysplasia, 526
  for neutropenia, 518, 1662, 1672t
  for stem cell mobilization, 540, 541
Financial abuse, of elderly, 16, 70
Financial planning, advance, for dementia patients, 60
Finasteride (5-alpha-reductase inhibitor)
  for androgenetic (male pattern) alopecia, 159
  for benign prostatic hyperplasia, 973t, 974, 974–975
  for hirsutism/virilization, 781, 1198
Fine-needle aspiration biopsy/cytology
  for breast lump evaluation/management, 743–744, 744, 745. *See also* Breast, biopsy of
  in lung cancer, 1609, 1612
  thyroid
    in thyroid nodules/cancer, 1121t, 1138t, 1139
    in thyroiditis, 1136
Fingernails, disorders of. *See* Nail disorders
Fingers. *See also under* Hand
  thromboangiitis obliterans (Buerger disease) involving, 480
Fingolimod
  adverse ophthalmic effects of, 178t
  for multiple sclerosis, 1024t, 1025
Firearms, prevention of injury/death caused by, 16
Firmagon. *See* Degarelix
First aid. *See also* Cardiopulmonary resuscitation
  in drowning, 1567

First-degree burn, 1568
First-degree heart block, 377, 399. *See also* Atrioventricular (heart) block
Fish oil/omega-3 fatty acids
  platelet function affected by, 558t
  preventable disease/deaths associated with low intake of, 3t
Fish (seafood) poisoning, **1603–1604**, 1604t
Fish tapeworm *(D latum)*, **1535**, 1536
  vitamin B$_{12}$ deficiency and, 506–507, 1535
Fistula in ano, 673
Fistulas
  in Crohn disease, 652, 653, 654
  in diverticulitis, 663, 664
  perianal, 673
  perilymphatic, 204, 211t, 212
FIT. *See* Fecal immunochemical test
Fitz-Hugh and Curtis syndrome, 778
5q– syndrome, 525, 526
Fixed drug eruptions, 162t
Flagyl. *See* Metronidazole
Flail leaflet, mitral valve prolapse and, 340
Flame (clothing) burns, 1570
Flash (arcing) burns, 1570
Flatus, **587**
Flaviviruses, encephalitis caused by, 1388
Flavobacterium species. *See* Elizabethkingia (Chryseobacterium/ Flavobacterium) species
Flea-borne endemic (murine) typhus, 1429t, **1430–1431**
Flea rickettsiosis, California, 1429t
Fleas
  in plague transmission, 1474
  in rickettsial disease transmission, 1429t
  skin lesions caused by, 151
Flecainide, 381, 382t
  for atrial fibrillation, 382t, 393
  overdose/toxicity of, 382t, 384
  for supraventricular tachycardia, 382t, 386
"Fleeting blindness" (amaurosis fugax), 188–189, 477
FleetsPhospho-soda. *See* Sodium phosphate enema
Flexible sigmoidoscopy. *See* Sigmoidoscopy
Flexor (decorticate) posturing, 1027
Flibanserin, for hypoactive sexual desire disorder, 782, 1064, 1206
Flolan. *See* Epoprostenol
Floppy iris/eye syndrome, 183
  cataract surgery and, alpha-blockers/ alpha-1a-blockers causing, 183, 464, 974
"Floppy" mitral valve. *See* Mitral valve prolapse
Flower cells, HTLV infections, 1396
Floxin. *See* Ofloxacin
FLT3 gene/inhibitors, in acute myeloid leukemia, 527, 529
Flu. *See* Influenza
Flu shots. *See* Influenza virus vaccine
Fluarix, 1414t. *See also* Influenza virus vaccine

Flublok, 1322t, 1413, 1415t. See also
Influenza virus vaccine
Flucelvax, 1414t. See also Influenza virus
vaccine
Fluconazole, 1559t
for candidiasis
cutaneous, 133
endocarditis, 1548
esophageal, 611, 1338t, 1341, 1548
funguria, 1548
invasive disease, 1548
oral, 226, 1341, 1548
vulvovaginal, 133, 767, 1338t, 1344,
1548
for coccidioidomycosis, 1550, 1551
for cryptococcal meningitis, 1337t,
1553, 1554
for onychomycosis, 161
prophylactic, 1292
for tinea versicolor, 115
Flucytosine, 1559t
for cryptococcal meningitis, 1337t,
1340, 1553–1554
Fludara. See Fludarabine
Fludarabine, 1664t
autoimmune hemolytic anemia caused
by, 514
for chronic lymphocytic leukemia, 530
Fludrocortisone
for adrenal insufficiency/Addison
disease, 1171–1172
for autonomic dysfunction/diabetic
neuropathy, 1035
for hyporeninemic hypoaldosteronism,
906t, 908
Fluid and electrolyte disorders, 884–903,
892t. See also specific
electrolyte
assessment of, 884–885, 885t
in drowning, 1567
genetic disorders and, 892t
management/replacement guidelines
and, 911–912, 911t
Fluid management/hydration, 911–912,
911t. See also specific disorder
and Water/fluid intake
in ARDS, 321
in burns, 1569
for diabetic ketoacidosis, 1247
for diarrhea/gastroenteritis, 590, 911t,
1305, 1310
dilutional acidosis and, 907
for electric burn injury, 1570
in end-of-life care, 91
in frostbite, 1566
for heat exposure syndromes, 1562,
1563
for hypercalcemia, 898, 1156
for hyperglycemic hyperosmolar state,
1250
for hypernatremia, 890
for hyponatremia, 887, 888, 888–889
hypotension in poisoning/drug
overdose and, 1578
with hypotonic fluids, hyponatremia
and, 886, 887
in shock, 495
for tumor lysis syndrome/
hyperuricemia, 1660
in uric acid nephrolithiasis/
nephropathy, 952

urinary stone formation and, 962, 963,
964
water deficit calculation and, 890
Fluid volume alterations
hyperosmolality with and without, 891
metabolic alkalosis and, 909, 910
Flukes, infections caused by, 1532–1535.
See also specific type
blood flukes (schistosomiasis),
1532–1533
liver/lung/intestinal flukes, 1533–1535
FluLaval, 1414t. See also Influenza virus
vaccine
Flumazenil, for benzodiazepine overdose/
coma, 1055, 1578, 1581t,
1595
FluMist, 1322t. See also Influenza virus
vaccine
Flunisolide
for allergic rhinitis, 219
for asthma, 250t
Fluocinolone/fluocinolone implant, 97t
for diabetic macular edema, 190
Fluocinonide, 97t, 1341
Fluorescein
contaminated, 199
toxic/hypersensitivity reactions to, 199
Fluorescent treponemal antibody
absorption test. See FTA-ABS
test
Fluorometholone, for ophthalmic
disorders, 171t
Fluoroquinolones
adverse ophthalmic effects of, 178t
hypo- and hyperglycemia caused by,
1257
for pneumonia, 269t, 271, 1446
for traveler's diarrhea, 1310
Fluorouracil, 1664t
adverse ophthalmic effects of, 178t
for breast cancer, 751, 753
for colorectal cancer, 1639
for gastric adenocarcinoma, 1631
gastrointestinal toxicity (mucositis/
diarrhea) and, 1673
for wart removal, 142
Fluoxetine, 1078t, 1079–1081. See also
Serotonin-selective reuptake
inhibitors
breastfeeding and, 798t
for dementia, 1104
lithium interaction and, 1087t
for OCD, 1057
overdose/toxicity of, 1078t, 1606
during pregnancy, 1081
Fluoxymesterone, for aplastic anemia,
517
Fluphenazine, 1068, 1069t, 1071. See also
Antipsychotic drugs
enanthate or decanoate forms of, 1071
relative potency/side effects of, 1069t
for Tourette syndrome, 1018
Flupirtine, for Creutzfeldt-Jakob disease,
1394
Flurandrenolide, 98t
Flurazepam, 1054t, 1055, 1089
Flurbiprofen, 75t
for ophthalmic disorders, 168, 171t
Flutamide, 1669t
for hirsutism/virilization, 781, 1198
for prostate cancer, 1649t

Fluticasone
for allergic rhinitis, 219
for asthma, 250t
Fluticasone/salmeterol
for asthma, 249t
for COPD, 260
Fluvastatin, 355t, 1265t. See also Statins
Fluvirin, 1414t. See also Influenza virus
vaccine
Fluvoxamine, 1078t, 1079–1081. See also
Serotonin-selective reuptake
inhibitors
overdose/toxicity of, 1078t, 1606
during pregnancy, 1081
Fluzone/Fluzone High-Dose/Fluzone
Intradermal, 1413, 1414t.
See also Influenza virus
vaccine
Flying. See Air travel
FML/FML Forte/FML S.O.P. See
Fluorometholone
FMR1 gene, in fragile X mental
retardation, 1679
FNA cytology. See Fine-needle aspiration
biopsy/cytology
FOBT. See Fecal occult blood testing
Focal nodular hyperplasia of liver, 715,
716
telangiectatic, 716
Focal segmental glomerulosclerosis, 934t,
944
in HIV-associated nephropathy, 946
Focal (partial) seizures, 984, 984t. See also
Seizures
differential diagnosis of, 986
drug therapy for, 987–988t
schizophrenia differentiated from,
1068
transient ischemic attack differentiated
from, 986, 992
Focal torsion dystonia, 1016–1017
FODMAPS
celiac sensitivity and, 634
flatus and, 587
irritable bowel syndrome and, 646
Folate. See Folic acid
Foley catheter
health care (hospital)-associated
urinary tract infection and,
1293, 1294, 1295
in shock management, 495
FOLFIRI regimen, 1639, 1640
FOLFIRINOX regimen, 1625
FOLFOX regimen, 1639, 1640
Folic acid (folate), 508
antagonists/inhibition of synthesis of.
See also Methotrexate
in cancer chemotherapy, 1663t
for malaria, 1518–1519
deficiency of, 502, 508–509, 508t
in homocystinuria/
hyperhomocysteinemia,
1681
thrombocytopenia and, 548
vitamin B12 deficiency and, 507, 508,
509
supplementary, 508–509
for hemoglobin H disease, 506
for homocystinuria/
hyperhomocysteinemia,
1681

with methotrexate (leucovorin rescue), 108, 651, 837, 1671*t*, 1674
    in pregnancy, 508, 799, 801
Folinic acid (leucovorin)
    with methotrexate, 108, 651, 837, 1671*t*, 1674
    in toxoplasmosis treatment, 1337*t*, 1350, 1524
Follicle-stimulating hormone (FSH), 1109*t*
    in amenorrhea, 1199, 1200, 1200–1201, 1201
    deficiency of, 1108, 1109, 1189. *See also* Hypogonadism
    in hirsutism/virilization, 1197
    in hypogonadism, 1109, 1189, 1191
    for hypogonadism/infertility, 970, 1112
    hypopituitarism caused by defects in gene for, 1108
    in infertility workup, 784, 969–970
    in polycystic ovary syndrome, 781, 1196
    recombinant, for ovulation induction, 784–785, 1112
Follicular bronchiolitis, 267
Follicular lymphoma, 531, 532
    stem cell transplantation for, 533, 541
Folliculitis, **130–131**, 130*f*
    acne and, 127, 131
    eosinophilic, 130, 131, 1333
    in HIV infection/AIDS, 130, 1343
    steroid (steroid acne), 127, 130
Follitropins, for infertility, 1112
Fomepizole, for methanol or ethylene glycol poisoning, 908, 1581*t*, 1584*t*, 1599
Fomivirsen, 1365*t*
Fondaparinux, 563
    for acute coronary syndromes, 367*f*, 368
    coagulopathy caused by, 562
    for DVT/PE (venous thromboembolic disease), 568*t*, 570*t*
    for heparin-induced thrombocytopenia, 553
    for myocardial infarction, after fibrinolytic therapy, 375
Food
    allergy/intolerance to, **877**
        dyspepsia caused by, 578
        eosinophilic esophagitis caused by, 613
    antibiotic administration and, 1317
    aspiration of/"café coronary," 238, **306**
    contaminated. *See specific disease and* Food poisoning
    MAOI interactions and, 1082, 1082*t*
    withholding, in end-of-life care, 91
Food anaphylaxis, 877
Food poisoning, 1305, 1306–1307*t*
    botulism, **1046–1047**, 1306*t*, **1453–1454**
    Cyclospora causing, 1305
    listeriosis and, 588*t*, 589, 1457
    seafood contamination/toxicity and, **1603–1604**, 1604*t*
    vibrios causing, 588*t*, 1305, 1307*t*, 1472
Foot. *See* Feet
Foramen ovale, patent, **324–327**

Forced expiratory volume in one second (FEV$_1$). *See* Pulmonary function tests
Forced expiratory volume in one second/ forced vital capacity ratio (FEV$_1$/FVC ratio). *See* Pulmonary function tests
Forced vital capacity (FVC). *See* Pulmonary function tests
Foreign body
    aspiration of, 238. *See also* Aspiration
        retention and, **306**
    conjunctival/corneal, **196**, 196*f*
    in ear canal, **202**
    esophageal, **238**
    intraocular, **196**
    in trachea and bronchi, **238**
    in upper aerodigestive tract, **238**
Formication, stimulant abuse and, 1068
Formoterol
    for asthma, 249*t*, 251
        with budesonide, 249*t*
    for COPD, 260
Fortaz. *See* Ceftazidime
Forteo. *See* Teriparatide
Fortesta, 1192
Forxiga. *See* Dapagliflozin
Fosamax. *See* Alendronate
Fosamprenavir, 1351*t*, 1356, 1357. *See also* Antiretroviral therapy
    with ritonavir, 1357
Fosaprepitant, 582*t*, 583, 1673
Foscarnet, 1365*t*
    for CMV infection, 191, 1338*t*, 1365*t*, 1376
    for herpes simplex infections, 1338*t*, 1365*t*
    for herpes zoster/varicella infection, 121, 1365*t*, 1370
Fosfomycin, for urinary tract infection, 955
Fosinopril, 455*t*
    with hydrochlorothiazide, 456*t*
Fosphenytoin, 989
14-3-3 protein, in Jakob-Creutzfeldt disease, 1022, 1394
Fourth nerve paralysis, 194
Foxglove, toxicity of, 1594
FPN1 gene, in hemochromatosis, 708
Fractional excretion, 884, 917, 917*t*. *See also specific electrolyte*
Fractional flow reserve, in angina, 358
    coronary revascularization and, 358–359
Fracture-dislocation, spinal, 1031–1032
Fracture Risk Assessment tool (FRAX), 1160
Fractures. *See also specific type and under Bone*
    atypical, bisphosphonates causing, 1162
    corticosteroid use and, 1208–1209
    in diabetes, 1242
    in elderly, falls and, 63, 64, 1701, 1702
    estrogen replacement therapy affecting risk of, 796, 1202
    in hypercalcemia/hyperparathyroidism, 1153, 1155
    malabsorption and, 633*t*
    in metabolic bone disorders/renal osteodystrophy, 927

    in osteomalacia, 1165
    in osteoporosis, 1159
        prevention of, 11, 1702
    in Paget disease of bone, 1167
    pathologic. *See* Pathologic fractures
    thiazolidinedione use and, 1225
Fragile X mental retardation, **1679–1680**
Fragile-X tremor-ataxia syndrome, 1679
Fragility fractures. *See* Pathologic fractures
Frailty, in elderly, 56–57
    hypertension management and, 446, 467
Frambesia (yaws), 1312*t*, **1498**
Framingham score/projections, 353
Francisella tularensis (tularemia), **1473–1474**
Frataxin gene, in Friedreich ataxia, 1035
FRAX (Fracture Risk Assessment tool), 1160
Freckles (ephelides), **103**
Free thyroxine assay (FT$_4$), 1121*t*. *See also* Thyroxine
    in euthyroid sick syndrome, 1121
    in hyperthyroidism, 1127, 1128
        amiodarone-induced, 1125–1126, 1126, 1128
        pregnancy and, 816, 1127, 1128
        after treatment, 1130
    in hypopituitarism, 1110, 1111
    in hypothyroidism, 1110, 1120
        pregnancy and, 816
Free thyroxine index (FT$_4$I), in hyperthyroidism, 1127
Free triiodothyronine (FT$_3$), in hyperthyroidism, 1121*t*, 1127
Freons, toxicity of, 1602
Fresh-frozen plasma, transfusion of, 544. *See also* Plasma/plasma fractions/components, transfusion of
Fresh whole blood, transfusion of, 542. *See also* Transfusion
Friction rubs
    in chest pain evaluation, 28
    in pericarditis/effusion, 425, 427
    in pulmonary embolism, 296*t*
Fried rice, *Bacillus cereus* contamination of, 1305
Friedreich ataxia, 1035–1036
Frontal lobe lesions, 1003
Frontal sinusitis, 216
Frontotemporal dementias, 1019*t*, 1020, 1021
Frostbite, 1565, **1565–1566**
    Raynaud phenomenon and, 844
Frostnip, **1565**
Frovatriptan, for migraine headache, 978
Frozen packed red blood cells, transfusion of, 542. *See also* Transfusion
Frozen shoulder, **1691–1692**
Fructosamine, in diabetes mellitus, 1216
Fructose malabsorption, diarrhea caused by, 591
FSGS. *See* Focal segmental glomerulosclerosis
FSH. *See* Follicle-stimulating hormone
FT$_3$. *See* Free triiodothyronine
FT$_4$. *See* Free thyroxine assay
FT$_4$I. *See* Free thyroxine index

FTA-ABS test, 1490, 1490t
    on cerebrospinal fluid (CSF FTA-ABS), 1496
    in HIV infection/AIDS, 1348
FTD. See Frontotemporal dementias
FU. See Fluorouracil
Fucithalmic. See Fusidic acid
Fukuda test, 211
Full liquid diet, 1278
Fulminant ulcerative colitis, 660–661
Fulvestrant, 1670t
    for breast cancer, 754, 755, 755t, 756
Fumagillin, for microsporidiosis, 1529
Functional alimentary hypoglycemia, **1256**
"Functional" asthma, 246
Functional dyspepsia, 578, 579, 580, 625
Functional hyperventilation. See Hyperventilation
Functional hypopituitarism, 1109
Functional proteinuria, 913
Fundoplication
    for erosive esophagitis/GERD, 610
    with myotomy, for achalasia, 618
Fungal infections, **111–115, 1547–1560**.
        See also specific type
    drugs for, 98–99t, **1558–1560**, 1558–1559t. See also Antifungal agents
    in HIV infection/AIDS, rashes, 1343
    household molds and, 1558
    keratitis, **175**
    myocarditis in, 413t
    of nails, 160, **160–161**
    opportunistic, 1292, **1557–1558**
    superficial/skin, **111–115**, 111f, 112f, 113f. See also Tinea
        in HIV infection/AIDS, 1343
    systemic/invasive, **1547–1560**
    sinusitis, **218**
Fungemia
    in candidiasis, 132, 1547, 1548
    in coccidioidomycosis, 1550
Funguria, candidal (candiduria), 1547, 1548
FUO. See Fever, of unknown/ undetermined origin
Furazolidone, for giardiasis, 1531
Furosemide. See also Diuretics; Loop diuretics
    in acute tubular necrosis, 920
    for cirrhotic ascites, 701
    for heart failure, 406, 412
        infarct-related, 378
    for hypertension, 448, 450t
        in urgencies/emergencies, 470t, 471
    for pulmonary edema, 412
Furuncles/furunculosis, **152–154**, 1315t, 1443t, 1448
    in HIV infection/AIDS, 1343
Fusarium, in opportunistic infection, 1557
Fusidic acid, for ophthalmic disorders, 169t
Fusilev. See Levoleucovorin
Fusion inhibitors. See also Entry inhibitors
    enfuvirtide, 1352t, 1357
    resistance to, 1361
Fusobacteria/Fusobacterium necrophorum, 1441, 1442, 1478

Fuzeon. See Enfuvirtide
FVC (forced vital capacity). See Pulmonary function tests
FXTAS (fragile-X tremor-ataxia syndrome), 1679

G6PD deficiency. See Glucose-6-phosphate dehydrogenase (G6PD) deficiency
G20210A prothrombin mutation
    in hepatic vein obstruction (Budd-Chiari syndrome), 711
    in noncirrhotic portal hypertension, 714
GA (tabun) poisoning, 1601–1602
Gabapentin, 987t. See also Anticonvulsant therapy
    for anxiety, 1055, 1056
    for menopausal symptoms, 795, 1202
    for neuropathic pain/painful diabetic neuropathy, 83t, 84, 1035, 1240, 1340
    overdose/toxicity of, 987t, 1589
    for phobic disorders, 1056
    for seizures, 987t
GABHS. See Group A beta-hemolytic streptococcal infection
GAD. See Generalized anxiety disorder
GAD65 (glutamic acid decarboxylase 65) antibodies, in type 1 diabetes, 1211, 1211t, 1233
Gadolinium, nephrogenic systemic fibrosis caused by, 358, 952
Gail 2 model, for breast cancer risk, 738
Gait/gait disorders
    in elderly, **63–65**, 63t, 64t
    in syphilis, 1496
Galactomannan, in invasive aspergillosis, 1555
Galactorrhea, 1117–1118
Galactose-alpha-1,3-galactose (alpha-gal) hypersensitivity, 877
Galantamine, for dementia, 59, 1021, 1104
Gallaverdin phenomenon, 341
Gallbladder
    carcinoma of, 719, 1618
    cholesterolosis of, 717t, 719
    gangrene of, 719
    hydrops of, 719
    porcelain, 717t, 719
    stones in. See Cholelithiasis
    strawberry, 719
Gallium nitrate, for cancer-related hypercalcemia, 1660
Gallstone ileus, 717
Gallstones. See Cholelithiasis
Galvus. See Vildagliptin
Gamete intrafallopian transfer, 785
Gamma-butyrolactone, overdose/toxicity of, 1595
Gamma globulin, intravenous. See Intravenous immune globulin
Gamma-glutamyl transpeptidase (GGTP) levels, 676–677
    alcohol use disorder and, 1094
Gamma-hydroxybutyrate, overdose/ toxicity of, **1595**
    Cushing syndrome and, 1173, 1174

Gamma interferon release assays, in tuberculosis, 4, 279–280
    in HIV infection/AIDS, 280, 1336, 1348
    latent disease treatment and, 283
    musculoskeletal disease and, 872
    pleural fluid analysis for, 312
    in pregnant patient, 821
Gamma knife radiosurgery, for pituitary tumor, 1116
Gamma4 (Bart's) hemoglobin, 505
Gammopathy, monoclonal. See Monoclonal gammopathy
Gamolenic acid, for fibrocystic condition, 735
Ganciclovir, 1365t
    for CMV infection, 191, 1292, 1338t, 1365t, 1376
    for ophthalmic disorders, 167, 170t, 175, 1338t, 1376
Ganciclovir intravitreal implant, 191, 1338t, 1376
Ganfort. See Bimatoprost/timolol
Ganglioneuromas, in MEN, 1187t, 1188
Ganglioside antibodies, in Guillain-Barré syndrome, 1038
Gangrene
    acute streptococcal, cellulitis differentiated from, 492
    anaerobic infection and, 1479, 1480f
    bacterial synergistic, 1480
    of feet, 475, 1480f
        in diabetes mellitus, 1242
    of gallbladder, 719
    gas, 1312t, **1451–1452**
Gardasil. See Human papillomavirus (HPV) vaccine
Gardner syndrome
    epidermal inclusion cysts in, 154
    thyroid cancer and, 1141
Gardnerella infection (bacterial vaginosis), 767, 1302
    sexual violence (rape/sexual assault) and, 1302
Gas, gastrointestinal, **587**
Gas gangrene, 1312t, **1451–1452**
Gases, sniffing, 1101
Gasoline, sniffing, 1101
Gastrectomy
    for gastric adenocarcinoma, 1630
        prophylactic, 1629
    sleeve, for obesity, 1272
    vitamin B12 deficiency and, 506
Gastric acid/gastric contents
    aspiration of. See also Aspiration
        acute (Mendelson syndrome), **305–306**, 1294
        chronic, **306**
        pneumonia and, 273, 1294
    hypersecretion of, in Zollinger-Ellison syndrome/gastrinoma, 631, 632, 1185
    inhibition of secretion of. See Acid-antisecretory agents; Antacids; H2 receptor blocking drugs; Proton pump inhibitors
    reflux of. See Gastroesophageal reflux disease
Gastric banding/gastric bypass. See Bariatric surgery

Gastric cancer, 1624*t*, **1629–1633**
  adenocarcinoma, **1629–1632**
    H pylori infection and, 622, 1629, 1630
    pernicious anemia gastritis and, 622–623, 1629
  carcinoid tumors, **1633**
  dyspepsia in, 578
  familial adenomatous polyposis and, 667
  gastric ulcers and, 624–625, 629, 1630
  GI bleeding and, 595
  H pylori gastritis and, 622, 1629
  HNPCC/Lynch syndrome and, 668, 669
  lymphoma, 532, **1632–1633**
    H pylori infection and, 532, 622, 1632
  mesenchymal tumors, 1633
  pernicious anemia gastritis and, 622–623, 1629
Gastric emptying
  delayed. *See also* Gastroparesis
    antipsychotics causing, 1071
    in GERD, 607
    in scleroderma, 846
    in poisoning/drug overdose, 1581–1583
Gastric lavage, for poisoning/drug overdose, 1582
Gastric outlet obstruction
  in peptic ulcer disease, 624, **630–631**
  vomiting and, 580, 581, 581–582, 581*t*, 630–631
Gastric polyps, 667
Gastric surgery. *See also* Bariatric surgery
  hypoglycemia after, 1252, 1256
  for obesity, 1271–1272
Gastric ulcers, 623, 624, 626*t*, 627. *See also* Peptic ulcer disease
  gastric cancer and, 624–625, 629, 1630
  H pylori gastritis and, 622, 623
  refractory, 628–629, 1630
Gastric varices, noncirrhotic portal hypertension and, 713, 714
Gastrin
  D cells secreting, 1185
  hypersecretion of
    carcinoid tumors and, 1633
    in gastrinoma/Zollinger-Ellison syndrome, 631, 632, 1185. *See also* Gastrinoma
    in pernicious anemia gastritis, 622
Gastrinoma (Zollinger-Ellison syndrome), **631–632**, 1185, 1186
  carcinoid tumors and, 1633
  in MEN, 631, 632, 1185, 1186, 1188
  peptic ulcer disease and, 623, 629, 631, 1185
Gastritis, **619–623**. *See also* Gastropathy
  alcoholic, 620, 621
  in anisakiasis, 623
  atrophic
    gastric adenocarcinoma and, 622–623, 1629
    H pylori infection and, 622
    pernicious anemia and, 622–623
  erosive/hemorrhagic, **620–621**
    GI bleeding and, 620

H pylori, 621–622
  gastric cancer and, 622, 1629
  nonerosive/nonspecific, **621–622**
  NSAID, 620, 621
  in pernicious anemia, 622–623
  phlegmonous/necrotizing, 623
  stress, 319, 620, 620–621
Gastroenteritis, 1305–1308, 1306–1307*t*, 1315*t*. *See also specific cause and* Diarrhea
  appendicitis differentiated from, 642
  Escherichia coli, 588*t*, 589, 1305, **1470–1471**
  food-borne. *See* Food poisoning
  Guillain-Barré syndrome and, 1038
  irritable bowel syndrome and, 644, 1308
  in measles, 1379
  reactive arthritis and, 866
  salmonella, 588*t*, 589, 1305, 1307*t*, 1308, 1315*t*, 1342, **1469**
  viral, 588*t*, 589, 1305, 1342, **1424–1425**
Gastroenteropancreatic neuroendocrine tumors, **1185–1187**. *See also specific type and* Neuroendocrine tumors
  in MEN, 1185, 1187*t*, 1188, 1252
Gastroesophageal junction
  dysfunction of, in GERD, 606
  mucosal laceration of (Mallory-Weiss syndrome/tears), 582, 595, 596, **612–613**
  stricture at. *See* Esophagus, strictures of
Gastroesophageal reflux disease (GERD), **606–611**
  antipsychotics causing, 1071
  Barrett esophagus and, 608, 609, 1626
  chest pain in, 359, 619
  chronic gastric aspiration and, 306
  cough in, 19, 20, 20*t*, 21
  dyspepsia in, 578, 579, 580, 607
  erosive (reflux) esophagitis/GI bleeding and, 595, 606, 607, 610
  esophageal webs and rings and, 613
  extraesophageal manifestations of, 607, 609–610
  heartburn in, 605, 606, 607, 609
  into larynx (laryngopharyngeal reflux), 233
  peptic stricture and, 608–609
Gastrointestinal adenocarcinoma
  gastric, **1629–1632**
    H pylori infection and, 622, 1629, 1630
    pernicious anemia gastritis and, 622–623, 1629
  small intestine, **1634**
    Crohn disease and, 654
Gastrointestinal bleeding, **594–600**. *See also specific cause*
  abdominal aortic aneurysm repair and, 482
  acute
    lower, **597–599**
    upper, **594–597**
  from angioectasias, 595, 597
  anorectal disease causing, 598
  in cirrhosis, 595, 596, 614, 700
  colorectal cancer and, 598
  in Crohn disease, 654

  diverticular, 597, 598, 599, 662, **664**
  in erosive esophagitis, 595
  in erosive/hemorrhagic gastritis (gastropathy), 620
  gastric cancer and, 595
  from gastrointestinal/esophageal varices, 594–595, 614–617
  hemorrhoids causing, 598, 669
  hepatic encephalopathy and, 615, 616, 703
  in hereditary hemorrhagic telangiectasia, 1684
  iron deficiency and, 500, 501, 599, 600
  Mallory-Weiss syndrome/tears and, 582, 595, 596, 612
  NSAIDs and, 74, 621, 829
  occult, 599, **600**
  in peptic ulcer disease, 594, 596, 624, **629–630**
  polypectomy and, 598, 666
  in portal hypertension/portal hypertensive gastropathy, 594–595, 621
  prophylaxis against after fibrinolytic therapy for STEMI, 375
  rebleeding and, 596, 614
  small bowel, **599–600**
  in stress gastritis, 620, 621
Gastrointestinal carcinoids, 1185, 1186, **1634–1636**
  gastric, **1633**
  small intestine, 1185, 1186, 1634–1636
Gastrointestinal fluid losses, replacement guidelines for, 911*t*
Gastrointestinal gas, **587**
Gastrointestinal irritant-type mushroom poisoning, 1600*t*
Gastrointestinal lymphoma
  gastric, 532, **1632–1633**
    H pylori infection and, 532, 622, 1632
  small intestine, **1634**
    Crohn disease and, 654, 1634
Gastrointestinal mesenchymal tumors, **1633–1634**
  small intestinal sarcoma and, **1636**
Gastrointestinal stromal tumors (GISTs), 1633–1634
Gastrointestinal system, **578–673**. *See also specific structure and under Intestinal*
  anorectal diseases, **669–673**
  decontamination of, in poisoning/drug overdose, **1581–1583**
  disorders of, **578–673**. *See also specific disorder and cause*
    adverse ophthalmic effects of drugs used in, 177*t*
    in anthrax, 1455, 1456
    bleeding. *See* Gastrointestinal bleeding
    cancer, **1626–1644**
    chemotherapy-induced, **1673**
    in CMV infection, 1374–1375, 1375
    colorectal diseases, **643–669**
    constipation, **583–587**, 584*t*, 585*t*
    diarrhea, **587–594**, 588*t*, 590*f*, 593*f*, 1305–1308, 1306–1307*t*, 1309–1310
    dyspepsia, **578–580**

Gastrointestinal system, disorders of (*Cont.*):
  enteral nutritional support and, 1281, 1281f, 1282
  esophageal disorders, **604–619**, 605t
  functional
    dyspepsia, 578, 579, 580
    irritable bowel syndrome, **643–647**
  gastric and duodenal disorders, **619–632**
  gastrointestinal gas, **587**
  hiccups (singultus), **583**
  in HIV infection/AIDS, 1341–1342
  in hypercalcemia/hyperparathyroidism, 1153
  motility. *See* Motility disorders
  nausea and vomiting, **580–583**, 581t, 582t
  peritoneal disease, **600–604**, 601t
  in pheochromocytoma/paraganglioma, 1180t
  pregnancy and, **823**
  small intestinal disease, **632–643**, 633t
  in syphilis, 1495
  thrombocytopenia caused by drugs used in, 555t
  in uremia, 924t
  Kaposi sarcoma involving, 146, 1636
  obstruction of. *See* Intestinal obstruction
Gastroparesis, **640–641**
  in diabetes, 640, 641, 1240
    hypoglycemia and, 641, 1237
    pregnancy and, 1244
  vomiting and, 580, 581, 581t, 582, 640
Gastropathy, **619–623**. *See also* Gastritis
  erosive/hemorrhagic, **620–621**
  in HIV infection/AIDS, 1342
  portal hypertensive, 620, 621. *See also* Portal hypertension
  GI bleeding and, 594–595, 621
Gastroplasty. *See* Bariatric surgery
Gastrostomies, 1281–1282. *See also* Enteral nutritional support
Gatifloxacin
  hypo- and hyperglycemia caused by, 1257
  for ophthalmic disorders, 169t
Gaucher cells, 1680
Gaucher disease, **1680**
Gazyva. *See* Obinutuzumab
GB (sarin) poisoning, 1601–1602
GBL (gamma-butyrolactone), overdose/toxicity of, 1595
GBM antibodies. *See* Anti-glomerular basement membrane antibodies
GBP (gastric bypass). *See* Bariatric surgery
GCS. *See* Glasgow Coma Scale
G-CSF (granulocyte colony-stimulating factor). *See* Filgrastim
GD (soman) poisoning, 1601–1602
Gefitinib, 1667t
  for lung cancer, 1612
Gemcitabine, 1664t
  for breast cancer, 757
  for lung cancer, 1612

Gemfibrozil, 1265, 1265t
  in combination therapy, 1266
  in HIV infection/AIDS, 1356
Gemifloxacin, for pneumonia, 269t, 271, 275t
Gemzar. *See* Gemcitabine
Gender identity disorder/gender dysphoria, 1062–1063, 1063–1064
Gene therapy
  for hemophilia, 558
  for parkinsonism, 1014
Generalized anxiety disorder, 1053, 1054–1055
Generalized seizures, 984–985, 984t. *See also* Seizures
  differential diagnosis of, 986
  drug therapy for, 987–988t
Genetic disorders. *See* Hereditary disorders
Genetic instability, in colorectal cancer/HNPCC/Lynch syndrome, 665, 668, 1637
Genetic testing/counseling. *See also specific disorder and* Prenatal testing
  for cancer susceptibility genes/cancer screening
    APC/MUTYH mutations/familial adenomatous polyposis and, 667
    breast cancer and, 738
    colorectal cancer and, 667, 668, 669
    HNPCC/Lynch syndrome and, 668, 669
  for Duchenne muscular dystrophy, 1047
  for hemochromatosis, 708, 709
  for Huntington disease, 1015
  for hypophosphatasia, 1165
  for male infertility, 970
  for medullary thyroid carcinoma, 1141
  for MEN, 1141, 1187, 1188
  for pheochromocytoma/paraganglioma, 1182
  for recurrent (habitual) abortion, 805
  in sickle cell syndromes, 511
  prenatal, 800
Genital herpes, **118–120**, 1363. *See also* Herpes simplex infection
  anorectal involvement and, 119, 671
  during pregnancy/neonatal/congenital infection, **823**, 1363–1364, 1366
Genital ulcers, 1302
  adenoviruses causing, 1421
  in Behçet syndrome, 861–862
  in chancroid, 1476
  in granuloma inguinale, 1477
  herpetic. *See* Genital herpes
  in lymphogranuloma venereum, 1485
  STDs causing, 1302
  in syphilis (chancre), 1488–1489, 1489f, 1489t, 1491
Genital warts. *See* Venereal (genital) warts
Genitalia, ambiguous, 1170
Genitourinary disorders, **953–976**. *See also specific cause or structure affected*

  benign prostatic hyperplasia, **971–976**, 971t, 973f, 973t, 974t
  cancer, **1644–1657**
  hematuria in, **953–954**
  infections, **954–960**, 955t, 957t
    anaerobic, in women, **1479**
  interstitial cystitis, **960–961**
  male erectile/sexual dysfunction, **965–968**
  male infertility, **968–971**, 969f
  ulcers. *See* Genital ulcers
  in uremia, 924t
  urinary incontinence, **65–67**
  urinary stone disease, **961–965**, 962t
Genitourinary syndrome of menopause, 43
Gentamicin. *See also* Aminoglycosides
  for endocarditis, 1461, 1461–1462, 1462
  for ophthalmic disorders, 169t
  for pneumonia, 269t, 271, 275t
  for urinary tract infection, 955t
Gentian violet, for candidal skin infection/mastitis, 133
Genvoya (tenofovir/elvitegravir/cobicistat/emtricitabine), 1354t, 1355, 1358, 1359t, 1360
Geodon. *See* Ziprasidone
"Geographic" age-related macular degeneration, 185
GEP-NETs. *See* Gastroenteropancreatic neuroendocrine tumors
GERD. *See* Gastroesophageal reflux disease
Geriatric Depression Scale, 61
Geriatric medicine/disorders, **55–71**. *See also* Age/aging; Older adults
  assessment of older adult and, **55–57**, 56f, 56t, 57t
  management of common problems and, **57–71**. *See also specific problem*
  principles of care and, **55**
Germ cell tumors, testicular, **1655–1657**
  bone marrow/stem cell transplantation for, 540
  gynecomastia and, 1195
Germline mutations/testing
  in breast cancer, 738
  in colorectal cancer/HNPCC/Lynch syndrome, 666, 668–669, 1637
  in pheochromocytoma/paraganglioma, 1179, 1180
  in thyroid cancer, 1141
Gerstmann syndrome, 1003
Gerstmann-Sträussler-Scheinker syndrome (GSS), 1394
Gestational breast cancer, 745–747
Gestational diabetes, 800, 817–818, 817t. *See also* Diabetes mellitus
Gestational hyperthyroidism. *See* Hyperthyroidism (thyrotoxicosis), during pregnancy
Gestational thrombocytopenia, **555–556**
Gestational trophoblastic disease, **807–808**, 1624t
  hyperthyroidism and, 807, 1126
"Geste antagoniste," 1016

Gestodene, in oral contraceptives, thromboembolism and, 786
gFOBT (guaiac-based fecal occult blood tests), 15, 1641. See also Fecal occult blood testing
GFR. See Glomerular filtration rate
GGTP levels. See Gamma-glutamyl transpeptidase (GGTP) levels
GH. See Growth hormone
GHB (gamma-hydroxybutyrate), overdose/toxicity of, **1595**
    Cushing syndrome and, 1173, 1174
Ghon complex, in tuberculosis, 279
GHRH. See Growth hormone–releasing hormone
Giant cell (temporal/cranial) arteritis, **853–855**
    fever/FUO caused by, 854, 1288
    ischemic optic neuropathy in, 192, 854
    retinal artery occlusion and, 187, 188
Giant cell myocarditis, 413, 413t, 414
Giant cell thyroiditis. See Subacute (de Quervain) thyroiditis
Giardia lamblia/intestinalis/duodenalis (giardiasis), 588t, 589, 592, 1305, 1342, **1530–1531**
Gibbus deformity, 872
Gigantism, **1114–1116**
Gilbert syndrome, 674, 675t
Gilles de la Tourette syndrome, **1017–1018**
    OCD and, 1018, 1057
Gilotrif. See Afatinib
Gingivitis/gingivostomatitis. See also Stomatitis
    herpes, 118, **227**, 1363
    in HIV infection/AIDS, 1341
    necrotizing ulcerative, **226**
Ginkgo, toxicity of, 1593
Ginseng, toxicity of, 1593
GIP1. See Glucose-dependent insulinotropic polypeptide
GISTs. See Gastrointestinal stromal tumors
Gitelman syndrome, 892t
Glanders, 1312t
Glanzmann thrombasthenia, 556
Glasgow alcoholic hepatitis score, 695
Glasgow Coma Scale, 1029, 1029t, 1031
Glatiramer, for multiple sclerosis, 1024, 1024t
Glaucoma
    acute angle-closure, 166t, **176–179**
        antipsychotics precipitating, 1071
        pupillary dilation and, 166t, 176, 198
    chronic, **179–181**
        angle-closure, 179, 180, 180–181
    in diabetes mellitus, 1238
    facial pain caused by, 983
    neovascular (rubeotic), 186
        after retinal vein occlusion, 186, 187
    treatment of, 172–173t, 176, 180–181
Gleason grading system/score, for prostate cancer, 1647, 1650
    CAPRA assessment tool and, 1650, 1650t
Gleevec. See Imatinib
Glenya. See Fingolimod
GLI-similar 3 mutation, in diabetes, 1212
Gliadin antibodies, in celiac disease, 634
Gliclazide, 1221t, 1223

Glimepiride, 1221t, 1223
    with pioglitazone, 1228
    with rosiglitazone, 1228
Glioblastoma multiforme, 1004t, 1624t
Gliomas, 1003, 1005
    brainstem, 1004t, 1005
    spinal, 1006
Glipizide, 1221t, 1223
    with metformin, 1228
GLIS 3 mutation, in diabetes, 1212
Glitazones. See Thiazolidinediones
Globe index, in primary biliary cholangitis/cirrhosis, 707
Globin gene/globin chain synthesis
    in sickle cell syndromes, 511, 512
    in thalassemias, 503
Glomerular diseases, 924t, **932–943**, 932f, 933t, 934t, 935f
    nephritic spectrum, 932, 932f, 933t, **934–941**, 935f. See also specific type and Glomerulonephritis
    nephrotic spectrum, 932–933, 932f, 934t, **941–943**. See also specific type and Nephrotic syndrome
Glomerular filtration rate/estimated glomerular filtration rate (GFR/eGFR), 914–915
    alkalosis in alkali administration and, 909
Glomerular hematuria, 914, 932f
Glomerular proteinuria, 914
Glomerulonephritis, 917t, **922–923**, 933t, 934t, 935f
    acute kidney injury caused by, 917t, **922–923**
    anti-glomerular basement membrane (anti-GBM), 304, 922, 933t, 935f, **939**
    crescentic, 933t, 935f, 938
    cryoglobulin-associated, 860, 933t, 935f, **939**
    in eosinophilic granulomatosis with polyangiitis (Churg-Strauss syndrome), 933t, 935f, 938
    in Goodpasture syndrome, 304, 922, 933t, 935f, **939**
    in granulomatosis with polyangiitis (Wegener granulomatosis), 304, 858, 922, 933t, 935f, 938
    in Henoch-Schönlein purpura, 861, 933t, **937–938**, 938f
    hepatitis C infection and, 683, 933t, 940
    IgA nephropathy, 933t, 935f, **937**
    immune-complex, 922, 935f, 940
    in lupus/SLE, 839t, 840, 841, 933t, 935f, **940–941**
    membranoproliferative, 933t, 935f, **939–940**
    in microscopic polyangiitis, 859, 860, 922, 935f
    nephritic presentation of, 932, 932f, 933t, **934–941**, 935f
    nephrotic spectrum presentation of, 932–933, 932f, 934t, **941–943**
    pauci-immune (ANCA-associated), 858, 922, 933t, 935f, **938–939**
    postinfectious, 933t, 935f, **936–937**
    rapidly progressive, 932, 932f

serologic testing in, 933t, 935f, 936
streptococcal pharyngitis and, 936, 1441
Glomerulonephropathies. See also Glomerulonephritis; Nephropathy
    hepatitis C infection and, 683, 933t, 940
    membranoproliferative, 933t, 934t, 935f, **939–940**
        hepatitis C and, 683, 933t, 940
Glomerulopathies. See also Glomerulonephritis
    C3, **939–940**
    sickle cell, 951
Glomerulosclerosis
    in diabetic nephropathy, 945
    focal segmental, 934t, **944**
        in HIV-associated nephropathy, 946
Glomus tumors (tympanicum/jugulare), 207
    tinnitus and, 207, 209
Glossitis, **226**
Glossodynia, **226**
Glossopharyngeal neuralgia, **982**
    chemotherapy-induced, 1674
    earache in, 207
Glottic (true vocal fold) cancer, 235, 236
GLP-1. See Glucagon-like peptide 1
GLP-1 receptor agonists. See Glucagon-like peptide 1 (GLP-1) receptor agonists
Glucagon
    A cells secreting, 1185
    for beta-blocker overdose/toxicity, 1578, 1591
    contraindications to use of in pheochromocytoma, 1182
    for hypoglycemia, 1237
    impaired response to, hypoglycemia and, 1237
    tumors secreting, 1185, 1213
Glucagon emergency kit, 1237
Glucagon-like peptide 1 (GLP-1), 1225, 1226
    hypoglycemia caused by tumors secreting, 1256
    in postprandial hypoglycemia, 1256
Glucagon-like peptide 1 (GLP-1) receptor agonists, 1221–1222t, 1226–1227, 1235f, 1236
    for postprandial hypoglycemia after gastric surgery, 1256
Glucagon stimulation test, 1110
Glucagonoma syndrome, 1185
Glucagonomas, 1185
    in MEN, 1188
Glucan levels, in *Pneumocystis* pneumonia, 1336
Glucocerebrosidase, in Gaucher disease, 1680
Glucocorticoid deficiency, familial, 1169. See also Adrenal insufficiency
Glucocorticoid-remediable hyperaldosteronism, 441–442, 892t. See also Aldosteronism
Glucocorticoid replacement, for adrenal insufficiency/Addison disease, 1171
    after pituitary surgery, 1175, 1176

Glucocorticoid-secreting tumors, 1213
Glucokinase gene defect, in MODY, 1211t, 1212
Glucophage/Glucophage XR. See Metformin
Glucosamine/glucosamine sulfate plus chondroitin, in osteoarthritis, 829, 1714
Glucose. See also Glucose tolerance/intolerance
  ascitic fluid, 602, 603
  blood levels of. See also Hyperglycemia; Hypoglycemia
    in alcoholic ketoacidosis, 906
    in diabetes mellitus, 1214–1215, 1215t
      acceptable, 1236
      control of. See Glycemic control in diabetes
      hospitalization/surgery and, 53, 1243–1244
      pregnancy and, 800, 817–818, 817t
      self/continuous-monitoring of, 1216–1217, 1217, 1233, 1234
        in pregnant patient, 818, 1217
    in diabetic ketoacidosis, 1246, 1246t, 1247
    in functional alimentary hypoglycemia, 1256
    hemoglobin A_{1c} levels and, 1215–1216, 1215t
    in hyperglycemic hyperosmolar state, 1246t, 1249, 1250
    in insulinoma, 1185, 1253, 1253t, 1254
    monitoring/management of during surgery, 53, 1243–1244
    normal values for, 1215, 1215t
    prebreakfast hyperglycemia and, 1234, 1234t
    testing, 1215, 1215t
      in pregnancy, 800, 817, 817t
  cerebrospinal fluid, 1297t
  fatal hypophosphatemia and, 900
  for hypoglycemia, 1237
    in drug overdose, 1581t, 1595
  pleural fluid, 312, 313t
  for porphyria, 1036, 1676
  in urine. See Glucosuria/glycosuria
  Wernicke encephalopathy/Wernicke-Korsakoff syndrome and, 694, 908, 1026, 1095
Glucose-dependent insulinotropic polypeptide (GIP1), 1225
Glucose-6-phosphate dehydrogenase (G6PD) deficiency, **510–511**
  dapsone therapy and, 511, 1291, 1350
  rasburicase therapy and, 511
  sulfasalazine therapy and, 837
Glucose tolerance/intolerance, 1215, 1215t. See also Diabetes mellitus
  in diabetes mellitus, 1215, 1215t
  endocrine tumors and, 1213
  impaired, 1215, 1215t
  lithium affecting, 1086
  normal values for, 1215, 1215t
  prediabetes and, 1215, 1215t, 1218
  in pregnancy, 800, 817, 817t

testing, 1215, 1215t
  in pregnancy, 800, 817, 817t
Glucosidase inhibitors, 1221t, 1225
  overdose/toxicity of, 1225
Glucosuria/glycosuria, 1214
  in diabetes mellitus, 1214
    hyperglycemic hyperosmolar state and, 1246t, 1249–1250
  nondiabetic (renal), 1214
Glucotrol/Glucotrol XL. See Glipizide
Glucovance. See Glyburide, with metformin
Glutamic acid decarboxylase, in gene therapy for parkinsonism, 1014
Glutamic acid decarboxylase 65 (GAD65) antibodies, in type 1 diabetes, 1211, 1211t, 1233
Glutathione reductase, in riboflavin deficiency, 1275
Gluten, in celiac disease/dermatitis herpetiformis, 123, 632
Gluten enteropathy. See Celiac disease
Gluten-free diet, for celiac disease/dermatitis herpetiformis, 123, 634
Glyburide, 1221t, 1222–1223
  with metformin, 1228
Glycated (glycosylated) hemoglobin. See Hemoglobin A_1/A_{1c}
Glycemic control in diabetes
  acceptable/target levels of, 1236
    hospitalization/surgery and, 1244
    older patients and, 1233
  angina and, 361–362
  blood glucose self/continuous-monitoring in, 1216–1217, 1217, 1233, 1234
    in pregnant patient, 818, 1217
  clinical studies in evaluation of, 1217–1219
  complications rate and, clinical studies of, 1217–1219
  estrogen replacement therapy affecting, 1203
  exercise/activity and, 1233
  fructosamine measurements and, 1216
  glycated hemoglobin (HbA_{1c}) measurements and, 1215–1216, 1217–1218. See also Hemoglobin A_1/A_{1c}
  intensive insulin therapy for. See Insulin therapy, intensive
  nephropathy development/progression and, 945, 1218, 1219, 1238
  neuropathy development/progression and, 1217, 1218, 1219
  pregnancy and, 817, 818, 1244
  retinopathy development/progression and, 189, 1218, 1219
  self/continuous-monitoring of blood glucose and, 1216–1217, 1217, 1233, 1234
    in pregnant patient, 818, 1217
  surgery and, 53, 1243–1244, 1243t
  vascular disorders and, 1217, 1218, 1219
Glycemic index, 1219
Glycohemoglobins. See Hemoglobin A_1/A_{1c}

Glycoprotein Ib/IX, in Bernard-Soulier syndrome, 556
Glycoprotein IIb/IIIa receptors
  drugs blocking
    for acute coronary syndromes/STEMI, 367–368, 367f
    PCI and, 362, 373
    platelet function affected by, 558t
  Glanzmann thrombasthenia and, 556
Glycoprotein B vaccine, for CMV infection, 1376
Glycosuria. See Glucosuria/glycosuria
Glycosylated (glycated) hemoglobin. See Hemoglobin A_1/A_{1c}
Glycyrrhetinic/glycyrrhizinic acid, hypertension/aldosteronism and, 442, 1178
Glynase. See Glyburide
Glyset. See Miglitol
Glyxambi. See Empagliflozin, with linagliptin
GM-CSF (granulocyte macrophage colony-stimulating factor). See Sargramostim
GN. See Glomerulonephritis
GnRH analogs. See Gonadotropin-releasing hormone (GnRH) analogs
Goeckerman regimen, for psoriasis, 108
Goiter
  endemic, **1148–1149**
  fetal, 1132
  hyperthyroidism and, 1137, 1138
  hypothyroidism/cretinism and, 1119, 1132
  lithium causing, 1086
  multinodular (nodular), **1137–1140**, 1138t
    in MEN, 1188
    toxic, 1125, 1131
  substernal/retrosternal, 1120–1121, 1138, 1148
Gold salts, adverse ophthalmic effects of, 179t
Golfer's elbow, 1697
Golimumab. See also Anti-TNF agents
  for inflammatory bowel disease/ulcerative colitis, 651–652, 660
  for rheumatoid arthritis, 837–838
GoLYTELY. See Polyethylene glycol
Gonadal dysgenesis. See Turner syndrome
Gonadotropin-releasing hormone (GnRH)
  deficiency/low pulse frequency of, in amenorrhea, 1199, 1200, 1200–1201
  hypopituitarism caused by defects in gene for, 1108
Gonadotropin-releasing hormone (GnRH) analogs. See also Luteinizing hormone-releasing hormone (LHRH) analogs
  for abnormal uterine bleeding, 763
  for breast cancer, 755
  for endometriosis, 766, 776
  for hyperandrogenism, 1199
  hypogonadism caused by, 1111
  for infertility, 1112

Gonadotropins
    deficiency of, 1109. *See also*
        Hypogonadism
    in amenorrhea, 1199
    human chorionic (hCG). *See* Human
        chorionic gonadotropin
    human menopausal (hMG), for
        ovulation induction, 784–785
    for hypogonadotropic hypogonadism,
        970, 1111–1112, 1193
Gonococcal infections/gonorrhea, 1311*t*,
    1475–1476
    anorectal involvement and, 670, 1475
    arthritis and, **868–869**, 1314*t*, 1475,
        1476
        reactive arthritis differentiated from,
            866, 869, 1476
    chlamydial coinfection and, 1486
    conjunctivitis, **167**, 1475
    diarrhea and, 588*t*, 589
    disseminated disease and, 1475, 1476
    drug resistant, 1476
    epididymitis in, 960, 1316*t*
    pelvic infection/PID, 778, 1316*t*, 1475,
        1476
    pharyngitis in, 1475
    during pregnancy, 799, 800, **823**
    prevention and, 1476
    screening for
        prenatal, 799, 800, 823
        in STD patients, 1302
        in women, 799, 800, 823
    sexual violence (rape/sexual assault)
        and, 793, 794, 1302
    urethritis and, 1316*t*, 1475, 1476
    in women, 799, 800, 823
Goodpasture syndrome, 304, 922, **939**
    alveolar hemorrhage in, 304
    glomerulonephritis in, 304, 922, 933*t*,
        935*f*, **939**
Gordon syndrome, 892*t*
Goserelin, 1670*t*. *See also* Luteinizing
        hormone-releasing hormone
        (LHRH) analogs
    for breast cancer, 755*t*
    for prostate cancer, 1649, 1649*t*
GOT. *See* Aspartate aminotransferase
Gottron papules, 848
Gottron sign, 848
Gout/gouty arthritis, 826, **829–834**, 830*t*,
        831*f*, 832*t*
    in diabetes, 1242
    kidney disease and, 830, **952**
    nongonococcal acute bacterial (septic)
        arthritis differentiated from,
        867
    rheumatoid arthritis differentiated
        from, 831, 836
    saturnine, in lead poisoning, 831, 948
    in transplant patient, 833
gp120, HIV vaccine development and,
    1347
GPT. *See* Alanine aminotransferase
GRACE Risk Score, 369, 380
Gradenigo syndrome, 206
Graft enteric fistula, after abdominal
        aortic aneurysm repair, 482
Graft-versus-host disease, transfusion-
        associated, 544
Graft-versus-host reaction, 541
Graft-versus-malignancy effect, 540, 541

Graham Steell murmur, 350
Gram-negative infections, 1311*t*,
        1311–1312*t*, **1463–1480**. *See
        also specific agent*
    bacteremia and sepsis, **1467–1468**
    folliculitis, 130, 131
Gram-positive infections, 1311*t*, 1312*t*,
        1441–1458. *See also specific
        agent*
Gramicidin/neomycin/polymyxin B, for
        ophthalmic disorders, 169*t*
Grand mal (tonic-clonic) seizures, 984*t*,
        985. *See also* Seizures
Grand mal (tonic-clonic) status
        epilepticus, 984*t*, 985,
        989–990
Granisetron, 582, 582*t*, 1672. *See also*
        Antiemetics
Granular urinary casts, 913, 914*t*
Granulocyte colony-stimulating factor
        (G-CSF). *See* Filgrastim
Granulocyte count
    chemotherapy dosage modification
        and, 1672*t*
    infections and, 1290
Granulocyte macrophage colony-
        stimulating factor
        (GM-CSF). *See*
        Sargramostim
Granulocytic anaplasmosis/ehrlichiosis,
        1429*t*, 1435, 1436
    Lyme disease coinfection and, 1436,
        1504
Granulocytopenia. *See also* Neutropenia
    infections and, 1290
Granuloma. *See also* Granulomatosis;
        Granulomatous disorders
    arytenoid cartilage, 234–235
    hepatic, drugs/toxins causing, 697
    inguinale, **1477**
    lethal midline, 223
    in sarcoidosis, 292, 293
    swimming pool, 1482
Granulomatosis
    eosinophilic, with polyangiitis
        (Churg-Strauss syndrome),
        304
        leukotriene modifiers for asthma
            and, 251
        pulmonary involvement in, 304
        renal involvement in, 933*t*, 935*f*, 938
    infantisepticum, 1457
    with polyangiitis (Wegener
        granulomatosis), 304,
        857–859, 857*f*
        autoantibodies/ANCA in, 840*t*, 857,
            858, 922, 933*t*, 935*f*, 938
        microscopic polyangiitis
            differentiated from, 858, 860
        nose and paranasal sinus
            involvement in, **223–224**,
            858
        pulmonary involvement in, 304, 857,
            858
        renal involvement in, 304, 857, 858,
            922, 933*t*, 935*f*, 938
        rheumatoid arthritis differentiated
            from, 836, 858
Granulomatous disorders. *See also specific
        type and* Granuloma;
        Granulomatosis

fever/FUO and, 1287
hypercalcemia in, 897, 1156
meningitis, 1297*t*
nasal involvement in, **222–224**
neck masses, **239**
thyroiditis. *See* Subacute (de Quervain)
        thyroiditis
Graves dermopathy (pretibial
        myxedema), 1124, 1127,
        1133
Graves disease, 1124–1125, 1127, 1128,
        1133–1134. *See also*
        Hyperthyroidism
    eye disease and, **194–195**, 1124, 1127,
        1129, 1130, 1132–1133
    in pregnancy, 816, 1126, 1127,
        1131–1132
    thyroid antibodies/TSH receptor
        antibody in, 1124, 1128
    transient neonatal, 1127
    treatment of, 195, 1129–1133
Graves ophthalmopathy/orbitopathy/
        exophthalmos, **194–195**,
        1124, 1127, 1129, 1130,
        1132–1133
    RAI treatment for hyperthyroidism
        and, 195, 1127, 1130, 1132
Gray platelet syndrome, 556
Grazoprevir, for hepatitis C, 690, 690*t*
Greta. *See* Azarcon
Grief reaction/grieving, 94, 1074
Grind (patellar) test, 1713
Grip (handgrip), heart murmurs affected
        by, 335*t*
Grippe, summer, 1426
Griseofulvin, for onychomycosis, 160
Ground itch, 1539
Group A beta-hemolytic streptococcal
        infection, 1311*t*,
        1443–1444
    cellulitis, 137, 138, 1315*t*, 1442–1443,
        1443*t*
    endocarditis, 1443, 1461
    erysipelas, 136, 137, 1315*t*, 1442–1443,
        1443*t*
    gangrene, cellulitis differentiated from,
        492
    glomerulonephritis and, 936
    necrotizing fasciitis, 1444
        cellulitis differentiated from, 138,
            492, 1444
    pharyngitis, 227, 228*f*, 1315*t*,
        1441–1442. *See also*
        Pharyngitis, streptococcal
    pneumonia and empyema, 1443
    rheumatic fever and, 229, 422, 424,
        1441, 1442
    scarlet fever, 1441, 1444
    skin infections, 1315*t*, **1442–1443**,
        1443*t*
Group B streptococcal infection, 1311*t*,
        1444
    arthritis, 867
    endocarditis, 1461
    meningitis, 1314*t*, 1444
    in pregnancy/neonate, 800–801,
        820–821, 1444
Group C streptococcal infection, 1311*t*,
        1444
    endocarditis, 1461
Group D streptococcal infection, 1444

Group G streptococcal infection, 1311t, 1444
 endocarditis, 1461
Growth factors. See also Filgrastim; Sargramostim
 for chemotherapy-induced toxicity, 1662, 1671–1672t
 for neutropenia, 518
 for stem cell mobilization, 540
Growth hormone (GH), 1109t
 deficiency of, 1108, 1109, 1110, 1111
 excess of, acromegaly and gigantism caused by, 1114
 replacement therapy with, 1110, 1112
  for HIV wasting, 1335
  during pregnancy, 1112
  for Turner syndrome, 1208
 tumors secreting, 1114, 1115, 1116, 1199, 1213
 prolactin cosecretion and, 1117
Growth hormone–releasing hormone (GHRH), ectopic secretion of, in acromegaly, 1114
Growth hormone stimulation tests, 1110
GSS. See Gerstmann-Sträussler-Scheinker syndrome
GTP cyclohydrolase I, mutation in gene for, in dystonia, 1016
Guaiac testing, 15, 1641. See also Fecal occult blood testing
Guanabenz, 464
 overdose/toxicity of, 464, 1592
Guanadrel, for hypertension, 364
Guanarito virus, 1399
Guanethidine
 for hypertension, 364
 MAOI interactions and, 1083t
Guanfacine, 462t, 464
 for migraine prophylaxis, 979t
 overdose/toxicity of, 462t, 464, 979t, 1592
 for Tourette syndrome, 1018
Guanidine, for myasthenic (Lambert-Eaton) syndrome, 1046
Guarana, toxicity of, 1593
Guargum, 585t
Guillain-Barré syndrome (acute idiopathic polyneuropathy), 1038–1039
 dysautonomia in, 990, 1038
 after herpes zoster, 1368
 influenza vaccine and, 1416
 poliomyelitis differentiated from, 1383
 yellow fever vaccination and, 1327
 Zika virus infection and, 1406
Gum disease. See Gingivitis
Gummas
 in endemic syphilis, 1499
 in syphilis, 1489t, 1494, 1495, 1495f
 in yaws, 1498
Gun-related injury/death, prevention of, 16
Guselkumab, for psoriasis, 108
Gut. See Gastrointestinal system
Gut dialysis (repeat-dose charcoal), 1583
Guttate psoriasis, 107. See also Psoriasis
GVH. See Graft-versus-host reaction
GVHD. See Graft-versus-host disease
GVM. See Graft-versus-malignancy effect

Gynecologic disorders, 762–796. See also specific disorder
 appendicitis differentiated from, 642
 diagnostic procedures used in, 763t
 in HIV infection/AIDS, 1344–1345
 in infertility workup, 783
Gynecomastia, 1194–1196, 1195t
 breast cancer and, 760, 1194–1195
 in Klinefelter syndrome, 1190, 1195, 1682
 testicular tumors causing, 1195
 testosterone replacement therapy causing, 1193, 1195
 testosterone replacement therapy for, 1195
Gypsy moths, skin lesions caused by, 151
Gyromitra (monomethylhydrazine) mushroom poisoning, 1600, 1600t

H₁ receptor blocking drugs. See Antihistamines
H₂ receptor blocking drugs
 after fibrinolytic therapy for STEMI, 375
 for GERD, 609
 for laryngopharyngeal reflux, 233
 for peptic ulcer disease, 625, 626t, 627
 antiplatelet therapy and, 628
 for stress gastritis, 319, 620, 620–621
H1N1 seasonal influenza, 1410, 1411, 1412, 1413, 1416. See also Influenza
 drug resistance and, 1412
 prevention of, 1413–1416, 1414–1415t. See also Influenza virus vaccine
H3N2 influenza, 1413. See also Influenza resistance to, 1412
H5N1 avian influenza, 1417–1418. See also Influenza
H5N1 influenza virus vaccine, 1418
H5N2 avian influenza, 1417
H5N8 avian influenza, 1417
H7 avian influenza, 1417, 1418
H9N2 avian influenza, 1417
H63D mutation, in hemochromatosis, 708, 709
H275Y mutation, oseltamivir resistance and, 1412
H1069Q mutation, in Wilson disease, 710
H pylori infection. See Helicobacter pylori infection
HAART (highly active antiretroviral therapy). See Antiretroviral therapy
"Habit cough" (tic cough), 21
Habitual (recurrent) abortion, 805
HACE. See High-altitude cerebral edema
HACEK organisms, endocarditis caused by, 1458, 1462
HAEM. See Herpes-associated erythema multiforme
Haemophilus, 1311t, 1466
 aphrophilus (Aggregatibacter aphrophilus). See HACEK organisms
 ducreyi, 1476
 influenzae, 1315t, 1466
  pneumonia caused by, 268t, 1466
  in HIV infection/AIDS, 1336

Haemophilus influenzae type b (Hib) vaccine, 1320t, 1321t, 1325t
 adverse effects/contraindications and, 1328t
Hair
 excess of. See Hirsutism
 loss of, 158–159. See also Alopecia
 chemotherapy-induced, 1673
 in women, 159
Hair analysis, in toxicology screening, 1092
Hair cells, hearing loss and, 200
Hairy cell leukemia, 1622t
 aplastic anemia differentiated from, 516–517
 rheumatologic manifestations of, 875
Hairy leukoplakia, 224, 225f, 1341
Halcion. See Triazolam
Haldol. See Haloperidol
Hallucinations/hallucinosis. See also specific cause
 alcoholic (organic), 1093, 1095
 intracranial tumors causing, 1003, 1005
 in narcolepsy, 1090
 psychedelic drug use/hallucinogens and, 1099, 1598
 in psychotic major depression, 1075
 in schizophrenia/psychotic disorders, 1066, 1067
 substance-induced, 1099, 1103, 1598
Hallucinogenic mushroom poisoning, 1598, 1600t
Hallucinogens, 1598
Hallucinosis. See Hallucinations/hallucinosis
Halo sign
 in invasive aspergillosis, 1555
 reverse, in mucormycosis, 1556
Halobetasol, 97t
Halofantrine, 1515t, 1520
Haloperidol, 1068, 1069t, 1070, 1071. See also Antipsychotic drugs
 for aggressive/violent behavior, 1091
 for alcoholic hallucinosis, 1095
 antidepressant drug interactions and, 1083t
 for bipolar disease/mania, 1085
 decanoate form of, 1071
 for delirium, 62, 87, 1103
 for dementia, 59, 1104
 for Huntington disease, 1015
 for opioid-induced nausea and vomiting, 83
 overdose/toxicity of, 1069t, 1589–1590
 ophthalmic, 177t
 for psychedelic/hallucinogen abuse/toxicity, 1099, 1598
 for Tourette syndrome, 1018
HAM. See Human T cell lymphotropic/leukemia virus (HTLV-1/HTLV-2), myelopathy caused by
Hamartoma, as solitary pulmonary nodule, 287
Hamartomatous polyposis syndromes, 667–668
Hamilton scale, assessment of suicide risk, 1077
Hamman-Rich syndrome (acute interstitial pneumonia/AIP), 290, 291t

HAMP gene, in hemochromatosis, 708
Hampton hump, 296
Hand
    complex regional pain syndrome and, 874
    in immersion syndrome, 1565
Hand eczema, vesiculobullous (pompholyx), **121–122**, 122*f*
    tinea differentiated from, 114, 122
Hand-foot-mouth disease
    coxsackieviruses causing, 1426
        herpes stomatitis differentiated from, 227
    enterovirus 71 causing, 1427, 1428
Hand-foot syndrome (acral erythema), chemotherapy-induced, 1673
Hand sanitizers, in infection control, 1295
Hand washing, in infection control, 648, 1295
Handgrip, heart murmurs affected by, 335*t*
Hansen disease (leprosy), 1312*t*, **1484–1485**
    neuropathy associated with, 1037, 1484
Hantaan virus, 1403, 1404
Hantavirus pulmonary syndrome, 1403, 1403–1404
Hantaviruses, 1399, **1403–1404**
HAP. *See* Hospital-acquired pneumonia
HAPE. *See* High-altitude pulmonary edema
HAPS (harmless acute pancreatitis score), 727
Haptoglobin, in hemolytic anemia, 509
Harmful use (alcohol), 17. *See also* Alcohol use disorder
Harmless acute pancreatitis score (HAPS), 727
Harris–Benedict equation, 1282
Hartley-Dunhill operation, 1130
Hashimoto (chronic lymphocytic/ autoimmune) thyroiditis, 1134–1135, 1135, 1135–1136, 1136
    hepatitis C and, 1120, 1134
    hyperthyroidism and, 1136
    hypothyroidism and, 1119, 1134–1135, 1136
    pregnancy/postpartum, 816, 1125, 1131, 1133
    thyroid antibodies in, 1134, 1135
Hashitoxicosis (painless sporadic thyroiditis), 1125, 1135, 1136. *See also* Hashimoto (chronic lymphocytic/ autoimmune) thyroiditis
HAV. *See* Hepatitis A virus
Havrix. *See* Hepatitis A vaccine
Hawkins impingement sign, 1685, 1687*t*
Hay fever. *See* Allergic rhinitis
Hb. *See* Hemoglobin
HbA$_1$/A$_{1c}$. *See* Hemoglobin A$_1$/A$_{1c}$
HbA$_2$. *See* Hemoglobin A$_2$
HbcAg, 679
    antibody to (anti-HBc), 680–681, 680*f*, 681*t*, 687
        screening blood for, 543, 681
HbCO. *See* Carboxyhemoglobin levels
HBeAg, 680*f*, 681, 681*t*, 687–688

antibody to (anti-HBe), 680*f*, 681, 681*t*, 687–688
    chronic hepatitis B and, 687, 687–688
HBeAg-negative chronic hepatitis B, 687
HbF. *See* Hemoglobin F
HBIG. *See* Hepatitis B immune globulin
HBsAg, 679, 680, 680*f*, 681*t*, 687
    antibody to (anti-HBs), 680, 680*f*, 681*t*
    inactive carrier state, 687
    maternal carrier state/transmission to newborn and, 681, 799, 822
    vaccination recommendations and, 681, 822
    screening blood for, 543, 681
HBV. *See* Hepatitis B virus
HCAP. *See* Health care–associated pneumonia
HCC. *See* Hepatocellular carcinoma
hCG. *See* Human chorionic gonadotropin
HCM (hypertrophic cardiomyopathy). *See* Cardiomyopathy
HCO$_3^-$. *See* Bicarbonate
Hct. *See* Hematocrit
HCTZ. *See* Hydrochlorothiazide
HCV. *See* Hepatitis C virus
HDAg, 684, 687
    antibody to (anti-HDV), 684, 687
HDCV (human diploid cell) rabies vaccine, 1326, 1387
HDL. *See* High-density lipoproteins/ cholesterol
HDL disorders. *See* Huntington disease-like (HDL) disorders
HDV. *See* Hepatitis D virus
Head injury, **1029–1031**, 1029*t*, 1030*t*
    cerebral/subdural/subarachnoid hemorrhage and, 998, 1030–1031, 1030*t*
    cognitive disorders/delirium and, 1029, 1031, 1102*t*
    coma or stupor caused by, 1029, 1029*t*, 1246*t*
    in drowning, 1567
    headache associated with, **980**
    hearing loss associated with, 208
    olfactory dysfunction and, 220
    seizures associated with, 983, 1031
    vertigo associated with, 212, 213
Head lice, 149–150
Head and neck cancer, 1623*t*
    lymphoma, **240**
    metastatic, **239–240**
    squamous cell carcinoma of larynx, **235–237**
Head and neck infections
    actinomycosis, 1480–1481
    anaerobic, **1478**
    deep neck infections and, **230**
    Lyme disease and, **239**
    masses caused by, **239**
Head-up tilt table testing, in syncope, 401
Headache, **39–42**, 40*t*, **977–981**, 979*t*. *See also specific type and* Migraine headache
    acute, **39–42**, 40*t*, 977
    brain tumors causing, 40, **980**
    chronic, 977
    oral contraceptive use and, 786
    in subarachnoid hemorrhage, 40, 41, 981, 998

Health care (hospital)-associated infections, **1293–1296**
    burn injury and, 1569
    cirrhosis and, 701
    coagulase-negative staphylococci causing, 1450
    fever/FUO and, 1287
    meningitis, 1298, 1299
    pneumonia, **272–274**, 273*t*, 275*t*, 1314*t*. *See also* Pneumonia
    prevention of, 1294, 1295–1296
    scabies, 148, 149
    sinusitis/bacterial rhinosinusitis, 216
    in transplant recipient, 1290–1291
Health care–associated pneumonia, **272–274**, 273*t*, 275*t*
Health care providers
    HIV transmission risk and, 1332, 1346–1347
    HSV transmission prevention and, 1366
    immunization recommendations for, 1321*t*
    influenza vaccination and, 1322*t*
    MMR vaccination and, 1321*t*, 1323*t*
    zoster transmission prevention and, 1370
Health care proxy. *See* Advance care planning/advance directives
Health maintenance/disease prevention, **1–18**, 2*t*, 3*t*. *See also specific disease*
    adherence and, 1–2
    approach to patient and, **1–2**
    immunization and, 3–5, **1319–1327**, 1320–1325*t*, 1328–1329*t*
    principles of care and, 2
Hearing aids/hearing amplification, 70, 201
Hearing evaluation, 200–201
Hearing loss, **200–201**, 201*t*. *See also specific type and cause*
    autoimmune, 209
    barotrauma causing, 204
    in chronic otitis media, 205
    conductive, 200, 201
    diabetes and (maternally inherited diabetes and deafness), 1212
    in elderly (presbyacusis), **70**, 200, 208
    eustachian tube dysfunction and, 200, 203
    in glomus tumors, 207
    hereditary, 208
    in HIV infection/AIDS, 214
    long QT syndrome and, 398
    neural, 200
    noise trauma causing, 201, 208
    ossicular chain disruption causing, 200, 207
    otosclerosis and, 200, 206–207
    ototoxicity and, 208. *See also* Ototoxicity
    physical trauma causing, 207, 208
    sensory/sensorineural, 200, 201, **207–209**
    sudden, 200, 201, 208
    tinnitus and, 209
    vertigo/vestibular disorders and, 210, 211, 211*t*, 212
    vestibular schwannoma (acoustic neuroma) causing, 211*t*, 213

Hearing rehabilitation, 70
Heart, **322–438**. *See also under Cardiac; Coronary; Myocardial and Cardiovascular disorders; Heart disease*
examination of
in athlete screening, 437, 437t
in cardiomyopathy, 415, 416t, 419, 421
in heart failure, 403–404
in myocardial infarction, 370–371
"holiday," 388
in hypertension, 10, 445
myxedema, 1120
sarcoidosis involving, 292, 293
traumatic injury of, **434**
sudden death of athlete and, 436
tumors of, **433–434**
Heart block. *See* Atrioventricular (heart) block
Heart disease, **322–438**. *See also specific disorder*
acute heart failure/pulmonary edema, 403, **411–412**
in alkaptonuria, 1677, 1678
amyloidosis and, 421–422, 539
anthracycline-induced, 414–415, 1674–1675
dexrazoxane for, 415, 1671t
aspirin/chemoprevention for, 6t, 10–11, 355. *See also* Lipid-lowering therapy
in diabetes, 1241–1242
in athletes, screening for, **436–437**, 437t, 438t
bradycardias, **384**, **399–402**
cardiomyopathies, **415–422**, 416t, 420f
peripartum, 420
cardiorenal syndrome and, 923
in Chagas disease, 1509, 1510
cholesterol/lipoproteins in, 10, 353, **1259–1260**
lowering levels of. *See* Lipid-lowering therapy
screening tests for levels of, 6t, 10, 1261–1262
in women/older adults, 1261, 1262
conduction disturbances, **399–402**
congenital, **322–331**
pregnancy and, 819
coronary (atherosclerotic CAD/ ischemic), **352–381**. *See also* Coronary heart disease
deaths attributable to, 2t
in diabetes mellitus, 1241–1242
in Down syndrome, 1678
endocarditis/endocarditis prophylaxis and, 1458, 1459
during pregnancy, **436**, 819
heart failure, **402–412**, 405f. *See also* Heart (cardiac) failure
in HIV infection/AIDS, 1345, 1356
homocysteine/hyperhomocysteinemia and, 1681
hypertension/hypertension management and, 6t, 10, 356, 360f, 362, 439, 440, 443–444, 446, 447f, 448t, 464
in hyperthyroidism, 1127, 1133
hypertriglyceridemia and, 1259

in hypothyroidism, 403, 1120, 1122
immunization recommendations in, 1321t
influenza and, 1412
in Kawasaki disease, 1439
lipid disorders and, 10, 353, **1259–1260**
in Lyme disease, 425, 1502, 1505, 1505t
metabolic syndrome and, 353
metastatic, **433–434**
myocarditis, **413–415**, 413t
neoplastic, **433–434**
pericardial disorders and, **424–429**
perioperative evaluation/management and, **45–48**, 46t, 47f, 47t
in pheochromocytoma/paraganglioma, 1180, 1180t, 1181, 1182
pregnancy and, **434–436**, 819
prevention of, **5–11**, 6t, 8–9t, 9t, 353–355, 354f, 355t, 1259, 1260. *See also specific risk or cause*
cholesterol screening and, 1261–1262
lipid-lowering therapy and, **1262–1266**, 1264t, 1265t. *See also* Lipid-lowering therapy
pulmonary hypertension and, 302, 303, **429–433**, 430t, 431t, 432f
rate and rhythm disturbances, **381–398**, 382–383t. *See also* Arrhythmias
rheumatic/rheumatic fever and, **422–424**, 423t
risk/risk stratification for, 5–6, 352–353, 354f, 361–362
lipoproteins/lipid fractions and, 353, 1259–1260
in sarcoidosis, 292, 293
seizure differential and, 986
in SLE, 840
spondylitic, 863
surgery in patient with, **45–48**, 46t, 47f, 47t
thiazolidinedione use and, 1224
traumatic, **434**
sudden death of athlete and, 437
valvular, **331–351**, 332–334t, 335t, 352t. *See also* Valvular heart disease
Heart (cardiac) failure, **402–412**, 405f
ACE inhibitors for, 405f, 406, 406–407, 410–411
hypertension and, 449t, 454
acute/pulmonary edema, 403, **411–412**
angiotensin II receptor blockers for, 405f, 407, 410–411
hypertension and, 449t, 459
in aortic regurgitation, 346
in aortic stenosis, 342
arrhythmias in, 403, 404, 409
antiarrhythmic therapy for, 409
asthma/wheezing caused by ("cardiac asthma"), 242
in atrial septal defect, 325
beta-blocker therapy and, 375, 405f, 407–408, 409, 454
hypertension and, 449t, 454
biventricular pacing (resynchronization) for, 405f, 409–410

cardiac transplantation for, 410
cardiomyopathy and, 402–403, 415, 416, 417, 420f, 422
cardiorenal syndrome and, 923
case management in, 410
chemotherapy-induced, 414, 415
chronic kidney disease and, 404, 923, 926
cirrhosis and, 700
classification of, 403
in coarctation of aorta, 324
combination therapies in management of, 409
contraindicated treatments and, 409
coronary heart disease/acute coronary syndromes and, 358, 365, 370, 377–378, 410
coronary revascularization for, 410, 411
cough in, 19, 20
in coxsackievirus myocarditis, 1426
diet in management of, 410
digitalis glycosides for, 408
diuretic therapy for, 405f, 406, 410
hypertension and, 449t
ejection fraction preserved in, treatment and, 410–411
ejection fraction reduced in, treatment and, 404–410, 405f
eplerenone for, 406, 407
hypertension/hypertension management and, 10, 444, 449t
in hypertensive emergency, 469t
in hyperthyroidism, 403, 1127, 1133
hyponatremia in, 887
in hypothyroidism/myxedema, 403, 1120
implantable cardioverter defibrillators for, 405f, 409
in infectious myocarditis, 413, 414
ivabradine for, 405f, 409
liver in, **712–713**
myocardial infarction and, 370, 377–378
nonpharmacologic management of, 409–410, 411
palliative care in, 410
in patent ductus arteriosus, 330
perioperative evaluation/management and, 47–48
pharmacologic management of, 405f, 406–409, 410–411
pleural effusion in, 312, 403
postoperative pulmonary complications and, 49
in pregnancy/postpartum period (peripartum cardiomyopathy), 420, **435**, 436, 819
pulmonary edema in, 403, **411–412**
pulmonary hypertension and, 302, 303, 430, 430t, 431
in pulmonary valve stenosis, 322, 323
refeeding in protein–energy malnutrition and, 1269
reversible causes of, correction of, 406, 410
saxagliptin use and, 1227
shock and. *See* Cardiogenic shock
in SLE, 840

spironolactone for, 406, 407, 411
statin therapy in, 409
surgical interventions in, 410
in tetralogy of Fallot, 329
thiamine deficiency and, 1274
thiazolidinedione use and, 1225
in tricuspid regurgitation, 348, 349
in tricuspid stenosis, 348
vasodilator therapy for, 408
in ventricular septal defect, 327, 328
Heart fatty acid binding protein, in acute
        coronary syndromes/STEMI
        /chest pain evaluation, 28
HEART (History, Electrocardiogram,
        Age, Risk Factors, Troponin)
        risk score, 27
Heart-lung transplant, for cystic fibrosis,
        266
Heart murmurs, 332–333t
    in aortic regurgitation, 332–333t, 346
    in aortic stenosis, 332–333t, 335t, 341
    in atrial septal defect/patent foramen
        ovale, 325
    bedside maneuvers/interventions
        affecting, 335t
    in cardiomyopathy, 335t, 415, 419
    in coarctation of aorta, 324
    in endocarditis, 1459
    in mitral regurgitation, 332–333t, 335t,
        337
    in mitral stenosis, 332–333t, 335
    in mitral valve prolapse, 335t, 340
    in myocardial infarction, 371, 379
    in patent ductus arteriosus, 330
    in pulmonary valve regurgitation, 350
    in pulmonary valve stenosis, 322–323
    in rheumatic carditis, 423
    in tetralogy of Fallot, 329
    in tricuspid regurgitation, 332–333t,
        349
    in tricuspid stenosis, 332–333t, 348
    in ventricular septal defect, 327
Heart rate and rhythm, disturbances of,
        381–398, 382–383t. See also
        Arrhythmias
Heart sounds
    in aortic regurgitation, 332t, 346
    in aortic stenosis, 332t, 341
    in atrial septal defect, 325
    in hypertension, 445
    in mitral regurgitation, 332t, 337
    in mitral stenosis, 332t, 335
    in mitral valve prolapse, 340
    in myocardial infarction, 27t, 371
    in patent ductus arteriosus, 330
    in pulmonary embolism, 296t
    in pulmonary valve regurgitation, 350
    in pulmonary valve stenosis, 323
    in tetralogy of Fallot, 329
    in tricuspid regurgitation, 332t, 349
    in tricuspid stenosis, 332t
    in valvular heart disease, 332t
Heart transplantation, for heart failure, 410
Heart valves. See Prosthetic heart valves;
        Valve replacement; Valvular
        heart disease
Heartburn (pyrosis), 605, 606, 607, 609
Heartland virus, 1399
Heat, disorders caused by exposure to,
        1561, 1561–1563. See also
        Burns; Hyperthermia

cholinergic urticaria, 134
miliaria (heat rash), 131
Heat cramps, 1562
Heat exhaustion, 1562
Heat rash, 131
Heat stroke, 1562, 1563
Heat syncope/collapse, 1562
Heavy metals. See also specific type
    overdose/poisoning and, 1581t
    tubulointerstitial disease caused by,
        947, 948
Heberden nodes, 827, 828f
Heimlich maneuver, for foreign body
        removal, 238
Heinz bodies, in G6PD deficiency, 511
Helical (spiral) CT. See also Computed
        tomography
    in colorectal cancer screening (virtual
        colonoscopy), 15, 665, 1638,
        1642–1643
    in lung cancer screening, 14t, 15, 286,
        1611
    in pulmonary embolism, 23, 28
    in renal artery stenosis, 442, 931
Helicobacter pylori infection, 621–622,
        1311t
    dyspepsia and, 578, 579, 579–580, 580,
        622
    eradication therapy for, 625–627, 626t
        dyspepsia management and,
            579–580, 580
        gastric cancer/MALT lymphoma
            and, 622, 1632
        gastritis management and, 622
        peptic ulcer management and,
            625–627, 626t, 627
            NSAID-induced ulcers and, 627
            rebleeding prevention and, 630
            recurrence prevention and, 626t,
                627
    gastric cancer/MALT lymphoma and,
        532, 622, 1629, 1630, 1632
    gastritis, 621–622
        gastric cancer and, 622, 1629
    peptic ulcer disease and, 622, 623, 625,
        627
        NSAID use and, 624, 627
        rebleeding prevention and, 630
        refractory, 628
    testing for, 579, 622, 625, 627
        gastric cancer and, 622, 1630
Heller cardiomyotomy, for achalasia, 618
HELLP syndrome, 554
Helminthic infections, 1532–1536. See
        also specific type
    cestodes causing, 1535–1538
    myocarditis in, 413t
    nematodes causing
        filariasis, 1543–1546, 1543f
        intestinal, 592, 1538–1541
        invasive, 1541–1543, 1543f
    trematodes (flukes) causing,
        1532–1535
Helper-inducer T cells. See CD4 T cells
Helvella (monomethylhydrazine)
        mushroom poisoning, 1600
Hemagglutinin, influenza virus, 1410
Hemangioblastoma, cerebellar, 1003,
        1004t, 1005
Hemangioma, cavernous, of liver, 715
Hemarthroses, of knee, 1705

Hematemesis, 594, 620, 629
Hematin, for porphyria, 1036, 1677
Hematochezia, 598
    in lower GI bleeding, 597, 598
    in ulcer-related GI bleeding, 629
    in upper GI bleeding, 594, 598
Hematocrit. See also specific disorder
    in anemia, 499
    in myeloproliferative neoplasms, 520t
Hematogenous osteomyelitis, 870, 871,
        1449
Hematologic disorders, 499–545. See also
        specific type and Hemostasis
        disorders
    anemias, 499–517, 500t
    blood transfusions and, 541–545
    in chronic kidney disease, 928
    leukemias/myeloproliferative
        neoplasms, 519–531, 519t,
        520t
    lymphomas, 531–539, 532t
    neutropenia, 517–519, 518t
    perioperative evaluation/management
        and, 45, 46t, 51–52, 51t, 52t
    in preeclampsia-eclampsia, 809t
    in SLE, 839t
    stem cell transplantation and, 540–541
Hematoma
    auricular (cauliflower ear), 201
    myocardial, 434
    perianal, thrombosed hemorrhoid
        causing, 670
    septal, in nasal trauma, 222
    subdural. See Subdural hemorrhage/
        hematoma
Hematopoietic progenitor cell
        transplantation. See Bone
        marrow/stem cell
        transplantation
Hematopoietic stimulating factors. See
        Filgrastim; Growth factors;
        Sargramostim
Hematuria, 914t, 953–954. See also
        specific cause
    chemotherapy-induced bladder toxicity
        and, 1674
    in cystic kidney disease, 949, 949t,
        950
    dysuria and, 42
    glomerular, 914, 932f
    with hemoptysis, 25
    in polycystic kidney disease, 949, 949t,
        950
    after renal biopsy, 916
    synpharyngitic, 937
Hemianopia. See Visual field defects
Hemicranias, headache and, 980
Hemiplegic migraine, familial/sporadic,
        977
Hemobilia, 595
Hemoccult/Hemoccult SENSA. See Fecal
        occult blood testing
Hemochromatosis, 708–709
    adrenal insufficiency/Addison disease
        and, 1171
    cirrhosis and, 700, 708
    hepatocellular carcinoma and, 708,
        709, 1616
Hemodiafiltration, continuous
        venovenous, for poisoning/
        drug overdose, 1583

Hemodialysis, 930. *See also* Dialysis
  for end-stage renal disease, 930
  for heat stroke, 1563
  for hyperkalemia, 894, 895*t*
  immunization recommendations for
     patient receiving, 1321*t*
  iron deficiency and, 502
  nephrogenic systemic fibrosis and,
     952
  for poisoning/drug overdose,
     1582–1583, 1583*t*. *See also*
     specific drug/toxin
  pruritus associated with, 147
  surgery in patient receiving, 54
Hemodynamic status
  atrial fibrillation management and,
     389–390
  GI bleeding and, 595
  in myocardial infarction, 371
Hemoglobin
  in anemias, 499
  Bart's, 505
  glycated/glycosylated. *See* Hemoglobin
     A_1/A_{1c}
  nephrotoxicity/acute tubular necrosis
     and, 920
  in sickle cell syndromes, 511, 512, 512*t*.
     See also Sickle cell anemia/
     syndromes
  in thalassemias, 504, 504*t*, 505
Hemoglobin A, 504
  in beta-thalassemia syndromes, 504,
     504*t*, 505
  in sickle cell syndromes, 512, 512*t*
Hemoglobin A_1/A_{1c} (glycated/
     glycosylated hemoglobin)
  in diabetes mellitus, 1215–1216, 1215*t*,
     1233
    acceptable levels of, 1236
    diagnosis and, 1215–1216, 1215*t*
    glycemic control and, 1215–1216,
     1217–1218
    pregnancy and, 818, 1244
    normal values for, 1215*t*
Hemoglobin A_2, 504
  in beta-thalassemia syndromes, 504,
     504*t*, 505
  in sickle cell syndromes, 512, 512*t*
Hemoglobin AS genotype (sickle cell
     trait), 512*t*, **513**
Hemoglobin electrophoresis
  in prenatal care, 800
  in sickle cell syndromes, 512, 512*t*, 513
  in thalassemias, 504
Hemoglobin F (fetal hemoglobin), 504
  in beta-thalassemia syndromes, 504,
     504*t*, 505
  in sickle cell syndromes, 511, 512, 512*t*
Hemoglobin H/hemoglobin H disease,
     504, 504*t*, 505
Hemoglobin S, 511, 512, 512*t*
Hemoglobin SC disease, retinopathy in,
     191
Hemoglobin SS, in pregnancy, 815
Hemoglobinuria
  hemolytic anemia and, 509
  iron deficiency and, 500
  paroxysmal nocturnal, **509–510**
Hemojuvelin, in hemochromatosis, 708
Hemolymphatic disease, in African
     trypanosomiasis, 1507, 1508

Hemolytic anemias/hemolysis, 509, 509*t*.
     See also specific type or cause
  autoimmune, **513–515**
  in cold agglutinin disease, 515
  in G6PD deficiency, 510, 511
  microangiopathic, 550, 551
  in sickle cell syndromes, 511, 512
  in thalassemia, 503, 505
Hemolytic crises, in sickle cell disease,
     511, 512
Hemolytic disease of newborn, 801
Hemolytic streptococcus. *See specific type
     under* Group
Hemolytic transfusion reactions, 542–543
Hemolytic-uremic syndrome, 550–552,
     551*t*, 589
  E coli causing, 550, 551, 551*t*, 589, 1471
Hemopericardium, 434
Hemophagocytosis, 556
  lymphohistiocytosis (Epstein-Barr
     virus) and, 556, 1373
Hemophilia A and B, **557–559**, 559*t*
Hemophilia C (factor XI deficiency),
     559*t*, **560**
Hemoptysis, **25–26**
  in pulmonary embolism, 25, 296*t*
Hemorrhage. *See specific type or structure
     affected and* Bleeding
Hemorrhagic conjunctivitis
  coxsackievirus infection and, 167, 1426
  enterovirus 70 causing, 167, 1427
Hemorrhagic cystitis
  adenoviruses causing, 1421
  chemotherapy-induced, 1674
    mesna for, 1671*t*, 1674
Hemorrhagic fever with renal syndrome
     (HFRS), 1403, 1404
Hemorrhagic fevers, **1397–1406**. *See also
     specific type*
Hemorrhagic (erosive) gastritis. *See*
     Gastritis
Hemorrhagic pleural effusion, 312. *See
     also* Hemothorax
Hemorrhagic/hypovolemic shock, 493,
     494*t*, 495, 496
Hemorrhoidectomy, 670
Hemorrhoids, **669–670**
  bleeding and, 598, 669
  fecal soiling/incontinence and, 669,
     671
  pruritus ani caused by, 147
  thrombosed, 670
Hemosiderin, 499
  accumulation of, 708–709. *See also*
     Hemochromatosis
Hemosiderosis
  idiopathic pulmonary, 304
  transfusional, in thalassemia, 505
Hemostasis disorders, **546–577**, 547*t*. *See
     also specific type and*
     Bleeding
  antithrombotic therapy and, **563–577**
  in cirrhosis, 562, 704
  coagulation disorders, **557–577**, 559*t*,
     561*t*
  perioperative evaluation/management
     and, 45, 46*t*, 51
  platelet disorders, **546–557**, 547*t*, 549*f*,
     551*t*, 555*t*, 558*t*
Hemosuccus pancreaticus, 595
Hemothorax, 311, 312, 313

Hemotympanum, 204, 207
Henderson-Hasselbalch equation, 903
Henoch-Schönlein purpura, **861**, 933*t*,
     937–938, 938*f*
HepA. *See* Hepatitis A vaccine
HepB. *See* Hepatitis B vaccine
Hepacare. *See* Hepatitis B vaccine
Hepar lobatum, 1495
Heparin/low-molecular weight heparin,
     563, 571
  for acute arterial limb occlusion,
     476
  for acute coronary syndromes/STEMI,
     367*f*, 368, 373
    after fibrinolytic therapy, 375
  for antiphospholipid antibody
     syndrome, 805, 816, 842, 843
  in bridging anticoagulation, 51, 51*t*,
     351, 352*t*
  cardiac valve replacement and, 351,
     352*t*
  coagulopathy/bleeding caused by, 300,
     562
  for DIC, 554
  for DVT/PE (venous thromboembolic
     disease), 300, 568*t*, 570*t*, 571
  for hepatic vein obstruction (Budd-
     Chiari syndrome), 712
  hyperkalemia caused by, 894
  for intracranial venous thrombosis,
     1002
  in pregnant patient, 351, 352*t*, 805,
     816, 842, 843
  for superficial thrombophlebitis, 488
  thrombocytopenia caused by, **552–553**,
     553*t*, 555*t*
Heparin-associated antibody, 552
Heparin-induced thrombocytopenia,
     552–553, 553*t*, 555*t*
Hepatic abscess
  amebic, 1525, 1526, 1527, 1527*t*
  pyogenic, **714–715**
Hepatic adenoma. *See* Hepatocellular
     adenoma
Hepatic amebiasis, 1525, 1526, 1527,
     1527*t*
Hepatic biopsy. *See* Liver, biopsy of
Hepatic coagulopathy, **562**, 704
Hepatic cysts, hydatid, 1537
Hepatic disease. *See* Liver, disorders of
Hepatic encephalopathy, 700, 703–704
  in acute liver failure, 685, 686
  in cirrhosis, 700, 703–704
  GI bleeding/esophageal varices and,
     615, 616, 703
  protein-restricted diet for, 703, 1279
  surgical risk in patients with, 50
Hepatic failure. *See* Liver (hepatic) failure
Hepatic fibrosis
  in cirrhosis, 699, 700
  drugs/toxins causing, 697
  in hemochromatosis, 709
  methotrexate toxicity and, 837
  in nonalcoholic fatty liver disease, 698,
     699
  in primary sclerosing cholangitis, 723,
     724
Hepatic hydrothorax, 702, 704
Hepatic iminodiacetic acid (HIDA) scan,
     in cholecystitis, 719
Hepatic steatosis. *See* Fatty liver

Hepatic vein obstruction (Budd-Chiari syndrome), **711–712**
Hepatitis. *See also specific type*
  alcoholic, 693, 694
    postoperative complications associated with, 50
  autoimmune, **692–693**
  CMV, 1375
  drugs/toxins causing, 696–697
  fibrosing cholestatic, 688
  herpetic, 1364
  hypoxic, 712–713
  ischemic, 712–713
  postoperative complications associated with, 50
  in varicella zoster virus infection, 1369
  viral. *See also specific type*
    acute, **677–686**
    adenoviruses causing, 1421
    arthritis in, 870
    chronic, 682, 683f, 684, **686–691**
      pregnancy and, 683, 688, 822–823
    cirrhosis and, 682, 683, 684, 687, 688, 689
    in drug users, 678, 680, 682–683, 1304
    in HIV infection/AIDS, 680, 683, 687, 688
    liver cancer and, 682, 684, 687, 1616, 1617
    liver failure and, 685, 686
    postoperative complications associated with, 50
    pregnancy and, 681, 683, 688, 799, 800, **822–823**
    transfusion-associated, 543, 680, 681, 682, 683–684
Hepatitis A, **677–679**, 678f
  prevention/immunization and, 4, 678, 679. *See also* Hepatitis A vaccine
  screening for, in STD patients, 1302
Hepatitis A and B vaccine, 679, 1324t, 1325t
Hepatitis A immune globulin, 4, 679, 1326
  during pregnancy/for newborn, 802
Hepatitis A vaccine, 4, 678, 679, 1320t, 1321t, 1324t, 1326
  adverse effects/contraindications and, 1328t
  in immunocompromised host/HIV infection/AIDS, 679, 1321t, 1326
  during pregnancy, 802, 1321t
  for travelers, 679, 1324t, 1326
Hepatitis A virus (HAV), 677–678, 678f
  antibody to, 678, 678f
Hepatitis B, **679–682**, 680f, 681t
  acute, **679–682**, 680f, 681t
  antiretroviral agents for, 687–688
  arthritis in, 870
  cancer associated with, 682, 687, 1616, 1617
  chronic, 682, 687, **687–689**
    pregnancy and, 688, **822**
  cirrhosis and, 682, 687, 688
  hepatitis D (delta agent) and, 684, 687
  HIV infection/AIDS and, 680, 687, 688, 1341
  inactive carrier state, 687

maternal carrier state/transmission to newborn and, 681, 799, **822**
  vaccination/vaccination recommendations and, 681, 802, 822
  polyarteritis nodosa and, 856
  pregnancy and, 681, 688, 799, **822**
  prevention/immunization/screening and, 681–682, 1302, 1326. *See also* Hepatitis B vaccine
  in STD patients, 1302, 1324t, 1325t
  sexual violence (rape/sexual assault) and, 1302
  transfusion in transmission of/ screening blood for, 543, 680, 681
Hepatitis B core antigen (HBcAg), 679
  antibody to (anti-HBc), 680–681, 680f, 681t, 687
  screening blood for, 543, 681
Hepatitis B e antigen (HBeAg), 680f, 681, 681t, 687–688
  antibody to (anti-HBe), 680f, 681, 681t, 687–688
  chronic hepatitis B and, 687, 687–688
Hepatitis B e antigen (HBeAg)-negative chronic hepatitis B, 687
Hepatitis B immune globulin, 681
  during pregnancy/for newborn, 681, 822
Hepatitis B surface antigen (HBsAg), 679, 680, 680f, 681t, 687
  antibody to (anti-HBs), 680, 680f, 681t
  inactive carrier state, 687
  maternal carrier state/transmission to newborn and, 681, 799, 822
  vaccination recommendations and, 681, 802, 822
  screening blood for, 543, 681
Hepatitis B vaccine, 4, 680, 681–682, 1320t, 1321t, 1324–1325t, 1326
  adverse effects/contraindications and, 1328t
  in cancer prevention, 13, 682, 1617
  in immunocompromised host/HIV infection/AIDS, 5, 681, 682, 1321t, 1324t, 1325t, 1348–1349
  for newborn/pregnant patient, 681, 802, 822, 1321t
  in STD patients, 1302, 1324t, 1325t
  for travelers, 1326
Hepatitis B virus (HBV), 679–680
Hepatitis B virus DNA, 680f, 681, 687, 688
Hepatitis C, **682–684**, 683f
  acute, **682–684**, 683f
  antiviral agents for, 689–691, 690t
  arthritis in, 870
  cancer associated with, 684, 1616, 1617
  chronic, 683f, 684, 687, **689–691**, 690t
    pregnancy and, 683, **822–823**
  cirrhosis and, 683, 684, 689
  cryoglobulinemia and, 683, 691, 860, 860–861, 939, 940
  HIV infection/AIDS and, 683, 1341–1342
  immune thrombocytopenia in, 550
  postoperative complications associated with, 50

in pregnancy, 683, 800, **822–823**
  renal disease and, 683, 933t, **940**
  thyroiditis/hypothyroidism and, 1120, 1134
  transfusion in transmission of/ screening blood for, 543, 682, 683–684
Hepatitis C virus (HCV), 682
  antibodies to (anti-HCV), 683, 683f, 689
  screening blood for, 543, 683–684
Hepatitis C virus RNA, 683, 683f, 689
Hepatitis D, **684**
  acute, **684**, 687
  chronic, **687–689**
  hepatitis B and, 684, 687
  hepatocellular carcinoma and, 1616
Hepatitis D antigen (HDAg), 684, 687
  antibody to (anti-HDV), 684, 687
Hepatitis D virus (HDV/delta agent), 682, 684, 687
Hepatitis D virus RNA, 684, 687
Hepatitis E, **684**
Hepatitis E vaccine, 684
Hepatitis E virus (HEV), 682, 684
  antibody to (anti-HEV), 684
Hepatitis E virus RNA, 684
Hepatitis G virus (HGV/pegivirus), 682
Hepatobiliary cancers, **1616–1626**. *See also specific type*
Hepatobiliary CMV, 1375
Hepatoblastoma, 1616
Hepatocellular adenoma, 715–716
  hepatocellular carcinoma arising from, 1616
  oral contraceptive use and, 715, 716, 786
Hepatocellular carcinoma, 1608t, **1616–1618**, 1625t
  with cholangiocarcinoma, 1619
  cirrhosis and, 701, 705, 1616, 1617
  hemochromatosis and, 708, 709, 1616
  hepatitis and, 682, 684, 687, 1616, 1617
  hepatitis B vaccine in prevention of, 13, 682, 1617
  nonalcoholic fatty liver disease and, 699, 1616
  primary biliary cholangitis/cirrhosis and, 707
  pyogenic abscess and, 714–715
Hepatocellular disease. *See also* Cirrhosis; Liver, disorders of
  jaundice in, 674, 675t, 676t
Hepatocyte nuclear factor (HNF)
  hepatocellular adenomas and, 715, 716
  in MODY, 1211t, 1212
Hepatolenticular degeneration. *See* Wilson disease
Hepatopathy, ischemic, 712–713
Hepatopulmonary syndrome, 704
Hepatorenal syndrome, 702–703
Hepatosplenic candidiasis, 1547
Hepatotoxicity, **695–697**. *See also specific cause*
  of acetaminophen, 74, 685, 686, 1585, 1587f
  of anesthetics, 50
  of methotrexate, 108, 837
  in mushroom poisoning, 685–686, 686, 1600
  of nevirapine, 1355–1356

Hepatotoxicity (*Cont.*):
  of statins, 1264
  of thiazolidinediones, 1225
  of tuberculosis therapy, 4
Hepcidin, 499
  in anemia of chronic kidney disease, 928
  in anemia of inflammation, 502, 503
  in hemochromatosis, 708, 709
  in iron deficiency anemia, 499, 500, 501
Hepegivirus-1, 682
HER2 overexpression/*HER2* gene. *See also* Trastuzumab
  in breast cancer, 748–749, 752, 753
    in male, 760
    prognosis and, 750, 751, 751*t*, 758
    therapy and, 748–749, 751, 752, 753, 756
  in esophageal cancer, 1628
"Herbal ecstasy" (ephedrine), 1587
Herbal products, toxicity of, **1593–1594**, 1593*t*
Herbicide poisoning (cholinesterase inhibitors), 1580*t*, 1581*t*, **1601–1602**
Herceptin. *See* Trastuzumab
Herd immunity
  enterovirus infection and, 1427
  measles and, 1379
Hereditary amyloidosis (mutated transthyretin/TTR), 421, 422, 538
Hereditary angioedema, 879*t*
Hereditary cholestatic syndromes, 674, 675*t*
Hereditary colorectal cancer/polyposis syndromes, **666–669**, 1637. *See also specific disorder*
Hereditary/genetic disorders, **1676–1684**. *See also specific disorder*
  electrolyte metabolism disturbances and, 892*t*
Hereditary hearing loss, 208
Hereditary hemorrhagic telangiectasia, **1683–1684**
Hereditary leiomyoma-renal cell carcinoma, 1654
Hereditary motor and sensory neuropathy (HMSN), types I to, IV, 1035–1036
Hereditary nonpolyposis colon cancer (HNPCC/Lynch syndrome), **668–669**
  endometrial carcinoma and, 668, 669, 774
  pancreatic/periampullary carcinoma and, 1620
  ureteral/renal pelvis cancer and, 1653
Hereditary papillary renal cell carcinoma, 1654
Hernias
  hiatal, 606
    esophageal webs and rings and, 613
    GERD and, 606
  vaginal (pelvic organ prolapse), **777–778**
Herniated nucleus pulposus. *See* Nucleus pulposus, herniation of
Herniation syndromes

intracranial tumors causing, 1003, 1005
lumbar puncture and, 998, 1005, 1298, 1299
Heroin abuse, 1098, 1601
Herpangina
  coxsackievirus, 1426
  enterovirus 71, 1427
Herpes-associated erythema multiforme, 135, 136, 1364, 1366
Herpes genitalis. *See* Genital herpes
Herpes labialis (cold/fever sore), **118–120**, 119*f*, 1363. *See also* Herpes simplex infection
Herpes simplex infection, **118–120**, 119*f*, **1363–1366**, 1364*f*
  acyclovir prophylaxis/treatment and, 119, 170*t*, 175, 1291, 1338*t*, 1343, 1365*t*, 1366
  anorectal involvement and, 119, 671
  Bell palsy and, 1041, 1364, 1366
  chemoprophylaxis for, 119
  conjunctivitis, 167
  disseminated/generalized, 1364, 1366
    dermatitis in (eczema herpeticum), 105, 106, 1364, 1367*t*
  encephalitis, 1364, 1366
  erythema multiforme associated with, 135, 136, 1364, 1366
  esophagitis in, 611, 612, 1364, 1366
  gladiatorum, 119, 1363
  HIV infection/AIDS and, 192, 1338*t*, 1343, 1363
    esophageal, 611, 612, 1364, 1366
  keratitis, **175**, 1363, 1364, 1364–1366
  during pregnancy/neonatal/congenital infection, **823**, 1363–1364, 1366
  retinitis, 192, 1363
  stomatitis/gingivostomatitis in, 118, **227**, 1363
  treatment/prophylaxis/prevention and, 119, 1291, 1364–1366, 1366
  type 1, 118, 1363
  type 2, 119, 1363
Herpes stomatitis/gingivostomatitis, 118, **227**, 1363
Herpes zoster (shingles), **120–121**, 120*f*, **1366–1372**
  earache in, 207, 1369
  eye involvement and, **175**, 192, 1369, 1370
  facial involvement/Ramsay Hunt syndrome/Bell palsy and, 120, 214, 1041, 1369
  in immunocompromised host/HIV infection/AIDS, 120, 121, 192, 214, 1338*t*, 1343, 1370
  neuralgia after, 5, 120–121, 121, 175, **982**, 1369–1370, 1370
  pregnancy and, 821
  prevention and, 5, 121, 1371. *See also* Herpes zoster vaccine
Herpes zoster ophthalmicus, 121, **175**, 192, 1369, 1370
Herpes zoster oticus, 1369
Herpes zoster retinitis, 192
Herpes zoster vaccine, 5, 121, 1320*t*, 1321*t*, 1323*t*, 1371
  adverse effects/contraindications and, 1321*t*, 1329*t*

immunocompromised host/HIV infection/AIDS and, 5, 1321*t*, 1323*t*, 1343, 1349
Herpesviruses, **1363–1377**. *See also specific type under Human herpesvirus*
Herpetic whitlow, 119, 1363, 1364*f*
Heterophyes flukes, 1535
Heterotopic pregnancy, 806. *See also* Ectopic pregnancy
HEV. *See* Hepatitis E virus
Hexosaminidase deficiency, in juvenile spinal muscular atrophy, 1034
HFA inhalers. *See* Hydrofluoroalkane inhalers
HFE gene/protein, in hemochromatosis, 708, 709
HFMD. *See* Hand-foot-mouth disease
HFRS. *See* Hemorrhagic fever with renal syndrome
HGD gene, in alkaptonuria, 1678
hGH. *See* Human growth hormone
HGV. *See* Hepatitis G virus
HHT. *See* Hereditary hemorrhagic telangiectasia
HHV. *See* Human herpesviruses
5-HIAA. *See* 5-Hydroxyindoleacetic acid
Hiatal hernia, 606
  esophageal webs and rings and, 613
  GERD and, 606
Hibernation, myocardial, 353
Hiccups, **583**
HIDA scan, in cholecystitis, 719
Hidradenitis suppurativa (acne inversa), 153
HIF2A mutations, in pheochromocytoma/paraganglioma, 1180
High-altitude-associated neurologic conditions, **1574**
High-altitude cerebral edema (HACE), **1574**
High-altitude illness, **1573–1575**. *See also specific type*
  prevention of, 1575
High-altitude pulmonary edema (HAPE), **1574**
High (eversion) ankle sprain, 1715*t*, **1716–1717**
High blood pressure. *See* Hypertension
High-calcium diet, 1280
High-carbohydrate diet
  cholesterol lowering and, 1263
  in porphyria, 1036, 1676, 1677
High-density lipoproteins/cholesterol, 1259–1260
  cardiovascular/coronary heart disease and, 353, 1259–1260
    in women, 1262
  in diabetes mellitus, 1217
  diet affecting levels of, 1263
  estrogen replacement affecting, 1202
  raising levels of, 355, 1262
    fibric acid derivatives for, 1264–1265
    niacin for, 355, 1264
  screening tests for levels of, 1261, 1262
    in women, 1262
  thiazolidinediones affecting, 1224

High dose chemotherapy, with bone marrow/stem cell transplantation, 540. *See also* Bone marrow/stem cell transplantation; Chemotherapy
High-dose insulin euglycemic therapy for beta-blocker overdose/toxicity, 1591
for calcium channel blocker overdose/toxicity, 1578, 1591
High-fiber diet. *See* Fiber, dietary
High-potassium diet, 1280
High-sensitivity C-reactive protein (hs-CRP), coronary heart disease risk and, 1261–1262
Highly active antiretroviral therapy (HAART). *See* Antiretroviral therapy
Hill-Sachs lesions, 1690
Hill sign, 346
Hip, **1701–1704**, 1702*t*
arthritis of, **1703–1704**
back pain and, 1693
Hip fracture, 63, 64, 1159, **1701–1703**
atypical, bisphosphonate use and, 1162
estrogen replacement therapy affecting risk of, 796, 1202
Hip replacement
for arthritis, 829, 1703
DVT/PE (venous thromboembolic disease) prevention and, 298–300, 1703
for fracture, 1702
Hip resurfacing surgery, 1703
Hippocampal sclerosis, epilepsy/seizures caused by, 983
Hirschsprung disease, in MEN, 1188
Hirsutism, **1196–1199**
in congenital adrenal hyperplasia, 1169, 1170, 1196, 1197
in polycystic ovary syndrome, 780, 781, 1196
in porphyria, 123, 1197
testosterone replacement therapy in women and, 1206
Histamine, drugs blocking receptors for. *See* Antihistamines; H$_2$ receptor blocking drugs
Histiocytic necrotizing lymphadenitis (Kikuchi disease), 239
Histoplasma capsulatum (histoplasmosis), **1548–1549**
History, Electrocardiogram, Age, Risk Factors, Troponin (HEART) risk score, 27
Histrelin, for prostate cancer, 1649*t*
Histrionic (hysterical) personality disorder, 1065*t*
HIT. *See* Heparin-induced thrombocytopenia
HIV. *See also* HIV infection/AIDS
drug resistance and, 1347, 1350, 1360, 1361–1362, 1361*f*
drugs blocking entry of into cells (entry inhibitors), 1352*t*, 1357–1358
screening blood for antibody to, 543, 1332, 1347
serologic tests in identification of. *See* HIV testing

HIV-associated dementia, 1339
HIV-associated nephropathy, 934*t*, **946**
HIV infection/AIDS, **1330–1362**. *See also* Immunocompromised host
adenovirus infection and, 1420
adherence to therapy and, 1, 1360, 1360–1361, 1361*f*
adrenal insufficiency and, 1171, 1343
anal dysplasia/cancer and, 1344, 1644
arthritis in, 869, 1340
autoimmunity/allergic reactions/hypersensitivity in, 1332–1333
bacillary angiomatosis/bartonellosis in, 1343, 1477
biliary disease in, 1342
breastfeeding in transmission of, 1332, 1346
campylobacter/campylobacter-like organisms causing disease in, 1472
cancer associated with, 1330, 1331*t*, 1332, 1337–1338*t*, 1344
candidiasis in, 132, 192, 611, 1335, 1343
esophageal, 611, 1335, 1338*t*, 1341
oral (thrush), 226, 611, 1335, 1341
vulvovaginal, 1338*t*, 1344
CD4 T cells in. *See* CD4 T cells
CDC definitions and, 1330, 1331*t*
cerebral lymphoma in, 1004*t*, 1006, 1337*t*, 1339, 1344
Chagas disease and, 1509
cholangiopathy in, 1529
CIN/cervical cancer in, 771, 1344, 1345
clinical findings in, 1333–1334, 1333*f*, 1334*t*
CMV infections in, 611–612, 1291–1292, 1336–1338, 1338*t*, 1341, 1374–1375, 1375, 1376
esophagitis, 611–612, 1375
prophylaxis/treatment of, 191, 1291–1292, 1376
retinitis, 191–192, 1338*t*, 1341, 1374, 1375, 1376
coccidial and microsporidial infection in, 1342, 1528–1529, 1529, 1530
coccidioidomycosis in, 1550
complications of, 1335–1345. *See also* HIV infection/AIDS, infections in
prevention of, 1347–1349, 1348*t*, 1349–1350, 1349*t*
treatment of, 1337–1338*t*, 1350
coronary heart disease in, 1345, 1356
counseling and, 1345–1346, 1346
cryptococcosis/cryptococcal meningitis in, 1006, 1337*t*, 1340, 1553, 1554
cryptosporidiosis in, 592, 1342, 1528
dementia associated with, 1339
diarrhea/enterocolitis in, 588*t*, 589, 1335, 1342
differential diagnosis of, 1334
drug use and, 1304, 1332
endocrinologic manifestations of, 1342–1343
epidemiology of. *See* HIV infection/AIDS, transmission of

erythrovirus (parvovirus) infection in, 1422
esophagitis in, 611, 1341
fever/FUO and, 1287, 1288, 1335
folliculitis and, 130, 1343
functional assessment in definition of, 1330
fungal rashes in, 1343
gastrointestinal manifestations of, 1341–1342
gastropathy in, 1342
gynecologic manifestations of, 1344–1345
gynecomastia and, 1195
hairy leukoplakia in, 224, 225*f*, 1341
health care maintenance for patients with, 1347–1349, 1348*t*, 1349–1350, 1349*t*
hepatic disease/hepatitis in, 680, 683, 687, 688, 1341–1342
hepatitis A vaccine in, 679, 1321*t*
hepatitis B/hepatitis B vaccine in, 5, 681, 682, 1321*t*, 1324*t*, 1325*t*, 1349
hepatitis C in, 683, 1341–1342
herpes simplex infection and, 192, 1338*t*, 1343, 1363
acyclovir treatment/prophylaxis and, 1338*t*, 1343
esophagitis, 611, 612, 1364, 1366
herpes zoster/herpes zoster vaccine and, 5, 120, 121, 1321*t*, 1338*t*, 1343, 1349
histoplasmosis in, 1549
Hodgkin disease in, 1344
home tests for, 1334
hyperkalemia in, 894
hyponatremia in, 886
immune thrombocytopenia in, 550
immunization recommendations in, 4, 1319, 1321*t*, 1348–1349
incidence/prevalence of, 1332
infections in, 1330, 1331*t*, 1332. *See also specific type and* Opportunistic infections
antiretroviral therapy affecting, 1353
CD4 T cell levels and, 1333, 1333*f*, 1334, 1348*t*, 1349, 1350
prevention of, 1347–1349, 1348*t*, 1349–1350, 1349*t*
treatment of, 1337–1338*t*, 1350
inflammatory reactions (immune reconstitution syndromes) in, 191–192, 1345
influenza vaccination and, 5, 1321*t*, 1416
intracranial tumors in, **1006**
Kaposi sarcoma in, 146, 192, 214, 1332, 1338*t*, 1344
laboratory findings in, 1333–1334, 1334*t*
leishmaniasis and, 1511
listeriosis in, 1457
lymphadenopathy in, 239, 1333
eustachian tube dysfunction/serous otitis media and, 214
lymphoma in, 1004*t*, 1006, 1337*t*, 1338–1339, 1339, 1344
MAC infections in, 285, 1337*t*, 1482–1483
prevention and, 1334, 1350, 1483

HIV infection/AIDS (*Cont.*):
  malabsorption in, 1335, 1342
  malaria in, 1513, 1519
  measles/measles (MMR) vaccine in, 5, 1321*t*, 1349, 1380
  mental status/cognitive changes in, 1339
  molluscum contagiosum in, 142, 1343, 1423
  mucormycosis in, 218
  myelopathies in, 1340
  myopathy in, 869, 1049, 1340
  nausea and vomiting in, 1335
  needle-stick injury and, 1332, 1347
  nephropathy in, 934*t*, **946**
  neurologic manifestations of
    central, 1339–1340
    peripheral/neuropathy, 1340
  non-Hodgkin lymphoma in, 1337*t*, 1338–1339, 1339, 1344
  nontuberculous mycobacterial infection in, 285, 1336
  oral lesions in, 1341
  otologic manifestations of, **214**
  pathophysiology of, 1332–1333
  perinatal transmission of, 1332, 1346
  pneumonia in, 268*t*, 276, 1335–1336, 1337*t*, 1551, 1552, 1553. *See also Pneumocystis jirovecii* infection/pneumonia
    CD4 T cell count and, 1333, 1334, 1336, 1349
    immunization against. *See* Pneumococcal vaccine
  pneumonitis in, nonspecific interstitial, 1339
  in pregnancy, 799, 800, **822**, 1332, 1346
  prevention of. *See* HIV infection/AIDS, transmission of, prevention of
  prognosis of, 1330, 1350, 1362
  progressive multifocal leukoencephalopathy in, 1340, 1395
  psoriasis/psoriatic arthritis in, 869, 1340, 1344
  pulmonary manifestations of, 268*t*, 271, **276**, 1335–1339. *See also* HIV infection/AIDS, pneumonia in
  reactive arthritis and, 866, 869, 1340
  retinal disorders associated with, **191–192**
    CMV retinitis, 191–192, 1338*t*, 1341, 1374, 1375, 1376
  rheumatic manifestations of, **869–870**, 1340
  RSV infection in, 1409
  Salmonella infection in, 1342, 1469, 1470
  scabies in, 149
  screening for. *See* HIV testing
  seborrheic dermatitis in, 1343
  seizures in, 983
  sinusitis in, 218, 1339
  skin disorders in, 1343–1344
  spermicides/nonoxynol 9 and, 790, 1346
  staphylococcal skin infections in, 1343
  strongyloidiasis in, 1540

syphilis/syphilis testing and, 1348, 1489, 1492, **1497**
systemic complaints associated with, 1335
T cells in. *See* CD4 T cells
toxoplasmosis in, 192, 1006, 1337*t*, 1339, 1523, 1524
  prevention/chemoprophylaxis and, 1350, 1525
transmission of, 1330–1332
  bites in, 1300, 1301
  to fetus/newborn, 822, 1332, 1346
  health care providers and, 1332, 1346–1347
  prevention of, 4, 1345–1347
    blood screening/blood treatment and, 543, 1332, 1347
    condoms for, 4, 791, 1346
    postexposure prophylaxis and, 4, 1302, 1303, 1346
    preexposure prophylaxis and, 4, 1303, 1346
  sexual behavior and, 1330, 1346, 1349
  sexual violence (rape/sexual assault) and, 793, 793–794, 1302
  transfusions and, 543, 1332, 1347
treatment of, 1349–1362
  adjunctive treatments and, 1350
  antiretroviral therapy in, 1350–1362, 1351–1353*t*, 1354*t*, 1359–1360*t*, 1361*f*. *See also* Antiretroviral therapy
  opportunistic infections/ malignancies and, 1337–1338*t*, 1349–1350, 1349*t*
  prophylaxis and, 1347–1349, 1348*t*, 1349–1350, 1349*t*
  in pregnancy, 822
  tuberculosis and, 1336
tuberculin skin test in, 1336, 1347
tuberculosis in, 277, 278, 279, 282, 1336, 1347–1348
  ART affecting outcome and, 1353
  chemoprophylaxis/prevention and, 1347–1348, 1350
  drug-resistant disease and, 277, 1336
  drug use and, 1304
  intestinal involvement in, 643
  treatment of, 4, 282, 1336
vaccine development and, 1347
varicella zoster virus infection/varicella vaccine in, 5, 120, 121, 1321*t*, 1338*t*, 1343, 1349
weight loss in, 1335
Wernicke encephalopathy in, 1026
in women, 1332
xerosis in, 1344
yellow fever vaccine in, 1349, 1405
HIV integrase inhibitors, 1352–1353*t*, 1358
  in combinations, 1358
  resistance to, 1361, 1362
HIV painful articular syndrome, 869
HIV rapid antibody tests, 1302, 1334, 1334*t*
HIV retinopathy, 191, 1341
HIV testing, 4, 1302, 1333–1334, 1334*t*, 1345–1346
  in blood screening, 543, 1332, 1347

  after needle stick, 1347
  in pregnancy, 799, 800, 822, 1332, 1346
  after sexual violence (rape/sexual assault), 793–794, 1302
  in STD patients, 1302
  syphilis patients and, 1348, 1492, 1497
  transmission prevention and, 4, 1302, 1345–1346
  in women, 799, 800, 822
HIV viral load tests, 1334, 1334*t*
  antiretroviral therapy initiation/ monitoring and, 1350, 1360
  for blood screening, 1332
HIV wasting syndrome, 1335
Hives. *See* Urticaria
HJV gene, in hemochromatosis, 708
HLA. *See* Human leukocyte antigen
HLA-B alleles, drug-induced hypersensitivity and, 880
HMBS mutation, in acute intermittent porphyria, 1676
hMG. *See* Human menopausal gonadotropins
HMG-CoA reductase inhibitors. *See* Statins
HMSN. *See* Hereditary motor and sensory neuropathy
HNF (hepatocyte nuclear factor)
  hepatocellular adenomas and, 715, 716
  in MODY, 1211*t*, 1212
HNPCC. *See* Hereditary nonpolyposis colon cancer
Hoagland sign, 1372
Hoarseness, **232–233**
  laryngitis causing, 233
  laryngopharyngeal reflux causing, 233
  vocal folds and, 232
Hodgkin lymphoma, **533–534**, 1622*t*
  bone marrow/stem cell transplantation for, 534, 540
  fever/FUO and, 1288
  in HIV infection/AIDS, 1344
  of kidney, 1655
"Holiday heart," 388
Holosystolic murmurs. *See* Heart murmurs
Holter monitoring. *See* Ambulatory electrocardiographic monitoring
Homans sign, 296*t*
Home blood pressure monitoring, 439, 440*f*
Home hemodialysis, 930
Home HIV tests, 1334
Home oxygen therapy, 259–260, 260*t*
Homeostenosis. *See* Age/aging
Homocysteine, disorders of metabolism of, **1681**
  DVT/PE (venous thromboembolic disease) and, 575*t*, 1681
  stroke and, 996, 1681
Homocystinuria, 1681
Homogentisic acid oxidase deficiency, in alkaptonuria, 1677
Homonymous field defects. *See* Visual field defects
Homosexuality
  gonococcal arthritis and, 868
  hepatitis transmission and, 680, 683, 684

HIV infection/AIDS transmission risk and, 1330, 1346
immunization recommendations and, 1321*t*
STD transmission/prevention/ screening and, 1302
syphilis and, 1488, 1491
Honey, infant botulism and, 1454
Hookworm disease, **1539**
cutaneous larva migrans, **1542–1543,** 1543*f*
Hordeolum, **164–165**
Hormone receptor sites, in breast cancer, 748
in male, 760
prognosis and, 750, 751*t*, 758
treatment and, 748, 752, 753, 754–756, 755*t*
Hormone therapy. *See also* Estrogen (hormone) replacement therapy; Testosterone replacement therapy
for abnormal uterine bleeding, 763
adverse ophthalmic effects of, 178*t*
for breast cancer, 752, 753, 754–756, 755*t*
adjuvant/neoadjuvant, 750, 751, 752, 753
hormone receptor sites and, 748, 751, 752, 753, 754–756, 755*t*
in male, 760
for metastatic disease, 754–756, 755*t*, 760
in contraception, **789**
injections/implants, **788–789**
IUDs, 789
oral contraceptives, **785–788,** 787*t*, 788*t*
for endometriosis/pelvic pain, 765, 776
for erectile dysfunction, 967
for infertility, 970
for menopausal symptoms, 795–796
for osteoporosis prevention/ management, 795, 796, 1161
for prostate cancer, 1649, 1649–1650, 1649*t*
Horner syndrome (oculosympathetic paralysis)
in coma or stupor, 1027
headache and, 40, 979, 980
in lung cancer, 1609
Hospice care, 90–91. *See also* End of life, provision of care at
Hospital-acquired pneumonia, **272–274,** 273*t*, 275*t*, 1294, 1314*t*
Hospital-associated infections. *See* Health care (hospital)-associated infections
Hospitalization
for alcohol use disorders/withdrawal, 1095, 1097
for asthma, 242, 254, 255–257, 256*f*
community-acquired pneumonia and, 267, 269, 269*t*, 271, 271–272, 1314*t*
for COPD, 262
diabetes management during, 1243–1244, 1243*t*
fever/FUO and, 1287
immobility prevention/treatment and, 63

infections acquired during, **1293–1296.** *See also* Health care (hospital)-associated infections
for preeclampsia/eclampsia, 810
pressure ulcers and, 68–69, 68*t*
prolonged, 1105
psychiatric problems associated with, **1104–1107**
for schizophrenia/psychotic disorders, 1068
for suicidal patients, 1077
for tuberculosis, 281
Host defenses, impairment of. *See* Immunocompromised host
Hot environments, disorders caused by exposure to, **1561, 1561–1563**
Hot flushes
in menopause, 794, 795, 1201
estrogen replacement therapy for, 795, 1202
topical progesterone for, 1205
niacin causing, 1264, 1276
Hot soaks, for wart removal, 142
Hot tub (*Pseudomonas*) folliculitis, 130, 131
Household cleaning agents. *See* Caustic/ corrosive agents
Household molds, **1558**
Howell-Jolly bodies, in sickle cell anemia, 512
HPC (hematopoietic progenitor cell transplantation). *See* Bone marrow/stem cell transplantation
HPeV. *See* Human parechovirus infection
HPIVs. *See* Human parainfluenza viruses
HPS. *See* Hantavirus pulmonary syndrome
HPV-genotype–specific testing, 15
HPV/HPV vaccine. *See* Human papillomavirus; Human papillomavirus (HPV) vaccine
HRIG. *See* Human rabies immune globulin
HRT (hormone replacement therapy). *See* Estrogen (hormone) replacement therapy
HRV. *See* Rotavirus vaccines
hs-CRP. *See* High-sensitivity C-reactive protein
HSV-1. *See* Herpes simplex infection, type 1
HSV-2. *See* Herpes simplex infection, type 2
5-HT$_3$ receptor antagonists. *See* Serotonin 5-HT$_3$-receptor-blocking agents
HTLV. *See* Human T cell lymphotropic/ leukemia virus
Humalog. *See* Insulin lispro
Human bite wounds, **1300–1301**
anaerobic skin infections and, 1300, 1301
Human chorionic gonadotropin (hCG)
in amenorrhea, pregnancy and, 1200, 1201
for cryptorchism, 1194
in ectopic pregnancy, 797, 806

in gestational trophoblastic disease, 807, 808
hyperthyroidism and, 807, 1126
gynecomastia and, 1195
hyperthyroidism during pregnancy and, 1126, 1128
for hypogonadism/infertility, 970, 1112, 1193
for ovulation induction, 784, 1112
pregnancy tests and, 797
in spontaneous abortion, 804
testicular tumors producing, 1656
Human deoxyribonuclease (rhDNase), for cystic fibrosis, 265
Human diploid cell (HDCV) rabies vaccine, 1326, 1387
Human granulocytic anaplasmosis/ ehrlichiosis, 1429*t*, 1435, 1436
Lyme disease coinfection and, 1436, 1504
Human growth hormone, 1112. *See also* Growth hormone
Human herpesvirus 1 and 2. *See* Herpes simplex infection
Human herpesvirus 3. *See* Varicella zoster virus
Human herpesvirus 4. *See* Epstein-Barr virus
Human herpesvirus 6, **1377**
aphthous ulcers and, 226
Human herpesvirus 7, **1377**
Human herpesvirus 8 (Kaposi sarcoma- associated herpes virus), 146, 1332, **1377**
Human herpesviruses, **1363–1377.** *See also specific type*
Human immunodeficiency virus. *See* HIV
Human insulin, 1229, 1229*t*. *See also* Insulin therapy
Human interferons. *See specific type under* Interferon
Human leukocyte antigen (HLA)
in diabetes, 1210
drug hypersensitivity syndromes and, 880
Human leukocyte antigen (HLA) typing
for platelet transfusions, 544
for stem cell transplant, 540
Human menopausal gonadotropins (hMG), for ovulation induction, 784–785
Human metapneumovirus, 1409, 1410
Human monocytic ehrlichiosis, 1429*t*, 1435, 1435–1436
Human papillomavirus (HPV)
in anal cancer, 1344, 1643–1644
in CIN/cervical cancer, 769, 770, 771, 1344
screening for, 14*t*, 15, 769–770, 769*t*, 1345
vaccination in prevention and, 4, 13, 770, 772
genital types of. *See* Venereal (genital) warts
in laryngeal cancer, 235
nasal tumors (inverted papillomas) caused by, 223
recurrent respiratory (laryngeal) papillomas caused by, 234

Human papillomavirus (HPV) (*Cont.*):
vaccine for. *See* Human papillomavirus (HPV) vaccine
in vulvar carcinoma, 775
warts caused by, 141. *See also* Venereal (genital) warts
Human papillomavirus (HPV) DNA, testing for, 14*t*, 15, 770
Human papillomavirus (HPV) vaccine, 4, 141, 671, 768, 770, 1320*t*, 1321*t*, 1322–1323*t*
adverse effects/contraindications and, 1328*t*
cancer prevention and, 4, 13, 770, 1644
in immunocompromised host/HIV infection/AIDS, 1321*t*, 1323*t*
STD prevention and, 1302
Human papillomavirus (HPV) virus-like particle (VLP) vaccine, 4. *See also* Human papillomavirus (HPV) vaccine
Human parainfluenza viruses, 1409
Human parechovirus infection, **1428**
Human parvovirus B19 infection. *See* Erythrovirus (parvovirus B19) infection
Human pegivirus (hepatitis G virus/ HGV), 682
Human rabies immune globulin, 1387
Human T cell lymphotropic/leukemia virus (HTLV-1/HTLV-2), **1396–1397**
adult T cell lymphoma/leukemia caused by, 1396
myelopathy caused by, **1026**, 1396
scabies infection and, 149
transfusion in transmission of/ screening blood for, 543, 1396, 1397
"Humidifier" lung, 308*t*
Humira. *See* Adalimumab
Humoral immunity. *See also* Immunoglobulins
infections associated with defects in, 882, 883, 1290
Hungry bone syndrome, 1149, 1158
Hunter canal, femoral artery disease and, 473
Huntingtin gene, 1015
Huntington disease, **1014–1015**
parkinsonism differentiated from, 1012
Huntington disease-like (HDL) disorders, 1015
Hürthle cell thyroid carcinoma, 1141, 1143, 1147
HUS. *See* Hemolytic-uremic syndrome
Hutchinson sign, 1369, 1370
Hyaline casts, 914*t*
Hyaluronic acid injections, for osteoarthritis of knee, 1714
Hycamtin. *See* Topotecan
Hydatid disease/cysts, 1537–1538
Hydatidiform mole, **807–808**
hyperthyroidism and, 807, 1126
Hydralazine, 463*t*
for heart failure, 405*f*, 408, 408–409
for hypertension, 463*t*, 464
eclampsia and, 810
in urgencies/emergencies, 470*t*, 471
Hydration. *See* Fluid management/ hydration

Hydrea. *See* Hydroxyurea
Hydrocarbon toxicity/abuse, 1598, 1602
pneumonia/pneumonitis and, 306, 1602
Hydrocele, in filariasis, 1544
Hydrocephalus
intracranial tumor causing, 1001, 1005
normal pressure, 1021
in subarachnoid hemorrhage, 999
Hydrochlorothiazide, 448, 450*t*. *See also* Diuretics; Thiazide diuretics
in combination products, 451*t*, 452*t*, 453*t*, 455*t*, 456*t*, 457*t*, 458*t*
for heart failure, 406
lithium interactions and, 1086
Hydrocodone, 74, 78*t*, 82
in combination agents, 74, 80*t*
Hydrocortisone, 95, 96*t*. *See also* Corticosteroids
for acute adrenal crisis, 1172
after adrenal carcinoma surgery, 1176
for adrenal insufficiency/Addison disease, 1111, 1171
for inflammatory bowel disease/ ulcerative colitis, 650, 659, 660
after pituitary surgery, 1175
topical, 95, 96*t*
Hydrodistention, for interstitial cystitis diagnosis/treatment, 961
Hydro-Diuril. *See* Hydrochlorothiazide
Hydrofluoric acid burns, 1586, 1586–1587
Hydrofluoroalkane inhalers, for asthma therapy, 250*t*, 253*t*
Hydrogen breath test, for carbohydrate/ lactose intolerance, 591, 638
Hydrogen cyanide gas, poisoning caused by, 1592
Hydromorphone, 74, 78*t*
overdose/toxicity of, 1601
Hydronephrosis, in tubulointerstitial disease, 948
Hydrops
endolymphatic (Ménière disease), 211–212, 211*t*
fetalis, 505
of gallbladder, 719
Hydroquinone, for hyperpigmentation, 158
Hydrothorax, hepatic, 702, 704
Hydroxocobalamin, for cyanide poisoning, 1581*t*, 1593
Hydroxybutyrate/hydroxybutyric acid beta
in alcoholic ketoacidosis, 905
in diabetes mellitus/diabetic ketoacidosis, 905, 1214, 1246, 1247
in insulinoma, 1253, 1253*t*
gamma, overdose/toxicity of, **1595**
Cushing syndrome and, 1173, 1174
Hydroxychloroquine
adverse ophthalmic effects of, 178*t*, 179*t*, 837
for lichen planus, 145
for lupus/SLE, 116, 841
for porphyria cutanea tarda, 123
for rheumatoid arthritis, 837
5-Hydroxyindoleacetic acid (5-HIAA), carcinoids secreting, 1635

11-Hydroxylase/P450c11 deficiency, 1170, 1196
17-Hydroxylase/P450c17 deficiency, 1169, 1190, 1199
21-Hydroxylase/P450c21 deficiency, 1169, 1170, 1196, 1197, 1198
Hydroxymethylbilane synthase deficiency, in acute intermittent porphyria, 1676
Hydroxymethylglutaryl-coenzyme A (HMG-CoA) reductase inhibitors. *See* Statins
17-Hydroxyprogesterone
in amenorrhea, 1199
in hirsutism/virilization, 1197
3-beta-Hydroxysteroid dehydrogenase deficiency, amenorrhea in, 1199
11-beta-Hydroxysteroid dehydrogenase deficiency, hypertension and, 442
17-beta-Hydroxysteroid dehydrogenase-3 deficiency, 1196
5-Hydroxytryptamine-3 receptor antagonists. *See* Serotonin 5-HT$_3$-receptor-blocking agents
Hydroxyurea
in cancer chemotherapy, 1669*t*
for essential thrombocytosis, 522
for polycythemia, 520
for primary myelofibrosis, 523
Hydroxyzine, 95, 1054*t*. *See also* Antihistamines
for insomnia, 1054*t*, 1089
Hygiene hypothesis, in diabetes mellitus, 1211
Hygroton. *See* Chlorthalidone
Hymen, imperforate, 1199
Hymenolepis
diminuta (rodent tapeworm), 1535
nana (dwarf tapeworm), **1535**, 1536
Hyoscyamus niger, toxicity of, 1590
Hyperacusis, **210**
Hyperadrenergic syndrome
in hypertensive emergency, 469*t*
mitral valve prolapse and, 340
Hyperaldosteronism. *See* Aldosteronism
Hyperalgesia, opioid-induced, 82
Hyperalimentation. *See* Central vein nutritional support
Hyperandrogenism
acne and, 126
amenorrhea caused by, 1199, 1200–1201
in hirsutism/virilization, 1196, 1197, 1198
in polycystic ovary syndrome, 780, 1196
Hyperbaric oxygen therapy
for carbon monoxide poisoning, 1581*t*, 1584*t*, 1592
for dysbarism/decompression sickness, 1573
for high-altitude illness, 1574, 1575
Hyperbilirubinemia, 674, 675*t*. *See also* specific cause
Hypercalcemia, **897–899**, 898*t*. *See also* Hyperparathyroidism
artifactual, 1155

bisphosphonate use causing, 1156, 1162
bisphosphonates for, 898, 1157, 1660
calcium/vitamin D ingestion causing, 897, 898, 1156
cancer-related, 897, 898, 1155–1156, **1659–1660**
  breast cancer and, 742, 1659
  lung cancer and, 1609, 1659
differential diagnosis of, 1155–1156
hypercalciuria and, 898, 962t
hyperparathyroidism and, 897, 898, 1152–1159, 1154f
hypocalciuric/familial hypocalciuric, 892t, 898, 1156
hypoparathyroidism/hypocalcemia treatment and, 1152
immobilization, 1156
in kidney injury/renal failure/dialysis patients, 898
lithium use and, 1086
in myeloma, 535, 536, 1156
nonparathyroid, 1154f
in Paget disease of bone, 1167
parathyroid carcinoma causing, 1153, 1154
parathyroidectomy for, 1157–1158
during pregnancy, 1153
teriparatide contraindicated in, 1162–1163
vitamin D analogs causing, 108
Hypercalciuria, 898, 962t, 963–964. See also Calcium nephrolithiasis
hypercalcemia/hyperparathyroidism and, 898, 962t, 963–964, 1152–1153, 1154, 1156
hypocalcemia/hypoparathyroidism and, 897, 1150
hypomagnesemia and, 892t
Hypercalciuric calcium nephrolithiasis, 962t, 963–964
Hypercapnia. See Permissive hypercapnia; Respiratory acidosis
Hypercarotenosis, 1277
Hyperchloremic normal anion gap acidosis, 904, 904t, **906–907**, 906t, 908. See also Normal anion gap acidosis
alcoholic ketoacidosis and, 906
diabetic ketoacidosis and, 905, 1248
parenteral nutritional support and, 907, 1285t
Hypercholesterolemia, 1259–1260. See also Cholesterol; Lipid disorders
clinical presentations in, 1261
heart disease risk and, 10, 353, 1259–1260
in nephrotic syndrome, 942
preventable disease/deaths and, 3t
screening for, 6t, 10, **1261–1262**
  in women/older adults, 1261, 1262
treatment of, **1262–1266**, 1264t, 1265t. See also Lipid-lowering therapy
Hypercoagulability
in acute mesenteric vein occlusion, 480
in antiphospholipid syndrome, 815, 816, 841
in Behçet syndrome, 862
DVT/PE (venous thromboembolic disease) and, 295, 574, 575t

in hepatic vein obstruction (Budd-Chiari syndrome), 711
in nephrotic syndrome/nephrotic spectrum disorders, 942–943
in noncirrhotic portal hypertension, 713–714
pulmonary hypertension and, 302, 303, 430, 430t
stroke and, 996
Hypercortisolism, **1172–1177**. See also Cushing syndrome
Hyperemesis gravidarum, **803**
gestational trophoblastic disease and, 807
thyroid disorders and, 803, 1126
Wernicke encephalopathy and, 1026
Hypereosinophilic syndromes, 879t
Hypergastrinemia
carcinoid tumors and, 1633
in pernicious anemia gastritis, 622
Zollinger-Ellison syndrome (gastrinoma) and, 631, 632, 1185
Hyperglycemia, 1210. See also Diabetes mellitus
in alcoholic ketoacidosis, 906
antipsychotic drug use and, 1071–1072, 1072
coma caused by. See Diabetic coma
in diabetic ketoacidosis, 905, 1246, 1247
drugs for treatment of, 1220–1228, 1221–1222t, 1235–1236, 1235f. See also Antidiabetic agents; Glycemic control in diabetes; Insulin therapy
hospitalization/surgery and, 53, 1243–1244, 1243t
in hyperglycemic hyperosmolar state, 1246t, 1249, 1250
insulin deficiency/resistance and, 1210, 1213, 1213t
parenteral nutritional support and, 1285t
pentamidine-induced, 1257, 1552
prebreakfast, 1234, 1234t
in pregnancy, 800, 817–818, 817t
  congenital anomalies caused by, 818
preventable disease/deaths and, 3t
secondary, 1213, 1213t
Hyperglycemic coma. See Diabetic coma
Hyperglycemic hypcrosmolar state, 1214, 1245, 1246t, **1249–1251**
Hyperhomocysteinemia, 1681
DVT/PE (venous thromboembolic disease) and, 575t, 1681
stroke and, 996, 1681
Hyperinfection syndrome, in strongyloidiasis, 1540
Hyperinsulinemia
acne and, 127
factitious, 1253, 1253t
in insulin resistance syndrome, 1213
insulinoma causing, 1185
pentamidine causing, 1257
in polycystic ovary syndrome, 780, 1196
Hyperkalemia, 892t, **893–896**, 894t, 895t
adrenal insufficiency/Addison disease and, 893, 1170, 1171

antihypertensive drug therapy and, 454, 459, 893–894
in diabetic ketoacidosis, 1246, 1248
genetic disorders and, 892t
hyperglycemic hyperosmolar state and, 1250
renal disorders/failure and, 893, 894, 916, 926f
spurious/venipuncture technique and, 893, 894, 894t, 1178
in tubulointerstitial disease, 948
in tumor lysis syndrome, 1660
Hyperkalemic periodic paralysis, 892t, 1049
Hyperketonemia. See Ketones/ketone bodies/ketonemia/ketonuria
Hyperlipidemia. See also Lipid disorders/ lipids
antipsychotics and, 1071, 1071t
antiretroviral therapy causing, 1174, 1345
clinical presentation of, 1261, 1261f
in diabetes mellitus, 1217, 1261
estrogen replacement therapy and, 1202, 1203
exercise affecting, 1262
in nephrotic syndrome/nephrotic spectrum disorders, 942
treatment of. See Lipid-lowering therapy
Hyperlordosis, lumbar, 1692
Hypermagnesemia, **902–903**
in acute tubular necrosis/kidney injury, 920
eclampsia treatment and, 810, 901, 902–903
hypocalcemia/hypoparathyroidism and, 901, 903, 1150
Hypermetabolism
in burn injury, 1569
in HIV infection/AIDS, 1335
thyroid tests affected by, 1128
Hypermethioninemia, screening for, homocysteine disorders and, 1681
Hypernatremia, **889–891**
in diabetes insipidus, 890, 1114
Hypernatremic dehydration, enteral nutritional support and, 1284
Hyperosmolality (hyperosmolar disorders), **891**
hyperglycemia and (hyperglycemic hyperosmolar state), 1214, 1245, 1246t, **1249–1251**
hypernatremia and, 890
Hyperosmolar nonketotic dehydration, parenteral nutritional support and, 1285t
Hyperostosis, diffuse idiopathic skeletal (DISH), 864, 1242
Hyperoxaluric calcium nephrolithiasis, 963, 964
Hyperparathyroidism, **1152–1159**, 1154f. See also Hypercalcemia
asymptomatic, 1156, 1157
bisphosphonate use and, 1156, 1162
bone changes and, 927, 927f, 1153, 1154, 1155
chronic kidney disease and, 926f, 927, 927f, 1153, 1155, 1157

Hyperparathyroidism (*Cont.*):
  hypercalcemia and, 897, 898,
    1152–1159, 1154*f*
  hypercalciuria and, 962*t*, 963–964,
    1152–1153, 1154, 1156
  hypophosphatemia and, 898, 899, 1154
  in MEN, 1152, 1153, 1155, 1158, 1187,
    1188
  normocalcemic, 1153, 1154
  pancreatitis and, 731, 1155
  after parathyroidectomy, 1158
  parathyroidectomy for, 1157–1158
  during pregnancy, 1153–1154
  after RAI treatment for
    hyperthyroidism, 1130
Hyperparathyroidism-jaw tumor
    syndrome, 1152, 1153
Hyperpathia. *See also* Thalamic
    syndrome
  intracranial tumors causing, 1003
  neuropathy causing, 1035
  in stroke, 1003
Hyperphosphatemia, **901**, 901*t*
  in diabetic ketoacidosis, 1246
  hypercalcemia and, 898
  hypercalciuria and, 898
  in kidney disease, 901, 916, 920, 926*f*
    bone disorders and, 927, 927*f*
    hyperparathyroidism and, 1157
    hypocalcemia/hypoparathyroidism
      and, 896, 897, 1150
  parenteral nutritional support and,
    1285*t*
  in tumor lysis syndrome, 1660
Hyperpigmentation, 157, 157–158, 158.
    See also Pigmented skin
    lesions
  in adrenal insufficiency/Addison
    disease, 1168, 1170
  in alkaptonuria, 1677
  antipsychotics causing, 1072
  chemotherapy-induced, 1673
  drugs causing, 158, 163*t*
  nail, drugs causing, 160, 163*t*
  in tinea (pityriasis) versicolor, 114
Hyperplastic polyps, 665
Hyperprolactinemia, **1116–1119**, 1117*t*
  amenorrhea and, 1110, 1118, 1200, 1201
  hypogonadotropic hypogonadism and,
    1109, 1110, 1111, 1117
  infertility and, 784, 1117, 1118
  nipple discharge in, 736
Hyperreactio luteinalis, virilization and,
    1197
Hypersensitivity, 876–881, 879*t*. *See also*
    Allergies/allergic disorders/
    reactions
  delayed, 876, **878–881**
  drug-induced, 161, 163, **877, 880,
    880–881**. *See also* Drug
    allergy
    antimicrobials and, **1318–1319**
  in HIV infection/AIDS, 1332–1333
  immediate, 876, **876–878**, 879*t*
  myocarditis caused by, 413*t*, 414
  to transfusions, 543
  to ultraviolet radiation. *See*
    Photodermatitis
  visceral
    chest pain/discomfort and, 619
    irritable bowel syndrome and, 644

Hypersensitivity pneumonitis, **307–308**,
    308*t*
Hypersomnias, **1089–1090**
Hypertension, **439–471**
  in adrenal hyperplasia, 1169
  aldosteronism and, 441–442, 442–443,
    444, 1177
  aortic dissection and, 27, 444, 469*t*,
    484, 485
  assessment/diagnosis/screening and,
    6*t*, 10, **439–440**, 440*f*,
    444–445
  cardiovascular disease/risk factors/
    prevention and, 6*t*, **10**, 356,
    360*f*, 362, 439, 440, 443–444,
    446, 447*f*, 448*t*, 464
  cerebrovascular disease and, 444
  chronic kidney disease/renal failure
    and, 442, 444, 466, 923, 925,
    926, 926*f*
  in coarctation of aorta, 324, 443
  complications of untreated disease and,
    443–444
  in cystic kidney disease, 949*t*, 950
  dementia and, 444
  in diabetes mellitus/diabetic
    nephropathy, 446, 447*f*, 449*t*,
    464, 465, 466, 945–946
    ACE inhibitors for, 449*t*, 454, 465,
      466, 945, 1218, 1238–1239,
      1241
    antihypertensive therapy for, 446,
      447*f*, 449*t*, 464, 465, 466,
      945–946, 1218, 1236,
      1238–1239
    benefits of control of, 945, 1218,
      1236, 1238–1239
    calcium channel blocking agents
      and, 449*t*, 465, 466, 946,
      1218
  in elderly, 446, 467
  epistaxis and, 221
  essential, 441, 444
  etiology/classification of, 441–443,
    441*t*
  fibromuscular dysplasia/renal artery
    stenosis and, 442, 466, 931
  genetic factors in, 441–442
  in heart disease/failure, 6*t*, 10, 356,
    360*f*, 362, 439, 440, 443–444,
    446, 447*f*, 448*t*, 464
  intracerebral hemorrhage and, 444,
    468–469, 997, 998
  intracranial. *See* Intracranial
    hypertension
  malignant, 468. *See also* Hypertensive
    emergencies
  management of
    in blacks, 466–467, 466*t*
    cardiovascular/heart disease and, 10,
      360*f*, 362, 446, 447*f*, 448*t*,
      464
    in diabetic patients, 446, 447*f*, 449*t*,
      464, 465, 1236
    in elderly, 446, 467
    exercise/activity and, 441, 445, 446*t*
    follow-up and, 467
    heart failure and, 10, 449*t*
    kidney disease/renal failure and,
      449*t*, 466, 929
    in hypertensive emergency, 469*t*

lifestyle modifications/
      nonpharmacologic therapy
      and, 445–446, 446*t*
    pharmacologic, 446–448, 447*f*,
      448–467, 448*t*, 449*t*,
      450–451*t*, 452–453*t*,
      455–458*t*, 460–461*t*,
      462–463*t*, 465*f*, 466*t*. *See also*
      Antihypertensive drug
      therapy
    in urgencies/emergencies,
      468–469, 469–471, 469*t*, 470*t*
    preoperative, 48
    treatment thresholds and, 446, 447*f*,
      448*t*
  "masked," 439
  metabolic syndrome and, 441
  in nephritic syndrome, 936
  ocular. *See* Ocular hypertension
  oral contraceptive use and, 443, 786
  perioperative evaluation/management
    and, 48
  in pheochromocytoma, 443, 444, 469,
    469*t*, 1179, 1180, 1180*t*,
    1182, 1183
  in poisoning/drug overdose, **1579**
  in polycystic kidney disease, 949*t*, 950
  portal. *See* Portal hypertension
  portopulmonary, 704
  during pregnancy, 442, 443, 808–811,
    818–819. *See also*
    Preeclampsia-eclampsia
  prehypertension and, **440–441**, 447*f*
  preventable disease/deaths and, 3*t*
  primary essential, 441, 444
  pulmonary. *See* Pulmonary
    hypertension
  renal vascular, 442, 931–932
  resistant, **467–468**, 468*t*
  retinochoroidopathy/retinopathy in,
    190–191, 191*f*, 444, 445*f*
  secondary, 441–443
  sleep apnea and, 316, 441
  sodium restriction and, 441
  stroke/stroke prevention and, 6*t*, 10,
    444, 446–447, 464
    in emergencies/urgencies, 468, 469*t*
  "white coat," 439
Hypertension exacerbated in pregnancy,
    442
Hypertensive emergencies, **468–471**,
    469*t*, 470*t*
  blood pressure in, 439, 440*f*, 468
  in pheochromocytoma, 443, 469, 469*t*,
    1180, 1182
  with retinopathy, 190–191, 191*f*, 468
  in scleroderma, 846–847
Hypertensive encephalopathy, 444, 468
Hypertensive nephropathy, 468
Hypertensive urgencies, **468–471**, 470*t*.
    See also Hypertensive
    emergencies
  blood pressure in, 439, 440*f*, 468
Hyperthecosis. *See* Polycystic ovary
    syndrome
Hyperthermia, **34–36**, 1561. *See also*
    Fever; Heat; Serotonin
    syndrome
  antipsychotics causing. *See* Neuroleptic
    malignant syndrome
  malignant, 35, 1294, 1580

in poisoning/drug overdose, **1580–1581**. *See also* Serotonin syndrome

Hyperthermia therapy, for benign prostatic hyperplasia, 976

Hyperthyroidism (thyrotoxicosis), 1121*t*, **1124–1134**, 1125*t*. *See also* Graves disease
amiodarone-induced, 1124, 1125–1126, 1128, 1132
apathetic, 1126, 1133
atrial fibrillation in, 388, 389, 1127, 1133
cancer-related, 1126
cardiac disorders/failure and, 403, 1127, 1133
cardiomyopathy in, 417, 1133
eye disease associated with, 194–195, 1124, 1127
factitious, 1126
fetal, 816
in gestational trophoblastic disease, 807, 1126
goiter/thyroid nodules and, 1125, 1131, 1137, 1138
Hashimoto thyroiditis and, 1136
hypothyroidism treatment and, 1123
hypothyroidism after treatment for, 1119, 1130, 1134
iodine-induced (Jod-Basedow disease/ phenomenon), 1126
medication-induced, 1125–1126
after parathyroidectomy, 1158
periodic paralysis and, 1049, 1127, 1133
perioperative evaluation/management and, 53
pituitary tumor/hyperplasia causing, 1126
postpartum/postpartum thyroiditis and, 1125, 1131, 1133
during pregnancy, 816, 1126, 1127, 1131–1132
recombinant human thyroid- stimulating hormone (rhTSH) causing, 1126, 1145
struma ovarii and, 1126
subacute (de Quervain) thyroiditis and, 1119, 1125, 1128, 1131, 1135
subclinical, 1128, 1134
thyroid carcinoma and, 1126
thyroid testing in, 1121*t*, 1125*t*, 1127–1128
thyroiditis and, 1119, 1125, 1128, 1131, 1133, 1135, 1136
toxic adenoma/solitary nodule causing, 1125, 1131
TSH levels in, 1121*t*, 1124

Hypertonic hyponatremia, 885–886, 885*f*

Hypertonic saline, for hyponatremia, 888, 889

Hypertrichosis
lanuginosa, 1197
minoxidil therapy and, 1197
in porphyria, 123

Hypertriglyceridemia, 1259, **1266–1267**. *See also* Lipid disorders
clinical presentations in, 1261
diabetes mellitus and, 1214, 1217, 1261
estrogen replacement therapy causing, 1203

HIV infection/antiretroviral therapy and, 1356
in nephrotic syndrome, 942
nonalcoholic fatty liver disease and, 697
pancreatitis and, 726, 729, 1266

Hypertrophic cardiomyopathy. *See* Cardiomyopathy

Hypertrophic osteoarthropathy/ hypertrophic pulmonary osteoarthropathy, 875
rheumatoid arthritis differentiated from, 836

Hyperuricemia, 830, 830*t*, 831
asymptomatic, 831
cancer-related/chemotherapy-induced, 920, **1660**
in diabetes insipidus, 1113, 1114
in diabetes mellitus, 1242
in gout, 830, 830*t*, 831
kidney disease/acute tubular necrosis and, 830, 920, 952
in myeloma, 535, 536
in transplant patient, 833
urinary stone formation and, 830, 952, 964. *See also* Uric acid urinary stones

Hyperuricosuric calcium nephrolithiasis, 964

Hyperventilation, **316**
in metabolic/lactic acidosis, 1251
neurogenic, in coma or stupor, 316, 1027
respiratory alkalosis (hypocapnia) and, 316, 910, 911

Hyperviscosity, in Waldenström macroglobulinemia, 537, 538

Hypervitaminosis A, 1277

Hypervolemic hypernatremia, 890

Hypervolemic hypotonic hyponatremia, 885*f*, 887–888, 888

Hyphema, 197

Hypnagogic hallucinations. *See also* Hallucinations
in narcolepsy, 1090

Hypnosis, for menopausal symptoms, 1202

Hypnotic drugs. *See* Sedative-hypnotics

Hypoactive delirium, 61

Hypoactive sexual (hyposexual) desire disorder, 782, 1063, 1206

Hypoadrenalism. *See* Adrenal insufficiency

Hypoalbuminemia
ascites and, 601*t*
calcium levels and, 896
decreased anion gap in, 905
in nephrotic syndrome, 942
in protein-losing enteropathy, 643

Hypoaldosteronism
after adrenalectomy, 1178
hyporeninemic/in renal tubular acidosis, 906*t*, 907

Hypobaric hypoxia, 1573–1574. *See also* High-altitude illness
air travel emergencies and, 1576

Hypocalcemia, **896–897**, 896*t*
acute (hypoparathyroid tetany), 1151
bisphosphonate use and, 1150, 1162, 1168
differential diagnosis of, 1150

familial, 892*t*
hyper-/hypomagnesemia and, 896, 897, 901, 902, 903
hypercalciuria and, 897, 1150
hyperphosphatemia and, 896, 897
hypoalbuminemia and, 896
hypoparathyroidism and, 896, 897, 1149, 1150. *See also* Hypoparathyroidism
hypophosphatemia and, 896
in kidney disease, 896
bone disorders and, 927, 927*f*
after parathyroidectomy, 1151, 1158
postoperative, prophylaxis against, 1151
PTH resistance causing (congenital pseudohypoparathyroidism), 1151
tetany and, 896, 1151
after thyroidectomy, 1151

Hypocalciuria
hypercalcemia and (hypocalciuric hypercalcemia), 892*t*, 898, 1156
hypoparathyroidism and, 1154

Hypocapnia. *See* Respiratory alkalosis

Hypochloremia, in respiratory acidosis, 910

Hypochlorite solution
for organophosphate removal, 1602
for skin decontamination, 1581

Hypocholesterolemic drugs. *See* Lipid-lowering therapy

Hypochondriasis, 1058, 1060

Hypocitraturic calcium nephrolithiasis, 963, 964

Hypocomplementemia, in hepatitis C-related renal disease, 940

Hypocretin deficiency syndrome, 1089–1090

Hypogammaglobulinemia, 882–883
bronchiectasis and, 263
infections associated with, 882

Hypoglycemia, **1252–1258**, 1252*t*
alcohol-related, 1098, 1236, 1252, 1252*t*, 1258, 1594–1595
in alcoholic ketoacidosis, 906
altered awareness of, 1236, 1253
autoimmune, **1257**
chronic kidney disease/uremia and, 924, 929, 1237
coma caused by, 1028, 1245, 1246*t*
in poisoning/drug overdose, 1578
counterregulatory issues and, 1237, 1253
diabetes treatment and, 1220, 1223. *See also* Hypoglycemia, insulin- induced
drug-induced, 1252*t*, **1257–1258**
exercise-induced, 1233, 1237
factitious, 1253*t*, **1257**
fasting, 1252, 1252*t*
functional alimentary, **1256**
after gastric surgery, 1252, **1256**
glucagon response to, impaired, 1237
hypophosphatemia associated with treatment of, 900
in hypopituitarism, 1110
immunopathologic, 1252, 1252*t*

Hypoglycemia (*Cont.*):
  insulin-induced/intensive glycemic control and, 1218, 1236–1237, 1595
    hospitalization/surgery and, 1244
    older patients and, 1233
  insulin receptor antibodies causing, 1252, **1257**
  insulinoma causing, 1185, 1252–1255
  noninsulinoma pancreatogenous hypoglycemia syndrome (islet cell hyperplasia) causing, 1252, **1256**
  nonislet cell tumor, **1255–1256**
  occult diabetes and, 1252, **1257**
  pancreatic B cell tumors causing, 1185, **1252–1255**, 1253t, 1254t
  patient education and, 1233
  pentamidine-induced, 1257, 1552
  postprandial (reactive), 1252, 1252t, **1256–1257**
  surgery and, prevention of, 53
Hypoglycemic drugs, 1220–1228, 1221–1222t, 1235–1236, 1235f. *See also* Antidiabetic agents; Insulin therapy
  overdose/toxicity of, **1595–1596**
Hypoglycemic unawareness, 1236, 1253
Hypogonadism
  adrenal insufficiency/Addison disease and, 1169–1170
  age-related, 1190, 1191
  female
    amenorrhea in, 1109
    premature (premature menopause/ovarian failure), 794, 1201
    in Turner syndrome, 1207
  GH-secreting pituitary tumor causing, 1115
  in HIV infection/AIDS, 1342
  hypergonadotropic, 970, 1189t, 1190, 1191
  hypogonadotropic, 970, 1109, 1110, 1111, 1111–1112, 1189–1190, 1189t, 1191, 1193
    hyperprolactinemia and, 1109, 1110, 1111, 1117
    isolated/congenital, 1108, 1109
  in hypopituitarism, 1109
  male, **1189–1194**, 1189t
    infertility and, 969, 969–970, 1112
    sexual dysfunction and, 967
    osteoporosis and, 1159, 1161
Hypokalemia, **891–893**, 892t
  aldosteronism and, 891, 892, 1177
  diabetic ketoacidosis treatment and, 1248
  diuretics causing, 448, 892, 893
  genetic disorders and, 891, 892t
  hyperglycemic hyperosmolar state and, 1250
  hypomagnesemia and, 892, 893, 902
  in metabolic alkalosis, 909
  parenteral nutritional support and, 1285t
  renal tubular acidosis and, 908
Hypokalemic periodic paralysis, 892t, 1049
  in hyperthyroidism, 1049, 1127, 1133
Hypomagnesemia, **901–902**, 902t
  hypercalciuria and, 892t

hypocalcemia/hypoparathyroidism and, 896, 897, 901, 902, 1150
  hypokalemia and, 892, 893, 902
  parenteral nutritional support and, 1285t
Hypomagnesemia-hypercalciuria syndrome, 892t
Hypomania, 1075. *See also* Bipolar disorder; Mania
  in cyclothymic disorders, 1076
  schizophrenia and, 1066
Hyponatremia, **885–889**, 885f, 887t
  adrenal insufficiency/Addison disease and, 886, 1111, 1170, 1171
  in diabetic ketoacidosis, 1246
  dilutional, heat exposure syndromes and, 1562, 1563
  drugs causing, 886, 1588
  in hyperglycemic hyperosmolar state, 1250
  in hypopituitarism, 1110
  in hypothyroidism/myxedema, 886, 1110, 1122
  MDMA causing, 886, 1588
  after pituitary surgery, 1111, 1115, 1119, 1175
  polydipsia/beer potomania causing, 886, 887, 1067
  in porphyria, 1676
  in SIADH, 887, 888
  in subarachnoid hemorrhage, 999
Hypoparathyroidism, **1149–1159**, 1154f
  hyper-/hypomagnesemia and, 896
  hypocalcemia and, 896, 897, 1149, 1150
  hypocalciuria and, 1154
  in newborn, maternal hyperparathyroidism and, 1153–1154
  after parathyroidectomy, 1149, 1158, 1187
  during pregnancy, 1152
  tetany and, 1150, 1151
  after thyroid surgery, 1143, 1149
Hypophosphatasia, 1165, 1166
Hypophosphatemia, **899–900**, 899t, 1164–1165
  in diabetic ketoacidosis, 900, 1248
  hypercalcemia/hyperparathyroidism and, 898, 899, 1154
  hypercalciuria and, 898, 962t, 963
  in hyperglycemic hyperosmolar state, 1250
  hypocalcemia and, 896, 900
  osteomalacia/rickets and, 892t, 900, 1164–1165, 1164t, 1166
Hypophysitis, lymphocytic, 1108, 1111, 1112
Hypopigmentation, 157, 158
  in tinea (pityriasis) versicolor, 114
  in tuberous sclerosis, 1010
Hypopituitarism, **1108–1113**, 1109t
  acquired, 1108–1109
  as acromegaly/gigantism complication, 1115
  amenorrhea and, 1109, 1110, 1199, 1201
  congenital, 1108
  functional, 1109
  hypogonadism and, 1108, 1109, 1110, 1111

with mass lesions, 1108
  postoperative, 1116
  postpartum pituitary necrosis/Sheehan syndrome and, 1109
  without mass lesions, 1108–1109
Hypopnea, sleep, 316, 1089. *See also* Sleep apnea hypopnea
Hypoproteinemia, in nephrotic syndrome, 942
Hypoprothrombinemia
  in cirrhosis, 704
  factor II antibodies and, 561
Hypopyon
  in anterior uveitis, 181
  in Behçet syndrome, 862
Hyporeninemic hypoaldosteronism, 906t
  in renal tubular acidosis, 906t, 907
Hyposexual (hypoactive sexual) desire disorder, 782, 1063
Hyposmia, 220–221
  intracranial tumors causing, 220
  in Kallmann syndrome, 1109, 1199, 1200
Hypotension
  antipsychotics causing, 1071, 1589
  in diabetes mellitus, 1214
  dysautonomia (autonomic dysfunction) and, 990, 991
  MAOIs causing, 1082
  myocardial infarction and, 378
  orthostatic (postural). *See* Orthostatic (postural) hypotension
  palpitations and, 30
  pheochromocytoma removal and, 1182
  in poisoning/drug overdose, **1578–1579**
    beta-adrenergic blockers and, 1578, 1591
  in right ventricular infarction, 378–379
  in shock, 494–495
  tricyclic antidepressants causing, 1082
Hypotensive agents. *See* Antihypertensive drug therapy
Hypothalamic amenorrhea, 1109, 1199, 1200
Hypothalamic disorders, **1108–1119**
  amenorrhea caused by, 1109, 1199, 1200
  hypopituitarism and, 1108, 1110. *See also* Hypopituitarism
Hypothermia
  coma and, 1027, 1028, 1564, 1578
  drowning and, 1567
  of extremities, **1565–1566**
  in poisoning/drug overdose, **1578**
  systemic (accidental), **1563–1565**, 1564f
Hypothyroidism, **1119–1124**, 1121t, 1122t
  Addison disease and (Schmidt syndrome), 1169
  amiodarone-induced, 1120
  cardiac disorders/failure and, 403, 1120, 1122
  congenital/fetal, 816, 1132, 1148, 1149
  consumptive, 1119
  cretinism and, 1119, 1132, 1148, 1149
  fibromyalgia and, 873, 874
  goiter/thyroid nodules and, 1119, 1132, 1137, 1138

Hashimoto thyroiditis and, 1119,
    1134–1135, 1136
hepatitis C and, 1120
after hyperthyroidism treatment/
    thyroid surgery, 1119, 1130,
    1131, 1134
hyponatremia in, 886, 1110, 1122
lithium causing, 1086
perioperative evaluation/management
    and, 53
after pituitary surgery, 1175
postpartum thyroiditis and, 1125
during pregnancy, 816, 1119, 1121,
    1122, 1123
pubertal delay and, 1199
in subacute (de Quervain) thyroiditis,
    1119, 1125, 1135
subclinical, 1120
thyroid testing in, 1120, 1121t, 1122t
treatment of. See Levothyroxine
TSH deficiency/levels in, 1109, 1110,
    1111, 1119, 1120, 1123–1124
Hypotonic fluids, hyponatremia caused
    by, 886, 887
Hypotonic hyponatremia, 885f, 886–888
Hypoventilation
    obesity and (Pickwickian syndrome),
        315–316
    respiratory acidosis and, 910
Hypovolemic hypernatremia, 890
Hypovolemic hypotonic hyponatremia,
    885f, 886, 888
Hypovolemic/hemorrhagic shock, 493,
    494t, 495, 496
Hypoxemia. See Arterial blood gases
Hypoxia, hypobaric, 1573–1574. See also
    High-altitude illness
    air travel emergencies and, 1576
Hypoxic hepatitis, 712–713
Hypoxis rooperi, for benign prostatic
    hyperplasia, 975
Hysterectomy. See also Oophorectomy
    for abnormal uterine bleeding, 763
    for cervical carcinoma, 772
    for endometrial carcinoma, 774
    for endometriosis/pelvic pain, 766, 777
    estrogen replacement therapy and, 795
    for fibroid tumors, 773
    for gestational trophoblastic disease,
        807
    for morbidly adherent placenta/
        bleeding, 813
    for ovarian cancer, 780
    for postmenopausal bleeding, 764
    premature ovarian failure and, 1201
    prophylactic, in HNPCC/Lynch
        syndrome, 669
Hysterical (histrionic) personality
    disorder, 1065t
Hysterosalpingography, 763t
    in infertility workup, 783–784
Hysteroscopy, 763t
Hytrin. See Terazosin
Hyzaar. See Losartan, with
    hydrochlorothiazide

123I. See Radioiodine thyroid scans and
    uptake
123I-MIBG scanning, in
    pheochromocytoma/
    paraganglioma, 1182, 1184

131I. See Radioactive iodine; Radioiodine
    thyroid scans and uptake
131I-MIBG therapy, in
    pheochromocytoma/
    paraganglioma, 1184
131I tositumomab, for non-Hodgkin
    lymphoma, 532
IAA. See Insulin, antibodies to
IADLs. See Instrumental activities of
    daily living
Iatrogenic Creutzfeldt-Jakob disease,
    1394
Iatrogenic pneumothorax, 314
Ibandronate, 1161. See also
    Bisphosphonates
Ibotenic acid, poisoning with mushrooms
    containing, 1600t
Ibrance. See Palbociclib
Ibritumomab tiuxetan, for non-Hodgkin
    lymphoma, 532
Ibrutinib, 1667t
    for chronic lymphocytic leukemia, 530,
        530–531
    for Waldenström macroglobulinemia,
        538
Ibuprofen, 75t
    lithium interactions and, 1087t
    for pericarditis, 426
    platelet function affected by, 558t
Ibutilide, 381, 382t, 383t
    for atrial fibrillation, 382t, 383t, 389,
        393
    for atrial flutter, 382t, 383t, 394
ICA. See Islet cell antibodies
ICA-512 (tyrosine phosphatase IA2)
    antibodies, in type 1
    diabetes, 1211, 1211t, 1233
ICA (islet cell antibodies), in diabetes,
    1211, 1211t
ICD. See Implantable cardioverter
    defibrillator
iCJD. See Iatrogenic Creutzfeldt-Jakob
    disease
ICSI. See Intracytoplasmic sperm
    injection
Icteric leptospirosis (Weil syndrome),
    1501
Icterus. See Jaundice
Idamycin. See Idarubicin
Idarubicin, 1665t
    toxicity of, 1665t, 1674–1675
Idarucizumab, reversal of dabigatran and,
    393, 564, 566t, 1588
Idelalisib, 1668t
    for chronic lymphocytic leukemia,
        530–531
IDH1/IDH2 mutation, in acute myeloid
    leukemia, 527, 529
Idiopathic adulthood ductopenia, 724
Idiopathic brachial plexus neuropathy
    (neuralgic amyotrophy),
    1043
Idiopathic bronchiolitis obliterans with
    organizing pneumonia. See
    Cryptogenic organizing
    pneumonia/pneumonitis
Idiopathic CD4 lymphopenia syndrome,
    progressive multifocal
    leukoencephalopathy in, 1395
Idiopathic crescentic glomerulonephritis,
    933t, 935f, 938

Idiopathic duct-centric chronic
    pancreatitis, 731
Idiopathic inflammatory myopathies,
    847–850, 848f, 848t. See also
    Dermatomyositis;
    Polymyositis
Idiopathic interstitial pneumonias, 290,
    290t. See also Diffuse
    interstitial pneumonias
Idiopathic intracranial hypertension,
    1009
    headache and, 981
Idiopathic membranoproliferative
    glomerulonephritis, 933t,
    940. See also
    Membranoproliferative
    glomerulonephritis/
    glomerulonephropathy
Idiopathic midline destructive disease,
    223
Idiopathic polyneuropathy, acute. See
    Guillain-Barré syndrome
Idiopathic pulmonary fibrosis, 289, 292,
    292f
Idiopathic pulmonary hemosiderosis,
    304
Idiopathic (primary) pulmonary
    hypertension, 301–302, 429,
    430, 430t, 431, 431t, 432f,
    433
Idiopathic skeletal hyperostosis, diffuse
    (DISH), 864, 1242
Idiopathic torsion dystonia, 1015–1016
Idiosyncratic drug reactions, liver disease
    caused by, 696
Idioventricular rhythm, accelerated, 398
    in myocardial infarction, 377, 398
Idoxuridine, 1365t
Ifex. See Ifosfamide
IFNL3 (IL28B) gene, in hepatitis C, 683,
    689
Ifosfamide, 1663t
    hemorrhagic cystitis caused by, 1674
    mesna for, 1671t, 1674
IgA, selective deficiency of, 881–882,
    881t
IgA nephropathy (Berger disease), 933t,
    935f, 937
IgA tTG antibody, in celiac disease/
    dermatitis herpetiformis,
    123, 634
IgA vasculitis, 933t
IgE, in immediate hypersensitivity, 876
IGF-1. See Insulin-like growth factor-1
IGF-2. See Insulin-like growth factor-2
IgG
    intravenous. See Intravenous immune
        globulin
    in pancreatitis, 731, 732
IgG4-associated disease, 851–852
    cholangitis, 724
    pancreatitis, 731, 732, 851
IGIV. See Intravenous immune globulin
IgVH somatic mutation, in chronic
    lymphocytic leukemia, 530
IIV3/4 influenza vaccines, 1414t
IL. See under Interleukin
IL2RA/IL7RA genes, in multiple sclerosis,
    1023
IL28B (IFNL3) gene, in hepatitis C, 683,
    689

Ileitis/ileocolitis, in Crohn disease, 652, 653, 655
Ileum. *See also* Small intestine
  resection of, short bowel syndrome and, 637
Ileus
  antipsychotics causing, 1071
  gallstone, 717
  paralytic (acute/adynamic), **638–639**
Iliac arteries, atherosclerotic/occlusive disease of, **472–473**
Illicit drug use. *See* Substance use disorders
Illness, psychiatric problems associated with, **1104–1107**
  mood disorders/depression, 1076, 1105, 1106
Illness behaviors, abnormal, **1058–1060**
Illusions, in schizophrenia/psychotic disorders, 1067
Iloperidone, 1068, 1069t
  relative potency/side effects of, 1069t
Iloprost, for pulmonary hypertension, 303, 432f
Iluvien. *See* Fluocinolone/fluocinolone implant
Imaging. *See also specific disorder and under* Radiation
  radiation exposure/cancer risk and, 1571, 1572, 1607
Imatinib, 1668t
  for chronic myeloid leukemia, 524–525
  for gastrointestinal mesenchymal tumors, 1633, 1634
  levothyroxine therapy affected by, 1123
Imbalance. *See* Falls; Vertigo; Vestibular disorders
Imbruvica. *See* Ibrutinib
Imidazoles, topical, 98t. *See also specific agent*
Imiglucerase, for Gaucher disease, 1680
Imipenem
  for anaerobic infections, 1479, 1479t
  for anthrax, 1456t
  for pneumonia, 269t, 271, 275t
Imipramine, 1078t, 1081. *See also* Antidepressants
  adverse ophthalmic effects of, 178t
  for cataplexy, 1090
Imiquimod, for genital warts, 141, 768
Immediate hypersensitivity, 876, **876–878**, 879t
Immersion (trench) foot/hand, **1565**
Immobility
  DVT/PE (venous thromboembolic disease) and, 295, 298t
  in elderly, **62–63**
  hypercalcemia and, 1156
  pressure ulcers and, 68
  urinary incontinence and, 65
Immune alveolar hemorrhage, 304
Immune clearance hepatitis B, 687
Immune complex membranoproliferative glomerulonephritis, 922, 935f, 940
Immune complexes
  glomerulonephritis and, 922, 935f, 940
  membranous nephropathy and, 944
Immune globulin. *See specific type and* Intravenous immune globulin

Immune insulin resistance, 1237
Immune reconstitution inflammatory syndromes (IRIS), 191–192, 1345
  in cryptococcosis, 1553
  Kaposi sarcoma, 146, 1344
  progressive multifocal leukoencephalopathy and, 1395
Immune recovery uveitis, 192
Immune thrombocytopenia, **548–550**, 549f. *See also* Thrombocytopenia
Immune tolerant hepatitis B, 687
Immunity/immune response disorders. *See* Allergies/allergic disorders/reactions; Atopic disease; Autoimmune disorders; Immunodeficiency
Immunizations (vaccines), 3–5, **1319–1327**, 1320–1325t, 1328–1329t. *See also specific type*
  for HIV, 1347
  recommended types/schedules for, 3–5, 1320–1325t
  for adults, **1319–1326**, 1320–1325t
  in immunocompromised host/HIV infection/AIDS, 1319, 1321t, 1325t, 1348–1349
  for infants/children/adolescents, **1319**
  during pregnancy, **802–803**, 1319, 1321t
  for travelers, 4, **1326–1327**
  safety (adverse effects/contraindications) and, **1327**, 1328–1329t
Immunocompromised host. *See also* HIV infection/AIDS; Immunodeficiency
  adenovirus infection and, 1420
  aspergillosis in, 1292, 1554–1555
  bacillary angiomatosis/bartonellosis in, 1343, 1477
  bronchiectasis in, 263
  cancer-related infection and, 1008, 1661
  CMV infections in, 1291–1292, 1374–1375, 1375, 1376
  coccidial and microsporidial infection in, 1528–1529, 1529, 1530
  coccidioidomycosis in, 1550
  cryptococcosis in, 1553
  diarrhea in, 588t, 589, 592, 1305
  Elizabethkingia infections in, 1478
  erythrovirus (parvovirus) infection in, 1422
  fever/FUO and, 1288
    antimicrobial therapy and, 35, 518, 1293, 1296, 1314t, 1661
  gastritis in, 623
  herpes simplex infections in, 1291, 1364
  herpes zoster/herpes zoster vaccine in, 5, 120, 121, 1321t, 1323t, 1343, 1370
  herpetic stomatitis in, 227
  histoplasmosis in, 1549
  immunizations in, 4–5, 1321t, 1325t

  herpes zoster vaccine, 5, 1321t, 1323t, 1343
  HPV vaccine, 1321t, 1323t
  influenza virus vaccine, 5, 1321t
  MMR vaccine, 5, 1321t, 1349, 1380, 1385
  pneumococcal vaccine, 1321t, 1324t
  varicella vaccine, 1321t, 1371
  infections in, 882, 883, **1289–1293**. *See also* Opportunistic infections
  infectious esophagitis in, 611
  listeriosis in, 1457
  mold infections in, 1292, **1557–1558**
  mucormycosis in, 218
  Pneumocystis infections in, 1291, 1551, 1552, 1553
  progressive multifocal leukoencephalopathy and, 1340, 1395
  pulmonary infiltrates/pneumonia in, 268t, 271, **276**, 1335
  RSV infection in, 1409
  Salmonella bacteremia in, 1342, 1469, 1470
  scabies in, 149
  squamous cell carcinoma in, 144
  strongyloidiasis in, 1540
  toxoplasmosis in, 1523, 1524
  yellow fever vaccine and, 1327, 1405
Immunodeficiency, **881–883**, 881t. *See also* Immunocompromised host
  common variable, 881t, **882–883**
  in Epstein-Barr virus infection, 1373
  in HIV infection/AIDS, 1330, 1332. *See also* HIV infection/AIDS
  infections associated with, 882, 883, **1289–1293**. *See also* Opportunistic infections
  primary, in adults, **881–883**, 881t
  selective IgA, **881–882**, 881t
Immunoglobulins. *See also specific type under Ig and* Antibodies
  in common variable immunodeficiency, 882
  live virus vaccines and, 1326
Immunologic disorders, **881–883**, 881t. *See also* Allergies/allergic disorders/reactions; Atopic disease; Autoimmune disorders; Immunodeficiency
  cognitive disorders/delirium caused by, 1102t
Immunomodulating therapy. *See also* Immunotherapy
  adverse ophthalmic effects of, 178t
  for asthma, 250t, 251
  in cancer chemotherapy, 1665t
  for inflammatory bowel disease, 650–651
    with anti-TNF agents, 650–651, 651, 656
    Crohn disease, 656, 657
    ulcerative colitis, 659–660
  for ophthalmic disorders, 172t
  thrombocytopenia caused by, 555t
Immunopathologic hypoglycemia, 1252, 1252t
Immunoreactive insulin, in prebreakfast hyperglycemia, 1234t

Immunosuppressive therapy. *See also*
　　Immunocompromised host;
　　Immunomodulating therapy
　for aplastic anemia, 517, 547, 548
　for autoimmune hemolytic
　　anemia, 514
　fever/FUO and, 1288
　herpes simplex infection and, 1364
　hyperkalemia and, 894
　infections and, 1290, 1661. *See also*
　　Opportunistic infections
　Kaposi sarcoma complicating, 146
　for lupus nephritis/SLE, 841, 842, 941
　for myelodysplastic syndromes, 526
　for neuromyelitis optica, 1025
　for polyarteritis nodosa, 856
　thrombocytopenia caused by, 555*t*
　after transplant
　　immunization recommendations
　　　and, 1319–1326
　　infections and, 1290, 1290–1291
　　squamous cell carcinoma and, 144
　　stem cell transplantation and, 541
Immunotherapy. *See also*
　　Immunomodulating therapy
　for allergic rhinitis, 220
　for asthma, 250*t*, 251
　intravesical, for bladder cancer, 1652
　venom, 878
　in wart removal, 142
Impedance plethysmography/testing
　in esophageal disorders, 606, 607, 610
　in venous thrombosis/pulmonary
　　embolism, 297, 298
Imperforate hymen, 1199
Impetiginization, 125
Impetigo, **123–124**, 124*f*, 1315*t*,
　　1442–1443
　allergic contact dermatitis
　　differentiated from,
　　124, 125
　antibiotics for, 98*t*, 124, 1315*t*
　glomerulonephritis after, 936
　in HIV infection/AIDS, 1343
Impingement syndrome (subacromial),
　　1685–1689, 1687*t*
　rotator cuff tears and, 1685, 1689
Implanon, 789
Implantable cardioverter defibrillator
　for cardiomyopathy, 417
　for heart failure, 405*f*, 409
　for long QT syndrome, 398
　postinfarction, 380
　preoperative/prophylactic/surgery
　　and, 48
　for ventricular fibrillation/sudden
　　death, 398
　for ventricular tachycardia, 397
Impotence. *See* Erectile dysfunction/
　　impotence
Impulse conduction, disturbances of. *See*
　　Conduction disturbances
Impulse control disorders, 1090
　in dementia, 1103
In vitro fertilization, 785, 970
Inactivated enhanced-potency
　　poliovaccine (IPV/Salk
　　vaccine), 1326, 1383
　pregnancy and, 802
　for travelers, 1326, 1383
Inactive HBsAg carrier state, 687

Inactivity, physical. *See also* Exercise/
　　activity
　obesity and, 11, 12, 13, 1271
　preventable disease/deaths and, 3*t*, 6*t*,
　　11–12
Incentive spirometry, postoperative
　　pulmonary complication risk
　　reduction and, 50
Incidentalomas
　adrenal, 1175, 1178, 1179
　thyroid, 1136, 1137, 1138–1139
Inclusion body encephalitis, measles and,
　　1378
Inclusion body myositis, 849,
　　1048–1049
Inclusion conjunctivitis, **167**
Inclusion cysts, epidermal (EICs), **154**
　furuncles/carbuncles differentiated
　　from, 153, 154
Inclusion disease, CMV, in newborn,
　　1374, 1375, 1376
Incompetent cervix, 804
　cerclage/activity restriction for, 805
Incomplete abortion, 804, 804–805
Incontinence. *See* Fecal incontinence;
　　Urinary incontinence
Increased intracranial pressure. *See*
　　Intracranial hypertension
Incretins, for diabetes mellitus,
　　1225–1227
Indacaterol, for COPD, 260
Indapamide, 450*t*
　adverse ophthalmic effects of, 177*t*
Inderal/Inderal LA. *See* Propranolol
Indian tick typhus, 1429*t*
Indigestion. *See* Dyspepsia
Indinavir, 1351*t*, 1356. *See also*
　　Antiretroviral therapy
Indocin. *See* Indomethacin
Indolent lymphoma, 532
Indometh. *See* Indomethacin
Indomethacin, 75*t*
　adverse ophthalmic effects of, 179*t*
　for gout, 831
　lithium interactions and, 1087*t*
　in pain management, 75*t*
　for patent ductus arteriosus, 330
　for pericarditis, 426
　for preterm labor, 812
Industrial bronchitis, 308
Inevitable abortion, 804, 804–805
Infant. *See* Newborn
Infant botulism, 1454
Infarcts. *See specific type*
Infection/infectious diseases, **1287–1310**.
　　See also specific type or
　　system affected
　in acute leukemia, 528
　adrenal insufficiency/Addison disease
　　and, 1169
　anorectal, **670–671**
　antimicrobial therapy and, **1310–1319**,
　　1311–1313*t*, 1314*t*,
　　1315–1316*t*
　arthritis, **867–870**
　bacterial, **1441–1485**
　bite wounds and, **1300–1301**
　of bone. *See* Osteomyelitis
　burn injury and, 1569
　in cancer patients, **1661**. *See also*
　　Opportunistic infections

catheter-associated, 1285, 1290, 1291,
　　1294, 1295, 1296, 1317
chlamydial, 1313*t*, **1485–1487**
in cirrhosis, 701
cognitive disorders/delirium caused by,
　　1019, 1102*t*
diarrhea in, 588*t*, 589, 592, 598,
　　1305–1308, 1306–1307*t*,
　　1309–1310
in drug users, **1303–1304**. *See also*
　　Injection drug use,
　　infections and
dysphagia in, 605*t*
erythema nodosum associated with,
　　151–152
erythemas, **136–139**
esophagitis caused by, **611–612**
fever/FUO and, 1287, 1288
gastritis caused by, 623
glomerulonephritis and, 933*t*, 935*f*,
　　936–937
headache and, 40
health care-associated, **1293–1296**
helminthic, **1532–1536**
immunization against, 3–5,
　　1319–1327, 1320–1325*t*,
　　1328–1329*t*. *See also*
　　Immunizations
in immunocompromised host, 882,
　　883, **1289–1293**. *See also*
　　HIV infection/AIDS;
　　Opportunistic infections
　immunization recommendations
　　and, 1319–1326, 1321*t*
insulin requirements and, 1233
keratitis, **174–176**
mycotic
　superficial/skin, **111–115**, 111*f*, 112*f*,
　　113*f*. *See also* Tinea
　systemic invasive, **1547–1560**
myocarditis and, **413–414**, 413*t*
neuropathies associated with, **1037**
neutropenia and, 35, 517–518, 518,
　　1290
opportunistic. *See* Opportunistic
　　infections
during pregnancy, **820–825**
prevention of/vaccine-preventable,
　　3–5, 1319–1327,
　　1320–1325*t*, 1328–1329*t*,
　　1377–1385. *See also*
　　Immunizations
protozoal, **1507–1531**
reactive arthritis and, 865–866
rickettsial, 1313*t*, **1428–1438**, 1429*t*
seizures and, 983
sexually transmitted, **1301–1303**
shock associated with. *See* Sepsis/septic
　　shock
spirochetal, 1312*t*, **1488–1506**
surgical site, 1294–1295, 1295
　antibiotic prophylaxis for, 54
thrombocytopenia and, **556**
transfusion in transmission of,
　　543–544
travel and, **1308–1309, 1309–1310**
tuberinterstitial nephritis caused
　　by, 947*t*
viral, **1363–1428**, 1365*t*
Infection (struvite) urinary stones, 961,
　　962, 964

Infectious diseases. *See* Infection
Infectious mononucleosis. *See*
    Mononucleosis
Infectious (suppurative) thyroiditis, 1135,
    1136, 1137
Infective endocarditis. *See* Endocarditis,
    infective
Inferior vena cava filters/interruption, for
    pulmonary embolism, 301,
    576–577
Inferior vena cava sinus venosus defect,
    325
Infertility, 783–785, 968–971, 969f
    female, 783–785
        endometriosis and, 776, 784
        pelvic infection/PID and, 778
        in polycystic ovary syndrome, 780,
            781, 784
        hyperprolactinemia and, 784, 1117,
            1118
        in hypopituitarism, 1109, 1112. *See also*
            Hypogonadism
    male, 783, 968–971, 969f
        cryptorchism and, 1194
        in cystic fibrosis, 265, 969, 970
        hypogonadism and, 969
        in Klinefelter syndrome, 970, 1190,
            1682
    marijuana use and, 1100
Inflammasomes, NALP-3, in gout, 830
Inflammation. *See also specific type and*
        structure/systems affected
    anemia of, 502, 503
    in HIV infection/AIDS, 1345
Inflammatory adenoma of liver, 716
Inflammatory aneurysm, 481
Inflammatory bowel disease, 649–662.
        See also Crohn disease;
        Ulcerative colitis
    arthritis and, 653, 867
    colorectal cancer and, 654, 661, 1637
    diarrhea in, 592
    GI bleeding and, 598
    primary sclerosing cholangitis and,
        723–724
    social support for patient with, 652
Inflammatory breast carcinoma, 745.
        See also Breast cancer
Inflammatory eye disease, 166–174, 166t.
        See also Conjunctivitis;
        Uveitis
Inflammatory myopathy, idiopathic,
        847–850, 848f, 848t. *See also*
        Dermatomyositis;
        Polymyositis
Inflammatory pericarditis, acute,
        424–427, 425t. *See also*
        specific cause and Pericarditis
Inflammatory polyneuropathy, chronic,
        1039
Inflammatory skin nodules, 151–155.
        See also specific type
Infliximab. *See also* Anti-TNF agents
    for inflammatory bowel disease, 651
        Crohn disease, 656–657
        ulcerative colitis, 660, 661
    for psoriasis, 108
    for rheumatoid arthritis, 837–838
Influenza
    avian (H5N1 and analogs), 1417–1418
    deaths attributable to, 2t, 1411

drug resistance and, 1412
neuraminidase inhibitors (oseltamivir/
    zanamivir/peramivir) for,
    1365t, 1412–1413, 1418
    prophylactic, 1416, 1418
    resistance to, 1412–1413
pneumonia and, 269, 271, 1411, 1412
prevention of, 3, 1413–1416,
    1414–1415t, 1418. *See also*
    Influenza virus vaccine
    seasonal, 1410–1417, 1414–1415t
    H1N1, 1410, 1411, 1412, 1413, 1416
Influenza virus vaccine, 3, 1320t, 1321t,
    1322t, 1413–1416,
    1414–1415t
    adverse effects/contraindications and,
        1328t, 1416
    in asthma patients, 251
    avian (H5N1 and analogs) influenza
        and, 1418
    in cystic fibrosis, 266
    in immunocompromised host/HIV
        infection/AIDS, 5, 1321t,
        1416
    pneumonia prevention and, 271
    pregnancy and, 802, 1319, 1321t,
        1322t, 1413
Infraclavicular lymph nodes, in breast
        cancer, 742
Infraspinatus tendon, evaluation of, 1689
Infratentorial arteriovenous
        malformations, 1001
Infundibular stenosis, 322
Infusion pumps, insulin. *See* Insulin
        infusion pumps
Ingrown nails, 160
INH. *See* Isoniazid
Inhalation injury/smoke inhalation, 305
    corrosive acids and, 1587
    cyanide poisoning and, 24, 305
Inhalational anthrax, 1454, 1455, 1456
Inhaled insulin, 1229t, 1232
Inhalers
    for asthma therapy, 248, 250t, 251, 253t
    for COPD therapy, 260, 262
Inherited (hereditary/genetic) disorders,
        1676–1684. *See also specific*
        disorder
    electrolyte metabolism disturbances
        and, 892t
Injection drug use. *See also* Substance
        use disorders
    febrile patient and, 1304
    infections and, 1303–1304
        arthritis, 867, 1304
        clostridial infection/wound botulism
            and, 1303, 1454, 1601
        endocarditis, 1304, 1314t, 1458
        hepatitis, 678, 680, 682–683, 1304
        HIV infection/AIDS, 1304, 1332,
            1345, 1346, 1349
        osteomyelitis, 870, 1304
        skin infections, 1303, 1479–1480
Injury. *See* Trauma
Inkspot lentigines, 103
Inlyta. *See* Axitinib
Inner ear, 207–213, 210t, 211t
Innocent murmurs. *See* Heart murmurs
InnoPran XL. *See* Propranolol
Inocybe (muscarine) mushroom
        poisoning, 1600t

Inotropic agents. *See also* Digitalis/
        digitalis glycosides/digoxin
    in acute heart failure/pulmonary
        edema, 412
    for shock, 496
Insect bites/stings
    allergic reactions to, 878
    myocarditis caused by, 413t
    scorpion stings, 1605
    skin lesions caused by, 150
    spider bites, 1605
    urticaria caused by, 134
Insecticide poisoning (cholinesterase
        inhibitors), 1580t, 1581t,
        1601–1602
Insemination, artificial, 785, 970
Insomnia, 1088–1089
    drug therapy for, 1054t, 1089
    fatal familial, 1394
Inspra. *See* Eplerenone
Instability. *See also* Falls; Gait/gait
        disorders; Genetic instability
    shoulder, 1688t, 1690–1691
        atraumatic, 1690, 1691
Instrumental activities of daily living
        (IADLs), assessment of
        ability to perform, 55–56
Insulin. *See also* Insulin therapy
    antibodies to (IAA)
        in autoimmune/immunopathologic
            hypoglycemia, 1252, 1257
        in diabetes mellitus, 1211, 1211t,
            1233
        in immune insulin resistance, 1237
        insulin therapy causing, 1211,
            1237
    B cell tumors/insulinomas secreting,
        1185, 1252–1255, 1253t,
        1254t
    B cells secreting, 1185
    factitious hypoglycemia caused by
        administration of, 1253,
        1253t, 1257
    immunoreactive, in prebreakfast
        hyperglycemia, 1234t
    insensitivity to. *See* Insulin resistance/
        insensitivity
    in insulinoma diagnosis, 1253, 1253t,
        1254
    mutant, in diabetes mellitus, 1212
    receptors for. *See* Insulin receptors
    resistance to. *See* Insulin resistance/
        insensitivity
    waning levels of, prebreakfast
        hyperglycemia and, 1234,
        1234t
Insulin aspart, 1229, 1229t, 1230, 1231.
        See also Insulin therapy
    in mixtures/combination therapy,
        1229t, 1231, 1234t
    in pregnancy, 817, 1244
Insulin degludec, 1229, 1229t, 1230, 1231.
        See also Insulin therapy
    in mixtures/combination therapy,
        1229t, 1231, 1234t
    in pregnancy, 1244
Insulin detemir, 1229, 1229t, 1230, 1231,
        1233, 1234, 1234t. *See also*
        Insulin therapy
    overnight insulin levels and, 1234
    in pregnancy, 1244

Insulin gene, in diabetes mellitus, 1210, 1212
Insulin glargine, 1229, 1229t, 1230, 1231, 1233, 1234, 1234t. *See also* Insulin therapy
overnight insulin levels and, 1230, 1234
in pregnancy, 1230, 1244
Insulin glulisine, 1229, 1229t, 1230, 1231, 1234t. *See also* Insulin therapy
in pregnancy, 1244
Insulin infusion pumps, 1231–1232, 1234
continuous glucose monitoring and, 1217
ketoacidosis and, 1231, 1245, 1249
during pregnancy, 1244
rapidly acting analogs used in, 1230
surgery/hospitalization and, 1243t, 1244
Insulin-like growth factor-1 (IGF-1)
deficiency of, 1109
in GH deficiency/rhGH therapy, 1109, 1110
in GH excess, 1114, 1115
Insulin-like growth factor-2 (IGF-2), nonislet cell tumor hypoglycemia and, 1255
Insulin lispro, 1229, 1229t, 1230, 1231, 1233. *See also* Insulin therapy
in mixtures/combination therapy, 1229t, 1231, 1234t
in pregnancy, 817, 1244
Insulin pens, 1230, 1231
Insulin pumps. *See* Insulin infusion pumps
Insulin receptors
antibodies to
in diabetes mellitus, 1212
in hypoglycemia, 1252, **1257**
mutant, diabetes caused by, 1212
Insulin resistance/insensitivity, 1211t, 1213. *See also* Metabolic syndrome
acanthosis nigricans and, 1212, 1212f, 1214
acne and, 127
in diabetes, 1211t, 1212, 1213
diabetic ketoacidosis and, 1248, 1249
endocrine tumors causing, 1213
hyperglycemia and, 1213, 1213t
hypertension and, 441
immune, 1237
nonalcoholic fatty liver disease and, 697, 698
obesity and, 12, 1270
in polycystic ovary syndrome, 780, 781, 1196
during pregnancy, 817
Insulin syringes and needles, 1231
Insulin therapy, 1217–1218, 1228–1232, 1229t, 1233–1234, 1234t, 1236–1237
administration methods/regimens for, 1231–1232
allergy to, 1237
antidepressant drug interactions and, 1083t
anti-insulin antibodies and, 1211, 1237
bioavailability of preparations and, 1229, 1229t

chronic kidney disease affecting, 929
complications of, 1236–1237
continuous subcutaneous infusion (CSII) pumps in, 1231–1232, 1234. *See also* Insulin infusion pumps
for diabetic ketoacidosis, 1229, 1247–1248, 1249
transition to subcutaneous regimen and, 1249
exercise affecting, 1233
factitious hypoglycemia and, 1253, 1253t, 1257
with glucose. *See* High-dose insulin euglycemic therapy
for hospitalized patient, 53, 1243–1244, 1243t
for hyperglycemic hyperosmolar state, 1250
for hyperkalemia, 894, 895t
hypoglycemia and, 1218, 1236–1237, 1595
immunopathology of, 1237
inhalation for administration of, 1229t, 1232
injection sites for, 1231
rotation of, 1231, 1237
intensive, 1217–1219, 1233–1234, 1234t
acceptable levels of glycemic control and, 1236
angina and, 362
clinical studies of, 1217–1219
diabetic nephropathy development/ progression and, 1218, 1219
diabetic retinopathy development/ progression and, 1218, 1219
hospitalization/surgery and, 53, 1244
hypoglycemia and, 1236
hospitalization/surgery and, 1244
during pregnancy, 1244
self/continuous-monitoring of blood glucose and, 1216–1217, 1217, 1233, 1234
in pregnant patient, 818, 1217
in type 2 diabetics, 1218, 1236
lipodystrophy/lipoatrophy/ lipohypertrophy and, 1231, 1237
MAOI interactions and, 1083t
mixtures/combination therapy and, 1229t, 1230–1231
with oral antidiabetic agents, 1236
patient education/self-management and, 1233
postoperative, 1244
prebreakfast hyperglycemia and, 1234, 1234t
during pregnancy, 817, 1244
preparation types available, 1229–1231, 1229t
purified insulin and, 1229
self/continuous-monitoring of blood glucose and, 1216–1217, 1217, 1233, 1234
in pregnant patient, 818, 1217
surgery and, 53, 1229, 1243–1244, 1243t
for type 1 diabetics, 1217–1218, 1228–1232, 1229t, 1233–1234, 1234t, 1236–1237

hospitalization/surgery and, 1243, 1243t
for type 2 diabetics, 1218, 1230–1231, 1231–1232, 1235, 1235f, 1236
hospitalization/surgery and, 1243, 1243t
Insulinomas, 1185, 1252–1255, 1253t, 1254t. *See also* Islet cell tumors
hypoglycemia caused by, 1185, 1252–1255
localization of, 1186, 1254–1255
in MEN, 1185, 1188, 1253
Intal. *See* Cromolyn
Integrase inhibitors, for HIV infection/ AIDS, 1352–1353t, 1358
in combinations, 1358
resistance to, 1361, 1362
Integrilin. *See* Eptifibatide
Intelence. *See* Etravirine
Intensive care unit, patient in. *See* Critical illness
Intensive care unit psychosis, 1105
Intercostal neuritis, chest pain and, 359
Intercourse, sexual. *See* Sexual intercourse
Interdigital (toe web) tinea pedis, 113, 113f
cellulitis and, 113, 137
Interferon, depression caused by, 1076
Interferon-alpha/interferon alfa, 1365t. *See also* Peginterferon
for cancer chemotherapy, 1670t
for renal cell carcinoma, 1654
toxicity of, ophthalmic, 178t
Interferon-beta, for multiple sclerosis, 1024, 1024t
Interferon-gamma, autoantibodies against, immunodeficiency disorders caused by, 881
Interferon gamma release assays, in tuberculosis, 4, 279–280
HIV infection/AIDS and, 280, 1336, 1348
latent disease treatment and, 283
musculoskeletal disease and, 872
pleural fluid analysis and, 312
in pregnant patient, 821
Interleukin-1 (IL-1) inhibitors, for gout, 832
Interleukin-2 (IL-2), 1670t
for renal cell carcinoma, 1654
Interleukin-2 receptor alpha gene, in multiple sclerosis, 1023
Interleukin-6 (IL-6), in amiodarone-induced thyrotoxicosis, 1128
Interleukin-7 receptor alpha gene, in multiple sclerosis, 1023
Interleukin-8 (IL-8), in familial Mediterranean fever, 604
Interleukin-11 (IL-11), recombinant (oprelvekin), for chemotherapy-induced thrombocytopenia, 1662–1672
Interleukin-31 (IL-31), in pruritus, 146
Intermediate-acting insulin, 1229t. *See also* Insulin therapy; NPH insulin
mixed insulin preparations and, 1229t, 1231

Intermediate uveitis (pars planitis), 181. *See also* Uveitis

Intermittent claudication, 472

Intermittent positive-pressure breathing (IPPB), postoperative pulmonary complication risk reduction and, 50

Internal hordeolum, 164–165

Internal rotation, assessment of
  in hip fracture, 1701–1702
  rotator cuff strength and, 1686*t*, 1687*t*

International Staging System, for myeloma, 537

Interosseous nerve, anterior, lesion of, **1039–1040**

Interpersonal relationships
  disturbed, in schizophrenia/psychotic disorders, 1067
  social issues for terminally ill/dying patient and, 92, 92*t*

Interstitial cells of Cajal, gastrointestinal stromal tumors and, 1633

Interstitial cystitis/painful bladder syndrome, 43, **960–961**

Interstitial lung disease, **289–294**, 290*t*, 291*f*, 292*f*. *See also specific disorder*
  acute pneumonia (AIP), 290, 291*t*
  cryptogenic organizing pneumonia/ pneumonitis (COP/ bronchiolitis obliterans with organizing pneumonia/ BOOP), 267, 291*t*, 292
  diffuse pneumonias, **289–292**, 290*t*, 291*t*, 292*f*
  drug-related, 290*t*, 310*t*
  idiopathic pneumonia, 290, 290*t*
  methotrexate causing, 837
  in microscopic polyangiitis, 860
  nonspecific pneumonia (NSIP), 291*t*, 292
    in HIV infection/AIDS, 1339
  pulmonary alveolar proteinosis, **294**
  pulmonary hypertension and, 302, 303, 430, 430*t*
  respiratory bronchiolitis-associated (RB-ILD), 291*t*, 292
  respiratory failure caused by, 318*t*
  in rheumatoid arthritis, 835
  sarcoidosis, **292–293**, 293*f*
  usual pneumonia (UIP), 290, 291*t*

Interstitial nephritis, 917*t*, **921**
  in SLE, 840

Intertriginous area, seborrhea of, 110

Intertrigo, **118**
  tinea differentiated from, 113

Interventricular septum, rupture of, in myocardial infarction, 379

Intervertebral disk disorders. *See* Cervical spine/disk disease; Lumbar spine/disk disease; Sacral spine/disk disease

Interview (medical), 1–2

Intestinal adenocarcinoma, **1634**

Intestinal amebiasis, 588*t*, 589, 592, 1305, 1315*t*, 1342, 1525, 1526, 1526*f*, 1527*t*
  postdysenteric colitis and, 1526

Intestinal angina (visceral artery insufficiency), **479–480**

Intestinal bacterial overgrowth. *See* Bacterial overgrowth

Intestinal carcinoids, 1185, 1186, **1634–1636**

Intestinal disorders. *See* Gastrointestinal system, disorders of

Intestinal flukes, **1534–1535**

Intestinal ischemia, 479

Intestinal lymphoma, **1634**
  Crohn disease and, 654, 1634

Intestinal motility disorders. *See* Motility disorders

Intestinal nematode (roundworm) infections, 592, **1538–1541**

Intestinal obstruction. *See also* Motility disorders
  in acute colonic pseudo-obstruction (Ogilvie syndrome), 639–640
  in colorectal cancer, 1638, 1638*f*
  constipation and, 584, 584*t*
  in Crohn disease, 654
  gallstones causing, 717
  in gastric carcinoma, 1629–1630, 1631
  in gastroparesis/chronic intestinal pseudo-obstruction, 640–641
  vomiting and, 580, 581, 581–582, 581*t*

Intestinal sarcoma, **1636**

Intestinal schistosomiasis, 1532, 1533

Intestinal tuberculosis, **643**

Intestinal-type gastric cancer, 1629

Intimate partner (domestic) violence, 16, 1090–1091, 1091

Intoxication. *See also specific substance causing*
  acute alcohol, 1093, 1584*t*
    metabolic acidosis/osmolar gap and, 891, 1094, 1584
  cognitive disorders/delirium caused by, 1102*t*

Intra-abdominal sepsis. *See* Abdominal abscess/infection

Intracerebral hemorrhage, 994*t*, **997–998**, 1030*t*. *See also* Stroke
  arteriovenous malformations causing, 1000, 1001
  fibrinolytic therapy for myocardial infarction and, 374
  head injury causing, 998, 1030*t*
  hypertension and, 444, 468–469, 997, 998

Intracoronary stents. *See* Coronary stents

Intracranial abscess. *See* Brain abscess

Intracranial aneurysm, **1000**. *See also* Stroke
  in polycystic kidney disease, 950
  subarachnoid hemorrhage and, 998, 1000

Intracranial bleeding. *See* Intracerebral hemorrhage; Subarachnoid hemorrhage

Intracranial hypertension
  in cryptococcal meningitis, 1554
  head injury and, 1030
  headache and, 40, 981
  idiopathic (pseudotumor cerebri), **1009**
  in liver failure/hepatic encephalopathy, 685, 686
  optic disk swelling and (papilledema), 194
  in stroke, 996–997

in subarachnoid hemorrhage, 999
tumors causing, 1003. *See also* Intracranial masses/tumors

Intracranial masses/tumors, **1003–1006**, 1004*t*, 1624*t*
  abscess causing, **1007–1008**, 1298, 1299. *See also* Brain abscess
  coma or stupor caused by, 1028
  false localizing signs and, 1005
  headache caused by, 40, **980**
    cough headache and, 980
  in HIV infection/AIDS, 1006
  metastatic, **1006**
  ocular motor palsies and, 194
  primary, **1003–1006**, 1004*t*
  seizures caused by, 983, 1003
  vertigo caused by, 213

Intracranial venous thrombosis, **1002**. *See also* Stroke

Intracytoplasmic sperm injection (ICSI), 783, 785, 970

Intradermal tests, for drug hypersensitivity, 1318

Intraepidermal squamous cell carcinoma (Bowen disease), **118**

Intrahepatic cholestasis, 674, 675*t*
  of pregnancy, 674, 675*t*, **824–825**

Intrahepatic portosystemic shunts. *See* Transvenous (transjugular) intrahepatic portosystemic shunts

Intralesional triamcinolone, for acne, 128

Intralipid. *See* Intravenous fat

Intranasal testosterone gel, 1193

Intraocular foreign body, **196**

Intraocular hypertension. *See* Ocular hypertension

Intraocular inflammation. *See also* Conjunctivitis; Uveitis
  conjunctivitis, **166–174**, 166*t*
  uveitis, 166*t*, **181–182**, 182*f*

Intraocular lenses, 183
  for refractive error, 164

Intraocular pressure, elevated. *See* Elevated intraocular pressure

Intrauterine devices (IUDs), **789–790**, 789*t*
  for emergency/postcoital contraception, 789, 791
  levonorgestrel/progestin-releasing (levonorgestrel intrauterine system), 789
    for abnormal uterine bleeding, 763–764
    for endometriosis, 776
    in estrogen replacement therapy, 1205
    for postmenopausal bleeding, 764
  pelvic infection/PID and, 778, 790

Intrauterine insemination, 970

Intravascular abscesses (septic superficial thrombophlebitis), 488, 1314*t*. *See also* Septic thrombophlebitis

Intravascular heat exchange catheter systems, for heat stroke, 1563

Intravascular ultrasound, in angina, 358

Intravenous drug use. *See* Injection drug use

Intravenous fat
  for antidepressant overdose, 1606

for beta-blocker overdose, 1591
for calcium channel blocker overdose, 1591
for hypotension in drug overdose/toxicity, 1578
in nutritional support, 1283, 1284
Intravenous fluids. *See* Fluid management/hydration
Intravenous immune globulin
    for autoimmune hemolytic anemia, 514
    for cold agglutinin disease, 515
    for common variable immunodeficiency, 883
    for Guillain-Barré syndrome, 1038
    for immune thrombocytopenia, 549, 549f, 550
    for pemphigus, 140
Intravenous lines. *See* Catheters/intravenous lines
Intraventricular conduction defects, **400**
Intravesical chemotherapy, for bladder cancer, 1652
Intrinsic acute kidney injury, 917t, 918, 921. *See also specific cause*
Intrinsic factor, in pernicious anemia/gastritis, 622
Intubation. *See also* Airway management; Mechanical ventilation
    for burn injuries/smoke inhalation, 305, 1568–1569
    in comatose patient, 1577–1578
    conversion to tracheotomy and, 237
    before gastrointestinal decontamination for poisoning/drug overdose, 1582
    for respiratory failure, 318
Intussusception, adenoviruses causing, 1421
Invasive fungal sinusitis, **218**
Invasive mole, 807
Invasive nematode (roundworm) infections, **1541–1543**, 1543f
Invasive/invasive fibrous (Riedel) thyroiditis, 1135, 1137
Invega. *See* Paliperidone
Inverse pityriasis rosea, 109
Inverse psoriasis, 107
    tinea differentiated from, 113
Inversion ankle sprains, **1715–1716**, 1715t
Inverted papilloma, **223**
Invirase. *See* Saquinavir
Invokamet. *See* Canagliflozin, with metformin
Invokana. *See* Canagliflozin
Iodinated contrast agents, for hyperthyroidism/Graves disease, 1130
    thyroiditis and, 1124, 1137
Iodine
    deficiency of, **1148–1149**
    dietary/supplementary
        in goiter prevention/treatment, 1148, 1149
        Graves disease triggered by, 1124–1125
        restriction of for thyroid nodules/cancer/goiter, 1139, 1144
    thyroiditis and, 1134, 1149
    in hyperthyroidism, 1124–1125, 1126

in hypothyroidism, 1120
Jod-Basedow disease/phenomenon and, 1126
radioactive. *See* Radioactive iodine; Radioiodine thyroid scans and uptake
Iodine-123. *See* Radioiodine thyroid scans and uptake
Iodine-123 MIBG scanning, in pheochromocytoma/paraganglioma, 1182, 1184
Iodine-131. *See* Radioactive iodine; Radioiodine thyroid scans and uptake
Iodine-131 MIBG therapy, in pheochromocytoma/paraganglioma, 1184
Iodine-131 tositumomab, for non-Hodgkin lymphoma, 532
Iodized salt, goiter prevention/treatment and, 1149
Iodochlorhydroxyquin, adverse ophthalmic effects of, 178t
Iodoquinol, for amebiasis, 1526, 1527t
Ionizing radiation, 1571. *See also under Radiation*
    cancer risk and, 1571, 1572, 1607
    from medical imaging, 1572
Iontophoresis sweat test, in cystic fibrosis, 265
Iopanoic acid, for hyperthyroidism/Graves disease, 1130
    amiodarone-induced, 1132
    thyroiditis and, 1137
Iopidine. *See* Apraclonidine
Ipecac, for poisoning/drug overdose, 1582
IPF. *See* Idiopathic pulmonary fibrosis
Ipilimumab, 1666t
    hypophysitis/hypopituitarism caused by, 1108
iPledge, 128
Ipodate sodium, for hyperthyroidism/Graves disease, 1130
    amiodarone-induced, 1132
    thyroid crisis/storm and, 1133
    thyroiditis and, 1137
IPPB. *See* Intermittent positive-pressure breathing
Ipratropium
    adverse ophthalmic effects of, 177t
    for allergic/vasomotor rhinitis, 219
    for asthma, 252, 253t
        with albuterol, 253t
    for COPD, 260, 262
IPV. *See* Intimate partner (domestic) violence
IPV (inactivated poliovaccine/Salk vaccine), 1326, 1383
    pregnancy and, 802
    for travelers, 1326, 1383
Irbesartan/irbesartan with hydrochlorothiazide, 457t
Iressa. *See* Gefitinib
Iridodialysis, 197
Iridotomy/iridectomy, for glaucoma, 176, 180–181
Irinotecan/irinotecan liposome, 1665t
    for colorectal cancer, 1639
    diarrhea caused by, 1673
    for gastric adenocarcinoma, 1631

IRIS (immune reconstitution inflammatory syndromes), 191–192, 1345
    in cryptococcosis, 1553
    Kaposi sarcoma, 146, 1344
    progressive multifocal leukoencephalopathy and, 1395
Iris neovascularization, in retinal vein occlusion, 186
Iritis (anterior uveitis), 166t, 181, 181–182, 182
Iron
    accumulation of, in hemochromatosis, 708–709
    deficiency of/iron deficiency anemia, 499, **499–500**, 500t
        anemia of inflammation and, 503
        celiac disease and, 500, 634
        chronic disease/chronic kidney disease and, 502, 503, 928
        esophageal webs and (Plummer-Vinson syndrome), 501, 613
        GI bleeding and, 500, 501, 599, 600
        in idiopathic pulmonary hemosiderosis, 304
        during pregnancy, 500, 799, 801, 815
    foreign body of, 196, 196f
    nutritional support requirements and, 1282–1283
    overdose/toxicity of, 1581t, 1584t, **1596**. *See also* Hemosiderosis
    supplementary
        for iron deficiency anemia, 500, 501–502
        in chronic kidney disease, 928
        in pregnancy, 500, 799, 801, 815
Iron deficiency anemia. *See* Iron, deficiency of
Iron overload. *See also* Hemochromatosis; Hemosiderosis
    dysmetabolic, 698
Iron-refractory iron deficiency anemia, 501
Iron-restricted erythropoiesis, 502
Irritable bowel syndrome, **643–647**
    constipation in, 584, 584t, 644, 645, 646
    diarrhea in, 592, 644, 645, 646, 646–647
    postinfectious, 644, 1308
Irritant contact dermatitis, 124, 125
Irritative voiding symptoms, 42, 954, 971
Isavuconazole, 1559t, 1560
    for aspergillosis, 1555, 1560
    for mucormycosis, 1556, 1560
Ischemia
    brainstem, seizures differentiated from, 986
    critical limb, 475
    intestinal, 479
    mesenteric, 479
    myocardial. *See* Angina, pectoris; Coronary heart disease; Myocardial ischemia
    ocular, 188–189
    visceral, 479
Ischemia testing, noninvasive, preoperative, 45–46

Ischemic cardiomyopathy. *See*
Cardiomyopathy
Ischemic chest pain, 26–27, 27, 27*t*, 28,
356, 357. *See also* Angina
Ischemic colitis, 479, 598
Ischemic heart disease, **352–381**. *See also*
Angina, pectoris; Coronary
heart disease; Myocardial
ischemia
Ischemic hepatitis/hepatopathy, 712–713
Ischemic optic neuropathy, **192**
in giant cell arteritis, 192, 854
Ischemic priapism, 966
Ischemic rest pain
in thromboangiitis obliterans (Buerger
disease), 480
in tibial/pedal occlusive disease, 475
Isentress. *See* Raltegravir
Islet cell antibodies (ICA), in diabetes,
1211, 1211*t*
Islet cell tumors, 1185–1186, 1252–1255,
1253*t*, 1254*t*. *See also*
Insulinoma
carcinoma, functioning, 1255
hypoglycemia caused by, 1185,
1252–1255, 1253*t*, 1254*t*
Islet cells, pancreatic, 1185. *See also*
B cells
hyperplasia of (noninsulinoma
pancreatogenous
hypoglycemia syndrome),
1252, **1256**
neuroendocrine tumors arising in,
1185–1186, 1252–1255,
1253*t*, 1254*t*
transplantation of, for diabetes, 1232
Isoantibodies/isoagglutinins,
compatibility testing and,
542
Isolated hypogonadotropic
hypogonadism
congenital, 1108, 1109
normosmic, 1109
Isoniazid, 281*t*, 282*t*
benzodiazepine interactions and, 1056*t*
for MAC infections, 286
overdose/toxicity of, 281*t*, 1581*t*, **1596**
ophthalmic, 178*t*
pyridoxine (vitamin B₆) and, 282,
283, 821, 1276, 1348, 1581*t*,
1596
seizures and, 1580*t*, 1596
for tuberculosis, 281–282, 281*t*, 282*t*
in HIV infection/AIDS, 1348
in latent disease/prophylactic, 284,
1350
in pregnancy, 282, 283, 821–822
resistance and, 283
Isoniazid/rifampin, for tuberculosis,
282
in latent disease/prophylactic, 284
Isoniazid/rifampin/pyrazinamide, for
tuberculosis, 282
Isophane (NPH) insulin. *See* Insulin
therapy; NPH insulin
Isopropanol, osmolar gap affected by, 906
Isoproterenol, for ventricular tachycardia,
397
Isosorbide. *See also* Nitrates
for angina, 359
for heart failure, 405*f*, 408, 412

infarct-related, 378
for pulmonary edema, 412
Isospora belli (isosporiasis), 588*t*, 592,
1305, 1342, **1527–1530**
Isotonic hyponatremia, 885–886, 885*f*
Isotretinoin
for acne, 128
adverse ophthalmic effects of, 179*t*
for lupus, 116
for rosacea, 129
teratogenicity of, 128
Isradipine, 461*t*
for angina, 361
for hypertension, 459, 461*t*
overdose/toxicity of, 459, 461*t*, 1591
Istalol. *See* Timolol
Itch-scratch cycle. *See also* Pruritus
Itch-X-Gel. *See* Pramoxine
Itching. *See* Pruritus
Itchy red bump syndrome (eosinophilic
folliculitis), 130, 131, 1333
ITP. *See* Immune thrombocytopenia
Itraconazole, 1559*t*
for aspergillosis, 1555
for blastomycosis, 1556
for candidiasis, 226, 611, 1548
for coccidioidomycosis, 1551
for histoplasmosis, 1549
for onychomycosis, 161
for paracoccidioidomycosis, 1557
for sporotrichosis, 1557
for tinea infection, 112, 114
IUDs. *See* Intrauterine devices
Ivabradine
for angina, 361
for heart failure, 405*f*, 409
Ivacaftor, for cystic fibrosis, 266
IVC filters. *See* Inferior vena cava filters/
interruption
Ivermectin
for cutaneous larva migrans, 1543
for filariasis, 1544
for loiasis, 1546
for onchocerciasis, 1545
for pediculosis, 150
for rosacea, 129
for scabies, 149
for strongyloidiasis, 1540
for trichuriasis, 1539
IVF. *See* In vitro fertilization
IVIG. *See* Intravenous immune globulin
IVUS. *See* Intravascular ultrasound
Ixabepilone, 1665*t*
for breast cancer, 757
Ixazomib, 1666*t*
Ixekizumab, for psoriasis, 108
Ixempra. *See* Ixabepilone

J wave, in hypothermia, 1564, 1564*f*
JAK2 inhibitors
for polycythemia vera, 520
for primary myelofibrosis, 523
for psoriasis, 108
JAK2 mutation
in essential thrombocytosis, 521
in hepatic vein obstruction
(Budd-Chiari syndrome),
711
in mesenteric vein occlusion, 480
in noncirrhotic portal hypertension,
714

in polycythemia, 519, 520, 521
in primary myelofibrosis, 522, 523
JAK3 inhibitor, for rheumatoid arthritis,
837
Jakob-Creutzfeldt disease, 1022,
1393–1394
myoclonus in, 1017
parkinsonism and, 1012
Jamestown Canyon virus, 1388
Janeway lesions, in endocarditis, 1459
Janumet. *See* Sitagliptin, with metformin
Janus kinase. *See under* JAK
Januvia. *See* Sitagliptin
Japanese B encephalitis, 1388, **1390–1391**
immunization against, 1327, 1391
Jardiance. *See* Empagliflozin
Jarisch-Herxheimer reaction
in leptospirosis, 1501
in relapsing fever, 1499
in syphilis, 1492
Jaundice (icterus), **674–677**, 675*t*.
See also specific cause
cholestatic, 674, 675*t*
antipsychotics causing, 1072
leptospirosis with (Weil syndrome),
1501
obstructive, 674, 674–676, 675*t*, 676*t*,
721
travel and, 1309
Jaw
osteonecrosis of, bisphosphonate use
and, 11, 875, 1162
tumors of, hyperparathyroidism and,
1152, 1153
Jaw pain, in acute coronary syndromes/
angina, 982
JC virus (John Cunningham virus/JCV),
progressive multifocal
leukoencephalopathy caused
by, 1395
natalizumab and, 652, 1024, 1395
Jejunostomies, 1281–1282. *See also*
Enteral nutritional support
Jentadueto. *See* Linagliptin, with
metformin
Jervell-Lange-Nielsen syndrome, 398
Jetrea. *See* Ocriplasmin
Jevtana. *See* Cabazitaxel
Jinteli, 1204
Jo-1 antibody, in polymyositis/
dermatomyositis, 840*t*, 848,
848*t*
Jock itch, **112–113**
Jod-Basedow disease/phenomenon
(iodine-induced
hyperthyroidism), 1126. *See
also* Graves disease;
Hyperthyroidism
John Cunningham virus. *See* JC virus
Joint fluid examination, 826, 827*t*, 828*t*.
See also specific disorder
Joints
Charcot. *See* Charcot joint
in decompression sickness, 1573
in diabetes, 1242
disorders/inflammation of. *See also
specific cause*
degenerative, **826–829**, 828*f*. *See also*
Arthritis; Osteoarthritis
infectious, **867–870**
palindromic, **875**

pattern of, 826, 827t
in rheumatoid arthritis, 834–835,
      835f
in SLE, 839t, 840
replacement of, 829. See also specific
      joint
coagulase-negative staphylococcal
      infection and, 1451
DVT/PE (venous thromboembolic
      disease) prevention and,
      298–300, 1703
nongonococcal acute bacterial
      (septic) arthritis and, 868
tuberculosis of, 283, **872**
Jones criteria, for rheumatic fever, 422,
      422–423, 423t
Jublia. See Efinaconazole
"Jump rope septum," 325
Junctional nevi, 101
Junctional rhythm, atrioventricular, **395**
Junctophilin-3, gene for, in Huntington
      disease-like disorders, 1015
Junin virus, 1399, 1400
Juvenile nephronophthisis-medullary
      cystic disease, 949t, **951**
Juvenile polyposis, familial, 667
Juvenile spinal muscular atrophy, 1034

K⁺. See Potassium
K-ras/KRAS gene/mutations
      colorectal cancer and, 665, 1637, 1639,
            1640
      gallbladder cancer and, 1618
      lung cancer and, 1612
      pancreatic/periampullary carcinoma
            and, 1621, 1625
K103N mutation, antiretroviral resistance
      and, 1355, 1360
Kadcyla. See Ado-trastuzumab emtansine
Kadian. See Morphine
Kala azar. See Visceral leishmaniasis
Kaletra. See Lopinavir/r
Kallmann syndrome, 1108, 1199, 1200
Kalydeco. See Ivacaftor
Kaolin pneumoconiosis, 307t
Kaposi sarcoma, **146**, 1332, 1338t, 1344,
      1625t
      chemotherapy for, 146, 1338t, 1344,
            1625t
      conjunctival, 192
      cutaneous, **146**
      ear involvement in, 214
      in HIV infection/AIDS, 146, 192, 214,
            1332, 1338t, 1344
      intestinal/visceral, 146, 1636
      oral, 1344
      pulmonary, 146, 1338
      virus causing, 146, 1377, 1636
Kaposi sarcoma-associated herpes virus
      (human herpesvirus 8), 146,
      1332, **1377**, 1636
Kaposi sarcoma–immune reconstitution
      inflammatory syndrome,
      146, 1344
Kappa amyloid, 539
Kasabach-Merritt syndrome, 715
Katayama syndrome, 1532
Kattan nomogram, for prostate cancer
      assessment, 1650
Kava, toxicity of, 1593
Kawasaki disease, 1367t, **1438–1440**

Kayexalate. See Sodium polystyrene
      sulfonate
Kayser-Fleischer ring, in Wilson disease,
      710, 710f
Kazano. See Alogliptin, with metformin
KCNE3 gene, in periodic paralysis, 1049
KCNJ2 gene, in periodic paralysis, 1049
Keflex. See Cephalexin
Kegel exercises, 66, 67, 777
Kent bundles, in preexcitation
      syndromes, 387
Kenya tick typhus, 1429t
Kepivance. See Palifermin
Keratic precipitates, 181, 182f
Keratitis. See also Cornea, ulcers of
      acanthamoeba, **175–176**
      adenovirus, 167, 1421
      bacterial, **174–175**
      chemical, **198**
      contact lens wear and, 164, 174, 175
      exposure, 174
      fungal, **175**
      herpes simplex, **175**, 1363, 1364,
            1364–1366
      herpes zoster ophthalmicus, **175**
      infectious, **174–176**
      neurotrophic, 174, 175
      in onchocerciasis, 1545
      ultraviolet (actinic), **198**
Keratoconjunctivitis. See also specific
      agent causing and
      Conjunctivitis
      atopic, 168
      chlamydial, **167**
      epidemic
            adenovirus, 167, 1421
            coxsackievirus, 1426
      sicca (dry eye), **167–168**
            in Sjögren syndrome, 167, 850, 851
      vernal, 168
Keratoderma blennorrhagicum, in
      reactive arthritis, 866,
      866f
Keratolytic agents, for wart removal, 141
Keratomalacia, in vitamin A deficiency,
      1277
Keratopathy, band, in hypercalcemia/
      hyperparathyroidism, 1153
Keratoses
      actinic, **117–118**
            squamous cell carcinoma arising
                  from, 118, 144
      seborrheic, **103**, 103f
Kerlone. See Betaxolol
Kernig sign, 1464
Kerydin. See Tavaborole
Ketamine
      for anxiety/depression, 1082
            at end of life, 92
      in pain management, 84
Ketoacidemia, in diabetic ketoacidosis,
      1246–1247
Ketoacidosis
      alcoholic, 905–906
      diabetic, 905, 1214, **1245–1249**, 1246t.
            See also Diabetic ketoacidosis
Ketoconazole, 98t, 1559t
      in cancer chemotherapy, 1670t
      for candidiasis, 226
      for Cushing syndrome, 1176
      for prostate cancer, 1649, 1649t

for tinea versicolor, 114–115, 115
      topical, 98t
Ketones/ketone bodies/ketonemia/
      ketonuria
      in alcoholic ketoacidosis, 906
      in diabetes mellitus, 1213, 1214, 1233
      in diabetic ketoacidosis, 905, 1246,
            1246t, 1247
      in terminally ill/dying patient, 91
Ketoprofen, 76t
Ketorolac, 76t
      for ophthalmic disorders, 168, 171t
Ketosis, in diabetes mellitus, 1210. See
      also Diabetic ketoacidosis
17-Ketosteroid reductase deficiency, in
      hypogonadotropic
      hypogonadism, 1191
Ketotifen, for allergic eye disease, 168,
      171t
Keytruda. See Pembrolizumab
Kidney. See also under Renal and Kidney
      disease/injury
      acute injury of (acute renal failure),
            913, **916–923**, 917t. See also
            Acute kidney injury; Renal
            failure
      biopsy of, **915–916**. See also specific
            disorder and Renal biopsy
      calculus formation in. See
            Nephrolithiasis; Urinary
            stone disease
      cancer of, 1608t, 1624t, **1653**,
            1654–1655, **1655**
      chronic disease of, 913, **923–932**, 923t,
            924t, 925f, 925t, 926f, 927f.
            See also Chronic kidney
            disease
      cystic diseases of, 924t, **948–951**, 949t.
            See also Renal cysts
      disorders of, **913–952**. See also Kidney
            disease/injury
      in gout, 830, **952**
      infection of. See Pyelonephritis
      medullary cystic, 949t, **951**
      medullary sponge, 949t, **950–951**
      metastatic disease of, 1655
      in myeloma, 535, 536, 920, 951
      NSAIDs affecting, 74, 829
      in phosphate regulation, 899
      polycystic, **949–950**, 949t
      in preeclampsia-eclampsia, 809t
      toxic drug effects on. See
            Nephrotoxicity
      transplantation of. See Kidney
            transplantation
      tumors of, **1653**, **1654–1655**, **1655**.
            See also Kidney, cancer of
Kidney disease/injury, **913–952**.
            See also under Renal and
            Nephritis; Nephropathy;
            Nephrotoxicity
      acid-base disorders in, 892t, 906–907,
            906t, 908, 926f, 928. See also
            Renal tubular acidosis
      acute, 913, **916–923**, 917t. See also
            Acute kidney injury; Renal
            failure
            postoperative, 54, 54t
      aminoglycosides and, 919
      in amyloidosis, 538, 934t, **946**
      assessment of, **913–915**, 914t, 915t

Kidney disease/injury (*Cont.*):
biopsy in, **915–916**. *See also specific disorder and* Renal biopsy
cardiorenal syndrome and, **923**
cardiovascular disorders and, 404, 924*t*, 925–927
chronic, 913, **923–932**, 923*t*, 924*t*, 925*f*, 925*t*, 926*f*, 927*f*. *See also* Chronic kidney disease
cirrhosis and (hepatorenal syndrome), 702–703, 917
cystic, 924*t*, **948–951**, 949*t*. *See also* Renal cysts
deaths attributable to, 2*t*
diabetes insipidus and, 892*t*, 1113–1114
diabetes mellitus and, 923, 929, 934*t*, 942, 945–946, 1238, 1238–1239. *See also* Diabetic nephropathy
drug/medication use and, 924, 929
in eosinophilic granulomatosis with polyangiitis (Churg-Strauss syndrome), 933*t*, 935*f*, 938
GFR in, 914–915
glomerular, 924*t*, **932–943**, 932*f*, 933*t*, 934*t*, 935*f*
nephritic spectrum, 932, 932*f*, 933*t*, **934–941**, 935*f*
nephrotic spectrum, 932–933, 932*f*, 934*t*, **941–943**
in gout, 830, **952**
in granulomatosis with polyangiitis (Wegener granulomatosis), 304, 857, 858, 858–859, 922, 933*t*, 935*f*, 938
hantaviruses causing (hemorrhagic fever with renal syndrome), 1403, 1404
hematuria in, 914, 953
Henoch-Schönlein purpura and, 861, 933*t*, **937–938**, 938*f*
hepatitis C infection and, 683, 933*t*, 940
in HIV infection/AIDS, 934*t*, **946**
hypercalcemia/hyperparathyroidism and, 926*f*, 927, 927*f*, 1153, 1155, 1157
hyperkalemia and, 893, 894, 916, 920, 926, 926*f*, 928
hypermagnesemia and, 902, 903
hyperphosphatemia in, 901, 916, 920, 926*f*, 927, 927*f*
hypertension and, 442–443, 444, 466, 923, 925, 926, 926*f*
treatment of, 449*t*, 466, 929
in hypertensive emergency, 469*t*
hyperuricemia and, 830, 952
hypocalcemia and, 896, 927, 927*f*
hypomagnesemia treatment and, 902
hyponatremia in, 888
infection. *See* Pyelonephritis
intrinsic, 917*t*, 918, 921
lithium use and, 1086, 1597
mercury causing, 1598
methotrexate and, 837, 1674
in microscopic polyangiitis, 859, 860, 922, 935*f*
multisystem diseases and, **951–952**
in myeloma, 535, 536, 920, **951**

myoglobinuria/rhabdomyolysis and, 852, 919–920
nephritic spectrum, 932, 932*f*, 933*t*, **934–941**, 935*f*. *See also* Nephritic syndrome
nephrotic spectrum, 932–933, 932*f*, 934*t*. *See also* Nephrotic syndrome
glomerular, 932–933, 932*f*, 934*t*, **941–943**
in primary renal disorders, **943–945**
from systemic disorders, **945–946**
neurologic disorders and, 924*t*, 928–929
neuropathy associated with, 929, 1036
NSAIDs causing, 74, 829
pancreatitis and, 726, 728
perioperative evaluation/management and, **53–54**, 54*t*
in pheochromocytoma/paraganglioma, 1180*t*
in preeclampsia-eclampsia, 809*t*
proteinuria in, 913–914, 925
pruritus associated with, 147
in scleroderma, 846, 846–847
sickle cell syndromes and, **951**
in SLE, 839*t*, 840, 841, 933*t*, 935*f*, **940–941**
in spontaneous bacterial peritonitis, 603–604
in systemic fibrosis, 358, 952
in thrombotic microangiopathies, 550, 551, 551*t*
toxic drug effects and. *See* Nephrotoxicity
in tuberculosis, **951–952**
tubulointerstitial, 924*t*, **946–948**, 947*t*
in tumor lysis syndrome, 920, 1660
urinalysis in, 913
Kidney stones. *See* Nephrolithiasis; Urinary stone disease
Kidney transplantation, 930
adenovirus infection and, 1421
hypercalcemia after, 1153
hyperkalemia and, 894
for IgA nephropathy, 937
infections after, 1290
pancreas transplantation and, for diabetes, 1232
Kiesselbach plexus, epistaxis and, 221
KIF1B mutations, in pheochromocytoma/paraganglioma, 1180
Kikuchi disease, 239
Killip classification, 370
Kimmelstiel-Wilson nodules, 945
Kinase inhibitors. *See* Tyrosine kinase inhibitors
Kindling, in substance abuse disorders, 1092, 1100
Kingella species. *See* HACEK organisms
KIT mutations, in gastrointestinal stromal tumors, 1633
Klatskin (perihilar) tumors, 1618
Klebsiella/Klebsiella pneumoniae, 1311*t*, 1315*t*
fever/neutropenia/chemotherapy and, 1314*t*
pneumonia caused by, 268*t*
urinary tract infection caused by, 1314*t*, 1315*t*
Kleine-Levin syndrome, 1090

Klinefelter syndrome, 970, 1190, 1191, **1682**
gynecomastia in, 1190, 1195, 1682
Klonopin. *See* Clonazepam
Knee, **1704–1715**, 1705*t*, 1706–1709*t*
arthritis of, **1713–1715**
nongonococcal acute bacterial (septic), 867
bursitis of, 1700–1701
complex regional pain syndrome and, 874
meniscal injuries and, 1708–1709*t*, **1711–1712**
Knee pain, **1704–1705**, 1705*t*
anterior (patellofemoral pain), 1705*t*, **1712–1713**
Knee realignment surgery, 1714
Knee replacement, for arthritis, 829, 1714
Koebner phenomenon
in lichen planus, 145
in psoriasis, 107
KOH preparation, 111, 111*f*
Kombiglyze XR. *See* Saxagliptin, with metformin
Koplik spots, 1378
Korsakoff psychosis/syndrome, 694, **1026**, 1093, 1095, 1275
KPs. *See* Keratic precipitates
KRAS/K-ras gene/mutations
colorectal cancer and, 665, 1637, 1639, 1640
gallbladder cancer and, 1618
lung cancer and, 1612
pancreatic/periampullary carcinoma and, 1621, 1625
Krukenberg tumor, 1630
KSHV. *See* Kaposi sarcoma-associated herpes virus
KS-IRIS. *See* Kaposi sarcoma–immune reconstitution inflammatory syndrome
Kübler-Ross, emotional patterns in dying described by, 92
Kupffer cells, in cirrhosis, 700–701
Kuru, 1394
Kussmaul respirations, 22, 907
Kussmaul sign
in myocardial infarction, 371
in pericarditis, 428, 429
Kwashiorkor/kwashiorkor-like secondary protein–energy malnutrition, 1268
Kyphoplasty, in osteoporosis, 1163
Kyphosis, 1692
Kyprolis. *See* Carfilzomib

L-carnitine, for valproic acid overdose/toxicity, 1584*t*, 1589
La belle indifférence, 1058
La/SSB antibody, 840*t*
in lupus/SLE, 115, 840*t*
in Sjögren syndrome, 840*t*, 850
Labetalol, for hypertension, 452*t*
in aortic dissection, 469*t*, 485
eclampsia and, 810
pheochromocytoma/pheochromocytoma surgery and, 469, 469*t*, 1183
during pregnancy, 435, 818
in urgencies/emergencies, 468–469, 469, 469*t*, 470*t*

Labor and delivery
  in acute fatty liver of pregnancy, 824
  for cardiac patient, **436**
    endocarditis prophylaxis and, **436**
  for diabetic patient, 1244
  herpes simplex transmission during,
    823, 1364, 1366
  for HIV-positive patient, 822, 1332,
    1346
  induction of, after 41 weeks, 801
  in preeclampsia-eclampsia, 810
  preparation classes for, 799
  preterm, 800, **811–812**
Laboratory tests. *See* Diagnostic/
    laboratory tests
Labral tears, 1688*t*, 1690
Labyrinthine concussion, 211*t*, 212
Labyrinthine decompression sickness,
    1573
Labyrinthitis, 211*t*, 212
Lacerations
  cerebral, 1030*t*
  ocular, **197–198**, 197*f*
  scalp, 1029, 1031
Lachman test, 1705–1710, 1706*t*
Lac-Hydrin-Five, 100*t*
Lacosamide, 987*t*
Lacrimal apparatus, disorders of,
    164–166
Lacrimal sac infection (dacryocystitis),
    166
LaCrosse agent, California encephalitis
    caused by, 1388, 1389
Lactam antibiotics. *See* Beta-lactam
    antibiotics
Lactase deficiency, **637–638**. *See also*
    Lactose (milk) intolerance
Lactase enzyme replacement, 638
Lactate. *See* Lactic acid
Lactate dehydrogenase (LD/LDH)
  ascitic fluid, 602, 603
  pleural fluid, 312
  in *Pneumocystis* pneumonia, 1336
  in testicular cancer, 1656
Lactation/breastfeeding, **802**
  antituberculosis drug therapy during,
    283
  breast abscess and, 736
  breast cancer and, 745–747
  drug/medication use avoidance during,
    798*t*, **802**. *See also specific*
    agent
  HIV infection/AIDS transmission and,
    1332, 1346
  iron requirements/supplementation
    during, 500
  mastitis and, 133, 813–814
  oral contraceptive use and, 786
  progestin minipill and, 788
  radioactive iodine contraindicated
    during, 1130, 1145
  suppression of, **802**
  thyroid medication during, 1132
Lactic acid (lactate)
  in alcoholic ketoacidosis, 905, 906
  in lactic acidosis, 905, 1251
  normal values for, 905
Lactic acidosis, 905, **1251–1252**
  alcoholic ketoacidosis and, 905–906
  antiretroviral therapy causing, 1341,
    1360

diabetic coma and, 1245, 1246*t*, 1251
metformin causing, 1224, 1251, 1595
rewarming, 1564
Lactobacillus probiotics, for
    antibiotic-associated colitis,
    648
Lactose-free diet, 638
Lactose (milk) intolerance, 633*t*, **637–638**
  diarrhea caused by, 591, 638
  flatus caused by, 587, 638
Lactulose
  for constipation, 585*t*, 586
  for hepatic encephalopathy, 615, 703
Lacunar infarction, **993–995**, 994*t*.
    See also Stroke
LADA. *See* Latent autoimmune diabetes
    mellitus of adulthood
LAIV influenza vaccine, 1322*t*, 1413,
    1413–1416, 1415*t*. *See also*
    Influenza virus vaccine
Lambda amyloid, 539
Lambert-Eaton (myasthenic) syndrome,
    1008, **1046**, 1609
Lamisil. *See* Terbinafine
Lamivudine (3TC), 1351*t*, 1354, 1360. *See*
    also Antiretroviral therapy
  with abacavir (Epzicom), 1353, 1354,
    1354*t*
    plus darunavir and cobicistat,
      1360*t*
    plus darunavir and ritonavir, 1360*t*
  with abacavir and dolutegravir
      (Triumeq), 1354*t*, 1358,
      1359*t*, 1360
  for hepatitis B, 687–688, 1341, 1354
  prophylactic, transmission to fetus/
      newborn and, 1346
  resistance to, 688, 1361
  with zidovudine, 1353, 1353–1354
  with zidovudine and abacavir
      (Trizivir), 1354, 1354*t*
Lamotrigine, 987*t*, 1087
  for bipolar disease/mania, 1087
  overdose/toxicity of, 987*t*, 1087, 1589
  for seizures, 987*t*
  pregnancy and, 820
LAMP (loop-mediated isothermal
    amplification) tests
  in filariasis, 1544
  is loiasis, 1546
  in malaria, 1514
  in trypanosomiasis, 1508
Laninamivir, 1365*t*, 1412
Lanreotide
  for acromegaly/gigantism, 1116
  for gastroenteropancreatic
      neuroendocrine tumors,
      1186
Lansoprazole, 609, 625. *See also* Proton
    pump inhibitors
Lanthanum, for hyperphosphatemia, 901,
    927
Lantus. *See* Insulin glargine
Laparoscopy
  in ascites, 602
  for ectopic pregnancy, 806
  in gynecologic disorders, 763*t*
Lapatinib, 1668*t*
  for breast cancer, 756
LAR. *See* Lymphangitis, rickettsiosis
    associated with

Large cell carcinoma of lung, 1609.
    See also Lung cancer
Large-needle (core needle) biopsy, for
    breast lump evaluation, 743,
    744. *See also* Breast, biopsy
    of
Large-volume paracentesis. *See*
    Paracentesis
Large-volume thoracentesis. *See*
    Thoracentesis
Laron syndrome/dwarfism, 1109
Laropiprant, in combination
    lipid-lowering therapy, 1266
Larva migrans
  cutaneous, **1542–1543**, 1543*f*
  ocular, 1542
  visceral, 1542
Laryngeal carcinoma, **235–237**
  leukoplakia and, 235
Laryngeal leukoplakia, **235**
Laryngeal nerve, recurrent
  damage to during thyroid surgery,
      1143
  vocal fold paralysis caused by damage/
      lesions of, 237, 1143
Laryngeal papillomas, **233–234**
Laryngectomy, for laryngeal cancer, 235,
    236
Laryngitis, **233**
Laryngopharyngeal reflux, **233**. *See also*
    Gastroesophageal reflux
    disease
Laryngotracheitis, human parainfluenza
    virus causing, 1409
Larynx, **232–238**. *See also under*
    Laryngeal
  masses of, **234–237**
  papillomas of, **233–234**
Laser-induced prostatectomy,
    transurethral (TULIP), 975
Laser therapy
  for acne scars, 128
  for benign prostatic hyperplasia, 975
  for CIN/cervical cancer, 771
  for glaucoma, 176, 180–181
  for hirsutism, 1197
  for refractive errors, 164
  for wart removal/condylomata
      acuminata, 142, 768
Lasix. *See* Furosemide
Lasmiditan, for migraine, 41
Lassa fever, 1399, 1400
Lastacaft. *See* Alcaftadine
Latanoprost/latanoprost and timolol, for
    glaucoma/ocular
    hypertension, 173*t*
Late-onset preeclampsia-eclampsia, 810
Late preterm birth, 811
Latent autoimmune diabetes mellitus of
    adulthood (LADA), 1211,
    1235
Lateral collateral ligament, 1704, 1710
  injury of, 1707*t*, 1710–1711
Lateral epicondylosis, **1697–1698**
Lateral femoral cutaneous nerve lesions
    (meralgia paresthetica), 1040
Lateral meniscus, 1704
  injury of, 1708–1709*t*
Lateral sclerosis
  amyotrophic, 1033, 1034
  primary, 1033

Latisse. *See* Bimatoprost
Latrodectus antivenom, 1605
Latrodectus mactans (black widow spider), 150, 1605
Latuda. *See* Lurasidone
Lavage, gastric, for poisoning/drug overdose, 1582
Laxative abuse, 1101
　diarrhea caused by, 588*t*, 591
Laxatives, 585*t*, 586
　for irritable bowel syndrome, 646
　for opioid-induced constipation, 86, 586
LCHAD deficiency, acute fatty liver of pregnancy and, 697, 824
LCIS. *See* Lobular carcinoma in situ
LCL. *See* Lateral collateral ligament
LCM. *See* Lymphocytic choriomeningitis
LD. *See* Lactate dehydrogenase
LDCT. *See* Low-dose helical computed tomography
LDH. *See* Lactate dehydrogenase
LDL. *See* Low-density lipoproteins/cholesterol
Lead encephalopathy, 1597
　gasoline sniffing and, 1101
Lead nephropathy, 947, 948
Lead poisoning, 1581*t*, 1596–1597
　gasoline sniffing and, 1101
　gout and, 831, 948
　tubulointerstitial disease caused by, 947, 948
Ledipasvir, for hepatitis C, 689–690, 690*t*, 1341, 1342
Leflunomide, for rheumatoid arthritis, 837
Left ventricular aneurysm
　cardiac trauma and, 434
　myocardial infarction and, 379
Left ventricular angiography, in angina, 359
Left ventricular (LV) apical ballooning syndrome. *See* Tako-Tsubo (stress/catecholamine-induced) cardiomyopathy
Left ventricular assist devices
　for cardiogenic shock, 378
　for cardiomyopathy, 417
　for heart failure, 405*f*, 410
Left ventricular ejection fraction
　anthracycline administration and, 1675
　in aortic regurgitation, 346, 347*t*
　in aortic stenosis, 341, 342, 342*t*
　in cardiomyopathy, 415, 416, 417, 420*f*
　in heart failure
　　preserved, treatment and, 410–411
　　reduced, treatment and, 404–410, 405*f*
　in mitral regurgitation, 338*f*, 339
Left ventricular end-diastolic pressure, increased, in dyspnea, 22, 23, 23*t*
Left ventricular (left heart) failure/dysfunction, 402, 403. *See also* Heart (cardiac) failure
　in hypertensive emergency, 469*t*
　myocardial infarction and, 378, 380
　perioperative evaluation/management and, 47–48
　pulmonary hypertension and, 302, 303, 430, 430*t*

Left ventricular hypertrophy
　aortic dissection and, 485
　in athletes, 419
　　sudden death and, 437
　in cardiomyopathy, 418, 419, 421. *See also* Cardiomyopathy
　hypertensive, 444, 445
Leg. *See also under Lower extremity*
　acute arterial occlusion of, 476–477
Leg ulcers
　in polyarteritis nodosa, 856
　in venous insufficiency/varicose veins/lower extremity occlusive disease, 32, 33, 155–157, 156*f*, 489, 490
Legalon-SIL. *See* Silymarin
Legionella/Legionella pneumophila, 268*t*, 269, 1311*t*, 1314*t*, 1315*t*, 1466–1467
Legionnaires disease (legionella pneumonia/legionellosis), 268*t*, 269, 1311*t*, 1314*t*, 1315*t*, 1466–1467
Leiden mutation, DVT/PE (venous thromboembolic disease) and, 295
Leiomyoma-renal cell carcinoma, 1654
Leiomyomas
　gastrointestinal, 1633–1634
　of uterus (fibroid tumor), 772–774
Leiomyosarcoma
　gastrointestinal. *See* Gastrointestinal stromal tumor
　of uterus, 773
Leipzig criteria, for Wilson disease, 710
Leishmania (leishmaniasis), 1510–1512
　cutaneous, 1510, 1510–1511, 1511, 1511*f*, 1512
　　post-kala azar, 1510
　HIV infection/AIDS and, 1511
　mucocutaneous (espundia), 1510, 1511, 1512
　post-kala azar dermal, 1510
　recidivans, 1511
　visceral (kala azar), 1510, 1511, 1511–1512
　viscerotropic, 1510
Leishmanin skin test, 1511
Lemierre syndrome, 230, 1442, 1478
Lemtrada. *See* Alemtuzumab
Lenalidomide, 1665*t*
　for myelodysplastic syndromes, 526, 548
　for myeloma, 536
　for primary myelofibrosis, 523
Lens opacity. *See* Cataract
Lentigines, 103
Lentigo maligna melanoma, 103
Lenvatinib, 1668*t*
　for thyroid cancer, 1145
Lenvima. *See* Lenvatinib
Leprechaunism, 1211*t*, 1212
Lepromatous leprosy, 1037, 1484. *See also* Leprosy
Lepromin skin test, 1484
Leprosy (Hansen disease), 1312*t*, 1484–1485
　neuropathy associated with, 1037, 1484
Leptin/leptin receptor, in obesity, 1270
Leptomeningeal metastases (carcinomatous meningitis), 1006

Leptospira/Leptospira interrogans (leptospirosis), 1312*t*, 1500–1501
Lescol. *See* Fluvastatin
Lethal midline granuloma, 223
Letrozole, 755*t*, 1670*t*
　for breast cancer, 752, 755*t*, 756
　for endometriosis, 776
　for ovulation induction, 784
Leucovorin (folinic acid)
　with methotrexate, 108, 651, 837, 1671*t*, 1674
　in toxoplasmosis treatment, 1337*t*, 1350, 1524
Leukemias, 519–531, 519*t*, 520*t*
　acute, 527–529, 1622*t*. *See also specific type*
　　erythrovirus (parvovirus) infection in, 1422
　　lymphoblastic/lymphocytic (ALL), 527, 528, 529, 1622*t*
　　of mixed phenotype, 528
　　myeloid (AML), 519*t*, 527, 528, 528–529, 1622*t*
　　promyelocytic (APL), 527, 528
　　　DIC associated with, 528, 554
　adult T cell (ATL), 1396. *See also* Human T cell lymphotropic/leukemia virus
　aleukemic, 528
　aplastic anemia differentiated from, 516–517
　chronic, 1622*t*
　　lymphocytic (CLL), 529–531, 1622*t*
　　myeloid (CML), 519, 519*t*, 520*t*, 523–525, 1622*t*
　　myelomonocytic (CMML), 525
　　prolymphocytic, 530
　erythrovirus (parvovirus) infection in, 1422
　fever/FUO and, 1288
　hairy cell, 1622*t*
　incidence/mortality/risk of, 1608*t*
　infection in, 528
　plasma cell, 535
　rheumatologic manifestations of, 875
　secondary to chemotherapy or radiation therapy, 527
　stem cell transplants for, 525, 528–529, 529, 531, 540, 541
Leukemic arthritis, 875
Leukeran. *See* Chlorambucil
Leukine. *See* Sargramostim
Leukoagglutinin transfusion reactions, 543
　leukocyte-poor blood in prevention of, 542, 543
Leukocyte count. *See* White blood cell count
Leukocyte-poor blood, transfusion of, 542, 543. *See also* Transfusion
　CMV transmission and, 543–544
Leukocytes, pleural fluid, 313*t*
Leukocytoclastic vasculitis, cancer-related, 875
Leukoencephalopathy, progressive multifocal (PML), 1395–1396
　dimethyl fumarate causing, 1025
　in HIV infection/AIDS, 1340, 1395
　natalizumab and, 652, 1024, 1395

Leukoplakia
  hairy, 224, 225f, 1341
  laryngeal, **235**
  oral, 224, 224f, 1341
Leukoreduced blood, transfusion of, 542,
      543. *See also* Transfusion
  CMV transmission and, 543–544
Leukotriene modifiers
  for allergic rhinitis, 219
  for asthma, 247f, 249–250t, 251
Leuprolide, 1670t. *See also* Luteinizing
      hormone-releasing hormone
      (LHRH) analogs
  for abnormal uterine bleeding, 763
  for endometriosis, 776
  hypogonadotropic hypogonadism
      caused by, 1111
  for male infertility, 1112
  for prostate cancer, 1649, 1649t
Leustatin. *See* Cladribine
Levalbuterol, for asthma, 252, 253t
Levamisole-associated purpura, **860**
Levaquin. *See* Levofloxacin
Levatol. *See* Penbutolol
Levemir. *See* Insulin detemir
Levetiracetam, 987t
  overdose/toxicity of, 987t, 1589
  for seizures, 987t
    pregnancy and, 820
Levitra. *See* Vardenafil
Levo-Dromoran. *See* Levorphanol
Levobunolol, for glaucoma/ocular
      hypertension, 172t
Levocabastine, for allergic eye disease,
      168, 170t
Levodopa
  benzodiazepine interactions and,
      1056t
  MAOI interactions and, 1013, 1083t
  for parkinsonism, 1012–1013
    with carbidopa, 1012–1013
    with carbidopa and entacapone,
      1013, 1014
Levofloxacin. *See also* Fluoroquinolones
  for bacterial rhinosinusitis, 217t
  for ophthalmic disorders, 169t
  for pneumonia, 269t, 271, 275t, 1446
  for sinusitis in HIV infection/AIDS,
      1339
  for traveler's diarrhea, 1310
  for urinary tract infection, 955t
Levoleucovorin rescue, with
      methotrexate, 1671t
Levomilnacipran, 1078t, 1079–1081
Levonorgestrel. *See also* Levonorgestrel/
      progestin-releasing IUD
  for emergency/postcoital
      contraception, 791
  for menopausal symptoms, 795
  in oral contraceptives, 787t
  with transdermal estradiol, 795, 1204
Levonorgestrel/progestin-releasing IUD
      (levonorgestrel intrauterine
      system), 789
  for abnormal uterine bleeding,
      763–764
  for endometriosis, 776
  in estrogen replacement therapy, 1205
  for postmenopausal bleeding, 764
Levorphanol, 78t
Levothyroxine (thyroxine)

for hypothyroidism/myxedema, 1111,
      1122–1124
  in Hashimoto thyroiditis, 1136
  myxedema crisis and, 1122
  during pregnancy, 816, 1122, 1123
  for thyroid cancer, 1144
    follow-up and, 1146
    withdrawal and, 1145
  thyroid nodule evaluation/treatment
      and, 1138t, 1139
  after thyroidectomy, 1143
Levulose, for porphyria, 1036
Lewy bodies, dementia with, 59, 1019t,
      1021. *See also* Dementia
Lexapro. *See* Escitalopram
Lexiva. *See* Fosamprenavir
Leydig cell tumors/hyperplasia
  hyperandrogenism in women caused
      by, 1197
  hypogonadism and, 1190, 1191
LGV. *See* Lymphogranuloma venereum
LHRH analogs. *See* Luteinizing
      hormone-releasing hormone
      (LHRH) analogs
LHRH antagonist. *See* Luteinizing
      hormone-releasing hormone
      (LHRH) antagonist
Lialda. *See* Mesalamine
Libido, loss of, 966. *See also* Sexual
      dysfunction
  in chronic kidney disease, 929
  tricyclic antidepressants causing, 1082
Libman-Sacks endocarditis, in SLE, 840,
      843
Librium. *See* Chlordiazepoxide
Lice, **149–150**
  relapsing fever transmission and, 150,
      1499
  trench fever transmission and, 149,
      1477
  typhus transmission and, 149,
      1428–1431, 1429t
Lichen planus, **144–146**, 145f
  drugs causing eruptions similar to, 145,
      162t
  oral, 145, 224
  vulvovaginal, 145, 775
Lichen planus-like drug eruptions, 145,
      162t
Lichen sclerosus, vulvar, 775, 782
Lichenoid drug eruptions, 145, 162t
Lichtheimia (Absidia) infection, 218,
      1555–1556
Licorice, hypertension/aldosteronism
      and, 442, 1178
Lid. *See* Eyelids
Liddle syndrome, 442, 892t
Lidex. *See* Fluocinonide
Lidocaine, 382t. *See also* Lidocaine patch
  for arrhythmias, 381, 382t
    infarct-related, 377
    ventricular tachycardia, 397
  for cluster headache, 980
Lidocaine patch, for neuropathic pain/
      diabetic neuropathy, 83t, 84,
      1240
Lidoderm. *See* Lidocaine patch
Life expectancy
  assessment/prognosis of older adult
      and, 55, 56f, 56t, 57t
  prognosis at end of life and, 88

Life support
  basic, in drowning, 1567
  withdrawal/withholding, in end-of-life
      care, 91–92, 92t
    advance directives and, 90
Lifestyle
  colorectal cancer risk and, 1637–1638
  modifications of
    adherence and, 1
    in aortoiliac disease management,
      472–473
    in constipation management,
      585–586
    in GERD management, 609
    in hypertension management,
      445–446, 446t
    in menopausal symptom
      management, 1202
    in nonalcoholic fatty liver disease
      management, 698
    in obesity prevention/management,
      12–13, 1270–1271
    pain behavior and, 1060
  sedentary
    obesity and, 12, 13, 1270
    preventable disease/deaths and, 3t,
      6t, **11–12**
Lift off test, 1686t, 1689
Light, pupillary reaction to. *See* Pupillary
      reactions
Light chains
  in amyloidosis, 538, 539, 946
  in myeloma, 535, 535–536, 951
  in urine. *See* Bence Jones proteinuria
Light eruption, polymorphous (PMLE),
      154, 155
Light therapy. *See* Phototherapy
Lightning injuries, 1570
Ligneous (Riedel) thyroiditis, 1135, 1137
Lille model/score, in alcoholic liver
      disease, 695
Lily-of-the-valley, toxicity of, 1594
Limb. *See* Extremities
Limb-girdle (Erb) muscular dystrophy,
      849, 1047, 1048t
Limb loss. *See* Amputation
Limbic encephalitis, 1008
Linaclotide, 585t, 586
  for irritable bowel syndrome, 646
Linagliptin, 1222t, 1227
  with empagliflozin, 1228
  with metformin, 1227, 1228
Linear scleroderma, 846
Linezolid
  adverse ophthalmic effects of, 178t
  for enterococcal infection, 1444, 1445
  for pneumonia, 269t, 271, 275t
  for skin and soft tissue infections, 1448
Linitis plastica, 1629, 1630
Linoleic acid, in nutritional support,
      1283
Liothyronine. *See also* Thyroid hormone
  antidepressant drug augmentation and,
      1079
  for myxedema coma, 1122
Lipase
  in pancreatic enzyme supplements,
      732, 732t
  in pancreatitis, 726, 731
Lipedema, chronic venous insufficiency
      differentiated from, 489–490

Lipemia retinalis, 1261
  in diabetes mellitus, 1214
Lipid-based amphotericin B, 1558, 1558t
  for aspergillosis, 1555
  for blastomycosis, 1556
  for candidiasis, 1548
  for histoplasmosis, 1549
  for mucormycosis, 218, 1556
  prophylactic, 1292
  for sporotrichosis, 1557
Lipid disorders/lipids, 10, **1258–1267**.
         See also Fat; Lipoproteins
  antipsychotics affecting, 1071, 1071t
  antiretroviral therapy and, 1174, 1345
  cardiovascular/coronary heart disease
         and, 6t, **10**, **1259–1260**
  cholesterol lowering and, 10, 1259,
         1260, **1262–1266**, 1264t,
         1265t. *See also* Lipid-
         lowering therapy
  clinical presentations in, **1261**, 1261f
  in diabetes mellitus, 1217, 1261
  disorders affecting metabolism and,
         1261
  exercise affecting, 1262
  in nephrotic syndrome/nephrotic
         spectrum disorders, 942
  screening/treatment for, 6t, **10**,
         1261–1262, **1262–1266**,
         1264t, 1265t. *See also*
         Lipid-lowering therapy
  in women/older adults, 1261, 1262
  secondary conditions and, **1261**
  thiazolidinediones affecting, 1224
  triglycerides and, 1259, **1266–1267**
Lipid emulsion, intravenous. *See*
         Intravenous fat
Lipid fractions, coronary heart disease
         risk and, 353, **1259–1260**.
         See also Lipoproteins
Lipid-lowering therapy, 10, 353, 354f,
         355t, 1259, 1260, **1262–1266**,
         1264t, 1265t
  for cardiovascular/heart disease
         prevention, **10**, 353, 354f,
         355t, 1259, 1260, **1262–1266**,
         1264t, 1265t
    postinfarction, 380
  cholesterol screening and, 10, 1261,
         1262
  combination therapy and, 1266
  in diabetes, 1261
  diet and, 1263, 1279
  exercise/activity and, 1262
  high LDL cholesterol and, 10, 353,
         355t, 1260, **1262–1266**,
         1264t, 1265t
  high triglycerides and, 1265t, 1267
  in nephrotic syndrome, 942
  pharmacologic, 10, 353, 354f, 355t,
         1263–1266, 1264t, 1265t. *See*
         also specific type of therapy
         and Statins
    rhabdomyolysis/myopathy/myositis
         and, 848t, 849, 852
  selection of agents for, 1266
  therapeutic effects of, 353, **1260**
Lipid-modifying diets, 1262, 1263, 1279
Lipitor. *See* Atorvastatin
Lipoatrophic diabetes, 1211t
Lipoatrophy. *See* Lipodystrophy

Lipodermatosclerosis, 32
Lipodox. *See* Liposomal doxorubicin
Lipodystrophy/lipoatrophy
  familial partial, type I, 1174
  HIV infection/antiretroviral therapy
         and, 1174, 1353, 1354, 1355,
         1356
  at insulin injection sites, 1231, 1237
Lipohypertrophy, at insulin injection
         sites, 1231, 1237
Lipoid nephrosis (minimal change
         disease), 934t, **943**
Lipoid pneumonia, 306
Lipomas
  atrial septal, 433
  epidermal inclusion cysts differentiated
         from, 154
  in MEN, 1187t, 1188
Liponyssoides sanguineus mites. *See* Mites
Lipoproteins. *See also specific type and*
         Cholesterol
  coronary heart disease and, **1259–1260**
  in diabetes mellitus, 1217
  estrogen replacement affecting, 1202,
         1203
  lowering. *See* Lipid-lowering therapy
  screening tests for levels of, 6t, 10,
         1261–1262
    in women/older adults, 1261, 1262
  thiazolidinediones affecting, 1224
Liposomal amphotericin B, 1558t. *See*
         also Lipid-based
         amphotericin B
  for cryptococcal meningitis, 1337t,
         1340, 1553, 1554
  for histoplasmosis, 1549
  for leishmaniasis, 1511, 1512
Liposomal daunorubicin, 1665t. *See also*
         Daunorubicin/daunomycin
Liposomal doxorubicin, 1665t. *See also*
         Doxorubicin
  for Kaposi sarcoma, 146
Liposomal vincristine, 1664t. *See also*
         Vincristine
5-Lipoxygenase inhibitor, for asthma,
         250t, 251
Liquid artificial nutrition (tube feedings),
         1281–1282, 1281f. *See also*
         Enteral nutritional support
Liquid diets, clear and full, 1278
Liquid nitrogen. *See also* Cryotherapy
  for actinic keratoses, 118
  for wart removal/condylomata
         acuminata, 141, 768
Liraglutide, 1221t, 1226
  weight reduction and, 1226,
         1235, 1271
Lisinopril
  breastfeeding and, 798t
  for heart failure, 407
  for hypertension, 456t
    with hydrochlorothiazide, 456t
Lispro insulin. *See* Insulin lispro
Listeria monocytogenes (listeriosis), 588t,
         1312t, **1457–1458**
  diarrhea caused by, 588t, 589, 1457
  meningitis caused by, 1297t, 1314t,
         1457
Literacy (health), adherence and, 1
LITH gene, in cholelithiasis/gallstones,
         716

Lithium, 1084, 1085–1087, 1087t
  antidepressant drug augmentation/
         interaction and, 1079, 1083t
  for cluster headache prophylaxis, 980
  for depression, 1085
  drug interactions of, 1083t, 1086–1087,
         1087t
  overdose/toxicity of, 1086, 1584t,
         1597–1598
    hemodialysis for, 1583t, 1584t, 1597
    ophthalmic, 177t
    seizures and, 1580t
  pregnancy/breastfeeding and, 798t,
         1086
  thyroid disorders and, 1086
Lithium-induced delirium, 1086
Lithotripsy
  for cholelithiasis, 718
  for renal stones, 965
  for sialolithiasis, 232
  for ureteral stones, 965
Livalo. *See* Pitavastatin
Live attenuated influenza vaccine (LAIV),
         1322t, 1413, 1413–1416,
         1415t
Livedo reticularis/livedo racemosa, **863**
  antiphospholipid antibody syndrome
         and, 843, 863
  in polyarteritis nodosa, 856, 863
Liver
  anesthesia/surgery affecting function
         of, 50
  biopsy of, 677
    in alcoholic liver disease, 694
    in cirrhosis, 700
    in hemochromatosis, 708–709
    in hepatic vein obstruction
         (Budd-Chiari syndrome),
         712
    in hepatocellular carcinoma, 1617
    in HIV infection/AIDS, 1341
    in nonalcoholic fatty liver disease,
         698
    in primary sclerosing cholangitis,
         724
  cancer of, 1608t, **1616–1618**, 1625t
    with cholangiocarcinoma, 1619
    cirrhosis and, 701, 705, 1616, 1617
    hemochromatosis and, 708, 709, 1616
    hepatitis and, 682, 684, 687, 1616,
         1617
    hepatitis B vaccine in prevention of,
         13, 682, 1617
    nonalcoholic fatty liver disease and,
         699, 1616
    primary biliary cholangitis/cirrhosis
         and, 707
    pyogenic abscess and, 714–715
  cavernous hemangioma of, 715
  disorders of, **677–716**. *See also specific*
         disorder and under Hepatic
    acute liver failure, **685–686**
    alcoholic, **693–695**
    amebic abscess, 1525, 1526, 1527,
         1527t
    ascites in, 601, 601t
      shock liver/cardiogenic liver
         injury, 713
      spontaneous bacterial peritonitis
         and, 601, 602, 602–604, 702
    cirrhosis, **699–706**

in CMV infection, 1375
coagulopathy, **562**, 704
diagnosis of, 676–677, 676*t*
drug- and toxin-induced, **695–697**.
    See also Hepatotoxicity
esophageal varices and, 595, 596,
    614, 615, 616, 617
in fascioliasis, 1533
in heart failure, **712–713**
hemochromatosis, **708–709**
hepatic vein obstruction (Budd-
    Chiari syndrome), **711–712**
hepatitis. *See* Hepatitis
in HIV infection/AIDS, 680, 683,
    687, 688, 1341–1342
immunization recommendations in,
    1321*t*
jaundice in, 674, 675*t*, 676*t*
neoplastic. *See also* Liver, cancer of
    benign tumors, **715–716**
    drugs/toxins causing, 697
    oral contraceptive use and, 715,
        716, 786, 1616
nonalcoholic fatty liver disease,
    697–699. *See also* Fatty liver
noncirrhotic portal hypertension,
    713–714
parenteral nutritional support and,
    1285*t*
perioperative evaluation/
    management and, **50**
in preeclampsia-eclampsia, 809*t*
pregnancy and, **823**
primary biliary cholangitis (biliary
    cirrhosis), **706–707**
pruritus associated with, 147
pyogenic abscess, **714–715**
syphilis and, 1495
thiazolidinedione use and, 1225
Wilson disease (hepatolenticular
    degeneration), **709–711**,
    710*f*, **1017**
fatty. *See* Fatty liver
fibrosis of. *See* Hepatic fibrosis
focal nodular hyperplasia of, 715, 716
    telangiectatic, 716
hydatid cyst of, 1537
nodular regenerative hyperplasia of,
    noncirrhotic portal
    hypertension and, 713
nutmeg, 713
passive congestion of, 713
shock, 712–713
transplantation of, 704–705. *See also*
        specific disease and
    Transplantation
    for acute liver failure, 686
    adenovirus infection and, 1421
    alcoholic liver disease and, 695
    for autoimmune hepatitis, 693
    for cirrhosis, 704–705, 705
    esophageal varices and, 616
    for hepatic coagulopathy, 562
    for hepatic vein obstruction
        (Budd-Chiari syndrome),
        712
    for hepatocellular carcinoma, 1617
    for hepatopulmonary syndrome/
        portopulmonary
        hypertension, 704
    for hepatorenal syndrome, 703

in HIV infection/AIDS, 704, 1342
infections after, 1290
for mushroom poisoning, 1601
for nonalcoholic fatty liver disease,
    698
for primary biliary cholangitis/
    cirrhosis, 707
for primary sclerosing cholangitis,
    725
for Wilson disease, 711
Liver biochemical tests, 676–677, 676*t*
Liver cell adenoma. *See* Hepatocellular
        adenoma
Liver (hepatic) failure, **685–686**
    acetaminophen causing, 74, 685, 686,
        1585
    drugs/toxins causing, 685, 686
    fatty liver of pregnancy and, 685, 824
    herpetic, 1364
    HHV-6 causing, 1377
    in HIV infection/AIDS, 1341
    in mushroom poisoning, 685–686,
        686, 1600
    nefazodone causing, 1081
    thiazolidinedione use and, 1225
Liver flukes, **1533–1534**
Liver-kidney microsome type 1
        antibodies (anti-LKM1), in
        autoimmune hepatitis, 692
Liver-kidney transplantation, for cirrhosis
        with kidney failure, 704
Liver spots (solar lentigines), 103, 158
Livial. *See* Tibolone
Livostin. *See* Levocabastine
Lixivaptan, for hyponatremia/SIADH, 889
LKB1/STK11 mutation, pancreatic/
        periampullary carcinoma
        and, 1620
LMWH (low-molecular-weight heparin).
        See Heparin
Loa loa (loiasis), **1546**
Load and shift test, 1688*t*, 1690
Lobular carcinoma in situ, 748, 748*t*
Local anesthetics, for eye disorders,
        precautions for use of, **198**
Locked-in syndrome (de-efferented
        state), **1029**
Lodine. *See* Etodolac
Lodoxamide, for allergic eye disease, 168,
        170*t*
Loeys-Dietz syndrome, aortic disorders/
        aneurysm in, pregnancy and,
        435
Löffler syndrome, 294
Loiasis, **1546**
"Lone atrial fibrillation," 390
Long-acting insulin, 1229, 1229*t*, 1230.
        See also Insulin therapy
    in mixtures/combination therapy,
        1229*t*, 1231, 1233
    in pregnancy, 1230, 1244
Long-chain acyl coenzyme A
        dehydrogenase (LCHAD)
        deficiency, acute fatty liver of
        pregnancy and, 697, 824
Long QT syndrome, **398**. *See also* QT
        interval, long
    sudden death of athlete and, 437, 438*t*
Long-term care facilities
    norovirus infections and, 1305, 1425
    scabies outbreaks and, 148, 149

Lonsurf. *See* Trifluridine/tipiracil
Loop diuretics. *See also* Diuretics;
        Furosemide
    for acute tubular necrosis, 920
    adverse effects of, 448, 450*t*
    for cirrhotic ascites, 701
    for heart failure, 406, 412
        in chronic kidney disease, 926
    for hyperkalemia, 894, 895*t*
    for hypernatremia, 890
    for hypertension, 448, 450*t*
        in chronic kidney disease, 448, 466,
            926
        in urgencies/emergencies, 469*t*, 471
    hypokalemia caused by, 892
    hyponatremia caused by, 886
    ototoxicity of, 208
    for pericarditis, 429
    for pulmonary edema, 412
Loop excision, for CIN, 771
Loop-mediated isothermal amplification
        (LAMP) tests
    in filariasis, 1544
    in loiasis, 1546
    in malaria, 1514
    in trypanosomiasis, 1508
Loperamide, 590, 594. *See also*
        Antidiarrheal agents
    for chemotherapy-associated diarrhea,
        1673
    for Crohn disease, 655
    for diabetic diarrhea, 1240
    for fecal incontinence, 672
    for irritable bowel syndrome, 646
    for microscopic colitis, 662
    for short bowel syndrome, 637
    for traveler's diarrhea, 1310
    for ulcerative colitis, 659
Lopid. *See* Gemfibrozil
Lopinavir/r (lopinavir/ritonavir), 1352*t*,
        1357. *See also* Antiretroviral
        therapy
    prophylactic, transmission to fetus/
        newborn and, 1346
Lopressor. *See* Metoprolol
Loprox. *See* Ciclopirox
Loratadine. *See also* Antihistamines
    for allergic eye disease, 168–174
    for allergic rhinitis, 219
Lorazepam, 1054, 1054–1055, 1054*t*.
        See also Benzodiazepines
    for alcohol withdrawal, 1097,
        1097–1098
    with antipsychotics, 1070
    for anxiety/stress disorders, 1054,
        1054–1055, 1054*t*
    for chemotherapy-induced nausea and
        vomiting, 1673
    for delirium, 1103
    for insomnia, 1089
    overdose/toxicity of, 1594–1595
    for psychedelic/hallucinogen abuse/
        toxicity, 1099, 1598
    for seizures
        in eclampsia, 810
        in poisoning/drug overdose, 1580
        status epilepticus and, 989
Lorcaserin, for obesity, 13, 1271
    in type 2 diabetes, 1235
Lorcet. *See* Hydrocodone
Lordosis, 1692

Lortab. *See* Hydrocodone
Losartan, 457*t*, 459
    with hydrochlorothiazide, 457*t*
Lotemax. *See* Loteprednol
Lotensin/Lotensin HCT. *See* Benazepril
Loteprednol, for ophthalmic disorders,
        171*t*
Lotrel. *See* Benazepril
Louse. *See* Lice
Louse-borne relapsing fever, 150, 1499
Louse-borne typhus, epidemic, 150,
        1428–1430, 1429*t*
Lovastatin, 355*t*, 1260, 1263–1264, 1265*t*.
        See also Statins
    protease inhibitor interactions and,
        1356
    for thyroid cancer, 1145
Lovenox. *See* Enoxaparin
Low back pain, **1692–1694**, 1692*t*, 1693*t*.
        See also Back pain
Low-calorie diets, in obesity
        management, 1270, 1271
Low-cholesterol diet, 1263, 1279
Low-density lipoprotein receptor-related
        protein antibodies, in
        myasthenia gravis, 1045
Low-density lipoproteins/cholesterol,
        1259
    antiretroviral therapy affecting, 1356
    cardiovascular/coronary heart disease
        and, 6*t*, **10**, 353, 1259–1260,
        1261–1262
    in diabetes mellitus, 1217, 1241, 1261
    diet affecting, 1263
    lowering levels of, 10, 353, 354*f*, 355*t*,
        1260, **1262–1266**, 1264*t*,
        1265*t*. *See also* Lipid-
        lowering therapy
    screening tests for levels of, 6*t*, **10**,
        1261–1262
        in women, 1262
    tendinous xanthomas and, 1261
    thiazolidinediones affecting, 1224
Low-dose helical computed tomography
        (LDCT), in lung cancer
        screening, 14*t*, 15, 286,
        1611
Low-fat diet, 1263, 1279
    in diabetes/diabetes prevention,
        1218, 1219
    for pancreatitis, 729, 732
Low flow aortic stenosis, "paradoxical,"
        341, 342, 342*t*
Low gradient, low valve area, low output,
        normal LVEF aortic stenosis,
        341, 342, 342*t*
Low gradient severe aortic stenosis with
        low EF, 341, 342, 342*t*
Low-iodine diet, 1139, 1144
Low-molecular-weight heparin. *See*
        Heparin
Low-protein diet. *See* Protein-restricted
        diet
Low-salt diet. *See* Sodium-restricted diet
Low-saturated-fat diet, 1263, 1279
Low-sodium diet. *See* Sodium-restricted
        diet
Low vision. *See* Visual impairment/loss
Lower airway/respiratory tract disorders,
        241–242. *See also*
        Pneumonia

adenoviruses causing, 1421
    asthma differentiated from, 246
Lower esophageal sphincter, in GERD,
        606
Lower extremity edema, **32–34**, 33*t*
    in venous insufficiency, 32–34, 33*t*,
        489
    leg ulcers and, 32, 33, 156, 489, 490
Lower GI bleeding, **597–599**. *See also*
        Gastrointestinal bleeding
Lower leg/foot arteries, atherosclerotic/
        occlusive disease of, 475–476
    leg ulcers and, 32, 33, **155–157**, 156*f*,
        489, 490
    osteomyelitis and, 871
Lower motor neuron lesions. *See* Motor
        neuron diseases
Loxapine, 1069*t*, 1071
Loxitane. *See* Loxapine
Loxosceles laeta/reclusa (brown recluse
        spider), 150, 1605
Loxoscelism, 150
Lozol. *See* Indapamide
LRP4 antibodies, in myasthenia gravis,
        1045
LRRK2 gene, in parkinsonism, 1011
LSD, 1099, **1598**
Lubiprostone, 585*t*, 586
    for irritable bowel syndrome, 646
    for opioid-induced constipation, 86
Lubriderm, 100*t*
Lucentis. *See* Ranibizumab
Ludiomil. *See* Maprotiline
Ludwig angina, 230
Lues maligna, 1494
Lumbar hyperlordosis, 1692
Lumbar plexus/nerve lesions, 1045
Lumbar puncture. *See also* Cerebrospinal
        fluid analysis
    in CNS infection/brain abscess, 1298,
        1299
    headache after, 981
    in headache evaluation, 41
    herniation syndromes and, 998, 1005,
        1298, 1299
    neuroimaging and, 1298, 1299
    in syphilis, 1496, 1497
Lumbar spine/disk disease
    back pain and, **1692–1694**, 1692*t*,
        1693*t*
    disk herniation and, **1695**
    spinal stenosis and, 1694
Lumbosacral plexus/nerve lesions, **1045**
Lumbosacral spine disease. *See also*
        Lumbar spine/disk disease
    anogenital pruritus in, 147
    neurologic testing in, 1692*t*
Lumefantrine-artemether (Coartem/
        Riamet), 1515*t*, 1516*t*, 1517*t*,
        1519, 1520
Lumigan. *See* Bimatoprost
Lump (breast), 741–742, 741*f*, 742*f*, 743*f*,
        744*f*. *See also* Breast cancer
    biopsy in evaluation of, 740, 742–744,
        743*f*, 744*f*
    differential diagnosis of, 745
    fat necrosis causing, 736
    fibroadenoma, **735**
    in fibrocystic condition, 734
    in male, 760
    removal of. *See* Lumpectomy

Lumpectomy, 749, 749–750
    genetic mutations for breast cancer
        and, 739
    local recurrence and, 758
    for noninvasive (ductal/lobular)
        carcinoma, 748
    for phyllodes tumor, 735
    during pregnancy, 747
Lunesta. *See* Eszopiclone
Lung. *See also under Pulmonary and*
        Respiratory
    abscess of, **274–276**, 1478
        in coccidioidomycosis, 1550, 1551
    aspergilloma of, 1554, 1555
    blood supply of, 25
    cancer of. *See* Lung cancer
    collapse of. *See* Atelectasis
    fibrosis of. *See* Pulmonary fibrosis
    hydatid cyst of, 1537
    neuroendocrine tumors of, in MEN,
        1188
    radiation injury of, **309–310**
    toxic/chemical injury of
        aspiration and, 306, 1602
        occupational, 290*t*, **309**
        smoke inhalation and, 305
Lung biopsy
    in granulomatosis with polyangiitis,
        304, 858
    in interstitial (diffuse parenchymal)
        lung disease, 290–292
    in lung cancer, 1609, 1612, 1614
    in mesothelioma, 1615
    in sarcoidosis, 293
Lung cancer, **1608–1616**, 1608*t*, 1610*t*,
        1612*t*
    adenocarcinoma, 1609, 1612
    asbestosis and, 307, 309, 1608
    bronchioloalveolar cell
        (adenocarcinoma in situ),
        1609
    bronchogenic carcinoma, 1608,
        1608–1613, 1610*t*, 1612*t*
    granulomatosis with polyangiitis
        differentiated from, 858
    hemoptysis as predictor of, 25
    in HIV infection/AIDS, 1338, 1344
    hypercalcemia and, 1609, 1659
    incidence/risk/mortality of, 1608,
        1608*t*, 1612, 1612*t*, 1613
    inhaled insulin and, 1232
    in situ, 1609
    large cell, 1609
    mesothelioma, 309, **1614–1616**, 1623*t*
    metastatic disease, **1613–1614**
    myasthenic syndrome in, 1046, 1609
    non-Hodgkin lymphoma, 1338
    non–small cell, 1609, 1611–1612,
        1623*t*. *See also* Non–small
        cell lung cancer
    occupational exposures and, 13, **309**
    palliative therapy for, 1612, 1613
    paraneoplastic syndromes associated
        with, 1609
    prevention of/screening for, 14*t*, 15,
        286–287, 1611
    prognosis/survival rates for, 1612*t*,
        1613
    pulmonary function testing in,
        1610–1611
    SIADH in, 887, 1609

small cell, 1609, 1612–1613, 1612t, 1623t. *See also* Small cell carcinoma of lung
smoking/smoking cessation and, 7, 13, 1607, 1608
as cocarcinogen, 309
screening and, 14t, 15, 286, 1611
solitary pulmonary nodule and, 287
squamous cell carcinoma, 1608–1609, 1612
staging of, 1609–1610, 1610t
superior vena caval obstruction/ syndrome in, 491, 1609
treatment of, 1611–1613
Lung capacity, total (TLC). *See* Pulmonary function tests
Lung flukes *(Paragonimus)*, 1534
Lung injury, acute
ARDS as, **319–321**, 320t
transfusion-related, 544
Lung transplantation. *See also* Transplantation
adenovirus infection and, 1421
for COPD, 262
for cystic fibrosis, 266
for pulmonary hypertension, 303, 432f
Lung volume reduction surgery (LVRS), for COPD, 262
Lung volumes. *See* Pulmonary function tests
Lupron. *See* Leuprolide
Lupus anticoagulant, **562–563**, 841t, 843
in antiphospholipid antibody syndrome, 662–663, 815, 841, 841t, 843
in SLE, 562–563, 841, 841t
Lupus cerebritis, 841
Lupus erythematosus
autoantibodies in, 115, 839t, 840–841, 840t, 841t
discoid/subacute (chronic cutaneous), **115–116**, 839t, 840
drug-related, 115, 116, 162t, 310t, **842**
photosensitivity and, 115
systemic, **839–842**, 839t, 840t, 841t. *See also* Systemic lupus erythematosus
Lupus nephritis, 839t, 840, 841, 933t, 935f, **940–941**
Lupus panniculitis, 152, 840
Lupus pernio, 292, 293f
Lupus profundus, 840
Lurasidone, 1068, 1069t, 1070, 1071t
Luteinizing hormone (LH), 1109t
in amenorrhea, 1200, 1201
deficiency of, 1108, 1109, 1189–1190, 1189t. *See also* Hypogonadism
gynecomastia and, 1195
in hirsutism/virilization, 1197
in hypogonadism, 1109, 1110, 1189–1190, 1189t, 1191
hypopituitarism caused by defects in gene for, 1108
in infertility workup, 784, 969–970
in polycystic ovary syndrome, 781, 1196
Luteinizing hormone-releasing hormone (LHRH) analogs
in cancer chemotherapy, 1670t

for prostate cancer, 1649–1650, 1649t
for psychosexual disorders, 1063
Luteinizing hormone-releasing hormone (LHRH) antagonist, in cancer chemotherapy, 1670t
for prostate cancer, 1649–1650, 1649t
Luteoma of pregnancy, virilization and, 1197
Luvox. *See* Fluvoxamine
LVEDP. *See* Left ventricular end-diastolic pressure
LVEF. *See* Left ventricular ejection fraction
LVH. *See* Left ventricular hypertrophy
LVRS. *See* Lung volume reduction surgery
Lyme disease (Lyme borreliosis), 1312t, **1501–1506**, 1505t
anaplasmosis and, 1436, 1504
arthritis in, 1502–1503, 1505, 1505t
gonococcal arthritis differentiated from, 869
nongonococcal (septic) arthritis differentiated from, 867
rheumatoid arthritis differentiated from, 836
babesiosis and, 1504
CDC guidelines for laboratory evaluation of, 1503–1504
chronic (post-Lyme disease syndrome), 1504, 1505t
coinfections and, 1436, 1504
erythema migrans in, **136**, 137f, 1502, 1504, 1505t
facial palsy and, 1041, 1041f, 1502, 1504–1505, 1505t
head and neck manifestations of, **239**
myopericarditis in, 425, 1502, 1505, 1505t
neurologic disorders/neuropathy associated with, 1037, 1041, 1041f, 1502, 1503, 1504–1505, 1505t
during pregnancy, 1504, 1505
prevention of, 1504
serologic testing in, 1503–1504
treatment of, 1312t, 1504–1505, 1505t
Lyme urinary antigen test, 1503, 1504
Lymph nodes. *See specific nodes and* Lymphadenitis; Lymphadenopathy
Lymphadenectomy, selective (sentinel lymph node biopsy)
in breast cancer, 750, 750f
arm edema avoidance and, 759
timing of/neoadjuvant therapy and, 753–754
in melanoma, 104
Lymphadenitis, **491–492**. *See also specific cause*
in filariasis, 1543, 1543f, 1544
histiocytic necrotizing (Kikuchi disease), 239
mycobacterial (tuberculous and nontuberculous), **239**, 1345, **1482**
in plague, 1474
Lymphadenopathy. *See also specific cause*
autoimmune, 239
dermatopathic, 116

HIV, 239, 1333
eustachian tube dysfunction/serous otitis media and, 214
reactive cervical, **239**
tick-borne/Dermacentor-borne-necrosis-erythema-lymphadenopathy/ scalp eschar neck lymphadenopathy, 1429t, 1434
Lymphangitic carcinomatosis, 1613, 1614
Lymphangitis, **491–492**, 1315t
in filariasis, 1543, 1543f, 1544
rickettsiosis associated with, 1429t, 1434
Lymphatic channel diseases, **491–493**
Lymphatic filariasis, **1543–1544**, 1543f
Lymphedema, **492–493**, 493f
chronic venous insufficiency differentiated from, 489
Lymphoblastic lymphoma, 533
Lymphocytic choriomeningitis, **1392–1393**
Lymphocytic colitis, 662
Lymphocytic hypophysitis, 1108, 1111, 1112
Lymphocytic meningitis, benign recurrent (Mollaret meningitis), 1364
Lymphocytoma, borrelial, 1502
Lymphocytosis, diffuse infiltrative, 869
Lymphoepithelioma, nasopharyngeal, 223
Lymphogranuloma venereum, 671, **1485**
Lymphohistiocytosis, hemophagocytic, 1373
Lymphoma, **531–539**, 532t, 1608t, 1622t. *See also* Burkitt lymphoma; Hodgkin lymphoma; Non-Hodgkin lymphoma
aggressive, 533
B-cell. *See* B-cell lymphoma
classification of, 531–532, 532t
common variable immunodeficiency and, 882
cutaneous T-cell (mycosis fungoides), **116–117**
exfoliative dermatitis/erythroderma and, 117
"double-hit," 533
fever/FUO and, 1288
follicular, 531, 532
gastric, 532, **1632–1633**
H pylori infection and, 532, 622, 1632
head and neck, **240**
high-grade, 533
in HIV infection/AIDS, 1004t, 1006, 1337t, 1338–1339, 1339, 1344
of kidney, 1655
large cell (Richter syndrome), 530
lymphoblastic, 533
mantle cell, 533
marginal zone, 532
mucosa-associated lymphoid tissue (MALToma)
gastric, 532, 1632
H pylori infection and, 532, 622, 1632
intestinal, 1634
of thyroid, 1142, 1145, 1148

Lymphoma (*Cont.*):
nose and paranasal sinus involvement and, 223
pemphigus and, 139
primary cerebral/central nervous system, 533, 1004*t*, 1006, 1337*t*, 1339, 1344
primary effusion (body cavity), 1377
small intestine, **1634**
Crohn disease and, 654, 1634
small lymphocytic, 532
stem cell transplantation for, 532, 533, 540
T-cell. *See* Human T cell lymphotropic/leukemia virus; T-cell lymphoma
tacrolimus/pimecrolimus associated with, 105
testicular, 1657
of thyroid, 1142, 1145, 1148
Lymphopenia, idiopathic CD4, progressive multifocal leukoencephalopathy in, 1395
Lymphoproliferative disorder
posttransplant, 1288, 1373–1374
X-linked, Epstein-Barr infection and, 1373
Lynch syndrome (hereditary nonpolyposis colon cancer/HNPCC), **668–669**, 1637
endometrial carcinoma and, 668, 669, 774
pancreatic/periampullary carcinoma and, 1620
ureteral/renal pelvis cancer and, 1653
Lynparza. *See* Olaparib
Lysergic acid diethylamide (LSD), 1099, **1598**

M2 inhibitors (amantadine/rimantadine), influenza/influenza resistance and, 1365*t*, 1412, 1418
M184V mutation, antiretroviral resistance and, 1361, 1362
M918T mutation, medullary thyroid carcinoma and, 1148
M-protein, 535, 536
Ma huang, toxicity of, 1593
MAC infections. *See* Mycobacterium (mycobacterial infections), *avium* complex
Machupo virus, 1399, 1400
Macroglobulinemia
neuropathy associated with, 1037
Waldenström. *See* Waldenström macroglobulinemia
Macrolides. *See also specific agent and* Erythromycin
for pharyngitis, 229, 1442
for pneumonia, 269*t*, 270–271, 271
pneumonia resistant to, 269*t*, 270–271, 271
Macrophage activation syndrome, 839
Macroprolactin/macroprolactinemia/macroprolactinoma, 1117, 1118
Macropsia, intracranial tumors causing, 1003

MACS (Manchester Acute Coronary Syndromes) decision rule, in chest pain evaluation, 28
Macugen. *See* Pegaptanib
Macular degeneration, age-related, **185–186**
Maculopathy/macular edema
age-related, 185
diabetic, 190, 1238
in retinal vein occlusion, 186
thiazolidinedione use and, 1225
Mad cow disease (vCJD/bovine spongiform encephalopathy), 1394
Maddrey discriminant function index, in alcoholic liver disease, 694
MADH4 gene, in familial juvenile polyposis, 667
Maduromycosis (eumycetoma), **1557**
MAG. *See* Myelin-associated glycoprotein
Magnesium
calcium balance/hypocalcemia and, 896, 897, 901, 902
dietary/supplementary
for hypocalcemia/hypoparathyroidism/tetany, 897, 1151
for hypomagnesemia, 902
after parathyroidectomy, 1158
requirements for in nutritional support, 1282
disorders of concentration of, 892*t*, **901–903**, 902*t*. *See also* Hypermagnesemia; Hypomagnesemia
genetic disorders and, 892*t*
normal values for, 901
potassium balance/hypokalemia and, 891–892, 893, 902
urinary excretion of, in hypomagnesemia, 902
Magnesium-ammonium-phosphate (struvite) urinary stones, 961, 962, 964
Magnesium chloride. *See* Magnesium, dietary/supplementary
Magnesium citrate, for constipation/bowel cleansing, 585*t*, 586
Magnesium hydroxide, 585*t*, 586
Magnesium oxide. *See* Magnesium, dietary/supplementary
Magnesium salicylate, 76*t*
choline, 75*t*
Magnesium sulfate
for asthma, 254
for eclampsia, 810
hypermagnesemia and, 810, 901, 902–903
for hypomagnesemia, 902
for preterm labor, 812
Magnetic resonance angiography (MRA), in renal artery stenosis/renal vascular hypertension, 442, 931
Magnetic resonance cholangiopancreatography (MRCP), 677
in pregnant patient, 824
Magnetic resonance imaging (MRI). *See also specific disorder and* Neuroimaging

in breast cancer evaluation/screening, 15, 740, 742, 745
cardiac
in angina/chest pain, 28, 358
in cardiomyopathy, 416, 416*t*, 419
in heart failure, 404
in myocardial infarction, 371
in pericarditis/effusion, 426, 428, 429
in hyperparathyroidism, 1155
in hyperthyroidism, 1128
in pheochromocytoma/paraganglioma, 1182
in prostate cancer, 1645
in thyroid cancer evaluation/follow-up, 1142
Mahaim fibers, in preexcitation syndromes, 387
Maisonneuve fracture, 1716
Major depressive disorder, 1075, 1079. *See also* Depression
in older adults, 60–61
Makona virus, 1397
Malabsorption, 592, **632–638**, 633*t*. *See also specific disorder or cause*
bacterial overgrowth causing, 592, 594, **636–637**
in celiac disease, **632–635**
in Crohn disease, 654
diarrhea caused by, 588*t*, 591, 592, 633*t*
HIV infection/AIDS, 1335, 1342
in lactase deficiency, **637–638**
in scleroderma, 846
in short bowel syndrome, **637**
in Whipple disease, **635–636**
Malar rash
in dermatomyositis, 848, 848*f*
in SLE, 839*t*, 840
Malaria, **1512–1521**
cerebral, 1513
congenital, 1513, 1521
drug resistance in, 1515, 1516, 1517
G6PD deficiency and, 510–511
laboratory findings in, 1514, 1514*f*
non-falciparum, 1515
during pregnancy, 1513, 1521
treatment/chemoprophylaxis and, 802, 1521
prevention of, 1520–1521, 1520*t*. *See also* Antimalarial agents
self-treatment and, 1520
severe, 1513, 1516, 1517*t*, 1519, 1521
treatment of, 1514–1520, 1515*t*, 1516*t*, 1517*t*. *See also* Antimalarial agents
uncomplicated falciparum, 1515–1516, 1516*t*, 1517*t*, 1521
vaccine development and, 1520
Malarone (atovaquone-proguanil), 1515*t*, 1517*t*, 1519
for chemoprophylaxis, 1519, 1520, 1520*t*
self treatment and, 1520
Malassezia furfur
folliculitis caused by, 130, 131
seborrheic dermatitis in HIV caused by, 1343
tinea versicolor caused by, 114
Malathion lotion, for pediculosis, 150
Malathion poisoning, 1601–1602

Male breast
  carcinoma of, **760–761**
  disorders/enlargement of, **1194–1196**,
    1195t. *See also* Gynecomastia
Male erectile dysfunction. *See* Erectile
    dysfunction/impotence
Male infertility. *See* Infertility
Male pattern (androgenetic) alopecia,
    158–159
  in women, 159
Malignancy-related DIC, 553
Malignant ascites, 601, 601t, **604**, 1658,
    1659
Malignant effusions, 312, 312–313, 313t,
    425, 426, 426–427, 428,
    1658–1659. *See also specific*
    type
Malignant external otitis, 202
Malignant hypertension, 468. *See also*
    Hypertensive emergencies
Malignant hyperthermia, 35, 1294, 1580
Malignant melanoma. *See* Melanoma
Malignant neoplastic disease. *See* Cancer
Malignant pleural mesothelioma, 309,
    1614, 1615
Mallory hyalin, 697
Mallory/Mallory-Denk bodies, in
    alcoholic liver disease, 694
Mallory-Weiss syndrome/tears, 582, 595,
    596, 612
Malnutrition. *See also* Nutritional
    disorders
  neuropathy associated with, 1036
  protein–energy, **1268–1269**
Malocclusion (dental), facial pain and, 982
MALT lymphoma (MALToma)
  gastric, 532, 1632
    H pylori infection and, 532, 622,
      1632
  intestinal, 1634
  thyroid, 1142, 1145, 1148
Maltese crosses, 942
Mammographic localization biopsy, 744
Mammography, 14–15, 14t, 739–740,
    740–741, 742, 743f, 744f
  breast implants and, 737
  in breast lump evaluation, 14–15, 14t,
    739–740, 740–741, 742, 743f,
    744f
  computerized stereotactic guided core
    needle biopsy and, 744
  digital, 15, 740
  follow-up/cancer recurrence and, 758
  localization biopsy and, 744
  pregnancy and, 745
Mammoplasty, augmentation. *See* Breast
    implants
Manchester Acute Coronary Syndromes
    (MACS) decision rule, in
    chest pain evaluation, 28
Mania/manic episodes, 1074, 1075–1076,
    1084–1087, 1087t. *See also*
    Bipolar disorder
  drug therapy for, 1084–1087, 1087t
  ECT for, 1083
  lithium for, 1084, 1085–1087, 1087t
  prognosis for, 1087–1088
  schizophrenia and, 1066, 1067
  sleep-wake disorders and, 1088
Manic-depressive disorder. *See* Bipolar
    disorder

Manic psychosis, 1067
Mannitol
  for ciguatera poisoning, 1603
  lithium interactions and, 1087t
Manometry, esophageal, 606
  in motility disorders, 606, 618
Mansonella/Mansonella perstans, filariasis
    caused by, 1543, 1544
Mantle cell lymphoma, 533
  bone marrow/stem cell transplantation
    for, 533, 540
Mantoux test, 279, 280t. *See also*
    Tuberculin skin test
MAO inhibitors (MAOIs). *See*
    Monoamine oxidase
    inhibitors
Maple bark stripper's disease, 308t
Maprotiline, 1078t
Marasmus/marasmus-like secondary
    protein–energy malnutrition,
    1268
Maraviroc, 1352t, 1357–1358. *See also*
    Antiretroviral therapy
Marfan syndrome, **1682–1683**
  aortic disorders (dissection/aneurysm/
    regurgitation) in, 345, 346,
    1682, 1683
  pregnancy and, 435, 436, 1683
  mitral valve prolapse and, 340, 1682
  sudden death of athlete and, 436, 437
"Marginal blepharitis," 110, 165
Marginal zone lymphoma, 532
Marijuana, **1099–1100**
  for nausea and vomiting, 83, 87, 583.
    See also Dronabinol
  in HIV infection AIDS, 1335
  for neuropathic pain, 84
  for wasting, 1335
Marine-Lenhart syndrome, 1125
Marqibo. *See* Liposomal vincristine
MARS. *See* Molecular adsorbent
    recirculating system
Marshall scoring system, modified, in
    pancreatitis, 726
MASCC (Multinational Association for
    Supportive Care in Cancer)
    score, 35
Mask of pregnancy (melasma/chloasma),
    157, 158
"Masked hypertension," 439
Mast cell stabilizers/mediator inhibitors.
    See also Cromolyn;
    Nedocromil
  for allergic eye disease, 168, 170t,
    170–171t
  for allergic rhinitis, 220
  for asthma, 248–251, 249t
Mast cells, in allergic/pseudoallergic
    reactions, 876, 878
Mastalgia (breast pain), 734, 735, 741,
    745
Mastectomy, 749, 750
  arm edema after, 759
  breast reconstruction/implants after,
    737, 750, 759
  cancer recurrence and, 758, 759
  for inflammatory carcinoma, 745
  in male, 760
  for noninvasive (ductal/lobular)
    carcinoma, 748
  partial. *See* Lumpectomy

  for phyllodes tumor of breast, 735
  prophylactic, 738
Mastitis, puerperal, 133, **813–814**
Mastocytosis, 879t
Mastoiditis, 204, 206
Match test, 20
Maternally inherited diabetes and
    deafness (MIDD), 1212
Matulane. *See* Procarbazine
Maturity-onset diabetes of young
    (MODY), 1211t, 1212, 1235
Mavik. *See* Trandolapril
MAX mutations, in pheochromocytoma/
    paraganglioma, 1180
Maxillary sinusitis, 215
Maximum laryngeal height, in dyspnea/
    COPD, 22–23, 23t
Maxipime. *See* Cefepime
Maxzide. *See* Triamterene, with
    hydrochlorothiazide
May-Thurner syndrome, 32
Mayer-Rokitansky-Küster-Hauser
    syndrome, 1199
Mayo risk score, 707, 724
Maze procedure, 336
Mazzotti test, 1545
MC2R (melanocortin 2 receptor), familial
    glucocorticoid deficiency
    and, 1169
McConnell taping, for patellofemoral
    pain, 1713
McCune-Albright syndrome, 1114, 1189
MCKD1/MCKD2 genes, medullary
    sponge kidney and, 950
MCL. *See* Medial collateral ligament
McMurray test, 1708t, 1712
MCV. *See* Mean cell/corpuscular volume
MCV/MCV4 vaccine. *See* Meningococcal
    vaccine
MDA5 antibody, in polymyositis/
    dermatomyositis, 848t
MDIs. *See* Metered-dose inhalers
MDMA (methylenedioxy-
    methamphetamine), 1101,
    1587
  hyponatremia caused by, 886, 1588
  seizures caused by, 1580t
MDPV (methylenedioxypyrovalerone),
    1587
MDR. *See* Multidrug resistance
MDRTB. *See* Multidrug resistance, in
    tuberculosis
MDS. *See* Myelodysplastic syndromes
Meal replacement diets, 1270, 1271
Mean cell/corpuscular volume (MCV)
  in alcohol use disorder, 1094
  in anemia classification, 499, 500t.
    See also specific disorder
Measles (rubeola), 1367t, **1377–1380**
  atypical, 1367t
  prevention/immunization and, 1378,
    1379–1380. *See also* MMR
    (measles-mumps-rubella)
    vaccine
Measles encephalitis, 1378–1379
Measles immune globulin, 1379
Measles-mumps-rubella vaccine. *See*
    MMR (measles-mumps-
    rubella) vaccine
Measles-mumps-rubella-varicella vaccine
    (MMRV), 1371, 1379

Measles vaccine, 1323t, 1379–1380. *See also* MMR (measles-mumps-rubella) vaccine
Mebendazole
for ascariasis, 1538
for enterobiasis/pinworms, 1541
for hookworm disease, 1539
for hydatid disease, 1537
for trichinosis, 1542
for trichuriasis/whipworm, 1539
Mechanical ventilation
for ARDS, 320
for asthma, 257
complications of, 319
for COPD, 262
pneumonia and (ventilator-associated pneumonia), 272–274, 273t, 275t, 319, 1294
for respiratory failure, 319
tracheotomy for, 237–238
withdrawal of, in end-of-life care, 91–92, 92t
Mechanic's hands, 848
Mechlorethamine, 1663t
Meclizine, 583
Meclofenamate, 76t
Meclomen. *See* Meclofenamate
Medial collateral ligament, 1704, 1710
injury of, 1707t, 1710–1711
Medial epicondylosis, **1697–1698**
Medial meniscus, 1704
injury of, 1708–1709t
Median nerve compression, in carpal tunnel syndrome, 1698, 1699
Mediastinal masses, **288–289**
Mediastinal widening, drug-induced, 310t
Mediastinitis, in histoplasmosis, 1549
Mediastinoscopy, in lung cancer, 1609
Mediator inhibitors. *See* Mast cell stabilizers/mediator inhibitors
Medical cannabis. *See* Marijuana
Medical curettage, 763
Medical imaging. *See also specific disorder and under* Radiation
radiation exposure/cancer risk and, 1571, 1572, 1607
Medical interview, 1–2
Medical marijuana. *See* Marijuana
Medical (or Physician) Orders for Life-Sustaining Treatment (MOLST/POLST) forms, 90
Medication diversion, long-term opioid therapy and, 74, 85
Medication-induced lung disease, 290t, **309**, 310t
Medication overuse headache, **980**
Medications. *See also under* Drug
adherence to regimen for, 1–2
elderly patients and, 69
use of during pregnancy, 798t, 799
Medicinal herbs, toxicity of, **1593–1594**, 1593t
Mediterranean diet, 1262, 1263
Mediterranean fever, familial, **604**
Mediterranean spotted fever, 1429t, 1434
Medrol Dosepak. *See* Methylprednisolone
Medroxyprogesterone (DMPA)
for abnormal uterine bleeding, 763
for contraceptive injection, 788

for endometriosis, 776
in hormone replacement therapy, 795, 1204, 1205
for postmenopausal bleeding, 764
for premenstrual syndrome, 765
for psychosexual disorders, 1063
Medullary cystic kidney, 949t, **951**
Medullary sponge kidney, 949t, **950–951**
Medulloblastoma, 1004t
Mefenamic acid, 76t
for premenstrual syndrome, 765
Mefloquine, 1515t, 1517–1518, 1517t
with artesunate, 1516t, 1517, 1519
for chemoprophylaxis, 1517, 1517–1518, 1520, 1520t
rabies vaccination and, 1327
Megace. *See* Megestrol
Megacolon, toxic
acute colonic pseudo-obstruction (Ogilvie syndrome) differentiated from, 640
in ulcerative colitis, 660
Megaesophagus, 618
Megaloblastic anemia, 499, 500t
folic acid deficiency causing, 508
subacute combined degeneration of spinal cord and, 1026
vitamin B$_{12}$ deficiency causing, 507
fish tapeworm infection and, 506–507, 1535
Megestrol
for breast cancer, 755, 755t
in elderly, 67
for HIV wasting, 1335
Meglitinide analogs, 1221t, 1223
Meglumine antimonate, for leishmaniasis, 1511–1512
Meibomian gland
abscess of (internal hordeolum), 164–165
inflammation of
blepharitis and, 165
chalazion and, 165
Mekinist. *See* Trametinib
Melancholic depression, 1075, 1079. *See also* Depression
Melanocortin 2 receptor (MC2R), familial glucocorticoid deficiency and, 1169
Melanocyte-stimulating hormone, alpha (alpha-MSH), in adrenal insufficiency/Addison disease, 1168, 1170
Melanocytic nevi (normal moles), **101–102**, 101f
Melanoma, **103–104**, 104f, 1608t, 1625t
atypical nevi and, 102
blue nevi and, 102
familial, 102
pancreatic/periampullary carcinoma and, 1620
Melanosis, arsenical, 157
Melarsoprol, for African trypanosomiasis, 1508, 1508t
MELAS syndrome, 1049
Melasma (chloasma), 157, 158
MELD (Model for End-Stage Liver Disease) score, 705, 705t
in alcoholic liver disease/cirrhosis, 694, 695, 704, 705, 705t
hepatocellular carcinoma and, 1617

in liver failure/hepatic encephalopathy, 685
postoperative complications and, 50
Melena, 594, 598, 599, 629
Melioidosis, 1312t
Mellaril. *See* Thioridazine
Melody valve, 350
Meloxicam, 621
Melphalan, 1663t
Memantine, for dementia, 59, 1021, 1104
Membranoproliferative glomerulonephritis/glomerulonephropathy, 933t, 934t, 935f, **939–940**
hepatitis C and, 683, 933t, 940
Membranous nephropathy, 934t, **944–945**
hepatitis C infection and, 940
Memory impairment
in dementia/delirium, 57, 58, 1020, 1102
ECT and, 1083–1084
MEN. *See* Multiple endocrine neoplasia
MenACWY vaccine. *See* Meningococcal vaccine
Menarche, 1199
failure of. *See* Amenorrhea
MenB vaccines. *See* Meningococcal vaccine
Mendelson syndrome, **305–306**, 1294
Menest, 1204
Ménière disease (endolymphatic hydrops), 211–212, 211t
menin gene, in MEN 1, 1187
Meningeal irritation, noninfectious, 1298
Meningiomas, 1003, 1004t, 1005
Meningismus, 1298. *See also specific infection*
Meningitis, 1297–1298, 1297t. *See also* Meningoencephalitis
aseptic/viral, 1297t, 1298. *See also specific agent and* Aseptic meningitis
benign recurrent lymphocytic (Mollaret), 1364
carcinomatous (le[...]
metasta[...]
chronic, 1298
in coccidioidomy[...]
1550–1[...]
in Colorado tick [...]
coxsackieviruses [...]
cryptococcal, 10[...]
1553–[...]
CSF analysis in, [...]
echoviruses caus[...]
Elizabethkingia [...]
fungal, 1297t
H influenzae causing, 1311t, 1466
health care–associated, 1298, 1299
herpes simplex, 1364, 1366
in HIV infection/AIDS (cryptococcal), 1006, 1337t, 1340, 1553, 1554
leptospiral, 1500, 1501
in listeriosis, 1297t, 1314t, 1457
in Lyme disease, 1502, 1505
meningococcal, 1297t, 1314t, 1326, **1464–1466**
prevention/immunization and, 1326, 1465. *See also* Meningococcal vaccine
in mumps, 1380, 1381

otogenic, 206
in plague, 1474
pneumococcal, 1297t, 1299, 1314t, **1447**
prevention of. *See* Pneumococcal vaccine
in poliomyelitis (nonparalytic), 1382, 1383
purulent/bacterial, 1297, 1297t, 1299, 1314t
partially treated, 1298
in syphilis, 1489t, 1493, 1496
in toxocariasis, 1542
tuberculous, 283, **1483–1484**
Meningococcal (*Neisseria meningitidis*) infections, 1311t
meningitis, 1297t, 1314t, 1326, **1464–1466**
nasopharyngeal carriage and, 1464, 1465
prevention/immunization and. *See* Meningococcal vaccine
Meningococcal vaccine, 1320t, 1321t, 1325t, 1326, 1465
adverse effects/contraindications and, 1328t
in immunocompromised host/HIV infection/AIDS, 1321t, 1465
for travelers, 1325t, 1326
Meningococcemia, 1368t, 1464
adrenal crisis and (Waterhouse-Friderichsen syndrome), 1169
Meningoencephalitis, 1297t. *See also* Encephalitis; Meningitis
in African trypanosomiasis, 1507, 1508
travel and, 1309
Meningovascular syphilis, 1489t, 1496. *See also* Neurosyphilis
Meniscal cartilage, of knee, 1704, 1711
injuries/tears of, 1708–1709t, **1711–1712**
Menopause/menopausal syndrome, **794–796**
early and premature, 794, 1201
estrogen replacement therapy for. *See* Estrogen (hormone) replacement therapy
normal/typical, 1201
osteoporosis and, 795, 1160
surgical, 796, 1201
vaginal bleeding after. *See* Postmenopausal vaginal bleeding
Menorrhagia, 762
iron deficiency anemia and, 500
IUD use and, 790
Menostar, 1204
Menstruation/menstrual cycle, 762. *See also* Vaginal bleeding
abnormalities of, in polycystic ovary syndrome, 780, 1196
asthma associated with (catamenial asthma), 242
cessation of, 794, 1201. *See also* Amenorrhea; Menopause
failure to appear. *See* Amenorrhea
iron deficiency anemia and, 500
IUD affecting bleeding in, 790
pain associated with. *See* Dysmenorrhea

pneumothorax associated with (catamenial pneumothorax), 314
Mental retardation
in Down syndrome, 1678
fragile, X, **1679–1680**
Mental status, altered. *See also* Cognitive disorders
in HIV infection/AIDS, 1339
Mentax. *See* Butenafine
Mepacrine. *See* Quinacrine
Meperidine, 79t
MAOI interactions and, 1083t
for myocardial infarction, 375
overdose/toxicity of, 1601
Mephedrone, toxicity of, 1598
Meralgia paresthetica, **1040**
Mercaptopurine, 1664t
for inflammatory bowel disease, 650–651
with anti-TNF agents, 656–657
Crohn disease, 656, 657
ulcerative colitis, 659
thiopurine methyltransferase variants and, 651
Mercury poisoning, 1581t, **1598–1599**
marijuana use and, 1099
tubulointerstitial disease and, 947
Mericitabine, for hepatitis C, 691
Merlin gene, in neurofibromatosis, 1010
Meropenem
for anaerobic infections, 1479t
for pneumonia, 269t, 271
Merrem. *See* Meropenem
MERRF syndrome, 1049
MERS-CoV (Middle East respiratory syndrome–coronavirus), **1419–1420**
Mesalamine, for inflammatory bowel disease, 650
Crohn disease, 655
ulcerative colitis, 659
Mescaline, 1099, 1598
Mesenchymal tumors, gastrointestinal, **1633–1634**
Mesenteric adenitis, adenoviruses causing, 1421
Mesenteric ischemia/mesenteric artery occlusive disease, 479
Mesenteric vascular insufficiency, nonocclusive, 479
Mesenteric vasculitis
in polyarteritis nodosa, 856
in SLE, 840
Mesenteric vein occlusion, **480**
Mesial temporal sclerosis, epilepsy/ seizures caused by, 983
Mesna, for hemorrhagic cystitis, 1671t, 1674
Mesnex. *See* Mesna
Mesothelioma, **1614–1616**, 1623t
asbestos exposure and, 309, 1615
Metabolic acidosis, 903, **904–905**, 904t. *See also* specific type or cause
anion gap. *See* Anion gap/anion gap acidosis
drowning and, 1567
in kidney disease/renal failure, 906, 916, 928. *See also* Renal tubular acidosis

nephrolithiasis/nephrocalcinosis/ urolithiasis and, 906–907, 962
parenteral nutritional support and, 907, 1285t
in poisoning/drug overdose, 1584
corrosive acids and, 1586
with methanol or ethylene glycol, 906, 1584, 1599
with salicylates, 906, 1603
posthypocapnia, 907
respiratory alkalosis and, 907, 911
Metabolic alkalosis, 903, 904t, **908–910**, 910t. *See also* specific cause
alcoholic ketoacidosis and, 906
posthypercapnia, 909
respiratory acidosis and, 910
saline-responsive, 908–909, 909t, 910
saline-unresponsive, 909, 909t, 910
Metabolic bone disease, **1159–1168**. *See also* specific disorder
in chronic kidney disease (renal osteodystrophy), 927–928, 927f, 1153, 1155
Metabolic disturbances
antipsychotic drug use and, 1072
cognitive disorders/delirium caused by, 1102t
coma or stupor caused by, 1027, **1028**
dysphagia in, 605t
epilepsy and, 983
neuropathies associated with, **1036–1037**
nutritional support and, 1284, 1285, 1285t
in pheochromocytoma/paraganglioma, 1180t
Metabolic encephalopathy
cancer-related, 1008
coma or stupor caused by, 1028
Metabolic syndrome, 12, 353, 1213. *See also* Insulin resistance/ insensitivity
coronary heart disease and, 353
diabetes and, 1213
hepatocellular carcinoma and, 1616
hypertension and, 441
nonalcoholic fatty liver disease and, 697
obesity and, 12, 1270
polycystic ovary syndrome and, 780
Metaglip. *See* Glipizide, with metformin
Metagonimus flukes, 1535
Metanephrines, in pheochromocytoma/ paraganglioma, 1181, 1181–1182, 1181t
Metapneumovirus, human, 1409, 1410
Metaproterenol, for COPD, 260
Metered-dose inhalers
for asthma therapy, 248, 250t, 252, 253t, 255f
for COPD therapy, 260, 262
Metformin
antipsychotic drug-related weight gain and, 1072
for diabetes mellitus, 1221t, 1223–1224, 1235–1236, 1235f
in combination preparations/ regimens, 1223, 1224, 1227, 1228

Metformin, for diabetes mellitus (*Cont.*):
hospitalization/surgery and, 1243
with insulin, 1236
intensive therapy with, 1218
prevention and, 1218
for hirsutism/virilization, 1198
lactic acidosis and, 1224, 1251, 1595
for polycystic ovary syndrome, 781
Methadone, 74, 79*t*, 82
for heroin/opioid withdrawal/
maintenance, 17, 1098–1099,
1099
overdose/toxicity of, 82, 1601
for pain management, 74, 79*t*, 82
Methamphetamine, 17, 1100, 1587
Methanol poisoning, 1581*t*, 1584*t*, **1599**
anion gap/osmolar gap in, 891, 906,
1584, 1599
ethanol for, 908, 1581*t*, 1584*t*, 1599
hemodialysis for, 1583*t*, 1584*t*, 1599
Methazolamide
adverse ophthalmic effects of, 177*t*
for glaucoma/ocular hypertension, 180
Methcathinone, 1587
Methemoglobinemia, 1584*t*, **1599–1600**
Methergine, avoidance of with
antiretroviral therapy, 822
Methicillin-resistant *S aureus* (MRSA)
infections, 1311*t*, 1447–1448,
1448*f*
arthritis, 867
cellulitis, 138
community-acquired pneumonia, 269,
269*t*, 271
endocarditis, 1462
health care/hospital-associated,
1295–1296, 1296
in HIV infection/AIDS, 1343
impetigo, 124
mastitis, 814
nosocomial pneumonia, 273, 273*t*,
275*t*
skin/soft tissue infections, 1343,
1447–1448, 1448*f*
Methicillin-susceptible *S aureus* (MSSA)
infections, cellulitis, 138
Methimazole
autoimmune hypoglycemia and, 1257
for hyperthyroidism/Graves disease,
1129
amiodarone-induced, 1132
during pregnancy/lactation, 816,
1129, 1132
RAI therapy and, 1129, 1130
thyroid crisis/storm and, 1133
toxic multinodular goiter and, 1131
toxic solitary thyroid nodule and,
1131
Methionine, in homocystinuria/
hyperhomocysteinemia, 1681
Methocarbamol, for black widow spider
bites, 1605
Methotrexate, 1663*t*
for breast cancer, 751
for ectopic pregnancy, 806
for elective abortion, 792
folinic acid/leucovorin/levoleucovorin
rescue and, 108, 651, 837,
1671*t*, 1674
for granulomatosis with polyangiitis,
859

for inflammatory bowel/Crohn disease,
651, 656
with anti-TNF agents, 656–657
for psoriasis/psoriatic arthritis, 108,
865
for rheumatoid arthritis, 837
toxicity of, 108, 651, 837, 1663*t*, 1673,
1674
Methyl alcohol. *See* Methanol
Methyl salicylate. *See also* Salicylates
overdose/toxicity of, 1602–1603
Methylcellulose, 585*t*. *See also* Fiber,
dietary
Methylcobalamin, 507–508. *See also*
Vitamin B$_{12}$
Methyldopa, 462*t*
antidepressant drug interactions and,
1083*t*
for hypertension, 462*t*, 464
during pregnancy, 818
lithium interactions and, 1087*t*
MAOI interactions and, 1083*t*
overdose/toxicity of, 462*t*, 464, 1592
Methylene blue, for methemoglobinemia,
1584*t*, 1600
Methylenedioxymethamphetamine. *See*
MDMA
Methylenedioxypyrovalerone (MDPV),
1587
Methylnaltrexone, for opioid-induced
constipation, 86, 586
Methylphenidate
abuse/overdose of, 1100
for depression, 1082
Methylprednisolone. *See also*
Corticosteroids
for adrenal insufficiency/Addison
disease, 1111, 1171
for alcoholic liver disease, 694
for allergic contact dermatitis,
inappropriateness of, 126
for asthma, 249*t*, 252, 253*t*
for inflammatory bowel disease, 650
Crohn disease, 655–656
ulcerative colitis, 659, 660
for multiple sclerosis, 1024, 1024*t*
for nausea and vomiting, 582*t*
4-Methylpyrazole. *See* Fomepizole
Methyltestosterone
with estrogens, 1206
oral, for male hypogonadism, 1193
Methylxanthines, for asthma, 250*t*
Metipranolol, for glaucoma/ocular
hypertension, 172*t*
Metoclopramide
for dyspepsia, 580
for gastroparesis, 641
for migraine headache, 978
for nausea and vomiting, 83, 87,
582*t*
tardive dyskinesia caused by, 580
Metolazone
for acute tubular necrosis, 920
for heart failure, 406
for hypertension, 450*t*
Metoprolol, 382*t*, 453*t*
for acute coronary syndromes/STEMI,
368, 375
for arrhythmias, 382*t*
atrial fibrillation, 389
infarct-related, 377

supraventricular tachycardia, 382*t*,
386
for heart failure, 407–408, 454
for hypertension, 453*t*, 454
with hydrochlorothiazide, 453*t*
pheochromocytoma/
pheochromocytoma surgery
and, 1183
Metritis, **814**, 820. *See also* Endometritis
Metronidazole
for amebiasis, 1526, 1527, 1527*t*
for anaerobic infections, 1478, 1479,
1479*t*
pneumonia/lung abscess, 276
for antibiotic-associated colitis, 649
for bacterial vaginosis, 768
for Crohn disease, 655, 657
for giardiasis, 1530–1531
in *H pylori* eradication therapy, 626,
626*t*
for rosacea, 129
for trichomoniasis, 767–768, 1531
Metrorrhagia, 762
Metyrapone, for hypercortisolism, 1176
Metyrosine, for pheochromocytoma/
paraganglioma, 1184
Mevacor. *See* Lovastatin
Mexiletine, 381, 382*t*
MF59, in CMV vaccine, 1376
Mg. *See* Magnesium
MGUS. *See* Monoclonal gammopathy of
unknown significance
MHA-TP test, 1490*t*
MI. *See* Myocardial infarction
Mi-2 antibody, in polymyositis/
dermatomyositis, 848, 848*t*
Miacalcin. *See* Calcitonin
MIC (minimal inhibitory concentration),
1317
Micafungin, 1559*t*
for candidiasis, 1548
Micardis/Micardis HCT. *See* Telmisartan
Miconazole, 98*t*
for vulvovaginal candidiasis, 133, 767,
1548
Micro-Coombs test. *See* Coombs test
Microangiopathic hemolytic anemias,
550, 551
Microangiopathy
in diabetes mellitus, 1241
thrombotic, **550–552**, 551*t*
Microbes. *See* Infection/infectious
diseases
Microcephaly, Zika virus infection and,
1406, 1407
Microglobulin, beta-2, in amyloidosis,
538
Microlithiasis (biliary sludge), 717
pancreatitis and, 726, 728, 729
Micronase. *See* Glyburide
Micronor. *See* Norethindrone
Microprolactinoma, 1117, 1118, 1119
Micropsia, intracranial tumors causing,
1003
Microsatellite instability, in colorectal
cancer/HNPCC/Lynch
syndrome, 665, 668, 1637
Microscopic colitis, 588*t*, 592, **662**
Microscopic polyangiitis, **859–860**
glomerulonephritis and, 859, 860, 922,
935*f*, 938

granulomatosis with polyangiitis
differentiated from, 858, 860
Microscopic urinalysis, 913. *See also*
Urinalysis
Microsporidiosis, 588*t*, 592, 1342,
1527–1530
Microsporum infection, tinea corporis/
circinata caused by, 112
Microwave hyperthermia, 976
Microzide. *See* Hydrochlorothiazide
Micturition. *See* Voiding
Midazolam, 1054*t*
for seizures
in poisoning/drug overdose, 1580
status epilepticus and, 989, 989–990
MIDD (maternally inherited diabetes and
deafness), 1212
Middle cerebral artery occlusion, in
stroke, 995
Middle ear, **204–207**, 205*f*, 207*f*
infection of. *See* Otitis, media
neoplasia of, **207**
trauma to, **207**, 207*f*
Middle East respiratory
syndrome–coronavirus
(MERS-CoV), **1419–1420**
Midline malignant reticulosis, 223
Midodrine, for autonomic dysfunction/
diabetic neuropathy, 1035
Midostaurin, for acute myeloid leukemia,
529
Mifepristone (RU 486)
for elective abortion, 792
clostridial infection after, 1452
for psychotic depression, 1079
Miglitol, 1221*t*, 1225
overdose/toxicity of, 1225, 1595
Miglustat, for Gaucher disease, 1680
Migraine equivalent, 977
Migraine headache, 40, 40*t*, **977–979**, 979*t*
nausea and vomiting in, 40, 40*t*, 581*t*,
977, 978
oral contraceptive use and, 786
prophylactic treatment of, 978–979,
979*t*
transient ischemic attacks
differentiated from, 992
vertigo/dizziness and, 211, 211*t*, 213
Migrainous vertigo, 211, 211*t*, 213
Milan criteria, 1617
Mild cognitive impairment, 58, 1018
Miliaria, **131**
crystallina/pustulosa/rubra, 131
"Miliary" tuberculosis, 279, 283
Milk-alkali syndrome, 897, 898, 909
Milk intolerance. *See* Lactose (milk)
intolerance
Milk thistle (silymarin), for mushroom
poisoning, 685–686, 1601
Milker's nodules (paravaccinia), 1423
Miller Fisher syndrome, 1038
poliomyelitis and, 1383
Milnacipran, 1078*t*, 1079–1081
Milrinone, for acute heart failure/
pulmonary edema, 412
Miltefosine, for leishmaniasis, 1512
Mineral oil/mineral oil enema, for
constipation, 585*t*
Mineralocorticoid replacement therapy,
for adrenal insufficiency/
Addison disease, 1171–1172

Mineralocorticoids. *See also* Aldosterone
apparent excess of, 442, 892*t*
deficiency of, 1169–1170. *See also*
Adrenal insufficiency
hyperkalemia and, 893
Minerals
metabolism of, chronic kidney disease/
renal osteodystrophy and,
927–928, 927*f*
requirements for in nutritional
support, 1282–1283
"Mini-cog" screening, in dementia, 58,
1020
Mini-Mental State Examination, in
dementia, 1020, 1103
Minimal change disease, 934*t*, **943**
Minimal inhibitory concentration (MIC),
1317
Minimally conscious state, **1029**
Minimally invasive coronary artery
bypass surgery, 363
Minimally invasive prostate surgery,
975–976
Minipill (progestin), 787*t*, 788
Minipress. *See* Prazosin
Minivivelle, 1204
Minnesota tube, for esophageal varices,
615
Minocycline
for acne, 127
adverse ophthalmic effects of, 178*t*
for rosacea, 129
for skin and soft tissue infections, 1448
Minoxidil, 463*t*
for androgenetic (male pattern)
alopecia, 158–159
in women, 159, 1198
for hypertension, 463*t*, 464
Miotics, for glaucoma/ocular
hypertension, 172*t*
Mirabegron, for urinary incontinence, 66
Miralax. *See* Polyethylene glycol
Miravirsen, for hepatitis C, 691
Mirena IUD, 789
in estrogen replacement therapy,
1205
Mirizzi syndrome, 719
Mirtazapine, 61, 83, 1077, 1078*t*,
1079–1081
Miscarriage. *See* Abortion
Mismatch repair gene defects, in
colorectal cancer/HNPCC/
Lynch syndrome, 665,
668–669, 1637
Misoprostol
for elective abortion, 792
for missed abortion, 804
for peptic ulcer disease/NSAID toxicity
mitigation, 625, 626*t*
Missed abortion, 804
Mistreatment (elder), 16, **70–71**, 71*t*
Mitchell-Riley syndrome, 1212
Mites
bird and rodent, 151
in rickettsial disease transmission,
1429*t*, 1431, 1434
skin lesions and, 151
in stored products, 151
trombiculid, 151
Miticides, for scrub typhus prevention,
1432

Mitiglinide, 1221*t*, 1223
Mitochondrial DNA mutations
in diabetes mellitus, 1211*t*, 1212
myopathies associated with, **1049**
Mitochondrial myopathies, **1049**
Mitomycin, 1669*t*
Mitotane
for ACTH-secreting adrenal tumor/
adrenocortical carcinoma,
1175–1176, 1176
hypopituitarism caused by, 1108–1109
TSH affected by, 1108–1109, 1109,
1176
Mitoxantrone, 1669*t*
for multiple sclerosis, 1024*t*
Mitral clip, 339
Mitral regurgitation/insufficiency,
332–334*t*, **337–339**, 338*f*. *See
also* Valvular heart disease
interventions affecting murmur in,
335*t*
mitral valve prolapse and, 340
in myocardial infarction, 338*f*, 339
Mitral stenosis, **331–337**, 332–334*t*, 336*f*.
See also Valvular heart
disease
pregnancy and, 335
Mitral valve
degenerative disease of (mitral valve
prolapse), **339–340**
parachute, 331–335
repair/replacement of, 335, 336, 336*f*,
337, 338*f*, 339, 340. *See also*
Valve replacement
in rheumatic fever/heart disease, 331,
335, 336*f*, 422
traumatic rupture of, 434
Mitral valve prolapse ("floppy"/
myxomatous mitral valve),
339–340
interventions affecting murmur in,
335*t*
in Marfan syndrome, 340, 1682
mitral regurgitation and, 340
in polycystic kidney disease, 950
Mittelschmerz, appendicitis differentiated
from, 642
Mixed acid-base disorders, **903–904**
alcoholic ketoacidosis and, 905
Mixed sleep apnea, 316
MLH1 gene, in colorectal cancer/
HNPCC/Lynch syndrome,
665, 668, 1637
pancreatic/periampullary carcinoma
and, 1620
MLL gene, in acute lymphoblastic
leukemia, 527
MLL-PTD mutation, in acute myeloid
leukemia, 527
MMR (measles-mumps-rubella) vaccine,
1320*t*, 1323*t*, 1378, 1379,
1381, 1385
adverse effects/contraindications and,
1321*t*, 1328*t*, 1380, 1385
encephalitis and, 1378
in immunocompromised host/HIV
infection/AIDS, 5, 1321*t*,
1349, 1380, 1385
pregnancy and, 1321*t*, 1323*t*, 1380,
1385
undervaccination and, 1378

MMRV (measles-mumps-rubella-varicella) vaccine, 1371, 1379
MMSE. *See* Mini-Mental State Examination
Mobility, limited/reduced. *See* Immobility
Mobitz type I (Wenckebach) atrioventricular block, 377, 399
Mobitz type II atrioventricular block, 377, 399
MoCA© (Montreal Cognitive Assessment), in dementia screening, 58, 1020
Modafinil
    for multiple sclerosis, 1025
    for sleep-wake disorders, 1090
Model for End-Stage Liver Disease (MELD) score, 705, 705t
    in alcoholic liver disease/cirrhosis, 694, 695, 704, 705t
    hepatocellular carcinoma and, 1617
    in liver failure/hepatic encephalopathy, 685
    postoperative complications and, 50
Modified Duke criteria, for endocarditis, 1460
Modified Marshall scoring system, in pancreatitis, 726
Modified McMurray test, 1708t, 1712
MODY. *See* Maturity-onset diabetes of young
Moexipril/moexipril with hydrochlorothiazide, 456t
Mohs surgery
    for basal cell carcinoma, 143
    for eyelid tumors, 165–166
    for squamous cell carcinoma, 144
Moisturizers (skin)/emollients, 95, 99–100t
Molar pregnancy, **807–808**
    hyperthyroidism and, 807, 1126
Molds
    household, **1558**
    opportunistic infections caused by, 1292, **1557–1558**
Mole, hydatidiform. *See* Hydatidiform mole
Mole (skin). *See also* Nevi
    atypical (atypical nevus), **102**, 102f
    benign, 101, 101f
    changes in, melanoma and, 102, 104
    normal, **101–102**, 101f
Molecular adsorbent recirculating system (MARS), for hepatorenal syndrome, 703
Mollaret meningitis, 1364
Molluscum contagiosum, **142**, 142f, 1423
    in HIV infection/AIDS, 142, 1343, 1423
MOLST forms, 90
Mometasone
    inhaled, for asthma, 250t
    intranasal, for allergic rhinitis, 219
    topical, for skin disorders, 97t
Mönckeberg medial calcific sclerosis, 475
Monge disease, 1574, **1575**
Monkeypox, 1423–1424
Monoamine oxidase inhibitors (MAOIs), 1077, 1078t, 1082, 1082t, 1083t

drug/food interactions of, 1013, 1082, 1082t, 1083t
    serotonin syndrome and, 35, 1080
    overdose/toxicity of, 1078t, 1082
        ophthalmic, 177t
        suicidal, 1079
    for parkinsonism, 1013
    transdermal, 1078t, 1082
    withdrawal from, 1081
Monoclonal antibodies
    in cancer chemotherapy, 1666–1667t. *See also specific agent*
    for lipid modification/cardiovascular/heart disease prevention, 353
Monoclonal gammopathy of unknown significance (MGUS), 536
    amyloidosis and, 539
    neuropathy associated with, 1037
Monoclonal protein. *See also* Paraproteins
    in myeloma, 535, 535–536, 951
    in Waldenström macroglobulinemia, 537, 538
Monocular visual loss, transient, **188–189**
Monocytic ehrlichiosis, 1429t, 1435, 1435–1436
Monomethylhydrazine mushroom poisoning, 1600, 1600t
Mononeuritis multiplex, **1034–1039**. *See also* Polyneuropathies
    in diabetes, 1240
    in Lyme disease, 1502
    microscopic polyangiitis and, 860
    polyarteritis nodosa and, 856
Mononeuropathies, 1034, **1039–1041**. *See also* Neuropathies
    in diabetes, 1240. *See also* Diabetic neuropathy
    in HIV infection/AIDS, 1340
    in sarcoidosis, 1037
Mononucleosis
    CMV, 1373, 1374, 1375
    Epstein-Barr virus, 228, 1367t, **1372–1373**, 1372f
    pharyngitis in, 228, 1372, 1373
Mononucleosis-like syndrome, 1374, 1375
Monopost. *See* Latanoprost
Monopril/Monopril HCT. *See* Fosinopril
Montelukast
    for allergic rhinitis, 219
    for asthma, 249t, 251
    for urticaria, 134
Montenegro (leishmanin) skin test, 1511
Montgomery-Asberg rating scale, assessment of suicide risk and, 1077
Montreal Cognitive Assessment (MoCA©), in dementia screening, 58, 1020
Mood disorders, **1074–1088**. *See also* Depression; Mania
Moraxella/Moraxella catarrhalis infections, 1311t, 1315t, **1466**
    pneumonia, 268t, 1466
Morbidly adherent placenta (placenta accreta/increta/percreta), 813
Morbilliform skin disorders, 96t
Morganella, 1312t
Moricizine, toxicity of, 384
Morning sickness. *See* Vomiting, of pregnancy

Morphea, 846
Morphine, 74, 79t, 82
    for dyspnea, 86–87, 262
    for myocardial infarction, 375
    overdose/toxicity of, 1601
        ophthalmic, 177t
    for pulmonary edema, 378, 412
de Morsier syndrome (septo-optic dysplasia), 1108
Mosaicism
    Klinefelter syndrome and, 1190
    X chromosome
        premature menopause and, 1201
        Turner syndrome and, 1208
Mosquitoes/mosquito control
    chikungunya fever and, 1407, 1408
    dengue and, 1401, 1403
    encephalitis and, 1388, 1389, 1390
    filariasis and, 1543, 1544
    malaria and, 1513, 1520
    yellow fever and, 1404, 1405
    Zika virus infection and, 1388, 1406, 1407
Moths, skin lesions caused by, 151
Motility disorders. *See also specific disorder*
    esophageal, **617–619**
        chest pain in, 27, 359, 617, 618, 619
        dysphagia in, 605, 605t, 617, 618, 618–619
        in scleroderma, 846
    intestinal, **638–641**. *See also* Intestinal obstruction
        constipation and, 584, 584t
        diarrhea and, 588t, 592
        in irritable bowel syndrome, 644
        vomiting and, 580, 581t
Motivational interview, at-risk drinking and, 1094
Motor activity, in schizophrenia/psychotic disorders, 1067
Motor conduction velocity studies. *See* Conduction velocity studies
Motor neuron diseases, **1033–1034**
    spasticity and, 1025, 1033, 1034
Motor palsies, ocular, **194**
Motor vehicle accidents. *See* Automobile accidents
Motrin. *See* Ibuprofen
Mountain sickness
    acute (AMS), **1574**
    chronic (Monge disease), 1574, **1575**
    subacute, 1574, **1575**
Mouth. *See* Oral cavity
Movement disorders, **1010–1018**. *See also specific type*
    drug-induced, **1017**
    in Wilson disease, 710, **1017**
MoviPrep. *See* Polyethylene glycol
Moxalactam, platelet function affected by, 558t
Moxifloxacin
    for anaerobic infections, 1478, 1479, 1479t
    for bacterial rhinosinusitis, 217t
    for ophthalmic disorders, 169t
    for pneumonia, 269t, 271, 275t, 1446
6-MP. *See* Mercaptopurine
MPGN. *See* Membranoproliferative glomerulonephritis/glomerulonephropathy

MPL mutation
  in essential thrombocytosis, 521
  in primary myelofibrosis, 522, 523
MPO-ANCA. *See* Antineutrophil
    cytoplasmic antibody;
    Myeloperoxidase ANCA
MPSV4 vaccine. *See* Meningococcal
    vaccine
MRA. *See* Magnetic resonance
    angiography
MRCP. *See* Magnetic resonance
    cholangiopancreatography
MRI. *See* Magnetic resonance imaging
MRSA infections. *See* Methicillin-
    resistant *S aureus* (MRSA)
    infections
MS Contin. *See* Morphine
MSH2/MSH6 genes, in HNPCC/Lynch
    syndrome, 668
  pancreatic/periampullary carcinoma
    and, 1620
MSI. *See* Microsatellite instability
MSSA infections. *See* Methicillin-
    susceptible S aureus (MSSA)
    infections
mTOR inhibitors
  for breast cancer, 756
  for insulinoma, 1255
  for renal cell carcinoma, 1654–1655
MTX. *See* Methotrexate
Mucocutaneous (mucosal) candidiasis,
    132–133, 132*f*, 1547, 1548
Mucocutaneous herpes simplex, 1363
Mucocutaneous leishmaniasis (espundia),
    1510, 1511, 1512
Mucocutaneous lymph node syndrome
    (Kawasaki disease), 1367*t*,
    1438–1440
Mucocutaneous syphilis, 1489*t*, 1492,
    1493*f*
Mucomimetics, for dry eye, 168
Mucor infection, 218, 1555–1556
Mucormycosis, **1555–1556**
  rhinocerebral, 218, 1556
Mucosa-associated lymphoid tissue
    lymphoma. *See* MALT
    lymphoma
Mucosal biopsy
  in celiac disease, 634
  in diarrhea, 593
Mucosal protective agents, for peptic
    ulcer disease, 625
Mucositis, oral, chemotherapy-induced,
    1673
Mucous membranes
  diabetes mellitus affecting, 1242
  leishmaniasis involving, 1510, 1511,
    1512
  melanoma involving, 103
  syphilis involving, 1489*t*, 1492, 1494
"Muddy brown (granular) casts," 913,
    914*t*
MUGA (Multi Gated Acquisition) Scan
  in angina, 357
  anthracycline administration and,
    1675
Müllerian agenesis, amenorrhea and,
    1199
Multi Gated Acquisition (MUGA) Scan
  in angina, 357
  anthracycline administration and, 1675

Multibacillary (lepromatous) leprosy,
    1037, 1484. *See also* Leprosy
Multidrug resistance. *See also* Drug
    resistance
  health care-associated infections and,
    1294
  in tuberculosis, 277, 283, 1336
Multifocal atrial tachycardia, **395**
Multinational Association for Supportive
    Care in Cancer (MASCC)
    score, 35
Multinodular (nodular) goiter,
    1137–1140, 1138*t*. *See also*
    Goiter
  toxic, 1125, 1131
Multiple endocrine neoplasia (MEN),
    1187–1189, 1187*t*
  MEN 1 (Wermer syndrome), 1187,
    1187–1188, 1187*t*
    acromegaly in, 1114
    adrenal adenoma/hyperplasia in,
      1187*t*, 1188
    gastric carcinoids in, 1633
    gastrinomas in, 631, 632, 1185, 1188
    gastroenteropancreatic
      neuroendocrine tumors in,
      1185, 1187*t*, 1188, 1252
    hyperparathyroidism in, 1152, 1153,
      1155, 1158, 1187
    insulinoma in, 1185, 1188, 1253
    parathyroid adenoma/hyperplasia
      in, 1152, 1187*t*
    pituitary adenoma in, 1187*t*, 1188
    prolactinomas in, 1188
    thyroid adenoma in, 1187*t*, 1188
  MEN 2 (MEN 2A/Sipple syndrome),
    1187, 1187*t*, **1188**
    hyperparathyroidism in, 1152, 1153,
      1188
    medullary thyroid carcinoma in,
      1141, 1145, 1147, 1187*t*, 1188
    parathyroid adenoma/hyperplasia
      in, 1152, 1187*t*
    pheochromocytoma in, 1179, 1187*t*,
      1188
  MEN 3 (MEN 2B), 1187, 1187*t*, **1188**
    medullary thyroid carcinoma in,
      1141, 1145, 1147–1148,
      1187*t*, 1188
    pheochromocytoma in, 1179, 1187*t*,
      1188
  MEN 4, 1187, 1187*t*, **1189**
    acromegaly in, 1114
    parathyroid adenoma/hyperplasia
      in, 1152, 1187*t*, 1189
    pituitary adenoma in, 1189
Multiple gestation pregnancy
  assisted reproductive procedures and,
    785
  preterm labor/birth and, 812
Multiple marker screening, in Down
    syndrome, 1678
Multiple myeloma. *See* Myeloma
Multiple sclerosis, **1022–1025**, 1024*t*
  optic neuritis and, 193, 1023
  trigeminal neuralgia and, 981
  vertigo/hearing loss in, 211*t*, **214**
Multisystem atrophy (Shy-Drager
    syndrome)
  dysautonomia and, 990
  parkinsonism and, 1012

Multisystem crisis, pheochromocytoma,
    1180*t*, 1181, 1182
Multitarget DNA tests, in cancer
    screening/polyp detection,
    665, 1641–1642
Mumps, **1380–1382**, 1381*f*
  prevention/immunization and,
    1381–1382. *See also* MMR
    (measles-mumps-rubella)
    vaccine
Mumps vaccine, 1323*t*, 1381–1382. *See
    also* MMR (measles-
    mumps-rubella) vaccine
Munchausen by proxy, 1059
Munchausen syndrome, 1059
Mupirocin, 98*t*, 218, 1343
Mural thrombus, myocardial infarction
    and, 379
Murine (flea-borne) typhus, 1429*t*,
    1430–1431
Murmurs. *See* Heart murmurs
Murphy sign, in cholecystitis, 718
Murray Valley encephalitis, 1388
Muscarine, poisoning with mushrooms
    containing, 1600*t*
Muscimol, poisoning with mushrooms
    containing, 1600*t*
Muscle biopsy
  in inclusion body myositis, 849, 1048
  in polyarteritis nodosa, 856
  in polymyositis/dermatomyositis, 849
Muscle cysticercosis, 1536
Muscle-specific tyrosine kinase (MuSK)
    antibodies, in myasthenia
    gravis, 1045
Muscle wasting. *See also* Wasting
  in malabsorption, 633*t*
Muscle weakness. *See* Myopathies;
    Myositis; Paralysis
Muscles, disorders of. *See*
    Musculoskeletal disorders
Muscular dystrophies, **1047**, 1048*t*
Musculoskeletal disorders, **1685–1717**.
    See also specific type
  ankle injuries, **1715–1717**, 1715*t*
  in cysticercosis, 1536
  dysphagia in, 506*t*
  hip problems, **1701–1704**, 1702*t*
  knee problems, **1704–1715**, 1705*t*,
    1706–1709*t*
  in malabsorption, 633*t*
  shoulder problems, **1685–1692**,
    1686–1688*t*
  spine problems, **1692–1697**, 1692*t*,
    1693*t*, 1696*t*
  sports injuries and, **1685–1717**
  in syphilis, 1494
  in trichinosis, 1542
  upper extremity problems, **1697–1701**,
    1699*t*, 1700*f*
Musculoskeletal tuberculosis, **871–872**
Mushroom picker's disease, 308*t*
Mushroom poisoning, **1600–1601**, 1600*t*
  anticholinergic-type mushrooms and,
    1590
  hallucinogenic mushrooms and, 1598,
    1600*t*
  liver failure and, 685–686, 686, 1600
MuSK antibodies, in myasthenia gravis,
    1045
Musset sign, 346

Mustargen. *See* Mechlorethamine

Mutamycin. *See* Mitomycin

Mutism
  akinetic (persistent vegetative state), **1028**
  in schizophrenia/psychotic disorders, 1067

"Mutton-fat" keratic precipitates, 181, 182*f*

MUTYH mutation, in familial adenomatous polyposis, 667

Myasthenia gravis, **1045–1046**
  aminoglycosides contraindicated in, 1046, 1047
  ocular, 195, 1045

Myasthenic crisis, 1045

Myasthenic (Lambert-Eaton) syndrome, 1008, **1046**, 1609

MYC translocations, in non-Hodgkin lymphoma, 533

Mycetoma, **1557**

Mycobacterium (mycobacterial infections), 1312*t*, **1481–1485**
  abscessus, 285, 286, 1482
  avium complex (MAC), 285, 286, 1312*t*, 1337*t*
    diarrhea caused by, 588*t*, 592
    disseminated disease caused by, 285, **1482–1483**
    in HIV infection/AIDS, 285, 1337*t*, 1345, 1482–1483
      prophylaxis and, 1334, 1350, 1483
    lymphadenitis caused by, 1345, 1482
    pulmonary disease caused by, 285, 286, 1481–1482
  bovis
    BCG vaccine made from, 279, 284
    intestinal disease caused by, 643
    lymphadenitis caused by, 1482
  chelonae/chelonei, 286, 1312*t*, 1482
  fortuitum, 286, 1312*t*, 1482
  gordonae, 1482
  haemophilum, 1482
  kansasii, 285, 286, 1312*t*, 1482
  leprae, 1312*t*, 1484
  lymphadenitis, **239**, **1345**
  malmoense, 285, 1482
  marinum, 1482
  meningitis, 1297*t*
  nontuberculous (atypical), **1481–1483**.
        See also Nontuberculous atypical mycobacteria
    in HIV infection/AIDS, 285, 1336
    lymphadenitis/adenitis caused by, **239**, 1345
    pulmonary disease caused by, **284–286, 1481–1482**
    skin and soft tissue infections caused by, **1482**
  scrofulaceum, 1482
  szulgai, 1482
  tuberculosis, **277–284**, 277*t*, 278*t*, 279*f*, 280*t*, 281*t*, 282*t*, 1312*t*, 1483.
        See also Tuberculosis
    bone and joint disease caused by, 283, **871–872**
    intestinal disease caused by, **643**
    lymphadenitis caused by, **239**, 1482
    meningitis caused by, 283, **1483–1484**

pulmonary disease caused by, **277–284**, 277*t*, 278*t*, 279*f*, 280*t*, 281*t*, 282*t*
    resistant strains of, 277, 278, 278*t*, 282–283, 1336
  ulcerans, 1482
  xenopi, 285, 1482

Mycophenolate mofetil
  for lupus nephritis, 841, 941
  for neuromyelitis optica, 1025
  for pemphigus, 140
  for scleroderma, 847

Mycoplasma, 1313*t*
  genitalium, 1486
  pneumoniae, 1314*t*, 1315*t*
    pneumonia caused by, 268*t*, 1314*t*, 1315*t*
    Stevens-Johnson syndrome caused by, 135

Mycosis fungoides (cutaneous T-cell lymphoma), **116–117**
  exfoliative dermatitis/erythroderma and, 117

Mycotic aneurysms
  drug use and, 1304
  intracranial, 1000

Mycotic infections (mycoses), **1547–1560**. *See also* Fungal infections
  allergic bronchopulmonary, **264**, 879*t*
  drugs for management of, 98–99*t*, **1558–1560**, 1558–1559*t*. *See also* Antifungal agents
  superficial/skin, **111–115**, 111*f*, 112*f*, 113*f*. *See also* Tinea
  in HIV infection/AIDS, 1343

MYD88 mutation, in Waldenström macroglobulinemia, 538

Myelin-associated glycoprotein (MAG), neuropathy and, 1037

Myelinolysis, central pontine (cerebral osmotic demyelination), hyponatremia treatment and, 885, 888

Myelodysplastic syndromes, 519*t*, **525–527**
  platelet function/thrombocytopenia and, 546–547, 548, 558*t*
  rheumatologic manifestations of, 875
  stem cell transplantation for, 526–527, 541

Myelofibrosis (primary/idiopathic), 519*t*, 520*t*, **522–523**

Myeloid growth factors. *See* Filgrastim; Growth factors; Sargramostim

Myeloid leukemia. *See* Acute myeloid leukemia; Chronic myeloid leukemia

Myeloma, **535–537**, 1622*t*
  amyloidosis and, 535, 951
  hypercalcemia and, 535, 536, 1156
  kidney involvement in, 535, 536, 920, **951**
  neuropathy associated with, 1036
  "nonsecretory," 536
  stem cell transplantation for, 536, 539, 540

Myeloma kidney, 535, 536, 920, 951

Myelopathy. *See also specific cause*
  in cervical spondylosis, 1042

epidural/subdural hemorrhage causing, 1002
  HIV, 1340
  human T-cell leukemia virus (HTLV), **1026**, 1396
  in multiple sclerosis, 1023
  in subacute combined degeneration of spinal cord, 1026

Myeloperoxidase ANCA (MPO-ANCA).
        See also Antineutrophil cytoplasmic antibody
  in glomerulonephritis, 938
  in granulomatosis with polyangiitis, 858, 938
  in microscopic polyangiitis, 859, 860, 938

Myeloproliferative disorders, **519–531**, 519*t*, 520*t*. *See also* Leukemias
  platelets affected in, 520*t*, 558*t*
  rheumatologic manifestations of, 875

Myeloradiculopathy, in spinal dural arteriovenous fistulae, 1002–1003

Myelosuppressive therapy
  bone marrow/stem cell transplantation and, 540, 541
  infection and, 1290
  for polycythemia, 520

Myerson sign, 1012

Myleran. *See* Busulfan

Myocardial abscess, endocarditis and, 1458

Myocardial contusions/hematomas, 434

Myocardial dysfunction. *See also* Heart (cardiac) failure
  myocardial infarction and, 377–378

Myocardial hibernation, 353

Myocardial hypertrophy. *See* Cardiomyopathy

Myocardial infarction/ST-segment elevation myocardial infarction (STEMI), 26–27, 27, 27*t*, 28, 365, 369*t*, **370–381**, 372*f*, 373*t*. *See also* Coronary heart disease
  abdominal aortic aneurysm repair and, 482
  accelerated idioventricular rhythm and, 377, 398
  antihypertensive therapy and, 449*t*, 464
    in hypertensive emergency, 469*t*
  arrhythmias associated with, 370, 377
  aspirin/chemoprevention for, 6*t*, 10–11, 355, 371–372, 376
    in diabetes, 1241–1242
  biomarkers in, 371
  chest pain/discomfort in, 26–27, 27, 27*t*, 28, 370, 375
  cocaine abuse and, 365, 370, 414, 1100
  complications of, 376–379
  coronary artery trauma and, 434
  coronary vasospasm causing, 365, 370
  in diabetes mellitus, 1241
    glycemic/hypertension control and, 1218
  fibrinolytic therapy for, 372*f*, 373, 373*t*, 374–375
  PCI and, 372*f*, 373
  heart failure and, 370, 377–378
  hemodynamic status and, 371

influenza and, 1412
ischemia after, 376–377
mitral regurgitation and, 338f, 339
oral contraceptive use and, 786
painless, 370
perioperative, preoperative risk
    assessment/management
    and, 46–47, 47f, 47t
during pregnancy, 435
Q waves and, 27t, 371. *See also* Non-Q
    wave (non-ST elevation)
    infarction
reinfarction and, 375
revascularization/reperfusion and,
    362–363, 372–375, 372f,
    373t, 380–381
    postinfarction, 375, 380–381
    prophylactic/preoperative, 46–47
risk/risk stratification for, 5–6,
    352–353, 354f, 361–362
    postinfarction, 380
shock and, 371, 372f, 378, 494
sudden death and, 370, 397
thiazolidinedione use and, 1224
treatment of, 371–376, 372f, 373t
    postinfarction management and,
    379–381
ventricular fibrillation and, 370, 397,
    398
Myocardial ischemia, **352–381**. *See also*
    Angina; Coronary heart
    disease; Myocardial
    infarction
in acute coronary syndromes, 365, 366
chest pain/discomfort in, 26–27, 27,
    27t, 28, 356, 357. *See also*
    Angina; Myocardial
    infarction
    recurrent, 375, 376
cocaine abuse and, 365, 370, 414, 1100
hypertension management in, 360f,
    362, 469t
mitral regurgitation and, 338f, 339
postinfarction, 376–377
preoperative testing for, 45–46, 47f
vasospasm causing, 356, 364–365
Myocardial perfusion scintigraphy
in angina, 357
in myocardial infarction, 371
preoperative, 46
Myocardial rupture
infarction and, 379
traumatic, 434
Myocardial sarcoidosis, 292, 293
Myocardial stress imaging, in angina/
    chest pain evaluation, 28,
    357–358
Myocardial stunning, 353
Myocarditis, **413–415**, 413t
adenovirus infection and, 1421
in African trypanosomiasis, 1507
catecholamine, 1183
in Chagas disease, 1510
clozapine causing, 1072
coxsackievirus, 1426
diphtheritic, 1457
drug-induced/toxic, 413t, **414–415**
infectious, **413–414**, 413t
sudden death of athlete and, 414, 438t
Myoclonic epilepsy, ragged red fiber
    (MERRF) syndrome, 1049

Myoclonic seizures, 984t, 985. *See also*
    Seizures
drug therapy for, 988t
Myoclonus, **1017**
with opsoclonus, 1008
palatal, tinnitus and, 209
Myoglobin
in acute coronary syndromes/STEMI,
    366
in kidney disease/injury/
    rhabdomyolysis, 852,
    919–920
Myoglobinuria, 919–920
acute tubular necrosis/rhabdomyolysis
    and, 852, 919–920
Myomas (leiomyomas/fibroid tumors), of
    uterus, **772–774**
Myomectomy, for fibroid tumors, 773
Myonecrosis, clostridial (gas gangrene),
    1312t, **1451–1452**
Myopathies (myopathic disorders),
    1047–1049, 1048t
ART/zidovudine causing, 1049, 1340
HIV, 869, 1049, 1340
inflammatory, idiopathic, **847–850**,
    848f, 848t. *See also*
    Dermatomyositis;
    Polymyositis
lipid-lowering therapy/statins causing,
    1264
mitochondrial, **1049**
nucleoside reverse transcriptase
    inhibitor-associated, 869,
    1340
Myopathy, encephalopathy, lactic
    acidosis, and stroke-like
    episodes (MELAS), 1049
Myopericarditis. *See also* Pericarditis
Borrelia burgdorferi/Lyme disease
    causing, 425, 1502, 1505,
    1505t
Myopia (nearsightedness), reduction of
    rate of progression of, 164
Myosin heavy chain, genes coding for, in
    hypertrophic
    cardiomyopathy, 418
Myositis, **847–850**, 848f, 848t. *See also*
    Dermatomyositis;
    Polymyositis
autoantibodies in, 848, 848t
in HIV infection/AIDS, 869
HMG-CoA reductase inhibitors
    (statins) causing, 848t, 849,
    1264
inclusion body, 849, **1048–1049**
Myotomy
for achalasia, 618
    per oral endoscopic (POEM), 618
for Zenker diverticulum, 614
Myotomy–myomectomy, 419
Myotonia/myotonic dystrophy,
    1047–1048, 1048t
congenita, **1048**
Myotonin-protein kinase, in myotonic
    dystrophy, 1048t
Myringotomy, 205
Myxedema, **1119–1124**. *See also*
    Hypothyroidism
pretibial (Graves dermopathy), 1124,
    1127, 1133
Myxedema coma, 1120, 1122

Myxedema crisis, 1121–1122, 1122
Myxedema heart, 1120
Myxedema madness, 1120, 1121
Myxoma, atrial, 433
    fever/FUO and, 1288
Myxomatous mitral valve. *See* Mitral
    valve prolapse

N-methyl-D-aspartate (NMDA) receptor
    antibodies, encephalitis and,
    1008
N-terminal proBNP (NT-proBNP)
in aortic regurgitation, 346
in aortic stenosis, 342
in cardiomyopathy, 415
in heart failure, 23, 404
    ascites and, 713
Na⁺. *See* Sodium
NAAT-TB/NAAT-R. *See* Nucleic acid
    amplification testing
Nabumetone, 76t
Nadolol, 453t
with bendroflumethazide, 453t
for esophageal varices, prevention of
    rebleeding and, 616
NAEPP (National Asthma Education and
    Prevention Program),
    asthma diagnosis/
    management and, 243f, 244t,
    246–248, 247f, 248–257,
    250t, 253–254t, 255f, 256f
Nafarelin
for abnormal uterine bleeding, 763
for endometriosis, 776
Nafcillin
for endocarditis, 1462
platelet function affected by, 558t
for skin and soft tissue infections,
    1443, 1443t, 1448
NAFLD. *See* Nonalcoholic fatty liver
    disease
NAFLD Fibrosis Score, 698
Naftifine, 99t
Naftin. *See* Naftifine
Nail disorders, **159–161**, 160f
candidal infection, 132f, 133, 159
chemotherapy-induced, 1673
hyperpigmentation, drugs causing,
    160, 163t
pitting/stippling, 160
    in psoriasis, 107, 107f, 160, 865
in Raynaud phenomenon, 844
tinea unguium (onychomycosis), 160,
    160–161
Nailbed capillary pulsations (Quincke
    pulses), 346
Nalfon. *See* Fenoprofen
Nalmefene, for opioid overdose, 1581t
Naloxegol, for opioid-induced
    constipation, 86
Naloxone, 1098
for coma, 1027, 1578
for heroin/opioid overdose/withdrawal,
    85–86, 1578, 1581t, 1601
NALP-3 inflammasomes, in gout, 830
Naltrexone
for alcohol use disorder, 17, 694, 1095
with bupropion, for obesity, 1271
    in type 2 diabetes, 1235
for heroin/opioid withdrawal, 1099
Naphazoline, overdose/toxicity of, 1592

Naprosyn. *See* Naproxen
Naproxen, 76t
    for gout, 831
Napsin-A, in lung cancer, 1609
Naratriptan, for migraine headache, 978
Narcissistic personality disorder, 1065t
Narcolepsy, 1089–1090
Narcotic (opioid) antagonists, 1099. *See also* Naloxone
    for heroin/opioid overdose/withdrawal, 85–86, 1099, 1578, 1581t, 1601
    for opioid-induced constipation, 86, 586
Narcotics. *See also* Opioids/opioid analgesics
    abuse of, 1098–1099
        narcotic antagonists/naloxone for, 85–86, 1099, 1578, 1581t, 1601
Nardil. *See* Phenelzine
Narrowband UVB (NB-UVB) therapy. *See also* Phototherapy
    for lichen planus, 145
    for psoriasis, 108
Nasal bleeding. *See* Epistaxis
Nasal CPAP, for sleep apnea, 317
Nasal gel, testosterone, 1193
Nasal polyps, **222**
    allergic rhinitis and, 219, 222
Nasal pyramid, fracture of, 222
Nasal septoplasty, for sleep apnea, 317
Nasal sinuses. *See* Paranasal sinuses
Nasal trauma, **222**
    epistaxis and, 221, 222
Nasal tumors, **222–224**
    benign, **222–223**
    malignant, **223**
Nasal vestibulitis, **218**
NASH. *See* Nonalcoholic steatohepatitis
Nasolacrimal duct obstruction
    congenital, 166
    dacryocystitis and, 166
Nasopharynx, malignant tumors of, **223**
    Epstein-Barr virus and, 223
    serous otitis media and, 203, 223
Natacyn. *See* Natamycin
Natalizumab
    for inflammatory bowel/Crohn disease, 652
    for multiple sclerosis, 1024, 1024t
    progressive multifocal leukoencephalopathy caused by, 652, 1024, 1395
Natamycin, for ophthalmic disorders, 170t, 175
Nateglinide, 1221t, 1223, 1236
    factitious hypoglycemia and, 1253t, 1257
Natesto. *See* Testosterone nasal gel
National Asthma Education and Prevention Program (NAEPP), asthma diagnosis/management and, 243f, 244t, 246–248, 247f, 248–257, 250t, 253–254t, 255f, 256f
National Surgical Quality Improvement Program (NSQIP) risk assessment tool, 45, 49
Native DNA, antibodies to, 840t, 841t

Natriuretic peptide
    atrial, in senile amyloidosis, 538
    B-type (BNP/beta)
        in aortic regurgitation, 346
        in aortic stenosis, 342
        in cardiomyopathy, 415, 435
        in dyspnea, 23
        in heart failure, 23, 404
            ascites and, 713
        recombinant. *See* Nesiritide
Nausea and vomiting, **87**, **580–583**, 581t, 582t. *See also specific cause*
    chemotherapy-induced, 87, 580, 581t, 582, 582t, **1672–1673**
    drugs for management of. *See* Antiemetics
    in HIV infection/AIDS, 1335
    hyponatremia caused by, 886
    in intestinal obstruction, 580, 581, 581–582, 581t
    in migraine, 40, 40t, 581t, 977, 978
    opioid-induced, 83, 580
    palliation of, **87**
    in pregnancy, 580, **803**, 823
        in gestational trophoblastic disease, 807
    Wernicke encephalopathy and, 1026
Navane. *See* Thiothixene
Navelbine. *See* Vinorelbine
NB-UVB therapy. *See* Narrowband UVB (NB-UVB) therapy
Near-infrared autofluorescence spectroscopy, during parathyroidectomy, 1158
Nearsightedness, reduction of rate of progression of, 164
Nebido. *See* Testosterone undecanoate
Nebivolol, 449, 453t, 454, 464
Nebulizer therapy
    for asthma, 248, 252, 253t, 255f, 256f
    for COPD, 260, 262
Necator americanus, 1539
Necitumumab, 1666t
Neck
    infections of
        anaerobic, **1478**
        deep, **230**
        masses caused by, **239**
    masses in, **238–240**. *See also* Head and neck cancer
        congenital lesions in adults, **238–239**
        infectious and inflammatory, **239**
        lymphoma, **240**
        metastatic, **239–240**
        thyroid. *See* Thyroid cancer; Thyroid nodules
Neck fractures/injury, 1696
    cervical vertigo and, 213
    head trauma and, 1029
Neck pain, **1696–1697**, 1696t
    disk-related, **1042**, 1043–1044f, 1696
Necrobiosis lipoidica diabeticorum, 1242
Necrolysis, toxic epidermal, 135–136
    drugs causing, 135, 136, 161, 162t, 163
    herpes simplex infection and, 1364
Necrosis-erythema-lymphadenopathy, Dermacentor-borne/scalp eschar neck lymphadenopathy/tick-borne lymphadenopathy, 1429t, 1434

Necrotizing cellulitis, synergistic, 1480
Necrotizing fasciitis
    anaerobes causing, 1480
    cellulitis differentiated from, 138, 492, 1444
    staphylococcal, 1448
    streptococcal, 492, 1444
Necrotizing (phlegmonous) gastritis, 623
Necrotizing lymphadenitis, histiocytic (Kikuchi disease), 239
Necrotizing pancreatitis, 726, 727, 728, 729, 729–730, 730
Necrotizing pneumonia, 275, 276
Necrotizing ulcerative gingivitis, **226**
Nedocromil
    for allergic eye disease, 168, 170t
    for allergic rhinitis, 219
    for asthma, 247f, 248–251, 249t
Needle ablation of prostate, transurethral (TUNA), 976
Needle-stick injury
    Ebola viral disease transmission and, 1398
    HIV infection/AIDS transmission and, 1332, 1347
Neer impingement sign, 1685, 1687t
Nefazodone, 1078t, 1079–1081
Neglect/abuse, of elderly, 16, **70–71**, 71t
Negri/Negri-like bodies, 1386, 1387
Neighborhood reaction, 1297t, 1298
Neisseria
    gonorrhoeae, 588t, 1311t, 1475. *See also* Gonococcal infections
        resistant strains of, 1476
    meningitidis, 1311t. *See also* Meningococcal (*Neisseria meningitidis*) infections
        resistant strains of, 1465
Nelfinavir, 1352t, 1357. *See also* Antiretroviral therapy
Nelson syndrome, 1175, 1176, 1176–1177
Nematode infections. *See also specific type*
    filariasis, **1543–1546**, 1543f
    intestinal, 592, **1538–1541**
    invasive, **1541–1543**, 1543f
Neoadjuvant chemotherapy. *See also* Chemotherapy
    for bladder cancer, 1652–1653
    for breast cancer, 749, 752, 753–754
    for colorectal cancer, 1639–1640, 1640
    for esophageal cancer, 1627
    for lung cancer, 1611
Neologisms, in schizophrenia/psychotic disorders, 1067
Neomycin/polymyxin B/gramicidin, for ophthalmic disorders, 169t
Neonatal Graves disease, transient, 1127
Neonate. *See* Newborn
Neoplasia. *See* Cancer
Neoplastic pericarditis/effusion, 425, 426, 426–427
Neorickettsia sennetsu, 1435
Neosporin. *See* Neomycin/polymyxin B/gramicidin
Neostigmine
    for acute colonic pseudo-obstruction (Ogilvie syndrome), 640
    adverse ophthalmic effects of, 177t
    for myasthenia gravis, 1045–1046
Neovascular age-related macular degeneration, 185

Neovascular (rubeotic) glaucoma, 186
Neovascularization
    iris
        in diabetes mellitus, 1238
        in retinal vein occlusion, 186
    retinal
        in diabetic retinopathy, 190, 1238
        in retinal vein occlusion, 186
Nepafenac, for ophthalmic disorders, 168,
        171*t*
Nephritic spectrum glomerular diseases,
        932, 932*f*, 933*t*, **934–941**,
        935*f*. *See also*
        Glomerulonephritis
Nephritic syndrome, 932, 932*f*, 936. *See
        also specific cause and*
        Glomerulonephritis
Nephritis. *See also* Glomerulonephritis
    deaths attributable to, 2*t*
    interstitial, 917*t*, **921**
    lupus, 839*t*, 840, 841, 933*t*, 935*f*,
        940–941
    penicillin causing, 1318
    tubulointerstitial, 924*t*, 946*t*
Nephrocalcinosis
    in hypercalcemia/hyperparathyroidism,
        1153, 1157
    hypoparathyroidism treatment causing,
        1150
    in renal tubular acidosis, 906–907
Nephrogenic diabetes insipidus. *See*
        Diabetes insipidus,
        nephrogenic
Nephrogenic fibrosing dermopathy, 846
Nephrogenic systemic fibrosis,
        358, **952**
Nephrolithiasis (kidney stones), 950, 962.
        See also Urinary stone
        disease
    calcium, 961, 962, 962*t*, 963–964
    calcium supplementation and, 963,
        964, 1161
    in Crohn disease, 653
    cystine, 961, 962, 964
    hyperparathyroidism and, 963–964,
        1153, 1155, 1157
    in polycystic kidney disease, 949, 950
    probenecid use and, 833
    in renal tubular acidosis, 906–907, 962
    in short bowel syndrome, 637
    struvite, 961, 962, 964
    uric acid, 830, 952, 961, 962, 964
        probenecid use and, 833
Nephronophthisis, juvenile, **951**
Nephropathia epidemica, 1403, 1404
Nephropathy
    analgesic, 947, 948
    Balkan, ureteral/renal pelvis cancer
        and, 1653
    contrast, 919
    diabetic, 934*t*, 942, **945–946**,
        1238–1239
        glycemic control affecting
            development/progression of,
            945, 1218, 1219, 1238
    HIV-associated, 934*t*, **946**
    hypertensive, 468
    IgA (Berger disease), 933*t*, 935*f*, **937**
    lead, 947, 948
    membranous. *See* Membranous
        nephropathy
    obstructive, chronic kidney disease
        caused by, 924*t*
    reflux, 947, 948
    urate/uric acid, 830, 952
Nephrosclerosis, hypertension causing,
        440
Nephrosis
    deaths attributable to, 2*t*
    lipoid (minimal change disease), 934*t*,
        943
Nephrotic spectrum diseases, 932–933,
        932*f*, 934*t*
    glomerular, 932–933, 932*f*, 934*t*,
        941–943. *See also* Nephrotic
        syndrome
    in primary renal disorders, **943–944**
    from systemic disorders, **945–946**
Nephrotic syndrome, 932*f*, 933, 942. *See
        also specific cause*
    deaths attributable to, 2*t*
    in diabetes mellitus, 1239. *See also*
        Diabetic nephropathy
    focal segmental glomerulosclerosis
        and, 944
    HIV-associated nephropathy and, 946
    hyponatremia in, 888
    lipid abnormalities and, 942
    membranous nephropathy and, 944
    minimal change disease and, 943
    in renal amyloidosis, 946
Nephrotoxicity. *See also specific agent*
    acute kidney injury and, 919–920
        acute tubular necrosis, 919–920
        interstitial nephritis, 921
    of aminoglycosides, 919
    of cisplatin, 1675
    of mercury, 1598
    of methotrexate, 837
    of NSAIDs, 74
    of radiographic contrast media, 919
Neprilysin inhibitor, for heart failure,
        405*f*, 407
Neptazane. *See* Methazolamide
Nerve agents, for chemical warfare,
        1601–1602
    skin decontamination after exposure
        to, 1581
Nerve biopsy, in polyarteritis nodosa,
        856
Nerve conduction velocity studies. *See*
        Conduction velocity studies
Nervous system. *See under* Neurologic
Nesina. *See* Alogliptin
Nesiritide, for acute heart failure/
        pulmonary edema, 412
Neulasta. *See* Pegfilgrastim
Neupogen. *See* Filgrastim
Neural foraminal stenosis, 1696
Neural hearing loss, 200. *See also* Hearing
        loss
Neuralgia
    glossopharyngeal, **982**
        chemotherapy-induced, 1674
        earache in, 207
    postherpetic, 5, 120–121, 121, 175,
        982, 1369–1370, 1370
    trigeminal, **981–982**
Neuralgic amyotrophy (idiopathic
        brachial plexus neuropathy),
        1043
Neuraminidase, influenza virus, 1410
    Neuraminidase inhibitors (oseltamivir/
        zanamivir/peramivir), 1365*t*,
        1412–1413, 1418
    prophylactic, 1416
    resistance to, 1412–1413
Neuritis
    intercostal, chest pain and, 359
    optic, **193**
        in multiple sclerosis, 193, 1023
        in neuromyelitis optica, 193, 1025
Neuroblastoma, 1624*t*
Neurocutaneous diseases, **1009–1010**,
        1010*f*
Neurocysticercosis, 1536
Neurodegenerative disease, head injury
        and, 1031
Neuroendocrine tumors. *See also specific
        type*
    diarrhea and, 594
    extrapancreatic, 1188
    gastrinoma differential diagnosis and,
        632
    gastroenteropancreatic, **1185–1187**
    lung, 1188
    nonfunctioning, 1185
    pancreatic, 1185–1186, 1620
    thymic, 1188
Neurofibromas, 1003, 1010, 1010*f*
Neurofibromatosis, **1010**, 1010*f*
    type 1, 1010
        gastroenteropancreatic
            neuroendocrine tumors in,
            1185
        pheochromocytoma/paraganglioma
            in, 1179–1180
    type 2/vestibular schwannoma (eighth
        nerve tumors/acoustic
        neuroma) and, 213, 1010
NEUROG3 mutation, in diabetes,
        1212
Neurogenic arthropathy (Charcot joint),
        875
    in diabetes mellitus, 875, 1239
    in tabes dorsalis, 875, 1496, 1496*f*
Neurogenic claudication, in spinal
        stenosis, 1694
Neurogenic hyperventilation, in coma or
        stupor, 316, 1027
Neurogenic shock, 494, 494*t*, 495
Neuroglycopenia, hypoglycemia and,
        1236, 1258
Neuroimaging
    in brain abscess, 1007, 1298, 1299
    in dementia, 58, 1020
    in head injury, 1030
    in headache, 40, 40*t*, 41
    in intracranial tumors, 1005
    lumbar puncture and, 1298, 1299
    in multiple sclerosis, 1023
    in schizophrenia/psychotic disorders,
        1067
    in stroke, 995–996, 998, 999, 1000,
        1001. *See also specific cause*
    in transient ischemic attacks, 992
Neurokinin receptor antagonists, for
        nausea and vomiting, 582*t*,
        583
    chemotherapy induced, 582, 582*t*, 583,
        1673
Neurokinin receptors, in nausea and
        vomiting, 580, 1672

Neuroleptic malignant syndrome, 35, 36, 1072, 1580, 1589, 1590
Neuroleptics. *See* Antipsychotic drugs
Neurologic disorders, **977–1049**. *See also specific cause and Neuropathies*
  adverse ophthalmic effects of drugs used in, 177–178t
  in Behçet syndrome, 862
  cancer-related, **1008–1009**
  in chikungunya fever, 1407
  in chronic kidney disease/uremia, 924t, 928–929
  CMV causing, 1375
  coxsackieviruses causing, 1426
  cryptococcal, 1553, 1553–1554
  drowning and, 1567
  dysphagia in, 605t
  herpes simplex infection, 1364, 1366
  in high-altitude illness, **1574**
  in HIV infection/AIDS, 1339–1340
  in hypercalcemia/hyperparathyroidism, 898, 1153
  infection, **1296–1300**, 1297t. *See also* Encephalitis; Meningitis
    anaerobic, **1478–1479**
    otitis media and, 206
  in Kawasaki disease, 1439
  in leprosy, 1484
  in Lyme disease, 1037, 1041, 1041f, 1502, 1503, 1504–1505, 1505t
  measles/measles vaccination causing, 1378–1379
  nausea and vomiting and, 580, 581, 581t
  nonmetastatic complications of cancer, **1008–1009**
  in pheochromocytoma/paraganglioma, 1180t
  postoperative, **52–53**, 52t
  in preeclampsia-eclampsia, 809t
  primary angiitis and, **862–863**
  respiratory failure caused by, 318t
  SIADH caused by, 887, 887t
  in SLE, 839t, 840, 841
  in syphilis, 1316t, 1489t, **1495–1497**, 1496f. *See also* Neurosyphilis
  in thrombotic microangiopathy, 551, 551t
  in toxocariasis, 1542
  in varicella zoster virus infection, 1369
  vertigo/vestibular disorders and, 210t, 211, 211t, 213, 213–214
  vitamin B_{12} deficiency causing, 507
  in Wilson disease, 710
Neurologic evaluation
  preoperative, **52–53**, 52t
  in spine disorders, 1692t, 1696, 1696t
Neuroma/neurinoma. *See also* Neurofibromatosis
  acoustic. *See* Acoustic neuroma/neurinoma
  mucosal, in MEN, 1188
  plexiform, 1010
Neuromodulation, for angina, 363
Neuromuscular/neuromuscular transmission disorders, **1045–1047**. *See also specific disorder*
  dysphagia in, 605, 605t

in hypercalcemia/hyperparathyroidism, 1153
respiratory failure caused by, 318t
in uremia, 924t
Neuromyelitis optica (Devic disease/syndrome), **1025**
  optic neuritis in, 193, 1025
Neuron-specific enolase, in Jakob-Creutzfeldt disease, 1022
Neuronal nicotinic acetylcholine receptor antibodies, in dysautonomia, 990
Neuronitis, vestibular, 211t, 212
Neuronopathy, cancer-related, 1008
Neuropathic bladder, 1035
  chemotherapy-induced, 1674
Neuropathic pain, **83–84**, 83t, 1035. *See also* Neuropathies
  in diabetes, 1239, 1239–1240
Neuropathies, **1034–1042**. *See also specific cause or type*
  acute motor axonal/acute motor and sensory axonal (AMAN/AMSAN), 1038. *See also* Guillain-Barré syndrome
  alcoholism and, 1036, 1039
  in amyloidosis, 1037
  antiretroviral agents causing, 1340
  autonomic. *See* Autonomic neuropathy
  brachial plexus, **1042–1043**
  cancer-related, **1037–1038**
  chemotherapy-induced, 1674
  in chronic kidney disease/uremia, 929, 1036
  cisplatin-induced, 1675
  in critically ill patient, **1037**
  in cryoglobulinemia, 860
  diabetic, 1036, 1239–1241, 1239f. *See also* Diabetic neuropathy
  didanosine therapy and, 1340, 1353, 1355
  diphtheritic, 1037, 1457
  dysautonomia and, 990
  entrapment/compression, 1037, 1039
  facial, **1041**, 1041f. *See also* Facial neuropathy/paralysis/palsy
  hereditary motor and sensory (HMSN), types I to IV, 1035–1036
  in HIV infection/AIDS, 1340
  infectious/inflammatory disease and, **1037**
  inherited, **1035–1036**
  in leprosy, 1037, 1484
  in Lyme disease, 1037, 1041, 1041f, 1502, 1503, 1504–1505, 1505t
  metabolic/systemic disease and, **1036–1037**
  in microscopic polyangiitis, 860
  nutritional, 1036. *See also specific nutrient*
  optic
    inflammatory (optic neuritis), **193**
      in multiple sclerosis, 193, 1023
      in neuromyelitis optica, 193, 1025
    ischemic, **192**
      giant cell arteritis and, 192, 854
    in paraproteinemias, 1036–1037
  peripheral, **1034–1042**. *See also specific type*

in polyarteritis nodosa, 856
in porphyria, 1036, 1676
in rheumatoid arthritis, 835, 1037
in sarcoidosis, 1037
stavudine therapy and, 1340
in thiamine deficiency, 1036, 1275
toxic, 1037
vincristine-induced, 1674
vitamin B_6 causing, 507, 1276
Neuropsychological assessment, in dementia, 1020
Neuroses, Sunday, 1053
Neurosyphilis, 1316t, 1489t, **1495–1497**, 1496f
  in HIV infection/AIDS, 1348, 1497
  treatment/treatment failures and, 1316t, 1491t, 1496–1497
Neurotoxicity. *See also* Neurologic disorders
  of cisplatin, 1675
  opioid-induced, 82
  peripheral neuropathies and, 1037
  of snake venom, 1604
Neurotransmitters. *See specific type*
Neurotrophic keratitis, 174, 175
Neurotropic disease
  viral, **1386–1397**. *See also specific disorder*
  yellow fever vaccine-associated, 1327, 1405
Neutral protamine Hagedorn (NPH) insulin. *See* Insulin therapy; NPH insulin
Neutral protamine lispro (NPL) insulin. *See* Insulin therapy; NPL insulin
Neutralizing antibodies, immunodeficiency disorders caused by, 881
Neutrocytic ascites, 601–602, 603
Neutrogena, 100t
Neutropenia, **517–519**, 518t
  antibiotic prophylaxis/therapy in, 518, 1292, 1293
  autoimmune, 518
  cancer chemotherapy causing, 35, 518, 1290, 1662
  cyclic, 518
  fever/FUO and, 518, 1287, 1288
    antimicrobial therapy and, 35, 518, 1293, 1296, 1314t, 1661
  infections and, 35, 517–518, 518, 1290
    in cancer patients, 1661
    prevention/treatment and, 35, 518, 1292
  pulmonary infiltrates in, 276
Neutrophil count. *See also* Neutropenia
  ascitic fluid, 601–602, 603, 604
  normal, 517
Neutrophil elastase gene mutations, in neutropenia, 518
Neutroval. *See* Tbo-filgrastim
Nevanac. *See* Nepafenac
Nevi. *See also* Mole (skin)
  atypical (dysplastic), **102**, 102f
  blue, **102–103**, 102f
  compound, 101, 101f
  junctional, 101
  melanocytic, **101–102**, 101f
Nevirapine, 1351t, 1355–1356. *See also* Antiretroviral therapy

Nevus. *See* Nevi
New (novel) anticoagulants. *See* Direct-acting oral anticoagulants
New World cutaneous leishmaniasis, 1510, 1510–1511, 1512
Newborn/infant
    antiretroviral therapy for, 1332, 1346
    chikungunya fever in, 1407
    chlamydial infection in, 823
    CMV infection/inclusion disease in, 1374, 1375, 1376
    coxsackievirus infection in, 1426
    dengue in, 1402
    gonococcal infection in, 823
    Graves disease (transient) in, 1127
    group B streptococcal infection and, 800–801, 820, 1444
    hemolytic disease of, 801
    hepatitis B transmission/vaccine and, 4, 680, 681, 822
    hepatitis C transmission and, 822–823
    herpes simplex infection and, 823, 1363–1364, 1366
    HIV transmission to, 822, 1332, 1346
    hypercalcemia/hyperparathyroidism in, 1153–1154
    hypocalcemia/tetany in, 1154
    hypoparathyroidism in, 1153
    immunization recommendations and, **1319**
    listeriosis in (granulomatosis infantisepticum), 1457
    malaria/malaria prophylaxis in, 1513, 1521
    parechovirus infection in, 1428
    pneumocystosis in, 1551
    rubella infection and, 1384, 1385
    syphilis in (congenital syphilis), 823, 1488, **1497–1498**
        penicillin treatment in maternal disease and, 1497
    toxoplasmosis in, 799, 1523, 1523–1524
    varicella in, 821
    Zika virus testing in, 1406
Nexavar. *See* Sorafenib
Nexplanon, 789
NF1/NF2 genes, in neurofibromatosis, 1010
NF-kappa-B, in myeloma, 535
NH₃. *See* Ammonia
Niacin (vitamin B₃)
    deficiency of, **1275–1276**
    for lipid modification, 355, 1263, 1264, 1265*t*, 1266, 1275–1276
    side effects/toxicity of, 1264, **1276**
Niacinamide, 1276. *See also* Niacin
Niaspan. *See* Niacin
Nicardipine, 461*t*
    for angina, 361
    for hypertension, 459, 461*t*
        pheochromocytoma/ pheochromocytoma surgery and, 469, 469*t*, 1183
        in urgencies/emergencies, 468–469, 469, 469*t*, 470*t*
    overdose/toxicity of, 459, 461*t*, 1591
Niclosamide, for tapeworm infection, 1536

Nicotinamide. *See also* Niacin
    for niacin deficiency, 1276
Nicotine/nicotine replacement therapy, 7. *See also* Smoking
    during pregnancy, 799
Nicotinic acid. *See* Niacin
Nifediac. *See* Nifedipine
Nifedical. *See* Nifedipine
Nifedipine, 461*t*. *See also* Calcium channel blocking drugs
    for angina, 361
    for high-altitude illness treatment/ prevention, 1575
    for hypertension, 459, 461*t*
        in urgencies/emergencies, 470*t*, 471
    for interstitial cystitis, 961
    overdose/toxicity of, 459, 461*t*, 1591
    pheochromocytoma/ pheochromocytoma surgery and, 1183
    for preterm labor, 812
Nifurtimox
    for African trypanosomiasis, 1508, 1508*t*
    for American trypanosomiasis/Chagas disease, 1509, 1510
Night blindness, in vitamin A deficiency, 1277
Nikolsky sign, 139
Nil disease (minimal change disease), 934*t*, **943**
Nilandron. *See* Nilutamide
Nilotinib, 1668*t*
    for chronic myeloid leukemia, 524–525
Nilutamide, 1669*t*
Nimodipine. *See also* Calcium channel blocking drugs
    overdose/toxicity of, 1591
    for vasospasm in subarachnoid hemorrhage, 999
Ninlaro. *See* Ixazomib
Nintedanib, for idiopathic pulmonary fibrosis, 292
Nipah virus, 1409
Nipent. *See* Pentostatin
NIPHS. *See* Noninsulinoma pancreatogenous hypoglycemia syndrome
Nipple, Paget disease of, 118, 118*f*, 745
Nipple discharge, **735–736**, 736*t*
    in breast cancer, 736, 736*t*
    in male, 760
    in fibrocystic breast condition, 734, 736, 736*t*
    in hyperprolactinemia, 736
NIPPV. *See* Noninvasive positive-pressure ventilation
Nipride. *See* Nitroprusside
Nisoldipine, 461*t*
    for angina, 361
    for hypertension, 459, 461*t*
    overdose/toxicity of, 459, 461*t*, 1591
Nitazoxanide
    for cryptosporidiosis, 1529
    for giardiasis, 1531
Nithiodote, 1593
Nitisinone, for alkaptonuria, 1678
Nitrates. *See also* Nitroglycerin
    for acute coronary syndromes/STEMI, 368, 375

    for angina
        for acute attack, 359, 360*f*
        prophylactic/longer acting, 359
    for heart failure, 408, 412
        infarct-related, 378
    phosphodiesterase inhibitor/sildenafil contraindications and, 375, 967, 1064, 1241
    for pulmonary edema, 412
Nitrendipine, for hypertension, 464
Nitric oxide, in erection, 966
Nitrites
    for cyanide poisoning, 1581*t*, 1593
    methemoglobinemia caused by, 1599
Nitrobenzene, methemoglobinemia caused by, 1599
Nitrofurantoin
    G6PD deficiency and, 511
    for urinary tract infection, 954, 955, 955*t*
Nitrogen, liquid. *See* Liquid nitrogen
Nitrogen balance, nutritional support and, 1285
Nitrogen mustards, in cancer chemotherapy, 1663*t*
Nitrogen oxide gases, methemoglobinemia caused by, 1599
Nitroglycerin. *See also* Nitrates
    for acute coronary syndromes/STEMI, 368, 375
    for angina
        for acute attack, 359, 360*f*
        in diagnosis, 356
        prophylactic administration of, 359
    for heart failure, 408, 412
        infarct-related, 378
    for hypertensive urgencies/ emergencies, 469*t*, 470*t*, 471
    phosphodiesterase inhibitor/sildenafil contraindications and, 375, 967, 1064, 1241
    for pulmonary edema, 412
Nitroimidazole, in *H pylori* eradication therapy, 626
Nitropress. *See* Nitroprusside
Nitroprusside
    for cardiogenic shock, 378
    cyanide poisoning caused by, 1592
    for heart failure, 408
        infarct-related, 378
    for hypertension
        in aortic dissection, 469*t*, 485
        pheochromocytoma surgery and, 1183
        in urgencies/emergencies, 469, 469*t*, 470*t*, 471
Nivolumab, 1666*t*
    for lung cancer, 1612
    for renal cell carcinoma, 1655
Nix. *See* Permethrin
Nizatidine, 609. *See also* H₂ receptor blocking drugs
Nizoral. *See* Ketoconazole
Njovera (endemic syphilis), **1498–1499**
NK-cell lymphoma, 531, 532*t*
    Epstein-Barr virus and, 1373, 1374
    nose and paranasal sinus involvement and, 223
NK₁ receptor antagonists, for nausea and vomiting, 582*t*, 583
    chemotherapy-induced, 583, 1673

NK$_1$ receptors, in nausea and vomiting, 580, 1672
NMDA receptors, cancer-related encephalitis and, 1008
NMO-IgG, in neuromyelitis optica, 1025
NMS. *See* Neuroleptic malignant syndrome
NNRTIs. *See* Nonnucleoside reverse transcriptase inhibitors
No-added-salt diet, 1279
Nocardia asteroides/brasiliensis (nocardiosis), 1312*t*, **1481**
Nodular goiter. *See* Multinodular (nodular) goiter
Nodular malignant melanoma, 103
Nodular regenerative hyperplasia, noncirrhotic portal hypertension and, 713
Nodules
  milker's (paravaccinia), 1423
  pulmonary
    in metastatic disease, 1613, 1614
    solitary, **287–288**
  rheumatoid, 835, 835*f*
    in coal workers (Caplan syndrome), 307
    gouty tophi differentiated from, 831, 836
  skin, 96*t*. *See also specific type*
    inflammatory, **151–155**
    violaceous to purple, **144–146**
  subcutaneous. *See* Subcutaneous nodules
  thyroid, **1137–1140**, 1138*t*. *See also* Goiter; Thyroid cancer; Thyroid nodules
  vocal fold, 234
Noise trauma
  hearing loss caused by, 201, 208
  tympanic membrane perforation and, 207
Nolvadex. *See* Tamoxifen
Non-ABCDE hepatitis, transfusion-associated, 682
Nonadherence/adherence, 1–2. *See also specific disorder*
  elderly patients and, 69
Non–albinism-associated storage pool disease, 556–557
Nonalcoholic fatty liver disease (NAFLD), **697–699**. *See also* Fatty liver
  cirrhosis and, 697, 698, 699
  hepatocellular carcinoma and, 699, 1616
Nonalcoholic steatohepatitis (NASH), 697, 698, 699
Nonarteritic anterior ischemic optic neuropathy, 192
Nonbacterial folliculitis, 130
Nonbacterial prostatitis, 957*t*, **958–959**
Noncancer pain, chronic (CNCP), 1060–1062, 1061*f*
  management of, 72–73, 82, **84–86**, 1061–1062
Noncirrhotic portal hypertension, **713–714**
Non-clostridial crepitant cellulitis, 1480
Noncompliance/compliance (nonadherence/adherence), 1–2. *See also specific disorder*
  elderly patients and, 69

Nonconvulsive status epilepticus, 990
Non-determined leukoencephalopathy, 1395
Nondiabetic (renal) glycosuria, 1214
Nonendocrine tumors, in MEN, 1188
Nonepileptic seizure, psychogenic (PNES), 986, 1058
Nonerosive/nonspecific gastritis, **621–622**
Nonexertional (classic) heat stroke, 1562
Non-falciparum malaria, 1515
Nonfamilial adenomatous and serrated polyps, **665–666**
Nonfluent/agrammatic variant primary progressive aphasia, 1019*t*
Nongonococcal acute bacterial (septic) arthritis, **867–868**, 1314*t*
  in drug users, 867, 1304
Non-group A streptococcal infections, **1444**
Non-Hodgkin lymphoma, **531–533**, 532*t*, 1622*t*. *See also* Lymphoma
  bone marrow/stem cell transplantation for, 533, 540
  classification of, 531–532, 532*t*
  fever/FUO and, 1288
  gastric, 532, 1632
  in HIV infection/AIDS, 1337*t*, 1338–1339, 1339, 1344
  kidney involved in, 1655
  pemphigus and, 139
  small intestine, 1634
Noninsulinoma pancreatogenous hypoglycemia syndrome (islet cell hyperplasia), 1252, **1256**
Noninsulinomas, localization of, 1186, 1254–1255
Noninvasive ischemia testing, preoperative, 45–46, 47*f*
Noninvasive positive-pressure ventilation (NIPPV)
  for COPD, 262
  for pulmonary edema, 412
  for respiratory failure, 318
Nonionizing radiation, 1571
Nonislet cell tumor hypoglycemia, **1255–1256**
Nonketotic hyperglycemic hyperosmolar coma (hyperglycemic hyperosmolar state), 1214, 1245, 1246*t*, **1249–1251**
Non-myeloablative allogeneic stem cell transplantation, 540, 541. *See also* Bone marrow/stem cell transplantation
Nonnucleoside polymerase inhibitors, for hepatitis C, 690, 690*t*
Nonnucleoside reverse transcriptase inhibitors (NNRTIs), 1351*t*, 1355–1356. *See also* Antiretroviral therapy
  antituberculous drug interactions and, 282
  oral contraceptive drug interaction and, 786
  resistance to, 1355, 1360, 1362
Nonocclusive mesenteric vascular insufficiency, 479
Nonoxynol-9, 790
  HIV infection/AIDS and, 790, 1346

Nonparalytic poliomyelitis, 1382, 1383
Nonparoxysmal junctional tachycardia, 395
Nonproliferative retinopathy, 189, 189–190, 189*f*, 190, 1238
Non-Q wave (non-ST elevation) infarction, 26–27, 27, 27*t*, 28, **365–370**, 367*f*, 369*t*, 371. *See also* Myocardial infarction; Non–ST-segment elevation syndromes
  fibrinolytic/thrombolytic therapy contraindicated in, 366, 372
Non-rapid eye movement (non-REM) sleep, 1088
Nonscarring alopecia, 158, 158–159
"Nonsecretory myeloma," 536
Nonseminomas, 1655, 1656, 1657
Non-sexually transmitted epididymitis, 955*t*, 960
Non-sexually transmitted treponematoses, **1498–1499**
Non–small cell lung cancer, 1609, 1611–1612, 1623*t*. *See also* Lung cancer
  pulmonary function testing in, 1610–1611
  staging of, 1610, 1610*t*
  treatment of, 1611–1612
Nonspecific interstitial pneumonia (NSIP), 291*t*, 292
  in HIV infection/AIDS, 1339
Non–ST-segment elevation syndromes (NSTEMI), **365–370**, 367*f*, 369*t*. *See also* Acute coronary syndromes
  angiography/revascularization in, 369, 369*t*. *See also* Revascularization procedures
  fibrinolytic/thrombolytic therapy contraindicated in, 366, 372
  postinfarction ischemia and, 376–377
Nonsteroidal anti-inflammatory drug (NSAID) exacerbated respiratory disease, **878**
Nonsteroidal anti-inflammatory drugs (NSAIDs), 74, 75–76*t*. *See also specific agent*
  for abnormal uterine bleeding, 763
  acute kidney injury and, 74, 829, 917
  in analgesic nephropathy, 947
  for ankylosing spondylitis, 864
  cardiovascular complications and, 621, 624, 829
  in colorectal cancer prevention, 1637
  COX-1/COX-2 affected by, 624, 828
  for endometriosis/pelvic pain, 765, 765–766, 776
  gastrointestinal side effects (bleeding/gastritis/gastropathy) and, 74, 620, 621, 624, 829
  for gout, 831
  hypertension and, 441
  hyponatremia caused by, 886
  for ophthalmic disorders, 168, 171*t*, 199
  for osteoarthritis, 828–829, 1714
  for pain management, **74**, 75–76*t*
    with opioid analgesics, 74
  in peptic ulcer disease, 623, 624, 829
    bleeding control and, 629–630

H pylori infection/eradication therapy and, 624, 627
misoprostol coadministration and, 626*t*
prevention and, 626*t*, 627
proton pump inhibitors for, 626*t*, 627, 627–628, 829
risk reduction and, 628
for pericarditis, 426
platelet function affected by, 558*t*, 829
pompholyx-like eruption caused by, 122
for psoriatic arthritis, 865
renal toxicity of, 74, 829
respiratory disease associated with sensitivity to, **878**
for rheumatoid arthritis, 836
topical, 74, 98*t*, 829
tubulointerstitial nephritis caused by, 947*t*
Nonstreptococcal exudative pharyngitis, 1421
Nonsustained ventricular tachycardia, 381, 397
Nontreponemal antigen tests, for syphilis, 1489, 1489–1490, 1490*t*
Nontuberculous (atypical) mycobacteria (NTM), **1481–1483**
in HIV infection/AIDS, 285, 1336
lymphadenitis/adenitis caused by, **239**, 1345
MAC infections. *See Mycobacterium* (mycobacterial infections), *avium* complex
pulmonary disease caused by, **284–286**, **1481–1482**
skin and soft tissue infections caused by, **1482**
Norelgestromin, in transdermal contraceptive patch, 789
Norepinephrine
for hypotension/shock, 496, 497
cardiogenic, 378, 497
in tricyclic antidepressant overdose, 1578
in pheochromocytoma/paraganglioma, 1179
Norepinephrine reuptake inhibitors, with opioid agonists, 80–81*t*
Norethindrone
for abnormal uterine bleeding, 763
for endometriosis, 776
in hormone replacement therapy, 795, 1204
in oral contraceptives, 787*t*, 788
with oral estrogens, 1204
for postmenopausal bleeding, 764
in progestin minipill, 788
with transdermal estradiol, 1204
Norfloxacin. *See also* Fluoroquinolones
for ophthalmic disorders, 169*t*
for urinary tract infection, 955*t*
Norgestimate
in estrogen replacement therapy, 1204
in oral contraceptives, 787*t*
for hirsutism/virilization, 1198
Norgestrel, in oral contraceptives, 787*t*
Normal anion gap acidosis, 904, 904*t*, **906–907**, 906*t*, 908
alcoholic ketoacidosis and, 906

diabetic ketoacidosis and, 905, 1248
dilutional, 907
parenteral nutritional support and, 907, 1285*t*
posthypocapnia, 907
renal disease/renal tubular acidosis and, 892*t*, 906–907, 906*t*, 908
tubulointerstitial disease and, 948
urinary anion gap in assessment of, 906, 906*t*, 907
Normal flora
Actinomyces as, 1480
anaerobic bacteria as, 1478
coagulase-negative staphylococci as, 1450
opportunistic infections caused by, 1290
Normal pressure hydrocephalus, 1021
Normetanephrine, in pheochromocytoma, 1181
Normocalcemic hyperparathyroidism, 1153, 1154
Normochloremic metabolic (increased anion gap) acidosis, 904*t*, **905–906**, 907–908, 1584
Normokalemic periodic paralysis, 1049
Normosmic isolated hypogonadotropic hypogonadism, 1109
Noroviruses, acute diarrhea/food poisoning caused by, 588*t*, 1305, 1307*t*, 1425
Norpramin. *See* Desipramine
Norprolac. *See* Quinagolide
Nor-QD. *See* Norethindrone
North Asian tick typhus, 1434
Norton score, for pressure ulcers, 68
Nortriptyline, 1078*t*, 1081. *See also* Antidepressants
for neuropathic pain/diabetic neuropathy, 83*t*, 1239–1240
Norvasc. *See* Amlodipine
Norvir. *See* Ritonavir
Norwalk virus, gastroenteritis caused by, 1425
Nose, **214–224**. *See also under Nasal*
in granulomatosis with polyangiitis, **223–224**, 858
infections of, **214–218**, 217*t*. *See also* Rhinosinusitis; Sinusitis
inflammatory disease of, **223–224**
in sarcoidosis, **223**, 293*f*
traumatic injury of, **222**
tumors/granulomatous disease of, **222–224**
Nosebleed. *See* Epistaxis
Nosocomial infections. *See* Health care (hospital)-associated infections
Nosocomial pneumonia, **272–274**, 273*t*, 275*t*, 1294, 1314*t*
Notch 1, in aortic stenosis, 341
Novantrone. *See* Mitoxantrone
Novel (new) anticoagulants. *See* Direct-acting oral anticoagulants
Novolin. *See also* Insulin therapy
Novolog. *See* Insulin aspart
NPH1/NPH2/NPH3 genes, in juvenile nephronophthisis-medullary cystic disease, 951

NPH insulin, 1229, 1229*t*, 1230, 1231, 1234. *See also* Insulin therapy
in mixtures/combination therapy, 1229*t*, 1231, 1234, 1236
in pregnancy, 817, 1244
NPL insulin, 1231. *See also* Insulin therapy
in mixtures/combination therapy, 1229*t*, 1231
NPM1 mutation, in acute myeloid leukemia, 527
NPPV. *See* Noninvasive positive-pressure ventilation
NREM sleep, 1088
NRTIs. *See* Nucleoside reverse transcriptase inhibitors
NS3/4A protease inhibitors, for hepatitis C, 689, 690, 690*t*, 691
NS5A inhibitors, for hepatitis C, 689–690, 690, 690*t*, 691
NS5B nonnucleos(t)ide polymerase inhibitors, for hepatitis C, 690*t*, 691
NS5B nucleos(t)ide polymerase inhibitor, for hepatitis C, 690*t*, 691
NSAIDs. *See* Nonsteroidal anti-inflammatory drugs
NSCLC. *See* Non-small cell lung cancer
NSIP. *See* Nonspecific interstitial pneumonia
nsNSAID (nonselective NSAIDs). *See* Nonsteroidal anti-inflammatory drugs
NSQIP (National Surgical Quality Improvement Program) risk assessment tool, 45, 49
NSVT. *See* Nonsustained ventricular tachycardia
NTM. *See* Nontuberculous (atypical) mycobacteria
NTZ. *See* Nitazoxanide
Nuclear bleeding scans, in GI bleeding, 598–599
Nuclear bone scanning. *See* Bone scanning
Nuclear factor-kappa B ligand (RANKL)
denosumab mechanism of action and, 1162
in myeloma, 535
Nuclear technology/medicine, radiation exposure and, 1571, 1572
Nuclear transcription factor mutations, in MODY, 1211*t*, 1212
Nucleic acid amplification testing (NAAT-TB/NAAT-R)
in STDs, 1302
in tuberculosis, 278–279, 278*t*
Nucleophosmin 1 (*NPM1*) mutation, in acute myeloid leukemia, 527
Nucleoside polymerase inhibitors, for hepatitis C, 690, 690*t*
Nucleoside reverse transcriptase inhibitors (NRTIs), 1351*t*, 1353–1355. *See also* Antiretroviral therapy
in combinations, 1353, 1358
for hepatitis B, 687–688
lactic acidosis caused by, 1341
myopathy associated with use of, 869, 1340
resistance to, 1362

Nucleotide reverse transcriptase inhibitor, 1351*t*, 1354–1355. *See also* Antiretroviral therapy
  for hepatitis B, 687–688
Nucleus pulposus, herniation of
  cervical, **1042**, 1043–1044*f*
  lumbar/sacral, 1695
Nucynta/Nucynta ER. *See* Tapentadol
NuLYTE. *See* Polyethylene glycol
Nursing (breastfeeding). *See* Lactation
Nursing homes
  norovirus infections and, 1305, 1425
  scabies outbreaks and, 148, 149
Nutcracker esophagus, 619
Nutmeg liver, 713
Nutrients. *See also* Diet; Nutritional disorders; Nutritional support
  diets restricting, **1279**
  diets supplementing, **1280**
  requirements for in nutritional support, **1282–1283**
Nutrition. *See also* Diet; Nutrients; Nutritional disorders; Nutritional support
  in Crohn disease, 655
  in end-of-life care, 91
  in pregnancy, 799, **801**
  preventable disease/deaths and, 3*t*, 6*t*
Nutritional disorders, **1268–1286**. *See also* Eating disorders; Malnutrition; Obesity/overweight
  cognitive disorders/delirium caused by, 1102*t*
  neuropathy associated with, 1036. *See also specific type*
  thrombocytopenia associated with, **548**
Nutritional support, **1280–1286**, 1281*f*, 1283*t*, 1284*t*, 1285*t*. *See also specific type*
  in alcoholic liver disease, 694
  in anorexia nervosa, 1273
  in burn injury, 1569
  in Crohn disease, 655
  in elderly/dementia/end-of-life care, 67, 91
  in HIV infection/AIDS, 1335
  indications for, **1281**
  methods for, 1281–1282, 1281*f*
  nutritional requirements and, **1282–1283**
  in pancreatitis, 729
  patient monitoring during, **1285–1286**
  for protein–energy malnutrition, 1269
  in short bowel syndrome, 637
  in ulcerative colitis, 660
Nutropin Depot. *See* Recombinant human growth hormone
NuvaRing, 1205
Nystagmus
  in coma or stupor, 1027
  in vertigo, 211, 213
Nystatin, for candidiasis
  balanitis and, 133
  cutaneous, 133
  oral, 226
  vulvovaginal, 133, 767

Obesity/overweight, **1269–1272**
  asthma and, 242
  bulimia nervosa and, 1274
  cancer risk and, 12, 13
  cholelithiasis/gallstones and, 716
  coronary heart disease and, 353
  in Cushing syndrome, 1173, 1174
  definition of/measurements in, 12, 1269–1270
  in diabetes mellitus, 1212, 1214, 1218, 1219, 1235
  diet/eating behavior changes and, 12, 13, 1270
  exercise/activity and, 11, 12, 13, 1270–1271
  genetic factors in, 1270
  GERD and, 606, 609
  GH deficiency and, 1109, 1110
  in hypertension, 441, 445, 446*t*
  hypogonadotropic hypogonadism and, 1109, 1193
  hypothalamic damage causing, 1111
  hypoventilation and (Pickwickian syndrome), **315–316**
  insulin resistance and, 12, 1270
  medical conditions/evaluation and, 1270
  medications in management of, 13, 1271
  nonalcoholic fatty liver disease and, 697, 698
  oral contraceptive use and, 788
  osteoarthritis and, 827, 828
  in polycystic ovary syndrome, 780, 781, 1196
  postoperative pulmonary complications and, 49
  preventable disease/deaths and, 3*t*, 6*t*, **12–13**
  psoriasis and, 107
  treatment of, 12–13, 1270–1272. *See also* Bariatric surgery
    in diabetes, 1235
  weight gain in pregnancy and, 801
Obesity-hypoventilation syndrome (Pickwickian syndrome), **315–316**
Obinutuzumab, 1666*t*
  for chronic lymphocytic leukemia, 530
Obliterative bronchiolitis, 266. *See also* Bronchiolitis
Obliterative portal venopathy, 713
O'Brien test, 1688*t*, 1690
Obsessions, 1057. *See also* Obsessive-compulsive disorder
Obsessive-compulsive disorder (OCD), **1057–1058**
  panic disorder and, 1053
  Tourette syndrome and, 1018, 1057
Obsessive-compulsive disorder spectrum, 1057
Obsessive-compulsive personality disorder, 1065*t*
Obstetrics/obstetric disorders, **797–825**. *See also* Pregnancy
  adverse ophthalmic effects of drugs used in, 178*t*
Obstructive jaundice, 674, 674–676, 675*t*, 676*t*, 721

Obstructive lung disease. *See* Airway disorders, obstruction; Chronic obstructive pulmonary disease
Obstructive nephropathy, chronic kidney disease caused by, 924*t*
Obstructive pancreatitis, 731
Obstructive shock, 494, 494*t*, 495
Obstructive sleep apnea hypopnea, 230, 231, 316, **316–317**, 1089
  obesity-hypoventilation syndrome and, 316
  postoperative pulmonary complications and, 49
Obstructive uropathy
  acute kidney injury caused by, 918
  tubulointerstitial disease caused by, 947, 948
Obstructive voiding symptoms, 970
Obturator sign, in appendicitis, 641, 642
Occipital lobe lesions, 1005
Occlusive dressings
  corticosteroid use and, 95, 117
  for cutaneous lupus, 115
  for leg ulcers, 156
  for wart removal, 141
Occult diabetes, 1252, **1257**
Occult GI bleeding, 599, **600**. *See also* Fecal occult blood testing; Gastrointestinal bleeding
Occupational asthma, 242, 308
Occupational pulmonary diseases, 290*t*, **306–309**, 307*t*, 308*t*. *See also specific disorder*
Occupational radiation exposure, 1572
OCD. *See* Obsessive-compulsive disorder
OCD spectrum, 1057
Ochronosis, 1677
Ocriplasmin
  for diabetic macular edema, 190
  for retinal detachment, 184
Octreotide
  for carcinoid syndrome, 1636
  for diarrhea, 594, 1342
  for gastric carcinoid tumors, 1633
  in gastroenteropancreatic neuroendocrine tumor localization, 1186
  for gastroenteropancreatic neuroendocrine tumors, 1186
  for GH-secreting tumor/acromegaly/ gigantism, 1116
  for GI bleeding/esophageal varices, 597, 615
  for nausea and vomiting, 87
  for pheochromocytoma/paraganglioma identification, 1182
  for short bowel syndrome, 637
  for sulfonylurea overdose/ hypoglycemia, 1581*t*, 1595
Ocudose. *See* Timolol
Ocuflox. *See* Ofloxacin
Ocular contusions, **197**
Ocular disease. *See* Eye, disorders of
Ocular examination. *See* Eye, examination of
Ocular hemorrhages
  eye injuries and, 197
  vitreous, **184–185**, 184*f*

Ocular hypertension, 180. *See also*
    Glaucoma
  in chronic glaucoma, 180
    treatment of, 172–173*t*
Ocular lacerations, **197–198**, 197*f*
Ocular larva migrans, 1542
Ocular medications. *See* Ophthalmic
    medications
Ocular melanoma, 103
Ocular motor palsies, **194**
Ocular movements. *See* Eye (extraocular)
    movements
Ocular myasthenia gravis, 195, 1045
Ocular transient ischemic attack,
    188–189
Ocular trauma, **196–198**, 196*f*, 197*f*
Oculocephalic reflex, in coma or stupor,
    1027
Oculomotor response, in coma or stupor,
    1027
Oculopharyngeal muscular dystrophy,
    1048*t*
Oculosympathetic paralysis. *See* Horner
    syndrome
Oculovestibular reflex, in coma or stupor,
    1027
Oddi, sphincter of. *See* Sphincter of Oddi
Odontogenic infections. *See also* Dental
    disorders
  deep neck infections and, 230
Odor identification/discrimination/
    threshold, disorders of,
    220–221
  intracranial tumors causing, 220
  in Kallmann syndrome, 1109, 1199,
    1200
Odynophagia, 229, 605
  in esophageal cancer, 1626
OEP. *See* Oil of evening primrose
Ofatumumab, 1666*t*
Ofloxacin. *See also* Fluoroquinolones
  for ophthalmic disorders, 169*t*
  for traveler's diarrhea, 1310
Ogilvie syndrome, **639–640**
Oil of evening primrose (OEP), for
    fibrocystic condition, 735
Oka/Merck VZV vaccine. *See* Herpes
    zoster vaccine
Olanzapine, 1068, 1069*t*, 1070, 1071,
    1071*t*, 1072, 1073. *See also*
    Antipsychotic drugs
  for aggressive/violent patient, 1091
  for bipolar disease/mania, 1085
  for depression, 1079, 1083
  diabetes and, 1072, 1213
  overdose/toxicity/side effects of, 1069*t*,
    1071*t*, 1072, 1589–1590
  ophthalmic, 177*t*
  for psychedelic/hallucinogenic abuse/
    toxicity, 1099, 1598
Olaparib, 1669*t*
Old World cutaneous leishmaniasis, 1510,
    1510–1511, 1512
Older adults, **55–71**. *See also specific
    disorder affecting*
  abuse/mistreatment/neglect and, 16,
    70–71, 71*t*
  advance directives and, 90
  anemia in, 502, 503
  assessment of, **55–57**, 56*f*, 56*t*, 57*t*
  benzodiazepine use in, 1055

  delirium in, **61–62**
    at end of life, 87
  dementia in, **57–60**. *See also* Dementia
  depressed, **60–61**. *See also* Depression
  dialysis in, 929, 930
  drug use (pharmacotherapy/
      polypharmacy) and, **69**
    falls and, 64, 64*t*
    urinary incontinence and, 65
  falls/gait disorders and, **63–65**, 63*t*, 64*t*,
      1701, 1702
  fecal incontinence and, 671
  fever/FUO in, 1287
  frail, 56–57
    hypertension management and, 446,
      467
  functional assessment/screening for,
      55–56
  hearing impairment in, **70**
  heart failure in, 402
  hypertension/hypertension
      management and, 446,
      467
  immobility and, **62–63**
  insomnia/insomnia management in,
      1089
  pressure ulcers in, **68–69**, 68*t*
  principles of care of, **55**
  prognosis/life expectancy and, 55, 56*f*,
      56*t*, 57*t*
  self neglect and, **70–71**, 71*t*
  urinary incontinence and, **65–67**
  values/preferences and, 55
  vision impairment in, **69–70**
  weight loss in, 35, **67**
Oleander, toxicity of, 1594
Olecranon bursitis, 1700–1701, 1700*f*
Olestra, diarrhea caused by, 591
Olfactory dysfunction, **220–221**
  intracranial tumors causing, 220
  in Kallmann syndrome, 1109, 1199,
      1200
Oligodendroglioma, 1004*t*
Oligomenorrhea, 762
Oligozoospermia, 969, 969*f*, 1112
  Y chromosome microdeletions
      causing, 970
Oliguria, 913, 917–918. *See also specific
      cause*
Olmesartan/olmesartan HCTZ/
      olmesartan with amlodipine,
      457*t*
Olopatadine, for allergic eye disease, 168,
      171*t*
Olsalazine, for inflammatory bowel
      disease, 650
Omacetaxine mepesuccinate, 1669*t*
Omalizumab
  for asthma, 247*f*, 250*t*, 251
  for urticaria, 134
Ombitasvir, for hepatitis C, 690*t*, 691,
      1341, 1342
Omega-3 fatty acids/fish oil
  in cardiovascular/heart disease
      prevention, 355
  platelet function affected by, 558*t*
  preventable disease/deaths associated
      with low intake of, 3*t*
Omeprazole, 609, 625. *See also* Proton
      pump inhibitors
On-off phenomenon, 1012

Onabotulinum toxin A, for urinary
    incontinence, 66
Onchocerca volvulus (onchocerciasis/river
    blindness), **1545–1546**
Oncocytoma, of kidney, 1655
Oncovin. *See* Vincristine
Ondansetron, 83, 582, 582*t*, 1672. *See also*
    Antiemetics
  for irritable bowel syndrome, 647
One-leg standing extension test, 1692
Onglyza. *See* Saxagliptin
Onivyde. *See* Irinotecan/irinotecan
    liposome
Onycholysis, 159, 160
Onychomycosis (tinea unguium), 160,
    160–161
Oophorectomy (salpingo-oophorectomy)/
    ovarian ablation
  in breast cancer prevention/treatment,
    738, 754, 755
  for endometrial carcinoma, 774
  for hirsutism/virilization, 1197
  for ovarian cancer, 779, 780
  prophylactic, 738, 779
    in HNPCC/Lynch syndrome, 669
  surgical menopause and, 796, 1201
Oophoritis, in mumps, 1381
Opana/Opana ER. *See* Oxymorphone
Opdivo. *See* Nivolumab
Open-angle glaucoma, chronic, **179–180**
Open biopsy, for breast lump evaluation,
    744. *See also* Breast, biopsy
    of
Open can test, 1686*t*, 1689
Ophthalmia neonatorum, 823
Ophthalmic artery occlusion, in stroke,
    995
Ophthalmic medications, 169–173*t*, 198
  adverse effects of, **199**
  contaminated, 199
  precautions for use of, **198–199**
  systemic effects of, **199**
  toxic and hypersensitivity reactions to,
    168, **199**
Ophthalmia, sympathetic, 181
Ophthalmopathy, Graves, **194–195**, 1124,
    1127, 1129, 1130, 1132–1133
  RAI treatment for hyperthyroidism
    and, 195, 1127, 1130, 1132
Ophthalmoplegic migraine, 978
Opiates. *See also* Opioids/opioid
    analgesics
  overdose/abuse of, **1601**
Opioid (narcotic) antagonists, 1099. *See
    also* Naloxone
  for heroin/opioid overdose/withdrawal,
    85–86, 1099, 1578, 1581*t*,
    1601
  for opioid-induced constipation, 86,
    586
Opioid-receptor antagonist laxatives, 86,
    586
Opioid Risk Tool, 85
Opioids/opioid analgesics, 73–74, **74–83**,
    77–81*t*, **84–86**. *See also
    specific agent*
  addiction and, 73, 85
  for chronic/chronic noncancer pain,
    82, **84–86**
  in combination products, 74, 80*t*, 82
  constipation caused by, 82, 86, 586

Opioids/opioid analgesics (*Cont.*):
dependency and, 73, 85
for diarrhea, 590, 594
diversion of medication and, 74, 85
for dyspnea, 86–87
in end-of-life care, 73–74
for myocardial infarction, 375
nausea and vomiting caused by, 83, 580
for neuropathic pain, 77–81*t*, 83, 1035
overdose/abuse of, 17, 73–74, 85–86,
    1098–1099, 1581*t*, **1601**
    management of, 85–86, 1098–1099
    narcotic antagonists/naloxone for,
      85–86, 1099, 1578, 1581*t*,
      1601
    pain management and, 17, 73–74, 85
during pregnancy, 799
pseudo-addiction and, 74
receptors for, in nausea and vomiting,
    580
tolerance and, 73, 82, 1098
withdrawal and, 1098–1099
Opisthorchis felineus/viverrini
    (opisthorchiasis), **1534**
cholangiocarcinoma and, 1534, 1619
Opium, tincture of, for diarrhea, 594
Opportunistic infections, 882, 883,
    1289–1293. *See also specific*
    type
in cancer patients, **1661**
fungi/molds causing, 1292, **1557–1558**
in HIV infection/AIDS, 1330, 1331*t*,
    1332
    antiretroviral therapy affecting, 1353
    CD4 T cell counts and, 1333, 1333*f*,
      1334, 1348*t*, 1349, 1350
    prevention of, 1347–1349, 1348*t*,
      1349–1350, 1349*t*
    treatment of, 1337–1338*t*, 1350
immunization recommendations and,
    4–5, 1321*t*, 1325*t*
prevention of, 1291–1292
in transplant recipients, 1290–1291
treatment of, 1292–1293
Oprelvekin, for chemotherapy-induced
    thrombocytopenia,
    1662–1672
Opsoclonus/myoclonus, 1008
Optic atrophy, 193
Optic disk
crowded, 194
    ischemic optic neuropathy and, 192
cupping of, in chronic glaucoma, 179,
    180
drusen of, 194
swelling of, **193–194**
Optic neuritis, **193**
in multiple sclerosis, 193, 1023
in neuromyelitis optica, 193, 1025
Optic neuropathy
inflammatory (optic neuritis), **193**
    in multiple sclerosis, 193, 1023
    in neuromyelitis optica, 193, 1025
ischemic, **192**
    in giant cell arteritis, 192, 854
OptiPranolol. *See* Metipranolol
Optivar. *See* Azelastine
OPV (oral/Sabin polio vaccine), 1383
IPV booster and, 1326
Oragrafin. *See* Ipodate sodium
Oral allergy syndrome, 877

Oral cavity, **224–231**
anaerobic flora of, 1478
    pneumonia/lung abscess and, 275,
      1478
bullous pemphigoid involving, 140
cancer of, 224, 225, 225*f*, 1608*t*
    incidence/mortality/risk of, 1608*t*
candidiasis involving (thrush),
    225–226, 225*f*
    esophagitis and, 611, 1547
    in HIV infection/AIDS, 226, 1335,
      1341
erythroplakia involving, 224
    in HIV infection/AIDS, 1341
leukoplakia involving, 224, 224*f*, 1341
lichen planus involving, 145, 224
pemphigus involving, 139
ulcerative lesions of, **226–227**
    in Behçet syndrome, 861, 862
    chemotherapy-induced, 1673
    in HIV infection/AIDS, 1341
Oral contraceptives, **785–788**, 787*t*, 788*t*
for abnormal uterine bleeding, 763
benzodiazepine interactions and, 1056*t*
breast cancer risk and, 738, 786
combined, 785–788, 787*t*, 788*t*
contraindications/adverse effects of,
    786–788, 788*t*
depression associated with use of, 786,
    1076
drug interactions and, 786
for emergency/postcoital
    contraception, 791
endometrial hyperplasia/carcinoma
    and, 774, 786
for endometriosis/pelvic pain, 765, 776
hepatocellular adenoma/liver tumors
    associated with, 715, 716,
    786, 1616
for hirsutism/virilization, 1198
for hormone replacement therapy,
    1204
melasma (chloasma) caused by, 157
nipple discharge caused by, 736
ovarian cancer risk and, 786
for premenstrual syndrome, 765
progestin minipill, 787*t*, 788
selection of, 785–786, 787*t*
Oral glucose tolerance test. *See* Glucose
    tolerance/intolerance
Oral hypoglycemic agents. *See*
    Antidiabetic agents
Oral nutritional supplements, 1281
for elderly, 67
Oral polio vaccine (OPV/Sabin vaccine),
    1383
IPV booster and, 1326
Oramorph. *See* Morphine
Orbital abscess, bacterial rhinosinusitis
    and, 217
Orbital cellulitis, **195**
bacterial rhinosinusitis and, 195, 217
Orbital floor, blowout fracture of, 197
Orbitopathy, Graves, **194–195**, 1124,
    1127, 1129, 1130, 1132–1133
    RAI treatment for hyperthyroidism
      and, 195, 1127, 1130, 1132
Orchiectomy
for intra-abdominal testes, 1194
for prostate cancer, 1649*t*, 1650
for testicular cancer, 1656, 1657

Orchiopexy/orchidopexy, 1194
infertility/testicular cancer risk and,
    1194, 1655
Orchitis
in filariasis, 1544
mumps, 1380–1381, 1381
Orellanine, *Cortinarius* mushroom
    poisoning and, 1600*t*
Orexin receptor antagonists, dual
    (DORAs), for sleep-wake
    disorders, 1089
Orf, 1423
Organ of Corti, hearing loss caused by
    disorders of, 200
Organ donation, 93–94. *See also*
    Transplantation
Organ failure, anemia of, 502, 503
Organ transplantation. *See specific type*
    and Transplantation
Organic brain syndrome. *See* Cognitive
    disorders; Delirium;
    Dementia
Organic (alcoholic) hallucinosis, 1093,
    1095
Organic personality syndrome, 1103
Organophosphate poisoning, 1580*t*,
    1581*t*, 1601–1602
Orgasm, 1062
loss of/orgasmic dysfunction. *See also*
    Sexual dysfunction
    antidepressants causing, 1079, 1082
    antipsychotics causing, 1071
    in female, 782, 1063
Oriental spotted fever, 1434
Orientia tsutsugamushi, 1429*t*, 1431
Orinase. *See* Tolbutamide
Oritavancin, for staphylococcal skin
    infections, 1448
Orlistat, for obesity, 1271
in type 2 diabetes, 1235
Ornithosis (psittacosis), 1313*t*,
    1486–1487
Oromandibular dystonia, 1016
Oropharyngeal anthrax, 1455
Oropharyngeal dysphagia, 605, 605*t*. *See*
    also Dysphagia
Oropharyngeal secretions, aspiration of,
    anaerobic pleuropulmonary
    infection and, 275, 1478
Orthodromic reentrant tachycardia, 387
Orthokeratology, 164
Orthopedics, **1685–1717**. *See also*
    Musculoskeletal disorders
Orthophosphates, for hypercalciuria, 963
Orthopox virus, novel, 1424
Orthostatic (postural) hypotension
antipsychotics causing, 1071, 1589
in diabetes mellitus, 1214
dysautonomia (autonomic
    dysfunction) and, 990, 991,
    1035
falls and, 64, 64*t*
heat syncope/collapse and, 1562
MAOIs causing, 1082
syncope and, 401
tricyclic antidepressants causing, 1082
Orthostatic proteinuria, 913–914
Orudis. *See* Ketoprofen
Oruvail. *See* Ketoprofen
Osborn wave, in hypothermia, 1564,
    1564*f*

OsCal (calcium carbonate). *See* Calcium, dietary/supplementary
Oseltamivir, 1365*t*, 1412, 1418
   prophylactic, 1416, 1418
   resistance to, 1412
Oseni. *See* Alogliptin, with pioglitazone
Osimertinib, 1668*t*
   for lung cancer, 1612
Osler nodes, in endocarditis, 1459, 1459*f*
Osler sign, 444
Osler triad, 1445
Osler-Weber-Rendu syndrome (hereditary hemorrhagic telangiectasia), **1683–1684**
Osmolality
   fecal/stool, 591
   serum, 884
      in diabetic ketoacidosis, 1246
      in hyperglycemic hyperosmolar state, 1250
   urine, 917*t*
      in hypernatremia, 890
Osmolar/osmol gap, 884, **891**
   calculation of, 1584*t*
   in poisoning/drug overdose, 1584, 1584*t*
      alcohol toxicity and, 891, 1094, 1584
      methanol or ethylene glycol toxicity and, 891, 906, 1584, 1599
Osmolarity, 884
Osmostat, reset, hyponatremia caused by, 887, 888
Osmotic diarrhea, 588*t*, 591, 593. *See also* Diarrhea
Osmotic diuretics, lithium interactions and, 1087*t*
Osmotic gap, stool, 591, 593
Osmotic laxatives, 585*t*, 586
Ospemifene, 1206
Osphena. *See* Ospemifene
Ossicular disruption, hearing loss and, 200, 207
Osteitis condensans ilii, 864
Osteitis deformans (Paget disease of bone), **1166–1168**
Osteitis fibrosa cystica, 927, 1153
Osteoarthritis, **826–829**, 828*f*. *See also specific joint affected and* Arthritis
   arthroplasty/joint replacement for, 829. *See also specific joint*
   coagulase-negative staphylococcal infection and, 1451
   of cervical spine, 1696, 1697
   glucosamine/chondroitin for, 829, 1714
   of hip, **1703–1704**
   of knee, **1713–1715**
   rheumatoid arthritis differentiated from, 828, 836
   spinal stenosis and, 1694
Osteoarthropathy, hypertrophic pulmonary. *See* Hypertrophic osteoarthropathy
Osteodystrophy, renal, 927–928, 927*f*, 1153, 1155
Osteogenic sarcoma. *See* Osteosarcoma
Osteoma, ear canal, **202–203**
Osteomalacia, 927, **1163–1166**, 1164*t*
   hypophosphatemic, 892*t*, 900, 1164–1165, 1164*t*, 1166

osteopenia/osteoporosis and, 1159, 1161, 1165
   tumor-induced, 1165
Osteomyelitis, **870–871**, 1314*t*, **1449**
   acute pyogenic, **870–871**
   bacterial rhinosinusitis and, 217
   in drug users, 870, 1304
   epidural/epidural abscess and, 870, 871, 1449
   of skull base (malignant external otitis), 202
   staphylococcal, 870, 1314*t*, **1449**
   vertebral, 870, 871, 1449
Osteonecrosis, **875–876**
   corticosteroid use and, 875
   in HIV infection/AIDS, 1340
   of jaw, bisphosphonate use and, 11, 875, 1162
Osteopenia, 1160, 1163. *See also* Osteoporosis
   bisphosphonates for, 1161
   in HIV infection/AIDS, 1340
Osteophytes, in diffuse idiopathic skeletal hyperostosis, 864
Osteoporosis, **11**, 795, **1159–1163**, 1159*t*
   circumscripta, 1167
   corticosteroid therapy and, 650, 1160, 1208–1209
   fractures/bone pain and, 1159
      of hip, 1701
      prevention of, 11, 1702
   in HIV infection/AIDS, 1340
   hyperthyroidism and, 1127
   hypogonadism and, 1159, 1161, 1191
   osteomalacia with, 1159, 1161, 1165
   postmenopausal, 795, 1160
   prevention/treatment of, **11**, 795, 1160–1163, 1702
      bisphosphonates in, 11, 1161–1162, 1702
      calcium in, 11, 795, 1161, 1280, 1702
         milk-alkali syndrome and, 897, 898
      estrogen replacement therapy in, 795, 796, 1161, 1202
      exercise/activity and, 11, 795, 1160
      selective estrogen receptor modulators in, 1163
      surgery and, 1163
      vitamin D in, 11, 795, 1702
Osteoprotegerin, in myeloma, 535
Osteosarcoma (osteogenic sarcoma), 1624*t*
   Paget disease of bone and, 1167
   teriparatide and, 1162
Osteosclerosis, vertebral (rugger jersey spine), 1155
Ostium primum/secundum atrial septal defects, 325, 326
Otalgia. *See* Earache
Otic barotrauma. *See* Barotrauma
Otic drops
   for cerumen removal, 201
   for external otitis, 202
   ototoxic, perforated tympanic membrane and, 208
Otitis
   external/malignant external, **202**
   H influenzae causing, 1311*t*, 1315*t*, 1466
   media, 1315*t*

   acute, **204–205**
   chronic, **205–206**, 205*f*
   complications of, 205–206, 205*f*
   hearing loss and, 200
   in HIV infection/AIDS, 214
   serous, **203–204**
      in HIV infection/AIDS, 214
      nasopharyngeal carcinoma and, 203, 223
Otoconia, vertigo associated with, 212
Otogenic meningitis, 206
Otosclerosis, 200, **206–207**
Ototoxicity, 208, 211*t*
   of aminoglycosides, 208
   of cisplatin, 208, 1675
   hearing loss and, 208
Ottawa Ankle Rules, 1716
Ottawa subarachnoid hemorrhage clinical decision rule, 41
Ovarian ablation. *See* Oophorectomy
Ovarian cancer/tumors, **779–780**, 1623*t*
   dermatomyositis and, 849
   estrogen replacement therapy and, 1203, 1204
   genetic mutations associated with, 779. *See also BRCA1/BRCA2* genes
   HNPCC/Lynch syndrome and, 669
   hirsutism/virilization caused by, 1196, 1197
   malignant ascites and, 604
   palmar fasciitis and, 875
   prevention of, 779
      oral contraceptive use and, 786
      screening and, 779
   thyroid tissue in (struma ovarii), 1126
Ovarian cyst, 780. *See also* Ovarian cancer/tumors
   appendicitis differentiated from, 642
   in gestational trophoblastic disease, 807
Ovarian failure, 794, 1199. *See also* Amenorrhea; Menopause
   in Turner syndrome, 1207
Ovarian tumor antigen. *See* CA 125
Ovaries, polycystic. *See* Polycystic ovary syndrome
Over-the-counter drugs, use/abuse of, 1101
   stimulants and, 1587
Overflow incontinence
   fecal, 586, 671
   urinary, 66, 67
"Overlap syndrome," 692
Overload proteinuria, 914
Overt small bowel bleeding, 599
Overweight. *See* Obesity/overweight
Ovide. *See* Malathion
Ovulation
   awareness of, contraception based on, **791**
   evaluation of in infertility workup, 783, 784
   induction of for infertility, 784–785
      in polycystic ovary syndrome, 781
Ovulation predictor kits, 783
Ovulatory abnormal uterine bleeding (AUB-O), 762, 763
Owl's eye inclusions, in CMV infection, 1376

Oxacillin
    for endocarditis, 1462
    for skin and soft tissue infections, 1448
Oxalate, dietary, urinary stone formation and, 963, 964
Oxaliplatin, 1663t
    for colorectal cancer, 1639
Oxandrolone, for HIVS wasting, 1335
Oxantel pamoate, for trichuriasis/whipworm, 1539
Oxaprozin, 76t
Oxazepam, 1054t
    overdose/toxicity of, 1594–1595
Oxcarbazepine, 987t, 1087. See also Anticonvulsant therapy
    for bipolar disease/mania, 1087
    overdose/toxicity of, 987t, 1087
    for seizures, 987t
        pregnancy and, 820
Oxiconazole, 99t
Oximetry. See Pulse oximetry/CO-oximetry
Oxistat. See Oxiconazole
Oxitriptan, for myoclonus, 1017
Oxprenolol, overdose/toxicity of, 1591
Oxybate. See Gamma-hydroxybutyrate
Oxybutynin, for urinary incontinence, 66
Oxycodone, 74, 79t, 82
    breastfeeding and, 798t
    in combination agents, 80t
    overdose/toxicity of, 1601
Oxycontin. See Oxycodone
Oxygen, partial pressure of. See Arterial blood gases
Oxygen saturation. See Arterial blood gases; Pulse oximetry
Oxygen therapy
    adverse ophthalmic effects of, 177t
    for ARDS, 320
    for asthma exacerbation, 254, 256f
    for carbon monoxide poisoning, 1581t, 1584t, 1592
    for COPD, 259–260, 260t, 262
    for drowning, 1567
    for dysbarism/decompression sickness, 1573
    for headache, 41, 980
    for high-altitude illness, 1574, 1575
    home, 259–260, 260t
    hyperbaric. See Hyperbaric oxygen therapy
    for methemoglobinemia, 1600
    for pulmonary edema, 412
    for pulmonary hypertension, 303, 431, 432f
    for respiratory failure, 318
    for smoke inhalation, 305
    surgical site infection prevention and, 54
    transtracheal, 260
Oxyhemoglobin saturation. See Arterial blood gases; Pulse oximetry
OxyIR. See Oxycodone
Oxymetazoline, overdose/toxicity of, 1592
Oxymorphone, 80t
Oxytocin, 1109t
Oxyuriasis. See Pinworm infection
Ozurdex. See Dexamethasone implant

P2Y$_{12}$ inhibitors
    for acute coronary syndromes/STEMI, 361, 366–368, 372, 376
    perioperative discontinuation of, 368
P16/CDKN2A mutations, pancreatic/periampullary carcinoma and, 1620
p24 antigen assay, in blood screening, 543
P40, in squamous cell carcinoma of lung, 1608–1609
P53 mutations. See also TP53 mutations
    in breast cancer, 738
    in colorectal cancer, 1637
P63, in squamous cell carcinoma of lung, 1608–1609
P450 aromatase (P450arom) deficiency, amenorrhea in, 1199
P450c11 deficiency, 1170, 1196
P450c17 deficiency, 1169, 1190, 1199
P450c21 deficiency, 1169, 1170, 1196, 1197, 1198
Pacemaker, 400
    for atrioventricular block, 377, 400
    for cardiomyopathy, 417, 419, 420f
    for heart failure, 405f, 409–410
    preoperative/prophylactic/surgery and, 48
    for sick sinus syndrome, 399
    for syncope, 402
    for ventricular tachycardia, 397
Pacemaker syndrome, 400
Packed red blood cells, transfusion of, 542. See also Transfusion
    autologous, 542
    frozen, 542
Paclitaxel, 1664t
    for breast cancer, 751, 753, 757
    coronary stents eluting, 362
    neuropathy caused by, 1674
    protein-bound, 1665t
Paco$_2$. See Arterial blood gases; Pulse oximetry
Pacritinib, for primary myelofibrosis, 523
PAD. See Peripheral arterial disease
Padua Risk Score, 567t, 569
Paecilomyces, in opportunistic infection, 1557
Paget carcinoma of breast, 118, 118f, 745
Paget disease, 118, 118f
    of bone, 1166–1168
    extramammary, 118
    mammary. See Paget carcinoma of breast
PAH. See Pulmonary arterial hypertension
Pain/pain disorders. See also specific type and Pain management
    assessment scales for, 72–73, 73t
    chronic/chronic noncancer (CNCP), 1060–1062, 1061f
        management of, 72–73, 82, 84–86, 1061–1062
    at end of life, 73–74
    hyponatremia caused by, 886
    neuropathic, 83–84, 83t, 1035. See also Neuropathies
        in diabetes, 1239, 1239–1240
    otic. See Earache
    response to, in coma or stupor, 1027
    somatic symptom disorder with, 1059
    treatment of. See Pain management

"Pain contracts," 85
Pain, energy, and general activity (PEG) tracking measure, 85
Pain management, 72–86. See also specific disorder and Analgesia/analgesics
    assessment scales and, 72–73, 73t
    back pain and, 1693–1694
    barriers to good care and, 73–74
    for burn injury, 1569
    chronic pain and, 72–73, 82, 1061–1062
    for electrical burns, 1571
    at end of life, 73–74
    nonpharmacologic, 86, 1061–1062, 1062
    pharmacologic, 74–84, 75–76t, 77–81t, 83t, 1062
        acetaminophen/NSAIDs/coxibs (COX-2 inhibitors), 74, 75–76t
        adjuvant, 84
        for neuropathic pain, 83–84, 83t
        opioids, 74–83, 77–81t, 84–86
    prescription drug abuse and, 17, 73–74, 85
    principles of, 72–73, 73t
    in seriously ill/dying patient, 73–74
Painful bladder syndrome (interstitial cystitis), 43, 960–961
Painful diabetic neuropathy, 1239, 1239–1240
Painful intercourse (dyspareunia), 782, 782–783
Painless myocardial infarction, 370
Painless postpartum thyroiditis, 1135
Painless sporadic thyroiditis (hashitoxicosis), 1125, 1135, 1136
PAIR (percutaneous aspiration/injection/reaspiration), for hydatid cysts, 1537–1538
Palatal myoclonus, tinnitus and, 209
Palbociclib, 1668t
    for breast cancer, 756
Palifermin, for chemotherapy-induced mucositis, 1671t, 1673
Palindromic rheumatism, 875
Paliperidone, 1068, 1069t, 1070, 1071, 1071t
    adverse ophthalmic effects of, 177t, 183
Palivizumab, 1365t
    for RSV prophylaxis, 1410
Palliative care, 72–94. See also specific disorder
    definition and scope of, 72
    at end of life, 88–94. See also End of life, provision of care at
    symptom management and
        constipation, 86
        delirium and agitation, 87
        dyspnea, 86–87
        fatigue, 87
        nausea and vomiting, 87
        pain, 72–86. See also Pain management
Palliative care institutions, 90–91. See also End of life, provision of care at
Palliative Performance Scale, prognosis at end of life and, 88

PALM-COEIN system, 762
Palmar fasciitis, cancer and, 875
Palms
    tinea of, **113–114**
    vesiculobullous dermatitis of
        (pompholyx), **121–122**, 122*f*
        tinea differentiated from, 114, 122
Palonosetron, 582, 582*t*, 1672, 1673. *See
        also* Antiemetics
Palpitations, **30–32**, 30*t*. *See also specific
        cause*
Palsies. *See specific type and* Paralysis/
        palsies
Paludrine. *See* Proguanil
2-PAM. *See* Pralidoxime
Pamelor. *See* Nortriptyline
Pamidronate, 1162. *See also*
        Bisphosphonates
    adverse ophthalmic effects of, 179*t*
    in breast cancer management, 754
    for chemotherapy-induced toxicity/
        bone pain, 1671*t*
    for hypercalcemia/
        hyperparathyroidism, 1157,
        1660
    for osteoporosis prevention/
        management, 1162
        corticosteroid use and, 1209
Panacinar bibasilar emphysema, 259. *See
        also* Emphysema
Panbronchiolitis, diffuse, 267
Pancreas
    cancer of, 1608*t*, **1620–1626**, 1624*t*
        cystic, 1620–1621, 1621, 1625
        GI bleeding and, 595
        incidence/mortality/risk of, 1608*t*,
            1620
        pancreatitis and, 731, 732, 733, 1620
    diseases of, **725–733**. *See also specific
        type and* Pancreatitis
        diabetes/hyperglycemia and, 731,
            1211*t*. *See also* Diabetes
            mellitus
        dyspepsia and, 578
        vomiting and, 581*t*, 582
    divisum, 726, 729
    functioning/neuroendocrine tumors
        of, 1185–1186
    hypoglycemia caused by, 1185,
        1252–1255, 1253*t*, 1254*t*
    pseudocysts of, 728, 730
        ascites and, 728
        cystic carcinoma and, 1620, 1625
        infected (pancreatic abscess), 728,
            730
    transplantation of, for diabetes
        mellitus, 1232
Pancreatectomy, 733
    diabetes/hyperglycemia and,
        733, 1213
    islet transplantation after, 1232
Pancreatic abscess, 728, 730
Pancreatic ascites, 602, 728
Pancreatic cystadenoma, 1620–1621,
        1621, 1625
Pancreatic duct
    ascites caused by disruption of, 728
    calculus formation in
        (pancreaticolithiasis), 731
Pancreatic duodenal homeobox (PDX1),
        in MODY, 1211*t*

Pancreatic enzyme supplements, 732,
        732*t*
Pancreatic islets, 1185. *See also* B cells,
        pancreatic
    hyperplasia of (noninsulinoma
        pancreatogenous
        hypoglycemia syndrome),
        1252, **1256**
    transplantation of, for diabetes, 1232
    tumors of. *See* Islet cell tumors
Pancreatic neuroendocrine tumors,
        1185–1186
    nonfunctioning, 1185
Pancreatic polypeptide
    F cells secreting, 1185
    pancreatic neuroendocrine tumors
        secreting, 1185, 1188
Pancreatic pseudocysts, 728, 730
    ascites and, 728
    cystic carcinoma and, 1620, 1625
    infected (pancreatic abscess),
        728, 730
Pancreatic secretory trypsin inhibitory
        (*PSTI*) gene, in pancreatitis,
        731
Pancreatic transcription factor mutations,
        in diabetes, 1212–1213
Pancreaticolithiasis, 731
Pancreatitis
    acute, **725–730**, 727*t*
    antidiabetic agents associated with,
        1226, 1227
    ascites in, 602, 728
    autoimmune, 731
    biliary/biliary stricture, 723, 725–726,
        726, 728, 729, 732
    cholelithiasis/cholecystitis and,
        725–726, 727, 729
    chronic, 728, **730–733**, 732*t*
        tumefactive, 731
    cystic fibrosis and, 265, 731, 732
    diabetes/hyperglycemia and, 728, 730,
        731, 1213
    didanosine causing, 1355
    hereditary, 731, 732
    hypercalcemia/hyperparathyroidism
        and, 731, 1155
    hypertriglyceridemia and, 726, 729,
        1266
    hypocalcemia/hypoparathyroidism
        and, 896, 1150
    in mumps, 1381
    necrotizing, 726, 727, 728, 729,
        729–730, 730
    obstructive, 731
    pancreatic/periampullary carcinoma
        and, 731, 732, 733, 1620
    pleural effusion in, 313*t*
    post-ERCP, 677, 729
        in pregnant patient, 824
    sphincter of Oddi dysfunction and,
        720, 726, 728, 729
    tropical, 731
Pancytopenia, 516, 516*t*
    in acute leukemia, 528
    in aplastic anemia, 516, 516*t*
    methotrexate causing, 837
    thiourea therapy causing, 1129
Panencephalitis, subacute sclerosing,
        1378
    myoclonus in, 1017

Panhypergammaglobulinemia,
        bronchiectasis and, 263
Panhypogammaglobulinemia, 882–883
    bronchiectasis and, 263
    infections associated with, 882
Panhypopituitarism, 1109, 1110,
        1111–1112
Panic disorders/panic attacks, 1053,
        1055–1056
    chest pain/discomfort in, 29, 619
    drug therapy in, 1055–1056
    OCD and, 1053
    palpitations in, 30, 31
    PTSD and, 1052
    seizures differentiated from, 986
    sleep, 1053
Panitumumab, 1666*t*
    for colorectal cancer, 1639, 1640
Panniculitis
    lupus, 152, 840
    sclerosing, 138
Panobinostat, 1669*t*
Pansinusitis, 215, 216
Pantoprazole, 609, 625. *See also* Proton
        pump inhibitors
Panuveitis, 181. *See also* Uveitis
Pao$_2$. *See* Arterial blood gases; Pulse
        oximetry
Papanicolaou smear (Pap smear),
        769–770, 769*t*
    anal, 1344
    in cancer screening, 14*t*, 15, 769–770,
        769*t*, 772
    in CIN, 769–770, 769*t*, 771
    in endometrial carcinoma, 774
    in HIV infection/AIDS, 1345
    for pregnant patient, 800
    for sexual violence (rape/sexual
        assault) victim, 793
    in STD patients, 1302
Papaverine, for erectile dysfunction
        diagnosis/treatment, 967
    in diabetes, 1241
Papillary muscle dysfunction/rupture
    mitral regurgitation and, 339
    mitral stenosis and, 331
    myocardial infarction and, 379
Papillary stenosis, in HIV infection/
        AIDS, 1342
Papilledema, 194
Papillitis, 193
Papillomas
    intraductal, nipple discharge and, 736
    inverted, **223**
    recurrent respiratory (laryngeal),
        233–234
Papillomaviruses. *See* Human
        papillomavirus
Papillopathy, diabetic, 192
PAPP-A (pregnancy-associated plasma
        protein-A), testing for, 800
Papular acne, 127–128
Papular urticaria, 134
Papules, 96*t*, **140–144**
    violaceous to purple, **144–146**
Paracentesis
    in ascites, 601–602, 604, 1659
        in cirrhosis, 701, 701–702
    large-volume, 604, 701, 1659
    in spontaneous bacterial peritonitis,
        603, 702

Paracetamol, 75t, 1585. *See also* Acetaminophen
in analgesic nephropathy, 947
Parachute mitral valve, 331–335
Paracoccidioides brasiliensis (paracoccidioidomycosis), **1556–1557**
Paradoxic aciduria, in metabolic alkalosis, 909
Paradoxic embolism, transient ischemic attack and, 991
Paradoxic pulse. *See* Pulsus paradoxus
Paradoxic sleep, 1088
"Paradoxical" low flow aortic stenosis, 341, 342, 342t
Paraganglioma, **1179–1184**, 1180t, 1181t
familial, 1180
metastatic, 1183–1184, 1184
Paragonimus/Paragonimus westermani (paragonimiasis), **1534**
Parainfluenza viruses, 1409
Paralysis/palsies. *See also specific type or structure affected*
acute flaccid, 1383
coxsackievirus infection and, 1426
enterovirus 71 causing, 1427
in conversion disorder, 1058
facial/Bell palsy, **1041**, 1041f
herpes simplex/varicella zoster infection and, 120, 214, 1041, 1364, 1366, 1369
ocular motor, **194**
periodic. *See* Periodic paralysis
in poliomyelitis, 1382, 1383
progressive supranuclear, parkinsonism differentiated from, 1012
sleep, in narcolepsy, 1090
spinal cord infarction and, 1002
spinal trauma and, 1031–1032
after thoracic aneurysm repair, 483
in tick-borne encephalitis, 1391, 1392
vocal fold, **237**
thyroid surgery and, 237, 1143
Paralytic (adynamic) ileus, **638–639**
Paralytic shellfish poisoning, 1603, 1604t
Paramalignant pleural effusion, 312
Paramyxovirus respiratory infections, **1409–1410**
Paranasal sinuses, **214–224**
in granulomatosis with polyangiitis, **223–224**, 858
infections of, **214–218**, 217t. *See also* Rhinosinusitis; Sinusitis
inflammatory disease of, **223–224**
malignant tumors of, **223**
in sarcoidosis, **223**
Paraneoplastic cerebellar degeneration, 1008
Paraneoplastic pemphigus, 139
Paraneoplastic syndromes. *See specific type*
Paranoid delusions/paranoia, 1066
in alcoholic (organic) hallucinosis, 1093
in psychotic major depression, 1075
Paranoid personality disorder, 1065t
Paraparesis, spastic
in cervical spondylosis, 1042
tropical, 1396
Paraphilias (sexual arousal disorders), 1062, 1063–1064
in female, 782

Paraplatin. *See* Carboplatin
Paraplegia. *See also* Paralysis
after spinal trauma, 1031–1032
after thoracic aneurysm repair, 483
Parapneumonic pleural effusion, 311, 312, 313–314, 313t
in community-acquired/pneumococcal disease, 1445, 1446
Paraproteins
in amyloidosis, 538, 539
in myeloma, 535, 535–536, 951
neuropathy associated with, 1036–1037
in Waldenström macroglobulinemia, 537, 538
Parasitic infections, diarrhea in, 588t, 592
Parasomnias, 1090
Parathar. *See* Teriparatide
Parathion poisoning, 1601–1602
Parathyroid gland
disorders of, **1149–1159**. *See also* Hyperparathyroidism; Hypoparathyroidism
adenoma/hyperplasia, 1152, 1158
in MEN, 1152, 1187t
resorptive hypercalciuria caused by, 963–964
carcinoma, 1153, 1154, 1158
resection of, 1157–1158. *See also* Parathyroidectomy
thyroid surgery affecting, 1143
transplantation of tissue from, for hypoparathyroidism, 1152
Parathyroid hormone (PTH), 1149. *See also* Hyperparathyroidism; Hypoparathyroidism
bisphosphonates affecting, 1156, 1162
calcium balance/imbalance and, 896, 1149, 1152–1153, 1154, 1154f
in hypercalcemia/hyperparathyroidism, 897, 898, 1152, 1154
in hypercalciuria, 962t, 963–964, 1152–1153, 1156
for hypocalcemia/hypoparathyroidism, 1152
in hypophosphatemia, 900
magnesium imbalances and, 896, 901, 902
in metabolic bone disorders/renal osteodystrophy, 927, 927–928, 927f, 1153
after parathyroidectomy, 1158
phosphate balance/imbalances and, 899
recombinant human (rhPTH). *See also* Teriparatide
for hypocalcemia/hypoparathyroidism, 1152
resistance to, in pseudohypoparathyroidism, 1151
Parathyroid hormone-related protein (PTHrP)
in cancer-related hypercalcemia, 897, 898, 1155, 1156
in hypophosphatemia, 900
Parathyroidectomy, 1157–1158
hypoparathyroidism/hypocalcemia after, 1149, 1158
in MEN 1, 1158, 1187
tetany after, 1158
Paravaccinia, 1423

Paravertebral abscess, in spinal tuberculosis, 872
Parechovirus infection, **1428**
Parenchymal lung disease
diffuse, **289–294**, 290t, 291t, 292f. *See also specific disorder and* Interstitial lung disease
pulmonary hypertension and, 302, 303, 430, 430t
respiratory failure caused by, 318t
Parenteral fluids. *See* Fluid management/ hydration
Parenteral nutritional support, 911–912, 1281f, 1282. *See also* Nutritional support
acidosis and, 907, 1285t
in burn injury, 1569
complications of, **1284–1285**, 1285t
for Crohn disease, 655
diabetes management/insulin therapy and, 1244
in end-of-life care, 91
in HIV infection/AIDS, 1335
in pancreatitis, 729
patient monitoring during, 1285–1286
for protein–energy malnutrition, 1269
for short bowel syndrome, 637
solutions for, **1284**, 1284t
Paresis (general), in syphilis, 1489t, 1496
Paresthesias
chemotherapy-induced, 1674, 1675
in diabetes mellitus, 1214
in malabsorption, 633t
Paricalcitol, for hyperparathyroidism, 1157
Parietal lobe lesions, 1003–1005
Paris criteria, for autoimmune hepatitis, 692
Paritaprevir, for hepatitis C, 690t, 691, 1341, 1342
Parkin gene, in parkinsonism, 1011
Parkinsonism, **1011–1014**
drug-induced, 1011, 1017
Wilson disease and, 710, 1012
Parkland formula, 1569
Parnate. *See* Tranylcypromine
Paromomycin
for amebiasis, 1526, 1527t
for cryptosporidiosis, 1529
for giardiasis, 1531
for leishmaniasis, 1512
Paronychia, 153
candidal, 132, 132f, 133
staphylococcal, 153
Parotid glands. *See also* Salivary glands
chronic inflammatory/infiltrative disorders affecting, 232
in mumps, 1380, 1381, 1381f
sialadenitis affecting, 231
tumors of, 232
Parotitis, in mumps, 1380, 1381, 1381f
Paroxetine, 1078t, 1079–1081. *See also* Serotonin-selective reuptake inhibitors
overdose/toxicity of, 1078t, 1606
ophthalmic, 177t
for PTSD, 1052
Paroxysmal atrial fibrillation, recurrent, 388, 394
Paroxysmal nocturnal hemoglobinuria, **509–510**

Paroxysmal supraventricular tachycardia, **385–387**

Pars planitis (intermediate uveitis), 181. *See also* Uveitis

Partial mole, 807

Partial seizures. *See* Focal (partial) seizures

Partner abuse (domestic violence), 16, 1090–1091, 1091

Parvovirus B19 gene, 1422

Parvovirus B19 infection. *See* Erythrovirus (parvovirus B19) infection

PAS. *See* Aminosalicylic acid

Pasireotide, for Cushing disease, 1176

Passive smoking (environmental tobacco smoke), health hazards of, 7
  cancer, 1608
  during pregnancy, 799

Pasteurella species, in animal bite infections, 1300

Patanol. *See* Olopatadine

Patch pump, insulin (electronic/ mechanical), 1231, 1231–1232

Patella, 1704

Patellar apprehension sign, 1709*t*, 1712–1713

Patellar grind test, 1713

Patellar tracking disorders, knee pain and, 1704, 1712

Patellofemoral joint, 1712

Patellofemoral joint test, 1709*t*

Patellofemoral pain/syndrome, 1709*t*, **1712–1713**

Patent ductus arteriosus, **330–331**, 331*t*

Patent foramen ovale, **324–327**

Pathergy phenomenon, in Behçet syndrome, 862

Pathologic fractures. *See also* Fractures
  of hip, 1701, 1702
  in hypercalcemia/hyperparathyroidism, 1153, 1155
  malabsorption and, 633*t*
  in osteomalacia, 1165
  in osteoporosis, 1159

Patient adherence/nonadherence (compliance/ noncompliance), 1–2. *See also specific disorder*
  elderly patients and, 69

Patient Health Questionnaire-9
  assessment of suicide risk and, 1077
  in elderly, 61

Patient interview, 1–2

Patient-provider agreements ("pain contracts"), 85

Patient surrogate, Durable Power of Attorney for Health Care, 90

Patient values/preferences, assessing in older adult, 55

Patiromer, for hyperkalemia, 894

Patulous eustachian tube, 203

Paucibacillary (tuberculoid) leprosy, 1037, 1484. *See also* Leprosy

Pauci-immune (ANCA-associated) glomerulonephritis, 858, 922, 933*t*, 935*f*, **938–939**

PAX-4 (Arg133Trp) mutation, in idiopathic type 1 diabetes mellitus, 1211

PAX8-PPARγ mutations, in thyroid cancer, 1139

Paxil. *See* Paroxetine

Pazopanib, 1668*t*

Pb. *See* Lead

PBC. *See* Primary biliary cholangitis/ cirrhosis

PBG. *See* Porphobilinogen

PCEC (purified chick embryo cell culture) rabies vaccine, 1326, 1387

PCI. *See* Percutaneous coronary intervention

PCL. *See* Posterior cruciate ligament

Pco$_2$. *See* Arterial blood gases; Pulse oximetry

PCOS. *See* Polycystic ovary syndrome

PCP. *See* Phencyclidine

PCR. *See* Polymerase chain reaction

PCSK9 (proprotein convertase subtilisin/ kexin type 9) inhibitors, for lipid modification/ cardiovascular/heart disease prevention, 353, 1266

PCV/PCV13 (pneumococcal conjugate vaccine). *See* Pneumococcal vaccine

PD-1 (programmed cell-death-1) inhibitors, for lung cancer, 1612

PDA. *See* Patent ductus arteriosus

PDE-5 inhibitors. *See* Phosphodiesterase inhibitors

PDGF. *See* Platelet-derived growth factor

PDX1, in MODY, 1211*t*

PE (pulmonary embolism). *See* Pulmonary venous thromboembolism

PE severity index (PESI), 571, 571*t*

Peak expiratory flow (PEF), in asthma, 244*f*, 245*t*, 246, 251, 252, 254, 255*f*, 256*f*

Pedal arteries, atherosclerotic/occlusive disease of, **475–476**

Pediculosis (capitis/corporis/pubis), **149–150**
  relapsing fever transmission and, 150, 1499
  trench fever and, 150, 1477
  typhus and, 150

Pediculus humanus var *capitis*/var *corporis*, 149. *See also* Pediculosis

PEF. *See* Peak expiratory flow

PEG. *See* Pain, energy, and general activity (PEG) tracking measure; Polyethylene glycol

Pegaptanib
  for age-related macular degeneration, 185
  for chronic macular edema in retinal vein occlusion, 186
  for diabetic macular edema, 190

Pegfilgrastim, for chemotherapy-induced toxicity, 1662, 1672*t*

Peginterferon. *See also* Interferon-alpha/ interferon alfa
  for essential thrombocytosis, 522
  for hepatitis B, 688
  for hepatitis C, 684, 689

for hepatitis D, 688
  for polycythemia, 520–521

Pegivirus (hepatitis G virus/HGV), 682

Pegloticase, for hyperuricemia/gout, 832, 833

Pegvisomant, for acromegaly/gigantism, 1116

Pelger-Huet abnormality, 526

Peliosis hepatis, 1477
  drugs/toxins causing, 697

Pellagra, 154, 1186, 1275–1276

Pelvic abscess, anaerobic, 1479

Pelvic appendicitis, 642

Pelvic floor dyssynergia, 584, 584*t*, 585

Pelvic floor muscle (Kegel) exercises, 66, 67

Pelvic inflammatory disease (PID)/pelvic infection, **778–779**, 1316*t*. *See also* Endometritis; Salpingitis
  in actinomycosis, 1480
  anaerobic, 778, 1316*t*, 1479
  chlamydial, 778, 1313*t*, 1316*t*, 1486
  gonococcal, 778, 1316*t*, 1475, 1476
  in HIV infection/AIDS, 1345
  IUDs and, 778, 790

Pelvic organ prolapse, **777–778**

Pelvic pain, chronic. *See also specific cause*
  in female, **765–766**, 776
  in male (nonbacterial prostatitis), 957*t*, **958–959**

Pembrolizumab, 1666*t*
  for lung cancer, 1612

Pemetrexed, 1663*t*
  for lung cancer, 1612

Pemirolast, for allergic eye disease, 168, 170*t*

Pemphigoid, bullous, **140**

Pemphigus, **139–140**, 139*f*
  foliaceus/erythematosus, 139
  paraneoplastic, 139
  vulgaris/vegetans, 139

Pen injectors, for insulin administration, 1230, 1231

Penbutolol, 453*t*

Penciclovir, 1365*t*. *See also* Famciclovir

Penicillamine
  adverse ophthalmic effects of, 179*t*
  for Wilson disease, 710–711

Penicillin. *See also specific disorder used in*
  allergy to, 877, 1318
  for anaerobic pleuropulmonary infection, 276, 1478
  for anthrax, 1456*t*
  for endocarditis, 1461, 1462
  for group B streptococcal infection prophylaxis in pregnancy, 800, 1444
  for Lyme disease, 1501, 1505, 1505*t*
  for non-sexually transmitted treponematoses, 1498
  for pharyngitis, 229, 1442
  platelet function affected by, 558*t*
  pneumococcal resistance and, 1446
  for pneumonia/lung abscess, 270, 1446
  for rheumatic fever, 424
  for streptococcal skin infections, 1443
  for syphilis. *See* Syphilis

Penicillin skin testing, 1318
Penile discharge. *See* Urethral discharge
Penile prostheses, 967–968
    in diabetes, 1241
Penlac. *See* Ciclopirox
Pentalogy of Fallot, 328
Pentamidine
    for African trypanosomiasis, 1508, 1508*t*
    blood glucose levels affected by
        (hyper-/hypoglycemia),
        1257, 1552
    for *P jirovecii* infection, 1337*t*, 1349*t*,
        1552
    pneumothorax and, 314
Pentasa. *See* Mesalamine
Pentavalent antimonials, for
        leishmaniasis, 1511–1512,
        1512
Pentobarbital, for status epilepticus, 990
Pentosan, for interstitial cystitis, 961
Pentostatin, 1664*t*
Pentoxifylline
    for alcoholic liver disease, 694
    for leg ulcers, 156
Peptic stricture of esophagus, 605*t*,
        608–609. *See also* Esophagus,
        strictures of
Peptic ulcer disease, **623–631**, 626*t*
    abdominal pain/dyspepsia in, 578, 624,
        625
    complications of, **629–631**
        risk reduction and, 628
    gastric outlet obstruction and, 624,
        630–631
    GI bleeding in, 594, 596, 624, **629–630**
    H pylori-associated, 623, 625, 625–627,
        626*t*, 627, 628, 630
        gastritis and, 622, 623
    herpes simplex infection and, 1364
    NSAID-induced, 623, 624, 626*t*, 627,
        627–628, 629–630, 829
    pharmacologic/medical management
        of, 625–629, 626*t*
    refractory, 628–629
    silent, 624
    ulcer perforation and, **630**
    Zollinger-Ellison syndrome
        (gastrinoma) and, 623, 629,
        631, 1185
Pepto-Bismol. *See* Bismuth compounds
Peptostreptococci, 1478, 1479
Per oral endoscopic myotomy (POEM),
        for achalasia, 618
Peramivir, 1365*t*, 1412, 1413, 1418
Perampanel, 987*t*
Percent free PSA, 1646
Perceptual distortions. *See also* Delirium
    in schizophrenia/psychotic disorders,
        1067
Percocet. *See* Oxycodone
Percodan. *See* Oxycodone
Percutaneous aspiration/injection/
        reaspiration (PAIR), for
        hydatid cysts, 1537–1538
Percutaneous balloon valvuloplasty. *See*
        Valvuloplasty
Percutaneous coronary intervention
        (PCI), 362–363
    for acute coronary syndromes/STEMI,
        362–363, 369*t*, 372–374,
        372*f*, 376

    for angina, 362–363
    antiplatelet therapy and, 373, 374
    CABG compared with, 362–363
    prophylactic/preoperative, 46–47
    thrombotic events and, 362,
        373, 374
Percutaneous dilatational tracheotomy,
        237
Percutaneous transhepatic
        cholangiography (PTC), 677
Percutaneous transluminal coronary
        angioplasty (PTCA). *See*
        Angioplasty, coronary;
        Percutaneous coronary
        intervention
Percutaneous valvuloplasty. *See*
        Valvuloplasty
Perennial rhinitis, 219
Perforation
    in appendicitis, 642
        pregnancy and, 825
    of colonic diverticula (diverticulitis),
        663
    ulcer, **630**
Performance anxiety, 1053, 1076
Perfusion scans
    lung. *See* Ventilation-perfusion scans
    myocardial. *See* Myocardial perfusion
        scintigraphy
Periampullary/ampullary carcinoma,
        1620–1626, 1634
Perianal cellophane tape test, in
        enterobiasis/pinworms,
        1541
Perianal disease. *See also* Anorectal
        disorders
    abscesses and fistulas, 673
    anal cancer, 1344, 1624*t*, **1643–1644**
    in Crohn disease, 652, 653, 654
    fissures, 672–673
    hematoma, thrombosed hemorrhoid
        causing, 670
    herpetic, 119, 671
    warts, 141, 141*f*, 671, 768. *See also*
        Venereal (genital) warts
Perianal pruritus. *See* Anogenital/perianal
        pruritus
Pericardial disease, **424–429**, 425*t*
    in SLE, 840
    tumors, 433. *See also* Mesothelioma
Pericardial effusions, **427–428**. *See also*
        Pericarditis
    malignant/neoplastic, 425, 426,
        426–427, 428, 1658, 1659
    in pneumococcal pneumonia, 1445,
        1446
Pericardial friction rub
    in chest pain evaluation, 28
    in pericarditis/effusion, 425, 427
Pericardial injury, pericarditis caused by,
        425
Pericardial "knock," 428
Pericardial tamponade. *See* Tamponade
Pericarditis
    acute inflammatory, **424–427**, 425*t*
    bacterial, 425, 426
    chest pain in, 27, 425
    constrictive, **428–429**
        cardiac cirrhosis and, 700
        restrictive cardiomyopathy
            differentiated from, 421, 429

    coxsackieviruses causing, 424, 1426
    effusion/tamponade and, 28, 378, 425,
        426, 427–428, 1658
    effusive-constrictive, 428
    myocardial infarction and, 378, 379,
        425
    neoplastic, 425, 426, 426–427
    pneumococcal, 1445, 1446
    postmyocardial infarction/
        postcardiotomy (Dressler
        syndrome), 379, 425, 426
    radiation, 425, 427
    tuberculous, 424–425, 425, 426
    uremic, 425, 426, 924, 926–927
    viral, 424, 425–426
Perichondritis, 201. *See also*
        Polychondritis
Perihepatitis, Fitz-Hugh and Curtis
        syndrome and, 778
Perihilar (Klatskin) tumors, 1618
Perilymphatic fistula, 204, 211*t*, 212
Perindopril
    with amlodipine, 456*t*
    in cardiovascular/heart disease
        prevention, 355
    for hypertension, 456*t*
Periodic limb movement disorder, 1090
Periodic paralysis, **1049**
    hyperkalemic, 892*t*, 1049
    hypokalemic, 892*t*, 1049
        in hyperthyroidism, 1049, 1127,
            1133
    normokalemic, 1049
Periodontal disease
    anaerobic, 1478
        pneumonia and, 275, 1478
    in HIV infection/AIDS, 1341
Perioperative management. *See*
        Preoperative evaluation/
        perioperative management
Periorbitopathy, prostaglandin-associated,
        180
Peripartum cardiomyopathy, 420
Peripartum period, complications of,
        813–814
Peripheral arterial disease, **472–480**. *See
        also specific artery and*
        Atherosclerosis
Peripheral artery aneurysms, **483–484**
Peripheral intravenous lines, infection/
        infection prevention and,
        1294, 1295, 1317
Peripheral nerve tumor, mononeuropathy
        caused by, 1039
Peripheral neuropathies, **1034–1042**. *See
        also specific type and*
        Neuropathies
    cancer-related/chemotherapy-induced,
        1037–1038, 1674
    diabetic, 1239–1240, 1239*f*. *See also*
        Diabetic neuropathy
    in HIV infection/AIDS, 1340
    in porphyria, 1036, 1676
Peripheral pulses. *See* Pulses
Peripheral T-cell lymphomas, 533
Peripheral vascular disease. *See* Vascular
        disorders
Peripheral vein nutritional support,
        1281*f*, 1282. *See also*
        Nutritional support
    solutions for, 1284

Peripheral vestibular disease, 210–211, 210t, 211–213
Perirectal abscess, in Crohn disease, 652, 653, 654
Peristalsis, disorders of. *See* Motility disorders
Peritoneal carcinomatosis, 604
Peritoneal dialysis, 930. *See also* Dialysis
  for end-stage renal disease, 930
  for hyperkalemia, 895t
Peritoneum
  diseases of, **600–604**, 601t. *See also specific type and* Ascites; Peritonitis
  nausea and vomiting in, 581t
Peritonitis, 1314t
  ascitic fluid analysis in, 602, 603
  bacterial/spontaneous bacterial, 601, 602, **602–604**, 702
  dialysis and, 930
  diverticulitis and, 663, 664
  in familial Mediterranean fever, 604
  peptic ulcer perforation and, 630
  perforated appendicitis and, 642
  pregnancy and, 825
  secondary, 603
Peritonsillar abscess/cellulitis, **229**
Peritrochanteric hip fracture, 1702. *See also* Hip fracture
Periungual lesions, malignant, 160
Periungual warts, 141
Perjeta. *See* Pertuzumab
PERK mutation, in diabetes, 1212–1213
Permethrin
  for pediculosis, 150
  for scabies, 149
Permissive hypercapnia, for asthma, 257
Permitil. *See* Fluphenazine
Pernicious anemia, 506
  carcinoid tumors and, 622, 1633
  gastritis and, 622–623
  subacute combined degeneration of spinal cord and, 1026
Peroneal (fibular) nerve, common, injury to, **1040**
Peroxisome proliferator-activated receptor alpha (PPAR-alpha) agonists, for lipid modification, 1264–1265
Peroxisome proliferator-activated receptor gamma (PPAR-gamma)
  thiazolidinediones affecting, 1224
  thyroid cancer and, 1139
Perphenazine, 1068, 1069t, 1070
  relative potency/side effects of, 1069t
Persistent anovulation. *See* Polycystic ovary syndrome
Persistent vegetative state, **1028**
Personal relationships, social issues for terminally ill/dying patient and, 92, 92t
Personality changes
  due to general medical condition, 1103
  in syphilis, 1489t, 1496
Personality disorders, **1064–1066**, 1065t
Perspiration. *See* Sweating
Pertussis (whooping cough), 19, 21, **1463–1464**
  prevention/immunization and, 4, 1464. *See also* Pertussis vaccine

Pertussis vaccine, with diphtheria and tetanus toxoids (DTaP/Tdap vaccines), 4, 1320t, 1321t, 1322t, 1329t, 1453, 1453t, 1457, 1464. *See also* Tetanus and diphtheria toxoids and pertussis vaccines
Pertuzumab, 1667t
  for breast cancer, 752, 753, 756
Pes anserine bursa/bursitis, 1704
PESI (pulmonary embolism severity index), 571, 571t
Pesticide poisoning (cholinesterase inhibitors), 1580t, 1581t, **1601–1602**
Pestiviruses, gastroenteritis caused by, 1424
PET. *See* Positron emission tomography
Petit mal (absence) seizures, 984–985, 984t. *See also* Seizures
  drug therapy for, 988t
Petroleum products, toxicity/abuse of, 1101, **1602**
  aspiration and, 306, 1602
Petrous apicitis, 206
Peutz-Jeghers syndrome, 667
  pancreatic/periampullary carcinoma and, 1620
Peyronie disease, 966, 968, 1186
PFO. *See* Patent foramen ovale
PFTs. *See* Pulmonary function tests
PGA. *See* Polyglandular autoimmune syndrome
PGI$_2$. *See* Prostacyclin
pH
  in acid-base disorders, 903. *See also specific type*
  in alcoholic ketoacidosis, 905
  in diabetic ketoacidosis, 1246, 1247
  in drowning, 1567
  esophageal, monitoring, 606, 607, 609–610
  gastric, nosocomial pneumonia and, 273
  in metabolic acidosis, 907
  in metabolic alkalosis, 910
  pharyngeal, monitoring, 233
  pleural fluid, 312
  in respiratory acidosis, 910
  in respiratory alkalosis, 911
  urine, 962
    manipulation of in poisoning/drug overdose, 1582
    normal, 962
    in normal anion gap/renal tubular acidosis, 906, 906t, 907
    stone disease and, 962, 964
  vaginal, 766
Phaeohyphomycosis, 1558
Phalen sign, in carpal tunnel syndrome, 1699, 1699t
Pharmaceuticals. *See under* Drug
Pharmacogenetic tests, in dermatitis medicamentosa prediction, 161
Pharyngeal cancer, incidence/mortality/risk of, 1608t
Pharyngeal dysphagia, 605. *See also* Dysphagia
Pharyngitis, **227–229**, 228f, 1315t, **1441–1442**
  antibiotics for, 227, 229, 1442

differential diagnosis of, 228, 1373, 1441–1442
  in diphtheria, 228, 1441, 1456, 1457
  Fusobacterium necrophorum, 1441, 1442, 1478
  gonococcal, 1475
  in mononucleosis, 228, 1372, 1373
  nonstreptococcal exudative (adenovirus), 1421
  streptococcal, 227, 228f, 1315t, **1441–1442**
    eruptive (guttate) psoriasis after, 107
    glomerulonephritis and, 936, 1441
    rheumatic fever and, 229, 422, 424, 1441, 1442
Pharyngoconjunctival fever, 167, 1421
Pharynx, **224–231**
PHD2 mutations, in pheochromocytoma/paraganglioma, 1180
Phenacetin, in analgesic nephropathy, 947
Phenazopyridine
  methemoglobinemia caused by, 1599
  for urinary tract infection, 955
Phencyclidine, **1099**, 1598
  aggressive/violent/psychotic behavior caused by, 1068, 1090, 1099
Phenelzine, 1078t
  overdose/toxicity of, 1078t
Phenobarbital, 987t, 1054t
  for anxiety, 1054t
  overdose/toxicity of, 987t
    hemodialysis for, 1583t
  for seizures, 987t
    in poisoning/drug overdose, 1580
    status epilepticus, 989
Phenothiazines, 1068. *See also* Antipsychotic drugs
  overdose/toxicity of, 1589–1590
  ophthalmic, 177t
Phenoxybenzamine, pheochromocytoma/pheochromocytoma surgery and, 1183
Phentermine/topiramate, for obesity, 1271
  in type 2 diabetes, 1235
Phentolamine
  for erectile dysfunction diagnosis/treatment, 967
  in diabetes, 1241
  for hypertensive urgencies/emergencies, 469, 469t
D-Phenylalanine derivatives
  abuse of, 1099
  for diabetes mellitus, 1221t, 1223
Phenylbutazone
  adverse ophthalmic effects of, 179t
  lithium interactions and, 1087t
Phenytoin, 987t
  antidepressant drug interactions and, 1083t
  overdose/toxicity of, 987t, 1589
  ophthalmic, 177t
  for seizures, 987t
    pregnancy and, 820
    status epilepticus and, 989
Pheochromocytoma, **1179–1184**, 1180t, 1181t
  beta-blocker use in, 454
  hypertension in, 443, 444, 469, 469t, 1179, 1180t, 1182, 1183
  in MEN, 1179, 1187t, 1188
  metastatic, 1183, 1183–1184, 1184

Pheochromocytoma multisystem crisis, 1180*t*, 1181, 1182
Pheochromocytomatosis, 1183, 1184
PHEX endopeptidase, mutation in gene encoding, in osteomalacia/rickets, 1165
PHF6 mutation, in acute myeloid leukemia, 527
Philadelphia chromosome, 519
  in acute lymphoblastic leukemia, 527, 529
  in chronic myeloid leukemia, 519, 523, 524
Phimosis, in chancroid, 1476
Phlebitis. *See* Thrombophlebitis
Phlebotomy
  for hemochromatosis, 709
  for polycythemia, 520
  for porphyria cutanea tarda, 123
  potassium levels affected by fist clench during, 893, 894*t*, 1178
Phlegmon
  in Crohn disease, 653
  in neck infection, 230
Phlegmonous (necrotizing) gastritis, 623
Phobic disorders/phobias, 1053, 1056
Phonophobia, in migraine, 40, 40*t*
Phosphate. *See* Phosphorus/phosphate
Phosphate enema, 585*t*
Phosphatonin (fibroblast growth factor-23), 899, 927, 1164–1165, 1165
Phosphaturia
  hyperparathyroidism and, 1154
  hypophosphatemia and, 900
Phosphodiesterase inhibitors
  adverse ophthalmic effects of, 177*t*
  for asthma, 251
  for benign prostatic hyperplasia, 974, 974*t*
  for erectile dysfunction, 967, 1064
    antidepressant-induced, 1064, 1079
    in diabetes, 1241
  for high-altitude illness treatment/prevention, 1575
  nitrate/nitroglycerin contraindications and, 375, 967, 1064, 1241
  for pulmonary hypertension, 303
Phospholipase A2 receptor, in membranous nephropathy, 944, 945
Phosphorus/phosphate
  calcium metabolism and, 896, 897, 899
  in calcium nephrolithiasis/hypercalciuria, 898, 962*t*, 963
  deficiency of, 1164–1165. *See also* Hypophosphatemia
    in osteomalacia/rickets, 892*t*, 900, 1164–1165, 1164*t*
  dietary/supplementary
    for diabetic ketoacidosis, 1248
    for hyperglycemic hyperosmolar state, 1250
    for hypophosphatemia, 900, 1166
    requirements for in nutritional support, 1282
    restriction of in chronic kidney disease, 927, 929

disorders of concentration/metabolism of, 892*t*, **899–901**, 899*t*, 901*t*. *See also* Hyperphosphatemia; Hypophosphatemia
  in chronic kidney disease/renal osteodystrophy, 926*f*, 927, 927*f*
  genetic disorders and, 892*t*, 1164–1165
  in hypercalcemia/hyperparathyroidism, 898
  in hypocalcemia/hypoparathyroidism, 896, 897, 1150
  parathyroid hormone affecting, 899
  urinary excretion of. *See* Phosphaturia
Photoallergy, 154, 155. *See also* Photodermatitis
Photochemotherapy. *See also* Psoralen plus ultraviolet A (PUVA) therapy
  for psoriasis, 108
Photodermatitis, 96*t*, **154–155**
  chemotherapy-induced, 1673
  drugs causing, 154, 155, 162*t*
Photoepilation, for hirsutism, 1197
Photophobia, in migraine, 40, 40*t*
Photosensitive epilepsy, 985
Photosensitivity
  contact, 154. *See also* Photodermatitis
  drugs causing, 154, 155, 162*t*
    antipsychotics, 1072
Phototherapy
  for lichen planus, 145
  for major depression with seasonal onset, 1084
  for psoriasis, 108, 1344
Phototoxicity, 154, 155. *See also* Photodermatitis
Photovaporization of prostate (PVP), 975
PHQ-9. *See* Patient Health Questionnaire-9
Phthirus pubis, 149
Phyllodes tumor of breast, 735
Physical abuse. *See* Abuse
Physical activity. *See* Exercise/activity
Physical inactivity. *See* Inactivity
Physical instability. *See* Falls; Gait/gait disorders; Instability
Physician (or Medical) Orders for Life-Sustaining Treatment (POLST/MOLST) forms, 90
Physiologic drug dependence, 1092. *See also* Substance use disorders
  in opioid therapy, 73, 85
Physostigmine, for atropine/anticholinergic overdose, 1581*t*, 1590, 1598
Phytanic acid metabolism, in Refsum disease, 1036
Phytonadione
  for anticoagulant overdose, 1588
  for hepatic coagulopathy, 704
  for vitamin K deficiency, 562
Phytotherapy, for benign prostatic hyperplasia, 975
PI. *See* Protease inhibitors
Pickwickian syndrome (obesity-hypoventilation syndrome), **315–316**
PID. *See* Pelvic inflammatory disease
Piebaldism, 157

"Pigeon-breeder's disease" (bird-fancier's lung), 308*t*
Pigmentary skin disorders, **157–158**, 157*f. See also* Hyperpigmentation; Hypopigmentation; Pigmented skin lesions
  drugs causing, 158, 163*t*
  in hypercarotenosis, 1277
Pigmented basal cell carcinoma, 143
Pigmented skin lesions, 96*t*, **101–104**. *See also specific type*
PIK3A mutations, in thyroid cancer, 1139
Pill-induced esophagitis, **612**
Pilocarpine
  for glaucoma/ocular hypertension, 172*t*, 180
  for radiation-induced xerostomia, 1671*t*
Pilocarpine iontophoresis sweat test, in cystic fibrosis, 265
Pilopine/Pilopine HS. *See* Pilocarpine
Pimecrolimus, 98*t*
  for atopic dermatitis, 105
  T-cell lymphoma and, 105
Pimozide, for Tourette syndrome, 1018
Pindolol, 453*t*
  for aggressive/violent behavior, 1091
  for angina, 359–361
  for hypertension, 453*t*
Pineal tumor, 1004*t*
Pinguecula/pinguecuitis, **174**
"Pink puffers," 257, 258*t*
PINK1 gene, in parkinsonism, 1011
Pinta, **1498**
Pinworm infection, **1540–1541**
  anogenital pruritus and, 147, 148, 1541
Pioglitazone, 1221*t*, 1224–1225, 1235*f*, 1236
  with glimepiride, 1228
  with insulin, 1236
  with metformin, 1228
  overdose/toxicity of, 1235*f*, 1595
Piperacillin-tazobactam
  for anaerobic infections, 1479, 1479*t*
  for pneumonia, 269*t*, 271, 275*t*
Piperaquine, 1515*t*, 1516
  with dihydroartemisinin, 1516, 1516*t*, 1517*t*, 1519, 1521
Pipracil. *See* Piperacillin
Pirbuterol, for asthma, 252, 253*t*
Pirfenidone, for idiopathic pulmonary fibrosis, 292
Piroxicam, 76*t*
Pit viper envenomation, 1604
Pitavastatin, 355*t*, 1265*t*
Pitting (nail), 160
  in psoriasis, 107, 107*f*, 160, 865
Pituitary adenoma, 1108
  ACTH-secreting, 1173, 1174, 1175, 1176
  diabetes insipidus and, 1113
  GH-secreting (acromegaly/gigantism), 1114, 1115, 1116
  hypopituitarism caused by, 1108, 1112
  in MEN, 1187*t*, 1188, 1189
  Nelson syndrome and, 1175, 1176, 1176–1177
  prolactin-secreting, 1117, 1118, 1118–1119, 1199

surgical resection/removal of, 1112,
        1115–1116, 1118–1119, 1175,
        1176
    thyrotrophe (TSH-secreting), 1126
Pituitary apoplexy, 1111
Pituitary Cushing disease, 1173, 1174,
        1175, 1176
Pituitary gland
    destruction/necrosis of
        adrenal crisis caused by, 1169
        postpartum hemorrhage causing
            (Sheehan syndrome), 1109
    disorders of, 1108–1119, 1109t
        acromegaly/gigantism, 1114–1116
        amenorrhea caused by, 1109, 1110,
            1199, 1200
        anterior hypopituitarism,
            1108–1113, 1109t
        diabetes insipidus, 1109, 1113–1114.
            See also Diabetes insipidus
        hyperprolactinemia, 1116–1119,
            1117t
    hormones produced by, 1109t
    hyperplasia of, thyrotrophe, 1126
    in hypothyroidism, 1109, 1110, 1111
    tumors of, 1111. See also Pituitary
        adenoma
        amenorrhea caused by, 1199, 1200
Pituitary surgery/microsurgery, 1112,
        1115–1116, 1118–1119
Pityriasis
    rosea, 109–110, 109f
        drugs causing eruptions similar to,
            109, 163t
    rubra pilaris, 117
    versicolor (tinea versicolor), 114–115
Pityrosporum ovale. See Malassezia furfur
Pivot shift test, knee stability/ACL injury
        and, 1706t, 1709
"Pizza-pie" retinopathy, in CMV
        infection, 1375
PKD1/PKD2 mutations, 949, 950
PKR-like ER kinase, mutation in gene for,
        in diabetes, 1212–1213
PLA₂R (phospholipase A2 receptor), in
        membranous nephropathy,
        944, 945
Placenta
    morbidly adherent (placenta accreta/
        increta/percreta), 813
    previa, 813
    Zika virus testing on, 1406
Placental abruption, 812, 813
Placental site trophoblastic tumor, 807
Plague, 1312t, 1474–1475
    chemoprophylaxis for, 1326, 1474
Plan B, for emergency/postcoital
        contraception, 791
Plantar nerves, compressive lesions of,
        1041
Plantar warts, 141, 142
Plaque psoriasis, 107. See also Psoriasis
Plasma/plasma fractions/components,
        transfusion of, 544. See also
        Transfusion
    for anticoagulant overdose, 1588
    for bleeding disorders, 544
    for DIC, 554
    for thrombotic microangiopathies,
        551–552
Plasma cell leukemia, 535

Plasma cells, in myeloma, 535
Plasma chromogranin A (CgA) screening
        test. See Chromogranin A
Plasma renin activity
    in adrenal insufficiency/Addison
        disease, 1170
    in aldosteronism, 442, 1178
Plasmacytomas, 535. See also Myeloma
Plasmodium, 1513–1521, 1514f. See also
        Malaria
    falciparum, 1513–1521, 1514f, 1515t,
        1516t, 1517t, 1520t
        uncomplicated infection caused by,
            1515–1516, 1516t, 1517t
    knowlesi, 1513
    malariae, 1513–1521, 1514f, 1517t
    ovale, 1513–1521, 1514f, 1515t, 1517t,
        1520t
    vivax, 1513–1521, 1514f, 1515t, 1517t,
        1520t
Platelet count
    chemotherapy affecting, 548
        dosage modification and, 1672t
    cyclic oscillations of (cyclic
        thrombocytopenia), 548
    desired ranges for, 547t
    in myeloproliferative neoplasms, 520t
    in thrombocytosis, 521
    transfusion and, 544
Platelet-derived growth factor
        (becaplermin), for diabetic
        foot ulcers, 156, 1239
Platelet disorders, 546–557, 547t, 549f,
        551t, 553t, 554t, 555t, 558t
    acquired, 557, 558f
    congenital, 556–557
    qualitative, 556–557, 558t
    quantitative
        decreased platelet production
            causing, 546–548, 547t
        increased platelet destruction
            causing, 547t, 548–555
    thrombocytopenia, 546–556, 547t,
        549f, 551t, 553t, 554t, 555t.
        See also Thrombocytopenia
Platelet factor 4 (PF4)-heparin antibody,
        552
Platelet glycoprotein IIb/IIIa receptors.
        See Glycoprotein IIb/IIIa
        receptors
Platelet-inhibiting agents. See Antiplatelet
        therapy
Platelet transfusion, 544. See also
        Transfusion
    contraindications to in thrombotic
        microangiopathy, 552
    for myelodysplastic syndrome, 548
Platelets. See also Platelet disorders
    aspirin/NSAIDs affecting function of,
        558t, 829
    autoantibodies against. See Antiplatelet
        antibody
    in Bernard-Soulier syndrome, 556
    in chronic kidney disease/uremia,
        558t
    drugs inhibiting. See Antiplatelet
        therapy
    in Glanzmann thrombasthenia, 556
    in myeloproliferative neoplasms, 520t,
        558t
    sequestration of in spleen, 547t, 555

in storage pool disease, 556
    in von Willebrand disease, 560
Platinol. See Cisplatin
Platinum analogs/platinum-based
        chemotherapy, 1663t. See
        also Cisplatin
    for lung cancer, 1612
    toxicity of, 1675
    for triple negative breast cancer, 753
Platypnea orthodeoxia, 325, 325–326
    in cirrhosis, 704
Plavix. See Clopidogrel
Pleconaril, in enterovirus meningitis,
        1426
Plenadren, for adrenal insufficiency/
        Addison disease, 1171
Plendil. See Felodipine
Plerixafor, for stem cell mobilization, 540
Plesiomonas, diarrhea caused by, 588t,
        592
Plethysmography, impedance
    in esophageal disorders, 606, 607, 610
    in venous thrombosis/pulmonary
        embolism, 297, 298
Pleural diseases, 311–315, 311t, 313t. See
        also Pulmonary disorders
    occupational, 309
    respiratory failure caused by, 318t
Pleural effusions, 311–314, 311t, 313t
    asbestos causing, 309
    drug-induced, 310t
    in heart failure, 312, 403
    in lung cancer, 312, 1609
    malignant, 312, 312–313, 313t, 1658,
        1659
    in mesothelioma, 1615
    paramalignant, 312
    parapneumonic, 311, 312, 313–314,
        313t
        in community-acquired/
            pneumococcal disease, 1445,
            1446
    rheumatoid, 313t
    tuberculous, 279, 312, 313t
Pleural fluid analysis, 311–312
    in lung cancer, 312, 313t, 1609
    mesothelioma, 1615
    in pneumonia, 270, 274, 312
Pleural friction rub, in pulmonary
        embolism, 296t
Pleural mesothelioma/malignant pleural
        mesothelioma, 309, 1614,
        1615
Pleuritis/pleuritic chest pain, 22, 27, 27t
Pleurodesis, for malignant pleural
        effusion, 313, 1659
Pleurodynia, epidemic, 1426
Pleuropulmonary infection, anaerobic,
        268t, 1478
Plexiform neuroma, 1010
Plexopathy (diabetic amyotrophy), 1036
Plummer disease (toxic adenoma of
        thyroid), 1125, 1131
    in MEN, 1187t, 1188
Plummer-Vinson syndrome, 501
PMDD. See Premenstrual dysphoric
        disorder
PML. See Progressive multifocal
        leukoencephalopathy
PML-RAR-alpha fusion gene, 527
PMLE. See Polymorphous light eruption

PMS. *See* Premenstrual syndrome/
    tension
PMS2 genes, in HNPCC/Lynch
    syndrome, 668
PNES. *See* Psychogenic nonepileptic
    seizure
pNET. *See* Pancreatic neuroendocrine
    tumors
Pneumatic dilation, for achalasia, 618. *See
    also* Esophageal dilation
Pneumococcal (*Streptococcus
    pneumoniae*) infections,
    1311*t*, 1315*t*, **1445–1447**
  brain abscess, 1314*t*
  drug resistance and, 270–271, 271,
    1316, 1446
  endocarditis, 1445, 1446, 1461
  immunization against. *See*
    Pneumococcal vaccine
  meningitis, 1297*t*, 1299, 1314*t*, **1447**
  pericarditis, 1445, 1446
  pneumonia, 268, 268*t*, 269–270,
    270–271, 271, 1314*t*, 1315*t*,
    1443, **1445–1446**
    in HIV infection/AIDS, 1336
    influenza and, 1412
Pneumococcal vaccine, 3, 1320*t*,
    1323–1324*t*
  adverse effects/contraindications and,
    1239*t*
  for asthma patients, 251
  in cystic fibrosis, 266
  in immunocompromised host/HIV
    infection/AIDS, 5, 1321*t*,
    1324*t*
  in pneumonia prevention, 271
  pregnancy and, 802, 1321*t*
Pneumoconioses, **306–307**, 307*t*
*Pneumocystis carinii. See Pneumocystis
    jirovecii* infection/pneumonia
Pneumocystis jirovecii infection/
    pneumonia
    (pneumocystosis), 268*t*,
    1335–1336, 1337*t*, 1349,
    1349*t*, 1350, **1551–1553**
  CD4 T cell count and, 1333, 1334,
    1336, 1349, 1552
  pentamidine treatment/
    chemoprophylaxis and,
    1337*t*, 1349*t*, 1552
  pneumothorax and, 314, 315
Pneumomediastinum, pneumothorax
    and, 315
Pneumonia, 20*t*, **267–276**, 268*t*, 269*t*,
    273*t*, 275*t*, 1314*t*, 1315*t*. *See
    also specific cause and*
    Pneumonitis
  acute interstitial (AIP), 290, 291*t*
  adenovirus, 1421
  anaerobic, 268*t*, **274–276**, 1314*t*, 1315*t*,
    1478
  in aspergillosis, 1555
  aspiration, 275, 1294, 1315*t*. *See also*
    Aspiration
    in anaerobic infections, 275, 1315*t*,
    1478
    drug use and, 1304
    gastric contents and, 273,
    1294
    toxic materials and, 306, 1602
  bronchial obstruction and, 242

bronchiolitis obliterans and (BOOP/
    cryptogenic organizing
    pneumonia/pneumonitis/
    COP), 267, 291*t*, 292
  chlamydial, 268*t*, 1314*t*, 1315*t*, 1487
  CMV, 1375, 1376
    in HIV infection/AIDS, 1336–1338
  in coccidioidomycosis, 1550, 1551
  community-acquired, **267–272**, 269*t*,
    1314*t*
  cryptococcal, 1553
  cryptogenic organizing (COP/
    bronchiolitis obliterans with
    organizing pneumonia/
    BOOP), 267, 291*t*, 292
  deaths attributable to, 2*t*, 267
  diffuse interstitial, **289–292**, 290*t*, 291*t*,
    292*f*
  eosinophilic, 294
  Escherichia coli causing, 268*t*
  Haemophilus influenzae causing, 268*t*,
    1466
  herpes simplex, 1364
  in histoplasmosis, 1549
  hospitalized patient with, 267, 269,
    269*t*, 271, 271–272, 1314*t*
  in immunocompromised host/HIV
    infection/AIDS, 268*t*, 271,
    276, 1291, 1335–1336, 1337*t*,
    1551, 1552, 1553. *See also
    Pneumocystis jirovecii*
    infection/pneumonia
    CD4 T cell count and, 1333, 1334,
    1336, 1349
  influenza and, 269, 271, 1411, 1412
  Klebsiella pneumoniae causing, 268*t*
  Legionnaires, 268*t*, 269, 1311*t*, 1314*t*,
    1315*t*, 1466–1467
  in leptospirosis, 1501
  lipoid, 306
  in measles, 1379
  mercury causing, 1598, 1598–1599
  Moraxella catarrhalis causing, 268*t*,
    1466
  mycobacterial, 1314*t*
  Mycoplasma pneumoniae causing, 268*t*,
    1314*t*, 1315*t*
  necrotizing, 275, 276
  nonspecific interstitial (NSIP), 291*t*,
    292
    in HIV infection/AIDS, 1339
  nosocomial (hospital-acquired/
    ventilator/health care-
    associated), **272–274**, 273*t*,
    275*t*, 319, 1294, 1314*t*
  plague, 1474
  pleural effusion in (parapneumonic
    pleural effusion), 311, 312,
    313–314, 313*t*
    in community-acquired/
    pneumococcal disease, 1445,
    1446
  pneumococcal/streptococcal, 268, 268*t*,
    269–270, 270–271, 271,
    1314*t*, 1315*t*, 1443,
    1445–1446
    immunization against. *See*
    Pneumococcal vaccine
  *Pneumocystis. See Pneumocystis
    jirovecii* infection/pneumonia
  postoperative, 1314*t*

Pseudomonas aeruginosa causing, 268*t*,
    269*t*, 271, 273, 275*t*
  RSV, 1409
  staphylococcal, 268*t*, 269, 273, 273*t*,
    1314*t*
  treatment of
    anaerobic infection, 276, 1478
    community-acquired disease, 269*t*,
    270–271, 1314*t*
    nosocomial disease, 274, 275*t*, 1314*t*
    in tularemia, 1473
    usual interstitial (UIP), 290, 291*t*
    varicella zoster virus, 1369
    during pregnancy, 821
  viral, 268
Pneumonia Severity Index (PSI), 272
Pneumonitis. *See also* Pneumonia
  acute gastric aspiration causing,
    305–306, 1294
  CMV, 1375, 1376
  cryptogenic organizing (COP/
    bronchiolitis obliterans with
    organizing pneumonia/
    BOOP), 267, 291*t*, 292
  in H1N1 seasonal influenza, 1411
  hydrocarbon/petroleum distillates/
    solvents causing, 306, 1602
  hypersensitivity, **307–308**, 308*t*
  interstitial
    drug-induced, 290*t*, 310*t*
    in HIV infection/AIDS, 1339
  mercury causing, 1598–1599
  methotrexate causing, 837
  radiation, **310**
  toxoplasmic, in HIV infection/AIDS,
    1523
Pneumoplasty, reduction, for COPD, 262
Pneumothorax, **314–315**
  in COPD, 259, 314
  in HIV infection/AIDS, 314, 315
  in *Pneumocystis* pneumonia, 314, 315
  spontaneous, **314–315**
Pneumovax. *See* Pneumococcal vaccine
PNH. *See* Paroxysmal nocturnal
    hemoglobinuria
Po₂. *See* Arterial blood gases; Pulse
    oximetry
Podagra, 830
Podophyllum resin (podophyllin/
    podofilox), for genital warts,
    141, 768
POEM (per oral endoscopic myotomy),
    for achalasia, 618
Poison control centers, 1577
Poison ivy/oak/sumac, 124, 125, 125*f*. *See
    also* Contact dermatitis
    urticaria and, 134
Poisoning/drug overdose, **1577–1606**. *See
    also specific drug or agent*
  abdominal radiographs in, 1585
  anion gap in, 1584. *See also* Anion gap/
    anion gap acidosis
  antidotes for, **1581**, 1581*t*
  arrhythmias in, **1579–1580**, 1579*t*
  assessment of danger and, 1577
  coma caused by, 1246*t*, **1577–1578**
  diagnosis of, **1583–1585**, 1584*t*
  eye decontamination in, **1581**
  gastrointestinal decontamination in,
    1581–1583
  hypertension in, **1579**

hyperthermia in, **1580–1581**
hypotension in, **1578–1579**
hypothermia in, **1578**
initial evaluation in, 1577
laboratory tests in, 1584–1585, 1584*t*
osmol gap in, 1584, 1584*t*
patient observation and, 1577
physical examination in, 1583–1584
seizures in, **1580**, 1580*t*
skin decontamination in, **1581**
toxicology screen in, 1584–1585, 1584*t*
Poisonous mushrooms, **1600–1601**, 1600*t*
anticholinergic-type, 1590
hallucinogenic mushrooms and, 1598,
1600*t*
liver failure and, 685–686, 686, 1600
Poisonous snakes, 1581*t*, **1604–1605**
Poliomyelitis, **1382–1384**
prevention/immunization and, 1326,
1383. *See also* Poliovirus
vaccine
vaccine-associated, 1326, 1383
Poliosis, uveitis in, 181
Poliovirus vaccine, 1326, 1383
in immunocompromised host/HIV
infection/AIDS, 5, 1383
pregnancy and, 802
for travelers, 1326, 1383
vaccine-associated disease and, 1326,
1383
Pollen-associated food allergy syndrome,
877
POLST forms, 90
Polyangiitis
with granulomatosis. *See*
Granulomatosis, with
polyangiitis
microscopic. *See* Microscopic
polyangiitis
Polyarteritis. *See also* Arteritis
glomerulonephritis in, 933*t*
neuropathy associated with, 856,
1037
nodosa, 152, **855–857**
livedo reticularis/racemosa and, 856,
863
Polyarthralgia/polyarthritis. *See* Arthritis/
arthralgia
Polycarbophil, 585*t*. *See also* Fiber,
dietary
Polychondritis, relapsing, 201, **861**
Polycystic kidney disease, **949–950**, 949*t*
Polycystic ovary syndrome, **780–781**,
1196
amenorrhea in, 780, 1196, 1199,
1200–1201
hirsutism in, 780, 781, 1196
infertility and, 780, 781, 784
Polycythemia/polycythemia vera,
519–521, 519*t*, 520*t*, 1623*t*
hepatic vein obstruction/Budd-Chiari
syndrome, 711
hypertension and, 441
spurious, 520
Polydipsia/thirst
in diabetes insipidus, 1113
in diabetes mellitus, 1213, 1214
hyponatremia caused by, 886, 887,
1067
psychogenic, 1067
hyponatremia caused by, 887, 1067

in schizophrenia/psychotic disorders,
1067
Polyendocrinopathy-candidiasis-
ectodermal dystrophy,
autoimmune, 1149, 1169. *See
also* Polyglandular
autoimmune syndrome
Polyethylene glycol/PEG 3350
for constipation/preoperative bowel
cleansing, 585*t*, 586
for whole bowel irrigation, 1582
Polyglandular autoimmune syndrome,
1149, 1169
adrenal insufficiency/Addison disease
in, 1169
autoimmune hepatitis in, 692
Hashimoto thyroiditis in, 1135
hypoparathyroidism in, 1149
Polymenorrhea, 762
Polymerase chain reaction (PCR) testing.
See also Reverse
transcriptase-polymerase
chain reaction testing
on cerebrospinal fluid, 1299
in Lyme disease, 1504
in poliomyelitis, 1382
in syphilis, 1489, 1491
for Zika virus, 1406
Polymerase inhibitors, for hepatitis C,
690–691, 690*t*, 691
Polymorphic reticulosis, 223
Polymorphic ventricular tachycardia, 397
Polymorphonuclear neutrophil count. *See*
Neutrophil count
Polymorphous light eruption (PMLE),
154, 155
Polymyalgia rheumatica, **853–855**
polymyositis differentiated from, 849
rheumatoid arthritis differentiated
from, 836
Polymyositis, 840*t*, **847–850**, 848*t*
Polymyxin/bacitracin, for ophthalmic
disorders, 169*t*
Polymyxin B/gramicidin/neomycin, for
ophthalmic disorders, 169*t*
Polymyxin B/trimethoprim sulfate, for
ophthalmic disorders, 169*t*
Polyneuropathies, **1034–1039**. *See also
specific type and*
Neuropathies
acute idiopathic. *See* Guillain-Barré
syndrome
cancer-related, 1037–1038
chronic inflammatory, **1039**
in critically ill patients, 1037
in diabetes, 1036, 1239–1240, 1239*f*.
See also Diabetic neuropathy
in HIV infection/AIDS, 1340
in Lyme disease, 1037, 1502
in polyarteritis nodosa, 856, 1037
in rheumatoid arthritis, 835, 1037
in sarcoidosis, 1037
toxic, 1037
Polypectomy, colonoscopic, 666
GI bleeding after, 598, 666
Polyphagia with weight loss, in diabetes
mellitus, 1214
Polypharmacy, in elderly, **69**
falls and, 64, 64*t*
urinary incontinence and, 65
Polypoid corditis, 234

Polyps/polyposis
adenomatous, 665. *See also*
Adenomatous polyps
familial, **666–667**, 1637, 1640. *See
also* Familial adenomatous
polyposis
nonfamilial, **665–666**
cervical, **768**
of colon, **665–666**
colorectal cancer and, 665, 666,
666–669, 1637, 1640
GI bleeding and, 598, 666
screening for, 15, 665–666,
1642–1643
gastric, 667
hamartomatous, **667–668**
hereditary, **666–669**
in HNPCC/Lynch syndrome, 668
hyperplastic, 665
juvenile familial, 667
nasal, **222**
allergic rhinitis and, 219, 222
nonneoplastic, 665
serrated, 665, **665–666**
submucosal, 665
vocal fold, 234
Polyradiculoneuropathy/
polyradiculopathy
in Guillain-Barré syndrome, 1038
in HIV infection/AIDS, 1340
in Lyme disease, 1037, 1502
Polysomnography
preoperative, 49
in snoring/sleep apnea, 231, 317
Polysporin. *See* Bacitracin/polymyxin
Polystyrene sulfonate, for hyperkalemia,
894–895, 895*t*
Polysurgery (surgery proneness), 1105
somatic symptom disorder and, 1058
Polytrim. *See* Polymyxin B/trimethoprim
sulfate
Polyuria. *See also specific cause*
in diabetes insipidus, 1113
in diabetes mellitus, 1213, 1214
in hypercalcemia, 898
Pomalidomide, 1665*t*
for myeloma, 536
for primary myelofibrosis, 523
Pomalyst. *See* Pomalidomide
Pomeroy tubal resection, 792
Pompholyx (vesiculobullous hand
eczema/dermatitis of palms
and soles), **121–122**, 122*f*
tinea differentiated from, 114, 122
Ponatinib, for chronic myeloid leukemia,
525
Poncet disease, 872
Ponstel. *See* Mefenamic acid
Pool (swimming pool) granuloma, 1482
Popliteal arteries
acute occlusion of, 476
aneurysms of, 484
atherosclerotic/occlusive disease of,
473–475
Popliteal (Baker) cyst, 1700, 1701, 1704
ruptured, lower extremity edema and,
32, 1701
Porcelain gallbladder, 717*t*, 719
Pork, trichinosis and, 1541
Pork tapeworm (*T solium*), **1535**, 1536
cysticercosis and, 1535, 1536–1537

Porphobilinogen, in porphyria, 1676
Porphyria
    acute intermittent, 1036, **1676–1677**, 1677*t*
    cutanea tarda, **122–123**, 123*f*, 154
        hirsutism/virilization and, 123, 1197
        sun exposure and, 123
    peripheral nerve involvement in, 1036, 1676
    variegate, 1036
Portal cavernoma, 713
Portal decompression, for esophageal varices, 615–616
Portal hypertension
    ascites in, 600, 601, 601*t*, 604
    cirrhosis and, 614, 699, 700, 701, 705
    esophageal varices and, 594–595, 614
    GI bleeding in, 594–595
    noncirrhotic, **713–714**
Portal hypertensive gastropathy, 620, 621. *See also* Portal hypertension
    GI bleeding and, 594–595, 621
Portal vein thrombosis, noncirrhotic portal hypertension and, 713, 714
Portal venopathy, obliterative, 713
Portopulmonary hypertension, 704
Portosplenomesenteric venous thrombosis, in pancreatitis, 728
Portosystemic shunts
    emergency/surgical, for esophageal varices, 616
        rebleeding prevention and, 616
    transvenous (transjugular). *See* Transvenous (transjugular) intrahepatic portosystemic shunts
Portrazza. *See* Necitumumab
Posaconazole, 1559*t*, 1560
    for aspergillosis, 1555
    for mucormycosis, 1556
    prophylactic, 1292
Positioning vertigo, benign paroxysmal (BPPV), 211*t*, 212
Positive inotropic agents. *See* Inotropic agents
Positron emission tomography (PET)
    in angina, 358
    in dementia, 1020
    in pheochromocytoma/paraganglioma, 1182
    in solitary pulmonary nodule, 287–288
    in thyroid cancer evaluation/follow-up, 1142–1143, 1147
    in thyroiditis, 1136
"Post-capillary" pulmonary hypertension, 302, 303
Postcardiotomy/postmyocardial infarction pericarditis (Dressler syndrome), 379, 425, 426
Postcholecystectomy syndrome, **720**
Postcoital/emergency contraception, 785, **791**
    IUD for, 789, 791
    for sexual violence (rape/sexual assault) victim, 791, 793, 794, 1302
Postdysenteric colitis, 1526
Postencephalitic parkinsonism, 1011

Postencephalitic syndrome, tick-borne encephalitis and, 1392
Postepileptic automatism, 985
Posterior blepharitis, 165
Posterior cerebral artery occlusion, in stroke, 995
Posterior cruciate ligament (PCL), 1704
    injury of, 1708*t*, **1711**
Posterior drawer sign/test, 1708*t*, 1711
Posterior inferior cerebellar artery obstruction, in stroke, 995
Posterior ischemic optic neuropathy, 192
Posterior nasal cavity, epistaxis originating in, 221
Posterior uveitis, 181, 182. *See also* Uveitis
Postgonococcal urethritis/cervicitis, 1486. *See also* Chlamydia (chlamydial infections)
Postherpetic neuralgia, 5, 120–121, 121, 175, **982**, 1369–1370, 1370
Posthypercapnia alkalosis, 909
Posthypocapnia acidosis, 907
Postinfarction ischemia/angina, 376–377
Postinfectious glomerulonephritis, 933*t*, 935*f*, **936–937**
Postinfectious irritable bowel syndrome, 644, 1308
Post-inflammatory hyperpigmentation, 157–158, 158
Post-kala azar dermal leishmaniasis, 1510
Post-Lyme disease syndrome, 1504, 1505*t*
Postmenopausal osteoporosis. *See* Osteoporosis
Postmenopausal vaginal bleeding, **764**
    endometrial carcinoma and, 764, 774
Postmicturition syncope, 401
Postmyocardial infarction/ postcardiotomy pericarditis (Dressler syndrome), 379, 425, 426
Postnasal drip, cough caused by, 19, 20, 20*t*, 21
Postoperative fever, 1294–1295
Postoperative hyponatremia, 886
    pituitary surgery and, 1111, 1115, 1119, 1175
Postoperative ileus, 638
Postoperative infection, 1294–1295
    antibiotic prophylaxis of, 54
Postpartum depression, 1075
Postpartum hemorrhage, pituitary gland necrosis caused by (Sheehan syndrome), 1109
Postpartum infection
    anaerobic, 1479
    C sordellii causing, 1452
    mastitis, 133, **813–814**
    pelvic, 814, 820
Postpartum preeclampsia-eclampsia, 810
Postpartum psychosis, 1075
Postpartum thyroiditis, 816, 1125, 1131, 1133, 1135
Postphlebitic syndrome, 32
Postpoliomyelitis syndrome, 1383
Postpolypectomy hemorrhage, 598, 666
Postpolypectomy surveillance, 666
Postprandial (reactive) hypoglycemia, 1252, 1252*t*, **1256–1257**. *See also* Hypoglycemia

Postrenal acute kidney injury/azotemia, 916, 917*t*, 918. *See also* Acute kidney injury
Postsurgical anxiety states, 1105, 1106
Post-thrombotic syndrome, 487, 489
    compression stockings in prevention of, 576
Posttransfusion purpura (PTP), **555**
Posttransplant lymphoproliferative disorder, 1288, 1373–1374
Posttraumatic epilepsy/seizure disorder, 983, 1031
Posttraumatic headache, **980**, 1031
Posttraumatic stress disorder, 1051–1052
    self-treatment and, 1092
    sexual/intimate partner violence and, 793
Posttraumatic syringomyelia, 1032
Posttraumatic vertigo, 212
Postural hypotension. *See* Orthostatic (postural) hypotension
Postural instability. *See* Falls; Gait/gait disorders; Instability
Postural tremor, drug-induced, 1017
Potassium
    aldosterone/aldosteronism and, 891, 892, 1177, 1178
    dietary/replacement, 1280
        for diabetic ketoacidosis, 1248
        in fluid management, 911, 911*t*
        for hyperglycemic hyperosmolar state, 1250
    hypertension and, 441, 445
    for hypocitraturic calcium nephrolithiasis, 964
    for hypokalemia, 893
    requirements for in nutritional support, 1282
    restriction of in chronic kidney disease, 928, 929
    disorders of concentration of, **891–896**, 892*t*, 894*t*, 895*t*. *See also* Hyperkalemia; Hypokalemia
    in acidosis, 906, 906*t*, 907
    genetic disorders and, 892*t*
    periodic paralysis and, 892*t*, 1049
    venipuncture technique affecting, 893, 894, 894*t*, 1178
Potassium channel blocking drugs, for arrhythmias, 381, 382–383*t*
Potassium chloride. *See* Potassium, dietary/replacement
Potassium citrate
    for hypocitraturic calcium nephrolithiasis, 964
    for urinary stone disease, 961
Potassium concentration gradient, transtubular (TTKG), 893
Potassium iodide
    in table salt, goiter prevention/ treatment and, 1149
    for thyroid crisis/storm, 1133
    before thyroid surgery, 1131
Potassium-sparing diuretics. *See* Diuretics
Potomania, beer, hyponatremia caused by, 887
Pott disease (spinal tuberculosis), **871–872**
Pott puffy tumor, 217
Potts shunt, for tetralogy of Fallot, 329
Pouchitis, 661

Poultry, avian influenza and, 1417, 1418
Powassan encephalitis/agent, 1388, 1391
Power of attorney, durable
    for finance matters (DPOAF), 60
    for health care, 90
Poxvirus infections, **1423–1424.** *See also specific type*
PPAR-alpha. *See* Peroxisome proliferator-activated receptor alpha
PPAR-gamma. *See* Peroxisome proliferator-activated receptor gamma
PPD (purified protein derivative) test, 279, 280t. *See also* Tuberculin skin test
PPSV/PPSV23. *See* Pneumococcal vaccine
PPV (pneumococcal polysaccharide vaccine). *See* Pneumococcal vaccine
PR3-ANCA. *See* Antineutrophil cytoplasmic antibody; Proteinase-3 ANCA
PRA. *See* Plasma renin activity
Prader-Willi syndrome, 1108, 1109
Pralidoxime, for cholinesterase inhibitor (anticholinesterase) poisoning, 1581t, 1602
PrameGel. *See* Pramoxine
Pramipexole, for parkinsonism, 1013
Pramlintide, 1222t, 1228
    overdose/toxicity of, 1228, 1595
Pramosone. *See* Hydrocortisone; Pramoxine
Pramoxine, 95, 99t, 148
Prandi-Met. *See* Repaglinide, with metformin
Prandin. *See* Repaglinide
Prasugrel, 366–367, 371
    postinfarction, 380
Pravachol. *See* Pravastatin
Pravastatin, 355t, 1260, 1263–1264. *See also* Statins
    in HIV infection/AIDS, 1356
    in older patients, 1262
Prax. *See* Pramoxine
Praziquantel
    for clonorchiasis/opisthorchiasis, 1534
    for cysticercosis, 1536
    for intestinal flukes, 1535
    for paragonimiasis, 1534
    for schistosomiasis, 1533
    for tapeworm infections, 1536
Prazosin, 462t
    adverse ophthalmic effects of, 183
    for benign prostatic hyperplasia, 974, 974t
    for hypertension, 459–464, 462t
    for PTSD, 1052
Pre-Gen Plus. *See* Multitarget DNA tests
Prebreakfast hyperglycemia, 1234, 1234t
Precholecystectomy syndrome, **720**
Precose. *See* Acarbose
Pred Mild. *See* Prednisolone
Prediabetes (impaired glucose tolerance), 1215, 1215t, 1218
    occult diabetes and, 1252, 1257
Prednicarbate, 97t
Prednisolone
    for asthma, 249t, 253t
    for ophthalmic disorders, 171–172t

Prednisone. *See also specific disease and* Corticosteroids
    for adhesive capsulitis (frozen shoulder), 1692
    for adrenal insufficiency/Addison disease, 1111, 1171
    for amiodarone-induced hyperthyroidism, 1132
    for aspergillosis, 1555
    for asthma, 249t, 252, 253t
    for autoimmune hemolytic anemia, 514
    for autoimmune hepatitis, 692–693
    for chronic inflammatory polyneuropathy, 1039
    for cluster headache prophylaxis, 980
    for contact dermatitis, 126
    for erythema nodosum leprosum, 1484
    for giant cell arteritis, 188, 854, 855
    for granulomatosis with polyangiitis, 859
    for immune thrombocytopenia, 549f, 550
    for inflammatory bowel disease, 650
        Crohn disease, 655–656
        ulcerative colitis, 659
    for lumbar disk herniation, 1695
    for minimal change disease, 943
    for multiple sclerosis, 1024, 1024t
    for myasthenic (Lambert-Eaton) syndrome, 1046
    for pericarditis, 426
    for *Pneumocystis* infection, 1336, 1337t, 1552
    for polymyalgia rheumatica, 854
    for prostate cancer, 1649t
    for reversal reaction (leprosy), 1485
    for SLE, 841, 842
Preeclampsia-eclampsia, 443, **808–811,** 809t, 818
    antihypertensive therapy in, 810
        in hypertensive emergency, 469t
    diabetes and, 1244
    headache and, 40
    hypermagnesemia associated with treatment of, 810, 901, 902–903
    late-onset (postpartum), 810
    in molar pregnancy, 807
Preexcitation syndromes, 31, 385, **387–388**
Prefest, 1204
Pregabalin, 987t
    for neuropathic pain/diabetic neuropathy, 83t, 84, 1035, 1240
    overdose/toxicity of, 987t
    for seizures, 987t
Pregnancy, **797–825**
    acne treatment and, 128
    adrenal insufficiency/Addison disease and, 1170, 1171
    adverse ophthalmic effects of drugs used in, 178t
    alcohol use during, 799, 1094
    amenorrhea (primary/secondary) caused by, 1200, 1201
    anemia during, **814–815**
    antidepressant use during, 1081
    antiphospholipid antibody syndrome and, 805, **815–816,** 841, 842, 843

antipsychotic drug use during, 1072
appendicitis during, 642, **825**
asthma during, **819–820**
biliary tract disorders of, **823**
bleeding during, 547t
    third-trimester, **812–813**
breast cancer and, 745–747, 758, 759–760
cardiomyopathy of (peripartum cardiomyopathy), 420, **435**
chikungunya fever and, 1407
Chlamydia trachomatis infection and, 799, 800, **823,** 1486
cholelithiasis/cholecystitis during, 717, **823–824**
cholestasis of, 674, 675t, **824–825**
chorioamnionitis/metritis and, **814,** 820
in chronic kidney disease, 929
CMV infection during, 1374, 1375, 1376
complications of
    cardiovascular, **435–436,** 819
    during first and second trimesters, **803–808**
    infectious, **820–825**
    medical conditions, **814–820**
    peripartum, **813–814**
    during second and third trimesters, **808–814**
coxsackievirus infection during, neonatal myocarditis and, 1426
dengue and, 1402
depression after (postpartum depression), 1075
diabetes insipidus and, 1113, 1114
diabetes mellitus and, 800, **817–818,** 817t, 1244
diagnosis/differential diagnosis of, **797–798**
drug/medication use avoidance during, 798t, 799. *See also specific agent*
ECT during, 1083
ectopic, **805–807**
    appendicitis differentiated from, 642
    hCG levels in, 797, 806
    IUDs and, 790
    minipill use and, 788
    PID and, 778
endocarditis prophylaxis and, **436,** 819
erythrovirus (parvovirus) infection in, 1422
fatty liver of (hepatic steatosis), 697, **824**
    liver failure and, 685, 824
fever during, 34
folic acid deficiency/supplementation during, 508, 799, 801
gastrointestinal disorders of, **823**
genital warts/wart removal and, 141, 768
glucosuria and, 1214
gonorrhea and, 799, 800, **823**
group B streptococcal infection and, 800–801, **820–821,** 1444
growth hormone replacement during, 1112
heart disease and, **434–436,** 819
hemolytic disease of newborn and, 801

Pregnancy (*Cont.*):
hepatitis B and, 681, 688, 799, **822**
vaccination/vaccination
recommendations and, 681,
802, 822, 1321*t*
hepatitis C and, 683, 800, **822–823**
hepatitis E and, 684
herpes infection during, **823**,
1363–1364, 1366
HHV-6 or HHV-7 infection during,
1377
HIV infection/AIDS in, 799, 800, **822**,
1332, 1346
HPV vaccine and, 1323*t*
hyperaldosteronism during, 1178, 1179
hypercalcemia/hyperparathyroidism
during, 1153–1154
hypercortisolism and, 1174
hypertension and, 442, 443, 808–811,
818–819. *See also*
Preeclampsia-eclampsia
hyperthyroidism/Graves disease
during, 816, 1126, 1127,
1131–1132
hypoparathyroidism during, 1152
hypothyroidism/hypothyroidism
treatment during, 816, 1119,
1121, 1122, 1123
immune thrombocytopenia associated
with, 550
immunizations during, **802–803**, 1319,
1321*t*
influenza/influenza vaccination and,
802, 1319, 1321*t*, 1322*t*, 1413
iodine deficiency and, 1148
iron requirements/deficiency anemia
during, 500, 799, 801, 815
IUDs and, 789–790
Kawasaki disease and, 1439
lactation and, **802**. *See also* Lactation
listeriosis during, 1457
liver disorders of, **823**
luteoma of, virilization and, 1197
Lyme disease and, 1504, 1505
lymphocytic choriomeningitis and,
1392, 1393
malaria/malaria treatment/
chemoprophylaxis during,
802, 1521
with artemisinins, 1519, 1521
manifestations of, 797
mask of (melasma/chloasma), 157, 158
measles/measles vaccine and, 1321*t*,
1380
mitral stenosis and, 335
MMR vaccination and, 1321*t*, 1323*t*,
1380, 1385
molar (hydatidiform mole), **807–808**
hyperthyroidism and, 807, 1126
multiple gestation
assisted reproductive procedures
and, 785
preterm labor/birth and, 812
nutrition in, 799, **801**
parathyroidectomy during, 1157
pheochromocytoma/paraganglioma
and, 1180*t*
polycystic ovary syndrome and, 780,
781
preeclampsia-eclampsia in, 443,
808–811, 809*t*, 818

hypermagnesemia associated with
treatment of, 810, 901,
902–903
prenatal care and, **798–801**, 798*t*
preterm labor/birth and, 800, **811–812**
prolactinoma/hyperprolactinemia in,
1117, 1118, 1119
prosthetic heart valves and, 351, 352*t*,
819
pulmonary hypertension as
contraindication to, 431,
432*f*, 434
Q fever during, 1436, 1437, 1438
rabies vaccination during, 1387
radiation exposure during, 799
radioactive iodine contraindicated in,
816, 1130, 1131, 1131–1132,
1145
Rhesus alloimmunization (Rh
incompatibility) and, 799,
800, **801**. *See also* Rh$_o$ (D)
immune globulin
rubella exposure/rubella vaccination
and, 1321*t*, 1384, 1384–1385,
1385
scabies/scabies treatment and, 149
screening tests in, 799–801
seizures/seizure treatment and, **820**
in eclampsia, 808, 809, 810
sexually transmitted disorders and, **823**
sickle cell anemia and, 800, 815
smoking during, 799
syphilis/syphilis testing and, 799, 800,
823, 1318, 1488, 1491,
1491–1492, **1497**
termination of
by delivery. *See also* Labor and
delivery
in acute fatty liver of pregnancy,
824
in preeclampsia-eclampsia, 810
by elective abortion. *See* Abortion,
elective/induced
by recurrent (habitual) abortion, **805**
by spontaneous abortion, **803–805**
thrombocytopenia during, 550,
555–556
thyroid disease and, **816–817**
hyperemesis gravidarum and, 803,
1126
hyperthyroidism, 816, 1126, 1127,
1131–1132
hypothyroidism, 816, 1119, 1121,
1122, 1123
thyroid cancer treatment and, 1144
thyroiditis, 816, 1125, 1131, 1133,
1135
toxoplasmosis during, 799, 1523,
1523–1524, 1524
travel and, **802–803**, 1576
traveler's diarrhea during, 802, 1310
trophoblastic disease and, **807–808**,
1624*t*
tuberculosis/tuberculosis screening
and treatment during, 282,
283, 800, **821–822**
of unknown location, 797
urinary tract infection during, 42, **820**
varicella (chickenpox)/varicella vaccine
during, 802, **821**, 1321*t*,
1322*t*, 1369, 1371

virilization during, 1197, 1198
vomiting of, 580, **803**, 823
gestational trophoblastic disease
and, 807
Wernicke encephalopathy and, 1026
von Willebrand disease and, 560
weight gain recommendations and, 801
yellow fever vaccination and, 1327,
1405
Zika virus infection and, 1390, 1406,
1407
Pregnancy-associated plasma protein-A
(PAPP-A), testing for, 800
Pregnancy tests, 797. *See also* Human
chorionic gonadotropin
in amenorrhea, 1200, 1201
in ectopic pregnancy, 797, 806
for sexual violence (rape/sexual
assault) victim, 793, 794
in spontaneous abortion, 804
Prehn sign, 960
Prehypertension, **440–441**, 447*f*
"Preleukemia," 525. *See also*
Myelodysplastic syndromes
Premarin/Premarin cream/Premarin
vaginal, 1204, 1205
Premature beats/contractions. *See* Atrial
(supraventricular) premature
beats; Ventricular premature
beats
Premature ejaculation, 966, 1063. *See also*
Erectile dysfunction/
impotence
Premature menopause/ovarian failure,
794, 1201
in Turner syndrome, 1207
Prematurity. *See* Preterm labor/birth
Premenopausal bleeding
abnormal, **762–764**
in polycystic ovary syndrome, 780,
1196
normal menstrual, 762. *See also*
Menstruation; Vaginal
bleeding
Premenstrual dysphoric disorder,
764–765, 1075
Premenstrual syndrome/tension,
764–765
Premixed insulins, 1229*t*, 1231
Premphase, 1204
Prempro, 1204
Prenatal care, **798–801**, 798*t*
Prenatal depression, 1081
Prenatal testing/diagnosis, 799–801. *See*
also specific disorder and
Genetic testing
Prenatal vitamins, 799, 801
Preoperative evaluation/perioperative
management, **45–54**. *See also*
specific type of disorder
adverse ophthalmic effects of agents
used in, 177*t*
antibiotic prophylaxis and, 54
asymptomatic patient and, **45**
cardiovascular disorders and, **45–48**,
46*t*, 47*f*, 47*t*
endocrine disorders and, **53**
hematologic disorders and, 45, 46*t*,
51–52, 51*t*, 52*t*
kidney disease and, **53–54**, 54*t*
liver disease and, **50**

neurologic disorders and, 52–53, 52t
pulmonary disorders in non-lung
    resection surgery and,
    49–50, 49t
Prepatellar bursae/bursitis, 1700–1701,
    1704
Prerenal acute kidney injury/azotemia,
    916, 917–918, 917t. See also
    Acute kidney injury
Presbyacusis (hearing impairment in
    elderly), 70, 200, 208
Presbyopia, 69
Prescription drug abuse, 17, 73–74, 85.
    See also Substance use
    disorders
Preservatives/preservative-free eye drops,
    172t, 173t, 199
    for glaucoma, 172t, 173t, 180
    toxic/hypersensitivity reactions and,
        168, 199
Pressure ulcers, 68–69, 68t
Presurgical anxiety states, 1105
Preterm labor/birth, 800, 811–812
Pretibial myxedema (Graves
    dermopathy), 1124, 1127,
    1133
Preventive care, 1–18, 2t, 3t. See also
    specific disease
    adherence and, 1–2
    approach to patient and, 1–2
    immunization and, 3–5, 1319–1327,
        1320–1325t, 1328–1329t
    principles of care and, 2
Prevnar-13. See Pneumococcal vaccine
Prevor, for alkali eye injury, 1587
Prevotella/Prevotella melaninogenica,
    1311t, 1478
Prezcobix. See Darunavir, with cobicistat
Prezista/Norvir. See Darunavir, with
    ritonavir
Priapism (prolonged painful erection),
    966
    erectile dysfunction therapy causing,
        966, 967
    trazodone causing, 1082, 1089
Prickly heat, 131
Primaquine
    G6PD deficiency and, 511, 1515, 1518,
        1552
    for malaria, 1515, 1515t, 1517t, 1518
        chemoprophylaxis, 1518, 1520,
            1520t
    for P jirovecii infection, 1337t, 1350,
        1552
Primary angiitis of central nervous
    system, 862–863
Primary biliary cholangitis/cirrhosis, 700,
    706–707
    autoimmune hepatitis and, 692
Primary cerebral/central nervous system
    lymphoma, 533, 1004t, 1006,
    1337t, 1339, 1344
Primary effusion (body cavity)
    lymphoma, 1377
Primary lateral sclerosis, 1033
Primary (idiopathic) pulmonary
    hypertension, 301–302, 429,
    430, 430t, 431, 431t, 432f,
    433
Primary sclerosing cholangitis, 723–725
    autoimmune hepatitis and, 692

cholangiocarcinoma and, 724, 725,
    1619
in HIV infection/AIDS, 1342
Primaxin. See Imipenem
Primidone, 987t
Primrose oil (oil of evening primrose/
    OEP), for fibrocystic
    condition, 735
Prinivil. See Lisinopril
Prinzide. See Lisinopril, for hypertension,
    with hydrochlorothiazide
Prinzmetal (variant) angina, 365
Prion diseases, 1393–1395
    Creutzfeldt-Jakob disease, 1022,
        1393–1394
    Huntington disease-like disorders and,
        1015
Prion protein/prion protein mutations,
    1393, 1394
Pristiq. See Desvenlafaxine
PRKAR1A mutation, in Carney complex,
    1175
PRNP gene
    in Huntington disease-like disorders,
        1015
    in Jakob-Creutzfeldt disease, 1022
Pro-IGF-2, nonislet cell tumor
    hypoglycemia and, 1255
Probenecid
    allopurinol interactions and, 833
    for gout, 832, 833
Probiotics
    for antibiotic-associated colitis, 648
    for flatus, 587
    for irritable bowel syndrome, 647
    for pouchitis, 661
    for ulcerative colitis, 660
Problem drinking. See Alcohol use
    disorder; At-risk (problem)
    drinking
Procainamide, 382t
    antidepressant drug interactions and,
        1083t
    for arrhythmias, 381, 382t
        infarct-related, 377
        supraventricular tachycardia, 386
        ventricular tachycardia, 397
    overdose/toxicity of, 382t
Procarbazine, 1663t
    antidepressant drug interactions and,
        1083t
Procardia. See Nifedipine
Prochieve, 1205
Prochlorperazine. See also Antiemetics
    for migraine headache, 978
    for nausea and vomiting, 83, 582t, 583,
        1673
    overdose/toxicity of, 1589–1590
Procollagen, in nephrogenic systemic
    fibrosis, 952
Procrit (epoetin alfa). See Erythropoietin
Proctitis, 670–671
    anorectal bleeding and, 598, 599
    chlamydial, 671
    diarrhea and, 589
    in gonorrhea, 670
    herpes simplex, 671, 1364, 1366
    HPV/condylomata acuminata
        and, 671
    in lymphogranuloma venereum, 671,
        1485

radiation, 598, 599
    in syphilis, 670
Proctoscopy, surveillance, in rectal
    cancer, 1640
Proctosigmoiditis, in ulcerative colitis,
    658, 659
Proctosigmoidoscopy. See Sigmoidoscopy
Prodromal schizophrenia, 1066
Profunda femoris artery, atherosclerotic/
    occlusive disease of, 474
Progesterone. See also Progestins
    ectopic pregnancy and, 806
    in estrogen replacement therapy, 1205
    pregnancy testing/viability and, 797,
        806
    for preterm labor prevention, 812
    receptors for, in breast cancer, 748
        prognosis and, 750, 758
        therapy and, 748, 754
    topical, 1205
Progestin minipill, 787t, 788
Progestin withdrawal test, in amenorrhea,
    1200, 1201
Progestins
    for abnormal uterine bleeding, 763
    adverse reactions to, 1204
    with contraceptive estradiol vaginal
        ring, 789, 1205
    for endometriosis, 776
    in estrogen replacement therapy, 795,
        1203, 1203–1204
        oral, 1205
        with oral estrogens, 1204
        with transdermal estradiol, 1204
    IUDs releasing, 789. See also
        Intrauterine devices
        in estrogen replacement therapy,
            1205
    long-acting (contraceptive injections/
        implants), 788–789
    in oral contraceptives, 786, 787t
        antiandrogenic, 1198
    for postmenopausal bleeding, 764
    for premenstrual syndrome, 765
Prognosis
    assessment of in older adult, 55, 56f,
        56t, 57t
    at end of life, 88
Programmed cell-death-1 (PD-1)
    inhibitors, for lung cancer,
    1612
Progressive bulbar palsy, 1033
Progressive disseminated histoplasmosis,
    1549
Progressive massive pulmonary fibrosis,
    307
Progressive multifocal
    leukoencephalopathy,
    1395–1396
    dimethyl fumarate causing, 1025
    in HIV infection/AIDS, 1340, 1395
    natalizumab and, 652, 1024, 1395
Progressive spinal muscular atrophy, 1033
Progressive supranuclear palsy,
    parkinsonism differentiated
    from, 1012
Proguanil-atovaquone (Malarone), 1515t,
    1517t, 1519
    for chemoprophylaxis, 1519, 1520,
        1520t
    self-treatment and, 1520

Proinsulin, in insulinoma, 1185, 1253, 1253t
PROKR2 mutation, hypogonadism and, 1189–1190
Prolactin (PRL), 1109t
  amenorrhea and, 1110, 1118, 1200, 1201
  cardiomyopathy of pregnancy and, 435, 1117
  deficiency of, 1108, 1110
  excess of. See also Hyperprolactinemia
  gynecomastia and, 1117, 1195
  hypogonadotropic hypogonadism and, 1109, 1110, 1111, 1117, 1191
  infertility and, 784, 970, 1117, 1118
  in psychogenic nonepileptic/ pseudoepileptic seizure identification, 986, 1058
  tumors secreting, 1117, 1199
Prolactinoma, 1117
  GH cosecretion and, 1117
  infertility and, 970, 1117, 1118
  in MEN, 1188
Proleukin. See Aldesleukin
Prolia. See Denosumab
Proliferative bronchiolitis, 266, 267. See also Bronchiolitis
Proliferative retinopathy, 189, 190, 1238
Prolixin. See Fluphenazine
Promethazine, 582t, 583. See also Antiemetics
  overdose/toxicity of, 1589–1590
Prometrium. See Progesterone
Pronator teres syndrome, **1039–1040**
Pronouncement (death), 93
Propafenone, 381, 382t
  for atrial fibrillation, 393
  overdose/toxicity of, 382t
  for supraventricular tachycardia, 382t, 386
Propamidine, for ophthalmic disorders, 169t
Propanil, methemoglobinemia caused by, 1599
Propecia. See Finasteride
Prophylactic antibiotics. See Antimicrobial chemoprophylaxis
Propionibacterium acnes, 126. See also Acne
  meningitis caused by, 1314t
Propofol, for seizures
  in poisoning/drug overdose, 1580
  in status epilepticus, 990
Propoxyphene
  benzodiazepine interactions and, 1056t
  overdose/toxicity of, 1601
Propranolol, 382t, 453t. See also Beta-adrenergic blocking drugs
  for aggressive/violent behavior, 1091
  antidepressant drug interactions and, 1083t
  for arrhythmias, 382t
    atrial fibrillation, 389
    supraventricular tachycardia, 386
  for esophageal varices, prevention of rebleeding and, 616
  for hypertension, 453t
    with hydrochlorothiazide, 453t

for hyperthyroidism/Graves disease, 1129
  amiodarone-induced, 1132
  preoperative, 1130–1131
  in thyroid crisis/storm, 1133
  thyroiditis and, 1131, 1137
  toxic multinodular goiter and, 1131
  toxic solitary thyroid nodule and, 1131
for migraine prophylaxis, 979t
  overdose/toxicity of, 382t, 979t, 1590–1591
Proprotein convertase subtilisin/kexin type 9 (PCSK9) inhibitors, for lipid modification/ cardiovascular/heart disease prevention, 353, 1266
Propylthiouracil, for hyperthyroidism/ Graves disease, 1129, 1130
  during pregnancy/lactation, 816, 1130, 1132
  RAI therapy and, 1130
  thyroid crisis/storm and, 1133
  toxic multinodular goiter and, 1131
  toxic solitary thyroid nodule and, 1131
ProQuad. See MMRV (measles-mumps-rubella-varicella) vaccine
Prosom. See Estazolam
Prosopagnosia, intracranial tumors causing, 1005
Prostacyclin/prostacyclin analogs, for pulmonary hypertension, 303, 431–433, 432f
Prostaglandin analogs. See also specific agent
  for glaucoma/ocular hypertension, 173t, 180
Prostaglandin-associated periorbitopathy, 180
Prostaglandins
  for erectile dysfunction diagnosis/ treatment, 967
  hyponatremia caused by, 886
  NSAIDs affecting, 828
Prostate cancer, 1608t, 1624t, **1644–1651**, 1647f, 1649t, 1650t
  hormone therapy for, 1624t, 1649, 1649–1650, 1649t
  incidence/risk/mortality of, 1608t, 1644, 1650–1651, 1650t
  localized, 1648
  locally/regionally advanced, 1649
  metastatic, 1649–1650
  pathology/staging of, 1647
    CAPRA score and, 1650, 1650t
  screening for, 14t, 15, 1645, 1646–1647, 1646t, 1647f
  surgery for, 1648
  testosterone replacement therapy and, 1191–1192, 1193
Prostate gland
  benign hyperplasia of, **971–976**, 971t, 973f, 973t, 974t. See also Benign prostatic hyperplasia
  biopsy of, 1645, 1647f, 1650t
  cancer of. See Prostate cancer
  inflammation/infection of. See Prostatitis
Prostate-specific antigen (PSA), 1645, 1646t
  in benign prostatic hyperplasia, 972
  in prostate cancer, 1645, 1646t

in CAPRA assessment tool, 1650, 1650t
  screening and, 14t, 15, 1645, 1646–1647, 1646t, 1647f
Prostate-specific antigen (PSA) velocity, in cancer screening, 1646, 1647f
Prostatectomy, 975, 1648
  for benign prostatic hyperplasia, 973f, 973t, 975
  for prostate cancer, 1648
Prostatitis
  acute bacterial, 955t, **957**, 957t
  chronic bacterial, 955t, 957t, **958**
  gonococcal, 1475
  nonbacterial, 957, **958–959**
Prostatodynia, 957t, **959**
Prosthetic heart valves, 350–351. See also Valve replacement
  anticoagulation therapy and, 337, 343, **350–351**, 352t
  coagulase-negative staphylococcal infection and, 1450, 1451
  endocarditis and, 337, 1458, 1461. See also Endocarditis
  anticoagulation and, 352t, 1463
  pregnant patient and, 351, 352t, 819
Protamine, for heparin neutralization, 562
Protease, in pancreatic enzyme supplements, 732t
Protease inhibitors, 1351–1352t, 1356–1357. See also Antiretroviral therapy
  antituberculous drug interactions and, 282, 1336, 1356
  for hepatitis C, 689, 690, 690t, 691
  lipid abnormalities caused by, 1356
  resistance to, 1362
  ritonavir-boosted, 1356
    oral contraceptive drug interaction and, 786
Proteasome inhibitors, in cancer chemotherapy, 1665–1666t
Protein
  ascitic fluid, 602, 603, 604
  cerebrospinal fluid, 1297t
  dietary, 1279
    chronic kidney disease/nephrotic syndrome/nephrotic spectrum disorders and, 928, 929, 942, 1279
    deficiency of (protein–energy malnutrition), **1268–1269**
    requirements for in nutritional support, 1282
    restriction of. See Protein-restricted diet
    urinary stone formation and, 962, 963
  pleural fluid, 312
  urinary, 913–914. See also Proteinuria
    ratio of to urinary creatinine, 914
Protein-bound paclitaxel, 1665t. See also Paclitaxel
Protein C
  activated, resistance to, DVT/PE (venous thromboembolic disease) and, 295, 575t
  deficiency of, 575t

Protein-calorie undernutrition (protein–energy malnutrition), **1268–1269**
Protein/creatinine urinary concentration, 914. *See also* Proteinuria
Protein–energy malnutrition, **1268–1269**
Protein-losing enteropathy, **643**
in measles, 1379
in Whipple disease, 635
Protein-restricted diet, 1279
in acute tubular necrosis, 920
for chronic kidney disease/nephrotic syndrome/nephrotic spectrum disorders, 928, 929, 942, 1279
in diabetes, 1238
for hepatic encephalopathy, 703, 1279
for urinary stones, 962, 963
Protein S, deficiency of, DVT/PE (venous thromboembolic disease) and, 575t
Proteinaceous infectious particles, 1393. *See also* Prion diseases
Proteinase-3 ANCA (PR3-ANCA). *See also* Antineutrophil cytoplasmic antibody
in glomerulonephritis, 938
in granulomatosis with polyangiitis, 858, 938
Proteinosis, pulmonary alveolar, **294**
Proteinuria, 913–914, 925. *See also specific cause*
Bence Jones. *See* Bence Jones proteinuria
in nephrotic syndrome/nephrotic spectrum disease, 932f, 933, 942
in preeclampsia-eclampsia, 808, 809t
Proteus/Proteus miribilis/vulgaris, 1312t, 1315t
Prothrombin (factor II), acquired antibodies to, **561**
Prothrombin gene mutation, DVT/PE (venous thromboembolic disease) and, 575t
Prothrombin time
in DIC, 554
in liver disease/jaundice, 676t, 694
normal values for, 676t
Proton beam therapy, for pituitary adenoma, 1116
Proton pump inhibitors
adverse effects of, 609, 625
atazanavir and, 1357
for Barrett esophagus, 608, 609
clopidogrel interaction/coadministration and, 628
for dyspepsia, 579, 580, 621
for eosinophilic esophagitis, 613
for esophageal motility disorders, 619
after fibrinolytic therapy for STEMI, 375
for GERD/esophagitis, 609, 610, 619
in *H pylori* eradication therapy, 626, 626t, 627
H pylori test results affected by, 622, 625
hypomagnesemia and, 902
hypoparathyroidism/hypocalcemia and, 1150
interstitial nephritis caused by, 921

for laryngopharyngeal reflux, 233
for NSAID gastritis/toxicity mitigation, 74, 621, 626t, 627, 627–628, 829
for peptic ulcer disease, 621, 625, 626t, 627, 627–628
bleeding management and, 596–597, 628, 629–630
prevention and, 626t, 627, 630
for stress gastritis, 319, 620, 621
for Zollinger-Ellison syndrome/gastrinoma, 632, 1186
Protopam. *See* Pralidoxime
Protopic. *See* Tacrolimus, topical
Protozoal infections, **1507–1531**. *See also specific type*
diarrhea in, 588t, 592, 1305, 1342
myocarditis in, 413t
Protriptyline, 1078t
Provenge. *See* Sipuleucel-T
Provera. *See* Progesterone
Providencia, 1312t
Proximal renal tubular acidosis, 892t, 906t, 907. *See also* Renal tubular acidosis
genetic defects associated with, 892t
tubulointerstitial disease and, 948
Prozac. *See* Fluoxetine
Prozone phenomenon, 1490
PrP[C]/PrP[Sc], in prion disease, 1393, 1394
PRSS1 gene, in chronic pancreatitis, 731
Prurigo, actinic, 154
Pruritus (itching), 96t, **146–147**. *See also specific cause and* Anogenital/perianal pruritus
ani, 147, 148
in chronic kidney disease/uremia, 147
in decompression sickness (skin bends), 1573
drugs for
systemic, 95–100
topical, 95
of ear canal, **202**
in hypercalcemia/hyperparathyroidism, 1153
jaundice and, 674
vulvae, 147
PRV. *See* Rotavirus vaccines
PSA. *See* Prostate-specific antigen
PSA free fraction, 1646
Pseudallescheria boydii (Scedosporium apiospermum), in opportunistic infection, 1557
Pseudoachalasia, 617
Pseudo-addiction, pain management and, 74
Pseudoallergic reactions, **878**, 879t
Pseudoaneurysm
femoral artery, 484
GI bleeding and, 595
myocardial rupture and, 379
Pseudobacteremia, 1295
Pseudobulbar palsy, 1033
Pseudo-Cushing syndrome, 1174
Pseudocysts, pancreatic, 728, 730
ascites and, 728
cystic carcinoma and, 1620, 1625
infected (pancreatic abscess), 728, 730
Pseudodementia (depression and dementia), 57, 61, 1103

Pseudoephedrine, MAOI interactions and, 1083t
Pseudoepileptic seizures. *See* Psychogenic nonepileptic seizure
Pseudofolliculitis, 130
Pseudogout, 826, 831, 834
nongonococcal acute bacterial (septic) arthritis differentiated from, 867
Pseudogynecomastia, 1194
Pseudohermaphroditism, 1169, 1199–1200
Pseudohyperkalemia, 893, 894t
Pseudohyperphosphatemia, 901t
Pseudohypoaldosteronism, types I and II, 892t
Pseudohyponatremia, 886, 888
Pseudohypoparathyroidism, **1149–1152**, 1154f. *See also* Hypoparathyroidism
congenital, 1151
Pseudomembranous colitis, 648. *See also* Colitis, antibiotic-associated
Pseudomonas aeruginosa, 1312t
fever/neutropenia/chemotherapy and, 1314t
hot tub folliculitis caused by, 130, 131
malignant external otitis caused by, 202
pneumonia caused by, 268t, 269t, 271, 273, 275t
in HIV infection/AIDS, 1336
urinary tract infection caused by, 1314t
Pseudo-obstruction, intestinal
acute (Ogilvie syndrome), **639–640**
chronic, **640–641**
Pseudo-papilledema, 194
Pseudoporphyria, 123
Pseudorheumatoid arthritis, 834, 836
Pseudoseizures. *See* Psychogenic nonepileptic seizure
Pseudoseptic arthritis, 867
Pseudothrombocytopenia, **556**
"Pseudothrombophlebitis," 32
Pseudotumor cerebri, **1009**
headache and, 981
PSI (Pneumonia Severity Index), 272
Psilocybin, 1099, 1600t
Psilocybe mushroom poisoning and, 1600t
Psittacosis (ornithosis), 1313t, **1486–1487**
Psoas sign, in appendicitis, 641, 642
Psoralen plus ultraviolet A (PUVA) therapy. *See also* Phototherapy
for lichen planus, 145
for psoriasis/psoriatic arthritis, 108, 865
Psoriasiform eruptions, drugs causing, 163t
Psoriasis, **106–109**, 107f
arthritis and, 107, **864–865**
atopic dermatitis differentiated from, 105, 107
drugs causing, 107, 163t
exfoliative dermatitis and (erythrodermic psoriasis), 107, 117
in HIV infection/AIDS, 869, 1344
nonalcoholic fatty liver disease and, 697
tinea differentiated from, 111–112, 113, 114

Psoriatic arthritis, 107, **864–865**
in HIV infection/AIDS, 869, 1340
Psoriatic erythroderma, 107, 117
Psoriatic spondylitis, 865
PSS1 mutation, pancreatic/periampullary carcinoma and, 1620
PSTI gene, in chronic pancreatitis, 731
Psychedelic drug abuse, **1099**, 1598
Psychiatric/psychologic disorders, **1050–1107**. *See also specific type*
asthma differentiated from, 246
chest pain/discomfort and, 29, 619
cognitive impairment and, 1019–1020
in elderly, urinary incontinence and, 65
fatigue/chronic fatigue and, 37, 38, 39
hospitalization and illness and, **1104–1107**
hyponatremia and, 887
intentional drug/poison ingestion and, 1577
irritable bowel syndrome and, 644, 645, 646, 647
palpitations and, 30, 31
in pheochromocytoma/paraganglioma, 1180*t*
thyroxine levels in, 1128
vomiting and, 580, 581, 581*t*
in Wilson disease, 710
"Psychogenic cough" (somatic cough syndrome), 21
Psychogenic nonepileptic seizure (PNES/pseudoepileptic seizure), 986, 1058
Psychogenic polydipsia, 1067
hyponatremia caused by, 887, 1067
Psychologic challenges, for terminally ill/dying patient, 92
Psychologic disorders. *See* Psychiatric/psychologic disorders
Psychologic drug dependence, 1092. *See also* Substance use disorders
Psychopathic (antisocial) personality disorder, 1064, 1065*t*, 1066
Psychosexual disorders, **1062–1064**
sexual dysfunction and, 966, 966–967, 967, 1063, 1064. *See also* Sexual dysfunction
Psychotic depression, 1066, 1067, 1070, 1075, 1079
Psychotic disorders (psychoses), **1066–1074**. *See also* Schizophrenia
alcohol use disorder and, 1092, 1094
alcohol withdrawal and (delirium tremens), 1093
alcoholic (organic) hallucinosis, 1093, 1095
brief, 1067
delusions and, 1066
depression and, 1066, 1067, 1070, 1075, 1079
differential diagnosis of, 1067–1068
drug-induced/toxic, 1068
drug therapy for, 1068–1073, 1069*t*, 1071*t. See also* Antipsychotic drugs
in hypothyroidism (myxedema madness), 1120, 1121
intensive care unit, 1105
Korsakoff, 694, **1026**, 1093, 1095, 1275

manic, 1067
phencyclidine use/abuse and, 1068, 1099
postpartum, 1075
stimulant/cocaine abuse and, 1068, 1100
suicide risk and, 1068, 1077
Psychotic resolution, 1067
Psychotropic agents. *See also* Antianxiety drugs; Antidepressants; Antipsychotic drugs
for irritable bowel syndrome, 646, 647
thrombocytopenia caused by, 555*t*
Psyllium fiber, 585*t*, 1280. *See also* Fiber, dietary
PT. *See* Prothrombin time
PTC. *See* Percutaneous transhepatic cholangiography
PTCA (percutaneous transluminal coronary angioplasty). *See* Angioplasty, coronary; Percutaneous coronary intervention
PTEN multiple hamartoma syndrome (Cowden disease), 668
thyroid cancer and, 1137, 1141
Pteroylmonoglutamic acid. *See* Folic acid
Pterygium, **174**
PTF1A mutation, in diabetes, 1212
PTH. *See* Parathyroid hormone
PTHrP. *See* Parathyroid hormone-related protein
PTP. *See* Posttransfusion purpura
PTSD. *See* Posttraumatic stress disorder
Puberty
delayed/failure to enter, 1111, 1189, 1190, 1199
amenorrhea and, 1199
male hypogonadism and, 1189, 1190
Turner syndrome and, 1207
gynecomastia during, 1194, 1195
Pubic lice, 149–150. *See also* Lice
Puerperal mastitis, 133, **813–814**
Puffer fish poisoning, 1603, 1604*t*
Puffy tumor, Pott, 217
Pulmonary alveolar proteinosis, **294**
Pulmonary angiography, in pulmonary embolism, 298
helical CT, 23, 28, 296–297, 297*f*
Pulmonary arterial hypertension, **301–304**, **429–433**, 430*t*, 431*t*, 432*f. See also* Pulmonary hypertension
Pulmonary artery catheter, in shock management, 495
Pulmonary aspiration syndromes, **305–306**. *See also* Aspiration
Pulmonary circulation disorders, **294–305**
alveolar hemorrhage syndromes, **304–305**
pulmonary hypertension, **301–304**
respiratory failure caused by, 318*t*
thromboembolism, **294–301**, 296*t*, 297*f*, 298*t*, 299*f*, 299*t. See also* Pulmonary venous thromboembolism
vasculitis, **304**
Pulmonary cysts, hydatid, 1537
Pulmonary decompression sickness, 1573

Pulmonary disorders, **241–321**. *See also specific type and under Respiratory and Breathing*
acute respiratory distress syndrome (ARDS), **319–321**, 320*t*
acute respiratory failure, **317–319**, 318*t*
adverse ophthalmic effects of drugs used in, 177*t*
airway disorders, **241–267**
in anthrax, 1454, 1455, 1456
in aspergillosis, 264, 879*t*, 1554, 1555
aspirin (NSAID) sensitivity and, **878**
in blastomycosis, 1556
chronic. *See specific disorder and* Chronic obstructive pulmonary disease
circulatory, **294–305**
cocaine use/abuse and, 309, 1100
in coccidioidomycosis, 1550, 1551
cognitive disorders/delirium caused by, 1102*t*
cryptococcal, 1553
deaths attributable to, 2*t*
drug-induced, 290*t*, **309**, 310*t*
environmental, 290*t*, **305–310**
eosinophilic, **294**
in granulomatosis with polyangiitis, 304, 857, 858
H influenzae causing, 268*t*, 1311*t*, 1466
hantaviruses causing, 1403, 1403–1404
in histoplasmosis, 1549
in HIV infection/AIDS/immunocompromised host, **276**, 1335–1339. *See also* Pneumonia; Tuberculosis
immunization recommendations in, 1321*t*
infections, **267–286**, 290*t. See also specific cause*
adenovirus, 1421
anaerobic, 268*t*, 1478
Bordetella bronchiseptica causing, 1464
CMV, 1375, 1376
herpes simplex, 1364
infiltrates in immunocompromised host and, **276**, 1291, 1335
interstitial, 290*t*
mycobacterial
nontuberculous, **284–286**, **1481–1482**
tuberculosis, **277–284**, 277*t*, 278*t*, 279*f*, 280*t*, 281*t*, 282*t. See also* Tuberculosis
pneumonia, 20*t*, **267–276**. *See also* Pneumonia
viral, **1409–1420**
influenza and, 269, 271, 1411, 1412
interstitial (diffuse parenchymal), **289–294**, 290*t*, 291*t*, 292*f*
Kaposi sarcoma, 146, 1338
in measles, 1379
metastatic, **1613–1614**
in microscopic polyangiitis, 859, 860
neoplastic, **286–289**. *See also* Lung cancer
in nocardiosis, 1481
occupational, 290*t*, **306–309**, 307*t*, 308*t*
in paragonimiasis, 1534
perioperative evaluation/management/risk and, **49–50**, 49*t*

in pheochromocytoma/paraganglioma, 1180*t*

pleural diseases and, **311–315**, 311*t*, 313*t*

pulmonary hypertension and, 302, 303, 430, 430*t*

radiation causing, **309–310**

respiratory failure, **317–319**, 318*t*

SIADH caused by, 887, 887*t*

in SLE, 840

in syphilis, 1495

toxic. *See* Toxic lung injury

transfusion-related, 544

travel and, 1308, 1309

tropical pulmonary eosinophilia, 1544

in uremia, 924*t*

ventilation control disorders and, **315–319**

Pulmonary edema, **411–412**

cardiogenic, **411–412**

drug-induced, 310*t*

in heart failure, 403, **411–412**

high-altitude (HAPE), **1574**

in hypertensive emergency, treatment of, 469*t*

respiratory failure caused by, 318*t*

transfusion-related (transfusion-related acute lung injury), 544

Pulmonary embolectomy, for pulmonary embolism, 301

Pulmonary embolism. *See* Pulmonary venous thromboembolism

Pulmonary embolism severity index (PESI), 571, 571*t*

Pulmonary fibrosis

drug-induced, 310*t*

idiopathic, 289, 292*f*

progressive massive, 307

radiation causing, **310**

Pulmonary function tests

in asthma/asthma exacerbation, 243*f*, 244*t*, 245–246, 245*t*, 251, 252, 254, 255*f*, 256*f*

bronchial provocation testing and, 246

classification/management and, 243*f*, 244*t*, 245–246, 245*t*, 251, 252, 254, 255*f*, 256*f*

in COPD, 258, 258*t*

in cystic fibrosis, 265

lung cancer surgery and, 1610–1611

preoperative, 49

Pulmonary heart disease (cor pulmonale), in COPD, 258, 262

Pulmonary hemosiderosis, idiopathic, 304

Pulmonary hypertension, **301–304**, **429–433**, 430*t*, 431*t*, 432*f*. *See also specific cause and* Eisenmenger physiology

drug and toxin, 301–302, 430

in hyperthyroidism, 1127

in mitral regurgitation, 338

in mitral stenosis, 335, 336

pulmonary valve regurgitation and, 350

in scleroderma, 430, 431, 846, 847

Pulmonary infarction, pleural effusion in, 313*t*

Pulmonary infiltrates. *See also* Pneumonia

drugs causing, 310*t*

in immunocompromised host/HIV infection/AIDS, **276**, 1291, 1335

travel and, 1308, 1309

Pulmonary nodules

in metastatic disease, 1613, 1614

solitary, **287–288**

Pulmonary osteoarthropathy, hypertrophic. *See* Hypertrophic osteoarthropathy

Pulmonary overinflation syndrome, 1572–1573

Pulmonary radiation fibrosis, **310**

Pulmonary rehabilitation, for COPD, 261

Pulmonary-renal syndromes, 844, 845

Pulmonary thromboembolism. *See* Pulmonary venous thromboembolism

Pulmonary tuberculosis, **277–284**, 277*t*, 278*t*, 279*f*, 280*t*, 281*t*, 282*t*. *See also* Tuberculosis

Pulmonary valve

repair/replacement of, 323, 350. *See also* Valve replacement

in rheumatic fever/heart disease, 422

Pulmonary valve regurgitation, 323, 329, **349–350**

Pulmonary valve stenosis, **322–323**

Pulmonary vasculitis, **304**

asthma differentiated from, 246

Pulmonary veno-occlusive disease, pulmonary hypertension and, 302, 303, 430, 430*t*, 431

Pulmonary venous hypertension, 302. *See also* Pulmonary hypertension

Pulmonary venous thromboembolism, **294–301**, 296*t*, 297*f*, 298*t*, 299*f*, 299*t*

anticoagulation for, 300, 569–576, 570*t*, 571*t*, 572*t*, 573*t*, 574*t*, 575*t*

in Behçet syndrome, 862

chest pain/discomfort in, 26, 27, 28, 295, 296*t*

in granulomatosis with polyangiitis, 857

hemoptysis in, 25, 296*t*

in nephrotic syndrome/nephrotic spectrum disorders, 943

nonpharmacologic measures in, 301, 576–577

prevention of, 298–300, 567–569, 567*t*, 568*t*, 569*t*

contraindications to, 569, 569*t*

pulmonary hypertension and, 302, 303, 430, 430*t*

risk/risk stratification for, 295, 296*t*, 298, 298*t*, 299*f*, 299*t*, 567–568, 567*t*, 569–571, 571*t*, 573–574, 574*t*, 575*t*

septic, 1478

in drug users, 1304

thrombolytic therapy for, 300–301, 576, 576*t*

venous thrombosis and, 294, 295, 297. *See also* Deep venous thrombosis; Venous thromboembolic disease

Pulmonary ventilation-perfusion scans. *See* Ventilation-perfusion scans

Pulmonic regurgitation. *See* Pulmonary valve regurgitation

Pulmonic stenosis. *See* Pulmonary valve stenosis

Pulsatile tinnitus, 209

in glomus tumors, 207, 209

Pulse generators, pacemaker, 400

Pulse oximetry/CO-oximetry. *See also* Arterial blood gases

in carbon monoxide poisoning, 24, 1592

in dyspnea evaluation, 24

in methemoglobinemia, 1599

Pulses, in hypertension, 445

Pulsus paradoxus, 427, 428

asthma exacerbation and, 245*t*

Pulvinar sign, 1394

Pupillary dilation

acute angle-closure glaucoma and, 166*t*, 176, 198

precautions in, **198**

Pupillary reactions, in coma or stupor, 1027

Pure autonomic failure, 990

Pure red cell aplasia, in erythrovirus (parvovirus) infection, 1422

Pure white cell aplasia, 518

Purgatives, for constipation/preoperative bowel cleansing, 585*t*, 586

Purified chick embryo cell culture (PCEC) rabies vaccine, 1326, 1387

Purified insulin, 1229. *See also* Insulin therapy

Purified protein derivative (PPD) test, 279, 280*t*. *See also* Tuberculin skin test

Purine analogs, in cancer chemotherapy, 1663–1664*t*

Purines, dietary

in hyperuricemia/gout, 832, 832*t*

in urinary stone formation, 963, 964

Purinethol. *See* Mercaptopurine

Purpura

cancer-related, 875

in cryoglobulinemia, 860, 939

fulminans, 553

Henoch-Schönlein, **861**, 933*t*, **937–938**, 938*f*

levamisole-associated, **860**

posttransfusion, **555**

thrombotic thrombocytopenic, 550–552, 551*t*. *See also* Thrombocytopenia

diarrhea and, 1471

Purulent meningitis, 1297, 1297*t*, 1299

Push enteroscopy, in GI/small bowel bleeding, 599

Pustular psoriasis, 107

Pustular skin disorders, 96*t*, **126–128**. *See also specific type*

Puumala virus, 1403, 1404

PUVA therapy. *See also* Phototherapy

for lichen planus, 145

for psoriasis/psoriatic arthritis, 108, 865

PVCs (premature ventricular contractions). *See* Ventricular premature beats

PVP. *See* Photovaporization of prostate
Pyelonephritis, 42, 955t, **956–957**, 1314t, 1315t
  emphysematous, 956
  during pregnancy, 820
Pygeum africanum, for benign prostatic hyperplasia, 975
Pylephlebitis
  noncirrhotic portal hypertension and, 713
  perforated appendicitis and, 642
Pyoderma
  in pediculosis, 150
  in scabies, 149
Pyogenic arthritis (nongonococcal acute bacterial/septic) arthritis, **867–868**, 1314t
  in drug users, 867, 1304
Pyogenic cholangitis, 721
Pyogenic hepatic abscess, **714–715**
Pyogenic osteomyelitis, acute, **870–871**
Pyrantel pamoate
  for ascariasis, 1538
  for enterobiasis/pinworms, 1541
Pyrazinamide, 281–282, 281t, 282–283, 282t
  contraindications to in pregnancy, 282, 283
Pyrazinamide/isoniazid/rifampin, for tuberculosis, 282
Pyridium. *See* Phenazopyridine
Pyridostigmine, for myasthenia gravis, 1045–1046
Pyridoxine (vitamin B$_6$)
  deficiency of, **1276**
  homocystinuria/hyperhomocysteinemia and, 1681
  isoniazid overdose/toxicity and, 282, 283, 821, 1276, 1348, 1581t, 1596
  toxicity of, **1276**
  for vomiting during pregnancy, 583, 803
Pyrimethamine
  for isosporiasis, 1529
  for malaria, with sulfadoxine (Fansidar), 1515t, 1519
    with amodiaquine, 1519, 1521
    with artesunate, 1516t, 1519
    for chemoprophylaxis, 1519
      in pregnancy/infants, 1521
    resistance to, 1515
    for uncomplicated falciparum disease, 1515
  for toxoplasmosis treatment/prophylaxis, 1337t, 1339, 1350, 1524, 1525
Pyrimidine analogs, in cancer chemotherapy, 1664t
Pyrogenic erythrotoxin (erythrogenic toxin), 1444
Pyronaridine, 1515t, 1516–1517
  with artesunate, 1515t, 1516t, 1517, 1519
Pyrophosphate (technetium-99m) scintigraphy, in myocardial infarction, 371
Pyrosis (heartburn), 605, 606, 607, 609
Pyuria, 913
  sterile, 951

Q fever, 1429t, **1436–1438**
Q fever vaccine, 1438
Q waves, in myocardial infarction, 27t, 366, 371. *See also* Myocardial infarction; Non-Q wave (non-ST elevation) infarction
Qinghaosu/qinghaosu derivatives. *See* Artemisinins
QRisk2 calculator, 446
QRS complex. *See also* Electrocardiogram
  wide, in poisoning/drug toxicity, 1579, 1579t
    antidepressants in, 1579, 1606, 1606f
    antipsychotics in, 1589
    beta-adrenergic blockers, 1591
Qsymia. *See* Phentermine/topiramate
QT interval. *See also* Electrocardiogram
  long, **398**
    in poisoning/drug toxicity, 1579, 1579t
      antiarrhythmic agents in, 398
      antidepressants in, 398, 1606
      antipsychotics in, 1071, 1071t, 1589, 1590
      opiates/opioids and, 1601
      quinine/quinidine in, 1518
      ranolazine and, 361
    sudden death of athlete and, 437, 438t
  short, in cancer-related hypercalcemia, 1659
Quad screen, in prenatal testing, 800
Quadrantanopia. *See* Visual field defects
Quadriplegia. *See also* Paralysis
  after spinal trauma, 1031–1032
Quadrivalent influenza vaccines, 1322t, 1413, 1414t, 1415t. *See also* Influenza virus vaccine
Quality of life
  assessment of for older adult, 55–56
  decision-making at end of life and, 90
  palliative care and, 72, 88, 90
QuantiFERON. *See* Interferon gamma release assays
Quantitative pilocarpine iontophoresis sweat test, in cystic fibrosis, 265
Quazepam, 1054t
Quebec platelet disorder, 557
Queensland tick typhus, 1429t, 1434
Questran. *See* Cholestyramine
Quetiapine, 1068–1070, 1069t, 1071t. *See also* Antipsychotic drugs
  for bipolar disease/mania, 1085
  for delirium, 62
  for dementia, 1021
  for depression, 1083
  for Huntington disease, 1015
  overdose/toxicity/side effects of, 1069t, 1071t, 1589–1590
Quinacrine, for lupus, 116
Quinagolide, for hyperprolactinemia, 1118
Quinapril/quinapril with hydrochlorothiazide, 456t
Quincke pulses, 346
Quinidine
  antidepressant drug interactions and, 1083t
  for arrhythmias, 381, 382t

  for malaria, 1515t, 1517t, 1518
    severe disease and, 1516, 1517t, 1518
    overdose/toxicity of, 382t, 1518
Quinine, for malaria, 1515, 1515t, 1517t, 1518
  adverse ophthalmic effects of, 178t
  self-treatment and, 1520
  severe disease and, 1516, 1517t, 1518
Quinsy (peritonsillar abscess), **229**
Quinupristin/dalfopristin, for E faecium infection, 1444, 1445
Quixin. *See* Levofloxacin

R 364D, tick typhus caused by, 1434
R-CHOP regimen, 532, 533
R-CVP regimen, 532
R-EPOCH regimen, 533, 1337t, 1344
Rabeprazole, 609, 625. *See also* Proton pump inhibitors
Rabies, **1386–1388**
  bite injuries and, 1300, 1301, 1386, 1387
  prevention/immunization and, 1326–1327, 1387–1388. *See also* Rabies vaccine
Rabies antiserum, 1387
Rabies immune globulin, 1387
Rabies vaccine, 1326–1327, 1387–1388
  adsorbed, 1326
  in animal population, 1386
  antimalarial drugs/chloroquine and, 1326–1327, 1388
  postexposure, 1386, 1387
  preexposure, 1326–1327, 1387–1388
  for travelers, 1326–1327, 1387
Rabson-Mendenhall syndrome, 1211t
Raccoon roundworm (*Baylisascaris procyonis*), visceral larva migrans caused by, 1542
Raccoon sign, 1029
Racemose cysticercosis, 1536
Radial nerve lesions, **1040**
Radiation exposure/reactions, **1571–1572**. *See also* Radiation therapy
  acute, 1571
  cancer risk and, 1571, 1572, 1607
  lung injury caused by, **309–310**
  from medical imaging, 1571
  occupational/environmental, 1572
  during pregnancy, 799
  thyroid cancer risk and, 1140–1141
  thyroiditis risk and, 1134
  vomiting and, 581t
Radiation fibrosis, pulmonary, **310**
Radiation pericarditis, 425, 427
Radiation pneumonitis, **310**
Radiation proctitis, 598, 599
Radiation syndrome, acute (radiation sickness), 1571
Radiation therapy. *See also* Radiation exposure/reactions
  for acromegaly/gigantism, 1116
  for bladder cancer, 1652
  for breast cancer, 749, 750, 754
    arm edema and, 759
    breast implants and, 737
    local recurrence and, 750, 758, 759
    in male, 760
    pregnancy and, 747
  cancer risks and, 1571, 1572

with chemotherapy. *See* Chemoradiation therapy
for esophageal cancer, 1627, 1628
for gliomas, 1005
in gynecomastia, 1195
for laryngeal cancer, 236
leukemia and, 527
for lung cancer, 1612, 1613
lung injury and, **309–310**
for lymphoma, 1337*t*, 1339, 1344
pericarditis caused by, 425, 427
pneumonitis and, **310**
for prostate cancer, 1648, 1649
pulmonary fibrosis and, **310**
for spinal tumors/cord compression, 1007, 1658
thrombocytopenia and, **548**
for thyroid cancer, 1145
thyroid cancer risk and, 1140–1141
Radiculopathy, cervical, 1696
Radioactive iodine. *See also* Radioiodine thyroid scans and uptake
for goiter, 1130, 1131, 1140
for hyperthyroidism/Graves disease, 1130
amiodarone-induced, 1132
hypothyroidism after, 1130, 1134
methimazole/thiourea treatment and, 1129, 1130
ophthalmopathy flares and, 195, 1127, 1130, 1132
toxic multinodular goiter, 1131, 1140
toxic solitary thyroid nodule and, 1131
side effects/contraindications to, 1130, 1145
pregnancy and, 816, 1130, 1131, 1131–1132, 1145
for thyroid cancer treatment/follow-up, 1144–1145
for thyroid nodules, 1131, 1140
for thyroid scanning. *See* Radioiodine thyroid scans and uptake
Radiocontrast media. *See* Contrast media
Radiofrequency ablation techniques
for arrhythmias, 384. *See also specific arrhythmia*
for Barrett epithelium, 608
for benign prostatic hyperplasia (TUNA), 976
for cardiomyopathy, 419, 420*f*
Radioiodine. *See* Radioactive iodine
Radioiodine thyroid scans and uptake. *See also* Radioactive iodine
in goiter, 1148
in hyperthyroidism/Graves disease, 1121*t*, 1128
amiodarone-induced disease and, 1128
in nodule evaluation, 1121*t*, 1138, 1138*t*
in thyroid cancer, 1141*t*, 1142
differential diagnosis and, 1143
follow-up and, 1146, 1146–1147
in thyroiditis, 1136
Radionuclide angiography
in angina, 357
in heart failure, 404
Radiosurgery, stereotactic, for pituitary adenoma, 1116, 1119, 1175
Radiotherapy. *See* Radiation therapy

Radium-223 dichloride, for bone metastases, 1671*t*
Radon, lung cancer associated with exposure to, 309, 1608
RADT. *See* Rapid antigen/rapid antigen detection testing
RAEB. *See* Refractory anemia with excess blasts
Raf-kinase inhibitors, for renal cell carcinoma, 1654–1655
Rage attacks, seizures differentiated from, 986
Ragged red fibers, in mitochondrial myopathies, 1049
Rai classification, for chronic lymphocytic leukemia, 530
RAI scans, thyroid. *See* Radioiodine thyroid scans and uptake
Rales. *See* Crackles
Raloxifene
breast cancer prevention and, 739
for gynecomastia, 1195
hypercalcemia/hyperparathyroidism and, 1157
for osteoporosis, 1163, 1205–1206
Raltegravir, 1352*t*, 1358. *See also* Antiretroviral therapy
after needle stick, 1347
prophylactic, 1346
with Truvada (emtricitabine and tenofovir [TDF]), 1358, 1359*t*
Ramelteon, 1054*t*, 1089
for delirium at end of life, 87
Ramipril
in cardiovascular/heart disease prevention, 355
for heart failure, 407
for hypertension, 454, 456*t*
diabetes and, 454
Ramosetron, 1672, 1673. *See also* Antiemetics
Ramsay Hunt syndrome, 214, 1369, 1370
Ramucirumab, 1667*t*
for gastric adenocarcinoma, 1631
Range of motion testing
ankle injuries and, 1715*t*
back pain and, 1692, 1693
hip disorders and, 1702*t*
neck pain and, 1696*t*
wrist disorders and, 1699*t*
Ranibizumab
for age-related macular degeneration, 185
for chronic macular edema in retinal vein occlusion, 186
for diabetic macular edema, 190
Ranitidine, 609. *See also* H₂ receptor blocking drugs
for nausea and vomiting, 87
RANK/RANKL
denosumab mechanism of action and, 1162
in myeloma, 535
Ranke complex, in tuberculosis, 279
Radionuclide angiography, stereotactic
Ranolazine, for angina, 360*f*, 361
Ranson criteria, 726, 727*t*
Rapamycin inhibitor, for breast cancer, 756
Rape/rape trauma syndrome, 792–794. *See also* Sexual violence

statutory, 793
STD transmission and, 1302
Rapid antigen/rapid antigen detection testing (RADT)
in community-acquired pneumonia, 269–270
in malaria, 1514
in pharyngitis, 228, 1441
Rapid cyclers, in bipolar disorder, 1076
lithium use and, 1085
Rapid detoxification, for heroin/opioid withdrawal, 17–18, 1099
Rapid eye movement (REM) sleep, 1088
Rapid eye movement (REM) sleep behavior disorder, 1090
Rapid HIV antibody tests, 1302, 1334, 1334*t*
Rapid plasma reagin test. *See* RPR test
Rapid treponemal tests, 1490–1491
Rapidly acting insulin analogs, 1229, 1229*t*, 1230. *See also* Insulin therapy
in mixtures/combination therapy, 1229*t*, 1231, 1233, 1234*t*
in pregnancy, 1244
in pumps, 1230
Rapidly progressive glomerulonephritis, 932, 932*f*
RAS mutations, in thyroid cancer, 1139
Rasagiline, for parkinsonism, 1013
Rasburicase
G6PD deficiency and, 511
for tumor lysis syndrome/hyperuricemia, 920, 1660, 1671*t*
Rashes. *See also specific type or cause and* Skin disorders
acute exanthems, 1367–1368*t*, **1421–1424**
chemotherapy-induced, 1673–1674
in dermatomyositis, 848, 848*f*
drugs causing (dermatitis medicamentosa), **161–163**, 162–163*t*, **880**
drug-induced hypersensitivity syndrome and, 161, 163, 880
penicillin/ampicillin, 1318
fungal, **111–115**, 111*f*, 112*f*, 113*f*
in HIV infection/AIDS, 1343
heat causing (miliaria), **131**
photodistributed (photodermatitis), 96*t*, **154–155**. *See also* Photodermatitis
in SLE, 839*t*, 840
travel and, 1308, 1309
Rat-bite fever, **1500**
Rat poison, anticoagulant toxicity and, 1588
Rate control
for atrial fibrillation, 389, 390
in cardiomyopathy, 417
cardioversion compared with, 393–394
for atrial flutter, 394
Rathke cleft cyst, 1112
Rattlesnake envenomation, 1604
Rauwolfia derivatives, antidepressant drug interactions and, 1083*t*
Raxibacumab, for anthrax, 1456
Raynaud disease, 844

Raynaud phenomenon, **843–845**, 844*t*
  Buerger disease (thromboangiitis obliterans) and, 844
  scleroderma and, 844, 845, 846
  SLE and, 840
RB-ILD. *See* Respiratory bronchiolitis-associated interstitial lung disease
RBC. *See* Erythrocyte count
RCRI (Revised Cardiac Risk Index), 45, 46*t*
Reactivated chronic hepatitis B, 687
Reactive arthritis (Reiter syndrome), **865–866**, 866*f*
  gonococcal arthritis differentiated from, 866, 869, 1476
  HIV infection/AIDS and, 866, 869, 1340
Reactive cervical lymphadenopathy, **239**
Reactive erythemas, **133–136**, 134*f*, 135*f*
Reactive (postprandial) hypoglycemia, 1252, 1252*t*, **1256–1257**. *See also* Hypoglycemia
Reactive thrombocytosis, 521
Rebif. *See* Interferon-beta
Rebound headache, analgesic, **980**
Recall. *See* Memory
Recklinghausen disease (neurofibromatosis), 1010
  gastroenteropancreatic neuroendocrine tumors in, 1185
  pheochromocytoma/paraganglioma in, 1179–1180
Reclast. *See* Zoledronate/zoledronic acid
Recombinant follicle-stimulating hormone (FSH), for ovulation induction, 784–785
Recombinant growth factors. *See* Growth factors
Recombinant human deoxyribonuclease (rhDNase), for cystic fibrosis, 265
Recombinant human growth hormone (rhGH), 1112
Recombinant human parathyroid hormone (rhPTH). *See also* Teriparatide
  for hypocalcemia/hypoparathyroidism, 1152
Recombinant human thyroid-stimulating hormone (rhTSH), RAI therapy/follow-up for thyroid cancer and, 1144–1145, 1146–1147
  hyperthyroidism and, 1126, 1145
Recombinant influenza vaccine (RIV/RIV3), 1322*t*, 1413, 1415*t*
Recombinant tissue plasminogen activator. *See* Alteplase
Recombivax-HB. *See* Hepatitis B vaccine
Recompression. *See also* Hyperbaric oxygen therapy
  for dysbarism/decompression sickness, 204, 1573
  for high-altitude illness, 1575
Reconstructive surgery
  after mastectomy, 737, 750, 759
    local recurrence and, 737, 759
  vascular. *See* Bypass grafting
Recrudescent epidemic typhus (Brill-Zinsser disease), 1430

Recruitment, in cochlear dysfunction, 210
Rectal bleeding, 598. *See also* Gastrointestinal bleeding
  hemorrhoids causing, 598, 669
  in ulcerative colitis, 598
Rectal carcinoids, 1635
Rectal examination
  cauda equina syndrome and, 1693
  in prostate cancer screening/diagnosis, 1646, 1646*t*, 1647*f*
Rectal prolapse, 669
Rectal (Blumer) shelf, 1630
Rectal temperature. *See* Core body temperature
Rectal ulcer, GI bleeding caused by, 598
Rectocele, 777
Rectovaginal fistulas, in Crohn disease, 653, 654
Rectum. *See also under* Rectal
  cancer of, 1608*t*, 1624*t*, 1638, 1639, 1640. *See also* Colorectal cancer
    adjuvant/neoadjuvant therapy for, 1640
    surgical excision and, 1639
  disorders of, **643–669**. *See also* Anorectal disorders
    gonococcal infection, 670, 1475
Recurrent (habitual) abortion, **805**
Recurrent laryngeal nerve
  damage to during thyroid surgery, 1143
  vocal fold paralysis caused by damage/lesions of, 237, 1143
Recurrent paroxysmal atrial fibrillation, 388, 394
Recurrent respiratory papillomatosis, **233–234**
Red blood cells. *See under Red cell* and Erythrocytes
Red bugs, skin lesions caused by, 151
Red cell aplasia, pure, in erythrovirus (parvovirus) infection, 1422
Red cell casts, 913, 914*t*
Red cell count, in pleural fluid, 313*t*
Red cell transfusions, **541–544**. *See also specific type and* Transfusion
Red man syndrome, 878, 879*t*
Reduced-intensity allogeneic stem cell transplantation, 540, 541. *See also* Bone marrow/stem cell transplantation
Reductase inhibitors. *See also* Finasteride
  for benign prostatic hyperplasia, 973*t*, 974
Reduction pneumoplasty, for COPD, 262
Reed-Sternberg cells, 533
Reentry
  atrial fibrillation/flutter and, 387, 394, 395
  in supraventricular tachycardia, 385, 387–388
  in ventricular premature beats, 396
  in ventricular tachycardia, 396
Refeeding
  fatal hypophosphatemia and, 900
  for protein–energy malnutrition, 1269
Refeeding edema, 1269
Reflex sympathetic dystrophy (complex regional pain syndrome), **874–875**

Reflux
  gastroesophageal. *See* Gastroesophageal reflux disease
  laryngopharyngeal, **233**
  venous. *See* Venous reflux
  vesicoureteral, tubulointerstitial disease caused by, 947, 948
Reflux esophagitis. *See* Esophagitis
Reflux nephropathy, 947, 948
Refractive errors, **164**
  in elderly, 69
Refractive surgery, 164
Refractory anemia, 525
Refractory anemia with excess blasts (RAEB), 525, 527
Refractory atrial fibrillation, 394
Refractory ulcers, 628–629
  gastric cancer and, 629, 1630
  Zollinger-Ellison syndrome (gastrinoma) and, 629, 631
Refsum disease, 1036
Regional poison control centers, 1577
Regorafenib, 1668*t*
  for colorectal cancer, 1640
  for gastrointestinal mesenchymal tumors, 1634
Regranex. *See* Becaplermin; Platelet-derived growth factor
Regular insulin, 1229, 1229*t*. *See also* Insulin therapy
  for diabetic ketoacidosis, 1229, 1247–1248
  in mixtures/combination therapy, 1229*t*, 1231, 1236
  in pregnancy, 817, 1244
Regurgitation, 580
  in GERD, 607
Rehydration. *See* Fluid management/hydration
Reinke edema, 234
Reiter syndrome. *See* Reactive arthritis
Relafen. *See* Nabumetone
Relapsing fever, 1312*t*, **1499**
Relapsing polychondritis, 201, **861**
Relapsing-remitting multiple sclerosis, 1023
REM sleep, 1088
REM sleep behavior disorder, 1090
Remeron. *See* Mirtazapine
Remicade. *See* Infliximab
Remitting seronegative synovitis with non-pitting edema, 875
Remnant ablation (thyroid), 1144
Renal amyloidosis, 934*t*, **946**
Renal angiography/arteriography, in renal artery stenosis/renal vascular hypertension, 442, 931
Renal artery stenosis, **931–932**
  hypertension caused by, 442, 466, 931–932
  renal hypoperfusion/acute kidney injury and, 917, 931
Renal biopsy, **915–916**. *See also specific disorder*
  in focal segmental glomerulosclerosis, 944
  in nephritic spectrum disorders, 936
  in nephrotic syndrome/nephrotic spectrum disorders, 942

Renal calculi, 962, 965. *See also*
    Nephrolithiasis; Urinary
    stone disease
Renal cell carcinoma, 1608t, 1624t,
    1654–1655
Renal colic/pain, urinary stones causing,
    962
Renal cysts, 924t, **948–951**, 949t
    acquired, 949t
    in autosomal dominant polycystic
        kidney disease, 949–950,
        949t
    complex, 949
    infected, 950
    in juvenile nephronophthisis-
        medullary cystic kidney, 951
    in medullary cystic kidney, 949t, 951
    in medullary sponge kidney, 949t,
        950–951
    simple/solitary, **949**, 949t
Renal disorders. *See* Kidney disease/
    injury
Renal failure. *See also* Acute kidney
    injury; Chronic kidney
    disease; Kidney disease/
    injury; Uremia
    acute, 913, **916–923**, 917t. *See also*
        Acute kidney injury
    chronic, 913, **923–932**, 923t, 924t, 925f,
        925t, 926f, 927f. *See also*
        Chronic kidney disease
    in cystic kidney disease, 949t
    dialysis for. *See* Dialysis
    immunization recommendations in,
        1321t
    intrinsic, 917t, 918, 921
    in myeloma, 535, 536
    myoglobinuria/rhabdomyolysis and,
        852, 919–920
    postoperative, 54, 54t
    transplantation for. *See* Kidney
        transplantation
Renal failure type (beta-2-microglobulin)
    amyloidosis, 538
Renal (nondiabetic) glycosuria, 1214
Renal hypercalciuria, 962t, 964
Renal imaging, in dysuria evaluation, 43
Renal osteodystrophy, 927–928, 927f,
    1153, 1155
Renal pelvis, cancer of, 1608t, **1653**
Renal salt wasting, 886
    in subarachnoid hemorrhage, 999
Renal transplantation. *See* Kidney
    transplantation
Renal tubular acidosis, 892t, 906–907,
    906t, 908
    genetic defects associated with, 892t
    hyperkalemia in, 894, 948
    nephrolithiasis/nephrocalcinosis/
        urolithiasis and, 906–907,
        962
    in tubulointerstitial disease, 948
    urinary anion gap in, 906, 906t, 907
Renal tubular cell casts, 913, 914t
Renal tubular necrosis, acute, 852, 917t,
    918–921
    in pancreatitis, 728
    rhabdomyolysis and, 852, 920
Renal vascular hypertension, 442,
    931–932. *See also*
    Hypertension

Renin activity
    in adrenal insufficiency/Addison
        disease, 1170
    in aldosteronism, 442, 1178
Renin-angiotensin-aldosterone system.
    See also Aldosterone
    in hypertension, 441–442, 442–443,
        454, 466, 1177
    inhibitors of, 449t, 454, 454–459,
        455–458t, 459. *See also*
        Angiotensin II receptor
        blocking agents;
        Angiotensin-converting
        enzyme (ACE) inhibitors;
        Renin inhibitors
Renin inhibitors, 455t. *See also*
        Angiotensin II receptor
        blocking agents;
        Angiotensin-converting
        enzyme (ACE) inhibitors
    for heart failure, 406–407, 410–411
    for hypertension, 454, 455t
        in chronic kidney disease/renal
            failure, 466
        in combination regimen, 464–465,
            465f
        in diabetes, 466
Renova. *See* Tretinoin
Repaglinide, 1221t, 1223, 1236
    factitious hypoglycemia and, 1253t,
        1257
    with metformin, 1223, 1228
Repeat-dose charcoal, 1583
Reperfusion therapy. *See also*
        Revascularization procedures
    for myocardial infarction, 372–375,
        372f, 373t
        fibrinolytic therapy, 372f, 373, 373t,
            374–375
        percutaneous coronary intervention
            (PCI), 369t, 372–374, 372f
Replens, 1202
Rescriptor. *See* Delavirdine
Rescue collapse, 1564
Rescula. *See* Unoprostone
Reserpine, 463t
    depression caused by, 463t, 464,
        1076
    for Huntington disease, 1015
    for hypertension, 463t, 464
    MAOI interactions and, 1083t
Reset osmostat, hyponatremia caused by,
    887, 888
Residual volume (RV). *See* Pulmonary
    function tests
Resin T₃/T₄ uptake, in hyperthyroidism,
    1127
    pregnancy and, 1128
Resistance, microbial. *See* Drug resistance
Resistance testing, in antiretroviral
    therapy, 1350, 1360,
    1361–1362
Resistant hypertension, **467–468**, 468t
Reslizumab, for asthma, 251
Resolution, psychotic, 1067
Resolution stage of sexual activity, 1062
Resorptive hypercalciuria, 962t,
    963–964
Resource allocation, principles of care
    and, 2
Respiration. *See* Breathing; Ventilation

Respiratory acidosis (hypercapnia), 903,
    904t, **910**. *See also specific*
    cause
    in asthma, 245
    metabolic alkalosis and, 909
    permissive, for asthma, 257
    respiratory failure and, 317–318, 910
Respiratory alkalosis (hypocapnia), 903,
    904t, **910–911**, 911t. *See also*
    specific cause
    alcoholic ketoacidosis and, 906
    in asthma, 245
    in hyperventilation syndromes, 316,
        910, 911
    mechanical ventilation and, 319
    metabolic acidosis and, 907, 911
    salicylate overdose/toxicity and,
        1603
Respiratory bronchiolitis, 267
Respiratory bronchiolitis-associated
    interstitial lung disease
    (RB-ILD), 291t, 292
Respiratory depression, opioid therapy/
    pain relief and, 83
Respiratory disorders. *See* Pulmonary
    disorders
Respiratory distress syndrome, acute. *See*
    Acute respiratory distress
    syndrome
Respiratory drugs, adverse ophthalmic
    effects of, 177t
Respiratory failure, **317–319**, 318t. *See*
    also Acute respiratory
    distress syndrome
    acidosis in, 317–318, 910
    asthma and, 25, 245t, 255–257, 256f
    in burn injury, 1569
    in COPD, 262
    in drowning, 1567
    drug-induced, 310t
    in Middle East respiratory syndrome,
        1420
    postoperative, 49–50, 49t
    smoke inhalation and, 305
    tracheotomy for, 237–238
Respiratory injection, of
    methylprednisolone, for
    asthma, 254t
Respiratory papillomatosis, recurrent,
    233–234
Respiratory syncytial virus (RSV),
    1409–1410
    bronchiolitis caused by, 266,
        1409–1410, 1410
Respiratory tract infection. *See*
    Pulmonary disorders,
    infections
Rest. *See also* Bed rest; Immobility
    requirements for during pregnancy,
        799
Rest pain
    in thromboangiitis obliterans
        (Buerger disease), 480
    in tibial/pedal occlusive disease, 475
Restasis. *See* Cyclosporine
Restenosis, with PCI, 362
Restless legs syndrome, **1017**
Restlessness, terminal (terminal
    delirium), 87, 1103
Reston virus, 1397
Restoril. *See* Temazepam

Restrictive cardiomyopathy. *See* Cardiomyopathy
RESTV. *See* Reston virus
Resurfacing surgery, hip, 1703
Resuscitation. *See* Cardiopulmonary resuscitation
Resynchronization (biventricular pacing). *See also* Pacemaker
  for cardiomyopathy, 417, 419
  for heart failure, 405f, 409–410
ret oncogene
  in medullary thyroid carcinoma, 1141, 1145
  in MEN, 1141, 1145, 1188
  in pheochromocytoma/paraganglioma, 1182
RET/PTC mutations, in thyroid cancer, 1139
Retardation. *See* Mental retardation
Retention, urinary. *See* Urinary retention
Reteplase, for myocardial infarction, 373t, 374
Reticulocytopenia, in anemia classification, 499, 500t
Reticulocytosis, in anemia classification, 499, 500t
Reticulosis, polymorphic (midline malignant), 223
Retigabine, adverse ophthalmic effects of, 177t
Retin-A/Retin A Micro. *See* Tretinoin
Retina
  detachment of, **183–184**
  in hypertension, **190–191**, 191f, 444, 445f
  systemic diseases affecting, **189–192**, 189f, 191f. *See also specific disorder*
Retinal arteries, in hypertension, 444, 445f
Retinal artery occlusions
  central and branch, **187–188**, 187f
  stroke and, 995
Retinal neovascularization
  in diabetic retinopathy, 190, 1238
  in retinal vein occlusion, 186
Retinal tears, detachment and, 183
Retinal vasculitis, 181. *See also* Uveitis
Retinal vein occlusions, central and branch, **186–187**
Retinitis
  in bartonellosis, 1477
  CMV, 191–192, 1338t, 1341, 1374, 1375, 1376
    herpetic (acute retinal necrosis), 192, 1363
Retinochoroiditis, toxoplasmic, 192, 1522, 1523
Retinochoroidopathy, hypertensive, **190–191**, 191f, 444, 445f
Retinoic acid. *See also* Tretinoin
  acute promyelocytic leukemia and, 527
Retinoids. *See also specific agent and* Vitamin A
  for acne, 127, 128
  adverse ophthalmic effects of, 179t
  for psoriasis, 108
  with PUVA (re-PUVA), for lichen planus, 145
Retinopathy
  antipsychotics causing, 1072

diabetic, **189–190**, 189f, 1238
  glycemic control affecting development/progression of, 189, 1218, 1219
  HIV, 191, 1341
  hypertensive, 190–191, 191f, 444, 445f
  "pizza-pie," in CMV infection, 1375
  sickle cell, 191
Retisert. *See* Fluocinolone/fluocinolone implant
Retrobulbar optic neuritis, 193
Retrocecal appendicitis, 641–642, 642
Retrograde ejaculation, 966, 1063. *See also* Erectile dysfunction/impotence
  antidepressants causing, 1079
  in infertility, 970
Retroileal appendicitis, 642
Retropharyngeal abscess, 1442
Retrovir. *See* Zidovudine
Revascularization procedures. *See also specific type and* Bypass grafting
  for acute arterial limb occlusion, 476–477
  for aortoiliac occlusive disease, 473
  coronary, 362–363. *See also* Reperfusion therapy
    for angina, 358–359, 360f, 362–363
    emergent, traumatic injury and, 434
    for heart failure, 410, 411
    for myocardial infarction, 362–363, 380–381
    prophylactic/preoperative, 46–47
  for femoral/popliteal occlusive disease, 474
  for intestinal ischemia, 479
  for tibial/pedal occlusive disease, 475
Reversal reactions, in leprosy, 1484, 1485
Reverse transcriptase inhibitors. *See* Nonnucleoside reverse transcriptase inhibitors; Nucleoside reverse transcriptase inhibitors; Nucleotide reverse transcriptase inhibitor
Reverse transcriptase-polymerase chain reaction testing. *See also specific disorder*
  for Ebola virus, 1398
  for measles, 1378
  for rabies, 1386
  for tick-borne encephalitis, 1392
  for Zika virus, 1406
Revised Atlanta classification, in pancreatitis, 727, 728
Revised Cardiac Risk Index (RCRI), 45, 46t
Revlimid. *See* Lenalidomide
Rewarming
  for frostbite, 1566
  for frostnip/chilblain, 1565
  for immersion syndrome, 1565
  for systemic hypothermia, 1564–1565
Rewarming shock, 1564
Reyataz. *See* Atazanavir
Reye syndrome, 1412
  aspirin use and, 74, 1369, 1371, 1412
  varicella zoster virus infection/vaccine and, 1369
Reynolds pentad, 721

Rezulin. *See* Troglitazone
RF. *See* Rheumatoid factor
RFX6 mutation, in diabetes, 1212
Rh$_o$ (D) immune globulin, 800, 801
  after delivery, 801
  after ectopic pregnancy, 801, 806
  after elective abortion, 791, 801
  prenatal screening for/administration of, 799, 800, 801
  after spontaneous abortion, 801, 804
Rh incompatibility, 799, 800, **801**. *See also* Rh$_o$ (D) immune globulin
  testing for, 542, 799, 800
Rh typing
  compatibility testing for transfusion and, 542
  during pregnancy, 799, 800
Rhabdomyolysis, **852–853**
  acute tubular necrosis and, 852, 920
  statins causing, 852, 1264
Rhabdomyoma, cardiac, 433
rhDNase, for cystic fibrosis, 265
Rhegmatogenous retinal detachment, 183–184
Rhesus alloimmunization (Rh incompatibility), 799, 800, **801**. *See also* Rh$_o$ (D) immune globulin
  testing for, 542, 799, 800
Rheumatic carditis/valvulitis, 422, 422–423, 423t, 424
  endocarditis/endocarditis prophylaxis and, 1458
Rheumatic fever, **422–424**, 423t
  arthritis in, 422, 423
    gonococcal arthritis differentiated from, 869
    nongonococcal acute bacterial (septic) arthritis differentiated from, 867
    rheumatoid arthritis differentiated from, 836
  prevention and, 424, 1442
  streptococcal infection and, 229, 422, 424, 1441, 1442
Rheumatic heart disease, 422–424, 423t
  endocarditis/endocarditis prophylaxis and, 1458
Rheumatism, palindromic, **875**
Rheumatoid arthritis, 35f, **834–838**, 840t,
  in coal workers (Caplan syndrome), 307
  CPPD and (pseudorheumatoid arthritis), 834, 836
  differential diagnosis of, 836
    ankylosing spondylitis and, 836, 864
    gouty/tophaceous arthritis and, 831, 836
    granulomatosis with polyangiitis and, 836, 858
    nongonococcal acute bacterial (septic) arthritis and, 867
    osteoarthritis and, 828, 836
    viral arthritis and, 870
  neuropathies associated with, 835, 1037
Rheumatoid factor, 835, 840t
  cryoglobulinemia and, 860, 939
  in polymyositis/dermatomyositis, 840t, 848

in rheumatoid arthritis, 835, 840*t*
in Sjögren syndrome, 840*t*, 850
Rheumatoid nodules, 835, 835*f*
in coal workers (Caplan syndrome), 307
gouty tophi differentiated from, 831, 836
Rheumatoid pleural effusion, 313*t*
Rheumatologic disorders, **826–876**. *See also specific disorder*
adverse ophthalmic effects of drugs used in, 179*t*
autoantibodies in, 840*t*
cancer and, **875**
dysphagia in, 605*t*
HIV infection/AIDS and, **869–870**, 1340
rhGH. *See* Recombinant human growth hormone
Rhinitis
allergic (hay fever), **218–220**
conjunctivitis and, 168
nasal polyps and, 219, 222
medicamentosa, 215
nasopharyngeal/paranasal sinus cancer and, 223
perennial, 219
vasomotor, 219
Rhinocerebral mucormycosis, 218, 1556
Rhinosinusitis
acute bacterial, **215–218**, 217*t*. *See also* Sinusitis
hospital-associated, 216
nasopharyngeal/paranasal sinus cancer and, 223
orbital cellulitis and, 195, 217
acute viral (common cold), **214–215**, 1420–1421
Rhizopus infection, 218, 1555–1556
Rhodococcus equi, pneumonia in HIV infection/AIDS caused by, 1336
rhPTH. *See* Recombinant human parathyroid hormone
rhTSH. *See* Recombinant human thyroid-stimulating hormone
Riamet (artemether-lumefantrine/Coartem), 1515*t*, 1516*t*, 1517*t*, 1519, 1520
Ribavirin, 1365*t*
for hemorrhagic fevers, 1400
for hepatitis C, 684, 689, 690, 1342
for influenza, 1365*t*
for RSV infection, 1365*t*, 1410
Ribociclib, for breast cancer, 756
Riboflavin (vitamin B₂)
deficiency of, **1275**
for migraine prophylaxis, 979*t*
Rice, *Bacillus cereus* contamination of, 1305
Rice water stool, in cholera, 1471
Richter syndrome, 530
Rickets, 1164
hypophosphatemic (vitamin D-resistant), 892*t*, 1164–1165, 1166
vitamin D-dependent, 1164
Rickettsia (rickettsial diseases), 1313*t*, **1428–1438**, 1429*t*. *See also specific disease*
364D, 1434

aeschlimannii, 1434
africae, 1429*t*, 1434
akari, 1429*t*, 1434
australis, 1429*t*, 1434
conorii, 1429*t*, 1434
felis, 1429*t*, 1435
helvetica, 1434
japonica, 1434
lymphangitis-associated, 1429*t*, 1434
massiliae, 1433, 1434
monacensis, 1434
myocarditis in, 413*t*
parkeri, 1433, 1434
phillipi, 1433
prowazekii, 1428, 1429, 1429–1430, 1429*t*, 1430
raoultii, 1429*t*, 1434
rickettsii, 1429*t*, 1433
sibirica, 1429*t*, 1434
mongolitimonae, 1429*t*, 1434
slovaca, 1429*t*, 1434
typhi, 1429*t*, 1430, 1431
Rickettsial fever (tick typhus), **1434–1435**
Rickettsialpox, 1429*t*, **1434**
Rickettsiosis
California flea, 1429*t*
lymphangitis-associated, 1429*t*, 1434
spotted fever, 1434
Riedel thyroiditis/struma, 1135, 1137
Rifabutin
adverse ophthalmic effects of, 178*t*
antiretroviral agent interactions and, 282, 1336
for MAC infection, 286, 1337*t*, 1482
Rifamate. *See* Rifampin/isoniazid
Rifampin, 281*t*, 282*t*
for anthrax, 1456*t*
antiretroviral agent interactions and, 282, 1336, 1356
benzodiazepine interactions and, 1056*t*
for endocarditis, 1461, 1462
for leprosy, 1484
for MAC infection, 286, 1482
for tuberculosis, 281–282, 281*t*, 282–283, 282*t*
in HIV infection/AIDS, 1336
in latent disease/prophylactic, 284
in pregnancy, 282, 283, 821
resistance and, 283
Rifampin/isoniazid, for tuberculosis, 282
in latent disease/prophylactic, 284
Rifampin/isoniazid/pyrazinamide, for tuberculosis, 282
Rifapentine, for tuberculosis, 281*t*
in latent disease/prophylactic, 284
Rifater. *See* Rifampin/isoniazid/pyrazinamide
Rifaximin
for Crohn disease, 655
for hepatic encephalopathy, 703
for irritable bowel syndrome, 647
for rosacea, 129
for traveler's diarrhea, 591, 1310
Rift Valley fever, 1399, 1400
Right middle lobe syndrome, **288**
Right ventricle
double-chambered, 322
double outlet, 328
Right ventricular (right heart) failure, 402, 403. *See also* Heart (cardiac) failure

Right ventricular infarction, 378–379
Rigidity, in parkinsonism, 1012
Rilonacept, for gout, 832
Rilpivirine, 1351*t*, 1355. *See also* Antiretroviral therapy
with tenofovir (TDF) and emtricitabine (Complera), 1354*t*, 1355, 1359*t*
Riluzole, for amyotrophic lateral sclerosis, 1034
Rimantadine, influenza/influenza resistance and, 1365*t*, 1412, 1418
Rimexolone, for ophthalmic disorders, 172*t*
Ring shadow sign, 948
Ring X chromosome, in Turner syndrome, 1207
Ringworm. *See* Tinea
Rinne test, 200
RIPA. *See* Ristocetin-induced platelet aggregation
Risedronate, 1161. *See also* Bisphosphonates
for osteoporosis prevention/management, 1161
Risky drinking. *See* At-risk (problem) drinking
Risperdal. *See* Risperidone
Risperidone, 1068, 1069*t*, 1070, 1071, 1071*t*. *See also* Antipsychotic drugs
for aggressive/violent behavior, 1091
for bipolar disease/mania, 1085
for delirium at end of life, 87
overdose/toxicity/side effects of, 1069*t*, 1071*t*, 1589–1590
ophthalmic, 177*t*, 183
for psychedelic/hallucinogen abuse/toxicity, 1099
Ristocetin-induced platelet aggregation, in von Willebrand disease, 560, 561*t*
Ritonavir, 1352*t*, 1356, 1356–1357. *See also* Antiretroviral therapy
with atazanavir, 1357
plus Truvada (emtricitabine and tenofovir [TDF]), 1359*t*
with darunavir, 1352*t*, 1357
plus Epzicom (abacavir/lamivudine), 1360*t*
plus Truvada (emtricitabine/tenofovir [TDF]), 1359*t*
with fosamprenavir, 1357
for hepatitis C, 691, 1341, 1342
with indinavir, 1356
with lopinavir (lopinavir/r), 1352*t*, 1357
for protease inhibitor boosting, 1356, 1357
with tipranavir, 1352*t*, 1357
Rituxan. *See* Rituximab
Rituximab, 1667*t*
for autoimmune hemolytic anemia, 514
for chronic lymphocytic leukemia, 530, 531
for cold agglutinin disease, 515
for granulomatosis with polyangiitis, 859

Rituximab (*Cont.*):
  for immune thrombocytopenia, 549–550, 549*f*, 550
  influenza vaccine and, 1413
  for microscopic polyangiitis, 860
  for neuromyelitis optica, 1025
  for non-Hodgkin lymphoma, 532, 1337*t*
  for pemphigus, 140
  progressive multifocal leukoencephalopathy caused by, 1395
  for rheumatoid arthritis, 838
  for SLE, 841
  for thrombotic microangiopathies, 552
  for Waldenström macroglobulinemia, 538
RIV/RIV3 (recombinant influenza vaccine), 1322*t*, 1413, 1415*t*
Rivaroxaban, 564, 565–566*t*, 567, 573
  for atrial fibrillation/stroke prevention, 391–393, 391*t*, 545*t*, 564
  for DVT/PE (venous thromboembolic disease), 564, 565*t*, 568*t*, 570*t*, 573
  overdose/toxicity of, 564, 566*t*, 1588
  perioperative management of, 52*t*, 566*t*
  for transient ischemic attacks, 993
Rivastigmine
  for dementia, 59, 1021, 1104
  for parkinsonism, 1014
River blindness (onchocerciasis), **1545–1546**
Rizatriptan, for migraine headache, 978
RMSF. *See* Rocky Mountain spotted fever
RNA
  hepatitis C virus, 683, 683*f*, 689
  hepatitis D virus, 684, 687
  hepatitis E virus, 684
Ro/SSA antibody, 840*t*
  in lupus/SLE, 115, 840*t*
  in Sjögren syndrome, 840*t*, 850
Rocaltrol. *See* Calcitriol
Rocephin. *See* Ceftriaxone
Rocky Mountain spotted fever, 1368*t*, 1429*t*, **1432–1434**, 1433*f*
Rodent tapeworm (*H diminuta*), 1535
Rodenticide poisoning, anticoagulant toxicity and, 1588
Rolapitant, 582*t*, 583, 1673
Romaña sign, 1509
Romano-Ward syndrome, 398
Romberg testing, 211
Romiplostim
  for myelodysplastic syndromes, 526, 548
  for thrombocytopenia chemotherapy-induced, 548, 1672 immune, 549*f*, 550
Ropinirole, for parkinsonism, 1013
ROS-1 tyrosine kinase inhibitor, for lung cancer, 1612
ROS1 rearranged lung cancer, 1612
Rosacea, **128–129**, 129*f*
  acne differentiated from, 127, 129
  steroid, 128
Rose spots, in enteric (typhoid) fever, 1468
Rosemont criteria, for chronic pancreatitis, 731

Roseola infantum (exanthema subitum), 1367*t*, 1377
Rosiglitazone, 1221*t*, 1224–1225
  with glimepiride, 1228
  with metformin, 1228
  overdose/toxicity of, 1595
Ross procedure, postoperative pulmonary valve stenosis and, 322, 350
Rosuvastatin, 355*t*, 1263–1264, 1265*t*. *See also* Statins
  in HIV infection/AIDS, 1356
RotaTeq. *See* Rotavirus vaccines
Rotation. *See* External rotation; Internal rotation
Rotator cuff tears, 1686–1687*t*, **1689–1690**
  impingement syndrome and, 1685, 1689
  shoulder dislocation and, 1690
  strength testing and, 1686–1687*t*, 1689
Rotatrix. *See* Rotavirus vaccines
Rotavac. *See* Rotavirus vaccines
Rotavin-M1. *See* Rotavirus vaccines
Rotavirus vaccines, 1424–1425
Rotaviruses, diarrhea/gastroenteritis caused by, 588*t*, 1305, 1307*t*, 1424, 1425
Roth spots, 191
  in endocarditis, 1459
Rotigotine, for parkinsonism, 1013
Rotor syndrome, 675*t*
Rotterdam score, 712
Rouleaux formation
  in myeloma, 535
  in Waldenström macroglobulinemia, 537
Roundworm infections. *See also specific type*
  filariasis, **1543–1546**, 1543*f*
  intestinal, 592, **1538–1541**
  invasive, **1541–1543**, 1543*f*
  visceral larva migrans caused by, 1542
Roux-en-Y gastric bypass. *See* Bariatric surgery
Rowasa. *See* Mesalamine
Roxanol. *See* Morphine
Roxicodone. *See* Oxycodone
Royal Free Hospital score, in cirrhosis, 705
Rozerem. *See* Ramelteon
RP. *See* Raynaud phenomenon
RPGN. *See* Rapidly progressive glomerulonephritis
RPR test, 1489–1490, 1490*t*
  in HIV infection/AIDS, 1348
RS3PE (remitting seronegative synovitis with non-pitting edema), 875
RSV. *See* Respiratory syncytial virus
RT-PCR. *See* Reverse transcriptase-polymerase chain reaction
RTA. *See* Renal tubular acidosis
rtPA (recombinant tissue plasminogen activator). *See* Alteplase; Tissue plasminogen activator
RTS, S vaccine, for malaria, 1520
RT$_3$U. *See* Resin T$_3$/T$_4$ uptake
RU 486. *See* Mifepristone
Rubber band ligation. *See* Banding
Rubella, 1368*t*, **1384–1385**
  arthritis and, 870, 1384, 1385

  during pregnancy/congenital, 1384, 1384–1385, 1385
  prevention/immunization and, 1384, 1385. *See also* MMR (measles-mumps-rubella) vaccine
Rubella virus vaccine, 1323*t*, 1385. *See also* MMR (measles-mumps-rubella) vaccine
Rubeola. *See* Measles
Rubeotic (neovascular) glaucoma, 186
Rufen. *See* Ibuprofen
Rufinamide, 988*t*
Rugger jersey spine, 1155
Rule of nines, 1568, 1568*f*
  for topical corticosteroid calculation, 95
Rumination, 580
Runner's knee (patellofemoral pain), 1709*t*, **1712–1713**
RUNX1/RUNX1T1 protein, in acute myeloid leukemia, 527
Russell viper venom clotting time, 841, 843
Rust ring, 196, 196*f*
Ruxolitinib
  for polycythemia vera, 520
  for primary myelofibrosis, 523
RVA (rabies vaccine adsorbed), 1326
RVVT. *See* Russell viper venom clotting time
RYGB (roux-en-Y gastric bypass). *See* Bariatric surgery

S stage sleep, 1088
SAAG. *See* Serum-ascites albumin gradient
Sabia virus, 1399
Sabin-Feldman dye test, in toxoplasmosis, 1523
Sabin vaccine (oral/OPV poliovaccine), 1383
  IPV booster and, 1326
Saccular (berry) aneurysm, 998, 1000. *See also* Intracranial aneurysm
Sacral plexus/nerve lesions, 1045
Sacral spine/disk disease. *See also* Spine
  back pain and, **1692–1694**, 1692*t*, 1693*t*
Sacroiliac joint/sacroiliitis, in ankylosing spondylitis, 864
Sacubitril/valsartan, for heart failure, 407
SAD. *See* Seasonal affective disorder
Saddle nose deformity
  in granulomatosis with polyangiitis, 857
  nasal trauma and, 222
SAE antibodies, in polymyositis/dermatomyositis, 848*t*
Safer sex
  in herpes simplex infection prevention, 119, 1366
  in HIV infection/AIDS prevention, 1345, 1346, 1349
  in syphilis prevention, 1491
Saflutan. *See* Tafluprost
Sag sign, 1708*t*, 1711
Salagen. *See* Pilocarpine
Salbutamol, adverse ophthalmic effects of, 177*t*

Salicylates. *See also* Aspirin
  overdose/toxicity of, 1584*t*, **1602–1603**
    alkali therapy for, 1582, 1584*t*, 1603
    anion gap/osmolar gap in, 906, 1603
    hemodialysis for, 1583*t*, 1584*t*, 1603
    ophthalmic, 179*t*
    platelet function affected by, 558*t*, 829
  for rheumatic fever/heart disease,
      423–424
Salicylic acid preparations, for wart
      removal, 141
Saline, 911*t*. *See also* Fluid management/
      hydration
  contrast media nephrotoxicity
      mediated by, 919
  dilutional acidosis and, 907
Saline breast prostheses. *See* Breast
      implants
Saline infusion sonohysterography, 763*t*
Saline purgatives. *See* Purgatives
Saline-responsive metabolic alkalosis,
      908–909, 909*t*, 910
Saline-unresponsive metabolic alkalosis,
      909, 909*t*, 910
Salivary cortisol, in Cushing syndrome
      diagnosis, 1174
Salivary glands, **231–232**
  infiltrative disorders of, **232**
  inflammatory disorders of
    acute, **231–232**
    chronic, **232**
    in mumps, 1380, 1381
  tumors of, **232**
Salivary stones (sialolithiasis), **231–232**
Salk vaccine (inactivated/IPV
      poliovaccine), 1326, 1383
  pregnancy and, 802
  for travelers, 1326, 1383
Salmeterol
  for asthma, 249*t*, 251
  for COPD, 260
  for high-altitude illness prevention,
      1575
Salmeterol-fluticasone
  for asthma, 249*t*
  for COPD, 260
Salmon calcitonin. *See* Calcitonin
Salmonella enterica subsp *enterica*
      (salmonellosis), **1468–1470**
  bacteremia caused by, 1308, 1312*t*,
      1468, **1470**
  choleraesuis, 1468
  diarrhea/enterocolitis/gastroenteritis
      caused by, 588*t*, 589, 1305,
      1307*t*, 1308, 1315*t*, 1342,
      1469
  drug resistance and, 1469, 1470
  enteric (typhoid) fever caused by,
      1468–1469
  typhi, 1468
  typhimurium, 1468
Salpingitis, **778–779**. *See also* Pelvic
      inflammatory disease
  appendicitis differentiated from, 642
  chlamydial, 1486
  gonococcal, 1475
  tuberculous, 778
Salpingo-oophorectomy. *See*
      Oophorectomy
Salt restriction. *See* Sodium-restricted
      diet

Salt tablets, contraindications to in heat
      exposure syndromes, 1562,
      1563
Salt wasting
  in adrenal hyperplasia, 1169, 1170,
      1197
  cerebral, 886, 888
  renal, 886
  in subarachnoid hemorrhage,
      999
Salvia divinorum, toxicity of, 1598
Samter triad, 222, 878
Sandostatin. *See* Octreotide
Sao$_2$ (oxygen saturation). *See* Arterial
      blood gases; Pulse oximetry
SAPE (sentinel acute pancreatitis event),
      731
Saphenous vein
  superficial thrombophlebitis of, 488
  varicose, 486, 487
Saphris. *See* Asenapine
Saquinavir, 1352*t*, 1356. *See also*
      Antiretroviral therapy
  with ritonavir, 1356
Sarafem. *See* Fluoxetine
Sarcocystis bovihominis/suihominis
      (sarcocystosis), **1527–1530**
Sarcoidosis, 223, **292–293**, 293*f*
  arthritis in, **872–873**
  hypercalcemia/hypercalciuria in, 897,
      1156
  neuropathy associated with, 1037
  nose and paranasal sinus involvement
      and, **223**, 293*f*
  optic neuritis in, 193
  pulmonary involvement and,
      292–293
Sarcoma. *See also specific type*
  soft tissue, 1625*t*
Sarcopenia, 56
Sarcoptes scabiei infection, **148–149**, 148*f*.
      See also Scabies
Sargramostim (GM-CSF)
  for aplastic anemia, 517
  for chemotherapy-induced toxicity,
      1672*t*
  for HIV infection/AIDS, 1350
  for neutropenia, 518
Sarin (GB) poisoning, 1601–1602
Sarna. *See* Camphor/menthol
      preparations
Satavaptan, for hyponatremia/SIADH,
      889
Saturday night palsy, 1039, 1040
Saturnine gout, in lead poisoning, 831,
      948
Savella. *See* Milnacipran
Saw palmetto, for benign prostatic
      hyperplasia, 975
Saxagliptin, 1222*t*, 1227
  with metformin, 1227, 1228
Saxenda. *See* Liraglutide
Saxitoxin, paralytic shellfish poisoning
      caused by, 1604*t*
Sb. *See* Stibogluconate
Scabies, **148–149**, 148*f*
  exfoliative dermatitis/erythroderma
      and, 117
  tinea differentiated from, 114
Scaling skin disorders, 96*t*, **104–118**. *See
      also specific type*

Scalp
  allergic contact dermatitis involving,
      125
  injuries of, 1029, 1031
  in pediculosis, 149, 150
  pemphigus involving, 139
  psoriasis of, 107, 108, 110
  seborrhea of, 110
Scalpicin. *See* Hydrocortisone
Scarlet fever, 1368*t*, 1441, 1444
Scarring (cicatricial) alopecias, 158, 159
SCC. *See* Squamous cell carcinoma
Scedosporium apiospermum/prolificans, in
      opportunistic infections, 1557
Schatzki rings, 605*t*, 613–614
Schirmer test, 850
*Schistosoma guineensis/haematobium/
      intercalatum/japonicum/
      mansoni/mekongi*
      (schistosomiasis), **1532–1533**
Schizoaffective disorder, 1066
Schizoid personality disorder, 1065*t*
Schizophrenia/schizophrenia spectrum
      disorders, **1066–1074**. *See
      also* Psychotic disorders
  depression and, 1066, 1067
  differential diagnosis of, 1067–1068
  drug-induced/toxic, 1068
  drug therapy for, 1068–1073, 1069*t*,
      1071*t*. *See also* Antipsychotic
      drugs
  ECT for, 1070, 1072, 1083
  positive and negative symptoms in,
      1066
    antipsychotics affecting, 1068–1070,
      1070
  prodromal, 1066
  suicidality and, 1068, 1077
Schizophreniform disorders, 1066–1067
Schizotypal personality disorder, 1065*t*,
      1066
Schmidt syndrome, 1169
Schneiderian papillomas, 223
Schwannoma
  gastrointestinal, 1633–1634
  vestibular (acoustic neuroma/
      neurinoma/eighth nerve
      tumor), 211*t*, **213–214**,
      1004*t*, 1005
  in neurofibromatosis, 213, 1010
Sciatic nerve palsy, **1040**
Sciatica, 1695. *See also* Back pain
Scintigraphy. *See specific type*
sCJD. *See* Sporadic Creutzfeldt-Jakob
      disease
SCL-70 (scleroderma) antibody, 840*t*, 846
SCLC. *See* Small cell carcinoma of lung
SCLE. *See* Subacute cutaneous lupus
      erythematosus
Sclera, lacerations of, 197–198, 197*f*
Scleritis, in granulomatosis with
      polyangiitis, 857, 857*f*
Scleroderma (systemic sclerosis), 840*t*,
      845–847
  dysphagia in, 605*t*
  limited. *See* CREST syndrome
  linear, 846
  pulmonary hypertension in, 430, 431,
      846, 847
  Raynaud phenomenon and, 844, 845,
      846

Scleroderma (anti-SCL-70) antibody, 840*t*, 846

Scleroderma renal crisis, 846, 846–847

Scleromyxedema, 846

Sclerosing panniculitis, 138

Sclerotherapy
for esophageal varices, 615
for GI bleeding, 596
for hemorrhoids, 670
for varicose veins, 487

SCN1A gene, in familial hemiplegic migraine, 977

SCN4A gene, in periodic paralysis, 1049

Scoliosis, 1692
neck pain and, 1696

Scombroid poisoning, 1603, 1604*t*

Scopolamine
for nausea and vomiting, 87, 583
overdose/toxicity of, 1101, 1590

Scorpion stings, **1605**
myocarditis caused by, 413*t*

"Screamer's nodules," 234

Screening tests. *See specific type and disorder and* Genetic testing; Prenatal testing

Scrofula, 239, **1482**

Scrotal mass. *See* Testicular cancer

Scrotal pruritus, 147, 148

Scrotal swelling, in filariasis, 1544

Scrub typhus, 1429*t*, **1431–1432**

Scuba/deep sea diving
dysbarism/decompression sickness and, 204, 1572–1573
eustachian tube dysfunction/otic barotrauma and, 203, 204

Scurvy, 1277

SDH (succinate dehydrogenase) mutations, in pheochromocytoma/ paraganglioma, 1179, 1180, 1182

Seafood, preventable disease/deaths associated with low intake of, 3*t*

Seafood poisonings, **1603–1604**, 1604*t*

Seasonal affective disorder, 1075, 1079, 1084

Seasonal influenza, **1410–1417**, 1414–1415*t*. *See also* Influenza

Seborrheic dermatitis, **110–111**, 110*f*
atopic dermatitis differentiated from, 105
in HIV infection/AIDS, 1343
pityriasis rosea differentiated from, 109
tinea differentiated from, 113

Seborrheic keratoses, **103**, 103*f*

Second-degree burn, 1568

Second-degree heart block, 377, 399. *See also* Atrioventricular (heart) block

Second-hand smoke. *See* Passive smoking

Second impact syndrome, 1030

Secretory diarrhea, 588*t*, 592, 594. *See also* Diarrhea

Sectral. *See* Acebutolol

Secukinumab, for psoriasis, 108

Sedative-hypnotics, 1054*t*
antidepressant drugs and, 1078*t*, 1083*t*
overdose/toxicity of, **1594**
sleep cycle affected by, 1054*t*, 1088–1089

Sedentary lifestyle. *See* Lifestyle, sedentary

Segmental myoclonus, 1017

Segond fracture, 1709

Seizures, **983–990**, 984*t*, 987–988*t*. *See also specific type and* Epilepsy; Status epilepticus
absence (petit mal), 984–985, 984*t*
alcohol withdrawal, 989, 1093, 1098
antidepressant use and, 1082, 1580*t*, 1590, 1606
antipsychotic use and, 1072
atonic (epileptic drop attacks), 984*t*, 985
cerebral arteriovenous malformations causing, 1001
classification of, 983–985, 984*t*
clonic, 984*t*, 985
cognitive disorders/delirium and, 983, 1102*t*
deep brain/thalamic stimulation for, 989
degenerative disorders and, 983
differential diagnosis of, 985–986
drug therapy for, 986–989, 987–988*t*. *See also* Anticonvulsant therapy
flumazenil use and, 1578, 1595
focal, 984, 984*t*
generalized, 984–985, 984*t*
in hypocalcemia, 897
hysterical, 986, 1058
infection/infectious diseases and, 983
intracranial tumors causing, 983, 1003
isoniazid causing, 1580*t*, 1596
myoclonic, 984*t*, 985
panic disorder differentiated from, 986
in poisoning/drug overdose, **1580**, 1580*t*
posttraumatic, 983, 1031
during pregnancy, **820**
eclampsia and, 808, 809, 810
psychogenic nonepileptic (pseudoepileptic), 986, 1058
schizophrenia differentiated from, 1068
serial, 985
solitary, 989
surgical management of, 989
theophylline use and, 1580*t*, 1605
tonic, 984*t*, 985
tonic-clonic (grand mal), 984*t*, 985
transient ischemic attacks differentiated from, 986, 992
vagal nerve stimulation for, 989
vascular disorders and, 983

Selective estrogen receptor modulators (SERMs), 1205–1206. *See also* Tamoxifen
in breast cancer prevention/treatment, 739, 755*t*
in cancer chemotherapy, 1669–1670*t*
estrogen replacement therapy, 1205–1206
for gynecomastia, 1195
for osteoporosis, 1163

Selective immunoglobulin A deficiency, **881–882**, 881*t*

Selective serotonin reuptake inhibitors. *See* Serotonin-selective reuptake inhibitors

Selegiline
overdose/toxicity of, 1078*t*
for parkinsonism, 1013
transdermal, 1078*t*, 1082

Selenium, for tinea versicolor, 114

Self-care
assessment of ability to manage, 55–56
asthma management and, 246–248
clinician, providing end-of-life care and, 89
diabetes management and, 1233

Self-examination, breast, breast lump identification/cancer screening and, 14*t*, 740

Self-monitoring of blood glucose
in diabetes mellitus, 1216–1217, 1233, 1234
prebreakfast hyperglycemia and, 1234
in pregnant patient, 818
in functional alimentary hypoglycemia diagnosis, 1256
in insulinoma diagnosis, 1253–1254

Self-mutilation, 1059

Self neglect, in elderly, **70–71**, 71*t*

Self-treatment, malaria prophylaxis and, 1520

Selzentry. *See* Maraviroc

Semantic variant primary progressive aphasia, 1019*t*

Semen analysis
in infertility workup, 783, 968, 969, 969*f*
in Klinefelter syndrome, 1190

Semicircular canal dehiscence, vertigo and, 213

Seminal emission, loss of (anejaculation), 966, 1063. *See also* Erectile dysfunction/impotence

Seminomas, 1655, 1656, 1657

SEN-V virus, 682

Sengstaken-Blakemore tube, for esophageal varices, 615

Senile amyloidosis, 538

Senile freckles. *See* Lentigines

Senna, 585*t*, 586

Sennetsu fever, 1435

SENSA tests. *See* Fecal occult blood testing

Sensorimotor peripheral neuropathy. *See* Neuropathies

Sensory conduction velocity studies. *See* Conduction velocity studies

Sensory/sensorineural hearing loss, 200, 201, **207–209**. *See also* Hearing loss
sudden, 200, 201, 208

Sensory neuronopathy, cancer-related, 1008

Sentinel acute pancreatitis event (SAPE), 731

Sentinel loop, in pancreatitis, 727

Sentinel lymph node biopsy
in breast cancer, 750, 750*f*
arm edema avoidance and, 759
timing of/neoadjuvant therapy and, 753–754
in melanoma, 104

Sentinel pile, 672

Seoul virus, 1403

Sepsis/septic shock, 494, 494t, 495, 497. *See also* Bacteremia; Infection/infectious diseases
ARDS and, 320
bleeding and, 547t
catheter-related, 1285, 1290, 1291, 1294, 1295
contaminated blood transfusion causing, 543
corticosteroid use in, 497
DIC and, 553
E coli causing, 1311t
early goal-directed therapy of, 496
gram-negative, **1467–1468**
in listeriosis, 1457
in pyelonephritis, 956
thrombocytopenia and, **556**
vibrios causing, 1312t, 1472
Septal hematoma, in nasal trauma, 222
Septal hypertrophy, asymmetric, 418
Septic (nongonococcal acute bacterial) arthritis, **867–868**, 1314t
in drug users, 867, 1304
Septic bursitis, 1700
Septic thrombophlebitis, 488, 1314t
anaerobic infections and, 1314t, 1478
catheter-associated infection and, 488, 1295, 1314t
in drug user, 1304
perforated appendicitis and, 642
portal vein, noncirrhotic portal hypertension and, 713
sigmoid sinus/otitis media and, 206
Septic transfusion reaction, 543
Septo-optic dysplasia (de Morsier syndrome), 1108
Septoplasty, nasal, for sleep apnea, 317
Septra. *See* Trimethoprim-sulfamethoxazole
Sequential organ failure assessment (SOFA) score
in liver failure, 685
in pancreatitis, 726
Sequoiosis, 308t
Serax. *See* Oxazepam
Serial seizures, 985. *See also* Seizures
Serine protease 1 (*PRSS1*) gene, in chronic pancreatitis, 731
Serine protease inhibitor (*SPINK1*) gene, in chronic pancreatitis, 731
Serine protease inhibitors, for hepatitis C, 689, 690, 690t, 691
Serine threonine kinase, gene for, in Peutz-Jeghers syndrome, 667
SERMs. *See* Selective estrogen receptor modulators
Seronegative spondyloarthropathies, **863–867**. *See also specific type*
rheumatoid arthritis differentiated from, 836, 864
Seronegative synovitis, remitting, with non-pitting edema, 875
Seroquel. *See* Quetiapine
Serotonin receptor agonists, for irritable bowel syndrome, 646–647
Serotonin 5-HT$_3$ receptors, in nausea and vomiting, 580, 1672
Serotonin 5-HT$_3$-receptor-blocking agents. *See also* Serotonin-selective reuptake inhibitors

for irritable bowel syndrome, 646–647
for nausea and vomiting, 582, 582t
chemotherapy-induced, 582, 582t, 1672–1673, 1673
Serotonin-selective reuptake inhibitors (SSRIs), 1078t, 1079–1081
for anxiety/stress disorders, 1055, 1055–1056, 1056
for dementia, 1021
for depression, 1077, 1078t, 1079–1081
in elderly, 61
for hot flushes/menopausal symptoms, 795, 1202
hyponatremia caused by, 886
for irritable bowel syndrome, 646
MAOI interaction and, 1083t
for OCD, 1057
overdose/toxicity of, 1078t, 1079–1081, 1580
ophthalmic, 177t
suicidal, 1077
for panic disorders/attacks, 1055, 1055–1056, 1056
for personality disorders, 1065
for phobic disorders, 1056
platelet function affected by, 558t
during pregnancy, 1081
for premenstrual syndrome, 765
for psychosexual disorders, 1063, 1064
for PTSD, 1052
serotonin syndrome caused by, 35, 1080, 1580
sexual side effects of, 1079
withdrawal from, 1080–1081
Serotonin (serotonin-selective) norepinephrine reuptake inhibitors (SNRIs/SSNRIs), 1078t, 1079–1081
for anxiety/stress disorders, 1054, 1055, 1056
for depression, 1077, 1078t, 1079–1081
MAOI interaction and, 1083t
for neuropathic pain, 83t, 84, 1079
overdose/toxicity of, 1078t, 1079–1081
ophthalmic, 177t
for phobic disorders, 1056
withdrawal from, 1080–1081
Serotonin syndrome, 35, 36, 1080, 1580, 1606
Serous otitis media, **203–204**
in HIV infection/AIDS, 214
nasopharyngeal carcinoma and, 203, 223
Serous retinal detachment, 183, 184
Serrated polyps/adenomas, 665, **665–666**
colorectal cancer and, 665, 666, 1637, 1640
Serratia, 1312t
Sertaconazole, 99t
Sertoli cell tumors, gynecomastia and, 1195
Sertoli cells, hypogonadism and, 1190
Sertraline, 61, 1077, 1078t, 1079–1081. *See also* Serotonin-selective reuptake inhibitors
in cardiovascular disease, 1080
levothyroxine therapy affected by, 1123
overdose/toxicity of, 1078t, 1606
ophthalmic, 177t
for panic attacks, 1055

during pregnancy, 1081
for PTSD, 1052
Serum-ascites albumin gradient (SAAG), 601t, 602, 604, 701. *See also* Ascites
in shock liver/cardiogenic liver injury, 713
Serum eye drops, for dry eye, 168
Serum osmolality, 884. *See also* Osmolality
Serum sickness/serum-sickness-like syndromes, 879t
penicillin allergy causing, 1318
urticarial vasculitis in, 134
Serzone. *See* Nefazodone
Sessile serrated polyps, 665
Sestamibi scintigraphy
in hyperparathyroidism, 1155
in hyperthyroidism, 1128
Sevelamer, for hyperphosphatemia, 901, 927
Severe fever with thrombocytopenia syndrome, 1399
Sex chromosomes. *See* X chromosome; Y chromosome
Sex steroid replacement therapy. *See* Estrogen (hormone) replacement therapy; Testosterone replacement therapy
Sexual arousal disorders, 1062, 1063–1064. *See also* Sexual dysfunction
in female, 782
Sexual assault. *See* Sexual violence
Sexual behavior. *See also* Sexually transmitted diseases
gonococcal arthritis and, 868
hepatitis/hepatitis vaccination and, 680, 683, 684, 1326
HIV infection/AIDS and, 1330, 1346, 1349
postexposure prophylaxis and, 4, 1303, 1346
preexposure prophylaxis and, 4, 1303, 1346
STDs and, 4, 1302
syphilis and, 1488, 1491
Zika virus transmission and, 1406
Sexual desire disorders, 1063, 1064
in female, 782, 1064
Sexual dysfunction
drugs causing, 966
antidepressants, 1064, 1079, 1082
antipsychotics, 1071
lithium, 1086
in female, **781–783**
in male, **965–968**. *See also* Erectile dysfunction/impotence
psychologic/psychosexual, 966, 966–967, 967, 1063, 1064
Sexual identity, disorders of, 1062–1063, 1063–1064
Sexual intercourse
HIV infection/AIDS transmission and, 1330, 1346
postexposure prophylaxis and, 1303, 1346
painful (dyspareunia), 782, 782–783
unlawful (statutory rape), 793

Sexual intercourse (*Cont.*):
  unprotected, emergency/postcoital
      contraception and, 791
    IUD for, 789
    sexual violence (rape/sexual assault)
        and, 791, 793, 794, 1302
Sexual pain disorders, in female, 782,
      782–783
Sexual violence (rape/sexual assault),
      792–794
  gamma-hydroxybutyrate ("date rape"
      drug) use and, 1595
  STDs and, 793–794, 1302
Sexually transmitted diseases,
      1301–1303. *See also specific*
      disease
  drug use and, 1304
  epididymitis, 955t, 959–960, 1316t
  HIV testing in patients with, 1302
  during pregnancy, **823**
  prevention of, 4, 1302–1303. *See also*
      Condoms
  reactive arthritis and, 866
  screening for, 1302–1303
  sexual violence (rape/sexual assault)
      and, 793–794, 1302
  syphilis/syphilis testing and, 1488,
      1491
  Zika virus infection as, 1406
Sézary cells, in cutaneous T-cell
      lymphoma (mycosis
      fungoides), 116
Sézary syndrome, 116
  exfoliative dermatitis/erythroderma
      and, 117
SFTS. *See* Severe fever with
      thrombocytopenia
      syndrome
SGLT2 gene, in nondiabetic (renal)
      glycosuria, 1214
SGLT2 inhibitors, 1222t, 1227–1228,
      1235f, 1236
SGOT. *See* Aspartate aminotransferase
SGPT. *See* Alanine aminotransferase
Shagreen patches, in tuberous sclerosis,
      1010
Shared epitope, in rheumatoid arthritis,
      834
Shaver disease, 307t
Shawl sign, 848
Sheehan syndrome, 1109
Sheep liver fluke, 1533–1534
Shift work sleep disorder, 1090
Shiga-toxin–mediated HUS, 550, 551,
      551t, 589
Shiga-toxin–producing *E coli*, 589, 1305,
      1306t, 1470–1471. *See also*
      Escherichia coli O157:H7
  hemolytic-uremic syndrome caused by,
      550, 551, 551t, 589, 1471
Shigella dysenteriae/flexneri/sonnei
      (shigellosis/bacillary
      dysentery), 588t, 589, 1305,
      1307t, 1312t, 1315t, 1342,
      1470
Shin spots, diabetic, 1242
Shingles. *See* Herpes zoster
Shiny corner sign, 864
Shock, **493–498**, 494t
  anaphylactic. *See* Anaphylaxis/
      anaphylactic shock

cardiogenic, 371, 372f, 378, 493–494,
      494t, 495, 497
  dengue, 1401, 1402
  distributive, 494, 494t, 495, 496–497,
      497
  in heat stroke, 1563
  hypovolemic/hemorrhagic, 493, 494t,
      495
  in infectious myocarditis, 414
  in myocardial infarction, 378, 494
  neurogenic, 494, 494t, 495
  obstructive, 494, 494t, 495
  pheochromocytoma/
      pheochromocytoma removal
      and, 1182
  rewarming, 1564
  septic. *See* Sepsis/septic shock
  vasodilatory (distributive), 494, 494t,
      495, 496–497, 497
Shock liver, 712–713
Shock wave lithotripsy
  for renal stones, 965
  for ureteral stones, 965
Short-acting insulin, 1229–1230, 1229t.
      See also Insulin therapy
Short bowel syndrome, **637**
Short stature
  in GH deficiency, 1109
  in Turner syndrome, 1207, 1208
Shortness of breath. *See* Dyspnea
Shoulder, **1685–1692**, 1686–1688t
  dislocated/unstable, 1688t, **1690–1691**
    atraumatic, 1690, 1691
  frozen (adhesive capsulitis),
      1691–1692
  rotator cuff tears and, 1686–1687t,
      1689–1690
  subacromial impingement syndrome
      and, **1685–1689**, 1687t
Shoulder apprehension test, 1688t, 1690
Shoulder-hand syndrome, 874
Shoulder stability/instability, 1688t,
      1690–1691
  atraumatic dislocation and, 1690, 1691
SHOX gene, in Turner syndrome, 1208
Shunt procedures, portosystemic. *See*
      Portosystemic shunts
Shy-Drager syndrome (multisystem
      atrophy)
  dysautonomia and, 990
  parkinsonism and, 1012
SIADH. *See* Syndrome of inappropriate
      ADH secretion
Sialadenitis, **231**
Sialolithiasis, **231–232**
Siberian/Siberian Asian tick typhus,
      1429t, 1434
Sick role, chronic pain disorders and,
      1060
Sick sinus syndrome, **399**
Sickle cell anemia/syndromes, **511–513**,
      512t
  genetic/prenatal/screening testing for,
      511, 800
  osteomyelitis and, 870
  in pregnancy, 800, 815
  renal dysfunction associated with, **951**
Sickle cell glomerulopathy, 951
Sickle cell retinopathy, 191
Sickle cell trait, 512t, **513**
Sickle thalassemia, 512, 512t, **513**

Siderosis, 307t
"Sigmoid esophagus," 617
Sigmoid sinus thrombosis, otitis media
      and, 206
Sigmoidoscopy
  in antibiotic-associated colitis, 648
  in cancer screening/polyp
      identification, 14t, 15, 1642
  in GI bleeding, 598
  in ulcerative colitis, 658
Signal recognition particle (SRP)
      antibody, in polymyositis/
      dermatomyositis, 848, 848t
Significant others. *See* Family/significant
      others
SIL. *See* Squamous intraepithelial lesions
Sildenafil
  adverse ophthalmic effects of, 177t
  for erectile dysfunction diagnosis/
      treatment, 967, 1064
    antidepressant-induced, 1064, 1079
    in diabetes, 1241
  for high-altitude illness treatment/
      prevention, 1575
  nitrate/nitroglycerin contraindications
      and, 375, 967, 1064, 1241
Silent thyroiditis, 1125, 1131, 1135. *See*
      also Subacute (de Quervain)
      thyroiditis
Silent ulcers, 624
Silibinin/silymarin, for mushroom
      poisoning, 685–686, 1601
Silicone gel breast implants. *See* Breast
      implants
Silicosis, 307, 307t
Silo-filler's disease, 309
Silodosin
  adverse ophthalmic effects of, 183
  for benign prostatic hyperplasia, 974t
Siltuximab, 1667t
Silymarin/silibinin, for mushroom
      poisoning, 685–686, 1601
Simbrinza. *See* Brimonidine/
      brinzolamide
Simeprevir, for hepatitis C, 689, 690t, 691,
      1342
Simple drug eruptions, 161
Simple partial seizures (focal seizures
      without impairment of
      consciousness), 984, 984t.
      See also Seizures
Simple/solitary renal cysts, **949**, 949t
Simultagnosia, intracranial tumors
      causing, 1005
Simvastatin, 353, 355t, 1264, 1265t. *See*
      also Statins
  in combination therapy, 1266
  for polycystic ovary syndrome, 1198
  protease inhibitor interactions and,
      1356
Sin Nombre virus, 1403
Sinemet. *See* Carbidopa/levodopa
Sinequan. *See* Doxepin
"Singer's nodules," 234
Single photon emission computed
      tomography (SPECT)
  in angina, 358
  in hyperparathyroidism, 1155
  in thyroid cancer follow-up, 1146
  in Zollinger-Ellison syndrome/
      gastrinoma, 632

Singultus (hiccups), **583**
Sinoatrial exit block (sick sinus
    syndrome), **399**
Sinonasal inflammatory disease, **223–224**
Sinus arrest (sick sinus syndrome), **399**
Sinus arrhythmia, **384**
Sinus bradycardia, **384**. *See also*
    Bradycardia/
    bradyarrhythmias
    in myocardial infarction, 370, 377
    persistent (sick sinus syndrome), **399**
    in poisoning/drug overdose, 1579*t*
Sinus tachycardia, **384–385**. *See also*
    Tachycardia/tachyarrhythmia
    hyperthyroidism, 1127, 1133
    in myocardial infarction, 370
    in poisoning/drug overdose, 1579*t*
Sinus venosus atrial septal defect, 325
Sinuses. *See* Paranasal sinuses
Sinusitis, **214–215**, **215–218**, 217*t*, 1315*t*
    in aspergillosis, 218, 1555
    bacterial, **215–218**, 217*t*, 1315*t*. *See*
        also Rhinosinusitis, acute
        bacterial
    fungal/molds causing, **218**
    Haemophilus causing, 1466
    in HIV infection/AIDS, 218, 1339
    hospital-associated, 216
    invasive fungal, **218**
    in mucormycosis, 218, 1556
    nasopharyngeal/paranasal sinus cancer
        and, 223
    orbital cellulitis and, 195, 217
    viral (common cold), **214–215**,
        1420–1421
Sinusoidal obstruction syndrome, 697,
    711–712
Sipple syndrome. *See* Multiple endocrine
    neoplasia (MEN), MEN 2
Sipuleucel-T, 1670*t*
    for prostate cancer, 1650
Sirolimus, 362, 1213
SIRS. *See* Systemic inflammatory
    response syndrome
Sister Joseph/Sister Mary Joseph nodule,
    1621, 1630
Sitagliptin, 1222*t*, 1227
    with metformin, 1227, 1228
    overdose/toxicity of, 1227, 1595
Siti (endemic syphilis), **1498–1499**
Situational (stress and adjustment)
    disorders, **1050–1051**. *See*
        also Adjustment (situational)
        disorders
Sixth disease (exanthema subitum),
    1367*t*, 1377
Sixth nerve paralysis, 194
Sjögren syndrome, 840*t*, **850–851**
SJS. *See* Stevens-Johnson syndrome
SJS/TEN overlap. *See* Stevens-Johnson
    syndrome/toxic epidermal
    necrolysis (SJS/TEN) overlap
Skeletal hyperostosis, diffuse idiopathic
    (DISH), 864, 1242
Skeletal system disorders. *See* Bone;
    Musculoskeletal disorders
Skin
    anaerobic flora of, 1478
    biopsy of, in polyarteritis nodosa, 856
    caustic/corrosive injuries of, 1581,
        1586–1587, 1587

in chronic venous insufficiency, 32, 33,
    489, 489*f*
decontamination of, **1581**
    for caustic/corrosive burns, 1581,
        1586–1587, 1587
disorders of. *See specific type and* Skin
    cancer; Skin disorders
dry, emollients for, 95, 99–100*t*
hardening of. *See* Scleroderma
preoperative preparation of, in
    infection control, 1295
Skin bends, 1573
Skin cancer. *See also specific type*
    basal cell carcinoma, **143**, 143*f*
    ear involvement and, 201
    eyelid involvement and, 165–166
    melanoma, **103–104**, 104*f*, 1625*t*
    squamous cell carcinoma, **144**, 144*f*
    sun exposure/avoidance and, 13,
        100–101, 143, 144
Skin disorders, **95–163**, 96*t*. *See also*
    under Cutaneous and
    Dermatitis
    anaerobic infections, **1479–1480**, 1480*f*
    anthrax, 1454, 1455, 1456
    arthropod infestations, **150–151**
    in Behçet syndrome, 862
    in blastomycosis, 1556
    blistering (bullous), 96*t*, **139–140**
    cancer. *See* Skin cancer
    candidal, **132–133**, 132*f*, 1343
    in Chagas disease (chagoma), 1509
    chemotherapy causing, **1673–1674**
    in coccidioidomycosis, 1550, 1551
    cryptococcal, 1553
    cystic, 96*t*
    in diabetes mellitus, 1214, 1242
    in drug users, 1303
    drugs causing (dermatitis
        medicamentosa/drug
        eruption), **161–163**,
        162–163*t*, **880**
        as complication of topical therapy,
            101
        drug-induced hypersensitivity
            syndrome and, 161, 163, 880
    in electrical burns, 1570, 1570–1571
    epidermal inclusion cysts, **154**
    erosive, 96*t*
    erythemas, 96*t*
    in frostbite, 1566
    in frostnip/chilblain, 1565
    fungal infections, **111–115**, 111*f*, 112*f*,
        113*f*. *See also* Tinea
        in HIV infection/AIDS, 1343
    in gonococcal arthritis, 1475, 1476
    in Henoch-Schönlein purpura, 861,
        937, 938*f*
    in HIV infection/AIDS, 1343–1344
    in leishmaniasis, 1510, 1510–1511, 1511*f*
    in leprosy, 1484
    in Lyme disease, **136**, 137*f*, 1502, 1503,
        1504, 1505*t*
    morbilliform, 96*t*
    in mycetoma, 1557
    mycobacterial infections, **1482**
    in niacin deficiency, 1276
    in nocardiosis, 1481
    nodules, 96*t*
        inflammatory, **151–155**
        violaceous to purple, **144–146**

in onchocerciasis, 1545
papules, 96*t*, **140–144**
    violaceous to purple, **144–146**
in paracoccidioidomycosis, 1556
in pheochromocytoma/paraganglioma,
    1180*f*
photodermatitis, 96*t*, **154–155**. *See also*
    Photodermatitis
pigmentary, **157–158**, 157*f*. *See also*
    Hyperpigmentation;
    Hypopigmentation
    drugs causing, 158, 163*t*
    in hypercarotenosis, 1277
pigmented lesions, 96*t*, **101–104**
    in polyarteritis nodosa, 856
pruritus (itching) and, 96*t*, **146–147**.
    See also specific cause
pustular, 96*t*, **126–128**
    in sarcoidosis, 292, 293*f*
scaling, 96*t*, **104–118**
    in schistosomiasis, 1532
    in sporotrichosis, 1557
staphylococcal infections, 1443, 1443*t*,
    1447–1449, 1448*f*
    in HIV infection/AIDS, 1343
streptococcal infections, **1442–1443**,
    1443*t*
in syphilis, 1489*t*, 1492–1493, 1493*f*.
    See also Chancre; Gummas
treatment of, **95–101**, 96–100*t*
    adverse ophthalmic effects of drugs
        in, 179*t*
    complications of, 101
ulcers, 96*t*, **155–157**, 156*f*
    in diabetes, 156, 475, 476, 1239
    in paracoccidioidomycosis, 1556
    in polyarteritis, 856
    pressure, **68–69**, 68*t*
    in tibial/pedal occlusive disease, 475,
        476
    venous insufficiency/varicose veins/
        lower extremity occlusive
        disease and, 32, 33, **155–157**,
        156*f*, 489, 490. *See also*
        Venous insufficiency/stasis
    in uremia, 924*t*
vesicular, 96*t*, **118–123**
weeping/crusted, 96*t*, **123–126**
    drying agents for, 95
Skin test anergy
    in HIV infection/AIDS, 1336, 1348
    measles causing, 1379
    tuberculin skin test and, 279
Skin testing, for drug allergies, 877,
    1318
Skull
    fracture of, 1029, 1031. *See also* Head
        injury
        vertigo caused by, 212
    in Paget disease of bone, 1167
Skull base tumors, vocal fold paralysis
    caused by, 237
Skyla IUD, 789
SLE. *See* Systemic lupus erythematosus
Sleep, 1088
    abnormal behaviors during
        (parasomnias), **1090**
    age-related changes in, 1088
    breathing disorders and, 230–231, **316**,
        1089. *See also* Sleep apnea
        hypopnea

Sleep (*Cont.*):
  disorders of, **1088–1090**
  drugs for problems with, 1054*t*, 1089
Sleep apnea hypopnea, 230, 231, 316, **316–317**, 1089
  hypertension and, 316, 441
  in obesity-hypoventilation syndrome, 316
  obstructive, 230, 231, 316, **316–317**, 1089
  in polycystic ovary syndrome, 1196
  postoperative pulmonary complications and, 49
  pulmonary hypertension and, 302, 316, 430, 431
  testosterone replacement therapy and, 1193
Sleep attacks, in narcolepsy, 1089–1090
Sleep hygiene, 1089
Sleep panic attacks, 1053
Sleep paralysis, in narcolepsy, 1090
Sleep-wake disorders, **1088–1090**
Sleepiness, excessive, **1089–1090**
Sleeping sickness, **1507–1508**, 1508*t*
Sleeve gastrectomy, for obesity, 1272
Slow colonic transit, constipation and, 584, 584*t*
Sm antibody, in lupus/SLE, 115, 840*t*, 841, 841*t*
SMA. *See* Spinal muscular atrophy
SMAD4 mutation, in hereditary hemorrhagic telangiectasia, 1684
Small cell carcinoma of lung, 1609, 1612–1613, 1612*t*, 1623*t*. *See also* Lung cancer
  myasthenic syndrome and, 1046, 1609
  paraneoplastic syndromes associated with, 1609
  staging of, 1610
  treatment of, 1612–1613, 1612*t*
Small intestine. *See also under* Intestinal
  adenocarcinomas in, **1634**
    Crohn disease and, 654
  bacterial overgrowth in, 636–637. *See also* Bacterial overgrowth
  biopsy of, in celiac disease, 634
  carcinoid tumors in, 1185, 1186, **1634–1636**
  disorders of, **632–643**
    appendicitis, **641–643**
    malabsorption, **632–638**, 633*t*
    malignant tumors, **1634–1636**
    motility disorders, **638–641**. *See also* Intestinal obstruction
    protein-losing enteropathy, **643**
    tuberculosis, **643**
  familial adenomatous polyposis and, 667
  lymphomas in, **1634**
    Crohn disease and, 654, 1634
  resection of, short bowel syndrome and, 637
  sarcomas in, **1636**
Small intestine push enteroscopy, in GI/small bowel bleeding, 599
Small intestine transplantation, for short bowel syndrome, 637
Small lymphocytic lymphoma, 532
Smallpox (variola), 1368*t*, 1423
Smallpox (variola) vaccination, 1423

Smell, dysfunction in sense of, **220–221**
  intracranial tumors causing, 220
  in Kallmann syndrome, 1109, 1199, 1200
Smith antibody, in lupus/SLE, 115, 840*t*, 841, 841*t*
SMN (survival motor neuron) gene, in spinal muscular atrophies, 1033
Smoke inhalation, **305**
  burn injuries and, 305, 1568
  carbon monoxide poisoning and, 305, 1591
  corrosive acids and, 1587
  cyanide poisoning and, 24, 305
Smoking/tobacco use/smoking cessation, 6*t*, **7–9**, 8–9*t*, 9*t*
  in aortoiliac disease, 473
  asbestosis and, 307, 309
  cancer and, 7, 13, 1607. *See also specific type*
    bladder cancer, 1651
    laryngeal cancer, 235
    lung cancer, 7, 13, 1607, 1608
      screening for, 14*t*, 15, 286, 1611
    pancreatic/periampullary carcinoma and, 1620
    renal cell carcinoma and, 1654
  in COPD, 7, 257, 259
  coronary heart disease and, 6*t*, 7, 353
  Crohn disease and, 653
  environmental exposure and. *See* Passive smoking
  health hazards and, 7
  hypertension and, 441
  pancreatitis and, 730, 731
  pneumothorax and, 314, 315
  postoperative pulmonary complications and, 49
  during pregnancy, 799
  preventable disease/deaths and, 3*t*, 6*t*, 7
  sleep-wake disorders and, 1088
  thromboangiitis obliterans (Buerger disease) and, 480
  thyroid eye disease flares and, 195
  ulcerative colitis and, 658, 723–724
  vocal fold changes and, 234, 235
Smoldering multiple myeloma, 535, 536
Snake bites, 1581*t*, **1604–1605**
  myocarditis caused by, 413*t*
Sneddon syndrome, 863
Sniffing (solvents/gases), 1101, 1598, 1602
Snip biopsy, for wart removal, 141–142
Snoring, **230–231**
  in sleep apnea hypopnea, 230, 231, 316
"Snow blindness," 198
SNRIs. *See* Serotonin (serotonin-selective) norepinephrine reuptake inhibitors
Social behavior, in schizophrenia/psychotic disorders, 1067
Social challenges, for terminally ill/dying patient, 92, 92*t*
Social phobias, 1053, 1056
Sodium
  dietary, 1279
    hypertension and, 441, 445, 446*t*
    preventable disease/deaths associated with high intake of, 3*t*

requirements for in nutritional support, 1282
  restriction of. *See* Sodium-restricted diet
  urinary stone formation and, 962, 963
disorders of concentration of, **885–891**, 885*f*, 887*t*. *See also* Hypernatremia; Hyponatremia
  in fluid management, 911*t*. *See also* Saline
  in hyponatremia treatment, 888, 888–889
Sodium bicarbonate. *See* Bicarbonate
Sodium channel blocking drugs, for arrhythmias, 381, 382*t*
Sodium deficit, calculation of, 889
Sodium-glucose cotransporter (*SGLT2*) gene, in nondiabetic (renal) glycosuria, 1214
Sodium-glucose cotransporter (SGLT2) inhibitors, 1222*t*, 1227–1228, 1235*f*, 1236
Sodium ipodate. *See* Ipodate sodium
Sodium nitrite, for cyanide poisoning, 1581*t*, 1593
Sodium nitroprusside. *See* Nitroprusside
Sodium oxybate. *See* Gamma-hydroxybutyrate
Sodium phosphate enema, 585*t*
Sodium polystyrene sulfonate, for hyperkalemia, 894–895, 895*t*
Sodium-restricted diet, 1279
  for chronic kidney disease, 926, 929
  in cirrhosis, 701
  for heart failure, 410
  for hypertension, 441, 445, 446*t*, 926
  for nephrotic syndrome/nephrotic spectrum disorders, 942
  for urinary stones, 962, 963
Sodium stibogluconate (antimony), for leishmaniasis, 1511–1512
Sodium sulfacetamide. *See* Sulfacetamide
Sodium thiosulfate, for cyanide poisoning, 1581*t*, 1593
SOFA score
  in liver failure, 685
  in pancreatitis, 726
Sofosbuvir, for hepatitis C, 689–690, 690*t*, 691, 1341, 1342
Soft diet, 1278–1279
Soft tissue infections, 1443*t*. *See also* Skin disorders
  anaerobic, **1479–1480**, 1480*f*
  in coccidioidomycosis, 1550, 1551
  mycobacterial, **1482**
  osteomyelitis caused by, 870–871
  staphylococcal, 1443*t*
  streptococcal, 1443*t*
Soft tissue sarcoma, 1625*t*
Solar lentigines (liver spots), 103, 158
Soles of feet
  tinea of, **113–114**, 113*f*
  vesiculobullous dermatitis of (pompholyx), **121–122**
    tinea differentiated from, 114, 122
Solitary pulmonary nodule, **287–288**
  metastatic disease and, 1614
Solitary/simple renal cysts, **949**, 949*t*
Solitary seizures, 989

Solitary thyroid nodule, toxic (thyroid adenoma), 1125, 1131
  in MEN, 1187t, 1188
Soluble liver antigen antibodies, in autoimmune hepatitis, 692, 693
Solvents, toxicity/abuse of, **1101**, 1598, 1602
Soma. *See* Carisoprodol
Soman (GD) poisoning, 1601–1602
Somatic cough syndrome ("psychogenic cough"), 21
Somatic symptom disorders (abnormal illness behaviors), **1058–1060**
  with predominant pain, 1059
Somatization disorders. *See* Somatic symptom disorders
Somatostatin/somatostatin analogs. *See also* Octreotide
  D cells secreting, 1185
  for esophageal varices, 615
  for gastroenteropancreatic neuroendocrine tumors, 1186, 1635
  for GH-secreting tumors/acromegaly/gigantism, 1116
  tumors secreting, 1185
Somatostatin receptor scintigraphy
  in ACTH-secreting tumors, 1174
  in gastroenteropancreatic neuroendocrine tumors, 1186
  for pheochromocytoma/paraganglioma identification, 1182
  in Zollinger-Ellison syndrome/gastrinoma, 632
Somatostatinomas, 1185, 1185–1186
  in MEN, 1188
Somatropin, 1112
Somatuline. *See* Lanreotide
Somnolence, excessive, **1089–1090**
Somogyi effect, 1234, 1234t
Sonata. *See* Zaleplon
SONIC staging system, in hepatic encephalopathy, 703
Sonography. *See* Ultrasonography
Sonohysterography, saline infusion, 763t
Sorafenib, 1668t
  for hepatocellular carcinoma, 1617–1618
  thyroiditis caused by, 1126
Sorbitol
  for constipation, 585t, 586
  diarrhea caused by, 591
Sore throat. *See* Pharyngitis
Sorivudine, for herpes zoster, 1370
Sotalol, 381, 382t, 383t
  for atrial fibrillation, 382t, 383t, 393
  for supraventricular tachycardia, 386
  toxicity of, 383t, 384
  for ventricular tachycardia, 382t, 383t
South African tick fever, 1429t
South American blastomycosis, **1556–1557**
Southern tick-associated rash illness (STARI), 1502
Spasmodic torticollis, 1016
Spastic paraparesis
  in cervical spondylosis, 1042
  tropical, 1396

Spasticity, **1025–1026**
  motor neuron lesions and, 1025, 1033, 1034
  spinal trauma and, 1031–1032
SPECT. *See* Single photon emission computed tomography
Spectazole. *See* Econazole
Sperm analysis, in infertility workup, 783, 968, 969, 969f
Spermatogenesis, 968
  hormone therapy for improvement of, 1112
  radioiodine therapy affecting, 1145
Spermicide, 790
  HIV infection/AIDS and, 790, 1346
  use with condom and, 791
Sphenoid sinusitis, 215–216
Spherocytes, in autoimmune hemolytic anemia, 514
Sphincter of Oddi dysfunction, 720
  pancreatitis and, 720, 726, 728, 729
Sphingolipid, in Gaucher disease, 1680
Spider bites, 150, **1605**
  myocarditis caused by, 413t
Spinal cord
  cavitation of (syringomyelia), **1032**
  compression of
    spinal trauma causing, 1031, 1032
    tumors causing, 1007, **1657–1658**
  dural arteriovenous fistulae of, 1002–1003
  epidural/subdural hemorrhage and, 1002
  infarction of, 1002, 1031
  lesions/tumors of, **1006–1007**
    cord compression by, 1007, **1657–1658**
    syringomyelia and, 1032
  subacute combined degeneration of, **1026**
  traumatic injury of, **1031–1032**
    drowning and, 1567
    head injury and, 1030
    syringomyelia and, 1032
  vascular diseases of, **1002–1003**
  vasculitis of (primary angiitis of central nervous system), **862–863**
Spinal cord stimulation, for angina, 363
Spinal dural arteriovenous fistulae, 1002–1003
Spinal muscular atrophy
  juvenile, 1034
  progressive, 1033
Spinal poliomyelitis, 1382
Spinal (neurogenic) shock, 494, 494t, 495
Spinal stenosis, **1694**
Spinal surgery
  for back pain, 1693–1694
  for lumbar disc herniation, 1695
  for spinal stenosis, 1694
Spinal tumors. *See* Spinal cord, lesions/tumors of
Spine. *See also* Spinal cord
  bamboo, 864
  disorders of, **1692–1697**, 1692t, 1693t, 1696t
    anogenital pruritus and, 147
    back pain and, **1692–1694**, 1692t, 1693t. *See also* Back pain
  cervical disk herniation, **1042**, 1043–1044f, 1696

  chest pain and, 359
  fractures, 1031–1032
  infection. *See* Vertebral osteomyelitis
  lumbar disk herniation, **1695**
  neck pain and, **1042**, 1043–1044f
  neurologic testing in, 1692t, 1696t
  stenosis, **1694**
  tuberculosis (Pott disease), **871–872**
  tumors. *See* Spinal cord, lesions/tumors of
  in Paget disease of bone, 1167
SPINK1 gene, in chronic pancreatitis, 731
Spinocerebellar degeneration, in vitamin E deficiency, 1025
Spinosad, for pediculosis, 150
Spiral (helical) CT. *See* Computed tomography; Helical (spiral) CT
Spiramycin, for toxoplasmosis during pregnancy, 1524
Spirillum minus, 1500
Spiritual challenges, for terminally ill/dying patient, 92–93, 93t
Spirochetal infections, 1312t, **1488–1506**. *See also specific type*
  anaerobic, 1478
  meningitis caused by, 1297t
  myocarditis in, 413t
  non-sexually transmitted, **1498–1499**
  syphilis, 1312t, 1316t, **1488–1498**
Spirometry. *See also* Pulmonary function tests
  in asthma/asthma exacerbation, 243f, 244t, 245–246, 245t, 251, 252, 254, 255f, 256f
  in COPD, 258, 258t
  in cough, 21
  in cystic fibrosis, 265
  incentive, postoperative pulmonary complication risk reduction and, 50
  lung cancer surgery and, 1610–1611
Spironolactone
  for adrenal hyperplasia, 1179
  for cirrhotic ascites, 701
  for heart failure, 406, 407, 411
    infarct-related, 376
  for hirsutism/virilization, 781, 1198
  for hypertension, 450t, 459
    with hydrochlorothiazide, 451t
  lithium interactions and, 1086, 1087t
Spirulina, toxicity of, 1593
Spleen, platelet sequestration in, 547t, **555**
Splenectomy, babesiosis and, 1522
Splenic vein thrombosis, noncirrhotic portal hypertension and, 713, 714
Splinter hemorrhages, in endocarditis, 1459, 1459f
Spondylitic heart disease, 863
Spondylitis
  alkaptonuria and, 1677
  ankylosing, **863–864**
  inflammatory bowel disease and, 867
  psoriatic, 865
Spondyloarthropathies, seronegative, **863–867**. *See also specific type*
  rheumatoid arthritis differentiated from, 836, 864

Spondylosis, cervical, **1042**
Spongiform encephalopathies/spongiosis (prion diseases), **1393–1395**
Spontaneous abortion, **803–805**
  in antiphospholipid antibody syndrome, 805, 815, 816, 841, 842, 843
  with IUD in place, 789–790
Spontaneous bacterial peritonitis, **602–604**, 702
Spontaneous fractures. *See* Pathologic fractures
Spontaneous pneumothorax, **314–315**. *See also* Pneumothorax
Spontaneous subarachnoid hemorrhage, 994*t*, **998–1000**. *See also* Subarachnoid hemorrhage
Spoon nails, 160
Sporadic Creutzfeldt-Jakob disease, 1394
Sporadic thyroiditis, painless (hashitoxicosis), 1125, 1135, 1136
Sporanox. *See* Itraconazole
Sporothrix schenckii (sporotrichosis), **1557**
Sports medicine, **1685–1717**. *See also* Musculoskeletal disorders
Spotted fever rickettsiosis, 1434
Spotted fevers, 1429*t*, **1432–1435**
Spousal abuse (domestic violence), 16, 1090–1091, 1091
Sprains, ankle, **1715–1717**, 1715*t*
  eversion (high), 1715*t*, **1716–1717**
  inversion, **1715–1716**, 1715*t*
Sprue, celiac. *See* Celiac disease
Sprycel. *See* Dasatinib
Spurling test, 1696, 1696*t*
Sputum/sputum examination
  blood found on (hemoptysis), **25–26**
  in lung cancer, 1609
  in nontuberculous mycobacterial infection, 285
  in pneumonia, 267, 268*t*, 269, 270, 274
  in solitary pulmonary nodule, 288
  in tuberculosis, 277, 277–278, 278*t*
SQSTM1 mutations, in Paget disease of bone, 1167
Squamous cell carcinoma
  of anus, 1643–1644
    in HIV infection/AIDS, 1344, 1644
  of bladder, 1651
  cervical, 771
  of ear canal, 203
  of esophagus, 1626
  intraepidermal (Bowen disease), **118**
  of larynx, **235–237**
    leukoplakia and, 235
  of lung, 1608–1609, 1612
  nasopharyngeal, 223, 1373
    inverted/schneiderian papillomas and, 223
  oral, 224, 225, 225*f*
  of skin, **144**, 144*f*
    actinic keratoses and, 118, 144
  of vulva, 775
Squamous intraepithelial lesions (SIL), 769*t*, 770
"Square-root" sign, 429
Squaric acid dibutylester, for wart removal, 142
Squatting, heart murmurs affected by, 335*t*

SRP antibody, in polymyositis/dermatomyositis, 848, 848*t*
SRS. *See* Somatostatin receptor scintigraphy
SRY gene, in testicular dysgenesis, 1190
SS-A/Ro antibody, 840*t*
  in lupus/SLE, 115, 840*t*
  in Sjögren syndrome, 840*t*, 850
SS-B/La antibody, 840*t*
  in lupus/SLE, 115, 840*t*
  in Sjögren syndrome, 840*t*, 850
SSc. *See* Scleroderma
SSI. *See* Surgical site infection
SSNRIs. *See* Serotonin (serotonin-selective) norepinephrine reuptake inhibitors
SSPE. *See* Subacute sclerosing panencephalitis
SSRIs. *See* Serotonin-selective reuptake inhibitors
St. Louis encephalitis, 1388
ST segment changes. *See also* Electrocardiogram
  in acute coronary syndromes/myocardial infarction, 27, 27*t*, 28, 366, 371. *See also* Myocardial infarction
  in angina, 356
ST-segment elevation myocardial infarction (STEMI), 26–27, 27, 27*t*, 28, 365, 369*t*, **370–381**, 372*f*, 373*t*. *See also* Myocardial infarction
Staggers, 1573
Stalevo. *See* Entacapone, with levodopa and carbidopa
Standing, heart murmurs affected by, 335*t*
Stanford V regimen, 534
Stannosis, 307*t*
Staphylococcus (staphylococcal infections), 1314*t*, **1447–1451**
  abscesses, 152, 1343, 1443*t*, 1447, 1448, 1448*f*
  arthritis, 867, 1314*t*
  atopic dermatitis and, 105, 106
  aureus, 1314*t*, 1315*t*, **1447–1451**
    methicillin-resistant (MRSA). *See* Community-associated methicillin-resistant *S aureus*; Methicillin-resistant *S aureus* (MRSA) infections
  bacteremia, **1449–1450**
  breast abscess/mastitis, 736, 813, 814
  carrier state and, **218**, 1447
    folliculitis and, 130–131
    furunculosis and, 153
    impetigo and, 124
    nasal vestibulitis and, 218
    surgical site infection associated with, 54, 1295
  cellulitis, 137, 138, 1315*t*, 1443*t*
  coagulase-negative, **1450–1451**
    endocarditis, 1450, 1458, 1462
  cohnii, 1450
  cystitis, 1315*t*
  diarrhea/food poisoning/gastroenteritis, 588*t*, 589, 1305, 1306*t*
  drug resistance and. *See* Methicillin-resistant *S aureus* (MRSA) infections

  endocarditis, 1314*t*, 1449, 1450, 1458, 1462, 1463
  epidermidis, 1450
  fever/neutropenia/chemotherapy and, 1314*t*
  folliculitis and, 130–131, 1343, 1448
  furunculosis/carbuncles and, 153, 1315*t*, 1343, 1443*t*, 1448, 1448*f*
  haemolyticus, 1450
  hominis, 1450
  impetigo, 124, 1343
  mastitis, 736, 813, 814
  meningitis, 1314*t*
  methicillin-resistant (MRSA). *See* Methicillin-resistant *S aureus* (MRSA) infections
  nasal vestibulitis, **218**
  non-penicillinase-producing, 1311*t*
  osteomyelitis, 870, 1314*t*, **1449**
  penicillinase-producing, 1311*t*
  pneumonia, 268*t*, 269, 273, 273*t*, 1314*t*
  saccharolyticus, 1450
  saprophyticus, 1315*t*, 1450
  septic thrombophlebitis, 488, 1314*t*
  of skin and soft tissues, 1443, 1443*t*, **1447–1449**, 1448*f*
    in HIV infection/AIDS, 1343
  toxic shock syndrome, **1450**, 1450*f*
  warnerii, 1450
STARI. *See* Southern tick-associated rash illness
Starlix. *See* Nateglinide
Starvation (protein–energy malnutrition), **1268–1269**
Stasis dermatitis, 33. *See also* Venous insufficiency/stasis
  cellulitis differentiated from, 138
  leg ulcers and, 156, 156*f*
Statins (HMG-CoA reductase inhibitors), 1263–1266, 1264*t*, 1265*t*
  adverse ophthalmic effects of, 177*t*
  in aortic stenosis, 342
  hepatotoxicity and, 1264
  high-, moderate, low-intensity, 353, 354*f*, 355*t*, 1263, 1264*t*
  for lipid modification/cardiovascular/heart disease prevention, 10, 353, 354*f*, 355*t*, 360*f*, 447, 1260, 1261, 1262, 1263–1266, 1264*t*, 1265*t*. *See also* Lipid-lowering therapy
  acute coronary syndromes and, 369, 1260
  cholesterol screening and, 1261, 1262
  combination therapy and, 1266
  heart failure and, 409
  in HIV infection/AIDS, 1356
  hypertension and, 447
  in older patients, 1262
  postinfarction, 369, 380
  in women, 1262
  perioperative, 46, 369
  for renal artery stenosis/renal vascular hypertension, 442
  rhabdomyolysis/myopathy/myositis caused by, 848*t*, 849, 852, 1264
Statoconia, detached, vertigo associated with, 212

Status epilepticus, 984t, 985
  alcohol withdrawal and, 989
  nonconvulsive, 990
  in theophylline overdose, 1605
  tonic-clonic, 985, 989–990
Statutory rape, 793
Stauffer syndrome, 1654
Stavudine (d4T), 1351t, 1353, 1355, 1360.
    See also Antiretroviral
    therapy
  lactic acidosis caused by, 1341, 1360
  lipid abnormalities caused by, 1345,
    1353, 1356
  neuropathy caused by, 1340
  resistance to, 1361
STDs. See Sexually transmitted diseases
Steatohepatitis, nonalcoholic (NASH),
    697, 698, 699
Steatorrhea, 633t. See also
    Malabsorption
  somatostatinoma and, 1185–1186
Steatosis, hepatic. See Fatty liver
STEC. See Shiga-toxin producing E coli
Stein-Leventhal syndrome. See Polycystic
    ovary syndrome
Stelara. See Ustekinumab
Stelazine. See Trifluoperazine
Stem cell disorders
  aplastic anemia, 516–517, 516t
  leukemias/myeloproliferative
    neoplasms, 519–531, 519t,
    520t
  multiple myeloma, 535–537
  paroxysmal nocturnal hemoglobinuria,
    509–510
Stem cell transplantation, 540–541. See
    also Bone marrow/stem cell
    transplantation
STEMI. See Myocardial infarction
"STEMI equivalent," 371
Steno-2 study, 1218–1219
Stensen duct, calculus formation in,
    231–232
Stent thrombosis, 362, 368, 373
  antiplatelet therapy for prevention of,
    362, 368, 373, 374, 376
Stents/stent grafts ("covered stents"). See
    also Endovascular surgery/
    prostheses
  for abdominal aortic aneurysm, 482
  carotid, 478
  coronary, 362–363. See also
    Percutaneous coronary
    intervention
    antiplatelet therapy for patient with,
      362, 373, 374
    preoperative/perioperative risks and,
      46–47
    thrombotic events and, 362, 368,
      373, 374, 376
  for renal artery stenosis/renal vascular
    hypertension, 442, 932
Stereotactic guided core needle biopsies,
    in breast cancer, 744
Stereotactic radiosurgery, for pituitary
    adenoma, 1116, 1119, 1175
Stereotypy, stimulant abuse and, 1068
Sterile pyuria, 951
Sterility. See Infertility
Sterilization, for birth control, 792
Steroid acne/folliculitis, 127, 130

Steroid-resistant nephrotic syndrome,
    943, 944
Steroid rosacea, 128
Steroidogenic enzyme defects
  amenorrhea and, 1199
  hirsutism/virilization and, 1196
Steroids. See Anabolic steroids;
    Corticosteroids
Stevens-Johnson syndrome, 135–136,
    135f
  drugs causing, 135, 136, 161, 162t, 163
  herpes simplex infection and, 1364
Stevens-Johnson syndrome/toxic
    epidermal necrolysis (SJS/
    TEN) overlap, 135
  drugs causing, 135–136, 161, 162t,
    163
Stibogluconate (antimony), for
    leishmaniasis, 1511–1512
Still disease, 838–839
Stimson procedure, 1690
Stimulant laxatives, 585t, 586
Stimulants
  abuse of, 1100, 1587–1588
    aggressive/violent/psychotic
      behavior and, 1068, 1090
    kindling and, 1092, 1100
    OTC medications and, 1587
  for dementia-related apathy, 1022
  for depression, 1077, 1082
  depression associated with withdrawal
    of, 1076
  for narcolepsy, 1090
Stings. See Insect bites/stings
Stippling (nail), 160
  in psoriasis, 107, 107f, 160, 865
Stivarga. See Regorafenib
STK11/LKB1 mutation, pancreatic/
    periampullary carcinoma
    and, 1620
Stomach disorders, 619–632. See also
    under Gastric and
    Gastrointestinal and Gastritis
  cancer, 1624t, 1629–1633. See also
    Gastric cancer
  in syphilis, 1495
Stomatitis
  herpes, 118, 227
  ulcerative (aphthous ulcers), 226–227,
    227f
    in Behçet syndrome, 861, 862
    in HIV infection/AIDS, 1341
Stool
  analysis of. See also Fecal occult blood
    testing
    in cancer screening/polyp
      identification, 14t, 15,
      1641–1642
    in diarrhea, 589, 592–593, 593, 648,
      1305, 1342
  blood in. See Diarrhea, bloody;
    Dysentery; Fecal occult
    blood testing
  impacted. See Fecal impaction
  incontinence of, 671–672. See also
    Fecal incontinence
  rice water, in cholera, 1471
Stool osmolality, 591
Stool softeners/surfactants, 585t
STOP questionnaire, 49
Storage pool disease, 556, 556–557

Straight leg raise test, 1693
Strawberry cervix, in Trichomonas
    vaginalis vaginitis, 767, 767f
Strawberry gallbladder, 719
Strength testing
  ankle, 1715t
  hip, 1702t
  shoulder/rotator cuff, 1686–1687t,
    1689
Strep throat. See Pharyngitis,
    streptococcal
Streptobacillary fever, rat-bite fever
    differentiated from, 1500
Streptobacillus moniliformis, 1500
Streptococcus (streptococcal infections),
    1311t, 1315t, 1441–1444
  abdominal infection, 1314t
  arthritis, 867, 1443
  brain abscess, 1314t
  cellulitis, 137, 138, 1315t, 1442–1443,
    1443t
  empyema, 1443
  endocarditis, 1314t, 1444, 1458,
    1461–1462
  erysipelas, 136, 137, 1315t, 1442–1443,
    1443t
  gallolyticus (bovis), 1444
    endocarditis caused by, 1444, 1462
  gangrene, cellulitis differentiated from,
    492
  glomerulonephritis after, 936
  group A. See Group A beta-hemolytic
    streptococcal infection
  group B. See Group B streptococcal
    infection
  impetigo, 124, 1315t, 1442–1443
  necrotizing fasciitis, 1444
    cellulitis differentiated from, 138,
      492, 1444
  non-group A, 1444
  otitis, 1315t
  pharyngitis. See Pharyngitis,
    streptococcal
  pneumonia, 268, 268t, 269–270,
    270–271, 271, 1314t, 1315t,
    1443
  pneumoniae (pneumococcal
    infections), 1311t, 1315t,
    1445–1446. See also
    Pneumococcal (Streptococcus
    pneumoniae) infections
    drug resistance and, 270–271, 271,
      1316, 1446
  pyogenes. See Group A beta-hemolytic
    streptococcal infection
  rheumatic fever and, 229, 422, 424,
    1441, 1442
  of skin, 1442–1443, 1443t
  toxic shock syndrome caused by,
    1444
  viridans, 1311t, 1444
    endocarditis caused by, 1314t, 1444,
      1458, 1461
Streptococcus thermophilus probiotic, for
    antibiotic-associated colitis,
    648
Streptokinase. See also Fibrinolytic
    therapy; Thrombolytic
    therapy
  for myocardial infarction, 373t, 374
  for pulmonary embolism, 300–301

Streptomycin, 281t. *See also*
        Aminoglycosides
    adverse ophthalmic effects of, 178t
    for MAC infection, 286
    for tuberculosis, 281t, 282, 283
        contraindications to in pregnancy,
            283
Stress cardiomyopathy. *See* Tako-Tsubo
        (stress/catecholamine-
        induced) cardiomyopathy
Stress disorders (psychiatric/psychologic),
        1050–1051
    depression and, 1050, 1052, 1053, 1075
    irritable bowel syndrome and, 644,
        645, 646, 647
    suicide and, 1076
    trauma and, **1051–1052**. *See also*
        Posttraumatic stress disorder
Stress echocardiography. *See*
        Echocardiography/Doppler
Stress fractures. *See* Pathologic fractures
Stress gastritis/ulcers, 319, 620, 620–621
Stress incontinence, 66, 67
Stress testing. *See also* Exercise testing
    in angina/chest pain evaluation, 28,
        357
    in athlete screening, 437
    postinfarction, 380
    preoperative, 46
Striae distensae, 1174
Striant. *See* Testosterone buccal tablets
Stribild (tenofovir/emtricitabine/
        elvitegravir/cobicistat), 1354t,
        1355, 1358, 1359t, 1360
Stridor, **232–233**
Stroke, **993–1003**, 994t
    in antiphospholipid antibody
        syndrome, 843, 995
    arteriovenous malformations causing,
        1000–1001
    aspirin/chemoprevention for, 6t,
        10–11, 997
    atrial fibrillation and, 388, 389t, 390,
        390t, 996
        anticoagulation in management/
            prevention of, 388, 389t, 390,
            390–393, 390t, 391t, 392f
    carotid intervention causing, 478
    carotid occlusion causing, 477–478,
        991, 993, 994t, 995
    cerebral infarct causing, 994t, **995–997**
    cerebrovascular occlusive disease
        causing, 477–478
    coma caused by, 995, 999, 1027, 1246t
    in endocarditis, 1459
    estrogen replacement therapy and, 796,
        1202, 1203, 1204
    hemorrhagic, 994t, 997–1003
        hypertension/hypertension
            management and, 444,
            468–469, 469t, 997, 998
    hypertension/hypertension
        management and, 6t, 10, 444,
        446–447, 449t, 464, 468–469,
        469t
        in emergencies/urgencies, 468–469,
            469t
    hypopituitarism and, 1108
    intracerebral hemorrhage causing,
        994t, **997–998**
    intracranial aneurysm causing, **1000**

intracranial venous thrombosis
        causing, **1002**
    ischemic (infarcts), 477, 994–997, 994t
        hypertension/hypertension
            management and, 444, 468,
            469t
        lacunar infarct causing, **933–935**, 994t
        oral contraceptive use and, 786
        patent foramen ovale and, 326
        postoperative, 52
        prevention of, **5–11**, 6t, 8–9t, 9t
        risk factors in, 5–6, 389t, 390–391, 390t
        seizures and, 983
        spinal cord vascular disease and,
            1002–1003
        subarachnoid hemorrhage causing,
            994t, **998–1000**
        transient ischemic attacks and, 477,
            992
        in varicella zoster infection, 1369, 1370
        vertebrobasilar occlusion causing, 994t,
            995
Stroke (heat), 1562, 1563
Stromal tumors (gastrointestinal stromal
        tumor/GIST), 1633–1634
Strongyloides fulleborni/stercoralis
        (strongyloidiasis), 588t, 592,
        1539–1540
Struma ovarii, 1126
Struvite urinary stones, 961, 962, 964
Strychnine poisoning, seizures caused by,
        1580t
Stunning, myocardial, 353
Stupor, **1026–1029**. *See also* Coma
Sturge-Weber syndrome, **1010**
Sty (external hordeolum), 164–165
Subacromial impingement syndrome,
        1685–1689, 1687t
    rotator cuff tears and, 1685, 1689
Subacute combined degeneration of
        spinal cord, **1026**
Subacute cutaneous lupus erythematosus
        (SCLE), 115–116, 839t, 840
Subacute lymphocytic thyroiditis (silent
        thyroiditis), 1125, 1131, 1135
Subacute measles encephalitis, 1378–1379
Subacute mountain sickness, 1574, **1575**
Subacute sclerosing panencephalitis, 1378
    myoclonus in, 1017
Subacute (de Quervain) thyroiditis, 1125,
        1128, 1131, 1135, 1136–1137
    hypothyroid phase in, 1119, 1125, 1135
Subarachnoid hemorrhage, 994t,
        998–1000. *See also* Stroke
    arteriovenous malformations/fistulae
        causing
        intracranial, 998, 1001
        spinal, 1002
    head injury and, 998
    headache in, 40, 41, 981, 998
    hypertension/hypertension
        management and, 468–469
    intracranial aneurysms causing, 998,
        1000
    oral contraceptive use and, 786
Subareolar abscess, 736–737, 737f
    nipple discharge in, 736
Subclavian steal syndrome, 992
Subclinical hyperthyroidism, 1128, 1134
Subclinical hypothyroidism, 1120
Subclinical thyroiditis, 1134

Subcutaneous insulin infusion,
        continuous, 1231–1232,
        1234. *See also* Insulin
        infusion pumps
Subcutaneous nodules
    in erythema nodosum, 151, 152, 152f
    in nocardiosis, 1481
    in rheumatic fever, 422, 423, 423t
    in rheumatoid arthritis, 835, 835f
        in coal workers (Caplan syndrome),
            307
        gouty tophi differentiated from, 831,
            836
    in sporotrichosis, 1557
Subdural hemorrhage/hematoma
    cerebral, 1030–1031, 1030t
    falls in elderly and, 64
    spinal, 1002
Suberosis, 308t
Submandibular glands. *See also* Salivary
        glands
    sialadenitis affecting, 231
    tumors of, 232
Submersion injury (drowning),
        1566–1567
Subscapularis tendon
    tears of, 1689
    testing strength of, 1686t, 1687t, 1689
Substance use disorders, **16–18**,
        1092–1101, 1096–1097f. *See
        also specific type and*
        Injection drug use
    aggressive/violent behavior and, 1068,
        1090, 1093
    cognitive disorders/delirium caused by
        withdrawal and, 1102t
    concerns about, pain management and,
        17, 73–74, 85
    febrile patient and, 1304
    hallucinations/hallucinosis caused by,
        1099, 1103
    HIV infection/AIDS and, 1304, 1332,
        1345, 1346, 1349
    infections and, **1303–1304**. *See also*
        Injection drug use, infections
        and
    overdoses. *See* Poisoning/drug
        overdose
    pregnancy and, 799
    prevention of/screening tests for,
        16–18, 18t
    PTSD and, 1052
    seizures and, 983, 985
    septic arthritis and, 867, 1304
    toxicology screen in, 1585
Subtalar tilt test, 1715–1716, 1715t
Subtentorial lesions. *See also* Brainstem
    coma or stupor caused by, 1028
Subungual lesions, malignant, 160
Succimer (DMSA)
    for arsenic poisoning, 1590
    for lead poisoning, 1597
    for mercury poisoning, 1599
Succinate dehydrogenase *(SDH)*
        mutations, in
        pheochromocytoma/
        paraganglioma, 1179, 1180,
        1182
Succinylcholine
    lithium interactions and, 1087t
    MAOI interactions and, 1083t

Succussion splash, in gastric outlet obstruction, 581, 631
Sucralfate
    for stress gastritis, 319, 621
    ventilator-associated pneumonia incidence affected by, 273
Sudan virus, 1397
Sudden death, **397–398**
    aborted, driving recommendations and, **402**
    of athlete, 436–437, 437t, 438t
        cardiomyopathy causing, 421, 436, 437, 438t
    cardiomyopathy and, 421
    myocardial infarction and, 370, 397
    ventricular fibrillation causing, **397–398**
    ventricular premature beats and, 395
    ventricular tachycardia and, 397
Sudden sensory hearing loss, 200, 201, 208
Sudeck atrophy, 874
SUDV. See Sudan virus
Suicide, 1076–1077
    acetaminophen overdose/liver failure and, 685
    alcohol use disorder and, 1076, 1093
    antidepressant overdose and, 1077, 1079
    carbon monoxide poisoning and, 1591
    chronic pain and, 1062
    deaths attributable to, 2t
    depression associated with hospitalization/illness and, 1076, 1077, 1106
    dispensing medications and, 1077, 1079
    intentional drug/poison ingestions and, 1577, 1591, 1606
    in older adults, 61
    panic disorder and, 1053
    personality disorders and, 1065
    schizophrenia/psychotic disorders/ antipsychotic drug use and, 1068, 1072, 1077
Sular. See Nisoldipine
Sulconazole, 99t
Sulfacetamide, for ophthalmic disorders, 169t
Sulfadiazine, for toxoplasmosis, 1337t, 1339, 1524
Sulfadoxine-pyrimethamine (Fansidar), 1515t, 1519
    with amodiaquine, 1519, 1521
    with artesunate, 1516t, 1519
    for chemoprophylaxis, 1519
        in pregnancy/infants, 1521
    resistance to, 1515
    for uncomplicated falciparum disease, 1515
Sulfamethoxazole-trimethoprim. See Trimethoprim-sulfamethoxazole
Sulfasalazine
    for ankylosing spondylitis, 864
    for inflammatory bowel disease/ ulcerative colitis, 650, 659
    for rheumatoid arthritis, 837
Sulfonamides, adverse ophthalmic effects of, 178t
Sulfonylureas, 1220–1223, 1221t, 1235f, 1236. See also specific agent

hypoglycemia and, 1220, 1236, 1595
    factitious, 1253, 1253t, 1257
    intensive therapy with, 1218
    MAOI interactions and, 1083t
    overdose/toxicity of, 1220, 1236, 1581t, 1595
    safety and, 1228
Sulfur-sodium sulfacetamide, for rosacea, 129
Sulindac, 76t
    for familial adenomatous polyposis, 667
    in pain management, 76t
Sumatriptan
    for cluster headache, 980
    for migraine headache, 978
Summer grippe, 1426
Sun exposure. See Ultraviolet light/ sunlight
Sunday neuroses, 1053
"Sundowning," 1103
Sunitinib, 1668t
    for gastroenteropancreatic neuroendocrine tumors, 1186
    for gastrointestinal mesenchymal tumors, 1634
    for pheochromocytoma/ paraganglioma, 1184
    for thyroid cancer, 1145
    thyroiditis caused by, 1126
Sunscreens, 100–101. See also Ultraviolet light/sunlight
    in cancer prevention, 13, 100–101
    in hyperpigmentation management, 158
    for lupus/SLE, 115, 841
    photodermatitis and, 154, 155
    for rosacea, 129
"Super-severe aortic stenosis," 341, 342t
Superficial femoral artery, atherosclerotic/occlusive disease of, 473–475
Superficial spreading melanoma, 103, 104
Superficial venous thrombophlebitis, **487–488**
Superior semicircular canal dehiscence, vertigo and, 213
Superior vena cava sinus venosus defect, 325
Superior vena caval obstruction/ syndrome, **490–491**, 1609
Superwarfarins, poisoning caused by, 1588
Supplements, dietary. See Dietary supplements
Suppurative sialadenitis, 231
Suppurative (infectious) thyroiditis, 1135, 1136, 1137
Supraclavicular lymph nodes, in breast cancer, 741, 742
Supraglottic carcinoma, 235, 236
Supraglottitis (epiglottitis), **234**
    Haemophilus causing, 234, 1466
Supranuclear palsy, progressive, parkinsonism differentiated from, 1012
Supraspinatus tendon
    testing strength of, 1686t, 1689
    torn, 1689
Supratentorial arteriovenous malformations, 1001

Supratentorial mass lesion, coma or stupor caused by, 1028
Supraventricular beats
    aberrantly conducted, differentiation of from ventricular beats, 385, 396
    premature. See Atrial (supraventricular) premature beats
Supraventricular tachycardia, 381
    accessory atrioventricular pathways causing, 385, **387–388**
    with bradyarrhythmia ("tachy-brady syndrome"), 399
    catheter ablation of, 384, 386
    in myocardial infarction, 377
    palpitations in, 30, 31
    paroxysmal, **385–387**
    treatment/prevention of, 382–383t, 385–386
Suramin, for African trypanosomiasis, 1508, 1508t
Surfer's ear, 203
Surgery. See also specific disorder
    antibiotic prophylaxis and, **54**
    anticoagulation discontinuation and, 51–52, 51t, 52t, 368, 392–393
    anticoagulation for prosthetic heart valve and, **350–351**, 352t
    anxiety before/after, 1105, 1106
    bowel cleansing before, 585t, 586
    in cardiac patient, preoperative risk assessment/reduction and, **45–48**, 46t, 47f, 47t
    in diabetic patient, 53, 1243–1244, 1243t
    fever after, 1294–1295
    hyponatremia after, 886
        pituitary surgery, 1111, 1115, 1119, 1175
    ileus after, 638
    liver function and, 50
    patient evaluation/management and, **45–54**. See also Preoperative evaluation/perioperative management
Surgery proneness (polysurgery), 1105
    somatic symptom disorders and, 1058
Surgical menopause, 796
Surgical site infection, 1294–1295, 1295
    prevention/antibiotic prophylaxis of, **54**, 1295
Surmontil. See Trimipramine
Surrogate, Durable Power of Attorney for Health Care, 90
Surveillance. See Watchful waiting/ surveillance
Survival motor neuron (SMN) gene, in spinal muscular atrophies, 1033
Susceptibility testing. See Drug resistance; Drug susceptibility testing
Sustained ventricular tachycardia, 397
Sustiva. See Efavirenz
Sutent. See Sunitinib
Suvorexant, 1054t, 1089
Swallowing disorders. See Dysphagia; Odynophagia
Swan-neck deformity, 838, 840
Sweat chloride test, in cystic fibrosis, 266

Sweating, fluid loss in, replacement guidelines for, 911t
Sweeteners, artificial, for diabetics, 1219
Swimmer's ear, 202
Swimmer's itch, 1532
Swimming pool granuloma, 1482
Swine-origin influenza A (pandemic H1N1), 1411. *See also* H1N1 seasonal influenza
SWL. *See* Shock wave lithotripsy
Sycosis, **130–131**
Sydenham chorea, 422, 423, 423t, 1015
Sylvant. *See* Siltuximab
Symlin. *See* Pramlintide
Sympathetic inhibitors, peripheral, for hypertension, 363t, 464
Sympathetic ophthalmia, 181
Sympatho-adrenal response, hypoglycemia and, 1237
Sympatholytic agents, 462t
for alcohol detoxification/withdrawal, 17
for hypertension, 462t, 464
in urgencies/emergencies, 470t
overdose/toxicity of, 462t, 464, **1592**
Sympatholytic syndrome, 1583
Sympathomimetic agents
adverse ophthalmic effects of, 177t
antidepressant drug interactions and, 1083t
for glaucoma/ocular hypertension, 172t
MAOI interactions and, 1083t
Sympathomimetic effects/syndrome, 1583
Symptom evaluation/management, **19–44**, 38f, 44f. *See also specific symptom*
Synaptobrevin, in tetanus, 1452
Syncope/near syncope, **400–402**
in aortic stenosis, 341, 342
cardiogenic, 401
driving recommendations and, **402**
dysautonomia (autonomic dysfunction) and, 401, 990, 991
heat, 1562
palpitations and, 30
seizures differentiated from, 986
vasodepressor/vasovagal, 401
Syndesmophytes
in ankylosing spondylitis, 864
in psoriatic spondylitis, 865
Syndrome X, 365, 1213. *See also* Insulin resistance/insensitivity; Metabolic syndrome
Syndrome of apparent mineralocorticoid excess, 442, 892t
Syndrome of inappropriate ADH secretion (SIADH), 887, 887t, 888
cancer-related, 887t
Synercid. *See* Quinupristin/dalfopristin
Synergistic necrotizing cellulitis, 1480
Syngeneic stem cell transplant, 541
Synjardy. *See* Empagliflozin, with metformin
Synovial fluid examination, 826, 827t, 828t. *See also specific disorder*
Synovitis, remitting seronegative, with non-pitting edema, 875

Synpharyngitic hematuria, 937
Synribo. *See* Omacetaxine mepesuccinate
Synthroid. *See* Levothyroxine
Syphilis, 1312t, 1316t, **1488–1498**
anorectal involvement and, 670
cerebrospinal fluid examination in, 1496
in HIV infection/AIDS, 1348, 1497
congenital, 823, 1488, **1497–1498**
penicillin treatment in maternal disease and, 1497
contact treatment and, 1492
course/prognosis of, **1488**
drug therapy for, 1312t, 1316t, 1491–1492, 1491t. *See also* Syphilis, penicillin for
HIV infection/AIDS and, 1497
Jarisch-Herxheimer reaction and, 1492
for neurosyphilis, 1316t, 1491t
early, 1316t, 1488, 1491t
endemic, **1498–1499**
follow-up care in, 1492
gummatous, 1489t, 1494, 1495f
HIV infection/AIDS and, 1348, 1489, 1492, **1497**
late (tertiary), 1488, 1489t, 1490t, 1491t, **1494–1495**, 1495f
latent, 1316t, 1491t, **1494**
early, 1316t, 1488, 1491t, 1494
late, 1316t, 1491t, 1494
meningovascular/meningitis, 1489t, 1493, 1496. *See also* Neurosyphilis
mucocutaneous, 1489t, 1492, 1493f
natural history of, **1488**, 1489t
neurologic involvement in, 1316t, 1489t, **1495–1497**, 1496f. *See also* Neurosyphilis
penicillin for, 1312t, 1316t, 1491–1492, 1491t
HIV infection/AIDS and, 1348, 1497
neurosyphilis and, 1316t, 1491t, 1496–1497
pregnancy and, 1318, 1491–1492, 1497
pityriasis rosea and, 109
pregnancy and, 799, 800, **823**, 1318, 1488, 1491, 1491–1492, **1497**
prevention of/screening for, 1489–1491, 1490t, 1491. *See also* Syphilis, serologic tests for
in HIV infection/AIDS, 1348, 1492, 1497
in pregnancy, 799, 800, 823, 1491, 1497
primary, 1488, **1488–1492**, 1489f, 1489t, 1490t, 1491t
public health measures in management of, 1488, 1492
secondary, 1488, 1489t, 1490t, 1491t, **1492–1494**, 1493f
serologic tests for, 1489–1491, 1490t. *See also specific test*
anticardiolipin/antiphospholipid antibody/lupus anticoagulant affecting, 841, 841t, 843
HIV infection/AIDS and, 1348, 1492, 1497
in neurosyphilis, 1496, 1497

in pregnant patient, 799, 800, 823, 1491, 1497
in STD patients, 1302, 1491
sexual violence (rape/sexual assault) and, 793, 794, 1302
treatment of, 1312t, 1316t, 1491–1492, 1491t, 1493–1494
failures and, 1492
uveitis in, 181, 1493
vertigo associated with, 211, 211t
Syringobulbia, 1032
Syringomyelia, **1032**
neurogenic arthropathy (Charcot joint) and, 875
Syrup of ipecac, for poisoning/drug overdose, 1582
Systemic fibrosing syndrome, Dupuytren contracture and, 1700
Systemic fibrosis, nephrogenic, 358, **952**
Systemic hypertension. *See* Hypertension
Systemic inflammatory response syndrome (SIRS), 494
in pancreatitis, 730
Systemic lupus erythematosus (SLE), **839–842**, 839t, 840t, 841t
arthritis in, 839t, 840
rheumatoid arthritis differentiated from, 836
autoantibodies in, 115, 839t, 840–841, 840t, 841t
drugs associated with, 162t, 310t, **842**
lupus anticoagulant/antiphospholipid antibody syndrome and, 562–563, 841, 841t, 842
renal involvement in, 839t, 840, 841, 933t, 935f, **940–941**
skin lesions in (discoid/subacute/chronic cutaneous lupus), **115–116**, 839t, 840
Systemic sclerosis, **845–847**. *See also* Scleroderma
Systolic blood pressure. *See also* Blood pressure
in hypertension, 439, 440f
treatment goals and, 446, 446–447. *See also* Antihypertensive drug therapy, goals of
in hypertensive urgencies/emergencies, 439, 440f, 468
in hypotension/shock, 494
in prehypertension, 440
Systolic heart failure, 402, 406. *See also* Heart (cardiac) failure
Systolic murmurs. *See* Heart murmurs

T_3. *See* Triiodothyronine
T_4. *See* Thyroxine
T315I mutation, in chronic myeloid leukemia, 525
T-cell gene rearrangement test, 116
T-cell lymphoma, 531, 533. *See also* Lymphoma; Non-Hodgkin lymphoma
adult (ATL), 1396. *See also* Human T-cell lymphotropic/leukemia virus
cutaneous (mycosis fungoides), **116–117**
exfoliative dermatitis/erythroderma and, 117
Epstein-Barr virus and, 1373, 1374

intestinal, 1634
nose and paranasal sinus involvement
and, 223
peripheral, 533
stem cell transplantation for, 533
tacrolimus/pimecrolimus associated
with, 105
T cell-mediated (delayed/type IV)
hypersensitivity, 876,
878–881
T cell tolerance genes, in type 1 diabetes,
1210–1211
T-DM1 (trastuzumab emtansine), 1666*t*
for breast cancer, 756
T helper cells. *See* CD4 T cells
T lymphocytes
defects in, common variable
immunodeficiency and, 882
in delayed hypersensitivity, 876,
878–881
in HIV infection/AIDS. *See* CD4
T cells
t-PA. *See* Tissue plasminogen activator
T pallidum hemagglutination (TPHA)
test, 1490
T pallidum particle agglutination (TPPA)
test, 1490, 1490*t*
T score, 1160
T-SPOT tests. *See* Interferon gamma
release assays
T waves. *See also* Electrocardiogram
in myocardial infarction, 371
T372R/YY1 mutation, in insulinoma,
1252
Tabes dorsalis, 1489*t*, 1496
neurogenic arthropathy (Charcot joint)
in, 875, 1496, 1496*f*
Tabun (GA) poisoning, 1601–1602
TAC regimen, 751
TACE. *See* Transarterial
chemoembolization (TACE)/
chemoinfusion (TACI)/
radioembolization (TARE)
Tâche noire, in tick typhus, 1434
"Tachy-brady syndrome," 399
Tachycardia/tachyarrhythmia, **384**. *See
also* Arrhythmias
accessory pathways causing, 385,
387–388
antidromic reentrant, 387
atrial, multifocal, **395**
AV nodal reentrant (AVNRT), 385
AV reciprocating (AVRT), 385, 387
driving recommendations
and, **402**
in hyperthyroidism, 1127, 1133
nonparoxysmal junctional, 395
orthodromic reentrant, 387
palpitations in, 30, 31
paroxysmal, **385–387**
in poisoning/drug overdose, 1579,
1579*t*
sinus. *See* Sinus tachycardia
supraventricular. *See under
Supraventricular*
treatment of, 382–383*t*
ventricular. *See under Ventricular*
TACI. *See* Transarterial
chemoembolization (TACE)/
chemoinfusion (TACI)/
radioembolization (TARE)

Tacrolimus, 98*t*
adverse ophthalmic effects of, 178*t*
hyperkalemia caused by, 894
insulin secretion affected by, 1213
topical, 98*t*
for anogenital pruritus, 148
for atopic dermatitis, 105
for lichen planus, 145
for ophthalmic disorders, 172*t*
T-cell lymphoma and, 105
Tadalafil
for benign prostatic hyperplasia, 974,
974*t*
for erectile dysfunction diagnosis/
treatment, 967, 1064
antidepressant-induced, 1064, 1079
in diabetes, 1241
for high-altitude illness treatment/
prevention, 1575
nitrate/nitroglycerin contraindications
and, 375, 967, 1064, 1241
Taenia
saginata (beef tapeworm), **1535**,
1536
solium (pork tapeworm), **1535**, 1536
cysticercosis and, 1535, 1536–1537
TAF. *See* Tenofovir
Tafenoquine, for malaria, 1515
Tafinlar. *See* Dabrafenib
Tafluprost, for glaucoma/ocular
hypertension, 173*t*
Tafluprost/timolol, for glaucoma/ocular
hypertension, 173*t*
TAFV. *See* Tai Forest virus
Tagrisso. *See* Osimertinib
Tai Forest virus, 1397
Takayasu arteritis, **855**
Tako-Tsubo (stress/catecholamine-
induced) cardiomyopathy/LV
apical ballooning, **417–418**
myocardial infarction mimicked by,
370, 418
pheochromocytoma and, 1181, 1182
Talcosis (talc exposure), 307*t*, 309
Talcott rules, 35
Tall stature
GH excess causing, 1114
in Klinefelter syndrome, 1190, 1682
in Marfan syndrome, 1682
Talofibular ligament, ankle sprains
involving, 1715
Tamm-Horsfall urinary mucoprotein, 913
Tamoxifen, 752, 755*t*, 1669*t*
adverse effects/risks of, 752, 755, 755*t*,
1669*t*
ophthalmic, 178*t*
for breast cancer, 752, 754, 755, 755*t*
in male, 760
as preventive agent, 738, 739
endometrial carcinoma and, 774
for GH-secreting tumor/acromegaly,
1116
for gynecomastia, 1195
for osteoporosis, 1163
for Riedel thyroiditis/struma, 1137
Tamponade, **427–428**
cancer-related, 1658
infarct-related, 378
in pericarditis/effusion, 28, 378, 425,
426, 427–428, 1658
in traumatic cardiac injury, 434

TAMs (thymidine analog mutations), in
antiretroviral resistance,
1361
Tamsulosin
adverse ophthalmic effects of, 177*t*, 183
for benign prostatic hyperplasia, 974,
974*t*
ureteral stone expulsion and, 965
Tanzeum. *See* Albiglutide
Tap water enema, 585*t*
Tapentadol, 80–81*t*
for neuropathic pain, 84
Tapeworm infections, **1535–1538**. *See
also* Cysticercosis;
Echinococcus
invasive, **1536–1538**
noninvasive, **1535–1536**
vitamin B_{12} deficiency in, 506–507
Taptiqom. *See* Tafluprost/timolol
TAR. *See* Thrombocytopenia-absent
radius syndrome
Tarceva. *See* Erlotinib
Tardive dyskinesia, 1073
Tardive dystonia, antipsychotics causing,
1072
TARE. *See* Transarterial
chemoembolization (TACE)/
chemoinfusion (TACI)/
radioembolization (TARE)
Target activity, in functional screening, 56
Targeted therapy, in cancer treatment,
1666–1668*t*
for breast cancer, 752, 754–756, 755*t*
Tarka. *See* Trandolapril/trandolapril with
verapamil
Tarsal tunnel syndrome, **1040–1041**
TAS-102 (trifluridine/tipiracil), 1669*t*
for colorectal cancer, 1640
Tasigna. *See* Nilotinib
Tau protein
in dementia, 1020, 1021, 1022
head injury and, 1031
in Jakob-Creutzfeldt disease, 1022,
1394
Tavaborole, 99*t*
for onychomycosis, 160
TAVR. *See* Transcatheter valve
replacement, for aortic
stenosis
tax gene, in adult T cell lymphoma/
leukemia, 1396
Taxanes, 1664–1665*t*
for breast cancer, 751, 753
during pregnancy, 747
for lung cancer, 1612
neuropathy caused by, 1674
Taxol. *See* Paclitaxel
Taxotere. *See* Docetaxel
Tay-Sachs disease, screening for, 800
Taztia. *See* Diltiazem
TBE. *See* Tick-borne encephalitis
TBG. *See* Thyroxine-binding globulin
TBI. *See* Traumatic brain injury
Tbo-filgrastim, for chemotherapy-
induced neutropenia, 1672*t*
3TC. *See* Lamivudine
TC regimen, 751
TCAs. *See* Tricyclic antidepressants
TcdA/TcdB toxins, in
antibiotic-associated/*C
difficile* colitis, 647

TCF7L2 gene, in type 2 diabetes, 1212
TCH regimen, 752
TCHP regimen, 753
Tcu380A IUD, 789
Td vaccine, 4, 1320t, 1321t, 1322t, 1329t, 1453, 1453t, 1457, 1464. *See also* Tetanus and diphtheria toxoids and pertussis vaccines
Tdap vaccine, 4, 1320t, 1321t, 1322t, 1329t, 1453, 1453t, 1457, 1464. *See also* Tetanus and diphtheria toxoids and pertussis vaccines
TDF. *See* Tenofovir
TDF/FTC. *See* Tenofovir (TDF/TAF), with emtricitabine
TdT. *See* Terminal deoxynucleotidyl transferase
Tears, artificial, for dry eye, 168
Techfidera. *See* Dimethyl fumarate
Technetium-99m scintigraphy
    in hyperparathyroidism, 1155
    in myocardial infarction, 371
    for red blood cell scanning, 598–599
    for thyroid scanning, 1121t, 1128
Technosphere inhaled insulin, 1229t, 1232
Tedizolid, for skin and soft tissue infections, 1448
Teduglutide, for short bowel syndrome, 637
TEE (transesophageal echocardiography). *See* Echocardiography/Doppler
Teeth, disorders of. *See* Dental disorders
Tekamlo. *See* Aliskiren, with amlodipine
Tekturna/Tekturna HCT. *See* Aliskiren
TEL-AML1 translocation, in acute lymphoblastic leukemia, 527
Telangiectasia
    GI bleeding and, 595, 598, 1684
    hereditary hemorrhagic, **1683–1684**
Telangiectatic focal nodular hyperplasia of liver, 716
Telaprevir, for hepatitis C, 689, 690t
Telavancin, for staphylococcal skin infections, 1448
Telbivudine, for hepatitis B, 687–688
Telepaque. *See* Iopanoic acid
Telmisartan, 457t
    with amlodipine, 458t
    with hydrochlorothiazide, 457t
Telogen effluvium, 159
Temazepam, 1054t, 1089
Temodar. *See* Temozolomide
Temovate. *See* Clobetasol
Temozolomide, 1663t
    diabetes insipidus and, 1113
    for gliomas, 1005
    for pheochromocytoma/paraganglioma, 1184
    for pituitary tumors/prolactinoma, 1119
Temperature. *See* Body temperature; Fever
Temporal (giant cell/cranial) arteritis. *See* Giant cell (temporal/cranial) arteritis
Temporal lobe herniation, intracranial tumors causing, 1003

Temporal lobe lesions, 1003
Temporal sclerosis, mesial, epilepsy/seizures caused by, 983
Temporomandibular joint dysfunction
    earache and, 207
    facial pain caused by, 982
Temsirolimus, 1668t
TEN. *See* Toxic epidermal necrolysis
Tendinopathy (tendinosis), upper extremity (lateral and medial epicondylosis), **1697–1698**
Tendinous xanthoma, 1261
Tenecteplase (TNK-t-PA)
    for myocardial infarction, 373t, 374
    for pulmonary embolism, 576t
Tenex. *See* Guanfacine
Tennis elbow, 1697
Tenofovir (TDF/TAF), 1351t, 1354–1355, 1360. *See also* Antiretroviral therapy
    with emtricitabine (Truvada), 1353, 1354t, 1355
        after needle stick, 1347
        plus atazanavir and cobicistat, 1359t
        plus atazanavir and ritonavir, 1359t
        plus darunavir and cobicistat, 1360t
        plus darunavir and ritonavir, 1359t
        plus dolutegravir, 1359t
        plus raltegravir, 1358, 1359t
        prophylactic, 4, 1346
    with emtricitabine and efavirenz (Atripla), 1354t, 1355, 1359t
    with emtricitabine and rilpivirine (Complera), 1354t, 1355, 1359t
    with emtricitabine/elvitegravir/cobicistat (Stribild [TDF] or Genvoya [TAF]), 1354t, 1355, 1358, 1359t, 1360
    for hepatitis B, 687–688, 1341, 1355
Tenoretic. *See* Atenolol, for hypertension, with chlorthalidone
Tenormin. *See* Atenolol
Tenosynovitis
    in chikungunya fever, 1407
    in gonococcal arthritis, 869, 1475
    in tuberculosis, 872
Tension pneumothorax, 314, 315
Tension-type headache, **979**
Teoptic. *See* Carteolol
Teratogenic drugs, 798t. *See also specific agent*
Teratoma, testicular, 1655, 1657
Teratozoospermia, 969f
Terazosin, 462t
    adverse ophthalmic effects of, 177t
    for benign prostatic hyperplasia, 974, 974t
    for hypertension, 459–464, 462t
Terbinafine, 99t, 1559t
    for onychomycosis, 161
    for sporotrichosis, 1557
    for tinea infection, 112, 114
Terbutaline
    for asthma/bronchospasm, 252
    for preterm labor, 812
Terconazole, for vulvovaginal candidiasis, 133, 767
Teres minor, evaluation of, 1689
Terfenadine, antidepressant drug interactions and, 1081, 1083t

Teriflunomide, for multiple sclerosis, 1024t
Teriparatide
    for bisphosphonate-related atypical fractures, 1162
    for osteoporosis, 1162–1163
        corticosteroid use and, 1209
Terlipressin, for GI bleeding/esophageal varices, 615
Terminal deoxynucleotidyl transferase (TdT), in acute lymphoblastic leukemia, 528
Terminal illness. *See* End of life
Terminal restlessness/delirium, 87, 1103
Terrorism. *See* Bioterrorism
TERT promoter mutations, in thyroid cancer, 1139
Testes
    diseases of, **1189–1194**, 1189t. *See also under* Testicular and Hypogonadism
    examination of in hypogonadism/infertility, 969, 1191
    masses/tumors of. *See* Testicular cancer
    retractile, 1194
    undescended (cryptorchism), **1194**
        testicular cancer and, 1190, 1194, 1655
Testicular cancer, 1624t, **1655–1657**
    bone marrow/stem cell transplantation for, 540
    cryptorchism and, 1190, 1194, 1655
    gynecomastia and, 1195
    screening for, 14t, 15
    secondary/metastatic, **1657**
Testicular dysgenesis, 1190
Testicular failure, 969, 1190, 1191. *See also* Hypogonadism
Testicular lymphoma, 1657
Testicular torsion, 960
Testim, 1192
Testis. *See* Testes
Testogel, 1192
Testopel. *See* Testosterone pellets
Testosterone. *See also* Androgens; Testosterone replacement therapy
    deficiency of, 1109, 1110, 1112, 1189–1194. *See also* Hypogonadism
    pseudohermaphroditism/amenorrhea and, 1199–1200
    in women, 1206
    excess of. *See* Hyperandrogenism
    in gynecomastia, 1195
    in hirsutism/virilization, 1197
    in hypogonadism, 1109, 1110, 1112, 1189, 1190, 1191
    in infertility, 969–970
    insensitivity/resistance to. *See* Androgen insensitivity/resistance
    normal values for, 1191
Testosterone buccal tablets, 1193
Testosterone cypionate, 1192, 1335
Testosterone deficiency syndrome, 1190–1191
Testosterone enanthate, 1193, 1335
Testosterone gels, 1192
    nasal, 1193
Testosterone pellets, 1192

Testosterone replacement therapy,
  1191–1193
 buccal, 1193
 for erectile dysfunction, 967
 for gynecomastia, 1195
 gynecomastia caused by, 1193
 for HIV wasting, 1335
 for hypogonadism, 1191–1193
 nasal gel, 1193
 oral, 1193
 for osteoporosis, 1161
 parenteral, 1192–1193
 topical gels, 1192
 transdermal, 1192
 in women, 1206
  vaginal, 795, 1206
Testosterone undecanoate,
  1192–1193
TET2 mutation
 in acute myeloid leukemia, 527
 in essential thrombocytosis, 521
Tetanospasmin, 1452
Tetanus, 1312*t*, **1452–1453**, 1453*t*
 prevention/immunization and, 4, 1453,
  1453*t*. *See also* Tetanus and
   diphtheria toxoids and
   pertussis vaccines
 bite wounds and, 1301
 burn injury and, 1569
 frostbite and, 1566
Tetanus-diphtheria 5-component
  acellular pertussis (Tdap)
  vaccine, 4, 1320*t*, 1321*t*,
  1322*t*, 1329*t*, 1453, 1453*t*,
  1457, 1464. *See also* Tetanus
  and diphtheria toxoids and
  pertussis vaccines
Tetanus-diphtheria toxoid (Td vaccine),
  4, 1320*t*, 1321*t*, 1322*t*, 1329*t*,
  1453, 1453*t*, 1457. *See also*
  Tetanus and diphtheria
  toxoids and pertussis
  vaccines
Tetanus and diphtheria toxoids and
  pertussis vaccines (DTaP/
  Tdap/Td vaccines), 4, 1320*t*,
  1321*t*, 1322*t*, 1329*t*, 1453,
  1453*t*, 1457, 1464
 adverse effects/contraindications and,
  1329*t*
 bite wounds and, 1301
 booster and, 4, 1320*t*, 1322*t*, 1453,
  1457, 1464
 burn injury and, 1569
 frostbite and, 1566
 in immunocompromised host/HIV
  infection/AIDS, 5, 1321*t*,
  1349
 pregnancy and, 802, 1319, 1321*t*,
  1322*t*, 1464
 Tdap replacing Td and, 4, 1320*t*, 1453,
  1464
Tetanus immune globulin, 1453, 1453*t*
Tetany
 in hypocalcemia/hypoparathyroidism,
  896, 897, 1150, 1151
 malabsorption and, 633*t*
 after parathyroidectomy, 1158
Tetrabenazine
 for Huntington disease, 1015
 for Tourette syndrome, 1018

Tetracycline
 adverse ophthalmic effects of, 178*t*
 for amebiasis, 1526, 1527*t*
 in *H pylori* eradication therapy, 626,
  626*t*
 for rosacea, 129
 for syphilis, 1491*t*
Tetrahydrocannabinol, 583, 1099. *See also*
  Dronabinol; Marijuana
Tetrahydrozoline, overdose/toxicity of,
  1592
Tetralogy of Fallot, **328–330**
Tetrodotoxin, puffer fish poisoning
  caused by, 1604*t*
Teveten/Teveten HCT. *See* Eprosartan
TFR2 (transferrin receptor 2) mutation,
  in hemochromatosis, 708
Tg. *See* Thyroglobulin
Tg (thyroglobulin) antibodies. *See*
  Antithyroid
   (antithyroglobulin/
   antithyroperoxidase)
   antibodies
TGF-beta. *See* Transforming growth
  factor beta
TGFBR1/TGFBR2 mutations, in Marfan
  syndrome, 1683
Thalamic stimulation
 for depression, 1084
 for parkinsonism, 1014
 for seizures, 989
Thalamic syndrome
 intracranial tumors causing, 1003
 posterior cerebral artery occlusion/
  stroke causing, 995
Thalassemias, **503–506**, 504*t*
 iron deficiency differentiated
  from, 501
 prenatal screening for, 800
 sickle, 512, 512*t*, **513**
Thalidomide
 for cancer chemotherapy, 1665*t*
 for erythema nodosum leprosum,
  1484, 1484–1485
 for lupus, 116
 for myeloma, 536
 neuropathy caused by, 1674
Thalitone. *See* Chlorthalidone
Thallium-201 scintigraphy
 in myocardial infarction, 371
 in thyroid cancer follow-up, 1147
Thalomid. *See* Thalidomide
THC (delta⁹-tetrahydrocannabinol). *See*
  Dronabinol; Marijuana
Theophylline, 251, 261
 for asthma, 247*f*, 250*t*, 251
 for COPD, 261, 262
 lithium interactions and, 1087*t*
 monitoring levels of, 251
 overdose/toxicity of, 251, 261, 1584*t*,
  1605–1606
  hemodialysis for, 1583*t*, 1584*t*, 1605
  seizures and, 1580*t*, 1605
Therapeutic abortion. *See* Abortion,
  elective/induced
Therapeutic diets, **1278–1280**. *See also*
  Diet; Nutrition
Thermal injury. *See* Burns
Thermoregulation, 1561, 1561–1562
 in burn injury, 1569
Thessaly test, 1709*t*, 1712

Thiabendazole
 for cutaneous larva migrans, 1543
 for strongyloidiasis, 1540
Thiamine (vitamin B₁)
 for alcohol withdrawal, 1095
 for coma, 1027, 1578
 deficiency of, **1274–1275**
  alcohol use/alcoholic ketoacidosis
   and, 905–906, 908, 1095,
   1274, 1578
  amnestic syndrome and, 1103
  neuropathy associated with, 1036,
   1275
  Wernicke encephalopathy/
   Wernicke-Korsakoff
   syndrome and, 1026, 1093,
   1275
 for Wernicke encephalopathy/
  Wernicke-Korsakoff
  syndrome/thiamine
  deficiency, 694, 908, 1026,
  1093, 1095, 1275
Thiazide diuretics. *See also* Diuretics
 for acute tubular necrosis, 920
 adverse effects of, 450*t*
  ophthalmic, 177*t*
 for heart failure, 406
  in chronic kidney disease, 926
 for hyperkalemia, 894
 for hypertension, 448, 450*t*, 464
  in chronic kidney disease, 448, 466,
   926
  in combination products, 451*t*, 452*t*,
   453*t*, 455*t*, 456*t*, 457*t*, 458*t*
  in combination regimens, 464–465,
   465*f*
 hyponatremia caused by, 886
 lithium interactions and, 1086, 1087*t*
Thiazolidinediones, 1221*t*, 1224–1225
 hospitalization/surgery and, 1243
 with insulin, 1224, 1236
 with metformin, 1224
 overdose/toxicity of, 1224–1225, 1595
  ophthalmic, 179*t*, 1225
Thienopyridines, platelet function
  affected by, 558*t*
Thiopurine methyltransferase variants,
  mercaptopurine therapy and,
  651
Thioridazine, overdose/toxicity of, 1589
 ophthalmic, 177*t*
Thiosulfate, for cyanide poisoning, 1581*t*,
  1593
Thiothixene, 1069*t*
 relative potency/side effects of, 1069*t*
Thioureas, for hyperthyroidism/Graves
  disease, 1129–1130
 during pregnancy/lactation, 816, 1129,
  1130, 1132
 preoperative, 1130
 thyroid crisis/storm and, 1133
 toxic multinodular goiter and, 1131
 toxic solitary thyroid nodule and, 1131
Thioxanthenes, 1068. *See also*
  Antipsychotic drugs
Third-degree burns, 1568
Third-degree (complete) heart block, 377,
  399, 399–400. *See also*
  Atrioventricular (heart)
  block
Third nerve paralysis, 194

Third-trimester bleeding, **812–813**

Thirst. *See* Polydipsia

Thoracentesis, 311. *See also* Pleural fluid
analysis
in lung cancer, 1609
in malignant pleural effusion, 313, 1659
in pneumonia, 270, 1446

Thoracic actinomycosis, 1480–1481

Thoracic aortic aneurysms, **482–483**

Thoracic carcinoid, in MEN, 1187*t*

Thoracic kyphosis, 1692

Thoracic outlet syndrome, **873**
chest pain and, 359
neck pain and, 873, 1696
Raynaud phenomenon and, 844

Thoracic spine disease, chest pain and,
359, 619

Thoracoscopic surgery, video-assisted
(VATS), for solitary
pulmonary nodule, 288

Thoracoscopy, in lung cancer, 1609

Thoracostomy, tube. *See* Tube
thoracostomy

Thoracotomy, in lung cancer, 1609

Thorazine. *See* Chlorpromazine

Thorotrast exposure, ureteral/renal pelvis
cancer and, 1653

Thought content, in schizophrenia/
psychotic disorders, 1067

"Thought stopping" technique, for OCD,
1057

THP regimen, 753

Threatened abortion, 804

Three-item word recall, in dementia
screening, 57–58

"3" sign, in coarctation of aorta, 324

"Thrifty" (*LITH*) gene, in cholelithiasis/
gallstones, 716

Throat, **224–231**

Throat culture, in pharyngitis,
228, 1441

Thrombasthenia, Glanzmann, 556

Thrombin inhibitors
for acute coronary syndromes, 368
for heparin-induced
thrombocytopenia, 552–553,
553*t*

Thromboangiitis obliterans (Buerger
disease), **480**
Raynaud disease/phenomenon and,
844

Thrombocytopenia, **546–556**, 547*t*, 549*f*,
551*t*, 553*t*, 554*t*, 555*t*. See
also specific cause
amegakaryocytic, 546
aplastic anemia and, 516, 517, 546,
547–548
with autoimmune hemolytic anemia
(Evans syndrome), 514
in bone marrow failure, **546–548**
in bone marrow infiltration, **548**
in cancer chemotherapy/irradiation,
548, 555*t*, 1662–1672
cyclic, **548**
decreased platelet production causing,
546–548, 547*t*
DIC and, 554
drug-induced, 552–553, 553*t*, **555**, 555*t*
gestational, **555–556**
heparin-induced, **552–553**, 553*t*, 555*t*
immune, **548–550**, 549*f*

increased platelet destruction causing,
547*t*, **548–555**
infection/sepsis-related, **556**
nutritional deficiencies and, **548**
platelet sequestration and, 547*t*, **555**
platelet transfusion for, 544, 549, 549*f*
in posttransfusion purpura (PTP), **555**
retinal/choroidal disease and, 191
with severe fever, 1399
in thrombotic microangiopathy, 550,
551, 551*t*
in von Willebrand disease type 2B, **555**

Thrombocytopenia-absent radius
syndrome, 546

Thrombocytosis
essential, 519*t*, 520*t*, **521–522**
reactive, 521

Thromboembolectomy
for acute arterial limb occlusion, 477
for stroke, 996

Thromboembolism. *See also* Embolism;
Thrombosis; Venous
thromboembolic disease
acute arterial limb occlusion caused by,
476–477
in antiphospholipid antibody
syndrome, 815, 816, 841, 843
in atrial fibrillation, 388
anticoagulation in prevention/
treatment of, 351, 352*t*, 388,
389, 389*f*, 390, 390–393,
390*t*, 391*t*, 392*f*
in atrial flutter, 395
in Behçet syndrome, 862
estrogen replacement therapy and,
1202, 1203
fever and, 1294
in granulomatosis with polyangiitis,
857
in heart failure, 409
in homocystinuria, 1681
in myocardial infarction, 370, 379
in nephrotic syndrome/nephrotic
spectrum disorders, 943
oral contraceptive use and, 786, 1198
during pregnancy, 435
air travel and, 1576
prosthetic heart valves and, 350–351,
352*t*
pulmonary. *See* Pulmonary venous
thromboembolism
pulmonary hypertension and, 302, 303,
430, 430*t*, 433

Thromboendarterectomy
carotid. *See* Carotid endarterectomy/
thromboendarterectomy
for femoral/popliteal occlusive disease,
474

Thrombolysis in Myocardial Infarction
(TIMI) risk score, 27, 369,
380

Thrombolytic therapy. *See also*
Fibrinolytic therapy
for acute arterial limb occlusion, 477
for DVT/PE (venous thromboembolic
disease), 300–301, 490, 576,
576*t*
for hepatic vein obstruction (Budd-
Chiari syndrome), 712
for retinal artery occlusion, 188
for stroke, 996

Thrombophilia. *See also*
Thromboembolism;
Thrombosis; Venous
thromboembolic disease
duration of anticoagulation and,
573–574, 574*t*, 575*t*

Thrombophlebitis. *See also* Deep venous
thrombosis; Thrombosis
oral contraceptive use and, 786
septic. *See* Septic thrombophlebitis
of superficial veins, **487–488**
varicosities and, 486, 487

Thrombopoietin, chemotherapy-induced
thrombocytopenia and, 1672

Thrombopoietin receptor agonists. *See
also* Eltrombopag;
Romiplostim
for immune thrombocytopenia, 549*f*,
550

Thrombosis, **546–577**. *See also*
Thromboembolism;
Thrombophlebitis
acute arterial limb occlusion caused by,
476
in antiphospholipid antibody
syndrome, 815, 816, 841, 843
in aortic aneurysm, 482
cavernous sinus, bacterial
rhinosinusitis and, 217
of deep veins. *See* Deep venous
thrombosis
in DIC, 553, 554
drugs in management of, **563–577**. *See
also* Antithrombotic therapy
in essential thrombocytosis, 521, 522
in granulomatosis with polyangiitis, 857
hemorrhoidal, 670
in heparin-induced thrombocytopenia,
552, 553
in homocystinuria, 1681
intracranial, **1002**. *See also* Stroke
in nephrotic syndrome/nephrotic
spectrum disorders, 943
peripheral arterial aneurysms and, 484
in polycythemia, 519
sigmoid sinus, otitis media and, 206
stent, 362, 368, 373
antiplatelet therapy for prevention
of, 362, 368, 373, 374, 376
venous. *See* Venous thromboembolic
disease

Thrombotic microangiopathy, **550–552**,
551*t*

Thrombotic thrombocytopenic purpura,
550–552, 551*t*
diarrhea and, 1471

Thrush (oral candidiasis), **225–226**, 225*f*
esophagitis and, 611, 1547
in HIV infection/AIDS, 226, 1335,
1341

"Thumb sign," 234

"Thunderclap headache," 40

Thymic neuroendocrine tumors, in
MEN, 1188

Thymidine analog mutations (TAMs), in
antiretroviral resistance,
1361

Thymoma, myasthenia gravis associated
with, 1045, 1046

Thyrogen. *See* Recombinant human
thyroid-stimulating hormone

Thyroglobulin
   antibodies to. *See* Antithyroid
      (antithyroglobulin/
      antithyroperoxidase)
      antibodies
   in thyroid cancer, 1142
      follow-up and, 1146
Thyroglossal duct cysts, **238–239**
Thyroid acropachy, 1127
Thyroid adenoma, toxic
   in MEN, 1187*t*, 1188
   multiple (toxic multinodular goiter),
      1125, 1131
   solitary (toxic solitary thyroid nodule),
      1125, 1131
Thyroid antibodies. *See* Antithyroid
      (antithyroglobulin/
      antithyroperoxidase)
      antibodies
Thyroid cancer, **1140–1148**, 1141*t*, 1143*t*,
      1608*t*, 1624*t*
   anaplastic/undifferentiated, 1141,
      1141*t*, 1142, 1145, 1148
   differentiated, 1140, 1143–1145, 1143*t*
   fine-needle aspiration biopsy and,
      1121*t*, 1138*t*, 1139
   follicular, 1140, 1141, 1141*t*, 1142,
      1143–1145, 1147
   follow-up care and, 1145–1147
   functioning, hyperthyroidism caused
      by, 1126
   lymphoma, 1142, 1145, 1148
   medullary, 1141, 1141*t*, 1142, 1145,
      1147–1148
      in MEN, 1141, 1145, 1147–1148,
      1187*t*, 1188
   metastatic, 1144, 1145
      follow-up and, 1145–1147
   microcarcinoma/microscopic/
      micropapillary, 1140, 1141
   papillary, 1140, 1140–1141, 1141*t*,
      1142, 1143–1145, 1143*t*, 1147
      follicular variant/mixed
         papillary-follicular, 1140,
         1147
   pregnancy and, 1144
   radiation exposure and, 1140–1141
   staging of, 1143, 1143*t*, 1147
   thyroid nodules and, 1137, 1139
   thyroid surgery for, 1143–1144, 1145
      radioactive iodine therapy after, 1144
   thyroid testing in, 1142
Thyroid crisis/storm, 1133
   perioperative, 53
   during pregnancy, 816, 1126
Thyroid cysts, 1138, 1139, 1140
Thyroid eye disease, **194–195**, 1124, 1127
Thyroid gland
   biopsy of, 1121*t*
      in thyroid nodules/cancer, 1121*t*,
         1131, 1138*t*, 1139
      in thyroiditis, 1136
   disorders of, **1119–1149**, 1121*t*. *See
      also* Hyperthyroidism;
      Hypothyroidism; Thyroiditis
      eye disease associated with,
      194–195, 1124, 1127
   in HIV infection/AIDS, 1343
   lithium causing, 1086
   neoplastic. *See* Thyroid cancer;
      Thyroid nodules

perioperative evaluation/
   management and, 53
pheochromocytoma/paraganglioma
   and, 1180*t*
during pregnancy, **816–817**, 1119,
   1121, 1122, 1123, 1126, 1127,
   1131–1132
   hyperemesis gravidarum and, 803,
      1126
thyroid testing in, 1121*t*. *See also*
   Thyroid testing
enlarged. *See* Goiter
examination of, in hyperthyroidism/
   Graves disease/thyroiditis,
   1127
infection of (infectious/suppurative
   thyroiditis), 1135, 1136,
   1137
nodular. *See* Multinodular (nodular)
   goiter; Thyroid cancer;
   Thyroid nodules
Thyroid hormone. *See also* Thyroxine;
   Triiodothyronine
antidepressant drug augmentation and,
   1079
excess/deficiency of. *See*
   Hyperthyroidism;
   Hypothyroidism
exogenous, excess ingestion of
   (thyrotoxicosis factitia),
   1126
replacement therapy with. *See*
   Levothyroxine
Thyroid incidentalomas, 1136, 1137,
   1138–1139
Thyroid microcarcinoma (microscopic/
   micropapillary), 1140,
   1141
Thyroid nodules, **1137–1140**, 1138*t*. *See
   also* Goiter; Thyroid cancer
cystic, 1138, 1139, 1140
incidentally discovered, 1136, 1137,
   1138–1139
solitary, toxic (thyroid adenoma), 1125,
   1131
   in MEN, 1187*t*, 1188
thyroid cancer and, 1137, 1139
thyroid testing in, 1121*t*, 1138, 1138*t*
Thyroid radioactive iodine uptake and
   scan. *See* Radioiodine
   thyroid scans and uptake
Thyroid remnant ablation, 1144
Thyroid-stimulating hormone (TSH/
   thyrotropin), 1121*t*
deficiency of, 1108, 1109, 1119
in euthyroid sick syndrome, 1121
fetal, 1132
in goiter, 1148
in hyperthyroidism, 1121*t*, 1124, 1125*t*,
   1127–1128
amiodarone-induced, 1128
pituitary adenoma/hyperplasia and,
   1126
pregnancy and, 816, 1126, 1128
in hypothyroidism, 1109, 1110, 1111,
   1119, 1120, 1121*t*, 1122*t*
amiodarone-induced, 1120
levothyroxine replacement and,
   1111, 1122, 1123–1124
pregnancy and, 816
pregnancy and, 816, 1126, 1128

recombinant human (rhTSH), RAI
   therapy/follow-up for thyroid
   cancer and, 1144–1145,
   1146–1147
hyperthyroidism and, 1126, 1145
reference/normal values for, 1120, 1123
suppression of. *See* Levothyroxine
   in thyroid nodules, 1138
   levothyroxine therapy and, 1139
   in thyroiditis, 1136
thyroxine suppression in thyroid
   cancer and, 1144
Thyroid-stimulating hormone receptor
   antibody. *See* Thyroid-
   stimulating
   immunoglobulins
Thyroid-stimulating immunoglobulins/
   TSH receptor antibodies
   (TSI/TSHrAb), in
   hyperthyroidism/Graves
   disease, 1124, 1128
amiodarone induced, 1125, 1126, 1128
during pregnancy, 1127
Thyroid storm. *See* Thyroid crisis/storm
Thyroid surgery/thyroidectomy
   for goiter, 1149
   for hyperthyroidism/Graves disease,
      1130–1131
      amiodarone-induced, 1132
      toxic multinodular goiter and, 1131
      toxic solitary thyroid nodule and,
         1131
   hypocalcemia after, 1151
   hypoparathyroidism after, 1143, 1149
   hypothyroidism after, 1119, 1130, 1131,
      1134
   during pregnancy, 1130, 1132
   for thyroid cancer, 1143–1144, 1145
      radioactive iodine treatment/
         follow-up after, 1144
   for thyroid nodules, 1131, 1139–1140
   vocal fold paralysis/recurrent laryngeal
      nerve damage and, 237, 1143
Thyroid testing, 1121*t*
   in hyperthyroidism, 1121*t*, 1125*t*,
      1127–1128
   in hypothyroidism, 1120, 1121*t*, 1122*t*
   pregnancy affecting, 816
   in thyroid cancer, 1142
   in thyroid nodules, 1121*t*, 1138, 1138*t*
   in thyroiditis, 1135–1136
Thyroid transcription factor-1 (TTF-1),
   in lung cancer, 1609
Thyroidectomy. *See* Thyroid surgery/
   thyroidectomy
Thyroiditis, **1134–1137**
   chronic lymphocytic. *See* Hashimoto
      (chronic lymphocytic/
      autoimmune) thyroiditis
   drugs causing, 1134
   Hashimoto. *See* Hashimoto (chronic
      lymphocytic/autoimmune)
      thyroiditis
   hepatitis C and, 1120, 1134
   hyperthyroidism/Graves disease and,
      1119, 1124, 1125, 1128, 1131,
      1133, 1135, 1136
   hypothyroidism and, 1119, 1125,
      1134–1135, 1136
   infectious (suppurative), 1135, 1136,
      1137

Thyroiditis (*Cont.*):
painless
postpartum, 1135
sporadic (hashitoxicosis), 1125,
1135, 1136
pregnancy/postpartum and, 816, 1125,
1131, 1133, 1135
Riedel, 1135, 1137
silent, 1125, 1131, 1135
sporadic (hashitoxicosis), 1125,
1136
subacute. *See* Subacute (de Quervain)
thyroiditis
subclinical, 1134
in Turner syndrome, 1134, 1207
Thyroperoxidase, antibodies against. *See*
Antithyroid
(antithyroglobulin/
antithyroperoxidase)
antibodies
Thyrotoxic hypokalemic periodic
paralysis, 1049, 1127,
1133
Thyrotoxicosis, 1121*t*, **1124–1134**, 1125*t*.
See also Hyperthyroidism
factitia, 1126
Thyrotrophe pituitary adenoma/
hyperplasia, 1126
Thyrotropin. *See* Thyroid-stimulating
hormone
Thyroxine (T$_4$)
in euthyroid sick syndrome, 1121
free. *See* Free thyroxine assay
in goiter, 1148
in hyperthyroidism, 1124, 1125*t*,
1127
amiodarone-induced, 1125–1126,
1126, 1128
pregnancy and, 816, 1127, 1128
thyroid cancer and, 1142
after treatment, 1130
in hypothyroidism, 1110, 1120,
1122*t*
amiodarone-induced, 1120
pregnancy and, 816, 1122,
1123
replacement therapy with. *See*
Levothyroxine
suppression of, 1111. *See also*
Levothyroxine
for thyroid cancer, 1144
uptake of (resin). *See* Resin T$_3$/T$_4$
uptake
Thyroxine-binding globulin (TBG)
in pregnancy, 1128
in thyroid crisis/storm, 1133
Thyroxine index, free (FT$_4$I). *See* Free
thyroxine index
Thyroxine-withdrawal stimulated [131]I
therapy, for thyroid cancer,
1145
TIA. *See* Transient ischemic attacks
Tiagabine, 987*t*
overdose/toxicity of, 987*t*, 1589
Tiazac. *See* Diltiazem
Tibial artery, atherosclerotic/occlusive
disease of, **475–476**
Tibial nerve, entrapment of (tarsal tunnel
syndrome), **1040–1041**
Tibiofibular ligament, in ankle sprains,
1716

TIBOLA/DEBONEL/SENLAT. *See*
Tick-borne
lymphadenopathy/
Dermacentor-
borne-necrosis-erythema-
lymphadenopathy/scalp
eschar neck
lymphadenopathy
Tibolone, 1206
Tic cough ("habit cough"), 21
Tic douloureux (trigeminal neuralgia),
981–982
chemotherapy-induced, 1674
Ticagrelor, for acute coronary syndromes/
STEMI, 361, 366, 367, 371
postinfarction, 380
proton pump interaction/
coadministration and, 628
Ticar. *See* Ticarcillin
Ticarcillin
for anaerobic infections, 1479
platelet function affected by, 558*t*
Tick bite fever, African, 1429*t*
Tick-borne encephalitis, 1388,
1391–1392
Tick-borne lymphadenopathy/
Dermacentor-borne-
necrosis-erythema-
lymphadenopathy/scalp
eschar neck
lymphadenopathy (TIBOLA/
DEBONEL/SENLAT), 1429*t*,
1434
Tick-borne relapsing fever, 1499
Tick fever, Colorado, **1408–1409**
Tick typhus, 1429*t*, **1434–1435**
Ticks
in babesiosis transmission, 1521, 1522
in hemorrhagic fever transmission,
1399
in Lyme disease transmission, 1502,
1504, 1505*t*
removal of, 1502
in rickettsial disease transmission,
1429*t*, 1433, 1434, 1435
skin lesions caused by, 151
Ticlopidine. *See also* Antiplatelet therapy
platelet function affected by, 558*t*
Tics, in Tourette syndrome, 1018
Tietze syndrome, 359
TIG. *See* Tetanus immune globulin
Tigecycline
for anaerobic infections, 1479
for staphylococcal skin infections, 1448
Tilt table testing
in dysautonomia, 991
in syncope, 401
TIMI (Thrombolysis in Myocardial
Infarction) risk score, 27,
369, 380
Timolol
for glaucoma/ocular hypertension,
172*t*
in combination agents, 173*t*
for systemic hypertension, 453*t*
Timoptic/Timoptic-XE/Timoptic GFS.
See Timolol
TIN. *See* Tubulointerstitial
nephritis-uveitis
Tincture of opium, for diarrhea, 594
in Crohn disease, 655

Tinea
corporis/circinata, **111–112**, 112*f*
cruris, **112–113**
manuum, **113–114**
pedis, 112, 112*f*, **113–114**, 114*f*
cellulitis and, 113, 137
pityriasis rosea differentiated from,
109, 112
profunda, furuncles/carbuncles
differentiated from, 153
unguium (onychomycosis), 160,
160–161
versicolor (pityriasis versicolor),
114–115
Tinel sign, in carpal tunnel syndrome,
1699, 1699*t*
Tinidazole
for amebiasis, 1526, 1527, 1527*t*
for bacterial vaginosis, 768
for giardiasis, 1530–1531
in *H pylori* eradication therapy, 626,
627
for trichomoniasis, 767–768, 1531
Tinnitus, **209–210**
in glomus tumors, 207, 209
vertigo/vestibular disorders and, 210,
211, 212
Tioconazole, for vulvovaginal candidiasis,
767
Tiotropium
for asthma, 249*t*, 251
for COPD, 260
Tipiracil/trifluridine, 1669*t*
for colorectal cancer, 1640
Tipranavir, 1357. *See also* Antiretroviral
therapy
with ritonavir, 1352*t*, 1357, 1360
TIPS. *See* Transvenous (transjugular)
intrahepatic portosystemic
shunts
Tirofiban
for acute coronary syndromes, 367*f*, 368
PCI and, 362
platelet function affected by, 558*t*
Tissue plasminogen activator (tPA/
alteplase), 373*t*, 374, 996. *See
also* Fibrinolytic therapy;
Thrombolytic therapy
for acute arterial limb occlusion, 477
for myocardial infarction, 373*t*, 374
for pulmonary embolism, 300–301,
576, 576*t*
for stroke, 996
Tissue transglutaminase. *See*
Transglutaminase
TIV influenza vaccine, 1413, 1416. *See
also* Influenza virus vaccine
Tivicay. *See* Dolutegravir
Tizanidine
overdose/toxicity of, 1026, 1592
for spasticity, 1026
TKM-Ebola, 1398
TLC (total lung capacity). *See* Pulmonary
function tests
TLS. *See* Tumor lysis syndrome
TMA. *See* Thrombotic microangiopathy
TMEM127 mutations, in
pheochromocytoma/
paraganglioma, 1180
TMP-SMZ. *See* Trimethoprim-
sulfamethoxazole

TMPRSS6 (transmembrane serine protease 6) gene, in iron-refractory iron deficiency anemia, 501
TNF. *See* Tumor necrosis factor
TNK-t-PA. *See* Tenecteplase
TNM staging classification, 1608. *See also specific type of cancer*
Tobacco use. *See* Smoking
Tobramycin. *See also* Aminoglycosides
    for ophthalmic disorders, 170t
    for pneumonia, 269t, 271, 275t
Tobrex. *See* Tobramycin
Tocilizumab
    for rheumatoid arthritis, 838
    for Still disease, 839
Tocolytics, 811–812
    adverse ophthalmic effects of, 178t
Toe web (interdigital) tinea pedis, 113, 113f
    cellulitis and, 113, 137
Toenails, disorders of. *See* Nail disorders
Toes, thromboangiitis obliterans (Buerger disease) involving, 480
Tofacitinib
    for psoriasis, 108
    for rheumatoid arthritis, 837
Tofranil. *See* Imipramine
Togaviruses, encephalitis caused by, 1388
Tolazamide, 1220, 1221t
Tolazoline, clonidine overdose and, 1592
Tolbutamide, 1220, 1221t
Tolcapone, for parkinsonism, 1013–1014
Tolectin. *See* Tolmetin
Tolerance (drug), 1092. *See also* Substance use disorders
    opioid, 73, 82, 1098
Tolinase. *See* Tolazamide
Toll-like receptors, in gout, 830
Tolmetin, 76t
Tolterodine, for urinary incontinence, 66
Toluene toxicity/abuse, 1101, 1598
    anion gap and, 906
Tolvaptan, for hyponatremia/SIADH, 889
Tonal tinnitus, 209
Tongue disorders (glossitis/glossodynia), **226**
Tonic-clonic (grand mal) seizures, 984t, 985. *See also* Seizures
Tonic-clonic status epilepticus, 985, 989–990
Tonic seizures, 984t, 985. *See also* Seizures
Tonicity, 884
Tonsillectomy/quinsy tonsillectomy, 229
Tonsillitis, **227–229**, 228f. *See also* Pharyngitis
Tooth disorders. *See* Dental disorders
Tophus (tophi)/tophaceous arthritis, 830, 831f, 833
    rheumatoid arthritis differentiated from, 831
Topical therapy. *See specific agent and disorder*
Topiramate, 987t
    for alcohol use disorder, 17
    for cluster headache prophylaxis, 980
    for migraine prophylaxis, 979t
    overdose/toxicity of, 979t, 987t, 1589
    ophthalmic, 178t
    with phentermine, for obesity, 1271

in type 2 diabetes, 1235
    for pseudotumor cerebri, 1009
    for seizures, 987t
    pregnancy and, 820
Topoisomerase inhibitors, in cancer chemotherapy, 1665t
Topotecan, 1665t
Toprol XL. *See* Metoprolol
Toradol. *See* Ketorolac
Toremifene, 755t, 1670t
    for breast cancer, 755t
Torisel. *See* Temsirolimus
Torsades de pointes, 396, 398
    in poisoning/drug toxicity, 1579t
    antiarrhythmics in, 396
    antidepressants in, 1606
    antipsychotics/phenothiazines in, 1071, 1590
    opiates/opioids and, 1601
Torsemide
    for heart failure, 406
    for hypertension, 450t
Torsion dystonia
    focal, **1016–1017**
    idiopathic, **1015–1016**
Torticollis, 1016
Tositumomab, for non-Hodgkin lymphoma, 532
Total body water. *See* Body water
Total lung capacity (TLC). *See* Pulmonary function tests
Total parenteral nutrition. *See* Central vein nutritional support
Total protein. *See* Protein
Tourette syndrome, **1017–1018**
    OCD and, 1018, 1057
Toxic adenoma
    multiple (toxic multinodular goiter), 1125, 1131
    solitary (toxic solitary thyroid nodule), 1125, 1131
    in MEN, 1187t, 1188
Toxic epidermal necrolysis, 135–136
    drugs causing, 135, 136, 161, 162t, 163
    herpes simplex infection and, 1364
Toxic lung injury
    aspiration and, 306, 1602
    occupational, 290t, **309**
    smoke inhalation and, 305
Toxic megacolon
    acute colonic pseudo-obstruction (Ogilvie syndrome) differentiated from, 640
    in ulcerative colitis, 660
Toxic-mold syndrome, 1558
Toxic multinodular goiter, 1125, 1131
Toxic myocarditis, 413t, **414–415**
Toxic neuropathies, 1037
Toxic psychosis, 1068
Toxic shock syndrome
    clostridial, **1452**
    diaphragm/cervical cap use and, 790
    staphylococcal, **1450**, 1450f
    streptococcal, 1444
Toxic solitary thyroid nodule (toxic adenoma), 1125, 1131
    in MEN, 1187t, 1188
Toxicology consultation (regional poison control center), 1577
Toxicology screen
    long-term opioid therapy and, 85

in poisoning/drug overdose, 1584–1585, 1584t
Toxicosis, T_3, 1127
Toxins. *See also* Poisoning/drug overdose
    anion gap affected by, 905, 906
    in *C difficile* colitis, 589, 647
    in diarrhea/food poisoning/ gastroenteritis, 588t, 589, 1305, 1306t, 1470, 1471
    liver disease caused by, **695–697**. *See also* Hepatotoxicity
    osmolar/osmol gap affected by, 1584, 1584t
    screening for, 1584–1585, 1584t
Toxocara canis/cati (toxocariasis), **1542**
Toxoplasma/Toxoplasma gondii (toxoplasmosis), **1522–1525**
    in HIV infection/AIDS, 192, 1006, 1337t, 1339, 1523, 1524
    prevention/chemoprophylaxis and, 1350, 1525
    during pregnancy/congenital, 799, 1523, 1523–1524, 1524
    retinitis caused by, 192, 1522, 1523
    uveitis caused by, 181, 1523
TP53 mutations. *See also P53* mutations
    in chronic lymphocytic leukemia, 530
    gallbladder cancer and, 1618
    hepatocellular carcinoma and, 1616
tPA. *See* Tissue plasminogen activator
TPHA test, 1490
TPMT. *See* Thiopurine methyltransferase
TPN (total parenteral nutrition). *See* Central vein nutritional support
TPPA test, 1490, 1490t
Trabeculectomy/laser trabeculoplasty, for glaucoma, 180
Trace elements, in nutritional support, 1283
Trachea
    foreign body in, **238**
    obstruction of, 241
    stenosis of, 241
Tracheal intubation. *See* Intubation; Mechanical ventilation
Tracheostomy/tracheotomy, **237–238**. *See also specific disorder*
    for obstructive sleep apnea, 317
Trachoma, **167**
Tractional retinal detachment, 183, 184
Traditional serrated adenoma, 665
Tradjenta. *See* Linagliptin
TRALI. *See* Transfusion-related acute lung injury
Tramadol, 81t
    for neuropathic pain, 83t, 84
    overdose/toxicity of, 1601
Trametinib, 1668t
Trandate. *See* Labetalol
Trandolapril/trandolapril with verapamil, 456t
Tranquilizers. *See specific agent and* Antipsychotic drugs
Trans fatty acids, preventable disease/ deaths caused by high intake of, 3t
Transarterial chemoembolization (TACE)/chemoinfusion (TACI)/radioembolization (TARE), for hepatocellular carcinoma, 1617

Transbronchial lung biopsy. *See* Lung biopsy
Transcatheter valve replacement
  for aortic stenosis, 342–344, 344*f*, 345*t*
  for tricuspid stenosis, 348
Transcranial magnetic stimulation, for depression, 1077, 1084
Transcutaneous valve replacement
  for aortic stenosis, 342–344, 344*f*, 345*t*
  for tricuspid stenosis, 348
Transdermal contraceptive patch, 789
Transdermal testosterone, 1192
Transesophageal echocardiography. *See* Echocardiography/Doppler
Transferrin
  in anemia of chronic disease, 503
  carbohydrate deficient, alcohol use disorder and, 1094
  in hemochromatosis, 708
  in iron deficiency anemia, 501, 503
Transferrin receptor 2 (*TFR2*) mutation, in hemochromatosis, 708
Transforming growth factor beta (TGF-beta), Marfan syndrome and, 1683
Transfusion (blood/blood products), **541–545**
  acute lung injury caused by, 544
  for anticoagulant overdose, 1588
  for aplastic anemia, 517
  in autoimmune hemolytic anemia, 514
  for bleeding disorders, **541–544**
  for chemotherapy-associated anemia, 1662
  contaminated blood and, 543
  for DIC, 554
  disease transmission and, 543–544
    donor screening programs and, 543–544
    hepatitis, 543, 680, 681, 682, 683–684
    HIV, 543, 1332, 1347
    HTLV, 543, 1396, 1397
  erythrovirus (parvovirus) infection and, 1422
  for fluid management/volume replacement, in shock, 496
  for GI bleeding/variceal hemorrhage, 595–596, 614–615
  graft-versus-host disease caused by, 544
  for myelodysplastic syndromes, 526
  preoperative, 51
  for primary myelofibrosis, 523
  purpura associated with, **555**
  for sickle cell anemia, 513
  for thalassemia, 504*t*, 505
  for thrombotic microangiopathies, 551–552
Transfusion graft-versus-host disease, 544
Transfusion reactions
  compatibility testing in prevention of, 542
  contaminated blood causing, 543
  hemolytic, 542–543
  hypersensitivity reactions, 543
  leukoagglutinin, 543
    leukocyte-poor blood in prevention of, 542, 543
Transfusion-related acute lung injury (TRALI), 544

Transglutaminase/tissue transglutaminase (tTG)
  in celiac disease/dermatitis herpetiformis, 123, 634
  in Hashimoto thyroiditis, 1136
Transient atrial fibrillation, 390
Transient autoimmune thyroiditis, postpartum, 816, 1125
Transient ischemic attacks, 477, 478, **991–993**
  atrial fibrillation and, 389*t*, 390, 390*t*, 477, 991, 993
  carotid, 477, 478, 991
  cerebrovascular occlusion/embolization and, 477, 478, 991, 993
  cocaine abuse and, 1100
  ocular, 188–189
  patent foramen ovale and, 326
  seizures differentiated from, 986, 992
  strokes/stroke risk and, 477, 992
  vertebrobasilar, 991
Transient monocular visual loss, **188–189**
Transient neonatal Graves disease, 1127
Transjugular intrahepatic portosystemic shunts. *See* Transvenous (transjugular) intrahepatic portosystemic shunts
Transketolase activity coefficient, in thiamine deficiency, 1275
Translocational hyponatremia, 888
Transmembrane serine protease 6 (*TMPRSS6*) gene, in iron-refractory iron deficiency anemia, 501
Transmissible spongiform encephalopathies (prion diseases), **1393–1395**
Transnasal positive-pressure ventilation, for COPD, 262
Transplantation. *See also specific type or organ and* Immunocompromised host
  fever/FUO and, 1288
  hyperkalemia and, 894
  hyperuricemia/gout and, 833
  immunization in recipients and, 1319–1326
  infections following, 1290, 1290–1291. *See also* Opportunistic infections
    adenoviruses causing, 1420, 1421
    CMV causing, 1291–1292, 1374, 1376
    fungal, 1288
    lymphocytic choriomeningitis virus causing, 1392–1393, 1393
    pneumonia, 276, 1290, 1291
    rabies causing, 1386
    toxoplasmosis, 1522, 1523
  lymphoproliferative disorder after, 1288, 1373–1374
  organ donation for, 93–94
  squamous cell carcinoma after, 144
Transsexualism, 1063, 1063–1064
Transthyretin (TTR) amyloidosis, 538
  cardiac, 421, 422
Transtracheal oxygen, for COPD, 260
Transtubular potassium concentration gradient (TTKG), 893
Transudates, pleural, 311, 311*t*, 312

Transurethral electrovaporization of prostate, 976
Transurethral incision of prostate (TUIP), 973*f*, 973*t*, 975
Transurethral laser-induced prostatectomy (TULIP), 975
Transurethral needle ablation of prostate (TUNA), 976
Transurethral resection of prostate (TURP), 973*f*, 973*t*, 975
Transurethral resection syndrome, 975
Transvenous (transjugular) intrahepatic portosystemic shunts (TIPS), 615–616, 702
  for cirrhotic ascites, 702
  for esophageal varices, 615–616
    in noncirrhotic portal hypertension, 714
    rebleeding prevention and, 616
  for GI bleeding, 597
  for hepatic vein obstruction (Budd-Chiari syndrome), 712
  for hepatorenal syndrome, 703
Tranxene. *See* Clorazepate
Tranylcypromine, 1078*t*
Trastuzumab, 752, 1667*t*
  for breast cancer, 750, 752, 753, 756
    during pregnancy, 747
  for gastric adenocarcinoma, 1631
  toxicity of, 1667*t*
    cardiac, 752
Trastuzumab emtansine, 1666*t*
  for breast cancer, 756
Trauma
  auricular (traumatic auricular hematoma), 201
  cardiac injury and, **434**
    sudden death of athlete and, 437
  cognitive disorders/delirium caused by, 1029, 1031, 1102*t*
  complex regional pain syndrome and, 874
  corneal, 166*t*
  deaths attributable to, 2*t*
  head injury and, **1029–1031**, 1029*t*, 1030*t*. *See also* Head injury
  headache associated with, **980**, 1031
  hearing loss associated with, 207, 208
  middle ear, **207**, 207*f*
  nasal, **222**
    epistaxis and, 221, 222
  ocular, **196–198**, 196*f*, 197*f*
  pneumothorax and, 314
  prevention of, **16**
  seizures caused by, 983, 1031
  spinal, **1031–1032**
    syringomyelia associated with, 1032
  stressor-related disorders and, **1051–1052**
    sexual violence (rape/sexual assault) and, 793, 794
  subarachnoid hemorrhage and, 998
  vertigo caused by, 212
Traumatic brain injury, 1029, 1030, 1031
Traumatic encephalopathy, chronic, 1031
Travatan/Travatan Z. *See* Travoprost
Travel. *See also* Air travel
  chikungunya fever and, 1407
  dengue and, 1401, 1402
  Ebola viral disease and, 1398

hepatitis A and, 678, 679, 1326
hepatitis B and, 1326
hepatitis E and, 684
immunizations recommended for, 4, **1326–1327**
infectious disease and, **1308–1309**
malaria and, 1513, 1514–1515, 1515–1516, 1520
during pregnancy, **802–803**, 1576
Zika virus infection and, 1406, 1407
Traveler's diarrhea, 589, 590, 1305, **1309–1310**
during pregnancy, 802, 1310
Traveler's thrombosis, 1576
Travoprost/travoprost and timolol, 173t
Trazodone, 1078t, 1079–1081. *See also* Antidepressants
for insomnia, 1089
in dementia, 1021
in PTSD, 1052
overdose/toxicity of, 1078t, 1606
priapism caused by, 1082, 1089
Treanda. *See* Bendamustine
Treatment refusal/withdrawal, 91–92, 92t
advance directives and, 90
Trelstar. *See* Triptorelin
Trematode (fluke) infections, **1532–1535**.
See also specific type
blood flukes (schistosomiasis), **1532–1533**
liver/lung/intestinal flukes, **1533–1535**
Tremor
benign essential (familial), **1010–1011**
drug-induced, 1017
fragile-X tremor-ataxia syndrome and, 1679
in parkinsonism, 1011, 1012
Trench fever, 1477
pediculosis and, 150, 1477
Trench (immersion) foot/hand, **1565**
Trench mouth (necrotizing ulcerative gingivitis), **226**
Trendelenburg test, 1702, 1702t
Treponema
non-sexually transmitted diseases caused by, **1498–1499**
pallidum, 1312t, 1488. *See also* Syphilis
carateum, 1498
endemicum, 1498
pertenue, 1312t, 1498
Treponemal antibody tests, 1489, 1490, 1490t
rapid, 1490–1491
Treprostinil, for pulmonary hypertension, 303, 431–433, 432f
Tretinoin. *See also* Retinoic acid
for acne, 127
adverse ophthalmic effects of, 179t
for cancer chemotherapy, 527, 1669t
teratogenicity of, 127
Trexall. *See* Methotrexate
Triad asthma (Samter triad), 222, 878
Triamcinolone, 97t. *See also* Corticosteroids
for acne, 128
for asthma, 250t
for chronic macular edema in retinal vein occlusion, 186
for cutaneous lupus, 115
for diabetic macular edema, 190

intra-articular injection of, 829, 832
topical, for skin disorders, 97t
Triamterene
for heart failure, 406
with hydrochlorothiazide, for hypertension, 451t
hyperkalemia caused by, 894
lithium interactions and, 1086, 1087t
Triazenes, in cancer chemotherapy, 1663t
Triazolam, 1054t, 1055, 1089
overdose/toxicity of, 1594–1595
Tribendimidine, for clonorchiasis/ opisthorchiasis, 1534
Tribenzor (olmesartan HCTZ and amlodipine). *See* Olmesartan
Trichinella/Trichinella spiralis (trichinosis/ trichinellosis), **1541–1542**
Trichloroethylene, toxicity of, 1598, 1602
Trichoderma longibrachiatum, in opportunistic infection, 1557
Trichomonas vaginalis vaginitis (trichomoniasis), 766–767, 767–768, 767f, 1302, **1531**
sexual violence (rape/sexual assault) and, 793, 1302
Trichophyton/Trichophyton rubrum
tinea corporis/circinata caused by, 111
tinea pedis caused by, 113
tinea unguium caused by, 160
Trichosporon, in opportunistic infection, 1557
Trichotillomania, 159
Trichuris dysentery syndrome, 1538
Trichuris trichiura (trichuriasis/ whipworm), **1538–1539**
Triclabendazole, for fascioliasis, 1533–1534
Tricor. *See* Fenofibrate/fenofibric acid
Tricuspid regurgitation, 332–334t, **348–349**. *See also* Valvular heart disease
heart failure in, 348, 349
Tricuspid stenosis, 332–334t, **347–348**. *See also* Valvular heart disease
Tricuspid valve
repair/replacement of, 348, 349. *See also* Valve replacement
in rheumatic fever/heart disease, 347, 422
Tricyclic antidepressants, 1077, 1078t, 1081–1082. *See also* Antidepressants
drug interactions of, 1083t
for neuropathic pain/painful diabetic neuropathy, 83, 83t, 1035
overdose/toxicity of, 1078t, 1082, 1590, **1606**
arrhythmias and, 1082, 1579, 1606, 1606f
hypotension and, 1082, 1578, 1606
ophthalmic, 178t
seizures and, 1082, 1580t, 1606
suicidal, 1077, 1079
withdrawal from, 1080–1081
Trientine, for Wilson disease, 711
Triferic. *See* Ferric pyrophosphate citrate
Trifluoperazine, 1068, 1069t
relative potency/side effects of, 1069t
Trifluridine, for herpes simplex keratitis, 170t, 175, 1365t

Trifluridine/tipiracil, 1669t
for colorectal cancer, 1640
Trigeminal cephalgias, 980
Trigeminal nerve
herpes zoster ophthalmicus and, 121, 175, 1369, 1370
postherpetic neuralgia and, 5, 120, 121, 175, 982
Trigeminal neuralgia (tic douloureux), **981–982**
chemotherapy-induced, 1674
Trigeminy, 396
Triglycerides, 1259, 1261, **1266–1267**. *See also* Hypertriglyceridemia
alcohol use disorder and, 1261
antiretroviral therapy/protease inhibitors affecting, 1356
diabetes mellitus and, 1214, 1217, 1261
lowering levels of, 1265t, 1267. *See also* Lipid-lowering therapy
thiazolidinediones affecting, 1224
Triiodothyronine (T₃)
free, 1121t
in hyperthyroidism, 1121t, 1124, 1125t, 1127, 1128
amiodarone-induced, 1126, 1128
pregnancy and, 1128
in hypothyroidism, 1122t, 1123
with levothyroxine, for hypothyroidism, 1122, 1123
uptake of (resin). *See* Resin T₃/T₄ uptake
Triiodothyronine (T₃) toxicosis, 1127
Trilafon. *See* Perphenazine
Trilasate. *See* Choline magnesium salicylate
Trilipix. *See* Fenofibrate/fenofibric acid
Trimethobenzamide, 582t. *See also* Antiemetics
Trimethoprim
hyperkalemia caused by, 894
for *P jirovecii* infection, 1337t, 1350, 1552
Trimethoprim/polymyxin B, for ophthalmic disorders, 169t
Trimethoprim-sulfamethoxazole
for bacterial rhinosinusitis, 217t
for cyclosporiasis, 1529
for isosporiasis, 1529
for malaria, 1519
for paracoccidioidomycosis, 1557
for *Pneumocystis* infection, 1291, 1336, 1337t, 1349t, 1552
resistance to, 1552
for skin and soft tissue infections, 1343, 1443t, 1448
for toxoplasmosis, 1337t, 1339, 1350, 1524, 1525
for urinary tract infection, 954, 955, 955t
Trimipramine, 1078t
Trinucleotide repeats
in fragile X mental retardation, 1679
in Friedreich ataxia, 1035
in Huntington disease, 1015
Triple A (Allgrove) syndrome, 1169, 1171, 1172
"Triple-negative" breast cancer, 749, 753, 756
Triptans
MAOI interactions and, 1083t
for migraine headache, 978

Triptorelin, 1670*t*
for prostate cancer, 1649*t*
Trisenox. *See* Arsenic trioxide
Trismus
in mumps, 1380
in tetanus, 1452
Trisomy 21 (Down syndrome),
1678–1679
prenatal screening for, 800, 1678
Triumeq (abacavir/lamivudine/
dolutegravir), 1354*t*, 1358,
1359*t*, 1360
Trivalent influenza vaccines, 1413, 1414*t*,
1415*t*. *See also* Influenza
virus vaccine
Trizivir (abacavir/lamivudine/
zidovudine), 1354, 1354*t*
Troglitazone, withdrawal of from market,
1225
Trombiculid mite larvae, skin lesions
caused by, 151
Tropheryma whipplei, 635
endocarditis caused by, 1462
Trophoblastic disease. *See* Gestational
trophoblastic disease
Tropical anhidrosis and asthenia, 131
Tropical pancreatitis, 731
Tropical pulmonary eosinophilia, 1544
Tropical spastic paraparesis, 1396
Tropisetron, 1672, 1672–1673. *See also*
Antiemetics
Troponins
in acute coronary syndromes/STEMI/
chest pain, 28, 366, 371
in heart failure, 404
in myocarditis, 414
Trousseau sign (carpal spasm)
in hypocalcemia/hypoparathyroidism,
897, 1150
in malabsorption, 633*t*
Trousseau syndrome, 553, 554
True vocal fold (glottic) cancer,
235, 236
Trulicity. *See* Dulaglutide
Trusopt. *See* Dorzolamide
TRUST ADP protocol, in acute coronary
syndromes/STEMI/chest
pain, 28
Truvada (tenofovir [TDF] with
emtricitabine), 1353, 1354*t*,
1355
with atazanavir and cobicistat, 1359*t*
with atazanavir and ritonavir, 1359*t*
with darunavir and cobicistat, 1360*t*
with darunavir and ritonavir, 1359*t*
with dolutegravir, 1359*t*
after needle stick, 1347
prophylactic, 4, 1346
with raltegravir, 1358, 1359*t*
Trypanosoma (trypanosomiasis)
African, **1507–1508**, 1508*t*
American (Chagas disease), 30,
1509–1510
achalasia and, 617
brucei gambiense/rhodesiense, 1507
cruzi, 1509
Trypsinogen gene mutations, in
pancreatitis, 731
TSE. *See* Transmissible spongiform
encephalopathies
TSH. *See* Thyroid-stimulating hormone

TSH receptor antibody (TSHrAb/TSH-R
Ab [stim]). *See* Thyroid-
stimulating
immunoglobulins
TSI. *See* Thyroid-stimulating
immunoglobulins
TSP. *See* Tropical spastic paraparesis
Tsutsugamushi fever (scrub typhus),
1429*t*, **1431–1432**
TT virus (TTV), 682
TT677 mutation
in hepatic vein obstruction (Budd-
Chiari syndrome), 711
in noncirrhotic portal hypertension,
714
TTF-1. *See* Thyroid transcription
factor-1
tTG. *See* Transglutaminase/tissue
transglutaminase
TTKG. *See* Transtubular potassium
concentration gradient
TTP. *See* Thrombotic thrombocytopenic
purpura
TTR (hereditary/wild-type) amyloidosis,
421, 422, 538
TTV. *See* TT virus
Tubal ligation/sterilization, 792
Tubal pregnancy, 806. *See also* Ectopic
pregnancy
Tube enterostomies, 1281–1282, 1281*f*.
See also Enteral nutritional
support
Tube feedings, 1281–1282, 1281*f*. *See also*
Enteral nutritional support
in elderly/dementia, 67, 91
Tube thoracostomy (chest tube drainage)
for anaerobic pleuropulmonary
disease, 276, 1478
for malignant pleural effusion, 313,
1659
for parapneumonic pleural effusion,
313–314, 1446
for pneumothorax, 315
Tuberculin skin test, 279, 280*t*
BCG vaccine affecting, 4, 279, 284
in HIV infection/AIDS, 1336, 1348
in intestinal tuberculosis, 643
latent disease treatment and, 283, 284
in musculoskeletal tuberculosis, 872
in pregnancy, 821
in tuberculous meningitis, 1483
Tuberculoid leprosy, 1037, 1484. *See also*
Leprosy
Tuberculoma, meningeal, 1483
Tuberculosis, **277–284**, 277*t*, 278*t*, 279*f*,
280*t*, 281*t*, 282*t*, 1312*t*, 1483
adrenal insufficiency/Addison disease
caused by, 1169, 1172
blood tests/interferon gamma release
assays in identification of, 4,
279–280
in HIV infection/AIDS, 280, 1336,
1348
latent disease treatment and, 283
musculoskeletal disease and, 872
bone and joint infection in, 283,
871–872
drug-resistant/multi-drug resistant/
extensively drug-resistant,
277, 278, 278*t*, 282–283, 284,
1336

directly observed therapy (DOT)
and, 281, 283
treatment of contacts and, 284
in drug users, 1304
extrapulmonary, 283. *See also specific
type or site*
in HIV infection/AIDS, 277, 278, 279,
282, 1336
ART affecting outcome and, 1353
chemoprophylaxis/prevention and,
1347–1348, 1350
drug-resistant disease and, 277, 1336
drug use and, 1304
intestinal involvement and, 643
IRIS and, 1345
treatment of, 4, 282, 1336
intestinal, **643**
latent, 277, 283–284
testing for, 279–280, 280*t*, 283
in pregnant patient, 800, 821
meningitis and, 283, **1483–1484**
musculoskeletal involvement and,
871–872
pericarditis and, 424–425, 425, 426
pleural effusion in, 279, 312, 313*t*
during pregnancy/lactation, 282, 283,
821–822
prevention/control of, 4, 283–284
HIV infection/AIDS and, 1347–
1348, 1350
primary, 277
progressive primary, 277
pulmonary, **277–284**, 277*t*, 278*t*, 279*f*,
280*t*, 281*t*, 282*t*
reactivation, 277
anti-TNF agents and, 652, 1292
renal manifestations of, **951–952**
reporting requirements and, 280
silicosis and, 307
skin test for. *See* Tuberculin skin test
spinal (Pott disease), **871–872**
treatment of contacts and, 284
treatment of, 4, 280–284, 281*t*, 282*t*.
See also Antituberculous
drugs
adherence/nonadherence and,
280–281, 283, 1336
Tuberculous arthritis, **872**
Tuberculous lymphadenitis, **239**
Tuberculous meningitis, 283, **1483–1484**
Tuberculous pericarditis, 424–425, 425,
426
Tuberculous salpingitis, 778
Tuberous sclerosis, **1010**
angiomyolipoma of kidney in, 1655
Tuberous sclerosis complex,
gastroenteropancreatic
neuroendocrine tumors in,
1185
Tubo-ovarian abscess, 779
anaerobic, 1479
appendicitis differentiated from, 642
Tubular acidosis. *See* Renal tubular
acidosis
Tubular necrosis, acute, 852, 917*t*,
918–921
in pancreatitis, 728
rhabdomyolysis and, 852, 920
Tubular proteinuria, 914
Tubulointerstitial diseases, 924*t*, **946–948**,
947*t*

acute, 946, 947*t*
chronic, **947–948**, 947*t*
Tubulointerstitial nephritis-uveitis, 947*t*
TUIP. *See* Transurethral incision of
     prostate
Tularemia, **1473–1474**
TULIP. *See* Transurethral laser-induced
     prostatectomy
Tumefactive chronic pancreatitis, 731
Tumor embolization, in lung cancer, 1613
Tumor-induced osteomalacia, 1165
Tumor lysis syndrome, 920, **1660**
Tumor necrosis factor (TNF/cachectin)
     agents inhibiting. *See* Anti-TNF agents
     in inflammatory bowel disease, 651
"Tumor plop," 433
Tumor suppressor gene mutations. *See*
     also specific type
     in breast cancer, 738
     in colorectal cancer, 665
Tums (calcium carbonate). *See* Calcium,
     dietary/supplementary
TUNA. *See* Transurethral needle ablation
     of prostate
Tungiasis *(Tunga penetrans)*, 151
Tuning fork tests, 200
Turcot syndrome, 667. *See also* Familial
     adenomatous polyposis
     thyroid cancer and, 1141
Turner syndrome (gonadal dysgenesis),
     1190, **1207–1208**, 1207*t*
     amenorrhea caused by, 1199, 1200,
         1208
     thyroiditis and, 1134, 1207
TURP. *See* Transurethral resection of
     prostate
12-lead ECG. *See* Electrocardiogram
Twinrix (hepatitis A and B vaccine), 679,
     1324*t*, 1325*t*
Twynsta. *See* Telmisartan, with
     amlodipine
Ty21a vaccine. *See* Typhoid vaccine
Tygacil. *See* Tigecycline
Tykerb. *See* Lapatinib
Tylenol. *See* Acetaminophen
Tylox. *See* Oxycodone
Tympanic membrane
     in acute otitis media, 204, 205
     cerumen removal and, 201
     in chronic otitis media, 205
     in eustachian tube dysfunction, 203
     in external otitis, 202
     ototoxic ear drops and, 208
     perforation of, 207, 208*f*
     in serous otitis media, 203–204
     underwater diving and, 204
Tympanocentesis, in otitis media, 205
Typhoid fever, **1468–1469**
     carrier state and, 1469
     prevention/immunization and, 1327,
         1469
Typhoid vaccine, 1327, 1469
Typhus, 1368*t*, **1428–1432**. *See also*
     specific type
Tyrosine kinase inhibitors, 1667–1668*t*
     for acute lymphoblastic leukemia, 529
     for chronic lymphocytic leukemia, 530
     for chronic myeloid leukemia, 524–525
     for gastrointestinal mesenchymal
         tumors, 1633, 1634
     for lung cancer, 1612

thyroid disorders and, 1126
toxicity of, 1673, 1673–1674
Tyrosine phosphatases IA2 (ICA-512)
     antibodies, in type 1
     diabetes, 1211, 1211*t*, 1233
Tysabri. *See* Natalizumab

U-Lactin, 100*t*
Uceris. *See* Budesonide
Udenafil, adverse ophthalmic effects of,
     177*t*
UDP. *See* Uridine diphosphate (UDP)
     glucuronosyl transferase
"Ugly duckling sign," 104
UIP. *See* Usual interstitial pneumonia
UKPDS (United Kingdom Prospective
     Diabetes Study), 1218, 1219,
     1236, 1245
Ulcer perforation, **630**
Ulcerative colitis, 649–650, **658–662**,
     658*t*. *See also* Inflammatory
     bowel disease
     arthritis in, 867
     colorectal cancer and, 661, 1637
     diarrhea in, 592, 658, 658*t*, 659
     fulminant, 660–661
     GI bleeding and, 598
     primary sclerosing cholangitis and,
         723–724
Ulcerative stomatitis. *See* Stomatitis,
     ulcerative
Ulcers. *See also* Peptic ulcer disease
     amebic, 1525, 1526, 1526*f*
     anal fissures, 672–673
     aphthous. *See* Aphthous ulcer
     Buruli, 1482
     contact, of arytenoid cartilage, 234–235
     corneal, **174**. *See also* Keratitis
         contact lens wear and, 164, 174
         in herpes simplex keratitis, 175,
             1363, 1364, 1364–1366
     genital/genitourinary. *See* Genital
         ulcers
     intraoral, **226–227**
         in Behçet syndrome, 861
         chemotherapy-induced, 1673
         in HIV infection/AIDS, 1341
     skin. *See* Skin disorders, ulcers
Ulipristal
     for emergency/postcoital
         contraception, 791
     for fibroid tumors, 773
Ulnar nerve lesions, **1040**
Ultram. *See* Tramadol
Ultrarapid detoxification, for heroin/
     opioid withdrawal, 1099
Ultrasonography/Doppler
     ultrasonography/duplex
     ultrasonography
     in abdominal aortic aneurysms, 7, 481
     in acute arterial limb occlusion, 476
     in aortoiliac occlusive disease, 472
     in ascites, 523
     in breast lump detection/evaluation,
         740, 742, 744
     in cerebrovascular occlusive disease,
         477
     in DVT/PE (venous thromboembolic
         disease), 33, 33*t*, 297
     in ectopic pregnancy, 806
     endoscopic, 677

in femoral/popliteal occlusive disease,
     474
in heart disease. *See* Echocardiography/
     Doppler
in hyperparathyroidism, 1155
intravascular, in angina, 358
in peripheral artery aneurysms, 484
during pregnancy, 800
     Zika virus infection and, 1406
in prostate cancer, 1645, 1646
in renal artery stenosis/renal vascular
     hypertension, 442, 445, 931
in spontaneous abortion, 804
in thyroid disorders
     hyperthyroidism, 1128
     thyroid cancer evaluation/follow-up,
         1142, 1146
     thyroid nodules, 1121*t*, 1138, 1138*t*
     thyroiditis, 1136
in tibial/pedal occlusive disease, 475
in varicose veins, 486, 487
Ultravate. *See* Halobetasol
Ultraviolet (actinic) keratitis, **198**
Ultraviolet light/sunlight
     actinic keratoses and, 117–118
     basal cell carcinoma and, 143
     cancer/cancer prevention and, 13,
         100–101, 143, 144
     corneal burns (ultraviolet/actinic
         keratitis) and, **198**
     herpes simplex recurrence and, 119
     hyperpigmentation and, 158
     lupus/SLE and, 115, 841
     photodermatitis and, 154, 155. *See also*
         Photodermatitis
     porphyria cutanea tarda and, 123
     with psoralen. *See* PUVA therapy
     rosacea and, 129
     squamous cell carcinoma and, 144
     sunscreens and, 100–101
     therapeutic. *See* Phototherapy
     vitamin D and, 1164, 1165
Umbilical cord blood, stem cells in, for
     transplantation, 540–541
Umeclidinum, for COPD, 260
Unasyn. *See* Ampicillin-sulbactam
Uncinate (temporal lobe) lesions, 1003
Undernutrition. *See* Malnutrition;
     Nutritional disorders
Underwater diving. *See* Scuba/deep sea
     diving
Undescended testes. *See* Cryptorchism
Unicuspid aortic valve, 341
Uniretic. *See* Moexipril/moexipril with
     hydrochlorothiazide
United Kingdom Prospective Diabetes
     Study (UKPDS), 1218, 1219,
     1236, 1245
Unithiol
     for arsenic poisoning, 1590
     for mercury poisoning, 1599
Univasc. *See* Moexipril
Universal precautions, 1295
     HIV infection/AIDS prevention and,
         1346–1347
Unlawful sexual intercourse (statutory
     rape), 793
Unoprostone, for glaucoma/ocular
     hypertension, 173*t*
Unstable angina. *See* Acute coronary
     syndromes

"Up and Go Test," 63
Upper airway cough syndrome (postnasal drip), 19, 20, 20*t*, 21
Upper airway/respiratory tract disorders, **241**
  asthma differentiated from, 246
  foreign body, 238, 241
  obstruction, 238, 241
  obstructive sleep apnea hypopnea, 230, 231
  thermal injury/smoke inhalation, 305
Upper endoscopy. *See* Endoscopy
Upper extremity musculoskeletal disorders, **1697–1701**, 1699*t*, 1700*f*
Upper GI bleeding, **594–597**. *See also* Gastrointestinal bleeding
Upper motor neuron lesions, spasticity and, 1025. *See also* Motor neuron diseases
Upper respiratory tract disorders. *See* Upper airway/respiratory tract disorders
UPPP. *See* Uvulopalatopharyngoplasty
Urates/urate crystals, 826. *See also* Uric acid
  in chronic urate nephropathy, 952
  in gout, 826, 830, 831
Urate lowering therapy, 832–833
Urate (uric acid) nephropathy, 830, 952
Urea
  lithium interactions and, 1087*t*
  topical, for skin disorders, 100*t*
Urea breath testing, in *H pylori* infection, 579, 622, 625
Urea clearance, 915
Urea nitrogen. *See* Blood urea nitrogen
Ureacin. *See* Urea
Ureaplasma urealyticum, 1486
Uremia/uremic syndrome, 916, 924–925, 924*t*, 926*f*. *See also* Hemolytic-uremic syndrome; Kidney disease/injury; Renal failure
  coma in diabetic patient and, 1246*t*
  neuropathy associated with, 929, 1036
  platelet function affected in, 558*t*
  pruritus in, 147
Uremic acidosis, 906
Uremic encephalopathy, 925, 928
Uremic fetor, 925
Uremic pericarditis, 425, 426, 924, 926–927
Ureter, cancer of, **1653**
Ureteral stones, 962, 965. *See also* Urinary stone disease
Ureterosigmoidostomy, normal anion gap acidosis and, 906
Urethra, incompetence/obstruction of, urinary incontinence and, 66, 67
Urethral discharge, STDs causing, 1302
  chlamydia, 1486
  gonorrhea, 1475
Urethral implant, for benign prostatic hyperplasia, 976
Urethritis, 1302, 1316*t*
  adenoviruses causing, 1421
  atrophic, urinary incontinence and, 43, 65
  chlamydial, 1313*t*, 1316*t*, **1486**

gonococcal, 1316*t*, 1475, 1476
  postgonococcal, 1486
  STDs causing, 1302, 1313*t*, 1316*t*
  Trichomonas causing, 1531
Urethrocele, 777
Urge incontinence, 65–66, 66
Urgencies, hypertensive, **468–471**, 469*t*, 470*t*. *See also* Hypertensive emergencies
  blood pressure in, 439, 440*f*, 468
Uric acid. *See also* Hyperuricemia
  calcium nephrolithiasis and, 964
  diuretics affecting, 448
  in gout, 830, 831, 952
    reducing levels of, 832–833
  kidney disease and, 830, 920, 948, 952
  in tumor lysis syndrome, 920, 1660
  uric acid nephrolithiasis/nephropathy and, 830, 952, 961, 962, 964
  probenecid use and, 833
Uric acid crystals. *See* Urates/urate crystals
Uric acid (urate) nephropathy, 830, 952
Uric acid urinary stones (calculi), 830, 952, 961, 962, 964
  probenecid use and, 833
Uricase, for hyperuricemia/gout, 832, 833
Uricosuric drugs, 832, 833
Uridine diphosphate (UDP) glucuronosyl transferase
  chronic pancreatitis and, 731
  hyperbilirubinemia and, 674
Urinalysis, 913. *See also specific disorder*
  for drug detection, 1092
    long-term opioid therapy and, 85
  in dysuria evaluation, 42–43, 44*f*
  in fluid and electrolyte disorders, 884
  in glomerulonephritis/nephritic spectrum disorders, 936
  in hematuria evaluation, 913, 914, 953
  in nephrotic spectrum disorders, 942
  in proteinuria evaluation, 913, 914
Urinary anion gap. *See also* Anion gap/ anion gap acidosis
  in normal anion gap/renal tubular acidosis, 906, 906*t*, 907
Urinary antigen testing
  in Lyme disease, 1503, 1504
  in pneumonia, 269–270
Urinary bladder. *See* Bladder
Urinary calculi. *See* Urinary stone disease
Urinary casts, 913, 914*t*. *See also specific type and specific disorder*
Urinary disorders. *See also specific type*
  adverse ophthalmic effects of drugs used in, 177*t*
Urinary free cortisol, in Cushing syndrome diagnosis, 1174
Urinary incontinence, **65–67**
  benign prostatic hyperplasia and, 66, 67
  in elderly, **65–67**
  estrogen replacement therapy and, 1203
Urinary retention, antipsychotics causing, 1071
Urinary schistosomiasis, 1532, 1533
Urinary stone disease, **961–965**, 962*t*. *See also* Nephrolithiasis
  calcium nephrolithiasis and, 961, 962
  calcium supplementation and, 963, 964, 1161
  Crohn disease and, 653

cystine stones and, 961, 962, 964
  hyperparathyroidism and, 963–964, 1153, 1155, 1157
  medical treatment/recurrence prevention and, 963–964
  metabolic evaluation and, 962
  in polycystic kidney disease, 949, 950
  in renal tubular acidosis, 906–907, 962
  struvite stones and, 961, 962, 964
  surgical treatment and, 964–965
  uric acid stones and, 830, 952, 961, 962, 964
    probenecid use and, 833
Urinary tract infection, 42–44, 44*f*, 1314*t*, 1315*t*. *See also* Cystitis; Pyelonephritis
  candidal, 1547, 1548
  dysuria and, 42–44, 44*f*
  E coli causing, 1311*t*, 1315*t*
  health care (hospital)-associated, 1293, 1294, 1295
  incontinence and, 65
  during pregnancy, 42, **820**
  struvite calculi and, 961, 962, 964
Urinary tract obstruction
  kidney injury and, 918, 924*t*
  stones causing, 962, 965
  tubulointerstitial disease caused by, 947, 948
Urinary urgency, 65
Urination. *See* Voiding
Urine
  acidification of, in poisoning/drug overdose, 1582
  alkalinization of
    for cystine calculi, 964
    in poisoning/drug overdose, 1582
    for salicylate toxicity, 1582, 1584*t*, 1603
    for uric acid calculi, 964
  candida in, 1547, 1548
  evaluation of. *See* Urinalysis
  ketones in. *See* Ketones/ketone bodies/ ketonemia/ketonuria
  pH of, 962
    manipulation of in poisoning/drug overdose, 1582
    normal, 962
    in normal anion gap/renal tubular acidosis, 906, 906*t*, 907
    stone disease and, 962, 964
Urine culture, in dysuria evaluation, 43, 44*f*
Urine drug testing. *See* Urinalysis, for drug detection
Urine output, incontinence in elderly and, 65
Urine protein-to-creatinine ratio, 914. *See also* Proteinuria
Urofollitropins, for male infertility, 1112
Urokinase. *See also* Thrombolytic therapy
  for pulmonary embolism, 300–301, 576*t*
Urolithiasis, **961–965**, 962*t*. *See also* Nephrolithiasis; Urinary stone disease
Urologic disorders, **953–976**. *See also* Genitourinary disorders
Uropathy, obstructive
  acute kidney injury caused by, 918
  tubulointerstitial disease caused by, 947, 948

Urosepsis, 42. *See also* Urinary tract
  infection
Urothelial cell carcinoma
  of bladder, 1651
  of ureter/renal pelvis, 1653
Ursodeoxycholic acid
  for cholelithiasis/gallstones, 718
  for intrahepatic cholestasis of
    pregnancy, 824
  for primary biliary cholangitis/
    cirrhosis, 707
  for primary sclerosing cholangitis,
    724–725
Urticaria, **133–135**, 134*f*
  drugs causing, 134, 162*t*
  insect bites/stings causing, 134
  transfusion causing, 543
Urticating hairs, skin lesions caused by,
  151
Ustekinumab, for psoriasis/psoriatic
  arthritis, 108, 865
Usual interstitial pneumonia (UIP), 290,
  291*t*
Uterine bleeding
  endometrial carcinoma and, 763, 764,
    774
  normal menstrual, 762. *See also*
    Menstruation
  postmenopausal, **764**
  during pregnancy, third-trimester,
    812–813
  premenopausal abnormal, **762–764**
Uterine tubes, interruption/ligation of,
  792
Uterus
  cancer of. *See* Endometrial carcinoma
  disorders of, amenorrhea in, 1199,
    1201
  gravid. *See* Pregnancy
  leiomyoma (fibroid tumor) of,
    772–774
  perforation of by IUD, 790
  peripartum infection of, 814
    C sordellii causing, 1452
UTI. *See* Urinary tract infection
UVA therapy, with psoralen. *See* PUVA
  therapy
UVB therapy. *See also* Phototherapy
  for lichen planus, 145
  for psoriasis, 108
Uveitis, 166*t*, **181–182**, 182*f*
  in ankylosing spondylitis, 863
  anterior (iritis), 166*t*, 181, 181–182,
    182
  in Behçet syndrome, 181, 862
  immune recovery, 192
  in leptospirosis, 1500
  posterior, 181, 182
  in reactive arthritis, 866
  in syphilis, 181, 1493
  toxoplasmic, 181, 1523
Uvulopalatopharyngoplasty, for sleep
  apnea/snoring, 231, 317

V1/V2 vasopressin receptors, in diabetes
  insipidus, 1113
V2 vasopressin receptor antagonists, for
  hyponatremia/SIADH, 889
V617F mutation. *See also JAK2* mutation
  in hepatic vein obstruction (Budd-
    Chiari syndrome), 711

  in noncirrhotic portal hypertension,
    714
  in polycythemia vera, 519
V-go insulin patch pump, 1231–1232
V/Q scans. *See* Ventilation-perfusion
  scans
vacA gene, in *H pylori* gastritis, 621
Vaccine-associated poliomyelitis, 1326,
  1383
Vaccine bacillus Calmette-Guérin. *See*
  BCG vaccine
Vaccine-preventable infections, 3–5,
  1319–1327, 1320–1325*t*,
  1328–1329*t*, **1377–1385**. *See
  also specific type*
Vaccines. *See specific type and*
  Immunization
Vaccinia, 1423
Vaccinia immunization, monkeypox
  prevention and, 1424
Vacuum erection device, 967
  in diabetes, 1241
VADT (Veteran Administration Diabetes
  Trial), 1219
Vagal nerve. *See* Vagus nerve
Vagal nerve stimulation
  for depression, 1084
  for seizures, 989
Vagifem, 1205
Vagina. *See also under Vaginal and*
  Vaginitis/vulvovaginitis
  anaerobic flora/infection of, 1478,
    1479
Vaginal atrophy. *See* Atrophic vaginitis
Vaginal bleeding
  in endometrial carcinoma, 763, 764,
    774
  normal menstrual, 762. *See also*
    Menstruation
  postmenopausal, **764**
  during pregnancy, third-trimester,
    812–813
  premenopausal abnormal, **762–764**
Vaginal discharge, 766, 1302. *See also*
  Vaginitis/vulvovaginitis
  STDs causing, 1302
Vaginal dryness. *See* Atrophic vaginitis
Vaginal estrogen, 795, 1205
  HRT risks and, 1203
Vaginal gels, progesterone, 1205
Vaginal hernias (pelvic organ prolapse),
  777–778
Vaginal ring
  contraceptive, 789, 1205
  for estrogen replacement therapy, 795,
    1202, 1205
Vaginal testosterone, 795, 1206
Vaginal warts, 768. *See also* Venereal
  (genital) warts
Vaginismus, 782, 782–783
Vaginitis/vulvovaginitis, **766–768**, 766*f*,
  767*f*. *See also* Vulvovaginal
  candidiasis
  atrophic. *See* Atrophic vaginitis
  dysuria and, 42, 44*f*
  gonococcal, 1475
  in lichen planus, 145, 775
  STDs causing, 1302
  Trichomonas vaginalis causing,
    766–767, 767–768, 767*f*,
    1302, 1531

Vaginosis, bacterial, 767, 768, 1302
  sexual violence (rape/sexual assault)
    and, 1302
Vagus nerve
  lesion/damage of, vocal fold paralysis
    and, 237
  stimulation of. *See* Vagal nerve
    stimulation
Valacyclovir, 1365*t*
  for herpes simplex infections, 119, 175,
    1338*t*, 1343, 1365*t*
  for herpes zoster/varicella infection,
    121, 175, 982, 1338*t*, 1343,
    1365*t*, 1370
  prophylactic/suppressive, 1343
Valeritas. *See* V-go insulin patch pump
Valganciclovir, 1365*t*
  for CMV infection, 191, 1291–1292,
    1338*t*, 1365*t*, 1376
Valgus stress test, 1707*t*, 1710
Valium. *See* Diazepam
Valproic acid/valproate, 987*t*, 988*t*, 1085
  for bipolar disease/mania, 1084, 1085
    lithium interactions and, 1087*t*
  for migraine prophylaxis, 979*t*, 1085
  overdose/toxicity of, 979*t*, 987*t*, 988*t*,
    1085, 1584*t*, 1589
    hemodialysis for, 1583*t*, 1584*t*, 1589
  pregnancy/breastfeeding/teratogenicity
    and, 798*t*, 820, 1085
  for seizures, 987*t*, 988*t*
    status epilepticus and, 989
Valsalva maneuver
  heart murmurs affected by, 335*t*
  paroxysmal supraventricular
    tachycardia interrupted by,
    386
Valsartan
  for heart failure, 407
    infarct-related, 376
    with sacubitril, 407
  for hypertension, 458*t*, 459
    with aliskiren, 458*t*
    with amlodipine, 458*t*
    with amlodipine and
      hydrochlorothiazide, 458*t*
    with hydrochlorothiazide, 458*t*
Valturna. *See* Aliskiren, with valsartan
Valve replacement. *See also* Prosthetic
    heart valves
  anticoagulation after, 337, 343,
    350–351, 352*t*
  endocarditis and, 352*t*, 1463
  pregnancy and, **351**, 352*t*
  for aortic regurgitation, 346–347, 347*t*
  for aortic stenosis, 342–344, 343*t*, 344*f*,
    345*t*
  coagulase-negative staphylococcal
    infection and, 1450, 1451
  for endocarditis, 1462
  for mitral regurgitation, 338*f*, 339
  for mitral stenosis, 336, 336*f*, 337
  in pregnant patient, 351, 352*t*, 819
  for pulmonary valve regurgitation, 350
  for pulmonary valve stenosis, 323
  in tetralogy of Fallot, 329
  for tricuspid regurgitation, 349
  for tricuspid stenosis, 348
Valves, cardiac. *See* Prosthetic heart
    valves; Valve replacement;
    Valvular heart disease

Valvular heart disease, **331–351**, 332–334t, 335t, 352t. *See also specific type*
in alkaptonuria, 1677, 1678
endocarditis/endocarditis prophylaxis and, 1458. *See also* Endocarditis
in Marfan syndrome, 1682, 1683
perioperative evaluation/management and, 48
pregnancy and, 351, 352t, 819
rheumatic fever/rheumatic heart disease and, 331, 335, 336f, 345, 347, 422–424, 423t
Valvular papillary fibroelastoma, 433
Valvular rupture, traumatic, 434
Valvulitis, rheumatic, 422
Valvuloplasty
for aortic stenosis, 343
for mitral stenosis, 335, 336, 336f
for pulmonary valve stenosis, 323
Vancocin. *See* Vancomycin
Vancomycin
for anthrax, 1456t
for antibiotic-associated colitis, 649
for endocarditis, 1461, 1462
for group B streptococcus prophylaxis in pregnancy, 800–801, 1444
for meningitis, 1297t
nephrotoxicity of, 919
for pneumonia, 269t, 271, 275t, 1446
red man syndrome caused by, 878, 879t
for skin and soft tissue infections, 1443, 1443t, 1448
Vandetanib, 1668t
for thyroid cancer, 1145
Vanicream, 95, 105
Vaniqua. *See* Eflornithine
Vantin. *See* Cefpodoxime
VAP. *See* Ventilator-associated pneumonia
Vaqta. *See* Hepatitis A vaccine
Vardenafil
for erectile dysfunction diagnosis/treatment, 967, 1064
antidepressant-induced, 1064, 1079
in diabetes, 1241
nitrate/nitroglycerin contraindications and, 375, 967, 1064, 1241
Varenicline, for smoking cessation, 7
Variant (Prinzmetal) angina, 365
Variant Creutzfeldt-Jakob disease, 1394. *See also* Creutzfeldt-Jakob disease
Varicella (chickenpox), **1366–1372**, 1368t, 1369f
during pregnancy/congenital, **821**, 1369
prevention/immunization and, 1370, 1371. *See also* Varicella vaccine
reactivation of, 120, 1368. *See also* Herpes zoster
Varicella vaccine, 5, 1320t, 1321t, 1322t, 1370, 1371
adverse effects/contraindications and, 1321t, 1329t
immunocompromised host/HIV infection/AIDS and, 1321t, 1371

postexposure, 1371
pregnancy and, 802, 1321t, 1322t, 1371
Varicella-zoster immune globulin, 1371
for newborn/during pregnancy, 821, 1371
Varicella zoster virus, 1367. *See also* Herpes zoster; Varicella
Bell palsy caused by, 1041, 1369
immunization against. *See* Herpes zoster vaccine; Varicella vaccine
pregnancy and, **821**, 1369
reactivation of, 5, 120, 1368. *See also* Herpes zoster
Varicella zoster virus vaccine. *See* Herpes zoster vaccine
Varicocele, 784, 969, 970
Varicose veins (varicosities/varices), **486–487**
esophageal. *See* Esophageal varices
GI bleeding from, 594–595, 614–617
portal hypertension/portal hypertensive gastropathy and, 594–595, 621
venous insufficiency/stasis and, 486, 489, 490
Variegate porphyria, 1036
Varilrix. *See* Varicella vaccine
Variola (smallpox), 1368t, 1423
Variola (smallpox) vaccination, 1423
VARIVAX. *See* Varicella vaccine
VariZIG. *See* Varicella-zoster immune globulin
Varus stress test, 1707t, 1710
Vas deferens
absence of, in cystic fibrosis/infertility, 265, 969, 970
obstruction of, in infertility, 970
Vasa previa, third-trimester bleeding caused by, 812
Vascular dementia, 57, 1019t. *See also* Dementia
Vascular disorders (vascular occlusion/anomalies), **472–491**. *See also specific type or vessel affected and* Vasculitis
arterial aneurysms, **480–486**
atherosclerotic, **472–480**
in diabetes mellitus, 1242
glycemic control and, 1217, 1218, 1219
hypertension control and, 446, 447f, 464, 465, 1217, 1218, 1219, 1236
tibial and pedal artery disease and, 475, 476
in drug user, 1304
erectile dysfunction and, 966, 967, 968
GI bleeding and, 595
glomerulonephritis and, 922, 924t
headache and, 40, 981
hepatic vein
Budd-Chiari syndrome, **711–712**
sinusoidal obstruction syndrome, 697, 711–712
homocysteine/hyperhomocysteinemia and, 1681
kidney disease and, 917, 923
nonatherosclerotic, **480**
osteomyelitis and, 871
in polycystic kidney disease, 950

in preeclampsia-eclampsia, 809t
pregnancy and, **435–436**
pulmonary hypertension and, 302, 303, 429–430, 430t
seizures caused by, 983
shock and, **493–498**, 494t
spinal cord, **1002–1003**
venous, **486–491**
vertigo caused by, **214**
Vascular endothelial growth factor (VEGF) inhibitors. *See* Anti-VEGF therapy
Vascular reconstruction. *See* Bypass grafting
Vasculitis, **853–863**, 853t. *See also specific disorder*
allergic, drugs causing, 162t
brain and spinal cord involvement and (primary angiitis of central nervous system), **862–863**
pulmonary, **304**
asthma differentiated from, 246
retinal, 181. *See also* Uveitis
in rheumatoid arthritis, 835
urticarial, 134
Vasculopathy. *See* Vascular disorders
Vasectomy, 792
Vaseretic. *See* Enalapril, for hypertension, with hydrochlorothiazide
Vasoactive drug therapy
for allergic eye disease, 168
for dysautonomia, 991
for erectile dysfunction diagnosis/treatment, 967
in diabetes, 1241
for esophageal varices, 615
for shock, 496–497
Vasoactive intestinal polypeptide, tumors secreting (VIPoma), 1185, 1186
in MEN, 1188
Vasodepressor syncope, 401
Vasodilator therapy
for heart failure, 408
for hypertension, 463t, 464
in urgencies/emergencies, 470t
Vasodilatory (distributive) shock, 494, 494t, 495, 496–497, 497
Vasomotor disorders
in menopause (hot flushes), 794, 795, 1201
estrogen replacement therapy for, 795, 1202
topical progesterone for, 1205
rhinitis, 219
syncope and ("common faint"), 401
Vaso-occlusive crises, in sickle cell syndromes, 512, 513
Vasopressin, 1109t. *See also* Antidiuretic hormone; Desmopressin
in diabetes insipidus, 1113
for shock, 497
Vasopressin antagonists, for hyponatremia/SIADH, 889
Vasopressin challenge test, in diabetes insipidus, 1113
Vasopressin V1/V2 receptors, in diabetes insipidus, 1113
Vasopressinase-induced diabetes insipidus, 1113, 1114

Vasospasm. *See also* Vasomotor disorders
  coronary, 356, **364–365**
  in pheochromocytoma/paraganglioma,
    1180*t*
  in Raynaud phenomenon, 845
  subarachnoid hemorrhage and, 999
Vasotec. *See* Enalapril; Enalaprilat
Vasovagal hypotension, syncope and
    ("common faint"), 401
Vater, ampulla of. *See* Ampulla of Vater
VATS. *See* Video-assisted thoracoscopic
    surgery
VC (vital capacity), forced (FVC). *See*
    Pulmonary function tests
vCJD. *See* Variant Creutzfeldt-Jakob
    disease
VDRL test, 1489–1490, 1490*t*
  on cerebrospinal fluid (CSF-VDRL),
    1496
  in HIV infection/AIDS, 1348
  for sexual violence (rape/sexual
    assault) victim, 793, 794
Vectibix. *See* Panitumumab
Vedolizumab, for inflammatory bowel
    disease, 652
  Crohn disease, 657
  ulcerative colitis, 660
Vegetarians/vegans, dietary vitamin B$_{12}$
    deficiency in, 506
Vegetative state, persistent, **1028**
VEGF Trap-Eye. *See* Aflibercept
Veins
  deep, thrombosis of. *See* Deep venous
    thrombosis
  disorders of, **486–491**. *See also under*
    Venous and Veno-occlusive
    disease
  superficial, thrombophlebitis involving,
    487–488
  varicose. *See* Varicose veins
Velban. *See* Vinblastine
Velcade. *See* Bortezomib
Velpatasvir, for hepatitis C, 690*t*, 691
Vemurafenib, 1668*t*
Vena cava, superior, obstruction of,
    490–491
Vena cava filters/interruption, for
    pulmonary embolism, 301,
    576–577
Venereal Disease Research Laboratory
    test. *See* VDRL test
Venereal infections. *See* Sexually
    transmitted diseases
Venereal (genital) warts, 140, 141–142,
    141*f*, **768**
  anal cancer and, 671, 1344, 1643–1644
  anorectal involvement and, 141, 141*f*,
    671, 768
  cervical/vaginal/vulvar, **768**
  HPV vaccination in prevention of, 141,
    671, 768
Venezuelan equine encephalitis, 1388, 1389
Venlafaxine, 1077, 1078*t*, 1079–1081
  for anxiety, 1055
  for menopausal symptoms, 795, 1202
  for migraine prophylaxis, 979*t*
  for neuropathic pain, 83*t*, 84, 1035
  overdose/toxicity of, 84, 979*t*, 1078*t*,
    1081, 1606
    ophthalmic, 177*t*
  during pregnancy, 1081

Venography
  in DVT/PE (venous thromboembolic
    disease), 298
  in superior vena caval obstruction, 491
Venomous insect bites/stings, 150
  allergic reaction to, 878
  myocarditis caused by, 413*t*
Venomous snake bites, 1581*t*, **1604–1605**
  myocarditis caused by, 413*t*
Veno-occlusive disease, hepatic
  Budd-Chiari syndrome, **711–712**
  sinusoidal obstruction syndrome, 697,
    711–712
Venous blood gases, in acid-base
    disorders, 903
Venous catheterization. *See* Catheters/
    intravenous lines
Venous disease, **486–491**. *See also specific*
    type and Veno-occlusive
    disease; Venous
    insufficiency/stasis
Venous insufficiency/stasis, **488–490**, 489*f*
  DVT/PE (venous thromboembolic
    disease) and, 32, 33, 33*t*, 295,
    488
  lower extremity disorders in
    cellulitis differentiated from, 138
    edema and, 32–34, 33*t*, 489
    ulcers and, 32, 33, **155–157**, 156*f*,
      489, 490
  varicose veins and, 486, 489, 489*f*, 490
Venous pressure
  central. *See* Central venous pressure
  in lower extremity, 32
Venous reflux
  in varicose veins, 486, 487
  in venous insufficiency, 488, 489, 490
Venous sinus thrombosis, 1008
Venous stasis. *See* Venous insufficiency/
    stasis
Venous thromboembolic disease. *See also*
    Deep venous thrombosis;
    Pulmonary venous
    thromboembolism
  air travel and, 33, 1576
  in antiphospholipid antibody
    syndrome, 815, 816, 841, 843
  in Behçet syndrome, 862
  chest pain/discomfort and, 26, 27, 28,
    295, 296*t*
  in essential thrombocytosis, 521
  estrogen replacement therapy and,
    1202, 1203
  fever and, 1294
  in granulomatosis with polyangiitis, 857
  in homocystinuria, 575*t*, 1681
  hypercoagulability and, 295
  intracranial, **1002**. *See also* Stroke
  lower extremity edema and, 32, 33, 33*t*
  in nephrotic syndrome/nephrotic
    spectrum disorders, 943
  oral contraceptive use and, 786, 1198
  prevention of, 298–300, 567–569, 567*t*,
    568*t*, 569*t*
    contraindications to, 569, 569*t*
    joint replacement surgery and,
      298–300, 1703
  risk/risk stratification and, 32, 33*t*, 295,
    296*t*, 298, 298*t*, 299*f*, 299*t*,
    567–568, 567*t*, 569–571,
    571*t*, 573–574, 574*t*, 575*t*

  treatment of, 569–577, 570*t*, 571*t*, 572*t*,
    573*t*, 574*t*, 575*t*, 576*t*
    anticoagulation in, 300, 569–576,
      570*t*, 571*t*, 572*t*, 573*t*, 574*t*,
      575*t*
    nonpharmacologic therapy in, 301,
      576–577
    thrombolytic therapy in, 300–301,
      576, 576*t*
Venous thrombophlebitis, superficial,
    487–488
Venous ultrasonography, in DVT/PE
    (venous thromboembolic
    disease), 33, 33*t*, 297
Venovenous hemodiafiltration,
    continuous, for poisoning/
    drug overdose, 1583
Ventilation
  disorders of control of, **315–319**. *See*
    also Hyperventilation;
    Hypoventilation
  mechanical. *See* Mechanical ventilation
  sleep-related disorders of, 230–231,
    316, 1089
Ventilation-perfusion scans
  in COPD, 258*t*
  in pulmonary embolism, 296, 297, 298,
    299*f*
Ventilator-associated pneumonia,
    272–274, 273*t*, 275*t*, 319,
    1294
Ventricular aneurysm
  cardiac trauma and, 434
  myocardial infarction and, 379
Ventricular arrhythmias. *See also specific*
    type
  catheter ablation of, 384
  differentiation of from aberrantly
    conducted supraventricular
    beats, 385, 396
  in myocardial infarction, 370, 377
  in poisoning/drug overdose, 1579,
    1579*t*
Ventricular assist devices
  for cardiogenic shock, 378
  for cardiomyopathy, 417
  for heart failure, 405*f*, 410
Ventricular dysfunction/failure. *See* Heart
    (cardiac) failure
Ventricular fibrillation, 381, **397–398**
  catheter ablation of, 384
  in myocardial infarction, 370, 397, 398
  prevention/treatment of, 382*t*, 397–398
  sudden death caused by, **397–398**
    in athlete, 437
Ventricular gallop. *See* Heart sounds
Ventricular hypertrophy
  aortic dissection and, 485
  in athletes, 419
    sudden death and, 437
  in cardiomyopathy, 418, 419, 421.
    See also Cardiomyopathy
  hypertensive, 444, 445
Ventricular premature beats (ventricular
    extrasystoles/premature
    ventricular contractions/
    PVCs), **395–396**
  in myocardial infarction, 377
  in poisoning/drug overdose, 1579*t*
  treatment of, 382*t*, 396
Ventricular rate control. *See* Rate control

Ventricular septal aneurysm, 327
Ventricular septal defect, **327–328**
Ventricular tachycardia, 381, **396–397**.
    See also Torsades de pointes
catheter ablation of, 384, 397
differentiation of from aberrantly
        conducted supraventricular
        beats, 385, 396
driving recommendations and, **402**
in myocardial infarction, 377, 396
palpitations and, 30, 31
in poisoning/drug overdose, 1579,
        1579*t*
prevention/treatment of, 382–383*t*,
        396–397
sudden death of athlete and, 437, 438*t*
Ventriculography, radionuclide, in
        cardiomyopathy, 416
Vepesid. *See* Etoposide
Verapamil, 383*t*, 460*t*. *See also* Calcium
        channel blocking drugs
for acute coronary syndromes, 368
for angina, 361
for arrhythmias, 383*t*
    atrial fibrillation, 389
    multifocal atrial tachycardia, 395
    supraventricular tachycardia, 383*t*,
        386
for cardiomyopathy, 419, 420*f*
for cluster headache prophylaxis, 980
for hypertension, 459, 460*t*
    with trandolapril, 456*t*
for insulin-secreting tumors, 1255
for migraine prophylaxis, 979*t*
overdose/toxicity of, 383*t*, 459, 460*t*,
        979*t*, 1591
Verbal utterances, in schizophrenia/
        psychotic disorders, 1067
Verbigeration, in schizophrenia/psychotic
        disorders, 1067
Verelan/Verelan PM. *See* Verapamil
Vernal keratoconjunctivitis, 168
Verner–Morrison syndrome, 1186
Verocell rabies vaccine, 1387
Verrucae (warts), **140–142**, 141*f*
venereal. *See* Venereal (genital) warts
Versed. *See* Midazolam
Vertebrae. *See* Spinal cord; Spine
Vertebral artery occlusion, in stroke, 995
Vertebral fracture, back pain caused by,
        1692
Vertebral osteomyelitis, 870, 871, 1449
injection drug use and, 870, 1304
Vertebral tuberculosis, 871–872
Vertebrobasilar insufficiency/obstruction
stroke caused by, 994*t*, 995
transient ischemic attacks caused by,
        991
vertigo caused by, 211*t*
Vertebroplasty, in osteoporosis, 1163
Vertigo, **210–213**, 210*t*, 211*t*
in audiovestibular disorders, 210–213,
        210*t*, 211*t*, 213–214
barotrauma causing, 204
benign paroxysmal positioning
        (BPPV), 211*t*, 212
central causes of, 210*t*, 211, 211*t*, 213,
        213–214
cervical, 213
in endolymphatic hydrops (Ménière
        disease), 211–212, 211*t*

in labyrinthitis, 211*t*, 212
migrainous, 211, 211*t*, 213
in multiple sclerosis, 211*t*, **214**
in perilymphatic fistula, 211*t*, 212
peripheral causes of, 210–211, 210*t*,
        211–213
in superior semicircular canal
        dehiscence, 213
traumatic, 212
vascular compromise causing, **214**
in vestibular neuronitis, 211*t*, 212
Very-low-calorie diets, in obesity
        management, 1271
Very-low-density lipoproteins/cholesterol,
        1259. *See also* Triglycerides
in coronary heart disease, 1259
lowering levels of. *See* Lipid-lowering
        therapy
Vesanoid. *See* Tretinoin
Vesicants, skin decontamination after
        exposure to, 1581
Vesicoureteral reflux, tubulointerstitial
        disease caused by, 947, 948
Vesicular dermatoses, 96*t*, **118–123**. *See*
        also specific type
Vesiculobullous hand eczema/dermatitis
        of palms and soles
        (pompholyx), **121–122**, 122*f*
tinea differentiated from, 114, 122
Vestibular disorders (vestibulopathy),
        210*t*, 211*t*, **213–214**
autoimmune hearing loss and, 209
central, 210*t*
nausea and vomiting caused by, 87,
        580, 581*t*
neuronitis, 211*t*, 212
peripheral, 210–211, 210*t*, 211–213
schwannoma. *See* Schwannoma,
        vestibular
vertigo in, 210–213, 210*t*, 211*t*,
        213–214. *See also* Vertigo
Vestibulitis
nasal, **218**
vulvar, 782
Veteran Administration Diabetes Trial
        (VADT), 1219
Vexol. *See* Rimexolone
VHL. *See* von Hippel-Lindau syndrome
VHL gene, in pheochromocytoma/
        paraganglioma, 1179, 1182
Vi capsular polysaccharide (Vi CPS)
        vaccine. *See* Typhoid vaccine
Viagra. *See* Sildenafil
Vibrio, 1312*t*, **1472**
    alginolyticus, 1472
    cholerae, 588*t*, 1305, 1307*t*, 1312*t*,
        1471. *See also* Cholera
    immunization against, 1326, 1471
    diarrhea/food poisoning caused by,
        588*t*, 589, 1305, 1307*t*, 1472
    parahaemolyticus, 588*t*, 1305, 1307*t*,
        1472
    vulnificus, 1472
Vicodin. *See* Hydrocodone
Victoza. *See* Liraglutide
Vidarabine, 1365*t*
Vidaza. *See* Azacitidine
Video-assisted thoracoscopic surgery
        (VATS)
in lung cancer, 1609
for solitary pulmonary nodule, 288

Videoesophagography, 605
Videx. *See* Didanosine
Vienna Prediction Model, 573
Vigabatrin, 988*t*
overdose/toxicity of, 988*t*, 1589
ophthalmic, 178*t*
Vigamox. *See* Moxifloxacin
Viibryd. *See* Vilazodone
Vilanterol, for COPD, 260
Vilazodone, 1077, 1078*t*, 1079–1081
Vildagliptin, 1222*t*, 1227
VIN. *See* Vulvar intraepithelial neoplasia
Vinblastine, 1664*t*
for Kaposi sarcoma, 146, 1338*t*
for renal cell carcinoma, 1654
Vinca alkaloids, 1664*t*
neuropathy caused by, 1674
Vincent angina (necrotizing ulcerative
        gingivitis), **226**
Vincristine, 1664*t*
adverse ophthalmic effects of, 178*t*
liposomal, 1664*t*
neuropathy caused by, 1674
Vinorelbine, 1664*t*
for lung cancer, 1612
Vioform. *See* Iodoquinol
Violaceous to purple papules/nodules,
        144–146
Violence, **1090–1092**. *See also* Rape
alcohol use disorder and, 1090, 1093
anabolic steroid use and, 1090, 1101
domestic, 16, 1090–1091, 1091
    elder abuse and, 16, **70–71**, 71*t*
    intimate partner, 16, 1090–1091,
        1091
phencyclidine use/abuse and, 1090, 1099
prevention of, **16**
sexual, **792–794**
VIPomas, 1185, 1186
in MEN, 1188
Viracept. *See* Nelfinavir
Viral diseases, **1363–1428**, 1365*t*. *See also*
        specific type
adenovirus, **1420–1421**
arthritis, **870**
conjunctivitis, **166–167**
diarrhea/gastroenteritis, 588*t*, 589,
        1305, 1342, **1424–1425**
drug therapy for, 1365*t*. *See also*
        Antiviral agents
enterovirus, **1425–1428**
exanthematous, 1367–1368*t*,
        1421–1424
hemorrhagic fevers, **1397–1406**
hepatitis. *See* Hepatitis
herpesvirus, **1363–1377**
meningitis. *See* Aseptic meningitis
myocarditis in, 413, 413*t*
neurotropic, **1386–1397**
pericarditis, 424, 425–426
respiratory, **1409–1420**
rhinosinusitis (common cold),
        214–215, 1420–1421
systemic, **1406–1409**
transfusion-associated, 543–544
tubulointerstitial nephritis and, 947*t*
vaccine-preventable, **1377–1385**
Viral load tests (HIV). *See* HIV viral
        load tests
Viramune. *See* Nevirapine
Virchow node, 1630

Virchow triad, 295
Viread. *See* Tenofovir
Viridans streptococci, 1311*t*, 1444
  endocarditis caused by, 1314*t*, 1444,
    1458, 1461
Virilization, **1196–1199**
Viroptic. *See* Trifluridine
Virtual colonoscopy, 15, 665, 1638,
    1642–1643
Viruses. *See* Viral diseases
Visceral artery insufficiency, **479–480**
Visceral hypersensitivity (heightened
    visceral nociception)
  chest pain/discomfort and, 619
  irritable bowel syndrome and, 644
Visceral ischemia, 479–480
Visceral larva migrans, 1542
Visceral leishmaniasis (kala azar), 1510,
    1511, 1511–1512
  dermal leishmaniasis after, 1510
  in HIV infection/AIDS, 1511
Viscerotropic disease
  leishmaniasis, 1510. *See also* Visceral
    leishmaniasis
  yellow fever vaccine-associated, 1327,
    1405
Visicol. *See* Sodium phosphate
Vision, impaired/blurred. *See* Visual
    impairment/loss
Visken. *See* Pindolol
Vismodegib, for basal cell carcinoma, 143
Vistaril. *See* Hydroxyzine
Visual acuity, reduced. *See* Visual
    impairment/loss
Visual field defects/loss. *See also* Visual
    impairment/loss
  in carotid territory occlusion, 995
  in glaucoma, 179, 180, 181
  in intracranial mass lesions, 1003, 1005
  in ischemic optic neuropathy, 192
  in optic neuritis, 193
  in retinal artery occlusion, 187
  in transient monocular visual loss,
    188–189
Visual impairment/loss. *See also specific*
    cause and Eye, disorders of;
    Visual field defects/loss
  in age-related macular degeneration, 185
  antipsychotics causing, 1071
  in cataract, 182, 183
  in diabetes, 189, 190, 1214, 1238. *See*
    also Diabetic retinopathy
  in elderly, **69–70**
  in giant cell arteritis, 854, 855
  in glaucoma, 176, 179, 180, 181
  in HIV infection/AIDS, 191–192, 1341.
    See also HIV infection/AIDS,
    retinal disorders associated
    with
  in methanol intoxication, 1599
  ocular trauma causing, 196
  onchocerciasis causing, 1545
  in optic neuritis, 193
  refractive errors causing, **164**
  in retinal artery occlusion, 187
  in retinal vein occlusion, 186
  in SJS/TEN, 136
  in trachoma, 167
  transient monocular, **188–189**
  in vitamin A deficiency, 1277
  in vitreous hemorrhage, 184

Visuospatial impairment, in dementia,
    1020
Vital capacity, forced (FVC). *See*
    Pulmonary function tests
Vitamin A
  deficiency of, **1277**
  toxicity of, **1277–1278**
    ophthalmic, 179*t*
Vitamin B₁. *See* Thiamine
Vitamin B₂. *See* Riboflavin
Vitamin B₃. *See* Niacin
Vitamin B₆ (pyridoxine)
  deficiency of, **1276**
  homocystinuria/
    hyperhomocysteinemia and,
    1681
  isoniazid overdose/toxicity and, 282,
    283, 821, 1276, 1348, 1581*t*,
    1596
  toxicity of, **1276**
  for vomiting during pregnancy, 583,
    803
Vitamin B₁₂ (cobalamin), 506
  deficiency of, **506–508**, 507*t*
    in bacterial overgrowth, 506, 636
    fish tapeworm infection and,
      506–507, 1535
    folic acid deficiency and, 507, 508,
      509
    homocystinuria/
      hyperhomocysteinemia and,
      1681
    neuropathy associated with, 507,
      1036
    in pernicious anemia gastritis, 622
    short bowel syndrome/ileal resection
      and, 506, 637
    subacute combined degeneration of
      spinal cord caused by, 1026
    thrombocytopenia associated with,
      548
  normal values for, 507
  supplemental, 507–508
    for homocystinuria/
      hyperhomocysteinemia,
      1681
    for short bowel syndrome, 637
    for subacute combined degeneration
      of spinal cord, 1026
Vitamin C (ascorbic acid)
  in chemoprevention, 11
  deficiency of, **1277**
  toxicity of, **1277**
Vitamin D
  adverse ophthalmic effects of, 179*t*
  deficiency of/resistance to, 1164, 1166
    in chronic kidney disease/renal
      osteodystrophy, 927, 927*f*
    in HIV infection/AIDS, 1340
    in hyperparathyroidism, 1154
    in hypocalcemia, 896
    in osteomalacia/rickets, 927, 1164,
      1164*t*, 1166
    in osteoporosis, 1160, 1161
  dietary/supplementary
    fall prevention and, 64, 64*t*
    hypercalcemia and, 898, 1156
    for hyperparathyroidism, 927, 1157
    for hypocalcemia/
      hypoparathyroidism/tetany,
      897, 1151, 1151–1152, 1151*t*

  for metabolic bone disorders/renal
    osteodystrophy, 927
  for osteomalacia, 1166
  for osteoporosis prevention/
    management, 11, 795, 1161,
    1702
  in hypercalciuria, 962*t*, 963
  hypophosphatemia/hypophosphatemic
    rickets and, 892*t*, 1164–1165,
    1166
  overproduction of, in hypercalcemia,
    897
  phosphate balance/imbalances and,
    899
Vitamin D₂ (ergocalciferol/ergosterol),
    1151–1152, 1151*t*. *See also*
    Vitamin D
  for hypoparathyroidism/tetany,
    1151–1152, 1151*t*
  for vitamin D deficiency/osteomalacia,
    1166
Vitamin D₃ (cholecalciferol), 1151*t*. *See*
    also Vitamin D
  for hypoparathyroidism/tetany, 1151*t*
  for vitamin D deficiency/osteoporosis/
    osteomalacia, 1161, 1166
Vitamin D analogs. *See also* Vitamin D
  for hyperparathyroidism, 1157
  for psoriasis, 108
Vitamin D-dependent rickets, 1164
Vitamin D-resistant (hypophosphatemic)
    rickets, 892*t*, 1164–1165,
    1166
Vitamin E
  in chemoprevention, 11
  deficiency of, **1025, 1278**
  toxicity of, **1278**
Vitamin K
  for anticoagulant overdose, 1588
  deficiency of, **562,** 704
  for esophageal varices, 615
  for hepatic coagulopathy, 704
Vitamin K antagonists, 563–564. *See also*
    Warfarin
  for atrial fibrillation/stroke prevention,
    391, 392, 392*f*
  after cardiac valve replacement, 351,
    352*t*
Vitamin K epoxide reductase complex
    (VKORC1), 562
  warfarin and, 572
Vitamin supplements, in HIV infection/
    AIDS, 1349
Vitamins. *See also specific vitamin*
  adverse ophthalmic effects of, 179*t*
  disorders of metabolism of,
    1274–1278
  prenatal, 799, 801
  requirements for in nutritional
    support, 1282, 1283
Vitekta. *See* Elvitegravir
Vitiligo, 157, 157*f*
  tinea versicolor differentiated from,
    114
Vitreous hemorrhage, **184–185,** 184*f*
Vivactil. *See* Protriptyline
Vivelle-Dot, 1204
VKA. *See* Vitamin K antagonists
VKORC1 (vitamin K epoxide reductase
    complex), 562
  warfarin and, 572

VLDL. *See* Very-low-density lipoproteins/
cholesterol
VLP vaccine, 4. *See also See also* Human
papillomavirus (HPV)
vaccine
Vocal fold cysts, 234
Vocal fold dysfunction syndrome, 241
Vocal fold nodules, 234
Vocal fold polyps, 234
Vocal folds
cancer of, 235, 236
in hoarseness, 232
leukoplakia of, **235**
paralysis of, **237**
thyroid surgery and, 237, 1143
traumatic lesions of, **234–235**
Vogelxo, 1192
Voglibose, 1221*t*, 1225
Vogt-Koyanagi-Harada syndrome, 181
Voice, abnormal, **232–233**
in laryngeal cancer, 235
laryngopharyngeal reflux causing, 233
in lung cancer, 1609
in vocal fold paralysis, 237
Voiding
dysfunctional, in prostatodynia, 959
increased. *See* Polyuria
involuntary. *See* Urinary incontinence
painful (dysuria), **42–44**, 44*f*
Voltage, in electrical injury, 1570
Voltaren/Voltaren-XR. *See* Diclofenac
Volume depletion
hypercalcemia and, 897, 898
saline-responsive metabolic alkalosis
and, 909, 910
Volume reduction surgery, for COPD, 262
Volume replacement. *See* Fluid
management/hydration
Volume status. *See also* Fluid and
electrolyte disorders; Fluid
management/hydration
diabetes insipidus and, 1114
diarrhea and, 589, 590
in drowning, 1567
hyper-/hyponatremia and, 885,
885–888, 885*f*, 888, 890
metabolic alkalosis and, 909, 910
pregnancy and, 819
weight change reflecting, 884
Volutrauma. *See also* Barotrauma
mechanical ventilation and, 319
Vomiting, 87, **580–583**, 581*t*, 582*t. See
also specific cause and*
Nausea and vomiting
induced, for poisoning/drug overdose,
1582
palliation of, **87**
of pregnancy, 580, **803**, 823
gestational trophoblastic disease
and, 807
Wernicke encephalopathy and, 1026
Vomiting center, 580
von Hippel-Lindau syndrome
gastroenteropancreatic neuroendocrine
tumors in, 1185
pheochromocytoma and, 1179, 1182
renal cell carcinoma in, 1654
von Recklinghausen disease. *See*
Recklinghausen disease
von Willebrand disease, 559*t*, **560**, 561*t*
type 2B, **555**, 560, 561*t*

von Willebrand factor, 560, 561*t*
in cryoprecipitate, 544
von Willebrand factor cleaving protease
(vWFCP/ADAMTS-13), in
thrombotic
thrombocytopenic purpura,
550, 551, 551*t*
von Willebrand factor concentrate, 559*t*,
560
von Willebrand factor-containing factor
VIII concentrate, 559*t*
von Willebrand factor receptor, in
Bernard-Soulier syndrome,
556
Vorapaxar, for angina, 361
Voriconazole, 1559*t*, 1560
for aspergillosis, 1555, 1560
for candidiasis, 226, 611, 1548, 1560
for ophthalmic disorders, 170*t*, 175
prophylactic, 1292
squamous cell carcinoma development
and, 144
Vorinostat, for myelodysplastic
syndromes, 526
Vortioxetine, 1077, 1078*t*, 1079–1081
Votrient. *See* Pazopanib
V/Q scans. *See* Ventilation-perfusion
scans
Vraylar. *See* Cariprazine
VSD. *See* Ventricular septal defect
VSL#3 probiotic
for irritable bowel syndrome, 647
for ulcerative colitis/pouchitis, 660, 661
VTE. *See* Venous thromboembolic
disease
Vulvar carcinoma, **775**
Vulvar dystrophy, 775
Vulvar intraepithelial neoplasia (VIN),
775
Vulvar vestibulitis, 782
Vulvar warts, 768. *See also* Venereal
(genital) warts
Vulvodynia, 782, 783
Vulvovaginal atrophy. *See* Atrophic
vaginitis
Vulvovaginal candidiasis, 133, 766, 766*f*,
767, 1302, 1547, 1548
in diabetes, 1214, 1242
in HIV infection/AIDS, 1338*t*, 1344
sexual violence (rape/sexual assault)
and, 1302
Vulvovaginitis. *See* Vaginitis
vWD. *See* von Willebrand disease
vWF. *See* von Willebrand factor
vWFCP. *See* von Willebrand factor
cleaving protease
VX poisoning, 1601–1602
VZIG. *See* Varicella zoster immune
globulin
VZV. *See* Varicella zoster virus
VZV syndrome, congenital, 821
VZV vaccine. *See* Herpes zoster vaccine

Waldenström macroglobulinemia,
537–538, 1623*t*
Warfarin, 563–564, 571–573, 572*t*, 573*t*,
574*t*
for antiphospholipid antibody
syndrome, 842, 843
for atrial fibrillation/stroke prevention,
391, 392

in hyperthyroidism, 1133
in mitral stenosis, 336
benzodiazepine interactions and, 1056*t*
cardiac valve replacement and, 351
coronary stents/STEMI and, 376
postinfarction, 376, 380
for DVT/PE (venous thromboembolic
disease), 300, 568*t*, 571–573,
572*t*, 573*t*, 574*t*
for heart failure, 409
for heparin-induced
thrombocytopenia, 552–553,
553*f*
for intracranial venous thrombosis,
1002
in nephrotic syndrome/nephrotic
spectrum disorders, 943
overdose/toxicity of, 300, 1588
perioperative management of, 51*t*, 351
pregnancy and, 351
for pulmonary hypertension, 431
switching to from DOAC, 566*t*
switching to DOAC from, 392, 566*t*
for transient ischemic attacks, 993
vitamin K epoxide reductase complex
(VKORC1) and, 572
Warts (verrucae), **140–142**, 141*f*
venereal. *See* Venereal (genital) warts
Washout time, in antidepressant drug
therapy, 1082
Wasting
in HIV infection/AIDS, 1335
in malabsorption, 633*t*
in protein-energy malnutrition, 1268
Watchful waiting/surveillance
for benign prostatic hyperplasia, 972,
973*f*, 973*t*
for prostate cancer, 1648, 1650
for testicular cancer, after orchiectomy,
1656
Water, body. *See* Body water
Water deficit, calculation of, 890
Water/fluid intake. *See also* Fluid
management/hydration
in diabetes insipidus, 1114
disorders of/inappropriate. *See also*
Psychogenic polydipsia
genetic disorders and, 892*t*
hypernatremia caused by, 890
hyponatremia caused by, 886, 887
replacement of/requirements for,
911–912, 1282
restriction of
for chronic kidney disease, 929
for hyponatremia, 888
urinary stone formation and, 962, 963,
964
Water-hammer pulse, 346
Water shifts, hyperosmolality with and
without, **891**
Waterhouse-Friderichsen syndrome, 1169
Waterston-Cooley shunt, for tetralogy of
Fallot, 329
WDHA, 1186
Weakness/muscle weakness. *See*
Myopathies; Myositis;
Paralysis
"Wearing off effect," with levodopa, 1012
Web space (interdigital) tinea pedis, 113,
113*f*
cellulitis and, 113, 137

Weber test, 200
Webs, esophageal. *See* Esophageal webs
Weeping/crusted skin lesions, 96*t*,
    123–126. *See also specific*
    type
    drying agents for, 95
Wegener granulomatosis. *See*
    Granulomatosis, with
    polyangiitis
Weight
    changes in. *See also* Weight gain;
        Weight loss
        water balance and, 884, 911
    exercise/activity in maintenance/
        reduction of, 11, 12, 13
    normal, 12
Weight gain. *See also* Obesity
    drugs causing
        antipsychotic agents, 1070, 1071,
            1071*t*, 1072
        thiazolidinediones, 1225
    prevention of, exercise/activity and, 11,
        12, 13
Weight loss (involuntary/unintended),
    36–37. *See also specific*
    disorder and Weight
    reduction
    in diabetes, 1214
        diabetic neuropathic cachexia and,
            1240
    in elderly, 35, **67**
    in HIV infection/AIDS, 1335
    malabsorption and, 633*t*
    in protein-energy malnutrition, 1268
    in Whipple disease, 635
Weight reduction
    exercise/activity in, 11, 12, 13,
        1270–1271
    for GERD, 609
    in hypertension management/
        prevention, 445, 446*t*
    for hypogonadotropic hypogonadism,
        1109, 1193
    in obesity, 12–13, 1270–1272
    for polycystic ovary syndrome, 781
    in psoriasis management, 107
    for sleep apnea/snoring, 231, 317
    for type 2 diabetes, 1235, 1235*f*
        liraglutide for, 1226, 1235
Weil syndrome, 1501
WelChol. *See* Colesevelam
Well syndrome, 1422
Wellbutrin. *See* Bupropion
Wells criteria/"Wells prediction rule," 23,
    25–26, 33
Wenckebach (Mobitz type I)
    atrioventricular block, 377,
    399
Wermer syndrome. *See* Multiple
    endocrine neoplasia (MEN),
    MEN 1
Wernicke aphasia, 995
Wernicke encephalopathy, 908, **1026**,
    1093, 1095, 1275
Wernicke-Korsakoff syndrome, 694, 908,
    1026, 1093, 1095, 1275
West African trypanosomiasis, 1507,
    1508, 1508*t*
West Nile virus/fever/encephalitis, 1388,
    1388–1389, 1389
    screening blood for virus causing, 543

Westermark sign, 296
Western blot assay, in HIV infection/
    AIDS, 1333, 1334, 1334*t*
Western (equine) encephalitis, 1388
Western subtype tick-borne encephalitis,
    1391
"Wet" age-related macular degeneration,
    185
Wet beriberi, 1274
WFS1 mutation, in Wolfram syndrome,
    1212
Wharton duct, calculus formation in,
    231–232
Wheals. *See* Urticaria
Wheat procedure, 347*t*
Wheezes
    in asthma, 242, 245, 245*t*
    in heart failure ("cardiac asthma"), 242
    in pulmonary embolism, 296*t*
Whiplash injuries, 1031, 1696
Whipple disease, **635–636**
    arthritis in, 635, 867
Whipple triad, 1253
Whipworm infections (trichuriasis),
    1538–1539
Whispered voice test, 70
White blood cell count (leukocyte count)
    ascitic fluid, 601–602, 603, 604
    cerebrospinal fluid, 1297*t*
    chemotherapy dosage modification
        and, 1672*t*
    joint fluid, 826, 827*t*, 828*t*
    in myeloproliferative neoplasms, 520*t*
    pleural fluid, 312, 313*t*
White blood cells. *See* Leukocytes
White cell aplasia, pure, 518
White cell casts, 913, 914*t*
"White coat" hypertension, 439
Whitewater Arroyo virus, 1399
Whitlow, herpetic, 119, 1363, 1364*f*
Whole blood. *See* Fresh whole blood
Whole bowel irrigation, for poisoning/
    drug overdose, 1582
Whooping cough. *See* Pertussis
Wickham striae, 145
Wide QRS complex. *See* QRS complex,
    wide
Wild-type TTR amyloidosis, 538
Wilson disease (hepatolenticular
    degeneration), **709–711**,
    710*f*, **1017**
    movement disorders/parkinsonism
        and, 710, 1012, **1017**
WinRho. *See* Anti-D
Winter acute respiratory disease, 1421
Winterbottom sign, 1507
Wiskott-Aldrich syndrome, 546
Withdrawal. *See also specific substance*
    cognitive disorders/delirium caused by,
        1102*t*
    seizures caused by, 989
Withdrawal response, in coma or stupor,
    1027
Withdrawal/withholding of curative
    effort, in terminally ill/dying
    patient, 91–92, 92*t*
    advance directives and, 90
Wolbachia bacteria, eradication of
    in filariasis, 1544
    in onchocerciasis, 1545
Wolcott-Rallison syndrome, 1212

Wolff-Parkinson-White syndrome, 31,
    387
    sudden death of athlete and, 437, 438*t*
Wolfram syndrome, 1113, 1212
Wood alcohol. *See* Methanol
Woody (Riedel) thyroiditis, 1135, 1137
Word-finding difficulty, in dementia,
    1020
Word recall, three-item, in dementia
    screening, 57–58
Wound botulism, 1454, 1601
Wound care
    for bite wounds, 1300
        rabies and, 1387
    for burn injuries, 1569
    for frostbite, 1566
    for lymphangitis/lymphadenitis, 492
    tetanus prophylaxis/treatment and,
        1453, 1453*t*
Wound infections
    clostridial
        botulism, 1454, 1601
        myonecrosis/gas gangrene, 1312*t*,
            1451–1452
        tetanus, 1312*t*, **1452–1453**, 1453*t*.
            See also Tetanus
    surgical site, 1294–1295
        antibiotic prophylaxis of, **54**
Wrestlers, epidemic herpes in (herpes
    gladiatorum), 119, 1363
Wrist
    in carpal tunnel syndrome, 1698–1699,
        1699*t*
    examination of, 1699*t*
Writer's cramp, 1016–1017
Wuchereria bancrofti, 1543, 1544

X chromosome
    fragile site on, 1679
    in Klinefelter syndrome, 1190, 1682
    in Turner syndrome, 1207, 1208
X chromosome mosaicism
    premature menopause and, 1201
    in Turner syndrome, 1208
X-inactive-specific transcriptase (XIST),
    in Klinefelter syndrome,
    1190
X-linked adrenoleukodystrophy, 1169,
    1171, 1172
X-linked hypophosphatemic rickets,
    1165, 1166
X-linked lymphoproliferative disorder,
    Epstein-Barr infection and,
    1373
X-ray studies. *See also specific disorder*
    and under Radiation
    radiation exposure/cancer risk and,
        1571, 1572, 1607
Xalacom. *See* Latanoprost/timolol
Xalatan. *See* Latanoprost
Xalkori. *See* Crizotinib
Xanax. *See* Alprazolam
Xanthine oxidase inhibitors, for gout,
    832, 833
Xanthogranulomatous cholecystitis, 719
Xanthomas
    eruptive, 1261, 1261*f*
        in diabetes, 1214, 1242, 1261, 1261*f*
    tendinous, 1261
Xeloda. *See* Capecitabine
Xenical. *See* Orlistat

Xerosis
in HIV infection/AIDS, 1344
in vitamin A deficiency, 1277
Xerostomia
antipsychotics causing, 1071
radiation-induced, pilocarpine for,
1671t
in Sjögren syndrome, 850, 851
Xgeva. *See* Denosumab
Xibrom. *See* Bromfenac
Xigduo. *See* Dapagliflozin, with
metformin
XIST. *See* X-inactive-specific
transcriptase
XO gonadal dysgenesis, 1207,
1207–1208, 1208
Xofigo. *See* Radium-223 dichloride
Xp-, in Turner syndrome, 1208
Xp11.2 translocation, in renal cell
carcinoma, 1654
Xq, in Turner syndrome, 1207
Xtandi. *See* Enzalutamide
XX karyotype, in Turner syndrome,
1208
XY gonadal dysgenesis/XY mosaicism,
1190, 1208. *See also* Turner
syndrome
XY karyotype
amenorrhea and, 1199–1200
hirsutism/virilization and, 1196
Xyloprim. *See* Allopurinol
Xyrem. *See* Gamma-hydroxybutyrate

Y chromosome, in Klinefelter syndrome,
1190
Y chromosome microdeletions, in male
infertility, 970
Yaws (frambesia), 1312t, **1498**
Yellow fever, **1404–1406**
prevention/immunization and, 1327,
1405
Yellow fever virus vaccine, 1327, 1405
Yersinia
enterocolitica, diarrhea/gastroenteritis
caused by, 588t, 589, 1305,
1307t
pestis, 1312t, 1474
Yervoy. *See* Ipilimumab
Yohimbine, toxicity of, 1593
Yttrium-90 ibritumomab tiuxetan, for
non-Hodgkin lymphoma,
532
YY1/T372R mutation, in insulinoma,
1252

Z score, 1160
Zaditor. *See* Ketotifen
Zafirlukast, for asthma, 250t, 251
Zaire ebolavirus, 1397
Zaleplon, 1054t, 1089
overdose/toxicity of, 1594–1595
Zaltrap. *See* Ziv-aflibercept

Zanamivir, 1365t, 1412, 1413, 1418
prophylactic, 1416
resistance to, 1413
ZAP-70, in chronic lymphocytic
leukemia, 530
Zaroxolyn. *See* Metolazone
Zarxio. *See* Filgrastim (G-CSF)/
filgrastim-sndz
Zebeta. *See* Bisoprolol
ZEBOV. *See* *Zaire ebolavirus*
Zelboraf. *See* Vemurafenib
Zenker diverticulum, **614**
Zerit. *See* Stavudine
Zestoretic. *See* Lisinopril, for
hypertension, with
hydrochlorothiazide
Zestril. *See* Lisinopril
Zeta-associated protein (ZAP-70), in
chronic lymphocytic
leukemia, 530
Zetia. *See* Ezetimibe
Ziac. *See* Bisoprolol, for hypertension,
with hydrochlorothiazide
Ziagen. *See* Abacavir
Zidovudine (AZT), 1351t, 1353,
1353–1354, 1360. *See also*
Antiretroviral therapy
with lamivudine, 1353, 1353–1354
with lamivudine and abacavir
(Trizivir), 1354, 1354t
myopathy caused by, 1049, 1340
for prevention of HIV transmission
to fetus/newborn, 822, 1346
postexposure/after needle stick, 1347
resistance to, 1361
Zika virus, **1406–1407**
encephalitis caused by, 1388, 1406
pregnancy and, 1390, 1406, 1407
Zika virus vaccine/vaccine development,
1407
Zileuton, for asthma, 247f, 250t, 251
Zinacef. *See* Cefuroxime
Zinc
parenteral nutritional support and,
1283, 1285t
toxicity of, 1593
for viral rhinosinusitis (common cold),
214
for Wilson disease, 711
Zinc transporter 8 (ZnT8) antibodies, in
type 1 diabetes, 1211, 1211t,
1233
Zinecard. *See* Dexrazoxane
Zioptan. *See* Tafluprost
Ziprasidone, 1068, 1069t, 1070, 1071t
for aggressive/violent patient, 1091
for hallucinogen overdose/toxicity,
1598
overdose/toxicity/side effects of, 1069t,
1071, 1071t, 1589–1590
Zirconium cyclosilicate, for
hyperkalemia, 894

Zirgan. *See* Ganciclovir
Zithromax. *See* Azithromycin
Ziv-aflibercept, 1669t
ZMapp, for Ebola viral disease, 1398
ZnT8 (zinc transporter 8) antibodies, in
type 1 diabetes, 1211, 1211t,
1233
Zocor. *See* Simvastatin
Zohydro. *See* Hydrocodone
Zoladex. *See* Goserelin
Zoledronate/zoledronic acid, 1161–1162,
1162. *See also*
Bisphosphonates
in breast cancer management, 754
for chemotherapy-induced toxicity/
bone pain, 1671t
for hypercalcemia/
hyperparathyroidism, 1157,
1660
for osteoporosis prevention/
management, 1161–1162,
1162
corticosteroid use and, 1209
for Paget disease of bone, 1168
for thyroid cancer bone metastases,
1145
Zollinger-Ellison syndrome (gastrinoma),
631–632, 1185, 1186
carcinoid tumors and, 1633
in MEN, 631, 632, 1185, 1186, 1188
peptic ulcer disease and, 623, 629, 631,
1185
Zolmitriptan
for cluster headache, 980
for migraine headache, 978
Zoloft. *See* Sertraline
Zolpidem, 1054t, 1089
for MAOI-induced insomnia, 1082
overdose/toxicity of, 1594–1595
sleep cycle affected by, 1088–1089
Zometa. *See* Zoledronate/zoledronic acid
Zonalon. *See* Doxepin
Zonisamide, 987t
overdose/toxicity of, 987t, 1589
ophthalmic, 178t
ZOSTAVAX. *See* Herpes zoster vaccine
Zoster. *See* Herpes zoster
Zoster ophthalmicus, 121, **175**, 192,
1369
Zoster oticus, 1369
Zoster sine herpete, 1370
Zoster vaccine. *See* Herpes zoster vaccine
Zostrix. *See* Capsaicin
Zosyn. *See* Piperacillin-tazobactam
Zotarolimus, 362
Zovirax. *See* Acyclovir
Zydelig. *See* Idelalisib
Zygote intrafallopian transfer, 785
Zykadia. *See* Ceritinib
Zymaxid. *See* Gatifloxacin
Zyprexa. *See* Olanzapine
Zytiga. *See* Abiraterone